中英文对照版

核心放射学：影像诊断图解教程

Core Radiology
A Visual Approach to Diagnostic Imaging

（第2版）

主　编　［美］孙夏萌(Ellen X. Sun)
　　　　［美］史君子(Junzi Shi)
　　　　［美］雅各布·C.马戴尔(Jacob C. Mandell)

主　译　王维平

副主译（按姓氏笔画排序）
丁铁钢　朱晓黎　杨　健　吴汉平　汪　晶
陈绍亮　郑葵葵　胡红杰　南海燕　贾中芝
唐　静　董伟华　程　瑾　舒晓军　谢双双

人民卫生出版社
·北　京·

图书在版编目（CIP）数据

核心放射学：影像诊断图解教程：汉英对照 /（美）孙夏萌（Ellen X. Sun），（美）史君子（Junzi Shi），（美）雅各布·C. 马戴尔（Jacob C. Mandell）主编；王维平主译. -- 北京 ：人民卫生出版社，2025. 4. -- ISBN 978-7-117-36401-0

Ⅰ. R445

中国国家版本馆 CIP 数据核字第 2024ER4234 号

图字：01-2022-5206号

核心放射学：影像诊断图解教程（中英文对照）
Hexin Fangshexue：Yingxiang Zhenduan Tujie Jiaocheng
（Zhongyingwen Duizhao）

主　　译： 王维平
出版发行： 人民卫生出版社（中继线 010-59780011）
地　　址： 北京市朝阳区潘家园南里 19 号
邮　　编： 100021
E - mail： pmph @ pmph.com
购书热线： 010-59787592　010-59787584　010-65264830
印　　刷： 三河市宏达印刷有限公司
经　　销： 新华书店
开　　本： 889 × 1194　1/16　**印张：** 85　**字数：** 3677 千字
版　　次： 2025 年 4 月第 1 版
印　　次： 2025 年 4 月第 1 次印刷
标准书号： ISBN 978-7-117-36401-0
定　　价： 898.00 元
打击盗版举报电话：010-59787491　E-mail：WQ @ pmph.com
质量问题联系电话：010-59787234　E-mail：zhiliang @ pmph.com
数字融合服务电话：4001118166　E-mail：zengzhi @ pmph.com

译　者

主　译　王维平　美国梅奥诊所

副主译（按姓氏笔画排序）

丁铁钢　美国麻省Good Samaritan医院
朱晓黎　苏州大学附属第一医院
杨　健　西安交通大学第一附属医院
吴汉平　美国Medical College of Georgia
汪　晶　华中科技大学同济医学院附属协和医院
陈绍亮　复旦大学中山医院
郑葵葵　温州医科大学附属第一医院
胡红杰　浙江大学医学院附属邵逸夫医院
南海燕　空军军医大学唐都医院
贾中芝　常州市第二人民医院
唐　静　四川大学华西医院
董伟华　海军军医大学第二附属医院
程　瑾　北京大学人民医院
舒晓军　兰州大学第一医院
谢双双　天津市第一中心医院

翻　译（按姓氏笔画排序）

于　千　于　瀛　马　聪　马宏星　王　玉　王　超　王亚玲　王苗苗　王草叶　王维平　王斯妮
毛志群　卞益同　卢　瞳　卢陈英　帅丹丹　吕霞飞　朱晓黎　仲斌演　全杰蓉　刘　进　刘杰克
祁　丽　许　倩　许长德　许棚棚　孙　欣　孙明菡　孙颖志　阳宁静　严承功　苏筱芮　李　西
李蓓蕾　杨　明　杨　晶　杨宏远　杨国威　杨学刚　杨喜彪　杨曦玥　吴　静　吴汉平　吴志远
吴艳艳　吴桂鹏　邱　伟　何　予　谷　涛　汪　晶　沈　琴　张　雯　张世军　张华为　张卓璐
张铁群　张秋丽　陈　穹　陈　珑　陈　娟　陈仰纯　陈丽舟　陈佳妮　陈珊珊　陈勇春　陈紫琪
陈榆舒　周　帆　周　璐　周大勇　郑　铤　郑葵葵　赵　振　赵　添　赵　赫　赵又瑾　胡立斌
南海燕　柏盈盈　费京乐　姚　旬　姚　骊　贺延莉　贺迎坤　骆永恒　聂　芳　贾中芝　高　杨
曹玉坤　常　娣　彭丹丹　彭程宇　彭新桂　蒋京真　韩　宇　韩世龙　程　瑾　程爱萍　舒胜雷
谢　弘　靳　勇　路　莉　管　婧　潘春树　薛　艺

审　校（按姓氏笔画排序）

丁宁宁　丁铁钢　马宏星　王　玉　王　伟　王　超　王　蓉　王苗苗　王维平　王斯妮　王焱钧
毛志群　卞益同　卢　阳　代　岳　朱晓黎　刘　哲　刘　莹　刘　慧　严承功　李华莉　李贤军
李超伦　杨　玲　杨　健　吴　静　吴汉平　邱　婷　汪　晶　张　雯　张月浪　张龙江　张卓璐
张铁群　张秋丽　张毅力　陈　穹　陈晓曦　郑丽丽　郑葵葵　赵　杰　赵　振　赵　赫　赵大兵
胡红杰　南海燕　姚　旬　贺延莉　贺迎坤　贾中芝　郭文君　唐　静　曹玉坤　常　娣　彭程宇
董　方　董伟华　韩曙光　程　瑾　程芝梅　程爱萍　舒胜雷　舒晓军　谢　弘　谢双双　楼海亚
楼敏超　赖　灿　雷子乔　路　莉　蔚　蓝　潘春树

各章翻译团队

1 胸部影像

章节负责人　南海燕

翻　译　孙颖志　南海燕　王维平　韩　宇　于　瀛

审　校　谢双双　贾中芝　吴汉平

总审校　南海燕　王维平

2 胃肠道影像

章节负责人　赵　振

翻　译　王亚玲　蒋京真　常　娣　聂　芳　彭丹丹　张世军　王　玉　赵　振　卢　瞳　柏盈盈

审　校　李超伦　程芝梅　常　娣　王　玉　赵　振

总审校　谢双双　王维平

3 泌尿生殖影像

章节负责人　程　瑾

翻　译　王斯妮　陈　穹　张卓璐　严承功　许　倩　全杰蓉　姚　旬　孙明菡　程　瑾　王维平

审　校　张月浪　杨　玲　董伟华　谢双双　贾中芝　王　玉　姚　旬　李华莉　张卓璐　王　蓉　邱　婷　韩曙光　代　岳　王斯妮　陈　穹　赵大兵　严承功

总审校　程　瑾　王维平

4 产科影像

章节负责人　吴艳艳

翻　译　吴艳艳

审　校　吴汉平　蔚　蓝　郑丽丽　程芝梅　贾中芝　楼海亚

总审校　王维平

5 乳腺影像

章节负责人　贺延莉　彭程宇

翻　译　王维平　阳宁静　彭程宇　贺延莉　王草叶　杨学刚

审　校　贺延莉　彭程宇　刘　莹　程芝梅　张毅力　刘　慧　路　莉　贾中芝

总审校　丁铁钢　王维平

6 核医学与分子影像

章节负责人　陈绍亮

翻　译　王维平　马宏星　李蓓蕾　程爱萍　陈仰纯　许长德

审　校　谢双双　吴汉平　贾中芝　程爱萍　卢　阳　马宏星　郑丽丽　程芝梅

总审校　王维平

7 心脏影像

章节负责人　汪　晶

翻　译　王维平　高　杨　杨　明　舒胜雷　孙　欣　杨宏远　曹玉坤　费京乐　汪　晶

审　校　谢双双　董伟华　贾中芝　舒胜雷　曹玉坤

总审校　汪　晶　胡红杰　王维平

8 血管影像

章节负责人　张龙江

翻　译　薛　艺　卢陈英　周　帆　谷　涛　陈　珑　许棚棚　吴汉平　贾中芝　全杰蓉

审　校　张龙江　贾中芝　董伟华

总审校　舒晓军　王维平

9 介入放射学

章节负责人　赵　赫

翻　译　李　西　吴志远　赵　赫　吴汉平　仲斌演　周大勇　胡立斌　朱晓黎　靳　勇　杨国威　韩世龙　张　雯

审　校　董伟华　吴汉平　程芝梅　朱晓黎　张　雯

总审校　赵　赫　王维平

10 神经影像：大脑

章节负责人　郑葵葵

翻　译　张铁群　贺迎坤　王苗苗　杨　晶　王维平　王草叶　张秋丽　王　超　潘春树　杨喜彪　陈勇春　吴　静

审　校　张月浪　王焱钧　潘春树　王苗苗　张秋丽　丁宁宁　王　伟　张铁群　程芝梅　吴　静　贺迎坤

总审校　郑葵葵　王维平

11 神经影像：头与颈

章节负责人　吴　静

翻　译　陈珊珊　骆永恒　管　婧　赵　添　沈　琴　郑葵葵　陈　娟　何　予　祁　丽　马　聪　吴　静

审　校　王　超　贾中芝　杨　健

总审校　郑葵葵　王维平

12 脊柱影像

章节负责人 杨 健

翻 译 王维平 卞益同

审 校 王焱钧 程芝梅 贾中芝 卞益同
楼敏超

总审校 杨 健 郑葵葵 王维平

13 骨骼与肌肉影像

章节负责人 唐 静

翻 译 姚 骊 吕霞飞 陈紫琪 陈丽舟
帅丹丹 刘杰克 杨曦玥 彭新桂
苏筱芮 赵又瑾 刘 进 张华为
陈榆舒

审 校 吴汉平 贾中芝

总审校 唐 静 王维平

14 小儿影像

章节负责人 赖 灿 郭文君

翻 译 周 璐 路 莉 谢 弘 陈佳妮
邱 伟 毛志群 吴桂鹏

审 校 赖 灿 贾中芝 程芝梅 郑葵葵
谢双双 程 瑾 丁宁宁 陈晓曦
路 莉 谢 弘 南海燕 毛志群

总审校 郭文君 王维平

15 影像物理

章节负责人 郑 铤

翻 译 于 千 郑 铤

审 校 吴汉平 董伟华 雷子乔 贾中芝
刘 哲 赵 杰 李贤军 王 玉

总审校 董 方 王维平

译者前言

《核心放射学：影像诊断图解教程》由哈佛大学住院医师团队倾力编撰，全面覆盖临床影像学的核心知识，包括常规放射诊断、超声、介入、核医学及放射物理等领域，体现了美国放射学委员会对住院医师培养的要求与指导方针，突显全面掌握影像学基础的重要性。自问世以来，本书迅速赢得放射影像住院医师的高度评价与广泛青睐。

自2017年第一版以中英文对照的形式出版以来，本书受到国内影像医学界的高度认可，成为住院医师学习与参考的重要教材。本书适用于医学影像各亚专业，中英文对照的编排形式不仅可帮助读者突破专业英语障碍，深入理解专业知识与术语，并提升医学英语的阅读和理解能力，还能拓宽视野，助力终身学习与自主提升。

原著第二版在第一版的基础上扩充了近三分之一的内容。翻译团队历经三年多潜心打磨，力求忠实于原文，从字句到段落皆追求精益求精，确保中文表达精准流畅，同时保留中英文对照的特色，使读者无论阅读中文还是英文，都能获得全面而专业的信息与知识。

本版翻译团队的大部分成员曾参与第一版翻译工作，他们现在已是影像医学各亚专业的青年专家与学者。在此，谨向每位译者致以诚挚的感谢！

本书旨在借鉴国际先进理念与经验，助力我国放射影像住院医师的规范化培训，为有志于投身医学影像事业的年轻医师奠定坚实的专业基础。我们期待本书能够帮助年轻医师在迈向医学影像领域的征途中，自信地站在国际前沿，为更多患者提供卓越的医疗服务，同时在国际舞台上展现中国医学影像的风采。

王维平

2025年1月

CONTRIBUTORS 编者

Ayaz Aghayev, MD
Staff Radiologist, Division of Cardiovascular Imaging,
Brigham and Women's Hospital
Instructor of Radiology,
Harvard Medical School

Sharath Bhagavatula, MD
Staff Radiologist, Abdominal Imaging and Intervention,
Brigham and Women's Hospital
Instructor of Radiology,
Harvard Medical School

Michael A. Buckner, MD
Resident in Radiology,
Brigham and Women's Hospital
Harvard Medical School

Leigh Casadaban, MD MS
Clinical Fellow in Interventional Radiology,
University of California, Los Angeles Medical Center
David Geffen School of Medicine

Francis Deng, MD
Resident in Radiology,
Massachusetts General Hospital
Harvard Medical School

Christine M. Denison, MD
Staff Radiologist, Division of Breast Imaging,
Brigham and Women's Hospital
Assistant Professor of Radiology,
Harvard Medical School

Madhvi Deol, MD
Resident in Radiology,
Brigham and Women's Hospital
Harvard Medical School

Khanant M. Desai, MD
Clinical Fellow in Interventional Radiology,
University of Virginia Medical Center

Sharmila Dorbala, MD
Director of Nuclear Cardiology,
Division of Cardiovascular Imaging,
Brigham and Women's Hospital
Associate Professor of Radiology,
Harvard Medical School

Mary C. Frates, MD
Assistant Director, Division of Ultrasound,
Brigham and Women's Hospital
Professor of Radiology,
Harvard Medical School

Michael P. George, MD
Staff Pediatric Radiologist,
Boston Children's Hospital
Instructor of Radiology,
Harvard Medical School

Colette Martin Glaser, MD
Resident in Radiology,
Brigham and Women's Hospital
Harvard Medical School

Robin Perlmutter-Goldenson, MD, MPH
Staff Radiologist, Division of Ultrasound,
Brigham and Women's Hospital
Assistant Professor of Radiology,
Harvard Medical School

Jeffrey P. Guenette, MD
Director of Head and Neck Imaging,
Division of Neuroradiology
Associate Program Director, Diagnostic Radiology Residency
Brigham and Women's Hospital
Assistant Professor of Radiology,
Harvard Medical School

Mark M. Hammer, MD
Thoracic Imaging Fellowship Director,
Brigham and Women's Hospital
Assistant Professor of Radiology,
Harvard Medical School

Raymond Y. Huang, MD, PhD
Assistant Division Chief, Division of Neuroradiology
Brigham and Women's Hospital
Associate Professor of Radiology
Harvard Medical School

Hyewon Hyun, MD
Program Director, Joint Program in Nuclear Medicine and Molecular Imaging,
Brigham and Women's Hospital
Assistant Professor of Radiology,
Harvard Medical School

Aaron Jen, MD
Resident in Radiology,
Brigham and Women's Hospital
Harvard Medical School

Khushboo Jhala, MD
Resident in Radiology,
Brigham and Women's Hospital
Harvard Medical School

Timothy P. Killoran, MD
Integrated and Independent Interventional Radiology Residency Director,
Brigham and Women's Hospital
Assistant Professor of Radiology,
Harvard Medical School

Regina Maria Koch, MD
Staff Radiologist, Interventional Radiology,
Brigham and Women's Hospital
Instructor of Radiology,
Harvard Medical School

Jose M. Lopez, MD, MBA
Resident in Radiology,
Brigham and Women's Hospital
Harvard Medical School

Yuntong Ma, MD
Resident in Radiology,
Brigham and Women's Hospital
Harvard Medical School

Fiona E. Malone, MD
Resident in Radiology,
Brigham and Women's Hospital
Harvard Medical School

Jacob Mandell, MD
Musculoskeletal Imaging and Intervention Fellowship Director,
Brigham and Women's Hospital
Assistant Professor of Radiology,
Harvard Medical School

Shanna A. Matalon, MD
Staff Radiologist, Division of Abdominal Imaging and Intervention,
Associate Program Director, Radiology Residency,
Brigham and Women's Hospital
Assistant Professor of Radiology,
Harvard Medical School

Shruti Mishra, MD
Resident in Radiology,
Brigham and Women's Hospital
Harvard Medical School

Nityanand Miskin, MD
Clinical Fellow in Neuroradiology,
Massachusetts General Hospital
Harvard Medical School

Steven Morales-Rivera, MD
Resident in Radiology,
Brigham and Women's Hospital
Harvard Medical School

Sanjay P. Prabhu, MBBS, DCH, FRCR
Staff Pediatric Neuroradiologist,
Director, Advanced Image Analysis Lab,
Medical Director, Imaging Informatics
Boston Children's Hospital
Assistant Professor of Radiology,
Harvard Medical School

Cory Robinson-Weiss, MD
Clinical Fellow in Abdominal Imaging,
Massachusetts General Hospital
Harvard Medical School

Christopher G. Sakellis, MD
Staff Radiologist, Division of Nuclear Medicine,
Brigham and Women's Hospital
Assistant Professor of Radiology,
Harvard Medical School

Junzi Shi, MD
Clinical Fellow in Musculoskeletal Radiology,
Brigham and Women's Hospital
Harvard Medical School

Daniel Souza, MD, MSc
Fellowship Program Director, Abdominal Imaging and Intervention,
Brigham and Women's Hospital
Instructor of Radiology,
Harvard Medical School

Ellen X. Sun, MD
Staff Radiologist, Division of Emergency Radiology,
Brigham and Women's Hospital
Instructor of Radiology,
Harvard Medical School

Michael L. Steigner,
Staff Radiologist, Division of Cardiovascular Imaging,
Brigham and Women's Hospital
Associate Professor of Radiology,
Harvard Medical School

Ngoc-Anh T. Tran, MD
Resident in Radiology,
Brigham and Women's Hospital
Harvard Medical School

CONTENTS

目录

1 Thoracic Imaging

Khushboo Jhala, Junzi Shi, Mark M. Hammer

1 胸部影像

Contents

目录

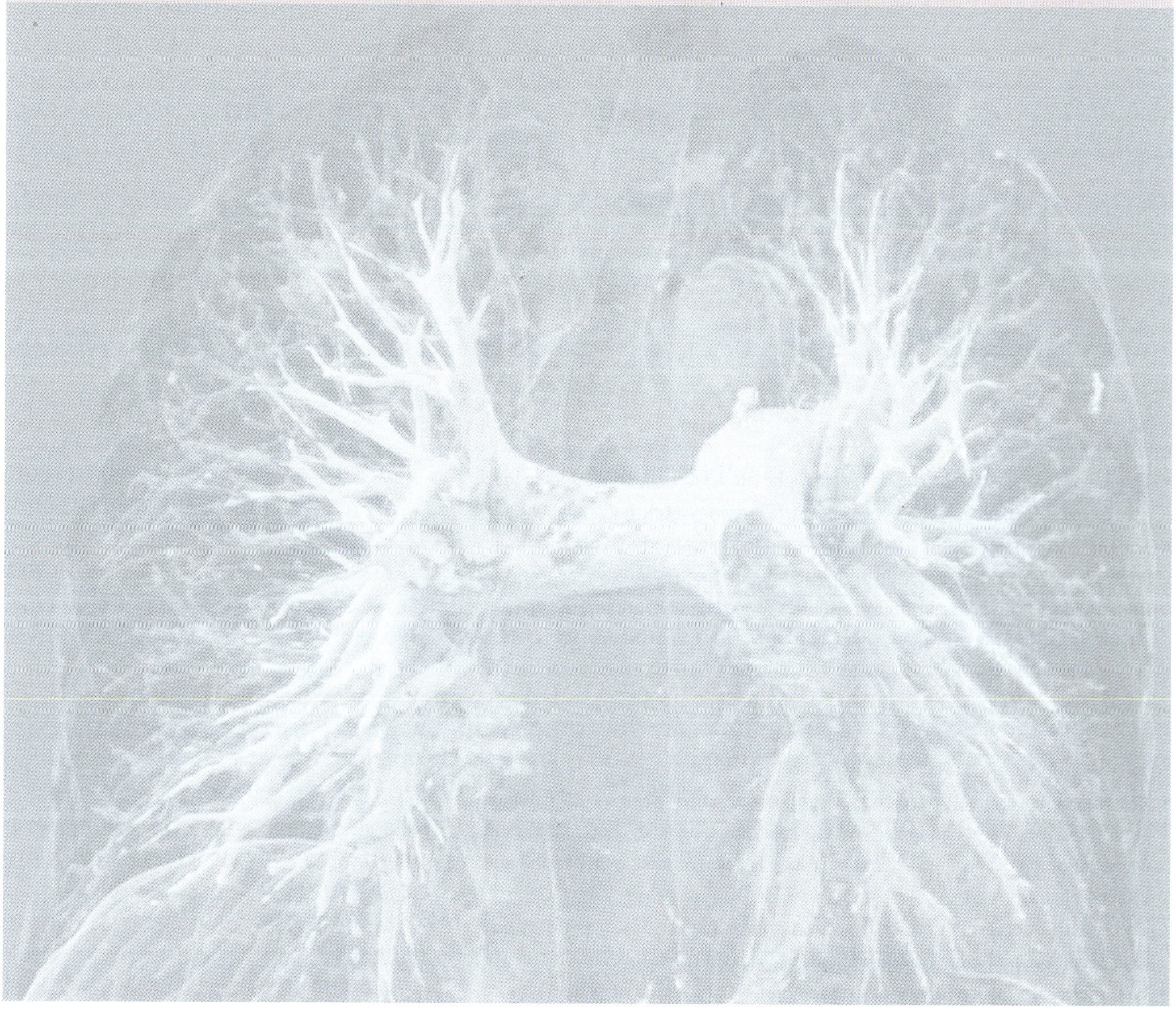

INTRODUCTORY CONCEPTS

概念介绍

ANATOMY

解剖

Lobar and segmental anatomy

肺叶和肺段解剖

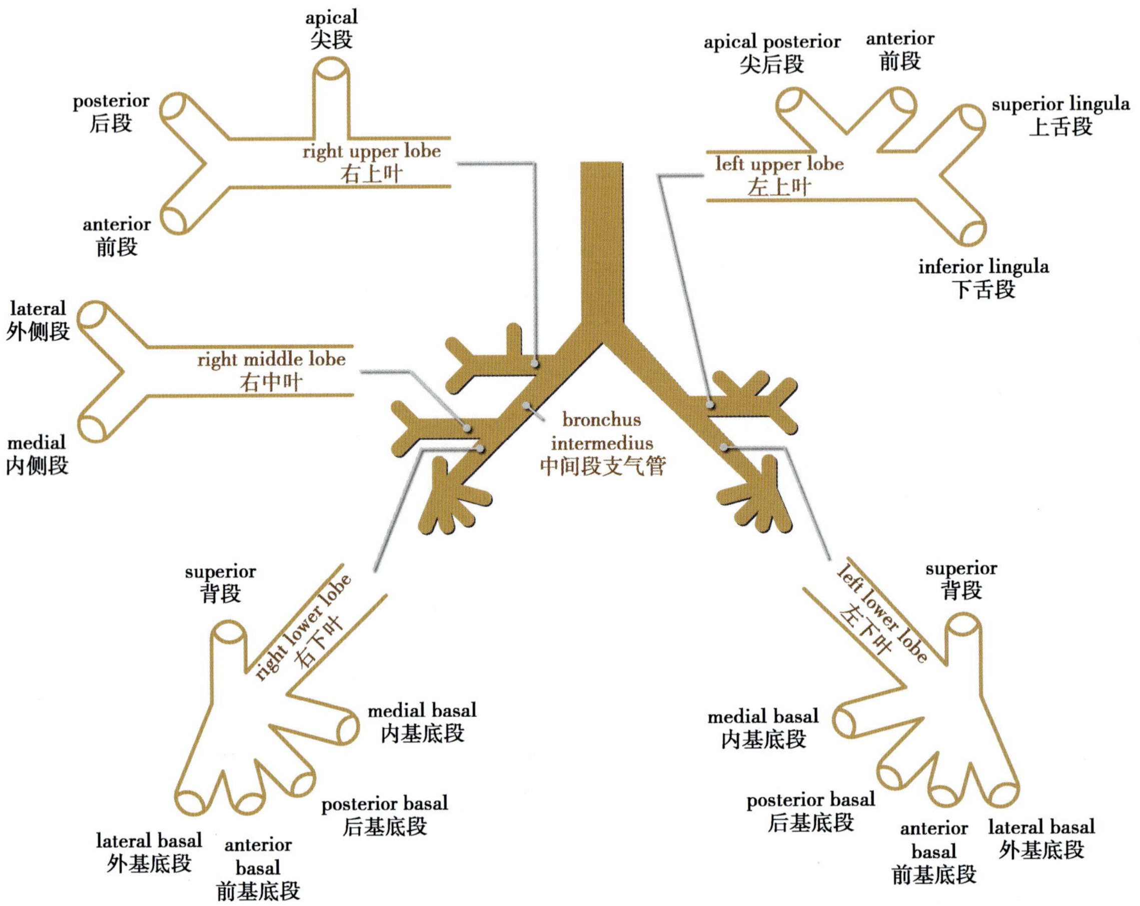

Interlobar fissures

- The minor fissure separates the right upper lobe (RUL) from the right middle lobe (RML) and is seen on both the frontal and lateral views as a fine horizontal line.
- The major (oblique) fissures are seen only on the lateral radiograph as oblique lines. However, if they are fluid-filled, the major fissures can be seen on the frontal view as concave curvilinear opacities in the lateral hemithorax.

  On the right, the major fissure separates the RUL and RML from the right lower lobe.

  On the left, the major fissure separates the left upper lobe (LUL) from the left lower lobe (LLL).

叶间裂

- 水平裂将右肺上叶(RUL)与右肺中叶(RML)分开，在正、侧位胸部X线影像上均显示为一条水平的细线。
- 斜裂仅见于侧位胸部X线影像，为一条斜线。然而，如果有叶间裂积液，斜裂也可在正位X线影像上呈现为一侧胸部的线样凹性致密影。

  在右肺，斜裂将右肺上叶、中叶与下叶分开。

  在左肺，斜裂将左肺上叶与下叶分开。

Accessory fissures

- The azygos fissure is an accessory fissure present in less than 1% of patients, seen in the presence of an azygos lobe. An azygos lobe is an anatomic variant where a portion of the apical right upper lobe is encased in its own parietal and visceral pleura.
- The superior accessory fissure is seen in approximately 5% of patients and separates the superior and basal segments of the right lower lobe.
- The inferior accessory fissure is seen in approximately 12% of patients, more

副裂

- 奇裂是一个副裂，发生率小于1%，见于有奇叶的患者。奇叶是一种解剖变异，为右肺尖的一部分肺组织被其脏层与壁层胸膜包绕而成。
- 上副裂见于约5%的患者，分隔右肺下叶背段和基底段。
- 下副裂见于约12%的患者，多见于右肺，将内

commonly in the right lung, and divides the medial basal segment from the other basal segments.

- The left minor fissure is present in approximately 8% of patients and separates the lingula from the left upper lobe.

Overview of Atelectasis

- Atelectasis is loss of lung volume due to decreased aeration. Atelectasis is synonymous with collapse. Atelectasis may be caused by bronchial obstruction, mucus plugging, or external compression (e.g., by small lung volumes or pleural effusions).
- Direct signs of atelectasis are from lobar volume loss and include:

Displacement of the fissures. Plate-like or triangular opacity from the collapsed lung itself.	Vascular crowding.

- Indirect signs of atelectasis are due to the effect of volume loss on adjacent structures and include:

Elevation of the diaphragm. Rib crowding on the side with volume loss. Mediastinal shift to the side with volume loss.	Overinflation of adjacent or contralateral lobes. Hilar displacement.

- Air bronchograms are *not* seen in atelectasis when the cause of the atelectasis is central bronchial obstruction, but air bronchograms can be seen in atelectasis caused by external compression.

Mechanisms of atelectasis

- **Obstructive** atelectasis occurs when alveolar gas is absorbed by blood circulating through alveolar capillaries but is not replaced by inspired air due to bronchial obstruction.

  Obstructive atelectasis can cause lobar atelectasis, which is complete collapse of a lobe, discussed on the following pages.

  Obstructive atelectasis occurs more quickly when the patient is breathing supplemental oxygen since oxygen is absorbed from the alveoli more rapidly than nitrogen.

  In children, airway obstruction is most often due to an aspirated foreign object. In contrast to adults, the affected side becomes hyperexpanded in children due to a ball-valve effect.

  Subsegmental atelectasis is a subtype of obstructive atelectasis commonly seen after surgery or general illness, due to mucus obstruction of the small airways.

- **Relaxation** (passive) atelectasis is caused by relaxation of lung adjacent to an intrathoracic lesion causing mass effect, such as a pleural effusion, pneumothorax, or pulmonary mass.
- **Adhesive** atelectasis is due to surfactant deficiency.

  Adhesive atelectasis is seen most commonly in neonatal respiratory distress syndrome, but can also be seen in acute respiratory distress syndrome (ARDS).

- **Cicatricial** atelectasis is volume loss from architectural distortion of lung parenchyma by fibrosis.

Lobar Atelectasis

- Lobar atelectasis is usually caused by central bronchial obstruction (obstructive atelectasis), which may be secondary to mucus plugging or an obstructing neoplasm.

基底段与其他基底段分开。

- 左侧水平裂约出现在8%的患者，将舌段与左肺上叶分开。

肺不张概述

- 肺不张是指由于通气下降引起的肺容积减少，不张与萎陷是同义词。肺不张可由支气管阻塞、黏液堵塞或外部压迫(如肺容量小或胸腔积液)引起。
- 肺不张的直接征象来自肺叶容积减少，包括：

叶间裂移位。 肺萎陷本身形成的片状或三角形密度增高影。	血管聚拢。

- 肺不张的间接征象来自肺容积减少对邻近结构的影响，包括：

横膈上抬。 患侧肋骨聚拢。 纵隔向患侧移位。	邻近肺叶或对侧肺过度膨胀。 肺门移位。

- 空气支气管征不出现在中央支气管阻塞引起的肺不张，但可见于外压性肺不张。

肺不张的机制

- **阻塞性**肺不张是由于肺泡内的气体被通过肺泡毛细血管循环的血液所吸收，但因支气管阻塞不能从吸入的空气中进行补充。

  阻塞性肺不张可导致肺叶不张，为一个肺叶的完全萎陷，将在下文讨论。

  阻塞性肺不张在辅助供氧的患者中发生更快，因为肺泡内的氧气比氮气吸收更快。

  在儿童，气道阻塞最常见的原因是吸入异物。与成人相比，儿童患侧肺会由于球阀效应而过度膨胀。

  亚段不张是阻塞性肺不张的一个亚型，常见于术后或全身性疾病，由小气道黏液阻塞引起。

- **松弛性**(被动性)肺不张是由胸内具有占位效应的病变造成邻近肺组织松弛而引起的不张，如胸腔积液、气胸或肺部肿块引起的肺不张。
- **粘连性**肺不张由肺泡表面活性物质缺乏导致。

  粘连性肺不张最常见于新生儿呼吸窘迫综合征，但也可见于急性呼吸窘迫综合征(ARDS)。

- **瘢痕性**肺不张是纤维化导致的肺实质结构扭曲所造成的肺容积减少。

肺叶不张

- 肺叶不张通常是由中央支气管阻塞(阻塞性肺不张)引起，可继发于黏液堵塞或阻塞性肿瘤。

  如果发生急性肺叶不张，黏液堵塞是最可能的

If the lobar atelectasis occurs acutely, mucus plugging is the most likely cause.

Mucus plugging is most common in the lower lobes, least common in the left upper lobe.

If lobar atelectasis is seen in an outpatient, an obstructing central tumor must be ruled out.

- Lobar atelectasis, or collapse of an entire lobe, has characteristic appearances depending on which of the five lobes is collapsed, as discussed on the following pages.

原因。

黏液堵塞最常见于肺的下叶，左肺上叶最少见。

如果肺叶不张见于门诊患者，必须排除阻塞性中央型肿瘤。

- 肺叶不张或整个肺叶的萎陷有特征性表现，取决于五个肺叶中的哪一个发生了萎陷，如下文所述。

Patterns of lobar atelectasis

肺叶不张的表现形式

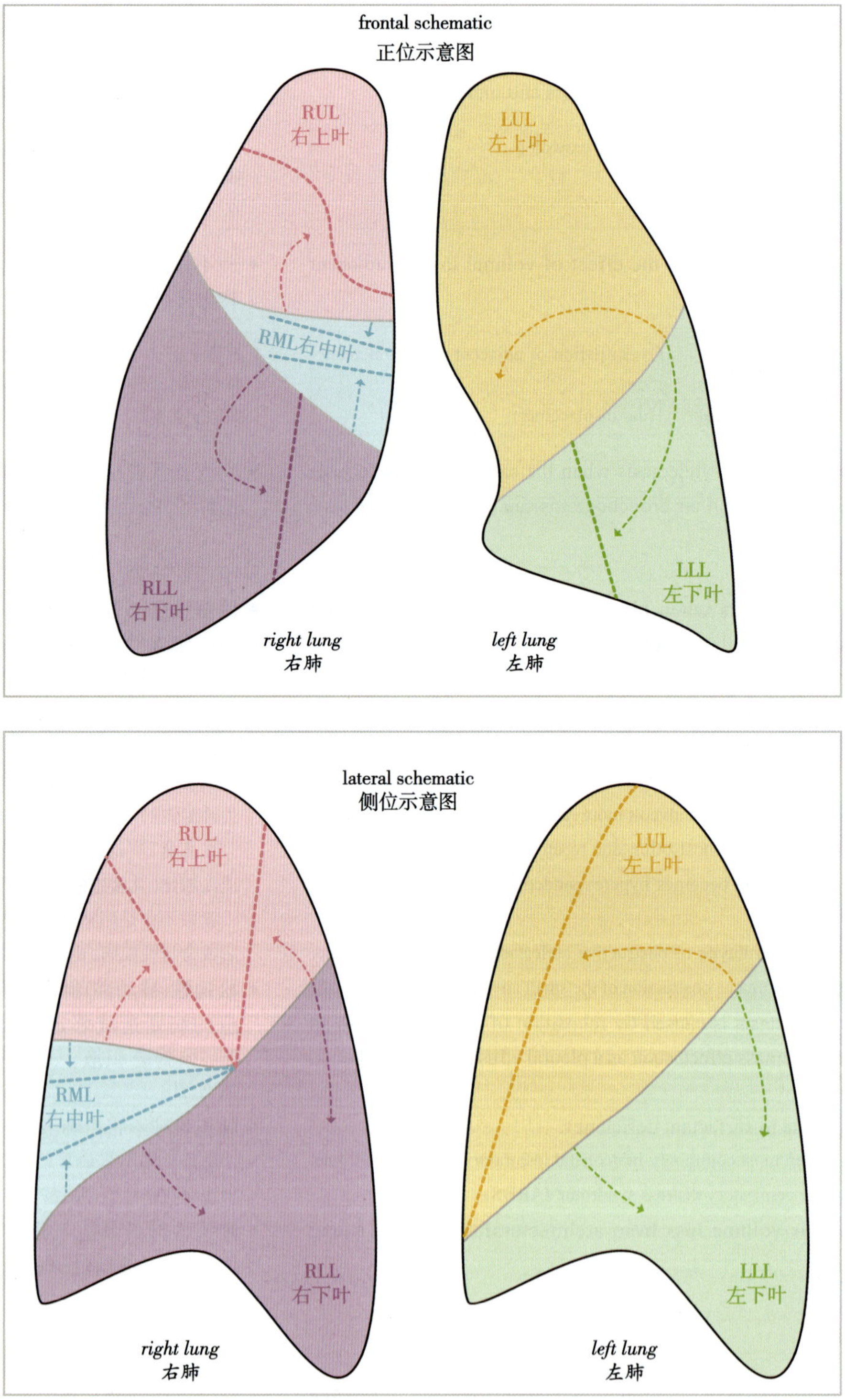

Illustration showing direction of collapse for each of the five lobes.
图示五个肺叶各自的萎陷方向。

Left upper lobe atelectasis

左肺上叶不张

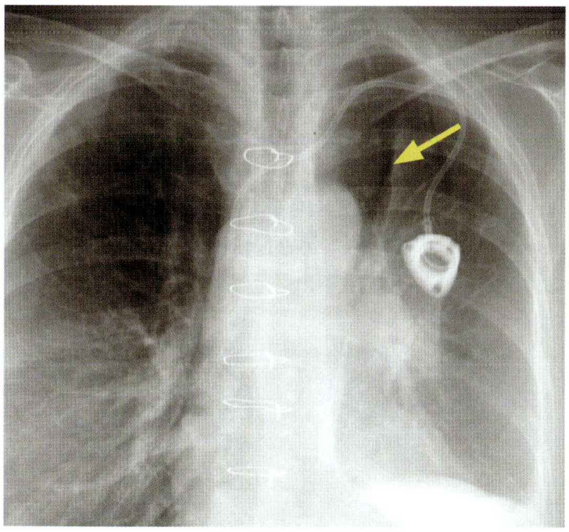
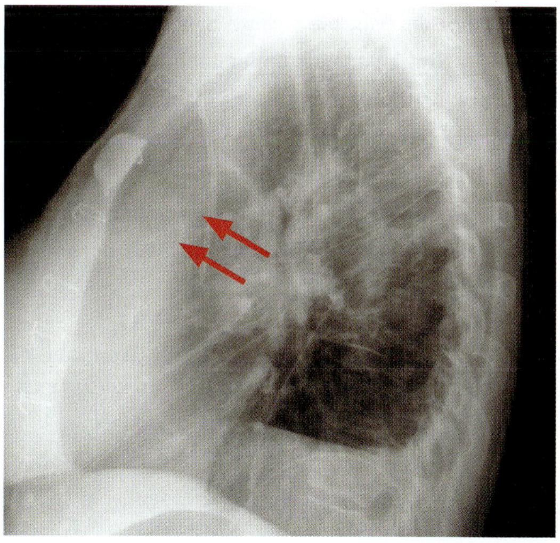

Left upper lobe collapse and *luftsichel sign*: Frontal radiograph (left image) shows veil-like opacity with obscured left cardiac margin, a characteristic finding of left upper lobe collapse on frontal view; note the crescent of air lateral to the aortic arch representing the *luftsichel sign* (yellow arrow). The lateral view (right image) shows the anterior displacement of the left major fissure and collapsed left upper lobe (red arrows).

左肺上叶萎陷和气镰征：正位X线影像(左图)显示面纱状阴影伴左心缘模糊，是左肺上叶萎陷在正位X线影像上的特征性表现；注意主动脉弓外侧的新月形气体影为气镰征(黄箭)。侧位X线影像(右图)显示左侧斜裂前移和左肺上叶萎陷(红箭)。

- Key imaging findings include the veil-like opacity on frontal radiograph, anterior displacement of major fissure and anterior collapsed lung on lateral radiograph.
- The *luftsichel* (*air-sickle* in German) *sign* is a crescent of air seen on the frontal radiograph, which represents the interface between the aorta and the hyperexpanded superior segment of the left lower lobe. However, this sign is not always present.
- It is important to recognize left upper lobe collapse and not mistake the left lung opacity for pneumonia or pleural effusion, since a mass obstructing the airway may be the cause of the lobar atelectasis.

- 主要影像学表现包括正位X线影像上的面纱状阴影、侧位X线影像上的斜裂前移和前部萎陷的肺。
- 气镰(德语中的“*Luftsichel*”意为空气镰刀的意思)征是正位X线影像上见到的新月形气体影，代表主动脉和过度膨胀的左肺下叶背段的交界面。然而，这种征象并不总是存在。
- 识别左肺上叶不张非常重要，不要将左肺面纱状阴影误认为肺炎或胸腔积液，因为阻塞气道的肿块可能是造成肺叶不张的原因。

Right upper lobe atelectasis

右肺上叶不张

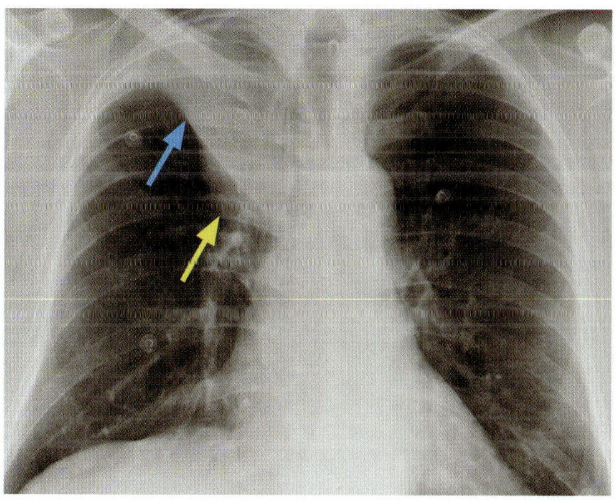
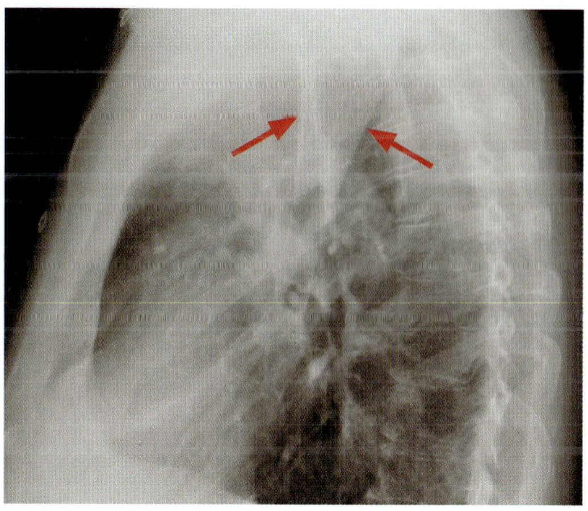

Right upper lobe collapse: Frontal radiograph (left image) shows a right upper lobe opacity with superior displacement of the minor fissure (blue arrow) and a convex mass (*Golden S sign*; yellow arrow). Lateral radiograph (right image) shows the wedge-shaped collapsed RUL projecting superiorly (red arrows).

右肺上叶不张：正位X线影像(左图)显示右肺上叶阴影伴水平裂上移(蓝箭)和一个隆凸肿块(Golden S征，黄箭)。侧位X线影像(右图)显示投影在上部的楔形不张的右上肺(红箭)。

- The *reverse S sign of Golden* is seen in right upper lobe collapse caused by an obstructing mass. The central convex margins of the mass form a reverse S. Although the sign describes a *reverse* S, it is also commonly known as the *Golden S sign*. Similar to left upper lobe collapse, a right upper lobe collapse should raise concern for an underlying malignancy in adults or mucus plugging, particularly common in children.
- The *juxtaphrenic peak sign* is a peridiaphragmatic triangular opacity caused by diaphragmatic traction from an inferior accessory fissure or an inferior pulmonary ligament, seen in upper lobe volume loss from any cause.

Left lower lobe atelectasis

- Golden反S征见于阻塞性肿块导致的右肺上叶不张。中央隆凸的肿块边缘形成反S形，此征象描述为反S，不过通常被称为Golden S征。与左肺上叶不张类似，右肺上叶不张在成人需考虑恶性肿瘤，在儿童则是黏液栓塞更为常见。
- 膈上尖峰征是膈旁三角形高密度影，为横膈被下副裂或下肺韧带牵拉所致，见于任何原因导致的上叶容积减少。

左肺下叶不张

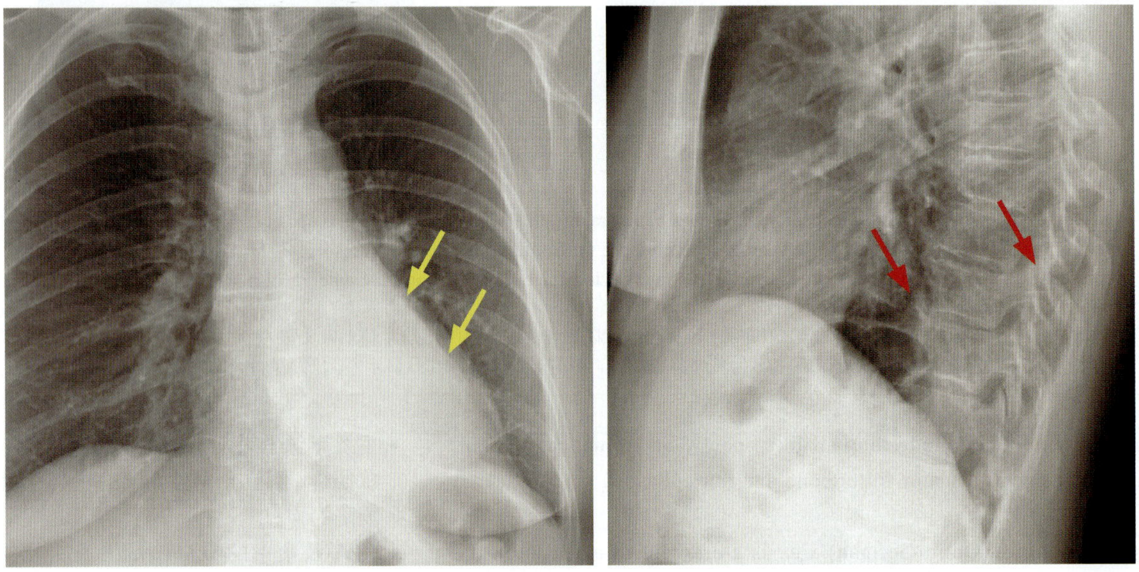

Left lower lobe collapse: Frontal radiographs demonstrate a triangular retrocardiac opacity representing the collapsed left lower lobe (yellow arrows). Lateral radiograph shows posterior hazy opacity (red arrows).
左肺下叶不张：正位X线影像(左图)显示有三角形心后高密度影，代表萎陷的左肺下叶(黄箭)。侧位X线影像(右图)显示后部模糊的高密度影(红箭)。

- Triangular retrocardiac opacity is the main imaging feature of left lower lobe collapse.
- The *flat waist sign* describes the flattening of the left heart border due to posterior shift of hilar structures and resultant cardiac rotation.

- 三角形心后高密度影是左肺下叶不张最主要的影像学特征。
- 平腰征指左心缘变平，由肺门结构后移引起的心脏旋转造成。

Right lower lobe atelectasis

右肺下叶不张

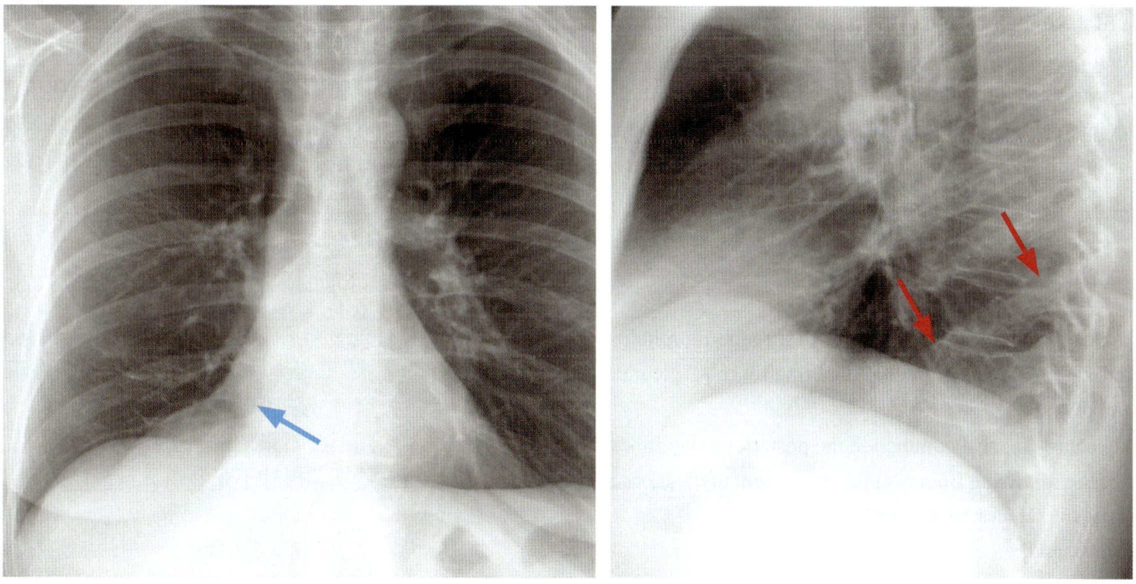

Right lower lobe collapse: Frontal radiograph shows a triangular opacity at the right lower zone with apex pointing towards the right hilum and obscuration of the medial right hemidiaphragm (blue arrow). Note there is preservation of the right heart border. Lateral radiograph shows a hazy posterior opacity of the collapsed right lower lobe (red arrows).
右肺下叶不张：正位X线影像显示右肺下野三角形高密度影，尖端指向肺门，右侧横膈内侧模糊(蓝箭)。注意右心缘不受累。侧位X线影像显示后部模糊的高密度影，是萎陷的右肺下叶(红箭)。

- Right lower lobe atelectasis is the mirror-image of left lower lobe atelectasis. Lower lobe collapse is not well-seen on lateral view since the lobes mostly collapse medially.
- The collapsed lower lobe appears as a triangular retrocardiac opacity.

- 右肺下叶不张是左肺下叶不张的镜像表现。下叶不张在侧位X线影像上显示不清，因为下叶大多向内侧萎陷。
- 不张的下叶表现为一个三角形心后高密度影。

Right middle lobe atelectasis

右肺中叶不张

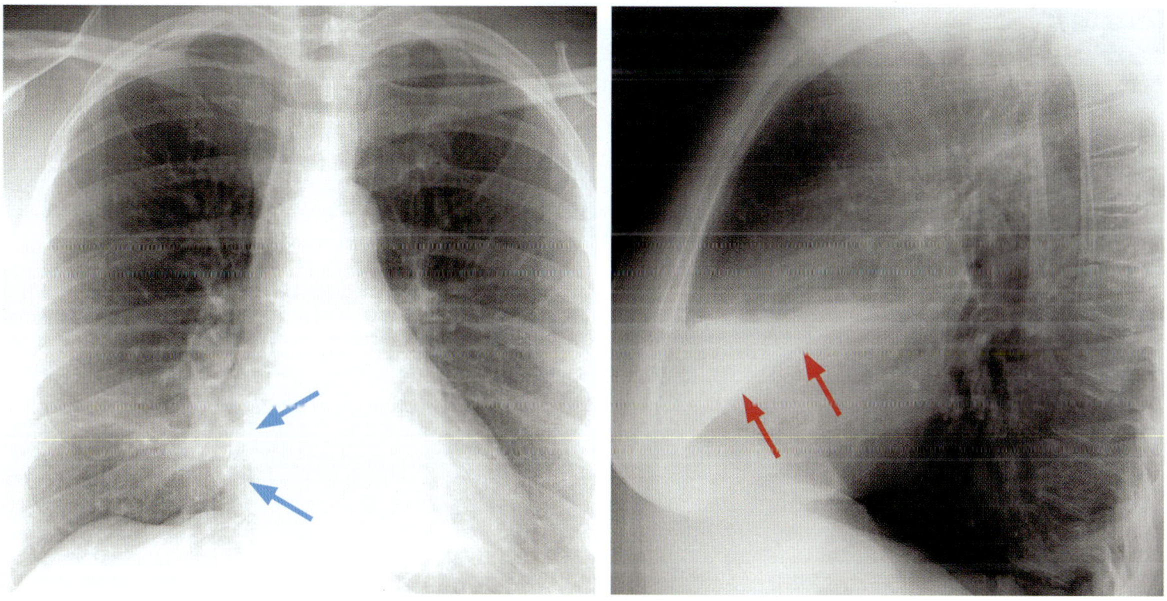

Right middle lobe atelectasis: Frontal chest radiograph shows an indistinct opacity in the right lung with focal silhouetting of the right heart border (blue arrows). There is elevation of the right hemidiaphragm due to volume loss. The lateral radiograph shows a triangular opacity (red arrow) projecting over the mid-heart representing the collapsed right middle lobe.
右肺中叶不张：正位胸部X线影像显示右肺模糊的密度增高影与右心缘局部分界不清(蓝箭)；右侧膈肌因右肺容积减少而抬高。侧位X线影像显示投射在心影中部一个三角形高密度影(红箭)，代表不张的右肺中叶。

- The findings of right middle lobe atelectasis can be subtle on the frontal radiograph. Silhouetting of the right heart border by the collapsed medial segment of the middle lobe may be the only clue. The lateral radiograph shows a triangular opacity anteriorly.
- Collapse of both right middle and lower lobes occurs from obstruction of the bronchus intermedius, and it causes obscuration of both the right heart border and right hemidiaphragm, with a linear superior margin directed towards the hilum.

- 右肺中叶不张在正位X线影像上表现不明显。唯一的线索可能是右肺中叶内侧段萎陷导致的右心缘模糊。侧位X线影像显示前部的三角形高密度影。
- 右肺中叶和下叶同时塌陷是由中间段支气管阻塞引起，这会导致右心缘和右半膈模糊，同时在影像上可见一个指向肺门的线样肺上缘。

Round atelectasis

- Round atelectasis is focal atelectasis with a round morphology that is *always* associated with an adjacent pleural abnormality (e.g., pleural effusion, pleural thickening or plaque).
- Round atelectasis is most common in the posterior lower lobes.
- All five of the following findings must be present to diagnose round atelectasis:
  1) Adjacent pleura must be abnormal.
  2) Opacity must be peripheral and in contact with the pleura.
  3) Opacity must be round or elliptical.
  4) Volume loss must be present in the affected lobe.
  5) Pulmonary vessels and bronchi leading into the opacity must be curved — this is the *comet tail sign*.

圆形肺不张

- 圆形肺不张是一个形态呈圆形的局灶性肺不张，总伴有邻近胸膜异常(如胸腔积液、胸膜增厚或胸膜斑块)。
- 圆形肺不张最常见于肺下叶的后部。
- 诊断圆形肺不张必须具备5个条件：
  1) 邻近胸膜必须异常。
  2) 高密度影必须位于外周并与胸膜接触。
  3) 高密度影必须为圆形或椭圆形。
  4) 受累肺叶必须有容积减少。
  5) 通向高密度影的肺血管和支气管必须是弯曲的——*彗星尾征*。

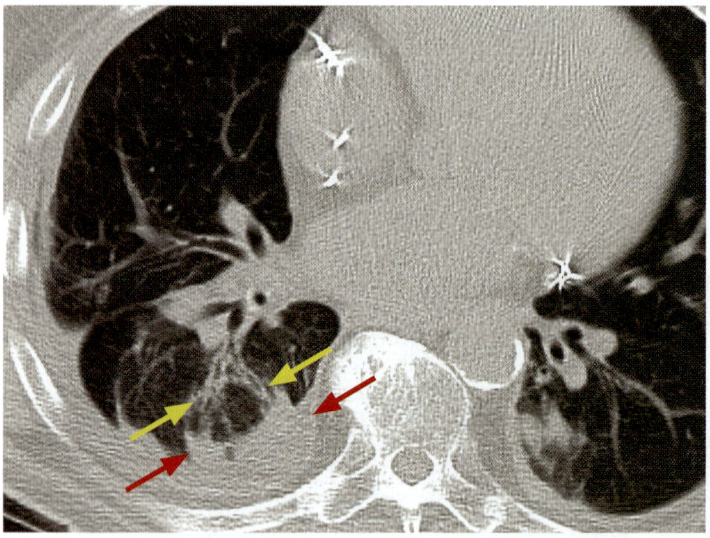

Round atelectasis: Noncontrast CT shows a rounded opacity in the medial right lower lobe (red arrows). This example meets all five criteria for round atelectasis including adjacent pleural abnormality (effusion), opacity in contact with the pleura, round shape, volume loss in the affected lobe, and the *comet tail sign* (yellow arrows) representing curved vessels and bronchi leading to the focus of round atelectasis.

圆形肺不张：平扫CT显示右肺下叶内侧圆形高密度影(红箭)。本例符合圆形肺不张的5个诊断标准，包括邻近胸膜异常(积液)、高密度影与胸膜接触、圆形、受累肺叶容积减少，以及*彗星尾征*(黄箭)，后者为弯曲的血管和支气管指向圆形肺不张的中心。

(翻译　孙颖志)

ESSENTIAL ANATOMY

基础解剖

Secondary pulmonary lobule (SPL)

次级肺小叶(SPL)

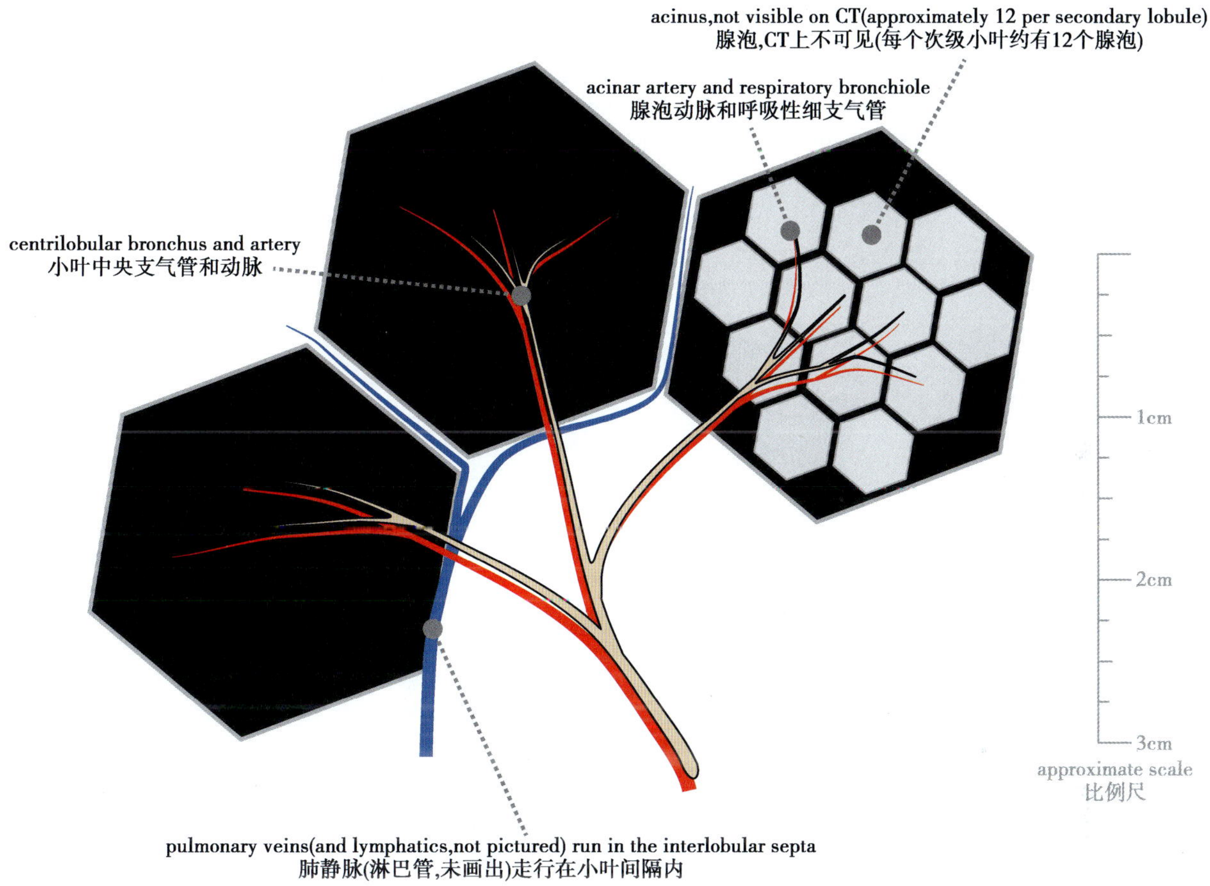

- The secondary pulmonary lobule (SPL) is the elemental unit of lung function.
- Each SPL contains a central artery (the aptly named centrilobular artery) and a central bronchus, each branching many times to ultimately produce acinar arteries and respiratory bronchioles.

  On CT, the centrilobular artery is often visible as a faint dot. The centrilobular bronchus is not normally visible.

  The acinus is the basic unit of gas exchange, containing several generations of branching respiratory bronchioles, alveolar ducts, and alveoli.

  There are generally 12 or fewer acini per secondary lobule.
- Pulmonary veins and lymphatics collect in the periphery of each SPL.
- Connective tissue, called interlobular septa, encases each SPL.

  Thickening of the interlobular septa can be seen on CT and suggests pathologic enlargement of either the venous or lymphatic spaces, as discussed on subsequent pages.
- Each SPL is between 1 and 2.5 cm in diameter.

- 次级肺小叶(SPL)是肺功能的基本单位。
- 每个SPL包含一条中央动脉(贴切地称之为小叶中央动脉)和一根中央支气管,二者经多次分支最终形成腺泡动脉和呼吸性细支气管。

  小叶中央动脉在CT上通常表现为一个浅淡的小点。小叶中央支气管在正常情况下看不到。

  腺泡是气体交换的基本单位,包含数个呼吸性细支气管的分支、肺泡管和肺泡。

  每个SPL通常含有12个或更少的腺泡。
- 肺静脉和淋巴管收集每个SPL外周的液体。
- 结缔组织,也被称为小叶间隔,包绕每个SPL。

  CT可以显示增厚的小叶间隔,提示静脉或淋巴管间隙病理性扩张,将在下文讨论。
- 每个SPL的直径在1.0~2.5cm。

Abnormalities of the Secondary Pulmonary Lobule

次级肺小叶异常

Consolidation and ground glass

- Consolidation and ground glass opacification are two very commonly seen patterns of lung disease caused by abnormal alveoli. The alveolar abnormality may represent either filling of the alveoli with fluid or incomplete alveolar aeration.
- Consolidation can be described on either a chest radiograph or CT, while ground glass is generally reserved for CT.
- Although consolidation often implies pneumonia, both consolidation and ground glass are nonspecific findings with a broad differential depending on chronicity (acute versus chronic) and distribution (focal versus patchy or diffuse).

实变和磨玻璃影

- 实变和磨玻璃影(GGO)是肺部疾病中两种很常见的表现，为异常肺泡所致。肺泡异常可能是肺泡被液体充填或肺泡通气不良。
- 实变既可用于描述胸部X线影像，也可用于描述CT表现，但磨玻璃影通常只用于CT。
- 实变通常是指肺炎，但实变与磨玻璃影均为非特异性表现，并有广泛的鉴别诊断，需要结合病程(急性或慢性)和分布(局灶性、斑片状或弥漫性)来考虑。

Consolidation

实变

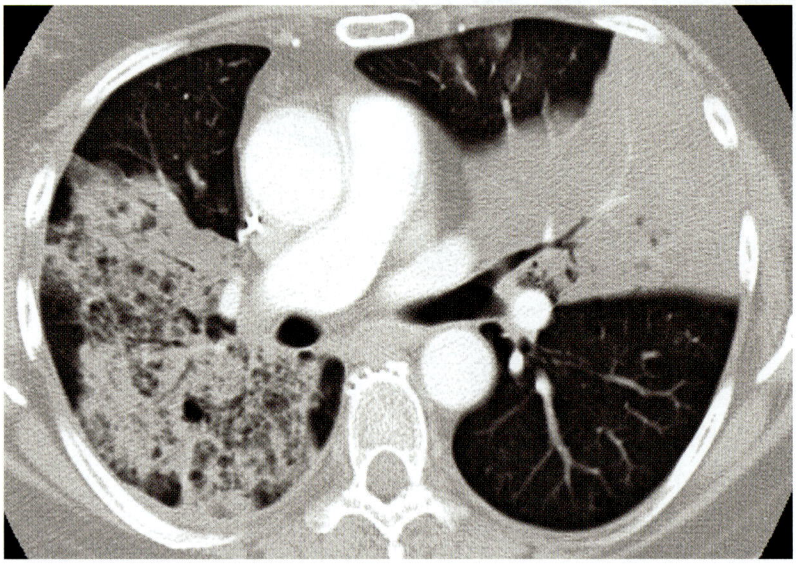

Consolidation: Contrast-enhanced CT shows bilateral consolidative opacities, more densely consolidated on the left. There are bilateral air bronchograms. Although these imaging findings are nonspecific, this was a case of multifocal consolidative adenocarcinoma.

实变：增强CT显示双肺实变影，左侧的实变更为致密。可见双侧支气管充气征。这些影像学表现是非特异性的，此病例为多灶性实性腺癌。

- Consolidation is histologically due to complete filling of affected alveoli (commonly remembered as *blood, pus, water,* or *cells*).
- Pulmonary vessels are **not** visible through the consolidation on an unenhanced CT.
- *Air bronchograms* are often present if the airway is patent. An air bronchogram represents a lucent air-filled bronchus (or bronchiole) seen within a consolidation.
- Consolidation causes silhouetting of adjacent structures on conventional radiography.
- **Acute consolidation** is most commonly due to pneumonia, but the differential includes:

Pneumonia (by far the most common cause of acute consolidation).
Aspiration, consolidation may appear heterogeneous from mucus plugging.
Pulmonary hemorrhage (primary pulmonary hemorrhage or aspiration of hemorrhage).
Adult respiratory distress syndrome (ARDS), which is noncardiogenic pulmonary edema seen in critically ill patients and thought to be due to increased capillary permeability.
Pulmonary edema may cause consolidation if severe.

- 实变在组织学上是由于受累肺泡被完全充填(常记为血、脓、水或细胞)。
- 平扫CT**不能**显示实变区的肺血管。
- 空气支气管征通常在气道通畅时出现，为透亮的空气充填了实变肺内的支气管(或细支气管)。
- 实变可导致X线影像上邻近结构发生轮廓改变。
- **急性实变**最常见的原因是肺炎，鉴别诊断包括：

肺炎(最为常见的急性实变原因)。
吸入，黏液栓可使实变不均匀。
肺出血(原发性肺出血或吸入非气道来源的出血)。
成人呼吸窘迫综合征(ARDS)，是一种见于重症患者的非心源性肺水肿，被认为是毛细血管渗透性增加所致。
肺水肿严重者可导致实变。

- The differential diagnosis of **chronic consolidation** includes:

> **Adenocarcinoma**, previously bronchioloalveolar carcinoma
> **Lymphoma**.
> **Organizing pneumonia**, which is a nonspecific response to injury characterized by granulation polyps which fill the distal airways, producing peripheral rounded and nodular consolidation.
> **Chronic eosinophilic pneumonia**, an inflammatory process characterized by eosinophils causing alveolar filling in an upper-lobe distribution.

- **慢性实变**的鉴别诊断包括：

> **腺癌**，曾称细支气管肺泡癌。
> **淋巴瘤**。
> **机化性肺炎**，是一种对损伤的非特异性反应，特征为肉芽肿性息肉充填远端气道，并产生外周的圆形和结节样实变。
> **慢性嗜酸性粒细胞性肺炎**，是一种以嗜酸性粒细胞为特征的炎症反应，导致上叶分布的肺泡填充。

Ground glass opacification (GGO)

磨玻璃影(GGO)

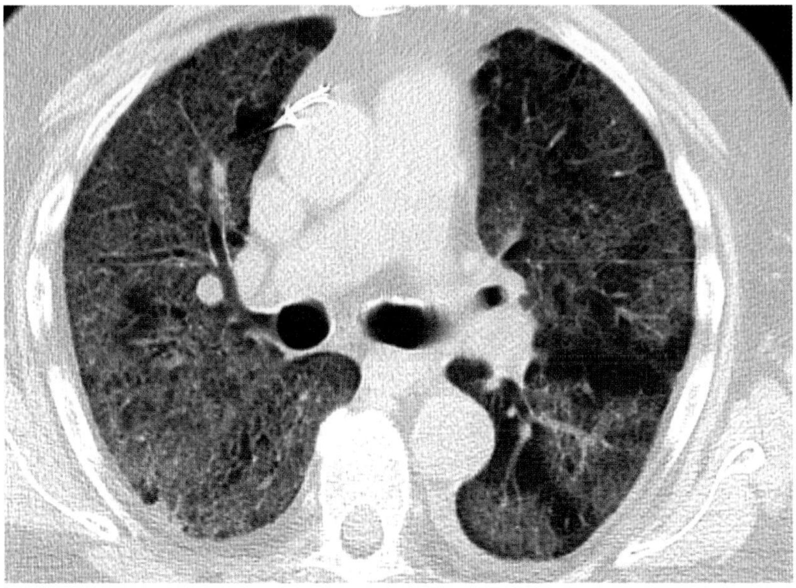

Ground glass opacification: Noncontrast CT shows diffuse ground glass opacification (GGO). The pulmonary architecture, including vasculature and bronchi, can be still seen, which is characteristic for GGO. Although these imaging findings are nonspecific, this was a case of acute respiratory distress syndrome (ARDS).

磨玻璃影：平扫CT显示弥漫性磨玻璃影。肺结构，包括血管和支气管仍可见，这是磨玻璃影的特征。这些影像学表现并非特异，本例患者为急性呼吸窘迫综合征(ARDS)。

- Ground glass opacification is histologically due to either partial filling of the alveoli (by blood, pus, water, or cells), alveolar wall thickening, or reduced aeration of alveoli (atelectasis).
- Ground glass is usually a term reserved for CT. CT shows a hazy, gauze-like opacity, through which pulmonary vessels are still visible.
- **Acute ground glass** opacification has a similar differential to acute consolidation, since many of the entities that initially cause partial airspace filling can progress to completely fill the airspaces later in the disease. The differential of acute ground glass includes:

> **Pulmonary edema**, which is usually central or dependent.
> **Pneumonia**. Unlike consolidation, ground glass is more commonly seen in atypical pneumonia such as viral or *Pneumocystis jiroveci* pneumonia.
> **Pulmonary hemorrhage**, seen as pure ground glass in acute phase, but subacute phase shows peripheral sparing and crazy paving.
> **Adult respiratory distress syndrome (ARDS)**.

- 磨玻璃影在组织学上可由肺泡部分充填(被血、脓、水或细胞)、肺泡壁增厚或肺泡通气不足(肺不张)所致。
- 磨玻璃影通常是CT的专用术语，表现为模糊、薄纱样影，透过磨玻璃影依然可见其中的肺血管。
- **急性磨玻璃影**与急性实变有相似的鉴别诊断，因为多种疾病最初引起的气腔部分充填可在晚期进展为全部充填。急性磨玻璃影的鉴别诊断包括：

> **肺水肿**，通常呈中心性或重力分布。
> **肺炎**。与实变不同，磨玻璃影更常见于非典型肺炎，如病毒性或耶氏肺孢子菌肺炎。
> **肺出血**，急性期为纯磨玻璃影，但亚急性期为外周不受累和铺路石征。
> **成人呼吸窘迫综合征(ARDS)**。

- **Chronic ground glass** opacification has a similar but broader differential diagnosis compared to chronic consolidation. In addition to all of the entities which may cause chronic consolidation, the differential diagnosis of chronic ground glass also includes:

- **慢性磨玻璃影**与慢性实变有类似的鉴别诊断，但需要鉴别的疾病更多。除了可引起实变的所有原因之外，慢性磨玻璃影的鉴别诊断还包括：

Lung adenocarcinoma, which can be focal or multifocal.
Organizing pneumonia, typically presenting as rounded, peripheral opacities.
Chronic eosinophilic pneumonia, usually with an upper-lobe predominance.
Interstitial lung disease, including desquamative interstitial pneumonia (DIP), nonspecific interstitial pneumonia (NSIP), and hypersensitivity pneumonitis (HP).
Hypersensitivity pneumonitis (HP) is a type Ⅲ hypersensitivity reaction to inhaled organic antigens. In the subacute phase there is ground glass, centrilobular nodules, and mosaic attenuation.

肺腺癌，可为局限或多灶。
机化性肺炎，典型表现为圆形、外周密度增高影。
慢性嗜酸性粒细胞性肺炎，常以上叶分布为主。
间质性肺疾病，包括脱屑性间质性肺炎(DIP)、非特异性间质性肺炎(NSIP)和过敏性肺炎(HP)。
HP是对吸入有机抗原产生的Ⅲ型变态反应。在亚急性期有磨玻璃影、小叶中心性结节和马赛克影。

Peripheral ground glass or consolidation

外周性磨玻璃影或实变

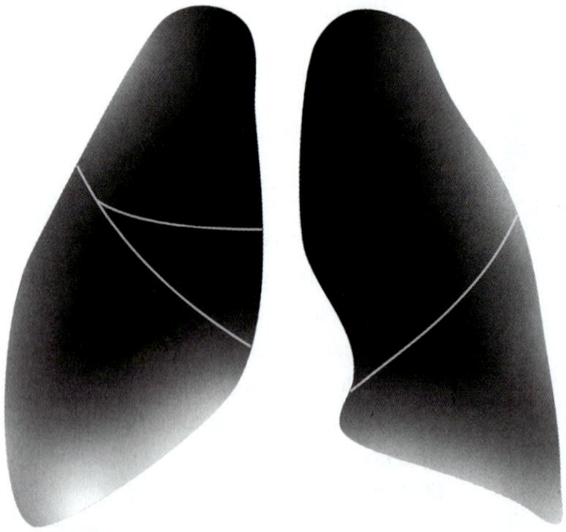

Coronal schematic demonstrates peripheral ground glass.
冠状示意图显示外周性磨玻璃影。

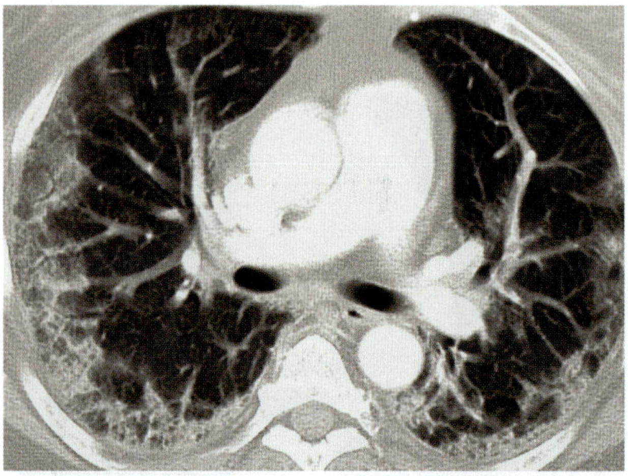

Axial CT shows peripheral and subpleural ground glass attenuation. This was a case of organizing pneumonia.
轴位CT显示外周和胸膜下的磨玻璃影。该病例为机化性肺炎。

- The differential diagnosis for **peripheral consolidation or ground glass** includes:

Organizing pneumonia.
Chronic eosinophilic pneumonia, typically with an upper lobe predominance.
Pulmonary infarction.

- **外周性实变或磨玻璃影**的鉴别诊断包括：

机化性肺炎。
慢性嗜酸性粒细胞性肺炎，通常以上叶分布为主。
肺梗死。

Interlobular septal thickening – smooth

小叶间隔增厚-平滑型

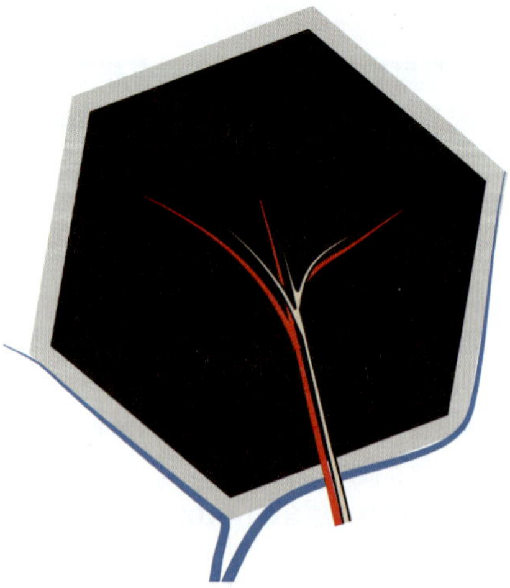

Schematic demonstrates smooth interlobular septal thickening.
示意图显示平滑的小叶间隔增厚。

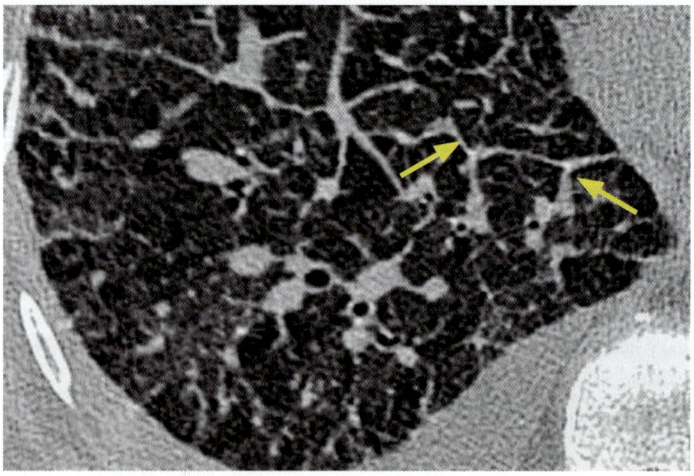

Smooth interlobular septal thickening: CT demonstrates smooth thickening of the interlobular septa (arrows) in pulmonary edema.
Courtesy Ritu R. Gill, MD, MPH, Brigham and Women's Hospital.
平滑的小叶间隔增厚：CT显示肺水肿时出现平滑增厚的小叶间隔(黄箭)。

- Conditions that dilate the pulmonary veins cause smooth interlobular septal thickening.
- By far the most common cause of **smooth interlobular septal thickening** is pulmonary edema; however, the differential diagnosis for smooth interlobular septal thickening is:

Pulmonary edema.
Lymphangitis carcinomatosis.

- 造成肺静脉扩张的各种原因均可导致平滑型小叶间隔增厚。
- **平滑型小叶间隔增厚**最常见的原因是肺水肿；鉴别诊断包括：

肺水肿。
癌性淋巴管炎。

Interlobular septal thickening – nodular, irregular, or asymmetric

小叶间隔增厚-结节样、不规则或不对称型

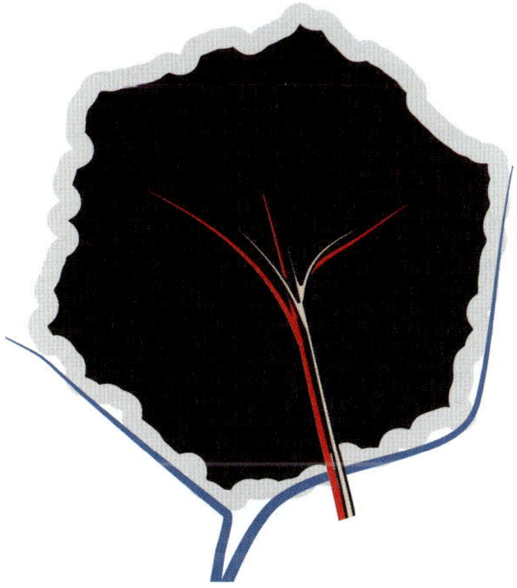

Schematic demonstrates irregular and nodular interlobular septal thickening.
示意图显示不规则和结节样小叶间隔增厚。

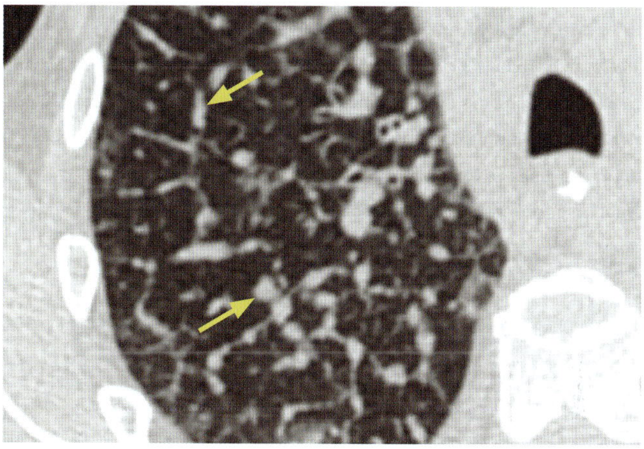

Axial CT shows a diffuse nodular septal thickening (yellow arrows). This was a case of lymphangitic carcinomatosis.
轴位CT显示弥漫性结节型小叶间隔增厚(黄箭)。该病例为淋巴管转移癌。

- **Nodular, irregular, or asymmetric septal thickening** tends to be caused by processes that infiltrate the peripheral lymphatics, most commonly by lymphangitic carcinomatosis and sarcoidosis:

Lymphangitic carcinomatosis is tumor spread through the lymphatics.
Sarcoidosis rarely causes septal thickening.

- **结节样、不规则或不对称型小叶间隔增厚**大多是外周淋巴管受侵，最常见的为淋巴管转移癌和结节病：

淋巴管转移癌是肿瘤通过淋巴管播散。
结节病偶尔导致小叶间隔增厚。

Crazy paving

铺路石征

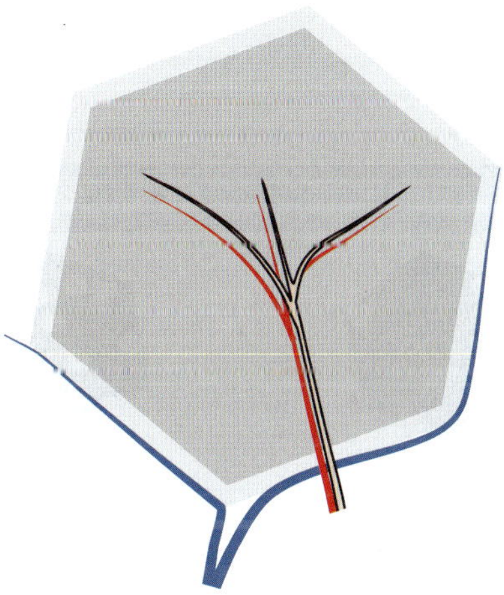

Schematic demonstrates interlobular septal thickening and ground glass opacification.
示意图显示小叶间隔增厚和磨玻璃影。

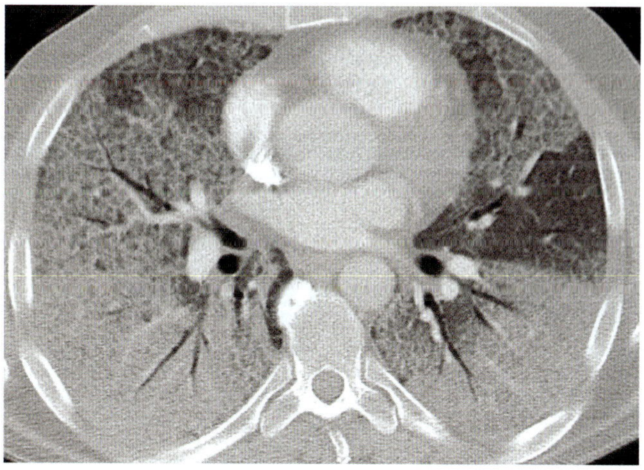

Axial CT shows interlobular septal thickening in regions of ground glass opacification, representing *crazy paving*. This was a case of alveolar proteinosis, the entity in which crazy paving was first described.
轴位CT显示小叶间隔增厚分布于磨玻璃影内，为*铺路石征*。该病例为肺泡蛋白沉积症，铺路石征首次用于描述这种疾病。

- *Crazy paving* describes interlobular septal thickening with superimposed ground glass opacification, which is thought to resemble the appearance of a stone path.
- Although nonspecific, this pattern was first described for alveolar proteinosis, where the ground glass opacification is caused by filling of alveoli by proteinaceous material and the interlobular septal thickening is caused by lymphatics taking up the same material.
- The differential diagnosis for **crazy paving** includes:

> **Pulmonary edema,** by far the most common cause.
> **Pulmonary hemorrhage.**
> **Acute respiratory distress syndrome.**
> **Pulmonary alveolar proteinosis (PAP),** an idiopathic disease characterized by alveolar filling by a proteinaceous substance. PAP is almost always seen with a crazy paving pattern.
> ***Pneumocystis jiroveci* pneumonia.**
> **Adenocarcinoma,** uncommon cause
> **Lipoid pneumonia,** an inflammatory pneumonia caused by reaction to aspirated lipids, uncommon cause.

- 铺路石征指增厚的小叶间隔重叠于磨玻璃影中，看起来像石头小路。
- 此为非特异性征象，首次被用于描述肺泡蛋白沉积症，其中的磨玻璃影是由于肺泡被蛋白质类物质充填，而小叶间隔增厚为淋巴管摄取了蛋白类物质的结果。
- **铺路石征**的鉴别诊断包括：

> **肺水肿**，最常见原因。
> **肺出血**。
> **急性呼吸窘迫综合征**。
> **肺泡蛋白沉积症(PAP)**，是一种特发性疾病，特征是肺泡内充满蛋白样物质。PAP几乎总是以铺路石模式出现。
> **耶氏肺孢子菌肺炎**。
> **腺癌**，不常见的原因。
> **类脂性肺炎**，是一种因吸入脂类物质引起的炎症性肺炎，属于不常见原因。

Approach to Multiple Micronodules

多发微结节诊断方法

Centrilobular	Tree-in-Bud (Form of centrilobular)	Perilymphatic	Random

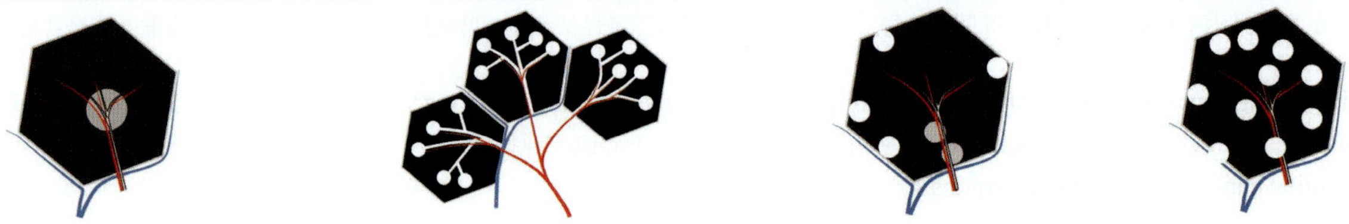

Centrilobular	Tree-in-Bud (Form of centrilobular)	Perilymphatic	Random
Viral pneumonia Hypersensitivity pneumonitis Aspiration Pulmonary capillary hemangiomatosis Metastatic calcification Occasionally, pulmonary edema	Infectious bronchiolitis: Mycobacterial infections Viral infections Bacterial pneumonia Aspiration Rarely, lymphangitic carcinomatosis and vascular abnormalities (endovascular metastases and pulmonary arterial aneurysms)	Sarcoidosis Pneumoconiosis Lymphangitic carcinomatosis	Hematogenous metastases Disseminated mycobacteria Disseminated fungal infections

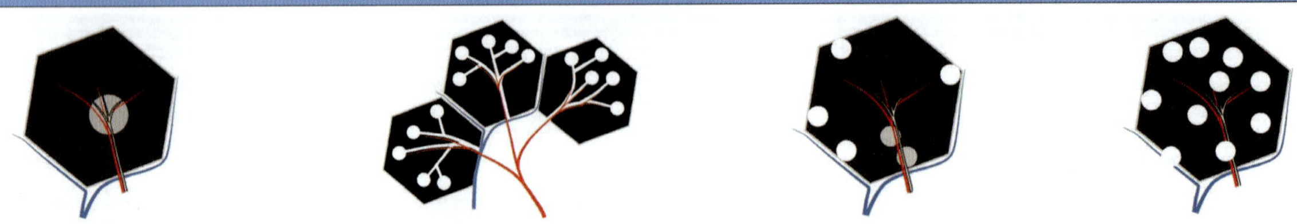

小叶中心	树芽征(小叶中心形式)	淋巴管周	随机
病毒性肺炎 过敏性肺炎 吸入 肺毛细血管瘤病 转移性钙化 偶尔肺水肿	感染性细支气管炎 分枝杆菌感染 病毒感染 细菌性肺炎 吸入 罕见，淋巴管转移癌和血管异常(血管内转移和肺动脉瘤)	结节病 肺尘埃沉着病 淋巴管转移癌	血行转移 播散性分枝杆菌感染 播散性真菌感染

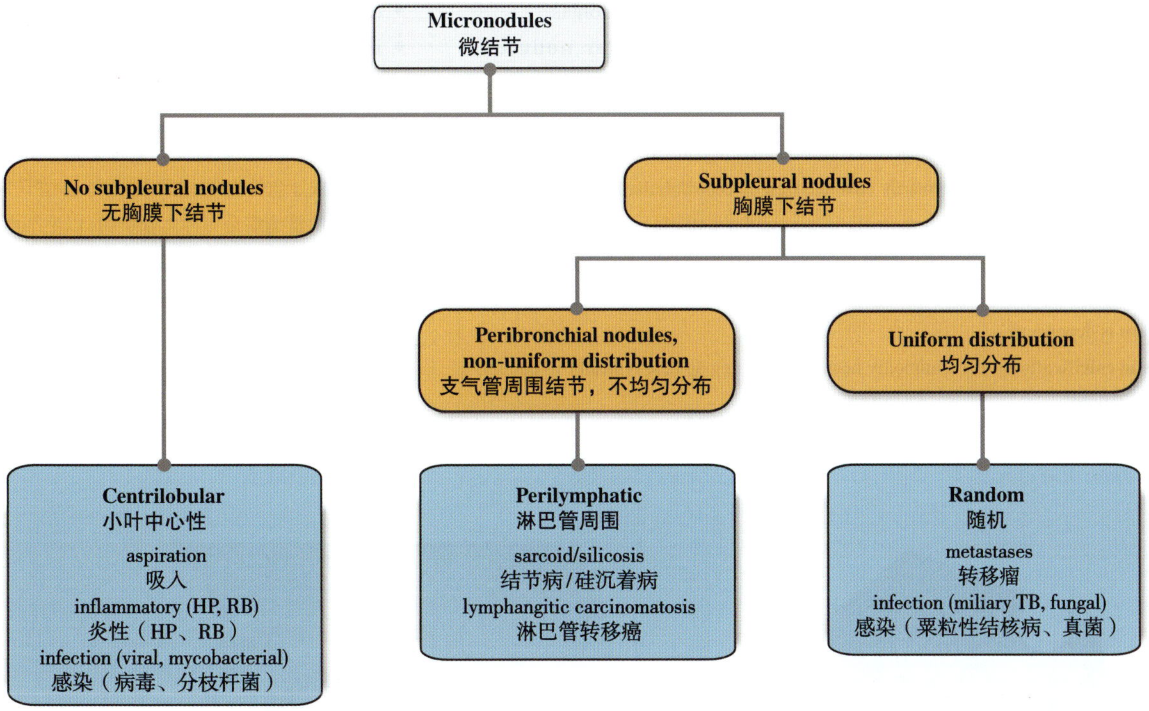

Centrilobular nodules

小叶中心结节

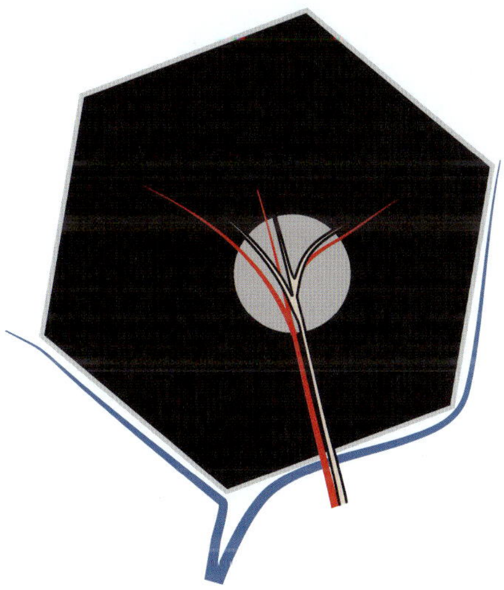

Schematic demonstrates a centrilobular nodule, located at the center of the pulmonary lobule.
示意图显示小叶中心结节，位于肺小叶的中央。

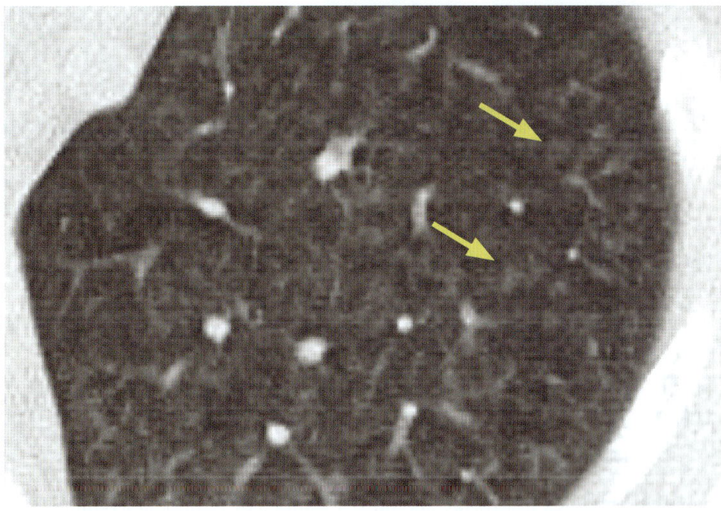

Axial CT demonstrates diffuse faint centrilobular opacities (arrows), none of which extend to the pleural surface, which is typical of a centrilobular distribution. This was a case of pulmonary capillary hemangiomatosis.
轴位CT显示弥漫性浅淡的小叶中心阴影(黄箭)无任何延伸至胸膜表面的迹象，呈典型的小叶中心分布。该例为肺毛细血管瘤病。

- Centrilobular nodules represent opacification of and around the centrilobular bronchiole (or less commonly the centrilobular artery) at the center of each secondary pulmonary lobule.
- On CT, multiple small nodules are seen in the centers of secondary pulmonary lobules. Centrilobular nodules never extend to the pleural surface. The nodules may be solid or of ground glass attenuation, and range in size from tiny up to a centimeter.
- Centrilobular nodules may be caused by infectious or inflammatory conditions.

- 小叶中心结节是小叶中心细支气管(或较少见的小叶中央动脉)及其周围密度增高，位于每个次级肺小叶的中心。
- CT表现为次级肺小叶中央的多发小结节。小叶中心结节不会扩展至胸膜的表面。结节可为实性或磨玻璃影，大小可从一个小点至1cm。
- 小叶中心结节可由感染或炎症引起。

- **Infectious** causes of **centrilobular nodules** include viral pneumonias.
- The most common **inflammatory** cause of **centrilobular nodules** is hypersensitivity pneumonitis (HP), an exposure-related lung disease.

- **感染性小叶中心结节**的病因包括病毒性肺炎。
- **炎症性小叶中心结节**最常见的原因是HP，一种与暴露相关的肺部疾病。

> **HP** is a type Ⅲ hypersensitivity reaction to an inhaled organic antigen. The acute or subacute presentation of HP is primarily characterized by centrilobular nodules.
> **Pulmonary capillary hemangiomatosis** is a vascular pathology characterized by abnormal capillary proliferation leading to pulmonary hypertension.
> **Viral pneumonias**.
> **Aspiration** is dependent.
> **Metastatic calcification** most commonly occurs in the lung apices, typically in patients with renal failure.

> **HP**是一种吸入有机抗原产生的Ⅲ型超敏反应。HP的急性或亚急性表现主要以小叶中心结节为特征。
> **肺毛细血管瘤病**是一种血管疾病，以毛细血管异常增生为特征，最终导致肺动脉高压。
> **病毒性肺炎**。
> **吸入**按重力分布。
> **转移性钙化**最常发生在肺尖，通常见于肾衰竭的患者。

Perilymphatic nodules

淋巴管周围结节

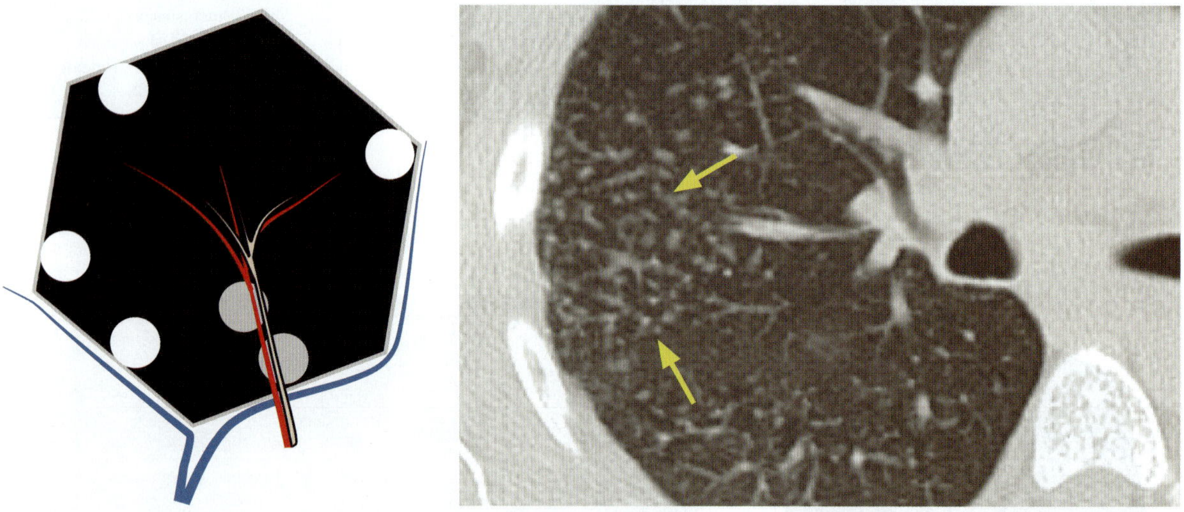

Perilymphatic nodules: Schematic of the secondary pulmonary lobule (left image) demonstrates gray nodules located along the bronchovascular bundle and white nodules located along the interlobular septa.
Axial CT (right image) demonstrates multiple subpleural nodules and nodules along the bronchovascular bundles (arrows). This was a case of sarcoidosis.
淋巴管周围结节：次级肺小叶示意图(左图)显示灰色结节沿支气管血管束分布，白色结节沿小叶间隔分布。
轴位CT(右图)显示多发胸膜下结节及沿支气管血管束分布的结节(黄箭)。该例为结节病。

- Perilymphatic nodules follow the anatomic locations of pulmonary lymphatics, which can be seen in three locations in the lung:
  1. Subpleural.
  2. Peribronchovascular.
  3. Septal (within the interlobular septa separating the secondary pulmonary lobules).
- Sarcoidosis is the most common cause of perilymphatic nodules, typically with an upper- lobe distribution. The nodules may become confluent creating the *galaxy sign* in which many tiny nodules surround a central lesion.

- 淋巴管周围结节沿肺淋巴管的解剖位置分布，可见于肺内三个位置：
  1. 胸膜下。
  2. 支气管血管周围。
  3. 间隔(在分隔次级肺小叶的小叶间隔内)。
- 结节病是淋巴管周围结节最常见的原因，通常分布在肺上叶。结节可融合形成星系征，即许多微小结节围绕在一个中央病灶的周围。

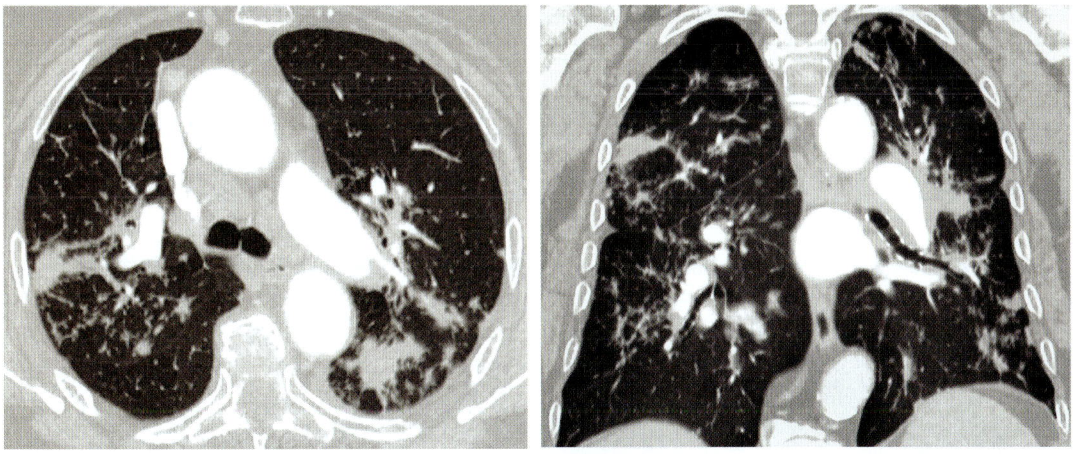

Pulmonary sarcoidosis with *galaxy sign*: Axial and coronal CT images demonstrate extensive upper-lobe predominant confluent perilymphatic nodules. The *galaxy sign* is most apparent on the axial image, where the confluent nodules appear like the confluence of stars forming a galaxy.
肺结节病伴*星系征*：轴位及冠状位CT显示大量上叶为主融合的淋巴管周围结节。*星系征*在轴位图像上最明显，融合的结节看起来像星星汇聚形成一个星系。

- The differential of **perilymphatic nodules** includes:

Sarcoidosis.
Pneumoconioses (silicosis and coal workers' pneumoconiosis) are reactions to inorganic dust inhalation. The imaging may look identical to sarcoidosis with perilymphatic nodules, but there is usually a history of exposure (e.g., a sandblaster who develops silicosis).
Lymphangitic carcinomatosis.

- **淋巴管周围结节**的鉴别诊断包括：

结节病。
肺尘埃沉着病（硅沉着病和煤矿工肺尘埃沉着病）是机体对吸入无机粉尘的反应。影像学表现可与结节病淋巴管周围结节相同，但通常有暴露史（如喷砂工发展为硅沉着病）。
淋巴管转移癌。

Random nodules

随机结节

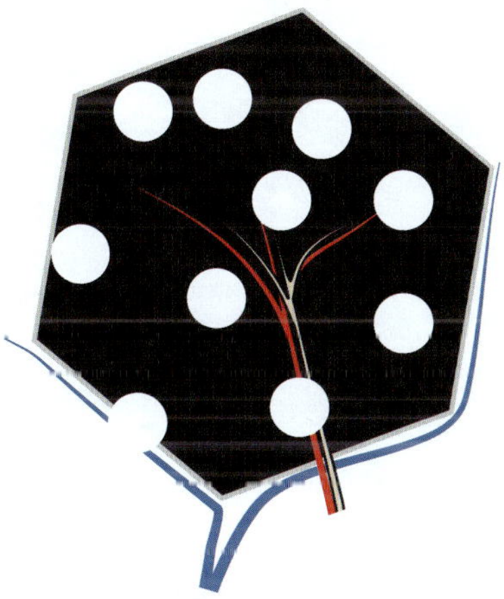

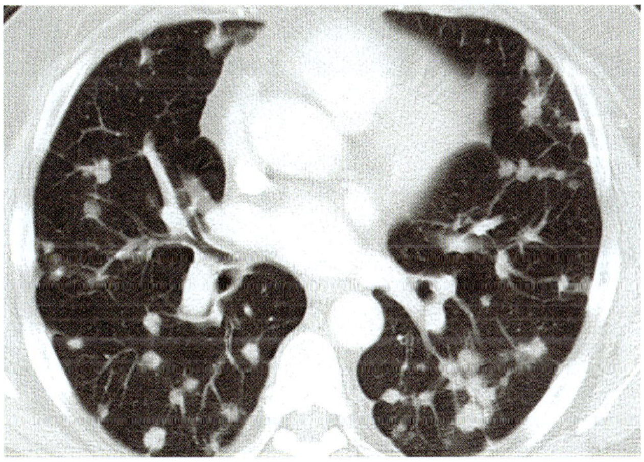

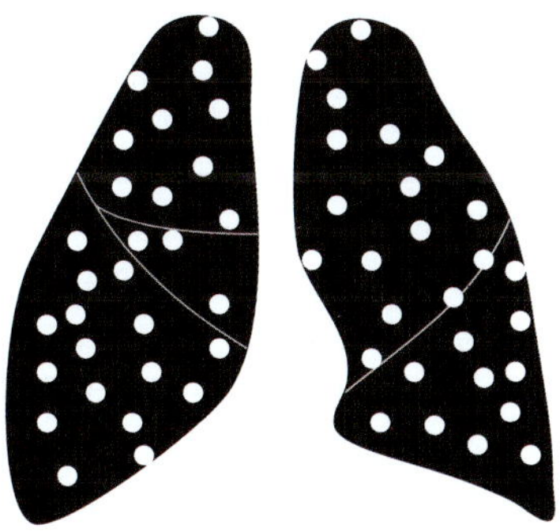

Random nodules:
Schematic of the secondary pulmonary lobule (top left image) demonstrates nodules distributed randomly throughout the SPL.
Schematic of the lungs (bottom left image) demonstrates nodules scattered randomly. Some of the nodules are in close contact with the pleural surface.
Axial CT (top right image) demonstrates multiple random nodules. Some of the nodules abut the pleural surface. This was a case of metastatic colon cancer.
随机结节：
次级肺小叶示意图（左上图）显示结节随机分布于整个SPL。
肺部示意图（左下图）显示结节随机分布，部分结节紧邻胸膜表面。
轴位CT（右上图）显示多发随机结节。一些结节紧贴胸膜表面。该例为转移性结肠癌。

- **Randomly distributed nodules** usually occur via hematogenous spread. The differential of random nodules includes:

Hematogenous metastases.
Disseminated mycobacteria.
Disseminated fungal infection.

- **随机分布结节**通常通过血行播散发生。随机结节的鉴别诊断包括：

血行转移肿瘤。
播散性分枝杆菌。
播散性真菌感染。

- A ***miliary* pattern** is innumerable tiny random nodules the size of millet seeds.

- **粟粒样分布**是无数像粟粒大小的微小随机结节。

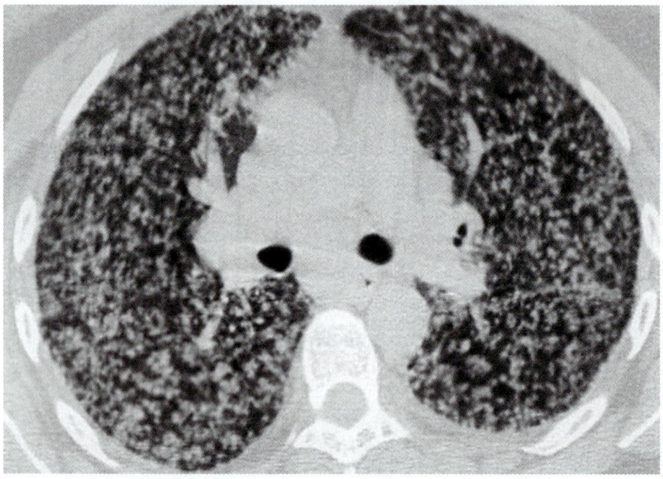

Miliary nodules: Axial CT shows innumerable tiny nodules distributed randomly throughout both lungs in a miliary pattern. This was a case of miliary tuberculosis.

Case courtesy Ritu R. Gill, MD, MPH, Brigham and Women's Hospital

粟粒样结节：轴位CT显示无数微小结节随机分布于两侧肺部，呈粟粒状。该例为粟粒性结核。

Tree-in-bud nodules

树芽样结节

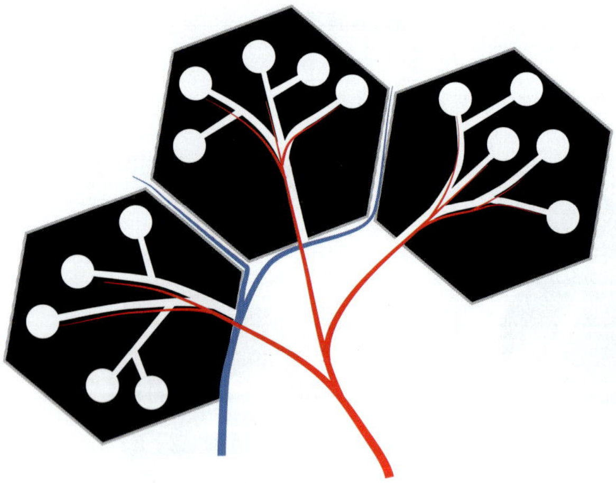

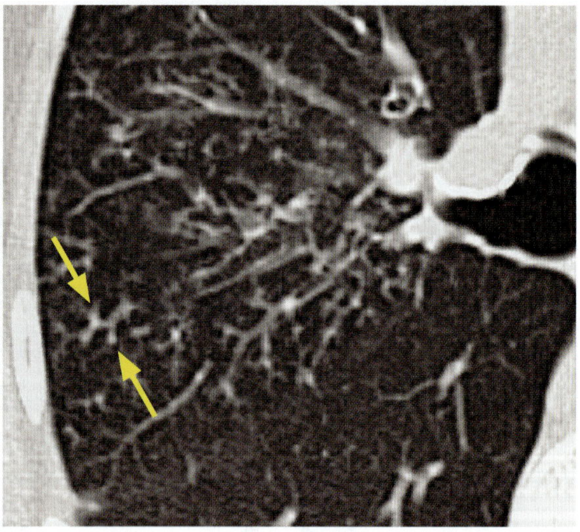

Schematic shows several nodules centered on an opacified small airway.

Tree-in-bud nodularity: Axial CT shows numerous small nodules (arrows) "budding" off of linear branching structures in the right middle lobe. This case was secondary to atypical mycobacteria.

示意图显示数个结节排列在不透明小气道的周围。

树芽样结节：轴位CT显示右肺中叶有大量小结节（黄箭）从线样分枝结构上"发芽"。该例为继发性非典型分枝杆菌感染。

- Tree-in-bud nodules are multiple small nodules connected to linear branching structures, which resemble a budding tree branch in springtime. The linear branching structures represent mucus-impacted bronchioles, which are normally invisible on CT, and the nodules represent impacted terminal bronchioles. Tree-in-bud nodules are due to mucus, pus, or fluid impacting bronchioles and terminal bronchioles.

- 树芽样结节是多发小结节与呈线样的分枝结构相连，类似于春天发芽的树枝。线样分枝结构代表被黏液阻塞的细支气管，正常情况下在CT上不可见，而结节代表阻塞的终末细支气管。树芽样结节由黏液、脓液或液体堵塞细支气管和终末细支气管所致。

- **Tree-in-bud nodules** are almost always associated with small airways infection or inflammation, such as endobronchial spread of tuberculosis.
- The differential of tree-in-bud nodules includes:

Mycobacterium tuberculosis and **atypical mycobacteria**.
Viral pneumonia.
Aspiration pneumonia.
Rarely, **lymphangitic carcinomatosis** and **vascular abnormalities** (endovascular metastases and pulmonary arterial aneurysms).

- **树芽样结节**几乎都与小气道感染有关，如支气管内播散型肺结核。
- 树芽样结节的鉴别诊断包括：

结核分枝杆菌和**非典型分枝杆菌感染**。
病毒性肺炎。
吸入性肺炎。
罕见，**淋巴管转移癌**和**血管异常**(血管内转移和肺动脉动脉瘤)。

CAVITARY AND CYSTIC LUNG DISEASE

空洞和囊性肺疾病

Solitary cavitary nodule/mass

孤立空洞性结节/肿块

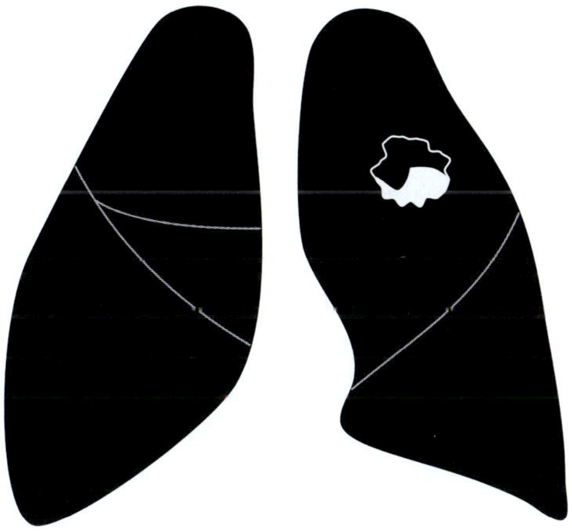

Coronal schematic demonstrates a single cavitary lesion.
冠状位示意图显示单个空洞性病变。

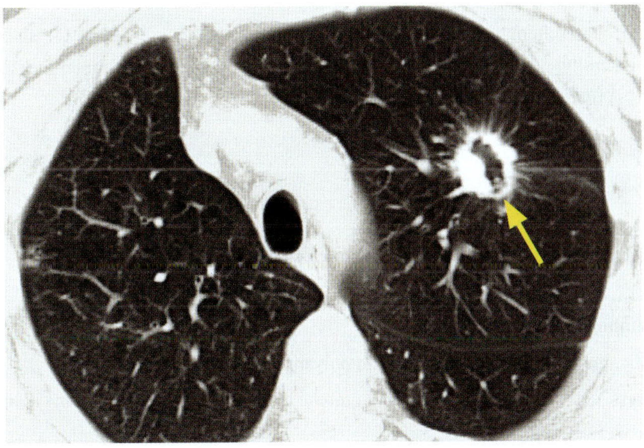

Axial CT shows a single spiculated cavitary lesion in the left upper lobe (arrow). This was a case of squamous cell carcinoma.
轴位CT显示左上叶单个毛刺状空洞性病变(黄箭)。该例为鳞状细胞癌。

- A cavitary lesion represents development of air within a pre-existing lesion (nodule, mass, or consolidation). It typically has a thick, irregular wall, often with a solid mural component. Although the findings of benign and malignant cavitary nodules overlap, a maximum wall thickness of ≤4 mm is usually benign and a wall thickness >15 mm is usually malignant. Spiculated margins also suggest malignancy.
- A **solitary cavitary lesion** is most likely cancer or infection.

Primary bronchogenic carcinoma. While both squamous cell and adenocarcinoma can cavitate, squamous cell cavitates more frequently. Small cell carcinoma is never known to cavitate.
Tuberculosis classically produces an upper-lobe cavitary consolidation.
Fungal pneumonia.
Cavitary bacterial pneumonia.

- 空洞性病变是指先前的病变(结节、肿块或实变)内出现了气体，通常具有厚实而不规则的壁，常伴有坚固的壁内成分。虽然良、恶性空洞性结节的表现相互重叠，但壁厚≤4mm往往为良性，而壁厚>15mm常为恶性。毛刺状边缘也提示恶性。
- **孤立的空洞性病变**最有可能是癌症或感染。

原发性支气管肺癌。鳞状细胞癌和腺癌均可形成空洞，但鳞状细胞癌更常见。小细胞肺癌从未报道有空洞。
肺结核常产生上叶空洞性实变。
真菌性肺炎。
空洞性细菌性肺炎。

Multiple cavitary nodules

多发空洞性结节

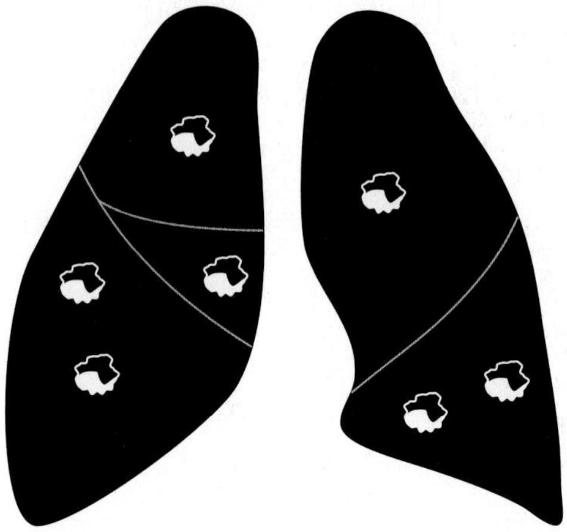

Coronal schematic shows numerous cavitary lesions bilaterally.
冠状位示意图显示双肺多发空洞性病变。

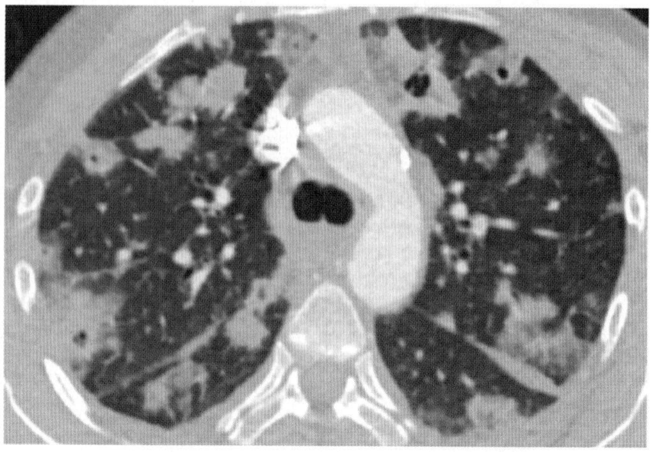

Axial CT shows numerous cavitary and non-cavitary lesions bilaterally, in a random distribution. This was a case of polysubstance abuse and septic emboli.
轴位CT显示双肺多发空洞和非空洞性病变，呈随机分布。这是一个滥用多种药物和有脓毒性栓子的病例。

- The differential diagnosis for **multiple cavitary lesions** includes:

Septic emboli, typically peripheral.
Vasculitis, including granulomatosis with polyangiitis (GPA).
Metastases, classically squamous cell carcinoma but any metastatic lesion can cavitate.

- **多发空洞性病变**的鉴别诊断包括：

脓毒性栓子，通常分布在外周。
血管炎，包括肉芽肿性多血管炎(GPA)。
转移瘤，典型如鳞状细胞癌，但任何转移性肿瘤都可能产生空洞。

Cystic lung diseases

囊性肺疾病

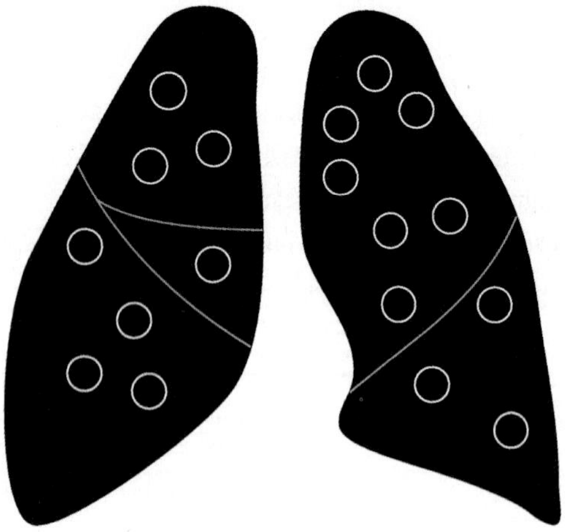

Coronal schematic shows numerous thin-walled cystic lesions bilaterally.
冠状位示意图示双肺多发薄壁囊性病变。

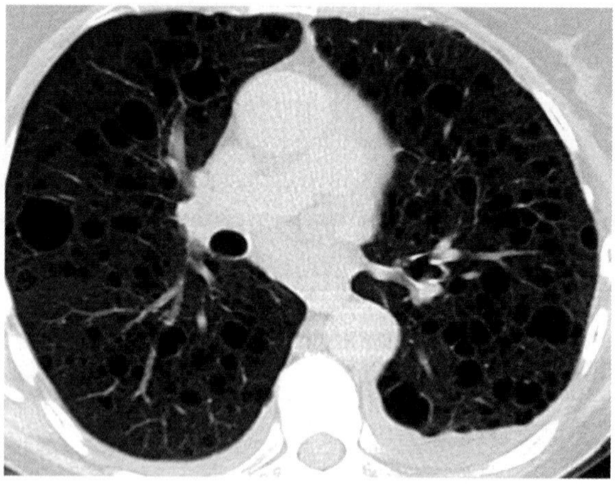

Axial CT shows bilateral thin-walled cysts that are of varying sizes but are predominantly regular in shape. There is a small left pleural effusion. This was a case of lymphangioleiomyomatosis.
轴位CT示双肺多发薄壁囊肿，大小不等但形状大多规则。左侧有少量胸腔积液。该病例为淋巴管平滑肌增生症。

- A cyst is an air-containing space with a thin wall. The differential diagnosis for **multiple lung cysts** includes:

- 囊肿是一个薄壁的含气结构。**多发性肺囊肿**的鉴别诊断包括：

Lymphangioleiomyomatosis (LAM), a diffuse cystic lung disease due to smooth muscle proliferation of the distal airways. LAM causes uniformly distributed, thin-walled cysts in a diffuse distribution. It may be associated with chylous effusion, as demonstrated in the above right case.

Pulmonary Langerhans cell histiocytosis, which features irregular cysts and nodules predominantly in the upper lungs.

Lymphoid interstitial pneumonia (LIP), a rare disease usually associated with Sjögren syndrome and characterized by lymphocytic infiltrate and multiple cysts.

Amyloid which appears similar to LIP.

Birt-Hogg-Dube syndrome which is an autosomal dominant genetic disorder characterized by renal tumors (most commonly chromophobe renal carcinoma and renal oncocytoma), and renal and pulmonary cysts. Spontaneous pneumothoraxes can occur as a sequela of pulmonary cysts.

***Pneumocystis jiroveci* pneumonia**, which features cysts in late-stage disease.

淋巴管平滑肌瘤病(LAM)，是一种弥漫性囊性肺疾病，由远端气道平滑肌增生所致。LAM产生均匀的薄壁囊肿，呈弥漫性分布。可伴有乳糜胸，如上图的右图所示。

肺朗格汉斯细胞组织细胞增生症，特征是上肺为主的不规则囊肿和结节。

淋巴细胞性间质性肺炎(LIP)，是一种罕见的疾病，常伴有干燥综合征，特征为淋巴细胞浸润和多发囊肿。

淀粉样变性的表现与LIP相似。

伯特-霍格-迪贝综合征是一种常染色体显性遗传疾病，以肾肿瘤(最常见的是嫌色细胞肾癌和肾嗜酸细胞腺瘤)、肾囊肿和肺囊肿为特征。自发性气胸可作为肺囊肿的后遗症发生。

耶氏肺孢子菌肺炎，其特点是疾病晚期出现囊肿。

- Of note, it is important to distinguish cysts from emphysema. The latter typically does not have walls and may have central vessels, whereas cysts classically do not have anything inside.
- The differential for **a single cyst** includes:

- 注意，区分囊肿和肺气肿非常重要。肺气肿通常没有壁但可有中央血管，而囊肿通常内部不含任何物质。
- **单发囊肿**的鉴别诊断包括：

Bulla. A bulla is an air-filled emphysematous space measuring >1 cm. A giant bulla occupies at least 30% of the volume of the thorax.

Bleb. A bleb is an air-filled cystic structure contiguous with the pleura measuring <1 cm. Rupture of a bleb is the most common cause of spontaneous pneumothorax.

Pneumatocele, which is an air-filled space caused by prior lung trauma or infection.

肺大疱，是一种由空气所充填的>1cm的气肿性腔隙。巨型肺大疱至少占胸腔容积的30%。

大疱，是紧邻胸膜、<1cm的含气囊性结构。大疱破裂是自发性气胸最常见的原因。

肺气囊，为含气间隙，由先前的肺创伤或感染引起。

Fibrotic Changes

纤维化改变

Lower lobe fibrotic changes

下叶纤维化改变

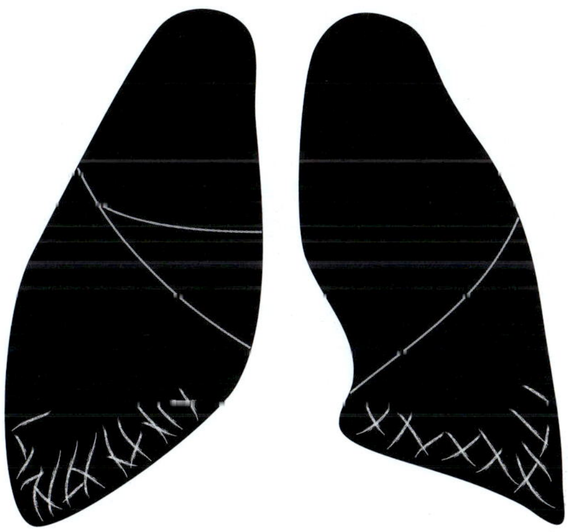

Coronal schematic shows basal-predominant fibrotic changes.
冠状位示意图显示以基底部为主的纤维化改变。

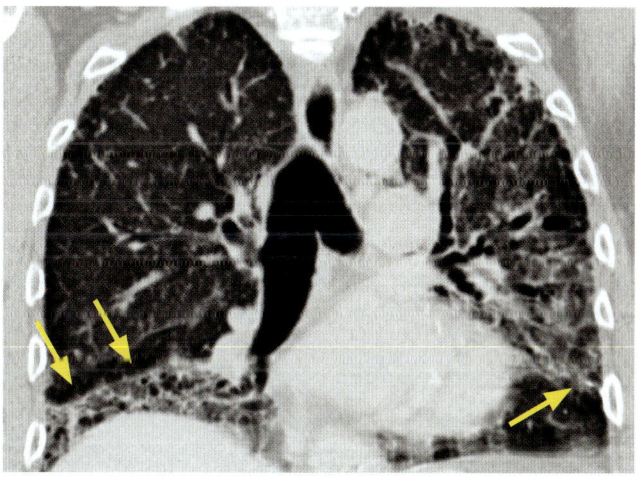

Coronal CT shows bibasilar fibrosis and honeycombing (arrows), with relative sparing of the upper lobes. This was a case of idiopathic pulmonary fibrosis.
冠状位CT显示双侧基底部纤维化和蜂窝状改变(黄箭)，上叶相对未受影响。这是一个特发性肺纤维化的病例。

- The differential diagnosis of basal-predominant fibrotic change includes:

Usual interstitial pneumonia (UIP) pattern. Idiopathic pulmonary fibrosis (IPF) is a clinical syndrome of progressive pulmonary fibrosis of unknown etiology and is the most common cause of basilar fibrosis. It almost always features basilar honeycombing.
Other causes of UIP pattern, including rheumatoid arthritis and asbestosis.
Nonspecific interstitial pneumonia (NSIP) is a lung response to injury commonly associated with collagen vascular disease and drug reaction. NSIP typically produces peribronchial reticulation and traction bronchiectasis. Ground glass may be present.

- 基底部为主的肺纤维化改变鉴别诊断包括：

普通型间质性肺炎(UIP)类，特发性肺纤维化(IPF)是一种病因不明的进行性肺纤维化的临床综合征，是基底部纤维化最常见的原因，几乎总是以基底部蜂窝为特征。
其他类型的UIP，包括类风湿性关节炎和石棉肺。
非特异性间质性肺炎(NSIP)是一种肺损伤反应，通常与胶原血管疾病和药物反应有关。NSIP通常产生支气管周围网格和牵拉性支气管扩张。可有磨玻璃影。

Upper lobe fibrotic changes

上叶纤维化改变

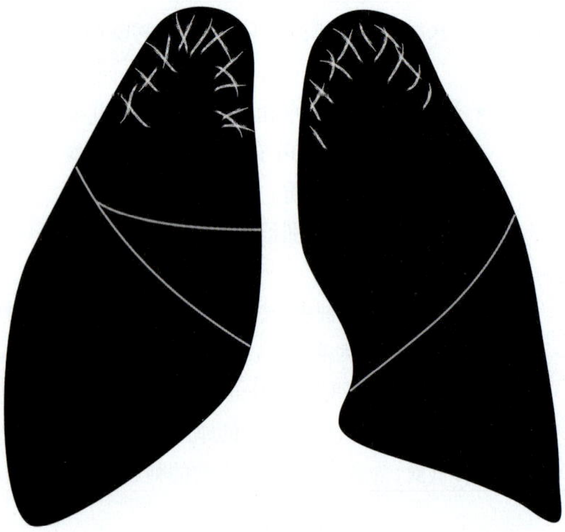

Coronal schematic shows fibrotic changes in the upper lobes.
冠状位示意图显示双肺上叶纤维化改变。

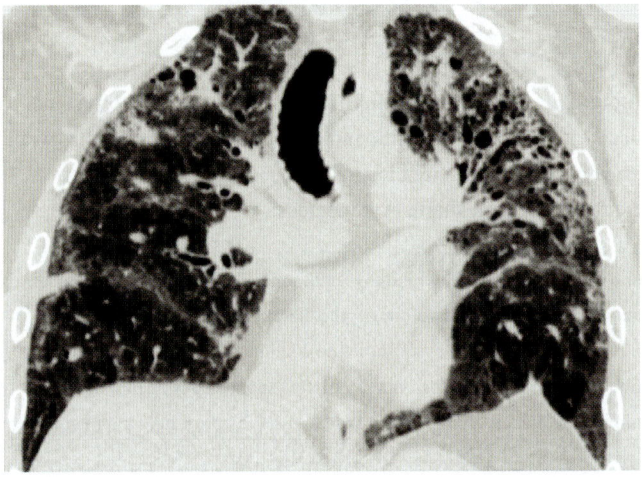

Coronal CT shows upper-lobe predominant subpleural fibrosis and traction bronchiectasis. A pathologic diagnosis was not established in this case.
冠状位CT显示上叶为主的胸膜下纤维化和牵拉性支气管扩张。该例无病理学诊断。

- Although IPF is the most common cause of pulmonary fibrosis, fibrosis primarily affecting the upper lobes is typically caused by an alternative diagnosis, such as:

End-stage sarcoidosis. Sarcoidosis is a disease that primarily affects the upper lobes. The late stage of sarcoidosis leads to upper-lobe predominant fibrosis.
Chronic hypersensitivity pneumonitis.
End-stage silicosis. The late stage of silicosis may lead to fibrosis with an upper lobe predominance.

- 虽然IPF是肺纤维化最常见的原因，但以累及肺上叶为主的纤维化通常由其他疾病引起，例如：

晚期结节病，结节病是一种主要累及上叶的疾病。晚期结节病会导致以上叶为主的纤维化。
慢性过敏性肺炎。
晚期硅沉着病，可导致上叶为主的纤维化。

(翻译　南海燕)

PULMONARY INFECTION

肺部感染

CLINICAL CLASSIFICATION OF PNEUMONIA

肺炎的临床分类

Community-acquired pneumonia (CAP)

- *S. pneumoniae* is the most common cause of community-acquired pneumonia

社区获得性肺炎(CAP)

- 肺炎链球菌是CAP最常见的原因。

(CAP).

- Atypical pneumonia, including *Mycoplasma*, viral, and *Chlamydia*, typically infects young and otherwise healthy patients.

  Mycoplasma has a varied appearance and can produce consolidation, areas of ground glass attenuation, centrilobular nodules, and tree-in-bud nodules.

- *Legionella* most commonly occurs in elderly smokers. Infections tend to be severe.
- Infection by *Klebsiella* and other gram-negatives occurs in alcoholics and aspirators.

  Klebsiella classically leads to voluminous inflammatory exudates causing the *bulging fissure sign*.

Hospital-acquired pneumonia (HAP)

- Hospital-acquired pneumonia (HAP) occurs in hospitalized patients and is due to aspiration of colonized secretions. HAP is caused by a wide variety of organisms, but the most important pathogens include MRSA and resistant gram-negatives including *Pseudomonas*.

Healthcare-associated pneumonia (HCAP)

- Healthcare-associated pneumonia is defined as pneumonia in a nursing home resident or in a patient with a >2 day hospitalization over the past 90 days. Pathogens are similar to HAP.

Ventilator-associated pneumonia (VAP)

- Ventilator-associated pneumonia is caused by infectious agents not present at the time mechanical ventilation was started. Most infections are polymicrobial and primarily involve gram-negative rods such as *Pseudomonas* and *Acinetobacter*.

Pneumonia in the immunocompromised patient

- Any of the above pathogens, plus opportunistic infections including *Pneumocystis*, fungi such as *Aspergillus*, *Nocardia*, CMV, etc., can be seen in immunocompromised patients.
- Different types of immunocompromise can lead to different infections. In particular, neutropenia predisposes to fungal pneumonia.

Radiographic Patterns of Infection

Lobar pneumonia

- Lobar pneumonia is consolidation of a single lobe. It is usually bacterial in origin and is the most common presentation of community-acquired pneumonia. The larger bronchi remain patent, causing air bronchograms.

Bronchopneumonia

- Bronchopneumonia is patchy peribronchial consolidation with air-space opacities, usually involving several lobes, and may be caused by both bacterial and viral pneumonias as well as aspiration.

Interstitial pneumonia

- Interstitial pneumonia is a misnomer, a finding on CXR that usually corresponds to ground glass on CT. Generally it can be caused by atypical (e.g., *Mycoplasma*, *Chlamydia*), viral, or *Pneumocystis* pneumonia.

Round pneumonia

- Round pneumonia is an infectious mass-like opacity seen in children, most commonly due to *S. pneumoniae*. Infection remains confined due to incomplete formation of pores of Kohn.

- 非典型肺炎，包括支原体、病毒和衣原体，通常感染年轻人和没有其他疾病的健康人。

  支原体肺炎影像学表现多样，可产生实变、磨玻璃密度区、小叶中心结节和树芽样结节。

- 军团菌最常见于老年吸烟患者，感染往往很严重。
- 克雷伯菌和其他革兰氏阴性菌感染发生在酗酒和误吸的患者。

  克雷伯菌通常会导致大量炎性渗出物，从而产生叶间裂膨隆征。

医院获得性肺炎(HAP)

- HAP发生在住院患者中，是由误吸含有寄生菌落的分泌物所致。HAP可由很多种微生物引起，但最重要的病原体是耐甲氧西林金黄色葡萄球菌(MRSA)和包括假单胞菌在内的耐药革兰氏阴性菌。

健康护理相关性肺炎(HCAP)

- HCAP的定义为：护理院患者或过去90天内曾在医院住院>2天所发生的肺炎；病原体与HAP相似。

呼吸机相关性肺炎(VAP)

- VAP指感染的病原体在开始使用机械通气时并不存在。大多数感染是多种微生物，主要涉及革兰氏阴性杆菌，如假单胞菌和不动杆菌。

免疫功能低下患者的肺炎

- 上述任何病原体及机会性感染，包括肺孢子菌、真菌如曲霉菌、诺卡菌、巨细胞病毒等，均可见于免疫功能低下的患者。
- 不同类型的免疫功能低下会导致不同的感染。尤其是中性粒细胞减少者易患真菌性肺炎。

感染的影像学表现方式

大叶性肺炎

- 大叶性肺炎是单个肺叶的实变。通常由细菌引起，是社区获得性肺炎最常见表现。较大的支气管仍然保持畅通，产生空气支气管征。

支气管肺炎

- 支气管肺炎是斑片状支气管周围实变伴气腔密度增高影，通常涉及多个肺叶，可由细菌性和病毒性肺炎及误吸引起。

间质性肺炎

- 间质性肺炎是一个不恰当的名词，在胸部X线影像上的发现往往与CT上的磨玻璃影相对应。通常可由非典型(如支原体、衣原体)、病毒性或肺孢子菌肺炎引起。

球形肺炎

- 球形肺炎是见于儿童的一种感染性肿块样的密度增高影，最常由肺炎链球菌引起。由于肺泡孔的形成不完全，感染范围有限。

Complications of Pneumonia

Pulmonary abscess

- Pulmonary abscess is necrosis of the lung parenchyma typically due to *Staphylococcus aureus*, *Pseudomonas*, or anaerobic bacteria.
- An air-fluid level is often present.
- An abscess is usually spherical, with equal dimensions on frontal and lateral views.

Empyema

- Empyema is infection within the pleural space.
- There are three stages in the development of an empyema:

  1) **Free-flowing exudative effusion**: Can be treated with needle aspiration or simple drain.

  2) **Development of fibrous strands**: Requires large-bore chest tube and fibrinolytic therapy.

  3) **Fluid becomes solid and jelly-like**: Usually requires surgery.

- Although pneumonia is often associated with a parapneumonic effusion, most pleural effusions associated with pneumonia are *not* empyema, but are instead a sterile effusion caused by increased capillary permeability.
- An empyema conforms to the shape of the pleural space, causing a longer air-fluid level on the lateral radiograph. This is in contrast to an abscess, discussed above, which typically is spherical and has the same dimensions on the frontal and lateral radiographs.
- The *split pleura sign* describes enhancing parietal and visceral pleura of an empyema seen on contrast-enhanced study.

肺炎的并发症

肺脓肿

- 肺脓肿是肺实质坏死，通常由金黄色葡萄球菌、假单胞菌或厌氧菌引起。
- 常出现气-液平面。
- 脓肿通常是球形的，其直径在正位和侧位上相同。

脓胸

- 脓胸是胸膜腔内的感染。
- 脓胸的发展分为三个阶段：

  1) **自由流动的渗出性积液**：可用针吸或单纯引流治疗。

  2) **纤维条索形成**：需要大口径胸腔引流管和纤溶治疗。

  3) **液体变成固体和果冻状**：通常需要手术。

- 尽管肺炎常伴发肺炎旁胸腔积液，但大多数与肺炎相关的胸腔积液不是脓胸，而是毛细血管通透性增加所致的无菌性积液。
- 脓胸的形状与胸膜腔一致，因而在侧位X线影像上出现更长的气-液平面。与上文讨论的脓肿不同，脓胸病灶通常呈球形，并且在正位和侧位X线影像上的大小相同。
- 胸膜分裂征是指脓胸处的壁胸膜和脏胸膜在增强扫描时都有强化。

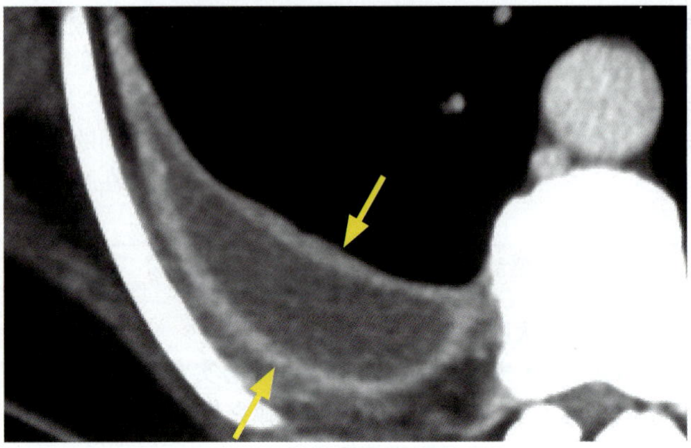

Split pleura sign: Contrast-enhanced CT shows enhancement of the thickened visceral and parietal pleural layers (arrows), which encase a pleural fluid collection.

The split pleura sign is seen in the majority of exudative effusions, although it is not specific. Similar findings can be seen in malignant effusion, mesothelioma, fibrothorax, and after talc pleurodesis.

Case courtesy Ritu R. Gill, MD, MPH, Brigham and Women's Hospital.

胸膜分裂征：增强CT显示增厚的脏胸膜和壁胸膜有强化(黄箭)，并包裹胸腔液体。

胸膜分裂征见于大多数渗出性积液，但不具特异性。类似的表现可见于恶性积液、间皮瘤、纤维胸和滑石粉胸膜固定术后。

Empyema necessitans

- Empyema necessitans is extension of an empyema to the chest wall, most commonly secondary to tuberculosis. Other causative organisms include *Actinomyces*.

Pneumatocele

- A pneumatocele is a thin-walled, gas-filled cyst that may be post-traumatic or develop as a sequela of pneumonia, typically from *Staphylococcus aureus* or *Pneumocystis*.

Bronchopleural fistula (BPF)

- Bronchopleural fistula (BPF) is an abnormal communication between the airway and the pleural space. It is caused by rupture of the visceral pleura. By far the most common cause of BPF is surgery; however, other etiologies include lung abscess, empyema, and trauma.

自溃性脓胸

- 自溃性脓胸是脓胸延伸至胸壁，最常继发于结核。其他致病微生物包括放线菌。

肺气囊

- 肺气囊是一种薄壁、充满气体的囊肿，可能是外伤或肺炎的后遗症发展而来，通常由金黄色葡萄球菌或肺孢子菌引起。

支气管胸膜瘘(BPF)

- 支气管胸膜瘘(BPF)是气道和胸膜腔之间的异常交通。它由脏胸膜破裂引起。BPF最常见的原因是手术；其他病因包括肺脓肿、脓胸和外伤。

- On imaging, new or increasing gas is present in a pleural effusion. A connection between the bronchial tree and the pleura is not always apparent, but is helpful when seen.
- The treatment of BPF is controversial and highly individualized.

- 在影像学上，胸腔积液中新增气体或原有气体增加。支气管树和胸膜之间的交通并不总是明显，但看到时会有所帮助。
- BPF的治疗存在争议且高度个体化。

TUBERCULOSIS (TB)

肺结核病(TB)

- Tuberculosis (TB), caused by *Mycobacterium tuberculosis,* remains an important disease despite remarkable progress in public health and antituberculous therapy over the past century. Tuberculosis remains a significant problem in developing countries. In the United States, TB is seen primarily in immigrant, institutionalized, and immunocompromised individuals.
- Initial exposure to TB can lead to two clinical outcomes:

  1) **Contained disease (90%)** results in calcified granulomas and/or calcified hilar lymph nodes. In a patient with normal immunity, the tuberculous bacilli are sequestered with a caseating granulomatous response.

  2) **Primary tuberculosis** results when the host cannot contain the organism. Primary tuberculosis is seen more commonly in children and immunocompromised patients.
- **Reactivation (post-primary)** TB is reactivation of a previously latent infection.

- 尽管在过去的一个世纪(20世纪以来)公共卫生和抗结核治疗方面取得了显著进展，但由结核分枝杆菌引起的结核病(TB)仍然是一种重要的疾病。TB在发展中国家仍然是一个重大问题。在美国，TB主要见于移民、收容机构居住者和免疫功能低下者。
- 初次接触结核会导致两种临床结果：

  1) **自限性疾病(90%)**导致钙化性肉芽肿和/或肺门淋巴结钙化。在免疫功能正常的患者，结核分枝杆菌被干酪样肉芽肿隔离。

  2) **原发性结核病**发生在宿主不能将微生物局限化时，更常见于儿童和免疫功能低下的患者。
- **复燃性(原发后)**TB是先前潜伏的感染被再次激活。

Primary tuberculosis

原发性结核病

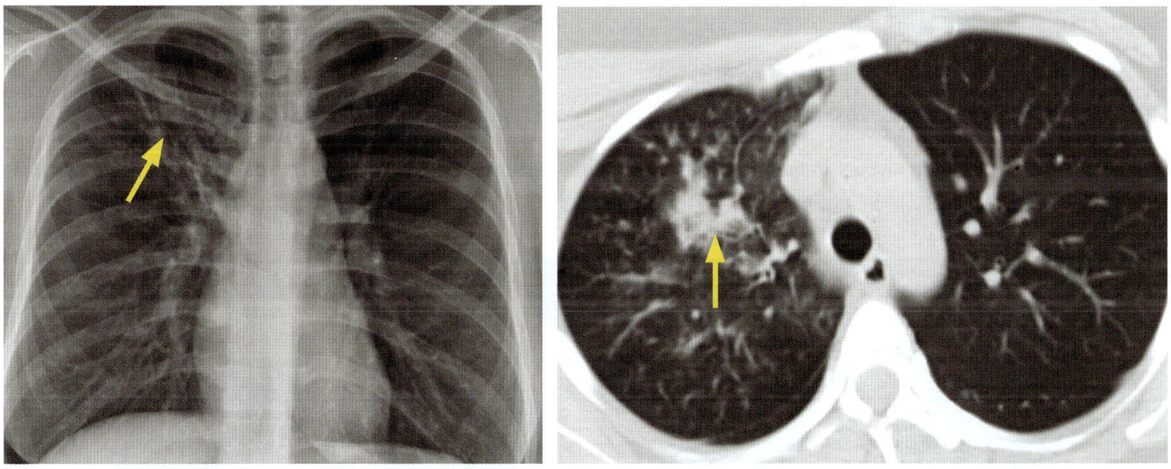

Primary TB. Chest radiograph (left image) shows a vague right upper lung opacity (arrow). CT shows a patchy opacification (arrow) in the lower portion of the right upper lobe with adjacent tree-in-bud nodularity. The patient's sputum grew *Mycobacterium tuberculosis.*
Case courtesy Ritu R. Gill, MD, MPH, Brigham and Women's Hospital.
原发性TB：胸部X线影像(左图)显示模糊的右上肺阴影(黄箭)。CT显示右肺上叶下部斑片状密度增高影(黄箭)伴邻近树芽结节。此患者的痰中有结核分枝杆菌生长。

- Primary TB represents infection from the first exposure to TB. Primary TB may involve the pulmonary parenchyma, the airways, and the pleura. Primary TB often causes adenopathy.
- As many as 15% of patients infected with primary TB have no radiographic changes and the imaging appearance of primary TB is nonspecific.
- The typical imaging manifestation of primary TB is lobar consolidation +/− pleural effusion and lymphadenopathy, although not all of these need to be present. Primary TB may occur in any lobe. Both primary and reactivation TB can also present as isolated pleural disease or miliary disease, see next section

- 原发性TB是指首次接触结核分枝杆菌而发生的感染，可能累及肺实质、气道和胸膜，常引起淋巴结肿大。
- 多达15%的原发性TB患者没有影像学上的改变，并且原发性TB的影像学表现无特异性。
- 原发性TB典型的影像学表现是肺叶实变+/−胸腔积液和淋巴结肿大，但这些表现并非全都会出现。原发性TB可发生在任何肺叶。原发性和复燃性TB也可以表现为孤立的胸膜

on miliary TB.

- Classic imaging findings are not always seen, but include:

  Ghon focus: Initial focus of parenchymal infection, usually located in the upper part of the lower lobe or the lower part of the upper lobe.

  Ranke complex: *Ghon focus* and lymphadenopathy.

- Cavitation is rare in primary TB, in contrast to reactivation TB.
- Adenopathy is common in primary TB, typically featuring central low-attenuation and peripheral enhancement, especially in children.

疾病或粟粒样病变，详见下文粟粒性结核。

- 典型的影像学表现并不总是出现，但包括：

  原发复合征(Ghon病灶)：肺实质感染的初始病灶，通常位于下叶上部或上叶的下部。

  Ranke复合体：Ghon病灶和淋巴结肿大。

- 空洞很少见于原发性TB，这与复燃性TB不同。
- 淋巴结肿大在原发性TB中很常见，通常表现为中央低密度和周边强化，尤其是在儿童。

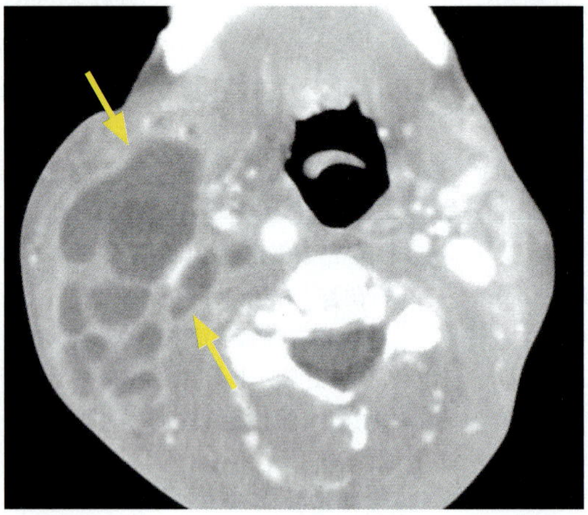

Tuberculous adenopathy: Contrast-enhanced neck CT shows marked right-sided adenopathy (arrows) with peripheral enhancement and central necrosis.

Case courtesy Ritu R. Gill, MD, MPH, Brigham and Women's Hospital.

结核性淋巴结肿大：颈部增强 CT显示明显的右侧淋巴结肿大(黄箭)，伴周边强化和中央坏死。

Reactivation (post-primary) tuberculosis

- Reactivation TB, also called post-primary TB, usually occurs in adolescents and adults and is caused by reactivation of a dormant infection acquired earlier in life. Clinical manifestations of reactivation TB include chronic cough, low-grade fever, hemoptysis, and night sweats.
- Reactivation TB most commonly occurs in the upper lobe apical and posterior segments and superior segments of the lower lobes.

复燃性(原发后)结核病

- 复燃性TB，也称为原发后TB，常见于青少年和成人，由早年感染而遗留的潜伏病灶激活所致。复燃性TB的临床表现包括慢性咳嗽、低热、咯血和盗汗。
- 复燃性TB最常见于上叶的尖段、后段和下叶背段。

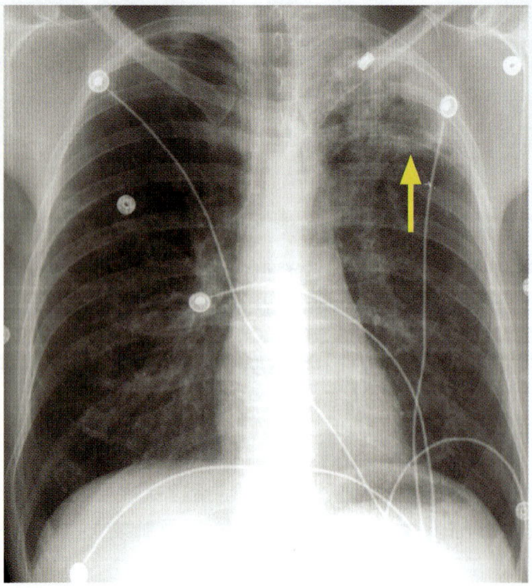

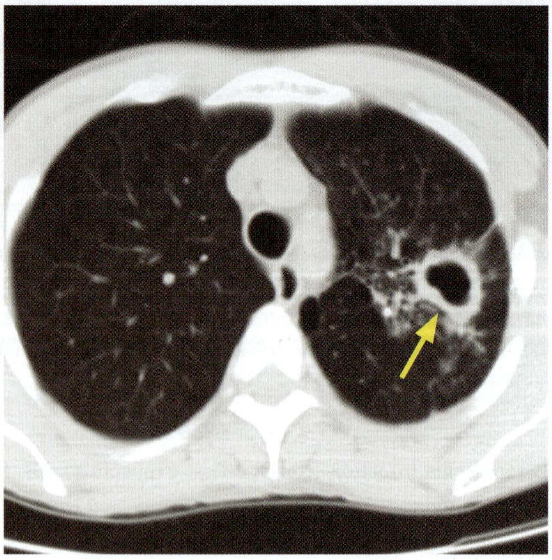

Reactivation TB: Frontal chest radiograph (left image) shows a cavitary lesion in the left upper lobe (arrow), confirmed by CT (arrow). There was no significant mediastinal adenopathy. The differential diagnosis of this appearance would include cavitary primary lung cancer, which would be expected to feature a thicker wall.

Case courtesy Michael Hanley, MD, University of Virginia Health System.

复燃性 TB：正位胸部X线影像(左图)显示左上叶一个空洞病灶(黄箭)，并得到CT(右图)证实(黄箭)，没有明显的纵隔淋巴结肿大。此影像学表现的鉴别诊断应包括空洞型原发性肺癌，特征是壁较厚。

- In an immunocompetent patient, the imaging hallmarks of reactivation TB are upper-lobe predominant consolidation with cavitation. Tree-in-bud nodules are common and suggest active **endobronchial spread**.
- Low-attenuation adenopathy is a common additional finding, seen more often in immunocompromised patients.
- A **tuberculoma** is a well-defined rounded opacity consisting of an encapsulating fibrous wall with central caseation, usually in the upper lobes.

- 在免疫功能正常的患者中，复燃性TB的影像学标志是上叶为主的实变伴空洞。树芽结节很常见，提示有活动性**支气管内播散**。
- 低密度淋巴结肿大是另一种常见的表现，更常见于免疫功能低下的患者。
- **结核瘤**是一种边界清楚的圆形阴影，由包裹性纤维壁和中央干酪样结构组成，通常在上叶。

Healed tuberculosis

痊愈后肺结核

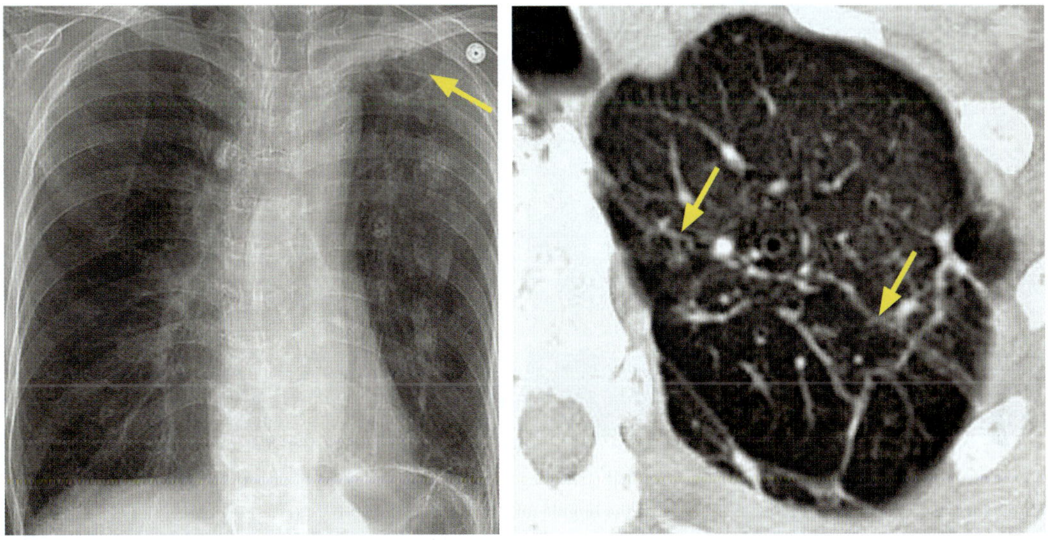

Healed TB: Radiograph shows scarring, volume loss, and superior hilar retraction (arrows). CT shows apical scarring. *Case courtesy Ritu R. Gill, MD, MPH, Brigham and Women's Hospital.*

痊愈后TB：X线影像(左图)显示瘢痕形成、肺容积减少和肺门向上牵拉(黄箭)。CT(右图)显示肺尖瘢痕。

- Healed TB is evident on radiography as apical scarring, usually with upper lobe volume loss and superior hilar retraction.
- Calcified granulomas may be present as well, which indicate containment of the initial infection by a delayed hypersensitivity response.

- 痊愈后TB在X线影像上表现为肺尖瘢痕，通常伴有上叶肺容积减少和肺门向上牵拉。
- 也可能存在钙化肉芽肿，这表明迟发性超敏反应使初始感染得到了控制。

Miliary tuberculosis

粟粒性肺结核

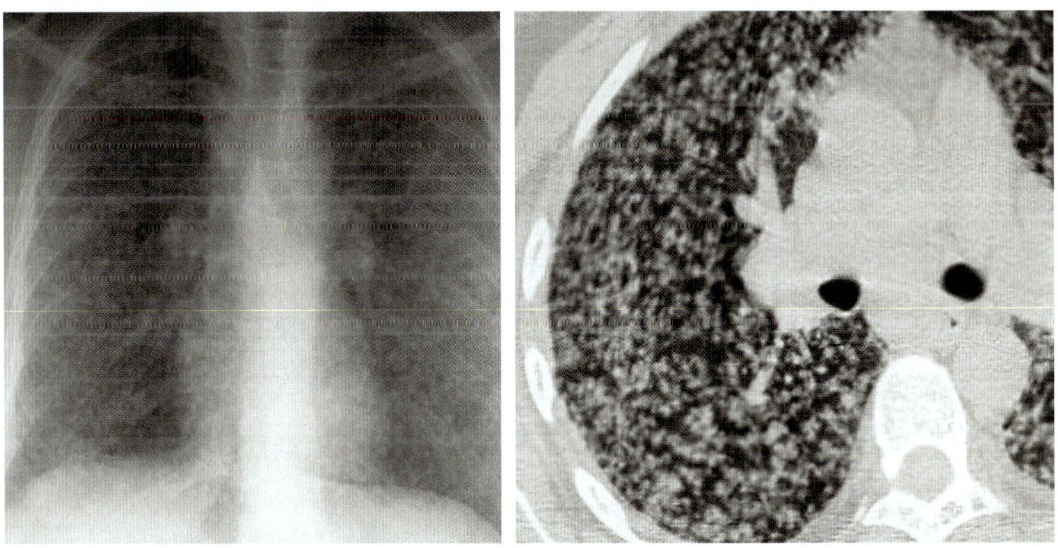

Miliary TB: Radiograph and CT show innumerable tiny nodules in a random pattern, reflecting hematogenous seeding of TB. *Case courtesy Ritu R. Gill, MD, MPH, Brigham and Women's Hospital.*

粟粒性TB：X线影像(左图)和CT(右图)显示无数随机分布的微小结节，反映TB的血行播散。

- Miliary TB is a diffuse random distribution of tiny nodules seen in hematogenously disseminated TB.
- Miliary TB can occur in primary or reactivation TB.

- 粟粒性TB是一种弥漫性随机分布的微小结节，见于血行播散性TB。
- 粟粒性TB可发生在原发性或复燃性TB。

ATYPICAL MYCOBACTERIA

非典型分枝杆菌

Atypical mycobacteria infection

非典型分枝杆菌感染

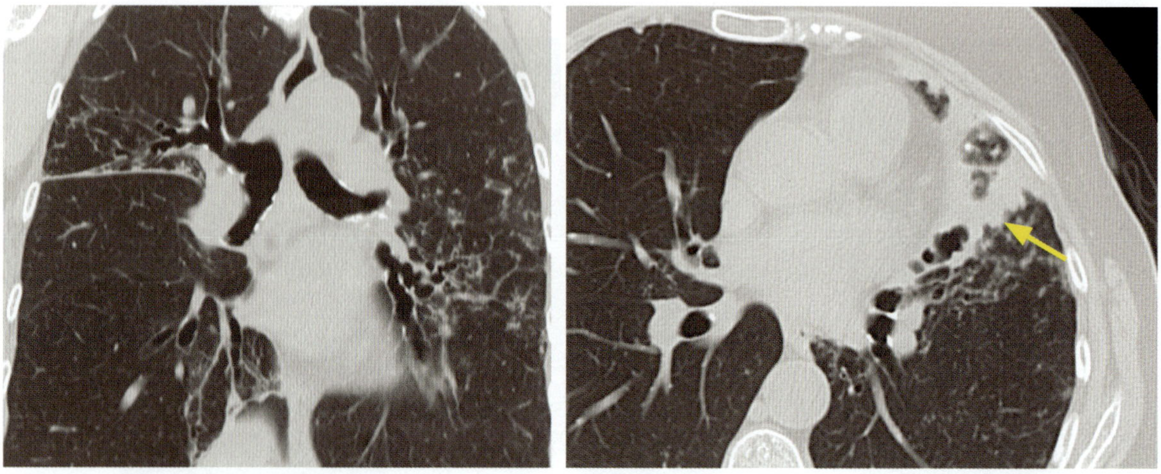

Mycobacterium avium intracellulare infection: Coronal (left image) and axial CT show right upper lobe and lingular tree-in-bud opacities and bronchiectasis, with more focal consolidation in the lingula (arrow).

鸟-胞内分枝杆菌感染：冠状位(左图)和轴位(右图)CT显示右肺上叶和左肺舌段树芽影和支气管扩张，在舌段有较多的局灶性实变(黄箭)。

- There are three types of atypical mycobacterial infection:
  (1) "Classic" or nodular cavitary form that simulates TB; typically seen in patients with chronic lung disease.
  (2) Non-classic or bronchiectatic form (more common).
  (3) Disseminated form, typically lymphadenopathy in immunocompromised patients (usually AIDS).
- The presentation of bronchiectatic atypical mycobacteria is an elderly woman with cough, low-grade fever, and weight loss, called **Lady Windermere syndrome**. *Mycobacterium avium intracellulare* and *M. kansasii* are the two most common organisms.
  Radiographic findings are bronchiectasis and tree-in-bud nodules, most common in the right middle lobe and lingula.

"Hot-tub" lung

- "Hot-tub" lung is a hypersensitivity pneumonitis in response to atypical mycobacteria, which are often found in hot tubs. There is no active infection and the typical patient is otherwise healthy. Imaging is similar to other causes of hypersensitivity pneumonitis, featuring centrilobular nodules.

- 非典型分枝杆菌感染分为三种类型：
  (1) 与结核相似的"经典"型或结节样空洞型；通常见于有慢性肺部疾病的患者。
  (2) 非经典型或支气管扩张型(较常见)。
  (3) 播散型，在免疫功能低下患者(通常是艾滋病)通常表现为淋巴结肿大。
- 支气管扩张型非典型分枝杆菌感染见于老年女性，表现为咳嗽、低热和体重减轻，故被称为**温夫人综合征**。鸟-胞内分枝杆菌和堪萨斯分枝杆菌是最常见的两种病原体。
  影像学表现为支气管扩张和树芽结节，最常见于右肺中叶和左肺上叶舌段。

"热浴"肺

- "热浴"肺是一种由非典型分枝杆菌引起的过敏性肺炎，在热水浴缸中常能够找到这种病菌。典型的病例通常没有活动性感染，且在其他方面表现正常。影像学表现与其他病因引起的过敏性肺炎相似，表现为小叶中心结节。

ENDEMIC FUNGI

地方性真菌

- Endemic fungi can cause pneumonia in normal individuals, with each subtype having a specific geographic distribution.

Histoplasma capsulatum

- *Histoplasma capsulatum* is localized to the Ohio and Mississippi river valleys, in soil contaminated with bat or bird guano.

- 地方性真菌可以在正常人引起肺炎，每种亚型都有其特定的地理分布。

荚膜组织胞浆菌属

- 荚膜组织胞浆菌在美国分布于俄亥俄州和密西西比河流域，存在于被蝙蝠或鸟粪污染的

- Acute infection usually produces nodules and lymphadenopathy.
- Chronic sequela of infection is a calcified granuloma. A less common radiologic manifestation is a pulmonary nodule (histoplasmoma), which can mimic a neoplasm.
- Fibrosing mediastinitis is a rare complication of *Histoplasma* infection of mediastinal lymph nodes leading to pulmonary venous obstruction, bronchial stenosis, and pulmonary artery stenosis. Affected lymph nodes tend to calcify.

土壤中。
- 急性感染通常会产生结节和淋巴结肿大。
- 慢性感染的后遗症为钙化性肉芽肿。较少见的一种影像学表现是肺结节(组织胞浆瘤)，可以与肿瘤相似。
- 纤维性纵隔炎是组织胞浆菌感染纵隔淋巴结的一种罕见并发症，可导致肺静脉阻塞、支气管狭窄和肺动脉狭窄。受累淋巴结常有钙化。

Coccidioides immitis and *Blastomyces dermatitidis*

- *Coccidioides immitis* is found in the southwestern United States and has a variety of radiologic appearances, including multifocal consolidation, multiple pulmonary nodules, and miliary nodules.
- *Blastomyces dermatitidis* is found in the central and southeastern United States. Infection is usually asymptomatic, but may present as flu-like illness that can progress to multifocal consolidation, ARDS, or miliary disease.

粗球孢子菌病和皮炎芽生菌病

- 粗球孢子菌病分布于美国西南部，具有多种影像学表现，包括多灶性实变、多发肺结节，以及粟粒样结节。
- 皮炎芽生菌病流行于美国中部和东南部。感染通常无症状，但可能表现为流感样症状，并可进展为多灶性实变、ARDS或粟粒性疾病。

Viral pneumonia

- In general, viral pneumonias have a large overlap with bacterial pneumonias in imaging appearance.
- Classic imaging findings on CT include centrilobular or tree-in-bud nodules, patchy ground glass opacities, and bronchopneumonia (peribronchial consolidations).

Severe acute respiratory syndrome coronavirus 2 (SARS-CoV-2)

- Severe acute respiratory syndrome coronavirus 2 SARS-CoV-2 (i.e., COVID-19) is a respiratory viral disease that became a pandemic in early 2020.
- Imaging findings are nonspecific, however bilateral, dependent, lower-lobe predominant ground glass opacities or consolidations are classic features.
- Pleural effusions, centrilobular nodules, and tree-in-bud nodules are typically not associated.

病毒性肺炎

- 一般而言，病毒性肺炎在影像学上的表现与细菌性肺炎有很大重叠。
- 典型的CT表现有小叶中心或树芽结节、斑片状磨玻璃影和支气管肺炎(支气管周围实变)。

严重急性呼吸综合征冠状病毒 2(SARS-CoV-2)

- SARS-CoV-2(即COVID-19，新型冠状病毒)是一种呼吸道病毒性疾病，并在2020年初开始大流行。
- 影像学表现无特异性，但常常以双肺、下垂部位、下叶为主的磨玻璃影或实变为特征。
- 通常不伴发胸腔积液、小叶中心结节和树芽结节。

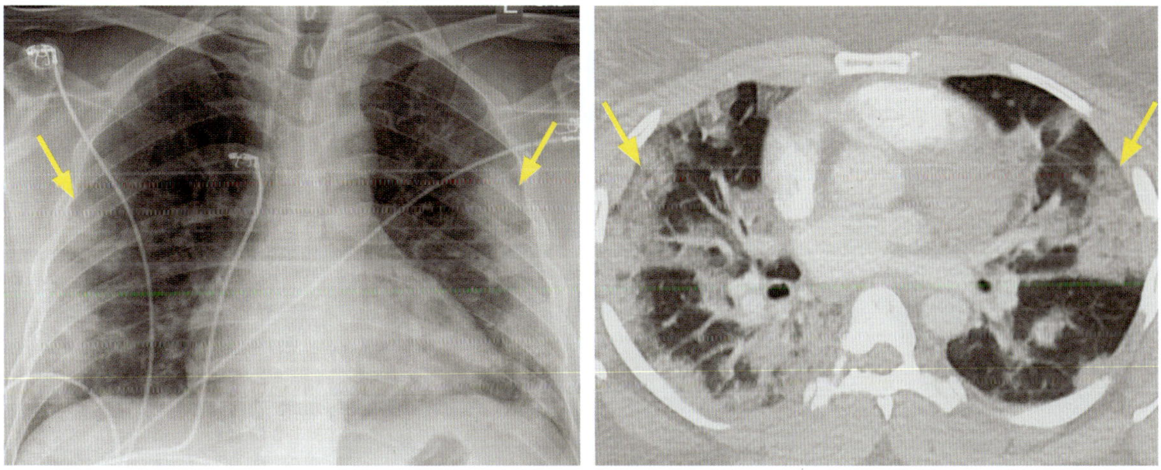

COVID-19 infection: Chest radiograph (left image) shows bilateral peripheral opacities (arrows). Chest CT (right) in a different patient shows peripheral ground glass and consolidations in both lungs (arrows).
新型冠状病毒感染：胸部X线影像(左图)显示双侧外周阴影(黄箭)。另一名患者的胸部CT(右图)显示双肺外周磨玻璃影和实变(黄箭)。

INFECTIONS IN THE IMMUNOCOMPROMISED

- Immunosuppressed patients are susceptible to the same organisms that infect immunocompetent patients; however, one must be aware of several additional opportunistic organisms that may present in the immunocompromised.
- An immunocompromised patient with a focal air space opacity is most likely to have a bacterial pneumonia (most commonly pneumococcus), but TB should also be considered if the CD4 count is low.
- In contrast, multifocal opacities have a wider differential diagnosis including *Pneumocystis* pneumonia and opportunistic fungal infection such as *Cryptococcus* or *Aspergillus*.

***Pneumocystis jiroveci* pneumonia**

- *Pneumocystis jiroveci* (previously called *Pneumocystis carinii*) is an opportunistic fungus that may cause pneumonia in individuals with CD4 counts <200 cells/cc or other T-cell deficiency (e.g., status post bone marrow transplant or solid organ transplant). The incidence of *Pneumocystis* pneumonia is decreasing due to routine antibiotic prophylaxis.

免疫功能低下者的感染

- 免疫抑制患者同样易感免疫功能正常患者所感染的病原体；但必须注意在免疫功能低下患者中可能出现的其他几种机会性微生物。
- 免疫功能低下患者出现局灶性气腔阴影最有可能是细菌性肺炎(最常见的是肺炎球菌)，但如果CD$_4$计数低，也应考虑TB。
- 相比之下，多灶性密度增高影有更广泛的鉴别诊断，包括肺孢子菌肺炎和机会性真菌感染，如隐球菌或曲霉菌。

耶氏肺孢子菌肺炎

- 耶氏肺孢子菌(旧称卡氏肺孢子菌)是一种机会性真菌，可在CD$_4$计数<200个细胞/mL或其他T细胞缺陷(如骨髓移植或实体器官移植后)的患者中引起肺炎。由于常规预防性抗生素的应用，肺孢子菌肺炎的发病率正在下降。

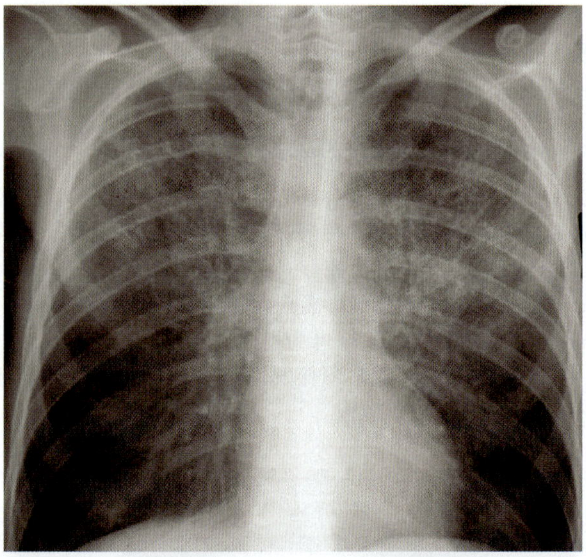

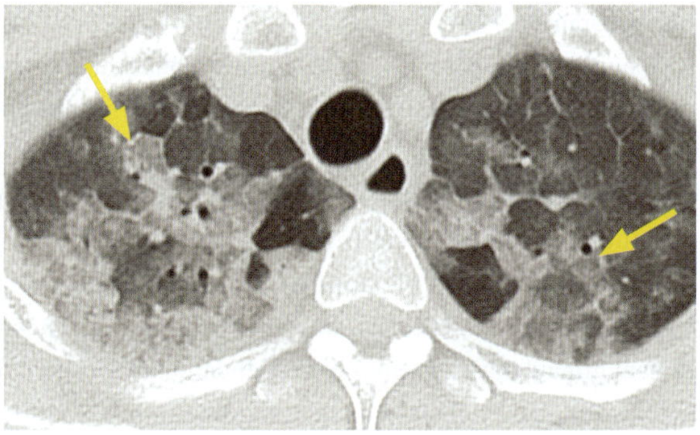

Pneumocystis pneumonia: Radiograph (top left image) shows multiple upper-lobe predominant airspace opacities. CT (top image) shows crazy paving (arrows), with confluent ground glass attenuation in the upper lobes.

肺孢子菌肺炎：X线影像(左上图)显示多发上叶为主的气腔阴影。CT(右上图)显示铺路石征(黄箭)，伴上叶融合的磨玻璃影。

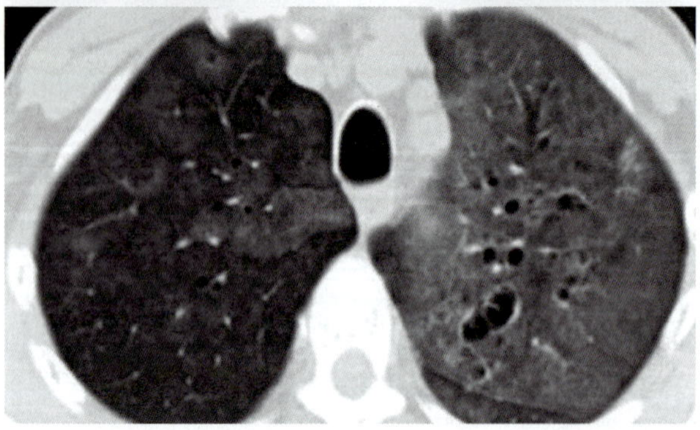

Axial CT in a different patient with *Pneumocystis* pneumonia (bottom left image) shows asymmetric ground glass opacification, with thin-walled cysts.

Cases courtesy Ritu R. Gill, MD, MPH, Brigham and Women's Hospital.

另一名肺孢子菌肺炎患者轴位CT(左下图)显示不对称的磨玻璃影，伴薄壁囊肿。

- Chest radiograph findings can be normal but a classic finding of *Pneumocystis* pneumonia is **bilateral perihilar (central) airspace opacities** with peripheral sparing.
- The classic CT appearance is **ground glass opacification**, sometimes with *crazy paving* (ground glass and thickening of the interlobular septa).
- A normal CT rules out *Pneumocystis* pneumonia; however, the disease can hide

- 胸部X线影像表现可以正常，但肺孢子菌肺炎的典型表现是**双侧肺门周围(中央性)气腔阴影**，周边不受累。
- 典型的CT表现是**磨玻璃影**，有时伴铺路石征(磨玻璃影和小叶间隔增厚)。
- CT影像正常可排除肺孢子菌肺炎；但胸部X

in a normal chest radiograph.

- *Pneumocystis* pneumonia has a propensity to cause upper lobe pneumatoceles particularly if untreated, which may predispose to pneumothorax or pneumomediastinum.

Cryptococcus neoformans

- *Cryptococcus* is an opportunistic organism and is the most common fungal infection in AIDS patients. Pulmonary infection usually coexists with cryptococcal meningitis.

  Typically CD4 count is less than 100 cells/cc in affected individuals.

- In the immunosuppressed, *Cryptococcus* can have a wide range of appearances ranging from ground glass attenuation to focal consolidation to cavitary nodules. *Cryptococcus* can also present as miliary disease, often associated with lymphadenopathy or effusions.

Aspergillus

Overview of Aspergillus

线影像可表现为正常。

- 肺孢子菌肺炎易引起上叶肺气囊，特别在未经治疗的患者，可导致气胸或纵隔气肿。

新型隐球菌

- 隐球菌是一种机会性微生物，是艾滋病患者中最常见的真菌感染。肺部感染通常与隐球菌性脑膜炎并存。

  感染患者的CD_4计数通常低于100个细胞/mL。

- 在免疫功能低下时，隐球菌的表现极具多样性，从磨玻璃影到实变，直至空洞性结节。隐球菌也可以表现为粟粒性疾病，常伴有淋巴结肿大或胸腔积液。

曲霉菌

曲霉菌概述

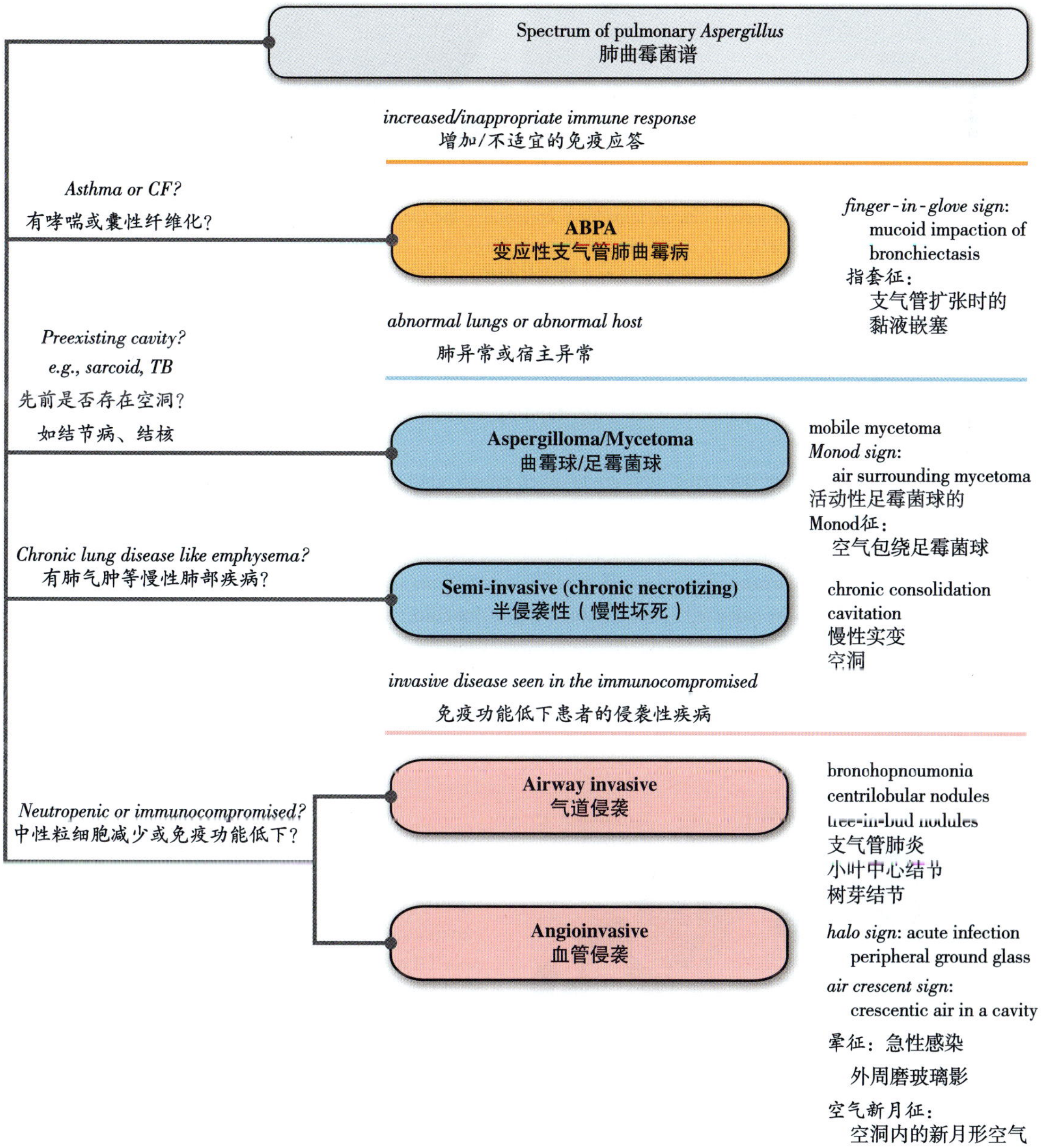

- *Aspergillus* is a ubiquitous soil fungus that manifests as five distinct categories of pulmonary disease. *Aspergillus* only affects those with abnormal immunity or preexisting pulmonary disease. Depending on the manifestation, the predisposing abnormality may include asthma, immunocompromised state, prior infection, or structural/congenital abnormality.

Allergic bronchopulmonary aspergillosis (ABPA)

- 曲霉菌是一种普遍存在的土壤真菌，可出现五种不同的肺部疾病。曲霉菌只影响免疫异常或原有肺部疾病的患者。根据临床表现，易感因素可包括哮喘、免疫抑制状态、既往感染或结构/先天性异常。

变应性支气管肺曲霉病(ABPA)

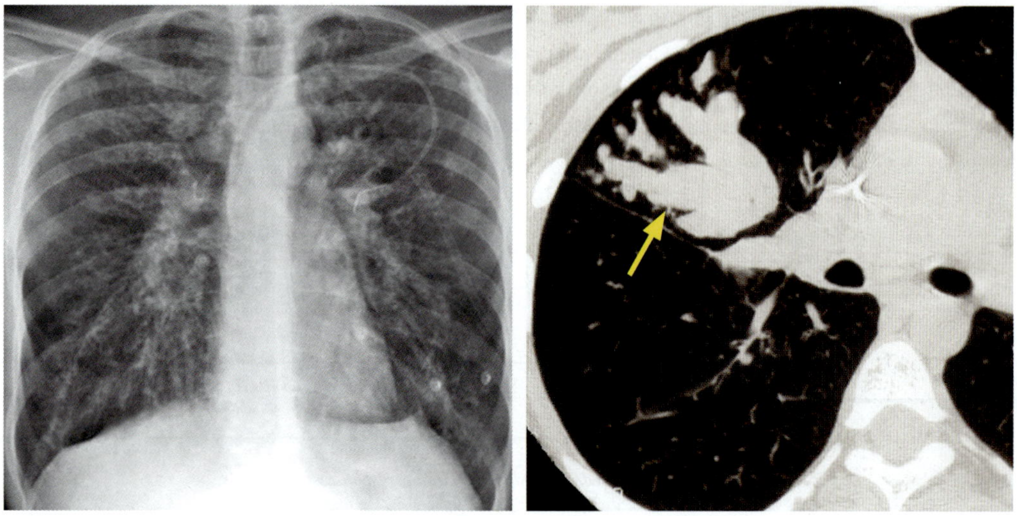

Finger-in-glove sign of ABPA: Chest radiograph shows upper-lobe predominant bronchiectasis with branching perihilar opacities. CT shows dense bronchial mucoid impaction representing the *finger-in-glove sign* (arrow).
Case courtesy Ritu R. Gill, MD, MPH, Brigham and Women's Hospital.
ABPA指套征：胸部X线影像(左图)显示上叶为主的支气管扩张伴肺门周围分支状阴影。CT(右图)显示高密度的支气管黏液嵌塞，为指套征(黄箭)。

- Allergic bronchopulmonary aspergillosis (ABPA) is a hypersensitivity reaction to aspergillus seen most commonly in patients with long-standing asthma. ABPA is not an infection.
- Patients present clinically with recurrent wheezing, low-grade fever, cough, and sputum production containing fragments of aspergillus hyphae. The diagnosis may be made using serum testing for aspergillus IgE.
- The key finding on CT is central bronchiectasis and mucoid impaction, which can be high attenuation or even calcified. This combination of mucoid impaction within bronchiectatic airways represents the *finger-in-glove sign*.

  The *finger-in-glove sign* is not specific to ABPA, however high attenuation mucus is a specific finding.

Saprophytic aspergillosis (aspergilloma)

- ABPA是一种对曲霉菌的超敏反应，最常见于长期哮喘的患者。ABPA不是感染。
- 患者在临床上表现为反复喘息、低热、咳嗽，痰中含有曲霉菌丝碎片。诊断可用血清检测曲霉菌免疫球蛋白E(IgE)。
- CT的主要表现是中央性支气管扩张和黏液嵌塞，后者可呈高密度甚至钙化。这种黏液嵌塞在扩张的支气管内的组合即为指套征。

  指套征不是ABPA特有的，但高密度黏液是一个特异性表现。

腐生性曲霉病(曲霉菌球)

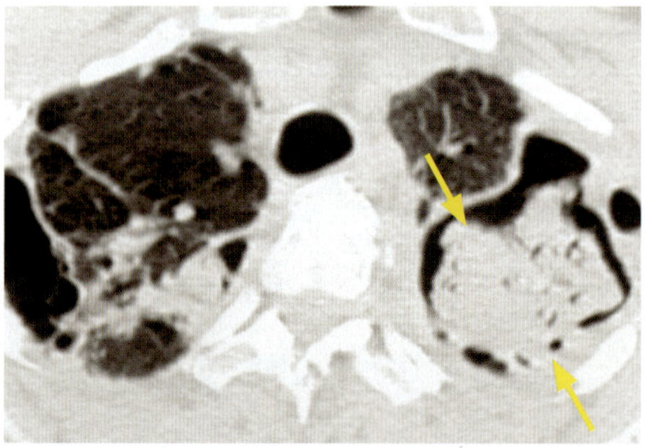

Aspergilloma and *Monod sign*: CT shows an irregular opacity (arrows) resting dependent within a left upper lobe cavity, representing an aspergilloma (arrows). The *Monod sign* is the curvilinear air surrounding the aspergilloma. This patient has prior TB with biapical scarring and left apical cavity.
Case courtesy Ritu R. Gill, MD, MPH, Brigham and Women's Hospital.
曲霉菌球和Monod征：CT显示不规则影(黄箭)位于左肺上叶空洞内的下垂位置，代表曲霉菌球(黄箭)。Monod征是曲霉菌球周围的曲线状空气影。该患者先前有TB伴双肺尖瘢痕和左肺尖空洞。

- An aspergilloma is a conglomeration of intertwined aspergillus fungal hyphae and cellular debris (a mycetoma or "fungus ball") in a *preexisting pulmonary cavity.*

  The aspergilloma is mobile and will shift position when the patient is imaged in a different position.

- The most common causes of a preexisting cavity are prior TB and sarcoidosis.

  Less common causes include congenital anomalies such as bronchogenic cyst or sequestration, and post-infectious/post-traumatic pneumatocele.

- If an aspergilloma is symptomatic, hemoptysis is the most common symptom. Treatment is embolization or resection rather than antifungal medication.
- When a crescent of air is seen outlining the mycetoma against the wall of the cavity, the correct term is *Monod sign*. The *air crescent sign* is reserved for angioinvasive aspergillus.

- 曲霉菌球是在原有的肺空洞内由曲霉菌丝和细胞碎片缠绕聚集而成(足菌肿或"真菌球")。

  曲霉菌球是可以移动的，当患者在不同体位成像时，曲霉菌球的位置会有改变。

- 最常导致空洞的原因是有TB和结节病史。

  较少见的原因包括先天性异常，如支气管囊肿或肺隔离症，以及感染/创伤后的肺气囊。

- 如果曲霉菌球出现症状，咯血最为常见。治疗采用栓塞或切除而不是抗真菌药物。
- 当看到新月形的空气围绕着空洞壁勾勒出真菌球体时，正确的术语应为Monod征。空气新月征用于血管侵袭性曲霉菌病。

Semi-invasive (chronic necrotizing) aspergillosis

- Semi-invasive aspergillosis is a necrotizing granulomatous inflammation (analogous in pathology to reactivation TB) in response to chronic aspergillus infection. Semi-invasive aspergillosis is seen in debilitated, diabetic, alcoholic, and COPD patients.
- Clinical symptoms include cough, chronic fever, and less commonly hemoptysis.
- On CT, there are segmental areas of consolidation, often with cavitation and pleural thickening, which progress slowly over months or years.

半侵袭性(慢性坏死性)曲霉菌病

- 半侵袭性曲霉菌病是针对慢性曲霉感染反应发生的一种坏死性肉芽肿性炎症(病理学上类似复燃性TB)。半侵袭性曲霉病见于虚弱、糖尿病、酗酒和慢性阻塞性肺疾病(COPD)患者。
- 临床症状包括咳嗽、慢性发热，偶尔咯血。
- CT表现为节段性实变区，常伴空洞和胸膜增厚，在数月或数年内缓慢进展。

Airway-invasive aspergillosis

- Airway-invasive aspergillosis is aspergillus infection deep to the airway epithelial cells. It is seen only in the immunocompromised, including neutropenic and AIDS patients.
- The spectrum of clinical disease ranges from bronchiolitis to bronchopneumonia.
- The main CT findings of airway-invasive aspergillosis are centrilobular and tree-in- bud nodules. When bronchopneumonia is present, radiograph and CT findings are indistinguishable from other causes of bronchopneumonia, such as *Staph. aureus*.

气道侵袭性曲霉菌病

- 气道侵袭性曲霉菌病是指曲霉菌进一步侵袭至气道上皮细胞。仅见于免疫功能低下的患者，包括中性粒细胞减少症和艾滋病患者。
- 临床表现从细支气管炎到支气管肺炎不等。
- 气道侵袭性曲霉菌病的主要CT表现是小叶中心型和树芽结节。当存在支气管肺炎时，X线影像和CT表现与其他原因的支气管肺炎无法区分，如金黄色葡萄球菌感染。

Angioinvasive aspergillosis

- Angioinvasive aspergillosis is an aggressive infection characterized by invasion and occlusion of arterioles and smaller pulmonary arteries by fungal hyphae. Angioinvasive aspergillosis is seen almost exclusively in neutropenic patients.
- The CT *halo sign* represents a halo of ground glass attenuation surrounding a consolidation. The ground glass corresponds to hemorrhage.

血管侵袭性曲霉菌病

- 血管侵袭性曲霉菌病是一种侵袭性感染，特征为真菌菌丝侵袭并阻塞小动脉和更小的肺动脉。血管侵袭性曲霉菌病几乎仅见于中性粒细胞减少的患者。
- CT晕征是指围绕实变区的磨玻璃影。磨玻璃影为出血所致。

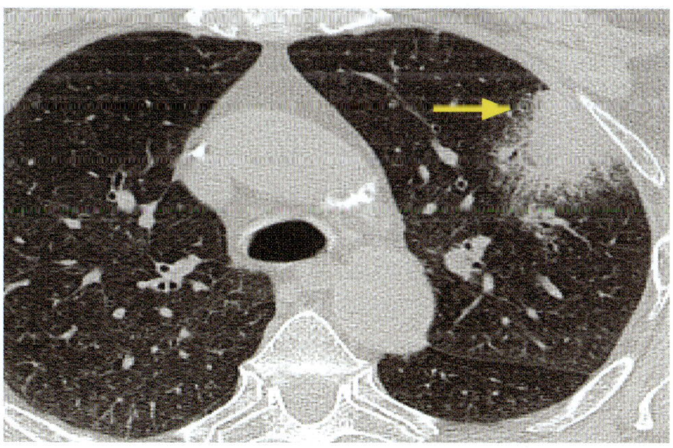

Halo sign: CT shows a left upper lobe mass with peripheral ground glass (yellow arrow), representing pulmonary hemorrhage.
Case courtesy Michael Hanley, MD, University of Virginia Health System.
晕征：CT显示左上叶肿块伴外周磨玻璃影(黄箭)，代表肺出血。

The *halo sign* is not specific to angioinvasive aspergillosis, and can also be seen in viral infection, granulomatosis with polyangiitis (GPA), Kaposi sarcoma, hemorrhagic metastasis, and others.

晕征不是血管侵袭性曲霉病所特有，也可见于病毒感染、肉芽肿性多血管炎(GPA)、卡波西肉瘤、出血性转移瘤等。

- The *air crescent sign* represents a crescent of air from retraction of infarcted lung and occurs with recovery of neutrophil counts. It a good prognostic sign as it indicates that the patient is in the recovery phase.

- 空气新月征代表梗死的肺组织回缩形成的新月形空气，出现时会伴随中性粒细胞计数恢复。这是一个预后良好的征象，因为它表明患者正处于恢复阶段。

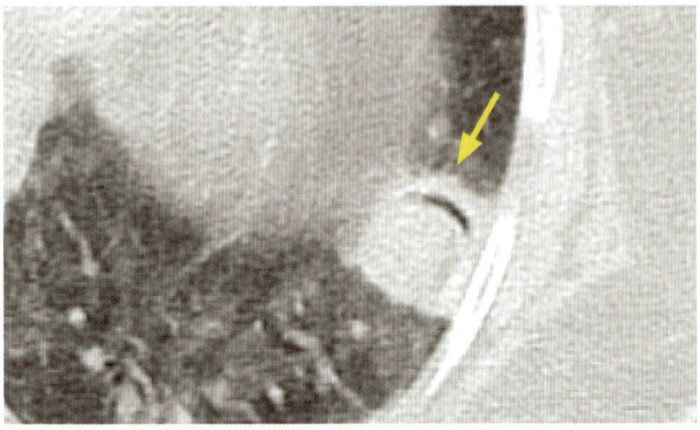

Air crescent sign: Noncontrast CT shows a lesion in the left lower lobe with a crescent-shaped air collection anteriorly (arrows).
空气新月征：平扫CT显示左肺下叶的病灶，前方有一处新月形的气体积聚(黄箭)。

(翻译　王维平)

PULMONARY EDEMA AND ICU IMAGING

肺水肿和ICU影像

PULMONARY EDEMA

肺水肿

Overview of pulmonary edema

肺水肿概述

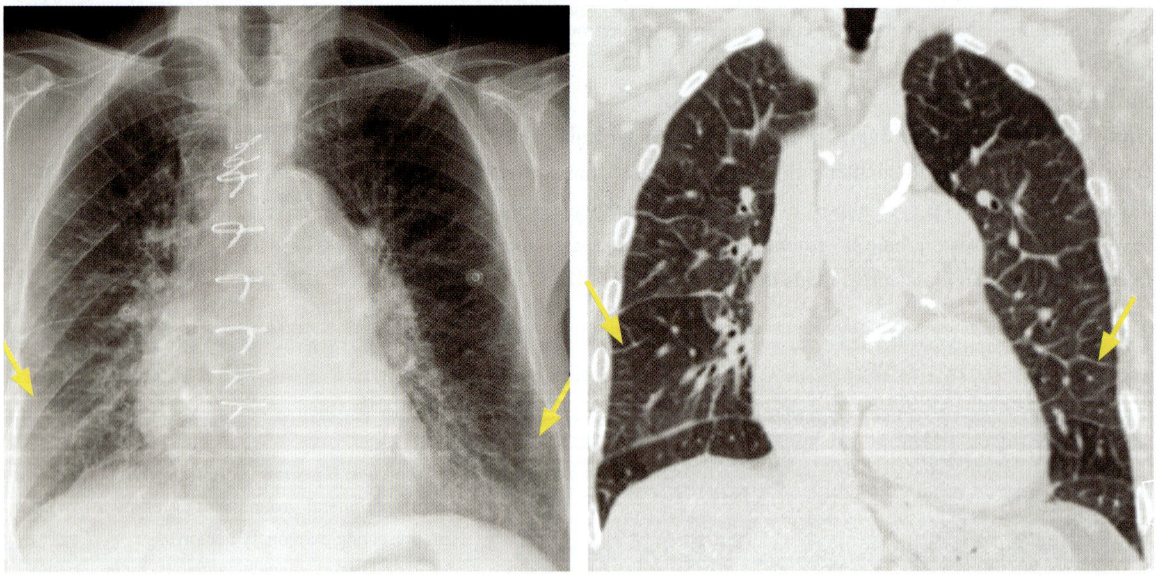

Mild pulmonary edema: Radiograph demonstrates moderate enlargement of the cardiac silhouette and sternotomy wires. There are increased interstitial markings with Kerley B lines (arrows). Chest CT shows smooth interlobular septal thickening (arrows), corresponding to the Kerley B lines seen on radiography. Mild geographic ground glass attenuation likely corresponds to early alveolar filling.
轻度肺水肿：X线影像显示心脏轮廓中度增大及胸骨金属缝合丝。肺间质纹理增加伴Kerley B线(黄箭)。胸部CT显示小叶间隔平滑性增厚(黄箭)，与X线影像上看到的Kerley B线相对应。轻微的地图样磨玻璃影可能为早期肺泡充盈。

- The radiographic severity of pulmonary edema typically progresses through three stages, corresponding to progressively increased pulmonary venous pressures.

- 影像学上肺水肿的严重程度通常经历三个阶段，对应于逐渐增加的肺静脉压力。

- **Vascular redistribution** is the first radiographic sign of increased pulmonary venous pressure. Imaging shows increased caliber of the upper lobe vessels compared to the lower lobe vessels.
- **Interstitial edema** is caused by increased fluid within the pulmonary veins, which surround the periphery of each secondary pulmonary lobule. On radiography, there are increased interstitial markings, indistinctness of the pulmonary vasculature, peribronchial cuffing, and Kerley B lines.

  Kerley B lines are seen at the peripheral lung and represent thickened interlobular septa.
- **Alveolar edema** is caused by filling of the alveoli with fluid. Edema typically has a perihilar (central) distribution. Pleural effusions and cardiomegaly are often present.
- CT findings of pulmonary edema include dependent or central ground glass opacification and interlobular septal thickening.
- Pulmonary edema is usually symmetric and dependent. A classic cause of asymmetric pulmonary edema is isolated right upper lobe pulmonary edema, caused by acute mitral regurgitation secondary to myocardial infarction and papillary muscle rupture.
- A complication of aggressive thoracentesis is **reexpansion pulmonary edema**, caused by rapid reexpansion of a lung in a state of collapse for more than three days.

- **血管再分布**是肺静脉压增高的第一个影像学征象。影像显示上叶血管的口径较下叶血管增粗。
- **间质性水肿**是由肺静脉内液体增多所引起，而肺静脉围绕每个次级肺小叶。在X线影像上，有肺间质纹理增加、肺血管模糊不清、支气管周围袖套和Kerley B线。

  Kerley B线见于肺的外周，代表增厚的小叶间隔。
- **肺泡性肺水肿**是由肺泡充满液体所致。水肿通常在肺门周围(中央)分布。常出现胸腔积液和心脏扩大。
- 肺水肿的CT表现包括下垂或中央部位磨玻璃影和小叶间隔增厚。
- 肺水肿通常呈对称性和下垂性分布。单侧肺水肿最常见的原因是孤立性右上叶肺水肿，这是由心肌梗死和乳头肌破裂引起的急性二尖瓣反流所致。
- 胸腔穿刺引流过度的一个并发症是**复张性肺水肿**，是由肺不张超过3天后被快速复张所致。

SUPPORT DEVICES

支持器材

Endotracheal tube

气管插管

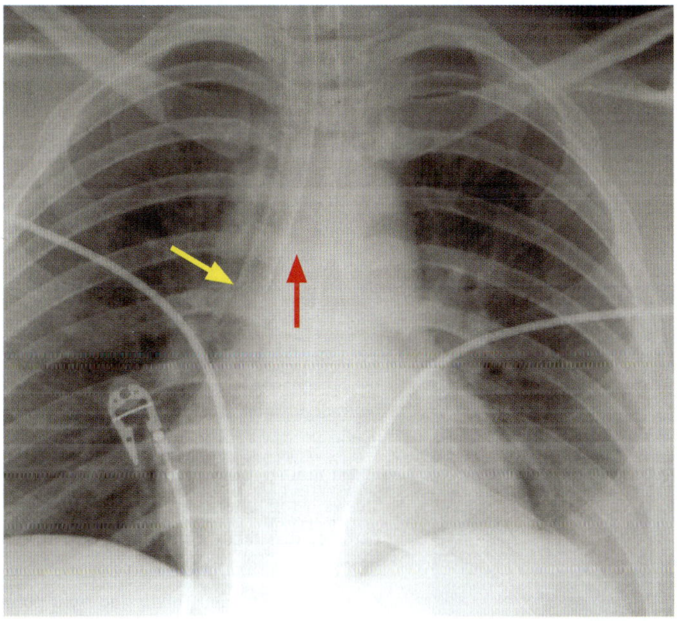

Right mainstem bronchus intubation: Chest radiograph shows the endotracheal tube terminating in the right mainstem bronchus (yellow arrow), a few centimeters distal to the carina (red arrow).

右主支气管插管：胸部X线影像显示气管插管末端进入右侧主支气管(黄箭)，在隆突下方约数厘米(红箭)。

- The endotracheal tube tip should be approximately 4–6 cm above the carina with the neck in neutral alignment. However, in situations with low pulmonary compliance (e.g., ARDS), a tip position closer to the carina may reduce barotrauma.
- Direct intubation of either the right or left mainstem bronchus (right mainstem bronchus far more common) is an emergent finding that can cause complete atelectasis of the un-intubated lung.

- 气管插管的尖端在颈部中立位时应位于隆突上方4~6cm。然而，在某些肺顺应性低的情况下(如ARDS)，尖端位置接近隆突可以减少气压伤。
- 插管直接进入右或左主支气管(右主支气管更为常见)是一个急症，可导致未插管侧肺完全性不张。

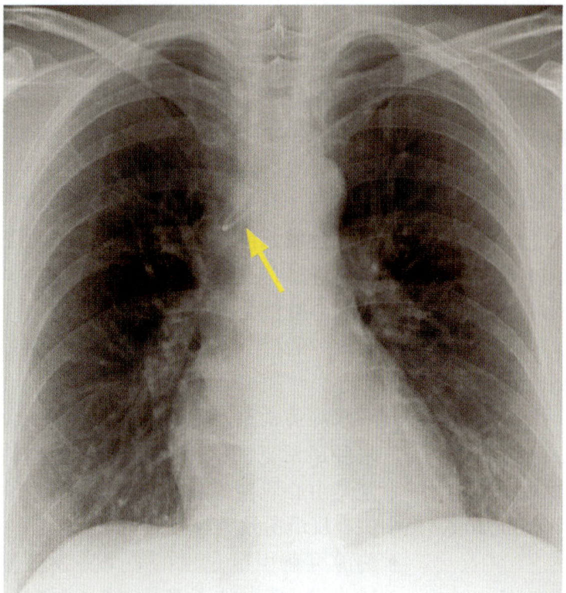

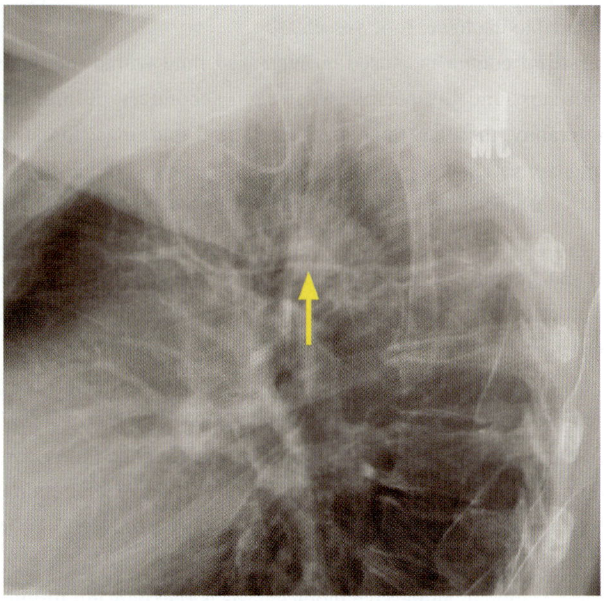

Peripherally inserted central catheter (PICC) in the azygous vein: Frontal radiograph shows a left-sided PICC coursing medially at the confluence of the brachiocephalic vein and the SVC (arrow). Lateral radiograph shows the PICC curves anteriorly before heading inferiorly and posteriorly into the azygous vein (arrow).

Case courtesy Beatrice Trotman-Dickenson, MD, Brigham and Women's Hospital.

经外周静脉穿刺中心静脉导管(PICC)位于奇静脉:正位X线影像显示左侧PICC在头臂静脉和上腔静脉(SVC)的汇合处向内走行(黄箭)。侧位X线影像显示 PICC 向前弯曲,然后向下向后进入奇静脉(黄箭)。

- The tip of a central venous catheter, including a PICC should be in lower SVC or the cavoatrial junction. Azygous malposition is seen in approximately 1% of bedside-placed PICCs. Azygous malposition is associated with increased risk of venous perforation and catheter-associated thrombosis, and repositioning is recommended.
- A dialysis catheter should be located in the right atrium.

- 中心静脉导管,包括PICC的尖端应位于SVC的下段或上腔静脉/右心房交界处。PICC误入奇静脉见于约 1%的床旁置管。奇静脉误置会增加静脉穿孔和导管相关性血栓形成的风险,建议重新调整位置。
- 血液透析导管应置于右心房内。

Pulmonary artery catheter | 肺动脉导管

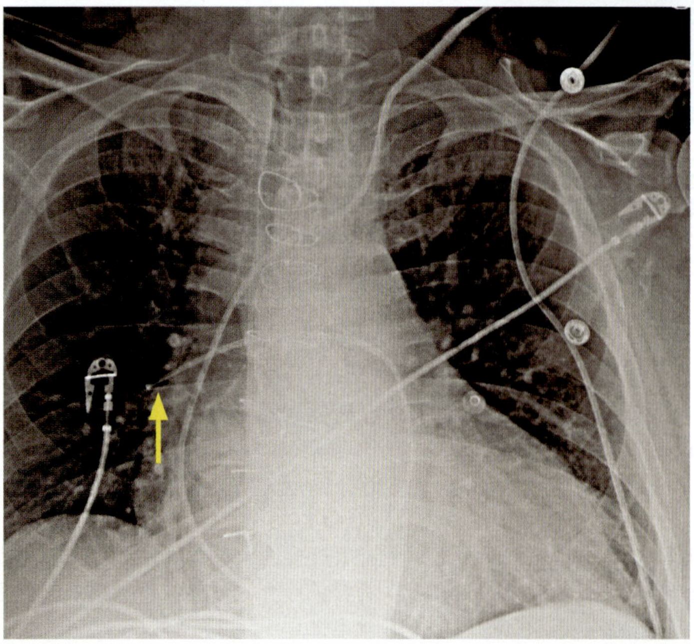

Normal position of a Swan-Ganz pulmonary artery catheter:

Chest radiograph with a sharpening filter applied shows a left internal jugular pulmonary artery catheter that takes a normal course through the SVC, right atrium, tricuspid valve, right ventricle, pulmonic valve, and finally the right pulmonary artery (arrow).

Swan-Ganz 肺动脉导管的正常位置:

胸部X线影像在经锐化滤镜调节后显示经左颈内静脉的肺动脉导管正常通过 SVC、右心房、三尖瓣、右心室、肺动脉瓣,最后到达右肺动脉(黄箭)。

- The tip of a Swan-Ganz pulmonary artery catheter should be in either the main, right, or left pulmonary artery.
- If the tip is distal to the proximal interlobar pulmonary artery, there is a risk of pulmonary artery rupture or pseudoaneurysm. Other complications of pulmonary artery catheter placement include intracardiac catheter knot and arrhythmia.

- 血流导向气囊导管的尖端应位于肺动脉、右肺动脉或左肺动脉。
- 如果尖端超越近端叶间肺动脉，则有造成肺动脉破裂或假性动脉瘤的风险。肺动脉导管放置的其他并发症包括心内导管打结和心律失常。

（翻译　王维平）

LUNG CANCER

肺癌

CLINICAL OVERVIEW OF LUNG CANCER

Epidemiology

- Lung cancer is the leading cause of cancer death in the United States.
- Including all stages and subtypes, the 5-year survival is 15%.

Risk factors for lung cancer

- Tobacco smoking is thought to cause 80–90% of lung cancers.

  Almost all cases of squamous cell and small cell carcinoma are seen in smokers.

  Adenocarcinoma is also associated with smoking, but primary bronchogenic carcinoma arising in a lifelong nonsmoker without history of secondhand exposure is almost always adenocarcinoma.
- Occupational and environmental exposures, including beryllium, radon, arsenic, etc., remain important risk factors for lung cancer. Asbestos exposure increases the risk of lung cancer by a factor of five, synergistic with smoking.
- Pulmonary fibrosis increases the risk of lung cancer by a factor of ten.
- Pulmonary scarring, such as from prior TB, also increases the risk of lung cancer.

肺癌临床概述

流行病学

- 在美国，肺癌是首位癌症致死的原因。
- 综合所有分期和亚型，肺癌的5年生存率为15%。

肺癌的风险因素

- 吸烟引起的肺癌占80%~90%。

  几乎所有的鳞状细胞癌和小细胞癌都见于吸烟的患者。

  腺癌也与吸烟有关，但终身不吸烟且无二手烟暴露史的原发性支气管肺癌几乎都是腺癌。
- 职业和环境暴露，包括铍、氡、砷等，仍然是肺癌的重要危险因素。接触石棉会使患肺癌的风险增加5倍，并与吸烟有协同作用。
- 肺纤维化会使罹患肺癌的风险增加10倍。
- 肺瘢痕，如既往结核感染，也会增加患肺癌的风险。

SOLITARY PULMONARY NODULE

Overview of the solitary pulmonary nodule

- A solitary pulmonary nodule is a well-defined round or oval lesion in the lung parenchyma measuring ≤30 mm. A lesion >30 mm is a mass.
- Differential diagnosis includes neoplastic, inflammatory, congenital etiologies.
- Common mimics on radiograph include nipple shadow, rib lesion, and summation of markings.

Solid pulmonary nodules

- Calcified nodules, including central, laminar, and diffuse calcification, are almost always benign.

  Popcorn calcification is suggestive of a pulmonary hamartoma, a benign tumor composed of connective tissue, muscle, fat, bone, and cartilage.
- Noncalcified nodules can be benign or malignant.

  Intra-lesional fat, suggestive of hamartoma or lipoid granuloma, is benign.
- Amorphous calcification is associated with malignancy (usually mucinous tumors)

孤立性肺结节

孤立性肺结节概述

- 孤立性肺结节是肺实质内≤30mm、边界清楚的圆形或椭圆形病灶。>30mm的病变称肿块。
- 鉴别诊断包括肿瘤、炎症、先天性疾病。
- X线影像上常见的假结节包括乳头阴影、肋骨病变和肺纹理重叠。

实性肺结节

- 钙化性结节，包括中央、分层和弥漫性钙化，几乎都属良性。

  爆米花样钙化提示肺错构瘤，一种由结缔组织、肌肉、脂肪、骨骼和软骨组成的良性肿瘤。
- 非钙化性结节既可为良性也可为恶性。

  病灶内脂肪为良性，提示错构瘤或脂质肉芽肿。
- 无定形钙化常与恶性肿瘤有关(通常为黏液性肿瘤)。

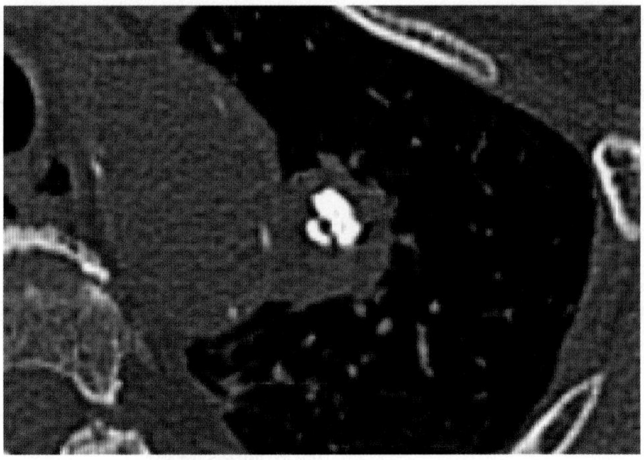

Noncontrast chest CT on bone windows shows a soft tissue mass with popcorn like calcifications in the left upper lobe, consistent with a benign hamartoma.
胸部CT平扫骨窗显示左肺上叶一个软组织肿块伴爆米花样钙化，符合良性错构瘤的改变。

Nodule morphology suggesting, but not diagnostic for, a benign etiology

Small nodules <3 mm have a 0.2% chance of being cancer and a 4–7 mm nodule is malignant in 2.7% of cases.
Oblong, polygonal, triangular, flat or geometric in shape, typically intrapulmonary lymph nodes.
Subpleural location.
Clustering of nodules suggests an infectious process.

形态学提示但不能诊断的良性结节

<3mm的小结节癌变的概率为0.2%，4~7mm的结节恶性的可能性为2.7%。
长方形、多边形、三角形、扁平或其他几何形状，通常为肺内淋巴结。
胸膜下结节。
成簇结节提示为感染性病变。

Nodule morphology suggesting malignancy

Large size is the single most important risk factor for malignancy, regardless of morphology: 0.8 to 3 cm nodules have 18% risk of being lung cancer and masses >3 cm have a high chance of being malignant.
Irregular edge or spiculated margins.

形态学提示为恶性的结节

体积大是恶性肿瘤最重要的单一风险因素，而不论其形态如何：0.8~3.0cm大小的结节其肺癌风险为18%，>3cm的肿块具有很高的恶性概率。
不规则边缘或毛刺。

Subsolid nodules

- Ground glass nodules (or mixed attenuation nodules containing both solid and ground glass) are more likely to be malignant than a solid nodule.
- A cavitary nodule or nodule containing small cystic spaces is suspicious for malignancy.

Follow-up of pulmonary nodule

- The 2017 Fleischner Society pulmonary nodule follow-up recommendations apply to noncalcified nodules in patients older than 35 without a history of malignancy.
- Risk factors for malignancy include older age, heavy smoking, emphysema, pulmonary fibrosis, and upper lobe location.
- Follow-up is not recommended for low risk patients with solitary or multiple pulmonary nodules <6 mm.
- Any interval nodule growth is suspicious. A 26% increase in diameter (for instance, from 1.0 to 1.26 cm) is a doubling in volume.

  Doubling time for lung cancers ranges from 42 days in very aggressive tumors to over 4 years in indolent lesions.
- A solid nodule with well-defined benign morphology that has not changed in size over two years is very likely, but not definitely, benign. Longer follow-up is recommended for subsolid nodules as these often represent indolent adenocarcinomas.
- A decrease in size of a suspicious nodule on a single follow-up study is not

亚实性结节

- 磨玻璃结节(或包含实性及磨玻璃密度的混合密度结节)较实性结节具有更高的恶性可能。
- 空洞性结节或结节含有小囊腔应怀疑恶性。

肺结节随访

- 2017年费莱舍尔学会的肺结节随访建议适用于年龄大于>35岁且无恶性肿瘤史的非钙化性结节患者。
- 恶性肿瘤的危险因素包括老年、大量吸烟、肺气肿、肺纤维化和位于上叶的结节。
- <6mm的单发或多发肺结节为低风险，不建议随访。
- 结节在任何随访期间出现增长都是可疑的。直径增加26%(如从1.0cm增加到1.26cm)意味着体积增大1倍。

  肺癌的倍增时间范围从极具侵袭性肿瘤的42天，到惰性病变的4年以上。
- 若实性结节具有明确的良性形态，且超过2年大小无变化，其良性的可能性很大，但并不绝对。建议对亚实性结节进行更长时间的随访，因为这些结节通常是惰性腺癌。

sufficient to establish a benign etiology.

Transient decrease in size of a malignant lesion can occur with collapse of aerated alveoli or fibrosis.

- 单次随访检查发现可疑结节体积缩小并不足以确定为良性。

恶性病变一过性缩小可由肺泡萎陷或纤维化所致。

HISTOLOGIC SUBTYPES OF LUNG CANCER

肺癌的组织学亚型

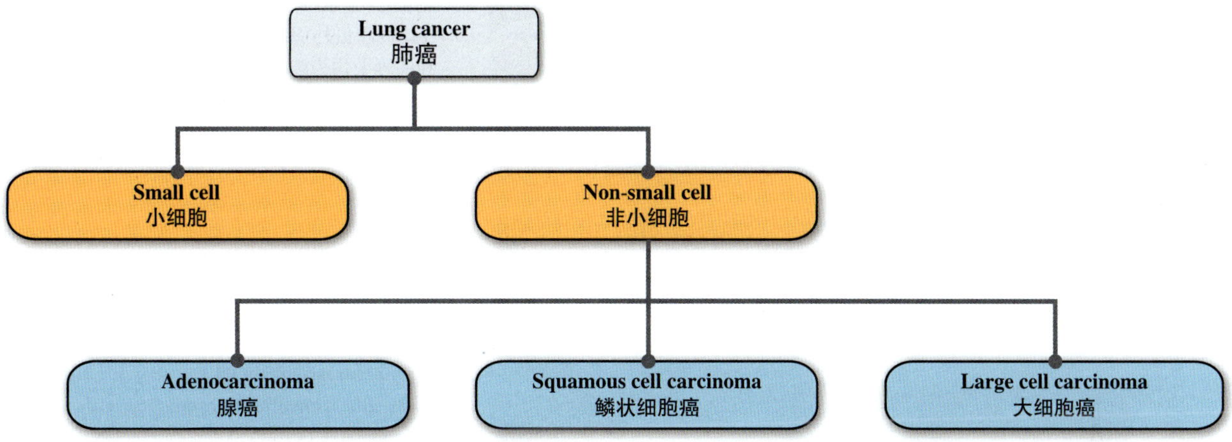

- Lung cancer can be thought of as two types: "small cell" and all other histologic types that are non-small cell, such as adenocarcinoma, squamous cell carcinoma, etc.
- Small cell is usually disseminated at diagnosis and has a much worse prognosis.

Adenocarcinoma

- Adenocarcinoma is the most common subtype of lung cancer. It is related to smoking, but less strongly than squamous cell.
- Cavitation can occur but is less commonly seen compared to squamous cell.
- The typical radiologic presentations of adenocarcinoma include:

  1. A solitary nodule with spiculated margins due to surrounding reactive fibrosis.
  2. Pure ground glass nodule or sub solid nodule with ground glass and solid components.
  3. Consolidative adenocarcinoma which may present as diffuse ground glass opacities or consolidation resembling airspace disease.
- In 2011, the IASLC/ATS/ERS classification removed the term "bronchioloalveolar carcinoma (BAC)" and introduced a new spectrum of adenocarcinoma subtypes.

- 肺癌被认为有两种类型："小细胞"型，以及所有其他组织学类型的非小细胞型，如腺癌、鳞状细胞癌等。
- 小细胞肺癌通常在确诊时已经播散，预后很差。

腺癌

- 腺癌是最常见的肺癌亚型。它与吸烟相关但没有鳞状细胞癌密切。
- 可出现空洞，但鳞状细胞癌更为常见。
- 腺癌的典型影像学表现包括：

  1. 单发结节，伴毛刺，为周边的纤维反应所致。
  2. 纯磨玻璃结节或伴磨玻璃和实性成分的亚实性结节。
  3. 实变性腺癌可表现为弥漫性磨玻璃影或实变类似肺泡病变。
- 2011年，IASLC/ATS/ERS分类法删除了"细支气管肺泡癌(BAC)"一词，并引入了一个新的腺癌亚型。

Pre-invasive lesions.

Atypical adenomatous hyperplasia (AAH).

Adenocarcinoma in-situ (AIS): non-mucinous, mucinous, mixed.

Minimally invasive adenocarcinoma (MIA): non-mucinous, mucinous, mixed.

Invasive adenocarcinomas: lepidic, acinar, papillary, micropapillary, or solid with mucin production.

侵袭前病变。

非典型腺瘤样增生(AAH)。

原位腺癌(AIS)：非-黏液型、黏液型、混合型。

微侵袭性腺癌(MIA)：非-黏液型、黏液型、混合型。

侵袭性腺癌：附壁型、腺泡型、乳头型、微乳头型，或实体型伴黏液生成。

- *Lepidic* growth is a spread of malignant cells using the alveolar walls as a scaffold.

The opposite of lepidic growth is *hilic* growth, demonstrated by most other forms of lung cancer, which describes cancer growth by invasion and destruction of lung parenchyma.

- 贴壁生长是恶性细胞以肺泡壁为支撑发生的播散。

与贴壁生长相对的是实体性生长，后者是大多数其他种类肺癌的生长方式，即肿瘤生长侵犯和破坏肺实质。

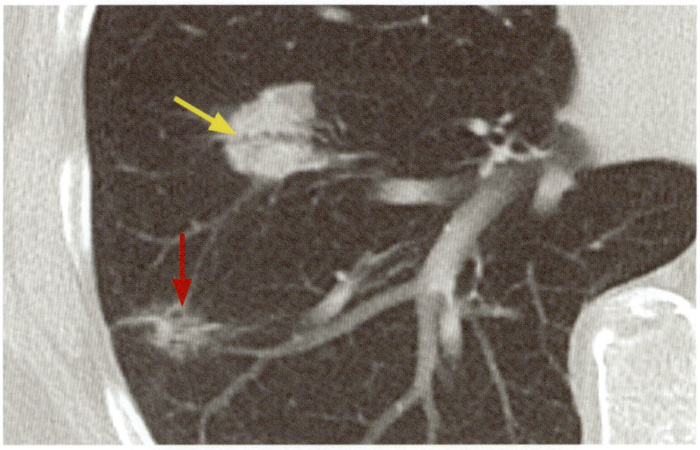

Axial CT shows a solid nodule with air bronchograms (yellow arrow) and a more peripheral ground glass nodule (red arrow), both shown to be adenocarcinoma subtypes on pathology.
轴位CT显示一个实性结节伴充气支气管征(黄箭)和更外周的磨玻璃结节(红箭),两者在病理上均为腺癌亚型。

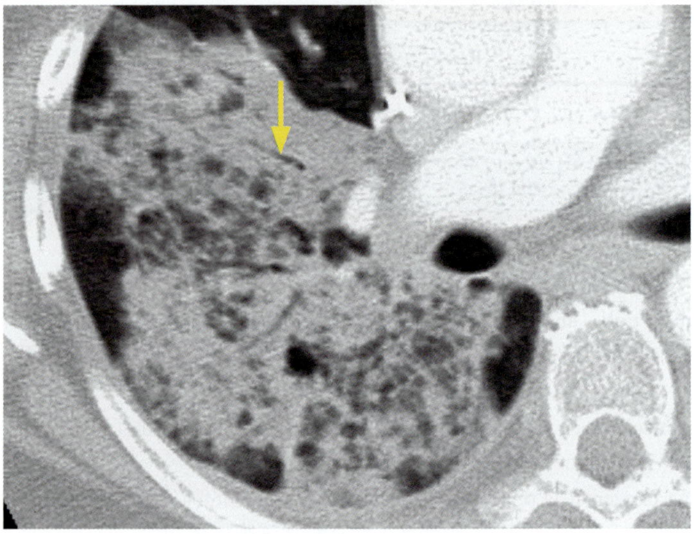

Axial contrast-enhanced CT shows a right lower lobe consolidative opacity with air bronchograms (arrow). Adenocarcinoma is an important differential consideration for chronic ground glass or consolidation.
轴位增强CT显示右肺下叶实变影伴充气支气管征(黄箭)。对于慢性磨玻璃影或实变影需要考虑的一个重要鉴别诊断是腺癌。

Squamous cell carcinoma (SCC)

鳞状细胞癌(SCC)

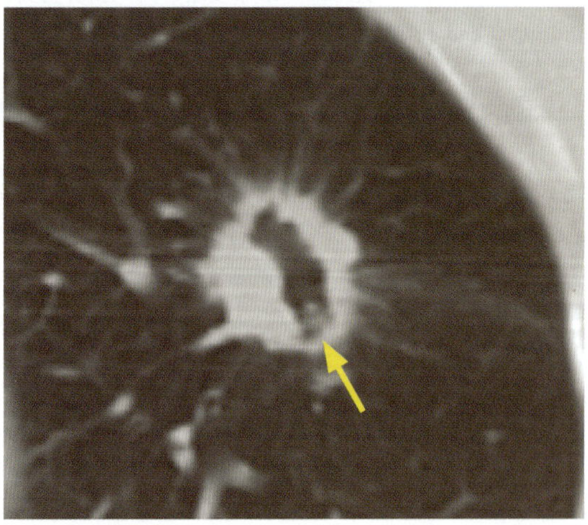

SCC: Axial CT shows a spiculated cavitary lesion (arrow), shown at pathology to be squamous cell carcinoma.
SCC:轴位CT显示毛刺样空洞性病变(黄箭),病理为SCC。

- Squamous cell carcinoma (SCC) is slightly less common today than adenocarcinoma. Prior to filtered cigarettes, SCC was more common.
- SCC most commonly presents as a spiculated nodule, just like adenocarcinoma. However, it can also present as an endobronchial or hilar lesion.
- The majority of SCC arise centrally from main, lobar, or segmental bronchi, where the tumor tends to cause symptoms early due to bronchial obstruction.

- 鳞状细胞癌(SCC)目前稍少于腺癌。在过滤嘴香烟出现之前,SCC更为常见。
- SCC最常见的表现为毛刺样结节,与腺癌类似。但它也可以出现支气管内或肺门的病变。
- 大多数SCC起源于中央的主支气管、叶或段支气管,因肿瘤堵塞支气管而往往在早期可出现症状。

- Common radiographic findings are lobar atelectasis, mucoid impaction, consolidation, and bronchiectasis. SCC has a propensity to cavitate.

- 常见的影像学表现为肺叶不张、黏液栓、实变和支气管扩张。SCC易发生空洞。

Small cell carcinoma

- Small cell carcinoma is the third most common lung cancer cell type (after adenocarcinoma and squamous cell). Neoplastic cells are of neuroendocrine origin and are associated with various paraneoplastic syndromes. Small cell carcinoma is strongly associated with smoking.
- Small cell usually presents as mediastinal or hilar lymphadenopathy, typically presenting as a large hilar or parahilar mass. Involvement of the SVC may cause SVC syndrome. Small cell rarely presents as a solitary pulmonary nodule.
- The primary tumor is usually not identified.
- For staging purposes, small cell is divided into limited-stage involving one hemithorax and extensive-stage disease. The limited-stage is treated with chemoradiation whereas the extensive-stage disease is treated with chemotherapy alone.

小细胞癌

- 小细胞癌是第三常见的肺癌类型(继腺癌和SCC之后)。肿瘤细胞为神经内分泌起源,且与多种副肿瘤综合征有关。小细胞癌与吸烟密切相关。
- 小细胞癌常表现为纵隔或肺门淋巴结肿大,通常表现为肺门或肺门旁肿块。SVC受累时可导致上腔静脉阻塞综合征。小细胞癌很少表现为孤立性肺结节。
- 常找不到原发肿瘤。
- 出于分期考虑,小细胞癌可分为累及单侧胸部的局限期,以及广泛期。局限期采用化疗合并放疗,而广泛期只有化疗。

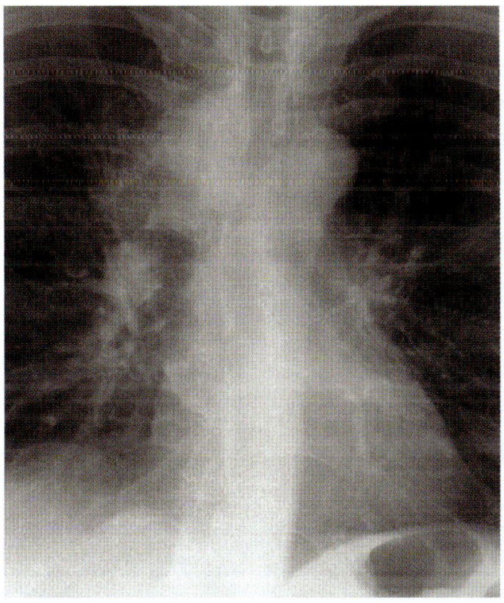

Radiograph
X线影像

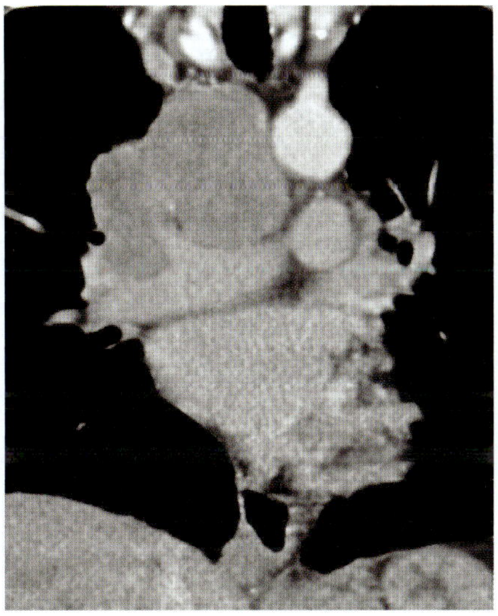

Coronal CT
冠状位CT

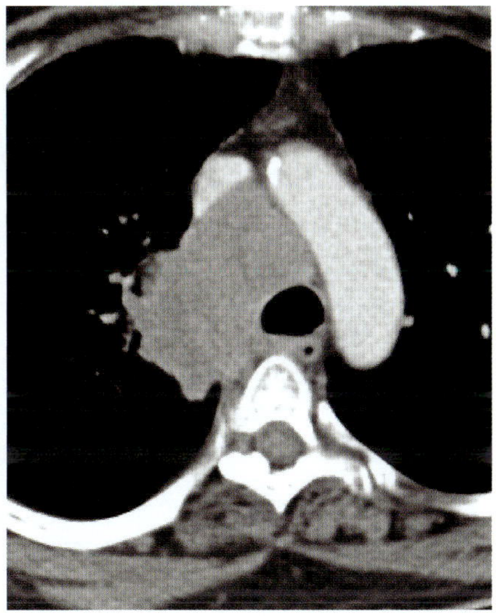

Axial CT
轴位CT

Small cell carcinoma: Chest radiograph shows a right paratracheal opacity which corresponds to mediastinal and hilar lymphadenopathy on CT. The lesion encases but does not significantly narrow the involved bronchi and main pulmonary artery.
小细胞癌:胸部X线影像显示气管右旁高密度影,与CT上纵隔及肺门淋巴结肿大相对应。病变包裹但未造成受累支气管和肺动脉主干明显狭窄。

Large cell carcinoma

- Large cell carcinoma often occurs in the lung periphery, where it presents as a large solid mass with irregular margins. Focal necrosis can be present.
- Histologically, large cell carcinoma is characterized by large nuclei and nucleoli with a moderate amount of cytoplasm.
- Large cell carcinoma can have rapid growth and early metastasis with overall poor prognosis.

大细胞癌

- 大细胞癌常发生在肺的外周,表现为一个大的实性肿块,其边缘不规则。可见灶状坏死。
- 组织学上,大细胞癌的特征是大的细胞核和核仁,伴中等量胞质。
- 大细胞癌生长迅速、转移早、预后差。

Carcinoid tumor

- Neoplastic carcinoid cells originate from neuroendocrine cells in the bronchial walls.
- Carcinoid tumor can either present as a pulmonary nodule (up to 20% of cases) or as an endobronchial lesion. The latter typically is located distal to the carina

类癌

- 类癌细胞起源于支气管壁内的神经内分泌细胞。
- 类癌可以表现为肺结节(高达20%的病例)或支气管腔内病变。后者通常位于隆突远端,

and may cause obstructive atelectasis.

- Carcinoid may be typical (low-grade) or the more aggressive atypical variant. Typical carcinoids without nodal or distant metastases have an excellent prognosis (92% 5-year survival). Atypical carcinoids tend to arise peripherally and have a worse prognosis.
- **Diffuse idiopathic pulmonary neuroendocrine cell hyperplasia (DIPNECH)** is an uncommon syndrome characterized by multiple foci of neuroendocrine hyperplasia or tumorlets (carcinoid foci <5 mm in size) and bronchiolitis obliterans as well as multiple carcinoid tumors. Radiologic presentation shows multiple pulmonary nodules with mosaic attenuation of the lungs secondary to air trapping from airflow obstruction.

可引起阻塞性肺不张。

- 类癌可为典型(低级别)或更具侵袭性的不典型变异型。典型类癌无淋巴结或远处转移，预后良好(5年生存率92%)。非典型类癌多起自肺的外周，预后较差。
- **弥漫性特发性肺神经内分泌细胞增生(DIPNECH)**是一种少见的以多灶性神经内分泌细胞增生或微小瘤(类癌灶<5mm)、闭塞性细支气管炎及多发性类癌为特征的综合征。影像学表现为多发肺结节伴马赛克密度，为气流阻塞引起的空气潴留所致。

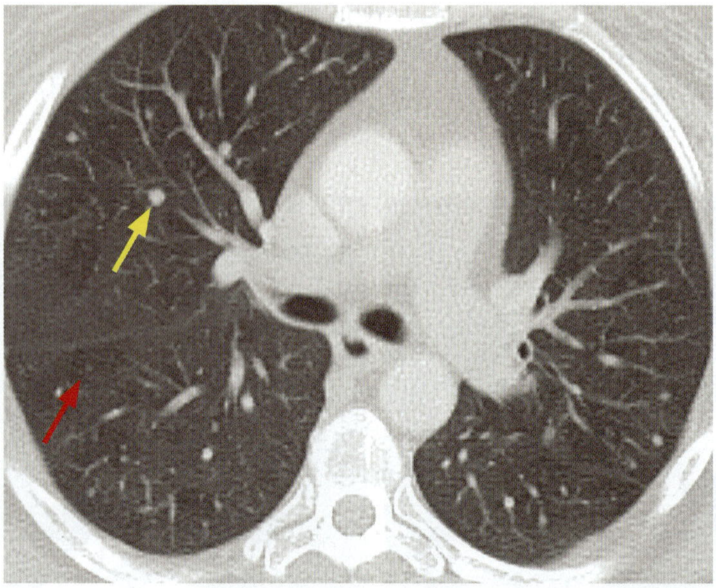

DIPNECH: Axial CT demonstrates several subcentimeter nodules (yellow arrow) and mosaic attenuation of the lungs (red arrow), in a case of diffuse idiopathic pulmonary neuroendocrine cell hyperplasia.

DIPNECH：一名弥漫性特发性肺神经内分泌细胞增生患者，轴位CT示多个毫米级大小的结节(黄箭)和双肺马赛克密度影(红箭)。

Pulmonary Lymphoma

肺淋巴瘤

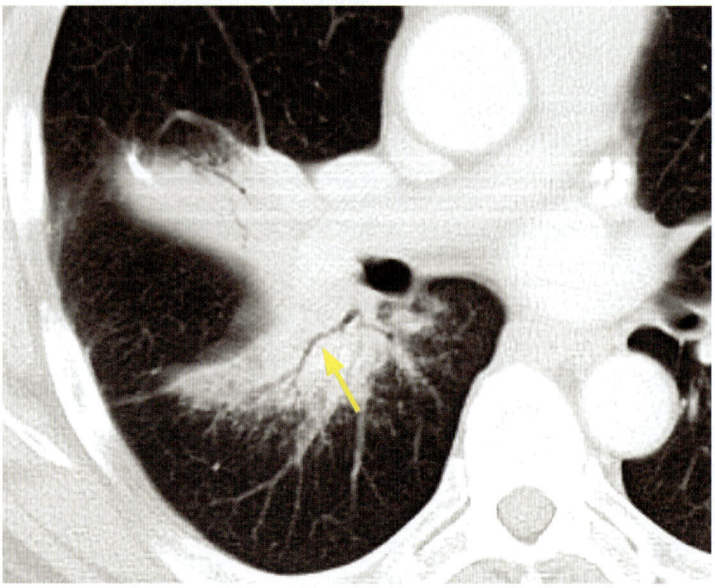

Pulmonary lymphoma: Axial CT demonstrates a region of dense consolidation involving the right upper and lower lobes with air bronchograms (arrow).

肺淋巴瘤：轴位CT示致密实变区累及右肺上下叶，伴充气支气管征(黄箭)。

- Primary pulmonary lymphoma is rare.

  Most commonly mucosa-associated lymphoid tissue lymphoma (MALToma), a form of extranodal B-cell lymphoma.

  Most common presentation is mass-like consolidations limited to the lung parenchyma without mediastinal nodal involvement.

  Pleural based masses, peribronchial or perivascular thickening, and interstitial infiltrates can also be present.

- Secondary pulmonary lymphoma is relatively common and includes manifestations of both Hodgkin disease and non-Hodgkin lymphoma.

  CT imaging features include lymphangitis, nodular, or consolidative pattern.

  Hodgkin disease presents as parenchymal involvement with lymphadenopathy as contiguous spread of disease and may cavitate.

- **Post-transplant lymphoproliferative disorder (PTLD)** presents as new pulmonary nodules in a patient after solid organ transplantation. Lymphadenopathy is often present.

- 原发性肺淋巴瘤很罕见。

  最常见的是黏膜相关淋巴组织淋巴瘤(MALToma),一种结外B细胞淋巴瘤。

  最常见的表现是局限于肺实质的肿块样实变,不累及纵隔淋巴结。

  以胸膜为基底的肿块、支气管周围或血管周围增厚,也可出现间质浸润。

- 继发性肺淋巴瘤相对常见,包括霍奇金淋巴瘤和非霍奇金淋巴瘤都可出现。

  CT影像学特征包括淋巴管炎、结节或实变。

  霍奇金淋巴瘤表现为实质受累伴淋巴结肿大,为连续播散性病变并可形成空洞。

- **移植后淋巴细胞增生性疾病(PTLD)**表现为实体器官移植后患者出现新的肺结节。常有淋巴结肿大。

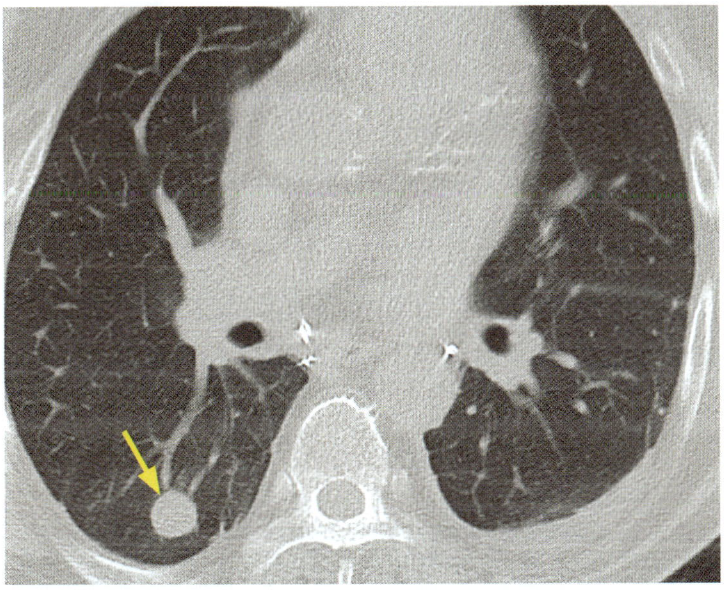

PTLD: Axial CT demonstrates a new nodule (arrow) in the right lower lobe in a patient 7 months following bilateral lung transplantation.
PTLD:轴位CT显示一名双侧肺移植术后7个月患者的右肺下叶新发结节(黄箭)。

This was biopsied, with pathology of post-transplant lymphoproliferative disorder.
活检病理结果为移植后淋巴细胞增生性病变。

Radiologic Presentation of Lung Cancer

Segmental or lobar atelectasis

- Atelectasis due to bronchial obstruction is a common presentation of lung cancer.
- Despite the presence of atelectasis, volume loss is variable, secondary to the volume- displacing effects of cells, mucus, and fluid.
- Obstructive pneumonia is a common presentation of lung cancer, caused by bronchial obstruction and parenchymal consolidation by inflammatory cells and lipid-laden macrophages.
- If two foci of atelectasis are present simultaneously that cannot be explained by a single endobronchial lesion, a benign process is much more likely.

Consolidation

- Consolidation that is indistinguishable from pneumonia can be seen with adenocarcinoma. Although adenocarcinoma and pneumonia may appear similar, adenocarcinoma is usually a non-resolving consolidation with (near) normal white blood cell count.

肺癌的影像学表现

肺段或肺叶不张

- 支气管阻塞导致的肺不张是肺癌的一个常见表现。
- 尽管有肺不张,但肺体积缩小的程度多变,取决于细胞、黏液和液体的体积替代效应。
- 阻塞性肺炎是肺癌的一个常见表现,由支气管阻塞和炎性细胞及载脂巨噬细胞所致的肺实变引起。
- 如果同时出现两处肺不张,且不能用单个支气管腔内病变来解释时,更可能是良性病变。

实变

- 与肺炎难以区分的实变可见于腺癌。虽然腺癌和肺炎的表现相似,但腺癌的实变通常不能消失且白细胞计数(接近)正常。

Hilar mass

肺门肿块

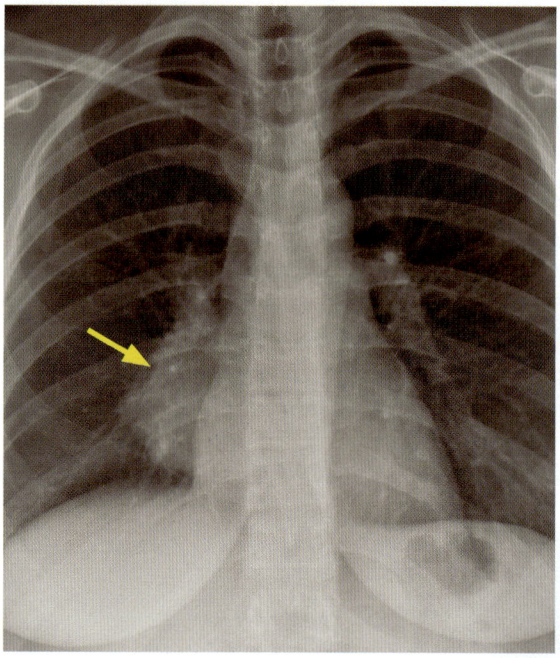

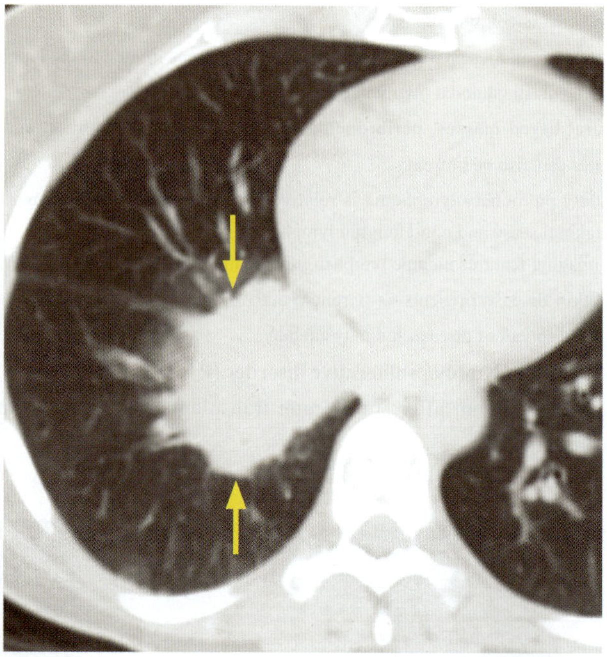

Lung cancer presenting as a hilar mass: Frontal radiograph (left image) shows a right paramediastinal opacity (arrow), which does not silhouette the right heart border. CT shows a large right infrahilar mass (arrows).

肺癌表现为肺门肿块：正位X线影像(左图)显示右纵隔旁高密度影(黄箭)，不掩盖右心缘轮廓。CT显示一个大的右肺门下肿块(黄箭)。

- A hilar mass is a common presentation of squamous cell and small cell carcinoma.
- Hilar enlargement may be due to a primary central tumor or nodal metastasis from a parenchymal neoplasm.
- Tumor may compress and narrow the bronchus.

- 肺门肿块是SCC和小细胞癌的一个常见表现。
- 肺门增大可能是由于原发性中央型肿瘤或肺实质肿瘤造成的淋巴结转移。
- 肿瘤可压迫并致支气管狭窄。

Superior sulcus tumor

肺上沟瘤

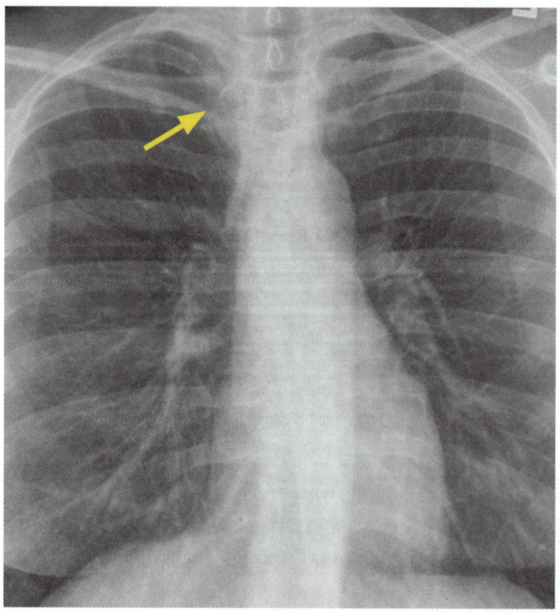

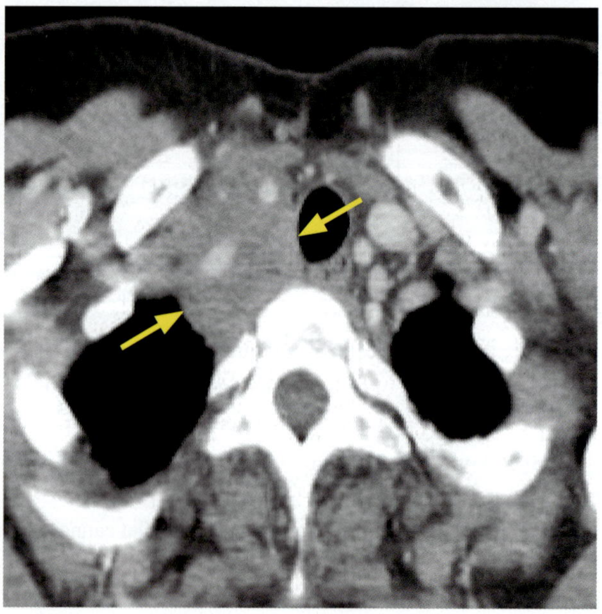

Superior sulcus tumor: Chest radiograph shows nearly imperceptible increased opacity in the right apex (arrow). A superior sulcus mass is clearly evident on CT (arrows), with encasement of the vasculature and effacement of the superior mediastinal fat.

Case courtesy Ritu R. Gill, MD, MPH, Brigham and Women's Hospital.

肺上沟瘤：胸部X线影像显示右肺尖(黄箭)几乎难以察觉的密度增高影。CT清晰显示肺上沟肿块(黄箭)，包绕血管，上纵隔脂肪消失。

- A superior sulcus tumor is a lung cancer occurring in the lung apex.
- A **Pancoast tumor** is a type of superior sulcus tumor with involvement of the sympathetic ganglia causing a Horner syndrome, with ipsilateral ptosis, miosis, and anhidrosis.
- A superior sulcus tumor is a stage T3 tumor. The staging of lung cancer is subsequently discussed.

Lymphangitic carcinomatosis

- 肺上沟瘤是发生在肺尖部的一种肺癌。
- **Pancoast瘤**是肺上沟瘤的一种类型，病变累及交感神经节，导致霍纳综合征，表现为同侧上睑下垂、瞳孔缩小和无汗。
- 肺上沟瘤是T_3期肿瘤。肺癌分期相关内容将在下文叙述。

淋巴管转移癌

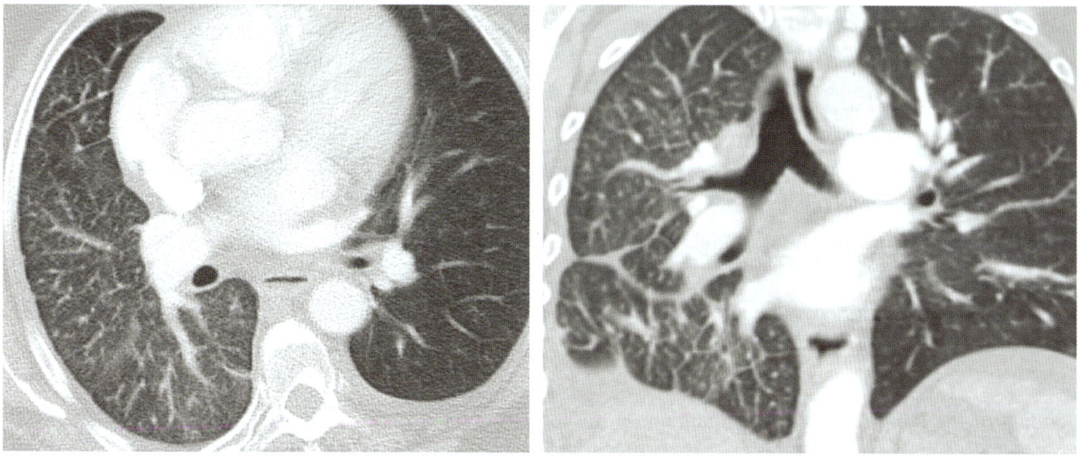

Lymphangitic carcinomatosis: Axial (left image) and coronal CT shows asymmetric, nodular septal thickening of the right lung in a patient with metastatic uterine sarcoma. Aside from a trace effusion, the left lung is clear.

Case courtesy Ritu R. Gill, MD, MPH, Brigham and Women's Hospital.

淋巴管转移癌：轴位(左图)和冠状位(右图)CT显示转移性子宫肉瘤患者右肺非对称性、结节状间隔增厚。除微量胸腔积液外，左肺正常。

- Lymphangitic carcinomatosis represents diffuse spread of neoplasm through the pulmonary lymphatics, typically seen in late-stage disease.
- On imaging, carcinomatosis manifests as smooth or nodular interlobular septal thickening, which is often asymmetric.

Pleural effusion

- Pleural effusions are relatively common in lung cancer, which may be due to lymphatic obstruction or pleural metastases.
- A *malignant* effusion is the presence of malignant cells within the effusion. A malignant effusion is an M1a lesion, which precludes curative resection. Not all effusions associated with lung cancer are malignant effusions, so cytologic evaluation is necessary.

- 淋巴管转移癌是指肿瘤通过肺淋巴管弥漫播散，常见于疾病晚期。
- 在影像学上，淋巴管转移癌表现为光滑或结节状小叶间隔增厚，通常是非对称的。

胸腔积液

- 胸腔积液在肺癌中较为常见，可能是由于淋巴阻塞或胸膜转移。
- 恶性胸腔积液是指积液中有恶性细胞。这是一种M_{1a}期病变，无法进行根治性切除。肺癌伴发的胸腔积液并非全都是恶性，因此需行细胞学检查。

STAGING OF LUNG CANCER

Overview of lung cancer staging

- The eighth edition of the TNM system, published in 2018, is based on data collected on over 77,000 patients with lung cancer from 1999 to 2010.
- The eighth edition re-categorizes tumor size by upstaging T-classifiers to reflect that survival is inversely proportional to every centimeter increase in size until 7 cm; at this point, the same prognosis as T4 disease is reached.
- Extrathoracic metastases that were classified as M1b in the seventh edition are further subcategorized into M1b (oligometastatic) and M1c (multiple metastases) in the eighth edition, to better define oligometastasis, which has a better prognosis and may benefit from more aggressive local therapy.

Treatment based on staging

- For early stages up to ⅡB and sometimes ⅢA, surgery is usually performed.

肺癌的分期

肺癌分期概述

- 2018年发布的第8版TNM系统是基于1999—2010年超过7.7万名肺癌患者收集的数据。
- 第8版通过上调T分类对应的肿瘤大小进行重新分类，以反映生存率与肿瘤每增加1cm成反比，直至7cm；一旦到达7cm，其预后与T_4相同。
- 在第7版中被归类为M_{1b}的胸外转移，在第8版中被进一步细分为M_{1b}(单灶转移)和M_{1c}(多灶转移)，以便引起对孤立转移的重视，因其预后较好，且可能受益于较为积极的局部治疗。

基于分期的治疗

- 对于≤ⅡB期的早期患者和某些ⅢA期患者，

Neoadjuvant or adjuvant chemotherapy and radiotherapy can be used.

- Stage ⅢB (N3 – contralateral or supraclavicular nodes; or T4/N2) is unresectable.
- Stage Ⅳ disease is generally not treated surgically unless there is a solitary adrenal or brain metastasis.

T (tumor)

- T1: Tumor ≤3 cm surrounded by lung or visceral pleura.
  T1a: Tumor ≤ 1 cm; T1b: >1 and ≤2 cm; T1c: >2 and ≤3 cm
- T2: Tumor >3 cm and ≤5 cm, or local invasion of the visceral pleura, or endobronchial lesions.
  T2a: >3 to ≤4 cm; T2b: >4 and ≤5 cm
- T3: Tumor >5 to ≤7 cm, or local invasion of chest wall, pericardium, phrenic nerve, or metastatic nodules in the same lobe
- T4: >7 cm, or invasion of mediastinum, diaphragm, heart, great vessels, recurrent laryngeal nerve, carina, trachea, esophagus, spine or separate tumor nodule in a different lobe in the ipsilateral lung

N (nodes)

- The color coding of the lymph nodes on the diagram on the following page represents the nodal staging of lung cancer for an example left-sided mass:

通常行手术治疗。也可应用新辅助治疗或辅助化疗和放疗。

- ⅢB期(N_3：对侧或锁骨上淋巴结；或T_4/N_2)不能手术切除。
- Ⅳ期一般不进行手术治疗，除非是孤立的肾上腺或脑转移瘤。

T(肿瘤)

- T_1：肿瘤≤3cm，被肺或脏胸膜包围。
  T_{1a}：肿瘤≤1cm；T_{1b}：>1cm且≤2cm；T_{1c}：>2cm且≤3cm
- T_2：肿瘤>3cm且≤5cm，或局部侵犯脏胸膜，或支气管内病变。
  T_{2a}：>3cm且≤4cm；T_{2b}：>4cm且≤5cm
- T_3：肿瘤>5cm且≤7cm，或局部侵犯胸壁、心包、膈神经，或有同一肺叶转移结节。
- T_4：>7cm，或侵犯纵隔、横膈、心脏、大血管、喉返神经、隆突、气管、食管、脊柱，或同侧不同肺叶内孤立肿瘤结节。

N(淋巴结)

- 下图中淋巴结的颜色编码代表了左侧肿块的肺癌淋巴结分期：

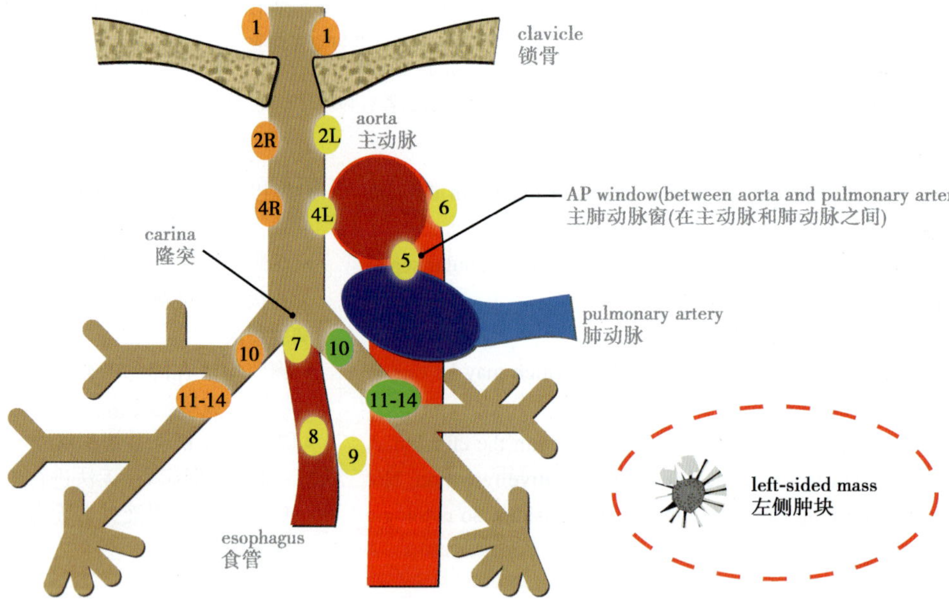

N1: ipsilateral hilar nodes and intrapulmonary nodes
10 - hilar
11 - interlobar (adjacent to interlobar bronchi)
12 - lobar (adjacent to lobar bronchi)
13 - segmental
14 - subsegmental

N2: ipsilateral mediastinal nodes
2 - upper paratracheal
3 - prevascular (anterior to aorta, not shown)
4 - paratracheal
5 - subaortic (AP window)
6 - paraaortic
7 - subcarinal
8 - paraesophageal
9 - pulmonary ligament

N3: 1 - supraclavicular nodes (any side)
any contralateral node
- the boundary between right and left for level 2 and 4 lymph nodes is set as the left lateral border of the trachea due to flow of lymphatic drainage.
- in this example of a left-sided primary, the right-sided nodes are drawn in orange to demonstrate N3 due to contralaterality

N_1：同侧肺门淋巴结和肺内淋巴结
10-肺门的
11-叶间的(邻近叶间支气管)
12-叶的(邻近叶支气管)
13-段的
14-亚段的

N_2：同侧纵隔淋巴结
2-上部气管旁
3-血管前(主动脉前，未示)
4-气管旁
5-主动脉下(主肺动脉窗)
6-主动脉旁
7-隆突下
8-食管旁
9-肺韧带

N_3：1-锁骨上淋巴结(任一侧)
任何对侧淋巴结
- 由于淋巴液引流原因，2组和4组左右分界设定为气管左缘
- 本例为左侧原发，根据对侧性原则，右侧淋巴结标注为橘色代表N_3期

- N0: No lymph node metastases.
- N1: Ipsilateral hilar or intrapulmonary lymph nodes (green in diagram above).
- N2: Ipsilateral mediastinal nodes (yellow in diagram above).
- N3: Contralateral mediastinal or hilar lymph nodes, or supraclavicular nodes on either side (orange in diagram above).

- N_0：无淋巴结转移。
- N_1：同侧肺门或肺内淋巴结(上方示意图中的绿色部分)。
- N_2：同侧纵隔淋巴结(上方示意图中的黄色部分)。
- N_3：对侧纵隔或肺门淋巴结，或任何一侧的锁骨上淋巴结(上方示意图中的橙色部分)。

M (metastasis)

- M0: No metastatic disease.
- M1a: Local thoracic metastatic disease.
    - Separate tumor nodule in contralateral lung
    - Malignant pleural or pericardial effusion
- M1b: Single extrathoracic metastasis, including single non-regional lymph node.
- M1c: Multiple extrathoracic metastases in one or more organs.

M(转移)

- M_0：无转移灶。
- M_{1a}：局限性胸部转移。
    - 对侧肺出现肿瘤结节
    - 恶性胸腔积液或心包积液
- M_{1b}：胸外孤立性转移灶，包括单个非区域淋巴结转移。
- M_{1c}：胸外一个或多个器官的多发性转移灶。

Example staging: Stage ⅢA

分期示例：ⅢA期

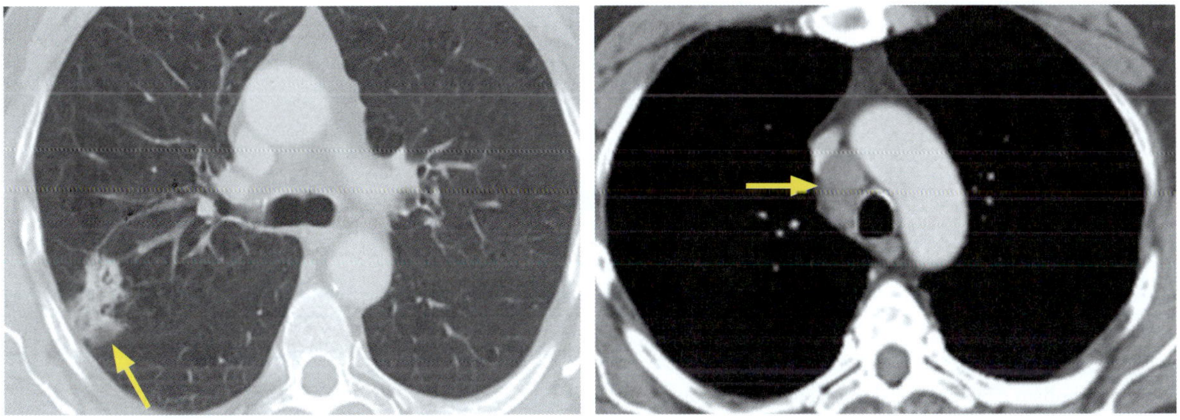

Stage ⅢA lung cancer: Axial CT in lung windows (left image) shows a right upper lobe peripheral mass (arrow) that abuts the pleura. There is diffuse centrilobular emphysema. Soft-tissue window CT shows ipsilateral right paratracheal adenopathy (arrow). The T staging is T2 (for size >3 cm) and the N staging is N2 for ipsilateral mediastinal nodes. The overall stage is therefore ⅢA and this tumor is resectable.
Case courtesy Ritu R. Gill, MD, MPH, Brigham and Women's Hospital.

ⅢA期肺癌：轴位CT肺窗(左图)显示右肺上叶外周一个与胸膜接壤的肿块(黄箭)。有弥漫性小叶中心性肺气肿。CT软组织窗示同侧气管右旁淋巴结肿大(黄箭)。T分期是T_2(大小>3cm)，N分期为N_2，因同侧纵隔淋巴结肿大。总分期为ⅢA期，手术可切除此肿瘤。

Example staging: Stage Ⅳ

分期示例：Ⅳ期

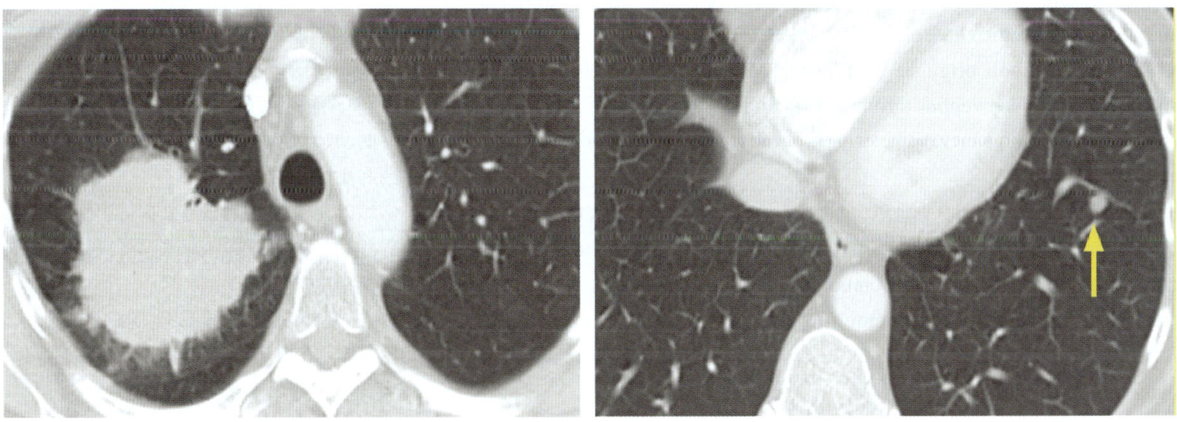

Stage Ⅳ lung cancer: Axial CT (left image) shows a dominant, spiculated right upper lobe T2 mass. More inferiorly (right image), a small contralateral nodule (arrow) is present. This nodule was determined to be malignant on follow-up, for an M staging of M1a and stage ⅣA disease.
Case courtesy Ritu R. Gill, MD, MPH, Brigham and Women's Hospital.

Ⅳ期肺癌：轴位CT(左图)显示右肺上叶一个巨大的毛刺状T_2期肿块。在肿块下方(右图)的对侧肺可见一个小结节(黄箭)。该结节经随访证实为恶性，所以M分期为M_{1a}，为ⅣA期肿瘤。

Example staging: Stage Ⅳ

分期示例：Ⅳ期

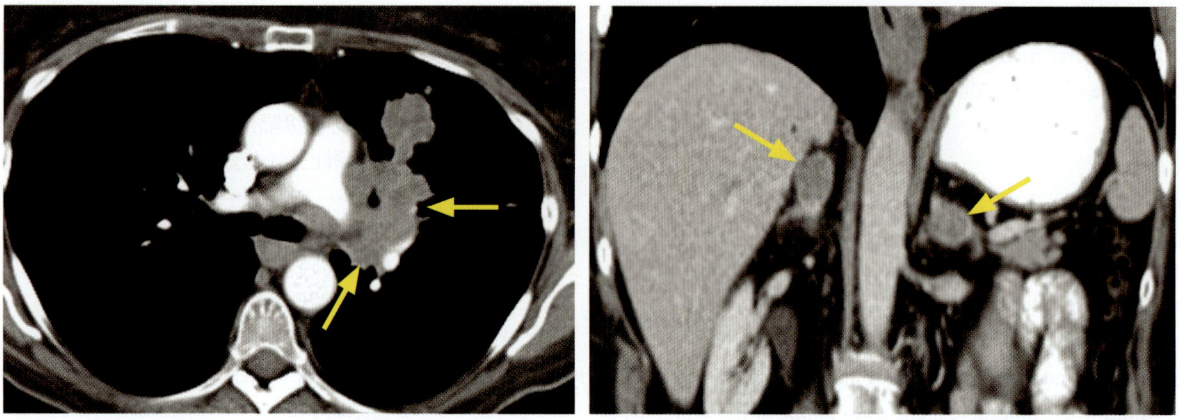

Stage Ⅳ lung cancer: Axial CT (left image) shows a left upper lobe mass with ipsilateral hilar adenopathy (arrows). Coronal CT through the upper abdomen shows bilateral adrenal masses (arrows), which were confirmed to be metastases (M1c), representing stage ⅣB disease. *Case courtesy Ritu R. Gill, MD, MPH, Brigham and Women's Hospital.*

Ⅳ期肺癌：轴位CT(左图)显示一个左肺上叶肿块伴同侧肺门淋巴结肿大(黄箭)。上腹部冠状位CT显示双侧肾上腺肿块(黄箭)，证实为转移瘤(M_{1c})，为ⅣB期肿瘤。

(翻译　韩宇)

PULMONARY VASCULAR DISEASE

肺血管疾病

PULMONARY EMBOLISM (PE)

肺栓塞(PE)

- Pulmonary embolism can be divided into acute and chronic subtypes

  Acute PE is associated with the typical symptoms of dyspnea, tachycardia, and pleuritic chest pain

  Chronic PE may be associated with pulmonary hypertension, further discussed in the next section.

- 肺栓塞可分为急性和慢性两种亚型。

  急性PE通常伴随呼吸困难、心动过速和胸膜性胸痛等典型的症状。

  慢性PE可能会引发肺高压，下一节将进一步讨论。

Acute Pulmonary Embolism

急性肺栓塞

Clinical diagnosis

临床诊断

- Diagnosis of pulmonary embolism (PE) can be challenging because the presenting symptoms are both common and nonspecific, including dyspnea, tachycardia, and pleuritic chest pain.
- Most pulmonary emboli originate in the deep veins of the thighs and pelvis. The risk factors for deep venous thrombosis include:

  Immobilization, malignancy, catheter use, obesity, oral contraceptive use, and thrombophilia.

  Approximately 25% of patients with PE do not have any identifiable risk factor.
- The Wells score assigns point values to clinical suspicion and various symptoms suggestive of pulmonary embolism.
- D-dimer is sensitive for thromboembolic disease and has a high negative predictive value, but is of little value in the typical inpatient population as there are many false positives.

- 诊断肺栓塞(PE)具有一定困难，因为其症状既常见又无特异性，包括呼吸困难、心动过速和胸膜性胸痛。
- 大多数肺栓子起源于大腿和盆腔的深静脉。深静脉血栓形成的风险因素包括：

  制动、恶性肿瘤、使用医用导管、肥胖、口服避孕药和血栓形成倾向。

  约25%的PE患者没有任何可识别的危险因素。
- Wells评分可对临床怀疑及各种提示有肺栓塞的症状进行打分。
- D-二聚体对血栓栓塞性疾病敏感，具有很高的阴性预测值，但对普通住院人群的价值不大，因为有很多假阳性情况。

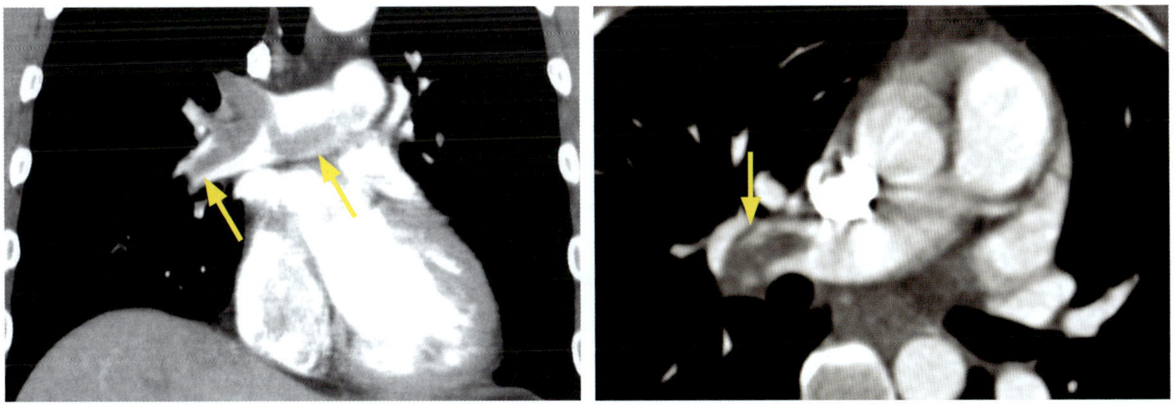

Pulmonary embolism: CT pulmonary angiogram shows a large, nearly-occlusive filling defect in the right main pulmonary artery (arrows) extending distally to the bifurcation.
肺栓塞：CT肺血管造影显示右肺动脉主干有一个大的充盈缺损(黄箭)，几乎造成完全性闭塞，并向远端延伸至分叉处。

- CT pulmonary angiogram is the most common method to image for PE, where an embolism is typically seen as a central intraluminal pulmonary artery filling defect. Pulmonary emboli tend to lodge at vessel bifurcations.
- Pulmonary infarction can be seen as peripheral wedge-shaped consolidations often with *reverse halo sign*.
- Pleural effusions often develop after several days. After congestive heart failure (CHF), parapneumonic effusion, and malignancy, pulmonary infarct is the fourth most common cause of pleural effusion.

Cardiac evaluation for acute pulmonary embolism

- In patients with acute PE, one should always examine the heart for imaging findings of right heart dysfunction which is associated with increased mortality. Findings of right heart strain include:
  - Bowing of the intraventricular septum to the left.
  - An elevated RV:LV ratio ≥1.
- Presence of right heart strain determines categorization of submassive versus massive PE.
  - Submassive PE shows RV enlargement on imaging or clinical signs of RV dysfunction.
  - Massive PE has systemic hypotension (<90 mmHg).

- CT肺血管造影是最常用的PE成像方法，栓塞通常表现为位于肺动脉管腔中央的充盈缺损。肺栓子常嵌顿在血管分叉处。
- 肺梗死可表现为肺外周楔形实变，通常伴有反晕征。
- 胸腔积液通常在数天后出现。继充血性心力衰竭(CHF)、肺炎旁积液和恶性肿瘤，肺梗死是第四常见的胸腔积液原因。

急性肺栓塞时的心脏评估

- 对于急性PE患者，必须检查心脏是否存在右心功能障碍的影像学表现，这与死亡率增加有关。右心劳损的表现有：
  - 室间隔向左弯曲。
  - 右心室(RV)：左心室(LV)比值升高≥1。
- 对PE进行大面积和次大面积分类取决于是否有右心劳损。
  - 次大面积 PE 在影像学上表现为 RV 扩大或临床有RV功能障碍的体征。
  - 大面积 PE 出现全身性低血压(<90mmHg)。

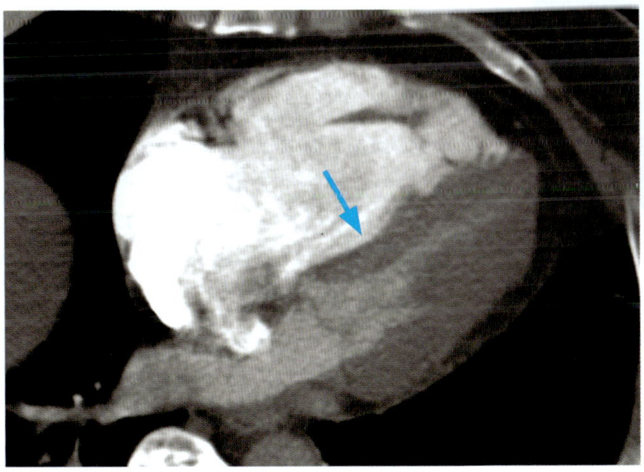

Axial CT demonstrates bowing of the interventricular septum to the left (arrow). The right ventricle is larger in diameter than the left ventricle. These are signs of right heart strain.
轴位CT显示室间隔向左弯曲(蓝箭)。右心室的直径大于左心室。此为右心劳损的征象。

Management of acute pulmonary embolism

Low risk PE (Non-massive): anticoagulation (AC) only or surveillance if isolated subsegmental PE with no proximal lower extremity DVT and low risk for recurrence.
Intermediate risk (Submassive): AC +/– intervention if more moderate to severe RV strain or any acute distress. Intervention includes systemic Ⅳ thrombolysis, mechanical thrombectomy and catheter-directed therapy.
High risk (Massive): AC + intervention. Intervention includes surgical embolectomy, systemic Ⅳ thrombolysis, mechanical thrombectomy and catheter-directed therapy.

急性肺栓塞的处理方法

低风险 PE(非大面积): 仅抗凝(AC)或监测，适用于孤立性亚段 PE 且无下肢近端深静脉血栓和低复发风险。
中度风险(次大面积): AC+/–干预，适用于中度至重度RV劳损或任何急性窘迫。 干预包括全身静脉溶栓、机械取栓和导管导向治疗。
高风险(大面积): AC+干预。 干预措施包括手术取栓、全身静脉溶栓、机械取栓和导管导向治疗。

Plain film evaluation of pulmonary embolism

- While a CT pulmonary angiogram is the standard tool to evaluate for pulmonary embolism, it is important to be aware of plain film findings that could suggest pulmonary embolism in case the diagnosis is not clinically suspected.
- The *Fleischner sign* describes widening of the pulmonary arteries due to clot.

评估肺栓塞的胸部X线影像

- 虽然 CT 肺血管造影是评估PE的标准方法，但认识胸部X线影像上的表现是重要的，可以在临床没有怀疑的情况下提示PE。
- 费莱舍尔征是指由血栓导致的肺动脉增宽。

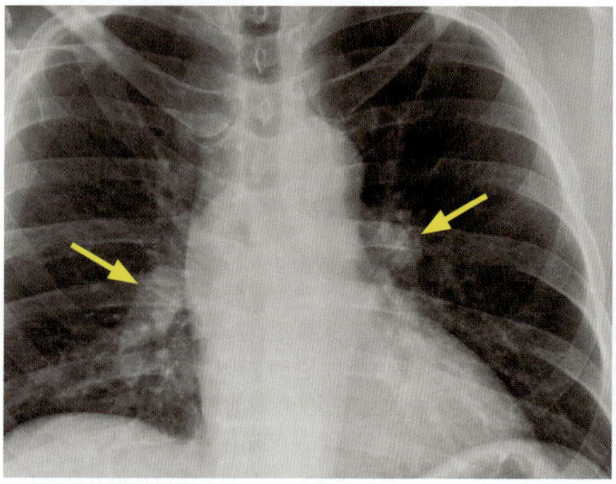

Current radiograph
当前的X线影像

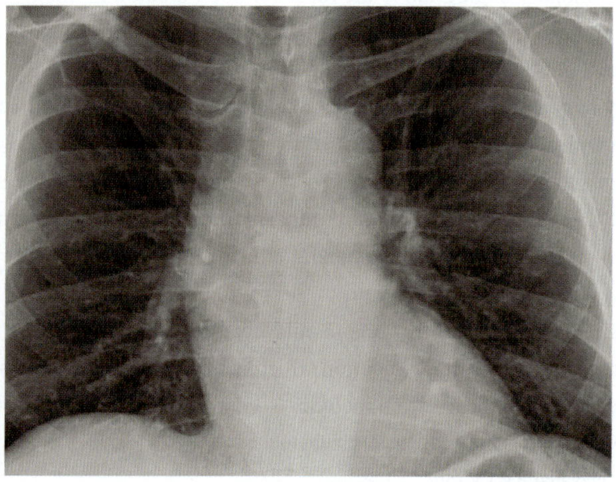

Prior radiograph
先前的X线影像

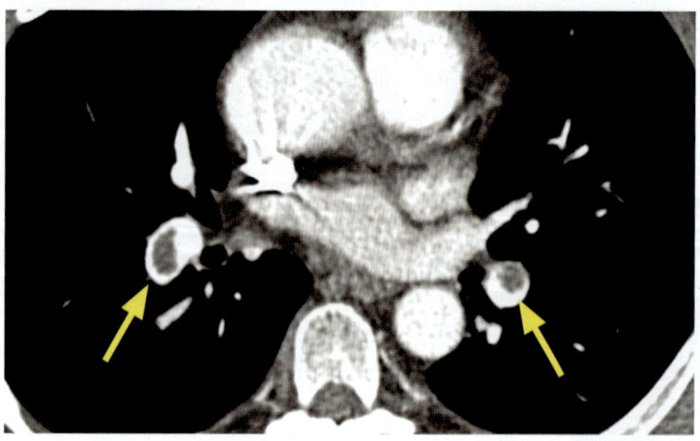

Fleischner sign: Current chest radiograph (top left image) shows relative enlargement of both pulmonary arteries (arrows), which is a new finding compared to the prior radiograph. Subsequently performed CT pulmonary angiogram (left image) shows bilateral pulmonary emboli (arrows).

Case courtesy Robert Gordon, MD, Brigham and Women's Hospital.

费莱舍尔征：当前的胸部X线影像(左上图)显示两侧肺动脉相对增粗(黄箭)，相比先前影像这是一个新的发现。随后CT肺血管造影(左图)显示双侧肺栓塞(黄箭)。

- *Hampton's hump* is a peripheral wedge-shaped opacity representing pulmonary infarct.
- *Westermark sign* is regional oligemia in the lung distal to the pulmonary artery thrombus.

- 汉普顿驼峰是一种肺外周楔形阴影，代表肺梗死。
- 韦斯特马克征是肺动脉血栓远端的肺呈低灌注区。

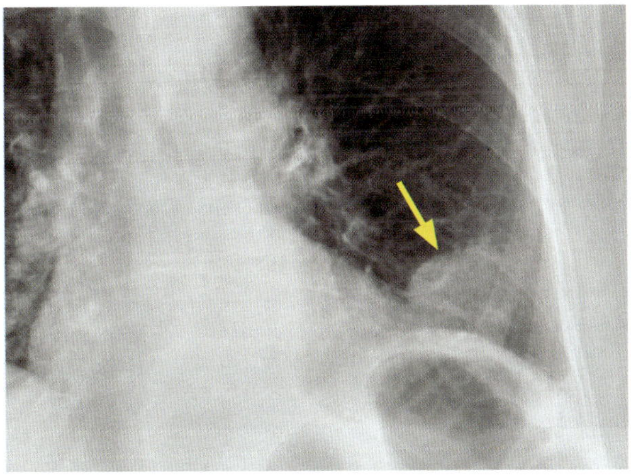

Rounded opacity (arrow) projecting over the lingula, representing Hampton's hump.
舌叶上突出圆形致密影(黄箭),代表汉普顿驼峰。

Chronic pulmonary embolism

Clinical diagnosis

- Chronic PEs present with signs and symptoms of pulmonary hypertension, including shortness of breath exacerbated with activity, fatigue, and chest pressure or pain.
- Note that not all patients with chronic PE develop pulmonary hypertension.

Imaging findings

慢性肺栓塞

临床诊断

- 慢性 PE 可出现肺高压的体征和症状,包括活动性气急、疲劳和胸部压迫感或疼痛。
- 注意,并非所有慢性PE患者都会出现肺高压。

影像学表现

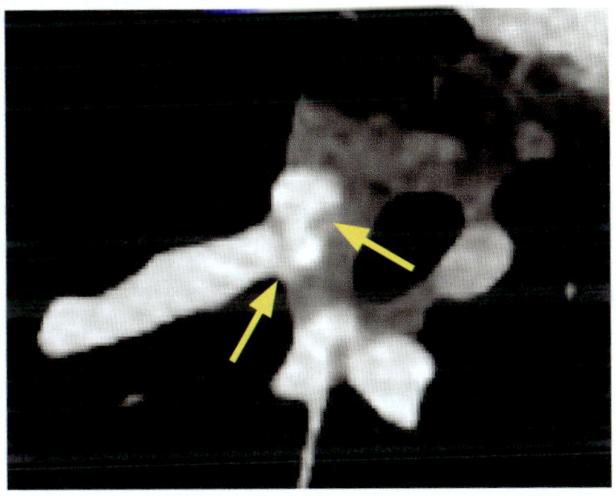

Axial CT demonstrates a subsegmental eccentric web, consistent with a chronic pulmonary embolism.
轴位 CT 显示亚段偏心性蹼样影,符合慢性肺栓塞。

- Chronic PEs present as eccentric filling defects, a web, or pruning of the pulmonary artery branches.
- Note that resolving acute PE will involute with eccentric filling defects or webs.
- Parenchymal signs include mosaic attenuation from altered perfusion and occasionally scarring.
- In these patients, it is important to look for signs of pulmonary hypertension which include:
  - Enlargement of the pulmonary artery when the PA to ascending aorta ratio is ≥ 1.
  - Right ventricular enlargement and hypertrophy.

Chronic thromboembolic pulmonary hypertension (CTEPH)

- CTEPH is the constellation of chronic PE and pulmonary HTN (subsequently discussed).
- Patients are often evaluated with V/Q scan and CTPA since each can miss defects.
- CT shows eccentric organized thrombi, pulmonary artery enlargement, mosaic attenuation and vascular pruning. V/Q scan shows segmental perfusion defects.

- 慢性PE表现为偏心性充盈缺损、呈蹼状或肺动脉分支修剪样改变。
- 注意,正在恢复的急性PE会形成偏心性充盈缺损或呈蹼状改变。
- 肺实质的征象包括因灌注改变所出现的马赛克样密度影,偶有瘢痕。
- 在这些患者中发现肺高压的征象很重要,包括:
  - 肺动脉扩张、肺动脉与升主动脉的比值≥1。
  - 右心室扩大和肥厚。

慢性血栓栓塞性肺高压(CTEPH)

- CTEPH 是慢性PE和肺动脉高压的集合(随后讨论)。
- 患者通常使用V/Q扫描和CTPA进行评估,因为每种检查都有可能遗漏缺损。
- CT可显示偏心性机化血栓、肺动脉增粗、马赛克密度影和血管分支样修剪。V/Q扫描可显示肺段性灌注缺损。

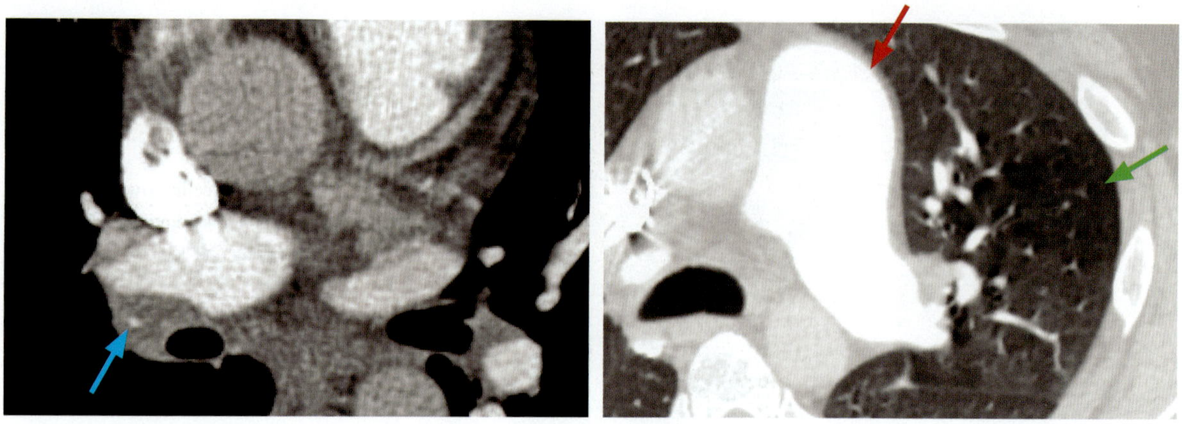

Contrast-enhanced CT axial images demonstrate extensive eccentric mural thrombi involving the distal right main pulmonary artery with foci of calcification (blue arrow). Lung-windows demonstrate enlarged pulmonary arterial trunk (red arrow) and mosaic attenuation of the lung parenchyma (green arrow).

轴位增强CT图像显示广泛的偏心附壁血栓，累及右肺动脉远端伴钙化灶(蓝箭)。肺窗显示肺动脉干增粗(红箭)及肺实质马赛克密度影(绿箭)。

Pitfalls of CT pulmonary angiogram

- Hilar lymph nodes and mucus-impacted bronchi may simulate PE.
- Unopacified pulmonary veins may simulate PE on a single CT slice; however, one may distinguish between a pulmonary artery and vein by tracing the vessel back to the heart.
- During the Valsalva maneuver, transient disruption of contrast bolus occurs when unopacified blood from the IVC enters the right atrium and is pumped into the lungs. This causes dense contrast to be seen in the SVC, no contrast in the pulmonary artery, and dense contrast in the aorta. On the other hand, late contrast timing would show less dense contrast in the SVC. This can be mitigated by a scan in expiration.
- Cardiac and respiratory motion artifacts can decrease image quality.

  Cardiac motion causes blurring of the left lower lobe pulmonary arteries, which may simulate small emboli. Respiratory motion decreases accuracy in evaluation of small pulmonary arteries.

CT肺血管造影的缺陷

- 肺门淋巴结和黏液堵塞支气管可能与PE相似。
- 无造影剂充盈的肺静脉在单个CT层面上可与PE混淆；但可以通过追踪血管回流入心脏以区分肺动脉与肺静脉。
- 在瓦尔萨尔瓦(Valsalva)动作期间，当IVC内不含造影剂的血液进入右心房并被泵入肺部时，会出现造影剂短暂中断，导致SVC内见高密度造影剂，肺动脉内无造影剂和主动脉内高密度造影剂。另一方面，采集时间延迟将淡化SVC中的造影剂。这可通过在呼气相时扫描解决。
- 心脏和呼吸运动伪影会降低图像质量。

  心脏运动导致左下叶肺动脉模糊，这可能会被误以为是小的栓子。呼吸运动会降低评估小口径肺动脉的准确性。

Pulmonary Hypertension

肺高压

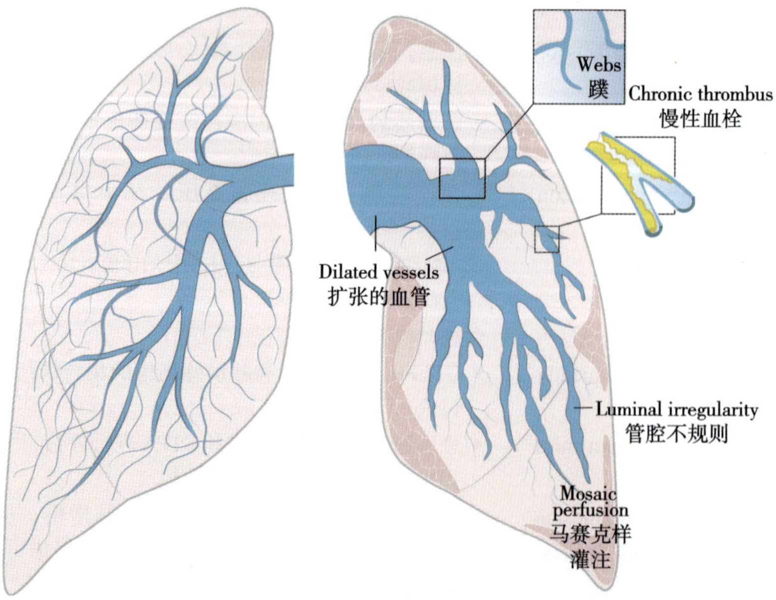

Illustration demonstrating the physiologic changes in pulmonary hypertension.

A normal lung is on the left and abnormal lung on the right. Key findings include dilated vessels with abrupt change in caliber or abrupt cut-off. Chronic eccentrically located pulmonary thrombus may be seen along the vessel walls. Webs, delicate ribbonlike structures attached to the vessel wall, are often seen in the setting of chronic pulmonary embolus. Mosaic perfusion of the lung parenchyma is due to heterogeneous perfusion.

示意图演示肺高压的生理变化。

右侧为一个正常肺，左侧为异常肺。关键征象包括扩张的血管口径突然变窄或突然中断。沿血管壁可见慢性偏心的肺血栓。蹼，是附着在血管壁上的纤细带状结构，常见于慢性肺栓塞。肺实质的马赛克灌注是由于灌注不均所致。

- The term *pulmonary hypertension* encompasses both pulmonary arterial and pulmonary venous hypertension. The term *pulmonary arterial hypertension* (PAH) is generally reserved for the WHO class 1 entities (primary pulmonary hypertension), discussed below.
- Pulmonary hypertension is pulmonary arterial systolic pressure ≥25 mm Hg at rest or ≥30 mm Hg during exercise. Elevated pulmonary venous pressures are present when pulmonary capillary wedge pressure (an approximation of pulmonary venous pressure) is ≥18 mm Hg.

- 肺高压一词包括肺动脉高压和肺静脉高压。肺动脉高压(PAH)一词通常只用于 WHO 1 类病变(原发性PAH),如下所述。
- PAH是指静息时肺动脉收缩压≥25mmHg或运动时≥30mmHg。当肺毛细血管楔压(肺静脉压的近似值)≥18mmHg时,即会出现肺静脉压升高。

Overview of pulmonary hypertension classification

- There are a number of causes of pulmonary hypertension including chronic thromboembolic disease, chronic respiratory disease, chronic heart disease, and idiopathic causes.
- The World Health Organization (WHO) clinical classification, based on the 2018 World Symposium on Pulmonary Hypertension, describes 5 groups of pulmonary hypertension.

肺高压分类概述

- 引起肺高压的原因很多,包括慢性血栓栓塞性疾病、慢性呼吸道疾病、慢性心脏病和特发性原因。
- 世界卫生组织(WHO)基于2018年世界肺高压研讨会内容,将肺高压临床分类归为5个组。

Group 1: **Pulmonary arterial hypertension (PAH).**
Primary pulmonary hypertension (PPH) may be idiopathic or familial.
Congenital left-to-right shunts, such as atrial septal defect (ASD) and ventricular septal defect (VSD), may cause PAH and shunt reversal (Eisenmenger syndrome).

Group 1′: **Pulmonary veno-occlusive disease (PVOD) and pulmonary capillary hemangiomatosis (PCH).**
PAH may be caused by pulmonary venous or capillary involvement.

Group 2: **Pulmonary venous hypertension.**
Left-sided heart disease (left atrial, left ventricular, or mitral/aortic valve disease may cause elevated pulmonary venous pressure in chronic disease).

Group 3: **Pulmonary hypertension associated with chronic hypoxemia.**
COPD, interstitial lung disease, and sleep apnea can cause pulmonary hypertension in chronic disease.

Group 4: **Pulmonary hypertension due to chronic thromboembolic disease.**

Group 5: **Pulmonary hypertension due to miscellaneous disorders.**
Sarcoidosis is a rare cause of pulmonary hypertension.
Compression of pulmonary vessels, which can be due to neoplasm, fibrosing mediastinitis, etc., may cause pulmonary hypertension.

第 1 组:**肺动脉高压(PAH)。**
原发性肺高压(PPH)可为特发性或家族性。
先天性左向右分流,如房间隔缺损(ASD)和室间隔缺损(VSD),可引起 PAH 和分流逆转(艾森门格综合征)。

第 1′组:**肺静脉闭塞性疾病(PVOD)和肺毛细血管瘤病(PCH)。**
PAH 可由肺静脉或毛细血管受累引起。

第 2 组:**肺静脉高压。**
左侧心脏疾病(慢性左心房、左心室或二尖瓣/主动脉瓣疾病可导致肺静脉压升高)。

第 3 组:**与慢性低氧血症相关的肺高压。**
COPD、间质性肺疾病和睡眠呼吸暂停慢性病变可引起肺高压。

第 4 组:**慢性血栓栓塞性疾病引起的肺高压。**

第 5 组:**由于其他疾病引起的肺高压。**
结节病是引起肺高压的一种罕见原因。
肺血管受压,可源自肿瘤、纤维性纵隔炎等,可导致肺高压。

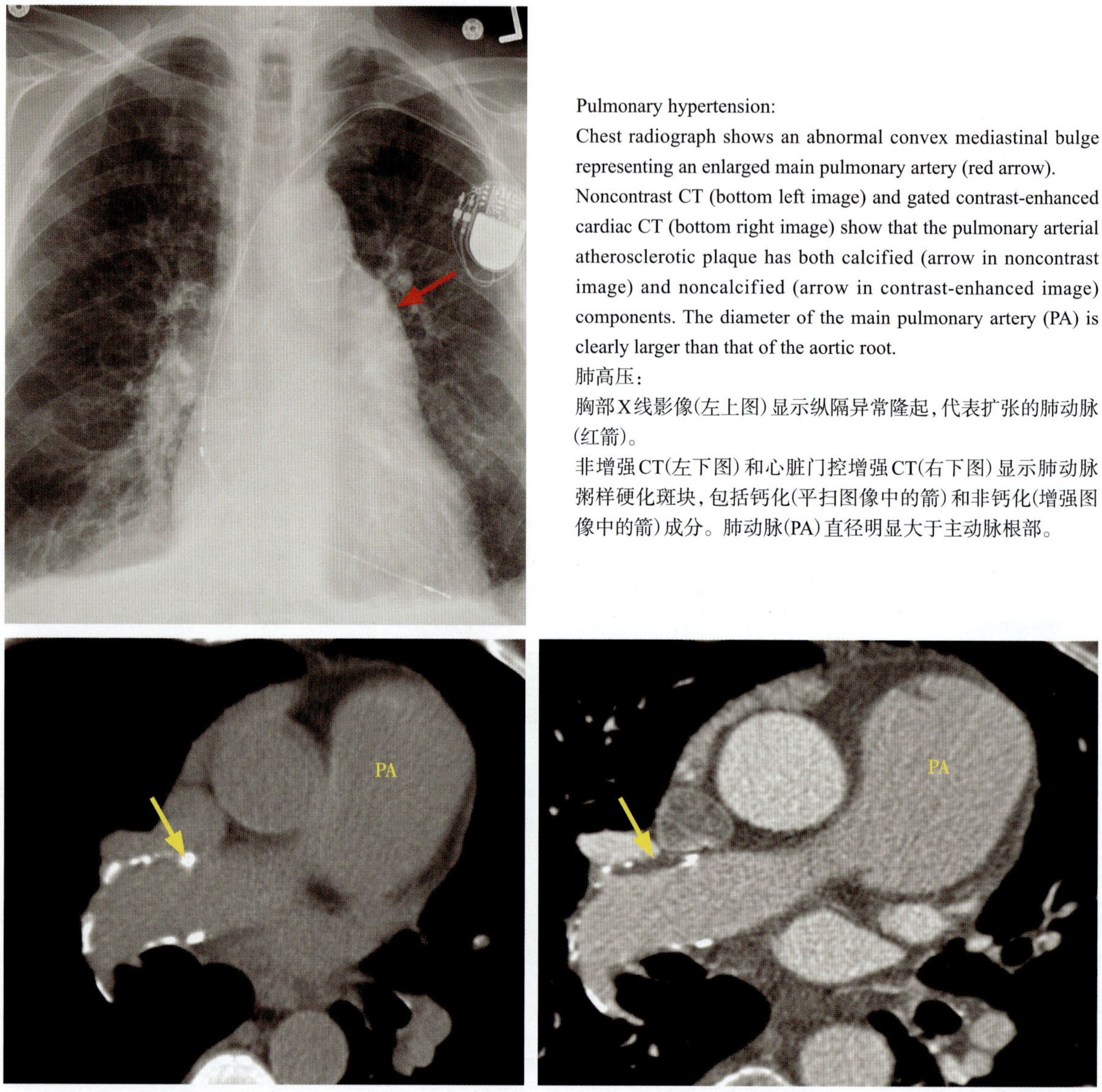

Pulmonary hypertension:
Chest radiograph shows an abnormal convex mediastinal bulge representing an enlarged main pulmonary artery (red arrow). Noncontrast CT (bottom left image) and gated contrast-enhanced cardiac CT (bottom right image) show that the pulmonary arterial atherosclerotic plaque has both calcified (arrow in noncontrast image) and noncalcified (arrow in contrast-enhanced image) components. The diameter of the main pulmonary artery (PA) is clearly larger than that of the aortic root.

肺高压：
胸部X线影像(左上图)显示纵隔异常隆起，代表扩张的肺动脉(红箭)。
非增强CT(左下图)和心脏门控增强CT(右下图)显示肺动脉粥样硬化斑块，包括钙化(平扫图像中的箭)和非钙化(增强图像中的箭)成分。肺动脉(PA)直径明显大于主动脉根部。

- A main pulmonary artery diameter ≥2.9 cm suggests the presence of pulmonary hypertension but is not highly sensitive or specific, and pulmonary hypertension may be present with a normal caliber pulmonary artery. A main pulmonary artery diameter larger than the aortic root diameter is also suggestive of pulmonary hypertension.
- Pulmonary artery wall calcifications are pathognomonic for chronic pulmonary artery hypertension typically seen due to shunts.
- Pulmonary hypertension may cause mosaic attenuation due to perfusion abnormalities, most commonly seen in chronic thromboembolic pulmonary hypertension (CTEPH).
- Pulmonary hypertension may be associated with ground glass centrilobular nodules, which may be cholesterol granulomas representing prior microhemorrhages. Centrilobular nodules may also be seen in PCH.
- An enlarged pulmonary artery can mimic a mediastinal mass. The *hilum convergence sign* is helpful to confirm that the apparent "mass" in fact represents the pulmonary artery. The *hilum convergence sign* describes the

- 肺动脉直径≥2.9cm提示有肺高压，但灵敏度或特异度不高，肺高压可出现在口径正常的肺动脉。肺动脉直径大于主动脉根部直径也提示肺高压。
- 肺动脉壁钙化可确诊为慢性肺动脉高压，后者通常由分流引起。
- 肺高压可能由于灌注异常导致马赛克样密度影，最常见于慢性血栓栓塞性肺高压(CTEPH)。
- 肺高压可能出现小叶中心磨玻璃结节，为先前微出血后形成的胆固醇性肉芽肿。小叶中心结节也可见于PCH。
- 扩张的肺动脉可以类似纵隔肿块。肺门汇聚征有助于确认看似"肿块"影的肺动脉。肺门汇聚征是指肺动脉分支在肺门汇聚成扩张的肺动脉的影像学表现。

appearance of hilar pulmonary artery branches converging into an enlarged pulmonary artery.

- In contrast, the *hilum overlay sign* describes the visualization of hilar vessels through a mass. It indicates that a mediastinal mass is present, which cannot be in the middle mediastinum.

Primary pulmonary hypertension (PPH) – WHO group 1, precapillary

- The pathologic hallmark of primary pulmonary hypertension (PPH) is the *plexiform lesion* in the wall of the muscular arteries, which is a focal disruption of the elastic lamina by an obstructing plexus of endothelial channels.
- PPH may be idiopathic (females > males) or familial (approximately 10% of cases).
- On imaging, there is typically enlargement of the main pulmonary arteries with rapidly tapering peripheral vessels.

Pulmonary hypertension due to left-to-right cardiac shunts – WHO group 1, precapillary

- Congenital left-to-right cardiac shunts, such as ventricular septal defect (VSD), atrial septal defect (ASD), and partial anomalous pulmonary venous return, cause increased flow through the pulmonary arterial bed. This chronically increased flow may eventually lead to irreversible vasculopathy characterized by pulmonary hypertension and reversal of the shunt, known as Eisenmenger syndrome.
- Imaging of PAH secondary to a congenital shunt is similar to that of PPH. There is enlargement of the central and main pulmonary arteries, with peripheral tapering. However, radiologists should look for the presence of an intracardiac or extracardiac shunt in any patient with unexplained pulmonary HTN.

Pulmonary veno-occlusive disease (PVOD) and pulmonary capillary hemangiomatosis (PCH) – WHO group 1, postcapillary

- PAH secondary to PVOD is caused by fibrotic obliteration of the pulmonary veins and venules. PVOD may be idiopathic but is associated with pregnancy, drugs (especially bleomycin), and bone marrow transplant.
- Imaging features interlobular septal thickening, patchy or centrilobular ground glass opacities, pulmonary arterial enlargement, mosaic attenuation, and pleural effusions.
- PCH is an entity that involves capillary proliferation leading to pulmonary hypertension in children and young adults.

Pulmonary venous hypertension – WHO group 2, postcapillary

- Left-sided cardiovascular disease leads to elevated pulmonary venous pressure, which is a cause of pulmonary hypertension.
- Most common etiologies are left ventricular systolic and diastolic dysfunction and valvular disease.

Pulmonary hypertension associated with hypoxemic lung disease – WHO group 3, precapillary

- COPD, sleep apnea, and interstitial lung disease can all lead to pulmonary hypertension.
- Chronic hypoxic vasoconstriction is thought to invoke vascular remodeling leading to hypertrophy of pulmonary arterial vascular smooth muscle and intimal thickening.
- Chronic lung disease can further contribute to obliteration of pulmonary microvasculature through emphysema and the perivascular fibrotic changes of pulmonary fibrosis.

- 相反，肺门覆盖征是指通过肿块可以看到穿过肺门的血管。此征象表明纵隔有肿块，但不位于中纵隔。

原发性肺高压(PPH) ——WHO第1组，毛细血管前

- PPH的病理性标志是肌性动脉壁出现丛状病变，这是由于内皮交通网的阻塞而导致了弹力层局灶性破坏。
- PPH 可能是特发性的(女性>男性)或家族性的(约10%的病例)。
- 在影像学上，典型表现为肺动脉扩张，伴外围血管迅速变细。

左向右心脏分流引起的肺高压——WHO 第 1 组，毛细血管前

- 先天性左向右心脏分流，如室间隔缺损(VSD)、房间隔缺损(ASD)和部分异常肺静脉回流，导致通过肺动脉床的血流增加。这种长期的血流增加最终可导致以肺高压和分流逆转为特征的不可逆性血管病变，称为艾森门格综合征。
- 继发于先天性分流的PAH的影像与PPH相似。表现为中央性肺动脉和肺动脉扩张，伴外周血管变细。然而，对于任何不明原因的肺HTN患者，放射科医师都应寻找是否存在心内或心外分流。

肺静脉闭塞性疾病(PVOD)和肺毛细血管瘤病(PCH) ——WHO 第 1 组，毛细血管后

- 继发于PVOD的PAH是肺静脉和小静脉纤维化闭塞。PVOD可能是特发性的，但与妊娠、药物(尤其是博来霉素)和骨髓移植有关。
- 影像学特征为小叶间隔增厚、斑片状或小叶中心磨玻璃影、肺动脉扩张、马赛克样影和胸腔积液。
- PCH 是一种由于毛细血管增生而导致儿童和年轻人肺高压的疾病。

肺静脉高压——WHO 第 2 组，毛细血管后

- 左侧心血管疾病导致肺静脉压升高，这是引起肺高压的一种原因。
- 最常见的病因是左心室收缩和舒张功能障碍，以及瓣膜疾病。

与低氧性肺病相关的肺高压——WHO 第 3 组，毛细血管前

- COPD、睡眠呼吸暂停和间质性肺疾病都可能导致肺高压。
- 慢性缺氧性血管收缩被认为可以引起血管重塑，从而导致肺动脉血管平滑肌肥大和内膜增厚。
- 慢性肺病可通过肺气肿和肺纤维化的血管周围纤维化改变进一步导致肺微血管闭塞。

Chronic thromboembolic pulmonary hypertension (CTEPH) – WHO group 4, precapillary

- Chronic occlusion of the pulmonary arterial bed can lead to pulmonary arterial hypertension, which is a complication affecting 1–5% of patients who develope acute pulmonary embolism (PE). Of note, many patients with CTEPH never had previously diagnosed acute PE.
- V/Q scan or CT pulmonary angiogram are typically done as part of the workup for new diagnosis of pulmonary HTN to rule out CTEPH.
- Features of chronic PE are described previously. Mosaic attenuation is typical.
- Treatment of CTEPH is surgical pulmonary thromboendarterectomy or balloon pulmonary angioplasty.

慢性血栓栓塞性肺高压(CTEPH)——WHO 第4组，毛细血管前

- 肺动脉床慢性阻塞可导致肺动脉高压，这是一种并发症，占急性肺栓塞(PE)患者的1%~5%。注意，许多 CTEPH 患者此前从未被诊断过急性PE。
- V/Q 扫描或 CT 肺血管造影通常作为新诊肺HTN检查的一部分，以排除CTEPH。
- 慢性 PE 的特征如前所述。典型表现为马赛克密度影。
- CTEPH 的治疗是外科肺血栓动脉内膜切除术或球囊肺血管成形术。

Fibrosing mediastinitis – WHO group 5, postcapillary

纤维性纵隔炎——WHO 第5组，毛细血管后

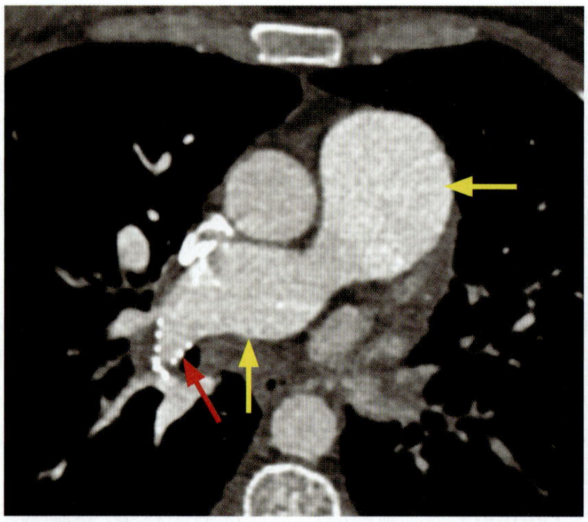

Axial CT
轴位CT

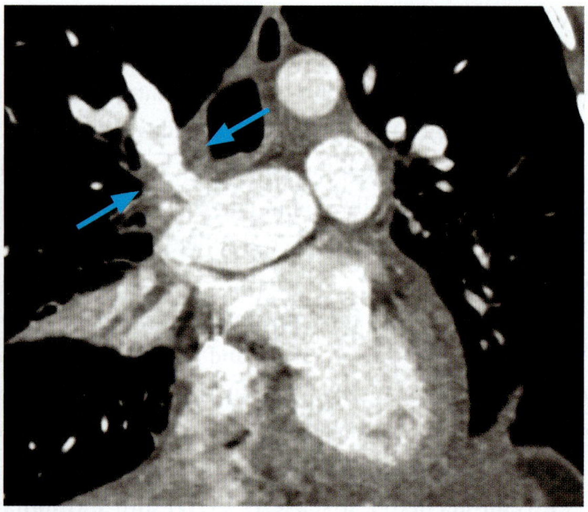

Coronal CT
冠状位CT

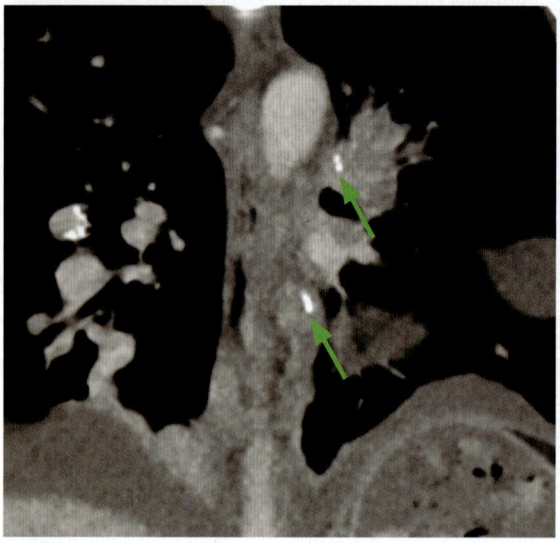

Coronal CT
冠状位CT

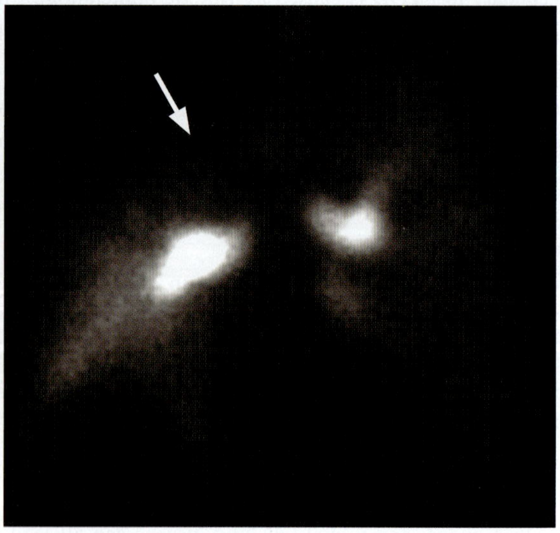

Nuclear medicine perfusion scan
核医学灌注扫描

Fibrosing mediastinitis: CT shows dilation of the main and right pulmonary arteries (yellow arrows). There is a partially imaged right lower lobe pulmonary artery stent (red arrow). Indistinct soft tissue (blue arrows) encases the right upper lobe pulmonary artery, which is narrowed and distally dilated. Mediastinal soft tissue with calcified lymph nodes (green arrows) can be seen posteriorly. Nuclear medicine perfusion scan shows markedly heterogeneous pulmonary perfusion, with near-absence of perfusion of the right upper lobe (white arrow).

纤维性纵隔炎：CT显示肺动脉及右肺动脉扩张(黄箭)。在右下叶肺动脉可见部分支架(红箭)。模糊的软组织影(蓝箭)包绕右上叶肺动脉，形成局部狭窄及远端扩张。后方可见纵隔软组织伴钙化淋巴结(绿箭)。核医学灌注扫描显示肺灌注明显不均匀，右上叶几乎没有灌注(白箭)。

- Progressive proliferation of fibrous tissue within the mediastinum may lead to encasement and compression of mediastinal structures. The most common causes of fibrosing mediastinitis are histoplasmosis and tuberculosis.
- Fibrous encasement of the pulmonary veins leads to permanent histological changes within the endothelial cells.
- Fibrosing mediastinitis may also encase the pulmonary arteries, creating a pre-capillary pulmonary hypertension.
- Imaging features of fibrosing mediastinitis include increased mediastinal soft tissue, often with calcified lymph nodes due to prior granulomatous infection.

- 纵隔内纤维组织进行性增生可导致纵隔结构被包绕和挤压。纤维性纵隔炎最常见的病因是组织胞浆菌病和肺结核。
- 肺静脉纤维包裹导致内皮细胞出现永久性组织学改变。
- 纤维性纵隔炎也可能包裹肺动脉，形成毛细血管前肺高压。
- 纤维性纵隔炎的影像学特征包括纵隔软组织增加，常伴有来自先前的肉芽肿感染而钙化的淋巴结。

（翻译　王维平）

DIFFUSE LUNG DISEASE

弥漫性肺疾病

INTERSTITIAL LUNG DISEASE

间质性肺疾病

Overview of interstitial lung disease

- Interstitial lung disease (ILD) may be idiopathic, or secondary to known insults which include drug toxicity, collagen vascular disease, or occupational exposure.

  A disease can only be classified as an idiopathic interstitial lung disease if there is no other explanation for the pathologic changes.
- Non-specific clinical symptoms of ILD consist of cough and dyspnea, however factors such as age, gender, risk factors, course of disease, and imaging features can help distinguish between the various entities.
- Histologically, the lung responds to injury by recruiting lymphocytes or macrophages, increasing inflammatory debris, and instigating a fibrotic reaction.
- There are eight entities which fall under ILD. The pathologic entities may have different clinical syndromes.

间质性肺疾病概述

- 间质性肺疾病（ILD）可能是特发性的，或继发于已知的损伤，包括药物毒性、胶原血管疾病或职业暴露。

  只有在用任何原因都无法解释病理改变的情况下，才能将疾病归类为特发性间质性肺疾病。
- ILD的非特异性临床症状包括咳嗽和呼吸困难，但如年龄、性别、危险因素、病程和影像学特征等因素可以帮助区分不同的疾病。
- 组织学上，肺通过募集淋巴细胞或巨噬细胞、增加炎症碎片并引发纤维化反应对损伤作出反应。
- 有八种疾病属于ILD。病理学改变可能有不同的临床综合征。

Histologic Pattern	Clinical Correlate	Main Imaging Findings
Usual interstitial pneumonia (UIP)	Idiopathic pulmonary fibrosis (IPF) Rheumatoid arthritis Asbestosis Drug toxicity	Basilar subpleural reticulation with honeycombing
Nonspecific interstitial pneumonia (NSIP)	Scleroderma Dermatomyositis Mixed connective tissue disease Drug toxicity	Peribronchial reticulation, traction bronchiectasis, +/– ground glass opacities
Organizing pneumonia	Cryptogenic organizing pneumonia (COP) – idiopathic Drug toxicity Connective tissue disorders, particularly SLE and dermatomyositis	Peripheral or peribronchial ground glass or consolidative opacities
Respiratory bronchiolitis (RB)	Smoking-related spectrum	Upper lobe centrilobular nodules
Desquamative interstitial pneumonia (DIP)	Smoking-related spectrum	Lower lung predominant ground glass
Lymphoid interstitial pneumonia (LIP)	Sjögren's syndrome Immune dysregulation including HIV and CVID	Nodules and cysts
Diffuse alveolar damage (DAD)	Acute interstitial pneumonia (AIP) Acute respiratory distress syndrome (ARDS) Transfusion-related acute lung injury (TRALI)	Diffuse airspace disease
Hypersensitivity pneumonitis (HP)	Hypersensitivity pneumonitis Drug toxicity	Acute: Extensive ground glass and air trapping Chronic: Ground glass, peribronchial fibrosis and air trapping, +/– upper lung predominant

Table showing types of interstitial lung disease.

组织学表现	相关的临床	主要的影像学表现
普通型间质性肺炎(UIP)	特发性肺纤维化(IPF) 类风湿关节炎 石棉肺 药物毒性	基底部胸膜下网状结构伴蜂窝样改变
非特异性间质性肺炎(NSIP)	硬皮病 皮肌炎 混合性结缔组织病 药物毒性	支气管周围网状结构,牵拉性支气管扩张,+/–磨玻璃影
机化性肺炎	隐源性机化性肺炎(COP)——特发性 药物毒性 结缔组织疾病,尤其是系统性红斑狼疮(SLE)和皮肌炎	外周或支气管周围磨玻璃影或实变影
呼吸性细支气管炎(RB)	吸烟相关系列	上叶小叶中心性结节
脱屑性间质性肺炎(DIP)	吸烟相关系列	下肺为主磨玻璃影
淋巴细胞性间质性肺炎(LIP)	干燥综合征 免疫失调,包括人类免疫缺陷病毒(HIV)和常见变异型免疫缺陷病(CVID)	结节和囊肿
弥漫性肺泡损伤(DAD)	急性间质性肺炎(AIP) 急性呼吸窘迫综合征(ARDS) 输血相关性急性肺损伤(TRALI)	弥漫性气腔疾病
过敏性肺炎(HP)	过敏性肺炎 药物毒性	急性:广泛的磨玻璃影和空气潴留 慢性:磨玻璃影、支气管周围纤维化和空气潴留,+/–上肺为主

表格概括了间质性肺疾病的类型。

Usual interstitial pneumonia (UIP)

- Idiopathic pulmonary fibrosis (IPF) is the clinical syndrome of UIP with unknown cause and is the most common cause of UIP. IPF has a much worse clinical outcome compared to secondary causes of UIP.

  The mean survival of IPF is not much different compared to lung cancer. Of all the interstitial pneumonias, only acute interstitial pneumonitis (AIP) has a worse prognosis.

  Clinical symptoms of IPF include dry cough and dyspnea.

  IPF usually affects male patients >50 years old, and typically smokers.

- Other triggers of lung injury that may result in a UIP pattern include:

  Collagen vascular disease (rheumatoid arthritis much more commonly than scleroderma).

  Drug toxicity.

  Asbestosis. An imaging clue to the presence of asbestosis is calcified plaques indicative of prior asbestos exposure.

- The pathology of UIP features interstitial fibroblastic foci and chronic alveolar inflammation with temporal and spatial heterogeneity.
- Early UIP features reticulation in the posterior subpleural lung bases.

普通型间质性肺炎(UIP)

- 特发性肺纤维化(IPF)是原因不明的UIP临床综合征,并且是UIP最常见的原因。IPF的临床转归远不及继发性UIP。

  IPF的平均生存率与肺癌相比没有太大差异。在所有间质性肺炎中,只有急性间质性肺炎(AIP)的预后较差。IPF的临床症状包括干咳和呼吸困难。

  IPF通常影响>50岁的男性患者,并且往往是吸烟者。

- 其他可导致UIP病变的肺损伤触发因素包括:

  胶原血管疾病(类风湿关节炎较硬皮病更常见)。

  药物毒性。

  石棉肺:存在石棉肺沉着病的影像学线索是钙化斑块,表明先前有石棉接触史。

- UIP的病理学特征为间质性成纤维细胞灶和慢性肺泡炎,伴有时-空异质性。
- 早期UIP的特征为肺底后部胸膜下网状结构。

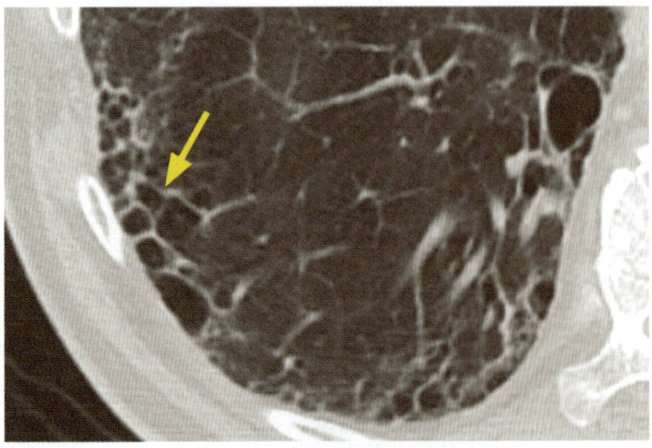

Noncontrast CT shows subpleural reticulations and honeycombing (arrow).
CT平扫显示胸膜下网状和蜂窝状结构(黄箭)。

- In later stages of UIP, traction bronchiectasis and subpleural honeycombing develop. The lung bases are the most severely affected.
- Surgical biopsy can be avoided if characteristic features, in particular peripheral basal location of reticulation, are present. The American Thoracic Society (ATS) developed updated guidelines in 2018 for how to characterize a UIP pattern on CT.

- 在UIP后期，会出现牵拉性支气管扩张和胸膜下蜂窝结构。肺底部受累最为严重。
- 当出现特征性表现，尤其是基底部的外周网状结构时，则可以避免手术活检。美国胸科学会(ATS)于2018年发布了关于如何在CT上确定UIP模式的最新指南。

ATS Guidelines on ILD Patterns

UIP	Probable UIP	Indeterminate for UIP	Alternative Diagnosis
1. Subpleural, basal predominance[†] 2. Reticulation 3. Honeycombing 4. Absence of inconsistent features	1. Subpleural, basal predominance 2. Reticulation 3. No honeycombing 4. Absence of inconsistent features	1. Very early fibrosis with subpleural+basal predominance OR 2. Atypical distribution but no findings to suggest alternative diagnosis	Any of: 1. Upper or mid-lung predominant* 2. Peribronchovascular predominant*,** 3. Predominant GGO*,** 4. Micronodules 5. Extensive mosaic/air trapping* 6. Nodules, consolidation, or cysts

*Suggests chronic HP **Suggests NSIP
[†]Diffuse or asymmetric allowed

2018 Update

ATS关于ILD模式的指南

普通型间质性肺炎	普通型间质性肺炎可能	普通型间质性肺炎不能确定	其他诊断
1. 胸膜下、基底部为主[†] 2. 网状结构 3. 蜂窝 4. 没有不一致的特征	1. 胸膜下、基底部为主 2. 网状结构 3. 无蜂窝 4. 没有不一致的特征	1. 极早期纤维化，以胸膜下+基底为主 或者 2. 非典型分布，但无征象支持其他诊断	以下任何 1. 上肺或中肺为主* 2. 支气管血管周围为主*,** 3. GGO为主*,** 4. 微结节 5. 广泛马赛克/空气潴留* 6. 结节、实变或囊肿

*提示慢性过敏性肺炎 **提示非特异性间质性肺炎
[†]可以弥漫或不对称

2018年更新

Nonspecific interstitial pneumonitis (NSIP)

非特异性间质性肺炎(NSIP)

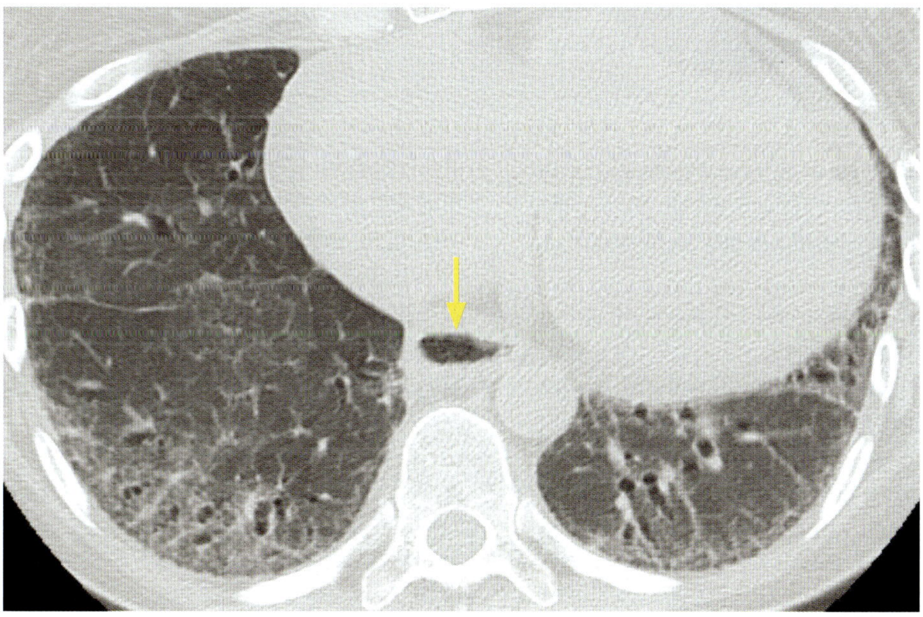

NSIP: Axial CT shows posterior basal predominant subpleural and peribronchial reticulation, mild ground glass attenuation, and mild traction bronchiectasis. This presentation likely represents the fibrotic subtype of NSIP. Esophageal dilation (arrow) is a clue to the presence of scleroderma, which is often associated with NSIP.
Case courtesy Ritu R. Gill, MD, MPH, Brigham and Women's Hospital.
NSIP：轴位CT显示以后基底部为主的胸膜下和支气管周围网状影，轻度磨玻璃影和轻度牵拉性支气管扩张。这种表现可能是NSIP的纤维化亚型。食管扩张(黄箭)提示硬皮病，后者常与NSIP相关。

- Nonspecific interstitial pneumonitis (NSIP) is both the name of the clinical syndrome and the corresponding pathologic diagnosis. Affected patients are typically younger (40–50 years old) compared to IPF. Symptoms are similar to IPF with chronic dry cough and dyspnea.
- NSIP has a better 5-year survival compared to IPF. Unlike IPF, NSIP does respond to steroids.
- NSIP is almost always associated with an underlying disease. NSIP is the most common pulmonary manifestation in patients with collagen vascular disease.

  NSIP may be associated with dermatomyositis, SLE, mixed connective tissue disease, and scleroderma.

  NSIP may also be caused by drug reaction.
- Histologically, NSIP features thickened alveolar septa from chronic inflammation – in contrast to IPF/UIP.
- An important imaging feature of NSIP is the presence of ground glass opacities (GGO) with peribronchial predominance which is a key feature to distinguish NSIP.
- A key imaging finding (not always seen but very specific) is sparing of immediate subpleural lung. This feature is NOT seen in UIP.
- Like UIP, NSIP tends to affect the lower lobes. Other diagnoses should be considered (e.g., chronic hypersensitivity pneumonitis or sarcoidosis) if there is primarily upper lobe disease.

- 非特异性间质性肺炎(NSIP)既是临床综合征的名称，也是相应的病理诊断。受累患者通常较IPF年轻(40~50岁)。症状与IPF相似，表现为慢性干咳和呼吸困难。
- NSIP患者的5年生存率高于IPF。与IPF不同，类固醇治疗对NSIP有效。
- NSIP几乎总是合并一种基础性疾病。NSIP是胶原血管病患者最常见的肺部表现。

  NSIP可能与皮肌炎、系统性红斑狼疮(SLE)、混合性结缔组织病和硬皮病相关。

  NSIP也可能由药物反应引起。
- 组织学上，NSIP的特征是慢性炎症导致的肺泡间隔增厚——这与IPF/UIP形成对比。
- NSIP的一个重要影像学特征是以支气管周围为主的磨玻璃影，这是区分NSIP的关键特征。
- 一个关键的影像学特征(并不总是可见，但非常特异)是紧邻胸膜下的肺组织不受累。这一特征在UIP中**看不到**。
- 与UIP相同，NSIP倾向于累及下叶。如果病变以上叶为主，应考虑其他诊断(如慢性过敏性肺炎或结节病)。

Organizing pneumonia (OP)

机化性肺炎(OP)

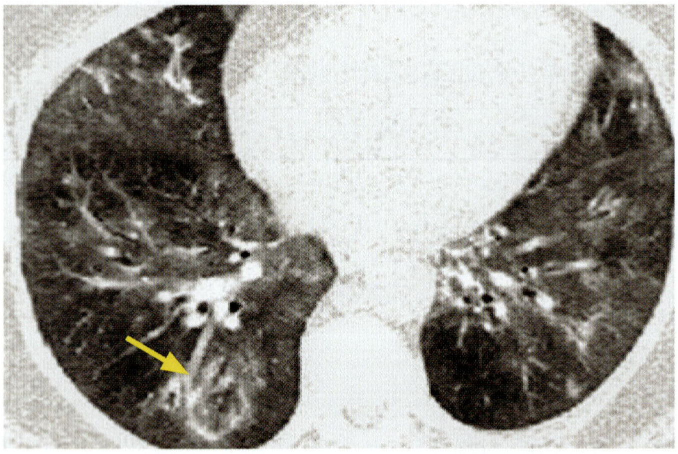

Axial CT shows patchy consolidative and ground glass opacities in a peribronchovascular distribution. There is a *reverse halo* or *atoll sign* in the right lower lobe (arrow), where a central lucency is surrounded by a peripheral opacity.

Case courtesy Seth Kligerman, MD, University of Maryland.

轴位CT显示斑片状实变影和磨玻璃影，沿支气管血管周围分布。右下叶可见*反晕征*或*环礁征*(黄箭)，其中央透亮区被外围的高密度影所包围。

- Organizing pneumonia is the histological pattern of alveolar inflammation with granulation tissue polyps that fill the distal airways and alveoli. OP may be a response to infection, drug reaction, or inhalation. OP may be idiopathic or related to connective tissue disease as well.
- Cryptogenic organizing pneumonia (COP) is idiopathic OP, previously called bronchiolitis obliterans organizing pneumonia (BOOP).
- COP clinically responds to steroids with a good prognosis and may resolve completely, although recurrences are common.
- CT shows consolidation or ground glass opacities in a peripheral and peribronchovascular distribution. The *reverse halo sign* (also known as the *atoll sign*) features a central lucency surrounded by a ground glass halo. *Reverse halo sign* is not specific but in the appropriate context is highly suggestive of OP.

  The *reverse halo sign* should not be confused with the *halo sign* that is typical of invasive aspergillus, which shows a central opacity with peripheral ground glass.

- 机化性肺炎(OP)在组织学上表现为肺泡炎症，伴远端气道和肺泡被肉芽组织息肉所填充。OP可能是一种对感染、药物或误吸的反应。OP也可能是特发性的或与结缔组织病有关。
- 隐源性机化性肺炎(COP)是特发性OP，过去称为闭塞性细支气管炎机化性肺炎(BOOP)。
- 临床上，类固醇治疗对COP有效，预后良好，且有可能完全缓解，但复发常见。
- CT显示分布于外周和支气管血管周围的实变影或磨玻璃影。*反晕征*(也称为*环礁征*)的特征是中央透亮，外围有磨玻璃影。*反晕征*不具特异性，但在适当的情况下可高度提示OP。

  *反晕征*不应与*晕征*相混淆，后者常见于侵袭性曲霉菌病，表现为中心高密度影伴周边磨玻璃影。

Respiratory bronchiolitis – interstitial lung disease (RB-ILD)

呼吸性细支气管炎-间质性肺病(RB-ILD)

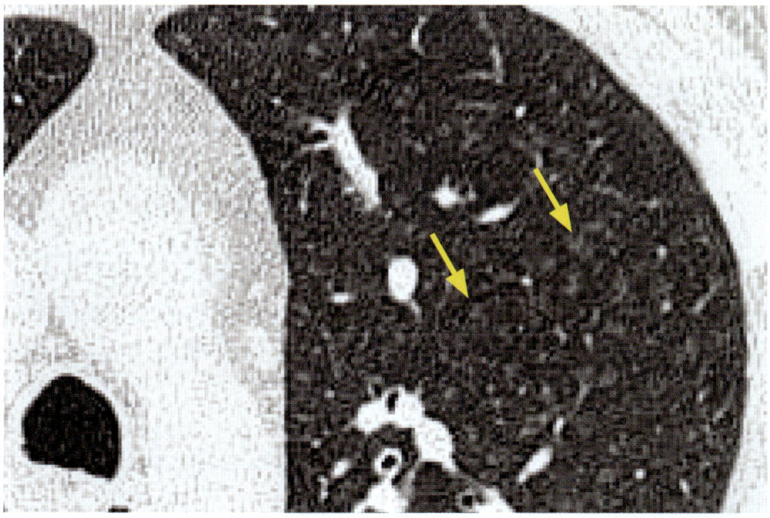

Axial CT shows innumerable subcentimeter centrilobular nodules of ground glass attenuation (arrows). None of the nodules extend to the pleural surface, which is typical of a centrilobular distribution. This was a case of respiratory bronchiolitis interstitial lung disease (RB-ILD).

轴位CT显示无数亚厘米的小叶中央磨玻璃结节(黄箭)。没有任何结节延伸至胸膜表面,这是典型的小叶中央分布方式。此病例为呼吸性细支气管炎-间质性肺疾病(RB-ILD)。

- Respiratory bronchiolitis – interstitial lung disease (RB-ILD) is both the clinical syndrome and the pathologic diagnosis of this smoking-related interstitial lung disease.
- Respiratory bronchiolitis (RB, without the ILD) is common in smokers, where pigmented macrophages are found in respiratory bronchioles. RB is usually asymptomatic, but if symptomatic (usually cough and shortness of breath), the clinical syndrome is called RB-ILD.
- Histologically, RB-ILD is characterized by sheets of macrophages filling the terminal airways, with relative sparing of the alveoli.
- The key imaging features of RB-ILD are centrilobular nodules in the lung apices.

- 呼吸性细支气管炎-间质性肺疾病(RB-ILD)既是临床综合征,也是吸烟相关间质性肺疾病的病理诊断。
- 呼吸性细支气管炎(RB,不伴ILD)在吸烟者中很常见,在呼吸性细支气管中可发现色素巨噬细胞。RB通常无症状,但如果有症状(通常是咳嗽和呼吸急促),其临床综合征称为RB-ILD。
- 组织学上,RB-ILD的特征是终末气道充满了巨噬细胞层,肺泡相对不受累。
- RB-ILD的关键影像学特征是肺尖小叶中心结节。

Desquamative interstitial pneumonia (DIP)

脱屑性间质性肺炎(DIP)

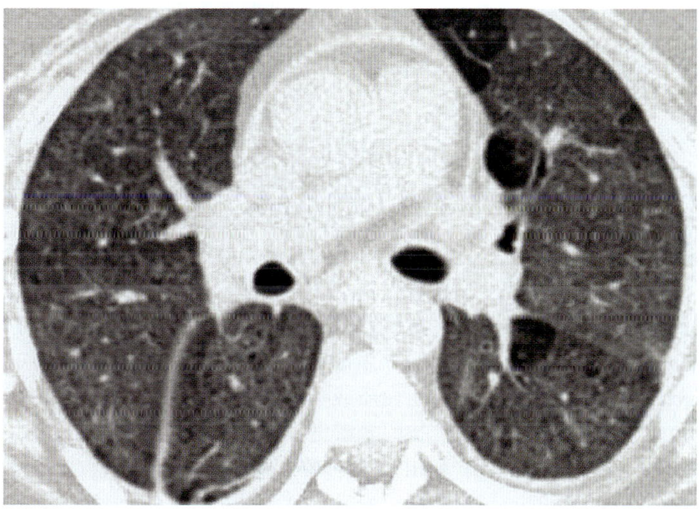

DIP: Axial CT shows extensive ground glass opacities. This is a nonspecific pattern.

Case courtesy Ritu R. Gill, MD, MPH, Brigham and Women's Hospital.

DIP:轴位CT显示广泛的磨玻璃影。这是一种非特异性表现。

- Like RB-ILD, desquamative interstitial pneumonia (DIP) is both the clinical syndrome and the pathologic diagnosis. Pathologically, RB, RB-ILD, and DIP represent a continuous spectrum of smoking-related lung disease.
- Like RB, brown-pigmented macrophages are involved in DIP; however, sheets of these abnormal macrophages also extend into the alveoli in DIP.
- Imaging of DIP shows diffuse basal-predominant ground glass opacification.

- 与RB-ILD相同,脱屑性间质性肺炎(DIP)既是临床综合征也是病理诊断。在病理学上,RB、RB-ILD和DIP代表了一个与吸烟相关的系列肺部病变。
- 与RB相同,棕色巨噬细胞也参与了DIP;但在DIP中,这些异常巨噬细胞层也延伸到肺泡。

Although the predominant abnormality is ground glass, a few cysts may also be present.

- DIP影像学表现为以基底部为主的弥漫性磨玻璃影。虽然主要的异常是磨玻璃影，但也可能存在一些囊肿。

Acute interstitial pneumonia (AIP)

急性间质性肺炎(AIP)

- Acute interstitial pneumonia (AIP), representing idiopathic diffuse alveolar damage (DAD), is the pathologic diagnosis seen in the clinical syndrome of acute respiratory distress syndrome (ARDS). Unlike the other ⅡPs, AIP is the only syndrome with an acute onset and has the worst prognosis.
- Two phases of AIP are recognized: early (exudative) and chronic (organizing).
- The **early (exudative) phase** features hyaline membranes, diffuse alveolar infiltration by immune cells, and noncardiogenic pulmonary edema.

- 急性间质性肺炎(AIP)代表特发性弥漫性肺泡损伤(DAD)，是急性呼吸窘迫综合征(ARDS)的病理学诊断。与其他特发性间质性肺炎不同，AIP是唯一一种急性起病的综合征，预后最差。
- AIP分为两个期：早期(渗出)和慢性期(机化)。
- **早期(渗出)**的特点是透明膜、免疫细胞弥漫性肺泡浸润和非心源性肺水肿。

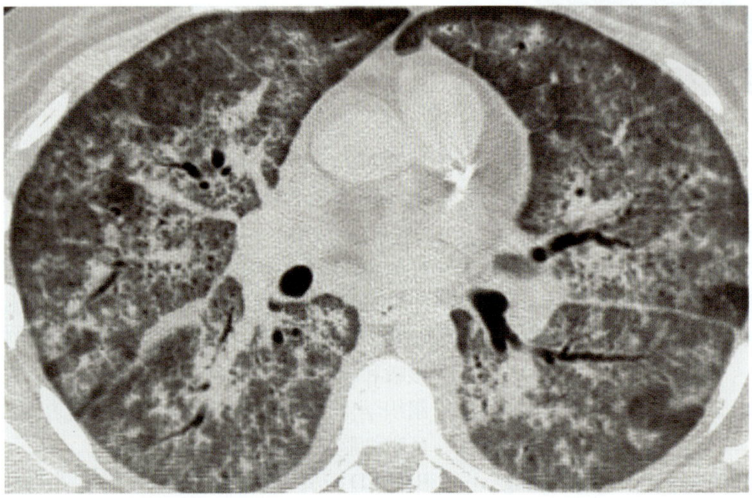

AIP (early or exudative phase):
Axial CT shows extensive geographic ground glass attenuation. This is a nonspecific pattern and may represent pulmonary edema, hemorrhage, infection, or ARDS/AIP.
Case courtesy Seth Kligerman, MD, University of Maryland.

AIP(早期或渗出期)：轴位CT显示广泛的地图样磨玻璃影。这种表现不具特异性，可能代表肺水肿、出血、感染或急性呼吸窘迫综合征(ARDS)/AIP。

- The **chronic (organizing) phase** features alveolar wall thickening due to granulation tissue. The chronic phase usually begins one week after the initial injury.
- On imaging, opacities coalesce with architectural distortion and bronchial dilation. These features will resolve over time, sometimes with residual fibrosis.

- **慢性(机化)期**的特点是肉芽组织导致的肺泡壁增厚。慢性期通常在初始损伤后一周开始。
- 影像学上，密度增高影融合在结构扭曲和支气管扩张中。这些特征会随着时间的推移而消退，有时残留纤维化。

ANTIGEN AND EXPOSURE-RELATED LUNG DISEASE

抗原和暴露相关的肺部疾病

- Most inhalational lung diseases predominantly affect the upper lobes because the lower lobes have more robust blood flow and lymphatic drainage.

- 大多数吸入性肺病主要影响上叶，因为下叶有更充足的血流和淋巴引流。

Hypersensitivity pneumonitis (HP)

过敏性肺炎(HP)

- Hypersensitivity pneumonitis (HP) is a common lung disease caused by a hypersensitivity reaction to inhaled organic antigens, such as bird proteins or thermophilic actinomycetes, although a history of antigen exposure is not elicited in about 1/3 of patients.
- HP is characterized by two clinical courses: acute/subacute and chronic. Chronic has progressive symptoms (+/– acute exacerbation) and fibrosis; acute/subacute may have recurrence but no fibrosis.
- **Acute/subacute** HP is characterized by inflammatory exudate filling the alveoli, which manifests on imaging as nonspecific ground glass or consolidation. Small, ill-defined centrilobular nodules and ground glass can also be seen.

  Mosaic attenuation (geographic areas of relative lucency) can be secondary to mosaic perfusion on inspiration and air trapping on expiration.

- 过敏性肺炎(HP)是一种常见的由吸入有机抗原产生超敏反应所引起的肺部疾病，如鸟类蛋白质或嗜热放线菌，但约1/3的患者找不到抗原暴露史。
- HP以两种临床病程为代表：急性/亚急性、慢性。慢性症状呈进行性(+/-急性加重)并有纤维化；急性/亚急性可复发但无纤维化。
- **急性/亚急性**HP的特点是炎性渗出物充满肺泡，在影像学上表现为非特异性的磨玻璃影或实变。也可见小而边界不清的小叶中心结节和磨玻璃影。

  马赛克样影(相对透亮的地图样区域)可能是由于吸气时的马赛克灌注和呼气时的空气滞留的缘故。

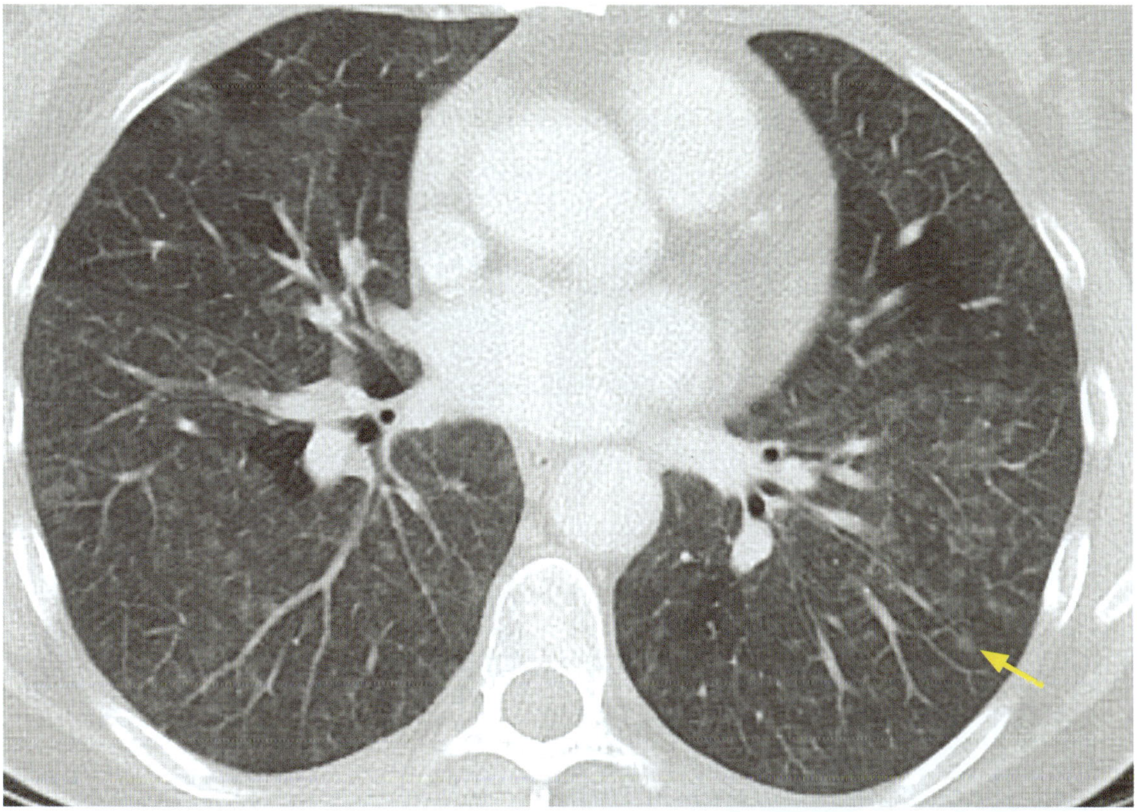

HP: Diffuse ground glass opacities affecting both lungs with mosaic attenuation. There are diffuse small centrilobular nodules (arrow). This was a case of acute/subacute HP.

HP：弥漫性磨玻璃影累及两肺并伴有马赛克样影。可见弥漫性小叶中心小结节(黄箭)。这是一个急性/亚急性HP病例。

- **Chronic** HP, from long-term exposure to the offending antigen, leads to pulmonary fibrosis, typically but not always upper-lobe predominant. Often the findings of acute/subacute disease, including centrilobular nodules, ground glass, and mosaic attenuation, may be superimposed.

  Symptoms may follow a chronic, progressive course or present as multiple exacerbations.

  The key feature of chronic HP, in either case, is fibrosis. Fibrosis is typically peribronchovascular.

  The *head-cheese sign* describes the combination of patchy ground glass and areas of lucency due to air trapping.

  Unlike IPF, honeycombing is not common in HP, but when present may involve the upper lobes.

- **慢性HP**，由于长期暴露于致病抗原会导致肺纤维化，通常以上叶为主，但不绝对。急性/亚急性HP的常见表现有小叶中心结节、磨玻璃影和马赛克样影，以上表现可有重叠。

  症状可能是慢性、进行性或表现为多次发作。

  无论哪种情况，慢性HP的关键特征都是纤维化。纤维化通常是在支气管血管周围。

  猪头肉冻征是指斑片状磨玻璃影兼空气潴留导致的透亮区。

  与IPF不同，蜂窝样改变在HP中并不常见，但出现时往往见于上叶。

Pneumoconioses

- A pneumoconiosis is a lung disease secondary to *inorganic* dust inhalation. In contrast, hypersensitivity pneumonitis is caused by *organic* dust inhalation.
- **Silicosis** and **coal workers pneumoconiosis (CWP)** are the two most common pneumoconioses. They have indistinguishable imaging findings even though they are due to different inhaled dusts and have different histologic findings. Imaging features also overlap with sarcoidosis.

  Silicosis is due to inhalation of silica dust, which miners may be exposed to.

  CWP is caused by inhalation of coal dust, which does not contain any silica.

  The most characteristic finding of *uncomplicated* disease is multiple upper-lobe predominant perilymphatic nodules.

  Eggshell lymph node calcifications are commonly seen in silicosis, less commonly in CWP.

尘肺病

- 尘肺病是一种继发于吸入无机粉尘的肺部疾病。相比之下，过敏性肺炎是由吸入有机粉尘所致。
- 硅沉着病(**矽肺**)和**煤工尘肺(CWP)**是最常见的两种尘肺病。两者在影像学上无法区分，尽管吸入的粉尘不同，组织学表现也不同。影像学表现与结节病也有重叠。

  矽肺由吸入二氧化硅粉尘引发，矿工可能有接触史。

  CWP由吸入煤尘引起，其中不含任何二氧化硅。

  在非复杂的病例，最具特征性的表现是以上叶为主的多发淋巴管周围结节。

  蛋壳样淋巴结钙化常见于矽肺，较少见于CWP。

Silicosis or CWP can become *complicated* with large conglomerate masses or **progressive massive fibrosis**.

矽肺或CWP可能变得复杂，可形成大的团块或**进行性大面积纤维化**。

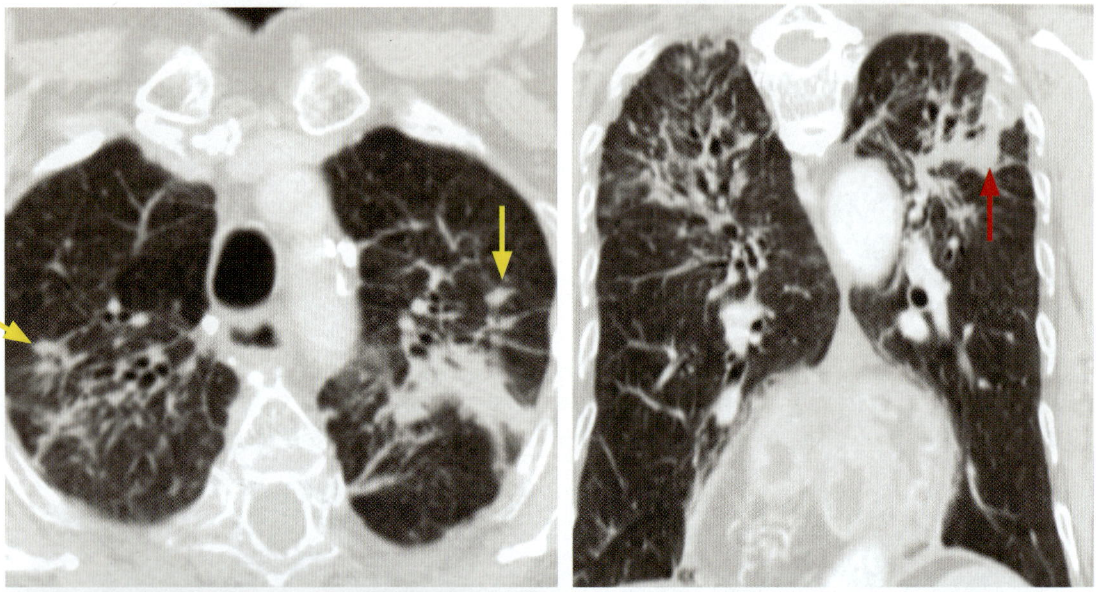

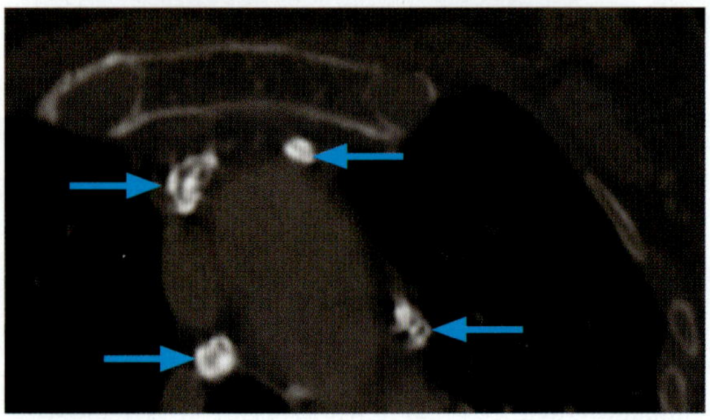

Silicosis complicated with progressive massive fibrosis: CT demonstrates upper lobe predominant fibrotic changes. There are perilymphatic nodules (yellow arrows) and a developing left upper lobe conglomerative mass (red arrow).
Egg-shell calcified lymph nodes are present in the mediastinum (blue arrows).
矽肺并发进行性大面积纤维化：CT显示上叶为主的纤维化改变。可见多个淋巴管周围结节(黄箭)和进展中的左上叶融合性肿块(红箭)。
纵隔内可见蛋壳样钙化淋巴结(蓝箭)。

Both silicosis and CWP confer an increased risk of TB.

Caplan syndrome is seen in patients with rheumatoid arthritis *and* either CWP or silicosis (more common in CWP) and represents necrobiotic rheumatoid nodules superimposed on the smaller centrilobular and subpleural nodules of the pneumoconiosis.

- **Asbestosis** is lung disease caused by inhalation of asbestos fibers. End-stage asbestosis can lead to pulmonary fibrosis with a UIP pathology.

Unlike the other inhalational lung diseases, asbestosis predominantly affects the lower lobes because the asbestos particles are too large to be removed by the alveolar macrophages and lymphatic system.

The radiographic/CT appearance and distribution of advanced asbestosis may be indistinguishable from IPF; however, an important clue seen in asbestosis is pleural thickening and plaques.

Even though pleural plaques (which may or may not be calcified) are due to asbestos exposure, they are not a component of asbestosis, do not lead to fibrosis, and are usually asymptomatic.

矽肺和CWP都会增加患结核病的风险。

卡普兰综合征见于类风湿关节炎和CWP或矽肺(更常见于CWP)患者，为坏死性类风湿结节叠加在尘肺病较小的小叶中心和胸膜下结节中。

- **石棉肺**是由吸入石棉纤维引起的肺部疾病。终末期石棉肺可以导致肺纤维化，病理表现为UIP。

与其他吸入性肺病不同，石棉肺主要累及下叶，因为石棉颗粒太大，无法被肺泡巨噬细胞和淋巴系统所清除。

晚期石棉肺的X线/CT表现和分布可能无法与IPF鉴别；然而，石棉肺的一条重要线索是胸膜增厚和斑块形成。

即使胸膜斑块(钙化或非钙化)是由于接触石棉引起的，但它们不是石棉肺的组成部分，不会导致纤维化，通常无症状。

Eosinophilic lung disease

- Eosinophilic lung disease is a spectrum of diseases that feature accumulation of eosinophils in the pulmonary airspaces and interstitium.

Simple pulmonary eosinophilia (Löffler syndrome)

- Simple pulmonary eosinophilia (also known as Löffler syndrome) is characterized by transient and *migratory* areas of focal consolidation, with an elevated eosinophil count in the peripheral smear.
- An identical appearance can be seen as a response to injury, especially with parasitic disease and drug reactions. The term *simple pulmonary eosinophilia* is reserved for idiopathic cases.

Chronic eosinophilic pneumonia

嗜酸性肺病

- 嗜酸性肺病是一系列以嗜酸性粒细胞在肺气腔和间质中积聚为特征的系列疾病。

单纯性肺嗜酸性粒细胞增多症(Löffler综合征)

- 单纯性肺嗜酸性粒细胞增多症(也称Löffler综合征)的特征是短暂性和迁移性局灶性实变区，伴外周涂片嗜酸性粒细胞计数升高。
- 相同的表现可见于损伤性反应，尤其是寄生虫病和药物反应。单纯性肺嗜酸性粒细胞增多症这一术语仅用于特发性病例。

慢性嗜酸性粒细胞性肺炎

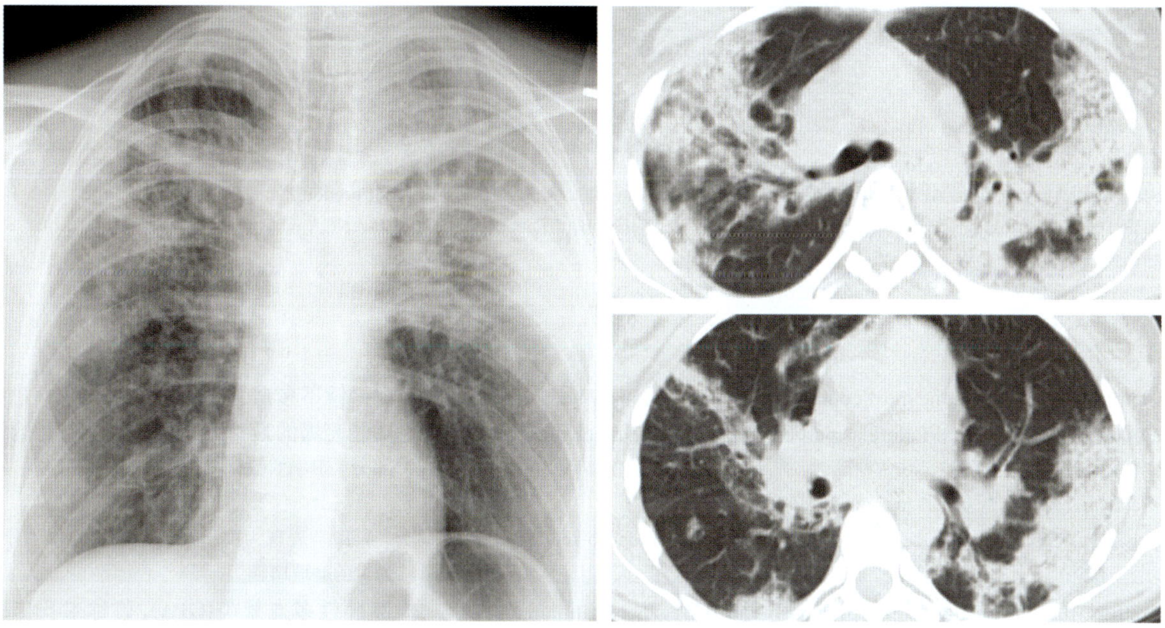

Chronic eosinophilic pneumonia: Chest radiograph demonstrates upper lobe and peripheral consolidation.
Axial CT shows bilateral patchy peripheral consolidative opacities.
Case courtesy Ritu R. Gill, MD, MPH, Brigham and Women's Hospital.
慢性嗜酸性粒细胞性肺炎：胸部X线影像显示上叶和外周实变。
轴位CT显示双侧斑片状外周实变影。

- Chronic eosinophilic pneumonia is an important consideration in the differential diagnosis of chronic consolidation. Chronic eosinophilic pneumonia causes extensive alveolar filling and interstitial infiltration with inflammatory eosinophils.
- Consolidation is patchy and *peripheral*, with an *upper lobe* predominance, in a *reverse batwing* configuration. Furthermore, consolidation may *cross fissures*, distinguishing it from COP. Chronic eosinophilic pneumonia is also much less common than COP.
- Compare to prior films for transient or changing infiltrates over time.
- Chronic eosinophilic pneumonia responds rapidly to steroids but relapse is common after steroid discontinuation. Patients almost always have peripheral blood eosinophilia.

- 在鉴别慢性实变时，慢性嗜酸性粒细胞性肺炎是一个重要的考虑因素。慢性嗜酸性粒细胞性肺炎会导致广泛的炎性嗜酸性粒细胞填充肺泡和间质浸润。
- 实变呈斑片状和外周性分布，以上叶为主，呈反向蝙蝠翼状。此外，实变可跨越肺裂，这与COP不同。同时，慢性嗜酸性粒细胞性肺炎较COP少得多。
- 对照过去的影像学表现可以判断浸润性改变是否为一过性或随时间而变化。
- 慢性嗜酸性粒细胞性肺炎对类固醇反应迅速，但停药后常见复发。患者几乎都有外周血嗜酸性粒细胞增高。

Pulmonary Vasculitis

- Pulmonary vasculitis includes a group of inflammatory conditions involving small vessels, large vessels, and granulomatous disease.
- Imaging manifestations include 1) alveolar hemorrhage and 2) nodular foci with cavitation.

肺血管炎

- 肺血管炎包括一组累及小血管和大血管的炎症，以及肉芽肿性疾病。
- 影像学表现包括：①肺泡出血；②有空洞的结节灶。

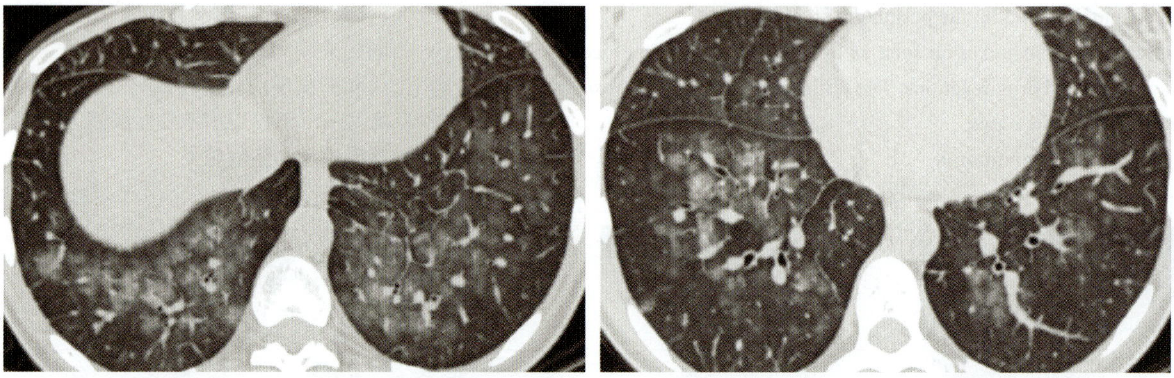

Alveolar hemorrhage due to ANCA-associated microscopic polyangiitis: Axial CT shows basal predominant central ground glass with associated mild interlobular septal thickening. This patient had renal insufficiency and had a P-ANCA positive vasculitis with alveolar hemorrhage.

ANCA相关的显微镜下多血管炎引起的肺泡出血：轴位CT显示以基底为主中央性磨玻璃影伴轻度小叶间隔增厚。该患者有肾功能不全及P-ANCA阳性血管炎伴肺泡出血。

- **Microscopic polyangiitis** is the most common cause of pulmonary hemorrhage with rapidly progressive renal failure as part of the pulmonary-renal syndrome. P-ANCA is positive.
  - Alveolar hemorrhage only occurs in about 20–30% of patients.
  - Imaging shows diffuse central-predominant ground glass opacities due to hemorrhage.

- **显微镜下多血管炎**是肺出血伴快速进行性肾功能衰竭的最常见原因，是肺-肾综合征的一部分。P-ANCA呈阳性。
  - 肺泡出血仅发生在20%~30%的患者。
  - 影像学表现为由出血导致的以弥漫性中央分布为主的磨玻璃影。

Granulomatosis with polyangiitis (GPA), previously called Wegener granulomatosis (WG)

- Granulomatosis with polyangiitis (GPA) is a systemic small-vessel vasculitis with a classic clinical triad of sinusitis, lung involvement, and renal insufficiency. C-ANCA is positive.
- In the upper airways, GPA may cause nasopharyngeal and eustachian tube obstruction. Involvement of the larynx and bronchi is common, leading to airway stenosis, most commonly subglottic.
- In the lungs, GPA may cause multiple nodules often with ground glass halo in the acute setting. The nodules may cavitate as well.

肉芽肿性多血管炎(GPA)，曾称韦氏肉芽肿病(WG)

- 肉芽肿性多血管炎(GPA)是一种系统性小血管炎，其典型的临床三联征为鼻窦炎、肺部受累和肾功能不全。抗中性粒细胞胞质抗体(C-ANCA)阳性。
- 在上呼吸道，GPA可能导致鼻咽和咽鼓管阻塞。喉和支气管受累很常见，导致气道狭窄，大多数位于声门下。
- 在肺部，GPA可导致多发结节，在急性期通常伴有磨玻璃影。结节也可有空洞。

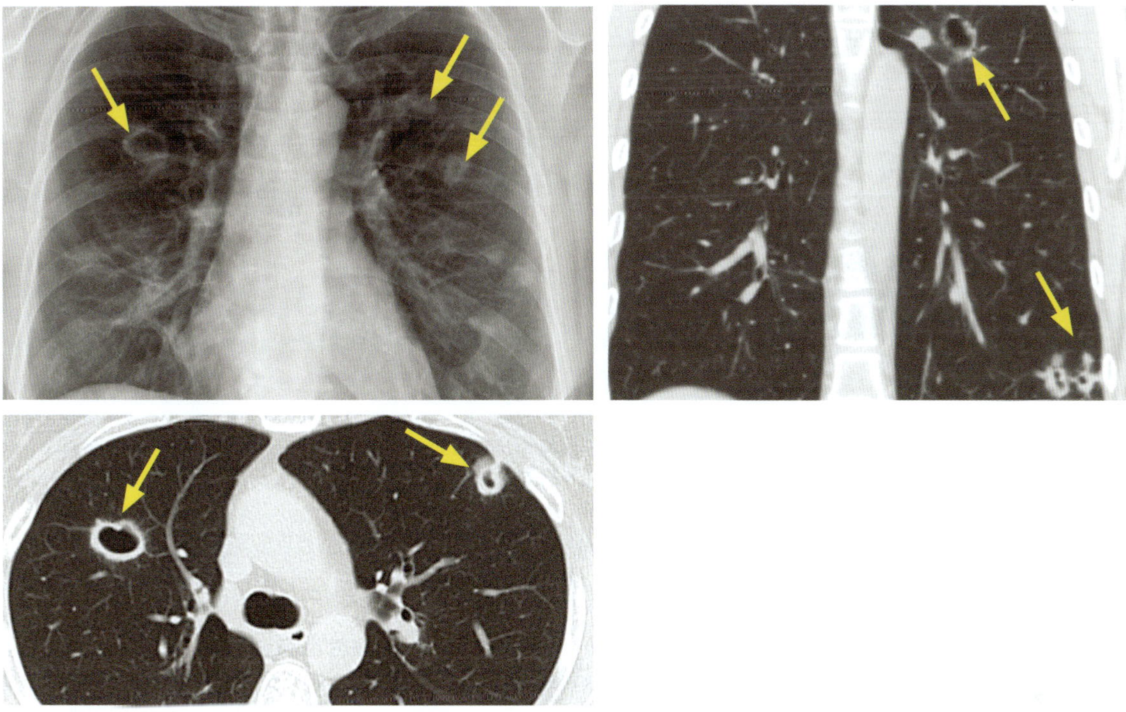

Chest radiograph shows numerous cavitary lesions bilaterally (arrows).
Coronal and axial CT confirms multiple thick-walled cavitary lesions (arrows). The primary differential consideration would be septic emboli; however, this patient was C-ANCA positive.
Case courtesy Ritu R. Gill, MD, MPH, Brigham and Women's Hospital.
胸部X线影像(左上图)显示双肺大量空洞性病变(黄箭)。
冠状和轴位CT(右上图,左下图)证实多发厚壁的空洞性病变(黄箭)。最主要的鉴别诊断是脓毒性栓子;然而,该患者C-ANCA为阳性。

IATROGENIC LUNG DISEASE

Drug toxicity

- The lung has a diverse but finite repertoire of responses to injury, including pulmonary edema (due to increased capillary permeability), ARDS, organizing pneumonia, eosinophilic pneumonia, bronchiolitis obliterans, pulmonary hemorrhage, NSIP, and UIP.
- Pulmonary drug reaction, most commonly to cytotoxic drugs, may elicit any of these injury responses.

Radiation lung injury

- Up to 40% of patients develop radiographic abnormalities after external radiotherapy, although most patients are asymptomatic. The radiographic abnormality is often but not always confined to the radiation port, usually with non-anatomic linear margins.

医源性肺部疾病

药物毒性

- 肺对损伤的反应多样但有限,包括肺水肿(由于毛细血管通透性增加)、急性呼吸窘迫综合征(ARDS)、机化性肺炎、嗜酸性粒细胞性肺炎、闭塞性细支气管炎、肺出血、NSIP和UIP。
- 肺部药物反应,其中最常见的是对细胞毒药物的反应,可能会引起其中任何一种损伤反应。

放射性肺损伤

- 多达40%的患者在接受体外放疗后出现影像学异常,但大多数患者并无症状。影像学异常通常但不总是局限于照射野,常有整齐的非解剖边缘。

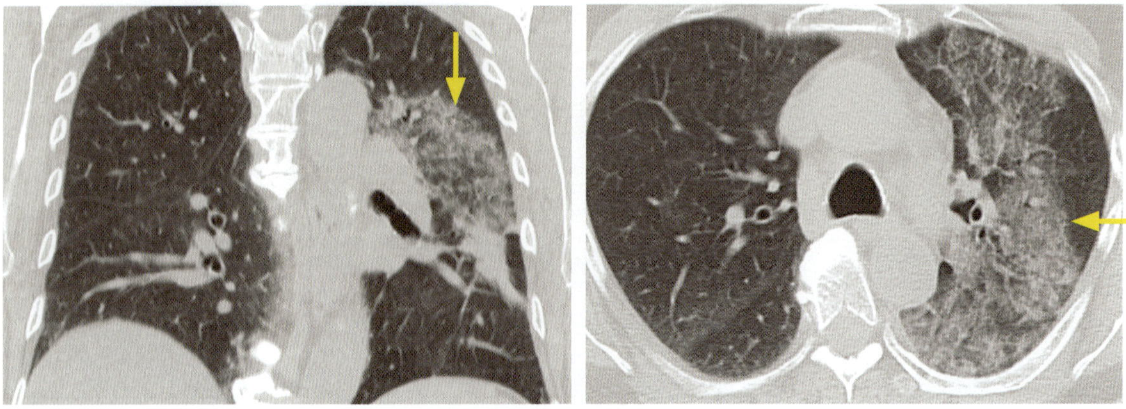

Acute radiation pneumonitis: Coronal and axial CT demonstrate geographic left upper lung ground glass (arrows) with non-anatomic superior and lateral linear margins. Radiation-associated findings may cross fissures.
Case courtesy Ritu R. Gill, MD, MPH, Brigham and Women's Hospital.
急性放射性肺炎：冠状位和轴位CT显示左上肺地图样的磨玻璃影(黄箭)，其上方和侧面为整齐的非解剖学边缘。辐射相关的表现可能会跨越肺裂。

- **Radiation pneumonitis** is the early stage of radiation injury, which can occur within one month of radiotherapy and is most severe 3–4 months after treatment. Radiation pneumonitis features ground glass centered on the radiation port, although extension out of the port is relatively common.
- **Radiation fibrosis** is the late stage of radiation injury. Fibrosis becomes apparent approximately 6–12 months after therapy. The key imaging finding is the distribution of fibrosis and traction bronchiectasis *within the radiation port*, although fibrosis may extend outside the port in 20%.

- **放射性肺炎**是放射性损伤的早期阶段，可在放疗后1个月内发生，治疗后3~4个月最严重。放射性肺炎的特征是以照射野为中心的磨玻璃影，但延伸至照射野外也相对常见。
- **放射性纤维化**是放射性损伤的晚期阶段。纤维化在治疗后6~12个月时变得明显。关键的影像学表现是纤维化和牵拉性支气管扩张分布在照射野内，但20%的纤维化可延伸至照射野外。

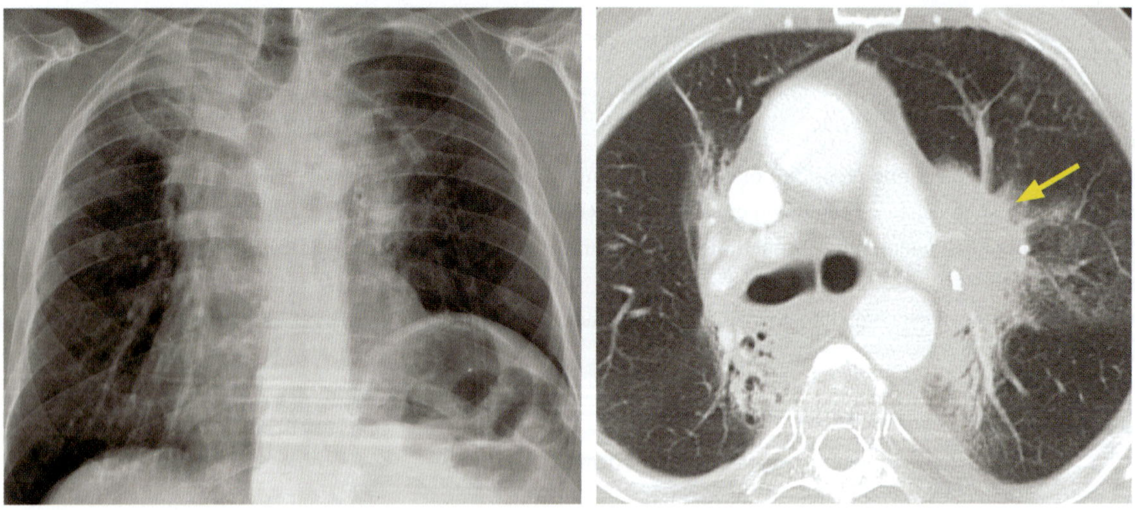

Radiation fibrosis: Chest radiograph and enhanced CT shows paramediastinal fibrotic changes within the radiation port. Despite radiation, the patient has persistent left mediastinal adenopathy (arrow).
放射性纤维化：胸部X线影像和增强CT显示照射野内的纵隔旁纤维化改变。尽管接受了放疗，患者仍有持续性左侧纵隔淋巴结肿大(黄箭)。

IDIOPATHIC SYSTEMIC DISEASES AFFECTING THE LUNGS

Sarcoidosis

- Sarcoidosis is an idiopathic systemic disorder of noncaseating granulomas that become coalescent to form nodules and masses throughout the body.

累及肺部的特发性全身性疾病

结节病

- 结节病是一种非干酪样肉芽肿的特发性全身性疾病，肉芽肿融合后形成的结节和肿块遍布全身。

- Pulmonary sarcoidosis may progress to pulmonary fibrosis. Unlike IPF (the most common cause of pulmonary fibrosis), the fibrotic changes of sarcoid have a mid and upper-lung predominance, similar to end-stage hypersensitivity pneumonitis.
- A historical staging system has been used for radiographic findings (not CT) in sarcoidosis; however, patients do not necessarily progress through the stages.

- 肺结节病可发展为肺纤维化。不同于IPF(肺纤维化最常见的原因),结节病的纤维化改变以中上肺为主,类似于终末期过敏性肺炎。
- 结节病在X线影像上的表现(而非CT)一直沿用旧的分期系统;然而,患者并不一定会按此分期顺序进展。

Stage 0: Normal radiograph.
Stage 1: Hilar or mediastinal adenopathy only, *without* lung changes.
Stage 2: Adenopathy *with* lung changes.
Stage 3: Diffuse lung disease *without* adenopathy
Stage 4: End-stage fibrosis.

0期: 胸部X线影像正常。
1期: 仅有肺门或纵隔淋巴结肿大,无肺部改变。
2期: 淋巴结肿大伴肺部改变。
3期: 弥漫性肺部疾病但无淋巴结肿大。
4期: 终末期纤维化。

- While the most common radiographic finding in sarcoidosis is *symmetric adenopathy*, sarcoid does NOT ALWAYS present with lymphadenopathy, and can be present without lymph node enlargement. Lymph nodes may contain stippled or eggshell calcification in up to 50%.

- 虽然结节病最常见的影像学表现是对称性淋巴结肿大,但结节病**并不总是**伴淋巴结肿大,也可无淋巴结肿大。高达50%的患者淋巴结可含有点状或蛋壳状钙化。

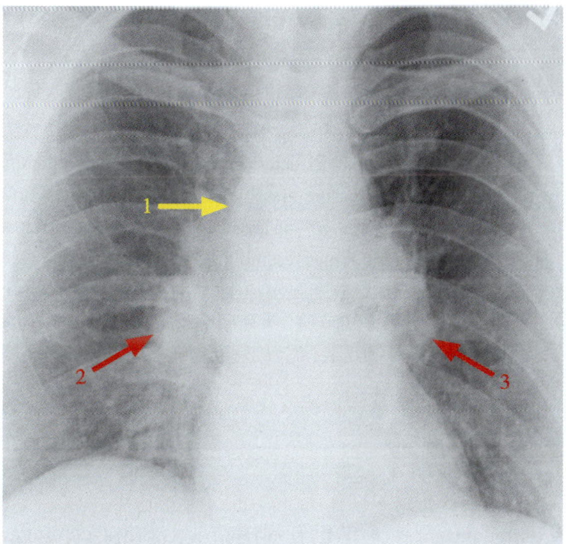

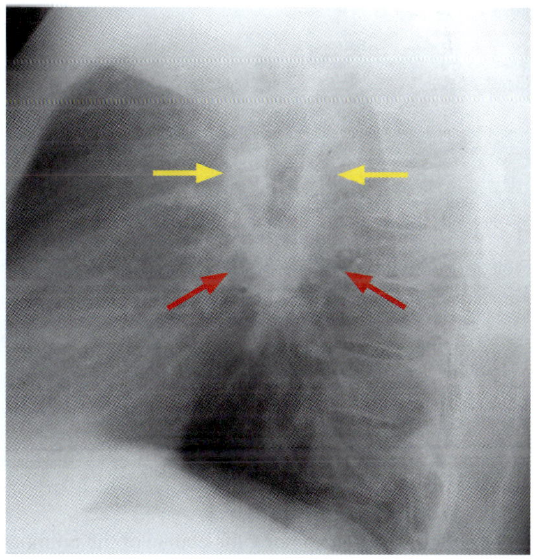

Stage 1 sarcoidosis: Frontal (left image) and lateral radiographs show symmetric adenopathy demonstrating the *1-2-3 sign*:
Right paratracheal adenopathy (yellow arrows, "1")
Right hilar adenopathy (red arrow, "2")
Left hilar adenopathy (red arrow, "3")
The lateral radiograph demonstrates the *donut sign* with adenopathy circumferentially encircling the airways (arrows).
The lung parenchyma is normal.
1期结节病:正位(左图)和侧位(右图)X线影像显示对称性淋巴结肿大,表现为1-2-3征:
右侧气管旁淋巴结肿大(黄箭,"1")
右肺门淋巴结肿大(红箭,"2")
左肺门淋巴结肿大(红箭,"3")
侧位X线影像显示甜甜圈征,肿大的淋巴结包绕气道(黄箭)。
肺实质正常。

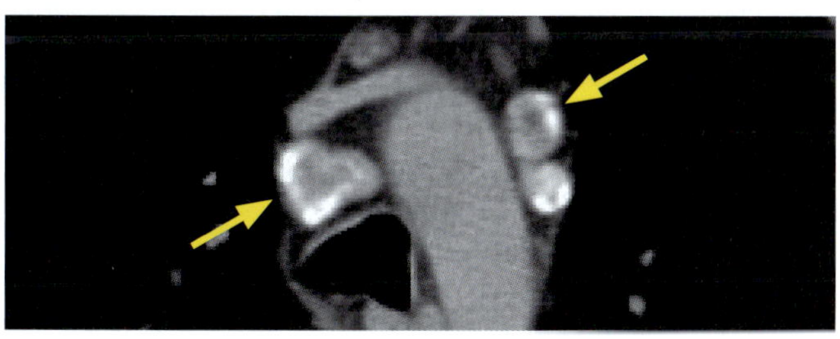

Sarcoidosis: Axial CT in a different patient shows peripherally-calcified ("eggshell") lymph nodes (arrows).
Case courtesy Ritu R. Gill, MD, MPH, Brigham and Women's Hospital.
结节病:另一名患者的轴位CT显示周围钙化("蛋壳")的淋巴结(黄箭)。

- The most common CT finding in sarcoidosis, in addition to adenopathy, is upper-lobe predominant *perilymphatic* nodules of variable sizes, representing sarcoid granulomas.

- 除淋巴结肿大外，结节病最常见的CT表现是以肺上叶为主的大小不一的淋巴管周围结节，代表结节性肉芽肿。

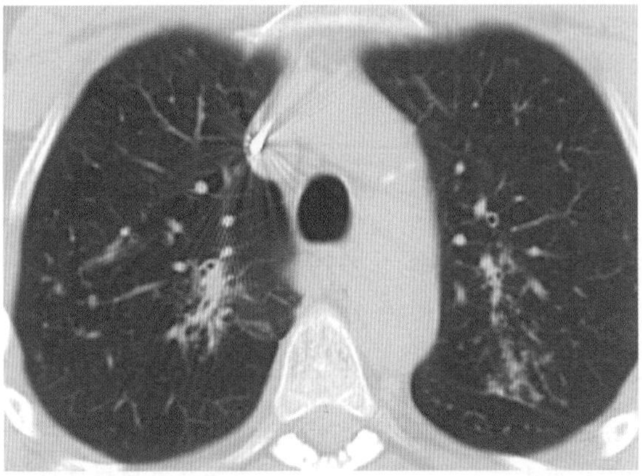

CT in a patient with sarcoidosis shows tiny peribronchovascular and fissural (subpleural) nodules in the bilateral upper lobes.
结节病患者的CT显示位于双肺上叶支气管血管周围和肺裂(胸膜下)的微小结节。

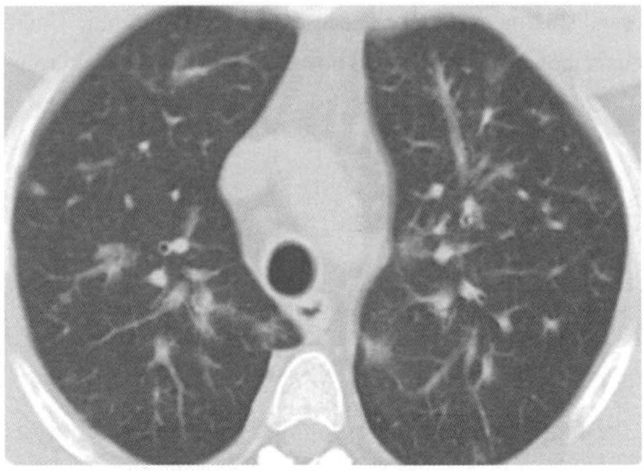

CT in a different patient with sarcoidosis shows slightly larger nodules in a peribronchovascular distribution.
另一名结节病患者的CT显示支气管血管周围分布稍大结节。

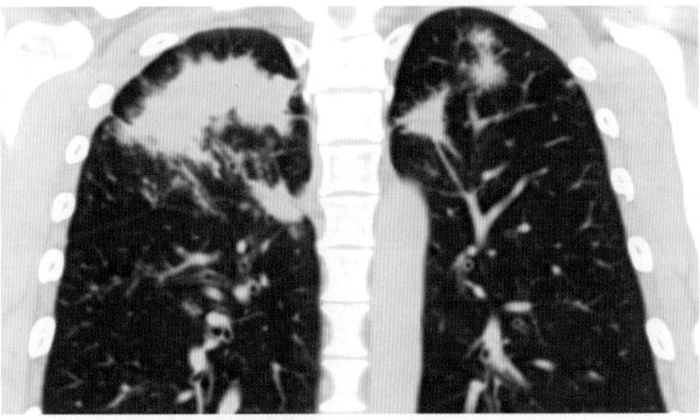

Coronal CT demonstrates upper- lobe predominant progressive massive fibrosis of sarcoid, with the *galaxy sign* – an area composed of numerous smaller granulomas resembling a galaxy.
冠状位CT显示以上叶为主的进行性大块纤维化性结节病，伴有*星系征*——由无数更小的肉芽肿组成，类似于星系。

- Perilymphatic nodules are found along the course of the pulmonary lymphatics, which are peribronchovascular, subpleural, and within the interlobular septa. Septal thickening may occur but is uncommon in sarcoid.
- Perilymphatic nodules may coalesce into a mass up to several centimeters in diameter. The *galaxy sign* is seen when small nodules are peripheral to a nodule or mass.
  - Nodules may occasionally be miliary.
  - Diffuse micronodules may simulate ground glass.
- Fibrotic sarcoid affects predominantly the upper lobes and can produce *progressive massive fibrosis* just as seen in pneumoconioses.
- Bronchial involvement may cause mosaic perfusion due to air trapping.
- Sarcoidosis may involve other organs, including the spleen, brain, and rarely bone.

- 淋巴管周围结节沿肺淋巴管走行，分布于支气管血管周围、胸膜下和小叶间隔内。可有间隔增厚，但在结节病中并不常见。
- 淋巴管周围结节可融合成一个直径达几厘米的肿块。当结节或肿块的周围出现多个小结节时，可见*星系征*。
  - 结节偶尔可呈粟粒状。
  - 弥漫的微小结节可类似磨玻璃影。
- 纤维化性结节病主要累及肺上叶，可像尘肺病一样导致*进行性大面积纤维化*。
- 支气管受累可因空气潴留导致马赛克样灌注。
- 结节病可能累及其他器官，包括脾、脑，但罕见累及骨骼。

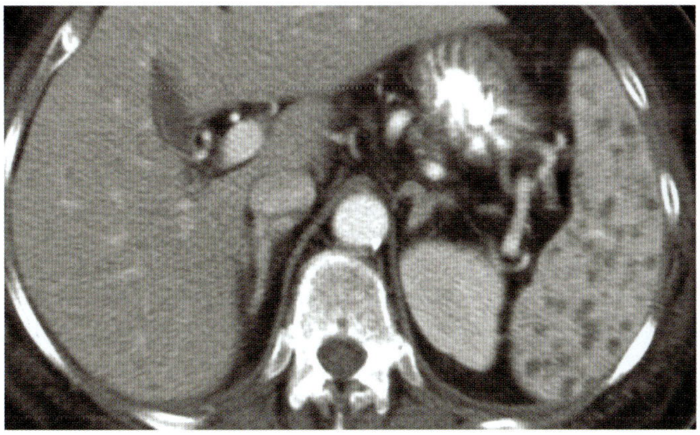

Axial contrast-enhanced CT through the liver and spleen in a patient with sarcoidosis shows innumerable small hypoattenuating splenic nodules.
Case courtesy Michael Hanley, MD, University of Virginia Health System.
结节病患者轴位增强CT经肝脾层面显示脾内无数微小的低密度结节。

Miscellaneous diffuse pulmonary disease

Pulmonary alveolar proteinosis (PAP)

- Pulmonary alveolar proteinosis (PAP) is an idiopathic disease causing filling of the alveoli with a proteinaceous lipid-rich material.
- On chest radiography, PAP may resemble pulmonary edema with perihilar opacification; however, the heart is normal in size in PAP and pleural effusions are not typically seen.
- The CT hallmark of PAP is the *crazy paving* pattern of smooth interlobular septal thickening in areas of patchy or geometric ground glass. Although initially described for PAP, the *crazy paving* pattern is not specific for PAP, as described at the beginning of the chapter.

其他弥漫性肺部疾病

肺泡蛋白沉积症(PAP)

- PAP是一种特发性疾病，导致肺泡充满了富含蛋白质的脂质物体。
- PAP在胸部X线影像上可类似于肺水肿伴肺门周围高密度影；但是，PAP患者的心脏大小正常，且通常无胸腔积液。
- PAP的CT特征是*铺路石征*，即在斑片样或地图样磨玻璃影区域内小叶间隔有平滑均匀的增厚。*铺路石征*最初用于描述PAP，但并非特异，如本章开头所述。

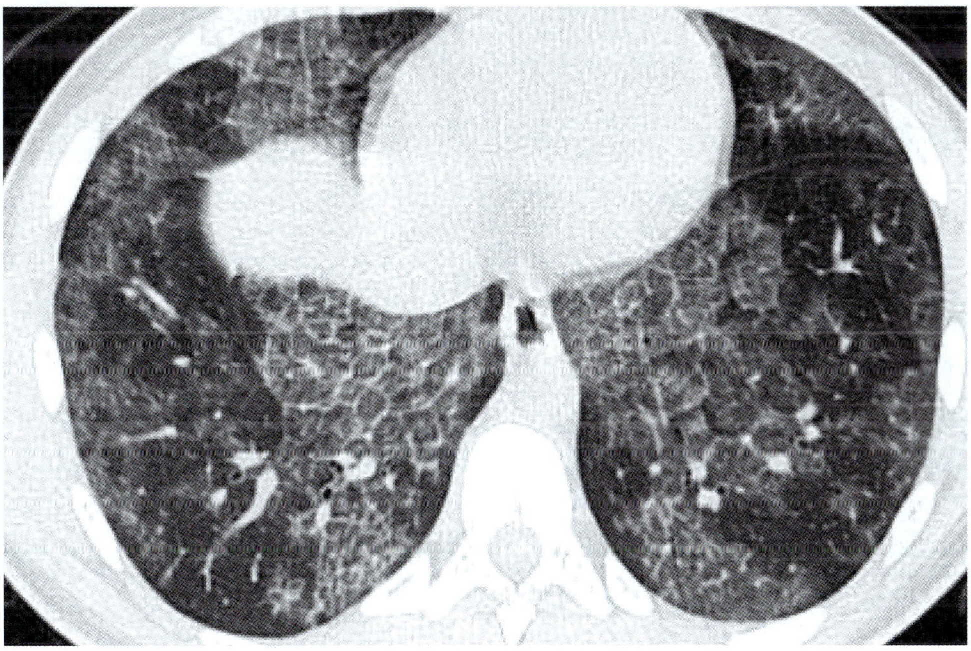

Pulmonary alveolar proteinosis: CT shows ground glass opacification with interlobular septal thickening representing the *crazy paving* pattern.
肺泡蛋白沉积症：CT显示磨玻璃影伴小叶间隔增厚，此为*铺路石征*。

- Patients with PAP are susceptible to superimposed infection, classically with *Nocardia*, which typically presents as a consolidation.
- Treatment of PAP is whole lung bronchoalveolar lavage.

- PAP患者易患多重感染，典型为诺卡菌感染，通常表现为实变。
- PAP的治疗方法是全肺支气管肺泡灌洗。

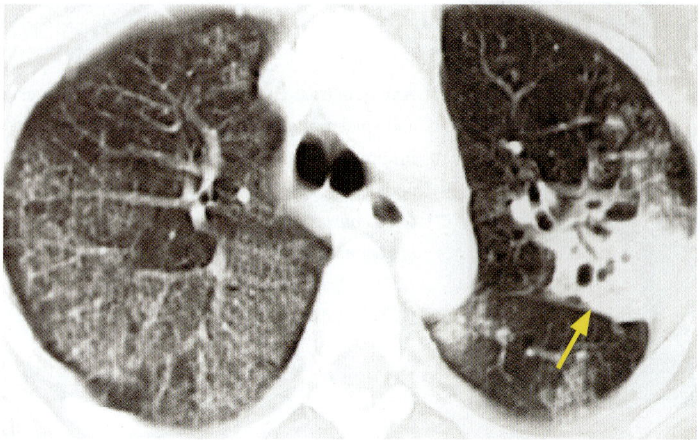

Pulmonary alveolar proteinosis with superimposed *Nocardia*:
CT shows bilateral *crazy paving* predominantly in the right lung, with a dense consolidative opacity in the left upper lobe (arrow) representing superimposed *Nocardia* pneumonia.
Case courtesy Ritu R. Gill, MD, MPH, Brigham and Women's Hospital.
肺泡蛋白沉积症合并诺卡菌感染：CT显示双侧铺路石征并以右肺为主，左上叶有一处致密的实变影(黄箭)，代表合并诺卡菌肺炎。

CYSTIC LUNG DISEASE

囊性肺部疾病

Pulmonary Langerhans cell histiocytosis (PLCH)

肺朗格汉斯细胞组织细胞增生症(PLCH)

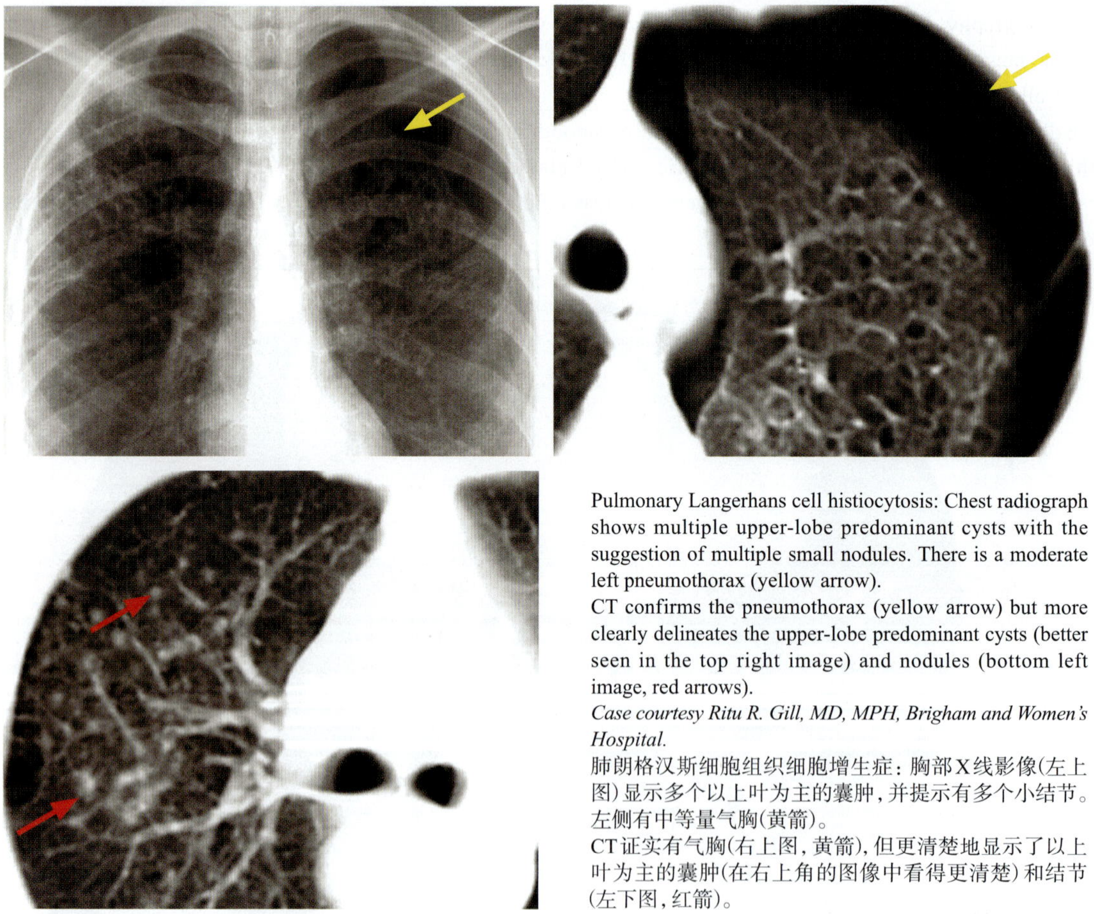

Pulmonary Langerhans cell histiocytosis: Chest radiograph shows multiple upper-lobe predominant cysts with the suggestion of multiple small nodules. There is a moderate left pneumothorax (yellow arrow).
CT confirms the pneumothorax (yellow arrow) but more clearly delineates the upper-lobe predominant cysts (better seen in the top right image) and nodules (bottom left image, red arrows).
Case courtesy Ritu R. Gill, MD, MPH, Brigham and Women's Hospital.
肺朗格汉斯细胞组织细胞增生症：胸部X线影像(左上图)显示多个以上叶为主的囊肿，并提示有多个小结节。左侧有中等量气胸(黄箭)。
CT证实有气胸(右上图，黄箭)，但更清楚地显示了以上叶为主的囊肿(在右上角的图像中看得更清楚)和结节(左下图，红箭)。

- Pulmonary Langerhans cell histiocytosis (PLCH) is a smoking-related lung disease – nearly 100% of adults with PLCH are smokers.

  The other smoking-related interstitial lung diseases (aside from emphysema) are RB-ILD and DIP.

  Multiple smoking-related lung diseases may be present simultaneously.
- PLCH may present as a spontaneous pneumothorax.
- Disease in adults is most often isolated to the lungs; however, lucent bone

- 肺朗格汉斯细胞组织细胞增生症(PLCH)是一种与吸烟有关的肺部疾病——几乎100%为吸烟的成年PLCH患者。

  其他与吸烟有关的间质性肺疾病(除肺气肿外)是RB-ILD和DIP。

  多种与吸烟有关的肺部疾病可以同时存在。
- PLCH可表现为自发性气胸。

lesions, diabetes insipidus from inflammation of the pituitary stalk (hypophysitis), and skin involvement can occasionally be seen.

- 成人发病最常局限在肺部。但偶尔可见溶骨性病变、垂体柄炎症(垂体炎)引起的尿崩症和皮肤受累。

> In addition to LCH, the differential diagnosis for diseases affecting the lungs and bones includes **malignancy**, **tuberculosis**, **fungal disease** (including Blastomycosis, Histoplasmosis, and Coccidiodomycosis), **sarcoidosis**, and **Gaucher disease** (pulmonary involvement is rare and may resemble DIP).

> 除LCH外，同时累及肺和骨骼的疾病鉴别诊断还包括**恶性肿瘤**、**结核病**、**真菌病**(包括芽生菌病、组织胞浆菌病和球孢子菌病)、**结节病**和**戈谢病**(肺部受累罕见，可类似于DIP)。

- The first detectable abnormality is nodules associated with airways. As the disease progresses, the nodules cavitate and resultant irregular cysts predominate.
- The natural progression is from nodules → cavitary nodules → irregular cysts.
- At any point in time, a patient may have nodules only; nodules + cysts; or cysts only.
- Radiographic and CT findings include upper-lobe predominant cysts and irregular peribronchovascular nodules, both sparing the costophrenic sulci.

  The *cheerio sign* in LCH refers to pulmonary nodules with a central lucent cavity supplied by a patent bronchus on CT imaging.
- Smoking cessation is critical for stopping the progression of PLCH. However, the cysts will not resolve.

- 最先可检测到的异常是与气道相关的结节。随着疾病进展，结节形成空洞并由此导致不规则囊肿成为主要表现。
- 自然进展是结节→空洞性结节→不规则囊肿。
- 在任何时间点，患者可以只有结节，或结节+囊肿，或仅有囊肿。
- X线影像和CT表现包括以上叶为主的囊肿和不规则的支气管血管周围结节，但双侧肋膈沟不受累。

  LCH中的*麦圈征*是指CT图像上肺结节具有中央透亮的空洞与未闭的支气管相通。
- 戒烟对阻止PLCH的进展至关重要，但囊肿不会消失。

Lymphangioleiomyomatosis (LAM)

淋巴管平滑肌瘤病(LAM)

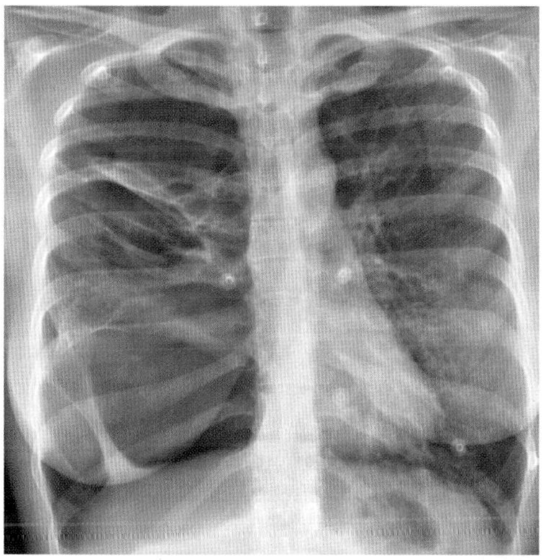

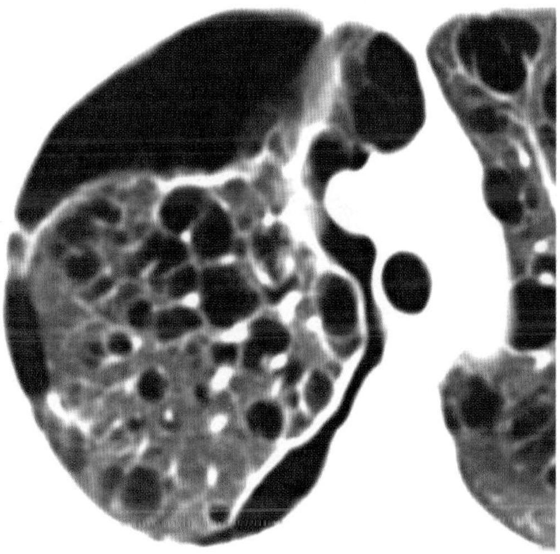

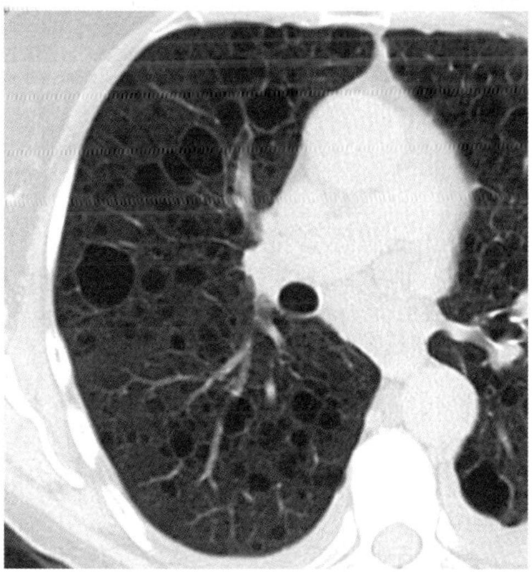

Two separate patients with lymphangioleiomyomatosis:
Patient 1 (top radiograph and top CT) has end-stage LAM with severe cystic change and moderate right pneumothorax.
Patient 2 (bottom left CT) shows a less severe stage of disease, with multiple smooth-walled cysts and bilateral pleural effusions. Although the pleural fluid was not sampled in this case, there is an association of LAM with chylous effusion.
Case courtesy Ritu R. Gill, MD, MPH, Brigham and Women's Hospital.

两名不同的淋巴管平滑肌瘤病患者：
患者1(上方两图，X线影像和CT)为晚期LAM伴有重度囊样改变和右侧中度气胸。
患者2(左下CT)显示疾病处于不太严重的阶段，可见多个光滑的薄壁囊肿和双侧胸腔积液。虽然该病例未采集胸腔积液，但LAM与乳糜胸相关。

- Lymphangioleiomyomatosis (LAM) is a diffuse cystic lung disease caused by bronchiolar obstruction and lung destruction due to proliferation of immature smooth muscle cells in small vessels, lymphatics, and bronchioles.
- Approximately 1% of patients with tuberous sclerosis (triad of seizures, mental retardation, and adenoma sebaceum) have LAM.
- Sporadic LAM is seen in women of childbearing age or older; the cysts do not disappear over time.
- The current treatment is mTOR inhibitors.
- LAM is associated with pneumothorax and chylous pleural effusion.
- CT of LAM shows numerous thin-walled lung cysts. In contrast to LCH, the cysts tend to be round and regular. Also, LAM affects the lungs diffusely while LCH is upper-lobe predominant.

- 淋巴管平滑肌瘤病(LAM)是一种由于未成熟平滑肌细胞在小血管、淋巴管和细支气管中增殖所导致的细支气管阻塞和肺破坏引起的弥漫性囊性肺病。
- 约1%的结节性硬化症患者(癫痫发作、智力低下和皮脂腺瘤)有LAM。
- 散发性LAM见于育龄期或育龄期以后的妇女;囊肿不会随时间消失。
- 当前的治疗是哺乳动物雷帕霉素靶蛋白(mammalian target of rapamycin, mTOR)抑制剂。
- LAM与气胸和乳糜胸相关。
- LAM在CT上表现为大量薄壁肺囊肿。与LCH相比,囊肿倾向于圆形而规则。此外,LAM弥漫性累及两肺,而LCH以上叶为主。

Lymphoid interstitial pneumonia (LIP)

- Lymphoid interstitial pneumonia (LIP) is both a clinical syndrome and the pathologic diagnosis. LIP is exceptionally rare as an isolated idiopathic disease and is most commonly associated with connective tissue disease (Sjögren syndrome), though also can be seen with HIV or CVID.
- The histologic hallmark of LIP is diffuse infiltration of the interstitium by lymphocytes and other immune cells, with resultant distortion of the alveoli.
- LIP imaging most commonly presents with cysts and nodules, though cysts alone, nodules alone, ground glass, or interlobular septal thickening may also be seen. The scattered thin- walled perivascular cysts are thought to be due to air trapping. LIP may be complicated by pneumothorax in advanced disease.

淋巴细胞性间质性肺炎(LIP)

- 淋巴细胞性间质性肺炎(LIP)既是一种临床综合征,也是一种病理诊断。LIP作为一种孤立的特发性疾病极为罕见,最常见的是与结缔组织病(干燥综合征)相关,但也可见于HIV或常见变异型免疫缺陷病。
- LIP的组织学特征是淋巴细胞和其他免疫细胞弥漫性浸润间质,从而导致肺泡变形。
- LIP影像学最常见的表现是囊肿和结节,但也可仅有囊肿、仅有结节,磨玻璃影或小叶间隔增厚也可见到。散在的血管周围薄壁囊肿被认为是由于空气潴留所致。晚期LIP可以并发气胸。

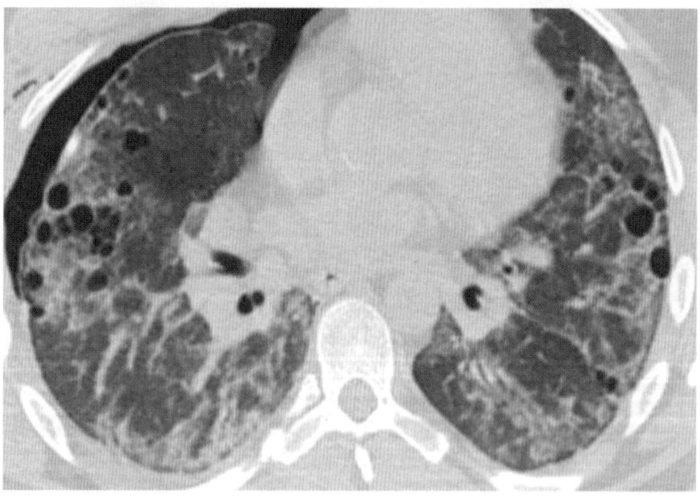

LIP: Unenhanced axial CT shows patchy ground glass opacities, scattered perivascular cysts, and a right-sided pneumothorax.
Case courtesy Ritu R. Gill, MD, MPH, Brigham and Women's Hospital.
LIP:平扫轴位CT显示斑片状磨玻璃影,散在的血管周围囊肿和右侧气胸。

Birt-Hogg Dube syndrome (BHD)

- Birt-Hogg-Dube syndrome (BHD) is an autosomal dominant genetic disorder caused by a mutation in the folliculin (FLCN) gene on chromosome 17p11.2.
- The syndrome is characterized by fibrofolliculomas (noncancerous skin lesions), renal tumors (most common chromophobe renal cell carcinoma and renal oncocytoma), and renal and pulmonary cysts. Spontaneous pneumothoraces can occur as sequelae of pulmonary cysts.
- Imaging findings include lower lung predominant cysts which are often subpleural or perivascular, with a polygonal or "floppy" shape.

伯特-霍格-迪贝综合征(BHD)

- 伯特-霍格-迪贝综合征(BHD)是一种常染色体显性遗传疾病,由位于17p11.2染色体上的卵泡素(*FLCN*)基因突变所致。
- 该综合征表现为纤维毛囊瘤(非癌性皮肤病变)、肾肿瘤(最常见的为肾嫌色细胞癌和肾嗜酸细胞瘤),以及肾囊肿和肺囊肿。自发性气胸为肺囊肿的并发症。
- 影像学表现包括以下肺为主的囊肿,通常位于胸膜下或血管周围，呈多边形或“松软”状。

Summary of cystic lung disease

Entity	Nodules	Pneumothorax	Pleural Effusion	Zonal Distribution	Number of Cysts
LAM	–	+/–	+/–	Diffuse	Many
PLCH	+/–	+/–	–	Upper	Few–Many
LIP	+/–	–	–	Lower	Few
BHD	–	+	–	Lower	Few

囊性肺病概括

病变名称	结节	气胸	胸腔积液	区域分布	囊肿数量
LAM	–	+/–	+/–	弥漫	多
PLCH	+/–	+/–	–	上肺	少~多
LIP	+/–	–	–	下肺	少
BHD	–	+	–	下肺	少

（翻译　王维平）

MEDIASTINUM

纵隔

ANATOMY OF THE MEDIASTINUM

纵隔解剖

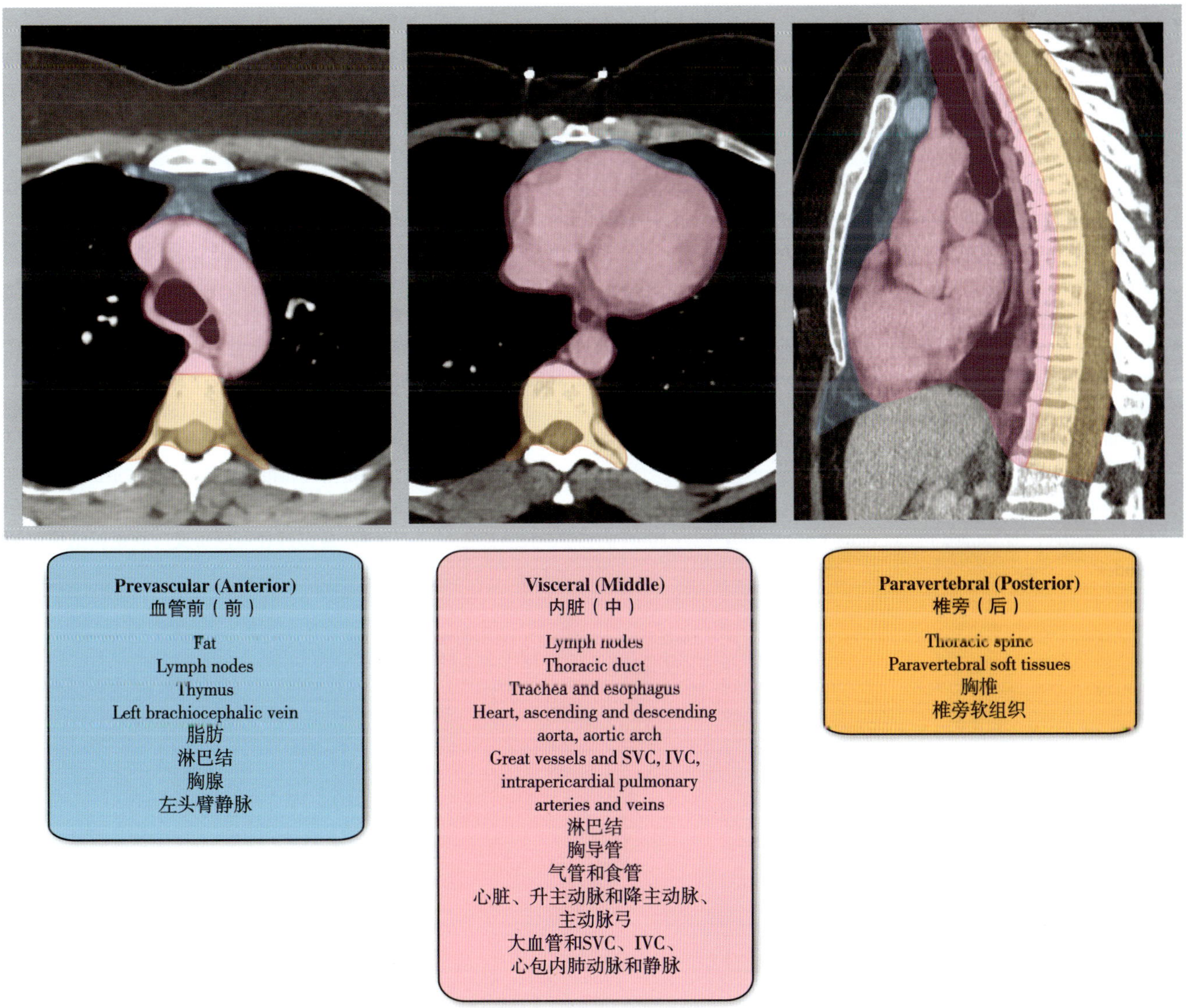

- Several methods have been proposed to divide the mediastinum. This text follows the International Thymic Malignancy Interest Group (ITMIG) method that has been accepted as a new standard.
- The mediastinum is divided into three arbitrary compartments to aid in the differential diagnosis of a mediastinal mass. However, there are no anatomic planes separating these divisions and disease can spread from one "compartment" to another.
- The three divisions are used to aid in the differential diagnosis of a mass and planning for biopsies and surgical procedures.

Prevascular compartment

- The prevascular compartment is bordered by (a) superiorly, the thoracic inlet; (b) inferiorly, the diaphragm; (c) anteriorly, the posterior border/cortex of the sternum; (d) laterally, the parietal mediastinal pleura; and (e) posteriorly, the anterior aspect of the pericardium.
- Essentially, it contains the thymus/thymic remnant.

Visceral compartment

- The boundaries include (a) superiorly, the thoracic inlet; (b) inferiorly, the diaphragm; (c) anteriorly, the posterior boundaries of the prevascular compartment; and (d) posteriorly, a vertical line connecting the thoracic vertebral bodies 1 cm posterior to its anterior margin.
- Essentially, it contains the heart, great vessels, trachea, and esophagus. Most lymph nodes are located in the middle mediastinum.
- The phrenic, vagus, and recurrent laryngeal nerves pass through the AP window within the visceral compartment.

Paravertebral compartment

- The anterior boundary of the paravertebral compartment is 1 cm posterior to the anterior vertebral body and the posterior boundary is a vertical line along the posterior margin of the chest wall at the lateral aspect of the transverse processes.

Lines, stripes, and interfaces

- Interfaces between anatomic structures in the lungs, mediastinum, and pleura may be displaced or thickened in the presence of a mediastinal mass or abnormality.

A "line" is a thin interface formed by tissue (typically <1 mm in thickness) with air on both sides.

A "stripe" is a thicker interface formed between air and adjacent soft tissue.

An "interface" is formed by the contact of two soft tissue structures of different densities.

- 纵隔的划分有多种。本文采用国际胸腺恶性肿瘤兴趣小组(ITMIG)方法，此为公认的新标准。
- 纵隔被人为划为三个区块，用以帮助鉴别纵隔内的肿块。然而，解剖学上并不存在这样的平面可以区分这些区块，而疾病可以从一个“区块”扩散到另一个“区块”。
- 该三个区块用于帮助鉴别肿块，以及规划活检和外科手术。

血管前区

- 血管前区(a)上界为胸廓入口；(b)下界为膈肌；(c)前界为胸骨后缘/皮质；(d)侧缘为纵隔胸膜壁层；(e)后界为心包前缘。
- 主要结构包含胸腺/胸腺残余。

内脏区

- 内脏区(a)上界为胸廓入口；(b)下界为膈肌；(c)前界是血管前区的后界；(d)后界为连接胸椎前缘后方1cm处的垂直线。
- 主要结构包含心脏、大血管、气管和食管。大多数淋巴结位于中纵隔。
- 膈神经、迷走神经和喉返神经通过内脏区的主肺动脉窗。

椎旁区

- 椎旁区的前界在椎体前缘后方1cm，后界是沿胸壁后缘在椎体横突外侧的垂线。

线、带和界面

- 出现纵隔肿块或异常时，肺、纵隔和胸膜的解剖结构之间的界面会发生移位或增厚。

“线”是由两侧含气的组织(通常厚度<1mm)所形成的菲薄界面。

“带”是空气和相邻软组织之间形成的一个较厚界面。

“界面”是由两种不同密度的软组织结构接触形成。

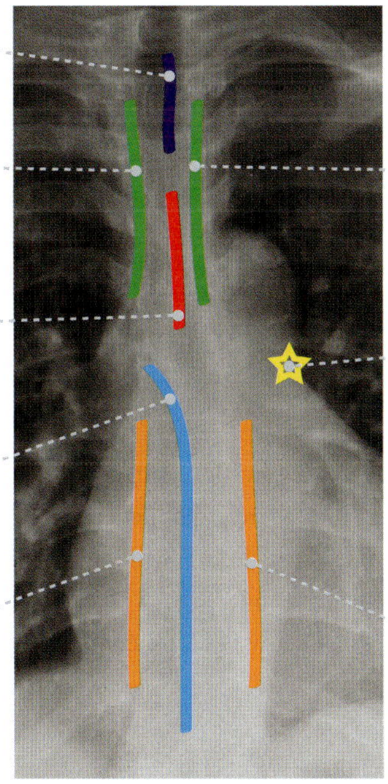

- The **anterior junction line** is formed by 4 layers of pleura (parietal and visceral pleura of each lung) at the anterior junction of the right and left lungs.

  On a frontal radiograph, the anterior junction line is a vertical line projecting over the superior two-thirds of the sternum.

  Abnormal convexity or displacement of this line suggests a prevascular mediastinal mass.

- The **posterior junction line** is also formed by 4 layers of pleura (parietal and visceral pleura of each lung), but at the posterior junction of the right and left lungs.

  On a frontal radiograph, the posterior junction line is a vertical line projecting through the trachea on the frontal view, more superior than the anterior junction line. Unlike the anterior junction line, the posterior junction line is seen above the clavicles because the posterior lungs extend more superiorly than the anterior lungs. It is much less commonly seen than the anterior junction line.

  Abnormal convexity or displacement of this line suggests a paravertebral mediastinal mass or aortic aneurysm.

- The **right and left paratracheal stripes** are formed by two layers of pleura where the medial aspect of each lung abuts the lateral wall of the trachea and intervening mediastinal fat.

  The right paratracheal stripe is the most commonly seen of these landmarks, seen in up to 97% of normal PA chest radiographs.

  Thickening of the right paratracheal stripe is most commonly due to a paratracheal mass (including adenopathy or thyroid or tracheal neoplasm).

  Thickening of the left paratracheal stripe has a similar differential. Note that the normal left subclavian reflection is a less dense stripe on the left of the trachea.

  Mediastinal hematoma should be considered in the setting of trauma.

- The **posterior tracheal stripe** or **tracheoesophageal stripe** is the only interface seen on the *lateral radiograph*, representing the interface of the posterior wall of the trachea with the two pleural layers of the medial right lung.

- The **right and left paraspinal lines** are actually interfaces but appear as lines due to Mach effect and are formed by two layers of pleura abutting the posterior chest wall.

  In contrast to the posterior junction line, the paraspinal lines are located inferiorly in

- **前联合线**在左右肺的前交界处由4层胸膜构成(每侧肺的壁胸膜和脏胸膜)。

  在正位X线影像上,前联合线是一条垂直线,投射在胸骨上2/3处。

  此线的异常突出或移位提示血管前纵隔肿块。

- **后联合线**也是由4层胸膜(每侧肺的壁胸膜和脏胸膜)构成,但位于右肺和左肺的后联合处。

  在正位X线影像上,后联合线是投射在气管上的一条垂直线,其位置高于前联合线。与前联合线不同,后联合线可见于锁骨的上方,因为后肺比前肺更向上延伸。但是后联合线要比前联合线少见得多。

  此线的异常突出或发生移位提示椎旁纵隔肿块或主动脉瘤。

- **左右气管旁带**由两层胸膜形成,每侧肺的内侧面紧靠气管的侧壁和中间的纵隔脂肪。

  右气管旁带是其中最为常见的标志,见于高达97%正常人的后前位胸部X线影像。

  右气管旁带增厚最常见的原因是气管旁肿块(包括淋巴结肿大或甲状腺或气管肿瘤)。

  左侧气管旁带增厚也有类似的鉴别诊断。注意,正常的左锁骨下反折为气管左侧较不致密的带影。

  在创伤情况下应考虑纵隔血肿。

- **后气管带或气管食管带**是在侧位X线影像上唯一能看到的界面,为气管后壁与右肺内侧两层胸膜的交界。

- **左右椎旁线**实际上是界面,但由于马赫效应而看起来像线,该线由两层胸膜紧贴后胸壁形成。

  与后联合线相比,椎旁线位于胸部下方,通常从第8肋骨到第12肋骨。

the thorax, typically from the eighth through twelfth ribs.

A paraspinal line abnormality suggests a paravertebral mediastinal mass, including hematoma, neurogenic tumor, aortic aneurysm, extramedullary hematopoiesis, esophageal mass, and osteophyte.

- The **azygoesophageal recess** is an interface formed by the contact of the posteromedial right lower lobe and the retrocardiac mediastinum.

The azygoesophageal recess extends from the subcarinal region to the diaphragm inferiorly.

Distortion of the azygoesophageal recess may be due to esophageal mass, hiatal hernia, left atrial enlargement, and adenopathy.

椎旁线异常提示椎旁纵隔肿块，包括血肿、神经源性肿瘤、主动脉瘤、髓外造血、食管肿块和骨赘。

- **奇食管隐窝**是右肺下叶后内侧与心后纵隔的接触界面。

奇食管隐窝从隆突下区域向下延伸至膈肌。

引起奇食管隐窝变形的原因可有食管肿块、食管裂孔疝、左心房增大和淋巴结肿大。

Aortopulmomary (AP) window

- The aortopulmonary (AP) window is a mediastinal space nestled underneath the aortic arch (which forms the superior, anterior, and posterior boundaries) and the top of the pulmonary artery. The medial border of the AP window is formed by the esophagus, trachea, and left mainstem bronchus.
- On a normal frontal radiograph, the AP window is a shallow concave contour below the aortic knob and above the pulmonary artery.
- Abnormal convexity (outwards bulging) of the AP window suggests a mass arising from or involving structures that normally live within the AP window, including:

> Lymph nodes: Adenopathy is the most common cause of an AP window abnormality.
> Left phrenic nerve: Injury may cause paralysis of the left hemidiaphragm.
> Recurrent laryngeal nerve: The AP window should be carefully evaluated in new-onset hoarseness, especially if associated with diaphragmatic paralysis.
> Left vagus nerve.
> Ligamentum arteriosum.
> Left bronchial arteries.
> Aortic aneurysm or traumatic injury of the aorta.

主肺动脉(AP)窗

- AP窗是位于主动脉弓(形成上界、前界和后界)下方和肺动脉上方的纵隔空间。AP窗的内侧边界由食管、气管和左主支气管组成。
- 在正常的正位X线影像上，AP窗是一个浅而凹陷的轮廓，位于主动脉结的下方和肺动脉的上方。
- AP窗异常凸出(向外膨出)提示肿块来自或累及位于AP窗内的正常结构，包括：

> 淋巴结：淋巴结肿大是AP窗异常的最常见原因。
> 左侧膈神经：损伤可能导致左侧膈肌麻痹。
> 喉返神经：对于新发声音嘶哑者，应仔细评估AP窗，特别是合并膈肌麻痹者。
> 左侧迷走神经。
> 动脉韧带。
> 左支气管动脉。
> 主动脉瘤或主动脉外伤。

Retrosternal clear space

- The retrosternal clear space is a normal area of lucency posterior to the sternum seen on the lateral radiograph. It correlates with the prevascular space on CT.
- Obliteration of the retrosternal clear space suggests a prevascular mediastinal mass, right ventricular dilation, or pulmonary artery enlargement.
- Increase in the retrosternal clear space can be seen in emphysema.

胸骨后间隙

- 胸骨后间隙是侧位X线影像上在胸骨后方的正常透亮区，与CT上的血管前间隙相对应。
- 胸骨后间隙消失提示血管前纵隔肿块、右心室扩张或肺动脉扩张。
- 胸骨后间隙增宽可见于肺气肿。

Left superior intercostal vein (LSIV)

- The left superior intercostal vein (LSIV) is a normal vein that is not often seen on radiography. When visible, the LSIV produces the *aortic nipple*, appearing as a small round shadow to the left of the aortic knob on the frontal radiograph.
- The LSIV may be dilated as a collateral pathway in SVC obstruction.

左上肋间静脉(LSIV)

- 左上肋间静脉(LSIV)是一条正常的静脉，在X线影像上不常见。如果出现，LSIV会产生*主动脉乳头样影*，即正位X线影像上显示主动脉结左侧的一个小圆形阴影。
- LSIV在SVC阻塞时可能扩张成为侧支通路。

Radiographic Localization of a Mediastinal Mass

Detection of an anterior mediastinal mass

- Deformation of the anterior junction line suggests a prevascular mediastinal mass. However, since the anterior junction line is not always seen, it is more common to infer the anterior location of a mass by preservation of the posterior lines in the presence of a mass.
- The *hilum overlay sign* is present on the frontal view if hilar vessels are visualized through the mass. It indicates that the mass cannot be in the visceral mediastinum. The mass may be anterior (more likely) or posterior.

纵隔肿块的放射影像学定位

前纵隔肿块的检测

- 前联合线变形提示前纵隔肿块。然而，由于前联合线并不总能被观察到，因此在有肿块的情况下，更常用后联合线的完整性来推测肿块是否位于前纵隔。
- *肺门重叠征*是指正位X线影像上见肺门血管从肿块中通过。这意味着肿块不可能位于内脏纵隔。肿块可位于前(更可能)或后纵隔。

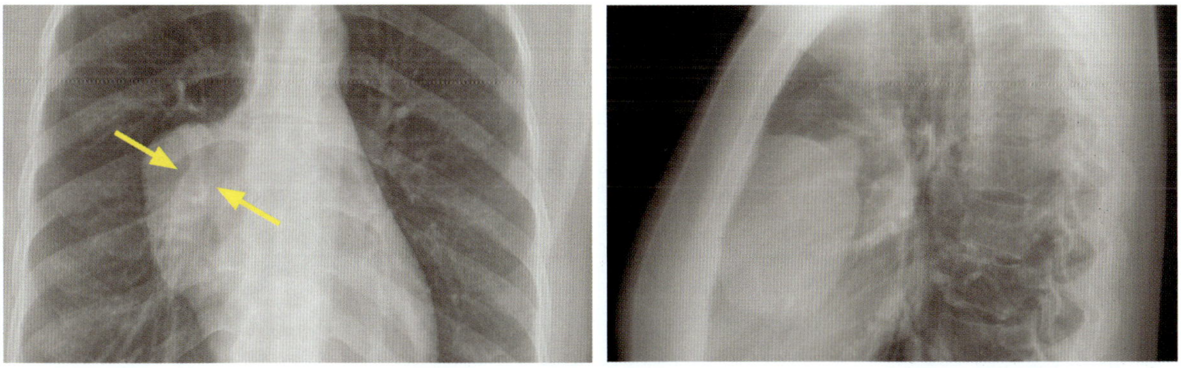

Anterior mediastinal mass: Frontal radiograph shows a right mediastinal mass with silhouetting of the right heart border. The right pulmonary artery is visible through the mass (arrows), representing the *hilum overlay sign* and indicating that the mass is not in the middle mediastinum. Lateral radiograph shows the mass in the retrosternal clear space, confirming its anterior mediastinal location. This was a teratoma.
前纵隔肿块：正位X线影像显示右侧纵隔肿块构成右心缘。可见右肺动脉穿过肿块(黄箭)，为肺门重叠征，表明肿块不在中纵隔内。侧位X线影像显示肿块位于胸骨后间隙，确认其前纵隔定位。这是一例畸胎瘤。

- Obliteration of the retrosternal clear space on the lateral radiograph is direct sign of prevascular mediastinal location.

- 侧位X线影像上胸骨后间隙消失是血管前纵隔定位的直接征象。

Detection of a middle mediastinal mass

- Distortion of the azygoesophageal recess, distortion of the posterior junction line, paratracheal stripes, or convexity of the AP window suggests a visceral compartment mediastinal mass.

中纵隔肿块的检测

- 奇食管隐窝变形、后联合线变形、气管旁带或AP窗突出提示内脏区纵隔肿块。

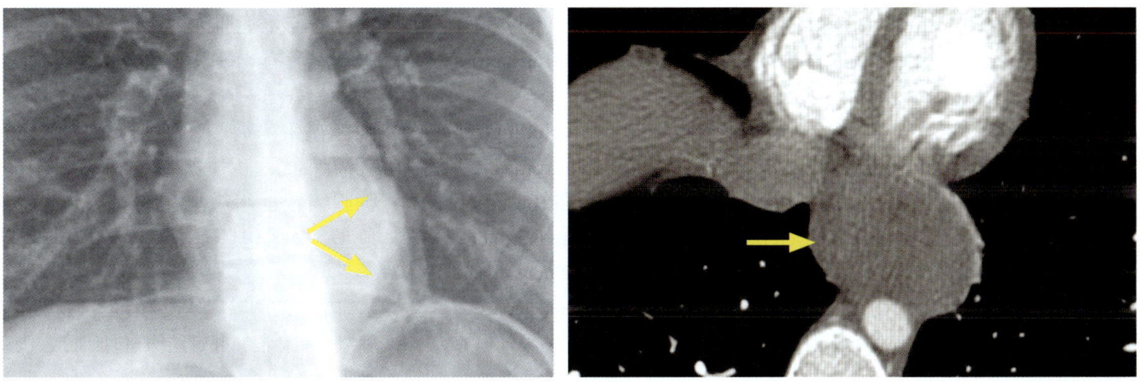

Displacement of the descending aortic stripe: Frontal chest radiograph (left) shows lateral displacement and bowing of the left para-aortic interface (arrows). Axial contrast-enhanced CT shows a nonenhancing homogeneous mass (arrow) effacing the esophagus. Although extremely rare, this was a liposarcoma.
降主动脉带移位：正位胸部X线影像(左图)显示主动脉左旁界面向外侧移位并弯曲(黄箭)。轴位增强CT(右图)显示均匀的非增强肿块(黄箭)并使食管消失。这是一例极为罕见的脂肪肉瘤。

Detection of a posterior mediastinal mass

- Distortion or displacement of the paraspinal lines suggests paravertebral disease.

后纵隔肿块的检测

- 椎旁线变形或移位提示椎旁疾病。

PREVASCULAR COMPARTMENT MEDIASTINAL MASS

Overview of prevascular mediastinal masses

- The differential diagnosis for a prevascular mediastinal mass includes:

Thymic epithelial neoplasm, such as thymoma if the pati ent is middle aged or older, or has a history of myasthenia gravis. Less common would be thymic carcinoma.
Germ cell tumor, including teratoma, if the pati ent is a young adult.
Lymphoma.
Thyroid goiter, only rarely in the anterior mediasti num.

血管前纵隔肿块

血管前纵隔肿块概述

- 血管前纵隔肿块的鉴别诊断包括：

胸腺上皮肿瘤，如果患者是中老年人，或有重症肌无力病史，则可能为胸腺瘤。较少见的是胸腺癌。
生殖细胞肿瘤，包括畸胎瘤，如果患者是年轻成人。
淋巴瘤。
甲状腺肿大，极少位于前纵隔。

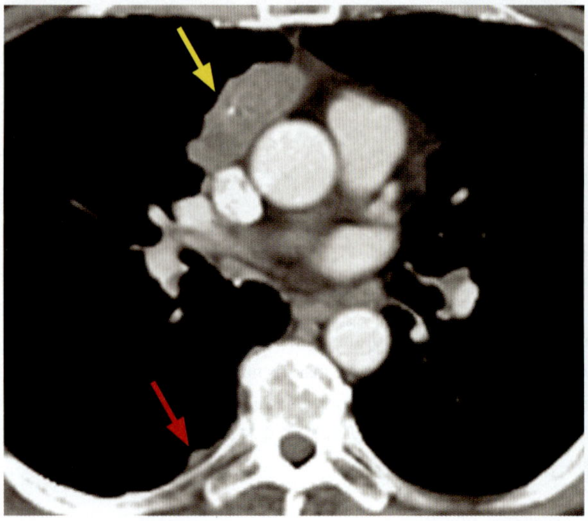

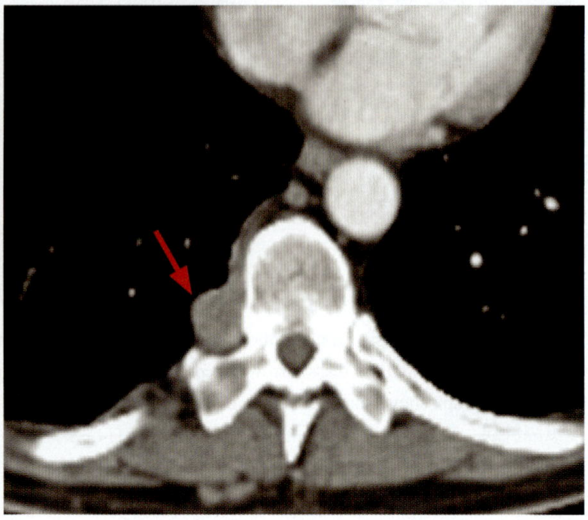

Invasive thymoma with drop metastasis: Contrast-enhanced CT shows a slightly heterogeneous mass with calcifications (yellow arrow) anterior to the aorta and SVC, with two pleural metastases (red arrows).

Case courtesy Ritu R. Gill, MD, MPH, Brigham and Women's Hospital.

侵袭性胸腺瘤伴脱落性转移：增强CT显示轻度不均匀强化的肿块伴钙化（黄箭）位于主动脉和SVC前方，伴两处胸膜转移瘤（红箭）。

- Thymoma is the most common primary tumor of the anterior mediastinum and typically occurs in middle-aged or older individuals, between 35 and 60 years.
- Thymoma is associated with myasthenia gravis (MG). Approximately 33% of patients with thymoma have MG, and 10% of patients with MG have a thymoma.
- In addition to MG, thymomas are associated with other diseases including red cell aplasia, hypogammaglobulinemia, and other paraneoplastic syndromes.
- Thymoma can be pathologically classified as low-risk or high-risk based on histology, and non-invasive or invasive based on whether the capsule is intact.

  Approximately 30% of thymomas are invasive. If invasive, the tumor may invade adjacent structures including the airways, chest wall, great vessels, and phrenic nerves.

  Elevation of a hemidiaphragm is suggestive of phrenic nerve invasion.
- Thymomas are generally lobulated masses in the anterior mediastinum, often off-center. They may calcify or develop necrosis.
- *Drop metastases* from invasive thymoma spread along pleural and pericardial surfaces.
- Hematogenous metastases are uncommon given that thymomas tend to be indolent tumors with local recurrence.

- 胸腺瘤是前纵隔最常见的原发性肿瘤，通常发生于35~60岁的中老年人。
- 胸腺瘤与重症肌无力（MG）有关。约33%的胸腺瘤患者有MG，10%的MG患者有胸腺瘤。
- 除了MG，胸腺瘤还与其他疾病有关，包括红细胞再生障碍、低丙种球蛋白血症和其他副肿瘤综合征。
- 胸腺瘤根据组织学在病理上分为低危型或高危型，根据包膜是否完整分为非侵袭性或侵袭性。

  约30%的胸腺瘤是侵袭性的。如果是侵袭性的，肿瘤可能会侵犯邻近结构，包括气道、胸壁、大血管和膈神经。

  一侧膈肌抬高提示膈神经受侵。
- 胸腺瘤通常是位于前纵隔的分叶状肿块，常呈偏心性。可钙化或发生坏死。
- 侵袭性胸腺瘤的脱落性转移沿胸膜和心包表面播散。
- 血行转移不常见，因为胸腺瘤往往是局部复发的惰性肿瘤。

Less common thymic lesions

- **Thymic carcinoma**

  Unlike thymoma, thymic carcinoma is histologically malignant, very aggressive, and often metastasizes hematogenously to lungs, liver, brain, and bone. Prognosis is poor.

  Distinction between invasive thymoma and thymic carcinoma is difficult by imaging alone.
- **Thymic cyst**

  A thymic cyst may be secondary to radiation therapy (e.g., administered to treat Hodgkin disease), associated with AIDS or Sjögren's syndrome (especially when multilocular), or congenital arising from remnants of the thymopharyngeal duct. A congenital thymic cyst may occur anywhere along the course of thymic descent from the

较少见的胸腺病变

- **胸腺癌**

  与胸腺瘤不同，胸腺癌在组织学上是恶性的，极具侵袭性，且常通过血行转移至肺、肝、脑和骨骼；预后差。

  侵袭性胸腺瘤和胸腺癌单从影像学上很难区分。
- **胸腺囊肿**

  胸腺囊肿可能继发于放疗（如用于治疗霍奇金淋巴瘤），可与艾滋病或干燥综合征（尤其是多房性囊肿）相关，或为起源于胸腺咽管残留的先天性囊肿。先天性胸腺囊肿可发生在胸腺从颈部下降过程中

neck, but most commonly in the prevascular mediastinum.

CT shows a simple fluid-attenuation cyst in the prevascular mediastinum, typically centrally located. It may measure greater than simple fluid if it contains proteinaceous or hemorrhagic contents. Cystic nature can be confirmed with MRI.

- **Thymolipoma**

Thymolipoma is a benign fat-containing lesion with interspersed soft tissue. It may become quite large and drape over the mediastinum.

- **Thymic hyperplasia**

Thymic hyperplasia appears as diffuse symmetric gland enlargement without focal mass.

True thymic hyperplasia is a reaction to systemic stressors such as radiation therapy, burns, chemotherapy, and steroids.

Lymphoid hyperplasia is associated with myasthenia gravis, SLE, RA, scleroderma, and Grave's disease.

的任何位置，但最常见于血管前纵隔。

CT显示血管前纵隔内一个单纯液性密度的囊肿，通常位于前纵隔的中央。如囊肿含有蛋白质或出血性内容物，其密度可高于纯液体。囊肿性质可用MRI确认。

- **胸腺脂肪瘤**

胸腺脂肪瘤是一种良性含脂质的散在软组织病变。胸腺脂肪瘤可以长得很大并覆盖纵隔。

- **胸腺增生**

胸腺增生表现为弥漫性对称性腺体肿大，无局灶性肿块。

真正的胸腺增生是一种对全身性应激的反应，如放疗、烧伤、化疗、类固醇。

淋巴样增生与重症肌无力、SLE、风湿性关节炎(RA)、硬皮病和格雷夫斯病有关。

Germ cell tumor (GCT)

- Several different types of GCTs may arise in the prevascular mediastinum from primitive germ cell elements.
- **Teratoma** is the most common mediastinal germ cell tumor, usually encapsulated and often predominantly cystic in nature, but fat and calcification are common. A fat/fluid level is specific for teratoma, but is not commonly seen. Teratoma can rarely be malignant, especially if there is a large soft tissue component.

生殖细胞肿瘤(GCT)

- 数种不同类型的生殖细胞肿瘤(GCT)可起源于血管前纵隔的原始生殖细胞。
- **畸胎瘤**是最常见的纵隔GCT，通常有包膜并以囊性为主，但脂肪和钙化很常见。脂/液平为畸胎瘤特有，但并不常见。畸胎瘤偶可为恶性，尤其是当有较多软组织成分时。

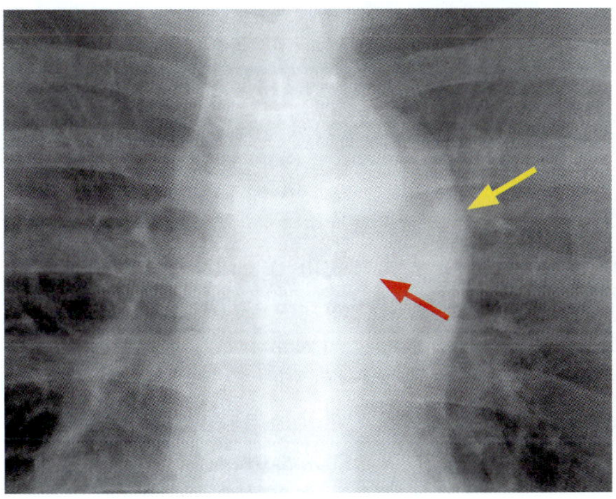

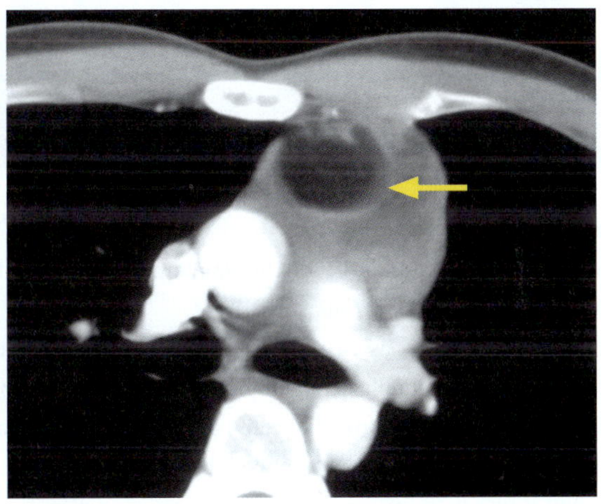

Teratoma: Chest radiograph shows an extra mediastinal contour (yellow arrow) lateral to the aortic arch (red arrow). Because the mass does not silhouette the aorta it cannot be in the middle mediastinum. On CT there is a mediastinal mass containing a large focus of fat (yellow arrow) likely representing a benign teratoma.

Case courtesy Ritu R. Gill, MD, MPH, Brigham and Women's Hospital

畸胎瘤：胸部X线影像(左图)显示外凸的纵隔轮廓(黄箭)，位于主动脉弓的外侧(红箭)；因为肿块没有勾勒出主动脉的轮廓，所以它不可能位于中纵隔。CT(右图)显示一个纵隔肿块，内含大块脂肪(黄箭)，可能为良性畸胎瘤。

- **Seminoma** is the most common *malignant* prevascular mediastinal germ cell tumor. It occurs almost exclusively in men 10 to 39 years old. Pleural effusions are rare but pulmonary metastases are relatively common.
- **Malignant GCT** occurs almost exclusively in males. There is a higher incidence of mediastinal GCT in Klinefelter syndrome.

- **精原细胞瘤**是血管前纵隔最常见的恶性GCT，几乎只发生在10~39岁的男性。胸腔积液罕见，但肺转移相对常见。
- **恶性GCT**几乎只发生在男性。纵隔GCT在克兰费尔特综合征患者中的发生率较高。

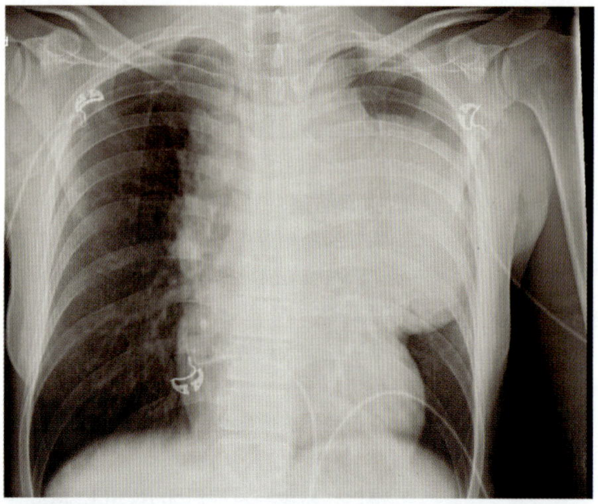

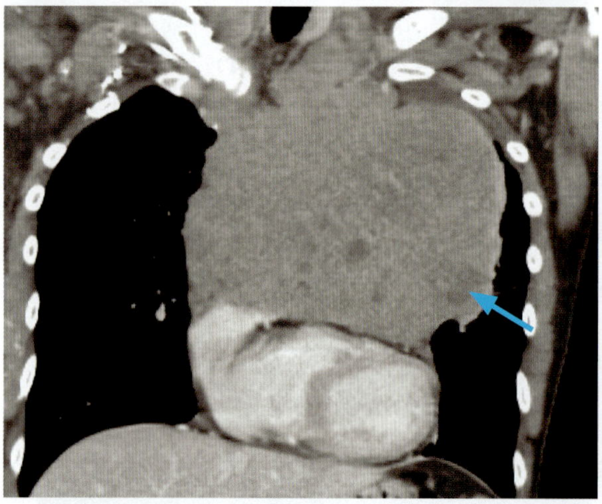

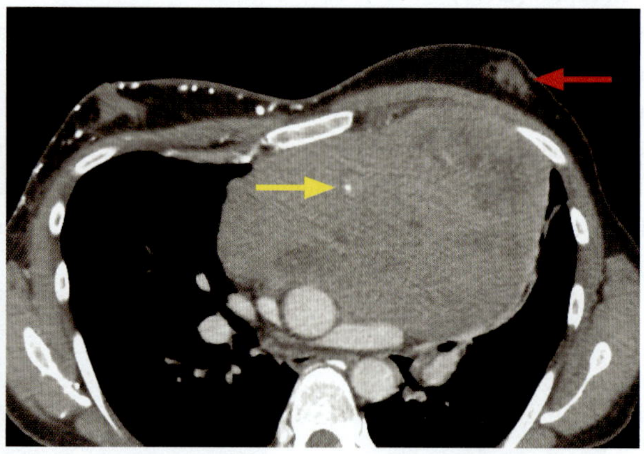

Malignant germ cell tumor with mixed pathology:
Chest radiograph (top left) in a 39-year-old male shows a large soft tissue mass overlying the upper mediastinum. Coronal CT chest image (top right) shows a large heterogeneous mass in the visceral compartment with low density components (blue arrow). Axial CT image (bottom right) demonstrates calcification (yellow arrow) and gynecomastia bilaterally (red arrow). Pathology showed mixed components of teratoma, high grade sarcoma, and leiomyosarcomatous differentiation.

混合性恶性生殖细胞肿瘤：
一名39岁男性患者的胸部X线影像(左上图)显示一个巨大软组织肿块占据上纵隔。冠状位CT胸部影像(左下图)显示一个位于血管前纵隔的巨大而不均匀的肿块，内含低密度成分(蓝箭)。轴位CT影像(右下图)显示钙化(黄箭)和双侧乳房发育(红箭)。病理示畸胎瘤、高级别肉瘤和平滑肌肉瘤样分化的混合成分。

Lymphoma

- Both Hodgkin disease and non-Hodgkin lymphoma are important differential considerations for an anterior mediastinal mass.
- Lymphoma often presents as an aggressive, invasive mass. There is usually associated mediastinal lymphadenopathy which can be in the prevascular or visceral compartments. In particular, internal mammary lymphadenopathy is very highly associated with mediastinal lymphomas.
- Calcification is rare in untreated lymphoma but common after treatment.

淋巴瘤

- 霍奇金淋巴瘤和非霍奇金淋巴瘤都是前纵隔肿块需要考虑的重要鉴别诊断。
- 淋巴瘤通常表现为恶性、侵袭性肿块。通常伴有纵隔淋巴结肿大，可位于前纵隔或中纵隔。尤其是内乳淋巴结肿大与纵隔淋巴瘤的关系非常密切。
- 钙化在未经治疗的淋巴瘤中罕见，但在治疗后很常见。

Visceral Compartment Mediastinal Mass

Adenopathy

- Lymphadenopathy is an important cause of a middle mediastinal mass on radiography, etiologies of which include malignant and non-malignant causes.
- Lymph node calcification, low attenuation, and avid enhancement are unusual features for lymphoma. An alternative diagnosis should be considered if these imaging findings are seen.
- Eggshell calcification of lymph nodes is often present in silicosis and coal worker's pneumoconiosis, less commonly in sarcoidosis. Given the greater prevalence of sarcoidosis, however, eggshell calcification may be seen more commonly in sarcoid overall.
- Dense calcification within a lymph node can be seen in sarcoidosis or as a sequela of prior granulomatous disease.

内脏纵隔肿块

淋巴结肿大

- 淋巴结肿大是放射影像学上中纵隔肿块的重要原因之一，包括恶性和非恶性两种。
- 淋巴瘤不常出现淋巴结钙化、密度减低和显著强化，如果出现这些影像学表现，应考虑其他诊断。
- 淋巴结蛋壳样钙化常见于矽肺和煤工尘肺，结节病少见。然而，鉴于结节病的患病率更高，蛋壳样钙化更有可能是结节病。
- 淋巴结内致密钙化可见于结节病或既往肉芽肿性疾病的后遗症。
- 低密度淋巴结虽然非特异，但应怀疑活动性

- Low attenuation lymph nodes, while nonspecific, should raise concern for active TB. Low attenuation lymph nodes can also be seen in fungal infection such as histoplasmosis, lymphoma, and metastatic disease.
- Hemorrhagic high-attenuation lymph nodes can be seen in anthrax inhalation as part of hemorrhagic lymphadenitis and mediastinitis.
- Avid lymph node enhancement can be seen in Castleman disease, sarcoidosis, TB, and vascular metastases. Avidly enhancing metastases include:

Renal cell carcinoma. Thyroid carcinoma. Lung carcinoma.	Sarcoma. Melanoma.

结核病。低密度淋巴结也可见于真菌感染(如组织胞浆菌病)、淋巴瘤和转移性疾病。

- 出血性高密度淋巴结可见于吸入性炭疽，作为出血性淋巴结炎和纵隔炎的一部分。
- 淋巴结显著强化可见于卡斯尔曼病、结节病、结核，以及血行转移。显著强化的转移瘤包括：

肾细胞癌。 甲状腺癌。 肺癌。	肉瘤。 黑色素瘤。

Castleman disease

- **Castleman disease**, also known as **angiofollicular lymph node hyperplasia**, is a cause of highly vascular thoracic lymph node enlargement. The key imaging feature is avidly enhancing lymph nodes.
- Unicentric Castleman disease is seen as a single enlarged lymph node in children or young adults. Surgical resection is usually curative.
- Multicentric Castleman disease is almost always seen in patients with AIDS associated with HHV8. Multicentric disease often results in systemic illness including fever, anemia, and lymphoma. It is typically treated with chemotherapy.

卡斯尔曼病

- **卡斯尔曼病**，也称为**血管滤泡性淋巴结增生**，是高度血管化胸腔淋巴结肿大的一个原因。关键影像学特征是淋巴结显著强化。
- 单中心卡斯尔曼病表现为儿童或年轻人的单个淋巴结肿大，手术切除通常可治愈。
- 多中心卡斯尔曼病几乎总是出现在与人类疱疹病毒8(HHV 8)相关的艾滋病患者中。多中心疾病常导致全身性表现，包括发热、贫血和淋巴瘤；通常采用化疗进行治疗。

Epicardial fat pad

心外膜脂肪垫

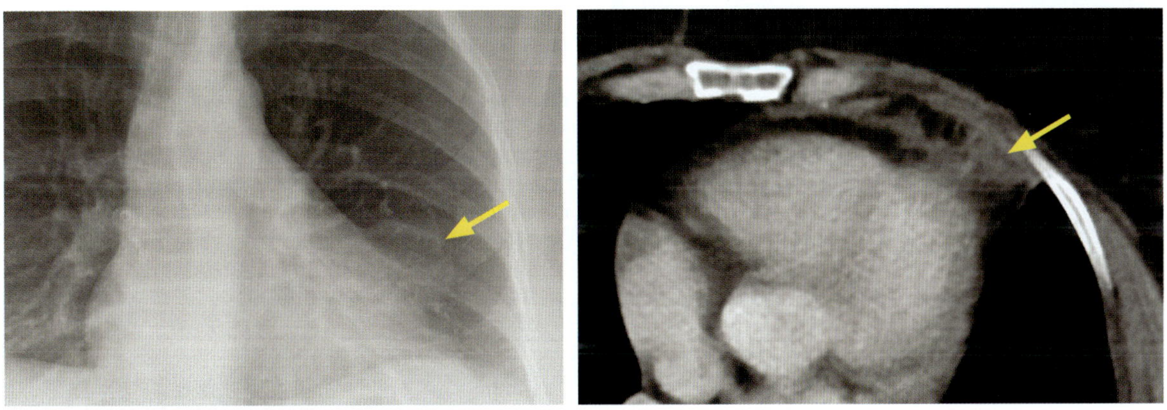

Epicardial fat infarct: Radiograph shows hazy opacity overlying the left heart border (arrow). Axial CT image shows fat stranding and edema of the left epicardial fat pad in keeping with infarct.

心外膜脂肪梗死：X线影像(左图)显示重叠于左心缘模糊阴影(黄箭)。轴位CT图像(右图)显示左心外膜脂肪垫条索影和水肿，与梗死表现一致。

- A prominent epicardial fat pad silhouettes the cardiac border on a frontal radiograph and may simulate cardiomegaly.

Pericardial cyst

- A pericardial cyst is a benign cystic lesion thought to be congenital. Most are located at the right cardiophrenic angle (between the heart and the diaphragm).
- Imaging shows a cystic lesion abutting the pericardium, which may change in shape on subsequent studies.

Cardiac masses

- Cardiac masses can be intracavitary, valvular, intramural, or epicardial/pericardial.
- Composition of the mass, behavior at the margins, and enhancement characteristics are important diagnostic imaging features, as further discussed in the Cardiac chapter.

- 正位X线影像上明显的心外脂肪垫构成心缘，并且可类似心脏肥大。

心包囊肿

- 心包囊肿是一种被认为是先天性的良性囊性病变。大多数位于右心膈角(心脏和横膈之间)。
- 影像学显示囊性病变紧贴心包，其形状可能会在随访中有所改变。

心脏肿块

- 心脏肿块可以位于心腔内、瓣膜、壁内或心外膜/心包。
- 肿块构成、边缘表现和增强特性是影像学诊断的重要特征，将在心脏章节中进一步讨论。

Thyroid lesion

甲状腺病变

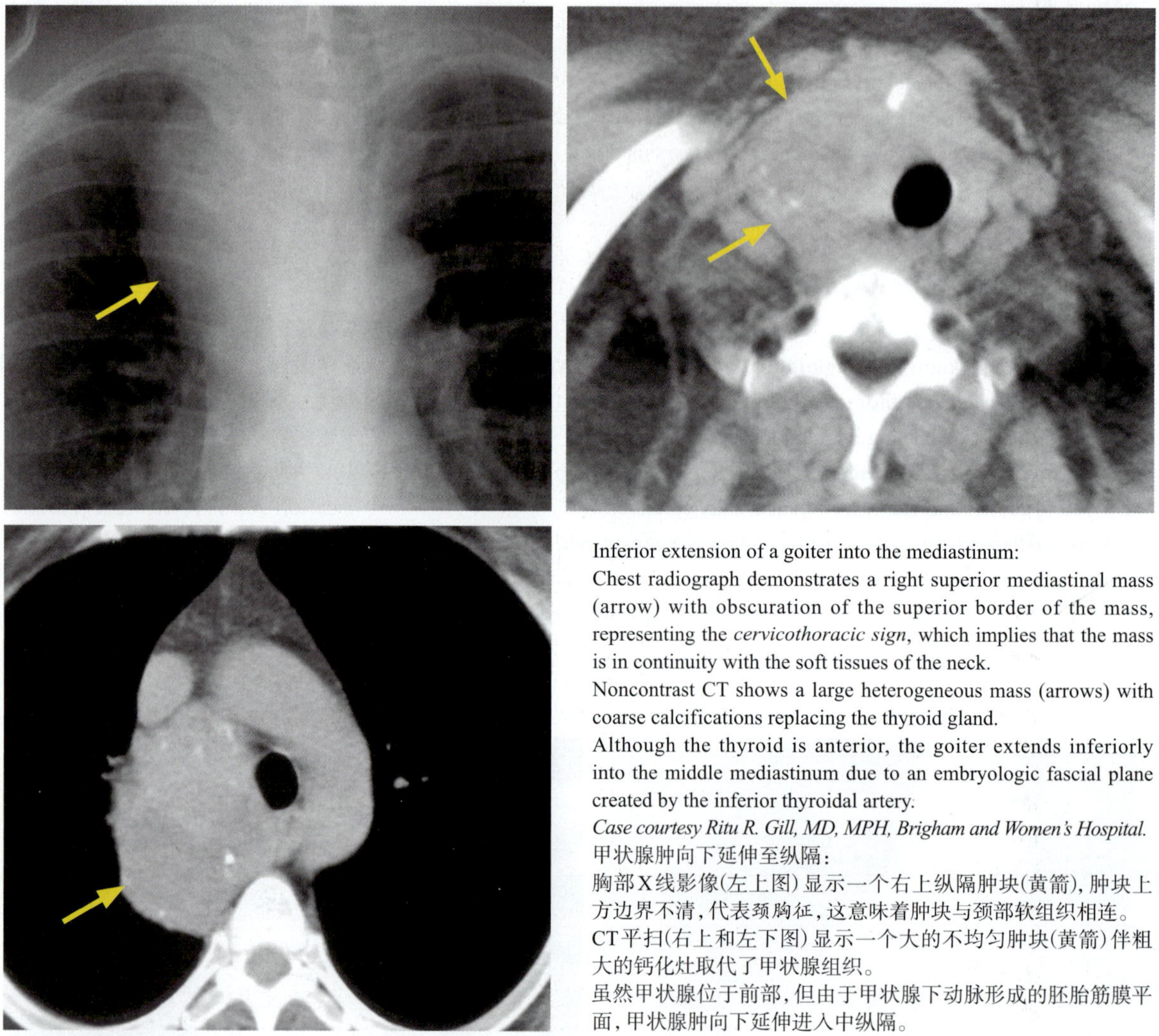

Inferior extension of a goiter into the mediastinum:
Chest radiograph demonstrates a right superior mediastinal mass (arrow) with obscuration of the superior border of the mass, representing the *cervicothoracic sign*, which implies that the mass is in continuity with the soft tissues of the neck.
Noncontrast CT shows a large heterogeneous mass (arrows) with coarse calcifications replacing the thyroid gland.
Although the thyroid is anterior, the goiter extends inferiorly into the middle mediastinum due to an embryologic fascial plane created by the inferior thyroidal artery.
Case courtesy Ritu R. Gill, MD, MPH, Brigham and Women's Hospital.
甲状腺肿向下延伸至纵隔：
胸部X线影像(左上图)显示一个右上纵隔肿块(黄箭)，肿块上方边界不清，代表颈胸征，这意味着肿块与颈部软组织相连。
CT平扫(右上和左下图)显示一个大的不均匀肿块(黄箭)伴粗大的钙化灶取代了甲状腺组织。
虽然甲状腺位于前部，但由于甲状腺下动脉形成的胚胎筋膜平面，甲状腺肿向下延伸进入中纵隔。

- Benign and malignant thyroid masses may extend into the mediastinum, including goiter, thyroid neoplasm, and an enlarged gland due to thyroiditis.
- The key to diagnosis is to show continuity superiorly with the thyroid.

- 良性和恶性甲状腺肿块均可能延伸到纵隔，其中包括甲状腺肿、甲状腺肿瘤，以及由于甲状腺炎引起的腺体肿大。
- 诊断的关键依据是向上连续到甲状腺。

Ascending aortic, aortic arch, or descending aortic aneurysm

- An abnormality of the ascending aorta or aortic arch may appear as a mediastinal mass on radiography.

升主动脉、主动脉弓或降主动脉动脉瘤

- 升主动脉或主动脉弓的异常在X线影像上可表现为纵隔肿块。

Enlarged pulmonary artery (PA)

- An enlarged pulmonary artery (PA) can simulate a mass on a chest radiograph. As previously discussed, the *hilum convergence sign* can help distinguish between an enlarged PA and a mediastinal mass. The hilum convergence sign shows the peripheral pulmonary arteries converging into the "mass" if the mass represents an enlarged pulmonary artery.

肺动脉(PA)扩张

- 肺动脉(PA)扩张在胸部X线影像上可以类似于肿块。如前所述，肺门汇聚征有助于区分扩张的PA和纵隔肿块。肺门汇聚征显示外周肺动脉汇入"肿块"，而此肿块则代表扩张的肺动脉。

Hiatal hernia

食管裂孔疝

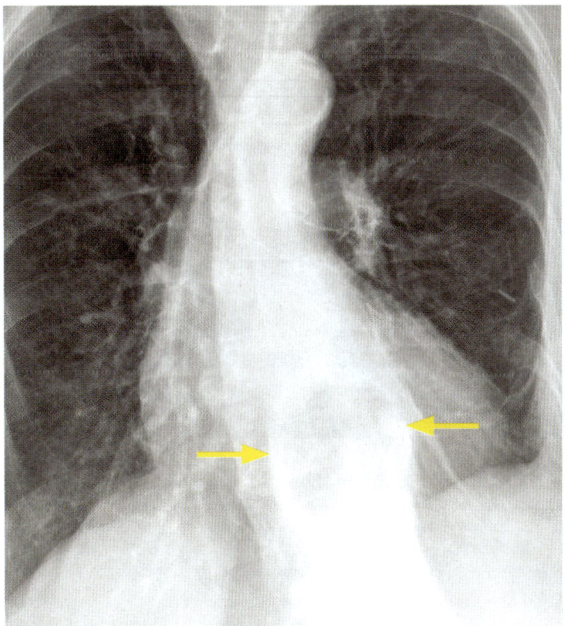

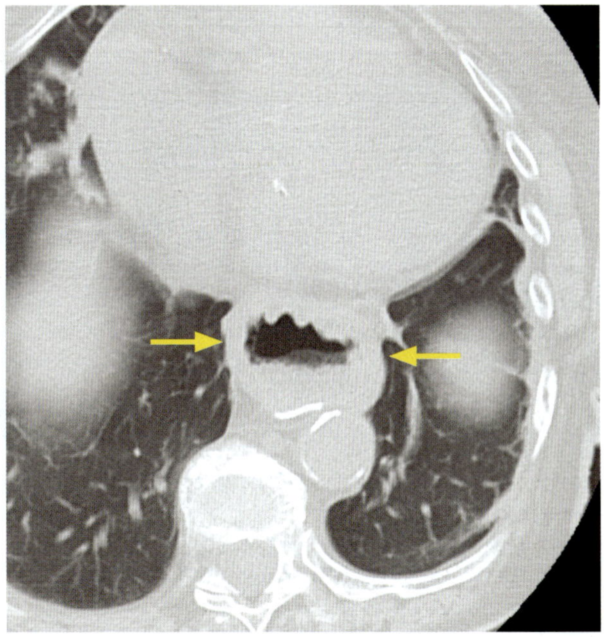

Hiatal hernia: Frontal radiograph shows a retrocardiac lucency (arrows), which was confirmed to be a moderate-sized hiatal hernia on CT (arrows).

食管裂孔疝：正位X线影像(左图)显示一个心后透亮区(黄箭)，CT(右图)证实为一个中等大小的食管裂孔疝(黄箭)。

- A hiatal hernia is protrusion of a portion of the stomach through the esophageal hiatus. The esophageal hiatus is an elliptical opening in the diaphragm just to the left of midline.
- On radiography, air or an air-fluid level is often present above the diaphragm.

Morgagni hernia

- Morgagni hernia is a diaphragmatic hernia through the foramen of Morgagni that occurs anteriorly where the two hemidiaphragms meet, containing omental fat and often bowel. The contents of a Morgagni hernia typically fall to the right.
- An anterior mediastinal mass in contact with the diaphragm containing bowel gas is diagnostic for a Morgagni hernia.
- If bowel gas is absent, a key to diagnosis on CT is the detection of omental vessels in the mass that can be traced into the upper abdomen.

Esophageal neoplasm

- A focal esophageal lesion is concerning for adenocarcinoma or squamous cell carcinoma. Esophageal carcinoma can present on radiography as abnormal convexity of the azygoesophageal recess, mediastinal widening, or a retrotracheal mass.
- Benign mesenchymal esophageal tumors include fibrovascular polyp, leiomyoma, fibroma, or lipoma.

Foregut duplication cyst

- Foregut duplication cysts include bronchogenic cysts, esophageal duplication cysts, and neurenteric cysts. Although often low attenuation, internal heterogeneity can be due to hemorrhagic or proteinaceous components or superinfection.

Bronchogenic cysts can arise from any mediastinal compartment, but they most commonly arise near the carina in the visceral compartment (typically in right paratracheal space, subcarinal space, or hila). The lesion's thin walls may enhance or

- 食管裂孔疝是胃的一部分通过食管裂孔突出。食管裂孔是横膈中线左侧的椭圆形开口。
- 在X线影像上，膈肌的上方经常出现气体或气-液平面。

先天性胸骨后膈疝(Morgagni疝)

- Morgagni疝是通过Morgagni孔的膈疝，发生的位置是两侧膈肌汇合的前方，包含网膜脂肪，更多为肠管。Morgagni疝的内容物通常在右侧。
- 前纵隔肿块与横膈接触并包含肠气可诊断为Morgagni疝。
- 如果未见肠道气体，CT诊断的关键是发现肿块内的网膜血管，其可以追溯到上腹部。

食管肿瘤

- 局灶性食管病变应考虑腺癌或鳞状细胞癌。食管癌在X线影像上可表现为奇食管隐窝异常突出、纵隔增宽或气管后肿块。
- 良性间叶性食管肿瘤包括纤维血管息肉、平滑肌瘤、纤维瘤或脂肪瘤。

前肠重复囊肿

- 前肠重复囊肿包括支气管囊肿、食管重复囊肿和神经管原肠囊肿。尽管通常为低密度影，但内部不均质可由出血或蛋白质成分或合并感染所致。

支气管囊肿可起源于纵隔的任何部位，但最常见于内脏纵隔的气管分叉附近(通常位于右侧气管旁间隙、隆突下间隙或肺门)。病灶的薄壁可出现强化

have intrinsic calcifications.

Esophageal duplication cysts are adjacent to the esophagus.

或有内部钙化。

食管重复囊肿与食管相邻。

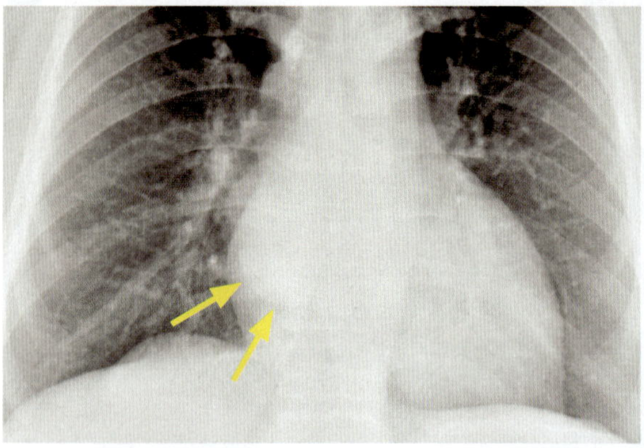

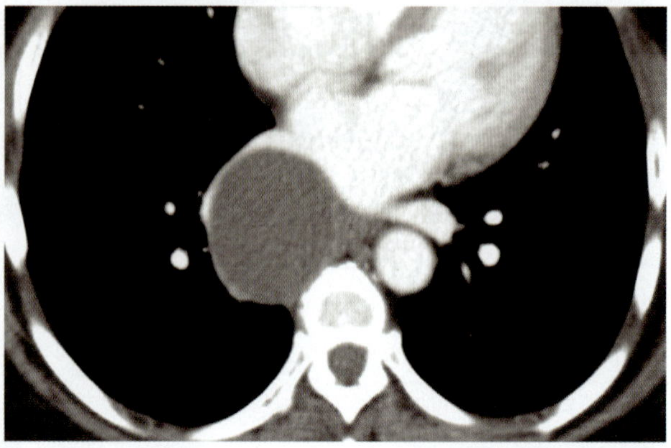

Bronchogenic cyst: Frontal radiograph shows a subtle opacity overlying the right heart (arrows), shown to be a fluid attenuation lesion adjacent to the esophagus on CT.

Case courtesy Darryl Sneag, MD, Brigham and Women's Hospital.

支气管囊肿：正位X线影像(左图)显示一个不明显的阴影重叠于右心(黄箭)，CT(右图)显示邻近食管液体密度病灶。

Paraganglioma

- Cardiac or aortopulmonary paragangliomas can present as a visceral compartment mediastinal mass, arising from phrenic, vagus, and recurrent laryngeal nerves.
- A paraganglioma or extra-adrenal pheochromocytoma is a highly vascular neuroendocrine tumor that originates from embryonic neural crest cells of the peripheral nervous system. It can be sympathetic or parasympathetic. A visceral compartment mediastinal paraganglioma tends to be parasympathetic in origin.
- Malignancy can occur in up to 10% of extra-adrenal pheochromocytomas. They can be functioning or non-functioning.
- CT appearance is of a hypervascular mass with robust feeding arteries. There may be internal heterogeneity representing necrosis.
- MRI shows a T1 intermediate, T2 hyperintense mass with homogeneous enhancement.

副神经节瘤

- 心脏或主-肺动脉副神经节瘤可表现为内脏纵隔肿块，起源于膈神经、迷走神经和喉返神经。
- 副神经节瘤或肾上腺外嗜铬细胞瘤是一种高度血管化的神经内分泌肿瘤，起源于周围神经系统的胚胎神经嵴细胞，可以来源于交感神经或副交感神经。内脏纵隔副神经节瘤往往起源于副交感神经。
- 高达10%肾上腺外嗜铬细胞瘤为恶性。它们可以是有功能的或无功能的。
- CT表现为一个富血供的肿块，具有丰富的供血动脉。肿块内部可能不均质，代表坏死。
- MRI显示T_1等信号、T_2高信号肿块，均匀强化。

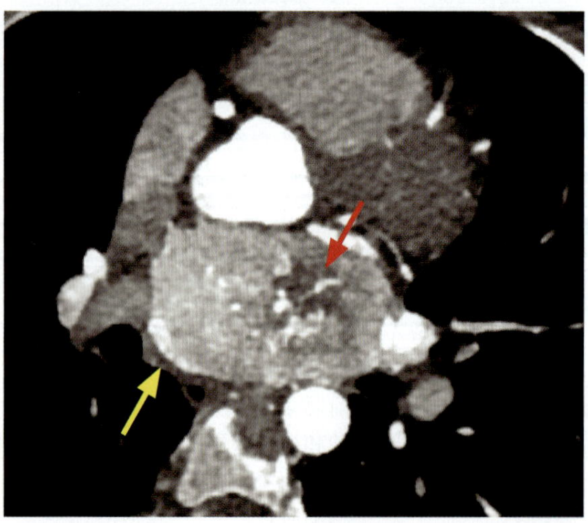

Contrast enhanced axial CT shows a hypervascular mediastinal mass (yellow arrow) with central areas of necrosis (red arrow) directly abutting the borders of the ascending and descending thoracic aorta just above the level of the pulmonary veins, consistent with a parasympathetic paraganglioma.

轴位增强CT显示一个富血供纵隔肿块(黄箭)伴中央坏死区(红箭)，紧邻肺静脉水平上方的升主动脉和降主动脉的边缘，符合副交感神经副神经节瘤。

Paravertebral Compartment Mediastinal Mass

Neurogenic tumor

- A neurogenic tumor may arise from either a peripheral nerve or the sympathetic ganglia. Most adult tumors are peripheral nerve sheath tumors and the vast majority of tumors in children are of sympathetic ganglionic origin. Overall, neurogenic tumors are the most common paravertebral compartment mediastinal masses.
- Imaging features typically show a smooth round mass. Benign pressure erosion of adjacent ribs, vertebrae, and enlargement of neuroforamina may occur.
- Interval growth of a neurogenic tumor with regions of internal heterogeneity should raise concern for transformation to **malignant peripheral nerve sheath tumor**.
- Peripheral nerve tumors (more common in adults) include:

> **Schwannoma** (most common), **neurofibroma**, and **malignant peripheral nerve sheath tumor**.

椎旁区纵隔肿块

神经源性肿瘤

- 神经源性肿瘤可起源于外周神经或交感神经节。大多数成人的肿瘤为外周神经鞘瘤，而绝大多数儿童的肿瘤起源于交感神经节。总体而言，神经源性肿瘤是最常见的椎旁区纵隔肿块。
- 影像学表现通常为光滑的圆形肿块。可出现邻近肋骨、椎体的良性压迫吸收，以及神经孔扩大。
- 间隔生长的神经源性肿瘤伴内部异质性区域者应警惕**恶性外周神经鞘瘤**。
- 外周神经肿瘤(更常见于成人)包括：

> **神经鞘瘤**(最常见)、**神经纤维瘤**和**恶性外周神经鞘瘤**。

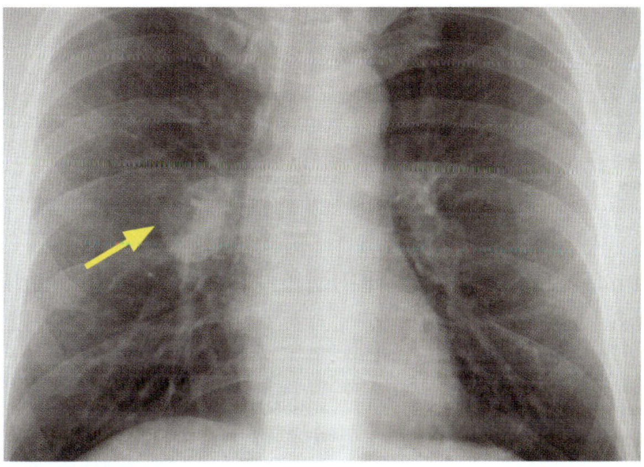

Frontal radiograph
正位X线影像

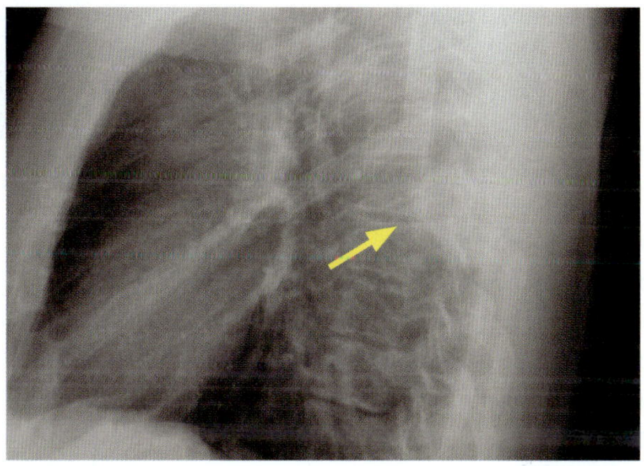

Lateral radiograph
侧位X线影像

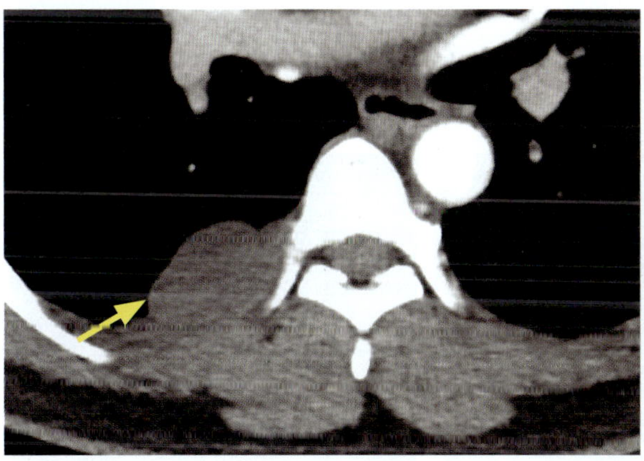

Axial CT with contrast
轴位增强CT

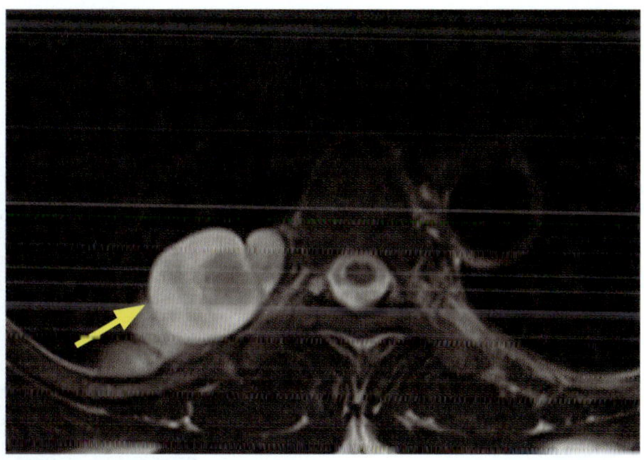

Axial T2-weighted MRI
轴位T_2加权MRI

Schwannoma: Frontal radiograph shows a round opacity overlying the right hilum with the hilum overlay sign (arrow) corresponding to a paravertebral abnormality on lateral radiograph. CT shows a low density lesion without significant enhancement. MRI shows heterogeneous T2 hyperintense signal within the cystic lesion in keeping with a schwannoma.

神经鞘瘤：正位X线影像显示一个圆形阴影重叠于右肺门，为肺门重叠征(黄箭)，对应于侧位X线影像上的椎旁异常。CT表现为低密度病灶，无明显强化。MRI显示囊性病变内不均匀T_2高信号，符合神经鞘瘤。

- Sympathetic ganglion tumors (more common in children/young adults) include:

- 交感神经节肿瘤(更常见于儿童/年轻人)包括：

Ganglioneuroma (most common), a benign tumor of sympathetic ganglion cells.
Neuroblastoma, a malignant tumor of ganglion cells seen in early childhood.
Ganglioneuroblastoma, intermediate in histology between ganglioneuroma and neuroblastoma, seen in older children than neuroblastoma.

节细胞神经瘤(最常见),交感神经节细胞的良性肿瘤。
神经母细胞瘤,一种见于幼儿期的神经节细胞恶性肿瘤。
节细胞神经母细胞瘤,组织学上介于节细胞神经瘤和神经母细胞瘤之间,比神经节细胞瘤发病儿童的年龄稍长。

- Paragangliomas can arise in the paravertebral compartment from spinal, intercostal, or sympathetic nerves.

- 副神经节瘤可起源于椎旁区的脊神经、肋间神经或交感神经。

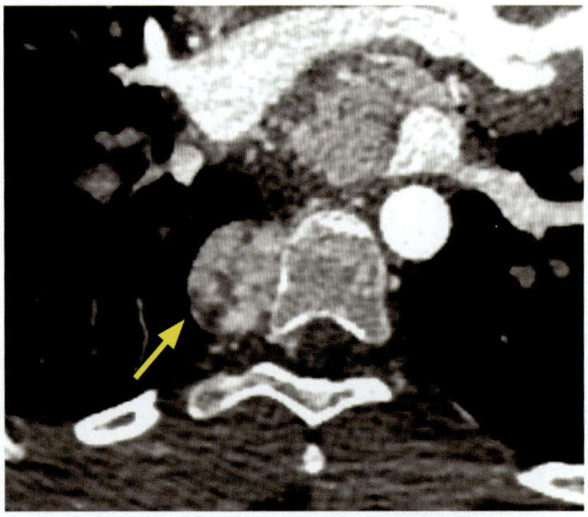

Contrast enhanced axial CT shows a paravertebral hypervascular mass with heterogeneous areas of necrosis (arrow) consistent with a paraganglioma along the sympathetic chain.
轴位增强CT显示椎旁富血供肿块伴不均匀坏死区(黄箭),符合沿交感神经链走行的副神经节瘤。

Extramedullary hematopoiesis

- Extramedullary hematopoiesis presents as soft tissue paravertebral masses in patients with severe hereditary anemias including thalassemia and sickle cell anemia.
- On imaging, lobulated soft tissue masses are typically bilateral and inferior to T6. They may contain internal fat.

Intrathoracic meningocele

- An intrathoracic or lateral meningocele is herniation of the leptomeninges through either an intervertebral foramen or a defect in the vertebral body. Lateral meningocele is associated with neurofibromatosis.

Paraspinal abscess

髓外造血

- 在严重的遗传性贫血(包括地中海贫血和镰状细胞贫血)患者中,髓外造血表现为椎旁软组织肿块。
- 影像学上,分叶状软组织肿块通常为双侧性,位于T_6下方。可含有内部脂肪。

胸腔内脊膜膨出

- 胸腔内或侧方脊膜膨出是软脊膜通过椎间孔或椎体缺损疝出。侧方脊膜膨出与神经纤维瘤病相关。

椎旁脓肿

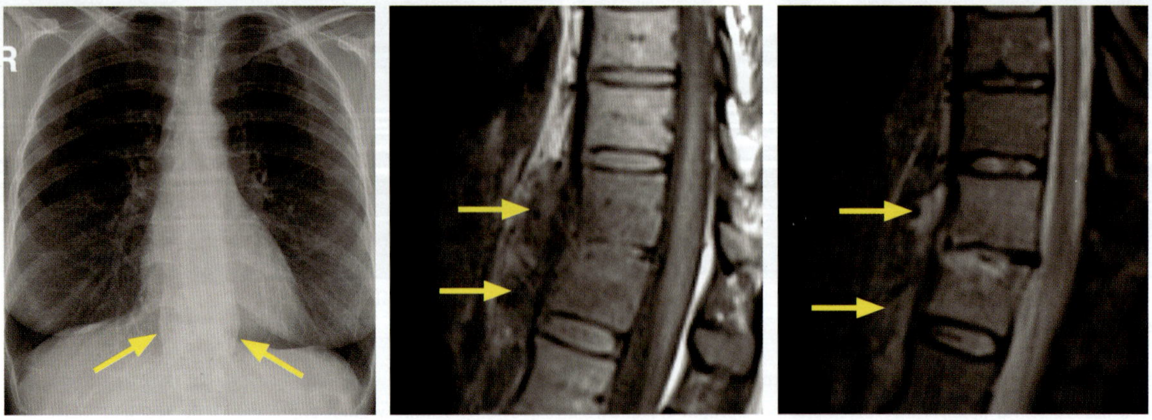

Osteomyelitis and paraspinal phlegmon: Radiograph shows displacement of the bilateral paraspinal lines (arrows). Sagittal T1- (middle image) and T2-weighted MRI (right image) shows loss of Disc space height and marrow edema in two adjacent lower thoracic vertebral bodies. There is associated paraspinal phlegmonous change (arrows), which caused the paraspinal line displacement on radiography.
骨髓炎和椎旁蜂窝织炎:X线影像(左图)显示双侧椎旁线移位(黄箭)。矢状位T_1(中图)和T_2加权(右图)MRI显示椎间盘高度丢失和两个相邻的下胸椎体的骨髓水肿。伴有椎旁蜂窝织炎的改变(黄箭),导致X线影像上的椎旁线移位。

- A clue to vertebral body pathology on radiography may be paraspinal line displacement.

- 在X线影像上椎体病变的一个诊断线索可能是椎旁线移位。

（翻译　王维平）

AIRWAYS

气道

MULTIFOCAL OR DIFFUSE NON-NEOPLASTIC TRACHEAL STENOSIS/WALL THICKENING

多灶性或弥漫性非肿瘤性气管狭窄/管壁增厚

Overview of non-neoplastic diffuse tracheal disease

弥漫性非肿瘤性气管疾病概述

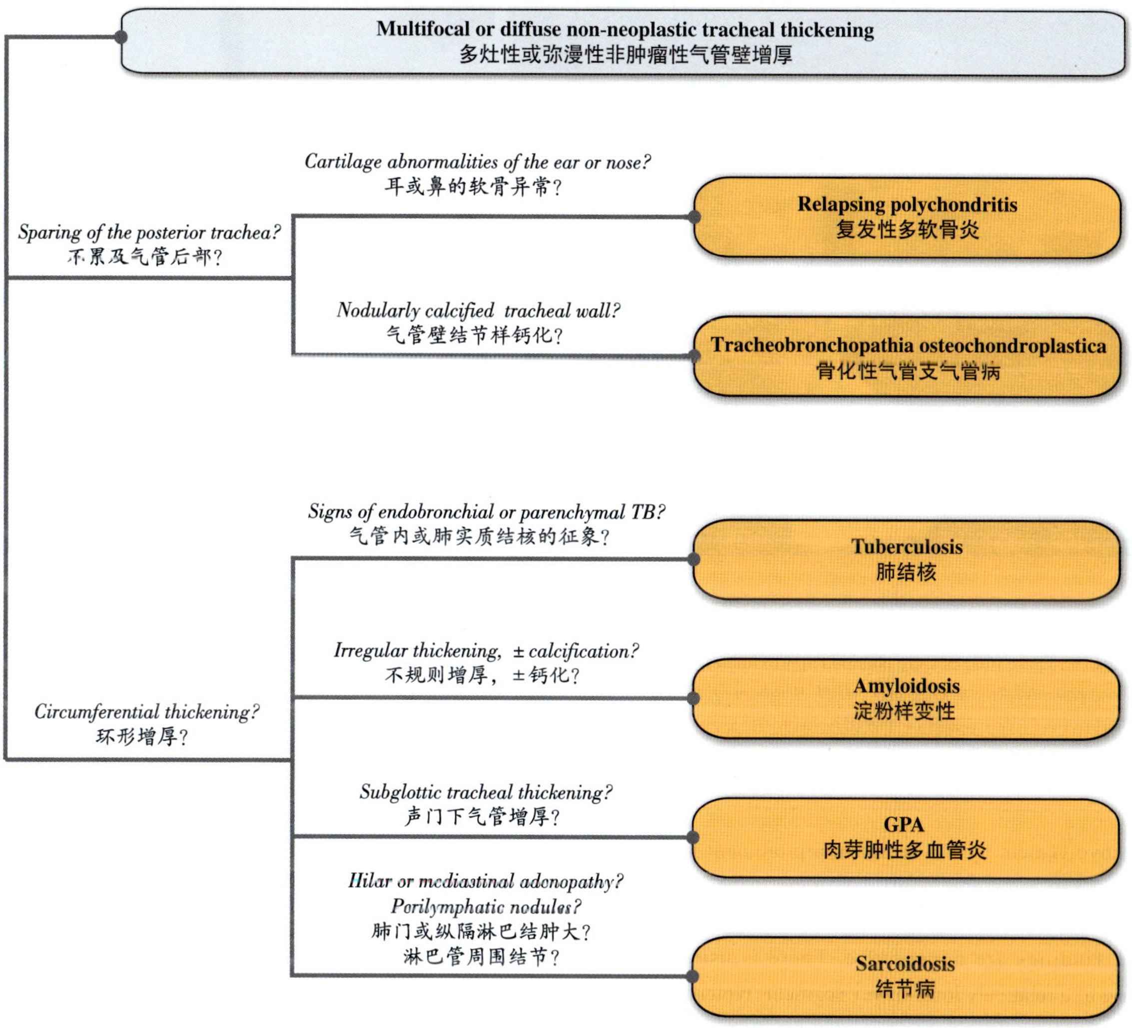

Relapsing polychondritis

- Relapsing polychondritis is a multisystemic disease of unknown etiology characterized by recurrent inflammation of cartilaginous structures. The nose, ear, joints, larynx, trachea, and bronchi can be affected, with airway involvement seen in 50% of patients.

  The larynx and subglottic trachea are the most common sites of airway involvement.
- Relapsing polychondritis usually occurs in middle-aged women.
- On cross-sectional imaging, there is smooth tracheal/bronchial wall thickening, with *sparing of the posterior membranous* trachea.

复发性多软骨炎

- 复发性多软骨炎是一种病因未明的多系统疾病，其特点是软骨结构反复发炎。鼻、耳、关节、喉、气管和支气管均可以受累，约50%的患者可见气道受累。

  喉和声门下气管是气道最易受累的部位。
- 复发性多软骨炎通常发生在中年女性。
- 在横断面图像上表现为气管/支气管壁均匀增厚，但气管后膜部不受累。

The tracheal cartilage is an incomplete ring, with no cartilage in the posterior membranous portion.

气管软骨是不完整的环，其后膜部没有软骨。

- There is often increased attenuation of the airway wall, ranging from subtly increased attenuation to frank calcification. Tracheomalacia (expiratory collapse of the trachea) is commonly present.

- 常见气道壁密度增高，可以从轻微的密度增高到明显的钙化。常出现气管软化(呼气时气管塌陷)。

Tracheobronchopathia osteochondroplastica (TPO)

骨化性气管支气管病(TPO)

- Tracheobronchopathia osteochondroplastica (TPO) is a benign condition of multiple submucosal osteocartilaginous nodules along the tracheal walls that appear as coarse calcifications, with sparing of the posterior membranous trachea.

- 骨化性气管支气管病(TPO)是一种良性疾病，表现为多发的粗糙黏膜下骨软骨钙化性结节，结节沿气管壁分布但不累及气管后膜部。

Tuberculosis

结核

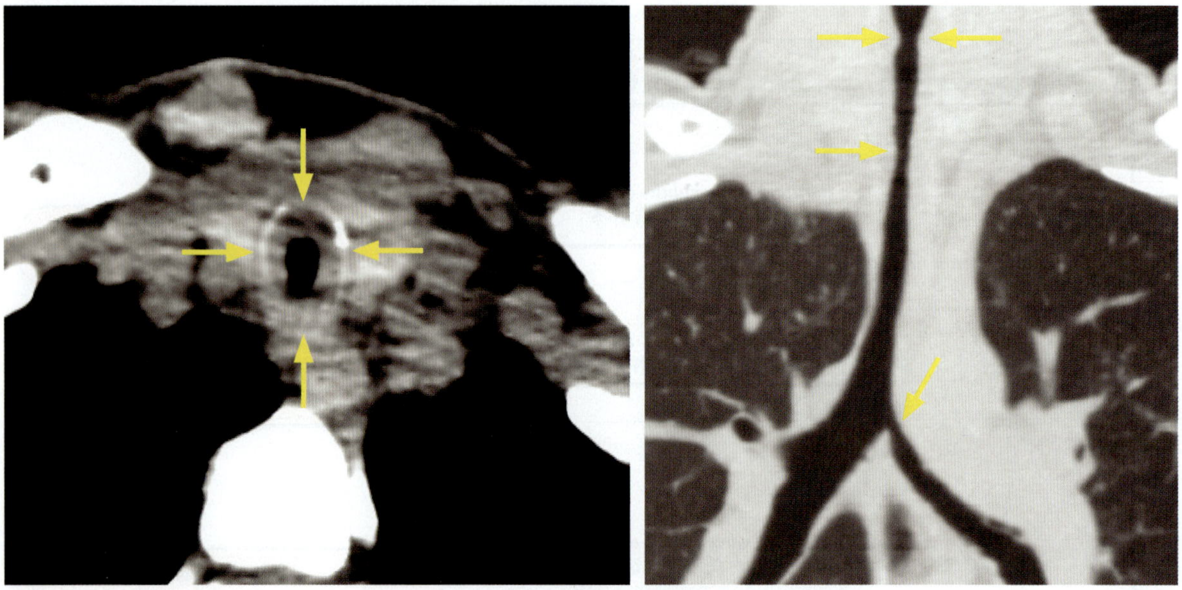

Tracheal tuberculosis: Axial CT in soft-tissue window through the upper trachea (left image) shows circumferential tracheal thickening (arrows). Coronal curved-multiplanar reformation (right image) shows multifocal tracheal stenosis (arrows) and left mainstem bronchus stenosis. These images were obtained approximately one month after treatment for active post-primary TB.

Case courtesy Ritu R. Gill, MD, MPH, Brigham and Women's Hospital.

气管结核：气管上部轴位CT软组织窗(左图)显示气管壁环形增厚(黄箭)。冠状位曲面多平面重建(右图)显示多灶性气管狭窄(黄箭)和左主支气管狭窄。这是活动性原发后肺结核病治疗约1个月后的图像。

- Airway involvement by TB occurs in a prominent minority of patients with pulmonary TB, most commonly involving the distal trachea and proximal bronchi.
- Imaging findings are nonspecific. There is usually smooth concentric narrowing of a relatively long airway segment (typically >3 cm).

- 极少数肺结核患者累及气道，而气管远端和支气管近端是最常受累的部位。
- 影像学表现无特异性。常表现为光滑的向心性狭窄，累及一段相对较长的气道(通常>3cm)。

Amyloidosis

淀粉样变性

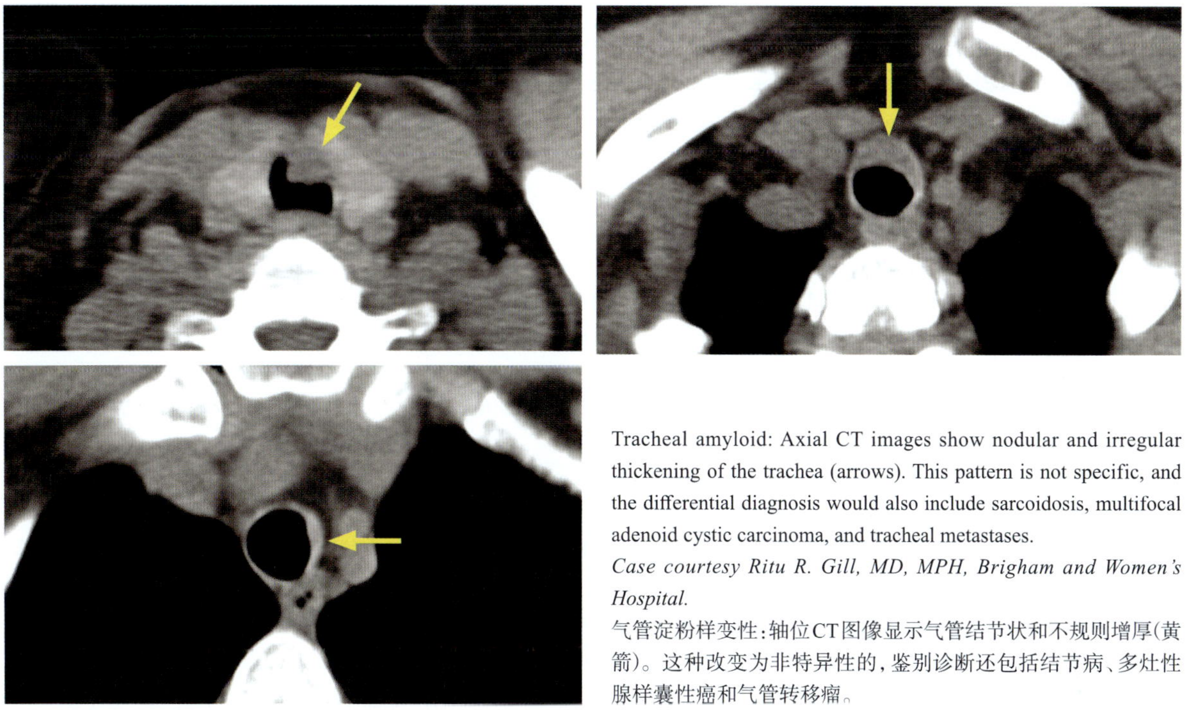

Tracheal amyloid: Axial CT images show nodular and irregular thickening of the trachea (arrows). This pattern is not specific, and the differential diagnosis would also include sarcoidosis, multifocal adenoid cystic carcinoma, and tracheal metastases.

Case courtesy Ritu R. Gill, MD, MPH, Brigham and Women's Hospital.

气管淀粉样变性：轴位CT图像显示气管结节状和不规则增厚(黄箭)。这种改变为非特异性的，鉴别诊断还包括结节病、多灶性腺样囊性癌和气管转移瘤。

- Amyloidosis causes irregular narrowing of the airways due to submucosal amyloid deposition, which may be calcified. Involvement may be mass-like or segmental. Tracheal amyloidosis is very rare.
- The posterior membranous trachea is not spared.

- 淀粉样变性会导致气道不规则狭窄，这是由黏膜下淀粉样物质沉积所致，这些沉积物可发生钙化。受累部位可表现为肿块样或节段性改变。气管淀粉样变性非常罕见。
- 气管后膜部同样受累。

Granulomatosis with polyangiitis (GPA)

- Large airway involvement is seen in approximately 20% of patients with GPA, most commonly manifesting as subglottic tracheal stenosis with circumferential mucosal thickening.
- The posterior membranous trachea is not spared. Calcifications are not seen.

肉芽肿性多血管炎(GPA)

- 约20%的肉芽肿性多血管炎(GPA)患者有大气道受累，最常见的表现是声门下气管狭窄伴环周黏膜增厚。
- 气管后膜部同样受累，无钙化。

Sarcoidosis

- Tracheal involvement by sarcoid is rare and usually seen in advanced disease. Tracheal sarcoid has a variable appearance ranging from smooth stenosis to a nodular or mass-like appearance.
- The posterior membranous trachea is not spared.

结节病

- 结节病极少累及气管，通常出现在疾病的晚期。气管结节病的表现多样，从光滑性狭窄到结节或肿块样表现均可出现。
- 气管后膜部同样受累。

LARGE AIRWAYS

大气道

Bronchiectasis

- Bronchiectasis is progressive, irreversible dilation of cartilage-containing bronchi.
- Three etiologies of bronchiectasis have been described, with a final common pathway of mucus plugging, superimposed bacterial colonization, and inflammatory response.

支气管扩张

- 支气管扩张为含软骨支气管出现进行性、不可逆性的扩张。
- 支气管扩张有以下三种原因，并有共同的转归：黏液栓、并发异常菌落生长和炎症反应。

Bronchial wall injury, typically from infection or inflammation.
Bronchial lumen obstruction.
Traction from adjacent fibrosis.

支气管壁损伤，通常为感染或炎症。
支气管管腔阻塞。
邻近纤维化牵拉。

- Morphologic classification of bronchiectasis is most useful as a rough gauge of severity.

Cylindrical bronchiectasis (least severe): Mild bronchial dilation.
Varicose bronchiectasis (moderately severe): Bronchi may become beaded and irregular.
Cystic bronchiectasis (most severe): Bronchi are markedly enlarged and ballooned.

- Radiographic findings depend on severity. In mild cases only *tram tracks* may be visible, representing thickened bronchial walls causing parallel radiopaque lines resembling tram tracks. In more severe cases there can be extensive cystic change.
- CT findings include the *signet ring sign*, which describes a dilated bronchus adjacent to a normal pulmonary artery branch.

  Normally each bronchus should be approximately the same size as the adjacent pulmonary artery branch.

  Other CT findings of bronchiectasis include lack of bronchial tapering, bronchial wall thickening, and mucus-filled bronchi. Often, adjacent tree-in-bud nodules are present, likely representing associated small-airways infection.
- Traction bronchiectasis occurs secondary to lung fibrosis (see earlier discussion of ILD).
- Patterns of primary bronchiectasis can be divided into lung zones and central to peripheral distribution:

Upper lung: cystic fibrosis, ABPA.
Mid lung: atypical mycobacteria.
Lower lung: chronic aspiration, post-infectious, immotile cilia, immunodeficiency.

Central: ABPA, Mounier-Kuhn (tracheobronchomegaly).
Mid-order bronchi: Williams-Campbell (fourth to sixth order bronchi).

- **Chronic aspiration** is the most common cause of bronchiectasis.

- 支气管扩张形态学分类是粗略评估病情严重程度最有用的方法。

柱状支气管扩张(最轻):支气管轻度扩张。
静脉曲张型支气管扩张(中等):支气管呈串珠状和不规则形状。
囊状支气管扩张(最重):支气管明显扩大和出现气球样改变。

- X线影像表现取决于疾病的严重程度。轻症只能看到*轨道征*,为支气管壁增厚所形成的轨道样平行的不透亮线。较为严重病例可出现广泛的囊性变。
- CT表现包括*印戒征*,形容扩张的支气管紧邻一条正常的肺动脉分支。

  正常情况下,支气管管径的大小应与邻近的肺动脉分支大致相同。

  支气管扩张的其他CT表现包括支气管缺乏逐渐变细的形态、支气管壁增厚、支气管被黏液填塞。病变周围常出现树芽状结节,可能代表相应的小气道感染。
- 牵拉性支气管扩张继发于肺纤维化(见前文关于ILD的讨论)。
- 支气管扩张可分为肺区,以及从中央到外周两大主要分布方式:

上肺:囊性纤维化、ABPA。
中肺:非典型分枝杆菌。
下肺:慢性吸入、感染后、无纤毛运动、免疫缺陷。

中央型:ABPA、莫-昆二氏综合征(巨气管支气管症)。
中等级别支气管:威-坎二氏综合征(第4~6级支气管)。

- **慢性吸入**是支气管扩张最常见的原因。

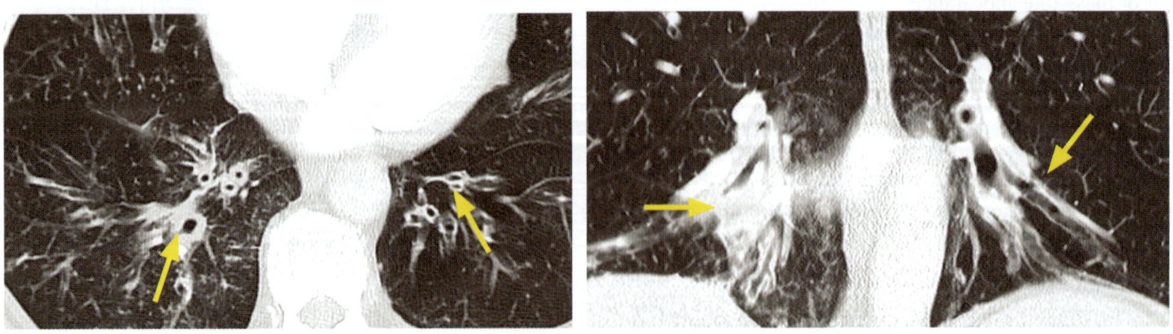

Bronchiectasis from chronic aspiration: Axial and coronal CT show bronchial wall thickening in the bilateral lower lobes due to dependent aspiration (arrows).
慢性吸入导致的支气管扩张:轴位和冠状位CT显示双肺下叶支气管壁增厚(黄箭),为吸入后按重力分布。

- Bronchocentric infections, such as **tuberculosis** and **atypical mycobacteria.**

- 支气管中心性感染，如**肺结核**和**非典型分枝杆菌**感染。

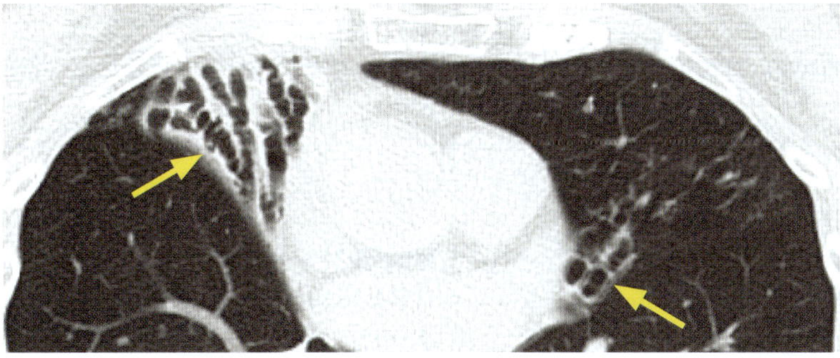

Bronchiectasis of the right middle lobe and lingula (arrows) due to *Mycobacterium avium intracellulare* infection.
右肺中叶和舌段支气管扩张(黄箭)，由胞内鸟分枝杆菌感染所致。

- Ineffective clearing of secretions – **cystic fibrosis** and **Kartagener** (primary ciliary dyskinesia).

- 分泌物清除障碍——**囊性纤维化**和**卡塔格内综合征**(一种原发性纤毛运动不良症)。

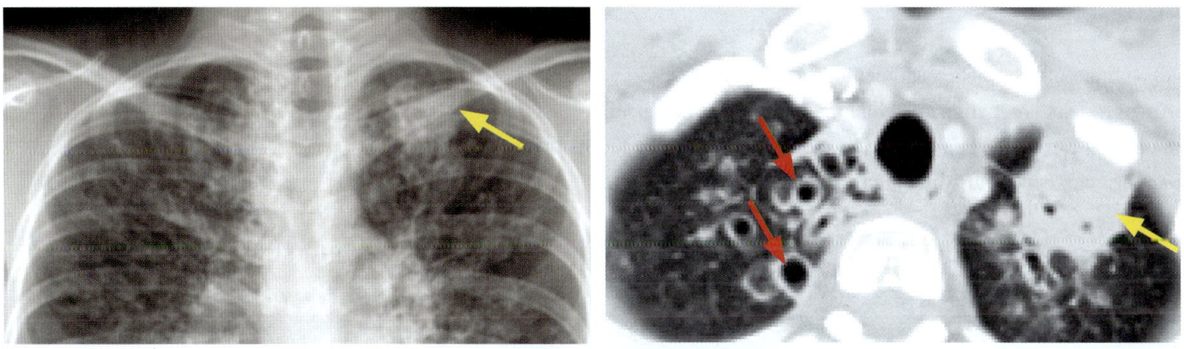

Bronchiectasis from cystic fibrosis with superimposed pneumonia: Radiograph shows upper-lobe bronchiectasis with a focal left upper lobe opacity (yellow arrow). CT confirms bronchiectasis (red arrows) and a left upper lobe consolidation (yellow arrow), representing pneumonia.
由囊性纤维化造成的支气管扩张合并肺炎：X线影像(左图)显示上叶支气管扩张伴左肺上叶局灶高密度影(黄箭)。CT(右图)确诊为支气管扩张(红箭)和左肺上叶实变(黄箭)，为肺炎。

- Congenital connective tissue disorders – **Mounier-Kuhn** (a connective tissue disorder causing tracheobronchomegaly leading to recurrent pneumonia), or **Williams-Campbell** (a rare disorder of the fourth to sixth mid-order bronchial cartilage, which may be congenital or acquired as a sequela of viral infection).

- 先天性结缔组织病——**莫-昆二氏综合征**(一种结缔组织疾病，可引起气管支气管巨大症并导致复发性肺炎)，或**威-坎二氏综合征**(一种罕见的第4~6级中等支气管软骨异常，可为先天性或后天病毒感染的后遗症)。

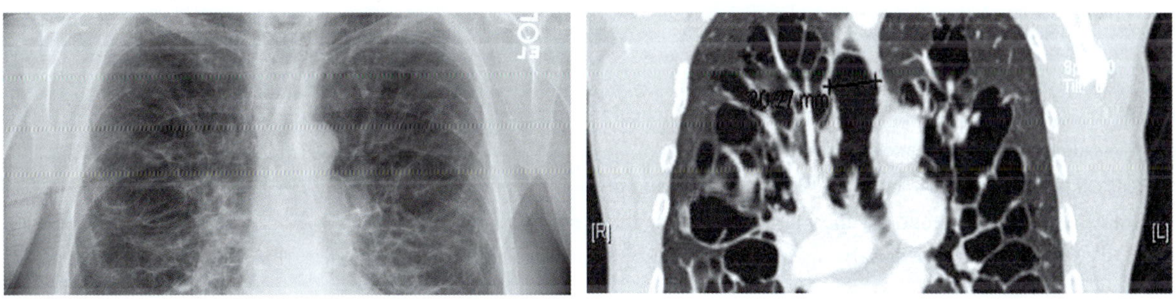

Mounier-Kuhn: Chest radiograph (left image) shows severe diffuse bronchiectasis. CT shows tracheal dilation (calipers) up to 3 cm and severe cystic bronchiectasis.
莫-昆二氏综合征：胸部X线影像(左图)显示严重的弥漫性支气管扩张。CT显示气管扩张(标尺)高达3cm和严重的囊状支气管扩张。

Broncholithiasis

- Broncholithiasis is a rare disorder of calcified/ossified material within the bronchial lumen, caused by erosion of an adjacent calcified granulomatous lymph node.
- Broncholithiasis clinically presents with nonproductive cough, hemoptysis, and air trapping.

支气管结石症

- 支气管结石症是一种罕见病，表现为支气管腔内出现钙化/骨化物质，为支气管壁被邻近的钙化肉芽肿性淋巴结侵蚀所致。
- 支气管结石症临床表现为干咳、咯血、空气潴留。

Focal non-neoplastic tracheal stenosis/wall thickening

局灶性非肿瘤性气管狭窄/管壁增厚

Intubation/tracheostomy

- There is approximately 1% risk of tracheal stenosis after intubation, but approximately 30% risk of stenosis after long-standing tracheostomy.

Rare causes of focal tracheal stenosis

- Extremely uncommon causes of focal tracheal stenosis include Behçet and Crohn disease.

气管插管/气管造口术

- 气管插管后发生气管狭窄的风险约为1%，但长期气管造口术后出现狭窄的风险则约为30%。

局部气管狭窄的罕见原因

- 极其罕见的局部气管狭窄的原因包括白塞综合征和克罗恩病。

Airway tumors

气道肿瘤

- Primary tumors of the trachea and central bronchi are rare. In adults, the vast majority of tumors are malignant, while in children most are benign.
- Squamous cell carcinoma and adenoid cystic carcinoma are by far the two most common primary central airway tumors in adults.

- 气管与中央支气管的原发肿瘤罕见。在成人，绝大多数肿瘤为恶性的，但在儿童则多为良性。
- 鳞状细胞癌和腺样囊性癌是成人最常见的两种原发性中央气道肿瘤。

Squamous cell carcinoma (SCC)

鳞状细胞癌(SCC)

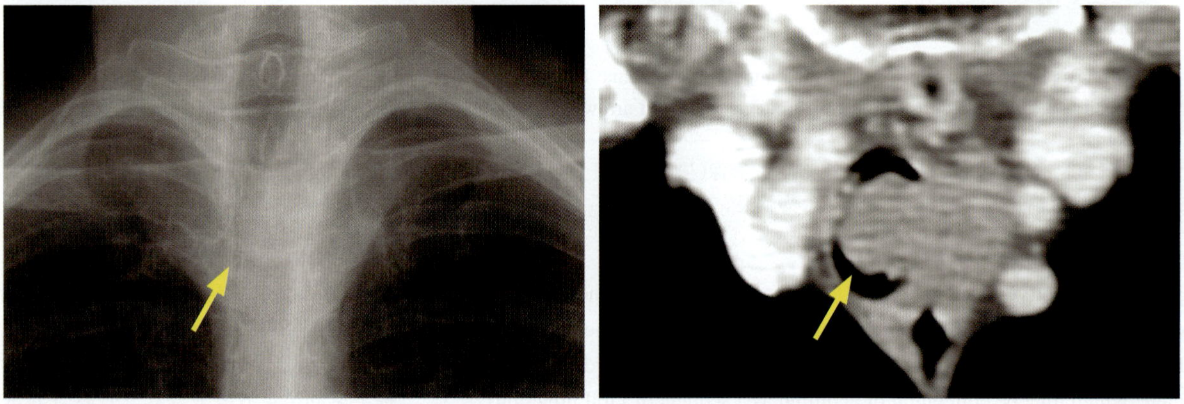

Endotracheal squamous cell carcinoma: Radiograph shows a tracheal luminal narrowing (arrow) at the level of the thoracic inlet. On CT there is an eccentric enhancing mass invading the left tracheal wall and markedly narrowing the tracheal lumen (arrow).
气管内鳞状细胞癌：X线影像显示胸腔入口处的气管腔狭窄(黄箭)。CT显示一个侵及气管左侧壁的偏心性肿块，有强化，且气管腔明显变窄(黄箭)。

- Squamous cell carcinoma is the most common primary tracheal malignancy. It is strongly associated with cigarette smoking.
- The typical CT appearance of tracheal squamous cell carcinoma is a polypoid intraluminal mass. The contours of the mass can be irregular, smooth, or lobulated. The tumor can occasionally invade into the esophagus, causing tracheoesophageal fistula.

- 鳞状细胞癌是最常见的原发性气管恶性肿瘤。它与吸烟密切相关。
- 气管鳞状细胞癌在CT上的典型表现为腔内息肉状肿块。肿块边缘可为不规则、光滑或呈分叶状。肿瘤偶尔可侵及食管，形成气管食管瘘。

Adenoid cystic carcinoma (ACC)

腺样囊性癌(ACC)

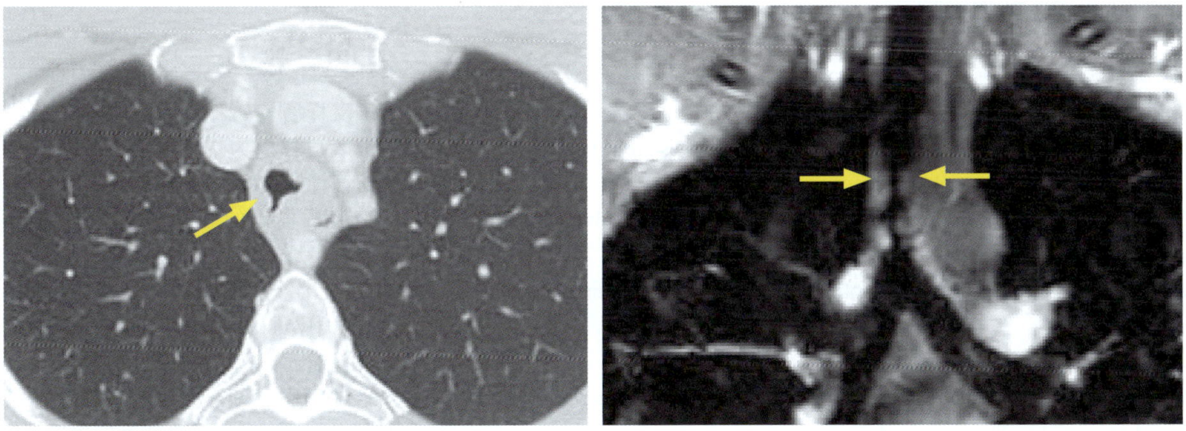

Tracheal adenoid cystic carcinoma: CT (left image) shows irregular circumferential tracheal thickening (arrow). Post-contrast coronal T1-weighted MRI (right image) shows an enhancing nodular mass extending into the tracheal lumen (arrows). *Case courtesy Ritu R. Gill, MD, MPH, Brigham and Women's Hospital.*

气管腺样囊性癌：CT(左图)显示气管不规则环形增厚(黄箭)。MRI冠状位增强T_1加权(右图)显示一个强化的结节样肿块突入气管腔(黄箭)。

- Adenoid cystic carcinoma (ACC) is a relatively low grade malignancy that usually affects patients in their forties, a decade or two younger than the typical SCC patient. It is not associated with cigarette smoking.
- ACC has a propensity for perineural and submucosal spread. It may spread over a long segment of the trachea, complicating the ability to resect the lesion.
- The typical CT appearance of ACC is a submucosal mass that infiltrates the tracheal wall and surrounding mediastinal fat. ACC may also present as circumferential tracheal or bronchial thickening causing airway stenosis.

- 腺样囊性癌(ACC)是一种恶性程度相对较低的肿瘤，通常发生于40多岁的成人，较鳞状细胞癌的患者年轻10~20岁，与吸烟无关。
- ACC易沿神经周围和黏膜下蔓延。它可能累及长段气管，增加了病变的切除难度。
- ACC的典型CT表现为黏膜下肿块，浸润气管壁和周围纵隔脂肪。ACC也可表现为气管或支气管环形增厚从而导致气道狭窄。

Carcinoid

类癌

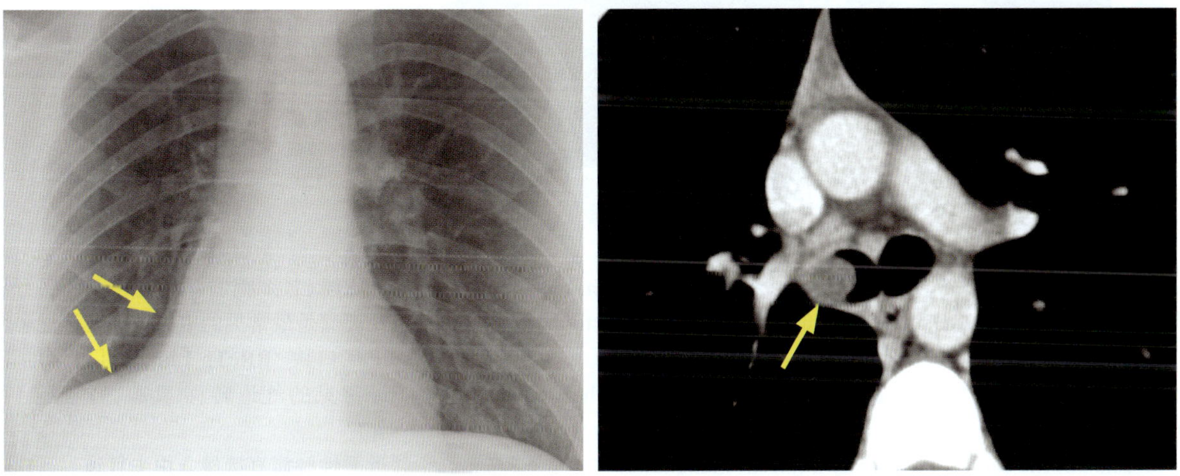

Endobronchial carcinoid: Chest radiograph shows right lower lobe atelectasis (arrows) and volume loss. Axial contrast-enhanced CT shows a mildly enhancing well-circumscribed endobronchial mass (arrow) in the right mainstem bronchus just distal to the carina.

支气管内类癌：胸部X线影像显示右下叶肺不张(黄箭)和肺体积减小。轴位增强CT显示在隆突远端右主支气管内有一个轻度强化、边界清楚的肿块(黄箭)。

- Carcinoid almost always occurs distal to the carina.
- CT shows an endoluminal bronchial mass that may calcify and often enhances avidly. Note that carcinoid tumors tend to have a larger extrinsic component than endobronchial component.

- 类癌几乎都发生在隆突的远端。
- CT显示为一个支气管腔内肿块，可钙化，常有显著强化。注意，类癌在支气管外的部分往往比支气管腔内部分更大。

In addition to carcinoid, the differential diagnosis of an enhancing endobronchial mass includes **mucoepidermoid carcinoma** and very rare entities such as **hemangioma** and **glomus tumor**.

除了类癌，支气管内强化肿块的鉴别诊断还包括**黏液表皮样癌**和一些非常罕见的疾病，如**血管瘤**和**血管球瘤**。

Mucoepidermoid carcinoma

- Mucoepidermoid carcinoma is a rare tumor that originates from tiny salivary glands lining the tracheobronchial tree.
- Mucoepidermoid carcinoma tends to affect younger patients than adenoid cystic carcinoma.
- CT appearance is a round or oval endobronchial mass, indistinguishable from carcinoid.

黏液表皮样癌

- 黏液表皮样癌为一种罕见的肿瘤，起源于气管支气管树表面的微小唾液腺。
- 黏液表皮样癌的好发年龄通常低于腺样囊性癌。
- CT表现为支气管内一个圆形或卵圆形的肿块，与类癌难以区分。

Tracheal lymphoma

- Tracheal lymphoma is rare. It is usually associated with mucosa-associated lymphoid tissue (MALT), a low-grade malignancy.

气管淋巴瘤

- 气管淋巴瘤罕见，通常与黏膜相关淋巴组织(MALT)有关，是一种低级别的恶性肿瘤。

Endobronchial metastasis

支气管内转移

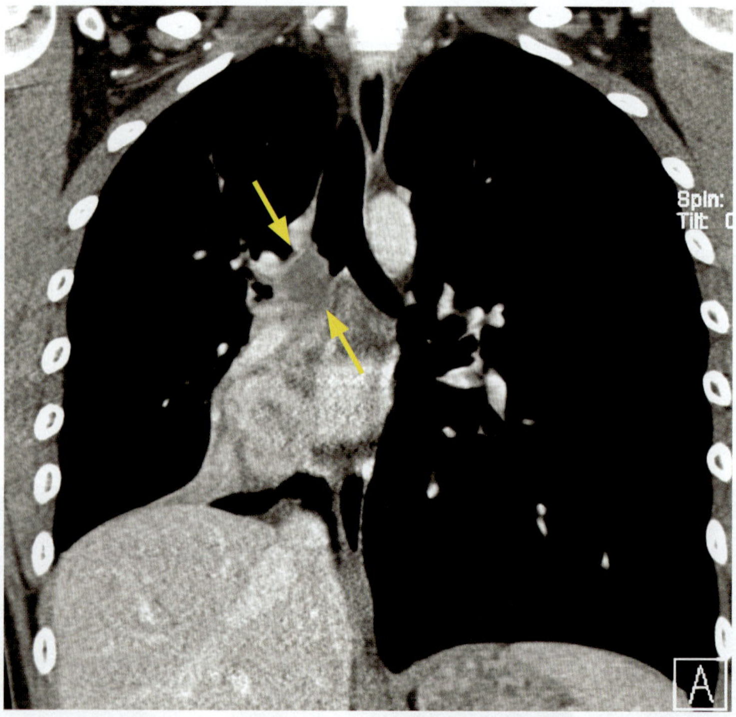

Endobronchial metastasis:
Coronal contrast-enhanced CT demonstrates a heterogeneously enhancing mass, which invades the right mainstem bronchus (arrows). This was a spindle-cell carcinoma, but the imaging appearance is nonspecific.
支气管内转移：冠状位增强CT显示不均匀强化肿块侵入右主支气管(黄箭)。此为梭形细胞癌，但影像学表现没有特异性。

- Breast cancer, renal cell carcinoma, thyroid cancer, lung cancer, melanoma, and sarcoma are the most common malignancies to metastasize to the central airways.
- The mnemonic **BReTh Lung** may be helpful to remember the four most common airway metastases (breast, renal cell, thyroid, and lung).

- 乳腺癌、肾细胞癌、甲状腺癌、肺癌、黑色素瘤及肉瘤是最常见的中央气道转移性恶性肿瘤。
- 记忆口诀"**BReTh Lung**"可以帮助记忆4种最常见的气道转移(乳腺、肾细胞、甲状腺、肺)。

Direct invasion of the central airways by adjacent malignancy

- Direct central airway invasion occurs more commonly than endobronchial metastases. Aggressive laryngeal, thyroid, esophageal, and lung cancer may cause direct airway invasion.

邻近恶性肿瘤直接侵入中央气道

- 中央气道直接受侵较支气管内转移更为常见。恶性程度高的喉癌、甲状腺癌、食管癌和肺癌都可以直接侵犯气道。

Benign endobronchial lesions

- **Papilloma** is a benign but potentially pre-malignant lesion that may transform into carcinoma. Suspected papillomas are typically closely followed.

  A single papilloma is usually caused by chronic irritation.

  Multiple papillomas (laryngotracheal papillomatosis) is caused by HPV, which may be acquired at birth. Distribution is usually centered in the larynx, with tracheobronchial

良性支气管内病变

- **乳头状瘤**是一种良性但可能转化为癌的潜在癌前病变。怀疑为乳头状瘤者通常需密切随访。

  单发乳头状瘤多由慢性刺激引起。

  多发乳头状瘤(喉气管乳头状瘤病)由人乳头状瘤

involvement in 1–5% of cases.

Papillomas may spread to the lungs, where they will form multiple cavitary nodules with dependent distribution.

- **Chondroma** is a benign cartilaginous tumor that rarely may occur in the airways.
- Other benign endobronchial lesions include schwannoma, adenoma, hamartoma, hemangioma, lipoma, and leiomyoma.

病毒(HPV)引起，可能在出生时被感染。分布多集中在喉部，1%~5%的病例累及气管支气管。

乳头状瘤可扩散至肺，可形成多发空洞性结节并按重力分布。

- **软骨瘤**是一种良性软骨肿瘤，极少发生于气道。
- 其他良性支气管内病变包括施万细胞瘤、腺瘤、错构瘤、血管瘤、脂肪瘤和平滑肌瘤。

Emphysema

- Emphysema is the destruction of alveolar walls resulting in irreversible enlargement of the distal airspaces.
- Elastase is produced by alveolar macrophages and neutrophils, both of which are increased in smokers. Elastase is a powerful destructive enzyme which functions in the host defense mechanism, but excess elastase can be highly harmful to the native tissues. Alpha-1- antitrypsin normally neutralizes elastase. Either a surplus of elastase (in smoking-related emphysema) or insufficient neutralizing enzyme (in alpha-1-antitrypsin deficiency) can cause lung destruction and resultant emphysema.

肺气肿

- 肺气肿是肺泡壁受损导致远端气腔出现不可逆扩张。
- 弹性蛋白酶由肺泡巨噬细胞和中性粒细胞产生，而吸烟者中这两种细胞均有增加。弹性蛋白酶是一种破坏性很强的酶，在宿主的防御机制中发挥作用。但过多的弹性蛋白酶会对自体组织造成严重损害。α1-抗胰蛋白酶正常情况下会中和弹性蛋白酶。弹性蛋白酶过多(吸烟相关肺气肿)或中和酶不足(α1-抗胰蛋白酶缺乏)均会导致肺组织破坏并引起肺气肿。

Centrilobular emphysema

小叶中央型肺气肿

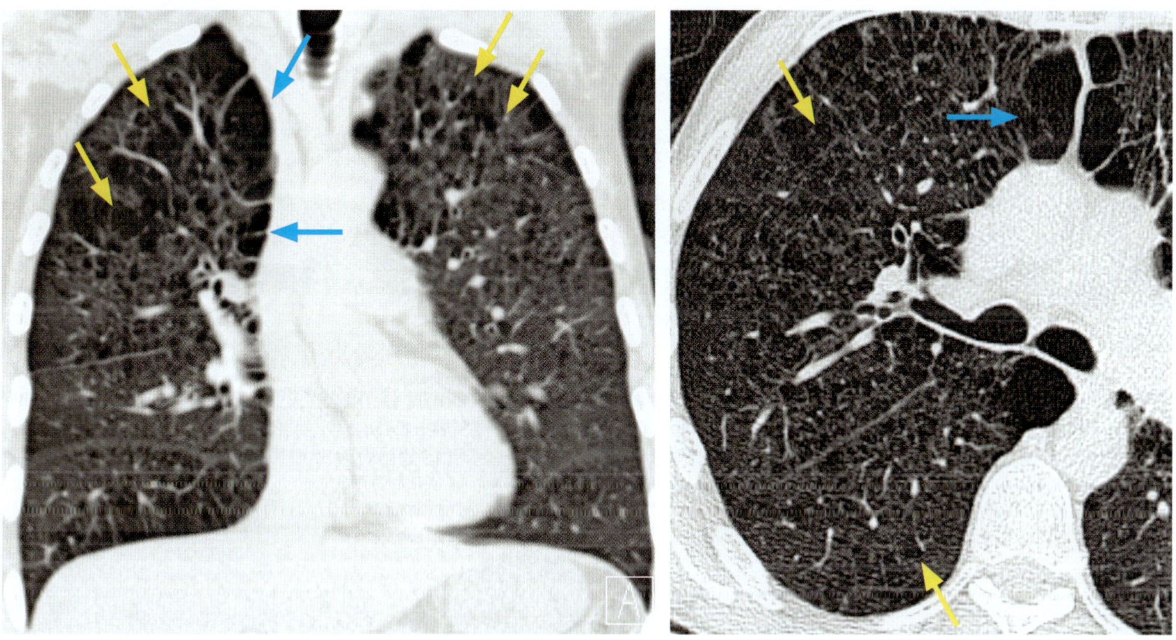

Centrilobular and paraseptal emphysema: Coronal (left image) and axial CT demonstrates both centrilobular and paraseptal emphysema. Centrilobular emphysema is predominant in the upper lobes (yellow arrows) and paraseptal emphysema is seen anteromedially (blue arrows).

小叶中央型及间隔旁型肺气肿：冠状位(左图)和轴位CT(右图)显示小叶中央型和间隔旁型肺气肿。小叶中央型肺气肿主要位于上叶(黄箭)，而间隔旁型肺气肿则见于前内侧(蓝箭)。

- Centrilobular emphysema is a smoking-related lung disease.
- Centrilobular emphysema predominantly affects the upper lobes. Like RB-ILD, another smoking-related lung disease, centrilobular emphysema primarily affects the center of the secondary pulmonary lobule.

All smoking-related lung disease (RB, RB-ILD, DIP, PLCH, and emphysema) may

- 小叶中央型肺气肿是一种与吸烟相关的肺部疾病。
- 小叶中央型肺气肿主要累及肺上叶。与另一种吸烟相关肺疾病RB-ILD相似，小叶中央型肺气肿主要累及次级肺小叶的中央。

be within the same spectrum of disease caused by macrophage-mediated inflammation in reaction to inhaled particles and toxins.

所有吸烟相关性肺疾病(RB、RB-ILD、DIP、PLCH和肺气肿)可能属于同一疾病谱，为巨噬细胞对吸入的颗粒物和毒素所介导的炎症反应所致。

Paraseptal emphysema

- Paraseptal emphysema is usually seen in combination with other forms of emphysema. It is also usually smoking related.
- Paraseptal emphysema is subpleural in location and may predispose to pneumothorax.

间隔旁型肺气肿

- 间隔旁型肺气肿通常与其他类型的肺气肿合并存在。此病也与吸烟有关。
- 间隔旁型肺气肿位于胸膜下，易造成气胸。

Panacinar (panlobular) emphysema

- Panacinar (also called panlobular) emphysema affects the entire acinus diffusely throughout the lung. The emphysematous changes are usually more severe at the lung bases.
- Alpha-1-antitrypsin deficiency is the main cause of panacinar emphysema.

全腺泡(全小叶)型肺气肿

- 全腺泡(又称全小叶)型肺气肿累及整个肺腺泡，弥漫分布于全肺。肺气肿改变通常在肺基底部更加严重。
- α1-抗胰蛋白酶缺乏是全腺泡型肺气肿的主要原因。

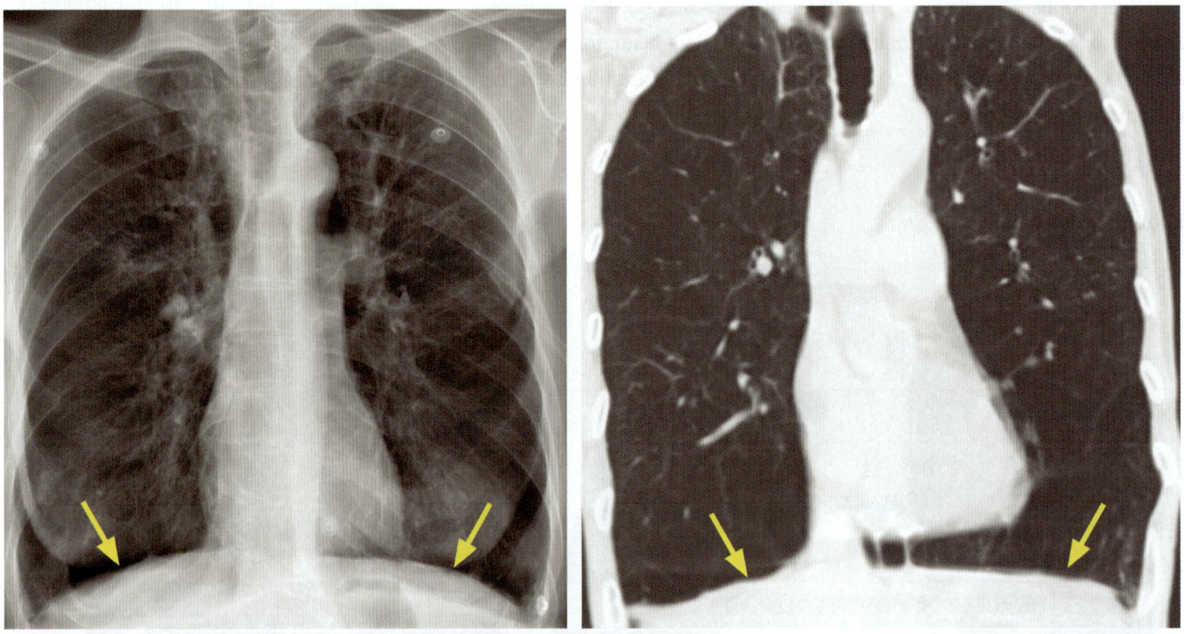

Panacinar emphysema due to alpha-1-antitrypsin deficiency: Frontal radiograph and coronal CT show diffuse emphysematous changes most severely affecting the lower lobes, with flattening of the diaphragms (arrows).

α1-抗胰蛋白酶缺乏导致的全腺泡型肺气肿：正位X线影像和冠状位CT显示弥漫的肺气肿改变，以双肺下叶为著，伴横膈变平(黄箭)。

（翻译　于瀛）

PLEURA

胸膜

PLEURAL MALIGNANCY

胸膜恶性肿瘤

Metastatic disease

- Metastatic disease is the most common cause of pleural malignancy.
- Lung and breast cancer, gastrointestinal and genitourinary adenocarcinoma, and invasive thymoma can metastasize to the pleura.

转移性疾病

- 转移瘤是胸膜恶性肿瘤最常见的原因。
- 肺癌和乳腺癌、胃肠道和泌尿生殖系统腺癌，以及侵袭性胸腺瘤都可转移到胸膜。

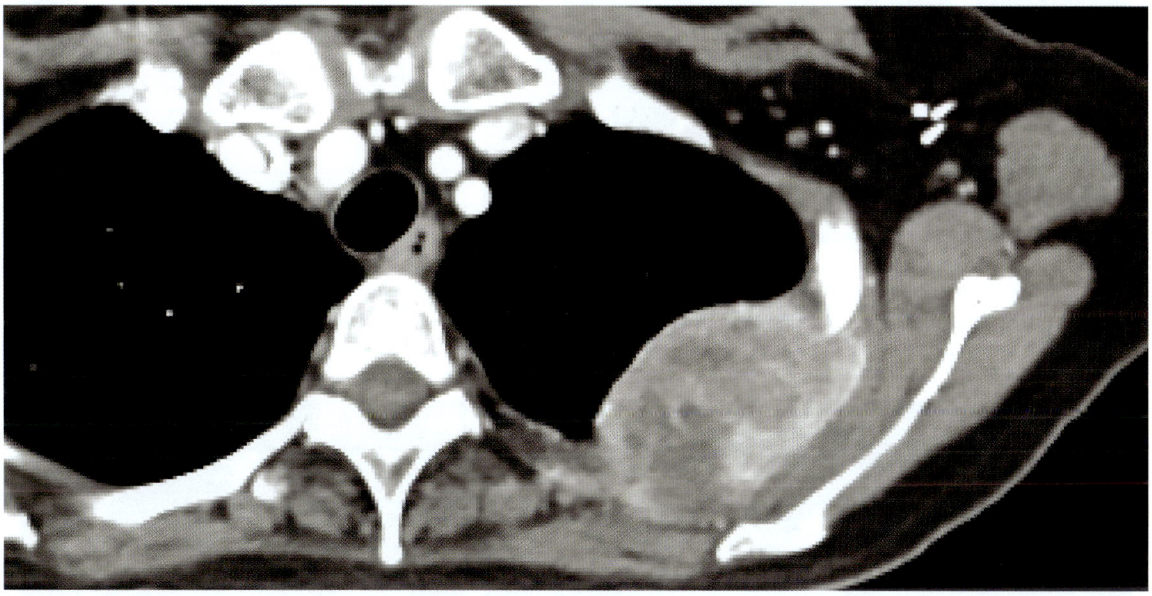

Chest wall metastases: Axial CT image shows a heterogeneously enhancing mass invading the chest wall and adjacent pleural of the left lung. This was a case of breast cancer metastasis.
胸壁转移瘤：轴位CT图像显示一个强化不均匀的肿块，累及胸壁及邻近左肺胸膜。这是一例乳腺癌转移。

Features to help differentiate malignant pleural effusions

- Unexplained recurrent pleural effusions should raise suspicion for underlying malignancy regardless of associated visualized pleural nodularity.
- The split pleura sign is characteristic of an empyema, formed by fibrin coating both parietal and visceral pleuras resulting in in-growth of blood vessels. Although rare, empyema can be seen in lung cancer.
- Features of malignant effusion include:

Nodular pleural thickening.
Large or recurrent effusion without etiology.
Thickening of mediastinal (medial) pleura.

有助于鉴别恶性胸腔积液的征象

- 不明原因的顽固性胸腔积液都需怀疑恶性肿瘤的可能，无论是否有可见的胸膜结节。
- 胸膜分裂征是脓胸的特征，由覆盖壁胸膜和脏胸膜的纤维蛋白导致形成血管内生。脓胸也可见于肺癌，但少见。
- 恶性积液的特征包括：

结节性胸膜增厚。
无原因的大量或顽固性积液。
纵隔(内侧)胸膜增厚。

Multiple myeloma/plasmacytoma

- Osseous metastases may have soft tissue components that are extrapleural, which may secondarily invade the pleura.

多发性骨髓瘤/浆细胞瘤

- 骨转移瘤可有软组织成分，这些成分位于胸膜外，可继发侵犯胸膜。

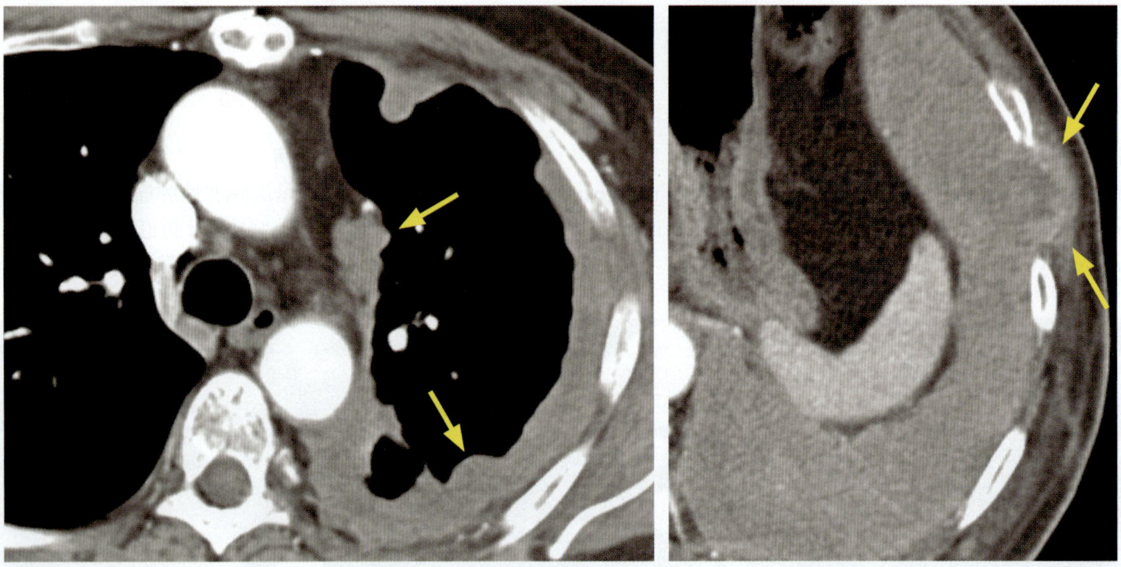

Mesothelioma: Contrast-enhanced CT through the thorax (left image) shows extensive nodular pleural thickening of the left hemithorax (arrows). Images through the upper abdomen show extensive soft tissue abnormality with invasion of the chest wall (arrows).
间皮瘤：胸部增强CT(左图)显示左侧胸膜弥漫性结节状增厚(黄箭)。上腹部图像(右图)显示广泛的软组织异常并侵犯胸壁(黄箭)。

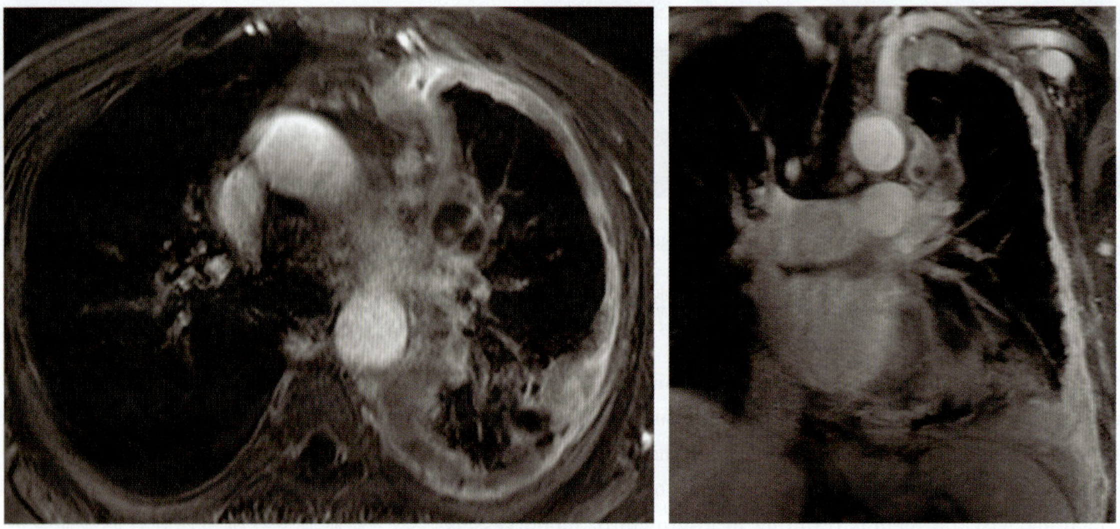

Mesothelioma (in different patient from above): Axial (left image) and coronal T1-weighted post-contrast fat- suppressed MR images demonstrate circumferential nodular thickening of the left pleura.
间皮瘤(与上图患者不同)：轴位(左图)和冠状位(右图)T_1加权增强后脂肪抑制MRI显示左侧胸膜环周结节状增厚。

- Mesothelioma is a highly aggressive neoplasm arising from the pleura. Most cases are due to prior asbestos exposure, with a latency of >20 years.
- The epithelial subtype is more common and has a slightly better prognosis. Sarcomatoid and mixed subtypes are more aggressive.
- CT of mesothelioma typically shows nodular concentric pleural thickening, often with an associated pleural effusion.
- The role of surgery is evolving, with the goal to resect all visible tumor. Trimodality therapy involving surgery, intraoperative heated chemotherapy, and radiation has been shown to provide benefit for a subset of patients.

Fibrous tumor of the pleura (FTP)

- Fibrous tumor of the pleura (FTP), also known as **solitary fibrous tumor**, is a focal pleural mass not related to asbestos or mesothelioma. It is not mesothelial

- 间皮瘤为起源于胸膜的高度侵袭性肿瘤。多数病例既往有石棉接触史，潜伏期至少20年。
- 上皮型间皮瘤更为常见且预后稍好；肉瘤样型和混合型更具侵袭性。
- 间皮瘤的典型CT表现为结节状向心性胸膜增厚，常伴有胸腔积液。
- 手术的作用在不断发展，目标是切除所有可见的肿瘤。三联疗法包括手术、术中热化疗和放疗，已证实对部分患者有效。

胸膜纤维性肿瘤(FTP)

- 胸膜纤维性肿瘤(FTP)又称**孤立性纤维性肿瘤**，是一种局灶性的胸膜肿块，与石棉或间皮

in origin.

瘤无关，并非起源于间皮细胞。

- Approximately 20–30% of FTP are malignant, so all are excised. Malignant potential is determined by number of mitoses seen at pathology.
- FTP may be associated with hypoglycemia or hypertrophic pulmonary osteoarthropathy, although these associated conditions are uncommon (5%).
- FTP may be pedunculated. A pleural based mass that changes position is suggestive of FTP. FTP tends to have low FDG uptake on PET.

- 约20%~30%的FTP是恶性的，所以均需切除。恶性潜能取决于病理上有丝分裂的数目。
- FTP可能与低血糖症和肥大性肺性骨关节病相关，尽管这些相关疾病并不常见(5%)。
- FTP可有蒂。位置可变化的胸膜肿块提示FTP。FTP在PET上氟代脱氧葡萄糖(FDG)的摄取较低。

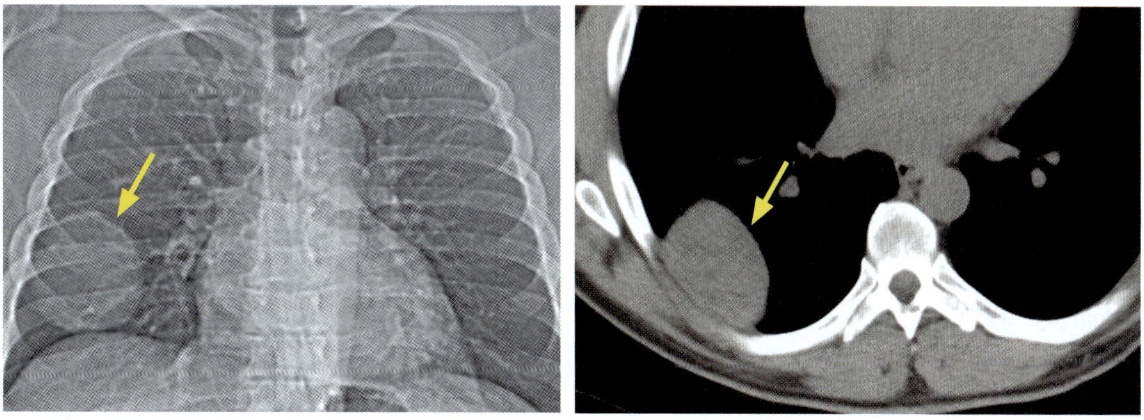

Fibrous tumor of the pleura: CT topogram (left image) shows a round opacity (arrow) with a circumscribed medial margin and indistinct lateral margin, suggesting a pleural-based mass. CT confirms that the mass (arrow) is pleural-based, with a broad attachment to the pleura.
Case courtesy Ritu R. Gill, MD, MPH, Brigham and Women's Hospital.
胸膜纤维性肿瘤：CT定位图(左图)显示一个圆形高密度影(黄箭)，其内侧缘边界清晰而外侧缘模糊，提示胸膜肿块。CT证实该肿块(黄箭)来自胸膜，广泛附着在胸膜之上。

Pleural effusion

Transudate

- A transudative effusion is caused by systemic or local imbalances in hydrostatic and oncotic forces. Common causes include systemic low-protein states, heart failure, and nephrotic syndrome.

Exudate

- An exudative effusion is distinguished from a transudate by thoracentesis. There are no reliable imaging features to distinguish between transudative and exudative effusions.
- The presence of an exudate implies pleural disease causing increased permeability of pleural capillaries, which may be due to:

> **Pneumonia** with parapneumonic effusion, **empyema**, or **tuberculous** pleuritis.
> **Mesothelioma** or pleural **metastasis**.
> **Rheumatoid arthritis** or other collagen vascular diseases.

Chylothorax

- A chylothorax is a pleural effusion consisting of intestinal lymph, most commonly caused by iatrogenic injury, less commonly neoplastic obstruction of the thoracic duct. Chylothorax is also associated with lymphangioleiomyomatosis (LAM).
- The thoracic duct originates at the cisterna chyli in the upper abdomen and drains into the left brachiocephalic or subclavian vein.

胸腔积液

漏出液

- 漏出液是由于全身或局部流体静力学和胶体渗透压不平衡所致。常见的原因为全身性低蛋白血症、心力衰竭和肾病综合征。

渗出液

- 可以通过胸腔穿刺术鉴别渗出液与漏出液。没有可靠的影像学特征来区分漏出液和渗出液。
- 出现渗出液提示胸膜疾病导致胸膜毛细血管通透性增加，可能的原因有：

> **肺炎**伴肺炎旁积液、**脓胸**或**结核**性胸膜炎。
> **间皮瘤**或胸膜**转移瘤**。
> **类风湿关节炎**或其他胶原血管病。

乳糜胸

- 乳糜胸是一种由肠道淋巴液组成的胸腔积液，最常见的原因为医源性损伤，其次为肿瘤性胸导管阻塞。乳糜胸也与淋巴管平滑肌瘤病(LAM)有关。
- 胸导管起源于上腹部的乳糜池，引流入左侧头臂静脉或锁骨下静脉。

（翻译　于瀛）

2 Gastrointestinal Imaging

2 胃肠道影像

Cory Robinson-Weiss, Fiona E. Malone, Ellen X. Sun, Junzi Shi, Khushboo Jhala, Shanna A. Matalon

Contents

目录

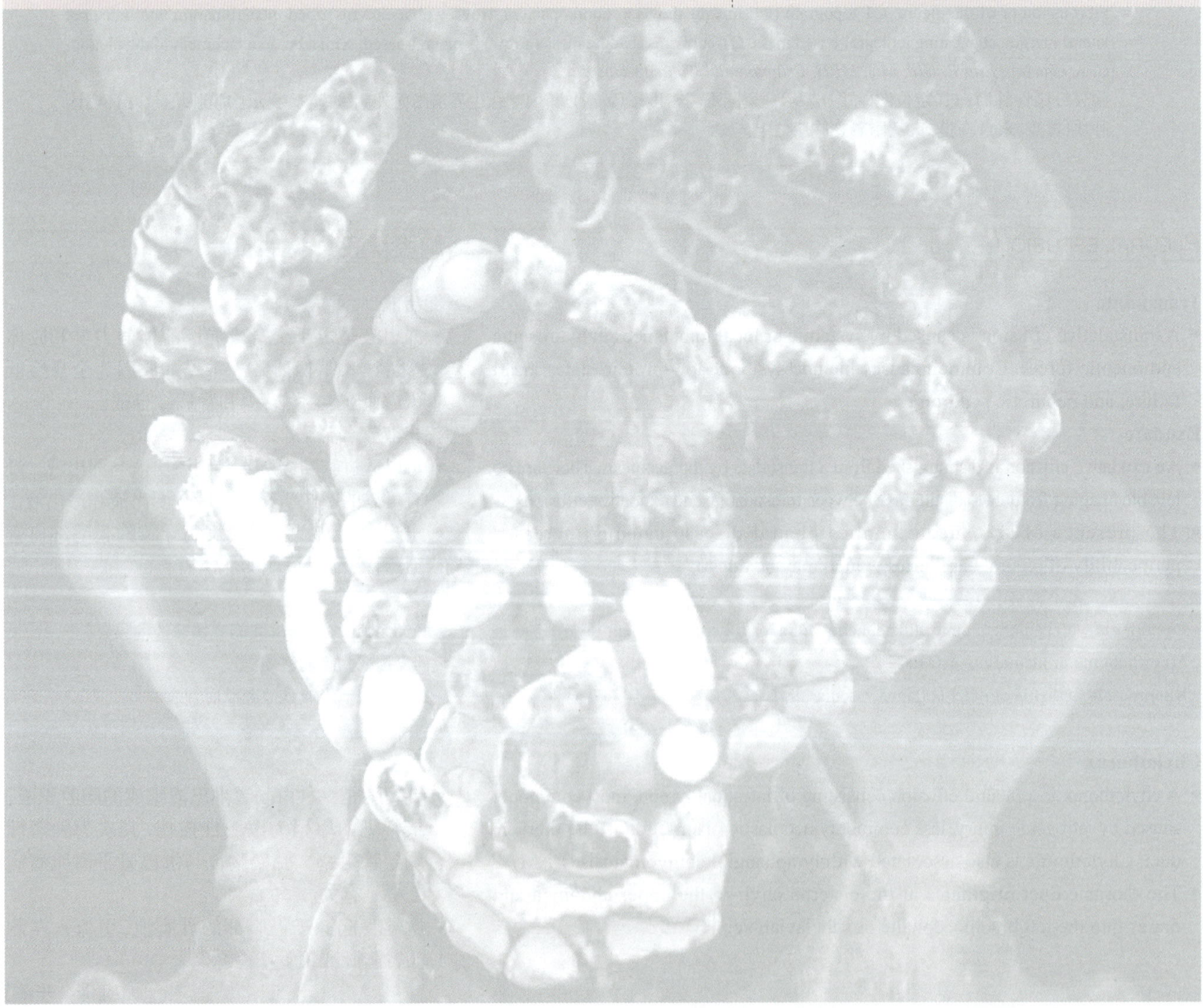

LIVER

肝脏

LIVER ANATOMY

- The Couinaud classification divides the liver into eight segments. Because each segment is self-contained with its own vascular inflow, outflow, and biliary drainage, an individual segment can be completely resected without disturbing the other segments.
- Numbering of hepatic segments is clockwise when looking at a frontal/coronal view.

肝脏解剖

- Couinaud分段法将肝脏分为8段。由于每一个肝段都有独立的动脉、静脉和胆道引流系统，所以切除一个完整的肝段不影响其他肝段。
- 在正面或冠状面视图上按顺时针方向进行肝段编号。

1 (caudate) not visible in frontal view
1（尾状叶）在正面看不到

*typically segments 6 and 7 are posterior and not visible on the frontal view.
*肝6、7段通常位于后方，在正面看不到。

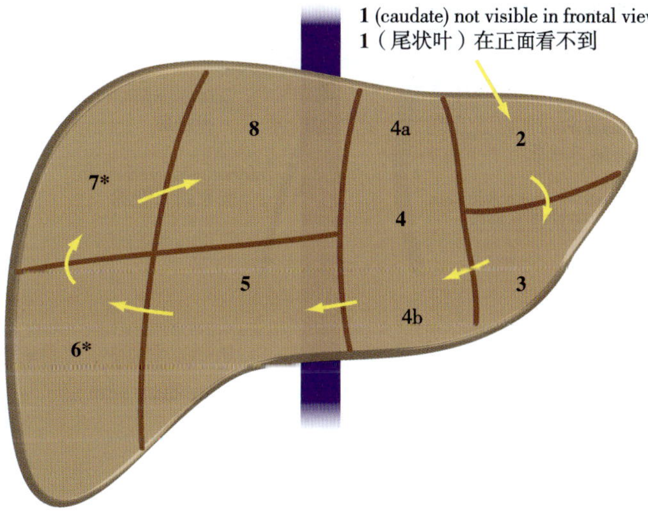

The portal veins divide the superior from inferior segments, while the hepatic veins form the segmental borders in the axial plane. The middle hepatic vein divides the left (segments 2–4) from right (segments 5–8) lobes of the liver.
门静脉将肝段分为上、下段，肝静脉在轴位平面上形成肝段的边界。
肝中静脉将肝脏分为左叶(2~4段)和右叶(5~8段)。

axial view above the portal veins
门静脉上方的轴位图

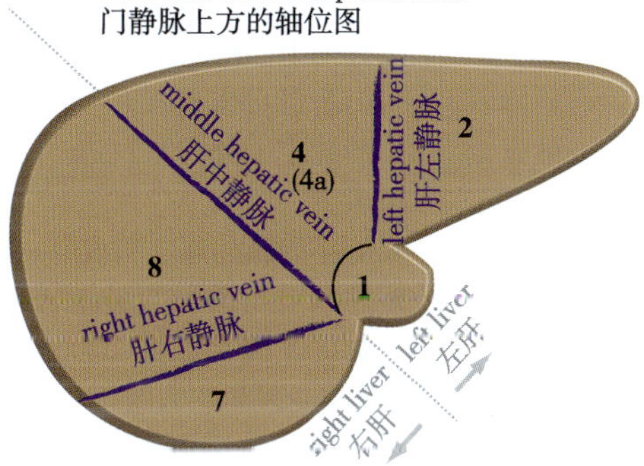

coronal view
冠状位图

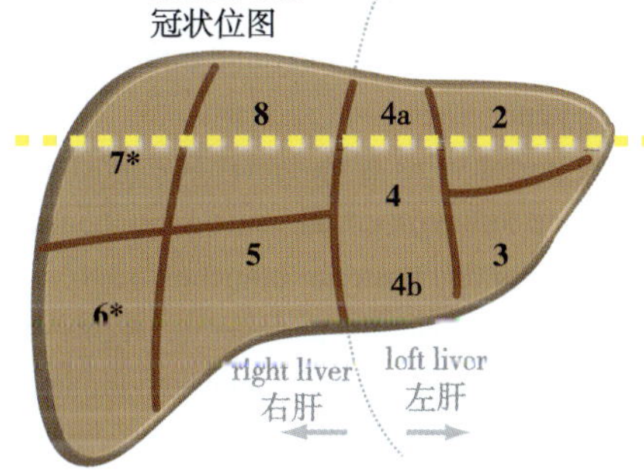

axial view below the portal veins
门静脉下方轴位图

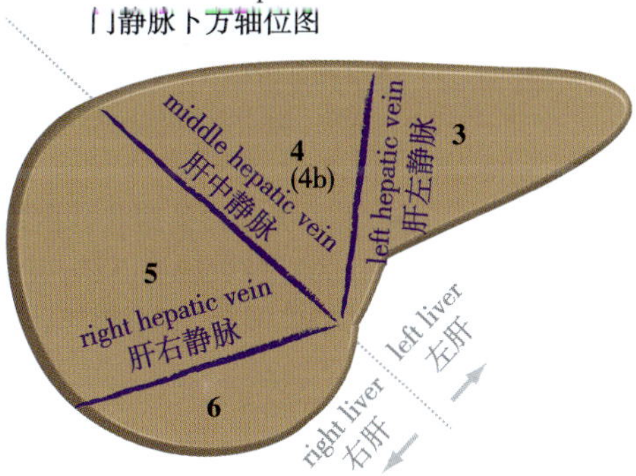

coronal view
冠状位图

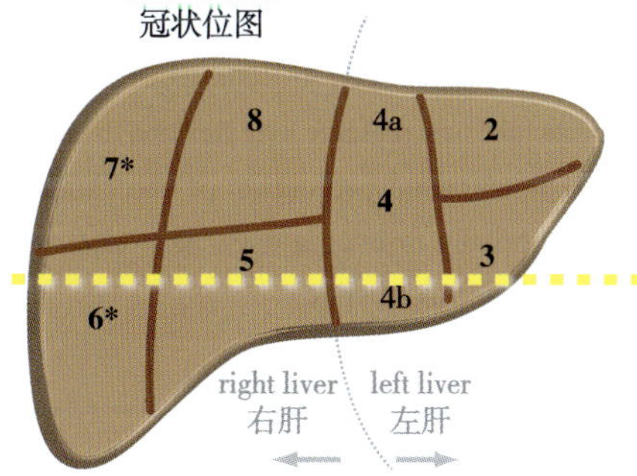

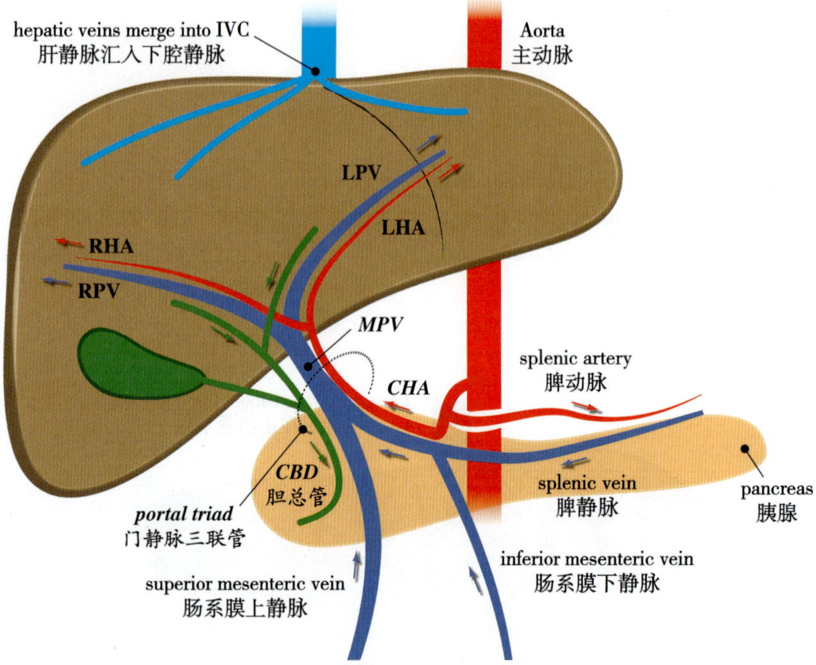

RHA = right hepatic artery
RHA = 肝右动脉
LHA = left hepatic artery
LHA = 肝左动脉
CHA = common hepatic artery
CHA = 肝总动脉
RPV = right portal vein
RPV = 门静脉右支
LPV = left portal vein
LPV = 门静脉左支
MPV = main portal vein
MPV = 门静脉主干

- Each hepatic segment features its own:

  Central portal triad made up of a portal vein, hepatic artery, and bile duct, with peripheral venous drainage to the hepatic veins and ultimately the IVC.
- Mnemonic for remembering the segments:

  Superior segments, from left to right: 2, 4, 8, 7, 1 (caudate). 2 doubled is 4; 4 doubled is 8; 8 minus 1 is 7.

  Inferior segments, from left to right: 3, 4, 5, 6.
- Segments 2, 3, and 4 are in the left lobe of the liver.
- Segments 5, 6, 7, 8 are in the right lobe of the liver.
- The left and right main portal veins divide the superior from the inferior segments and continue to branch superiorly and inferiorly before terminating in the center of each segment.
- The branching of the portal veins is variable. The most common pattern is a bifurcation into right and left main portal veins, with the right main portal vein then branching into anterior and posterior branches.
- Small hepatic vein tributaries mark the peripheral margins of each segment.
- The caudate lobe drains directly to the IVC, not into the hepatic veins. For this reason, the caudate lobe is often not affected in early cirrhosis since the direct drainage to the IVC spares the caudate from increased venous pressures due to portal hypertension. This leads to compensatory hypertrophy of the caudate lobe, which is a typical morphologic change of early cirrhosis.

  Similarly, direct venous drainage to the IVC allows the caudate lobe to bypass the increased hepatic venous pressures seen in Budd-Chiari syndrome. Compensatory hypertrophy of the caudate lobe may preserve liver function in these patients.
- The papillary process is a medial projection of the caudate lobe and can be mistaken for lymphadenopathy or even a mass as it may appear separate from the medial process on a single axial slice.

- 每一个肝段都有独自的特征：

  门静脉、肝动脉、胆管构成门静脉三联管，而外周肝静脉引流到肝静脉，最终汇入下腔静脉。
- 肝段简易记忆法：

  上段，从左至右：2、4、8、7、1(尾状叶)。2的倍数是4；4的倍数是8；8减1是7。

  下段，从左至右：3、4、5、6。
- 2、3、4段位于肝左叶。
- 5、6、7、8段位于肝右叶。
- 门静脉左、右主干将肝分为上、下段，后者继续向上、下发出分支并终止于各肝段的中央。
- 门静脉分支有多种变异。最常见的类型为门静脉主干分为左、右支，门静脉右支又分为前、后支。
- 肝小静脉的属支构成每一肝段的边界。
- 尾状叶的静脉直接汇入下腔静脉，而非肝静脉。正因为如此，尾状叶在肝硬化早期不受影响，因为它直接汇入下腔静脉，可使其免受门静脉高压造成静脉压力升高的影响，导致尾状叶代偿性肥大，此为肝硬化早期的特征性形态改变。

  同样的道理，在布-加综合征患者中，由于尾状叶血流直接汇入下腔静脉，避免了肝静脉压力增高的影响。尾状叶代偿性肥大使这些患者的肝功能维持正常。
- 乳头状突起是尾状叶的内侧突起，可能被误认为是肿大的淋巴结，甚至是肿块，因为在某些轴位图上，它可能与肝内侧面是分开的。

IMAGING OF THE LIVER

Liver CT

- A "routine" contrast-enhanced abdominal CT is acquired in the portal venous phase of enhancement, obtained 70 seconds following intravenous contrast administration.
- In the portal venous phase, the portal veins should be fully opacified and contrast should also be seen in the hepatic veins. The liver should be homogeneously enhancing, allowing detection of attenuation alterations and/or morphologic changes of diffuse liver disease, such as hepatic steatosis and cirrhosis. As most metastatic tumors are not hypervascular (with a few notable exceptions, which will be subsequently discussed), liver metastases can also generally be detected on the portal venous phase as hypoattenuating masses. Of note, some breast cancers may rarely be isoattenuating on the portal venous phase and may be more conspicuous on unenhanced CT.
- Most benign and malignant primary liver masses are hypervascular and thus are most conspicuous in the late arterial phase of enhancement (~45 seconds). If the patient has a known hypervascular primary malignancy, both a late arterial phase and portal venous phase may be obtained for metastatic workup and restaging. If the patient has a suspected primary liver mass (such as hemangioma, focal nodular hyperplasia, hepatocellular carcinoma), a multiphase CT or MRI may be obtained, usually including a noncontrast, arterial phase, portal venous phase and delayed phase.

Liver MRI

- Compared to CT, MRI of the liver has superior lesion-to-liver contrast.
- MRI also does not impart ionizing radiation, allowing for dynamic post-contrast imaging in multiple phases without any penalty in radiation exposure to the patient. In- and out- of-phase gradient imaging allows for detection of intracytoplasmic lipid, which is seen in hepatic steatosis and may be seen within certain masses, including hepatocellular carcinoma (HCC) and adenomas. Diffusion-weighted imaging is useful for detection of metastatic lesions.
- MRI Contrast agents:

  Extracellular agents pass through the intravascular system and interstitium similarly to CT contrast.

  Gadobutrol (Gadavist) is a commonly used extracellular contrast agent that is 90% excreted through the renal system.

  Combined extracellular/hepatobiliary agents pass through the intravascular system and interstitium similarly to CT contrast, but are partially excreted through the biliary system. Gadoxetic acid disodium (Eovist) is 50% excreted through the biliary system and 50% through the renal system. Indications for use include evaluation for metastatic lesions and focal nodular hyperplasia (FNH).

肝脏影像

肝脏CT

- "常规" 腹部增强CT应在门静脉期采集，一般是静脉注入造影剂后70秒进行。
- 在门静脉期，门静脉应该完全被造影剂所充盈，同时，肝静脉内也应见到造影剂。肝脏应呈均匀性强化，这样可以使弥漫性肝病时的密度改变和/或形态学变化得以显现，如肝脂肪变性和肝硬化。大多数转移瘤不是富血供(除了小部分情况例外，下文讨论)，因而它们通常在门静脉期表现为低密度肿块。注意，极少数乳腺癌肝转移瘤在门静脉期为等密度，但在平扫CT图像上可能更为明显。
- 大多数良性和恶性原发性肝脏肿瘤是富血供的，因而在动脉晚期(约45秒)显示最明显。若患者已知有富血供的原发恶性肿瘤，动脉晚期和门静脉期图像都需要采集，以发现转移灶和进行重新分期。若患者怀疑有原发性肝脏肿瘤(如血管瘤、局灶性结节增生、肝细胞癌)则可以进行多期CT或MRI检查，通常包括平扫、动脉期、门静脉期和延迟期。

肝脏MRI

- 与CT相比，肝脏MRI具有更好的病灶与肝脏的对比度。
- MRI没有辐射，允许进行多期动态增强扫描而不对患者构成辐射威胁。同相位、反相位梯度成像可用于检测肝细胞内脂肪，如肝脂肪变性和某些特定肿瘤，包括肝细胞癌(HCC)和腺瘤。弥散加权成像有利于发现转移性病变。
- MRI造影剂(对比剂)

  细胞外造影剂能够进入血管内和间质内，与CT造影剂类似。

  钆布醇(Gadavist)是一种常用的细胞外造影剂，其中90%由肾脏排泄。

  细胞外兼肝胆造影剂能够进入血管内和间质内，与CT造影剂类似，但部分由胆道系统排泄。钆塞酸二钠(Eovist)通过胆道系统排泄50%，其余50%通过肾脏排泄。适应证包括评估转移性病变和局灶性结节增生(FNH)。

	Hepatobiliary Contrast Agent	Mechanism	Indications
Gadolinium-based, combined extracellular/hepatobiliary agents	Gadoxetic acid disodium (Eovist)	Taken up by liver in the delayed phase 50% biliary excretion	Differentiating FNH and adenoma (FNH is iso to hyperintense) Hepatic metastases (uptake excludes a metastasis from nonliver primary)
	Gadobenate dimeglumine (MultiHance)	Only 5% taken up by the liver, requires 1 hour delay	Now mainly used in pelvic, cardiac and MSK imaging
Iron oxide- based	Ferumoxides or ferumoxytol	Particles trapped by Kupffer cells and reduce T2 relaxivity, making liver or spleen dark on T2	Adjunct for detection of HCC

肝胆造影剂		机制	适应证
钆基 细胞外/肝胆共同排泄制剂	钆塞酸二钠(Eovist)	经胆道排泄在延迟期被肝脏摄取50%	鉴别局灶性结节增生(FNH)和腺瘤(FNH呈等高信号) 肝转移瘤(病灶摄取则排除非肝脏原发)
	钆苯酸葡胺(MultiHance)	只有5%被肝脏摄取,须延迟1小时	主要用于盆腔、心脏及肌骨成像
氧化铁基	氧化铁或纳米氧化铁	颗粒被库普弗细胞捕获,T_2弛豫时间降低,导致肝脏或脾脏在T_2加权上呈低信号	辅助检测肝细胞癌(HCC)

Liver ultrasound

- Ultrasound of the liver is often used to evaluate patients with abnormal LFTs, as it can identify biliary pathology and diffuse parenchymal processes. Ultrasound is commonly used as a screening tool for HCC in high-risk patients given its relatively low cost and lack of ionizing radiation. Characterization of hepatic masses, however, requires further workup with cross-sectional imaging.
- Hepatic Doppler ultrasound is a valuable tool for determining abnormal blood flow to, within, or from the liver and can also be utilized to evaluate transplants and TIPS.

肝脏超声

- 肝脏超声常用于评估肝功能异常的患者,可以用于识别胆道病变和弥漫性肝病变。超声常用于筛查有较高HCC风险的患者,因其成本相对较低且无电离辐射。然而,若要明确肝脏肿块的特征,则需要进一步行横断面影像学检查。
- 肝脏多普勒是一种有价值的工具,可用于评估肝脏的异常血流,包括流向、流经或流出肝脏的情况,同时也可用于评估肝移植和经颈静脉肝内门体分流术。

DIFFUSE PARENCHYMAL LIVER DISEASE

Hepatic steatosis

- Nonalcoholic fatty liver disease can be divided into steatosis and steatosis with associated inflammatory activity (steatohepatitis). Overall, greater than 25% of the population is afflicted with nonalcoholic fatty liver disease (NAFLD) and approximately 5% have steatohepatitis. Ultimately, steatohepatitis may progress to cirrhosis.
- Common patterns of hepatic steatosis include diffuse, focal (commonly seen in the gallbladder fossa and periportal spaces), geographic, and nodular.
- Ultrasound shows a diffuse increase in hepatic echogenicity relative to the right kidney. Normally, the liver and kidney should have the same echogenicity. Hepatic steatosis also causes increased sound attenuation, leading to poor visualization of deeper structures.

肝脏弥漫性疾病

肝脂肪变性(脂肪肝)

- 非酒精性脂肪肝可分为脂肪变性和伴随炎症活动的脂肪变性(脂肪性肝炎)。总体来说,超过25%的人群患有非酒精性脂肪肝(NAFLD),以及约5%的人患有脂肪性肝炎。脂肪性肝炎最终可进展为肝硬化。
- 肝脂肪变性常见的类型包括弥漫性、局灶性(常见于胆囊窝和门静脉周围间隙)、地图形和结节样。
- 超声表现为肝脏回声相对于右肾呈弥漫性增强。正常情况下,肝和肾应具有相同的回声。肝脂肪变性还会导致回声衰减增强,深部结构显示较差。

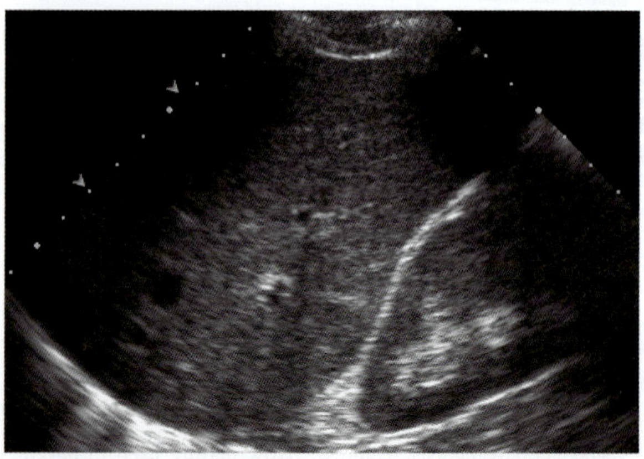

Normal liver: Ultrasound of the liver and kidney shows the normal isoechoic appearance of liver relative to renal cortex.
正常肝脏:肝脏和肾脏超声显示为肝脏相对于肾皮质呈正常的等回声。

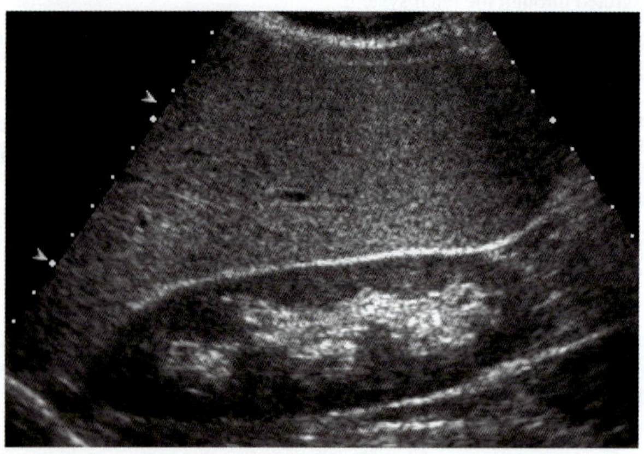

Hepatic steatosis: Ultrasound in a different patient shows diffusely increased echogenicity of the liver when compared to the renal cortex.
肝脂肪变性:另一名患者超声显示肝脏相对于肾皮质回声增强。

- CT shows decreased attenuation relative to the spleen.

  On unenhanced CT, the liver should be slightly hyperattenuating relative to the spleen. The traditional teaching is that steatosis is present if the liver attenuates at least 10 Hounsfield units (HU) less than the spleen, although new work suggests that even a single HU of relative hypoattenuation compared to the spleen may represent hepatic steatosis.

  On contrast-enhanced CT, evaluation of hepatic steatosis is less reliable compared to unenhanced CT due to different contrast uptake rates of the liver and the spleen. However, the liver is considered diffusely hypoattenuating if it attenuates at least 25 HU less than the spleen in the portal venous phase.

- MRI can determine if steatosis is present and can provide a rough gauge as to its severity. In- and out-of-phase MRI imaging can more accurately quantify the degree of steatosis, although liver biopsy is the gold standard and best evaluates for the presence of steatohepatitis and early fibrotic change.

- 肝脏CT的密度低于脾。

  在平扫CT上，肝脏相对于脾呈略高密度。传统的肝脂肪变性的教学标准是肝脏密度低于脾至少10HU，而新的研究提示，即使肝脏较脾的密度低1HU也可能是肝脂肪变性。

  增强CT评估肝脂肪变性的可靠性不及平扫CT，是由于肝脏和脾对造影剂的摄取率不同。然而，如果在门静脉期肝脏密度低于脾25HU以上，则可认为肝脏密度呈弥漫性降低。

- MRI可以确定是否存在肝脂肪变性，且可以对严重程度进行粗略评估。MRI的同相位、反相位成像可以更准确地量化肝脂肪变性的程度，而肝脏活检依然是判断脂肪性肝炎和早期纤维化的“金标准”和最佳评估方式。

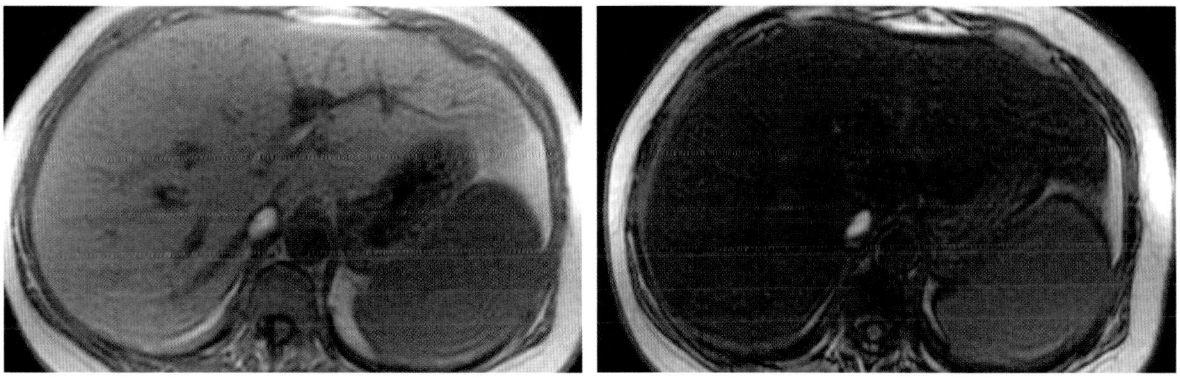

Diffuse hepatic steatosis: In- (left image) and out-of-phase (right image) images demonstrate diffuse signal loss of the liver parenchyma on out-of-phase images. When water-protons and fat-protons are present in the same MR voxel, the fat and water signals are summed in the in-phase images and subtracted in the out-of-phase images, leading to decrease in signal (hypointensity).

Case courtesy Cheryl Sadow, MD, Brigham and Women's Hospital.

弥漫性肝脂肪变性：同相位(左图)和反相位(右图)图像，显示肝实质在反相位图像上弥漫性信号降低。当水质子与脂肪质子出现在同一个磁共振体素时，水与脂肪信号在同相位图像上相加，而在反相位图像上相减(低信号)。

- Variations in portal venous supply may cause geographic regions that are affected to a greater or lesser degree by fatty change. **Focal fat** does not have any mass effect, vessels characteristically run through it, and it tends to occur in the following typical locations and distributions:

  Gallbladder fossa (drained by gallbladder vein).

  Subcapsular (along the falciform ligament).

  Periportal.

  Focal fat may also be nodular and dispersed throughout the liver.

- Ultrasound would demonstrate hyperechoic lesions, which would be hypoattenuating on CT and demonstrate drop in signal intensity on out-of-phase dual-phase GRE on MRI.

- 门静脉供血变异可导致肝脏各区域的脂肪变性程度有所不同。**局灶性脂肪**变性无占位效应，血管穿过为其特征，以下是典型的部位和分布区域：

  胆囊窝(胆囊静脉引流)。

  包膜下(沿肝镰状韧带)。

  门静脉周围。

  局灶性脂肪肝也可以呈结节状并散在分布于整个肝脏。

- 超声表现为高回声病变，而相应的区域在CT上表现为低密度，并在双相GRE MRI反相位图像上表现为信号强度降低。

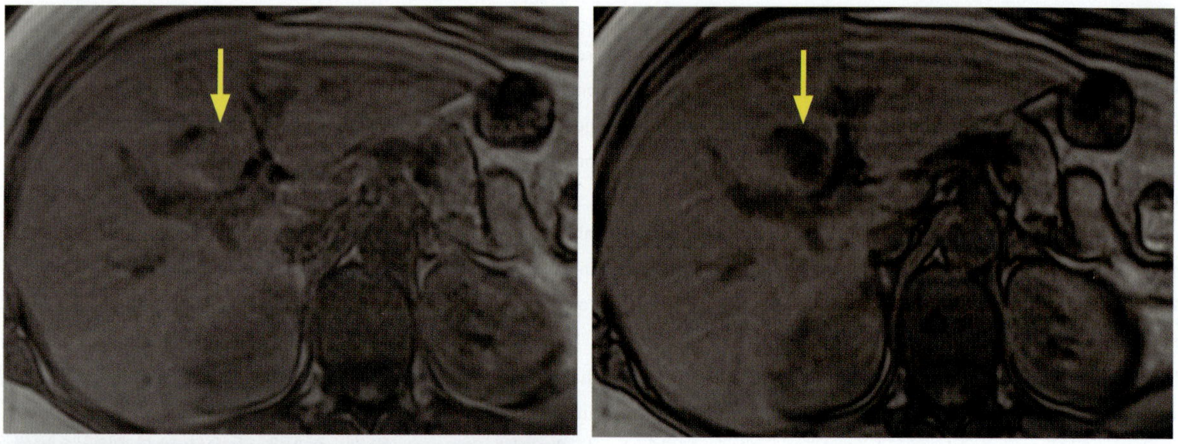

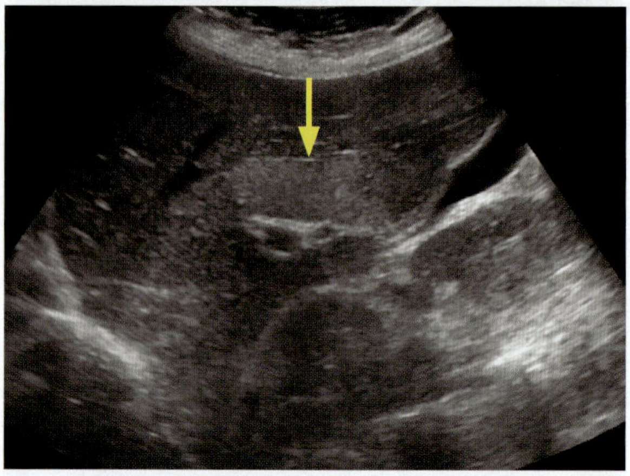

Focal fat on MRI and ultrasound:

A masslike region in hepatic segment 4 (arrows) demonstrates signal loss on out-of-phase image (top right) relative to in-phase image (top left), and has a vessel coursing through it (not well seen here), consistent with focal fat.

Grayscale ultrasound (bottom left image) in a different patient shows an echogenic mass (arrow) in the medial left hepatic lobe. This was also found to represent focal fat.

局灶性脂肪肝的MRI和超声图像：

位于肝脏4段内的肿块样病变(黄箭)在反相位图像上(右上图)相对于同相位图像(左上图)呈信号降低，并有一条血管穿过(此处显示不清)，符合局灶性脂肪肝。

另一名患者的超声灰阶图(左下图)显示肝左内叶高回声肿块(黄箭)。这也是局灶性脂肪肝。

Hepatic iron overload

- Regardless of the etiology, the iron-overloaded liver is hypointense on all MRI sequences relative to the paraspinal muscles as an internal control, and there is signal dropout on in- phase images.
- There are two pathways to excess hepatic iron accumulation, as described below.
- **Primary hemochromatosis** is the most common cause of iron overload, due to a genetic defect causing increased iron absorption through the GI tract.

  Excess iron is deposited in **hepatocytes** (not the Kupffer cells that make up the intrahepatic reticuloendothelial system or RES), pancreas, myocardium, skin, and joints. Excess iron in hepatocytes can cause cirrhosis.

  Liver and pancreas are markedly T2 hypointense and show signal dropout on in-phase images. The spleen and bone marrow are normal since the RES is not involved.

  Treatment of primary hemochromatosis is phlebotomy.

肝脏铁过载

- 不论何种病因，肝脏铁过载在所有MRI序列上相对于脊柱旁肌肉都呈低信号，并在同相位图像上信号降低。
- 肝脏铁过多沉积有两种途径，如下所述。
- **原发性血色素沉着病**是造成铁过载最常见的原因，由于遗传缺陷导致胃肠道吸收铁增加。

  过量的铁沉积在**肝细胞**(而不是构成肝内网状内皮系统的库普弗细胞)、胰腺、心肌、皮肤和关节。肝细胞铁过载可引起肝硬化。

  肝脏和胰腺呈显著的T_2低信号，同相位图像表现为信号降低。脾和骨髓正常，因网状内皮系统不受累。

  原发性血色素沉着病的治疗方法是静脉抽血。

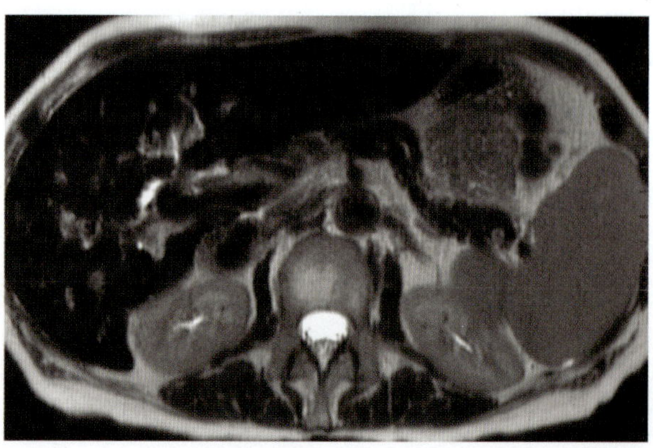

Primary hemochromatosis: Axial T2-weighted MRI demonstrates diffuse low T2 signal in the liver and pancreas with associated signal loss on in-phase imaging (not shown).

原发性血色素沉着病：轴位T_2加权MRI显示肝脏和胰腺呈弥漫性T_2低信号，并伴同相位成像信号降低(未显示)。

- **Secondary hemochromatosis** is usually seen in diseases that cause **hemosiderosis**, where excess iron accumulates within the **RES**. This may be due to frequent blood transfusions or defective erythrocytosis. Treatment of hemosiderosis is with iron chelators, not phlebotomy.

The RES has a large capacity for iron. Therefore, iron stored in the RES is generally not harmful and the liver is normal in morphology without cirrhosis. However, when the RES becomes overwhelmed with iron, the hepatocytes begin to store the excess. Just as in primary hemochromatosis, hepatocyte iron uptake may lead to cirrhosis.

MRI imaging of hemosiderosis demonstrates hypointense liver on conventional MRI sequences and signal drop on in-phase images, as in hemochromatosis. Additionally, the spleen and bone marrow will also appear hypointense due to increased iron stores throughout the entire reticuloendothelial system. The pancreas is spared.

- **继发性血色素沉着病**通常见于引起**含铁血黄素沉着症**的疾病，其过量的铁积聚于网状内皮系统内。原因可能是频繁输血或有缺陷的红细胞增多。治疗含铁血黄素沉着症使用铁螯合剂，而不是静脉抽血。

网状内皮系统储存铁的能力很强。所以，贮存在网状内皮系统内的铁通常没有危害，而且肝脏的形态也是正常的，没有肝硬化。然而，当网状内皮系统内出现铁过载时，肝细胞会开始储存多余的铁，就如原发性血色素沉着病，肝细胞吸收铁而可能导致肝硬化。

在常规MRI序列上含铁血黄素沉着症患者肝脏呈低信号，在同相位图像上信号减低，如血色素沉着病。此外，脾和骨髓也会因整个网状内皮系统的铁储存增加而出现低信号。但胰腺信号正常。

Primary = Pancreas
Secondary = Spleen

原发性=胰腺
继发性=脾

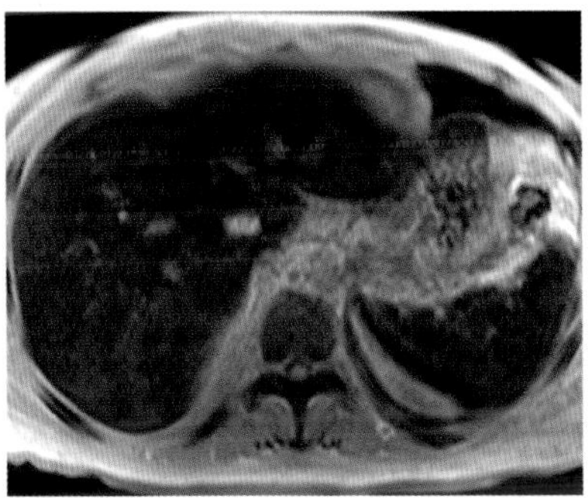

In-phase MRI
同相位MRI

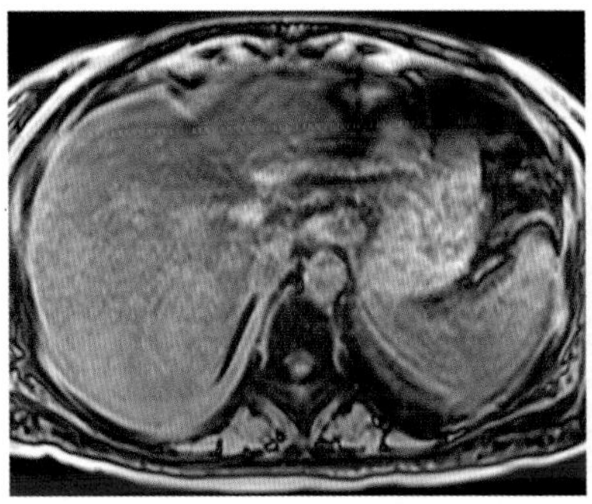

Out-of-phase MRI
反相位MRI

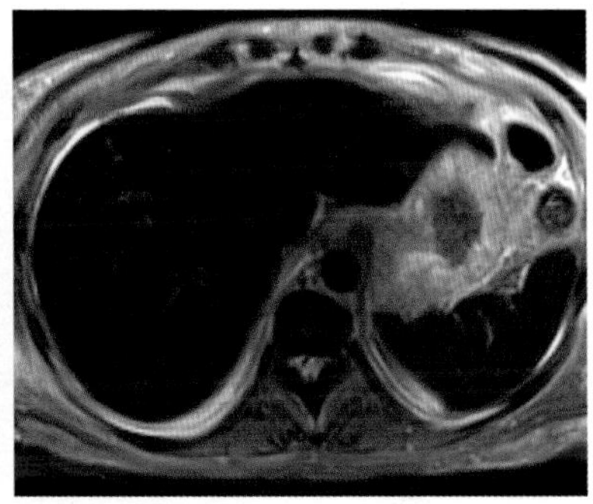

T2-weighted MRI
T_2加权MRI

Secondary hemochromatosis: Multisequence MRI shows diffuse low T2 signal in the liver and spleen with associated signal loss on in-phase imaging compared to out-of-phase imaging, consistent with iron deposition from hemosiderosis in this patient with transfusion-dependent anemia.
继发性血色素沉着病：多序列MRI显示肝脏和脾呈弥漫性T_2低信号，且肝、脾信号在同相位较反相位呈低信号，符合含铁黄素沉着的表现，此患者为输血依赖性贫血。

Amyloid

- Abnormal extracellular deposition of amyloid protein in the liver can cause focal or diffuse areas of decreased attenuation on CT imaging.

Wilson disease

- Wilson disease causes high levels of copper to accumulate in the basal ganglia, cornea, and liver due to an autosomal recessive genetic defect. The liver may be hyperattenuating on CT with multiple nodules, eventually leading to hepatomegaly and cirrhosis.

Variations in CT attenuation

- **Hypoattenuating** liver: The liver is generally considered hypoattenuating if it attenuates less than the spleen on an unenhanced CT.

Fatty liver (hepatic steatosis) is by far the most common cause of a diffusely hypoattenuating liver.
Hepatic amyloid is rare and may cause either focal or diffuse hepatic hypoattenuation.

淀粉样变性

- 淀粉样蛋白质在肝细胞外异常沉积可导致肝脏在CT图像上呈局限性或弥漫性密度降低。

肝豆状核变性(威尔逊病)

- 威尔逊病为常染色体隐性遗传性疾病，导致铜在基底节、眼角膜和肝脏过度积聚。肝脏可表现为CT密度增高并见多发结节，最终导致肝脏肿大和肝硬化。

CT密度的变化

- **低密度**肝脏：肝脏在CT平扫上若密度低于脾则通常被认为是低密度。

肝脂肪变性(脂肪肝)是肝实质弥漫性密度降低最常见的原因。
肝淀粉样变性很罕见，并可引起局灶性或弥漫性肝密度降低。

- **Hyperattenuating** liver: The normal unenhanced attenuation of the liver is 30 to 60 HU. An absolute attenuation greater than 75 HU is considered hyperattenuating.

> **Iron overload** is by far the most common cause of a hyperattenuating liver.
> **Medications** (e.g., amiodarone, gold, and methotrexate).
> **Wilson disease** (Copper overload).
> **Glycogen excess**.

- **高密度**肝脏：正常平扫肝脏的密度为30~60HU。若绝对密度高于75HU则被认为是高密度。

> **铁过载**是最常见的导致肝脏密度增高的原因。
> **药物**，如胺碘酮、金和甲氨蝶呤。
> **威尔逊病**(铜过载)。
> **糖原过剩**。

Cirrhosis

Etiology and pathology

- Cirrhosis is the replacement of functioning hepatocytes with dysfunctional fibrotic tissue, caused by repeated cycles of injury and repair. Etiologies include metabolic (alcohol, steatohepatitis, hemochromatosis, or Wilson disease), infectious (chronic hepatitis B or C), or inflammatory (primary biliary cirrhosis or primary sclerosing cholangitis). The hallmarks of cirrhosis are disorganized attempted regeneration in the form of nodules and fibrosis.

肝硬化

病因和病理

- 肝硬化是由于肝脏在反复的损伤和修复过程中，正常功能的肝细胞被异常功能的纤维化组织所替代。病因包括代谢性(酗酒、脂肪性肝炎、血色素沉着病或威尔逊病)、感染性(慢性乙型或丙型肝炎)或炎症性(原发性胆汁性肝硬化或原发性硬化性胆管炎)。肝硬化的标志是无规律再生而形成结节和纤维化。

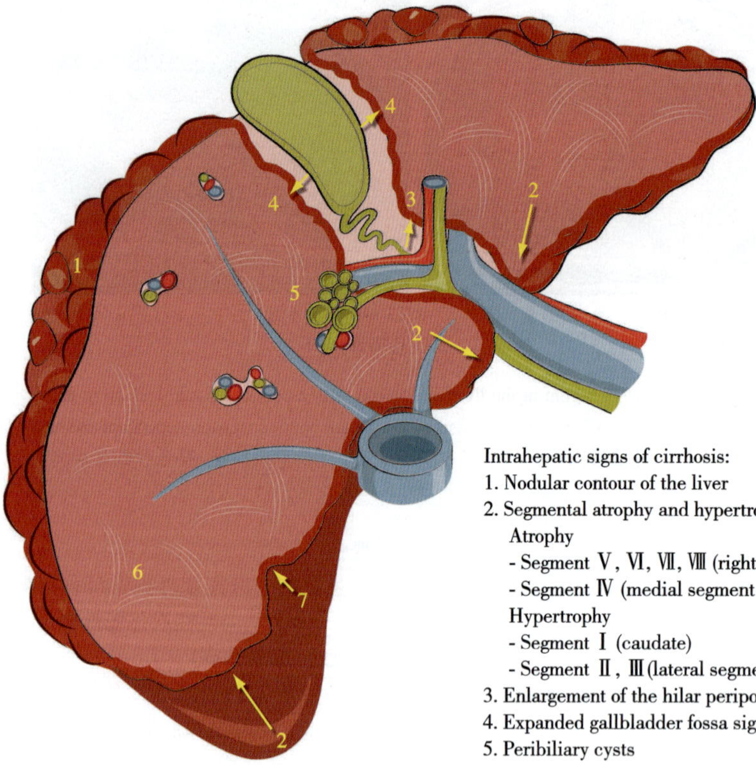

Intrahepatic signs of cirrhosis:
1. Nodular contour of the liver
2. Segmental atrophy and hypertrophy
   Atrophy
   - Segment Ⅴ, Ⅵ, Ⅶ, Ⅷ (right lobe)
   - Segment Ⅳ (medial segment of the left lobe)
   Hypertrophy
   - Segment Ⅰ (caudate)
   - Segment Ⅱ, Ⅲ (lateral segment of the left lobe)
3. Enlargement of the hilar periportal space
4. Expanded gallbladder fossa sign
5. Peribiliary cysts
6. Intrahepatic fibrosis
7. Right posterior hepatic notch sign
8. Iron deposition (not shown)

肝硬化的肝内表现：
1. 结节状肝脏轮廓
2. 肝段萎缩和增生
   萎缩
   - Ⅴ、Ⅵ、Ⅶ、Ⅷ段（右叶）
   - Ⅳ段（左叶内侧段）
   增生
   - Ⅰ段（尾状叶）
   - Ⅱ、Ⅲ段（左叶外侧段）
3. 门静脉周围间隙增大
4. 胆囊窝扩大征
5. 胆管周围囊肿
6. 肝内纤维化
7. 肝右后叶切迹征
8. 铁沉积（未展示）

Early signs of cirrhosis

- One of the earliest signs of cirrhosis is expansion of the periportal spaces. Atrophy of the medial segment of the left hepatic lobe in early cirrhosis causes increased fat anterior to the right main portal vein.
- Enlargement of caudate lobe is a specific sign of cirrhosis. Specifically, a caudate to right lobe size ratio of >0.65 highly suggests cirrhosis. As discussed

肝硬化的早期征象

- 肝硬化的早期表现之一是门静脉周围间隙扩大。早期肝硬化肝左叶内侧段的萎缩导致门静脉右支主干前方脂肪组织增加。
- 尾状叶增大是肝硬化的特异性表现。具体来说，尾状叶与肝右叶之比大于0.65时高度提

previously, the caudate drains directly to the IVC, not via the hepatic veins, which is initially protective against cirrhosis.

- The *empty gallbladder fossa sign* results when hepatic parenchyma surrounding the gallbladder is replaced with periportal fat.

示肝硬化。如前所述，尾状叶直接回流到下腔静脉，不通过肝静脉，这在最初具有防止肝硬化的作用。

- 空胆囊窝征是由于胆囊周围的肝实质被门静脉周围脂肪代替所致。

Secondary manifestations of cirrhosis

- Portal hypertension causes splenomegaly and formation of portosystemic collaterals/ varices, including recanalization of the paraumbilical vein.

  Gamna-Gandy bodies are splenic microhemorrhages secondary to portal hypertension. These appear as tiny echogenic foci on US, tiny hypo- or hyperattenuating foci on CT, and tiny hypointense foci on in-phase MRI. This is discussed further later in the chapter.

- Gallbladder wall thickening is due to hypoalbuminemia and resultant edema.
- Micronodular cirrhosis causes cirrhotic nodules less than 3 mm in size and is usually associated with alcoholism.
- Macronodular cirrhosis features larger nodules (>3 mm) separated by wide scars and fibrous septae. Macronodular cirrhosis is caused by fulminant viral hepatitis which does not uniformly affect the liver.

肝硬化的继发性表现

- 门静脉高压引起脾大，门-体侧支循环形成和静脉曲张，包括副脐静脉再通。

  Gamna-Gandy小体是继发于门静脉高压的脾实质微小出血灶。这些病灶超声表现为微小的回声灶，CT表现为微小的低或高密度，MRI同相位图像表现为微小的低信号灶。这将在本章后文进一步讨论。

- 胆囊壁增厚是由低蛋白血症引发的水肿所致。
- 微小结节性肝硬化是指肝硬化结节小于3mm，通常与酗酒有关。
- 大结节性肝硬化是以较大的结节（>3mm）为特征，由宽大的瘢痕和纤维将它们隔开。大结节性肝硬化是由暴发性病毒性肝炎引起的，而这种肝炎对肝脏的影响并不均匀。

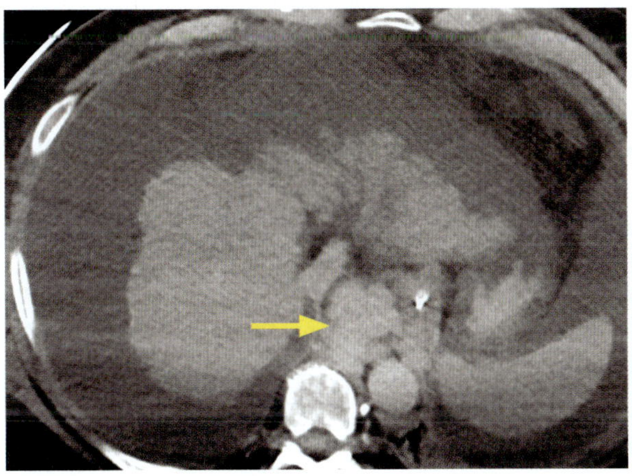

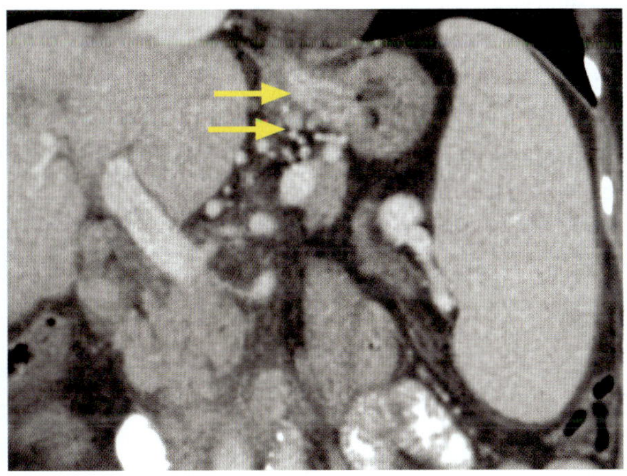

Patient 1 (left image): Axial contrast-enhanced CT shows cirrhotic morphology of the liver with large volume ascites and large esophageal varices (arrow).

Patient 2 (right image): Coronal contrast-enhanced CT shows splenomegaly and small gastric varices (arrows), consistent with sequelae of portal hypertension.

患者1(左图)：轴位增强CT显示肝硬化的形态，并伴有大量腹水和食管静脉曲张(黄箭)。

患者2(右图)：冠状位增强CT显示脾大和小胃底静脉曲张(黄箭)，为门静脉高压的后遗症。

Imaging of cirrhosis

- The typical appearance of cirrhosis is segmental atrophy and hypertrophy with nodular contour and parenchyma.

肝硬化影像学表现

- 肝硬化的典型表现是肝段萎缩与增生，伴结节状轮廓和实质改变。

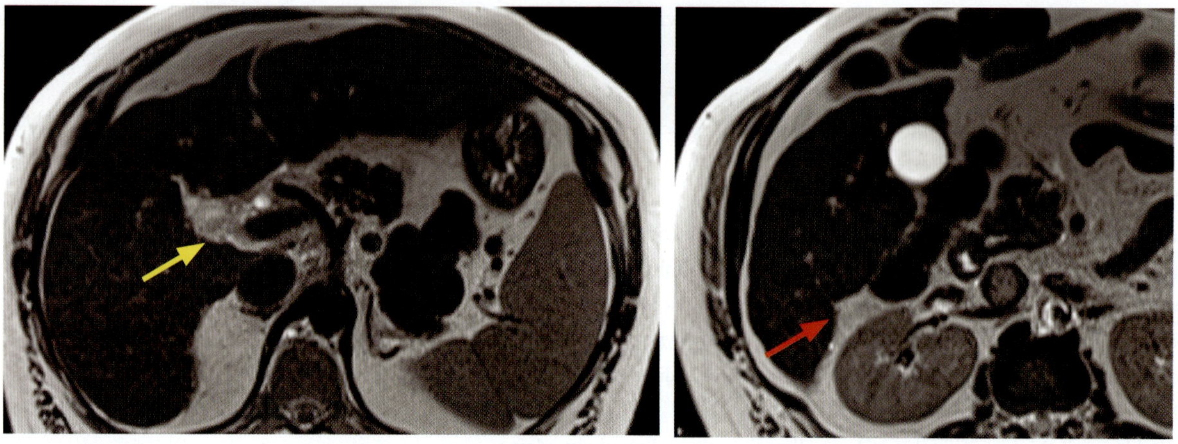

Axial T2-weighted MR images show nodular contour of the liver with hypertrophy of the left lobe, atrophy of the right lobe, widened periportal space (yellow arrow), and *right posterior hepatic notch sign* (red arrow) in keeping with cirrhosis. This patient had a history of hepatitis C.

轴位T_2加权MRI显示肝脏结节状轮廓、左叶增大、右叶萎缩、门静脉周围间隙增宽(黄箭)、*肝右后叶切迹征*(红箭)。该患者有丙型肝炎病史。

- Ultrasound appearance is a coarse, heterogeneous liver echotexture with a nodular contour.
- **MR elastography** is a non-invasive technique in which the patient wears a device resting over their right hepatic lobe which transmits mechanical waves at a fixed frequency, typically 60 Hertz. A phase-contrast pulse sequence with motion-encoding gradients is obtained to measure micron-level tissue deformation in response to the stimulus. Liver stiffness in kPa is measured by drawing ROI on the elastogram images.
- **Sonoelastography** is also a non-invasive way to grade the degree of fibrosis in chronic liver disease. Subtypes include shear-wave elastography and strain elastography.

- 超声表现为粗糙、不均匀的肝脏回声，伴有结节状轮廓。
- **磁共振弹性成像**是一种非创伤性技术，患者腹部肝右叶区域佩戴一个装置，以固定频率传输机械波，频率通常为60Hz。获取带有运动编码梯度的一个相位脉冲序列，用于测量微米级组织对刺激的反应。通过在弹性图像上绘制感兴趣区(ROI)来测量肝脏硬度。
- **超声弹性成像**也是一种无创伤性评估慢性肝病纤维化程度的方法，分为剪切波弹性成像和应变弹性成像。

Malignant hepatic masses

恶性肝肿瘤

Pathway to hepatocellular carcinoma

肝细胞癌(HCC)的演变过程

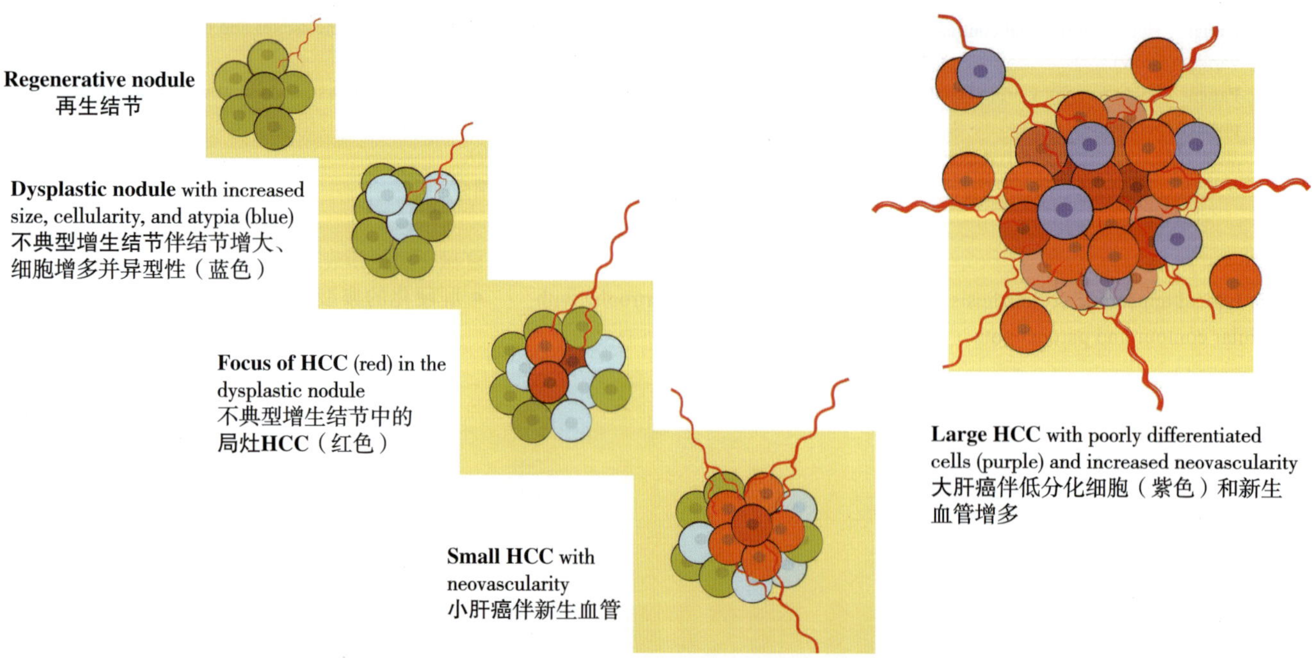

- In the setting of cirrhosis, hepatocellular carcinoma (HCC) is thought to develop in a sequence from regenerative nodule → dysplastic nodule → HCC. Regenerative and dysplastic nodules cannot be reliably differentiated on imaging. High-grade dysplastic nodules cannot be reliably differentiated from well-differentiated HCC.
- **Regenerative nodule**: A regenerative nodule is completely supplied by the portal vein and is not premalignant. A regenerative nodule should *not* enhance in the arterial phase.

  Most regenerative nodules show low signal intensity on T2-weighted images, with variable signal intensity on T1-weighted images. Rarely, a regenerative nodule may be hyperintense on T1-weighted images due to glycogen deposition.

  On contrast-enhanced MRI, most regenerative nodules enhance to the same (or slightly less) degree as the adjacent hepatic parenchyma.
- **Dysplastic nodule**: Unlike a regenerative nodule, a dysplastic nodule is premalignant. However, most dysplastic nodules do not demonstrate arterial phase enhancement (unless high grade), since blood supply is still from the portal vein.

  Dysplastic nodules are variable in signal intensity on T1-weighted images. Most dysplastic nodules are hypointense on T2-weighted images, although high-grade dysplastic nodules may be T2 hyperintense.

  Contrast-enhanced MRI shows low-grade dysplastic nodules to be isoenhancing relative to liver and thus indistinguishable from regenerative nodules. High-grade dysplastic nodules can demonstrate arterial enhancement and may be indistinguishable from well-differentiated HCC.
- A **siderotic nodule** is an iron-rich regenerative or dysplastic nodule. A siderotic nodule is hypointense on T1 and T2*-weighted images (including in-phase GRE images) and hyperattenuating on CT. A siderotic nodule is rarely, if ever, malignant.

Hepatocellular carcinoma (HCC)

- 在肝硬化的情况下，肝细胞癌(HCC)被认为是从再生结节 → 不典型增生结节 → HCC 的顺序中发展而来。在影像学上，再生结节很难与低级别不典型增生结节进行可靠区分。高级别不典型增生结节不能与分化良好的HCC进行有效区分。
- **再生结节**：再生结节完全由门静脉供血，并非癌前病变。再生结节不会在动脉期强化。

  大多数再生结节在T_2加权上呈低信号，而在T_1加权上的信号强度不定。罕见的情况下，当再生结节内有糖原沉积时，在T_1加权上可呈高信号。

  在增强MRI上，大多数再生结节的强化程度与邻近的肝实质相同(或略低)。
- **不典型增生结节**：与再生结节不同，不典型增生结节是癌前病变。然而大多数不典型增生结节在动脉期无强化(除非为高级别结节)，这是由于其血供仍然来自门静脉。

  不典型增生结节在T_1加权上的信号强度不定。多数不典型增生结节在T_2加权上呈低信号，而高级别不典型增生结节可以表现为T_2加权高信号。

  增强MRI显示低级别不典型增生结节与肝实质的强化程度相同，因此无法与再生结节相鉴别。高级别不典型增生结节可呈动脉期强化，难以与分化良好的HCC相鉴别。
- **铁质沉着结节**为富含铁的再生结节或不典型增生结节。铁质沉着结节在T_1和T_2*加权(包括同相位GRE图像)上均呈低信号，在CT上呈高密度。铁质沉着性结节罕见，一旦出现，则为恶性。

肝细胞癌(HCC)

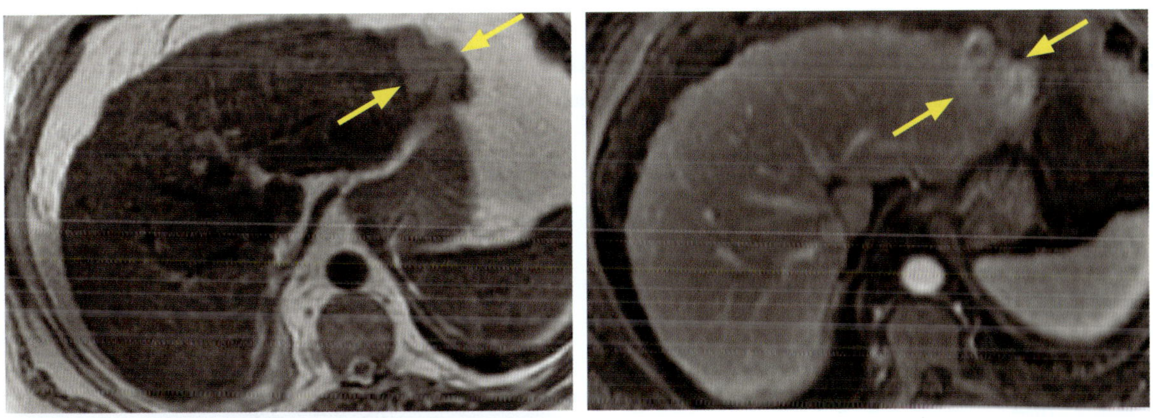

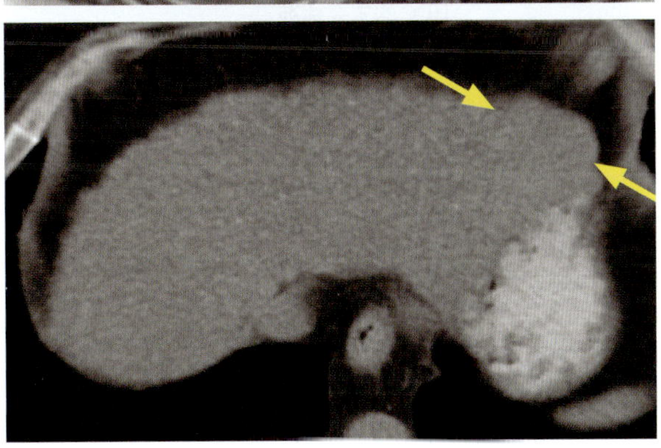

HCC in a cirrhotic liver: T2-weighted (top left image) and T1-weighted post-contrast late arterial phase (top right image) MRI shows a nodular external contour of the liver, consistent with cirrhosis. There is a T2 hyperintense, hypervascular mass in hepatic segment 2 (arrows), representing HCC.

Unenhanced CT (left image) shows the mass to be isoattenuating and barely perceptible (arrows).

Case courtesy Cheryl Sadow, MD, Brigham and Women's Hospital.

肝硬化伴HCC：MRI T_2加权(左上图)和增强后动脉晚期T_1加权(右上图)显示肝脏轮廓呈结节状外突，为肝硬化的表现。肝S_2段(黄箭)可见一处T_2加权高信号和富血供的肿块，代表HCC。

CT平扫(左下图)显示肿块呈等密度，很难被发现(黄箭)。

- Hepatocellular carcinoma is the most common primary liver tumor. Cirrhosis is the major risk factor for development of HCC, with other risk factors including chronic viral hepatitis (hepatitis B) and fatty liver disease. A hypervascular liver mass in a patient with cirrhosis or chronic hepatitis is HCC until proven otherwise.
- Alpha-feto protein (AFP) is elevated in approximately 75% of cases of HCC.
- Patients with cirrhosis or chronic viral hepatitis are regularly screened for HCC with serum α -fetoprotein levels and imaging, typically ultrasound or MRI.

  Ultrasound is not very sensitive to detect small HCC in end-stage cirrhotic livers. The aim is to detect single HCC foci measuring less than 20 mm in diameter, characterized by a better prognosis and exhibiting less than 20% risk of hematogenous spread.

  HCC has a variety of ultrasound appearances – therefore, a mass in a cirrhotic liver is considered HCC until proven otherwise. High Doppler flow may be present, especially at the periphery of the mass, due to arteriovenous shunting.
- The classic CT or MRI appearance of HCC is an encapsulated mass that enhances on arterial phase and washes out on portal venous phase with an enhancing capsule. HCC may be difficult to detect on non-contrast or portal venous phase CT. On unenhanced MRI, HCC is characteristically slightly hyperintense on T2-weighted images relative to surrounding liver and may show restricted diffusion.

  The *nodule in a nodule* appearance describes an enhancing nodule within a dysplastic nodule and represents an early HCC.
- HCC is often locally invasive and tends to invade into the portal and hepatic veins, IVC, and bile ducts. In contrast, cholangiocarcinoma and metastases to the liver are much less likely to do so.

  The portal veins should always be carefully evaluated in the presence of a hepatic mass. Internal Doppler flow or enhancement within a venous clot suggests a tumor-in-vein.
- **LI-RADS** is an imaging reporting and classification system for HCC on CT and MRI which is an indication of the relative risk of HCC ranging from LR-1 (favoring benignity) to LR-5 (favoring malignancy). This is used only in people with risk factors for HCC (chronic hepatitis infections, cirrhosis, but not cirrhosis due to cardiac or vascular etiologies). The 2018 version describes major and ancillary criteria: the major imaging criteria lead to the assignment of the LI-RADS score, while the ancillary findings may be used as tie breakers.

Major criteria for HCC:

- Arterial enhancement.
- Non-peripheral washout on portal venous and delayed phases.
- Enhancing capsule/pseudocapsule seen in portal venous or delayed phases.
- Threshold growth with diameter increase of >50% in <6 months.

Ancillary findings favoring HCC include non-enhancing capsule, nodule-in-nodule architecture, mosaic architecture, fat in mass, blood products in mass.

- Treatment options for HCC include partial hepatectomy, orthotopic liver transplantation, radiation therapy, percutaneous ablation, and transcatheter embolization.

- 肝细胞癌(HCC)是最常见的原发性肝肿瘤。肝硬化是发生HCC的主要危险因素，其他危险因素包括慢性病毒性肝炎(乙型肝炎)和肝脂肪变性。在肝硬化或慢性肝炎患者中出现富血供肿块即可认为是HCC，直到被证实为其他病变。
- 约75%的HCC患者有甲胎蛋白(AFP)的升高。
- 肝硬化或慢性病毒性肝炎患者需要定期进行血清甲胎蛋白测量及影像学检查以筛查HCC，通常进行超声或MRI检查。

  超声对检测晚期肝硬化中的小肝癌并不十分敏感，其用途是识别直径小于20mm的单个HCC病灶，这类病灶通常具有更好的预后，并且血行转移的风险低于20%。

  HCC在超声上表现多样，因此，在有肝硬化背景下出现的肝肿块首先应被看作是HCC，直到被证实为其他病变。由于动静脉分流，可出现高速多普勒血流，特别是在肿块的周围。
- HCC的典型CT或MRI表现为具有包膜的肿块，在动脉期强化，门静脉期廓清。HCC在CT平扫或门静脉期可能很难被发现。在平扫MRI中，典型的HCC在T_2加权上较周围肝实质呈稍高信号，并可能表现为弥散受限。

  结中结的表现是指不典型增生结节中出现强化结节，代表早期HCC。
- HCC通常具有局部侵袭性，常侵犯门静脉、肝静脉、下腔静脉和胆管。相反，胆管癌和肝脏转移瘤很少出现局部侵犯。

  当存在肝肿块时，必须仔细评估门静脉。静脉血栓内出现多普勒血流或有强化则提示肿瘤侵犯了静脉。
- **LI-RADS**是一种CT和MRI对HCC的影像学报告和分类系统，用于评估HCC的相对风险，从LR-1(倾向于良性)到LR-5(倾向于恶性)不等。该系统只适用于有HCC危险因素的人群(包括慢性肝炎、肝硬化，但不适合心源性或血管源性病因导致的肝硬化)。2018版制定了主要标准和辅助标准：主要标准用于确定LI-RADS评分，辅助标准可以用作决策的补充依据。

HCC的**主要标准**

- 动脉期强化。
- 门静脉及延迟期非周边廓清。
- 门静脉或延迟期可见强化包膜/假包膜。
- 6个月内直径增长阈值>50%。

支持HCC的**辅助征象**包括无强化的包膜、结中结征、马赛克征、肿瘤内脂肪组织，以及肿瘤内出血。

- HCC的治疗方法包括部分肝切除、原位肝移植、放疗、经皮消融术，以及经导管栓塞术。

Fibrolamellar HCC

纤维板层样肝癌

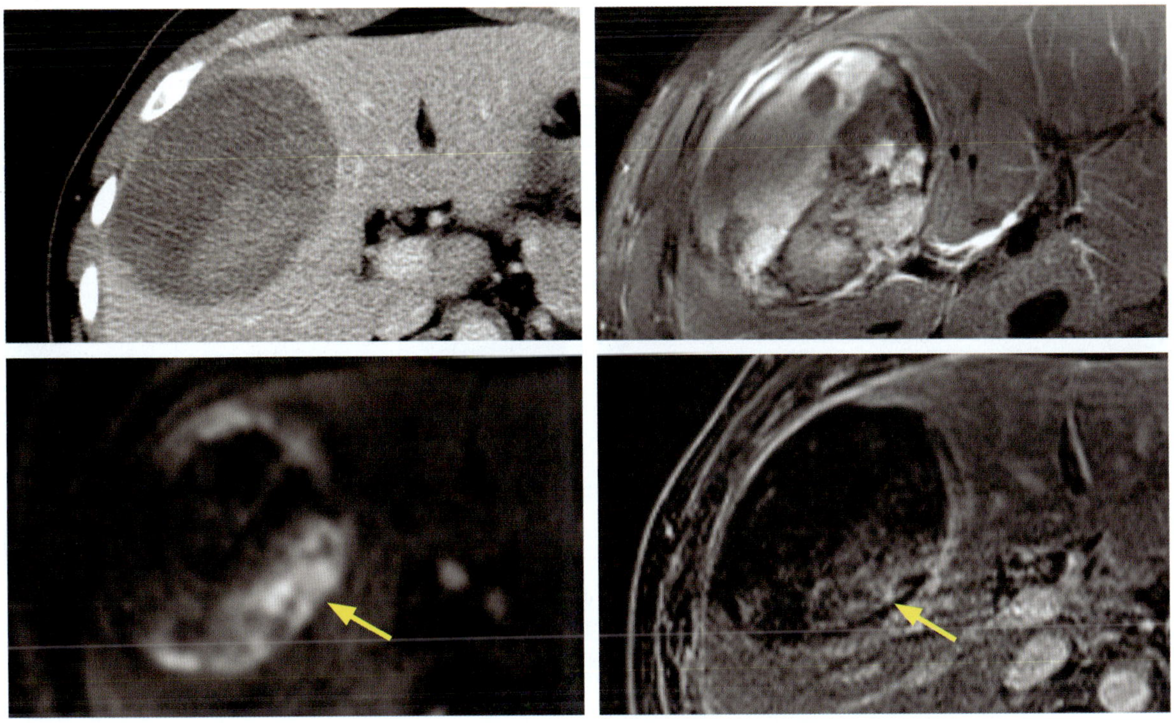

Fibrolamellar HCC: Axial CT (top left image) shows a heterogeneous lesion corresponding to heterogeneous signal on T2-weighted MRI (top right). DWI (bottom left) and post-contrast (bottom right) images show hypercellular enhancing components within the mass (arrows).

纤维板层样肝癌：轴位CT(左上图)显示一个不均匀密度肿块，与T_2加权MRI上的信号不均匀相对应(右上图)。弥散加权(左下图)和增强后(右下图)图像显示肿块内富细胞并有强化成分(黄箭)。

- Fibrolamellar carcinoma is a rare subtype of HCC that occurs in young patients without cirrhosis. The tumor tends to be large when diagnosed but has a better prognosis than typical HCC. Unlike in conventional HCC, AFP is not elevated.
- On imaging, fibrolamellar HCC is a large, heterogeneous liver mass. A fibrotic central scar is classic, which is hypointense on T1- and T2-weighted MRI images (in contrast, focal nodular hyperplasia features a T2 hyperintense scar that enhances late). Capsular retraction may be seen in 10%.
- Unlike HCC, the fibrolamellar subtype does not have a capsule, although there may be a pseudocapsule of peripherally compressed normal hepatic tissue.

- 纤维板层样肝癌是罕见的HCC亚型，见于无肝硬化的年轻患者。肿瘤的体积通常在就诊时较大，但其预后通常好于HCC。与常规的HCC不同，AFP不升高。
- 在影像学上，纤维板层HCC表现为大而不均质的肿块。纤维样中心瘢痕为典型表现，其在T_1及T_2加权上均呈低信号(相反，局灶性结节性增生的特征为T_2加权上高信号的瘢痕并呈延迟强化)。包膜回缩见于10%的患者。
- 与HCC不同，纤维板层亚型没有包膜，但有时可见到假包膜，为外周正常肝组织受压所致。

Mass-forming cholangiocarcinoma

- One of three recognized subtypes of intrahepatic cholangiocarcinomas and usually presents as large and relatively well-defined hepatic mass with lobulated margins and demonstrates delayed/progressive enhancement.
- They are often associated with peripheral biliary dilatation and although biliary in origin, must be considered in the differential for a hepatic mass.

肿块型胆管细胞癌

- 此为已知肝内胆管癌的三个亚型之一，通常为大而边界相对清晰的肝实质性肿块，具有分叶状边缘，并表现出延迟/渐进性强化。
- 常伴有外周胆管扩张，虽然起源于胆管，但在肝脏肿块的鉴别诊断中必须加以考虑。

Hepatic metastases

- Metastatic disease to the liver is far more common than primary HCC.
- Although metastases are supplied by branches of the hepatic artery induced by tumoral angiogenesis, most metastases are hypovascular and best appreciated on portal venous phase (in contrast to HCC, which is hypervascular and best visualized on late arterial phase).
- On MRI, metastatic lesions tend to be hypointense on T1-weighted images and hyperintense on T2-weighted images. Blood products and melanin (seen in

肝转移瘤

- 肝转移瘤比原发性肝癌更常见。
- 肝转移瘤血供来自肝动脉分支，但这些血管是由肿瘤诱导而产生的新生血管，而大多数转移瘤是乏血供的，且门静脉期显示最佳(相反，HCC是富血供的，在动脉晚期显示最佳)。
- 在MRI上，转移瘤在T_1加权上呈低信号，在T_2加权上呈高信号。血液成分和黑色素(在黑色

melanoma metastases) are T1 hyperintense.

- Metastases can have a variable ultrasound appearance, although the classic finding is a hypoechoic rim producing a target sign. If an incidental liver mass is seen on ultrasound, further characterization by MRI is recommended.

素瘤肝转移中可见)为T_1加权高信号。

- 转移瘤的超声表现多样,但典型的表现是低回声环产生的靶征。如果在超声检查中偶然发现肝脏肿块,建议采用MRI进一步检查。

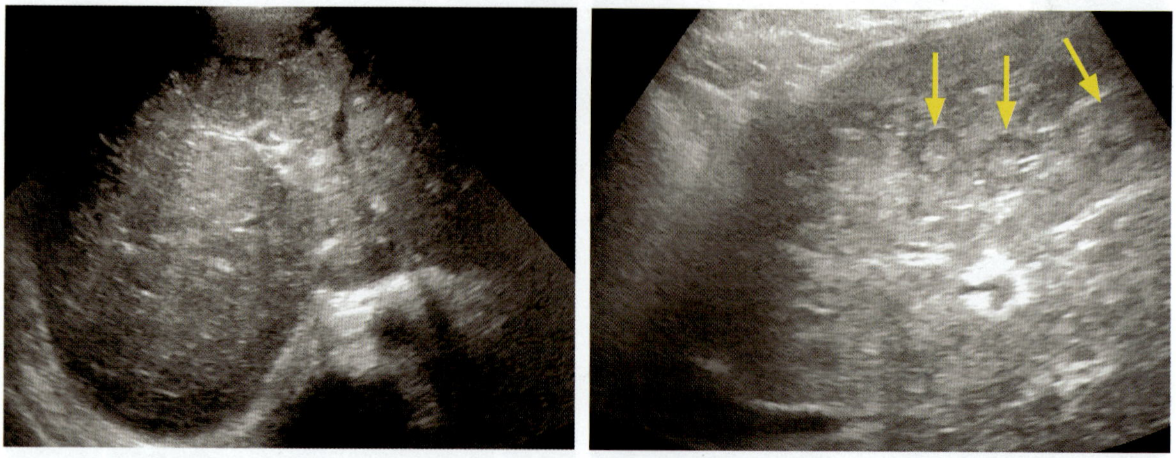

Innumerable liver metastasis on ultrasound, initially difficult to see due to technique: Initial scanning with a low-frequency vector probe (left image) demonstrates a coarsened hepatic echotexture without definite mass. This appearance may mimic cirrhosis. When a higher frequency curved probe is used (right image), innumerable target lesions (arrows) become apparent, consistent with innumerable hepatic metastases.

Case courtesy Julie Ritner, MD, Brigham and Women's Hospital, Boston.

无数肝转移灶在最初的扫描时由于技术原因难以看清:使用低频矢量探头(左图)初步扫查显示肝脏回声变粗,但无明确肿块。这种表现类似肝硬化。当使用高频弯曲探头(右图)时,大量靶本病灶(黄箭)变得清晰可见,符合多发肝转移瘤的表现。

- **Hypovascular** hepatic metastases include:

Breast.	Lung.
Pancreas.	Lymphoma.

- **Hypervascular** hepatic metastases include (mnemonic = MRCT):

Melanoma.	Carcinoid / Choriocarcinoma.
Renal cell carcinoma.	Thyroid.

- **Calcified** hepatic metastases include:

Mucinous cancers (including colon, gastric, ovarian).
Osteosarcoma.
Treated lymphoma.

- **Cystic** hepatic metastases include:

Ovarian cystadenocarcinoma.
Gastrointestinal sarcoma.

- **Pseudocirrhosis** describes the macronodular liver contour resulting from multiple scirrhous hepatic metastases with capsular retraction, mimicking cirrhosis. Although termed "pseudo", these patients may have similar physiologic consequences of cirrhosis including portal hypertension. Treated breast cancer is the most common cause of this appearance.

- **乏血管**性肝转移瘤包括:

乳腺癌。	肺癌。
胰腺癌。	淋巴瘤。

- **富血管**肝转移瘤包括(记忆诀窍"MRCT")

黑色素瘤(**M**)。	类癌/绒毛膜癌(**C**)。
肾细胞癌(**R**)。	甲状腺癌(**T**)。

- **钙化性**肝转移瘤包括:

黏液性癌(包括结肠、胃、卵巢)。
骨肉瘤。
治疗后淋巴瘤。

- **囊性**肝转移瘤包括:

卵巢囊腺癌。
胃肠道肉瘤。

- **假性肝硬化**是指多发性硬化性肝转移瘤导致的肝脏轮廓呈巨大结节样改变伴肝包膜回缩,类似肝硬化。虽然被称为"假性",但这些患者可能会出现与肝硬化相似的生理后果,如门静脉高压。治疗后的乳腺癌肝转移最常出现这样的表现。

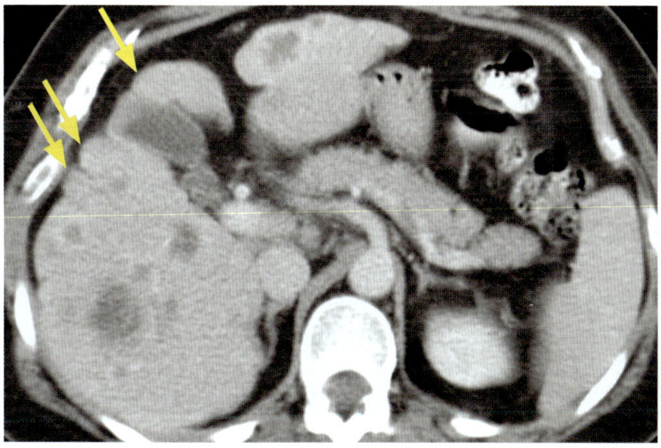

Pseudocirrhosis due to multiple treated breast cancer metastases:
Contrast-enhanced CT shows numerous hypoattenuating hepatic lesions with a markedly nodular external hepatic contour (arrows) that resembles cirrhosis.
Liver function in this patient remained normal.
乳腺癌转移瘤反复治疗后出现的假性肝硬化：
增强CT显示大量肝内低密度病灶，伴有明显的肝脏轮廓结节状改变(黄箭)，类似肝硬化。该患者肝功能仍然正常。

Hepatic lymphoma

肝淋巴瘤

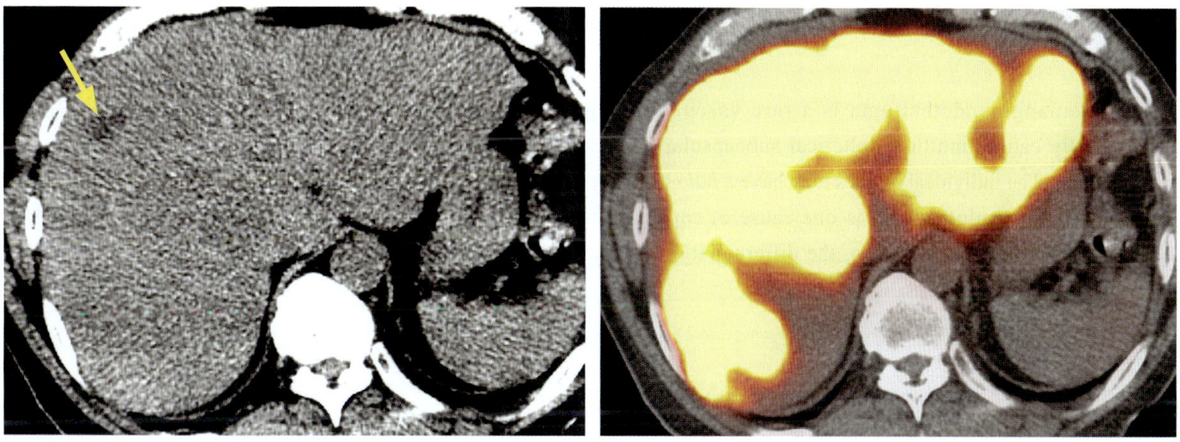

PET/CT demonstrates a single defined low density hepatic lesion (arrow, left image) and more diffuse low density changes of the liver parenchyma with remarkable FDG avidity (right image), in this patient with biopsy proven hepatic lymphoma.
PET/CT显示一处明确的低密度肝脏病灶(黄箭，左图)，以及较为广泛的肝实质密度降低伴显著FDG摄取(右图)，此患者活检证实为肝淋巴瘤。

- Primary hepatic lymphoma is very rare and may present as a single mass or multiple masses. They tend to be infiltrative and preserve hepatic vasculature.
- Lymphomatous involvement of the liver tends to be secondary to systemic disease, with associated splenomegaly and lymphadenopathy.
- On ultrasound, lymphoma tends to be hypoechoic and may have the target sign typical of metastases.
- On CT and MRI, lymphoma is hypoenhancing and tends to show restricted diffusion on MRI.

- 原发性肝淋巴瘤非常罕见，可表现为单个或多个肿块。病变具有浸润性，但肝血管系统不受侵犯。
- 肝脏淋巴瘤通常继发于系统性疾病，并伴脾肿大和淋巴结肿大。
- 淋巴瘤的超声表现多为低回声，并可能具有转移灶典型的靶征。
- 在CT和MRI上，淋巴瘤呈低强化，并在MRI显示弥散受限。

Post transplant lymphoproliferative disorder (PTLD)

- PTLD appears as a mass with a variable and nonspecific appearance. Therefore, it is important to mention PTLD if a liver mass is seen in a transplant patient. This is discussed further later in the chapter.

移植后淋巴增生性疾病(PTLD)

- PTLD的肿块外观多变且无特异性。因此，在肝移植患者发现肝肿块时必须注意PTLD。这将在本章后文进一步讨论。

Epithelioid hemangioendothelioma

上皮样血管内皮瘤

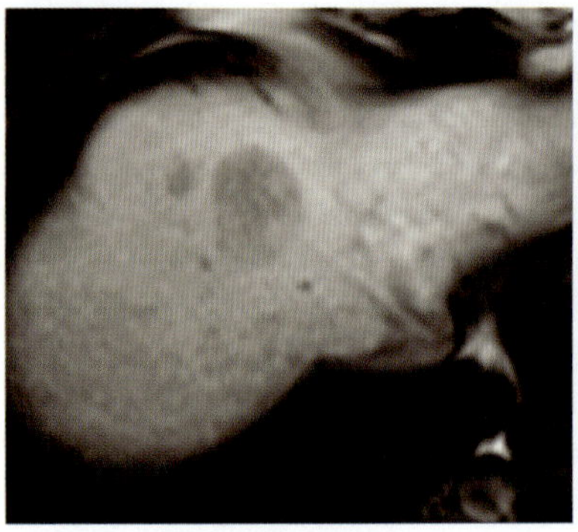

Precontrast T1-weighted MRI
平扫T_1加权MRI

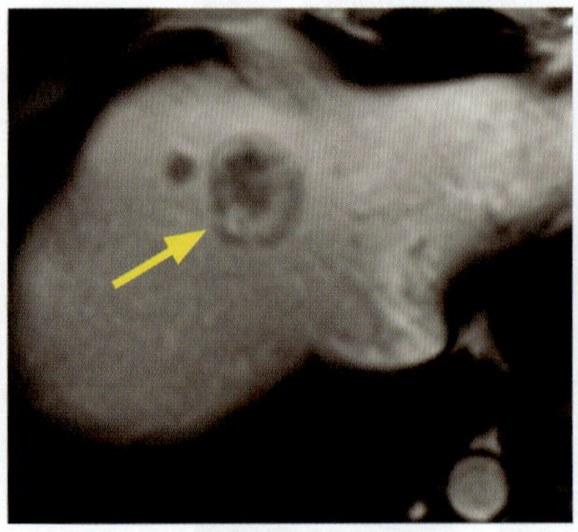

Post-contrast T1-weighted MRI
增强T_1加权MRI

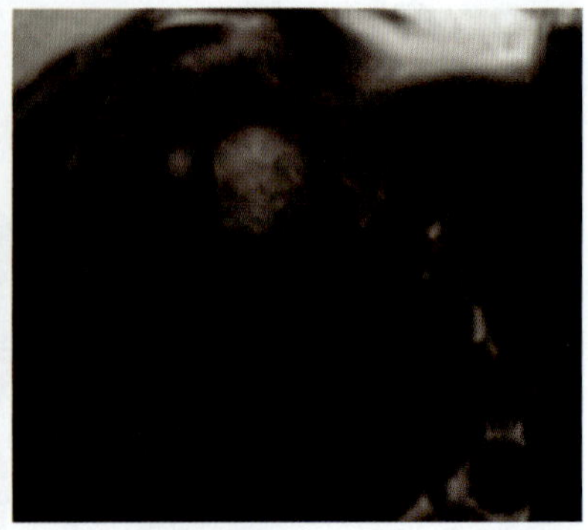

T2-weighted MRI
T_2加权MRI

Multisequence MRI shows multiple T1 hypointense, T2 hyperintense hepatic lesions with peripheral *target pattern* enhancement (arrow), predominant peripheral distribution, and associated capsular retraction (not shown).
多序列MRI显示多发T_1加权低信号、T_2加权高信号肝脏病变，边缘靶环样强化(黄箭)，主要分布在外周，伴包膜回缩(未显示)。

- Epithelioid hemangioendothelioma is a rare vascular malignancy that characteristically causes multiple spherical subcapsular masses which can become confluent. The individual masses may have a *halo* or *target* appearance.
- Epithelioid hemangioendothelioma is one cause of capsular retraction. As summarized at the end of this section, the differential of capsular retraction includes:

- 上皮样血管内皮瘤是一种罕见的血管恶性肿瘤，以多发球形包膜下肿块为特征，肿块可融合。单个肿块可以有晕或靶样的表现。
- 上皮样血管内皮瘤是引起包膜回缩的原因之一。如本节最后所述，包膜回缩征的鉴别诊断包括：

Mass-forming cholangiocarcinoma.
Fibrolamellar HCC (seen in 10% of cases of fibrolamellar HCC).
Epithelioid hemangioendothelioma.
Pseudocirrhosis (macronodular liver contour with capsular retraction due to treated metastases).
Confluent hepatic fibrosis (wedge-shaped fibrosis that may be seen in cirrhosis).

肿块样胆管癌。
纤维板层HCC(见于10%的纤维板层HCC)。
上皮样血管内皮瘤。
假性肝硬化(结节状肝脏轮廓和肝包膜回缩征见于治疗后肝转移瘤)。
融合性肝纤维化(肝硬化时可见楔形纤维化)。

Benign Liver Masses

良性肝脏肿块

Hemangioma

血管瘤

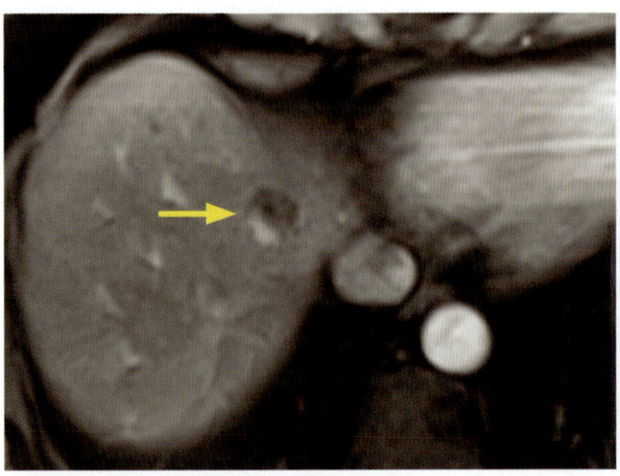

Early arterial post-contrast T1-weighted MRI
增强动脉早期T_1加权MRI

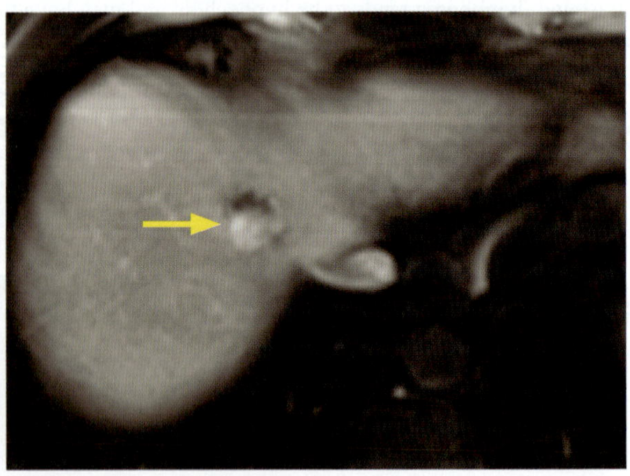

Portal venous post-contrast T1-weighted MRI
增强门静脉期T_1加权MRI

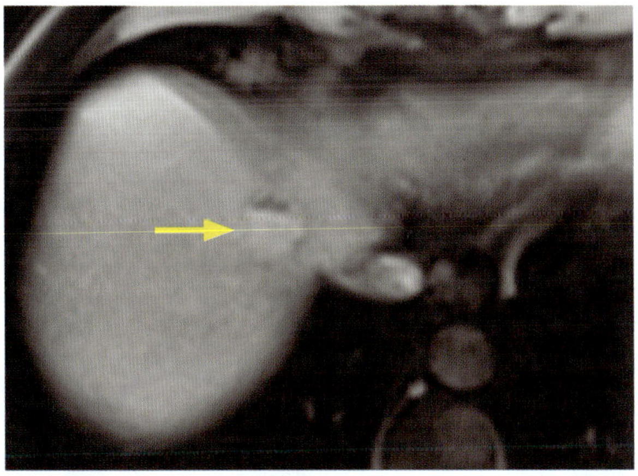

Delayed post-contrast T1-weighted MRI
增强延迟期T_1加权MRI

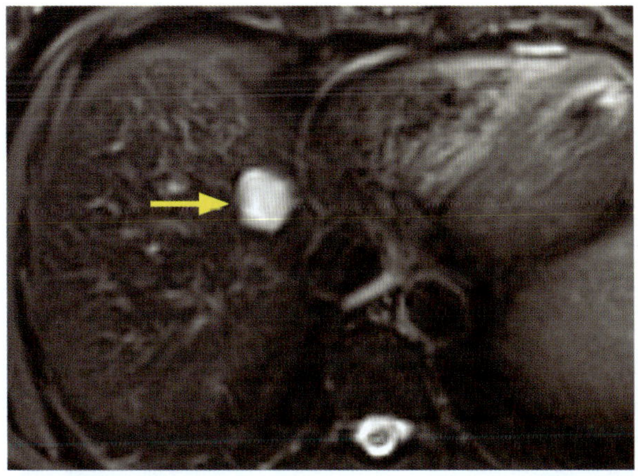

T2-weighted MRI
T_2加权MRI

Hemangioma: Dynamic contrast-enhanced T1-weighted MRI (early arterial top left image to delayed bottom left image) shows a segment 8 lesion (yellow arrows) demonstrating peripheral discontinuous nodular enhancement. There is progressively increasing centripetal enhancement towards the center of the lesion on delayed images. The signal intensity of the peripheral enhancement is similar to that of the aorta.

The hemangioma is hyperintense on the T2-weighted image (bottom right image).

肝血管瘤：动态增强T_1加权MRI(左上动脉早期图像至左下延迟期)显示一处位于肝8段的病灶(黄箭),其边缘呈非连续性结节样强化。在延迟期呈向中心渐进性填充。周围增强的信号强度与主动脉相同。

血管瘤在T_2加权上呈高信号(右下图)。

- Hepatic cavernous hemangioma is the most common benign hepatic neoplasm. It is composed of disorganized endothelial cell-lined pockets of blood vessels, supplied by a peripheral branch of the hepatic artery.
- Hemangioma is more common in females and uncommon in cirrhosis. When a known hemangioma is sequentially followed in a patient with early cirrhosis, the hemangioma involutes as the liver becomes more cirrhotic.
- Hemangioma may range in size from <1 cm to >10 cm. **Giant hemangiomas** tend to have a non-enhancing central area representing cystic degeneration.
- On CT and MRI, a virtually pathognomonic imaging feature is peripheral discontinuous progressive nodular enhancement. The degree of enhancement should match the blood pool on all images and demonstrate gradual centripetal fill-in on later phases.
- The noncontrast CT appearance is not helpful, as a hemangioma appears as a nonspecific hypoattenuating liver mass.
- On MRI, hemangiomas are typically T2 hyperintense and become even more hyperintense on T2-fat saturated images compared to conventional T2-weighted images.
- The classic ultrasound appearance is a circumscribed, homogeneously echogenic mass with no flow on color Doppler. Posterior acoustic enhancement may be present. If a solitary, classic-appearing hemangioma is seen on ultrasound and the patient has an otherwise normal-appearing liver, normal LFTs, no known malignancy or risk factors for HCC, and is asymptomatic, then no further workup is required.

A hypoechoic halo (*target sign*) should never be seen – this finding suggests malignancy. Ultrasound appearance of hemangioma can be confusing in a patient with underlying fatty liver and may appear relatively hypoechoic compared to the background of echogenic fatty liver.

Any heterogeneity or atypical ultrasound findings should prompt consideration of an alternative diagnosis such as hyperechoic HCC or metastatic disease (even in the absence

- 肝海绵状血管瘤是最常见的良性肝脏肿瘤，是由血窦内衬以无序的内皮细胞所组成，由肝动脉的外周分支供血。
- 血管瘤较常见于女性，但肝硬化中不多见。如果对早期肝硬化患者的血管瘤进行跟踪随访，血管瘤将随着肝硬化的进展而逐渐退化。
- 肝血管瘤可以小到不足1cm，也可以大于10cm。**巨型肝血管瘤**的中央区域通常不强化，为囊性变。
- 在CT和MRI上，几乎具有病理诊断意义的影像学表现为周边非连续性、渐进性结节样强化。强化程度应与所有血池图像相同，并在后期呈渐进性向心填充。
- 平扫CT对诊断没有帮助，因肝血管瘤表现为非特异性低密度肝肿块。
- 在MRI上，血管瘤呈典型的T_2高信号，而脂肪抑制T_2加权信号高于常规T_2加权。
- 典型的超声表现为边界清晰、回声均匀的肿块，彩色多普勒显示无血流。可出现后部回声增强。如果超声检查为一个孤立的典型血管瘤，且肝脏外形正常、肝功能正常、无恶性肿瘤史或HCC危险因素，以及无症状，则无须进一步检查。

不应看到低回声晕(靶征)，此为可疑恶性肿瘤征象。肝脂肪变性患者的血管瘤超声表现不确定，可能相对于肝脂肪变性的超声背景呈低回声。

对任何不均质肿块或非典型的超声表现都应考虑其他诊断，如高回声的HCC或转移性病灶(即使

of a halo). In a patient with cirrhosis or any known primary malignancy, further workup (MRI or CT) is usually warranted.

没有晕征)。对于肝硬化或任何已知有原发性恶性肿瘤患者，进一步检查(MRI或CT)通常是必要的。

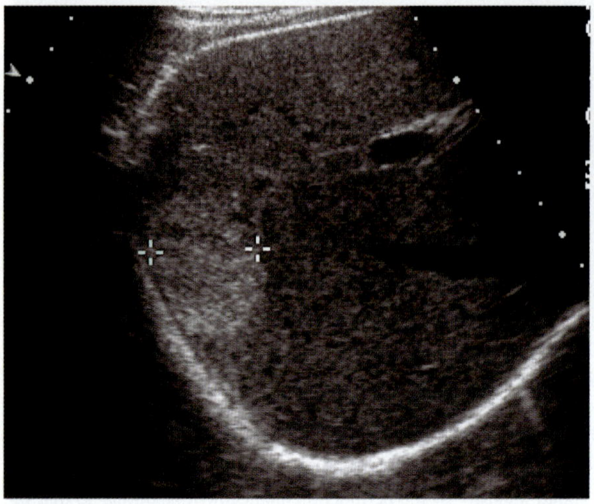

Cavernous hemangioma: Transverse ultrasound through the right lobe of the liver demonstrates a circumscribed slightly heterogeneous echogenic mass (calipers) with mild posterior acoustic enhancement.
海绵状血管瘤：肝右叶横切面超声显示界限分明但回声稍不均匀的肿块(卡尺)，后部有轻微回声增强。

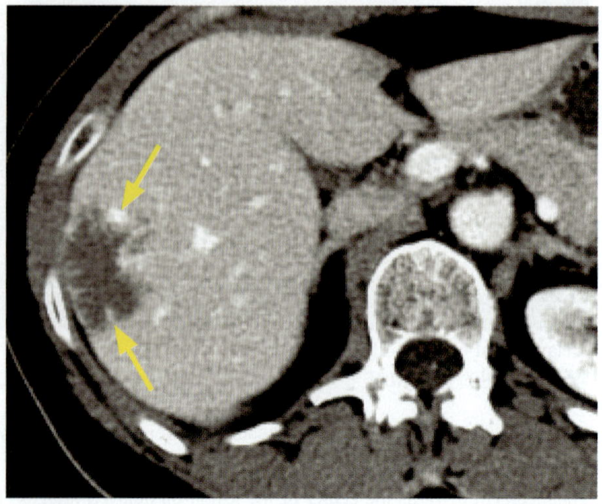

Portal venous phase axial contrast-enhanced CT demonstrates a hypoattenuating lesion with peripheral discontinuous nodular enhancement (arrows), typical of a hemangioma.
门静脉期轴位增强CT显示低密度病变伴周围非连续性结节样强化，为典型的血管瘤。

Case courtesy Julie Ritner, MD, Brigham and Women's Hospital, Boston.

Focal nodular hyperplasia (FNH)

- Focal nodular hyperplasia (FNH) is a hamartoma consisting of disorganized liver tissue with no malignant potential.
- It is more common in women and is not associated with oral contraceptives.
- FNH is called a *stealth lesion* because it resembles background liver parenchyma on all modalities, except arterial phase imaging due to vascular supply.
- Approximately 15% of FNH have a characteristic central scar consisting of biliary ductules and venules which does not contain fibrotic tissue and therefore is not a true scar.
- FNH does not have a capsule.
- MRI with Eovist contrast is the most useful imaging modality to diagnose FNH. FNH typically is isointense to liver on all MRI sequences, except it is arterially hyperenhancing and will show retained Eovist enhancement iso- or hyper-intense relative to liver in the hepatobiliary phase (20 minutes after contrast administration) due to the presence of hepatocytes and biliary ductules. The central scar will show delayed enhancement with extracellular contrast agents (such as Gadavist), but will not enhance with Eovist.

局灶性结节增生(FNH)

- 局灶性结节增生(FNH)是一种由结构紊乱的肝组织构成的错构瘤，无恶性潜能。
- 此病在女性中更常见，与口服避孕药无关。
- FNH被称为隐性病变，因为它与周围肝实质除在动脉期因血管血供而表现不同外，其余所有的影像学表现均相似。
- 约15%的FNH具有特征性的中央瘢痕，它们由胆管和小静脉组成，不含纤维组织，因此不是真正的瘢痕。
- FNH不具有包膜。
- 使用钆塞酸二钠增强MRI是诊断FNH最有用的影像学方法。FNH在所有MRI序列上通常与肝脏呈等信号，不包括在动脉期增强时出现明显亮度增强，以及在肝胆期(造影剂注射后20分钟)由于存在肝细胞和胆小管，会显示出相对于肝脏保留Eovist增强，呈等或高信号强度。中央瘢痕在使用细胞外造影剂(如钆布醇)时会出现延迟增强，但在使用钆塞酸二钠时则不会。

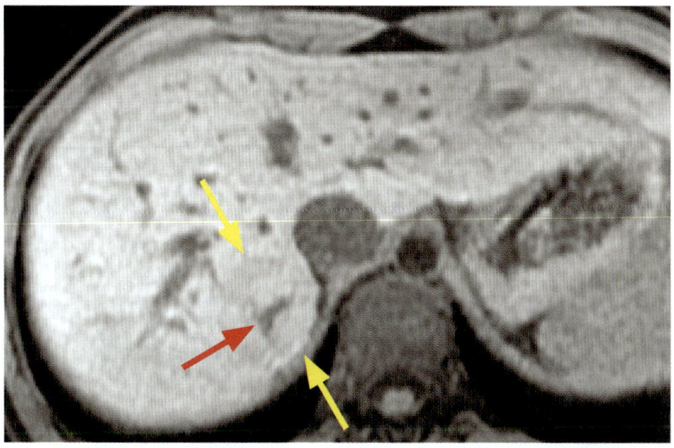

T1-weighted fat-saturated MRI
T_1 加权脂肪饱和MRI

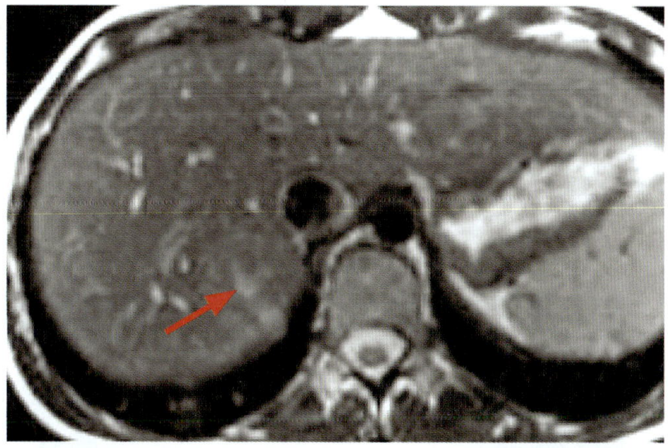

T2-weighted MRI
T_2 加权MRI

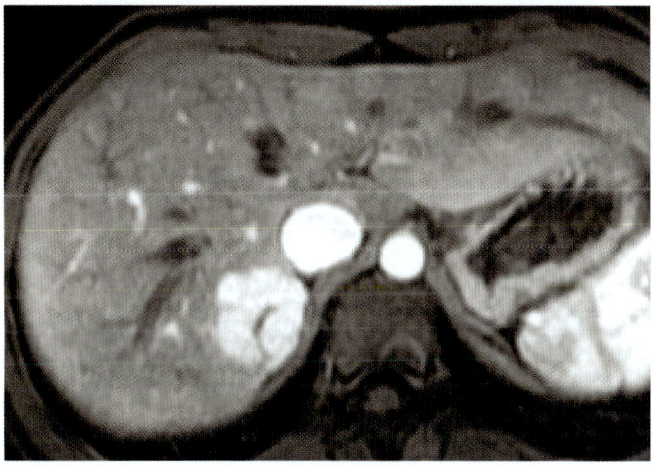

Late arterial post-contrast T1-weighted fat-sat MRI
增强动脉晚期 T_1 加权脂肪饱和MRI

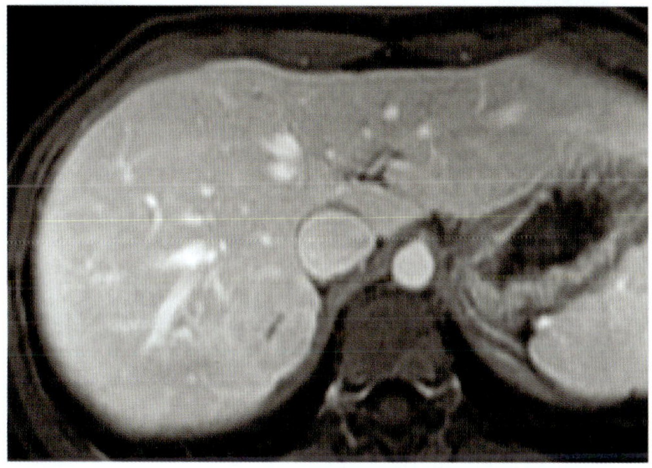

Portal venous post-contrast T1-weighted fat-sat MRI
增强门静脉期 T_1 加权脂肪饱和MRI

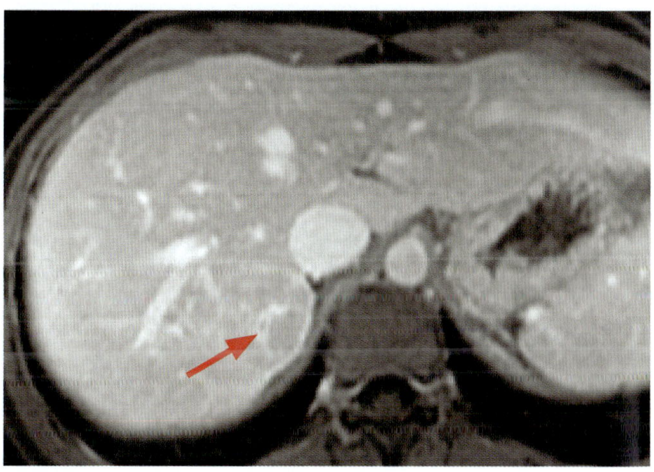

Delayed post-contrast T1-weighted fat-sat MRI
增强延迟期T_1加权脂肪饱和MRI

Focal nodular hyperplasia: T1-weighted MRI shows a barely perceptible mass in the right liver (yellow arrows) with a central low intensity scar (red arrow).
The mass is T2 isointense with the subtle suggestion of T2 hyperintense central scar (red arrow).
Arterial phase of enhancement shows avid enhancement with non-enhancement of the scar.
The mass washes out immediately on portal venous phase, with no change in intensity of the scar.
Delayed T1-weighted image shows late enhancement of the central scar (red arrow).
Case courtesy of Cheryl Sadow, MD, Brigham and Women's Hospital
局灶性结节增生：T_1 加权MRI显示在肝右叶有一个几乎察觉不到的肿块(黄箭)，伴中央低信号瘢痕(红箭)。
肿块在T_2加权呈等信号，并可见不明显的高信号中央瘢痕(红箭)。
增强扫描动脉期有明显强化，而中央瘢痕无强化。
肿块在门静脉期已迅速廓清，而中央瘢痕信号无明显改变。
延迟期T_1加权可见中央瘢痕延迟强化(红箭)。

- FNH can be difficult to see on noncontrast or portal venous phase CT as it typically matches the parenchymal attenuation. On a multiphase contrast-enhanced CT, there will be bright and homogeneous arterial enhancement with the exception of the central scar, and the portal venous phase will often show only the unenhanced scar, which enhances late (~5 minutes).
- Ultrasound findings are nonspecific. The central scar is rarely seen on ultrasound, and even when it is, this finding can be seen in other lesions,

- FNH很难在CT平扫或增强CT门静脉期被看到，因为它通常与肝实质密度相似。在多期增强CT上，病灶在动脉期呈明显均匀强化(除外中央瘢痕)，门静脉期往往只能看到无强化的瘢痕(但延迟达5分钟时可显示瘢痕)。
- 超声检查无特异性。中心瘢痕在超声上很少见，即便能看到，该征象也可见于其他病灶，

including HCC, giant hemangioma, or adenoma. Doppler findings of FNH include a *spoke-wheel* configuration of arterial vessels.

包括HCC、巨大血管瘤或腺瘤。FNH的多普勒成像表现为动脉血管的轮辐征。

- Kupffer cells and bile ductules are both present so nuclear medicine studies can be utilized to confirm the diagnosis. Kupffer cells may be confirmed by a sulfur colloid study (1/3 of the time) and bile duct cells can be visualized on a HIDA scan.

- FNH同时含有库普弗细胞和胆管，因此可利用核医学检查确诊。库普弗细胞可通过硫胶体显像证实(1/3为阳性)，而胆管细胞可使用肝胆亚氨基二乙酸(HIDA)扫描显示。

Hepatic adenoma

肝腺瘤

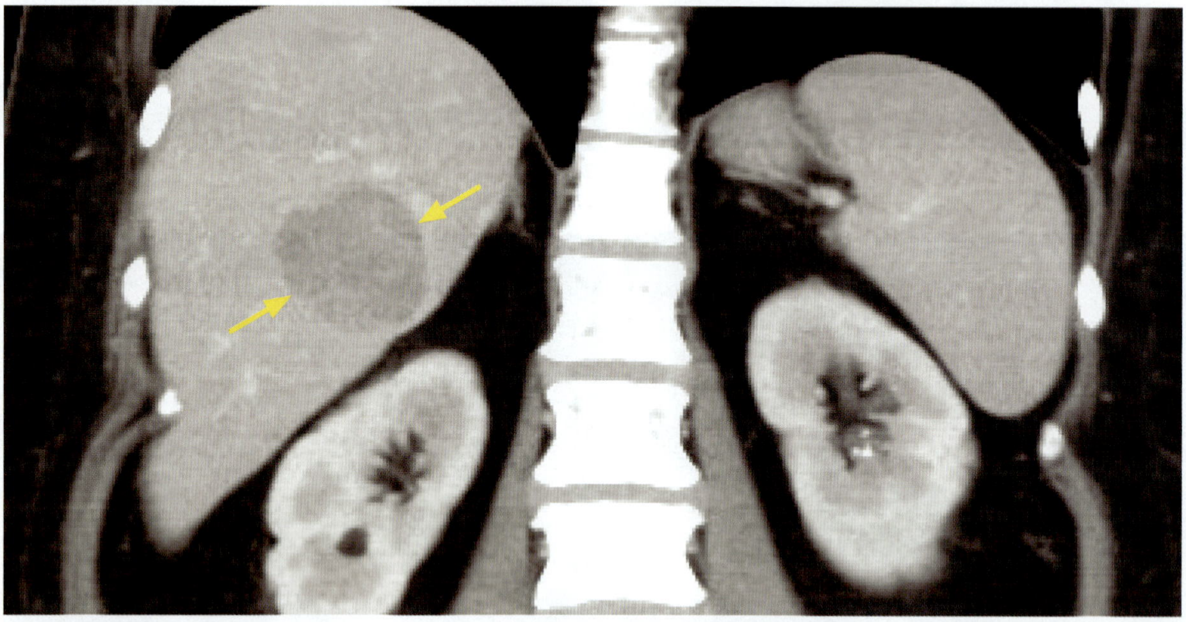

Coronal portal venous phase contrast-enhanced CT demonstrates a heterogeneously enhancing hypoattenuating mass (arrows) in the liver, which is a nonspecific appearance.

冠状位增强CT门静脉期可见肝内一个强化不均匀的低密度肿块(黄箭)，影像学表现不具有特异性。

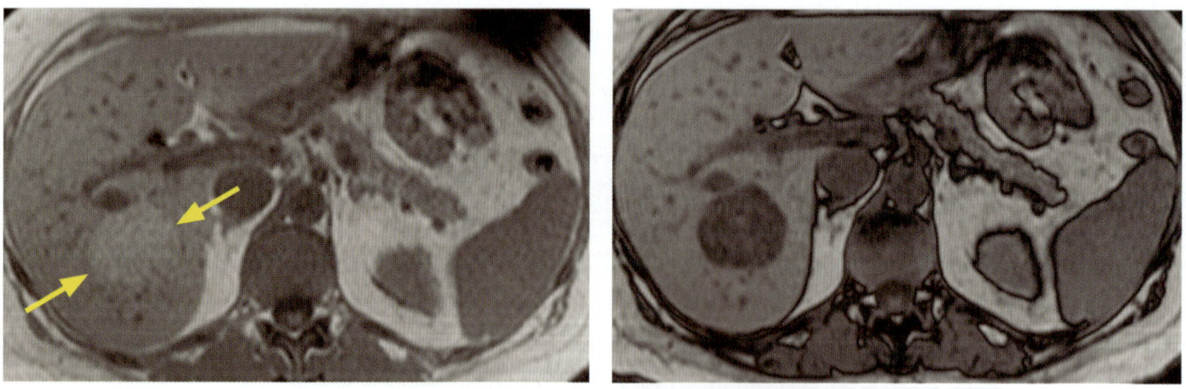

In- (left image) and out-of-phase (right image) MRI shows a mass in the right lobe of the liver (arrows) that demonstrates signal loss on out-of-phase images, consistent with a lesion containing intracellular lipid.

Case courtesy Cheryl Sadow, MD, Brigham and Women's Hospital.

同相位(左图)和反相位(右图)MRI显示一个肝右叶肿块(黄箭)，其反相位信号降低，表明病灶内含有细胞内脂肪。

- Hepatic adenoma is a benign hepatic neoplasm containing hepatocytes, scattered Kupffer cells, and no bile ducts.

  The absence of bile ducts makes a nuclear medicine HIDA scan a useful test to distinguish between focal nodular hyperplasia (which contains bile ducts and would be positive on HIDA) verses a hepatic adenoma, which does not contain bile ducts and will show a paucity of uptake on HIDA.

- Adenomas are much more common in females, especially with prolonged

- 肝腺瘤是良性肝肿瘤，内含肝细胞和散在的库普弗细胞，但无胆管。

  因为不含胆管，核医学HIDA扫描有助于鉴别局灶性结节增生(含胆管且在HIDA扫描中呈阳性)和肝腺瘤(不含胆管且在HIDA扫描中呈阴性)。

- 腺瘤多见于女性，尤其是长期使用口服避孕药者。当出现在男性时，则可能与使用合成

oral contraceptive use. When seen in males, adenoma may be associated with anabolic steroid use. Other associations include collagen vascular disease and type Ⅰ glycogen storage disease (von Gierke's disease).

- There are four histologic subtypes with varied imaging findings.

Inflammatory: Most common, has the highest bleeding risk.
HNF-alpha 1 mutated: Second most common, characterized by multiple adenomas, associated with FAP and von Gierke's.
Beta-catenin mutated: Least common, seen in men on anabolic steroids, has the highest risk of malignant transformation.
Unclassified.

- Adenomas have a relatively high risk of hemorrhage, which is often the presenting symptom. For this reason, incidentally discovered adenomas >5 cm are usually resected.
- Adenomas are supplied by the hepatic artery and thus tend to be hypervascular on arterial phase. Some subtypes (inflammatory) may demonstrate intralesional fat which on MRI will demonstrate T1 hyperintensity and signal loss on out-of-phase images. Adenomas may be difficult to differentiate from other hypervascular liver lesions in the absence of fat or hemorrhage.
- As stated above, each subtype has slightly different imaging features, making confident imaging diagnosis somewhat difficult and often requiring tissue sampling for confirmation.

Adenomas are typically circumscribed masses with arterial hyperenhancement, becoming iso- or hypo- to liver on portal venous and delayed phase imaging. They may appear heterogeneous due to fat or hemorrhagic content. A fibrous pseudocapsule may be present, which tends to enhance late.

- There are no specific ultrasound features to distinguish an adenoma from other hepatic masses. An adenoma may be hyperechoic, isoechoic, or hypoechoic relative to normal liver.
- Nuclear medicine is not usually helpful to differentiate adenoma from other liver masses. Adenomas are usually photopenic on Tc-99m sulfur colloid scintigraphy (in contrast to FNH), but not always. There is usually lack of uptake on a HIDA scan due to the absence of biliary ductules.

Other fat-containing hepatic lesions

- In addition to adenomas, other fat-containing lesions in the liver include lipoma (very rare), angiomyolipoma, and pseudolipoma of the Glisson's capsule.

Biliary cystadenoma/cystadenocarcinoma

- Biliary cystadenoma is a benign cystic mass lined with biliary-type epithelium.
- Although benign, most are surgically resected since malignant transformation to cystadenocarcinoma may occur.
- These typically appear as a multiseptated cystic mass on all imaging modalities. Cystadenoma and cystadenocarcinoma are not easily differentiated on imaging. Mural nodules should be regarded with suspicion for malignant transformation to cystadenocarcinoma.
- This is further discussed under "Biliary Neoplasia" later in the chapter.

代谢类固醇有关。其他相关因素包括胶原血管疾病和糖原贮积症Ⅰ型(冯・基尔克病)。

- 共有四种组织学亚型,其影像学表现多样。

炎症:最常见,出血风险最高。
HNF-α1突变:次常见,以多发腺瘤为特征,与家族性腺瘤样息肉病(FAP)和糖原贮积症Ⅰ型相关。
β-连环蛋白突变:最少见,见于服用合成代谢类固醇的男性,恶性转化的风险最高。
未分类。

- 腺瘤具有相对较高的出血风险,且往往是其首发症状。因此,偶然发现的腺瘤如直径>5cm通常需要进行手术切除。
- 腺瘤由肝动脉供血,因此在动脉期表现为富血供。某些亚型(炎症型)可能内含脂肪,故在T_1加权MRI上表现为高信号,在反相位图像上呈低信号。腺瘤若不含脂肪或发生出血,可能难以与其他富血供肝脏病变进行鉴别。
- 如上所述,每个亚型的影像学特征都略有不同,因而作出明确的影像学诊断比较困难,往往需要进行组织活检进行确诊。

腺瘤通常是边界清楚的肿块,动脉期有明显强化,在门静脉期和延迟期对于肝组织呈等密度或低密度。腺瘤可能表现为不均质肿块,为病灶内脂肪或出血成分所致。可出现纤维性假包膜,在延迟期可见强化。

- 超声缺乏特殊的征象可用于鉴别腺瘤与其他肝脏肿块。腺瘤相对于正常肝脏可呈高回声、等回声或低回声。
- 核医学通常对鉴别腺瘤与其他肝脏肿块没有帮助。腺瘤通常在^{99m}Tc硫胶体闪烁显像上呈阴性(与FNH相反),但也有例外。HIDA扫描通常没有摄取,因其缺乏胆管结构。

其他含脂肪的肝脏病变

- 除腺瘤外,其他肝脏含脂肪的病变包括脂肪瘤(非常罕见)、血管平滑肌脂肪瘤和格利森鞘假性脂肪瘤。

胆管囊腺瘤/囊腺癌

- 胆管囊腺瘤是良性囊状肿块,内衬胆道样上皮。
- 虽属良性,但大部分需要手术切除,因其可能恶变为囊腺癌。
- 在所有影像学检查中,它们大多表现为多分隔囊性肿块。囊腺瘤和囊腺癌在影像学上不易鉴别。若出现壁结节应视为恶变。
- "胆道肿瘤"将在本章后文进一步讨论。

Enhancement patterns of common hepatic masses

	Arterial phase	Portal venous phase	Delayed phase
HCC	↑	↓	↓
FNH	↑	iso	iso
Hepatic adenoma	↑	↓	↓
Hypervascular metastasis	↑ or iso	↓ or iso	↓ or iso
Non-hypervascular metastasis	↓	↓	↓

常见肝肿块的强化模式

	动脉期	门静脉期	延迟期
肝细胞癌	↑	↓	↓
局灶性结节增生	↑	相等	相等
肝腺瘤	↑	↓	↓
肝脏转移瘤	↑或相等	↓或相等	↓或相等
乏血供转移瘤	↓	↓	↓

Hepatic infection

肝脏感染

Viral hepatitis

病毒性肝炎

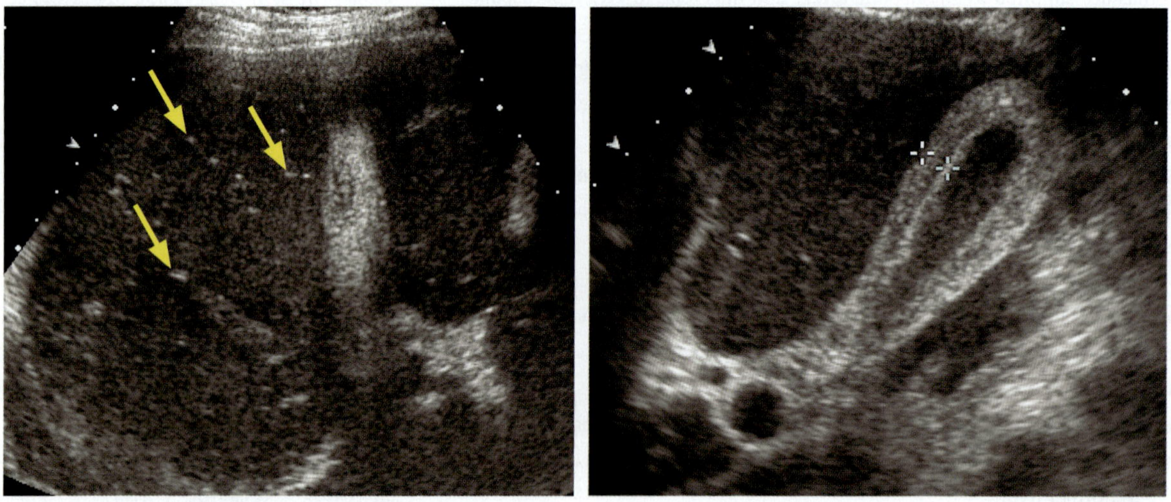

Viral hepatitis: Sagittal image of the liver (left image) demonstrates increased echogenicity of the portal triads appearing as numerous echogenic dots (arrows) that produce a *starry sky* appearance. Sagittal view of the gallbladder in the same patient (right image) shows marked diffuse gallbladder wall thickening (calipers), which is commonly seen in acute hepatitis.

Case courtesy Julie Ritner, MD, Brigham and Women's Hospital, Boston.

病毒性肝炎：肝脏矢状切面(左图)显示门静脉三联征回声增强，表现为多发点状高回声(黄箭)形成星系样改变。同一名患者胆囊矢状切面(右图)显示胆囊壁弥漫性增厚(卡尺)，是急性肝炎的常见表现。

- Viral hepatitis is infection of the liver by a hepatotropic virus. Hepatitis B and C cause chronic disease.
- The most common imaging finding is of a normal liver. When imaging is abnormal, the most common findings are periportal edema (*starry sky* pattern of increased portal triad echogenicity on ultrasound; fluid on both sides of the portal vein on CT and MRI) and gallbladder wall thickening/edema.

- 病毒性肝炎是由一种嗜肝病毒引起的肝脏感染；乙型和丙型肝炎会引起慢性疾病。
- 最常见的影像学表现是肝脏无明显异常。当出现影像学异常时，最常见的是门静脉周围水肿(*星系征*，超声上门静脉三联征回声增强，CT和MRI显示门静脉两侧积液)和胆囊壁增厚/水肿。

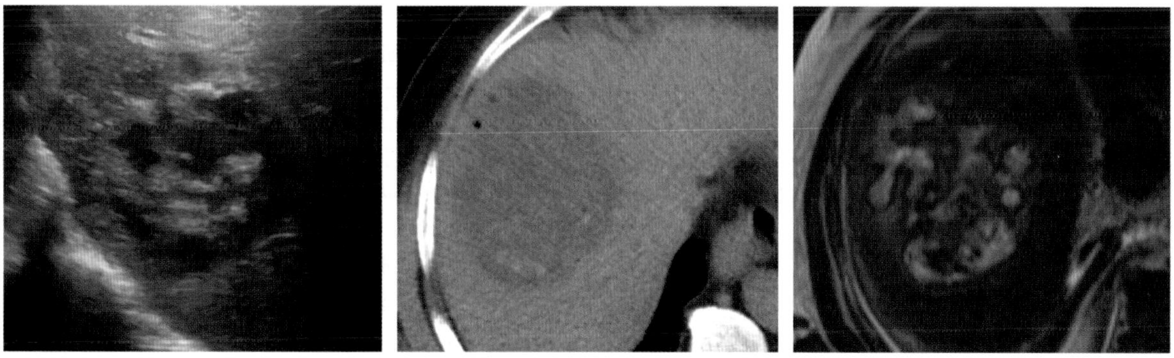

Grayscale ultrasound 灰阶超声 | Unenhanced CT 平扫CT | T2-weighted MRI T_2加权MRI

Ultrasound (left image) shows a heterogeneously hypoechoic lesion corresponding to a hypodense lesion with foci of gas on noncontrast CT (middle image). This lesion was heterogeneously T2 hyperintense on MRI (right image) with enhancement and restricted diffusion (not shown).

超声(左图)显示一个不均匀的低回声病变，在相应的病灶部位平扫CT呈低密度伴气泡(中图)。该病变在MRI上呈不均匀T_2高信号(右图)，并可见强化和弥散受限(未显示)。

- **Hepatic abscess** is most commonly caused by a bowel process and resultant infectious nidus carried through the portal system to the liver. Common causes include diverticulitis, appendicitis, Crohn's disease, and bowel surgery. *E. coli* is the most common causative organism.
- Imaging features of hepatic abscess may mimic metastasis, appearing as a ring-enhancing mass on CT and MRI. Reactive perilesional hyperenhancement may be present. On MRI, there is typically also central T2 hyperintensity and restricted diffusion.
- On ultrasound, infection starts as an ill-defined area of altered echogenicity (phlegmon stage) which evolves into a well-defined hypoechoic structure with internal echoes (mature abscess).
- **Cholangitic abscess** can be seen with bacterial cholangitis, or may occur in patients with biliary stents, prior sphincterotomies or hepaticojejunostomies due to gastrointestinal reflux into the biliary tree.

- **肝脓肿**最常见的原因是肠道病变所引起的感染性病灶通过门静脉系统播散到肝脏。常见的病因包括憩室炎、阑尾炎、克罗恩病和肠道手术。大肠埃希菌是最常见的致病菌。
- 肝脓肿的影像学表现可类似于肝转移瘤，在CT和MRI上表现为环形强化的肿块。病灶周围可出现反应性高强化。在MRI上，病灶中央呈典型的T_2高信号和弥散受限。
- 在超声上，感染最初表现为边界不清的回声增强区(蜂窝织炎期)，然后演变为一个边界清楚的内部低回声病灶(成熟脓肿)。
- **胆管脓肿**可见于细菌性胆管炎，也可能发生在胆道支架植入、括约肌切开术或肝空肠吻合手术史的患者，原因是胃肠反流进入胆道。

Tuberculosis (TB)

- Tuberculosis (TB) causes granulomatous hepatitis, usually secondary to hematogenous spread from primary pulmonary TB.
- Lesions may be micro- or macronodular (rare), with multiple small hypoechoic hypoenhancing nodules or larger mass-like areas which demonstrate variable enhancement. These findings are often accompanied by hepatosplenomegaly.

结核病(TB)

- 结核病(TB)可引起肉芽肿性肝炎，通常继发于原发性肺结核的血行播散。
- 病变可以是小结节或大结节(罕见)，有多个小的低回声、低强化结节或较大肿块样区域，其强化方式不定。这些表现常伴有肝脾肿大。

Fungal infection

- Hepatic fungal infections typically show punctate, hypoenhancing microabscesses on CT and MRI and tiny hypoechoic lesions on ultrasound. Lesions are T2 hyperintense and restrict diffusion on MRI. Prior asymptomatic exposure and/or treated disease may show punctate, echogenic calcifications/granulomas.

真菌感染

- 肝脏真菌感染在CT和MRI上通常表现为点状低强化的微小脓肿，而在超声上则为很小的低回声病变。病变在MRI上呈T_2高信号且弥散受限。既往无症状性暴露和/或治疗后的TB可表现为点状钙化样或肉芽肿样回声。

Histoplasmosis

- Histoplasmosis is another form of granulomatous hepatitis secondary to the endemic fungus *Histoplasma capsulatum* which is most commonly found in the Ohio and Mississippi river valleys. It is more common in immunocompromised patients but can be seen in immunocompetent patients as well.
- Hepatic involvement is usually secondary to spread from pulmonary

组织胞浆菌病

- 组织胞浆菌病是另一种形式的肉芽肿性肝炎，继发于地方性真菌荚膜组织胞浆菌病，在美国，这种菌在俄亥俄州和密西西比河流域最常见。该病常见于免疫功能低下的患者，但也可发生于免疫功能正常的患者。

histoplasmosis. In addition to the typical imaging findings of fungal infections, hepatosplenomegaly and hypoattenuating lymph nodes may also be seen.

- 肝脏受累通常来自肺组织胞浆菌病的扩散。除真菌感染的典型影像学表现外，还可见到肝脾肿大和低密度的淋巴结。

Pneumocystis jiroveci

- Hepatic *Pneumocystis jiroveci* is seen in disseminated disease in the severely immunocompromised. Hepatic infection is classically secondary to the use of inhaled pentamidine to treat pulmonary *Pneumocystis* pneumonia, as pentamidine is not absorbed systemically and thus would not prevent hepatic infection.

肺孢子虫病

- 肝脏肺孢子虫病见于免疫功能严重受损且有扩散的患者。肝脏感染通常继发于吸入喷他脒治疗肺孢子虫肺炎，因为喷他脒不被吸收进入全身而不能预防肝脏感染。

Candidiasis

- Systemic candida infection is almost always seen in immunocompromised patients and may seed the liver (and commonly the spleen as well).

念珠菌病

- 系统性念珠菌感染几乎总是见于免疫功能低下的患者，并可能播散到肝脏(脾也同样常见)。

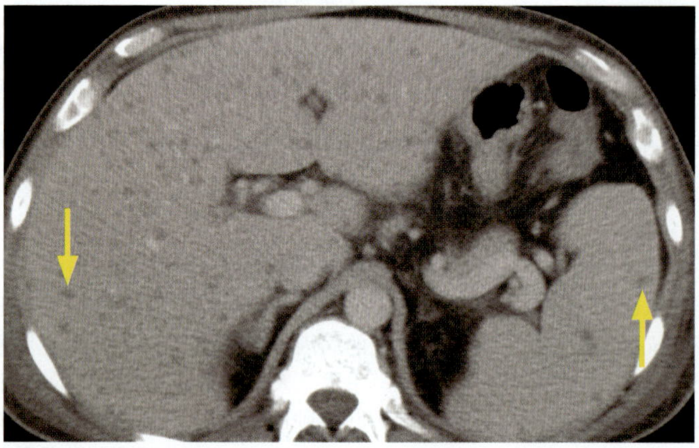

Noncontrast CT shows innumerable tiny hypoattenuating lesions scattered throughout the liver and spleen (arrows), representing candidal microabscesses in a bone marrow transplant patient with fungemia.
平扫CT肝脏和脾脏显示无数微小低密度病灶(黄箭)分布于整个肝脏和脾脏，为念珠菌性微脓肿，为一名并发真菌血症的骨髓移植患者。

Echinococcal disease

- Hepatic echinococcosis is caused by ingestion of the eggs of *Echinococcus granulosus*, which is endemic in the Mediterranean basin and associated with sheep-raising. Echinococcal eggs can develop into hydatid cysts.

包虫病(棘球蚴病)

- 肝包虫病是由于摄入细粒棘球绦虫虫卵引起的，是流行于地中海盆地的一种地方性疾病，与饲养羊有关。细粒棘球绦虫虫卵可发育成包虫囊。

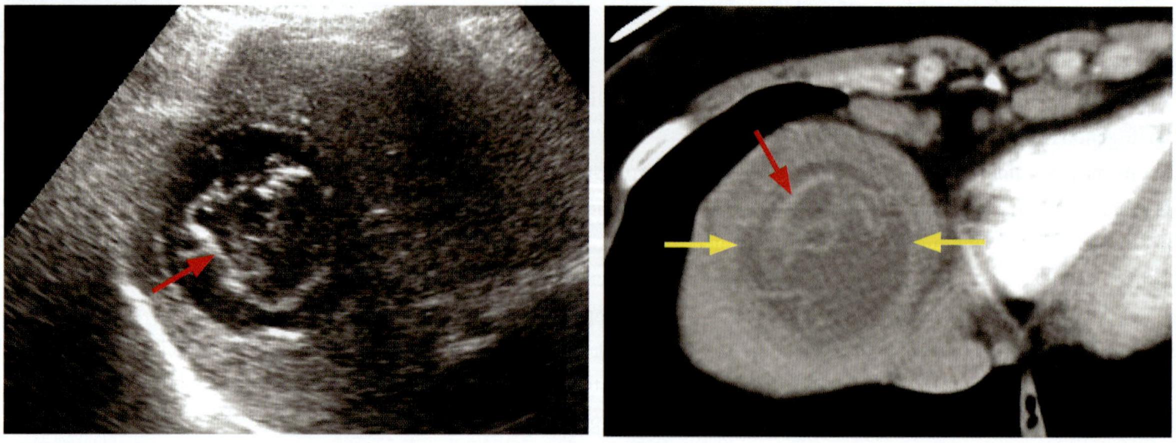

Hepatic echinococcus: Ultrasound (left image) shows a complex, primarily hypoechoic mass in the superior aspect of the liver containing a hyperechoic undulating membrane (red arrow). Contrast-enhanced CT (right image) shows a fluid-attenuating cystic mass (yellow arrows) containing an undulating membrane (red arrow).
Case courtesy Cheryl Sadow, MD, Brigham and Women's Hospital.
肝包虫病：超声(左图)显示肝顶有一个低回声为主的混杂回声肿块，内包含高回声的波状膜(红箭)。增强CT(右图)显示一个液性密度肿块(黄箭)，内含波状膜(红箭)。

- On CT and MRI, a hydatid cyst is a well-defined hypoenhancing cystic mass featuring a characteristic floating membrane or an associated daughter cyst. Peripheral calcification may be seen on CT.
- Classic ultrasound appearance is a large liver cyst with numerous peripheral daughter cysts.

  A highly suggestive finding is the change in position of daughter cysts as the patient is repositioned.

  The *water-lily sign* is an undulating membrane within the hydatid cyst.

  Hydatid sand is a fine sediment caused by separation of the membranes from the endocyst.
- There is a theoretical risk of anaphylaxis with peritoneal spillage of cyst fluid, although these are often biopsied and drained uneventfully. Medical treatment is albendazole or mebendazole.

Amebic abscess

- Amebic abscess is caused by *Entamoeba histolytica*. A near-universal presenting symptom is pain, seen in 99% of patients. The most common location is near the dome of the right lobe.
- On imaging, an amebic abscess is indistinguishable from a pyogenic abscess.
- Antimicrobial therapy is usually sufficient treatment, and drainage is rarely necessary.

- 包虫囊在CT和MRI上呈边界清楚的低强化囊性肿块，具有典型的漂浮膜或子囊。CT可能显示外周钙化。
- 典型的超声表现是大的肝内囊性灶伴多发周围子囊。

  高度提示肝包虫病的表现是子囊位置随着患者体位的改变而发生变化。

  水上浮莲征是包虫囊内的波状膜。

  包虫砂是一种细小的沉积物，为内囊脱落的膜。
- 理论上，包虫囊液流入腹腔有发生过敏反应的风险，但活检和引流包虫囊通常没有任何意外。药物治疗用阿苯达唑或甲苯达唑。

阿米巴脓肿

- 阿米巴脓肿是由阿米巴原虫引起的。99%的患者临床症状表现为疼痛。最常见的部位是肝右叶膈顶附近。
- 阿米巴脓肿在影像学上与化脓性脓肿难以区分。
- 抗阿米巴药物通常是有效的治疗方法，极少需要引流。

CYSTIC LIVER DISEASE

Imaging simple cysts

- On all imaging modalities, simple hepatic cysts are characterized by a round or oval, well- circumscribed, thin/nearly imperceptible wall. A few thin septa may be seen.
- On ultrasound, a simple cyst is anechoic, shows posterior acoustic enhancement, and demonstrates no internal vascularity on Doppler.
- CT shows homogeneous low attenuation (0–20 HU) and no contrast enhancement.
- MRI shows low T1, high T2 signal intensity and no contrast enhancement.

Biliary hamartomas (von Meyenburg complexes)

- Biliary hamartomas are small, benign cystic lesions which do not communicate with the biliary tree and are caused by embryologic failure of normal bile duct formation.
- Biliary hamartomas tend to be smaller and more irregularly shaped than simple cysts.
- Small biliary hamartomas may actually appear echogenic on ultrasound.

Autosomal dominant polycystic liver disease (ADPLD)

- 40% of patients with autosomal dominant polycystic kidney disease (ADPKD) have a similar disease process in the liver, called ADPLD. Even in severe disease, hepatic failure is rare.
- On imaging, there are innumerable non-enhancing simple cysts throughout the liver.

von Hippel-Lindau (VHL)

- Von Hippel-Lindau (VHL) syndrome results from mutation in the VHL gene and is characterized by benign and malignant tumors in many organs. Within the liver, there are often innumerable simple cysts.

囊性肝脏病变

单纯肝囊肿的影像学表现

- 在所有影像学检查中，单纯肝囊肿的特征是圆形或椭圆形、边界清楚、壁薄或几乎无法辨认的薄壁。可以有少量薄的分隔。
- 单纯肝囊肿超声表现为无回声，后部有回声增强，并且多普勒显示内部无血流。
- CT表现为均匀低密度(0~20HU)，无强化。
- MRI表现为T_1低信号、T_2高信号，无强化。

胆道错构瘤(von Meyenburg complexes)

- 胆道错构瘤是小的良性囊性病变，与胆道分支不相通，是胚胎发育过程中正常胆道形成障碍所致。
- 胆道错构瘤通常小于单纯囊肿，且形态不规则。
- 小的胆道错构瘤在超声上可能出现高回声。

常染色体显性多囊肝病(ADPLD)

- 约40%的常染色体显性多囊肾病(ADPKD)患者会在肝脏出现相似的疾病，被称为ADPLD。即使非常严重，肝衰竭也很少见。
- 影像学上，肝脏布满无数无强化的单纯性囊肿。

希佩尔-林道病(von Hippel-Lindau disease, VHL)

- 希佩尔-林道病(VHL)是由*VHL*基因突变引起的，以多器官良性和恶性肿瘤为特征。在肝脏表现为无数单纯性囊肿。

COMMON IMAGING PATTERNS OF LIVER LESIONS

Multicystic

Multiple simple cyst or biliary hamartomas.
Caroli disease (saccular dilation of the intrahepatic bile ducts).
ADPLD (associated with ADPKD).
VHL.

Cystic with internal echoes on ultrasound

Simple cyst with internal hemorrhage or superimposed infection.
Abscess.
Hematoma.
Necrotic or cystic metastasis.

Hyperenhancing lesions

FNH.
Adenoma.
HCC.
Hemangioma (especially flash-filling subtype).
Hypervascular metastases.

Fat-containing

Focal fat.
Adenoma.
HCC.
Angiomyolipoma, lipoma, pseudolipoma of the Glisson's capsule (rare).

Hemorrhagic

Adenoma.
HCC.
Metastases.

Central scar

FNH.
Fibrolamellar HCC.
Giant hemangioma.

Calcified

Mucinous metastases.
Osteosarcoma metastases.
Biliary cystadenoma/cystadenocarcinoma.

Hepatic capsular retraction

Mass-forming cholangiocarcinoma.
Fibrolamellar HCC.
Epithelioid hemangioendothelioma.
Pseudocirrhosis (treated metastases).
Confluent hepatic fibrosis (wedge-shaped fibrosis that may be seen in cirrhosis).

肝脏病变的常见影像学表现

多囊

多发单纯性囊肿或胆道错构瘤。
卡罗利病(肝内胆管囊状扩张)。
ADPLD(合并ADPKD)。
VHL。

囊内超声有内部回声

单纯囊肿伴内出血或合并感染。
脓肿。
血肿。
坏死或囊性转移。

高回声病灶

局灶性结节增生。
腺瘤。
肝细胞癌。
血管瘤(尤其是快速充盈型)。
富血供转移瘤。

含脂病灶

局限性脂肪。
腺瘤。
肝细胞癌。
血管平滑肌脂肪瘤、脂肪瘤、格利森鞘假脂肪瘤(罕见)。

出血性

腺瘤。
肝细胞癌。
转移瘤。

中央瘢痕

局灶性结节增生。
纤维板层样肝癌。
肝巨大血管瘤。

钙化

黏液性转移瘤。
骨肉瘤转移。
胆管囊腺瘤/囊腺癌。

肝包膜回缩征

肿块型胆管癌。
纤维板层样肝细胞癌。
上皮样血管内皮瘤。
假性肝硬化(转移瘤治疗后)。
融合性肝纤维化(肝硬化中可见楔形纤维化)。

LIVER TRAUMA

Overview of liver trauma

- The liver is the second most commonly injured solid organ due to blunt trauma, second to the spleen.
- The 2018 revised organ injury scale (OIS) for liver published by the American Association for the Surgery of Trauma (AAST) includes imaging, operative, and pathologic criteria for grading injury. The final AAST grade assigned is based on the highest of the three criteria.
- The imaging criteria is based on CT findings and is more commonly used by radiologists. It is similar to the organ injury scale for splenic trauma.

肝外伤

肝外伤概述

- 肝脏是钝性外伤中第二常见受损的实质器官，仅次于脾。
- 美国创伤外科协会(AAST)于2018年发布了修订版的肝脏损伤量表(OIS)，其中包括影像学、手术和病理损伤分级标准，最终的AAST评分是基于上述三个标准中最高的一个。
- 影像学标准以CT为准，较常被放射科医生采用。这与脾外伤的脏器损伤量表相似。

American Association for the Surgery of Trauma liver injury scale (imaging criteria)

AAST liver injury scale

- Grade Ⅰ:
  Subcapsular hematoma <10% liver surface.
  Superficial laceration <1 cm deep.
- Grade Ⅱ:
  Subcapsular hematoma 10–50% liver surface.
  Intraparenchymal hematoma <10 cm in size.
  Laceration 1–3 cm deep.
- Grade Ⅲ:
  Subcapsular hematoma >50% liver surface.
  Ruptured subcapsular/intraparenchymal hematoma.
  Laceration >3 cm deep.
  Any intraparenchymal vascular injury (i.e., pseudoaneurysm or AV fistula) or contained active bleeding.
- Grade Ⅳ:
  Laceration involving 25–75% of one hepatic lobe.
  Extraparenchymal extension of active bleeding into the peritoneum.
- Grade Ⅴ:
  Laceration or destruction >75% of one hepatic lobe.
  Injury to retrohepatic IVC or central hepatic veins.

- When multiple injuries are present, advance one grade up to a grade Ⅲ.
- AAST grading system is limited for assessment of biliary injury. If injury to the biliary system is suspected, nuclear medicine HIDA scan is often needed to demonstrate an active bile leak. MRI with hepatobiliary agent such as Eovist may also be helpful.

美国创伤外科协会肝损伤量表(影像学标准)

AAST肝脏损伤量表

- Ⅰ级:
  肝被膜下血肿<10%肝表面。
  浅表撕裂伤,深度<1cm。
- Ⅱ级:
  肝被膜下血肿占10%~50%肝表面。
  实质内血肿直径<10cm。
  撕裂深度1~3cm。
- Ⅲ级:
  肝被膜下血肿>50%肝表面。
  被膜下破裂/实质内血肿。
  撕裂深度>3cm。
  任何实质内血管损伤(如假性动脉瘤或动静脉瘘)或包裹性活动性出血。
- Ⅳ级:
  撕裂伤累及肝叶的25%~75%。
  活动性出血延伸到实质外并进入腹腔。
- Ⅴ级:
  撕裂或损毁累及肝叶>75%。
  损伤累及肝后的下腔静脉或中央肝静脉。

- 当出现多处损伤时,级别上升1~3级。
- AAST分级系统对胆道损伤的评估有限。如果怀疑胆道系统受伤,通常需要核医学HIDA扫描来证实活动性胆汁瘘。MRI采用肝胆造影剂(如钆塞酸二钠)也可能有帮助。

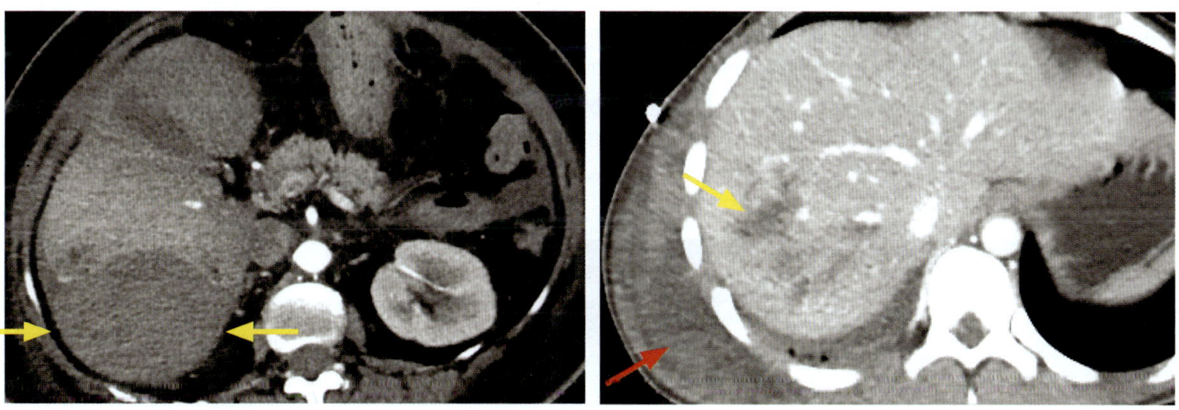

Left image: CT angiogram axial image demonstrates a large subcapsular hematoma (yellow arrows) along the right hepatic lobe with no evidence of active extravasation.

Right image: Portal venous phase CT axial image shows hypodense geographic/linear regions (yellow arrow) in the right hepatic lobe, indicating hepatic lacerations. Note the large right chest wall hematoma (red arrow).

左图:轴位CT血管造影显示沿肝右叶的被膜下有一个大血肿(黄箭),但无活动性造影剂外渗。

右图:轴位门静脉期CT图像显示肝右叶有一处呈低密度的地图样或线样区域(黄箭),提示肝撕裂伤。注意右胸壁有一个巨大血肿(红箭)。

LIVER TRANSPLANT

Surgical candidates

- The **Milan criteria** is used to assess appropriateness of liver transplantation in those with HCC or cirrhosis. To be considered for orthotopic liver transplantation, one must have:

  Single tumor <5 cm or up to three tumors, each with diameter <3 cm.

肝移植

手术适应证

- **米兰标准**用于评估HCC或肝硬化患者是否适合肝移植。考虑全肝移植,必须具备:

  单个肿瘤直径<5cm,或最多3个肿瘤,且每个直径<3cm。

No extrahepatic involvement.

No major vascular involvement.

未累及肝外组织。

无大血管受累。

Post-operative appearance

- Normal findings may include periportal edema, minimal ascites, right-sided pleural effusion, and a small perihepatic hematoma.

手术后的表现

- 正常表现包括门静脉周围水肿、少量腹水、右侧胸腔积液和肝周小血肿。

Complications

- **Vascular**: Hepatic artery thrombosis is the most common vascular complication. Others include hepatic artery stenosis and pseudoaneurysm, IVC or hepatic vein stenosis or thrombosis and portal vein stenosis or thrombosis.
- **Biliary**: Ductal stricture is the most common biliary complication. Leaks and obstruction due to choledocholithiasis are also possible.
- **Other** complications include hematoma, abscess, hepatitis, splenic infarct, recurrent malignancy or primary sclerosing cholangitis (depending on the indication for transplant) and **post-transplant lymphoproliferative disorder (PTLD)**.

PTLD is a type of lymphoma caused by Epstein-Barr virus which can arise after solid organ or bone marrow transplant. Patients with renal transplants are at particular risk. PTLD may occur anywhere, regardless of which organ was transplanted. Treatment is reduction/withdrawal of immunosuppression. PTLD appears as a mass with a variable and nonspecific appearance.

并发症

- **血管**：肝动脉血栓形成是最常见的血管并发症。其他包括肝动脉狭窄和假性动脉瘤、下腔静脉或肝静脉狭窄或血栓形成，以及门静脉狭窄或血栓形成。
- **胆道**：胆管狭窄是最常见的胆道并发症。胆道结石所致的胆漏和梗阻也可能发生。
- **其他**并发症包括血肿、脓肿、肝炎、脾梗死、恶性肿瘤复发或原发性硬化性胆管炎复发(取决于移植适应证)和**移植后淋巴增生性疾病(PTLD)**。

PTLD是一种由EB病毒引起的淋巴瘤，可发生在实体器官或骨髓移植后，肾移植患者尤其危险。PTLD可发生在任何部位，与所移植的器官无关。治疗方法是减少或撤除免疫抑制。PTLD表现为肝脏肿块，外形多变且无特异性。

Vascular liver disease

肝血管性疾病

Budd-Chiari

- Budd-Chiari is hepatic venous outflow obstruction, which can be thrombotic or non-thrombotic. Thrombotic Budd-Chiari may be due to hypercoagulative states including hematological disorders, pregnancy, oral contraceptive use, malignancy, infection, and trauma. It is very rare to have primary Budd-Chiari due to congenital hepatic vein anomaly, as pictured below.

布-加综合征

- 布-加综合征是指肝静脉回流受阻，可以是血栓性或非血栓性。血栓性布-加综合征可能为高凝状态所致，包括血液系统疾病、怀孕、口服避孕药、恶性肿瘤、感染，以及创伤。罕见的原发性布-加综合征为先天性肝静脉发育异常所致，如下图所示。

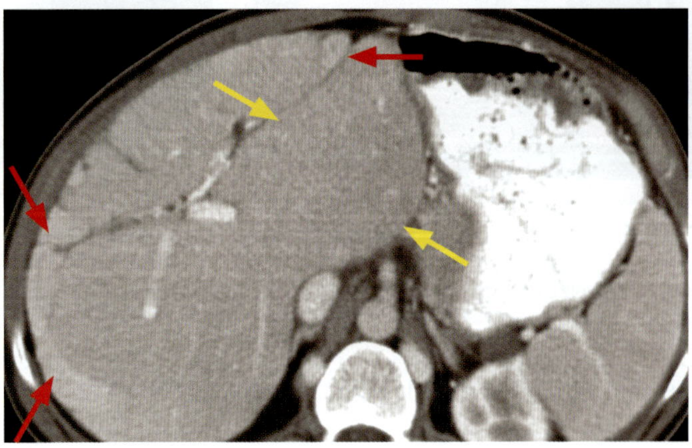

Congenital Budd-Chiari: Axial contrast- enhanced CT shows massive enlargement of the caudate lobe (yellow arrows) and the right posterior segment. There is atrophy of the left lobe and right anterior segments of the liver. Collateral venous drainage in the periphery of the liver is seen as geographic peripheral hyperenhancement (red arrows). The causative congenital hepatic vein anomaly is not visualized at this level.

Case courtesy Cheryl Sadow, MD, Brigham and Women's Hospital.

先天性布-加综合征：轴位增强CT显示肝尾状叶(黄箭)及右后段肥大。肝左叶和右前段萎缩。肝周多发侧支静脉引流呈地图样边缘强化(红箭)。引起本病的先天性肝静脉异常未在此层面显示。

- Acute Budd-Chiari presents with the clinical triad of hepatomegaly, ascites, and abdominal pain.
- Vascular findings include lack of Doppler flow or contrast within hepatic veins, thrombus in the hepatic veins/IVC, and the formation of collateral vessels which appear as a *spider web* on venography.
- Acute intraparenchymal findings include an edematous, mottled liver (*nutmeg liver*) with sparing of the caudate lobe. As discussed above, the caudate is often

- 急性布-加综合征表现为临床三联征：肝大、腹水和腹痛。
- 血管表现包括肝静脉内无多普勒血流或造影剂、肝静脉/下腔静脉血栓，以及侧支血管形成，在静脉造影上表现为蜘蛛网征。
- 急性期肝实质表现包括肝实质水肿、花斑状肝(肉豆蔻肝)，但不累及尾状叶。如前所述，

spared as it drains directly into the IVC. *Flip-flop enhancement* may be seen, with early central enhancement and delayed peripheral enhancement.

- Chronic findings are marked by progressive liver failure, with caudate lobe hypertrophy and atrophy of peripheral liver with prominent regenerative nodules.

Veno-occlusive disease

- Veno-occlusive disease (VOD) is destruction of small hepatic vessels secondary to toxin exposure, with patent hepatic veins. VOD is often seen in patients after stem cell transplant and exposure to certain chemotherapy agents.
- Imaging findings are nonspecific. In the acute phase, periportal edema, narrowing of the hepatic veins, hepatomegaly, heterogeneous hepatic enhancement, gallbladder wall edema and ascites have been reported. Liver Doppler may show decreased velocity or reversal of flow in the portal veins. In contrast to Budd-Chiari, the caudate lobe is not spared. The findings in chronic disease are similar to those of cirrhosis.
- Differential diagnosis in patients after stem cell transplant includes graft-versus-host disease (GVHD). Veno-occlusive disease is more likely if the right hepatic vein diameter is <0.45 cm while GVHD is more likely if there is associated small bowel wall thickening.

Peliosis hepatis

- Peliosis hepatis is a rare benign disorder of sinusoidal dilatation and formation of blood- filled lacunae.
- It is often idiopathic but may occur due to certain medications (including steroids, oral contraceptives, tamoxifen and methotrexate), immune disorders (including HIV, immunosuppression post-transplant) and infections (including HIV, TB, *Bartonella*).
- CT and MRI show early central enhancement with delayed centrifugal enhancement. Ultrasound may show a non-specific hyperechoic mass.

Cardiac hepatopathy

- Cardiac hepatopathy is passive hepatic congestion from cardiac surgery, heart failure, constrictive pericarditis, or right-sided valvular disease, which may ultimately lead to cirrhosis.
- Imaging findings include enlarged hepatic veins and IVC, with reflux of intravenous contrast from the right atrium into the IVC and hepatic veins. The liver is typically enlarged and demonstrates mottled enhancement (*nutmeg liver*). Ascites is usually present.

尾状叶正常是因为它直接引流至下腔静脉。影像学上可见翻转性增强，伴早期中央强化和延迟周边强化。

- 慢性期表现为进行性肝衰竭、尾状叶肥大、周围性肝萎缩，且伴有显著的再生结节。

静脉闭塞性疾病(VOD)

- 静脉闭塞性疾病(VOD)是继发于中毒后的肝小血管受损，而肝静脉是通畅的。VOD常见于干细胞移植和某些化疗药物使用后的患者。
- 影像学表现无特异性。有报道急性期可见门静脉周围水肿、肝静脉狭窄、肝大、肝实质不均匀强化，胆囊壁水肿和腹水等。肝脏多普勒可显示门静脉流速下降或出现反向流动。与布-加综合征不同，尾状叶同时受累。慢性期表现类似于肝硬化。
- 干细胞移植后患者的鉴别诊断包括移植物抗宿主病(GVHD)。如果肝右静脉直径<0.45cm，则更可能是静脉闭塞性疾病，而GVHD则更有可能合并小肠壁增厚。

肝紫癜症

- 肝紫癜症是一种罕见的良性疾病，表现为肝窦扩张并形成充满血液的腔隙。
- 该病通常是特发性的，但也可能由于某些药物所致(包括类固醇、口服避孕药、他莫昔芬和甲氨蝶呤)、免疫紊乱(包括人类免疫缺陷病毒感染、移植后免疫抑制)和感染(包括人类免疫缺陷病毒感染、结核病、巴尔通体)。
- CT和MRI显示早期中央强化伴延迟的离心性强化。超声可显示非特异性高回声肿块。

心源性肝病

- 心源性肝病为被动性肝充血，其原因有心脏手术、心脏衰竭、缩窄性心包炎或右心瓣膜性疾病，最终可导致肝硬化。
- 影像学表现包括肝静脉和下腔静脉增宽，静脉内造影剂从右心房反流至下腔静脉和肝静脉。肝脏通常表现为肿大并呈斑点状强化(肉豆蔻肝)。常合并腹水。

(翻译　王亚玲)

Hepatic Doppler

肝脏多普勒

Normal anatomy and Doppler waveforms

正常解剖和多普勒波形

normal = *hepatopetal* flow (towards the liver)
正常=向肝血流（朝向肝脏）
hepatic arteries and portal veins flow in the same direction
肝动脉与门静脉的血流方向相同

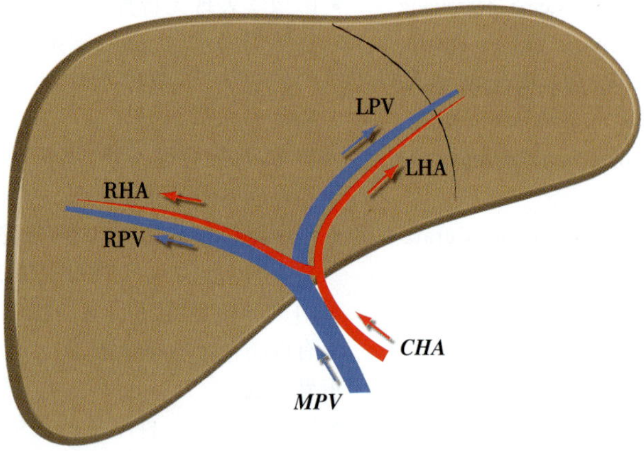

RHA = right hepatic artery
RHA = 肝右动脉
LHA = left hepatic artery
LHA = 肝左动脉
CHA = common hepatic artery
CHA = 肝总动脉
RPV = right portal vein
RPV = 门静脉右支
LPV = left portal vein
LPV = 门静脉左支
MPV = main portal vein
MPV = 门静脉主干

- The normal **hepatic artery** waveform is pulsatile and towards the liver, called *hepatopedal* flow (-pedal = toward).

- 正常**肝动脉**的波形呈搏动性的向肝血流频谱，简称向肝(hepatopedal)血流(-pedal=朝向)。

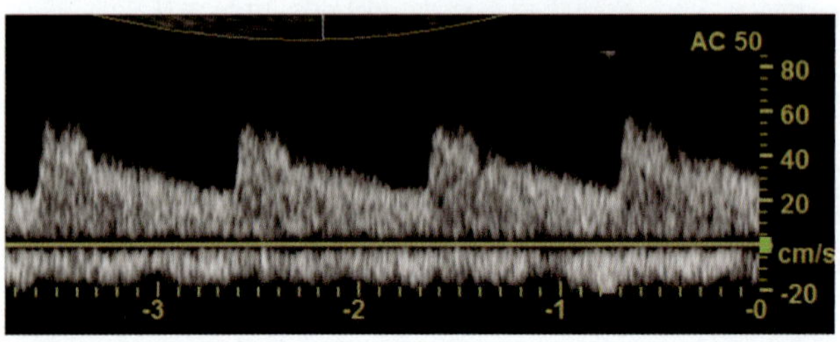

Normal hepatic artery waveform:
Doppler tracing shows a pulsatile waveform, above the baseline, indicating hepatopedal flow. The peak height corresponds to the peak systolic velocity while the trough corresponds to end-diastolic velocity. A typical resistive index (RI) is 0.55–0.7.
RI is calculated by (peak systolic velocity – end diastolic velocity) / peak systolic velocity.
正常肝动脉波形：
频谱多普勒呈搏动性波形，位于基线上方，提示向肝血流。波峰与收缩期峰值速度对应，而波谷则与舒张末期速度对应。典型的阻力指数(RI)为0.55~0.70。
RI计算方法：(收缩期峰值速度－舒张末期速度)/收缩期峰值速度。

- The normal **portal vein** waveform is above the baseline (*hepatopedal*) and gently undulating (*phasic*) with velocity ranging from 16–40 cm/sec.
- The **hepatic veins** feed into the IVC and the right side of the heart. The spectral Doppler waveform is pulsatile and representative of changes during the cardiac cycle, though with the majority of blood flowing antegrade (away from the liver and towards the heart). The normal hepatic venous waveform has four distinct components: The A, S, V and D waves.

- 正常**门静脉**频谱位于基线上方(向肝)，呈轻微波动(相位)，流速在16~40cm/s。
- **肝静脉**汇入下腔静脉，然后至右心。多普勒频谱呈波动性，且随心动周期呈典型改变，其中大部分为顺行血流(从肝脏流向心脏)。正常肝静脉波形包括A波、S波、V波和D波四个部分。

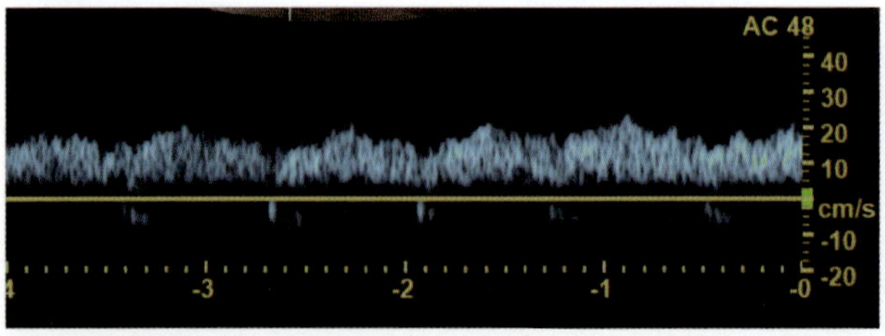

Normal portal vein waveform.
正常门静脉波形

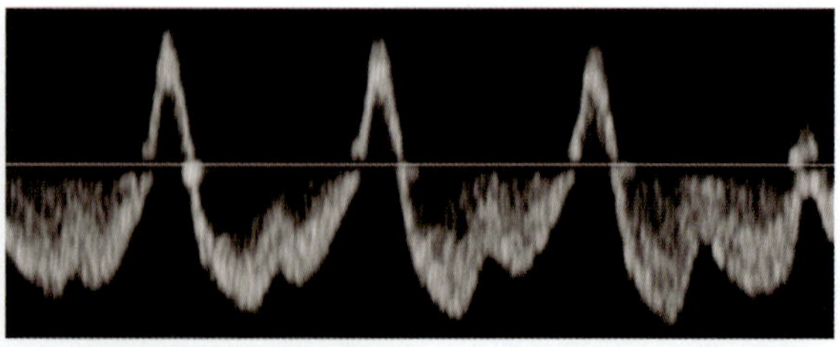

Normal hepatic vein waveform.
正常肝静脉波形

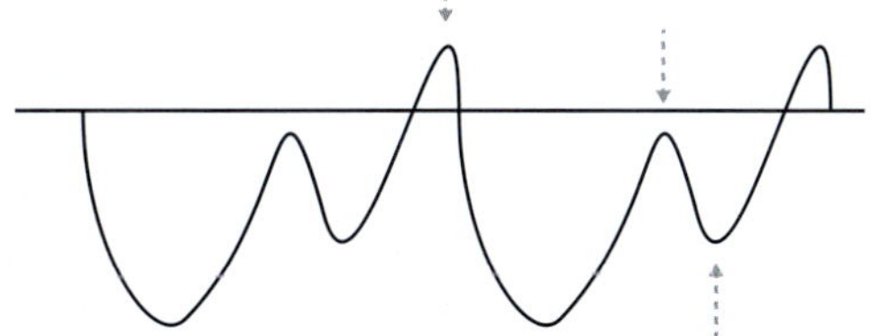

A-wave: Atrial contraction, during which blood is forced retrograde (away from the heart) into the liver.

A 波：心房收缩，此时血液因压力逆行(离开心脏)进入肝脏。

S-wave: Ventricular systole, during which a large volume of blood returns to the right atrium.

S 波：心室收缩，此时大量血液返回右心房。

V-wave: Atrial overfilling, followed by tricuspid valve opening (peak of the V-wave) and early ventricular diastolic filling of the right ventricle.

V 波：心房过度充盈，随后三尖瓣打开(V 波峰值)和右心室舒张早期充盈。

D-wave: Continued filling of the right ventricle during ventricular diastole, during which a smaller volume of blood returns to the right atrium.

D 波：心室舒张期右心室持续充盈，伴少许血液反流入右心房。

PORTAL VEIN PATHOLOGIES

Portal venous pulsatility

While the normal portal venous waveform may be gently undulating (described as phasic), a pulsatile portal venous waveform is abnormal. The differential diagnosis for a pulsatile portal venous waveform includes tricuspid regurgitation and right-sided heart failure.

Portal vein thrombosis

- Thrombosis of the portal vein can be bland (simple thrombosis) or may be due to tumor invasion.
- Bland portal vein thrombus can be caused by a hypercoagulable state or may be due to local inflammation from pancreatitis or hepatitis.

  In infants, omphalitis or dehydration may also lead to portal vein thrombosis.
- Tumor thrombus is most commonly caused by HCC and is referred to as "tumor-in-vein".

门静脉病变

门静脉搏动

- 正常门静脉频谱呈轻微波动(称为相位)，若出现搏动性门静脉频谱则为异常，此时需要与三尖瓣反流和右心衰竭相鉴别。

门静脉栓子

- 门静脉栓子可以是单纯的(只含血栓)，也可以是肿瘤侵袭引起的癌栓。
- 单纯的门静脉血栓可由高凝状态引起，也可由胰腺炎或肝炎所致局部炎症引起。

  在婴儿中，脐带炎症或脱水也可以导致门静脉血栓形成。
- 肿瘤性栓子最常由肝细胞癌引起，称为"癌栓"。

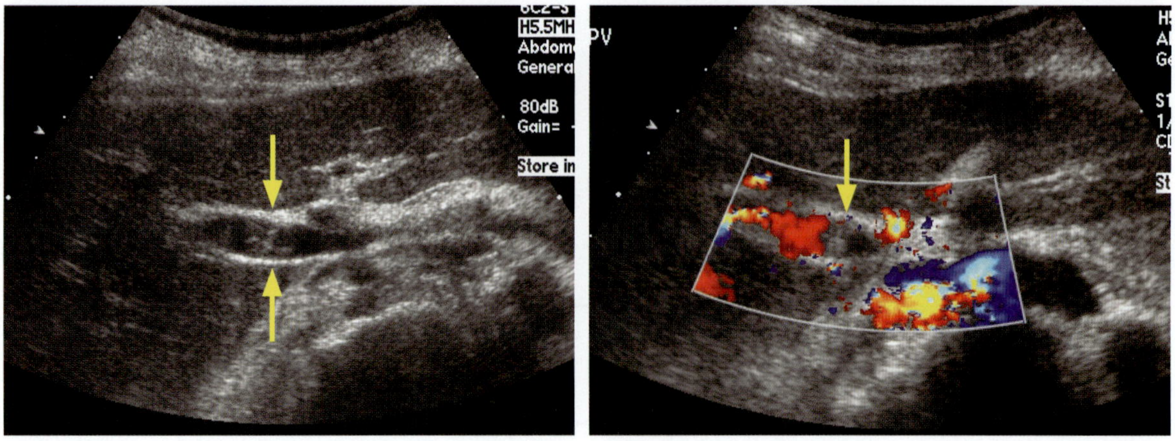

Grayscale transverse image of the porta hepatis shows echogenic debris within the main portal vein (arrows). Color Doppler confirms partial portal vein thrombosis with lack of flow in the proximal portal vein (arrow).

Case courtesy Julie Ritner, MD, Brigham and Women's Hospital, Boston.

肝门区横切面灰阶图像显示门静脉主干内呈碎片样回声(黄箭)。彩色多普勒证实部分门静脉血栓形成，门静脉近端未见血流信号充盈(黄箭)。

- Ultrasound of portal vein thrombosis shows lack of portal venous flow, often with echogenic thrombus within the portal vein.

  Expansion/enlargement of the portal vein can be seen with either bland or tumor thrombus.

  On color Doppler, flow within the thrombus suggests tumor thrombus.
- One potential pitfall to be aware of is slow (<16 cm/sec) or stagnant portal venous flow in the presence of portal hypertension, which may mimic portal vein thrombosis.
- Long-standing portal vein thrombosis leads to *cavernous transformation* of the portal vein, characterized by formation of multiple small periportal collateral vessels.

- 门静脉血栓在超声上表现为门静脉内血流信号缺失，常伴门静脉内血栓回声。

  门静脉扩张/增粗可见于单纯血栓或肿瘤性癌栓。

  在彩色多普勒超声上检测栓子内有血流信号则提示癌栓。
- 需要注意，当门静脉高压时，门静脉的血流会变缓(<16cm/s)或淤滞，此时与门静脉血栓的表现相似。
- 长期的门静脉血栓可导致门静脉海绵样变，特征为门静脉周围多条侧支血管形成。

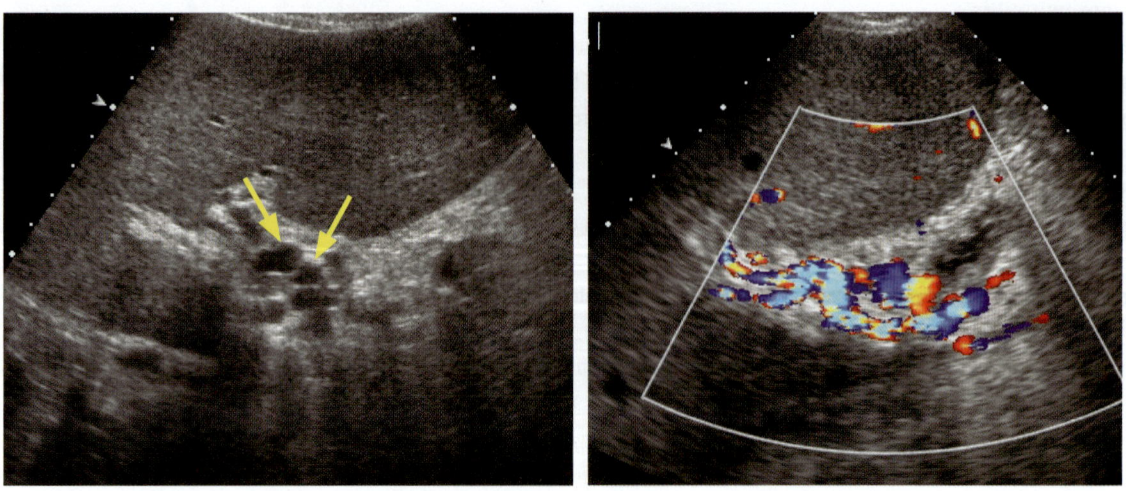

Cavernous transformation of the portal vein: Grayscale transverse image of the porta hepatis shows numerous tubular hypoechoic structures in the expected location of the portal vein (arrows). Color Doppler (right image) demonstrates flow within these collateral vessels, with no identifiable portal vein.

Case courtesy Julie Ritner, MD, Brigham and Women's Hospital, Boston

门静脉海绵样变性：在肝门横切面的灰阶图像中，可以看到在预期的门静脉位置有许多管状低回声结构(箭头)。彩色多普勒图像(右图)显示这些侧支血管内有血流，但无法识别门静脉。

Portal venous gas

门静脉积气

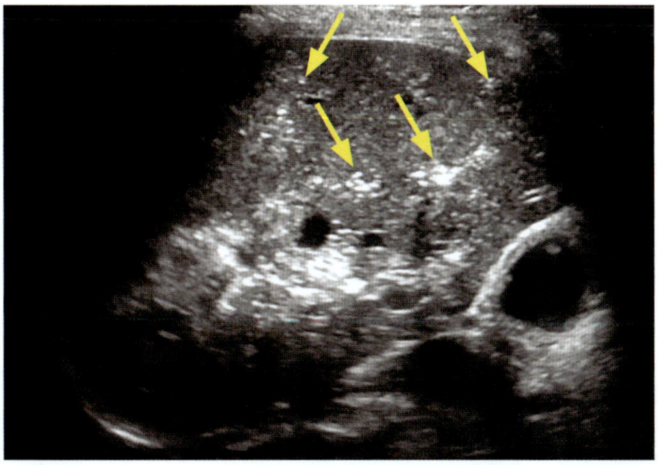

Portal venous gas: Grayscale ultrasound through the liver shows numerous tiny echogenic foci (arrows) in a branching pattern throughout the liver, extending to the periphery.

Case courtesy Julie Ritner, MD, Brigham and Women's Hospital, Boston.

门静脉积气：灰阶超声显示肝脏有许多微小的强回声灶(黄箭)，呈分支状分布，并向外周延伸。

- Portal venous gas is due to bowel ischemia/infarction until proven otherwise. If the cause of the portal venous gas is unknown, CT should be performed emergently.
- Grayscale ultrasound shows *peripheral* branching echogenic foci that may be transient or seen to change position on cine clips. Spectral Doppler of the portal vein features numerous characteristic spikes.
- In contrast to portal venous gas, pneumobilia tends to be more central (discussed later in the chapter).

Portal hypertension

- Portal hypertension is increased pressure of the portal venous system. Etiology is classified in relation to the hepatic capillary bed as pre-sinusoidal, sinusoidal, or post-sinusoidal:

  Pre-sinusoidal: Insult is proximal to the hepatic parenchyma, such as portal vein thrombosis.

  Sinusoidal: Insult is hepatic in origin, such as cirrhosis.

  Post-sinusoidal: Insult is beyond the liver, such as Budd-Chiari (hepatic vein thrombosis) or IVC thrombosis.
- Portal hypertension is defined as a direct portal venous pressure of >5 mm Hg greater than IVC pressure, although the portal venous pressure is not measured directly.
- Ultimately, when portal venous pressure is higher than forward pressure, the portal venous flow may decrease below 16 cm/sec or reverse (called *hepatofugal*; -fugal = away, same Latin root as fugitive), which is diagnostic for portal hypertension.

- 门静脉积气一般是由肠缺血/梗死引起，如门静脉积气原因不明，应紧急进行CT检查。
- 灰阶超声显示门静脉外周分支内强回声病灶，动态观察呈一过性或随体位改变。门静脉频谱具有大量毛刺状的特征。
- 与门静脉积气相反，胆道积气往往聚集在肝门附近(在本章后文讨论)。

门静脉高压

- 门静脉高压是指门静脉系统内的压力升高。病因学分类根据其与肝毛细血管床的关系分为窦前性、窦性或窦后性：

  窦前性：病变位于肝实质前，如门静脉血栓形成。

  窦性：肝实质受侵，如肝硬化。

  窦后性：肝后病变，如布-加综合征(肝静脉血栓)或下腔静脉血栓形成。
- 门静脉高压定义为直接门静脉压>5mmHg，但通常不直接测量。
- 当门静脉压力最终高于向肝的压力时，门静脉的流速可降至16cm/s以下，甚至反流(称为肝逆流；-fugal = away，和“fugitive”的拉丁词根相同)，此时可诊断门静脉高压。

reversed = *hepatofugal* flow
反向血流=离肝血流
hepatic arteries and portal veins flow in opposite directions
肝动脉和门静脉的血流方向相反

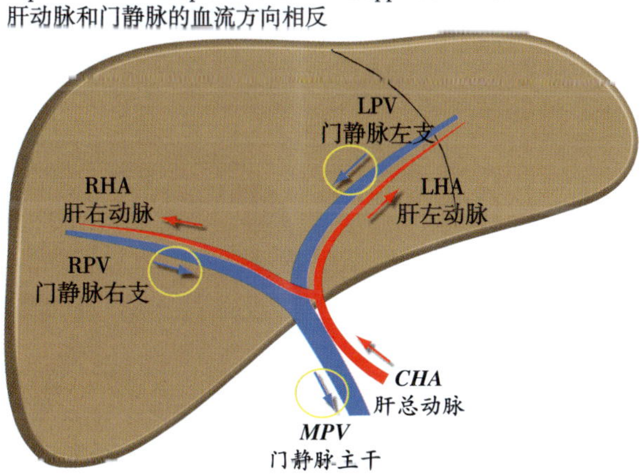

- In addition to slow flow or flow reversal, there are several secondary findings of portal hypertension:

Dilated portal vein (13 mm is the maximal normal diameter in quiet respiration).

Splenomegaly.

Gamna-Gandy bodies.

Varices.

Portosystemic shunts (most commonly gastroesophageal, paraumbilical, or splenorenal). Note that an isolated portosystemic shunt may not be caused by portal hypertension. For instance, isolated obstruction of the splenic vein from pancreatitis-related thrombosis or neoplasm may lead to a shunt. However, a recanalized paraumbilical vein is diagnostic of portal hypertension.

- 除了血流缓慢或反向，还有其他门静脉高压的继发征象：

门静脉增宽(平静呼吸时的正常直径上限为13mm)。

脾大。

含铁结节。

静脉曲张。

门静脉系统分流(最常见的胃食管、脐旁或脾肾分流)。注意，孤立的门静脉系统分流不一定由门静脉高压引起，如胰腺炎导致的血栓形成或肿瘤引起的孤立性脾静脉阻塞。但当出现脐静脉重新开放时即可诊断为门静脉高压。

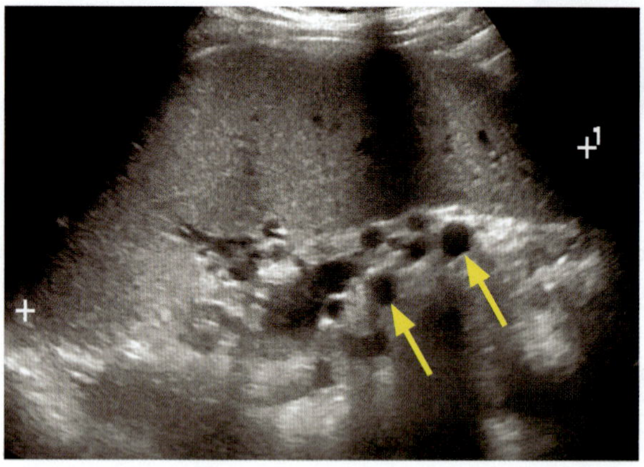

Splenomegaly and splenic varices: Sagittal ultrasound in the left upper quadrant shows an enlarged spleen (calipers) measuring 15 cm in craniocaudal dimension. There are numerous tubular hypoechoic structures (arrows) at the splenic hilum representing varices.
脾大及脾静脉曲张：左上腹矢状切面超声显示脾大(卡尺)，上下径15cm。脾门区多发管状低回声(黄箭)，为曲张的静脉。

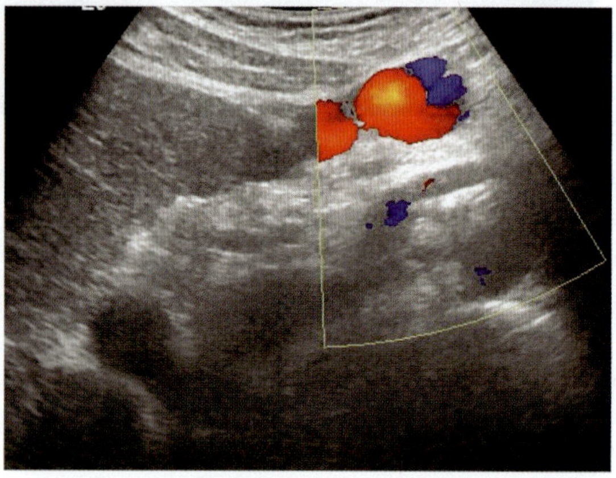

Transverse Doppler ultrasound of the left lobe of the liver shows a recanalized umbilical vein, which is considered diagnostic of portal hypertension.
横切面肝左叶多普勒超声显示脐静脉再通，可诊断为门静脉高压。

Transjugular intrahepatic portosystemic shunt (TIPS)

- Portal hypertension (and reversal of portal flow) can be treated with a transjugular intrahepatic portosystemic shunt (TIPS), which connects a branch of the portal vein to a systemic hepatic vein.
- Ultrasound is used for surveillance of TIPS patency, starting with a post-procedure baseline. Routine follow-up is performed according to the following schedule: in 1 month, every 3 months for the first year, and then every 6 to 12 months.
- Flow in a patent TIPS will be towards the hepatic veins, and flow in the portal veins will be towards the TIPS. Therefore, flow in the main portal vein will be hepatopetal and flow in the right and left portal veins will be hepatofugal (highlighted below with yellow circles).

经颈静脉肝内门体分流术(TIPS)

- 门静脉高压(和门静脉反流)可以通过TIPS治疗，将门静脉分支连接到体循环的肝静脉。
- 超声用于随访TIPS支架的通畅情况，以术后超声检查作为基线。常规随访时间为术后第1个月进行一次，第1年每3个月一次，以后每6~12个月一次。
- 血流在一个通畅的TIPS中是流向肝静脉的方向，而门静脉中的流向则是朝着TIPS。因此门静脉主干的血流是向肝的，而门静脉左右支的血流是远离肝的(下图中用黄色圆圈标出)。

Patent TIPS:
blood flows through TIPS to hepatic veins
RPV and LPV have reversed flow (toward TIPS)
MPV has hepatopetal flow (toward TIPS)
通畅的TIPS：
血流通过TIPS流向肝静脉
门静脉左右支为反向血流（流向TIPS）
门静脉主干为向肝血流（流向TIPS）

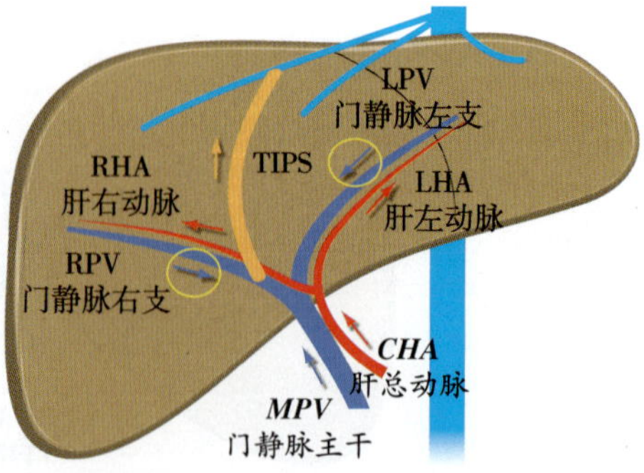

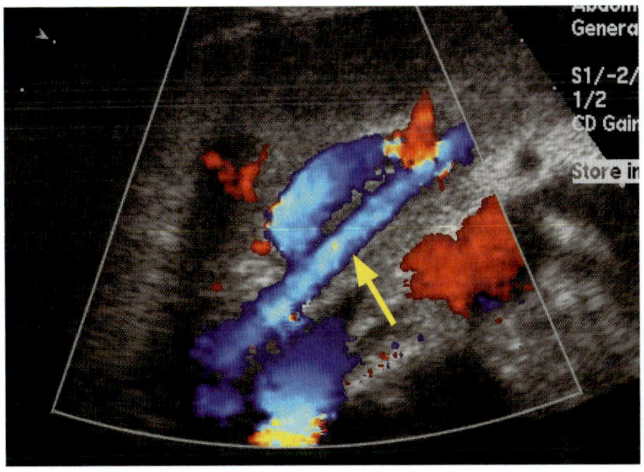

Patent TIPS: Color Doppler of the porta hepatis including the proximal TIPS shows flow within the TIPS (yellow arrow).

Case courtesy Julie Ritner, MD, Brigham and Women's Hospital, Boston.

通畅的TIPS：彩色多普勒显示肝门包括近端TIPS内的血流(黄箭)。

- US can evaluate for stenosis of the TIPS.

- 超声可以评估TIPS狭窄。

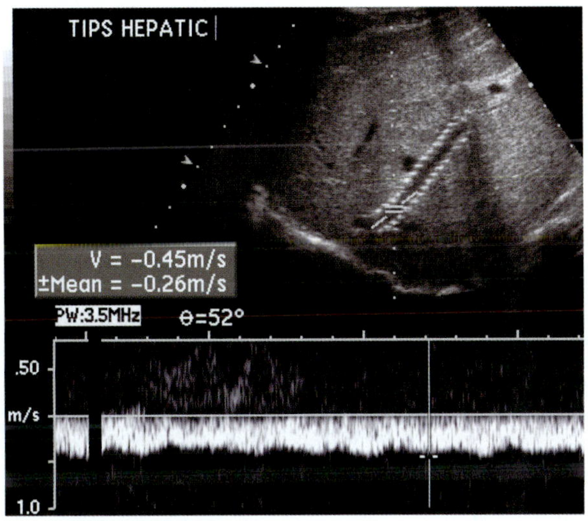

TIPS stenosis: Spectral Doppler of a TIPS shows a velocity of 45 cm/sec, indicative of stenosis due to slow flow.

Case courtesy Julie Ritner, MD, Brigham and Women's Hospital, Boston

TIPS狭窄：频谱多普勒显示TIPS内血流速度为45cm/s，提示狭窄引起血流缓慢。

High intra-TIPS velocity >190 cm/sec or low intra-TIPS velocity of <90 cm/sec suggests stenosis.

Intra-TIPS velocity change of ± >50 cm/sec since the baseline study is also concerning for stenosis.

Low main portal vein velocity (<30 cm/sec) suggests TIPS stenosis.

- If the TIPS becomes occluded, the right and left portal vein will "re-reverse" and become hepatopetal.

当TIPS内血流速度>190cm/s或TIPS内血流速度<90cm/s提示有狭窄。

与术后第一次超声检查相比，TIPS内流速变化>50cm/s也提示可能有狭窄。

当门静脉主干流速<30cm/s提示TIPS狭窄。

- 如果TIPS闭塞，门静脉左右支会"再次反转"，成为向肝血流。

Occluded TIPS:
no blood flow through TIPS
RPV and LPV have "re-reversed":
  now have hepatopetal flow (away from TIPS)
MPV has hepatopetal flow (towards occluded TIPS)
TIPS闭塞：
无血流通过TIPS
门静脉右支和左支"再次反转"：
  成为向肝血流（远离TIPS）
门静脉主干为向肝血流（流向闭塞的TIPS）

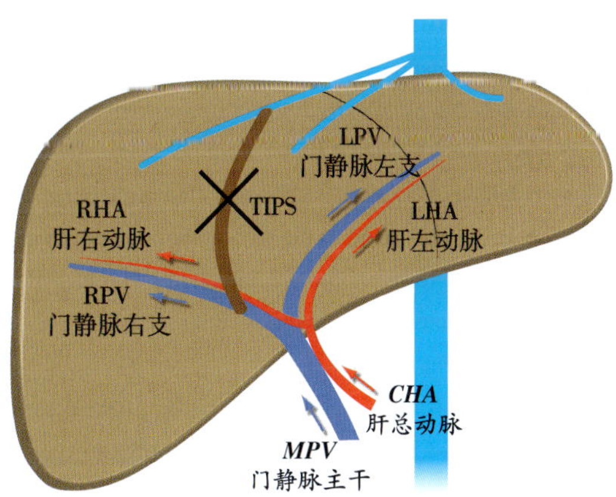

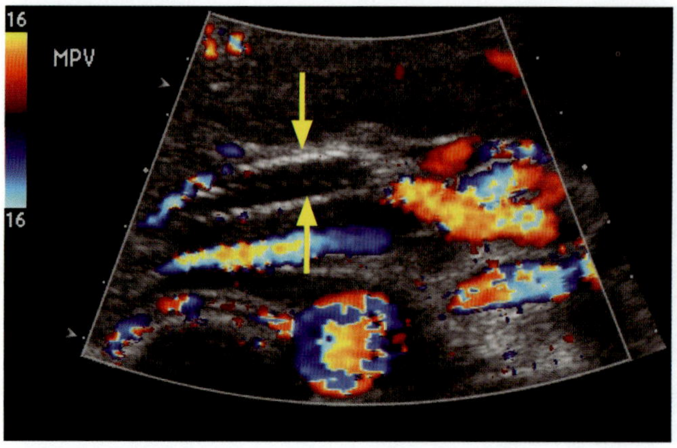

TIPS occlusion: Color Doppler of the porta hepatis including the proximal TIPS shows complete absence of flow within the TIPS (arrows).

Case courtesy Julie Ritner, MD, Brigham and Women's Hospital, Boston

TIPS闭塞：彩色多普勒显示肝门区包括近端TIPS内血流信号完全缺失(黄箭)。

Hepatic vein pathologies

肝静脉病变

Increased hepatic vein pulsatility

- Increased hepatic vein pulsatility is caused by a right-sided cardiac abnormality, either right-sided heart failure or tricuspid regurgitation. Both conditions are characterized by accentuated A- and V-waves due to increased retrograde flow during atrial systole.

肝静脉搏动性增加

- 肝静脉搏动增强是由右侧心脏异常引起，见于右心衰竭或三尖瓣反流。两者的特征都表现为心房收缩期反向血流增加所引起增强的A波和V波。

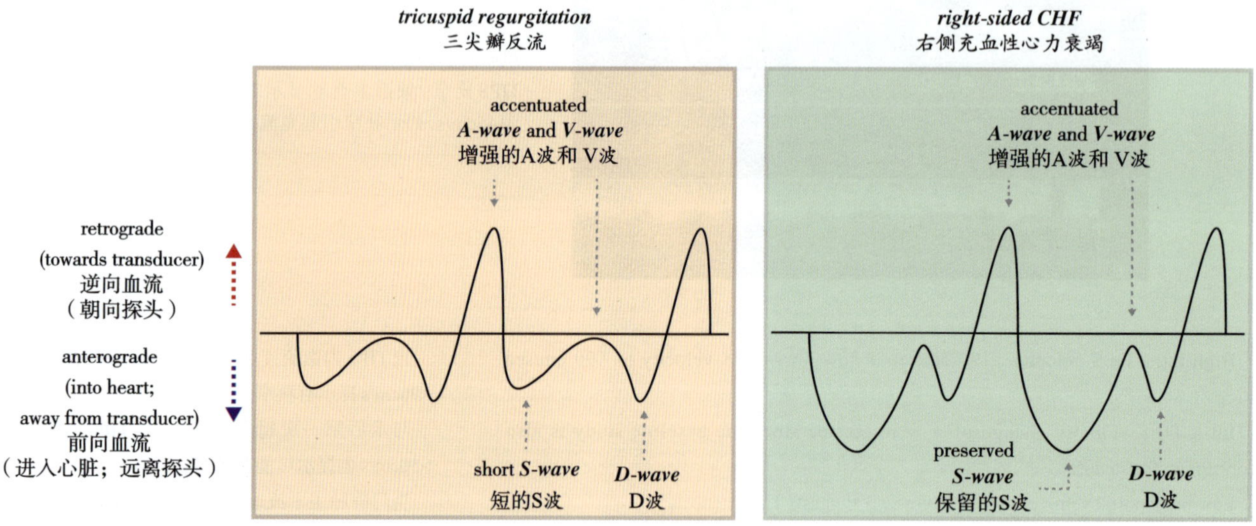

Tricuspid regurgitation: Normally, the tricuspid valve closes at the beginning of ventricular systole (the beginning of the S-wave), allowing for filling of the right atrium (S-wave). In tricuspid regurgitation, there is less or even reversed antegrade flow into the right atrium during ventricular systole, resulting in a prominent A-wave and decreased or even retrograde S wave.

Right-sided heart failure: Waveform is affected by too much blood volume in the right side of the cardiovascular system, including the right atrium, resulting in tall A- and V-waves due to increased right atrial pressure; however, in contrast to tricuspid regurgitation, the S-wave is normal since the tricuspid valve remains competent.

三尖瓣反流：正常情况下，三尖瓣在心室收缩开始时关闭(S波开始)，使右心房充盈(S波)。当三尖瓣反流时，心室收缩期流入右心房的血流较少，甚至逆行，导致A波突出，S波减低，甚至反向。

右心衰竭：波形受右侧心血管系统血容量过多影响，包括右心房，如心房压增加可引起A波和V波增高；而与三尖瓣反流不同的是S波正常，此时三尖瓣保持功能正常。

Decreased hepatic vein pulsatility

- Decreased hepatic vein pulsatility due to hepatic vein narrowing or compression is seen in cirrhosis, Budd-Chiari (hepatic vein thrombosis), and hepatic veno-occlusive disease.

肝静脉搏动性降低

- 肝静脉搏动性降低是由肝静脉狭窄或受压所致，见于肝硬化、布-加综合征(肝静脉栓子)和肝静脉闭塞性病变。

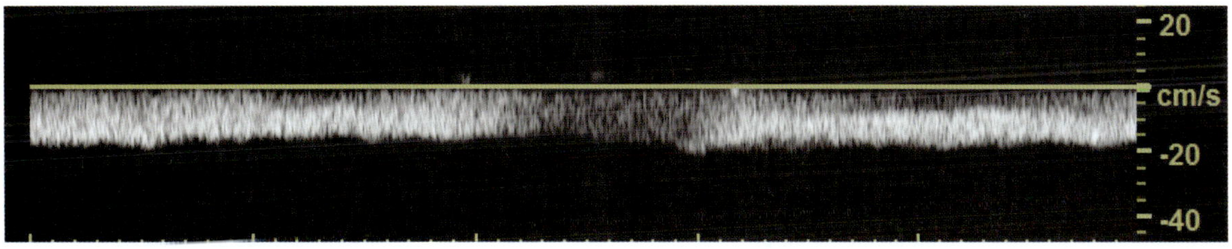

Flattened hepatic vein waveform thought to be due to chemotherapy-related liver injury and/or fatty liver.
平坦的肝静脉波形被认为与化疗相关的肝损伤和/或肝脂肪变性。

（翻译　蒋京真）

Biliary Imaging

胆道影像

Anatomy

解剖

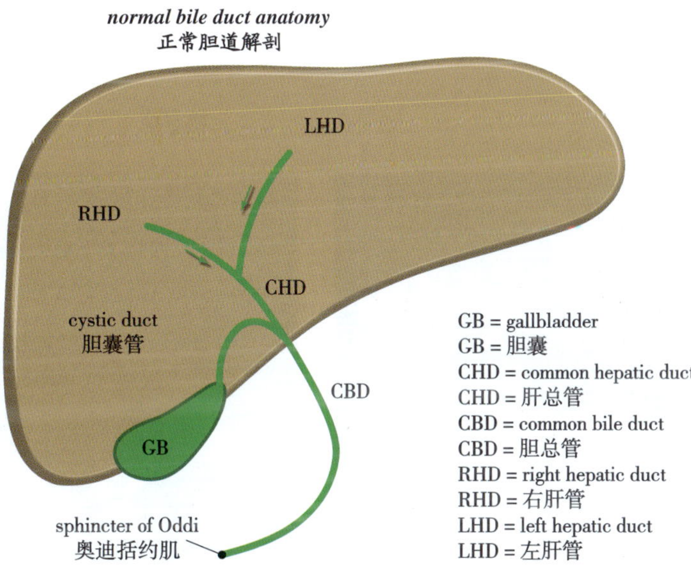

- Sagittal view of the normal porta hepatis on CT and ultrasound:

- 矢状位CT与超声的正常肝门图像：

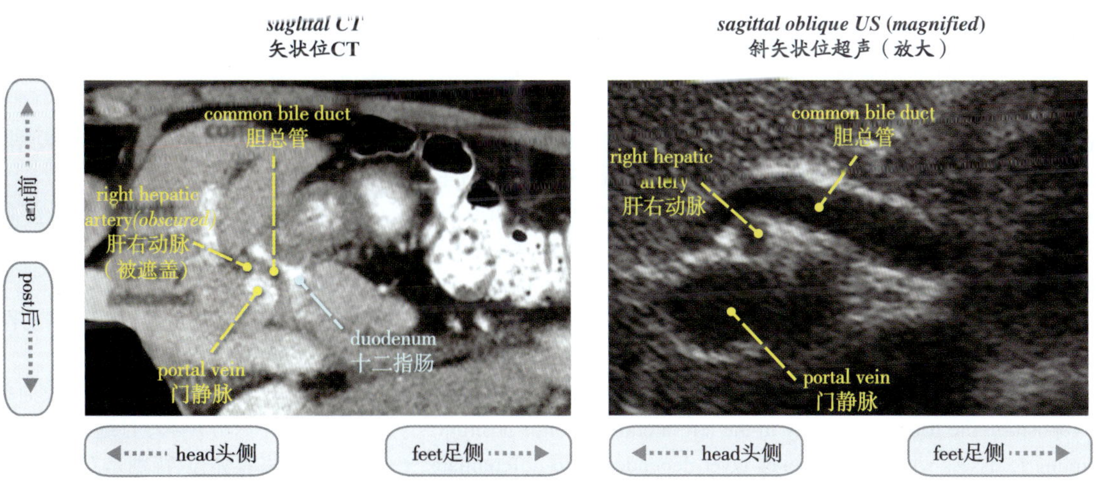

Biliary anatomical variants

Low insertion of cystic duct

- With a low insertion of the cystic duct, the surgeon may misidentify the common duct as the cystic duct if the patient undergoes cholecystectomy, possibly leading to inadvertent common duct ligation.

Aberrant right posterior duct

- An aberrant right posterior duct is only important if the patient is a right hepatic lobe liver donor, as the two right hepatic ducts need to be anastomosed separately in the recipient.

Long common channel

- A long common channel is also known as pancreaticobiliary maljunction where the union of the CBD and pancreatic duct occurs outside the duodenal wall to form a long common channel (>15 mm). It may occur with or without biliary dilatation.
- This entity may be associated with choledochal cyst, bile duct stricture, and increased risk of biliary cancer.

胆道解剖变异

胆囊管低位汇合

- 胆囊管开口较低的患者在接受胆囊切除术时，外科医生有可能将胆总管误认为是胆囊管，从而有可能导致误扎胆总管。

迷走右后肝管

- 迷走右后肝管仅对肝移植右叶供体有重要意义，因为两条右肝管需要与受体分别进行吻合。

超长合流管

- 超长合流管也被称为胰胆管汇合异常，为胆总管和胰管在十二指肠壁的外侧汇合而形成一个长的管道（>15mm）。胆道是否发生扩张不定。
- 这一变异可能与胆总管囊肿、胆管狭窄和胆管癌风险增加有关。

Gallstones and cholecystitis

Cholelithiasis

胆囊结石和胆囊炎

胆石症

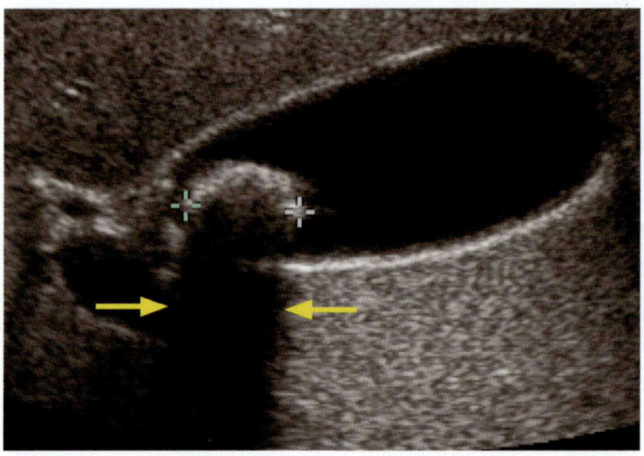

Single gallstone: Sagittal ultrasound of the gallbladder shows an echogenic gallstone (calipers) in the gallbladder neck, with posterior acoustic shadowing (arrows).
单发胆囊结石：胆囊矢状切面超声扫查显示胆囊颈部有一颗强回声胆囊结石（卡尺），后方伴有声影（黄箭）。

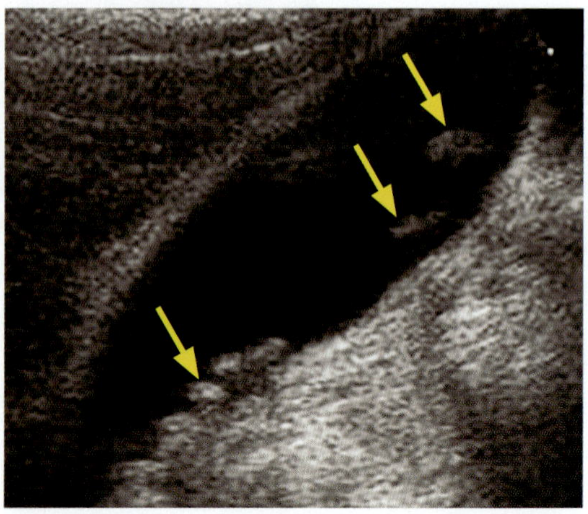

Multiple small gallstones: Sagittal ultrasound of the gallbladder in a different patient shows multiple small shadowing gallstones (arrows).
多发胆囊小结石：另一名患者的胆囊矢状切面超声显示多发小胆囊结石伴有声影（黄箭）。

- Cholelithiasis is a gallbladder stone or stones, without associated inflammation.
- The classic clinical presentation of symptomatic cholelithiasis is colicky right upper quadrant pain after eating a fatty meal, but it is common to see gallstones incidentally in asymptomatic patients.
- Risk factors for developing gallstones include female sex, obesity, pregnancy, middle age, and diabetes.
- The ultrasound diagnosis of gallstones is usually straightforward. Stones are echogenic with posterior acoustic shadowing and are usually mobile. It is often helpful to reposition the patient (typically in the left lateral decubitus position) while scanning to assess whether the stones layer dependently to differentiate stones from polyps or other masses.

- 胆石症是指胆囊内单发或多发结石，未并发炎症。
- 胆石症的典型临床表现是进食高脂肪餐后右上腹绞痛，但胆结石更常发生在无症状的患者。
- 发生胆囊结石的危险因素包括女性、肥胖、妊娠、中年和糖尿病。
- 胆囊结石的超声诊断通常比较简单。结石为高回声伴后方声影，且通常有移动性。检查时改变患者体位（特别是左侧卧位）有助于评估结石是否按重力的方向向下运动，以区分

- A gallbladder completely full of stones can be more challenging to identify. The *wall-echo- shadow (WES) sign* describes a gallbladder full of multiple stones (or one giant stone).

结实与息肉或其他肿块。

- 识别一个充满结石的胆囊可能有一定困难。*囊壁-回声-声影三合征*(WES)是指一个胆囊充满了很多结石(或单个巨大结石)的超声征象。

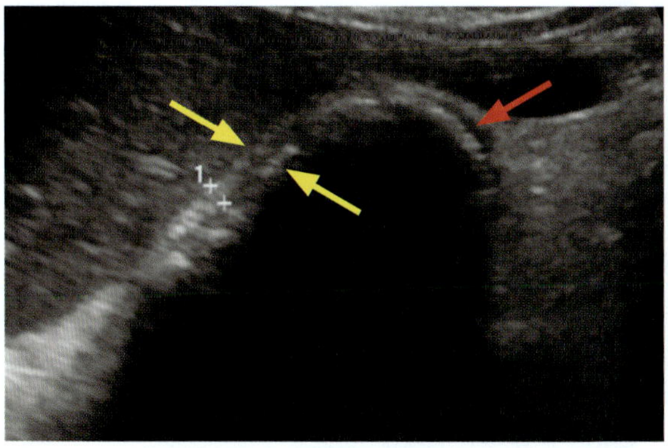

Wall-echo-shadow sign on ultrasound: Two parallel echogenic arcs represent the gallbladder wall and leading edge of the stone (yellow arrows), with an intervening thin layer of hypoechoic bile (red arrow). The gallstones cast a prominent shadow, obscuring evaluation of the remainder of the gallbladder wall, as in this image.

超声囊壁-回声-声影三合征：两条平行的回声弧代表胆囊壁和结石边缘(黄箭)，中间有一薄层低回声胆汁(红箭)。如图所示，结石投射出明显的声影，使胆囊壁的其余部分模糊不清。

- The differential diagnosis of echogenic material within the gallbladder includes:

Gallstone(s) (echogenic, mobile, shadowing).
Gallbladder sludge (echogenic, mobile, non-shadowing).
Gallbladder polyp (echogenic, non-mobile, non-shadowing, often attached to the gallbladder wall via a stalk, may be vascular).
Hyperplastic cholecystoses (echogenic, non-mobile, multiple polyps).
Porcelain gallbladder (echogenic wall, shadowing).
Adjacent bowel (echogenic wall, dirty shadowing).

- 胆囊内回声物体的鉴别诊断包括：

胆囊结石(回声、移动、声影)。
胆囊泥沙沉积(回声、移动、无声影)。
胆囊息肉(回声、无移动、无声影，常带蒂附着于胆囊壁，可有血供)。
增生性胆囊病(回声、无移动、多发息肉)。
瓷化胆囊(回声壁、伴声影)。
邻近肠道(回声壁、浑浊声影)。

Acute calculus cholecystitis

- Acute calculus cholecystitis is inflammation of the gallbladder due to an obstructing gallstone impacting the gallbladder neck or cystic duct.
- Patients typically present with right upper quadrant (RUQ) pain and fever.

急性结石性胆囊炎

- 急性结石性胆囊炎是由于胆结石阻塞胆囊颈或胆囊管所引起的胆囊炎症。
- 患者通常表现为右上象限(RUQ)腹痛和发热。

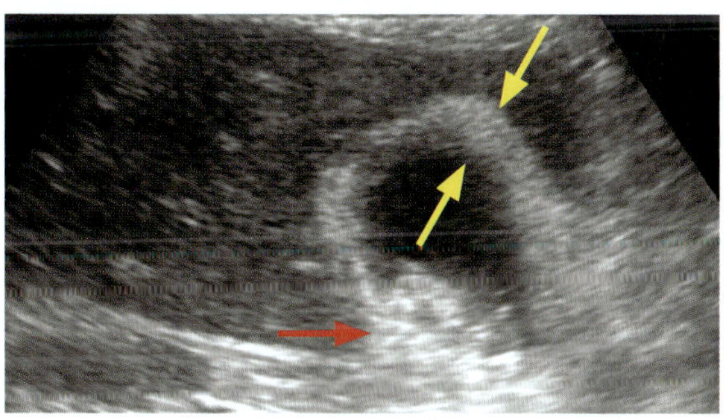

Acute calculus cholecystitis: Oblique sagittal ultrasound through the gallbladder demonstrates a thickened, echogenic gallbladder wall (arrows). The gallbladder contains numerous echogenic gallstones (red arrow).

急性胆石性胆囊炎：斜矢状切面超声显示胆囊壁增厚并呈高回声(黄箭)。胆囊内有大量高回声的胆囊结石(红箭)。

- Ultrasound is the first-line evaluation of suspected acute cholecystitis.
- There is no sonographic finding that is 100% specific for acute cholecystitis. However, gallstones are seen >90% of the time and a positive sonographic Murphy's sign (RUQ pain with pressure from the transducer during inspiration) also has a high positive predictive value. Other findings include:

Gallbladder wall thickening >3 mm.
Distended gallbladder >4 cm in diameter.
Pericholecystic fluid or inflammatory changes in the pericholecystic fat.
Color Doppler showing **hyperemic gallbladder wall**.

- 超声是评估疑似有急性胆囊炎的首选方法。
- 超声检查对诊断急性胆囊炎的特异度并不是100%。但是，超声可以发现>90%的胆囊结石，并且超声墨菲征阳性(吸气时探头按压引起右上腹痛)具有很高的阳性预测价值。其他发现包括：

胆囊壁增厚>3mm。
胆囊扩张>4cm(直径)。
胆囊周围积液或囊周围脂肪炎性改变。
彩色多普勒显示**胆囊壁充血**。

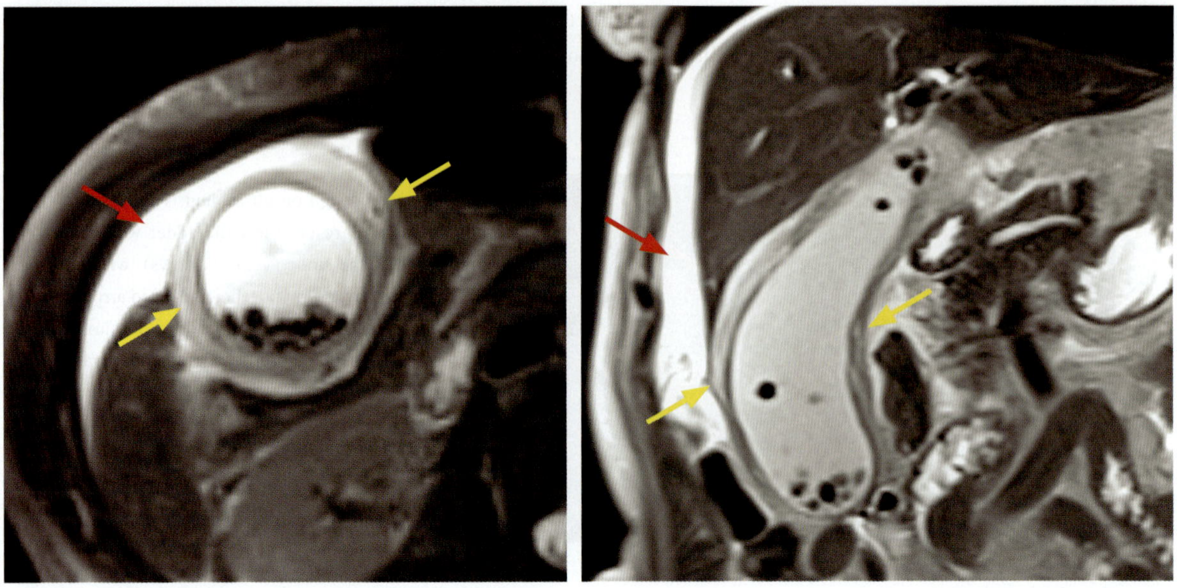

Axial and coronal T2 MRI shows gallbladder wall edema (yellow arrows), perihepatic and pericholecystic fluid (red arrows), and small T2 hypointense stones within a distended gallbladder.

Case courtesy Felipe Boschini Franco MD, Brigham and Women's Hospital.

轴位和冠状位 T_2 MRI 显示胆囊壁水肿(黄箭),肝周和胆囊周围积液(红箭),以及肿大的胆囊腔内有多个 T_2 低信号的小结石。

- Complications of acute cholecystitis are rare but serious and include:

Emphysematous cholecystitis.
Gangrenous cholecystitis.
Gallbladder perforation.

- Surgical treatment of uncomplicated acute calculous cholecystitis is cholecystectomy. In patients who are not good surgical candidates, a temporizing percutaneous cholecystostomy tube can be placed prior to definitive surgical cholecystectomy.

Acalculous cholecystitis

- Acalculous cholecystitis is cholecystitis without gallstones, typically seen in very sick patients such as those in the ICU, thought to be due to bile stasis and hypoperfusion. Risk factors include sepsis, prolonged total parenteral nutrition, and trauma.
- The ultrasound appearance is similar to that of acute cholecystitis, but without the presence of an obstructing stone. Since many patients are ventilated or obtunded, it's often not possible to evaluate for sonographic Murphy's sign.
- Treatment of acalculous cholecystitis is typically percutaneous cholecystostomy by interventional radiology. Unlike the treatment of calculous cholecystitis, cholecystostomy is often the definitive therapy.

Emphysematous cholecystitis

- Emphysematous cholecystitis is a severe complication of acute cholecystitis caused by gas- forming bacteria. It is rare but elderly diabetic patients are more susceptible.
- On imaging, gas may be present either within the lumen or the wall of the gallbladder.
- Treatment of emphysematous cholecystitis is most often emergent cholecystectomy or cholecystostomy in patients with a very high surgical risk.

- 急性胆囊炎的并发症很少见,但很严重,包括:

气肿性胆囊炎。
坏疽性胆囊炎。
胆囊穿孔。

- 外科治疗无合并症的急性结石性胆囊炎的方法是胆囊切除术。对于不适合手术的患者,可以在外科胆囊切除术之前放置临时经皮胆囊造瘘管。

非结石性胆囊炎

- 非结石性胆囊炎是一种无胆囊结石的胆囊炎,常见于重症患者,如ICU的患者,可能是由于胆汁淤积和灌注不良导致。危险因素包括败血症、长期全肠外营养和创伤。
- 超声表现与急性胆囊炎相似,但无梗阻性结石。由于许多患者是气管插管或呈昏迷状态,因此通常无法评估超声墨菲征。
- 治疗非结石性胆囊炎常采用介入学方法进行经皮胆囊造瘘术。与治疗结石性胆囊炎不同,胆囊造瘘术通常是根治性疗法。

气肿性胆囊炎

- 气肿性胆囊炎是急性胆囊炎的一种严重并发症,由产气菌所致。这种情况较为罕见,但易发生于老年糖尿病患者。
- 影像学上,气体可出现在胆囊腔内或胆囊壁。
- 治疗气肿性胆囊炎最常用的方法是急诊胆囊切除术,而对于手术风险高的患者,可以采用胆囊造瘘术。

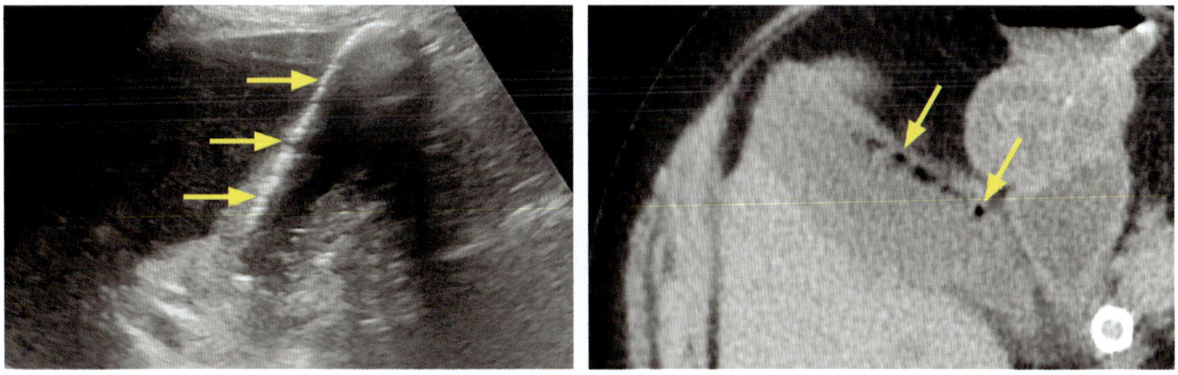

Grayscale ultrasound (left image) shows diffuse echogenic foci within the gallbladder wall corresponding to intramural foci of gas on axial CT (right image; arrows).
灰阶超声(左图)显示胆囊壁弥漫性高回声灶，与轴位CT胆囊壁内的气体灶相对应(右图；黄箭)。

Gangrenous cholecystitis

- Gangrenous cholecystitis is due to increased intraluminal pressure, leading to gallbladder wall ischemia and necrosis with high risk for gallbladder perforation.
- On imaging, gallbladder wall thickening may be notably asymmetric and intraluminal membranes may be present.
- Treatment is emergent cholecystectomy or cholecystostomy.

坏疽性胆囊炎

- 坏疽性胆囊炎是指由于胆囊腔内压力升高，导致胆囊壁缺血和坏死，并增加胆囊穿孔的风险。
- 在影像学上，胆囊壁增厚并可能呈明显不对称，或出现囊腔内膜状物。
- 治疗方法是急诊胆囊切除术或胆囊造瘘术。

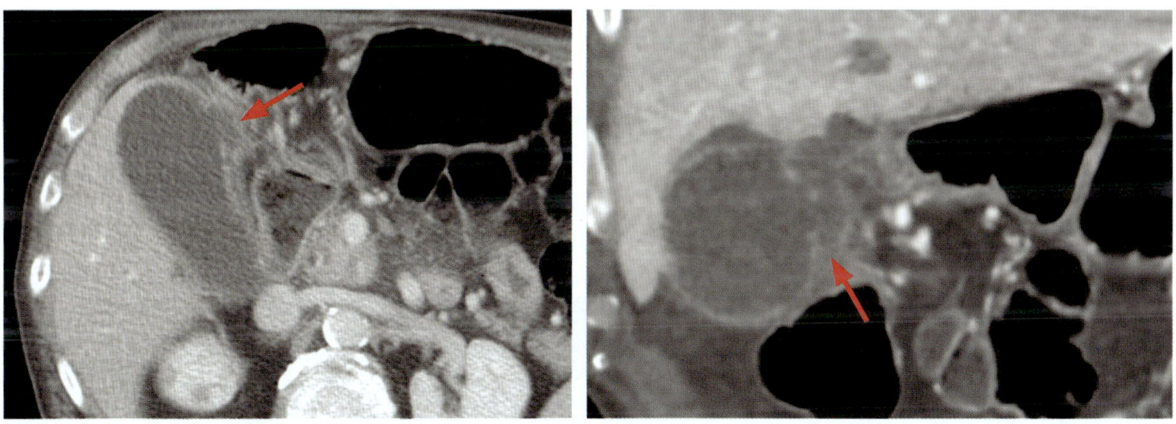

Axial and coronal contrast-enhanced CT shows gallbladder wall edema and pericholecystic fluid. There is discontinuous mucosal enhancement of the medial gallbladder wall (red arrow) due to necrosis and perforation with spillage of contents into the right subhepatic space.
轴位及冠状位增强CT显示胆囊壁水肿及囊周积液。胆囊内侧壁强化的黏膜连续性中断(红箭)，为坏死和穿孔所致，并有内容物溢出至右肝下间隙。

Gallbladder perforation

- Acute gallbladder perforation has a very high mortality due to generalized bile peritonitis. Subacute perforation may lead to a pericholecystic abscess and chronic perforation may cause a cholecystoenteric fistula.

胆囊穿孔

- 急性胆囊穿孔易引起广泛的胆汁性腹膜炎，因此具有很高的死亡率。亚急性穿孔可能导致胆囊周围脓肿，而慢性穿孔可能导致胆囊肠瘘。

Porcelain gallbladder

瓷化胆囊

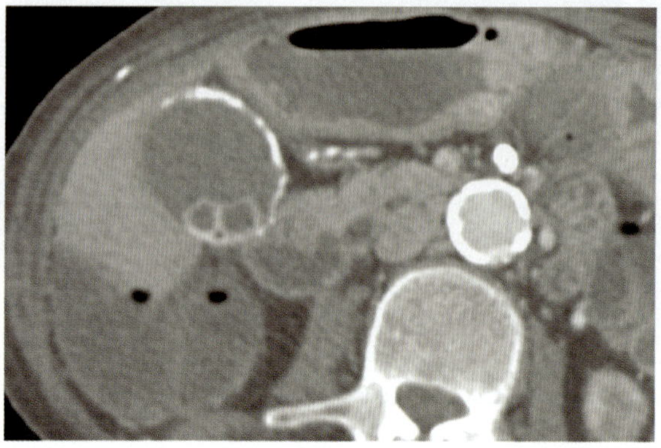

Axial contrast-enhanced CT demonstrates a calcified gallbladder wall consistent with porcelain gallbladder, and multiple peripherally calcified gallstones.
轴位增强CT显示胆囊壁钙化，符合瓷化胆囊的表现，另有多个位于周边的胆囊结石。

- Porcelain gallbladder describes a peripherally calcified gallbladder wall, thought to be a sequela of chronic cholecystitis due to either chronic irritation from supersaturated bile or repeated bouts of gallbladder obstruction.
- Porcelain gallbladder is associated with a (somewhat controversial) increased risk of gallbladder carcinoma. Historically, prophylactic cholecystectomy was the standard of care; however, some advocate for observation in asymptomatic patients.
- On ultrasound, the gallbladder wall is echogenic and gallstones are almost always present.
- The differential diagnosis of an echogenic gallbladder wall includes:

> Porcelain gallbladder.
> A gallbladder packed full of stones (which will feature the *wall-echo-shadow sign*).
> Emphysematous cholecystitis (intramural gas will have dirty shadowing).
> Adjacent bowel confused for gallbladder (bowel wall, echogenic gas with dirty shadowing).

- 瓷化胆囊是指胆囊周壁钙化，可能为慢性胆囊炎的后遗症，是由浓缩胆汁的慢性刺激或反复发作的胆囊梗阻所致。
- 瓷化胆囊有增加胆囊癌发生率的风险(尚有争议)。预防性胆囊切除术是既往治疗瓷化胆囊的标准方法；但现在主张对无症状患者进行随访观察。
- 在超声检查中，胆囊壁呈高回声，并总是合并有胆囊结石。
- 胆囊壁回声增高的鉴别诊断包括：

> 瓷化胆囊。
> 胆囊充满结石(其特征是*囊壁-回声-声影征*)。
> 气肿性胆囊炎(囊壁内气体会有浑浊声影)。
> 与胆囊混淆的邻近肠道(肠壁，气体回声伴浑浊声影)。

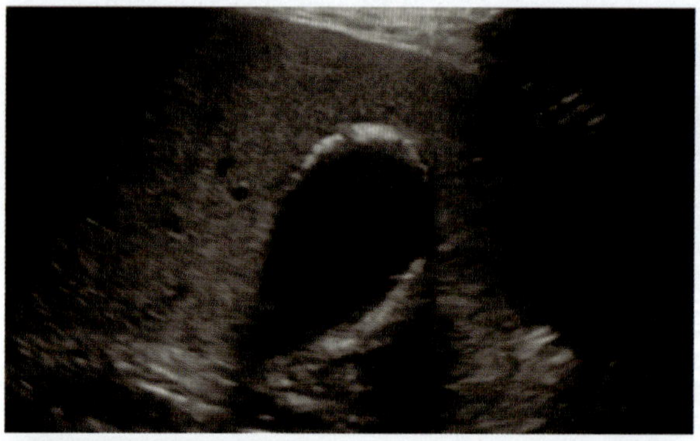

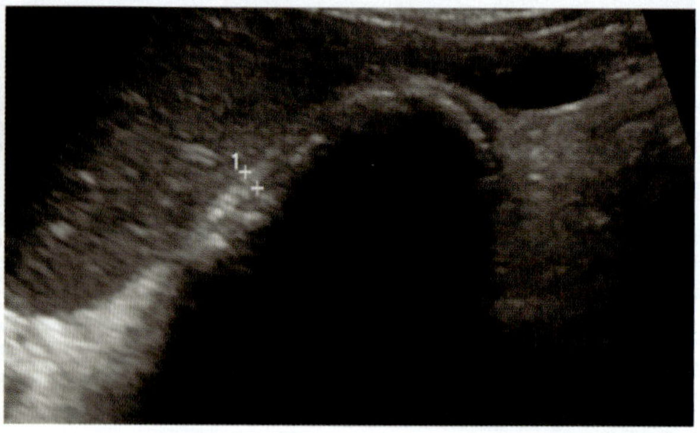

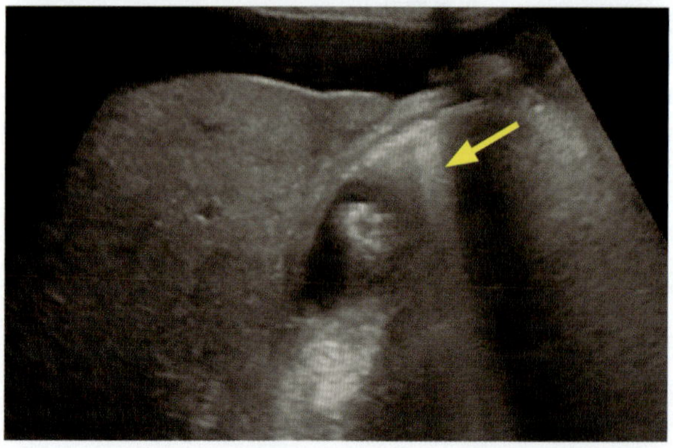

Different etiologies of an echogenic gallbladder wall in three different patients:
Top left image shows a porcelain gallbladder with associated posterior acoustic shadowing.
Top right image demonstrates the *wall-echo-shadow sign* described earlier in the chapter.
Bottom left image shows gallstones and dirty shadowing (yellow arrow) representing gas in the gallbladder, in this patient following biliary stent placement.
三名不同病因患者的胆囊壁回声增强：
左上图为瓷化胆囊伴后方声影。
右上图为本章前文描述的*囊壁-回声-声影征*。
左下图显示胆道支架置入术后复查患者的胆囊结石和浑浊声影(黄箭)，后者代表胆囊内的气体。

Courvoisier gallbladder | **库瓦西耶胆囊**

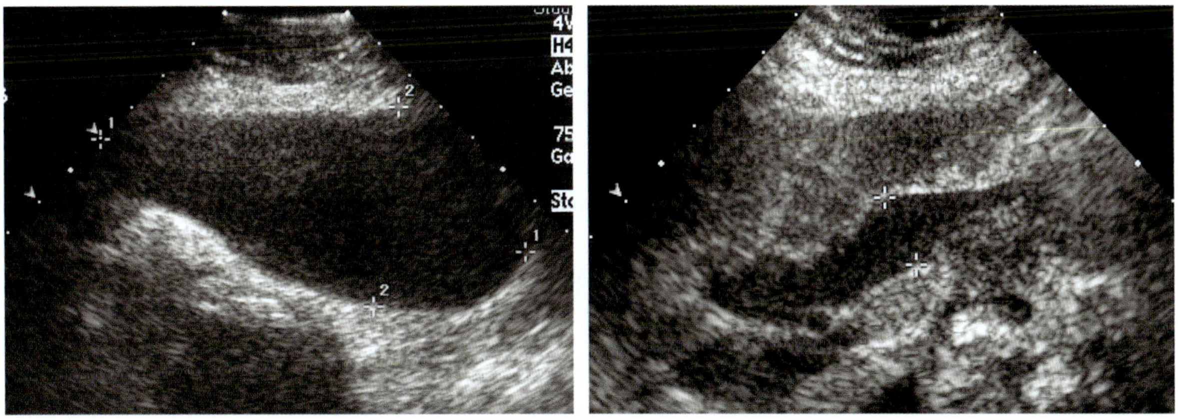

Sagittal ultrasound of the gallbladder (left image, marked with calipers) demonstrates a massively distended gallbladder. The common bile duct (right image, indicated by calipers) is also distended due to chronic malignant obstruction.

Case courtesy Julie Ritner, MD, Brigham and Women's Hospital.

胆囊矢状切面超声(左图，卡尺所示)显示胆囊极度扩张。胆总管(右图，卡尺所示)也因慢性恶性梗阻而扩张。

- The Courvoisier gallbladder refers to a markedly dilated gallbladder (originally described as being so large to be directly palpable on physical exam) from malignant obstruction of the common bile duct.
- A markedly distended gallbladder without acute cholecystitis implies chronic obstruction of either the cystic duct (when seen in isolation) or the common bile duct (when seen in combination with dilation of the common bile duct and intrahepatic biliary dilation).

- 库瓦西耶胆囊是继发于恶性胆总管梗阻而出现的胆囊极度扩张(最初是指体检时触及增大的胆囊)。
- 胆囊明显扩张而无急性胆囊炎的表现意味着胆囊管(孤立时)或胆总管(合并胆总管扩张和肝内胆管扩张)出现慢性梗阻。

HYPERPLASTIC CHOLECYSTOSES

胆囊增生性疾病

Overview of hyperplastic cholecystoses

- The hyperplastic cholecystoses are a spectrum of non-neoplastic proliferative disorders caused by deposition of cholesterol-laden macrophages within the wall of the gallbladder. The cholecystoses range from abnormalities of the gallbladder wall (adenomyomatosis and strawberry gallbladder) to gallbladder polyps extending into the lumen.

胆囊增生性疾病概述

- 胆囊增生性疾病是一类非肿瘤性增殖性疾病，由胆囊壁内沉积吞噬胆固醇的巨噬细胞所致。胆囊增生性疾病包括从胆囊壁的异常(胆囊腺肌症和草莓样胆囊)至胆囊腔内的胆囊息肉的一系列病变。

Adenomyomatosis

胆囊腺肌症(胆囊腺肌瘤)

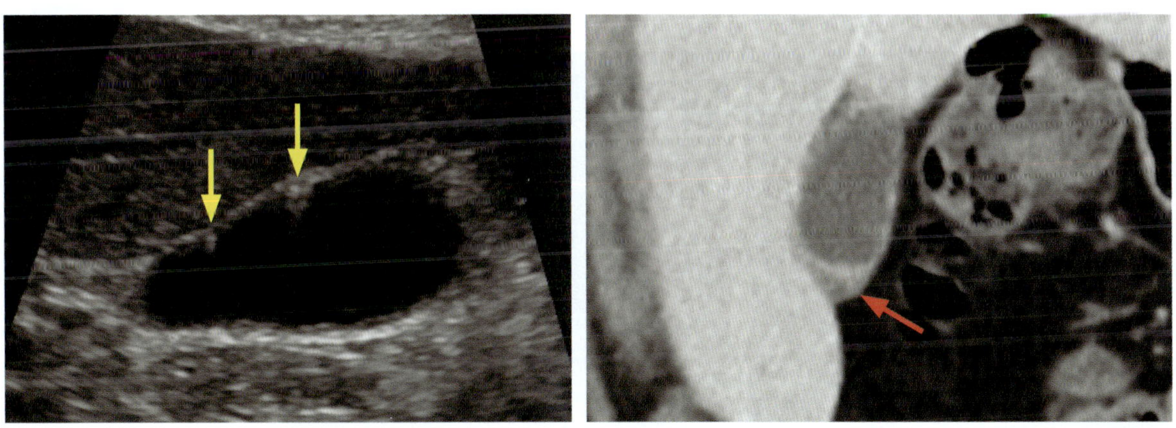

Ultrasound shows multiple echogenic foci in the gallbladder wall that demonstrate comet tail artifact (yellow arrows). Coronal CT image shows focal wall thickening in the gallbladder fundus with enhancement (red arrow) consistent with adenomyomatosis.

超声(左图)显示胆囊壁多处高回声灶，并可见彗星尾征(黄箭)。冠状位CT(右图)显示胆囊底部局灶性壁增厚并强化(红箭)，符合胆囊腺肌症。

- Adenomyomatosis is cholesterol deposition in mural Rokitansky-Aschoff sinuses.

  It is important not to confuse with adenomyosis of the uterus: It may be helpful to remember that there are three **L**'s in gallbladder, and adenomyomatosis is a **l**onger word than adenomyosis. Another way to remember is that "gallbladder" is a longer word than "uterus".
- Adenomyomatosis is often seen in the gallbladder fundus but can be diffuse or focal. It can be difficult to differentiate focal adenomyomatosis from malignancy.
- The ultrasound hallmark of adenomyomatosis is the *comet-tail* artifact due to reflections off tiny crystals seen in a focally thickened and echogenic gallbladder wall.
- The typical MRI appearance of adenomyomatosis is focal, bubbly T2 hyperintense thickening along the gallbladder fundus.

- 胆囊腺肌症是胆固醇沉积在囊壁的罗-阿窦内。

  注意不要与子宫腺肌病混淆：记住"gallbladder"(胆囊)中有三个"L"，"adenomyomatosis"(胆囊腺肌症)是一个比"adenomyosis"(子宫腺肌病)更长的单词。另一种记忆的方法是"胆囊"的英文单词比"子宫"要长。
- 胆囊腺肌症常见于胆囊的底部，可呈弥漫性或局灶性。局灶性胆囊腺肌症有时很难与恶性肿瘤区分。
- 胆囊腺肌症的超声特征是*彗星尾样伪影*，这是由于位于局灶性增厚且回声增强的胆囊壁中的微小晶体造成的反射。
- 胆囊腺肌症的典型MRI表现是胆囊底部呈局灶性、泡状T_2高信号。

Gallbladder polyps

- Most gallbladder polyps are benign cholesterol polyps that are part of the hyperplastic cholecystosis spectrum. Rarely (<5%), polyps may be premalignant adenomas.
- Gallbladder polyps are usually incidental and asymptomatic, but may cause right upper quadrant pain or even cholecystitis if they obstruct the cystic duct.
- The following characteristics, known as the *six S's*, increase the risk for a polyp being malignant:

胆囊息肉

- 大多数胆囊息肉是良性胆固醇息肉，属于胆囊增生性疾病谱中的一种。仅有很少(<5%)的息肉可能是癌前病变。
- 胆囊息肉通常是偶然发现且无症状，但当阻塞胆囊管时可引起右上腹疼痛，甚至胆囊炎。
- 以下特征被称为6个"S"，会增加息肉恶变的风险：

> **S**ize >10 mm or rapid growth. As a caveat, ultrasound has limited sensitivity and specificity in detecting small polyps (<10 mm), especially in the presence of gallstones.
>
> **S**ingle: A solitary polyp is more suspicious for malignancy. In contrast, benign cholesterol polyps tend to be multiple.
>
> **S**essile (broad-based): Sessile morphology is suspicious. A polyp is more likely benign if pedunculated.
>
> **S**tones: The presence of stones may induce chronic inflammation, which can predispose towards malignancy.
>
> Primary **S**clerosing cholangitis increases risk of malignancy.
>
> **S**ixty (age) or greater.

> 尺寸(Size)：>10mm或快速增长。值得注意的是，超声在检测小息肉(<10mm)时的灵敏度和特异度有限，尤其是在存在胆结石的情况下。
>
> 单发(Single)：单发息肉为恶性肿瘤的可疑程度更高。相反，良性胆固醇息肉往往呈多发。
>
> 宽基底(Sessile)：具有宽基底形态者可疑。如果息肉带蒂，则更可能为良性。
>
> 结石(Stone)：结石可以诱发慢性炎症，从而增加恶性肿瘤风险。
>
> 硬化(Sclerosing)：原发性硬化性胆管炎会增加恶性肿瘤的风险。
>
> 60岁(Sixty)：年龄60岁以上。

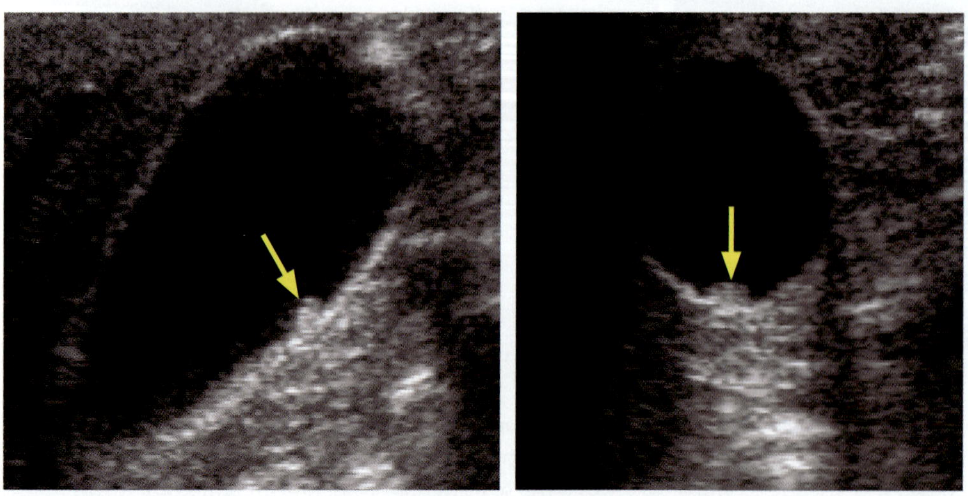

Gallbladder polyp: Sagittal and transverse views of the gallbladder show a small non-shadowing echogenic lesion (arrows). After repositioning the patient, this was shown to be non- mobile.

胆囊息肉：矢状切面(左图)与横切面(右图)胆囊图像显示一个小的无声影病变(黄箭)。患者体位改变之后，此病变无移动性。

- In patients with several of these high-risk features, cholecystectomy should be considered in the presence of a polyp greater than 10 mm in size.
- The typical ultrasound appearance of a polyp is a non- mobile, non-shadowing polypoid or sessile lesion extending from the wall into the lumen of the gallbladder. There may be vascular flow in the stalk.
- The main differential consideration is adherent sludge, which will not have any vascular flow.

- 对于具有上述几种高危特征的患者，如果息肉大于10mm，则应考虑行胆囊切除术。
- 息肉的典型超声表现是无移动性、无声影的息肉样或从囊壁突向胆囊腔内的带蒂病灶。蒂部可能有血流。
- 主要的鉴别诊断是黏附性沉积物，其内没有任何血流。

Gallbladder: Common imaging patterns

胆囊：常见的影像学表现

Diffuse gallbladder wall thickening >3 mm (common causes in bold)

弥漫性胆囊壁增厚>3mm(常见原因用黑体字标记)

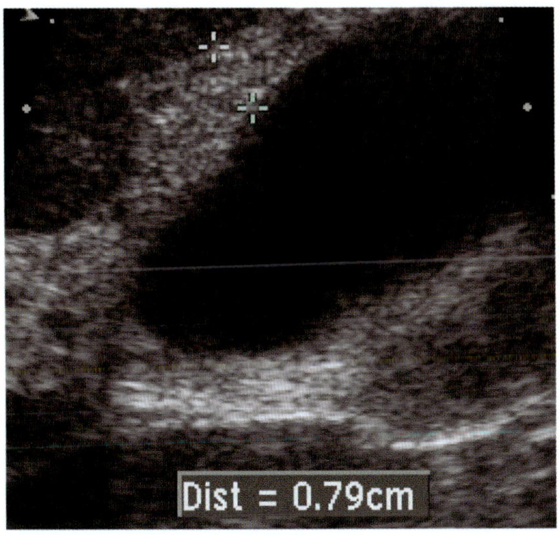

Sagittal ultrasound of the gallbladder shows diffuse wall thickening to 8 mm (calipers). In this case, the wall thickening was due to cirrhosis and resultant hypoproteinemia.
胆囊矢状切面超声显示胆囊壁弥漫性增厚至8mm(卡尺)。本例胆囊壁增厚为肝硬化和低蛋白血症所致。

- Fluid-overload/edematous states:
  - **Cirrhosis:** Hypoalbuminemia leads to diffuse gallbladder wall thickening.
  - **Congestive heart failure.**
  - Protein-wasting nephropathy.
- Inflammatory/infectious:
  - **Cholecystitis**, usually with associated cholelithiasis.
  - **Hepatitis.**
  - Pancreatitis.
- Infiltrative neoplastic disease:
  - Gallbladder carcinoma.
  - Metastases to gallbladder (rare)
- Post-prandial state.

Focal gallbladder wall thickening (common causes in bold)

- Hyperplastic cholecystoses: **Adenomyomatosis** and **cholesterol polyp**.
- Vascular: **Varices.**

- 容量负荷过多/水肿状态：
  - **肝硬化**：低蛋白血症导致弥漫性胆囊壁增厚。
  - **充血性心力衰竭**。
  - 低蛋白血症性肾病。
- 炎症/感染：
  - **胆囊炎**，通常伴有胆石症。
  - **肝炎**。
  - 胰腺炎。
- 浸润性肿瘤疾病：
  - 胆囊癌。
  - 胆囊转移癌(罕见)。
- 餐后状态。

局灶性胆囊壁增厚(常见原因用黑体字标记)

- 胆囊增生性疾病：**胆囊腺肌症**和**胆固醇息肉**。
- 血管：**静脉曲张**。

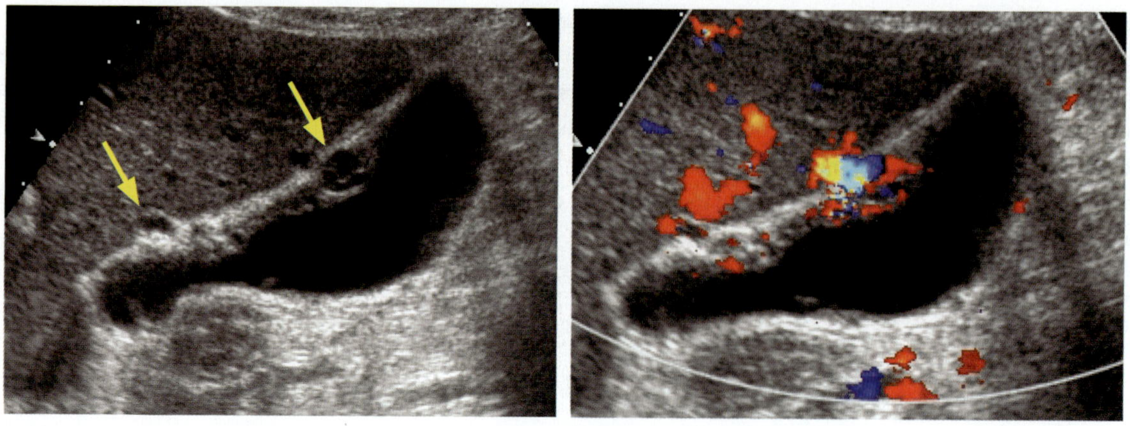

Gallbladder varices due to portal hypertension: Sagittal grayscale ultrasound of the gallbladder (left image) demonstrates several hypoechoic, cystic-appearing structures within the gallbladder wall (arrows). Color Doppler (right image) confirms the vascular etiology.
Case courtesy Julie Ritner, MD, Brigham and Women's Hospital.
门静脉高压导致胆囊静脉曲张：胆囊矢状切面灰阶超声图像(左图)显示胆囊壁内数个低回声的囊状结构(黄箭)。彩色多普勒(右图)被证实为血管。

- Neoplastic disease:
  - Adenomatous polyp.
  - Gallbladder carcinoma.
  - Adjacent hepatic tumor.
  - Metastases (rare).

Non-shadowing "mass" in the gallbladder lumen

- Tumefactive sludge (mobile).
- Blood/pus (mobile).
- Gallbladder polyp (immobile).
- Gallbladder carcinoma (immobile).

Echogenic gallbladder wall

- Porcelain gallbladder.
- Gallbladder full of stones (*wall-echo-shadow sign*).
- Emphysematous cholecystitis.

- 肿瘤性疾病：
  - 腺瘤样息肉。
  - 胆囊癌。
  - 邻近的肝脏肿瘤。
  - 转移癌(罕见)。

胆囊腔内无声影"肿块"

- 泥沙样沉积物(可移动)。
- 血块/脓液(可移动)。
- 胆囊息肉(不可移动)。
- 胆囊癌(不可移动)。

胆囊壁高回声

- 瓷化胆囊。
- 充满型胆囊结石(囊壁-回声-声影征)。
- 气肿性胆囊炎。

Magnetic Resonance Cholangiopancreatography (MRCP)

磁共振胰胆管成像(MRCP)

Magnetic resonance cholangiopancreatography (MRCP) overview

磁共振胰胆管成像(MRCP)概述

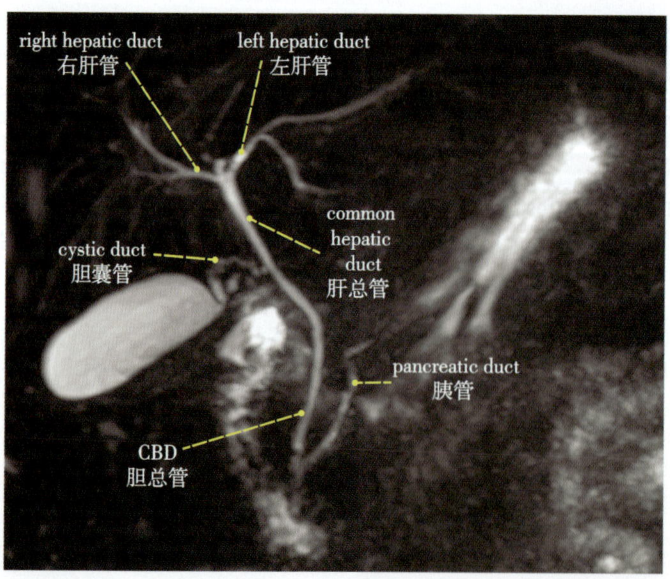

- Magnetic resonance cholangiopancreatography (MRCP) involves specific sequences of an abdominal MRI acquired to image the biliary tree, utilizing heavily T2-weighted sequences that increase the contrast between T2 hyperintense stationary fluid in the biliary tract and the surrounding structures.
- Sequences with intermediate T2-weighting (TE 80–100 ms) are best suited for visualization of the biliary ductal system and surrounding tissue, in particular to evaluate extraluminal structures.
- Fast spin echo sequences are most commonly used for MRCP acquisition. Various techniques can be employed to optimize imaging including breath-hold sequences and respiratory-triggered sequences.
- Advantages of MRCP over endoscopic retrograde cholangiopancreatography (ERCP) include:

MRCP is noninvasive. It does not require sedation. It has ability to visualize surrounding anatomy.

- Disadvantages of MRCP compared to ERCP include:

MRCP cannot simultaneously diagnose and treat abnormalities.

- Contrast-enhanced MRCP can also be performed with fat-saturated T1-weighted imaging after injection of gadolinium contrast agents that have biliary excretion, such as gadoxetic acid disodium (Eovist). These agents shorten T1 relaxation, resulting in T1 hyperintense biliary fluid, but require at least a 20-minute delay prior to imaging to allow time for biliary excretion.

- 磁共振胰胆管成像(MRCP)采用特定的腹部MRI序列对胆道进行成像，采用重T_2加权序列，以增加胆道内呈T_2高信号的潴留液体与其周围结构之间的对比。
- 中等T_2加权序列(TE 80~100毫秒)最适合显示胆管系统和周围组织，特别是评估腔外结构。
- 快速自旋回波序列是最常用的MRCP采集序列。可采用多种技术优化MRCP图像质量，包括屏气序列和呼吸触发序列。
- MRCP较内镜逆行胰胆管成像(ERCP)的优势包括：

MRCP为无创。 无须麻醉镇静。 可以显示周围的解剖结构。

- MRCP与ERCP相比的劣势包括：

MRCP不能同时进行诊断和治疗。

- 对比增强MRCP可以在注射由胆道排泄的钆造影剂后，如钆塞酸二钠，采用脂肪饱和T_1加权序列进行。造影剂可以缩短T_1，导致胆汁呈T_1高信号，但在成像前至少需要等待20分钟，以便造影剂排泄至胆道。

CHOLEDOCHAL CYSTS

胆管囊肿

Overview and Todani classification of choledochal cysts

胆管囊肿概述及Todani分型

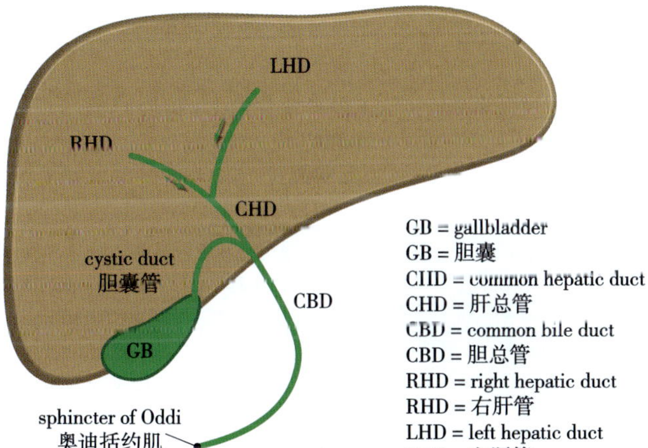

Type I choledochal cyst: Fusiform common bile duct dilation
Ⅰ型胆管囊肿：梭形胆总管扩张

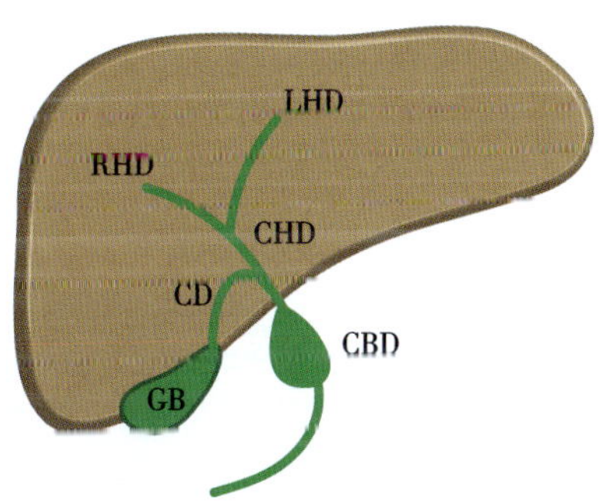

Most common, ~50% of choledochal cysts
最常见，高达50%的胆管囊肿

Type Ⅱ choledochal cyst: Extrahepatic saccular dilation
Ⅱ型胆管囊肿：肝外胆管囊状扩张

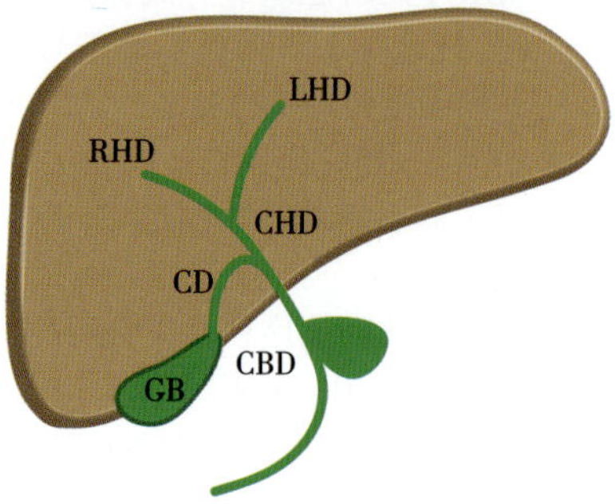

Type Ⅲ choledochal cyst: Dilation of intraduodenal bile duct
Ⅲ型胆管囊肿：十二指肠壁内段胆总管扩张

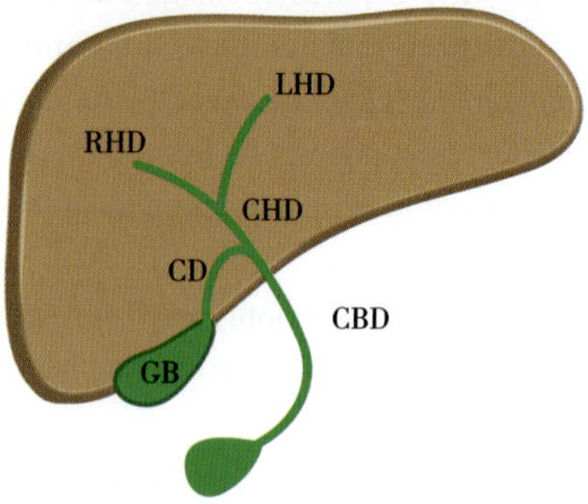

Type Ⅳ choledochal cyst: Multiple segments dilated
Ⅳ型胆管囊肿：多发节段扩张

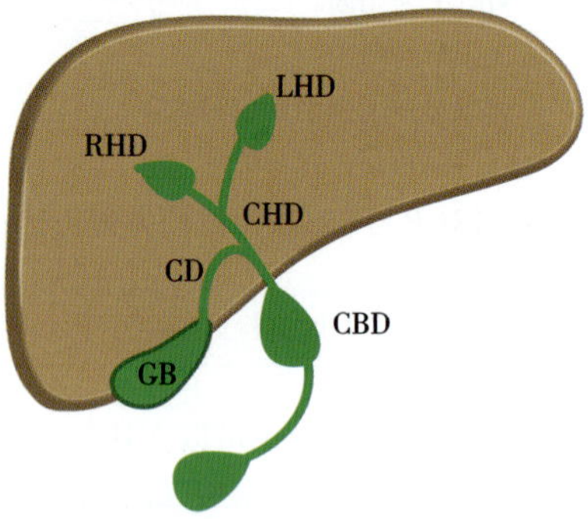

Type ⅣA: Intra- and extrahepatic dilation (pictured)
Type ⅣB: Extrahepatic dilation only
ⅣA型：肝内、外胆管扩张（图示）
ⅣB型：仅为肝外胆管扩张

Type Ⅴ choledochal cyst: Intrahepatic dilation = Caroli disease
Ⅴ型胆管囊肿：肝内胆管扩张=卡罗利病

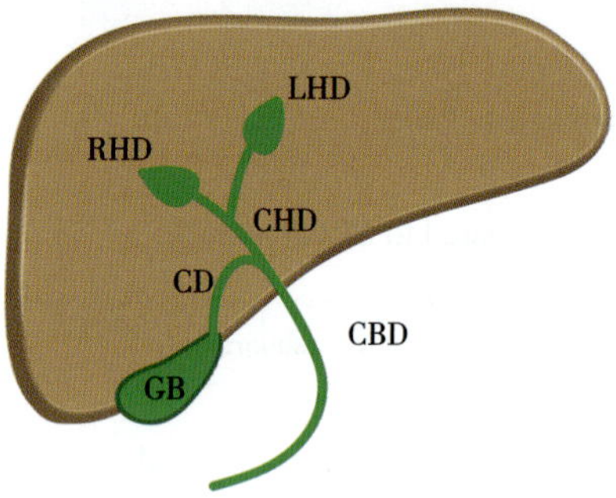

- Choledochal cysts represent a heterogeneous group of diseases with a common end pathway of intrahepatic or extrahepatic biliary ductal dilation. The Todani system divides the cysts into types Ⅰ–Ⅴ based on their number, distribution, and morphology.
- Most choledochal cysts are diagnosed in childhood, but less commonly may be a new diagnosis for an adult. Clinically, choledochal cysts can present with nonspecific abdominal pain or may be found incidentally. Choledochal cysts are often resected due to increased cholangiocarcinoma risk, which can be as high as 25%.
- In contrast to biliary hamartomas, choledochal cysts *do* communicate with the biliary tree.

- 胆管囊肿是一组由不同原因引起疾病，其共同的终末表现为肝内或肝外胆管扩张。Todani分类系统根据囊肿的数量、分布和形态将其分为Ⅰ～Ⅴ型。
- 大多数胆管囊肿在儿童时期就得到诊断，而成人较少为首发诊断。临床上，胆管囊肿可表现为非特异性腹痛或被偶然发现。胆管囊肿通常需要行手术切除，因其胆管癌的风险可高达25%。
- 与胆道错构瘤不同，胆管囊肿与胆管系统是相通的。

Type Ⅰ choledochal cyst

Ⅰ型胆管囊肿

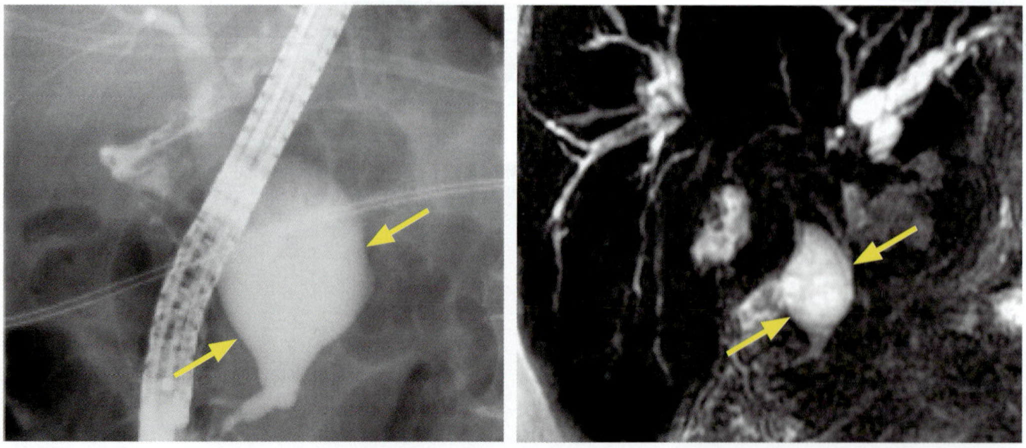

Type Ⅰ choledochal cyst: ERCP (left image) and thick-slab coronal MRCP heavily T2-weighted sequence (right image) shows a fusiform dilation of common bile duct (arrows).

Ⅰ型胆管囊肿：ERCP(左图)和厚层冠状位MRCP重T_2加权序列(右图)显示胆总管呈梭形扩张(黄箭)。

- A type Ⅰ choledochal cyst, representing fusiform dilation of the common bile duct, is the most common type of extrahepatic cyst.

Caroli disease (Type Ⅴ choledochal cysts)

- Caroli disease represents saccular dilation of the intrahepatic bile ducts, which may be segmental or diffuse. Caroli disease may be associated with polycystic kidneys.
- **Caroli syndrome** is Caroli disease plus hepatic fibrosis.
- The *central-dot sign* describes the small branches of the portal vein and hepatic artery bridging the dilated bile ducts, which look like a central dot on contrast-enhanced CT.

- Ⅰ型胆管囊肿为胆总管梭形扩张，是最常见的肝外胆管囊肿。

卡罗利病(Ⅴ型胆管囊肿)

- 卡罗利病为肝内胆管呈囊状扩张，可呈节段性或弥漫性。卡罗利病可能与多囊肾有关。
- **卡罗利综合征**是卡罗利病合并肝纤维化。
- 中心点征是指门静脉和肝动脉的小分支跨过扩张的胆管，在CT增强图像上看起来像一个中心点。

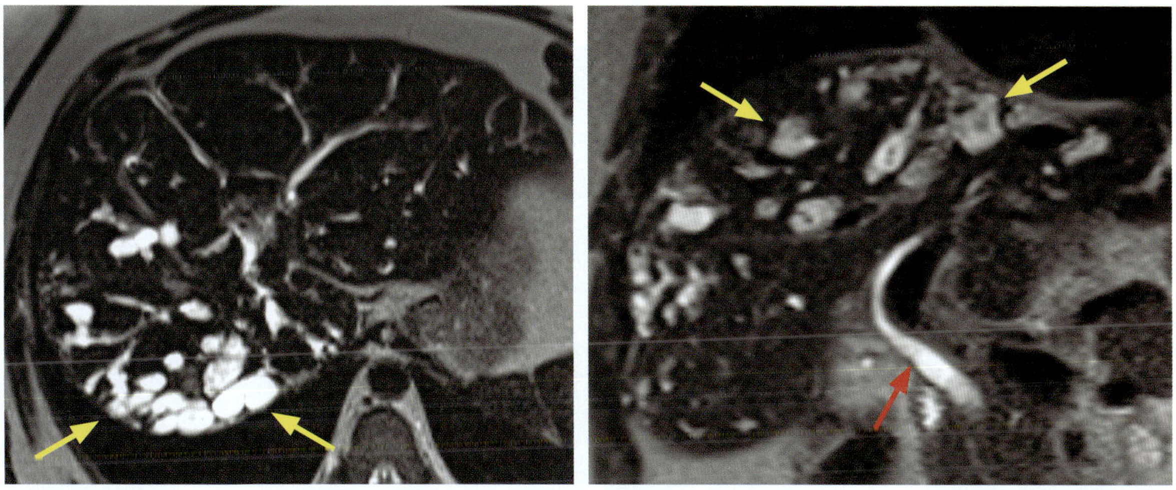

Axial and coronal T2-weighted MRI images demonstrate dilated intrahepatic bile ducts (arrows) throughout the liver consistent with Caroli disease. The common bile duct (red arrow) is normal caliber.

轴位和冠状位T_2加权MRI显示肝内胆管扩张(黄箭)弥漫分布于整个肝脏，符合卡罗利病的表现。胆总管(红箭)直径正常。

Bile Duct Pathology

胆管病变

Choledocholithiasis

胆总管结石

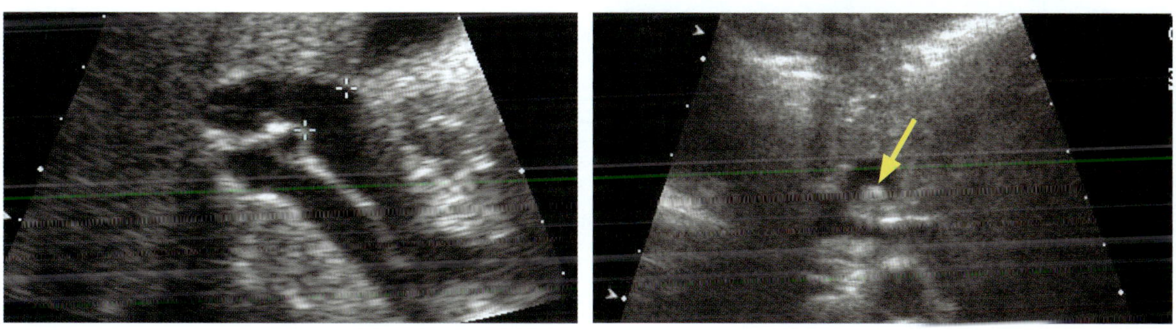

Choledocholithiasis: Sagittal ultrasound (left image) of the porta hepatis demonstrates common bile duct dilation (calipers) to 1.1 cm. Transverse scan (right image) through the region of the head of the pancreas shows an echogenic gallstone within the distal common bile duct (arrow).

胆总管结石：肝门部矢状切面超声(左图)显示胆总管扩张(卡尺)至1.1cm。胰头部横切面超声(右图)显示胆总管远端(黄箭)有结石回声。

- Choledocholithiasis is a stone in the common bile duct, generally treated with ERCP.
- Patients may be asymptomatic, but more often have right upper quadrant pain, nausea, vomiting and cholestatic pattern of LFT abnormalities secondary to obstructed bile outflow.

- 胆总管结石是指结石位于胆总管内，通常采用ERCP进行治疗。
- 患者可能无症状，但更常表现为右上腹疼痛、恶心、呕吐和胆汁淤积，以及继发于胆汁流出受阻而出现的肝功能异常。

Mirizzi syndrome

- Mirizzi syndrome is inflammation and external compression of the common hepatic duct (CHD) caused by a stone in the adjacent cystic duct. It is essential for the surgeon to know about preoperatively because the CHD may be mistakenly ligated instead of the cystic duct. Additionally, inflammation can cause the gallstone to erode into the CHD and cause a cholecystocholedochal fistula and biliary obstruction.
- On ultrasound, a stone is typically impacted in the distal cystic duct and the CHD is dilated. The cystic duct tends to run in parallel with the CHD.

米里齐综合征

- 米里齐综合征是由胆囊管中的结石引起邻近肝总管(CHD)的炎症和外部受压。术前了解这一点对于外科医生很重要，因为肝总管可能会被误扎，而非结扎胆囊管。此外，炎症可导致胆结石侵入到肝总管内，从而导致胆囊肝总管瘘和胆道梗阻。
- 在超声影像上，结石通常嵌顿在胆囊管的远端，并且肝总管是扩张的。胆囊管往往与肝总管平行。

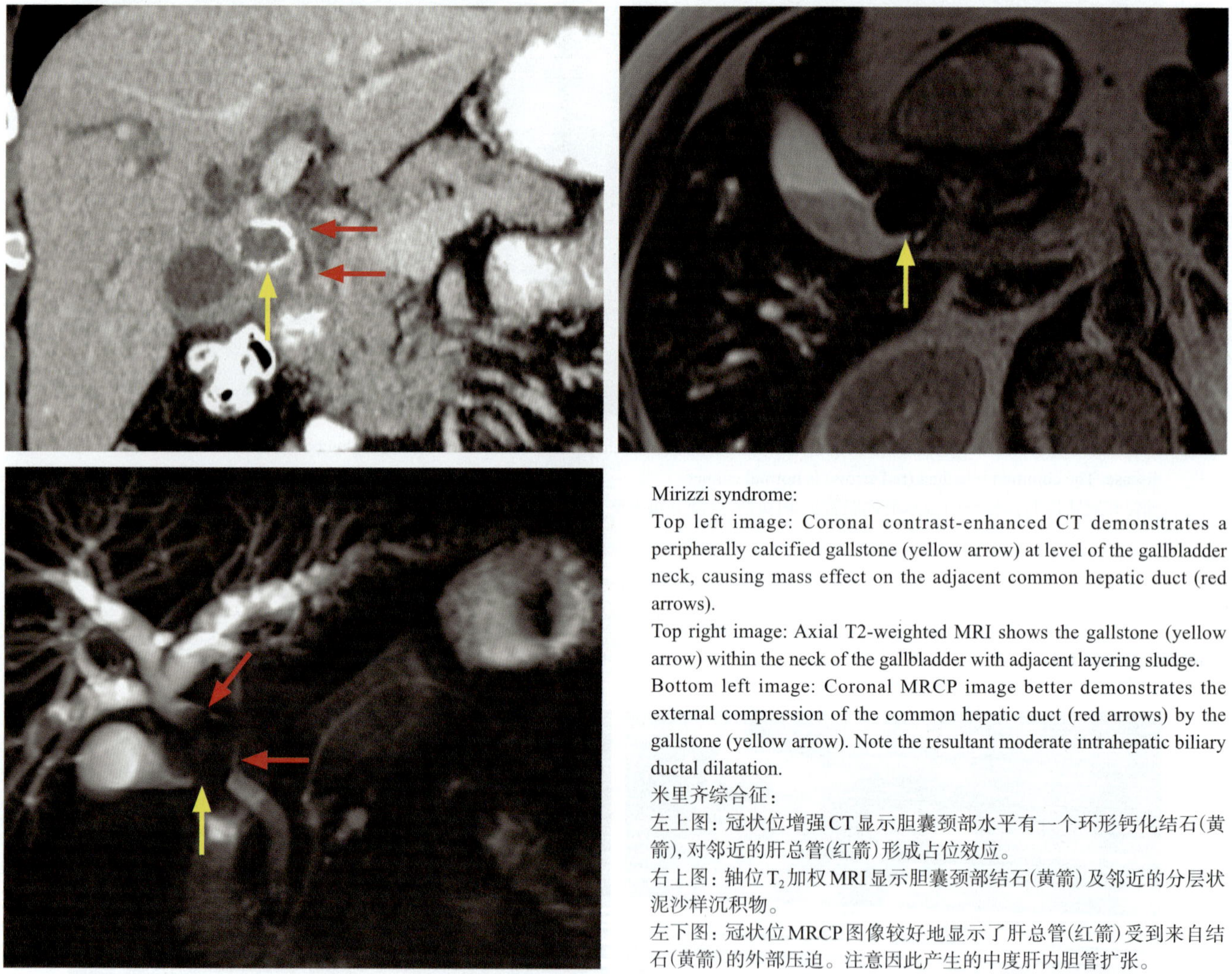

Mirizzi syndrome:
Top left image: Coronal contrast-enhanced CT demonstrates a peripherally calcified gallstone (yellow arrow) at level of the gallbladder neck, causing mass effect on the adjacent common hepatic duct (red arrows).
Top right image: Axial T2-weighted MRI shows the gallstone (yellow arrow) within the neck of the gallbladder with adjacent layering sludge.
Bottom left image: Coronal MRCP image better demonstrates the external compression of the common hepatic duct (red arrows) by the gallstone (yellow arrow). Note the resultant moderate intrahepatic biliary ductal dilatation.
米里齐综合征：
左上图：冠状位增强CT显示胆囊颈部水平有一个环形钙化结石(黄箭)，对邻近的肝总管(红箭)形成占位效应。
右上图：轴位T_2加权MRI显示胆囊颈部结石(黄箭)及邻近的分层状泥沙样沉积物。
左下图：冠状位MRCP图像较好地显示了肝总管(红箭)受到来自结石(黄箭)的外部压迫。注意因此产生的中度肝内胆管扩张。

Pneumobilia

- Pneumobilia is air in the biliary tree. It is commonly seen after sphincterotomy or biliary-to-enteric anastomosis, but rarely may be due to cholecystoenteric fistula or emphysematous cholecystitis.

胆管积气

- 胆管积气是指胆道内出现气体。常见于括约肌切开术或胆-肠吻合术后，较少见于胆肠瘘或气肿性胆囊炎。

Modality	Pneumobilia	Portal venous gas
CT/MRI	• Branching gas • Seen more centrally	• Branching gas • Extends to liver periphery
Ultrasound	• Branching echogenic foci with dirty shadowing	• Branching echogenic foci with dirty shadowing • Causes "spiky" spectral Doppler waveform

*Gas can be difficult to visualize by MRI; gas is T1 and T2 hypointense and causes "blooming" (more prominent low signal) on in-phase images.

成像方式	胆管积气	门静脉积气
CT/MRI	• 分支内气体 • 常见中心性分布	• 分支内气体 • 延伸至肝脏周边
超声	• 分支内局造性回声增高伴浑浊声影	• 分支内局灶性回声伴浑浊声影 • 引起"尖峰"样多普勒波形

*气体在MRI上显示较为困难；气体在T_1和T_2上均呈低信号，且在同相位图像上会产生"磁敏感伪影"(更明显的低信号)。

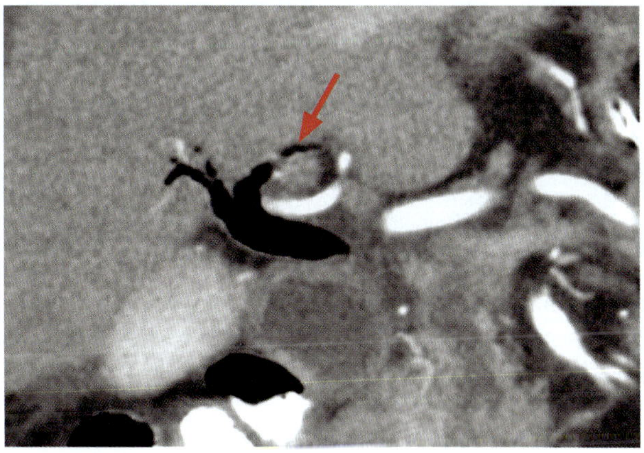

Pneumobilia (central).
肝内胆管积气(中央性分布)。

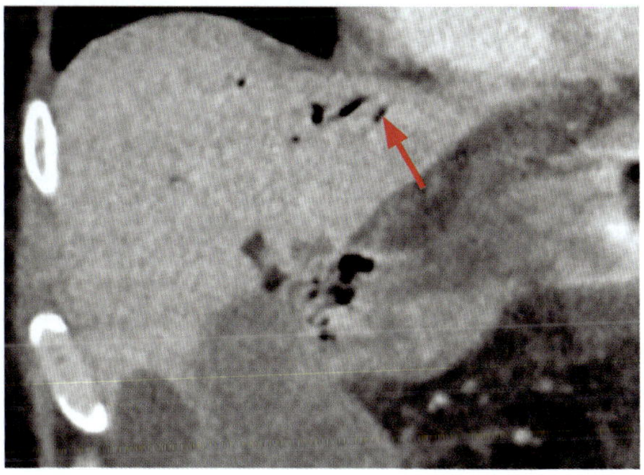

Portal venous gas (peripheral).
门静脉积气(外周性分布)。

Biliary ductal dilation

- A rule of thumb for assessing the common bile duct (CBD) diameter is to assume that the CBD should be 6 mm or less before age 60, but may still be normal if 1 mm larger per decade after that age. For example, an 8 mm duct in an 80-year-old patient may be considered normal.

  Some sources, however, suggest very small differences with age (mean duct diameter of 3.6 mm for 60-year-old patients and 4.0 mm for 85-year-old patients).

  For the hepatic ducts, >2 mm in size or >40% of the adjacent portal vein diameter is abnormal.
- The common bile duct is often mildly dilated in patients who have undergone cholecystectomy, usually 10 mm or less.
- In general, malignancy causes more prominent ductal dilation than benign disease.

胆管扩张

- 评估胆总管直径大小的一个经验法则是，60岁之前胆总管直径一般≤6mm，60岁之后，每10年增加1mm属于正常。例如，一个80岁的患者胆总管直径为8mm时，可认为是正常。

  然而，某些资料表明年龄的差异非常小(60岁患者的平均直径为3.6mm，85岁患者的平均直径为4.0mm)。

  肝管直径大于2mm或大于邻近门静脉直径的40%时则为异常。
- 胆囊切除术后的患者胆总管常呈轻度扩张，大多≤10mm。
- 一般而言，恶性肿瘤比良性疾病引起的胆管扩张更加明显。

Ascending cholangitis

逆行性胆管炎

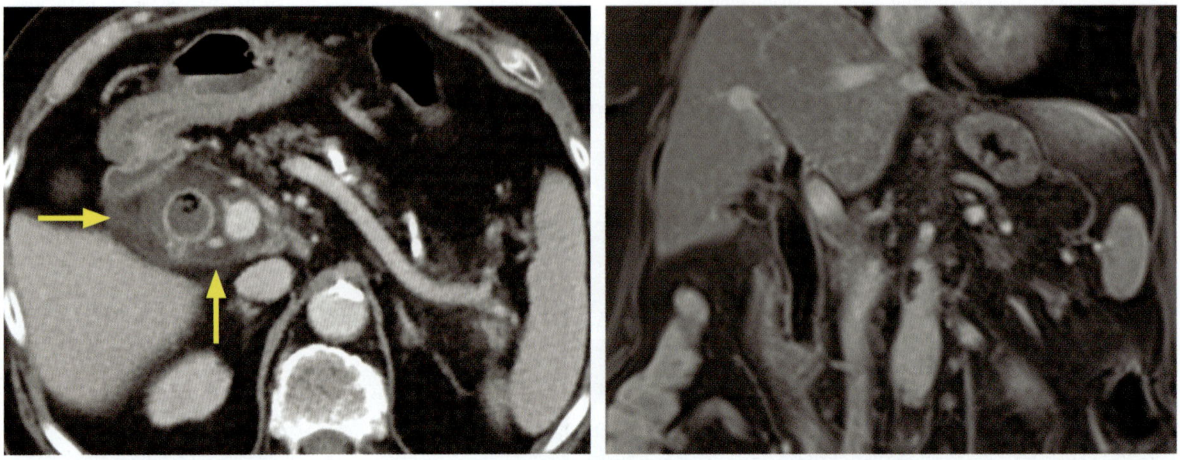

Axial contrast-enhanced CT (left image) demonstrates fat stranding and edema around the common bile duct (arrows), which is dilated, with wall thickening and enhancement and contains small amount of intraluminal gas (patient has a history of sphincterotomy). Subsequent coronal post-contrast T1-weighted MRI (right image) also shows common bile duct wall thickening and hyperenhancement. These findings are highly suspicious for cholangitis.

轴位增强CT(左图)显示胆总管周围脂肪密度异常和水肿(黄箭),胆总管扩张及管壁增厚与强化,腔内含少量气体(患者有括约肌切开手术史)。随后的冠状位增强T_1加权MRI(右图)也显示胆总管壁增厚和强化。这些发现可高度怀疑为胆管炎。

- Obstruction of the biliary tree, most commonly due to choledocholithiasis, may cause ascending cholangitis, which presents with the clinical triad of fever, abdominal pain, and jaundice (*Charcot's triad*).
- Imaging may be completely normal, although when abnormal, the key findings are hyperenhancement and thickening of the walls of the bile ducts, often with intraluminal debris and/or choledocholithiasis.

- 胆道系统梗阻最常由胆总管结石所致,可能会引起逆行性胆管炎,在临床上表现为发热、腹痛和黄疸三联征(查科三联征)。
- 影像学检查可能完全正常,但异常时,主要表现为胆管壁强化与增厚,通常伴有管腔内碎片和/或胆总管结石。

Primary sclerosing cholangitis (PSC)

原发性硬化性胆管炎(PSC)

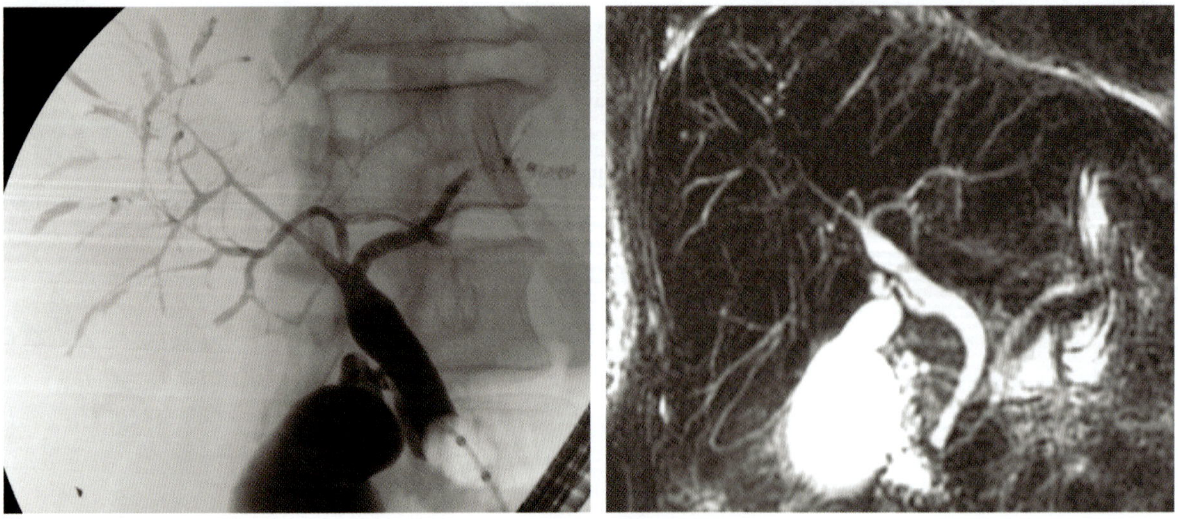

Primary sclerosing cholangitis: ERCP (left image) and thick-slab coronal MRCP heavily T2-weighted sequence (right image), show a beaded, irregular appearance to the intrahepatic bile ducts.

Case courtesy Cheryl Sadow, MD, Brigham and Women's Hospital.

原发性硬化性胆管炎:ERCP(左图)和厚层冠状位MRCP重T_2加权序列(右图)显示肝内胆管呈串珠状、不规则改变。

- Primary sclerosing cholangitis (PSC) is idiopathic inflammation and destruction of bile ducts.
- PSC is associated with ulcerative colitis (UC) and to a lesser extent, Crohn's disease, and is more common in males.

  Most (75%) patients with PSC have UC, while only a few (4–5%) of patients with UC have PSC.
- Biliary imaging shows a characteristic beaded, irregular appearance of the common bile duct and intrahepatic bile ducts.
- PSC appearance is similar to that of AIDS cholangiopathy, although cholangitis in HIV/AIDS patients is more commonly associated with papillary stenosis.
- Long-term complications of PSC include cirrhosis (often seen with prominent caudate lobe hypertrophy), cholangiocarcinoma, and recurrent biliary infections. Cross-sectional imaging is better at evaluating for these complications compared to ERCP.

- 原发性硬化性胆管炎(PSC)是一种不明原因的特发性胆管炎症和破坏性疾病。
- PSC与溃疡性结肠炎(UC)相关，少数与克罗恩病相关，且多见于男性。

  大多数(75%)PSC患者合并UC，而仅有少数(4%~5%)UC患者有PSC。
- 胆管成像显示胆总管和肝内胆管呈典型的串珠状、不规则改变。
- PSC的表现与获得性免疫缺陷综合征(AIDS)胆管病类似，而HIV感染者/AIDS患者发生的胆管炎更常伴发十二指肠乳头狭窄。
- PSC的长期并发症包括肝硬化(常伴有明显的尾状叶增大)、胆管癌和复发性胆道感染。在评估这些并发症方面，断层图像优于ERCP。

Primary biliary cirrhosis (PBC)

- Primary biliary cirrhosis (PBC) is inflammation and destruction of smaller bile ducts. Compared to PSC, PBC usually affects middle-aged women and often presents with pruritus.
- Similar to PSC, chronic PBC can lead to hepatic cirrhosis, often with prominent caudate lobe hypertrophy.

原发性胆汁性肝硬化(PBC)

- 原发性胆汁性肝硬化(PBC)是小胆管的炎症与破坏。与PSC相比，PBC多见于中年女性，且常表现为皮肤瘙痒。
- 与PSC类似，慢性PBC可导致肝硬化，常伴有明显的尾状叶增大。

AIDS cholangitis (AIDS cholangiopathy)

- Patients with acquired immunodeficiency syndrome are susceptible to biliary infection with *Cryptosporidium* and CMV, which clinically present with right upper quadrant pain, fever, and elevated LFTs.
- The imaging of AIDS cholangitis appears nearly identical to PSC, with multiple strictures and a beaded appearance of the bile ducts. A distinguishing feature of AIDS cholangitis is *papillary stenosis*, which is not typically seen in PSC.

AIDS胆管炎(AIDS胆管病)

- 获得性免疫缺陷综合征患者易患隐孢子虫和巨细胞病毒(CMV)引起的胆道感染，临床表现为右上腹疼痛、发热和肝功能指标升高。
- AIDS胆管炎的影像学表现与PSC几乎完全相同，为多发胆管狭窄和串珠样改变。AIDS胆管炎较为特殊的表现是十二指肠乳头狭窄，而PSC并不常见。

Recurrent pyogenic cholangitis (oriental cholangiohepatitis)

- Recurrent pyogenic cholangitis, also known as oriental cholangiohepatitis, is thought to be caused by the parasite *Clonorchis sinensis*, which leads to pigment stone formation, biliary stasis, and cholangitis. Nutritional deficiency may also play a role. The disease is typically observed in patients from Southeast Asia.
- Clinically, patients present with recurrent jaundice and fevers.
- Recurrent pyogenic cholangitis features an imaging triad of:
  1) Pneumobilia.
  2) Lamellated bile duct filling defects.
  3) Intrahepatic and extrahepatic bile duct dilation and strictures.
- Patients with recurrent pyogenic cholangitis have an increased risk of cholangiocarcinoma.

复发性化脓性胆管炎(东方胆管肝炎)

- 复发性化脓性胆管炎，又称为东方胆管性肝炎，被认为是由华支睾吸虫(Clonorchis sinensis)所致，可导致色素性结石形成、胆汁淤积和胆管炎。营养不良也可能是其中的一个原因。该病患者主要来自东南亚。
- 患者临床表现为反复黄疸和发热。
- 复发性化脓性胆管炎的影像学三联征：
  1) 胆道积气。
  2) 板层状胆管内充盈缺损。
  3) 肝内与肝外胆管扩张和狭窄。
- 对于反复发作的化脓性胆管炎患者，其患胆管癌的风险增加。

Biliary cystadenoma/cystadenocarcinoma

胆管囊腺瘤和囊腺癌

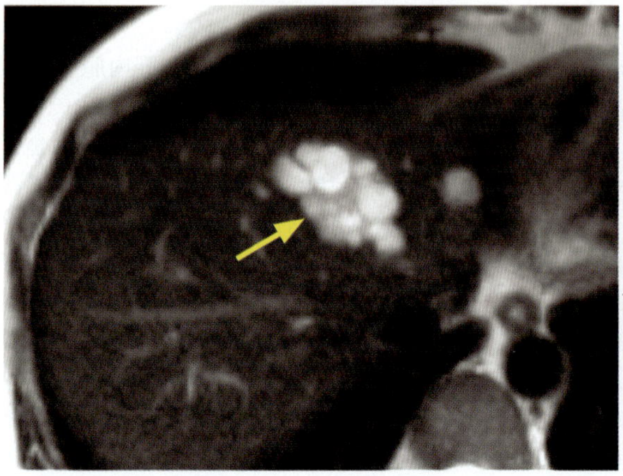

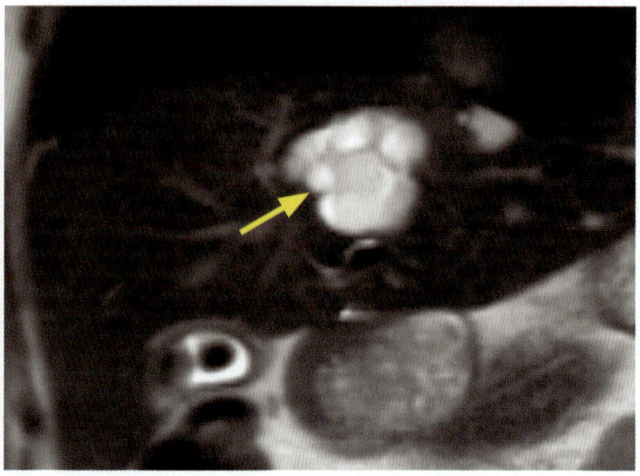

Axial (left image) and coronal T2-weighted (right) images demonstrate multiseptated T2 hyperintense lesion in segment Ⅳ consistent with a biliary cystadenoma. There is also a small adjacent cystic lesion in segment Ⅱ that may be an additional biliary cystadenoma or hepatic cyst.

轴位(左图)和冠状位T_2加权(右图)图像显示肝脏Ⅳ段一处多房性T_2高信号病灶，符合胆管囊腺瘤。肝脏Ⅱ段也有一个小的近囊性病灶，可能是另一个胆管囊腺瘤或肝囊肿。

- Biliary cystadenoma is a benign cystic neoplasm occurring predominantly in middle-aged women. Biliary cystadenoma may be quite large at presentation and cause nonspecific symptoms such as abdominal pain, nausea, vomiting, and obstructive jaundice.
- Biliary cystadenoma does not communicate with the biliary system.
- On imaging, biliary cystadenoma appears as a large, multiloculated, cystic mass. The presence of septations distinguishes cystadenoma from a simple cyst. The septations may mimic an echinococcal cyst. In contrast to hepatic abscess or necrotic metastasis, a thick enhancing wall is not a feature of cystadenoma.
- Due to risk of malignant degeneration to biliary cystadenocarcinoma (occurs in up to 15% of patients), resection is often pursued. The presence of frank invasion into adjacent liver, a large solid component or thick calcification should raise concern for cystadenocarcinoma.

- 胆管囊腺瘤是一种良性囊性肿瘤，主要发生于中年女性。胆管囊腺瘤在发病时通常比较大，会产生一些非特异性症状，如腹痛、恶心、呕吐和梗阻性黄疸。
- 胆管囊腺瘤与胆管系统不相通。
- 在影像学上，胆管囊腺瘤表现为一个大的、多房性的囊性肿块。如有分隔可对囊腺瘤与单纯性囊肿进行鉴别。分隔可类似于包虫囊肿。与肝脓肿或坏死性转移瘤不同，增强的厚壁不是囊腺瘤的特征。
- 由于胆管囊腺癌存在恶变风险(出现在高达15%的患者)，通常需要尽快切除。如果邻近有明显的肝脏浸润，或出现大的实性成分或厚的钙化，需要警惕恶变为囊腺癌的可能。

Cholangiocarcinoma

- Cholangiocarcinoma is a highly malignant tumor of the biliary ductal epithelium and is the second most common primary hepatic mass.
- It classically presents with painless jaundice. Most cases of cholangiocarcinoma are sporadic, although key risk factors include chronic biliary disease (in the United States) and liver fluke infection (in the Far East).
- There are three main subtypes:

  Mass forming cholangiocarcinoma.

  Periductal cholangiocarcinoma: most often at the confluence of the right and left hepatic biliary ducts (known as **Klatskin tumor**).

  Intraductal cholangiocarcinoma: has variable imaging appearance.

胆管癌

- 胆管癌是胆管上皮的高度恶性肿瘤，是第二常见的肝脏原发肿瘤。
- 典型表现为无痛性黄疸。大多数胆管癌病例是散发的，但主要的危险因素包括慢性胆道疾病(美国)和肝吸虫感染(远东地区)。
- 共有三种主要亚型：

  肿块形成型胆管癌。

  导管周围型胆管癌：最常见于左右肝管汇合处(被称为**克拉茨金瘤**)。

  导管内型胆管癌：影像学表现多样。

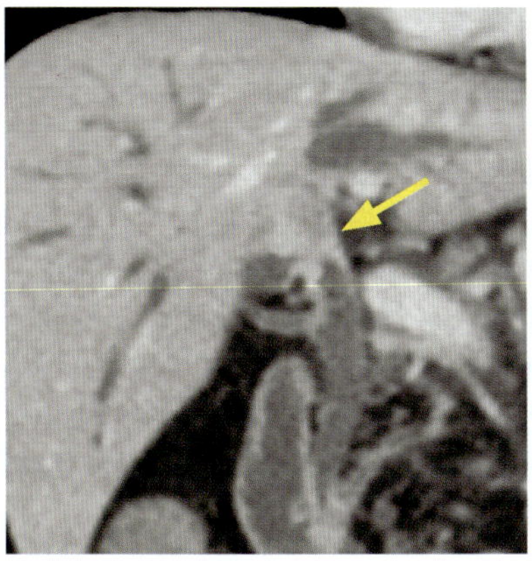

Contrast-enhanced CT
增强CT

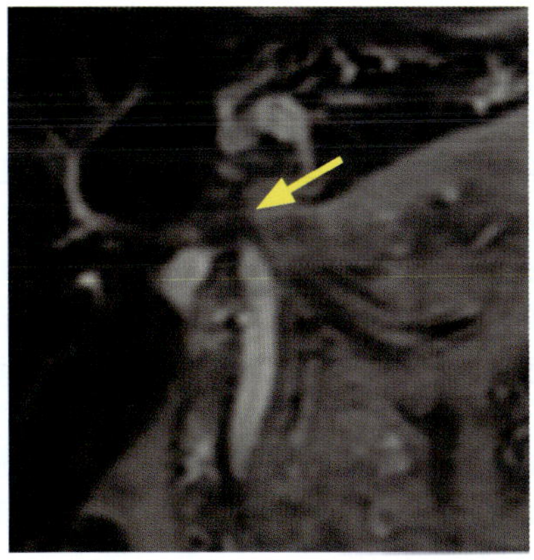

T2-weighted MRI
T_2加权MRI

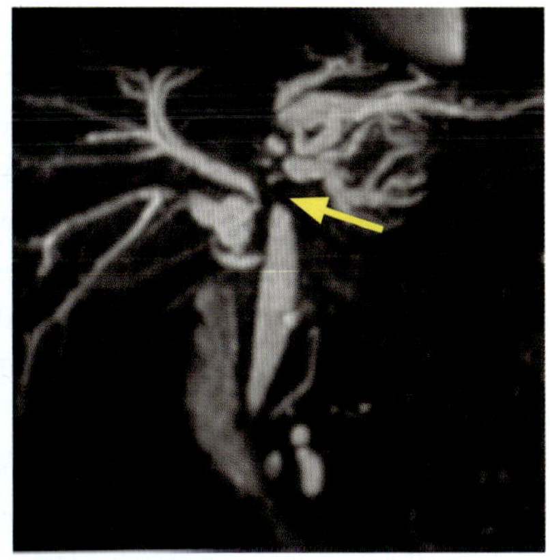

MRCP MIP image
MRCP MIP成像

Klatskin tumor: Coronal contrast-enhanced CT and T2-weighted MRI show an enhancing, mildly T2 hyperintense tumor (arrows) at the common hepatic duct bifurcation, resulting in moderate intrahepatic biliary ductal dilatation.
克拉茨金瘤：冠状位增强CT和T_2加权MRI显示肝总管分叉处有一个强化的、T_2稍高信号的肿瘤(黄箭)，导致肝内胆管中度扩张。

- Cholangiocarcinoma tends to obstruct bile ducts and lead to intrahepatic ductal dilation and capsular retraction. Eventually, the obstruction may lead to lobar atrophy.
- Risk factors for development of cholangiocarcinoma include:

- 胆管癌容易阻塞胆管，并导致肝内胆管扩张和肝包膜回缩。最终，梗阻可能会导致肝叶萎缩。
- 诱发胆管癌的危险因素包括：

Choledochal cyst(s).
Primary sclerosing cholangitis.
Familial adenomatous polyposis syndrome.
Clonorchis sinensis infection.
Thorium dioxide (alpha-emitter contrast agent), not used since the 1950s. Thorium dioxide is also associated with angiosarcoma and HCC.

胆总管囊肿。
原发性硬化性胆管炎。
家族性腺瘤型息肉综合征。
中华睾吸虫感染。
二氧化钍(含α射线造影剂)，自20世纪50年代起已停用。二氧化钍也与血管肉瘤和肝细胞癌的发生有关。

Primary gallbladder carcinoma

原发性胆囊癌

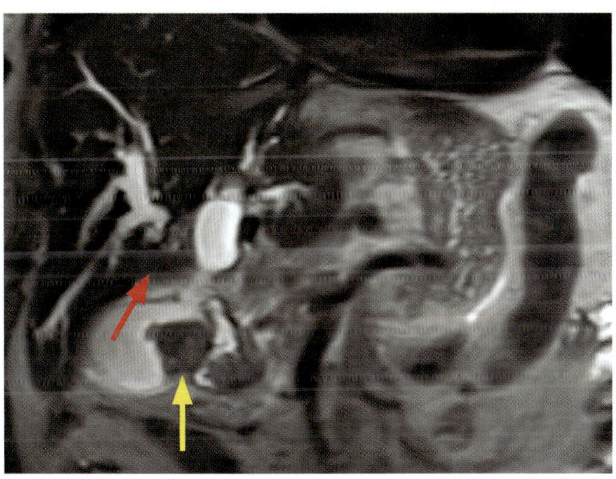

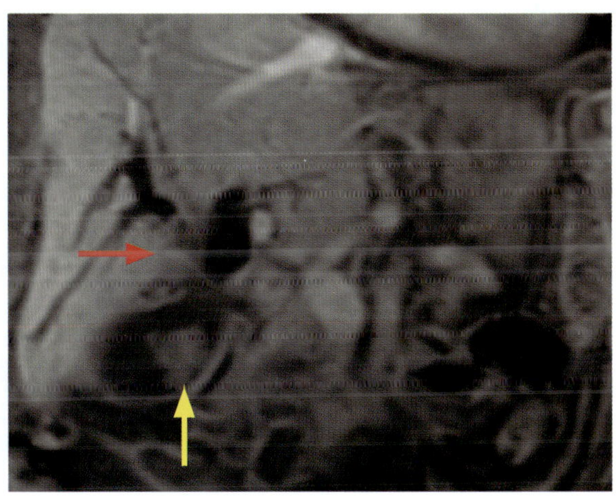

Coronal T2-weighted (left image) and post-contrast T1-weighted (right image) MRI demonstrates an intraluminal enhancing mass within the gallbladder (yellow arrows) and an associated porta hepatis mass (red arrows) resulting in severe intra- and extrahepatic biliary ductal dilatation. Pathology upon resection showed gallbladder carcinoma with metastatic pancreaticoduodenal lymph node.
冠状位T_2加权(左图)和增强T_1加权(右图)MRI显示胆囊腔内有一个强化肿块(黄箭)，邻近肝门亦可见一个肿块(红箭)，并引起肝内外胆管显著扩张。切除后病理检查结果显示为胆囊癌伴胰十二指肠淋巴结转移。

- Gallbladder cancer is a rare malignancy with a poor prognosis. A typical clinical presentation may include right upper quadrant pain, weight loss, and jaundice.
- Gallstones and concomitant chronic cholecystitis are typically present. Porcelain gallbladder, a result of chronic cholecystitis, is thought to be a risk factor for gallbladder cancer, although this is controversial.
- Gallbladder carcinoma most commonly presents as a scirrhous infiltrating mass that invades through the gallbladder wall into the liver. Less commonly, gallbladder carcinoma may appear as a polypoid mass. Very rarely it can present as focal mural thickening.
- Tumor spread is via direct extension into the liver, although lymphatic and hematogenous metastases are also common. Prognosis is generally poor, although small polypoid lesions may undergo curative resection.
- Risk factors for development of gallbladder cancer include:

> Gallstones and chronic cholecystitis.
> Porcelain gallbladder (somewhat controversial).
> Primary sclerosing cholangitis.
> Inflammatory bowel disease (ulcerative colitis more frequently than Crohn's disease).
> Adenomatous polyp >10 mm or with multiple risk factors, as described above.

Gallbladder metastases

- Metastases to the gallbladder are uncommon.
- Hepatocellular carcinoma can spread directly to the gallbladder through the bile ducts.
- Melanoma can spread hematogenously to the gallbladder mucosa.

- 胆囊癌是一种罕见的恶性肿瘤，预后较差。典型的临床表现包括右上腹痛、体重减轻和黄疸。
- 胆囊癌通常会同时存在胆结石和慢性胆囊炎。瓷化胆囊由慢性胆囊炎发展而来，被认为是胆囊癌的危险因素，但目前尚有争议。
- 胆囊癌最常见的表现是硬化性浸润性肿块，通过胆囊壁侵犯肝脏。胆囊癌较少见的表现为息肉样肿块。极少表现为局灶性内壁增厚。
- 肿瘤通过直接侵犯肝脏进行播散，但淋巴转移和血行转移也很常见。虽然小的息肉样病变可行根治性切除，但胆囊癌的预后通常较差。
- 诱发胆囊癌的危险因素包括：

> 胆囊结石和慢性胆囊炎。
> 瓷化胆囊(尚有争议)。
> 原发性硬化性胆管炎。
> 炎症性肠病(溃疡性结肠炎比克罗恩病更常见)。
> 腺瘤性息肉>10mm或合并多种危险因素，如上所述。

胆囊转移瘤

- 胆囊转移瘤不常见。
- HCC可通过胆管直接扩散至胆囊。
- 黑色素瘤可通过血行播散至胆囊黏膜。

(翻译　常娣)

PANCREAS

Normal ductal anatomy

- Normally, the main pancreatic duct drains to the major papilla (the ampulla of Vater) through the duct of Wirsung, while the duct of Santorini drains to the minor papilla.

  The sphincter of Oddi is a circular band of muscle encircling the ampulla of Vater.

胰腺

正常胰管解剖

- 正常情况下，主胰管通过Wirsung管引流至大乳头(肝胰壶腹)，而副胰管(Santorini管)引流至小乳头。

  奥迪括约肌是环绕肝胰壶腹的环形平滑肌带。

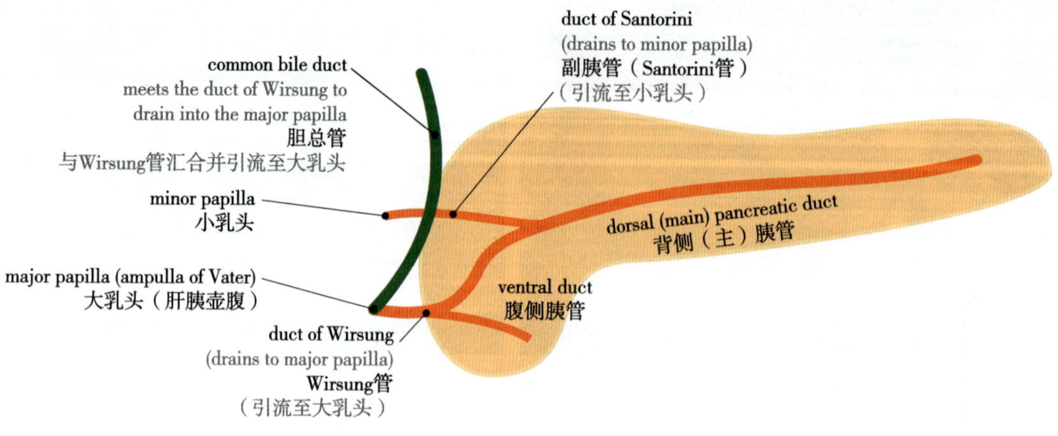

- Mnemonic for normal anatomy: Santorini is superior and drains to small (minor) papilla.
- The following anatomy is *always* constant, regardless of whether an anomaly is present:

- 正常解剖记忆法："Santorini is superior and drains to small(minor)papilla"，副胰管(Santorini管)位于上方并引流至小乳头。
- 以下解剖结构总是固定的，不受变异影响：

1) The common bile duct always drains to the major papilla where it meets the duct of Wirsung.
2) The dorsal pancreatic duct always drains the pancreatic tail.
3) The duct of Santorini always drains to the minor papilla.

1) 胆总管总是引流至大乳头并在此与Wirsung管汇合。
2) 背侧(主)胰管总是引流胰腺的尾部。
3) 副胰管(Santorini管)总是引流至小乳头。

CONGENITAL PANCREATIC ANOMALIES

先天性胰腺异常

Pancreas divisum

- Pancreas divisum is the most common congenital pancreatic ductal anomaly. It is caused by failure of fusion of the ventral and dorsal pancreatic ducts. The ventral duct (Wirsung) only drains the ventral portion of the pancreas while the dorsal portion (majority) of the exocrine gland output is drained through the smaller duct of Santorini into the minor papilla.

胰腺分裂

- 胰腺分裂是最常见的先天性胰腺导管异常，是由腹侧和背侧胰管未能融合所致。Wirsung管只引流腹侧部分的胰腺，而背侧(大部分)胰腺外分泌腺的产物通过较小的副胰管(Santorini管)引流至小乳头。

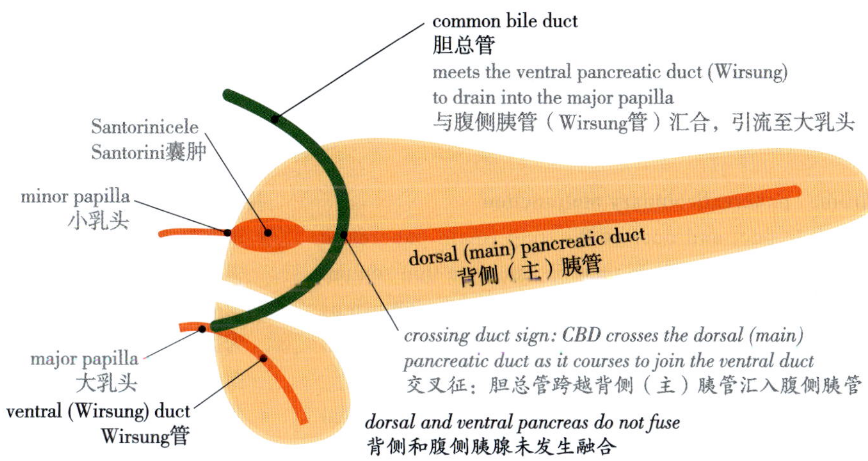

- Pancreas divisum increases the risk for pancreatitis due to the inability of the minor papilla to adequately drain the majority of the pancreatic parenchyma.
- Treatment is sphincterotomy or stenting.
- The *crossing duct sign* describes the common bile duct crossing over the main duct to join the duct of Wirsung.

- 胰腺分裂增加了胰腺炎的风险，因小乳头不能完全引流胰腺的大部分实质。
- 治疗方式是括约肌切开术或支架植入。
- 交叉征是指胆总管跨越主胰管汇入Wirsung管。

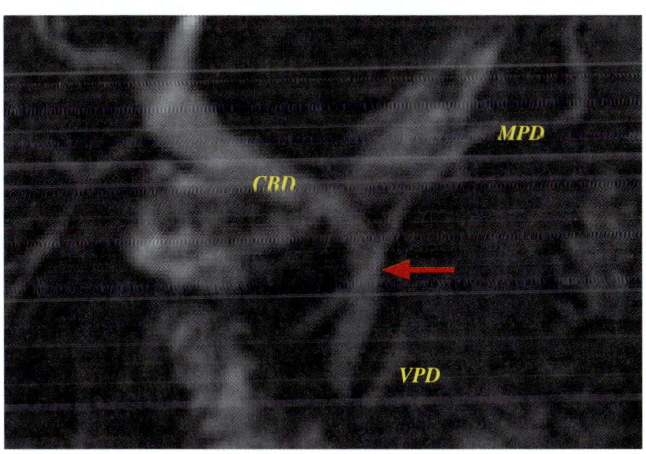

Crossing duct sign of pancreas divisum: Thick-slab coronal MRCP heavily T2- weighted sequence shows the common bile duct (CBD) crossing the main pancreatic duct (MPD) at the arrow.
The CBD courses towards the ventral pancreatic duct (VPD) to empty into the major papilla. The main/dorsal pancreatic duct drains separately into the minor papilla.
Case courtesy Cheryl Sadow, MD, Brigham and Women's Hospital.
胰腺分裂交叉征：厚层冠状位MRCP重T_2加权序列显示胆总管(CBD)在红箭所示部位跨越主胰管(MPD)。CBD与腹侧胰管(VPD)汇合并引流至大乳头。主/背侧胰管单独引流至小乳头。

Annular pancreas

- Annular pancreas is a rare congenital anomaly where a portion of the pancreas encircles the duodenum, secondary to incomplete rotation of the ventral pancreatic bud.

环状胰腺

- 环状胰腺是一种罕见的先天性异常，为部分胰腺包绕十二指肠，是腹侧胰芽不完全旋转所致。

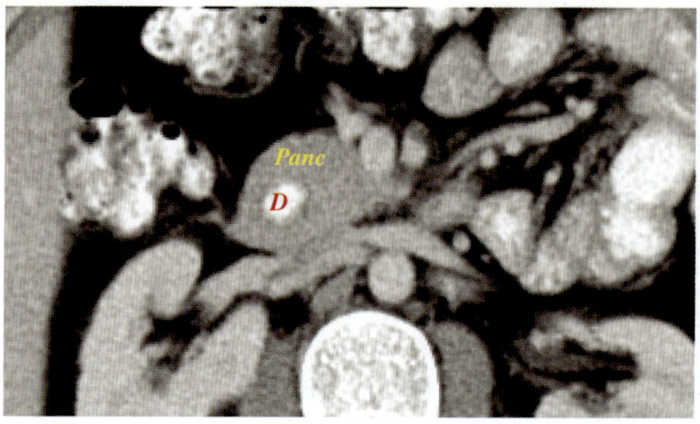

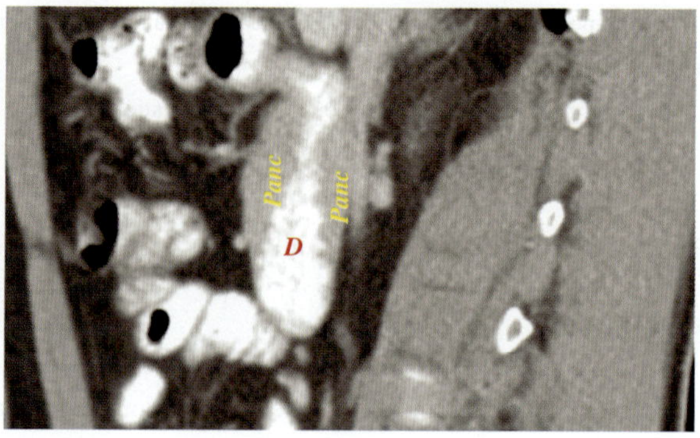

Annular pancreas: Axial (left image) and sagittal (right image) contrast-enhanced CT shows circumferential encircling of the pancreas (Panc) around the duodenum (D), which is filled with oral contrast.
Case courtesy Cheryl Sadow, MD, Brigham and Women's Hospital.
环状胰腺：轴位(左图)和矢状位(右图)增强CT显示胰腺(Panc)环绕口服造影剂所充盈的十二指肠(D处)。

- In a neonate, it presents with duodenal obstruction and is in the differential for the *double bubble sign* (discussed further in the "Pediatrics" chapter). In an adult, annular pancreas can cause pancreatitis, peptic ulcer disease, and duodenal obstruction.

Common channel syndrome / pancreaticobiliary maljunction

- Normally the common bile duct and duct of Wirsung (main pancreatic duct) both drain to the major papilla, where there is usually a thin septum separating these two systems. In common channel syndrome, also known as pancreaticobiliary maljunction, this septum is absent, allowing reflux between the two systems.
- Common channel syndrome may predispose to choledochal webs, choledochal cysts, pancreatitis and cholangiocarcinoma.

- 在新生儿中，环状胰腺可表现为十二指肠梗阻，是"双泡征"(这部分将在小儿影像章节讨论)的鉴别诊断之一。在成人中，环状胰腺可能导致胰腺炎、消化道溃疡，以及十二指肠梗阻。

共管综合征/胰胆管汇合异常

- 正常情况下胆总管和Wirsung管(主胰管)共同引流至大乳头，但通常会有薄的分隔在大乳头处将这两套系统分开。共管综合征也被称为胰胆管汇合异常，是指由于这层分隔缺失而使两套系统之间出现反流。
- 共管综合征可能引起胆总管蹼、胆总管囊肿、胰腺炎和胆管癌。

Pancreatitis

- Pancreatitis is inflammation of the pancreas, which may be due to a variety of etiologies that share a final common pathway of premature activation of pancreatic enzymes and resultant autodigestion of pancreatic parenchyma.
- Pancreatitis may range in severity from mild self-limited disease to necrotizing infection resulting in multiorgan failure and death.

Ultrasound role of imaging

- Ultrasound is useful in the initial evaluation of clinically suspected acute pancreatitis to evaluate for gallstones, choledocholithiasis or biliary obstruction.
- Ultrasound has limited utility in evaluating complications of pancreatitis such as pancreatic necrosis or peripancreatic fluid collections.

CT protocol and role of imaging

- Imaging of pancreatitis is ideally performed in the pancreatic phase (late arterial; ~40 seconds after contrast injection when the pancreatic parenchyma is maximally enhancing), which is the optimal time to detect subtle areas of decreased enhancement suggestive of necrosis.
- CT may be helpful when the clinical presentation is equivocal for pancreatitis, a patient is critically ill or worsening over time, to assess for severity, detect complications, and guide treatment.
- CT imaging is *not* indicated in patients with clinical diagnosis of mild acute pancreatitis, especially if they are improving. CT imaging may be negative or show a mildly edematous pancreas in these cases.

胰腺炎

- 胰腺炎是胰腺发炎，可由多种因素所致，其最终的共同发病机制为胰酶过早被激活并导致胰腺实质自体消化。
- 胰腺炎的严重程度可从轻度的自限性疾病到坏死性感染，可引起多器官衰竭和死亡。

超声影像价值

- 超声用于初步评估临床上疑似急性胰腺炎，了解是否有胆囊结石、胆总管结石或胆道梗阻。
- 超声在评估胰腺炎的并发症方面有局限性，如胰腺坏死或胰腺周围积液。

CT扫描方法及影像价值

- 胰腺炎的最佳成像期为胰腺实质期(动脉晚期；造影剂注射约40秒后胰腺实质达到最大强化)，此期是发现轻微强化减低区域(提示胰腺坏死)的最敏感时期。
- 对于临床表现不明确的胰腺炎，CT可能有助于在患者病情危重或病程加重时评估其严重程度、发现并发症，以及指导治疗。
- CT不适用于临床诊断为轻度急性胰腺炎的患者，尤其是正处于恢复期的患者。CT影像在这些病例中可能呈阴性，或显示为胰腺轻度水肿。

MR protocol and role of imaging

- MRI is indicated for evaluation of etiology (i.e., choledocholithiasis), edema, necrosis, associated neoplasm, and the pancreatic duct.
- Different sequences in MRI with MRCP assess for the following pancreatic abnormalities:

MR Sequence	Can evaluate for
T2-weighted fat saturation	Edema and fluid collections
MRCP	Biliary tree and pancreatic duct
Pre-contrast T1-weighted	Pancreatic parenchymal bulk and signal (normally, pancreas should be the brightest organ)
T1 post-contrast at 30, 60, and 90 seconds	Pancreatic parenchymal enhancement, vascular complications and fluid collections
Subtraction	Best to evaluate for pancreatic necrosis

MR扫描方法及影像价值

- MRI适用于评估胰腺炎的病因(如胆总管结石)、水肿、坏死、合并肿瘤,以及胰管情况。
- 评估以下胰腺异常的不同MRI序列和MRCP:

MR序列	可用于评估
T_2加权脂肪抑制	水肿和积液
磁共振胰胆管成像(MRCP)	胆道和胰管
增强前T_1加权	胰腺实质体积和信号(正常情况下,胰腺应该是最亮的器官)
增强后T_1加权(30秒、60秒、90秒)	胰腺实质强化,血管并发症和液体积聚
减影	评估胰腺坏死最佳

Acute pancreatitis

急性胰腺炎

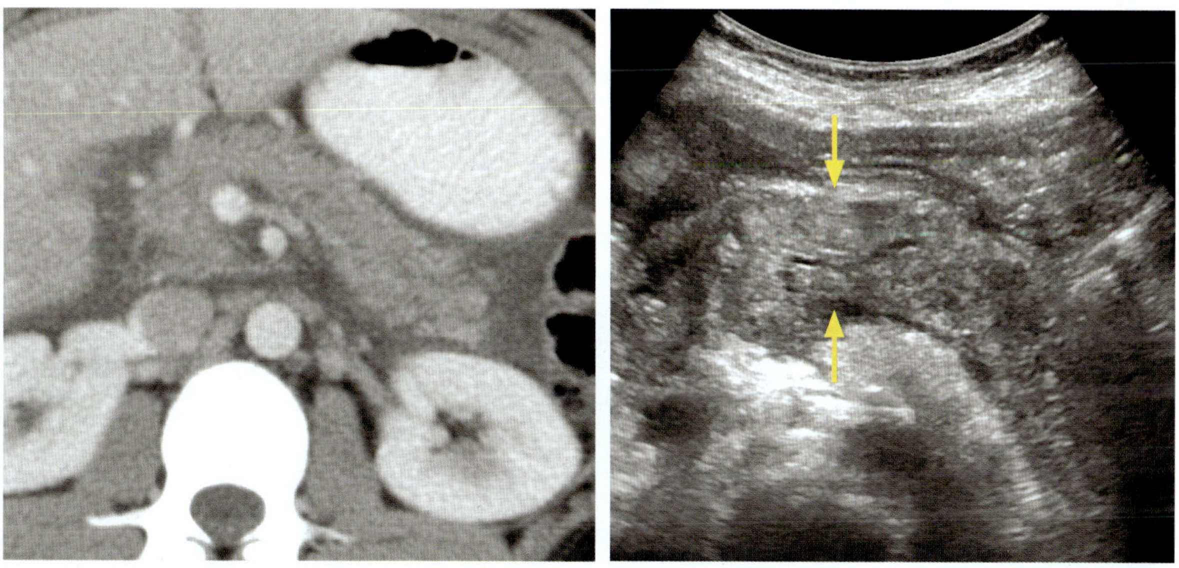

Acute pancreatitis on CT and ultrasound:
Contrast-enhanced axial CT (left image) demonstrates diffuse pancreatic enlargement and peripancreatic edema. The pancreatic parenchyma enhances uniformly, without evidence for necrosis.
Transverse ultrasound (right image) of the head and body of the pancreas shows a diffusely enlarged, heterogeneous pancreas (arrows) due to pancreatic edema.
Ultrasound case courtesy Julie Ritner, MD, Brigham and Women's Hospital, Boston.
急性胰腺炎的CT和超声图像:
轴位增强CT(左图)显示弥漫性胰腺增大和胰周水肿。胰腺实质均匀强化,没有坏死征象。胰头和胰体部横切面超声(右图)显示胰腺水肿造成的弥漫性胰腺增大及胰腺回声不均匀。

- Acute pancreatitis is most commonly caused by alcohol use or an obstructing gallstone.
- There are two morphologic subtypes:
  1. Interstitial edematous pancreatitis
  2. Necrotizing pancreatitis
- Acute pancreatitis can be classified either with the Balthazar grading system or by the CT severity index.
- Pancreatic and peripancreatic complications of pancreatitis:

- 急性胰腺炎最常见的原因是饮酒和阻塞性胆结石。
- 形态学上有两种亚型:
  1. 间质水肿性胰腺炎。
  2. 坏死性胰腺炎。
- 急性胰腺炎分级既可以按照Balthazar分级系统,也可以按照CT严重指数。
- 胰腺炎的胰腺和胰周并发症:

< 4 weeks	> 4 weeks
Acute peripancreatic fluid collection: Non-encapsulated fluid collection.	**Pseudocyst**: Encapsulated fluid collection. A pancreatic pseudocyst is a collection of pancreatic enzymes and fluid enclosed by a fibrous wall lacking an epithelial lining. The fibrous wall usually takes about 4–6 weeks to mature.
Acute necrotic collection: Non-encapsulated collection containing heterogeneous material.	**Walled-off necrosis**: Encapsulated heterogeneous, non-liquified collection with thick walls.

<4周	>4周
急性胰周积液：非包裹性积液	**假性囊肿**：包裹性积液。胰腺假性囊肿是胰酶和液体被包裹在无上皮衬里的纤维壁内。纤维壁通常需要4~6周才能成熟。
急性坏死性积液：非包裹性液体，内含非均质物质。	**包裹性坏死**：被厚壁包裹的非均质、非液性物质。

- Any of the above collections may be sterile or infected. The presence of gas suggests infection, but the absence of gas does not exclude infection.
- Extra-pancreatic complications:

  Perihilar renal inflammation, which may lead to venous compression or thrombosis.

  Bowel involvement, may see ileus or even a fistula, often to the transverse colon or duodenum.
- Secondary inflammation of adjacent vessels can cause vascular complications:

  Pseudoaneurysm, due to erosion, most commonly of the splenic artery or gastroduodenal artery and may result in hemorrhage.

  Venous thrombosis, most commonly splenic vein thrombosis, which may lead to portal hypertension.

- 以上任何一种积液都可能是无菌性的或感染性的。出现气体提示感染，但是没有气体不能排除感染。
- 胰腺外并发症：

  肾门周围炎症可能导致静脉受压或血栓形成。

  肠道受累，可见肠梗阻甚至瘘管，常发生于横结肠或十二指肠。
- 邻近血管的继发性炎症可引起血管并发症：

  假性动脉瘤，由侵蚀所致，最常见于脾动脉或胃十二指肠动脉，并可导致出血。

  静脉血栓形成，脾静脉血栓最常见，可能会导致门静脉高压。

Chronic pancreatitis

慢性胰腺炎

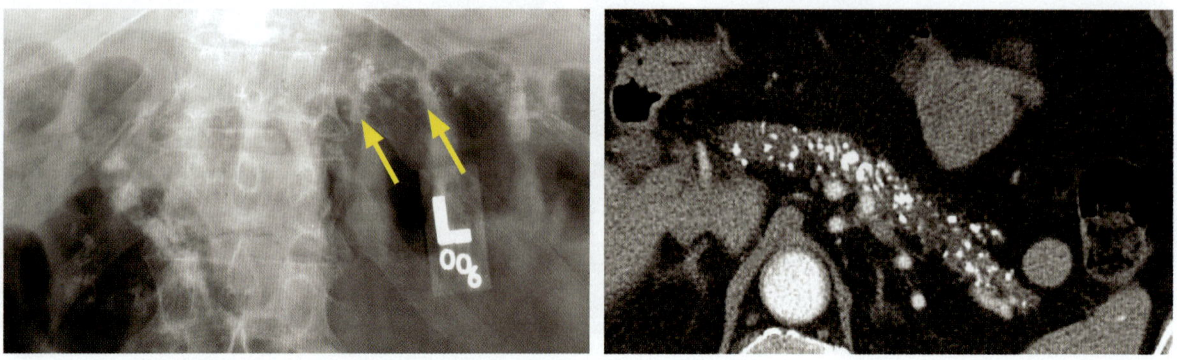

Abdominal radiograph (left image) and contrast-enhanced axial CT (right image) show numerous coarse calcifications in the pancreas (arrows).

腹部X线影像(左图)和轴位增强CT(右图)显示胰腺内大量粗大的钙化灶(黄箭)。

- Chronic pancreatitis, most commonly from long-term alcohol abuse, causes irreversible pancreatic damage. A much less common cause of chronic pancreatitis is pancreas divisum.
- The classic appearance of chronic pancreatitis is an atrophied gland, with diffuse calcifications and a dilated and beaded distal pancreatic duct.

  Calcifications in the distribution of the pancreatic duct are pathognomonic for chronic pancreatitis.

  Splenic artery calcifications are commonly seen in this region and can be mistaken for pancreatic calcifications; check to see if they follow the course of a vessel.

- 慢性胰腺炎最常见的原因是长期酗酒，导致不可逆的胰腺损伤；较为少见的原因是胰腺分裂。
- 慢性胰腺炎的典型表现是腺体萎缩伴弥漫性钙化，远端胰管扩张且呈串珠状。

  钙化灶沿胰管分布可以确诊慢性胰腺炎。

  脾动脉钙化常见于此区域，有可能被误诊为胰腺钙化；需观察它们是否沿血管分布。

Groove pancreatitis

- Groove pancreatitis is an uncommon form of focal pancreatitis located in the groove between the head of the pancreas, duodenum, and common bile duct. Groove pancreatitis usually affects young men who are heavy drinkers. The main differential consideration is adenocarcinoma of the head of the pancreas.

沟槽状胰腺炎

- 沟槽状胰腺炎是一种不常见的局灶性胰腺炎，位于胰头、十二指肠和胆总管之间的沟槽。沟槽状胰腺炎常发生于大量饮酒的年轻男性。主要的鉴别诊断是胰头的腺癌。

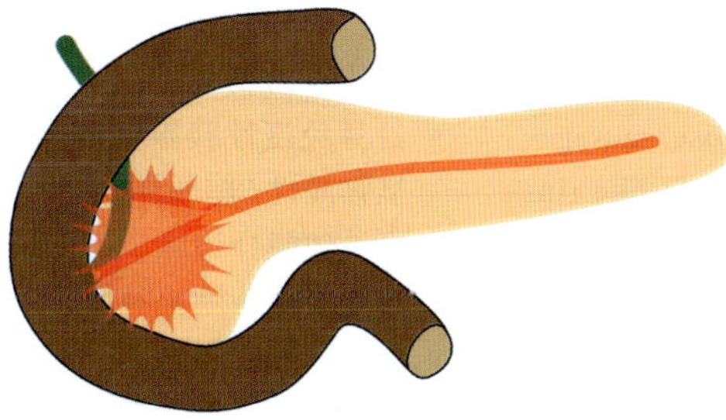

Illustration demonstrates inflammation within the groove between the head of the pancreas, duodenum, and common bile duct.
示意图显示位于胰头、十二指肠和胆总管之间沟槽内的炎症。

- The histopathologic hallmark is fibrosis in the pancreaticoduodenal groove. Chronic inflammation of the duodenum can cause duodenal stenosis or cystic change of the duodenal wall. Duodenal thickening and cystic change are often apparent on imaging with cystic change best appreciated on MRI.

- 组织病理学上的标志性改变是胰十二指肠沟槽处纤维化。十二指肠慢性炎症可引起不同程度的十二指肠狭窄或十二指肠壁囊性变。十二指肠壁增厚及囊性变在影像学检查通常较为明显，而MRI对囊性变显示最佳。

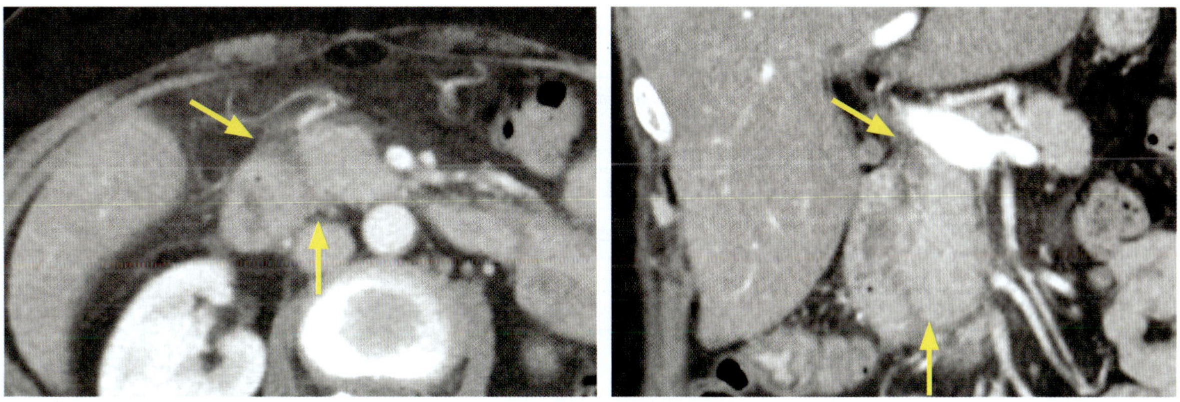

Groove pancreatitis: Axial (left image) and coronal (right image) contrast-enhanced CT shows fat stranding in the pancreaticoduodenal groove (arrows) between the second portion of the duodenum and pancreatic head.
沟槽胰腺炎：轴位(左图)和冠状位(右图)增强CT显示在十二指肠降段与胰头之间的胰十二指肠沟(黄箭)内的脂肪条索密度影。

Autoimmune pancreatitis

自身免疫性胰腺炎

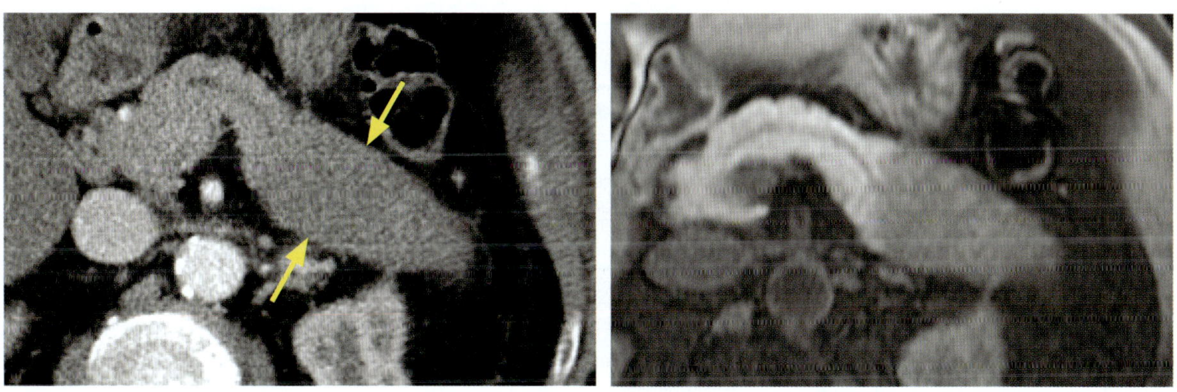

Segmental autoimmune pancreatitis: Contrast-enhanced axial CT (left image) shows a segmental region of low attenuation enlargement of the pancreatic tail and body (arrows), with loss of the normal ductal architecture.
T1-weighted unenhanced MRI (right image) shows a corresponding segmental loss of the normal T1- hyperintense pancreatic signal, with effacement of the pancreatic duct in the affected body and tail.
The differential diagnosis for this appearance would include pancreatic lymphoma, less likely pancreatic adenocarcinoma as there is no ductal dilation.
Case courtesy Cheryl Sadow, MD, Brigham and Women's Hospital.
节段性自身免疫性胰腺炎：轴位增强CT(左图)显示胰腺尾部和体部增大并呈节段性低密度影(黄箭)，正常胰管结构消失。
平扫T_1加权MRI(右图)显示相应节段内正常胰腺的T_1加权高信号缺失，伴有体尾部胰管消失。
这种表现的鉴别诊断应包括胰腺淋巴瘤，胰腺癌可能性较小(因节段性自身免疫性胰腺炎不伴有胰管扩张)。

- Autoimmune pancreatitis is the pancreatic manifestation of *IgG4*-related sclerosing disease.
- The typical imaging appearance of autoimmune pancreatitis is diffuse, sausage-like enlargement of the pancreas with loss of lobulation. A capsule-like rim may be seen. The appearance can also be focal or multifocal, which may mimic a pancreatic mass.
- Treatment is with steroids, which can lead to a complete resolution.

Immunotherapy-related changes

- Immunotherapy can lead to episodes of pancreatitis (which may be clinically occult) and can result in pancreatic atrophy.

- 自身免疫性胰腺炎是IgG4相关的硬化性疾病在胰腺的表现。
- 自身免疫性胰腺炎的典型影像学表现是胰腺呈弥漫性“腊肠样”增大，以及小叶结构消失。可见包膜样边缘。病变可呈局灶性或多灶性，可能类似于胰腺肿块。
- 治疗采用类固醇，可完全治愈。

免疫治疗相关的改变

- 免疫治疗可引起胰腺炎发作(可能是临床隐匿性的)而导致胰腺萎缩。

OVERVIEW OF PANCREATIC NEOPLASMS

胰腺肿瘤概述

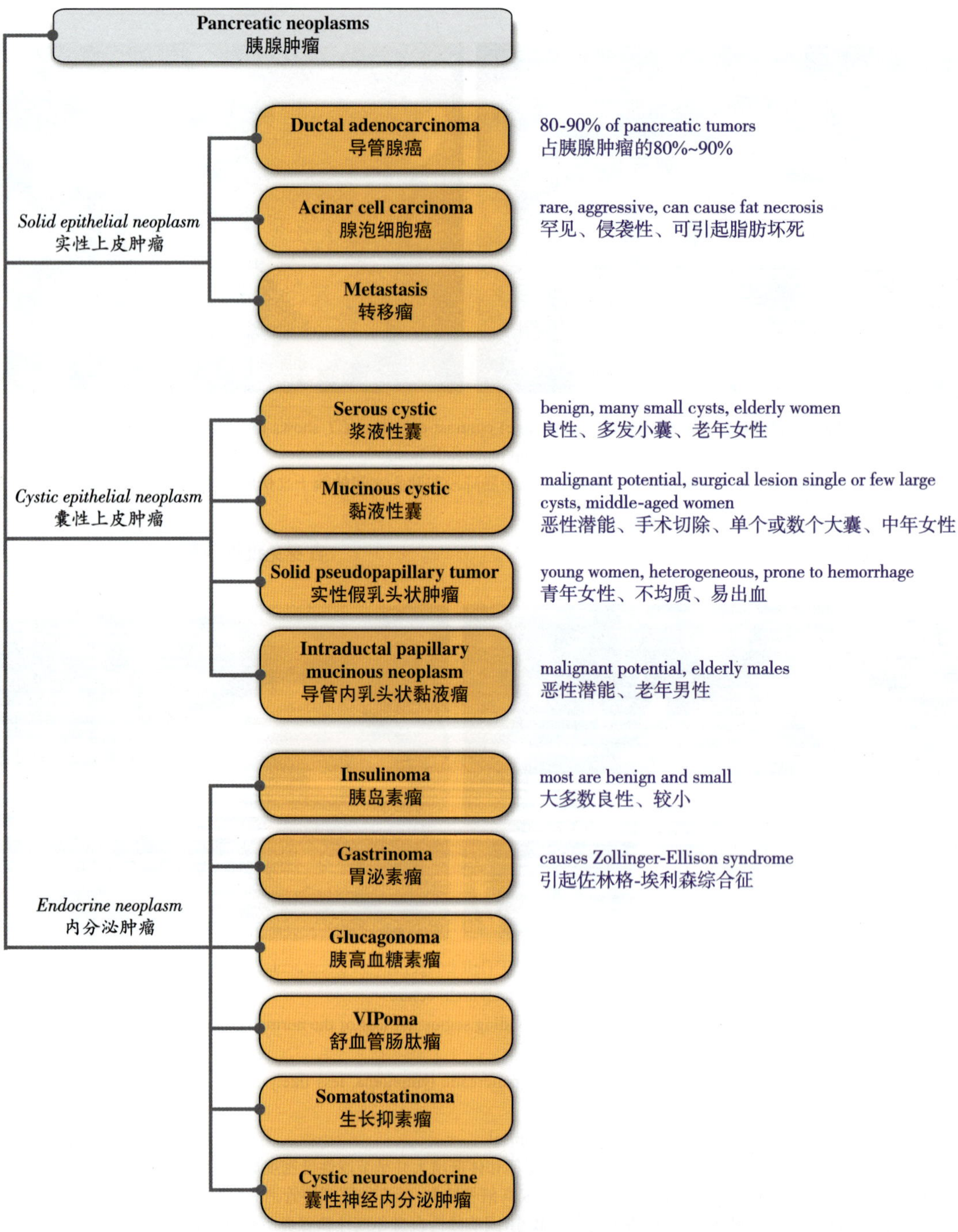

Adenocarcinoma (ductal adenocarcinoma)

腺癌(导管腺癌)

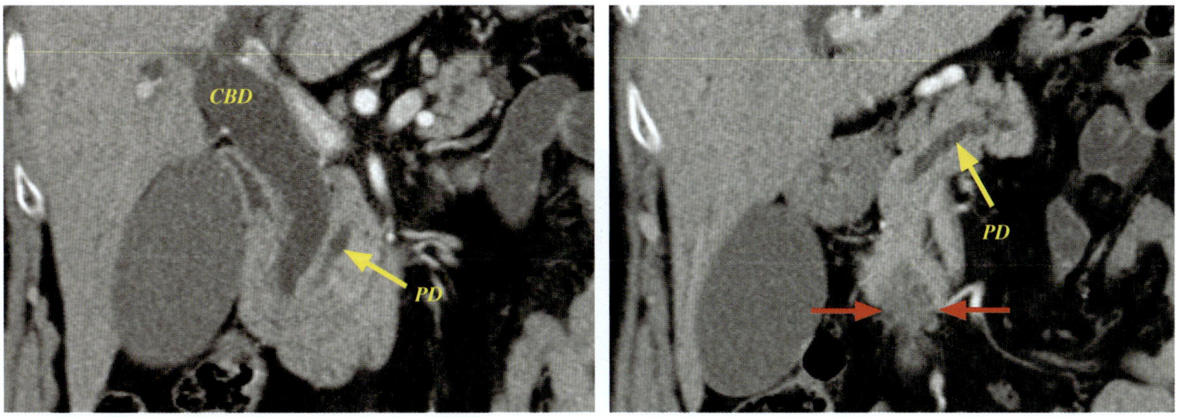

Pancreatic adenocarcinoma of the head causing the *double duct sign*: Two coronal images from a contrast-enhanced CT show marked dilation of the common bile duct (CBD), moderate dilation of the pancreatic duct (PD), and the obstructing, ill-defined hypoattenuating mass in the pancreatic head (red arrows).

胰头腺癌所致的双管征：两幅冠状位增强CT显示显著扩张的胆总管(CBD)、中度扩张的胰管(PD)，以及胰头部边界不清的低密度肿块(红箭)。

- Pancreatic ductal adenocarcinoma accounts for 80–90% of all pancreatic tumors. It is typically seen in patients over age 60, with a slight male predominance. Risk factors include smoking, alcohol use, chronic pancreatitis, and family history of pancreatic adenocarcinoma.
- A pancreatic mass protocol CT includes early arterial phase, late arterial phase (pancreatic phase), and portal venous phase images. The late arterial phase (pancreatic parenchymal phase) has the greatest conspicuity for detecting the hypoenhancing tumor against the background enhancing pancreas.
- The most common location for a tumor to arise is the pancreatic head where it often causes ductal obstruction. Pancreatic adenocarcinoma is usually hypoenhancing relative to pancreatic parenchyma and results in upstream (towards the tail) ductal dilatation and parenchymal atrophy. The *double duct sign* describes dilation of both the pancreatic duct and the CBD due to obstruction by the pancreatic head mass.
- Since pancreatic adenocarcinoma is almost always associated with a dilated pancreatic duct, an alternative diagnosis should be strongly considered if there is a pancreatic mass with no ductal dilation, such as:

Autoimmune pancreatitis. Groove pancreatitis. Cystic pancreatic tumor. Neuroendocrine tumor.	Duodenal gastrointestinal stromal tumor (GIST). Peripancreatic lymph node. Pancreatic metastasis (e.g., renal cell, thyroid, or melanoma). Lymphoma.

- Conversely, if a dilated pancreatic duct or *double duct sign* is present but no mass is visible, one should still be suspicious for pancreatic adenocarcinoma. Approximately 10% of lesions will be isoattenuating relative to pancreas and/or difficult to visualize on a portal venous phase CT and thus extremely difficult to detect.
- When evaluating whether a pancreatic neoplasm is resectable, it is important to evaluate for any vascular variants and to determine tumor involvement of the nearby vessels. SMA (including first jejunal branch), SMV, portal vein, celiac

- 胰腺导管腺癌占所有胰腺肿瘤的80%~90%。主要见于60岁以上的患者，男性稍多见。危险因素包括吸烟、饮酒、慢性胰腺炎和胰腺腺癌家族史。
- 胰腺肿瘤的CT扫描方案包括动脉早期、动脉晚期(胰腺实质期)和门静脉期图像。在动脉晚期(胰腺实质期)，低强化的肿瘤病灶在胰腺强化的背景下显示最为明显。
- 肿瘤最常发生的位置是胰头，并常引起胰管梗阻。胰腺癌相对于胰腺实质通常为低强化，引起上游(胰尾方向)胰管扩张和胰腺实质萎缩。双管征是指胰头肿块导致的胰管和胆总管同时扩张。
- 由于胰腺腺癌几乎均伴有胰管扩张，因此，如果存在胰腺肿块而不伴有胰管扩张，需要重点考虑其他诊断，例如：

自身免疫性胰腺炎。 沟槽状胰腺炎。 囊性胰腺肿瘤。 神经内分泌肿瘤。	十二指肠胃肠道间质瘤(GIST)。 胰腺周围淋巴结。 胰腺转移瘤(如肾细胞癌、甲状腺癌或黑色素瘤)。 淋巴瘤。

- 相反，如果只有胰管扩张或双管征阳性却未见肿块，仍需怀疑胰腺腺癌。约10%的病变与胰腺实质呈等密度，和/或难以在增强CT门静脉期显示，因此肿瘤检测极其困难。
- 在判断胰腺肿瘤是否可以切除时，评估血管变异和肿瘤对邻近血管的侵犯非常重要：肠系膜上动脉(包括第一空肠分支)、肠系膜上静脉、门静脉、腹腔干、肝总动脉和脾动脉。

axis, common hepatic artery, and splenic artery.

Abutment: <180° circumferential contact with vessel.

Encasement: >180° circumferential contact and/or deformation of the vessel.

- Limited extension to the duodenum, distal stomach, or CBD does not preclude resection, as these structures are resected during a Whipple procedure.

毗邻：肿瘤与血管接触面<180°周长。

包绕：肿瘤与血管接触面>180°周长和/或血管变形。

- 当侵犯仅限于十二指肠、胃远端或胆总管时并不排除手术切除，因为这些结构在行胰十二指肠切除术时会被切除。

Acinar cell carcinoma

腺泡细胞癌

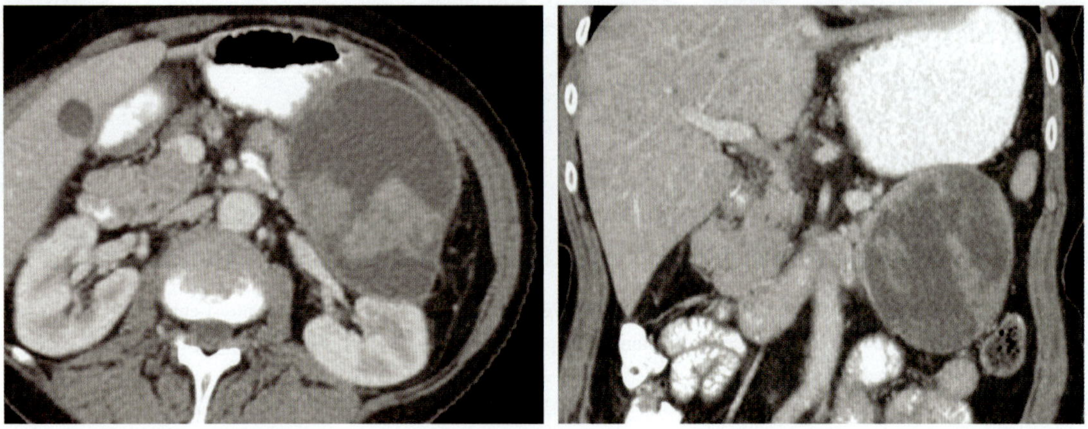

Acinar cell carcinoma: Axial (left image) and coronal (right image) contrast-enhanced CT shows a large pancreatic tail mass with mixed soft tissue and fluid attenuation and surrounding fat stranding. The mass effaces and possibly invades the greater curvature of the stomach and left kidney.

腺泡细胞癌：轴位(左图)和冠状位(右图)增强CT显示胰尾部一个大的肿块，呈囊实混合密度，并可见周围脂肪条索影。肿块压迫且可能侵犯胃大弯及左肾。

- Acinar cell carcinoma is a rare, aggressive variant of pancreatic adenocarcinoma, exclusively seen in *elderly males*.
- The malignant cells produce a large amount of lipase which leads to the clinical triad of lipase hypersecretion syndrome: subcutaneous fat necrosis, bone infarcts causing polyarthralgias, and eosinophilia.

- 腺泡细胞癌是一种少见的、具侵袭性的胰腺腺癌变异，仅见于*老年男性*。
- 恶性肿瘤细胞产生大量的脂肪酶而引起临床三联征，即脂肪酶高分泌综合征：皮下脂肪坏死、骨梗死引起的多关节痛，以及嗜酸性粒细胞增多症。

Cystic Pancreatic Epithelial Neoplasms

囊性胰腺上皮肿瘤

Solid pseudopapillary tumor (SPT)

实性假乳头状肿瘤(SPT)

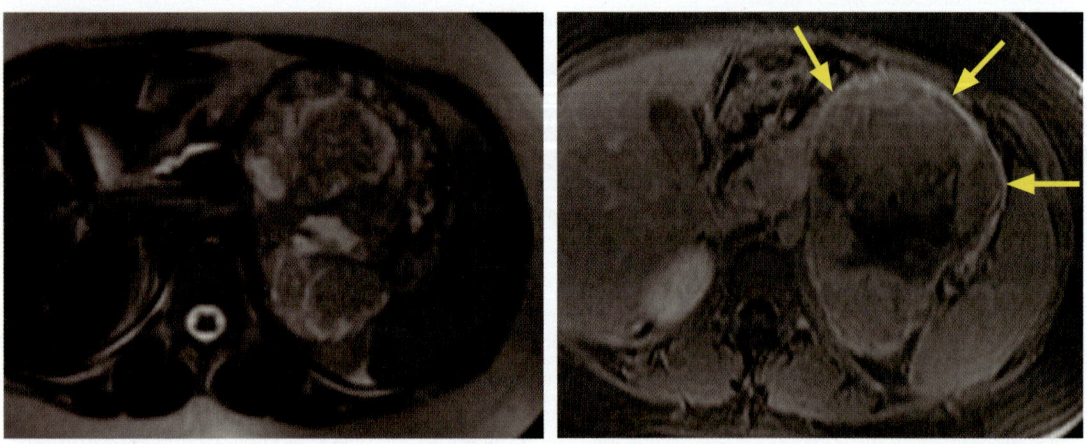

Solid pseudopapillary tumor: Axial T2-weighted (left image) and post-contrast T1-weighted (right image) MRI demonstrates a mixed solid and cystic lesion arising from the tail of the pancreas with heterogeneous internal enhancement and a T2 hypointense, enhancing capsule (arrows).

实性假乳头状肿瘤：轴位T_2加权(左图)和增强T_1加权(右图)MRI显示胰尾部一个囊实混杂性肿块，内部强化不均匀，以及呈T_2低信号的强化包膜(黄箭)。

- Solid pseudopapillary tumor (SPT), formerly known as solid and papillary epithelial neoplasm (SPEN), occurs in young women and children and is nicknamed the *daughter* tumor. It may rarely cause abdominal pain but is often asymptomatic. It is more often located in the tail.
- It has a low malignant potential and is typically resected.
- On imaging, SPT appears as a large mass with heterogeneous solid and cystic areas. Hemorrhage is typical. SPT features a capsule, the only other pancreatic tumor with a capsule is mucinous cystic neoplasm (MCN) (below).

- 实性假乳头状肿瘤(SPT),曾称实性乳头状上皮肿瘤(SPEN),发生于年轻女性和儿童,也称女儿瘤。它偶尔可以引起腹痛,但通常无症状。病变常位于胰腺尾部。
- 具有低度恶变潜能,通常进行手术切除。
- 在影像上,SPT表现为一个大的肿块伴不均匀实性及囊性区域。常有出血。SPT以包膜为特征,其他具有包膜的胰腺肿瘤只有黏液性囊性肿瘤(MCN)(见下文)。

Mucinous cystic neoplasm (MCN)

黏液性囊性肿瘤

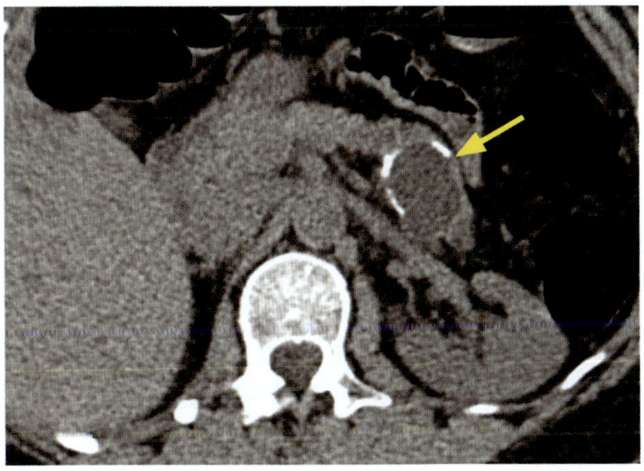

Mucinous cystic neoplasm: Axial unenhanced CT shows a cystic, peripherally calcified mass in the tail of the pancreas (arrow). Pathology at resection showed borderline malignancy.

Case courtesy Cheryl Sadow, MD, Brigham and Women's Hospital.

黏液性囊性肿瘤:轴位平扫CT显示胰尾部一个囊性的、边缘钙化的肿块(黄箭),术后病理为临界恶性肿瘤。

- Mucinous cystic neoplasm affects middle-aged women and has therefore been nicknamed the *mother* tumor.
- It is benign but does have malignant potential, so treatment is typically resection.
- The tumor consists of a single or a few large cysts (<6 cysts that are >2 cm) and typically occurs in the pancreatic body and tail.
- MCN has a capsule. When calcifications are seen, they tend to be peripheral.

- 黏液性囊性肿瘤发生于中年女性,因此也称妈妈瘤。
- 该瘤虽为良性,但具有恶性潜能,治疗通常为手术切除。
- 肿瘤由单个或数个大的囊肿(<6个,>2cm的囊肿)组成,通常发生于胰腺体部或尾部。
- 黏液性囊性肿瘤有包膜,钙化通常位于外周。

Serous cystadenoma

浆液性囊腺瘤

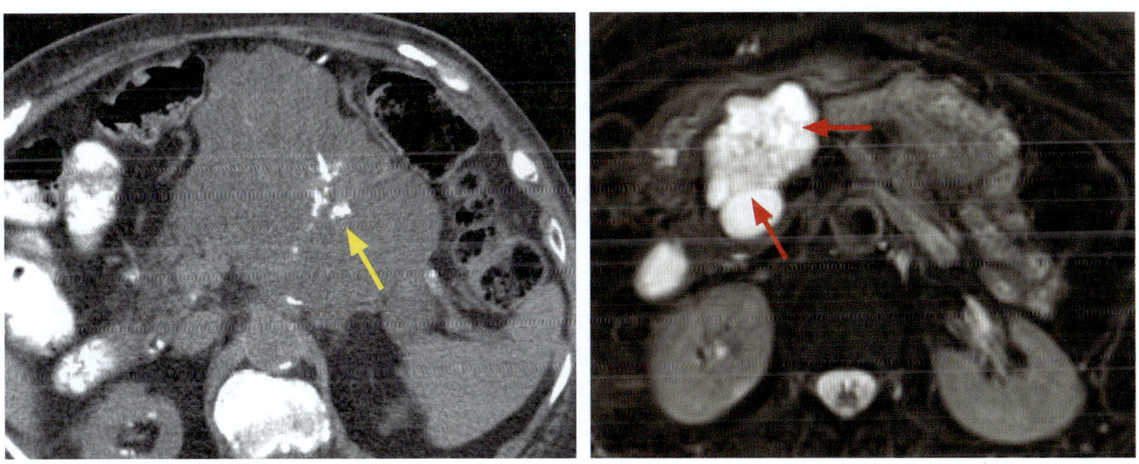

Serous cystadenoma in two different patients:

Axial oral-contrast-only CT (left image) shows a large multicystic pancreatic mass containing central stellate calcification (yellow arrow). Axial T2-weighted MRI (right image) shows a T2 hyperintensity multicystic mass in the pancreatic head with innumerable thin internal septations (red arrows).

Left case courtesy Cheryl Sadow, MD, Brigham and Women's Hospital.

两名不同患者的浆液性囊腺瘤:

口服造影剂后轴位CT(左图)显示一个大的多囊性胰腺肿块,内见中心放射状钙化灶(黄箭)。轴位T_2加权MRI(右图)显示胰头部一个T_2高信号的多囊性肿块,内见大量纤细的间隔(红箭)。

- Serous cystadenoma is a benign tumor that occurs in elderly women and has been nicknamed the *grandmother* tumor.
- Serous cystadenoma consists of many small cysts (>6 cysts that are <2 cm) that can appear as a *"bunch of grapes"* or may have a solid appearance on CT due to apposition of many cyst walls. MRI is useful to show the cystic nature of the lesion.
- Classic imaging feature is a central enhancing scar with stellate calcification.

Comparison of solid pseudopapillary tumor, mucinous cystic neoplasm, and serous cystadenoma

Tumor	Age	Mnemonic	Features
Solid pseudopapillary tumor (SPT)	Daughter	"SPry, goes to spin class"	+ capsule cystic and solid
Mucinous cystic neoplasm (MCN)	Mother	"Motherly"	+ capsule cystic
Serous cystadenoma	Grandmother	"SEnile"	SEntral (central) enhancing scar with stellate calcification; *"bunch of grapes"*

Intraductal papillary mucinous neoplasm (IPMN)

- Intraductal papillary mucinous neoplasm (IPMN) occurs most commonly in elderly males and is nicknamed the *grandfather* tumor, although these tumors exhibit the greatest age and sex variability of the cystic pancreatic neoplasms.
- IPMNs are considered premalignant neoplasms and also increase the risk of developing a primary pancreatic adenocarcinoma, so these lesions are followed to ensure stability.
- IPMNs may arise from the main pancreatic duct (MPD) or a side branch. The main duct and mixed-type IPMNs have greater malignant potential.

- 浆液性囊性腺瘤是一种发生在老年女性的良性肿瘤，也称奶奶瘤。
- 肿瘤由许多小的囊肿（>6个，<2cm的囊肿）构成，CT可表现为"葡萄串"样或由于许多囊肿壁相互紧贴形成的类似实性的肿块。MRI对显示病灶的囊性特征有帮助。
- 典型影像学特征是中心强化的瘢痕伴放射状钙化。

实性假乳头状肿瘤、黏液性囊性肿瘤、浆液性囊腺瘤的区别

肿瘤	年龄	记忆诀窍	特征
实性假乳头状肿瘤(SPT)	女儿	"Spry, goes to spin clas"	有包膜，囊性和实性
黏液性囊性肿瘤(MCN)	妈妈	"Motherly"	有包膜，囊性
浆液性囊性腺瘤	奶奶	"Senile"	中心强化瘢痕伴放射状钙化，"葡萄串"

导管内乳头状黏液瘤(IPMN)

- 导管内乳头状黏液瘤(IPMN)最常发生于老年男性，因此也称爷爷瘤，但这些肿瘤中，囊性胰腺肿瘤发病年龄和性别上表现出极大的差异。
- IPMN被认为是癌前病变，也会增加罹患原发性胰腺癌的风险，因此对这些病变需进行随访以确保其稳定性。
- IPMN可能起源于主胰管(MPD)或胰管的分支。主胰管型和混合型IPMN具有较大的恶性潜能。

	Main duct IPMN	Branch duct IPMN	Mixed type
Definition	Segmental or diffuse dilatation of MPD >5 mm	Cysts >5 mm communicating with the MPD	Meets criteria for both main duct and branch duct type
Illustration	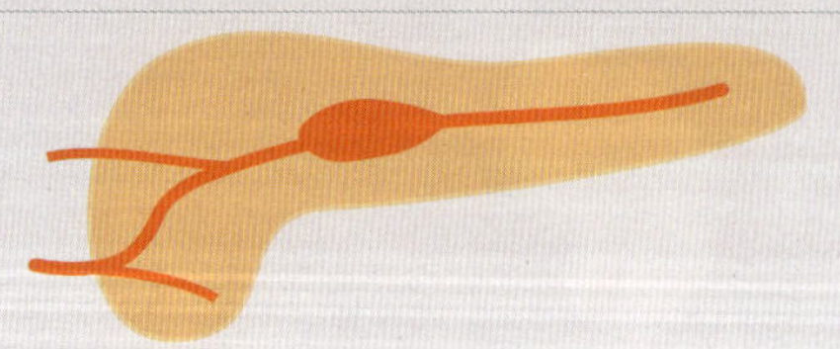	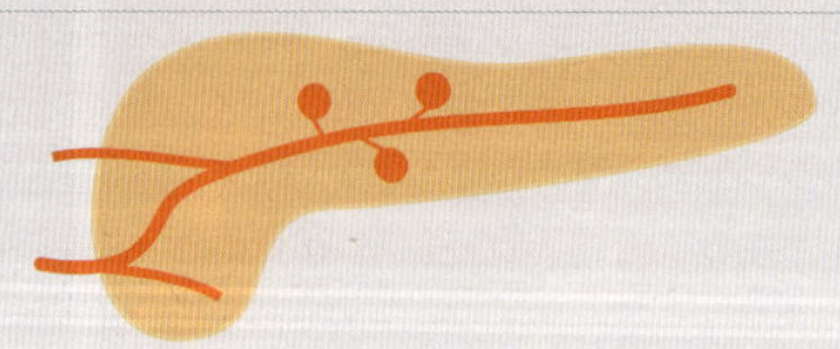	

	主胰管型IPMN	分支胰管型IPMN	混合型
定义	节段性或弥漫性主胰管扩张>5mm	囊性灶>5mm并与主胰管相通	符合主胰管型和分支胰管型IPMN标准
示意图	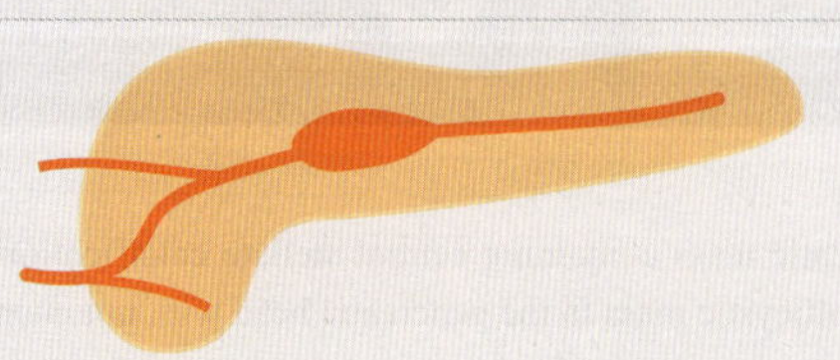	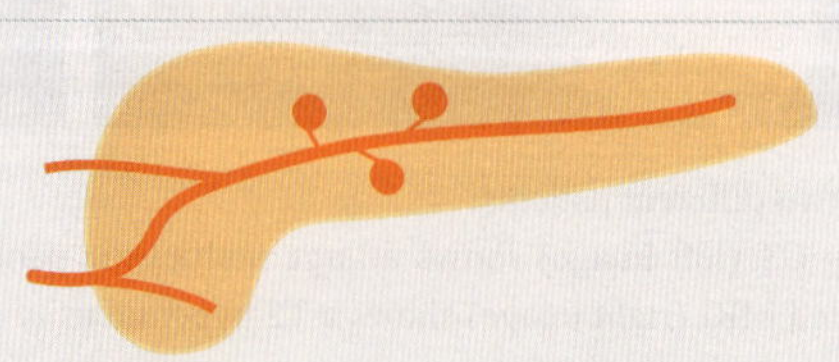	

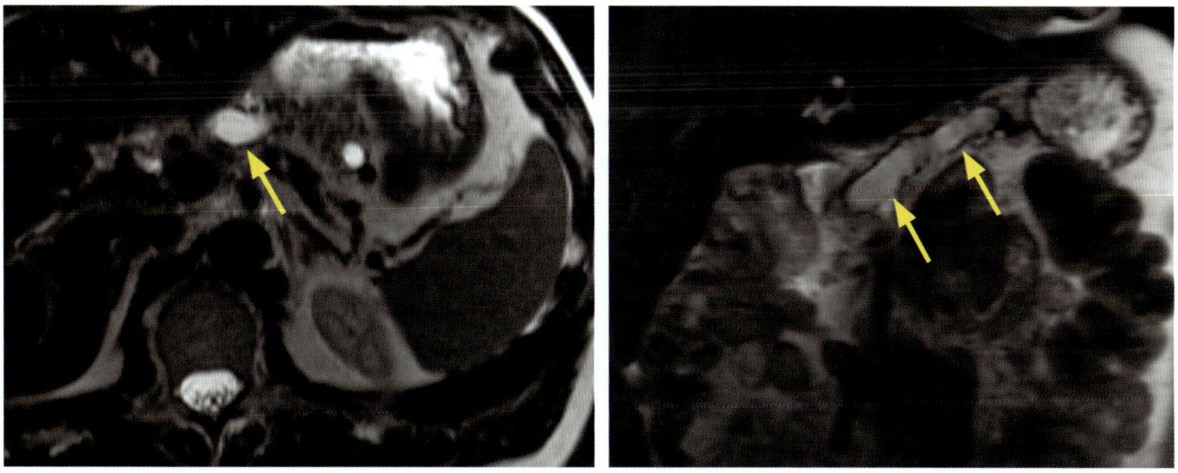

Main duct IPMN: Axial (left image) and coronal (right image) T2-weighted MRI in a patient with history of chronic pancreatitis shows pancreatic atrophy and main duct dilation (arrows). This was found on pathology to be a main duct IPMN.

主胰管型IPMN：轴位(左图)和冠状位(右图)T_2加权MRI显示一个慢性胰腺炎患者胰腺萎缩，主胰管扩张(黄箭)。病理显示为主胰管型IPMN。

- The Fukuoka consensus guidelines (2017) for IPMNs and MCNs recommend imaging with CT or MRI for cysts greater than 5 mm. Further evaluation with either endoscopic ultrasound (EUS) or resection is recommended based on the following imaging features:

- Fukuoka共识指南(2017)建议，若IPMN和MCN的囊肿大于5mm，需进行CT或MRI检查。如果发现以下影像学特征，建议行超声内镜(EUS)进一步评估或手术切除：

Worrisome features (should be evaluated by EUS)
- Cyst ≥3 cm
- Enhancing mural nodule <5 mm
- Thickened enhanced cyst walls
- MPD 5–9 mm
- Abrupt change in the MPD caliber with distal parenchymal atrophy
- Lymphadenopathy
- Elevated CA 19-9
- Rapid rate of cyst growth >5 mm over two years

High-risk stigmata (should undergo resection without further testing)
- Obstructive jaundice
- Enhancing mural nodule ≥5 mm
- MPD ≥10 mm

可疑表现(推荐行EUS进一步评估)
- 囊肿≥3cm
- 强化壁结节<5mm
- 囊肿壁增厚强化
- MPD 5~9mm
- MPD管径突然变化伴远端胰腺实质萎缩
- 淋巴结肿大
- CA19-9升高
- 囊肿快速生长，2年内增长>5mm

高危表现(应该进行手术切除，无须行其他检查)
- 梗阻性黄疸
- 强化壁结节≥5mm
- MPD≥10mm

Pancreatic endocrine neoplasms

胰腺内分泌肿瘤

Overview

- Pancreatic neuroendocrine tumors may be hyperfunctioning or non-hyperfunctioning.
- Hyperfunctioning tumors come to clinical attention due to symptoms of endocrine excess.
- Non-hyperfunctioning tumors tend to be larger at diagnosis. These tumors may undergo cystic change and should be considered in the differential of a cystic pancreatic neoplasm. There is often central necrosis and calcification in these large tumors as well.
- Pancreatic endocrine tumors tend to be hypervascular and are best seen in the late arterial phase. Most are solid unless very large in size. A hypervascular liver mass with an associated pancreatic mass is most likely a metastatic lesion

概述

- 胰腺内分泌肿瘤分为有功能性肿瘤和无功能性肿瘤
- 有功能性肿瘤由于内分泌过度所引发的症状而引起临床注意。
- 无功能性肿瘤在确诊时往往体积已经较大。这些肿瘤可以发生囊变，因而在诊断胰腺囊性肿瘤时应将其列入鉴别诊断。这些较大的肿瘤常出现中央坏死和钙化。
- 胰腺内分泌肿瘤通常是富血供的，并在动脉晚期显示最佳。大部分是实性的，除非体积很大。一个富血供的肝脏肿瘤同时伴有胰腺肿块很

from a pancreatic endocrine neoplasm.

Insulinoma

- Insulinoma is the most common pancreatic endocrine tumor. Due to symptoms of hypoglycemia, insulinomas tend to present early and have the best prognosis of all neuroendocrine tumors with only 10% demonstrating malignant behavior.
- The *Whipple triad* describes the clinical symptoms of insulinoma: Hypoglycemia, clinical symptoms of hypoglycemia, and alleviation of symptoms after administration of glucose.

Gastrinoma

- Gastrinoma is the second most common pancreatic endocrine tumor. Liver metastases are present at the time of diagnosis in 60% of patients.
- **Zollinger-Ellison syndrome** is a clinical syndrome that occurs secondary to a gastrinoma. Hypersecretion of gastrin leads to gastritis, diarrhea, peptic ulcer disease and even gastroesophageal reflux disease.
- Gastrinoma is associated with **multiple endocrine neoplasia (MEN) type 1** and in this case tends to be multiple and located in the duodenum rather than the pancreas.
- The **gastrinoma triangle** describes the typical location of gastrinomas in an area bounded by the junction of the cystic duct and CBD, the duodenum inferiorly, and the neck/body of the pancreas medially.
- High gastrin levels can lead to formation of carcinoid tumors in the stomach, which may regress after the gastrinoma is resected.

有可能是来自胰腺内分泌肿瘤的转移病灶。

胰岛素瘤

- 胰岛素瘤是最常见的胰腺内分泌肿瘤。由于低血糖症状，胰岛素瘤往往在早期就能被发现，并在所有的内分泌肿瘤中预后最好，仅有10%表现为恶性。
- 惠普尔三联征是指胰岛素瘤的临床症状：低血糖、低血糖所致的临床症状，以及给予葡萄糖后的症状缓解。

胃泌素瘤

- 胃泌素瘤是第二常见的胰腺内分泌肿瘤。在确诊时，60%的患者已经有肝转移。
- **佐林格-埃利森综合征**是继发于胃泌素瘤的一种临床综合征。胃泌素过度分泌会导致胃炎、腹泻、消化道溃疡，甚至胃食管反流病。
- 胃泌素瘤与**多发性内分泌瘤病(MEN)1型**有关，当出现这种情况时，胃泌素瘤往往为多发且位于十二指肠，而非胰腺。
- **胃泌素瘤三角**是指胃泌素瘤的典型发生部位，其外侧边界为胆囊管和胆总管、下方为十二指肠，内侧为胰的颈部/体部。
- 高胃泌素水平可能导致在胃发生类癌，在胃泌素瘤切除后类癌可消失。

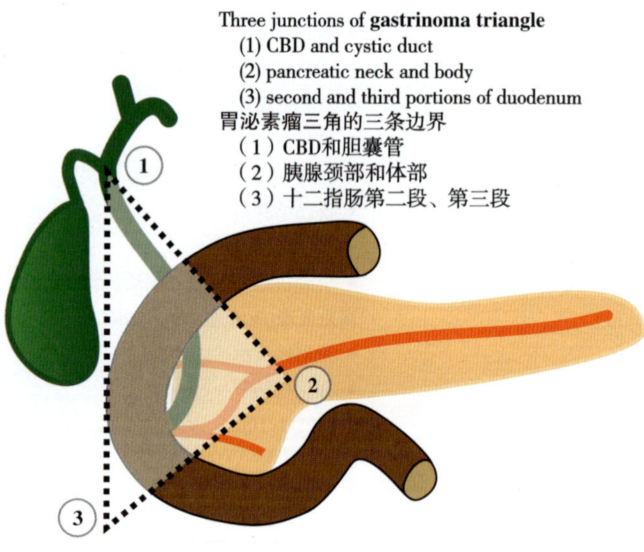

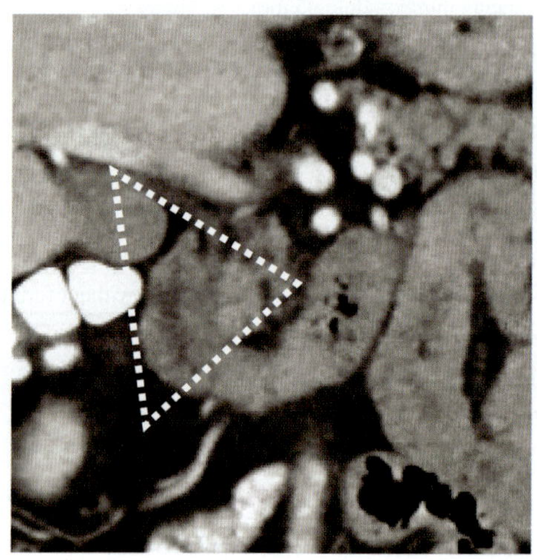

Other pancreatic endocrine tumors

- **Glucagonoma** is the third most common pancreatic endocrine tumor. Patients may present with migratory rash, diabetes, and glossitis. They have a high rate of malignant behavior (~80%) and 50–60% have liver metastases at diagnosis. Prognosis is poor.
- **VIPoma** (Vasoactive Intestinal Peptide) is a rare pancreatic endocrine tumor. Patients may present with profuse watery diarrhea and hypokalemia. Most are malignant and 60–80% have liver metastases at diagnosis.
- **Somatostatinoma** is very rare. Patients may present with abdominal pain, diarrhea and impaired glucose tolerance. 50–75% of patients have liver or lymph node metastases at diagnosis.

其他胰腺内分泌肿瘤

- **胰高血糖素瘤**是第三常见的胰腺内分泌肿瘤。患者可表现为迁徙性皮疹、糖尿病和舌炎。该肿瘤的恶性行为发生率很高(约80%)，50%~60%确诊时已有肝转移。预后很差。
- 舒血管肠肽瘤(**VIPoma**)是一种少见的胰腺内分泌肿瘤。患者可出现大量水样腹泻和低血钾。该肿瘤大多数为恶性，60%~80%在确诊时已有肝转移。
- **生长抑素瘤**非常少见。患者可能出现腹痛、腹泻和糖耐量受损。50%~75%确诊时已经出现肝或淋巴结转移。

Systemic diseases that affect the pancreas

Pancreatic lymphoma

- B-cell lymphoma is the most common subtype of lymphoma to affect the pancreas. There is almost always associated adenopathy and multiorgan involvement by the time the pancreas is involved.
- The typical imaging appearance is of a homogeneously, diffusely enlarged gland without ductal dilatation, with associated lymphadenopathy. More aggressive types of lymphoma may show heterogeneity/central necrosis.

von Hippel-Lindau

- von Hippel-Lindau is an inherited multisystemic disease which confers increased risk of multiple malignancies and leads to formation of cysts in various organs including the pancreas.
- Pancreatic neoplasms seen in von Hippel-Lindau include serous cystadenoma and pancreatic neuroendocrine tumors.

Cystic fibrosis (CF)

累及胰腺的系统性疾病

胰腺淋巴瘤

- B细胞淋巴瘤是最常累及胰腺的淋巴瘤亚型。当胰腺受累时，几乎总伴有淋巴结肿大和多器官受累。
- 典型影像学表现为胰腺呈均匀性弥漫性肿大，无胰管扩张，伴有淋巴结肿大。侵袭性淋巴瘤可能表现为不均质/中央性坏死。

希佩尔-林道病(VHL)

- 希佩尔-林道病(VHL)是一种遗传性多系统疾病，此类患者罹患多种恶性肿瘤的风险增高，且会在多器官形成囊肿，包括胰腺。
- 发生于VHL中的胰腺肿瘤包括浆液性囊腺瘤和胰腺神经内分泌肿瘤。

囊性纤维化(CF)

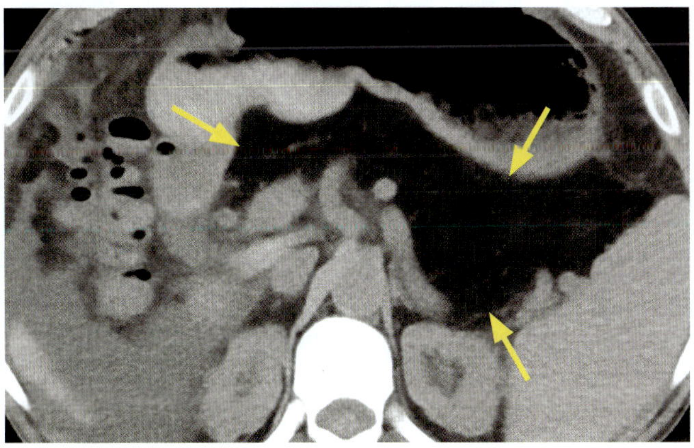

Axial unenhanced CT in a patient with cystic fibrosis shows complete fatty replacement of the pancreas (arrows).
一名囊性纤维化患者的轴位平扫CT显示胰腺(黄箭)完全被脂肪所替代。

- Cystic fibrosis (CF) is the most common cause of childhood pancreatic atrophy.
- CF can cause either fatty atrophy of the pancreas or pancreatic cystosis (diffuse replacement of the pancreas with innumerable cysts).

Schwachman-Diamond

- Schwachman-Diamond is a rare inherited disorder characterized by diffuse fatty replacement of the pancreas, resultant pancreatic exocrine insufficiency, neutropenia, and bone dysplasia.
- Schwachman-Diamond is the second-most common cause of childhood pancreatic atrophy.

Obesity and exogenous steroid use

- Both obesity and steroids can cause fatty atrophy of the pancreas.

- 囊性纤维化(CF)是儿童胰腺萎缩最常见的原因。
- CF可引起胰腺脂肪性萎缩，或引起胰腺囊性化(胰腺被无数囊肿所取代)。

施-戴综合征

- 施-戴综合征是一种少见的遗传性疾病，特点为胰腺广泛被脂肪组织替代，导致胰腺外分泌不足、中性粒细胞减少和骨发育不良。
- 施-戴综合征是儿童胰腺萎缩第二常见的原因。

肥胖和使用外源性类固醇

- 肥胖和类固醇均能引起胰腺脂肪性萎缩。

Miscellaneous Pancreatic Lesions

胰腺其他病变

Intrapancreatic accessory spleen

胰腺内副脾

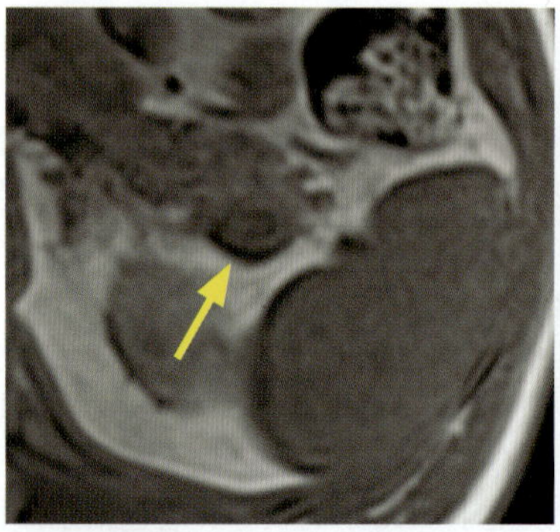

In-phase MRI
同相位MRI

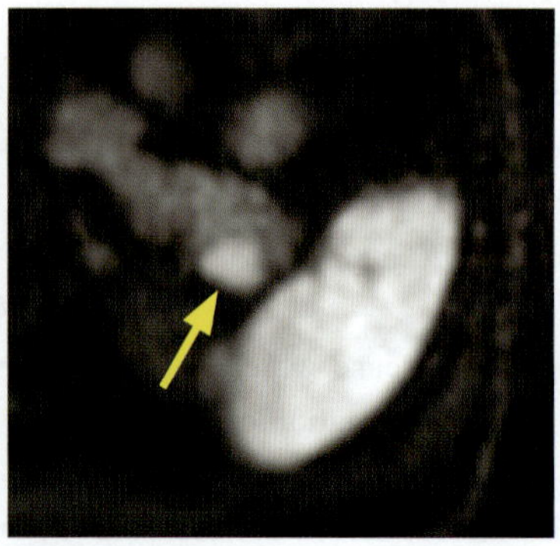

DWI
弥散加权成像(DWI)

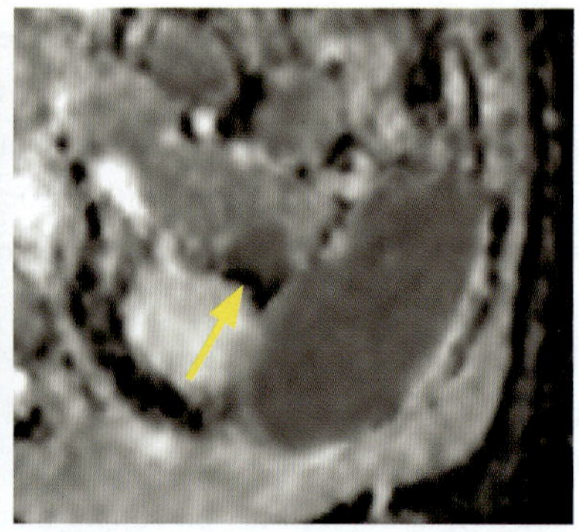

ADC
表观弥散系数成像(ADC)

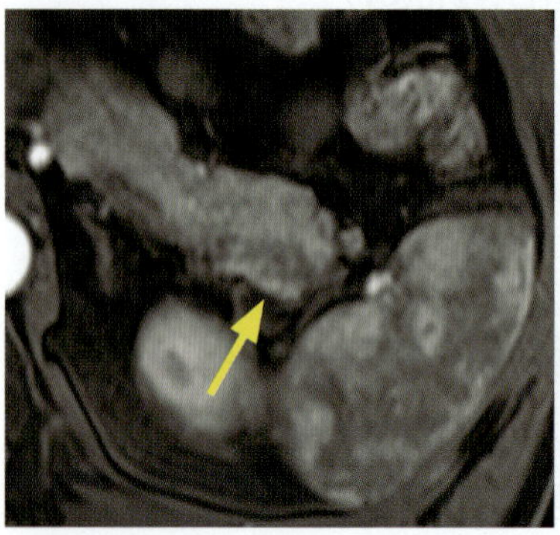

Arterial phase T1-weighted
动脉期T_1加权

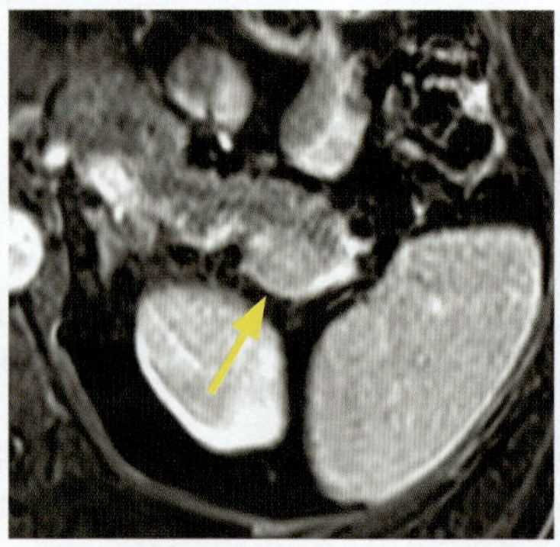

Portal venous phase T1-weighted
门静脉期T_1加权

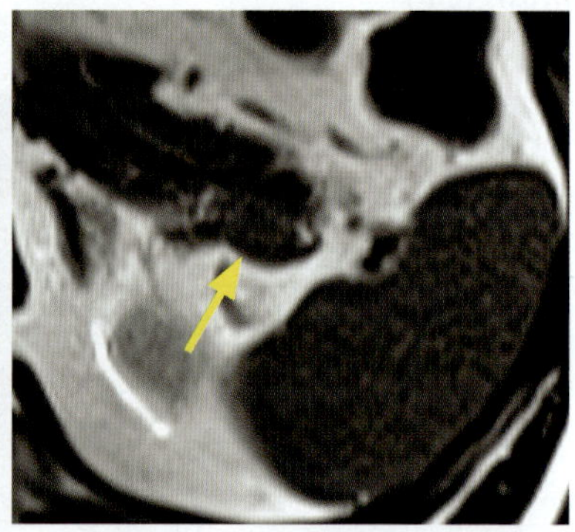

T2-weighted
T_2加权

Axial MRI images show a T1 hypointense, mildly T2 hyperintense mass in the pancreatic tail (arrows) that completely follows splenic signal intensity on all sequences, consistent with intrapancreatic accessory spleen.
轴位MRI显示位于胰尾的一个T_1低信号、T_2稍高信号肿块(黄箭),其所有序列的信号均与脾脏一致,符合胰腺内副脾。

- Intrapancreatic accessory spleen is a benign mimic of a hypervascular pancreatic neoplasm.
- On imaging, an intrapancreatic spleen typically is a small (1–3 cm), well-defined mass usually found in the pancreatic tail. It follows the density, signal intensity, and enhancement of the spleen on all CT and MRI sequences.
- MRI is usually diagnostic. Either technetium-99m sulfur colloid or technetium-99m damaged-RBC scintigraphy can confirm the diagnosis in ambiguous cases.

- 胰腺内副脾是良性病变,其表现类似于一个富血供的胰腺肿瘤。
- 胰腺内副脾在影像学上通常表现为一个小(1~3cm)而边界清晰的团块,常位于胰腺尾部。它在所有CT和MRI序列上的密度、信号强度和强化方式均与脾脏一致。
- MRI通常可以进行诊断。在疑似病例中,^{99m}Tc-硫胶体或^{99m}Tc-红细胞闪烁显像可用于确诊。

Pancreas: Common Imaging Patterns

Hypervascular lesions	Cystic lesions
Neuroendocrine tumor.	Cystic fibrosis.
Metastases (usually renal cell carcinoma).	von Hippel-Lindau.
Intrapancreatic accessory spleen.	Pseudocyst.
Pseudoaneurysm (often seen after pancreatitis).	IPMN.
	SPT, MCN, and serous cystadenoma.

胰腺:常见的影像学表现

富血供病变	囊性病变
神经内分泌肿瘤。	囊性纤维化。
转移瘤(肾细胞癌常见)。	希佩尔-林道病。
胰腺内副脾。	假性囊肿。
假性动脉瘤(常见于胰腺炎后)。	胰腺导管内乳头状黏液瘤。
	实性假乳头状肿瘤、黏液性囊性肿瘤和浆液性囊腺瘤。

Diffuse enlargement

Diffuse enlargement
Acute pancreatitis. IgG4-mediated autoimmune pancreatitis. Immunotherapy-related changes. Lymphoma.

Atrophy

Atrophy
Age-related. Immunotherapy-related changes. Chronic pancreatitis. Metabolic syndrome.

Fatty infiltration

Fatty infiltration
Cystic fibrosis. Exogenous steroids. Obesity. Schwachman-Diamond syndrome.

弥漫性增大

弥漫性增大
急性胰腺炎。 IgG4相关自身免疫性胰腺炎。 免疫治疗相关改变。 淋巴瘤。

萎缩

萎缩
年龄相关改变。 免疫治疗相关改变。 慢性胰腺炎。 代谢综合征。

脂肪浸润

脂肪浸润
囊性纤维化。 外源性类固醇。 肥胖。 施-戴综合征。

（翻译　聂芳）

SPLEEN

CONGENITAL SPLENIC VARIATIONS AND ANOMALIES

Splenule (accessory spleen)

- Also called an accessory spleen, a splenule is a focus of normal splenic tissue separate from the main body of the spleen due to embryologic failure of fusion of the splenic anlage. The most common location is the splenic hilum.
- Although usually an incidental finding, the presence of a splenule does have significance in certain clinical settings. For instance, splenectomy for consumptive thrombocytopenia may not be curative if there is sufficient unresected accessory splenic tissue present. A splenule may be mistaken for a lymph node or mass when in an unusual location. As previously discussed, an intrapancreatic splenule may be mistaken for a hypervascular pancreatic mass.
- A splenule should follow splenic tissue on all MRI sequences. If in doubt, a Tc-99m sulfur colloid scan or a heat-damaged Tc-99m RBC scan can be confirmatory.

Polysplenia syndrome

- Polysplenia syndrome is a spectrum of anatomic disorders characterized by some degree of visceral heterotaxia in addition to multiple discrete foci of splenic tissue. Multiple spleens may be located on the right or left but are always on the same side as the stomach.
- Polysplenia is usually associated with severe congenital cardiac anomalies. Most patients die in early childhood, but a few may have only minor cardiac defects and polysplenia may be incidentally discovered in adulthood.
- Polysplenia is associated with venous anomalies including interruption of the IVC with azygos or hemiazygos continuation. A less common association is a preduodenal portal vein.

Wandering spleen

- A wandering spleen is a normal spleen with abnormal laxity or absence of its fixed ligamentous attachments.
- Wandering spleen may present clinically as an abdominal mass or may cause acute abdominal pain secondary to torsion.

脾脏

先天性脾变异和异常

副脾(accessory spleen)

- 副脾(splenule)，英文又称“accessory spleen”，是游离于脾主体之外的一块正常脾组织，是由于胚胎时期脾芽未能融合所致。最常见的位置是脾门。
- 副脾通常是一种偶然发现，但它在某些情况下具有一定的临床意义。例如，在脾切除术治疗脾亢进引起的血小板减少时，如果未切除足够的副脾组织则不能获得痊愈。当副脾位于不常见的位置时，可被误认为淋巴结或肿块。如前所述，胰腺内的副脾可能会被误认为富血供的胰腺肿块。
- 副脾在所有MRI序列上应与脾的表现一致。如有怀疑，可行^{99m}Tc-硫胶体扫描或热变性^{99m}Tc-红细胞扫描进行确诊。

多脾综合征

- 多脾综合征是指一系列的解剖学异常，特征为一定程度的内脏异位外加多发散在的局灶性脾组织。多发脾可位于右侧或左侧，但总是位于胃的同侧。
- 多脾通常与严重的先天性心脏发育异常相关。大多数患者死于幼儿期，但少数仅患有轻微D的心脏缺陷，到成年可能会偶然发现多脾。
- 多脾与静脉发育异常相关，包括下腔静脉中断伴奇静脉或半奇静脉交通。较少见的一个相关发现是门静脉位于十二指肠的前方。

游走脾

- 游走脾是正常的脾，但有异常松动或韧带缺乏固定的部位。
- 游走脾在临床上可以表现为腹部肿块或由于扭转而导致急性腹痛。

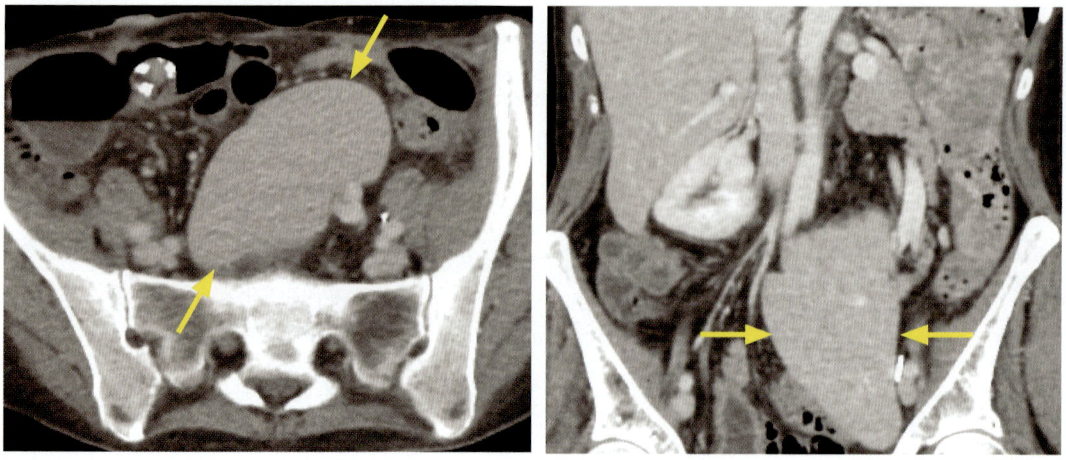

Axial (left image) and coronal (right image) contrast-enhanced CT demonstrates a normal sized spleen (arrows) in the left pelvis, consistent with wandering spleen. There are no findings to suggest torsion.
轴位(左图)和冠状位(右图)增强CT显示位于盆腔左侧的一个正常大小的脾(黄箭),符合游走脾诊断。无扭转表现。

OVERVIEW OF SPLENIC LESIONS

脾病变概述

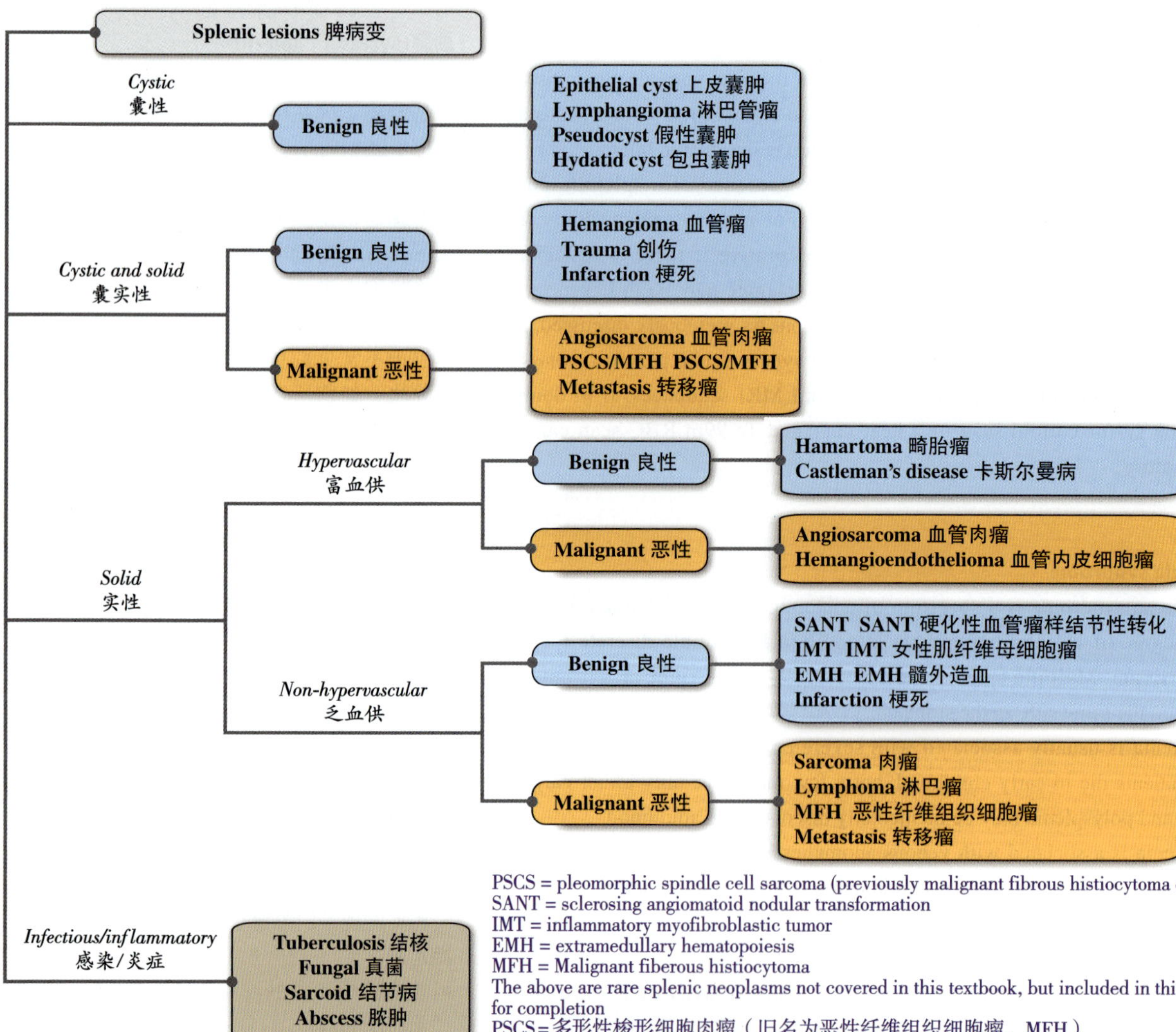

PSCS = pleomorphic spindle cell sarcoma (previously malignant fibrous histiocytoma or MFH)
SANT = sclerosing angiomatoid nodular transformation
IMT = inflammatory myofibroblastic tumor
EMH = extramedullary hematopoiesis
MFH = Malignant fiberous histiocytoma
The above are rare splenic neoplasms not covered in this textbook, but included in this list for completion
PSCS=多形性梭形细胞肉瘤（旧名为恶性纤维组织细胞瘤，MFH）
SANT=硬化性血管瘤样结节性转化
IMT=炎性肌纤维母细胞瘤
EMH=髓外造血
MFH=恶性纤维组织细胞瘤
上述罕见脾肿瘤不在本书编写内容之列，但归纳入此图表内作为全面介绍

Cystic splenic lesions

囊性脾病变

- Cystic lesions in the spleen are overwhelmingly benign in nature.

- 脾的囊性病变绝大部分属于良性。

Congenital true (epithelial) cyst

先天性真性(上皮)囊肿

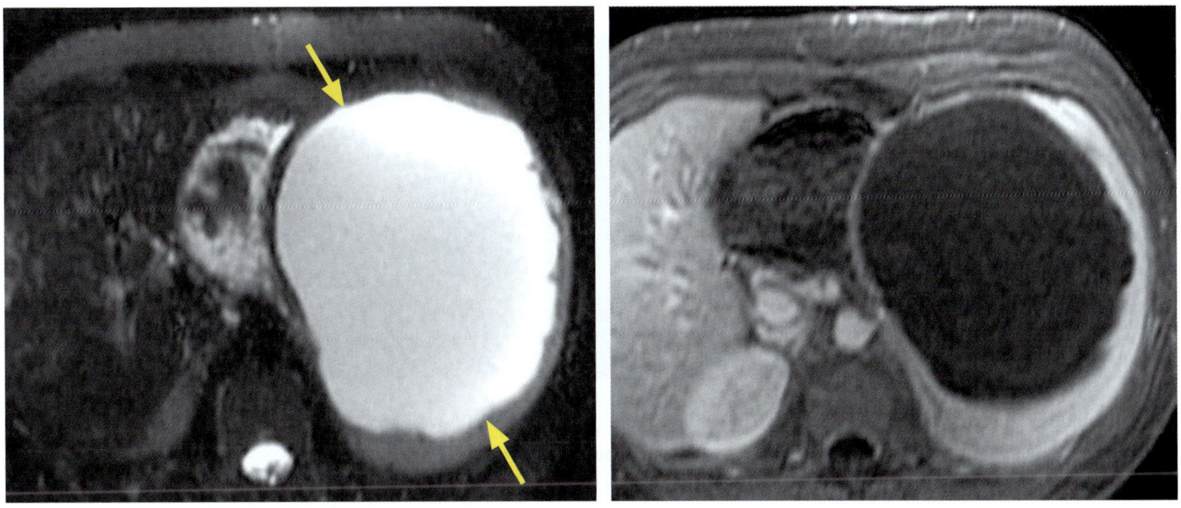

Splenic epithelial cyst: T2-weighted MRI with fat saturation (left image) and enhanced T1-weighted MRI (right image) shows a large T2 hyperintense, T1 hypointense, non-enhancing structure (arrows) replacing nearly the entire splenic parenchyma.
Case courtesy Cheryl Sadow, MD, Brigham and Women's Hospital.
脾上皮性囊肿：脂肪抑制T_2加权(左图)和增强T_1加权MRI(右图)可见一个巨大的T_2高信号、T_1低信号、无强化的结构(黄箭)，几乎占据了整个脾实质。

- A congenital true cyst is defined as having an epithelial lining. Interestingly, a splenic epithelial cyst may cause elevation of tumor markers including *CA19-9, CA125,* and *CEA*, despite its completely benign nature.
- Unlike a post-traumatic pseudocyst, a true cyst may have septations, but mural calcification is uncommon.

- 按照定义，先天性真性囊肿须内衬上皮细胞。有意思的是，脾上皮性囊肿虽然在本质上完全属于良性，但会引起CA19-9、CA125和CEA等肿瘤标志物升高。
- 与创伤后假性囊肿不同，真性囊肿可能有分隔，但囊壁钙化不常见。

Post-traumatic pseudocyst

- A post-traumatic pseudocyst is the end result of evolution of a splenic hematoma.
- Unlike a true (epithelial) splenic cyst, the periphery of a pseudocyst is not cellular but made of fibrotic tissue and septations are uncommon but there may be mural calcifications.
- On imaging, a post-traumatic pseudocyst appears as a well-circumscribed, fluid-density lesion with no peripheral enhancement.

创伤后假性囊肿

- 创伤后假性囊肿是脾血肿演变的最终结果。
- 与真性(上皮)脾囊肿不同，假性脾囊肿的边缘不是由细胞，而是由纤维组织所构成，分隔不常见，但可能有附壁钙化。
- 影像学上，创伤后假性囊肿表现为边界清晰、液性密度病灶，并且无周边强化。

Intrasplenic pancreatic pseudocyst

- A post-pancreatitis pancreatic pseudocyst involving the tail of the pancreas may extend into the spleen.
- Unlike a true congenital cyst, it lacks an epithelial lining and histology more closely resembles a post-traumatic pseudocyst.
- Splenic rupture has been reported in some cases of intrasplenic post-pancreatitis pseudocysts.

脾内胰腺假性囊肿

- 胰腺炎并发的假性囊肿累及胰尾时可能会蔓延至脾。
- 与真性先天性囊肿不同，该囊肿缺乏上皮内衬，并在组织学上更类似于创伤后假性囊肿。
- 有报道，部分继发于胰腺炎并发的脾内胰腺假性囊肿病例可发生脾破裂。

Lymphangioma

- Splenic lymphangioma is a rare, benign neoplasm usually diagnosed in childhood, which may be solitary or multiple.
- Lymphangioma features a classic imaging appearance of a multilocular cystic structure with thin septations. Post-contrast images may show septal enhancement.

淋巴管瘤

- 脾淋巴管瘤是一种罕见的良性肿瘤，通常发生在儿童，可以单发也可以为多发。
- 淋巴管瘤典型的影像学特征为多房囊性结构伴薄的分隔，增强后图像可显示分隔有强化。

Benign non-cystic splenic lesions

良性非囊性脾病变

- If a mass is found in the spleen and the patient has no history of widespread malignancy or symptoms referred to the left upper quadrant, the mass is most likely benign.

- 如果脾内发现一个肿块，且患者没有广泛恶性肿瘤转移的病史，或左上腹缺乏相关的症状，那么该肿块很可能是良性的。

Hemangioma

血管瘤

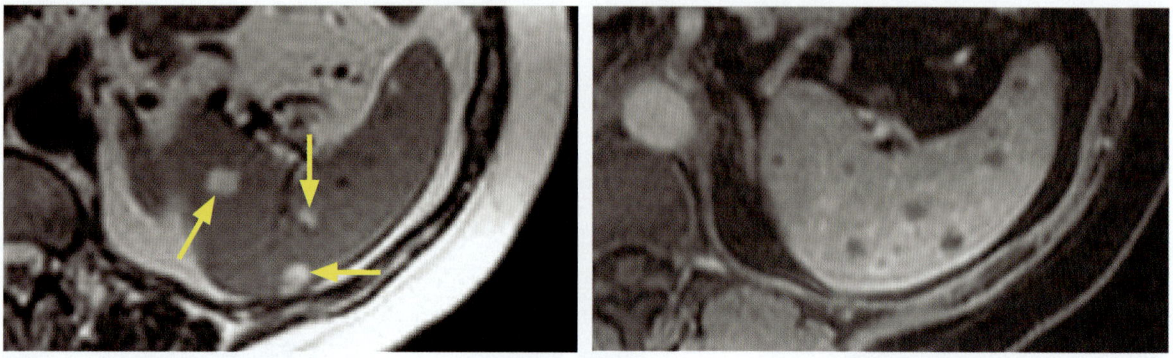

Multiple splenic hemangiomas: T2-weighted (left image) and post-contrast T1-weighted (right image) MRI shows multiple T2 hyperintense splenic lesions (arrows) that demonstrate subtle peripheral enhancement.

多发脾血管瘤：T_2加权(左图)及增强T_1加权(右图)MRI显示多发T_2高信号的脾病灶(黄箭)，并有轻度周边强化。

- Hemangioma is the most common benign splenic neoplasm. They may be solitary or multiple and they tend to be small.
- Splenic hemangiomas are associated with **Kasabach-Merritt syndrome** (anemia, thrombocytopenia, and consumptive coagulopathy) and **Klippel-Trenaunay-Weber syndrome** (cutaneous hemangiomas, varicose veins, and extremity hypertrophy). These visceral hemangiomatosis syndromes are usually associated with phleboliths.
- On CT, hemangiomas are typically iso- or hypoattenuating pre-contrast and hyperenhancing. On MR, hemangiomas are typically hyperintense on T2-weighted images and may enhance peripherally or homogeneously. However, the classic pattern of discontinuous nodular enhancement seen in hepatic hemangiomas is uncommon.
- Nuclear medicine scintigraphy with Tc-99m labeled red blood cells would show increased activity within the lesion on delayed images. In contrast, Tc-99m sulfur colloid scanning may show either increased or decreased activity.

- 血管瘤是最常见的脾良性肿瘤。它们可以单发或多发，病灶大多偏小。
- 脾血管瘤与**卡萨巴赫-梅里特综合征**(贫血、血小板减少症和消耗性凝血病)和**血管骨肥大综合征**(皮肤血管瘤、静脉曲张和肢端肥大症)相关。这些内脏血管瘤病综合征通常与静脉结石相关。
- 血管瘤在CT图像上的典型表现为平扫呈等或低密度，增强后呈高密度。在MRI图像上，血管瘤的典型表现为T_2加权高信号，也可呈周边强化或均匀强化。然而，在脾血管瘤中很少看到肝脏血管瘤中那样典型的、不连续的结节样强化。
- 用^{99m}Tc-标记红细胞进行核医学闪烁显像，在延迟图像中会显示病变部位活性增加。相比之下，^{99m}Tc-硫胶体扫描可能出现活性增加或减少。

Hamartoma

错构瘤

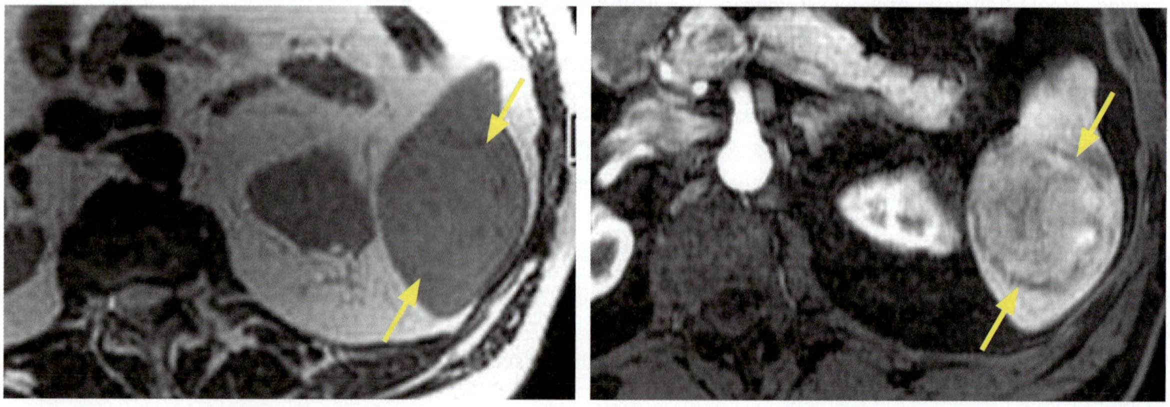

Splenic hamartoma: T2-weighted (left image) and arterial-phase enhanced T1-weighted (right image) MRI shows a vague T2 isointense splenic mass (arrows) that enhances heterogeneously.

脾错构瘤：T_2加权(左图)和动脉期增强T_1加权(右图)MRI可见一个模糊的T_2等信号脾肿块(黄箭)，增强后呈不均匀强化。

- Splenic hamartoma is a rare, benign lesion composed of malformed red pulp elements. It may be associated with tuberous sclerosis.
- Splenic hamartoma is typically a well-circumscribed, iso- or hypoattenuating mass on unenhanced CT that enhances heterogeneously after contrast administration.
- On MRI, a hamartoma is iso- to slightly hyperintense on T2-weighted images, featuring heterogeneous early enhancement and relatively homogeneous delayed enhancement.

- 脾错构瘤是一种罕见的良性病变，由畸形的红髓成分组成。它可能与结节性硬化症相关。
- 脾错构瘤在CT平扫的典型表现为边界清晰的等或低密度肿块，增强后呈不均匀强化。
- MRI上，错构瘤在T_2加权呈等至稍高信号，表现为早期呈不均匀强化，延迟强化相对均匀。

INFLAMMATORY SPLENIC LESIONS

脾的炎性病变

Sarcoidosis

- Sarcoidosis is a systemic disease of unknown etiology characterized histologically by multiple nodules composed of noncaseating granulomas.
- When sarcoidosis involves the spleen, splenomegaly is the most common presenting finding, often associated with hepatomegaly and lymphadenopathy.
- Less commonly, sarcoidosis may involve the spleen in a multinodular pattern with numerous hypoattenuating 1–3 cm lesions demonstrating essentially no enhancement.

  These nodules are formed by coalescent sarcoid granulomas and have low signal on all MRI sequences.

  Sarcoid nodules are most conspicuous on T2-weighted images and early-phase post-contrast T1-weighted images. On the post-contrast images, the nonenhancing nodules will stand out against the avidly enhancing splenic parenchyma.
- Imaging appearance is generally indistinguishable from splenic lymphoma.

结节病

- 结节病是一种病因不明的系统性疾病，在组织学上以非干酪样肉芽肿所形成的多发结节灶为特征。
- 当结节病累及脾时，脾大是最常见的表现，通常还伴有肝大和淋巴结肿大。
- 较少情况下，结节病可以呈多发结节的形式累及脾，表现为大量1~3cm大小的低密度结节，基本无强化。

  这些结节由结节样肉芽肿融合而成，在所有MRI序列上均为低信号。

  结节病结节在T_2加权及增强后早期T_1加权上最为明显。在增强图像上，非强化的结节在明显强化的脾实质背景衬托下会显得非常清晰。
- 影像学表现通常难以与脾淋巴瘤相鉴别。

Inflammatory pseudotumor

- Splenic inflammatory pseudotumor is a rare focal collection of immune cells and associated inflammatory exudate of unclear etiology. Patients often have constitutional symptoms including fever and malaise.
- Inflammatory pseudotumor has a variable and nonspecific imaging appearance, but a typical presentation is of a well-circumscribed, heterogeneously enhancing mass.

炎性假瘤

- 脾的炎性假瘤是一种罕见的免疫细胞堆积形成的局灶性病变，与原因不明的炎性渗出有关。患者通常会有全身症状，包括发热和不适。
- 炎性假瘤有多种影像学表现，但无特异性，常见的典型表现为一个边界清晰、不均匀强化的肿块。

SPLENIC INFECTION

脾感染

Pyogenic abscess

细菌性脓肿

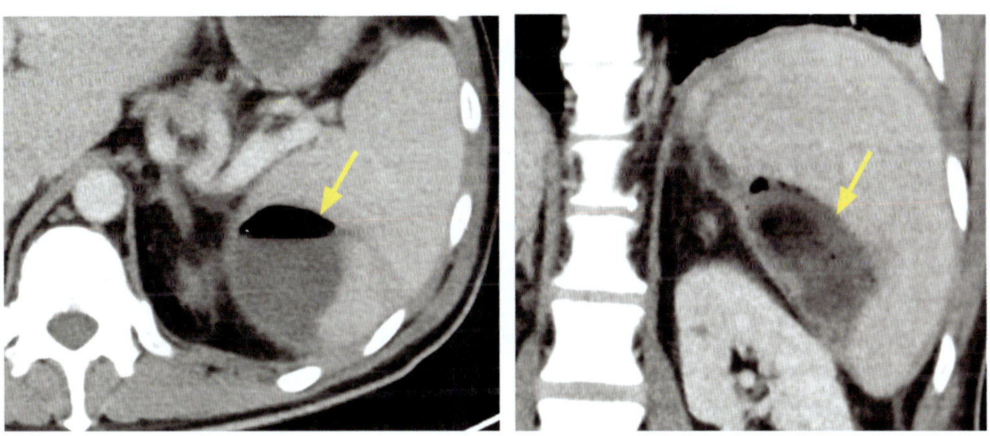

Axial and coronal contrast-enhanced CT of the abdomen demonstrates a heterogeneous gas-containing fluid collection (arrows) within the medial spleen with irregular wall thickening and surrounding perisplenic stranding. This was a case of *Staph. aureus* pyogenic splenic abscess that was subsequently drained percutaneously.

轴位和冠状位腹部增强CT显示脾内侧有一处密度不均的含气积液(黄箭)，伴不规则壁增厚及脾周条纹影。这是一名金黄色葡萄球菌脓肿病例，随后进行了经皮穿刺引流术。

- Splenic bacterial abscesses are uncommon and usually seen in immunocompromised patients. A solitary abscess is much more likely to be bacterial. In contrast, multifocal small abscesses are more likely to be fungal.
- On CT, a bacterial abscess usually has an irregular, enhancing wall. Gas is not usually seen but is highly specific for a bacterial abscess when present.
- A characteristic ultrasound finding is the *wheel within a wheel* or *bull's-eye* appearance, which describes concentric hyperechoic and hypoechoic rings surrounding the abscess.
- Treatment is CT- or ultrasound-guided percutaneous drainage in addition to antibiotics.

Fungal abscess

- Splenic fungal abscesses are typically multiple and small, usually <1 cm in size. Almost all patients with splenic fungal abscesses are immunocompromised.
- The most common causative agents include *Candida*, *Aspergillus*, and *Cryptococcus*, all of which have a common appearance of multiple tiny hypoattenuating foci on CT.
- Splenic *Pneumocystis jiroveci* (formerly known as *Pneumocystis carinii*) infection is rare, almost always seen in advanced AIDS, and has a classic appearance of multiple calcified splenic lesions.

Echinococcal cyst

- Splenic involvement of *Echinococcus granulosus* infection is unusual, seen in only 1–3% of echinococcal infections, and is almost always associated with infection of other organs as well.
- An echinococcal cyst is a true cyst with a cellular lining. As with echinococcal abscesses elsewhere, characteristic imaging findings are a cystic lesion with internal undulating membrane and daughter cysts.

- 细菌性脾脓肿不常见，通常发生于免疫功能不全的患者。孤立性脓肿大多为细菌性；相反，多发小脓肿更可能为真菌所致。
- CT上，细菌性脓肿通常有一层不规则、可强化的壁。气体并不常见，而一旦出现，则对诊断细菌性脓肿具有高度特异性。
- 超声的典型表现为双轮征或牛眼征，即中央高回声和脓肿周围低回声所组成的同心环。
- 治疗为CT或超声引导下经皮穿刺引流加抗生素。

真菌性脓肿

- 真菌性脾脓肿通常是多发的小病灶，大多<1cm。几乎所有真菌性脾脓肿患者都有免疫功能低下。
- 最常见的病原体包括念珠菌、曲霉菌和隐球菌，在CT上均表现为多发微小低密度灶。
- 脾耶氏肺孢子虫(曾称卡氏肺孢子虫)感染罕见，几乎都见于晚期艾滋病，其典型表现为多发脾钙化灶。

包虫囊肿

- 脾感染细粒棘球绦虫并不常见，仅见于1%~3%感染的患者，并且几乎都伴有其他器官感染。
- 包虫囊肿是真性囊肿，内衬有细胞。与其他部位的包虫脓肿类似，影像学特征性的表现为囊性病灶内可见波浪状的膜及子囊。

Malignant splenic lesions

Splenic lymphoma

- Splenic lymphoma is the most common splenic malignancy.
- Primary splenic lymphoma is rare, accounting for less than 1% of all cases of lymphoma, and usually presents as a solitary hypovascular mass. In contrast to splenic hamartoma or metastatic disease, primary splenic lymphoma may extend beyond the splenic capsule and involve adjacent organs.
- Secondary splenic involvement of systemic lymphoma is much more common. Four imaging presentations have been described, depending on the size of the lymphomatous masses:

> Miliary masses, in which discrete tiny masses may be difficult to see.
> Multiple small- to moderate-sized masses.
> One large mass.
> Splenomegaly without discrete mass.

- Conspicuity is highest on post-contrast T1-weighted images, where the involved portion of the spleen tends to be *hypoenhancing*.
- On ultrasound, lymphoma may appear cystic, but color Doppler shows internal flow.

恶性脾病变

脾淋巴瘤

- 脾淋巴瘤是最常见的脾恶性肿瘤。
- 原发性脾淋巴瘤罕见，在所有淋巴瘤病例中不到1%，通常表现为一个孤立的乏血供肿块。与脾错构瘤或转移瘤不同，原发性脾淋巴瘤可突破脾包膜并累及邻近器官。
- 继发于系统性淋巴瘤的脾病变更为常见。影像学表现有四种，取决于淋巴瘤肿块的大小：

> 粟粒状结节，散在的微小结节，可能不易发现。
> 小到中等大小的多发肿块。
> 单个大的肿块。
> 脾大无明显的肿块。

- 病灶在T_1加权增强图像上最明显，受累部分的脾呈低强化。
- 超声上，淋巴瘤可能呈囊性，但彩色多普勒超声显示内部有血流存在。

Splenic metastasis

脾转移瘤

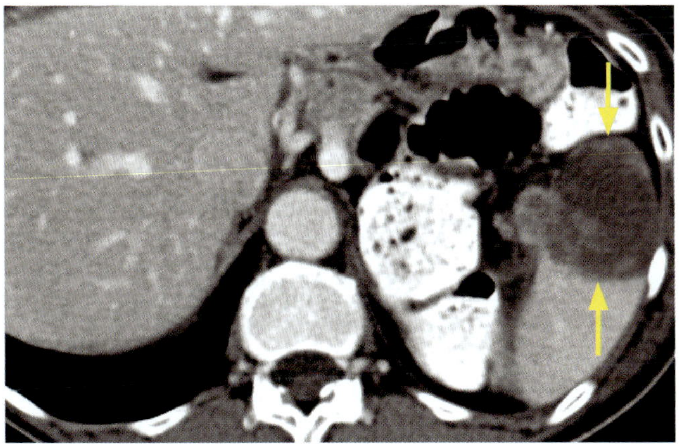

Splenic metastasis from lung cancer: Contrast-enhanced axial CT shows a hypoattenuating, irregular mass in the inferior anterior aspect of the spleen (arrows) demonstrating wispy, heterogeneous enhancement.
Case courtesy Cheryl Sadow, MD, Brigham and Women's Hospital.
肺癌脾转移：轴位增强CT显示在脾前下部可见一个低密度、不规则的肿块(黄箭)，并有轻微不均匀强化。

- Splenic metastases may be solitary or multiple, cystic or solid. However, metastases to the spleen are rare, occurring in 2–9% of cancer patients. Most patients with splenic metastases already have confirmed widespread disease.

  Isolated splenic metastases are seen in only 5% of patients with metastatic involvement of the spleen.
- Theories for the low rate of splenic metastases include the antineoplastic properties of lymphoid-rich splenic tissue and lack of afferent lymphatics available to bring tumor cells into the spleen.
- The most common primary tumors known to metastasize to the spleen include breast, lung, ovarian, and melanoma. Ovarian cancer and melanoma typically cause cystic metastasis.
- Calcification is rare unless the primary is a mucinous adenocarcinoma.

- 脾转移瘤可以单发或多发，呈囊性或实性。然而，肿瘤转移至脾较为罕见，在癌症患者中的发生率为2%~9%。大多数脾转移瘤的患者已经有广泛转移。

  孤立性脾转移瘤只占脾转移瘤患者的5%。
- 脾转移瘤发生率低的假说包括富含淋巴的脾组织具有抗肿瘤作用，以及入脾淋巴管缺乏而使得癌细胞无法进入脾。
- 最常转移至脾的原发肿瘤有乳腺癌、肺癌、卵巢癌及黑色素瘤。卵巢癌和黑色素瘤通常为囊性转移灶。
- 钙化罕见，除非原发肿瘤为黏液腺癌。

Angiosarcoma

- Angiosarcoma is a rare, extremely aggressive malignancy, with a 20% 6-month survival.
- Unlike hepatic angiosarcoma, the associations with Thorotrast, vinyl chloride, and arsenic have not been well-established.
- Angiosarcoma usually presents as a large, heterogeneous mass that may completely replace the normal spleen. Enhancement is variable and heterogeneous.

血管肉瘤

- 血管肉瘤是一种罕见的、极具侵袭性的恶性肿瘤，6个月生存率为20%。
- 与肝脏血管肉瘤不同，它与氧化钍胶体、氯乙烯及砷之间的相关性并不明确。
- 血管肉瘤常表现为大而不均质的肿块，并可能完全取代正常脾。强化方式多变且不均匀。

MISCELLANEOUS SPLENIC LESIONS

其他脾病变

Splenic infarct

脾梗死

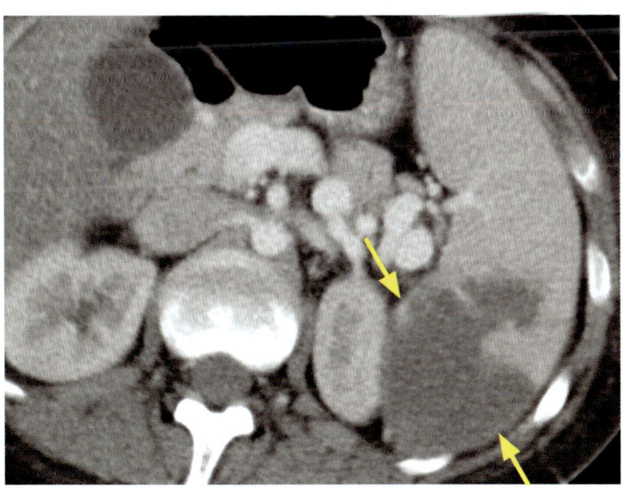

Axial contrast-enhanced CT shows a posterior peripheral wedge-shaped region of splenic non-enhancement (arrows), consistent with infarct.
Case courtesy Cheryl Sadow, MD, Brigham and Women's Hospital.
轴位增强CT显示脾后部外周楔形无强化区(黄箭)，提示脾梗死。

- Splenic infarcts are most commonly due to emboli (in older patients) and thrombosis (in younger patients with hematologic disease).
- Splenic infarct classically manifests as a wedge-shaped peripheral region of nonenhancement, but a more heterogeneous, mass-like appearance can also be seen.
- On MR, the affected regions may be T1 hyperintense if acute and hemorrhagic, while chronic infarcts are T1 hypointense and T2 hyperintense.
- Lack of enhancement of the entire spleen should raise the concern for complete infarction, possibly due to a wandering spleen with torsion.

- 脾梗死最常见为栓子(见于老年人)或血栓形成(见于有血液系统疾病的年轻人)。
- 脾梗死的典型表现为外周无强化的楔形区，但也可见到较不均匀的肿块样改变。
- MRI上，如果是急性期或出血性，受累区域在T_1加权上可呈高信号，而慢性梗死呈T_1加权低信号、T_2加权高信号。
- 若整个脾无强化，要考虑完全性脾梗死，可能是游走的脾蒂发生了扭转。

Gamna-Gandy bodies

- Gamna-Gandy bodies are multiple tiny foci of hemosiderin deposition and are a sequela of portal hypertension.
- Other signs of portal hypertension and cirrhosis are usually apparent on imaging, such as splenomegaly, varices, recanalized umbilical vein, ascites, and a nodular liver contour.
- The hemosiderin deposits demonstrate low signal on all sequences. On in- and out-of-phase gradient-echo sequences, the longer TE of the in-phase images demonstrates *blooming* (relatively decreased signal on in-phase images), due to longer dephasing time and exaggeration of T2* effect.

Gamna-Gandy小体(铁质沉着结节)

- Gamna-Gandy小体是多发含铁血黄素的微小沉着灶，为门静脉高压的后遗症。
- 其他门静脉高压和肝硬化的征象在影像学上通常很明显，如脾大、静脉曲张、脐静脉再通、腹水和结节状肝轮廓改变。
- 含铁血黄素沉着在所有序列上均为低信号。在同相位、反相位梯度回波序列上，更长回波时间的同相位图像会出现开花样(放大)效应(同相位上信号相对减低)，为延长的反相位时间和放大的T_2*效应所致。

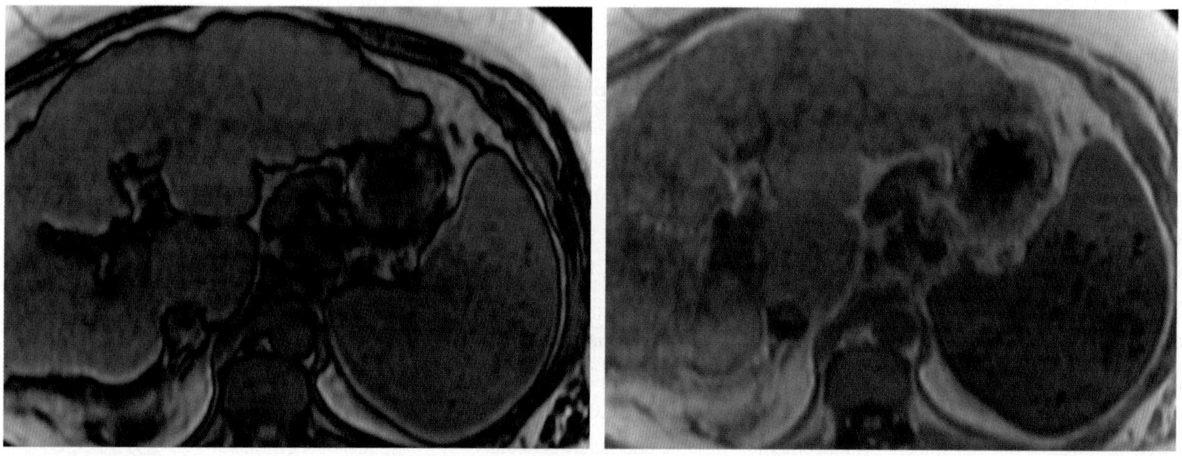

Axial in- and out-of-phase gradient echo MRI shows numerous low signal foci in the spleen which demonstrate *blooming* on in-phase imaging (right image) compared to out-of-phase imaging (left image), representing Gamna-Gandy bodies. Note cirrhotic morphology of the liver (nodular contour, widened fissures, multiple regenerative nodules).

轴位同相位、反相位MRI显示脾内大量局部低信号，同相位图像(右图)相对于反相位图像(左图)上的病灶呈开花样(放大)效应，提示为Gamna-Gandy小体。注意肝硬化的形态改变(结节样轮廓、肝裂增宽、多发再生结节)

Gaucher disease

- Gaucher disease is an autosomal recessive deficiency of glucocerebrosidase, leading to accumulation of glucocerebrosides in the reticuloendothelial system.
- Splenic manifestations of Gaucher disease include splenomegaly (almost always) and multiple splenic nodules (seen in one-third of Gaucher patients).
- Associated bony findings seen in Gaucher disease include the characteristic *Erlenmeyer flask* deformity of the distal femurs, femoral head avascular necrosis, and *H-shaped* vertebral bodies from endplate avascular necrosis.

戈谢病

- 戈谢病是一种葡萄糖脑苷脂酶缺乏的常染色体隐性疾病，导致网状内皮系统内积聚葡萄糖脑苷脂酶。
- 戈谢病的脾表现包括脾大(几乎都有)和多发脾结节(见于1/3戈谢病的患者)。
- 戈谢病相关的骨骼表现包括特征性的股骨远端锥形烧瓶样畸形、股骨头缺血性坏死和椎体终板缺血性坏死所致的椎体“H”形改变。

Splenic Trauma

Overview of splenic trauma

- The spleen is the most commonly injured abdominal organ in blunt trauma.
- Splenectomy dramatically increases the risk of subsequent sepsis, which has driven the trend towards splenic preservation and conservative management of splenic trauma.
- The spleen must be evaluated for injury in the portal venous phase, as physiologic heterogeneous enhancement in the arterial phase can both mask and mimic injury.
- A splenic hematoma is a focal collection of blood (hypoattenuating relative to enhanced spleen and hyperattenuating relative to unenhanced spleen), usually subcapsular in location. Less commonly, a hematoma may be intraparenchymal, where it is irregular in shape.
- A splenic laceration can only be well seen on a contrast-enhanced study, where it appears as a linear or branching area of decreased attenuation.
- Active contrast extravasation due to vessel injury appears as an area of increased attenuation (initially iso-enhancing to the arterial blood pool), which continues to increase in size or attenuation on delayed scanning due to pooling of extravasated blood.
- In contrast to active extravasation, pseudoaneurysm and arteriovenous (AV) fistula are contained vascular injuries that also initially appear as a focal area of increased attenuation, but do not increase in size on delayed scanning.

A pseudoaneurysm is caused by injury to the intima and media of the arterial wall and is essentially a rupture contained only by the adventitia. There is a high chance of rupture without treatment.

A traumatic AV fistula is indistinguishable from pseudoaneurysm by CT and is due to injury of an artery and the adjacent vein. Splenic arteriography is the only way to differentiate pseudoaneurysm from arteriovenous fistula.

American Association for the Surgery of Trauma organ injury scale for spleen

- The 2018 revision of the AAST spleen injury scale takes into consideration the extent of injury seen on CT imaging, at operation, or on pathologic specimen. The highest-grade assessment represents the final grade assigned.
- The revision incorporates vascular injury seen on CT including active bleeding, pseudoaneurysm, and AV fistula as defined above.
- The CT imaging criteria is similar to that used for liver trauma.

AAST spleen injury scale

- Grade Ⅰ:
  Subcapsular hematoma <10% spleen surface.
  Tear of splenic capsule or superficial laceration <1 cm deep.
- Grade Ⅱ:
  Subcapsular hematoma 10–50% spleen surface.
  Intraparenchymal hematoma <5 cm in size.
  Laceration 1–3 cm deep.
- Grade Ⅲ:
  Subcapsular hematoma >50% spleen surface.
  Ruptured subcapsular/intraparenchymal hematoma.
  Laceration >3 cm deep.
- Grade Ⅳ:
  Any intraparenchymal vascular injury (i.e., pseudoaneurysm or AV fistula) or contained active bleeding.
  Laceration involving central splenic vessels resulting in >25% devascularization.
- Grade Ⅴ:
  Extraparenchymal extension of active bleeding into the peritoneum.
  Shattered spleen.

脾外伤

脾外伤概述

- 脾是发生腹部钝性创伤时最常受损的器官。
- 脾切除会明显增加继发性败血症的风险，所以创伤后应尽量保留脾而采取保守治疗。
- 评估脾必须在门静脉期进行，因为动脉期脾会出现生理性不均匀强化，从而掩盖损伤或影像类似于损伤。
- 脾血肿是局灶性血液积聚(相对于强化后的脾呈低密度，相对于无强化的脾呈高密度)，通常位于包膜下。少见情况下，血肿可能位于实质内，呈不规则形。
- 脾撕裂可能仅在增强检查时才能清楚显示，表现为线样或分支状密度降低区。
- 血管损伤引起的活动性造影剂外渗可表现为区域性密度增高(初始与动脉血池呈等密度)，在延迟扫描时因持续性出血，该区域会进一步增大。
- 与活动性出血相反，假性动脉瘤和动静脉瘘是包裹性的血管损伤，最初也表现为境界清晰的密度增高区，但是延迟扫描病灶不会增大。

假性动脉瘤为动脉壁的内膜和中膜受损，本质上是血管撕裂后仅有外膜包裹。如不进行治疗，破裂的概率很高。

创伤性动静脉瘘在CT上与假性动脉瘤无法区分，为动脉及其邻近的静脉共同损伤所致。脾动脉造影是区分假性动脉瘤和动静脉瘘的唯一方法。

美国创伤外科协会(AAST)脾损伤分级指标

- 2018美国创伤外科协会(AAST)脾损伤分级指标修订版将CT影像、手术探查及病理切片所显示的损伤范围进行综合考虑。最终的级别认定基于最高的评分。
- 修订版整合了CT所显示的血管损伤，包括了之前描述的活动性出血、假性动脉瘤和动静脉瘘。
- CT影像评分标准与肝脏创伤相似。

AAST脾损伤分级

- Ⅰ级：
  包膜下血肿范围占脾表面积<10%。
  脾包膜撕裂，或表面撕裂深度<1cm。
- Ⅱ级：
  包膜下血肿范围为脾表面积的10%~50%。
  实质内血肿大小<5cm。
  撕裂深度1~3cm。
- Ⅲ级：
  包膜下血肿范围>50%脾表面积。
  包膜下/实质内血肿破裂。
  撕裂深度>3cm。
- Ⅳ级：
  任何实质内血管损伤(如假性动脉瘤和动静脉瘘)或活动性出血。
  撕裂伤累及脾中央血管，导致血流量减少>25%。
- Ⅴ级：
  活动性出血向实质外延伸至腹腔。
  脾碎裂。

- When multiple injuries are present, advance one grade up to a grade Ⅲ.

- 合并多发损伤时，将等级提高一级至最高Ⅲ级。

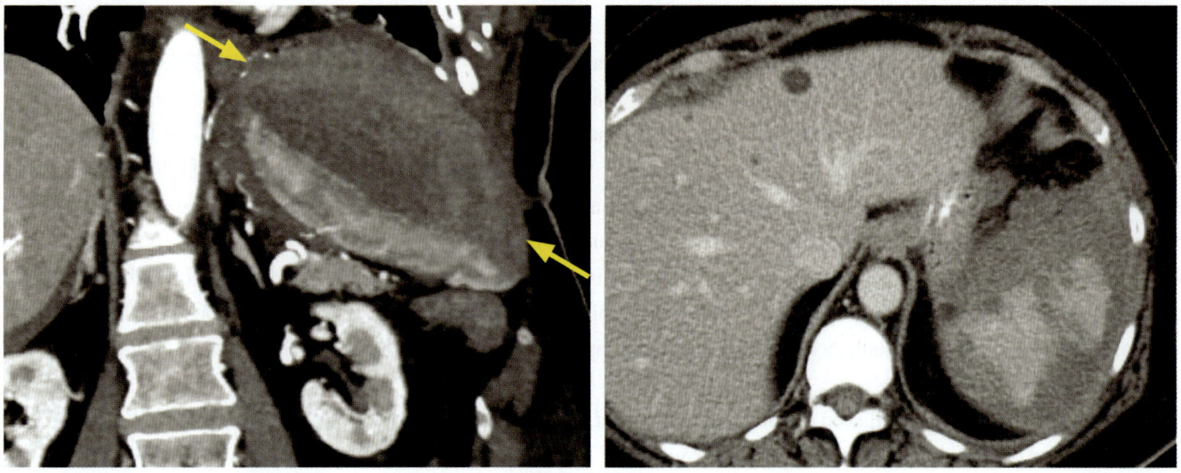

Left image: Coronal contrast-enhanced CT demonstrates a large subcapsular hematoma (arrows) compressing the spleen, without evidence of active extravasation, in keeping with grade Ⅲ splenic injury.
Right image: Axial contrast-enhanced CT shows a shattered spleen (grade Ⅴ) with surrounding hematoma.
左图：冠状位增强CT显示一个大的包膜下血肿(黄箭)并压迫脾，无活动性出血，判定为Ⅲ级脾损伤。
右图：轴位增强CT显示破碎的脾(Ⅴ级)，伴周围血肿形成。

Common imaging patterns of splenic disease

Splenic calcification

Granulomatous disease (calcifications may be scattered or diffuse).
Infarct (remote).
Hematoma.
Calcified splenic artery aneurysm.

Cystic splenic lesion (on ultrasound, color Doppler should always be used to exclude a vascular etiology)

Epithelial cyst.
Splenic artery aneurysm or pseudoaneurysm.
Hematoma.
Abscess.
Pancreatic pseudocyst.

Hypervascular or hyperechoic splenic lesion

Hemangioma (can also be hypoechoic).
Hamartoma.
Lymphangioma.
Angiosarcoma.

Hypovascular or hypoechoic splenic lesion

Laceration (in the setting of trauma).
Abscess.
Lymphoma.
Sarcoidosis.
Metastasis.
Infarct (tends to be peripheral).
Extramedullary hematopoiesis.

脾疾病常见的影像学表现

脾钙化灶

肉芽肿性病变(钙化可能散在或弥漫分布)。
梗死(陈旧性)。
血肿。
脾动脉瘤壁钙化。

囊性脾病变(超声检查时，应使用彩色多普勒排除血管性病因)

上皮囊肿。
脾动脉瘤或假性动脉瘤。
血肿。
脓肿。
胰腺假性囊肿。

富血管或高回声脾病变

血管瘤(也可以是低回声)。
错构瘤。
淋巴管瘤。
血管肉瘤。

乏血管或低回声脾病变

撕裂伤(外伤)。
脓肿。
淋巴瘤。
结节病。
转移。
梗死(倾向于外周)。
髓外造血。

Splenomegaly (defined as >14 cm in sagittal plane)

Mild to moderate splenomegaly:

- **Portal hypertension** (most common).
- Infection.
- AIDS.

Moderate to marked splenomegaly:

- Leukemia/lymphoma.
- Infectious mononucleosis.

Massive splenomegaly:

- Myelofibrosis.

脾大(矢状面长径>14cm)

轻度至中度脾大：

- **门静脉高压**(最常见)。
- 感染。
- 艾滋病。

中度至显著脾大：

- 白血病/淋巴瘤。
- 传染性单核细胞增多症。

重度脾大：

- 骨髓纤维化。

(翻译　彭丹丹)

ESOPHAGUS

食管

ANATOMY

Pharynx

- **Nasopharynx**: Extends from the base of the skull to the soft palate.
- **Oropharynx**: Located behind the mouth and extends from the uvula to the hyoid bone.
- **Hypopharynx**: Extends from the hyoid bone to the cricopharyngeus muscle, which is located at the lower end of the cricoid cartilage, usually between C5–6.

Esophagus

- The cricopharyngeus muscle is the upper esophageal sphincter and demarcates the transition between the hypopharynx superiorly and the cervical esophagus.
- The esophagus extends from the neck to the gastroesophageal junction. The distal esophagus passes through the diaphragmatic hiatus at approximately T10.
- The three anatomic rings of the distal esophagus are the A (muscular), B (mucosal), and C (diaphragmatic impression) rings.

解剖

咽部

- **鼻咽部**：自颅底延伸至软腭。
- **口咽部**：位于口腔后方，自悬雍垂延伸至舌骨。
- **喉咽部**：自舌骨延伸至环咽肌，后者位于环状软骨的下端，通常在C_5~C_6。

食管

- 环咽肌为食管上括约肌，是下咽上方与颈段食管过渡的标志。
- 食管自颈部延伸至胃食管交界处。远端食管在约T_{10}水平穿过膈肌裂孔。
- 食管远端有三个解剖环，分别为A环(肌环)、B环(黏膜环)和C环(膈压迹环)。

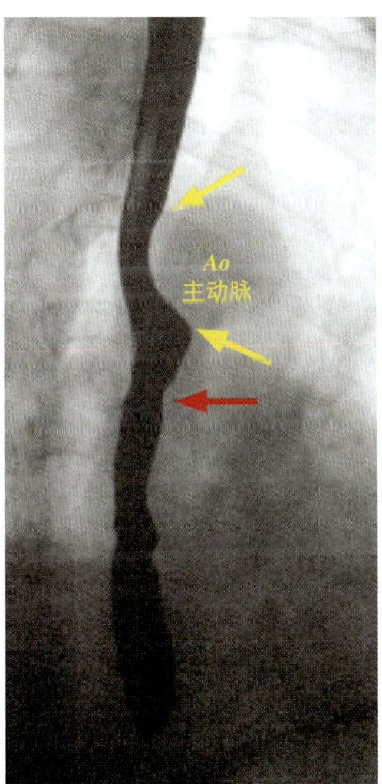

Double-contrast barium swallow showing normal impressions on the esophagus by the aortic arch (Ao, yellow arrows) and left mainstem bronchus (red arrow).
气钡双重对比造影显示来自主动脉弓(黄箭)和左主支气管(红箭)对食管产生的正常压迹。

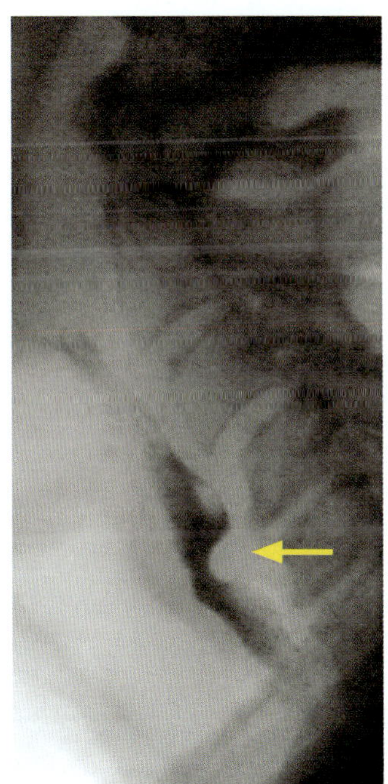

Single-contrast barium speech and swallow study demonstrates a prominent cricopharyngeus muscle (arrow) on sagittal view, forming a smooth posterior indentation on the esophagus at level of C5.
侧位单一钡餐和吞咽检查显示突起的环咽肌(黄箭)，在C_5水平食管后部形成平滑的凹痕。

Imaging the Esophagus

Overview of esophageal imaging

- The primary imaging modality for evaluating the esophagus is fluoroscopy, which allows for anatomic and function evaluation.
- A **double-contrast** esophagram utilizes barium and gas-forming crystals to simultaneously distend the esophagus and coat the mucosa with radiopaque contrast. The dynamic nature of the study also allows for evaluation of reflux and motility disorders.
- A **single-contrast** esophagram may be used when you are evaluating for a post-operative leak (performed with water-soluble contrast rather than barium) or if a patient cannot tolerate the gas-forming crystals.
- Barium is the contrast agent of choice unless there is concern for an esophageal leak, in that case water-soluble contrast is preferred. If the patient has a significant aspiration risk, however, high osmolality water-soluble contrast should be avoided (due to risk of pneumonitis).
- If an esophageal malignancy has been diagnosed, PET/CT may be used to stage for locoregional lymph nodes and metastatic disease, and endoscopic ultrasound is utilized for evaluating the depth of the lesion (T stage) and the presence of local lymph nodes.
- CT and MRI have a limited role in evaluation of primary esophageal pathology.

食管成像

食管影像学概述

- 评估食管的最基本成像方式是透视，可以对解剖和功能进行评估。
- **双重对比**食管造影利用钡剂和产气结晶颗粒使食管扩张的同时将不透射线的造影剂涂于黏膜。该检查的动态属性还能对反流和运动障碍进行评估。
- **单一造影剂**食管造影可用于评估术后渗漏(使用水溶性造影剂而不是钡造影剂)，或患者不能耐受产气结晶颗粒时。
- 首选钡剂，若怀疑有食管漏，应改用水溶性造影剂。如果患者有明显的误吸风险，则应避免使用高渗性水溶性造影剂(由于肺炎的风险)。
- 如果已诊断为食管恶性肿瘤，PET/CT可用于对局部淋巴结和转移性病变进行分期，并利用内镜超声评估病变的深度(T分期)和局部淋巴结。
- CT和MRI对原发性食管病变的评估作用有限。

Esophageal Rings and Webs

Esophageal web

- An esophageal web is a thin anterior infolding/indentation, usually occurring in the anterior cervical esophagus, which is often asymptomatic but may be a cause of dysphagia if it significantly narrows the lumen. There is a controversial association with anemia (Plummer- Vinson syndrome) and carcinoma of the upper esophagus.

Schatzki ring

食管环及食管蹼

食管蹼

- 食管蹼是食管前壁一层薄内折/压迹，通常发生在颈椎前的食管，一般无症状，但如果引起食管腔明显变窄，可能成为吞咽困难的原因之一。食管蹼与贫血(缺铁性吞咽困难综合征)和上段食管癌之间的关系尚存在争议。

Schatzki环(下食管括约肌环)

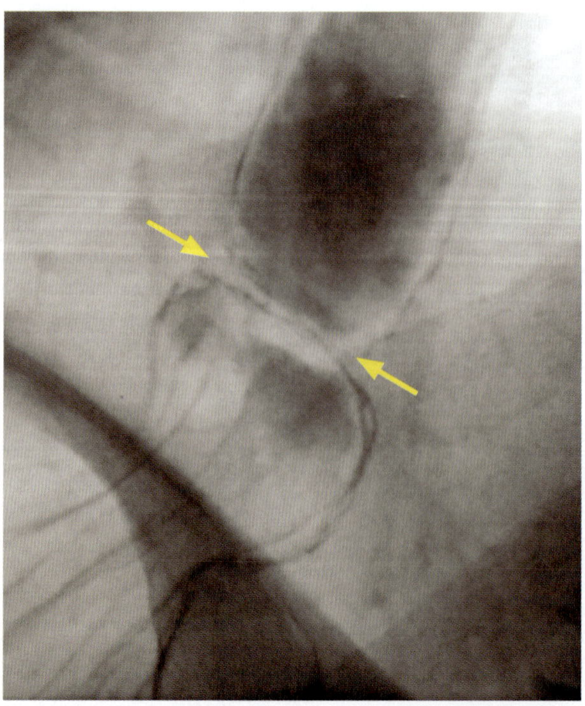

Schatzki ring: Double-contrast barium swallow in a patient with dysphagia shows a circumferential narrowing (arrows) at the gastroesophageal junction, associated with a small hiatal hernia.

Case courtesy Cheryl Sadow, MD, Brigham and Women's Hospital.

Schatzki环：吞咽困难患者气钡双重吞咽造影显示胃食管交界处环状狭窄(黄箭)，并伴有小裂孔疝。

- A Schatzki ring is a focal pathologic narrowing of the B (mucosal) ring of the distal esophagus less than 13 mm causing intermittent dysphagia.

  Asymptomatic narrowing of the B ring is referred to as a lower esophageal ring.
- The key imaging feature is focal, thin, circumferential constriction near the GE junction, almost always associated with a hiatal hernia, best seen in the RAO/prone position. An upper GI study is more sensitive than endoscopy for diagnosis.

  On an esophagram or an upper GI study, most symptomatic rings do not allow passage of a 13 mm barium tablet.
- The differential of circumferential esophageal constriction includes:

> Focal stricture.
> Muscular esophageal ring above the GE junction (also known as an A ring).
> Esophageal cancer (associated with irregular mucosal contour and an *apple-core* appearance).
> Esophageal web (rarely circumferential, usually in cervical esophagus).

- Schatzki环是指远端食管的B(黏膜)环呈局部病理性狭窄，直径小于13mm，导致间歇性吞咽困难。

  无症状的B环狭窄被称为下食管环。
- 关键的影像学特征是近胃食管交界处的局部、菲薄的环形缩窄，几乎都伴食管裂孔疝，右前斜/俯卧位显示最好。上消化道造影比内镜检查对诊断更敏感。

  在食管或上消化道造影中，大多数有症状的Schatzki环无法容纳直径为13mm的钡片通过。
- 环状食管缩窄的鉴别诊断包括：

> 局部缩窄。
> 胃食管交界处上方的食管肌环(也被称为A环)。
> 食管癌(伴有不规则的黏膜轮廓和苹果核外观)。
> 食管蹼(环状罕见，通常位于颈段食管)。

Esophagitis

Reflux (peptic) esophagitis

- Reflux (peptic) esophagitis is caused by gastroesophageal reflux leading to the exposure of the esophageal mucosa to acidic gastric secretions, which may lead to distal ulcerations and eventual stricture as well as the development of Barrett's esophagus.
- Peptic esophagitis is most commonly caused by an incompetent lower esophageal sphincter but may also be seen in:

  Zollinger-Ellison syndrome, due to increased acid production.

  Scleroderma, due to gastroesophageal sphincter fibrosis and resultant incompetence.
- Fluoroscopic findings of reflux esophagitis are usually seen in the distal esophagus and are best demonstrated on double-contrast images. These findings include:

  Mucosal granularity.

  Thickened folds.

  Erosions (may be solitary or multiple, typically on posterior wall).

  Strictures.

食管炎

反流性(消化性)食管炎

- 反流性(消化性)食管炎是由于胃食管反流导致食管黏膜直接接触酸性胃分泌物，从而可导致远端食管溃疡，并最终形成狭窄并发展为巴雷特食管。
- 消化性食管炎最常见的原因是食管下括约肌功能不全，但也可见于：

  佐林格-埃利森综合征(胃泌素瘤)，由于胃酸产生过多所致。

  硬皮病，胃食管括约肌纤维化并导致功能不全。
- 透视下反流性食管炎的表现通常在食管的远端，气钡双重对比造影显示最佳。这些表现包括：

  颗粒样黏膜。

  皱襞增粗。

  溃疡(可单发或多发，典型位于后壁)。

  狭窄。

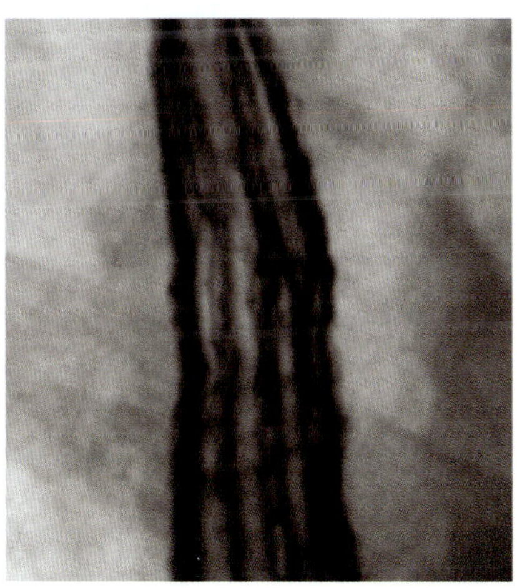

Thickened esophageal folds in reflux esophagitis.
反流性食管炎时出现的食管皱襞增厚。

Barrett's esophagus

巴雷特食管

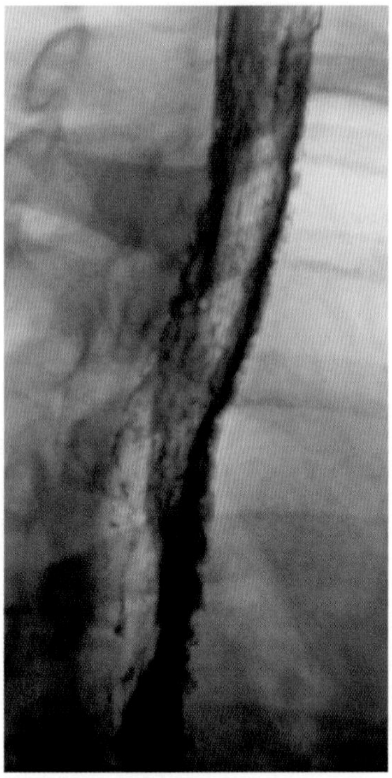

Candida esophagitis: Spot image from double-contrast esophagram shows a diffuse, shaggy appearance to the entire visualized esophagus, consistent with severe candida esophagitis. *Case courtesy of Cheryl Sadow, MD, Brigham and Women's Hospital.*

念珠菌性食管炎：双重对比食管点片显示食管呈弥漫、粗糙的外观，与重度念珠菌性食管炎一致。

- An important long-term sequela of peptic esophagitis is Barrett's esophagus, which is metaplasia of normal squamous epithelium to gastric-type adenomatous mucosa. Barrett's esophagus is a precursor lesion to esophageal adenocarcinoma.
- Nearly 10% of patients with reflux esophagitis may have some adenomatous metaplasia.
- On double-contrast fluoroscopy, Barrett's esophagus demonstrates a reticular (web-like) mucosal pattern, often with a segmental stricture in the mid-esophagus.
- Barrett's esophagus is often associated with esophageal stricture, which is abnormally high in location compared to a peptic stricture.

- 消化性食管炎的一个重要远期后遗症是巴雷特食管，即正常鳞状上皮化生为胃型腺瘤样黏膜。巴雷特食管是食管癌的一种癌前病变。
- 约10%的反流性食管炎患者可能会有一定程度的腺瘤样化生。
- 巴雷特食管在气钡双重对比造影上，黏膜呈网状(蜘蛛网)结构，常在食管的中部有一段狭窄。
- 巴雷特食管通常伴有食管狭窄，与消化性狭窄相比，其位置异常高。

Infectious esophagitis

- Although radiographic distinction between types of infections has been described, endoscopy and biopsy are typically performed in clinical practice to differentiate.
- **Esophageal candidiasis** can present as a spectrum from scattered plaque-like lesions in mild disease to very shaggy-appearing esophagus in severe cases.
- **Herpes esophagitis** typically causes small, discrete ulcerations scattered randomly throughout the esophagus.
- **CMV/HIV esophagitis** characteristically causes a large, flat, ovoid ulcer.

感染性食管炎

- 尽管有报道采用影像学检查区分不同类型的感染，但实际临床通常使用内镜和活检。
- **食管念珠菌感染**可有一系列不同的表现，从病情较轻的散在斑块样病变到严重病例中的极度毛糙的食管。
- **疱疹性食管炎**通常导致小而离散的溃疡，随机散布于整个食管。
- **CMV/HIV食管炎**的典型表现为大而扁平的卵圆形溃疡。

Medication esophagitis

- Medication-induced esophagitis occurs secondary to pills being stuck in areas of relative narrowing, classically at level of aortic arch or distal esophagus, resulting in erosions.

药物性食管炎

- 药物引起的食管炎继发于药片卡在相对狭窄的区域，进而导致溃烂，典型的部位是主动脉弓水平或食管的远端。

Crohn's esophagitis

- Crohn's esophagitis is very rare and is usually seen in the setting of severe disease throughout the small bowel and colon.
- Aphthous ulcers (discrete ulcers surrounded by mounds of edema) may become confluent.

克罗恩食管炎

- 克罗恩食管炎非常罕见，常出现在病变严重并累及所有小肠及结肠的情况下。
- 鹅口疮样溃疡(散在溃疡周边环以丘形水肿)可相互融合。

Eosinophilic esophagitis

- Eosinophilic esophagitis is an idiopathic inflammatory disorder characterized by activation of eosinophils within the wall of the esophagus leading to strictures, webs, and spasm. This often presents with food impaction.
- The appearance is of concentric mucosal ring-like strictures.

Chemotherapy-associated mucositis

- Certain chemotherapy agents can cause oropharyngeal mucositis, which may extend to the esophagus. This can lead to severe odynodysphagia, subsequent dehydration and malnutrition.
- While the condition is usually self-limited, it can last weeks to months.

嗜酸性食管炎

- 嗜酸性食管炎是一种特发性炎症性疾病，特征是食管壁内嗜酸性粒细胞的活化导致狭窄、食管蹼和痉挛。常表现为食物嵌塞。
- 外观为黏膜同心性环状狭窄。

化疗相关黏膜炎

- 某些化疗药物可引起口咽黏膜炎，可能延伸至食管。这会导致严重的吞咽困难，随后引起脱水和营养不良。
- 尽管这种情况通常是自限性的，但可持续数周到数月。

Esophageal strictures

Peptic stricture

- As previously discussed, a peptic stricture is secondary to chronic reflux.
- Peptic strictures are located distally, usually just above GE junction, and may be focal or involve a longer segment of the esophagus. Fibrosis can cause esophageal shortening, leading to a hiatal hernia as the stomach is pulled into the thorax.

Barrett's esophagus stricture

- A Barrett's stricture typically occurs in the mid-esophagus above the metaplastic adenomatous transition because adenomatous tissue is acid-resistant and therefore unaffected by gastric secretions.

Malignant stricture (due to esophageal carcinoma)

食管狭窄

消化性狭窄

- 如前所述，消化性狭窄继发于慢性反流。
- 消化性狭窄位于食管的远端，通常在胃食管交界处的稍上方，可以为局灶性或累及一段较长的食管。纤维化可引起食管缩短，当胃被拉入胸腔时可导致食管裂孔疝。

巴雷特食管狭窄

- 巴雷特食管狭窄通常发生在腺瘤样化生移行区上方的中段食管，这是因为腺瘤样组织耐酸，因此不受胃分泌物影响。

恶性狭窄(食管癌所致)

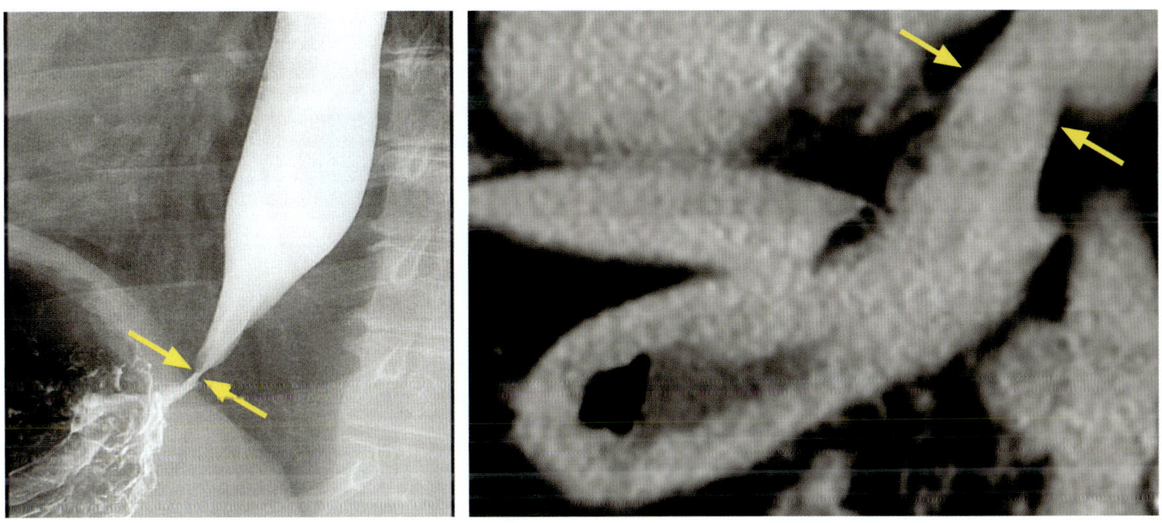

Barium swallow (left image) demonstrates abrupt narrowing (arrows) of the distal esophagus with subtle mucosal irregularity. Sagittal CT (right image) shows mass-like soft tissue thickening in the same region.
钡餐(左图)显示食管远端陡然狭窄(黄箭)，伴有不太明显的黏膜不规则。矢状位CT(右图)显示同一区域肿块样软组织增厚。

- The key imaging finding is irregular narrowing with shouldered margins (*apple-core* appearance).

Caustic stricture / nasogastric tube stricture

- Both caustic strictures and strictures secondary to nasogastric tube placement are typically long, smooth, and narrow.
- Strictures develop 1–3 months after the causative event.
- Caustic strictures are associated with an increased risk of cancer with a long lag time of up to 20 years after the initial insult. Caustic strictures are usually

- 主要影像学表现为不规则狭窄伴肩状边缘(苹果核表现)。

腐蚀性狭窄/鼻饲管狭窄

- 腐蚀性狭窄和鼻饲管插入后引起的狭窄通常都为长而光整的狭窄。
- 狭窄出现在诱发事件后的1~3个月。
- 腐蚀性狭窄者患癌的风险升高，其潜伏期长，可在初始受损后20年出现。腐蚀性狭窄通常

longer than peptic strictures.

Radiation stricture

- Like caustic strictures, radiation strictures are long, smooth and narrow and occur in the radiation field.
- It generally requires more than 50 Gy of radiation to cause an esophageal stricture.
- Acute radiation esophagitis occurs 1–4 weeks after radiation therapy. Radiation strictures develop later, about 4–8 months after radiation.

Extrinsic compression from mediastinal adenopathy

- Cross-sectional imaging with CT or MRI is best to evaluate if extrinsic compression is suspected.

较消化性狭窄长。

放射性狭窄

- 与腐蚀性狭窄类似，放射性狭窄长而平滑，并发生在照射区域。
- 辐射剂量通常需要超过50Gy时才会引起食管狭窄。
- 急性放射性食管炎发生在放疗后的1~4周。放射性狭窄则较晚发生，在放疗后的4~8个月。

纵隔淋巴结肿大引起的外部压迫

- 使用CT或MRI进行轴位成像是评估是否存在外源性压迫的最佳方法。

Evaluation of Esophageal Masses

- Masses arising from the mucosa, submucosa, and extrinsic to the esophagus produce characteristic effects on the esophagus, which are usually able to be seen on imaging.
- Lesions arising from the mucosa create an *acute* angle relative to the adjacent wall, whereas the submucosal lesions create an *obtuse* angle as demonstrated below.

食管肿块的评估

- 起源于黏膜、黏膜下层和食管外的肿块会对食管产生特征性影响，而这些影响通常在影像学上有所反映。
- 起源于黏膜的病变与相邻管壁形成一个锐角，而黏膜下病变则形成一个钝角，如下所示。

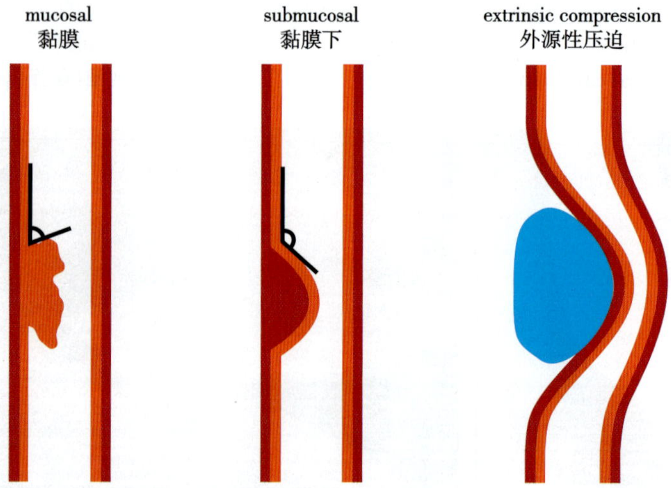

Benign Esophageal Masses

Mesenchymal tumor

- Benign mesenchymal tumors are the most common *submucosal* esophageal tumors and include leiomyoma, lipoma, hemangioma, and others. Leiomyomas are the most common. On a barium swallow, a mesenchymal tumor typically appears as smooth, round, submucosal filling defect.
- Compared to esophageal leiomyomas, esophageal gastrointestinal stromal tumors (GIST) are rare and may be benign or malignant. In contrast, GISTs are more common than leiomyomas in the stomach.

Adenoma

- An esophageal adenoma is a benign mucosal lesion with malignant potential, usually arising within Barrett's esophagus and appears as a filling defect (most <1.5 cm in size) with acute margins on esophagram.

良性食管肿瘤

间叶性肿瘤

- 良性间叶性肿瘤是最常见的食管黏膜下肿瘤，包括平滑肌瘤、脂肪瘤、血管瘤等，其中平滑肌瘤最常见。钡餐检查中，间叶性肿瘤通常表现为光滑圆形的黏膜下充盈缺损。
- 与食管平滑肌瘤相比，食管的胃肠道间质瘤(GIST)罕见，可为良性也可为恶性。相比之下，胃的GIST比平滑肌瘤更常见。

腺瘤

- 食管腺瘤是一种良性黏膜病变，有恶变潜能，通常发生于巴雷特食管，食管造影上表现为呈锐角的充盈缺损(大部分直径<1.5cm)。

Fibrovascular polyp

- A fibrovascular polyp is a pedunculated mass composed of mesenchymal elements with a significant fatty component. In contrast to an esophageal adenoma, there is no malignant potential.
- Fibrovascular polyps usually occur in the cervical esophagus where they gradually elongate. Clinical presentation can be dramatic with regurgitation of a fleshy mass.
- CT is usually diagnostic demonstrating an intralesional fatty component.

纤维血管性息肉

- 纤维血管性息肉是一个带蒂的肿块，由间叶组织和丰富的脂肪成分构成。与食管腺瘤不同，无恶变潜能。
- 纤维血管性息肉常出现在颈段食管，并在此被逐渐拉长。临床表现有时极其夸张：可呕出一团鲜肉。
- CT通常可以进行诊断，表现为病灶内含脂肪成分。

Inflammatory polyp

- An inflammatory polyp is a non-neoplastic, enlarged gastric mucosal fold that protrudes up into the lower esophagus. Inflammatory polyps are almost always associated with reflux and must be contiguous with a gastric fold.

炎性息肉

- 炎性息肉是非肿瘤性的、增大的胃皱襞并向上突入食管的下段。炎性息肉几乎均与反流有关，且都与胃皱襞相连。

Varices

静脉曲张

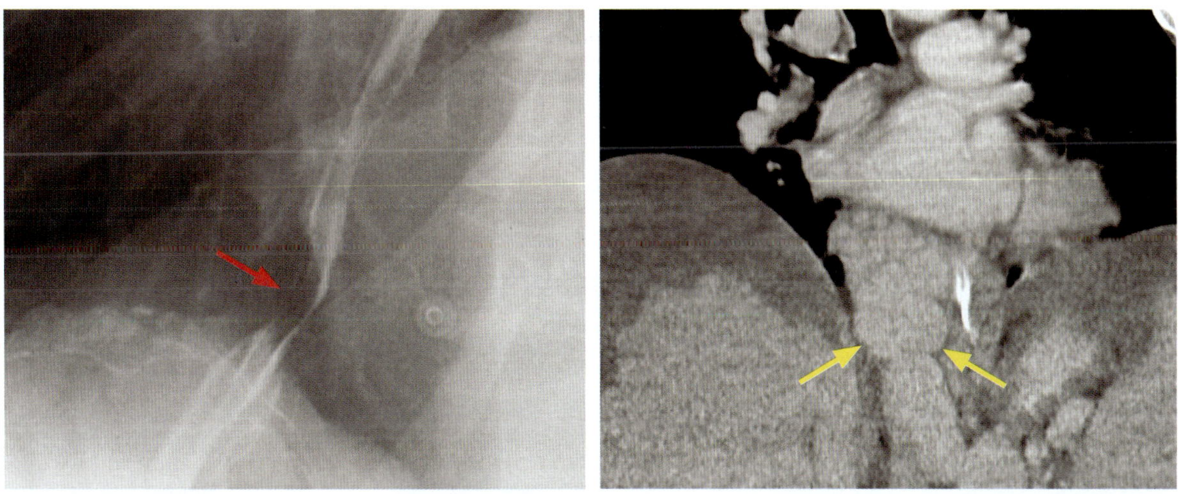

Barium esophagram (left image) demonstrates oblique extrinsic impression along the left anterolateral distal esophagus (red arrow). Coronal contrast-enhanced CT (right image) demonstrates extensive bulky esophageal varices. Note this patient also has cirrhotic liver with ascites, presumably the etiology of portal hypertension.

食管钡餐造影(左图)显示远端食管沿左前外侧的斜形外部压迹(红箭)。冠状位增强CT(右图)显示广泛的大块食管静脉曲张。注意该患者还伴有肝硬化和腹水，原因可能是门静脉高压。

- Varices can usually be distinguished from a solid mass on fluoroscopy since varices change in size and shape with peristalsis and Valsalva maneuver. However, thrombosed varices may mimic a tumor.
- *Uphill* varices are most common, due to portal hypertension, affecting the distal esophagus.

  Blood flows "uphill" from the portal vein → left gastric (coronary vein) → periesophageal venous plexus → azygos/hemiazygos collaterals → SVC.
- *Downhill* varices are less common, due to superior vena cava obstruction, usually affecting the proximal esophagus.

  Enlarged collateral vessels include the supreme intercostal veins (drain the first intercostal space), bronchial veins, and inferior thyroidal veins.

- 在透视上静脉曲张通常可与实性肿块进行区分，因静脉曲张随食管蠕动或瓦尔萨尔瓦动作可改变大小和形状。但是，栓塞后的静脉曲张可类似于肿瘤。
- 上行性静脉曲张，由门静脉高压所致，累及远端食管。

  血流自门静脉上行→胃左(冠状静脉)静脉→食管周围静脉丛→奇/半奇静脉丛→上腔静脉。
- 下行性静脉曲张较少见，为上腔静脉阻塞所致，通常累及近端食管。

  增粗的侧支血管包括最上肋间静脉(引流第一肋间隙)、支气管静脉和甲状腺下静脉等。

Foregut duplication cysts

- **Esophageal duplication cysts** are lined with squamous epithelium, have a smooth muscle wall, and are usually in the posterior mediastinum. They may be either extrinsic to the esophagus or submucosal; the latter is impossible to differentiate from a leiomyoma by esophagram.

前肠重复囊肿

- **食管重复囊肿**内衬鳞状上皮，具有光滑的肌壁，且通常位于后纵隔，既可位于食管外，也可以位于黏膜下，后者在食管造影时无法与平滑肌瘤相鉴别。

- **Bronchogenic cysts** are lined by respiratory epithelium and are usually in the middle mediastinum. They are generally indistinguishable from an esophageal duplication cyst on esophagram and CT.
- **Neurenteric cysts** are associated with vertebral body anomalies.

Esophageal foreign body

- A radiopaque esophageal foreign body is best visualized with a lateral radiograph or CT.
- Bony foreign objects usually get stuck in the cervical esophagus.
- Meat impaction usually occurs at the gastroesophageal junction. There is a risk of esophageal perforation from transmural ischemia if the food bolus is impacted for >24 hours. Most cases of food bolus impaction are treated with endoscopic removal of the impacted food.

- **支气管源性囊肿**内衬呼吸道上皮并通常位于中纵隔，在食管造影和CT上通常无法与食管重复囊肿相鉴别。
- **神经肠源性囊肿**与椎体异常相关。

食管异物

- 不透射线的食管异物的最佳显示方式是侧位X线影像或CT。
- 骨性异物通常卡在食管的颈段。
- 食物嵌顿通常发生于胃食管交界处。食物团嵌顿超过24小时可造成透壁性缺血而增加发生食管穿孔的风险。大多数病例可以用内镜清除嵌顿的食物。

MALIGNANT ESOPHAGEAL MASSES

恶性食管肿瘤

Esophageal carcinoma

食管癌

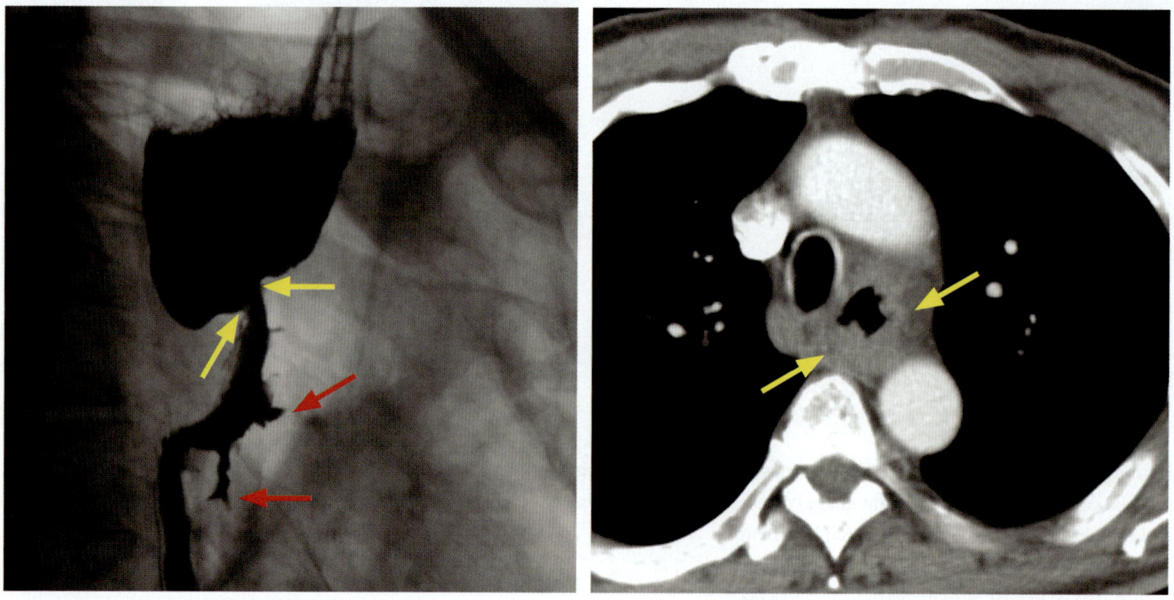

Esophageal carcinoma: Oblique fluoroscopic spot image from a barium swallow (left image) shows an irregular stricture (yellow arrows) with proximal dilation of the esophagus. Two linear ulcerations (red arrows) project into the mural mass.
Contrast-enhanced axial CT (right image) shows irregular thickening of the esophagus (arrows).
Case courtesy of Cheryl Sadow, MD, Brigham and Women's Hospital
食管癌：斜位钡餐透视点片(左图)显示近段食管不规则狭窄(黄箭)及狭窄上方的食管扩张。两个线样溃疡(红箭)突入壁内的肿块。
轴位增强CT(右图)显示食管不规则增厚(黄箭)。

- Esophageal carcinoma has a broad range of appearances. Early esophageal cancer may be apparent on barium swallow as a plaque-like lesion, polypoid lesion, or focal irregularity of the esophageal wall. A classic appearance of advanced esophageal carcinoma is a mass causing a stricture with a "shouldered" edge and irregular contour (*apple-core* appearance).

  The uncommon varicoid appearance can be confused with varices, but the tumor does not change shape with peristaltic waves as varices typically do.
- Esophageal carcinoma may be squamous cell carcinoma (SCC) or adenocarcinoma. These cannot be reliably differentiated by imaging, although SCC tends to involve the upper or mid-esophagus and adenocarcinoma typically involves the distal esophagus and may extend into the stomach.
- SCC is most commonly due to smoking and alcohol. Less common risk factors

- 食管癌的表现极其多样。早期食管癌在钡餐中可能表现为斑块样或息肉样病变，或食管壁局灶性不规整。进展期食管癌的典型表现为肿块所致的狭窄，具有“肩膀状”边和不规则的轮廓(苹果核表现)。

  少见的静脉曲张样表现可与静脉曲张混淆，但肿瘤并不会因蠕动波而改变形状，而静脉曲张则通常都有改变。
- 食管癌可以是鳞状细胞癌(SCC)或腺癌，它们在影像学上不能进行可靠区分，尽管SCC倾向于累及食管的上段或中段，而腺癌通常累及食管的远端并可以蔓延至胃部。

include celiac disease, Plummer-Vinson syndrome, achalasia, and human papilloma virus (more commonly causes laryngeal SCC).

- Adenocarcinoma usually arises from Barrett's esophagus and is due to chronic reflux. The incidence has been rising in recent years.

- SCC最常由吸烟和酗酒引起。少见的危险因素包括乳糜泻、缺铁性吞咽困难综合征、贲门失弛症及人乳头状瘤病毒(更常引起喉部SCC)。
- 腺癌常起源于巴雷特食管，为慢性反流所致，其发病率近年来持续上升。

Metastasis

- Direct invasion of the esophagus is most commonly from gastric, lung, or breast primaries. Hematogenous spread is very rare.
- Most often, mediastinal lymph node metastases will be prominent. The mid-esophagus is most commonly affected due to its proximity to mediastinal lymph nodes.

转移

- 最常直接侵犯食管的原发肿瘤来自胃、肺或乳腺。血行播散非常罕见。
- 大多数情况下，纵隔淋巴结已经有明显移转。中段食管最常受累，因此处与纵隔淋巴结距离很近。

Lymphoma

- Esophageal lymphoma is often indistinguishable from primary esophageal cancer.

淋巴瘤

- 食管淋巴瘤通常无法与原发性食管癌进行鉴别。

Malignant gastrointestinal stromal tumors

- Malignant GIST is a submucosal mesenchymal tumor which tends to be bulkier and more irregular than the benign variant.

恶性胃肠道间质瘤

- 恶性胃肠道间质瘤是一种黏膜下间质肿瘤，与良性相比体积往往更大且更不规则。

Esophageal motility disorders

食管运动障碍

Contraction waves

收缩波

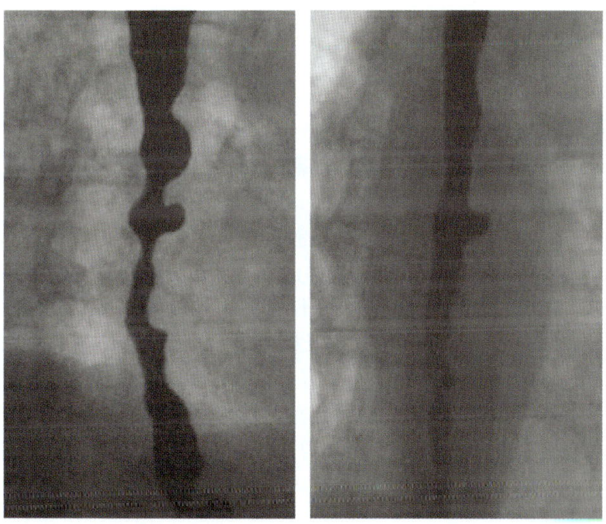

In the left image, tertiary contractions result in moderate delay of contrast passage during the primary swallow, with subsequent reflux of contrast (right image).
左图显示三级收缩波在初始吞咽过程中引起造影剂通过中度延迟，随后有造影剂反流(右图)。

- A primary contraction wave is a normal, physiologic wave initiated by a swallow.
- A secondary contraction wave is a normal, physiologic wave initiated by a bolus in the esophagus.
- A tertiary wave is a non-propulsive contraction that does not result in esophageal clearing. Tertiary contractions are seen more commonly in the elderly.

- 初级收缩波是正常的、由吞咽动作引发的生理性波型。
- 次级收缩波是由食管内食团引发的一种正常的生理性收缩波。
- 三级波是一种无推动作用的收缩，并不引起食管清除作用。三级收缩波更常见于老年人。

Achalasia

贲门失迟症

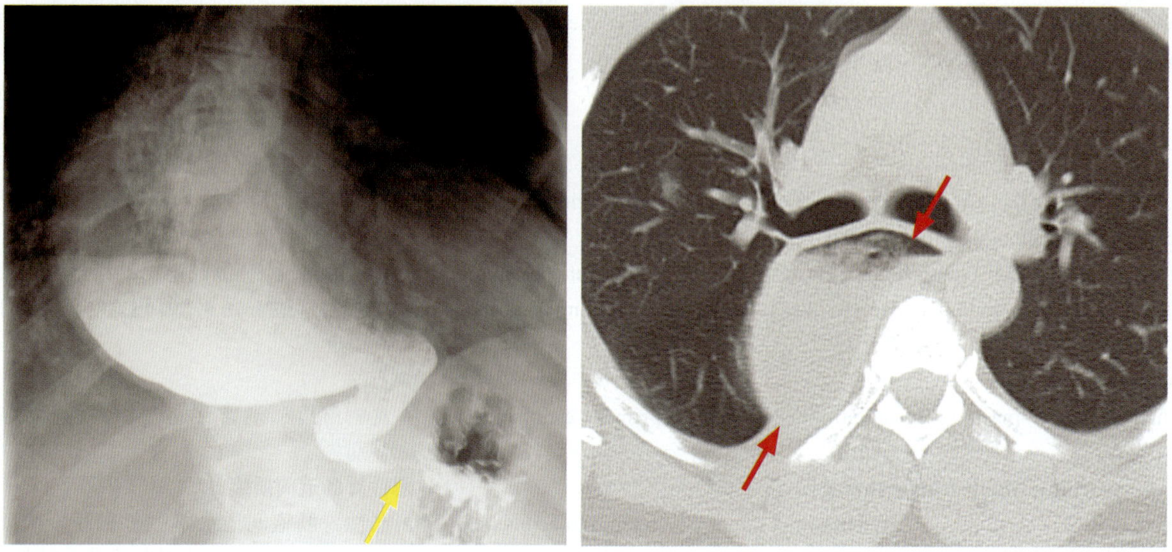

Achalasia: Fluoroscopic spot image from an upper GI series (left image) shows a markedly dilated esophagus terminating in a *bird's beak* (yellow arrow) at the GE junction, due to failure of the distal esophageal sphincter to relax. Axial non-contrast CT confirms the markedly dilated, debris-filled esophagus (red arrows).
贲门失弛症：上消化道造影透视点片(左图)显示明显扩张的食管，以鸟嘴样(黄箭)止于胃食管交界处，为末端食管括约肌不能松弛所致。轴位平扫CT(右图)证实食管显著扩张，充满食糜(红箭)。

- Achalasia is a motility disorder resulting from the inability of the distal esophagus to relax because of abnormal myenteric ganglia in the Auerbach plexus. **Vigorous achalasia** is a less severe form of achalasia consisting of repetitive non-propulsive contractions.
- Chagas disease causes a secondary achalasia that is indistinguishable radiographically from primary achalasia.
- Complications of chronic achalasia include esophageal cancer, which has a lag period of at least 20 years, and candidal infection from stasis.
- The classic imaging appearance of achalasia is a massively dilated esophagus with a *bird's beak* stricture near the gastroesophageal junction.
- Treatment options include physical disruption of the lower esophageal sphincter by pneumatic dilatation, surgical myotomy (Heller myotomy), or peroral endoscopic myotomy (POEM), and pharmacologic interventions such as botulinum toxin injection.
- **Pseudoachalasia** is caused by an obstructing gastroesophageal junction cancer mimicking primary achalasia. These can be differentiated on fluoroscopy because in achalasia there is eventual transient relaxation of the narrowing when the patient stands but the fixed obstruction of pseudoachalasia will not relax with standing.

- 贲门失弛症是由于肌间神经丛中的肠肌层神经节异常导致食管远端不能放松而引起的一种运动障碍。**强力型痉挛性贲门失弛症(一种早期的形式)**是一种程度相对较轻的贲门失弛症，表现为反复而无推动作用的食管收缩。
- 美洲锥虫病引起的继发性贲门失弛症在影像学上无法与原发性贲门失弛症相鉴别。
- 慢性贲门失弛症的并发症包括食管癌(潜伏期至少20年)，以及积食所致的念珠菌感染。
- 贲门失弛症的典型影像表现是食管显著扩张，并在胃食管连接处附近出现的鸟嘴样狭窄。
- 治疗方案包括通过气囊扩张对低段食管括约肌进行物理性破坏、外科肌切开术(黑勒贲门肌切开术)或经口内镜肌切开术(POEM)，以及注射肉毒毒素等药物干预。
- **假性贲门失弛症**是由胃食管交界处的癌症所致，类似于原发性失弛缓的梗阻。该病可通过透视鉴别，因为贲门失弛症患者站立时最终可见狭窄处有一过性松弛，而在假性贲门失弛症患者中，固定的梗阻不会在站立位时发生松动。

Scleroderma

- Scleroderma is a systemic disease involving excess collagen deposition in multiple tissues.
- The esophagus is involved in 80% of patients with scleroderma, producing lack of peristalsis of the distal 2/3 of the esophagus due to smooth muscle atrophy and fibrosis, which leads to marked esophageal dilation.
- Secondary candidiasis or aspiration pneumonia can result from prolonged

硬皮病

- 硬皮病是一种全身性疾病，涉及胶原在多个组织中过量沉积。
- 约80%的硬皮病患者累及食管，由于平滑肌萎缩和纤维化会导致食管远端2/3缺乏蠕动，从而导致食管明显扩张。
- 长期食管淤滞可引起继发性念珠菌病或吸入

esophageal stasis.

- The esophageal dilation is often apparent before the typical skin changes of scleroderma become evident.

Diffuse esophageal spasm

性肺炎。

- 食管扩张通常在硬皮病的典型皮肤变化显现之前就已经明显。

弥漫性食管痉挛

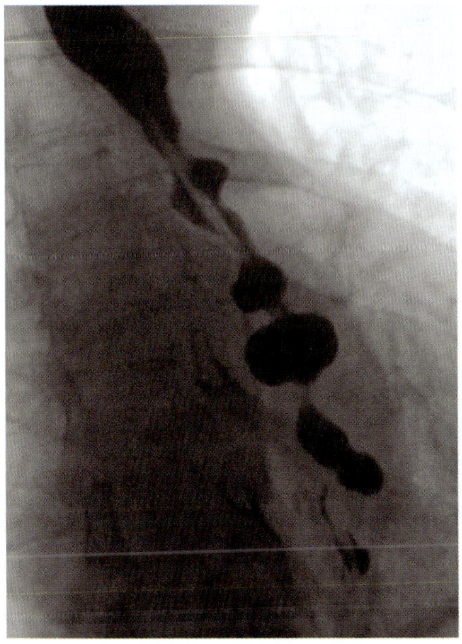

Single-contrast esophagram demonstrates delayed passage of barium through the esophagus, with multiple tertiary contractions in a corkscrew configuration, and subsequent esophageal reflux (not shown).
单一钡餐食管造影显示钡剂通过食管延迟，出现多个螺旋状三级收缩波，随后出现食管反流(未展示)。

- Diffuse esophageal spasm is a clinical syndrome of chest pain or dysphagia caused by repetitive, non-propulsive esophageal contractions. The non-propulsive contractions have a characteristic appearance on barium swallow leading to the descriptive name of *corkscrew esophagus*.

- 弥漫性食管痉挛是一种表现为胸痛或吞咽困难的临床综合征，由重复而无推动作用的食管收缩所致。无推动作用的收缩在钡餐透视上有特征性的表现，被描述为*螺旋样食管*。

ESOPHAGEAL DIVERTICULA

食管憩室

Types of diverticula

憩室类型

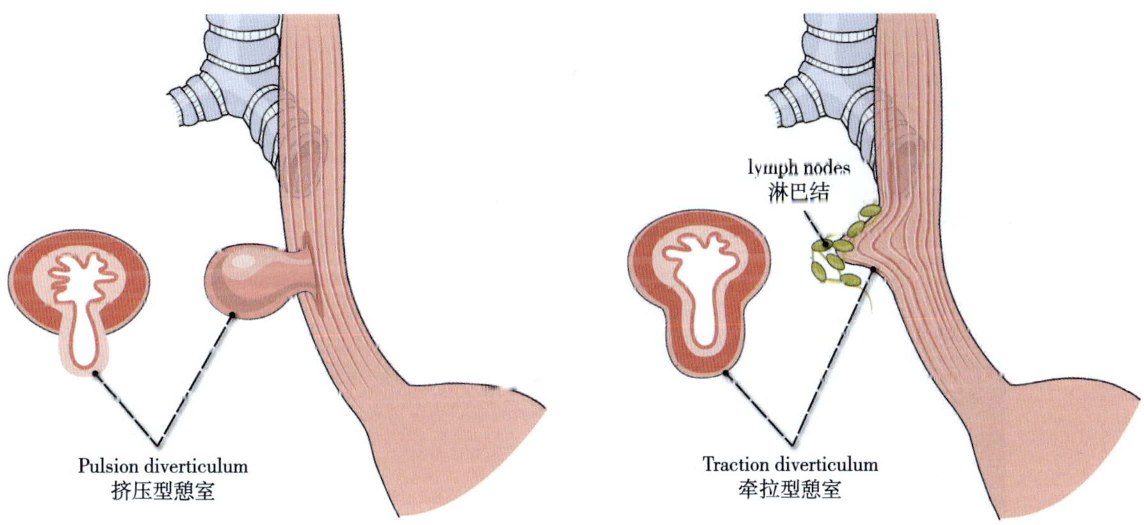

- **Pulsion diverticula** are caused by increased esophageal pressure, they usually occur near the GE junction, and comprise nearly all diverticula seen in the United States.
- **Traction diverticula** are caused by external traction by mediastinal inflammation adhering to the esophagus with associated lymphadenopathy, usually in the

- **挤压型憩室**是因食管内压力增加所致，通常发生在胃食管交界处附近，几乎所有在美国见到的憩室均为此型。
- **牵拉型憩室**是由食管外纵隔炎症及相关的淋巴结病变与食管粘连牵拉所致，通常在食管

mid-esophagus. They occurred in the past when TB and other infections were more prevalent and are rarely seen today.

中部。在过去结核病和其他感染疾病流行时该类型较为普遍，而现在很少见到。

Zenker diverticulum

咽食管憩室

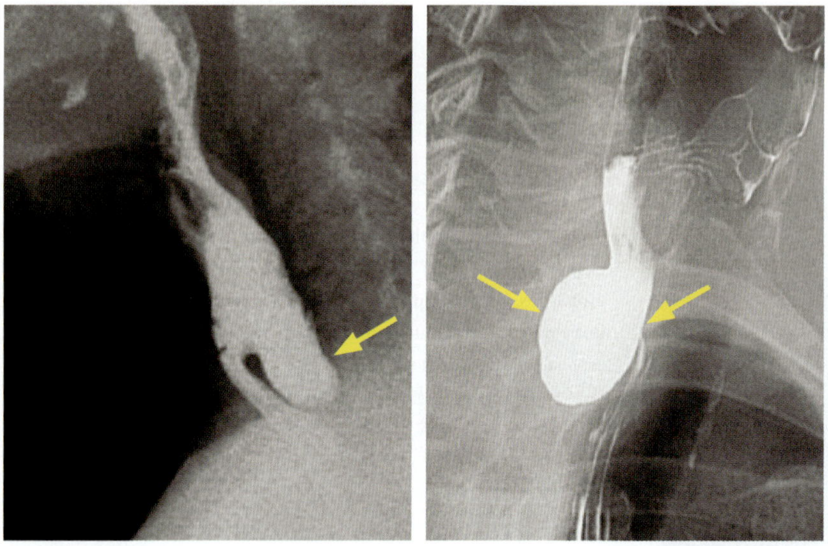

Lateral and right anterior oblique barium esophagram images demonstrate contrast filling a blind-ending pouch (arrows) arising posteriorly from the pharyngoesophageal junction at level of C5, in keeping with a Zenker diverticulum.

食管侧位和右前斜位钡餐造影显示在C_5水平咽食管连接处后方的一个充满造影剂的盲袋(黄箭)，此为咽食管憩室。

- Zenker diverticulum is caused by failure of the cricopharyngeus muscle to relax, leading to elevated hypopharyngeal pressure and resultant outpouching.
- Symptoms of a Zenker diverticulum include halitosis, aspiration, and regurgitation of undigested food.
- A Zenker diverticulum is located in the hypopharynx, just above the upper esophageal sphincter (cricopharyngeus muscle) and is posteriorly protruding. The cricopharyngeus muscle is usually hypertrophied.
- A Zenker diverticulum is best seen on a lateral view.

- 咽食管憩室是由于环咽肌不能松弛而导致下咽压力升高，继而发生膨出。
- 咽食管憩室的症状包括口臭、误吸入及未消化食物的反流。
- 咽食管憩室位于下咽，直接与上食管括约肌(环咽肌)的上方相邻并向后突出；环咽肌通常肥大。
- 咽食管憩室最好在侧位上进行观察。

Killian-Jamieson (KJ) diverticulum

Killian-Jamieson(KJ)憩室

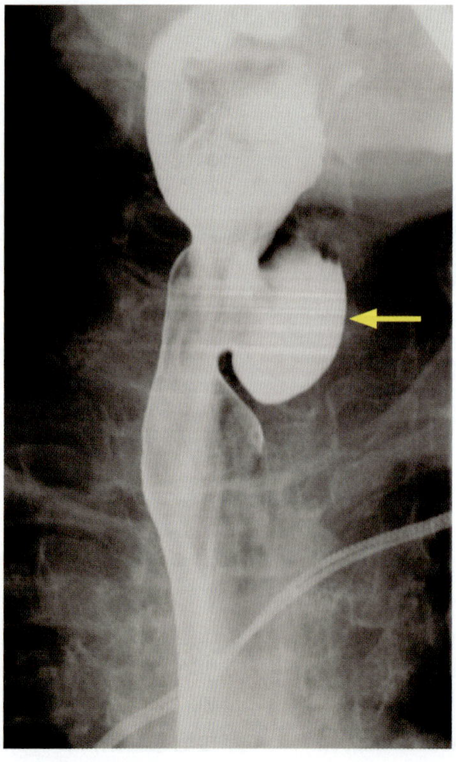

Frontal view from a barium esophagram shows a 3 cm Killian-Jamieson diverticulum on the left (arrow).

正位食管钡餐造影显示位于左侧的一个3cm的KJ憩室(黄箭)。

- A Killian-Jamieson (KJ) diverticulum is located in the proximal cervical esophagus, at the Killian-Jamieson space, which is an area of weakness below the attachment of the cricopharyngeus muscle.
- A KJ diverticulum protrudes anterolaterally, best seen on the AP view and is more often bilateral.
- KJ diverticula are less commonly seen than a Zenker's diverticulum. Both are false diverticula. In contrast to a true diverticulum, a false diverticulum does not involve the muscular or adventitial layers.

Pseudodiverticulosis

- Pseudodiverticulosis is the imaging finding of multiple tiny outpouchings into the esophageal lumen caused by dilated submucosal glands from chronic reflux esophagitis. These submucosal glands are analogous to the Rokitansky-Aschoff sinuses of the gallbladder.
- Pseudodiverticulosis is often associated with a smooth stricture in the mid/upper esophagus, which may cause symptoms.
- Candida is frequently cultured, but infection is not believed to be the causal factor.

- Killian-Jamieson (KJ)憩室位于颈段食管近端的Killian-Jamieson区，此为环咽肌附着处下方的薄弱区。
- KJ憩室向前外侧突出，常为双侧，在正位观察最佳。
- KJ憩室较咽食管憩室少见，两者都属于假性憩室。与真性憩室相比，假性憩室不累及食管肌层或外膜层。

假憩室病

- 假憩室病影像学表现为向食管腔内多发微小的突起，为慢性反流性食管炎造成的黏膜下腺体增大所致。这些黏膜下腺体类似于胆囊的罗-阿窦。
- 假憩室病通常伴发中/上段食管的平滑狭窄，并可能引起症状。
- 常可以培养出念珠菌，但感染并不被认为是一种致病因素。

MISCELLANEOUS ESOPHAGEAL DISORDERS

其他食管疾病

Feline esophagus

猫食管

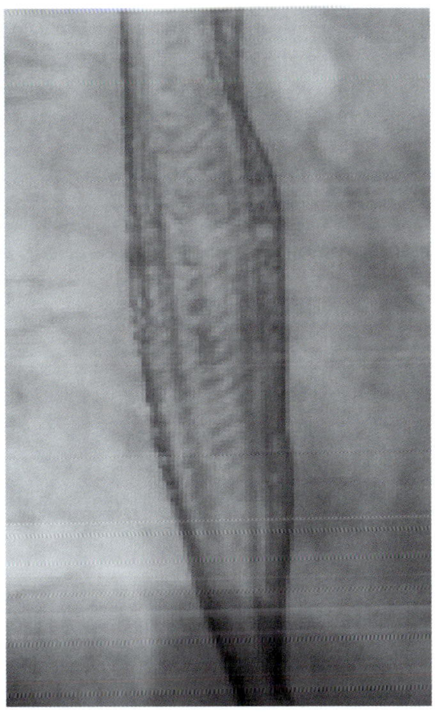

Feline esophagus: Spot image from double-contrast esophagram shows characteristic multiple transverse folds in the lower esophagus.
Case courtesy Cheryl Sadow, MD, Brigham and Women's Hospital.
猫食管：食管气钡双重造影点片显示下段食管典型的多发横行皱襞。

- Feline esophagus is thought to be a normal variant characterized by multiple thin transverse esophageal folds.
- There is a controversial association with esophagitis, where the incidence of esophagitis may be increased in the presence of feline esophagus.
- Compared to eosinophilic esophagitis, the circumferential folds in feline esophagus are thinner.

- 猫食管可能是一种正常变异，特征为多发、菲薄的横向食管皱襞。
- 与食管炎的关系尚存在争议，但在有猫食管时食管炎的发病概率会增加。
- 与嗜酸性食管炎相比，猫食管的环状皱襞较薄。

Aberrant right subclavian artery　迷走右锁骨下动脉

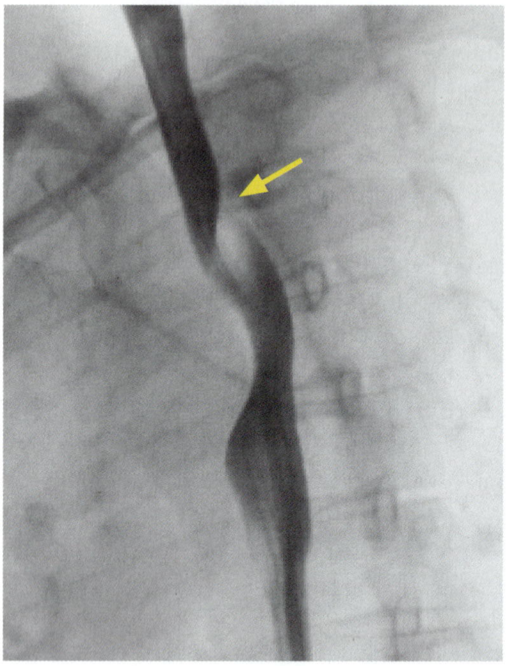

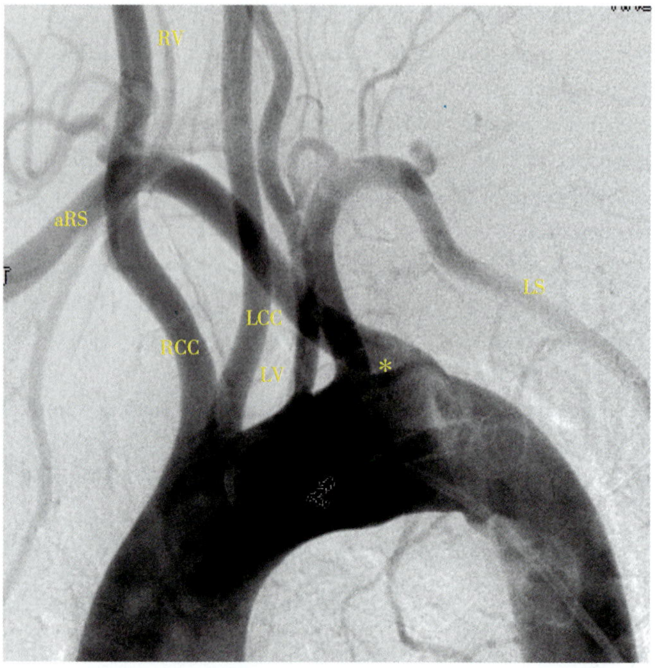

Aberrant right subclavian artery: Oblique single-contrast barium esophagram (left image) demonstrates a smooth posterior indentation of the proximal thoracic esophagus (arrow). Aortogram in the same patient (right image) demonstrates the aberrant right subclavian artery (aRS, * at origin) crossing midline before heading towards the right arm. This patient has an additional aortic branching anomaly, with the left vertebral artery (LV) arising directly from the aorta. The right vertebral artery (RV), arising from the aberrant right subclavian, is hypoplastic. The right and left common carotid arteries (RCC and LCC), and left subclavian (LS) are normal.

Case courtesy Cheryl Sadow, MD, Brigham and Women's Hospital.

迷走锁骨下动脉：斜位单一钡餐食管造影(左图)见胸段食管近端的后方有一个光滑的压迹(黄箭)。同一名患者的主动脉造影(右图)可见迷走右锁骨下动脉(aRS，*为起始部)跨越中线汇入右侧头臂干。该患者还存在另一处主动脉分支异常，即左椎动脉(LV)直接发自于主动脉。右椎动脉(RV)起自迷走右锁骨下动脉，且发育不良。右侧和左侧颈总动脉(RCC和LCC)，和左锁骨下动脉(LS)正常。

- Aberrant right subclavian artery (with a normal left arch) is seen in approximately 1% of patients and is almost always asymptomatic. The aberrant right subclavian artery travels posterior to the esophagus, where it may rarely produce dysphagia.
- On an upper GI study, the resultant posterior esophageal indentation is always smooth.

- 迷走右锁骨下动脉(伴有正常的左位主动脉弓)约见于1%的患者，几乎都无症状。迷走右锁骨下动脉穿过食管后方，偶可引起吞咽困难。
- 在上消化道造影中，相关的食管后方压迹通常是光滑的。

(翻译　张世军)

STOMACH

胃

ANATOMY

解剖

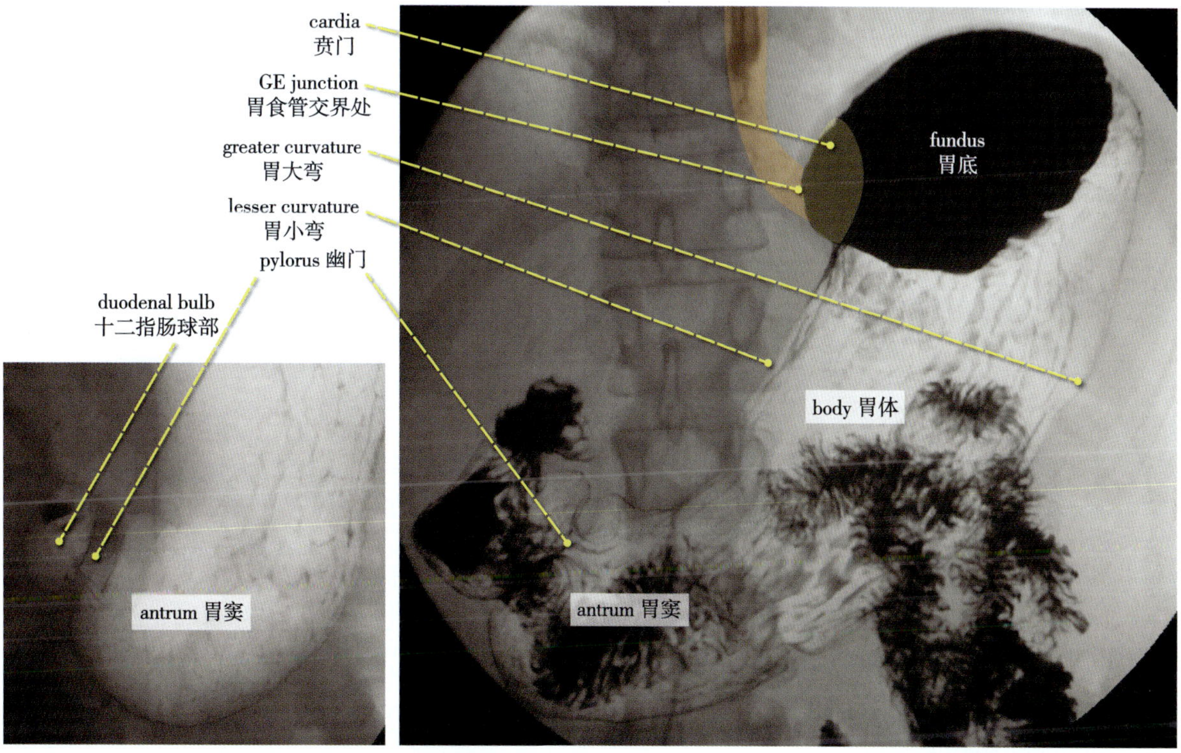

HIATAL HERNIAS

Hiatal hernias

- A hiatal hernia is present when abdominal contents herniate up through the esophageal hiatus into the posterior mediastinum and gastric folds are seen above the diaphragm. There are four types of hiatal hernias, which are managed differently.
- The Society of American Gastrointestinal and Endoscopic Surgeons (SAGES) 2013 guidelines do not recommend surgery for type Ⅰ hernia in the absence of reflux disease. However, all symptomatic paraesophageal hiatal hernias (types Ⅱ–Ⅳ) should be repaired, particularly with acute obstructive symptoms or volvulus.
- **Type Ⅰ–Sliding hiatal hernia** (most common). A sliding hiatal hernia is present when the gastroesophageal junction (GEJ) slides up into the posterior mediastinum and gastric folds are seen above the diaphragm.
- **Type Ⅱ–Paraesophageal with GEJ in normal position** (least common). A type Ⅱ hiatal hernia is herniation of the gastric fundus, with a normally positioned GEJ (below diaphragm).
- **Type Ⅲ–Paraesophageal with GEJ above the diaphragm** (second most common). In a type Ⅱ hiatal hernia, both the GEJ and fundus/body of the stomach protrude into the lower mediastinum.
- **Type Ⅳ–Associated with herniation of other organs above the diaphragm.** A type Ⅳ hiatal hernia is displacement of the stomach and other organs (spleen, pancreas, small bowel, colon) above the diaphragm.

食管裂孔疝

食管裂孔疝

- 食管裂孔疝是指腹腔内容物通过食管裂孔向上突入后纵隔，胃皱襞见于膈肌的上方。有四种类型的食管裂孔疝，它们的处理方法各不相同。
- 美国胃肠内镜和外科学会(SAGES)2013年的指南不建议对无反流的Ⅰ型食管裂孔疝进行手术。但是，对所有有症状的食管旁裂孔疝(Ⅱ~Ⅳ型)都应该进行修补，尤其是患者出现急性梗阻症状或扭转。
- **Ⅰ型——滑动型食管裂孔疝**(最常见)：滑动型食管裂孔疝是指胃食管交界处向上滑入后纵隔，以及胃皱襞位于膈肌的上方。
- **Ⅱ型——食管旁型伴胃食管交界处位置正常**(最少见)：Ⅱ型食管裂孔疝是胃底疝，胃食管交界处位置正常(位于膈下)。
- **Ⅲ型——食管旁型伴胃食管交界处位于膈上**(第二常见)：发生Ⅱ型食管裂孔疝时，胃食管交界处和胃底/胃体都突入下纵隔。
- **Ⅳ型——伴有其他器官疝入膈肌的上方**：Ⅳ型食管裂孔疝是指胃和其他器官(脾、胰腺、小肠、结肠)位于膈肌之上。

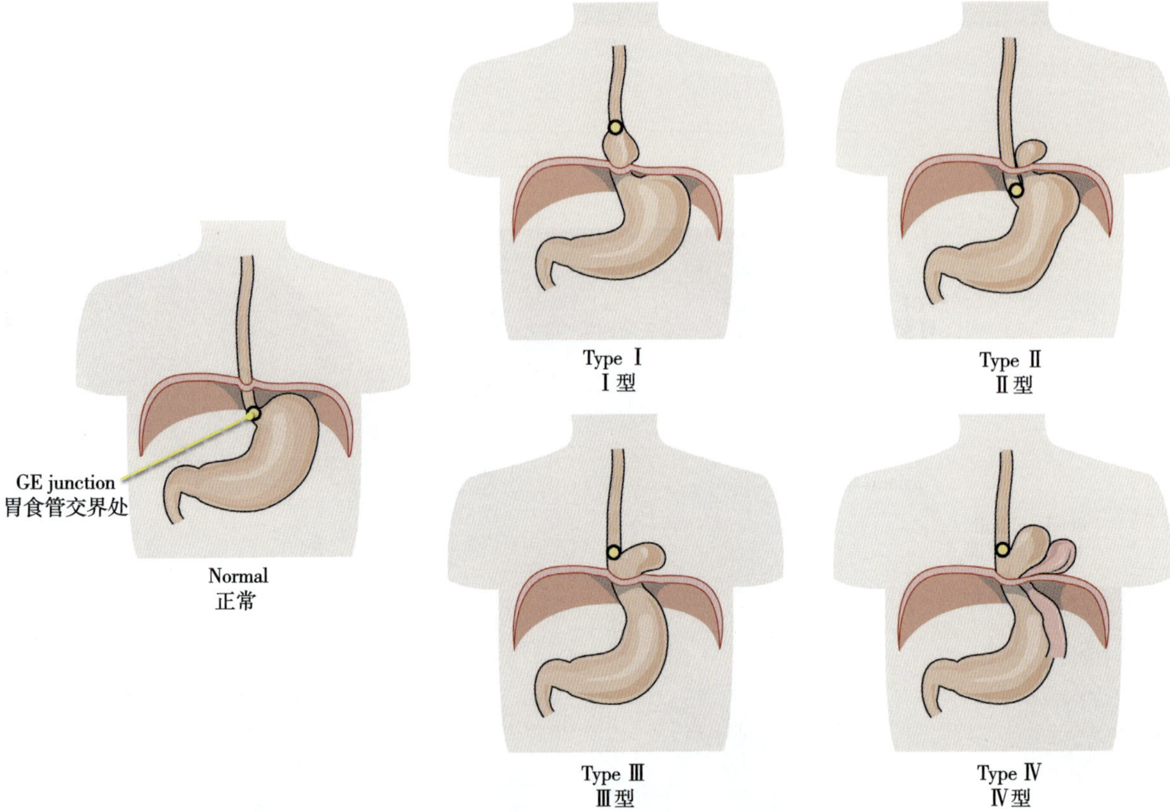

Illustration demonstrates the four types of hiatal hernias.
四种类型的食管裂孔疝示意图。

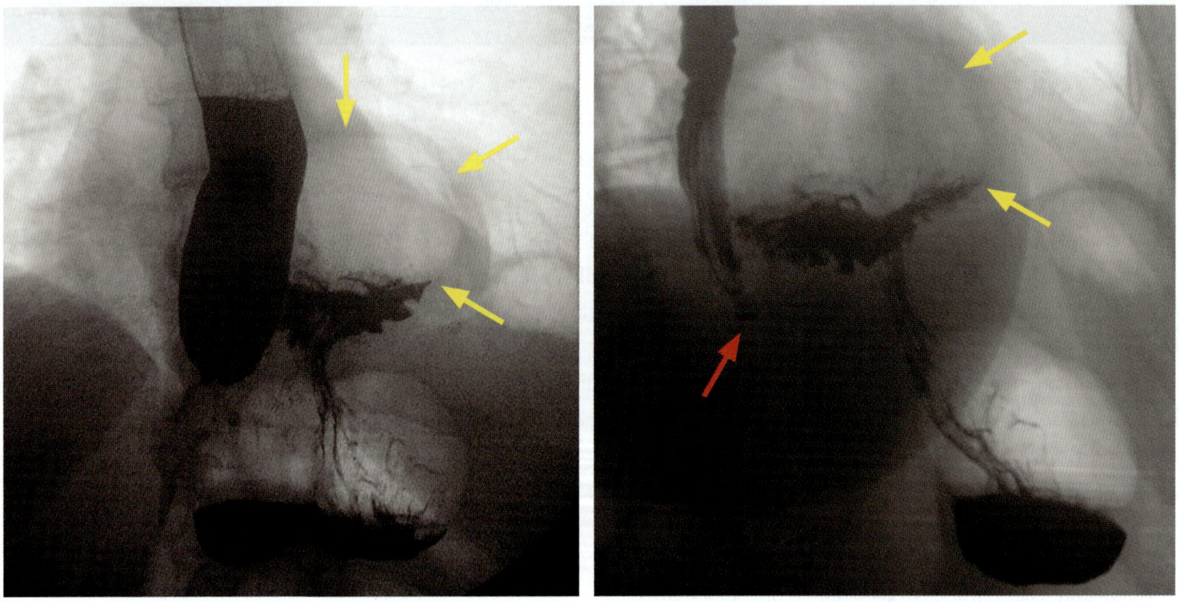

Paraesophageal hernia: Frontal and oblique single-contrast barium upper GI study shows intrathoracic herniation of the gastric fundus (yellow arrows), consistent with a recurrent paraesophageal hernia in this patient with prior history of hernia repair. The GE junction (red arrow) remains below the diaphragm, consistent with a type Ⅱ hiatal hernia.
食管旁型疝：正位(左图)和斜位(右图)上消化道单对比钡餐造影显示胃底疝入胸腔内(黄箭)，此患者有疝修补史，符合食管旁疝复发。GE交界处(红箭)仍位于膈肌下方，符合Ⅱ型食管裂孔疝的特点。

Gastric volvulus

- Gastric volvulus occurs when the stomach twists on its mesentery by at least 180 degrees and results in bowel obstruction or ischemia. The stomach may be

胃扭转

- 胃沿肠系膜扭转至少180°并导致肠梗阻或缺血时，称为胃扭转。胃可以部分或全部位于

partly or entirely above the diaphragm.

- If the stomach is twisted but without obstruction or ischemia, it is referred to as gastric "rotation."
- *Organoaxial* rotation/volvulus is when the stomach rotates on its long-axis.
- *Mesenteroaxial* rotation/volvulus is when the stomach rotates on its short-axis.
- Most commonly occurs in the setting of a paraesophageal hernia or trauma.

膈肌的上方。

- 如果出现胃扭曲，但没有梗阻或缺血，则称为胃“旋转”。
- 器官轴旋转/扭转是指胃在其长轴上旋转。
- 肠系膜轴旋转/扭转是指胃在其短轴上旋转。
- 在有食管旁疝时或外伤的情况下最常出现。

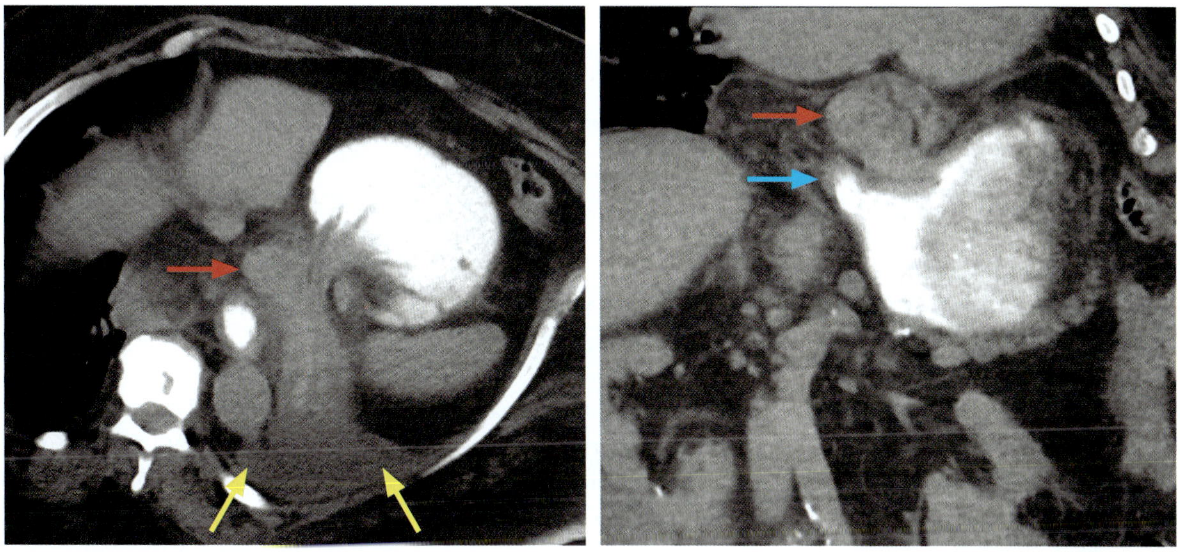

Gastric volvulus: Axial (left image) and coronal (right image) oral contrast only CT shows mesenteroaxial gastric volvulus with the distal stomach (yellow arrows) located in the chest through a large hiatal hernia.
The gastroduodenal junction (red arrow) appears to be cranial to the gastroesophageal junction (blue arrow). Enteric contrast is pooled in the proximal stomach with reflux into the esophagus; no contrast is seen distal to the stomach.
胃扭转：轴位(左图)和冠状位(右图)口服造影剂CT显示肠系膜轴位胃扭转，胃远端(黄箭)通过扩大的裂孔疝入胸腔。
胃十二指肠连接处(红箭)位于胃食管交界处(蓝箭)的上方。肠内造影剂潴留在胃的近端，并反流进入食管；胃远端未见造影剂。

THICKENED GASTRIC FOLDS

- Thickened gastric folds are most commonly due to inflammatory gastritis, which characteristically produces smooth fold thickening.
- Nodular fold thickening is suggestive of neoplasm, either gastric lymphoma or submucosal carcinoma (which may be primary gastric or metastatic).

胃皱襞增厚

- 胃皱襞增厚最常见于炎症性胃炎，产生具有特征性的光滑而增厚的皱襞。
- 结节状的胃皱襞增厚提示肿瘤、胃淋巴瘤或黏膜下癌肿(可能是原发于胃或转移)。

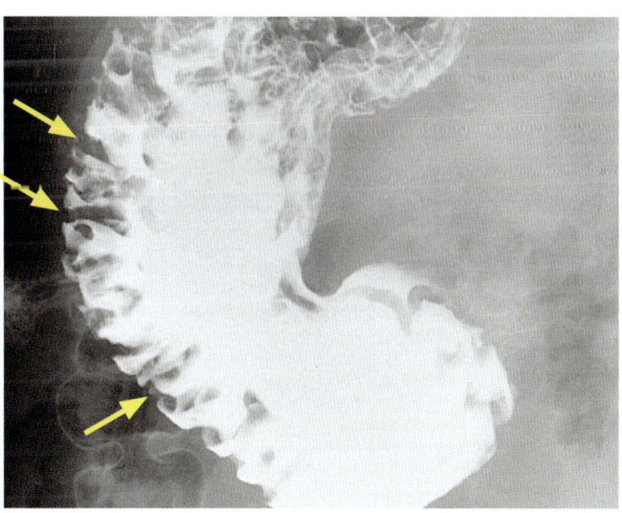

Contrast filling thickened gastric folds (arrows) on a double contrast barium study, thought to represent gastritis in this patient.
气钡双重造影显示造影剂填充增厚的胃皱襞(黄箭)，此为胃炎患者。

***Helicobacter pylori* gastritis**

- *Helicobacter pylori* is a major cause of gastritis, gastric ulcers, and duodenal ulcers.

Zollinger-Ellison (ZE) syndrome

- Zollinger-Ellison (ZE) is gastrin over-production from a gastrinoma, which is a neuroendocrine tumor located in the duodenum or pancreas that has a 50% rate of malignancy. ZE features elevated gastrin level and a paradoxical increase in gastrin after secretin administration.
- 25% of patients with gastrinoma have multiple endocrine neoplasia (MEN) type 1.

  MEN-1 consists of parathyroid adenoma, pituitary adenoma, and pancreatic islet cell tumors.

Eosinophilic gastritis

- Eosinophilic gastritis is characterized by thickened folds in the stomach and small bowel in a patient with a history of atopy.

Ménétrier disease (hypertrophic gastropathy)

- Ménétrier disease is a protein-losing enteropathy that is often a diagnosis of exclusion. It usually affects the proximal stomach and is pathologically characterized by replacement of parietal cells by hyperplastic epithelial cells, leading to achlorhydria.
- Ménétrier disease has a controversial association with gastric carcinoma.

Crohn's disease

- The stomach is rarely an isolated site of involvement by Crohn's disease. Usually the distal half of the stomach is affected.
- Typical imaging features include thickened folds and mural ulcers most commonly affecting the antrum with eventual tubular stenosis of the antrum leading to the characteristic *ram's horn* appearance.

  Differential diagnosis of the *ram's horn* appearance is sarcoid, Crohn's disease, and treated ulcer disease.

Other causes of thickened gastric folds

- Gastric varices (from portal hypertension), sarcoidosis, gastric lymphoma, and submucosal carcinoma are non-inflammatory causes of thickened gastric folds.

GASTRIC POLYPS

Hyperplastic polyp (inflammatory polyp)

- A hyperplastic polyp, also known as an inflammatory polyp, is a cystic dilation of a gastric gland that develops in response to chronic inflammation, often associated with *H. pylori* infection. Hyperplastic polyps are almost always benign, with very rare cases of malignant transformation having been reported.

幽门螺杆菌胃炎

- 幽门螺杆菌是造成胃炎、胃溃疡及十二指肠溃疡的主要原因。

佐林格-埃利森综合征

- 佐林格-埃利森综合征由胃泌素瘤过度分泌胃泌素引起，是位于十二指肠或胰腺的一种神经内分泌肿瘤，恶性概率为50%。佐林格-埃利森综合征的特征性表现为胃泌素水平升高，并且在给予促胰液素后出现胃泌素水平反常性增高。
- 约25%的胃泌素瘤患者伴有1型多发性内分泌瘤病(MEN-1)。

  MEN-1包括甲状旁腺腺瘤、垂体腺瘤，以及胰岛细胞瘤。

嗜酸性粒细胞性胃炎

- 嗜酸性粒细胞性胃炎的特征性表现为胃及小肠皱襞增厚，见于有特应性变态反应史的患者。

Ménétrier病(肥厚性胃炎)

- Ménétrier病是一种蛋白丢失性肠道病，通常是一种排除性诊断。该病通常累及近端胃组织，病理学上以壁细胞被增生的上皮细胞所替代为特征，最终导致胃酸缺乏症。
- Ménétrier病与胃癌之间的关系仍存在争议。

克罗恩病

- 罕见情况下胃是克罗恩病的唯一发病器官。通常累及胃远端的一半。
- 典型的影像学特征包括胃皱襞增厚和黏膜溃疡，最常见于胃窦部，最终导致胃窦管状狭窄，形成特征性的羊角样外观。

  羊角样外观的鉴别诊断包括类癌、克罗恩病和溃疡病治疗后。

其他造成胃皱襞增厚的疾病

- 胃静脉曲张(门静脉高压所致)、结节病、胃淋巴瘤，以及黏膜下癌都是胃皱襞增厚的非炎症性原因。

胃息肉

增生性息肉(炎性息肉)

- 增生性息肉，又称炎性息肉，是由于慢性炎症刺激造成的胃腺体囊性扩张，通常与幽门螺杆菌感染相关。增生性息肉几乎都是良性的，恶变报道极为罕见。

Fundic gland polyps

胃底腺息肉

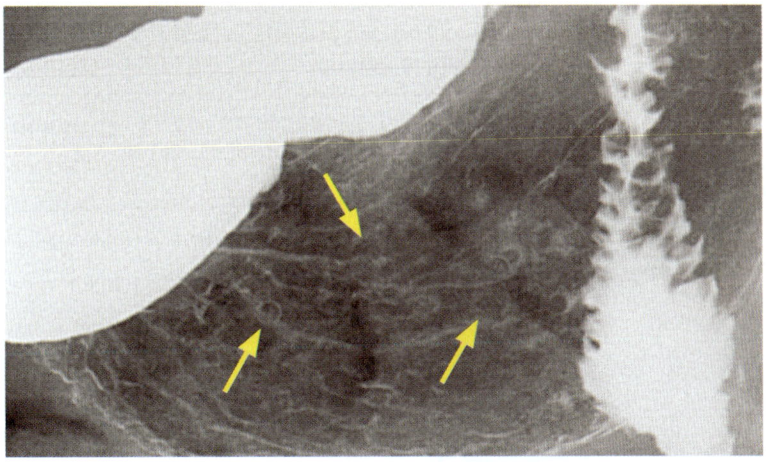

Double-contrast barium study demonstrates a few small, round, well-circumscribed radiolucent filling defects (arrows) within the greater curvature of the stomach, consistent with gastric polyps seen on patient's prior endoscopy.

气钡双重造影检查显示胃大弯侧有一些小的、圆形、边界清楚的低密度充盈缺损(黄箭),与患者既往内镜检查发现的胃息肉一致。

- Fundic gland polyps are associated with proton pump inhibitor use, but may also occur in polyposis syndromes such as familial adenomatous polyposis (FAP). Fundic gland polyps have a rare malignant potential, which is more common in patients with FAP.

- 胃底腺息肉与使用质子泵抑制剂相关,但也可见于息肉综合征,如家族性腺瘤样息肉病。胃底腺息肉罕见恶变,多见于家族性腺瘤样息肉病。

Adenomatous polyp

- An adenomatous polyp is a neoplastic polyp with malignant potential. There is an elevated risk of malignant transformation to adenocarcinoma with increased size, villous contour and the presence of cellular dysplasia. There is an association with atrophic gastritis.
- Adenomatous polyps are usually solitary but may be multiple.
- They are usually treated with endoscopic biopsy and polypectomy.

腺瘤样息肉

- 腺瘤样息肉是一种有恶变潜能的肿瘤样息肉。恶变风险增高与体积增大、绒毛样轮廓或细胞异型增生有关。可合并萎缩性胃炎。
- 腺瘤样息肉通常单发,但也可多发。
- 通常使用内镜进行活检和息肉切除术进行治疗。

Hamartomatous polyp

- Hamartomatous polyps are benign polyps usually associated with syndromes such as Peutz- Jeghers, juvenile polyposis, and Cronkhite-Canada syndromes.

错构瘤性息肉

- 错构瘤性息肉为良性息肉,常与综合征相关,如波伊茨-耶格综合征、青少年多发息肉征和卡纳达-克朗凯特综合征。

GASTRIC ULCERS

胃溃疡

Benign gastric ulcer

- Although less commonly encountered in the modern era of proton pump inhibitors and *Helicobacter pylori* treatment, benign gastric ulcers tend to have typical imaging findings:

Radiating gastric folds are smooth and symmetric.
Ulcer extends beyond the normal contour of the gastric lumen (deep).
The *Hampton line* represents nonulcerated acid-resistant mucosa surrounding the ulcer crater.
Most benign ulcers occur along the lesser curvature of the stomach, although benign ulcers associated with aspirin ingestion can occur in the greater curvature and antrum, which are dependent locations.

良性胃溃疡

- 由于使用质子泵抑制剂和抗幽门螺杆菌治疗的普及,良性胃溃疡在当今已经不是很常见,但它具有一些典型的影像学表现:

光滑、对称的放射样胃皱襞。
溃疡延伸至正常胃腔轮廓之外(深)。
Hampton 线为沿溃疡口周边的非溃疡性耐酸黏膜。
良性胃溃疡大多发生于胃小弯侧,而与服用阿司匹林相关的良性溃疡可发生于胃大弯和胃窦重心下方的位置。

Gastric carcinoma

- Gastric carcinoma may present with malignant ulceration, which can usually be distinguished from a benign ulcer by the following features:

Asymmetric ulcer crater, with surrounding nodular tissue.
Abrupt transition between normal gastric wall and surrounding tissue.

胃癌

- 胃癌可表现为恶性溃疡,以下征象通常可以帮助与良性溃疡区分:

非对称性的溃疡口伴周围结节样组织。
正常胃壁与周围组织之间交界分明。

Ulcer crater does *not* project beyond the expected location of gastric wall (shallow).

The *Carman meniscus sign* is considered pathognomonic for tumor. It describes the splaying open of a large, flat malignant ulcer when compression is applied.

溃疡口不突出于胃壁(阴影)轮廓之外。

Carman半月征被认为是对胃癌诊断具有病理学意义的征象。具体表现为对恶性溃疡施压时，溃疡口变得大而扁平。

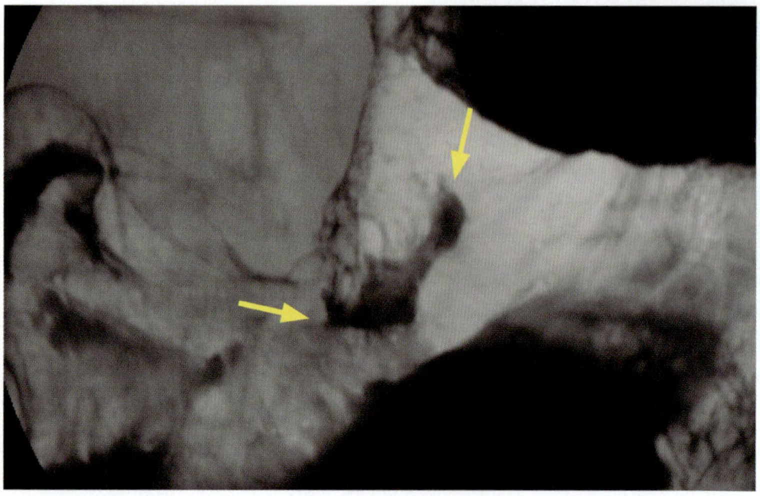

Carmen meniscus sign (arrows) of a malignant gastric ulcer on double-contrast barium study.

气钡双重造影检查显示恶性胃溃疡的Carman半月征(黄箭)。

BENIGN GASTRIC MASSES

良性胃肿瘤

Gastrointestinal stromal tumor (GIST) (benign)

胃肠道间质瘤(GIST)(良性)

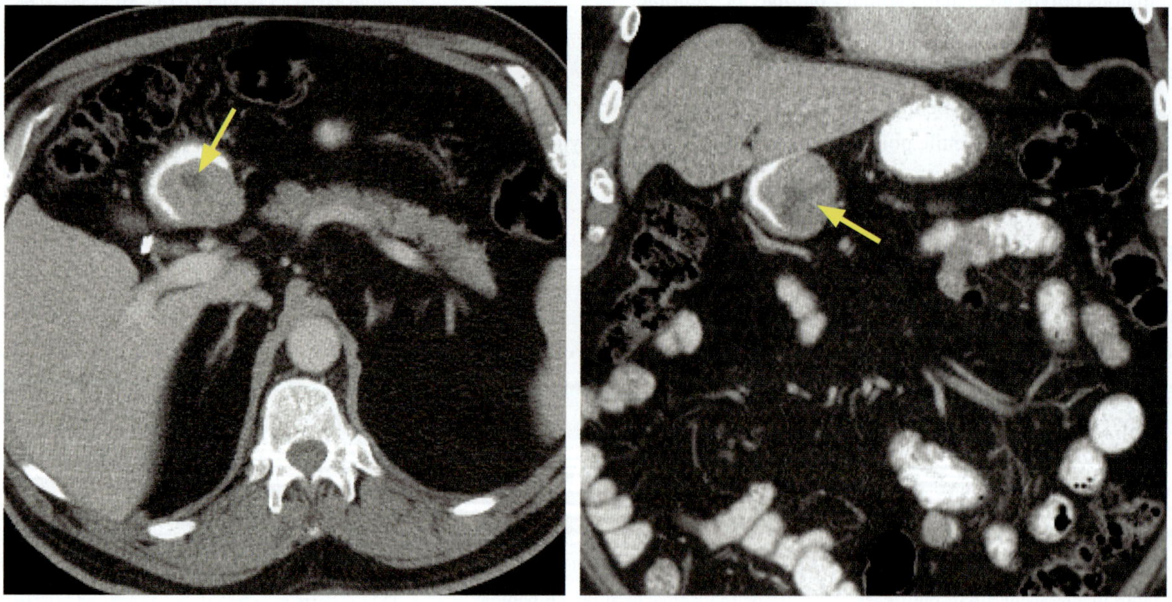

Submucosal GIST: Axial (left image) and coronal (right image) contrast-enhanced CT shows a well-circumscribed, relatively homogeneous mass with a central focus of necrosis (arrows), located in the submucosal posterior wall of the gastric antrum. Incidental cholecystectomy clips are seen on the axial CT.

Case courtesy Cheryl Sadow, MD, Brigham and Women's Hospital.

黏膜下胃肠道间质瘤：轴位(左图)和冠状位(右图)增强CT显示位于胃窦后壁黏膜下一个边界光整、相对均质但伴有中央区坏死的肿块(黄箭)。在轴位CT上可见胆囊切除术后的金属夹。

- Gastrointestinal stromal tumor (GIST) is the most common submucosal gastric tumor and may be benign or malignant. While GIST may occur anywhere in the GI tract, the stomach is the most common location. The tumor arises from

- 胃肠道间质瘤是最常见的胃黏膜下肿瘤，可以是良性或恶性。胃肠道间质瘤可以起源于胃肠道的任何部位，但胃是最常见的部位。肿瘤起

the interstitial cells of Cajal, which are pacemaker cells that drive peristalsis.

- Risk of malignancy is determined by size and number of mitoses. Regardless of size and number of mitoses, gastric GIST is less likely to be malignant compared to similar-sized GISTs in the duodenum, jejunum/ileum, or rectum.
- Small gastric GISTs are usually asymptomatic but may be a cause of melena.
- On imaging, a smooth endoluminal surface is characteristic due to its submucosal location. Larger tumors tend to become exophytic, or less commonly to invade/ulcerate into the mucosa and cause melena.
- The differential diagnosis of a **submucosal gastric mass** includes:

Mesenchymal tumors (GIST, fibroma, lipoma, neurofibromas, etc).	Carcinoid. Ectopic pancreatic rest.

Lipoma

- A lipoma is a benign, submucosal, mesenchymal neoplasm. At fluoroscopy, a gastric lipoma is indistinguishable from a GIST. Fatty attenuation on CT is diagnostic of a lipoma.

Ectopic pancreatic rest

- An ectopic pancreatic rest is a focus of heterotopic pancreatic tissue in the gastric submucosa. The ectopic tissue is susceptible to pancreatic diseases, including pancreatitis and carcinoma.
- On imaging, the classic appearance is an umbilicated submucosal nodule, with the umbilication representing a focus of normal epithelium. The ulceration is not always seen, in which case imaging will show a nonspecific submucosal gastric mass.

MALIGNANT GASTRIC MASSES

Gastric adenocarcinoma

源于卡哈尔间质细胞，是胃肠蠕动的起搏细胞。

- 恶变的风险取决于肿瘤大小和有丝分裂数目。无论大小和有丝分裂的数目，发生在胃的胃肠道间质瘤比同样大小，但发生于十二指肠、空肠/回肠或直肠的胃肠道间质瘤恶变率要低。
- 小的胃肠道间质瘤通常是无症状的，也可能会引起黑便。
- 在影像学上，腔内表面光滑为其特征性表现，这是因为肿瘤起源于黏膜下。大的肿瘤往往呈外生性生长，较少情况下可侵犯或引发黏膜溃疡，以及黑便。
- **胃黏膜下肿瘤**的鉴别诊断包括：

间叶组织肿瘤（胃肠道间质瘤、纤维瘤、脂肪瘤、神经纤维瘤等）。	类癌。 异位胰腺。

脂肪瘤

- 脂肪瘤是一种良性、黏膜下的间叶源性肿瘤。在透视检查时，胃脂肪瘤难以与胃肠道间质瘤区分。CT上的脂肪密度是诊断脂肪瘤的依据。

异位胰腺残余

- 异位胰腺残余是发生于胃黏膜下层的局灶性异位的胰腺。异位的胰腺组织易并发病变，包括胰腺炎和胰腺癌。
- 在影像学上，典型的表现为肚脐样的黏膜下结节，而脐部则代表局部正常的上皮细胞。溃疡并非总能看到，影像学上显示为一个非特异性的胃黏膜下肿块。

恶性胃肿瘤

胃腺癌

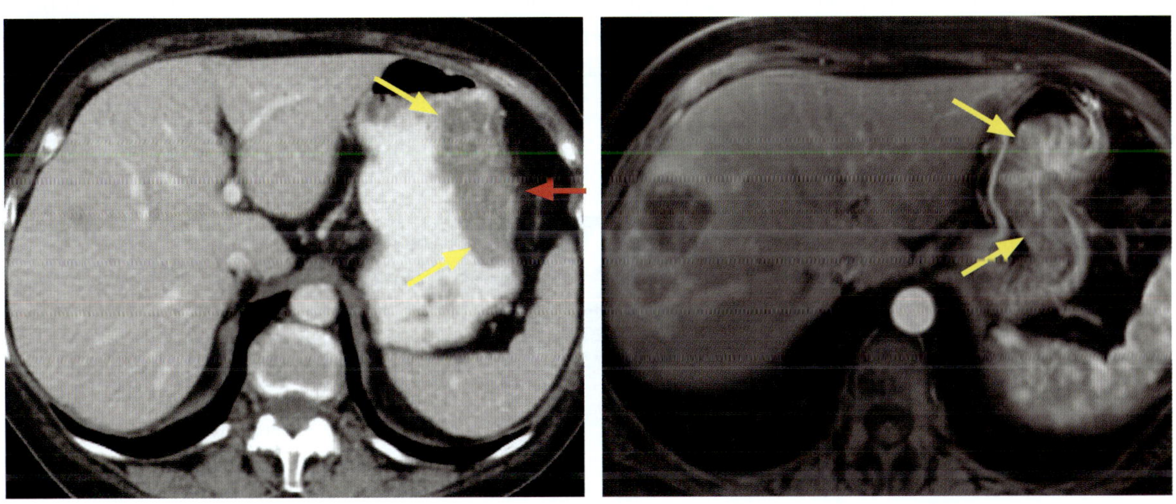

Gastric adenocarcinoma with hepatic metastases: Axial contrast-enhanced CT (left image) shows a mucosal- based hypoattenuating mass (yellow arrows) along the greater curvature of stomach protruding into the gastric lumen, with likely transmural extension (red arrow). On axial post-contrast T1-weighted MRI (right image) performed at a later time point, the gastric mass demonstrates heterogeneous enhancement. Also present are hypoenhancing hepatic metastases which are less well seen on the prior CT.

胃腺癌伴肝转移：轴位增强CT（左图）显示胃大弯侧一个起源于黏膜并突入胃腔的低密度肿块（黄箭），有壁外延伸的可能（红箭）。在此之后的轴位增强T_1加权MRI（右图）上，胃肿块呈不均匀强化。同时还显示低强化的肝转移，这在之前的CT上并不明显。

- Gastric adenocarcinoma may present either as a focal mass, malignant ulcer, or diffuse wall thickening (*linitis plastica*). Gastric cancer is generally caused by chronic inflammation, with specific risk factors including:

Ingestion of polycyclic hydrocarbons and nitrosamines (from processed meats). Atrophic gastritis.	Pernicious anemia. Post-subtotal gastrectomy.

- 胃腺癌既可以表现为局部肿块，也可以表现为恶性溃疡，或弥漫性胃壁增厚(皮革胃)。胃癌通常由慢性炎症引起，与其相关的危险因素包括：

摄取多环碳氢化合物和亚硝胺(来自加工过的肉类)。 萎缩性胃炎。	恶性贫血。 胃次全切除术后。

- Lymphatic spread occurs along the lesser curvature → the gastrohepatic ligament and the greater curvature.
- A **Krukenberg tumor** is classically described as metastatic spread of gastric carcinoma to the ovary; however, the term has also been used to describe any mucinous metastasis to the ovary.

- 淋巴转移的途径是沿着胃小弯到肝胃韧带再到胃大弯。
- **克鲁肯贝格瘤**通常是指胃癌转移播散到卵巢；但这个术语也被用来描述任何转移到卵巢的黏液癌。

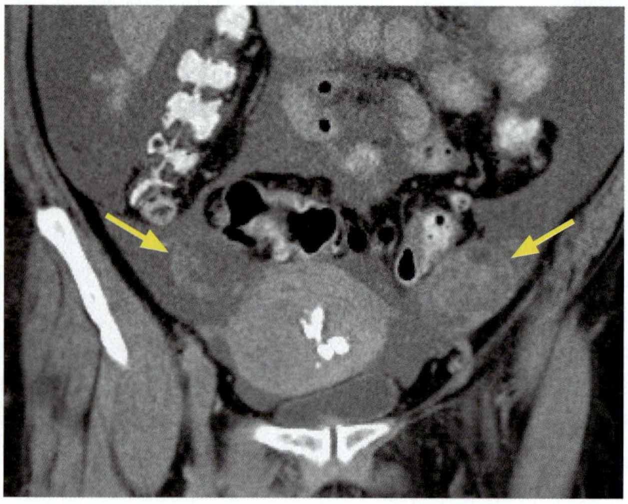

Krukenberg tumors of the ovaries from gastric cancer:
Coronal contrast-enhanced CT shows bilateral adnexal masses (arrows), representing ovarian metastases. Moderate ascites is present.
Case courtesy Cheryl Sadow, MD, Brigham and Women's Hospital.
胃癌播散到卵巢的克鲁肯贝格瘤：
冠状位增强CT显示双侧附件肿物(黄箭)，提示卵巢转移癌。有中等量腹水。

GIST (malignant)

- Malignant GISTs tend to be larger than benign GISTs, often reaching sizes of >10 cm, with central necrosis. Although the tumor originates in the submucosa, it can be difficult to determine the site of origin of large tumors as they may become very large and exophytic and may ulcerate into the mucosa.

胃肠道间质瘤(恶性)

- 恶性胃肠道间质瘤的瘤体一般大于良性胃肠道间质瘤，通常直径超过10cm，伴有中央坏死。尽管肿瘤起源于黏膜下，但大的肿瘤很难确定其起源部位，这是由于该类肿瘤体积巨大且呈外生性生长，并可能穿透黏膜。

Lymphoma

淋巴瘤

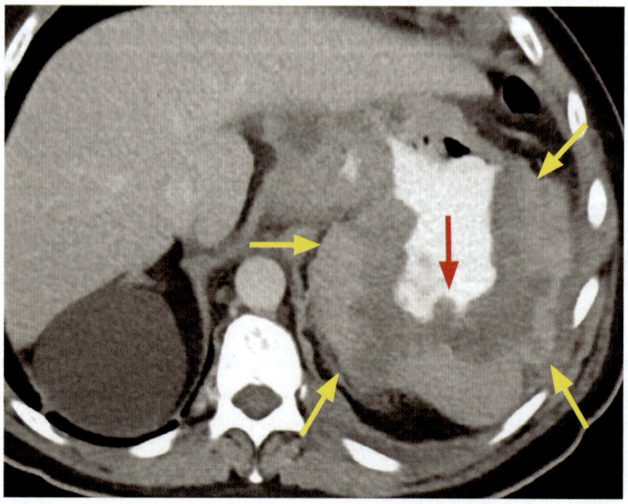

Gastric lymphoma:
Axial contrast-enhanced CT demonstrates a large, lobular partially necrotic mass (yellow arrows) in the left upper quadrant, that appears to directly communicate with and invade the gastric fundus, with oral contrast seen pooling within the necrotic portions of the lesion (red arrow). The mass also invades the spleen.
Biopsy showed diffuse large B-cell lymphoma.
胃淋巴瘤：
轴位增强CT显示左上腹可见一个大的、分叶状、部分坏死肿块(黄箭)，肿块似乎直接与胃底相连并侵犯胃底，口服造影剂聚集于病变的坏死部分(红箭)。肿块还侵犯脾。活检显示为弥漫大B细胞淋巴瘤。

- Gastric lymphoma can have a wide variety of presentations. If solitary, lymphoma can mimic gastric carcinoma or a large malignant GIST. To differentiate between lymphoma and gastric carcinoma, the pattern of adenopathy can be helpful. In gastric cancer, adenopathy at or below the level of the renal hila is uncommon, but in lymphoma it occurs in 1/3 of patients.
- The stomach is a common extranodal site for non-Hodgkin lymphoma.

- 胃淋巴瘤有多种不同的表现。若为单发，淋巴瘤可以类似于胃癌或一个大的恶性胃肠道间质瘤。鉴别淋巴瘤和胃癌时，确认淋巴结肿大的方式可以有所帮助。在胃癌中，肾门及其以下平面的淋巴结肿大不常见，但见于1/3的淋巴瘤患者中。
- 胃是非霍奇金淋巴结瘤常见的结外发生部位。

Metastases

- Metastatic disease to the stomach is rare. Breast, lung, and melanoma are the most common primary malignancies to metastasize to the stomach.

转移癌

- 转移到胃的肿瘤比较罕见。乳腺癌、肺癌和黑色素瘤为最常见的可转移到胃的原发恶性肿瘤。

Overview of Common Gastric Surgeries

常见胃手术概述

Fundoplication

胃底折叠术

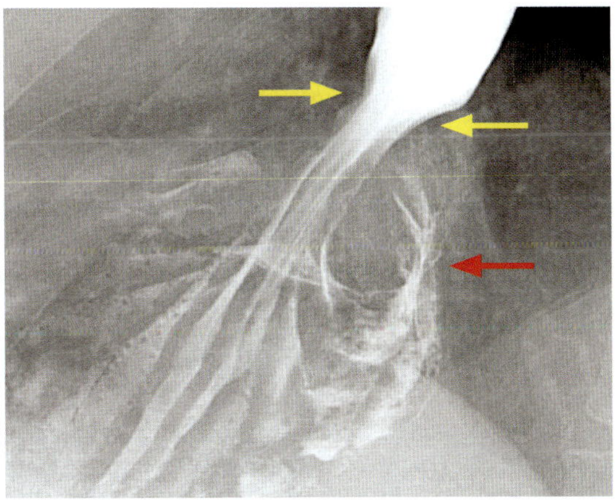

Double-contrast barium study demonstrates expected extrinsic impression on the distal esophagus (yellow arrows) secondary to Nissen fundoplication. Small amount of contrast filling the intact wrap is within normal limits (red arrow).

气钡双重造影检查显示Nissen胃底折叠术后在食管远端出现相应(手术)位置的外源性压迹(黄箭)。少量的造影剂充填完整的包绕部分属正常现象(红箭)。

- Fundoplication is a form of antireflux surgery used for cases refractory to medical management as well as for treatment of symptomatic hiatal or paraesophageal hernias.
- Fundoplication involves surgically wrapping the gastric fundus around the distal esophagus, reinforcing the lower esophageal sphincter. Types of fundoplication are listed below:

  Nissen: a 360° wrap, posteriorly.

  Dor: a 180° wrap, anteriorly.

  Toupet: a 270° wrap, posteriorly.
- Complications include slippage, disruption and overly tight and long fundoplications which manifest as dysphagia.

- 胃底折叠术是一种抗反流手术，用于治疗药物难治性反流病，以及治疗有症状的裂孔或食管旁疝。
- 胃底折叠术是通过手术将胃底环绕在食管远端周围，以强化食管下括约肌。胃底折叠术的类型如下：

  Nissen胃底折叠术：从后方360°包绕。

  Dor胃底折叠术：从前方180°包绕。

  Toupet胃底折叠术：从后方270°包绕。
- 并发症包括滑脱、缝合断裂、折叠过紧和过长，表现为吞咽困难。

Bariatric surgeries

- **Sleeve gastrectomy** is the most common bariatric surgery procedure and involves resecting the greater curvature of the stomach, leaving only a small residual gastric pouch.
- **Gastric banding** is surgical placement of an adjustable silicone device around the stomach to reduce the volume of the stomach, with a port placed in the subcutaneous tissues of the abdomen.

减肥手术

- **袖状胃切除术**是最常见的减肥手术，涉及切除胃大弯，仅留下一小部分胃袋。
- **胃束带**是通过手术，环绕胃周植入一种可调节的硅胶材料，以减少胃的容积，端口置于腹部的皮下组织。

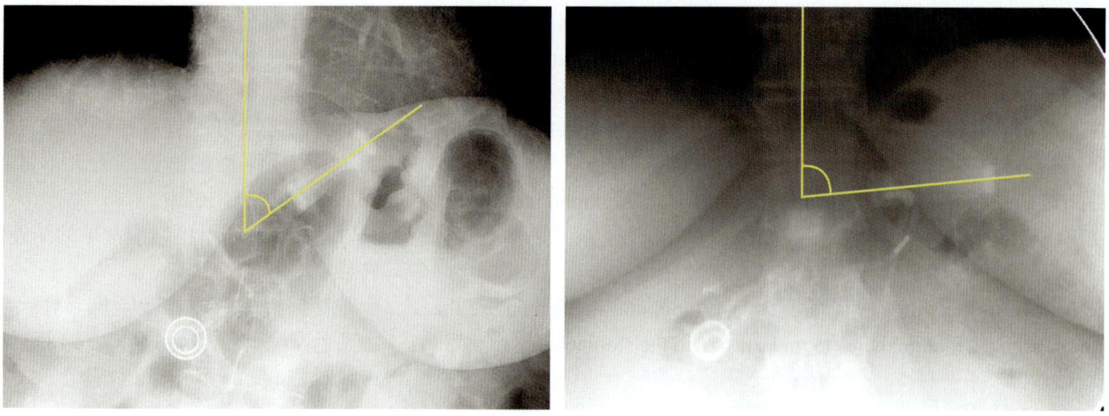

Normal versus slipped gastric band: Left frontal fluoroscopic image shows a normal phi angle of 54° (normal is 4-58°) formed by the gastric band profile and vertical axis of the spine. Right fluoroscopic image shows a slipped band with a phi angle of 87°.
正常和滑动的胃束带：左侧正位图像显示由胃束带轮廓和脊柱纵轴形成的φ夹角为54°（正常为4°~58°）。右侧图像显示束带滑动形成的φ夹角为87°。

- **Roux-en-Y gastric bypass** (RYGB) is described on the subsequent page.

- **鲁氏Y形胃旁路术(RYGB)**

Postoperative anatomy of Roux-en-Y gastric bypass (RYGB)

鲁氏Y形胃旁路术(RYGB)的术后解剖结构

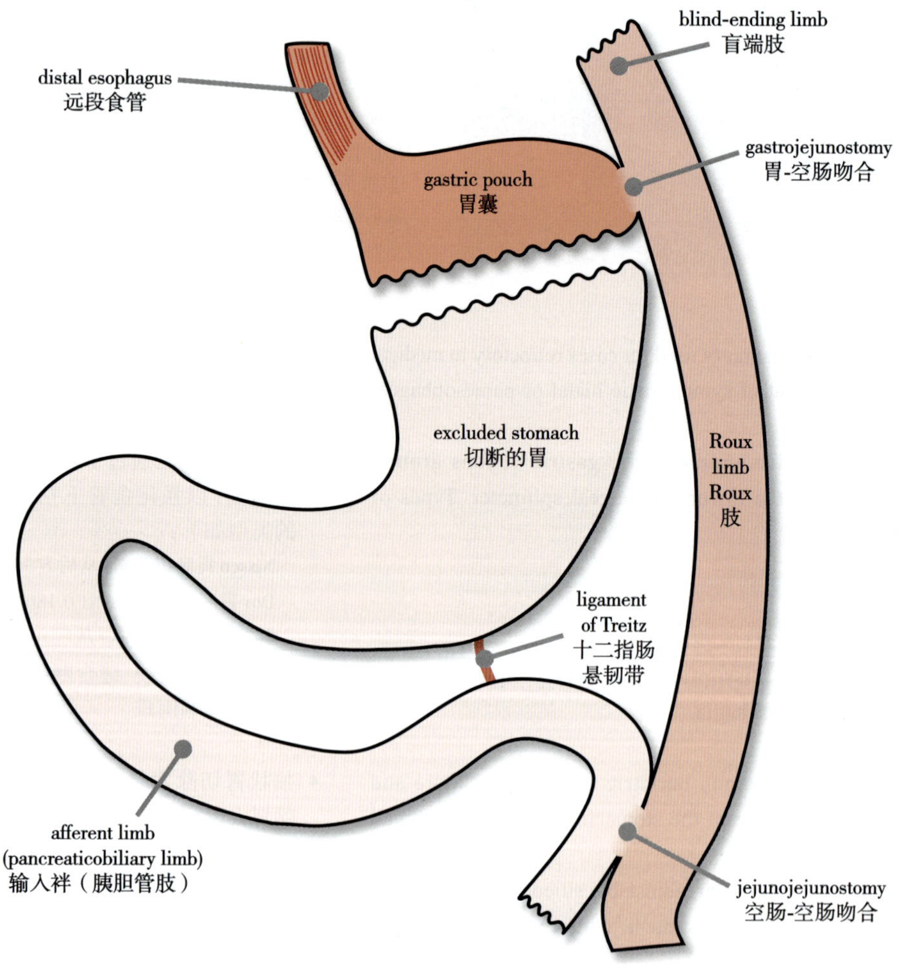

- In order to evaluate for and accurately describe complications of RYGB surgery, it is important to be familiar with the procedure and normal postsurgical anatomy.
- A small gastric pouch is created with a volume of approximately 15–30 mL by

- 为了评估及准确描述鲁氏Y形胃旁路术的术后并发症，熟悉手术和术后正常解剖很重要。
- 用手术形成一个容量为15~30ml的小胃囊，将远端的胃组织排出在食物消化路径上。

excluding the distal stomach from the path of food.

- The Roux limb is created by transecting the jejunum approximately 35–45 cm distal to the ligament of Treitz, then bringing it up to be anastomosed to the gastric pouch via a narrow gastrojejunostomy stoma.
- The current favored approach for placement of the Roux limb is antecolic (in front of the transverse colon). The Roux limb used to be placed retrocolic, which required the creation of a surgical defect through the transverse mesocolon (mesentery of the transverse colon). A retrocolic Roux limb has a higher risk of a transmesocolic hernia due to the defect in the transverse mesocolon.

  Although the antecolic approach is now more commonly performed, there are many patients who have previously undergone a retrocolic approach.
- A distal side-to-side jejunojejunostomy is created to connect the pancreaticobiliary limb to the jejunum.
- The RYGB leads to weight loss both from early satiety (due to small size of the gastric pouch) and malabsorption (due to surgical bypass of the proximal jejunum).

- 手术在距十二指肠悬韧带远端35~45cm处切断空肠形成Roux肢，并将其上提，通过一个狭小的胃空肠吻合口使其与残留胃囊达到解剖学吻合。
- 目前比较流行的方法是将Roux肢置于结肠前(位于横结肠前方)。过去，Roux肢置于结肠后，这就需要在横结肠系膜(mesentery of the transverse colon)处做一个手术开口。结肠后Roux肢具有较高的结肠系膜疝的发生风险，这是因为横结肠系膜局部缺损。

  尽管目前普遍采用结肠前术式，但有很多患者在过去接受了结肠后术式。
- 远端空肠-空肠侧侧吻合术是将胰胆管肢与空肠连接起来。
- 鲁氏Y形胃旁路术导致体重下降是由于早期的饱腹感(由于胃囊体积较小)和吸收不良所致(由于近端空肠的手术旁路)。

Complications of Roux-en-Y Surgery

Postoperative leak

- Postoperative leak is usually diagnosed by 10 days after surgery.
- An upper GI study with water-soluble contrast is the study of choice if a leak is suspected.
- Leaks may arise from the gastric pouch or blind-ending jejunal limb. It is rare for a leak to arise from the distal jejunojejunostomy.

Gastrogastric fistula

鲁氏Y形手术并发症

术后渗漏

- 术后渗漏通常于术后10天得到诊断。
- 怀疑渗漏时应选择水溶性造影剂进行上消化道造影。
- 渗漏可发生于胃囊或空肠肢的盲端。发生在远端空肠-空肠的吻合口的渗漏很少见。

胃-胃瘘管

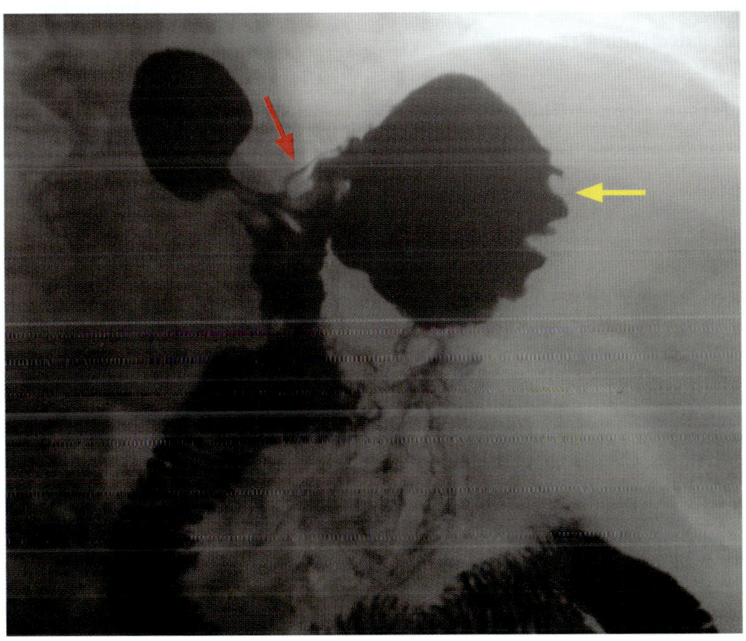

Single contrast upper GI study in a patient status post Roux-en-Y gastric bypass shows prompt contrast filling of the excluded stomach (yellow arrow) via a gastrogastric fistula at the superior aspect of the gastric suture line (red arrow).
鲁氏Y形胃旁路术后患者的单一对比上消化道造影显示造影剂通过胃缝合线上方的胃-胃瘘管(红箭)迅速充填被隔离的胃(黄箭)。

- A gastrogastric fistula is a communication between the gastric pouch and the excluded stomach, which may be an early or late complication of RYGB. Imaging findings include gas and fluid (or enteric contrast, if given) within the excluded stomach on CT or upper GI study.
- A gastrogastric fistula may be a cause of inadequate weight loss or recurrent weight gain.

- 胃-胃瘘管是指胃囊与远端被切断胃之间存在交通，可以是鲁氏Y形胃旁路术术后早期或晚期的并发症。影像学表现包括CT或上消化道造影可见切除胃腔内有积气或积液(给予造影剂后可见肠道显影)。
- 胃-胃瘘管可能是造成体重下降不足或肥胖复

发的原因。

Small bowel obstruction (SBO)

- Early SBO in the acute postoperative period is most often due to edema or hematoma at the gastrojejunostomy or jejunojejunostomy.

  With a retrocolic Roux limb, edema at the transverse mesocolon defect may also cause obstruction. Treatment is usually conservative, with most cases resolving as the edema and/or hematoma resolves.

- Late presentation of SBO may be due to internal hernia (more common with laparoscopic surgery) or adhesions (more common with open surgery).

小肠梗阻(SBO)

- 术后急性发生的早期小肠梗阻(SBO)最常继发于胃-空肠吻合处或空肠-空肠吻合处发生的水肿或血肿。

  在结肠后Roux肢手术，横结肠系膜缺损处发生的水肿也会引起梗阻。一般采用保守治疗，多数病例的症状会随水肿和/或血肿的消退而得到缓解。

- 迟发性小肠梗阻可能是由于内疝(更常见于腹腔镜下手术)或粘连(更常见于开腹手术)所致。

Afferent loop syndrome

- Intermittent partial or complete mechanical obstruction of the afferent limb is seen in up to 13% of patients both in acute (<7 days postoperative) or chronic (>7 days postoperative) phase.
- Fluoroscopy would not show this complication, as the afferent limb does not usually opacify with contrast (unless there is reflux from the jejunojejunostomy). CT would show dilated, fluid-filled afferent/pancreaticobiliary limb.

输入袢综合征

- 输入袢间歇性部分或完全机械性梗阻在急性期(术后<7天)或慢性期(术后7天)患者中都高达13%。
- 透视检查不能显示这种并发症，因为输入袢通常无造影剂充填(除非有空肠-空肠吻合口反流)。CT表现为扩张的、充满液体的输入袢/胰胆管肢。

Internal hernia

- Laparoscopic Roux-en-Y procedures are associated with a higher rate of internal hernias (seen in 2.5% of laparoscopic procedures) compared to open procedures (0.5%). Internal hernias can be difficult to diagnose, both clinically and by imaging.
- Internal hernias usually present within two years of bypass and are the most common cause of SBO after a laparoscopic Roux-en-Y.

  Internal hernias may also present as mesenteric and bowel edema without obstruction.

- Most RYGB-associated internal hernias occur in three characteristic locations.
- The surgically created defect in the mesentery of the transverse colon is the most common site (the **transmesocolic** hernia), associated with a retrocolic Roux limb.
- Less common sites of internal hernia include **Peterson's space** (located between the mesentery of the Roux limb and the transverse mesocolon) and the **mesenteric defect created by the jejunojejunostomy**.
- Imaging features of internal hernia include swirling of the mesentery, a mushroom shape of the mesentery, and/or the presence of small bowel loops posterior to the superior mesenteric artery.

腹内疝

- 腹腔镜下鲁氏Y形胃旁路术后腹内疝的发生率(见于2.5%的腹腔镜手术患者)高于开腹手术患者(0.5%)。内疝诊断可能比较困难，无论是根据临床症状还是影像学表现。
- 腹内疝通常发生于旁路术后2年内，是腹腔镜下鲁氏Y形胃旁路术后小肠梗阻最常见的原因。

  内疝也可表现为肠系膜及肠管水肿而无梗阻。

- 大多数鲁氏Y形胃旁路术相关性腹内疝发生在三个经典的部位。
- 手术造成的横结肠系膜缺损处最常发生(肠系膜疝)，这与结肠后Roux肢相关。
- 较少见的腹内疝发生部位包括**Peterson间隙**(位于Roux肢系膜和横结肠系膜之间)和**空肠-空肠吻合术造成的肠系膜缺损处**。
- 腹内疝的影像学特征包括肠系膜扭转、蘑菇状肠系膜和/或肠系膜上动脉后方出现小肠肠袢。

Stomal stenosis

- Narrowing of the gastrojejunostomy stoma may occur in up to 10% of patients, leading to dilation of the gastric pouch and distal esophagus. Stomal stenosis is usually treated with endoscopic dilation.
- Narrowing of the distal jejunojejunostomy is less common and usually requires surgery.

吻合口狭窄

- 近10%的患者会发生胃-空肠吻合口狭窄，导致胃囊和远端食管扩张。吻合口狭窄的治疗方法通常是内镜扩张。
- 远端空肠-空肠吻合口狭窄较少见，通常需要手术治疗。

Marginal ulcers

- The jejunal mucosa adjacent to the gastrojejunal anastomosis is susceptible to gastric secretions, which can cause marginal ulcers in up to 3% of patients.
- A marginal ulcer is diagnosed by upper GI as a thickening and small outpouching of a gastric fold.
- Treatment is conservative.

吻合口溃疡

- 邻近胃-空肠吻合处的空肠黏膜易受胃分泌物的损害，导致近3%的患者发生吻合口溃疡。
- 吻合口溃疡可通过上消化道造影诊断，表现为胃皱襞增厚和小的囊袋样突出。
- 治疗采用保守疗法。

(翻译　王玉)

SMALL BOWEL

SMALL BOWEL ANATOMY

- The duodenum has 4 parts: superior (D1), descending (D2), horizontal/transverse (D3) and ascending (D4).
- Valvulae conniventes (also known as plicae circulares) are the circumferential small bowel folds.

  In contrast, colonic haustra are not circumferential.
- The superior mesenteric artery (SMA) supplies both the jejunum and ileum while the duodenum receives blood from branches of the celiac axis.
- A common small bowel mesentery anchors the jejunum and ileum to the posterior abdominal wall.
- The jejunum features larger, closer together folds and larger villi compared to the ileum.
- The Ligament of Treitz (suspensory muscle of the duodenum) is a thin muscle located at the junction of duodenum and the jejunum and serves as the divider between the upper and lower GI tract. This becomes clinically relevant when trying to localize the source of GI bleeding. It is not directly visualized by imaging, but can be indirectly located at the distant edge of the ascending (fourth) portion of the duodenum.

  An upper GI bleed is defined as occurring proximal to the Ligament of Treitz.

  A lower GI bleed occurs distally to the Ligament of Treitz.

SMALL BOWEL OBSTRUCTION (SBO)

- Small bowel obstruction (SBO) is common and most often due to adhesions from prior surgery or hernia. Neoplasm, stricture, and intussusception are less common causes.

Radiographic evaluation of small bowel obstruction

- An abdominal radiograph is often the initial imaging evaluation for suspected obstruction.
- Radiographic findings of SBO include small bowel distention >3 cm. Multiple air-fluid levels at different heights may be seen on the upright view. In addition, the lack of gas in the colon is especially suggestive of obstruction.
- Differential diagnosis of dilated loops of small bowel on plain radiographs include:

  Post-operative adynamic ileus (recent history of surgery, will often see gas in the colon).

  Focal ileus related to inflammatory process (pancreatitis, enteritis, bowel dilatation may be focal near the location of inflammation).

  Ileus due to ascites: Ascites often compresses the ascending and descending colon and rectum as these structures are not on a mesentery. However, gas in the transverse colon and sigmoid colon is still apparent. Small bowel may be medialized.
- A potential pitfall may be in a patient with a total colectomy or a bowel diversion where no gas will be seen in the colon and the small bowel caliber may be greater than normal by necessity.

CT imaging of small bowel obstruction

- CT is highly sensitive and specific for diagnosis of SBO. Small bowel distention ≥3 cm with a focal/discrete transition point to collapsed bowel is highly specific for a SBO.

小肠

小肠解剖

- 十二指肠有4个部分：球部(D_1)、降部(D_2)、水平/横部(D_3)和升部(D_4)。
- 环状襞(又称环状皱襞)是环形的小肠褶皱。

  相比之下，结肠袋不是环形的。
- 肠系膜上动脉(SMA)同时供应空肠及回肠，而十二指肠接受来自腹腔干分支的血液。
- 小肠系膜将空肠和回肠共同固定于后腹壁。
- 空肠较回肠更为突出的特点是肠皱襞大、褶皱更紧密，肠绒毛也较大。
- 十二指肠悬韧带(十二指肠悬肌)是位于十二指肠和空肠交界处的薄层肌肉，是上消化道和下消化道之间的分界。这对于定位消化道出血的来源具有临床意义。虽然不能在影像上直接进行观察，但可以间接地将十二指肠悬韧带定位于十二指肠升部(第四段)远端的边缘。

  上消化道出血发生在十二指肠悬韧带上游。

  下消化道出血发生在十二指肠悬韧带下游。

小肠梗阻(SBO)

- 小肠梗阻(SBO)比较常见，而且通常为先前手术造成的粘连或疝所致。肿瘤、狭窄及肠套叠是较少见的病因。

小肠梗阻的X线表现：

- 疑有小肠梗阻时，腹部X线影像通常是首选的影像学检查方法。
- 小肠梗阻的影像学表现包括：小肠扩张>3cm。站立位可见呈阶梯状的多发气-液平面。另外，结肠内缺乏气体高度提示有梗阻。
- 腹部影像上小肠袢扩张的鉴别诊断有：

  术后麻痹性肠梗阻(近期手术史，结肠内常可见气体)。

  与炎症相关的局灶性肠梗阻(如胰腺炎、肠炎，局部肠道扩张可能在炎症的附近出现)。

  腹水所致的肠梗阻：腹水常压迫升结肠、降结肠及直肠，因这些结构不附着在肠系膜上。但气体在横结肠及乙状结肠内仍潴留明显。小肠可能受压向内侧移位。
- 一个潜在的误判是在行全结肠切除术或肠改道的患者，他们的结肠中看不到气体，而小肠的直径可能大于正常数值。

小肠梗阻的CT表现

- CT诊断小肠梗阻具有很高的灵敏度和特异度。小肠肠腔扩张≥3cm并可见一个局灶/明确的小肠萎陷的转折点对诊断小肠梗阻具有

- Benefits of CT include confirmation of diagnosis of SBO, visualization of the etiology and assessment of complications of obstruction such as ischemia or strangulation.
- It is important to approach the interpretation of an obstruction in a systematic way.
- **First**, look for the transition point to decompressed bowel to determine the cause.
- **Second**, always determine if the obstruction is *simple* or *closed-loop* (see below). A closed- loop obstruction is a *never miss* diagnosis as there is very high risk for bowel ischemia and therefore, severe morbidity and mortality.
- **Third**, evaluate for signs of ischemia or impending ischemia, which include (in rough order of severity):

> **Engorged mesenteric vessels.**
> **Mesenteric edema.**
> **Ascites surrounding the bowel** or **inter-loop fluid**, due to increased capillary permeability.
> **Wall thickening**, due to submucosal edema.
> **Lack of bowel wall enhancement**, due to vasoconstriction or underperfusion. Note that the presence or absence of bowel wall enhancement can only be assessed if positive oral contrast was not given.
> **Pneumatosis intestinalis**, which is gas in the bowel wall due to necrosis. Pneumatosis produces multiple small locules of gas seen circumferentially in the bowel wall.

- In addition to small bowel distention >3 cm and a transition point to decompressed bowel, an additional helpful CT finding of SBO is the *small bowel feces sign,* which describes particulate feculent material mixed with gas bubbles in the small bowel that resembles the CT appearance of stool.

  The small bowel feces sign is often seen just proximal to the transition point and is helpful to localize the site of transition.

  The sign may be especially helpful in subacute or partial obstruction, which can otherwise be difficult to diagnose.

  The sign is thought to be due to bacterial overgrowth and undigested food.

高度特异性。

- CT的优势包括确诊小肠梗阻、显示梗阻原因，以及评估梗阻的并发症，如缺血或绞窄。
- 掌握系统性分析肠梗阻的方法非常重要：
- **第一**，寻找肠道萎陷的转折点以确定梗阻的原因。
- **第二**，必须判断肠梗阻为单纯性还是闭袢性（见下文）。闭袢性肠梗阻是一个不可漏诊的病变，因其发生小肠缺血的风险非常高，因而有严重的合并症和极高的死亡率。
- **第三**，评价缺血或即将发生缺血的征象，包括（按严重程度大概排序）：

> **肠系膜血管充盈肿胀。**
> **肠系膜水肿。**
> **腹水包绕肠管或肠袢内积液**，为毛细血管通透性增高所致。
> **肠壁增厚**，由于黏膜下水肿导致。
> **肠壁无强化**，由于血管收缩或灌注不足所致。注意，判断是否有肠壁强化只能在未服用口服阳性造影剂的情况下进行。
> **肠壁积气**，由于肠壁坏死而造成肠壁内积气。积气造成多发小气泡沿小肠壁四周分布。

- 除了小肠肠腔扩张>3cm和肠腔塌陷的转折点，另一个有用的CT小肠梗阻的征象为小肠积粪征，即小肠内出现颗粒状粪便物与气泡混合物，类似于粪便在CT上的表现。

  小肠积粪征常见于转折点的近端，并有助于对转折点的定位。

  此征象在亚急性或部分性肠梗阻时可能特别有用，否则诊断较为困难。

  此征象被认为是由于细菌增殖和尚未消化的食物所致。

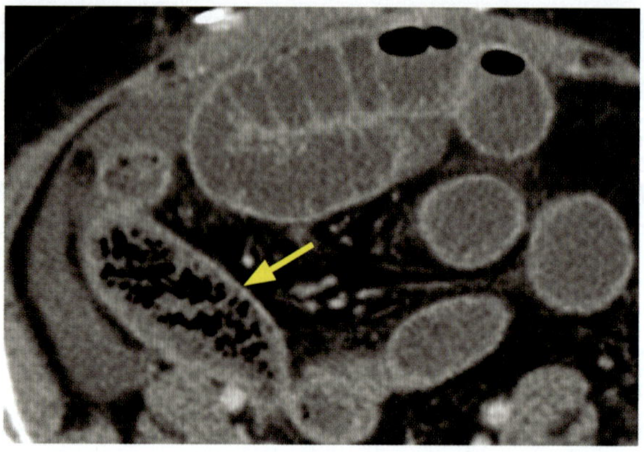

Small bowel feces sign: Axial CT shows an obstruction. A loop of small bowel in the right lower quadrant (arrow) demonstrates numerous gas locules and particulate material in the small bowel.
小肠积粪征：轴位CT显示小肠梗阻。右下腹的一段小肠内（黄箭）可见无数气泡影和颗粒样物质。

Closed-loop obstruction

闭袢性肠梗阻

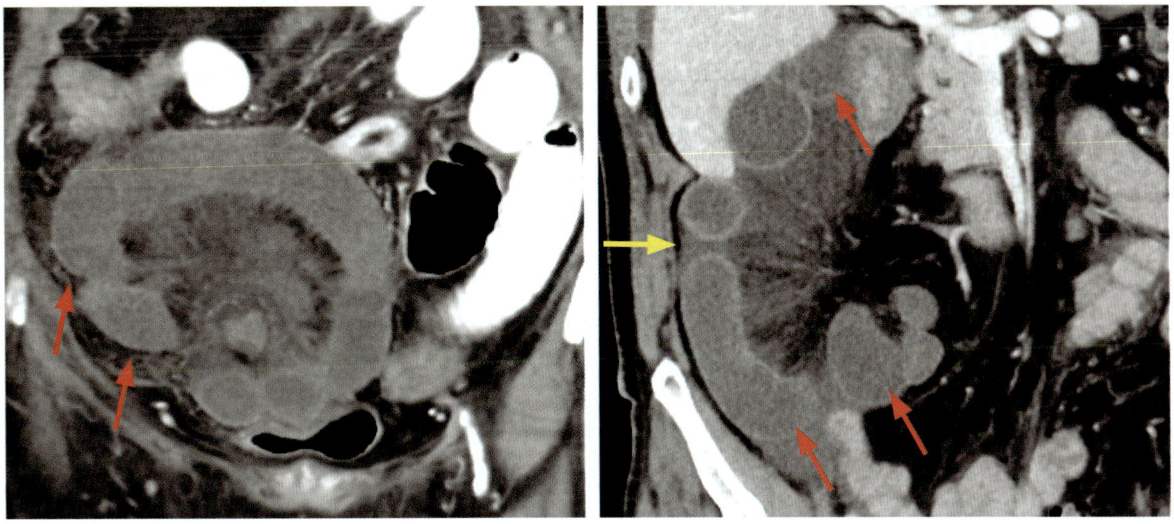

Closed-loop obstruction in two different patients: Note the similar C-shape configuration of dilated small bowel loops with associated swirling of the mesentery, mesenteric edema, and inter-loop fluid (yellow arrow). There is segmental bowel wall hypoenhancement (red arrows) when compared to adjacent normally enhancing bowel loops, concerning for ischemia.
两名不同患者的闭袢性肠梗阻：注意扩张的小肠袢具有相似的"C"形结构，伴有肠系膜旋转、肠系膜水肿和袢间积液(黄箭)。节段性肠壁(红箭)的强化程度低于相邻正常强化的肠袢，考虑有缺血。

- Closed-loop obstruction is a surgical emergency that may lead to bowel ischemia. Closed-loop obstruction represents obstruction of both the efferent and afferent segments of a single loop of bowel. Closed-loop obstruction is almost always seen in association with small bowel volvulus, which may be due to adhesions or internal hernia.
- CT imaging features include the *whirl sign* due to twisting of mesenteric vessels seen in volvulus. Other CT findings include a U-or C-shaped distribution of the distended bowel loops with radially oriented vessels. Mesenteric edema is often present.

- 闭袢性肠梗阻是外科急症，可导致肠缺血。闭袢性肠梗阻是指一段肠管的输入袢和输出袢均发生梗阻。闭袢性肠梗阻几乎总合并小肠扭转，可能为粘连或内疝所致。
- CT影像学特征包括漩涡征，为肠扭转时被扭转的肠系膜血管。其他CT表现包括：扩张的肠袢呈"U"形或"C"形分布，其肠系膜血管呈放射状排列。肠系膜水肿常见。

Obstruction due to adhesions

粘连性肠梗阻

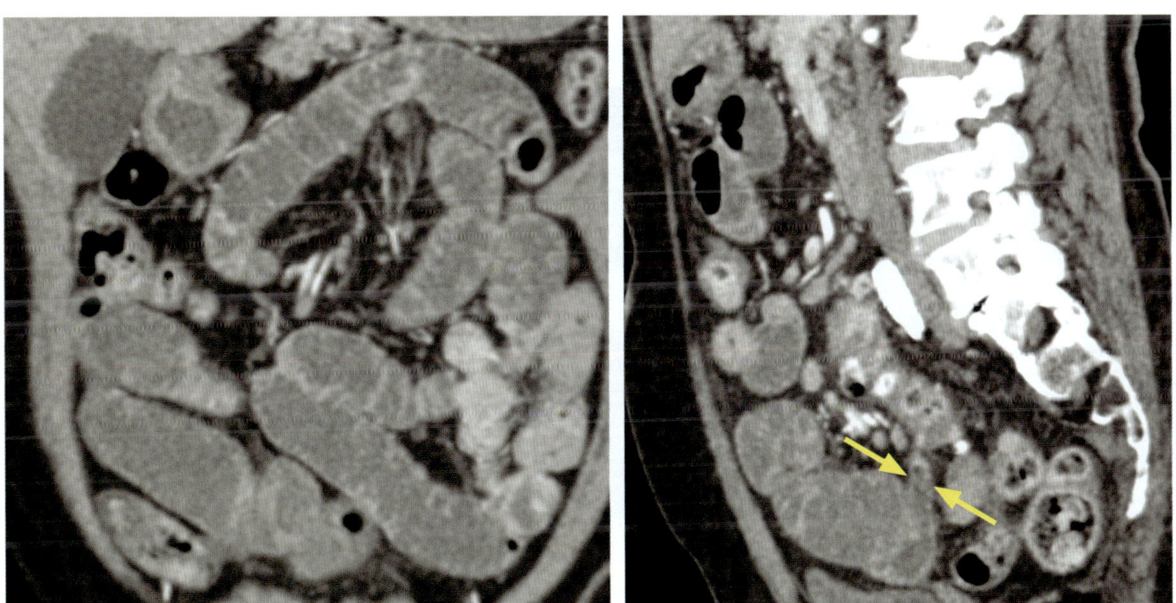

Small bowel obstruction due to adhesions: Coronal (left image) and sagittal CT (right image) shows multiple dilated, fluid-filled loops of small bowel. A transition point is located in the midline pelvis (arrows on sagittal image), with no obstructing mass or evidence of hernia.
粘连性小肠梗阻：冠状位(左图)及矢状位(右图)CT显示多个扩张和充满积液的小肠肠管。转折点位于盆腔中线(矢状位，箭)，未见梗阻性肿块或疝的征象。

- Adhesions from prior surgery or intra-peritoneal inflammatory process are the most common cause of SBO. The vast majority of patients with SBO due to adhesions have had prior abdominal surgery.
- Adhesions are an imaging diagnosis of exclusion as they are not directly visualized by imaging. On CT, a transition point is seen, but no alternative cause for the transition (e.g., no mass or hernia, etc.) is identified.
- In the absence of signs of impending ischemia, this is usually managed non-operatively with nasogastric tube decompression and bowel rest.

- 既往手术或腹腔内炎症造成的粘连是小肠梗阻最常见的病因。绝大多数因粘连而发生肠梗阻的患者之前都做过腹部手术。
- 粘连是影像学上的一种排除性诊断，因为它们不能在图像上直接显示。CT可见转折点，但无明显造成转折的原因(如无肿瘤或疝等)。
- 在没有明显缺血迹象的情况下，通常采用鼻胃管减压和肠道休息进行保守治疗。

Obstruction due to external hernia

- Protrusion of bowel through an abdominal wall defect is the second most common cause of SBO. Approximately 75% of external hernias occur in the groin, with the majority being inguinal hernias.
- The term *strangulation* refers to ischemia due to vascular compromise by the hernia.
- The term *incarceration* refers to a hernia that cannot be reduced and is a physical exam finding, not an imaging finding.
- An **inguinal hernia** may be either indirect or direct, depending on the relation of the hernia to the inferior epigastric vessels.

腹外疝性肠梗阻

- 肠管通过腹壁疝出是小肠梗阻的第二常见病因。约75%腹外疝发生于腹股沟区，大部分为腹股沟疝。
- 绞窄是指由于疝引起血管供血障碍而造成的缺血。
- 嵌顿是指无法复位的疝，这是一种体格检查发现，而不是影像学的表现。
- **腹股沟疝**根据疝囊与腹壁下血管的关系，分为斜疝及直疝：

Indirect: Indirect inguinal hernia is the most common type and is more common in males. The neck of the hernia is lateral to the inferior epigastric vessels. Hernia contents travel with the spermatic cord, often *into the scrotum*. Indirect inguinal hernias are considered congenital due to a patent processus vaginalis.

Direct: The neck of a direct inguinal hernia is medial to the inferior epigastric vessels, protruding through a weak area in the anterior abdominal wall (Hesselbach's triangle). The hernia contents *do not go into the scrotum*. These are considered acquired and may be caused by increased intra-abdominal pressure, such as obesity, COPD and chronic constipation.

斜疝：腹股沟斜疝是最常见的类型，多发于男性。疝囊颈位于腹壁下血管的外侧。疝内容物穿过精索，常疝入阴囊。腹股沟斜疝被认为是先天性的，为内环闭合不良所致。

直疝：腹股沟直疝的囊颈位于腹壁下血管的内侧，疝内容物通过前腹壁薄弱区疝出(海氏三角)。疝内容物不进入阴囊。直疝被认为是后天性的，可能由腹内压增加引起，如肥胖、慢性阻塞性肺疾病和慢性便秘。

When an inguinal hernia contains the appendix, it is called an **Amyand hernia**.
When it contains a Meckel's diverticulum, it is called a **Littre hernia**.

当腹股沟疝含有阑尾时，被称为**Amyand疝**。
当包含梅克尔憩室时，则称为**憩室疝**。

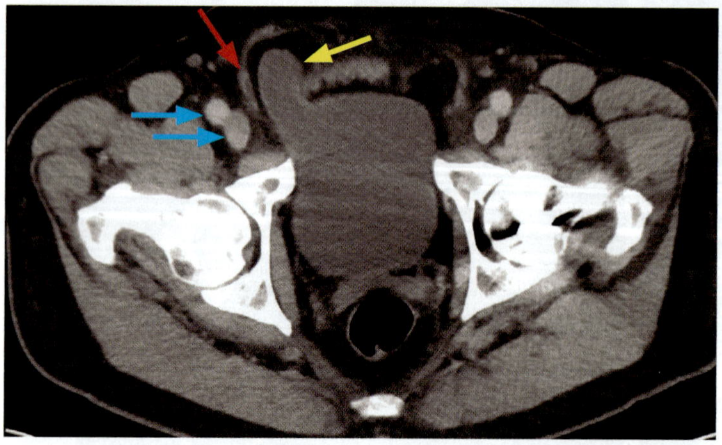

Direct inguinal hernia:
Axial contrast-enhanced CT shows a direct inguinal hernia on the right containing a portion of the urinary bladder (yellow arrow). Note the right inferior epigastric vessels and inguinal canal contents (red arrow) are displaced laterally and compressed by the hernia. The right common femoral artery and vein are normal in caliber (blue arrows).
腹股沟直疝：
轴位增强CT显示右侧腹股沟直疝，内含部分膀胱(黄箭)。注意右侧腹壁下血管和腹股沟管的内容物(红箭)向外侧移位并被疝压迫。右股总动脉和静脉直径正常(蓝箭)。

- In an **obturator hernia**, bowel herniates through the obturator canal. Obturator hernias are almost always seen in elderly women due to pelvic floor laxity.

The key imaging finding is bowel located between the pectineus and obturator muscles.

It is important to correctly diagnose an obturator hernia preoperatively. An obturator

- **闭孔疝**是肠道从闭孔管中疝出。闭孔疝几乎都见于老年女性，为盆底结构松弛所致。

关键的影像学表现为肠管位于耻骨肌与闭孔肌之间。

术前正确诊断闭孔疝十分重要。闭孔疝的手术方

hernia requires a different surgery from inguinal hernia and has an especially high morbidity and mortality if incarcerated.

式与腹股沟疝完全不同，若发生嵌顿，合并症发生率与死亡率极高。

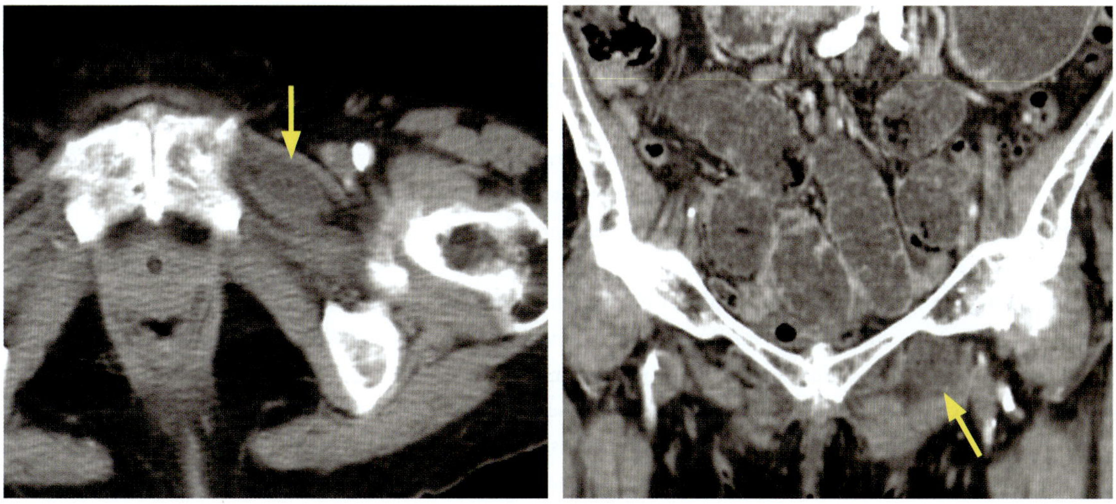

Obturator hernia: Axial (left image) and coronal (right image) contrast-enhanced CT demonstrates herniation of a bowel loop (arrows) through the left obturator canal, between the obturator and pectineus muscles, with a resultant upstream SBO.
闭孔疝：轴位(左图)和冠状位(右图)增强CT显示一段疝出的肠袢(黄箭)穿过左侧闭孔管，位于闭孔肌和耻骨肌之间，并导致上游小肠梗阻。

- **Ventral hernia** is often due to prior laparotomy or other abdominal surgery.
- **Femoral hernia** is a protrusion into the femoral canal posterior and inferior to the inguinal ligament. When it contains the appendix, it is called **De Garengeot hernia**. In addition to location below the inguinal ligament, it can be differentiated from an inguinal hernia by its tendency to compress the adjacent femoral vein.

- **腹壁疝**常由之前的开腹手术或其他腹部手术所致。
- **股疝**是在股管后腹股沟韧带下方的突起。当它包含阑尾时，就被称为**De Garengeot疝**。除位于腹股沟韧带下方外，与腹股沟疝的区别在于其倾向于压迫邻近的股静脉。

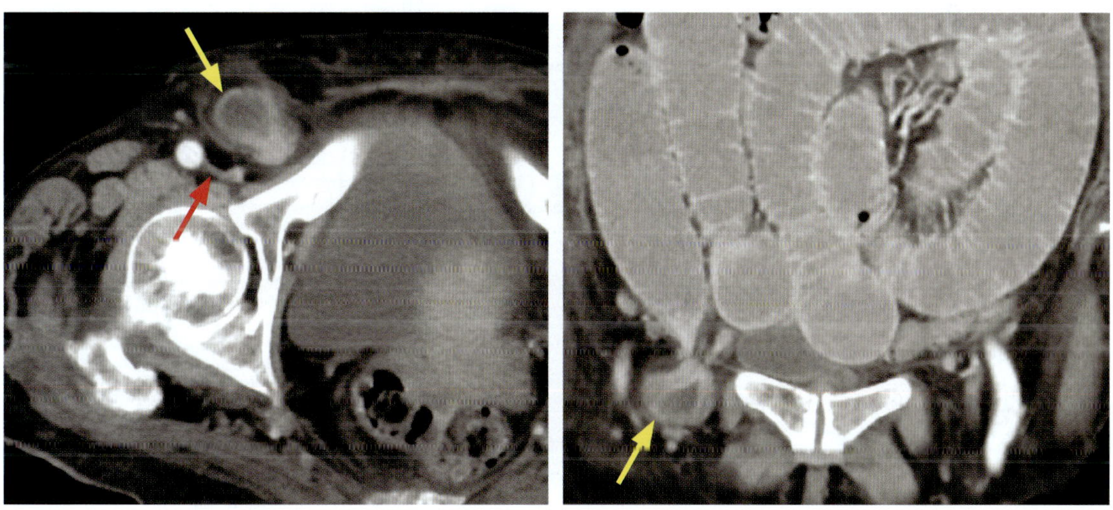

Femoral hernia: Axial (left image) and coronal (right image) contrast-enhanced CT shows herniation of a short segment of small bowel into the right femoral canal (yellow arrows), causing upstream SBO. Note the right femoral vein (red arrow) is compressed by the hernia.
股疝：轴位(左图)和冠状位(右图)增强CT显示一段短的小肠疝入右侧股管(黄箭)，引起上游小肠梗阻。注意右股静脉(红箭)被疝压迫。

- **Spigelian hernia** is a lateral ventral hernia that occurs at the semilunar line (between the rectus abdominis and lateral oblique muscles). It is associated

- **半月线疝**是发生在半月线(腹直肌和侧面腹斜肌之间)的侧腹壁疝，与男性婴儿的同侧隐睾

with ipsilateral cryptorchidism amongst male infants due to failure of development of a gubernaculum.

- **Richter hernia** can occur in any of the above hernias and occurs when only the antimesenteric portion of the bowel wall is herniated. These hernias are more likely to result in strangulation than obstruction.

Obstruction due to internal hernia

- Protrusion of bowel through a defect or opening in the peritoneal cavity or mesentery is a relatively uncommon cause of SBO. Internal hernias carry a high rate of volvulus. If volvulus is present, the *whirl sign* may be visible.
- Many different subtypes may be seen including transmesenteric, paraduodenal, and foramen of Winslow among others.
- **Transmesenteric hernia** is a broad category of bowel herniation through defects in any of the three true mesenteries (small bowel mesentery, transverse mesocolon, and sigmoid mesentery). The most common type of transmesenteric hernia is the **transmesocolic** hernia due to a defect in the transverse mesocolon (mesentery of the transverse colon). Transmesocolic hernia is seen most commonly post Roux-en-Y gastric bypass or biliary- enteric anastomosis from liver transplant.
- **Paraduodenal hernia** was previously the most common internal hernia (prior to the rise in gastric bypass surgery). Paraduodenal hernias are congenital anomalies, due to embryologic failure of mesenteric fusion and resultant mesenteric defect. They more commonly occur on the left and are associated with abnormal intestinal rotation.

症有关，是引带发育不良所致。

- **肠壁疝**可发生在上述任何一种疝中，但其疝内容物只包含肠系膜对侧的肠壁。这些疝更可能导致绞窄而不是梗阻。

由腹内疝引起的肠梗阻

- 肠管从腹膜或肠系膜的缺损或开口处疝出是小肠梗阻相对少见的原因。腹内疝合并肠扭转的概率很高。如果存在肠扭转，则可能会看到漩涡征。
- 可以见到多个不同种类的亚型，其中包括经肠系膜、十二指肠旁和网膜孔等。
- **肠系膜疝**是一大类通过肠系膜缺损的肠疝，包括以下三个中任意一个真性肠系膜(小肠系膜、横结肠系膜和乙状结肠系膜)。最常见的肠系膜疝是**横结肠系膜疝**，是由于横结肠系膜缺损所致。横结肠系膜疝最常见于鲁氏Y形胃旁路术或肝移植的胆-肠吻合术后。
- **十二指肠旁疝**曾经是最常见的腹内疝(在胃旁路手术开展之前)。十二指肠旁疝是先天性异常，是由于胚胎期肠系膜融合障碍造成肠系膜缺损所致。最常发生于左侧，与肠旋转异常相关。

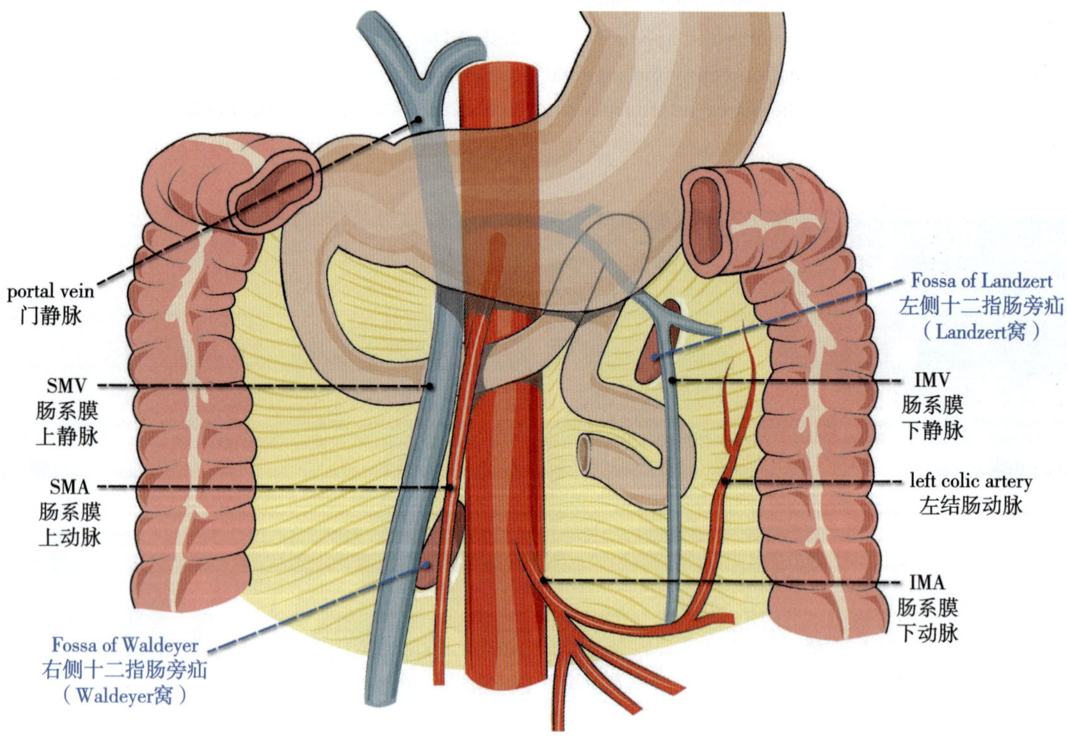

Illustration demonstrating the anatomy most relevant to paraduodenal hernia. Note the fossa of Landzert (**left** paraduodenal hernia) and fossa of Waldeyer (**right** paraduodenal hernia).
示意图显示与十二指肠旁疝最相关的解剖结构。注意Landzert窝(**左侧**十二指肠旁疝)和Waldeyer窝(**右侧**十二指肠旁疝)。

In the more common **left** paraduodenal hernia, the bowel can herniate through a mesenteric defect named *fossa of Landzert*, located to the left of the ascending (fourth portion) duodenum, behind the IMV.

在较为常见的左侧十二指肠旁疝中，肠管可通过一个称为Landzert窝的肠系膜缺损疝出，Landzert窝位于十二指肠升部(第四段)的左侧，IMV后方。

The key imaging finding is a cluster of small bowel loops between the pancreas and stomach.

关键的影像学表现为一团小肠肠袢位于胃与胰腺之间。

In a **right** paraduodenal hernia, the bowel and mesentery containing iliocolic, right colic, middle colic arteries herniate through the *fossa of Waldeyer*, a mesenteric defect located behind the SMA and SMV.

在**右侧**十二指肠旁疝中，肠和肠系膜包含髂结肠动脉、右结肠动脉和中结肠动脉通过Waldeyer窝疝出，肠系膜缺损位于SMA和SMV的后方。

- **Foramen of Winslow hernia**: The foramen of Winslow is the communication between the lesser sac and the greater peritoneal cavity. The key imaging features of a foramen of Winslow hernia are dilated loops of bowel in the lesser sac and presence of mesentery and/or bowel loops between the IVC and main portal vein.

- **网膜孔(Winslow孔)疝**：网膜孔是沟通小网膜囊与大腹膜腔之间的通道。网膜孔疝最关键的影像学表现为小网膜囊中有扩张的肠袢，且肠系膜出现在下腔静脉与门静脉主干之间。

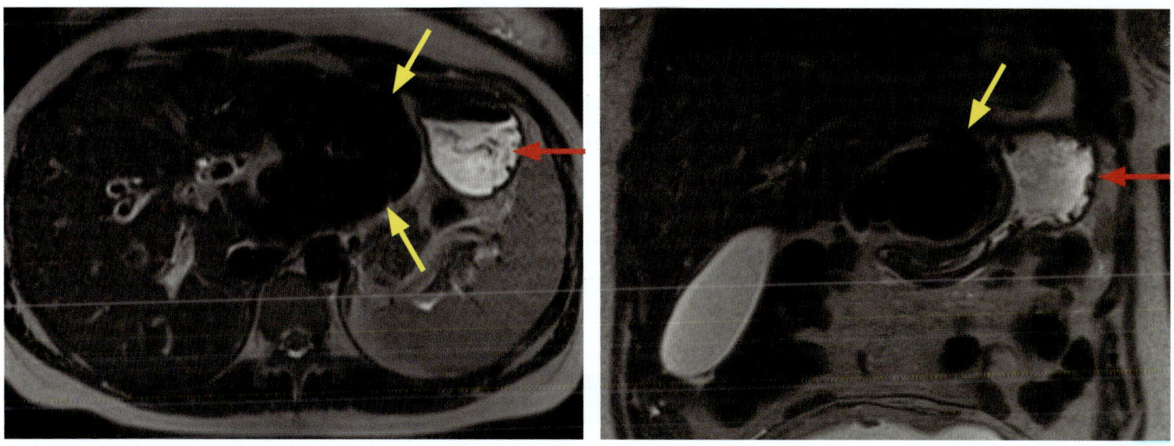

Foramen of Winslow hernia: Axial (left image) and coronal (right image) T2-weighted MRI shows unusual configuration of the right hemicolon (yellow arrows), which extends into the lesser sac through the foramen of Winslow, displacing the stomach laterally (red arrows). There is no evidence of colonic wall thickening or pericolonic edema.

网膜孔疝：轴位(左图)和冠状位(右图)T_2加权MRI显示右半结肠的结构异常(黄箭)，其通过网膜孔疝入小网膜囊，而胃受压向外侧移位(红箭)。无结肠壁增厚或结肠周围水肿的迹象。

Obstruction due to neoplasm

- A mass intrinsic to the bowel or compression from an extrinsic mass may cause SBO. An extrinsic mass is usually straightforward to diagnose by CT.
- Although the presence of an intraluminal mass may be more difficult to detect on CT, clues to the presence of an intrinsic mass include irregular bowel wall thickening and/or regional lymphadenopathy.
- Primary small bowel neoplasm causing intrinsic bowel obstruction may be due to adenocarcinoma, GIST, and carcinoid. Metastatic causes of intrinsic bowel neoplasm include melanoma, ovarian, and lung cancer. Melanoma is known to cause intussusception.
- Lymphoma is generally a "soft" tumor and rarely causes obstruction. *Aneurysmal* dilatation of the small bowel wall is a classic appearance, but presentation is highly variable.

肿瘤性肠梗阻

- 来自肠道内、外肿瘤的压迫可造成小肠梗阻。肠外肿瘤在CT上通常比较容易进行诊断。
- 肠腔内肿瘤在CT上可能相对困难，但某些线索可以提示存在肠腔内的肿瘤，如肠壁不规则增厚和/或区域淋巴结肿大。
- 可造成肠梗阻的原发性小肠肿瘤包括腺癌、胃肠道间质瘤及类癌。肠腔内转移性肿瘤包括黑色素瘤、卵巢癌及肺癌。黑色素瘤可造成肠套叠。
- 淋巴瘤通常为"软"性肿瘤，极少导致肠梗阻。小肠壁呈动脉瘤样扩张为其典型表现，但表现形式多样化。

Obstruction due to intussusception

肠套叠性肠梗阻

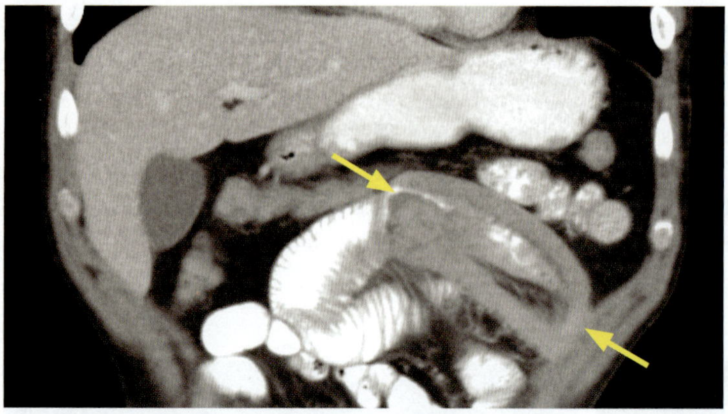

Intussusception causing small bowel obstruction: Coronal contrast-enhanced CT demonstrates a segmental jejunojejunal intussusception (arrows), causing an early or partial proximal small bowel obstruction. This was a case of metastatic melanoma (metastatic lesion not visualized on this image).
肠套叠导致的小肠梗阻：
冠状位增强CT显示一段空肠与空肠套叠(黄箭)，并导致早期或不完全性近端小肠梗阻。此病例为转移性黑色素瘤(转移病灶在图中未显示)。

- While transient intussusceptions are a common incidental finding, an intussusception causing obstruction should raise suspicion for an underlying lesion and prompt surgery.
- Transient small bowel intussusceptions tend to be short segments without wall thickening or upstream obstruction, while malignant intussusceptions involve longer segments with associated wall thickening and upstream obstruction.

- 一过性肠套叠通常是一种意外发现，肠套叠造成肠梗阻时应该警惕有潜在的病变并需要及时手术。
- 一过性小肠肠套叠涉及较短的肠段，不伴有肠壁增厚或上游梗阻，而恶性肠套叠累及较长的肠段，伴有肠壁增厚及上游梗阻。

Obstruction due to Crohn's disease

克罗恩病导致的肠梗阻

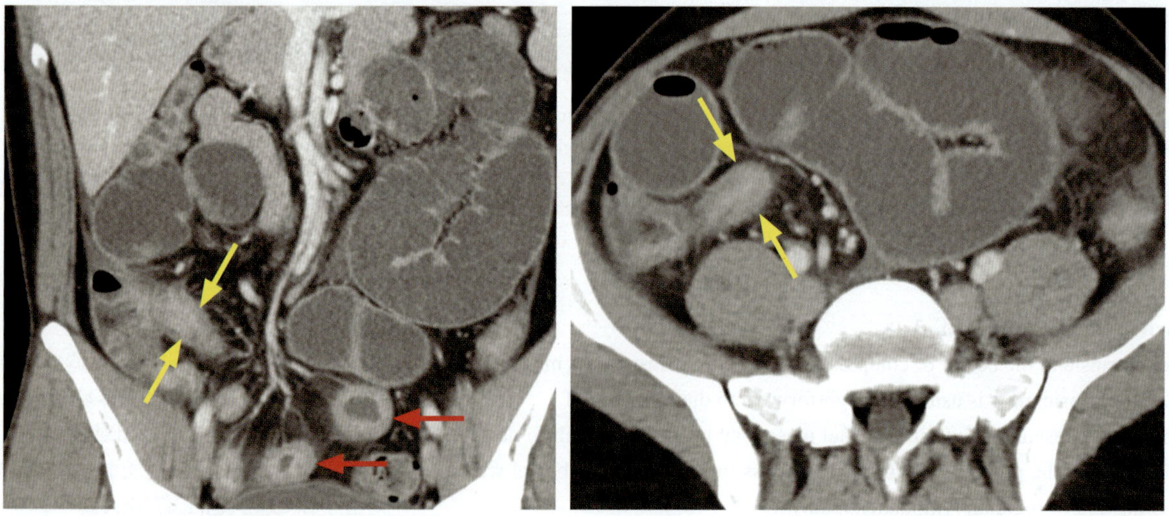

Obstruction due to Crohn's ileitis: Coronal (left image) and axial contrast-enhanced CT shows dilated loops of proximal small bowel. The terminal ileum (yellow arrows) and several loops of distal ileum (red arrows) are thickened, reflecting enteritis.
克罗恩回肠炎导致的肠梗阻：冠状位(左图)及轴位(右图)增强CT显示小肠近端肠管扩张。回肠末端(黄箭)及部分远端回肠(红箭)肠壁增厚，提示肠炎。

- Stricturing disease or active inflammation resulting in luminal narrowing is an important cause of bowel obstruction in Crohn's disease. Crohn's disease is discussed below.

- 狭窄性病变或活动性肠炎是克罗恩病引起肠梗阻的重要病因。克罗恩病将在下文进行讨论。

Obstruction due to gallstone

- **Gallstone ileus**, which is actually misnomer, is a subtype of SBO due to a gallstone, which has eroded from gallbladder into the duodenum, causing the classic *Rigler's triad* of pneumobilia (from cholecystoduodenal fistula), SBO, and ectopic gallstone within the small bowel.
- **Bouveret syndrome** is a proximal form of gallstone ileus due to impaction of the gallstone in the pylorus or proximal duodenum.

胆石性肠梗阻

- **胆石性肠梗阻**实际上是一个不恰当的名词，它是由胆囊结石引起小肠梗阻的一个亚型，为胆结石侵蚀胆囊进入十二指肠肠腔，导致典型的Rigler三联征，即胆道积气(由于胆囊-十二指肠瘘)、小肠梗阻，以及小肠内异位的胆囊结石。
- **Bouveret综合征**是一种发生在近端的胆石性肠梗阻，胆囊结石嵌顿在幽门或近端十二指肠。

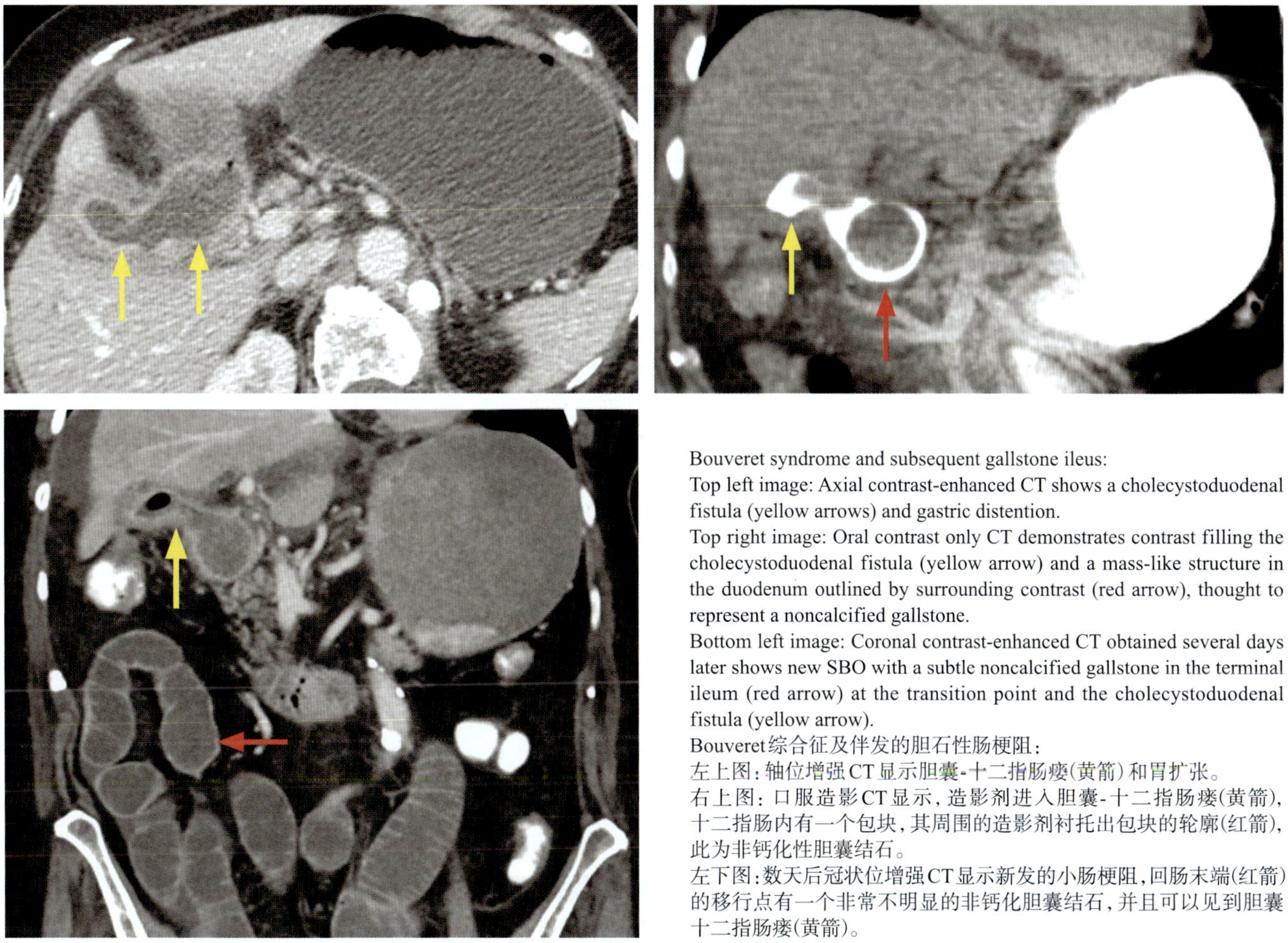

Bouveret syndrome and subsequent gallstone ileus:
Top left image: Axial contrast-enhanced CT shows a cholecystoduodenal fistula (yellow arrows) and gastric distention.
Top right image: Oral contrast only CT demonstrates contrast filling the cholecystoduodenal fistula (yellow arrow) and a mass-like structure in the duodenum outlined by surrounding contrast (red arrow), thought to represent a noncalcified gallstone.
Bottom left image: Coronal contrast-enhanced CT obtained several days later shows new SBO with a subtle noncalcified gallstone in the terminal ileum (red arrow) at the transition point and the cholecystoduodenal fistula (yellow arrow).
Bouveret综合征及伴发的胆石性肠梗阻：
左上图：轴位增强CT显示胆囊-十二指肠瘘（黄箭）和胃扩张。
右上图：口服造影CT显示，造影剂进入胆囊-十二指肠瘘（黄箭），十二指肠内有一个包块，其周围的造影剂衬托出包块的轮廓（红箭），此为非钙化性胆囊结石。
左下图：数天后冠状位增强CT显示新发的小肠梗阻，回肠末端（红箭）的移行点有一个非常不明显的非钙化胆囊结石，并且可以见到胆囊十二指肠瘘（黄箭）。

Enteritis

- Enteritis is inflammation of the small bowel. The most common CT manifestation of enteritis is bowel wall thickening. Mesenteric stranding or free fluid may also be present.

Crohn's disease

- Crohn's disease is a chronic granulomatous inflammatory condition which may affect any part of the GI tract from the mouth to the anus, though most commonly involves the terminal ileum. Bowel involvement is discontinuous, with characteristic skip lesions with intervening normal GI tract.
- The earliest histologic changes occur in the submucosa, seen on imaging as aphthous ulcers due to lymphoid hyperplasia and lymphedema.
- There are three phenotypes that may exist independently or may coexist. Imaging findings include:

Active inflammation: Mural hyperenhancement, intramural edema, mural ulcerations.
Stricturing disease: Luminal narrowing with upstream dilatation.
Penetrating disease*: Sinus tracts, simple fistulas, complex fistulas, inflammatory mass, abscess.

*Perianal disease is not considered penetrating disease.

- Endoscopy and barium fluoroscopy (small bowel follow-through, enteroclysis,

肠炎

- 肠炎是指小肠的炎症，在CT上最常见的表现为肠壁增厚，也可以有肠系膜水肿或游离液体。

克罗恩病

- 克罗恩病是慢性肉芽肿性炎性病变，可累及从口腔到肛门的胃肠道的任意部分，但最常累及的是回肠末端。受累肠道呈间断性分布，且病变跳跃分布于正常肠道之间为特征。
- 最早的组织学改变发生于黏膜下层，影像学表现为鹅口疮样溃疡，为淋巴样增生及淋巴水肿所致。
- 共有三种表型，可以单独存在，也可以共存。影像学表现包括：

活动性炎症：肠壁高强化，肠壁水肿，肠壁溃疡。
狭窄性疾病：肠腔狭窄伴上游肠管扩张。
穿透性疾病*：窦道、单纯性瘘管、复合性瘘管、炎性肿块、脓肿。

*肛周疾病不属于穿透性疾病。

- 内镜及X线钡剂造影（小肠动态造影、小肠灌

and barium enema) have historically been the modalities to evaluate Crohn's disease. CT and MR enterography are now the exams of choice.

The advantages of CT and MRI are the ability to evaluate the entire bowel wall (not just the mucosa), presence of extraintestinal complications, and the vasculature.

The disadvantages of CT and MRI compared to fluoroscopy and endoscopy are reduced spatial resolution and limited sensitivity for detecting subtle early signs of disease.

- The most common imaging findings on all modalities are wall thickening and inflammatory changes of the terminal ileum.
- Fluoroscopic findings include thickened, nodular folds in the affected regions of small bowel, luminal narrowing, mucosal ulceration, and separation of bowel loops (due to fibrofatty proliferation). The typical *cobblestone* appearance seen on endoscopy and fluoroscopy is a result of crisscrossing deep ulcerations.
- CT/MRI findings of Crohn's disease include:

  Creeping fat describes widely separated loops of bowel due to fibrofatty proliferation.

  Comb sign describes engorged vasa recta (mesenteric blood vessels) adjacent to an inflamed bowel loop.

  Pseudosacculation describes the bulging appearance along the antimesenteric border which is spared compared to the fibrotic and shortened mesenteric side.

  Restricted diffusion, when seen with other findings of active inflammation, indicates more severe disease.
- There is an increased risk of developing adenocarcinoma so close attention should be paid for any nodular thickening of the bowel wall.

肠造影及钡剂灌肠）是传统的克罗恩病检查方法。CT及肠道MRI是现在的检查手段。

CT及MRI的优势是能够评估整个肠壁（不只是黏膜）、肠外并发症及血管结构。

相对于肠镜及X线肠道造影检查，CT和MRI的主要缺点是空间分辨率低，对病变早期不明显的征象敏感性有限。

- 在所有影像学检查方法中常见的影像学表现是回肠末端肠壁增厚及炎症性改变。
- 透视检查表现包括受累区域的小肠壁增厚、结节状皱襞、管腔狭窄、黏膜溃疡，以及小肠肠袢分离（由于纤维脂肪增生）。肠镜及透视下典型的*鹅卵石征*是由于交错的深溃疡所致。
- 克罗恩病的CT/MRI表现包括：

  爬行样脂肪：由于纤维脂肪增生而广泛分离的肠袢。

  梳齿征：发炎肠袢附近的直血管（肠系膜血管）肿胀。

  假性积聚征：肠系膜对侧的肠管边缘隆起，较肠系膜侧的纤维化和缩短未受侵。

  弥散受限：当与其他活动性炎症表现同时出现时，表明疾病更为严重。
- 发生腺癌的风险增加，因此应密切注意肠壁的结节状增厚。

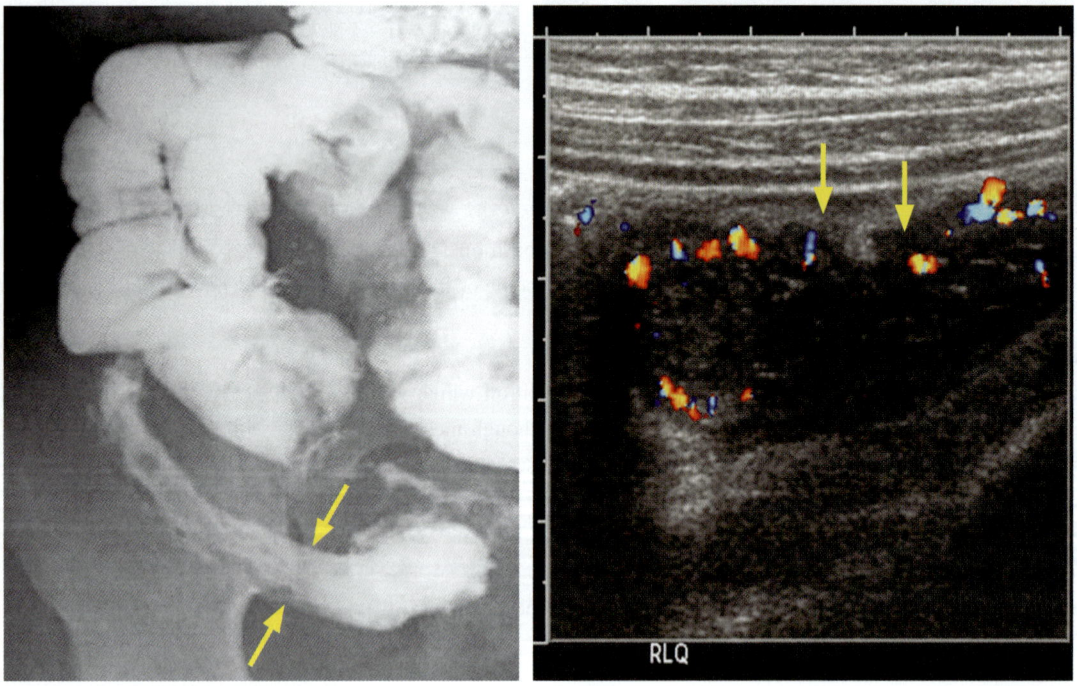

Crohn's disease (terminal ileitis): Small bowel follow-through (left image) shows terminal ileum nodular fold thickening, mucosal ulceration, and separation of the terminal ileum (arrows) from adjacent loops of small bowel.

Right lower quadrant color Doppler ultrasound (right image) in the same patient demonstrates the nodular fold thickening (arrows) and hyperemic wall.

Case courtesy Michael Callahan, MD, Boston Children's Hospital.

克罗恩病（末端回肠炎）：小肠动态造影（左图）可见回肠末端呈结节状皱襞增厚、黏膜溃疡，以及回肠末端（黄箭）与邻近小肠肠袢分离。

同一名患者右下腹彩色多普勒超声（右图）显示小肠皱襞结节状增厚（黄箭）和肠壁充血。

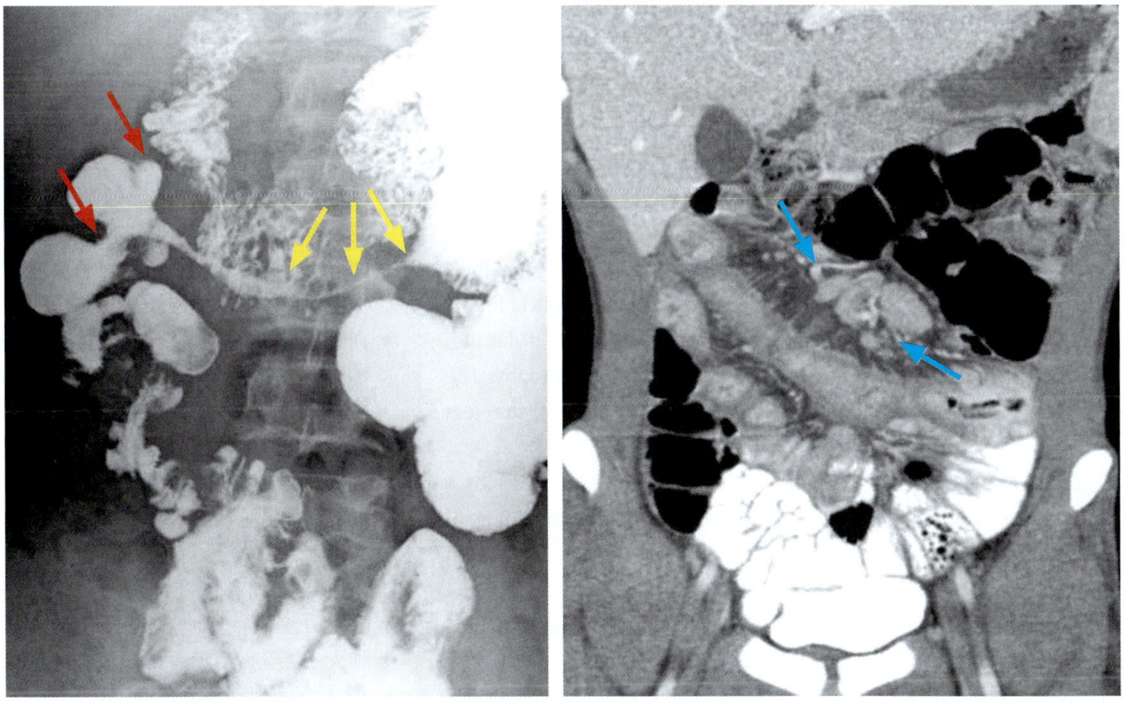

Crohn's disease with stricturing disease: Small bowel follow-through (left image) shows the *string sign* (yellow arrows) representing segmental stricture in a loop of distal ileum, with a few small antimesenteric *pseudosacculations* (red arrows). Contrast-enhanced CT (right image) shows bowel wall thickening and fibrofatty mesenteric changes (blue arrows), known by pathologists and surgeons as *creeping fat*.

Case courtesy Michael Callahan, MD, Boston Children's Hospital.

克罗恩病合并狭窄性病变：小肠动态显影(左图)显示串珠征(黄箭)，为远段回肠袢节段性狭窄，并可见多个肠系膜对侧缘假性憩室样改变(红箭)。冠状位增强CT(右图)显示肠壁增厚和肠系膜纤维脂肪样改变(蓝箭)，病理科医生和外科医生称之为爬行样脂肪。

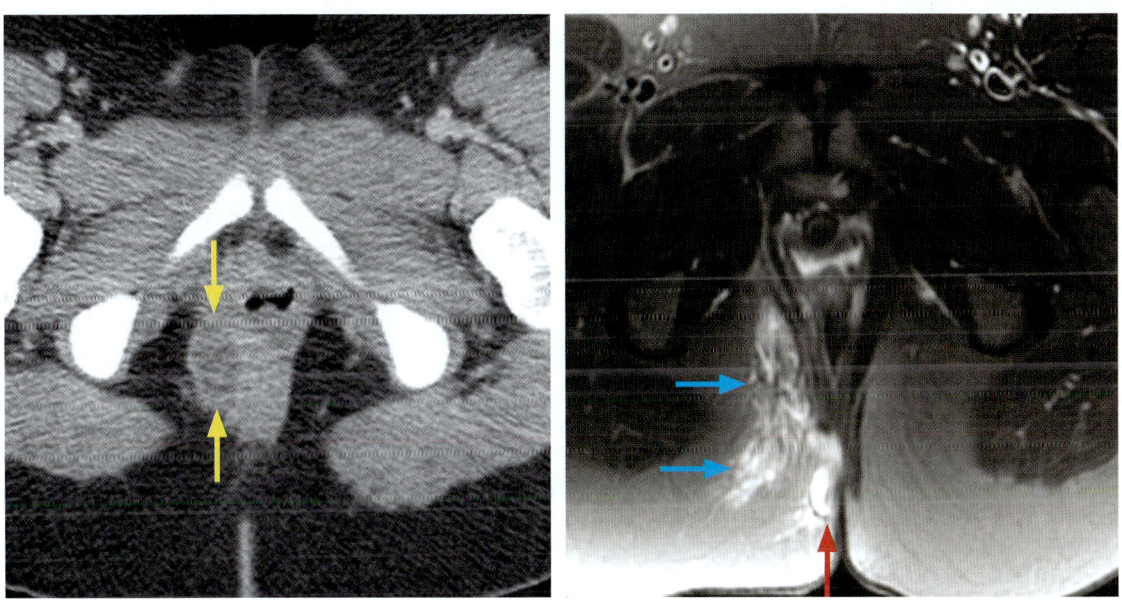

Perirectal abscess and enterocutaneous fistula secondary to Crohn's disease: Contrast-enhanced CT (left image) shows a peripherally enhancing fluid collection to the right of the rectum (yellow arrows).

T2-weighted MRI (right image) shows the distal portion of an enterocutaneous fistula extending to the skin surface (red arrow). There is marked subcutaneous edema (blue arrows) extending into the subcutaneous tissues of the right buttock.

Case courtesy Michael Callahan, MD, Boston Children's Hospital.

继发于克罗恩病的直肠周围脓肿及肠-皮肤窦道：轴位增强CT(左图)显示直肠右侧周边强化的积液(黄箭)。

T_2加权MRI(右图)显示肠-皮肤窦道的远端通向皮肤表面(红箭)。皮下可见明显的水肿(蓝箭)并延伸至右侧臀部皮下组织。

Celiac disease (sprue, gluten-sensitive enteropathy)

- Celiac disease, also known as sprue and gluten-sensitive enteropathy, is an autoimmune, proximal enteritis caused by a T-cell-mediated immune response triggered by antigens in ingested gluten.
- The primary sites of involvement are the duodenum and jejunum.
- The most characteristic imaging finding of celiac disease is reversal of jejunal and ileal fold patterns. Normally, the jejunum has more and closer together folds compared to the ileum. However, in celiac disease, the loss of jejunal folds due to villous atrophy causes a compensatory increase in the number of ileal folds.
- Fluoroscopy small bowel follow-through may show *flocculations* of barium due to lack of contrast adhesion to the bowel wall due to villous atrophy. The *moulage* (French for casting) refers to a cast-like appearance of the featureless jejunum.
- The CT findings of celiac disease include dilated, fluid-filled bowel loops, often with intra- luminal *flocculations* of enteric contrast. Reversal of jejunal and ileal fold patterns may be seen. Contrast can be seen both insinuated between the small bowel folds and centrally within the bowel, with a peripheral layer of low-attenuation secretions. Other CT findings of celiac disease include mesenteric adenopathy and engorgement of mesenteric vessels.
- Unlike with other causes of enteritis, diffuse bowel wall thickening and ascites are less common.
- An important complication of celiac disease is small bowel **T-cell lymphoma**, which may manifest as an exophytic mass, circumferential bowel wall thickening, or enlarged mesenteric lymph nodes.
- Other complications of celiac disease include:

> **Intussusception**, thought to be due to uncoordinated peristalsis, without a lead-point mass.
>
> **Pneumatosis intestinalis**, thought to be due to dissection of intraluminal gas through the inflamed bowel wall. Pneumatosis in the setting of celiac disease is not thought to reflect bowel ischemia.
>
> **Splenic atrophy.**
>
> Increased risk of **venous thromboembolism**.
>
> Lab abnormalities include anemia (secondary to malabsorption), leukopenia, and immunoglobulin deficiency. Skin abnormalities include the characteristic dermatitis herpetiformis rash.
>
> **Cavitating mesenteric lymph node syndrome** (CMLNS) is a very rare complication of celiac disease. The central portion of affected lymph nodes become low attenuation due to liquid necrosis. CMLNS is thought to be highly specific for celiac disease when seen in combination with villous atrophy and splenic atrophy. The differential diagnosis of low attenuation mesenteric lymph nodes includes TB, Whipple disease, treated lymphoma, and CMLNS.

Infectious enteritis

- Several bacterial, viral, and fungal organisms may cause enteritis.
- *Yersinia* and TB have a propensity to affect the terminal ileum, mimicking Crohn's disease.
- *Salmonella* is the most common cause of food-born gastroenteritis and causes segmental distal small bowel thickening on CT and segmental nodular thickened folds on fluoroscopy.

Whipple disease

- Whipple disease is due to infection by *Tropheryma whippelii,* which manifests

乳糜泻(口炎性腹泻，麸质敏感性肠病)

- 乳糜泻，又名口炎性腹泻或**麸质**敏感性肠病，是一种自身免疫性近端肠炎，为摄入的麸质抗原而引发的T细胞介导的免疫反应所致。
- 主要受累部位为十二指肠及空肠。
- 乳糜泻最具特征性的影像学表现为空肠和回肠皱襞形态反转。正常情况下，空肠皱襞较回肠多且密。但在乳糜泻患者中，因绒毛萎缩空肠皱襞的减少造成回肠皱襞代偿性增多。
- 在钡餐透视小肠动态造影检查时，由于绒毛萎缩，钡剂不易附着于肠壁而形成*絮状凝结*。Moulage征(Moulage在法语中表示铸造)指无空肠特征的铸型外观。
- 乳糜泻CT表现为小肠肠袢扩张与积液，常可见肠腔内的造影剂呈*絮状凝结*。可见空肠和回肠黏膜皱襞形态反转。造影剂迂回分布于小肠皱襞间和肠腔的中心，其外周有一层低密度分泌物。其他CT表现包括肠系膜淋巴结肿大，以及肠系膜血管肿胀。
- 与其他病因引起的肠炎不同，该病中弥漫性肠壁增厚及腹腔积液少见。
- 乳糜泻的一个重要并发症是小肠**T细胞淋巴瘤**，可表现为小肠外的肿块、肠壁环状增厚或肠系膜淋巴结增大。
- 其他并发症包括：

> **肠套叠**：可能是肠蠕动不协调所致，一般无诱发梗阻的肿块。
>
> **肠壁积气**：可能是由于肠腔内气体撕裂炎性的肠壁所致，乳糜泻发生的肠壁积气并不代表其反映了肠壁缺血。
>
> **脾萎缩**。
>
> **静脉血栓性栓塞**风险增加。
>
> 实验室检查异常包括：贫血(继发于吸收不良)、白细胞减少及免疫球蛋白缺乏。皮肤异常包括特征性疱疹样皮炎皮疹。
>
> **空泡肠系膜淋巴结综合征**(CMLNS)为乳糜泻的一种极为罕见的并发症。受累淋巴结的中央部位由于液化坏死而密度降低。CMLNS伴发绒毛萎缩和脾脏萎缩被认为对乳糜泻诊断有高度的特异性。低密度肠系膜淋巴结的鉴别诊断包括结核、惠普尔病、治疗后淋巴瘤及CMLNS。

感染性肠炎

- 某些细菌、病毒及真菌等病原体可引起肠炎。
- 耶尔森菌及结核分枝杆菌感染好发于回肠末端，表现类似于克罗恩病。
- 沙门菌是食源性胃肠炎中最常见的病原体，CT表现为远端小肠节段性肠壁增厚，肠道X线透视表现为小肠皱襞节段性、结节性增厚。

惠普尔病

- 惠普尔病是由于惠普尔养障体(一种革兰氏阳

in the GI tract as malabsorption and abdominal pain. Whipple disease may cause arthralgias and increased skin pigmentation.

- Whipple disease characteristically causes low attenuation adenopathy that may appear similar to the cavitating mesenteric lymph node syndrome seen in celiac disease.
- Radiographically, Whipple disease causes thickening and nodularity of duodenal and proximal small bowel folds. In contrast to celiac disease, there is typically no hypersecretion.

Radiation enteritis

性菌)感染所致，胃肠道症状表现为吸收不良及腹痛。惠普尔病可引起关节痛及皮肤色素沉着。

- 惠普尔病可以引起特征性的低密度淋巴结肿大，表现类似于乳糜泻中的CMLNS。
- 在影像学上，惠普尔病会导致十二指肠及近端小肠皱襞增厚和结节状改变。相对于乳糜泻，惠普尔病通常无过多肠道分泌。

放射性肠炎

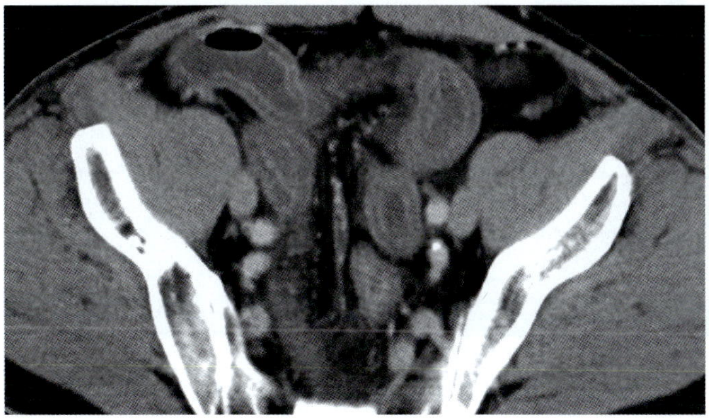

Axial contrast-enhanced CT shows wall thickening of the distal ileum, most prominent in the deep pelvis, with hyperenhancement of the inner mucosa and mesenteric vessel engorgement.
Although the findings are nonspecific, given the patient had recently completed radiation to the pelvis, this likely represents radiation enteritis.
轴位增强CT可见远端回肠壁增厚，盆腔深部最明显，黏膜高强化，肠系膜血管肿胀。虽然表现是非特异性的，但如果患者近期进行了盆腔放疗，则很可能为放射性肠炎。

- Long-term effects of radiation to the pelvis include adhesive and fibrotic changes to the mesentery and small bowel.
- Clues to the diagnosis of radiation enteritis include a history of radiation therapy and regional involvement of bowel loops not confined to a vascular territory and matching the radiation field.
- Imaging findings include mural thickening and mucosal hyperenhancement (in the acute stages) with narrowing of the lumen (in the later stages). Radiation enteritis may be a cause of SBO.

- 盆腔放疗的长期效应包括肠系膜和小肠出现粘连和纤维化改变。
- 诊断放射性肠炎的依据包括放疗病史和肠袢区域性受累范围并不局限于血管分布区域，但与放疗范围吻合。
- 影像学表现为受累节段肠壁增厚、黏膜明显强化(急性期)并伴有肠腔狭窄(晚期)。放射性肠炎可导致小肠梗阻。

OTHER DISEASES OF THE SMALL BOWEL

Scleroderma

- Scleroderma is a systemic disease characterized by the deposition of collagen into multiple internal organs and the skin.
- The primary insult in the GI tract in scleroderma is impaired motility due to replacement of the muscular layers with collagen, which leads to slowed transit and subsequent bacterial overgrowth, progressive dilation, and pseudo-obstruction.
- Radiographic findings are *sacculations* on the antimesenteric border (side opposite where the mesentery attaches) and a *hidebound bowel* due to thin, straight bowel folds stacked together.

其他小肠疾病

硬皮病

- 硬皮病是以胶原沉积在多个内脏器官及皮肤为特征的一种系统性疾病。
- 硬皮病对胃肠道最主要的损害是降低胃肠运动能力，这是由于肠壁肌层被胶原所取代，从而导致胃肠排空减慢、继发性菌群过度生长、肠道进行性扩张，以及假性肠梗阻。
- 影像学表现包括肠系膜对侧缘憩室形成，并可见肠道绷紧征，表现为受累肠段变薄变直并聚集。

Graft versus host disease (GVHD)

移植物抗宿主病(GVHD)

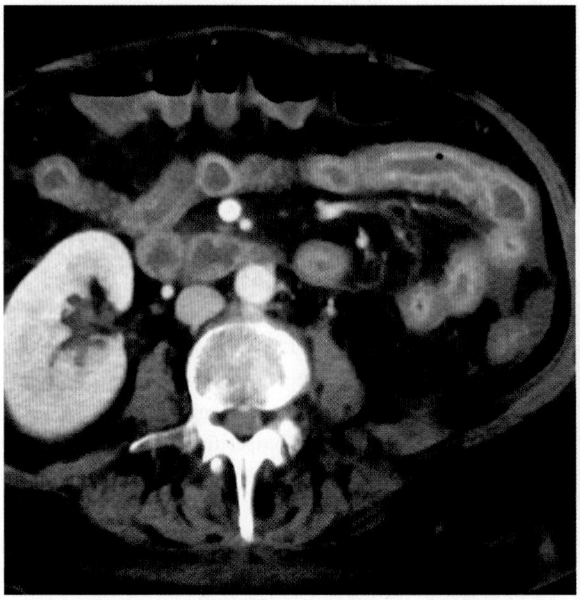

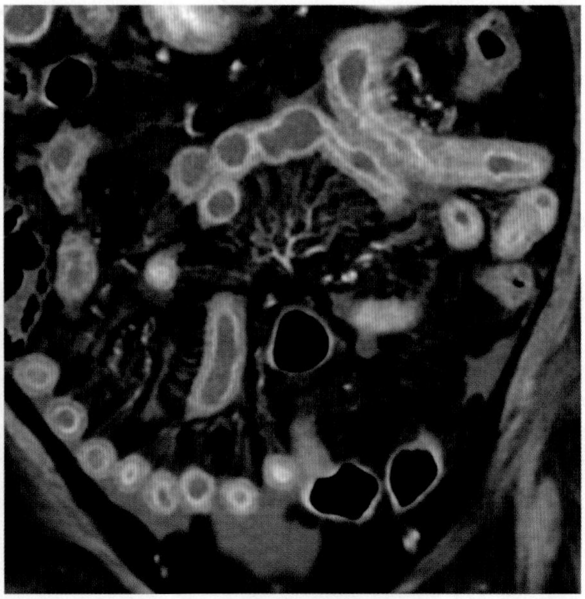

Axial (left image) and coronal (right image) contrast-enhanced CT shows diffuse wall thickening and mucosal hyperenhancement of jejunal and ileal loops, with associated mesenteric stranding and small volume ascites.
轴位(左图)和冠状位(右图)增强CT显示空肠和回肠壁弥漫性增厚和黏膜过度强化,并伴有肠系膜渗出和少量腹水。

- Graft versus host disease (GVHD) is a complication of bone marrow transplantation. The skin, liver, and GI tract are most commonly affected.
- CT/MRI findings of GVHD include wall thickening with mucosal hyperenhancement and effacement of the normal small bowel fold pattern. The classic small bowel follow-through finding is the *ribbon bowel* (due to diffuse luminal narrowing by bowel wall thickening).

Intestinal angioedema

- Intestinal angioedema is a rare condition in which submucosal edema occurs secondary to extravasation of protein from vasculature. It may be seen with ACE inhibitor or angiotensin Ⅱ receptor blockers use and hereditary C1-inhibitor deficiency.
- Imaging findings include thickening of the bowel submucosa with possible straightening of bowel loops, mesenteric edema, and ascites.

- 移植物抗宿主病(GVHD)是骨髓移植的一种并发症。最常累及皮肤、肝脏及胃肠道。
- GVHD在CT/MRI上表现为肠壁增厚,黏膜高度强化,正常小肠皱襞消失。典型的小肠动态造影表现为丝带状肠(由于肠壁增厚导致弥漫性管腔狭窄)。

肠道血管性水肿

- 肠道血管性水肿是一种罕见的情况,是因蛋白质从血管外渗而产生的黏膜下水肿。还可见于使用血管紧张素转化酶抑制剂或血管紧张素Ⅱ受体阻滞剂和遗传性C1抑制剂缺乏。
- 影像学表现包括肠黏膜下层增厚,并可能伴有肠袢伸直、肠系膜水肿和腹水。

APPENDIX

阑尾

Appendicitis

阑尾炎

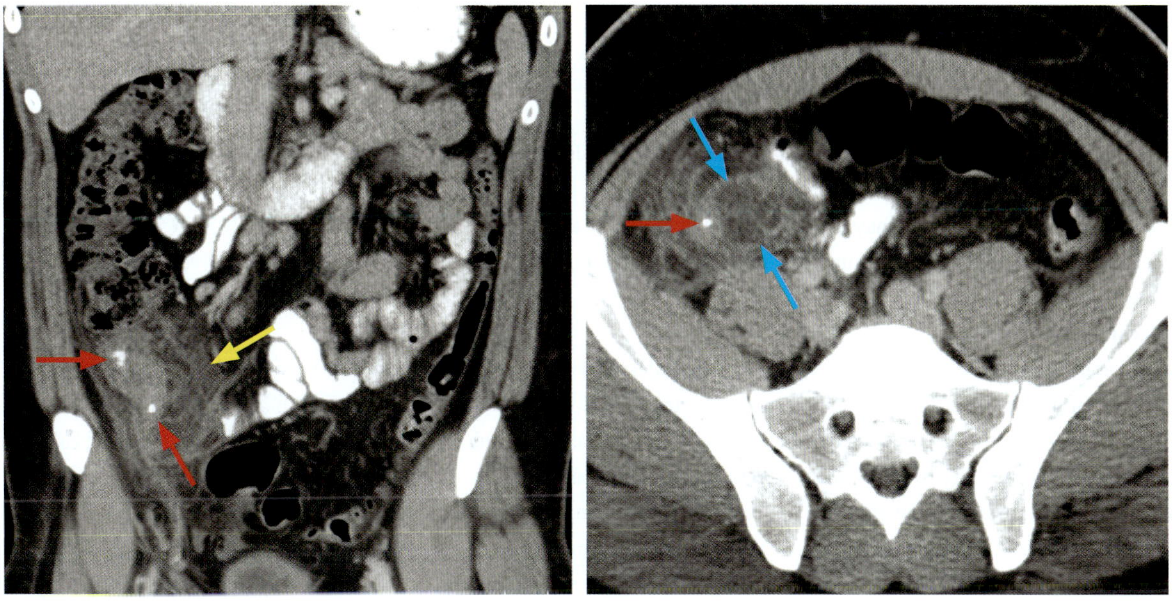

Appendicitis: Coronal (left image) and axial (right image) contrast-enhanced CT shows a large focus of inflammatory stranding centered around the appendix in the right lower quadrant (yellow arrow). The margins of the appendix itself are indistinct and there is the suggestion of an early fluid collection (blue arrows). Note the two appendicoliths within the appendix (red arrows).

阑尾炎：冠状位(左图)和轴位(右图)增强CT显示右下腹阑尾周围一处炎性渗出的大病灶(黄箭)。阑尾边缘模糊不清，提示早期积液(蓝箭)。注意阑尾内的两块阑尾石(红箭)。

- Appendicitis is the most common cause of acute abdomen. Acute inflammation of the appendix is thought to be due to obstruction of the appendiceal lumen by an appendicolith, fecal debris, or a mass, leading to venous congestion, mural ischemia, and bacterial translocation.
- Appendicitis represents a spectrum of severity ranging from tip appendicitis (inflammation isolated to the distal appendix) to gangrenous/perforated appendicitis with abscess if the disease is not diagnosed until late.
- For an adult with RLQ (right lower quadrant) pain and suspected appendicitis, CT is the preferred imaging modality. For a pediatric patient, ultrasound is first line. For pregnant women, ultrasound or MRI may be the most appropriate.
- Imaging of appendicitis relies on direct and indirect imaging findings.
- **Direct findings of appendicitis** are due to abnormalities of the appendix itself:

- 阑尾炎是急腹症中最常见的原因。阑尾急性发炎被认为是由于粪石、粪便碎块或肿块阻塞阑尾腔所致，从而导致静脉淤血、肠壁缺血和肠道细菌易位(出现在肠道外)。
- 阑尾炎包括了一系列不同严重程度的病变，从阑尾尖端发炎(阑尾远端孤立的炎症)到晚期的坏疽性/穿孔性阑尾炎伴脓肿。
- 对于有右下腹疼痛和疑似阑尾炎的成人，CT是首选的成像方式。对于儿科患者，超声是首选。对于孕妇，超声或MRI可能最合适。
- 阑尾炎的影像学诊断依靠直接和间接影像学表现。
- **阑尾炎的直接影像学表现**与阑尾本身异常有关：

Distended, fluid-filled appendix: 6 mm is used as cutoff for normal diameter of the appendix, although there is wide normal variability and 6 mm is from the ultrasound literature using compression. A normal appendix distended with air can measure >6 mm; therefore, some authors advocate using caution with a numeric cutoff in an otherwise normal-appearing appendix filled with air or enteric contrast.

Appendiceal wall-thickening or hyperenhancement.

Appendicolith, which may be a cause of luminal obstruction; however, appendicoliths are commonly seen without associated appendicitis.

阑尾肿胀、积液：6mm是正常阑尾直径的上限，尽管个体差异很大，但超声相关文献采用压迫后>6mm为异常；因此，一些研究者主张，对于一个充满空气或肠内造影剂的正常阑尾，要谨慎使用数字作为阈值来进行解释。

阑尾壁增厚或高强化。

阑尾石，可能是阑尾腔阻塞的原因；然而，阑尾石通常不伴有阑尾炎。

- **Indirect findings of appendicitis** are due to the spread of inflammation to adjacent sites:

Periappendiceal fat stranding.	Hydroureter.
Cecal wall thickening.	Small bowel ileus.

- On ultrasound, the key sonographic finding is a tubular, blind-ending, non-compressible structure in the right lower quadrant measuring >6 mm in diameter. It is generally necessary to use graded compression to evaluate for compressibility.

  Secondary findings of appendicitis can be evaluated by ultrasound, including free fluid and periappendicular abscess.
- Chronic or recurrent appendicitis may cause clinical symptoms of appendicitis for weeks to even years and is often misdiagnosed. Imaging findings are very similar to those of acute appendicitis.

Appendiceal neoplasms

- Appendiceal neoplasms are uncommon (0.5–1.0% of appendectomy specimens) and most often present as acute appendicitis secondary to luminal obstruction (50%) by the mass itself. They may also present as intussusception, increasing abdominal girth, GI bleeding, and secondary genitourinary complications.
- **Carcinoid** is the most common primary appendiceal neoplasm but is not as often detected on imaging. It is typically small and may be mass-like or demonstrate a diffuse infiltrative pattern. Carcinoid syndrome is present in only 5% of patients.

- **阑尾炎的间接影像学表现**与炎症扩散到邻近部位有关：

阑尾周围脂肪渗出。	输尿管积水。
盲肠壁增厚。	小肠梗阻。

- 超声检查的关键征象是右下腹呈管状、盲端、不可压缩的结构，直径>6mm。一般需要用分级压缩法来评估压缩性。

  超声也可以评估阑尾炎的继发表现，包括游离液体和阑尾周围脓肿。
- 慢性或复发性阑尾炎引起的阑尾炎症状在临床可长达数周甚至数年，并常被误诊。影像学表现与急性阑尾炎非常相似。

阑尾肿瘤

- 阑尾肿瘤不常见(占阑尾切除术标本的0.5%~1.0%)，最常表现为肿块阻塞管腔(50%)导致的继发性急性阑尾炎。还可能表现为肠套叠、腹围增加、胃肠道出血和继发性泌尿生殖系统并发症。
- **类癌**是最常见的原发性阑尾肿瘤，但在影像上常不被发现。它通常很小，可能呈肿块状或呈弥漫性浸润。只有5%的患者存在类癌综合征。

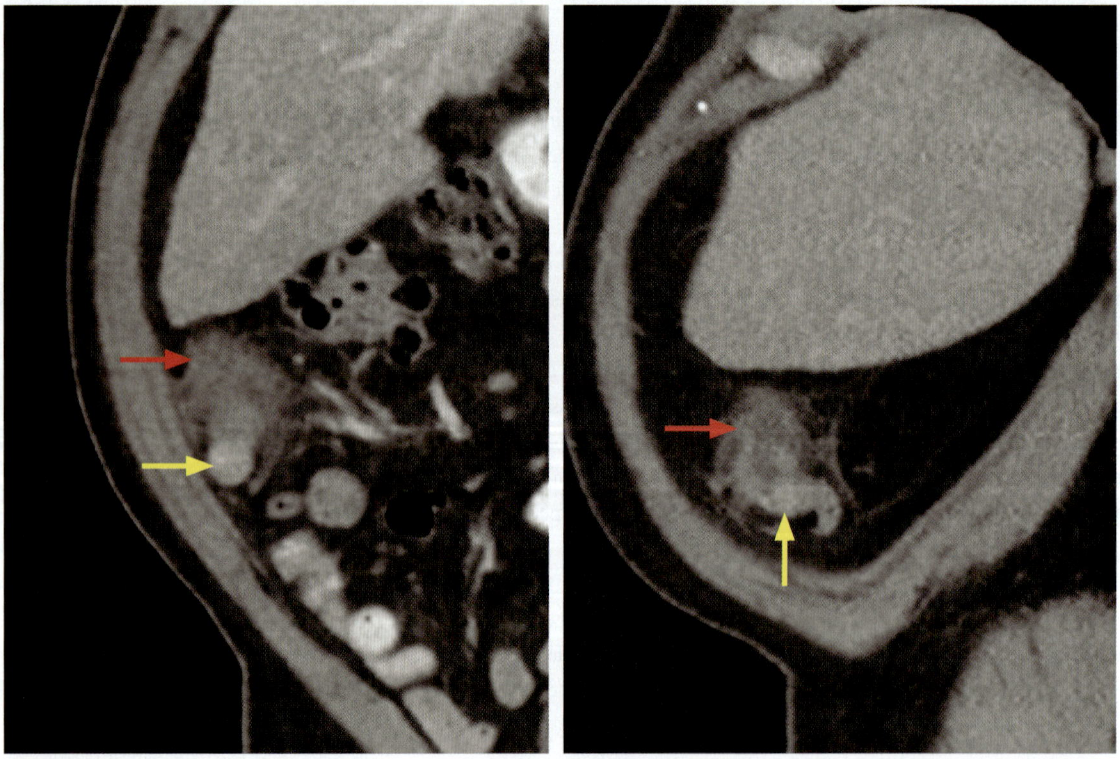

Appendiceal carcinoid: Coronal (left image) and sagittal (right image) contrast-enhanced CT demonstrates a round enhancing appendiceal mass (yellow arrows) with associated dilatation and perforation of the appendiceal tip (red arrows). Patient underwent appendectomy with surgical pathology showing appendiceal carcinoid tumor.

阑尾类癌：冠状位(左图)和矢状位(右图)增强CT显示一个圆形强化的阑尾肿物(黄箭)，伴阑尾尖部扩张和穿孔(红箭)。患者行阑尾切除术，手术病理示阑尾类癌。

- **Mucinous neoplasms** include a spectrum of entities ranging from mucocele, to low-grade mucinous neoplasm to mucinous adenocarcinoma. Pseudomyxoma peritonei may be a complication. Imaging most often shows a dilated, fluid-filled appendix, possibly with a soft tissue mass. If curvilinear mural calcification is present, the specificity is increased.

- **黏液性肿瘤**包括黏液囊肿、低级别黏液性肿瘤和黏液腺癌。腹膜假性黏液瘤可能是一种并发症。最常见的影像学表现为阑尾扩张并充满液体，可伴有软组织肿块。如果存在曲线状壁钙化，则诊断特异性增加。

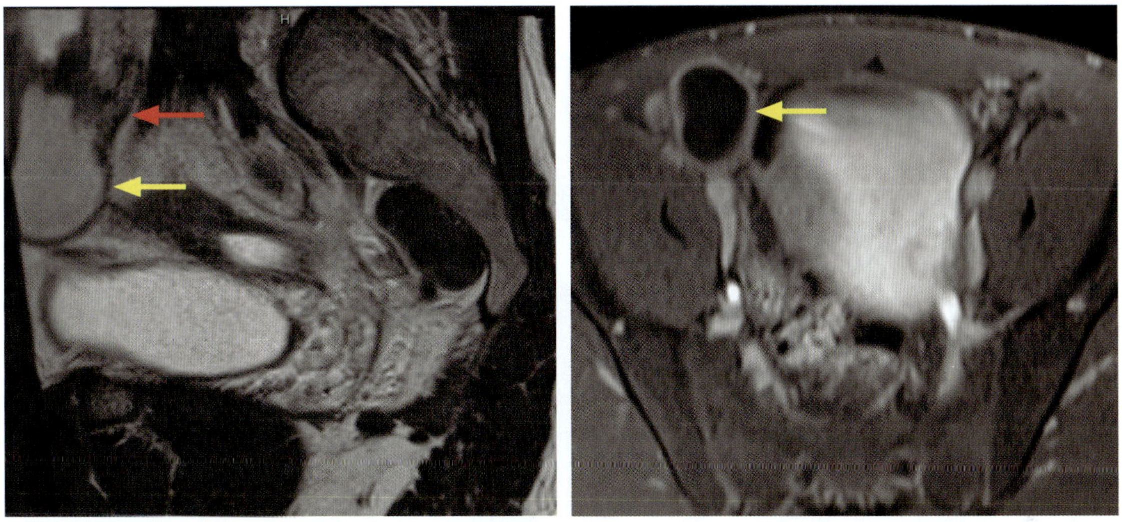

Appendiceal mucocele. Sagittal T2-weighted (left image) and axial post-contrast T1-weighted (right image) MRI demonstrates a homogeneously T2 hyperintense, nonenhancing lesion (yellow arrows) arising from the tip of the appendix (red arrow).
阑尾黏液囊肿：矢状位T_2加权(左图)和轴位增强T_1加权(右图)MRI显示阑尾尖部(红箭)出现均匀T_2高信号、无强化的病变(黄箭)。

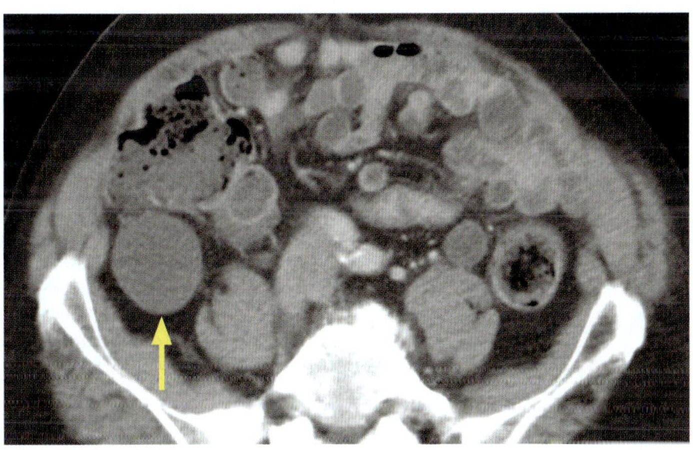

Axial contrast-enhanced CT image shows a well circumscribed, fluid filled structure arising from the base of the cecum with no significant solid component (arrow), found on pathology to be a low grade appendiceal mucinous neoplasm.
轴位增强CT显示盲肠底部边界清楚、充满液体的结构，无明显的实性成分(黄箭)，病理诊断为低级别阑尾黏液性肿瘤。

- **Non-mucinous adenocarcinoma** is much less common. If seen on imaging, it appears as a soft tissue mass, not associated with a mucocele.

- **非黏液腺癌**不常见。在影像学上表现为软组织肿块，与黏液囊肿无关。

（翻译　赵振）

Large Bowel

大肠

Anatomy

解剖

- Branches of the SMA and IMA supply the colon as depicted in the diagram below.
- The ascending and descending colon are secondarily retroperitoneal structures.

- 肠系膜上动脉(SMA)和肠系膜下动脉(IMA)的分支供应结肠，如下方示意图所示。
- 升结肠和降结肠均为腹膜间位器官。横结肠

The transverse and sigmoid colons are intraperitoneal. The upper to mid rectum is partially covered by peritoneum; the lower third is extraperitoneal and surrounded by mesorectal fascia.

和乙状结肠属于腹膜内位器官。直肠上段和中段被部分腹膜所覆盖；而直肠下1/3段位于腹膜外，由直肠系膜筋膜所包绕。

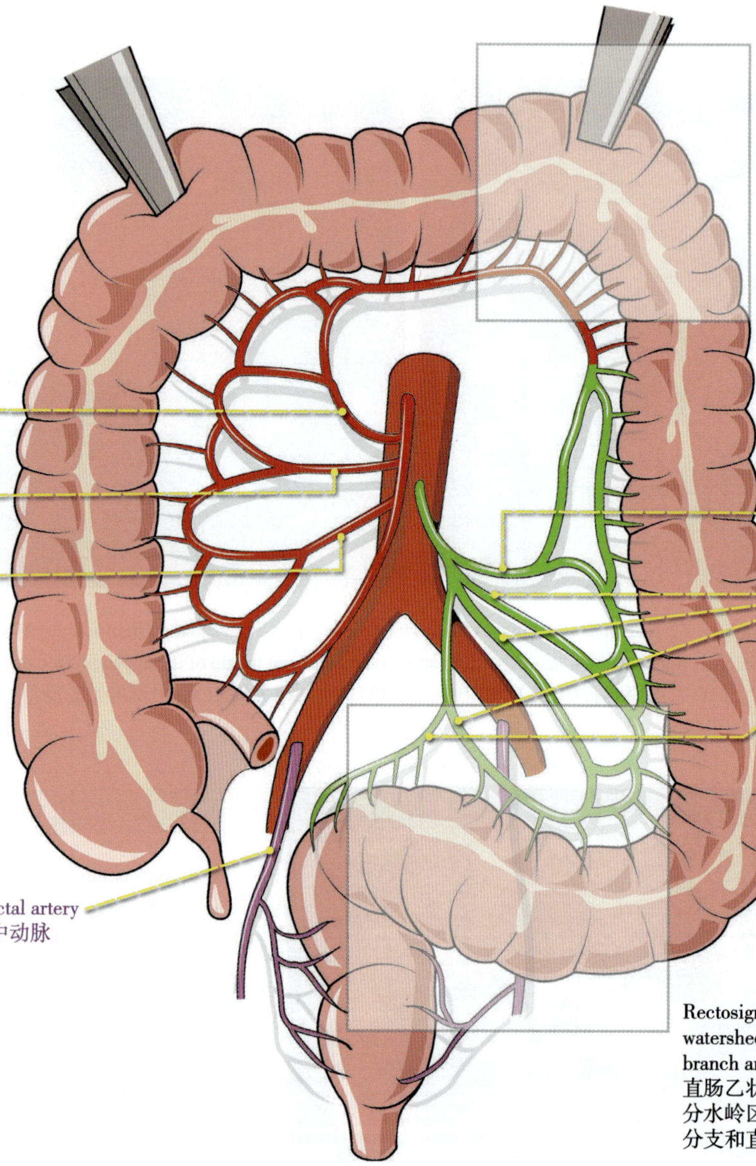

Colitis

结肠炎

Overview of colitis

结肠炎概述

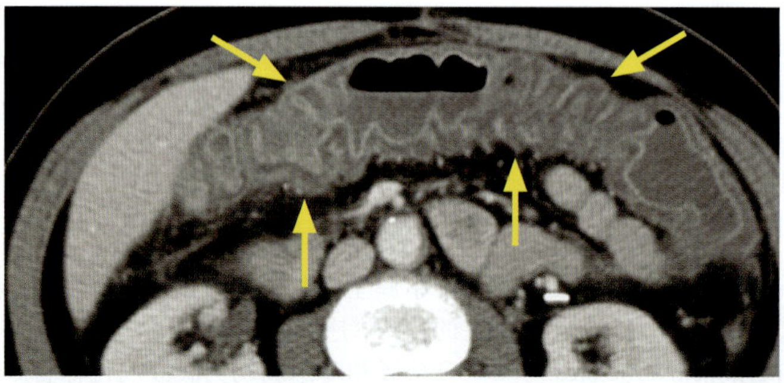

Pan colitis: Contrast-enhanced CT shows severe mural thickening of the entire visualized colon (arrows) with mucosal hyperenhancement. Although nonspecific, this was a case of pseudomembranous colitis.

全结肠炎：增强CT显示所有可见的结肠壁重度增厚，伴黏膜高度强化(黄箭)。虽然不具特异性，但该患者为伪膜性结肠炎。

- Colitis is inflammation of the colon that may be caused by several unrelated etiologies, often with overlapping imaging findings.
- The primary imaging feature of colitis is wall thickening. Generally, a full clinical evaluation, stool studies, and sometimes colonic biopsy are required for a definitive diagnosis of the causative etiology.

- 结肠炎为结肠的炎症病变，可以由数个不相关的病因所致，影像学表现常有重叠。
- 结肠炎最主要的影像学特征是肠壁增厚。一般来说，对结肠炎确切的病因诊断需要进行全面的临床评估、粪便检查，有时还需要进行结肠活检。

Ischemic colitis

- Colonic ischemia can be caused by acute arterial thrombus, chronic arterial stenosis, low- flow states (e.g., congestive heart failure), and venous thrombosis.
- The splenic flexure is the watershed region between the superior and inferior mesenteric arteries and is especially susceptible to ischemia in low-flow states.
- The rectum is supplied by a dual blood supply and is almost never affected by ischemia. The superior rectal artery (terminal branch of the IMA) and the inferior and middle rectal arteries (arising from the internal iliac artery anterior division) form perirectal collaterals.
- CT findings suggestive of ischemic colitis are segmental thickening of the affected colon in a vascular distribution, with sparing of the rectum.

  If arterial thromboembolic disease is suspected, one should evaluate for the presence of aortic atherosclerotic disease or a left atrial thrombus in the setting of atrial fibrillation.

  If chronic arterial stenosis is suspected, one should evaluate for atherosclerosis of the mesenteric vessels.

缺血性结肠炎

- 结肠缺血可由以下原因所致：急性动脉血栓、慢性动脉狭窄、低血流状态(如充血性心力衰竭)和静脉血栓形成。
- 脾曲是肠系膜上动脉和肠系膜下动脉供血的分水岭区域，极易在低血流状态时发生缺血。
- 直肠有双重血供，几乎从不发生缺血。直肠上动脉(肠系膜下动脉终末分支)和直肠下动脉、直肠中动脉(起于髂内动脉的前分支)形成直肠周围侧支循环。
- 可疑缺血性结肠炎的CT表现是受累结肠壁呈节段性增厚，并以血管走行分布，而直肠不受累。

  如果怀疑有动脉血栓栓塞性疾病，应检查是否有动脉粥样硬化性疾病，或心房颤动患者是否存在左心房血栓。

  如果怀疑有慢性动脉狭窄，应检查肠系膜血管是否有动脉粥样硬化。

Infectious colitis

- Infectious colitis can be bacterial, mycobacterial, viral, fungal, or amebic. There is significant overlap in the clinical presentation and imaging findings of the various pathogens.
- In general, infectious colitis features pericolonic stranding and ascites in addition to the colonic wall thickening seen in all forms of colitis.
- *Yersinia, Salmonella,* and colonic TB tend to affect the right colon. TB is known to involve the ileocecal valve, resulting in a desmoplastic reaction that mimics Crohn's disease.
- *E. coli*, CMV, and *C. difficile* colitis (discussed below) most commonly cause pancolitis.

感染性结肠炎

- 感染性结肠炎可由细菌、分枝杆菌、病毒、真菌或阿米巴所致。各种病原体引起的临床表现和影像学表现均有显著重叠。
- 一般来说，感染性结肠炎的特征包括结肠周围炎性条纹影和腹腔积液，以及其他所有类型结肠炎均可见到的结肠壁增厚。
- 耶尔森菌、沙门菌和结肠结核常累及右侧结肠。结核通常累及回盲瓣，导致结缔组织增生反应，与克罗恩病类似。
- 大肠埃希菌、巨细胞病毒和艰难梭菌(后文讨论)最常引起全结肠炎。

Pseudomembranous colitis (*C. difficile* colitis)

- Pseudomembranous colitis is an especially prevalent form of infectious colitis caused by overgrowth of *Clostridium difficile*, most commonly due to alteration in colonic bacterial flora after antibiotic use. Pseudomembranous colitis may also occur without a history of antibiotics, especially in hospitalized or nursing home patients. Severely immunocompromised patients' status post bone marrow or solid organ transplant is also at risk.
- Key imaging finding is marked thickening of the colonic wall, typically with involvement of the entire colon (pancolitis). The *accordion sign* describes severe colonic wall thickening combined with undulation of enhancing inner mucosa. It signifies severe colonic edema but is not specific to *C. difficile*. *Thumbprinting* is a fluoroscopic finding of thickened haustra and is also due to edema.

伪膜性结肠炎(艰难梭菌结肠炎)

- 伪膜性结肠炎是一种极其流行的感染性结肠炎，为艰难梭菌过度繁殖所致，最常见的原因是使用抗生素后引起的结肠菌群失调。伪膜性结肠炎也可以发生在无抗生素使用史的患者，尤其是住院或养老院的患者。骨髓或实体器官移植后免疫功能严重受损的患者也处于高危状态。
- 关键的影像学表现是结肠壁明显增厚，通常累及全结肠(全结肠炎)。手风琴征是指严重结肠壁增厚并伴有波浪状强化的内层黏膜。此征象提示结肠严重水肿，但并非为艰难梭菌的特异表现。拇指印征是透视下增厚的结肠袋的一种表现，同样为水肿所致。

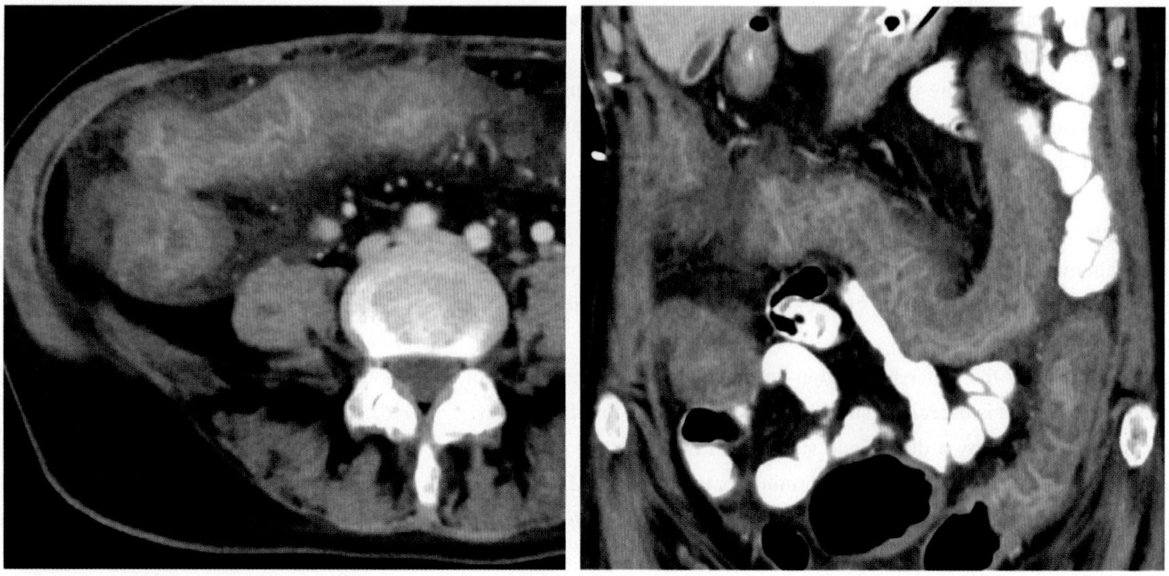

Axial (left image) and coronal (right image) contrast-enhanced CT demonstrates diffuse bowel wall edema and mucosal enhancement of the entire colon (*accordion sign*) with pericolonic stranding and mesenteric vasculature engorgement, consistent with pseudomembranous colitis in this patient with fever, leukocytosis, and a positive *C. diff.* culture.

轴位(左图)和冠状位(右图)增强CT显示全结肠弥漫肠壁水肿和黏膜强化(手风琴征),伴结肠周围条纹影和肠系膜血管充血,符合伪膜性结肠炎的表现,该患者有发热、白细胞升高,且艰难梭菌培养阳性。

Ulcerative colitis (UC)

- Ulcerative colitis (UC) is an idiopathic inflammatory bowel disease that begins distally in the rectum and spreads proximally in a continuous manner (unlike Crohn's disease, which features skip areas).

  Of note, it is possible for the rectum to appear normal with more proximal colonic involvement present if the patient has been treated with corticosteroid enemas.
- Patients with UC have an increased risk of primary sclerosing cholangitis, cholangiocarcinoma and colon cancer.
- Extra-abdominal manifestations of UC include sacroiliitis (symmetric, bilateral), iritis, erythema nodosum (tender red subcutaneous nodules), and pyoderma gangrenosum (cutaneous ulcers).
- UC does not extend more proximally than the cecum; however, **backwash ileitis** caused by reflux of inflammatory debris into the ileum may mimic Crohn's disease.

溃疡性结肠炎(UC)

- 溃疡性结肠炎(UC)是一种特发性炎症性肠病,始于直肠的远端,并向近端呈连续性扩展(而克罗恩病以跳跃式分布为特征)。

  需要注意,如果患者接受了皮质类固醇灌肠治疗,直肠可能表现为正常,但近端结肠的病变仍然存在。
- UC患者有增加原发性硬化性胆管炎、胆管细胞癌和结肠癌的风险。
- UC的腹外表现包括骶髂关节炎(双侧、对称)、虹膜炎、结节性红斑(柔软的红色皮下结节)和坏疽性脓皮病(皮肤溃疡)。
- UC不会累及盲肠近心端的肠管;但是,**反流性回肠炎**可类似于克罗恩病,为炎性碎片反流到回肠所致。

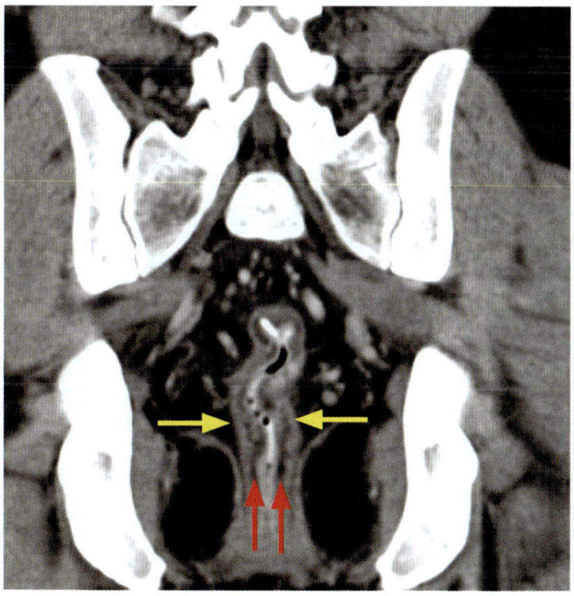

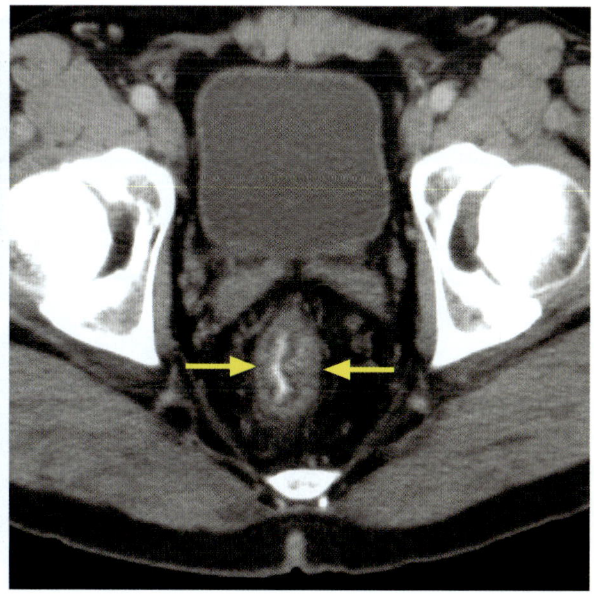

Chronic ulcerative colitis: Coronal (left image) and axial (right) contrast-enhanced CT shows continuous thickening of the rectal wall (yellow arrows) with submucosal fat deposition (red arrows).
慢性溃疡性结肠炎：冠状位(左图)和轴位(右图)增强CT显示延续性直肠壁增厚(黄箭)，伴有黏膜下脂肪沉积(红箭)。

- Imaging of ulcerative colitis features circumferential wall thickening with a granular mucosal pattern that is best seen on barium enema. Pseudopolyps may be present during bouts of acute inflammation and represent islands of normal mucosa surrounded by inflamed mucosa. A *collar-button* ulcer is nonspecific but represents mucosal ulceration undermined by submucosal extension.
- Chronic changes of ulcerative colitis include a featureless (ahaustral) and foreshortened *lead pipe colon*. As in Crohn's disease, submucosal fat deposition suggests chronic disease, as seen in the case above.
- **Toxic megacolon** is a severe complication of UC (and less commonly, Crohn's disease) caused by inflammation extending through the muscular layer. Imaging of toxic megacolon shows dilation of the colon to greater than 6 cm in association with adynamic ileus. Colonic perforation may occur, therefore colonoscopy is contraindicated in patients with suspected toxic megacolon.

- 溃疡性结肠炎的影像学特征是环形管壁增厚伴颗粒状黏膜，以钡灌肠观察最佳。假性息肉可以出现在急性炎症发作期，为正常黏膜岛被炎性黏膜环绕所致。衣领扣溃疡是一种非特异性征象，但意味着病变向黏膜下延伸而出现黏膜溃疡。
- 溃疡性结肠炎的慢性表现包括结肠无特征(无结肠袋性)且短缩呈铅管样。与克罗恩病类似，黏膜下脂肪沉积提示病变为慢性期，如上图病例所示。
- **中毒性巨结肠**是溃疡性结肠炎的一种严重并发症(较少见于克罗恩病)，为炎症延伸至肌层所致。中毒性巨结肠的影像学表现为结肠扩张超过6cm，伴有麻痹性肠梗阻。可能会发生结肠穿孔，因此对怀疑有中毒性巨结肠的患者禁忌进行结肠镜检查。

Typhlitis (neutropenic enterocolitis)

- Typhlitis is a necrotizing inflammatory colitis seen in the right colon and/or terminal ileum occurring in neutropenic patients.
- Imaging features may include cecal thickening, fat stranding, ileus or features of SBO, and even pneumatosis intestinalis. Low attenuation areas within the wall may represent edema or hemorrhage.

盲肠炎(中性粒细胞缺乏性肠炎)

- 盲肠炎是发生在右侧结肠和/或末端回肠的一种坏死性炎症性结肠炎，见于中性粒细胞减少的患者。
- 影像学特征包括盲肠壁增厚、脂肪条纹影、肠梗阻或小肠梗阻的特征，以及肠壁积气。肠壁内的低密度区域可能为水肿或出血。

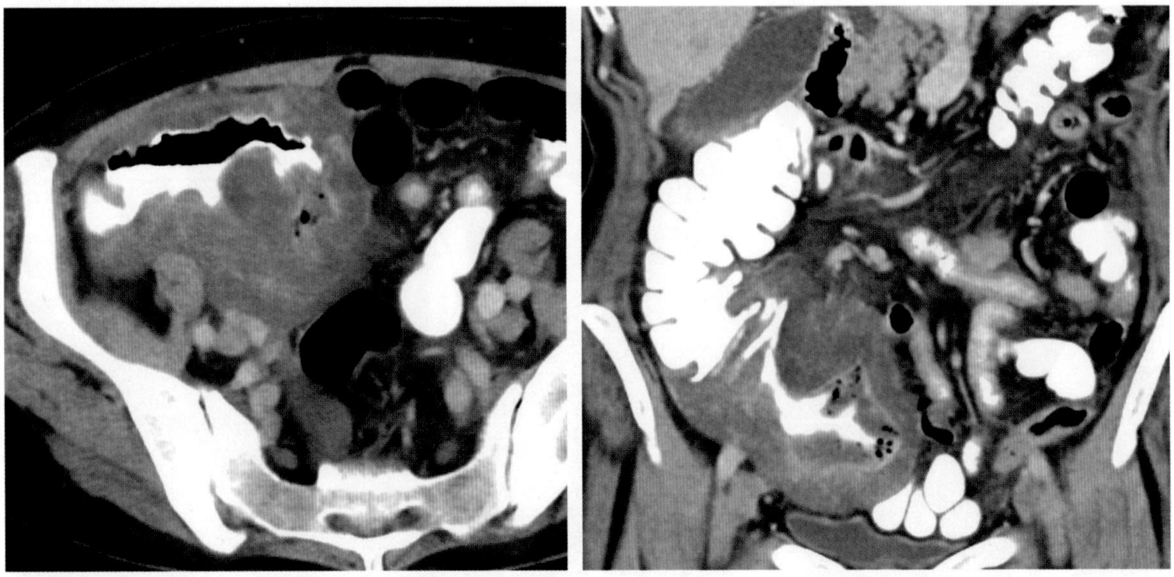

Axial (left image) and coronal (right) contrast-enhanced CT shows marked circumferential wall thickening of the cecum and proximal ascending colon, with associate pericolonic fat stranding, in a neutropenic patient.
轴位(左图)和冠状位(右图)增强CT显示盲肠和近端升结肠壁明显环形增厚，伴结肠周围脂肪条纹，此患者为中性粒细胞减少。

Immunotherapy-related colitis

- As immunotherapy and molecular targeted therapies become more common, more cases of drug-related colitis are being reported.
- Imaging findings of drug-related colitis can be very subtle and include mild, diffuse bowel wall thickening, vasa recta engorgement, and fluid-filled colonic distention. The most common culprit immunotherapy agents are ipilimumab and pembrolizumab.

免疫治疗相关性结肠炎

- 免疫治疗和分子靶向治疗越来越常见，而与药物相关的结肠炎的报道也越来越多。
- 药物相关的结肠炎在影像学上的表现可以很轻微，包括轻度弥漫性肠壁增厚、直小动脉充血、结肠扩张积液。最常见的此类免疫治疗药物是伊匹单抗和派姆单抗。

Stercoral colitis

积粪性结肠炎

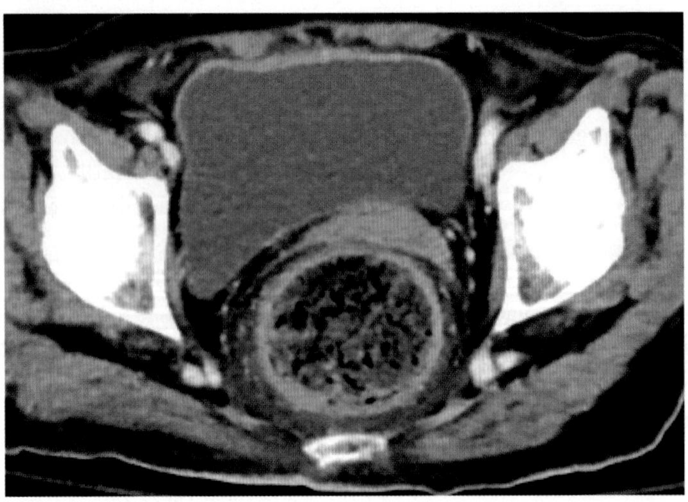

Stercoral colitis: Axial contrast-enhanced CT demonstrates a distended, stool-filled rectum with circumferential wall thickening and mesorectal fat stranding.
积粪性结肠炎：轴位增强CT显示直肠扩张、积粪，伴肠壁环形增厚和直肠系膜炎性脂肪条纹影。

- Stercoral colitis is focal inflammatory colitis caused by increased pressure on the bowel wall by impacted fecal material in the colon and/or rectum.
- It can lead to bowel wall ischemia, pressure ulceration (stercoral ulcer), and perforation.
- Imaging shows colonic distention by an intraluminal impacted fecal mass, with associated bowel wall thickening and pericolonic fat stranding.

- 积粪性结肠炎是局灶性炎症性结肠炎，由结肠和/或直肠内密实的粪便引起肠壁压力增高所致。
- 此病可导致肠壁缺血、压力性溃疡(粪性溃疡)、穿孔。
- 影像学表现为肠腔内密实的粪便团块导致结肠扩张，伴肠壁增厚和结肠周围脂肪条纹影。

OTHER ACUTE LARGE BOWEL PATHOLOGIES

其他急性大肠疾病

Diverticulitis

憩室炎

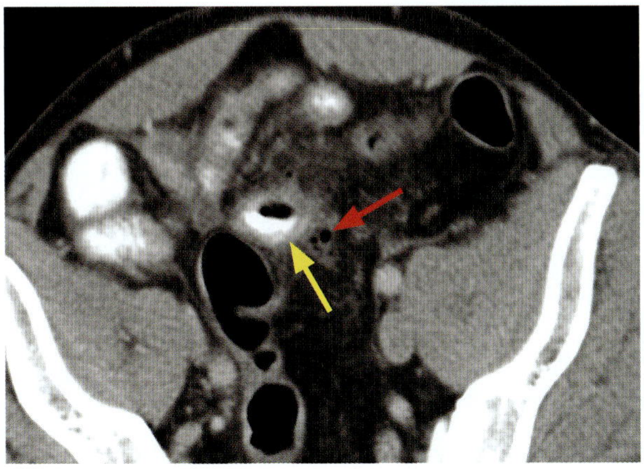

Complicated diverticulitis: Axial CT shows a large diverticulum arising from the sigmoid colon containing enteric contrast (yellow arrow), with surrounding mesenteric fat stranding. A few adjacent locules of extraluminal gas (red arrow) are present.

复杂性憩室炎：轴位CT可见起源于乙状结肠的含肠道造影剂的大憩室(黄箭)，伴有周围肠系膜脂肪条纹影。邻近肠腔外有数个气泡(红箭)。

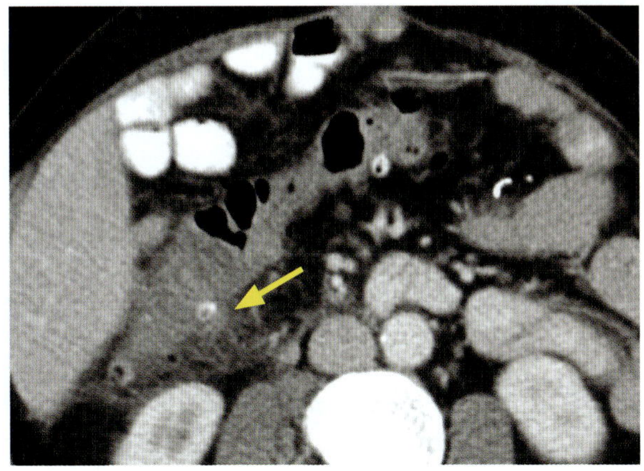

Uncomplicated diverticulitis: Axial CT in a different patient shows fat stranding surrounding a diverticulum at the hepatic flexure (arrow).

单纯性憩室炎：不同患者的轴位CT显示结肠肝曲憩室周围可见脂肪条纹影(黄箭)。

- Diverticulitis is acute inflammation of an obstructed colonic diverticulum, leading to diverticular wall ischemia and microperforation. CT is the primary modality for diagnosis, triage, and evaluation of severity and complications.
- **Uncomplicated diverticulitis** does not have any imaging evidence of bowel perforation (even though histopathologically, all diverticulitis is associated with bacterial translocation across the bowel wall/microperforation). CT findings of uncomplicated diverticulitis include short segment bowel wall thickening and pericolonic fat stranding, usually centered around a culprit diverticulum. Uncomplicated diverticulitis is typically treated conservatively.
- **Complicated diverticulitis** implies the presence of at least one of the following additional findings, including:

Pericolonic or hepatic abscess. Extraluminal air. Bowel obstruction.	Colonic fistula (colovesical fistula most common, apparent on imaging as gas in the bladder not explained by Foley catheter placement). Mesenteric venous thrombosis or septic thrombophlebitis.

- 憩室炎是结肠憩室阻塞后发生的急性炎症，导致憩室壁缺血和微穿孔。CT是憩室炎诊断、分类、评价严重程度和并发症的主要方法。
- **单纯性憩室炎**不具有任何肠穿孔的影像学征象(即便组织病理学上所有憩室炎均伴有细菌穿过肠壁出现移位/微穿孔)。单纯性憩室炎的CT表现包括短节段肠壁增厚和结肠周围脂肪条纹影，通常以发病憩室为中心。单纯性憩室炎通常采用保守治疗。
- **复杂性憩室炎**意味着至少存在下列一种附加条件，包括：

结肠周围或肝脓肿。 肠腔外气体。 肠梗阻。	结肠瘘(结肠膀胱瘘最常见，影像学显示膀胱内积气，但不能用插导尿管来解释)。 肠系膜静脉血栓或脓毒性血栓性静脉炎。

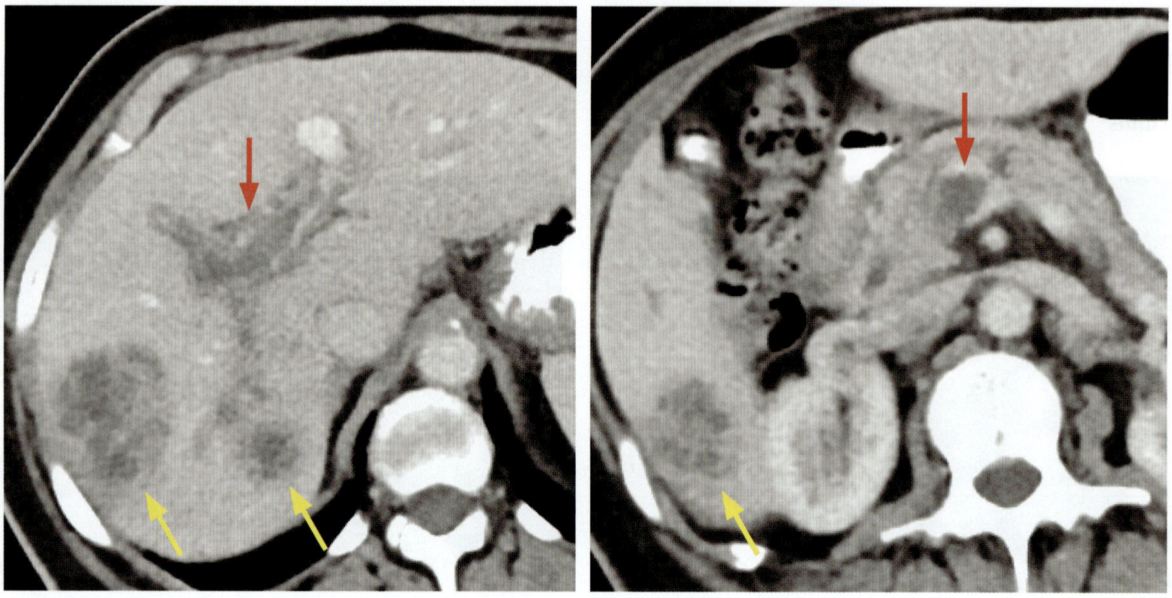

Diverticulitis complicated by septic thrombophlebitis and hepatic abscesses: Axial contrast-enhanced CT images show complex multiloculated hepatic lesions (yellow arrows). There are filling defects within the inferior mesenteric vein draining the site of diverticulitis (not shown), main portal vein and right portal vein (red arrows). The constellation of findings are consistent with diverticulitis complicated by ascending septic thrombophlebitis and hepatic abscesses.
憩室炎并发脓毒性血栓性静脉炎和肝脓肿：轴位增强CT显示复杂多房性肝脏病灶(黄箭)。可见多个静脉充盈缺损，包括憩室炎引流区肠系膜下静脉(图像未显示)、门静脉主干和右支(红箭)。这些表现符合憩室炎并发上行性脓毒性血栓性静脉炎和肝脓肿。

- Abscesses can usually be drained percutaneously with CT guidance.
- Pertinent positives to include in your report include the presence of extraluminal gas, fistula or abscess, or the clinical history of recurrent diverticulitis, as this may affect treatment algorithms.
- Due to the extensive colonic wall thickening that is sometimes seen, it can be difficult to distinguish acute diverticulitis from colon cancer. Depending on the level of certainty of diagnosis, some radiologists may recommend a follow-up CT or colonoscopy after resolution of the acute episode.

- 肝脓肿通常可以在CT引导下进行经皮引流。
- 诊断报告中应包括相关的阳性发现：肠腔外气体、瘘或脓肿、临床复发性憩室炎的病史，这些可能会影响治疗决策。
- 有时见到的广泛结肠壁增厚可能难以鉴别急性憩室炎或结肠癌。依据对诊断的把握程度，一些放射科医生推荐患者在急性发作好转后进行CT随访或结肠镜检查。

Epiploic appendagitis

肠脂垂炎

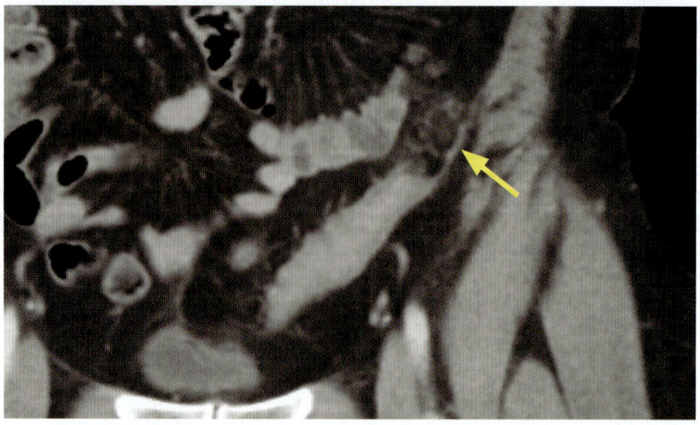

Epiploic appendagitis: Coronal contrast- enhanced CT demonstrates an oval circumscribed area of fat with central tiny hyperdense dot (*central dot sign*). There is mild surrounding inflammatory stranding and focal area of peritoneal thickening.
肠脂垂炎：冠状位增强CT显示一个边缘清楚的卵圆形脂肪区，其中央有一个高密度的微小点影(*中央点征*)。并可见周围轻度炎性脂肪条纹影和局部腹膜增厚。

- Epiploic appendagitis is a benign, clinical mimic of diverticulitis caused by torsion of a normal fatty tag (appendage) hanging from the colon.
- Epiploic appendagitis has a pathognomonic imaging appearance of an oval fat-attenuation lesion abutting a normal colonic wall, with mild associated fat stranding. The *central dot sign* refers to a central hyperdense dot in cross-section representing the thrombosed central vein of the epiploic appendage.

- 肠脂垂炎属于良性，临床与憩室炎类似，由悬挂于结肠上的正常脂肪垂(肠脂垂)扭转所致。
- 影像学上，具有病理性诊断意义的肠脂垂炎表现为紧邻正常结肠壁的卵圆形脂肪密度灶，伴周围轻度脂肪条纹样改变。**中央点征**为轴位图像上的中央高密度点，代表肠脂垂中央

- Treatment is with anti-inflammatories, *not* antibiotics or surgery.

静脉血栓形成。
- 治疗为抗炎，而非抗生素或手术治疗。

Colorectal Carcinoma

- Colorectal carcinoma (98% of which is adenocarcinoma) is the most common malignancy of the GI tract and the second most frequently diagnosed malignancy in adults, more commonly affecting older adults with a slight male predilection. They most often arise in the rectosigmoid region but can occur anywhere from cecum to rectum.
- Rare subtypes include mucinous carcinoma of the colon and neuroendocrine carcinoma.
- There are many risk factors and associated syndromes, some of which are discussed elsewhere in this chapter.

  Risk factors: inflammatory bowel disease, low fiber/high fat diets, obesity, prior radiation, and family history of colorectal cancer among others.

  Associated syndromes: FAP, Gardner and Turcot syndrome variants, Peutz-Jeghers, HNPCC.
- CT colonography is increasingly being used as a non-invasive alternative to colonoscopy for screening.
- Many patients are asymptomatic at diagnosis obtained by screening colonoscopy or CT colonography, but may present with imaging findings of obstruction or perforation. Non- imaging clinical findings may include melena or frank GI bleeding, iron deficiency-anemia or altered bowel habits, which people may dismiss as being related to diet or aging.
- CT is the modality most often used for staging of colorectal carcinoma and can demonstrate evidence of nodal involvement or metastases. Most carcinomas appear as soft tissue density masses that may narrow the bowel lumen and can ulcerate when they become large.
- MRI is used for locoregional staging of rectal cancer to evaluate for T and N stage.

结直肠癌

- 结直肠癌(98%为腺癌)是最常见的胃肠道恶性肿瘤，是成人第二常见的恶性肿瘤，多见于老年人，男性稍多发。最常起源于直肠乙状结肠区，但是盲肠至直肠的任何部位均可以发生。
- 罕见的亚型包括结肠黏液癌和神经内分泌癌。
- 有许多危险因素和相关综合征，其中一些内容在本章其他部分有所讨论。

  危险因素：炎症性肠病、低纤维/高脂肪饮食、肥胖、既往放疗、结直肠癌家族史等。

  相关综合征：家族性腺瘤样息肉病、加德纳综合征和特科特综合征变异型、波伊茨-耶格综合征、遗传性非息肉性结肠癌综合征。
- CT结肠造影正越来越多地作为一种非侵入性的方法替代结肠镜筛查。
- 许多患者在接受筛查性结肠镜或CT结肠造影时并无症状，但影像学上可出现梗阻或穿孔的表现。非影像学临床表现可能包括黑便或胃肠道出血、缺铁性贫血或排便习惯改变，而患者可能误认为与饮食或衰老有关。
- CT是最常用于结直肠癌分期的方法，可以显示淋巴结浸润或转移的征象。大多数肿瘤表现为软组织密度肿块，可使肠腔狭窄，而当肿瘤较大时可形成溃疡。
- MRI可用于直肠癌的局部分期，评估T和N分期。

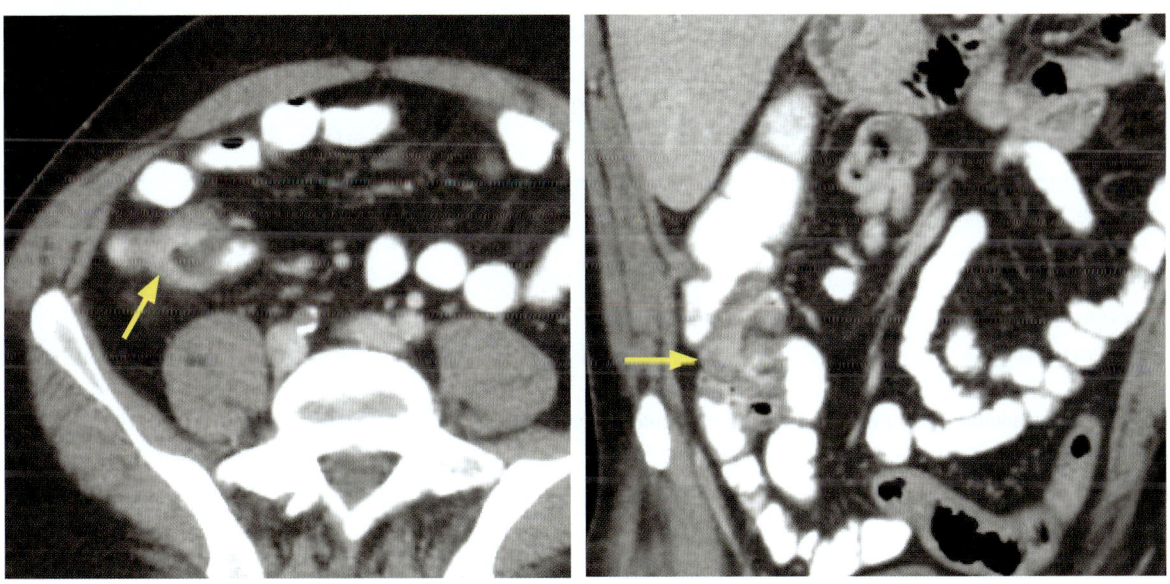

Axial (left image) and coronal (right image) contrast-enhanced CT demonstrates asymmetric wall thickening of the cecum at the level of the ileocecal valve with mass-like protrusion (arrows). Pathology on biopsy revealed adenocarcinoma.
轴位(左图)和冠状位(右图)增强CT显示回盲瓣层面盲肠壁不对称增厚，并有肿块样突出物(黄箭)。病理活检显示为腺癌。

Polyposis syndromes affecting the bowel

累及肠道的息肉综合征

Familial adenomatous polyposis (FAP)

家族性腺瘤样息肉病(FAP)

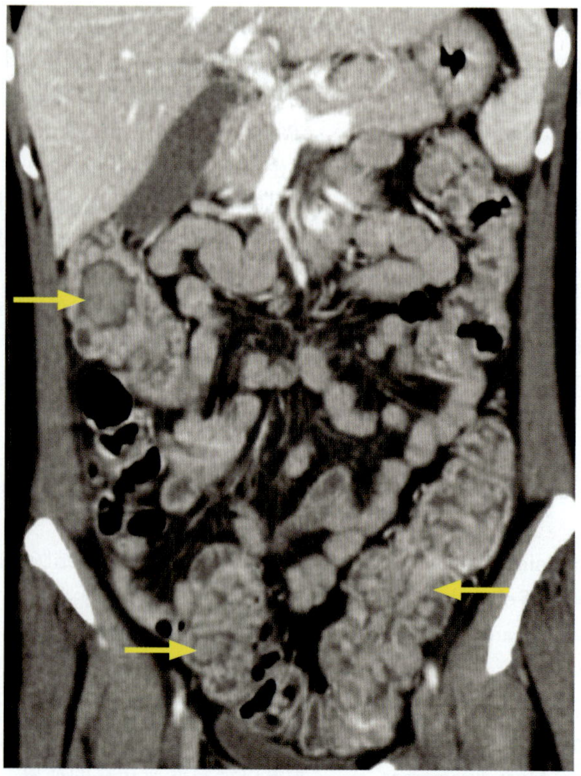

FAP: Coronal CT image demonstrates fluid-filled colon with innumerable polypoid enhancing lesions (arrows) seen throughout the ascending, transverse, descending, and sigmoid colon and into the rectum.

FAP：冠状位CT显示结肠积液伴无数息肉样强化病灶(黄箭)，分布于升结肠、横结肠、降结肠、乙状结肠和直肠。

- Familial adenomatous polyposis (FAP) is an autosomal-dominant syndrome featuring innumerable premalignant adenomatous polyps in the colon and to a lesser extent the small bowel. The risk of colon cancer is 100% with average onset of development at 39 years. Prophylactic colectomy is the standard of care to prevent colon cancer.
- Gastric polyps are also present, although the gastric polyps are hyperplastic and are not premalignant.
- **Gardner** syndrome is a variant of FAP. In addition to colon polyps, patients also have:

Desmoid tumors.
Osteomas.
Papillary thyroid cancer.
Epidermoid cysts.

Mnemonic: DOPE Gardner

- **Turcot** syndrome is another variant of FAP. In addition to colon polyps, patients also have CNS tumors (gliomas and medulloblastomas).

  Mnemonic: TURbans go over your head

- 家族性腺瘤样息肉病(FAP)是一种常染色体显性遗传综合征，以结肠大量癌前腺瘤样息肉为特征，较少情况下也可累及小肠。结肠癌风险为100%，平均发病年龄为39岁。预防性结肠切除术是防止结肠癌的标准治疗方法。
- 息肉也可发生在胃部，但胃息肉为过度增生并非癌前病变。
- 加德纳综合征是FAP的一种变异类型。除了结肠息肉，患者还有：

硬纤维性肿瘤(D)。
骨瘤(O)。
乳头状甲状腺癌(P)。
表皮样囊肿(E)。

英文记忆口诀：DOPE Gardner(DOPE花园)。

- **特科特综合征**是FAP的另一种变异类型。除结肠息肉外，患者同时有中枢神经系统肿瘤(胶质瘤和髓母细胞瘤)。

  英文记忆口诀："TURbansgo over your head"（头巾飞过头顶）。

Hereditary nonpolyposis colon cancer syndrome (HNPCC) = Lynch syndrome

- Hereditary nonpolyposis colon cancer (HNPCC) syndrome (also called Lynch syndrome) is an autosomal dominant polyposis syndrome caused by DNA mismatch repair, leading to colon cancer from microsatellite instability on a

遗传性非息肉性结肠癌综合征(HNPCC)=林奇综合征

- 遗传性非息肉性结肠癌综合征(HNPCC)(也称林奇综合征)是一种DNA错位修复导致的常

molecular level. Risk of colon cancer is less than with FAP. Similar to FAP, the colon polyps of HNPCC are adenomatous.

- HNPCC is associated with other cancers, including endometrial, gastric, small bowel, liver, and biliary malignancies.

Peutz-Jeghers

- Peutz-Jeghers is an autosomal dominant syndrome that features multiple hamartomatous pedunculated polyps, usually in the small bowel. These polyps may act as lead points and cause intussusception.
- Characteristic skin manifestations include perioral mucocutaneous blue/brown pigmented spots on the lips and gums.
- Peutz-Jeghers is associated with gynecologic neoplasms as well as gastric, duodenal, and colonic malignancies.

Cowden syndrome

- Cowden syndrome is an autosomal dominant syndrome of multiple hamartomatous polyps most commonly found in the skin and external mucous membranes, but also in the GI tract.
- Cowden syndrome is associated with an increased risk of thyroid cancer (usually follicular), as well as skin, oral, breast, and uterine malignancies.

Cronkhite-Canada

- Cronkhite-Canada is a non-inherited disorder (the only polyposis syndrome in this list that is not autosomal dominant) consisting of hamartomatous polyps throughout the GI tract.
- Cutaneous manifestations include abnormal skin pigmentation, alopecia, and onychodystrophy (malformation of the nails).

染色体显性遗传的息肉病综合征，是由于分子水平上的微卫星不稳定而导致的结肠癌。HNPCC患者罹患结肠癌的风险低于FAP。与FAP类似，HNPCC的结肠息肉为腺瘤性。

- HNPCC可伴发其他癌症，包括子宫内膜癌、胃癌、小肠癌、肝癌和胆道恶性肿瘤。

波伊茨-耶格综合征

- 波伊茨-耶格综合征是一种常染色体显性遗传综合征，以多发错构瘤样带蒂息肉为特征，通常位于小肠。这些息肉可作为触发点而导致肠套叠。
- 具有特征性的皮肤表现，包括嘴唇和牙龈的口周皮肤与黏膜的蓝色/棕色色素沉着斑。
- 波伊茨-耶格综合征可以并发妇科肿瘤，以及胃、十二指肠和结肠恶性肿瘤。

多发性错构瘤综合征

- 多发性错构瘤综合征是一种常染色体显性遗传综合征，表现为多发错构瘤样息肉，最常见于皮肤和外部黏膜，但也可见于胃肠道。
- 多发性错构瘤综合征患者具有增加罹患甲状腺癌(常为滤泡性)，以及皮肤、口、乳腺及子宫恶性肿瘤的风险。

卡纳达-克朗凯特综合征

- 卡纳达-克朗凯特综合征为一种非遗传性疾病(为所有介绍中唯一的非常染色体显性遗传的息肉病综合征)，表现为错构瘤样息肉累及整个胃肠道。
- 皮肤表现包括异常皮肤色素沉着、脱发和甲营养不良(指甲畸形)。

(翻译　卢瞳)

MESENTERY, PERITONEUM, AND OMENTUM

肠系膜、腹膜和网膜

ANATOMY

解剖

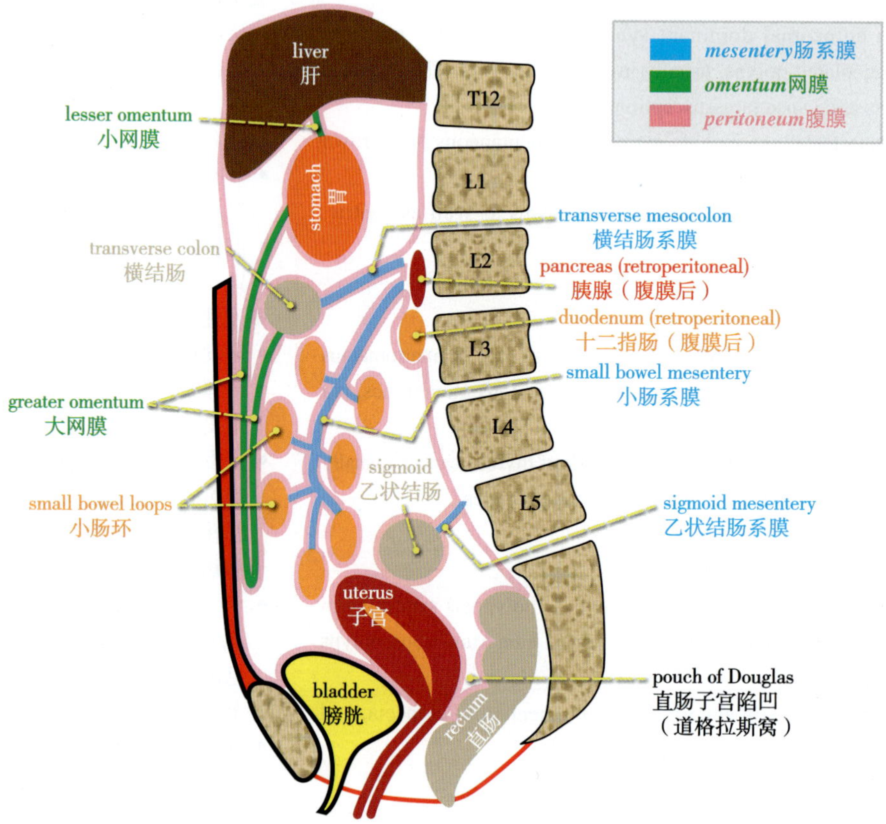

Peritoneum

- The peritoneum is a thin membrane consisting of a single layer of mesothelial cells that are supported by subserosal fat cells, lymphatic cells, and white blood cells.
- The visceral peritoneum lines the surface of organs, while the parietal peritoneum lines the outer walls of the peritoneal cavity.
- The most dependent portion of the peritoneal cavity (both supine and upright) is the retro- uterine space (pouch of Douglas) in women and the retrovesical space in men.

Mesentery

- There are three true mesenteries, each of which supply a portion of the bowel and connect to the posterior abdominal wall. Each mesentery consists of a network of blood vessels and lymphatics, sandwiched between layers of peritoneum.
- The three true mesenteries are:

> **Small bowel mesentery**: Supplies both the jejunum and ileum. Oriented obliquely from the ligament of Treitz in the left upper quadrant to the ileocecal junction in the right lower quadrant.
>
> **Transverse mesocolon**: Mesentery to the transverse colon, connecting the posterior transverse colon to the posterior abdominal wall.
>
> **Sigmoid mesentery**: Mesentery to the sigmoid colon.

腹膜

- 腹膜是由单层间皮细胞组成的薄层膜样结构，由浆膜下脂肪细胞、淋巴细胞及白细胞组成。
- 脏腹膜覆盖所有器官的表面，而壁腹膜位于腹膜腔的外壁。
- 腹膜腔的最低位置(包括仰卧位和立位)在女性为直肠子宫陷凹(道格拉斯窝)，在男性为膀胱后间隙。

肠系膜

- 真正的肠系膜有三个，它们各自支持一部分肠管并将其固定于后腹壁。每个肠系膜是由血管和淋巴管组成的网状结构，呈三明治样夹在两层腹膜的中间。
- 三个真性肠系膜为：

> **小肠系膜**：支持空肠和回肠。斜行走行于左上腹的十二指肠悬韧带至右下腹的回盲部之间。
>
> **横结肠系膜**：横结肠的系膜，将横结肠后壁固定至后腹壁。
>
> **乙状结肠系膜**：乙状结肠的系膜。

- The transverse mesocolon divides the peritoneal cavity into *supra*-mesocolic and *infra*-mesocolic compartments, the latter of which is divided into right and left infracolic recesses by the root of the small bowel mesentery.

Omentum

- The greater and lesser omentum are specialized mesenteries that attach to the stomach. The greater and lesser omentum do not connect to the posterior abdominal wall.

> **Greater omentum**: Large, drape-like mesentery in the anterior abdomen, which connects the stomach to the anterior aspect of the transverse colon.
> **Lesser omentum**: Connects stomach to liver.

Flow of peritoneal fluid

- Peritoneal fluid is constantly produced, circulated, and finally reabsorbed around the diaphragm, where it eventually drains into the thoracic duct.
- Peritoneal fluid preferentially travels in certain directions generally from the pelvis into the upper abdomen via the paracolic gutters (right over left) and pools in dependent recesses including the retrouterine (female)/retrovesical (male) recess, along the superior portion of the sigmoid mesocolon, the ileocolic region (root of the small bowel mesentery), the right paracolic gutter and in Morrison's pouch. As a result, these regions are the most prone to involvement of peritoneal and serosal metastases. Flow is limited anatomically in some locations like the falciform ligament on the right and the phrenicocolic ligament on the left.

"MISTY" MESENTERY

Overview of the "misty" mesentery

- As previously discussed, the abdominal mesenteries are fatty folds covered by peritoneum through which the arterial supply and venous and lymphatic drainage of the bowel run.
- The mesenteries themselves are not seen on CT because they are made primarily of fat and blend in with intra-abdominal fat. However, the vessels which course through the mesentery are normally seen.
- Infiltration of the mesentery by fluid, inflammatory cells, tumor, or fibrosis may increase the attenuation of the mesentery and cause the mesenteric vasculature to appear indistinct. These findings are often the first clue to certain pathologies.

Mesenteric edema

- Edema of the mesentery may be secondary to either systemic or intra-abdominal etiologies.
- Systemic causes of edema include congestive heart failure, low protein states, and third-spacing, all of which can lead to diffuse mesenteric edema.
- Focal mesenteric edema may be secondary to an intra-abdominal vascular cause, such as mesenteric vessel thrombosis, Budd-Chiari syndrome, or IVC obstruction. Abdominal vascular insults may cause bowel ischemia, which manifest on imaging as bowel wall thickening, pneumatosis, or mesenteric venous gas.

Mesenteric inflammation

- The most common cause of mesenteric inflammation in the upper abdomen is acute pancreatitis. However, any focal inflammatory process such as

- 横结肠系膜将腹腔分为结肠系膜上和结肠系膜下两个腔室，后者在小肠系膜根部分为右和左结肠下隐窝。

网膜

- 大网膜和小网膜是特殊的肠系膜，它们附着于胃。大网膜和小网膜与后腹壁不相连。

> **大网膜**：位于前腹部一个大的围裙样肠系膜，连接胃和横结肠的前部。
> **小网膜**：连接胃和肝脏。

腹腔的液体流动

- 腹腔液体在不断地产生与循环，最终在膈附近被吸收，并引流进入胸导管。
- 腹腔液体优先沿着某些特定的方向流动，通常是经结肠旁沟(右侧多于左侧)从骨盆流动至上腹部，液体聚集在一些低洼的隐窝，如子宫后(女性)/膀胱后(男性)隐窝，沿着乙状结肠系膜上部、回盲区(小肠系膜根部)、右侧结肠旁沟和Morrison窝流动。因此，这些地方最容易发生腹膜和浆膜转移。液体流动在某些位置受到解剖限制，如右侧的镰状韧带和左侧的膈结肠韧带。

"雾状"肠系膜

"雾状"肠系膜概述

- 如前所述，肠系膜为腹膜覆盖的脂肪皱褶，其中有供血动脉，以及引流肠管的静脉及淋巴管从中通过。
- CT无法显示肠系膜本身，因它们主要由脂肪组成并与腹腔脂肪相融合。但在正常情况下可以显示其内走行的血管。
- 当肠系膜被积液、炎症细胞、肿瘤或纤维化浸润时密度增高，导致肠系膜血管模糊不清。这些表现通常是相关病理改变的第一线索。

肠系膜水肿

- 肠系膜水肿可继发于系统性疾病或腹腔内病变。
- 引起水肿的系统性病因包括充血性心力衰竭、低蛋白状态及第三间隙，所有这些病因都可以引起弥漫性肠系膜水肿。
- 局灶性肠系膜水肿可继发于腹腔内血管性疾病，如肠系膜血管血栓形成、布-加综合征或下腔静脉梗阻。腹腔血管受损可能会导致肠缺血，在影像学上表现为肠壁增厚、肠壁积气或肠系膜静脉内出现气体。

肠系膜炎症

- 最常引起上腹部肠系膜炎症的病因为急性胰腺炎。然而，任何局灶性炎症性疾病(如阑尾

appendicitis, inflammatory bowel disease, and diverticulitis may cause local mesenteric inflammation leading to the *misty mesentery* appearance.

- Mesenteric panniculitis or sclerosing mesenteritis is a spectrum of idiopathic inflammatory conditions which may cause a diffuse *misty mesentery* or a mesenteric mass-like lesion with surrounding misty attenuation. This entity is discussed later in the mesenteric mass section.

Intra-abdominal hemorrhage

- Intra-abdominal hemorrhage tends to be localized to the area surrounding the culprit bleeding vessel unless the bleed is very large. Hemorrhage may be post-procedural, secondary to trauma, or due to anticoagulation.

Neoplastic infiltration

- Neoplastic infiltration of the mesentery may cause the *misty mesentery*. The most common tumor involving the mesentery is non-Hodgkin lymphoma, which typically also causes bulky adenopathy.
- Mesenteric involvement may be especially apparent after treatment, where the *misty mesentery* is limited to the portion of the mesentery that contains the treated lymph nodes.
- Other tumors which may involve the mesentery include carcinoid, pancreatic, colon, breast, GIST, and mesothelioma.

炎、炎症性肠病及憩室炎）均可引起局灶性肠系膜炎症，从而表现为雾状肠系膜。

- 肠系膜脂膜炎或硬化性肠系膜炎包括系列特发性炎症疾病，可以导致弥漫性雾状肠系膜或肠系膜肿瘤样病变伴周围雾状密度围绕。这一病变将在后文的肠系膜占位部分详细讨论。

腹腔内出血

- 腹腔内出血一般局限于出血血管的周围区域，除非出血量很大。出血可继发于手术、外伤或抗凝治疗。

肿瘤性浸润

- 肠系膜肿瘤性浸润可造成雾状肠系膜。最常累及肠系膜的肿瘤为非霍奇金淋巴瘤，通常也会引起明显的淋巴结肿大。
- 肠系膜受累在治疗后可能更为明显，雾状肠系膜局限于治疗后的淋巴结所在的肠系膜区域。
- 其他可能累及肠系膜的肿瘤包括类癌、胰腺癌、结肠癌、乳腺癌、胃肠道间质瘤及间皮瘤。

Mesenteric masses

Overview of mesenteric masses

- Primary mesenteric tumors are rare, although the mesentery is a relatively common site for metastasis. The differential diagnosis of a mesenteric mass includes:

Carcinoid. Desmoid tumor. Sclerosing mesenteritis.	Lymphoma. Metastasis.

Carcinoid

肠系膜占位

肠系膜占位概述

- 原发性肠系膜肿瘤罕见，但肠系膜是相对常见的转移部位。肠系膜肿瘤的鉴别诊断包括：

类癌。 硬纤维瘤。 硬化性肠系膜炎。	淋巴瘤。 转移瘤。

类癌

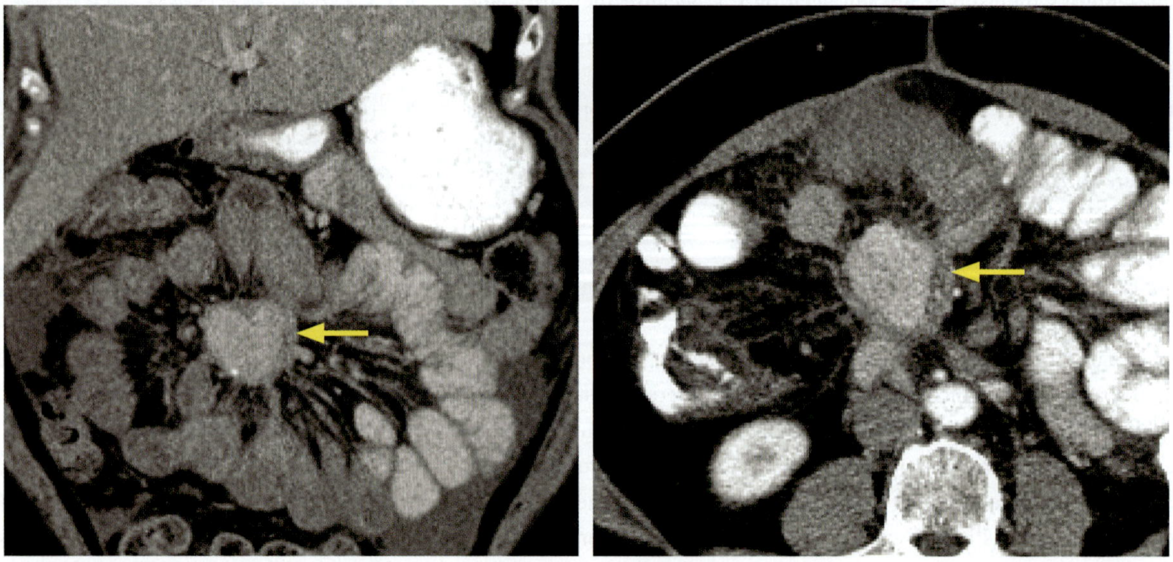

Carcinoid metastatic to the mesentery: Coronal (left image) and axial contrast-enhanced CT shows a hyperenhancing mesenteric mass (arrows) that contains a few tiny foci of calcification peripherally. There are numerous linear soft tissue strands radiating from the mass.
类癌转移至肠系膜：冠状位(左图)及轴位(右图)增强CT显示一个强化的肠系膜肿块(黄箭)，外周可见数个很小的钙化灶。有很多发自肿块的线样软组织密度影，呈放射状分布。

- Gastrointestinal carcinoid is uncommon compared to other GI malignancies but is the most common small bowel tumor. It typically occurs in the distal ileum.
- Carcinoid usually arises as an intraluminal mass and may spread secondarily to the mesentery either by direct extension or lymphatic spread. Up to 80% of carcinoids spread to the mesentery.
- A classic imaging appearance of mesenteric involvement is an enhancing soft-tissue mass with radiating linear bands extending into the mesenteric fat. Calcification is common.

The radiating linear bands do not represent infiltrative tumor but are the result of an intense desmoplastic reaction caused by the release of serotonin by the tumor.

- 胃肠道类癌相对于其他胃肠道恶性肿瘤较为少见，但却是最常见的小肠肿瘤。此肿瘤常发生在远端回肠。
- 类癌通常是起源于肠腔内的一个肿块，随后可以通过直接蔓延或淋巴结转移到肠系膜。高达80%的类癌有肠系膜转移。
- 典型的累及肠系膜的类癌影像学表现为强化的软组织肿块伴有放射状条索延伸到肠系膜脂肪。钙化常见。

放射状条索并不代表肿瘤浸润，而是由于肿瘤释放血清素所引起的强烈的结缔组织增生反应。

Desmoid tumor

硬纤维瘤

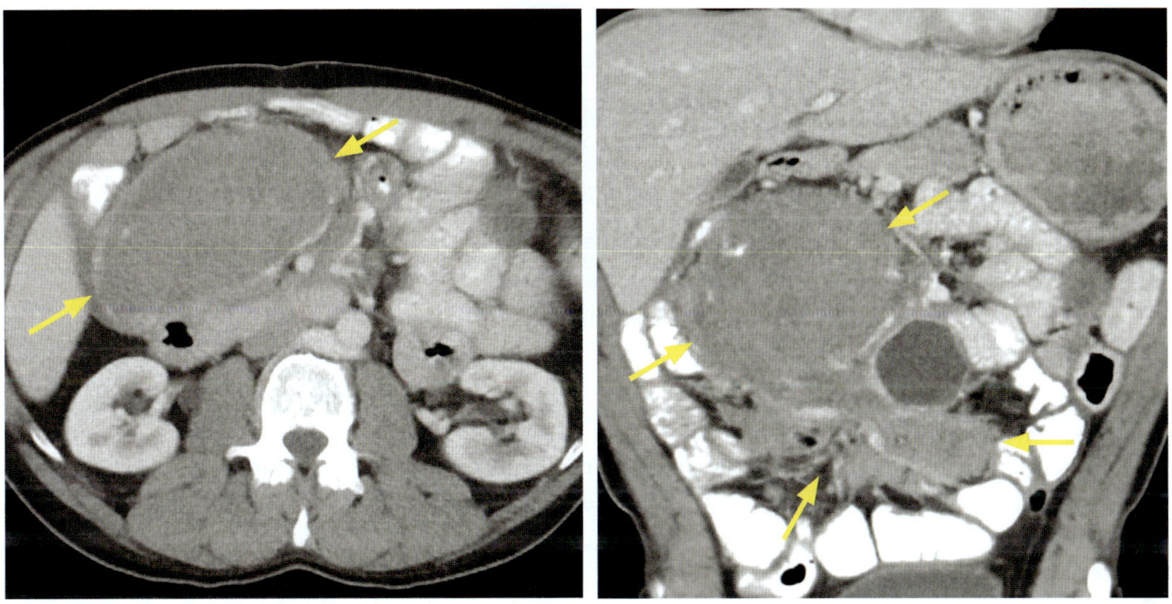

Desmoid tumor in a patient with Gardner's syndrome and status post proctocolectomy: Axial (left image) and coronal (right) CT shows a heterogeneous, infiltrative mesenteric mass (arrows) with central cystic component, consistent with a mesenteric desmoid. Note, no colon is seen on these images.

一名加德纳综合征患者在直肠切除术后的硬纤维瘤：轴位(左图)和冠状位(右图)CT显示一个不均质的、浸润性的肠系膜肿块(黄箭)，伴有中央囊性成分，符合肠系膜硬纤维瘤的表现。注意，图像未显示结肠。

- Desmoid tumor is a benign, but locally aggressive mass composed of proliferating fibrous tissue.
- Desmoid may be sporadic or may arise in post-operative and postpartum patients, but mesenteric desmoid tumors are more common in patients with Gardner syndrome (a variant of familial adenomatous polyposis).
- On CT, most desmoids are isoattenuating to muscle, but large tumors may show central necrosis. A characteristic imaging feature is strands of tissue radiating into the adjacent mesenteric fat, similar to mesenteric carcinoid and sclerosing mesenteritis.

- 硬纤维瘤是一种良性，但具有局部侵袭性的肿瘤，由增生的纤维组织构成。
- 硬纤维瘤可能是散发的，也可能出现在术后或产后的患者，但肠系膜硬纤维瘤更常见于加德纳综合征的患者(家族性腺瘤息肉病的一种变异)。
- 大多数硬纤维瘤在CT上与肌肉呈等密度，但大的肿瘤可以出现中央坏死。典型的影像学表现是条纹状组织呈放射状进入邻近肠系膜脂肪，与肠系膜类癌和硬化性肠系膜炎类似。

Sclerosing mesenteritis

- Sclerosing mesenteritis is a continuum of idiopathic disorders of the mesentery most commonly of the small bowel that can be divided into the three following stages.
- **Mesenteric lipodystrophy** is characterized by foamy macrophages replacing the mesenteric fat. Imaging may show subtle increased attenuation of the

硬化性肠系膜炎

- 硬化性肠系膜炎是一个系列的特发性肠系膜疾病，最常见于小肠，可分为以下三个阶段。
- **肠系膜脂肪营养不良**是以泡沫巨噬细胞取代肠系膜脂肪为特征。影像学可以表现为肠系膜密度轻微增高。

mesentery.

- **Mesenteric panniculitis** represents an infiltrate of immune cells that results in chronic inflammation. Imaging shows increased attenuation of the mesentery, referred to as *misty mesentery*, often associated with prominent mesenteric lymph nodes (<1 cm in short-axis). The lymph nodes may have a halo of preserved fat in a background of diffuse fat stranding referred to as a *fat ring sign*. Linear bands of soft tissue representing early fibrosis may be present.

- **肠系膜脂膜炎**是一种免疫细胞浸润导致的慢性炎症。影像学表现为肠系膜密度增高，称为*雾状肠系膜*，常伴有显著的肠系膜淋巴结(短径<1cm)。淋巴结周围可能有一圈残存的脂肪并以弥漫性脂肪条索为背景，此为*脂肪环征*。可能出现线样软组织条纹，为早期纤维化。

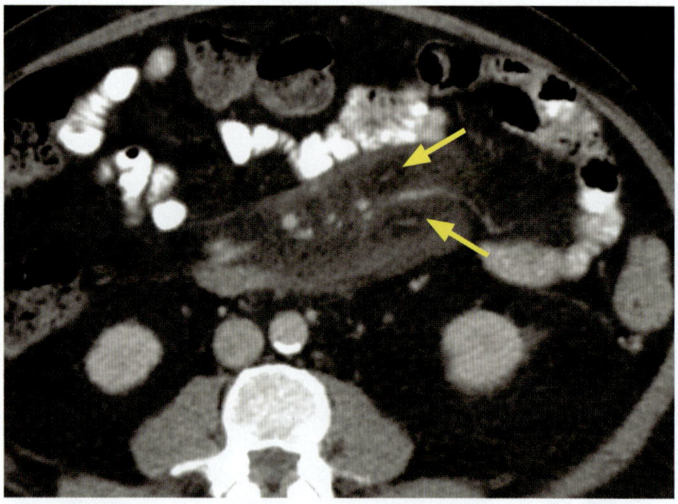

Mesenteric panniculitis: Axial contrast-enhanced CT shows *misty* soft tissue attenuation of the small bowel mesentery, with preservation of normal fat density surrounding the mesenteric vessels and mesenteric lymph nodes (*fat halo sign*) (arrows).

肠系膜脂膜炎：轴位增强CT显示小肠系膜*雾状*软组织密度影，但环绕肠系膜血管和肠系膜淋巴结的脂肪密度影仍为正常(*脂肪环征*)(黄箭)。

- **Retractile mesenteritis** is characterized by collagen deposition, fat necrosis and fibrosis leading to tissue retraction of the mesenteric root. CT shows a mass-like area of heterogeneously increased fat attenuation which may displace loops of bowel. Calcifications may be present, especially in any necrotic portions.

Mesenteric metastases and lymphoma

- In addition to carcinoid as described above, gastric, ovarian, breast, lung, pancreatic, biliary, colon cancer, and melanoma can metastasize to mesenteric lymph nodes.
- Mesenteric lymphoma can produce the *sandwich sign*, where the mesenteric fat and vessels (the sandwich filling) are engulfed on two sides by bulky lymphomatous masses (the bread).

- **回缩性肠系膜炎**是以胶原沉积、脂肪坏死和纤维化并导致肠系膜根部回缩为特征。CT表现为一个肿块样的脂肪密度不均匀增高的区域，可使肠袢移位。钙化可见，尤其是在任何坏死的部位。

肠系膜转移和淋巴瘤

- 除上文提到的类癌外，胃、卵巢、乳腺、肺、胰腺、胆道、结肠癌及黑色素瘤均可以转移到肠系膜淋巴结。
- 肠系膜淋巴瘤可形成典型的*三明治征*，即肠系膜脂肪和血管(三明治馅)被两侧明显肿大的淋巴瘤肿块(面包状)包绕。

OMENTAL DISEASE

Omental carcinomatosis

- The term *omental caking* describes the replacement of omental fat by tumor and fibrosis.

网膜病变

网膜癌病

- 网膜饼指的是网膜脂肪被肿瘤和纤维化取代。

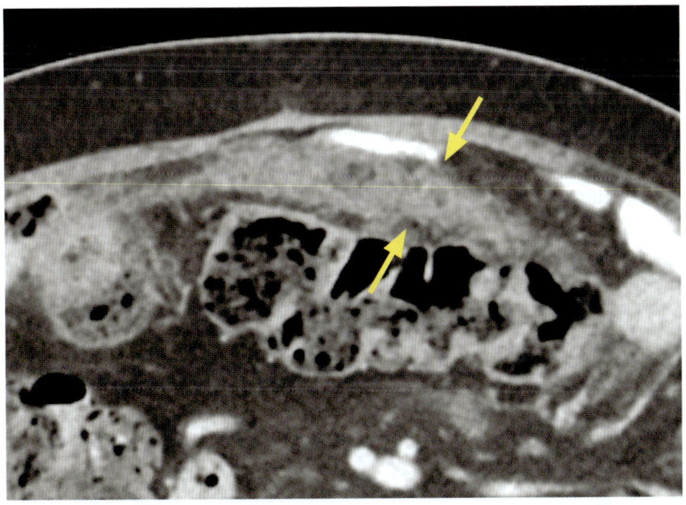

Contrast-enhanced CT axial image shows soft tissue thickening of the omentum (arrows) just beneath the anterior abdominal wall in keeping with biopsy-proven omental carcinomatosis from ovarian primary tumor.

轴位增强CT显示网膜软组织增厚(黄箭),位于前腹壁正后方,符合病理证实的卵巢原发肿瘤来源的网膜扩散。

Omental infarct

- Omental infarct is a rare cause of acute abdominal pain resulting from vascular compromise to the greater omentum which may be idiopathic, or secondary to recent surgery, trauma or related to omental inflammation. The idiopathic form occurs classically in the RLQ medial to the cecum/ascending colon while the secondary form occurs at the site of the initial insult.
- CT shows a circumscribed area of fat stranding, usually large (>5 cm), which may be accompanied by swirling of omental vessels and a hyperdense peripheral halo. Ultrasound may show a focal area of increased echogenicity in the omental fat.

网膜梗死

- 网膜梗死是一种少见的急性腹痛病因,由大网膜血管损伤引起,它可能是特发性的,或继发于近期手术、创伤,或与网膜炎症相关。特发性网膜梗死常发生在右下腹盲肠/升结肠内侧,而继发性网膜梗死发生在最初受伤的部位。
- CT表现为边界清晰的脂肪条索影,通常较大(>5cm),可以伴随网膜血管旋转和外周环状高密度晕。超声可能显示局灶性网膜脂肪回声增强区。

DIFFUSE PERITONEAL DISEASE

Peritoneal carcinomatosis

弥漫性腹膜疾病

腹膜转移癌

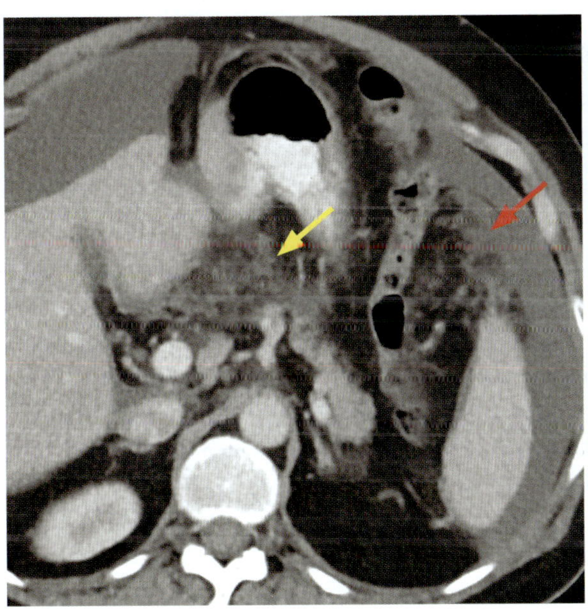

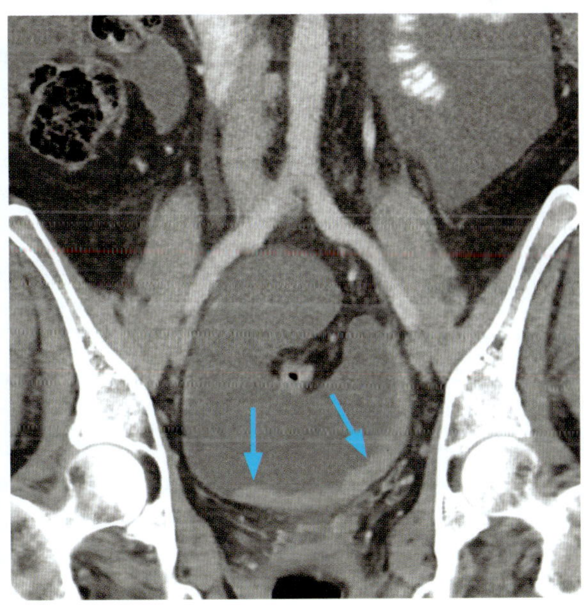

Axial and coronal contrast-enhanced CT demonstrate nodular mesenteric fat stranding (left image, yellow arrow), omental carcinomatosis (left image, red arrow) and nodular peritoneal thickening (right image), most prominent along the pelvic peritoneal reflection (blue arrows) consistent with peritoneal carcinomatosis.

轴位和冠状位增强CT显示结节状的肠系膜脂肪条索影(左图,黄箭)、网膜转移(左图,红箭)和结节状腹膜增厚(右图),主要沿着盆腔腹膜反折处(蓝箭),符合腹膜转移癌。

- Peritoneal carcinomatosis represents disseminated metastases to the peritoneal surface. It is often associated with omental carcinomatosis and serosal disease of intra-abdominal organs (such as liver, spleen and bowel).
- Mucinous adenocarcinoma is the most common tumor type to cause peritoneal carcinomatosis, but peritoneal carcinomatosis due to mucinous adenocarcinoma should not be confused with pseudomyxoma peritonei, discussed below.

- 腹膜转移癌是指转移癌沿腹膜的表面播散，常与网膜转移癌和腹腔内器官(如肝脏、脾脏和肠道)的浆膜病变有关。
- 黏液腺癌是引起腹膜转移癌最常见的肿瘤类型，但黏液腺癌引起的腹膜转移癌不应与腹膜假性黏液瘤混淆，如下所述。

Pseudomyxoma peritonei

腹膜假性黏液瘤

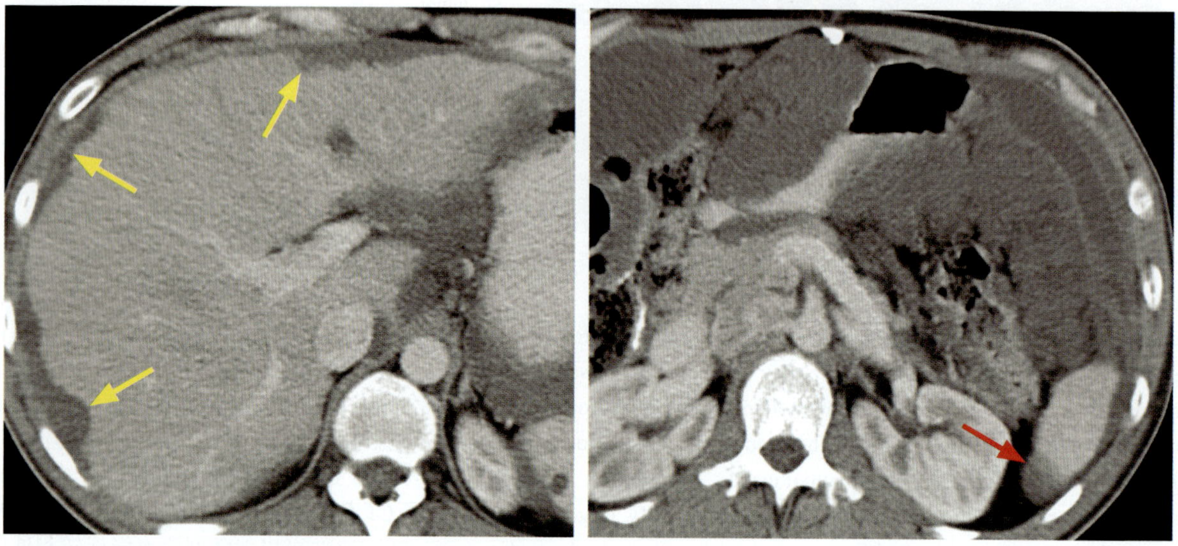

Pseudomyxoma peritonei: Axial contrast-enhanced CT through the liver (left image) shows scalloping of the hepatic capsule by low attenuation material (arrows). A lower image through the kidneys shows the lobulated, mucinous peritoneal material exerting mass effect on adjacent bowel loops. A splenic implant is also visible (red arrow).

Case courtesy Cheryl Sadow, MD, Brigham and Women's Hospital.

腹膜假性黏液瘤：轴位经肝层面的增强CT(左图)显示肝包膜呈低密度的扇贝形(黄箭)。下方经肾脏层面显示对邻近肠管产生占位效应的分叶状、黏液性腹水样物质。亦可见脾种植(红箭)。

- Pseudomyxoma peritonei is a low-grade malignancy characterized by copious amounts of mucus in the peritoneal cavity.
- Pseudomyxoma peritonei is most commonly due to a mucin-producing adenoma or adenocarcinoma of the appendix; however, it can also be seen with other mucinous tumors including gallbladder, pancreatic and ovarian.

  Pseudomyxoma peritonei is often associated with an ovarian mass (up to 30% of female patients), but it is thought that these are most often metastatic deposits rather than primary sites.
- Pseudomyxoma peritonei was previously thought to be produced by a benign appendiceal mucocele, which is now believed to occur much less commonly than originally thought.
- Tumor deposits tend to spread throughout the entire peritoneal cavity due to intraperitoneal fluid currents.
- Clinically, pseudomyxoma peritonei presents with recurrent mucinous ascites.
- CT shows lobular intraperitoneal material that is typically of slightly higher attenuation (5–20 HU) compared to fluid ascites and that may cause mass effect/scalloping of adjacent organs. Occasionally, mucus can be seen in the region of the appendix, but the flow of peritoneal contents tends to spread the mucinous ascites diffusely throughout the peritoneum.
- Treatment continues to evolve, but the best outcomes are primarily with surgical treatment and hyperthermic intraperitoneal chemotherapy lavage.

- 腹膜假性黏液瘤是一种低级别恶性肿瘤，以腹膜腔内大量的黏液为特征。
- 腹膜假性黏液瘤最常见的原因是产生黏蛋白的腺瘤或阑尾腺癌，也可以见于其他包括胆囊、胰腺和卵巢的黏液性肿瘤。

  腹膜假性黏液瘤通常与卵巢肿瘤有关(高达30%的女性患者)，但这被认为通常是来自种植转移，而不是原发部位。
- 腹膜假性黏液瘤过去被认为由良性的阑尾黏液囊肿引起，但现在认为这种发生率远小于之前的观点。
- 肿瘤种植因受腹膜腔内液体循环影响而易播散至整个腹膜腔。
- 腹膜假性黏液瘤在临床上表现为复发性黏液性腹水。
- CT呈分叶状腹水，通常比正常腹水的密度稍高(5~20HU)，可以造成占位效应/邻近器官扇贝样改变。偶然情况下，黏液可见于阑尾区，但腹膜腔的液体流动而容易将黏液性腹水弥漫播散至整个腹膜。
- 治疗方法在不断更新，但是手术及超热腹膜腔内化疗灌洗的预后最好。

(翻译　柏盈盈)

3 Genitourinary Imaging

Cory Robinson-Weiss, Madhvi Deol, Fiona E. Malone, Khushboo Jhala, Junzi Shi, Ellen X. Sun, Michael A. Buckner, Jose M. Lopez, Khanant M. Desai, Daniel Souza

3 泌尿生殖影像

Contents

目录

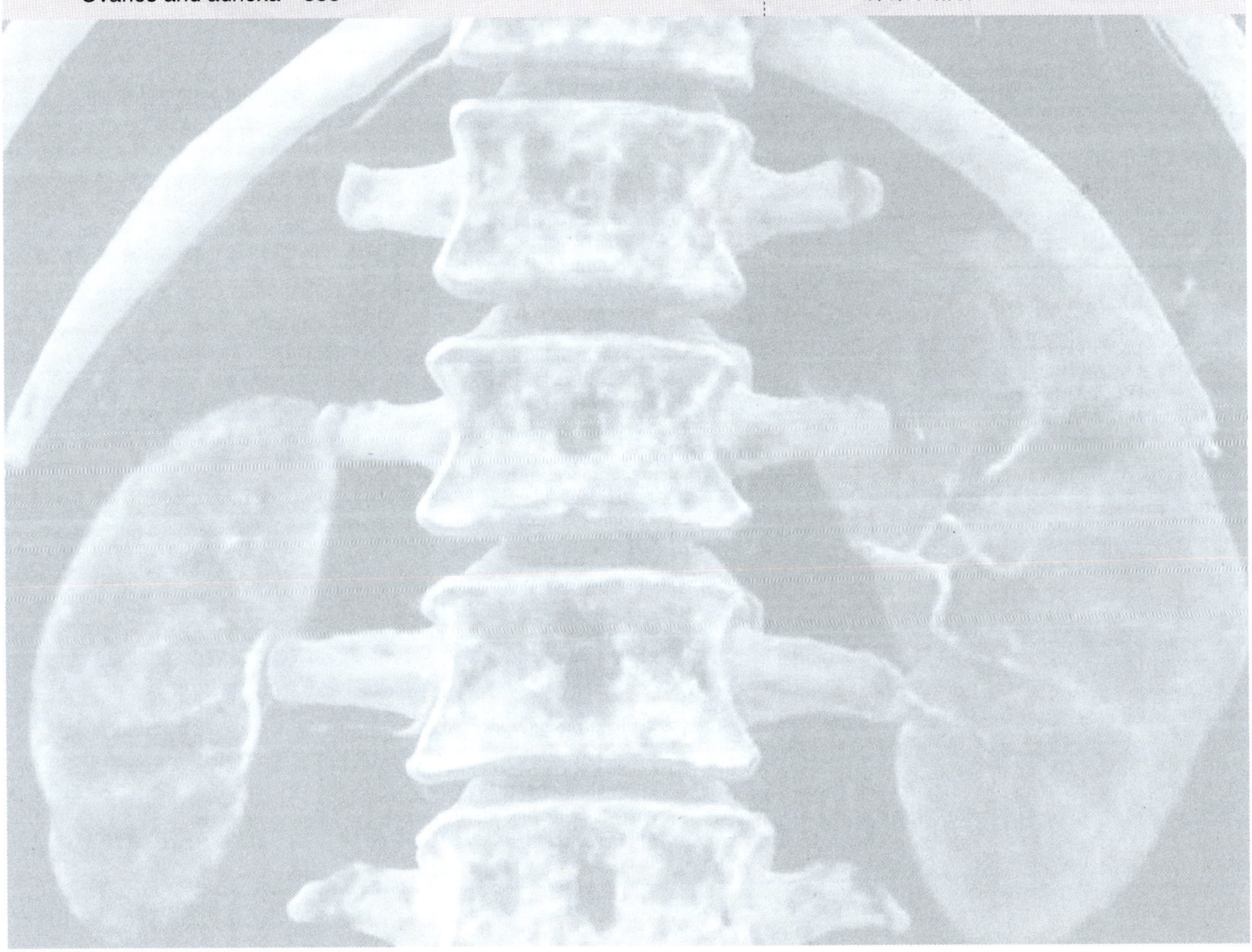

RETROPERITONEUM

腹膜后间隙

RETROPERITONEAL ANATOMY

腹膜后间隙解剖

- The retroperitoneum can be separated into three compartments by the anterior and posterior renal fascia and the lateroconal fascia.

- 腹膜后间隙以肾前筋膜、肾后筋膜和侧锥筋膜为界分为三个部分。

3 compartments of the retroperitoneum
腹膜后间隙的三个组成部分

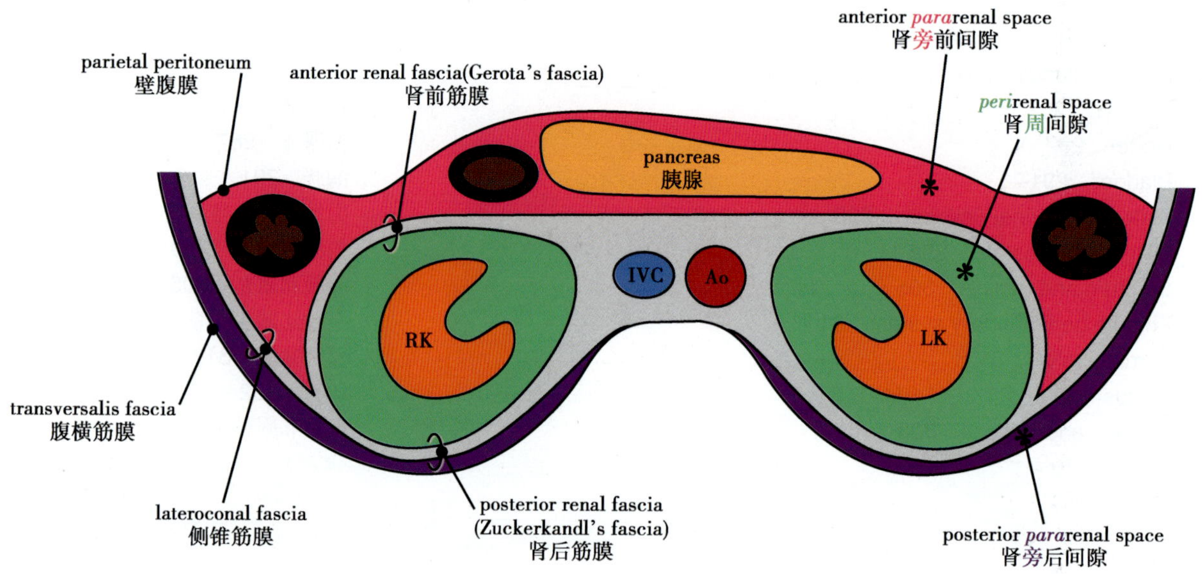

RK, right kidney
RK, 右肾
LK, left kidney
LK, 左肾
IVC, inferior vena cava
IVC, 下腔静脉
Ao, aorta
Ao, 主动脉

anterior pararenal space
肾旁前间隙
- ascending colon
- 升结肠
- descending colon
- 降结肠
- (second and third)duodenum
- (第2、3段)十二指肠
- pancreas
- 胰腺

perirenal space: surrounds each kidney
肾周间隙: 包绕每侧肾
- kidneys
- 肾
- proximal ureter
- 近端输尿管
- adrenals
- 肾上腺
- lots of fat
- 大量脂肪

posterior pararenal space
肾旁后间隙
- potential space,contains only fat
- 潜在腔隙,仅包含脂肪
- may become secondarily involved in inflammatory processes
- 可在炎症过程中继发受累

Liposarcoma

脂肪肉瘤

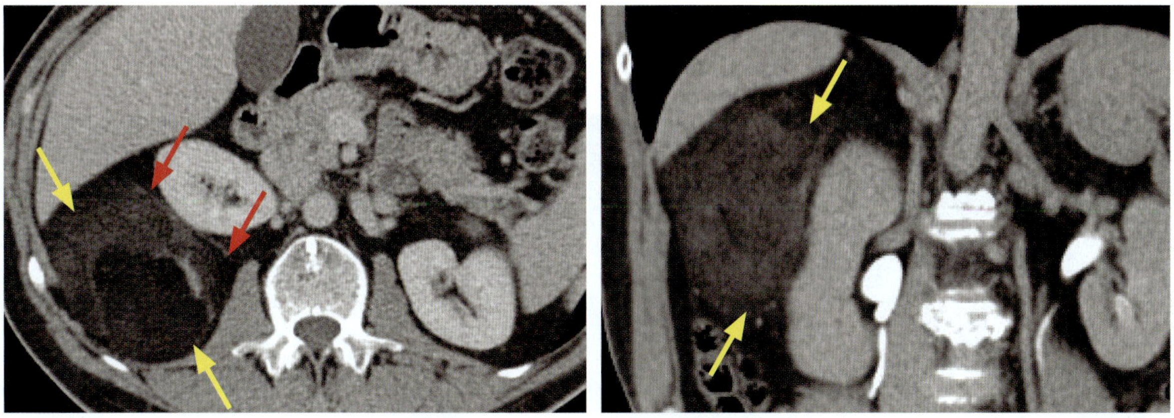

Retroperitoneal liposarcoma: Axial contrast-enhanced nephrographic phase (left image) and coronal excretory phase CT shows a predominantly fat-attenuation mass (yellow arrows) in the right posterior pararenal space, with Zuckerkandl's fascia (red arrows) separating the mass from the perirenal space. Pathology showed a well- differentiated adipocytic liposarcoma.
Case courtesy Cheryl Sadow, MD, Brigham and Women's Hospital.
腹膜后脂肪肉瘤：轴位增强肾实质期(左图)和冠状位排泄期CT显示右侧肾旁后间隙内一个以脂肪密度为主的肿块(黄箭)，肾后筋膜(红箭)将肿块与肾周间隙分开。病理显示为高分化脂肪细胞型脂肪肉瘤。

- Liposarcomas are the most common primary retroperitoneal malignant tumors; 10–15% of all liposarcomas arise from the retroperitoneum.
- Liposarcomas are divided into five histological groups. The well-differentiated subtype, mainly comprised of fat, is the most common and also least aggressive. The other subtypes, in order of increasing aggressiveness, include myxoid, round-cell, pleomorphic, and dedifferentiated.
- The more aggressive subtypes often have minimal macroscopic fat and may be indistinguishable from other soft tissue masses.

- 脂肪肉瘤是最常见的原发性腹膜后恶性肿瘤；10%~15%的脂肪肉瘤起源于腹膜后间隙。
- 脂肪肉瘤在组织学上分为五种亚型。高分化型主要由脂肪组成，是最常见且侵袭性最低的亚型；其他亚型按侵袭性递增的顺序分别为黏液型、圆形细胞型、多形型和去分化型。
- 侵袭性较高的亚型通常仅含少量肉眼可见的脂肪，且难以与其他软组织肿块相鉴别。

Retroperitoneal fibrosis

腹膜后纤维化

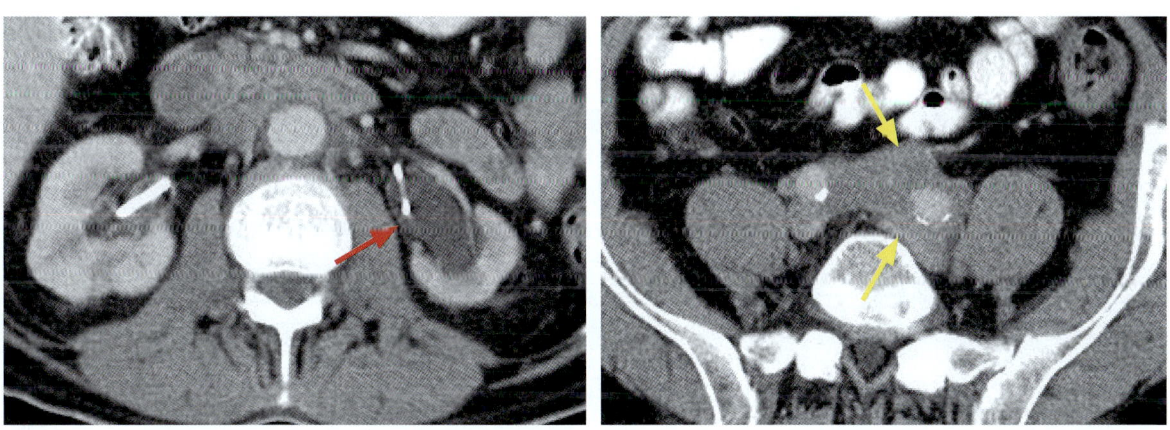

Retroperitoneal fibrosis: Axial contrast-enhanced CT through the kidneys (left image) shows bilateral nephroureteral stents and left hydronephrosis (red arrow). Axial image through the lower abdomen (right image) shows a soft tissue mass (yellow arrows) surrounding the common iliac arteries, with no significant narrowing of the vessels.
Case courtesy Cheryl Sadow, MD, Brigham and Women's Hospital.
腹膜后纤维化：肾脏轴位增强CT(左图)显示双侧肾盂输尿管支架和左侧肾盂积水(红箭)。下腹部轴位图像(右图)显示髂总动脉周围的软组织肿块(黄箭)，无明显血管狭窄。

- Retroperitoneal fibrosis is a rare inflammatory disorder associated with fibrosis deposition in the retroperitoneum, often leading to ureteral obstruction.
- Unlike malignant retroperitoneal lymphadenopathy, retroperitoneal fibrosis rarely displaces the aorta away from the spine.

- 腹膜后纤维化是一种罕见的炎性疾病，与腹膜后间隙过多的纤维沉积有关，常导致输尿管梗阻。
- 与腹膜后恶性淋巴结肿大不同，腹膜后纤维化极少对主动脉产生挤压而使其远离脊柱。

Retroperitoneal hematoma

腹膜后血肿

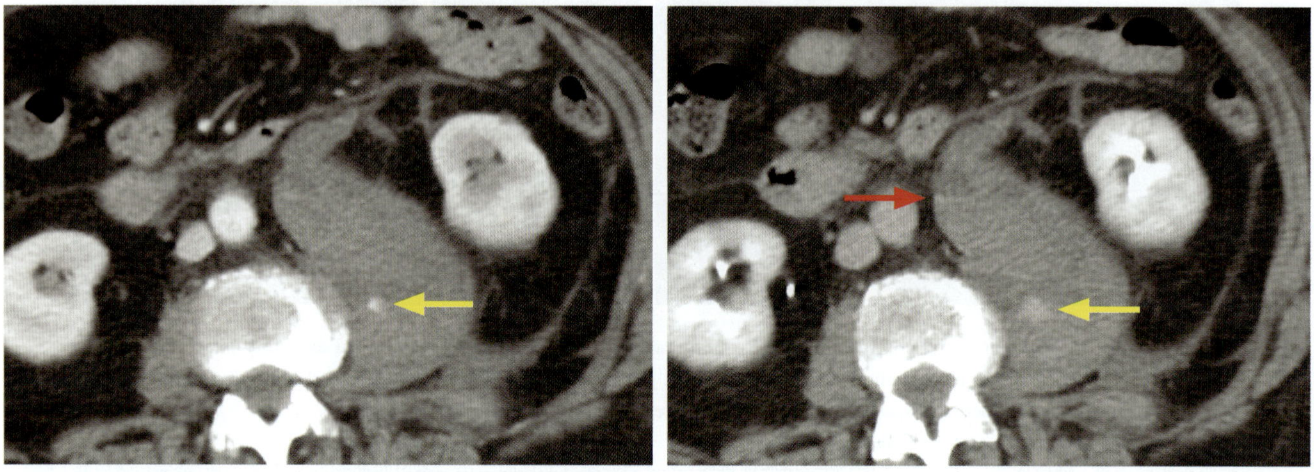

Retroperitoneal hematoma with active extravasation: Axial contrast-enhanced CT (left image) shows a heterogeneous isodense mass in the left paravertebral region indistinct from the left psoas, with anterior extension along the left perirenal space. A punctate hyperdensity (yellow arrow) is seen within the mass which demonstrates blush on delayed phase (right image; yellow arrow), representing active extravasation. Also seen is a subtle fluid-fluid level (*hematocrit effect*; red arrow). This patient was on anticoagulation.

腹膜后血肿伴活动性出血：轴位增强CT(左图)显示左侧椎旁区有一个混杂密度肿物，与左侧腰大肌分界不清，并沿左侧肾周间隙向前延伸。肿物内可见一个点状高密度影(黄箭)，且于延迟期(右图；黄箭)增大，代表活动性出血。另可见模糊的液-液平面(*血细胞比容效应*；红箭)。该患者曾接受过抗凝治疗。

- Retroperitoneal hemorrhage can occur in the setting of trauma, ruptured abdominal aortic aneurysm, renal masses (e.g., renal angiomyolipoma or hemorrhagic renal cyst), or as complication of femoral vascular access. Spontaneous retroperitoneal hemorrhage can occur in patients who are anticoagulated.

- 腹膜后血肿可出现于外伤、腹主动脉瘤破裂、肾脏肿块破裂(如肾血管平滑肌脂肪瘤或出血性肾囊肿)等情况，或为股血管穿刺的并发症。抗凝治疗的患者可发生自发性腹膜后出血。

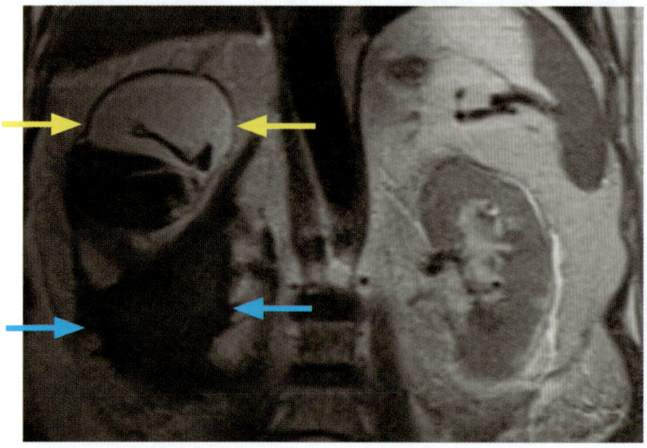

Coronal T2-weighted MRI
冠状位T_2加权MRI

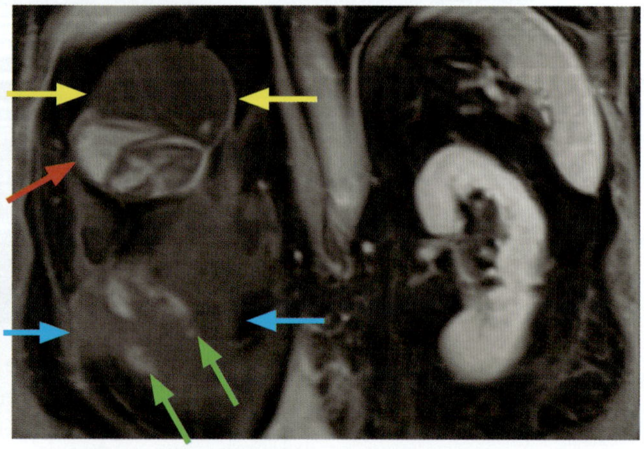

Coronal post-contrast T1-weighted MRI with fat supp.
冠状位增强T_1加权脂肪抑制MRI

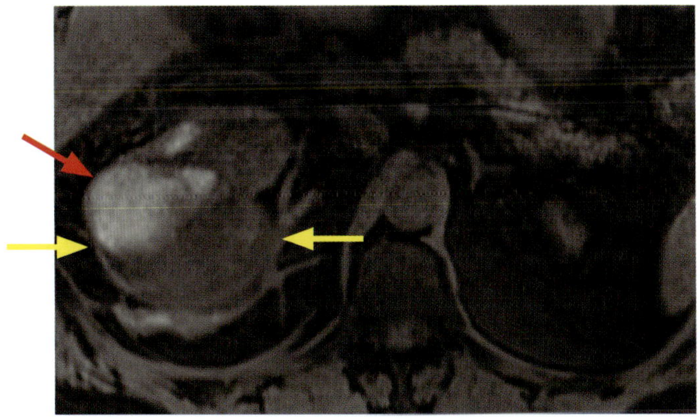

Axial pre-contrast T1-weighted MRI with fat supp.
轴位平扫T_1加权脂肪抑制MRI

Retroperitoneal hematoma due to ruptured hemorrhagic renal cyst: There is a complex cystic mass of the right upper pole (yellow arrows), with internal foci of hyperintense signal on T1-weighted images (red arrows), in keeping with blood products. There is a large retroperitoneal hematoma inferior to the right kidney (blue arrows) with foci of blood products (green arrows). Careful comparison of the pre-and post-contrast images and subtraction images (not shown) showed no enhancement. It is important not to confuse the regions of T1 shortening (bright signal) with active extravasation; such regions are due to methemoglobin in evolving blood products.
出血性肾囊肿破裂引起的腹膜后血肿：右肾上极见一个复杂的囊性肿物(黄箭)，病灶内部见多个T_1高信号区(红箭)，与血液成分信号一致。右肾下方见一个较大的腹膜后血肿(蓝箭)，内有血液成分(绿箭)。仔细比对增强前后图像及减影图像(未展示)未见强化。需强调勿将短T_1区域(高信号)与活动性出血相混淆；这些区域是由于血液中不断演变的高铁血红蛋白所致。

- Retroperitoneal bleeds may explain acute anemia in patients without an identifiable source of bleeding on physical exam.
- To assess for retroperitoneal bleed, noncontrast CT is a reasonable choice as an initial study to more rapidly image the patient. However, intravenous contrast can be helpful to diagnose active extravasation, especially if a large retroperitoneal hematoma is clinically suspected.

- 急性贫血患者在体检时找不到出血原因时应考虑腹膜后有出血的可能。
- CT平扫是评估腹膜后出血的一项快速、合理的初步检查。在此基础上，使用静脉造影剂有助于诊断活动性出血，尤其当临床上怀疑有腹膜后大血肿时。

（翻译　王斯妮）

ADRENAL GLANDS

肾上腺

ANATOMY

- The adrenal glands are inverted Y-shaped endocrine glands that mediate the stress response by releasing cortisol and catecholamines. The adrenal glands are also a site of secondary sex hormone synthesis and blood pressure regulation (with aldosterone).
- The adrenal glands have two distinct components, the cortex and medulla, with different embryological origins (the cortex is derived from mesothelium; the medulla is derived from neural crest). The cortex and medulla are susceptible to different diseases.
- The adrenal glands are often asymmetric with the left gland thicker than the right.

Adrenal cortex

- The adrenal cortex is the peripheral portion of the gland and is composed of three layers that synthesize distinct hormones derived from cholesterol.

解剖

- 肾上腺是一对倒“Y”形的内分泌腺体，它主要通过释放皮质醇和儿茶酚胺调节应激反应。肾上腺也是第二性征激素合成和血压调节(通过醛固酮)的部位。
- 肾上腺包括皮质和髓质两个组成部分，分别来自不同的胚胎起源(皮质来源于间皮；髓质来源于神经嵴)。皮质和髓质好发的疾病不同。
- 肾上腺通常不对称，左侧腺体厚于右侧。

肾上腺皮质

- 肾上腺皮质是腺体的外周部分，由三层组成，分别将胆固醇合成为不同的激素。

Zona glomerulosa (most superficial): Produces aldosterone.

Zona fasciculata: Produces glucocorticoids in response to pituitary adrenocorticotropic hormone (ACTH).

Zone reticularis (deepest; closest to the adrenal medulla): Produces androgens.

球状带(最表浅): 合成醛固酮。

束状带: 受垂体促肾上腺皮质激素(ACTH)调节产生糖皮质激素。

网状带(最深，最接近肾上腺髓质): 合成雄激素。

- Adrenal hyperplasia, adenoma, and cortical carcinoma are lesions that can be diagnosed on imaging.

- 影像学能够诊断的肾上腺皮质疾病包括肾上腺增生、腺瘤和皮质癌。

Adrenal medulla

- The medulla is the central inner portion of the adrenal gland and it is associated with catecholamine production (norepinephrine and epinephrine, derived from tyrosine).
- Masses that arise in the medulla include pheochromocytomas and neuroblastic tumors (ganglioneuroma, ganglioneuroblastoma, and neuroblastoma). Neuroblastoma is the most common extracranial solid tumor of childhood and is discussed in the pediatric imaging section.

肾上腺髓质

- 髓质是肾上腺的中央部分，它与儿茶酚胺(包括去甲肾上腺素和肾上腺素，二者均来自酪氨酸)的生成相关。
- 起源于肾上腺髓质的肿块包括嗜铬细胞瘤和成神经细胞性肿瘤(节细胞神经瘤、节细胞神经母细胞瘤和神经母细胞瘤)。神经母细胞瘤是儿童最常见的颅外实体肿瘤，具体将在儿科影像部分探讨。

Biochemical approach to adrenal lesions

- A patient may be suspected of having a hyperfunctioning adrenal lesion, based on clinical signs/symptoms or lab abnormalities. However, most incidental adrenal lesions are NOT hyperfunctioning.

Adrenal hyperfunction

- **Cushing syndrome** is caused by excess circulating cortisol by exogenous administration or endogenous production, as the result of pituitary (Cushing disease) or from non-pituitary disease, including idiopathic adrenal hyperplasia, adrenal adenoma, or ectopic/paraneoplastic ACTH (e.g., from small cell lung cancer).
- **Conn syndrome** is the result of excess aldosterone production, usually from an adrenal adenoma, resulting in hypertension and hypokalemia. Adenomas implicated in Conn syndrome are typically small and may be difficult to detect on CT. Localizing the side of excess hormone production with venous sampling may be a helpful diagnostic adjunct.
- **Adrenal cortical carcinoma** is a very rare adrenal malignancy that arises from the cortex and typically causes an increase in levels of all cortical adrenal hormones and their precursors.
- **Pheochromocytomas** usually arise from the adrenal medulla and can be associated with excess catecholamine production. This can result in episodic headaches, tachycardia, diaphoresis, and uncontrolled hypertension.

Adrenal hypofunction

- Substantial destruction of adrenal tissue is required to produce adrenal insufficiency.
- Though usually not an imaging diagnosis, **Addison disease** represents chronic adrenocortical insufficiency. It can be caused by autoimmune destruction of the adrenal glands or by prior infection.
- **Waterhouse-Friderichsen syndrome** is post-hemorrhagic adrenal failure secondary to Neisseria *meningitidis* bacteremia.
- **Idiopathic adrenal hemorrhage** is usually unilateral and rarely causes adrenal hypofunction.

肾上腺病变的生物化学

- 患者可能因临床体征/症状或实验室检查异常而被怀疑患有肾上腺功能亢进的病变。然而，大多数偶然发现的肾上腺病变并非功能亢进。

肾上腺功能亢进

- **库欣综合征**由循环皮质醇过多导致，如垂体(库欣病)或垂体外疾病，这些皮质醇可经外源性摄入或内源性产生，包括特发性肾上腺增生、肾上腺腺瘤或异位/副肿瘤性ACTH(如来源于小细胞肺癌等)。
- **原发性醛固酮增多症(康恩综合征)**是指醛固酮过度分泌从而导致高血压和低钾血症，常见于肾上腺腺瘤。导致原发性醛固酮增多症的腺瘤通常较小，CT可能很难发现。通过肾上腺静脉采血有助于确定过量产生激素的一侧。
- **肾上腺皮质癌**是一种非常罕见的起源于肾上腺皮质的恶性肿瘤，常导致各种肾上腺皮质激素及其前体水平升高。
- **嗜铬细胞瘤**通常起源于肾上腺髓质，并伴有儿茶酚胺的过量产生，可导致间歇性头痛、心动过速、出汗和恶性高血压。

肾上腺功能减退

- 双侧肾上腺组织被严重破坏后会出现肾上腺功能不全。
- **艾迪生病**表现为慢性肾上腺皮质功能不全，通常不是一个影像学上的诊断。它可能由肾上腺自身免疫破坏或既往感染所致。
- **暴发型脑膜炎球菌败血症(沃-弗综合征)**是继发于脑膜炎奈瑟菌菌血症后肾上腺出血所致的功能衰竭。
- **特发性肾上腺出血**常为单侧，极少导致肾上腺功能减退。

Imaging of Adrenal Adenoma and the Indeterminate Adrenal Mass

Adrenal adenoma

- Adrenal adenoma is a benign tumor of the adrenal cortex. Adenomas are usually incidental, but occasionally produce excess aldosterone that results in secondary hypertension (Conn syndrome). The majority of adrenal adenomas have two properties that allow for diagnosis by imaging: microscopic fat and/or rapid washout characteristics on contrast-enhanced CT.
- An adrenal protocol CT (described below) is the best imaging study to evaluate for the presence of an adrenal adenoma.

  An adrenal nodule with attenuation ≤10 Hounsfield units (HU) on noncontrast CT can be reliably diagnosed as adenoma; 70–80% of adenomas measure <10 HU on noncontrast CT.

  If a nodule measures >10 HU on noncontrast CT, IV contrast is administered to assess washout characteristics; 20–30% of adenomas measure >10 HU on noncontrast CT (lipid-poor adenoma).

  An adrenal adenoma has an absolute washout >60% or a relative washout >40%.
- If a nodule does not meet CT density or washout criteria for an adenoma, it is considered indeterminate. In practice, an indeterminate adrenal nodule in a patient without known malignancy most likely represents a lipid-poor adenoma and advanced imaging is usually not required.
- If diagnosis is required for further management (e.g., in a lung cancer patient without known metastatic disease), further workup is based on lesion size, history of malignancy, and availability of prior imaging. In some cases, FDG PET/CT and adrenal mass biopsy can be helpful.
- A **collision tumor** represents co-existence of two tumors within an adrenal mass, such as metastasis within an adrenal adenoma or myelolipoma.

肾上腺腺瘤与不确定性肾上腺肿块的影像

肾上腺腺瘤

- 肾上腺腺瘤是肾上腺皮质的一种良性肿瘤。腺瘤常为偶然发现，但也可能因产生过量的醛固酮而导致继发性高血压(原发性醛固酮增多症)。大多数肾上腺腺瘤在影像学上具有两个特征，可协助诊断：微小脂肪灶和/或增强CT上显示造影剂快速廓清的特征。
- 肾上腺CT(见下文)是评估肾上腺腺瘤的最佳影像学方法。

  若一个肾上腺结节的平扫CT值≤10HU，则诊断为腺瘤的可能性较大；70%~80%的腺瘤平扫CT值<10HU。

  若一个结节平扫CT值>10HU，则需静脉注射造影剂以获得廓清特征；20%~30%的腺瘤平扫CT值>10HU(乏脂性腺瘤)。

  肾上腺腺瘤的绝对廓清率>60%或相对廓清率>40%。
- 若结节不符合腺瘤的CT值或廓清标准，则被视为不确定性。在临床上，若患者无恶性肿瘤病史，则该不确定性肾上腺结节最可能为乏脂性肾上腺腺瘤，通常不需要行进一步影像学检查。
- 若需要进一步诊断(如未发现有转移灶的肺癌患者)，则后续评估应根据病变大小、恶性肿瘤史和既往影像学检查而定。在某些情况下，氟代脱氧葡萄糖(FDG)正电子发射计算机体层显像(PET/CT)和肾上腺肿块活检有助于诊断。
- **碰撞瘤**是指同一个肾上腺肿物内同时存在2种肿瘤，例如，在肾上腺腺瘤或髓样脂肪瘤内出现转移性肿瘤。

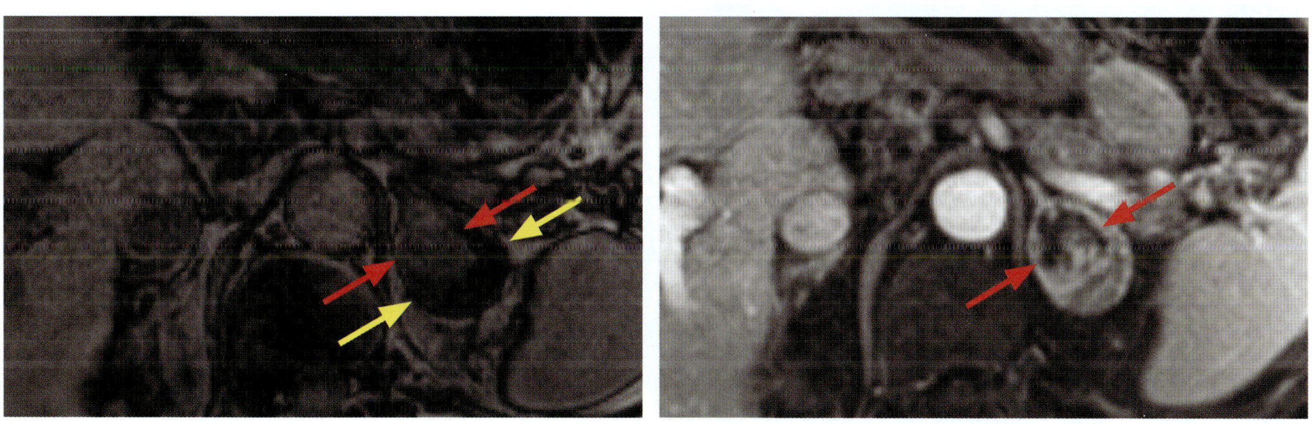

Collision tumor: There is a left adrenal mass. Opposed phase MRI (left image) shows a crescentic lesion posterolaterally with signal drop-out (yellow arrows), in keeping with an adrenal adenoma. There is an additional lesion located anteromedially (red arrows), which does not demonstrate signal drop-out on opposed phase imaging, and which shows central necrosis with enhancement on post-contrast imaging (right image).

碰撞瘤：左肾上腺肿块。反相位MRI(左图)显示病灶后外侧呈新月形信号减低区(黄箭)，符合肾上腺腺瘤的诊断。前内侧有一个稍高信号病灶(红箭)，反相位未显示信号下降，而增强后显示强化伴中央坏死(右图)。

If an "adenoma" appears heterogeneous or shows an interval increase in size, then a collision tumor should be considered in patients with a known primary malignancy, even if a portion of the lesion attenuates <10 HU.

CT imaging: Adrenal washout CT

- Typically, adrenal adenomas demonstrate rapid washout characteristics, while adrenal metastases demonstrate slow washout (<60% absolute washout; <40% relative washout).
- The adrenal protocol study consists of three phases: unenhanced, enhanced (60 seconds post-injection), and delayed (15 minutes post-injection).
- If an adrenal nodule measures <10 HU on noncontrast CT, adrenal adenoma is diagnosed and the exam is terminated. If the nodule measures >10 HU on noncontrast CT, IV contrast is administered and enhanced plus delayed imaging is obtained.

- **>60% absolute washout is diagnostic of adenoma.**

$$\%\ \text{washout} = \frac{E-D}{E-U} = \frac{\text{enhanced attenuation} - \text{delayed attenuation}}{\text{enhanced attenuation} - \text{unenhanced attenuation}}$$

若一个"腺瘤"显示密度不均或发现有阶段性增大，且患者存在原发肿瘤病史，即使一部分病变的CT值<10HU，也需要考虑碰撞瘤。

CT成像：肾上腺廓清CT

- 典型的肾上腺腺瘤具有快速廓清的特征，而肾上腺转移瘤表现为缓慢廓清(绝对廓清率<60%，相对廓清率<40%)。
- 肾上腺扫描方案包括3个时相：平扫、增强(注射造影剂后60秒)和延迟相(注射造影剂后15分钟)。
- 若肾上腺结节平扫<10HU，可诊断为肾上腺腺瘤，不需要进一步检查。若肾上腺结节平扫>10HU，则需静脉注射造影剂获得增强和延迟影像。
- **绝对廓清率>60%可以诊断为腺瘤。**

$$\text{廓清率} = \frac{E-D}{E-U} = \frac{\text{强化密度} - \text{延迟密度}}{\text{强化密度} - \text{平扫密度}}$$

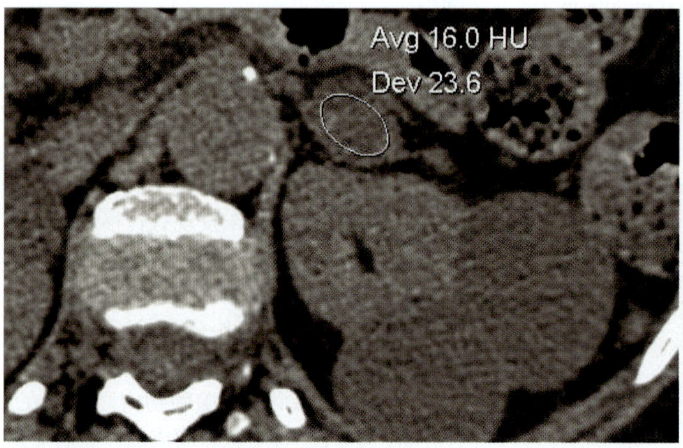

Unenhanced (precontrast) phase
平扫(增强前)

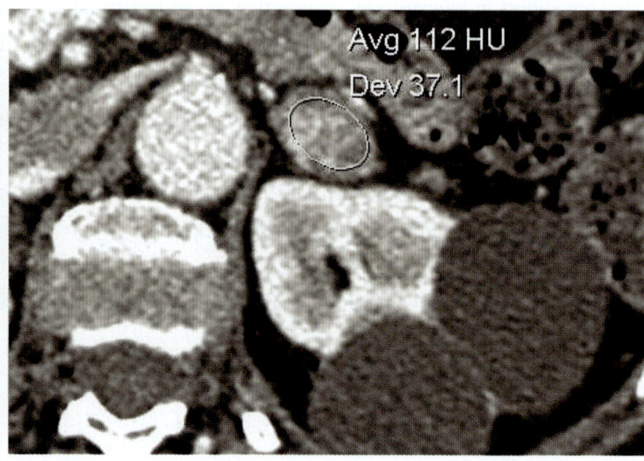

60-second contrast-enhanced phase (adrenal parenchymal phase)
增强后60秒(肾上腺实质期)

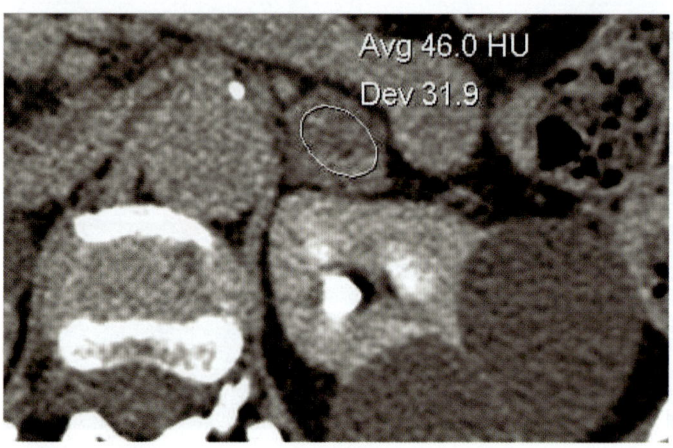

15-minute delay washout
15分钟延迟廓清

Axial unenhanced, enhanced, and delayed images from adrenal washout protocol CT show an adrenal nodule measuring 16 HU, 112 HU, and 46 HU, respectively.

Using the washout formula E – D/E – U: (112 – 46) / (112 – 16) = 69% washout, >60% washout is diagnostic of an adenoma.

Note is made of two large simple cysts of the left kidney.

Case courtesy Cheryl Sadow, MD, Brigham and Women's Hospital.

肾上腺廓清轴位平扫、增强和延迟相CT显示一个肾上腺结节，CT值分别为16HU、112HU和46HU。

采用廓清率计算公式(E–D)/(E–U)：(112–46)/(112–16)=69%，廓清率>60%，诊断为腺瘤。

注意左肾有2个大的单纯性肾囊肿。

- If unenhanced CT images are unavailable, relative washout calculation can still be performed by using the formula below.
>40% relative washout is diagnostic of adenoma:

$$\textbf{\% relative washout} = \frac{\mathbf{E-D}}{\mathbf{E}} = \frac{\text{enhanced attenuation} - \text{delayed attenuation}}{\text{enhanced attenuation}}$$

- 若无CT平扫，仍可用以下公式计算相对廓清率。
相对廓清率>40%可以诊断为腺瘤：

$$\text{相对廓清率} = \frac{E-D}{E} = \frac{\text{强化密度}-\text{延迟密度}}{\text{强化密度}}$$

- In a patient with a known primary malignancy, lesions that do not demonstrate benign washout kinetics are suspicious for, but not diagnostic of, metastasis.

- 对一个已知有原发恶性肿瘤的患者，若病灶的廓清动力学不能证明是良性病变，需要怀疑，但不能诊断为转移性肿瘤。

MRI adrenal imaging: Chemical shift imaging = in and out of phase imaging

- Lipid-rich adenomas contain intracytoplasmic lipid. MRI can detect even small amounts of intracytoplasmic lipid that may be undetectable by CT. MRI takes advantage of the fact that protons resonate at different frequencies in fat and in water.

  Chemical shift imaging consists of paired GRE images obtained at different echo times (TEs): in-phase (IP) and out-of-phase (OOP). When fat and water are contained within the same voxel, OOP images will show a drop in signal intensity when compared to IP, due to cancellation effect caused by fat and water protons being in "opposite direction" (out of phase). Adenomas suppress on OOP images, while metastases generally do not.

肾上腺MRI：化学位移成像=同反相位成像

- 富含脂质的腺瘤含有胞质内脂质。MRI可以检测到少量CT检测不到的胞质内脂质，其主要原理是利用了水和脂肪内质子共振频率的差异。

  化学位移成像为包括不同回波时间(TEs)的成对梯度回波序列(GRE)图像：同相位(IP)和反相位(OOP)。当脂肪和水包含在同一体素内时，因为脂肪和水质子处于"相反方向"(反相位)而产生抵消作用，因而反相位图像的信号丢失(较同相位图像而言)。腺瘤在反相位图像上受抑制，而转移灶一般不会受抑制。

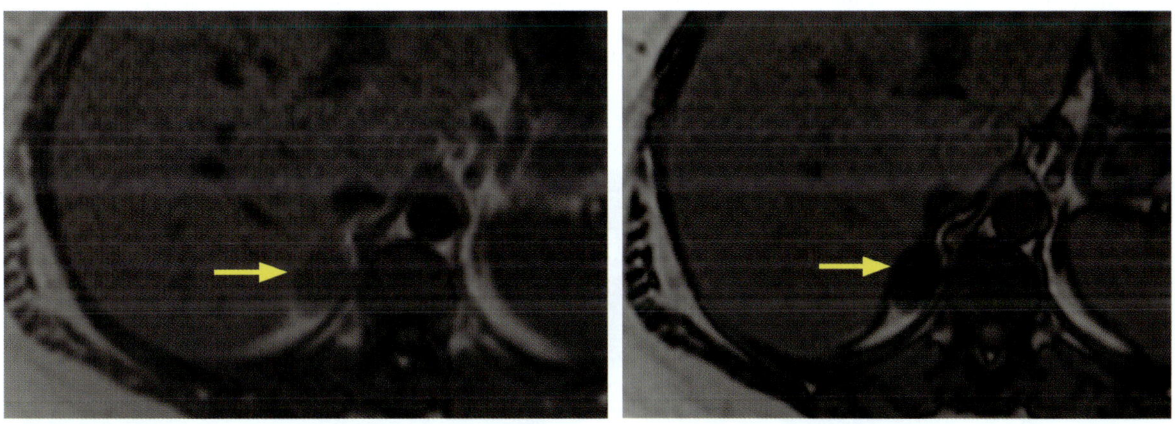

Axial MRI demonstrates signal dropout in a right adrenal mass (arrows) on OOP (right image) compared to IP (left image), consistent with a lipid-rich adenoma.
轴位MRI显示右侧肾上腺肿块在反相位图像(黄箭)中的信号较同相位(左图)有丢失，与富脂腺瘤一致。

- Some malignant adrenal masses may rarely contain intracytoplasmic lipid and lose signal on out-of-phase images:

Well-differentiated adrenocortical carcinoma (very rare).
Metastatic clear cell renal cell carcinoma (RCC).
Metastatic hepatocellular carcinoma (HCC).
Liposarcoma (typically a predominantly fatty mass that is rarely confused with adrenal adenoma).

- 在罕见的情况下，一些恶性肾上腺肿块也可能含有胞质内脂质，因而在反相位图像上出现信号丢失：

分化良好的肾上腺皮质癌(非常罕见)。
转移性肾透明细胞癌(RCC)。
转移性肝细胞癌(HCC)。
脂肪肉瘤(通常为以脂肪为主的肿块，极少与肾上腺腺瘤产生混淆)。

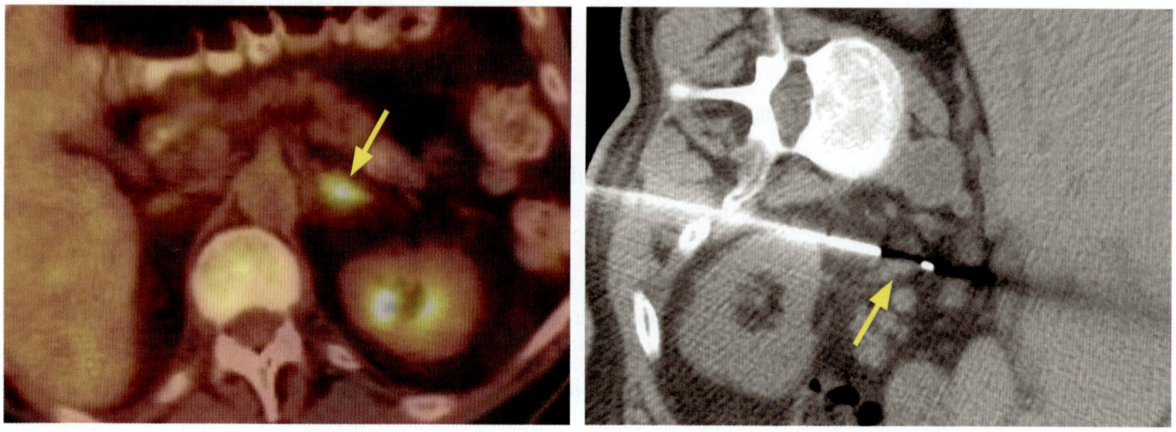

Adrenal biopsy: Fused axial PET-CT (left image) in a patient with lung cancer and indeterminate adrenal mass demonstrates an FDG-avid left adrenal mass (yellow arrow). Intraprocedural image from a CT-guided left adrenal biopsy with the patient decubitus demonstrates the deployed tract of the biopsy needle traversing the mass (yellow arrow). Pathology was metastatic lung cancer.
肾上腺活检：一名肺癌患者的轴位PET/CT融合图像(左图)显示左肾上腺有一个性质待定的肿块呈FDG高摄取(黄箭)。患者侧卧位，在CT引导下左侧肾上腺活检术中图像显示活检针穿过肿块(黄箭)。病理报告为肺癌转移。

- Percutaneous adrenal mass biopsy is a safe procedure often performed under CT guidance. It is very accurate in providing definitive diagnosis.
- Biopsy is indicated for an adrenal mass that remains indeterminate after comprehensive imaging workup, particularly in the context of underlying malignancy.

- 经皮肾上腺肿块活检是一种安全的手术，常在CT引导下进行，可获得准确的诊断。
- 活检适用于综合影像学检查后仍不能定性的肾上腺肿块，特别是有已知恶性肿瘤的患者。

Myelolipoma

髓样脂肪瘤

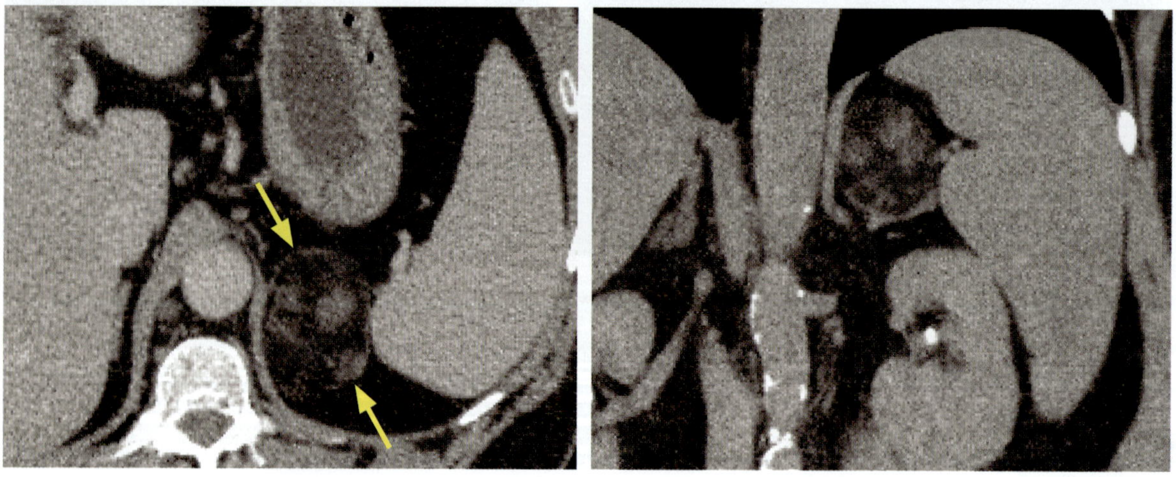

Adrenal myelolipoma: Axial (left image) and coronal (right image) CT shows a predominantly fatty mass with a few circumscribed foci of soft-tissue attenuation in the left adrenal (arrows). The mass is clearly distinct from the kidney, as best seen on the coronal image.
Case courtesy Cheryl Sadow, MD, Brigham and Women's Hospital.
肾上腺髓样脂肪瘤。轴位(左图)和冠状位(右图)CT显示左侧肾上腺有一个以脂肪为主的肿块，其内有一些边界清楚的局灶性软组织密度影(黄箭)。肿块与肾脏分界清楚，冠状位显示最佳。

- An adrenal myelolipoma is a benign neoplasm consisting of myeloid cells (i.e., erythrocyte precursors – *not* “myo” as in muscle) and fat cells. In rare cases, they can be extra-adrenal and are pathologically indistinguishable from extramedullary hematopoiesis, which occurs in patients with hematologic disorders.

- 肾上腺髓样脂肪瘤是一种良性肿瘤，由髓样细胞(如红细胞前体——不是肌肉里的“肌”)和脂肪细胞组成。在罕见的病例中，它可以发生在肾上腺外并且在病理上难以与髓外造血区分，后者发生在血液病患者中。

- An adrenal mass with macroscopic (gross) fat is virtually diagnostic of a myelolipoma. It is usually an incidental finding and can be large (>4 cm) at the time of diagnosis. There are few reports of adrenocortical carcinoma and metastatic carcinoma with macroscopic fat, but these cases are very rare. A retroperitoneal liposarcoma may mimic a myelolipoma, although liposarcoma typically presents as a large mass that may displace, rather than arise from, the adrenal.
- An adrenal myelolipoma should not be confused with a *renal angiomyolipoma* (AML). These two entities are unrelated, although they do have similar names, are located in adjacent organs, and are both diagnosed by the presence of macroscopic fat.

Adrenal cyst

- Adrenal cysts are relatively uncommon but have typical imaging characteristics of benign cysts that occur elsewhere in the body: internal fluid content with thin, smooth, non-enhancing wall).
- **Endothelial adrenal cysts** are the most common (45%) type and may be lymphatic or angiomatous in origin.
- **Pseudocysts** secondary to adrenal hemorrhage represent 39% of adrenal cysts and lack an epithelial lining. Peripheral calcification may be present.
- **Epithelial cysts** are rare, comprising only 9% of adrenal cysts.
- Occasionally an adrenal cyst may have a complex appearance and can be difficult to differentiate from a cystic/necrotic neoplasm. In such a case, percutaneous aspiration or surgical resection may be considered.
- Small, asymptomatic, simple cysts can be ignored. A cyst may rarely grow so large as to cause symptoms, such as dull pain or compression of the stomach/duodenum, but these cases are very uncommon.
- Very rarely, hydatid disease may affect the adrenal glands, typically producing a complex cystic lesion with an internal membrane.

Malignant (or Potentially Malignant) Adrenal Masses

Pheochromocytoma: Potentially malignant

- 在肾上腺肿块中若发现肉眼能够分辨的脂肪，则基本可以诊断为髓样脂肪瘤，常为偶然发现并在诊断时可以很大(>4cm)。少数文献报道肾上腺皮质癌和转移癌会出现肉眼可见的脂肪成分，但这些病例罕见。腹膜后脂肪肉瘤可类似于肾上腺髓样脂肪瘤，但脂肪肉瘤通常表现为一个巨大的肿块并可以使肾上腺移位，而不是起源于肾上腺。
- 肾上腺髓样脂肪瘤不应与*肾血管平滑肌脂肪瘤*(AML)相混淆，这是两种互不相关的疾病，尽管其名称相似，都位于邻近的器官，且都需要存在肉眼可见的脂肪进行诊断。

肾上腺囊肿

- 肾上腺囊肿相对少见，但具备其他部位良性囊肿的典型影像学特征：内为液体成分伴有薄而光滑、无强化的囊壁。
- **内皮性肾上腺囊肿**是最常见(45%)的类型，可起源于淋巴管或血管。
- **假性囊肿**继发于肾上腺出血，占肾上腺囊肿的39%，无内衬上皮细胞。周边可出现钙化。
- **上皮囊肿**非常罕见，只占肾上腺囊肿的9%。
- 肾上腺囊肿偶尔有复杂的表现，可能难以与囊性/坏死性肿瘤相鉴别。在这种情况下，应考虑经皮穿刺抽吸或手术切除。
- 小而无症状的单纯性囊肿可以忽略。囊肿偶可长得很大且引起临床症状，如钝痛或压迫胃/十二指肠，这种情况非常少见。
- 极罕见情况下，棘球蚴病可累及肾上腺，通常形成一个复杂的囊性病灶，伴有内膜。

恶性(或潜在恶性)肾上腺肿瘤

嗜铬细胞瘤：潜在恶性

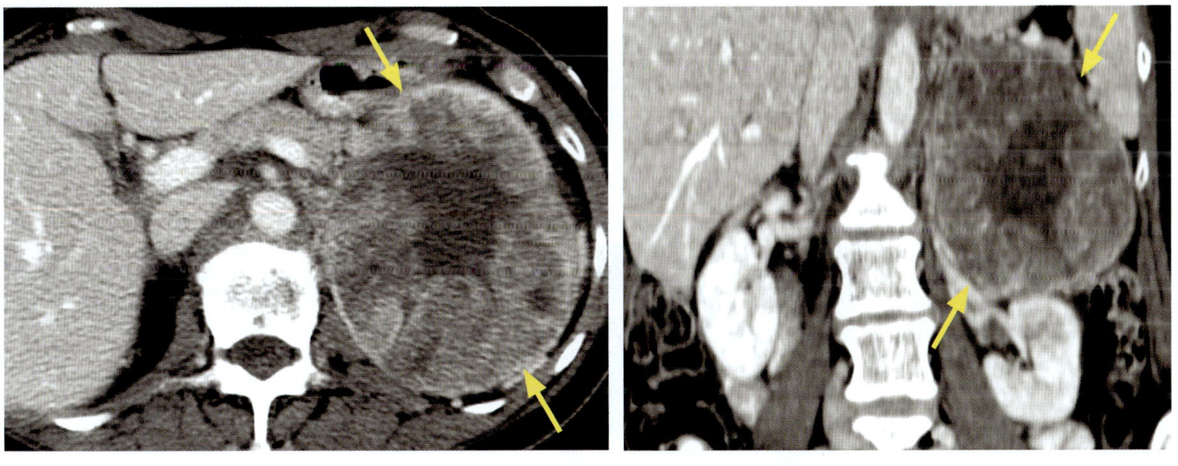

Pheochromocytoma: Contrast-enhanced axial (left image) and coronal (right image) CT shows a large, heterogeneous mass (arrows) with central necrosis arising superior to the left kidney. The extra-renal origin is best appreciated on the coronal image.

嗜铬细胞瘤：轴位(左图)和冠状位(右图)增强CT显示一个起源于左肾上方大而不均的肿块(黄箭)，伴中央坏死。其肾外起源在冠状位图像上最易辨认。

- A pheochromocytoma (intra-adrenal paraganglioma) is a neuroendocrine tumor that typically originates from the adrenal medulla. Pheochromocytomas are composed of chromaffin cells that secrete catecholamines and can cause uncontrolled secondary hypertension and episodic headaches/diaphoresis. Approximately 90% of these tumors are benign.
- Pheochromocytomas can be large and heterogeneous due to areas of necrosis, hemorrhage, and occasionally calcification. On CT, they demonstrate avid enhancement. On MRI, they demonstrate marked T2 hyperintensity (*light bulb sign*) and avid enhancement with variable washout kinetics.
- Nuclear medicine Iodine-123 MIBG or Indium-111 pentetreotide scintigraphy, Gallium-68 DOTATATE PET/CT, or contrast-enhanced MRI can be used for detection of extra-adrenal pheochromocytoma, such as in the context of metastatic workup in patients with hereditary conditions that increase risk of developing pheochromocytoma (see below).
- Pheochromocytoma/paragangliomas are associated with several syndromes:

Multiple endocrine neoplasia (MEN) 2A and 2B: Typically bilateral intra-adrenal pheochromocytomas.
von Hippel-Lindau.
Neurofibromatosis type 1.
Carney's triad (gastric leiomyosarcoma, pulmonary chondroma, and paragangliomas)
Hereditary paraganglioma-pheochromocytoma syndrome: SDHD gene mutation, paragangliomas and pheochromocytomas (50% risk of malignant pheochromocytomas).

- The most common site of an extra-adrenal paraganglioma is the organ of Zuckerkandl, located along the aortic bifurcation to the level of the bladder. Although rare, when the bladder is involved, it can produce a distinctive clinical presentation of post-micturition syncope (syncope after urination).
- Paragangliomas of the head and neck are generally called glomus tumors and may be associated with the tympanic membrane (glomus tympanicum), the jugular foramen (glomus jugulare), the carotid body (called a carotid body tumor), or the vagus nerve (glomus vagale).
- In theory, pheochromocytoma/paragangliomas should be diagnosed by urine/plasma catecholamines and metanephrines, with imaging reserved for localization and staging. In clinical practice, when patients have suspected pheochromocytoma (such as refractory hypertension), CT is often used as the first line imaging test to rule out an adrenal mass.

- 嗜铬细胞瘤(肾上腺内副神经节瘤)是一种神经内分泌肿瘤，通常起源于肾上腺髓质。嗜铬细胞瘤包含分泌儿茶酚胺的嗜铬细胞，可引起继发性恶性高血压和间歇性头痛/大汗。大约90%该类肿瘤为良性。
- 嗜铬细胞瘤可能大而不均质，为部分区域坏死、出血和偶发钙化所致。CT表现为明显强化。MRI表现为显著的T_2高信号(*灯泡征*)和明显强化，但廓清动力学多变。
- 核医学 ^{123}I-MIBG、^{111}In-喷曲肽闪烁显像、^{68}Ga-DOTATATE PET/CT、增强MRI可用于检测肾上腺外嗜铬细胞瘤，如对有可增加嗜铬细胞瘤风险遗传性疾病的患者进行排查(见下文)。
- 嗜铬细胞瘤/副神经节瘤与多个综合征有关：

多发性内分泌瘤病(MEN)2A和2B：通常为双侧肾上腺内嗜铬细胞瘤。
脑视网膜血管瘤病(希佩尔-林道病，VHL)。
神经纤维瘤病1型。
卡尼三联征(胃平滑肌肉瘤、肺软骨瘤和副神经节瘤)。
遗传性副神经节瘤-嗜铬细胞瘤综合征：*SDHD*基因突变，副神经节瘤和嗜铬细胞瘤(恶性嗜铬细胞瘤的风险为50%)。

- 肾上腺外副神经节瘤最常见的部位为Zuckerkandl器官(主动脉旁体)，沿主动脉分叉分布至膀胱水平。尽管罕见，但当膀胱受累时，可出现排尿后晕厥的特殊临床表现。
- 头颈部副神经节瘤通常被称为血管球瘤，并可发生在鼓膜(鼓室血管球瘤)、颈静脉孔(颈静脉球瘤)、颈动脉体(颈动脉体瘤)或迷走神经(迷走神经球瘤)。
- 理论上，嗜铬细胞瘤/副神经节瘤应通过检测尿/血浆儿茶酚胺和甲氧基肾上腺素水平进行诊断，影像学检查仅用于定位和分期。在临床实际中，当患者被怀疑有嗜铬细胞瘤(如顽固性高血压)时，CT常作为一线影像学检查方法，以除外肾上腺肿物。

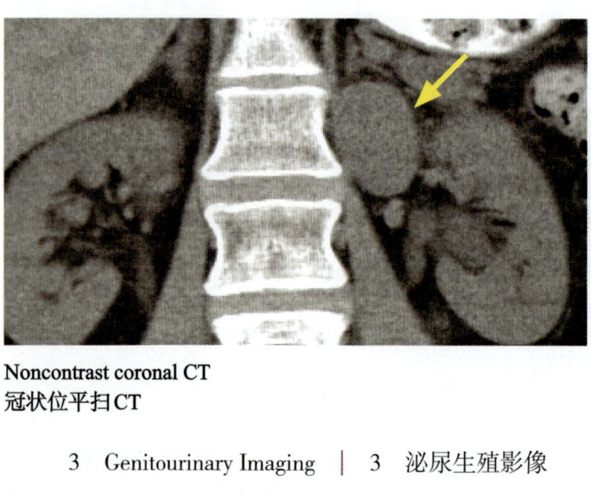

Noncontrast coronal CT
冠状位平扫CT

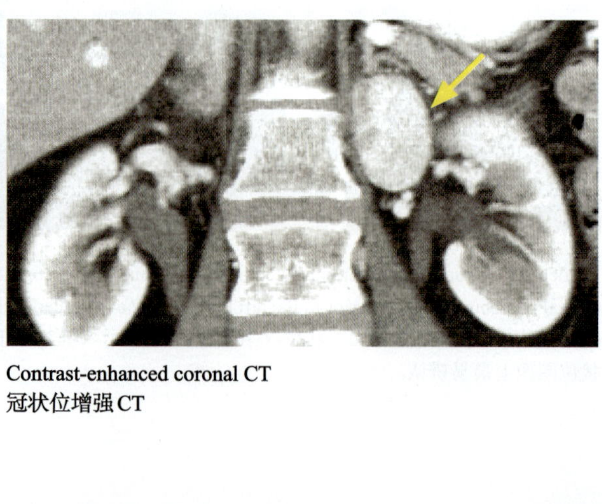

Contrast-enhanced coronal CT
冠状位增强CT

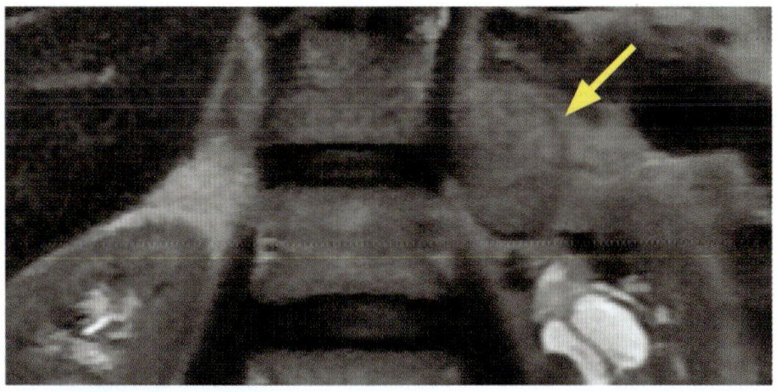

Coronal T2-weighted MRI
冠状位T_2加权MRI

Pheochromocytoma in a different patient:
Multiphase CT shows an avidly enhancing left adrenal mass (arrows).
This mass demonstrates heterogeneous T2 hyperintensity on MRI (*light bulb sign*).
另一名患者的嗜铬细胞瘤：多期CT显示一个明显强化的左肾上腺肿块(黄箭)。
该肿块在MRI上表现为混杂T_2高信号(灯泡征)。

Adrenal cortical carcinoma

肾上腺皮质癌

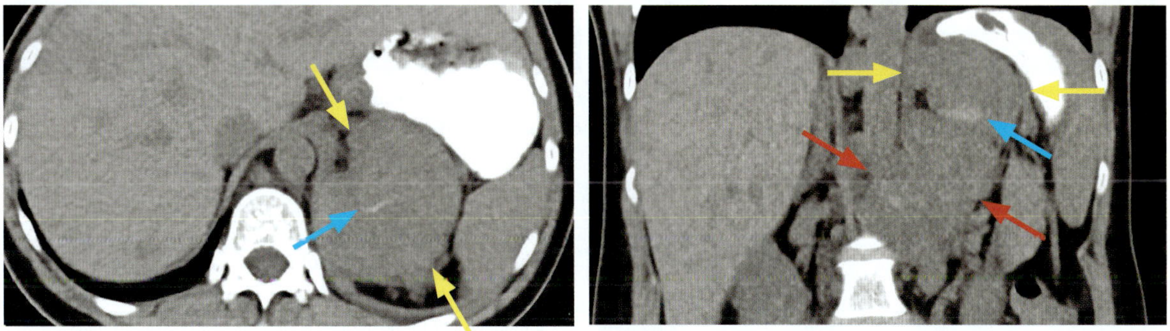

Adrenal cortical carcinoma: Axial (left image) and coronal noncontrast CT demonstrates a large, complex mass replacing the left adrenal gland (yellow arrows). The mass is contiguous with a conglomerate of retroperitoneal lymph nodes (red arrows) encasing the aorta, seen on the coronal image. Small intratumoral linear hyperattenuating region (blue arrows) may represent tumoral mineralization or hemorrhage.
肾上腺皮质癌：轴位(左图)和冠状位(右图)平扫CT显示一个大的复杂性肿块(黄箭)并取代了左肾上腺。在冠状位上，肿块与包裹主动脉的腹膜后淋巴结(红箭)相邻。肿块内小的条片状高密度区(蓝箭)可能为肿瘤钙化或出血。

- Adrenal cortical carcinoma is a very rare malignancy, with a prevalence of approximately 1/1,000,000. Approximately 66% are functional, producing a disordered array of hormones that may manifest as Cushing syndrome, hyperaldosteronism, and virilization.
- Adrenal cortical carcinoma usually presents as a large and heterogeneous mass on imaging studies. Internal necrosis and hemorrhage are typical features.

- 肾上腺皮质癌是一种非常罕见的恶性肿瘤，发病率约1/1 000 000。约66%为功能性肿瘤，产生一系列激素功能紊乱，表现为库欣综合征、高醛固酮血症和男性化。
- 肾上腺皮质癌的影像学表现常为大而不均质的肿块，内部坏死和出血为特征性表现。

Metastasis

- Autopsy studies show that adrenal metastases are present in >25% of patients with a known primary malignancy. Lung cancer and melanoma are the most common adrenal primaries. As discussed earlier, washout study can distinguish metastasis from adenoma.

转移瘤

- 尸检显示，超过25%的已知原发恶性肿瘤患者存在肾上腺转移瘤。肺癌和黑色素瘤是最常见转移到肾上腺的原发肿瘤。如前所述，强化廓清可区分腺瘤和转移瘤。

Lymphoma

- Primary adrenal lymphoma is rare, but should be suspected in the context of splenomegaly and/or lymphadenopathy.

淋巴瘤

- 原发性肾上腺淋巴瘤罕见，但在脾大和/或淋巴结肿大时应怀疑。

DIFFUSE ADRENAL DISORDERS

弥漫性肾上腺病变

Adrenal hyperplasia

- Adrenal hyperplasia is caused by a prolonged stress response or ectopic ACTH secretion.

肾上腺增生

- 肾上腺增生是由于长期应激反应或异位ACTH分泌所致。

Adrenal hemorrhage

- Adrenal hemorrhage can be spontaneous but, in adults, is usually due to anticoagulation or an underlying malignancy.

肾上腺出血

- 肾上腺出血可为自发性，但在成人，常源于抗凝治疗或存在恶性肿瘤。

- Hemorrhage may appear mass-like and is often heterogeneous on CT, but does not enhance on postcontrast images. When prior imaging is available, it should be suspected in the event of rapid onset of an adrenal mass. In this context, follow-up imaging can be helpful to confirm resolution and/or interval decrease in size.

- 出血可类似于肿块，CT常表现为混杂密度，但无强化。若与既往的影像比较，肾上腺肿块迅速出现应怀疑为肾上腺出血。此种情况下，影像学随访能够帮助确定肿块消失和/或逐渐缩小。

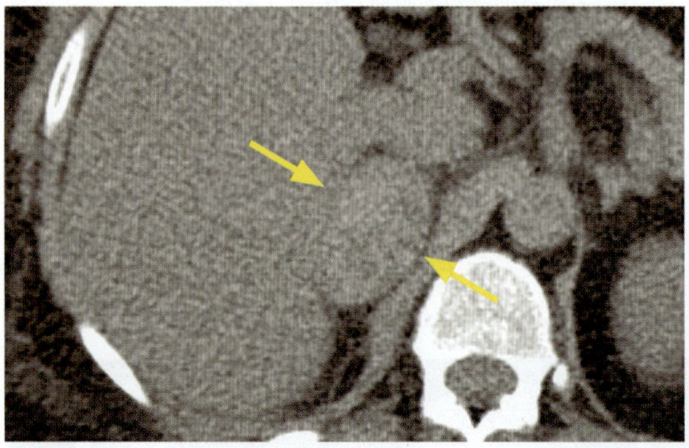

Noncontrast axial CT
轴位平扫CT

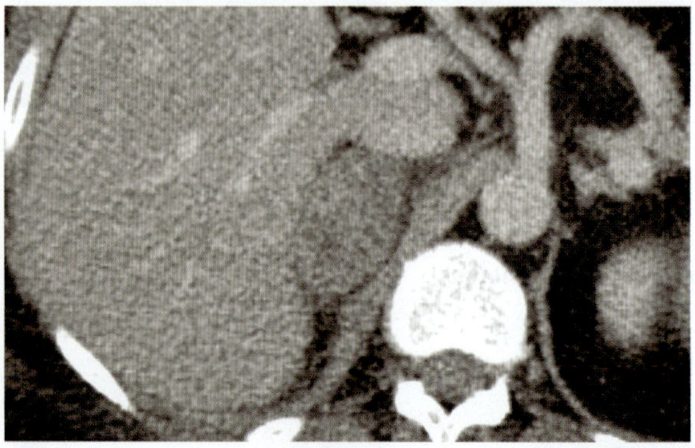

60-second delay postcontrast axial CT
60秒延迟轴位增强

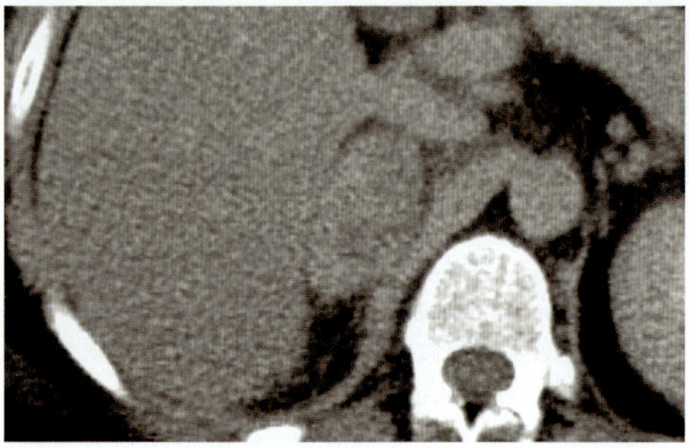

15-minute delay washout axial CT
15分钟延迟廓清轴位CT

Adrenal hemorrhage:
Multiphase adrenal protocol CT demonstrates a heterogeneous right adrenal mass (arrows) that does not demonstrate enhancement on postcontrast images (46 HU on all phases). This mass is new compared to imaging from only two weeks prior (not shown).
肾上腺出血：肾上腺多期增强CT显示右肾上腺非强化肿块(黄箭)，CT值在三期显像中均为46HU。
与2周前图像(未展示)比较，该肿块为新发。

Adrenal calcification

肾上腺钙化

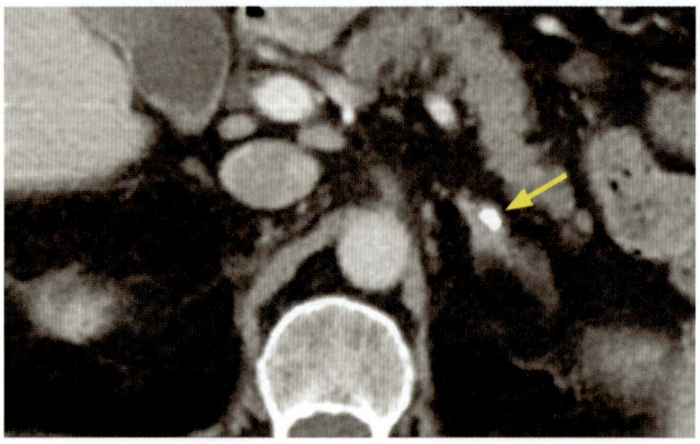

Axial contrast-enhanced CT shows a coarse calcification in the left adrenal gland (arrow), which may be due to remote hemorrhage or prior granulomatous disease.
轴位增强CT显示左侧肾上腺粗糙钙化(黄箭)，可能源于陈旧性出血或既往肉芽肿性疾病。

- Adrenal calcifications are not infrequent but rarely cause adrenal hypofunction. Adrenal calcifications can be due to hemorrhage, granulomatosis with polyangiitis, tuberculosis, and histoplasmosis.

- 肾上腺钙化并不少见，但很少引起肾上腺功能减退。肾上腺钙化可由出血、肉芽肿性多血管炎、结核和组织胞浆菌病引起。

(翻译　陈穹)

KIDNEYS

RENAL IMAGING PATTERNS

Sonographic appearance of kidneys

- **Grayscale ultrasound** (US) is used to assess the renal parenchyma (masses, scarring, calcification), to evaluate for stones, and to evaluate for hydronephrosis. The proximal ureter can also be seen in some patients allowing for evaluation of proximal hydroureter.
- **Color Doppler** can be used to evaluate the main renal arteries for pathology (renal artery stenosis, aneurysms) or for donation evaluation. Evaluation of the main renal vein can be conducted to assess for clots or tumor thrombus. Renal Doppler can also be used to assess the smaller intra-parenchymal vessels and calculate the resistive index (non-specific, suggests a number of entities including ureteral obstruction and intrinsic renal disease).
- **Contrast-enhanced US** (CEUS): Contrast-enhanced ultrasound permits evaluation of microvascular blood flow in real time, which is too small to detect by color Doppler. Among other things, it can be used to detect subtle solid renal masses and better characterize complex cystic masses. Of note, US contrast agents do not affect renal function and can be useful in patients with CKD.

肾

肾脏成像方式

肾脏超声影像表现

- **灰阶超声**(US)用于评估肾实质(肿块、瘢痕、钙化)、结石和肾盂积水。部分患者可显示近端输尿管，可用于评估近端输尿管积水。
- **彩色多普勒**主要用于评估肾动脉主干的病变(肾动脉狭窄、动脉瘤)或评估肾移植供体。对于肾静脉主干，则主要用于评估血栓或瘤栓。肾脏多普勒也可用于评估肾实质内较小的血管并计算阻力指数(非特异性，可提示多种疾病，包括输尿管梗阻和肾源性疾病)。
- **超声造影**(CEUS)：超声可实时评估微血管血流，这些血管过于细小而无法用多普勒检测。此外，该方法可用于发现不明显的肾脏实性肿块，更好地显示复杂的囊性肿块。值得一提的是，超声造影剂不影响肾功能，因而可用于慢性肾病(CKD)的患者。

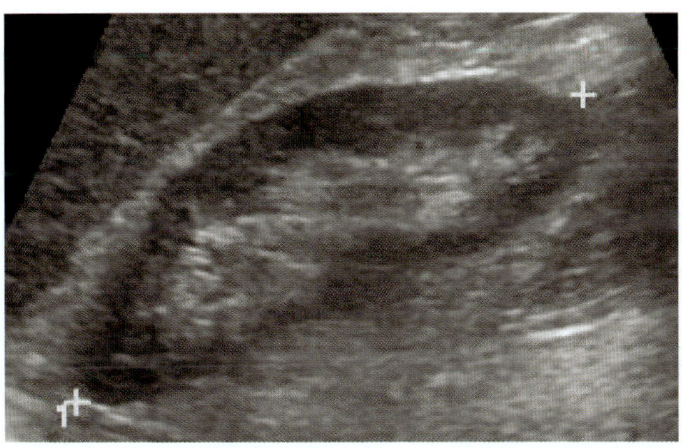

Sagittal grayscale ultrasound of a normal right kidney. The renal cortex is normally isoechoic to the hepatic parenchyma. Medullary pyramids are seen as hypoechoic triangles bordering to the renal sinus. The renal sinus is surrounded by hyperechoic fat. The major and minor calyces are usually not apparent unless hydronephrosis is present.

正常右肾矢状切面灰阶超声。肾皮质回声通常与肝实质相同。肾髓质是邻近肾窦的三角形低回声区。肾窦被高回声脂肪包绕。如无肾盂积水，肾大盏和肾小盏通常不显示。

Diffusely increased echogenicity

- Echogenic kidneys are most commonly due to medical renal disease, such as diabetic nephropathy, glomerulosclerosis, acute tubular necrosis, etc.
- HIV nephropathy can cause bilateral enlarged and echogenic kidneys.

Focally increased echogenicity

- Focal increase in echogenicity can be caused by renal lesions or areas containing fat, calcium, and air.

differential of echogenic renal mass

- Angiomyolipoma (AML). An echogenic renal mass is suggestive of AML (due to internal fat content), particularly when isoechoic to the sinus fat.
- Renal calculus.
- Milk of calcium, caused by crystals precipitating out of supersaturated solution.
- Sloughed papilla, secondary to papillary necrosis, may appear as an echogenic mass in the collecting system (often calcified).
- Intrarenal gas (e.g., infection, recent nephrostomy tube placement).
- Malignant neoplasm (atypical appearance).

弥漫性回声增强

- 肾脏回声增强最常见的原因是内科肾脏疾病，如糖尿病肾病、肾小球硬化、急性肾小管坏死等。
- HIV肾病可导致双侧肾脏增大和回声增强。

局部回声增强

- 局部回声增强的原因可为肾脏病灶或局部含有脂肪、钙化和空气。

肾脏强回声肿块的鉴别

- 血管平滑肌脂肪瘤(AML)：回声增强的肾脏肿块常提示AML(因内部含有脂肪)，特别是当其回声与肾窦脂肪相等时。
- 肾结石。
- 钙乳：由过饱和溶液中沉淀出的晶体引起。
- 脱落的肾乳头：继发于肾乳头坏死，可表现为集合系统中的强回声团块(常有钙化)。
- 肾内气体(如感染、近期放置肾造瘘管)。
- 恶性肿瘤(不典型表现)。

CT/MR imaging appearance of kidneys

- On standard abdominopelvic CT, conducted in portal venous phase (70 seconds post-injection), the renal parenchyma is relatively homogeneous (similar to nephrographic phase as described below), but can show more corticomedullary differentiation depending on the exact timing of image acquisition post-injection.
- **Phases of contrast in renal/ureteral imaging:**

> **Noncontrast:** Unenhanced imaging is used to assess for intralesional fat, renal stones, parenchymal calcifications, and hemorrhage. It also provides baseline attenuation of renal lesions.
> **Arterial phase** (20–40 seconds post-injection) imaging can be performed to evaluate the renal vasculature, primarily for surgical planning. In this phase, there is significant corticomedullary differentiation.
> The **nephrographic phase** (100 seconds post-injection) is used to evaluate the renal parenchyma (neoplasm, scarring, inflammation). In this phase, the renal parenchyma appears homogeneous.
> The **excretory phase** (8–15 minutes post-injection, depending on protocol) is used to assess for urothelial abnormalities (calyceal diverticulum, papillary necrosis, tumors, stricture). Lasix can be used to maximize contrast excretion. This phase can obscure ureteral stones.

肾脏CT/MR影像表现

- 标准的腹盆腔CT是在门静脉期进行采集(注射造影剂70秒后),此时肾实质密度相对均匀(与下述肾实质期类似),但随后肾皮质、髓质之间密度的差异程度取决于注射造影剂后采集图像的确切时间。
- **肾脏/输尿管的增强扫描时相**

> **平扫:**为非强化图像,用于评估病灶内脂肪、肾结石、实质钙化及出血,也能提供肾脏病灶的基线CT值。
> **动脉期**(注射造影剂20~40秒后)图像可评估肾血管结构,主要用于制订手术计划。皮质、髓质密度差异在该期显著。
> **肾实质期**(注射造影剂100秒后)图像用于评估肾实质(肿瘤、瘢痕、炎症)。肾实质在该期密度均匀。
> **排泄期**(注射造影剂8~15分钟后)用于评估尿路上皮异常(肾盏憩室、肾乳头坏死、肿瘤、狭窄)。呋塞米(速尿)可用于加速造影剂排泄。输尿管结石在该期可被掩盖。

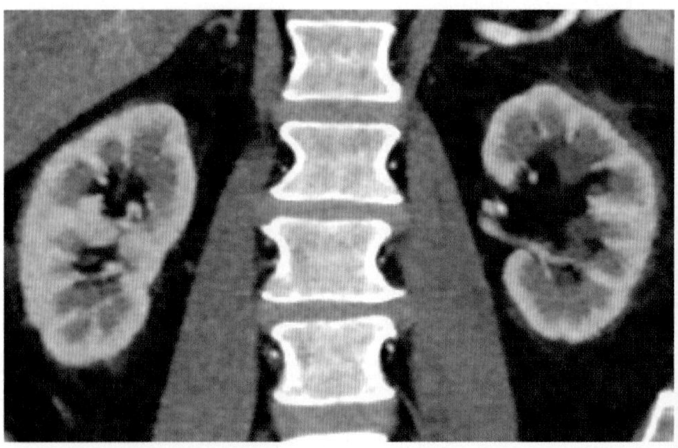

CT arterial/corticomedullary phase.
CT动脉/皮髓质期。

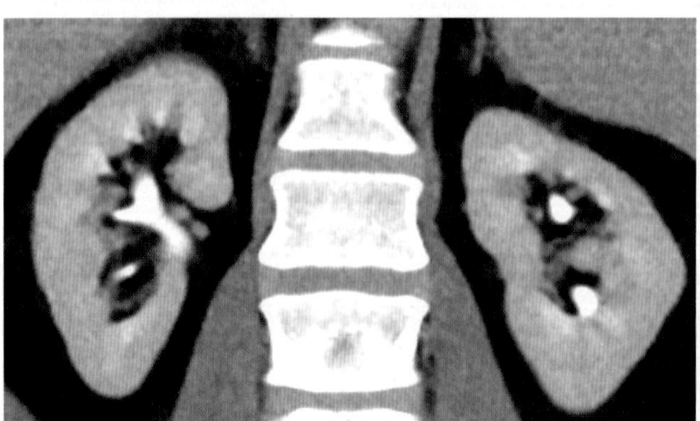

CT nephrographic phase.
CT肾实质期。

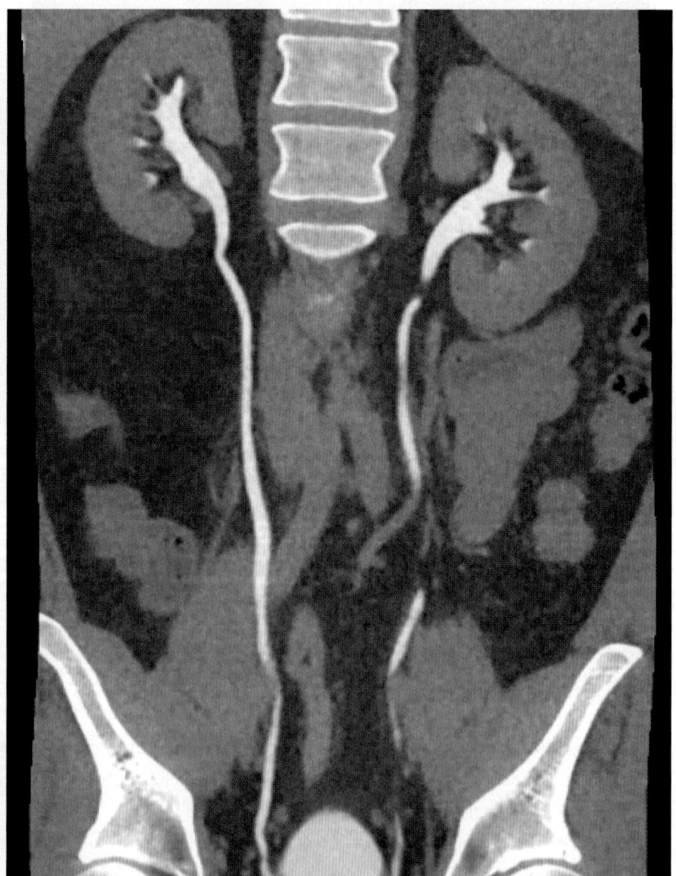

CT excretory phase.
CT排泄期。

Absent nephrogram

- An absent nephrogram describes the absence of normal renal parenchymal enhancement in the renal fossa, historically seen on plain film urography but also can apply to CT urography.
- Differential for a unilateral absent nephrogram includes renal agenesis, ectopic kidney, surgically absent kidney, or an abnormal kidney that is present but does not enhance. The latter can be caused by acute renal artery/vein occlusion, chronic ureteral obstruction, congenital or acquired renal disease resulting in nonfunctioning nephrons.

Delayed, prolonged (hyperdense), and persistent nephrograms

- A unilateral **delayed** nephrogram describes slow renal parenchymal uptake of intravenous contrast compared to the normal contralateral kidney.
- A unilateral **prolonged** or **hyperdense** nephrogram refers to diffusely increased density of the kidney relative to the contralateral side, with prolonged parenchymal enhancement and delayed urine excretion.
- The term **bilateral persistent nephrogram** is used when both kidneys retain intravenous contrast material longer than three minutes and there is delayed urine excretion. Causes include systemic hypotension, acute tubular necrosis, bilateral obstructive uropathy, contrast nephropathy, and myeloma kidney.

肾脏不显影

- 肾脏不显影是指肾窝内未见正常强化的肾实质；曾用于X线尿路造影，但也适用于CT尿路造影。
- 单侧肾脏不显影的鉴别诊断包括肾发育不全、异位肾、外科肾切除或有肾脏但无强化的异常肾。后者可能是由急性肾动脉/静脉阻塞、慢性输尿管梗阻、先天性或后天性肾病疾病引起，导致肾单位无法正常功能。

肾显影延迟、延长(高密度)和持续显影

- 单侧肾显影**延迟**是指一侧肾实质摄取造影剂慢于对侧正常肾脏。
- 单侧肾显影**延长(高密度)**是指较对侧肾脏弥漫性密度增高，伴肾实质持续强化和尿液排泄延迟。
- **双侧肾持续显影**是指双肾造影剂的滞留时间超过3分钟并且尿液排泄延迟。原因包括全身性低血压、急性肾小管坏死、双侧尿路梗阻、造影剂肾病，以及骨髓瘤肾病。

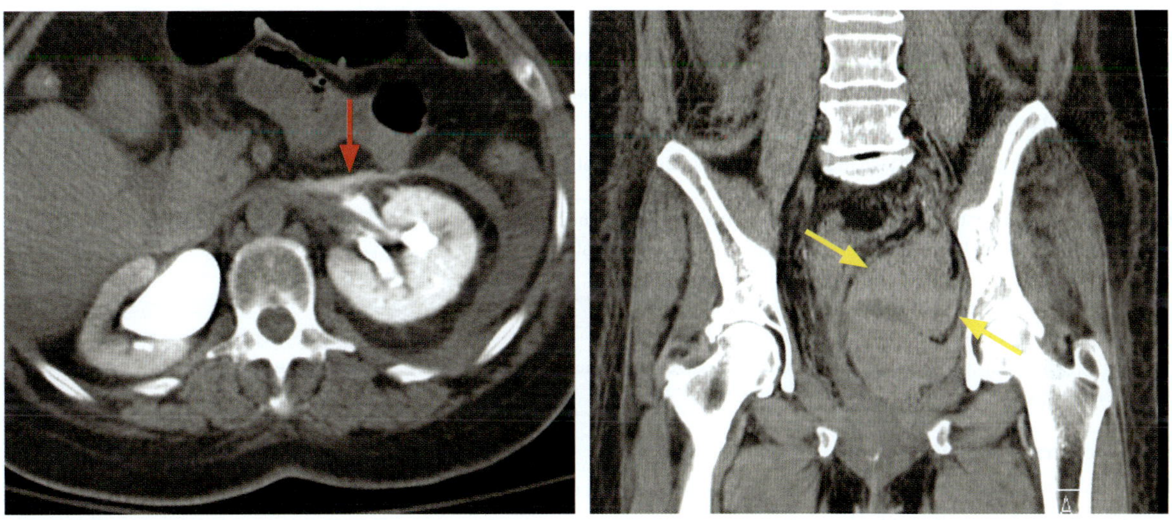

Bilateral persistent nephrogram due to obstruction: Unenhanced CT through the kidneys performed several hours after cardiac catheterization shows bilateral left > right persistent nephrogram and densely opacified urine in the proximal collecting system. There is contrast extravasation due to forniceal rupture (red arrow), consistent with distal obstruction. Coronal image from the same study shows the large left-sided pelvic hematoma (yellow arrows) compressing and displacing the bladder.

由梗阻引起的双侧肾持续显影：心导管术后数小时肾脏平扫CT显示双侧肾脏(左侧>右侧)持续显影，以及在近端集合系统中的高密度尿液。穹隆破裂引起尿液溢出(红箭)，符合远端梗阻。同一检查的冠状位显示盆腔左侧血肿(黄箭)，膀胱受压并移位。

- Differential diagnoses for these imaging patterns are listed below.

Unilateral delayed nephrogram:	Unilateral prolonged (hyperdense) nephrogram:
Acute ureteral obstruction.	Acute ureteral obstruction.
Renal artery stenosis.	Renal artery stenosis.
Renal vein thrombosis/compression.	Renal vein thrombosis/compression.
Acute pyelonephritis.	

Bilateral persistent nephrogram:	
Systemic hypotension.	Acute urate nephropathy.
Acute tubular necrosis.	Proteinuria (e.g., myeloma kidney).
Contrast nephropathy.	Bilateral obstructive uropathy.

- 影像学表现的鉴别诊断如下：

单侧肾显影延迟：	单侧肾显影延长(高密度)：
急性输尿管梗阻。	急性输尿管梗阻。
肾动脉狭窄。	肾动脉狭窄。
肾静脉血栓/压迫。	肾静脉血栓/压迫。
急性肾盂肾炎。	

双肾持续显影：	
全身性低血压。	急性肾小管坏死。
急性高尿酸性肾病。	蛋白尿(如多发性骨髓瘤肾)。
造影剂肾病。	双侧梗阻性尿路病变。

Striated nephrogram

条纹肾图

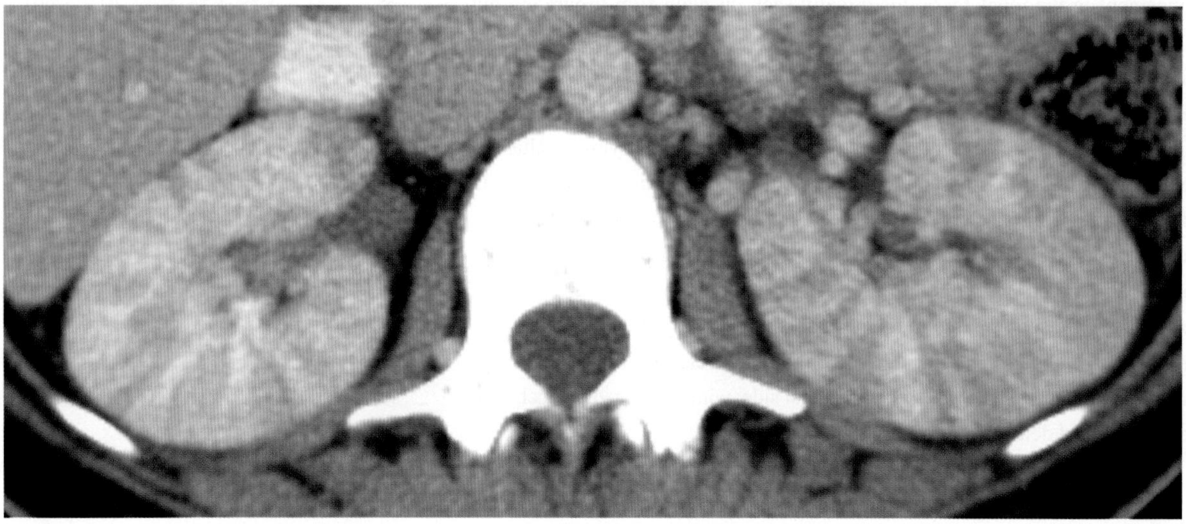

Axial contrast-enhanced CT shows bilateral striated nephrogram due to pyelonephritis.
轴位增强CT示肾盂肾炎致双侧条纹肾图。

- A striated nephrogram describes alternating linear bands of low and high enhancement in a radial pattern through the corticomedullary layers of the kidney following IV contrast administration.
- A striated nephrogram is a nonspecific pattern and can be seen in a number of pathologies:

Unilateral striated nephrogram:	Bilateral striated nephrograms:
Acute urinary obstruction (unilateral).	Acute urinary obstruction (bilateral).
Acute pyelonephritis.	Acute pyelonephritis.
Renal infarct.	Acute tubular necrosis.
Renal vein thrombosis or vasculitis.	Hypotension.
Renal contusion (typically focal).	Autosomal recessive polycystic kidney disease (ARPKD).
Acute radiation therapy.	

- 条纹肾图是指静脉注射造影剂后在肾皮质、髓质出现的放射状密度高低交替的强化带。
- 条纹肾图为非特异性征象，可见于多种病变：

单侧条纹肾图：	双侧条纹肾图：
急性尿路梗阻（单侧）。	急性尿路梗阻（双侧）。
急性肾盂肾炎。	急性肾盂肾炎。
肾梗死。	急性肾小管坏死。
肾静脉血栓或血管炎。	低血压。
肾挫伤（典型者为局灶性）。	常染色体隐性遗传多囊肾病（ARPKD）。
急性放疗损伤。	

Extracalyceal contrast material

- Papillary necrosis, medullary sponge kidney/tubular ectasia, and calyceal diverticulum may cause contrast to be seen beyond calyces on excretory phase images.
- **Tubular ectasia** causes paintbrush-like streaks of contrast that extend from the papillae into the tubules on excretory urogram. **Medullary sponge kidney** is tubular ectasia with associated calcifications of the renal medullary pyramids.
- **Calyceal diverticulum** is an outpouching of the collecting system into the corticomedullary region. Dependent sediment or multiple small stones may be present.
- **Papillary necrosis,** discussed later in this chapter, may also cause extracalyceal contrast.

肾盏造影剂外溢

- 肾乳头坏死、髓质海绵肾/肾小管扩张和肾盏憩室可导致排泄期图像中肾盏外出现造影剂。
- **肾小管扩张**时，排泄性尿路造影可见画笔样条状造影剂，从肾乳头向肾小管延伸。**髓质海绵肾**为肾小管扩张伴肾髓质锥体钙化。
- **肾盏憩室**是集合系统突入皮髓质交界区，可见重力性沉积物或多发小结石。
- 本章后文将讨论**乳头状坏死**也可导致造影剂肾盏外溢。

Unilateral renal enlargement

- The differential diagnosis of a unilateral enlarged kidney includes:

Pyelonephritis.
Acute ureteral obstruction.
Renal vein thrombosis.
Compensatory hypertrophy.

单侧肾脏增大

- 单侧肾脏增大的鉴别诊断包括：

肾盂肾炎。
急性输尿管梗阻。
肾静脉血栓。
代偿性肥大。

RENAL ANOMALIES AND NORMAL VARIANTS

肾脏先天异常及正常变异

Renal anomalies

肾脏先天异常

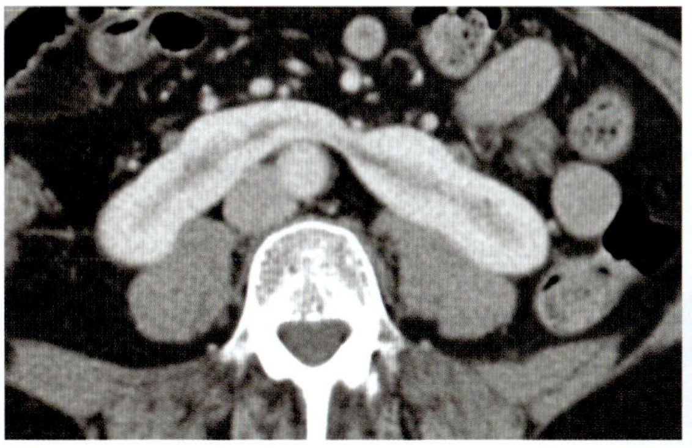

Horseshoe kidney.
马蹄肾。

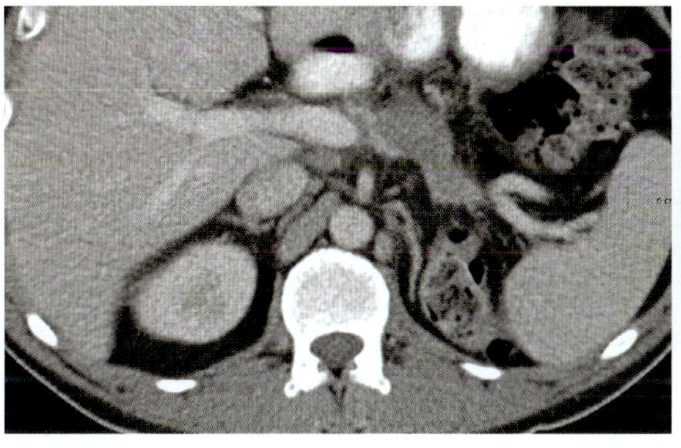

Congenital left renal agenesis.
先天性左肾发育不良。

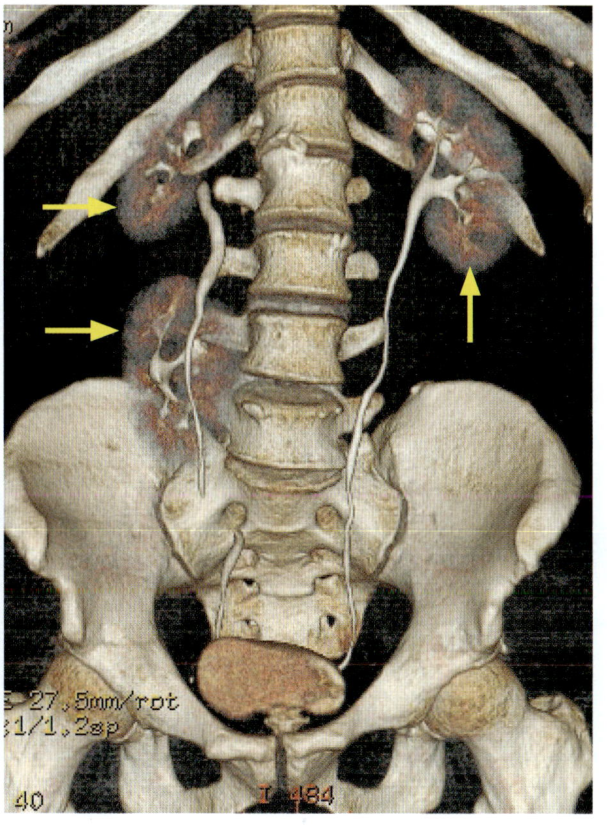

Three kidneys (arrows).
三个肾(黄箭)。

- **Horseshoe kidney:** two kidneys connected anteriorly across midline.
- **Crossed fused renal ectopia:** two kidneys located on the same side of the body (and at least partially fused), with normal insertion of both ureters in the bladder.
- **Unilateral renal agenesis:** a single hypertrophied kidney is present. Bilateral renal agenesis is not compatible with life.
- In very rare cases, one or two **(accessory) supernumerary** kidney(s) can be found. **Duplicated collecting system:** upper and lower moieties are drained by separate ureters.

  Weigert Meyer rule:

  Upper pole ureter has an ectopic insertion on the bladder (usually medial and inferior), often resulting in ureterocele and obstruction (Mnemonic: upper obstructs).

  Lower pole ureter has a normal insertion on the bladder, often associated with reflux (Mnemonic: lower refluxes).

- **马蹄肾：**两侧肾脏在脊柱前方融合。
- **交叉融合异位肾：**两个肾脏位于身体同一侧(且至少有部分融合)，两侧输尿管均正常汇入膀胱。
- **单侧肾发育不全：**出现单个增大的肾脏。双侧肾发育不全则无法存活。
- 在极为罕见的情况下，可能会发现1个或2个**(额外)多余的肾**。
- **集合系统重复畸形：**上、下两半肾分别由单独的输尿管引流。

  Weigert-Meyer规则：

  上极输尿管异位汇入膀胱(通常位于内侧和下方)，常导致输尿管膨出和梗阻(记忆诀窍："上梗阻")。

  下极输尿管正常汇入膀胱，常伴反流(记忆诀窍："下反流")。

Normal variants (renal pseudotumors)

正常变异(肾脏假性肿瘤)

- Renal pseudotumors are normal variations of renal morphology that may mimic a renal mass.
- **Hypertrophied column of Bertin:** The columns (septa) of Bertin are normal structures that anchor the renal cortex to the hilum, and create the separations

- 肾脏假性肿瘤是肾脏在形态学上的正常变异，可类似于肾脏肿块。
- **肾柱肥大：**肾柱(间隔)是将肾皮质固定于肾门的正常结构，在肾锥体间形成分隔。当肾柱

between the renal pyramids. When hypertrophied, the columns of Bertin may mimic a renal mass.

- **Persistent fetal lobation/lobulation:** In normal fetal development, the fetal kidneys are divided into discrete lobes. Occasionally, these lobulations persist into adulthood, producing an indentation of the renal cortex. This indentation can cause an adjacent focal bulge that simulates a renal mass. This pseudomass can usually be distinguished from a true mass by the presence of septa of Bertin on either side.
- **Dromedary hump:** focal bulge seen at the lateral left kidney, may be secondary to compression of the superolateral kidney by the spleen.

肥大时，可类似于肾肿块。

- **胚胎期持续分叶/叶状结构：**在正常胎儿发育过程中，胎肾分离成明显的分叶结构。偶尔，这些叶状结构会持续至成年，导致肾皮质凹陷。这种凹陷可能导致邻近的组织局部隆起而类似于肾肿块。若观察到双侧均存在肾柱间隔，通常可以把这种假性肿块与真性肾肿块进行区分。
- **驼峰征：**左肾外侧可见局灶性隆起，可能继发于脾脏对肾上外侧的压迫。

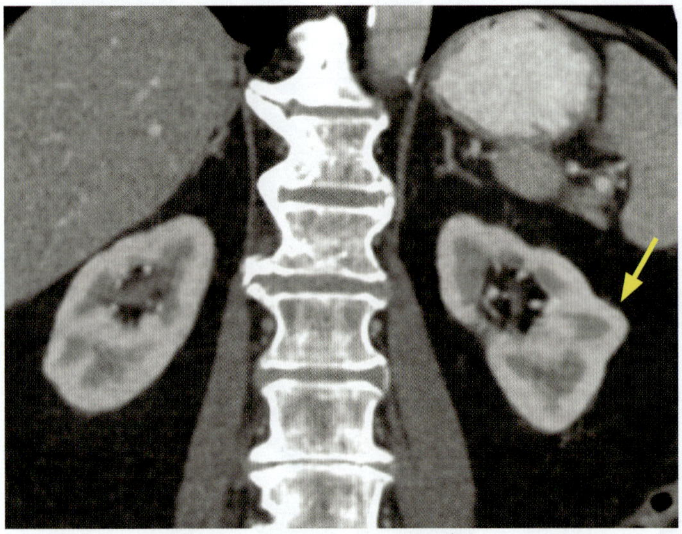

Dromedary hump:
Coronal contrast-enhanced CT of a patient being evaluated for a left renal interpolar mass found on ultrasound. Imaging reveals a left dromedary hump (arrow).
驼峰征：一名患者因超声示左肾中部肿块而行CT检查。冠状位增强CT显示左肾外侧驼峰征。

Nephrocalcinosis, cortical and papillary necrosis

肾钙质沉积症、皮质和乳头坏死

Medullary nephrocalcinosis

肾髓质钙沉积症

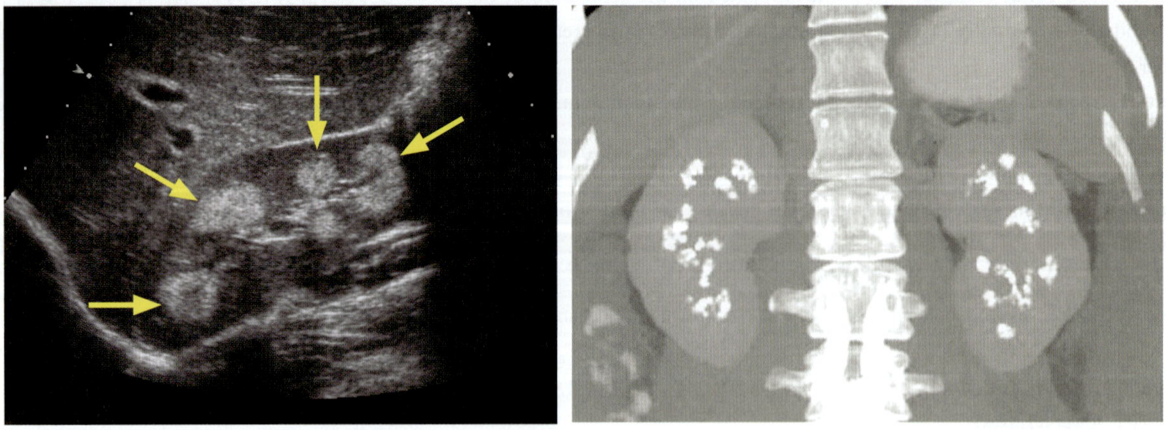

Medullary nephrocalcinosis: Sagittal ultrasound through the right kidney (left image) shows diffusely echogenic renal pyramids (arrows). Coronal CT MIP in bone windows (right image) in a different patient demonstrates symmetric amorphous renal medullary calcification bilaterally.
Ultrasound case courtesy Julie Ritner, MD, Brigham and Women's Hospital.
肾髓质钙沉积症：右肾矢状切面超声(左图)显示肾锥体呈弥漫性高回声(黄箭)。另一位患者的冠状位CT骨窗重建(右图)显示双肾对称性无定形髓质钙沉积。

- Medullary nephrocalcinosis represents calcification of the renal medullary pyramids, caused by any disease entity that leads to hypercalcemia and hypercalciuria.
- Patients usually have preserved renal function.

differential of medullary nephrocalcinosis

- Hyperparathyroidism is the most common cause of medullary nephrocalcinosis.
- Sarcoidosis (hypercalcemia).
- Type 1 renal tubular acidosis (distal type).
- Medullary sponge kidney is caused by ectatic tubules in the medullary pyramids that can lead to stasis and stone formation.
- Papillary necrosis.
- In children, treatment with furosemide (Lasix) can lead to medullary nephrocalcinosis.

- 肾髓质钙沉积症是指肾髓质锥体的钙化，任何原因引起的高钙血症和高钙尿症都可导致肾髓质钙沉积症。
- 患者通常保留正常的肾功能。

肾髓质钙沉积症的鉴别

- 甲状旁腺功能亢进症是肾髓质钙沉积症最常见的原因。
- 结节病(高钙血症)。
- Ⅰ型肾小管酸中毒(远端型)。
- 髓质海绵肾，肾锥体内的肾小管扩张可导致瘀滞和结石形成。
- 肾乳头坏死。
- 儿童应用呋塞米治疗可导致肾髓质钙沉积症。

Cortical nephrocalcinosis

肾皮质钙化症

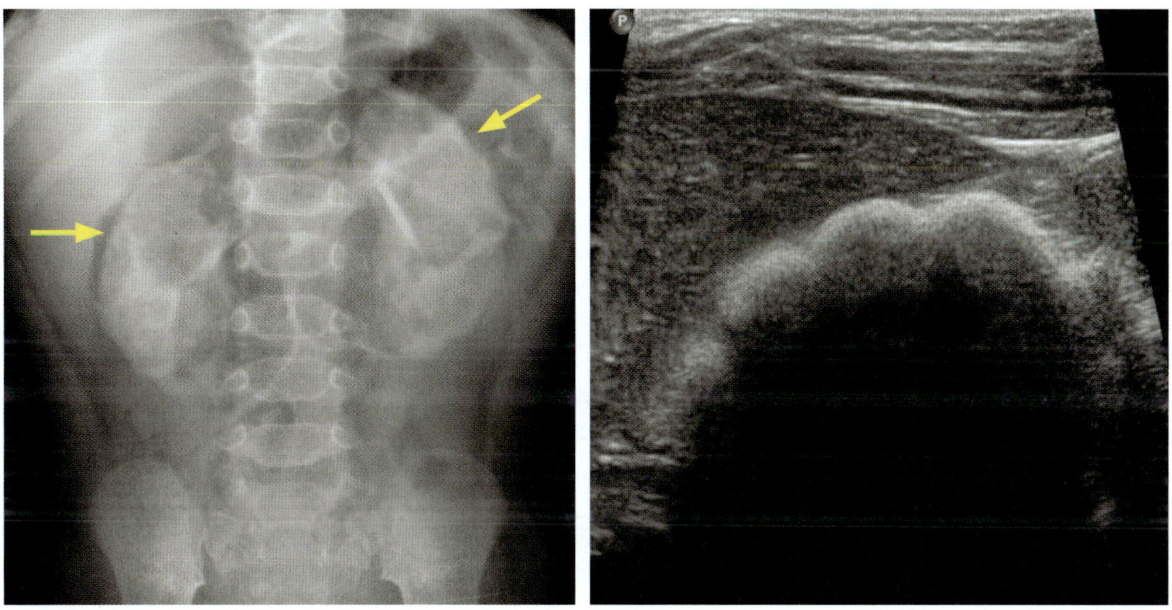

Cortical nephrocalcinosis in a child: Abdominal radiograph shows dense cortical calcification of the kidneys (arrows). Ultrasound shows densely calcified and shadowing renal cortex, obscuring the renal parenchyma.
Case courtesy Michael Hanley, MD, University of Virginia Health System.
儿童肾皮质钙化症：腹部X线影像显示肾脏有致密的皮质钙化(黄箭)。超声显示肾皮质有致密钙化和声影，使肾实质显影模糊。

- Cortical nephrocalcinosis is dystrophic peripheral calcification of the renal cortex, with sparing of the medullary pyramids. This entity is much less common than medullary nephrocalcinosis and it is usually due to diffuse cortical injury.
- Causes of cortical nephrocalcinosis include:

Acute cortical necrosis. **Chronic glomerulonephritis.** **Chronic transplant rejection.**	**Hyperoxaluria.** **Alport syndrome** (hereditary nephropathy and deafness). **Autosomal recessive polycystic kidney disease.**

- 肾皮质钙化症是肾皮质外周区发生萎缩性钙化，不累及肾髓质锥体。该病远比肾髓质钙化症要少见，通常是由于皮质广泛损伤引起。
- 导致肾皮质钙化症的原因包括：

急性肾皮质坏死。 **慢性肾小球肾炎。** **移植肾慢性排斥。**	**高草酸盐尿症。** **奥尔波特综合征**(遗传性肾病和耳聋综合征)。 **常染色体隐性多囊肾病。**

Cortical necrosis

皮质坏死

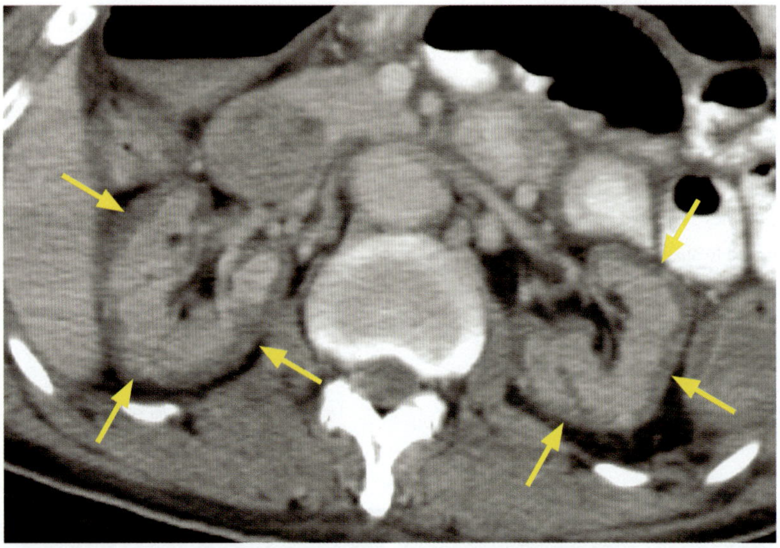

Cortical necrosis: Contrast-enhanced axial CT shows lack of enhancement of the renal cortices bilaterally (arrows).
肾皮质坏死：轴位增强CT显示双侧肾皮质无强化(黄箭)。

- Cortical necrosis is a rare form of renal injury resulting from acute ischemia in setting of small vessel vasospasm or systemic hypotension. Predisposing factors include hemolyticuremic syndrome and thrombotic microangiopathy. Chronic renal failure develops in up to 50% of patients.
- On CT, there is lack of enhancement of the renal cortex with preservation of medullary enhancement. Cortical necrosis may lead to cortical nephrocalcinosis.

Papillary necrosis

- Papillary necrosis is necrosis and sloughing of renal papillary tissue, which clinically can cause gross hematuria and may lead to chronic renal insufficiency.
- There are numerous causes of papillary necrosis, most commonly NSAIDs, sickle cell anemia, diabetes, and renal vein thrombosis. The commonly used POSTCARD mnemonic may be helpful to remember all causes:

Pyelonephritis.	**C**irrhosis.
Obstruction.	**A**nalgesics (NSAIDS).
Sickle cell disease.	**R**enal vein thrombosis.
Tuberculosis.	**D**iabetes mellitus.

- On ultrasound, the kidneys may show focal areas of increased papillary echogenicity.
- On the excretory phase of CT urography, papillary necrosis causes pooling of contrast in the papillary regions adjacent to the calyces. The calyces may appear club-shape or saccular in morphology. Filling defects representing sloughed papilla may be seen in the calyces, renal pelvis, or ureter.

- 肾皮质坏死是一种罕见的，由小血管痉挛或全身性低血压造成肾脏急性缺血而引起的损伤。诱发因素包括溶血性尿毒综合征和血栓性微血管病。高达50%的患者将发展为慢性肾衰竭。
- CT表现为肾皮质无强化，但肾髓质仍有强化。肾皮质坏死可致肾皮质钙化症。

肾乳头坏死

- 肾乳头坏死为肾乳头组织坏死和脱落，临床上可引起肉眼血尿，并可导致慢性肾功能不全。
- 导致肾乳头坏死的原因很多，最常见的有非甾体抗炎药、镰状细胞贫血、糖尿病和肾静脉血栓形成。常使用“POSTCARD”帮助记忆所有的病因：

肾盂肾炎(**P**)。	肝硬化(**C**)。
梗阻(**O**)。	非甾体抗炎药(**A**)。
镰状细胞贫血(**S**)。	肾静脉血栓(**R**)。
结核(**T**)。	糖尿病(**D**)。

- 在超声检查中，肾脏可出现局部乳头区域回声增强。
- 在CT尿路造影的排泄期，肾乳头坏死会导致造影剂在肾盏相邻的乳头区域内聚集。肾盏的形态可以呈棒状或囊状。在肾盏、肾盂或输尿管中可见到充盈缺损，为脱落的乳头。

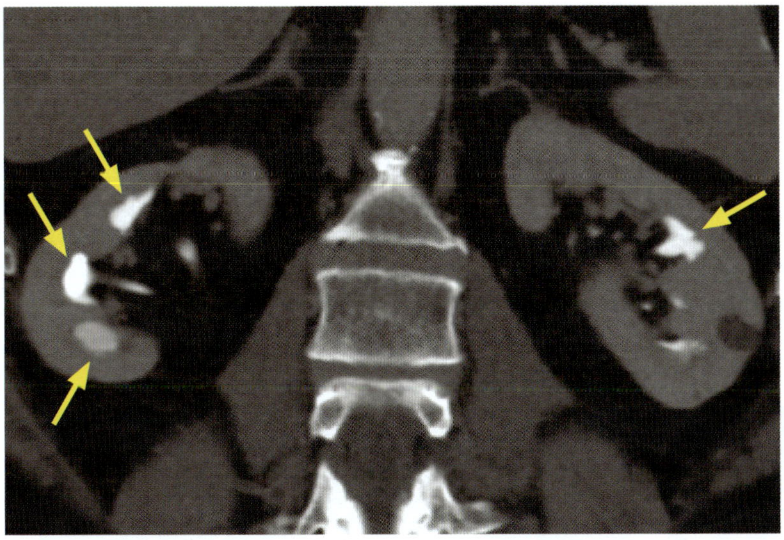

Papillary necrosis: Coronal excretory phase CT urography shows bilateral blunted, rounded calyces (arrows).

肾乳头坏死：冠状位CT尿路造影排泄期显示双侧圆钝的肾盏(黄箭)。

- Three classic signs of papillary necrosis include the *ball on tee sign*, *lobster claw sign* (not to be confused with the *bear paw sign* of xanthogranulomatous pyelonephritis), and *signet ring sign*, which describe patterns of papillary excavation.

  The *ball on tee sign* describes contrast filling a central papilla.

  The *lobster claw sign* describes contrast filling only the periphery of the papilla.

  The *signet ring sign* describes contrast surrounding the sloughed papilla.

- 肾乳头坏死的三个典型征象包括杆上球征、龙虾爪征(勿与黄色肉芽肿性肾盂肾炎的熊掌征混淆)和印戒征，这些征象用于描述肾乳头坏死后的空洞形状。

  杆上球征代表造影剂填充肾乳头中央。

  龙虾爪征代表造影剂仅填充肾乳头外周。

  印戒征代表造影剂环绕在脱落的肾乳头周围。

Renal trauma

肾外伤

Organ Injury Scale (OIS) -American Association for the Surgery of Trauma (AAST)

- The OIS scale from the AAST is the most commonly used system for classifying renal trauma. It was initially a surgical classification, but now encompasses findings from CT imaging, operative report, and pathology. The highest injury among the three is assigned the final AAST grade. The OIS was updated in 2018 to include vascular injuries.

OIS/AAST grading of renal trauma

- **Grade I:** by far the most common type of renal injury (95%) and describes a renal contusion or subcapsular hematoma. Treatment is conservative.
- **Grade Ⅱ:** superficial laceration (≤1 cm) or perinephric hematoma confined to Gerota's fascia, without urinary extravasation. Treatment is conservative.
- **Grade Ⅲ:** deeper laceration (>1 cm), without urinary extravasation; any injury in the presence of renal vascular injury or active bleeding contained within Gerota's fascia. Treatment is typically conservative.

  A potential pitfall of a grade Ⅲ injury is that a clot at the collecting system may prevent urinary extravasation initially, but urinary extravasation may occur later as the clot lyses from urinary urokinase.
- **Grade IV:** deep laceration which extends into the collecting system (causing urinary extravasation), renal pelvis laceration or complete disruption of the ureteropelvic junction, segmental renal artery/vein injury, vascular thrombosis resulting in segmental or complete kidney infarction, or active bleeding beyond Gerota's fascia. Vascular grade IV injury can be treated with endovascular embolization or stenting.
- **Grade V:** most severe injury and includes main renal artery/vein laceration or avulsion of the renal hilum, devascularized kidney with active bleeding, or shattered kidney. Treatment is variable but typically surgical.

器官损伤分级(OIS)——美国创伤外科协会(AAST)

- AAST的OIS是最常用的肾外伤分级系统。其最初是一种外科分级，但目前包括CT影像、手术及病理分级。三者中的最高级别被定义为AAST最终分级。OIS 2018年更新版还包括了血管损伤。

肾脏外伤AAST的OIS

- **Ⅰ级损伤：**是目前最为常见的肾脏损伤(95%)，包括肾挫伤和包膜下血肿。采用保守治疗。
- **Ⅱ级损伤：**浅表性撕裂(≤1cm)，或局限于肾前筋膜内的肾周血肿但无尿外渗。采用保守治疗。
- **Ⅲ级损伤：**深度撕裂(>1cm)(无尿外渗)，包括任何累及肾血管的损伤或局限于肾前筋膜内的活动性出血。多数采用保守治疗。

  Ⅲ级损伤分级的一个潜在缺陷是早期集合系统血凝块会阻止尿外渗，晚期血凝块被尿激酶溶解后则可能会出现尿外渗。
- **Ⅳ级损伤：**深度撕裂至集合系统(导致尿外渗)，肾盂撕裂或肾盂输尿管交界区完全破裂，节段性肾动脉/静脉损伤，血管内血栓形成导致节段性或完全性肾梗死，或有肾前筋膜外活动性出血。血管的Ⅳ级损伤可通过血管内栓塞或支架植入进行治疗。
- **Ⅴ级损伤：**是最严重的损伤，包括肾动脉/静脉主干撕裂或肾门撕脱、肾血管断流伴活动性出血或肾碎裂。治疗方法多样，但通常为外科治疗。

CT description of renal trauma

- Renal vascular injury described in the 2018 OIS update is defined as renal artery pseudoaneurysm or arteriovenous (AV) fistula. Both appear on imaging as a hyperattenuating focus with density similar to the aorta, that decreases in attenuation on delayed phase.
- In contrast, active bleeding appears as focal or diffuse vascular contrast that increases in attenuation and/or size with delayed phase imaging.
- Traumatic renal artery thrombosis occurs with tearing of the intima, initiating thrombosis. There is permanent loss of renal function after approximately two hours of ischemia.

肾外伤的CT描述

- 在2018年OIS更新版中，肾血管损伤被定义为肾假性动脉瘤或肾动-静脉瘘。两者在影像上都表现为与主动脉密度类似的局部病灶，密度在延迟期降低。
- 相反，活动性出血表现为局灶性或弥漫性血管密度影，其密度和/或范围会随着延迟而增加。
- 外伤性肾动脉血栓常由内膜撕裂引起。缺血约2小时后肾功能将永久丧失。

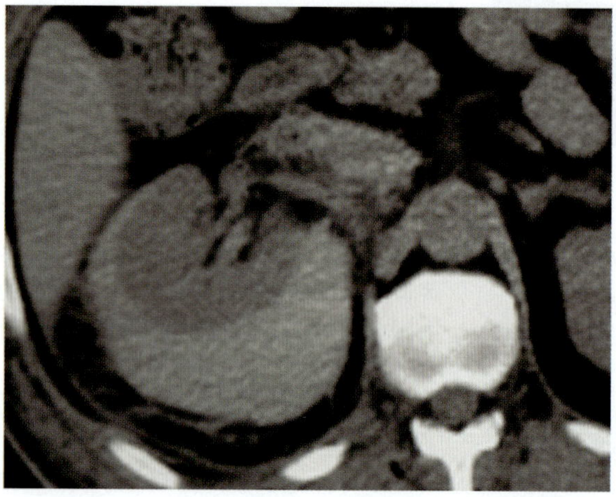

Axial unenhanced CT demonstrates a hyperdense subcapsular renal hematoma on the right. This is considered AAST grade I injury.
轴位CT平扫显示右肾包膜下高密度血肿，符合AAST Ⅰ级损伤。

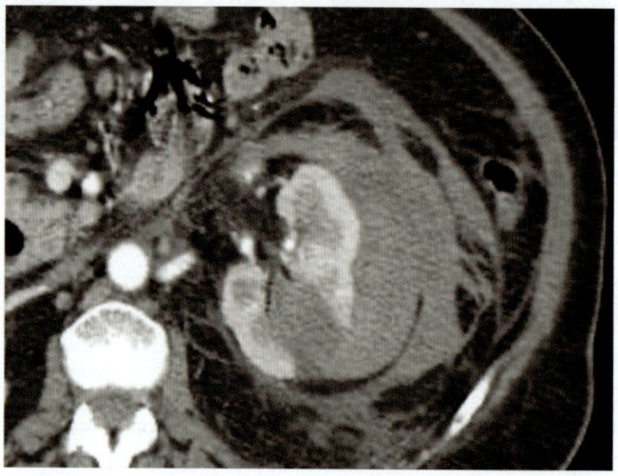

Axial contrast-enhanced CT shows AAST grade Ⅲ renal injury with deep laceration, subcapsular and perirenal hematoma. There is no injury to the collecting system.
轴位增强CT显示AAST Ⅲ级肾损伤，包括深部撕裂、包膜下和肾周血肿。集合系统无损伤。

Page kidney

- A Page kidney (named after the doctor who performed experiments wrapping animal kidneys with cellophane) is a rare cause of secondary hypertension due to extrinsic compression of the kidney by a subcapsular collection (hematoma/urinoma), usually following trauma.
- A subscapular hematoma compresses the renal parenchyma and decreases its blood flow. Altered hemodynamics induce increased renin secretion, which can lead to hypertension. It usually takes several months for hypertension to develop.
- Imaging shows a subcapsular hematoma causing deformation and flattening of the kidney.
- Percutaneous drainage of the hematoma may be effective treatment.

Page 肾

- Page肾(以一位用玻璃纸包裹动物肾脏进行实验的医生命名)是一种罕见引起继发性高血压的原因，为包膜下液体聚集(血肿/尿性囊肿)对肾脏产生外部压迫所致，通常继发于肾外伤。
- 包膜下血肿压迫肾实质使其血供减少。肾脏血流动力学改变引起肾素分泌增加，从而导致高血压。高血压发展的时间一般需几个月。
- 影像学表现为包膜下血肿导致的肾脏变形和扁平。
- 经皮穿刺引流血肿的方法可能有效。

Hydronephrosis, urinary obstruction, and stones

Common causes of hydronephrosis

Obstructive (more common):	Non-obstructive:
Obstructing calculus is the most common cause. Ureteral or bladder malignancy. External compression of the ureter by a mass or retroperitoneal fibrosis.	Vesicoureteral reflux: congenital or acquired (post-procedural or post-treatment). Pregnancy (usually right > left).

肾盂积水、尿路梗阻和结石

肾盂积水的常见原因

梗阻性(较常见):	非梗阻性:
梗阻性结石是最常见的原因。 输尿管或膀胱恶性肿瘤。 肿块或腹膜后纤维化对输尿管的外部压迫。	膀胱输尿管反流：先天性或获得性(术后或治疗后)。 妊娠(通常是右侧>左侧)。

Stones

- Nephro/ureterolithiasis is a common problem that presents with renal colic. Hematuria is usually present, but may be absent if the stone is completely obstructing.
- Calcium-containing stones (calcium oxalate plus phosphate, pure calcium oxalate, or pure calcium phosphate) represent 73% of urinary stones.
- Urinary stones can also be comprised of uric acid, xanthine, matrix (mucin), pure struvite, and indinavir (seen in HIV patients on antiretroviral therapy).

结石

- 肾/输尿管结石是导致肾绞痛的常见原因，通常伴有血尿，但结石造成完全梗阻时可无血尿。
- 含钙结石(草酸钙加磷酸盐、纯草酸钙或纯磷酸钙)占尿路结石的73%。
- 尿路结石也可能由尿酸、黄嘌呤、基质(黏蛋白)、纯磷酸铵镁和茚地那韦(Indinavir)(见于接受抗反转录病毒治疗的HIV患者)组成。

Radiographic evaluation of stones

- Calcium-stones are radiopaque.
- Stones comprised of uric acid, xanthine, matrix, pure struvite, or indinavir are radiolucent.

结石的影像学表现

- 含钙结石不透射线。
- 射线可透过由尿酸、黄嘌呤、基质、纯磷酸铵镁和茚地那韦组成的结石。

CT evaluation of stones

- Most stones are radiopaque on CT, except for indinavir and matrix stones (rare).

结石的CT表现

- 除茚地那韦结石和基质结石(罕见)外，几乎所有的肾结石在CT上都是不透射线的。

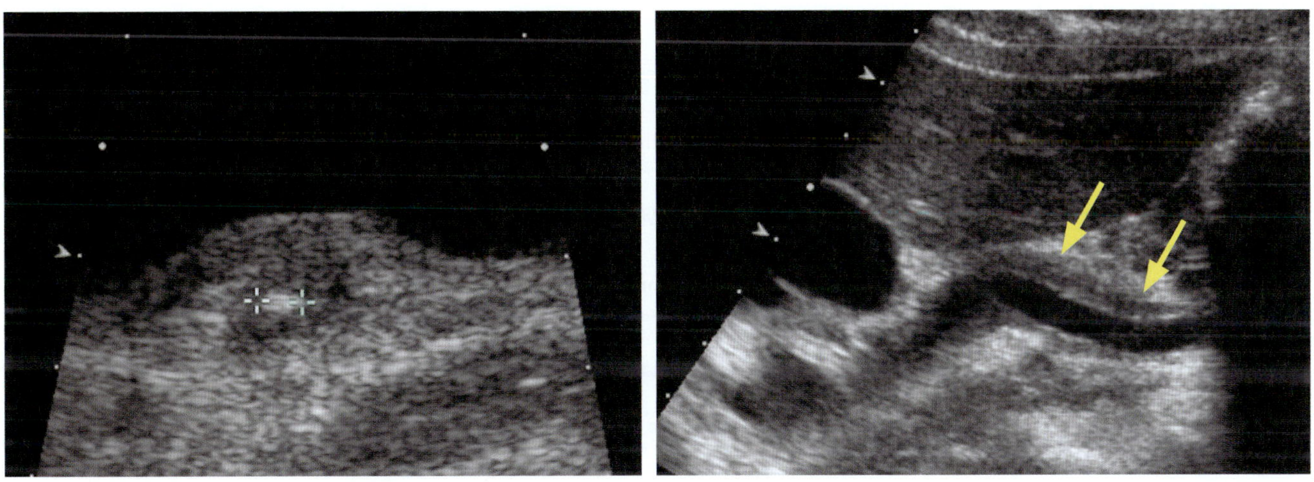

Indinavir stone: Transverse grayscale ultrasound of the bladder shows a 4 mm non-shadowing stone (calipers on left image) at the right ureterovesical junction (UVJ). There is upstream mild right hydroureteronephrosis and urothelial thickening (right image; arrows). No radiopaque stone was seen on CT performed two days prior to this ultrasound (CT not shown).

茚地那韦结石：膀胱的横切面灰阶超声显示右侧输尿管膀胱交界处(UVJ)有一个4mm的无声影结石(左图的卡尺)。上游右侧输尿管轻度积水伴尿路上皮增厚(右图，黄箭)。在超声检查2天前进行的CT检查未显示不透射线的结石(CT图像未展示)。

- Dual-energy CT can be used to differentiate the chemical composition of urinary stones, and in turn, provide useful information for clinical management.
- The *soft tissue rim sign* helps to distinguish a phlebolith from a ureteral stone. The presence of a small amount of soft tissue surrounding the calcification, thought to represent the edematous ureteral wall, favors a ureteral stone.
- Secondary signs of ureteral obstruction include ipsilateral hydronephrosis and perinephric stranding.

- 双能CT可用于区分尿路结石的化学成分，进而为临床诊治提供有用的信息。
- 软组织环状征能够帮助鉴别静脉石和输尿管结石。钙化灶周围出现少量软组织被认为是水肿的输尿管壁，提示为输尿管结石。
- 输尿管梗阻的继发征象包括同侧肾盂积水和肾周条索样改变。

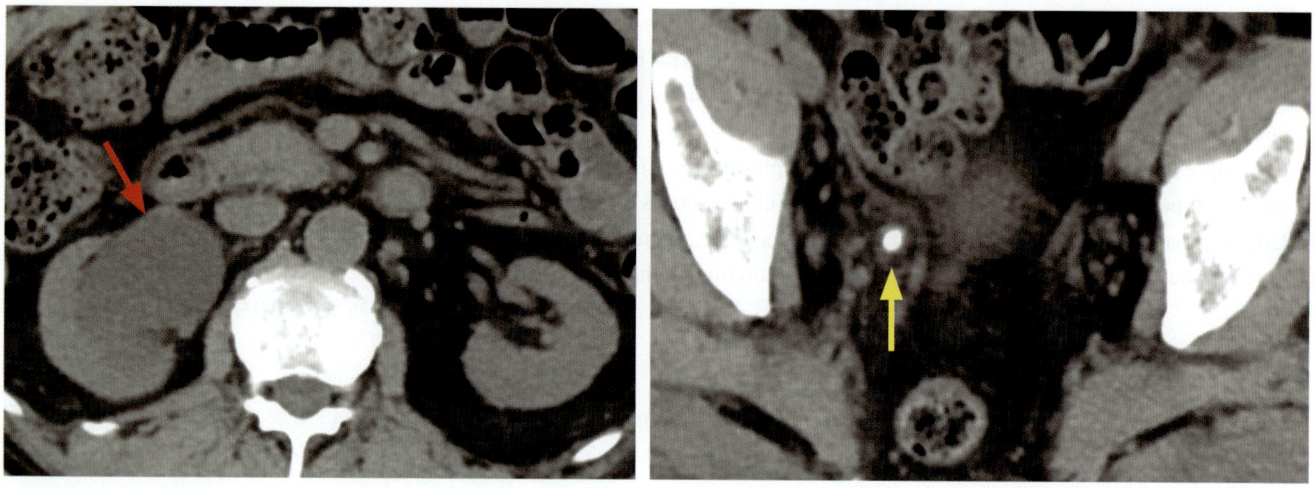

Right obstructive uropathy caused by a distal ureteral stone: Noncontrast axial CT through the kidneys (left image) shows unilateral right hydronephrosis (red arrow). Axial image through the pelvis shows a calcification along the expected course of the right ureter (yellow arrow) demonstrating the *soft tissue rim sign*, with a faint halo of soft tissue surrounding the calculus.
由输尿管末端结石引起的右侧梗阻性尿路病：轴位平扫CT(左图)显示右侧肾盂积水(红箭)。轴位盆腔图像显示一个钙化灶位于右侧输尿管的走行位置(黄箭)，表现为软组织环状征，即结石周围浅淡的软组织晕。

Sonographic evaluation of stones and hydronephrosis

- Ultrasound is a fast and inexpensive way to evaluate for nephrolithiasis and hydronephrosis.
- An echogenic shadowing focus in the kidney, ureter or bladder is suspicious for a stone, particularly when associated with *twinkling artifact*.
- After diagnosing a renal or ureteral calculus, assess for the presence of hydronephrosis and perinephric fluid.
- **Resistive index (RI)** may be helpful in diagnosing obstruction.

  RI can be elevated in acute obstruction.

  It is calculated with pulse-width Doppler of the renal segmental or arcuate arteries.

  RI = (PSV–EDV)/PSV

  PSV = peak systolic velocity

  EDV = end-diastolic velocity

  Higher resistive indices correlate with higher resistance.

  With no diastolic flow, RI = PSV/PSV = 1

  Reversal of diastolic flow technically causes RI >1, although in such cases RI is not measured.

  A RI of >0.7 on the affected side, or a difference of >0.1 between kidneys, suggests acute obstruction. Bilateral elevated RIs (>0.7) are nonspecific and can be due to any number of medical renal processes. RI is not used to diagnose chronic obstruction.
- **Ureteral jets** may help diagnose hydronephrosis but are controversial. A ureteral jet is flow of urine into the bladder as seen by color Doppler.

  Flow from the kidney to the bladder would be completely eliminated in complete obstruction, so theoretically the presence of a ureteral jet excludes complete obstruction. However, ureteral jets are commonly seen even with stones, and jets are often *absent* in normal patients.

结石、肾盂积水的超声表现

- 超声是一种快速且经济的评估肾结石和肾盂积水的方法。
- 在肾、输尿管或膀胱内发现高回声团时，应怀疑结石，尤其是伴闪烁伪像时。
- 诊断肾脏或输尿管结石后，还应检查是否伴有肾盂积水和肾周积液。
- **阻力指数(RI)**有助于诊断梗阻。

  肾RI可在急性梗阻时升高。

  肾RI由肾段动脉或弓状动脉的脉冲多普勒计算得出。

  RI=(PSV–EDV)/PSV

  PSV=收缩期峰值流速

  EDV=舒张末期流速

  阻力越大，RI越高。

  没有舒张期血流时，RI=PSV/PSV=1

  舒张期血流反向会导致RI>1，但此时不测量RI。

  患侧肾脏RI>0.7或双肾RI之差>0.1提示急性梗阻。双侧肾脏RI升高(>0.7)没有特异性，可因多种肾脏病变所致。RI不用于诊断慢性梗阻。
- **输尿管喷射**有助于诊断肾盂积水，但尚有争议。输尿管喷射在彩色多普勒上显示尿液进入膀胱。

  完全性梗阻时肾脏产生的尿液无法进入膀胱，因而从理论上讲，存在输尿管喷射可排除完全性梗阻。但是，在结石患者中常可见输尿管喷射，而正常人中常无喷射。

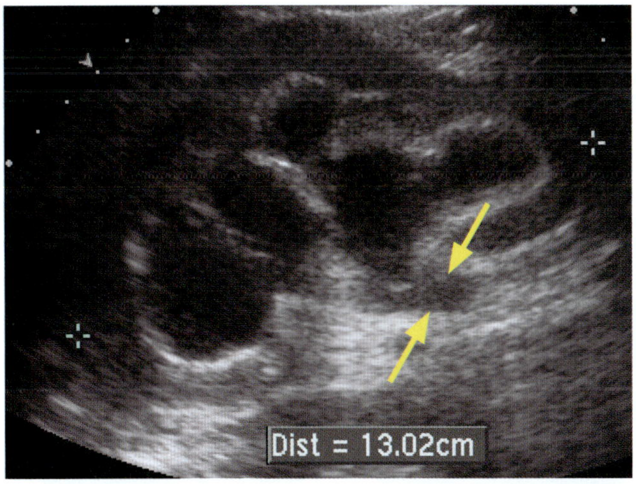

Sagittal grayscale ultrasound of the left kidney shows marked hydroureteronephrosis (arrows show dilation of the proximal ureter and filling defect in the ureter which may represents stones or blood product).
左肾矢状切面灰阶超声见明显的肾盂输尿管积水(黄箭所示近端输尿管扩张和输尿管充盈缺损,充盈缺损可能为结石或血液成分)。

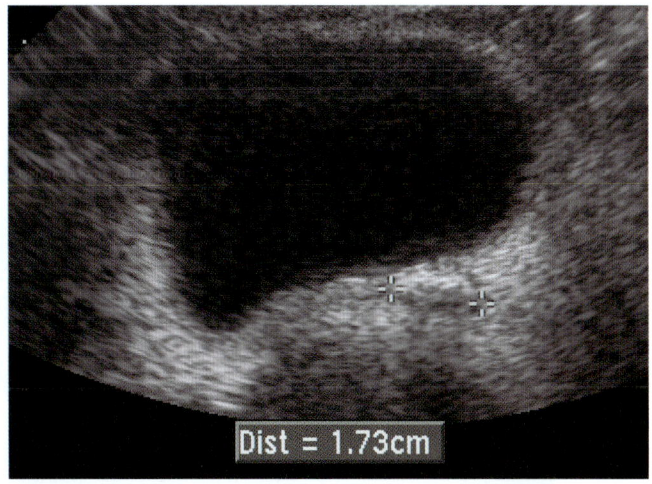

Transverse view of the bladder in the same patient shows a 17 mm shadowing left UVJ stone (calipers).
同一名患者膀胱横切面显示左侧输尿管膀胱交界处有一个17mm声影的结石(卡尺)。

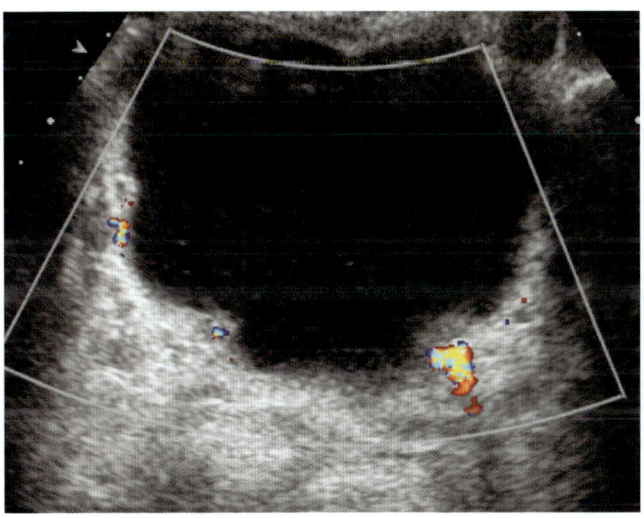

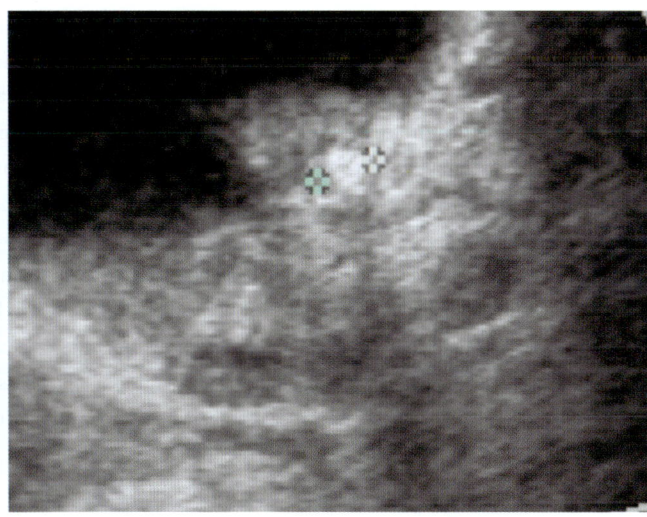

Transverse grayscale ultrasound of the bladder (left image) in a different patient from above shows *twinkling artifact* and posterior shadowing associated with a left UVJ stone (calipers on right image).
另一名患者的膀胱横切面(左图)灰阶图像显示左侧输尿管膀胱交界处结石的闪烁伪像及其后方声影(右图卡尺)。

Pitfalls in diagnosing hydronephrosis

- Obstruction without hydronephrosis can occur in cases of very acute obstruction, severe dehydration, or obstruction with ruptured fornix (results in decompression of the renal pelvis and perinephric fluid).
- Outside of non-obstructive causes described above, hydronephrosis without obstruction can be seen in patients with a recently passed stone (or radiolucent stone).
- Hydronephrosis can be difficult to distinguish from renal sinus cysts (peri- and parapelvic cysts). On imaging, renal sinus cysts will show a single or multiple discrete cystic lesions that do not communicate with each other. In true hydronephrosis, the dilated fluid-filled spaces are contiguous.

影像诊断肾盂积水的局限性

- 超急性梗阻、严重脱水或梗阻合并穹隆破裂(导致肾盂和肾周积液减压)时,虽有梗阻但可无肾盂积水表现。
- 除上述非梗阻性原因外,有肾盂积水但未见梗阻的现象可发生于近期排出结石(或可透射线的结石)的患者。
- 肾盂积水有时难以与多发性肾窦囊肿(肾盂旁及肾盂周围囊肿)相鉴别。影像学上,肾窦囊肿可表现为单个囊肿或多个互不相通的独立囊肿。而真正的肾盂积水,充满液体的扩张区域是相互连通的。

Pyelonephritis

肾盂肾炎

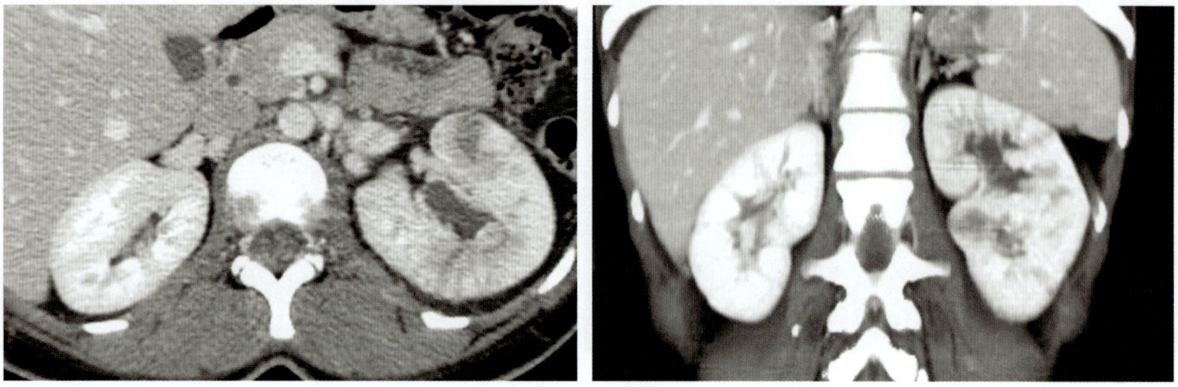

Pyelonephritis: Axial (left image) and coronal (right image) contrast-enhanced CT demonstrates an enlarged left kidney with delayed and striated nephrogram. These imaging features are nonspecific but are compatible with acute pyelonephritis given patient's clinical symptoms and positive urinalysis.

肾盂肾炎：轴位(左图)和冠状位(右图)增强CT显示左侧肾脏增大、延迟显像，以及条纹影。这些影像学表现无特异性，但结合患者的临床症状和阳性尿液结果，与急性肾盂肾炎相符合。

- Pyelonephritis is infection of renal parenchyma and is the most common bacterial infection of the kidney. Infection typically ascends from the bladder.
- CT imaging findings of pyelonephritis can be nonspecific, and the kidneys can appear normal in up to 75% of cases. Additional imaging patterns include unilateral kidney enlargement, wedge-shaped or striated regions of decreased enhancement, and perinephric stranding. The urothelium may also be thickened and hyperenhancing.
- Focal pyelonephritis (previously called focal lobar nephronia) may mimic a renal mass.
- On ultrasound, the classic appearance of focal pyelonephritis is a hypoechoic mass (or masses) with low-amplitude echoes that disrupts the corticomedullary junction. A distinct wall is lacking. Mild hydronephrosis can be seen on the affected side, thought to be due to a bacterial endotoxin causing reduced peristalsis, and should not be confused with obstructive uropathy.

- 肾盂肾炎是肾实质感染，最常见的为肾脏细菌性感染。通常为膀胱逆行感染所致。
- 肾盂肾炎的CT影像无特异性，高达75%病例的影像学表现正常。异常影像学表现包括单侧肾脏增大、楔形或条纹状的强化减低区，以及肾周条索样影；尿路上皮也可增厚并有明显强化。
- 局灶性肾盂肾炎(过去称为“局灶性大叶性肾病”)可类似于肾脏肿块。
- 典型的超声表现为单个(或多个)低回声肿块，低回声使皮髓质交界不清，无明确的边界。患侧可见轻度肾盂积水，被认为是由于细菌内毒素导致蠕动减少所致，不应与梗阻性尿路病混淆。

Pyonephrosis

肾盂积脓

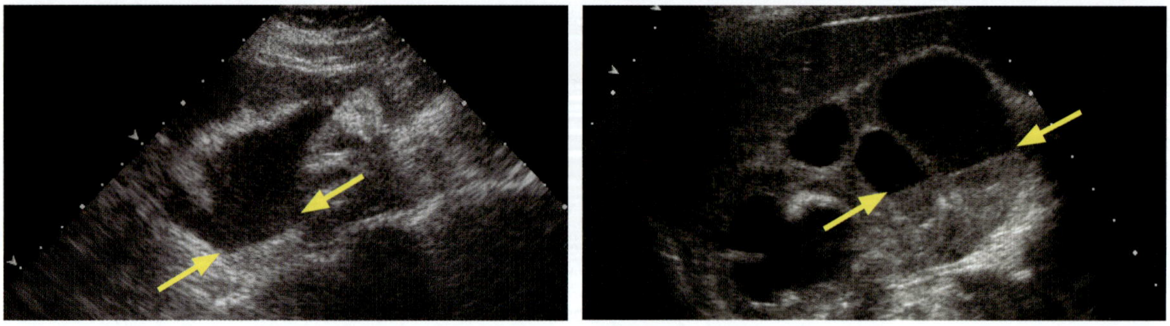

Pyonephrosis due to malpositioned nephroureteral stent: Initial ultrasound (left image) shows moderate hydronephrosis with a subtle echogenic dependent fluid-debris level (arrows). Low-level echoes are present within the collecting system. The nephroureteral stent is not visualized.
Subsequent ultrasound less than 12 hours later (right image) shows marked progression of hydronephrosis, a much larger fluid-debris level (arrows), and low level internal echoes within the dilated collecting system. Scanning of the distal ureter (not shown) revealed a malpositioned nephroureteral stent as the cause of obstruction. *Case courtesy Julie Ritner*, MD, *Brigham and Women's Hospital.*

肾输尿管支架位置不当引起的肾盂积脓：初始超声(左图)显示中度肾盂积水，其内可见模糊的体位性(下垂性)液体-碎片平面回声(黄箭)。集合系统呈低回声，未见肾输尿管支架。
12小时内的重复超声检查(右图)显示肾盂积水显著增加，液体-碎片平面明显扩大(黄箭)，以及扩张的集合系统内的内部低回声。远端输尿管扫查(未展示)显示肾输尿管支架异位，为导致梗阻的原因。

- Pyonephrosis is the infection of an obstructed collecting system and is colloquially referred to as "pus under pressure." Treatment is emergent relief of obstruction, either with percutaneous nephrostomy or ureteral stent.
- Ultrasound shows nonshadowing echogenic material within a dilated collecting system. A fluid-fluid level may be present.

Renal abscess

- Renal abscess is a focal necrotic parenchymal infection with a defined wall within the kidney that most commonly results from coalescence of small microabscesses in the setting of acute bacterial pyelonephritis. An abscess may simulate a cystic renal mass.
- Urinalysis may be negative in up to 30% of the time if the infection does not involve the collecting system.
- Ultrasound shows a fluid-filled mass with a distinct thick wall, which may be multiloculated.
- Small abscesses (<3 cm) often undergo a trial of conservative medical therapy, while larger abscesses typically undergo percutaneous drainage.

Emphysematous pyelonephritis

- 肾盂积脓是集合系统梗阻导致的感染，俗称"受压脓液"，属于外科急症。治疗方法为紧急解除梗阻，可行经皮肾造瘘术或放置输尿管支架。
- 超声显示扩张的集合系统内出现无阴影的回声物质，可出现液-液平面。

肾脓肿

- 肾脓肿是局部肾实质感染性坏死并有明确的囊壁，最常见于急性细菌性肾盂肾炎时微小脓肿的融合。脓肿可类似于囊性肾肿块。
- 若感染未侵犯到集合系统，尿检阴性率可达30%。
- 超声表现为肾内有充满液体的肿块并具有清晰的囊壁，可以为多房。
- 小脓肿(<3cm)一般采用内科保守治疗，较大脓肿一般需要经皮引流。

气肿性肾盂肾炎

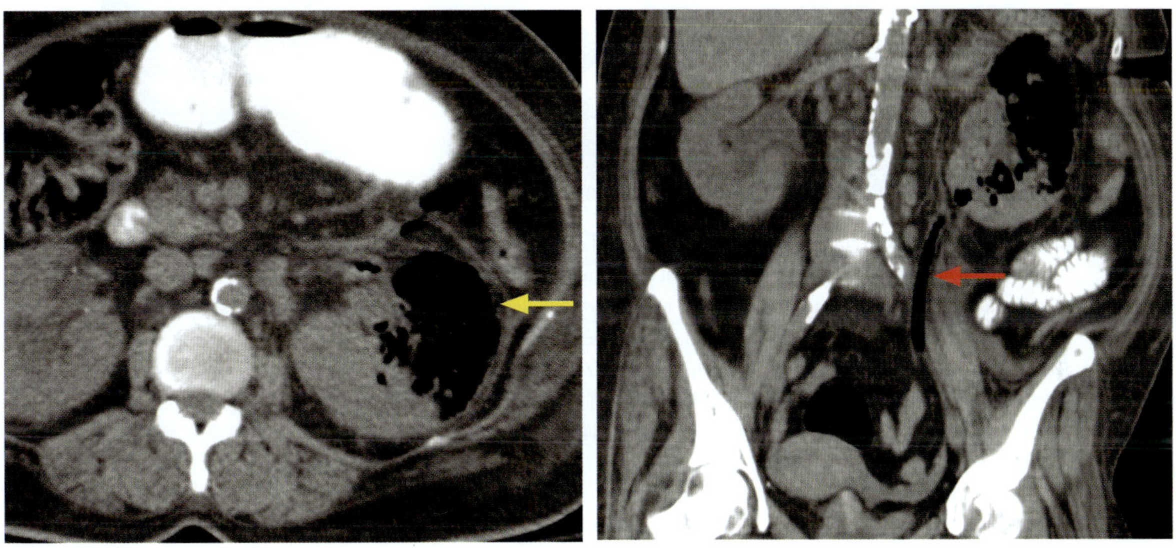

Emphysematous pyelonephritis: Axial (left image) and coronal CT with oral contrast only shows gas replacing the superior and lateral aspect of the left kidney (yellow arrow). There is gas extending into the left ureter, best seen on the coronal (red arrow).

气肿性肾盂肾炎：轴位和冠状位口服造影剂后CT显示左肾的上外侧被气体取代(左图，黄箭)。气体延伸至左侧输尿管，冠状位显示最佳(右图，红箭)。

- Emphysematous pyelonephritis is a complication of acute pyelonephritis characterized by replacement of renal parenchyma by gas. It is caused by gas-forming organisms, most commonly *E. coli*. Emphysematous pyelonephritis is almost exclusively seen in diabetic or immunocompromised individuals.
- Emphysematous pyelonephritis is a surgical emergency requiring broad-spectrum antibiotics and emergent nephrectomy. Mortality can reach 40%.
- Ultrasound shows high-amplitude echoes in the renal parenchyma representing gas locules with posterior dirty acoustic shadowing.

Renal tuberculosis

- *Mycobacterium tuberculosis* infection of the renal parenchyma results from hematogenous dissemination. Active pulmonary TB is present in approximately 10%.

- 气肿性肾盂肾炎是急性肾盂肾炎的并发症，特征为肾实质被积气所替代。该病由产气微生物引起，多为大肠杆菌。气肿性肾盂肾炎几乎只见于患糖尿病或免疫力低下的人群。
- 气肿性肾盂肾炎是外科急症，需给予广谱抗生素和紧急肾切除。该病死亡概率高达40%。
- 超声表现为肾实质内高回声，为局部气体聚集，其后方伴浑浊声影。

肾结核

- 肾实质结核分枝杆菌感染由血行播散导致，约10%的肾结核患者有活动性肺结核。

- Although initial renal TB infection typically involves both kidneys, chronic changes tend to be unilateral.
- Imaging findings are characterized by focal cavitary renal lesions with calcification. In addition, scarring, papillary necrosis, and infundibular strictures can be seen.
- End-stage renal TB produces auto nephrectomy and the characteristic *putty kidney* appearance, which represents an atrophic, calcified kidney.

- 肾感染结核最初多为双侧，但慢性结核往往为单侧。
- 影像学特征是肾局灶性空洞病变伴有钙化。此外，还可见瘢痕、肾乳头坏死，以及漏斗部狭窄。
- 晚期肾结核会形成肾自截，呈特征性油灰肾，为肾脏萎缩、钙化的结果。

Xanthogranulomatous pyelonephritis

黄色肉芽肿性肾盂肾炎

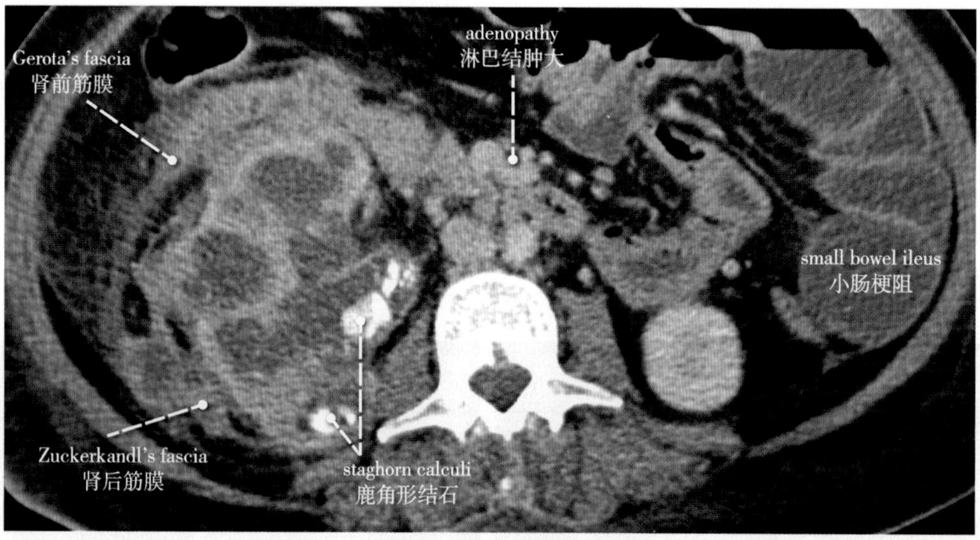

Xanthogranulomatous pyelonephritis: Contrast-enhanced CT shows a massively enlarged, poorly enhancing right kidney with dilated and distorted calyces. Several staghorn calculi are present. There is thickening of Zuckerkandl's and Gerota's fascia, perinephric stranding, and retroperitoneal adenopathy. The partially visualized small bowel in the left hemiabdomen is dilated secondary to ileus from perirenal inflammation.

Case courtesy Shreya Sood, MD, Brigham and Women's Hospital.

黄色肉芽肿性肾盂肾炎：增强CT显示右肾极度增大，强化差，伴肾盂肾盏扩张和扭曲。可见一些鹿角形结石，并可见肾后筋膜和肾前筋膜增厚、肾周条索样改变及腹膜后淋巴结肿大。左侧腹部可见部分小肠扩张，由肾周炎症引起的肠梗阻造成。

- Xanthogranulomatous pyelonephritis (XGP) is a chronic renal infection due to obstructing staghorn calculi, leading to replacement of renal parenchyma with fibrofatty inflammatory tissue.
- *Proteus mirabilis* and *Escherichia coli* are the two most common organisms.
- The clinical presentation of XGP includes flank pain and nonspecific constitutional symptoms, such as fever and weight loss. Anemia and hematuria are also common.
- XGP can be diffuse (85%) or localized. The localized form, also known as "tumefactive XGP," may mimic a renal mass.
- CT is the primary modality for imaging, which demonstrates fatty replacement of the renal parenchyma, marked perinephric inflammatory stranding, and staghorn calculi. The *bear paw sign* represents the configuration of the hypoattenuating fibrofatty masses arranged in a radial pattern, reminiscent of a bear's paw.
- Complications include perinephric abscess and fistula formation. Treatment is nephrectomy.
- Primary differential considerations include acute obstructing calculus with pyonephrosis or renal/transitional neoplasm with calcification.

- 黄色肉芽肿性肾盂肾炎(XGP)是一种由梗阻性鹿角形肾结石引起的慢性肾感染，导致肾实质被纤维脂肪炎性组织代替。
- 变形杆菌和大肠杆菌是两种最常见的病原体。
- XGP的临床表现为季肋部痛和非特异性的全身症状，如发热和体重下降。贫血和血尿也常见。
- XGP可为弥漫型(85%)或局限型，其中局限型也被称为"肿瘤型XGP"，可类似于肾脏肿块。
- CT是XGP的主要影像诊断方法，表现为肾实质被脂肪代替，肾周明显炎性条索样改变，以及鹿角形肾结石。熊掌征代表呈放射状分布的低密度纤维脂肪肿块，形如熊掌。
- 并发症包括肾周脓肿和瘘管形成。治疗方法为肾切除。
- 主要的鉴别诊断包括急性梗阻性结石伴肾盂积脓，或肾脏/移行细胞肿瘤伴钙化。

HIV-associated nephropathy

- HIV virus may directly infect the kidney to produce HIV nephropathy, most commonly resulting in focal segmental glomerulosclerosis (FSGS). HIV nephropathy clinically presents with nephritic renal failure.
- The kidneys are characteristically echogenic. **Enlarged echogenic** kidneys are specific for HIV nephropathy, although the kidneys are enlarged only about 20% of the time.

HIV相关的肾病

- HIV可直接感染肾实质而导致HIV肾病，最常导致局灶性节段性肾小球硬化症(FSGS)。HIV肾病的临床表现为肾衰竭。
- HIV肾病以高回声为特征。**大而有高回声**的肾脏是HIV肾病的特异性表现，但肾脏增大仅见于20%的患者。

DIAGNOSTIC APPROACH TO A RENAL MASS

Ultrasound of a renal mass

- *Ultrasound is particularly useful for the initial evaluation of a cystic renal mass.*
- Color Doppler should be utilized to evaluate for internal blood flow. Color Doppler is also useful to distinguish a cystic mass from a renal artery aneurysm since they appear similar in grayscale.

CT of a renal mass

- *CT is useful for the evaluation of both cystic and solid renal masses.*
- A **renal mass protocol CT** consists of at least three CT phases, each providing different types of information to aid in evaluation.
- **Unenhanced** phase: quantify baseline attenuation and evaluate for intralesional fat and calcifications.
- **Nephrographic** phase (100 second delay): evaluate for enhancement by comparing to the unenhanced images.
- **Excretory** phase (8 minute delay): helpful to show the relationship of a renal mass to the collection system for surgical planning, and to diagnose mimics of cystic renal masses.

  The delayed excretory phase can distinguish between hydronephrosis (will show dense opacification in the pyelographic phase) versus renal sinus cysts (will not opacify).

  Reflux nephropathy may cause a dilated calyx that can simulate a cystic renal mass on the nephrographic phase. The excretory phase would show opacification of the dilated calyx.

  The excretory phase is also useful to demonstrate a calyceal diverticulum.
- Although not done routinely, an arterial phase can be performed for presurgical planning.

MRI of a renal mass

- *MRI is particularly useful for the evaluation of solid renal masses. MRI can provide information about internal fat and fluid content, as well as enhancement.* Further details are provided in the solid renal mass section.
- MRI plays a limited role in the evaluation of a cystic renal mass. However, given the increased general use of MRI, the new 2019 Bosniak classification formally incorporates MRI into its classification. This is discussed further below.
- Calcifications are harder to detect with MRI.

Evaluating enhancement of a renal mass (CT and MRI)

- The presence of enhancement is the most important characteristic to diagnose a solid renal mass, but intralesional fat is almost always diagnostic of benign angiomyolipoma. A non-fat-containing renal mass can still be benign, particularly when small (<1 cm), but the risk of malignancy increases with increasing mass size (>3 cm).

肾脏肿块的诊断方法

肾脏肿块的超声检查

- *超声对囊性肾脏肿块的初步评估具有重要价值。*
- 应使用彩色多普勒来评估内部血流。彩色多普勒能够区分囊性肿块和肾动脉瘤，而两者在灰阶图像中表现相似。

肾脏肿块的CT检查

- *CT可用于评估囊性和实性肾脏肿块。*
- **肾脏肿块的CT检查方案**至少包括3个期相，每个期相提供不同类型的信息有助于评估。
- **平扫：**量化基线密度(CT值)并评估病灶内脂肪和钙化。
- **肾实质期**(100秒延迟)：通过比较平扫图像以评估强化程度。
- **排泄期**(8分钟延迟)：显示肾脏肿块与集合系统之间的关系以制订手术计划，并用以诊断类囊样肾脏肿块。

  延迟排泄期可用于鉴别肾盂积水(在肾盂期呈高密度影)和肾窦囊肿(无强化)。

  反流性肾病可导致肾盏扩张，在肾实质期可类似于一个囊性肾肿块。排泄期可以看到扩张的肾盏内充填造影剂。

  排泄期对显示肾盂憩室也有帮助。
- 动脉期扫描并非常规，但可用于制订术前计划。

肾脏肿块的MRI检查

- *MRI对于评估实性肾肿块非常有价值。MRI可提供病灶内部脂肪、液体，以及强化的信息。*更多细节将在实体肾肿块部分讨论。
- MRI在评估囊性肾肿块方面的作用有限。然而，鉴于MRI的应用已普遍增加，2019年Bosniak新分类正式将MRI表现纳入了分类标准。相关内容将在下文进一步讨论。
- MRI难以识别钙化。

评估肾脏肿块的强化(CT和MRI)

- 强化是诊断肾脏实性肿块最重要的特征，而病灶内若含脂肪，几乎都可以诊断为良性血管平滑肌脂肪瘤。不含脂肪的肾脏肿块仍有可能为良性，尤其是小病灶(<1cm)，但随着肿块大小的增加(>3cm)，恶性风险也随之增加。

- On CT, enhancement is quantified as the *absolute* increase in Hounsfield units on postcontrast images, compared to pre-contrast:

<10 HU: No enhancement.	10–19 HU: Equivocal enhancement.	≥20 HU: Definite enhancement.

- On MRI, enhancement is quantified as the *percent* increase in signal intensity as measured on postcontrast images:

<15%: No enhancement.	15–19%: Equivocal enhancement.	≥20%: Definite enhancement.

- Lesions are considered "too small to characterize" if the lesion diameter is smaller than twice the slice thickness. For instance, using 3 mm slices, a lesion less than 6 mm cannot be accurately characterized based on attenuation or enhancement.

Biopsy of a renal mass

- After full imaging workup is complete, there are several well-accepted indications for percutaneous renal mass biopsy:

> To distinguish renal cell carcinoma from metastasis in a patient with a known primary.
> To distinguish between renal infection and cystic neoplasm.
> To definitively diagnose a hyperdense, homogeneously enhancing mass (after MRI has been performed), as it may represent a benign angiomyolipoma with minimal fat versus a renal cell carcinoma.
> To definitively diagnose a suspicious renal mass in patient with multiple comorbidities for whom nephrectomy would be high risk.
> To definitely diagnose malignancy and subtype in unresectable disease to guide treatment. To ensure correct tissue diagnosis prior to renal mass ablation or stereotactic radiotherapy.
> To provide definite diagnosis in patients with multiple or bilateral renal masses.
> To provide definite diagnosis in a renal mass that is in a solitary (or transplant) kidney.
> To exclude benign neoplasm in small renal masses (<4 cm), as 20% of solid renal masses are benign, and proportion increases among smaller masses.

Cystic renal masses

Overview of Bosniak classification of cystic renal masses

- The 2019 Bosniak classification for cystic renal masses was updated from 2012 to incorporate MRI, formalize definitions, and reclassify additional masses as lower risk. The Bosniak system risk-stratifies cystic renal masses, with increasing risk for malignancy (RCC) with each subsequent category. Classification is based on morphology, and thus MRI criteria generally mirror those of CT. Calcification plays a limited role in classification.
- MRI frequently upgrades Bosniak criteria due to higher sensitivity for detecting features including septations. MRI can also provide more accuate characterization of enhancement and is most useful to distinguish a Bosniak ⅡF lesion from a Bosniak Ⅲ lesion (which can impact management). MRI is not obscured by calcification which also permits easier lesion evaluation.
- Risk stratification of cystic renal mass based on Bosniak classification:

- CT检查时，强化定量为增强前、后CT值的绝对值之差：

<10HU：无强化。	10~19HU：可疑强化。	≥20HU：强化。

- MRI检查时，强化定量为增强前、后图像上测量的信号强度所增加的百分比：

<15%：无强化。	15%~19%：可疑强化。	≥20%：强化。

- 如果病变直径小于两个横断面的厚度，则可将此称为"太小而不能定性"。例如，在使用3mm层厚的情况下，小于6mm的病灶不能使用衰减密度或增强来对其精确定性。

肾脏肿块活检

- 在所有影像学检查完成后，公认的经皮肾脏穿刺活检的指征为：

> 在已知原发肿瘤病史的患者中，鉴别肾细胞癌和肾转移。
> 鉴别肾脏感染和囊性肿瘤。
> 明确诊断高密度、均匀强化肿块(完成MRI扫描后)，如含少量脂肪的良性血管平滑肌脂肪瘤或肾细胞癌。
> 明确诊断有多种合并症而肾切除术风险很高的患者中的可疑肾脏肿块。
> 明确诊断不可切除的恶性病变及其亚型，以指导治疗。确保肾脏肿块消融或立体定位放射治疗之前获得正确的组织学诊断。
> 明确诊断多个或双侧肾脏肿块。
> 明确诊断孤立(或移植)肾脏肿块。
> 排除肾脏小肿块(<4cm)中的良性肿瘤，因20%的肾实质肿块为良性，且肿块越小良性比例越高。

囊性肾肿块

Bosniak囊性肾肿块分级概述

- 2019年Bosniak囊性肾肿块分级在2012版的基础上进行了以下更新：纳入MRI分级标准、明确定义，并将其他肿块重新分级为更低风险。Bosniak系统对囊性肾肿块进行了风险分层，其每个后续类别的恶性风险(如RCC)都有所增加。分类基于形态学，因此MRI标准基本类似CT标准。钙化在分类中的作用有限。
- MRI常可提高Bosniak级别，因其对一些特征(包括分隔)的检测具更高的灵敏度。MRI还可提供更准确的增强特征，对于区分Bosniak ⅡF和Bosniak Ⅲ级病变(可能影响治疗方式)最具价值。MRI不受钙化影响，可使病变评估更加容易。
- 基于Bosniak分级的囊性肾肿块的风险分层：

Category Ⅰ and Ⅱ: <1% risk of malignancy. No follow-up necessary.

Category ⅡF: 0-38% risk of malignancy. Imaging follow-up is needed; any morphologic change or new enhancement would be concerning for malignancy.

Category Ⅲ: ~50% risk of malignancy but range varies by studies. Concern for malignancy, but may be benign (e.g., infection, multilocular cystic nephroma). Management varies from imaging follow-up to surgical excision (if without comorbidities).

Category Ⅳ: ~90% risk of malignancy. Surgical excision is required unless significant comorbidities.

Ⅰ和Ⅱ级：<1%的恶性肿瘤风险。不需要随访。

ⅡF级：0~38%的恶性肿瘤风险。需要影像随访；出现任何形态学变化或新的强化时，应怀疑为恶性肿瘤。

Ⅲ级：约50%的恶性肿瘤风险，但不同研究结果不一致。需考虑恶性肿瘤，但也可能为良性(如感染、多房囊性肾瘤)。从影像学随访到手术切除，其诊疗方法不同(在没有合并症的情况下)。

Ⅳ级：高达90%的恶性肿瘤风险。除非有严重的合并症，否则都应手术切除。

Summary of 2019 Bosniak classification of cystic renal masses

Category Ⅰ

Cystic (water-attenuation/intensity) mass with a thin (≤2 mm) smooth wall which may enhance. No septa or calcifications. Practically, this classification is never used; this lesion is usually called a simple renal cyst.

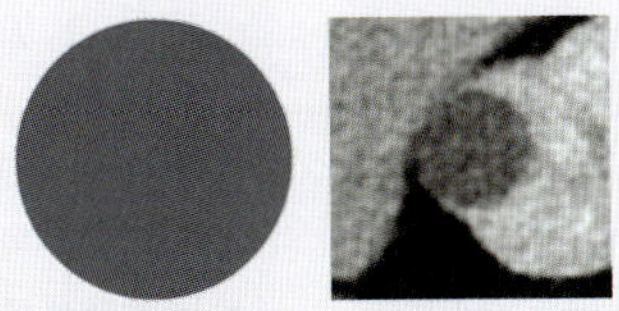

Bosniak Ⅰ

Category Ⅱ

Six proposed Bosniak subtypes can be distilled to these rules:

- **Non**enhancing (excludes thin septa/wall, which may enhance).
- <4 septa with thickness ≤2 mm.
- Proteinaceous/hemorrhagic cysts (nonenhancing, homogeneous, hyperattenuating ≥70 HU or intrinsically T1 hyperintense) ≤3 cm in size.
- Homogeneous low-attenuation masses too small to characterize.

Any violation gets upgraded.

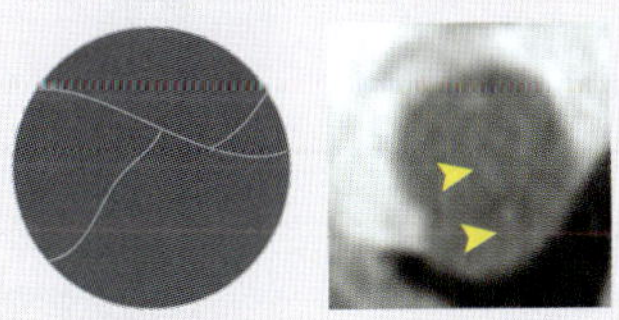

Bosniak Ⅱ

Category ⅡF

Cystic mass violating any of the above rules but less than Category Ⅲ falls here.

Note that Ca++ is no longer included, as this isolated feature has little predictive value.

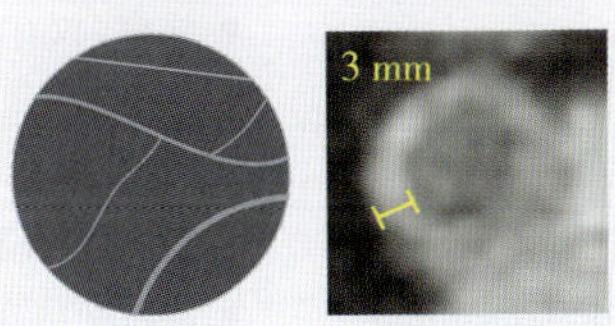

Bosniak ⅡF

Category Ⅲ

Any enhancing **thick** (≥4 mm) septation/wall.

Any enhancing **irregular** protrusion with obtuse margins, ≤3 mm) septation/wall.

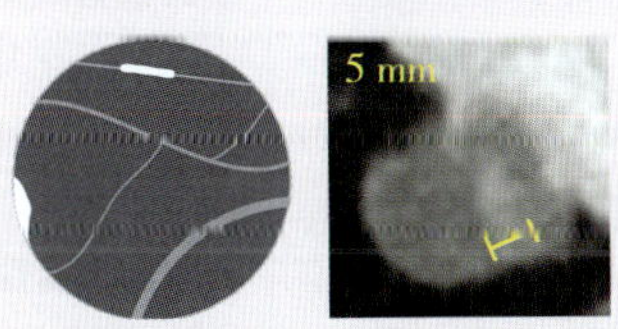

Bosniak Ⅲ

Category Ⅳ

Any **enhancing nodule** with acute margins irrespective of size.

Any **enhancing nodule** ≥4 mm with obtuse margins.

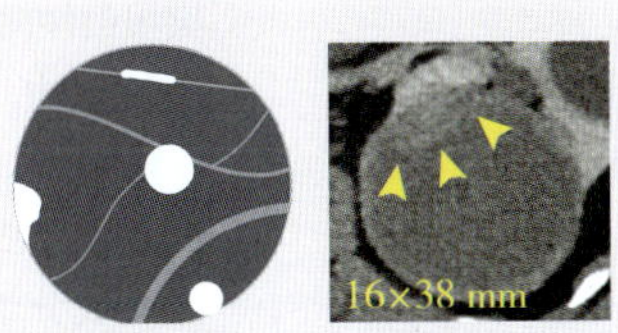

Bosniak Ⅳ

2019年Bosniak囊性肾肿块分级总结

Ⅰ级

囊性(水样密度/信号)肿块，壁薄(≤2mm)、光滑，囊壁可强化。无分隔或钙化。该分类实际上从未被使用过，此类病变通常被称为单纯肾囊肿。

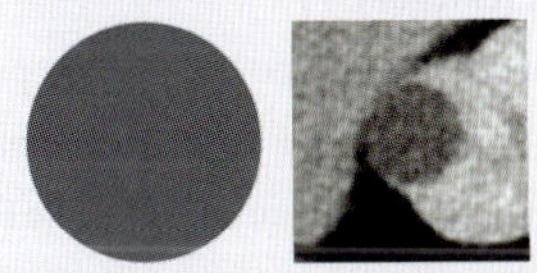

Bosniak Ⅰ

Ⅱ级

按以下标准提议出6种Bosniak亚型：

- **无**强化(不包括可能强化的薄的分隔/壁)。
- 分隔<4个，其厚度≤2mm。
- 蛋白质/出血性囊肿(无强化、均质、高密度≥70HU或T_1高信号)，大小≤3cm。
- 过小而无法评估的均匀低密度肿块。

超出任何标准都将升级。

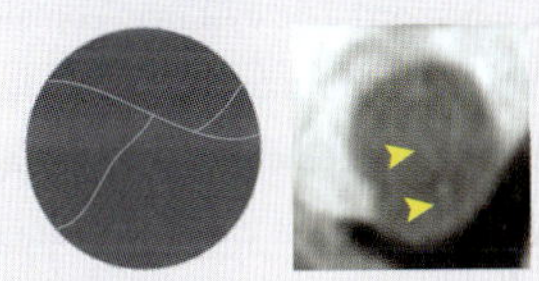

Bosniak Ⅱ

ⅡF级

超出上述任何标准，但又未达到Ⅲ级标准的**囊性**肿块属于此类。

注意，不再包括钙化，因为该孤立的特征几乎无预测价值。

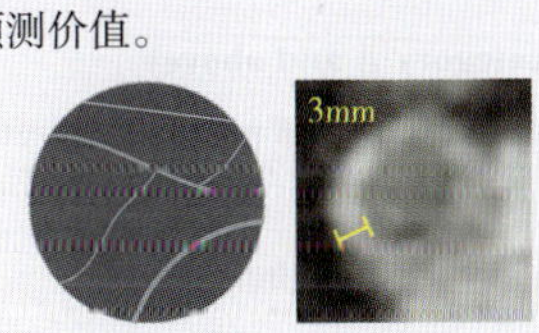

Bosniak ⅡF

Ⅲ级

任何强化的**厚壁**(≥4mm)或分隔。

任何壁或分隔强化且**不规则**(出现≤3mm的钝角凸起)

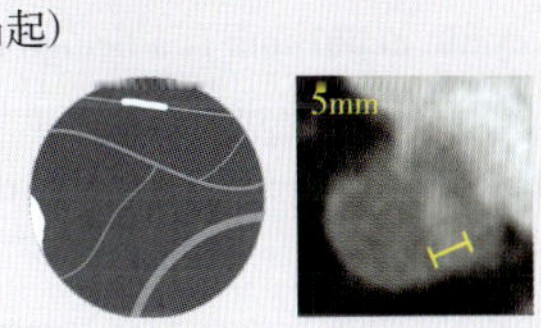

Bosniak Ⅲ

Ⅳ级

任意大小的与囊壁或分隔呈锐角的**强化结节**。

任何≥4mm的与囊壁或分隔呈钝角的**强化结节**。

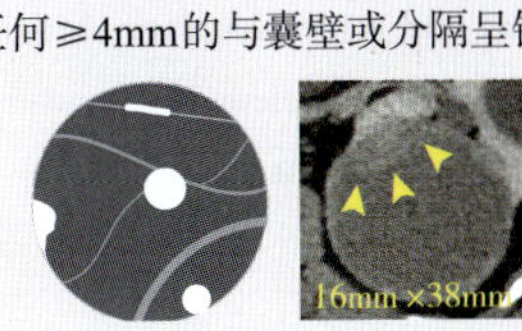

Bosniak Ⅳ

Differential diagnosis of cystic renal masses

Simple renal cyst (Bosniak category Ⅰ)

- Simple renal cysts are very common, found in approximately 50% of patients over age 50. A simple renal cyst is an incidental lesion that requires no follow-up, even when large.
- A simple renal cyst should have the sonographic hallmarks of a simple cyst, featuring an imperceptible thin wall, anechoic internal contents, and posterior through transmission.
- Harmonic imaging can be helpful in confirming the diagnosis of simple renal cyst by eliminating artifactual low-level internal echoes.
- On CT, a simple cyst should attenuate close to 0 HU (and must be < 20 HU), not contain any enhancing components, and have a thin imperceptible wall.
- On MRI, a simple cyst must be hypointense on T1-weighted images, hyperintense on T2-weighted images, and not contain any enhancing component.

Renal sinus cyst (category Ⅰ)

- Cysts in the renal sinus may be classified as parapelvic and peripelvic cysts.
- A **parapelvic** cyst is a renal cortical cyst that herniates into the renal sinus and is usually solitary. These cysts are usually large but solitary.
- **Peripelvic** cysts are secondary to lymphatic obstruction and are often small and multiple.
- When multiple renal sinus cysts are present (usually peripelvic cysts), the appearance may mimic hydronephrosis. In contrast to hydronephrosis, renal sinus cysts are not contiguous with each other and will not contain excreted contrast on delayed imaging.

Hyperdense cyst (category Ⅱ)

- On ultrasound, a hemorrhagic cyst may contain low-level echoes or layers of echoes.
- On noncontrast CT, hemorrhagic cysts are homogeneous and hyperattenuating (>70 HU). The main differential includes a proteinaceous cyst (debris).
- Note that a hyperdense cyst cannot be diagnosed on postcontrast imaging alone because it cannot be distinguished from an enhancing renal mass (unless dual energy CT is used).

Renal abscess (category Ⅱ and above)

- A renal abscess is a contained purulent collection within the kidney. It is described in the renal infection section.

Neoplasm (category ⅡF and above)

- **Cystic renal cell carcinoma:** Although renal cell carcinoma most commonly presents as a solid renal mass, it can also manifest as a complex cystic mass. Worrisome ultrasound findings include thick septa, irregular wall thickening, and a mural nodule.
- **Multilocular cystic nephroma** is a benign cystic neoplasm with enhancing septa that occurs in a bimodal age distribution in baby boys and middle-aged women. A characteristic but nonspecific feature is the propensity to herniate into the renal pelvis, causing hydronephrosis.

  In adults, multilocular cystic nephroma can be indistinguishable from cystic RCC.

  In children, multilocular cystic nephroma can be indistinguishable from cystic Wilms tumor.
- **Mixed epithelial and stromal tumor (MEST)** is a benign neoplasm composed of epithelial and mesenchymal elements, typically found in middle-aged women. MEST may appear as either a solid or cystic mass.

囊性肾肿块鉴别诊断

单纯肾囊肿(Bosniak Ⅰ级)(以下均为Bosniak分级)

- 单纯肾囊肿极为常见，50岁以上者发生率约50%。单纯肾囊肿是一个偶然发现的病变，即使体积较大也不需要随访。
- 单纯肾囊肿应具有单纯囊肿的超声特征：不易辨认的薄壁，内部无回声，后方回声增强。
- 谐波成像可以排除内部低回声伪影，有助于确诊单纯性囊肿。
- 在CT上，单纯肾囊肿的密度应接近0(须<20HU)，不含任何强化成分，有一层不易察觉的薄壁。
- 在MRI上，单纯肾囊肿必须是T_1加权图像为低信号，T_2加权图像为高信号，且不含任何强化成分。

肾窦囊肿(Ⅰ级)

- 肾窦囊肿可分为肾盂旁囊肿和肾盂周围囊肿。
- **肾盂旁**囊肿是肾皮质囊肿疝入肾窦后形成，这类囊肿通常大且单发。
- **肾盂周围**囊肿继发于淋巴梗阻，通常体积小且多发。
- 当存在多个肾窦囊肿(通常为肾盂周围囊肿)时，其外观可能类似于肾盂积水。与肾盂积水不同的是，肾窦囊肿彼此不相通，且在延迟期不含排出的造影剂。

高密度囊肿(Ⅱ级)

- 在超声上，出血性囊肿可能呈低回声或分层状回声。
- 在平扫CT图像上，出血性囊肿呈均匀高密度(>70HU)。主要鉴别包括含有蛋白成分的囊肿(碎片)。
- 注意，仅有增强后的图像不能对高密度囊肿进行诊断，因其不能与强化的肾肿块区分(除非使用双能CT)。

肾脓肿(Ⅱ级及以上)

- 肾脓肿是肾内的脓液聚集。详见肾脏感染部分。

肿瘤(ⅡF级及以上)

- **囊性肾细胞癌**：尽管肾细胞癌大多为实性肿物，但也可呈复杂的囊性病灶。超声上可疑恶性的特征包括分隔较厚、囊壁不规则增厚，以及囊壁结节。
- **多房性囊性肾瘤**是一种良性囊性肿瘤，具有强化的分隔，在男婴和中年女性中呈双峰样年龄分布。一个典型而非特异性的特征是具有向肾盂突出的倾向，可导致肾盂积水。

  在成人中，多房囊性肾瘤与囊性RCC无法区分。

  在儿童中，多房囊性肾瘤与囊性肾母细胞瘤无法区分。
- **混合性上皮间质肿瘤(MEST)**是一种由上皮和间质成分组成的良性肿瘤，常见于中年女性。MEST可表现为实性或囊性肿块。

MULTICYSTIC RENAL DISEASE

多囊肾病

Autosomal dominant polycystic kidney disease (ADPKD)

常染色体显性遗传多囊肾病(ADPKD)

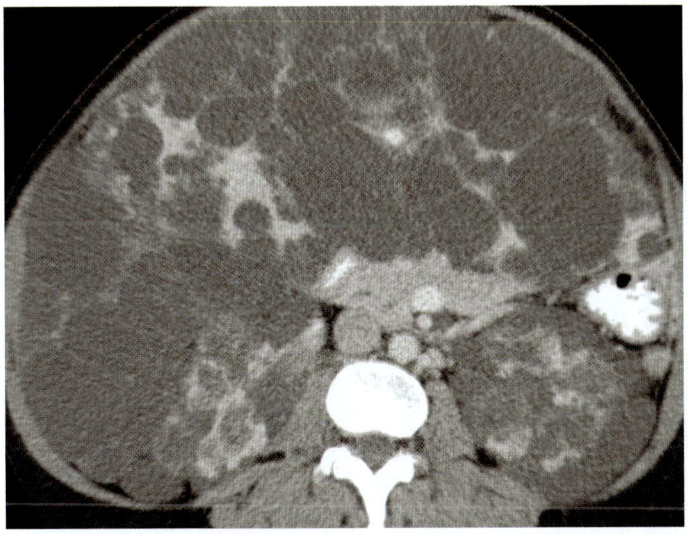

ADPKD: Axial enhanced CT shows bilateral enlarged kidneys with innumerable renal cysts of mixed attenuation. The liver is also enlarged and contains innumerable fluid attenuation cysts.
轴位增强CT显示双侧肾脏增大并含无数混合密度的肾囊肿。肝脏亦增大且含无数个液体密度的囊肿。

- Autosomal dominant polycystic kidney disease (ADPKD) features bilaterally enlarged kidneys with multiple large renal cysts. Patients present with progressive renal failure in their third to fourth decades. The kidneys are sometimes palpable from enlargement and patients may display secondary hypertension and hematuria (nephrolithiasis vs. rupture of a renal cyst into the collecting system). Approximately 70% of patients have multiple hepatic cysts and 15% of patients have saccular cerebral aneurysms.
- ADPKD is responsible for 10% of patients on long-term dialysis.
- On imaging, the kidneys are markedly enlarged and feature multiple cysts of varying attenuation (or signal intensity on MRI) due to hemorrhage.
- ADPKD is not known to increase the risk of renal cell carcinoma, though some authors propose that there is a slightly increased risk. Renal cell carcinoma associated with ADPKD tends to occur at a younger age and is more often bilateral, multifocal, and sarcomatoid.

- 常染色体显性遗传多囊肾病(ADPKD)的特点是双侧肾脏增大，合并多发大囊肿。患者在30~40岁时出现进行性肾衰竭。肾脏因增大而有时可被触及，患者可出现继发性高血压和血尿(肾结石或肾囊肿破裂入集合系统)。约70%的患者合并多囊肝，15%的患者伴囊状脑动脉瘤。
- ADPKD在长期透析患者中占10%。
- 影像学上，肾脏显著增大，特征为因出血而导致的不同密度(或信号)的多发囊肿。
- ADPKD是否会增加肾细胞癌的风险尚不明确，但一些研究者认为风险略有增加。肾细胞癌在ADPKD患者中往往在年轻时发病，常为双侧、多个病灶，以及肉瘤样分化。

Autosomal recessive polycystic kidney disease (ARPKD)

- Autosomal recessive polycystic kidney disease (ARPKD) features enlarged kidneys with innumerable tiny renal cysts. ARPKD is a diagnosis of infancy and has a poor prognosis. If the child survives infancy, hepatic fibrosis usually develops.
- ARPKD presents in utero as enlarged echogenic kidneys (the cysts are too small to be individually resolved by ultrasound).

常染色体隐性遗传多囊肾病(ARPKD)

- 常染色体隐性遗传多囊肾病(ARPKD)的特点是肾脏增大伴无数微小的肾囊肿。ARPKD通常在婴儿期确诊，预后较差。若患儿在婴儿期得以存活，常会发生肝纤维化。
- ARPKD在子宫内表现为肾脏增大伴回声增强(囊肿太小，无法通过超声分辨)。

Acquired cystic kidney disease (due to end-stage kidney disease)

- Patients on long-term dialysis often develop many small renal cysts superimposed upon atrophic kidneys.
- Dialysis-associated cystic renal disease portends an increased risk of renal cell carcinoma (~2–3% prevalence, compared to 1/10,000 prevalence in the general population).

获得性肾囊肿病(为终末期肾病所致)

- 长期透析的患者通常会在肾萎缩的基础上形成许多小囊肿。
- 透析相关的囊性肾病有增加肾细胞癌的风险(患病率约为2%~3%，普通人群为1/10 000)。

Localized cystic renal disease

- This is characterized by benign, slowly progressive proliferation of cysts, typically within a normal functioning kidney and asymptomatic. It is always unilateral, and usually affects only part of the kidney. No imaging follow-up or treatment required.

局限性囊性肾病

- 局限性囊性肾病特征为良性、缓慢进展的囊肿，肾功能常正常且无症状。单侧发病，仅影响肾脏的一部分。不需要影像学随访或治疗。

Lithium nephropathy

- Lithium nephropathy is related to long-term lithium use and can present as nephrogenic diabetes insipidus or chronic renal insufficiency.
- The classic imaging appearance is numerous scattered uniform microcysts in bilateral normal-sized kidneys. On ultrasound, these small cysts usually appear as punctate echogenic foci. CT may show calcification within the cysts. MRI is most sensitive and shows tiny nonenhancing fluid intensity cysts in the renal cortex and medulla.

锂肾病

- 锂肾病与长期使用锂有关，可表现为肾源性尿崩症或慢性肾功能不全。
- 典型影像学表现为双侧正常大小的肾脏内分布着含无数均匀的微囊肿。在超声上，这些微囊肿通常表现为点状高回声病灶。CT可显示囊肿内钙化。MRI对该病最敏感，可显示肾皮质和髓质中微小的非强化液体信号囊肿。

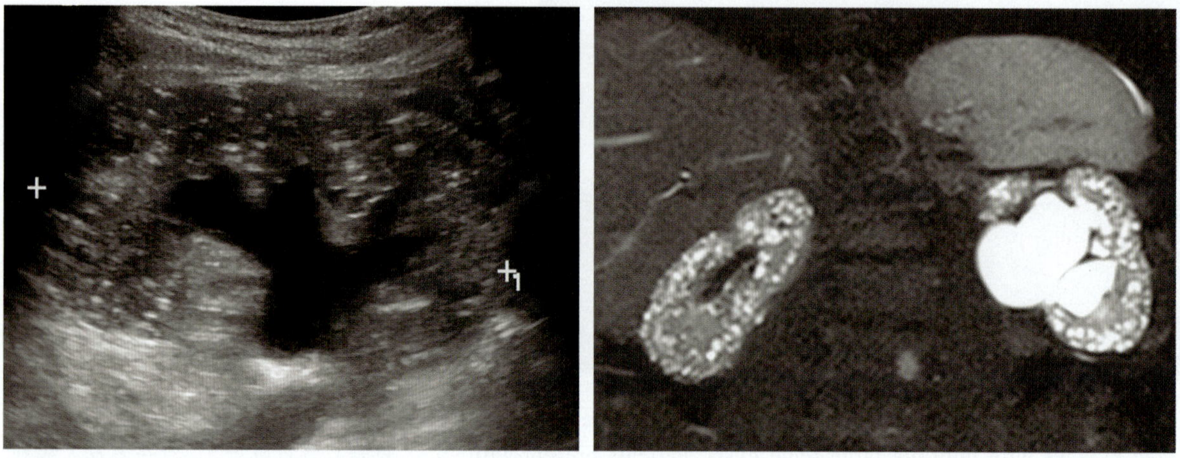

Sagittal grayscale ultrasound of the left kidney (left image) demonstrates multiple tiny echogenic foci in the renal parenchyma and moderate hydronephrosis. Coronal T2-weighted MRI (right image) shows numerous microcysts in bilateral kidneys, consistent with lithium nephropathy in this patient on long-term lithium therapy. Again seen is left hydronephrosis.

左肾矢状切面灰阶超声(左图)显示肾实质中有多个微小的强回声灶和中度肾盂积水。冠状位T_2加权MRI(右图)显示双侧肾脏多发微囊肿，与该患者长期锂治疗的锂肾病相符。同时可见左侧肾盂积水。

Solid Renal Masses – Malignant

- The likelihood of malignancy in a solid renal mass increases with lesion size. Roughly 50% of solid renal masses <1 cm are benign, whereas 75% of renal masses >3 cm are malignant.
- In the presence of a solid renal mass, the renal veins must be carefully evaluated for tumor thrombus and extension.

Renal cell carcinoma (RCC)

肾脏实性肿块——恶性

- 实性肾脏肿块的恶性概率随着病灶增大而增加。约50% <1cm的肾肿块为良性，而75% >3cm的肾肿块为恶性。
- 如发现实性肾肿块，必须仔细评估肾静脉是否有癌栓和受侵。

肾细胞癌(RCC)

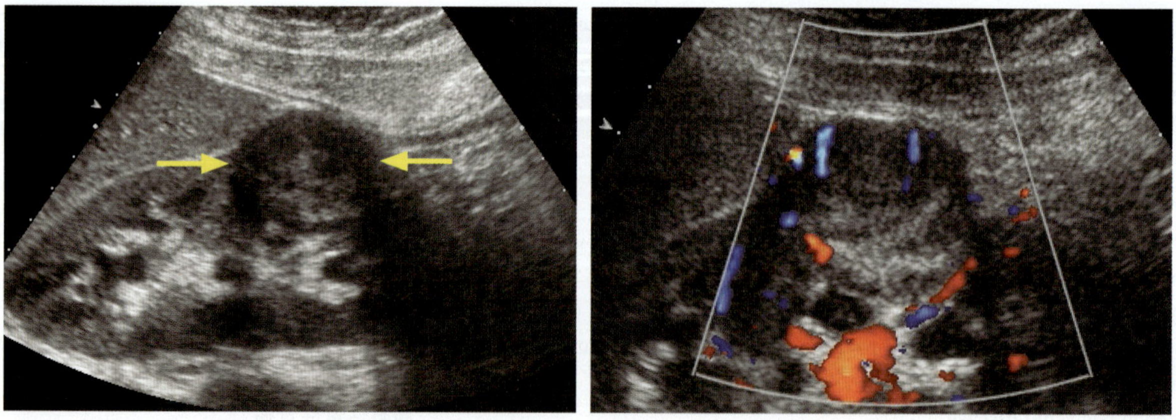

Renal cell carcinoma: Sagittal ultrasound through the kidney shows a hypoechoic solid mass (arrows) with heterogeneous echotexture in the interpolar region. The mass demonstrates vascularity on color Doppler (right image).

Case courtesy Julie Ritner, MD, Brigham and Women's Hospital.

肾细胞癌：经肾脏矢状切面超声显示肾中极有一个低回声实性肿块(左图，黄箭)，其内部回声不均。彩色多普勒显示肿块内有血管分布(右图)。

- Renal cell carcinoma (RCC) is the most common solid renal mass and arises from renal tubular epithelium. It represents 2–3% of all cancers. Risk factors include smoking, acquired cystic kidney disease, von Hippel-Lindau (VHL), and tuberous sclerosis.
- RCC has a propensity for venous invasion, which significantly alters surgical approach.
- Staging of RCC is based on the Robson system, which characterizes fascial extension and vascular/lymph node involvement. Stages Ⅰ–Ⅲ are usually resectable, although the surgical approach may need to be altered for venous invasion (stages ⅢA and ⅢC).
- On ultrasound, RCC is usually isoechoic to renal cortex, but can be hypo-or hyperechoic. If hyperechoic (mimicking AML), imaging features such as a hypoechoic rim and intratumoral cystic changes favor RCC. Color and spectral Doppler are helpful in differentiating bland renal vein thrombus (which would not be stage ⅢA) from tumor thrombus. Tumor thrombus will have color Doppler flow with an arterial waveform.

- 肾细胞癌(RCC)是最常见的肾实性肿块，起源于肾小管上皮细胞，占所有癌症的2%~3%。危险因素包括吸烟、获得性囊性肾脏疾病、VHL和结节性硬化。
- RCC有侵犯静脉的倾向，对手术方案有明显影响。
- RCC分期采用Robson系统，根据筋膜侵犯和血管/淋巴结累及情况进行确定。Ⅰ~Ⅲ期通常可手术切除，但手术方法可因静脉受侵程度而有所不同(ⅢA期和ⅢC期)。
- RCC在超声上常表现为与肾皮质一致的等回声，但有时也可呈低回声或高回声。如为高回声(类似于AML)，当出现低回声晕征和肿瘤内部囊性变等影像学特征，则支持肾细胞癌(RCC)的诊断。彩色和频谱多普勒有助于鉴别肾静脉血栓(不属于ⅢA期)和癌栓。癌栓内有彩色多普勒血流信号及动脉波形。

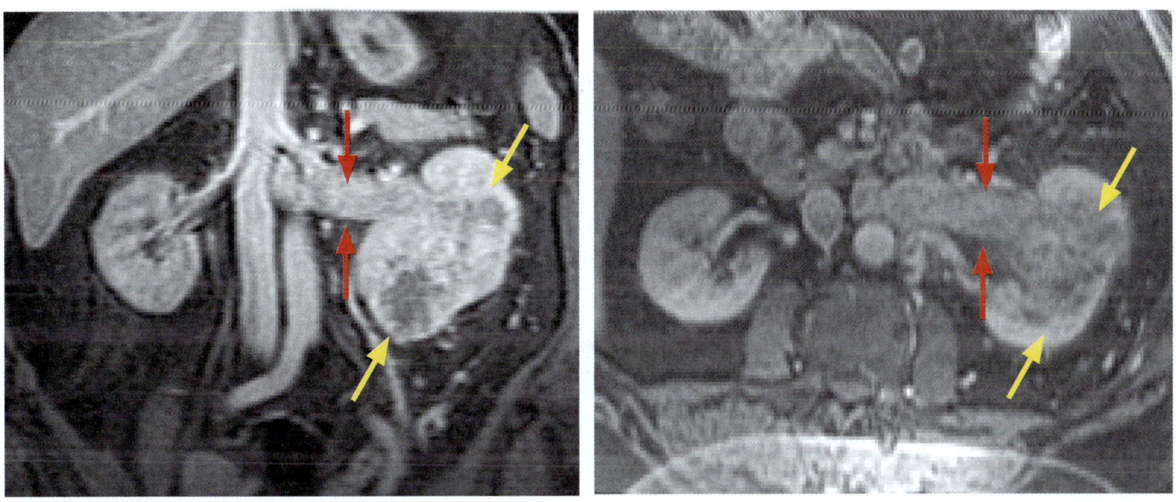

Renal cell carcinoma, stage 3A: Coronal (left image) and axial postcontrast fat-suppressed T1-weighted MRI (right image) shows a heterogeneously enhancing mass (yellow arrows) replacing and expanding most of the left kidney. Contiguous to the mass there is expansion and heterogeneous enhancement of the left renal vein (red arrows), representing tumor thrombus and extension of the renal carcinoma into the renal vein.

肾细胞癌(RCC)ⅢA期：冠状位(左图)和轴位增强后脂肪抑制T_1加权MRI(右图)显示一个增强不均匀的肿块(黄箭)，占据并取代了左肾的大部。与肿块相邻的左肾静脉有扩张和不均匀强化(红箭)，代表癌栓形成和肾癌累及肾静脉。

- **Clear cell** RCC is the most common subtype (~75%), with 5 year survival of ~55%.

  Clear cell RCC tends to enhance more avidly than the less common subtypes. Clear cell can be sporadic or associated with Von Hippel-Lindau.

  MRI shows T2 hyperintense signal with marked enhancement.
- **Papillary** RCC is a hypovascular subtype, with a 5-year survival of 80–90%.

  Papillary RCC tends to enhance only mildly due to its hypovascularity.

  A renal "adenoma" is frequently seen on autopsy specimens and is a papillary carcinoma ≤5 mm. MRI shows T2 hypointensity with mild enhancement.
- **Chromophobe** is the subtype with the best prognosis, featuring a 90% 5-year survival.

- **透明细胞**RCC是最常见的亚型(约75%)，5年生存率约为55%。

  肾透明细胞癌较其他不常见的亚型强化更加明显。透明细胞癌可以散发或见于VHL。

  MRI示T_2高信号及显著强化。
- **乳头状**RCC是一种乏血供亚型，5年生存率为80%~90%。

  乳头状RCC因其乏血供而仅有轻微强化。

  肾脏"腺瘤"常见于尸检标本，为≤5mm的乳头状癌。MRI为T_2低信号伴轻度强化。
- **嫌色细胞**型是预后最好的亚型，5年生存率达90%。

- **Sarcomatoid** differentiation can occur with subtypes above, resembling sarcoma with an aggressive behavior and poor prognosis.
- The enhancement kinetics can help differentiate the subtypes of RCC.

- **肉瘤样**变可发生在上述各亚型，类似于肉瘤的侵袭性和不良预后。
- 强化曲线可帮助区分RCC亚型。

Enhancement intensity of RCC subtypes
RCC亚型强化程度

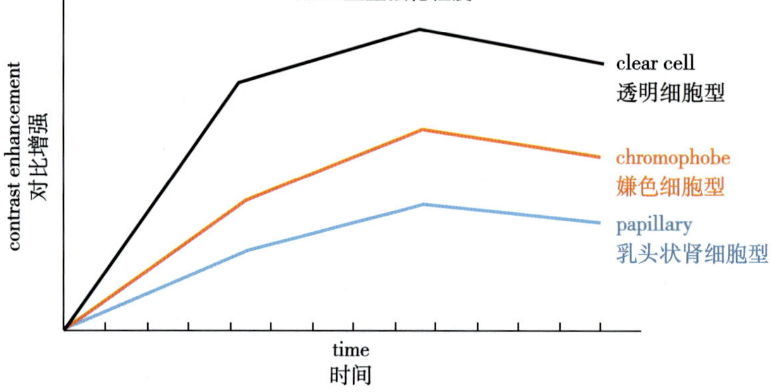

Enhancement characteristics of RCC subtypes: Clear cell RCC enhancement is the most rapid and highest over time, thus they may retain contrast on delayed images. Papillary RCC has relatively little enhancement.

RCC亚型的强化特征：透明细胞型RCC的强化最快且最高，因此在延迟图像上可能仍有造影剂滞留。乳头状RCC的强化程度相对较低。

Renal medullary carcinoma

- Medullary carcinoma is an infiltrative, extremely aggressive neoplasm, with a mean survival of 15 months, not helped by chemotherapy.
- On CT, it is seen as an ill-defined, infiltrative, hypovascular central renal mass. Necrosis and hemorrhage are common.
- Mostly affects young adult males with sickle cell trait. The imaging appearance is similar to renal transitional cell carcinoma, which occurs in an older population.

肾髓样癌

- 髓样癌是一种浸润性肿瘤，极具侵袭性，该病的平均生存期为15个月，化疗无效。
- CT表现为边界不清、浸润性、乏血供的中央型肾肿块。坏死和出血常见。
- 主要影响携带镰状细胞性状的年轻成年男性。影像学表现与肾脏移行细胞癌类似，而后者通常发生在年龄较大的患者中。

Collecting duct carcinoma

- Collecting duct carcinoma is rare. It shares features with renal medullary carcinoma and also has a poor prognosis.

集合管癌

- 集合管癌罕见，与肾髓样癌具有相同的特征，并且预后也很差。

Renal lymphoma

- Renal lymphoma (most commonly high-grade B-cell) may disseminate hematogenously or spread directly from the retroperitoneum to the kidney. Primary renal lymphoma is very rare and of uncertain origin as there is no native lymphoid tissue within the kidney.
- The most common imaging presentation of renal lymphoma is multiple hypoechoic renal masses. Retroperitoneal adenopathy is usually present. A solitary mass is an uncommon presentation. Diffuse lymphomatous infiltration producing nephromegaly is relatively rare.
- Renal involvement of lymphoma has several patterns of disease:

Multiple lymphomatous masses (most common pattern; seen in 50% of cases of renal lymphoma).
Solitary renal mass.
Diffuse lymphomatous infiltration, causing nephromegaly.
Direct extension of retroperitoneal disease.

肾淋巴瘤

- 肾淋巴瘤(最常见的为高级别B细胞)可经血行播散或直接从腹膜后扩散至肾脏。原发性肾淋巴瘤非常罕见且起源不明，因为肾内没有原生淋巴组织。
- 肾淋巴瘤最常见的影像学表现是多发性低回声肿块。腹膜后常见肿大淋巴结，孤立性肿块并不常见。引起肾肿大的弥漫性淋巴瘤浸润相对少见。
- 淋巴瘤肾脏受累有几种形式：

多发性淋巴瘤样肿块(最常见的类型，见于50%的肾淋巴瘤病例)。
孤立肾肿块。
弥漫性淋巴瘤样浸润，导致肾肿大。
腹膜后病变直接扩散。

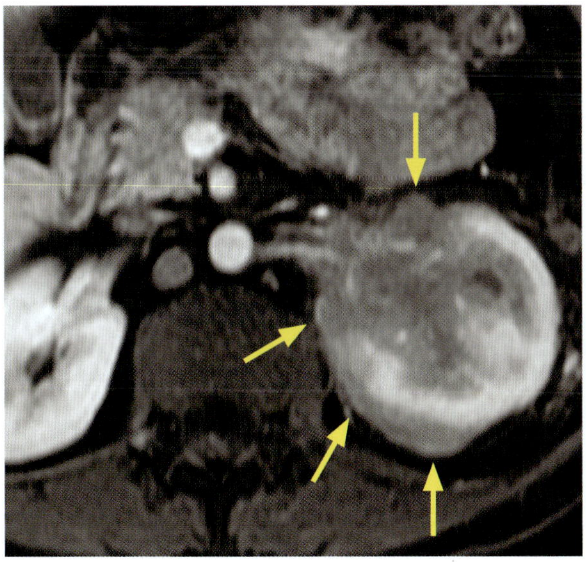

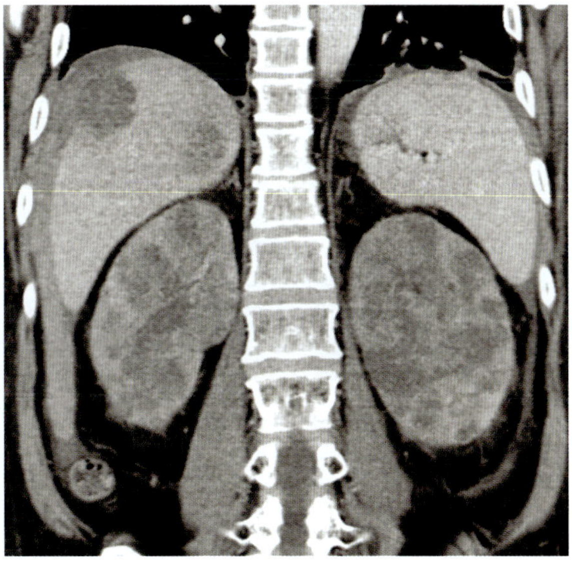

Two patterns of lymphoma involving the kidneys:

Axial contrast-enhanced T1-weighted MRI (left image) shows hypoenhancing soft tissue mass infiltrating the left kidney and perirenal region, and encasing the renal hilum/vessels (arrows).

Coronal contrast-enhanced CT (right image) shows multiple masses in bilateral kidneys and the liver, as well as enhancing soft tissue in the perihepatic region, all representing lymphomatous involvement.

淋巴瘤侵犯肾脏的两种方式：

轴位增强T_1加权MRI(左图)显示强化不明显的浸润性软组织肿块，累及左肾和肾周区域，并包裹肾门/血管(黄箭)。

冠状位增强CT(右图)显示双侧肾脏和肝脏有多发肿块，以及肝周区域的软组织强化，均为淋巴瘤所致。

SOLID RENAL MASSES – BENIGN

肾脏实性肿块——良性

Angiomyolipoma (AML)

血管平滑肌脂肪瘤(AML)

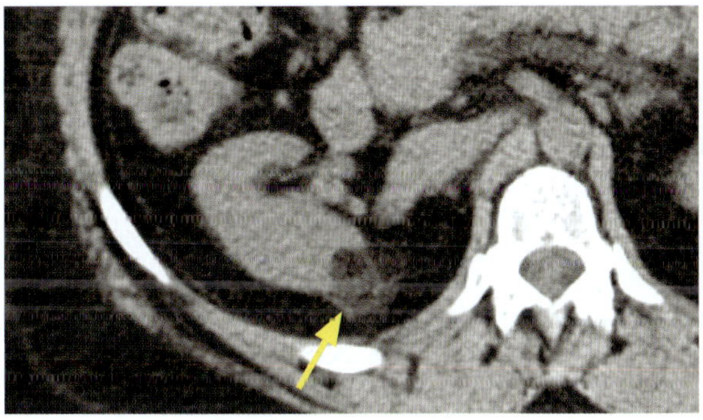

Axial noncontrast CT shows an exophytic mass (arrow) in the right kidney containing macroscopic fat. There are a few linear strands of soft tissue within the lesion.

轴位平扫CT显示右肾有一个外生性肿块(黄箭)，其中含有宏观的脂肪。病变内有一些线性软组织条纹影。

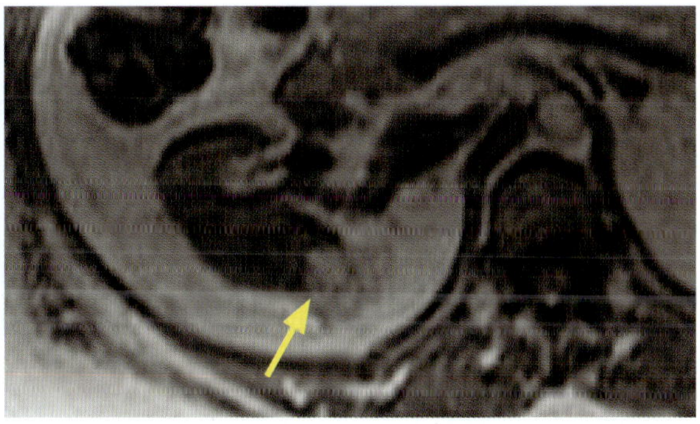

Axial T1-weighted MRI shows that the lesion is predominantly isointense to intra-abdominal fat.

轴位T_1加权MRI显示病变信号基本与腹腔内脂肪相等。

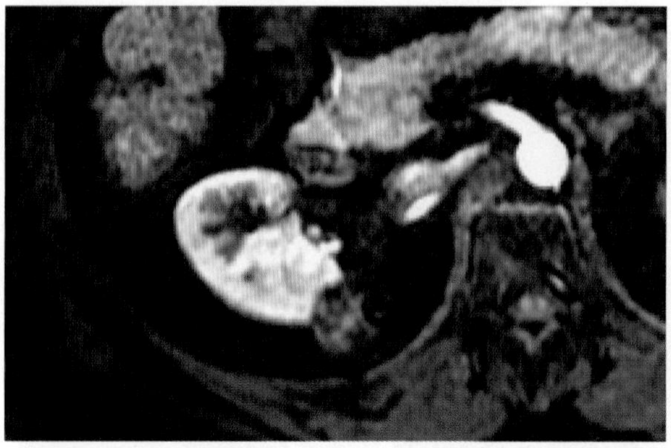

Axial early arterial postcontrast T1-weighted fat suppressed image shows slight enhancement of the soft tissue components.
轴位动脉早期增强T_1加权脂肪抑制图像显示软组织成分略有增强。

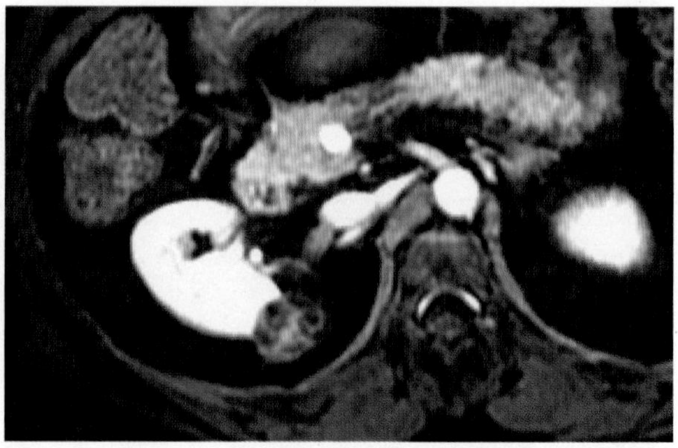

Late arterial postcontrast T1-weighted fat suppressed image shows more prominent enhancement of the soft tissue components of the lesion.
动脉晚期增强T_1加权脂肪抑制显示病变内软组织成分增强更加明显。

- Angiomyolipoma (AML) is a benign hamartoma made up of blood vessels (angio), smooth muscle (myo), and fat (lipoma). AMLs are the most common benign renal neoplasm. Most occur sporadically (unilateral and solitary), but 40% are associated with tuberous sclerosis (typically multiple and bilateral).
- Although benign, when AMLs are >4 cm in size, there is an increased risk of hemorrhage due to microaneurysm rupture within the vascular components of the AML.
- The presence of macroscopic fat in a non-calcified renal lesion is diagnostic of AML. The nonfat-containing portion enhances avidly and homogeneously. Calcification is rare in AMLs and should raise suspicion for RCC with macroscopic fat.
- On ultrasound, AML is echogenic due to the fat component. There is considerable overlap between the ultrasound appearance of AML and RCC. About one-third of AML demonstrate shadowing, which is a specific finding for AML.
- On MRI, the fat component will follow retroperitoneal fat on all sequences and will saturate out on fat-saturated sequences. The muscle component will be T2 hypointense. Intracytoplasmic lipid is not a feature of AML, so there should be no significant signal drop-out on dual-echo in- and out-of-phase images on MRI.
- 4% of AMLs lack macroscopic fat and appear as hyperdense enhancing mass on CT. In such cases, MRI can be helpful. A T2 *hyper*intense mass is suggestive of clear cell RCC or less likely oncocytoma. A T2 *hypo*intense mass may represent a fat-poor AML or papillary RCC, thus biopsy is usually recommended for definitive diagnosis. In rare cases, RCC with macroscopic fat has been described.

- 血管平滑肌脂肪瘤(AML)是一种良性错构瘤，由血管、平滑肌和脂肪组成。AML是最常见的良性肾肿瘤。大多数呈散发(单侧和单发)，但40%与结节性硬化有关(典型为多发和双侧)。
- AML虽为良性，但当大小>4cm时，因AML血管成分中的微动脉瘤破裂，出血的风险会增加。
- 无钙化的肾脏病灶中存在肉眼可见的脂肪是AML的诊断依据。不含脂肪的部分呈明显而均匀的强化。钙化在AML中很罕见，否则应怀疑为含脂肪RCC的可能。
- AML因存在脂肪成分而在超声上表现为回声增强。AML和RCC的超声表现存在很大重叠。约1/3的AML伴有声影，为AML的一个特异性征象。
- 在MRI图像上，肿块内的脂肪成分在所有序列上与腹膜后间隙的脂肪信号一致，且脂肪抑制序列上信号减低。肌肉成分为T_2低信号。胞质内脂质并非AML的特征性表现，因此在MRI的双回波同反相位图像上不应有明显的信号丢失。
- 约4%的AML不含宏观脂肪并在CT上表现为高密度的强化肿块。此时，MRI对这种情况有所帮助。T_2高信号的肿块常提示透明细胞RCC或可能性较低的嗜酸细胞瘤。T_2低信号肿块可能代表乏脂AML或乳头状RCC，因此通常需要活检以明确诊断。罕见情况下，RCC内有宏观脂肪。

Oncocytoma

肾嗜酸细胞瘤

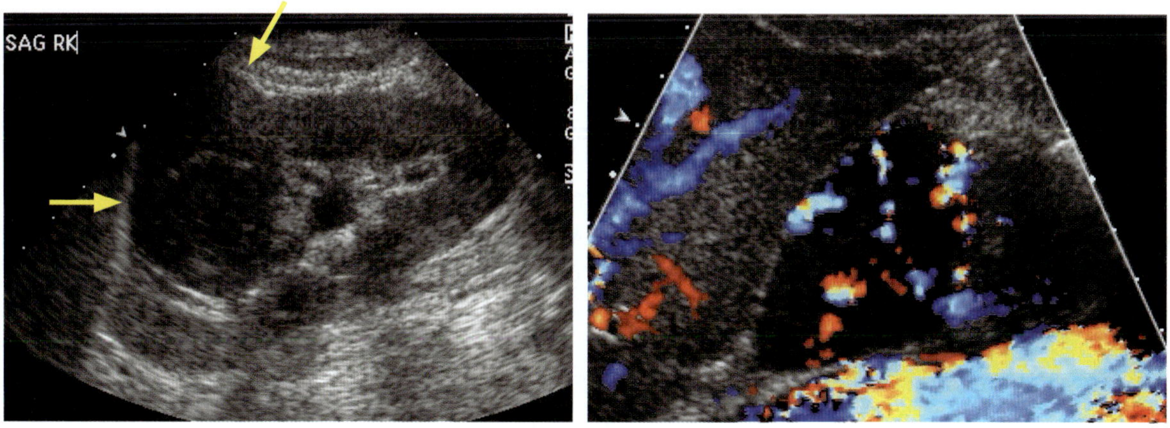

Oncocytoma: Sagittal ultrasound through the right kidney (left image) demonstrates an exophytic solid renal mass (arrows) that is isoechoic to cortex. Color Doppler suggests a *spoke-wheel* pattern of vascularity.

Case courtesy Julie Ritner, MD, Brigham and Women's Hospital.

肾嗜酸细胞瘤：右肾矢状切面超声(左图)显示一个外生性的实性肿物(黄箭)，以及肾皮质等回声。彩色多普勒(右图)显示血管呈轮辐状分布。

- Oncocytoma is a benign renal tumor arising from tubular cells. Due to significant imaging overlap with RCC, oncocytomas are usually biopsied or surgically resected.
- On ultrasound, oncocytoma is indistinguishable from RCC. It has variable echogenicity. A spoke-wheel vascular pattern is sometimes seen on color Doppler.
- On CT/MRI, certain features can *suggest* oncocytoma, but cannot reliably differentiate it from RCC. Features suggestive of oncocytoma include homogeneous enhancement and a central scar. The *segmental enhancement inversion sign* can be a more specific feature, referring to a "flip-flop" of enhancement of the tumor and central scar on early and late phases.

- 肾嗜酸细胞瘤是一种肾脏良性肿瘤，起源于肾小管细胞。嗜酸细胞瘤的影像学表现与RCC十分相似，因而常需要活检或手术切除。
- 肾嗜酸细胞瘤超声图像上无法与RCC进行鉴别。肾嗜酸细胞瘤回声表现多变，在彩色多普勒上有时可见轮辐状血流信号。
- 在CT/MRI上，某些特征可提示肾嗜酸细胞瘤，但不能可靠地将其与RCC进行区分。提示嗜酸细胞瘤的特征包括均匀强化和中央瘢痕。节段性增强反转征可能是一种更为特殊的特征，是指肿瘤和中央瘢痕在早期和晚期强化时呈"反转"现象。

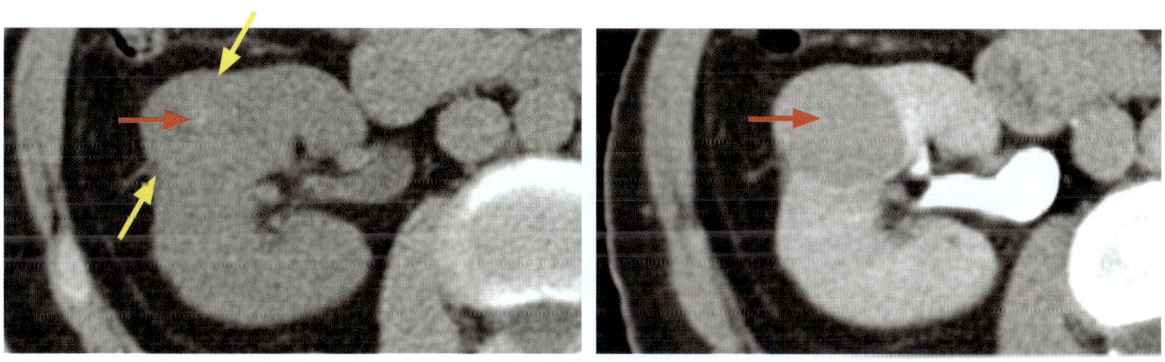

Oncocytoma: Noncontrast CT (left image) shows an isodense renal mass (yellow arrows) containing a central punctate focus of hyperattenuation (red arrow). The contrast-enhanced excretory phase CT (right image) demonstrates that the mass enhances. There is a faint suggestion of a central focus of non-enhancement (red arrows), corresponding to a central scar.

肾嗜酸细胞瘤：平扫CT(左图)显示一个等密度肾脏肿块(黄箭)，中心含点状高密度影(红箭)。增强CT排泄期(右图)显示肿块有强化，中央似有非强化灶(红箭)，对应于中央瘢痕。

- Diagnosis can be confirmed with percutaneous biopsy. Of note, oncocytic cells can be found in the rare chromophobe RCC subtype. However, pathologists can usually distinguish oncocytoma from the more common clear cell and papillary RCC subtypes.

- 经皮活检可确诊。注意，嗜酸细胞可见于罕见的RCC嫌色细胞Ⅲ型，但病理医生通常能将嗜酸细胞瘤与较为较常见的透明细胞和乳头状RCC进行区分。

Non-neoplastic solid renal masses

- When evaluating a potential renal mass, it's critical to exclude non-neoplastic etiologies with mass-like appearance.
- **Infection**, especially focal pyelonephritis, can mimic a solid renal mass. Renal abscess may be difficult to differentiate on imaging from a cystic renal cell carcinoma. Follow-up imaging is usually performed to confirm resolution following treatment with antibiotics.
- **Renal arteriovenous malformation** (AVM) will avidly enhance and can mimic a hypervascular renal mass. One clue to the presence of an AVM would be asymmetric enhancement of the renal vein on the affected side, due to early shunting of venous blood.

非肿瘤性实性肾脏肿块

- 评估一个潜在的肾脏肿块时，应首先排除具有肿块样外观的非肿瘤性病变。
- **感染**，尤其是局灶性肾盂肾炎，可与实性肾肿块的表现相似。肾脓肿在影像上可能难以与囊性RCC鉴别。通常会进行影像学随访，以确认在抗生素治疗后病变的消退情况。
- **肾动静脉畸形(AVM)**呈明显增强，可类似于富血供的肾肿瘤。提示AVM的一条线索是非对称性患侧肾静脉增强，为静脉早期分流所致。

SYNDROMES WITH RENAL MASSES (ALL HAVE INCREASED RIS OF RCC)

伴有肾脏肿块的综合征(均增加RCC的风险)

von Hippel-Lindau (VHL)

- von Hippel-Lindau (VHL) is an autosomal dominant multi-organ syndrome caused by a mutation in the VHL tumor suppressor gene on chromosome 3, which leads to cysts and neoplasms in multiple organs.
- The primary manifestation of VHL in the genitourinary system is multiple bilateral renal cell carcinomas, most commonly the clear cell subtype.
- Other genitourinary manifestations of VHL include multifocal pheochromocytoma and renal cysts.
- Central nervous system manifestations of VHL include hemangioblastoma of the brainstem, cerebellum, or spinal cord.
- Pancreatic and hepatic manifestations include malignant neuroendocrine pancreatic tumor, pancreatic serous cystadenoma (a benign neoplasm), and pancreatic/hepatic cysts.

希佩尔-林道病(VHL)

- 希佩尔-林道病(VHL)是一种由3号染色体的VHL抑癌基因突变引起的常染色体显性多器官综合征，可导致多器官出现囊肿和肿瘤。
- VHL在泌尿生殖系统的主要表现是双侧多发RCC，透明细胞亚型最常见。
- VHL的其他泌尿生殖系统表现包括多发嗜铬细胞瘤和肾囊肿。
- VHL的中枢神经系统表现包括脑干、小脑或脊髓的血管母细胞瘤。
- 胰腺和肝脏的表现包括胰腺恶性神经内分泌肿瘤、胰腺浆液性囊腺瘤(良性肿瘤)和胰腺/肝脏囊肿。

Birt-Hogg-Dubé

- Birt-Hogg-Dubé is an autosomal dominant syndrome (mutation of BHD gene on chromosome 17p) of dermatologic lesions, cystic lung disease, and multiple renal oncocytomas, renal cell carcinomas (chromophobe subtype), and hybrid chromophobe RCC-oncocytoma tumors.

伯特-霍格-迪贝综合征

- 伯特-霍格-迪贝综合征是一种常染色体显性遗传综合征(染色体17p上的*BHD*基因突变)，包括皮肤病变、肺囊性疾病和多发肾嗜酸细胞瘤、RCC(嫌色细胞亚型)、混合性嫌色细胞RCC-嗜酸细胞瘤。

Tuberous sclerosis (TS)

结节性硬化症(TS)

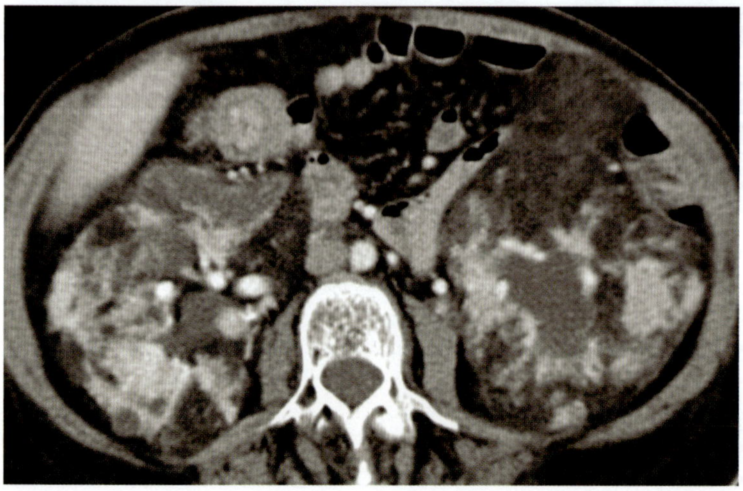

Axial contrast-enhanced CT shows multiple bilateral fat-containing renal masses, compatible with AMLs in this patient with known tuberous sclerosis.

轴位增强CT显示双侧多发含脂肪的肾脏肿块，与该患者已知结节性硬化症所伴发的AML相符。

- Tuberous sclerosis (TS) is an autosomal dominant neurocutaneous disease caused by a tumor suppressor gene mutation. It manifests clinically with seizures, developmental delay, and (mostly) benign tumors in multiple organ systems.
- The most common renal manifestation of TS is multiple bilateral renal angiomyolipomas (AMLs). Approximately 50% of patients with TS will have at least one AML.
- Renal cysts can be seen in ~25%.
- The relative risk of renal cell carcinoma is increased in patients with TS, which occurs in approximately 2–3% of patients. Diagnosis of renal cell carcinoma is complicated by the abnormal kidneys that may have multiple cysts and/or AMLs.
- In the heart, the most common neoplasm is a rhabdomyoma. A cardiac rhabdomyoma may be present during fetal life and can be detected by fetal ultrasound.
- In the lung, a process of smooth muscle proliferation identical to lymphangioleiomyomatosis can occur, causing cystic replacement of lung parenchyma. It has been suggested that the abnormal smooth muscle in the lung in patients with TS represents genetically identical metastatic smooth muscle from a renal angiomyolipoma.

Hereditary papillary RCC (HPRCC)

- HPRCC is an autosomal dominant syndrome that presents with multiple, bilateral papillary RCCs. It is associated with mutations in the MET gene.

Hereditary leiomyomatosis and RCC (HLRCC)

- HLRCC is an autosomal hereditary syndrome characterized by the development of multiple RCCs, uterine and cutaneous leiomyomas, and adrenal hyperplasia. The most commonly seen renal cancer subtype is papillary RCC.

Sickle cell trait

- Sickle cell is associated with medullary renal carcinoma.

Comparison of syndromes with renal masses

von Hippel-Lindau	Birt-Hogg-Dubé	Tuberous sclerosis	Hereditary papillary RCC	HLRCC	Sickle cell trait
Clear cell RCCs Renal cysts	Chromophobe RCCs Oncocytomas	Slightly increased risk of RCC Bilateral AMLs Renal cysts	Papillary RCCs	Multiple renal cancer subtypes, papillary most common	Medullary RCCs

Imaging of Renal Transplant

Approach to renal transplant

- The transplanted kidney is implanted in the right > left iliac fossa. It is easily evaluated by ultrasound due to its superficial location. Usually, a single kidney is transplanted, but en-bloc transplant of both kidneys into the recipient can be occasionally performed (i.e., pediatric donor kidneys to an adult recipient).
- The goal of ultrasound evaluation after renal transplant is to determine whether there is a treatable surgical or vascular complication. Ultrasound cannot reliably differentiate between the various causes of parenchymal rejection, but it is useful to guide percutaneous biopsy for definite diagnosis.
- An elevated RI (>0.7) suggests renal dysfunction, but this finding is nonspecific.

- 结节性硬化症(TS)是一种常染色体显性遗传性神经皮肤性疾病，为肿瘤抑制基因突变所致。临床表现为癫痫、发育延迟和多器官良性肿瘤(大部分)。
- TS最常见的肾脏表现是双侧多发血管平滑肌脂肪瘤(AML)。约50%的TS患者至少有一个AML。
- 约25%的患者有肾囊肿。
- RCC在结节性硬化症患者中的发生风险相对增加，为2%~3%。多发囊肿和/或AML等肾脏异常会增加RCC诊断的难度。
- 在心脏，最常发生的肿瘤是横纹肌瘤。心脏横纹肌瘤可能在胎儿时发生，胎儿超声可帮助检测。
- 在肺部，可出现与淋巴管平滑肌瘤病一样的平滑肌增殖，导致肺实质囊性化。有人认为，TS患者肺内异常的平滑肌在基因上与肾脏血管平滑肌脂肪瘤转移中的平滑肌完全一致。

遗传性乳头状肾细胞癌(HPRCC)

- 遗传性乳头状肾细胞癌(HPRCC)是一种常染色体显性遗传综合征，表现为双侧多发乳头状RCC。它与*MET*基因的突变有关。

遗传性平滑肌瘤病及RCC综合征(HLRCC)

- HLRCC是一种常染色体遗传性综合征，特征为多发RCC、子宫和皮肤平滑肌瘤，以及肾上腺增生。最常见的肾癌亚型是乳头状RCC。

镰状细胞性状

- 镰状细胞性状与肾髓样癌相关。

伴有肾脏肿块的综合征比较

希佩尔-林道病(VHL)	伯特-霍格-迪贝综合征	结节性硬化症	遗传性乳头状肾细胞癌(HPRCC)	遗传性平滑肌瘤病及RCC综合征(HLRCC)	镰状细胞性状
透明细胞RCC 肾囊肿	嫌色细胞RCC 嗜酸细胞瘤	RCC风险略有增加 双侧多发血管平滑肌脂肪瘤(AML) 肾囊肿	乳头状RCC	多种肾癌亚型，其中乳头状最常见	髓样RCC

肾移植影像

肾移植概要

- 移植肾植入髂窝，右侧较左侧常见。因其位置表浅，易行超声评估。通常行单个肾脏移植，但偶尔也可将两个肾脏一起移植到受体(即将儿童供体双肾移植至一个成人受体)。
- 肾移植后超声检查的目的是发现有无可治疗的外科或血管并发症。超声不能可靠地区分各种实质的排斥反应，但有助于引导经皮活检以明确诊断。
- RI升高(>0.7)提示肾功能异常，但无特异性。

Surgical complications following renal transplant

肾移植后的外科并发症

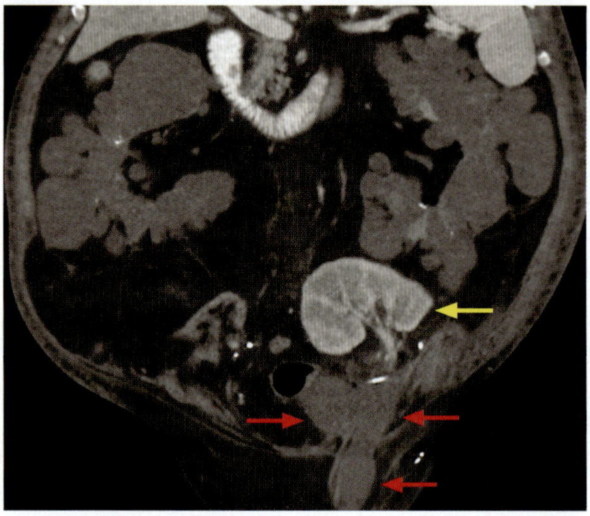

Coronal contrast-enhanced CT shows a transplant kidney in the left lower quadrant (yellow arrow) and native bilateral polycystic kidneys. There is a loculated fluid collection inferior to the transplant kidney which tracks into a left inguinal hernia (red arrows). Differential for this collection includes a seroma, urinoma, or lymphocele.

冠状位增强CT显示左下腹出现移植肾(黄箭)和自体双侧多囊肾。移植肾下方可见局限性液体聚集,并延伸至左侧腹股沟疝内(红箭)。该积液的鉴别诊断包括浆液囊肿、尿性囊肿和淋巴管囊肿。

- **Ureteral obstruction** is apparent on ultrasound as hydronephrosis.
- **Fluid collection** (blood, pus, urine) is highly dependent on timing:
  Immediately postoperative: Hematoma.
  1–2 weeks postoperative: Urinoma.
  3–4 weeks postoperative: Abscess.
  2nd month and beyond: Lymphocele.

Vascular complications following renal transplant

- **Renal vein thrombosis:** The renal *artery* Doppler may show reversal of diastolic flow.
- **Renal artery stenosis:** Elevated flow velocities are seen at the site of stenosis, with a *parvus et tardus* waveform distal to the stenosis. Usually takes several weeks to months to develop.
- **Pseudoaneurysm** is usually due to renal biopsy.

Medical complications following renal transplant

- Medical complications generally cannot be differentiated on ultrasound. Biopsy is necessary for diagnosis, although the time elapsed since the transplant may be a helpful clue.
- Hyperacute rejection: Occurs in first few hours after transplant.
  Hyperacute rejection is very rare, and is due to ABO blood type incompatibility.
- Acute tubular necrosis (ATN): Occurs in the immediate few postoperative days.
  ATN is usually a sequela of pre-implantation ischemia.
- Acute rejection: Occurs within three months of transplant.
- Chronic rejection: Occurs after three months of transplant.
- Drug toxicity may be caused by cyclosporine, which is nephrotoxic.

Post-transplant lymphoproliferative disorder (PTLD)

- Post-transplant lymphoproliferative disorder (PTLD) is a type of lymphoma that is thought to be due to immune suppression and Epstein-Barr virus proliferation.
- PTLD can arise anywhere in the body. Any new mass in any organ in a transplant patient should raise concern for potential PTLD.
- Ultrasound of renal PTLD will show an amorphous hypoechoic mass which may simulate a fluid collection on grayscale images. Unlike fluid, PTLD will demonstrate Doppler flow.

- **输尿管梗阻**在超声上表现为肾盂积水。
- **积液**(血液、脓液、尿液)与术后时间密切相关:
  术后即刻:血肿。
  术后1~2周:尿性囊肿。
  术后3~4周:脓肿。
  术后第2个月或以上:淋巴管囊肿。

肾移植后血管并发症

- **肾静脉血栓:**肾动脉多普勒检查可显示舒张期反向血流。
- **肾动脉狭窄:**可见狭窄处血流速度增快,狭窄远端出现小慢波。多在术后数周至数月出现。
- **假性动脉瘤**通常为肾活检所致。

肾移植后内科并发症

- 内科并发症通常不能用超声进行鉴别。明确诊断需要进行活检,移植术后的发病时间只能作为线索。
- 超急性排斥反应:发生在移植后的数小时内。
  超急性排斥反应非常罕见,为ABO血型不相容所致。
- 急性肾小管坏死(ATN):发生在术后数天内。
  ATN一般是肾植入前缺血所致。
- 急性排斥反应:发生在移植后3个月之内。
- 慢性排斥反应:发生在移植3个月之后。
- 药物毒性可能是由具有肾毒性的环孢素引起。

移植后淋巴增殖性疾病(PTLD)

- 移植后淋巴增殖性疾病(PTLD)是淋巴瘤的一个类型,可能是由免疫抑制和EB病毒增殖所致。
- PTLD可发生于人体的任何部位。移植患者的任何脏器出现任何新的肿块都应考虑PTLD的可能。
- 肾脏PTLD的超声表现为形态不规则的低回声团块,灰阶超声表现与积液相似。与积液不同,PTLD的内部有多普勒血流信号。

(翻译　张卓璐)

Ureter

Overview of ureteral imaging

CT urography (CTU) indications and protocol

- The goal of CT urography (CTU) is to evaluate the kidneys, ureters and bladder. The key to successful imaging is to opacify and optimally distend the ureters and bladder.
- One of the most common indications for CTU is the evaluation of hematuria. Hematuria may be caused by a urinary tract calculus, renal mass (e.g., renal cell carcinoma), and urothelial tumor (e.g., transitional cell carcinoma).
- Protocols vary by institution. Typically, patients are given 900 mL of water PO and either 250 mL of IV saline or 10 mg of IV furosemide to optimally distend the ureters and bladder.
- In adults ≥35 years of age, CTU is performed as a three-phase exam:

  Unenhanced CT of the abdomen and pelvis.

  Nephrographic phase through the kidneys (100 seconds after IV contrast administration).

  Excretory phase of the abdomen and pelvis (15 minutes after IV contrast).
- A split-bolus (dual-phase) technique decreases radiation exposure in patients under age 35:

  Unenhanced CT of the abdomen and pelvis.

  Combined nephrographic/excretory phase (8 minutes delay after first IV contrast bolus and 100 seconds after the second bolus).

Malignant ureteral disease

Transitional cell carcinoma (TCC)

输尿管

输尿管影像概述

CT尿路造影(CTU)的适应证和检查方法

- CT尿路造影(CTU)的目的是评估肾、输尿管及膀胱。影像成功的关键是让造影剂充盈并最大限度地扩张输尿管及膀胱。
- CTU最常见的适应证是评估血尿。血尿可由尿路结石、肾脏肿瘤(如RCC)或尿路上皮肿瘤(如移行细胞癌)引起。
- 检查方法因所在医院不同而有差异。通常的做法为:患者口服900mL饮用水,之后静脉注射250mL生理盐水或10mg呋塞米,使输尿管和膀胱得以最大充盈。
- 对35岁及以上的成人患者,CTU需做3期扫描:

  CT腹部和盆腔平扫。

  肾实质期肾脏扫描(静脉注射造影剂后100秒)。

  排泄期腹部和盆腔扫描(静脉注射造影剂后15分钟)。
- 对35岁以下的患者,进行分次团注法(双期)以降低辐射剂量:

  CT腹部和盆腔平扫。

  肾实质期/排泄期联合扫描(第1次团注造影剂后延迟8分钟及第2次团注造影剂后延迟100秒)。

恶性输尿管疾病

移行细胞癌(TCC)

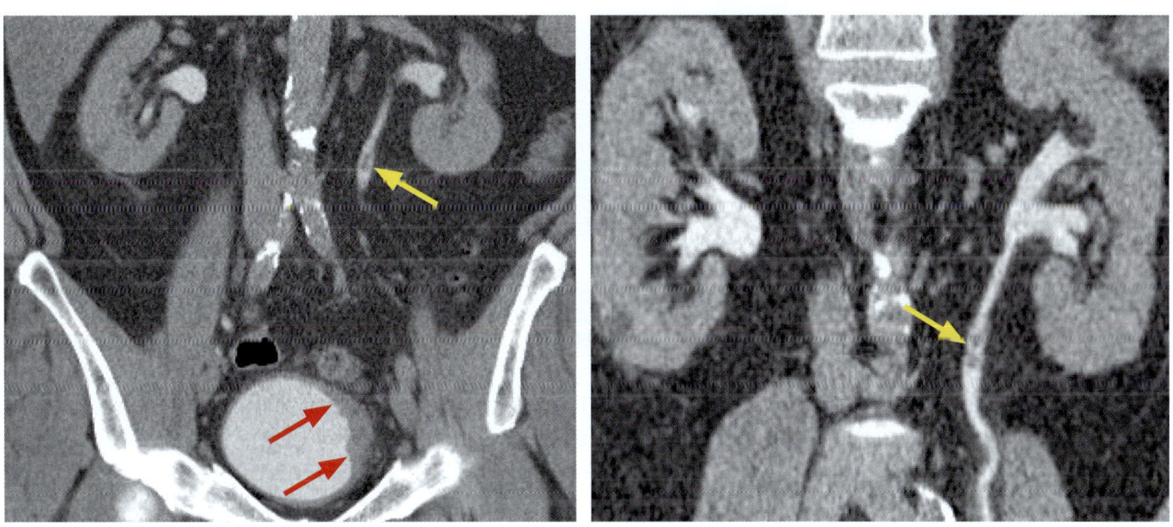

Multifocal transitional cell carcinoma: Coronal CT (left image) from the excretory phase of a CT urogram shows a sessile mass within the left lateral aspect of the bladder (red arrows) and a filling defect within the proximal left ureter (yellow arrow). Curved multiplanar reformation from the same study (right image) better shows the proximal ureteral filling defect (arrow).

Case courtesy Cheryl Sadow, MD, Brigham and Women's Hospital.

多发移行细胞癌:冠状位排泄期CT尿路造影(左图)显示膀胱左侧有无蒂肿块(红箭)及左侧近端输尿管内有充盈缺损(黄箭)。同一病例的曲面重建(右图)更好地显示了近端输尿管充盈缺损(黄箭)。

- Although upper tract malignancy is relatively rare, transitional cell carcinoma (TCC) is the most common ureteral neoplasm.
- The typical CTU appearance is of a single short segment of wall thickening, stricture, or filling defect at the excretory phase. However, multiple filling defects may be seen in 40%. Given the propensity of TCC for multifocal disease, the bladder should be evaluated for a synchronous mass.

- 上尿路恶性肿瘤相对罕见，但移行细胞癌(TCC)是其中最常见的输尿管肿瘤。
- 典型的CTU表现为排泄期一小段输尿管壁增厚、狭窄或充盈缺损；但多发充盈缺损可见于40%的病例。鉴于TCC有多发的倾向，应对膀胱进行检查以排除同步性肿瘤。

Benign ureteral masses

输尿管良性肿块

Fibroepithelial polyp

- Fibroepithelial polyp is the most common benign tumor of the ureter. It typically affects the proximal ureter. Fibroepithelial polyp features a long stalk and can be large. They usually appear as an elongated smooth tubular lesion. CTU best shows the lesion on the coronal images in the excretory phase. Transurethral excision is the treatment of choice.

Urothelial papilloma

- Urothelial papilloma is a rare benign neoplasm that may involve the bladder or ureter. The mass may become quite large and mimic a malignancy.

Inverted papilloma

- Inverted papilloma is a benign mass with a central core of urothelium.

输尿管纤维上皮息肉

- 纤维上皮息肉是输尿管最常见的良性肿瘤，常累及近段输尿管。纤维上皮息肉的特征是呈长柄状，且可能会很大，通常表现为长而光滑的管状病变。病变在排泄期冠状位CTU的图像显示最佳。治疗采用经尿道切除术。

尿路上皮乳头状瘤

- 尿路上皮乳头状瘤是一种罕见的良性肿瘤，可累及输尿管或膀胱。肿块可变得很大而类似于恶性肿瘤。

内翻性乳头状瘤

- 内翻性乳头状瘤是一种良性肿瘤，其中央核心为尿路上皮。

Inflammatory and infectious ureteral disease

炎症和感染性输尿管疾病

Ureteritis cystica

囊性输尿管炎

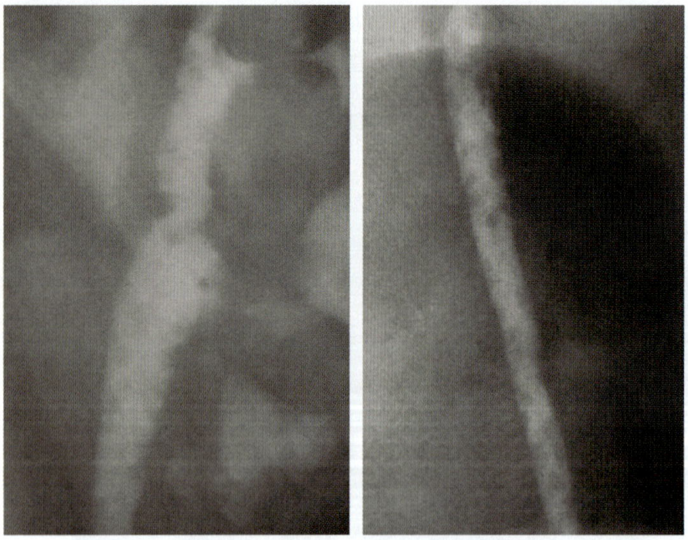

Pyeloureteritis cystica:
Frontal projection intravenous pyelogram shows multiple small nodular filling defects along the renal pelvis (left image) and ureter (right image).
囊性肾盂输尿管炎：
正位静脉肾盂造影显示多个沿肾盂(左图)和输尿管(右图)分布的小结节状充盈缺损。

- Ureteritis cystica is a benign response to chronic urinary tract inflammation, such as chronic infection or stone disease. Several small subepithelial cysts can be found unilaterally in the proximal third of the ureter and renal pelvis. Ureteritis cystica does not have any malignant potential.
- Imaging characteristically shows multiple tiny filling defects in the ureter.
- The same disease entity can affect the renal pelvis (called **pyelitis cystica**) and bladder (called **cystitis cystica**).

Leukoplakia (squamous metaplasia)

- Leukoplakia, also known as squamous metaplasia, is a rare urothelial inflammatory condition named for the characteristic white patch that it produces. Leukoplakia is not

- 囊性输尿管炎是慢性尿路炎症(如慢性感染或结石)引起的一种良性反应。可在单侧近段输尿管(上1/3)及肾盂内发现多个上皮下小囊肿。囊性输尿管炎无任何恶性倾向。
- 影像学特征为输尿管多发微小充盈缺损。
- 同一病变可累及肾盂(称为**囊性肾盂炎**)和膀胱(称为**囊性膀胱炎**)。

黏膜白斑病(鳞状上皮化生)

- 黏膜白斑病又称鳞状上皮化生，是一种罕见的尿路上皮炎性病变，命名来自其特征性的

thought to be premalignant when the renal collecting system is involved, although there is an association between squamous cell carcinoma and bladder leukoplakia.

- Imaging shows a flat mass or focal thickening of the renal pelvic or ureteral wall that may produce a characteristic *corduroy* appearance.

Malacoplakia

- Malacoplakia (*soft plaque*) is a rare chronic inflammatory granulomatous condition associated with chronic urinary tract infection (usually *Escherichia coli*) that is typically seen in middle-age women. It is not premalignant. The bladder is the most frequently involved organ, followed by the renal parenchyma, upper urinary tract, and urethra.
- Imaging shows multiple flat filling defects that characteristically involve the distal ureter and/or bladder.

Ureteral tuberculosis

- Multifocal ureteral stenoses are suggestive of ureteral tuberculosis, even more so if there is also evidence of renal tuberculosis (parenchymal calcification and scarring) and/or bladder tuberculosis (small capacity bladder with a thickened wall).

Differential diagnosis of a ureteral filling defect

- *The primary concern of a ureteral filling defect on CT urography is ureteral malignancy.*

differential of ureteral filling defect		
	• **Ureteral malignancy**, of which transitional cell carcinoma is by far the most common. • Ureteral calculus, which is almost always visible on pre-contrast images. • Blood clot. • Malacoplakia (multiple flat defects).	• Leukoplakia. • Infectious debris (e.g., a mycetoma). • Sloughed renal papilla. • Benign ureteral mass (e.g., fibroepithelial polyp).

Structural ureteral lesions

Ureteropelvic junction obstruction (UPJ obstruction)

白斑。黏膜白斑病累及肾脏集合系统时并不被认为是一种癌前病变，尽管鳞状细胞癌与膀胱黏膜白斑有相关性。

- 影像学表现为肾盂或输尿管壁内有扁平的肿块或局限性增厚，可产生灯芯绒样外观。

软化斑

- 软化斑(软斑)是一种罕见的慢性炎症性肉芽肿，与慢性尿路感染(常为大肠杆菌)有关，常见于中年妇女。软化斑不是癌前病变。膀胱是最常受累的器官，其次是肾脏、上尿路和尿道。
- 影像学表现为多发扁平的充盈缺损，以累及远端输尿管和/或膀胱为特征。

输尿管结核

- 多发局灶性输尿管狭窄提示输尿管结核，尤其合并肾结核(肾实质钙化和瘢痕)和/或膀胱结核(膀胱挛缩伴壁增厚)的迹象时可能性更大。

输尿管充盈缺损的鉴别诊断

- *CT输尿管造影显示输尿管充盈缺损时应首先考虑输尿管恶性肿瘤。*

输尿管充盈缺损的鉴别诊断		
	• **输尿管恶性肿瘤**，其中移行细胞癌最为常见。 • 输尿管结石，几乎在平扫图像上都可看到。 • 血凝块。 • 软化斑(多发扁平充盈缺损)。	• 黏膜白斑病。 • 感染碎片(如足菌肿)。 • 脱落的肾乳头。 • 良性输尿管肿块(如纤维上皮息肉)。

输尿管结构性病变

肾盂输尿管交界区(UPJ)梗阻

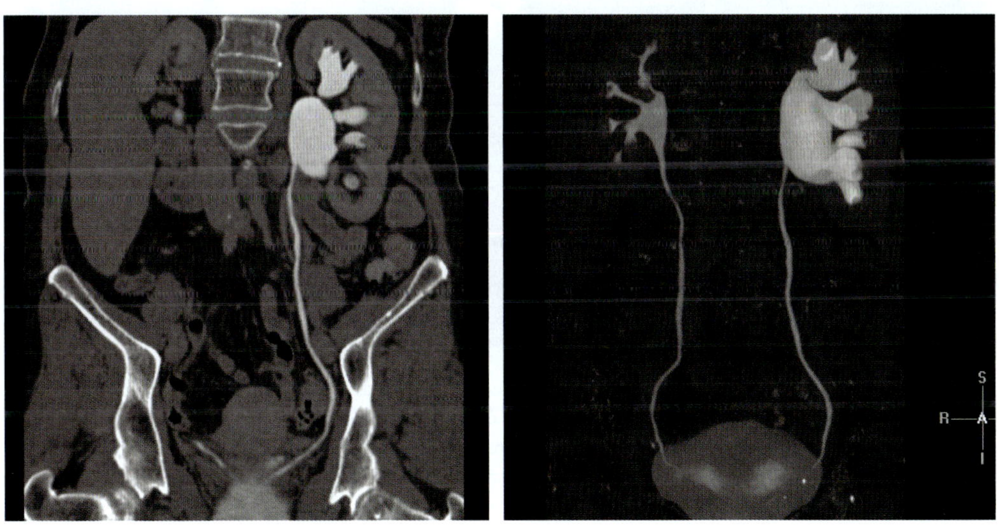

Coronal excretory phase CT and maximum intensity projection image show moderate left hydronephrosis without hydroureter, thought to represent primary UPJ obstruction.

冠状位排泄期CT和最大密度投影显示左侧中度肾盂积水，无输尿管积水，可能为原发性UPJ梗阻。

- Obstruction of the ureteropelvic junction (UPJ) can be either primary or secondary to infection, stones, or prior surgery.
- Primary UPJ obstruction may be due to a congenital aperistaltic segment of ureter, high insertion of the ureter on the renal pelvis, or crossing vessels causing extrinsic compression.
- The key imaging finding is a dilated renal pelvis with a normal caliber ureter.

- 肾盂输尿管交界区(UPJ)梗阻可以是原发或继发于感染、结石或手术后。
- 原发性UPJ梗阻可能是由于先天性无节段性输尿管蠕动、输尿管与肾盂交接处的位置过高或血管跨越肾盂引起的外压性梗阻导致。
- 关键的影像学表现是肾盂扩张但输尿管的直径正常。

Ureterocele

- An ureterocele is a focal dilation of the most distal portion of the ureter which protrudes into the bladder (*cobra head sign*). An ureterocele may be orthotopic or ectopic.
- An **orthotopic ureterocele** is seen with a normally inserting ureter, and is seen most commonly in adults. Orthotopic ureteroceles are also known as *simple*, *adult-type*, and *intravesicular* ureteroceles. Orthotopic ureteroceles are usually asymptomatic.
- An **ectopic ureterocele** is seen in the setting of a duplicated collecting system, with ectopic insertion of the upper pole ureter into the bladder (Weigert-Meyer rule), and is usually diagnosed in children.
- A **pseudoureterocele** represents intussusception of the distal ureter into the bladder, which may be due to tumor, radiation cystitis, or vesicoureteral junction stone.

输尿管囊肿

- 输尿管囊肿是输尿管末端的局限性扩张，并向膀胱内突出(蛇头征)。输尿管囊肿可为原位或异位。
- **原位输尿管囊肿**的输尿管开口正常，最常见于成人。原位输尿管囊肿又称为单纯性、成人型、膀胱内输尿管囊肿。原位输尿管囊肿常无症状。
- **异位输尿管囊肿**见于双重集合系统，上极输尿管异位汇入膀胱(Weigert-Meyer规则)，常在儿童期得到诊断。
- **假性输尿管囊肿**为远端输尿管发生套叠进入膀胱，可能为肿瘤、放射性膀胱炎或膀胱输尿管交界处结石所致。

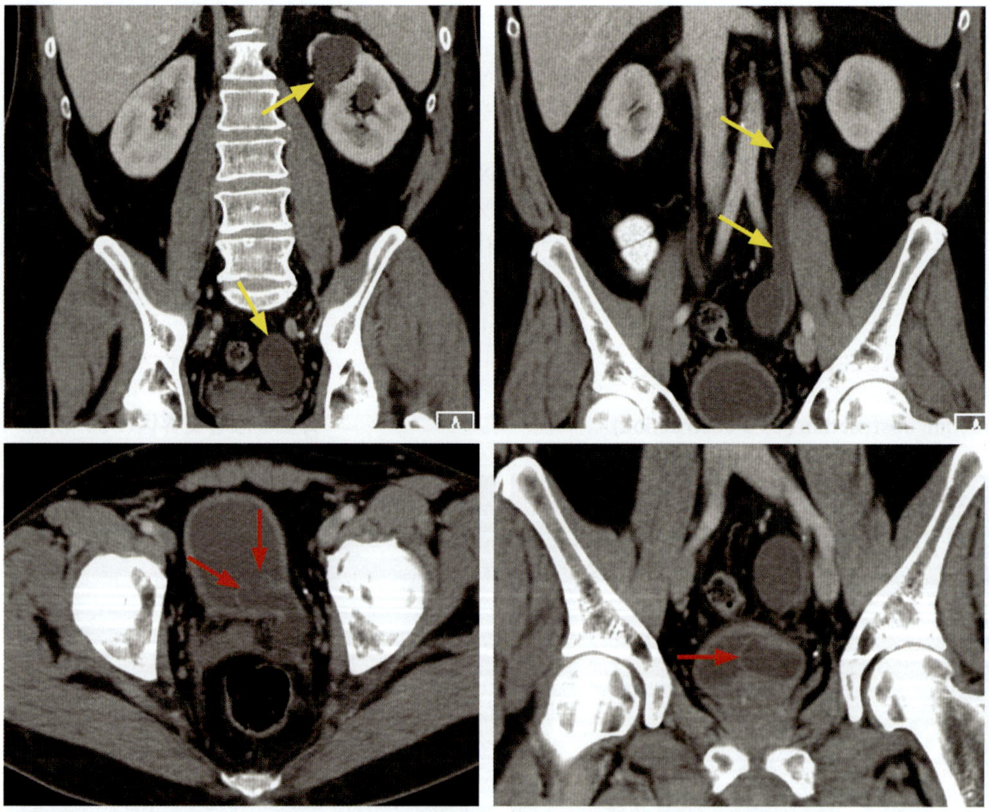

Duplicated ureter with ureterocele: Coronal contrast-enhanced CT (top images) show a duplicated left ureter. There is hydronephrosis of the upper pole moiety and marked dilation of the upper pole ureter (yellow arrows). Axial (bottom left image) and coronal (bottom right image) CT show the dilated ureter terminating within a ureterocele (red arrows). The dilated upper pole ureter inserts slightly posteriorly relative to the lower pole ureter (not shown) and represents an ectopic ureterocele.
Case courtesy Cheryl Sadow, MD, Brigham and Women's Hospital.
重复输尿管伴输尿管囊肿：冠状位增强CT(上两图)显示左侧重复输尿管，上极肾盂积水及输尿管明显扩张(黄箭)。轴位(左下图)和冠状位(右下图)CT显示扩张的输尿管终止在输尿管囊肿内(红箭)。扩张的上极输尿管较下极输尿管在稍靠后的部位进入膀胱(未展示)，此为异位输尿管囊肿。

(翻译　张卓璐)

BLADDER

膀胱

Bladder stones

- Risk factors for bladder stones include urinary stasis (most often bladder outlet obstruction) and chronic inflammation (e.g., from infection or foreign body).
- An off-midline bladder stone should raise concern for a bladder mass or enlarged prostate which displaces the bladder stone, or a stone within a ureterocele or a bladder diverticulum.

膀胱结石

- 膀胱结石的危险因素包括尿潴留(最常见于膀胱出口阻塞)和慢性炎症(如感染或异物引起的)。
- 偏离中线的膀胱结石应怀疑是否因膀胱肿块或增大的前列腺导致结石移位，或结石位于输尿管囊肿或膀胱憩室内。

Bladder transitional cell carcinoma (TCC)

膀胱移行细胞癌(TCC)

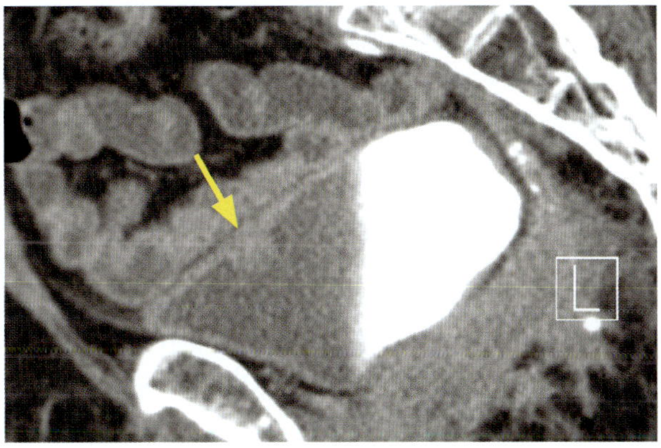

Sagittal CT in the excretory phase shows excreted contrast opacifying the posterior half of the bladder. There is a mass (arrow) arising in the superior bladder wall in the unopacified portion of the bladder. Bladder masses can be extremely subtle without complete bladder opacification.

矢状位CT排泄期显示造影剂充盈膀胱的后半部分。在无造影剂充盈的部分可见起源于膀胱上壁的肿块(黄箭)。膀胱未被造影剂完全充盈，膀胱肿块可能极其隐蔽而不易观察。

- Transitional cell carcinoma is by far the most common bladder cancer.
- TCC typically presents with painless hematuria, more commonly seen in older males with risk factors such as smoking and aromatic amines.
- Bladder cancer spreads through the wall of the bladder. Organ-confined disease can be divided into non-muscle-invasive (70%; typically resected endoscopically) and muscle-invasive (25%; typically treated with radical cystectomy/nodal dissection).
- Metastatic bladder cancer (5%) is treated with systemic therapy.
- If bladder cancer is clinically suspected in the context of macroscopic hematuria, cystoscopy and urine cytology are warranted regardless if a lesion is detected on CT urogram.

- 膀胱移行细胞癌(TCC)为最常见的膀胱癌。
- TCC通常表现为无痛性血尿，常见于吸烟或有芳香胺接触史的老年男性。
- 膀胱癌通过膀胱壁进行播散。局限性膀胱癌可分为非肌层浸润型(70%；通常行内镜下切除)和肌层浸润型(25%；通常行根治性膀胱切除术/淋巴结清扫术)。
- 转移性膀胱癌(5%)需进行系统治疗。
- 临床因肉眼血尿怀疑膀胱癌时，无论CT尿路造影是否检测到病变，都需行膀胱镜检查和尿细胞学检查。

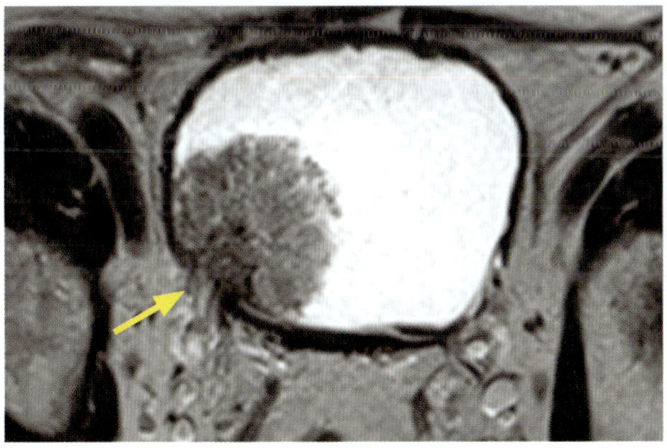

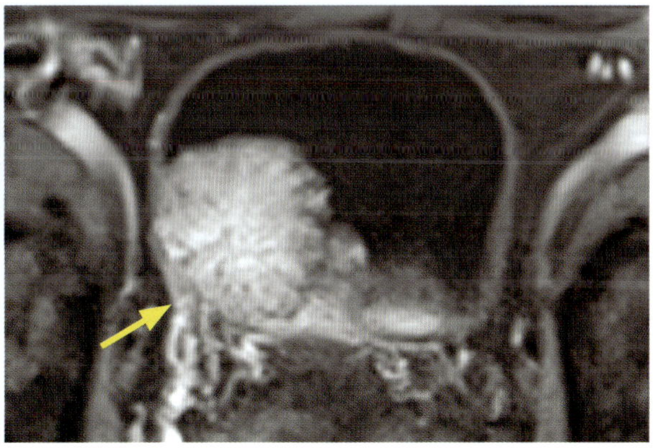

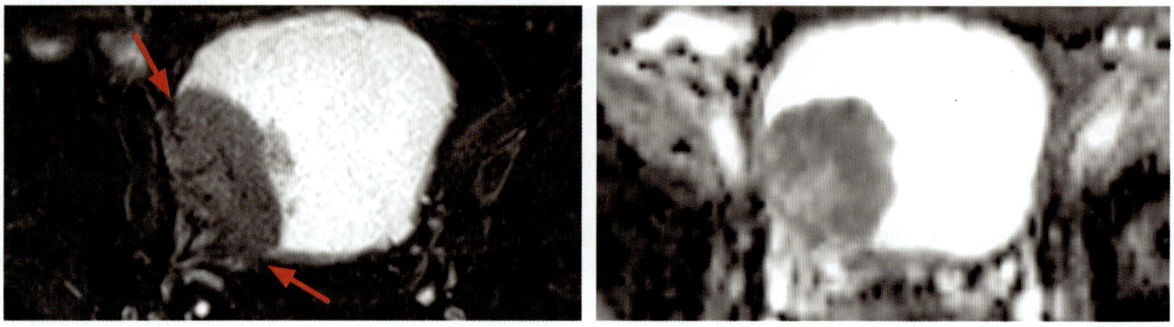

MRI Axial T2 (top left image) shows polypoidal mass arising from the right posterolateral bladder wall with a T2 hypointense stalk (yellow arrows). Axial T1 post-contrast (top right image) shows avidly enhancing mass with feeding vessels from the right internal iliac artery branches. ADC (bottom right image) show restricted diffusion of the "cap" of the tumor rather than the stalk. T2 with fat sat (bottom left) is key as it shows T2 intermediate signal involving the bladder wall and invading the muscularis propria (red arrows), **stage Ⅱb disease**.
轴位T_2加权MRI(左上图)显示膀胱右后外侧壁的息肉状肿块，具有T_2低信号蒂(黄箭)。增强T_1加权(右上图)显示肿块明显强化和来自右侧髂内动脉分支的供血血管。ADC图(右下图)显示肿瘤"帽"部呈扩散受限，而蒂部无扩散受限。脂肪抑制T_2序列(左下图)是关键，显示T_2中等信号侵及膀胱壁并侵入固有肌层(红箭)，**因此为Ⅱb期**。

Bladder adenocarcinoma

- Adenocarcinoma of the bladder is rare but it is usually associated with an urachal remnant.
- The fetal urachus extends from the bladder dome to the umbilicus. It should be obliterated after birth, but may persist as a urachal anomaly (discussed in the Pediatric imaging section).

膀胱腺癌

- 膀胱腺癌罕见，但常与残留脐尿管相关。
- 胎儿脐尿管从膀胱顶部延伸至脐。脐尿管在出生后应消失，若持续存在即为脐尿管异常(将在儿科影像部分讨论)。

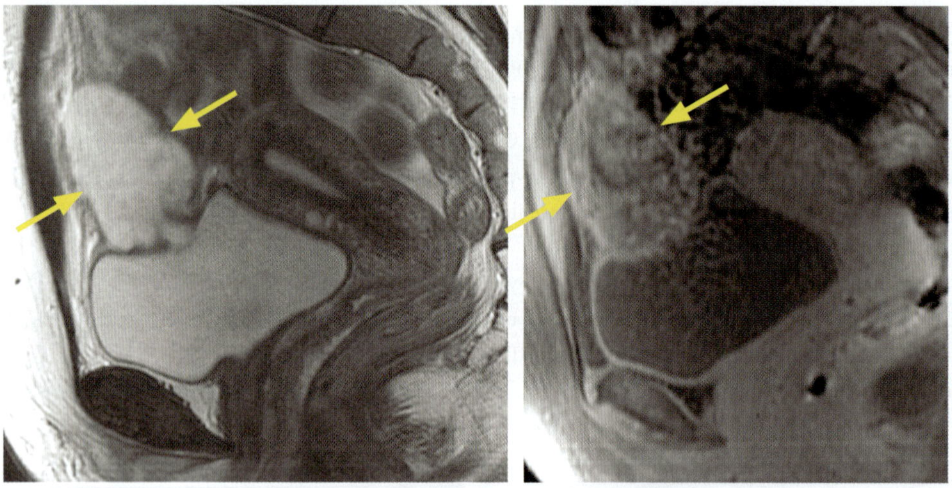

Urachal adenocarcinoma: Sagittal T2-weighted (left image) and sagittal postcontrast fat suppressed T1-weighted MRI (right image) shows an irregular, T2 hyperintense, avidly enhancing mass directly superior to the bladder (arrows). The mass connects to both the bladder and the umbilicus (not shown).
Case courtesy Cheryl Sadow, MD, Brigham and Women's Hospital.
脐尿管腺癌：矢状位T_2加权(左图)和矢状位增强脂肪抑制T_1加权 MRI(右图)显示一个紧贴膀胱上方的不规则肿块(黄箭)，呈T_2高信号并显著强化。此肿块连接膀胱和脐部(未展示)。

Bladder trauma

- CT cystography/cystogram is the standard test to evaluate for suspected bladder rupture.
- Full distension of the bladder is needed to evaluate for bladder rupture. Delayed imaging of an intravenous contrast study with opacification of excreted urine

膀胱创伤

- CT膀胱摄影术/膀胱造影是评估可疑膀胱破裂的标准检查方法。
- 评估膀胱破裂时需将膀胱完全充盈。静脉注射造影剂后延迟尿路显影的方法不够敏感，

is not sensitive enough, as it does not adequately distend the bladder, and is not the standard of care.

- To perform a CT cystogram, a total volume of at least 300 mL (or as much as the patient can tolerate) of dilute water-soluble contrast (50 mL of IV contrast mixed in 500 mL of warm saline) is instilled into the bladder by gravity, with the bag raised 40 cm above the bladder.
- Male patients with bladder injury may have associated urethral injury. If there is blood at the urethral meatus or if there is gross hematuria, a retrograde urethrogram should be performed prior to Foley catheter placement.
- Bladder injury can be classified as extraperitoneal (most common), intraperitoneal, or combined.

因造影剂不能充分扩张膀胱，所以不是标准的检查方法。

- 行CT膀胱造影时，需将至少300mL(或患者可以忍受的最大量)稀释的水溶性造影剂(50mL造影剂与500mL温生理盐水混合)通过重力作用灌入膀胱，可将输液袋抬高至膀胱上方40cm处。
- 男性患者在膀胱损伤时可能伴发尿道损伤。如有尿道口出血或肉眼血尿，在插入导尿管前应行逆行尿道造影。
- 膀胱损伤可分为腹腔外(最常见)、腹腔内或腹腔内外联合损伤。

Extraperitoneal bladder rupture

腹腔外膀胱破裂

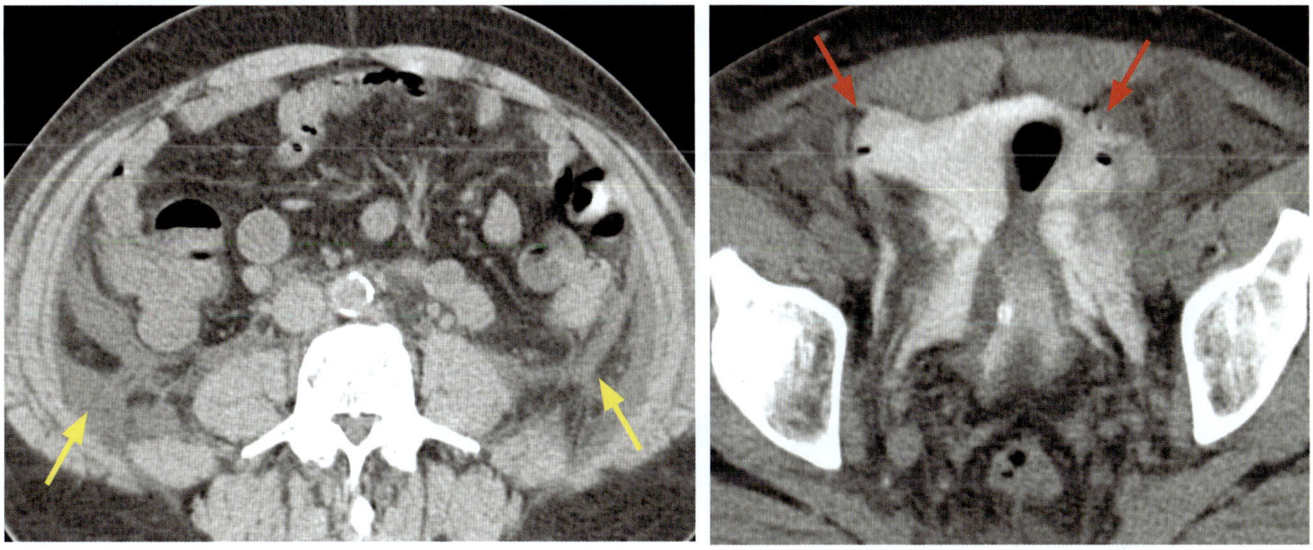

Unenhanced CT (left image) shows fluid stranding within the retroperitoneum (yellow arrows). There is no fluid between loops of bowel. CT cystogram (right image) shows the *molar tooth sign* of extravasated contrast anterior to and lateral to the bladder. There are few extra-luminal foci of gas (red arrows) within this extra-peritoneal contrast collection. *Case courtesy Cheryl Sadow, MD, Brigham and Women's Hospital.*

平扫CT(左图)显示腹膜后有液体渗出(黄箭)，肠袢之间未见积液。CT膀胱造影(右图)显示膀胱的前方与两侧有造影剂溢出而形成的*磨牙征*，腹膜外的造影剂中可见少许气泡(红箭)。

- Extraperitoneal bladder rupture is defined as rupture of the bladder outside of the peritoneal space. Extraperitoneal bladder rupture is at least twice as common as intraperitoneal rupture.
- Extraperitoneal bladder rupture is more commonly associated with pelvic fractures compared to intraperitoneal rupture. It is typically caused by direct laceration of the bladder by a bone fragment.
- The *molar tooth sign* describes the characteristic inverted U appearance of extravasated contrast in the extraperitoneal space of Retzius, which mimics a molar tooth.
- Extraperitoneal bladder rupture is typically managed conservatively, by placement of a urinary catheter.

- 腹腔外膀胱破裂指膀胱破裂位于腹膜外间隙。腹腔外膀胱破裂发生率至少是腹腔内膀胱破裂的2倍。
- 与腹腔内破裂相比，腹腔外膀胱破裂更常见于骨盆骨折，常由骨折碎片直接撕裂膀胱所致。
- *磨牙征*是指特征性的“反U”形造影剂外溢，并积聚于腹膜外耻骨后间隙，类似于“磨牙”。
- 腹腔外膀胱破裂通常行保守治疗，即放置导尿管。

Intraperitoneal bladder rupture

腹腔内膀胱破裂

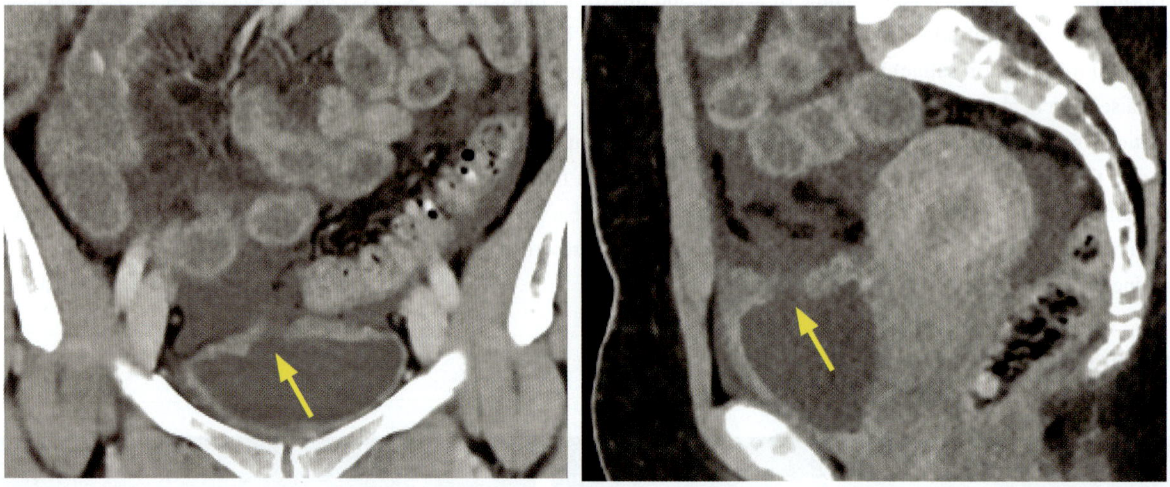

Coronal and sagittal contrast-enhanced CT demonstrates a focal wall defect at the bladder dome (arrows) and intraperitoneal fluid interdigitated between loops of bowel.
冠状位和矢状位增强CT显示膀胱顶部有局部壁缺损(黄箭)和肠袢之间的腹腔内液体积聚。

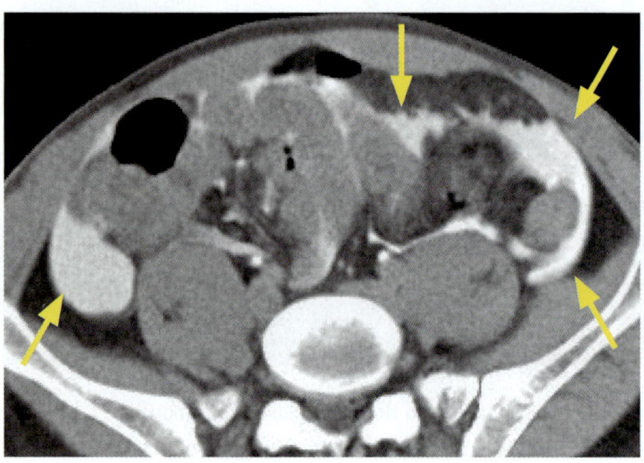

Axial CT cystogram in another patient shows intraperitoneal contrast extravasation (arrows) between numerous loops of bowel, diagnostic of an intraperitoneal bladder rupture.
另一名患者轴位CT膀胱造影显示腹腔内多个肠袢间有外渗的造影剂(黄箭),可诊断为腹腔内膀胱破裂。

- Intraperitoneal bladder rupture occurs with disruption of the bladder dome and peritoneum, causing resultant extravasation of urine into the peritoneal space.
- The mechanism of intraperitoneal bladder rupture is thought to be through pressure forces on a full bladder causing bursting at the dome into the peritoneum.
- The pathognomonic imaging finding on CT cystogram is intraperitoneal contrast interdigitating between loops of bowel.
- Intraperitoneal bladder rupture is typically treated surgically.

- 腹腔内膀胱破裂见于膀胱穹隆和腹膜出现破裂,造成尿液外渗至腹膜腔。
- 腹腔内膀胱破裂的机制可能是压力作用于完全充盈的膀胱,引起膀胱穹隆破裂,尿液进入腹腔。
- 具有诊断价值的CT膀胱造影征象为腹腔内造影剂交错出现在肠袢间。
- 腹腔内膀胱破裂常需通过手术进行治疗。

(翻译　张卓璐)

MALE GENITOURINARY SYSTEM

男性泌尿生殖系统

MALE URETHRAL ANATOMY

男性尿道解剖

***posterior urethra* 后尿道**

prostatic urethra 尿道前列腺部
site of TURP 经尿道前列腺切除术的部位
membranous urethra 尿道膜部

***anterior urethra* 前尿道**

bulbous urethra 尿道球部
site of gonococcal stricture 淋病性狭窄的部位
penile urethra 尿道阴茎部
site of post-catheter stricture 插管后狭窄的部位

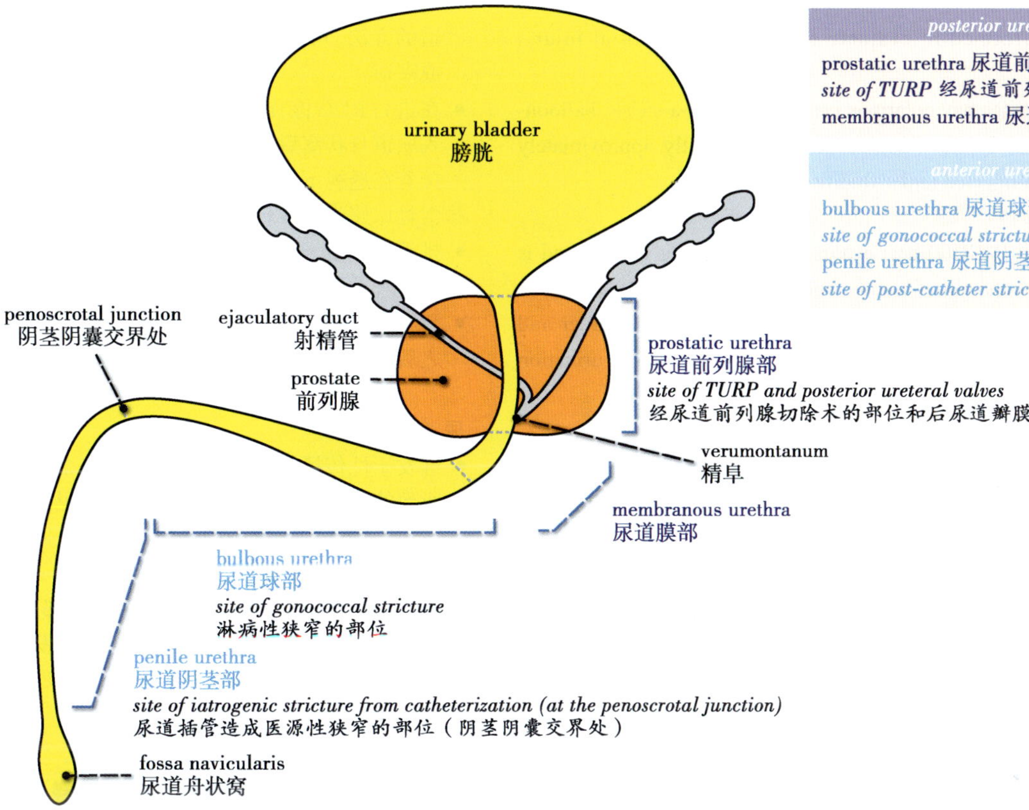

posterior urethra：
后尿道
prostatic urethra
尿道前列腺部
membranous urethra
尿道膜部

anterior urethra：
前尿道
bulbous urethra
尿道球部
penile urethra
尿道阴茎部

Prostatic urethra (posterior urethra)

- The prostatic urethra is lined with transitional epithelium.
- The verumontanum is a prominent ridge of smooth muscle in the posterior portion of the prostatic urethra and the site of the paired ejaculatory duct orifices. The verumontanum is also the site of obstruction in posterior urethral valves in children. The prostatic utricle is a Müllerian duct derivative and is the blind-ending male homologue of the uterus and vagina, which is also located at the verumontanum.

Membranous urethra (posterior urethra)

- The membranous urethra is the shortest, least mobile urethral segment.
- The membranous urethra is contained within the urogenital diaphragm, which contains the external urethral sphincter and the paired Cowper's glands.

Bulbous urethra (anterior urethra)

- The bulbar urethra is the site of drainage of Cowper's (or bulbourethral) glands.

Penile urethra (anterior urethra)

- The penile urethra is the longest urethral segment, lined with squamous epithelium.
- The distal portion of the penile urethra is dilated at the glans penis. This dilation is called the fossa navicularis.
- The glands of Littré are small mucous glands of the penile urethra. Normally, small ducts would be occluded by balloon during a retrograde urethrogram, and

尿道前列腺部(后尿道)

- 尿道前列腺部内衬移行上皮。
- 精阜是尿道前列腺部后壁平滑肌的隆起部分，是一对射精管的开口位置。精阜也是儿童后尿道瓣膜梗阻的位置。前列腺小囊也位于精阜，是米勒管的残留物，相当于子宫和阴道在男性的同源盲端。

尿道膜部(后尿道)

- 尿道膜部是尿道最短、最固定的部位。
- 尿道膜部位于尿生殖膈内，包括尿道外括约肌和一对尿道球腺。

尿道球部(前尿道)

- 尿道球部是尿道球腺(又称Cowper腺)开口的位置。

尿道海绵体部(前尿道)

- 尿道海绵体部是尿道中最长的部分，衬有鳞状上皮。
- 尿道海绵体部的远段在阴茎头处膨大，此膨大被称为舟状窝。
- 尿道腺是尿道海绵体部的小黏液腺。正常情况下，逆行尿路造影时小导管被球囊封闭，因

therefore would not opacify with injected contrast. The glands of Littré tend to opacify more prominently when inflamed in the setting of urethritis.

而无造影剂充填。尿道炎时，尿道腺可因炎症而出现更加明显的强化。

IMAGING OF THE MALE URETHRA

男性尿道影像

Retrograde urethrogram (RUG)

- Retrograde urethrogram (RUG) provides excellent evaluation of the anterior urethra and may be performed to evaluate for suspected urethral injury, stricture, or fistula.
- To perform a RUG, the fossa navicularis is cannulated with a sterile balloon-tipped catheter that is inflated with 1–2 mL saline. Subsequently, approximately 10 mL of contrast is hand-injected under fluoroscopy.

Voiding cystourethrogram (VCUG)

- Voiding cystourethrogram (VCUG) best evaluates the posterior urethra and is typically performed for evaluation of bladder and voiding function.
- To perform a VCUG, a Foley catheter is sterilely placed in the bladder and subsequently contrast is instilled into the bladder. The patient initiates urination during fluoroscopy.

逆行尿路造影(RUG)

- 逆行尿路造影(RUG)是一个极好的评估前尿道的方法，可用于评估可疑的尿道损伤、狭窄或窦道。
- 在进行RUG检查时，将消毒后的球囊导管插入尿道舟状窝后用1~2mL生理盐水扩张球囊。接着在透视下手动注射约10mL造影剂。

排泄性尿路造影(VCUG)

- 排泄性尿路造影(VCUG)是评估后尿道的最佳检查手段，通常用于检查膀胱的排空功能。
- 行VCUG检查时，将无菌福莱导管插入膀胱，之后灌注造影剂。患者在透视下开始排尿。

Urethral stricture

- Urethral strictures secondary to sexually transmitted disease (most commonly chronic urethritis from *Neisseria gonorrhoeae*) occur most commonly in the bulbous urethra. A complication of chronic urethral infection is a periurethral abscess, which may result in a urethroperineal fistula.
- Post-traumatic saddle injury strictures also tend to occur in the bulbous urethra.
- In contrast, an iatrogenic stricture from a Foley catheter tends to occur in the penile urethra at the penile-scrotal junction.

尿道狭窄

- 继发于性传播性疾病(最常见为淋病奈瑟球菌所致的慢性尿道炎)的尿道狭窄最常见于尿道球部。慢性尿路感染的并发症之一是尿道周围脓肿，可导致尿道会阴瘘。
- 骑跨伤导致的狭窄也常发生于尿道球部。
- 相反，福莱导管所致的医源性狭窄常发生于尿道海绵体部的阴茎阴囊交界处。

Urethral trauma

尿道外伤

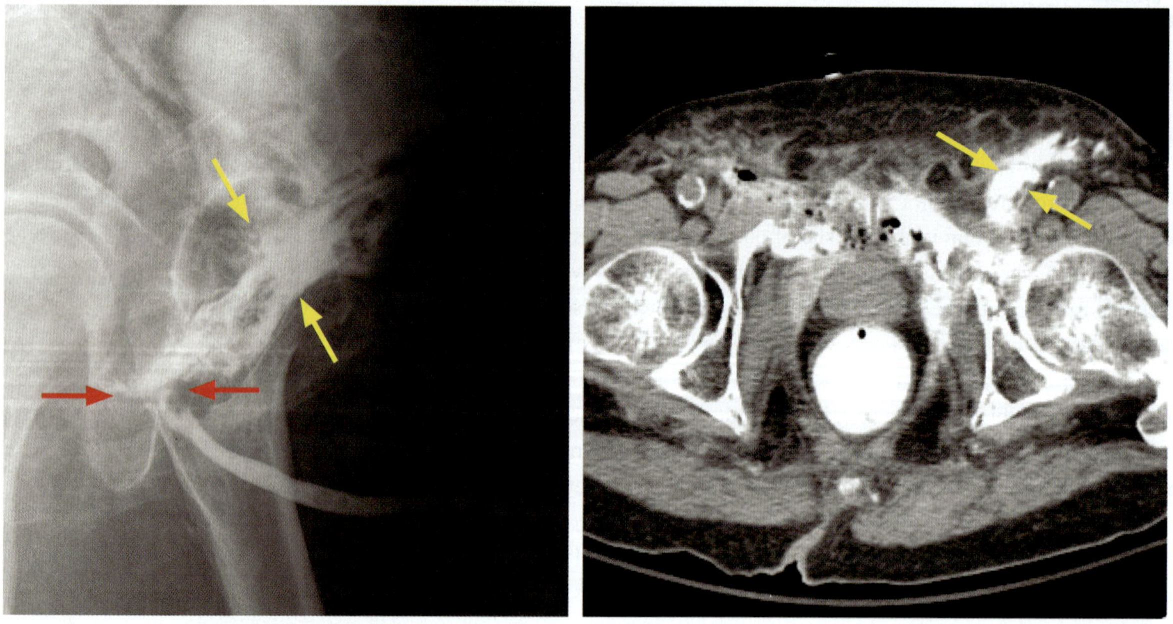

Type Ⅲ urethral injury: Retrograde urethrogram (left image) shows free extravasation of contrast (arrows) at the bulbomembranous urethra (red arrows). Post-RUG CT shows the excreted contrast in the left inguinal space (arrows) and the deep pelvis. Pelvic fractures and gas from a projectile tract are partially seen.

Case courtesy Cheryl Sadow, MD, Brigham and Women's Hospital.

Ⅲ型尿道损伤：逆行尿路造影(RUG)(左图)显示尿道球、膜部(红箭)游离外渗的造影剂(黄箭)。RUG后CT(右图)显示左侧腹股沟间隙(黄箭)及骨盆深部外渗的造影剂。同时观察到子弹贯穿路径上的骨盆骨折及气体。

- In the setting of trauma, if there is blood at the meatus, painful urination, or inability to void, a RUG should be performed emergently to exclude an urethral injury. If confirmed, a suprapubic catheter is typically placed.
- There are five types of urethral injury. Type Ⅲ, pictured above, is the most common, with disruption of the urogenital diaphragm and rupture of the bulbomembranous urethra with contrast extravasating both into the pelvis and out into the perineum.

- 创伤后出现尿道口出血、排尿疼痛，或无法排尿时，应立即行RUG检查以排除尿道损伤。一旦确诊，应常规进行耻骨上膀胱插管引流。
- 尿道损伤共分为5型，上图所示的Ⅲ型最为常见，会伴有尿生殖膈破裂和尿道球部、膜部断裂。在Ⅲ型损伤中造影剂会向内渗入骨盆，向外渗入会阴。

PENILE ABNORMALITIES

阴茎异常

Normal anatomy

正常解剖

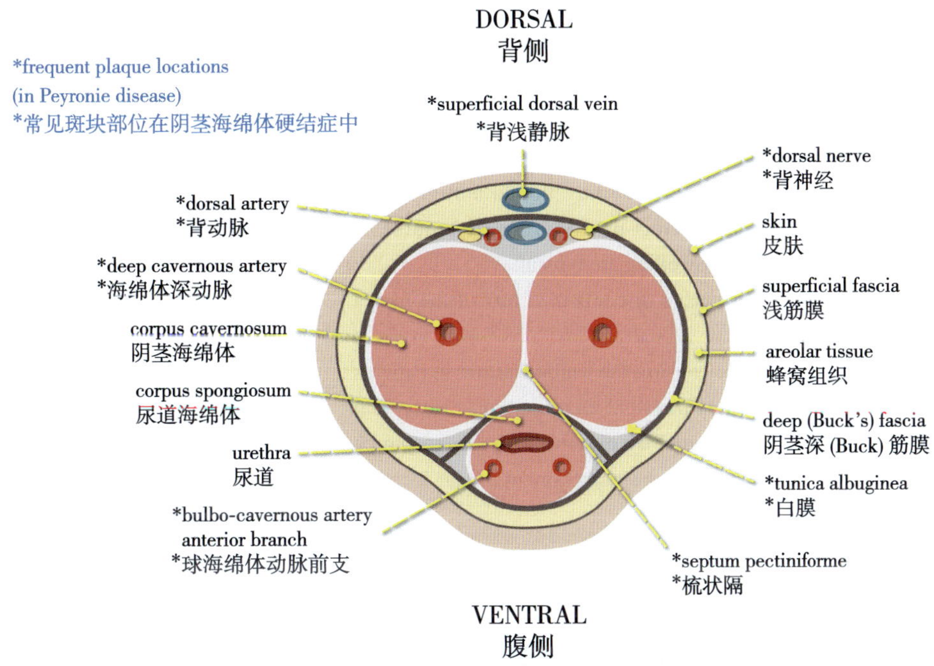

Peyronie disease

- Peyronie disease is an acquired condition associated with penile deformity and shortening of the penis that can lead to sexual dysfunction. A dorsal curvature is common, usually at the distal 1/3. It is caused by (palpable) plaque formation in the tunica albuginea and corpus cavernosum. The etiology is unclear but possibly associated with abnormal response to repetitive microtrauma, collagen vascular disease, or advancing age.
- Peyronie disease has an acute phase that can last for 12–18 months, associated with pain and sometimes flaccidity during intercourse. In the chronic phase, penile deformity is most commonly dorsal curvature (77%) or lateral curvature (20%). Surgical intervention is indicated in cases of severe bending or shortening of the penis, and typically deferred until the chronic phase, to minimize theoretical recurrence of fibrosis.
- Ultrasound is highly sensitive for penile plaques (which appear as localized echogenic thickening of the tunica albuginea) and calcifications. Plaques are most often seen on the dorsal surface (70%) or midshaft (42%).
- MRI can be used in more complex cases for surgical planning, and better characterizes abnormal penile curvature. Plaques can be seen as focal areas of T1 and T2 hypointense thickening, but calcifications are difficult to see on MRI. CT has limited role in evaluation.

阴茎海绵体硬结症

- 阴茎海绵体硬结症是一种后天获得性疾病，伴有阴茎畸形和阴茎缩短，可导致性功能障碍。阴茎背部常呈弯曲，多在远端1/3处，是由白膜和阴茎海绵体中形成的(可触及)瘢痕所致。病因尚不明确，但可能与重复性微创伤、胶原血管疾病或高龄引起的异常反应有关。
- 阴茎海绵体硬结症的急性期可持续12~18个月，伴随性交时疼痛和勃起无力。在慢性期，阴茎畸形以背曲(77%)或侧曲(20%)最为常见。手术干预适用于阴茎严重弯曲或缩短的情况，通常应推迟至慢性期进行，以减少理论上的纤维化复发。
- 超声对阴茎瘢痕(表现为局限性白膜高回声)和钙化高度敏感。瘢痕最常见于背侧表面(70%)或中段(42%)。
- MRI可用于较为复杂病例的术前计划，以便更好地显示阴茎弯曲异常。瘢痕在T_1和T_2上呈局灶性增厚的低信号，但MRI很难显示钙化灶。CT的评估价值有限。

Penile carcinoma

- Penile cancer is relatively rare; squamous cell carcinoma (SCC) accounts for >95% of primary penile neoplasms and typically occurs in the glans penis.
- Spread of penile cancer typically occurs via lymphatics and varies depending on the location of the primary lesion: skin of penis and prepuce to superficial inguinal nodes; glans penis to deep inguinal and external iliac nodes. The Buck fascia acts as a barrier for corporal invasion and hematogenous spread.
- Two staging systems are used: TNM (most commonly) or Jackson classification. Important components of staging include invasion into the shaft/corpora and metastatic lymphadenopathy.
- Lower stage (Ⅰ/Ⅱ disease) is usually curable with local resection with or without partial penectomy. High stage disease often requires palliative treatment.

阴茎癌

- 阴茎癌相对罕见；鳞状细胞癌(SCC)占原发性阴茎肿瘤的95%以上，通常发生在阴茎头。
- 阴茎癌常通过淋巴管发生扩散，并随原发病变的位置不同而有所不同：阴茎皮肤和包皮病变可转移至腹股沟浅淋巴结；阴茎头病变则转移至腹股沟深部和髂外淋巴结。阴茎深筋膜在防止肿瘤向体部侵犯和血行扩散的过程中起屏障作用。
- 分期系统有两种：TNM(最常用)或Jackson分级。分期的重要依据包括是否侵犯阴茎体和淋巴结转移。
- 早期(Ⅰ/Ⅱ期病变)经局部切除或联合部分阴茎切除后通常可治愈。晚期病变常需姑息治疗。

Penile fracture

- Penile fracture is a urologic emergency. It is defined as rupture (usually unilateral) of a corpus cavernosum and surrounding tunica albuginea. It is usually caused by external force on an erect penis during intercourse. A cracking sensation, severe pain, and rapid swelling are typical.
- Surgical repair is recommended for suspected or confirmed tear of the tunica albuginea and/or with urethral injury.
- Imaging (US or MRI) may be required to confirm the penile fracture in patients with severe pain/swelling that precludes physical examination, or atypical presentation. Penile fracture is demonstrated by discontinuity of the tunica albuginea. MRI is more sensitive and provides best assessment of tear location and extent.

阴茎折断

- 阴茎折断是泌尿外科急症，定义为阴茎海绵体(通常为单侧)及其周围白膜破裂。常见的原因为性交时勃起的阴茎受到强烈的外作用力。典型的症状是撕裂感、剧烈疼痛和快速肿胀。
- 对于怀疑或确诊的白膜撕裂和/或尿道损伤，应进行手术修复。
- 影像学检查(超声或MRI)适用于确诊因严重疼痛/肿胀而无法接受体格检查或症状不典型的阴茎折断的患者。阴茎折断表现为白膜不连续。MRI较为敏感，能很好地评估撕裂的位置和范围。

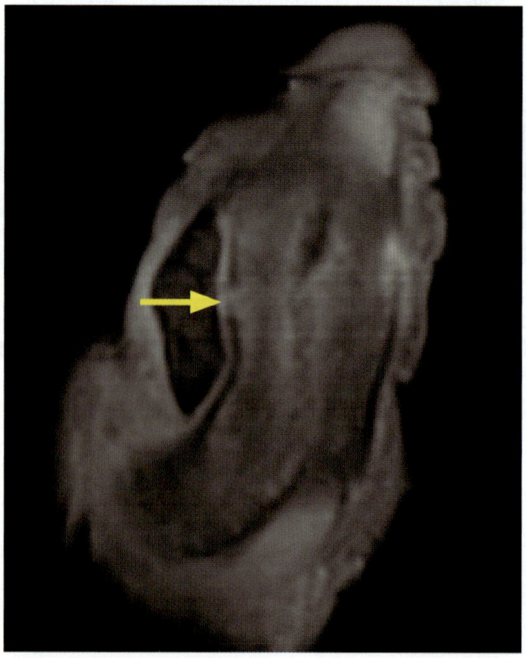

Sagittal oblique T2-weighted fat-suppressed MRI shows penile fracture with focal disruption of the tunica albuginea (arrow) along the right lateral border.
斜矢状位T_2加权脂肪抑制MRI显示阴茎折断，白膜(黄箭)沿着右侧边缘局限性中断。

(翻译　严承功)

MRI OF THE PROSTATE

前列腺MRI

Prostate anatomy

前列腺解剖

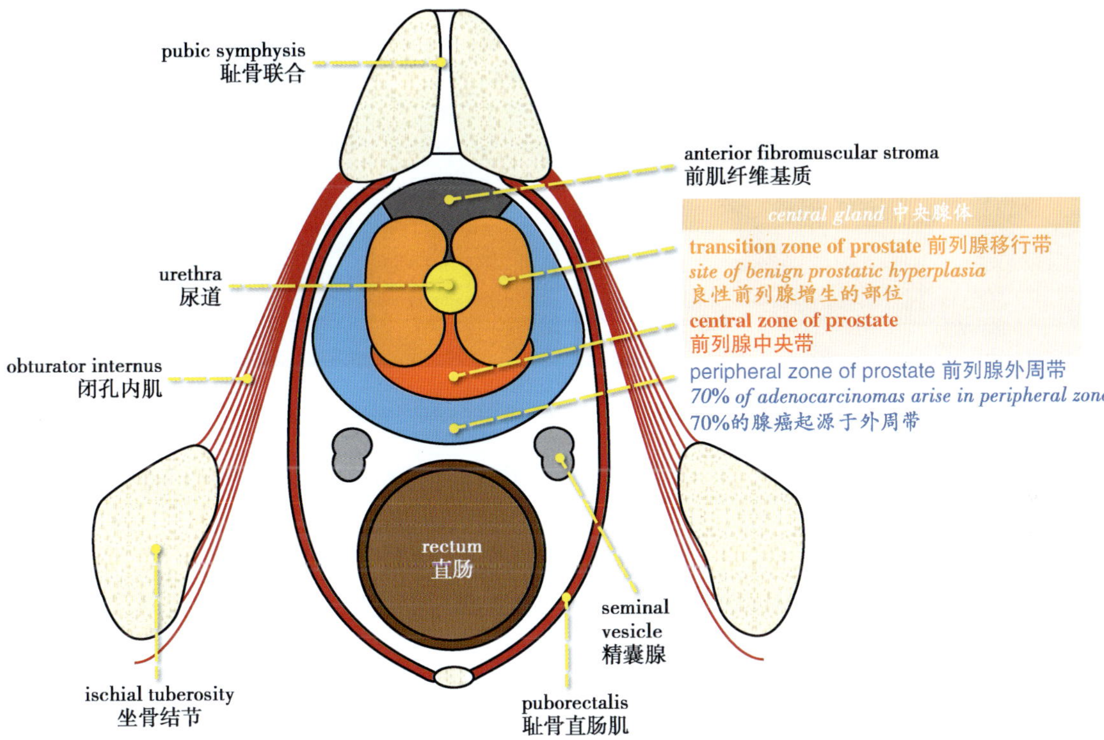

- The prostate consists of the **peripheral zone (PZ), central zone (CZ), transitional zone (TZ) and the anterior fibromuscular stroma (AFM).**
- In younger men, the central gland is composed mostly of the central zone; however, the transition zone enlarges as benign prostatic hyperplasia develops. These changes result in the central gland becoming predominantly composed of transition zone in older males.

- 前列腺由**外周带(PZ)、中央带(CZ)、移行带(TZ)和前肌纤维基质(AFM)**组成。
- 在年轻男性，中央腺体主要由中央带组成；而移行带随着良性前列腺增生而逐渐增大。这些变化导致老年男性的中央腺体主要由移行带组成。

Seminal vesicles (SV)

- The seminal vesicles (SV) produce and secrete seminal fluid (50–80% of ejaculate volume).
- The seminal vesicles are located posterior to the bladder/distal ureters and superior to the prostate gland, joining the distal portion of the vas deferens to form the ejaculatory duct, which in turn drains into the prostatic urethra.
- On MRI, they are seen as fluid-containing structures with thin septa. They show high signal on T2-weighted imaging and low signal on T1-weighted imaging.
- Bilateral SV agenesis is seen in 60–70% of patients with cystic fibrosis, likely related to luminal obstruction by thick secretions. These patients have normal kidneys.
- Congenital SV cysts or SV hypoplasia are often associated with other GU anomalies (e.g., ipsilateral renal agenesis, ADPKD).

精囊(SV)

- 精囊(SV)产生并分泌精液(占射精量的50%~80%)。
- 精囊位于膀胱/远端输尿管的后方、前列腺的上方，与输精管的远端汇合形成射精管，后者开口于尿道前列腺部。
- 精囊在MRI上表现为内含纤薄分隔的液性结构。在T_2加权上为高信号，在T_1加权上为低信号。
- 双侧SV发育不全见于60%~70%的囊性纤维化患者，可能与黏稠的分泌物阻塞管腔有关。这些患者的肾脏正常。
- 先天性SV囊肿或SV发育不全通常与其他泌尿生殖系统异常相关(如同侧肾发育不全、常染色体显性遗传多囊肾病)。

Utricle cyst

前列腺小囊囊肿

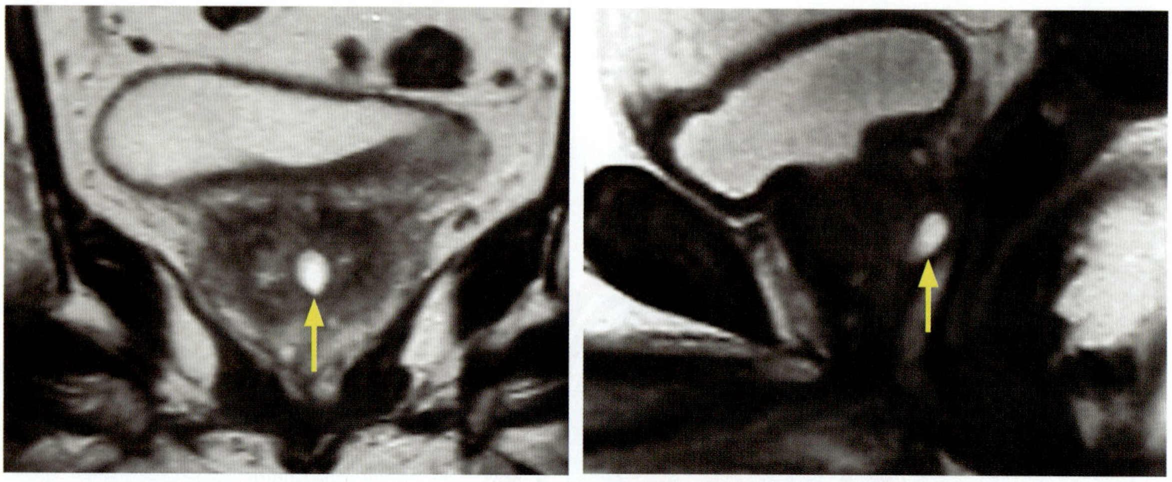

Coronal (left image) and sagittal (right image) T2-weighted MRI show a midline cystic lesion in the prostate, at the posterior aspect of the urethra, consistent with a prostatic utricle cyst (arrows).

冠状位(左图)和矢状位(右图)T_2加权MRI显示前列腺中线处有一个囊性病变，位于尿道的后部，为前列腺小囊囊肿(黄箭)。

- An utricle cyst is a midline cystic structure within the prostate, usually located posterior to the urethra. Utricle cysts communicate freely with the urethra and can result in post-void dribbling.
- Utricle cysts are remnants of the Müllerian duct system and are associated with hypospadias. They are always midline and diagnosed in younger patients (10–20 years of age) whereas Müllerian duct cysts occur in 30–40-year-old patients and can be found anywhere along the path of regression from scrotum to utricle.
- On ultrasound, a utricle cyst is seen as midline anechoic cyst posterior to the prostatic urethra. On MRI, they demonstrate high signal on T2-weighted imaging, but can have variable signal if they develop superimposed infection or hemorrhage.

- 前列腺小囊是一个位于前列腺中线的囊性结构，通常在尿道的后方。若前列腺小囊与尿道相通，可导致尿后滴沥。
- 前列腺小囊是米勒管系统的残留，与尿道下裂有关，它们总是位于中线，并发生于年轻的患者(10~20岁)；而米勒管囊肿发生在30~40岁患者，可见于阴囊到前列腺小囊退化途径上的任何一处。
- 前列腺小囊超声表现为前列腺尿道后方中线处的无回声囊肿。在MRI上，T_2加权显示为高信号，但若合并感染或出血，则信号多变。

Prostatitis

- Bacterial prostatitis is fairly common (prevalence of 10%) and can manifest as acute or chronic disease. Fluctuating PSA levels or decreasing PSA levels with antibiotic therapy raises suspicion for prostatitis.
- Acute bacterial prostatitis is less common and typically presents with local (painful urination, hematuria) and systemic (fever, malaise) symptoms. It usually occurs in young men from intra-prostatic reflux of infected urine, but can occur following instrumentation (e.g., biopsy).
- Chronic bacterial prostatitis usually occurs in older men with undertreated/recurrent acute prostatitis or lower urinary tract obstruction. Chronic prostatitis is more indolent and presents with local symptoms only.
- Prostatitis can be diffuse or focal and typically occurs within the peripheral zone. On MRI, regions of T2 hypointense signal and mild-moderate diffusion restriction are due to inflammatory cellular infiltrates. Both prostatitis and prostate cancer show increased and early enhancement. Compared to prostate cancer, chronic prostatitis shows less diffusion restriction.
- Another type of prostatitis, granulomatous prostatitis, is usually idiopathic and self-limited.

前列腺炎

- 细菌性前列腺炎相当常见(患病率为10%)，可呈急性或慢性表现。PSA水平波动或使用抗生素治疗后PSA水平下降可怀疑前列腺炎。
- 急性细菌性前列腺炎较少见，常有局部(尿痛、血尿)和全身(发热、不适)症状。该病常见于年轻男性，由感染的尿液反流进入前列腺所致，但也可能发生于器械检查之后(如活检)。
- 慢性细菌性前列腺炎常见于老年男性，由治疗不当/急性前列腺炎反复发作，或下尿路梗阻所致。慢性前列腺炎较为隐匿，仅有局部症状。
- 前列腺炎可为弥漫性或局灶性，通常局限于外周带。MRI上呈T_2低信号和轻中度扩散受限，为炎性细胞浸润所致。前列腺炎和前列腺癌均表现为强化增强和早期强化。慢性前列腺炎扩散受限程度较前列腺癌低。
- 另一种类型的前列腺炎，即肉芽肿性前列腺炎，通常为特发性且有自限性。

Prostate Cancer

Overview of prostate cancer imaging

- Most prostate cancers (90%) occur in the peripheral zone.
- Histologically, prostate cancers are classified by the Gleason scale (1–5) where the first number is the predominant pattern and the second number is the secondary pattern.
- The most important goal of MRI is to distinguish between surgical and nonsurgical disease. Cancer that is contained within the gland (tumor stage T2) is generally amenable to radical prostatectomy, while cancer that has spread outside of the gland is typically treated non-surgically (e.g., anti-androgen and radiation therapy).
- MRI may not detect all prostate cancers: low Gleason (<7) grade prostate cancers are typically not detectable; some cancers are not T2 hypointense; central zone cancers are difficult to detect on T2-weighted images; and cancer conspicuity is decreased if the peripheral zone is not T2 hyperintense due to underlying disease, such as chronic prostatitis.
- Pitfalls of imaging include prostatitis and involutional changes from androgen-deprivation therapy which may appear as abnormal T2 hypointense lesions.
- Post-biopsy normal prostatic tissue is T1 hyperintense due to high concentration of citrate that causes more bleeding (following image, yellow arrows). Neoplastic tissue does not produce as much citrate and will bleed less, resulting in the *hemorrhage exclusion sign* (red arrows).

前列腺癌

前列腺癌影像概述

- 大多数前列腺癌(90%)发生在外周带。
- 组织学上，前列腺癌按Gleason评分(1~5级)进行分类，其中第一个数字代表主要成分，第二个数字代表次要成分。
- MRI最重要的目的是区分病变是否可以进行手术治疗。肿瘤局限于腺体内(肿瘤分期为T_2期)一般可以进行根治性前列腺切除术；如果累及腺体以外，则通常进行非手术治疗(如抗雄激素治疗及放疗)。
- MRI不能发现所有的前列腺癌：Gleason低级别(<7分)的前列腺癌通常无法被发现；一些肿瘤在T_2加权图像上并不呈低信号；中央带的前列腺癌很难在T_2加权图像上显示；当外周带因基础疾病(如慢性前列腺炎)而不呈T_2高信号时，其癌症的显示能力就会降低。
- 影像学(MRI)的缺点：前列腺炎和去雄性激素治疗引起的退化改变可能表现为异常的T_2低信号病变。
- 正常的前列腺组织在活检后呈T_1高信号，这是由于高浓度的柠檬酸盐会引起出血增加(下图，黄箭)。肿瘤组织不会产生很多柠檬酸盐，因此出血较少，导致出血排除征(红箭)。

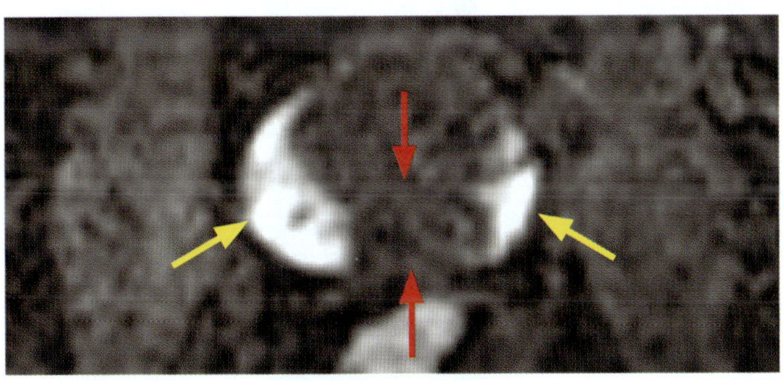

Post-biopsy T1-weighted post-contrast MR with fat suppression demonstrates T1 hyperintense bleeding within normal prostatic tissue peripherally (yellow arrows). Prostate cancer (red arrows) does not bleed, resulting in the *hemorrhage exclusion sign.*

活检后增强T_1加权脂肪抑制MRI显示正常外周前列腺组织T_1高信号出血区(黄箭)。前列腺癌内(红箭)无出血，导致出血排除征。

- Prostate cancer typically shows: (1) restricted diffusion with high signal on high B-value DWI and low signal on ADC, (2) low T2 signal, and (3) early enhancement relative to the surrounding peripheral zone.

  DWI assessment is usually qualitative, not quantitative, but active research is under way to determine thresholds for ADC value(s).
- MRI spectroscopy of prostate cancer may show elevated choline and depressed citrate peaks compared to normal prostate, but it is not routinely performed in most centers.

Prostate Imaging Reporting and Data System (PI-RADS)

- Prostate Imaging Reporting and Data System (PI-RADS) was designed to provide a global standard for reporting and interpreting multiparametric prostate MRI. Using PI-RADS system improves communication of clinically significant cancer, increases confidence in benign disease and dormant malignancies, and reduces unnecessary biopsies and treatments.

- 典型的前列腺癌表现：扩散受限，高b值DWI高信号，ADC低信号；T_2低信号；强化早于周围的外周带。

  DWI评估通常是定性，而非定量，但确定ADC阈值的研究正在进行中。
- 与正常前列腺比较，前列腺癌的MRI波谱特征为胆碱峰升高和柠檬酸盐峰降低，但大多数医疗中心并不常规进行此项检查。

前列腺影像报告和数据系统(PI-RADS)

- 前列腺影像报告和数据系统(PI-RADS)是为全球标准化报告和解读多参数前列腺MRI而设计的。通过使用PI-RADS系统，可改善对有临床意义癌症的沟通，增加对良性疾病和潜在恶性肿瘤诊断的信心，以及减少不必要的活检和治疗。

- Assignment of a PI-RADS score (last updated 2019 v2.1) is based on MRI findings only. PSA or clinical findings are not included. The likelihood of clinically significant cancer is reported on a scale of 1–5, with a progressively increased likelihood with increasing score:

- PI-RADS分类(最新更新2019 v2.1)仅根据MRI表现。PSA或临床发现不包括在内。根据临床意义前列腺癌的可能性按1~5个等级进行报告，等级增加，其可能性也随之增加：

PI-RADS 1: Clinically significant cancer is highly unlikely (0%).
PI-RADS 2: Clinically significant cancer is unlikely (10%).
PI-RADS 3: Equivocal (16–20%).
PI-RADS 4: Clinically significant cancer is likely (21–86%).
PI-RADS 5: Clinically significant cancer is highly likely (93%).

PI-RADS 1：临床意义前列腺癌极不可能(0)。
PI-RADS 2：临床意义前列腺癌不太可能(10%)。
PI-RADS 3：可疑(16%~20%)。
PI-RADS 4：临床意义前列腺癌很有可能(21%~86%)。
PI-RADS 5：临床意义前列腺癌高度可能(93%)。

- PI-RADS assessment is based on T2-weighted images (T2WI), diffusion weighted images (ADC/DWI), and dynamic contrast imaging (DCE). PI-RADS category assignment is weighted to a specific sequence according to zonal anatomy.

- PI-RADS评估依据病变在T_2加权成像(T_2WI)、扩散加权成像(ADC/DWI)和动态增强成像(DCE)的表现。PI-RADS分类则是根据不同解剖分区采用特定的序列进行评分。

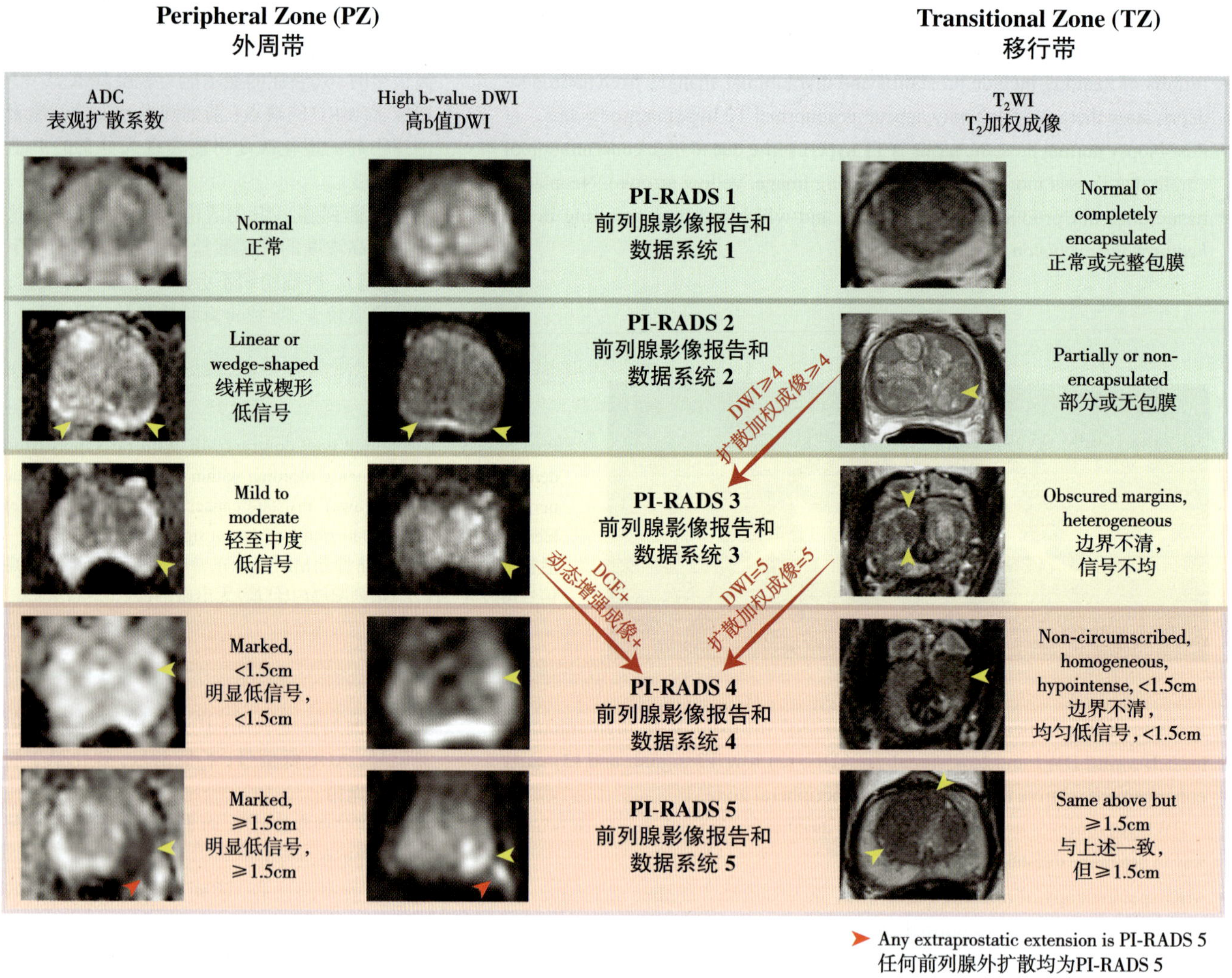

- For **transitional zone (TZ) lesions**, T2WI should be used to assign a PI-RADS category, but it is correlated to ADC/DWI. Transitional zone lesions are measured on T2WI.
- For **peripheral zone (PZ) lesions**, ADC/DWI should be used to assign a PI-RADS category, but it is correlated to T2WI. Peripheral zone lesions are measured on ADC images.

- 对于**移行带(TZ)病变**，PI-RADS分类应依据T_2加权，但应与ADC/DWI相对应。在T_2加权上测量移行带病变。
- 对于**外周带(PZ)病变**，PI-RADS分类应依据ADC/DWI，但应与T_2加权相对应。在ADC图像上测量外周带病变。

- DCE can act as a "tie-breaker" for peripheral zone lesions when ADC/DWI characteristics are equivocal for malignancy (a score of 3). An equivocal peripheral zone lesion should be upgraded to PI-RADS 4 if DCE is positive.
- If a transitional zone lesion has a T2WI score of 2 or 3, correlation with DWI imaging characteristics is required. A high DWI score (see table above) would upgrade the lesion.
- For both PZ and TZ lesions, any extraprostatic extension makes the lesion PI-RADS 5. Evaluation of the tumor margin should be performed in three planes. If the tumor is contiguous with the prostatic capsule, it has a higher risk of extracapsular invasion. The neurovascular bundles should be carefully examined where they abut the peripheral zone posterolaterally.
- Studies have shown that PI-RADS score correlated with Gleason score ≥3 + 4 disease, whereas Gleason <4 disease generally does not have a MRI correlate.
- Note that PI-RADS does not address the use of MRI for detection of suspected recurrent prostate cancer following therapy, progression during surveillance, or use of MRI for evaluating other parts of the body involved with prostate cancer.

Prostate cancer staging

- Prostate cancer uses the TNM staging system.

T: If the tumor is confined within the prostate or extends beyond the capsule (involvement of seminal vesicles or neurovascular bundle). If there is tumor fixation or invasion into other adjacent structures (e.g., bladder, rectum).

N: Metastasis to regional lymph nodes (pelvic, hypogastric, sacral, internal and external iliac).

M: Non-regional lymph node involvement (aortic, common iliac, inguinal, and supraclavicular), bone, and distant organ involvement.

- MRI can help determine N or M status, although PET/CT or CT is more commonly used for nodal staging. If PSA is high or there is suspicion for metastasis, a bone scan is usually performed to evaluate for osteoblastic bone metastasis.
- Staging example: T2a prostate cancer, which can be treated with radical prostatectomy.

- 当外周带的病变在ADC/DWI上的表现不能确定为恶性时(得分为3分)，DCE可作为"决定性因素"。若DCE为阳性，可疑的外周带病变则升级为PI-RADS 4。
- 若移行带病变的T_2加权评分为2分或3分，则需要结合DWI影像学特征。DWI评分高(见上表)则应升高病变级别。
- 对于外周和移行带病变，出现任何前列腺外的病变即为PI-RADS 5。评估肿瘤边缘应在三个平面上进行。如果肿瘤与前列腺包膜相邻，则包膜外浸润的风险较高。对于外周带后外侧的病变，应仔细检查紧邻的神经血管束。
- 研究表明，PI-RADS评分与Gleason评分≥(3+4)的疾病相关，而Gleason<4分的疾病通常与MRI无相关性。
- 注意，PI-RADS评分并不适用于前列腺癌治疗后对复发检测、肿瘤进展随访或对其他部位前列腺癌的评估。

前列腺癌分期

- 前列腺癌使用TNM分期系统。

T: 肿瘤是否局限在前列腺内或延伸到包膜外(累及精囊或神经血管束)。肿瘤是否固定或侵入其他邻近结构(如膀胱、直肠)。

N: 区域性淋巴结转移(盆腔、下腹部、骶部、髂内外)。

M: 非区域性淋巴结受累(主动脉、髂总、腹股沟和锁骨上)、骨和远处器官受累。

- MRI有助于确定N或M分期，但PET/CT或CT更常用于淋巴结分期。如果PSA升高或怀疑有转移，通常使用骨扫描以评估是否有骨转移。
- 分期举例：T_{2a}期前列腺癌，可以行根治性前列腺癌切除术进行治疗。

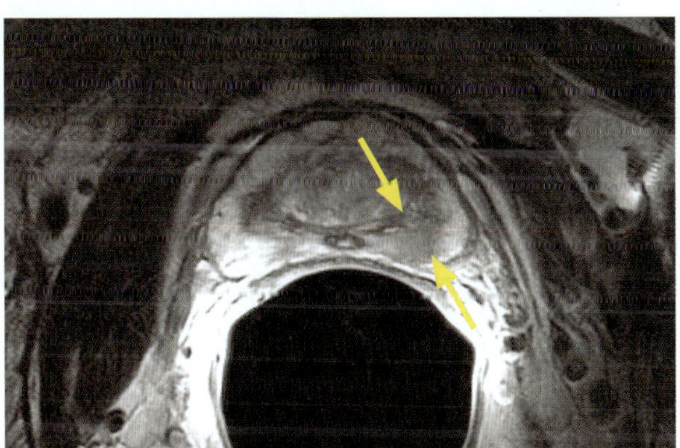

Axial T2-weighted MRI with an endorectal coil in place shows a focus of hypointensity within the posterior left peripheral zone (arrows), representing the site of cancer. There is no extraglandular extension.

轴位T_2加权直肠线圈MRI显示前列腺左后方的外周带(黄箭)有一个局灶性低信号，为癌灶。

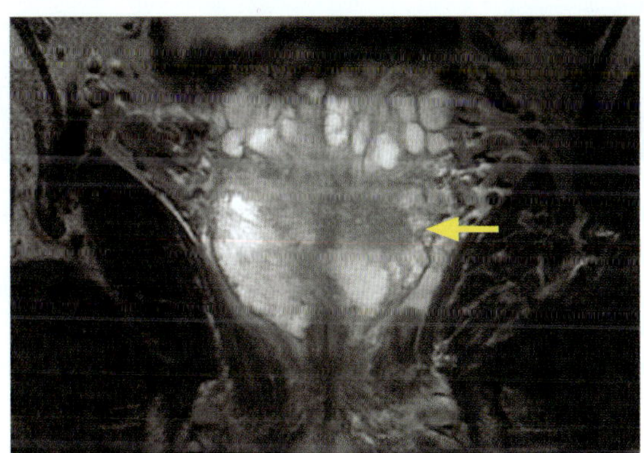

Coronal T2-weighted image through the posterior portion of the gland shows the tumor as a focal region of T2 hypointensity (arrow) in the peripheral zone.

此例并无腺体外的侵犯。经前列腺腺体后部的冠状位T_2加权显示肿瘤位于外周带，表现为局灶性T_2低信号(黄箭)。

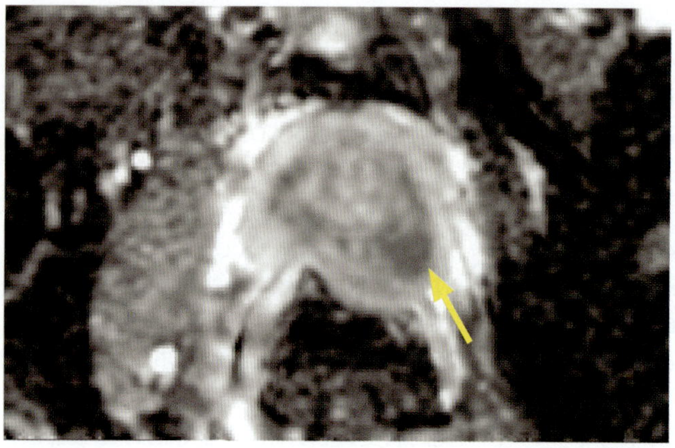

Axial ADC map shows that the tumor features restricted diffusion (arrow; dark on the ADC map).
轴位ADC图显示肿瘤呈扩散受限(黄箭；在ADC图上为黑色)。

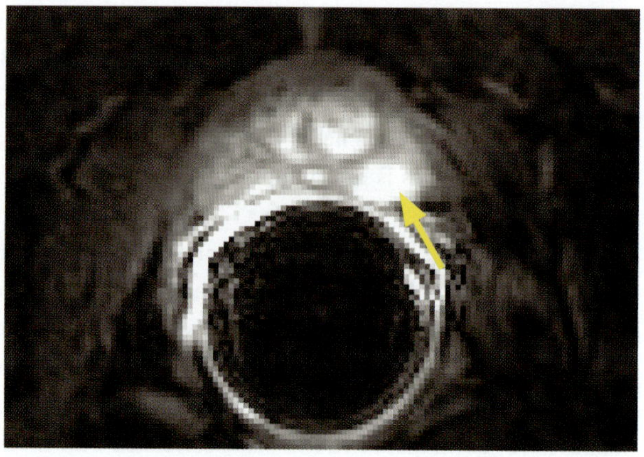

Axial early-phase dynamic gradient-echo contrast-enhanced MRI shows relative hyperenhancement of the prostate cancer (arrow).
轴位早期增强MRI动态梯度回波显示前列腺癌相对显著强化(黄箭)。

In this case, the focus of prostate cancer is entirely confined within the gland. The tumor involves less than one-half of one lobe for a stage of T2a. Because the tumor is so small, the advanced techniques of diffusion and dynamic contrast enhancement are helpful to increase specificity.
在本例中，前列腺癌病灶完全局限于腺体中。肿瘤累及不到单叶的50%，分期为T_{2a}期。由于肿瘤比较小，一些先进的技术(如扩散加权成像及动态增强成像)有助于增加诊断的特异度。

- Staging example: T3b N1 prostate cancer, which is typically treated nonsurgically.

- 分期举例：$T_{3b}N_1$期前列腺癌，通常采用非手术治疗。

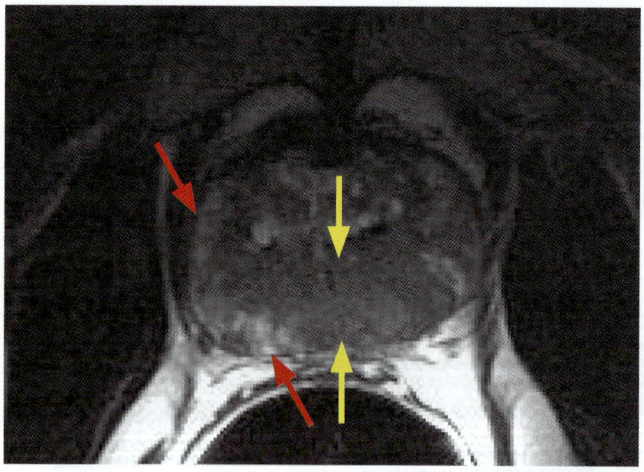

Axial T2 (with endorectal coil) of the prostate mid-gland shows near-complete replacement of the normal T2 hyperintense peripheral zone with a T2 hypointense mass (yellow arrows). There is some residual normal peripheral zone on the right (red arrows).
经前列腺中部轴位T_2加权(应用直肠线圈)MRI显示正常T_2高信号的外周带几乎完全被T_2低信号的肿块所取代(黄箭)。右侧尚残留一些正常前列腺外周带组织(红箭)。

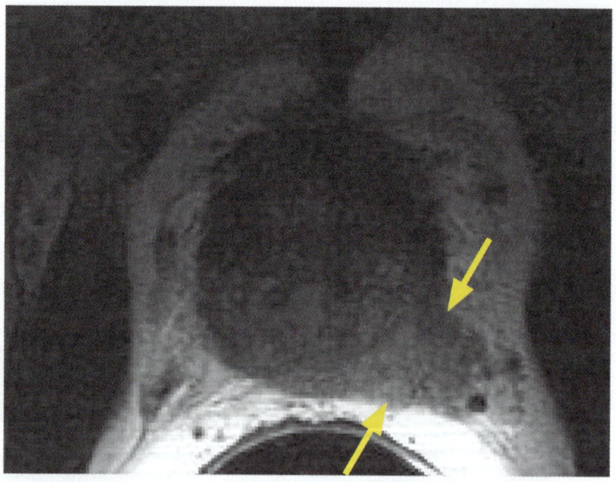

Axial T2 slightly more inferiorly shows left extra-glandular spread (arrows) with engulfment of the left seminal vesicle.
稍下方轴位T_2加权显示癌肿向左侧腺体外侵犯(黄箭)，与左侧精囊腺分界不清。

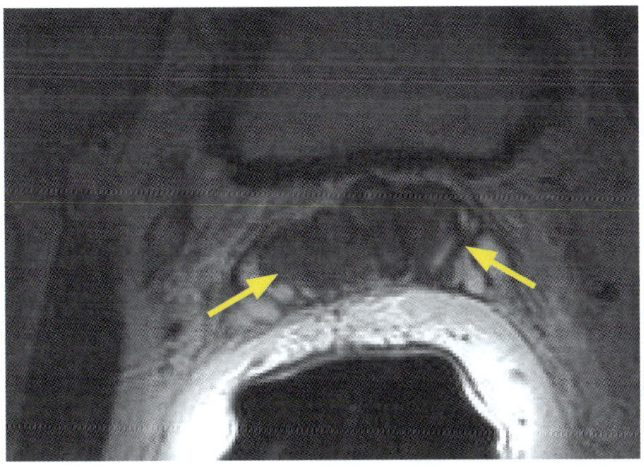

Axial T2 through the base of the bladder superior to the prostate shows abnormal T2 hypointensity in the medial aspect of both seminal vesicles (arrows).
轴位经膀胱底部、前列腺上方T_2加权显示双侧精囊腺内侧部分异常T_2低信号(黄箭)。

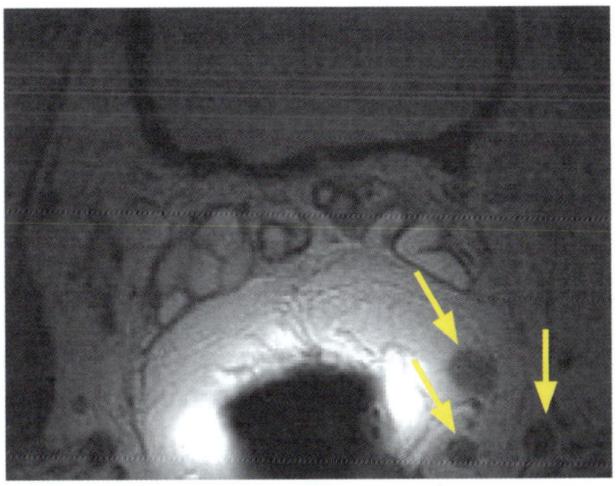

Axial T2 demonstrates several regional lymph nodes (arrows).
轴位T_2加权显示数个区域性淋巴结(黄箭)。

In this case, the tumor involves most of the peripheral zone of both lobes and clearly demonstrates extra-glandular spread, making the tumor T3. Because the tumor invades the seminal vesicles it is T3b: If it only extended out of the capsule, but the seminal vesicles were preserved, it would be T3a.

The presence of regional lymph nodes is N1.

Advanced MRI techniques would not add much in this case because the anatomic imaging demonstrates malignant behavior.

Prostate cancer staging cases courtesy Cheryl Sadow, MD, Brigham and Women's Hospital.

在本病例中,肿瘤累及了前列腺两侧叶大部分外周带,而且清楚显示了腺体外播散,属T_3期。由于肿瘤侵犯了精囊腺,分期为T_{3b}期;如果肿瘤仅突破前列腺包膜,而并没有累及精囊腺,则分期为T_{3a}期。

出现区域淋巴结为N_1期。

由于此病例的解剖学影像已经显示了明确的恶性行为,因此其他先进的MRI技术并无更多帮助。

(翻译　许倩)

SCROTUM AND TESTICLE

SCROTAL ANATOMY

Testicle

- The testes produce sperm and androgens.
- The testicle is an oval shaped structure with a homogeneous echogenicity on ultrasound.

Epididymis

- The epididymis carries sperm away from the testicle to the vas deferens.
- The epididymis is composed of head, body, and tail. The head may measure up to 10 mm.
- The epididymis is normally hypoechoic and has less blood flow compared to the testicle.

Rete testis

- The rete testis is a network of tubules that carries sperm from the seminiferous tubules in the testicle towards the epididymis. It transports and concentrates sperm.

Mediastinum testis

- The mediastinum testis is fibrous tissue in the hilum of the testicle, from which fibrous septa radiate towards the testicular periphery. It provides structural support to the rete testis.

阴囊和睾丸

阴囊解剖

睾丸

- 睾丸产生精子和雄激素。
- 睾丸为椭圆形结构,超声上回声均匀。

附睾

- 附睾将精子从睾丸输送到输精管。
- 附睾分头、体、尾三部分。附睾头直径可达10mm。
- 正常附睾呈低回声,与睾丸相比血供较少。

睾丸网

- 睾丸网是将精子从睾丸内的生精小管输送到附睾的管道网络,其功能是运输和聚集精子。

睾丸纵隔

- 睾丸纵隔为睾丸门处的纤维组织,纤维隔自睾丸门向睾丸外周呈放射状分布。睾丸纵隔为睾丸网提供结构性支持。

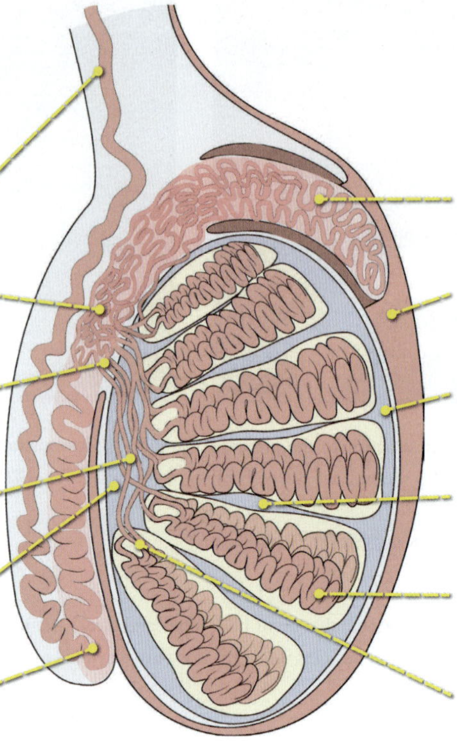

VASCULAR DISEASE OF THE TESTIS

Testicular torsion

- Testicular torsion is twisting of the testicle around the spermatic cord and the vascular pedicle. Torsion presents with acute scrotal pain and is a surgical emergency.
- Torsion may lead to irreversible testicular infarction if not de-torsed within a few hours.

  De-torsion within 6 hours has an excellent prognosis.

  De-torsion after 24 hours has a poor prognosis for testicular salvage.

睾丸血管性疾病

睾丸扭转

- 睾丸扭转指睾丸围绕精索和血管蒂发生了扭转。扭转表现为急性睾丸疼痛，是外科急症。
- 若数小时内未解除扭转，睾丸可发生不可逆性梗死。

  若6小时内解除扭转，则预后良好。

  若24小时后解除扭转，则睾丸存活的可能性低。

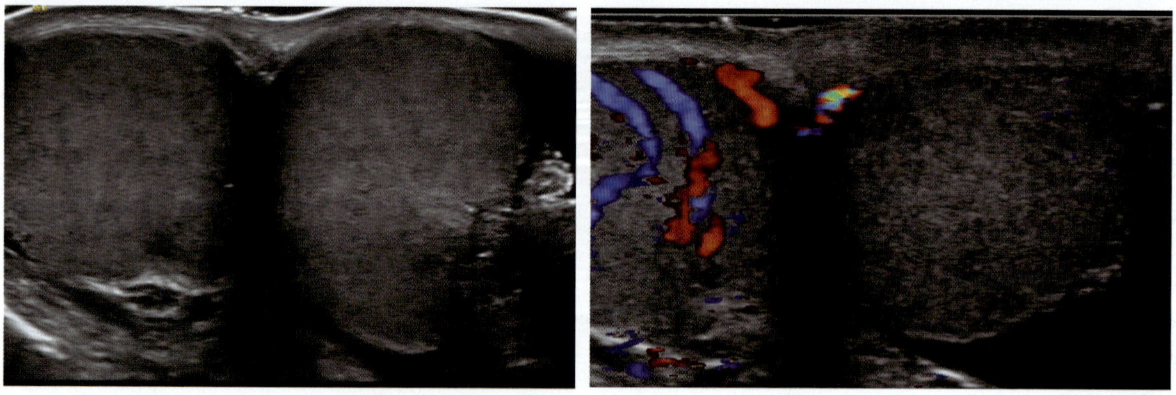

Transverse grayscale ultrasound (left image) shows slight enlargement of the left testis relative to the right. There is an absence of arterial or venous flow within the left testis on color Doppler (right image), consistent with testicular torsion.
横切面灰阶超声(左图)显示左侧睾丸较右侧轻微增大。彩色多普勒(右图)显示左侧睾丸内无动、静脉血流，符合睾丸扭转。

- The *bell-clapper deformity* predisposes to torsion due to a small testicular bare area. The bare area is the testicular attachment site and normally prevents the testicle from rotation.
- Ultrasound findings of torsion are dependent on the time elapsed since torsion:

Hyperacute (within a few hours): Ultrasound shows a hyperechoic and shadowing *torsion knot* of twisted epididymis and spermatic cord, with no blood flow in the affected testicle.
Acute (between a few hours and 24 hours): Affected testicle is enlarged and heterogeneous.
Missed torsion (>24 hours): Affected testicle is enlarged and mottled, with scrotal skin thickening and increased flow in the scrotal wall. A complex or septated hydrocele may be present.

- 铃锤样畸形使睾丸的裸区变小，容易发生睾丸扭转。裸区为睾丸的附着点，在正常情况下可防止睾丸发生旋转。
- 睾丸扭转的超声表现取决于发生扭转后所经历的时间：

超急性期(数小时内)：扭转的附睾和精索在超声上表现为高回声的*扭曲结节*，受累的睾丸内无血流信号。
急性期(数小时到24小时)：扭转的睾丸增大，回声不均匀。
过期扭转(>24小时)：扭转的睾丸增大，且呈斑点状，伴有阴囊皮肤增厚及阴囊壁血流信号增加。可见混合性或有分隔的睾丸鞘膜积液。

Segmental infarction

- Segmental infarction is a focal testicular infarction which can be due to microvascular thrombosis from acute inflammation, vasculitis, or sickle cell disease.
- Patients are typically in their thirties and present with acute pain which may mimic epididymitis or torsion clinically.
- The typical appearance of infarction is a wedge-shaped hypoechoic area with no flow on Doppler.
- The primary differential consideration of infarction is a hypovascular tumor. Infarcted tissue may undergo necrosis, making differentiation from tumor even more difficult. MRI may be helpful to distinguish infarction from tumor in ambiguous cases to potentially spare the patient from unnecessary orchiectomy.

节段性梗死

- 节段性梗死是一种局部睾丸梗死，由急性炎症、血管炎或镰状细胞贫血时的微血栓所致。
- 患者多为30多岁，表现为急性睾丸疼痛，临床表现类似于附睾炎或睾丸扭转。
- 超声上梗死灶的典型表现为楔形低回声区，内无多普勒血流信号。
- 梗死的主要鉴别诊断是乏血供肿瘤。梗死灶可发生坏死，导致与肿瘤鉴别更加困难。MRI有助于在模棱两可的病例中区分梗死或肿瘤，从而避免误切睾丸。

Scrotal trauma

Scrotal hematoma

- The sonographic appearance of an acute scrotal hematoma is an echogenic, extra-testicular mass with no Doppler flow. When large, the hematoma can compress the testicle.
- When the hematoma evolves into a complex, multiseptated mass-like lesion, the distinction between the extra-testicular hematoma and the testicle may become difficult. Proper distinction is necessary to avoid mistaking the hematoma for a testicular mass.

Testicular hematoma

阴囊外伤

阴囊血肿

- 急性阴囊血肿在超声上表现为睾丸外回声增强的肿块，无多普勒血流信号。当血肿增大时会挤压睾丸。
- 当血肿演变为复杂的多分隔的肿块样病变时，睾丸外血肿与睾丸本身的区分可能会非常困难。必须进行适当鉴别，以免将血肿误诊为睾丸肿块。

睾丸血肿

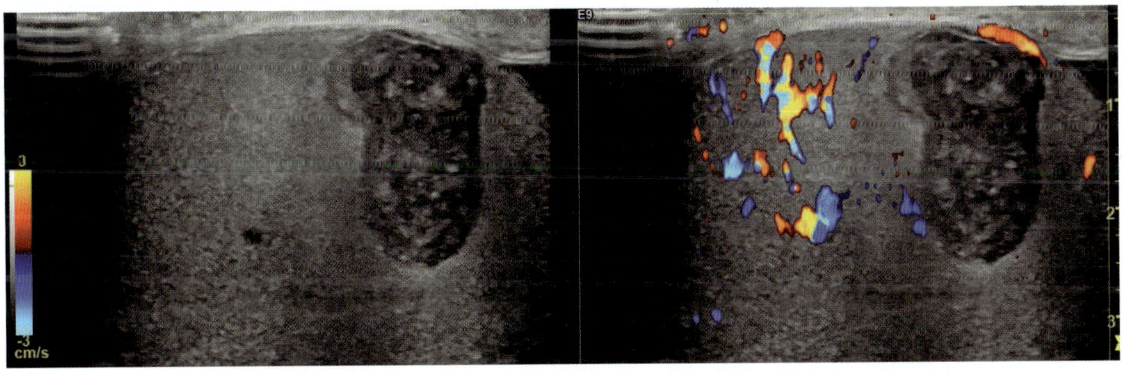

Testicular hematoma: Sagittal grayscale ultrasound (left image) shows a heterogeneous hypoechoic mass within the testicle, which has no internal Doppler flow (right image). Given recent trauma, this was thought to represent a hematoma. Follow up ultrasound (not shown) demonstrated decrease in size of the hematoma.
睾丸血肿：矢状切面灰阶超声(左图)显示睾丸内不均匀低回声肿块，内部无多普勒血流(右图)。结合近期创伤史，考虑为血肿。超声随访(未展示)显示血肿缩小。

- Testicular hematoma produces a peripheral hypoechoic lesion that may mimic tumor.
- Even with a history of trauma, a suspicious testicular lesion requires further evaluation to exclude malignancy, typically with a short-term follow-up.

Testicular rupture

- Testicular rupture causes capsule disruption, often with protrusion of testicular parenchyma through the defect. Rupture is often associated with a testicular hematoma or contusion.
- Prompt diagnosis is critical, as testicular viability is dependent upon timely repacking of the seminiferous tubules back inside the capsule.
- Testicular rupture results in disruption of the blood-testis barrier and may be associated with future infertility due to the formation of anti-spermatozoa antibodies.

- 睾丸血肿表现为睾丸外周有低回声灶，可类似于肿瘤。
- 即使有外伤史，对可疑的睾丸病灶仍需进一步检查以除外恶性肿瘤，通常为短期随访。

睾丸破裂

- 睾丸破裂会导致包膜撕裂，睾丸实质常由缺损处向外突出。破裂常合并睾丸血肿或挫伤。
- 及时诊断至关重要，因为睾丸能否存活取决于是否及时将生精小管重新置入包膜内。
- 睾丸破裂可导致血睾屏障受损，可因产生抗精子抗体而继发不育。

Scrotal infection

阴囊感染

Epididymitis

附睾炎

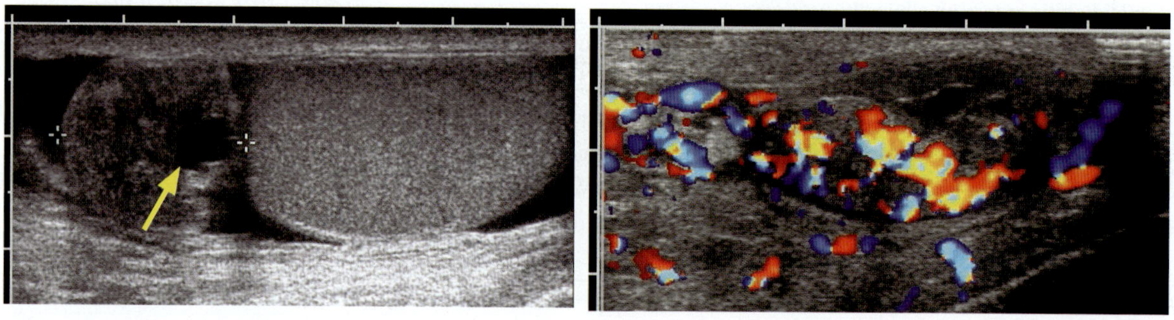

Epididymitis: Sagittal grayscale ultrasound (left image) of the testicle and epididymis shows a markedly enlarged epididymis measuring 1.7 cm (calipers). Incidental note is made of an epididymal cyst (arrow).
The testicle has a normal sonographic appearance. Transverse color Doppler of the epididymis (right image) demonstrates markedly increased flow.
Case courtesy Julie Ritner, MD, Brigham and Women's Hospital.
附睾炎：睾丸和附睾矢状切面灰阶超声(左图)显示附睾明显增大，测量约1.7cm(卡尺处)。意外发现为附睾囊肿(黄箭)。
睾丸超声呈正常表现。附睾横切面彩色多普勒(右图)显示血流量显著增加。

- Epididymitis is infection of the epididymis, almost always ascending from the urinary tract.
- The classic clinical presentation of epididymitis is acute unilateral scrotal pain.
- A key ultrasound finding of epididymitis is an enlarged epididymis with increased color Doppler flow relative to the testicle. An associated hydrocele may be present, which often contains low-level echoes.
- The main differential based on clinical presentation is testicular torsion, which would demonstrate decreased testicular blood flow. In contrast, epididymitis features normal testicular blood flow.

Epididymo-orchitis

- Epididymo-orchitis is infection which has spread from the epididymis to the testicle.
- Epididymo-orchitis has a similar ultrasound appearance to epididymitis, but blood flow to the testicle will also be increased.
- Infection and secondary inflammation can cause venous hypertension, which is a risk factor for focal testicular ischemia.

- 附睾炎是附睾发生的感染，几乎均源于泌尿道的上行感染。
- 附睾炎的典型临床表现为急性单侧阴囊疼痛。
- 附睾炎的超声图像主要表现为附睾增大，彩色多普勒血流信号相对高于睾丸。可并发鞘膜积液，常为低回声。
- 主要的临床鉴别诊断是睾丸扭转，睾丸扭转表现为睾丸血供减少；相反，附睾炎的特征是睾丸血供正常。

附睾-睾丸炎

- 附睾-睾丸炎为附睾炎扩散到睾丸。
- 附睾-睾丸炎与附睾炎超声表现相似，但睾丸血供也会增加。
- 感染和继发炎症可致静脉压力增高，增加睾丸局部缺血的风险。

Fournier gangrene

富尼埃坏疽

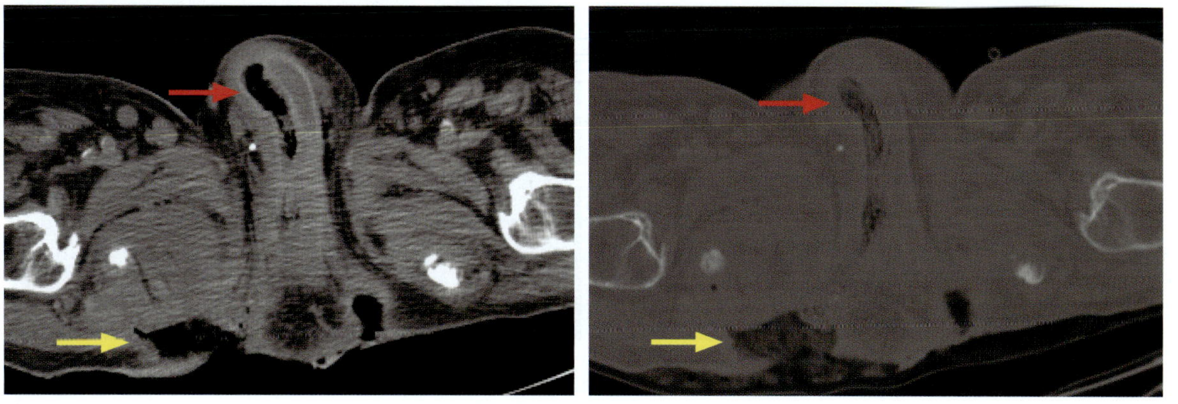

Fournier gangrene: Axial unenhanced CT shows a right ischial decubitus ulcer (yellow arrows) and soft tissue gas (better seen on bone window, right image; red arrows) in the right perineum tracking along the lateral margin of the penile base.
富尼埃坏疽：轴位平扫CT(左图)显示右侧坐骨部压疮溃疡(黄箭)和右侧会阴部沿阴茎根部外侧边缘分布的软组织积气(骨窗显示更佳，右图；红箭)。

- Fournier gangrene is necrotizing fasciitis of the scrotum and perineum, a highly morbid and surgically emergent condition.
- Infection is usually polymicrobial.
- The key imaging finding is the presence of subcutaneous gas, often evaluated with CT. The appearance on ultrasound is of multiple echogenic foci in the subcutaneous tissues with *dirty* posterior shadowing.

- 富尼埃坏疽是阴囊和会阴部的坏死性筋膜炎，为高危病变，需外科紧急处理。
- 感染常由多种微生物引起。
- 主要的影像学发现为皮下积气，常使用CT进行评估。超声表现为皮下软组织内多发局灶性回声增强，伴有不洁的后方声影。

TESTICULAR MASSES

Approach to a testicular mass

- **Intratesticular** masses are usually **malignant** (90–95%). Conversely, most **extratesticular** masses are benign in an adult, although a pediatric mass in this location may be malignant.
- The retroperitoneum should always be evaluated if an intratesticular mass is seen. Likewise, if retroperitoneal adenopathy is seen in a reproductive-age male, the testicles should always be examined.
- Most scrotal masses are hypoechoic relative to normal testicular parenchyma.
- On Doppler ultrasound, most masses will have increased vascularity with high diastolic flow, producing a low resistance waveform.

Malignant germ cell tumor (GCT): Seminoma

- Seminoma is the most common testicular malignancy. It has a favorable prognosis.
- Seminoma typically occurs in middle-aged men and it accounts for about half of all GCTs. It is usually more homogeneous than nonseminomatous germ cell tumors (NSGCT). It tends to be uniformly hypoechoic on ultrasound. Uncommonly, hCG may be elevated.

The spermatocytic subtype of seminoma occurs in slightly older men (mid-fifties) and has excellent prognosis with orchiectomy only. Tumor markers are not elevated.

睾丸肿块

睾丸肿块的诊断方法

- **睾丸内**肿块常为**恶性**(90%~95%)。相反，成人的**睾丸外**肿块大多为良性，儿童则有可能为恶性。
- 如发现睾丸内肿块，必须检查腹膜后间隙。同样，生育期男性若发现腹膜后淋巴结肿大，必须对睾丸进行检查。
- 多数阴囊肿块相对于正常睾丸实质为低回声。
- 多普勒超声检查时，多数肿块血运增加，伴舒张期高血流，从而产生低阻频谱。

恶性生殖细胞肿瘤(GCT)：精原细胞瘤

- 精原细胞瘤是最常见的睾丸恶性肿瘤，但预后较好。
- 精原细胞瘤常发生于中年男性，约占所有生殖细胞肿瘤的50%。回声通常比非精原生殖细胞瘤(NSGCT)更均匀。超声上倾向于均匀的低回声。少数患者有人绒毛膜促性腺激素(hCG)增高。

精原细胞瘤的精母细胞瘤亚型发生于年龄较长的男性(50多岁)，预后较好，只需切除睾丸。肿瘤标志物不升高。

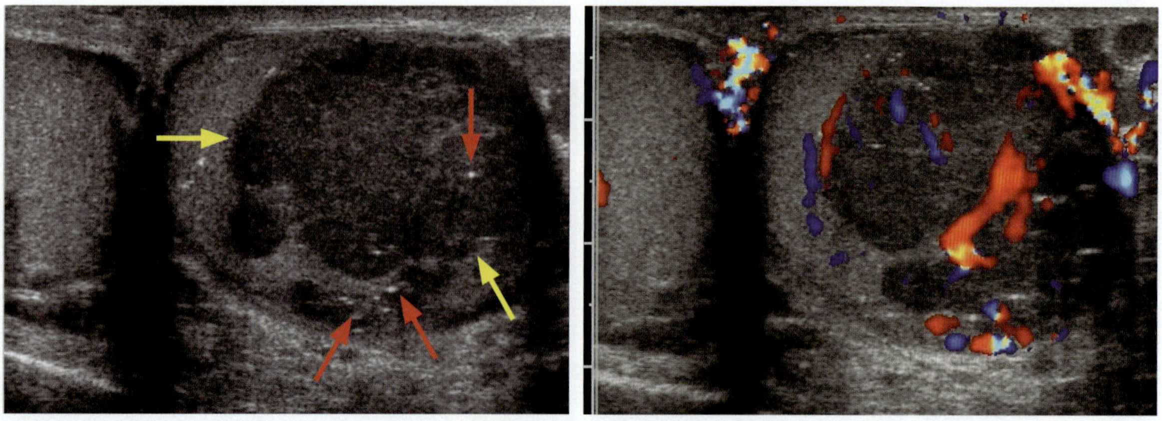

Seminoma: Grayscale (left image) and color Doppler show a heterogeneous hypoechoic vascular mass (yellow arrows) in the left testis. Note the presence of numerous tiny echogenic foci (red arrows) representing microlithiasis.

Case courtesy Julie Ritner, MD, Brigham and Women's Hospital.

精原细胞瘤：灰阶超声(左图)和彩色多普勒显示左侧睾丸内有不均匀的低回声血管性肿块(黄箭)。注意，肿块内许多微小回声灶(红箭)为微结石症。

Malignant germ cell tumors: Nonseminomatous germ cell tumors (NSGCT)

- Nonseminomatous germ cell tumors (NSGCT) include embryonal carcinoma, teratoma, yolk sac tumor, choriocarcinoma, and mixed subtypes.

  Mixed germ cell tumor is the most common NSGCT, and is the second most common primary testicular malignancy after seminoma (about 1/3). The most common components of mixed NSGCT are embryonal carcinoma and teratoma. It may contain elements of seminoma

  Embryonal cell carcinoma in its pure form is rare and in adults is typically seen as a component of mixed germ cell tumors. The infantile form, called endodermal sinus tumor or yolk sac tumor, is the most common testicular tumor of infancy. AFP is elevated.

  Teratoma is rare in its pure form in adults, but is seen in 50% of mixed NSGCT. Teratoma is classified as mature, immature, and malignant. In adults, teratomas are usually malignant. In children, teratomas are usually benign, with the mature subtype most commonly seen.

  Choriocarcinoma is the most aggressive and rare NSGCT. Choriocarcinoma metastasizes early, especially to brain and lung. Metastases tend to be hemorrhagic. hCG is always elevated and gynecomastia may result from elevated chorionic gonadotropins.

- NSGCT generally occur in younger patients compared to seminomas, typically in young men in their twenties and thirties. NSGCT tend to be more aggressive than seminomas. Local invasion into the tunica albuginea and visceral metastases are common.
- A heterogeneous testicular mass which contains solid and cystic components and coarse calcification is a typical appearance for a NSGCT. It is not possible to distinguish the various subtypes of NSGCT on ultrasound.

恶性生殖细胞肿瘤：非精原生殖细胞瘤(NSGCT)

- 非精原生殖细胞瘤(NSGCT)包括胚胎性癌、畸胎瘤、卵黄囊瘤、绒毛膜癌及混合亚型。

  混合型生殖细胞瘤：是最常见的NSGCT，是仅次于精原细胞瘤的第二大原发性睾丸恶性肿瘤(约占1/3)。混合型生殖细胞瘤最常见的组成成分是胚胎癌和畸胎瘤。也可含精原细胞瘤的成分。

  胚胎细胞癌：单纯胚胎细胞癌罕见，在成人中通常是混合型生殖细胞瘤的一个组成部分。婴儿型，也称为内胚窦瘤或卵黄囊瘤，是最常见的婴儿睾丸肿瘤，伴有甲胎蛋白升高。

  畸胎瘤：单纯畸胎瘤成人罕见，但可见于50%的混合型NSGCT。畸胎瘤分为三类亚型：成熟型、未成熟型和恶性型。成人畸胎瘤通常为恶性，儿童畸胎瘤则通常为良性，成熟型亚型最为常见。

  绒毛膜癌：是最具侵袭性的、罕见的NSGCT。很早发生转移，尤其是脑转移和肺转移，转移灶有出血倾向。该病患者hCG总会升高，可致男性乳腺发育。

- 与精原细胞瘤相比，NSGCT的发病年龄较小，多为20~30岁的青年男性。NSGCT通常比精原细胞瘤更具侵袭性，常见局部白膜侵袭和远处脏器转移。
- NSGCT的典型超声表现为囊实混合性团块，伴粗大钙化。超声无法区分不同亚型的NSGCT。

Burnt-out germ cell tumor

- *Burnt-out* germ cell tumor is a primary testicular neoplasm that is no longer viable in the testicle even though there is often viable metastatic disease, especially retroperitoneal.
- In the testicle, focal calcification with posterior shadowing is characteristic. A mass may or may not be present.
- Treatment is orchiectomy in addition to systemic chemotherapy.

无活性生殖细胞肿瘤

- 无活性生殖细胞肿瘤是一种原发的睾丸肿瘤，睾丸内原发灶已不再具有活性，但远处的转移灶有活性，尤其是腹膜后。
- 典型超声图像为睾丸局限性钙化灶伴后方声影。肿块可有可无。
- 治疗方法为睾丸切除术加全身化疗。

Testicular microlithiasis

- Testicular microlithiasis is the presence of multiple punctate intratesticular

睾丸微石症

- 睾丸微石症是指睾丸内出现多发点状钙化灶。

calcifications.

- There is a controversial association between microlithiasis and testicular neoplasm. While the overall absolute risk for developing testicular cancer remains very small in the presence of microlithiasis, the relative risk may be increased.
- Current guidelines do not support screening by ultrasound or tumor markers, but patients with microlithiasis may perform self-examinations and be seen in follow-up as needed.
- At least 5 microcalcifications must be present per image to be called microlithiasis. If there are less than 5 microcalcifications the term *limited microlithiasis* is used.
- Microlithiasis can produce a *starry sky* appearance if calcifications are numerous.

  In the liver, hepatitis can cause a *starry sky* appearance due to increased echogenicity of the portal triads.

- 微石症与睾丸肿瘤之间的相关性目前仍存在争议。睾丸微石症患者罹患睾丸恶性肿瘤的绝对风险很低，但相对风险可能会增加。
- 目前的指南不支持使用超声或肿瘤标志物进行筛查，但有睾丸微石症的患者可行自我检查和必要的随访。
- 诊断微石症需在单幅图像发现5个以上的微钙化。如少于5个，则称为*局限性微石症*。
- 当出现无数钙化灶时，微石症可表现为*星空征*。

  肝炎时由于汇管区回声增强，也可表现为*星空征*。

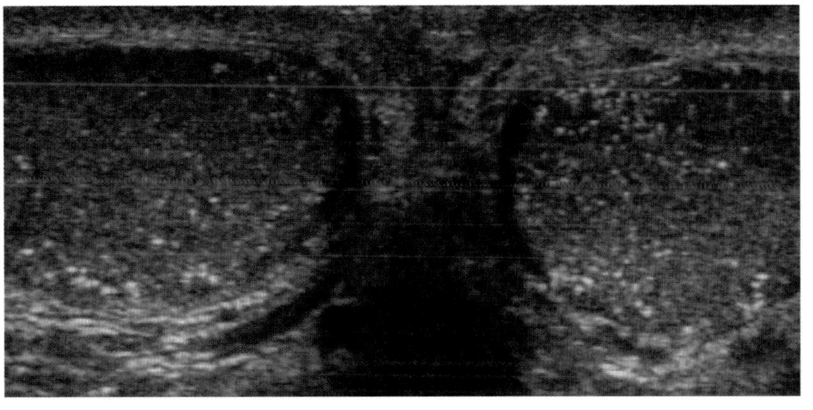

Transverse grayscale ultrasound shows numerous echogenic foci within both testes, consistent with microlithiasis.
横切面灰阶超声显示双侧睾丸内有无数强回声灶，为微石症。

Testicular metastases

- The most common metastases to the testicles are leukemia and lymphoma, as the relevant chemotherapeutic agents do not cross the blood-testis barrier.
- Hematologic malignancies typically present in older patients, tend to be bilateral, and may be infiltrative with diffuse testicular enlargement.

Benign testicular tumors

- An **epidermoid** is a keratin-filled cyst with a distinctive *onion skin* appearance of concentric alternating rings of hypo-and hyperechogenicity. If suspected, local excision is performed instead of the standard orchiectomy typically performed for presumed malignant masses.
- **Sex cord-stromal tumors** are 90% benign but are sonographically indistinguishable from malignant tumors. Orchiectomy is therefore the standard treatment.

  Leydig cell tumor can present with gynecomastia due to estrogen secretion.

  Sertoli cell tumor is associated with Peutz-Jeghers and Klinefelter syndromes.

睾丸转移性肿瘤

- 睾丸最常见的转移性肿瘤是白血病和淋巴瘤，因为相关的化疗药物不能通过血睾屏障。
- 恶性血液病常发生于老年人，多为双侧，可浸润而致睾丸弥漫性肿大。

良性睾丸肿瘤

- **表皮样囊肿**是一个充满角蛋白的囊腔，有很特殊的“洋葱皮”样外观，为高、低回声同心交替的结果。若考虑该诊断，可行局部病灶切除术，这不同于恶性肿块时需要进行的标准睾丸切除术。
- 约90%的**性索间质肿瘤**为良性，但超声无法将其与恶性肿瘤相鉴别。睾丸切除术为标准的治疗方案。

  睾丸间质肿瘤可引起男性乳腺发育，为分泌雌激素所致。

  睾丸支持细胞瘤与黑斑息肉病与克兰费尔特综合征相关。

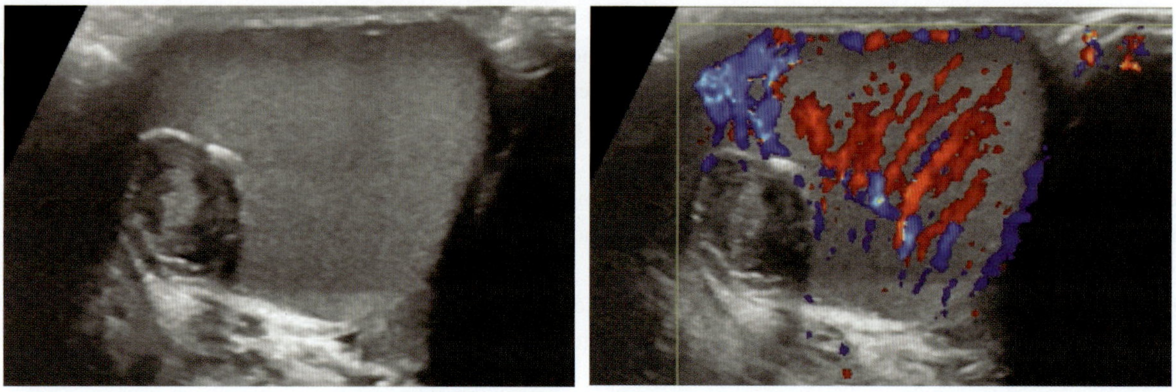

Testicular epidermoid: Transverse grayscale ultrasound (left image) demonstrates a circumscribed, encapsulated mass in the testicle with peripheral calcification and *onion skin* appearance. There is no demonstrable Doppler flow within the mass (right image).
睾丸表皮样囊肿：横切面灰阶超声(左图)显示睾丸内有边界清晰的包裹性肿块，伴周边钙化和洋葱皮样外观。肿块内无多普勒血流信号(右图)。

Sarcoidosis

- Sarcoidosis may involve either the testis, the epididymis, or both. Scrotal involvement is rare, but presents clinically as painless scrotal enlargement.
- The ultrasound appearance of testicular sarcoid is indistinguishable from a solid malignant mass. If sarcoidosis is suggested by clinical history, the testicular mass must be biopsied to exclude malignancy. Without tissue pathology, a mass cannot be assumed to be sarcoid.

Benign testicular tumor mimics

- Congenital adrenal rests are embryologic remnants of adrenal tissue trapped within the testis. These are typically seen in newborns with congenital adrenal hyperplasia.

  Adrenal rests appear as *bilateral* hypoechoic masses and classically enlarge with ACTH exposure.
- Polyorchidism/supernumerary testis: An extra testicle has an identical imaging appearance to normal testicular parenchyma.

  Extranumerary testes carry a slightly increased risk of torsion and testicular cancer.

结节病

- 结节病可累及睾丸或附睾，或两者同时受累。阴囊结节病罕见，临床表现为无痛性阴囊肿大。
- 睾丸结节病的超声表现无法与实质性恶性肿瘤相鉴别。若临床怀疑有结节病，须对睾丸肿块行活检以排除恶性可能。不能在缺乏组织病理结果的情况下将肿块假定为结节病。

睾丸良性肿瘤样病变

- 先天性肾上腺残留是胚胎时期的肾上腺组织遗留在睾丸内。常见于先天性肾上腺增生的新生儿。

  肾上腺残留表现为双侧低回声肿块，典型的表现为促肾上腺皮质激素可使其增大。
- 多睾症/多余睾丸：多余的睾丸在声像上的表现与正常睾丸相同。

  多余睾丸发生扭转和恶性肿瘤的风险略增加。

Extra-testicular masses

- In contrast to intratesticular masses, **extratesticular** masses are usually **benign**. Up to 16% of extratesticular masses may be malignant, however, and ultrasound cannot reliably differentiate benign from malignant masses.

Benign extratesticular masses

- Spermatic cord lipoma is the most common extratesticular neoplasm overall.
- Benign adenomatoid tumor of the tunica albuginea is the most common epididymal neoplasm.

睾丸外肿物

- 与睾丸内肿块不同，**睾丸外**肿块通常为**良性**。但近16%睾丸外肿块可能为恶性，超声无法准确鉴别良恶性。

良性睾丸外肿物

- 精索脂肪瘤是最常见的睾丸外肿物。
- 白膜的良性腺瘤样瘤是最常见的附睾肿瘤。

The "-celes" and cystic lesions

Hydrocele

- A hydrocele is excess fluid in the scrotum surrounding the testicle. Most are asymptomatic.
- A hydrocele may be congenital (due to patent processus vaginalis in utero or infancy), idiopathic, or post-inflammatory. Regardless of etiology, there is never fluid at the bare area where the testicle is attached to the tunica vaginalis.

"积液"和囊性病变

睾丸鞘膜积液

- 睾丸鞘膜积液是指阴囊内、睾丸周围有过量的液体。大多无症状。
- 睾丸鞘膜积液可为先天性(由宫内或婴儿期鞘状突未闭引起)，也可为特发性，或为炎症后反应。无论何种病因，积液不应出现在裸区，即睾丸附着于鞘状突的部位。

Hematocele

- A hematocele is blood in the scrotum due to trauma or torsion.

睾丸血性鞘膜积液

- 睾丸血性鞘膜积液是由外伤或睾丸扭转导致的阴囊内积血。

Varicocele

精索静脉曲张

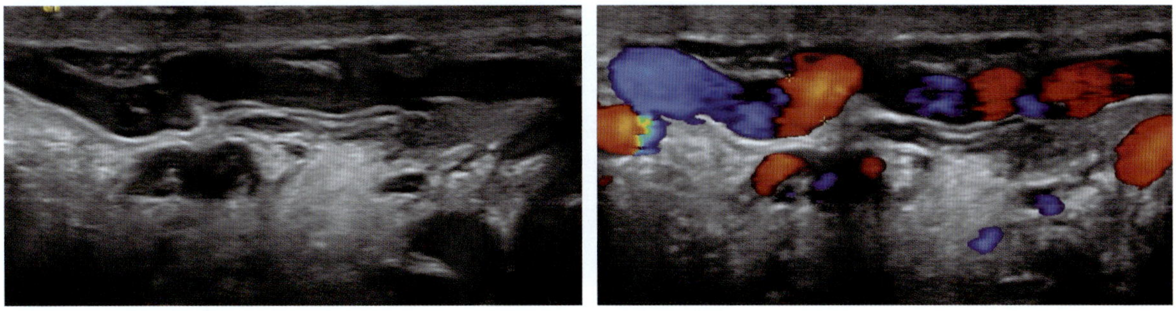

Varicocele: Transverse grayscale ultrasound of the left scrotum (left image) shows dilated serpiginous vessels posterior to the left testis, which demonstrate increased Doppler flow with Valsalva maneuver (right image).
精索静脉曲张：左侧阴囊横切面灰阶超声(左图)显示左侧睾丸后方迂曲扩张血管，瓦尔萨尔瓦动作时多普勒血流增加(右图)。

- A varicocele is a dilated venous pampiniform plexus in the scrotum.
- A primary varicocele is due to incompetent valves of the internal spermatic vein. A secondary (reactive) varicocele is due to increased venous pressure caused by obstruction, usually caused by retroperitoneal mass.
- Varicocele is a common cause of infertility, seen in up to 40–75% of males presenting to an infertility clinic.
- Varicoceles are much more common on the left, as the left testicular vein drains into the left renal vein at straight angle, whereas the right testicular vein drains directly into the infrarenal IVC. 85% of varicoceles are left-sided and 15% are bilateral. *An isolated right-sided varicocele should prompt a search for a right-sided retroperitoneal mass.*
- On ultrasound, varicoceles appear as multiple tubular and serpentine anechoic structures >2–3 mm in diameter in the region of the upper pole of the testis and epididymal head. The varicoceles follow the spermatic cord into the inguinal canal and can be compressed by the transducer. Careful optimization of Doppler parameters shows the slow venous flow within the varicocele.

- 精索静脉曲张是阴囊内蔓状静脉丛迂曲扩张。
- 原发性精索静脉曲张由精索内静脉瓣功能不全引起。继发性(反应性)精索静脉曲张则为梗阻后引起的静脉压力升高所致，梗阻常由腹膜后肿块导致。
- 精索静脉曲张是引起不育的常见病因，见于高达40%~75%的男性不育门诊患者。
- 左侧精索静脉曲张更常见，因为左侧睾丸静脉以直角汇入左肾静脉。而右侧睾丸静脉则直接汇入肾下下腔静脉。左侧精索静脉曲张占85%，双侧发病为15%。*若仅有右侧精索静脉曲张，需及时寻找有无右侧腹膜后肿块。*
- 超声上精索静脉曲张表现为睾丸上极和附睾头多发迂曲小管状无回声结构，直径大于2~3mm。曲张静脉沿精索走行至腹股沟管，探头加压可闭合。仔细调节和优化多普勒参数可显示管腔内低速静脉血流信号。

Epididymal cysts and spermatocele

- A spermatocele is cystic dilation of the epididymis filled with spermatozoa, usually occurring in the epididymal head, but potentially occurring anywhere in the epididymis. Classic ultrasound appearance is an epididymal cyst with internal low-level mobile echoes.
- A simple epididymal cyst and a spermatocele cannot be reliably distinguished by ultrasound.

附睾囊肿和精液囊肿

- 精液囊肿是附睾的囊性扩张，内部充满精子，常见于附睾头部，但也可发生于附睾任何部位。典型超声表现为附睾内的囊性病变，内见低水平移动性回声。
- 超声不能将单纯性附睾囊肿和精液囊肿进行有效区分。

Simple testicular cyst

- A simple testicular cyst meets sonographic criteria for a simple cyst (smooth posterior wall, imperceptible wall thickness, completely anechoic, posterior through transmission).

睾丸单纯性囊肿

- 睾丸单纯性囊肿符合单纯性囊肿的超声诊断标准(后壁光滑、囊壁薄、完全无回声、后方回声增强)。

Tubular ectasia of rete testis

睾丸网管状扩张

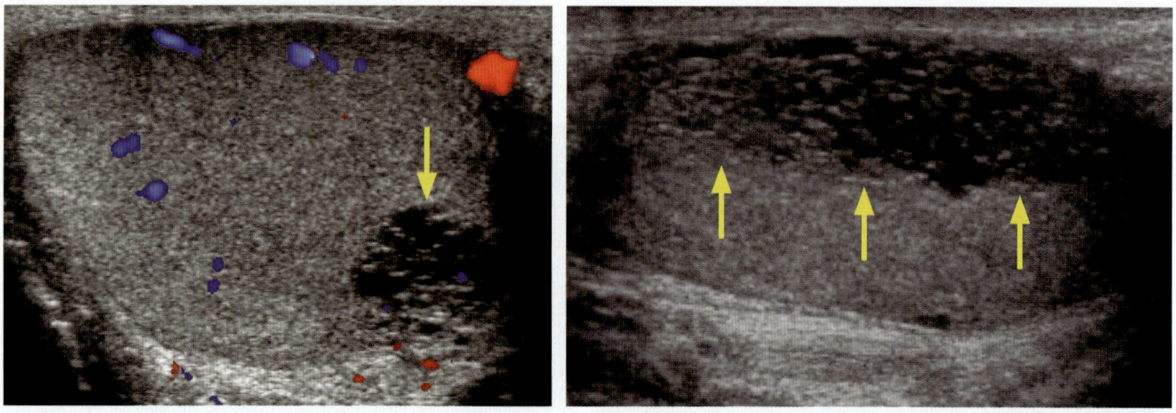

Transverse color Doppler ultrasound of the right testicle (left image) shows cystic dilation at the mediastinum testes (arrow). There is no flow within the lesion. This appearance is highly suggestive of tubular ectasia, although an avascular mass may rarely have a similar appearance.
Sagittal ultrasound (right image) shows elongation of the cystic dilation (arrows) along the mediastinum testes, which is confirmatory for tubular ectasia.
右侧睾丸横切面彩色多普勒图像(左图)显示睾丸纵隔处囊状扩张(黄箭),内部未见血流信号。这一表现高度提示睾丸网管状扩张,但极少数无血供肿块也可有相似的表现。
矢状切面(右图)显示囊状扩张(黄箭)沿睾丸纵隔呈纵向分布,可确诊为睾丸网管状扩张。

- Tubular ectasia of the rete testis is nonpalpable, asymptomatic, cystic dilation of the tubules at the mediastinum testes caused by epididymal obstruction. Tubular ectasia is often accompanied by an epididymal cyst or spermatocele. Tubular ectasia of the rete testis is common in older patients and may be bilateral.
- Imaging shows numerous tiny dilated structures in the region of the mediastinum testis, often seen in conjunction with an epididymal cyst/spermatocele.
- Tubular ectasia is benign and no treatment is necessary.

Tunical cyst

- The tunica albuginea is the capsule overlying the testis. A cyst of the tunica albuginea presents as a palpable superficial nodule that resembles a BB. No treatment is necessary.
- Ultrasound shows a typically small, simple, extra-testicular cyst.

- 睾丸网管状扩张是睾丸纵隔处的小管呈囊状扩张,不可触及且无症状,为附睾梗阻所致。它常合并附睾囊肿或精液囊肿。睾丸网管状扩张常见于老年男性,可双侧发病。
- 影像学表现为睾丸纵隔区无数细小扩张的管状结构,常合并附睾囊肿或精液囊肿。
- 睾丸网管状扩张是良性病变,无须治疗。

鞘膜囊肿

- 白膜是覆盖于睾丸表面的包膜。鞘膜囊肿表现为可触及的表浅结节,与“BB弹”相似,无须治疗。
- 典型的超声表现为睾丸外的单纯性小囊肿。

(翻译　全杰荣)

Female Genitourinary System

女性泌尿生殖系统

Female Urethra

女性尿道

Anatomy

- The female urethra is much shorter than the male urethra. Unlike the male urethra, the female urethra is not divided into discrete segments. The proximal third of the urethra is lined by transitional epithelium, while the distal portion of the urethra is lined with a stratified squamous epithelium.

Urethral diverticulum

- Urethral diverticulum presents clinically with post-void dribbling, urethral pain, and dyspareunia. Often, however, the symptoms may be vague and nonspecific.
- Diverticula are thought to arise from glandular dilation caused by inflammation and chronic infection of the paraurethral glands of Skene.

解剖

- 女性尿道远短于男性。与男性尿道不同,女性尿道无明确分段。尿道近段1/3覆盖移行上皮,而远段则覆盖复层鳞状上皮。

尿道憩室

- 尿道憩室临床表现为排尿后滴沥、尿道疼痛和性交痛。然而,这些症状通常不明确且非特异。
- 憩室被认为是由尿道旁腺的炎症和慢性感染所致的腺体扩张。

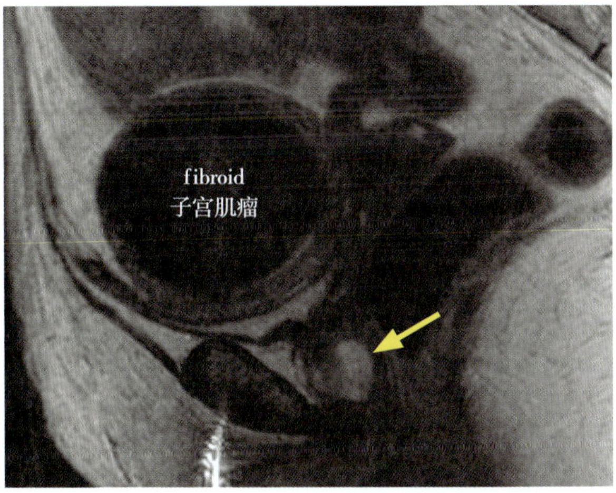

Midline sagittal T2-weighted MRI shows a rounded, hyperintense structure (arrow) in the region of the urethra, representing a urethral diverticulum. There is incidentally a large intramural fibroid.
正中矢状位T2加权MRI显示尿道区一个圆形(黄箭)的高信号结构,为尿道憩室。另见一个大的肌壁间子宫肌瘤。

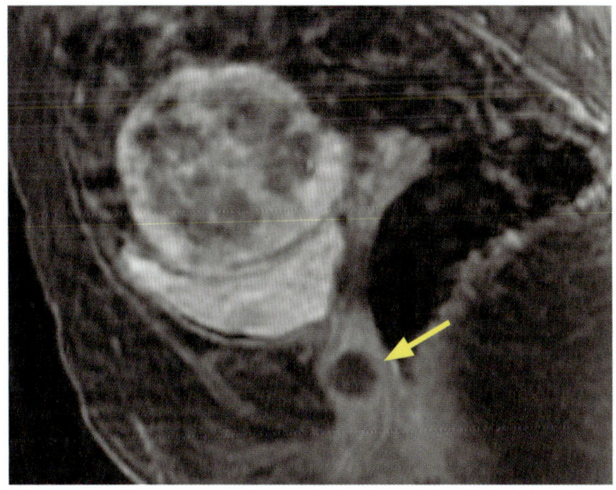

Postcontrast sagittal T1-weighted image shows no enhancement within or surrounding the diverticulum (arrow).
增强后矢状位T_1加权显示憩室内或周围无强化(黄箭)。

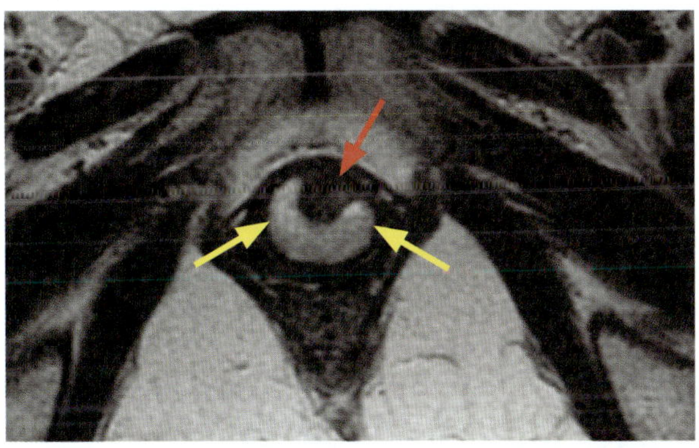

Axial T2-weighted image shows that the urethral diverticulum is U-shaped (yellow arrows) surrounding the normal decompressed urethra (red arrow).
轴位T_2加权显示尿道憩室呈"U"形(黄箭),并包绕正常减压的尿道(红箭)。

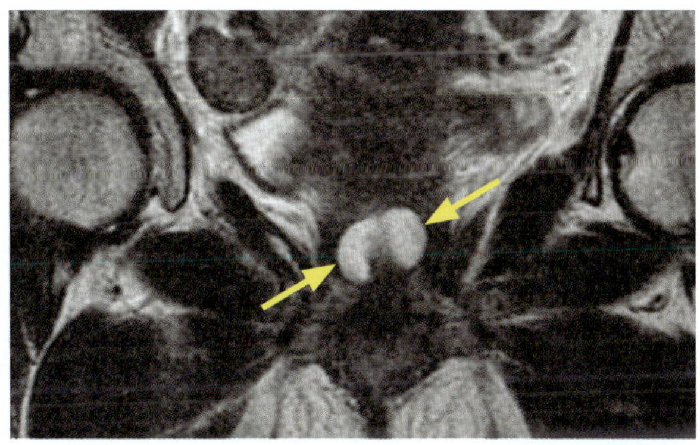

Coronal T2-weighted image again shows the urethral diverticulum as a lobulated focus of T2 hyperintensity (arrows) in the region of the urethra.
冠状位T_2加权也显示尿道憩室为尿道区一个呈分叶状的T_2高信号病灶(黄箭)。

- On imaging, urethral diverticulum appears as a periurethral cystic lesion that typically arises from the posterolateral urethra and wraps around the urethra circumferentially with a classic *saddlebag* or *U-shaped* morphology.
- Urethral diverticula are prone to develop calculi due to urinary stasis.
- Very rarely, adenocarcinoma may develop within a urethral diverticulum.

- 尿道憩室在影像学上表现为尿道周围囊性病变,通常发生在尿道的后外侧,并环状包绕尿道形成一个典型的鞍包或"U"形结构。
- 尿道憩室可因尿潴留而容易形成结石。
- 极罕见情况下,尿道憩室内可发生腺癌。

Vagina: Anatomy and Imaging

Anatomy

- The vagina is a 8–10 cm fibromuscular organ consisting of the vaginal orifice, vault, and the anterior, posterior, and lateral fornices.
- The posterior fornix is covered by the peritoneum of the rectouterine pouch (Pouch of Douglas).
- The vagina is supported by the levator ani, transverse cervical ligament, pubocervical ligament, uterosacral ligament, and perineal body.
- The **paraurethral glands of Skene** are paired anterior glands on either side of the urethral opening. They are homologous to the male prostate and secrete mucus at the external meatus.

阴道:解剖和影像

解剖

- 阴道是一个8~10cm的肌肉纤维器官,由阴道口、穹隆顶、前穹隆、后穹隆和侧穹隆组成。
- 后穹隆被**直肠子宫陷凹**的腹膜所覆盖。
- 阴道由肛提肌、宫颈横韧带、耻骨宫颈韧带、子宫骶韧带和会阴体支撑。
- **尿道旁腺**是一对阴道前壁的腺体,开口于尿道的两侧,相当于男性前列腺,在外生殖道分泌黏液。

- The **Bartholin glands** are posterior paired pea-sized structures on either side of the vaginal opening as part of the vulva. They are analogous to the bulbourethral (Cowper) glands in the male and secrete lubricating fluid.
- **Arterial supply:** vagina, uterine, internal pudendal and middle rectal arteries (internal iliac artery branches).
- **Venous drainage:** into internal iliac veins.
- **Lymphatic drainage** is divided in thirds.

  The upper third drains to the external iliac nodes.

  The middle third drains to the internal iliac and sacral nodes.

  The lower third drains to superficial inguinal and perirectal nodes.

Imaging of the vagina

- MRI imaging is the modality of choice for imaging of the distal urethra and distal vagina at the introitus. Self-administered intra-vaginal ultrasound gel may improve visualization on MRI but is not always used.

- **前庭大腺**是位于阴道口两侧后部的一对豌豆大小的结构，是外阴的一部分，相当于男性的尿道球腺，分泌润滑液。
- **动脉供应：**阴道、子宫、阴部内动脉和直肠中动脉(髂内动脉分支)。
- **静脉引流：**汇入髂内静脉。
- **淋巴引流**分为三部分。

  上1/3引流至髂外淋巴结。

  中1/3引流至髂内淋巴结和骶淋巴结。

  下1/3引流至腹股沟浅淋巴结和直肠周围淋巴结。

阴道影像

- MRI是尿道远端和阴道远端阴道口成像的首选方式。让患者自行在阴道内注入超声凝胶可改善MRI的显示效果，但并不常用。

Benign vaginal lesions

阴道良性病变

Retention cysts of the vagina

阴道潴留囊肿

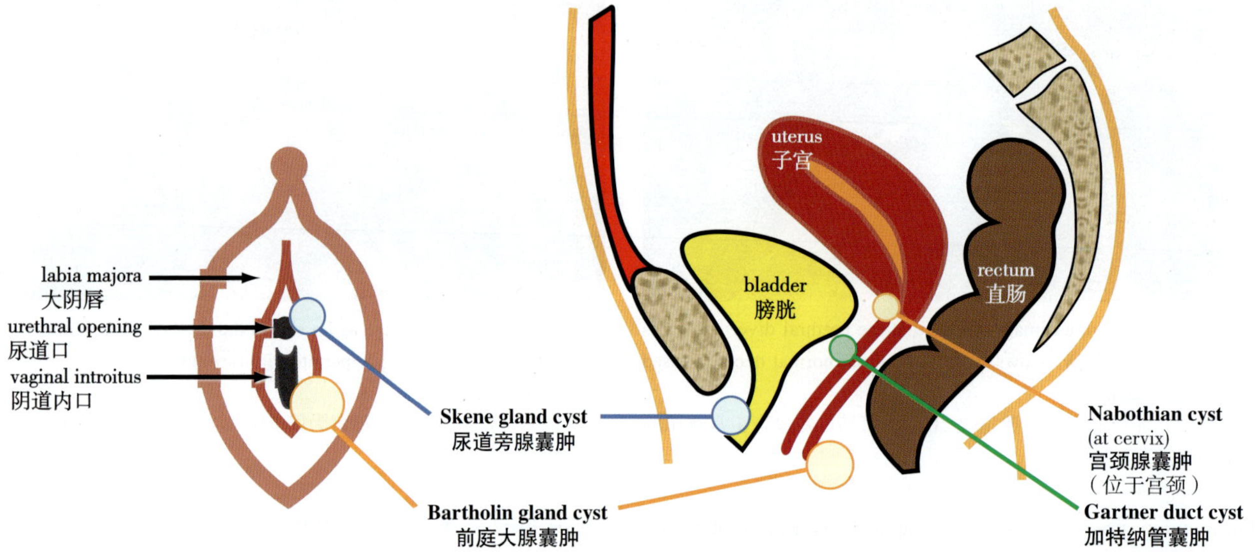

- Periurethral cysts is a general category of cystic lesions around the urethra and vagina. They are usually asymptomatic, often seen incidentally on MRI. These secretory retention cysts can become large or infected and cause pain. Location is the key to differentiation, as summarized in the illustration above and the details on the following page.

- 尿道周围囊肿是尿道和阴道周围囊性病变的总称。它们通常无症状，多为MRI上的偶然发现。分泌液潴留时囊肿可变大或继发感染，从而引起疼痛。正如前文图示，囊肿部位是鉴别的关键，将在下文中详述。

Skene duct cysts (paraurethral duct cyst): Retenti on cysts due to obstructi on or in flammati on of the paraurethral ducts. They are typically located anterior, near midline and below the level of pubic symphysis. MRI shows T2 hyperintense signal if uncomplicated, but hemorrhage may cause fluid-fluid levels.

Gartner duct cysts: Retenti on cysts arising from the embryologic remnants of the mesonephric (Wolffi an) duct. They are found in the anterolateral vaginal wall, above the level of pubic symphysis. MRI and US oft en detect Gartner duct cysts incidentally.

尿道旁(腺)导管囊肿：是由于尿道旁(腺)导管阻塞或炎症而形成的潴留性囊肿。常位于前方近中线、耻骨联合的下方。单纯囊肿在MRI上呈T_2高信号，出血时可出现液-液平面。

加特纳管囊肿：胚胎发育过程中残余的中肾(Wolffian)管形成的囊肿。位于阴道前侧壁，耻骨联合的上方。加特纳管囊肿常为MRI与超声检查时的偶然发现。

Bartholin gland cysts: Retenti on cysts due to obstructi on of the Bartholin duct by prior infecti on or trauma resulti ng in stenosis, stone, or thick mucus and retained secreti ons. They are found in the inferior third of the vagina at the posterolateral vaginal wall, below the level of pubic symphysis and associated with the labia majora. Superinfecti on of the cysts may occur. MRI signal characteristi cs depend on protein content of the cyst resulti ng in variable T1 and heterogeneous T2 signal.

Nabothian cysts are located at the cervix and are due to occlusion of cervical glands.

前庭大腺囊肿：是由前庭大腺导管阻塞所致的潴留性囊肿，原因包括既往感染或创伤导致的狭窄、结石或黏稠的黏液和残留的分泌物。囊肿位于阴道下1/3的后侧壁，耻骨联合水平以下，并与大阴唇相连。囊肿可发生感染。MRI信号特征取决于囊肿内蛋白质的成分，相应会出现T_1信号多变和T_2信号不均匀。

宫颈腺囊肿：位于宫颈，由宫颈腺阻塞所致。

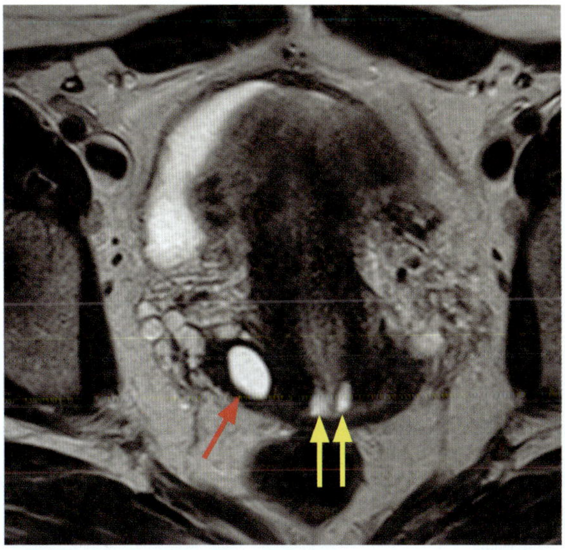

Axial T2-weighted MRI shows two Nabothian cysts (yellow arrows) within the cervical stroma, and a right Gartner duct cyst (red arrow) along the right anterolateral aspect of the superior vagina.
轴位T_2加权MRI显示两个位于宫颈间质内的宫颈腺囊肿(黄箭)，以及一个位于阴道上段右前侧壁的加特纳管囊肿(红箭)。

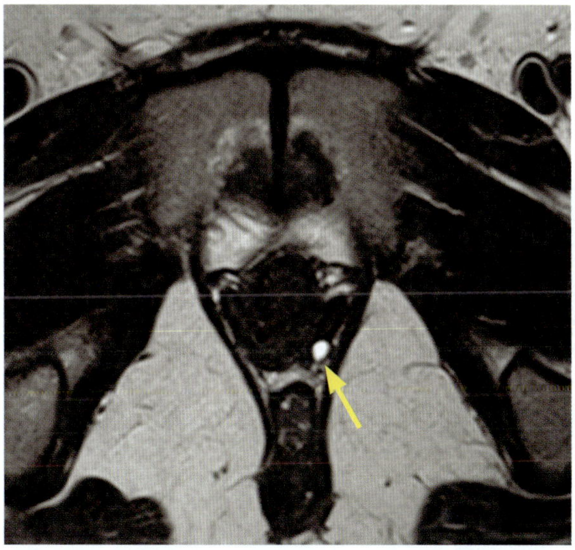

Axial T2-weighted MRI at level of the inferior margin of pubic symphysis demonstrates a Bartholin gland cyst (arrow) along the left posterolateral aspect of the inferior vagina.
轴位T_2加权MRI显示耻骨联合下缘水平的前庭大腺囊肿(黄箭)，位于阴道下段左后侧壁。

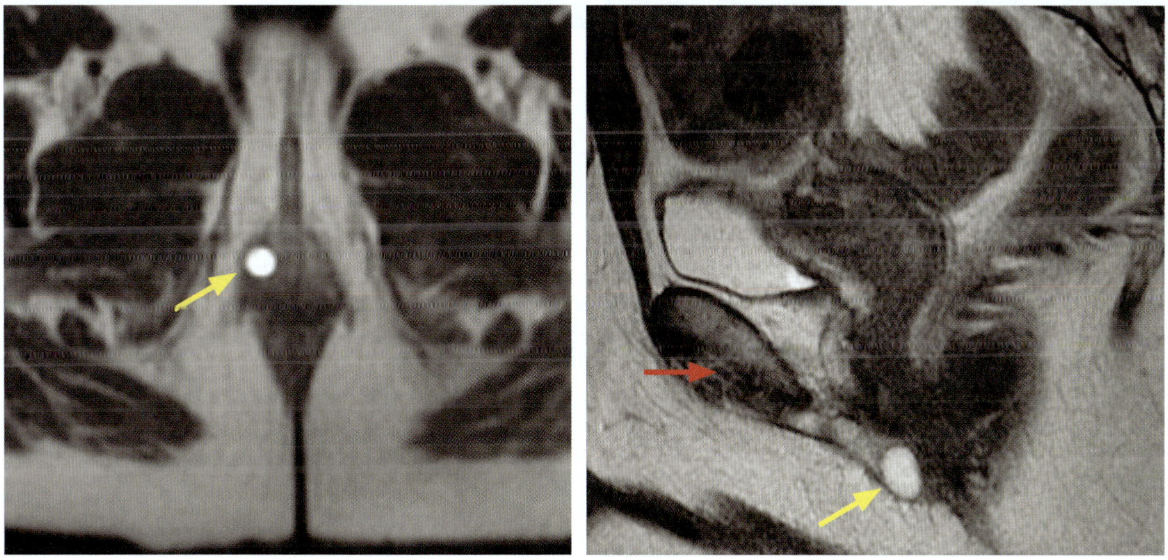

Axial and sagittal T2-weighted MRI images show a paraurethral (Skene) duct cyst (yellow arrows) located at the right lateral aspect of the urethral meatus and inferior to the pubic symphysis (red arrow).
轴位和矢状位T_2加权MRI显示尿道旁(腺)导管囊肿(黄箭)，位于尿道口右侧，耻骨联合下方水平(红箭)。

Fistulas involving the vagina

- **Anovaginal fistula** can arise from Crohn's disease, obstetric trauma, pelvic floor surgery, and radiation therapy. Gas and feces passed through the vagina can cause recurrent vaginal infections.
- **Urethrovaginal fistula** can occur after excision for urethral diverticulum, resulting in urinary incontinence.
- **Vesicovaginal fistula** represents a significant morbidity in female urology and occurs most commonly in the setting of obstructed childbirth or after urologic or pelvic surgery.
- On MRI imaging, sagittal plane is the most reliable plane for visualization of fistulas.
- Real-time fluoroscopic evaluation can be useful tools to characterize fistulas. Depending on location and organs involved, contrast can be injected into the relevant space to assess for abnormal extravasation.

阴道瘘

- **肛门阴道瘘**的原因包括克罗恩病、产科创伤、盆底手术和放射治疗。气体和粪便进入阴道可导致反复阴道感染。
- **尿道阴道瘘**可发生于尿道憩室切除术后，可出现尿失禁。
- **膀胱阴道瘘**是女性泌尿外科发病率较高的疾病，最常见于难产、泌尿外科或盆腔手术后。
- 在MRI中，矢状位是显示瘘管最可靠的平面。
- 实时X线透视检查可作为评估瘘管特征的有效工具。根据所累及的位置和器官，可以将造影剂注射到相应部位，以评估异常外渗。

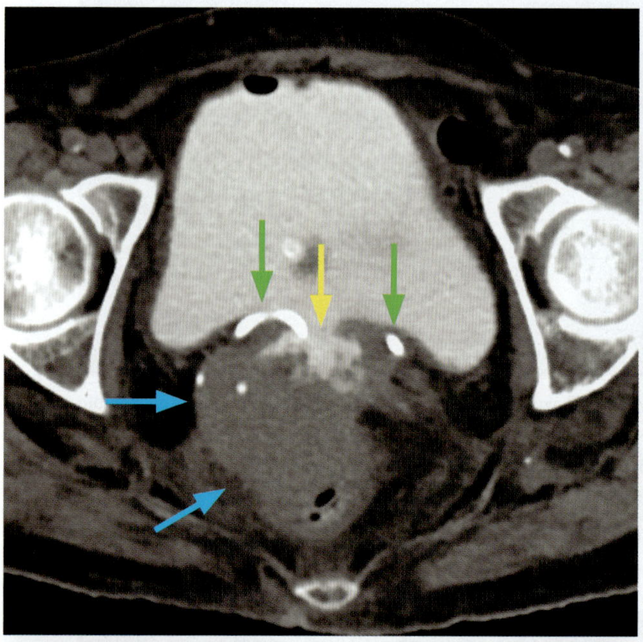

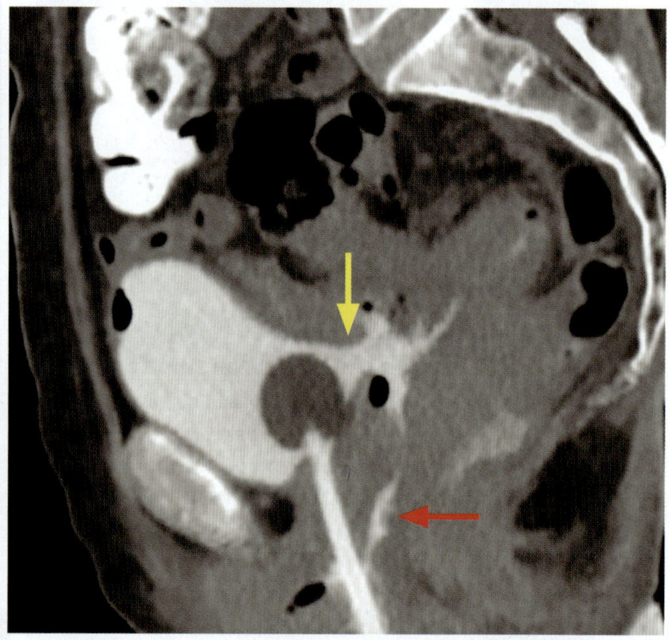

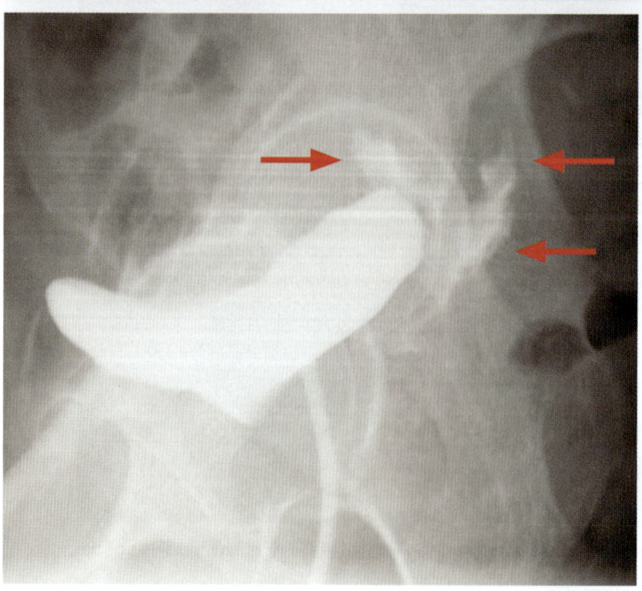

Vesicovaginal fistula in a patient with locally advanced rectal cancer:
Axial (left image) and sagittal (right image) CT cystogram demonstrates a fistulous connection between the bladder and upper vagina (yellow arrows). Contrast is seen in the mid to lower vagina (red arrow). Note the infiltrative rectal mass involving the vagina (blue arrows). Also seen are bilateral ureteral stents; the right ureteral stents traverse the vesicovaginal fistula (green arrows). A foley catheter is present in the bladder.
Sagittal spot image on follow-up fluoroscopic cystogram by contrast filling the upper vagina and vaginal fornices (red arrows) extravasating through the fistula.

局部进展期直肠癌患者并发的膀胱阴道瘘：
轴位(左上图)和矢状位(右上图)CT膀胱造影显示膀胱和阴道上段之间有瘘管相通(黄箭)。阴道中下段可见造影剂(红箭)。注意，浸润性直肠肿块累及阴道(蓝箭)。同时可见双侧输尿管支架；右侧输尿管支架穿过膀胱阴道瘘(绿箭)。膀胱内有导尿管。
后续矢状位X线透视膀胱造影局部图像(左下图)显示造影剂通过瘘管外渗至阴道上段和阴道穹隆(红箭)。

Malignant vaginal disease

Vaginal cancer

- **Squamous cell carcinoma of the vagina** accounts for 80–85% of primary vaginal malignancies and usually presents in older women. It is associated with HPV similar to SCC of the cervix.
- **Adenocarcinoma of the vagina** presents in younger women (15% of vaginal malignancies) and can arise from vaginal adenosis.
- **Clear cell carcinoma of the vagina** is rare and associated with previous diethylstilbestrol (DES) exposure. These patients will often have a "T-shaped" uterus, described later in the uterine malformations section.
- **Primary vaginal melanoma** is rare and most commonly presents in postmenopausal women. It has an aggressive course.
- Vaginal sarcoma presents as **rhabomyosarcoma** in the pediatric population. This is the most common vaginal tumor in children. It has a bimodal distribution, usually ages 2–6 and 14–18.

Vulvar cancer

- Vulvar cancer commonly involves the labia majora and minora, accounting for up to 5% of female genital tract malignancies with peak age 65–70 years old.

Metastasis

- Metastasis to the vagina can occur from the upper genital tract or the GI tract.
- Metastasis located in the upper 1/3 of the vagina (typically anterior) is usually from the upper genital tract. Metastasis located in the lower 1/3 (typically posterior) is usually from the GI tract.

阴道恶性疾病

阴道癌

- **阴道鳞状细胞癌**占原发性阴道恶性肿瘤的80%~85%，多见于老年女性。与HPV有关，类似于宫颈鳞状细胞癌。
- **阴道腺癌**见于年轻女性(占阴道恶性肿瘤的15%)，可由阴道腺病引起。
- **阴道透明细胞癌**罕见，且与既往己烯雌酚(DES)暴露有关。此类患者通常会伴随“T”形子宫，相关内容将在下文子宫畸形部分讨论。
- **原发性阴道黑色素瘤**罕见，最常见于绝经后妇女。侵袭性高。
- 儿童阴道肉瘤通常为**横纹肌肉瘤**。为儿童最常见的阴道肿瘤，具有双峰分布，通常为2~6岁和14~18岁。

外阴癌

- 外阴癌通常累及大阴唇和小阴唇，占女性生殖道恶性肿瘤的5%，发病高峰年龄为65~70岁。

转移癌

- 阴道转移可源自上生殖道或胃肠道。
- 位于阴道上1/3(常为前壁)的转移通常来自上生殖道。位于阴道下1/3(常为后壁)的转移通常来自胃肠道。

(翻译　姚旬)

Female pelvis

Anatomy

True and false pelvis

- The linea terminalis is a bony landmark separating the true (inferior) pelvis from the false (superior) pelvis. The linea terminalis is a composite of the arcuate line of the ilium, the iliopectineal line, and the pubic crest.
- Normally, the uterus and ovaries are in the true pelvis.
- The dome of a full bladder extends into the false pelvis, pushing small bowel out of the true pelvis. The bladder acts as a sonographic window into the true pelvis.

女性盆腔

解剖

真、假骨盆

- 髂耻线是真(下部)假(上部)骨盆的骨性分界标志，由髂骨的弓状线、髂耻线和耻骨嵴组成。
- 正常情况下，子宫和卵巢位于真骨盆。
- 膀胱充盈后其圆顶会延伸到假骨盆，并将小肠推出真骨盆。超声检查时以膀胱作为真骨盆的透声窗。

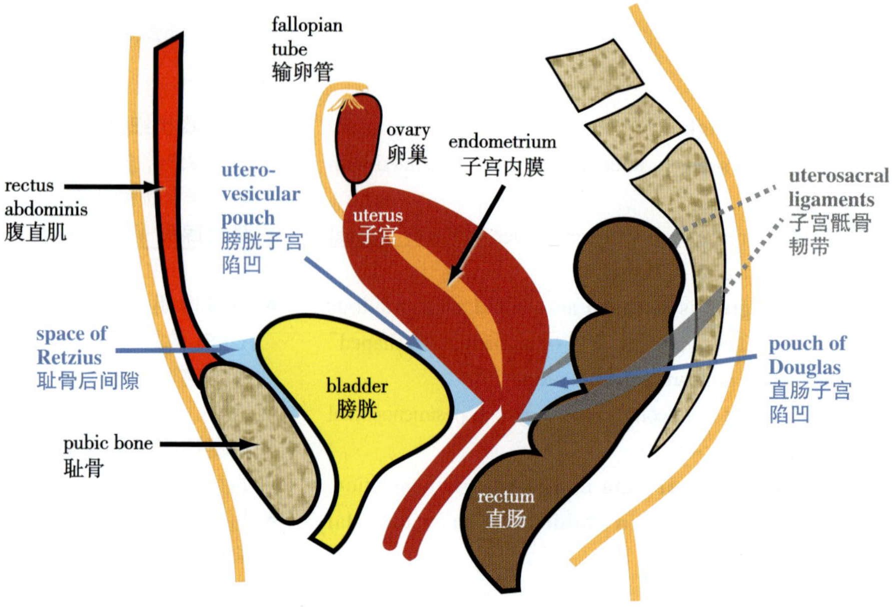

Space of Retzius

- The space of Retzius is an extraperitoneal potential space between the pubic symphysis and the bladder.
- A mass in the space of Retzius (such as a hematoma) can displace the bladder posteriorly.
- In contrast, pelvic or abdominal masses will displace the bladder inferiorly or anteriorly.

Uterovesicular space

- Intraperitoneal space created by double folding of peritoneum between the anterior surface of the uterus and the bladder.
- Inferior to this space, the cervix is attached to the posterior edge of the bladder by the parametrium.

Rectouterine pouch (of Douglas)

- Intraperitoneal space created by double folding of peritoneum between the posterior surface of the uterus and the rectum.
- Also known as the cul de sac, this is the most dependent portion of the peritoneal cavity.

耻骨后间隙

- 耻骨后间隙是位于腹膜外的潜在间隙，位于耻骨联合和膀胱之间。
- 位于耻骨后间隙的包块(如血肿)可使膀胱向后移位。
- 相反，盆腔或腹腔包块则将膀胱向下或向前推移。

子宫膀胱间隙

- 为子宫前表面和膀胱之间由双层腹膜反折形成的腹膜内空间。
- 在该间隙下方，子宫颈通过宫旁腹膜与膀胱后缘相连。

直肠子宫陷凹

- 为子宫后表面和直肠之间的双层腹膜反折形成的腹膜内空间。
- 也称为"袋底"，是腹膜腔的最底部。

Imaging the pelvis

Ultrasound of the female pelvis

- Both transabdominal and transvaginal imaging can be used for pelvic evaluation. In general, transvaginal ultrasound provides better resolution due to closer proximity to the internal organs.
- Transabdominal and transvaginal imaging is usually performed sequentially. Transabdominal imaging is conducted first because it is less invasive and can sometimes provide more comprehensive and sufficient diagnostic information. Transabdominal imaging requires a full bladder to provide an acoustic window for visualization of deep pelvic structures. Prior to transvaginal ultrasound, the bladder should be emptied to minimize discomfort and improve visualization.
- The sagittal scan plane is rotated 90 degrees between transabdominal and endovaginal orientation. The patient typically empties her bladder prior to endovaginal scanning.

盆腔影像

女性盆腔超声检查

- 经腹和经阴道超声都可用于评估盆腔。一般来说，经阴道超声因更接近内部器官而能提供更好的图像分辨率。
- 经腹和经阴道超声常按顺序进行，先进行经腹超声，因其侵害性小，有时可提供更全面和充分的诊断信息。经腹超声需膀胱充盈，以提供一个声学窗口来显示盆腔深部结构；而在经阴道超声检查之前，应排空膀胱，以减少患者不适并提高可视性。
- 经腹与经阴道扫查的矢状切面之间需要旋转90°。阴道内扫查前患者常需排空膀胱。

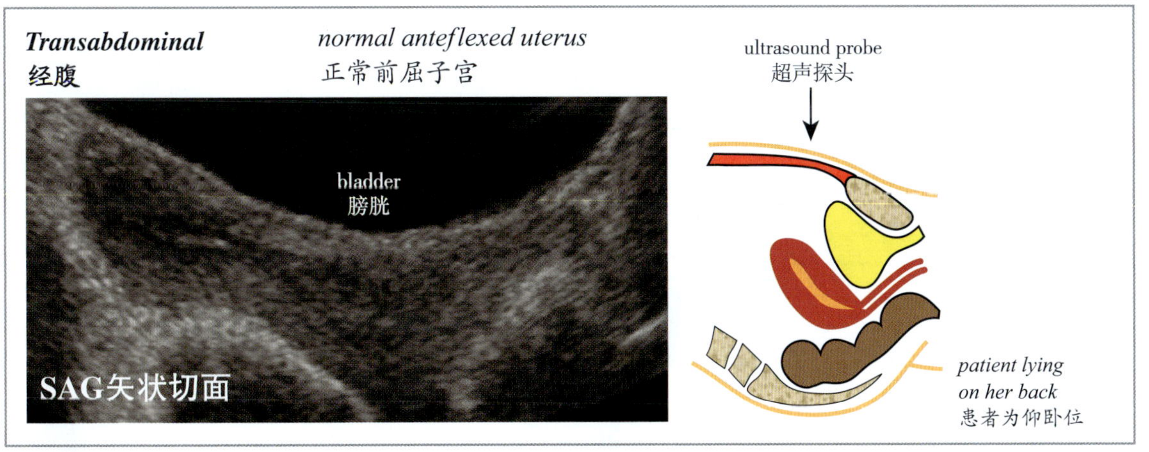

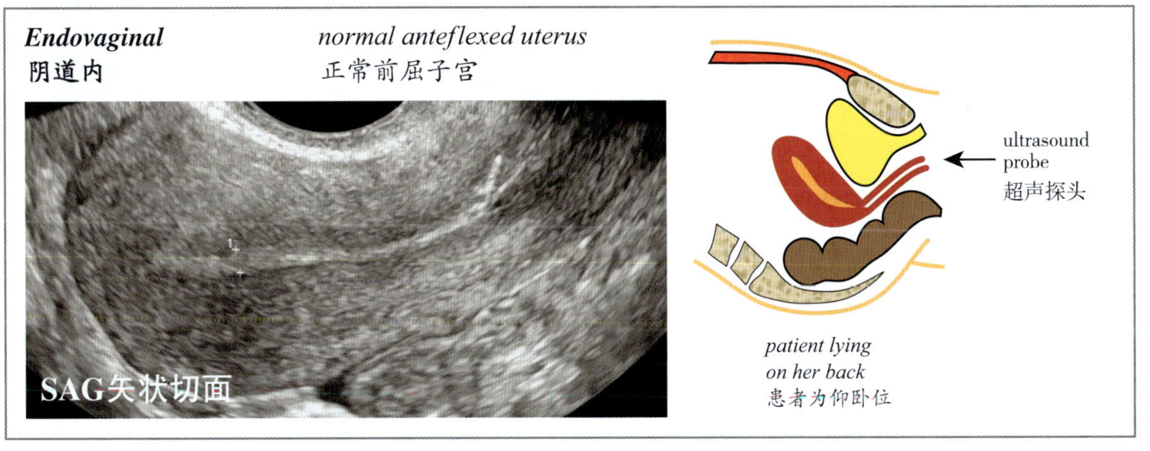

MRI of the female pelvis

- MRI provides the greatest anatomic detail in pelvic imaging and is used for diagnostic evaluation in challenging or indeterminate cases on the previously mentioned modalities.
- MRI can also permit evaluation of adjacent structures and assessment for pelvic lymphadenopathy.

女性盆腔的MRI

- MRI在盆腔影像中可提供最佳的软组织分辨力，可对前述检查方法中有困难或不能确定的病例进行诊断性评估。
- MRI还可以评估邻近结构及盆腔淋巴结。

CT of the female pelvis

- CT has overall low sensitivity in the evaluation of pelvic disorders, but can be used in staging of pelvic tumors to assess for metastatic disease.

女性盆腔的CT

- CT在评估盆腔疾病中的总体敏感性较低，但可用于评估转移性疾病，以利于盆腔肿瘤分期。

Hysterosalpingogram

- Hysterosalpingogram (HSG) is commonly used during evaluation of infertility. Pregnancy should be excluded prior to the exam.
- Using a speculum, a catheter is placed into the uterine cervix. Contrast is injected under fluoroscopy into the uterine cavity to evaluate uterine contour (early filling) and fallopian tubes (late filling).
- The uterus can be evaluated for congenital anomalies and acquired filling defects (e.g., polyps or endometrial cancer).
- Contrast should enter the fallopian tubes and spill freely into the peritoneum. If free spill is not seen from a fallopian tube, it is likely occluded. If occlusion is caused by tubal spasm, slow continued injection will subsequently opacify the tube.

子宫输卵管造影

- 子宫输卵管造影(HSG)常用于评估不孕症。检查前应除外怀孕。
- 通过阴道窥器将导管插入宫颈。在透视下将造影剂注入宫腔，以评估子宫轮廓(早期充盈)和输卵管(晚期充盈)。
- 可评估子宫是否存在先天性发育异常和后天性充盈缺损(如息肉或子宫内膜癌)。
- 造影剂应进入输卵管并自由弥散至腹腔。若输卵管末端未见造影剂溢出，则可能发生阻塞。若阻塞是由输卵管痉挛引起，则缓慢持续注射会使输卵管显影。

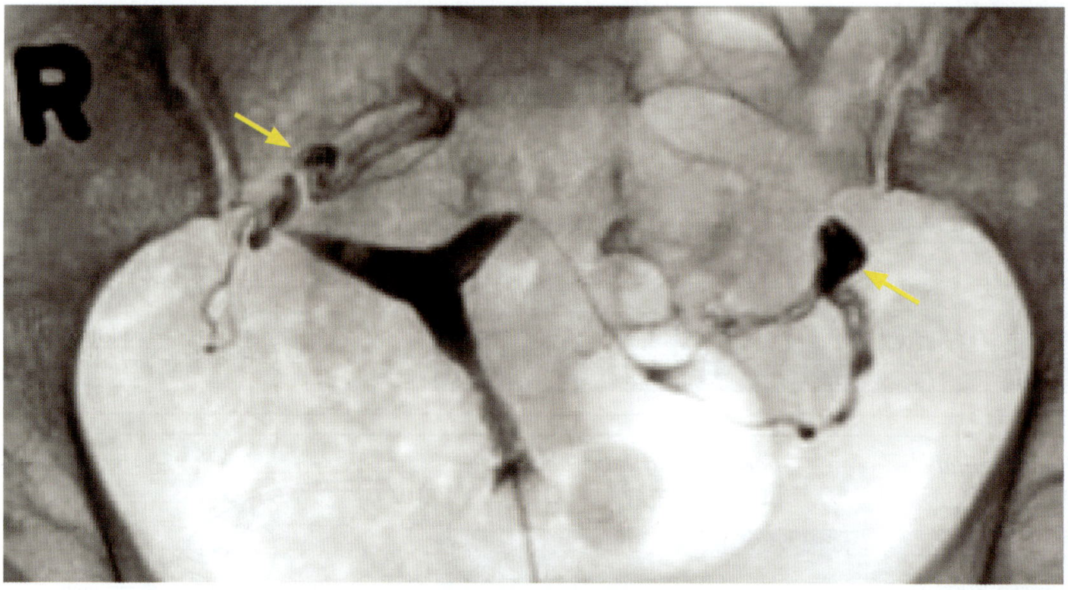

Normal bilateral intraperitoneal spill of contrast on hysterosalpingogram (arrows), indicating patency of both fallopian tubes.
子宫输卵管造影显示造影剂溢出至腹腔两侧(黄箭),表明双侧输卵管通畅。

- Sometimes, contrast is seen spilling into the peritoneum, but remains localized (loculated). Loculated peritoneal contrast is suggestive of pelvic adhesions, which can be seen in pelvic inflammatory disorder.

- 有时可见造影剂溢出到腹腔,但无弥散(局部积聚)。腹腔内局部造影剂积聚提示盆腔粘连,可见于盆腔炎性疾病。

(翻译 姚旬)

UTERUS

子宫

ANATOMY

- Normal segments of the uterus include: fundus (superior to the ostia of fallopian tubes), body (upper 2/3, superior boundary is the fundus), cervix (lower 1/3), and isthmus (junction of body and cervix).

Normal variant uterine positions

- "Version" of the uterus refers to angle between the cervix and the vagina.
- "Flexion" of the uterus refers to angle between the body and the cervix.
- About 20 degrees of uterine anteflexion is normal. As the bladder fills, the degree of anteflexion decreases.
- Retroversion of the uterus may cause poor visualization of the uterine fundus transabdominally.
- Retroflexion of the uterus may cause even poorer visualization of the fundus and can mimic an intramural fibroid.

解剖

- 正常子宫包括宫底(位于输卵管开口上方)、宫体(上2/3,上界为宫底)、宫颈(下1/3)和峡部(宫体和宫颈的连接段)。

子宫位置正常变异

- 子宫的"倾"是指宫颈和阴道之间的角度。
- 子宫的"屈"是指宫体与宫颈之间的角度。
- 子宫前屈20°为正常。当膀胱充盈时,前屈的角度减小。
- 子宫后倾不利于经腹超声观察宫底。
- 子宫后屈可能导致对子宫底部的观察更差,并可有类似壁内子宫肌瘤的表现。

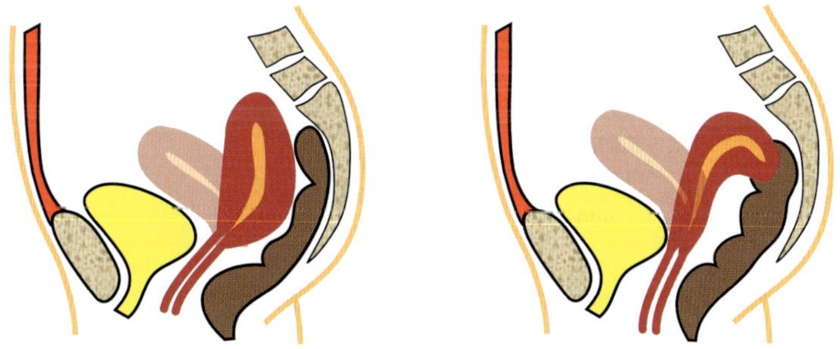

Normal T2 zonal anatomy

- T2-weighted MRI sequence can distinguish the three layers of the uterus.
- **Endometrial stripe:** T2 hyperintense (glandular).
- **Junctional zone** (first zone of myometrium): T2 hypointense.

  The T2 hypointense signal is due to the extremely compact smooth muscle.

  Normal junctional zone should measure ≤12 mm: Thickening of the junctional zone is seen in adenomyosis.
- **Outer myometrium:** Relatively T2 hypointense, although less so than junctional zone.

正常子宫 T_2 分区解剖

- T_2 加权 MRI 可识别子宫三层解剖结构。
- **内膜层：**T_2 高信号(腺体)。
- **结合带**(子宫肌层第一区)：T_2 低信号。

  T_2 低信号是因为结合带为非常致密的平滑肌。

  正常结合带厚度应≤12mm：厚度增加见于腺肌病。
- **外肌层：**T_2 相对低信号，但稍高于结合带。

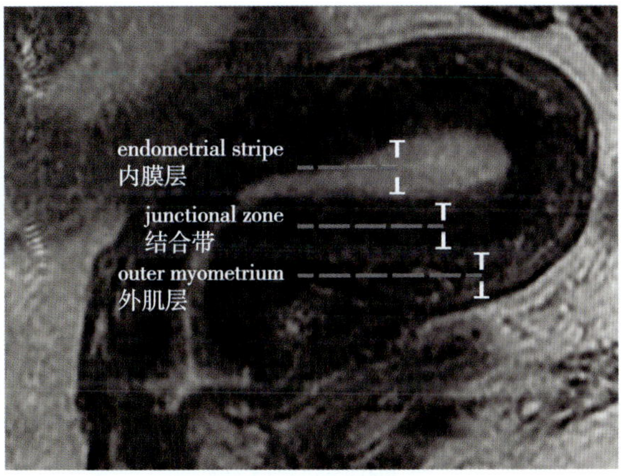

Normal sagittal T2 zonal anatomy of the uterus.
Case courtesy Cheryl Sadow, MD, Brigham and Women's Hospital.
正常子宫矢状位 T_2 解剖。

Endometrium

Endometrial thickness

- The thickest portion of the endometrium should be measured transvaginally in the sagittal orientation. Information about the last menstrual period is critical to adequately evaluate the endometrium. Ideally, the endometrium should be measured in the *menstrual* phase.
- Endometrial fluid is not included in the measurement: If endometrial fluid is present, the flanking endometrium is measured and the two components are summed.

子宫内膜

子宫内膜的厚度

- 测量子宫内膜最厚部位需在矢状位经阴道进行。末次月经的信息对准确评估子宫内膜状态至关重要。测量子宫内膜最好是在月经期。
- 宫腔积液不应计算在内：如有积液，应分别测量单层子宫内膜厚度，再将两者相加。

Days 天数/天	Phase in menstrual cycle 月经周期	Endometrial thickness 内膜厚度/mm	Ultrasound findings 超声表现	Illustration 示意图
1~4	**Menstrual** **月经期**	<4	Thin, echogenic line 纤细的条带回声	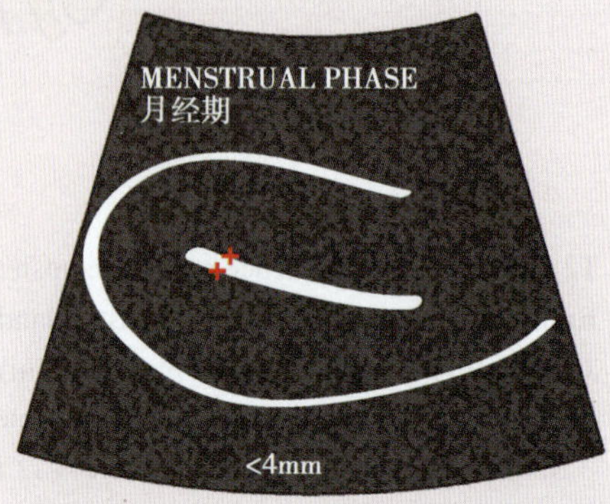
5~9	**Early proliferative** **增殖早期**	4~8	—	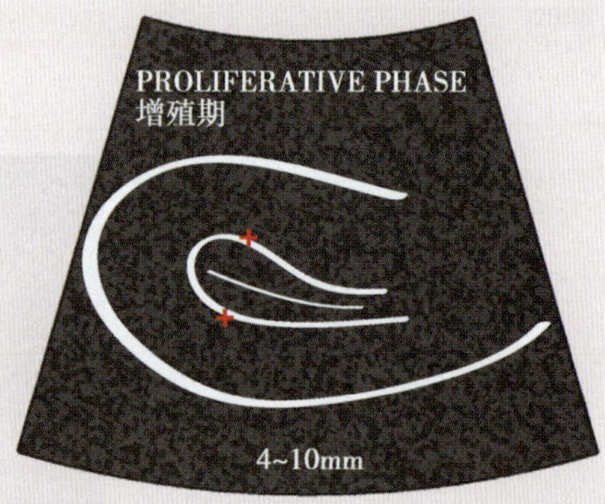
10~14	**Late proliferative** (peri-ovulatory) Estrogen effects dominate, increasing functional zone thickness. **增殖晚期**(近排卵期) 雌激素效应明显，使功能区的厚度增加	6~10	Classic trilaminar appearance, with hypoechoic zone between the linear echogenic collapsed endometrial cavity and the thicker peripheral echogenic endometrium. 典型的三线征，塌陷宫腔线和增厚的内膜外缘之间呈低回声区	
15~28	**Secretory** Progesterone effects dominate, causing further thickening of the functional layer. The functional zone becomes soft and edematous as the spiral arteries become tortuous. **分泌期** 孕激素效应明显，使内膜功能层进一步增厚、变软、肿胀，并伴随螺旋动脉更加弯曲	7~14	The endometrium reaches maximum thickness and echogenicity (becomes isoechoic relative to the basal layer). 内膜厚度最大，回声最强(相对于基底层变成等回声)	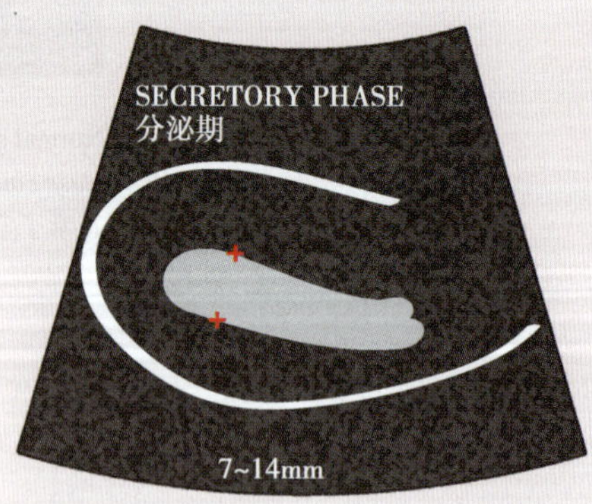

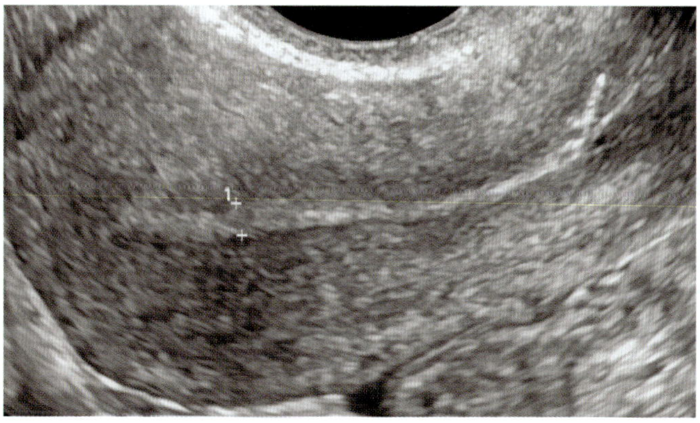

Thin, linear endometrium during menstrual phase.
月经期，子宫内膜薄、呈线状。

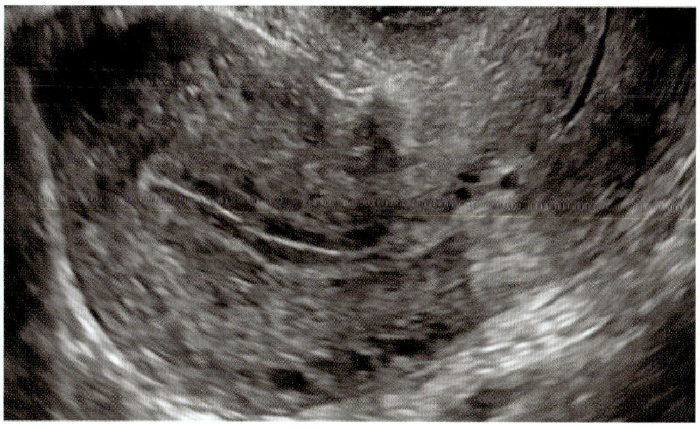

Trilaminar endometrium during proliferative phase.
增殖期，子宫内膜呈三线征。

BENIGN ENDOMETRIAL PATHOLOGY

Endometrial polyp

- An endometrial polyp can cause mucous discharge or irregular vaginal bleeding between cycles. Most endometrial polyps are benign, but larger polyps (>1.5 cm) occurring in postmenopausal patients may have malignant potential.
- Ultrasound shows a focal nodular area of endometrial thickening, often with a feeding vessel or internal flow by Doppler. A polyp is more definitively diagnosed by sonohysterogram, where saline is instilled into the uterus prior to transvaginal ultrasound.

Endometrial hyperplasia/metaplasia

- Endometrial hyperplasia refers to abnormal proliferation of the endometrial glands and stroma. It can be seen in all age groups. It typically presents as abnormal uterine bleeding.
- Hyperplasia occurs due to unopposed estrogen stimulation, and can have various causes (obesity, polycystic ovary syndrome, pregnancy, estrogen-secreting ovarian tumors, and tamoxifen).
- Endometrial hyperplasia is typically diagnosed by ultrasound. The imaging findings are nonspecific but can include smooth endometrial thickening and/or cystic changes. Hyperplasia, metaplasia, or carcinoma cannot be reliably distinguished by imaging.

In premenopausal women, evaluation is based on clinical symptoms, in particular, abnormal uterine bleeding. Endometrial thickness varies with the menstrual cycle and is a poor predictor for endometrial pathology.

In post-menopausal women, endometrial thickness in combination with clinical picture (symptoms, medications) can prompt further workup including biopsy and/or hysteroscopy. Refer to the chart below for more detail.

良性子宫内膜病变

子宫内膜息肉

- 子宫内膜息肉可引起黏液性分泌物增多或非月经期的不规则阴道出血。多数子宫内膜息肉为良性病变，但绝经后患者出现较大息肉(>1.5cm)则有恶变可能。
- 超声表现为局部结节样内膜增厚，彩色多普勒可见供血血管或内部血流。经阴道宫腔超声造影更易确诊息肉，在经阴道超声前需将生理盐水灌入宫腔。

子宫内膜增生/化生

- 子宫内膜增生是指子宫内膜腺体和间质的异常增生。可见于任何年龄。通常表现为异常子宫出血。
- 增生是因雌激素刺激未受抑制所致，原因有多种(肥胖、多囊卵巢综合征、妊娠、分泌雌激素的卵巢肿瘤和服用他莫昔芬)。
- 子宫内膜增生通常使用超声进行诊断。影像学表现无特异性，可包括平滑的子宫内膜增厚和/或囊性改变。影像学无法可靠地鉴别增生、化生或癌变。

在绝经前妇女中，评估基于临床症状，尤其是异常子宫出血。子宫内膜厚度随月经周期而变化，因而不能作为一个预测子宫内膜病变的指标。

在绝经后妇女中，需结合子宫内膜厚度与临床表现(症状、药物)及时做进一步检查，包括活检和/或宫腔镜检查。更多相关详细信息见下图。

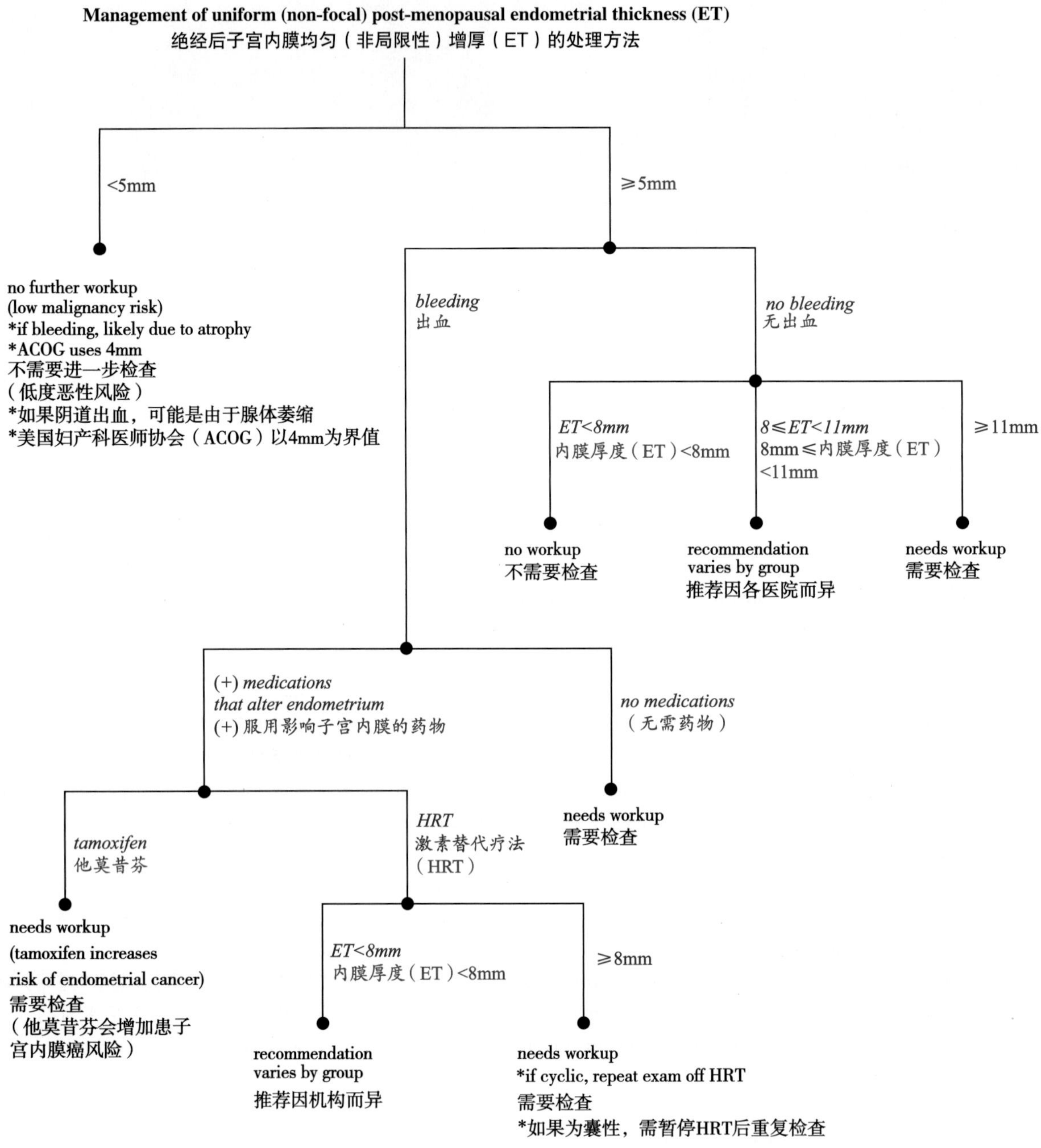

*The ET cutoff for further workup of post-menopausal bleeding varies by institution. For example, American College of Obstetricians and Gynecologists (ACOG) use 4 mm instead of 5 mm.

The above management approach can only be used if the *entire* endometrial lining is visualized.

Focal endometrial thickening requires workup regardless of thickness.

*关于绝经后出血进一步检查的子宫内膜厚度(ET)的临界值，因各医院而异。例如，美国妇产科学会(ACOG)推荐用4mm而不是5mm。

只有当整个子宫内膜线可见时，才能使用上述方案。

对于局限性子宫内膜增厚，无论厚度如何，都需要进行检查。

ENDOMETRIAL CANCER

子宫内膜癌

Endometrial carcinoma overview

子宫内膜癌概述

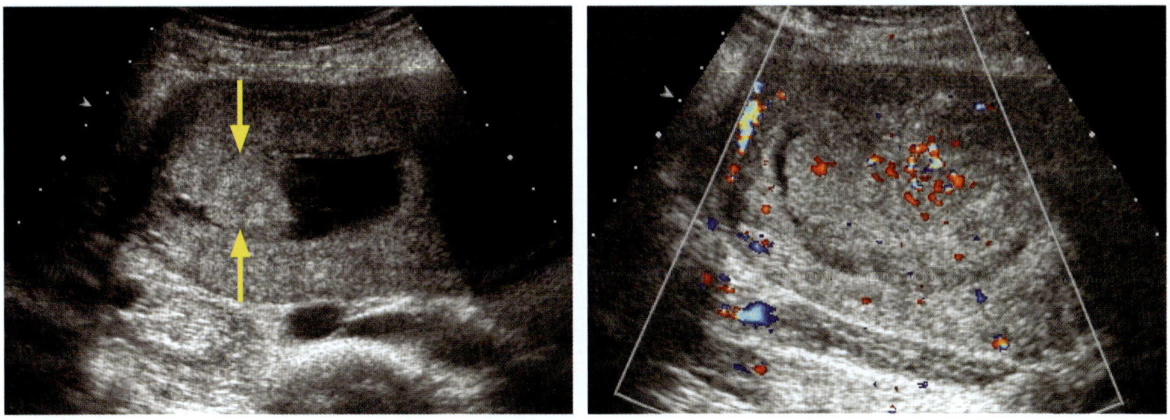

Endometrial cancer: Grayscale ultrasound of the uterus (left image) shows a mildly echogenic, irregular endometrial mass (arrows). Fluid in the endometrial canal has likely accumulated due to cervical stenosis. Color Doppler shows vascularity within the mass.
Case courtesy Julie Ritner, MD, Brigham and Women's Hospital.
子宫内膜癌：子宫灰阶超声(左图)显示一个轻度回声和不规则的内膜肿块(黄箭)。子宫腔内有积液，可能由宫颈狭窄所致。彩色多普勒显示肿块内有血管床。

- Endometrial carcinoma is the most common female gynecologic malignancy and is thought to be caused by prolonged estrogen exposure. Specific risk factors include nulliparity, hormone replacement therapy (HRT), and tamoxifen.
- Over 95% of endometrial carcinoma presents with postmenopausal bleeding. The average endometrial thickness of patients with endometrial carcinoma is 21 mm.
- In patients with postmenopausal bleeding, endometrial thickness ≥5 mm requires further workup (usually biopsy and/or hysteroscopy). If endometrial thickness <5 mm, this most likely represents endometrial atrophy.

  For patients on HRT, postmenopausal bleeding with endometrial thickness ≥8 mm requires further workup. This cutoff accounts for effects of HRT on endometrial proliferation. If HRT is given cyclically, imaging should be repeated when patient is off HRT.
- Without bleeding, endometrium thickness ≥8–11 mm (based on source) requires workup.
- Although uncommonly seen in the absence of bleeding, the finding most suggestive of endometrial carcinoma is the presence of ill-defined margins separating the endometrium and the myometrium.

Staging of endometrial carcinoma

- MRI can be used for staging once endometrial carcinoma is confirmed by histologic sampling.
- Staging of endometrial carcinoma is based on the International Federation of Gynecology and Obstetrics (FIGO) system, which characterizes extent of disease based on involvement of the cervix, vagina, uterine serosa, adnexa, adjacent bladder/bowel, inguinal lymph nodes, and/or distant metastases.
- The presence (and extent) of myometrial invasion is key for staging purposes. In a premenopausal patient, an intact junctional zone confirms no myometrial invasion. The junctional zone cannot be distinguished in post-menopausal patients.
- The depth of myometrial invasion highly correlates with the presence of lymph node metastasis.

- 子宫内膜癌是最常见的妇科恶性肿瘤，被认为是由于长期雌激素暴露所引起。具体风险因素包括未生育、激素替代疗法(HRT)和使用他莫昔芬。
- 超过95%的子宫内膜癌表现为绝经后阴道出血。子宫内膜癌的平均内膜厚度为21mm。
- 对于绝经后出血患者，子宫内膜厚度≥5mm时需进一步检查(通常是活检和/或宫腔镜检查)。若子宫内膜厚度<5mm，最可能的原因是子宫内膜萎缩。

  对于接受HRT的患者，子宫内膜厚度≥8mm的绝经后出血需进一步检查。该临界值考虑了HRT对子宫内膜增生的影响。若患者周期性地接受HRT，应停止HRT后重复检查。
- 无阴道出血时，子宫内膜厚度在8~11mm或以上(基于文献)时需要检查。
- 最能提示子宫内膜癌的表现是子宫内膜和肌层间分界不清，但这种情况在无出血时不常见。

子宫内膜癌的分期

- MRI用于组织病理学确诊后对子宫内膜癌进行分期。
- 子宫内膜癌的分期基于国际妇产科联盟(FIGO)系统，根据病灶是否累及宫颈、阴道、子宫浆膜、附件、邻近膀胱/肠道、腹股沟淋巴结和/或是否为远处转移来进行分期。
- 肌层侵犯情况(及深度)是分期的关键。在绝经前的患者中，如有完整的结合带则说明未侵犯肌层。但结合带在绝经后患者中无法被辨认。
- 肌层侵犯深度与淋巴结转移有高度相关性。

- Postcontrast images demonstrate the tumor with the highest conspicuity, as endometrial cancer enhances less avidly than the surrounding myometrium.

- 肿瘤在增强后的图像上显示最明显，因肿瘤强化弱于周围的肌层。

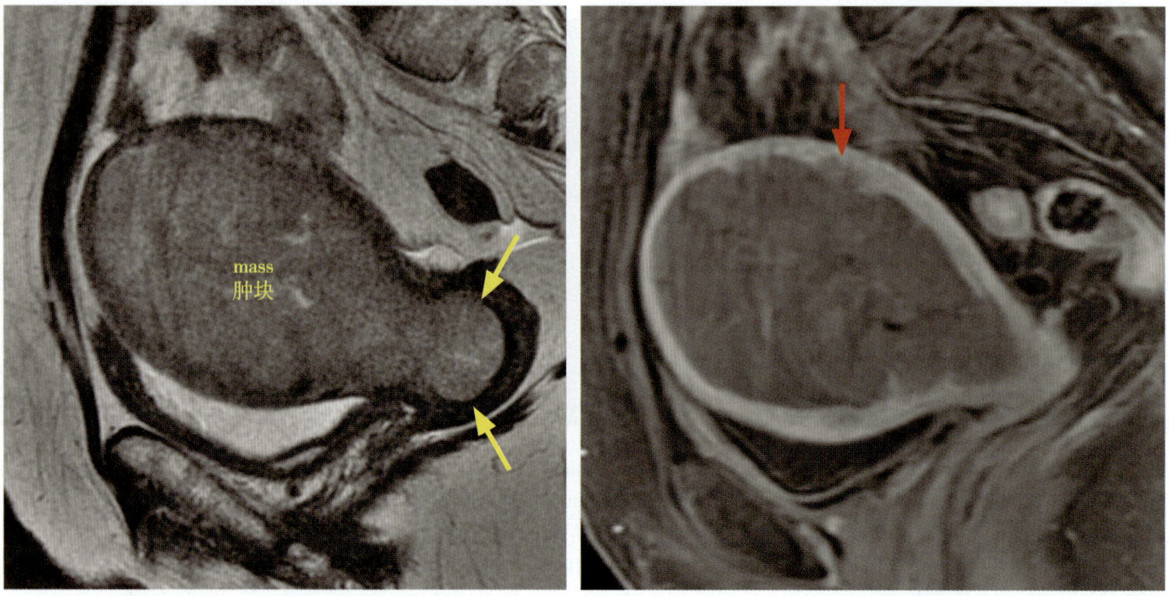

Endometrial carcinoma, stage IB:
Sagittal T2-weighted MRI (left image) shows a large mass distending the endometrial canal and invading into the myometrium, and protruding into the cervix (yellow arrows). No definite cervical stromal invasion is seen.
Sagittal postcontrast fat-suppressed T1-weighted MRI (right image) shows that the mass is relatively hypoenhancing relative to the myometrium. The extent of myometrial invasion is best appreciated, with foci of invasion extending >50% of the myometrial wall (red arrow).
Case courtesy Cheryl Sadow, MD, Brigham and Women's Hospital.
子宫内膜癌，ⅠB期：
矢状位T_2加权MRI(左图)显示一个大肿块使宫腔扩张伴肌层受侵，并突入宫颈(黄箭)。未见明确的宫颈基质侵犯。
矢状位增强后脂肪抑制T_1加权MRI(右图)显示肿块强化低于肌层。增强后肌层受侵清晰可见，局部肌层受侵厚度超过50%(红箭)。

Other diseases of the endometrium/endometrial cavity

Endometrial fluid

- Trace amount of fluid in the endometrial canal can be normal finding, particularly in premenopausal patients (e.g., menses). Larger amount of fluid is always abnormal, and it can be due to spontaneous abortion.
- In a postmenopausal woman, endometrial fluid can be due to cervical stenosis, and a careful evaluation for cervical malignancy should be performed.

Infection

- **Endometritis** is inflammation or infection of the endometrium, commonly seen postpartum.

  Imaging findings are often normal in uncomplicated cases. Gas in the uterus >3 weeks post delivery is suspicious for endometritis. Other less specific features include an enlarged (and tender) uterus, associated with endometrial thickening. Note that gas in the uterus can be found up to three weeks postpartum (seen in 7% of normal cases).
- **Pyometra** (pus within the uterus) is very rare and usually due to outflow obstruction, usually due to cervical malignancy – which needs to be excluded – but untreated endometritis is another potential cause.

Hemorrhage

- Intrauterine hemorrhage can occur for a variety of reasons in both the gravid and non-gravid uterus. In the non-gravid uterus (outside of menstruation), it

其他子宫内膜/宫腔疾病

宫腔积液

- 微量宫腔内液体可为正常，尤其是在绝经前患者中(如月经期)。大量积液通常为异常，可由自然流产引起。
- 绝经后妇女，宫腔积液可能继发于宫颈狭窄，此时应进行细致检查以排除宫颈恶性病变。

感染

- **子宫内膜炎**是指子宫内膜的炎症或感染，常见于产后。

  无合并症时影像学表现多为正常。若产后3周有宫腔积气，需怀疑子宫内膜炎。该病的非特异性征象包括子宫增大(和压痛)伴子宫内膜增厚。注意，产后3周内宫腔亦可观察到积气(可见于7%的正常病例)。
- **子宫积脓**(宫腔积脓)极罕见，常由流出道梗阻所致，多为宫颈恶性肿瘤，应加以排除，而未经治疗的子宫内膜炎是另一个潜在原因。

出血

- 子宫内出血有各种原因，可出现于妊娠和非妊娠期。在非妊娠期子宫(月经期外)中可见

may be seen with endometrial polyps, endometrial hyperplasia, endometrial carcinoma, and fibroids.

- If a patient has had a recent miscarriage or dilation and curettage, blood clot (nonvascular) should be distinguished from retained products of conception (vascular). This is further explained within the Obstetrics chapter.

于子宫内膜息肉、子宫内膜增生、子宫内膜癌和子宫肌瘤。

- 若患者近期有流产或刮宫史，应区分血块(非血管性)与妊娠残留产物(血管性)。具体将在产科影像章节中进一步解释。

Ectopic Endometrium

异位子宫内膜

Endometriosis

子宫内膜异位症

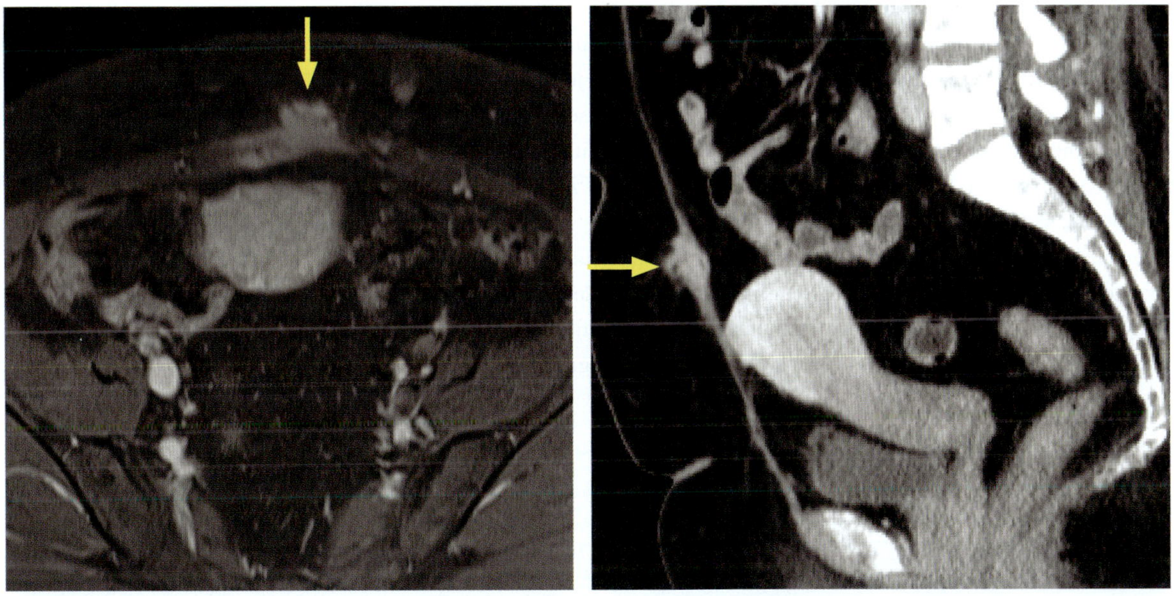

Axial postcontrast fat-suppressed T1-weighted MRI (left image) and sagittal postcontrast CT (right image) demonstrate an irregular enhancing lesion within the anterior abdominal wall involving the rectus abdominis (arrows). This was a biopsy-proven endometriosis within a Caesarian section scar (termed "scar endometriosis").

轴位增强后脂肪抑制T_1加权MRI(左图)和矢状位增强后CT(右图)显示前腹壁有一个不规则强化病灶，累及腹直肌(黄箭)。经活检证实为剖宫产瘢痕内的子宫内膜异位症(称为"瘢痕子宫内膜异位症")。

- Endometriosis is ectopic endometrial tissue outside of the endometrial cavity. Endometriosis has three main forms including superficial masses/implants, ovarian endometriomas, and deep infiltration endometriosis.
- The most common sites of endometriosis include the ovaries, followed by the myometrium (adenomyosis), ligaments and peritoneal surfaces of the anterior, posterior, and middle pelvic compartments. Less common sites of endometriosis include surgical scars (post Caesarean section, myomectomy), or even rarely within organs outside of the pelvis, such as the liver surface, lungs and brain.
- Pelvic endometriosis can manifest in three main forms.

  Superficial lesions: non-invasive implants, which are typically small and not visible on MRI.

  Ovarian endometrioma: typically seen as T2 hypointense, T1 hyperintense lesions on MRI.

  Deep (or solid) infiltrating type: defined by invasion of endometrial glands and stroma at least 5 mm beyond the peritoneal surface.
- Endometrioma is described in more detail later under the Ovarian section.

- 子宫内膜异位症指子宫内膜组织异位至子宫内膜腔外。子宫内膜异位症有3种主要形式：浅表肿块/植入、卵巢子宫内膜异位囊肿，以及深部浸润型子宫内膜异位症。
- 子宫内膜异位症最常见的部位为卵巢，其次是子宫肌层(子宫腺肌病)，韧带和前、后、中盆腔的腹膜表面。不常见的子宫内膜异位症部位包括手术瘢痕(剖宫产术、子宫肌瘤切除术后)，在极少数情况下甚至可发生在盆腔以外的器官，如肝表面、肺和大脑。
- 盆腔子宫内膜异位症可有三种主要表现形式。

  浅表病变：非侵入性植入，通常较小，在MRI上不可见。

  卵巢子宫内膜异位囊肿：典型的MRI表现为T_2低信号，T_1高信号。

  深部(或实性)浸润型：指子宫内膜腺体和间质的浸润深度至少5mm。
- 子宫内膜异位瘤(巧克力囊肿)将在下文卵巢部分详细描述。

Benign Myometrial Pathology

Adenomyosis

- Adenomyosis refers to ectopic endometrial tissue within the myometrium (endometriosis interna). In contrast to endometriosis, the ectopic endometrial tissue seen in adenomyosis is nonfunctioning, and it does not respond to cyclic ovarian hormones.
- Most patients are asymptomatic. But classic clinical presentation includes dysmenorrhea, menorrhagia, dyspareunia, infertility, and chronic pelvic pain.
- Ultrasound shows an enlarged uterus with heterogeneous myometrium, without focal mass. Multiple subendometrial cysts or echogenic foci can be found. There is often loss of differentiation of the endometrial-myometrial junction.
- On MRI, adenomyosis is best seen on T2-weighted images as diffuse (or focal) thickening of the junctional zone (>12 mm), often associated with multiple small T2 hyperintense foci. Borderline thickening of the junctional zone (8–12 mm) may be due to adenomyosis, but not diagnostic.
- Focal adenomyosis may mimic leiomyoma, appearing as more focal T1 and T2 hypointense signal. Although imaging features may overlap, leiomyomas typically show well-defined margins, no relationship to the junctional zone, mass effect (lobular external uterine contour), and more homogeneous T2 hypointense signal.

良性子宫肌层病变

腺肌病

- 子宫腺肌病是子宫内膜组织异位于子宫肌层内(子宫内子宫内膜异位症)。与子宫内膜异位症不同，腺肌病中的异位子宫内膜组织不具有功能，对周期性卵巢激素无反应。
- 大多数患者无症状。但典型的临床表现包括痛经、月经过多、性交痛、不孕，以及慢性盆腔疼痛。
- 超声显示子宫增大，子宫肌层回声不均匀，无局灶性肿块。可见多个子宫内膜下囊肿或强回声灶。子宫内膜与肌层间界限常不清。
- MRI上，子宫腺肌病在T_2加权图像上显示最为清晰，表现为结合带弥漫性(或局灶性)增厚(>12mm)，常伴多发点状T_2高信号。结合带的临界增厚(8~12mm)可能为腺肌病所致，但不能用于确诊腺肌病。
- 局灶性腺肌病可类似于平滑肌瘤，表现为局限性T_1和T_2加权低信号。尽管影像学表现可重叠，但平滑肌瘤通常有清晰的边界、与结合带无关、具有占位效应(子宫轮廓外突)，以及更均匀的T_2低信号。

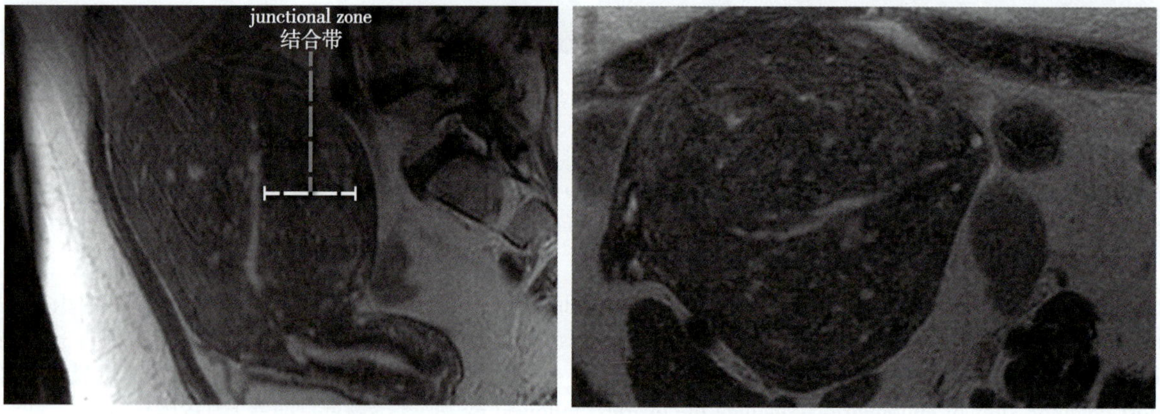

Adenomyosis: Sagittal (left) and axial T2 MRI of the uterus shows a markedly thickened junctional zone containing numerous T2 hyperintense foci.

Case courtesy Cheryl Sadow, MD, Brigham and Women's Hospital.

子宫腺肌病：子宫矢状位(左)和轴位T_2加权MRI显示结合带明显增厚并含有大量T_2高信号病灶。

Fibroid (leiomyoma)

- Fibroids are extremely common benign tumors of smooth muscle seen in 25% of white women, 50% of black women over age 30, and 40% of reproductive-age women.
- A **lipoleiomyoma** is a variant of fibroid which contains fat and is echogenic on US.
- Fibroids can be found in several locations:

  Intramural: located within the myometrium; most common location.

  Submucosal: directly underneath the endometrial mucosa and may bulge into the endometrial canal.

子宫肌瘤(平滑肌瘤)

- 子宫肌瘤是极其常见的良性平滑肌肿瘤，见于25%的白种人女性、50%的30岁以上黑人女性和40%的育龄期女性。
- **脂肪平滑肌瘤**是子宫肌瘤的一种变异，其内含有脂肪组织并在超声上呈高回声。
- 子宫肌瘤可见于多个部位：

  肌壁间：位于肌层，是最常发生的部位。

  黏膜下：位于子宫黏膜下，可隆起进入宫腔。

A submucosal fibroid can be resected hysteroscopically if >50% of the fibroid is intraluminal.

An intracavitary fibroid is a variant which is located nearly entirely within the endometrial cavity.

Subserosal: directly underneath the outer uterine serosa. A subserosal fibroid may simulate an adnexal mass if pedunculated, but Doppler will show blood supply coming from the uterus.

Cervical: rare, may simulate cervical cancer.

- The typical ultrasound appearance of a fibroid is a slightly heterogeneous, hypoechoic uterine mass with linear bands of shadowing.

  Calcification is often seen.

  May undergo cystic degeneration and appear as an anechoic mass with posterior through-transmission.

若黏膜下平滑肌瘤瘤体的50%以上位于宫腔内，可用宫腔镜进行切除。

宫腔内平滑肌瘤是黏膜下肌瘤的变异，其瘤体几乎完全位于宫腔内。

浆膜下：位于子宫浆膜下。有蒂的浆膜下平滑肌瘤可与附件肿块相似，但多普勒超声可显示其血供来自子宫。

宫颈：少见，可与宫颈癌相似。

- 典型的子宫平滑肌瘤超声表现为略不均匀的低回声肿块，内部有条带样声影。

  钙化很常见。

  可出现囊性变，表现为无回声肿块，伴后方回声增强。

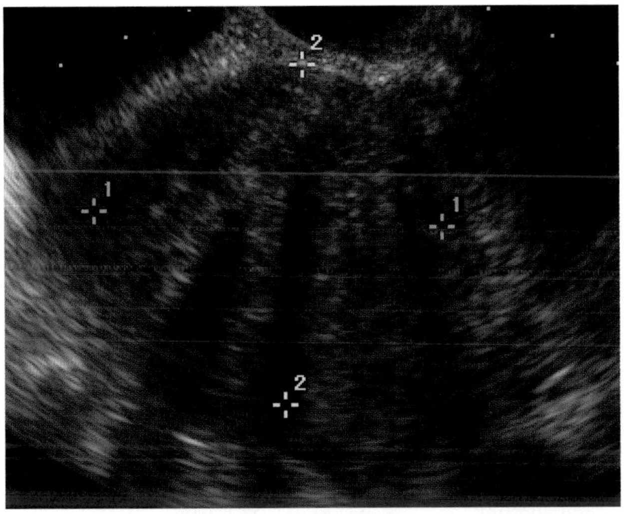

Fibroid: Ultrasound shows a hypoechoic myometrial mass (calipers) with linear bands of shadowing.
子宫肌瘤：超声显示肌层一个低回声肿块(卡尺)，内部有条带样声影。

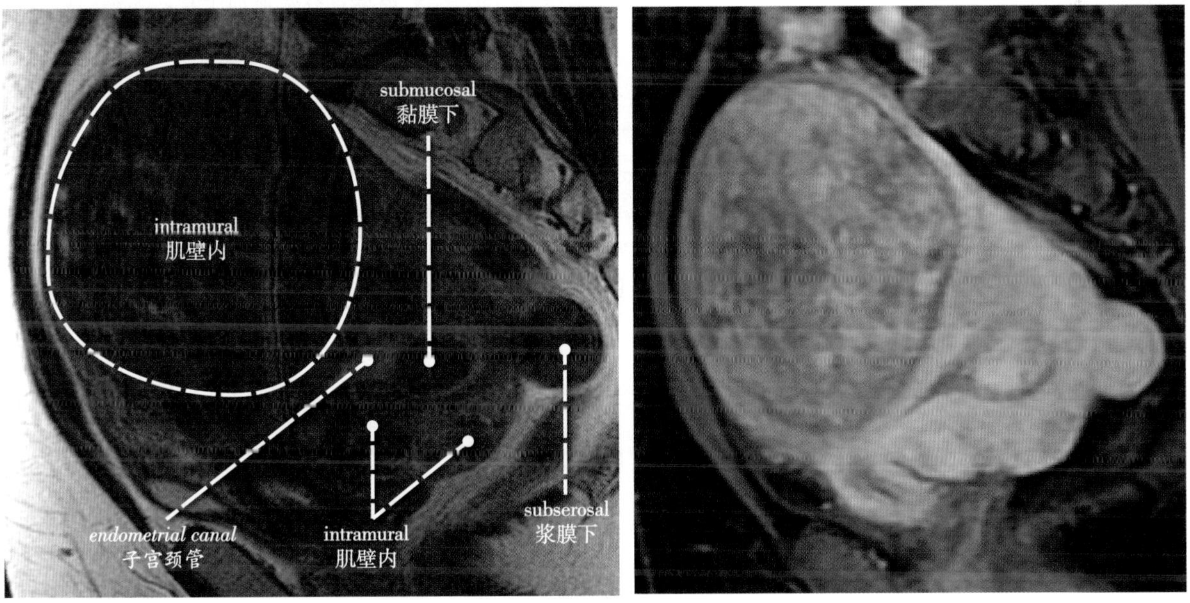

Submucosal, subserosal, and intramural fibroids: Sagittal T2-weighted (left image) and postcontrast sagittal T1-weighted fat suppressed MRI shows numerous fibroids, with the largest a dominant intramural fibroid. There are other smaller intramural fibroids, in addition to single submucosal and subserosal fibroids.

Case courtesy Cheryl Sadow, MD, Brigham and Women's Hospital.

黏膜下、浆膜下和肌壁内肌瘤，矢状位T_2加权(左图)和增强后T_1加权脂肪抑制MRI显示多发肌瘤，最大的位于肌壁内。除黏膜下和浆膜下各有一个肌瘤，肌壁内还有许多小肌瘤。

- On MRI, leiomyomas are T2 hypointense due to the presence of compact smooth muscle but up to 2/3 of leiomyomas show some form of degeneration.

  Internal cystic or myxoid degeneration may increase T2 signal heterogeneously.

  Red (carneous) degeneration due to hemorrhagic infarction, often during pregnancy or following oral contraceptive pill (OCP) use, may appear T1 hyperintense.
- Calcifications are common and can be seen in up to 25% of cases.
- MRI is often performed for treatment planning prior to uterine artery embolization (UAE). Hemorrhagic or necrotic leiomyomas are not treated effectively by UAE. Surgical myomectomy or hysterectomy would be the preferred treatment in these cases.

  Additionally, there is less chance of UAE success if an ovarian-uterine artery anastomosis is present.

MALIGNANT MYOMETRIAL PATHOLOGY

Leiomyosarcoma

- Uterine leiomyosarcoma is very rare and may arise de-novo or from malignant degeneration of a fibroid.
- A "funny looking fibroid" is much more likely to be a benign inhomogeneous fibroid rather than a leiomyosarcoma, but rapid growth should raise suspicion.
- Although signal heterogeneity, restricted diffusion, internal hemorrhage, and ill-defined contour have been described in leiomyosarcomas, imaging cannot reliably differentiate between leiomyoma and leiomyosarcoma. In the absence of obvious malignant features (such as local invasion or regional metastases), an unusual-looking fibroid is overwhelmingly likely to represent a degenerating benign fibroid rather than a leiomyosarcoma.
- Tamoxifen increases the risk of leiomyosarcoma in addition to endometrial carcinoma.

CONGENITAL UTERINE MALFORMATIONS

- Uterine malformations are caused by abnormal development of the paired Müllerian ducts, which normally fuse during embryogenesis. A septate uterus is the most common congenital abnormality, followed by bicornuate uterus.
- These anomalies increase the risk of infertility or recurrent pregnancy loss because the uterine cavity is abnormal in size (often small, multiple) or morphology.
- Congenital uterine abnormalities are associated with urinary tract abnormalities such as renal ectopia or agenesis.
- The American Society of Reproductive Medicine classifies Müllerian duct anomalies. Class I is uterine agenesis/hypoplasia; Class Ⅱ is a unicornuate uterus, and classes Ⅲ through Ⅶ represent the anomalies discussed below.

Normal uterus	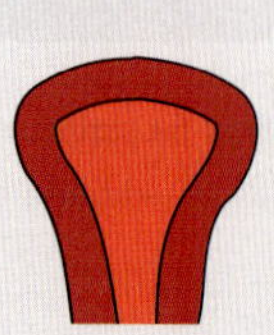	• The normal uterus is shaped like a pear. • The endometrial cavity changes with the menstrual cycle. • The fundus of the endometrium should be smooth without thickening or protrusion.

- 子宫肌瘤在MRI上表现为T_2低信号，为致密的平滑肌所致，但高达2/3的肌瘤会表现出某种形式的变性。

  内部出现囊变或黏液变性可使T_2信号不均匀增高。

  红色(坏死性)变性继发于出血性梗死，通常发生在妊娠期间或使用口服避孕药(OCP)后，可出现T_1高信号。
- 钙化很常见，见于多达25%的病例。
- MRI常用于制订子宫动脉栓塞术(UAE)的术前计划。UAE对出血性或坏死性平滑肌瘤的疗效不佳。此类肌瘤的治疗应首选肌瘤切除术或子宫切除术。此外，当存在卵巢-子宫动脉吻合时，UAE的成功率会降低。

恶性子宫肌层病变

子宫平滑肌肉瘤

- 子宫平滑肌肉瘤非常罕见，可以原发或由子宫肌瘤恶变而来。
- 一个“外形奇怪的子宫肌瘤”更有可能为良性、不均质的子宫平滑肌瘤，而非子宫平滑肌肉瘤，但当其快速生长时应警惕恶变。
- 尽管平滑肌肉瘤会出现信号不均、扩散受限、内部出血和边界模糊，但影像学仍无法可靠地对平滑肌瘤和平滑肌肉瘤进行鉴别。如无明确的恶性征象(如侵犯邻近结构或转移)，即便瘤体的表现特殊，其良性肌瘤退变的可能性仍远高于平滑肌肉瘤。
- 他莫昔芬除增加子宫内膜癌的患病风险外，也会增加子宫平滑肌肉瘤的患病风险。

先天性子宫畸形

- 子宫畸形是由于双侧副中肾管发育异常所致，正常情况下双侧副中肾管应在胚胎期相互融合。纵隔子宫是最常见的先天性畸形，其次是双角子宫。
- 畸形会增加不孕或习惯性流产的风险，因为子宫腔的大小(常较小或有多个腔)或形态有异常。
- 先天性子宫畸形可合并泌尿道畸形，如异位肾或肾发育不全。
- 美国生殖医学协会对副中肾管畸形进行了分类：Ⅰ型是子宫不发育/发育不全；Ⅱ型是单角子宫；Ⅲ~Ⅶ型讨论如下：

正常子宫	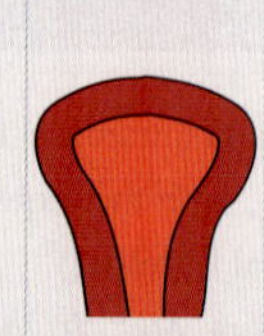	• 正常子宫呈梨形。 • 子宫内膜腔随着月经周期而变化。 • 子宫底部的内膜应该是光滑的，没有增厚或突出。

continued

Arcuate uterus (class VI)	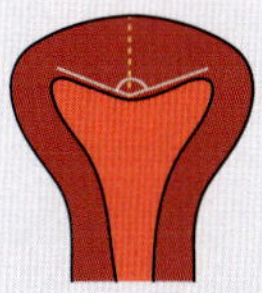		• Small indentation of the fundal surface of the endometrial cavity, with indentation depth <10 mm and angle >90 degrees. • There is no division of the uterine horns and external fundal contour is convex. This isconsidered along a spectrum with septate uterus. • Usually incidental and asymptomatic, and rarely associated with pregnancy loss, arcuate uterus is often considered a normal variant rather than an anomaly. Treatment is almost always conservative.
Septate uterus (class V)	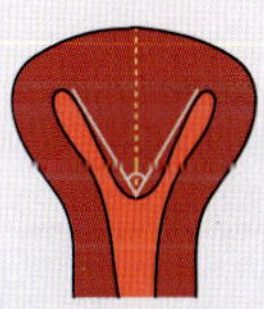	Failed resorption of inter-Müllerian septa	• Two uterine cavities, divided by a fibrous or muscular septum (>15 mm indentation depth, angle <90 degrees). External fundal contour is convex. • Most likely of all uterine anomalies to be implicated in pregnancy loss since the fibrous septal tissue or myometrium is relatively avascular. • Metroplasty (resection of the septum) can be performed hysteroscopically if the septum is fibrous, or transabdominally if the septum is muscular.
Bicornuate uterus (class IV)	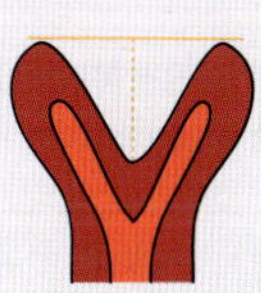	Parti al failure of Müllerian duct fusion	• Two uterine fundi with shared lower uterine segment; can have one cervix (bicornis unicollis) or two cervices (bicornis bicollis). • In contrast to a septate uterus, bicornuate uterus has a concave external fundal contour which pinches inwards > 15 mm. • If treated, metroplasty must be performed transabdominally.
Didelphys uterus (class Ⅲ)	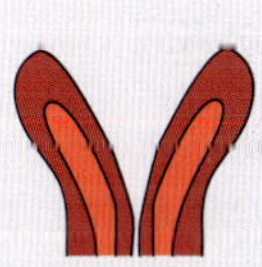	Complete failure of Müllerian duct fusion	• Two completely separate uteri and cervices, with complete endometrium, myometrium and serosal surfaces on each side. • 75% have a vaginal septum.
DES uterus (class Ⅶ)	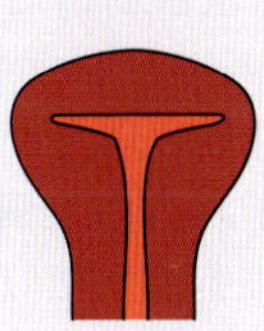		• In utero exposure to diethylsti lbestrol (DES) causes the fetus to develop classic imaging appearance of hypoplasti c uterus with a T-shaped endometrial contour. It is associated with an increased risk of clear cell vaginal cancer. • DES has not been used since the 1970s.

续表

弓形子宫（Ⅵ型）	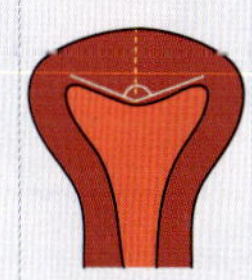		• 子宫底部的内膜有小凹陷，深度<10mm，角度>90°。 • 子宫角无分离，宫底外轮廓是外凸形的。与纵隔子宫类似。 • 常偶然发现且无症状，极少与流产相关，弓形子宫通常被认为是正常变异而非畸形。选择保守治疗。
纵隔子宫（Ⅴ型）	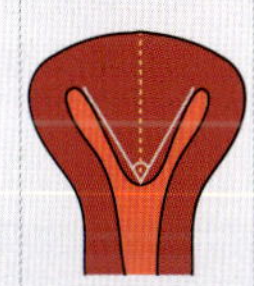	副中肾管内间隔吸收不全	• 有两个宫腔，被纤维间隔或肌性间隔分开(凹陷深度>15mm，角度<90°)。宫底外轮廓是外凸形的。 • 是最有可能发生妊娠失败的子宫畸形，因为纤维或肌性的间隔相对无血供。 • 如纵隔为纤维性，可通过宫腔镜进行子宫成形术(纵隔切除)治疗；如为肌性纵隔，可使用经腹手术予以治疗。
双角子宫（Ⅳ型）	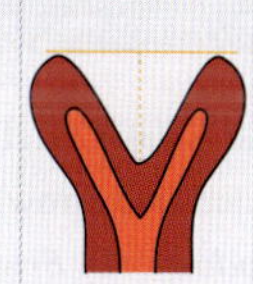	副中肾管部分未融合	• 双角子宫有两个子宫底部和一个共同的子宫下段；可以有一个宫颈(双角单宫颈子宫)或两个宫颈(双角双宫颈子宫)。 • 与纵隔子宫不同的是，双角子宫的宫底外轮廓向内凹陷超过15mm。 • 若需治疗，须行经腹子宫成形术。
双子宫（Ⅲ型）	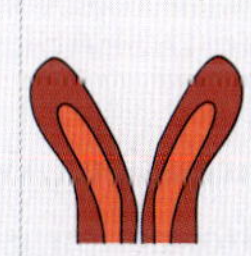	副中肾管完全未融合	• 两个完全分离的子宫和宫颈，但两边都有完整的子宫内膜、肌层，以及浆膜面。 • 75%有阴道隔膜。
己烯雌酚(DES)子宫（Ⅶ型）	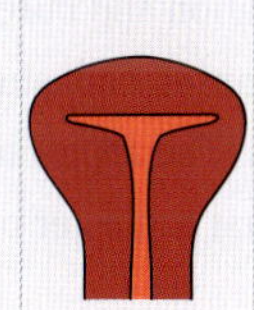	—	• 胎儿宫内DES暴露可引起胎儿子宫发育不全，典型影像学表现为宫腔呈“T”形改变。其与阴道透明细胞癌的风险增加有关。 • DES自20世纪70年代起已被停止使用。

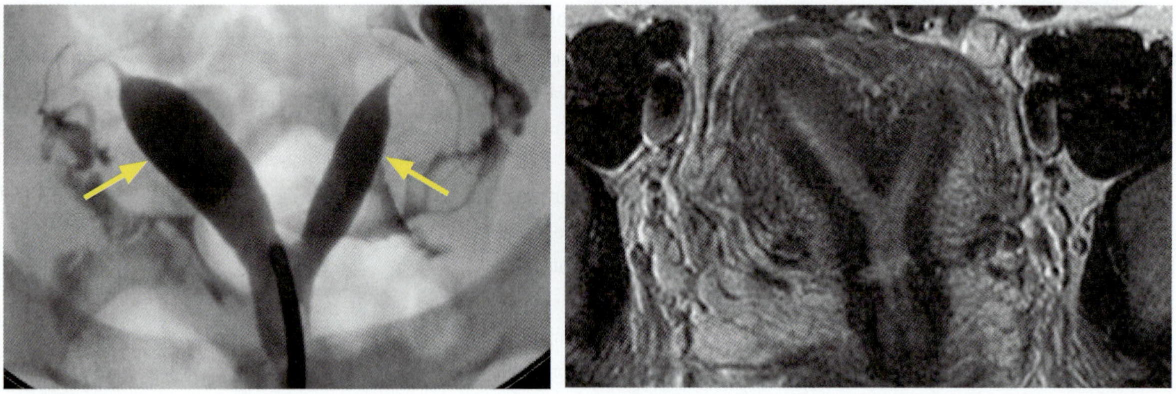

Septate uterus: Hysterosalpingogram (left image) shows a common lower endometrial cavity which splits to form two separate endometrial cavities (yellow arrows). HSG appearance may correspond to either a septate or bicornuate uterus. Bilateral intraperitoneal spillage of contrast confirms tubal patency.

Axial T2 MRI (right image) reidentifies the two endometrial cavities and provides further information about the external fundal contour, which is normal (convex) and diagnostic of septate uterus.

纵隔子宫：输卵管子宫造影(左图)示子宫的下方有一个共同的宫腔，其上方分隔为两个宫腔(黄箭)。输卵管子宫造影的表现可以是纵隔子宫或双角子宫。双侧腹腔内造影剂溢出证实输卵管通畅。

轴位 T_2 加权MRI(右图)显示有两个宫腔，并提供宫底正常的(外突形的)外侧轮廓信息，可诊断为纵隔子宫。

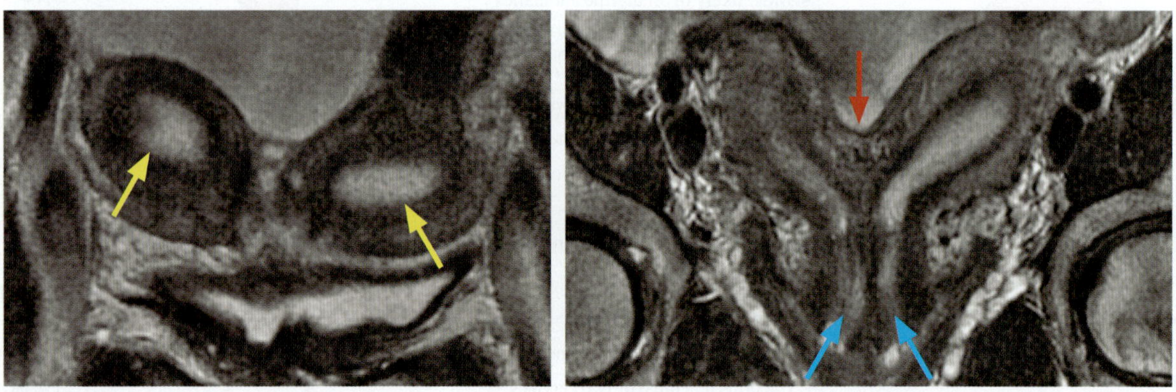

Bicornuate bicollis uterus: Axial T2 (left image) and coronal T2 (right image) show two separate endometrial canals (yellow arrows) with a definite external fundal cleft (red arrow). There are two separate cervices (bicollis; blue arrows) that share a common myometrium.

Cases courtesy Cheryl Sadow, MD, Brigham and Women's Hospital.

双角双宫颈子宫：轴位(左图)和冠状位(右图) T_2 加权显示两个独立的宫腔(黄箭)，宫底有一个明显的裂隙(红箭)。可见两个宫颈(双宫颈，蓝箭)共有一个肌层。

MISCELLANEOUS UTERINE DISEASE

Uterine arteriovenous malformation (AVM)

- Uterine arteriovenous malformation is caused by abnormal communication between the uterine arterial branches and draining myometrial venous plexus. It may be congenital (very rare) or acquired (post-traumatic, infection, or iatrogenic, such as post dilation and curettage (D&C)).
- Grayscale and color Doppler can show an enlarged, heterogeneous, and multicystic-appearing uterus. The appearance is similar to gestational trophoblastic disease (discussed in the first trimester of pregnancy section), but with negative β-hCG.

其他子宫疾病

子宫动静脉畸形(AVM)

- 子宫动静脉畸形(AVM)是由于子宫动脉分支与引流的子宫肌层静脉丛之间出现的异常交通。子宫动静脉畸形可为先天性(非常罕见)，也可为后天获得性(包括创伤后、感染，或医源性如刮宫术后)。
- 灰阶超声和彩色多普勒表现为子宫体积增大、回声不均匀，以及子宫内多发囊性病变。该表现与妊娠期滋养细胞疾病相似(将在早期妊娠部分讨论)，但β-hCG阴性。

INTERVENTION/POST-SURGICAL CHANGE

Intrauterine device (IUD)

干预/术后改变

宫内节育器(IUD)

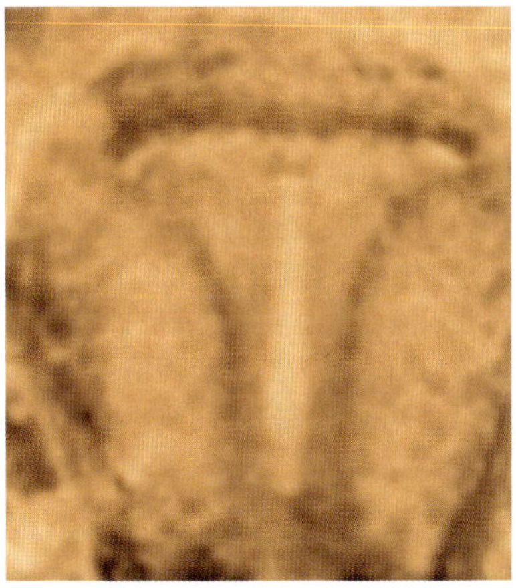

3D ultrasound shows normal position of IUD within the endometrial cavity.
三维超声显示宫腔内有一个正常位置的宫内节育器。

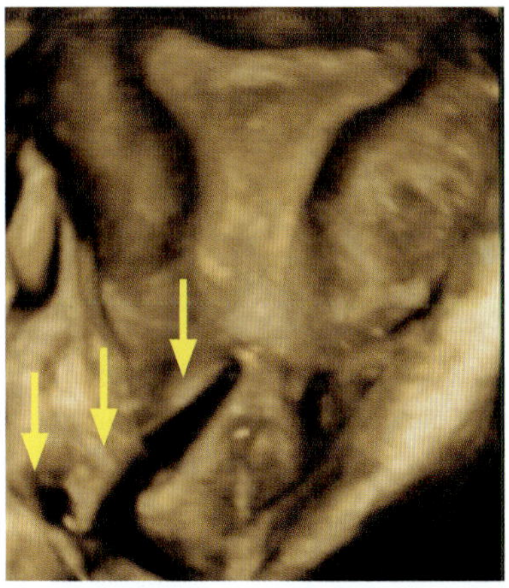

Malpositioned and malrotated IUD (arrows) within the lower uterine segment/cervix.
子宫下段/宫颈内异常位置和异常旋转的宫内节育器(黄箭)。

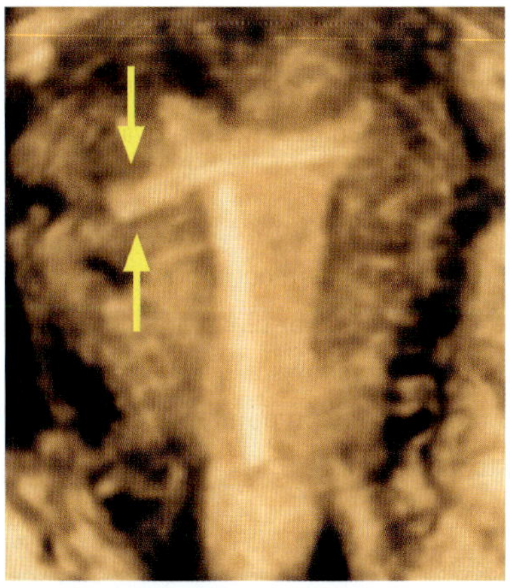

Right arm of the IUD is embedded within the myometrium (arrows).
宫内节育器的右臂嵌入子宫肌层(黄箭)。

- The ultrasound appearance of an intrauterine device (IUD) is dependent on the type of IUD:

  Hormonal plastic IUD (delivers progesterone): Shadowing structure in endometrial canal.

  Copper IUD: Highly echogenic.
- Complications of IUD are overall rare and include:

  Malpositioning.

  Infection: Increased risk of infection with prolonged IUD use, especially actinomycosis.

  Ectopic pregnancy: When pregnancy occurs in the presence of an IUD, there is increased risk for ectopic pregnancy.

  Uterine perforation (extremely rare).

Post Caesarean section complications

- **Bladder-flap hematoma** is a rare complication of a low-transverse Caesarean section, where a postsurgical hematoma forms in the vesicouterine space (between the posterior bladder and the anterior uterus).

  Ultrasound of a bladder-flap hematoma will show a complex mass posterior to the bladder.
- **Subfascial hematoma** is also a rare complication of Caesarean section due to extraperitoneal hemorrhage within the prevesical space (anterior to the bladder).

  Ultrasound shows a complex mass anterior to the bladder.
- It is important to distinguish a subfascial hematoma from a bladder-flap hematoma, as the surgical approach for repair is different.

- 宫内节育器(IUD)的超声表现取决于节育器的类型：

  激素塑料型IUD(释放孕酮)：宫腔内后方伴声影结构。

  铜制IUD：高回声。
- IUD的并发症总体上很少见，包括：

  位置异常。

  感染：长期使用IUD可增加感染风险，尤其是放线菌病。

  异位妊娠：使用IUD的情形下发生妊娠时，宫外孕的风险增加。

  子宫穿孔(非常罕见)。

剖宫产术后并发症

- **膀胱瓣血肿**是低位横切口剖宫产导致的罕见并发症，术后形成的血肿位于膀胱子宫间隙(膀胱的后方，子宫的前方)。

  膀胱瓣血肿在超声上为膀胱后方的一个混合性包块。
- **筋膜下血肿**也是一种罕见的剖宫产后并发症，为腹膜外出血至膀胱前间隙(位于膀胱的前方)。

  超声检查显示一个位于膀胱前方的混合性包块。
- 区分膀胱瓣血肿和筋膜下血肿非常重要，因两者手术修补方法不同。

MRI OF THE CERVIX

Normal cervical T2 zonal anatomy

- **Endocervix:** T2 hyperintense due to mucin, analogous to uterine endometrium.

宫颈MRI

正常宫颈T_2分区解剖

- **宫颈管：**T_2高信号，为有黏液所致，类似于子宫内膜。

- **Cervical mucosa:** T2 intermediate.
- **Inner cervical stroma:** Very T2 hypointense, analogous to the uterine junctional zone. Unlike the uterine junctional zone, however, the decreased T2 signal is due to compact fibrous tissue, not smooth muscle. The superior aspect of the inner cervical stroma is continuous with junctional zone of uterus.

Cervical carcinoma

- Cervical carcinoma is the third most common gynecologic malignancy. There has been a steep decline in prevalence over the past 50 years due to screening with Pap smears.
- Ultrasound may show a hypoechoic or isoechoic soft tissue mass involving the cervix with/ without intratumoral necrosis. The endometrial cavity may be distended by fluid or blood products due to cervical obstruction.
- MRI typically shows a T2 intermediate to hyperintense signal mass replacing the normally T2 hypointense cervical stroma. Enhancement is variable on postcontrast images.

- **宫颈黏膜：**T_2等信号。
- **宫颈内层基质：**T_2极低信号，类似于子宫结合带。宫颈基质低信号由致密的纤维组织而非结合带中的平滑肌层所致。宫颈上部的内层基质与子宫的结合带相连。

宫颈癌

- 宫颈癌是妇科的第三常见肿瘤。过去50年来（译者注：1941年以来）由于宫颈涂片的应用，其患病率明显降低。
- 超声表现为累及宫颈的低回声或等回声软组织肿块，伴或不伴瘤内坏死。宫颈出口受阻后宫腔积液或出血可造成宫腔扩张。
- 典型的MRI表现为T_2等至高信号的肿块取代了T_2低信号的正常宫颈间质。增强影像学表现多样。

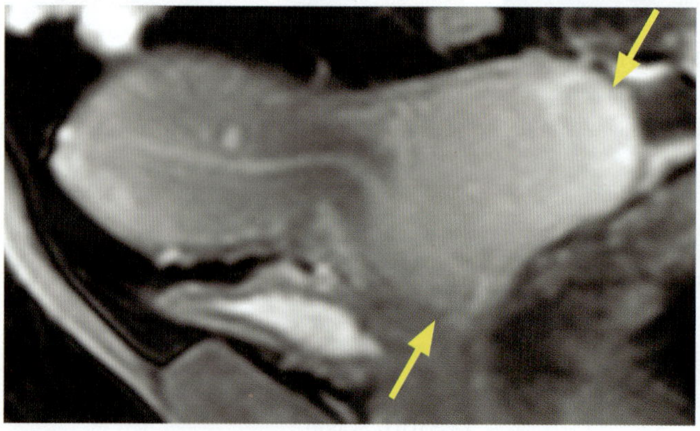

Sagittal T1-weighted MRI with fat saturation
矢状位T_1加权脂肪抑制MRI

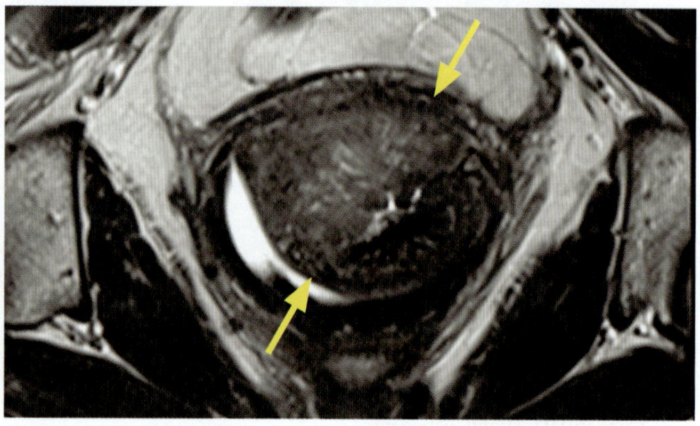

Coronal T2-weighted MRI
冠状位T_2加权MRI

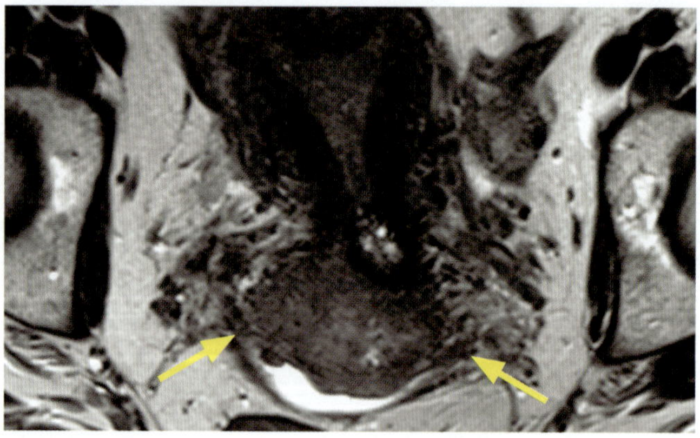

Axial T2-weighted MRI
轴位T_2加权MRI

Local cervical cancer:
MRI images show a heterogeneous, T2 intermediate cervical mass with well circumscribed margins.
Although the mass abuts neurovascular bundles and the parametrium, there is no evidence of parametrial invasion. This mass was treated with chemoradiation.
局限性宫颈癌：
MRI显示宫颈有一个不均匀的T_2等信号肿块，边界清楚。
尽管肿块毗邻神经血管束和宫旁，但无宫旁侵犯迹象。此患者接受了放射治疗和化学治疗。

- A cervical mass >1.5 cm should be evaluated by MRI for staging. The cervical stroma is the key landmark in the staging of cervical cancer: If tumor extends through the cervical stroma into the **parametrium**, the cancer is stage **ⅡB** and treatment is typically non-surgical (“ⅡB or not ⅡB”). Other key findings to note are involvement of bladder or rectum, which denotes stage IV disease (if shown to extend to the mucosal surface with cystoscopy or endoscopy).

- 宫颈肿块超过1.5cm时，需行MRI分期。宫颈基质是宫颈癌分期的重要标志：如肿瘤侵犯宫颈基质至宫旁，则为ⅡB期；通常使用非手术治疗（“ⅡB期或非ⅡB期”）。其他观察要点包括膀胱或直肠是否受侵，若受侵则为Ⅳ期（可通过膀胱镜或肠内镜检查发现黏膜表面受侵）。

- Staging of cervical carcinoma is based on the FIGO (International Federation of Gynecology and Obstetrics) system, which characterizes extent of disease based on involvement of the uterus, vagina (upper 2/3 versus lower 1/3), parametrium, pelvic sidewall, adjacent bladder and rectum, pelvic lymph nodes, and/or distant metastases.

- 宫颈癌按国际妇产科联盟(FIGO)系统进行分期，该系统的依据是病灶是否累及子宫、阴道(上2/3与下1/3)、宫旁、盆腔侧壁、邻近膀胱和直肠、盆腔淋巴结和/或远处转移。

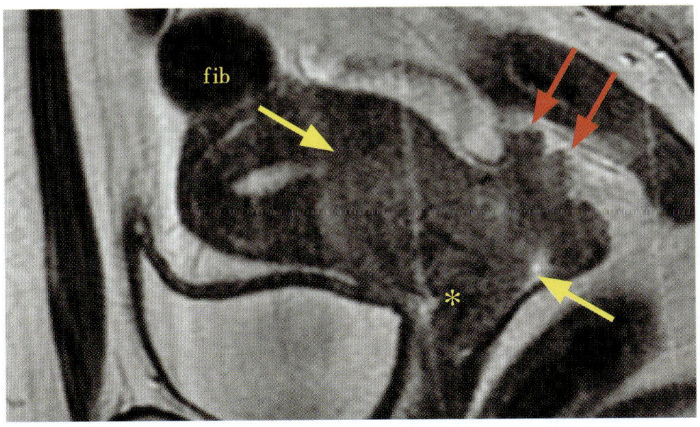

Sagittal T2-weighted MRI
矢状位 T_2 加权MRI

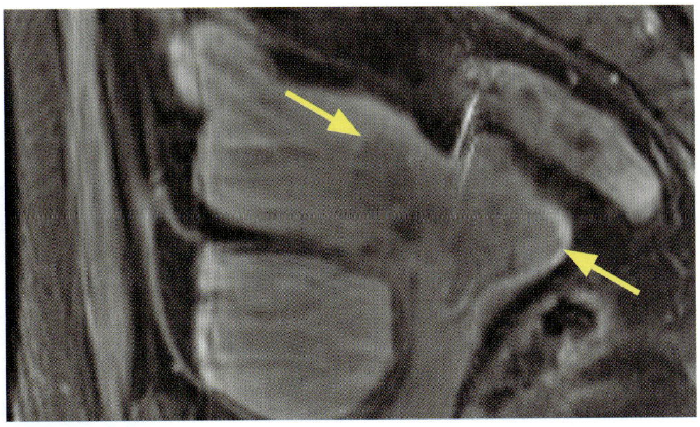

Sagittal T1-weighted MRI with fat saturation.
矢状位 T_1 加权脂肪抑制MRI

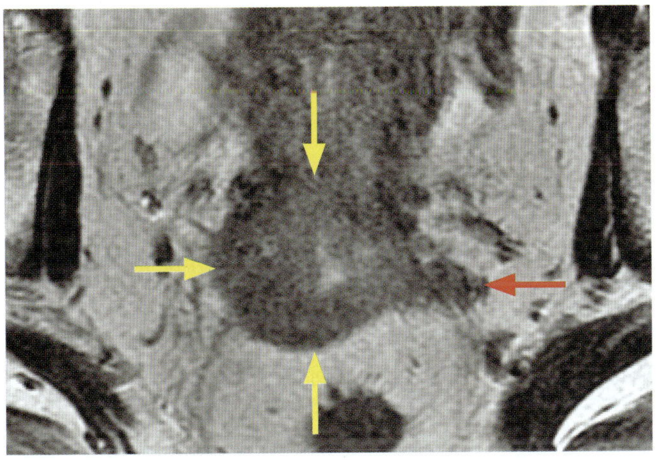

Axial T2-weighted MRI
轴位 T_2 加权MRI

Cervical carcinoma, stage ⅡB:
MRI images show an ill-defined, hyperintense mass (yellow arrows) centered at the cervix, with invasion into the lower uterine segment and the anterior vaginal fornix (*). There is nodular parametrial invasion (red arrows). A subserosal fibroid (fib) is present.
The mass enhances heterogeneously (top right image). The axial (left image) shows near complete circumferential cervical involvement (yellow arrows) and left parametrial spread (red arrow).
Case courtesy Cheryl Sadow, MD, Brigham and Women's Hospital.
宫颈癌ⅡB期：
MRI显示一个中心位于宫颈的高信号肿块(黄箭)，边界模糊，侵犯子宫体下段及阴道前穹隆(左上图，*处)。宫旁结节状侵犯(红箭)。浆膜下有一个肌瘤(fib)。
肿块强化不均匀(右上图)。轴位(左下图)显示宫颈全周受侵(黄箭)和左侧宫旁受侵(红箭)。

Adenoma malignum

- Adenoma malignum is a rare subtype of well-differentiated mucinous adenocarcinoma of the cervix. It has an unfavorable prognosis due to peritoneal dissemination in early stage and poor response to radiation and chemotherapy.
- Classic imaging appearance is a multicystic mass (cluster of cysts) with solid components that extends from the endocervical glands to deep cervical stroma.
- Associations with Peutz-Jeghers syndrome and mucinous ovarian neoplasms have been reported.

恶性腺瘤

- 恶性腺瘤是宫颈高分化黏液腺癌的一种罕见亚型。预后不良，因为该疾病早期即可发生腹膜播散，且对放疗和化疗反应差。
- 典型的影像学表现是多发囊性肿块(簇状囊肿)伴有实性成分，从宫颈管腺体延伸到深部宫颈间质。
- 根据文献报道，恶性腺瘤与波伊茨-耶格综合征及黏液性卵巢肿瘤有关。

(翻译　孙明菡　程瑾)

Ovaries and Adnexa

Anatomy and Physiology

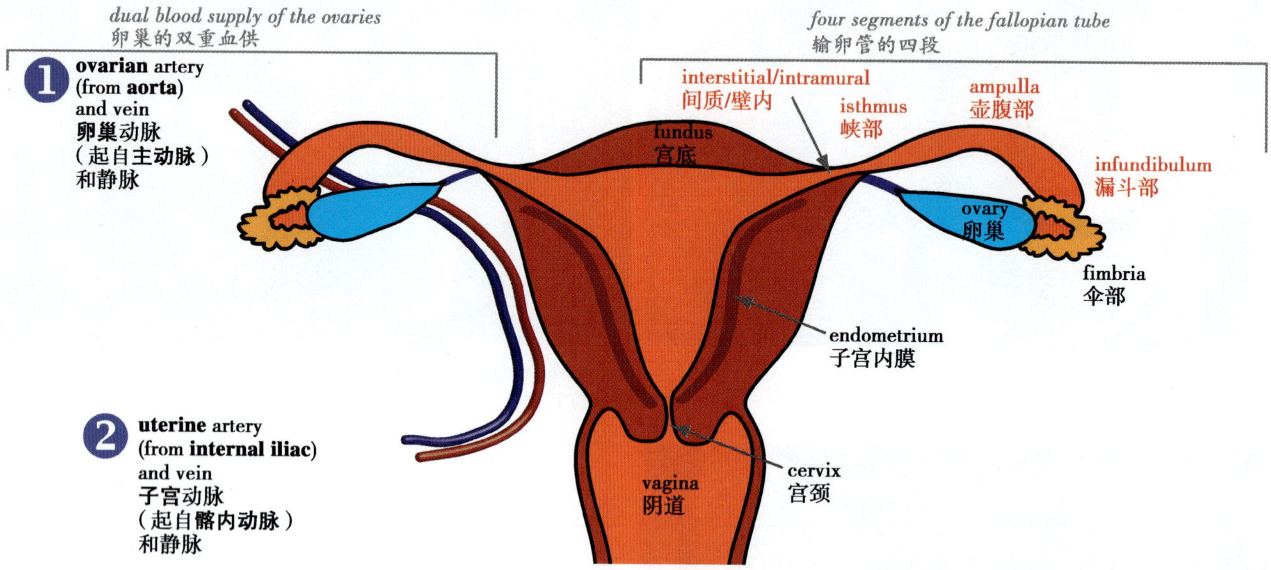

- There is a dual blood supply to the ovary:
  The ovarian artery comes directly off the aorta to supply the lateral aspect of the ovary.
  A branch of the uterine artery arises from the internal iliac artery to supply the medial aspect of the ovary.
- The fallopian tube is divided into four segments, from proximal to distal:
  Interstitial (intramural) is the narrowest segment.
  Isthmus.
  Ampulla.
  Infundibulum.

Cyclical changes in the ovaries

- Day 5–7 of the menstrual cycle: Multiple Graafian follicles become apparent in the ovary (these are <3 cm in diameter).
- Day 8–13: One (or more) dominant follicles arise.
- Day 14: **Ovulation.** Physiologic bleeding occurs into the follicle at the time of ovulation, at which point the follicle is called the corpus hemorrhagicum. After ovulation, the corpus hemorrhagicum becomes the corpus luteum.
- Day 15–20: The corpus luteum retains fluid over the next 4–5 days to reach a maximal size of approximately 3 cm.
- Day 20–28. If pregnancy doesn't occur, the corpus luteum involutes to become the corpus albicans, which cannot be seen by ultrasound.
- If pregnancy occurs, the corpus luteum develops into a gland secreting β-hCG. A prominent corpus luteum may be mistaken for an ectopic pregnancy due to its similar appearance. However, an ectopic pregnancy will only very rarely be in the ovary.

卵巢和附件

解剖和生理功能

- 卵巢有双重血液供应：
  起自主动脉的卵巢动脉供应卵巢外侧。
  起自髂内动脉的子宫动脉卵巢分支供应卵巢内侧。
- 输卵管由近至远分为四段：
  间质部(壁内部)为最狭窄的部分。
  峡部。
  壶腹部。
  漏斗部。

卵巢的周期性改变

- 月经周期第5~7天：卵巢内出现多个明显的成熟卵泡(直径<3cm)。
- 第8~13天：出现一个(或数个)优势卵泡。
- 第14天：**排卵**。排卵时卵泡内出现生理性出血，此时的卵泡被称为血体。排卵后，血体演变成黄体。
- 第15~20天：黄体在此后的4~5天继续潴留液体，最大直径可达约3cm。
- 第20~28天：如未受孕，黄体内陷萎缩成为白体，超声不能显示。
- 如受孕，黄体发展为可分泌β-hCG的腺体。增大的黄体可能会被误诊为异位妊娠，因其外形相似。但异位妊娠发生在卵巢的情况非常罕见。

ADNEXAL TORSION

Adnexal torsion

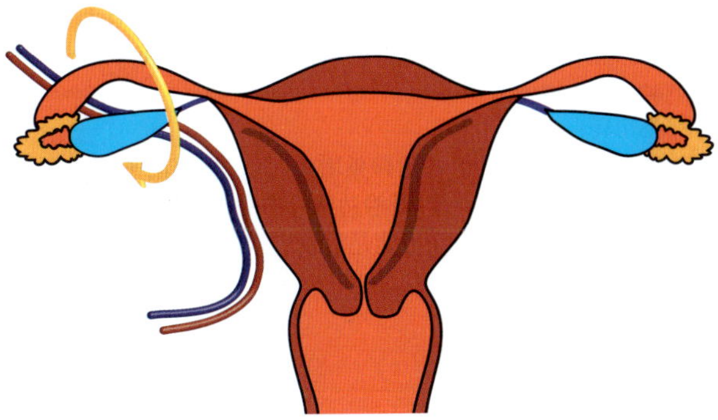

Diagram demonstrates dual blood supply of the ovary, with the yellow curved arrow representing adnexal torsion.
示意图显示卵巢双重血供，黄色弯曲箭代表附件扭转。

- Adnexal torsion results from twisting of the ovarian vascular pedicle. This results in pain and potential vascular compromise to the ovary.
- Acute pain is usually localized to the affected side. Pain may be episodic, especially if the torsion is intermittent. Torsion occurs mainly in reproductive-age women, and commonly occurs in pregnancy. Torsion occurs more commonly on the right side due to the position of the sigmoid colon, which inhibits free rotation of the left adnexa. Torsion may clinically mimic appendicitis.
- The ovary may be predisposed to torsion by a lead-point adnexal mass, particularly if large, most commonly an ovarian dermoid.
- Because of the dual blood supply to the ovary (lateral from the ovarian vessels off the aorta, and medial from the uterine vessels from the internal iliac), flow may still be detectable by color Doppler, even with torsion. Intermittent ovarian torsion and detorsion may also explain detectable color Doppler flow in these cases.
- Classic ultrasound features of ovarian torsion in a patient with acute pelvic pain includes an enlarged, edematous ovary with abnormal Doppler, and free fluid. Twisting ("swirling") of the vascular pedicle (*whirlpool sign*) is very specific, but not often seen. Less specific but most common features include:

  Enlarged ovary >4 cm in diameter.

  Unusual position of affected ovary, which may be even found on the contralateral side.

  Follicles pushed to the periphery of the ovary.

  Free fluid in the pelvis.

  Variable Doppler findings: Lack of flow is not always seen and usually indicates necrosis or infarction. Other Doppler findings include normal or intermittent flow, absent or reversed arterial diastolic flow on spectral imaging.
- MRI and CT features of ovarian torsion are similar to the ultrasound findings. The most common (but nonspecific) finding is an enlarged ovary > 4 cm in diameter. The follicles may be peripherally displaced due to central hemorrhage and edema. Twisting of the ovarian pedicle is uncommonly seen, but is pathognomonic for torsion when identified.

附件扭转

附件扭转

- 附件扭转是由于卵巢血管蒂发生扭转所致。可导致腹痛并影响卵巢血供。
- 急性疼痛常位于患侧。疼痛可呈阵发性，尤其是间歇性的扭转。扭转主要发生在育龄妇女，妊娠时多见。附件扭转以右侧多见，因左侧附件的自由转动会受到乙状结肠的限制。扭转在临床上可能与阑尾炎的表现类似。
- 附件肿物可促发卵巢扭转，尤其是肿物较大时，最常见为皮样囊肿。
- 卵巢具有双重血供(外侧供应来自主动脉发出的卵巢动脉，内侧来自髂内动脉发出的子宫动脉)，因此，即使发生扭转，彩色多普勒仍能检测到卵巢血流。间歇性扭转和复位也可解释为何这些病例能够检测到彩色多普勒血流。
- 卵巢扭转致急性盆腔疼痛患者的典型超声表现有卵巢增大、水肿、异常多普勒，以及盆腔游离积液。血管蒂扭曲("漩涡征")是非常特异的征象，但并不常见。常见但特异性较低的征象包括：

  卵巢增大，直径超过4cm。

  患侧卵巢位置异常，甚至可出现在对侧。

  卵泡被挤压至卵巢边缘。

  盆腔游离积液。

  多普勒表现多样：并非都能观察到缺乏血流的情况，但通常这会提示组织坏死或梗死。其他还包括正常或间歇性血流、消失或反向的舒张期动脉血流频谱。
- 卵巢扭转的MRI和CT表现与超声类似。最常见(但不特异)的表现为卵巢增大(直径>4cm)、卵泡因卵巢中央出血和水肿而被挤压至外周。卵巢蒂扭曲少见，不过一旦发现便具有病理学诊断意义。

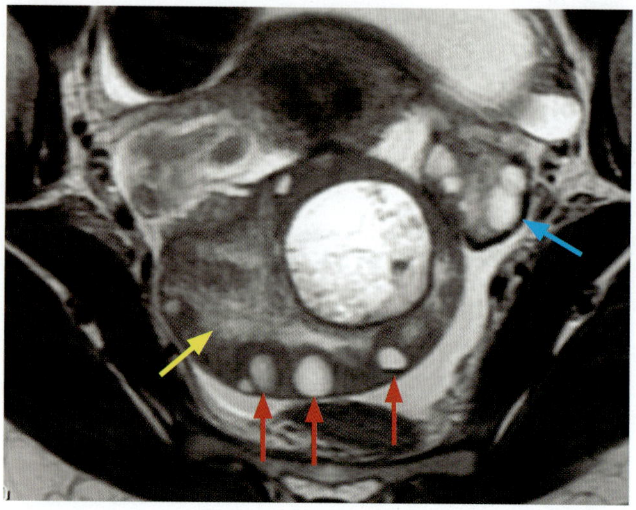

Ovarian torsion:

Axial T2-weighted MRI demonstrates an enlarged right ovary that is displaced into the pouch of Douglas. Note the edematous central stroma (yellow arrow) and peripherally distributed small follicles (red arrows). The heterogeneously T2 hyperintense lesion within the right ovary may have been the lead-point. Note the partially imaged, normalized left ovary (blue arrow).

卵巢扭转：

轴位T_2加权MRI显示右侧卵巢增大，并占据直肠子宫陷凹。注意卵巢中央基质水肿（黄箭）及沿边缘分布的小卵泡（红箭）。右侧卵巢内的混杂T_2高信号病灶可能是促发因素。左侧正常卵巢（蓝箭）有部分显示。

Overview of ovarian masses

卵巢肿块概述

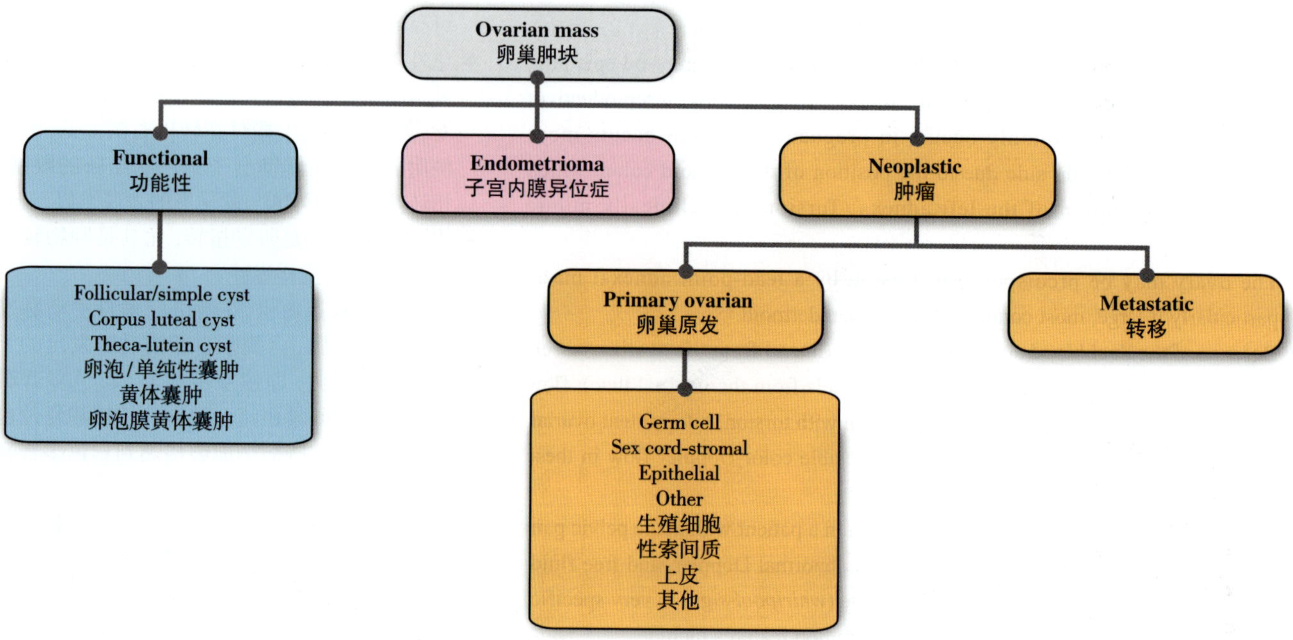

Functional ovarian cysts

Overview of functional ovarian cysts

- Functional cysts include follicular cysts, corpus luteal cysts, and theca lutein cysts.
- A **follicular cyst** (usually called a simple cyst), results from failed ovulation of the dominant follicle(s). The dominant follicle continues to grow in size and is considered a follicular cyst when >3 cm.

  A simple ovarian cyst is a round or oval anechoic structure with smooth and imperceptibly thin walls, posterior acoustic enhancement, and lack of worrisome features such as solid components, septations, or internal flow on color Doppler.
- A **corpus luteal cyst** results from failed involution of the corpus luteum. Like the follicular cyst, it can continue to grow in size and must be >3 cm for diagnosis.

  A corpus luteal cyst can have variable appearances, but will often look like a complex

功能性卵巢囊肿

功能性卵巢囊肿概述

- 功能性囊肿包括卵泡囊肿、黄体囊肿和卵泡膜黄体囊肿。
- **卵泡囊肿**（通常被称为单纯囊肿）为优势卵泡未能排卵所致。优势卵泡持续增大，当其直径>3cm时被认为是卵泡囊肿。

  卵巢单纯囊肿呈圆形或椭圆形无回声结构，具有光滑且不易察觉的薄壁，伴后方声影增强，且无可疑恶性征象，如实性成分、分隔或内部彩色多普勒血流。
- **黄体囊肿**是黄体未能萎缩退化的结果。类似于卵泡囊肿，可持续增大，但直径必须大于3cm时才能诊断。

ovarian cyst. High diastolic flow is often present, which can also be seen in ovarian cancer.

- **Theca lutein cysts** are often multiple and arise from elevated hCG. They can be seen in molar pregnancy, multiple gestations, or infertility patients on gonadotropins or clomiphene.
- A **hemorrhagic cyst** is most often the result of hemorrhage into a functional cyst, most commonly a corpus luteum. Ultrasound findings can be suggestive, although a complex cyst should be followed-up at least once to ensure resolution.

  An acutely hemorrhagic cyst may be hyperechoic and potentially mimic a solid mass, but will usually show posterior enhancement. As the clot dissolves, the internal echo pattern becomes more complex to produce characteristic web-like internal echoes. Retractile mural clot features concave margins and absent Doppler flow. In contrast, a solid mural nodule features a convex margin and internal flow

黄体囊肿表现多样，但通常类似于一个复杂的卵巢囊肿。常出现舒张期血流增加，但此征象也可见于卵巢癌。

- 卵泡膜黄体囊肿常多发，由hCG增高引起。可见于葡萄胎妊娠、多胎妊娠，或使用促性腺激素或氯米芬治疗的不孕症患者。
- **出血性囊肿**是功能性囊肿内部出血，最常见于黄体。超声检查可提示诊断，但对于复杂性囊肿，应至少随访一次，以确保囊肿消退。

  急性出血性囊肿可表现为强回声，可类似实性肿块，但通常后方有回声增强效应。随着血块溶解，囊肿内部回声杂乱，表现为特征性的网格样内部回声。囊壁因血块回缩而表现为边缘向内凹陷，内部无血流信号。相反，囊壁的实性结节则表现为边缘向外突起，并且内部有血流信号。

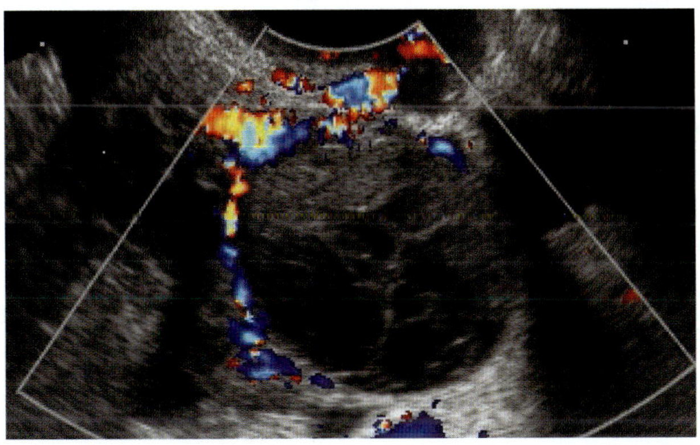

Hemorrhagic cyst:
Transvaginal color Doppler of an ovary shows a large complex ovarian cyst containing web-like internal echoes, with no flow on color Doppler. Follow-up ultrasound confirmed resolution of the mass.

出血性囊肿：
经阴道彩色多普勒显示卵巢内一个大的复杂性囊性肿块，内部可见网格样回声，但无彩色多普勒血流信号。超声随访证实囊肿消失。

- The Society of Radiologists in Ultrasound (SRU) published a consensus in 2010 regarding management of asymptomatic ovarian and adnexal cysts imaged at ultrasound, which was updated in 2019.
- Simple cysts do not confer any increased risk of ovarian cancer, presuming the cyst can be completely visualized and reliably characterized.
- Simple ovarian cysts should be followed if >7 cm in premenopausal women, or >5 cm in postmenopausal women per updated 2019 SRU consensus criteria.
- On follow-up exams, regardless of menopausal status:

  A cyst stable in size for two years can be considered benign and no further imaging follow-up needed.

  A cyst that decreases in size on follow-up (by >10–15%) in average linear dimension can be considered benign and no further follow-up needed.

- 超声放射医师学会(SRU)在2010年发表了无症状卵巢和附件囊肿的超声检查共识，并于2019年更新。
- 单纯囊肿不会增加患卵巢癌的风险，但前提是必须要看到完整的囊肿结构和特征。
- 根据2019 SRU更新的共识标准，对于绝经前>7cm，或绝经后>5cm的单纯卵巢囊肿，应进行随访。
- 在随访检查中，不论绝经状态：

  若囊肿大小稳定超过2年则考虑为良性，不需要进一步影像随访。

  在随访过程中囊肿体积平均线性测量值减少(>10%~15%)则为良性，不需要进一步随访。

Physiologic simple cyst (in a premenopausal patient)

SRU consensus (premenopausal)

- Cysts ≤3 cm do not need to be described in the report, and there is no need for follow-up.
- Cysts >3 and ≤5 cm should be mentioned in the report and described as benign, with no follow-up necessary.
- Cysts >5 cm should be described.
  If superior visualization and confidence AND ≤7 cm, no follow-up is needed.
  If standard visualization or confidence OR >7 cm, follow-up should be performed in 2–6 or 6–12 months.
    2–6 months: Early follow-up if proper characterization desired.
    6–12 months: To assess growth.

生理性单纯囊肿(绝经前期患者)

SRU共识(绝经前期)

- 卵巢囊肿≤3cm时，不需要在报告中描述，也不需要进行随访。
- 卵巢囊肿>3cm但≤5cm时，需在报告中提及并描述为良性，不需要随访。
- 卵巢囊肿>5cm应进行描述。
  如果显示非常清晰并诊断明确，同时≤7cm，不需要随访。
  如果显示较清晰或诊断较明确，或>7cm，应在2~6个月内或6~12个月内随访。
    2~6个月：对相关特征进行早期随访。
    6~12个月：用于评估生长情况。

Postmenopausal simple ovarian cyst

SRU consensus (postmenopausal)

- Cysts ≤1 cm are considered normal and do not need to be reported or followed.
- Cysts >1 cm and ≤3 cm are almost certainly benign, but should be described to document. No follow-up is needed.
- Cysts >3 cm should be described.
  If superior visualization and confidence AND ≤5 cm, no follow-up is needed.
  If standard visualization or confidence OR >5 cm, follow-up should be performed in 3–6 or 6–12 months.
  - 3–6 months: Early follow-up if proper characterization desired.
  - 6–12 months: To assess growth.

Hemorrhagic cyst

- In both pre-and post-menopausal women, hemorrhagic cysts >5 cm should undergo shortterm follow-up US (6–12 weeks) to ensure resolution. If it does not resolve, the diagnosis of endometrioma is considered.

Cyst with indeterminate, but probably benign, characteristics

- These include cysts with features that are suggestive, but not sufficient to allow a confident diagnosis of hemorrhagic cyst, endometrioma, or dermoid.

- In women of reproductive age or women in early menopause, follow-up US within 6–12 weeks is suggested for resolution of a lesion to confirm that it is a hemorrhagic cyst. If unchanged, then continued follow-up is to be considered. If follow-up imaging does not confirm an endometrioma or dermoid, surgical evaluation is recommended.
- In post-menopausal women, surgical evaluation is considered.

ENDOMETRIOMA

- Endometriomas, also referred to as endometriotic cysts, represent ectopic endometrial tissue implanted on the adnexa. As endometrial tissue is hormonally responsive, an endometrioma may be composed of blood products of varying ages (*chocolate cyst*).
- They can be solitary but bilateral ovarian involvement is common (30–50%) and increases specificity for the diagnosis of endometriosis.
- Endometriomas can rupture as a result of rapid growth, particularly during pregnancy, which can lead to acute pelvic pain and hemoperitoneum. They can lead to adhesions, tethering of bowel loops, and obliteration of the fat planes. Another rare complication is malignant degeneration into endometrioid or less commonly clear cell subtypes of ovarian cancer.
- On ultrasound, an endometrioma may represent as a well-defined complex cyst with homogeneous low-level internal echoes and posterior acoustic enhancement. Occasionally an endometrioma may appear similar to a neoplasm.

绝经后卵巢单纯囊肿

SRU共识(绝经后期)

- 囊肿<1cm为正常，不需要报告或随访。
- 囊肿>1cm但<3cm几乎都为良性，但应描述记录。不需要随访。
- 囊肿>3cm时，需要描述。
  如果显示非常清晰并诊断明确，同时≤5cm，不需要随访。
  如果显示较清晰或诊断较明确，或>5cm，应在3~6个月内或6~12个月内随访。
  - 3~6个月：对相关特征进行早期随访。
  - 6~12个月：用于评估生长。

出血性囊肿

- 无论是绝经前还是绝经后的妇女，如出血性囊肿>5cm则应行短期(6~12周)超声随访以确认消退。否则应考虑子宫内膜异位症。

不确定但可能为良性囊肿的特征

- 此类囊肿具备提示性特征，但不足以诊断为出血性囊肿、子宫内膜异位症或皮样囊肿。

- 对于育龄期或绝经早期妇女，建议6~12周内进行超声随诊以确定出血性囊肿发生消退。如无变化，则考虑继续随诊。如随诊图像仍不能确定为内膜异位或皮样囊肿，则建议进行外科评估。
- 绝经后妇女，建议外科评估。

子宫内膜异位瘤

- 子宫内膜异位瘤，也称子宫内膜异位囊肿，为子宫内膜组织异位种植于附件。由于子宫内膜组织受激素影响，病灶内含有新旧不一的出血成分(*巧克力囊肿*)。
- 子宫内膜异位瘤可单发，但双侧更常见(30%~50%)，该特点可提高对子宫内膜异位症诊断的特异性。
- 子宫内膜异位瘤快速生长可发生破裂，尤其在妊娠期，可导致急性盆腔疼痛和腹腔出血。可引起肠管粘连和栓系，以及脂肪间隙消失。另一种少见的并发症是恶变为卵巢的子宫内膜样癌，或更少见的透明细胞癌。
- 子宫内膜异位瘤超声表现为边界清楚的复杂性囊肿，内为均质低回声并伴有后方声影增强。偶可与肿瘤的表现相似。

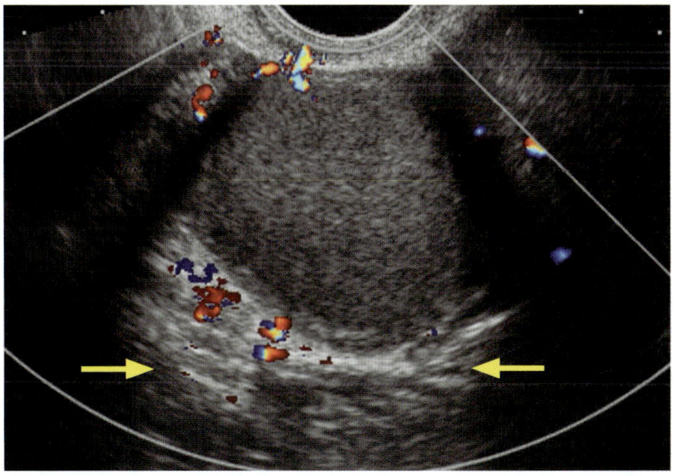

Endometrioma on ultrasound:
Coronal grayscale ultrasound demonstrates a right ovarian mass with uniform low-level internal echoes, posterior acoustic enhancement (arrows), and no internal flow on color Doppler.
子宫内膜异位症超声检查：
冠状切面灰阶超声显示右侧卵巢内均匀低回声肿物，伴有后方回声增强(黄箭)，内部无彩色多普勒血流。

- MRI typically shows multiple T1 hyperintense masses (due to hemorrhagic content) which demonstrate signal gradient ("shading") on T2-weighted images. Endometriomas – unlike dermoids – do not suppress on fat-saturated sequences. Less commonly, endometriosis may appear hyperintense on both T1-and T2-weighted images.

  Tiny hemorrhagic endometrial implants may be apparent as hyperintense foci on T1-weighted images.
- Laparoscopy is the gold standard for the diagnosis of suspected endometriosis, with implants appearing as small areas of tissue distortion with hemorrhagic spots or large masses with associated adhesions.

- 典型的MRI表现为T_1加权上多发高信号肿块(内部出血)，T_2加权上信号呈阶梯状("阴影")。子宫内膜异位症与皮样囊肿不同，前者在脂肪抑制序列信号并不被抑制。少数情况下，子宫内膜异位症在T_1和T_2加权上均为高信号。

  小的出血性子宫内膜异位病灶可能在T_1加权上仅表现为局灶性高信号灶。
- 腹腔镜是诊断疑似子宫内膜异位症的"金标准"，种植灶表现为小片区域组织变形伴出血点或大片粘连性的肿块。

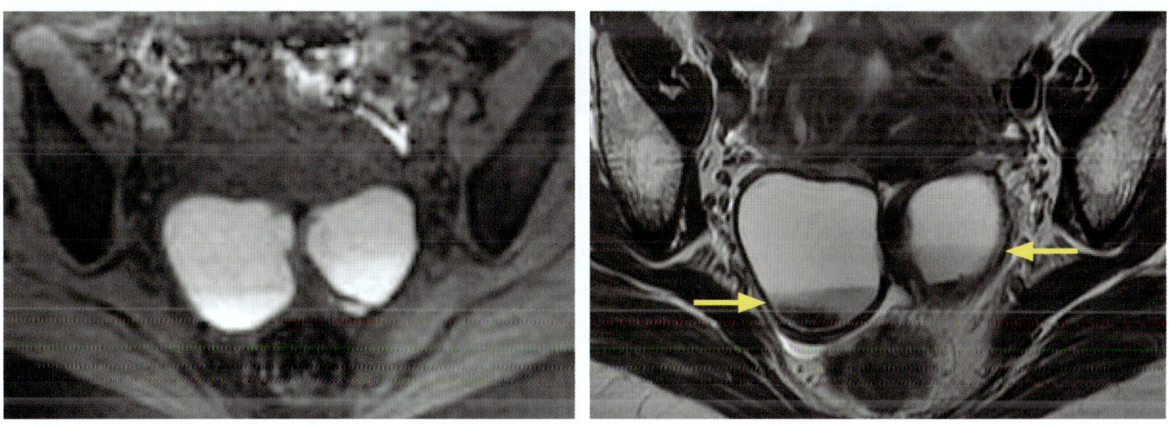

Endometriomas on MRI: Axial fat-suppressed T1-weighted MRI (left image) shows bilateral T1 hyperintense ovarian lesions in direct contact (*kissing ovaries sign*). The T2-weighted axial MRI (right image) demonstrates characteristic dependent shading (arrows). *Case courtesy Cheryl Sadow, MD, Brigham and Women's Hospital.*
子宫内膜异位症MRI：轴位脂肪抑制T_1加权MRI(左图)显示双侧卵巢内T_1高信号病灶，彼此紧邻(卵巢对吻征)。轴位T_2加权MRI(右图)显示有特征性的重力分布性阴影(黄箭)。

Ovarian neoplasms

- Ovarian neoplasms include a large group of benign and malignant tumors that can be classified based on where they originate in the ovary. 80% of ovarian masses are benign.
- The three histologic types of primary ovarian neoplasm include epithelial neoplasm, germ cell tumor, and sex cord-stromal tumor.

卵巢肿瘤

- 卵巢肿瘤包括一组广泛的良、恶性肿瘤，分类可根据卵巢组织的起源。约80%的卵巢肿瘤为良性。
- 原发性卵巢肿瘤的三种组织学类型包括上皮性肿瘤、生殖细胞肿瘤和性索间质肿瘤。

- **Surface epithelial** tumors account for 70% of ovarian neoplasms overall and >90% of ovarian cancers.
- **Germ cell** tumors include mature cystic teratomas (dermoid) and dysgerminomas. *Struma ovarii* is a subtype of teratoma that is composed of mature, functioning thyroid tissue.
- **Sex cord-stromal** tumors include fibroma, thecoma, and fibrothecoma.

  Meigs syndrome is the triad of benign ovarian fibroma, ascites, and right pleural effusion.

  Tumors containing thecal cells produce estrogen and may cause endometrial carcinoma.
- The Ovarian-Adnexal Reporting and Data System (O-RADS) provides risk stratification for ovarian and adnexal lesions on ultrasound and MRI. It divides lesions into five categories from normal ovary (1) to high risk (>50% chance of malignancy based on ultrasound, or ~90% risk of malignancy based on MRI).

- **表面上皮**肿瘤占所有卵巢肿瘤的70%，在卵巢癌中占90%以上。
- **生殖细胞**肿瘤包括成熟囊性畸胎瘤(皮样囊肿)和无性细胞瘤。卵巢甲状腺肿是畸胎瘤的一个亚型，由成熟并具有功能的甲状腺组织构成。
- **性索间质**肿瘤包括纤维瘤、卵泡膜细胞瘤和纤维卵泡膜细胞瘤。

  梅格斯综合征是一个三联征，包括良性卵巢纤维瘤、腹水和右侧胸腔积液。

  含有纤维卵泡膜细胞的肿瘤可产生雌激素，可引起子宫内膜癌。
- 卵巢附件影像报告和数据系统(O-RADS)提供了超声和MRI上卵巢和附件病变的风险分层标准。它将病变分为五类，从正常卵巢(1级)到高度风险(5级，超声提示恶性可能性>50%，或MRI提示恶性可能性高达90%)。

Dermoid cyst (mature cystic teratoma)

皮样囊肿(成熟囊性畸胎瘤)

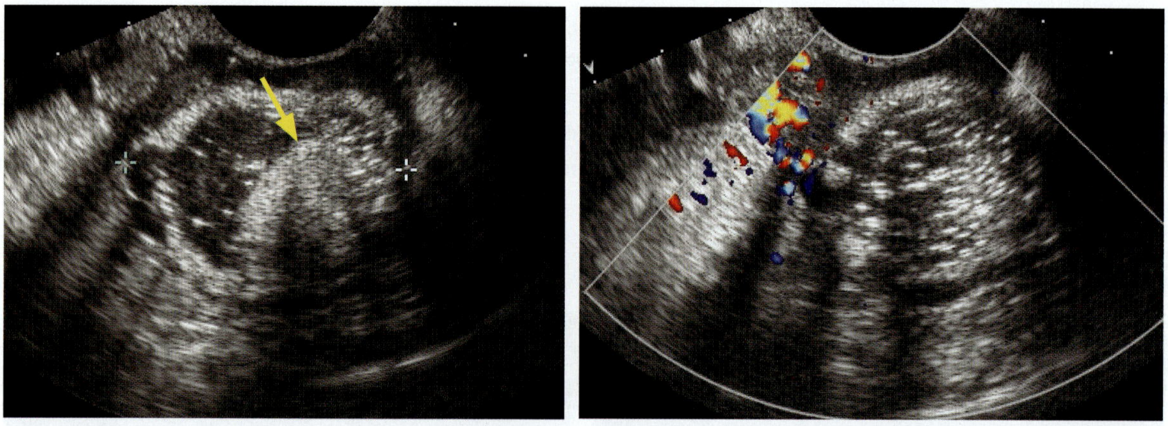

Dermoid cyst: Grayscale ultrasound image of the right ovary (left image) shows a complex ovarian cyst with a densely echogenic, shadowing focus centrally representing the Rokitansky nodule (arrow). Color Doppler shows the *dot-dash* sign, echogenic shadowing, and no significant internal Doppler flow.

皮样囊肿：右侧卵巢灰阶超声(左图)显示一个复杂性卵巢囊肿，内有密集高回声，中央有声影，其为Rokitansky结节(黄箭)。彩色多普勒显示点线征及声影，但无显著的内部多普勒血流。

- Dermoid cyst, also called a mature cystic teratoma, is the most common ovarian neoplasm. Technically, a *teratoma* contains all three primitive germ cell layers, while a *dermoid cyst* may contain only two. In general use, however, these terms are interchangeable.
- Malignant transformation is very rare and typically occurs in postmenopausal patients. Another rare complication is intraperitoneal rupture leading to acute peritonitis.
- A dermoid cyst can act as a lead point for adnexal torsion particularly when large (>4 cm).
- The classic ultrasound appearance of a dermoid cyst is a complex ovarian cyst with an echogenic *Rokitansky* nodule, which is a solid nodule projecting into the cyst cavity, from which hair or teeth may arise. The imaging appearance can be variable, however, and other common imaging features include:

  The *dot-dash* pattern describes interrupted echogenic lines thought to be produced by keratin fibers.

- 皮样囊肿也称成熟囊性畸胎瘤，是最常见的卵巢肿瘤。严格来讲，畸胎瘤应包含三层原始生殖细胞，而皮样囊肿可能仅包含两层。然而，这些术语常被相互混用。
- 恶变非常罕见，通常发生于绝经后患者。另一个罕见的并发症为腹膜腔内破裂导致急性腹膜炎。
- 皮样囊肿可促发附件扭转，尤其是体积较大者(>4cm)。
- 皮样囊肿的典型超声表现为卵巢复杂囊肿，内可见高回声的Rokitansky结节，即为伸向囊腔的实性结节，毛发或牙齿从该处生长。但其影像学特征多变，其他常见征象有：

  点线征：不连续的线样高回声，可能为角蛋白纤维所致。

The *tip of* the iceberg sign describes obscuration of the deeper contents due to high-attenuation material.

- CT and MRI typically show a heterogeneous unilocular cystic structure with coarse calcification, corresponding to sebaceous material, hair follicles, and fat. A Rokitansky nodule may or may not be seen.

  Less commonly, a dermoid cyst may appear as a solid hyperdense or fat-density mass.

- Both endometriomas and teratomas are predominantly hyperintense on T1-weighted images due to their blood and fat content, respectively. Distinction can be made by using the fat-suppressed imaging sequences. Teratoma will show signal loss on the fat-suppressed images, due to internal macroscopic fat, while an endometrioma will not.

冰山一角征：由于衰减明显，深层结构显示不清。

- CT或MRI的典型表现为混杂单房囊性结构，伴有粗大钙化，对应皮脂腺组织、毛囊和脂肪。有或无Rokitansky结节。

  少见情况下，皮样囊肿可表现为实性高密度或脂肪密度肿块。

- 子宫内膜异位囊肿和畸胎瘤分别因出血和脂肪而在T_1加权上呈高信号。可通过脂肪抑制图像鉴别。畸胎瘤由于内有大块脂肪，在脂肪抑制图像上信号减低，但子宫内膜异位囊肿无此表现。

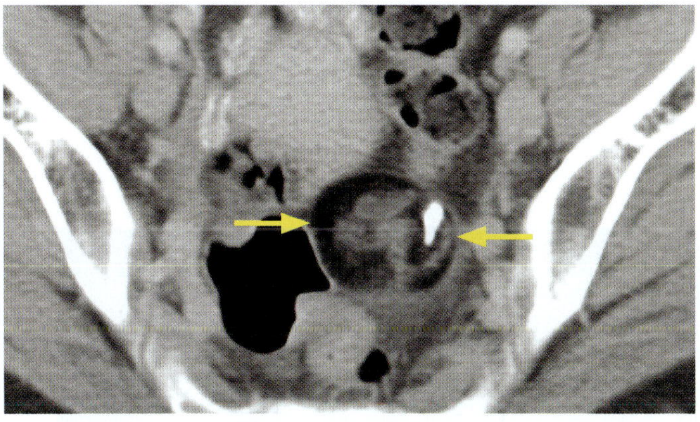

Dermoid causing ovarian torsion:
Axial contrast-enhanced CT demonstrates abnormal location of the right ovary which is displaced to the left adnexa. The lead-point is a right ovarian mass (arrows) containing fat, soft tissue, and calcification.
表皮样囊肿导致卵巢扭转：
轴位增强CT显示右侧卵巢异位至左附件区。触发点为右卵巢肿物(黄箭)，内含脂肪、软组织及钙化。

Ovarian cancer

- Ovarian cancer is the tenth most common female malignancy, but ranks fifth in cancer deaths among women as it often presents at a late stage.
- Ovarian cancer may be **epithelial**, **germ cell**, **sex cord-stromal**, or **metastatic** in origin.
- Approximately 90% of malignant tumors are of epithelial origin. Serous tumors are the most common epithelial subtype, followed by mucinous, endometrioid, and clear cell.

  Serous cystadenocarcinomas are frequently bilateral and typically appear as mixed solid and cystic masses. The solid portions demonstrate avid enhancement. There is often concomitant ascites.

  Mucinous cystadenocarcinomas are large, most commonly unilateral, and occur in older patients compared to serous cystadenocarcinomas. Mucinous cystadenocarcinoma typically presents as a multiloculated cystic mass containing mucin-rich T1 hyperintense fluid.

  Clear cell carcinoma and less commonly **endometrioid carcinoma** are associated with endometriosis.

- Malignant **germ cell** tumors occur in younger patients and include dysgerminoma, endodermal sinus tumor, and immature teratoma.
- **Metastases** to the ovary are uncommon but may result from gastric cancer, colon cancer, pancreatic cancer, breast cancer, and melanoma. Metastases are often bilateral.

  A **Krukenberg tumor** is an ovarian metastasis of a mucin-producing tumor, typically gastric or colonic adenocarcinoma.

  Endometrial cancer may also metastasize to the ovaries.

- Ultrasound findings suggestive of a malignant ovarian mass include:

卵巢癌

- 卵巢癌的发生率在所有女性恶性肿瘤中居第十位，但在女性恶性肿瘤相关死亡率中排名第5位，因其发现时通常已为晚期。
- 卵巢癌的来源可为**上皮**、**生殖细胞**、**性索间质细胞**或**转移**。
- 约90%的恶性肿瘤起源于上皮。浆液性肿瘤是最常见的上皮性肿瘤亚型，然后为黏液性、子宫内膜样和透明细胞型。

  浆液性囊腺癌通常为双侧囊实混合性肿块，实性成分有明显强化，常伴腹水。

  黏液性囊腺癌体积较大，常为单侧，相对于浆液性囊腺癌发病年龄更大。典型的黏液性囊腺癌表现为多房囊性肿块，内含丰富的黏液，呈T_1高信号。

  透明细胞癌和少见的子宫内膜样癌与子宫内膜异位症有关。

- 恶性**生殖细胞瘤**好发于年轻患者，包括无性细胞瘤、内胚窦瘤和未成熟畸胎瘤。
- **转移性**卵巢肿瘤不常见，可来自胃癌、结肠癌、胰腺癌、乳腺癌和恶性黑色素瘤。转移性肿瘤多为双侧。

  克鲁肯贝格瘤是一种产生黏液的卵巢转移肿瘤，常来源于胃和结肠腺癌。

  子宫内膜癌也可以转移至卵巢。

- 超声提示为卵巢恶性肿块的征象有：

Mural nodule.
Thick or irregular walls or septae.
Solid components.
High flow on color Doppler.
Presence of ascites.
Papillary projecti ons.

- MRI is used to characterize indeterminate adnexal masses, rather than for staging.
- Features suggesting malignancy include a large size (>10 cm), solid enhancing component(s), internal necrosis, ascites, or peritoneal nodularity, although no finding is 100% specific.
- Staging of ovarian carcinoma is based on the FIGO (International Federation of Gynecology and Obstetrics) system. It characterizes extent of disease based on involvement of the ovaries (one or two), fallopian tubes, uterus, pelvic intraperitoneal tissues, retroperitoneal lymph nodes, malignant cells in peritoneal washings, and/or peritoneal or distant metastasis.
- MRI is highly sensitive to detect peritoneal implants, which occur most commonly in the pouch of Douglas, paracolic gutters, bowel surface, greater omentum, and liver surface.

附壁结节。
厚壁或不规则囊壁或有分隔。
实性成分。
彩色多普勒显示高血流。
出现腹水。
乳头样突起。

- MRI主要用于评估不能定性的卵巢肿块，而非用于分期。
- 提示为恶性的征象包括巨大(>10cm)、实性强化成分、内部坏死、腹水或腹膜结节，但均无100%的特异性。
- 卵巢癌根据国际妇产科联盟(FIGO)系统进行分期。该系统的依据是肿瘤累及范围，包括卵巢(单侧或双侧)、输卵管、子宫、盆部腹膜腔内组织、腹膜后淋巴结、腹腔灌洗液中的恶性细胞，和/或腹膜或远处转移。
- MRI对发现腹膜种植具有高度敏感性，腹膜种植最常发生于直肠子宫陷凹、结肠旁沟、肠管表面、大网膜及肝脏表面。

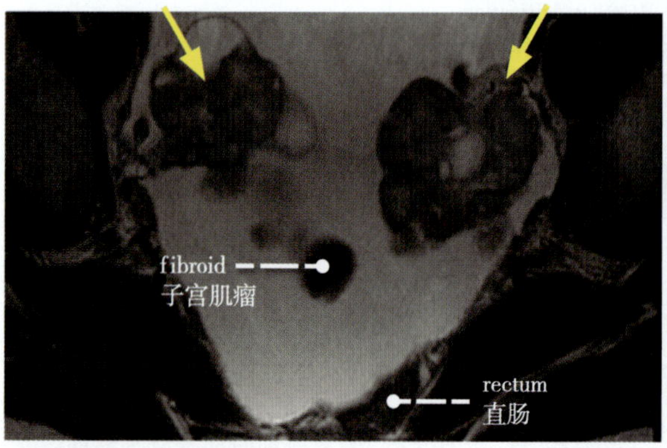

Axial T2-weighted fat suppressed MRI
轴位 T_2 加权脂肪抑制MRI

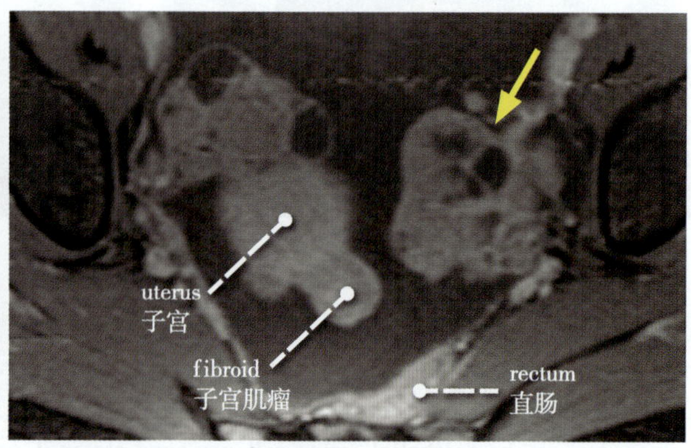

Axial postcontrast T1-weighted fat suppressed MRI
轴位增强后 T_1 加权脂肪抑制MRI

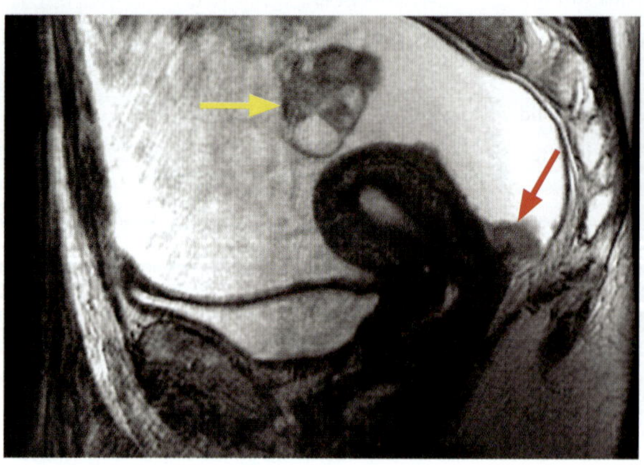
Sagittal T2-weighted fat suppressed MRI
矢状位 T_2 加权脂肪抑制MRI

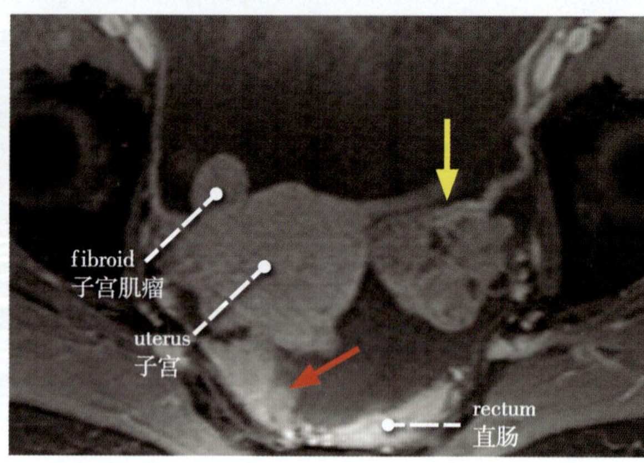

Axial postcontrast T1-weighted fat suppressed MRI
轴位增强后 T_1 加权脂肪抑制MRI

Ovarian cancer with peritoneal carcinomatosis: MRI shows bilateral enhancing adnexal masses (yellow arrows). There are enhancing peritoneal implants in the pouch of Douglas posterior to the uterus (red arrows). The uterus contains several T2 hypointense enhancing fibroids. This histology was papillary serous carcinoma.

Case courtesy Cheryl Sadow, MD, Brigham and Women's Hospital.

卵巢癌伴腹膜转移：MRI显示强化的双侧附件肿块(黄箭)。子宫后方的直肠子宫陷凹内有强化的腹膜种植灶(红箭)。子宫含数个 T_2 低信号增强肌瘤。组织学诊断为乳头状浆液性癌。

(翻译　孙明菡　程瑾)

Ovarian hyperstimulation syndrome (OHSS)

卵巢过度刺激综合征(OHSS)

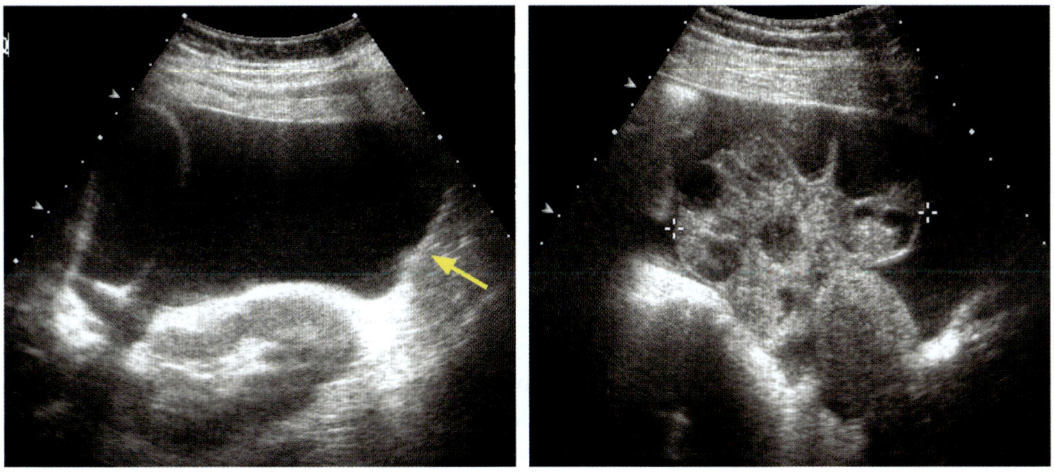

Ovarian hyperstimulation syndrome: Sagittal grayscale ultrasound of the right upper quadrant (left image) shows a large amount of ascites (arrow). Right lower quadrant ultrasound (right image) shows a markedly enlarged ovary (calipers measure greater than 8 cm), with numerous enlarged follicles. The patient was receiving infertility treatment.
卵巢过度刺激综合征:右上腹矢状切面灰阶超声(左图)显示大量腹水(黄箭)。右下腹超声(右图)显示卵巢明显增大(卡尺测量>8cm),伴大量增大的卵泡。患者曾接受过不孕症治疗。

- Ovarian hyperstimulation syndrome (OHSS) is a complication of infertility treatment, thought to be due to vascular endothelial growth factor (VEGF) dysregulation causing capillary leak.
- The criteria for diagnosis of OHSS include abdominal pain, bilateral and symmetric *spoke-wheel* enlargement of the ovaries (>5 cm), and presence of either ascites or hydrothorax. At least one additional laboratory or clinical symptom must be met, including elevated hematocrit (≥45%), elevated WBC (>15,000), elevated LFTs, acute renal failure, or dyspnea.
- OHSS increases the risk of ovarian torsion and ectopic pregnancy, and it can lead to coagulopathy, hypovolemia, and shock.

- **卵巢过度刺激综合征(OHSS)**是治疗不孕症的一个并发症,被认为是由血管内皮生长因子(VEGF)失调导致毛细血管渗漏所致。
- OHSS的诊断标准包括腹痛、双侧卵巢呈对称性辐轮样增大(>5cm),并存在腹水或胸腔积液。至少还必须满足一项额外的实验室检查或临床症状,包括血细胞比容升高(≥45%)、WBC升高(>15 000/μL)、LFT升高、急性肾衰竭或呼吸困难。
- OHSS会增加卵巢扭转和异位妊娠的风险,并可能导致凝血功能障碍、低血容量,以及休克。

Polycystic ovarian syndrome (PCOS)

多囊卵巢综合征(PCOS)

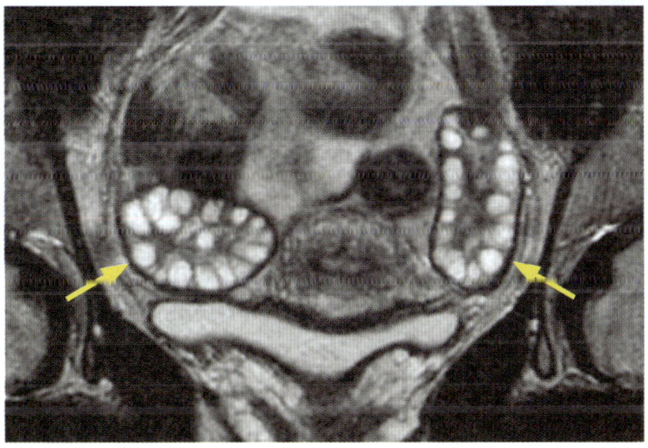

PCOS: Coronal T2 MRI shows enlarged ovaries with multiple peripherally located small follicles, in the classic *string of pearls* configuration (arrows).
PCOS:冠状位T_2 MRI显示增大的卵巢伴位于外周的多发小卵泡,呈典型的串珠样结构(黄箭)。

- Polycystic ovarian syndrome is a clinical syndrome of obesity, insulin resistance, anovulation, and hirsutism secondary to excess androgens.
- Ultrasound criteria include >12 small follicles (most often arranged around the periphery of the ovary), none greater than 9 mm in diameter, and an ovarian volume >10 mL. Ovarian volume is calculated by multiplying the diameters in

- **多囊卵巢综合征(PCOS)**是一种临床综合征,包括肥胖、胰岛素抵抗、无排卵和继发于雄激素过多的多毛症。
- 超声标准包括>12个小卵泡(最常排列在卵巢周边),直径均不超过9mm,卵巢体积>10mL。

three orthogonal planes by 0.52.

- The ovarian stroma is typically very vascular when evaluated by color Doppler.
- A differential consideration includes normal ovaries under the influence of oral contraceptives, although contraceptives will not increase the vascularity of the ovary.

卵巢体积是通过将3个正交平面的直径乘积与0.52相乘而计算得出。

- 卵巢间质在彩色多普勒上通常显示非常丰富的血运。
- 鉴别诊断应考虑口服避孕药对正常卵巢的影响，但避孕药不会增加卵巢的血运。

Adnexal cystic lesions

Paraovarian cyst

- A paraovarian cyst is a simple cyst separate from the ovary, thought to be developmental in origin.
- Paraovarian cysts are considered normal if <5 cm.
- The main differential is an ovarian cyst. Ovarian cysts should be reported (and followed) if >3 cm, while paraovarian cysts do not need to be followed unless >5 cm. Transvaginal ultrasound can help confirm extra-ovarian location via gentle pressure by the transducer, which displaces it away from the ovary.

Peritoneal inclusion cyst

- A peritoneal inclusion cyst is a septated fluid collection formed by adhesions, almost always related to prior surgery. The ovary is closely associated with the peritoneal inclusion cyst, either trapped within or adjacent to it.
- It is important *not* to recommend surgery for treatment of a peritoneal inclusion cyst, as it is benign, and further surgery may create additional adhesions.
- The main differential of a peritoneal inclusion cyst is a cystadenoma, which has thick septations and tends to exert mass effect.

Dilated fallopian tube

- The fallopian tube may become distended due to infection, inflammation, or traction from pelvic adhesions.
- A **hydrosalpinx** is a fluid-filled fallopian tube lacking internal echoes. Ultrasound shows a dilated, anechoic, paraovarian tubular structure with incomplete septations that represent infolding of the tubular walls.

附件囊性病变

卵巢旁囊肿

- 卵巢旁囊肿是从卵巢分离出来的单纯囊肿，被认为来源于发育过程的异常。
- 卵巢旁囊肿通常<5cm。
- 主要的鉴别诊断是卵巢囊肿。卵巢囊肿如果>3cm应进行报告(并随访)，而卵巢旁囊肿则不需要随访，除非>5cm。经阴道超声可以通过将探头轻轻压迫使囊肿远离卵巢从而帮助确认其位于卵巢外。

腹膜包涵囊肿

- 腹膜包涵囊肿是由粘连形成的有分隔的液体聚集，几乎都与之前的手术有关。卵巢与腹膜包涵囊肿密切相关，或被包裹在其中，或与之邻近。
- 必须牢记，对腹膜包涵囊肿不应推荐手术治疗，因为它是良性病变，而进一步的手术可能会产生更多粘连。
- 腹膜包涵囊肿的主要鉴别诊断是囊腺瘤，后者有厚的间隔并容易产生占位效应。

输卵管扩张

- 输卵管可能因感染、炎症或盆腔粘连的牵拉而扩张。
- **输卵管积水**是指输卵管充满了液体，无内部回声。超声显示为一个扩张、无回声、卵巢旁的管状结构，有不完全的分隔，为管壁内折所致。

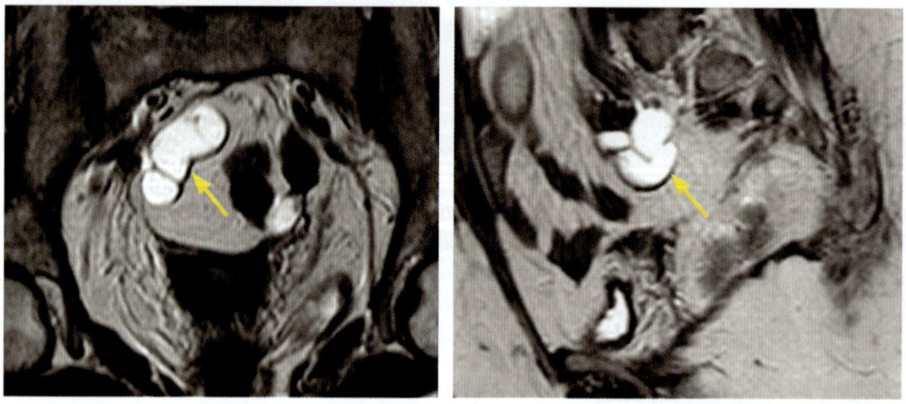

Coronal (left image) and sagittal (right image) T2-weighted MRI show a tubular T2 hyperintense structure in the right adnexa (arrows) that did not enhance on postcontrast images (not shown), consistent with hydrosalpinx.

MRI冠状位(左图)和矢状位(右图)T_2加权MRI显示右侧附件一个管状T_2高信号结构(黄箭)，但在增强后(未展示)无强化，符合输卵管积水的表现。

- **Hematosalpinx** is a blood-filled fallopian tube that can be seen in the setting of a ruptured ectopic pregnancy or endometriosis. Imaging will show internal echoes within the dilated tube.
- **Pyosalpinx** is a pus-filled fallopian tube resulting from pelvic inflammatory disease. As in hematosalpinx, imaging will show internal echoes within the dilated tube.

- **输卵管积血**是指血液充满了输卵管，可见于异位妊娠破裂或子宫内膜异位症。影像学检查显示扩张的输卵管内存在内部回声。
- **输卵管脓肿**是由盆腔炎症引起输卵管内积脓。与输卵管积血相同，影像学检查显示扩张的输卵管内存在内部回声。

(翻译　王维平)

4 Obstetrical Imaging

Ellen X. Sun, Junzi Shi, Robin Perlmutter-Goldenson, Mary C. Frates

4 产科影像

Contents

目录

FIRST TRIMESTER PREGNANCY

IMAGING OF THE EARLY PREGNANCY

Gestational sac

- The gestational sac is first seen at **5 weeks** of gestational age by transvaginal ultrasound (TVUS). A gestational sac is usually seen transvaginally if the β-hCG is greater than 2000 mIU/mL. However, use caution when using this discriminatory value as there are exceptions such as in multiple gestations.
- **With a positive pregnancy test and normal adnexae, any round or oval fluid collection in the uterus is overwhelmingly likely to represent a very early intrauterine pregnancy (IUP).**
- The mean sac diameter (MSD) is the average diameter of the gestational sac measured in three orthogonal planes (L×W×H)/3). The MSD is not routinely measured but may be helpful in assessing viability.

  If the MSD measures 8 mm by TVUS, a yolk sac should be visible. If a yolk sac is not present, the pregnancy is unlikely to be successful.

  If the MSD measures 16 mm, a live embryo should be visible. If an embryo is not seen when the MSD is 16–24 mm, the pregnancy is suspicious for but not diagnostic of failed pregnancy.

  If the MSD measures 25 mm or greater and no embryo is seen, it is diagnostic of failed pregnancy.
- A **subchorionic hematoma** is a complication of early pregnancy caused by bleeding of the chorionic attachment.

  A small subchorionic hematoma adjacent to the gestational sac is of no clinical significance.

  In general, as size of the subchorionic hematoma increases, the risk of pregnancy loss increases. However, the extent of the gestational sac surrounded by hematoma is more predictive of pregnancy loss than volume of the hematoma.

Yolk sac

- The yolk sac is normally seen by **5.5 weeks**.
- An abnormally large (>5 mm) yolk sac increases the risk of failed pregnancy.

Embryo and heartbeat

- The embryo is first visualized adjacent to the yolk sac by about **6 weeks**, at which time the heartbeat is present as a flickering motion.

早期妊娠

早期妊娠影像

妊娠囊

- 妊娠囊最早可在孕龄**5周**时经阴道超声(TVUS)进行观察。如果β-hCG>2 000mIU/mL，通常经阴道可见妊娠囊。但在使用该临界值时需谨慎，因为有例外情况，如多胎妊娠。
- **当妊娠试验呈阳性，附件正常时，子宫内任何圆形或椭圆形的液性暗区都极有可能代表非常早期的宫内妊娠(IUP)。**
- 妊娠囊平均直径(MSD)是在3个垂直切面测得的平均值。MSD并不常规测量，但可能有助于评估存活能力。

  如果经阴道超声测量的MSD为8mm，则应该看到卵黄囊。若卵黄囊缺失，妊娠就不太可能成功。

  如果MSD为16mm，则应该看到一个活的胚胎。如果MSD为16~24mm时未见胚胎，则妊娠可疑，但不能诊断妊娠失败。

  如果MSD为25mm或以上，且未见胚胎，则诊断为妊娠失败。
- **绒毛膜下血肿**是由绒毛膜附着物出血引起的早期妊娠并发症。

  在妊娠囊附近的小范围绒毛膜下血肿不具任何临床意义。

  一般来说，随着绒毛膜下血肿增加，妊娠失败的风险也随之增加。然而，妊娠囊周围血肿涉及的范围比血肿体积更能预测妊娠失败。

卵黄囊

- 在正常情况下可以在妊娠第**5.5周**时看到卵黄囊。
- 若卵黄囊异常增大(直径>5mm)，妊娠失败的风险增加。

胚胎和(原始)胎心搏动

- 胚胎大约在妊娠**6周**时首先出现在卵黄囊附近，此时胎儿心跳以闪烁运动的形式出现。

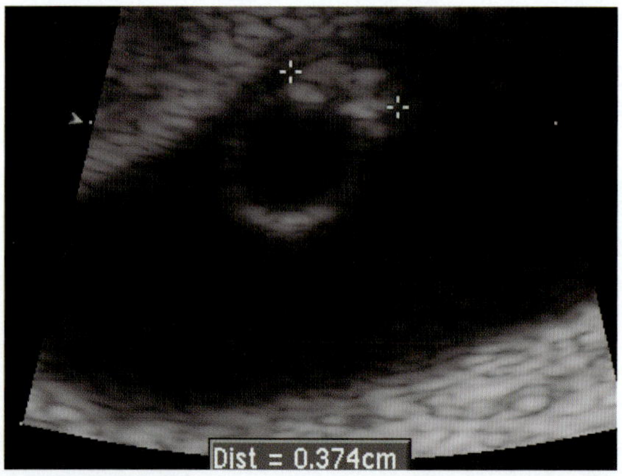

Normal embryo (measuring 3.7 mm) and yolk sac. This embryo had normal heart rate of 112 bpm.
正常胚胎(测值3.7mm)和卵黄囊。该胚胎心率正常，为112次/min。

- It is unusual to see an embryo with a measurable crown-rump length (CRL) but without a heartbeat. No heartbeat with a CRL <7 mm is suspicious for, though not diagnostic of, failed pregnancy.
- No heartbeat with a CRL ≥7 mm is diagnostic of failed pregnancy.
- If the early heart rate is less than 90 bpm, there is very little chance that the pregnancy will be successful. There is no such thing as a "too fast" heart rate. In fact, embryos with a faster heart rate have the highest chance of normal outcome.

  If the CRL is ≤4 mm, ≤90 bpm is considered slow and ≥100 is normal.

  If the CRL is ≥5 mm, ≤110 bpm is considered slow and ≥120 is normal.
- Heart rate is measured using M-mode.

- 当看到胚胎并可测量其顶臀长(CRL)时，如没有心管搏动是异常的。当CRL<7mm且无心管搏动时，妊娠失败可疑，但不能确诊妊娠失败。
- CRL≥7mm且无心管搏动可诊断为妊娠失败。
- 若早期胎儿心率<90 次/min，其妊娠成功的机会很小。早期妊娠时并无心率"过快"一说，事实上胚胎心率越快则正常的可能性越大。

  若CRL≤4mm，心率≤90 次/min为过缓，≥100 次/min为正常。

  若CRL≥5mm，心率≤110 次/min为过缓，≥120 次/min为正常。
- M型超声测量心率

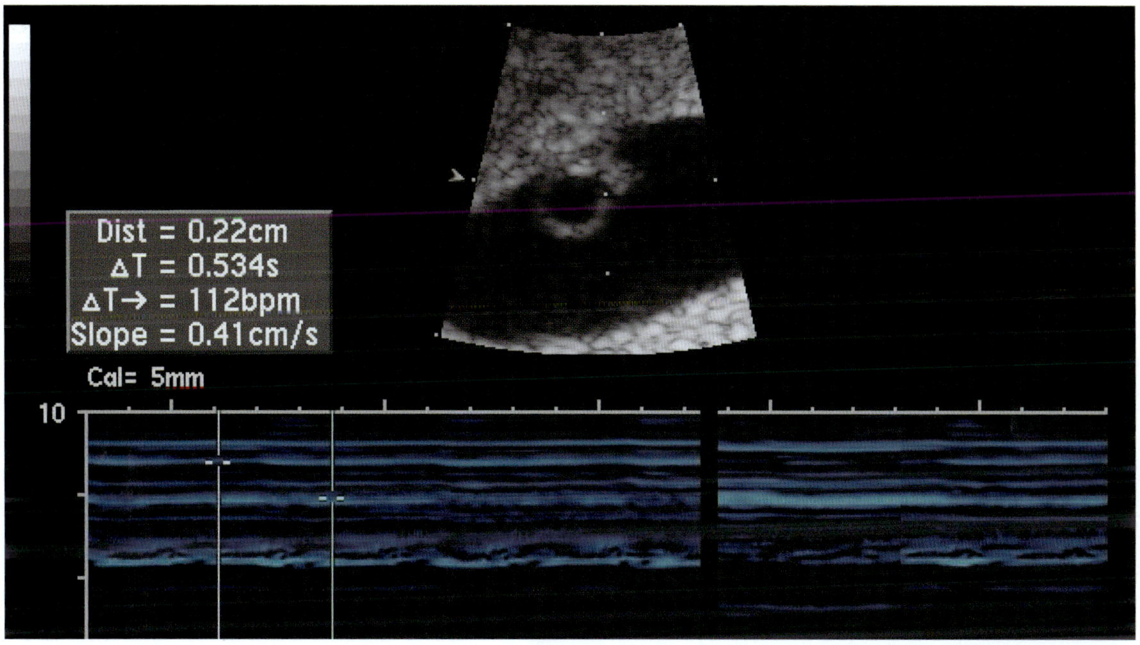

Normal heart rate:
mode shows a calculated heart rate of 112 bpm, which is normal in this 6-week embryo with a 3 mm crown-rump length.
正常心率：
M型超声显示的胚胎心率为112 次/min，此为正常6周的胚胎心率，顶臀长为3mm。

Amnion

- The amnion is visible by TVUS beginning around 7 weeks.

羊膜

- 羊膜约在妊娠7周时可被经阴道超声观察到。

Pregnancy dating

Dating convention

- Gestational age is calculated from the first day of the last menstrual cycle, *not* from conception. Therefore, a "six week" pregnancy has really only existed for four weeks. For IVF patients with a precisely known implantation date, two weeks are added to be consistent with the dating of spontaneous pregnancies.

Assigning gestational age

- Between 5 and 6 weeks gestation, gestational age is determined based on three typical appearances of the early pregnancy.

孕期计算

常规孕龄计算法

- 孕龄是从末次月经周期的第一天开始计算，而不是从受孕开始计算。因此"6周"妊娠实际只有4周。体外受精者的受精时间明确，加上2周即相当于自然妊娠孕龄。

确定孕龄

- 孕龄可在妊娠5~6周时根据早期妊娠时的三个典型表现进行确定。

Gestational sac only: 5.0 weeks.
Gestational sac with a yolk sac, but without an embryo: 5.5 weeks.
Gestational sac with an embryo <3 mm and heartbeat: 6 weeks.

仅有妊娠囊：5周。
有妊娠囊和卵黄囊，但无胚胎：5.5周。
妊娠囊伴胚胎<3mm及心管搏动：6周。

- For embryos ≥3 mm in length, the CRL is used to assign gestational age using established reference tables. The CRL can be used to estimate gestational age up to 12 weeks. After 12 weeks, dating is estimated using multiple fetal measurements.
- The only ways to reliably know a precise gestational age are if a previous ultrasound was performed to establish dating, or the patient underwent in vitro fertilization with a known embryo transfer date.

- 胚胎≥3mm时，将测得的CRL通过已建立的参考值来确定孕龄。CRL适用于确定妊娠12周内的孕龄。12周以后的孕龄确定需采用多种胎儿测量指标。
- 确定孕龄唯一可靠的方法是先前有明确的超声检查日期，或患者接受体外受精并有已知的胚胎移植日期。

Early Pregnancy Prognosis

早期妊娠的转归

- The following sonographic findings are **diagnostic of failed pregnancy:**

Crown–rump length ≥7 mm with no heartbeat.
Mean sac diameter ≥25 mm with no embryo.
No embryo with heartbeat ≥2 weeks after a scan that showed a gestational sac without a yolk sac.
No embryo with heartbeat ≥11 days after a scan that showed a gestational sac *with* a yolk sac.

- 以下超声表现可**诊断妊娠失败：**

顶臀长≥7mm，无心管搏动。
妊娠囊平均直径≥25mm，无胚胎。
妊娠囊内无卵黄囊，妊娠2周后仍未见有心管搏动的胚胎。
妊娠囊内可见卵黄囊，妊娠11天后仍未见有心管搏动的胚胎。

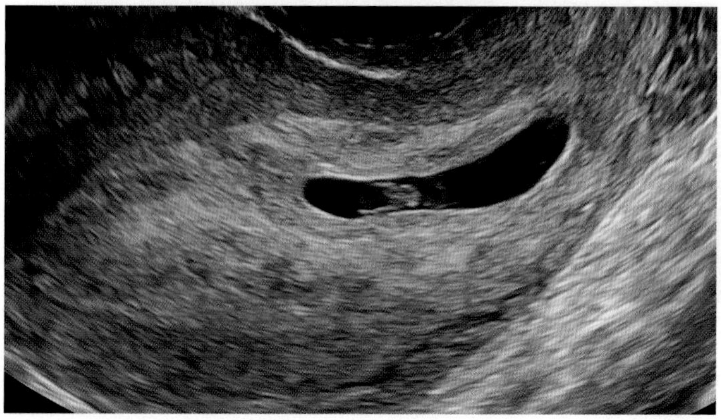

Sagittal grayscale ultrasound shows a flattened intrauterine gestational sac with yolk sac and a 7 mm embryo but no heartbeat in the lower uterine segment. These findings are diagnostic of failed pregnancy in this patient who presented with heavy vaginal bleeding.
矢状切面灰阶超声显示宫腔下段有一个扁平的妊娠囊，可见卵黄囊和一个直径7mm的胚胎，但无心管搏动，这些声像表现可以诊断妊娠失败，该患者因阴道大量出血而就诊。

- The following findings are **suspicious for, but not diagnostic of, failed pregnancy:**

Crown–rump length <7 mm with no heartbeat.
Mean sac diameter of 16–24 mm with a yolk sac but no embryo.
An empty amnion with yolk sac and no embryo.
Small gestational sac relative to the embryo (<5 mm difference between the MSD and CRL).

- 以下表现**可疑妊娠失败，但不能确诊：**

顶臀长<7mm，无心管搏动。
妊娠囊平均直径16~24mm，有卵黄囊但无胚胎。
有一个空的羊膜，有卵黄囊，无胚胎。
胚胎相对妊娠囊偏小(MSD和CRL之差<5mm)。

- **Other worrisome findings** which increase the risk of a spontaneous pregnancy loss even in the presence of a heartbeat:

Bradycardia <90 bpm.
Irregular heartbeat.
Enlarged yolk sac >5 mm.
Lagging embryo size relative to gestational age.
Sliding gestational sac.
Subchorionic hematoma surrounding >50% the circumference of the gestational sac.

- **其他的不良征兆**，即使有心管搏动也会增加自然流产的风险：

心动过缓，心率<90次/min。
心管搏动不规则。
卵黄囊增大>5mm。
胚胎大小相对滞后于孕龄。
妊娠囊移位。
妊娠囊周围绒毛膜下血肿>50%妊娠囊周长。

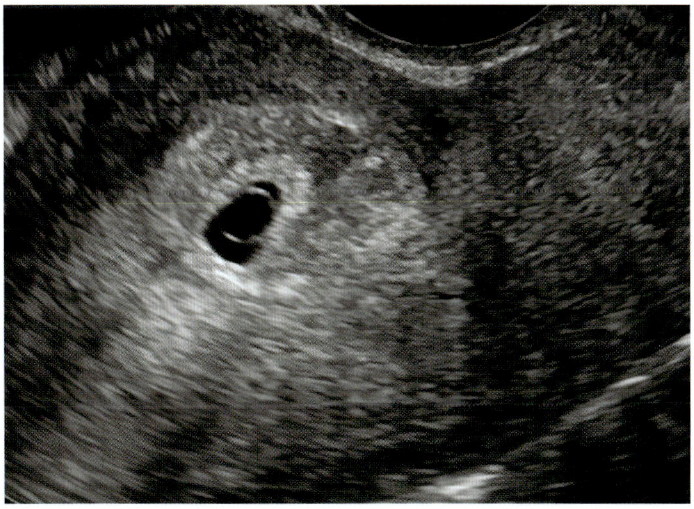

Sagittal grayscale ultrasound shows an intrauterine gestational sac with an enlarged yolk sac, a worrisome finding.
矢状切面灰阶超声显示一个宫内妊娠囊和增大的卵黄囊，此为一个不良的征兆。

Ectopic pregnancy

异位妊娠

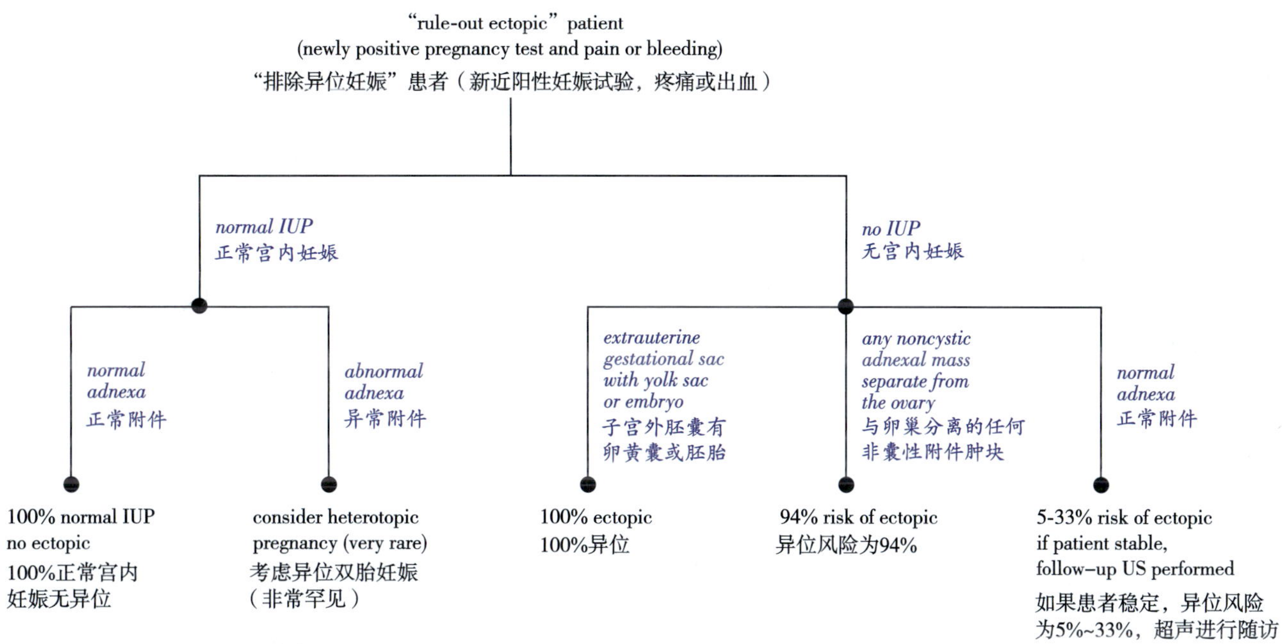

Overview of ectopic pregnancy

- Ectopic pregnancy is defined as pregnancy outside of the endometrial cavity. Hemorrhage and resultant hypovolemic shock may be life-threatening to the mother.
- The classic clinical presentation of ectopic pregnancy is a positive pregnancy test, vaginal bleeding, pelvic pain, and tender adnexal mass. This presentation is seen in less than 50% of patients.

Risk stratification

- Any woman with a newly positive pregnancy test and either pain or bleeding is classified as a *rule-out ectopic* or *clinically suspected ectopic* patient.
- A *rule-out ectopic* patient may have an intrauterine pregnancy (IUP), ectopic pregnancy, or spontaneous abortion. The IUP may be normal, abnormal, or too early to detect.

异位妊娠概述

- 异位妊娠是指妊娠位于宫腔之外。出血和低血容量性休克可危及孕妇生命。
- 典型的临床表现包括妊娠试验阳性、阴道出血、盆腔疼痛和触痛性附件肿块。这些表现只见于不到50%的患者。

风险分层

- 任何妇女有新出现的妊娠试验阳性，且伴有疼痛或阴道出血，均应归为异位妊娠待排或临床可疑异位妊娠。
- 异位妊娠待排患者可能为宫内妊娠、异位妊娠或自发流产。宫内妊娠可能为正常、异常或因时间太早而不能确定。

- The role of imaging is to determine if an IUP is present and to evaluate the common locations (especially the adnexae) where an ectopic may potentially be found.

- 影像学检查的作用在于确定是否为宫内妊娠，并对常见的异位妊娠多发位置(尤其是附件)进行检查。

Definite diagnoses are the exception

确诊即为排除法

- It is often not possible to definitively diagnose ectopic pregnancy, except when an extrauterine gestational sac containing either yolk sac or embryo is seen.
- Any extra-ovarian adnexal mass in the absence of an IUP is highly suspicious for ectopic pregnancy.
- A suspected ectopic pregnancy should prompt careful clinical management and close imaging follow-up. Meanwhile, any round or oval cystic space in the endometrium is likely to represent a gestational sac.

- 异位妊娠往往并不能明确诊断，除非看到一个宫外含有卵黄囊或胚胎的妊娠囊。
- 没有宫内妊娠的任何卵巢之外的附件肿块都应高度怀疑异位妊娠。
- 一旦怀疑异位妊娠，应立即进行仔细的临床处置和密切的影像学随访。同时，子宫内任何圆形或椭圆形的囊性暗区都可能是妊娠囊。

Ectopic location

异位妊娠的位置

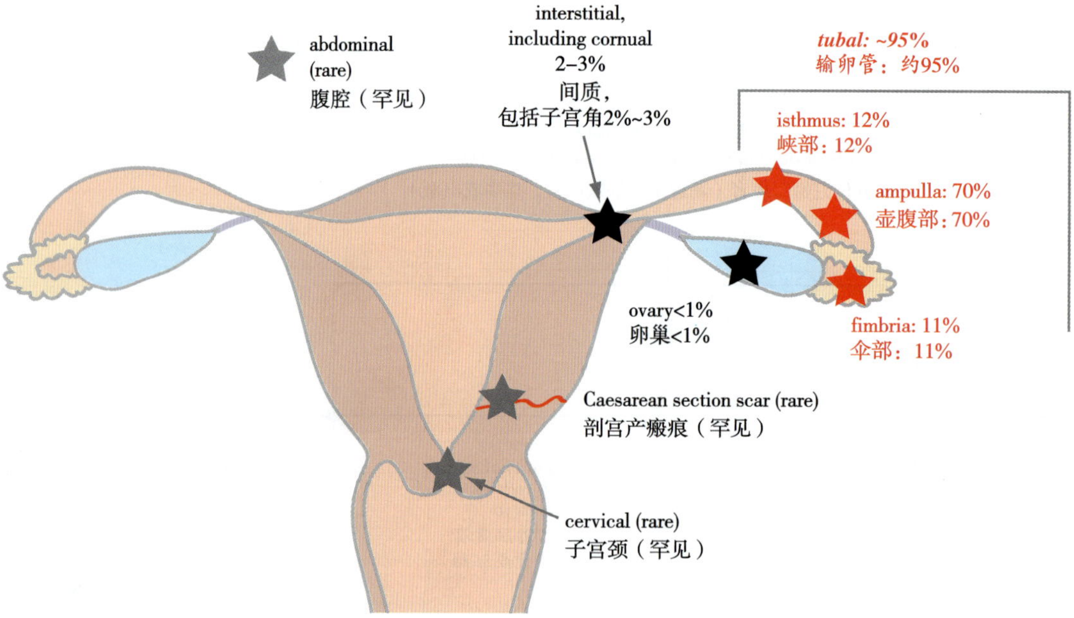

- Most (~95%) ectopic pregnancies occur in the fallopian tube, with the ampullary segment being the most common site.
- It is rare for an ectopic pregnancy to be in the ovary (<1% of all ectopics).
- An especially dangerous location for an ectopic pregnancy is the interstitial (intrauterine) portion of the fallopian tube, because of the lack of early symptoms. An **interstitial ectopic** carries an especially high risk of catastrophic hemorrhage due to its propensity for delayed uterine rupture and proximity to the ovarian vessels.

  Ultrasound of an interstitial ectopic shows absent myometrium along the lateral edge. The *interstitial line sign* represents a thin, echogenic line extending from the endometrial canal to the center of the interstitial ectopic mass. This echogenic line is thought to represent the medial, nondistended interstitial portion of the tube.

- A **heterotopic pregnancy** is a simultaneous IUP and ectopic pregnancy. Patients undergoing assisted reproductive techniques are at increased risk for heterotopic pregnancy. In these patients, the adnexae must be carefully evaluated even in the presence of an IUP.

- 绝大多数(约95%)异位妊娠发生在输卵管，而壶腹部是最常见的部位。
- 位于卵巢的异位妊娠罕见(<1%所有异位妊娠)。
- 最具危险的异位妊娠部位是输卵管间质部(包括宫角部)，因其缺乏早期症状。由于有延迟破裂的倾向并靠近卵巢血管，**间质部异位妊娠有极高的致命性大出血风险。**

  间质部妊娠的超声表现为妊娠囊的外侧缘缺乏子宫肌层。间质线征是指细小的线样高回声从宫腔延伸至间质异位妊娠团块的中央，该回声线被认为是位于内侧未扩张的输卵管间质部。

- **异位双胎妊娠**是指同时发生宫内和宫外妊娠。接受辅助生殖技术的患者发生异位双胎妊娠的风险会增加，在这些患者中，即使存在宫内妊娠，也必须仔细检查附件。

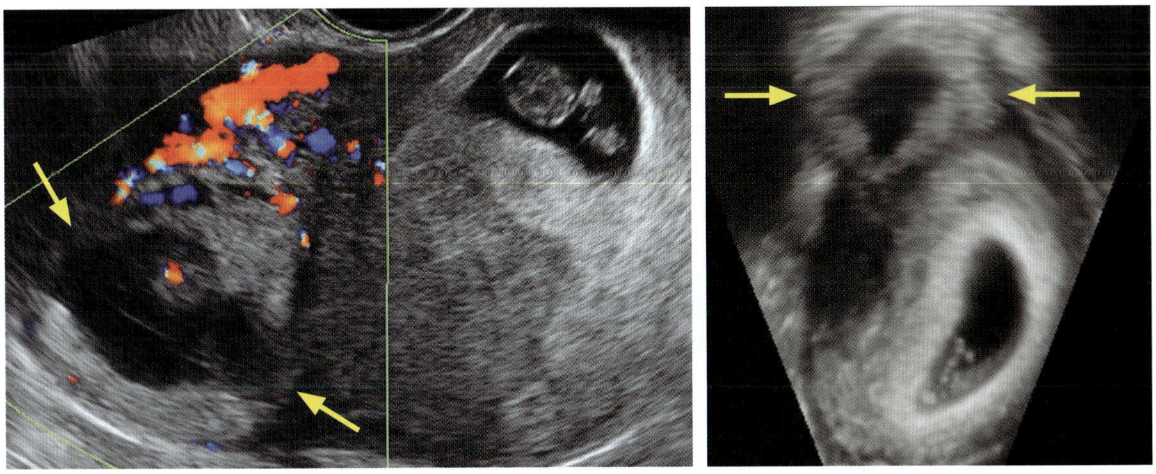

Heterotopic pregnancy: Transverse grayscale ultrasound with Doppler overlay (left image) demonstrates a normal intrauterine pregnancy and a second, eccentrically located gestational sac (arrows) with live embryo abutting the left adnexa, possibly within a rudimentary uterine horn or cornua. This is better depicted on the 3D rendering on the right. A cornual pregnancy was confirmed on laparoscopy.
异位妊娠：子宫横切面灰阶超声及彩色多普勒(左图)显示正常宫内妊娠和第二个偏心的、毗邻左侧附件的、有活胚胎的妊娠囊(黄箭)，可能位于残角或宫角部。右图三维超声显示效果更好。经腹腔镜检查证实为子宫角部妊娠。

- Ectopic pregnancy may also occur (rarely) in a prior myomectomy scar, in the cervix, or in the abdomen. When in the abdomen, the ectopic pregnancy can become large before causing symptoms.

- 异位妊娠也可发生于既往剖宫产切口的瘢痕处、宫颈或腹腔(均罕见)。发生于腹腔的异位妊娠可长到很大才引起症状。

Imaging findings of tubal ectopic pregnancy

输卵管异位妊娠的影像学表现

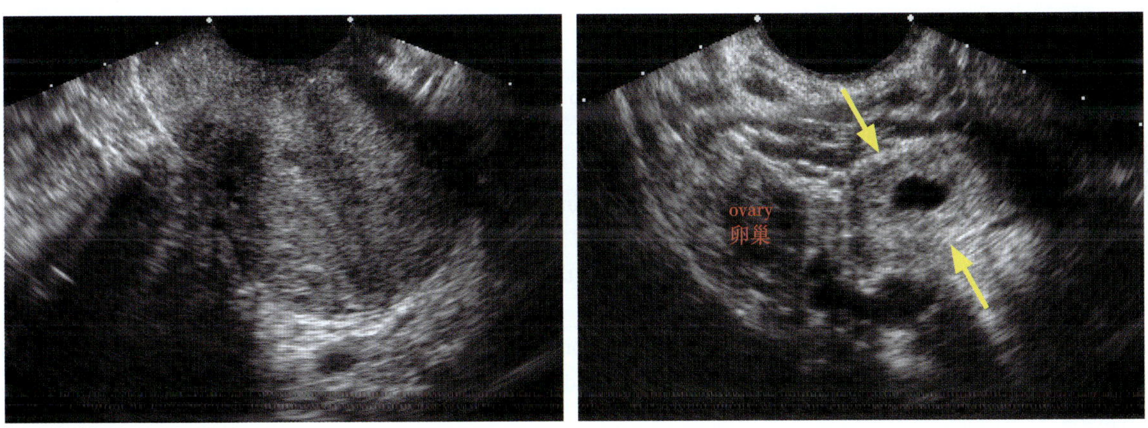

Adnexal ectopic: Sagittal grayscale endovaginal ultrasound of the uterus (left image) shows a normal uterus, with no evidence of intrauterine pregnancy. Ultrasound of the adnexa (right image) shows an adnexal ring (yellow arrows), discrete from the normal ovary. In a patient with a suspected ectopic, the presence of an adnexal ring and no intrauterine pregnancy has a 95% positive predictive value of being an ectopic pregnancy.
Case courtesy Julie Ritner, MD, Brigham and Women's Hospital.
附件异位妊娠：子宫矢状切面阴道灰阶超声(左图)显示正常子宫，未见宫内妊娠。附件区超声(右图)显示一个环形结构(黄箭)，与正常卵巢分界明显。在有可疑异位妊娠时，若出现附件环形结构但未见宫内妊娠征象，其异位妊娠的阳性预测值为95%。

- Tubal ectopic pregnancy can have the following imaging appearances:

1. Absence of an IUP.
2. Extrauterine gestational sac separate from the ovary which can present as a tubal ring or adnexal ring. The presence of yolk sac, embryo, and cardiac activity is variable.
3. Ill-defined, inhomogeneous adnexal mass separate from the ovary.
4. Pelvic free fluid only.

- 输卵管异位妊娠可有以下影像学表现：

1. 未见宫内妊娠。
2. 宫外妊娠囊与卵巢分离，可表现为输卵管环或附件环。卵黄囊、胚胎和心管搏动情况可有可无。
3. 边界不清，内回声不均的卵巢旁附件肿块。
4. 仅有盆腔游离积液。

- In the absence of an IUP, an extrauterine gestational sac and tubal/adnexal ring have high positive predictive values for ectopic pregnancy (>95%).
- An extrauterine gestational sac with yolk sac or embryo (with or without heartbeat) has a 100% positive predictive value of being an ectopic.
- The nonspecific *ring of fire sign* describes increased peripheral color Doppler flow surrounding an adnexal mass. This sign is rarely helpful as it can be seen in both ectopic pregnancy and corpus luteum.
- In a *rule-out ectopic* patient, an ovarian mass is almost always a corpus luteum rather than an ectopic pregnancy unless a definite embryo or yolk sac is identified. In contrast, an extra-ovarian mass is highly concerning for an ectopic. When an adnexal mass is seen, it is helpful to gently apply pressure with the ultrasound probe and assess for movement of the mass separate from the ovary to identify its true location.

- 未见到宫内妊娠时，宫外妊娠囊和输卵管/附件环形结构对异位妊娠有很高的阳性预测值(>95%)。
- 伴有卵黄囊或胚胎(有或无胎心)的宫外妊娠囊，其异位妊娠的阳性预测值为100%。
- 非特异的火环征是指附件肿块周围彩色多普勒血流信号增加。此征象极少对诊断有帮助，它既可见于异位妊娠，也可见于黄体。
- 对于一位异位妊娠待排的患者，卵巢内肿块几乎都是黄体而非异位妊娠，除非确切看到胚胎和卵黄囊；相反，卵巢外的肿块应该高度怀疑异位妊娠。当看到一个附件肿块时，可用超声探头轻轻加压并观察肿块是否能够与卵巢分离，以此来帮助确定其真实位置。

Following serial hCG

动态随访 hCG

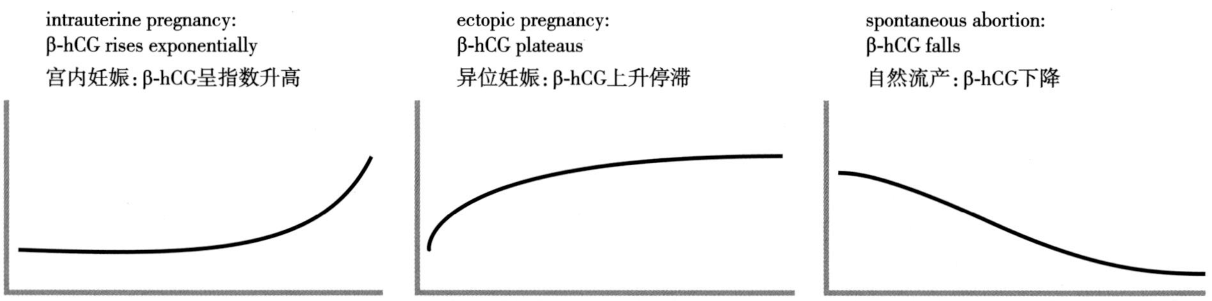

- The pattern of β-hCG levels over time may be a helpful adjunct to imaging in following-up the *rule-out* ectopic patient.

Caesarian section scar implantation

- Caesarean section scar is typically located in the low anterior uterine segment. Implantation of the embryo at this location is not considered an ectopic pregnancy due to being within the uterus. However, this condition is life-threatening.
- Abnormal endometrium at the scar results in invasion of the myometrium by the trophoblastic tissue, leading to high risk of placenta accreta and associated uterine rupture.

- β-hCG的动态变化特征可以辅助影像随访排除异位妊娠。

剖宫产切口着床

- 剖宫产瘢痕通常位于子宫前下段，该位置属于子宫内，因而植入胚胎不被认为是异位妊娠。但这种情况会危及生命。
- 瘢痕处的异常子宫内膜会导致滋养层组织侵入子宫肌层，可致胎盘植入的风险增高及子宫破裂。

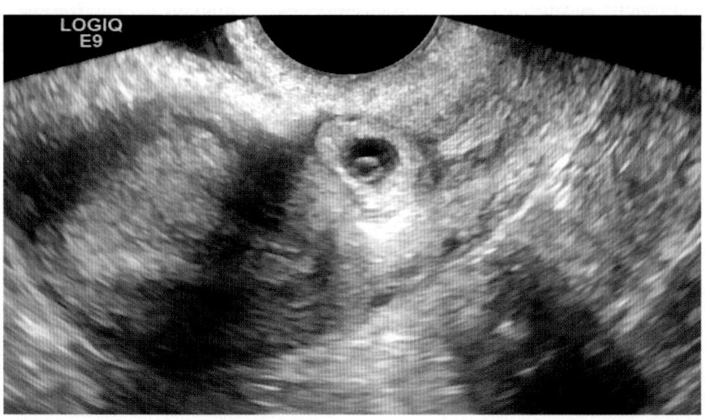

Sagittal grayscale ultrasound of the uterus demonstrates a gestational sac with yolk sac in the anterior lower uterine segment, centered at the site of a prior C-section scar.

子宫矢状切面灰阶超声显示子宫前下段有一个含有卵黄囊的妊娠囊，位于先前剖宫产瘢痕的中央。

MISCELLANEOUS FIRST TRIMESTER DISORDERS

其他早期妊娠异常

Gestational trophoblastic disease

- Gestational trophoblastic disease results from abnormal neoplastic overgrowth of the placental trophoblast and includes a spectrum of benign and malignant entities.
- There are three stages of gestational trophoblastic disease: complete hydatidiform mole, invasive mole, and choriocarcinoma.
- **Complete hydatidiform mole** does not contain any fetal parts. It is caused by loss of the egg's DNA prior to fertilization by the sperm and has a diploid karyotype of 46,XX (most commonly) or 46,XY. A complete mole may become invasive and progress to metastatic choriocarcinoma.
- The classic clinical presentation of molar pregnancy is hyperemesis, markedly elevated β-hCG, and an enlarged uterus. The patient may also present with painless vaginal bleeding.
- On ultrasound, molar disease causes uterine enlargement with a classic heterogeneous and multicystic bunch of grapes appearance. Visualization of fetal parts suggests a partial mole (see below).

妊娠滋养细胞疾病

- 妊娠期滋养细胞疾病是胎盘滋养层细胞呈肿瘤样过度生长所致，包括一系列良性和恶性的病变。
- 妊娠期滋养细胞疾病有3个阶段：完全性葡萄胎、侵袭性葡萄胎和绒毛膜癌。
- **完全性葡萄胎**不含任何胎儿成分。它是由于卵子受精前失去DNA所致，核型为二倍体：46，XX(最常见)或46，XY。完全性葡萄胎可具侵袭性并可进展成转移性绒毛膜癌。
- 葡萄胎的典型临床表现是剧吐、β-hCG显著升高、子宫增大。患者也可能出现无痛性阴道出血。
- 超声可见葡萄胎引起子宫增大，呈典型的不均匀及多囊"葡萄串"样改变。若见部分胎儿结构，则提示为部分性葡萄胎(见下文)。

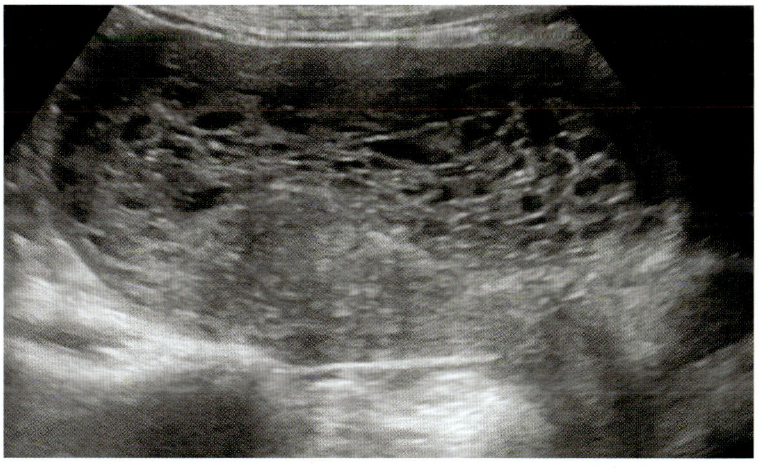

Sagittal grayscale ultrasound of the uterus demonstrates a large multicystic mass with internal vascularity (Doppler not shown) in the endometrial cavity. The appearance is consistent with gestational trophoblastic disease.

子宫矢状切面灰阶超声显示宫腔内有一个大的多囊样肿块，内有血管分布(未展示多普勒)。其外观符合妊娠期滋养层疾病。

- Molar pregnancy is associated with theca lutein cysts in the ovaries, which arise in response to elevated β-hCG.
- Treatment of a molar pregnancy is endometrial suction curettage and close follow-up of serum hCG levels for 6 months.
- **Invasive mole** is characterized by trophoblastic proliferation invading into the myometrium or (rarely) beyond the uterus. Diagnosis is made with color Doppler showing abnormal blood flow in myometrium.
- **Choriocarcinoma** is a rare malignant trophoblastic disease which may occur after a hydatidiform mole, normal pregnancy, ectopic or failed pregnancy. Diagnosis is made based on the presence of metastatic disease.
- **Partial hydatidiform mole** is a triploid pregnancy. It is usually caused by two sperm fertilizing the same egg and results in the triploid karyotype of 69,XXX, 69,XXY, or 69,XYY. Partial mole is less likely to progress to choriocarcinoma. A triploid pregnancy has severe fetal anomalies and an abnormal placenta. The imaging appearance of the placenta mimics a complete mole.

- 葡萄胎常伴发卵巢黄素囊肿，这是由β hCG升高引起的。
- 葡萄胎的治疗方法是对子宫内膜进行抽吸性刮宫，并密切监测血清hCG水平6个月。
- **侵袭性葡萄胎**的特征是滋养层增生侵入子宫肌层或(罕见情况下)突破子宫。诊断依据为彩色多普勒出现子宫肌层血流异常。
- **绒毛膜癌**是一种罕见的恶性滋养细胞疾病，可发生在葡萄胎、正常妊娠、异位妊娠或流产后。诊断依据为是否存在转移。
- **部分性葡萄胎**是一种三倍体妊娠。它通常由两个精子与同一卵子受精引起，导致三倍体核型为69，XXX、69，XXY或69，XYY。部分性葡萄胎发展为绒毛膜癌的可能性较小。三倍体妊娠有严重的胎儿异常和胎盘异常，胎盘的声像表现类似于完全性葡萄胎。

Retained products of conception (RPOC)

胎物残留(RPOC)

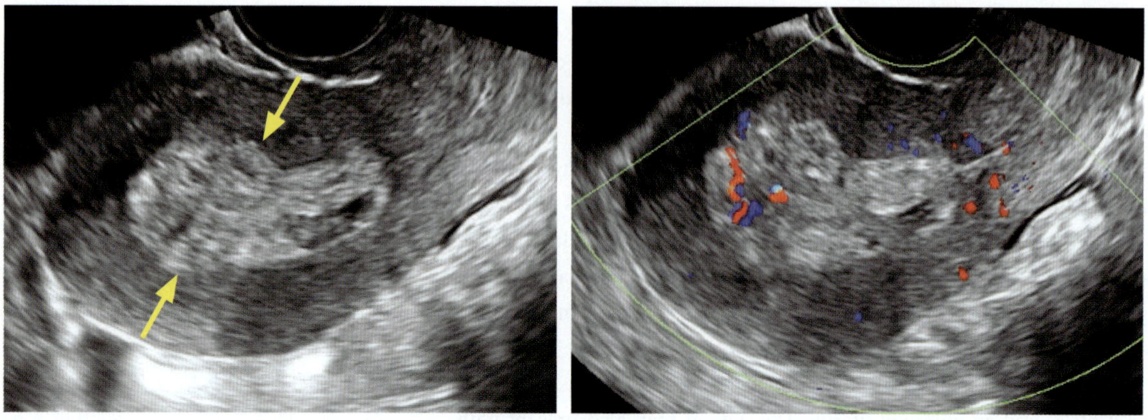

Retained products of conception: Sagittal grayscale ultrasound through the uterus demonstrates an echogenic mass within the endometrial cavity (arrows). Color Doppler shows vascularity within the mass. These imaging findings are highly suggestive of RPOC. Retained products of conception were proven at curettage.

Case courtesy Julie Ritner, MD, Brigham and Women's Hospital.

胎物残留：子宫矢状切面灰阶超声显示宫内有高回声肿块(黄箭)。彩色多普勒显示肿块内有血流信号，这些声像表现高度提示为胎物残留。受孕残留物须由诊刮术确诊。

- Retained products of conception (RPOC) is placental or fetal tissue that remains in the uterus after delivery, miscarriage, or termination.
- Untreated RPOC can lead to continued maternal bleeding and endometritis.
- The sonographic findings of an endometrial blood clot and RPOC can overlap. However an endometrial mass, with or without Doppler flow, in the appropriate clinical context is strongly suggestive of RPOC.
- A linear endometrium without blood flow has a high negative predictive value and is highly unlikely to contain RPOC.

- 胎物残留(RPOC)是指在分娩、流产或终止妊娠后残留在子宫内的胎盘或胎儿组织。
- 若RPOC未得到治疗，可导致母体持续出血或子宫内膜炎。
- 宫内血凝块和胎物残留在超声图像上的表现有部分重叠。然而，对于子宫内膜的肿块，不论其有无血流信号，如果有相应的临床病史都高度提示RPOC。
- 呈线状且不含血流的子宫内膜具有很高的阴性预测值，RPOC的可能性非常低。

MULTIPLE GESTATIONS AND PLACENTATION

- The placentation type (chorionicity and amnionicity) substantially affects the risk for pregnancy complications and influences how closely the pregnancy should be followed. The placentation should always be stated when first describing a multiple gestation.
- The **zygosity** (number of fertilized eggs) cannot be determined by ultrasound. Monozygotic twins can have any placentation type, depending on when the developing zygote splits. Dizygotic twins, however, are always diamniotic/dichorionic, and only dizygotic twins can be different sexes.
  - Monozygotic ("identical") twins arise from a single egg fertilized with a single sperm.
  - Dizygotic ("fraternal") twins arise from two individually fertilized eggs.
- **For the purposes of imaging and pregnancy management, chorionicity and amnionicity are utilized rather than zygosity.**
- **Chorionicity** is the number of placentas.
  - Monochorionic twins share a single placenta.
  - Dichorionic twins have separate placentas.

多胎妊娠和胎盘形成

- 胎盘的类型(绒毛膜性和羊膜囊性)在很大程度上决定了妊娠并发症的风险，并决定对妊娠期随访的密切程度。在报告多胎妊娠时必须对胎盘的类型进行描述。
- **合子性(受精卵数量)(zygosity)**并不能够用超声进行确定。单卵双胎可出现在任何胎盘类型中，这取决于受精卵分裂的时间。但双卵双胎常为双绒毛膜性/双羊膜囊性，而且只有双卵双胎可以有不同的性别。
  - 单卵双胎(同卵双生)起源于同一受精卵。
  - 双卵双胎(异卵双生)起源于两个不同的受精卵。
- **为了使影像学和妊娠处理更加方便，应使用绒毛膜特性和羊膜特性，而不是受精卵数进行描述。**
- **绒毛膜特性**是指胎盘的数量。
  - 单绒毛膜双胎共用一个胎盘。
  - 双绒毛膜双胎各自有一个胎盘。

- **Amnionicity** is the number of amnions.

  Monoamniotic twins share a single amniotic sac and must therefore share the placenta.

  Diamniotic twins each have a separate amniotic sac and may or may not share their placenta.

  The number of amniotic sacs usually correlates with the number of yolk sacs.
- By convention, chorionicity is stated before the amnionicity when stating the placentation. For instance, the abbreviation mono/di refers to monochorionic/diamniotic twins.

- **羊膜特性**是指羊膜囊的个数。

  单羊膜囊双胎共用一个羊膜囊，因此必须共用一个胎盘。

  双羊膜囊双胎各自有一个单独的羊膜囊，可能共享也可能不共享胎盘。

  羊膜囊的数量通常与卵黄囊的数量有关。
- 按照惯例，描述胎盘类型时应首先描述绒毛膜特性，然后是羊膜囊特性。例如，缩写“单绒/双羊”表示单绒毛膜/双羊膜囊双胎。

Overview of complications by placentation type

- The more that the twins share, the greater the risk of complications.
- Di/di twins have an increased risk of premature delivery and low birth weight compared to singleton gestations.
- Mono/di twins have an increased risk of complications related to a shared placenta, including twin-twin transfusion, acardiac twin syndrome, and twin embolization.
- In addition to being at risk for the same complications as mono/di twins, mono/mono twins are also at risk for cord entanglement and being conjoined.

不同胎盘类型的并发症概述

- 双胎共享的胎盘越多，并发症风险越大。
- 双绒/双羊双胎发生早产和低出生体重的风险高于单胎。
- 单绒/双羊双胎共用一个胎盘的相关并发症风险增大，包括双胎间输血、无心双胎综合征，以及双胎栓塞。
- 单绒/单羊双胎除了有单绒/双羊同样的并发症风险外，还有脐带缠绕和连体的风险。

Early counting of multiple gestations

- If two separate gestational sacs are identified, the placentation is di/di. The zygosity is indeterminate.

  Although dizygotic twins are always di/di, early splitting of a single fertilized egg can also lead to di/di monozygotic twins.
- If a single gestational sac contains two yolk sacs, the placentation is mono/di, and the twins are monozygotic.

早期确立多胎妊娠

- 如果两个独立的妊娠囊完全相同，则胎盘的类型为双绒/双羊。受精卵个数不能确定。

  虽然双卵双胎均为双绒/双羊，但是单个受精卵在早期分裂也可形成双绒/双羊。
- 如果一个妊娠囊内包含两个卵黄囊，胎膜类型为单绒/双羊，则是单卵双胎。

Dizygotic (“fraternal”) twins

- Dizygotic twins result when two eggs are each fertilized by a different sperm.
- Dizygotic twins are always dichorionic/diamniotic.

双卵双胎

- 2个卵子分别与2个精子受精则形成双卵双胎。
- 双卵双胎均为双绒/双羊。

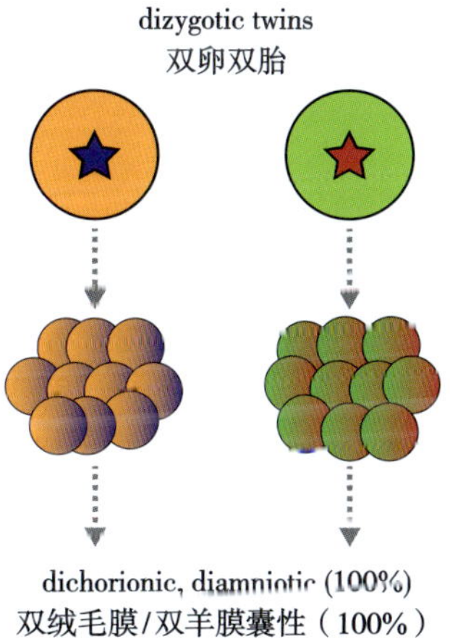

Monozygotic (“identical”) twins

单卵双胎(完全相同)

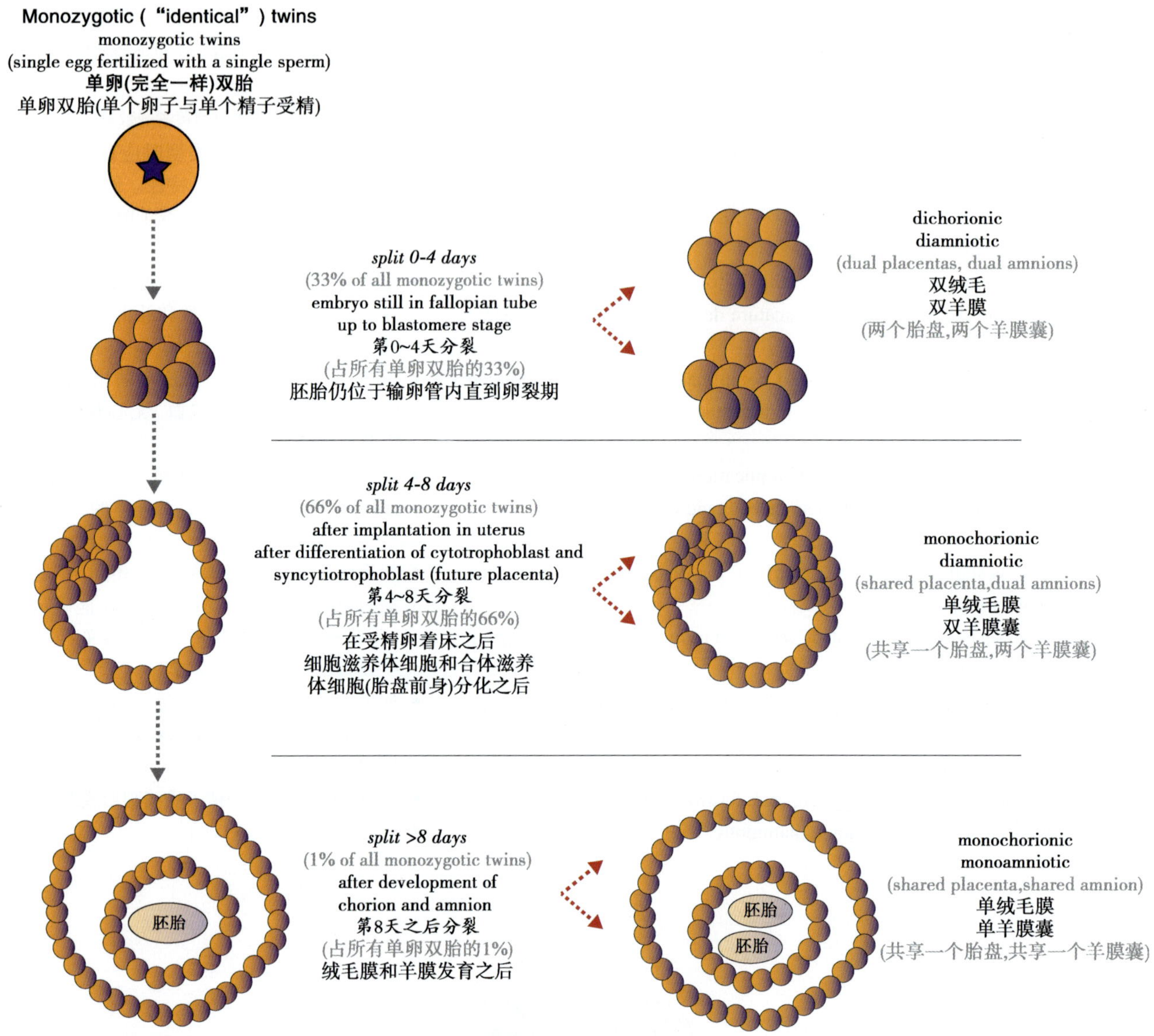

- Monozygotic twins are the result of splitting of the blastocyst or embryo, formed by fertilization of a single egg by a single sperm. Although “identical” monozygotic twins are always the same sex, they may not be identical phenotypically due to local differences in the uterine and placental environment.
- **33% split early** (0–4 days), before formation of either the placenta or amnion, leading to **dichorionic/diamniotic twins.**
- **66% split intermediate** (4–8 days), after formation of the placenta but before the amnion has developed), leading to **monochorionic/diamniotic twins.**
- **1% split late** (>8 days), after formation of the chorion and amnion, leading to **monochorionic/monoamniotic** twins. Very late splitting may result in conjoined twins, which are always monochorionic/monoamniotic.

- 单卵双胎是由一个卵子与一个精子受精形成胚泡或胚胎后分裂形成。同卵双胎均为相同性别，但由于宫内位置和胎盘环境不同，其表型并不完全相同。
- **早期分裂**(0~<4天)占33%，发生在绒毛膜和羊膜形成前，形成**双绒/双羊双胎**。
- **中期分裂**(4~8天)占66%，发生在绒毛膜形成后，但在羊膜形成前，形成**单绒/双羊双胎**。
- **晚期分裂**(>8天)占1%，发生在绒毛膜和羊膜形成后，**形成单绒/单羊双胎**。很晚期的分裂可导致连体双胎，且总是单绒/单羊。

Di/di (dichorionic/diamniotic) twins

- Di/di twins each have a separate placenta and amniotic sac.
- On ultrasound, two placentas can usually be separately identified in the second trimester.
- The inter-twin membrane will be relatively thick as there are two layers of chorion and two layers of amnion separating each twin.

双绒/双羊双胎

- 双绒/双羊双胎各自有一个胎盘和羊膜囊。
- 超声上，两个独立的胎盘通常在妊娠中期可以辨认。
- 胎儿间的隔膜相对较厚，由两层绒毛膜和两层羊膜组成，并将两胎儿分隔开来。

- In the second and third trimesters, the thickness of the inter-twin membrane is less reliable to determine chorionicity because the membrane becomes thinner as gestation progresses.
- The *twin peak sign* (also called *lambda sign*) represents a triangle-shaped placental infolding at the interface of the placenta and the thick inter-twin membrane that is seen in di/di twins. The *twin peak sign* is most useful when it is difficult to distinguish two placentas.
- If the twins are different sexes, they must be dizygotic twins, which are always di/di.

- 在妊娠中晚期，双胎间隔膜的厚度难以作为判定绒毛膜性的可靠根据，因其随妊娠进展而愈发变薄。
- 双峰征(或称λ征)是指两胎盘与较厚隔膜交界处向内凹陷所形成的三角，可见于双绒/双羊双胎。双峰征在鉴别是否有两个胎盘遇到困难时最有价值。
- 若两胎儿性别不同，则一定为双卵双胎，且总是为双绒/双羊双胎。

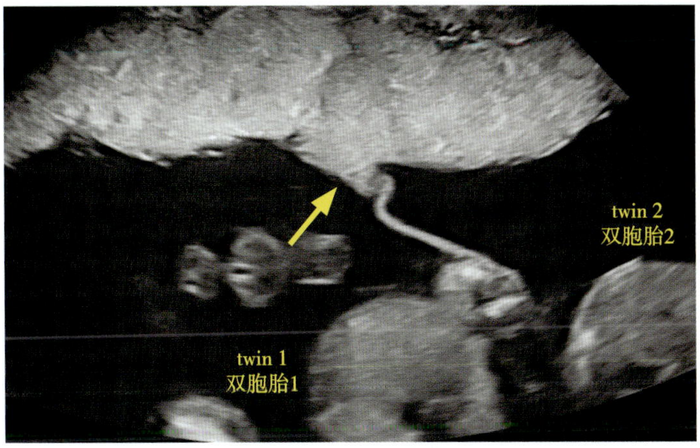

Grayscale ultrasound demonstrates the *twin peak* or *lambda sign* (arrow) seen with dichorionic/diamniotic twins, where the inter-twin membrane is thickened at the placental junction and tapers to a point, resulting in a triangular morphology.
灰阶超声显示双绒/双羊双胎的双峰征或λ征(黄箭)，双胎间膜在胎盘连接处增厚并逐渐变细到一个点，形成三角形。

Mono/di (monochorionic/diamniotic) twins

- Mono/di twins share a placenta, but have separate amniotic sacs.
- The shared placenta is usually apparent on ultrasound in the second trimester.
- The inter-twin membrane is thin, as it is composed of only two layers of amnion. This membrane meets the placenta in a *T-shape* configuration.

单绒/双羊双胎

- 单绒/双羊双胎共享一个胎盘，但有各自的羊膜囊。
- 在妊娠中期，共享的胎盘在超声上通常比较明显。
- 胎间隔膜纤薄，因只含有两层羊膜。此膜与胎盘融合处呈“T”形。

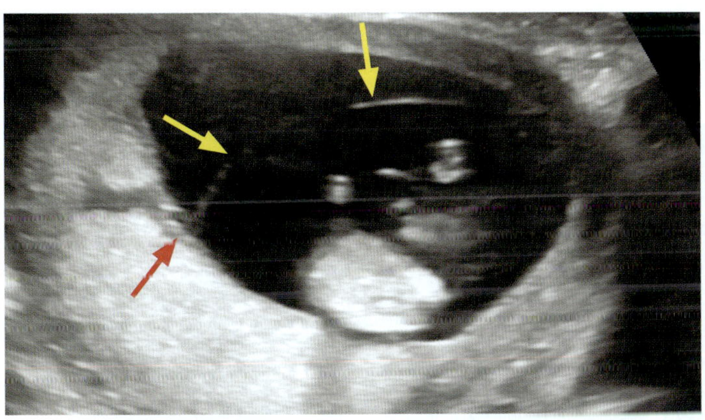

Grayscale ultrasound of monochorionic/diamniotic twins shows a thin inter-twin membrane (yellow arrows) which inserts on the placenta in a *T-shape* configuration (red arrow).
灰阶超声显示单绒/双羊双胎中纤薄的膜(黄箭)，并以“T”形结构止于胎盘(红箭)。

Mono/mono (monochorionic/monoamniotic) twins

- Mono/mono twins share both a placenta and a single amniotic sac with no intervening membrane between the twins. Intertwined cords are diagnostic of mono/mono placentation when seen.
- Isolated lack of visualization of an inter-twin membrane is not sufficient to diagnose mono/ mono twins. If no inter-twin membrane (or intertwining cord) is seen, then the amnionicity cannot be determined. Because mono/mono twins are so rare, it is more common to have mono/di twins with non-visualization of the inter-twin membrane.

单绒/单羊双胎

- 单绒/单羊双胎共享一个胎盘和羊膜囊，无胎儿间隔膜。若见脐带相互缠绕则可诊断单绒/单羊双胎。
- 若双胎间隔膜缺如为唯一的发现，则尚不足以诊断单绒/单羊双胎。若双胎间未见隔膜(或脐带缠绕)，羊膜囊的属性也无法确定。由于单绒/单羊双胎非常少，双胎间无隔膜通常是单绒/双羊双胎。

Conjoined twins

- Conjoined twins are caused by late (>13 days) incomplete division of embryo.

连体双胎

- 连体双胎是由于胚胎晚期(>13天)不完全分裂所致。

Complications of monochorionic twins

单绒毛膜双胎的并发症

Twin embolization syndrome

- When one monochorionic twin dies in utero, the surviving twin is at risk for twin embolization syndrome, which can cause CNS, gastrointestinal, or renal infarcts.
- In general, prognosis for a surviving monochorionic twin is very poor when one twin dies in utero. In contrast, prognosis is generally good for a surviving dichorionic twin when one twin dies in utero.

双胎栓塞综合征

- 当单绒毛膜双胎中的其中一个死于宫内时，存活的另一个胎儿则有罹患双胎栓塞综合征的风险，此综合征可导致中枢神经系统、胃肠道或肾梗死。
- 一般来说，当单绒毛膜双胎其中之一死于宫内时，另一个胎儿的预后非常差。相反，当双绒毛膜双胎之一死于宫内时，另一个胎儿的预后通常是良好的。

Twin-twin transfusion syndrome (TTTS)

- Twin-twin transfusion syndrome (TTTS) is a complication of monochorionic twins (either mono- or diamniotic) and is the result of abnormal vascular communications in the single shared placenta, with disproportionate blood flow between the fetuses.
- The **donor** twin transfers excess blood flow to the **recipient** twin. The donor twin is small and has oligohydramnios. The recipient twin is larger and has polyhydramnios.
- There are three criteria to diagnose TTTS by ultrasound:

> 1) Single shared placenta (monochorionic).
> 2) Disproportionate fetal sizes, with at least 25% discrepancy.
> 3) Disproportionate amniotic fluid, with the small twin having oligohydramnios and the large twin having polyhydramnios.

- There is a spectrum of severities of TTTS. In the earliest stages, the donor twin's bladder is still visible and amniotic fluid discrepancy is mild. Later stages are marked by absent bladder, marked fluid discrepancy, fetal hydrops or death.

双胎输血综合征(TTTS)

- 双胎输血综合征(TTTS)是单绒毛膜双胎(可以是单羊或双羊)的并发症，是单一共用胎盘出现血管交通异常，导致胎儿之间的血流量不成比例。
- **供血**胎儿将更多的血流输送给**受血**胎儿。供血胎儿小且羊水过少，受血胎儿大且羊水过多。
- 超声诊断TTTS有三条标准：

> 1) 共享一个胎盘(单绒毛膜性)。
> 2) 胎儿大小不成比例，差异至少为25%。
> 3) 羊水量不成比例，小胎儿羊水量过少，大胎儿羊水量过多。

- TTTS的严重程度存在差异。早期超声可见供血胎儿的膀胱，羊水的差异轻微。晚期以膀胱缺失为标志、羊水差异显著、胎儿水肿或死亡。

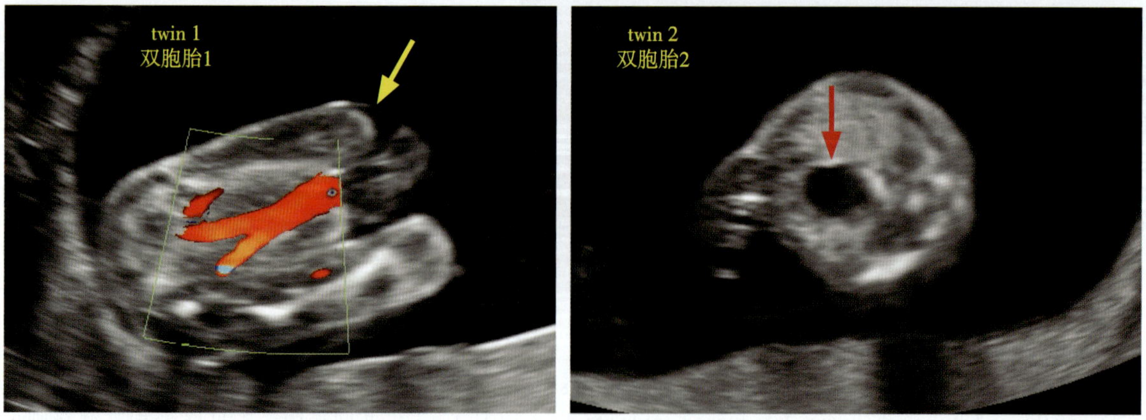

Ultrasound of monochorionic/diamniotic twins: Grayscale image with Doppler overlay (left) of twin #1 at level of the pelvis shows normal appearance of two umbilical arteries, but no visualization of the bladder. Twin #1 also has moderate oligohydramnios with the amnionic membrane "stuck" to the body (yellow arrow), and size discrepancy by gestational age. Twin #2 (right image) has a large bladder (red arrow) and mild polyhydramnios. These findings are suggestive for twin-twin transfusion syndrome.

单绒/双羊双胎超声：双胞胎1盆腔平面彩色多普勒超声图像(左图)显示2个脐动脉表现正常，但未见膀胱；双胞胎1也有中度羊水过少，羊膜"粘"在身体上(黄箭)，且大小与孕龄不一致。双胞胎2(右图)有一个较大的膀胱(红箭)和轻度羊水过多。这些表现提示了双胎输血综合征。

- A **stuck** twin describes severe oligohydramnios in the donor (small) twin. A stuck twin has so little amniotic fluid that the amnion is wrapped around the twin like shrink wrap.
- Treatment options of TTTS include laser ablation of placental arteriovenous connections, therapeutic amniocentesis from the recipient (large, poly) twin, or selective coagulation of the umbilical cord of the less viable twin.

Acardiac twin

- 一个**被裹住**的双胎是指供血(小的)胎儿羊水严重过少。由于羊水太少以至于羊膜包裹住了胎儿,像缩小的包裹。
- 治疗TTTS可选择激光消融胎盘动静脉瘘、对受血(较大)胎儿进行治疗性羊水穿刺,或选择性结扎存活可能性小的胎儿脐带。

无心双胎

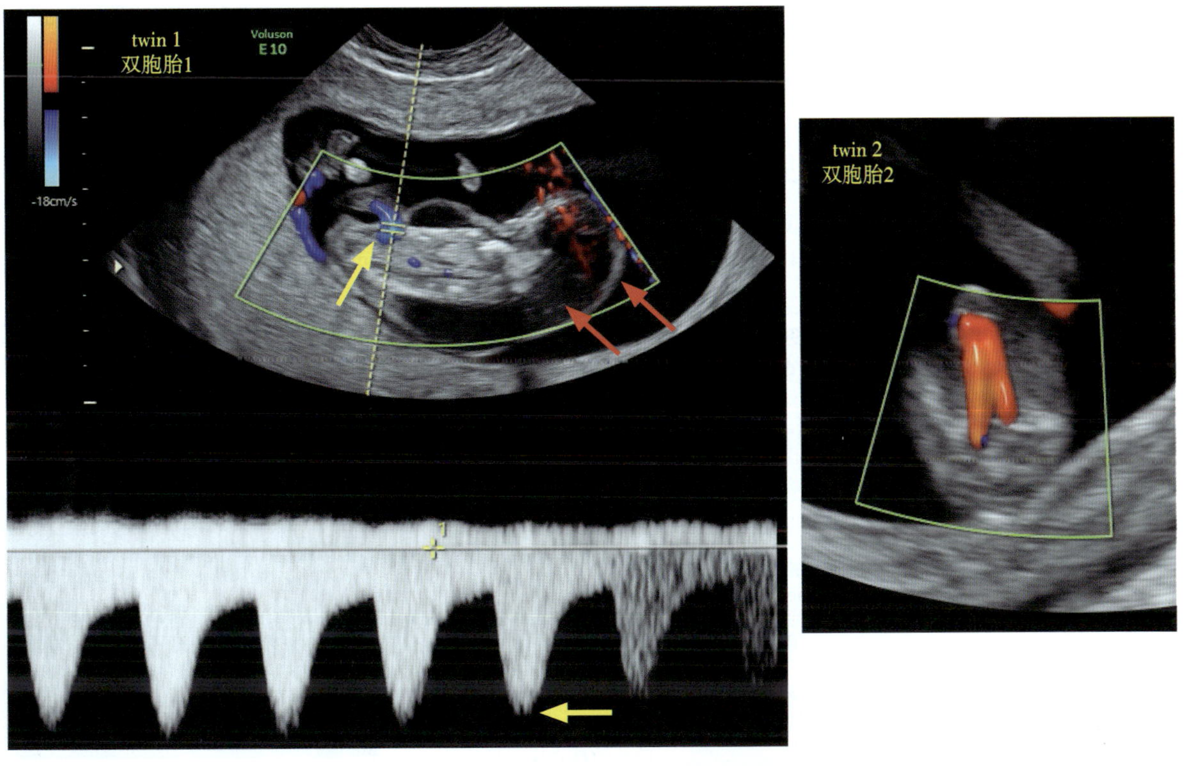

Acardiac twin:
Grayscale ultrasound with Doppler overlay of monochorionic/diamniotic twins:
Color Doppler and waveform (left image) demonstrates reversed flow in the umbilical vessels of the acardiac (recipient) twin, with arterial flow into the fetus (yellow arrows) and venous flow towards the placenta (not shown). Also note diffuse body wall edema (red arrows).
Color Doppler of the donor twin (right image) shows normal umbilical arterial flow out of the fetus.
无心双胎:
单绒/双羊双胞胎的灰阶叠加多普勒超声表现:
彩色多普勒和频谱(左图)显示无心(受血)胎儿的脐血反向流动,其动脉流向胎儿(黄箭),静脉流向胎盘(未展示),同时可见弥漫性体壁水肿(红箭)。
彩色多普勒显示供血胎儿(右图)脐动脉血流正常。

- Acardiac twinning, also called **twin reversed arterial perfusion (TRAP) sequence**, is a severe variant that occurs when there is arterial-arterial communication in the shared placenta, causing reversed umbilical arterial flow in the recipient, acardiac twin. Similar to TTTS, acardiac twinning is a complication of monochorionic twins (either mono-or diamniotic).
- In acardiac twins, the donor fetus supplies circulation to itself and an acardiac twin, which has rudimentary or no development of structures above the thorax.
- Doppler of the umbilical arteries and vein shows reversed direction of flow in the acardiac twin.

- 无心双胎,也称**双胎反向动脉灌注(TRAP)**,是一种在共享胎盘时出现的动脉-动脉交通的严重变异,会导致受血胎儿(即无心胎儿)脐动脉血流逆转。与TTTS一样,无心双胎也发生在单绒毛膜双胎(可以是单羊或双羊)。
- 在无心双胎中,供血胎儿给自身和无心胎儿供血。无心胎儿胸部以上结构发育不全或未发育。
- 多普勒可显示无心胎儿的脐动脉静脉呈反向血流。

Normally, the umbilical arteries carry deoxygenated blood *out* of the fetus, pumped by the fetal heart. In the acardiac twin, the umbilical arteries carry nutrient-depleted, poorly-oxygenated blood *into* the fetus, pumped by the donor twin's heart. Doppler of the acardiac twin's umbilical arteries show an arterial waveform going into the fetus.
Normally, the umbilical vein carries oxygenated blood *into* the fetus, from the placenta. In the acardiac twin, the umbilical vein carries deoxygenated blood out of the fetus, still pumped by the donor heart. Doppler of the acardiac twin's umbilical vein shows a venous waveform going out of the fetus.
The entire circulation of both twins is maintained by the single donor fetus.

正常情况下，胎心通过脐动脉将含氧量低的血液带出胎儿。在无心双胎中，供血胎儿通过脐动脉将无营养物质、低氧的血液输送到胎儿体内。多普勒显示无心胎儿的脐动脉血流方向朝向胎儿。
正常情况下，脐静脉从胎盘将高氧含量血输送到胎儿体内。在无心畸形双胎中，无心胎儿脐静脉则是运送低氧含量的血离开胎儿。多普勒显示无心胎儿脐静脉血流方向背离胎儿。
两个双胞胎的循环都是由一个供血胎儿来维持。

- Treatment is coagulation of the acardiac twin's umbilical cord.

- 治疗方法为凝固无心胎儿的脐带。

Evaluation of the First Trimester Embryo

- The first trimester embryo is too small for a complete fetal survey; however, a few key anatomic structures can be identified and evaluated.

Crown-rump length (CRL)

- The crown-rump length (CRL) is used to assign gestational age from 6–12 weeks. Measuring the CRL is straightforward in the first trimester as the fetus cannot flex or extend the neck.

Nuchal translucency

评估早期妊娠胚胎

- 早期妊娠时的胚胎过小，无法进行全面评估，但可对部分重要解剖结构进行确认和评估。

胚胎顶臀长(CRL)

- 胚胎顶臀长(CRL)用于6~12周的孕龄评估。CRL在妊娠早期时易于测量，因此时胎儿颈部无法弯曲和伸展。

颈项透明层

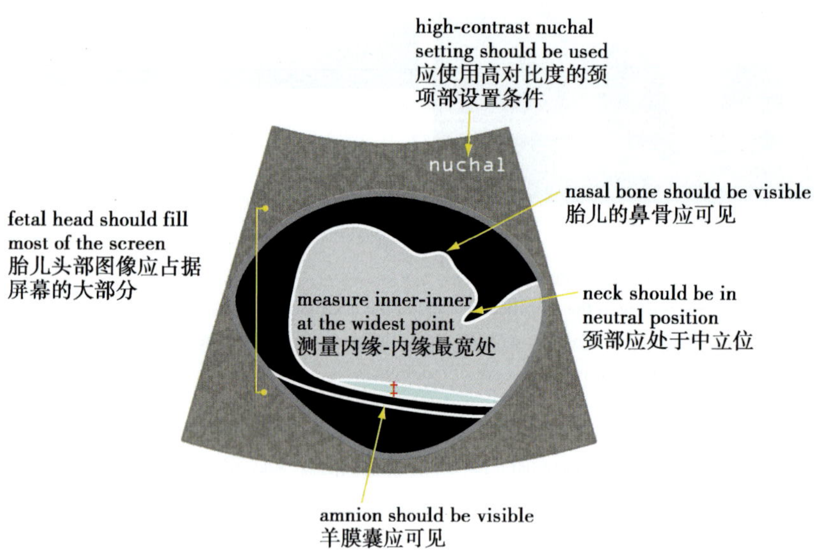

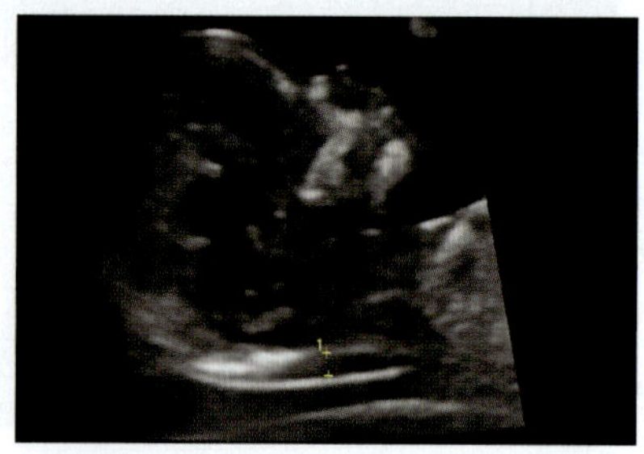

Normal nuchal translucency.
正常的颈项透明层

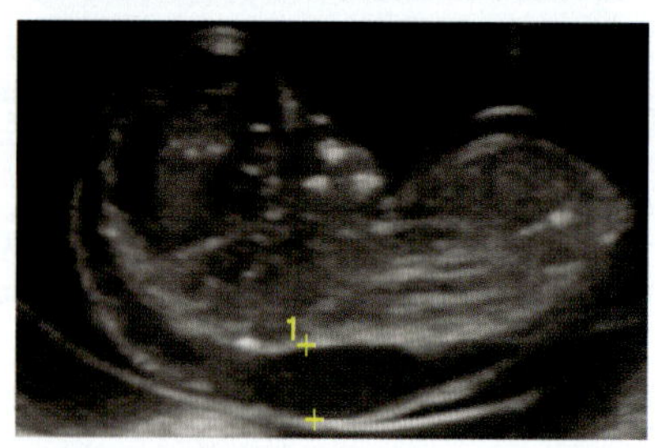

Thickened nuchal translucency.
增厚的颈项透明层

- Increased thickness of the nuchal translucency is associated with increased risk of Down syndrome and other chromosomal abnormalities. With a fixed false-positive rate of 5%, nuchal translucency alone can detect approximately 2/3 of cases of trisomy 21.
- The nuchal translucency must be measured properly to obtain an accurate value.
- Nuchal translucency is measured at 11–14 weeks, when CRL is between 45 and 85 mm. Measurement is adjusted for gestational age and combined with maternal serum testing to calculate an overall risk of aneuploidy.

- 颈项透明层厚度增加与唐氏综合征和其他染色体异常的风险增加有关。由于假阳性率固定在5%，仅颈项透明层异常就可以检测到约2/3的21-三体病例。
- 必须采用正确的测量方法才能保证颈项透明层测量值的准确性。
- 测量颈项透明层应在妊娠11~14周时进行，此时的CRL为45~85mm。测量结果根据孕龄进行调整，并结合母体血清试验来计算非整倍体的总体风险。

- Regardless of gestational age correction, a nuchal translucency ≥3 mm is associated with a 6-fold increased risk of aneuploidy and alone warrants further diagnostic workup.
- An abnormally thickened nuchal translucency can also indicate congenital heart disease in an euploid fetus.

Prosencephalon and rhombencephalon

- By 8 weeks, the forebrain (prosencephalon) can be distinguished from the hindbrain (rhombencephalon). Both prosencephalon and rhombencephalon are hypoechoic, although the rhombencephalon is much more prominent. Absence of these structures may be the earliest finding of anencephaly.

- 无论是否对孕龄进行矫正，若颈项透明层厚度≥3mm，非整倍体风险便会增加6倍，需要做进一步诊断性检查。
- 颈项透明层异常增厚也可提示整倍体胎儿的先天性心脏病。

前脑和后脑

- 妊娠第8周，前脑可以与后脑加以区分。前脑与后脑均表现为低回声，但后脑更为明显。如缺乏这些结构，可能是无脑畸形的最早期表现。

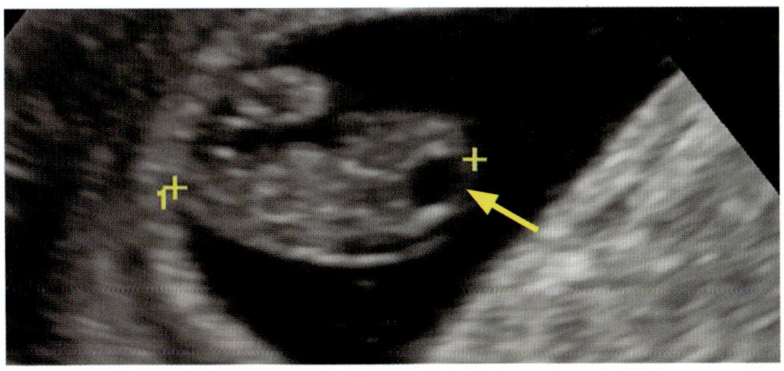

Grayscale ultrasound of an embryo (calipers) show a normal hypoechoic/anechoic rhombencephalon (arrow).
胚胎灰阶超声(卡尺)显示后脑呈正常的低回声/无回声(黄箭)。

Ventral abdominal wall

- The midgut normally herniates through the ventral abdominal wall in the first trimester. During this herniation, the midgut rotates 270 degrees around the axis of the superior mesenteric artery (SMA).
- **Physiologic midgut herniation is usually complete by 12–13 weeks.** Therefore, a pathologic ventral wall defect, such as omphalocele or gastroschisis, is generally not diagnosed before 13 weeks.
- It is common to see some fullness at the base of the umbilical cord before 13 weeks, which usually represents physiologic midgut herniation. If the fullness is especially prominent (≥7 mm) then it may be prudent to bring the patient back for a follow-up at 13 weeks to evaluate for a true ventral wall defect.

前腹壁

- 正常情况下，胎儿中肠在妊娠的早期从前腹壁疝出。在此期间，中肠以肠系膜上动脉(SMA)为轴旋转270°。
- **生理性中肠疝通常在妊娠12~13周结束。**因此，病理性前腹壁缺损不能在妊娠13周前进行诊断，如脐膨出或腹壁裂。
- 在妊娠13周前，常能见到脐带基部有些饱满，大多为生理性中肠疝所致。如果饱满非常明显(≥7mm)则最好在妊娠13周后复诊随访，以确认是否为真正的腹壁缺失。

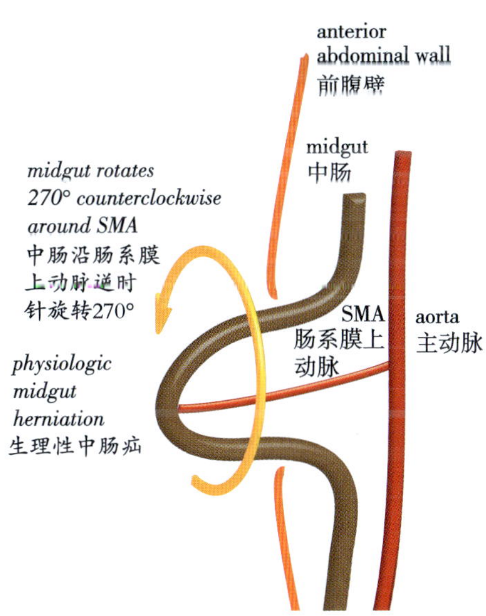

Normal early fetal anatomy (11–14 weeks)

- At 11–14 weeks gestation, following structures should be assessed when possible: falx cerebri, stomach, bladder, ventral abdominal wall, and the presence of four extremities.

正常早期胎儿解剖(妊娠11~14周)

- 在妊娠11~14周时，应尽可能对大脑镰、胃、膀胱、前腹壁和四肢进行评估。

SECOND AND THIRD TRIMESTERS

中期及晚期妊娠

SECOND AND THIRD TRIMESTER MEASUREMENTS

中期及晚期妊娠测量

Head measurements

- The **biparietal diameter** (BPD) is measured from the outer edge of the skull closest to the transducer to the inner edge of the skull farthest from the transducer.

  The plane of measurement is at the level of the thalami and cavum septum pellucidum. The skull should be completely visualized all the way around.

  The corrected BPD incorporates the occipital frontal diameter (OFD) and a correction factor.

- The **occipital frontal diameter** (OFD) is measured from the middle of the frontal skull to the middle of the occipital skull.

  The measurement plane is the same used to measure the BPD, at the level of the thalami and cavum septum pellucidum.

头部测量

- **双顶径(BPD)**是测量从颅骨最靠近超声探头的外缘到离超声探头最远颅骨的内缘的距离。

  测量平面为丘脑和透明隔腔水平。颅骨的任何部分都必须显示完整。

  计算校正后的双顶径应包括枕额径(OFD)和校正因子。

- **枕额径(OFD)**是测量从额骨中部到枕骨中部的距离。

  测量平面和双顶径平面一样，为丘脑和透明隔腔水平。

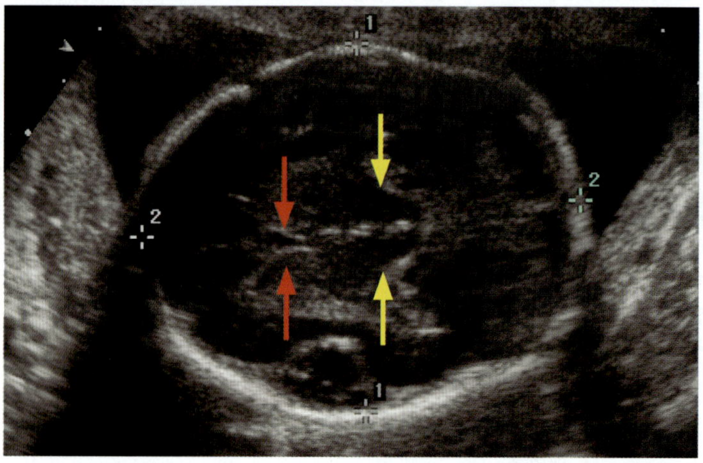

The scanning plane for head measurements is at the level of the thalami (yellow arrows) and cavum septum pellucidum (red arrows).

The BPD (calipers marked 1) is measured from outer edge to inner edge of calvarium.

The OFD (calipers marked 2) is measured from middle to middle edge of calvarium.

Case courtesy Carol Benson, MD, Brigham and Women's Hospital.

头部测量的扫查平面为丘脑(黄箭)和透明隔腔(红箭)水平。

测量BPD(卡尺1)是从颅骨的外缘到内缘。

测量OFD(卡尺2)是从前颅骨中点到后颅骨中点。

Abdomen measurements

- The abdominal diameter is measured from outer skin-to-skin in AP and transverse at the level of the intrahepatic umbilical vein, portal vein, and fetal stomach.
- Ideally, the abdomen should be round, with less than 1 cm difference between the AP and transverse measurements. The entire circumference of the skin should be well visualized.
- The best measurements are often obtained if the anterior-posterior axis of the fetal abdomen is angled approximately 45 degrees so that the artifacts from the spine are minimized.

腹部测量

- 测量腹部的前后径和横径以肝内脐静脉、门静脉和胎儿胃泡为水平，从外层皮肤到皮肤之间的距离。
- 腹部在理想的情况下应为圆形，前后径和横径之差<1cm。整个皮肤轮廓应清晰显示。
- 当胎儿腹部的前后轴约呈45°倾斜时，通常可以获得最好的测量经线，此时脊柱的伪影不明显。

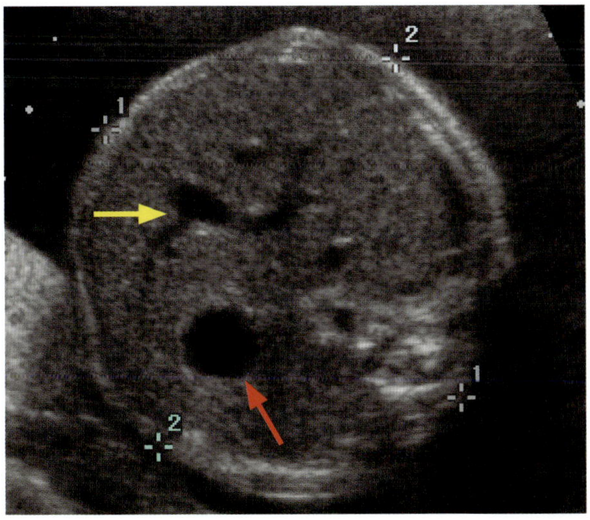

The scanning plane for abdominal diameter is at the junction of the umbilical vein and portal vein (yellow arrow). The stomach (red arrow) should be visualized. Note how the anterior-posterior axis of the abdomen is angled approximately 45 degrees to minimize artifacts from the spine.
Case courtesy Carol Benson, MD, Brigham and Women's Hospital.
腹部径线扫查以脐静脉与门静脉交界处(黄箭)为平面，该平面应该看到胃泡(红箭)。注意，腹部的前后轴线约呈45°倾斜，以此减少脊柱伪影的影响。

Femur length

- The femur length is most accurately measured when the femur is closest to the transducer, perpendicular to the sound beam.

股骨长径

- 股骨长径测量最准确的方法是股骨与探头的距离最近且与声束垂直。

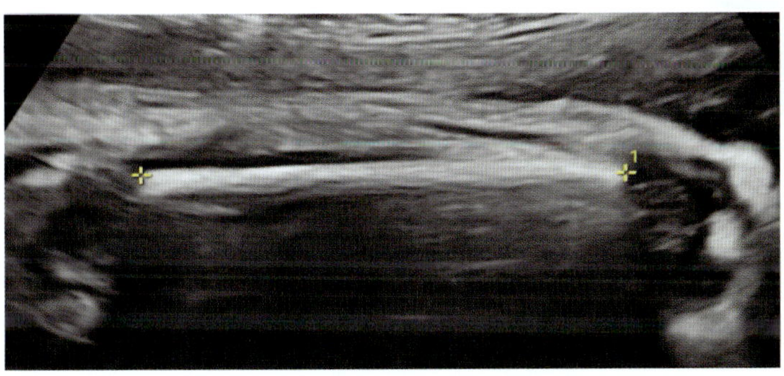

Grayscale ultrasound demonstrating femur length measurement (calipers).
灰阶超声测量股骨长度(卡尺)。

Amniotic fluid assessment

- The amount of amniotic fluid should always be subjectively assessed. There are three options for assessing amniotic fluid volume.
  1. Subjective assessment only.
  2. Deepest vertical pocket of fluid is measured in cm.
  3. Amniotic fluid index.
- To quantify the amniotic fluid index (AFI) between 16–42 weeks, the largest vertical pocket of fluid is measured (in cm) in each of the four quadrants and summed. AFI varies with gestational age. In borderline cases, the subjective assessment should take precedent. Some references state that an AFI between 7 and 25 is normal, but these cutoffs vary.

  Oligohydramnios: AFI ≤6.3 cm is ≤2.5th percentile. Peaks at 24 weeks: 9.0 cm = 2.5th percentile.

  Polyhydramnios: AFI ≥19.2 cm is ≥97.5th percentile. Peaks at 36 weeks: 27.9 cm = 97.5th percentile.

羊水测量

- 羊水量应始终是主观性的评估。评估羊水量有三种方法。
  1. 仅为主观评估。
  2. 垂直测量羊水最深处深度(cm)。
  3. 羊水指数。
- 妊娠16~42周时的羊水指数(AFI)定量方法为，分别测量四个象限羊水的最大液体积聚的垂直径线(cm)，然后取其和。AFI随孕周而变化。处于临界值的病例应以主观评价为主。一些参考文献认为AFI在7~25cm为正常，但这些分界值存在差异。

  羊水过少： AFI≤6.3cm为≤第2.5百分位。24周的峰值：9.0cm=第2.5百分位。

  羊水过多： AFI≥19.2cm为≥第97.5百分位。36周的峰值：27.9cm=第97.5百分位。

Nuchal fold (second trimester only)

- A thickened nuchal fold is the most sensitive and specific ultrasound finding to suggest Down syndrome.
- The nuchal fold is measured in the axial plane at the level of the posterior fossa.

颈部皮肤皱褶(只在妊娠中期)

- 颈部皮肤皱褶增厚是超声提示唐氏综合征最具有灵敏度和特异度的征象。
- 与颈项透明层不同，测量颈部皮肤皱褶在中期妊娠的后期进行，并在颅后窝的横切面进行。

- The nuchal fold is only measured from **16–20 weeks.**
  <5 mm is normal.
  5–5.9 mm is borderline.
  ⩾6 mm is a major marker for Trisomy 21.
- A very thick nuchal fold may represent a cystic hygroma, which is associated with Turner syndrome (45,X).

- 颈部皮肤皱褶只在**16~20周进行**测量。
  <5mm为正常。
  5.0~5.9mm为临界值。
  >6mm为21-三体的主要指标。
- 非常厚的颈部皮肤皱褶可能为水囊状淋巴管瘤，与特纳综合征(45，X)相关。

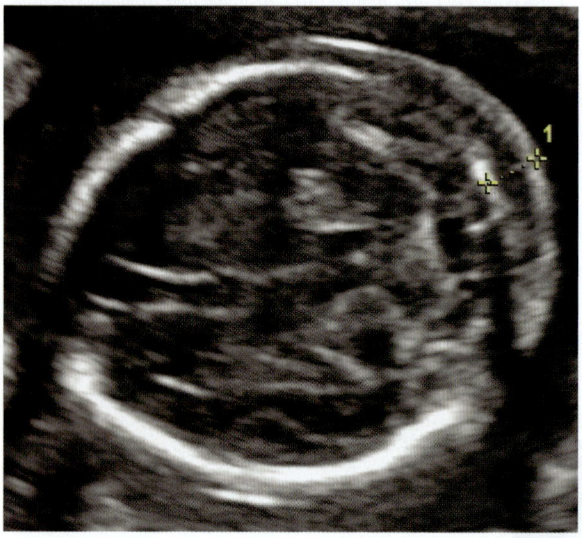

Ultrasound of a 20-week fetus at the level of the brain and posterior fossa demonstrates a thickened nuchal fold >6 mm (calipers).
Case courtesy Beryl Benacerraf, MD, Diagnostic Ultrasound Associates, Boston.
超声图像显示妊娠20周胎儿大脑颅后窝平面的颈部皮肤皱褶增厚>6mm(卡尺)。

EVALUATION OF THE CERVIX IN SECOND AND THIRD TRIMESTERS

中期和晚期妊娠宫颈评估

Cervical shortening

宫颈缩短

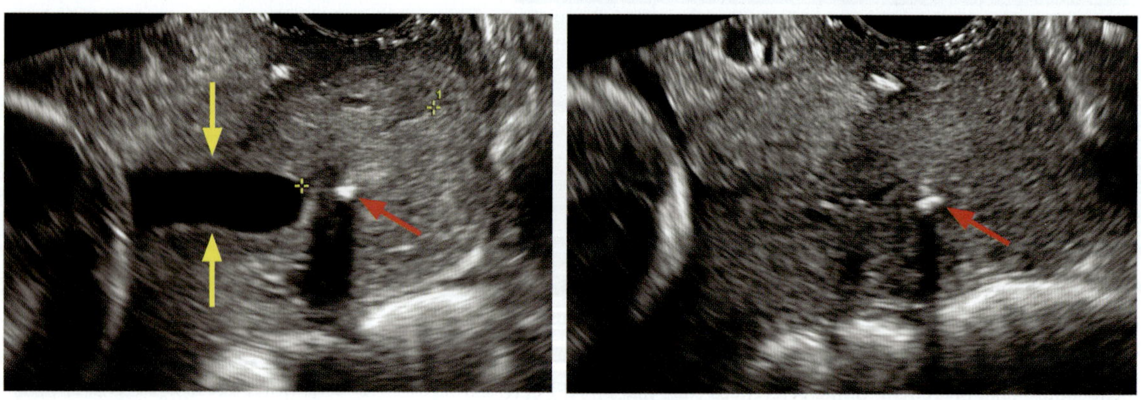

Transvaginal grayscale ultrasound (left image) shows a shortened cervix (calipers) measuring 2.2 cm in length, with U-shaped funneling (yellow arrows). The right image is taken at a different time point during the same scan and shows false elongation of the cervix due to uterine contractions. Note cerclage wire with associated posterior acoustic shadowing (red arrows).
经阴道灰阶超声(左图)显示子宫颈缩短(卡尺)，长度为2.2cm，呈"U"形的漏斗状(黄箭)。右图是在同一次检查时不同时间点获得的图像，显示因子宫收缩导致宫颈假性延长，注意伴后方声影的环扎线(红箭)。

- Shortening of the cervix is a risk factor for pre-term delivery. **A cervical length <3 cm is abnormal**. If there is any uncertainty about cervical length, a transvaginal ultrasound should be obtained.
  A potential pitfall is false elongation of the cervix due to distended bladder or uterine contractions.
- The presence of cervical funneling (change in shape) is an ancillary finding.

- 宫颈缩短是早产的危险因素。**宫颈长度<3cm为异常**。若对宫颈长度有任何不确定，应进行阴道超声检查。
  潜在的子宫颈假性延长可能是因为膀胱扩张或子宫收缩。
- 出现宫颈漏斗(形状改变)是一个辅助性发现。

The mnemonic ***t**rust **y**our **v**aginal **u**ltrasound* can be used to remember the sequence of cervical funneling. A **T**-shaped cervix is normal. As funneling progresses, the cervix resembles **Y**, **V**, and **U** shapes.

- Prior to viability (24 weeks), treatment is cervical cerclage. After 24 weeks, treatment tends to be conservative (bedrest) due to concern for membrane rupture with any procedure.

可用“TYVU”（**t**rust **y**our **v**aginal **u**ltrasound）来记忆漏斗状宫颈的发生顺序。宫颈正常为“**T**”形，随漏斗状改变进一步发展，宫颈逐渐类似于“**Y**”“**V**”和“**U**”形。

- 在胎儿可以存活(妊娠24周)之前，治疗方法选择宫颈环扎术。在妊娠24周后倾向于保守治疗(卧床)，因任何手术均可以造成胎膜破裂。

UMBILICAL CORD

- The normal umbilical cord has two umbilical arteries and a single umbilical vein.

脐带

- 正常的脐带有两条脐动脉和一条脐静脉。

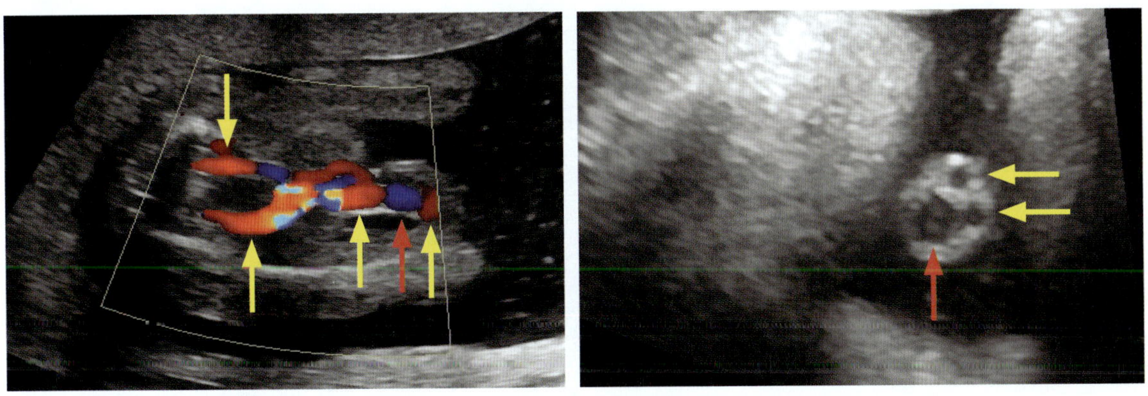

Grayscale ultrasound with Doppler overlay (left image) of the fetal pelvis demonstrates a three-vessel umbilical cord. Ultrasound of a different patient (right image) shows the normal appearance of the three-vessel cord on transverse view. Yellow arrows point to the two arteries, red arrow to the single vein.
胎儿盆腔灰阶超声(左图)显示三条血管的脐带。另一名患者的超声检查(右图)横切面显示三支血管外观正常。黄箭指向两条动脉，红箭指向一条静脉。

- Normal systolic/diastolic ratio of the umbilical artery waveform depends on the gestational age. Reference table should be consulted.
- The umbilical artery should always have antegrade diastolic flow. Absent or reversed flow is a major indication of significant fetal stress.

Two vessel umbilical cord (single umbilical artery)

- A single umbilical artery is associated with an increased incidence of fetal anomalies and growth restriction.
- There is an increased incidence of a single umbilical artery in trisomies 13 and 18.

- 脐带动脉频谱的正常收缩压/舒张压比值取决于孕龄。应查阅相关参考表。
- 脐带动脉应始终存在舒张期前向血流信号。舒张期血流消失或反向是胎儿宫内窘迫的主要征象。

两条血管的脐带(单条脐动脉)

- 单条脐动脉与胎儿异常和胎儿生长受限的发生率增加相关。
- 13-三体和18-三体中，单条脐动脉的发病率增加。

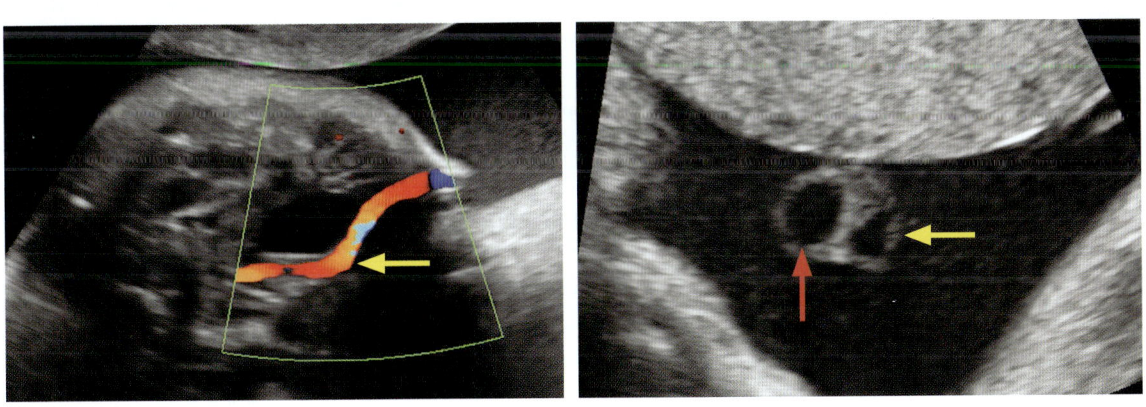

Grayscale ultrasound with Doppler overlay (left image) of the fetal abdomen demonstrates a single umbilical artery (yellow arrows). Transverse view of the umbilical cord (right image) shows two vessels. The red arrow points to the umbilical vein.
胎儿腹部多普勒超声(左图)显示单条脐动脉(黄箭)。脐带横切面(右图)显示两条血管，红箭指的是脐静脉。

Marginal/velamentous cord insertion

- **Marginal insertion** is eccentric insertion of the umbilical cord at the margin of the placenta.
- **Velamentous insertion** is when the umbilical cord inserts outside the margin of the placenta, into the free membranes where it is not protected by Wharton's jelly. Velamentous cord insertion is at risk for vasa previa as subsequently described.

Vasa previa

- Vasa previa is the traversing of fetal placental vessels across the internal cervical os, which can be caused by velamentous insertion or a placental succenturiate lobe (discussed below).

脐带边缘性/帆状附着

- **脐带边缘性附着**是指脐带终止于胎盘的边缘而非中央。
- **脐带帆状附着**是指脐带插入胎盘边缘外侧的游离胎膜，后者不受华通胶保护。脐带帆状附着有发生前置血管的风险，将在下文讨论。

前置血管

- 前置血管是指胎盘血管跨越宫颈内口，可由脐带帆状附着或副胎盘引起(下文讨论)。

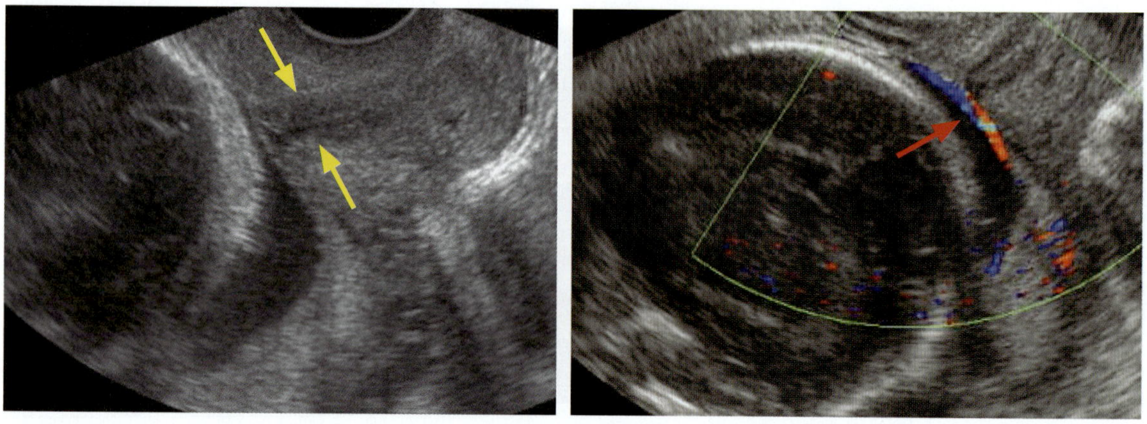

Vesa previa: Grayscale ultrasound (left image) in region of the fetal head and cervix demonstrates the position of the endocervical canal (yellow arrows). Although the grayscale image appeared normal, color Doppler shows a placental vessel (red arrow) traversing the internal cervical os. Spectral Doppler (not shown) confirmed presence of a fetal arterial vessel.
Case courtesy Beryl Benacerraf, MD, Diagnostic Ultrasound Associates, Boston.
灰阶超声(左图)经胎儿头部与宫颈切面显示宫颈的位置(黄箭)。虽然灰阶图像表现正常，但彩色多普勒发现胎盘血管(红箭)横跨宫颈内口。频谱多普勒(未展示)确认为胎儿动脉血管。

Amniotic fluid

Overview of fetal amniotic fluid

- Amniotic fluid surrounds the fetus and is required for normal development of multiple organ systems, including the lungs.
- It is produced primarily by the fetal genitourinary tract and is excreted by the fetus as urine. A small amount is also produced by the fetal lungs and nasopharyngeal cavities.
- Amniotic fluid is absorbed primarily by fetal swallowing and passage of fluid through the GI tract.
- Assessment of amniotic fluid volume is discussed earlier in the chapter.

Oligohydramnios

- Oligohydramnios is too little amniotic fluid.
- Most commonly, oligohydramnios is associated with intrauterine growth restriction (IUGR) without a fetal structural anomaly.
- When severe, oligohydramnios results in pulmonary hypoplasia. It may also lead to **Potter sequence**, a constellation of findings including facial dysmorphism, club feet, and musculoskeletal contractures due to diminished intrauterine space.
- Although malformations are relatively uncommon, the genitourinary system must be carefully evaluated in the setting of oligohydramnios. Genitourinary anomalies that may lead to oligohydramnios include:

羊水

胎儿羊水概述

- 羊水包围胎儿，这是众多器官系统正常发育所必需的，包括两肺。
- 羊水主要来自胎儿的泌尿生殖道，为胎儿排泄的尿液。少部分羊水来自胎儿肺和鼻咽腔。
- 羊水主要通过胎儿吞咽然后液体通过胃肠道来吸收。
- 对羊水量的评估已在本章的前文进行了讨论。

羊水过少

- 羊水过少是指羊水量过少。
- 羊水过少通常合并胎儿宫内发育受限(IUGR)但并无结构异常。
- 当羊水严重过少时，会导致肺发育不全。也可能导致**波特后遗症**，表现为因宫内空间减少所致的一系列症状，包括面部畸形、畸形足和肌肉骨骼挛缩。
- 尽管畸形并不常见，但合并羊水过少时应对泌尿生殖系统进行仔细检查。可导致羊水过少的泌尿生殖系统异常包括：

Renal agenesis – fatal if bilateral.
Congenital bladder outlet obstruction, including posterior urethral valves.
Bilateral ureteropelvic junction obstructions.
Renal dysplasias, including autosomal recessive polycystic kidney disease (ARPKD).

肾功能发育不全——双侧为致命。
先天性膀胱出口梗阻，包括后尿道瓣膜。
双侧肾盂输尿管交界处梗阻。
肾发育不良，包括常染色体隐性遗传多囊肾病(APPKD)。

Polyhydramnios

- Polyhydramnios is too much amniotic fluid.
- Greater than half of cases of polyhydramnios are idiopathic, with a normal fetus. The remainder may be associated with chromosomal abnormalities, diabetes, or structural defects (primarily of the gastrointestinal tract), including:

羊水过多

- 羊水过多是指羊水量过多。
- 超过半数的羊水过多是特发性的，但胎儿正常。其他可能与染色体异常、糖尿病或结构缺陷(主要是胃肠道)相关，包括：

Primary upper GI obstruction or atresia, such as laryngeal, esophageal or duodenal atresia.
Secondary obstruction, due to diaphragmatic hernia, gastroschisis, or omphalocele.
Severe CNS anomalies (which often cause disorders in swallowing).
Monochorionic twin syndromes, such as twin-twin transfusion syndrome (one twin polyhydramnios and one twin oligohydramnios).
Placental abnormalities, such as chorioangioma.

原发性上消化道梗阻或闭锁，如喉、食管或十二指肠闭锁。
由膈肌疝、腹裂或脐膨出所致的继发性梗阻。
严重的中枢神经系统异常(常导致吞咽异常)。
单绒毛膜双胎综合征，如双胎输血综合征(双胞胎中，一个羊水过多，另一个羊水过少)。
胎盘异常，如绒毛膜血管瘤。

Placenta

Placental embryology, physiology, and morphology

- The placenta is formed by fetal chorion and maternal decidualized endometrium.
- The mature placental circulation allows exchange of oxygen and nutrients between maternal and fetal vessels through a membrane, although the blood does not admix.
- Placental location should be accessed in every patient.
- A **succenturiate lobe** is an island of placental tissue separate from the main placenta, connected to the main placenta by blood vessels. Patients with succenturiate lobe have an increased incidence of velamentous cord insertion and retained products of conception.

Placenta previa

- Placental position is assessed starting in the second trimester. If there is uncertainty about placental position with relationship to the cervix, transvaginal evaluation should be performed.
- **Normal** placental position is greater than 2 cm from the internal os.
- **Low-lying placenta** is ≤2 cm from the internal os. Majority of low-lying placentas will resolve by the third trimester due to placental migration.
- In **placenta previa**, the placenta covers the internal cervical os. Patients typically present with painless vaginal bleeding in the second trimester. Placenta previa is seen in approximately 0.5–1% of deliveries and requires a Caesarean section for safe delivery.

  A potential pitfall is over-diagnosis in the second trimester due to uterine contractions or overfilling of the maternal bladder.

Placental abruption

- Placental abruption is premature separation of the placenta from its uterine attachment. Patients most commonly present with pain. On physical exam, blood may be present in the vaginal canal.
- There is an increased incidence of abruption in maternal hypertension, drug

胎盘

胎盘的胚胎学、生理学和形态学

- 胎盘是由胎儿的绒毛膜和母体蜕膜化的子宫内膜所形成。
- 成熟的胎盘循环允许母体和胎儿血管之间通过膜交换氧气和营养物质，但不发生血液混合。
- 对每个患者都应该检查胎盘的位置。
- **副胎盘**是与主胎盘分离的孤立性胎盘组织，通过血管与主胎盘相连。副胎盘患者出现帆状胎盘和产后胎物残留的概率增加。

前置胎盘

- 评估胎盘的位置应从妊娠中期开始。如果胎盘位置与子宫颈的关系不明确，应进行经阴道超声检查。
- **正常胎盘**的位置应距离宫颈内口>2cm。
- **低置胎盘**是指胎盘下缘距离宫颈内口≤2cm。大多数低置胎盘随胎盘迁移而在妊娠晚期消失。
- 在**前置胎盘**中，胎盘覆盖宫颈内口。患者通常在妊娠中期出现无痛性阴道出血。前置胎盘占生产总量的0.5%~1.0%，需要剖宫产才能安全分娩。

  妊娠中期子宫收缩或母亲膀胱过度充盈也可表现为前置胎盘，易导致过度诊断。

胎盘早剥

- 胎盘早剥是指胎盘与子宫附着处过早分离。患者最常表现为疼痛。在体格检查时，阴道内可能有血液。
- 胎盘早剥的发生率在妊娠高血压、药物滥用、

abuse, trauma, or rapid decompression of a distended uterus (e.g., from a large-volume amniocentesis).

- Placental abruption can have variable ultrasound findings and may appear normal. Therefore, a negative ultrasound cannot exclude abruption. When visible, ultrasound shows a hematoma, which can be subchorionic (most commonly), retroplacental, or pre-placental.
- Acute abruption may be especially challenging to diagnose on imaging as the hematoma is isoechoic to placenta.

创伤或膨胀子宫的快速减压(如大容量羊膜穿刺术)中增加。

- 胎盘早剥的超声表现多变,并可能为正常。因此,阴性超声不能排除胎盘早剥。当超声阳性并表现为血肿时,可以是绒毛膜下(最常见的)、胎盘后或胎盘前的血肿。
- 超声诊断急性胎盘早剥可能极其困难,因为血肿的回声与胎盘相同。

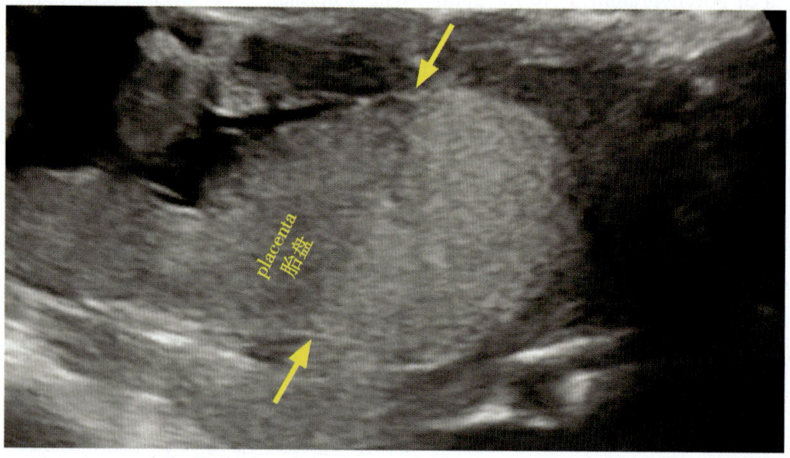

Acute retroplacental abruption:
Ultrasound of the placenta shows a subtle, minimally hyperechoic retroplacental hematoma (arrows at placental/hematoma interface), nearly isoechoic to placenta. Acute retroplacental hematoma can be very difficult to identify. Realtime scanning or review of cine loops may be helpful.
Case courtesy Julie Ritner, MD, Brigham and Women's Hospital.
急性胎盘后早剥:
胎盘超声显示一个不明显的稍高回声胎盘后血肿(黄箭所示为胎盘和血肿交界),几乎与胎盘回声相同。急性胎盘后血肿可能极难被发现。实时扫查或回顾录像可能有帮助。

- Chronic abruption features hypoechoic blood products within or around the placenta.

- 慢性早剥的特征是胎盘内及胎盘周围的低回声血液衍生物。

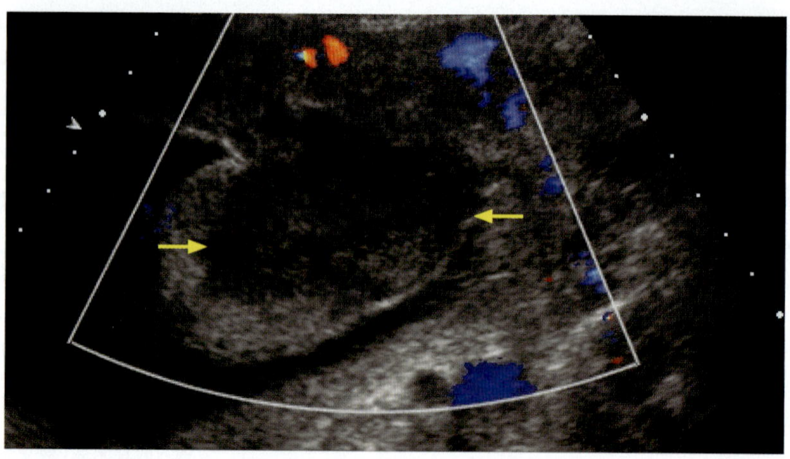

Chronic abruption:
Ultrasound of the placenta shows a heterogeneous, primarily hypoechoic preplacental hematoma (arrows), which lacks Doppler flow.
Case courtesy Julie Ritner, MD, Brigham and Women's Hospital.
慢性胎盘早剥:
超声显示胎盘前方出现不均匀、以低回声为主的血肿(黄箭),内部未见血流信号。

Placenta accreta spectrum

- Placenta accreta spectrum is abnormally tenacious or deep attachment of the placenta into the myometrium, carrying a risk of hemorrhage at the time of placental separation.
- Accreta is thought to be caused by uterine scarring (which may be secondary to prior Caesarean section, dilation and curettage, endometritis, or adenomyosis) and resultant endometrial deficiency. It is especially important to consider accreta if an anterior placenta is present with a history of prior Caesarean section. Other predisposing conditions include placenta previa, advanced maternal age, and multiparity.
- Ultrasound findings of accreta include prominent irregular vascular lacunar spaces within the placenta and thinning or absence of the myometrium underlying the placenta. The presence of a *moth-eaten* placenta with vascular lacunar spaces near the bladder is highly specific for accreta.
- Placenta accreta is an umbrella term that describes three degrees of placental attachment/invasion. Confusingly, the term "placenta accreta" also describes one of the specific three degrees.
- In **placenta accreta**, the placenta attaches deeply into the myometrium. Ultrasound shows thinning or absence of the normal hypoechoic subplacental myometrium.
- In **placenta increta**, the placenta invades into the myometrium to the serosa.
- In **placenta percreta**, placenta penetrates through the serosa to invade other structures. A focal bulge in the uterine wall is seen.

胎盘植入的种类

- 胎盘植入是胎盘与子宫肌层异常附着过紧或过深所致，由此导致胎盘分离时出血风险增加。
- 胎盘植入可能是由瘢痕(可能继发于剖宫产、刮宫术、子宫内膜炎或子宫腺肌病)所致，并引起子宫内膜缺陷。如果胎盘位于前壁且有剖宫产史，必须考虑是否有胎盘植入。其他易感因素包括前置胎盘、高龄、多次生产。
- 胎盘植入的超声表现有胎盘内明显的不规则血管腔隙和子宫肌层变薄或消失。若出现虫蚀样胎盘并且在邻近膀胱处有血管腔隙，对诊断胎盘植入具有高度特异性。
- 胎盘植入是一个概括性术语，用以描述三种不同程度的胎盘附着/侵入。令人混淆的是，术语"placenta accrete"同时被用来描述三种不同程度中的任一种。
- **胎盘粘连**，胎盘与子宫肌层附着紧密，超声显示胎盘下方正常子宫肌层的低回声带变薄或消失。
- **胎盘植入**，胎盘侵入子宫肌层内到达浆膜层。
- **穿透性胎盘植入**，胎盘穿过子宫浆膜层侵入其他结构，在子宫壁可见一个局灶性隆起。

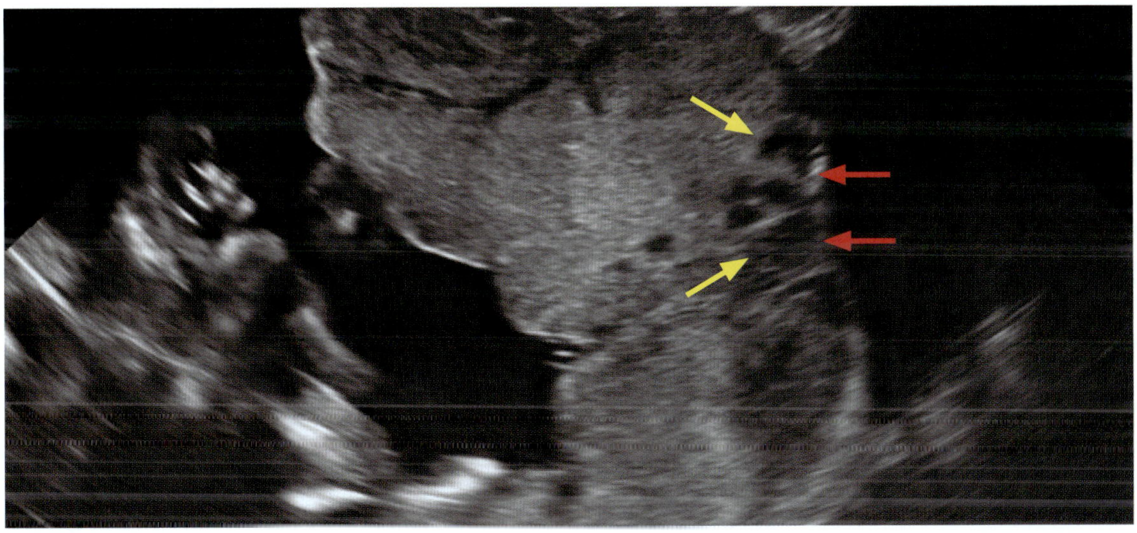

Placenta percreta: Sagittal ultrasound of the uterus shows cystic spaces (yellow arrows) within the inferior placenta abutting the bladder, consistent with vascular lacunae. There is thinning of the myometrium at the placental/bladder interface (red arrows).
穿透性胎盘植入：宫颈矢状切面超声显示在胎盘下缘紧贴膀胱处有一个囊性结构(黄箭)，为血管腔隙。胎盘/膀胱界面的子宫肌层变薄(红箭)。

Placental chorioangioma

- Chorioangioma is the most common benign tumor of the placenta.
- It is associated with hydrops, congenital abnormalities, hemolytic anemia, polyhydramnios, intrauterine growth restriction, and intrauterine fetal death.
- On ultrasound, chorioangioma appears as a hypoechoic, rounded mass in the placenta with anechoic cystic areas and low resistance flow representing enlarged vascular channels.

胎盘绒毛膜血管瘤

- 绒毛膜血管瘤是胎盘中最常见的良性肿瘤。
- 绒毛膜血管瘤与胎儿水肿、胎儿先天性异常、胎儿溶血性贫血、羊水过多、胎儿宫内生长受限和宫内胎儿死亡有关。
- 绒毛膜血管瘤在超声上表现为胎盘内圆形低回声肿块，团块伴无回声囊性暗区，血流阻力低，表明团块内部血管增宽。

FETAL HYDROPS

胎儿水肿

Overview of hydrops

胎儿水肿概述

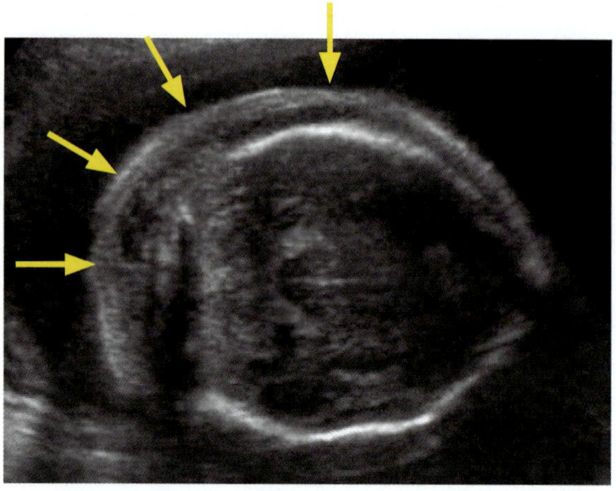

Fetal hydrops:
Transverse ultrasound of a fetal head shows diffuse skin thickening of the scalp (arrows). Polyhydramnios is also present (although incompletely seen on this single image).
Case courtesy Beryl Benacerraf, MD, Diagnostic Ultrasound Associates, Boston.
胎儿水肿：
胎儿头部横切面超声显示皮肤呈弥漫性增厚(黄箭)，同时还有羊水过多(此图未完全展示)。

- Hydrops is a fluid-overload state characterized by at least two of the following: ascites, pleural or pericardial effusion, skin thickening, polyhydramnios, and placental enlargement.
- Hydrops may be classified as immune or non-immune. Prognosis is variable but tends to be poor for non-immune hydrops.

- 水肿是液体过多的一种状态，至少包含以下2项特征：腹水、胸腔积液或心包积液、皮肤水肿、羊水过多和胎盘增大。
- 水肿可分为免疫性和非免疫性，预后不尽相同，但非免疫性水肿的预后往往较差。

Immune hydrops

- Immune-mediated hydrops is fetal hemolytic anemia caused by prior maternal exposure to fetal antigens, by far most commonly the Rh antigen.
- Prognosis is good if treated with intrauterine or peripartum fetal blood transfusions.

免疫性水肿

- 免疫介导性水肿是由于母体曾暴露于胎儿抗原从而导致胎儿发生溶血性贫血，最常见的为Rh抗原。
- 若进行宫内或围产期胎儿输血则预后良好。

Non-immune hydrops

- Non-immune hydrops can be due to a diverse array of causes, most of which lead to a common pathway of extracellular fluid overload. Prognosis of non-immune hydrops tends to be poor, as the primary cause is often not effectively treatable.
- Common etiologies include:

非免疫性水肿

- 非免疫性水肿的病因很多，其中大多数以造成细胞外液过多为共同路径。非免疫性水肿的预后往往较差，因其原发病因常无法得到有效治疗。
- 常见病因包括：

> Cardiac arrhythmias.
> Extra-cardiac shunt, including vein of Galen malformation, hepatic hemangioendothelioma, twin-twin transfusion syndrome, and sacrococcygeal teratoma, all of which may lead to high-output cardiac failure.
> Infectious, especially Parvovirus B19 and TORCH infections, due to fetal aplastic anemia which is diagnosed by elevated middle cerebral artery velocity and treated with percutaneous fetal blood transfusions.
> Intrathoracic masses.

> 心律失常。
> 心外分流，包括大脑大静脉畸形、肝血管内皮瘤、双胎输血综合征，以及骶尾畸胎瘤，这些都会导致高输出量性心力衰竭。
> 感染，尤其是细小病毒B19和TORCH感染，会导致胎儿再生障碍性贫血，后者表现出大脑中动脉流速升高即可做出诊断，治疗为经皮胎儿输血。
> 胸腔内肿块。

Fetal ascites

- When seen with other abnormalities, ascites is a criterion for diagnosis of hydrops.
- Isolated fetal ascites may be due to urinary obstruction and resultant calyceal or bladder rupture, or bowel rupture and resultant meconium peritonitis.

胎儿腹水

- 当合并有其他异常时，腹水是诊断胎儿水肿的一项标准。
- 孤立性腹水可由尿路梗阻引发肾盏或膀胱破裂，或肠破裂和由此引发的胎粪性腹膜炎导致。

Fetal pleural effusion

- Fetal pleural effusion (usually bilateral) is a criterion for diagnosis of hydrops.

胎儿胸腔积液

- 胎儿胸腔积液(通常为双侧)是诊断胎儿水肿的一项标准。

- When seen in isolation (not a component of hydrops or due to any other abnormality), fetal pleural effusion is most commonly a chylothorax. Fetal chylothorax is due to thoracic duct or lymphatic malformation. Prenatally and at birth the pleural fluid is clear, but after the baby begins to feed it becomes chylous (white-colored).
- Fetal pleural effusions can also be seen in Noonan, Turner, or Down syndromes.

- 当出现孤立性胸腔积液(不是胎儿水肿的一个组成部分或由其他异常疾病所致)时，最常见病因是先天性乳糜胸，胎儿乳糜胸是由于胸导管或淋巴管畸形所致。胎儿产前和出生时的胸腔积液透明，婴儿开始进食后则变为乳糜性(白色)。
- 胎儿胸腔积液也可见于努南综合征、特纳综合征或唐氏综合征。

Fetal brain

胎儿大脑

Ventriculomegaly

脑室扩张

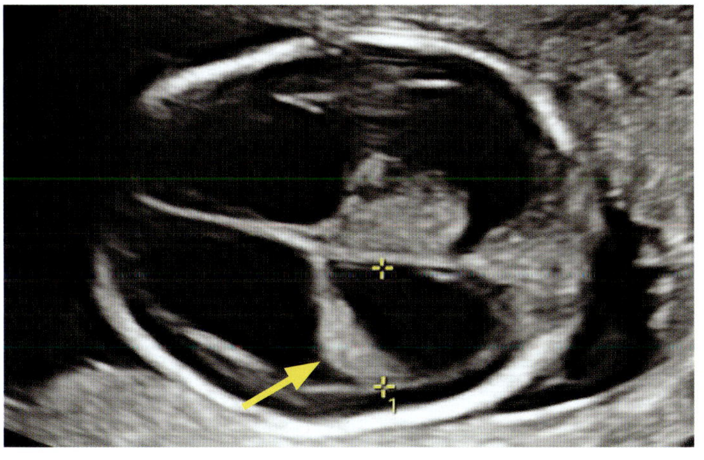

Transverse ultrasound of the fetal head shows severe symmetrical dilation of the lateral ventricles, with the calipers measuring 14 mm. Regardless of the gestational age, the lateral ventricles should always measure <10 mm. Note the dangling choroid (arrow).

胎儿颅脑横切面超声显示双侧侧脑室呈对称性极度扩张，卡尺测量为14mm。不论任何胎龄，侧脑室宽度都应始终<10mm。注意悬挂的脉络丛(黄箭)。

- Ventriculomegaly is enlargement of the cerebral ventricles. The term hydrocephalus is usually avoided because it implies ventriculomegaly due to obstruction.
- Throughout gestation, **the lateral ventricles should each measure less than 10 mm when measured at the atrium.** The atrium is the confluence of the lateral ventricle, temporal horn, and occipital horn. The normal choroid plexus has a rounded border in this location.

  Mild ventriculomegaly: 10–12 mm; moderate: 12–15 mm; marked: >15 mm.
- Normally, the choroid plexus fills the lateral ventricle. The *dangling choroid sign* represents the dependent drooping of choroid plexus seen in ventriculomegaly.

  Ventriculomegaly may be present even in a ventricle measuring <10 mm if there is >3 mm of fluid between the medial margin of the ventricle and the choroid.
- Ventriculomegaly is a sign that something else is wrong, with a diverse array of etiologies:

Primary CNS structural (aqueductal stenosis, Dandy Walker, Chiari Ⅱ, holoprosencephaly, agenesis of the corpus callosum).
Genetic (trisomies 13 and 18).
Destructive (due to infecti on, hemorrhage, or infarct).
Idiopathic.

- 脑室扩张是指脑室增大。应避免使用“脑积水”这一术语，因它是指由梗阻所致的脑室增大。
- 在整个妊娠期中，**侧脑室在中庭位置所测得的值都应该<10mm。**中庭为侧脑室、颞角与枕角的交会处。正常脉络丛在中庭的部位呈圆形。

  脑室轻度扩张：10~12mm；中度扩张：>12~15mm；显著扩张：>15mm。
- 正常情况下，脉络丛充填侧脑室。脉络丛悬挂征为脑室扩张时看到其内的脉络丛下垂。

  若脑室内侧缘与脉络丛之间积液厚度>3mm，即使脑室测值<10mm，也可存在脑室扩张。
- 脑室扩张提示有异常，其中的病因有很多：

原发性中枢神经系统结构畸形(中脑导水管梗阻、丹迪-沃克畸形、基亚里Ⅱ型畸形、全前脑畸形、胼胝体发育不良)。
遗传性(13-三体和18-三体)。
损毁性(感染、出血、梗死所致)。
特发性。

Anencephaly

无脑畸形

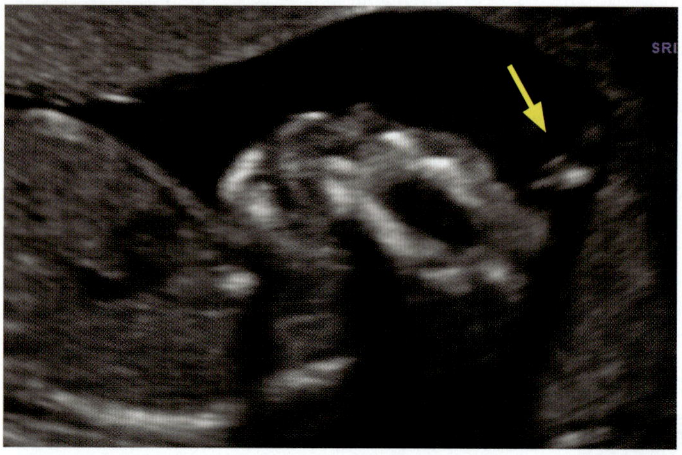

Anencephaly:
Sagittal paramedian 17-week fetal ultrasound through the head and thorax shows lack of calvarium above the level of the orbits. Echogenic foci superior to the anencephalic head likely represent angiomatous stroma (arrow).
Case courtesy Beryl Benacerraf, MD, Diagnostic Ultrasound Associates, Boston.
无脑畸形：妊娠17周胎儿旁正中经头部和胸腔矢状切面显示眼眶平面以上的颅骨缺失。头部上方的高回声灶可能为血管瘤样基质(黄箭)。

- Anencephaly is a lethal anomaly with complete lack of development of the calvarium and destruction of the fetal cerebral cortex and calvarium above the orbits due to toxins in the amniotic fluid. Anencephaly may cause polyhydramnios due to impairment in swallowing.
- AFP is elevated in anencephaly, due to direct exposure of neural tissue to the amniotic fluid.
- **Angiomatous stroma** is residual neural-type tissue that may be tethered above the head and may be confused with an encephalocele.
- The differential of anencephaly is amniotic band syndrome, which is typically asymmetric.

- 无脑畸形是一种致死性异常，表现为胎儿颅骨发育完全缺失，以及胎儿大脑皮层和眼眶上方的颅骨损毁，原因是羊水中的毒素。无脑畸形胎儿可因吞咽障碍而导致羊水过多。
- 甲胎蛋白在无脑畸形胎儿中会升高，因神经组织直接暴露于羊水中。
- **血管瘤样基质**是残留的神经样组织，其拴在胎儿的头部，可能与脑膨出相混淆。
- 无脑畸形需要与羊膜带综合征进行鉴别，后者通常为不对称的。

Cephalocele

- A **cephalocele** is a midline neural tube defect characterized by protrusion of intracranial structures outside of the calvarium. The occipital skull is the most common location.
- A **meningocele** contains only meninges. An **encephalocele** also contains neural tissue.
- In addition to cephalocele, the primary differential consideration of a mass posterior to the occipital skull is a cystic hygroma, which is a congenital lymphatic malformation and the most common fetal neck mass.

脑膨出

- **脑膨出**是正中神经管缺陷，特征为颅内结构突出于颅外。枕骨是最常发生的部位。
- **脑膜膨出**时仅涉及脑膜，**脑膨出**时还包括神经组织。
- 除了脑膨出，枕骨后方肿块的主要鉴别诊断为囊状水囊瘤，后者由先天性淋巴畸形所致，为胎儿最常见的颈部肿块。

Dandy Walker malformation

- Dandy Walker is a diverse spectrum of diseases characterized by hypogenesis of the cerebellar vermis and resultant fourth ventricular dilation.
- Dandy Walker is associated with agenesis of the corpus callosum.
- Differential diagnosis includes Blake's pouch cyst (embryological structure contiguous with the fourth ventricle that fails to regress) and mega cisterna magna (delayed fenestration of Blake's pouch) which are risk factors for associated anomalies but when isolated have an excellent prognosis, unlike Dandy Walker malformation and vermian hypoplasia.

丹迪-沃克畸形

- 丹迪-沃克畸形是一系列以小脑发育不良和第四脑室扩张为特征的疾病。
- 丹迪-沃克畸形与胼胝体发育不良相关。
- 鉴别诊断包括布莱克囊肿(与第四脑室相连的一个未退化的胚胎结构)和巨小脑延髓池(布莱克囊开孔延迟)，它们是相关异常的危险因素，但单独存在时预后良好，这一点不同于丹迪-沃克畸形和小脑蚓发育不全。

Chiari Ⅱ / Myelomeningocele

- Chiari Ⅱ is the combination of a small posterior fossa and a neural tube defect. By far the most common associated neural tube defect is a lumbar myelomeningocele. A myelomeningocele contains both neural elements and meninges.
- The *banana sign* describes the characteristic flattened cerebellar hemispheres in the small posterior fossa. The banana sign is very specific for Chiari Ⅱ.

基亚里Ⅱ型畸形/脊髓脊膜膨出

- 基亚里Ⅱ型畸形是颅后窝窄小合并神经管缺陷。合并神经管缺陷中最常见的为腰脊髓脊膜膨出。脊髓脊膜膨出中包含神经组织和脑脊膜。
- 香蕉征用以描述具有特征性的扁平小脑半球位于小的颅后窝。香蕉征是基亚里Ⅱ型畸形非常特异性的征象。

- The *lemon sign* describes flattening of the frontal bones, causing the calvarium to have the morphology of a lemon when seen axially. Unlike the banana sign, the lemon sign is not specific for Chiari Ⅱ.
- A myelomeningocele may be difficult to visualize by ultrasound but is presumed to be present if the brain is abnormal, as the brain abnormalities are more easily appreciated sonographically.

- 柠檬征用以描述扁平额骨导致颅骨在轴位的形状类似于柠檬。与香蕉征不同，柠檬征对基亚里Ⅱ型畸形不具特异性。
- 脊髓脊膜膨出可能很难在超声上进行观察，只能在大脑有异常时推测其有存在的可能，因为大脑异常更容易通过超声进行识别。

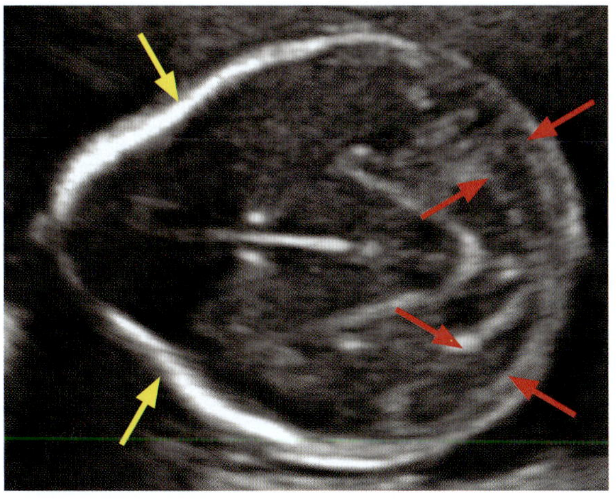

Fetal ultrasound through the brain and posterior fossa demonstrates the *banana* and *lemon* signs. There is flattening of the frontal bones (*lemon sign*, yellow arrows) and flattening of the cerebellar hemispheres (*banana sign*, red arrows). Although the *lemon sign* is nonspecific, the *banana sign* is very specific for Chiari Ⅱ.
经大脑及颅后窝胎儿超声显示香蕉征和柠檬征。额骨变扁平(柠檬征，黄箭)，小脑半球变扁平(香蕉征，红箭)。虽然柠檬征没有诊断特异性，但香蕉征对基亚里Ⅱ型畸形的诊断具有高度特异性。

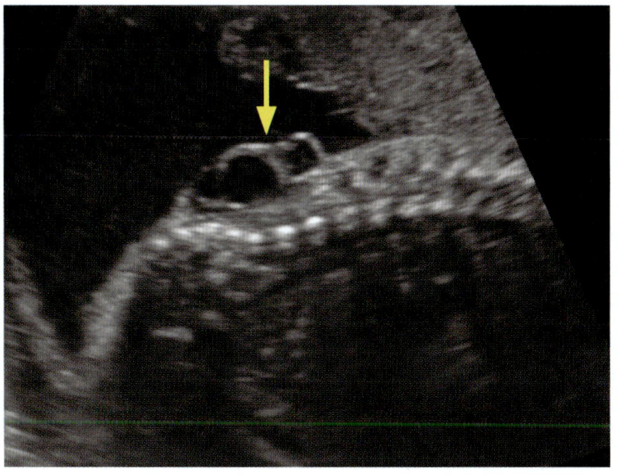

Sagittal ultrasound through the thoracolumbar spine in a different fetus shows a lumbar open neural tube defect (arrow) representing either a meningocele or myelomeningocele.
另一个胎儿矢状切面经胸腰椎超声图像显示腰椎开放性神经管缺损(黄箭)，为脊膜膨出或脊髓脊膜膨出。

Case courtesy Beryl Benacerraf, MD, Diagnostic Ultrasound Associates, Boston.

Holoprosencephaly

- Holoprosencephaly is failure of midline cleavage of the primitive prosencephalon in early embryologic development. The most severe form, *alobar* holoprosencephaly, leads to fused thalami and a single monoventricle that may communicate with a large dorsal cyst. Brain tissue surrounds the monoventricle, forming a characteristic *boomerang* shape.
- Holoprosencephaly is associated with trisomy 13, facial hypoplasias, and midline facial anomalies including clefts, hypotelorism/cyclopia, absent nose and proboscis.

全前脑畸形

- 全前脑畸形为胚胎发育早期原始前脑中线分裂障碍所致。最严重的类型为无叶全前脑畸形，会导致丘脑融合和单脑室，后者可与背侧一个较大囊肿相通。脑组织包绕单脑室，呈有特征性的飞镖形状。
- 全前脑畸形与13-三体、面部发育不全及面部中线畸形相关，包括唇腭裂、眼距低下/独眼、鼻缺如和长鼻畸形。

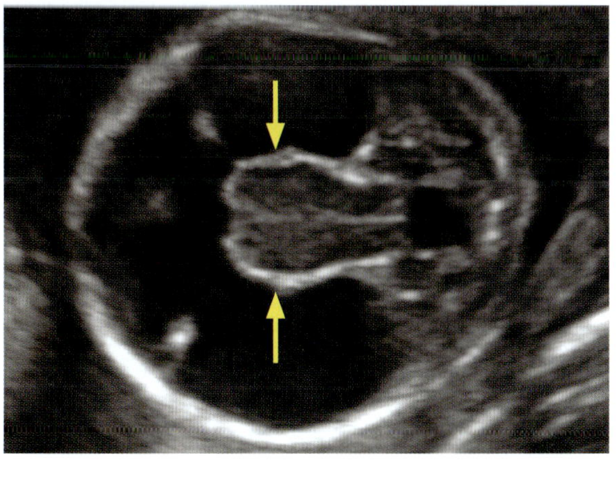

Oblique axial/coronal ultrasound through the posterior brain shows fused thalami across the midline (arrows). A large dorsal cyst is present, largely replacing the visualized supratentorial brain. No falx is seen.
Case courtesy Beryl Benacerraf, MD, Diagnostic Ultrasound Associates, Boston.
经后脑斜轴/冠状切面超声显示丘脑在中线融合(黄箭)。背侧有一个大的囊肿，取代了可见部分的幕上大脑。未见大脑镰。

Agenesis of the corpus callosum (ACC)

- Normal corpus callosum forms by 20 weeks gestational age from the body to the splenium. The rostrum forms last.
- Absence of the corpus callosum (ACC) can be a difficult diagnosis to make prenatally.
- Because the normal corpus callosum is not always visualized on ultrasound, it is often necessary to rely on secondary abnormal morphology of the ventricular system to diagnose absence of the corpus callosum.

胼胝体发育不良(ACC)

- 正常胼胝体在妊娠20周时已形成，从体部向压部方向进行，最后形成胼胝体的嘴部。
- 胼胝体发育不良(ACC)在产前很难得到诊断。
- 超声并不总是能够看到正常的胼胝体，因此通常需要依靠继发的脑室系统形态异常来诊断胼胝体缺失。

Absence of the cavum septum pellucidum is associated with ACC.

Abnormal teardrop morphology of the lateral ventricles with dilated occipital horns, known as **colpocephaly**, is associated with ACC. Colpocephaly is often seen together with ventriculomegaly.

Widely separated ventricular frontal horns and **parallel configuration** of the lateral ventricles both suggest ACC. This is sometimes referred as the *steer horn* or *Viking helmet* configuration.

A **midline interhemispheric cyst** may be present, representing superior herniation of the third ventricle.

透明隔腔缺失与ACC有关。

侧脑室泪滴状形态异常伴枕角扩大，称为**空洞脑**，与ACC有关。空洞脑畸形常伴有脑室扩大。

广泛扩张的脑室前角和侧脑室呈平行结构均提示ACC。这有时被称为反向喇叭或海盗头巾形态。

可能存在一个**中线半球间囊肿**，代表第三脑室上疝。

- A minority of fetuses with agenesis of the corpus callosum have trisomy 8, 13, or 18.

- 少数胼胝体发育不全的胎儿为8-三体、13-三体或18-三体。

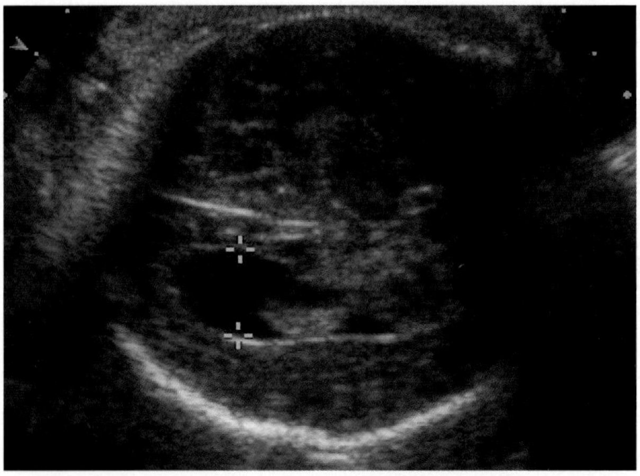

Transverse ultrasound through the fetal head shows ventriculomegaly and a colpocephalic configuration of the lateral ventricle with a dilated teardrop-shaped occipital horn (calipers). The ventricle is oriented parallel to the falx.

Case courtesy Beryl Benacerraf, MD, Diagnostic Ultrasound Associates, Boston.

胎儿头部横切面超声图像显示脑室扩张，以及侧脑室呈枕角扩张样的形态伴枕角泪滴样扩张(卡尺)。脑室与大脑镰平行。

Absence of the cavum septum pellucidum (CSP)

- The cavum septum pellucidum (CSP) should always be identified in a normal fetus.
- If the CSP is not seen, the primary consideration is agenesis of the corpus callosum, as the cavum septum pellucidum and corpus callosum are formed simultaneously.
- Uncommonly, the CSP may be absent in the presence of a normal corpus callosum. This may represent septo-optic dysplasia and fetal MRI should be recommended.

Hydranencephaly

- Hydranencephaly is complete cortical destruction due to infarct or infection. The brain parenchyma is obliterated and replaced by fluid. In most instances, this finding follows a previously normal fetal survey.
- The most common cause of hydranencephaly is in utero complete occlusion of both internal carotid arteries.
- In contrast to severe hydrocephalus, a cortical mantle is absent in hydranencephaly.
- In contrast to holoprosencephaly, a falx is typically visualized in hydranencephaly because it is supplied by the external carotid artery.

透明隔腔(CSP)缺失

- 正常胎儿总应看到透明隔腔(CSP)。
- 若未能发现CSP，首先考虑胼胝体发育不全，因为透明隔腔与胼胝体同时形成。
- 少数情况下，透明隔腔缺失但胼胝体正常。这可能提示中隔发育不良，应对胎儿进行MRI检查。

积水性无脑畸形

- 积水性无脑畸形是指胎儿脑皮质因梗死或感染遭到完全损毁，脑实质消失并被液体替代。在发现这一情况时，大多数先前的胎儿检查并无异常。
- 引起积水性无脑畸形最常见的病因是宫内胎儿大脑两侧颈内动脉完全闭塞。
- 与严重脑积水不同，积水性无脑畸形胎儿没有脑皮质。
- 与全前脑畸形不同，积水性无脑畸形胎儿通常可见大脑镰，因为它由颈外动脉供血。

Choroid plexus cyst

脉络丛囊肿

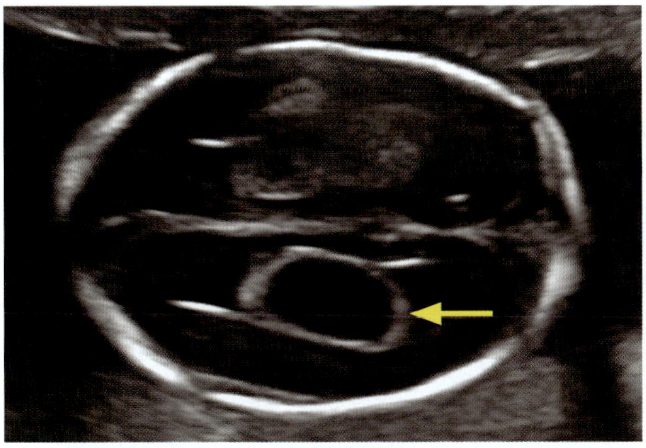

Transverse ultrasound of a fetal head shows a hypoechoic cyst (arrow) located within the echogenic, otherwise normal-appearing choroid.
胎儿头部横切面超声显示一个低回声囊肿(黄箭)位于除了高回声外看似正常的脉络膜内。

- Cysts within the choroid plexus are common. The vast majority of choroid plexus cysts are present in normal fetuses and resolve on follow-up scans. However, choroid plexus cysts are a hallmark of trisomy 18.
- Choroid plexus cysts can be considered an incidental finding in the absence of any other sonographic abnormality and with a normal maternal serum screen.
- A choroid plexus cyst appears on ultrasound as a discrete and round hypoechoic to anechoic lesion within the choroid plexus that is visible in two planes, and measures ≥3 mm in size.
- A potential mimicker of a choroid plexus cyst is the *spongy choroid*, which describes a heterogeneous echogenic choroid that is a normal variant.

- 脉络丛内的囊肿较为常见。大多数脉络丛囊肿见于正常胎儿，并在随访过程中消退。但是，脉络丛囊肿是18-三体的一个标志。
- 脉络丛囊肿被认为是一种偶然的良性发现，除非有其他超声异常及母体血清学异常。
- 脉络丛囊肿在超声上表现为脉络丛内有一个清楚的圆形低回声至无回声病变，并在两个平面上得到展示，直径≥3mm。
- 与脉络丛囊肿相似的病变是海绵状脉络丛，后者为不均质高回声脉络丛，是一种正常变异。

Vein of Galen malformation

大脑大静脉畸形

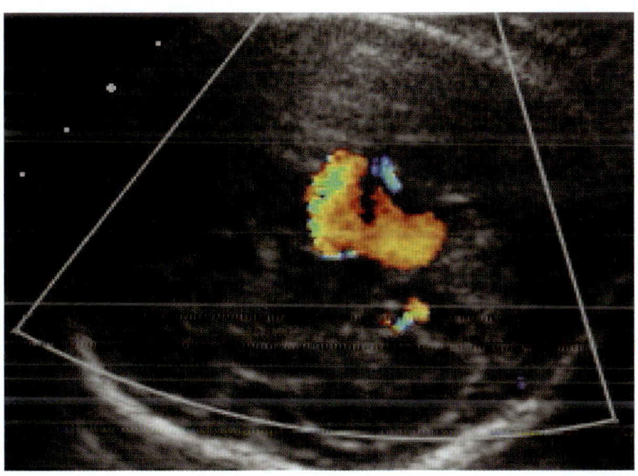

Color Doppler ultrasound of the fetal head shows an enlarged midline vascular structure representing a vein of Galen malformation.
Case courtesy Beryl Benacerraf, MD, Diagnostic Ultrasound Associates, Boston.
胎儿头部彩色多普勒超声显示位于中线的一个扩张的血管结构，为大脑大静脉畸形。

- Vein of Galen malformation is dilation of the vein of Galen (in the pineal region) caused by an arteriovenous fistula.
- Vein of Galen aneurysm is a shunt lesion which may cause high-output cardiac failure, leading to hydrops.

- 大脑大静脉畸形是指因动静脉瘘导致大脑大静脉(松果体区)扩张。
- 大脑大静脉动脉样瘤是一种分流性病变，可引起高输出量性心力衰竭，导致胎儿水肿。

FETAL SPINE

胎儿脊柱

Evaluation of the fetal spine

- In the normal fetal spine, three primary ossification centers are seen on transverse axial plane for each vertebra, one for the vertebral body (centrum) and one on either side for the posterior elements (neural arch).

胎儿脊柱评估

- 在正常胎儿脊柱中，每个椎体的横轴平面上有三个初级骨化中心，一个为椎体(中心)，另外两个分别位于后方(神经弓)各一侧。

- It is important to examine the entire spine, especially the caudal end, to assess for neural tube defects. The spinal level can be determined by identifying the last ossified vertebra (presumed to be S4 in the second trimester, and S5 in the third trimester).

- 评估神经管缺陷的关键是要检查整个脊柱，特别是尾端。脊柱水平可以通过确认最后一个骨化椎体来确定(通常，妊娠中期为S_4，妊娠晚期为S_5)。

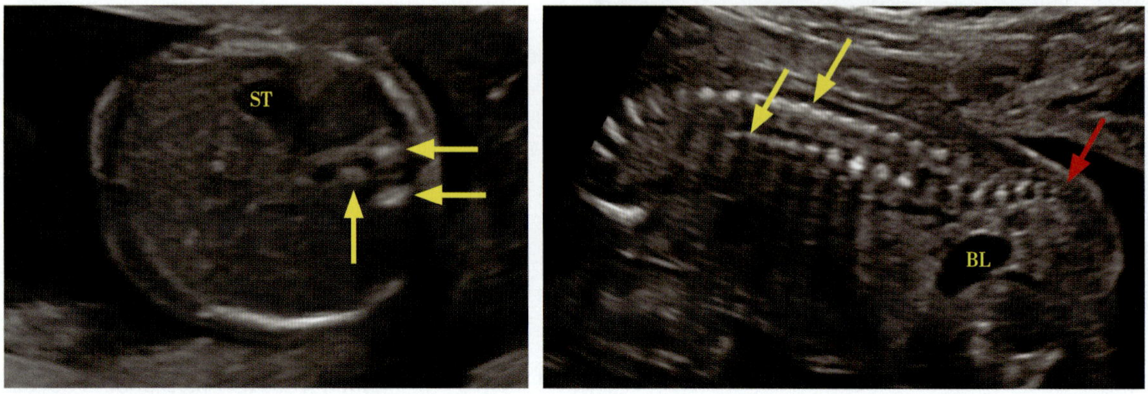

Transverse ultrasound through the fetal abdomen at level of the stomach (ST) shows the normal three ossification centers of the vertebra (yellow arrows). Sagittal ultrasound shows the normal fetal spine as two parallel echogenic lines (yellow arrows) that converge at the sacrum (red arrow). It is important to assess the integrity of the skin overlying the spine. "BL" denotes the bladder.
胎儿腹部(ST)经胃横切面超声显示椎体三个骨化中心(黄箭)。矢状切面超声显示正常胎儿脊柱为两条平行的回声线(黄箭)，汇聚于骶骨(红箭)。评估覆盖在脊柱的皮肤的完整性很重要。"BL"表示膀胱。

Spina dysraphism / Myelomeningocele

- Spinal dysraphism is a spectrum of congenital anomalies due to incomplete closure of the neural tube. When this results in a defect in the posterior neural arch, the term spina bifida is used.
- Meninges and neural tissue can protrude through the dorsal defect, resulting in meningocele (meninges only) and myelomeningocele (both meninges and neural tissue).
- Myelomeningocele is more common than meningocele and occurs most often in the lumbar spine, followed by the cervical spine. Determination of the spinal level is useful for outcome counseling.
- Imaging shows a cystic lesion protruding from the spinal canal at the midline back, with associated splaying of the vertebral pedicles/laminae and a dorsal skin defect.
- Other types of spinal dysraphism are discussed in the "Spine" chapter.

椎管闭合不全/脊髓脊膜膨出

- 椎管闭合不全是由于神经管不完全闭合而引起的一系列先天性异常。当这一异常导致后神经弓缺损时，则使用"脊柱裂"这个术语。
- 脊膜和神经组织可通过背侧缺损向外突出，导致脊膜膨出(仅为脊膜)和脊髓脊膜膨出(包括脊膜和神经组织)。
- 脊髓脊膜膨出比脊膜膨出更常见，最常发生于腰椎，其次是颈椎。确定脊柱水平有助于判断预后。
- 声像图显示突出的囊性病变位于椎管中线，伴有椎弓根/椎弓板的扩张和背侧皮肤缺损。
- 其他类型的脊柱发育不良将在"脊柱影像"一章中讨论。

Sacrococcygeal teratoma

骶尾骨畸胎瘤

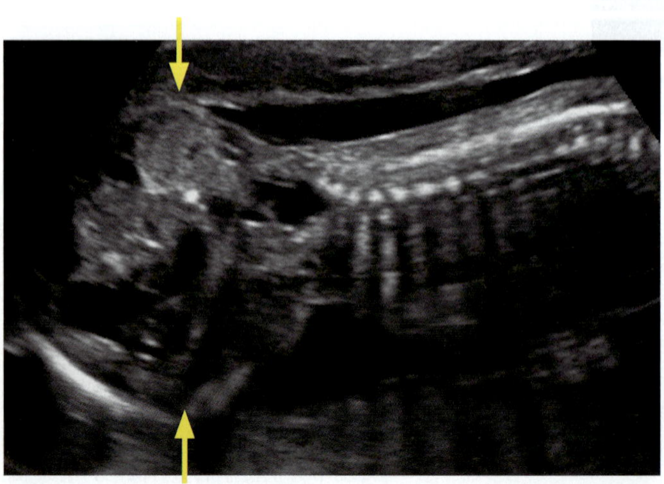

Sagittal ultrasound of the fetal torso and lumbosacral spine shows a large, heterogeneous, solid and cystic mass (arrows) arising from the sacrum/ coccyx.
In contrast to myelomeningocele, the lumbosacral spine demonstrates normal tapering and the overlying skin is intact.
Case courtesy Beryl Benacerraf, MD, Diagnostic Ultrasound Associates, Boston.
胎儿躯干和腰骶骨矢状切面超声显示一个起于骶骨/尾骨的大而不均匀、囊实混合性肿块(黄箭)。
与脊髓脊膜膨出相比较，腰骶椎表现为正常的逐渐变细，覆盖的皮肤完好无损。

- Sacrococcygeal teratoma is a germ cell tumor of the sacrum. It often presents prenatally as a mixed solid and cystic complex mass.
- Sacrococcygeal teratoma may be associated with high output cardiac failure.
- The other primary differential consideration for a distal fetal spinal mass is a myelomeningocele (Chiari Ⅱ). Assessing the brain will be useful as it is always abnormal with a myelomeningocele and normal with a sacrococcygeal teratoma.

- 骶尾骨畸胎瘤是骶骨的一种生殖细胞瘤，通常在产前表现为囊实混合性肿块。
- 骶尾骨畸胎瘤可能与高心输出量性心力衰竭有关。
- 胎儿远端脊柱肿块的另一个主要鉴别诊断是脊髓脊膜膨出(基亚里Ⅱ型畸形)。对大脑进行检查有助于鉴别，因脊髓脊膜膨出时的大脑总为异常，而骶尾部畸胎瘤时则为正常。

Fetal face

胎儿面部

Evaluation of the fetal face

- The fetal face should be examined for the presence of two orbits, normal nose and lips, nasal bone and a normal sized chin on sagittal profile view.

胎儿面部评估

- 胎儿面部矢状切面超声应检查是否存在两个眼眶、正常的鼻和口唇、鼻骨和正常大小的下巴。

Absent nasal bone

鼻骨缺失

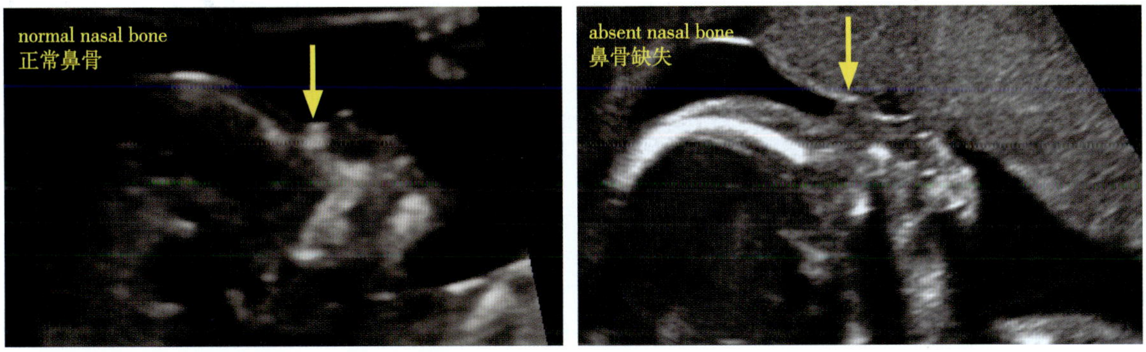

Sagittal ultrasound of the fetal profile showing normal nasal bone in one fetus (left image) and absence of the nasal bone in a different fetus (right image; arrows).
胎儿矢状切面超声显示一个胎儿的鼻骨正常(左图；黄箭)，另一个胎儿的鼻骨缺失(右图；黄箭)。

- A hypoplastic or absent nasal bone is associated with trisomy 21 if seen on first trimester ultrasound, and with aneuploidy if seen on second or third trimester ultrasound in patients with other markers of aneuploidy.

- 超声显示鼻骨发育不全或缺失在妊娠早期与21-三体相关，在妊娠中期或晚期超声检查中若发现其他整倍体标记，则与非整倍体异常相关。

Cleft lip and palate

- Facial clefts are associated with aneuploidy (including trisomies 13 and 18), cardiac and CNS anomalies, or less commonly present as an isolated finding. Discovery of a facial cleft should therefore prompt a search for additional structural abnormalities.
- On imaging, a linear defect is seen extending from the lip to the nostril (cleft lip), and may further extend through the alveolar ridge and palate (cleft lip and palate). The defect may be unilateral or bilateral.
- Large facial clefts may affect fetal swallowing and lead to polyhydramnios.

唇裂和腭裂

- 唇腭裂与非整倍体(包括13-三体和18-三体)、心脏和中枢神经系统异常有关，较少为孤立性表现。因此，一旦发现唇腭裂应该立即寻找是否有其他结构异常。
- 声像图上可见一个从唇部到鼻孔(唇裂)的线性缺陷，并可能进一步延伸至牙槽嵴和腭裂(唇裂和腭裂)。缺损可能为单侧或双侧。
- 大的面部裂口可能影响胎儿吞咽而导致羊水过多。

Micrognathia

- Micrognathia is hypoplasia of the mandible, resulting in a small chin. It can be an isolated finding or associated with other anomalies (e.g., trisomy 18) or syndromes.
- Severe micrognathia can impair fetal swallowing (leading to polyhydramnios), cause airway obstruction after birth (due to crowding of tongue in a small oral cavity) and difficulty in postnatal feeding.

小颌畸形

- 小颌畸形为下颌骨发育不全，导致小下巴。它可以是一个孤立的畸形，也可与其他异常(如18-三体)或综合征相关。
- 严重的小颌畸形可影响胎儿吞咽(导致羊水过多)，造成出生后气道阻塞(由于舌头被挤在一个小口腔内)和产后喂养困难。

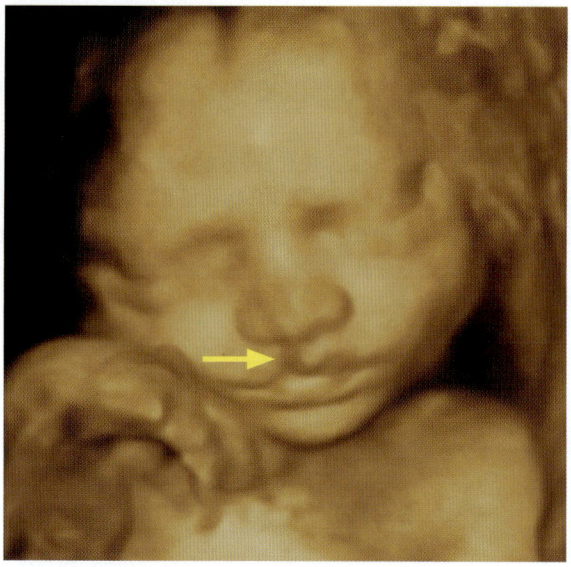

3D ultrasound of the fetal face shows a cleft lip (arrow).
Case courtesy Beryl Benacerraf, MD, Diagnostic Ultrasound Associates, Boston.
胎儿面部三维超声显示唇裂(黄箭)。

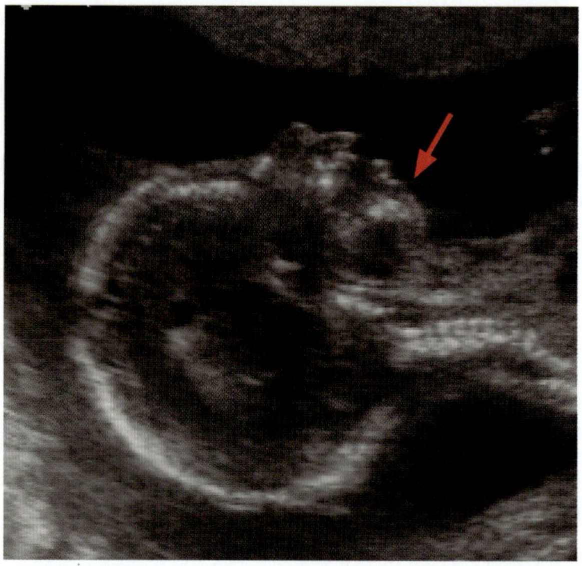

Sagittal ultrasound of the head (different fetus) shows micrognathia, or a small chin (arrow).
头部(另一个胎儿)矢状切面超声显示小颌,或“小下巴”(红箭)。

FETAL THORAX

Evaluation of the fetal thorax

- Abnormal position of the heart in the thorax is an important clue to the possible presence of a thoracic anomaly. Abnormal cardiac position or axis may be secondary to a thoracic mass lesion or unilateral pulmonary agenesis.

Congenital diaphragmatic hernia (CDH)

胎儿胸腔

评估胎儿胸腔

- 心脏位置异常是可能存在胸腔异常的一条重要线索。心脏位置或心轴异常可继发于胸腔肿块或肺脏发育不良。

先天性膈疝(CDH)

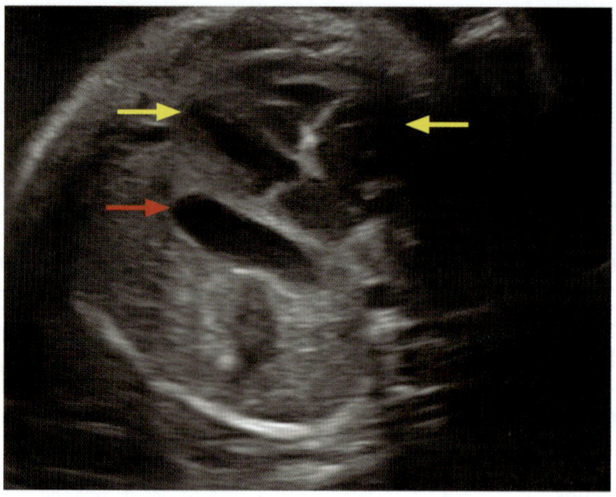

Congenital diaphragmatic hernia:
Grayscale transverse ultrasound through the fetal thorax demonstrates rightward displacement of the heart (yellow arrows) due to herniation of intra-abdominal content into the left hemithorax, including the stomach (red arrow).
先天性膈疝:
经胎儿胸部横切面灰阶超声显示心脏(黄箭)向右移位,原因是腹腔内容物(包括胃)(红箭)疝入左半胸。

- Congenital diaphragmatic hernia (CDH) is herniation of abdominal organs (most commonly bowel) into the thorax through a diaphragmatic defect. CDH is the most common cause of a fetal intrathoracic mass lesion.
- Most cases are isolated, although a prominent minority of fetuses have other anomalies, most commonly congenital heart disease.
- By far the most common location for CDH is the left posterior thorax, termed a Bochdalek hernia (mnemonic: “back to the left”). A Bochdalek hernia frequently displaces the heart to the right.

- 先天性膈疝(CDH)是指腹腔器官(最常为肠管)经有缺损的膈肌疝入胸腔,是最常见的胎儿胸腔肿块。
- 大多数为孤立性异常;但不少病例合并有其他异常,最常见的为先天性心脏病。
- 绝大多数CDH位于胸腔左后方,胸腹膜裂孔疝(记忆诀窍:“左后”)。胸腹膜裂孔疝常使心脏向右移位。

- When a CDH occurs on the right it is termed a Morgagni hernia. The diaphragmatic defect of a Morgagni hernia tends to be anterior, with the liver the most commonly herniated organ.
- The two classic prenatal findings of CDH are a cystic intrathoracic mass representing the stomach and/or bowel and nonvisualization of the stomach below the diaphragm.
- Complications of CHD include pulmonary hypoplasia, bowel obstruction with resultant polyhydramnios, and obstruction of venous return due to IVC compression, which may lead to ascites.

Bronchopulmonary foregut malformation

- Bronchopulmonary foregut malformations are a spectrum of congenital abnormalities of the fetal lungs and upper GI tract.
- **Congenital pulmonary airway malformation (CPAM)** is a hamartomatous proliferation of small airways which communicates with the bronchial tree. *Blood supply is from the pulmonary circulation*. CPAM was previously called congenital cystic adenomatoid malformation (CCAM).

  CPAM can be classified into three types based on the size of cysts (Type Ⅰ – large cysts; Type Ⅱ – small cysts; Type Ⅲ – tiny cysts too small to see on ultrasound). Today this classification is not used much anymore as prognosis is dependent on size of the entire lesion rather than the size of the individual cysts.

  CPAM is not associated with other anomalies (unlike CDH).

  Many CPAM decrease in size and may disappear on ultrasound, but remain apparent on CT or MRI.

- 如果CDH发生于胸腔的右侧则称先天性胸骨后膈疝。先天性胸骨后膈疝常发生于前方，肝脏为最常见的疝内器官。
- CDH两个最典型的超声特征是胸腔内囊样肿块代表胃和/或肠管，以及在横膈下方无胃泡。
- CDH的并发症包括肺脏发育不良、肠梗阻，以及由此并发的羊水过多，下腔静脉受压使静脉回流受阻而出现腹水。

支气管肺前肠畸形

- 支气管肺前肠畸形是一系列的先天性胎儿肺和上消化道异常。
- **先天性肺气道畸形(CPAM)**是指与支气管树相连的小气道呈错构瘤样增生，*血供来自肺循环*。CPAM的旧称为先天性囊腺瘤畸形(CCAM)。

  CPAM可根据囊肿大小分为三种类型(Ⅰ型：大囊肿；Ⅱ型：小囊肿；Ⅲ型：超声无法分辨的微小囊肿)。但目前这种分类方式已经不再流行，因为该病预后取决于整个病变的大小而不是单个囊肿的大小。

  CPAM不会并发其他异常(与CDH不同)。

  很多CPAM在超声上变小，甚至消失，但CT或MRI上依然明显。

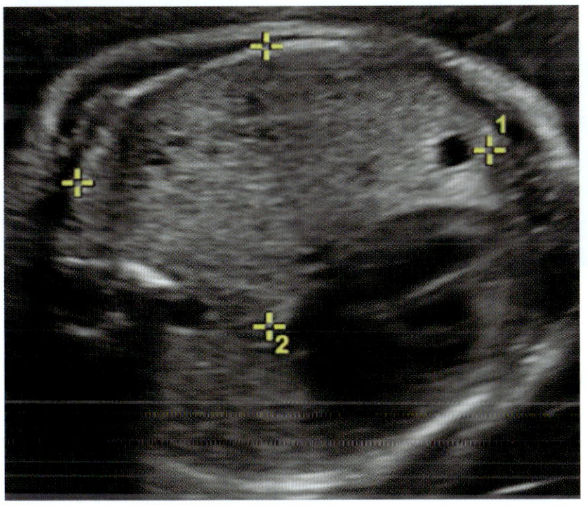

Transverse ultrasound through the fetal thorax shows a large echogenic mass (calipers) containing small cystic spaces in left hemithorax, displacing the heart to the right. This was found to be a CPAM following surgical resection.
胎儿胸部横切面超声显示一个大的回声肿块(卡尺)而左侧胸腔仅剩一个很小的囊性空间，心脏向右侧移位。手术证实为CPAM。

- **Sequestration** is aberrant lung tissue with a *systemic blood supply*, usually from the aorta. The most characteristic location of sequestration is the left lower lobe.

  Classic ultrasound appearance of sequestration is an echogenic mass at the left lung base. The sequestration may occasionally be subdiaphragmatic and simulate an adrenal mass.

  Systemic blood supply should be confirmed with color Doppler. In the absence of the Doppler findings, sequestration may be difficult to differentiate from CPAM. In contrast to the findings of CPAM, cysts are less common, there is less mass effect, and location is almost always in the lower lobes.

- Combination or hybrid CPAM/sequestration lesions are common at pathology.

- **肺隔离症**是指畸变的肺组织由*体循环供血*，通常为主动脉。肺隔离症最典型的位置是左下肺。

  典型肺隔离症的声像图表现为左肺基底部有一个高回声肿块。肺隔离症偶尔也会发生在膈下，与肾上腺肿块类似。

  体循环供血应采用彩色多普勒超声进行确定。若缺乏多普勒的征象，肺隔离症难以与CPAM相鉴别。与CPAM表现不同，肺隔离症很少见到囊肿，也很少有肿块效应，且其位置几乎都在肺的下叶。

- 肺隔离症合并CPAM在病理上很常见。

- Bronchogenic, gastrointestinal duplication, and neurenteric cysts almost always appear as solitary, simple cysts in the thoracic cavity on ultrasound.

- 支气管源囊肿、胃肠重复畸形，以及神经管原肠囊肿在超声上几乎均表现为孤立的单纯性囊肿。

Pulmonary hypoplasia

- Pulmonary hypoplasia is inadequate lung development. Hypoplasia can be due to a thoracic mass lesion (such as CDH), oligohydramnios, or a skeletal dysplasia affecting the ribs.
- It is important to evaluate the size of the fetal thorax in relation to the abdomen on coronal images. A small, *bell-shaped* fetal thorax suggests pulmonary hypoplasia. The normal heart appears enlarged relative to the small thorax.

肺发育不良

- 肺发育不良是指肺脏发育不完全。发育不良可继发于胸腔肿块(如CDH)、羊水过少或骨骼发育不良而累及肋骨。
- 评估胎儿冠状面胸腔和腹腔之间的大小关系非常重要。一个小而又呈钟形的胎儿胸腔提示肺脏发育不良。正常的心脏对于小胸腔显得相对增大。

Laryngeal or tracheal atresia

- Atresia of the upper airway, otherwise known as **congenital high airway obstruction syndrome (CHAOS)**, is lethal and may cause *bilateral enlarged echogenic lungs*.

喉或气管闭锁

- 上气道闭锁，也称**先天性高位气道阻塞综合征(CHAOS)**，是一种致死性病变，可引起双肺增大且回声增强。

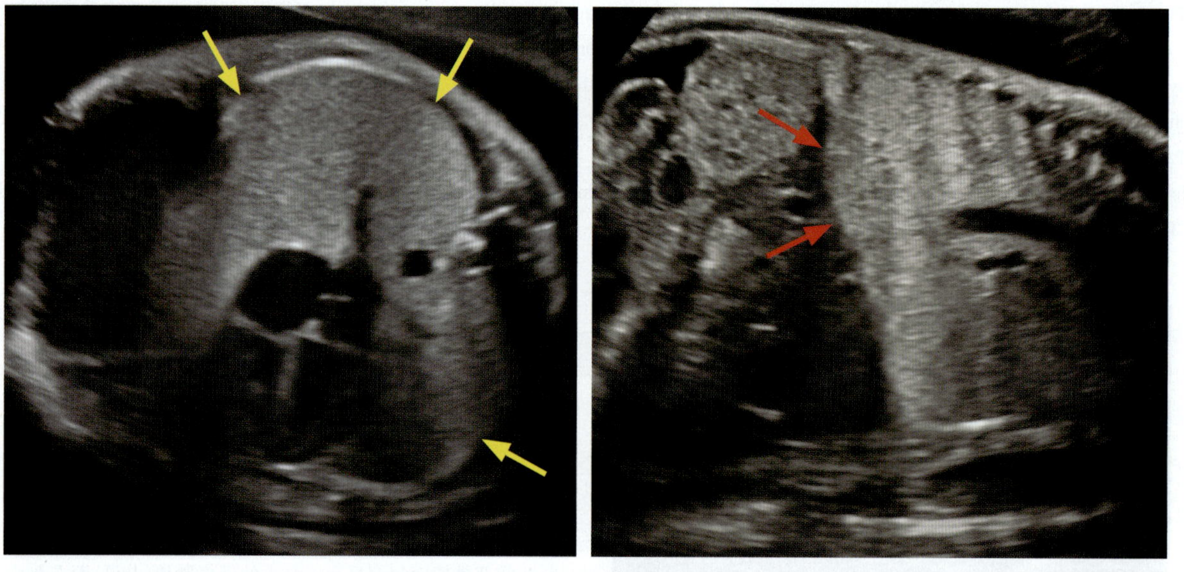

Transverse and sagittal ultrasound through the fetal thorax demonstrates symmetrically enlarged echogenic lungs (yellow arrows) flattening and inverting the hemidiaphragms (red arrows). There is large volume abdominal ascites, moderate polyhydramnios, and distended trachea and mainstem bronchi (not shown). Etiology was thought to be laryngeal web versus agenesis.

胎儿胸部横切面及矢状切面显示两肺对称性增大且回声增强(黄箭)，膈肌扁平甚至反转(红箭)。大量腹水，中度羊水过多，气管和主干支气管扩张(未展示)。病因可能是喉蹼或喉发育不全。

Fetal heart

Evaluation of the fetal heart

- When congenital heart disease (CHD) is identified on prenatal ultrasound, genetic analysis is always indicated because of the high association with aneuploidy.
- CHD is discussed in more detail under the "Pediatrics" chapter.
- Sonographic assessment of the fetal heart should include the following:

  Four-chamber **(4CH)** view.

  Left ventricular outflow tract **(LVOT)**.

  Right ventricular outflow tract **(RVOT)**.

  Three-vessel view, which depicts the main pulmonary artery-ductus arteriosus confluence, aortic arch, and SVC in one plane.

  Aortic arch, SVC, and **IVC.**

胎儿心脏

胎儿心脏评估

- 产前超声发现先天性心脏病(CHD)时需进行基因筛查，因为这与非整倍体异常高度相关。
- 先天性心脏病将在“小儿影像”一章进行详细讨论。
- 胎儿超声心脏评估应包括以下内容：

  四腔心切面(4CH)。

  左心室流出道(LVOT)。

  右心室流出道(RVOT)。

  三血管切面，此切面显示肺动脉-动脉导管汇合处、主动脉弓和上腔静脉(SVC)。

  主动脉弓，SVC和下腔静脉(IVC)。

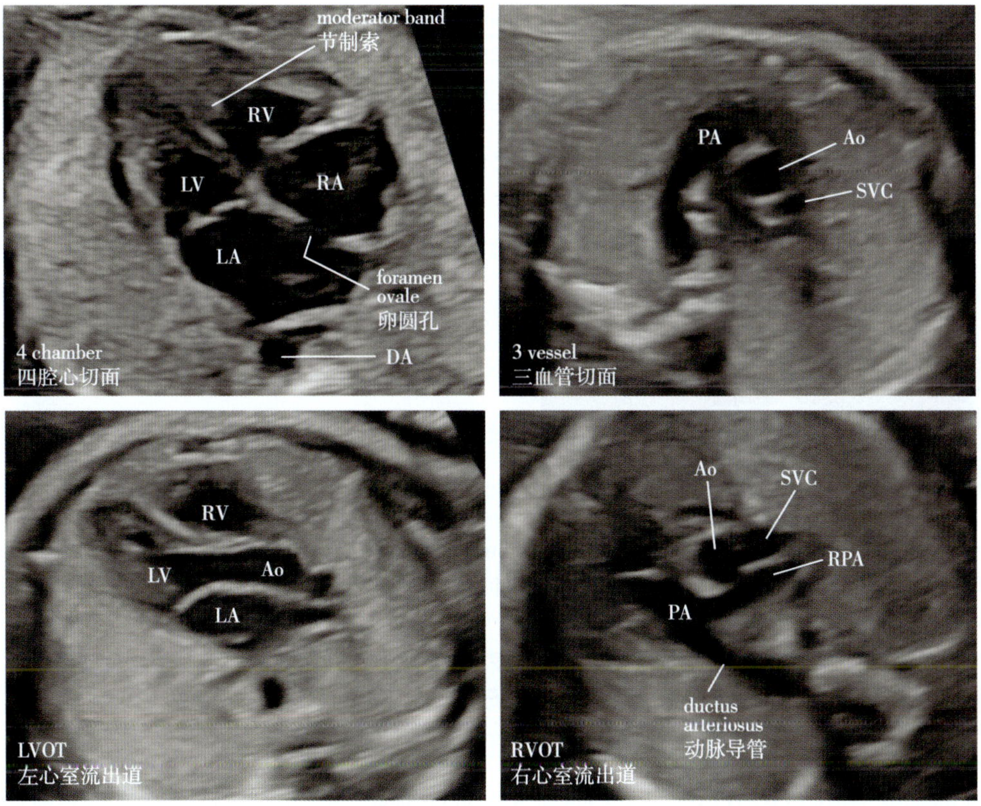

Four normal sonographic views of the fetal heart:
The morphologic right ventricle (RV) is characterized by the moderator band (which extends from the interventricular septum to the RV side wall) and tricuspid valve septal leaflet (which inserts onto the septum more anteriorly).
LV = left ventricle. LA = left atrium. RA = right atrium. Ao = ascending aorta. DA = descending aorta. PA = main pulmonary artery. RPA and LPA = right and left pulmonary arteries.
胎儿心脏正常四腔心切面超声图：
右心室(RV)的形态学特征是调节束(从室间隔延伸至右心室侧壁)和三尖瓣隔瓣等(更靠前插入室间隔)。
LV=左心室；LA=左心房；RA=右心房；Ao=升主动脉；DA=降主动脉；PA=肺动脉；RPA和LPA=左肺动脉和右肺动脉。

Ventricular septal defect (VSD)

- Ventricular septal defect (VSD) is the most common CHD. It may be isolated or associated with other structural cardiac anomalies.
- VSD is identified on prenatal ultrasound as a defect in the interventricular septum, best seen on four-chamber view, with bidirectional flow across the defect on color Doppler imaging.

Atrioventricular septal defect

室间隔缺损(VSD)

- 室间隔缺损(VSD)是最常见的先天性心脏病。它可以是单一病变或与其他心脏结构性异常有关。
- VSD在产前超声上表现为室间隔缺损，在四腔心切面上显示最佳，而彩色多普勒成像显示双向血流信号通过缺损。

房室间隔缺损

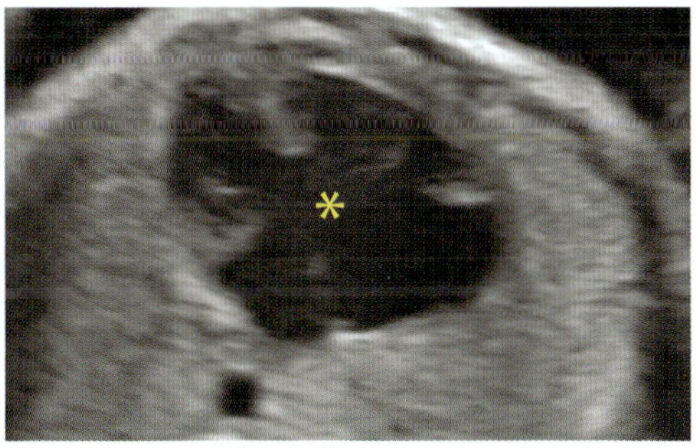

Transverse ultrasound through the fetal thorax shows a central hole (*) within the heart, consistent with an atrioventricular septal defect.
胎儿胸腔横切面显示心脏中央有一个缺损(*)，符合房室间隔缺损的诊断。

- Atrioventricular (AV) septal defect, also called endocardial cushion defect or AV canal defect, represents a spectrum of CHD resulting from deficiency in the AV junction. It is strongly associated with Down syndrome.

- 房室(AV)间隔缺损，也称为心内膜垫缺损或房室管缺损，为一系列由房室交界处缺损引起的先天性心脏病。它与唐氏综合征密切相关。

- Four-chamber view shows absent AV septum and a single common AV valve, resulting in the appearance of a central hole in the heart when the valve opens during diastole.

Tetralogy of Fallot (TOF)

- 四腔心切面显示房室间隔缺失，以及单一共用的房室瓣膜，导致在舒张期瓣膜打开时心脏出现一个中央孔。

法洛四联症(TOF)

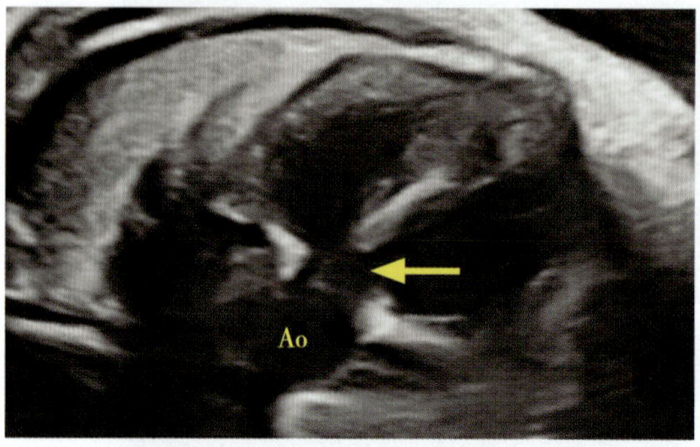

Transverse ultrasound through the fetal heart demonstrates an overriding, dilated aorta (Ao) and a subaortic VSD (arrow).
胎儿心脏横切面超声显示骑跨、扩张的主动脉(Ao)和主动脉下室间隔缺损(黄箭)。

- Tetralogy of Fallot (TOF) is characterized by a VSD, an overriding aorta, and a hypoplastic RVOT. The fourth component of the tetralogy, right ventricular hypertrophy, occurs postnatally.
- Fetal ultrasound shows the aorta overriding both ventricles and a subaortic VSD. The main pulmonary artery is usually small in caliber while the ascending aorta is dilated.

Transposition of the great arteries (TGA)

- Transposition of the great arteries (TGA) has a classic appearance on prenatal ultrasound.
- The ventricular outflow tract views show parallel orientation of the pulmonary trunk and ascending aorta, which normally cross at 90 degrees to each other.
- The three-vessel view shows only two vessels, the aorta and SVC. The 4-chamber view can be normal.
- TGA may or may not have an associated VSD.

- TOF以VSD、主动脉骑跨和RVOT发育不全为特征。四联症的第四个组成部分，即右心室肥厚发生在出生之后。
- 胎儿超声显示主动脉骑跨于两个心室和主动脉下室间隔缺损。肺动脉的主干通常较小，而升主动脉则会扩张。

大动脉转位(TGA)

- 大动脉转位(TGA)在产前超声检查中具有典型的声像表现。
- 心室流出道切面显示肺动脉干和升主动脉呈平行方向，而正常应为90°交叉。
- 三血管切面只显示两条血管，即主动脉和上腔静脉。四腔心切面可为正常。
- TGA不一定合并VSD。

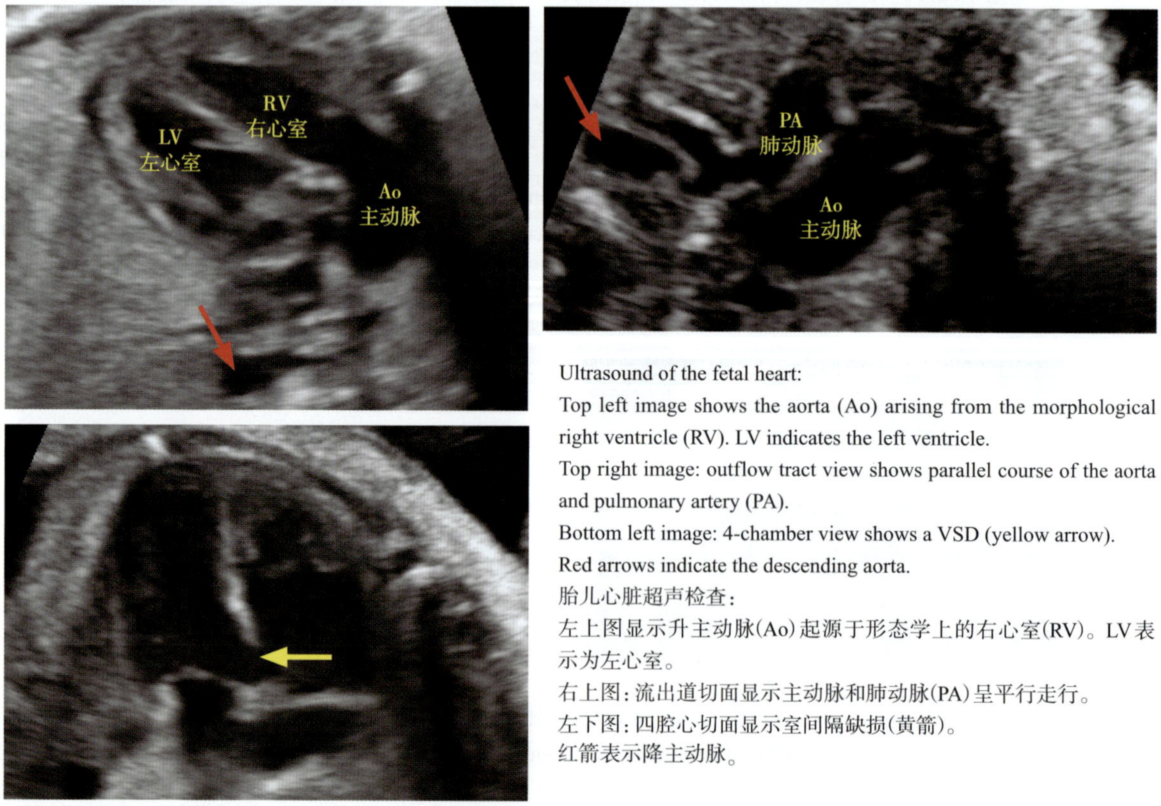

Ultrasound of the fetal heart:
Top left image shows the aorta (Ao) arising from the morphological right ventricle (RV). LV indicates the left ventricle.
Top right image: outflow tract view shows parallel course of the aorta and pulmonary artery (PA).
Bottom left image: 4-chamber view shows a VSD (yellow arrow).
Red arrows indicate the descending aorta.
胎儿心脏超声检查：
左上图显示升主动脉(Ao)起源于形态学上的右心室(RV)。LV表示为左心室。
右上图：流出道切面显示主动脉和肺动脉(PA)呈平行走行。
左下图：四腔心切面显示室间隔缺损(黄箭)。
红箭表示降主动脉。

FETAL ABDOMEN

- Anomalies of the fetal gastrointestinal tract may cause polyhydramnios due to disruption of swallowing or impaired absorption of swallowed amniotic fluid if the anomaly is proximal. The amniotic fluid volume is typically normal in abnormalities of the mid or distal GI tract.

Esophageal atresia

- Esophageal atresia is a blind-ending esophagus, due to incomplete division of the foregut in early embryologic development.
- Esophageal atresia is usually associated with a tracheoesophageal fistula.
- The classic ultrasound findings of esophageal atresia are polyhydramnios and an absent stomach bubble.

Duodenal atresia (DA)

胎儿腹部

- 胎儿近端消化道异常会引起吞咽功能受损或羊水吞咽后吸收障碍，可导致羊水过多。羊水量在中段或远段肠道异常时通常为正常。

食管闭锁

- 食管闭锁是指食管远端为盲端，由胚胎发育早期前肠不全分裂所致。
- 食管闭锁通常合并气管食管瘘。
- 食管闭锁的典型超声表现为羊水过多和胃泡消失。

十二指肠闭锁(DA)

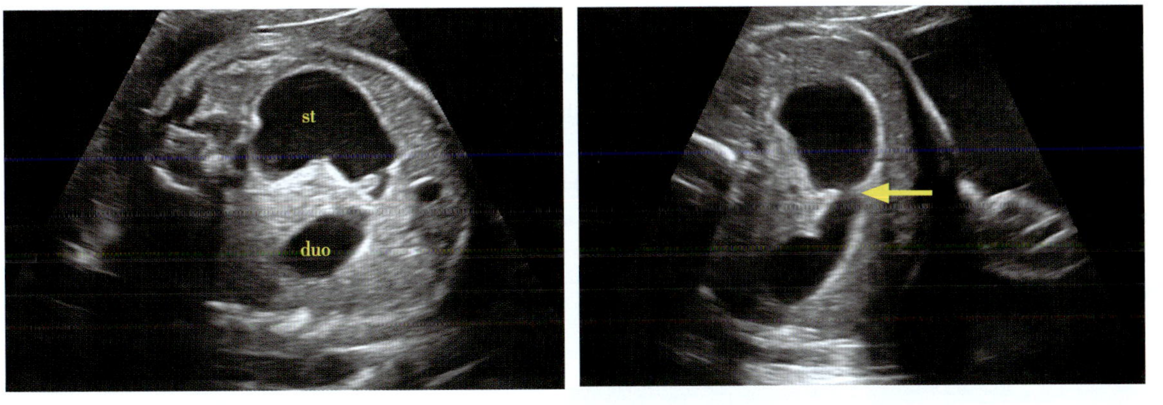

Two transverse ultrasound images through the fetal abdomen (left image) show the dilated stomach (st) and dilated proximal duodenum (duo) representing the double *bubble sign*. The image on the right confirms that these two dilated structures connect (arrow).

Case courtesy Julie Ritner, MD, Brigham and Women's Hospital.

经胎儿腹部横切面超声图像(左图)显示扩张的胃(st)及扩张的十二指肠近端(duo)，为双泡征。右图显示两个扩张的结构相互连通(黄箭)。

- Duodenal atresia (DA) causes duodenal obstruction from lack of recanalization of the duodenal lumen. Duodenal atresia is the most common cause of fetal duodenal obstruction.
- DA has a strong association with Down syndrome. If a *double bubble sign* is seen, a careful screen for additional findings of Down syndrome should be performed (e.g., thorough cardiac exam, nuchal fold if 16–20 weeks, etc).
- The classic appearance of DA is the *double bubble sign*, representing a dilated stomach and dilated proximal duodenum. The differential diagnosis of the double bubble sign includes duodenal web, stenosis, and annular pancreas.

Distal fetal bowel obstruction

- A distal fetal bowel obstruction may be structural or functional.
- Structural causes of distal bowel obstruction include jejunal atresia, ileal atresia, and anorectal malformation.

  Anorectal malformation is commonly associated with additional abnormalities, including the VACTERL association (vertebral, anorectal, cardiac, tracheoesophageal, renal, and limb anomalies).

- Functional bowel obstruction may be due to Hirschsprung disease or meconium ileus.

  Hirschsprung disease results in a functional obstruction due to absent distal enteric ganglion cells.

- 十二指肠闭锁(DA)性肠梗阻是由于十二指肠管腔未出现空泡化而导致的。十二指肠闭锁是胎儿十二指肠梗阻的最常见原因。
- DA与唐氏综合征有很强的关联性。若超声发现双泡征，则应仔细筛查是否有唐氏综合征的其他表现(如全面心脏扫查，在妊娠16~20周时行颈部褶皱检查等)。
- 典型的十二指肠闭锁表现为双泡征，代表扩张的胃和近端十二指肠。双泡征的鉴别诊断包括十二指肠蹼、狭窄和环状胰腺。

胎儿远端肠道梗阻

- 胎儿远端肠道梗阻可为结构性或功能性。
- 肠道远端梗阻的结构性原因包括空肠闭锁、回肠闭锁及直肠肛门畸形。

  直肠肛门畸形通常合并有其他畸形，包括VACTERL综合征[脊柱(V)、直肠肛门(A)、心脏(C)、气管食管(TE)、肾脏(R)和肢体畸形(L)]。

- 功能性梗阻可由先天性巨结肠或胎粪性肠梗阻造成。

  先天性巨结肠是由于远端肠管神经节细胞缺如导致的肠腔功能性梗阻。

Meconium ileus causes obstruction from impaction of meconium in the ileum. Nearly all infants with meconium ileus have cystic fibrosis; however, meconium ileus is rarely identified before the third trimester.

Fetal manifestations of meconium

- **Meconium ileus** is bowel obstruction caused by impacted meconium in a fetus with cystic fibrosis.
- **Meconium peritonitis** is peritoneal inflammation secondary to in utero bowel perforation (due to atresia or unknown cause) and resultant spillage of meconium into the peritoneal cavity. This leads to chemical peritonitis with ascites, peritoneal adhesions and, ultimately, dystrophic calcifications.
- **Meconium pseudocyst** is a cystic abdominal structure, often with peripheral calcification, representing a walled-off bowel perforation. It is a sequela of meconium peritonitis.

Hyperechoic small bowel

- Hyperechoic or echogenic bowel is a nonspecific finding that is associated with Down syndrome, TORCH infection, cystic fibrosis, and swallowing of blood products in the amniotic fluid. It may also be associated with intrauterine growth restriction.
- If the bowel is only mildly echogenic (less echogenic than bone) and no mass effect is present, this appearance may represent a normal variant.

Omphalocele

胎粪性肠梗阻是由于回肠内胎粪嵌顿导致的梗阻。几乎所有患胎粪性肠梗阻的胎儿都有囊性纤维化；但胎粪性肠梗阻极少能在妊娠晚期前被发现。

胎粪在胎儿的表现

- **胎粪性肠梗阻**是患有囊性纤维化的胎儿因胎粪嵌顿所造成的肠梗阻。
- **胎粪性腹膜炎**是指继发于宫内胎儿肠道穿孔(由于闭锁或不明原因)并导致胎粪泄漏进入腹腔所引起的腹膜炎症。这一过程会造成化学性腹膜炎、腹水、腹膜粘连，并最终出现营养不良性钙化。
- **胎粪性假性囊肿**为一种腹腔内囊性结构，周边常伴有钙化，为包裹性的肠道穿孔。这是胎粪性腹膜炎的一个后遗症。

高回声小肠

- 强回声或高回声小肠是一种非特异性表现，与唐氏综合征、TORCH感染、囊性纤维化，以及胎儿吞咽含有血液的羊水相关。它还可能与胎儿宫内生长受限有关。
- 如果肠道仅表现为轻度高回声(比骨骼回声低)，且不伴有肿块压迫效应，则可能属于一种正常变异。

脐膨出

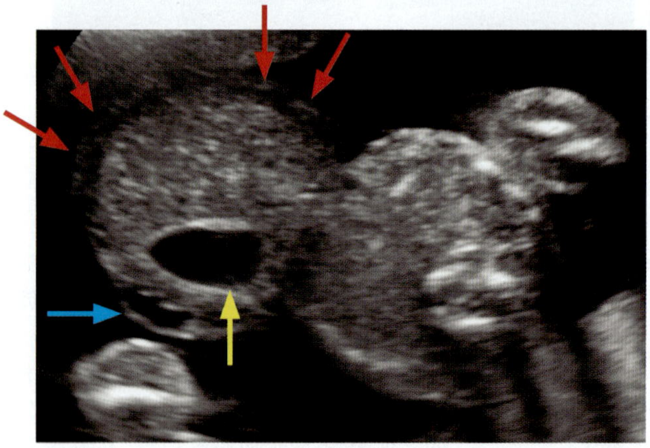

Omphalocele: Transverse ultrasound through the fetal abdomen shows herniation of intra-abdominal content including the stomach (yellow arrow) outside of the anterior abdominal wall, covered by a peritoneal membrane (red arrows). The umbilical cord (blue arrow) inserts onto the herniated sac.

脐膨出：胎儿腹部横切面超声显示腹腔内容物突出于前腹壁，其中包括胃(黄箭)，外层盖有腹膜(红箭)。脐带(蓝箭)终止于膨出的疝囊。

- Omphalocele, the most common anterior abdominal wall defect, is a midline defect with herniation of intra-abdominal contents resulting from disruption of the normal physiologic first trimester bowel herniation process. The herniated bowel is covered by a peritoneal membrane.
- The key to differentiate omphalocele from gastroschisis is the umbilical cord insertion site. In omphalocele, the umbilical cord inserts *centrally* at the base of the herniated sac.
- When small, omphaloceles may contain only bowel. Larger omphaloceles may also contain liver. The presence of liver in the omphalocele carries a better prognosis.
- Omphalocele is associated with other anomalies in 50–75% of cases, including cardiac anomalies, trisomies, and Beckwith-Wiedemann syndrome (a congenital overgrowth syndrome characterized by omphalocele, macroglossia, hemihypertrophy, and visceromegaly). Associated anomalies and aneuploidy are more likely if liver is not involved.

- 脐膨出是最常见的前腹壁缺损，是一种伴有腹腔内容物疝出的中线缺损，原因是早期妊娠中生理性肠扭转过程被中断。膨出的肠管被腹膜覆盖。
- 鉴别脐膨出与腹裂的关键是脐带附着的位置，脐膨出者脐带集中附着于膨出基底部的中央。
- 小的脐膨出可能只含有肠道，大的脐膨出可能还包括有肝脏。膨出物中包含肝脏者预后可能更好。
- 50%~75%的脐膨出病例合并其他异常，包括心脏异常、三倍体和贝-维综合征(一种先天性过度生长综合征，以脐膨出、巨舌症、半侧肥大、内脏巨大为特征)。如果不涉及肝脏，伴发相关异常和整倍体异常的可能性更大。

Gastroschisis

腹裂畸形

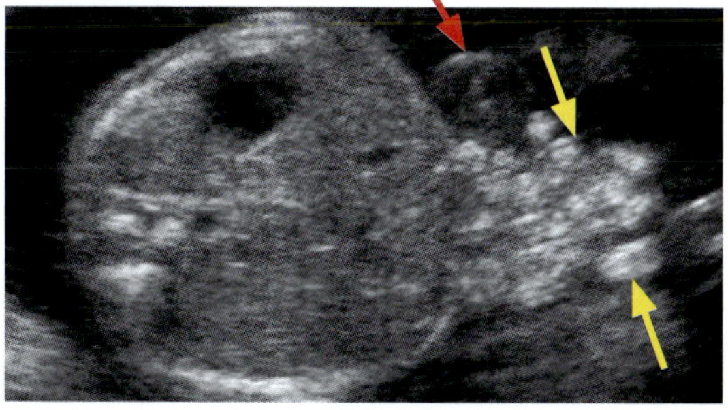

Gastroschisis: Transverse ultrasound through the fetal abdomen shows loops of bowel herniating outside of the anterior abdominal wall (yellow arrows), lateral to the normal midline cord insertion (red arrow). The bowel loops have a lobulated contour because there is no peritoneal covering.

腹裂畸形：经胎儿腹部横切面超声显示肠管从前腹壁(黄箭)疝出，脐带终止于正常中线的外侧(红箭)。肠袢因无腹膜覆盖而呈分叶状。

- Gastroschisis is a paraumbilical (usually right-sided) anterior abdominal wall defect, through which bowel herniates without a peritoneal covering. Gastroschisis is the second most common abdominal wall defect.
- Unlike omphalocele, gastroschisis is usually seen as an isolated anomaly.
- Gastroschisis is seen more commonly in very young (teenage) mothers and smokers, possibly related to a vascular insult.
- Prognosis is dependent on the degree of bowel injury.

Pentalogy of Cantrell

- Pentalogy of Cantrell is a rare disorder consisting of ectopia cordis (extra-thoracic heart), omphalocele, diaphragmatic defect, pericardial defect, and disruption of the sternum.

- 腹裂畸形是指脐旁腹前壁(常为右侧)缺损，肠管经此缺损疝出，无腹膜覆盖。腹裂畸形是第二常见的腹壁缺损。
- 与脐膨出不同，腹裂畸形多为孤立性异常。
- 腹裂畸形常见于非常年轻(青少年)的孕妇和吸烟者，可能与血管损伤有关。
- 预后取决于肠道损伤的程度。

坎特雷尔五联症

- 坎特雷尔五联症是一组罕见的畸形，包括心脏异位(胸外心)、脐膨出、膈肌缺损、心包缺损和胸骨异常。

Fetal Genitourinary

- Although oligohydramnios may be due to many causes, the complete genitourinary (GU) tract (kidneys, ureters, bladder, and urethra) should be carefully evaluated in every fetus with oligohydramnios.
- Oligohydramnios due to a fetal GU malformation can be divided into three categories:
  - Fetal hydronephrosis (obstructive uropathy).
  - Cystic renal disease.
  - Bilateral renal agenesis.
- If the fetal bladder is not visualized (an empty bladder is not visible on ultrasound) the cause of oligohydramnios is likely a renal anomaly, such as:
  - Bilateral multicystic dysplastic kidneys.
  - Bilateral renal agenesis.
  - Autosomal recessive polycystic kidney disease (ARPKD).
- Normal fetal kidneys grow approximately 1 mm per week of gestation. For instance, a 20-week fetus should have kidneys approximately 2 cm in length.

Fetal hydronephrosis overview

胎儿泌尿生殖系统

- 羊水过少的原因有很多，但发现有羊水过少时应全面检查每个胎儿的泌尿生殖道(包括肾脏、输尿管、膀胱和尿道)。
- 由胎儿泌尿生殖系统畸形引起的羊水过少可分为3类：
  - 胎儿肾盂积水(梗阻性尿路疾病)。
  - 囊性肾病。
  - 双侧肾脏发育不良。
- 若看不到胎儿膀胱(超声看不到无尿液的膀胱)，羊水过少的原因可能是肾脏异常，如：
  - 双侧多囊性肾发育不良。
  - 双侧肾缺如。
  - 常染色体隐性遗传多囊肾病(ARPKD)。
- 正常胎儿肾脏每周生长约1mm。例如，妊娠20周时胎儿肾脏长约2cm。

胎儿肾积水概述

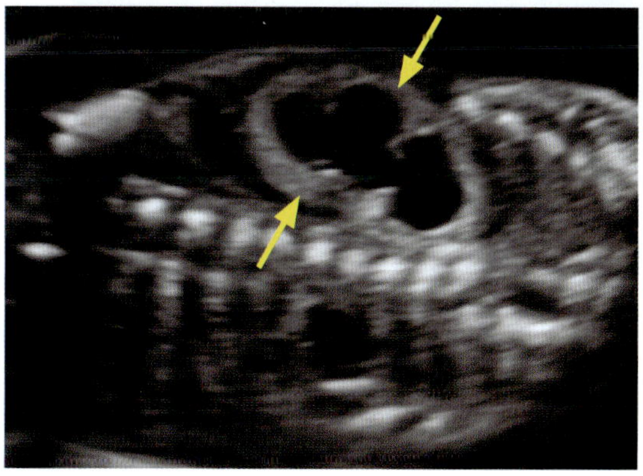

Coronal fetal ultrasound shows bilateral hydronephrosis, severe on the right (arrows). This fetus has trisomy 18, which is associated with hydronephrosis.

Case courtesy Beryl Benacerraf, MD, Diagnostic Ultrasound Associates, Boston.

胎儿冠状切面超声显示双侧肾盂积水，右侧更严重(黄箭)。此胎儿为18-三体综合征，合并肾盂积水。

- Screening for fetal hydronephrosis is routinely performed to evaluate for potentially treatable causes, such as obstruction or reflux, which may lead to progressive childhood kidney damage if undiagnosed.
- The anterior-posterior renal pelvis diameter (APRPD) is measured to assess for hydronephrosis. The accepted range of normal depends on gestational age. Less than 4 mm is always normal.
- Below is the 2014 consensus on classification of prenatal urinary tract dilation (UTD classification system):

> **Normal:** APRPD <4 mm less than 28 weeks; <7 mm at or after 28 weeks.
> **Possibly abnormal:** 4 to <7 mm less than 28 weeks; 7 to <10 mm at or after 28 weeks.
> **Abnormal**:** ≥7 mm less than 28 weeks; ≥10 mm at or after 28 weeks.
> **Any of the following is also considered **abnormal**, independent of the APRPD: peripheral calyceal dilation, abnormal renal parenchymal thickness or appearance, dilated ureter, abnormal bladder, oligohydramnios thought to be due to an urinary cause. These features should be assessed in every fetus.

- Hydronephrosis, hydroureter, and a **normal bladder** may be due to distal ureteral obstruction or reflux.

  Distal ureteral obstruction from **ectopic insertion of the ureter** into the bladder is often associated with the upper pole moiety of a duplicated collecting system. The most common ectopic insertion of an upper pole moiety is inferior and medial to the normally inserting lower pole ureter.

  A **ureterocele** is dilation of the intramural portion of the ureter, which balloons out into the bladder and causes a functional obstruction at the ureterovesicular junction. Ureterocele is also associated with ectopic insertion of the upper pole moiety of a duplicated system.

  Although not a physical obstruction, severe **vesicoureteral reflux** may cause hydronephrosis and hydroureter, but the bladder remains normal.
- Bladder outlet obstruction leads to hydronephrosis, hydroureter, and a **dilated bladder.**

  Posterior urethral valves are by far the most common cause of bladder outlet obstruction.

  Urethral atresia is a rare cause of bladder outlet obstruction.
- Hydronephrosis can lead to cystic renal dysplasia (increased echogenicity and cortical thinning), a sign of irreversible renal damage.

Posterior urethral valves

- 应常规进行超声筛查确认有无肾积水，以发现潜在可治疗的病因(如梗阻或反流)，若这些情况没有得到诊断，它们都可能使患儿的肾功能进一步受到损害。
- 评估肾盂积水应测量肾盂前后径(APRPD)，正常范围随孕周而不同，只要小于4mm均为正常。
- 以下是2014年产前尿路扩张分类的共识(UTD分类系统)：

> **正常：**妊娠28周内，APRPD<4mm；妊娠28周后，APRPD<7mm。
> **可疑异常：**妊娠28周内，APRPD 为4~< 7mm；妊娠28周后，APRPD 为7~<10 mm。
> **异常**：**妊娠28周内，APRPD≥7 mm；妊娠28周后，APRPD≥10 mm。
> **除APRPD外，以下任何一种情况也被认为是**异常**：外周肾盏扩张、肾实质厚度或外观异常、输尿管扩张、膀胱异常、尿路原因引起的羊水过少。应对每个胎儿的这些特征进行评估。

- 若发现肾盂积水和输尿管积水，但**膀胱正常**，则可能是由于输尿管远端梗阻或反流所致。

  因**输尿管异位插入**膀胱导致的输尿管远端梗阻常发生在重复集合系统的上极。上极部分最常见的异位插入点位于正常下极输尿管插入点的内下方。

  输尿管膨出是指输尿管内壁向膀胱呈球状膨出，导致输尿管膀胱连接处功能性梗阻。输尿管膨出也与重复肾上极异位插入有关。

  尽管是非机械性梗阻，严重的膀胱输尿管反流可致肾积水和输尿管积水，但膀胱正常。
- 膀胱出口梗阻导致肾盂积水、输尿管积水和**膀胱扩张**。

  后尿道瓣膜是导致膀胱出口梗阻最为常见的病因。

  尿道闭锁导致膀胱出口梗阻的情况较为罕见。
- 肾盂积水可导致囊性肾发育不良(回声增强和皮质变薄)，是一个不可逆性肾损害的标志。

后尿道瓣膜

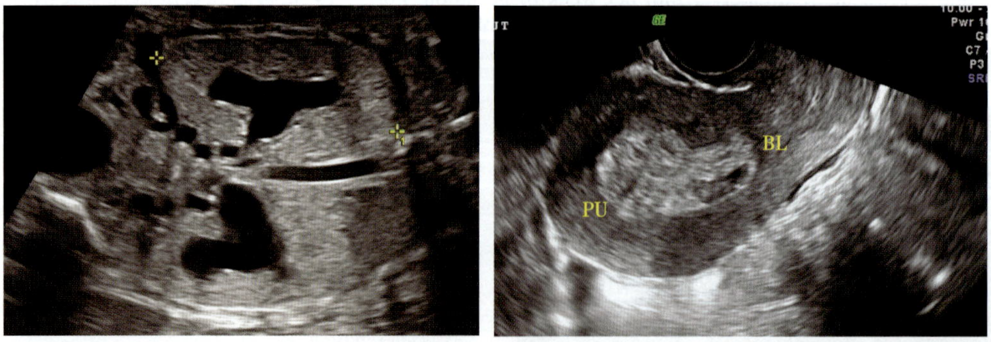

Coronal ultrasound through the fetal abdomen (left image) demonstrates bilateral hydronephrosis. Transverse ultrasound through the fetal pelvis (right image) shows dilated bladder (BL) and posterior urethra (PU) in a *keyhole* morphology. There is associated severe oligohydramnios (not shown).
胎儿腹部冠状切面超声检查(左图)显示双侧肾盂积水。经胎儿骨盆横切面超声(右图)显示膀胱(BL)和后尿道(PU)扩张呈锁孔形态。伴有严重羊水过少(未展示)。

- Posterior urethral valves are congenital obstructions of the posterior urethra due to a membranous flap in male fetuses.
- Ultrasound findings show severe dilation of the posterior urethra resulting in the *keyhole sign*. The bladder is typically enlarged and thickened. Bilateral severe hydroureteronephrosis and oligohydramnios are usually present.

- 后尿道瓣膜是男性胎儿由膜性皮瓣引起的先天性后尿道阻塞。
- 超声检查显示后尿道严重扩张，导致锁孔征。膀胱通常会增大且有膀胱壁增厚。通常有双侧严重输尿管肾盂积水和羊水过少。

Autosomal recessive polycystic kidney disease (ARPKD)

常染色体隐性遗传多囊肾病(ARPKD)

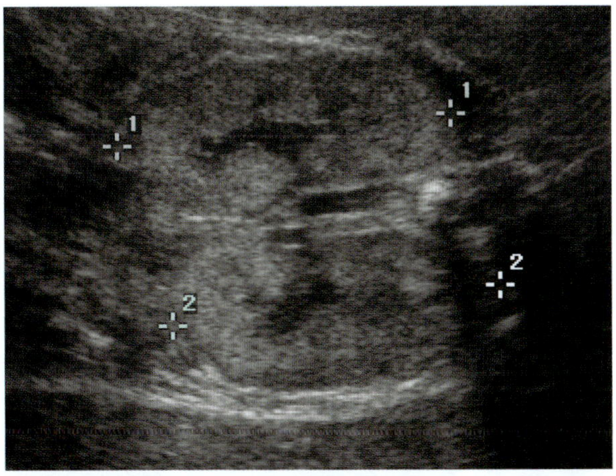

Transverse ultrasound through the fetal abdomen at the level of the kidneys shows massively enlarged and echogenic kidneys (calipers).
There is complete absence of surrounding amniotic fluid, consistent with severe oligohydramnios (not shown).
经胎儿腹部横切面超声显示肾脏巨型增大且回声增强(卡尺)。
周围的羊水完全缺失，符合严重羊水过少的表现(未展示)。

- Autosomal recessive polycystic kidney disease (ARPKD) is a congenital disorder of diffuse collecting tubule dilation, leading to innumerable tiny renal cysts which are too small to be resolved by sonography.
- Ultrasound findings include very large and echogenic kidneys and severe oligohydramnios, caused by markedly reduced renal function.
- Prognosis is poor. ARPKD is associated with pulmonary hypoplasia and Potter's syndrome in utero, and with hepatic fibrosis if the baby survives infancy.

- 常染色体隐性遗传多囊性肾病(ARPKD)是一种集合小管弥漫性扩张的先天性疾病，导致肾脏无数细小囊肿，但因囊肿过小超声无法分辨。
- 超声表现包括肾脏显著增大且回声增强，以及严重羊水过少，此为肾功显著降低所致。
- ARPKD预后差，它与宫内肺发育不良和波特综合征有关。若能存活到婴儿期，将合并肝纤维化。

Multicystic dysplastic kidney (MCDK)

多囊性肾发育不良(MCDK)

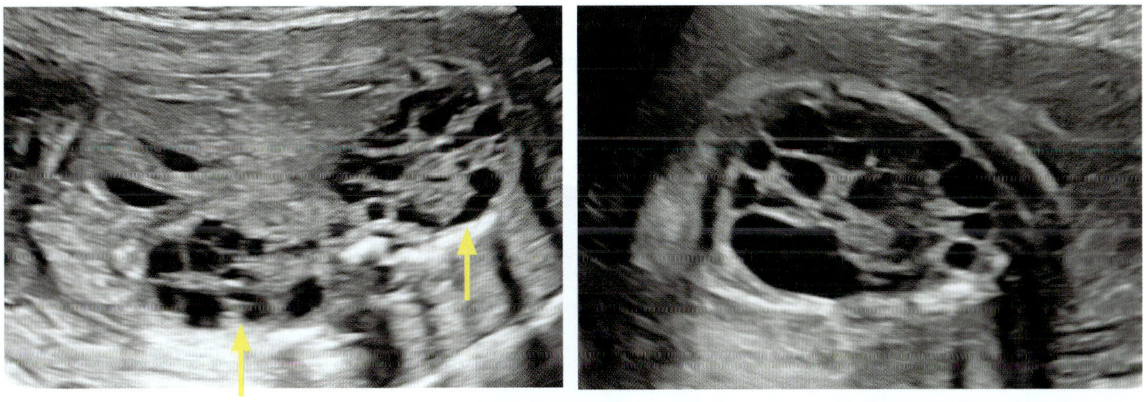

Transverse ultrasound through the fetal abdomen (left image) demonstrates bilateral enlarged and echogenic kidneys with multiple non-communicating cysts (arrows). On the right is a sagittal image of one of the kidneys.
经胎儿腹部横切面超声(左图)显示双侧肾脏增大和回声增强，并伴有多个非交通性囊肿(黄箭)。右图是其中一个肾脏的矢状切面图像。

- Multicystic dysplastic kidney (MCDK) is thought to be the end result of fetal obstructive uropathy.
- If MCDK is unilateral and there are no associated abnormalities, the prognosis is excellent. MCDK is fatal if bilateral, however.

- 多囊肾发育不良(MCDK)可能是胎儿梗阻性尿路疾病的最终结果。
- 若MCDK为单侧，且无其他相关异常，则预后很好。但双侧MCDK是致命的。

- MCDK may affect only the upper pole of an obstructed duplicated system.
- On imaging, multiple *non-communicating* cysts are interspersed with dysplastic renal parenchyma. In contrast to hydronephrosis, the cysts of MCDK do not connect to the collecting system.
- The natural history of MCDK is gradual involution which can occur pre- or post-natally.

- MCDK可只累及重复肾的上极部分。
- 超声表现为多个互不相连的囊肿分布于发育不良的肾实质内。与肾盂积水不同，这些囊肿不与集合系统相连。
- MCDK的自然进程是逐渐消退，可发生在产前或产后。

Fetal Musculoskeletal Imaging

胎儿肌肉骨骼影像

Clubfoot

足内翻畸形

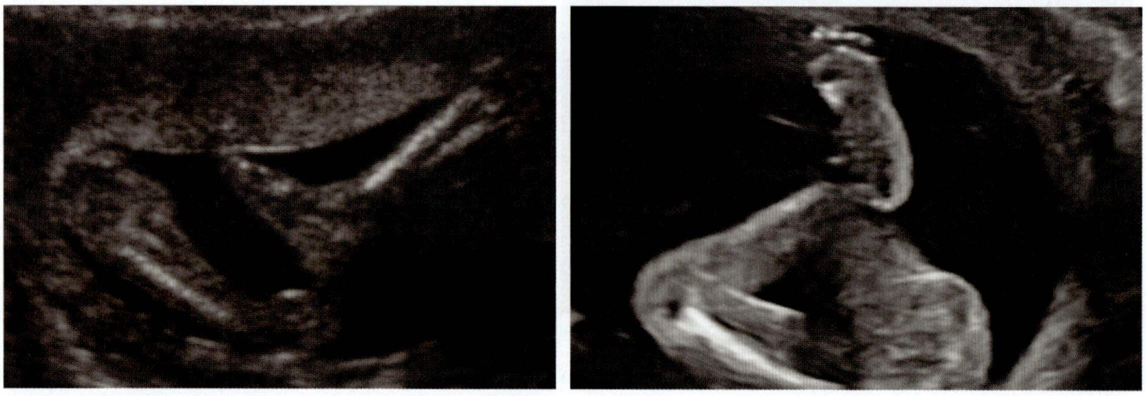

Left image shows normal foot-ankle relationship on grayscale ultrasound. Right image demonstrates a plantar flexed right foot with the sole seen at the same plane as the lower leg, consistent with clubfoot.
左图为足-踝在灰阶超声上的正常关系。右图显示右足跖屈，足底与小腿在同一平面，为足内翻。

- The ankle-foot relationship should be assessed in every fetus.
- Clubfoot (talipes equinovarus) is a congenital deformity of the ankle and foot in which the foot is fixed in plantar flexion, with the forefoot adducted and heel inverted.
- Clubfoot may be isolated or part of a syndrome. The presence of other structural abnormalities in a fetus with clubfoot warrants workup for an underlying genetic disorder.
- On ultrasound, the plantar surface of the foot is seen in the same plane as tibia and fibula.

- 每个胎儿都应该评估足-踝关系。
- 足内翻(马蹄内翻足)是一种先天性的踝关节和足部畸形，其特点是足跖屈固定，前脚掌内收，足跟内翻。
- 马蹄内翻足可能是孤立的，也可能是某一综合征的一部分。畸形足胎儿可能存在其他结构异常，需要检查潜在的遗传性疾病。
- 超声显示足底与胫骨、腓骨在同一平面。

Osteogenesis imperfecta (OI)

成骨不全症(OI)

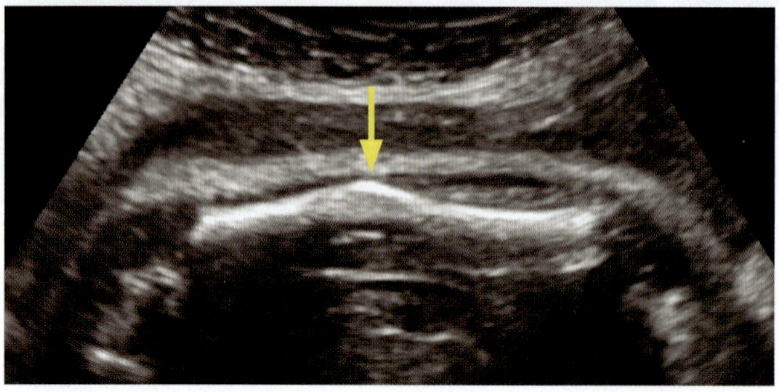

Osteogenesis imperfecta (non-fatal type): Third-trimester fetal survey shows an abnormal kinking (arrow) of the femur from prior in utero fracture. *Case courtesy Julie Ritner, MD, Brigham and Women's Hospital.*
成骨不全症(非致死型)：妊娠晚期胎儿检查显示股骨异常扭曲(黄箭)，为先前宫内骨折。

- Osteogenesis imperfecta (OI) is a spectrum of congenital bone anomalies characterized by multiple fractures due to abnormal type Ⅰ collagen. There are several types of OI, with type 2 being lethal. Type 2 can be diagnosed in the second trimester, but types 1, 3, and 4 are not typically diagnosed until the third trimester.

- 成骨不全症(OI)包括一系列先天性骨异常，以多发性骨折为特征，由1型胶原蛋白异常所致。有数种OI分类，其中2型为致死性。在妊娠中期可以诊断2型，但1型、3型和4型一般要到妊娠晚期才能诊断。

- OI causes severe shortening of the long bones (<3 SD below the mean). The long bones and ribs appear "wrinkled" due to multiple fractures. The thorax is usually small due to broken and structurally soft ribs.
- Unlike thanatophoric dysplasia, bony mineralization is decreased. Decreased calvarial mineralization causes the entire brain (including the nearfield) to be unusually well visualized.

Thanatophoric dysplasia

- Thanatophoric dysplasia is a lethal skeletal dysplasia with characteristic *telephone receiver* femurs, severe limb shortening and bowing, and rib shortening.
- Platyspondyly is characteristic, which is flattening of the ossified portions of the vertebral bodies.
- The classic *cloverleaf skull* is caused by protrusion of the frontal and temporal lobes.
- Bony mineralization is normal.

TRISOMIES AND SYNDROMES

- Fetal anomalies often occur in associations. For instance, omphalocele may be a *sentinel* finding that signifies the presence of trisomy 13, 18, or Beckwith-Wiedemann syndrome. If a sentinel finding is seen, a careful search should be performed for associated anomalies seen in trisomies and syndromes.

Trisomy 13 from head to toe

trisomy 13

- IUGR.
- Holoprosencephaly and midline facial anomalies (cleft lip and cyclops).
- Encephalocele.
- Congenital heart disease.
- Omphalocele.
- Horseshoe kidney.
- Polycystic kidneys.
- Polydactyly.

Trisomy 18 from head to toe

trisomy 18

- IUGR, especially in combination with polyhydramnios
- *Strawberry sign:* Inward bowing of the frontal bones creates a strawberry shape to the calvarium, with the tip of the strawberry projected anteriorly.
- Choroid plexus cysts.
- Micrognathia.
- Cardiac anomalies.
- Omphalocele.
- Congenital diaphragmatic hernia.
- Horseshoe kidney.
- Hydronephrosis.
- Clenched hand that never opens, with overlapping fingers.
- Rocker bott om feet.

- OI可导致长骨严重缩短(低于平均值3*SD*以上)。由于多发骨折,长骨和肋骨会出现"皱褶"样改变。由于肋骨骨折和软化,胸腔通常狭小。
- 与致死性侏儒不同,OI的骨钙化减少。由于颅骨钙化减少,导致整个大脑(包括近场)异常清晰可见。

致死性侏儒

- 致死性侏儒是一种致死性的骨发育不良,其特征有股骨呈电话听筒状、肢体严重缩短和弯曲,以及肋骨变短。
- 椎体扁平具有特征性,为椎体骨化部分呈扁平状。
- 典型的三叶草头颅是由于颅骨的额叶和颞叶突出所致。
- 骨的钙化正常。

三倍体畸形和综合征

- 胎儿畸形常出现关联性异常。例如,脐膨出可能是一种预警性的发现,意味着可能存在13-三体、18-三体或贝-维综合征。如果看到预警性的表现,需仔细寻找与三倍体畸形和综合征相关的异常。

13-三体的所有表现

13-三体

- 宫内发育迟缓(IUGR)。
- 全前脑畸形和面部中线畸形(唇腭裂和独眼畸形)。
- 脑膨出。
- 先天性心脏病。
- 脐膨出。
- 马蹄肾。
- 多囊肾。
- 多指畸形。

18-三体的所有表现

18-三体

- 宫内发育迟缓,尤其合并羊水过多。
- 草莓征:额骨内陷,形成尖端朝前的草莓样颅骨。
- 脉络丛囊肿。
- 面部唇裂和腭裂。
- 小颌畸形。
- 心脏畸形。
- 脐膨出。
- 先天性膈疝。
- 马蹄肾。
- 肾盂积水。
- 手掌紧握无法松开及重叠指。
- 摇篮底样足。

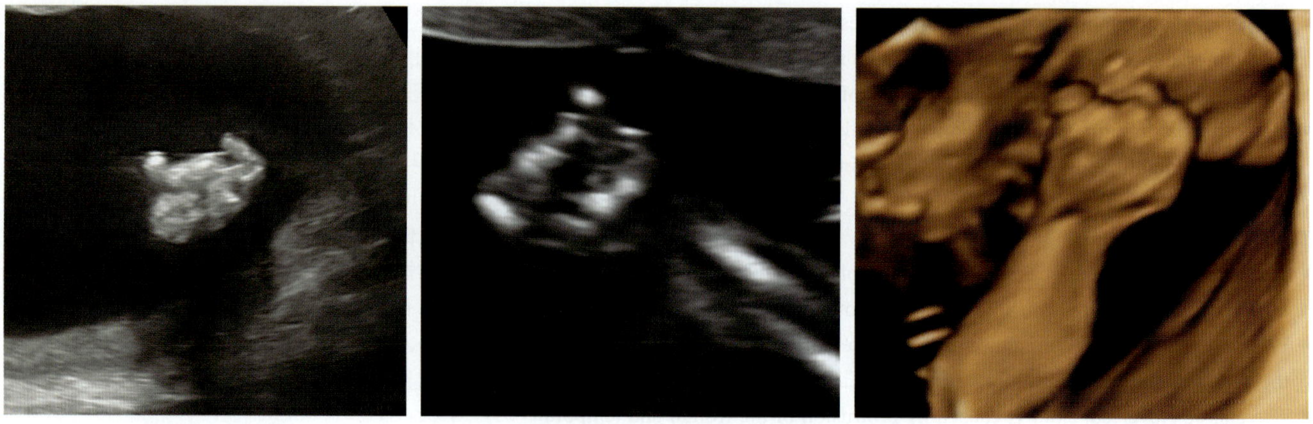

Left image: Clenched hand with overlapping fingers of a fetus with known trisomy 18. Ultrasound also showed severe IUGR and polyhydramnios.
Middle and right images: Clenched hand of a different fetus on grayscale ultrasound and 3D rendering.
左图：已知为18-三体胎儿的紧握手和重叠指。超声检查也发现有严重的IUGR和羊水过多。
中间和右侧图像：另一名胎儿握拳手的灰阶超声和三维超声表现。

Trisomy 21 (Down syndrome) from head to toe

trisomy 21

- *Increase in* **nuchal fold** *(>6 mm), measured between weeks 15 and 21, is the single most sensitive and specific ultrasound finding for trisomy 21.*
- *In contrast,* **nuchal translucency** *is measured earlier in the pregnancy (11–14) weeks, and is less specific for trisomy 21.*
- Absent/hypoplastic ossification of nasal bone.
- Cystic hygroma (although more common in Turner syndrome).
- Congenital heart disease: in particular VSD, endocardial cushion defect, and TOF.
- Echogenic intracardiac focus.
- Echogenic bowel.
- Duodenal atresia.
- Urinary tract dilatation.
- Shortened femur and humerus.
- Clinodactyly.
- Hypoplasia of the middle phalanx of the little finger.
- Sandal gap toes.

VACTERL

- VACTERL is a nonrandom association of multiple structural anomalies listed below.

VACTERL

- Vertebral segmentation anomalies.
- Anal atresia.
- Congenital heart disease, most commonly VSD.
- Tracheoesophageal fistula.
- Esophageal atresia.
- Renal anomalies.
- Limb defects, including radial ray malformation.

Beckwith-Wiedemann syndrome (BWS)

- Beckwith-Wiedemann syndrome (BWS) is a syndrome of overgrowth that carries an increased risk of childhood cancers. BWS is mostly sporadic, but 10–15% of cases follow an autosomal dominant inheritance.

21-三体(唐氏综合征)的所有表现

21-三体

- 颈后皮肤**皱褶**增厚(>6mm)，妊娠15~21周测量，为单项超声诊断21-三体最具灵敏度和特异度的征象。
- 相比之下，**颈部透明层**在妊娠早期(11~14周)进行测量，对于21-三体的特异性较低。
- 鼻骨骨化缺失/发育不良。
- 囊状水囊瘤(特纳综合征中更常见)。
- 先天性心脏病：尤其是室间隔缺损、心内膜垫缺损和法洛四联症。
- 心内局部回声增高。
- 肠管回声增高。
- 十二指肠闭锁。
- 尿路扩张。
- 股骨和肱骨缩短。
- 手指弯曲变形。
- 小指中节指骨发育不良。
- “凉鞋样”脚趾间隙增宽。

VACTERAL综合征

- VACTERAL综合征与下列多个结构异常有非随机关联。

VACTERAL

- 椎体分节异常。
- 肛门闭锁。
- 先天性心脏病，最常见的为VSD。
- 气管食管瘘。
- 食管闭锁。
- 肾异常。
- 肢体缺陷，包括桡骨畸形。

贝-维综合征(BWS)

- 贝-维综合征(BWS)为一种机体过度生长的综合征，可增加儿童肿瘤的风险。绝大多数为散发，但也有10%~15%的病例为常染色体显性遗传。

Beckwith-Wiedemann	
	• BWS increases the risk of developing Wilms tumor (the most common tumor in BWS), hepatoblastoma, and other childhood tumors. The standard of care is screening with abdominal ultrasound every three months until age 8. • Hemihypertrophy, organomegaly. • Macroglossia. • Omphalocele. • Perinatal hypoglycemia.

贝-维综合征	
	• BWS会增加儿童患肾母细胞瘤(BWS中最常见的肿瘤)、肝母细胞瘤和其他肿瘤的风险。标准的处理方法是每3个月进行一次腹部超声扫查，直至8岁。 • 偏侧肥大，器官巨大症。 • 巨舌症。 • 脐膨出。 • 围产期低血糖。

Meckel-Gruber

• Meckel-Gruber is an autosomal recessive multiorgan syndrome.

梅克尔-格鲁贝尔综合征

• 梅克尔-格鲁贝尔综合征是一种常染色体隐性遗传性多器官畸形综合征。

Meckel-Grubrer	
	• Encephalocele. • Polydactyly. • Renal dysplasia causing multiple tiny renal cysts, which appear as echogenic kidneys, analogous to ARPKD. • Severe oligohydramnios, which may hinder identification of the encephalocele and polydatyly

梅克尔-格鲁贝尔综合征	
	• 脑膨出。 • 多指畸形。 • 肾发育不良导致肾脏多发细小囊肿，表现为肾脏回声增高，类似于ARPKD。 • 严重羊水过少，这可能妨碍脑膨出和多指畸形的检出。

Amniotic band syndrome (ABS)/Limb body wall complex (LBWC)

• Fetal malformation in ABS/LBWC is caused by disruption of structures due to loss of amniotic fluid, vascular disruption, or genetic disruption. This spectrum is seen in 1 in 70 spontaneous abortions and 1 in 1300–2000 births.

• Presentation is variable and includes craniofacial defects, body wall defects, and amputation.

羊膜带综合征(ABS)/肢体-体壁综合征(LBWC)

• 羊膜带综合征(ABS)/肢体-体壁综合征(LBWC)中的胎儿畸形是由羊水缺失、血管破坏或基因破坏导致的结构性破坏所致。这一系列的异常在自发性流产胎儿中的发生率为1/70，新生儿中发生率为1/(1 300~2 000)。

• 表现多样，包括颅面缺损、体壁缺损和截肢。

（翻译　吴艳艳）

5 Breast Imaging

Aaron Jen, Ellen X. Sun, Christine M. Denison

Contents

5 乳腺影像

目录

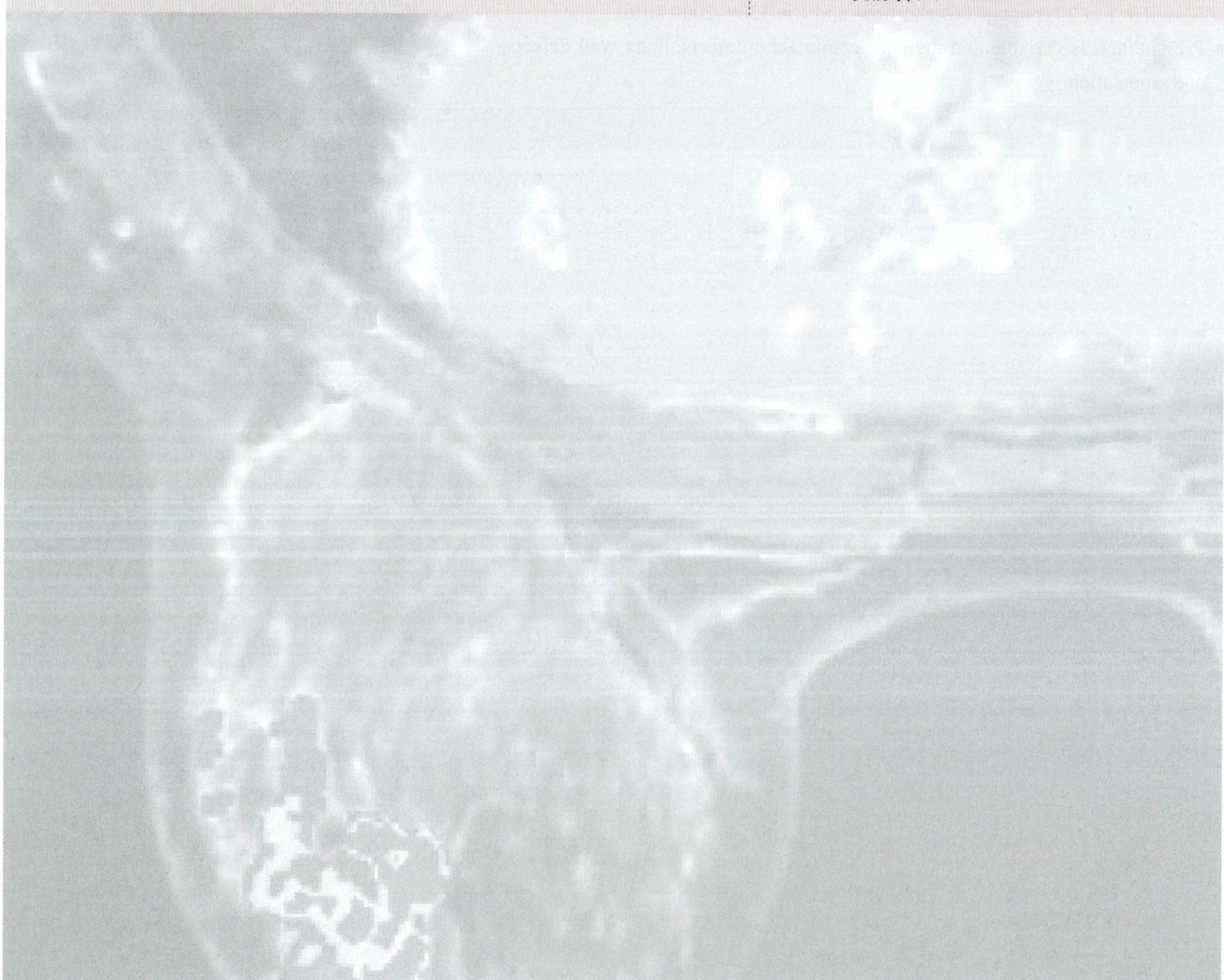

INTRODUCTION TO BREAST CANCER

Key facts and imaging modalities

- Breast cancer is the most common female cancer in the United States. The average woman has a one in eight chance of being diagnosed with breast cancer during her lifetime.
- **Mammography** is the first-line tool for detection of breast cancer. The sensitivity of screening mammography for detecting cancer has been estimated at between 68% and 90%. Diagnostic mammography has a higher sensitivity, up to 93%.

  Digital breast tomosynthesis (DBT) is becoming the standard of care for breast cancer screening and diagnostic imaging. Compared to digital mammography, DBT decreases recall rate and increases cancer detection rate.
- **Ultrasound** is a critical adjunct to diagnostic mammography, and an important tool in further evaluation of symptomatic patients when mammography is negative. Use of whole breast ultrasound as a supplemental screening tool (in addition to mammography) is more controversial; it can detect an additional 2–4 cancers per 1,000 women over mammography alone, but at the cost of increased intervention.

  Indications for breast ultrasound are characterization of palpable abnormalities, further characterization of mammographic findings, first-line evaluation of a breast abnormality in a young (under age 30), pregnant, or lactating woman, guidance for interventional procedures, and evaluation of breast implants. As mentioned above, it is also used in some settings as supplemental screening in women with dense breasts or those at high risk unable to undergo MRI surveillance.
- **MRI** is the most sensitive imaging modality for breast cancer detection and is the most definitive imaging modality in evaluation of implant integrity.

  Indications for breast MRI include screening in high-risk patients (greater than 20% lifetime risk of developing breast cancer), evaluation of extent of disease in a patient newly diagnosed with breast cancer, evaluation of neoadjuvant chemotherapy response, assessment for residual disease after positive surgical margins or for tumor recurrence after breast conserving treatment, evaluation for occult breast cancer in a patient with axillary metastases and for assessment of breast implants.

Pathway of invasive ductal breast cancer progression

- The current understanding of progression of ductal breast cancer is a multi step transformation from normal cells to flat epithelial atypia (FEA), to atypical ductal hyperplasia (ADH), to ductal carcinoma in situ (DCIS), to invasive ductal carcinoma (IDC).

乳腺癌概述

要点与成像方式

- 在美国，乳腺癌是女性最常见的癌症。平均有1/8的女性在她们的一生中可能被诊断为乳腺癌。
- **乳腺X线检查**是检测乳腺癌的首选方法。筛查性乳腺X线检查检测癌症的灵敏度估计为68%~90%。诊断性乳腺X线检查的灵敏度更高，可达93%。

  乳腺数字断层融合摄影(DBT)正在成为乳腺癌筛查和影像诊断的标准方法。与数字乳腺X线摄影相比，DBT可降低召回率并增加癌症的检出率。
- **超声**是诊断性乳腺X线检查的重要辅助手段，对于乳腺X线检查结果为阴性的有症状患者，它是进一步评估的重要工具。对整个乳房进行超声检查作为补充筛查工具(除了乳腺X线)存在很多争议，尽管每1 000名女性在乳腺X线检查后超声可额外检测出2~4例癌症，但同时也增加了干预的代价。

  乳腺超声的适应证包括对可触及的异常进行评估，对乳腺X线检查的发现进行定性，对年轻患者(30岁以下)、孕妇或哺乳期妇女乳腺异常进行初步评估，为介入手术提供引导，以及评估乳腺假体。如上所述，超声在某些情况下也用于对致密型乳腺或无法接受MRI检查的高危女性进行辅助筛查。
- **MRI**是检测乳腺癌最灵敏的影像学方法，也是评估乳腺假体完整性最可靠的方法。

  乳腺MRI的适应证包括筛查高风险患者(终身患乳腺癌的风险超过20%)，评估新诊断乳腺癌患者的病变范围，评估新辅助化疗的反应，评估手术切缘阳性残余病灶或乳腺保守治疗后肿瘤复发，评估有腋窝转移的隐匿性乳腺癌患者，以及评估乳腺假体。

乳腺浸润性导管癌的进展途径

- 目前认为，乳腺导管癌进展有多个步骤，从正常细胞转变为平坦型上皮不典型增生(FEA)、导管不典型增生(ADH)，然后为导管原位癌(DCIS)，直至浸润性导管癌(IDC)。

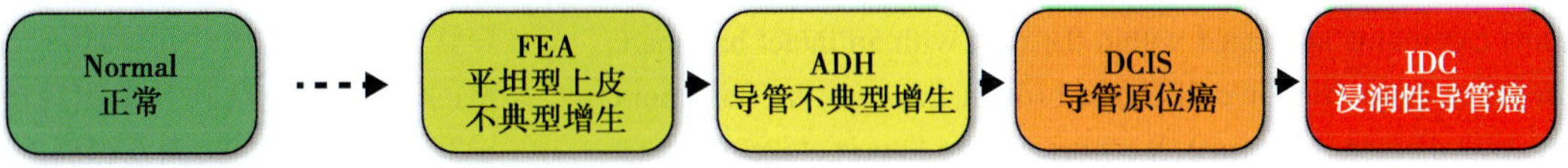

Although controversial, it has been suggested that some steps in this pathway may be reversible.
有人认为该途径中的某些步骤是可逆的，但存在争议。

- **FEA** is a low-grade form of atypia involving the breast acini; it is seen in 3–5% of core needle biopsies and usually presents as grouped amorphous or punctate calcifications.
- **ADH** is a proliferation of intraductal luminal cells and represents a greater degree of atypia, differing from DCIS only in extent or lack of certain architectural features. It is seen in 4–14% of core biopsies and also typically presents as calcifications.
- FEA and ADH are considered non-obligatory precursor lesions, meaning they sometimes, but not always, progress to ductal carcinoma in situ or invasive ductal cancer. Both increase a woman's risk for subsequent breast cancer, FEA, likely 3 times the general population and ADH 4–5 times the general population
- **Upstaging** (or upgrading) refers to the diagnosis of a higher grade malignant lesion (such as DCIS or IDC) following surgical excision than initially diagnosed by core needle biopsy.
- Management of the above high-risk lesions when identified at core needle biopsy is related to the upstage rate. For example, the upstage rate for ADH is relatively high (up to 20%), therefore surgical excision is recommended. The upstage rate for the other entities are still under investigation, and therefore different institutions may recommend excision versus surveillance.

- FEA是侵犯乳腺腺泡的一种低级别不典型增生；见于3%~5%的核芯针穿刺活检，通常表现为团簇状无定形钙化或点状钙化。
- ADH是导管内上皮细胞增殖，更大程度上代表不典型增生，与DCIS的区别仅在于增生的程度或缺乏某些结构特征。可见于4%~14%核芯针穿刺活检，通常也表现为钙化。
- FEA和ADH并非确定性的前驱病变，这意味着它们有时会出现，但并不一定会进展为导管原位癌或浸润性导管癌。两者都会增加女性患乳腺癌的风险，FEA者的风险可能是一般人群的3倍，而ADH者是一般人群的4~5倍。
- **升期**(或升级)是指手术切除后恶性病变(如DCIS或IDC)级别高于最初核芯针穿刺活检的结果。
- 核芯针穿刺活检发现上述高危病变的处理方法与级别上升率相关。如ADH级别上升率相对较高(高达20%)，因此建议手术切除。其他病变的升级率仍在研究之中，因此不同医院可能对上述病变的切除或随访给出不同的建议。

Risk factors for developing breast cancer

乳腺癌的危险因素

- The two most important risk factors for breast cancer are **female sex** and **advancing age**.
- Inherited ***BRCA1*** or ***BRCA2*** **mutation**. Women with an inherited mutationhave greater than50% chance (some believe as high as 80% chance) of developing breast cancer by age 80.
- **First degree relative with breast cancer**. In contrast, a non-first degree relative with postmenopausal breast cancer is not considered an increased risk.
- **Prior chest radiation** for Hodgkin or non-Hodgkin lymphoma.
- **Prior biopsy** result of one of the following **high-risk lesions**:
  Atypical lobular hyperplasia (ALH)
  Lobular carcinoma in situ (LCIS)
  Atypical ductal hyperplasia (ADH)
  Flat epithelial aplasia (FEA)
  Radial scar
  Intraductal papilloma/atypical papilloma
- **Long-term estrogen exposure**, such as early menarche, late menopause, late first pregnancy, nulliparity, or obesity (through increased estrogen production by adipocytes).

- 乳腺癌最重要的两个危险因素是女性**性别**和**年龄增长**。
- 遗传性***BRCA1***或***BRCA2*****基因突变**。具有遗传突变基因的女性到80岁时患乳腺癌的概率为50%(有些人认为高达80%)。
- **一级亲属罹患乳腺癌**。相比之下非一级亲属患绝经后乳腺癌并不增加风险。
- 曾因霍奇金或非霍奇金淋巴瘤接受过**胸部放疗**。
- 曾活检发现**以下任何一种高危病变**：
  小叶不典型增生(ALH)。
  小叶原位癌(LCIS)。
  导管不典型增生(ADH)。
  平坦型上皮不典型增生(FEA)。
  放射状瘢痕。
  导管内乳头状瘤/非典型乳头状瘤。
- **长期雌激素暴露**，如初潮早、绝经晚、高龄初次妊娠、未产或肥胖(脂肪细胞产生过量雌激素)。

Ductal carcinoma in situ (DCIS)

- DCIS represents carcinoma contained within the duct with an intact basement membrane in place (once tumor cells have broken through the basement membrane invasive disease is present). It represents the lowest stage of breast cancer, Stage 0.
- DCIS is the most frequent occult cancer detected mammographically, accounting for approximately 20% of new cancer diagnoses and usually presents mammographically as calcifications. Much less frequently DCIS presents as mammographic asymmetry, mass or architectural distortion. It is most often asymptomatic, but may present as nipple discharge, nipple changes or infrequently as a palpable mass.

导管原位癌(DCIS)

- 导管原位癌(DCIS)指肿瘤位于导管内并有完整的基底膜(一旦肿瘤细胞突破基底膜则为浸润性病变)。它代表乳腺癌的最低级别，即0期。
- DCIS是乳腺X线检查中最常见的隐匿性癌症，约占新诊断病例的20%，且在乳腺X线影像上通常表现为钙化。DCIS很少在乳腺X线影像上表现为不对称、肿块或结构扭曲。DCIS通常是无症状的，但也可能表现为乳头溢液、乳头改变，或偶尔表现为可触及的包块。

- On MRI, a pattern of linear or segmental, clumped enhancement is suspicious for DCIS.
- Pathologically, DCIS is graded as low, intermediate or high grade. High grade DCIS is more likely to progress to invasive disease if not adequately treated.

- 在MRI上，出现线样或节段样分布的成簇强化应怀疑DCIS。
- DCIS在病理学上分为低、中和高级别。高级别DCIS如果不经过适当的治疗更容易进展为浸润性病变。

Invasive ductal carcinoma (IDC)

- Breast cancer is a diverse spectrum of disease with varying histopathology and prognosis.
- The most common subtype of breast cancer is invasive ductal carcinoma (IDC), representing 70–80% of cases. It often presents as a palpable mass, with the classic associated mammographic appearance being an irregular mass with spiculated margins and associated pleomorphic calcifications.
- Basal-type breast carcinoma is a phenotype given to triple (ER, PR, and *HER2/neu*) negative carcinomas due to gene underexpression. This phenotype includes various morphologic types including medullary carcinoma and invasive carcinoma in the setting of *BRCA1* mutation. Although these tumors are usually high grade, basal-like breast carcinomas have been associated with favorable response to neoadjuvant chemotherapy.

浸润性导管癌(IDC)

- 乳腺癌是一类多样化的疾病，其组织病理学和预后有非常大的差异。
- 最常见的乳腺癌亚型是浸润性导管癌(IDC)，占70%~80%。它通常表现为可触及的包块，典型的乳腺X线影像表现为不规则肿块、边缘呈毛刺状，并伴有多形性钙化。
- 基底样乳腺癌是一种呈三阴性(ER、PR和HER2/neu)表型的癌症，为基因表达不足所致。这种表型有多种形态类型，包括*BRCA1*突变基础上的髓样癌和浸润性癌。虽然这些肿瘤通常是高级别的，但基底样乳腺癌对新辅助化疗有良好的反应。(译者注：ER，雌激素受体；PR，孕激素受体；HER2/neu，人类表皮生长因子受体2)

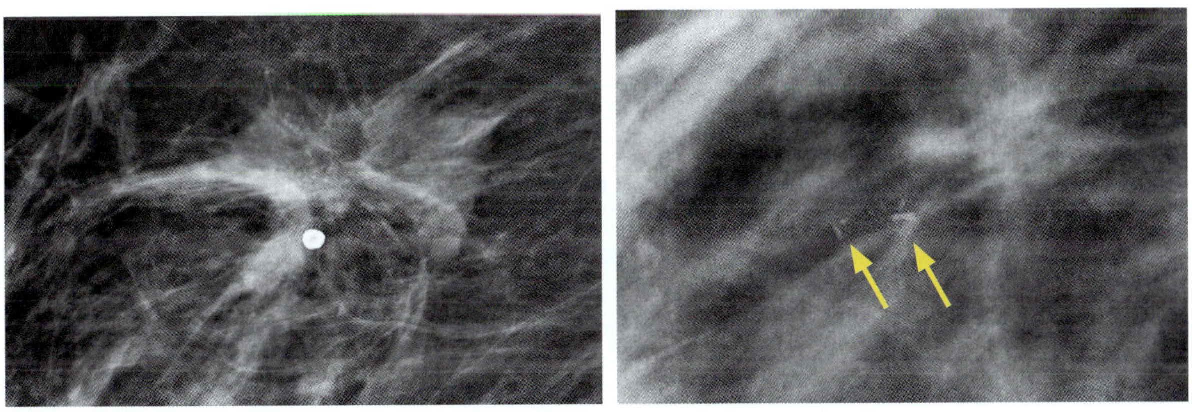

Left mammographic image shows an irregular mass with spiculated margins and associated calcifications (not well seen at this resolution); this was found to be invasive ductal carcinoma. Right mammographic image shows grouped calcifications (arrows) in the same breast at a separate location; biopsy showed DCIS.

左侧乳腺X线影像显示不规则肿块，伴毛刺样边缘和钙化(在此分辨率下不容易看清)；后证实为浸润性导管癌。右侧乳腺X线影像显示同一乳腺不同位置的簇状钙化(黄箭)；活检显示DCIS。

- Combined, a number of less common subtypes make up <10% of all breast cancers. Some of these special subtypes have better prognosis than IDC NOS (not otherwise specified).

- 其他不太常见的亚型在所有乳腺癌中的占比<10%。其中一些特殊亚型的预后优于非特殊型浸润性导管癌(未另作说明)。

special histologic subtypes of IDC with favorable prognosis

- **Tubular carcinoma** is a low-grade cancer that typically presents as architectural distortion or a small spiculated mass and accounts for <2% of invasive ductal cancers.
- **Mucinous carcinoma** (synonyms: colloid carcinoma, mucoid carcinoma, and gelatinous carcinoma) accounts for approximately 2% of breast cancers and is more common in older women. It often presents as a circumscribed mass on mammography. It can show acoustic enhancement on ultrasound and high T2 signal intensity on MRI, features which might cause it to be confused with a benign lesion.
- **Medullary carcinoma** accounts for <5% of breast cancer and is typically seen in younger women, often with *BRCA1* mutation. It frequently presents as a more circumscribed mass on mammography and ultrasound. Despite its classification as a basal-like triple negative breast cancer, medullary carcinoma has a favorable prognosis.
- **Encapsulated papillary carcinoma/solid papillary carcinoma** accounts for <2% of breast cancer and is most common in older women (average onset age 69.5 years). It may present clinically as a palpable mass or nipple discharge. It often appears mammographically as a round or oval mass with predominantly circumscribed margins. Ultrasound shows a complex cystic and solid mass in the setting of encapsulated papillary carcinoma.
- **Adenoid cystic carcinoma** is a variant of adenocarcinoma typically seen in the salivary gland, but very rarely occurs in the breast (<0.1% of all breast cancers). Mammographic appearances can include an irregular mass, distortion or asymmetry.

具有良好预后的IDC特殊组织学亚型

- **小管癌**是一种低级别癌症，通常表现为结构扭曲或小的毛刺状肿块，占浸润性导管癌的比例不到2%。
- **黏液癌**(同义词：胶样癌、黏液样癌和凝胶状癌）约占乳腺癌的2%，在老年女性中更常见。它通常在乳腺X线检查中表现为边界清楚的肿块。超声表现为后方回声增强，MRI检查表现为T_2高信号，这些特征可能会与良性病变混淆。
- **髓样癌**占乳腺癌的比例不到5%，多见于年轻女性，通常有*BRCA1*突变。它在乳腺X线和超声往往表现为边界非常清楚的肿块。尽管被归类为基底样三阴性乳腺癌，但髓样癌预后通常良好。
- **包裹性乳头状癌/实性乳头状癌**占乳腺癌的比例不到2%，最常见于老年女性(平均发病年龄69.5岁）。临床上表现为可触及的肿块或乳头溢液。乳腺X线影像常表现为边界清晰、圆形或椭圆形的肿块。超声显示为一个复杂的囊实性肿块。
- **腺样囊性癌**是腺癌的一种变异型，通常见于唾液腺，在乳腺中非常罕见(在所有乳腺癌中占比<0.1%)。乳腺X线影像表现可能包括不规则肿块、结构扭曲或不对称。

Invasive lobular carcinoma (ILC)

- Invasive lobular carcinoma (ILC) comprises approximately 5–10% of breast cancer cases.
- Compared to invasive ductal carcinoma, invasive lobular is typically much more difficult to diagnose mammographically and clinically due to its tendency to spread through the breast tissue without forming a discrete mass.
- ILC presents an imaging challenge due to its elusive appearance, which ranges from a one- view asymmetry to architectural distortion to a spiculated mass.

浸润性小叶癌(ILC)

- 浸润性小叶癌(ILC)占乳腺癌的5%~10%。
- 与浸润性导管癌相比，ILC通常更难通过乳腺X线检查进行诊断，因为临床上它倾向于随乳腺组织扩散而不形成一个明显的肿块。
- 由于ILC影像学表现多样，因此影像诊断较为困难，它可以表现为单个体位上的不对称、结构扭曲或毛刺状肿块。

Inflammatory carcinoma

- Inflammatory carcinoma is a very aggressive form of breast cancer that represents tumor invasion of dermal lymphatics; it carries a poor prognosis.
- Clinically, inflammatory carcinoma presents with breast erythema, edema, and firmness, often referred to as a *peau d'orange* or orange peel appearance.
- On mammography, the affected breast is larger and denser, with trabecular thickening and skin thickening. Occasionally, no discrete mass will be apparent. The primary differential consideration is mastitis, which can often be differentiated in the clinical setting.

炎性乳腺癌

- 炎性乳腺癌是一种极具侵袭性的乳腺癌，肿瘤侵入真皮淋巴管；预后很差。
- 临床上，炎性乳腺癌表现为乳房红斑、水肿和变硬，通常被称为"*Peau d'orange*"或橘皮样外观。
- 在乳腺X线检查中，患侧乳腺大而致密，伴有小梁和皮肤增厚。偶尔会出现不明确的肿块。初步鉴别诊断应考虑乳腺炎，而这往往可以通过临床表现进行区分。

Paget disease of the nipple

- Paget disease of the nipple is a form of DCIS that infiltrates the epidermis of the nipple.
- Clinically, Paget disease of the nipple presents with erythema, ulceration, and eczematoid changes of the nipple.

乳头佩吉特病

- 乳头佩吉特病是一种浸润乳头表皮的DCIS。
- 佩吉特病在临床上表现为乳头红斑、溃疡和湿疹样改变。

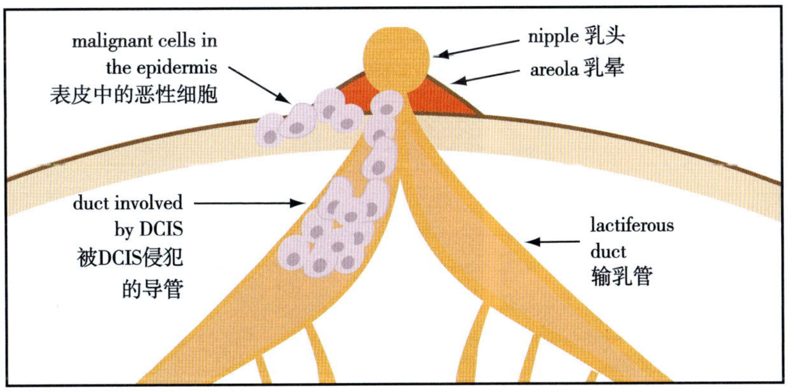

Breast cancer prognosis

- In non-metastatic invasive breast cancer, axillary lymph node status is the most important prognostic factor, with the absence of nodal involvement offering the highest likelihood of cure. Survival is progressively worse with increased number of involved axillary nodes.

  The primary method to detect axillary involvement is a surgical sentinel lymph node biopsy, with a sensitivity of 93%. Sentinel lymph node biopsy is not routinely performed for DCIS unless necrosis or microinvasive disease is present.

  Alternatively, surgical axillary lymph node dissection has a 99% sensitivity for detecting lymph node involvement. Lymph node dissection is performed if the sentinel lymph node is positive or not identified.

  Women with positive lymph nodes or with large tumors may benefit from neoadjuvant chemotherapy.

- The presence of tumor receptors affects prognosis. Patients with estrogen receptor (ER) and progesterone receptor (PR) positive tumors have longer disease-free survival.

  Cancers with *HER2/neu* overexpression may respond to the monoclonal antibody trastuzamab (brand name Herceptin) or tyrosine kinase inhibitors such as lapatinib.

- **Triple-negative** cancers are ER, PR, and *HER2/neu* negative, and the majority are biologically aggressive with poor prognosis. Triple-negative cancers account for the majority of breast cancers in patients with *BRCA1* mutation. On imaging, they may show features more typical of benign lesions despite their aggressive nature.

乳腺癌预后

- 在没有远处转移的浸润性乳腺癌中，腋窝淋巴结是否受累是最重要的预后因素，没有淋巴结受累的治愈可能性最高。随着受累腋窝淋巴结数量增加，患者生存率逐渐降低。

  检测腋窝是否受累的主要方法是前哨淋巴结手术活检，灵敏度为93%。对DCIS不进行常规前哨淋巴结活检，除非有坏死或存在微浸润性病变。

  另外，外科手术腋窝淋巴结清扫检测淋巴结的灵敏度为99%。如果前哨淋巴结阳性或不确定，则应进行淋巴结清扫。

  淋巴结阳性或肿瘤较大的女性可能会受益于新辅助化疗。

- 肿瘤的受体影响预后。雌激素受体(ER)和孕激素受体(PR)阳性的肿瘤患者无肿瘤生存期更长。

  *HER2/neu*过度表达的癌症可能对单克隆抗体曲妥珠单抗(品牌名称赫赛汀)或酪氨酸激酶抑制剂[如拉帕替尼]治疗有反应。

- **三阴性癌症**是指ER、PR和*HER2/neu*均为阴性，大多数生物学上具有侵袭性，预后差。三阴性癌症常见于*BRCA1*突变的患者。影像学上，它们可能具有良性病变的特征，但其在本质上具有侵袭性。

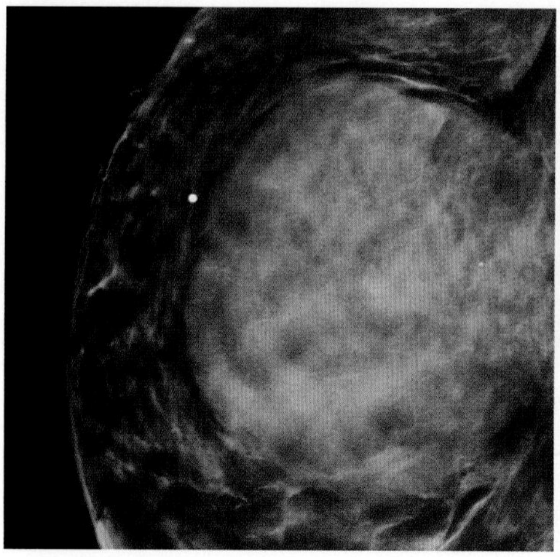

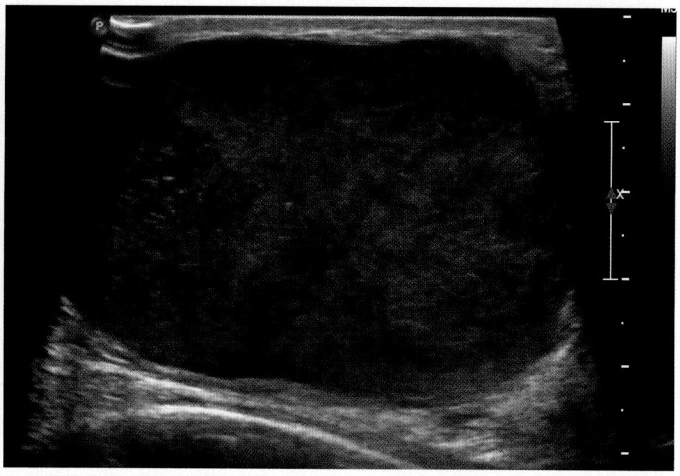

Tomosynthesis (left image) and targeted ultrasound (right image) show a large oval, circumscribed mass with heterogeneous echotexture and posterior acoustic enhancement (not shown). Although these are typically benign mammographic and sonographic features, this mass also demonstrated internal vascularity on Doppler imaging and had rapid growth per patient history, prompting a biopsy which showed triple-negative invasive ductal carcinoma.
断层融合影像(左图)和靶向超声(右图)显示一个大而边界清楚的卵圆形肿块,伴不均匀回声和后方声影增强(未展示)。尽管这是典型的良性病变的乳腺X线和超声特征,但该肿块在多普勒上还显示内部有血管分布且患者有肿块快速增长的病史,后续活检显示为三阴性浸润性导管癌。

(翻译　王维平)

INTRODUCTION TO BI-RADS

Overview

- The breast imaging and reporting data system (BI-RADS) is a system for standardizing mammography, ultrasound, and MRI reports that incorporates a strict lexicon, structured reporting, and clearly defined assessment categories. This text adheres to the terminology of the fifth edition of the BI-RADS atlas, which was released in 2013.
- All mammographic, ultrasound, and breast MRI findings and reports should closely adhere to the BI-RADS lexicon and assessment categories.

Structure of the mammographic report

- 1) History and indication for examination with patient risk factors stated.
- 2) List of comparison studies.
- 3) Description of the overall breast composition, using the following categories:

  The breasts are almost entirely fatty.

  There are scattered areas of fibroglandular density.

  The breasts are heterogeneously dense, which may obscure small masses.

  The breasts are extremely dense, which lowers the sensitivity of mammography.
- 4) A clear description of any significant findings, including location.
- 5) Overall impression, with BI-RADS assessment category and course of action when appropriate.

  Almost always, the course of action will be concordant with the BI-RADs assessment category. However, the fifth edition of BI-RADS allows the course of action to be separated from the assessment category in certain clinical situations. For example, the aspiration of a simple cyst designated as BI-RADS 2 to relieve patient pain. Additionally, a clinically suspected breast abscess or hematoma may be given a designation of BI-RADS 4, with the biopsy deferred for one month pending a repeat diagnostic evaluation.

BI-RADS简介

概述

- 乳腺影像和数据报告系统(BI-RADS)是一个对乳腺X线、超声和MRI报告进行标准化的系统,它采用严格的术语、结构化报告,对评估分类进行明确定义。本文遵循2013年发布的第五版BI-RADS图集的术语。
- 所有的乳腺X线、超声和MRI表现及报告应与BI-RADS术语和评估分类相一致。

乳腺X线影像报告结构

- 1) 描述患者的病史、检查的适应证和危险因素。
- 2) 列出可进行比较的既往检查。
- 3) 描述乳腺的总体构成,使用以下分类:

  乳腺几乎完全为脂肪组织。

  散在纤维腺体组织。

  乳腺密度不均,可掩盖小的肿块。

  乳腺极度致密,降低乳腺X线检查的灵敏度。
- 4) 任何重要发现都需要描述清楚,包括位置。
- 5) 总体印象,BI-RADS评估分类和在适当时机采取的干预措施。

  必须牢记,所采取的干预措施需要与BI-RADS评估类别一致。但是,第五版BI-RADS允许在某些临床情况下干预措施与评估分类不一致。例如,对一个BI-RADS 2类的单纯囊肿进行抽吸以减轻患者的疼痛。此外,临床怀疑的乳腺脓肿或血肿可能被评为BI-RADS 4类,活检推迟1个月等待重复诊断评估。

BI-RADS ASSESSMENT CATEGORIES

Category 0: Need additional imaging

- Additional imaging evaluation (such as spot compression, magnification, special mammographic views, or ultrasound) and/or prior mammograms are necessary before a final assessment can be assigned.
- Category 0 is only appropriate for screening. All diagnostic mammography must conclude with a final assessment from 1–6.

Category 1: Negative

- Breasts are normal.

Category 2: Benign

- A finding that is described but is definitely benign is BI-RADS 2.
- No additional workup or follow-up is needed.
- Examples: Vascular or other typically benign calcifications, simple breast cysts, intramammary lymph nodes.

Category 3: Probably benign

- A finding placed in BI-RADS 3 should have <2% risk of malignancy.
- It is necessary to conduct a complete diagnostic imaging evaluation using diagnostic views (e.g., spot compression magnification, etc.) and/or ultrasound before assigning a probably benign (BI-RADS 3) assessment. BI-RADS 3 is never appropriate for screening mammography.
- Three specific mammographic findings that may be appropriate for a BI-RADS 3 designation after complete diagnostic assessment include a circumscribed solid mass, focal asymmetry, and a single group of punctate calcifications.
- BI-RADS 3 should generally be reserved for baseline exams. If a comparison is available and a finding is new or increased but otherwise meets criteria for a probably benign assessment, then biopsy is usually appropriate. BI-RADS 3 is generally not supported for palpable lesions, although there are single institution studies suggesting that it is acceptable to assign appropriate palpable lesions as BI-RADS 3 after a full imaging workup.
- **Action required:** Short interval follow-up, typically 6 months. After 12 months of stability it is acceptable to lengthen the follow-up interval to one year. In general, if a benign-appearing lesion demonstrates two to three years of stability it can be considered benign (BI-RADS 2). Any interval change is suspicious and may warrant biopsy.

Category 4: Suspicious

- Findings are suspicious of malignancy, with a probability of being malignant >2% and <95%.
- Category 4 can be subdivided into Category 4A, 4B, and 4C, with 4A being least suspicious, and 4C being most suspicious.
- **Action required:** Biopsy.

Category 5: Highly suggestive of malignancy

- These lesions have a high probability (>95%) of being cancer. A lesion that a radiologist describes as "I'll eat my hat if that's not cancer!" should be classified as BI-RADS 5. The prototypical BI-RADS 5 cancer would be an irregular mass with spiculated margins and associated fine pleomorphic/fine

BI-RADS评估分类

0类：需补充影像

- 最终评估分类前需要额外的影像学资料(如局部加压、局部放大、特殊体位或超声)和/或既往乳腺X线影像。
- 0类仅适合于筛查。所有诊断性乳腺X线影像必须得出1~6类最终的评估结论。

1类：阴性

- 正常乳腺。

2类：良性

- 有病变但绝对是良性，应归为BI-RADS 2类。
- 无须进一步的检查和随访。
- 举例：血管或其他典型的良性钙化、单纯性乳腺囊肿、乳内淋巴结。

3类：可能良性

- 一个病变被定为BI-RADS 3类，其恶性肿瘤风险应小于2%。
- 把一个病变定为可能良性(BI-RADS 3类)之前，需要进行一套完整的诊断性影像检查，包括诊断性X线(如局部加压放大等)和/或超声检查。BI-RADS 3类绝不能用于筛查性乳腺X线检查的评估结论。
- 完成诊断性评估后，可能适合BI-RADS 3类的三种特定乳腺X线发现包括边界清晰的实性肿块、局灶性不对称和单组点状钙化。
- BI-RADS 3类通常用于初始检查。如果能够进行比较，而且病灶是新的或有所增大，其他条件又能满足良性可能的评估标准，活检作为下一步措施应该是合适的。BI-RADS 3类通常不适用于可触及的病变，但有多个单中心机构的研究提示，一个可触及的病变在进行了全套的影像检查后可以将其归为BI-RADS 3类。
- **采取措施：**短期随访，一般间隔6个月。稳定12个月后，可将随访间隔延长至1年。通常情况下，一个表现为良性的病灶若在2~3年内保持稳定，可将其考虑为良性(BI-RADS 2类)。随访间期出现的任何变化均为可疑并且需要活检确认。

4类：可疑恶性

- 对于可疑恶性的病变，其恶性概率>2%，但<95%。
- 4类可进一步分为4A、4B和4C 3个亚类，4A恶性可疑性最小，而4C可疑性最大。
- **采取措施：**活检。

5类：高度可疑恶性肿瘤

- 这类病变的癌症概率高(>95%)。如果一个病变被放射医师描述为"如果这不是癌症，我会吃掉我的帽子！"的时候，应归为BI-RADS 5类。典型的BI RADS 5类癌症应是带有边缘

linear-branching calcifications.

- **Action required:** Biopsy. Any pathologic result other than cancer would be discordant.

毛刺的不规则肿块，伴有多形性/细小线样分支状钙化。

- **采取措施：**活检。除癌症以外的任何病理结果都视为不一致。

Category 6: Known biopsy-proven malignancy

- This category is reserved for lesions identified on the imaging study with prior biopsy proof of malignancy. Typically, a plan of action is already in place.

6类：已证实的恶性肿瘤

- 这一分类用于已经被活检证实为恶性的影像学病灶。通常情况下，已经有了相应的处理方案。

（翻译　阳宁静　彭程宇）

MAMMOGRAPHY

乳腺X线检查

SCREENING MAMMOGRAPHY

- The goal of screening mammography is to detect pre-clinical breast cancer in asymptomatic women. Screening mammography detects 2 to 8 cancers per 1,000 women screened.
  Mammography has decreased sensitivity in women with dense breasts.
- Since 1990, the mortality from breast cancer has been steadily declining at a rate of approximately 2.2% per year, thought to be due to improvements in adjuvant therapy and screening mammography.
- The current standard recommendation in the United States is annual screening mammography beginning at age 40 for women at average risk for breast cancer, based on guidelines issued by multiple national organizations including the American College of Radiology (ACR) and Society of Breast Imaging (SBI).
- In contrast, while the American Cancer Society (ASC) and the US Preventative Services Task Force (USPSTF) agree that screening from age 40 reduces breast cancer mortality, both organizations recommend beginning to screen at a later age due to uncertain benefits versus risks in younger women.
- The ACS (2015) recommends annual screening mammography between ages 45–54 and biennial screening for age 55 or older. Women have the option to start annual screening at ages 40–44.
- The USPSTF (2009) recommends biennial mammography between ages 50–74. Decision to start screening at ages 40–49 should be made on an individual basis.
- The potential concerns for mammographic screening include a very small risk of inducing breast cancer from radiation exposure, and risks of over diagnosis including anxiety from false positives and unnecessary biopsies.
- Randomized control trials have shown that screening mammography can significantly reduce breast cancer mortality for women aged 40–74 by at least 20%.
- Computer modeling of breast cancer screening also showed that the greatest reduction in breast cancer specific mortality is achieved with screening mammography starting at age 40.
- There are varying recommendations on the age to stop screening, as listed below.

乳腺X线筛查

- 筛查性乳腺X线检查的目的是在无症状的女性中发现临床前乳腺癌。乳腺X线影像筛查可在每1 000名女性中发现2~8名乳腺癌患者。
  乳腺X线检查对致密型乳腺的女性灵敏度低。
- 自1990年以来，乳腺癌患者的病死率以每年约2.2%的速度逐渐下降，这可能与辅助治疗的改进和乳腺X线影像筛查有关。
- 根据美国放射学院（ACR）和乳腺影像协会（SBI）等多个全国性组织发布的相关指南，目前美国的标准建议是对具有乳腺癌平均风险的女性从40岁开始进行年度乳腺X线筛查。
- 尽管美国癌症协会（ASC）和美国预防服务工作组（USPSTF）认同从40岁开始筛查可降低乳腺癌致死概率，但却建议筛查应该在较晚的年龄开始，因为其对年轻女性的益处与风险还不确定。
- ACS（2015）建议45~54岁每年进行一次乳腺X线筛查，55岁或以上每2年进行一次筛查。40~44岁女性可以选择进行年度筛查。
- USPSTF（2009）建议50~74岁每2年进行一次乳腺X线检查。40~49岁应根据个人情况决定什么时候开始筛查。
- 筛查性乳腺X线检查的潜在弊端是辐射暴露带来的微小乳腺癌风险，以及过度诊断引起的焦虑（包括假阳性结果和不必要的活检）。
- 随机对照试验表明，乳腺X线检查可显著降低40~74岁女性乳腺癌患者的病死率，至少达20%。
- 计算机乳腺癌筛查模型也表明，从40岁开始进行乳腺X线筛查可最大程度降低乳腺癌患者的病死率。
- 停止筛查年龄的各种不同建议如下。

Current guidelines for screening mammography				
	Starting Age	**Frequency**	**Age to Stop**	**Comment**
ACR	40 or older	annual	continue as long as good health	
ACS	45–54	annual	continue as long as good health and life expectancy 10+ years left	option to start annual screening at age 40
	55 or older	biennial		
USPSTF	50–74	biennial	75	option to start at age 40

当前乳腺X线筛查指南				
	起始年龄/岁	**频率**	**停止年龄**	**建议**
ACR	≥40	每年	健康状况允许则继续	
ACS	45~54	每年	健康状况允许和预期寿命≥10年则继续	40岁开始选择性进行年度筛查
	≥55	每2年		
USPSTF	50~74	每2年	75岁	40岁开始选择性进行筛查

Routine screening mammographic views

常规乳腺X线摄影体位

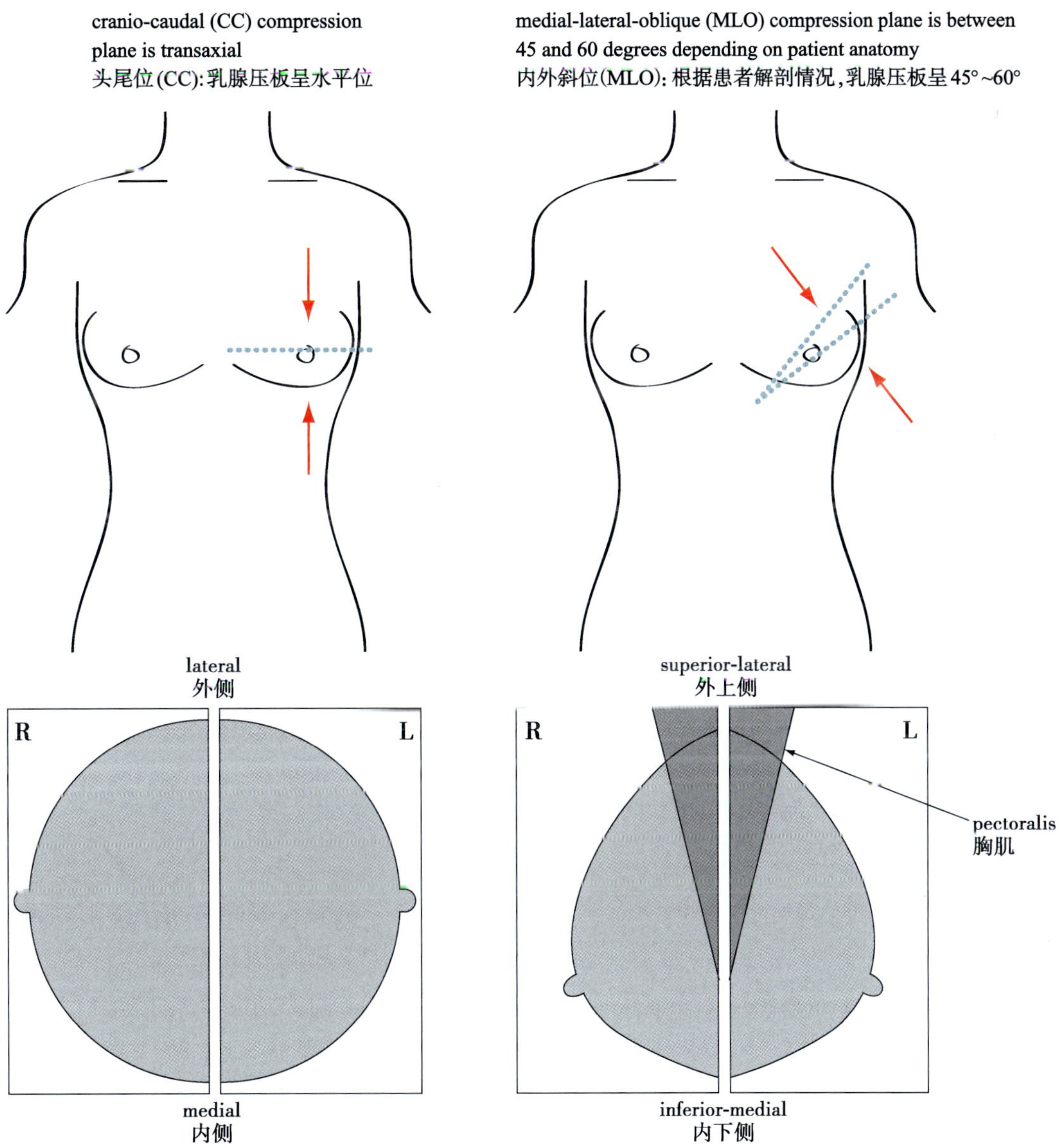

- The two standard mammographic views are cranio-caudal (CC) and medial-lateral-oblique (MLO).

- 两个标准的乳腺X线摄影体位是头尾位(CC)和内外斜位(MLO)。

- The cranio-caudal (CC) image plane is transaxial.
- The medial-lateral-oblique (MLO) image plane is approximately 45–60 degrees from the axial plane, paralleling the course of the pectoralis muscle heading into the axilla.

  The MLO view is ideal for screening, as it captures most of the breast tissue in a single view.

  Note that the superior-medial breast tissue may be excluded on the MLO view.
- At the technologist's discretion, additional views may be performed to assure complete imaging of all fibroglandular tissue:

  Cleavage view (CV) images the medial breast tissue of both breasts.

  The **exaggerated CC (XCC)** view pulls either lateral or medial tissue into the imaging detector.

Online and offline screening

- Typically, most screening mammography is interpreted **offline**, where a batch of exams is reviewed in bulk some time after the films were taken.
- **Online** screening, where women have mammography performed and then wait to get a final report from the radiologist, leads to more imaging being performed and more false- positives, with the same cancer detection rate.
- In contrast to screening mammography, all diagnostic mammography is performed "online" as a monitored exam with the patient staying for all possible imaging and the final results/ recommendations before leaving.

- CC位影像的平面为横轴位。
- MLO位影像的平面大概与横轴呈45°~60°，与胸大肌朝向腋窝的走行平行。

  MLO位是理想的筛查体位，因为这一体位包括了大部分的乳腺组织。

  注意，此体位可能会遗漏上内侧的乳腺组织。
- 技师应酌情考虑附加体位以确保图像包括所有的腺体纤维组织：

  乳沟位(CV)显示双侧乳腺内侧的组织。

  夸大头尾位(XCC)将内侧或外侧乳腺组织纳入图像探测器的范围内。

在线(患者在现场)和离线(患者不在现场)筛查

- 通常，大多数筛查性乳腺X线检查是在离线情况下解读的，即在拍摄胶片一段时间后，批量审查一组检查结果。
- 在线筛查中，女性进行乳腺X线检查后等待放射科医师提供最终报告，这会导致更多成像检查和更多的假阳性结果，而癌症检出率却是一样的。
- 与筛查性乳腺X线检查不同，所有诊断性乳腺X线检查都是"在线"进行的，作为监控检查，患者会在现场等候所有可能的成像结果，并在离开前得到最终检查结果和建议。

Diagnostic Mammography

Indications for diagnostic mammography

- Diagnostic mammography is usually performed for a breast problem (pain, lump, skin thickening, nipple discharge).
- Other indications for diagnostic mammography include annual mammography in an asymptomatic woman with a past history of breast cancer, short interval follow-up (following of BI-RADS 3 lesions), and evaluation of an abnormality found on screening mammogram.

Diagnostic mammography procedure

- Any mammographic abnormality is first localized in three-dimensional space, then worked-up with special problem-solving techniques, which are discussed later in this section.
- Often, ultrasound is added at the radiologist's discretion.
- Each patient waits until all imaging is completed before receiving a summary of the final interpretation and recommendations from the radiologist.

诊断性乳腺X线检查

诊断性乳腺X线检查的适应证

- 诊断性乳腺X线检查通常用来解决乳腺问题(疼痛、包块、皮肤增厚、乳头溢液)。
- 其他诊断性乳腺X线检查的适应证包括对有乳腺癌病史的无症状妇女进行年检、短期随访(BI-RADS 3类病灶)，以及评估在筛查性乳腺X线检查时发现的异常。

诊断性乳腺X线检查的方法

- 首先对任何乳腺X线检查图像上的异常进行三维定位，然后采取具体问题具体解决的方法，这将在本章后文进行讨论。
- 通常，超声检查会根据放射科医师的判断酌情添加。
- 每个患者在所有影像检查完毕前不能离开，直到放射科医师给出最终报告和建议。

Approach to Interpreting a Mammogram

Evaluate image quality and adequacy

- The first step in evaluating a mammogram is to determine if the study is technically adequate.
- There should be adequate tissue imaged on both the CC and MLO views. The posterior nipple line is a line drawn from the nipple to the pectoralis muscle – or edge of the film on the CC view if the pectoralis is not visualized. The posterior nipple lines drawn on the CC and MLO views should be within 1 cm of each other.

乳腺X线摄影图像的解读方法

评价图像质量和准确性

- 乳腺X线影像评价的第一步是确定技术上是否合格。
- CC位和MLO位应显示有足够的组织。乳头后线是从乳头后方至胸大肌的一条连线，或在胸大肌未显示时的乳头后方至CC位片边缘的一条线。在CC位和MLO位上所画的乳头后线的差别应小于1cm。

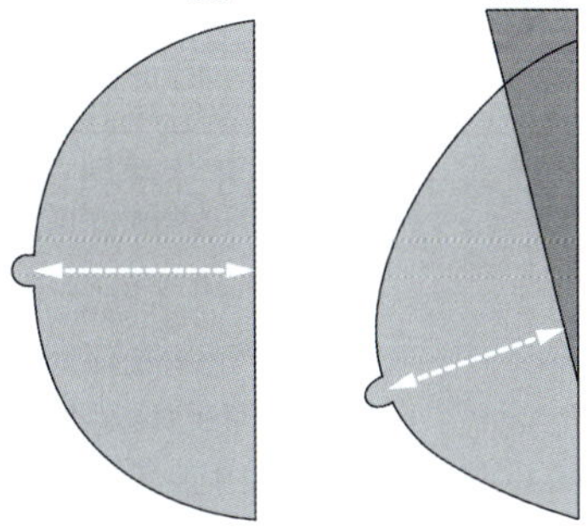

On the MLO view, the pectoral muscle should be convex anteriorly and visible at least to the level of the nipple.
在MLO位图像上，胸大肌应向前凸起并至少要达到乳头水平。

- The image must be free from blur and artifacts. The trabeculae should be sharp; if blur is present, then benign calcifications can be mistaken for suspicious amorphous calcifications, and subtle calcifications can be missed entirely.
- The nipple of each breast should be in profile in at least one view.

Compare each side

- Each projection should be globally compared side-to-side to evaluate for symmetry.

Evaluate and magnify each image

- Each image should be carefully evaluated for signs of malignancy. The mammographic signs of malignancy are mass, calcification, architectural distortion, and asymmetry. Calcifications are best viewed at 1∶1 or higher magnification, while architectural distortion is best seen when the whole breast is visualized.
- When viewing a digital mammogram, every portion of the image should be carefully evaluated at 1∶1 zoom.

Compare to prior studies

- Even if a study appears unremarkable at first glance, comparison to prior exams can often reveal a subtle progressive change. For instance, an apparent normal island of parenchymal tissue may be slowly growing and represent malignancy.
- In general, it is best to carefully compare the previous exam from at least two years prior, to appreciate slowly growing changes.

- 图像必须清晰且无伪影。小梁应锐利；如果图像模糊，良性钙化可能被误认为是可疑的无定形钙化，而不明显的钙化则可能被完全遗漏。
- 每侧乳腺的乳头至少在一个体位上显示它的轮廓。

双侧比较

- 每个体位应与对侧相应的体位进行大体比较以评价对称性。

评价和放大每幅图像

- 每幅图像应仔细评估恶性肿瘤的征象。乳腺X线影像的恶性征象包括肿块、钙化、结构扭曲和不对称性。钙化最好用1∶1或更大的放大倍率进行显示，结构扭曲最好在全乳图像中进行显示。
- 在观察数字化乳腺X线影像时，图像的每一部分应在1∶1的放大比例下进行仔细评估。

比较以往检查

- 即使初看一个检查并无异常，但与先前的检查进行对比常常可发现细微的进展变化。例如，一个看似正常的实质腺体岛组织可能在缓慢生长，这可能提示恶性肿瘤。
- 一般来说，最好仔细比较至少两年前的检查，以便发现缓慢的生长变化。

Fibroglandular Density

纤维腺体密度

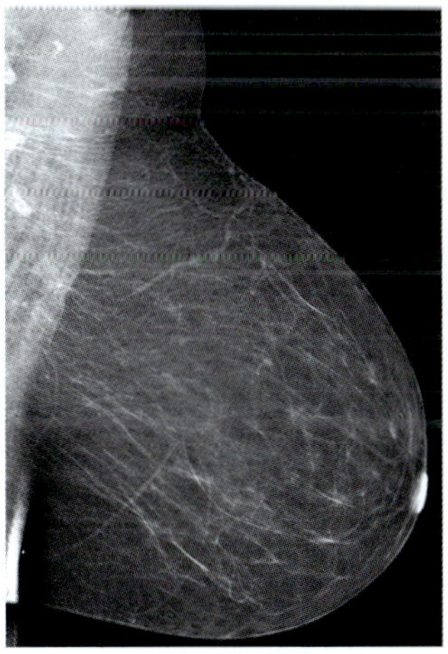

Almost entirely fatty
几乎完全为脂肪

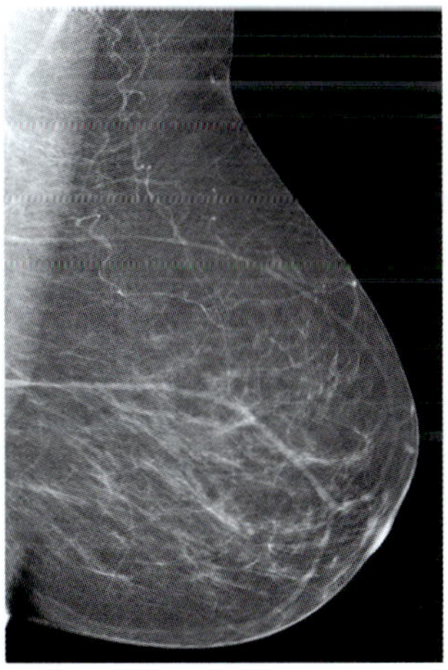

Scattered areas of fibroglandular density
散在纤维腺体密度

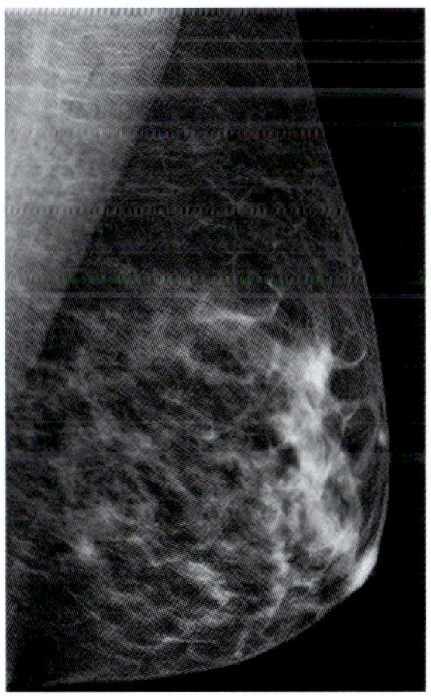

Heterogeneously dense, which may obscure small masses
不均质高密度，可掩盖小的肿块

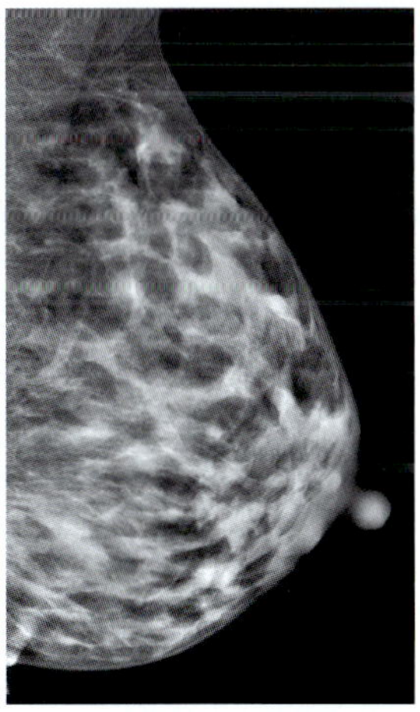

Extremely dense, which lowers the sensitivity of mammography
极度致密腺体，会降低乳腺X线检查的灵敏度

- In every mammographic report, the mammographic pattern of fibroglandular density should be characterized into one of the above descriptors.
- Women with dense fibroglandular tissue have an increased risk of developing breast cancer, and detection of early cancer can be obscured by the fibroglandular tissue. A woman with extremely dense breasts has a 5x relative risk of breast cancer compared to a woman with almost entirely fatty breasts.
- Bilateral interval increase in fibroglandular density is usually benign and may be caused either by hormonal effects or breast edema. A unilateral increase in fibroglandular density is worrisome for lymphatic obstruction, which may be malignant.
- Edema due to systemic causes, such as congestive heart failure, typically causes bilateral trabecular blurring and skin thickening.
- Hormone therapy may cause an increase in fibroglandular density, without skin thickening. Proliferation of cysts and fibrocystic change can be seen, even in postmenopausal women.
- Pregnancy, lactation, and weight loss may all cause an interval increase in fibroglandular density.

- 在每份乳腺X线报告中，纤维腺体密度特征必须按以上分类中的一种进行描述。
- 具有致密型纤维腺体组织的女性，乳腺癌患病风险会增加，且增加的纤维腺体组织密度会影响检出早期乳腺癌。一个乳房极度致密的女性，其患乳腺癌的相对风险是乳房几乎是完全脂肪型女性的5倍。
- 随访期间双侧纤维腺体密度增加通常为良性，可能由激素作用或乳房水肿所引起。单侧纤维腺体密度增加需要考虑淋巴管阻塞，并可能是恶性的。
- 由全身原因引起的水肿，如充血性心力衰竭，通常表现为双侧小梁模糊或皮肤增厚。
- 激素治疗可导致纤维腺体密度增加，但没有皮肤增厚。即使为绝经后女性，也可见囊肿增生和纤维囊性改变。
- 妊娠、哺乳和减肥都可能导致间歇性纤维腺体密度增加。

Skin thickening

- Unilateral skin thickening can be due to either benign or malignant causes. Similar to changes in fibroglandular density, bilateral skin thickening is usually benign and the result of a systemic process.

Skin thickening: Benign causes

- Radiation therapy (usually unilateral).
- Acute mastitis (usually unilateral).
- Skin inflammation (usually unilateral and focal).
- CHF (fluid overload), renal failure (fluid overload due to protein wasting), and liver failure (fluid overload due to hypoalbuminemia) may all produce unilateral or bilateral skin thickening.

Skin thickening: Malignant causes

- Inflammatory carcinoma, which represents invasion of dermal lymphatics by cancer. A mammographic mass may be present.
- Locally advanced carcinoma.
- Lymphatic obstruction from axillary adenopathy.

皮肤增厚

- 单侧皮肤增厚既可以是良性也可以是恶性的。与纤维腺体密度变化类似，双侧皮肤增厚通常是良性和系统性疾病所致。

皮肤增厚：良性原因

- 放射治疗(常为单侧)。
- 急性乳腺炎(常为单侧)。
- 皮肤炎症(常为单侧或局灶性)。
- 充血性心力衰竭(液体负荷过度)、肾衰竭(蛋白丢失所致液体过负荷)和肝衰竭(低蛋白血症导致液体过负荷)均可导致单侧或双侧皮肤增厚。

皮肤增厚：恶性原因

- 炎性癌，为癌症侵及真皮淋巴管。乳腺X线检查可见肿块。
- 局部癌症晚期。
- 腋窝淋巴结病变导致淋巴管阻塞。

BI-RADS lexicon for mammographic masses

Is the mass seen in more than one view?

- A mammographic **mass** is a space-occupying lesion with convex borders seen in two different projections. In contrast, an **asymmetry** is seen in one view only.

Evaluate past films: Is it new?

- There are many different descriptors to characterize a mammographic mass using the BI- RADS lexicon, but regardless of morphology, the presence of a new mass is suspicious and must be evaluated fully.
- Conversely, a malignant-looking mass should still be regarded with suspicion even if it hasn't changed. Slow growing carcinomas, such as tubular carcinoma, can stay stable for years.
- A stable mass with all benign features is almost always regarded as benign.

乳腺肿块的BI-RDAS术语

肿块见于一个以上的体位吗?

- 乳腺X线影像上的**肿块**是在两个不同体位上均具有边缘凸起的占位性病变。相比之下，**不对称**仅见于一个体位。

与过去的图像相比较：有新的变化吗?

- 使用BI-RADS术语可以对乳腺影像上的肿块特征进行各种不同的描述，但无论形态如何，一个新出现的肿块都是可疑的，必须进行充分评估。
- 相反，对于一个具有恶性外观的肿块，即使没有发生变化也要始终认为其可疑。生长缓慢的癌(如小管癌)可以多年保持稳定。
- 一个稳定并具有良性特征的肿块几乎可以视为良性。

Evaluate the margins, using the BI-RADS lexicon

使用BI-RADS术语评价病变边缘

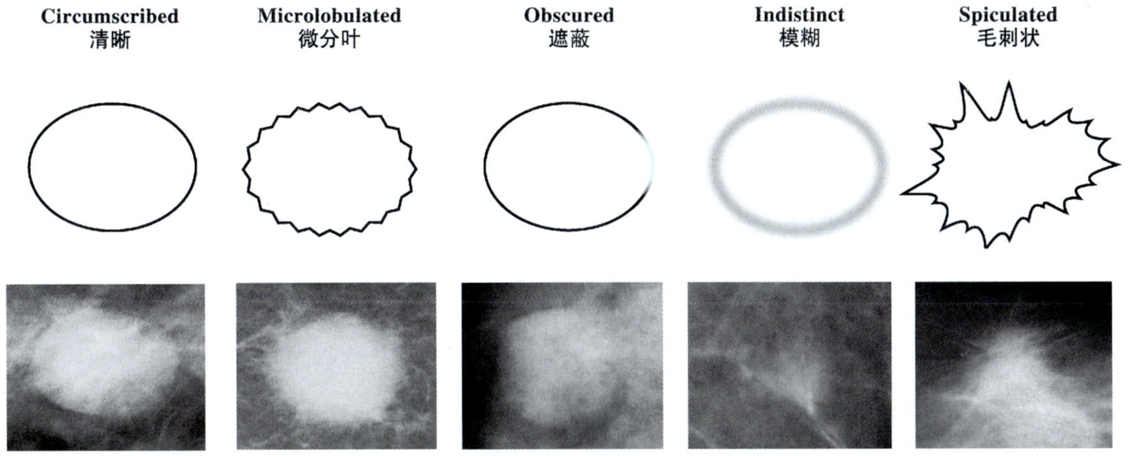

- Careful evaluation of the margins of a mammographic mass at the interface with surrounding tissue is key to stratifying the suspicion for malignancy. The five BI-RADS terms used to describe the margins are circumscribed, microlobulated, obscured, indistinct, and spiculated.
- **Circumscribed**: At least 75% of the margin must be well-defined, while the remainder may be obscured with overlying tissue.

  In general, unless a mass is new, a circumscribed mass is benign, and a non-circumscribed mass is suspicious. Of course, there are exceptions to this: abscesses can present with non-circumscribed margins and certain types of cancers can present with predominantly circumscribed margins.
- **Microlobulated**: A microlobulated mass has a finely irregular or serrated edge.
- **Obscured**: A margin is obscured if it is greater than 25% hidden by superimposed or adjacent normal tissue. The term "obscured" implies that the radiologist believes that the mass may be circumscribed, but the margin is hidden by overlying tissue.
- **Indistinct**: A poorly defined margin (or portion of the margin) raises concern that the lesion may be infiltrating.
- **Spiculated**: Linear densities radiate from a mass. A spiculated mass is malignant until proven otherwise.

- 仔细评价乳腺X线影像上肿块与周围组织的边界是对可疑恶性肿瘤进行分析的关键。五种描述边缘的BI-RADS术语分别为清晰、微分叶、遮蔽、模糊和毛刺状。
- **清晰：**至少75%的边缘必须是清晰的，而其余边缘可以因组织重叠而模糊。

  通常情况下，除非是新增病灶，否则边界清楚的肿块是良性的，而边界不清的肿块为可疑恶性。当然，也有例外情况：脓肿可表现为边界不清晰，而某些类型的癌症往往有清晰的边界。
- **微分叶：**微分叶肿块有细微的不规则或锯齿状边缘。
- **遮蔽：**如果肿块边缘25%以上有重叠或被邻近组织掩盖则为遮蔽。使用遮蔽一词意味着放射科医师相信肿块边界可能是清晰的，但其边缘被叠加的组织所遮挡。
- **模糊：**边缘（或部分边缘）不清可提示为浸润性病变。
- **毛刺状：**肿块发出放射状线样密度影。毛刺状肿块为恶性，除非证实为其他情况。

Describe the density

密度描述

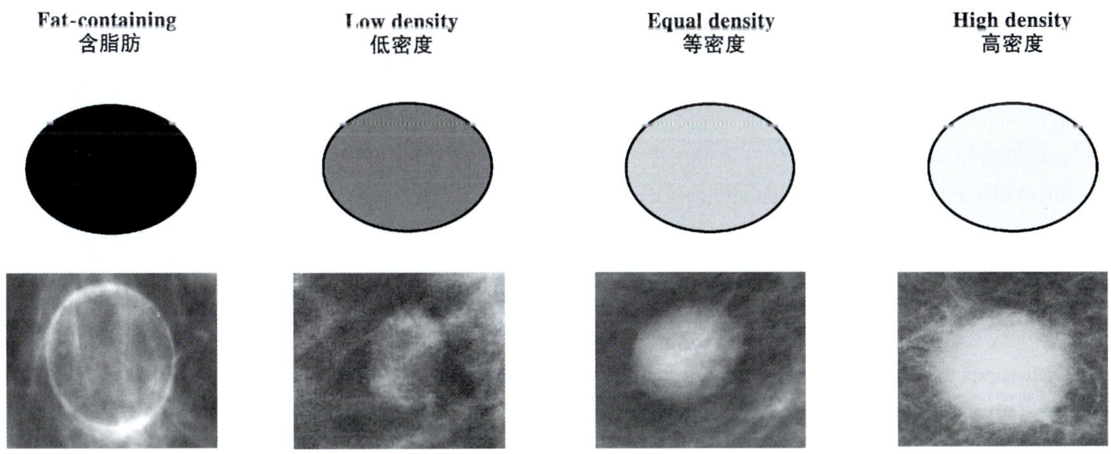

- Most breast cancers that form a visible mass are of equal or higher density than the surrounding fibroglandular tissue.
- The BI-RADS lexicon for density includes **fat-containing**, **low density**, **equal density**, and **high density**. A circumscribed fat-containing mass is benign.

- 大多数乳腺癌所形成的可见肿块与周围的纤维腺体组织呈等密度或高密度。
- 用来描述密度的BI-RADS术语包括“**含脂肪**、**低密度**、**等密度**、**高密度**”。一个边界清晰的透亮肿块是良性的。

Describe the shape

形状描述

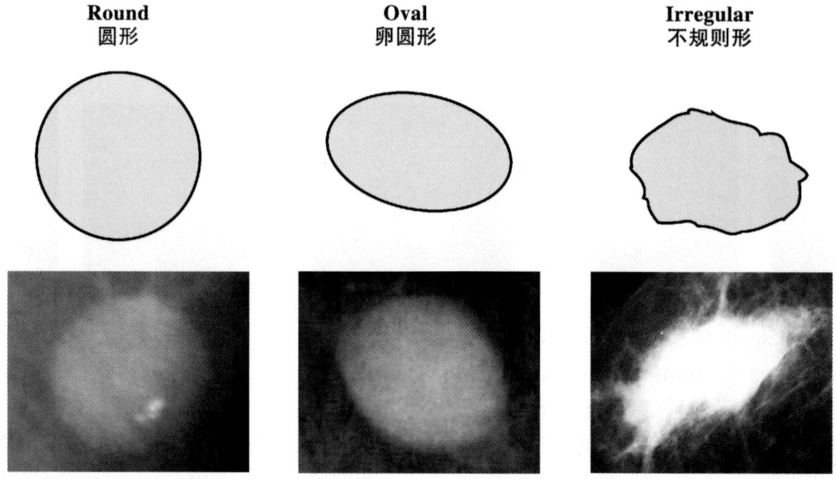

- The BI-RADS lexicon for shape includes **round**, **oval**, and **irregular**. Although malignancy may be any form, an irregular mass is most suspicious for malignancy. An oval-shaped mass may include up to two to three smooth lobulations.

Describe the location by naming the quadrant and (optionally) the depth

- The four quadrants of each breast are: Upper outer quadrant, upper inner quadrant, lower outer quadrant, and lower inner quadrant.
- When referring to the opposite breast, the *mirror opposite* quadrant is the contralateral quadrant with the same name. For instance, the upper outer quadrant of the left breast is the mirror opposite quadrant of the upper outer quadrant of the right breast.
- If *subareolar* or *axillary tail* are used to localize a lesion, then it is not necessary to specify a quadrant.
- Although clockface is used for ultrasound location, quadrant is preferred for mammography.
- Depth is commonly described as anterior (or shallow), middle, or posterior depth, separating the breast into thirds.

Measure the size

- Size is a poor predictor of malignancy, but changes in size determine if a lesion is growing.

Look for associated features

- **Architectural distortion** represents radiating linear densities emanating from a central point, without a definite mass visible. Architectural distortion is caused by tethering of the normal fibroglandular tissue and is highly concerning for a cancer, although there are some benign causes. If there is no history of surgery or trauma, biopsy is appropriate.
- **Microcalcifications** may be associated with malignant ductal calcification.
- **Skin retraction** is most commonly postsurgical but may be due to a desmoplastic tumor.
- **Nipple retraction** is tethering or angulation of the nipple. Retraction should

- BI-RADS术语对形状的描述包括**圆形**、**卵圆形**和**不规则形**。恶性肿瘤可以呈任何形状，但不规则的肿块恶性可能性最大。卵圆形肿块可包括2~3个光滑的分叶。

描述病变的位置：象限和深度(可选)

- 每个乳房有四个象限：外上、内上、外下和内下象限。
- 参照对侧乳房时，镜像象限与对侧象限同名。例如：左乳外上象限是右乳外上象限的镜像对侧象限。
- 如果使用*乳晕下*或*腋尾*来定位病变，则无须指定象限。
- 尽管超声使用钟表定位，但象限定位更适用于乳腺X线影像。
- 描述深度时，通常将乳房分为前部(或浅表)、中部及后部三部分。

测量大小

- 大小对恶性肿瘤的预测能力较差，但大小的变化可以判断病变是否正在生长。

寻找相关特征

- **结构扭曲**为从中心点向四周呈放射状样的线状密度影，但无明确可见的肿块。结构扭曲是因周围正常纤维腺体组织受到牵拉所致，高度可疑为恶性肿瘤，但需除外一些良性病变。如果无手术或创伤史，应考虑活检。
- **微钙化**可能与恶性导管钙化有关。
- **皮肤凹陷**最常见于手术后，也可见于促纤维增生性肿瘤。
- **乳头回缩**是乳头受到牵拉或出现成角。**回缩**

not be confused with inversion (where the whole nipple points inwards). Nipple inversion may be developmental, bilateral, and is not necessarily a sign of malignancy if stable.

- **Skin thickening** may represent edema or may be secondary to prior radiation therapy.
- **Trabecular thickening** represents thickening of the fibrous septa of the breast, which can be seen in edema or in patients who have received radiation therapy.
- **Axillary adenopathy** may be hyperplastic or malignant. Although it is normal for a few nodes to be present in the axilla, nodes with replacement of the normal fatty hilum may warrant evaluation, especially if new.

不应与反转(整个乳头向内)相混淆。乳头反转可能为发育异常所致,表现为双侧;如果乳头情况稳定,则不一定是恶性肿瘤的征象。

- **皮肤增厚**可能为水肿或继发于先前的放射治疗。
- **小梁增厚**为乳腺纤维间隔增厚,可见于水肿或接受过放射治疗的患者。
- **腋窝淋巴结肿大**可能是增生或恶性。存在数个腋窝淋巴结属于正常,但当淋巴结脂肪门消失,尤其为新发病灶时,则需要进行评估。

Example of BI-RADS terminology

BI-RDAS术语举例

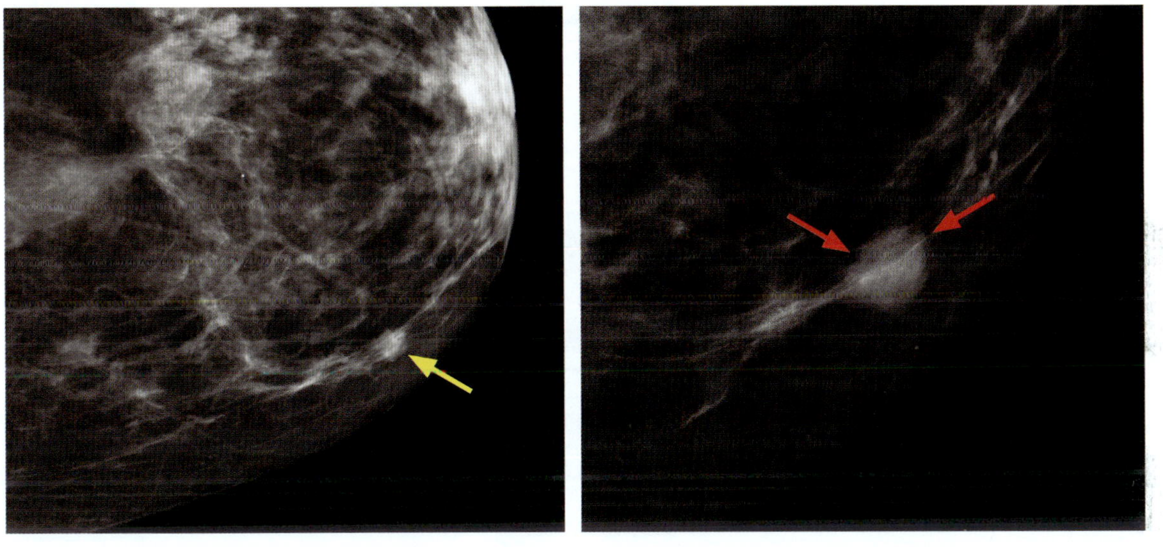

CC view mammogram (left image) shows an oval mass (yellow arrow) with partially obscured margins in the inner anterior breast. The mass is better evaluated on spot compression view (right image) and demonstrates microlobulated margins (red arrows). Biopsy of this mass revealed papilloma with carcinoma in situ.

乳腺X线CC位图像(左图)显示在乳腺内侧前部有一个边缘被部分遮蔽的椭圆形肿块(黄箭)。在点压视图(右图)上,该肿块显示更为清晰,可见边缘呈微小分叶(红箭)。对该肿块进行的活检结果显示为乳头状瘤伴原位癌。

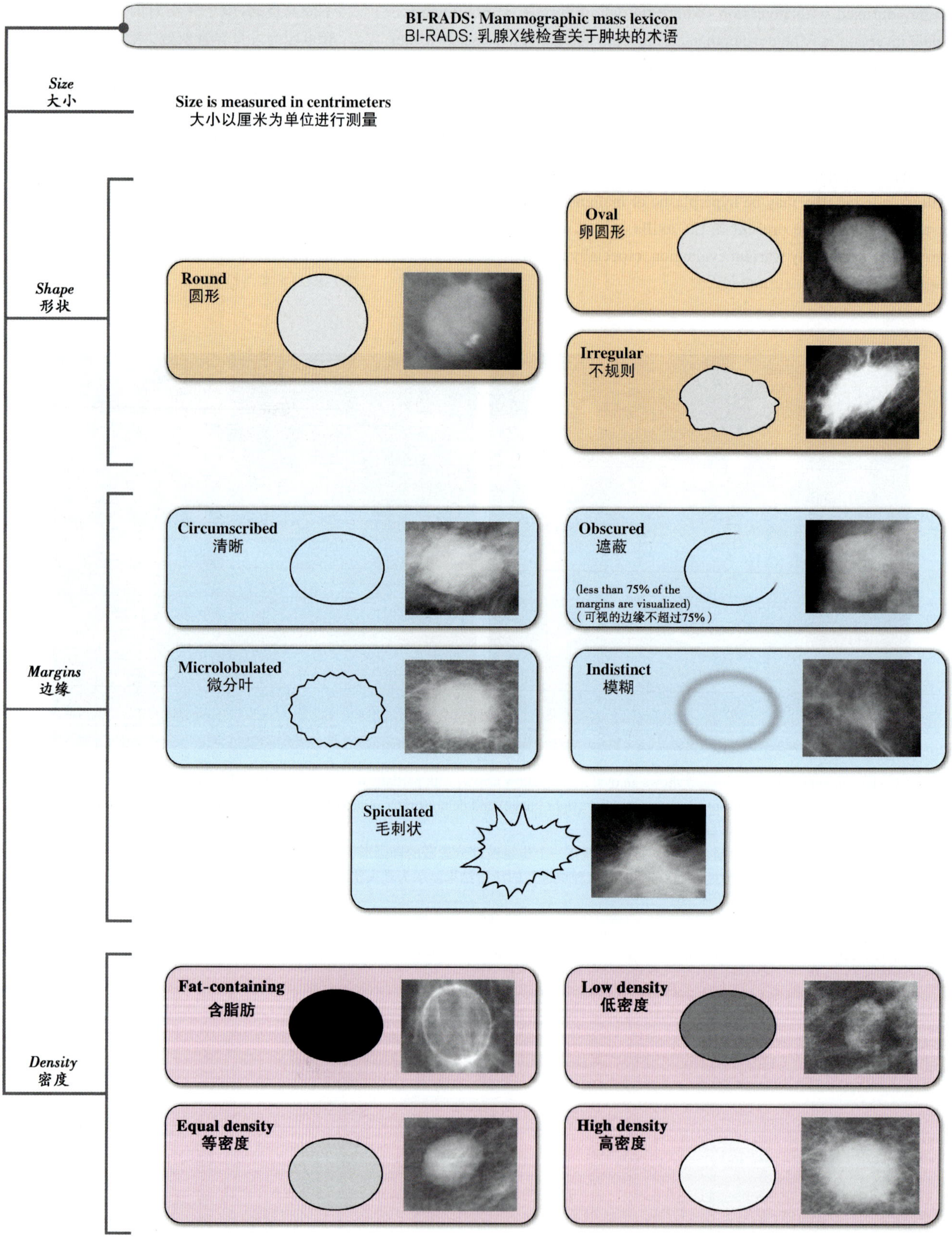
BI-RADS: Mammographic mass lexicon
BI-RADS: 乳腺X线检查关于肿块的术语
Size
大小
Size is measured in centrimeters
大小以厘米为单位进行测量
Shape
形状
Round
圆形
Oval
卵圆形
Irregular
不规则
Margins
边缘
Circumscribed
清晰
Obscured
遮蔽
(less than 75% of the margins are visualized)
（可视的边缘不超过75%）
Microlobulated
微分叶
Indistinct
模糊
Spiculated
毛刺状
Density
密度
Fat-containing
含脂肪
Low density
低密度
Equal density
等密度
High density
高密度

Overview of Mammographic Calcifications

Significance of mammographic calcifications

- Most mammograms will show calcifications, which are overwhelmingly likely to be benign. However, careful analysis of breast calcifications is essential. Abnormal calcification may be the earliest, and possibly the only, mammographic manifestation of cancer.
- When characterizing calcifications, **morphology** and **distribution** are essential.
- Certain types of calcifications can be definitively characterized as benign, while some are highly suspicious for malignancy. Other morphologies are indeterminate.

Mammographic technique

- It is almost always necessary to perform spot compression *magnification* to characterize calcifications as either indeterminate or suspicious for malignancy. In contrast, most types of benign calcification can be described on routine full-field views (an exception would be milk of calcium calcifications, which generally require a true lateral view with magnification).
- Magnification employs air-gap technique and a small (0.1 mm) focal spot.

乳腺X线影像钙化概述

乳腺钙化的意义

- 大多数乳腺X线影像会显示钙化灶，其中绝大多数可能是良性的。然而，仔细分析乳腺钙化是必不可少的。乳腺X线影像上的异常钙化可能是最早，也可能是唯一的恶性表现。
- 在描述钙化灶时，必须包括**形态**和**分布**。
- 某些类型的钙化可以确认为良性，而有些则高度怀疑恶性。其他形态为不确定性。

乳腺X线摄影技术

- 对于不确定或怀疑为恶性的钙化灶，几乎总是需要进行点压放大进行观察。相比之下，大多数良性钙化可以在常规全视野视图中进行观察(除外钙乳样钙化，它通常需要一张侧位放大图)。
- 放大采用空气间隙技术和小焦点(0.1mm)。

Typically Benign Calcifications (BI-RADS 2)

Skin calcifications

- Skin calcifications are associated with sweat glands, are usually punctate or lucent-centered, and are most common medially where the concentration of sweat glands is higher.
- A cluster of skin calcifications projecting over the breast may be confused for grouped calcifications in the breast itself. If skin calcifications are suspected, a tangential view should be performed by placing a BB directly over the calcifications in one view and then re-imaging with the BB in tangent. Calcifications which are in the skin should be seen in the dermis on the tangential view. Tomographic imaging can also help confirm whether or not calcifications lie within the skin.

Vascular calcifications

典型良性钙化(BI-RADS 2类)

皮肤钙化

- 皮肤钙化与汗腺相关，通常呈点状或中央透明，最常见于汗腺浓度较高的内侧。
- 投射在乳腺内的簇状皮肤钙化可能会与乳腺组织本身的钙化相混淆。如果怀疑皮肤钙化，需要获得切线位影像，先将“BB弹”标记直接置于钙化点的位置进行成像，然后在切线位置重新成像。皮肤钙化应该位于切线位的真皮层。断层成像也可以帮助确认钙化是否存在于皮肤内。

血管钙化

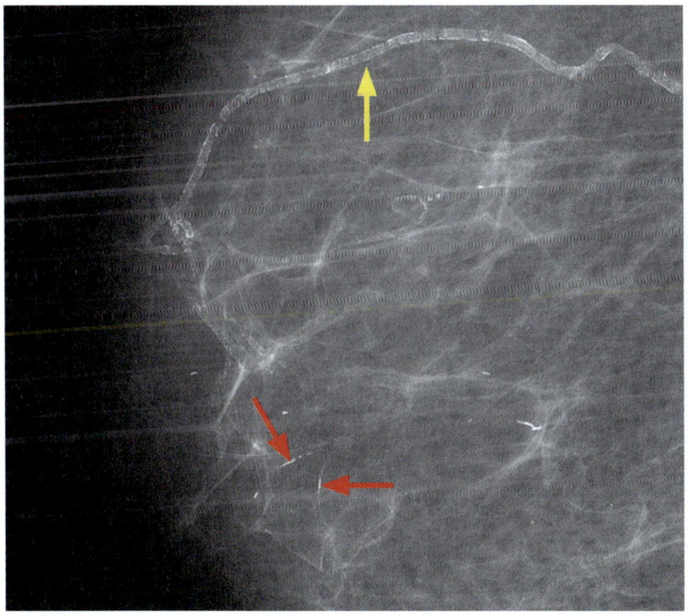

Vascular and secretory calcifications:
Arterial vascular calcifications are present in the upper portion of the image (yellow arrow), while large rod-like calcifications are present in the inferior portion of the image (red arrows).
Case courtesy Sughra Raza, MD, Brigham and Women's Hospital.
血管和分泌性钙化：
动脉血管钙化(黄箭)见于图像的上方，大的杆状钙化位于图像的下方(红箭)。

- Arterial vascular calcifications within the breast have a distinctive morphology and are typically not mentioned in the body of the report unless they are very extensive or the patient is very young.
- Early or incomplete vascular calcifications may pose a potential problem as they may appear similar to fine linear calcifications, which are suspicious.

Large rod-like calcifications

- Large rod-like calcifications are caused by secretory disease (also called plasma cell mastitis), which is a benign, inflammatory process seen in postmenopausal women.
- These calcifications follow a ductal pattern similar to DCIS, however they have a classic appearance which should not be confused with fine linear or fine-linear branching calcifications.

Coarse or "popcorn-like" calcifications

- 乳腺内的动脉血管壁钙化有着独特的形态结构，但通常不会在报告中提及，除非钙化异常广泛或患者非常年轻。
- 因早期或不完全性动脉钙化看起来与可疑的细小的线样钙化相似，可能会给诊断带来困难。

大的杆状钙化

- 大的杆状钙化由分泌性疾病引起(也被称为浆细胞性乳腺炎)，是一种见于绝经后妇女的良性炎性病变。
- 这些钙化与DCIS的导管分布模式类似，但其具有典型的表现，不应与细线状或细的分支状钙化灶相混淆。

粗糙的或"爆米花"样钙化

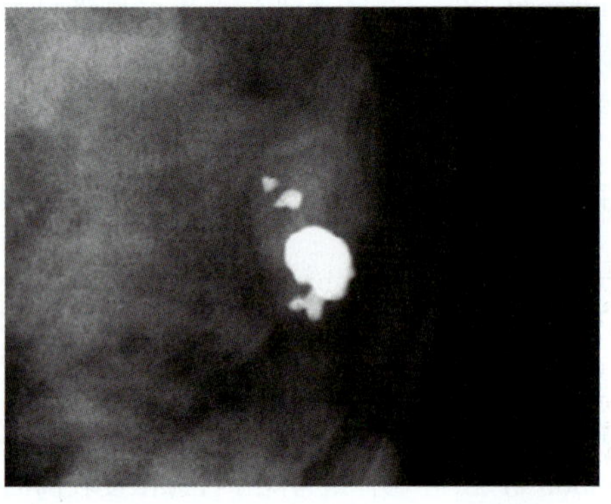

Mammogram shows a circumscribed, oval mass with associated "popcorn-like" calcifications, diagnostic of a hyalinizing fibroadenoma.
乳腺X线影像显示一个边界清晰的卵圆形肿块，伴有"爆米花"样钙化，可诊断为透明样变性纤维腺瘤。

- "Popcorn-like" calcifications are caused by an involuting or hyalinizing fibroadenoma.
- Not all fibroadenomas calcify. However, when calcification does occur, it starts as *peripheral* calcification and progresses to the classic chunky popcorn-like appearance.
- At an early stage, the small calcifications of a fibroadenoma may resemble those of cancer and prompt biopsy; however, a benign fibroadenoma can be diagnosed with confidence when the calcifications have the typical "popcorn-like" morphology.

Milk of calcium calcifications

- "爆米花"样钙化是纤维腺瘤退化或透明样变性的结果。
- 并不是所有的纤维腺瘤都会钙化。当钙化出现时，会先从周边开始，之后逐步发展为典型的粗短的"爆米花"样形态。
- 在早期阶段，纤维腺瘤内的小钙化可能会与癌症钙化相似并进行活检；然而，当出现典型的"爆米花"样钙化时可有把握诊断为良性纤维腺瘤。

钙乳样钙化

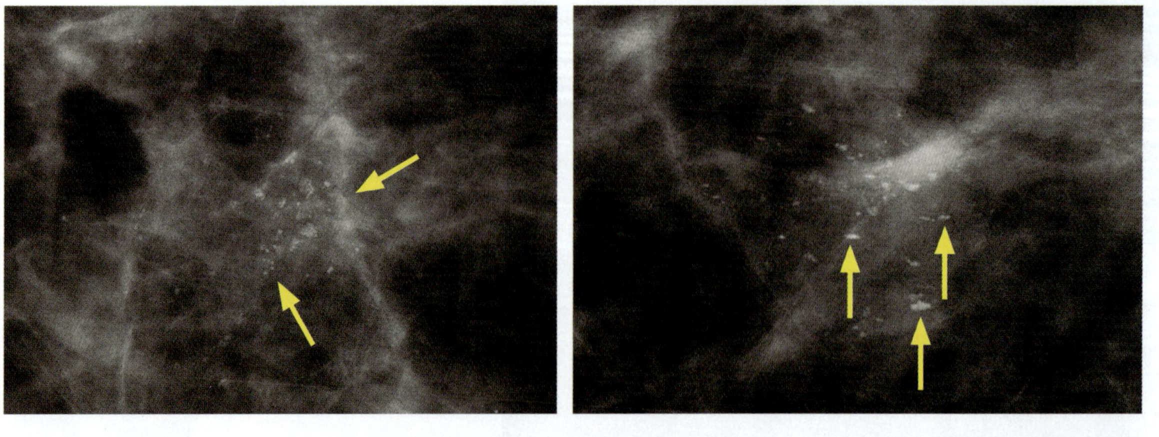

CC spot-magnification view (left image) shows amorphous calcifications (arrows). A true lateral spot- magnification view (right image) shows layering of the calcific sediment (arrows), diagnostic of milk of calcium.
点压放大CC位(左图)显示不定形状钙化(黄箭)。真侧位局部放大图像(右图)显示分层状钙化沉积(黄箭)，可诊断为钙乳样钙化。

- Milk of calcium represents free-floating calcium in tiny benign cysts.
- The most important feature of these calcifications is the apparent change in shape of the calcium particles between the CC and lateral projections.
- On the CC view the calcifications are often indistinct and appear as fuzzy, round, amorphous deposits. On the 90 degree lateral, they are more clearly defined, semilunar or crescent- shaped in morphology due to dependent layering.

- 钙乳样钙化是微小良性囊肿内的自由漂移钙。
- 这些钙化最重要的特点是钙化颗粒在CC位和侧位图像上发生明显的形态改变。
- 在CC位上，这些钙化经常边界不清，表现为模糊、圆形、无定形状沉积物。在90°侧位片上，由于沉积分层，它们的形态更加清晰，呈半月形或新月形。

Suture calcifications

缝线钙化

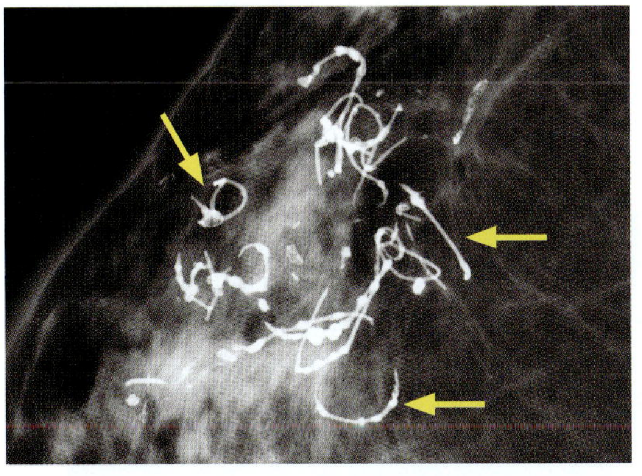

Curvilinear calcifications of variable lengths (arrows) represent calcified surgical suture material.
不同长度的曲线钙化(黄箭)为钙化的手术缝合线。

- Suture calcifications represent calcium deposited on suture material, usually after radiation therapy. Suture calcifications are uncommonly seen due to changes in modern surgical technique.

- 缝线钙化是缝合材料上沉积了钙，通常发生在放射治疗之后。缝线钙化在当代外科技术快速发展的今天已经不再常见。

Dystrophic calcifications

营养不良性钙化

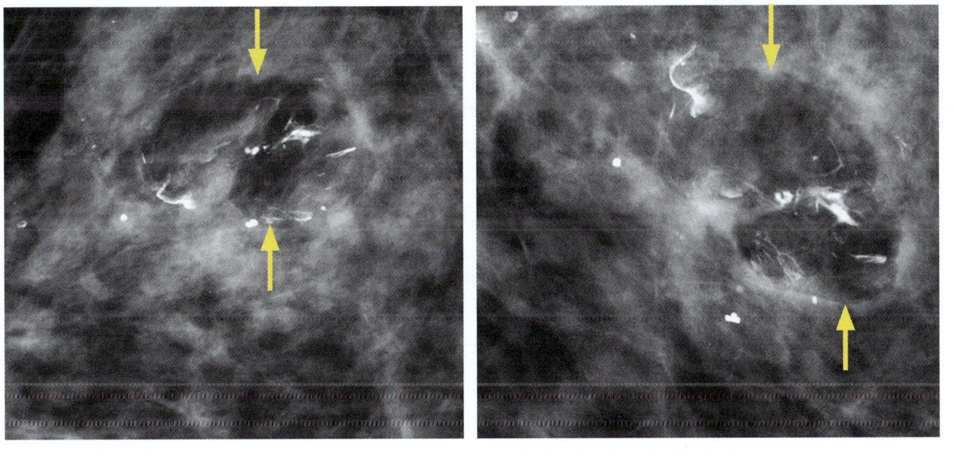

CC and MLO views show a lucent lesion with a bizarre whorled appearance and geometric calcifications (arrows), typical of fat necrosis.
CC位和MLO位图像显示一个透亮的病变，伴有奇异的轮状外观和几何型钙化(黄箭)，为典型的脂肪坏死。

- Dystrophic calcifications may occur as a sequela of surgery, biopsy, trauma, or irradiation.
- Usually the appearance of dystrophic calcification is distinctive, with coarse, irregular shapes often in association with areas of lucency (due to fat necrosis), but these may pose a diagnostic challenge when new or evolving.

- 营养不良性钙化可继发于外科手术、活检、外伤或放疗。
- 营养不良性钙化的外观通常很独特，表现为粗糙、不规则，常伴有透亮区(由于脂肪坏死)，但当这些钙化是新发或正在演变之中时，可能会给诊断带来困难。

Round and punctate calcifications

- Round and punctate calcifications are associated with various etiologies including fibrocystic change. The round shape is sometimes due to deposition in the small terminal acini of breast lobules. When diffusely or randomly distributed, round and punctate calcifications are considered benign.

圆形和点状钙化

- 圆形和点状钙化与多种病因有关，包括纤维囊性改变。圆形钙化有时是由于钙质沉积在乳腺小叶的末端腺泡中所致。弥漫性或随机分布的圆形和点状钙化被认为是良性的。

- When a round calcification is smaller than 0.5 mm, the term "punctate" is preferred.
- An isolated group of punctate calcifications on a baseline mammogram should be classified as BI-RADS 3 (discussed later in chapter).

Rim calcifications

- Fine peripheral calcification represents calcium deposited on the surface of a sphere, usually occurring in an area of fat necrosis or a cyst with calcified walls.
- Previous versions of BI-RADS described these calcifications as "lucent centered" or "eggshell."

- 当圆形钙化直径<0.5mm时，则用"点状"这一术语。
- 首次乳腺X线检查一组孤立的点状钙化应归为BI-RADS 3类(本章后文进行讨论)。

边缘钙化

- 细小的边缘钙化是指钙质沉积在球体表面，通常见于脂肪坏死区域或囊肿的壁钙化。
- BI-RADS早期版本有使用"透亮中心"或"蛋壳样"术语描述这些钙化。

Suspicious morphology calcifications (BI-RADS 4)

可疑钙化形态(BI-RADS 4类)

Amorphous calcifications

无定形钙化

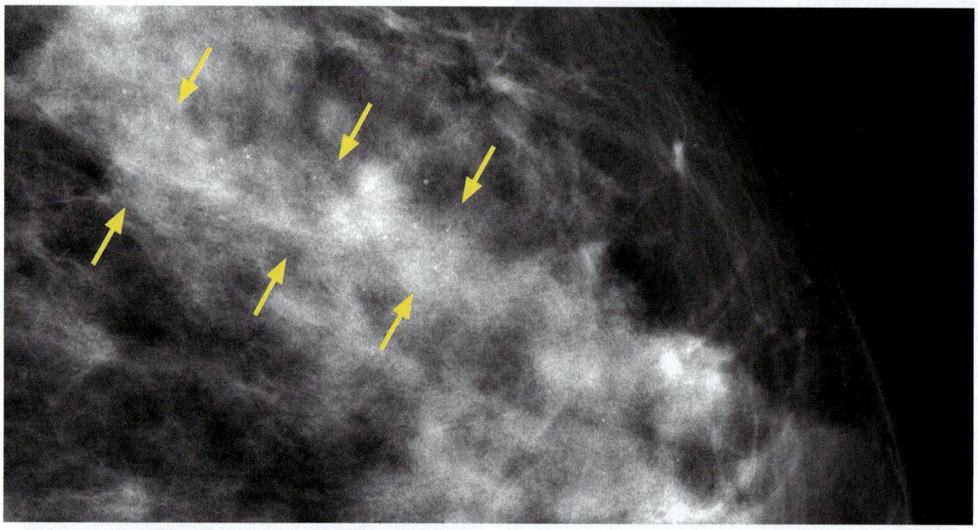

Numerous amorphous calcifications are present in a dense breast in a segmental distribution (arrows). This pattern is suspicious for malignancy and biopsy is warranted.
大量不定形钙化出现在一个致密的乳腺中并呈节段样分布(黄箭)。这种表现提示可疑恶性并需要进行活检。

- Amorphous calcifications are too small or hazy to ascertain their detailed morphologic appearance.
- Amorphous calcifications in a diffuse distribution are usually benign, although magnification views may be necessary to evaluate for any suspicious groups.
- Amorphous calcifications in a grouped, regional, linear, or segmental distribution are more suspicious and warrant biopsy. The positive predictive value of amorphous calcifications has been reported at 20%.

Coarse heterogeneous calcifications

- 无定形钙化通常太小或太模糊，以致不能明确其具体的形态学表现。
- 无定形钙化呈弥漫性分布通常是良性的，但对任何可疑的簇都需要进行放大评估。
- 无定形钙化以成簇、区域、线状或节段样分布则更为可疑并需要进行活检。无定形钙化的阳性预测值为20%。

粗糙不均质钙化

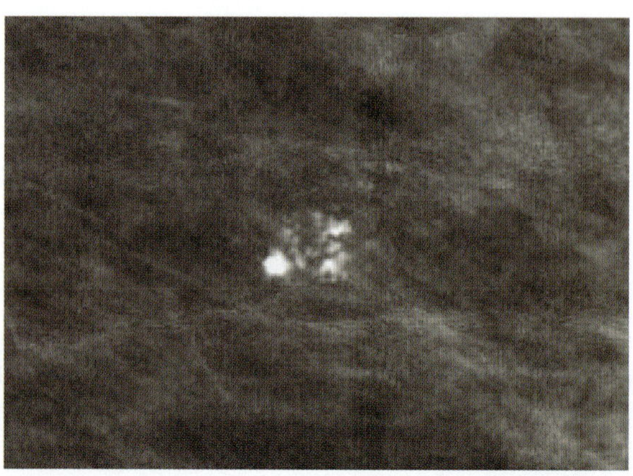

Coned-down image from a spot magnification mammogram shows a cluster of coarse heterogeneous calcifications. These are suspicious and biopsy is warranted.
局部加压放大的乳腺X线影像显示一簇粗糙不均质钙化。这种钙化可疑并需要活检。

- Coarse heterogeneous calcifications are irregular calcifications that are generally larger than 0.5 mm, but smaller than dystrophic calcifications.
- Evolving dystrophic calcifications or early calcifications associated with hyalinizing fibroadenomas or fat necrosis may appear as coarse heterogeneous calcifications and pose a diagnostic challenge.
- Coarse heterogeneous calcifications may be associated with malignancy and biopsy is warranted.

Fine pleomorphic calcifications

- 粗糙不均质钙化为不规则钙化，通常直径大于0.5mm，但小于营养不良性钙化。
- 进展中的营养不良性钙化、透明变性纤维腺瘤或脂肪坏死相关的早期钙化也可能为粗糙不均质，使其诊断变得困难。
- 粗糙不均质钙化可能与恶性相关，需要进行活检。

细小多形性钙化

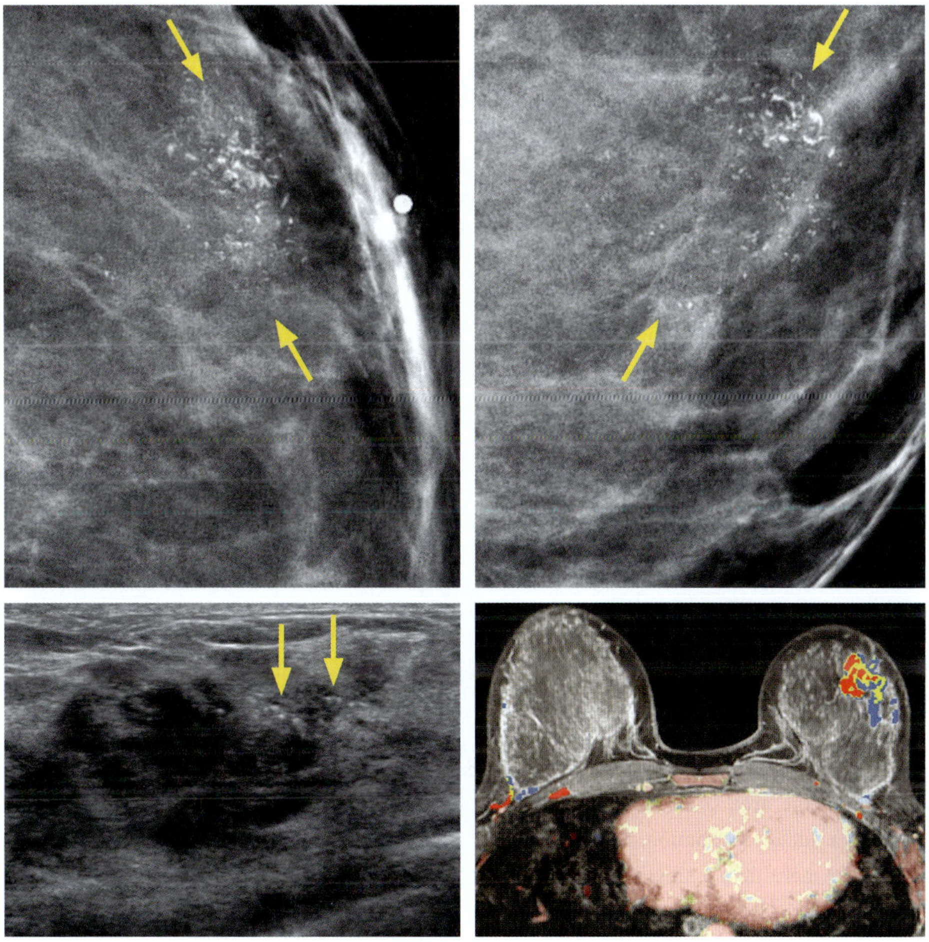

CC and MLO mammograms (top images) demonstrate a large group of fine pleomorphic calcifications (arrows). Ultrasound (bottom left image) shows an ill-defined hypoechoic mass, with the calcifications evident as punctate echogenic foci (arrows). Color CAD angiomap from the patient' s breast MRI shows the segmental, non-mass enhancement in a regional distribution in the left breast, with the red color map corresponding to malignant-type washout kinetics. This lesion is highly suspicious for malignancy (BI-RADS 5).

乳腺X线CC位和MLO位(上两图)显示大片成簇的细小多形性钙化(黄箭)。超声(左下图)显示一个边界不清的低回声肿块，伴有明显钙化的点状回声(黄箭)。磁共振彩色CAD血管图像(右下图)显示患者左侧乳腺内节段性、区域状分布非肿块样强化，图中红色区域与恶性的廓清血流动力学特征相符合。这一病变为高度恶性可疑(BI-RADS 5类)。

- By definition, fine pleomorphic calcifications vary in shape and size, producing a characteristic *dot-dash* appearance.
- Fine pleomorphic calcifications are highly suspicious for malignancy, most commonly seen in DCIS or invasive ductal carcinoma.
- When evaluating any group of calcifications, one should always ask, "can these be pleomorphic?" If so, biopsy should be obtained.

Fine linear or fine-linear branching calcifications

- Fine linear and fine-linear branching calcifications are highly suspicious for malignancy. Branching pattern suggests filling of the lumen of a duct system involved by DCIS.
- If fine linear or fine-linear branching calcifications are seen in a segmental distribution, BI- RADS 5 is appropriate (highly suggestive of malignancy).

- 根据定义，细小多形性钙化在形态和大小上不均一，产生一种具有特征性的"点-线"样表现。
- 细小多形性钙化为高度可疑恶性，最常见于DCIS或浸润性导管癌。
- 当发现任何成簇的钙化时，必须自问"这些钙化是多形性的吗？"如果是，则需要进行活检。

细线样或细线分支状钙化

- 细线或细线分支状钙化都是高度可疑恶性的征象。钙化分支状的形态提示钙质填充于DCIS所累及的导管系统。
- 如果在节段性分布中看到细线或细线状分支钙化，应归为BI-RADS 5类(高度提示恶性)。

Distribution of Calcium

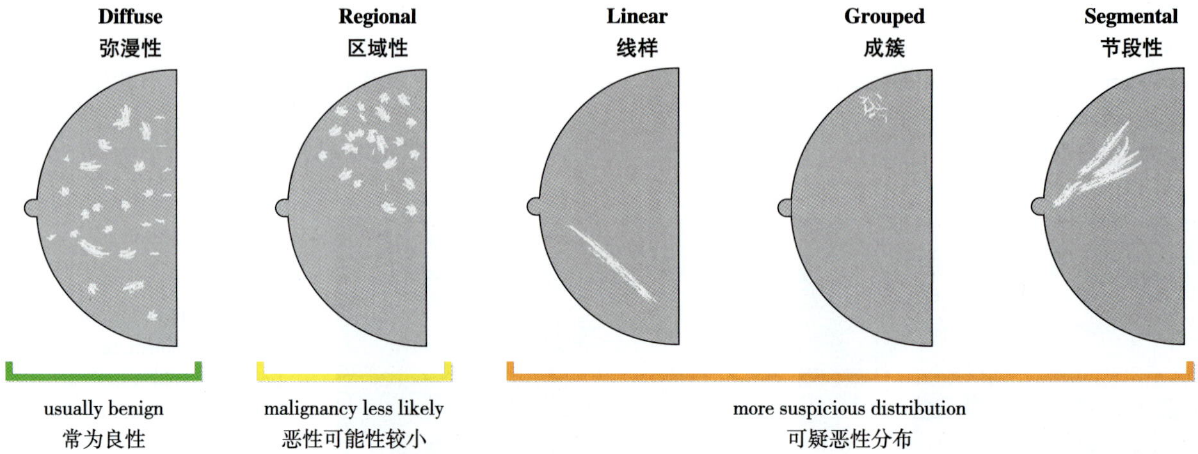

- The distribution of calcification can greatly affect the suspicion of malignancy.
- Although diffuse and regional calcifications are usually benign, the morphology of the calcifications in question is also important. A regional distribution of suspicious fine pleomorphic or fine-linear branching calcifications may represent cancer.
- Similarly, a more suspicious distribution (linear, grouped/clustered, or segmental) of calcifications with a typically benign morphology may warrant further workup.

Diffuse

- Diffuse calcifications are distributed randomly throughout the breast.
- Punctate and amorphous calcifications in a diffuse or scattered distribution are usually benign and often bilateral, typically associated with fibrocystic change or sclerosing adenosis.

Regional

- Regional calcifications are distributed in a large area (>2 cm in largest dimension) of breast tissue not conforming to a ductal distribution. Since this distribution may involve most of a quadrant or more than a single quadrant, malignancy is less likely.

Linear

- Linear calcifications are arrayed in a line.
- Linear distribution of calcifications elevates suspicion for malignancy as this suggests calcium deposits within a duct.
- Note that typically benign large rod-like calcifications are often linear in distribution.

Grouped

- Grouped calcifications are defined as at least five small calcifications located within 1 cm of each other, with the extent of the calcifications measuring <2 cm in size. Calcifications >2 cm in extent are considered regional in distribution, as described above.
- Grouped calcifications raise suspicion for malignancy.

Segmental

- Segmental calcifications suggest calcium deposited in a ductal system, which is worrisome.
- When the morphology is clearly secretory (rod-like), a segmental distribution can be benign.

钙化的分布

- 钙化的分布可以极大影响恶性的可疑程度。
- 尽管弥漫性钙化和区域性钙化通常是良性的，但是相应的钙化形态也非常重要。呈区域性分布但疑似细小多形性钙化或细线分支状钙化的可能是癌症。
- 同样，分布非常可疑(线样、成簇/簇状或节段性)的钙化，即便有典型的良性形态可能也需要进一步检查。

弥漫性

- 弥漫性钙化随机分布于整个乳房。
- 点状和不定形钙化呈弥漫或散在分布通常是良性的，尤其是双侧分布时，多见于纤维囊性改变或硬化性腺病。

区域性

- 区域性钙化分布在乳腺组织内一个较大的区域(>2cm)，但不是沿导管分布。这种分布可能占据整个象限或超过一个象限，其恶性的可能性比较小。

线样分布

- 线样钙化是指钙化呈线样排列。
- 线样分布的钙化增加了恶性的可疑度，提示钙化沉积于导管内。
- 注意，典型的良性大棒状钙化通常呈线样分布。

成簇状

- 成簇状钙化的定义是：直径1cm范围内至少5个微小钙化灶，钙化的范围<2cm。如上所述，范围>2cm的钙化称为区域分布。
- 成簇状钙化有恶性可疑。

节段性分布

- 节段性钙化提示钙化沉积在导管内，值得引起重视。
- 当分布的形态明显为分泌性(杆状)，其节段性钙化可以是良性的。

- When intermediate-suspicion (such as amorphous) or typically benign (such as round or punctate) calcifications are seen in a segmental distribution, concern should be raised for malignancy.

- 当中度可疑(如无定形)或典型的良性钙化(如圆形或点状钙化)呈节段性分布时，则应考虑有恶性可能。

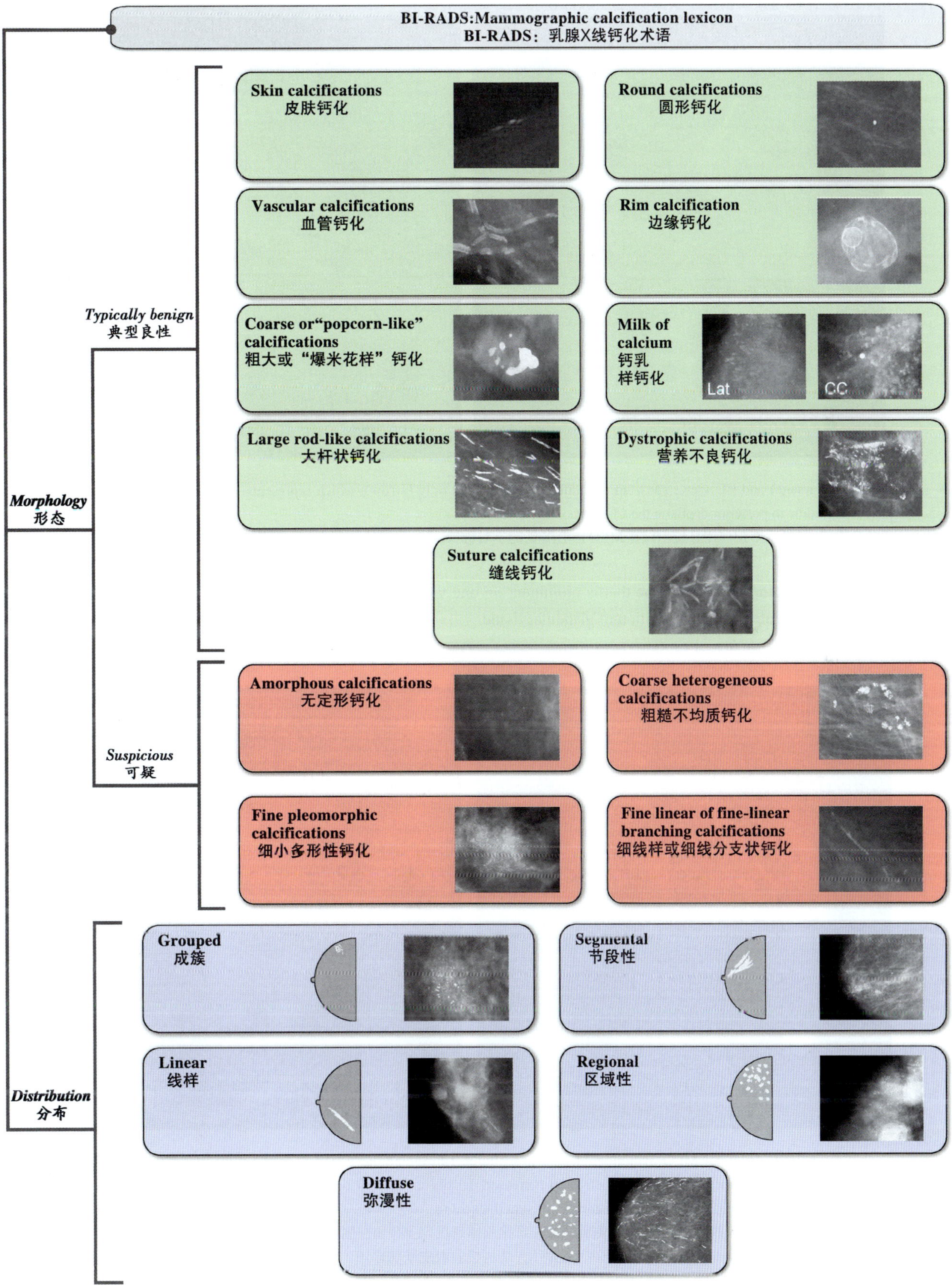

Asymmetry

不对称

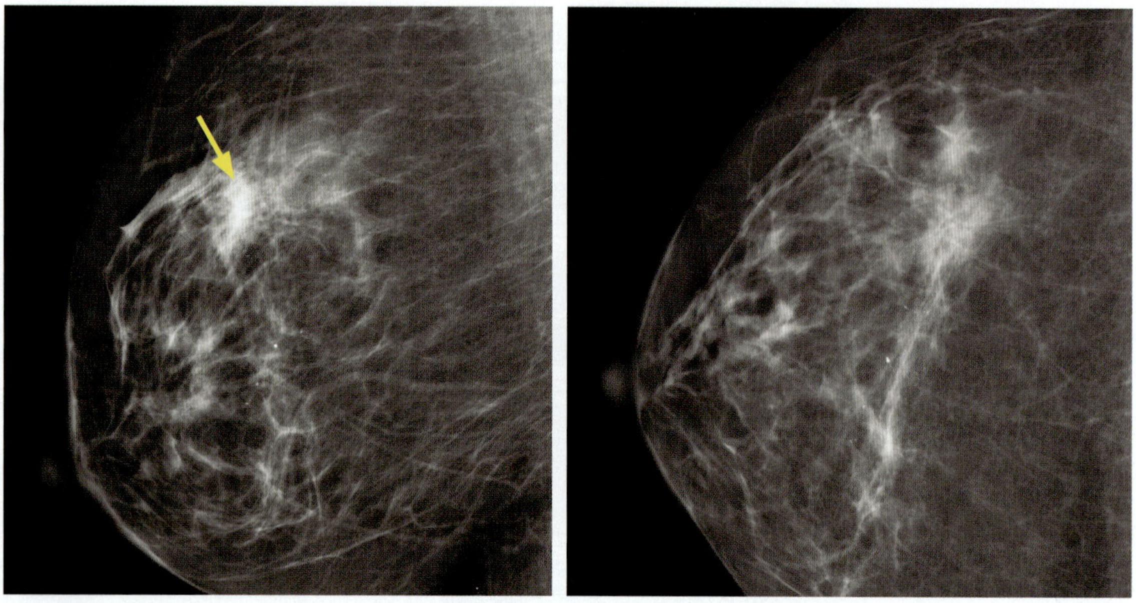

MLO (left image) and CC views show an asymmetry on the MLO only (arrow), which represents superposition of fibroglandular tissue at middle to posterior depth on the CC view.

MLO位(左图)和CC位(右图)显示仅在MLO位上可见的不对称(黄箭),为该体位的中、后部深处重叠的纤维腺体组织。

- An *asymmetry* is a region of breast tissue that is prominent on one view only and most commonly represents superposition of glandular tissue.

- 不对称是仅指在一个摄影体位图像上突显的乳腺组织致密区区域通常是重叠的腺体组织。

Global asymmetry

整体不对称

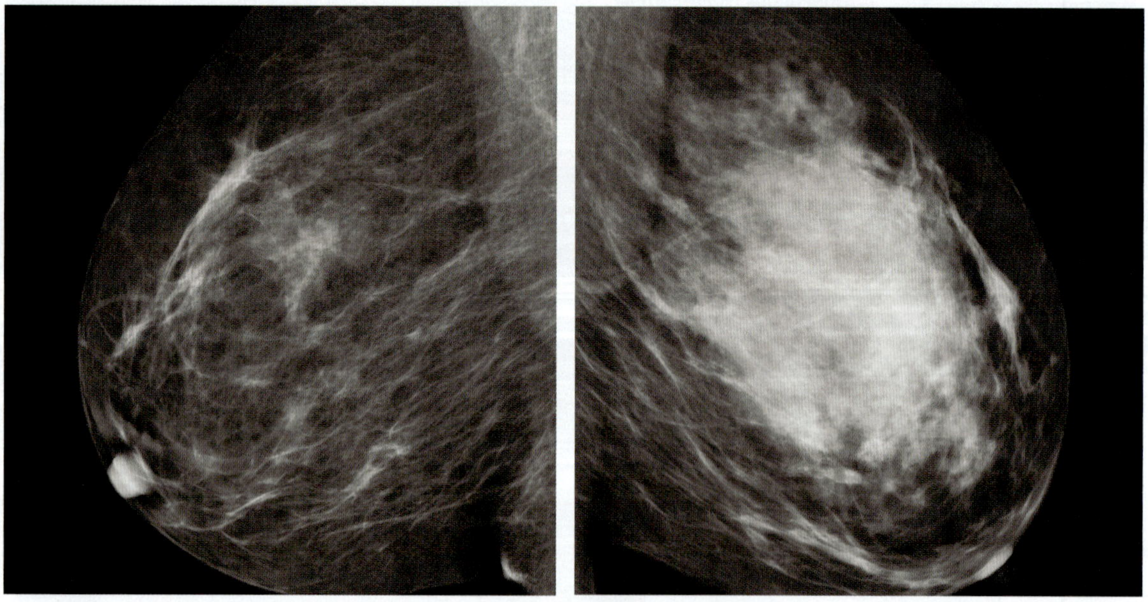

Global asymmetry: Bilateral MLO mammograms show scattered fibroglandular densities in the right breast (left image) and an extremely dense left breast, with the asymmetrically increased density on the left occupying more than one quadrant. There is no associated mass, calcification, architectural distortion, or skin thickening.

整体不对称：双侧乳腺X线MLO位显示右侧乳腺散在纤维腺体密度(左图)和左侧乳腺极其致密腺体密度(右图),不对称的密度增高超过了左乳一个象限的范围。没有伴随肿块、钙化、结构扭曲或皮肤增厚。

- *Global asymmetry* is an asymmetric amount or density of breast tissue involving the majority of one breast only, most commonly due to greater volume of parenchyma in one breast compared to the other. More than one quadrant must be involved.
- Although global asymmetry is usually a normal variant, further workup is warranted when associated with a concerning finding such as a mass, architectural distortion, skin thickening, or any palpable abnormality.

Focal asymmetry

- 整体不对称是指一侧乳房的腺体数量或密度与对侧不对称，可涉及该侧乳腺的大部分，最常见的原因是一侧乳房的实质体积大于另一侧。必须涉及一个象限以上。
- 整体不对称通常是一种正常变异，但当发现伴有肿块、结构扭曲、皮肤增厚或任何可触及的异常等，则需要进一步检查。

局部不对称

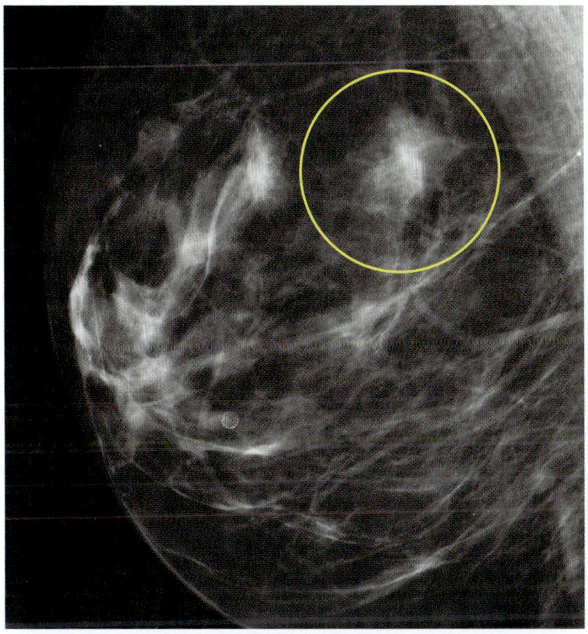

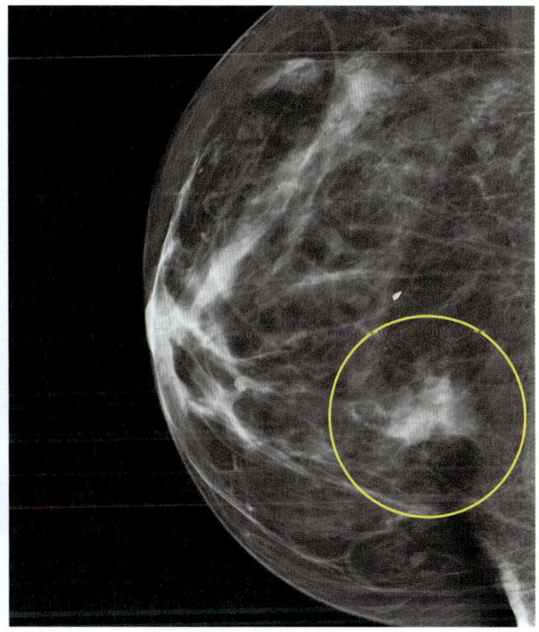

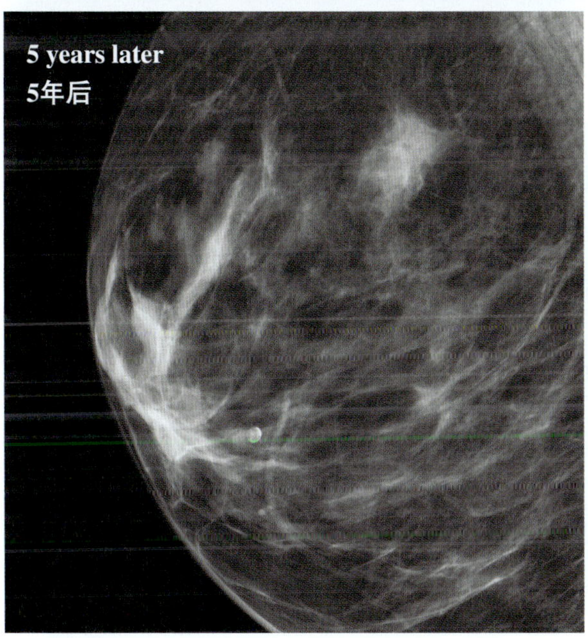

MLO and CC mammograms of the right breast (top images) show a focal asymmetry (circles) in the upper inner breast at posterior depth. This is stable at 5 years follow-up (left image, MLO view).
右乳乳腺X线检查MLO和CC位(上两图)显示乳房内上方后深部有一个局灶性不对称(圆圈内)。在5年随访中表现稳定(左下图，MLO位)。

- A *focal asymmetry* is an abnormality involving less than one quadrant seen on two views (in contrast to an asymmetry) but that does not meet the criteria for a mass. A mass will have distinct borders and convex contours, while a focal asymmetry will have concave contours.
- A focal asymmetry usually represents a prominent area of normal breast tissue,

- 局灶性不对称是指在两个摄影体位图像上看到的小于一个象限的异常(与仅见于一个体位的不对称不同)，但没有达到肿块的标准。肿块具有明显的边界和外凸形轮廓，而局灶性不对称具有内凹形轮廓。

particularly when there is interspersed fat, but further evaluation may be warranted.

- After a complete workup (including additional mammographic views with spot compression and targeted ultrasound), a nonpalpable focal asymmetry has <1% chance of being malignant and can be placed in BI-RADS 3 if seen on a baseline exam. The lesion can be called benign after two to three years of stability.

- 局灶性不对称通常为正常乳腺组织的局部重叠区域，特别是其内夹杂有脂肪，但也可能需要进行进一步评估。
- 在完成所有的检查后(包括点压片和靶向乳腺超声检查)，一个不可触及的局灶性不对称的恶性可能性<1%，若为初次检查可将其归类为BI-RADS 3类。若病变2~3年后仍稳定，则可认为是良性病变。

Developing asymmetry

新发现/进展性不对称

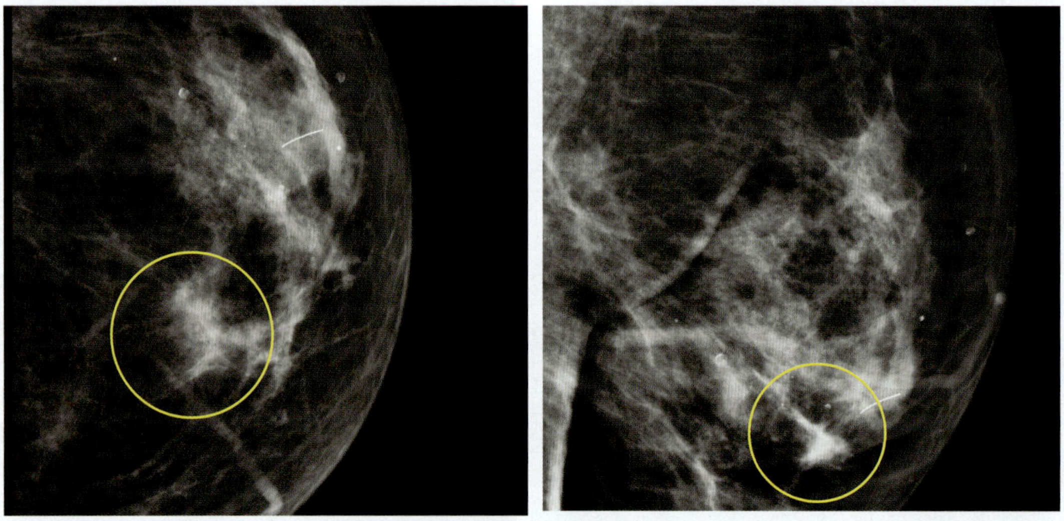

CC (top left) and MLO (top right) mammograms demonstrate a subtle new focal asymmetry (circles) in the lower inner breast that is best appreciated when compared to the prior year's study (below). Ultrasound (not shown) demonstrated an irregular shadowing mass.
乳腺X线CC位(左上)和MLO位(右上)显示位于乳腺内下方一个不明显的新的局灶性不对称(圆圈)，与1年前的检查(下两图)进行对照显得更为清楚。超声(未展示)显示一个不规则声影的肿块。

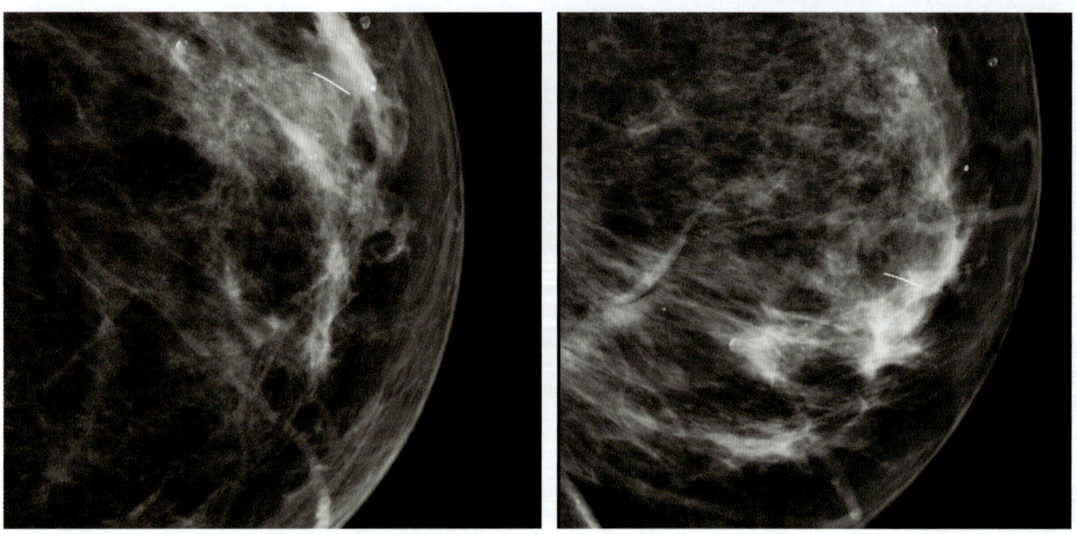

- A developing asymmetry is a focal asymmetry that is either new or increased in size.
- A developing asymmetry is a suspicious finding, shown to represent breast cancer in 12.8% of cases at screening mammography and in 26.7% of cases at diagnostic mammography.
- The initial step in the workup of a developing asymmetry is to determine if it is

- 进展性不对称是一个新的或增大的局灶性不对称。
- 进展性不对称是一种可疑发现，其乳腺癌的检出率在筛查性乳腺X线检查中为12.8%，在诊断性乳腺X线检查中为26.7%。
- 进展性不对称应首先明确是真实病变还是重

a true lesion or summation artifact. A typical mammographic workup includes spot compression views and/or repeating the standard views to confirm that the questioned asymmetry persists.

- After diagnostic evaluation confirms that the developing asymmetry is a true lesion that can be localized in three-dimensional space, then ultrasound is performed. A mass demonstrated sonographically can be targeted for biopsy, and if a benign correlate is seen (e.g., a simple cyst) then the developing asymmetry can be assessed as BI-RADS 2 (benign).
- If no sonographic correlate is seen for a true developing asymmetry then stereotactic biopsy is required, as the risk of cancer is greater than 2% despite the absence of a sonographic abnormality.
- MRI generally does not play a role in the standard evaluation of a developing asymmetry. Since a developing asymmetry is a suspicious mammographic finding, then the absence of an MRI correlate would not obviate the need for biopsy.

Architectural distortion

叠伪影。常规乳腺X线检查应包括局部点压和/或重复标准体位图，以确认不对称是一个确实存在的病变。

- 在诊断评估确认发展中的不对称是一个可以在三维空间中定位的真实病变后，进行超声检查。超声显示的肿块可以作为活检的目标，如果为良性病变(如单纯性囊肿)，则可以将进展性不对称列为BI-RADS 2类(良性)。
- 如果超声检查没有发现与进展性不对称相关的病变，则需要进行立体定向活检，因为即便超声没有异常，其癌症风险依然大于2%。
- MRI通常不作为一个标准的方法评估进展性不对称。因为进展性不对称仅为一个乳腺X线检查的可疑结果，所以MRI没有对应的阳性发现并不能避免活检。

结构扭曲

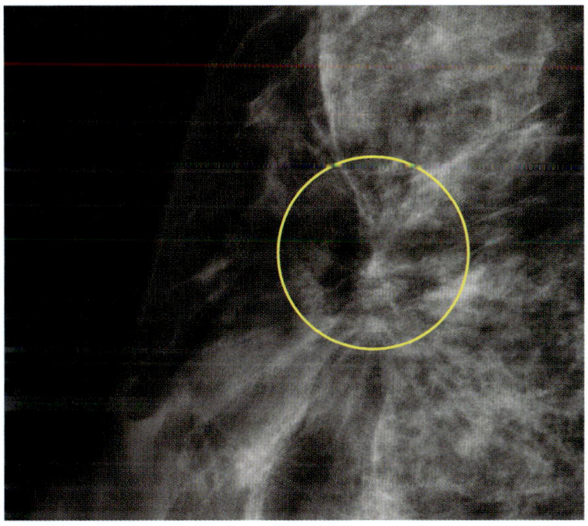

Patient A: Architectural distortion is caused by a scar from prior excisional biopsy (circle).
患者A：结构扭曲是由先前切除活检的瘢痕所致(黄圆圈)。

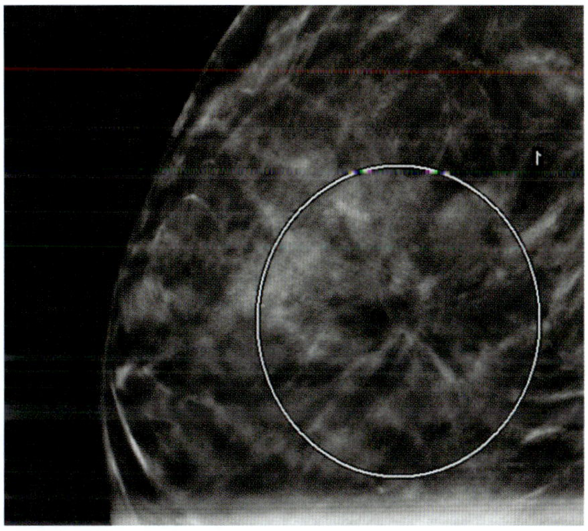

Patient B: Single slice from a mammographic tomogram shows architectural distortion (circle), which was invasive ductal carcinoma on biopsy.
患者B：乳腺X线断层中的一个单张图片显示结构扭曲(白圆圈)，活检示浸润性导管癌。

- Architectural distortion describes lines radiating from a central point with no central mass visible, producing tethering and indentation of the breast tissue.
- Architectural distortion is suspicious for malignancy. The differential for architectural distortion includes invasive malignancy, complex sclerosing lesion/radial scar, post-biopsy scar, and some forms of fibrocystic change such as sclerosing adenosis.

- 结构扭曲是指发现从中心向外的辐射状线条而没有可见的中央肿块，是因对乳腺组织的牵拉和压迫作用而产生。
- 结构扭曲为可疑恶性。其鉴别诊断包括侵袭性恶性肿瘤、复杂的硬化性病变/放射状瘢痕、活检后瘢痕和某些形式的纤维囊性改变，如硬化性腺病。

Mammographic workup and problem solving

Spot compression (with or without magnification)

- Spot compression is compression of a focal region of the breast, which allows for better compression and therefore better resolution. Spot compression is almost always the next step in evaluating a focal suspicious mammographic abnormality.
- Typically, for evaluation of calcifications, spot compression *magnification*

乳腺X线检查和解决问题的方法

点压影像(使用或不使用放大)

- 点压是针对乳腺的一个局部区域进行施压，通过压迫获得更好的分辨率。点压几乎是所有可疑乳腺X线检查的下一步评估方法。
- 评估钙化通常用点压放大。评估肿块或不对

is used. For evaluation of a mass or asymmetry, magnification is usually not needed. Note that areas of architectural distortion may actually appear less apparent on magnification views.

- If an apparent asymmetry "presses out" with focal compression, then the apparent abnormality more likely represents superimposition of normal pliable fibroglandular tissue. Often ultrasound will also be performed to further assure absence of any corresponding suspicious finding.
- If the abnormality does not significantly change shape when compressed, then it is suspicious and its margins could be further assessed on spot magnification views. Evaluation with ultrasound would also be warranted.
- A smaller compression device will allow more precise compression, with the downside of potentially losing landmarks in the surrounding parenchyma.
- Compared to full-field digital mammography, tomosynthesis has the advantage of improved lesion detection and characterization by reducing the effect of overlapping breast tissue. Tomosynthesis may decrease the need for additional diagnostic imaging such as spot compression.

XCC (exaggerated cranio-caudal)

- The lateral XCC (XCCL) pulls lateral breast tissue into the detector.
- The medial XCC (XCCM) pulls medial breast tissue into the detector.

Rolled views (CC variant)

- Rolled views are obtained by moving the top and bottom of the breast in opposite directions. Rolled CC views are helpful to localize a lesion that is seen on the CC view only.
- Two rolled views are typically obtained. One view is obtained with the top of the breast rolled medially (RCCM) and a second view with the top rolled laterally (RCCL).

  If a lesion moves medially with an RCCM view, then it's in the superior breast.

  If a lesion moves laterally with an RCCM view, then it's in the inferior breast.
- The lateral view can also be rolled, although this is less commonly performed.

Reduced compression

- Images with reduced compression can be obtained to image far posterior lesions that may "slip out" of the detector when full compression is applied.

True lateral view (ML or LM)

- A true lateral can be obtained in an ML (most commonly) or LM projection. In an ML view, the X-rays first travel through the medial breast, with the detector placed laterally. Conversely, the detector is medial in an LM projection. It is ideal to place the lesion in question closer to the detector if possible. For instance, a medial lesion is best imaged in an LM projection.
- The true lateral is used to diagnose milk of calcium. In addition to spot compression magnification, magnification spot views should also be obtained in the true lateral projection when milk of calcium is suspected.

  In the true lateral view, the precipitated calcium sinks to the bottom of the small cysts, where it is seen mammographically as tiny crescents (versus the fuzzy round appearance of the CC view).
- The true lateral view is helpful to triangulate a lesion seen in the MLO view but not CC.
- The true lateral can be helpful for planning a stereotactic procedure.

称性病灶则通常不需要放大。注意，在放大的图像上，结构扭曲的区域会显得不明显。

- 如果明显的不对称在局部施压后“消失”，那么这个大体上的异常更可能代表重叠的正常柔韧的纤维腺体组织。通常还需要进行超声检查，以确保没有任何相应的可疑发现。
- 如果异常区域在挤压时的形态没有明显变化则为可疑，需要对其边界在点片放大图上进行评估，还需要进行超声评估。
- 小的加压装置可以使加压更为精确，但缺点是可能会失去周围实质中的自然标志。
- 与全野数字乳腺X线相比，断层融合影像通过减少重叠乳腺组织的影响来提高对病变的检测和观察细节的优势。断层融合可以减少对额外诊断成像的需求，如点压影像。

夸大头尾位(XCC)

- 外侧夸大头尾位(XCCL)把乳腺外侧的腺体组织纳入摄影范围。
- 内侧夸大头尾位(XCCM)把乳腺内侧的腺体组织纳入摄影范围。

旋转位(变异的CC位)

- 旋转位是把乳腺上方和下方的组织朝相反方向牵拉后进行摄片。旋转CC位图像对只能在CC位图像上发现的病变的定位有帮助。
- 通常需要获得2种旋转位：一种是将乳腺的顶部朝内侧转动(RCCM)；另一种是将顶部朝外侧转动(RCCL)。

  如果病变在RCCM图像上向内侧移位，则病变位于乳腺的上方。

  如果病变在RCCM图像上向外侧移位，则病变位于乳腺的下方。
- 侧位图像也可以进行旋转，但并不常用。

部分加压

- 部分加压影像可以用于非常靠近后方的病变，因全力按压可能使病变“溜出”探测器检查范围。

真侧位像(ML或LM)

- 真侧位像可以用ML(最常见)或LM位的投影方法。在ML视图中，探测器置于外侧，X线首先穿过乳腺内侧；与之相反，LM视图时，探测器置于内侧。理想的情况是将病变尽量靠近探测器。例如，内侧病变的最佳成像体位为LM投影。
- 真侧位像用来诊断钙乳样钙化。此外，在怀疑乳样钙化时，应在真侧位进行局部加压放大或放大点片摄影。

  在真侧位片上，沉淀的钙质位于小囊肿的底部，呈微小的新月形(而在CC位显示为模糊的圆形)。
- 真侧位像有助于对MLO位显示而CC位未见的病变进行定位。
- 真侧位像可帮助制订立体定位手术计划。

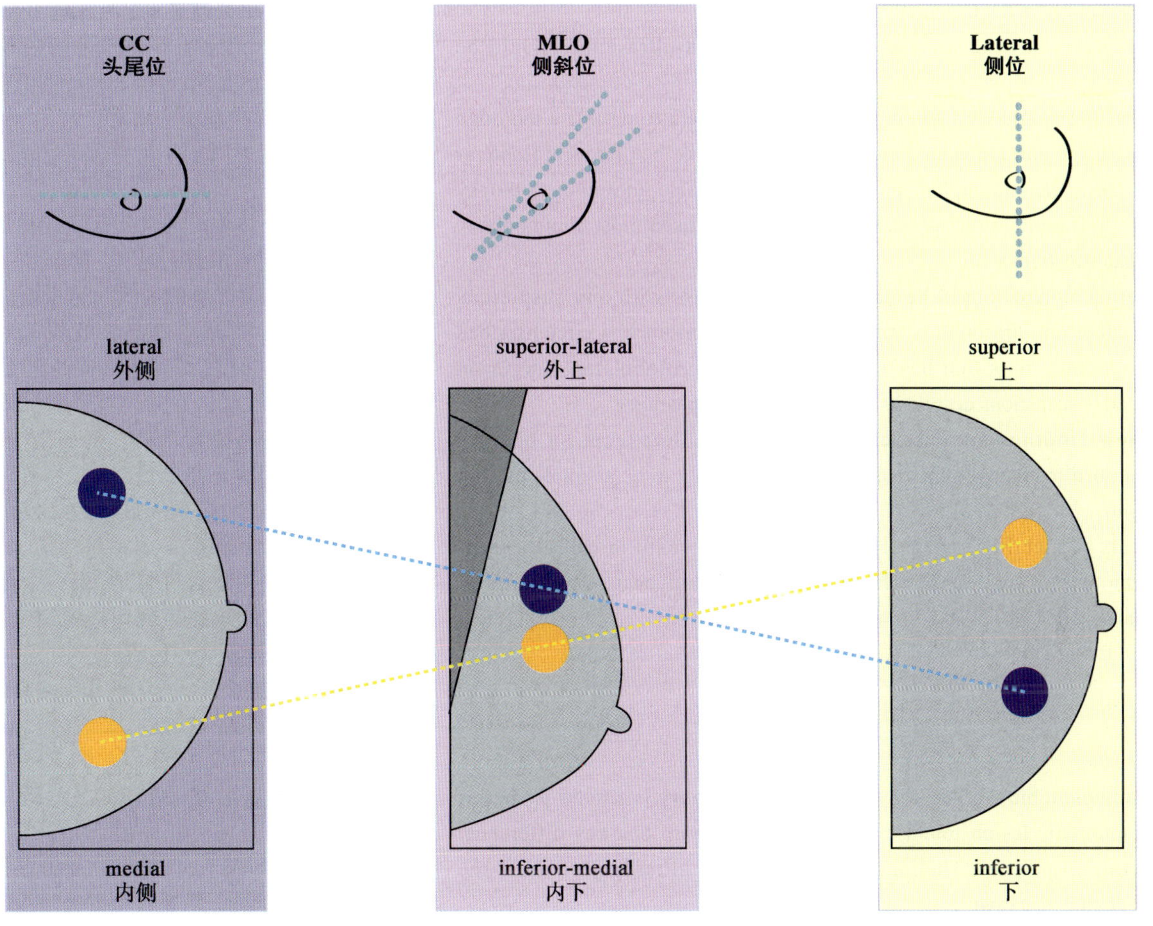

- A true lateral view is helpful to triangulate a lesion seen only on the MLO view.
- If the lesion rises on the lateral compared to the MLO, the lesion is located in the medial breast (**m**edial: **m**uffins rise). If the lesion sinks, it is lateral (**l**ateral: **l**ead sinks).

Working up a mass or focal asymmetry seen on screening mammography

- A screening mammogram *can only receive the BI-RADS 1, 2, or 0 assessments.* If screening mammogram findings are concerning, the patient is assessed as BI-RADS 0 and is recalled for additional evaluation.
- When the patient returns for the diagnostic workup, spot compression views of the area in question should be obtained. Altered projections or rolled views can also be used if necessary. If additional diagnostic mammographic views show only normal pliable fibroglandular tissue, then no further workup is needed (BI-RADS 1).
- If an abnormality persists on spot compression, then it needs to be localized on two orthogonal views. When correlating a lesion on two views, it is important to remember that the lesion should be located at approximately the same distance (within 1 cm) from the nipple on each view. This rule may prevent mistaken localization of different lesions on each projection.
- If the lesion is seen only on the MLO, a lateral view should be obtained to triangulate the lesion. A lesion seen on the MLO view but not the CC view may be located far laterally. An exaggerated CC lateral (XCCL) view can better image the far lateral tissue.

- 真侧位有助于对仅在MLO位上显示的病变进行定位。
- 如果病变在真侧位的位置相对于MLO位有所上升，则病变位于乳腺内侧；如果病变位置下降，则病变位于外侧。

筛查性乳腺X线上的肿块或局灶性不对称的处理方法

- 筛查性乳腺X线影像仅能提供BI-RADS 1类、2类或0类评估。如果乳腺X线筛查有可疑，则患者被归为BI-RADS 0类，并需要召回做进一步检查。
- 当患者回访接受诊断性检查时，应获取可疑区域的局部加压影像。如有必要，也可使用不同的投照或旋转体位。如果补充的诊断性乳腺X线检查显示为正常柔韧的纤维腺体组织，则无须进一步检查(BI-RADS 1类)。
- 如果一个异常在局部加压后仍然存在，则需要用两个呈正交的影像进行定位。当一个病变在两个体位上能够对应起来时，该病变在两个体位像上与乳头的距离也应大致相同(<1cm)。这个规则可防止在不同的体位上错误定位不同的病变。
- 如果病变仅见于MLO位，应获得侧位对其进

- A lesion seen only on the CC view may be in the upper-inner quadrant and not included in the MLO view. Rolled CC views are typically performed to localize lesions seen only in the CC view.
- Once a lesion is localized to a quadrant, targeted ultrasound should be performed.
- If a suspicious single-view finding still cannot be localized despite a thorough mammographic and ultrasound evaluation, MRI can be helpful as a problem-solving tool. Mammographic stereotactic biopsy is also an option to biopsy a one-view finding (although stereotactic biopsy is used most commonly to biopsy calcifications).
- In general, biopsy should be performed for a mass with any suspicious feature either on ultrasound or mammography. For instance, a circumscribed mammographic mass that has an indistinct or microlobulated margin on ultrasound is suspicious despite its mammographic appearance.
- Most new findings are suspicious, with a notable exception being a circumscribed mammographic mass shown definitively to be a simple cyst on ultrasound.
- Two years of stability is generally considered adequate to call a benign-appearing mass benign, although some institutions advocate three years of surveillance.

行三维定位。一个见于MLO位但CC位未显示的病变可能位于远外侧。外侧夸大头尾位(XCCLC)可更好地显示远外侧的组织。

- 一个仅在CC位上显示的病变可能位于内上象限而不包括在MLO位。旋转体位常用来定位仅在CC位上显示的病变。
- 当确定病变局限于某个象限后，需进行针对性超声检查。
- 如果仅一个体位上的可疑病变无法在乳腺X线和超声检查中进行定位，MRI是一个有用的针对性工具。乳腺X线立体定向活检也是对单个体位可疑病变进行诊断的一种选择(虽然立体定向活检更常用于活检钙化灶)。
- 通常情况下，任何在超声或乳腺X线上有可疑的肿块都应进行活检。例如，乳腺X线影像上表现为边缘清晰的肿块，尽管乳腺X线的表现为良性，但超声显示边缘模糊或呈微分叶时应视为可疑。
- 大多数新的发现是可疑的，但一个显著的例外是乳腺X线检查表现为边缘清晰的肿块，且超声明确显示为单纯囊肿。
- 肿块保持稳定2年，通常可认为是良性，但有些医院建议跟踪3年。

Palpable mass

- The mammographic workup for a palpable abnormality is similar to that of an asymptomatic lesion found on mammography, with one key difference: In general, all palpable findings are evaluated by ultrasound, even if the mammogram is negative.

可触及的肿块

- 乳腺X线检查的流程在可触及异常与无症状的乳腺X线异常是相同的，但有一个重要的差别：通常情况下，所有可触及的病变都需行超声检查，即便乳腺X线检查为阴性。

Mammographic Use of BI-RADS 3

- There is data to support the assignment of BI-RADS 3 in the following three situations, which are not definitively benign but have been shown to have less than 2% risk of cancer.

Circumscribed, benign-appearing solid mass

- A probably benign solid mass must meet certain mammographic criteria. Its shape must be round or oval, and its margins must be circumscribed. The mass cannot have any associated suspicious microcalcifications.
- Typically, any visible mammographic mass should also be evaluated with ultrasound. For a mass to be considered probably benign by ultrasound it must be oval (may have two or three smooth lobulations) with a visible echogenic capsule AND lack any malignant features, or must be uniformly hyperechoic AND lack any malignant features (see later section on ultrasound differentiation of benign and malignant solid masses). If both mammographic and sonographic criteria are met, a mass may be assigned BI-RADS 3.
- A probably benign solid mass that has demonstrated at least two years of stability can usually be considered benign (BI-RADS 2).
- Any interval growth or suspicious change in morphology should be recommended for biopsy.

BI-RADS 3类的乳腺X线检查应用

- 有数据支持将以下三种情况归为BI-RADS 3类，这些并非绝对为良性，但癌症的风险小于2%。

边界清晰、良性表现的实性肿块

- 一个可能为良性的实性肿块必须符合的乳腺X线影像标准：是圆形或卵圆形，边缘必须清晰；该肿块不能含有任何可疑的微小钙化。
- 通常，任何乳腺X线上所见肿块还应使用超声进行评估。超声上认为可能良性的肿块必须是卵圆形(可能有两个或三个光滑的分叶)，有包膜且不具备任何恶性特征，或必须是均匀的高回声并且没有任何恶性特征(参见下文超声良恶性实体肿块鉴别部分的内容)。如果同时满足乳腺X线检查和超声检查标准，则可将肿块判定为BI-RADS 3类。
- 一个可能是良性的实性肿块若至少2年没有变化，通常被认为是良性的(BI-RADS 2类)。
- 随访期有任何生长或可疑形态学变化都应建议活检。

Grouped punctate round calcifications

- Punctate calcifications are a subset of round calcifications that are <0.5 mm in size. It is usually necessary to use spot-compression magnification views to accurately characterize calcifications.
- Grouped punctate calcifications (≥5 calcifications/cm) on a baseline exam can be diagnosed as probably benign (BI-RADS 3). Note that the morphology must be clearly punctate or round, and the distribution must be in a group. For instance, a group of amorphous calcifications is indeterminate and usually warrants biopsy. Similarly, although rare, punctate or round calcifications in a linear or segmental distribution would be suspicious.

Focal asymmetry

- Assuming no ultrasound correlate is seen, a focal asymmetry seen on a baseline exam can be assessed as probably benign (BI-RADS 3) after a thorough imaging workup.

成簇点状圆形钙化

- 点状钙化是一种直径<0.5mm的圆形钙化的亚型。这种钙化通常需要使用局部加压放大才能对其特征进行准确描述。
- 基线检查中的成簇点状钙化(≥5个钙化灶/cm)可诊断为可能良性(BI-RADS 3类)。注意，形态学必须是清晰的点或圆，并且必须是成簇分布。例如，无定形的钙化簇是不确定的，通常需要活检。同样，虽然少见，点状或圆形钙化若呈线样或节段性分布则为可疑。

局灶性不对称

- 假如没有相应的超声发现，基线检查所见的局灶性不对称在经过全面的影像检查后可归为良性病变(BI-RADS 3类)。

（翻译　阳宁静）

BREAST ULTRASOUND

乳腺超声

ZONAL ANATOMY AND PATHOLOGY

区带解剖和病理学

Normal zonal anatomy

正常区带解剖

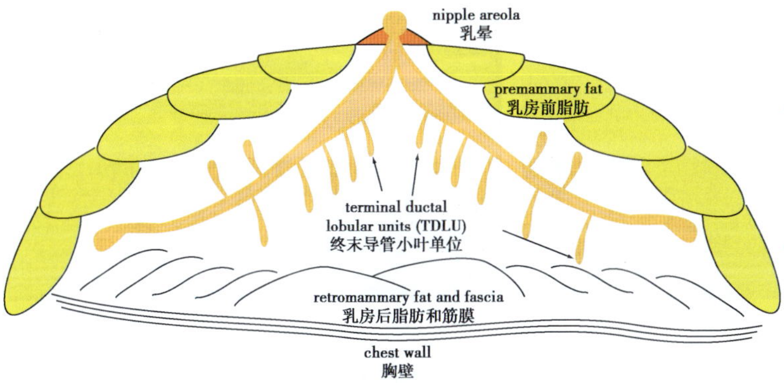

subcutaneous/premammary zone
mostly premammary fat
皮下/乳房前区
大部分为乳房前脂肪

mammary zone	***乳房区***
ducts/TDLUs	导管/终末导管小叶单位
fat	脂肪
fibrous tissue	纤维组织
Cooper's ligaments	Cooper韧带

retromammary zone
mostly fat
乳房后区
大部分为脂肪

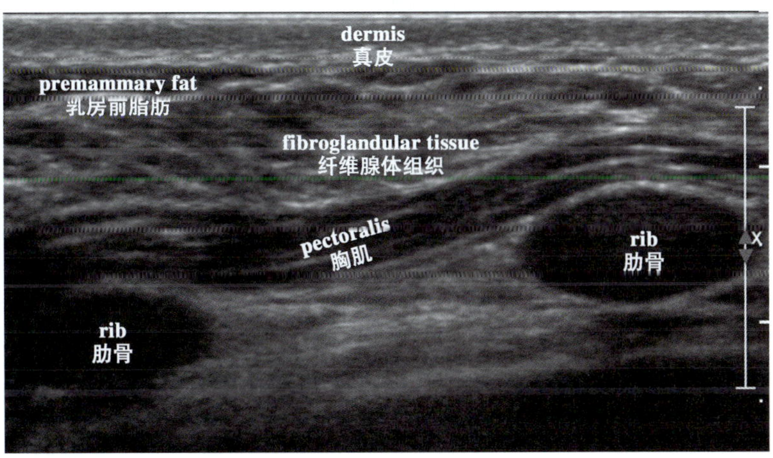

Subcutaneous zone and skin lesions

- The subcutaneous (premammary) zone of the breast contains skin and dermis, subcutaneous fat, and some suspensory Cooper's ligaments. Dermal lesions are almost always benign and include epidermal inclusion cysts and sebaceous cysts.

皮下区及皮肤病变

- 乳房皮下(乳房前)区的结构包括皮肤、真皮、皮下脂肪和部分乳房悬韧带。真皮病变几乎都是良性，包括表皮包涵囊肿和皮脂腺囊肿。

- **Epidermal inclusion cysts** have a true epidermal cell lining and arise either from plugging of a hair follicle by keratinous debris, or from traumatic epidermal implantation. They are the most common type of epithelial cyst. On ultrasound imaging, an epidermal inclusion cyst most often appears as a circumscribed lesion with variable internal echotexture ranging from anechoic to heterogeneous, depending on the amount of internal keratinous debris.
- **Sebaceous cysts** are associated with sebaceous ducts and share an epithelial lining with the sebaceous gland. They may be indistinguishable from epidermal inclusion cysts on clinical exam and ultrasound but are typically lucent on mammography due to the fatty sebum contents; the keratin debris contained in epidermal inclusion cysts, on the other hand, appears dense mammographically.
- A lesion can be confidently diagnosed as a benign epidermal inclusion cyst or sebaceous cyst when it is located completely within the echogenic dermis.
- When a lesion is not completely within the dermis, two clues can be helpful to establish **dermal origin**:

  1) Visualization of a claw of dermal tissue wrapping around the lesion (indicates the point at which the inclusion cyst interrupts the deep dermal layer).

  2) Visualization of a tract connecting the lesion to the epidermal skin surface.

- **表皮包涵囊肿**内衬真性表皮细胞，由于角质碎屑堵塞毛囊或外伤性表皮植入所致，是上皮囊肿最常见的类型。超声图像上，表皮包涵囊肿最常表现为一边缘清晰的病变，其内部回声特征取决于内部角质碎屑的含量，从无回声到不均匀回声。
- **皮脂腺囊肿**与皮脂腺导管相关，内衬的上皮与皮脂腺相同。临床和超声检查中可能与表皮包涵囊肿无法区分，但在乳腺X线影像上因其含脂肪而通常表现为透亮影；而表皮包涵囊肿含有角蛋白碎片，所以乳腺X线影像表现为致密影。
- 如果超声显示病变完全位于真皮层，则有把握诊断为良性表皮包涵囊肿或皮脂腺囊肿。
- 当病变不完全位于真皮内，有两条线索可以帮助确定是否起源于**真皮**：

  1) 可见真皮组织爪样包绕病灶(表示包涵囊肿于此处中断深层真皮层)。

  2) 可见连接病灶与表皮通道。

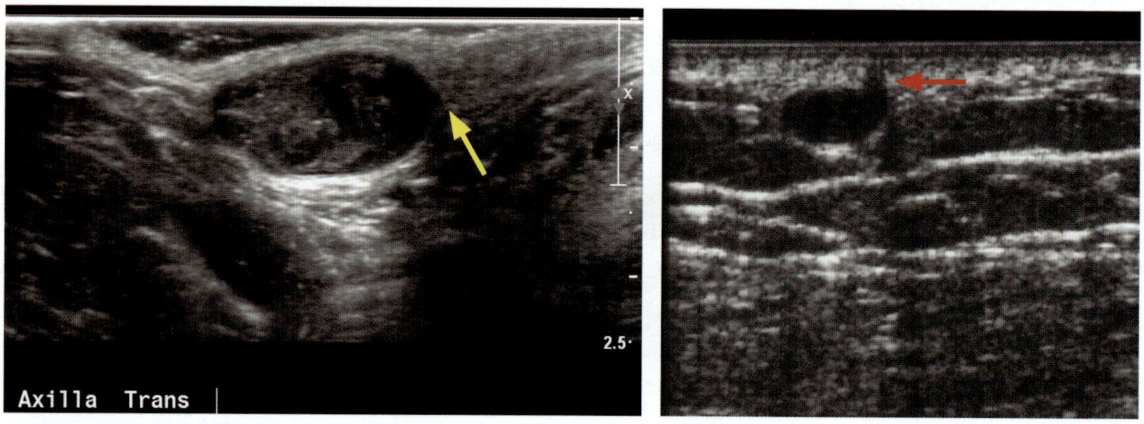

Epidermal inclusion cysts in two different patients:
Transverse ultrasound of the axilla (left image) demonstrates a heterogeneously hypoechoic, oval circumscribed mass partially situated in the dermis, as indicated by dermal tissue wrapping around the mass (*claw sign*, yellow arrow).
Ultrasound of a separate patient (right image) shows a hypoechoic lesion just deep to the epidermis with a tract connecting to the skin surface (red arrow).
来自两名患者的表皮包涵囊肿：
腋窝横切面超声(左图)显示一个不均匀的低回声、边缘清晰的椭圆形肿块，部分位于真皮中，其标志为真皮组织包裹肿块(爪征，黄箭)。
另一名患者的超声(右图)显示了一个低回声病变，位于表皮深处，并有连接到皮肤表面的通道(红箭)。

- Rupture of an epidermal inclusion cyst or sebaceous cyst can incite a severe inflammatory reaction, leading to chemical dermatitis. Therefore, core needle biopsy is to be avoided if epidermal inclusion cyst is suspected. If tissue sampling is felt to be indicated, surgical excision is preferable.
- In contrast, **lesions arising from the hypodermis** (subcutaneous fat) can include a broader range of pathologies, including papilloma, fibroadenoma, and breast cancer. It is therefore critical to identify the anatomic site of origin as best as possible.

- 表皮包涵囊肿或皮脂腺囊肿破裂可引发严重的炎症反应，导致化学性皮炎。因此，当怀疑表皮包涵囊肿时应避免核芯针穿刺活检。如果需要获得组织样本，最好进行手术切除。
- 相反，如果病变**起源于皮下组织**(皮下脂肪)，则包括的病变很广，如乳头状瘤、纤维腺瘤和乳腺癌。因此，病变的解剖起源至关重要，需尽最大可能进行识别。

Mammary zone

- The mammary zone is the site of most breast pathology and includes ducts

乳腺区

- 乳腺区是大多数乳腺病变的发源地，其结构

and terminal ductal lobular units (TDLUs), fat, fibrous tissue, and Cooper's ligaments.

包括导管、终末导管小叶单位、脂肪、纤维组织和乳房悬韧带。

Retromammary zone

- The retromammary zone is just superficial to pectoralis and contains fat and a few Cooper's ligaments.

乳腺后区

- 乳腺后区位于胸大肌的表面，此区域包含脂肪和部分乳房悬韧带。

Imaging fat in the breast

- Parenchymal breast fat is *hypoechoic*, unlike ultrasound imaging of fat elsewhere in the body.
- In contrast, fat in a lymph node hilum, fat in a lipoma, and fat necrosis may all appear *hyperechoic*.

乳腺内脂肪成像

- 乳腺实质内的脂肪为低回声，这与身体内其他部位的脂肪回声不同。
- 相反，淋巴结门、脂肪瘤内的脂肪及坏死的脂肪均表现为高回声。

Ultrasound Technique

超声技术

Scanning planes

- Ultrasound scanning can be performed in radial/antiradial or transverse/longitudinal planes.
- Radial/antiradial scanning has been advocated as superior because ductal anatomy is oriented radially.

扫查平面

- 超声扫查可以按放射状/弧线状或横向/纵向进行。
- 使用放射状/弧线状扫查是一种优先被提倡的方法，因为乳腺导管呈放射状分布。

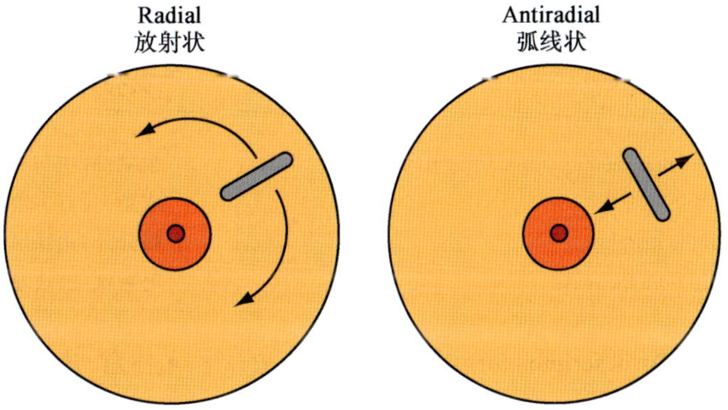

- Transverse/longitudinal orientation is less suited to the centripetal breast anatomy but is familiar from body ultrasound imaging.

- 横向/纵向平面不适合于向心性的乳腺解剖结构，但体部超声成像都使用这样的平面。

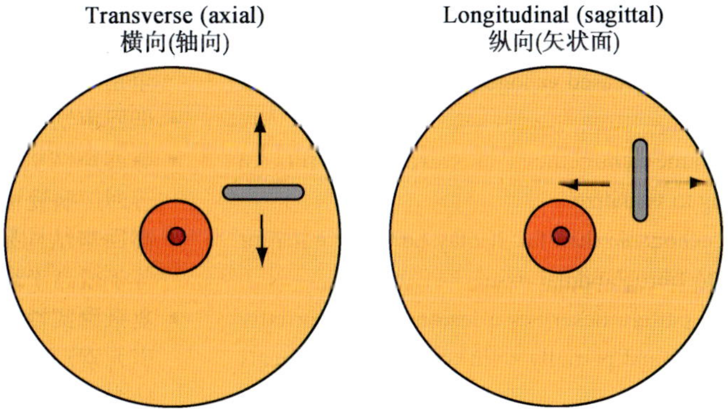

Annotation

- Full annotation is mandatory, including the side, the clock face position, the distance from the nipple, and the transducer orientation (radial/antiradial or transverse/longitudinal).
- Alternatively, some ultrasound systems allow graphical annotations. Documenting the distance from the nipple in addition to the graphic is recommended.

注释

- 必须做完整的注释，包括左右侧、钟面位置、与乳头的距离及探头方向(放射状/弧线状或横向/纵向)。
- 此外，某些超声系统允许影像注释。除了图片，建议记录与乳头间的距离。

BI-RADS LEXICON FOR ULTRASOUND MASSES

- Use of the BI-RADS lexicon allows one to stratify sonographic masses on a spectrum from benign to malignant based solely on the report wording.

Size and position

- A mass should be measured in all three orthogonal planes, with position labeled in terms of clockface and distance from the nipple.

Shape

- The BI-RADS lexicon for the shape of an ultrasound mass includes **round**, **oval**, and **irregular**, the same as for a mammographic mass.

Orientation

- The orientation of the long axis of a mass (relative to the skin) is unique to ultrasound.
- A mass that is **parallel** in orientation is more likely to be benign.
- In contrast, a **non-parallel** mass (known informally as "taller-than-wide") is oriented with the long axis vertical and is suspicious for malignancy. This finding is based on the propensity of a malignant process to violate tissue planes.

Margin

- Similar to mammography, benign masses are typically **circumscribed**.
- If the margins of a mass are not circumscribed, they can be characterized as **indistinct**, **angular**, **microlobulated**, or **spiculated**.

> **Indistinct**: No clear boundary between the mass and its surrounding tissue.
> **Angular**: Featuring sharp corners.
> **Microlobulated**: Serrated appearance of the margins.
> **Spiculated**: Linear projections emanating from the mass.

- Note that *obscured* is not a BI-RADs descriptor for ultrasound, only for mammography.

Echo pattern

- The echo pattern describes the internal texture of an ultrasound lesion. Most benign and malignant lesions are hypoechoic. The margins of a lesion are more reliable than the echogenicity in determining if a lesion has benign features.
- An **anechoic** structure has no internal echoes and most commonly (but not always) represents a simple cyst.
- A **hypoechoic** structure is defined as decreased echogenicity in comparison to the surrounding mammary fat.
- An **isoechoic** structure has the same echogenicity as surrounding fat. An isoechoic lesion can be challenging to visualize.
- A **hyperechoic** structure is more echogenic than fat. It may be either equal or greater in echogenicity compared to fibroglandular tissue.
- A **complex cystic and solid** echo pattern describes a lesion that is partially cystic (containing anechoic elements) and partially solid (containing elements of varying echogenicity).
- A **heterogeneous** echo pattern represents a combination of internal echogenicities.

Posterior features

- The posterior features of a lesion describe the attenuation characteristics of the sound beam deep to the lesion.
- Acoustic **enhancement** (also called posterior through-transmission) refers to a column of increased echogenicity posterior (deep) to the mass. Posterior enhancement is one of the characteristics of a simple cyst, although on its own

超声肿块的BI-RADS术语

- 使用BI-RADS词汇可以让人根据报告术语对超声上的肿块进行良恶性分类。

大小和位置

- 肿块应在三个正交平面进行测量，并需要标记钟面位置及与乳头之间的距离。

形态

- 超声肿块形态的BI-RADS术语包括**圆形、椭圆形**和**不规则形**，与乳腺X线检查相同。

方向性

- 肿块长轴的方向(相对于皮肤)是超声特有的。
- **平行**方向肿块的良性可能更大。
- 相反，一个**非平行**的肿块(非正式地称为"高大于宽")则为恶性可疑。这一发现是基于恶性肿瘤有破坏组织平面的倾向。

边缘

- 与乳腺X线影像相似，良性肿块的边缘通常是**清晰**的。
- 如果一个肿块的边缘不清，则可用**模糊、成角、微分叶**或**毛刺**进行描述。

> **模糊**：肿块与其周围组织之间没有明确的界限。
> **成角**：具有尖角。
> **微分叶**：边缘呈锯齿状。
> **毛刺状**：肿块发出线性凸起。

- 注意，*遮蔽*不是超声BI-RIADS的描述用语，仅适用于乳腺X线检查。

回声特征

- 回声特征是指病变内部在超声上的声像特征。大多数良性和恶性病变是低回声的。在确定病变的良恶性特征时，病变的边缘比回声更可靠。
- **无回声**结构不具内部回声，最常见于(并非完全是)单纯性囊肿。
- **低回声**结构定义为回声低于周围的乳腺脂肪。
- **等回声**结构是指回声与周围脂肪相同。一个等回声病变可能不易被发现。
- **高回声**结构是指回声高于周围脂肪。它可以等于或高于纤维腺体组织的回声。
- **复杂囊实性**回声模式是指部分囊性(包含无回声元素)和部分实性(包含不同回声的元素)的病变。
- **异质回声**是内部各种回声的组合。

病灶后部特征

- 病变后部特征用于描述位于病灶深处的声衰减特性。
- **回声增强**(也称穿透后增强)是指肿块后方(深部)有一束增强的回声。后方回声增强是单纯性囊肿的一个重要特征，但不为单纯性

posterior enhancement is not specific.

- **Shadowing** is attenuation of the sound beam as it passes through the lesion. Shadowing is associated with fibrosis, such as from a neoplastic desmoplastic reaction or surgical scar.
- If a lesion has **no posterior acoustic features**, then the echogenicity of the area immediately deep to the mass is the same as adjacent tissue.
- A lesion can also have a **combined pattern** of posterior acoustic features, such as a fibroadenoma containing a large, coarse, shadowing calcification.

囊肿所特有。

- 声影是指声波通过病变时的衰减现象。声影与纤维化有关，如由肿瘤间质反应或手术瘢痕引起的纤维化。
- 如果病灶**没有后部回声**，则该病灶后方紧邻的组织回声特性应与其周围组织相同。
- 同一病灶可存在**混合**后部回声特征，如纤维腺瘤有大而粗的钙化声影。

ULTRASOUND DIFFERENTIATION OF BENIGN AND MALIGNANT SOLID MASSES

- Certain ultrasound features are associated with benign or malignant lesions. In some circumstances, a solid mass that demonstrates only benign ultrasound findings may be classified as BI-RADS 3 and followed.

Ultrasound features of a benign mass

- *Lack of any malignant findings: If even a single malignant feature is present then a lesion is indeterminate or suspicious and should be biopsied.*
- Marked hyperechogenicity (relative to fat).
- Circumscribed margins.
- Parallel orientation to the skin (wider-than-tall; width:height >1.4).
- Oval shape.
- Few gentle lobulations
- Thin echogenic pseudocapsule.

Ultrasound features of a malignant mass

- Spiculated margins, which is the most specific sign of malignancy.
- Non-parallel (taller-than-wide) orientation, the second most specific sign.
- Angular or microlobulated margins.
- Posterior shadowing.
- Markedly hypoechoic echotexture.

Indeterminate ultrasound features

- The following features are not helpful in differentiating between benign or malignant masses: Lesion size, iso- or mild hypoechogenicity, posterior acoustic enhancement, and heterogeneous or homogeneous texture.

超声鉴别实性肿块的良恶性

- 一些超声特征与病灶的良恶性有关。在某些情况下，只具备良性超声特征的实性肿块可按照BI-RADS 3类进行分类和随访。

良性肿块的超声特征

- *没有任何恶性特征：即使只发现一个恶性特征，此病灶的性质即为不确定或可疑，应进行活检。*
- 明显的高回声(相对于脂肪)。
- 边缘清晰。
- 长轴与皮肤平行(宽大于高；宽：高>1.4)。
- 椭圆形。
- 少量光滑的分叶。
- 薄的假包膜。

恶性肿块的超声特征

- 毛刺状边缘，恶性肿瘤最特异的征象。
- 非平行方向(高大于宽)，是第二个最特异的征象。
- 成角或微分叶。
- 后方声影。
- 明显的低回声特征。

不具特征的超声表现

- 对于区别良恶性肿瘤没有帮助的特征包括病变大小、等回声或轻微低回声、后方回声增强、回声不均匀或均匀等。

ULTRASOUND USE OF BI-RADS 3

- It may be appropriate to place specific well-defined entities into the BI-RADS 3 (probably benign) category, with literature supporting less than 2% risk of cancer.
- Isolated **complicated cyst** containing low-level internal echoes, without solid component
- **Clustered microcysts** (discussed later in the chapter).
- **Oval, hypoechoic, circumscribed, parallel mass**, most likely a fibroadenoma.
- **Hyperechoic mass** with central hypoechogenicity, most likely fat necrosis. Note that if an oil cyst is seen at mammography this finding can be classified as benign.
- Additional BI-RADS 3 cases for which robust data does not exist include isolated shadowing without a mass, and architectural distortion thought to be due to a surgical scar.

BI-RADS 3类的超声应用

- 将超声上有以下典型表现的病变归为BI-RADS 3类(可能良性)，文献表明其癌症风险小于2%。
- 孤立的**复杂性囊肿**为内部低回声，无实性成分。
- **成簇的微囊肿**(本章后文进行讨论)。
- **卵圆形、低回声、边缘清晰、与长轴平行的肿块**，多数为纤维腺瘤。
- **高回声肿块伴**中央低回声，很可能是脂肪坏死。注意，如果乳腺X线影像看到油性囊肿，则该发现可归类为良性。
- 其他BI-RADS 3类情况尚没有可靠的数据支撑，其中包括孤立性声影不伴有肿块，以及手术瘢痕造成的结构扭曲。

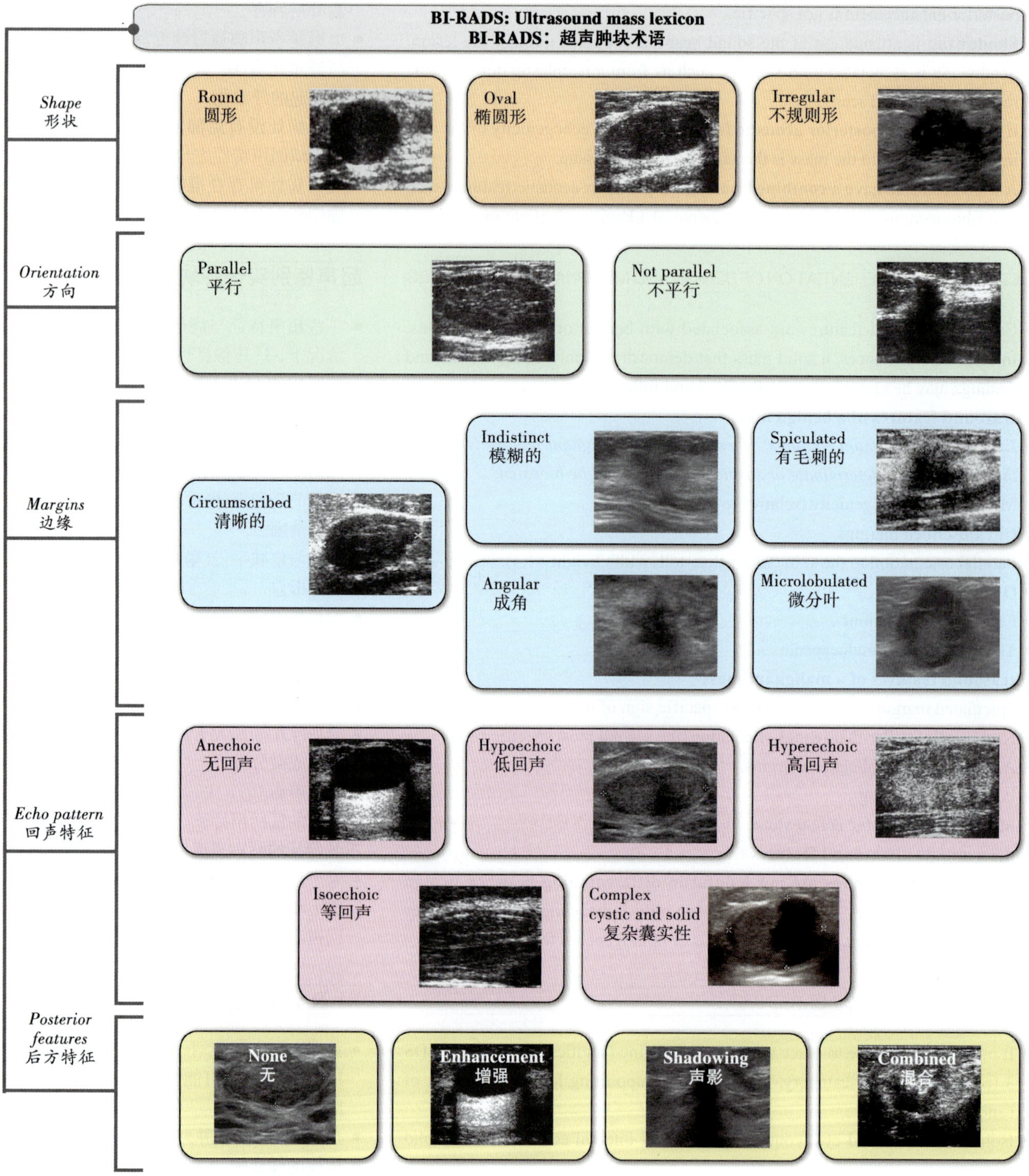

（翻译　阳宁静）

BREAST MRI

乳腺MRI

INTRODUCTION

前言

Overview of clinical role of breast MRI

- Breast MRI plays a complementary role to mammography in the evaluation of breast cancer.

乳腺MRI临床应用概述

- 在乳腺癌的评估中乳腺MRI是对乳腺X线检查的一种补充手段。

- Contrast-enhanced breast MRI features excellent soft tissue contrast and high sensitivity for the detection of cancer. Although the distinction between normal or benign structures and malignancy is often not apparent using standard T1- and T2-weighted sequences, the addition of dynamic contrast enhancement greatly increases the accuracy for detection of malignancy.
- One of the greatest challenges facing the evolving field of breast MRI is the overlap in imaging findings between benign and malignant lesions. Both tumors and benign lesions may enhance and may exhibit similar morphologic characteristics. Strategies such as the characterization of enhancement kinetic curves and development of a stringent BI-RADS lexicon help to tackle this problem.

  One relative weakness of MRI compared to mammography is the lack of sensitivity to microcalcifications. While some larger calcifications can be detected as susceptibility artifact, mammography is superior to MRI for detection of small calcifications.
- In clinical use to evaluate for breast cancer, standard 1.5 or 3 Tesla breast MRI has been shown to have very high negative predictive values and relatively low false positive rates.

- 乳腺增强MRI具有较好的软组织对比度，对肿瘤检测具有很高的灵敏度。虽然正常或良性结构与恶性组织结构在常规T_1和T_2加权序列中并不能很好地进行区分，但加入动态对比增强序列可以大大提高恶性肿瘤检测的准确性。
- 对正处在不断发展的乳腺MRI领域，人们所面临的最大挑战之一是良恶性病灶的影像学表现有重叠。良性与恶性病灶都可能强化，并出现类似的形态学特征。采用不同的策略，如分析动态强化曲线的特征和严格的BI-RADS定义，将有助于解决这个问题。

  相对于乳腺X线影像，MRI的一个不足之处是对微小钙化缺乏灵敏度。尽管有些较大的钙化灶在MRI图像上可因磁敏感伪影而被发现，但乳腺X线影像对于检测微小钙化的能力优于MRI。
- 在乳腺癌临床评估中，标准的1.5T或3T MR乳腺成像可以达到很高的阴性预测值及相对较低的假阳性率。

Breast MRI technique

- The risk stratification of an enhancing lesion involves separate evaluation of the lesion morphology (including morphologic description of the enhancement pattern) and the kinetic pattern of enhancement.
- Breast MRI is performed with the patient prone using a dedicated breast coil. Imaging of both breasts should be performed simultaneously unless the patient has had a previous mastectomy. Bilateral imaging is very helpful to distinguish background parenchymal enhancement from pathological enhancement.
- Standard sequences include T1- and T2-weighted images, with and without fat saturation. Essential to the breast MRI exam are the pre- and post-contrast images, which are typically obtained using fat saturation. Dynamic enhanced images are obtained sequentially to evaluate for enhancement over time.
- Intraductal fluid may be hyperintense on T1-weighted images, complicating the evaluation of enhancement. Post-processing is required to evaluate for true enhancement.
- The simplest form of post-processing is **subtraction**, where the dynamic post-contrast images are subtracted from the initial T1-weighted fat-saturated images.
- The **maximum-intensity projection (MIP)** image is a useful post-processing tool based on the subtraction images. A MIP highlights the brightest pixel along each parallel ray to create a volumetric data set where the enhancement can easily be seen in three-dimensional space.
- **Computer-aided detection (CAD)** is a helpful adjunct for analysis of contrast-enhanced MRI sequences. CAD allows creation of a color angiomap, assigning colors to different temporal patterns of enhancement and allowing further characterization of a lesion to help determine the level of suspicion for malignancy.

乳腺MRI技术

- 对一个强化病灶的危险等级分析包括评估病灶的形态(包括强化图像的形态学描述)及其动态强化曲线特征。
- 乳腺MRI检查时患者采用俯卧位，并使用乳腺专用线圈。除有乳房切除史外，两侧应同时成像。双侧乳腺成像对区别背景实质强化和病理性强化极有帮助。
- 标准的序列包括T_1加权和T_2加权成像，伴或不伴脂肪抑制。乳腺MRI检查的关键是要获取增强前后的图像，并通常采用脂肪抑制序列。动态增强成像需进行连续采集，以评估随时间变化的强化程度。
- 乳腺导管内的液体在T_1加权图像上可能呈高信号，这使分析强化状况变得复杂。需要进行后处理来评估真正的强化。
- 最简单的后处理方法是**减影**，即用动态增强后图像减去增强前T_1加权脂肪抑制图像。
- **最大密度投影(MIP)**是一个基于减影图像的有用的后处理工具。MIP突出显示每一平行线像素点中最亮的像素，产生一个容积数据，使强化的区域在三维空间中容易进行观察。
- **计算机辅助检测(CAD)**有助于分析对比增强MRI的各种序列。CAD可以生成彩色图谱，不同色彩对应不同时间的强化模式，并进一步显示病灶的特征，以帮助确定恶性的可疑程度。

INDICATIONS FOR BREAST MRI

Screening for breast cancer in women at increased risk

- Screening for cancer in high-risk patients is an accepted indication for breast MRI. High risk is defined as a 20% or greater lifetime risk of developing

乳腺MRI的适应证

对高风险女性进行乳腺癌筛查

- 对高风险女性进行乳腺癌筛查是一个被认可的乳腺MRI适应证。高风险是指一生中发生

breast cancer. There are several models for risk prediction taking into account family history, gene mutations, and exposures such as thoracic radiation (typically administered for treatment of lymphoma). *BRCA1* or *BRCA2* gene mutation carriers (or untested first-degree relatives of a confirmed carrier) are high risk, with 50–85% lifetime risk of developing breast cancer.

- MRI has been shown to detect occult breast cancer in 2–5% of high-risk women.

乳腺癌的概率≥20%。数个乳腺癌风险预测模型将以下几个因素考虑在内：家族史、基因突变及危险暴露，如胸部放射治疗(通常用于淋巴瘤的治疗)。*BRCA1*和*BRCA2*突变基因携带者(或未接受突变基因检测的直系亲属中有已知携带者)为高危人群，其一生中发生乳腺癌的风险达50%~85%。

- MRI可在2%~5%的高风险女性中发现隐匿性乳腺癌。

Staging of known cancer

- In patients with an established diagnosis of breast cancer, MRI can be helpful to evaluate the extent of disease and can change clinical management.
- The presence of two or more sites of cancer in one quadrant (**multifocal** disease) may preclude breast conservation, depending on the size of the breast. MRI has been reported to find additional cancer in the same quadrant in 1–20% of women.
- The presence of cancer in more than one quadrant (**multicentric** disease) usually requires mastectomy. Unsuspected multicentric disease was found by MRI in 2–24% of women.
- MRI can accurately measure tumor size and has the highest correlation with pathology specimens when compared to ultrasound or mammography, which tend to underestimate the true size.
- MRI can assess for the presence of enlarged or abnormal axillary lymph nodes.
- MRI can evaluate for pectoralis or intercostal muscle invasion.

已知癌症分期

- 对已确诊的乳腺癌患者，MRI有助于评估病灶的范围，并可能改变临床治疗决策。
- 一个象限出现2个或多处癌灶(**多发**病灶)可能排除保乳治疗，但取决于乳房的大小。据报道，MRI发现同一象限有额外的癌性病灶见于1%~20%的女性。
- 肿瘤出现在一个以上象限时(**多中心**病灶)，一般需要乳房切除术。在2%~24%的女性中，MRI发现未曾怀疑的多中心病灶。
- MRI能够准确测量肿瘤大小，并且与病理标本有最高的一致性，而超声和乳腺X线检查常低估肿瘤的真实大小。
- MRI可以评估是否存在肿大或异常的腋窝淋巴结。
- MRI可以评估胸肌或肋间肌的侵犯。

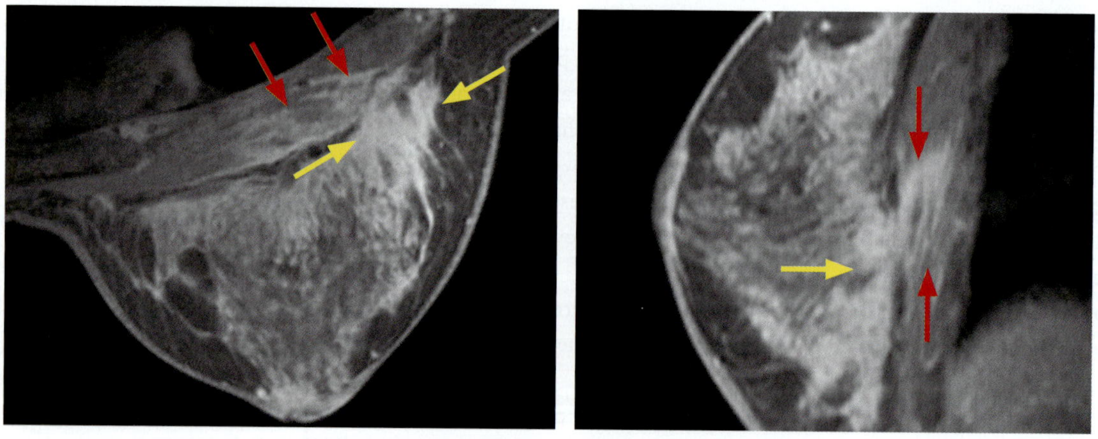

Pectoralis muscle invasion: Axial (left image) and sagittal contrast-enhanced fat-suppressed MRI shows an ill-defined enhancing mass (yellow arrows) in the far posterior breast with loss of normal fat plane separating the posterior fibroglandular tissue from the pectoralis muscle. There is associated abnormal enhancement of the pectoralis muscle itself (red arrows).
胸大肌受侵：轴位(左图)和矢状位(右图)增强后脂肪抑制MRI显示一处边界不清的强化病灶(黄箭)，位于乳房的后部较深处，而且乳房后缘的腺体组织与邻近胸大肌之间脂肪间隙消失。同时，胸大肌本身出现异常强化(红箭)。

Evaluation for recurrent or residual disease

- Breast conservation therapy combines lumpectomy with radiation therapy and is the treatment of choice for most early stage breast cancers. If resection margins after lumpectomy pathologically show remaining tumor, MRI can evaluate for the extent of residual disease, which may manifest as small nodular areas of enhancement around the lumpectomy site.
- Normal enhancement following lumpectomy can be seen for up to 18 months due to granulation tissue. Suspicious features include enhancement beyond 18

评估复发或残留病灶

- 保乳治疗是对病灶行局部切除手术并辅以放射治疗，是大多数早期乳腺癌的治疗方法。若病理显示手术切缘呈阳性，MRI可用于评估残留病灶的范围，表现为围绕病灶切除部位周围的小结节状强化灶。
- 乳房肿瘤切除术后因肉芽组织而出现强化可长达18个月，为正常反应。如果术后强化超

months or new enhancement after the initial post-operative enhancement has subsided.

- Breast MRI is also commonly performed following breast cancer treatment to evaluate for local recurrence or a metachronous primary in the ipsilateral or contralateral breast.
- Local recurrence rates at 15 years are 12% for women who received radiation and 36% for women who did not receive radiation.

过18个月或术后最初强化消退后再次出现强化，要警惕病灶复发。

- 乳腺MRI也常用于随访乳腺癌治疗后的患者，以评估同侧或对侧乳房的局部复发或其他的原发病灶。
- 接受放射治疗的女性在15年时的局部复发率为12%，而未接受者为36%。

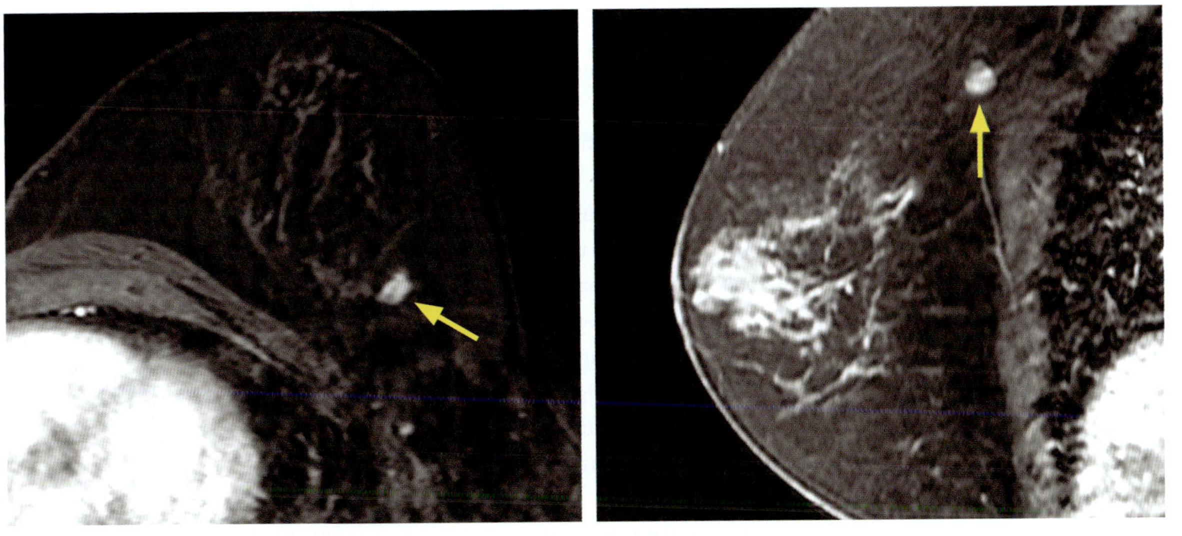

Contralateral second primary after mastectomy: Unilateral contrast-enhanced fat-saturated T1-weighted MRI of the left breast in a patient with previous mastectomy shows a new irregular, enhancing mass with irregular margins (arrows).

乳房切除术后对侧出现第二个原发病灶：左侧乳腺增强脂肪抑制T_1加权MRI显示一个新发、不规则及伴有强化的肿块(黄箭)，患者曾行乳房切除手术。

Evaluation of response to neoadjuvant chemotherapy

- Neoadjuvant therapy is employed to reduce the size of large tumors prior to resection. Follow-up MRI performed even after one or two cycles of chemotherapy can evaluate if the patient has responded to chemotherapy.
- Cytotoxic therapy may reduce tumor vascularity, which will often alter the enhancement kinetics of a lesion.
- After completion of neoadjuvant therapy, MRI can detect the location and extent of residual disease to guide surgical planning.

Diagnostic problem solving

- In certain situations, MRI can be useful for problem solving after a thorough mammographic and ultrasound workup remains indeterminate. For instance, an asymmetry that persists after spot compression but is not localizable on an orthogonal view or by ultrasound may be assessed by MRI.

Evaluation of silicone implants

- MRI has the highest sensitivity and specificity for evaluation of silicone implant rupture. Unlike the standard breast mass protocol, no gadolinium is administered for an implant evaluation and this exam does not evaluate for cancer.
- Saline implants are typically evaluated by physical exam, mammography, and ultrasound. MRI is not indicated.

对新辅助化疗反应的评估

- 新辅助化疗用于术前缩小肿瘤的体积。在1~2个化疗周期后用MRI进行随访能评估化疗是否对患者有效。
- 细胞毒性治疗可以减少肿瘤血管，因而通常会改变病灶的动力学强化特征。
- 完成新辅助化疗以后，MRI可以探查残留病灶的位置和范围以指导外科手术计划。

解决疑难诊断

- 在某些情况下，MRI可以帮助解决乳腺X线和超声检查后仍然不能确定的问题。例如，在局部加压后仍然存在的不对称影，但不能在正交位图像或超声上进行定位时，可用MRI进行评估。

硅胶假体评估

- MRI对硅胶假体破裂敏感度和特异度最高。不同于标准乳腺肿块检查操作规程，对假体的评估无须注射钆对比剂，此时检查目的不是评估肿瘤。
- 生理盐水假体通常采用体检、乳腺X线和超声进行评估。MRI不是适应证。

BI-RADS LEXICON FOR MRI MASSES

Overview of BI-RADS lexicon for MRI masses

- The mammographic and MRI lexicons have several terms in common to

MRI肿块的BI-RADS词汇

BI-RADS术语中有关MRI肿块的概述

- 在描述肿块形状和边缘时，乳腺X线影像和

describe mass shape and margin. However, since MRI incorporates dynamic contrast enhancement, new terminology was developed to describe a mass's internal pattern of enhancement.

- A **mass** is defined as a space-occupying lesion that displaces normal breast parenchyma.

Mass shape

- The MRI lexicon for mass shape is identical to that of mammography and ultrasound.
- **Round**: Spherical in shape.
- **Oval**: Elliptical or oblong in shape. May include two to three undulations in contour.
- **Irregular**: Uneven shape. An irregular shape is suspicious for malignancy.

Mass margin

- Evaluation of the margin of an enhancing mass is the MRI imaging feature most predictive of malignancy. The BI-RADS MRI lexicon for mass margin includes **circumscribed**, **irregular**, and **spiculated**. Unlike the mammography lexicon which uses the word irregular only to describe mass shape, irregular is used in the MRI lexicon as a description of both mass shape and mass margin. Circumscribed margins are more suggestive of benignity, while not circumscribed (irregular or spiculated) margins are more suspicious for malignancy. A mass with spiculated margins is thought to represent cancer 84–91% of the time.
- The shape and margin of a mass are best evaluated in the early postcontrast sequences. Progressive enhancement of the normal surrounding breast parenchyma on the subsequent postcontrast sequences may obscure the true margins of a mass.

Internal enhancement

- Several descriptive terms unique to breast MRI are used to describe the internal enhancement pattern within a mass.
- **Homogeneous** internal enhancement is uniform and can be seen in both benign and malignant lesions.
- **Heterogeneous** internal enhancement describes non-uniform enhancement within the lesion and is suspicious, especially in the presence of rim enhancement.
- **Rim enhancement** is a highly suspicious finding for cancer, representing malignancy in up to 84% of cases, although this finding is only seen in 16% of cancers. Potential pitfalls are a peripherally enhancing inflammatory cyst or fat necrosis, both of which can demonstrate rim enhancement and are discussed later in the chapter.
- **Dark internal septations** are highly specific for a benign fibroadenoma (>95% positive predictive value). A fibroadenoma will also typically be circumscribed and hyperintense on T2-weighted images. A hyalinizing fibroadenoma, typically seen in older women, rarely enhances.

MRI的有些术语是相同的。但是，MRI增加了动态对比增强，因而增加了新的术语用来描述肿块内部的强化方式。

- **肿块(mass)**被定义为取代正常乳腺实质的一个空间占位性病变。

肿块形状

- MRI描述肿块形状的术语与乳腺X线及超声完全一致。
- **圆形**：形状如球状。
- **卵圆形**：形状呈椭圆或长方形状。可能会出现2~3个波浪样的边缘。
- **不规则形**：凹凸不平，形态不规则为可疑恶性。

肿块边缘

- MRI在分析强化肿块的边缘时，其影像特征最具恶性预测性。描述肿块边缘的MRI BI-RADS术语包括**清晰**、**不规则**和**毛刺状**。不同于乳腺X线影像术语中“不规则”这个词仅用来描述肿块的形状，MRI术语中的“不规则”同时用来描述肿块的形状及边缘。边缘清晰常提示为良性，而边缘不清晰(不规则和毛刺状)更怀疑为恶性。具有毛刺状边缘肿块的癌症可能性为84%~91%。
- 评估肿块的边缘和形状最好用早期增强序列。后期增强序列因正常乳腺实质逐渐强化使得肿块真实边缘变得模糊。

内部强化

- 有数个乳腺MRI的术语专门用于描述肿块内部的强化方式。
- **均匀**内部强化是指病灶内部强化完全一致，可同时见于良性和恶性病灶。
- **不均匀**内部强化是指病灶内部强化不一致，疑为恶性，尤其是存在有边缘强化。
- **边缘强化**是一个高度可疑恶性的表现，恶性概率高达84%，但这一发现仅见于16%的癌症。可能带来的问题是炎性囊肿或脂肪坏死时的边缘有强化，两者都可以显示边缘强化，将在本章后文进行讨论。
- **低信号内部分隔**对良性纤维腺瘤有高特异度(阳性预测值>95%)。纤维腺瘤在T_2加权图像上的典型表现为边界清晰及高信号。透明样变性纤维腺瘤常发生在老年女性，极少出现强化。

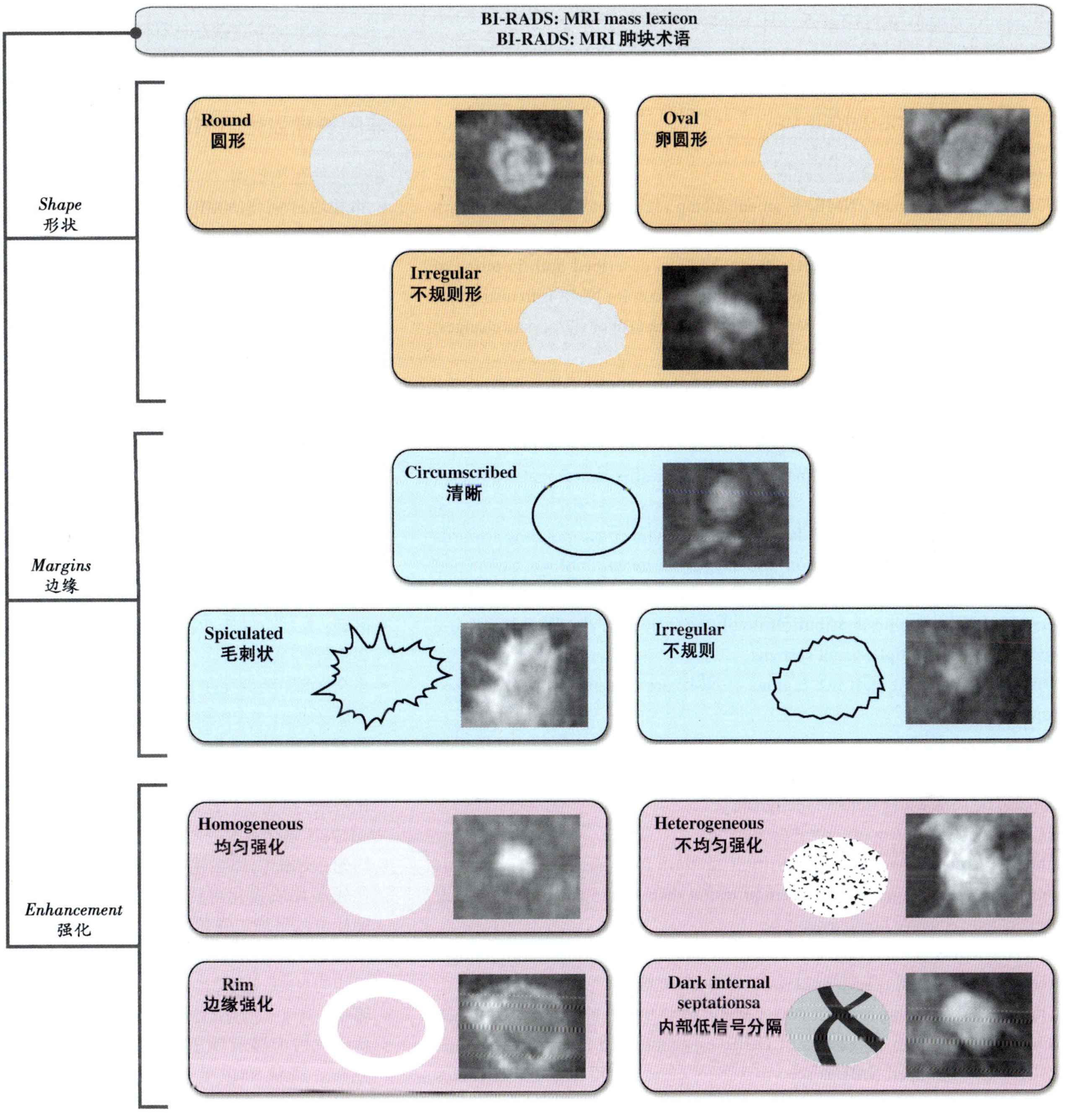

MRI FOCUS

- A **focus** is a small dot of enhancement **<5 mm** in size that does not have any mass effect or correlate on pre-contrast images. A focus is too small for accurate assessment of margins or internal enhancement characteristics.
- It can be difficult to differentiate a single focus from normal background parenchymal enhancement (BPE). Multiple bilateral enhancing foci may be due to BPE and are generally considered benign. Some authors advocate for assigning a conspicuous, isolated focus as BI- RADS 3.
- It is generally not possible to characterize enhancement kinetics of a focus by CAD due to its small size; however, if kinetics appear to be washout based

MRI点状灶

- **点状灶**是指**<5mm的小强化**点，无肿块占位效应，或相应部位在平扫上无异常。由于点状灶太小以至于无法准确评估其边缘或内部强化特征。
- 单个点状灶可能很难与正常背景实质强化(BPE)加以区分。双侧多发点状灶有可能为BPE所致，并通常被认为是良性的。部分学者提议将一个明显、孤立的点状灶归为BI-RADS 3类。

on manual measurements then suspicion should be raised. If a focus has any suspicious features, it should be described as a mass even if less than 5 mm.

- 由于其体积太小，通常不可能通过CAD分析点状灶的增强动力学特征；但若手工测量的动力学曲线显示有增强后流出时，则应怀疑为恶性。如果一个点状灶具有任何可疑特征，即使该病灶直径<5mm也应该被当作一个肿块。

NON-MASS ENHANCEMENT (NME)

Overview of non-mass enhancement

- Non-mass enhancement (NME) is an enhancing region that is not a mass or a focus.
- Similar to mammographic calcifications, NME is described both in terms of distribution and morphology. The purpose of the lexicon for NME is to distinguish between malignancy and benign parenchymal enhancement or fibrocystic changes.

NME distribution

- **Focal**: Distribution is <25% of a quadrant and contains interspersed fat/glandular tissue.
- **Linear**: The distribution is arranged in a line or branching pattern. Linear distribution is up to 26% malignant and can suggest enhancement associated with a duct.
- **Segmental**: Triangular-shaped distribution of enhancement pointing towards the nipple. Segmental distribution also suggests a ductal etiology. Segmental distribution is the most common distribution of DCIS (42% of DCIS cases).
- **Regional**: Geographic distribution involving at least a quadrant, implying involvement of multiple ductal systems.
- **Multiple regions**: At least two regions of NME are present, with interspersed normal tissue.
- **Diffuse**: Uniform NME is present throughout the breast. A diffuse distribution of NME may represent prominent background parenchymal enhancement, but can also be seen with extensive malignancy.

NME internal enhancement patterns

- **Homogeneous**: Enhancement intensity is uniform throughout the NME. This pattern is more suggestive of a benign lesion than heterogeneous, but small cancers may enhance homogeneously.
- **Heterogeneous**: Enhancement is confluent and non-uniform in morphology. Heterogeneous NME is seen in 21% of cases of DCIS.
- **Clumped**: Resembling a cobblestone pattern, or a "bunch of grapes." Clumped enhancement is most suggestive of DCIS, especially in a linear or segmental distribution. Clumped NME is seen in 51% of cases of DCIS and necessitates biopsy.
- **Clustered ring**: Thin rings of enhancing tissue surrounding the ducts. This is a suspicious pattern.

非肿块样强化(NME)

非肿块样强化概述

- 非肿块样强化(NME)指既不是肿块，也不是点状的强化区域。
- 与乳腺X线上的钙化类似，NME需要对分布和形态进行描述。使用NME术语的目的是区别恶性和良性乳腺实质强化或纤维囊性改变。

NME的分布

- **局灶**：分布小于1/4象限，并且夹杂散在脂肪及腺体组织。
- **线样**：分布排列成线状或树枝状。线样分布有高达26%恶性可能，并且提示强化与导管相关。
- **段样**：三角形强化区域，尖端指向乳头。段样分布常提示病变起源于导管，是DCIS最常见的分布类型(见于42%的DCIS)。
- **区域**：几何分布至少涉及一个象限，提示累及多个导管系统。
- **多个区域**：至少存在2个NME区域，并与正常组织交叉。
- **弥漫**：NME均匀分布于整个乳房组织内。弥漫性分布的NME可能为重度乳腺背景实质强化所致，也见于广泛的恶性病变。

NME内部强化方式

- **均匀**：NME内部强化程度均匀一致。这种强化较不均质强化更提示为良性病灶，但小的癌症也可呈均匀强化。
- **不均匀**：强化在形态上呈融合性，且不均匀。不均匀NME见于21%的DCIS病例。
- **簇状**：类似于铺路石样分布，或"葡萄串"。簇状强化最为提示DCIS，尤其是以线样或段样分布。簇状NME见于51%的DCIS病例，需要活检。
- **簇环状**：导管周围的强化组织呈细环状。此为可疑恶性的征象。

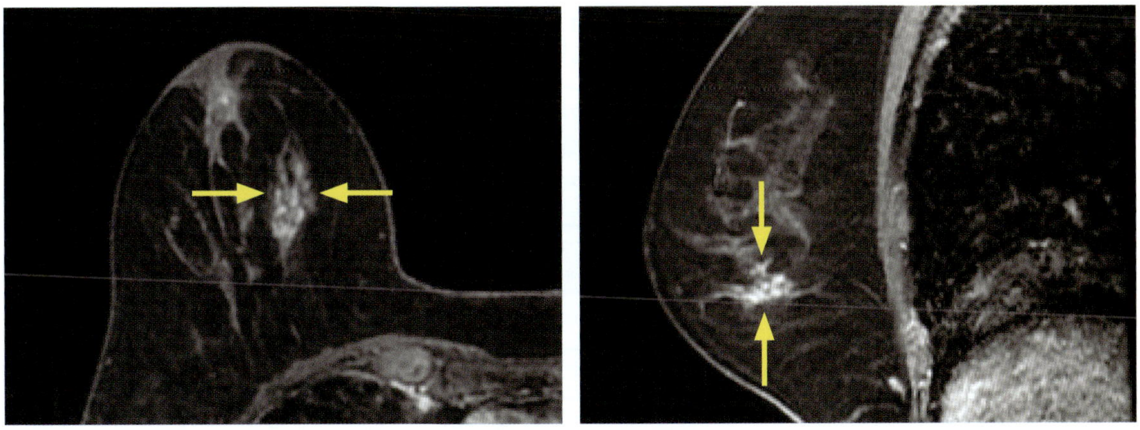

Non-mass enhancement suggestive of DCIS:
Axial (left image) and sagittal fat-saturated T1-weighted postcontrast images show an area of NME in the lower inner quadrant of the right breast (arrows) with clumped morphology and segmental distribution.
非肿块样强化提示DCIS：
轴位(左图)和矢状位(右图)增强脂肪抑制T_1加权显示右乳内下象限非肿块样强化区域(黄箭)，呈簇状和段样分布。

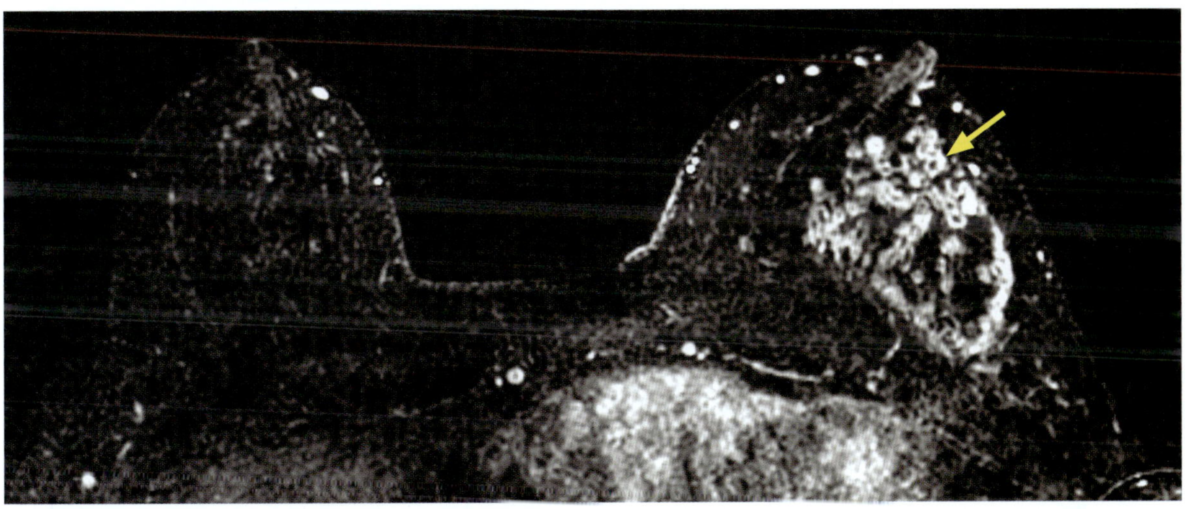

Clustered ring non mass enhancement in a patient with biopsy-proven high-grade DCIS of the left breast:
MRI subtraction image shows extensive NME in the left breast in a regional distribution, with clustered ring (arrow) and clumped internal enhancement patterns. No MRI evidence of malignancy is seen in the right breast.
患者左乳活检证实的成簇环状非肿块样强化为高级别DCIS：
MRI减影图像显示左乳区域性大面积NME，内部强化呈簇环状(黄箭)及簇状。右乳MRI未见恶性征象。

Summary of non-mass enhancement

非肿块样强化小结

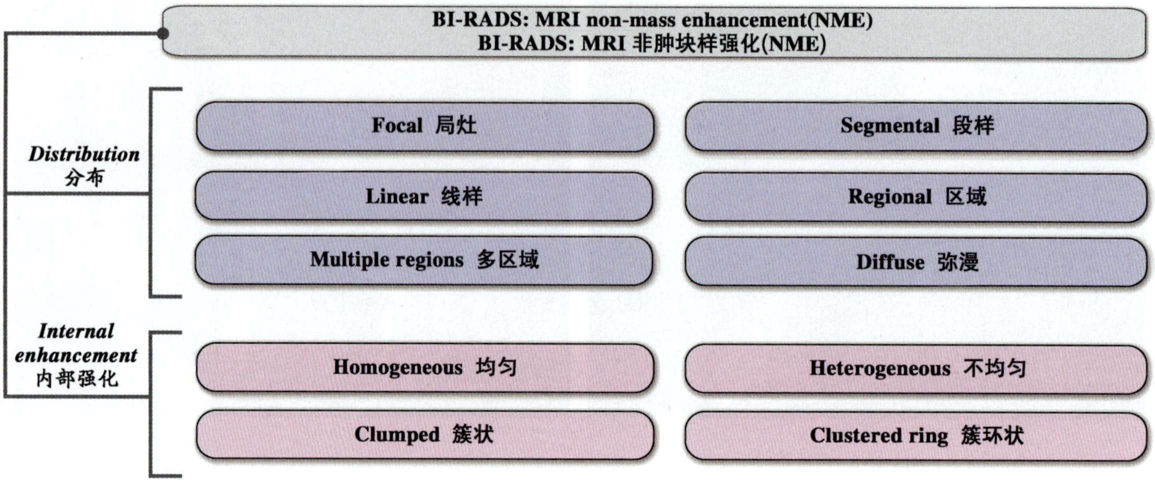

ENHANCEMENT KINETICS

动态增强曲线

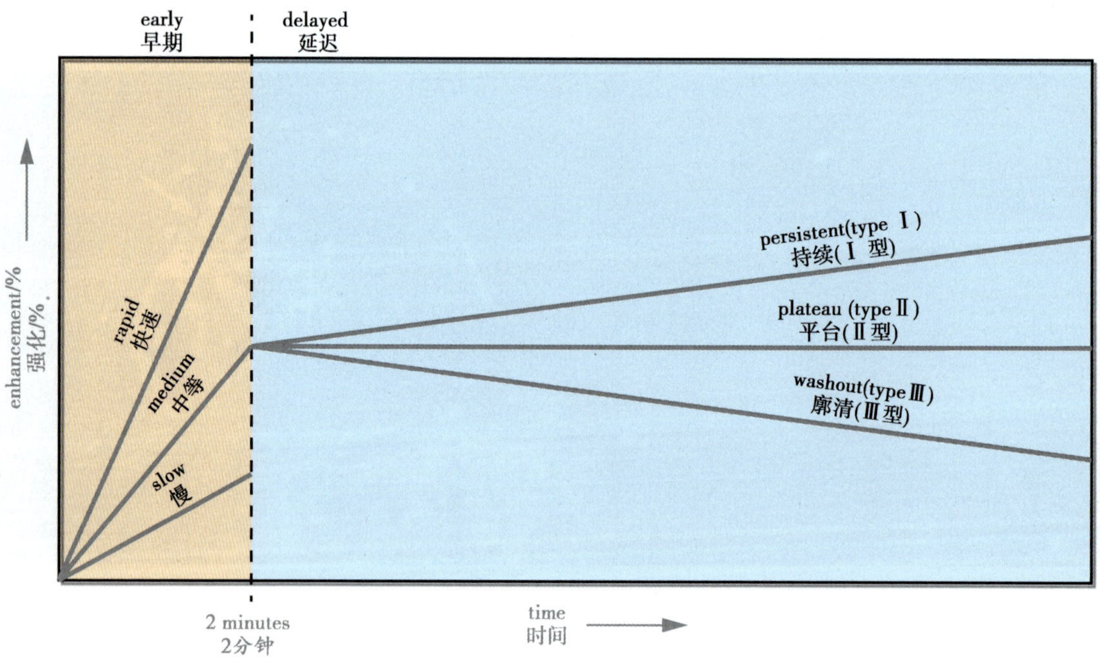

- Tumor angiogenesis and resultant capillary permeability would be theoretically expected to cause rapid enhancement and washout. This principle is the foundation for kinetic analysis in dynamic contrast-enhanced breast MRI.
- After repeated imaging of the breast at multiple time points (dynamic contrast-enhanced sequence), enhancement curves can be generated by plotting percent relative enhancement (compared to the unenhanced image) against time. The enhancement curve is divided into *early* (within the first two minutes) and *delayed* phases.
- Per the BI-RADS lexicon, the kinetics of **early** enhancement can be characterized as slow, medium, and rapid. A malignant lesion would be expected to have rapid early enhancement.
- Analysis of the **delayed** phase of enhancement allows one to further stratify

- 肿瘤血管生成及由此导致的毛细血管通透性增加理论上将导致快速强化和廓清。这一原理是乳腺MRI动态增强动力学分析的基础。
- 在多个时间点对乳腺进行重复成像(动态对比增强序列)后，可绘制出时间与相对增强百分数(与非强化图像相比)的增强曲线。增强曲线可以分为**早期**(最开始2分钟内)和**延迟期**。
- 按照BI-RADS的术语，**早期**强化的动力学特征可以分为缓慢、中等和快速。恶性病灶应该表现出早期快速增强。
- 分析**延迟期**强化可以对恶性风险做进一步分

the risk of malignancy. The three kinetic patterns of delayed enhancement are: Persistent (type Ⅰ), plateau (type Ⅱ), and washout (type Ⅲ).

- A **type Ⅰ (persistent)** curve shows continuously increasing (>10%) enhancement in the delayed phase. Although a type Ⅰ curve is associated with a benign finding in 83% of cases, up to 9% of malignant lesions may feature a type Ⅰ curve.
- A **type Ⅱ (plateau)** curve has an early rise in enhancement, but levels off (within 10%) in the delayed phase. A type Ⅱ curve is suspicious, although less strongly so than a type Ⅲ curve. Type Ⅱ curves have been reported to have a positive predictive value between 64–77%.
- A **type Ⅲ (washout)** curve has a >10% decrease in signal intensity in the delayed phase and is suspicious for malignancy. A type Ⅲ curve has a positive predictive value of 87–92%, but is seen in only 21% of malignant lesions. False positive benign lesions that may show washout kinetics include lymph nodes, adenosis, and papillomas.
- In the evaluation of a lesion, morphology is much more important than the pattern of enhancement. If a mass with malignant morphology (e.g., spiculated margins or rim enhancement) demonstrates type Ⅰ enhancement, it remains just as suspicious for cancer. Similarly, a small, circumscribed, reniform mass adjacent to a vessel with type Ⅲ kinetics is a typical appearance for a benign intramammary lymph node and should not be biopsied.

级。延迟强化的三种动力学类型为持续型(Ⅰ型)、平台型(Ⅱ型)和廓清型/增强后递减(Ⅲ型)。

- **Ⅰ型(持续型)**曲线为延迟期强化持续上升(>10%)。虽然Ⅰ型曲线出现在83%的良性病灶，但也有约9%的恶性病灶表现为Ⅰ型曲线。
- **Ⅱ型(平台型)**曲线有早期上升的强化，但延迟期下降(幅度波动在10%以内)。Ⅱ型曲线为可疑，但没有Ⅲ型的曲线可疑程度高。据报道，Ⅱ型曲线的阳性预测值为64%~77%。
- **Ⅲ型(廓清型)**曲线的信号强度在延迟期下降超过10%，为可疑恶性病变。Ⅲ型曲线的阳性预测值为87%~92%，但仅见于21%的恶性病灶。具有廓清型的血流动力学特征的良性假阳性病灶包括淋巴结、腺病和乳头状瘤。
- 在分析一个病灶时，形态学往往比增强的方式更加重要。如果一个具有恶性形态的肿块(如毛刺状边缘或环形强化)表现为Ⅰ型曲线，仍应怀疑为癌症。同样，一个小而边缘光滑，又毗邻血管的肾脏形态样肿块，即使其表现为Ⅲ型曲线，也还是一个良性乳内淋巴结的典型表现，应避免进行活检。

Interpreting Breast MRI

- The main component of breast MRI is the dynamic post-contrast images with post-processing to evaluate for the morphology, and kinetics of any enhancing mass, focus, or NME. Initial evaluation of the post-processed CAD angiomap or MIP images can give a global overview of any abnormal enhancement.
- T1-weighted images best show susceptibility artifact from biopsy clips or calcifications, and demonstrate hyperintense hemorrhagic cysts and proteinaceous ductal fluid.
- T2-weighted images can be helpful to confirm benignity in a lesion that appears morphologically benign on the post-contrast images. Although no specific BI-RADS nomenclature exists to describe T2 characteristics, T2 hyperintensity within the enhancing portion of a mass is suggestive of a benign lesion. For instance, in younger women, myxoid fibroadenomas are typically hyperintense on T2-weighted images.
- In isolation, T2 hyperintensity is not reliable for determining benignity. An important example is mucinous carcinoma, which is typically hyperintense on T2-weighted images.

乳腺MRI解读

- 乳腺MRI的主要组成部分是对动态对比增强图像进行后处理来评估强化的肿块、点状灶或NME的形态学和动力学特征。通过对CAD后处理血管图或MIP图像的初步分析可以得到一个异常强化的整体印象。
- T_1加权图像能很好地显示在活检时植入的(金属)定位夹或钙化所产生的磁敏感伪影，还能显示高信号的出血囊肿和富含蛋白质的导管内液体。
- T_2加权可以用来确定强化图像上形态学为良性的病灶是否确实是良性的。虽然没有特殊的BI-RADS术语来描述肿块在T_2序列上的信号特征，若肿块的增强区在T_2加权上呈现高信号特征则提示为良性病灶。例如，年轻女性的黏液性纤维腺瘤在T_2加权图像上通常表现为高信号。
- 仅用T_2加权高信号特征不足以判定为良性病灶。典型的例子为黏液癌，T_2加权图像上通常表现为高信号。

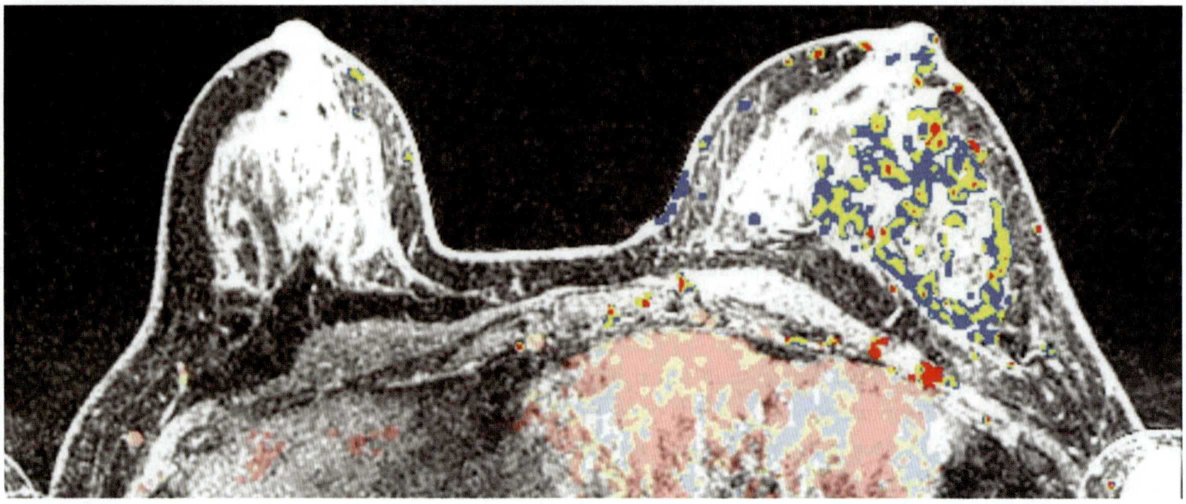

Contrast-enhanced MRI of a patient with biopsy-proven high-grade DCIS of the left breast: Post-processed color CAD angiomap shows extensive regional non-mass enhancement with suspicious enhancement kinetics (red and yellow colors).
活检证实患者左乳高级别DCIS的增强MRI：彩色CAD血管图像后处理显示广泛的区域性非肿块样强化，其增强动力学表现为可疑恶性(红色和黄色)。

BI-RADS CLASSIFICATION OF MASSES OR NME

- Classification should be determined based on morphology and enhancement kinetics. Note that a lesion with malignant morphology is suspicious regardless of enhancement curve.
- Mass or NME with a type Ⅰ kinetic curve and benign morphology:

  BI-RADS 2: Bilateral scattered foci of enhancement, without a dominant mass or suspicious focal NME.

  BI-RADS 3: Mass or NME with benign morphology and enhancement kinetics, and negative targeted ultrasound. In order for follow-up to be appropriate (rather than biopsy), the lesion must demonstrate only benign features on MRI. It is specifically these benign MRI features, rather than the negative targeted ultrasound, that allow a lesion to be classified as BI-RADS 3.

  BI-RADS 4: Solitary, dominant, or asymmetric NME in a high-risk patient.
- Mass or NME with type Ⅱ or Ⅲ kinetic curve and benign morphology:

  BI-RADS 4: A notable exception is a benign intramammary lymph node, which is typically located in the lateral breast adjacent to a vessel, and is reniform in shape.
- Mass or NME with type Ⅰ kinetics and malignant morphology is generally classified as BI- RADS 4.
- A mass or NME with a type Ⅱ–Ⅲ kinetic curve and malignant morphology may be classified as BI-RADS 4 or 5.

肿块或NME的BI-RADS分类

- 分类应根据形态学和增强动力学来确定。注意，无论强化曲线如何，具有恶性形态学特征的病灶都是可疑病灶。
- 肿块或NME具有Ⅰ型动力学曲线和良性形态特征：

  BI-RADS 2类：双侧散在点状强化灶，没有明显肿块或可疑的局灶性NME。

  BI-RADS 3类：肿块或NME具有良性形态和增强动力学特征，以及为靶病灶超声阴性。为了确保随访是恰当的(而不是活检)，病灶在MRI上的特征只能为良性。只有肿块具备这些良性的MRI特征，而不是阴性靶病灶超声检查结果，病灶才能被归入BI-RADS 3类。

  BI-RADS 4类：高危患者出现孤立的、明显的或不对称的NME。
- 肿块或NME具有Ⅱ型或Ⅲ型动力学曲线及良性形态特征：

  BI-RADS 4类：一个重要的例外是良性炎性淋巴结，它通常位于乳房的外侧，毗邻血管，呈肾形。
- 肿块或NME具有Ⅰ型动力学和恶性形态特征通常归为BI-RADS 4类。
- 肿块或NME具有Ⅱ~Ⅲ型动力学曲线和恶性形态特征应该归为BI-RADS 4类或5类。

(翻译　彭程宇)

BREAST MASSES

- Often a synthesis of the three major breast imaging modalities (mammography, ultrasound, MRI) is required to make a diagnosis. Therefore, a solid understanding of the previous sections and ways in which these modalities are

乳腺肿块

- 对乳腺进行诊断通常需要综合三种主要的成像方法(乳腺X线、超声、MRI)。因此，充分了解前文内容及应用这些成像方法，包括使用

used, including the appropriate BI-RADS terminology, is crucial.

- Commonly tested breast masses and their characteristic imaging features are described below.

恰当的BI-RADS术语至关重要。

- 常见的乳腺肿块及对它们的影像学特征描述如下。

FATTY MASSES

脂肪肿块

- All *entirely* fat-density circumscribed masses are benign (BI-RADS 2).

- 完全是脂肪密度且边缘清晰的任何肿块都是良性的(BI-RADS 2类)。

Lipoma

脂肪瘤

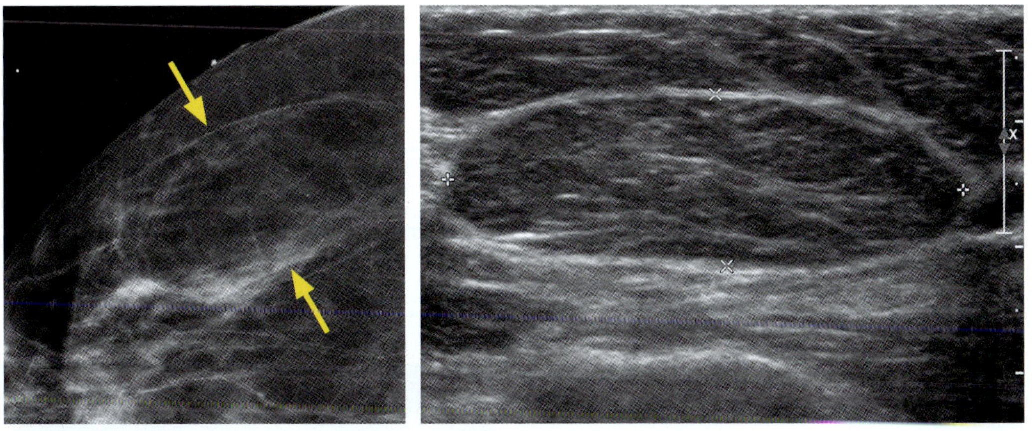

Lipoma: Mammogram shows a circumscribed oval mass that is almost entirely lucent (arrows). Ultrasound shows a circumscribed oval mass (calipers) with internal echotexture identical to the surrounding fat.

脂肪瘤：乳腺X线影像显示一个边缘清晰的椭圆形肿块，几乎完全透亮(黄箭)。超声显示一个边缘清晰的椭圆形肿块(卡尺)，其内部回声与周围脂肪相同。

- A lipoma is a benign lesion composed of mature adipocytes.
- Clinically, a lipoma may present as a palpable mass.
- Mammography is sufficient to make the diagnosis of a benign lipoma and will demonstrate a radiolucent mass that may have a thin discrete rim. In contrast to an oil cyst, a lipoma will not exhibit peripheral calcification.
- Ultrasound is not necessary when mammographic features are diagnostic, however, it may be utilized when a palpable lipoma is not clearly evident on mammography or in a very young, pregnant or male patient. A lipoma will appear as an oval isoechoic or hyperechoic mass with a circumscribed margin on ultrasound.

- 脂肪瘤是一种良性病变，由成熟的脂肪细胞所构成。
- 临床上脂肪瘤可表现为一个可触及的肿块。
- 乳腺X线检查完全可以对一个良性脂肪瘤做出诊断，其表现为射线穿透性的肿块并可能有一个清晰的薄边。与脂质囊肿不同，脂肪瘤不会出现边缘钙化。
- 如果乳腺X线征象足以诊断，则没有必要进一步做超声检查；但是，当可触及的脂肪瘤不能在乳腺X线影像上得到肯定时，或在非常年轻、妊娠妇女或男性患者中，可以使用超声检查。脂肪瘤在超声上表现为椭圆形的等回声或高回声肿块，其边缘清晰。

Oil cyst (fat necrosis)

脂质囊肿(脂肪坏死)

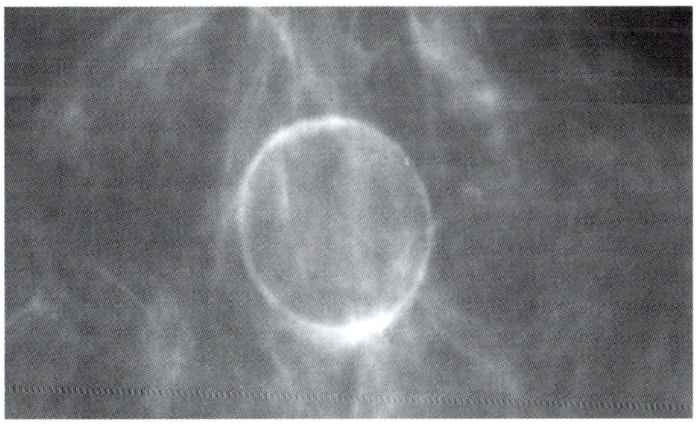

Mammogram shows a radiolucent mass with a fine peripherally calcified rim, consistent with an oil cyst.

乳腺X线影像显示一个低密度的肿块，伴以纤细的边缘钙化，符合脂质囊肿表现。

- An oil cyst is a form of fat necrosis and can occur post-trauma or surgery. Fat necrosis can have many imaging appearances, most commonly dystrophic calcification. The formation of an oil cyst following fat necrosis is less common but has a distinctive appearance.
- Mammography will demonstrate a circumscribed, lucent lesion that can peripherally calcify.
- When the mammographic appearance is diagnostic, ultrasound is not necessary, but will show a round or oval circumscribed mass. The entire spectrum of internal echogenicities are possible: anechoic, hypoechoic, hyperechoic, complex cystic and solid, or heterogeneous. If the wall of the oil cyst is fibrotic or calcified, there may be posterior acoustic shadowing.
- On MRI, an oil cyst will demonstrate internal fat signal, and may have rim enhancement.

- 脂质囊肿是脂肪坏死的一种形式，可发生于创伤或手术后。脂肪坏死可以有多种影像学表现，最常见的是营养不良性钙化。脂肪坏死后形成的脂质囊肿相对少见，但有非常独特的表现。
- 乳腺X线影像表现为边缘清晰的低密度病灶，可伴有边缘钙化。
- 当乳腺X线影像表现足以诊断时，超声检查是不必要的，超声显示为圆形或椭圆形、边缘清晰的肿块。各种内部回声都可能出现无回声、低回声、高回声、复杂囊实性或异质性。如果脂质囊肿的壁纤维化或钙化，可能出现后方声影。
- MRI上脂质囊肿表现为内部脂肪信号，并可有边缘强化。

Fat-containing circumscribed masses

- Like purely fatty masses, all fat-*containing* circumscribed masses are benign (BI-RADS 2).

Hamartoma (fibroadenolipoma)

边缘清晰的含脂肿块

- 与纯脂肪肿块一样，**含有**脂肪且边缘清晰的肿块，一般都是良性(BI-RADS 2类)

错构瘤(纤维腺脂肪瘤)

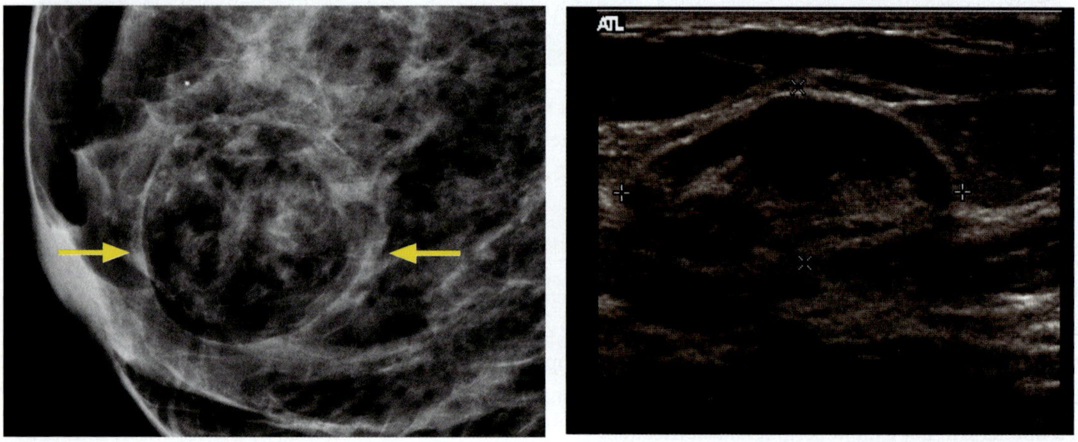

Mammogram (left image) demonstrates an oval mass containing fat and glandular elements, surrounded by a thin pseudocapsule (arrows). Ultrasound of the same area demonstrates an oval, heterogeneous echotexture hypoechoic and hyperechoic mass with circumscribed margins (calipers).

乳腺X线影像(左图)显示一个椭圆形的肿块，内含有脂肪及腺体组织，其周围有薄的假包膜(黄箭)。超声在同一区域显示一个椭圆形、边缘清晰、不均质的高、低混杂回声肿块(卡尺)。

- A hamartoma, also known as a fibroadenolipoma, is a benign mass containing fat and glandular tissue elements. It is often described as a "breast within a breast" as it is composed of the same elements as the normal breast, but in a focal area demarcated by a pseudocapsule.
- The classic mammographic appearance is an oval mass of mixed soft tissue and fat density with circumscribed margins. The surrounding pseudocapsule may be visible as a thin radiodense line when fat inside the lesion and outside the lesion are adjacent.
- Mammography is almost always diagnostic, but familiarity with the ultrasound appearance is important as it may be the first exam performed in younger patients presenting with a palpable hamartoma. At ultrasound, a hamartoma will be seen as an oval circumscribed heterogeneous echotexture (mixed hypoechoic and hyperechoic) lesion with a subtle thin echogenic pseudocapsule.

- 错构瘤，也被称为纤维腺脂肪瘤，是一种含有脂肪及腺体组织成分的良性肿块。它通常被描述为"乳房中的乳房"，因为它与正常乳房有相同的成分，但它的边缘为假包膜包裹的局灶组织。
- 典型乳腺X线影像表现为边缘清晰的椭圆形肿块，密度为混合软组织与脂肪。当病变内外的脂肪相邻时，可以看到包绕的假包膜呈一条纤细的高密度线。
- 乳腺X线几乎完全可以进行诊断，但熟悉超声表现很重要，因为这可能是年轻患者可触及错构瘤的首诊检查。在超声检查中，错构瘤表现为椭圆形、边缘清晰的不均匀回声(混合低回声和高回声)病变，伴有非常薄的假包膜回声。

- Because fibroglandular elements are present within a hamartoma, it is possible (but rare) for breast cancer to occur within a hamartoma. Any suspicious mass or calcifications within a hamartoma should be worked up.

Galactocele

- A galactocele is a cystic collection of milk that can present as a palpable mass in a lactating woman.
- On mammography, a galactocele typically appears as an oval mass with circumscribed margins. This may be soft tissue density, fat density or mixed density with a fat-fluid level. If a palpable mass in a lactating patient is fat density or has a *fat-fluid level* it is benign.

- 因为错构瘤有纤维腺体成分，所以有可能在错构瘤内发生乳腺癌(但罕见)。错构瘤内有任何可疑的肿块或钙化都应做进一步检查。

积乳囊肿

- 积乳囊肿是乳汁淤积成囊，表现为哺乳期女性出现可触及的乳房肿块。
- 积乳囊肿的典型乳腺X线影像表现为一个边缘清晰的椭圆形肿块。密度可能与软组织相等，也可为脂肪密度或混杂密度并伴有脂肪-液体平面。如果哺乳期患者的可触及肿块是脂肪密度或含有脂肪-液体**平面**，则为良性。

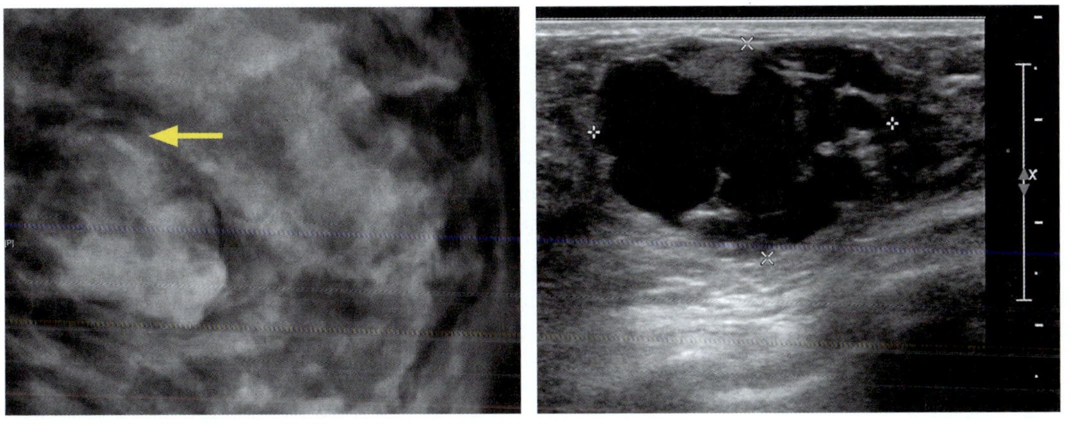

Mammogram (left image) shows a circumscribed, oval mass containing both high density and fat. A fat-fluid level (arrow) is specific for a galactocele. Ultrasound shows a complex cystic and solid mass (calipers).
乳腺X线影像(左图)显示一个边缘清晰、椭圆形肿块，内含高密度及脂肪影。脂肪-液体平面(黄箭)为积乳囊肿的一个独特的征象。超声(右图)显示一个复杂的囊实性肿块(卡尺)。

- On ultrasound, a galactocele may have a variable appearance. If ultrasound shows a hypoechoic, heterogeneous or complex cystic mass and mammography does not confirm fat to be present, aspiration or core biopsy is indicated. If aspiration is performed, the obtained fluid would be milky.

Intramammary lymph node

- 积乳囊肿在超声检查中可能有多种不同的表现。如果超声显示低回声、异质或复杂的囊性肿块，而乳腺X线检查又不能证实有脂肪，下一步需要抽吸或核芯针穿刺活检。如果进行抽吸，液体应该呈乳汁样。

乳腺内淋巴结

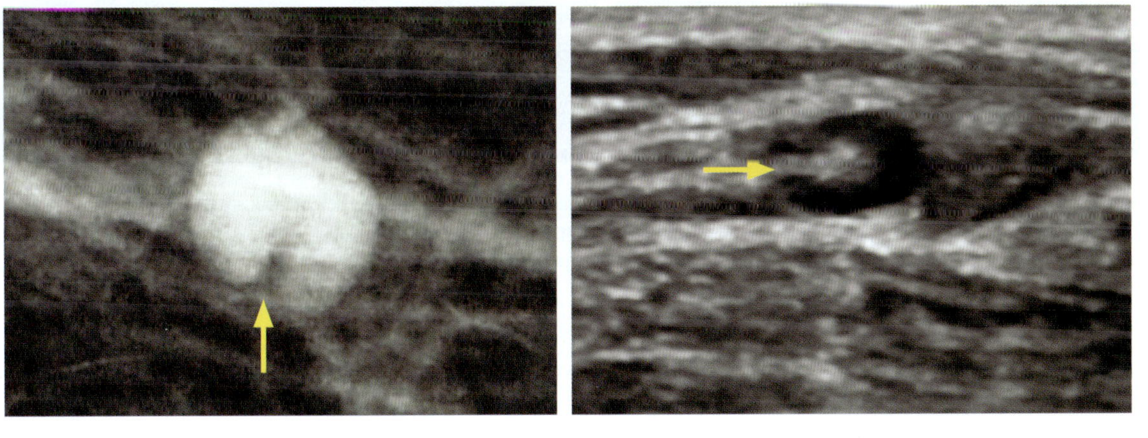

Mammogram (left image) shows a circumscribed, reniform mass (arrow), highly suggestive of an intramammary lymph node. Ultrasound (in a different patient) of an intramammary lymph node shows an oval, circumscribed mass with a central echogenic fatty hilum (arrow).
乳腺X线影像(左图)显示一个边缘清晰，呈肾形的肿块(黄箭)，高度提示乳内淋巴结。超声检查(不同患者，右图)乳腺内淋巴结显示一个椭圆形、边缘清晰的肿块，伴中央淋巴门脂肪回声(黄箭)。

- An intramammary lymph node is benign normal structure within the breast. The vast majority of intramammary lymph nodes occur in the upper outer quadrant. An adjacent vessel entering the fatty hilum can sometimes be seen, especially on tomographic imaging.
- On mammography, an intramammary lymph node should have a characteristic reniform shape with a fatty hilum (a lucent notch in the middle). If the hilum is not visible, a full workup should be performed including spot compression and/or ultrasound, particularly if location is atypical for an intramammary node.
- Typically, a normal intramammary lymph node with a fatty hilum can be diagnosed with confidence on mammography, but ultrasound can be useful as a problem-solving tool.
- Ultrasound will show a hypoechoic mass with central echogenicity that represents the fatty hilum. Color Doppler imaging would show vessels coursing into the hilum.
- Note that while normal intramammary lymph nodes are only sometimes seen within the breast, there are *almost always* lymph nodes present in the axilla. If there is unilateral axillary lymph node enlargement and/or abnormal morphology, concern should be raised for ipsilateral breast cancer. Bilateral enlarged axillary lymph nodes are unlikely to be caused by breast cancer and may be due to systemic inflammatory or neoplastic disease, such as collagen vascular disease or lymphoma.

- 乳腺内淋巴结是乳腺内的良性正常结构。绝大部分乳腺内淋巴结位于外上象限。有时可以看到邻近血管进入呈脂肪密度的淋巴门，断层图像更为清晰。
- 乳内淋巴结的乳腺X线影像表现为具有特征性的肾形并伴有脂肪密度的淋巴门(中央的低密度切迹)。如果没有观察到该淋巴门，则需要进行全面检查，包括局部加压点片或超声，特别要针对位置不典型的乳内淋巴结。
- 通常，带有脂肪门的正常乳腺内淋巴结在乳腺X线检查中可以明确诊断，但超声可作为解决疑难病例的辅助工具。
- 超声显示为低回声肿块，中央的高回声代表含有脂肪的淋巴门。彩色多普勒成像可以显示进入该淋巴门内的血管。
- 注意，乳腺内正常的淋巴结不多见，几乎都是腋窝淋巴结。如果发现单侧腋窝淋巴结增大或形态异常，应警惕同侧乳腺癌。两侧同时增大的腋窝淋巴结不大可能是由乳腺癌引起，常由系统性炎症或肿瘤性疾病导致，如胶原血管疾病或淋巴瘤。

CYSTIC BREAST LESIONS

- Note that it is not possible to reliably differentiate cystic versus solid lesions on mammography. However, a cyst may become less dense on spot compression owing to its compressibility.

Simple cyst

乳腺囊性病变

- 注意，乳腺X线检查不能有效区分囊性和实性病变。但是，囊性病变在加压点片上因其被压缩而密度变低。

单纯囊肿

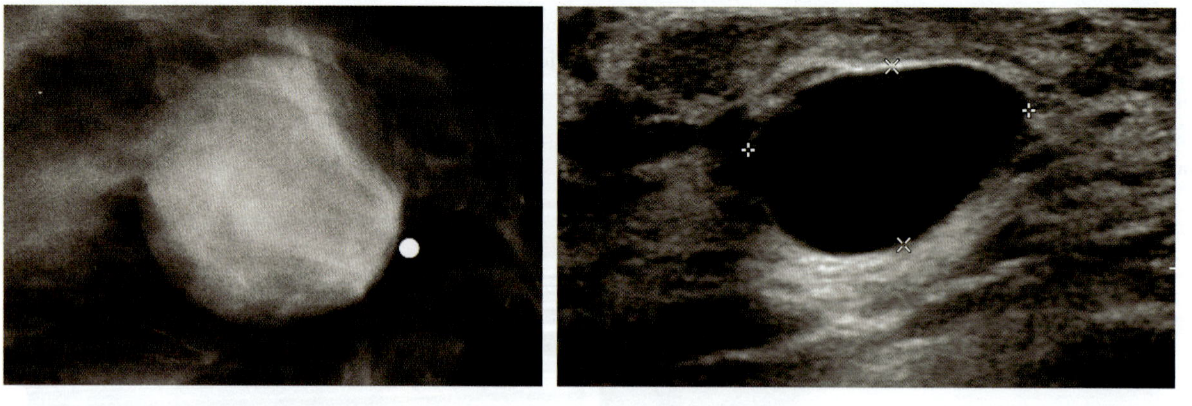

Simple cyst: Mammogram shows a circumscribed, round, isodense mass underlying a radiodense cutaneous marker. Ultrasound shows an anechoic, oval, circumscribed structure with an imperceptibly thin wall and posterior enhancement.

单纯囊肿：乳腺X线影像显示位于高密度的皮肤标记深层的一个边缘清晰、圆形、等密度肿块。超声显示为一个椭圆形、边缘清晰的无回声结构，伴有不易分辨的薄壁及后方声影增强。

- A simple cyst is a benign, fluid-filled structure that is round or oval in shape, with circumscribed margins and anechoic internal echo pattern. Two to three gentle lobulations may be present. A cyst features an imperceptibly thin wall and posterior through- transmission (posterior enhancement).
- A cyst that meets all the above criteria is benign and can be classified as BI-RADS 2.

- 单纯囊肿是一个良性，充满液体的圆形或椭圆形结构，其边缘清晰，内部无回声。可有2~3个光滑的分叶。囊肿的特点是不易分辨的薄壁及后方声影增强。
- 一个囊肿符合上述所有条件者为良性，可归为BI-RADS 2类。

- A simple cyst causing pain or discomfort may be aspirated.

Complicated cyst

- 若单纯囊肿引起疼痛或不适时可进行抽吸。

复杂囊肿

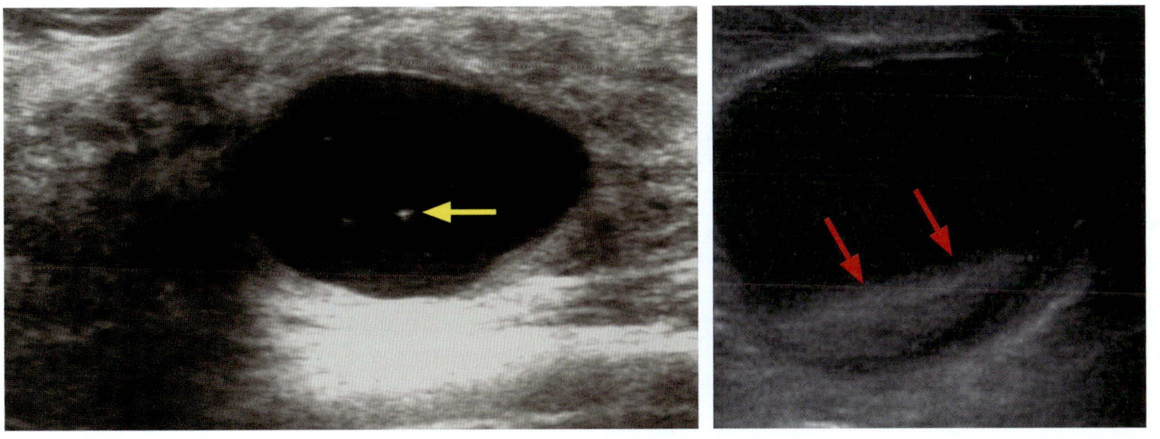

Complicated cysts in two different patients: The complicated cyst on the left features low-level internal echoes (yellow arrow), while the complicated cyst on the right demonstrates layering debris with a fluid level (red arrows).

两名不同患者的复杂囊肿：左图显示复杂囊肿内部呈低回声(黄箭)，而右图显示为分层碎片伴液平面(红箭)。

- A complicated cyst is a cyst that contains low-level internal echoes or layering debris, but otherwise meets criteria similar to a simple cyst.
- A complicated cyst is highly likely to be benign, with risk of malignancy below 2%. If solitary, a complicated cyst may be classified as probably benign (BI-RADS 3). If multiple and bilateral, it is reasonable to classify them as benign (BI-RADS 2).
- Occasionally, a complicated cyst may be difficult to differentiate from a solid mass with homogeneous internal echoes or may not meet all the required criteria. In such a case, aspiration or core biopsy is typically performed. If aspirated fluid is white, clear, or yellow, the fluid is presumed benign and discarded. Bloody fluid is sent for cytology.

Clustered microcysts

- 复杂囊肿内含低回声或含有分层碎片，其他特征与单纯囊肿类似。
- 复杂囊肿很大可能是良性的，恶性的风险低于2%。如果是单发，复杂囊肿可被归为可能良性(BI-RADS 3类)。如果是多发和双侧，则被归为良性(BI-RADS 2类)。
- 偶尔，复杂囊肿可能难以与内部回声均匀的实性肿块进行区分，或可能不满足所有标准。在这种情况下，通常需要进行抽吸或核芯针穿刺活检。如果抽吸液的液体呈白色、清亮或黄色，便可认为是良性的，无须进一步处理。血性液体需要送细胞学检查。

簇状微囊肿

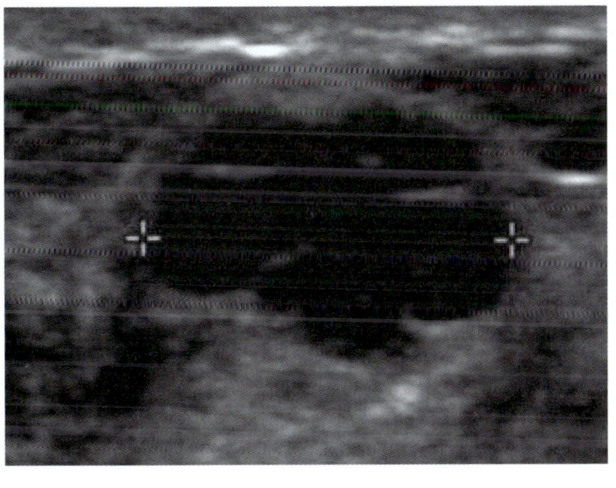

Clustered microcysts:
Ultrasound shows a cystic lesion (calipers) composed of several small 2–3 mm cysts with thin septations and no solid component.

簇状微囊肿：
超声显示一个囊性病变(卡尺)，由数个2~3mm大小的小囊组成，有薄的分隔，无实性成分。

- Thought to be due to apocrine metaplasia or fibrocystic change, clustered microcysts are composed of several adjacent tiny 2–5 mm cystic spaces separated by thin (<0.5 mm) septae.
- Clustered microcysts can be classified as BI-RADS 3 if well seen with no solid component and no associated internal vascularity.

- 簇状微囊肿可能是顶泌汗腺化生或纤维囊性改变所致，由数个相邻的2~5mm囊性立体结构组成并为薄壁所分隔(<0.5mm)。
- 如能确定簇状微囊肿没有实性成分和内部血管成分，则可归为BI-RADS 3类。

- Clustered microcysts may eventually evolve into a simple benign cyst.

- 簇状微囊肿最终可能演变成一个单纯的良性囊肿。

Complex cystic and solid mass

复杂囊实性肿块

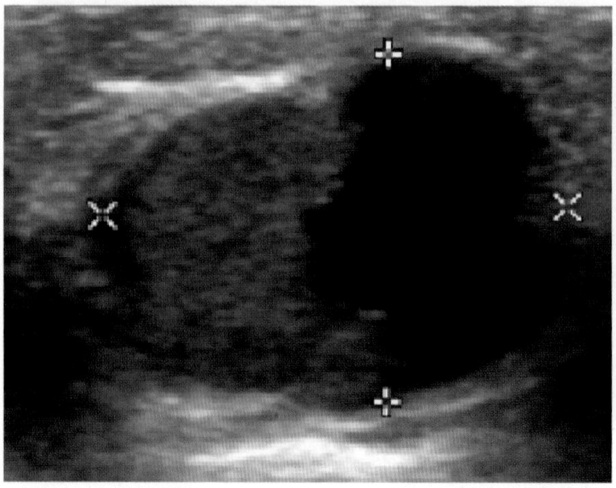

Ultrasound shows a mixed cystic and solid mass (calipers) with an irregular solid component (arrows). Although the mass is oval in shape and has circumscribed margins, the solid component makes this lesion suspicious for malignancy.

超声显示一个囊实混合性肿块(卡尺)，有不规则实性成分(黄箭)。尽管肿块是椭圆形并具有清晰的边缘，但实性成分使这个病变成为可疑恶性。

- The BI-RADS term *complex cystic and solid mass* describes a cyst with any solid feature, including thick walls or septations, or any solid or nodular element.
- A complex cystic and solid mass is a suspicious BI-RADS 4 lesion that should be biopsied. The solid component should be targeted with a core needle and a post-biopsy tissue marker should be placed.
- 36% of complex cystic and solid masses will be cancer upon biopsy.
- Malignancies that may present as a complex cystic and solid mass include DCIS, encapsulated papillary carcinoma, high grade phyllodes tumor, and invasive carcinoma with central necrosis (common for high grade triple negative breast cancers).
- Benign causes of a complex cystic and solid mass include papilloma, hematoma, abscess, fat necrosis, galactocele, and benign cyst with adherent debris.

- BI-RADS术语复杂囊实性肿块用来描述任何具有实性特征的囊肿，包括厚壁或分隔，或任何实性或结节成分。
- 复杂囊实性肿块是一种可疑BI-RADS 4类病变，应进行活检。对实性成分进行核芯针穿刺活检，并在活检部位放置标记。
- 约36%的复杂囊实性肿块活检时会被诊断为癌症。
- 恶性肿瘤有可能表现为复杂囊实性肿块，包括DCIS、包裹性乳头状癌、高级别分叶状肿瘤和伴有中央坏死的侵袭性癌(常见于高级别三阴性乳腺癌)。
- 良性的复杂囊实性肿块包括乳头状瘤、血肿、脓肿、脂肪坏死、积乳囊肿，以及伴有附壁碎片的良性囊肿。

Fibroadenoma

纤维腺瘤

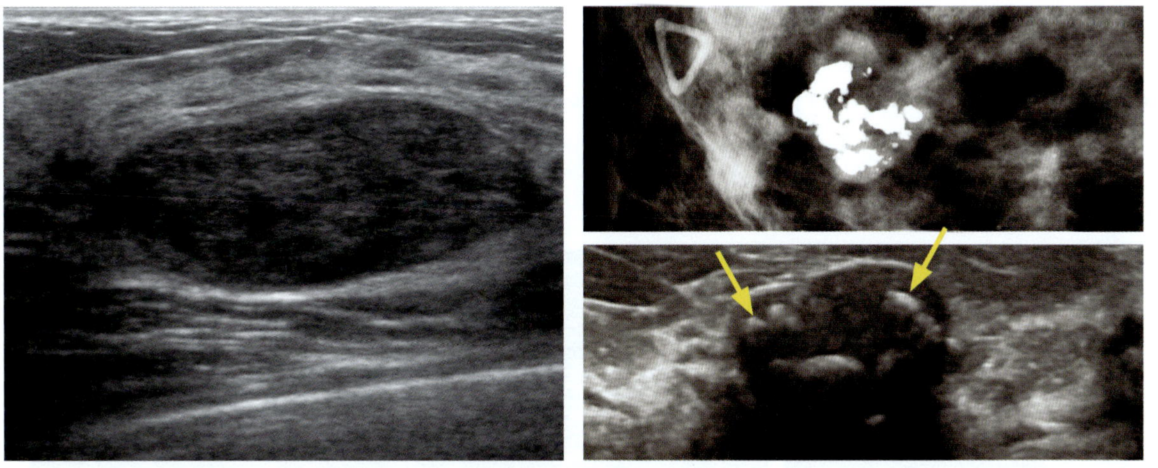

Two different patients with fibroadenomas: On the left is an ultrasound image demonstrating the typical appearance of a fibroadenoma in a young woman, as a circumscribed, oval, parallel, hypoechoic mass with mild posterior enhancement.

On the right is the characteristic mammographic appearance of a hyalinized fibroadenoma in an older woman (top right), as a circumscribed mass with coarse "popcorn-like" calcifications. This appearance is completely diagnostic and no further workup is necessary. Ultrasound (below right) was performed as this lesion was palpable, as evident by the triangular skin marker on the mammogram. Note the calcifications within the mass (arrows).

两名不同患者的纤维腺瘤：

左侧的超声图像为一名年轻女性患者的典型纤维腺瘤，表现为一个边缘清晰、椭圆形、长轴与皮肤表面平行的低回声肿块，伴有后方回声轻微增强。

右侧是一名老年女性患者典型的透明样变纤维腺瘤的乳腺X线影像(右上)，表现为边缘清晰的肿块，内含"爆米花"样钙化。这种表现具有诊断价值，无须进一步检查。因肿块可触及，该病例进行了超声检查(右下)，在乳腺X线图像有三角形标记为佐证，注意肿块内的钙化(黄箭)。

- Fibroadenoma is a benign neoplasm common in young women under age 35 and is the most frequent cause of a palpable breast mass in this age group.
- Clinically, a fibroadenoma will present as a firm, mobile mass.
- The classic mammographic appearance of a fibroadenoma is an oval, equal density circumscribed mass, although this imaging appearance is nonspecific. A hyalinizing fibroadenoma, typically seen in older women, has a definitively benign mammographic appearance containing coarse "popcorn-like" calcification.
- The typical ultrasound appearance of a fibroadenoma is an oval, circumscribed mass with homogeneous hypoechoic echotexture. Occasionally, a histologically benign fibroadenoma may have more suspicious features on ultrasound including irregular margins, heterogeneous internal echotexture, or shadowing, prompting biopsy in these cases.
- On MRI, fibroadenoma typically appears as an oval, circumscribed mass with iso- or hyperintense T2 signal and persistent (type Ⅰ) enhancement. Dark internal septations are specific for fibroadenoma.
- Masses presenting with imaging features typical of a fibroadenoma are often either followed (BI-RADS 3) or biopsied (BI-RADS 4), depending on the imaging characteristics and clinical context.
- If the following ultrasound features are met, the presumed fibroadenoma can be classified as BI-RADS 3, with a false negative rate of 0.5%:

  Ovoid shape, parallel orientation with a width to height ratio of >1.4 (wider-than-

- 纤维腺瘤是一种良性肿瘤，常见于35岁以下的年轻女性，为该年龄段最常见的可触及性包块。
- 纤维腺瘤在临床上表现为质韧、可活动的肿块。
- 纤维腺瘤典型的乳腺X线影像表现为椭圆形、等密度、边缘清晰的肿块，但这种表现并不具有特异性。透明样变的纤维腺瘤通常发生于老年女性，乳腺X线影像具有明确的良性表现，即含有粗大的"爆米花"样钙化。
- 纤维腺瘤的典型超声表现为椭圆形、边缘清晰的均匀低回声肿块。偶尔组织学上良性的纤维腺瘤在超声上的表现却可疑，包括边缘模糊，内部回声不均匀或阴影，从而需要对这些病例进行活检。
- 纤维腺瘤的典型MRI表现为椭圆形、边缘清晰的肿块，T_2WI呈等或高信号，持续性强化(Ⅰ型曲线)。内部低信号分隔为纤维腺瘤所特有的表现。
- 具有纤维腺瘤典型影像学特征的肿块需要根据影像学特征及临床表现进行随访(BI-RADS 3类)或活检(BI-RADS 4类)。
- 如果符合以下超声表现，该疑似纤维腺瘤可以被归为BI-RADS 3类，其假阴性率为0.5%。

tall).

All margins circumscribed.

Not highly hypoechoic.

- Variants of fibroadenoma include juvenile fibroadenoma and giant fibroadenoma.

A juvenile fibroadenoma is seen in adolescents and is characterized by very rapid growth.

A giant fibroadenoma is a fibroadenoma greater than 8 cm in size.

- Fibroadenoma may appear identical to a phyllodes tumor, especially when larger.

椭圆形，与皮肤平行且宽高比>1.4。

所有边缘都是清晰的。

不是极低回声。

- 变异的纤维腺瘤包括青少年纤维腺瘤和巨大纤维腺瘤。

青少年纤维腺瘤见于青少年，以快速生长为特征。

巨大纤维腺瘤指直径>8cm的纤维腺瘤。

- 纤维腺瘤可能与叶状肿瘤的表现完全一致，尤其当肿瘤较大时。

Epidermal inclusion cyst

表皮包涵囊肿

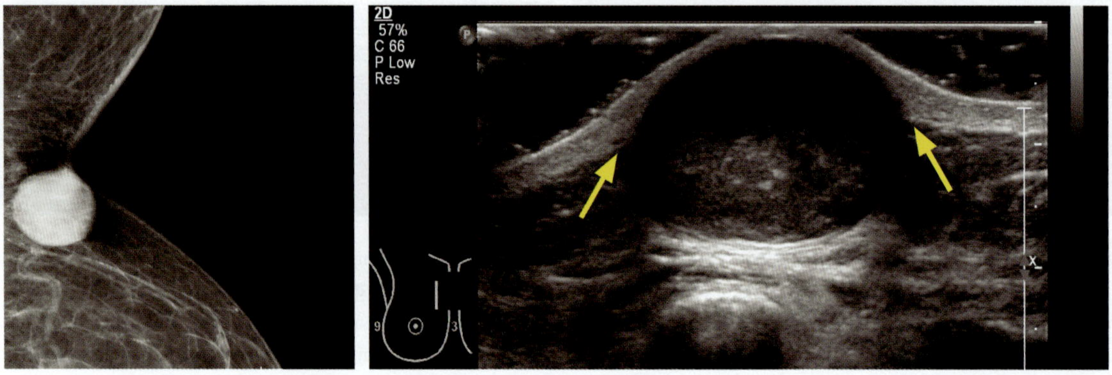

Cleavage view mammogram (left image) shows a round mass in the parasternal region. Targeted ultrasound demonstrates an oval hypoechoic lesion partially situated in the dermis with associated *claw sign* (arrows), consistent with an epidermal inclusion cyst.

乳沟位X线影像(左图)显示胸骨旁区有一个圆形肿块。超声显示一个椭圆形低回声病灶，部分位于真皮，伴爪征(黄箭)，为表皮包涵囊肿。

- Discussed earlier under the "Breast Ultrasound" section, an epidermal inclusion cyst can present as a round or oval mass on mammography, although it has a typical sonographic appearance.

Pseudoangiomatous stromal hyperplasia (PASH)

- Pseudoangiomatous stromal hyperplasia (PASH) is a benign entity of unknown etiology composed of stromal and myofibroblast proliferation, thought to be under hormonal control.
- On mammography and ultrasound, PASH appears as a round or oval noncalcified mass with circumscribed or indistinct margins. It can also present as an asymmetry or focal asymmetry.
- MRI features of PASH are nonspecific. However, the presence of high T2 signal slit-like spaces and cystic components favor a diagnosis of PASH. Persistent (type Ⅰ) enhancement pattern is often associated with PASH.
- PASH has no malignant potential. Growth and recurrence after excision are not uncommon. While clinical management of PASH remains controversial, most patients undergo follow-up imaging.

- 在本章“乳腺超声”中已经讨论过，表皮包涵囊肿具有典型的超声表现，但在乳腺X线检查中表现为圆形或椭圆形肿块。

假血管瘤样间质增生(PASH)

- 假血管瘤样间质增生(PASH)是一种病因不明的良性病变，由间质和肌成纤维细胞增生组成，可能是激素影响的结果。
- 在乳腺X线和超声检查中，PASH表现为圆形或椭圆形的非钙化肿块，边缘清晰或不清。也可表现为不对称或局灶性不对称。
- PASH的MRI表现缺乏特异性。但是，出现T_2高信号、裂隙样间隙和囊性成分有利于PASH的诊断。PASH通常表现为持续性强化(Ⅰ型曲线)。
- PASH无恶性潜能，但生长和切除后复发并不少见。临床上对PASH的治疗仍有争议，大多数患者都进行影像学随访。

Intraductal papilloma

导管内乳头状瘤

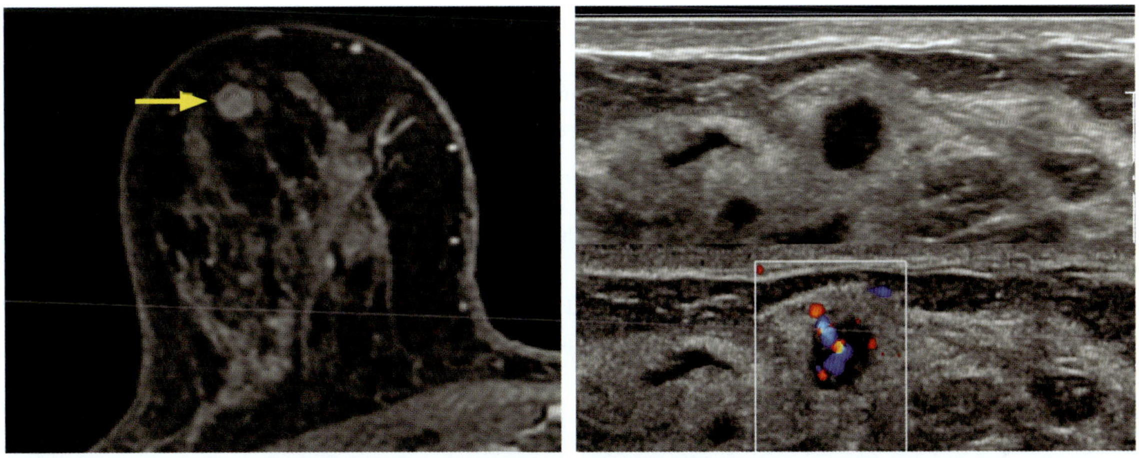

Axial MRI (left image) shows a round enhancing mass in the inner right breast at anterior depth (arrow). Targeted ultrasound (right images) of this region demonstrates an oval, hypoechoic mass with circumscribed margins and internal vascularity on Doppler. Biopsy revealed intraductal papilloma without atypia.
轴位MRI(左图)显示右乳内侧前方有一个圆形的强化肿块(黄箭)。超声显示(右图)该区域一个椭圆形的低回声肿块,边缘清晰,多普勒内部有血流。活检提示为导管内乳头状瘤,无异型性。

- A papilloma is a benign tumor of lactiferous ducts, usually seen in women between ages 30 and 50. Papillomas that occur in the larger retroareolar ducts are referred to as *solitary* papillomas. Those that occur in the terminal aspect of the duct system are referred to as *multiple* papillomas.
- Solitary papillomas are the most common cause of pathologic (bloody, serous, or serosanguinous) nipple discharge. They grow on a fibrovascular stalk and torsion of the stalk can cause pain and bleeding. Note that DCIS may also present with bloody nipple discharge.
- The mammographic appearance of a papilloma includes a round or oval, predominantly circumscribed mass, a tubular structure/focally dilated duct, and calcifications, either alone or in association with a mass or dilated duct.
- The majority of papillomas that present with nipple discharge are mammographically occult, but if visible on imaging are usually in the more anterior, retroareolar region.
- On ultrasound, a papilloma may appear as a round or oval hypoechoic or complex cystic mass. When causing nipple discharge, the papilloma may be evident as an isoechoic or hypoechoic mass in a fluid-filled duct.
- In patients presenting with nipple discharge with no visible findings on mammography or ultrasound, galactography or contrast-enhanced MRI may be utilized for further evaluation. Galactography can demonstrate a filling defect within the opacified discharging duct. MRI may show an intraductal enhancing mass with washout kinetics. The duct may be filled with fluid (T2 hyperintense) or blood (T1 hyperintense on pre-contrast). Papillomas may also present as an enhancing focus or round or oval mass, often with washout kinetics.
- Follow-up of biopsied benign papilloma (without atypia) is controversial. For papillomas with atypia or other suspicious features, surgical excision is recommended.

- 乳头状瘤是一种乳腺导管的良性肿瘤,通常见于30~50岁的女性。发生于乳晕后较大导管的乳头状瘤多为单发乳头状瘤,而发生在终末导管系统的则多为多发乳头状瘤。
- 单发导管内乳头状瘤是病理性乳头溢液最常见的原因(包括血性、浆液性、血性浆液性)。它们生长在纤维血管的蒂上,蒂扭转会导致疼痛及出血。注意,导管原位癌也会出现血性乳头溢液。
- 乳头状瘤的典型乳腺X线影像表现为圆形或椭圆形、大部分边缘清晰的肿块、管状结构/局部扩张的导管、钙化,以上征象可单独出现,或伴随肿块或扩张的导管。
- 大多数乳头状瘤伴乳头溢液的乳腺X线检查是阴性的,如果在影像学上可见,通常位于乳腺前部、乳晕后区域。
- 乳头状瘤的超声表现为圆形或椭圆形低回声或复杂囊性肿块。当有乳头溢液时,乳头状瘤可能表现等回声或低回声肿块位于被液体充盈的导管中。
- 当乳头溢液患者的乳腺X线及超声检查未发现病变,可采用乳管造影或MRI增强扫描做进一步评估。乳管造影可显示乳头溢液的导管内有充盈缺损。MRI可显示导管内强化肿块伴有廓清。导管中可能充满液体(T_2高信号)或血液(增强前T_1高信号)。乳头状瘤也可表现为灶状、圆形或椭圆形肿块样强化,动态扫描常见廓清。
- 对良性乳头状瘤(无异型性)进行活检随访存在争议。对于非典型性或存在其他可疑征象的乳头状瘤,建议手术切除。

Breast cancer

- It is uncommon for breast carcinoma to be circumscribed, but a new circumscribed mass must prompt suspicion especially in a post-menopausal woman.
- Several subtypes of breast cancer that can present as a round or oval, circumscribed mass on mammography include triple negative breast cancer, medullary, mucinous, and papillary carcinoma.

Metastasis

- A solitary metastasis to the breast is much more frequently seen than multiple metastases.
- A hematogenous metastasis most commonly presents as a circumscribed round mass.
- Melanoma and renal cell carcinoma have a propensity to metastasize to the breast.

乳腺癌

- 边缘清晰的乳腺癌不常见，但一个新发的边缘清晰的肿块应该引起怀疑，尤其是绝经后妇女。
- 乳腺癌的部分亚型在乳腺X线上可表现为圆形或椭圆形、边缘清晰的肿块，包括三阴性乳腺癌、髓质癌、黏液癌和乳头状癌。

转移瘤

- 乳腺单发转移瘤比多发转移瘤更常见。
- 血行转移瘤最常表现为边缘清晰的圆形肿块。
- 黑色素瘤和肾细胞癌有向乳房转移的倾向。

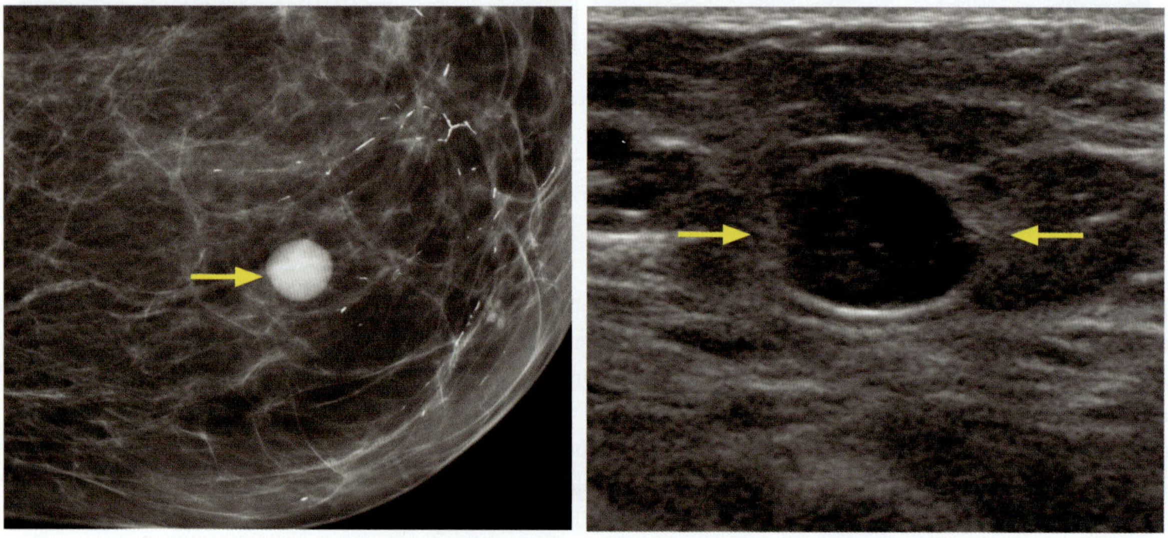

CC mammogram (left image) shows a high-density, round, circumscribed mass in the inner breast. Targeted ultrasound shows a complex cystic and solid mass with angular and indistinct margins (arrows). Biopsy revealed metastatic melanoma.

乳腺X线CC位(左图)显示一个圆形、边缘清晰的高密度肿块，位于乳腺内侧。超声显示一个复杂的囊实性肿块，边缘有棱角、模糊不清(黄箭)。活检证实为转移性黑色素瘤。

LARGE CIRCUMSCRIBED MASSES, GREATER THAN 3 CM

- Size is a poor predictor of malignancy for solid circumscribed masses; however, there are some specific entities that tend to be large on presentation.

Giant fibroadenoma

- A giant fibroadenoma is simply a large fibroadenoma >8 cm in size which is otherwise similar in appearance.
- A juvenile fibroadenoma is a rapidly growing fibroadenoma variant seen in adolescents, which may become giant.

Phyllodes tumor

- A phyllodes tumor (previously called cystosarcoma phyllodes) is a rare, rapidly growing tumor that is typically large when first detected.
- Phyllodes tumors tend to occur in an older population in comparison to fibroadenomas, typically in women age 40–50.
- The typical mammographic appearance of phyllodes tumor is a large, oval, circumscribed mass.
- The typical ultrasonographic appearance of phyllodes tumor is a circumscribed

大而边缘清晰的肿块，直径超过3cm

- 对于一个边缘清晰的实性肿块，大小是一个预测恶性程度较差的指标。因为有一些特殊病变的形态往往较大。

巨大纤维腺瘤

- 巨大纤维腺瘤是指直径超过8cm的纤维腺瘤，而其他方面的表现与纤维腺瘤相同。
- 青少年纤维腺瘤是见于青少年的一种快速生长的变异形纤维腺瘤，可以变得巨大。

叶状肿瘤

- 叶状肿瘤(以前称为叶状囊肉瘤)是一种罕见的、生长迅速的肿瘤，通常首次发现已经很大。
- 叶状肿瘤发病年龄比纤维腺瘤高，通常为40~50岁的女性。
- 叶状肿瘤典型的乳腺X线影像表现为大而呈椭圆形的边缘清晰的肿块。
- 叶状肿瘤的典型超声表现为边缘光滑的肿块，

mass with heterogeneous internal echotexture. The imaging differential of such a mass includes a large fibroadenoma or cancer.

- The majority of phyllodes tumors are benign, although approximately 25% are malignant and 20% of those may metastasize. Since imaging cannot distinguish between benign and malignant phyllodes, **treatment is wide surgical excision**. Incomplete excision leads to recurrence.

内部回声不均匀。这种肿块的影像学鉴别诊断包括大纤维腺瘤或癌。

- 大多数叶状肿瘤是良性的，但有约25%为恶性，其中的20%可能有转移。由于影像学不能区分良恶性叶状肿瘤，**治疗采用广泛手术切除**。不完全的切除常导致复发。

Lactating adenoma

泌乳性腺瘤

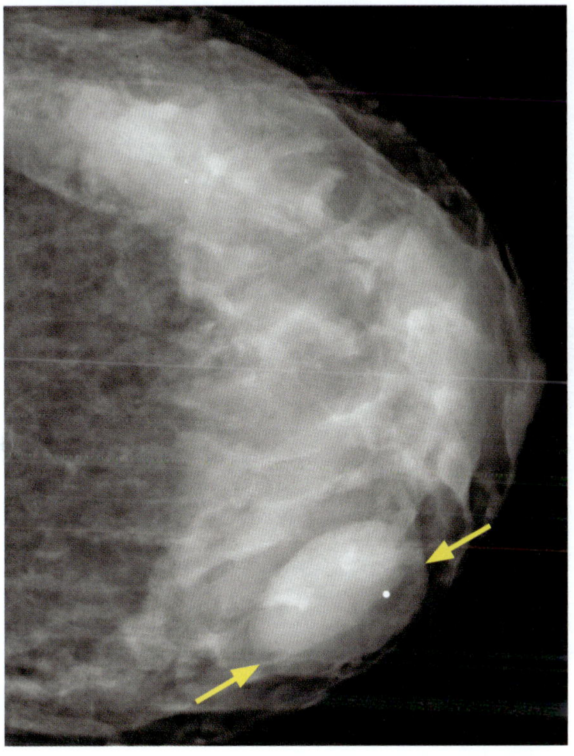

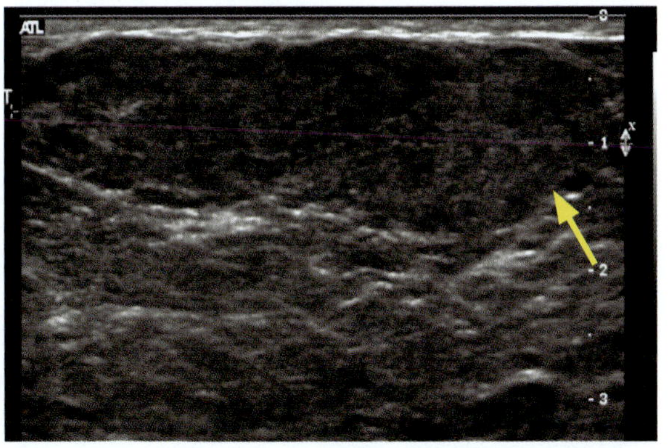

CC mammogram in a patient with diffusely dense breasts due to lactational change demonstrates a circumscribed, oval, isodense mass in the medial breast (arrows), marked with a BB.

Ultrasound demonstrates a large, circumscribed, oval, parallel, hypoechoic mass extending the entire width of the field of view (arrow).

乳腺X线CC位显示一名患者由泌乳导致的弥漫致密型乳腺，在乳腺的内侧(黄箭)见一个边缘清晰、椭圆形的等密度肿块，见"BB弹"标记。

超声显示一个大的、边缘清晰的、椭圆形、平行的低回声肿块占据整个视野横向宽度(黄箭)。

- Lactating adenomas are seen in the second or third trimester of pregnancy or the postpartum period.
- Patients present with a freely mobile mass, which may be tender if it has rapidly enlarged.
- A lactating adenoma is benign and does not need excision after biopsy. It regresses after the patient is no longer lactating.

- 泌乳性腺瘤见于中期妊娠或晚期妊娠或产后。
- 患者出现可活动性肿块，快速生长时可伴有触痛。
- 泌乳性腺瘤是良性的，活检后不需要行手术切除。肿块在患者停止哺乳后消退。

Hematoma/seroma

- Breast hematoma and seroma can be iatrogenic or post-traumatic. They appear as round or oval masses and should decrease in size over time.
- An acute hematoma may appear high-density on mammogram. On ultrasound, both hematoma and seroma should be fluid-filled, avascular, and may contain debris, fluid-fluid levels, or septa.

血肿/血清肿

- 乳腺血肿和血清肿可以是医源性或创伤性。表现为圆形或椭圆形的肿块，随着时间推移而体积减小。
- 急性血肿在乳腺X线检查中可能呈高密度。在超声检查中，血肿和血清肿都应该充满液体、无血管，有可能含有碎片、液-液平面或间隔。

Triple-negative breast cancer

- Triple-negative breast cancer typically presents with a larger size than other subtypes of breast cancer, and is associated with aggressive clinical course and poor outcome.

三阴性乳腺癌

- 三阴性乳腺癌的体积通常大于其他亚型的乳腺癌，临床病程具有侵袭性且预后差。

MULTIPLE BREAST MASSES

多发乳腺肿块

Multiple bilateral circumscribed breast masses

双侧多发、边缘清晰的乳腺肿块

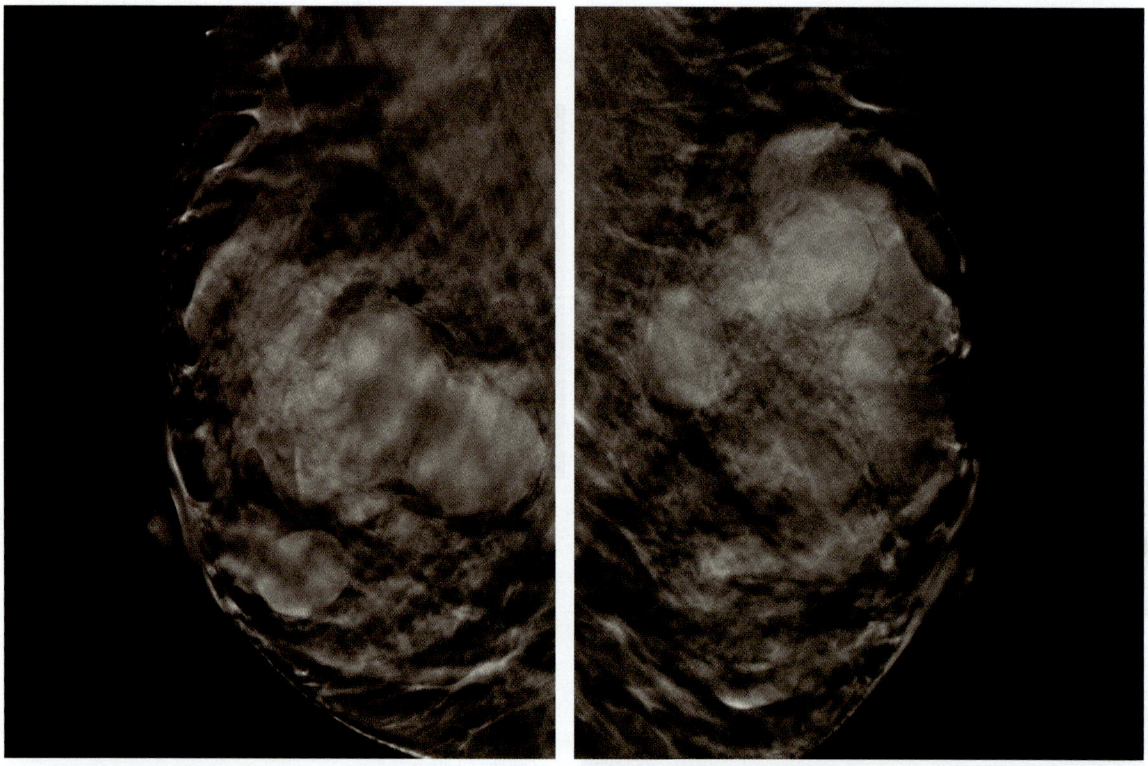

MLO view digital breast tomosynthesis images show multiple oval circumscribed masses in bilateral breasts. These were found to represent cysts on targeted ultrasound.

MLO位数字乳腺融合成像显示双侧乳腺多发椭圆形、边缘清晰的肿块。局部超声发现这些病变具有囊肿的表现。

- Multiple bilateral circumscribed breast masses are defined as at least three circumscribed masses, with at least one in each breast. None should have disproportionate size, density or margins in comparison to the others, have any associated suspicious findings or show interval growth when others remain stable. *Common underlying origin for these masses is multiple cysts or fibroadenomas.*
- Multiple bilateral circumscribed masses are seen in up to 1.7% of screening mammograms, and up to 6.2% of patients undergoing screening ultrasound.
- The interval cancer rate in setting of multiple bilateral circumscribed masses with the criteria detailed above has been shown to be between 0–0.14%. Therefore, if no concerning imaging features are present, multiple bilateral circumscribed breast masses can be classified as benign (BI-RADS 2). However, if any mass demonstrates suspicious features, such as spiculated or indistinct margins or increasing size, further workup is required.
- Criteria for management of multiple bilateral breast masses detected with MRI, contrast- enhanced mammography, or nuclear breast imaging have not yet been defined.

- 双侧多发、边缘清晰的乳腺肿块是指边缘清晰的肿块至少有三个，其中一侧乳腺至少有一个。它们之间的大小、密度或边缘没有不成比例，没有伴随任何可疑的征象，或随访间期个别有生长而其他肿块维持稳定。*这些肿块的常见原因是多发囊肿或纤维腺瘤。*
- 双侧多发、边缘清晰的乳腺肿块在筛查性乳腺X线检查时高达1.7%，而筛查性超声检查则高达6.2%。
- 根据上述详细的标准，双侧多发、边缘清晰的肿块随访癌变发生率在0~0.14%。因此，如果影像学上没有可疑的征象，此类肿块可归为良性(BI-RADS 2类)。但是，如果任何肿块表现出可疑征象，如毛刺、边缘模糊或体积增大，则需要进一步检查。
- 在MRI、对比增强乳腺X线或核医学检查中发现的双乳多发肿块的处理标准尚未明确。

Multiple intraductal papillomas

多发导管内乳头状瘤

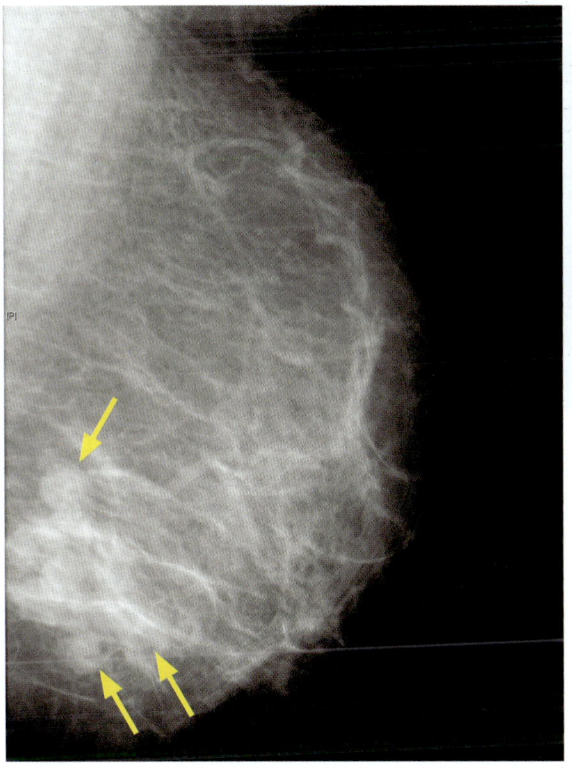

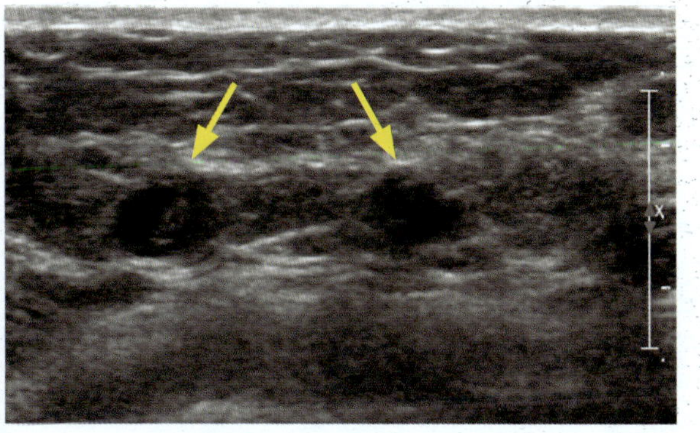

Multiple intraductal papillomas:
Mammogram shows numerous round, circumscribed masses (arrows) in the inferior breast on this MLO view.
Ultrasound shows two of these round, hypoechoic, indistinct masses on a single frame (arrows); multiple adjacent similar lesions were also present (not shown).
多发导管内乳头状瘤：
乳腺X线MLO位显示乳腺下方多个边缘清晰的圆形肿块(黄箭)。
超声图像显示其中两个圆形、边缘模糊的、低回声肿块(黄箭)，同时周围有多个类似的病灶(未展示)。

- Multiple intraductal papillomas tend to occur in younger patients compared to solitary papillomas. When multiple, papillomas tend to be more peripheral in location and bilateral. In contrast to solitary papillomas, multiple papillomas are infrequently associated with pathologic nipple discharge.
- Multiple intraductal papillomas confer slightly increased risk of breast cancer.
- Depending on the size of each of these multiple intraductal lesions, they may or may not be visible on imaging; therefore, the mammographic appearance may be a single or multiple round or oval circumscribed mass(es) located in the more peripheral breast. Given the ductal origin of these lesions, they may show a segmental distribution.
- Two similarly named entities have potentially confusing terminology.

  Papillomatosis is a term that is frequently mistaken with multiple intraductal papillomas. Papillomatosis represents microscopic foci of intraductal hyperplasia with a papillary architecture. It is a pathologic diagnosis rather than an imaging finding.

  Juvenile papillomatosis is a rare cause of a mass that resembles a fibroadenoma in adolescents or younger women up to age 40.

- 多发导管内乳头状瘤在年轻的患者较单发乳头状瘤更多见。当乳头状瘤呈多发时，更多出现在乳腺的外周，且为双侧。与单发乳头状瘤不同，多发乳头状瘤很少有病理性乳头溢液。
- 多发导管内乳头状瘤的乳腺癌风险略有增加。
- 多发导管内乳头状瘤在影像学上的表现取决于每个病变的大小，可见或不可见；因此，乳腺X线检查可能表现为乳腺外周单个或多个圆形或椭圆形、边缘清晰的肿块。由于这些病变起源于导管，它们可能呈节段样分布。
- 两个名称相似的疾病可能引起术语上混淆：

  乳头状瘤病常与多发导管内乳头状瘤混淆。乳头状瘤病指的是显微镜下导管内增生的微小病灶并伴有乳头状结构，是一个病理诊断而非影像学表现。

  青少年乳头状瘤病是一种罕见的类似纤维腺瘤的肿块，发生于青少年或40岁以下的年轻女性。

Ductal carcinoma in situ (DCIS)

- DCIS can present as multiple masses, typically in segmental distribution.

导管原位癌(DCIS)

- 导管原位癌(DCIS)可表现为多发肿块，通常呈节段样分布。

Metastasis

转移瘤

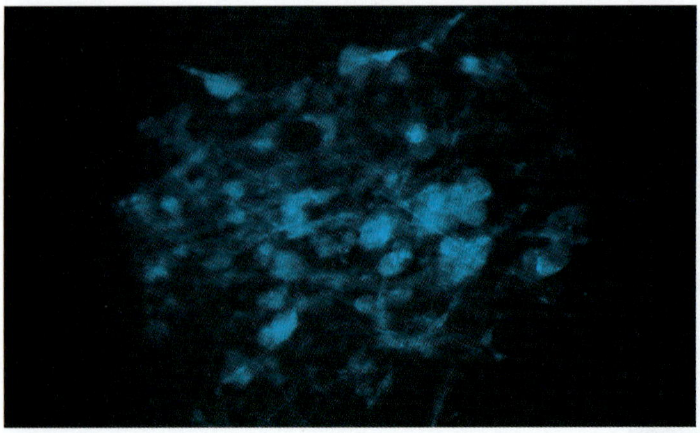

Biopsy-proven DCIS which presented as multiple masses in a segmental distribution on mammography.
活检证实的导管原位癌，乳腺X线影像显示呈节段样分布的多发肿块。

- Multiple new masses in a non- ductal distribution are concerning for hematogenous metastases from a non-breast primary, though this occurs less often than solitary metastasis.

- 多发新的肿块呈非导管分布应引起警惕，可能是非乳腺原发肿瘤的血行转移，但这种情况较单发转移少见。

Multiple skin lesions: neurofibromatosis

- Neurofibromatosis type 1 (NF1) is an autosomal dominant neurocutaneous disease that features pigmentary changes (e.g., café au lait spots and Lisch nodules) and neurofibromas.
- Cutaneous neurofibromas are the hallmarks of NF1, thought to arise from small nerve tributaries of the skin.
- On mammography, multiple cutaneous neurofibromas may appear as multiple skin masses outlined by air.

多发皮肤病变：神经纤维瘤病

- 神经纤维瘤病1型(NF1)是一种常染色体显性遗传神经上皮疾病，以皮肤色素变化(如咖啡牛奶斑和Lisch结节)和神经纤维瘤为主要表现。
- 皮肤神经纤维瘤是NF1的标志性特征，被认为来自皮肤神经末梢。
- 在乳腺X线检查中，多发皮肤神经纤维瘤可能表现为突出于皮肤表面的多发肿块。

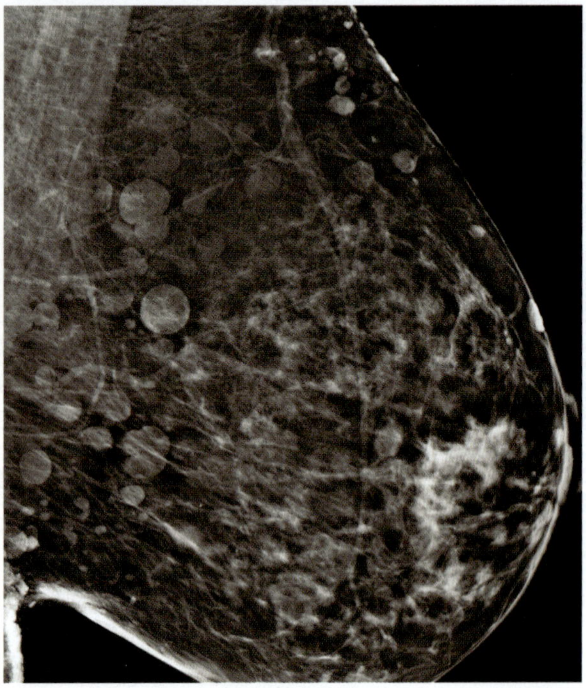

Mammogram shows multiple bilateral cutaneous masses consistent with known neurofibromatosis.
乳腺X线影像显示双侧多发皮肤肿块，符合已知的神经纤维瘤病。

Multiple skin lesions: steatocystoma multiplex

- Steatocystoma multiplex is a rare, autosomal dominant disease of multiple intradermal cysts containing sebum. When the skin over the breasts is involved, mammography shows innumerable fat- density masses.

多发皮肤病变：多发性皮脂腺囊肿

- 多发性皮脂腺囊肿是一种罕见的常染色体显性遗传疾病，为含有皮脂的多发皮内囊肿。当累及乳房皮肤时，乳腺X线影像显示无数的脂肪密度肿块。

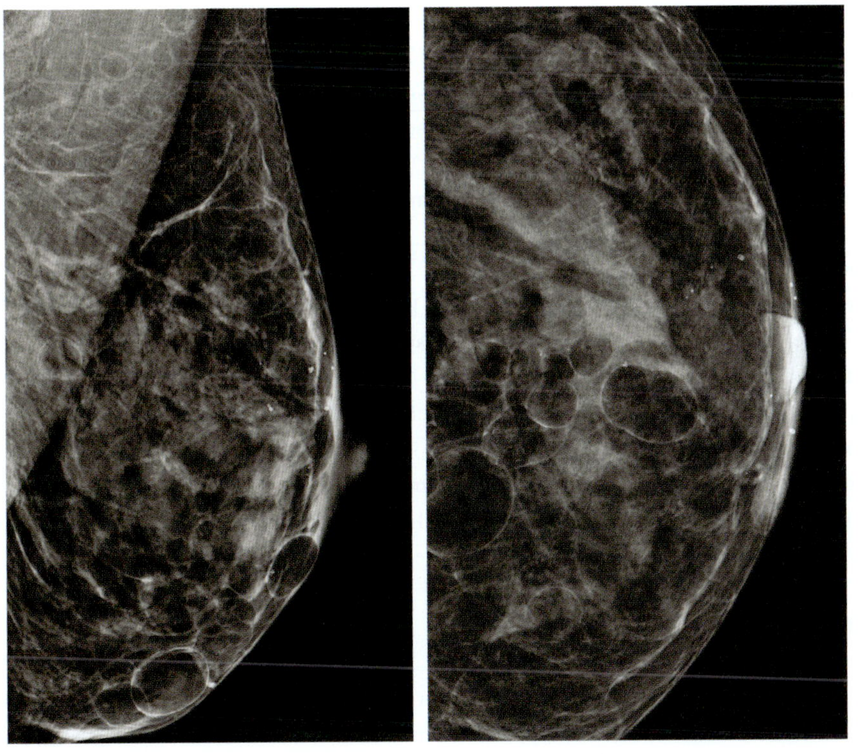

Patient with known diagnosis of steatocystoma multiplex: MLO and CC view mammograms show multiple subcutaneous fat-density masses in the left breast and axilla.
患者已确诊为多发性皮脂腺囊肿：乳腺X线MLO位及CC位影像显示左侧乳腺及腋窝有多个脂肪密度皮下肿块。

IRREGULAR/SPICULATED MASSES

不规则/毛刺样肿块

Invasive ductal carcinoma (IDC)

浸润性导管癌(IDC)

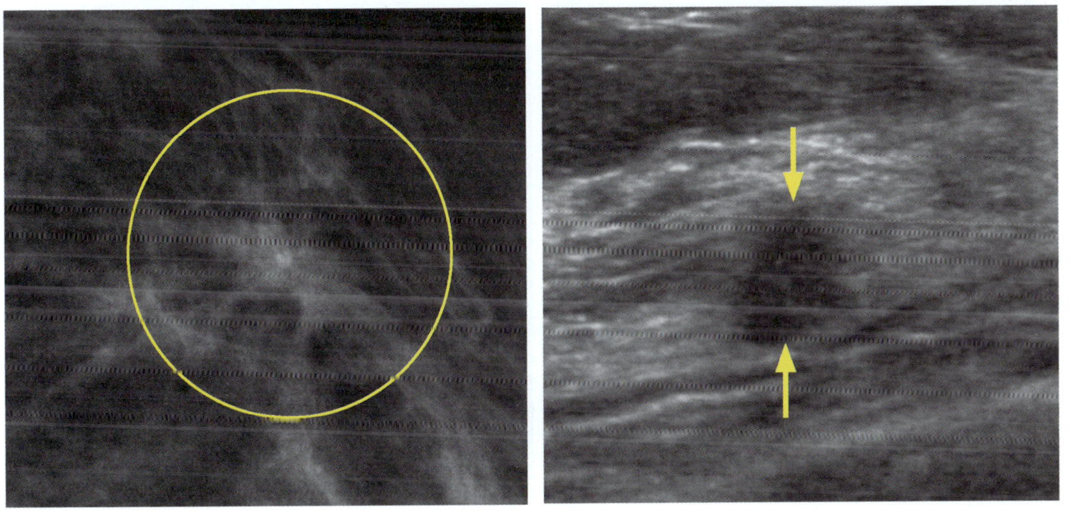

Invasive ductal cancer: Spot compression mammography (left image) demonstrates a high density, irregular mass with spiculated margins and associated architectural distortion (circle). Targeted ultrasound shows an irregular, hypoechoic mass (arrows) with indistinct margins and taller-than-wide orientation.
浸润性导管癌：乳腺点压影像(左图)显示一个高密度、不规则且有毛刺样边缘的肿块，伴腺体结构扭曲(圆圈)。局部超声显示一个不规则、低回声肿块(黄箭)，边缘模糊，高大于宽。

- Invasive ductal carcinoma (IDC) is the most common form of breast cancer. A typical mammographic appearance of IDC is a high density, spiculated mass.

- 浸润性导管癌(IDC)是乳腺癌最常见的类型。典型的IDC乳腺X线影像表现为高密度、毛刺

Malignant-type (e.g., pleomorphic or fine linear branching) calcifications may be present within the mass.

- It is important to remember that IDC can have a variable imaging appearance and may also present as a round mass, as isolated calcifications, as architectural distortion, or any combination of these findings.
- Subtypes of IDC carry different prognoses and are discussed earlier in the chapter.

Invasive lobular carcinoma (ILC)

- Invasive lobular carcinoma (ILC) represents approximately 10% of all breast cancers and can be challenging to diagnose, with a false-negative mammography rate as high as 21%. ILC tends to spread in an infiltrating pattern surrounding the glandular tissue, thus making its detection by mammogram or physical exam often quite difficult.
- The imaging appearance of ILC is variable. Similar to IDC, ILC may present as a mass (with or without spiculation) or subtle architectural distortion (which may be seen in one view only). In contrast to IDC, ILC rarely contains microcalcifications.
- ILC is more often multifocal or bilateral compared to IDC.

Tubular carcinoma

- Tubular carcinoma is a slow-growing subtype of IDC that typically presents as a small, spiculated mass. The imaging appearance may remain stable across several prior mammograms, which emphasizes the fact that a malignant-appearing finding must be fully evaluated even if stability is demonstrated.
- Prognosis of tubular carcinoma is more favorable compared to IDC NOS.

Radial scar (complex sclerosing lesion)

样肿块。肿块内可伴有恶性钙化(多形性或细线分支状)。

- 必须牢记，IDC的影像学表现多样，可表现为圆形肿块、孤立钙化、结构扭曲或以上任何表现的组合。
- IDC的亚型具有不同的预后，这在本章前文已经进行了讨论。

浸润性小叶癌(ILC)

- 浸润性小叶癌(ILC)约占所有乳腺癌的10%，诊断上有一定的困难，其乳腺X线影像的假阴性率可高达21%。ILC往往以浸润的方式向周围腺体组织扩散，从而不易被乳腺X线影像或体检所发现。
- ILC的影像学表现多变。与IDC相类似，ILC可能表现为肿块(伴或不伴毛刺)或轻微的结构扭曲(可能只出现在一个体位上)。与IDC相比，ILC很少含有微钙化。
- ILC往往表现为多发或双侧，这与IDC不同。

小管癌

- 小管癌是一种生长缓慢的IDC亚型，通常表现为一个小的、毛刺样肿块。影像学表现可能与以往多次乳腺X线检查保持不变，因而必须强调对于具有恶性表现的病变即使处于稳定状态也必须对其进行充分的评估。
- 小管癌的预后较IDC NOS(非特殊型)好。

放射状瘢痕(复杂硬化性病变)

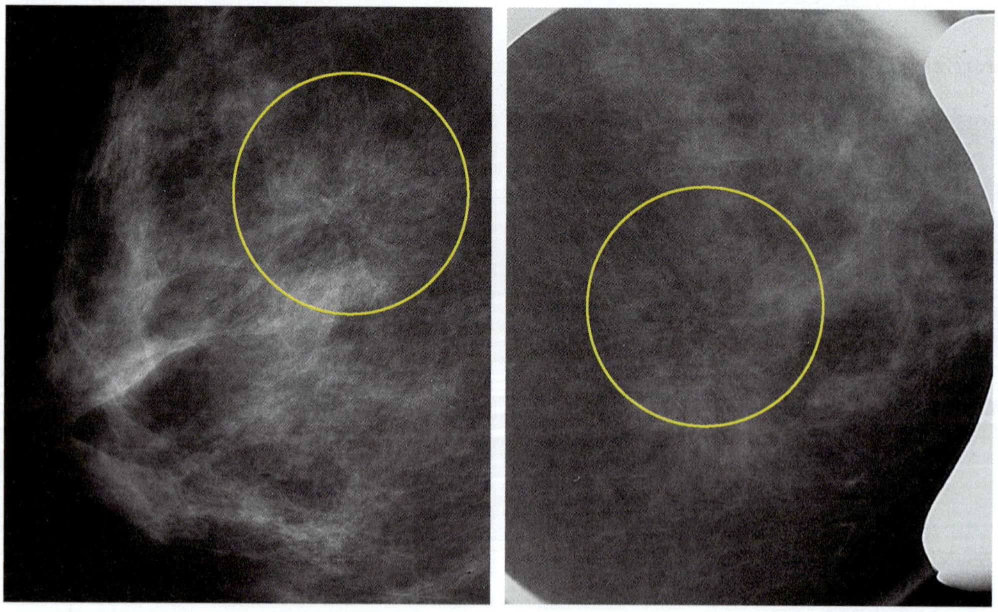

Radial scar: MLO mammogram (left image) shows subtle architectural distortion in the upper breast at middle to posterior depth (circle). Spot compression (right image) better shows architectural distortion (circle).

放射状瘢痕：乳腺X线MLO位影像(左图)显示乳腺上部的中后位置有轻微的腺体结构扭曲(圆圈)。加压局部影像(右图)较好显示了结构扭曲(圆圈)。

- A radial scar is a benign proliferative lesion of the breast. Despite the name, a radial scar has nothing to do with a post-traumatic or post-surgical scar. A complex sclerosing lesion is histologically identical to a radial scar, but is used

- 放射状瘢痕是一种乳腺的良性增生性病变。尽管听起来很像，但这一名称与创伤或术后瘢痕无关。放射状瘢痕与复杂的硬化性病变

to describe those that are larger (>1 cm).

- Histologically, a radial scar is characterized by adenosis, hyperplasia, and central atrophy resulting in pulling-in of adjacent tissue into a stellate pattern.
- The mammographic and ultrasound appearance of a radial scar may be identical to cancer, appearing as a spiculated mass or architectural distortion (sometimes with associated calcifications) on mammography and a hypoechoic shadowing mass on ultrasound. Radial scars can also show enhancement on MRI. Although the classic appearance of a radial scar on mammography is an area of architectural distortion with central lucency, this appearance is not diagnostically reliable, and biopsy is always warranted.
- Management of radial scars diagnosed by core needle biopsy remains controversial due to varying reported upgrade rates. The most common management is surgical excision.

Post-lumpectomy or post-excisional biopsy scar

- A post-surgical scar, either due to prior lumpectomy or excisional biopsy, may be indistinguishable on mammography from cancer in the absence of clinical history.
- Additional post-surgical changes are often present to aid in the diagnosis, including volume loss in the treated breast and skin retraction. Additionally, unlike recurrent tumor, a post- surgical scar should not get larger over time.
- If the patient was treated with radiation therapy, dystrophic calcification and skin thickening/retraction may also be present.

在组织学上是完全相同的，只是用于描述较大的病变(>1cm)。

- 放射状瘢痕在组织学上以腺病、增生、中央萎缩导致的邻近组织牵拉为特征。
- 放射状瘢痕与癌症在乳腺X线检查和超声上的表现可完全相同，即乳腺X线影像呈毛刺样肿块或结构扭曲(有时伴有钙化)，超声为低回声肿块。放射状瘢痕在MRI上也可出现强化。尽管放射状瘢痕的典型乳腺X线影像的表现是结构扭曲的区域伴中央低密度，但这一表现在诊断上并不可靠，活检是必要的。
- 因报道的恶变率有差异，如何处理核芯针穿刺活检后诊断的放射状瘢痕仍存在争议。最常见的方法是手术切除。

乳房肿瘤切除术或切除性活检术后的瘢痕

- 如果缺乏临床病史，肿瘤切除或切除性活检所造成的术后瘢痕可能在乳腺X线影像上无法与癌症区分。
- 其他的术后变化常可以帮助诊断，包括治疗后的乳房体积缩小和皮肤收缩。此外，与复发性肿瘤不同，术后瘢痕不会随着时间而增大。
- 如果患者曾接受过放疗，还可以出现营养不良性钙化和皮肤增厚/收缩。

AXILLARY MASS

腋窝肿块

Axillary lymphadenopathy

腋窝淋巴结病

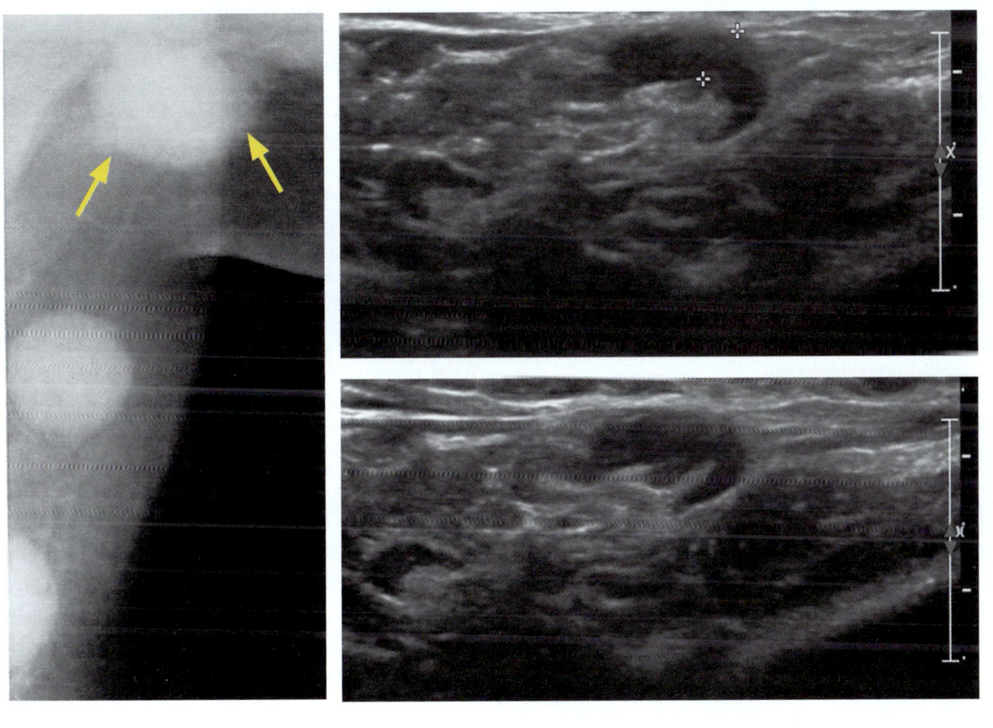

Malignant adenopathy: MLO mammogram (left image) shows numerous round, high density masses in the axilla, with the suggestion of indistinct margins of the superior-most mass (arrows). Ultrasound demonstrates several enlarged lymph nodes with asymmetrically thickened cortex measuring up to 1 cm (calipers).
恶性淋巴结增大：乳腺X线MLO位(左图)显示腋窝多发圆形、高密度肿块，最上方肿块边缘显示不清(黄箭)。超声显示多个增大淋巴结伴不对称皮质增厚达1cm(卡尺)。

- Unilaterally enlarged axillary lymph nodes are suspicious for breast cancer metastasis, although size alone is nonspecific for determining metastatic involvement.
- Sonographic features suspicious of lymph node metastasis include:

Round shape.	**Focal outwards cortical bulge.**
Thickened (>3 mm) cortex.	**Hilar indentation** or **obliteration of the**
Eccentrically thickened cortex.	**hilum** by thickened cortex.

- Bilateral adenopathy is more likely to be due to a systemic process, including collagen vascular disease, lymphoma, leukemia, metastases from nonbreast primary, and infection.

Breast mass in the axilla

- The axillary tail of Spence is normal extension of fibroglandular tissue into the axilla. Accessory breast tissue can also separately occur in the axilla. These can be mistaken as a mass on physical exam. Alternatively, any associated primary benign or malignant process of the breast can also occur here and present as a mass.

Skin lesions

- Epidermal inclusion cysts and sebaceous cysts (discussed in detail earlier in the chapter) are commonly seen in the axilla though they can occur anywhere. Another common location is the inframammary fold.

OTHER MALIGNANT DISEASE OF THE BREAST

Angiosarcoma

- 单侧腋窝淋巴结肿大应怀疑有乳腺癌转移，但其大小本身对转移不具备特异性。
- 可疑淋巴结转移的超声表现包括：

圆形。	**局灶皮质层外突。**
皮质层增厚(>3mm)。	**淋巴门凹陷或消失**继发
偏心性皮质层增厚。	于皮质层增厚。

- 双侧淋巴结增大源于系统性疾病的可能性更大，包括胶原血管疾病、淋巴瘤、白血病、非乳腺原发转移和感染。

腋窝的乳腺肿块

- Spence腋尾是纤维腺体组织向腋窝的正常延伸。副乳腺组织也可单独出现在腋窝。这些结构在查体时可能会被误认为是肿块。另外，任何与乳腺相关的原发良性或恶性病变也可在此处出现并表现为一个肿块。

皮肤病变

- 表皮包涵囊肿和皮脂腺囊肿(在本章前文已详述)常见于腋窝，但它们可以发生在其他任何部位。另一个常见部位是乳房下褶皱。

乳腺的其他恶性疾病

血管肉瘤

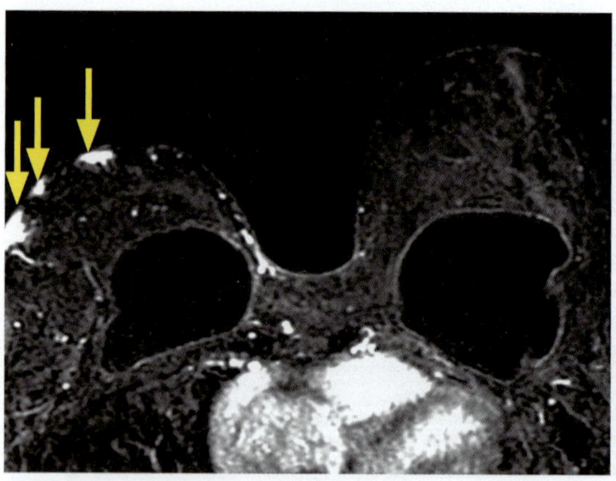

Axial post-contrast subtraction.
轴位增强后减影

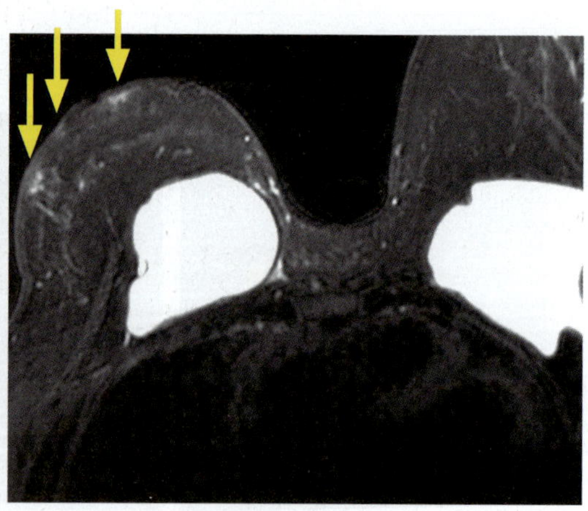

Axial T2-weighted image with fat suppression.
轴位脂肪抑制T_2加权成像

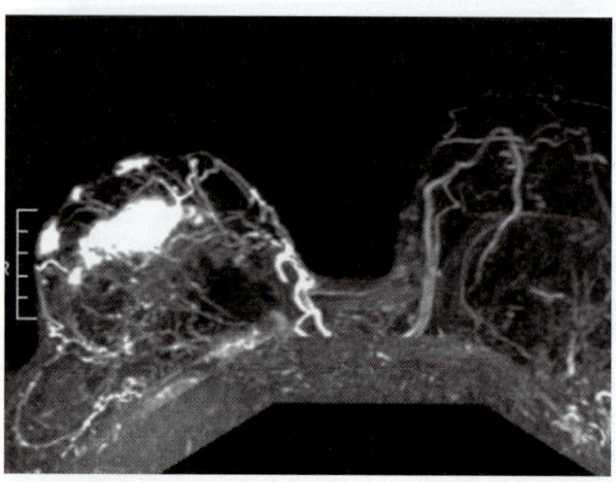

Maximum intensity projection(MIP).
最大密度投影(MIP)

Radiation-associated angiosarcoma: There are T2 hyperintense superficial nodular areas of enhancement in the right breast that are contiguous with the skin (arrows). MIP image shows the extent of the abnormality involving both the skin and the deeper tissues of the right breast. The patient was previously treated for breast cancer on the right and has bilateral implants.

Case courtesy Lorraine B. Smith, MD, Brigham and Women's Hospital.

辐射相关的血管肉瘤：右侧乳房浅表紧贴皮肤的多发T_2高信号的结节样强化区域(黄箭)。
MIP示异常病灶侵及右侧乳房的皮肤及深层组织。
患者曾接受右侧乳腺癌治疗及双侧乳房假体植入。

- Angiosarcoma of the breast is a rare and aggressive malignancy that may be primary in origin, or secondary to prior breast conservation therapy with radiation.

  Primary angiosarcoma arises in the breast parenchyma and can present as a palpable mass or diffuse breast enlargement without a mass.

  Radiation-associated angiosarcoma arises in the breast dermis and subcutis, presenting as areas of skin thickening and ecchymosis that can mimic bruising, thereby delaying diagnosis.
- Mammographic and ultrasound findings of radiation-associated angiosarcoma are nonspecific. On MRI, angiosarcoma is hyperintense on T2-weighted images and demonstrates intense enhancement.

Lymphoma
- The most common primary breast lymphoma is **diffuse large B-cell lymphoma**. Clinically, most breast lymphomas present as a palpable mass. Axillary adenopathy may be present.
- On mammography, lymphoma may present as a mass with indistinct margins. On ultrasound, lymphoma typically appears as a hypoechoic mass. In contrast to epithelial cancers such as invasive ductal carcinoma, calcifications are rarely seen in breast lymphoma.
- In a patient with a known diagnosis of lymphoma and a new breast mass, the primary consideration remains breast cancer. Histologic sampling is essential as lymphoma is treated with chemoradiation, not surgery.
- **Breast implant-associated anaplastic large cell lymphoma** is a rare primary T-cell lymphoma of the breast. It is most often seen with textured breast implants and classically presents as an effusion around the implant or residual fibrous capsule. Therefore, any new peri-implant effusion occurring more than 12 months following implant placement should prompt consideration for this rare entity.

- 乳房血管肉瘤是一种罕见的、具有侵袭性的恶性肿瘤，可能是原发的，或继发于保乳放射治疗。

  原发性血管肉瘤起源于乳腺实质，可表现为可触及的肿块或无肿块性弥漫性乳房增大。

  放射相关的血管肉瘤发生于乳房真皮层和皮下，表现为皮肤增厚和瘀斑，可类似挫伤因而延误诊断。
- 放射相关的血管肉瘤在乳腺X线和超声上的表现是非特异性的。乳房血管肉瘤在MRI上表现为T_2加权高信号，且明显强化。

淋巴瘤
- 最常见的原发性乳腺淋巴瘤是**弥漫性大B细胞淋巴瘤**。大多数乳腺淋巴瘤的临床表现为可触及的肿块，可伴有腋窝淋巴结肿大。
- 淋巴瘤的乳腺X线检查可能表现为边缘不清的肿块。超声检查中，淋巴瘤通常为低回声肿块。与上皮性癌(如浸润性导管癌)相比，钙化在乳腺淋巴瘤中罕见。
- 在已知的淋巴瘤患者中，新发的乳腺肿块首先要考虑乳腺癌。组织学活检至关重要，因为淋巴瘤多采用放化疗，而不是手术。
- **人工乳房植入相关的间变性大细胞淋巴瘤**是一种罕见的乳腺原发性T细胞淋巴瘤。它最常见于有假体植入的乳房，通常表现为假体周围积液或残余纤维囊。因此，在植入超过12个月后，假体周围出现任何新的积液均应立即考虑到这种罕见的情况。

(翻译　贺延莉)

BENIGN BREAST DISEASE

CYCLICAL AND PROLIFERATIVE BREAST DISEASE

Fibrocystic change
- Fibrocystic change is an essentially normal pattern of breast physiology.
- Clinically, fibrocystic change presents as cyclical breast pain, sometimes with a palpable lump. Fibrocystic change is almost always seen in pre menopausal women.
- Imaging findings are not specific and the diagnosis of fibrocystic change is never made based on imaging alone. Its only significance is that it may cause certain imaging abnormalities that instigate further workup, such as cysts and calcifications.

Sclerosing adenosis
- Sclerosing adenosis is a benign proliferative lesion caused by lobular hyperplasia and formation of fibrous tissue that distorts the glandular elements.
- Similar to fibrocystic change, the imaging importance of sclerosing adenosis is that it can mimic DCIS with microcalcifications.

良性乳腺病变

周期性和增生性乳腺疾病

纤维囊性改变
- 纤维囊性变在本质上是乳房的正常生理变化。
- 临床上，纤维囊性变表现为周期性乳房疼痛，有时伴有可触及的肿块。纤维囊性变几乎只见于绝经前的妇女。
- 影像学表现不具特异性，因而诊断纤维囊性变不能仅以影像为依据。其唯一的意义在于它可能会导致某些影像学表现异常，从而需要做进一步的检查，如囊肿和钙化。

硬化性腺病
- 硬化性腺病是一种良性增生性病变，由小叶增生和纤维组织形成所引起的腺体结构扭曲。
- 与纤维囊性变相似，硬化性腺病影像学上的重要意义在于它与伴有微小钙化的原位癌表现相似。

Infectious and Inflammatory Breast Disease

Mastitis

- Mastitis is infection of the breast, most commonly by *Staphylococcus aureus*. It is typically seen in nursing mothers (called lactational or puerperal mastitis) or in diabetic patients.
- Clinically, mastitis presents with breast pain, induration, and erythema. Treatment is antibiotics. If inadequately treated, mastitis can develop into a breast abscess.
- Imaging is usually not performed, unless symptoms persist after antibiotics. Mammography and ultrasound can show focal or diffuse skin thickening, breast edema, and adenopathy.
- The primary differential in this setting is inflammatory carcinoma. A skin punch biopsy can be performed if the two entities cannot be differentiated clinically or on imaging.

乳房感染和炎性疾病

乳腺炎

- 乳腺炎为乳房感染，病原菌通常为金黄色葡萄球菌。多发生于哺乳期的女性(称为哺乳期或产后乳腺炎)或糖尿病患者。
- 临床上，乳腺炎表现为乳房疼痛、硬结和红肿。治疗方法为用抗生素。如果处理不当，乳腺炎可以发展成乳房脓肿。
- 通常无须影像学检查，除非使用抗生素后症状依然没有缓解。乳腺X线或超声检查可显示局限性或弥漫性皮肤增厚、乳房水肿和淋巴结肿大。
- 主要的鉴别诊断是炎性乳腺癌。如果两者在临床或影像学上无法区分，可以进行经皮肤穿刺活检。

Breast abscess

乳房脓肿

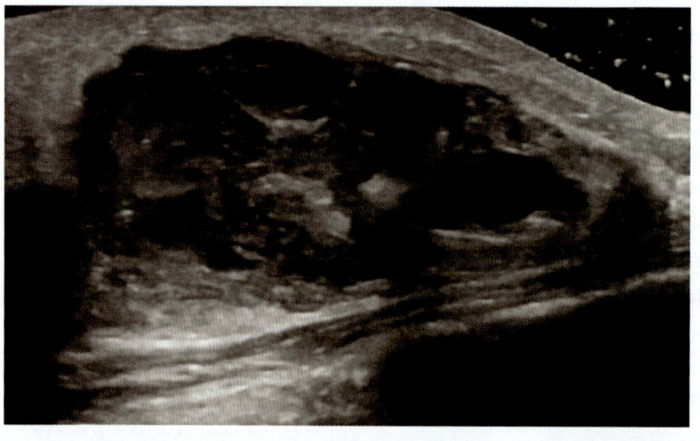

Targeted ultrasound in a lactating patient who presented with breast pain, skin erythema, and palpable lump concerning for abscess. Image shows a heterogeneous collection containing low level internal echoes and layering debris, with surrounding inflammatory changes including overlying skin thickening. Cultures from subsequent aspiration grew *S. auerus*.

对一名哺乳期临床表现为乳房疼痛、皮肤红斑和可触及肿块的可疑乳腺脓肿患者进行局部超声检查。图像显示一个含有内部低回声和分层碎片的异质集合，伴周围炎症改变和表面皮肤增厚。抽吸物培养发现有金黄色葡萄球菌生长。

- A breast abscess is a walled-off purulent collection, most commonly subareolar in location. Clinically, breast abscess presents with focal breast pain, erythema, fluctuance, and fever.
- On mammography, breast abscess can appear as a mass, asymmetry, or architectural distortion, with overlying skin thickening.
- Ultrasound often shows an oval or irregular mass with complex cystic and solid echotexture, indistinct margins and an echogenic halo. The periphery of the mass is often hypervascular.
- Treatment is ultrasound-guided aspiration in addition to antibiotics.

Idiopathic granulomatous mastitis

- Idiopathic granulomatous mastitis is a rare cause of breast inflammation that is more common in young reproductive age women who have previously lactated. Hormonal influences are felt to likely contribute. Although no infectious etiology is identified in many cases, a certain subset is felt to be due to indolent infection with *Corynebacterium* species.
- Granulomatous mastitis usually presents as one or more painful palpable breast masses. There may be associated skin erythema or nipple discharge.
- Mammography most often shows focal asymmetry or an irregular mass.
- On ultrasound there is usually an irregular mass or confluent masses with parallel orientation and hypoechoic or heterogeneous echotexture. In longstanding cases, fluid collections may be present.

- 乳房脓肿是一个边界不清的脓性液体聚集区，最常位于乳晕的周围。临床上它表现为局部乳房疼痛、红肿、波动感和发热。
- 乳腺X线影像可表现为肿块、不对称或结构扭曲，伴有皮肤增厚。
- 超声常显示为椭圆形或不规则形肿块，内部复杂的囊实性回声结构，边缘模糊，周围回声晕环。肿块的外围通常为富血供区。
- 治疗方法为抗生素治疗加超声引导下引流。

特发性肉芽肿性乳腺炎

- 特发性肉芽肿性乳腺炎是一种罕见的乳腺炎症，常发生于哺乳后的育龄期年轻女性。可能与激素的影响有关。大多情况下没有发现感染病因，但少部分是棒状杆菌隐性感染所致。
- 肉芽肿性乳腺炎通常表现为一个或多个伴有疼痛的可触及的乳房肿块。可能伴有皮肤红斑或乳头溢液。
- 乳腺X线最常显示为局灶性不对称或不规则的肿块。
- 超声常显示为平行方向的不规则肿块或融合肿块，低回声或不均匀回声。慢性病例中可

- Granulomatous mastitis shows enhancement on MRI and may present as segmental distribution NME.
- The imaging features of granulomatous mastitis may mimic breast cancer and biopsy is usually warranted. Treatment of idiopathic granulomatous mastitis can be challenging, and symptoms may be longstanding.

能存在积液。

- 肉芽肿性乳腺炎的增强MRI可表现为节段性分布的NME。
- 肉芽肿性乳腺炎的影像学特征可能与乳腺癌相似，通常需要进行活检。治疗特发性肉芽肿性乳腺炎具有挑战性，其症状可能较为顽固。

Periductal mastitis

- Periductal mastitis, also known as plasma cell mastitis, is caused by the irritating contents of intraductal lipids. It is seen in post-menopausal women and produces the classic mammographic appearance of large, rod-like secretory calcifications.

导管周围乳腺炎

- 导管周围乳腺炎，也称为浆细胞乳腺炎，由导管内脂质分泌物刺激引起。见于绝经后妇女，典型的乳腺X线影像表现为大的、呈棒状的分泌型钙化灶。

Diabetic mastopathy

糖尿病性乳腺病

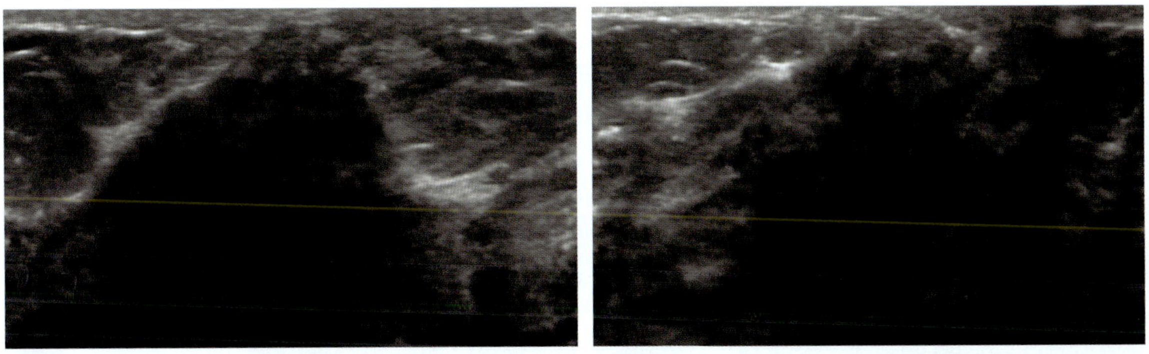

Targeted ultrasound of bilateral breasts in a patient with type 1 diabetes who presented with palpable bilateral subareolar masses. Images show irregular hypoechoic masses with posterior shadowing in the bilateral subareolar regions. Given similar appearances and patient history, these masses may represent diabetic mastopathy, however malignancy must be excluded. Patient underwent core needle biopsy of the right breast mass which confirmed diabetic mastopathy.

对一名临床表现为双侧乳晕下可触及肿块的1型糖尿病患者行双侧乳房局部超声检查。图像显示不规则的低回声肿块，伴双侧乳晕下区域后方阴影。鉴于相似的外观和病史，这些肿块可能为糖尿病性乳腺病，但必须排除恶性肿瘤。对患者右侧乳房肿块进行核芯针穿刺活检，结果证实为糖尿病性乳腺病。

- Diabetic mastopathy is a sequela of long-term insulin-dependent diabetes. An autoimmune reaction to matrix proteins from chronic hyperglycemia causes a firm and sometimes painful mass.
- On mammography, diabetic mastopathy can appear as an ill-defined, asymmetric density without microcalcifications or as architectural distortion.
- Ultrasound typically shows a hypoechoic mass or regional acoustic shadowing, mimicking the appearance of a scirrhous breast cancer.
- Because the mammographic and sonographic appearance can mimic breast cancer, core biopsy is required.

- 糖尿病性乳腺病是长期胰岛素依赖型糖尿病（1型糖尿病）的后遗症。慢性高血糖会导致对基质蛋白质的自体免疫反应，形成一个坚硬且有时会疼痛的包块。
- 糖尿病性乳腺病患者的乳腺X线影像可表现为边界不清且不含微小钙化的非对称性致密区。
- 超声通常呈低回声肿块或局限性声影区，类似于硬化型乳腺癌的表现。
- 因乳腺X线和超声表现可类似于乳腺癌，需要进行穿刺活检。

Mondor disease

蒙多病

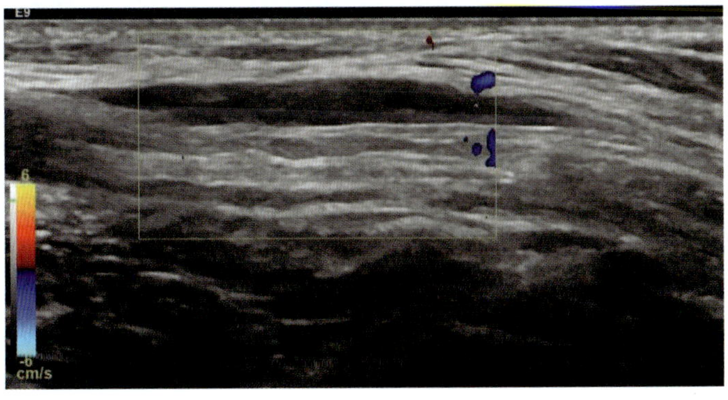

Ultrasound image with color Doppler shows a tubular hypoechoic mass without internal vascularity, likely a thrombosed superficial vessel.

彩色多普勒超声图像显示管状低回声肿块，无内部血管，可能为有血栓形成的浅表血管。

- Mondor disease is thrombophlebitis of a superficial vein of the breast, most commonly the thoracoepigastric vein.
- Clinically, Mondor disease presents with pain and tenderness in the region of the thrombosed vein. A cordlike, elongated superficial mass may be present.
- Ultrasound shows a dilated, "bead-like" tubular structure with no flow on color Doppler.

- 蒙多病是乳房浅表静脉的血栓性静脉炎，通常出现在胸腹壁静脉。
- 临床上，蒙多病表现为静脉血栓形成相应区域的疼痛和压痛。可能出现棒状或长条索状的浅表包块。
- 超声显示为扩张的、"念珠状" 的管状结构，彩色多普勒上无血流信号。

（翻译　王草叶）

NORMAL VARIANTS

正常变异

Sternalis muscle

胸骨肌

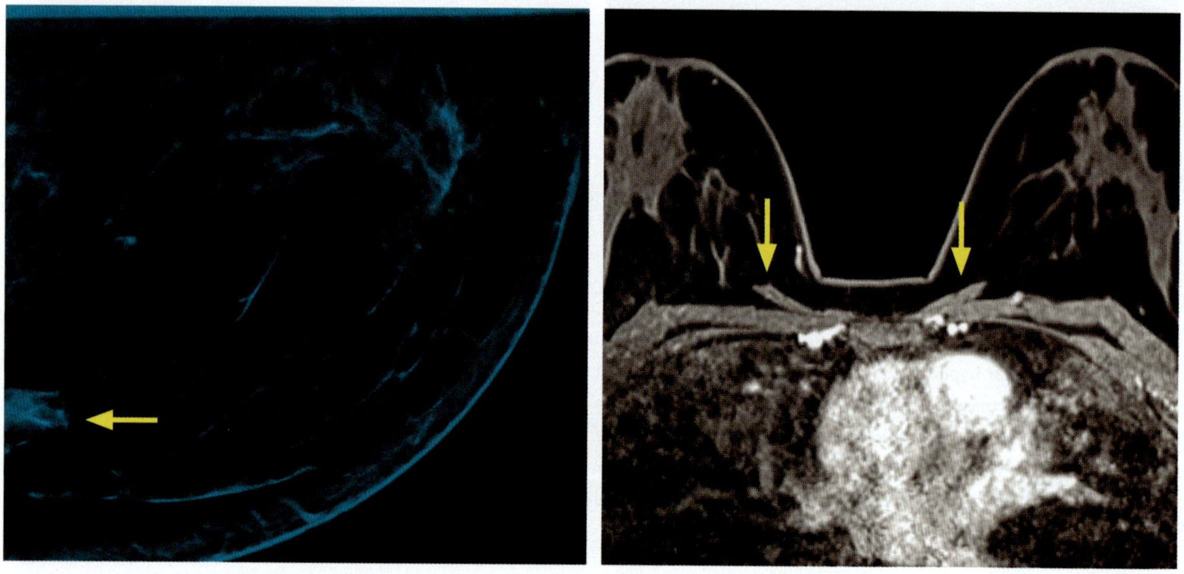

Mammogram shows an asymmetry in the far posterior medial left breast (arrow), seen on CC view only, that persists on spot compression view (left image). No corresponding abnormality was seen on ultrasound (not shown). Follow up MRI (right image) shows an accessory muscle lying anterior to the left pectoralis (arrow). A similar muscle is seen on the contralateral side. These represent bilateral sternalis muscles.

乳腺X线影像显示左侧乳腺后内侧不对称(黄箭)，仅见于CC位，点压后仍未消失(左图)。超声未见相应异常(未展示)。随后MRI(右图)显示左侧胸大肌前方的附属肌(黄箭)，对侧可见类似肌肉。这些发现为双侧胸骨肌。

- The sternalis muscle is a vertically oriented accessory parasternal chest wall muscle present in less than 10% of patients. It is either triangular or rounded in shape and seen only on the CC view medially at far-posterior depth. It is more commonly unilateral.
- The main differential consideration is a medial mass; however, the characteristic shape and lack of corresponding finding on the lateral or MLO views is usually sufficient to diagnose a sternalis muscle. MRI can be performed in ambiguous cases.

Accessory nipple (polythelia)

- An accessory nipple (polythelia) is seen in approximately 2% of neonates and may present on mammography as a rounded mass along the mammary crest.
- Physical exam is diagnostic.

Accessory breast tissue

- Accessory or ectopic breast tissue occurs in 2–6% of women and is most common in the axilla. It may be unilateral or bilateral.

- 胸骨肌是一块垂直的胸骨旁胸壁附属肌肉，见于不到10%的患者。它呈三角形或圆形，仅见于CC位内侧靠后的深部。单侧多见。
- 主要需与该病鉴别诊断的是位于内侧的肿块，但胸骨肌的形状特殊及在MLO位或侧位上缺乏相应的发现通常足以进行诊断。MRI可以用于诊断不明确的病例。

副乳头(多乳头)

- 副乳头(多乳头)约见于2%的新生儿，并在乳腺X线检查表现为沿着乳腺嵴生长的一个圆形肿块。
- 查体即可诊断。

副乳腺组织

- 副乳或异位乳腺组织出现在2%~6%的女性，多位于腋窝。可以是单侧或双侧。

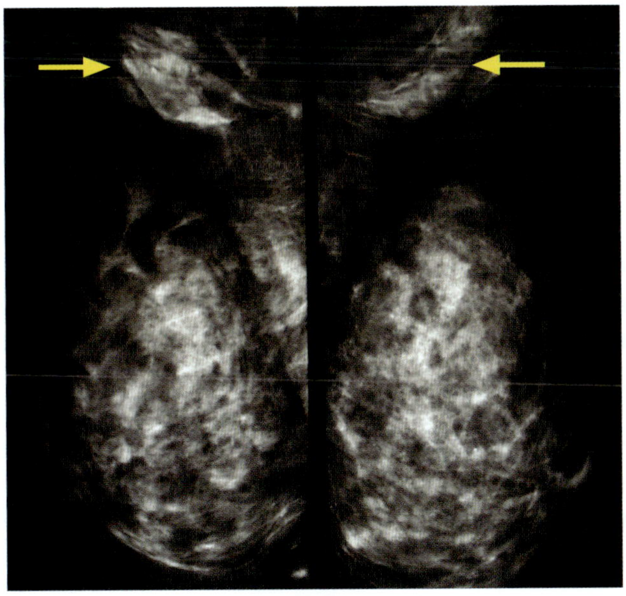

Mammogram shows accessory fibroglandular tissue in bilateral axillae (arrows).
乳腺X线影像显示双侧腋窝副纤维腺体组织(黄箭)

Poland syndrome

- Poland syndrome is a congenital disorder characterized by unilateral absence of the pectoralis major muscle, often associated with ipsilateral absence of breast tissue and syndactyly.

波伦综合征

- 波伦综合征是一种先天性疾病,以单侧胸大肌缺如为特征,常伴有同侧乳腺组织缺如及并指/趾畸形。

(翻译　贺延莉)

POSTSURGICAL IMAGING

IMAGING IMPLANTS

Overview of implants

- Implants can be used either for cosmetic reasons or for breast reconstruction after mastectomy. The two types of implants in common use are filled with either silicone or saline, although double lumen (inner silicone lumen and outer saline compartment) and other varieties of implants exist.
- Silicone implants are comprised of a silicone gel and come in pre-manufactured sizes. Saline implants contain a valve that allows filling of the implant during surgery.
- Regardless of the type of implant, a fibrous capsule is gradually formed as a reaction to the foreign body. The capsule may become calcified. Over time, the implant may partially herniate through the capsule without rupturing, causing a palpable contour deformity.
- Implants can be placed either behind the pectoralis (retropectoral) or directly in front of the pectoralis/behind the fibroglandular tissue (prepectoral/retroglandular).

Mammographic imaging of implants

- When implants are imaged with mammography, standard views are difficult to interpret because the high-attenuation implant can obscure breast tissue. Implant-displaced views (also called Eklund views) displace the implant posteriorly and pull the native breast tissue anteriorly to allow for improved compression and visualization of the breast tissue.
- A saline implant can be identified on mammography due to the presence

手术后影像

假体影像

假体简介

- 假体用于美容或乳腺切除术后对乳房进行重建。常用的两种假体分别为硅胶和生理盐水,此外还有双腔假体(内腔为硅胶、外腔为生理盐水)和其他类型的假体。
- 硅胶型假体由硅胶凝胶组成并提前塑形而成。生理盐水假体有一个阀门,通过这个阀门可以在手术中进行填注塑形。
- 不管哪种类型的假体都是外来物,其周围都会逐渐形成一层反应性纤维包膜。纤维包膜可能会形成钙化。随着时间推移,假体可能会部分从纤维包膜疝出(而假体本身并没有破裂),形成可以触摸到的轮廓变形。
- 假体可以植入至胸大肌的后方(胸大肌后型)或胸大肌的前方/纤维腺体组织的后方(胸大肌前型/腺体后型)。

乳腺假体的X线影像

- 对假体进行乳腺X线检查时,标准体位的图像较难评估乳腺组织,因为高密度的假体会妨碍对乳腺组织的观察。假体移动体位(又称Eklund体位)可将假体向后推,同时将正常乳腺组织向前牵拉,从而增加对自然乳腺组织的压迫,提高成像效果。

of its valve. Additionally, the wall of the implant will be denser than the center because the wall is made of silicone elastomer that is denser than saline.

- In contrast, a silicone implant will be uniformly dense, and no valve will be present.

- 生理盐水假体因有活瓣而在乳腺X线影像上可以进行确认。另外，假体壁的密度要高于中央区，因为假体的壁由硅胶组成，其密度高于生理盐水。
- 相比之下，硅胶假体的密度均匀，且没有活瓣。

Ultrasound imaging of implants

- While ultrasound probes designed specifically for breast imaging provide superior imaging of the breast tissue, they do not always allow sufficient penetration to fully evaluate a more posteriorly positioned implant. An ultrasound machine with multiple probe choices is therefore advantageous in the setting of implant evaluation.

假体的超声影像

- 为乳腺成像而设计的超声探头对于乳房组织可提供超清晰的影像，但它们并没有足够的穿透力来全面评估位于后方的假体。具有多种探头的超声仪则有利于对假体的评估。

MR imaging of silicone implants

- Specific MRI protocols allow for the evaluation of implants, including silicone-only and silicone-suppression sequences.
- MRI has a higher sensitivity and specificity for detecting silicone implant rupture than both mammogram and ultrasound.

硅胶假体的MRI

- 特定MRI扫描方案可以对假体进行评估，包括单纯硅胶和硅胶抑制序列。
- MRI对检测硅胶假体破裂较乳腺X线和超声两种检查具有较高的灵敏度和特异度。

Overview of implant rupture

假体破裂简介

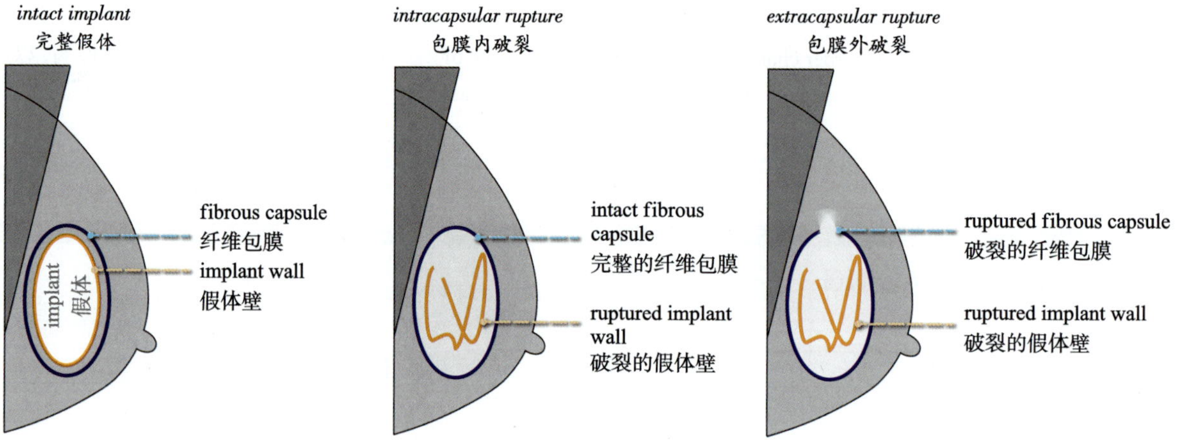

- Rupture of an implant can be contained within the fibrous capsule (intracapsular rupture) or may extend out of the fibrous capsule (extracapsular rupture).
- The distinction between intra- and extracapsular rupture is only important for silicone implants. The contents of a saline implant will leak out even if the fibrous capsule remains intact.

- 假体破裂后可以局限于纤维包膜内(纤维包膜内破裂)或突破纤维包膜(纤维包膜外破裂)。
- 鉴别包膜内和包膜外破裂仅对硅胶假体有意义。生理盐水假体即使纤维囊完整，其内容物也会漏出。

Intracapsular silicone implant rupture

- Intracapsular rupture of a silicone implant may manifest clinically as a subtle change in the implant contour but without significant change in the size or even shape of the breast. Rupture of a silicone implant can be challenging to diagnose clinically.
- Mammography is often normal, and ultrasound or MRI is usually necessary to diagnose silicone implant rupture.
- MRI of intracapsular silicone implant rupture can have several appearances:

纤维包膜内型硅胶植入体的假体破裂

- 硅胶假体发生纤维包膜内破裂后，临床可表现为轻微的假体轮廓改变，但没有明显的乳腺大小变化，甚至乳腺形状也没有明显改变。临床上诊断硅胶假体包膜内破裂会很困难。
- 乳腺X线检查常表现为正常，通常需要使用超声或MRI检查对硅胶假体破裂作出诊断。
- 纤维包膜内型硅胶假体破裂在MRI的表现有以下几种：

> *Linguine sign* is the most classic and describes the presence of multiple curvilinear lines representing the fragmented and collapsed elastomer shell that is floating within the intracapsular silicone.
> *Subcapsular line sign* describes a thin layer of silicone interposed between the implant shell and fibrous capsule.
> *Keyhole* and *teardrop signs* describe focal invagination of the implant shell due to leaked silicone outside the shell.

> 舌样征最经典，表现为多条曲线，代表漂浮包膜内碎裂和塌陷的胶状外壳。
> 包膜下线征指的是假体外壳和纤维囊之间一层薄薄的硅胶。
> 锁孔征和泪滴征是指由于假体外壳外的硅胶泄漏导致的局部假体外壳内陷。

- *Radial folds* are normal infoldings of the implant shell that can mimic implant rupture.
- Ultrasound of intracapsular silicone implant rupture may show segments of broken and collapsed implant shell floating within intracapsular silicone at various levels, termed the *stepladder sign*.

- 放射状折叠是假体外壳的正常内折，与假体破裂类似。
- 纤维包膜内型硅胶假体破裂在超声检查上可表现为破裂、坍塌的假体外壳碎片不同程度地漂浮于纤维包膜内硅胶中，称为阶梯征。

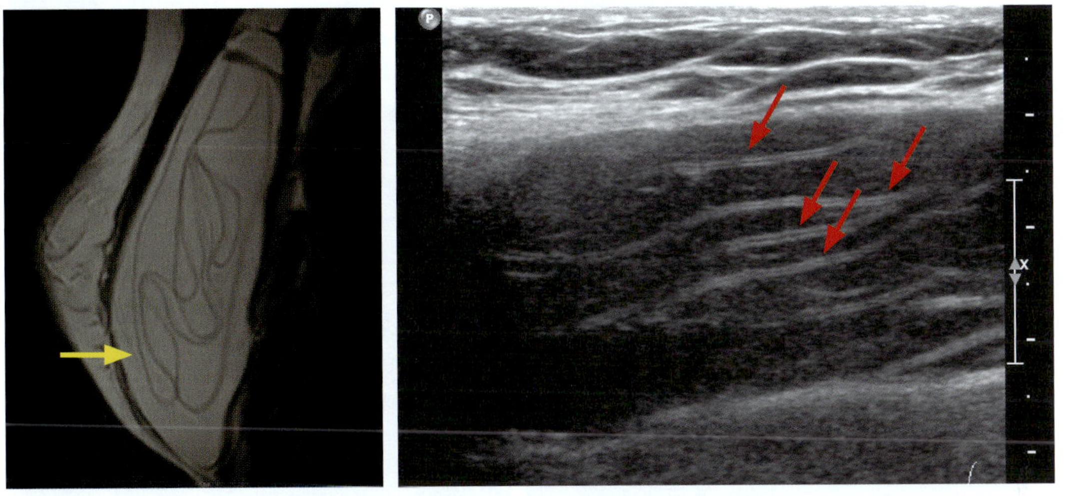

Left: Axial T2-weighted MRI of the left breast without fat saturation shows the curvilinear undulating contour of the disrupted and collapsed silicone implant shell (arrow), representing the *linguine sign*.
Right: Ultrasound shows a *stepladder* pattern of the echogenic silicone implant shell (arrows). The implant envelope is floating within a lake of fluid containing low-level internal echoes, representing silicone.
左图：左乳轴位T_2加权无脂肪抑制MRI显示硅胶植入物外壳破裂和塌陷的曲线样起伏轮廓(黄箭)，代表舌样征。
右图：超声显示呈阶梯状回声的硅胶假体外壳(红箭)。假体壁漂浮在内部为低回声的硅胶液体池中。

Extracapsular silicone implant rupture

- Extracapsular rupture of a silicone implant may be evident on mammography as high density silicone extending beyond the edge of the capsule into the breast parenchyma.

纤维包膜外型硅胶假体破裂

- 纤维包膜外型硅胶假体破裂在乳腺X线影像中可能表现为高密度的硅胶位于纤维包膜的外侧，并进入乳腺实质中。

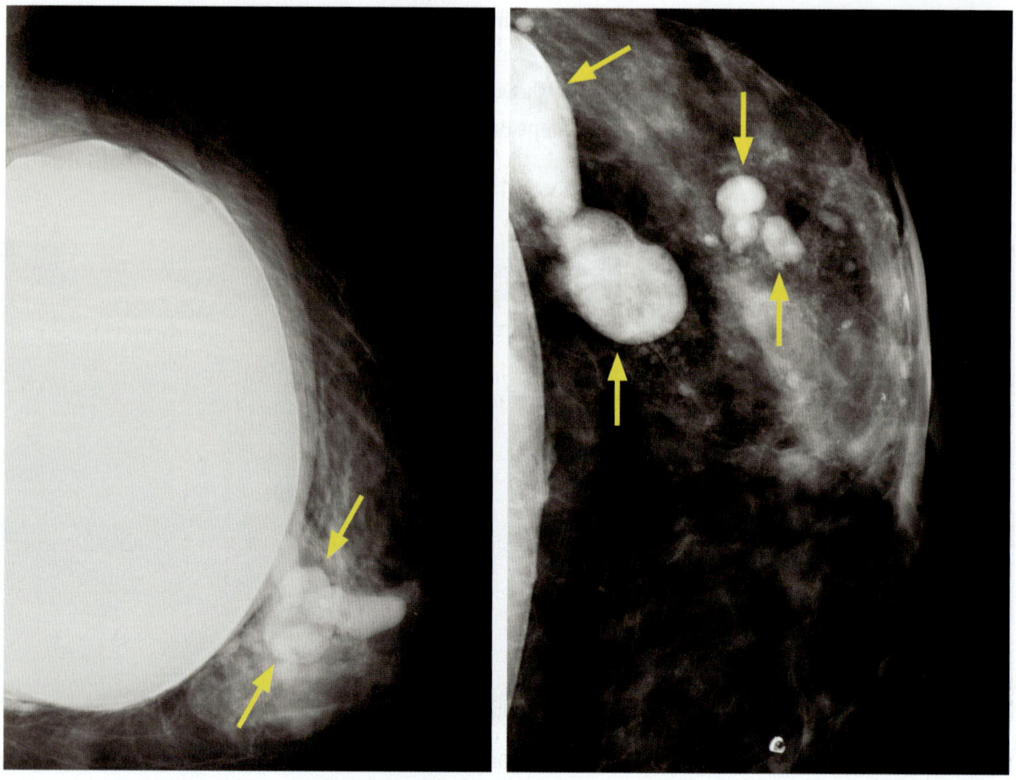

Extracapsular rupture: Standard MLO mammogram (left image) shows a retropectoral implant and frank extravasation of high density silicone into the breast parenchyma (arrows). The implant-displaced CC mammogram better shows the extent of the high density intraparenchymal silicone granulomas.
纤维包膜外型破裂：标准乳腺X线MLO位影像(左图)显示胸大肌后方一个假体和明显的高密度硅胶直接渗入乳腺实质(黄箭)。CC位影像(右图)更好地显示出乳腺实质内高密度硅胶肉芽肿。

- On ultrasound, extracapsular silicone rupture causes free silicone to appear in the breast parenchyma, which has a classic *snowstorm* appearance on ultrasound.
- Silicone uptake by regional nodes can occur with free silicone injection, extracapsular rupture and much less commonly with intracapsular rupture or *gel bleed* through an intact but weakened implant shell.

- 超声检查时，硅胶破出包膜外导致乳腺间质中有游离的硅胶，呈现为典型的暴风雪样改变。
- 局部淋巴结摄取硅胶可发生在注射游离硅胶、囊外破裂，以及较少见的囊内破裂或通过完整但脆弱的假体外壳发生胶溢出。

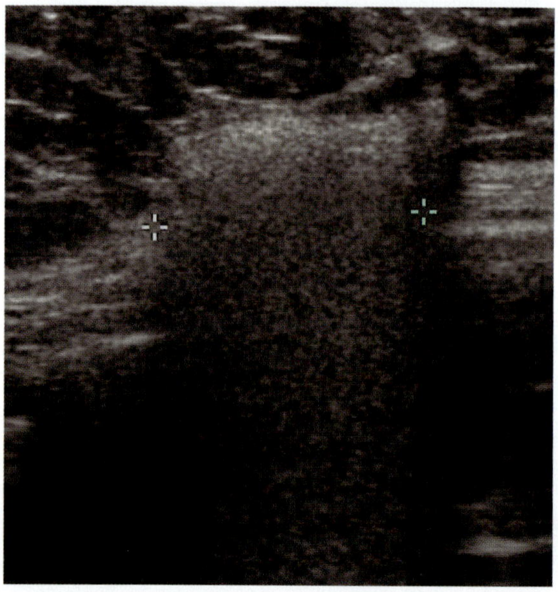

Ultrasound shows an echogenic, shadowing mass with a classic *snowstorm* appearance (calipers), suggestive of silicone granuloma from extracapsular rupture.
超声显示一个回声增强、有声影的肿块，并呈典型的暴风雪样表现(卡尺)，提示因硅胶纤维包膜外破裂后形成的肉芽肿。

Saline implant rupture

- Rupture of a saline implant is usually evident clinically. Rupture causes sudden collapse and resultant instantaneous decrease in breast size. The residual implant envelope folds in on itself and the saline is absorbed.

生理盐水型假体破裂

- 生理盐水型假体破裂后的临床表现通常比较明显，假体破裂后会导致乳腺形状突然塌陷，从而导致乳腺体积减小。残留假体薄膜自身折叠，而生理盐水则被吸收。

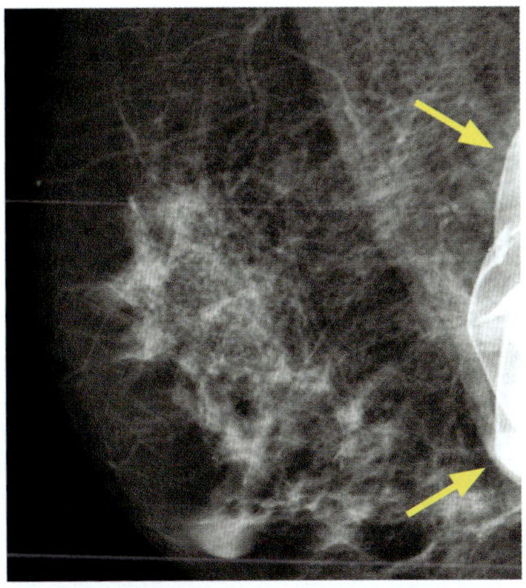

MLO mammogram partially shows a collapsed retropectoral saline implant (arrows) at the posterior aspect of the image.
MLO位乳腺X线影像显示胸大肌后方塌陷的生理盐水假体(黄箭)。

Reduction Mammoplasty

缩乳术

Reduction mammoplasty

缩乳术

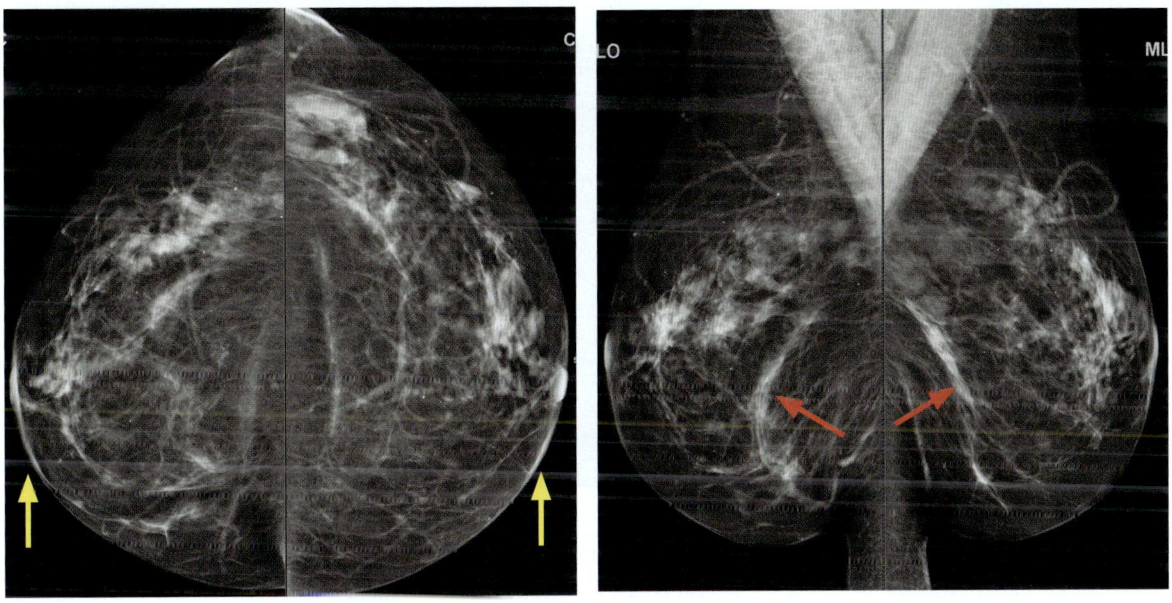

Reduction mammoplasty: Bilateral CC (left images) and MLO mammograms show subtle skin thickening of the lower medial breasts (yellow arrows). Symmetric distortion of the fibroglandular tissue (red arrows) in the lower breast is best seen on the MLO views. The nipples are superiorly displaced.
缩乳术：双侧乳腺CC位和MLO位影像显示乳腺下缘内侧轻微皮肤增厚改变(黄箭)。MLO位较好地显示乳腺下方对称性的纤维腺体组织扭曲(红箭)。乳头向上移位。

- Reduction mammoplasty is performed for aesthetic reasons or to reduce back pain caused by large breasts.
- The surgeon removes breast parenchyma and skin from the inferior breast and relocates the nipple to a more superior location.

- 缩乳术通常用于美容或减轻由于乳腺腺体过大引起的背痛。
- 外科医师通过切除乳腺下缘的部分乳腺腺体和皮肤，使乳头置于一个相对较高的位置。

- The mammographic findings of reduction mammoplasty include:

Elevation of the nipple. Redistribution of breast tissue to the lower breast. Curvilinear architectural distortion in the lower breast. Postsurgical skin thickening over the areola and lower breast. Fat necrosis, suture and dermal calcifications may be present.

- 缩乳术后的乳腺X线影像表现包括：

乳头抬高。 乳腺组织重新分布到乳腺下方。 乳腺下方的曲线状结构扭曲。 术后乳晕和乳腺下方皮肤增厚。 可能存在脂肪坏死、缝线和真皮钙化。

（翻译　彭程宇）

MALE BREAST DISEASE

男性乳腺疾病

Gynecomastia

男性乳房发育

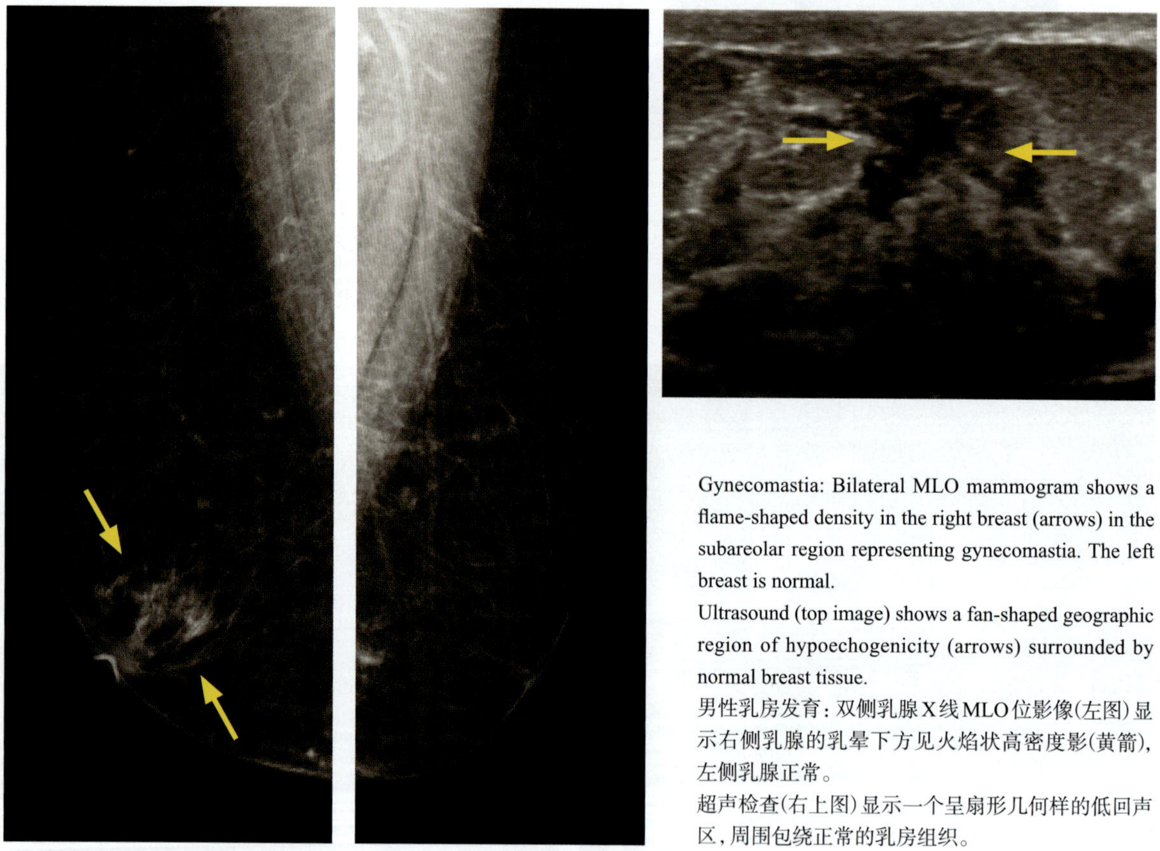

Gynecomastia: Bilateral MLO mammogram shows a flame-shaped density in the right breast (arrows) in the subareolar region representing gynecomastia. The left breast is normal.
Ultrasound (top image) shows a fan-shaped geographic region of hypoechogenicity (arrows) surrounded by normal breast tissue.

男性乳房发育：双侧乳腺X线MLO位影像(左图)显示右侧乳腺的乳晕下方见火焰状高密度影(黄箭)，左侧乳腺正常。
超声检查(右上图)显示一个呈扇形几何样的低回声区，周围包绕正常的乳房组织。

- Gynecomastia is the benign development of glandular tissue in a male. It is the most common diagnosis of males evaluated for a focal breast complaint and clinically presents with a subareolar palpable abnormality.
- Gynecomastia may be idiopathic or be due to cirrhosis, drugs (e.g., antihypertensives and antidepressants), marijuana, pituitary hormone dysfunction, or a hormone-producing tumor.
- The typical mammographic appearance is a flame-shaped or triangular subareolar density with interspersed fat. Mammography is usually diagnostic, but familiarity with the ultrasound appearance is also important as it may be the first exam performed in very young patients. Ultrasound often shows a hypoechoic or heterogeneous echotexture region centrally behind the nipple that is disc or fan shaped.

- 男性乳房发育即男性乳腺增生症，是男性乳腺腺体组织的良性发育，是男性因局部乳房不适及乳晕下触摸异常而就诊的最常见诊断。
- 男性乳房发育可能是特发，或由肝硬化、药物(降压药、抗抑郁药)、大麻、垂体激素功能紊乱、内分泌肿瘤等引起。
- 典型的乳腺X线影像表现为乳晕下一个火焰状或三角形的致密影，夹杂脂肪组织。乳腺X线检查常可以进行诊断，但熟悉超声表现也很重要，因为年轻患者的首次检查可能就是超声。超声通常显示乳头后的中央区有一个低回声或混合回声区，呈盘状或扇形。

Male breast cancer

男性乳腺癌

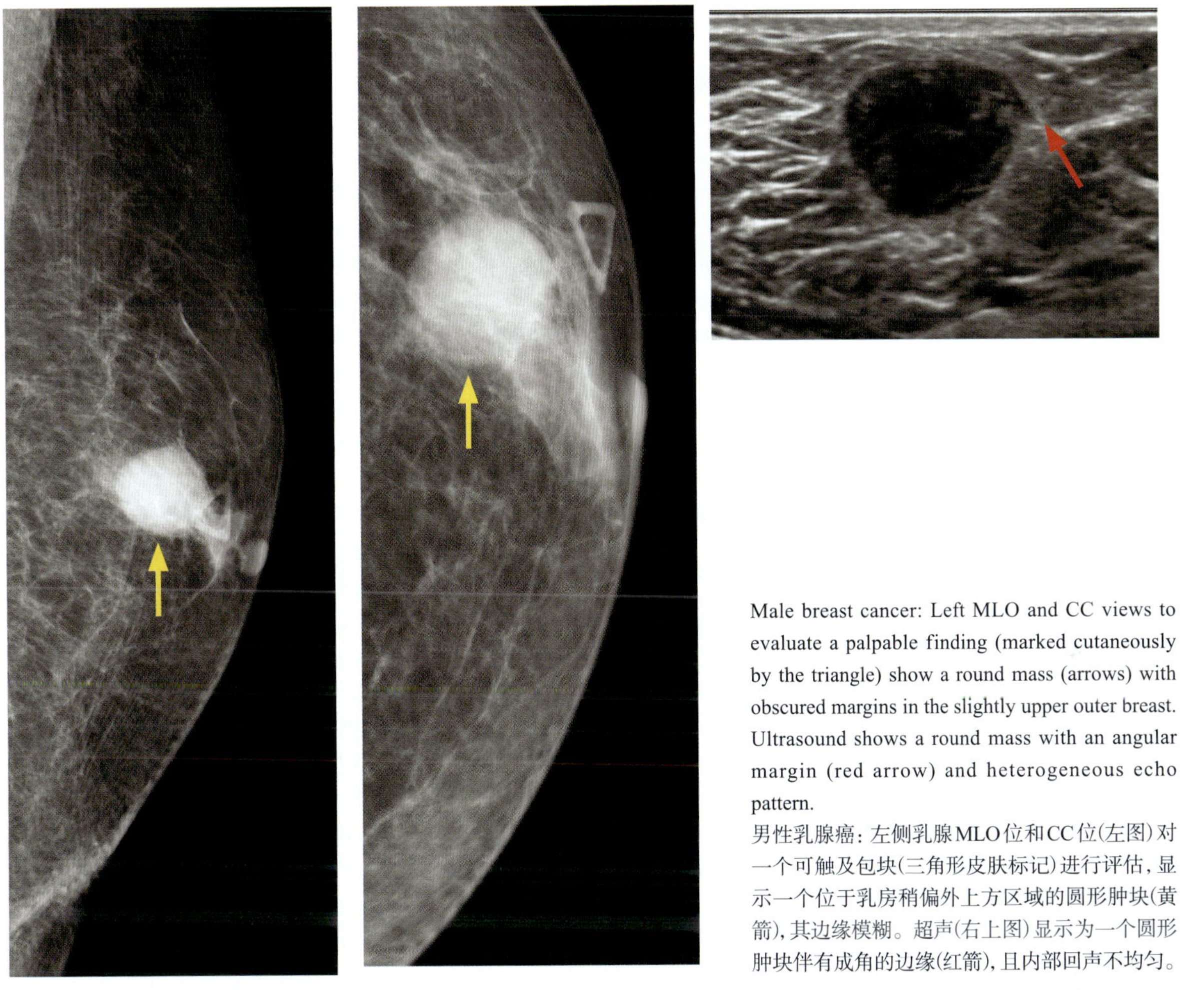

Male breast cancer: Left MLO and CC views to evaluate a palpable finding (marked cutaneously by the triangle) show a round mass (arrows) with obscured margins in the slightly upper outer breast. Ultrasound shows a round mass with an angular margin (red arrow) and heterogeneous echo pattern.

男性乳腺癌：左侧乳腺MLO位和CC位(左图)对一个可触及包块(三角形皮肤标记)进行评估，显示一个位于乳房稍偏外上方区域的圆形肿块(黄箭)，其边缘模糊。超声(右上图)显示为一个圆形肿块伴有成角的边缘(红箭)，且内部回声不均匀。

- Male breast cancer accounts for less than 1% of all breast cancers. It tends to affect men greater than 60 years of age and clinically presents as a palpable mass or less commonly, nipple discharge. Because the male breast lacks lobules, invasive ductal carcinoma is the most common pathological diagnosis in men.
- Risk factors include age, elevated estrogen levels (e.g., Klinefelter syndrome, liver disease, alcohol use, obesity), *BRCA2* mutation, family history, and radiation exposure.
- Most breast cancers in men present mammographically as a high density non calcified irregular mass. They are typically eccentric to the nipple or associated with nipple retraction if retroareolar. In contrast to the more vague, ill-defined hypoechoic area behind the nipple seen on ultrasound with gynecomastia, breast cancers most often present as discrete irregular hypoechoic masses with angular, microlobulated or spiculated margins.

- 男性乳腺癌在所有乳腺癌中的比例不到1%。主要见于60岁以上男性，临床表现为一个可触及的包块，偶有乳头泌乳。由于男性乳腺缺乏小叶，因此浸润性导管癌是最常见的病理类型。
- 危险因素包括年龄、过高的雌激素水平(如克兰费尔特综合征、肝病、饮酒和肥胖)，*BRCA2* 基因突变、家族史和辐射。
- 大多数男性乳腺癌乳腺X线影像表现为高密度非钙化的不规则形肿块。病变通常与乳头呈偏心，或伴有乳头回缩(如位于乳晕后)。与男性乳腺发育症超声所见的乳头后方模糊、没有明确边界的低回声区相比，乳腺癌最常表现为清晰但不规则的低回声肿块，边缘呈棱角状、微分叶状或毛刺状。

Benign male breast masses

- The most common benign breast mass in a male is a lipoma. Other very rare benign entities include myofibroblastoma, granular cell tumor, hemangioma and schwannoma.

男性乳腺良性肿块

- 男性最常见的乳腺良性肿块是脂肪瘤。其他良性肿块非常罕见，包括肌纤维母细胞瘤、颗粒细胞瘤、血管瘤和神经鞘瘤。

(翻译　杨学刚)

APPROACH TO THE SYMPTOMATIC BREAST

Breast pain

- Breast pain is common and experienced by up to 80% of women in their lifetime.
- Clinically significant breast pain is defined as **focal** and **non-cyclical**.
- For women under age 30, initial evaluation of clinically significant breast pain should be with ultrasound.
- For women aged 30 or older, initial evaluation of clinically significant breast pain can be performed with mammography or ultrasound.
- Imaging is not appropriate for the initial evaluation of non-clinically significant breast pain (non-focal, cyclical).
- MRI is never appropriate for the initial evaluation of breast pain.

Pathologic nipple discharge

- Pathologic nipple discharge is usually **unilateral**, **spontaneous**, and either **serous**, **bloody**, or **clear**. Causes include duct ectasia, intraductal papilloma, DCIS and invasive carcinoma.
- By contrast, physiologic nipple discharge is usually bilateral, non-spontaneous and milky, green, or yellow in color.
- For women under age 30, initial imaging evaluation of pathologic discharge should be with ultrasound.
- For women aged 30 or older and all men, initial evaluation of pathologic discharge should be with mammography and ultrasound, although ultrasound alone can be considered in women between ages 30–39.
- MRI is never appropriate for the initial evaluation of pathologic discharge but is increasingly utilized over galactography for further assessment of nipple discharge when mammography and ultrasound are negative.
- Imaging is not appropriate for the initial evaluation of physiologic discharge.

Palpable breast mass

- In women aged 40 or older, initial evaluation of a palpable breast mass should be with mammography. For further characterization of corresponding mammographic findings that are not clearly benign and if mammography is negative, ultrasound of the palpable abnormality should also be performed. Any suspicious finding should be biopsied.
- In women under age 30, initial evaluation should be performed with ultrasound. If ultrasound findings are suspicious, mammography should be considered for further workup and biopsy should be performed. If ultrasound is negative, mammography should be added if the clinical finding is striking; otherwise clinical follow-up is appropriate. For clearly benign or probably benign ultrasound findings in young women, further assessment with mammography is not necessary; ultrasound short interval follow-up or core biopsy should be performed for probably benign or low suspicion lesions.
- In women between ages 30 and 39, initial evaluation can be performed with ultrasound or mammography.
- In men under age 25, initial evaluation of an indeterminate breast mass (that is not classic for gynecomastia) should be with ultrasound.
- In men aged 25 or older, or at any age with physical exam suspicious for breast cancer, both mammography and ultrasound are appropriate initial imaging options.

乳腺症状的处理方法

乳腺疼痛

- 乳腺疼痛很常见，超过80%的女性在其一生中都有此经历。
- 临床有意义的乳腺疼痛定义为**局灶性**和**非周期性**疼痛。
- 对于30岁以下的女性，初始评估临床有意义的乳腺疼痛应使用超声。
- 对于30岁及以上的女性，初始评估临床有意义的乳腺疼痛可以采用乳腺X线或超声检查。
- 对于不具临床意义的乳腺疼痛(非局灶性、周期性)不适合采用影像学进行初始评估。
- MRI不应用于乳腺疼痛的初始评估。

病理性乳头溢液

- 病理性乳头溢液通常为**单侧**、**自发**、**浆液性**、**血性**或**透明**。原因包括导管扩张、导管内乳头状瘤、DCIS和浸润性癌。
- 相反，生理性乳头溢液通常为双侧、非自发、乳白色、绿色或黄色。
- 年龄在30岁以下的女性，对病理性乳头溢液的初始影像学评估应采用超声。
- 30岁及以上的女性和所有男性，病理性乳头溢液的初始评估应联合应用乳腺X线摄影及超声检查，30~39岁女性也可以考虑单独进行超声检查。
- MRI不应用于病理性乳头溢液的初始评估，但乳腺X线和超声检查呈阴性时，MRI正逐渐取代乳腺导管造影对乳头溢液做进一步评估。
- 影像学不适用于生理性乳头溢液的初始评估。

可触及的乳腺肿块

- 40岁及以上的女性，可触及的乳腺肿块初始评估应采用乳腺X线检查。如果乳腺X线影像的检查结果不能明确为良性，应对可触及的异常进行超声检查。任何可疑的发现都应做活检。
- 对于30岁以下的女性，应使用超声进行初步检查。如果超声检查结果可疑，应考虑进一步行X线检查和活检。如果超声检查为阴性但临床表现显著，应增加乳腺X线检查或进行临床随访。若年轻女性的超声检查结果明确为良性或可能良性，不需要进一步的乳腺X线检查；对于可能为良性或低度怀疑恶性的病变，应进行超声短期间隔随访或核芯针穿刺活检。
- 对30~39岁的女性，初始评估可以采用超声或乳腺X线检查。
- 25岁以下的男性，对于不确定的乳房肿块(不是典型的男性乳房发育症)的初步评估应选择超声。
- 年龄在25岁或以上任何年龄的男性体检若怀

- Benign appearing palpable breast cysts can be aspirated for symptomatic relief.

疑为乳腺癌，乳腺X线和超声都是合适的初始影像学检查方法。

- 良性可触及的乳腺囊肿可行抽吸术以缓解症状。

（翻译　彭程宇）

BREAST INTERVENTIONS

Overview of breast interventions

- Regardless of the method of biopsy, the radiologist must perform a radiology-pathology correlation of every case to ensure that the pathologic diagnosis is concordant with the imaging findings. Discordant findings should receive further workup, typically requiring repeat biopsy, either core or excisional. An example of a discordant finding is benign pathology (e.g., fragments of a fibroadenoma) for a highly suspicious, spiculated mass.

乳腺介入

乳腺介入概述

- 无论采用哪种活检方法，放射科医师都必须对每个病例进行放射-病理学对照，以确保病理诊断与影像学表现的一致性。如果结果不一致，应该做进一步检查，通常需要重复活检，即核芯针穿刺或手术切除取样。一个结果不一致的例子是：病理报告为良性(纤维腺瘤的碎片)但高度可疑的毛刺状肿块。

PERCUTANEOUS NEEDLE BIOPSY

Ultrasound-guided core needle biopsy

经皮穿刺针活检

超声引导下核芯针穿刺活检

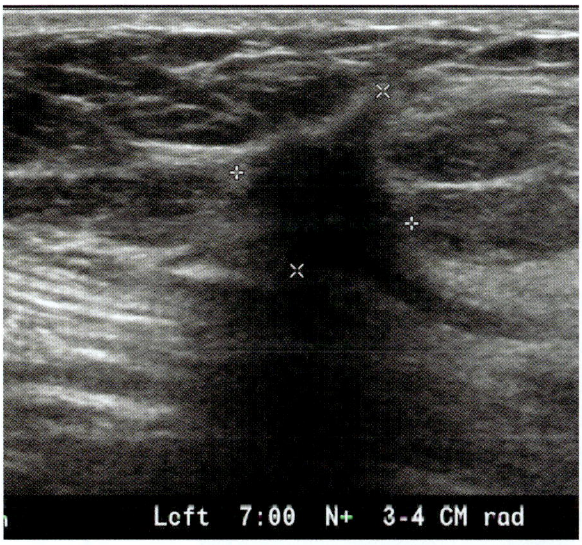

Pre-procedure ultrasound demonstrates a shadowing, spiculated mass (calipers) with taller-than-wide orientation that is highly suspicious.

穿刺前超声显示 个具有声影的毛刺状肿块(卡尺)，其高度大于宽度，高度可疑恶性。

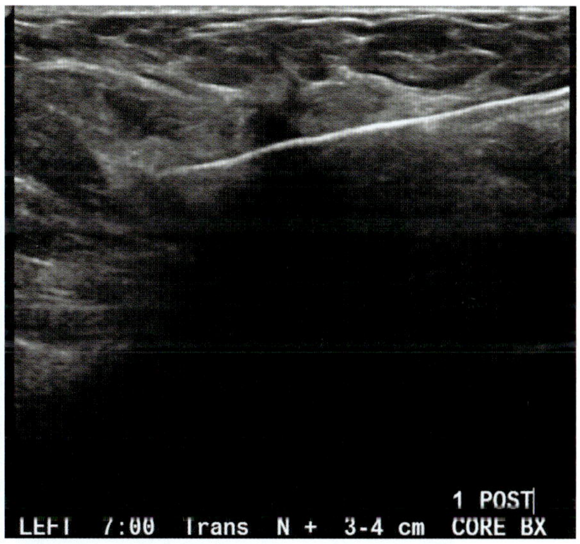

Post-fire image from an ultrasound-guided core needle biopsy shows the core needle traversing the lesion with an appropriate shallow angle of approach.

超声引导组织活检图像显示核芯针穿过，并与病灶形成 个适当的夹角。

- Ultrasound-guided core needle biopsy is the preferred approach for a lesion that is well seen on ultrasound. Ultrasound-guided biopsy using standard freehand technique and a 14-gauge spring-loaded needle is a highly accurate method to biopsy breast masses.
- Ultrasound-guided interventions are the most user-dependent and take time to master. Appropriate initial positioning of the patient and planning of the approach allows a smooth procedure. Some practitioners always hold the ultrasound probe in the non-dominant hand to allow the dominant hand control over the needle. Others take an ambidextrous approach.

- 若超声可以很好地显示病灶，则超声引导核芯针穿刺活检为首选方法。采用标准徒手技术和14G弹簧穿刺针是一种高度精确的超声引导下乳腺肿块活检方法。
- 超声引导的介入方法在很大程度上取决于操作者个人，并需花时间去掌握。一开始将患者置于合适的体位和进行术前计划可使穿刺过程变得顺利。部分医师习惯使用非优势手操作超声探头，使用优势手控制活检针；另外

- A lateral approach to the lesion is generally preferred. It is critical when performing an ultrasound-guided procedure to always keep the biopsy device parallel to the chest wall, or at a very shallow angle of obliquity. A standard breast biopsy needle advances approximately 2 cm when sampling. Far posterior lesions can be entered with the tip of the biopsy device and lifted anteriorly off the chest wall before sampling.
- Posterior lesions require a larger distance between the lesion and the entry site to maintain a nearly parallel biopsy needle course. Once an entry site is chosen, cutaneous and subcutaneous anesthesia is administered under ultrasound guidance and a small skin incision is made. Each needle pass should be documented and needle positioning within the target demonstrated in an orthogonal plane for at least 1–2 passes.
- After adequate sampling, a tissue marker is typically placed, and post-procedure mammography is performed to confirm marker position within the targeted lesion.

Ultrasound-guided cyst aspiration

- The technique for ultrasound-guided cyst aspiration is similar to that of a core needle biopsy. Instead of employing a spring-loaded biopsy gun, a standard syringe is attached to a 20- or 18-gauge needle and the targeted cyst is aspirated.
- The cyst aspirate should be sent for cytology if bloody or clear. Benign-appearing aspirate, which may be green, grey, yellow, or cloudy, may be discarded. Note that only benign-appearing cysts should be aspirated. A complex cystic and solid mass should be biopsied with a core device (with the solid component targeted).

Mammographic-guided stereotactic core biopsy

一部分医师则左右手均可操作。

- 外侧入路进入病灶较为常用。超声引导穿刺的关键是保持穿刺针与胸壁平行或形成非常小的夹角。标准的乳腺穿刺活检是在取材过程中将针推进2cm。对于较深位置的病灶，先将活检针的头端插入病灶，然后将病灶提起离开胸壁之后获取标本。
- 深部病灶需要病灶与进针点之间保持较大距离，使活检针的路径保持几乎平行状态。一旦选定穿刺点，在超声引导下进行皮肤及皮下组织局部浸润麻醉，并在皮肤切一个小口。记录每次进针，并在正交平面上证实穿刺针位于病灶内1~2次及以上。
- 获得满意取样后，通常将组织标记放在穿刺点，然后进行术后X线摄影以确定标记的位置位于靶病灶内。

超声引导下囊肿抽吸

- 超声引导的囊肿抽吸技术类似于核芯针穿刺活检。抽吸不用穿刺时的弹簧活检针，取而代之的是20G或18G的空心针，连接普通注射器后对囊肿进行抽吸。
- 凡是血性或透明的抽吸物均应送细胞学检查。良性的抽吸液可能是绿色、灰色、黄色或浑浊的，可以丢弃。需要注意，只有良性囊肿才进行抽吸。而复杂囊实性肿块应进行核芯针穿刺活检(实性成分作为目标)。

乳腺X线影像引导下立体定向活检

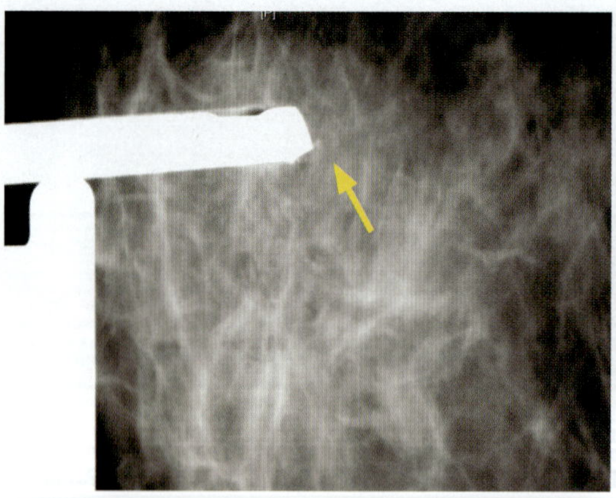

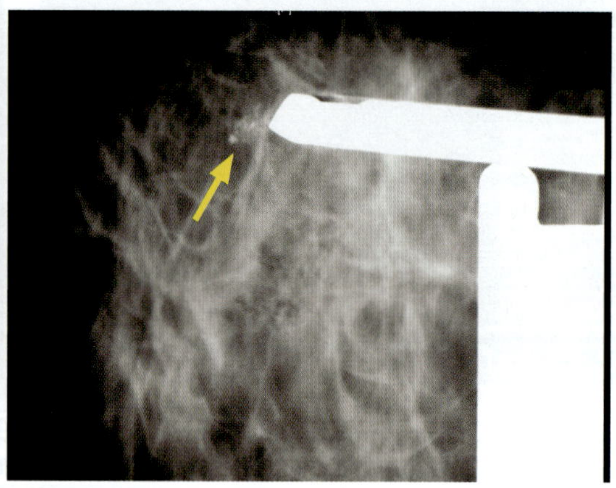

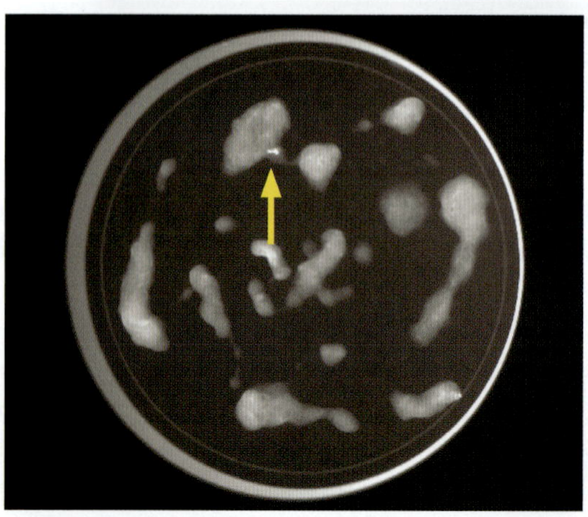

Stereotactic biopsy of calcifications:
Paired 15° oblique pre-fire images (top images) show the targeted calcifications (arrows) with appropriate position of the biopsy device.
Specimen radiograph confirms that the targeted calcifications are present within the specimen (arrow).
钙化灶立体定向活检：
核芯针穿刺活检前一对成15°的斜位X线影像(上两图)显示靶钙化灶(黄箭)和穿刺设备处于恰当的位置。
穿刺标本X线影像(左下图)确认标本内有靶钙化灶(黄箭)。

- Stereotactic guidance using 2D mammography is used most commonly to biopsy calcifications. Less commonly, a stereotactic approach can be used to sample a mammographic finding seen only in one view or a mammographic mass or architectural distortion not seen on ultrasound.
- Stereotactic biopsy tables can be prone or seated upright. The advantage of a prone table is elimination of risk from vasovagal syncope. The seated stereotactic apparatus is less expensive and may offer greater patient comfort. The breast is immobilized in compression during the entire procedure.
- Contraindications to stereotactic biopsy include a thin breast measuring <3 cm compressed (although petite needles are available to sample lesions in breasts as thin as 22 mm), far posterior or subareolar location, inability to be positioned on the stereotactic table, and uncontrolled coagulation abnormality.
- Paired stereo spot views of the target are obtained 15° to each side (30° apart) relative to the needle path. Once targeting is confirmed by the radiologist, the actual needle path in three-dimensional space is calculated by computer.
- Adequate local anesthesia is administered to the dermis and along the expected path of the biopsy needle (without imaging guidance) and a small skin incision is sometimes made at the biopsy needle entrance site (biopsy needles typically have extremely sharp tips and can be directly advanced through the skin).
- A vacuum-assisted biopsy needle (7- to 12-gauge options are available) is employed, and appropriate positioning is confirmed on the horizontal (x), vertical (y), and depth (z) axes. After the samples are obtained, the specimen must be radiographed to confirm that the targeted calcifications are present.
- Once the presence of calcification is confirmed in the sample, a marker clip is placed, and post-procedure two-view mammograms are obtained to confirm clip position. Often, small calcifications will be completely removed by the vacuum-assisted biopsy and correct position of the clip is essential if the lesion requires subsequent surgical treatment.

Tomosynthesis-guided stereotactic core biopsy

- Compared to traditional 2D mammography-guided stereotactic biopsy, tomosynthesis- guided core biopsy has the advantages of easier user operation, faster targeting given no need for the paired 15° stereo views, and facilitates the biopsy of asymmetries, focal asymmetries, or architectural distortions.
- One disadvantage is that subtle calcifications may be difficult to visualize on tomosynthesis images, which may necessitate conversion to a 2D mammography-guided stereotactic biopsy.
- Apart from the elimination of the paired stereo views, tomosynthesis-guided core biopsy follows similar steps to its 2D mammographic counterpart.

- 使用二维乳腺X线影像的立体定向引导最常用于钙化灶活检。少数情况下，立体定向活检也用于仅在单个乳腺X线影像体位中发现的异常，或超声未能显示的乳腺X线影像上的肿块或结构扭曲。
- 立体定向活检台可置于卧位或坐立位。卧位台的优点是可避免血管迷走神经性晕厥的风险。使用坐立位立体定位装置价格较低且能提高患者的舒适度。在整个过程中，乳房是加压固定的。
- 立体定位穿刺活检的禁忌证包括乳房过薄且厚度在加压后<3cm(虽然短小活检针可用于厚度低于22mm的乳腺病灶)、很深或乳晕下的病灶、不能固定于立体定向台及无法纠正的凝血功能异常。
- 拍摄一对与穿刺针路径呈15°（相隔30°）的立体局部影像，放射科医师一旦确认穿刺靶点后，由计算机算出实际三维空间的穿刺路径。
- 对真皮及活检针的预期路径(没有影像引导)给予充分的局部麻醉，有时在活检针入口处做一个小切口(活检针通常有非常锋利的尖端，可以直接穿过皮肤)。
- 采用负压辅助活检针(7~12号可供选择)，确定在水平(x)、垂直(y)和深度(z)轴上合适的位置。获得标本后，必须对标本进行X线摄影以确认存在靶钙化灶。
- 一旦确认活检标本中有钙化灶，在乳腺病灶处放置一个标记，之后拍摄两个体位的乳腺X线影像以确认标记的位置。小的钙化灶通常完全被负压活检针吸出，正确的标记夹位置对于病变的后续手术治疗极为重要。

断层融合影像引导的立体定向活检

- 与传统二维乳腺X线影像引导立体定向活检相比，断层融合影像引导的核芯针穿刺活检具有操作更简单、快速定位、不需要成对15°立体视图的优点，并有助于对不对称、局灶不对称或结构扭曲情况的活检。
- 断层融合影像的一个缺点是可能不易看到细微的钙化灶，这可能需要换用二维乳腺X线影像引导立体定向活检。
- 除省去成对立体视图之外，断层成像引导的活检与二维乳腺X线影像立体定位步骤相同。

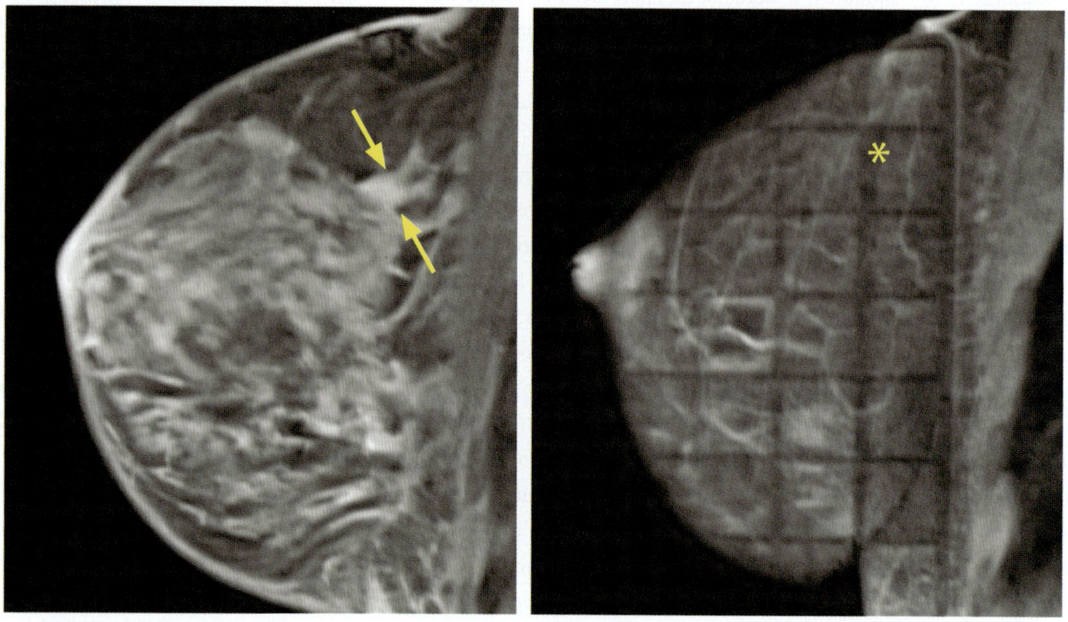

MR images obtained during an MRI-guided biopsy. Post-contrast image through the mid breast (left image) shows the targeted abnormal enhancement (arrows). The lesion is not very conspicuous because the patient had to be repositioned and delayed parenchymal enhancement partially obscures the lesion. The image on the right shows the grid applied to the lateral breast, and the star marks the position of the targeted lesion on the grid. Note that despite the sagittal orientation of these images, the patient is positioned prone.

MRI引导下活检术中获得的MRI图像。增强后图像(左图)显示乳腺中部异常强化的靶病灶(黄箭)。病灶不是很明显，因患者必须重新摆体位，且延迟实质强化部分掩盖了病灶。右图显示网格放置在乳房侧面，星号标记了网格中靶病灶的位置。注意，图像展示的是矢状位，患者是俯卧位。

- MRI-guided biopsy can be performed for lesions seen only on MRI. Given that MRI-guided biopsy is expensive and can be more uncomfortable for the patient, it is common to perform a second-look ultrasound targeted towards the MRI abnormality so that ultrasound-guided biopsy might be an option. A corresponding ultrasound finding is identified in 56–57% of cases, with masses and larger lesions being more likely to have a correlate than non-mass enhancement and smaller lesions.
- MRI-guided biopsy almost always requires intravenous gadolinium. Time is of the essence during the procedure because the lesion must be targeted before contrast washes out or the lesion becomes obscured by delayed parenchymal enhancement.
- The grid-coordinate method allows accurate biopsy of an abnormality seen only on MRI. This method is most analogous to a grid-based CT-guided biopsy elsewhere in the body.
- With the patient lying prone, a grid is applied to either the medial or lateral breast. A lateral approach is preferred whenever possible as it allows greater access to posterior tissues. After initial images are obtained, the targeted lesion is localized on the grid. Local anesthesia is administered without imaging guidance. During the biopsy, the core needle device is inserted exactly perpendicular to the breast to a pre-measured depth, similar to stereotactic biopsy. Multiple 9- to 11-gauge vacuum-assisted samples are obtained. Finally, a post-biopsy marker is deployed.

- MRI引导下活检只适用于在MRI上所显示的病灶。由于MRI引导下活检的费用昂贵且患者的舒适度差，对MRI发现的异常通常使用超声进行针对性重复检查，从而转为超声引导下活检。超声能发现56%~57%的对应病灶，肿块和较大病变的相关性较好，但非肿块性强化和较小的病变则不然。
- MRI引导下活检几乎总是需要静脉注射钆对比剂。手术过程中的时间把握非常重要，因为病灶必须在对比剂消退之前定位，否则病灶会因实质延迟强化而被掩盖。
- 网格坐标法可以帮助仅在MRI上显示的病灶进行精确活检。这一方法与身体其他部位网格CT引导下活检相似。
- 患者采取俯卧位，网格放在乳房的内侧或外侧。尽可能选择外侧，这样对深部组织进行活检较为容易。在获得初始图像后，将靶病灶定位在网格上。局部实施麻醉不需要影像引导。活检过程与立体定向活检类似，活检针必须精确垂直乳房插入到预先测量的深度。获得多条9~11G的穿刺标本。最后放置活检后标记。

PRE-OPERATIVE LESION LOCALIZATION

Radioactive seed localization

- Prior to excisional biopsy or lumpectomy, pre-operative localization of a breast lesion can be performed using an iodine-125 radioactive seed. Under either mammographic or ultrasound guidance, the seed is placed within or next to the targeted lesion. Its position is confirmed by orthogonal mammographic images. In the operating room, the surgeon uses a gamma probe to detect the radioactivity prior to excision.
- Radioactive seeds are increasingly utilized due to certain advantages over wire localization.

  Unlike wire localization which is restricted to the day of surgery, radioactive seed can be placed up to 5 days before surgery.

  There is more flexibility in approach for placement by the radiologist and choice for incision location by the surgeon, allowing potentially better cosmesis.

  Lack of external wires outside the skin surface leads to higher patient satisfaction, and less risk for wire migration or dislodgement.
- The main drawback of radioactive seeds is implementing the many safety requirements for their use. Additionally, if a seed is inaccurately positioned, it cannot be removed prior to surgery; a second seed must be placed to localize the targeted lesion, with both seeds removed during surgery. Radioseeds cannot currently be placed under MRI guidance as the pre-loaded radioseed needles and gamma probes used to check for deployment are not MRI compatible.

Wire localization

- Another option for pre-operative marking of a breast lesion is wire localization. The wire can be placed under mammographic, sonographic or MRI guidance (if an MRI compatible system is used).
- The shortest approach to the lesion should be used and an appropriate wire length should be chosen (typically 5, 7, or 9 cm).
- After the lumpectomy or excisional biopsy, specimen radiographs are obtained to confirm that the targeted lesion and the intact hook wire are contained within the specimen.

Steps in mammographic wire localization

外科术前病灶定位

放射性粒子定位

- 在切除活检或乳房肿瘤切除术之前，可以使用碘-125(^{125}I)放射性粒子对乳房病变进行术前定位。在乳腺X线或超声引导下，将^{125}I放射性粒子放在靶病灶内或病灶旁。其位置采用正交乳腺X线影像进行确认。在手术室，外科医师在切除前使用伽马探头探测放射性。
- 放射性粒子较金属导丝有更多的优势，故越来越多地被用于定位。

  与导丝定位仅限于当天手术不同，放射性粒子可以最早在手术前5天植入。

  放射科医师采用的植入路径和外科医师对切口位置的选择具有更大的灵活性，从而有可能达到较好的美容结果。

  皮肤表面不留导线可提高患者满意度，并降低金属勾线移动或脱落的风险。
- 放射性粒子的主要缺点是需要遵循许多安全上的规定。此外，如果粒子位置不准确，不能在手术前将其取出；必须放置第二颗粒子对靶病变进行定位，术中一起切掉这两颗粒子。放射性粒子目前不能在MRI引导下放置，因为用于装载放射性粒子的针和检测伽马射线的探头与MRI不兼容。

金属导丝定位

- 另一个术前标记乳腺病灶的方法是导丝定位。导丝植入可以用乳腺X线、超声或MRI引导(如果MRI兼容)。
- 应采用最短的路径入路，并选择长度合适的导丝(通常为5cm或7cm或9cm)。
- 在乳腺肿瘤切除术或切除活检后，对标本进行X线摄影以确认靶病变和完整的导丝在标本内。

乳腺X线影像引导下金属导丝定位步骤

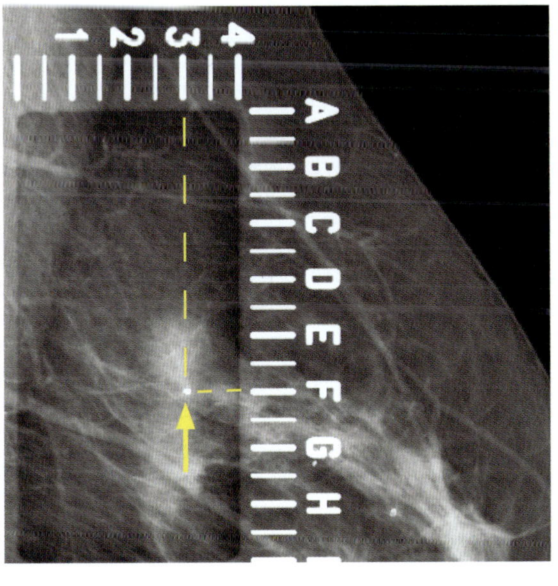

Step 1: Imaging is performed with the alphanumeric localization grid in place. The clip (arrow) is the target of the localization wire (F3 on the grid; dashed lines). The clip is associated with an ill-defined mass, which was previously biopsied as malignant.

第一步：获得由字母数字标尺的乳腺X线图像。定位夹(黄箭)作为定位导丝的靶点位置(栅格上的“F3”位置，虚线)。定位夹位于一个边界不清的肿块，该肿块先前活检为恶性。

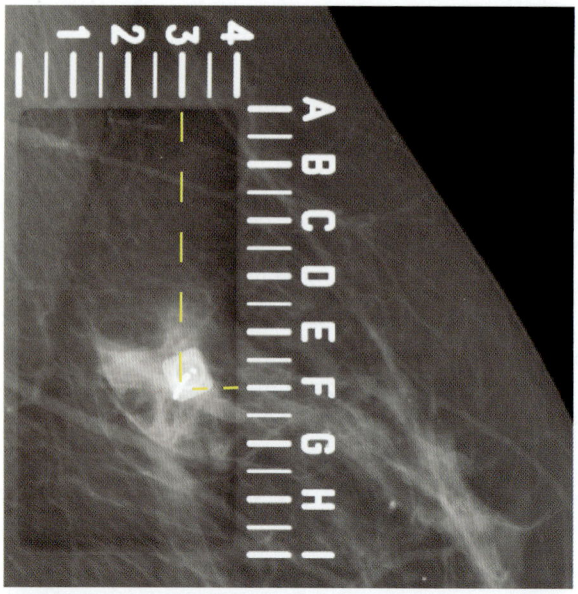

Step 2: After local anesthesia, the needle is inserted into the skin entry site based on the grid and advanced towards the target. Ideally the needle shaft should be exactly in-line with the x-ray beam.

第二步：局部麻醉后，根据网格标记定位，穿刺针经皮肤插入乳房。理想的进针路径应完全与X线束平行。

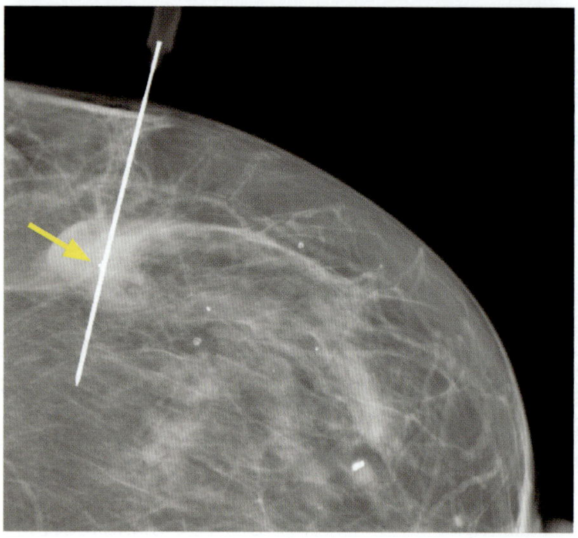

Step 3: Orthogonal imaging is obtained. If necessary, the needle can be advanced or pulled back. The mass is more evident on this orthogonal view. Note the clip location in the epicenter of the mass (arrow).

第三步：获取正交图像。如果需要，针可向前或后退。肿块在正交图像上显示更加清楚。注意定位夹位于肿块偏心的位置(黄箭)。

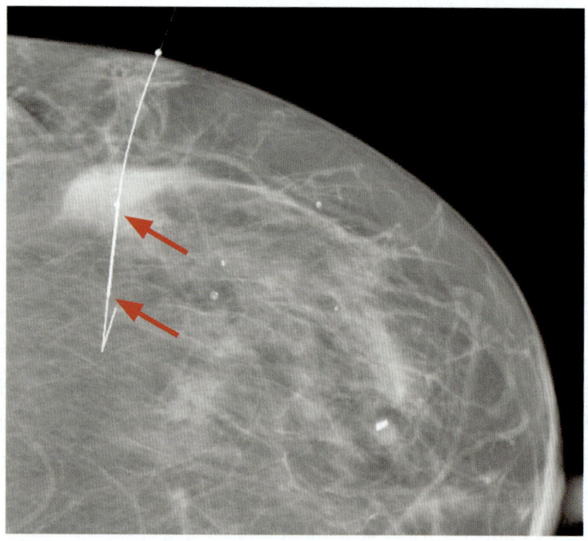

Step 4: Once satisfactory position is confirmed, the wire hook is unsheathed. Note the thickened distal segment (red arrows), which begins 1 cm from the hook and is 2 cm in length. The thickened segment gives the surgeon tactile feedback.

第四步：一旦确定满意的位置，移出导丝鞘。注意增粗的远段(红箭)距离钩1cm，总长2cm。此增粗段可提供给外科医师触觉反馈。

Other localization modalities

- Non-magnetic radioactive radar localization and magnetic seed localization are additional newer methods used for pre-operative localization.

Bracketing method

- When targeting a large area of breast tissue, two or more wires or seeds can be placed, to delineate the boundaries of the target. The surgeon can then remove the tissue in between and around the bracketing wires or seeds, to ensure excision of the targeted lesion in its entirety.

其他定位方式

- 非磁性放射性雷达定位和磁性粒子定位是用于术前定位的新方法。

病灶边界包裹法

- 当靶病灶是大面积的乳腺组织时，可放置两个或更多个导丝或粒子，以勾画出靶病灶的边界。然后，外科医师可以切除导丝或粒子间和周围的组织，以确保靶病灶被完整切除。

(翻译　杨学刚)

6 Nuclear and Molecular Imaging

Ellen X. Sun, Christopher G. Sakellis, Hyewon Hyun

Contents

6 核医学与分子影像

目录

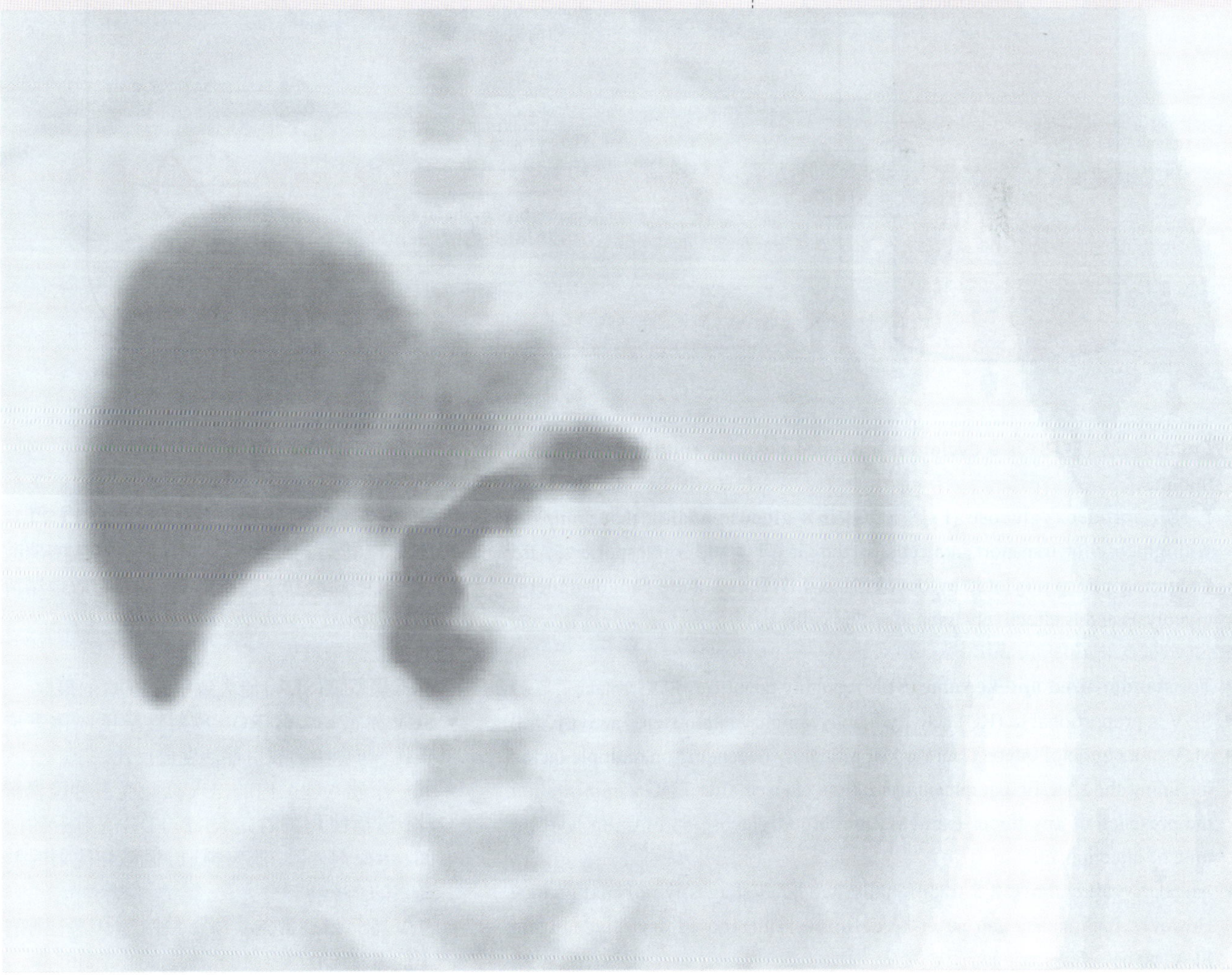

PET/CT

PET/CT

Basic positron emission tomography (PET) physics

- A positron emission tomography (PET) radiotracer emits a positron that travels a small local distance within the tissue. After meeting an electron, both the positron and electron annihilate and create two 511 keV photons travelling nearly 180 degrees apart.
- The two high-energy photons travelling in opposite directions are simultaneously detected by a circular ring of crystals, which can determine that the two photons arrived coincidentally.

正电子发射断层扫描(PET)的基础物理:

- 正电子发射断层扫描(PET)放射性示踪剂发射一个正电子,该正电子在组织内移行一小段距离。在遇到一个负电子后,正负两个电子发生湮灭辐射,产生两个方向近乎为180°的511keV的移动光子。
- 两个移动方向相反的高能光子同时被能确定两个光子同时到达的圆形晶体环所检测。

TECHNICAL CONSIDERATIONS OF F-18 FDG PET/CT

^{18}F-FDG PET/CT的技术考虑

Radiotracer: Fluorine-18 FDG

放射性示踪剂:^{18}F-氟代脱氧葡萄糖(^{18}F-FDG)

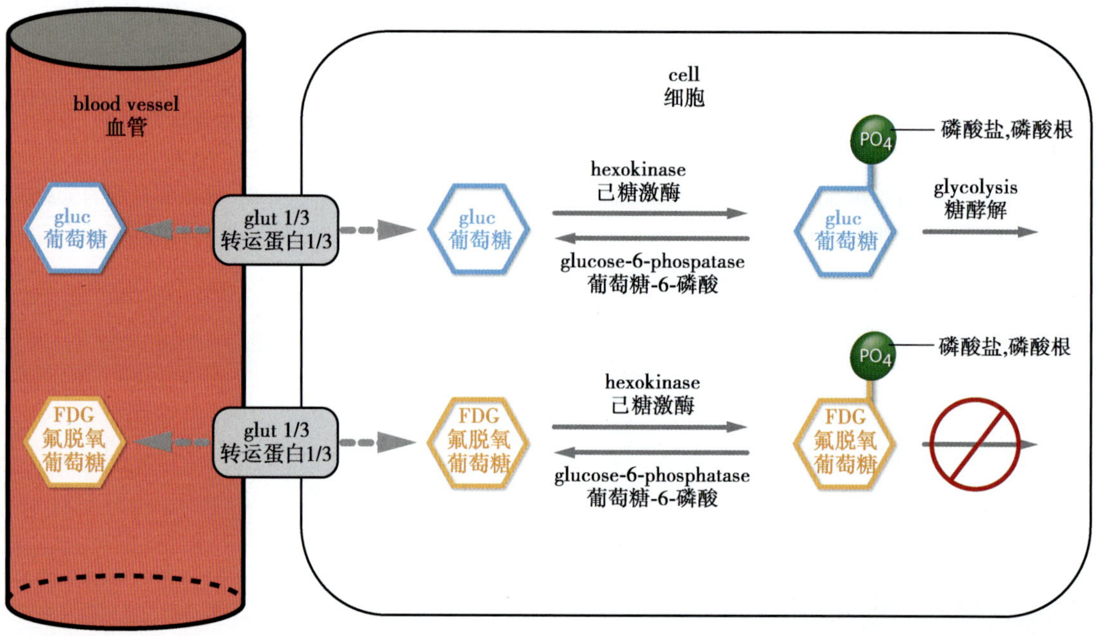

- Fluorine-18 (F-18) is a cyclotron-produced positron emitter, half-life 110 minutes.
- F-18-fluorodeoxyglucose (F-18 FDG) is a glucose analog that competes with glucose for transport into cells by the GLUT 1 and 3 transporters. After becoming phosphorylated by hexokinase, FDG-phosphate cannot undergo glycolysis and is effectively trapped within cells.

Radiotracer uptake quantification

- The **standardized uptake value (SUV)** roughly quantifies FDG uptake.
- SUV is proportional to (ROI activity * body weight)/administered activity.
- SUV of a region of interest can vary significantly depending on multiple factors including the specific equipment used, time elapsed after FDG administration, the presence of any tracer extravasation, blood glucose and insulin levels at time of injection, etc.
- An SUV value above 2.5 traditionally has been suggestive of malignancy. However, malignancy can never be definitively diagnosed or excluded using SUV as the sole criterion.

- ^{18}氟(^{18}F)为正电子发射体,半衰期为110分钟。
- ^{18}F-氟代脱氧葡萄糖(^{18}F-FDG)是葡萄糖类似物,它与葡萄糖竞争而被转运蛋白GLUT1和GLUT3转运到细胞内。一旦被己糖激酶磷酸化,FDG磷酸盐不能被酵解,从而有效地滞留在细胞内。

放射性示踪剂摄取的定量分析

- **标准摄取值(SUV)**能大致定量FDG的摄取。
- SUV和感兴趣区(ROI)放射性活度与体重成正比,与总给药放射性活度成反比。
- 同一个感兴趣区内的SUV变化受多种因素影响,包括使用的特定设备、FDG注射后的时间、示踪剂外溢、肌肉摄取、血糖和注射时胰岛素的水平等。
- SUV高于2.5通常提示为恶性肿瘤。但恶性肿瘤不能用SUV作为唯一的指标进行诊断和排除。

- Size threshold for lesion detection on FDG PET is 6 mm. For small lesions, the average SUV may be falsely low due to partial volume averaging; the maximum SUV is a better measure.
- An alternative approach to calculating SUV values is visual or quantitative assessment of FDG uptake relative to background activity in normal tissues (e.g., liver or cerebellum) or the mediastinal blood pool.

CT correlation

- Most modern PET studies are performed together with CT as a PET/CT. One important exception is in the pediatric population, where PET may be performed in isolation to reduce the risk of radiation exposure from CT.
- The CT exam is often performed with a lower dose than a diagnostic-quality CT. The CT protocol varies by institution (e.g., whether intravenous contrast is administered).
- The CT is used for anatomic localization and attenuation correction.
- Very dense retained oral contrast or dense metallic objects (such as joint prostheses) may cause artifactual FDG uptake due to miscalculation of attenuation correction.

Patient preparation

- The uptake of FDG in both normal and pathological tissues is dependent on the serum glucose and insulin levels.
- Elevated insulin levels will cause increased muscle uptake and decrease the sensitivity for detecting mildly FDG-avid lesions.
- Patients should be NPO for at least 4 hours to allow insulin to reach a basal level.

  In type 1 diabetes, imaging should be performed in the morning after an overnight fast. Insulin is not recommended.

  In type 2 diabetes, regular insulin should be held 2–4 hours prior to the study. Short-acting insulin can be used but is not recommended. There is no need to hold long-acting insulin and oral hypoglycemic medications such as Metformin, though the latter can increase bowel uptake.
- Blood glucose should be below 200 mg/dL, preferably below 150.

  Elevated serum glucose will result in decreased FDG uptake by tumors and the brain.
- The typical administered dose of F-18 FDG is 10–25 mCi. After intravenous injection, the patient should rest in a quiet room for 60 minutes before imaging.

  If the patient talks, the vocal cords may show FDG uptake.

  If the patient walks, the muscles may show FDG uptake.

Normal FDG distribution

- *Brain:* The brain has intense FDG uptake. Brains love sugar!

  Despite intense uptake, with appropriate windowing, excellent detail of the cortex, basal ganglia, and cerebellum can be seen.
- *Renal, ureters, and bladder:* FDG is concentrated in the urine, with very intense activity in the renal collecting system, ureters, and bladder. As a result, bladder is the **critical organ** (the body part most susceptible to radiation damage from a given isotope). Good hydration is recommended for clearance of radioactivity.
- *Salivary glands, tonsils, thyroid:* Mild to moderate symmetric uptake.
- *Liver:* Moderate, largely homogeneous uptake.
- *Bowel:* Diffuse mild to moderate uptake is normal. Focal uptake within the bowel, however, should be regarded with suspicion.

  Metformin can increase colonic, and to a lesser extent, small bowel FDG uptake and may mask a lesion.
- *Heart:* Uptake is often variable, depending on insulin/glucose levels and the patient's fasting state. The heart prefers fatty acids but will use glucose in the

- FDG PET检测病变大小的阈值为6mm。对于小病灶，平均SUV由于部分容积效应而有可能被低估；最大SUV则是一个较好的衡量标准。
- 另一种计算SUV的方法是采用视觉或定量评估FDG的摄取与正常组织的本底(如肝脏或小脑)或纵隔血池的相对比值。

与CT对应

- 大多数现代的PET检查与CT同时进行，即PET/CT。唯一重要的例外是小儿人群，只做PET检查可以降低CT带来的辐射风险。
- CT扫描通常采用低于诊断性CT的剂量。CT扫描的方法因不同医院而有所不同(如是否注射静脉造影剂等)。
- CT用于解剖定位和衰减校正。
- 残留很高密度的口服造影剂或高密度金属物体(如人工关节)可能会引起CT衰减校正计算错误，从而造成FDG摄取伪影。

患者准备

- 无论正常还是病变组织的FDG摄取都依赖于血清葡萄糖浓度和胰岛素水平。
- 胰岛素水平升高会导致肌肉摄取增加，因而会降低对检测轻度摄取PET病变的灵敏度。
- 患者至少禁食4小时，使胰岛素达到基础水平。

  对于1型糖尿病，检查应该在隔夜禁食后的早晨进行。不应使用胰岛素。

  对于2型糖尿病，在检查前2~4小时暂停使用常规胰岛素。可以使用短效胰岛素，但不推荐使用。无须暂停使用长效胰岛素和口服降糖药物，如二甲双胍，但后者可以增加肠道吸收。
- 血糖应低于200mg/dL，最好在150mg/dL以下。

  血糖升高会导致肿瘤和大脑对FDG摄取减少。
- ^{18}F-FDG的常规给药剂量为10~25mCi。静脉注射后，患者应安排在安静的房间内休息等待，60分钟后显像。

  如果患者讲话，可能会出现声带摄取FDG。

  如果患者走动，可能会出现肌肉摄取FDG。

正常FDG分布

- 脑：脑组织对FDG有强烈亲和性。"脑喜欢糖！"

  尽管高度摄取，只要合理选择窗位，可以清晰显示皮质、基底节和小脑的细节。
- 肾、输尿管和膀胱：FDG在尿液中浓集，肾脏集合系统、输尿管和膀胱可出现强烈放射性活性。因此，膀胱成为关键器官(最容易受到给定同位素辐射损伤的身体部位)。建议大量喝水以排出放射性物质。
- 唾液腺、扁桃体、甲状腺：轻度至中度对称性摄取。
- 肝脏：中度摄取，通常为均匀性摄取。
- 肠道：弥漫性轻度至中度摄取属于正常。局灶性肠道摄取应视为可疑。

  二甲双胍可以增加结肠摄取FDG并在一定程度上也会增加小肠摄取FDG，因而可能掩盖病灶。

postprandial state.

- *Muscles:* FDG uptake is normally low. However, elevated insulin levels or recent exercise can cause increased muscle uptake.
- *Brown fat:* **Brown fat** is metabolically active adipose tissue that can be found in the supraclavicular, axillary, mediastinal and paravertebral regions in adults that can be mildly to moderately FDG avid, especially if the patient is cold or after food intake.

- 心脏：摄取变异很大，取决于胰岛素/血糖水平，以及患者的空腹情况。心脏优先摄取脂肪酸，但在饱餐后会利用葡萄糖。
- 肌肉：肌肉摄取FDG通常较低。然而，当胰岛素水平升高或运动后不久会导致肌肉摄取增加。
- 棕色脂肪：**棕色脂肪**是代谢活跃的脂肪组织，在成人常见于锁骨上、腋窝、纵隔和椎旁区域，可为轻度至中度FDG摄取，特别是患者发冷时或进食后。

ONCOLOGIC INDICATIONS OF F-18 FDG PET/CT

^{18}F-FDG PET/CT的肿瘤适应证

Lung cancer

肺癌

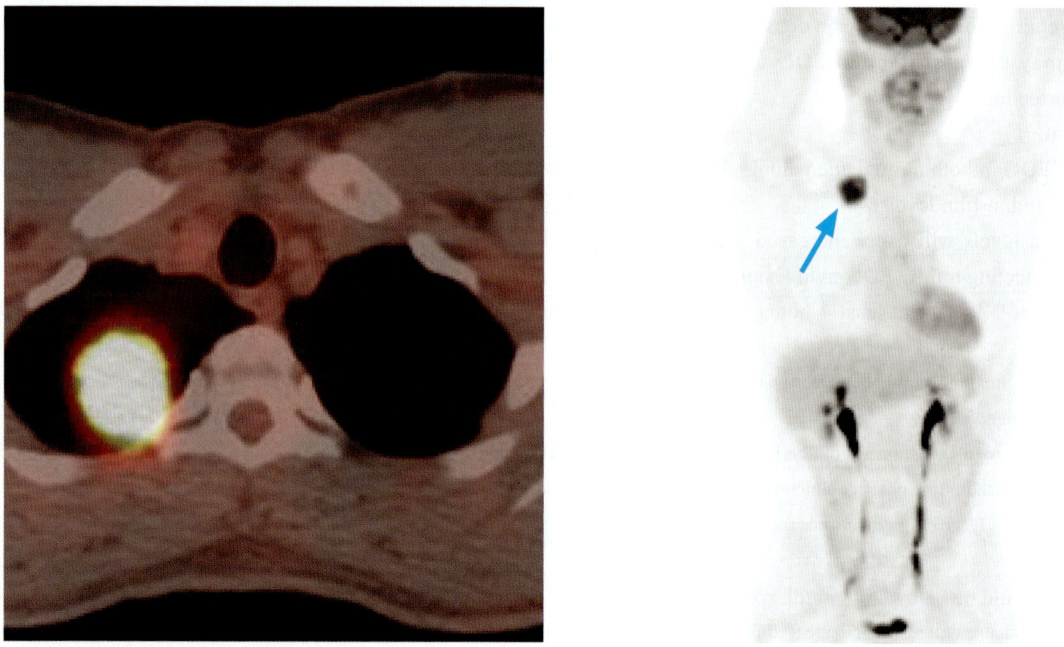

Lung cancer initial staging: Fused axial PET/CT (left image) and coronal PET MIP (right image) show an intensely FDG-avid right upper lobe mass (blue arrow) representing the patient's primary bronchogenic carcinoma. There were no enlarged or FDG-avid hilar or mediastinal lymph nodes, and no FDG-avid distant metastases. Also note normal biodistribution of FDG in the other organs.

肺癌初始分期：轴位PET/CT融合图像(左图)和冠状位PET MIP图像(右图)显示一个右肺上叶高FDG摄取肿块(蓝箭)为原发性支气管肺癌。无肿大或FDG摄取的纵隔和肺门淋巴结，也无远处摄取FDG的转移灶。另外，FDG在其他器官的生物学分布也正常。

- PET/CT plays a role both in the initial staging of patients with lung cancer, and in evaluating response to treatment.
- For initial staging, PET/CT is most useful in evaluating local tumor extension and searching for distant metastases. Approximately 10% of patients with a negative metastatic workup by CT will have PET evidence of metastasis.
- PET/CT also plays a role in the initial detection of mediastinal and hilar lymph nodes. Although PET is very sensitive for detecting malignant lymph nodes, it is not specific. Mediastinoscopy is the gold standard for lymph node staging. Given the lack of PET specificity, PET-positive mediastinal nodes must be followed by mediastinoscopy before potentially curative surgery is denied based solely on the PET.

- PET/CT对肺癌患者的初始分期和疗效评估都起着重要的作用。
- 在初始分期中，PET/CT最有价值的应用是评估局部病灶的侵袭范围和发现远处转移。约有10% CT检查转移阴性的患者在PET检查时发现有转移灶。
- PET/CT在筛选纵隔和肺门淋巴结中具有价值。虽然PET对检测恶性淋巴结非常敏感，但并不特异。纵隔镜检查是淋巴结分期的“金标准”。由于PET的特异性不足，对PET阳性的纵隔淋巴在考虑根治性手术前，必须进行纵隔镜检查已进行确认，不可完全依赖PET结果。

Solitary pulmonary nodule (SPN)

- Evaluation of a suspicious solitary pulmonary nodule (SPN) is an indication for PET/CT.
- Depending on the equipment used, 5–8 mm is typically the smallest size for a nodule that can be reliably evaluated by PET.
- The majority of malignant SPNs are FDG-avid. However, low-grade tumors such as lung adenocarcinoma or carcinoid may not be metabolically active and may be falsely negative on PET.
- Conversely, the majority of benign SPNs are not FDG-avid. Active granulomatous disease (including tuberculosis) may take up FDG, thus falsely positive on PET.
- It is never possible to definitively diagnose a nodule as benign or malignant based on SUV value alone.
- In general, if a nodule is not FDG-avid, short-term follow-up is reasonable. If the nodule is FDG-avid then biopsy or resection is preferred.

孤立性肺结节(SPN)

- 评估可疑的孤立性肺结节(SPN)是PET/CT的适应证之一。
- 根据所使用的仪器，5~8mm通常是PET能够对结节进行可靠评估的最小直径。
- 大多数恶性SPN会摄取FDG。然而，低度恶性肿瘤，如肺腺癌或类癌，可能由于代谢不活跃而出现PET假阴性。
- 相反，大多数良性SPN不摄取FDG。代谢活跃的肉芽肿性疾病(包括肺结核)可能会摄取FDG而呈PET假阳性。
- 确定结节的良恶性绝不能仅仅依靠SUV。
- 通常情况下，如果一个结节不摄取FDG，短期随访较为合理。如果结节有FDG摄取，则应该进行活检或手术切除。

Colon cancer

结肠癌

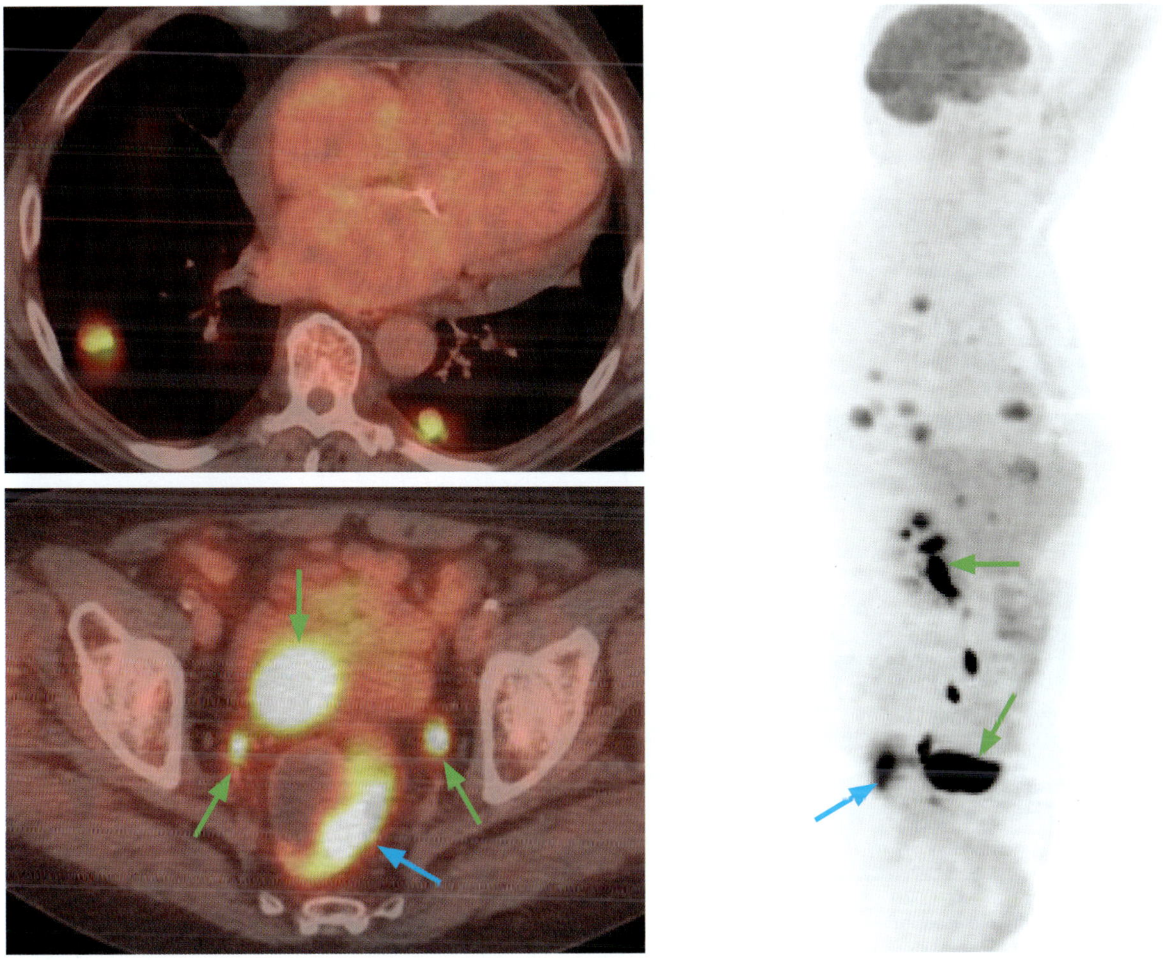

Metastatic rectosigmoid cancer: Fused axial PET/CT through the lungs (top left image), through the pelvis (bottom left image), and a sagittal PET MIP (right image) show the intensely FDG-avid primary rectosigmoid malignancy (blue arrows), with numerous pulmonary metastases. Note the physiologic intense activity in the renal collecting system, bladder and ureters (green arrows).
转移性直肠乙状结肠癌：经肺(左上图)和经盆腔(左下图)轴位PET/CT融合图像及矢状位PET MIP(右图)显示显著摄取FDG的原发性直肠乙状结肠恶性肿瘤(蓝箭)，伴有大量肺转移。注意肾脏集合系统、膀胱和输尿管内示踪剂的生理聚集(绿箭)。

- PET/CT has a limited role in determining local extent of colon cancer due to poor spatial resolution and physiologic bowel uptake, but it does play a primary

- PET/CT在确定结肠癌局部侵犯中的作用有限，这是因为受制于空间分辨率的限制和生理性

role in evaluating metastatic disease in colorectal malignancies. In particular, since an isolated hepatic metastasis can be resected or ablated, evaluation for extrahepatic metastases is a common indication for PET/CT.

肠道摄取的影响，但它对评估结直肠恶性肿瘤的转移具有重要的作用。尤其是一个孤立的肝脏转移性病灶可以进行切除或消融，因而评估肝外转移灶是PET/CT的一个常用适应证。

- After initial treatment, follow-up PET/CT is usually delayed approximately two months due to increased FDG uptake in the peritreatment period related to inflammation that can occur.

- 初次治疗后，PET/CT随访通常要在约2个月后进行，因为在围治疗期间的炎性反应也会使FDG摄取增高。

Head and neck cancer

头颈部肿瘤

- PET/CT is often used in the initial staging of head and neck squamous cell carcinoma, especially for evaluation of regional nodal metastases.
- Specificity for evaluating recurrent disease after chemoradiation is limited due to altered anatomy and inflammation from treatment. Usually post-treatment scans should be delayed 4 months after treatment.

- PET/CT常用于头颈部鳞状细胞癌的初始分期，特别是用来评估是否有局部淋巴结转移。
- 由于治疗后的解剖结构改变和炎症反应，评估放化疗后复发的特异度有限。通常治疗后扫描应该要延迟到治疗4个月后进行。

Thyroid cancer

甲状腺癌

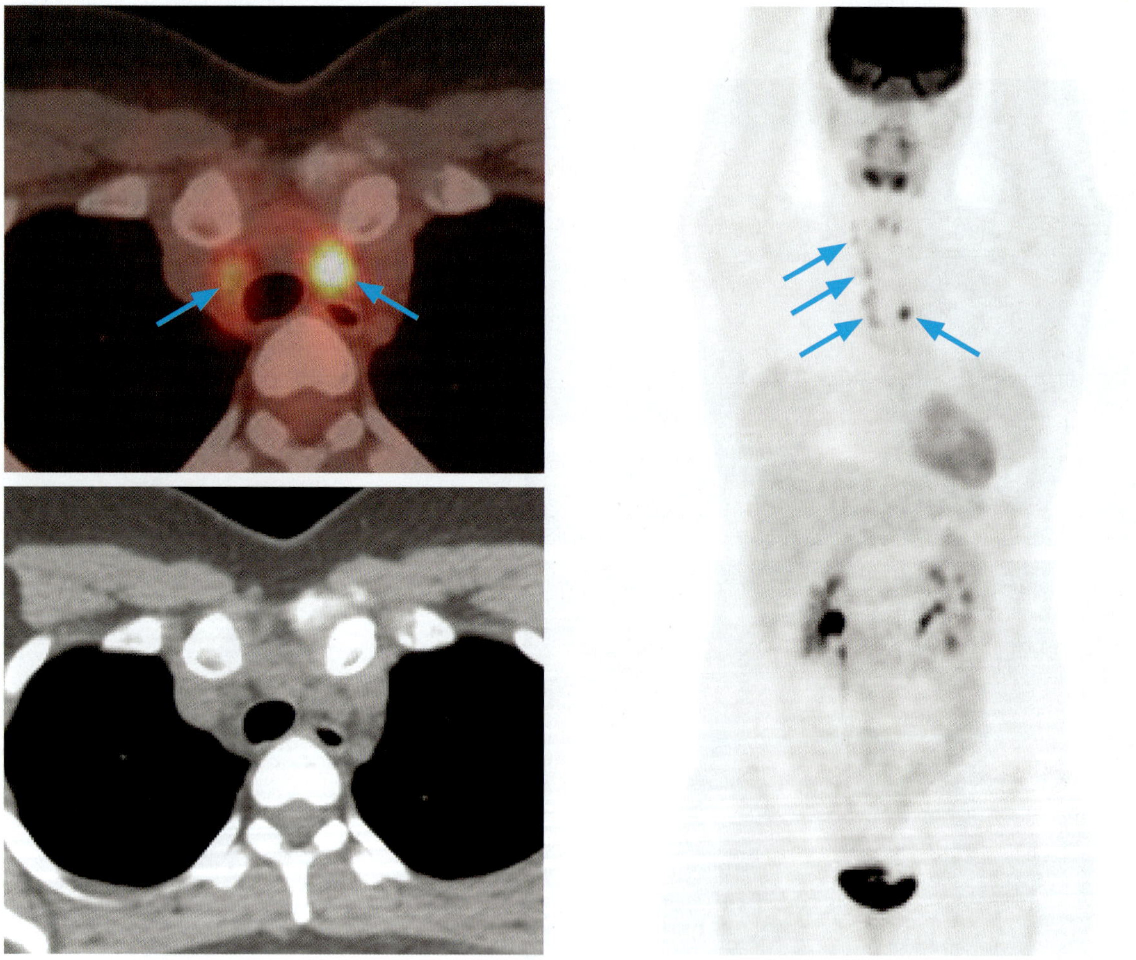

Iodine-resistant thyroid cancer: Fused axial PET/CT (top left image), non-contrast CT (bottom left image), and coronal PET MIP show several moderately FDG-avid right cervical and paratracheal lymph nodes and a single intensely FDG-avid left paratracheal node (arrows). There is symmetric physiologic salivary gland uptake seen on the coronal MIP. I-131 scan (not shown) was negative.

不摄取碘的甲状腺癌：轴位PET/CT融合图像(左上图)、CT平扫(左下图)和冠状位PET MIP(右图)显示数个中度摄取FDG的右侧颈部和气管旁淋巴结，以及一个高度摄取FDG的左侧气管旁淋巴结(蓝箭)。在冠状位MIP上可见对称的生理性唾液腺摄取。^{131}I显像呈阴性(未展示)。

- Undifferentiated or medullary thyroid cancers may not take up radioiodine but may be FDG avid. PET/CT is used in the clinical setting of a rising thyroglobulin level with negative whole-body radioiodine scans.

- 未分化或髓样甲状腺癌可能不摄取放射性碘，但可能会摄取FDG。PET/CT常用于临床上甲状腺球蛋白水平持续增高而放射性碘全身扫描阴性的患者。

Lymphoma

- PET/CT plays a key role in the staging and restaging of patients with lymphoma.
- Most histological types of lymphoma, including Hodgkin and non-Hodgkin lymphoma, are FDG-avid. Low-grade lymphomas, such as small lymphocytic and mantle cell lymphoma, however, tend to be less FDG-avid.
- Increased marrow uptake in lymphoma patients can be difficult to interpret. Diffuse marrow uptake may be due to granulocyte colony-stimulating factor (G-CSF) stimulation, rebound effect from chemotherapy, or malignant marrow infiltration. Focal increased uptake, however, is more likely to represent lymphoma.

淋巴瘤

- PET/CT在淋巴瘤患者的分期和再分期中发挥关键作用。
- 大多数组织类型的淋巴瘤都摄取FDG，包括霍奇金淋巴瘤和非霍奇金淋巴瘤。然而，一些低级别淋巴瘤，如小淋巴细胞性和套细胞淋巴瘤，为低FDG摄取。
- 淋巴瘤患者若出现骨髓FDG摄取增高则难以得出结论。弥漫性骨髓摄取可能是由于粒细胞集落刺激因子(G-CSF)的刺激、化疗后的反跳作用或恶性病变的骨髓浸润。但是，局灶性摄取增高多为淋巴瘤。

Breast cancer

- Although used in the staging and response to therapy of recurrent or stage Ⅳ breast cancer, standard PET/CT is not used to evaluate small nodal metastases.
- PET/CT is not routinely used for patients with stage Ⅰ–Ⅲ breast cancer.

乳腺癌

- 虽然PET/CT用于分期、评估疗效和Ⅳ期乳腺癌患者，但常规PET/CT并不用于评估小的结节性转移。
- PET/CT并不常规用于Ⅰ~Ⅲ期乳腺癌患者。

Esophageal cancer

食管癌

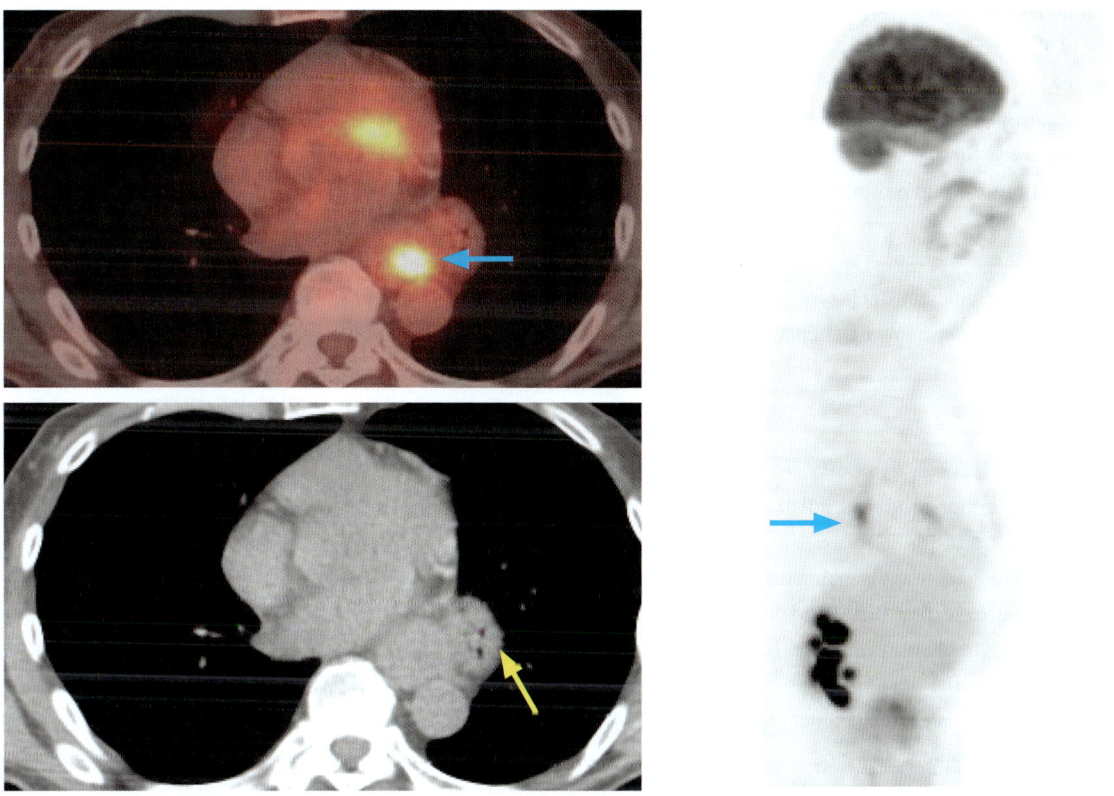

Non-metastatic esophageal cancer: Fused axial PET/CT (top left image) and sagittal PET MIP (right image) show a single focus of intense FDG uptake within the distal esophagus (blue arrows). Marked esophageal thickening is also apparent on the non-contrast CT (bottom left image). There is no evidence of metastatic disease. The focus of FDG uptake within the heart on the fused image is physiologic myocardial uptake. Note the presence of a small paraesophageal hernia (yellow arrow).

未转移食管癌：轴位PET/CT融合图像(左上图)及矢状位PET MIP(右图)显示位于食管远端一个局部FDG高度摄取病灶(蓝箭)。平扫CT显示食管壁显著增厚(左下图)。未见转移性病灶征象。在融合影像中心脏局部FDG摄取为心肌生理性摄取。注意有个小的食管旁疝(黄箭)。

- The primary role of PET/CT in the evaluation of esophageal cancer is to identify patients with stage Ⅳ disease who are not surgical candidates. PET/CT is limited for primary tumor staging of esophageal cancer, which is better assessed with endoscopic ultrasound.
- After initial neoadjuvant treatment, a decrease in FDG avidity by at least 30% suggests a more favorable prognosis. In contrast, those patients who do not show a decrease in FDG uptake can potentially be spared ineffective chemotherapy regimens.

- PET/CT在食管癌评估中的主要作用是除外不适合手术治疗的Ⅳ期患者。PET/CT对食管癌的初始肿瘤分期作用有限，而更好的评估方法是超声内镜。
- 在初期辅助治疗后，FDG摄取率降低30%以上者提示预后良好。相比之下，对FDG摄取没有降低的患者则可以避免使用无效的化疗方案。

CANCERS WHERE F-18 FDG PET/CT PLAYS A LIMITED ROLE

Hepatocellular carcinoma (HCC)

- Only 50% of HCCs can be imaged with FDG-PET due to relatively high levels of phosphatase compared to other cancers which dephosphorylates FDG and allows it to diffuse out of cells.

Renal cell carcinoma (RCC) and bladder cancer

- Only 50% of RCCs are FDG-avid, though PET may play a role in detecting metastatic disease.
- Detection of ureteral or bladder lesions is extremely limited due to surrounding high urinary FDG activity.

Prostate cancer

- Most prostate cancers have low FDG uptake.
- FDG-PET is reserved for assessing treatment response of bony metastases in aggressive castration-resistant prostate cancer and as a prognostic indicator.

Other tumors

- Well-differentiated or mucinous cell type tumors, lung adenocarcinoma, and carcinoid tumors tend to have low FDG uptake or are non-FDG-avid.

^{18}F-FDG PET/CT作用有限的肿瘤

肝细胞癌(HCC)

- 只有50%的肝细胞癌(HCC)能够在FDG PET图像上显示，因为HCC较其他肿瘤具有较高水平的磷酸酶，它可以使FDG去磷酸化而弥散出细胞。

肾细胞癌(RCC)和膀胱癌

- 只有50%的肾细胞癌(RCC)摄取FDG，但PET对探测RCC转移灶有一定的作用。
- PET在诊断输尿管或膀胱病变中的价值极其有限，因其周围有含高浓度FDG的尿液。

前列腺癌

- 大多数前列腺癌的FDG摄取量较低。
- FDG PET仅用于评估对性去势有顽固抵抗的前列腺癌的治疗反应，以及作为一项预后指标。

其他肿瘤

- 分化良好或黏液细胞型肿瘤、肺腺癌和类癌往往为FDG低摄取或无摄取。

OTHER TYPES OF PET/CT

Gallium-68 DOTATATE (GaTate)

- Gallium-68 is a generator-produced positron emitter with a half-life of 68 minutes.
- Ga-68 DOTATATE is a somatostatin analog that is used in the imaging of tumors with high somatostatin receptor (SSTR) expression, including neuroendocrine tumors, pheochromocytoma, paraganglioma, neuroblastoma, and meningioma.
- DOTATATE PET/CT is the new first-line diagnostic imaging modality for neuroendocrine tumors, replacing the older Octreoscan and MIBG scintigraphy (discussed later in this chapter).
- DOTATATE and FDG PET/CT are complementary exams, helping to identify both well-differentiated (high DOTATATE uptake) and poorly differentiated (high FDG uptake) tumors.

其他类型的PET/CT

^{68}镓-DOTATATE(GaTate)

- ^{68}镓(^{68}Ga)是加速器产生的发射正电子的元素，半衰期为68分钟。
- ^{68}Ga-DOTATATE是一种生长抑素类似物，用于生长抑素受体高表达(SSTR)的肿瘤成像，包括神经内分泌肿瘤、嗜铬细胞瘤、副神经节瘤、神经母细胞瘤和脑膜瘤。
- DOTATATE PET/CT是新的一线诊断神经内分泌肿瘤的影像示踪剂，取代了较旧的^{111}In-喷曲肽(奥曲肽)扫描和间碘苄胍(MIBG)闪烁显像(本章后文进行讨论)。
- DOTATATE和FDG PET/CT为互补检查，有助于识别高分化(高DOTATATE摄取)和低分化(高FDG摄取)的两种肿瘤。

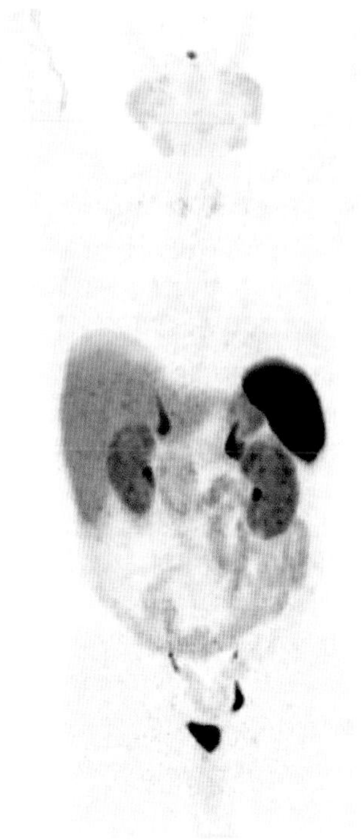

Coronal PET MIP shows physiologic distribution of Ga-68 DOTATATE. Note intense uptake in the spleen, followed by the adrenals, kidneys/bladder, pituitary, salivary glands, thyroid, liver, and bowel.

冠状位PET MIP显示生理性^{68}Ga-DOTATATE分布。注意，脾脏为强烈摄取，其次为肾上腺、肾脏/膀胱、垂体、唾液腺、甲状腺、肝脏和肠道。

PET agents for prostate cancer imaging

- Because of the limitation of FDG PET/CT in prostate cancer imaging, a number of alternative PET radiotracers have been developed in the past decade.
- **Carbon-11/F-18 choline** are biomarkers of cell membrane metabolism and are FDA-approved for imaging biochemically recurrent prostate cancer with high PSA levels, but are not in widespread use.
- **PSMA ligands** such as ProstaScint and Ga-68 PSMA target the prostate membrane specific antigen (PSMA) which is highly expressed in prostate cancer. PSMA PET/CT is highly sensitive for biochemically recurrent prostate cancer with low PSA levels, but is not yet FDA-approved.
- **F-18 fluciclovine (Axumin)** is an amino acid analog which targets amino acid transporters that are overexpressed in prostate cancer. Imaging is performed only minutes after injection of the tracer, which limits any significant urinary excretion. It is FDA-approved for detection of biochemically recurrent prostate cancer.
- **F-18 sodium fluoride** (F-18 NaF) is an analog of the hydroxyl group in hydroxyapatite bone crystals and a biomarker of osteoblastic activity. It is highly sensitive for the detection of prostate cancer bone metastases, but is not routinely used due to low specificity, high cost, and limited availability.

用于前列腺癌成像的PET试剂

- 由于FDG PET/CT在前列腺癌成像中的局限性，在过去十年中人们开发了多种替代PET的放射性示踪剂。
- **^{11}C/^{18}F-胆碱**是细胞膜代谢的生物标志物，并获得美国食品药品管理局(FDA)批准用于对前列腺特异性抗原(PSA)水平高的复发性前列腺癌进行生化成像，但并未广泛使用。
- **前列腺特异性膜抗原(PSMA)制剂**，如ProstaScint和^{68}Ga-PSMA针对PSMA，它们在前列腺癌中有高度表达。PSMA PET/CT对低水平PSA的生化性复发前列腺癌高度敏感，但尚未获得FDA批准。
- **^{18}F-fluciclovine(Axumin)**是一种氨基酸类似物，针对氨基酸转运蛋白并在前列腺癌中呈过度表达。成像在注射示踪剂仅数分钟后进行，这样就限制了其从尿中大量排泄。该类物质被FDA批准用于检测生化复发性前列腺癌。
- **^{18}F-氟化钠**(^{18}F NaF)是羟基磷灰石骨晶体中的羟基，为成骨细胞活性的生物标志物。它对检测前列腺癌骨转移非常敏感，但由于其特异度低、成本高和获取困难而不作为常规使用。

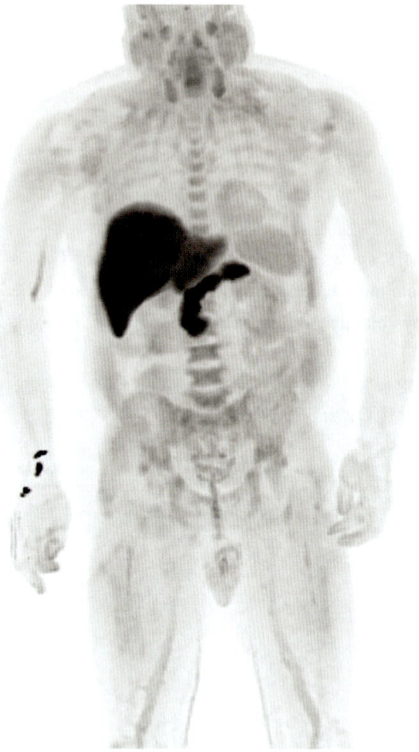

Coronal PET MIP shows normal distribution of F-18 fluciclovine. Note intense uptake in liver and pancreas, and variable uptake in muscles. Foci of uptake at the right arm represent the injection site.

冠状位PET MIP显示正常^{18}F-氟环素分布。注意，肝脏和胰腺为强烈摄取，肌肉摄取程度不同。右臂的数个局部摄取为注射点。

（翻译　王维平）

CEREBROVASCULAR

RADIOTRACERS

Tc-99m DTPA/Tc-99m pertechnetate

- Technetium-99m has a half-life of 6 hours and is used in the majority of nuclear imaging.
- Tc-99m DTPA and pertechnetate are transient perfusion agents. There is no uptake within the brain parenchyma as they do not cross intact blood-brain barrier. Activity is seen in the scalp, calvarium, subarachnoid spaces, major cerebral arteries and venous sinuses.
- Transient perfusion agents are reserved for planar imaging only and are now uncommonly used.

Tc-99m HMPAO/Tc-99m ECD

- Both HMPAO and ECD are lipophilic perfusion agents that cross the blood-brain barrier. To be retained in the cell, ECD is enzymatically modified. In contrast, HMPAO simply needs to be protonated to be trapped. Thus, ECD is only taken up by living cells while HMPAO uptake is a marker of perfusion. In the evaluation of subacute infarct, the phenomenon of luxury perfusion can cause HMPAO uptake to increase (due to increased perfusion), while ECD will show the true defect representing the infarct core.
- HMPAO and ECD show activity in the brain parenchyma, mainly gray matter.

脑血管

放射性示踪剂

^{99m}Tc-DTPA(二乙撑三胺五乙酸)/^{99m}TcO$_4$(高锝酸盐)

- ^{99m}锝(^{99m}Tc)的半衰期为6小时，用于大多数核素成像。
- ^{99m}Tc-DTPA和高锝酸盐是一过性的灌注显像剂。脑实质内没有摄取，因为它们不能穿过完整的血脑屏障。放射性分布来自头皮、颅骨、蛛网膜下腔、大脑的主要动脉和静脉窦。
- 一过性的灌注显像剂仅用于平面成像，目前已不常用。

^{99m}Tc-HMPAO(甲基丙二胺肟)/^{99m}Tc-ECD(双半胱乙酯)

- HMPAO和ECD都是亲脂性脑灌注显像剂，都可通过血脑屏障。ECD被酶修饰后滞留在脑细胞内。相比之下，HMPAO只需要质子化后就可滞留在脑细胞内。因而，ECD仅被活细胞摄取，而HMPAO摄取只代表有血液灌注。在评估亚急性脑梗死时，过度灌注现象会导致HMPAO摄取增加(由于增加了血流灌注)，而ECD所显示的真正缺损为脑梗死的核心区。
- HMPAO和ECD显示脑实质的放射性活动，主要是灰质。

- Of these two agents, ECD is generally preferred for brain imaging, because it has more rapid blood pool clearance, better shelf life, more accurate characterization of perfusion, and is only taken up by living cells.
- Both tracers are used for SPECT imaging.

Iodine-123 ioflupane (I-123 FP-CIT or DaTscan)

- Iodine-123 has a half-life of 13 hours. I-123 ioflupane is a cocaine analog that binds to the presynaptic dopamine transporter (DaT). It is used in SPECT imaging for the differentiation of essential tremor from parkinsonism.

Thallium-201

- Thallium-201 has a half-life of 73 hours and is used for SPECT imaging in the differentiation of tumor recurrence versus radiation necrosis. Thallium accumulates in viable tumor but not normal brain tissue.

PET agents

- F-18 FDG is the most common FDA-approved PET agent used for brain imaging.
- F-18 florbetapir, F-18 florbetaben and F-18 flutemetamol are FDA-approved PET agents for imaging of beta-amyloid.
- In 2020, F-18 flortaucipir was approved by FDA for tau imaging.
- Other PET radiotracers are emerging that target specific neuroreceptors (such as F-18-DOPA targeting the dopamine transporter).

- 这两种显像剂中，ECD通常首选用于脑显像，因为此显像剂的血池清除快、储存有效期长、更准确地反映灌注情况，并且只被存活细胞摄取。
- 两种示踪剂都用于SPECT显像。

^{123}I-ioflupane（^{123}I-FP-CIT或DaTscan或碘氟潘）

- ^{123}I的半衰期为13小时。^{123}I-ioflupane是一种可卡因类似物，与突触前多巴胺转运体(DaT)结合。它被用于SPECT显像，以鉴别原发性震颤和帕金森病。

^{201}Tl(铊)

- ^{201}Tl的半衰期为73小时，用于SPECT显像以区分肿瘤复发和辐射性坏死。Tl在有活性的肿瘤中浓聚，但并不被正常脑组织摄取。

PET显像剂

- ^{18}F-FDG是FDA批准的最常用的PET脑显像剂。
- ^{18}F-florbetapir、^{18}F-florbetaben和^{18}F-flutemamol是FDA批准的用于β-淀粉样蛋白成像的PET显像剂。
- 在2020年，^{18}F-flortaucipir被FDA批准用于微管相关蛋白显像。
- 以特定神经受体为靶点的其他PET放射示踪剂也正逐步出现(如靶点为多巴胺转运体的^{18}F-DOPA)。

RADIONUCLIDE IMAGING OF THE BRAIN

Evaluation of cerebral perfusion

- Cerebral perfusion reserve can be assessed with an **acetazolamide (Diamox) challenge**. Normally, cerebral blood flow increases after administration of 1 g Diamox, a carbonic anhydrase inhibitor that causes increased cerebral CO_2 concentration and thereby cerebrovascular vasodilation.
- Areas of the brain that already have maximized their autoregulatory mechanisms will not show an increase in perfusion after Diamox administration, and therefore will have relatively reduced activity compared to the rest of the brain. These areas are at risk for infarction.

放射性核素脑显像

评估脑血流灌注

- 脑血流灌注储备可用**乙酰唑胺(Diamox)负荷试验**进行评估。正常情况下，注射1g乙酰唑胺后可见脑血流灌注增加。乙酰唑胺是碳酸酐酶抑制剂，可导致脑CO_2浓度增加，从而使脑血管舒张。
- 当脑的某些区域自动调节机制发挥到极限时，静脉注射乙酰唑胺后不会增加脑血流灌注，因而放射性计数较其他脑区相对减少。这些区域有脑梗死的风险。

Brain death

脑死亡

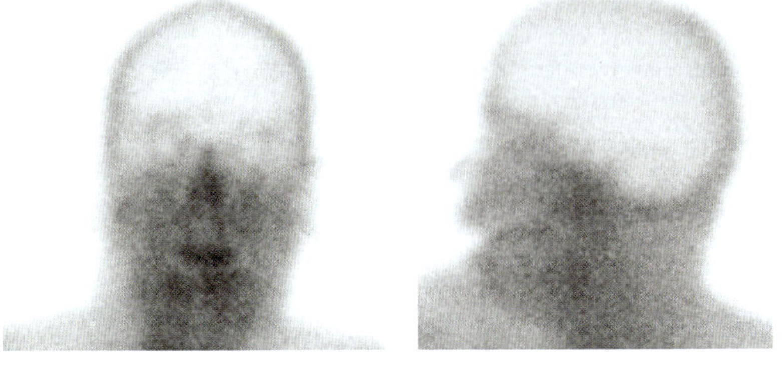

Frontal and lateral planar images following injection of Tc-99m HMPAO show absent intracranial uptake (*empty light bulb sign*) and increased perfusion in the face (particularly nasal region) and scalp. Absent cerebral perfusion is consistent with brain death in the proper clinical setting.

注射^{99m}Tc-HMPAO后的前位和侧位平面图像显示颅内无放射性摄取(空灯泡征)，面部(尤其是鼻)和头皮血流灌注增加。结合临床，脑灌注缺失等同于脑死亡。

- In brain death, intravenously injected radiotracer is unable to enter the cranial cavity due to increased intracranial pressure.
- SPECT imaging can be performed, either with HMPAO or ECD-labeled Tc-99m.
- Imaging shows absence of tracer perfusing the brain. The *hot-nose sign* represents increased collateral flow seen in brain death, but is not specific.

- 脑死亡后，静脉注射的放射性示踪剂因颅内压增高而不能进入颅内。
- 可以使用^{99m}T标记的HMPAO或ECD为示踪剂进行SPECT成像。
- 图像显示脑组织无示踪剂灌注。热鼻征代表脑死亡后有侧支循环增加，但并不具备特异性。

Dementia imaging

- Perfusion imaging with SPECT and glucose metabolism with PET are helpful in the early diagnosis of dementia based on parallel patterns.
- **Alzheimer disease** typically shows asymmetrically to symmetrically reduced perfusion (on SPECT) or hypometabolism (on FDG-PET) in the posterior cingulate gyrus and posterotemporal and parietal lobes, with sparing of the sensorimotor cortex, occipital lobes and deep nuclei. With further progression of disease, frontal lobes can also be involved.

痴呆显像

- 基于平行模式，联合SPECT灌注显像和PET糖代谢显像有助于早期痴呆的诊断。
- **阿尔茨海默病**通常表现为后扣带回、后颞叶和顶叶的对称或不对称灌注减少(SPECT)或代谢降低(FDG-PET)，但感觉运动皮层、枕叶和深部核团不受影响。随着病情的进一步发展，额叶也可受累。

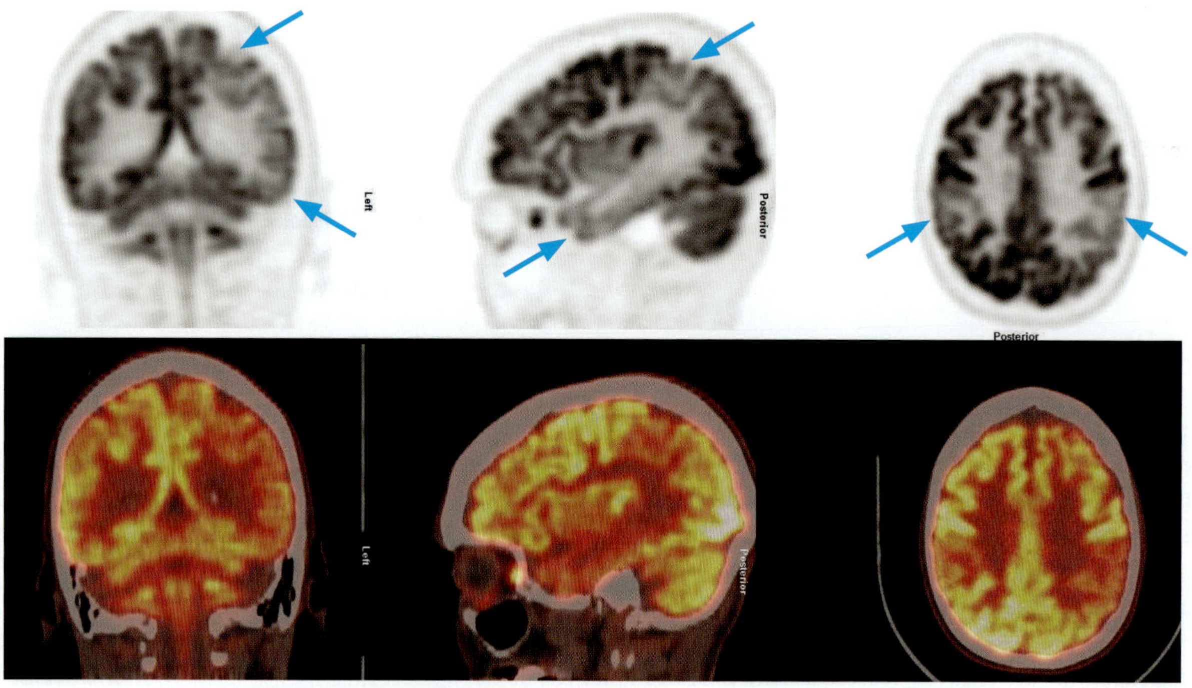

F-18 FDG PET and PET/CT overlay images of a patient with memory difficulties show hypometabolism predominantly in the parietal and temporal cortex (arrows), greater on the left. There is sparing of the sensorimotor cortex, occipital cortex, and deep nuclei (not shown). This pattern can be seen with Alzheimer disease in the appropriate clinical context. *Case courtesy Matthew Robertson, MD.*

一名记忆困难患者的^{18}F-FDG PET和PET/CT融合图像显示代谢降低，主要位于顶叶和颞叶皮质(蓝箭)，左侧更明显。感觉运动皮层、枕叶皮层和深部核团未受影响(未展示)。这种表现可见于有一定临床表现的阿尔茨海默病患者。

- **Lewy body dementia** appears similar to Alzheimer but also involves the occipital lobes.
- **Multi-infarct dementia** shows multiple asymmetric foci of decreased metabolism/perfusion.
- **Pick disease** (frontotemporal dementia) is characterized by decreased uptake in the frontal lobes and anterior portion of the temporal lobes.
- **Huntington disease** shows decreased uptake in the basal ganglia.
- **Parkinson disease** is characterized by decreased dopamine transporter density in the striatum on SPECT and PET, demonstrated with use of agents such as I-123 ioflupane (DaTscan) or F-18-DOPA.

- **路易体痴呆**的影像学表现与阿尔茨海默病相似，但还累及枕叶。
- **多发梗死性痴呆**表现为多发、不对称的低代谢/低灌注病灶。
- **皮克病**(额颞叶痴呆)的特征是额叶和颞叶的前部摄取减少。
- **亨廷顿病**显示基底神经节摄取减少。
- **帕金森病**SPECT和PET显像特征是纹状体中多巴胺转运体密度下降，显像剂为^{123}I-ioflupane或^{18}F-DOPA。

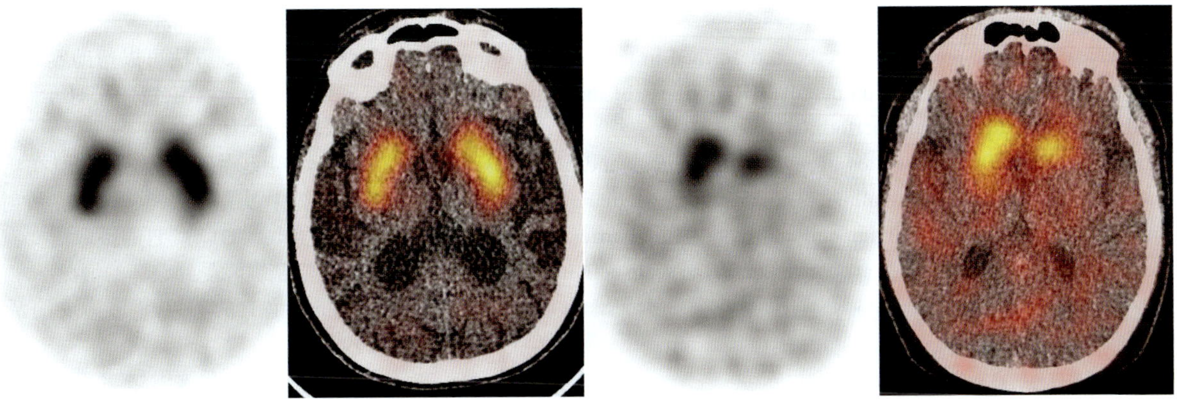

Normal versus abnormal I-123 ioflupane uptake on SPECT and SPECT/CT overlay: The left two images show normal symmetric comma-shaped activity in the caudate nucleus and putamen. The right two images show asymmetric and reduced activity in both striata, greater on the left, resulting in loss of the comma shape.

正常的与异常的^{123}I-ioflupane摄取SPECT和SPECT/CT融合图像：左侧两幅图像显示正常尾状核和壳核对称的逗号形状放射性分布。右侧两幅图像显示两侧纹状体放射性分布不对称及放射性摄取降低，左侧纹状体更明显，导致其放射性分布失去逗号形状。

Seizure imaging

- In general, blood perfusion and metabolism of seizure foci are increased during seizure (ictal imaging), and decreased between seizures (interictal imaging).
- Ictal perfusion SPECT with Tc-99m HMPAO or ECD is the most sensitive, but technically challenging to perform because the radiotracer must be injected during the seizure or within 30 seconds after the end of the seizure.
- Interictal PET with F-18 FDG is very sensitive in localizing partial complex seizures, which usually originate in the temporal lobe. Ictal PET is not possible due to slow FDG uptake.
- Extratemporal seizure focus is more difficult to localize. Ictal SPECT is the most sensitive.

癫痫显像

- 一般来说，癫痫灶在癫痫发作时的血流灌注和代谢增加(发作显像)，在癫痫发作的间隙时降低(发作间隙显像)。
- 发作期^{99m}Tc-HMPAO或^{99m}Tc-ECD灌注SPECT是最敏感的，但在技术上有一定困难，因为放射性示踪剂必须在发作期或于癫痫发作结束后30秒内注射完成。
- 发作间期^{18}F-FDG PET显像对定位复杂部分性癫痫发作非常敏感，通常起源于颞叶。由于FDG摄取缓慢，无法在急性发作期进行PET显像。
- 颞叶以外的癫痫灶较难定位。发作期SPECT最为敏感。

Crossed cerebellar diaschisis

- Crossed cerebellar diaschisis is a commonly encountered phenomenon in the presence of a supratentorial lesion (seen in tumors, stroke, and trauma), where the cerebellar hemisphere contralateral to the lesion shows decreased radiotracer uptake. This phenomenon is thought to be due to interruption of corticopontine-cerebellar pathways.

交叉性小脑失联络

- 交叉性小脑失联络是小脑幕上的病变经常遇到的一种现象(见于肿瘤、卒中和创伤)，其病灶对侧的小脑半球呈放射性示踪剂摄取减少。这种现象被认为是由皮质脑桥-小脑通路的中断所致。

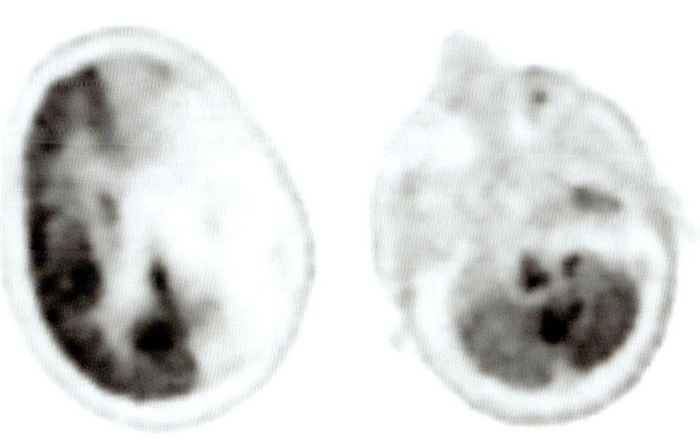

Axial F-18 FDG PET (left image) shows near absent glucose metabolism in the left cerebral hemisphere due to known encephalomalacia. Relatively decreased FDG uptake in the *right* cerebellum (right image) is consistent with crossed cerebellar diaschisis.

^{18}F-FDG PET轴位图像(左图)显示由于已知的脑软化症，左侧大脑半球几乎没有糖代谢。右侧小脑FDG摄取相对较低(右图)，与交叉性小脑失联络征一致。

Brain tumor recurrence versus radiation necrosis

- Several nuclear imaging protocols have been described in the differentiation of tumor recurrence versus radiation necrosis. Regardless of the radiotracer involved, fusion to MRI is usually performed.
- Thallium-201 generally accumulates in malignant gliomas and not in post-treatment granulation tissue (i.e., thallium is not taken up by radiation necrosis). Thallium-201 uptake requires a living cell and blood-brain barrier disruption. The degree of uptake can be graded in comparison to the scalp activity:

  Uptake <scalp is low; uptake between scalp and 2x scalp is moderate; and uptake >2x scalp is high.

脑肿瘤复发与放射性坏死

- 多种核医学检查方法可以帮助鉴别肿瘤复发与放射性坏死。无论使用哪种示踪剂，通常与MRI进行图像融合。
- ^{201}Tl通常聚集在恶性胶质瘤，但在治疗后的肉芽组织中没有聚集(也就是说，放射性坏死组织不摄取^{201}Tl)。^{201}Tl的摄取需要有活细胞并且在血脑屏障受到破坏的情况下才能发生。病灶摄取^{201}Tl的程度可与头皮的活性进行比较：

  摄取低于头皮为低度；摄取介于头皮与头皮的两倍之间为中度；摄取大于头皮的2倍为高度摄取。

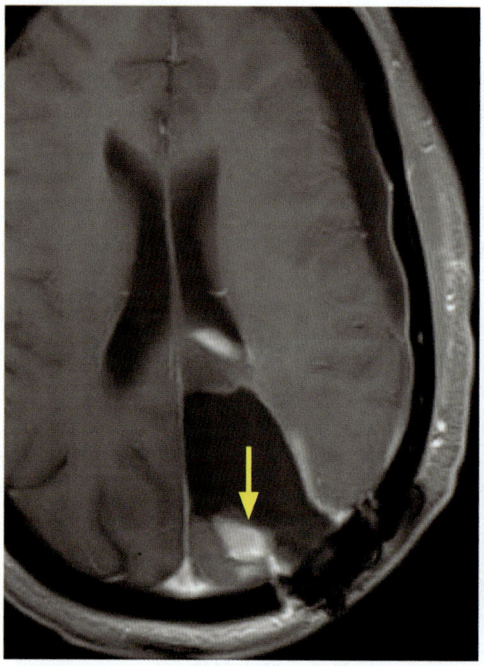

Axial T1-weighted post-contrast MRI shows a left parietal resection cavity with an enhancing nodule (arrow) along the posteromedial aspect of the resection cavity.

轴位增强T$_1$加权MRI 显示左侧顶叶切除后空腔的后内侧有一个强化的结节灶(黄箭)。

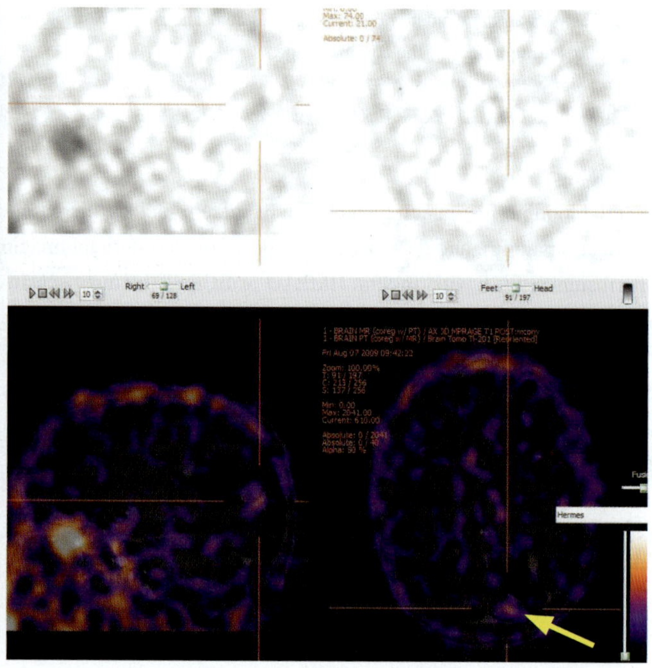

SPECT thallium-201 (top image, with 4.4 mCi administered) and fused SPECT-MRI (bottom image) show thallium uptake in the posteromedial aspect of the resection cavity correlating with the enhancing nodule seen on MRI (arrow). This pattern is suggestive of tumor recurrence.

^{201}Tl SPECT(上图，4.4 mCi ^{201}Tl)和融合SPECT-MRI(下图)显示切除后空腔的后内方有^{201}Tl摄取，与MRI扫描时的增强结节一致(黄箭)。这种影像学表现提示有肿瘤复发。

- Dual-phase F-18 FDG PET employs early and delayed imaging to evaluate a region of suspected tumor recurrence versus radiation necrosis. PET scanning is performed at 1 hour and 4 hours after the injection of the radiotracer. Dual phase PET has been shown to have increased accuracy for the assessment of recurrence versus post-treatment changes in metastatic disease compared to single-phase PET.

- 早期和延迟双相^{18}F-FDG PET显像用于评估可疑肿瘤复发或放射性坏死。PET显像是在注射药物后1小时和4小时进行。双相PET在评估肿瘤复发或治疗后改变时，其准确性高于单相PET显像。

Cerebrospinal fluid imaging

Radiotracer: Indium-111 DTPA

- Indium-111 has a half-life of 67 hours.
- In-111 DTPA is ideal for cerebrospinal fluid imaging because it is non-lipid soluble, not metabolized, and has a long half-life (CSF imaging may span

脑脊液(CSF)显像

放射性示踪剂：^{111}In-DTPA(^{111}铟-二乙撑三胺五乙酸)

- ^{111}铟(^{111}In)的半衰期为67小时。
- ^{111}In-DTPA是理想的脑脊液(CSF)显像剂，因为它是非脂溶性的，不被代谢，而且有很长的

several days). It is administered intrathecally by lumbar puncture.

- Normally, radiotracer should reach the basal cisterns by 1 hour, the sylvian and anterior interhemispheric cisterns by 2–6 hours, cerebral convexities by 12 hours, and the arachnoid villi in the sagittal sinus by 24 hours.
- Presence of radiotracer activity in the lateral ventricles is abnormal. Failure of radiotracer ascent over the cerebral convexities at 24 hours is also abnormal.

半衰期(可以连续数天进行CSF成像)。通过腰椎穿刺向鞘内注射给药。

- 正常情况下，放射性示踪剂在1小时内到达基底池，在2~6小时到达侧裂池和纵裂池前部，12小时到达大脑凸面，在24小时内到达矢状窦的蛛网膜绒毛。
- 侧脑室出现放射性示踪剂为异常。如24小时在大脑凸面未见放射性示踪剂同样为异常。

Radiotracer: Tc-99m DTPA

- Due to its short half-life (6 hours), Tc-99m DTPA is used for CSF studies that do not require prolonged imaging, including the evaluation of CSF leak and shunt patency.

放射性示踪剂：^{99m}Tc-DTPA(二乙撑三胺五乙酸)

- 由于^{99m}Tc-DTPA的半衰期短(6小时)，故仅用于短时间的CSF显像，包括评价CSF漏及其分流管的通畅情况。

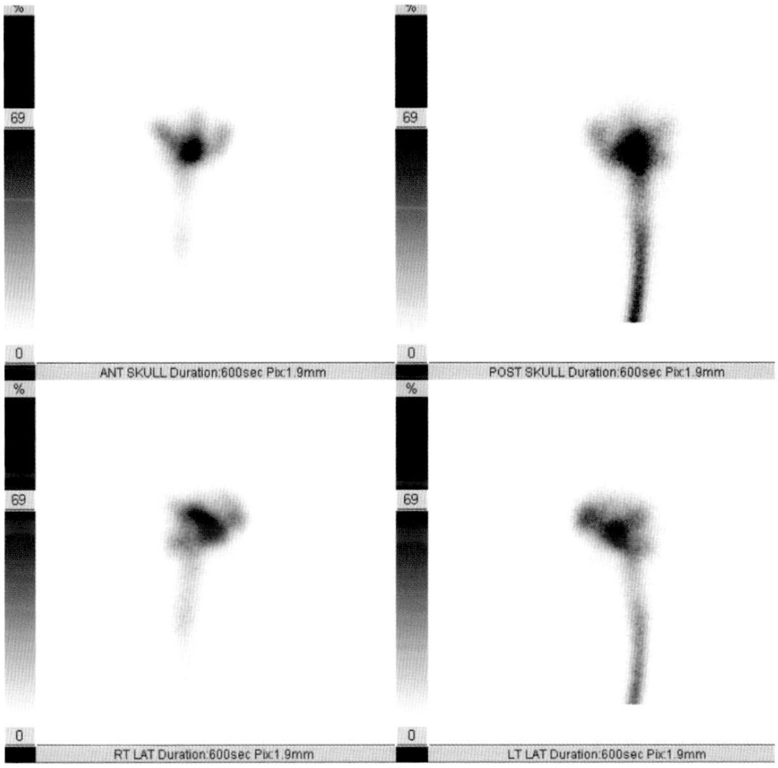

Normal cisternogram:
Planar images at different projections were obtained at 4 hours following intrathecal injection of 0.54 mCi In-111 DTPA. There is normal *trident appearance* of tracer activity in the sylvian and anterior interhemispheric cisterns. Activity is also present in the basilar cisterns and spinal canal.

正常脑池显像图：
在鞘内注射0.54mCi ^{111}In-DTPA 4小时后获取不同方位的平面图像。侧裂池和纵裂池前部正常示踪剂分布，呈三叉戟样形状。基底池和椎管中也有示踪剂。

Normal pressure hydrocephalus

- Radionuclide cisternography can be used to confirm suspected communicating hydrocephalus in patients with the classic clinical triad of normal pressure hydrocephalus (ataxia, incontinence, dementia), who would benefit from CSF shunting.
- Communicating hydrocephalus is characterized by early entry of radioactivity into the lateral ventricles within 6 hours, persistent intraventricular activity, and lack of activity over the cerebral convexities after 24–48 hours.

正常压力脑积水

- 放射性核素脑池造影可用于确认疑似交通性脑积水并具有典型临床三联征(共济失调、失禁、痴呆)的正常压力的脑积水患者。这些患者可以行CSF分流术而得到缓解。
- 交通性脑积水的特点是早期侧脑室内出现放射性示踪剂(6小时内)，并持续存在于脑室，但大脑的凸面在24~48小时后依然缺乏放射性分布。

CSF leak

- Common locations for CSF leak are the ear, paranasal sinuses, and nose.
- CSF leak can be identified by asymmetric activity in the region of the ears on frontal imaging, or activity in the nose on lateral imaging. Subtle leaks can only be detected by placing cotton pledgets in the area of concern, removing after several hours and counting the pledgets' activity relative to plasma activity.
- For spinal CSF leak, radioisotope cisternography shows diffusion of the tracer into the paraspinal extra-arachnoidal space. Correlation with MR or CT

CSF漏

- CSF漏的常见部位是耳、鼻窦和鼻。
- CSF漏在正位显像图上表现为双耳不对称性放射性分布，在侧位显像图上表现为鼻部有放射性分布。微量的渗漏只能通过在有怀疑的区域放置棉絮来检测，在几个小时后移除棉絮，并测量棉絮相对于血浆的放射性活度。
- 对于椎管CSF漏，放射性核素脑池显像可

myelography may show triangular CSF space expansion at nerve root sleeves. A common pitfall is perineural cysts which are discrete round lesions.

见示踪剂扩散到脊柱旁蛛网膜以外的空间。MRI或CT脊髓造影术可见相应部位神经根袖处的三角形CSF空间扩张。经常与之混淆的是神经周围囊肿，后者是非常清楚的圆形病灶。

Evaluation of CSF shunt patency

- Tc-99m DTPA or less commonly In-111 DTPA are injected into the shunt reservoir.
- If the distal limb of the shunt is patent, radiotracer activity should rapidly pass through the shunt catheter and into the peritoneal cavity or right atrium.
- Manual occlusion of the distal limb should normally show reflux of radiotracer into the ventricular system. This is not seen in the presence of proximal limb occlusion.

评估CSF分流导管通畅性

- 通常将^{99m}Tc-DTPA(较少使用^{111}In-DTPA)注射入分流导管的引流池内。
- 如果CSF分流导管的远端通畅，放射性示踪剂应该迅速通过分流导管进入腹腔或右心房。
- 人工阻塞CSF分流导管的远端后，通常应看到放射示踪剂回流进入脑室系统。这种现象在导管近端闭塞时不会出现。

(翻译　马宏星)

THYROID

甲状腺

RADIOTRACERS

放射性示踪剂

Iodine-131

- I-131 emits both beta particles and 364 keV gamma photons (only the gamma photons are used for imaging). The half-life is 8 days. I-131 is produced by fission in a nuclear reactor. It is administered orally.
- I-131 is ideal for therapy due to its high radiation dose to the thyroid and relatively low whole body dose. Indications include treatment of thyroid cancer status post thyroidectomy, and hyperthyroidism from Graves disease or multinodular goiter.

131碘(^{131}I)

- ^{131}I同时发射β粒子和364keV的γ光子(只有γ光子用于成像)。^{131}I半衰期为8天，为核反应裂变产生。口服给药。
- ^{131}I适用于治疗，因其对甲状腺的放射剂量高而对全身剂量相对较低。适应证包括甲状腺癌切除术后、格雷夫斯病或结节性甲状腺肿引起的甲状腺功能亢进。

Iodine-123

- I-123 decays by electron capture and emits 159 keV gamma photons. The half-life is 13 hours. I-123 is expensive because it is produced by cyclotron. It is administered orally.
- I-123 is the preferred radioisotope for thyroid imaging, as it can image in high detail and obtain thyroid uptake values.

123碘(^{123}I)

- ^{123}I衰减时俘获电子并产生159keV的γ光子，它的半衰期为13小时。^{123}I由回旋加速器生产，所以价格昂贵。口服给药。
- ^{123}I是一种优良的甲状腺显像核素，它能很好地显示细节，还能获取甲状腺对碘的摄取率。

Tc-99m pertechnetate

- Tc-99m emits 140 keV gamma photons, has a half-life of 6 hours, and is generator-produced.
- Unlike iodine, pertechnetate is trapped but not organified by the thyroid. After initial uptake it is released into the blood pool. Thyroid uptake is not routinely quantified with pertechnetate due to its rapid washout.
- Pertechnetate is an excellent alternative to I-123 for thyroid imaging because of its ready availability from generators, and its low patient dose which allows administration of higher doses and thereby permits quicker imaging with less motion artifact. It is administered intravenously.
- Because pertechnetate does not specifically localize to the thyroid, high background counts are typical. Only 1–5% of administered activity is taken up by the thyroid.
- In contrast to I-123, the salivary glands are well seen with pertechnetate.
- Tc-99m pertechnetate is preferred over I-123 when the patient has received recent intravenous iodinated contrast (iodine in contrast blocks thyroid uptake of additional iodine), when Ⅳ administration is necessary, or when a quick

99mTc高锝酸盐($^{99m}TcO_4$)

- ^{99m}Tc发射140keV的γ光子，半衰期为6小时，由发生器产生。
- 与碘不同，高锝酸盐被甲状腺摄取但不被有机化。在最初吸收后，它会释放到血池中。因快速洗脱，高锝酸盐不常规用于定量测定甲状腺摄取率。
- 高锝酸盐是一种很好的^{123}I甲状腺成像替代品，因为它随时可以从发生器获得、对患者的辐射低，因此允许给予较高的剂量，快速成像而减少了运动伪影。静脉注射给药。
- 高锝酸盐并不特异性地留在甲状腺，通常具有较高的本底计数。甲状腺摄取只占所给剂量的1%~5%。
- 与^{123}I不同，唾液腺在高锝酸盐显像时清晰可见。
- 当患者近期接受含碘的静脉造影剂(造影剂所

study is required.

含的碘会阻碍甲状腺摄取额外的碘)、必须静脉给药及需要快速得出研究结果时，^{99m}**TcO$_4$** 优于 ^{123}I。

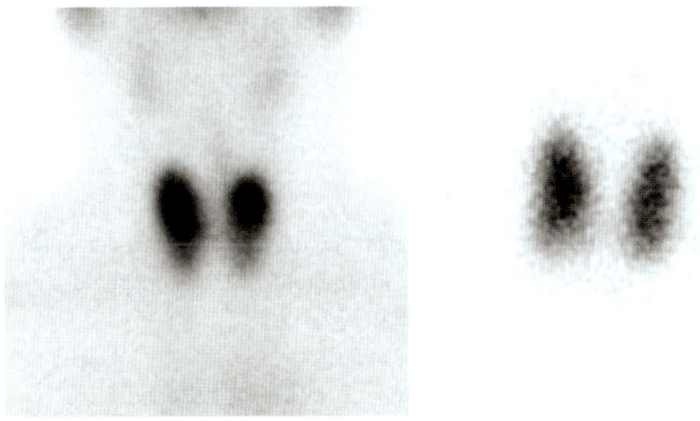

Tc-99m pertechnetate (left image) versus I-123 (right image) thyroid scans. Note, pertechnetate has higher background counts and physiologic uptake in salivary glands.

^{99m}TcO$_4$(左图)对比 ^{123}I(右图)甲状腺扫描。注意，高锝酸盐具有较高的本底计数和唾液腺的生理性摄取。

Patient preparation

- Patients undergoing I-123 or I-131 imaging/therapy must have non-suppressed TSH, which can be achieved by stopping exogenous thyroid hormone for 4 weeks, or by two intramuscular injections of recombinant TSH (rTSH).
- Patients who received intravenous iodinated contrast should wait one month before radioiodine imaging.

Pregnancy and breastfeeding

- All thyrotropic agents cross the placenta and I-131 is contraindicated in pregnancy. Fetal iodine is taken up beginning at 12 weeks of gestation.
- A breastfeeding mother who requires an I-131 ablative dose must stop breastfeeding permanently for the current child.
- For I-123, breastfeeding can be resumed two to three days after administration.
- For Tc-99m, breastfeeding can be resumed 12–24 hours after administration.

患者准备

- 对患者使用 ^{123}I 或 ^{131}I 成像/治疗时，TSH 必须处于未抑制状态，这可以通过停止外源性甲状腺激素 4 周，或肌内注射重组 TSH(rTSH)2 周来实现。
- 接受静脉含碘造影剂的患者应等待 1 个月后进行放射性碘成像。

妊娠和哺乳

- 所有促甲状腺制剂都会通过胎盘，因此妊娠者禁用 ^{131}I。胎儿在 12 周胎龄时开始吸收碘。
- 哺乳期妇女需要接受 ^{131}I 清扫剂量时，必须永久停止对当前孩子的母乳喂养。
- 哺乳期妇女接受 ^{123}I 后，给药 2~3 天后可以恢复母乳喂养。
- 哺乳期妇女接受 ^{99m}Tc 后，给药 12~24 小时后可以恢复母乳喂养。

DIAGNOSTIC INDICATIONS (I-123 OR TC-99M PERTECHNETATE)

Ectopic thyroid

- Either I-123 or Tc-99m can be used to localize suspected ectopic thyroid tissue.
- Lingual thyroid is ectopic thyroid tissue at the base of the tongue.
- Functional thyroid tissue may rarely be seen in an ovarian teratoma (struma ovarii).
- Retrosternal thyroid tissue is most often due to a substernal goiter.

Thyroid nodule

- Thyroid nodules are typically only imaged if the cytology is indeterminate.
- Hyperfunctioning nodules are almost always benign adenomas.
- Cold nodules have approximately 20% risk of malignancy, although the most common cold nodule (~70–75%) is a benign colloid cyst.
- A warm nodule usually represents a cold nodule with overlapping thyroid tissue.

  A warm nodule requires further investigation such as biopsy if oblique views are indeterminate.

诊断适应证(^{123}I 或 ^{99m} 高锝酸盐)

异位甲状腺

- 无论 ^{123}I 还是 ^{99m}Tc 都可用于对可疑异位甲状腺组织进行定位。
- 舌部甲状腺是位于舌根部的异位甲状腺组织。
- 功能性甲状腺组织偶尔会出现在卵巢畸胎瘤(卵巢甲状腺肿)。
- 胸骨后的甲状腺组织通常是胸骨后甲状腺肿。

甲状腺结节

- 甲状腺结节通常在细胞学检查不能明确诊断时才进行显像。
- 功能亢进的结节几乎总是良性腺瘤。
- 冷结节的恶性肿瘤风险约为20%，大多数冷结节(70%~75%)是良性胶样囊肿。
- 温结节常是一个冷结节与正常的甲状腺组织相重叠。

  如果斜位图像不能确定温结节性质的话，需要进一步检查，如活检。

- A discordant thyroid nodule is "hot" on Tc-99m and "cold" on I-123 as it has maintained the ability to trap pertechnetate but is unable to organify iodine. Biopsy is usually recommended as a discordant nodule may be malignant.

- 甲状腺结节不匹配是指结节在^{99m}Tc图像上是"热"的，而在^{123}I图像上是"冷"的，这是由于结节有摄取高锝酸盐的能力，却不能滞留碘。这种不匹配的结节可能是恶性的，通常建议活检。

Graves disease

格雷夫斯病(弥漫性毒性甲状腺肿)

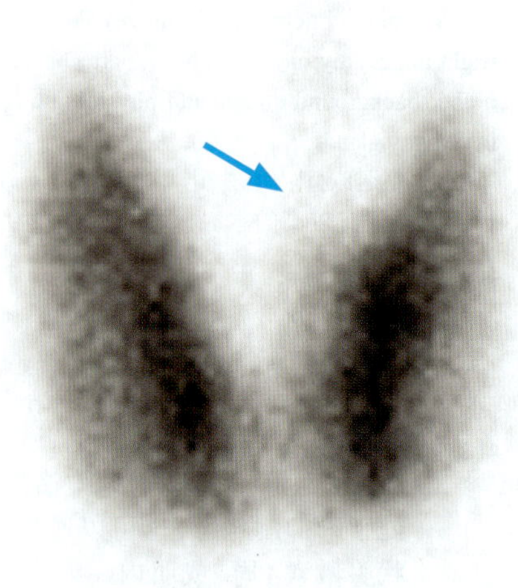

Graves disease on I-123 scan with 0.3 mCi I-123 NaI administered. There is diffuse uptake throughout the thyroid gland. A faint pyramidal lobe is present (arrow).
24-hour uptake is elevated at 56%.
格雷夫斯病在给予0.3mCi ^{123}I-NaI后获得^{123}I图像。
甲状腺呈弥漫性摄取。显示一个浅淡的锥体叶(蓝箭)。
24小时吸碘率高达56%。

- Graves disease is an autoimmune disorder characterized by hyperthyroidism, thyromegaly, homogeneously increased thyroid activity, and often a prominent pyramidal lobe.
- Both 6-hour and 24-hour **iodine uptake** are elevated.
  Normal 6-hour uptake is 6–18% and normal 24–hour uptake is 10–30%.
- Although usually an I-123 and a Tc-99m scan can be differentiated by the presence of salivary uptake with Tc-99m, in Graves disease this distinction is often not possible. In Graves disease, thyroid uptake can be so strong that the salivary glands are often not seen, causing a similar appearance with either radiotracer.
- Definitive treatment of Graves disease is I-131 radiotherapy or (less commonly) surgery. Antithyroid drugs (e.g., methimazole or propylthiouracil) are another option and may achieve a remission after one to two years of use.

- 格雷夫斯病是一种自身免疫性疾病，其特征是甲状腺功能亢进、甲状腺肿、甲状腺摄碘呈均匀性增加，锥体叶通常明显。
- 吸碘率在6小时和24小时均增高。
  正常6小时吸碘率为6%~18%，正常24小时为10%~30%。
- 通常可以通过是否有唾液腺摄取^{99m}Tc来区分^{123}I和^{99m}Tc扫描图像，但是在格雷夫斯病时几乎很难。格雷夫斯病时的甲状腺摄取功能非常强大，以致唾液腺往往不显影，导致这两种放射性示踪剂的图像很相似。
- 根治格雷夫斯病的方法是^{131}I放射治疗或手术(较少用)。抗甲状腺药物(如甲巯咪唑或丙基硫氧嘧啶)是另一种选择，需要经过1~2年治疗后才能达到缓解。

Toxic multinodular goiter (Plummer disease)

- Patients with toxic multinodular goiter are often middle-aged to elderly women and present with symptoms of hyperthyroidism.
- Thyroid scan shows an irregular, nodular thyroid contour and heterogeneous uptake corresponding to single or multiple hot nodules with suppression of the remaining normal functioning thyroid. Iodine uptake is elevated.
- Treatment options include medical therapy with antithyroid drugs for thyrotoxicosis, I-131 ablation, or thyroidectomy.
- Malignancy is relatively uncommon in a multinodular goiter. While a dominant cold nodule should undergo further investigation, smaller cold nodules are unlikely to be malignant.

毒性多结节性甲状腺肿(普卢默病)

- 毒性多结节性甲状腺肿患者多见于中老年妇女，表现为甲状腺功能亢进的症状。
- 甲状腺扫描显示甲状腺轮廓不规则并呈结节状，摄取不均匀与单个或多个热结节相对应，而其余正常功能的甲状腺受到抑制。碘摄取增加。
- 治疗选择包括使用抗甲状腺药物对甲状腺毒症进行内科治疗，^{131}I消融或甲状腺切除术。
- 多结节性甲状腺肿的恶变相对少见。对于大的冷结节应进一步检查，但较小的冷结节为恶性的可能不大。

Hashimoto thyroiditis

- Hashimoto thyroiditis is the most common inflammatory disease of the thyroid.
- Like Graves disease, Hashimoto thyroiditis also clinically presents with thyromegaly. In Hashimoto thyroiditis, however, thyroid hormone levels

桥本甲状腺炎

- 桥本甲状腺炎是最常见的甲状腺炎性疾病。
- 与格雷夫斯病一样，桥本甲状腺炎在临床上也可表现为甲状腺肿大。但是，桥本甲状腺

are variable depending on the disease stage. Most patients with Hashimoto thyroiditis are hypothyroid.

- Appearance on thyroid scan is variable, ranging from diffusely increased activity that resembles Graves disease to patchy uptake similar to a multinodular goiter. The patchiness is thought to be due to cold areas from infiltration by lymphocytes and lymphoid follicles.

炎的甲状腺激素水平在不同的疾病阶段变化很大。大多数桥本甲状腺炎患者会发生甲状腺功能减退。

- 甲状腺扫描表现也是多变的，包括从类似于格雷夫斯病那样的弥漫性摄取增高，或像结节性甲状腺肿那样的斑片状摄取。斑片状摄取通常被认为是由于淋巴细胞和淋巴滤泡浸润导致的冷区所致。

Subacute thyroiditis

亚急性甲状腺炎

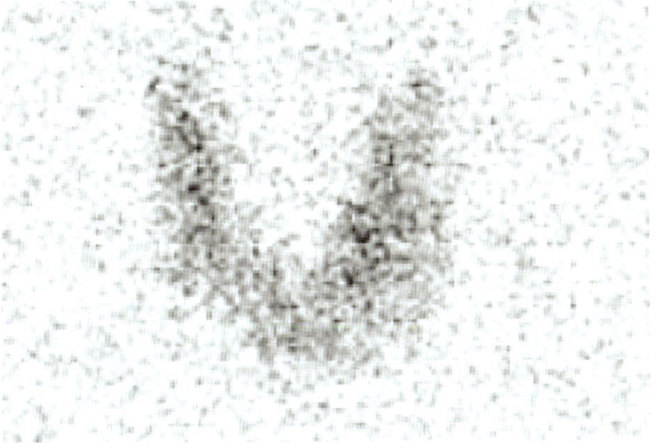

Subacute thyroiditis on I-123 scan with 0.22 mCi administered. There is diffusely low thyroid uptake with very low background to thyroid uptake ratio. 24-hour uptake was only 4.9%.

亚急性甲状腺炎在给予0.22mCi ^{123}I后所获得的显像。甲状腺呈普遍低摄取且本底与甲状腺摄取的比例非常低。24小时摄取率只有4.9%。

- The classical clinical presentation of subacute thyroiditis is a painful swollen gland, although many patients present with silent hyperthyroidism.
- Imaging shows decreased radiotracer uptake and a low 24-hour uptake.
- Subacute thyroiditis is typically a self-limited condition. Treatment is directed towards symptom control with nonsteroidal anti-inflammatory drugs or steroids in severe cases.

- 亚急性甲状腺炎的典型临床表现是甲状腺肿痛，但许多患者表现为无症状性甲状腺功能亢进。
- 影像显示放射性示踪剂摄取减少和24小时吸碘率降低。
- 亚急性甲状腺炎通常是自限性的。采用非甾体抗炎药进行对症治疗，严重病例可使用类固醇激素。

THERAPEUTIC INDICATIONS (I–131)

^{131}I的治疗适应证

Thyroid carcinoma, post-thyroidectomy

- Approximately one to two months after thyroidectomy, I-131 is administered to treat and simultaneously image residual and potential metastatic disease.
- Following thyroidectomy, thyroid replacement therapy is withheld to allow endogenous TSH to increase. This increases uptake of therapeutic I-131 by any residual or metastatic thyroid tissue. The goal TSH is 30–50 mIU/mL.
- The dosing of I-131 is dependent on the oncologic risk:

  Low-risk patient (tumor<1.5 cm, no invasion of thyroid capsule): ≤30 mCi I-131 administered.

  High-risk patient: 100–200 mCi I-131 administered.
- A new approach is a standard dose of 30 mCi for treatment of all T1, T2, and N1 cancers.
- Functioning lung or skeletal metastases require high doses of I-131, usually >200 mCi.
- To avoid or minimize the complication of irreversible pulmonary fibrosis, care is taken to limit the whole-body retention to 80 mCi at 48 hours after administration. To avoid bone marrow suppression, the absorbed dose to the blood is limited to 2 Gy.

甲状腺癌，甲状腺切除术后

- 甲状腺切除术后1~2个月左右，给予^{131}I治疗并同时对残留甲状腺和潜在转移病灶进行显像。
- 甲状腺切除术后，应停止甲状腺素替代治疗，以便使内源性TSH增高。这样可以使残留或转移性甲状腺癌组织增加对^{131}I的吸收。TSH要达到30~50mIU/mL。
- ^{131}I的剂量取决于肿瘤风险：

  低危患者(肿瘤<1.5cm，甲状腺被膜未受侵犯)：给予^{131}I≤30mCi。

  高危患者：给予^{131}I 100~200mCi。
- 一种新方法是给予30mCi的标准剂量治疗所有T1、T2和N1的甲状腺癌患者。
- 功能性肺或骨转移患者需要高剂量^{131}I，通常大于200mCi。
- 为了防止和减轻肺纤维化并发症，注意给药后48小时全身残余辐射剂量低于80mCi。为避免骨髓抑制，血液的吸收剂量局限于2Gy。

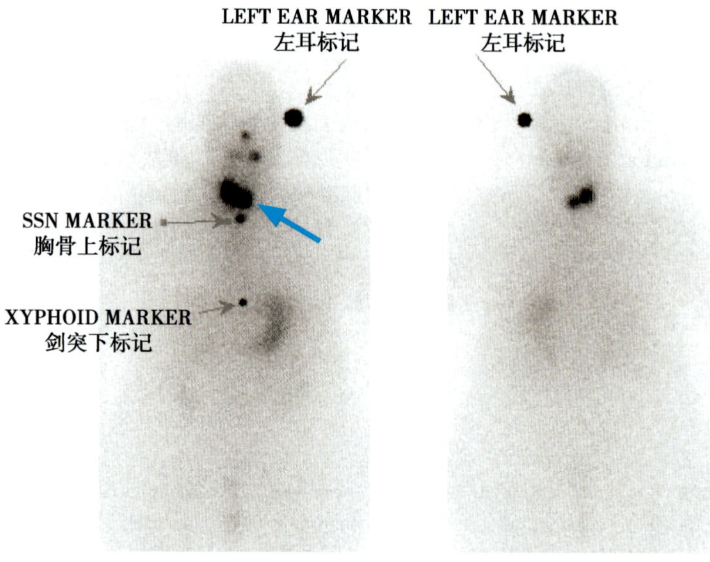

I-131 ablative therapy: 99 mCi I-131 administered orally 4 days prior to scanning. The gray arrows point to markers.
Anterior and posterior planar imaging shows a large focus of residual uptake in the thyroid bed (arrow) and mild symmetric salivary gland uptake. There is physiologic uptake in the stomach, bladder, and bowel.
^{131}I清扫治疗：口服99mCi ^{131}I 4天后进行扫描。灰箭所指为体外定位标记。
前位和后位平面显像显示甲状腺床区一个较大残留灶摄取(蓝箭)和对称性轻度唾液腺摄取。胃、膀胱和肠道有生理性摄取。

Thyroid carcinoma, post radioiodine therapy

- After ablation with I-131, patients with thyroid carcinoma are monitored by following thyroglobulin levels. If thyroglobulin levels rise, an I-123 scan is performed to evaluate for disease recurrence or metastasis. If the I-123 scan is positive, repeat I-131 radioiodine is administered for ablation. Note that the presence of anti-thyroglobulin antibodies precludes the ability to monitor the thyroglobulin levels.

Treatment of Graves disease

- I-131 is administered in a single oral dose to treat Graves disease. Contraindications to I-131 include pregnancy, lactation, and inability to comply with radiation safety guidelines.
- The dosing of I-131 for treatment of Graves varies by institution. Many endocrinologists advocate a calculated dose based on the estimated thyroid weight and 24-hour uptake, while another study has shown one of three fixed doses (up to 15 mCi) to be equally effective.
- Adequate dosing of I-131 can treat greater than 90% of patients with Graves disease.

Treatment of multinodular goiter

- I-131 can be used to reduce goiter size, especially in patients who choose not to undergo surgery. Compared to Graves disease, toxic multinodular goiter is more resistant to iodine radiotherapy, therefore requires a higher I-131 dose (20–30 mCi) and often multiple treatments.

Treatment of toxic/autonomous nodule

- Solitary toxic thyroid nodules can be successfully treated with 20–25 mCi of I-131.

甲状腺癌，放射性碘治疗后

- ^{131}I清扫治疗后，甲状腺癌患者可以通过监测甲状腺球蛋白水平进行随访。如果甲状腺球蛋白升高，则需行^{123}I扫描以评估复发或转移。如果^{123}I扫描阳性，则再次清扫。需要注意，如存在抗甲状腺球蛋白抗体，无法监测甲状腺球蛋白。

治疗格雷夫斯病

- 治疗格雷夫斯病需要一次性口服^{131}I。^{131}I治疗的禁忌证包括怀孕、哺乳期、无法遵守辐射安全要求的患者。
- 不同单位治疗格雷夫斯病所选用的^{131}I剂量不同。许多内分泌学家建议^{131}I剂量应基于甲状腺重量和24小时的吸碘率进行估算，而另一个研究使用了三种不同的固定剂量，其结果是等效的(其中一个高达15mCi)。
- 只要^{131}I剂量合适，90%以上的格雷夫斯病患者可以得到治疗。

毒性多结节性甲状腺肿的治疗

- ^{131}I可以用于缩小甲状腺肿，尤其适用于不愿意选择外科手术的患者。毒性多结节性甲状腺肿较格雷夫斯病对^{131}I的敏感性差，因而需要使用更高的^{131}I剂量(20~30mCi)，并且往往需要多次治疗。

毒性结节性甲状腺肿的治疗

- 孤立性毒性甲状腺结节可以使用20~25mCi的^{131}I成功地治疗。

(翻译　王维平)

PARATHYROID

甲状旁腺

RADIOTRACER

Tc-99m sestamibi

- Tc-99m sestamibi localizes to the mitochondria in parathyroid adenomas, hyperplastic parathyroids, normal thyroid tissue, and thyroid adenomas; however, thyroid activity decreases over time. It is *not* taken up by normal functioning parathyroid tissue.
- The same agent is used for nuclear cardiology and can also be taken up by malignancy, particularly breast and lung cancers.

放射性示踪剂

^{99m}Tc-甲氧基异丁基异腈(MIBI)

- ^{99m}Tc-MIBI可以被甲状旁腺腺瘤、增生性甲状旁腺、正常甲状腺组织和甲状腺腺瘤内的线粒体摄取；但甲状腺的放射性随时间而下降。^{99m}Tc-MIBI不被功能正常的甲状旁腺组织所摄取。
- 上述同一示踪剂用于核心脏病学，也可被恶性肿瘤所摄取，尤其是乳腺癌和肺癌。

INDICATIONS

Parathyroid adenoma

适应证

甲状旁腺腺瘤

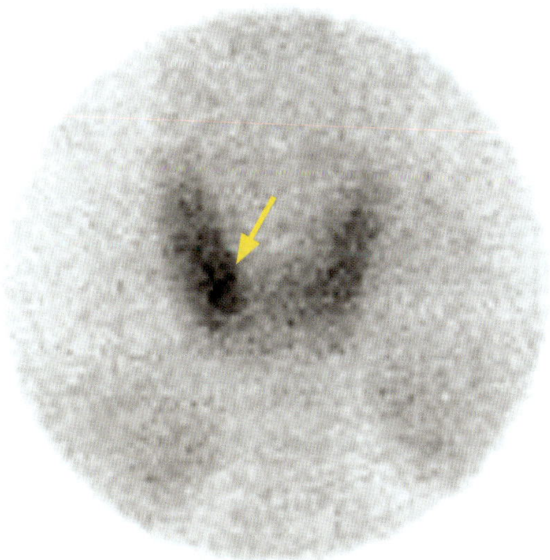

Early anterior pinhole image of the thyroid after the administration of 5 mCi Tc-99m sestamibi shows diffuse uptake throughout the thyroid, with a focal area of increased uptake (arrow) in the lower pole of the right lobe.
静脉注射5mCi ^{99m}Tc-MIBI后，早期前位针孔图像显示整个甲状腺呈弥漫性放射性摄取，其中右叶下极见局灶性放射性浓聚(黄箭)。

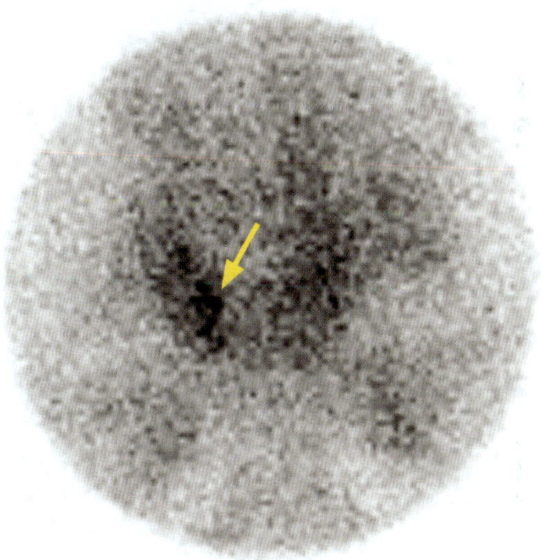

Delayed anterior pinhole image shows interval partial washout of Tc-99m sestamibi. There is a persistent focus of radiotracer uptake (arrow) in the right lower pole. A right inferior parathyroid adenoma was confirmed at surgery.
延迟前位针孔图像示甲状腺内^{99m}Tc-MIBI部分洗脱。甲状腺右叶下极见一个局部持续放射性浓聚(黄箭)。手术确诊右下甲状旁腺腺瘤。

- Dual-phase (early and delayed) imaging with Tc-99m sestamibi can localize a suspected parathyroid adenoma in a patient with elevated parathyroid hormone.
- A parathyroid adenoma shows increased uptake on early images and persistent retained activity on delayed images. In contrast, a thyroid adenoma will also initially show increased uptake but will then wash out on delayed images.
- Parathyroid tissue does *not* take up Tc-99m pertechnetate, which can be administered in indeterminate cases.
- SPECT/CT imaging is also frequently performed to provide more precise localization of uptake to aid in presurgical planning.

- ^{99m}Tc-MIBI双相(早期和延迟)显像可以对甲状旁腺素升高，并怀疑有甲状旁腺腺瘤的患者进行定位。
- 甲状旁腺腺瘤在早期图像中表现为放射性摄取增高，而在延迟图像中呈持续性放射性滞留。相比之下，甲状腺腺瘤早期也摄取增高，但在延迟图像中出现洗脱。
- $^{99m}TcO_4$不被甲状旁腺组织摄取，可用于无法确定的病例。
- SPECT/CT显像常用于摄取病灶的精确定位，以帮助制订外科术前计划。

(翻译　李蓓蕾)

GASTROINTESTINAL

胃肠道

LIVER–SPLEEN IMAGING

肝-脾显像

Radiotracer: Tc-99m sulfur colloid

- Sulfur colloid is taken up by reticuloendothelial cells, which are found in the liver, spleen, and bone marrow. Sulfur colloid is also taken up by Kupffer cells in the liver. Hepatic Kupffer cells make up only approximately 10% of the liver mass.
- 80–90% of sulfur colloid particles are taken up by the liver. Most of the remainder is taken up by the spleen, and a small amount taken up in the bone marrow. The bone marrow is not normally seen at typical windowing levels.
- Although Tc-99m has a physical half-life of 6 hours, sulfur colloid is rapidly cleared with a biologic half-life of 2–3 minutes.

放射性示踪剂：^{99m}Tc-硫胶体

- 硫胶体被肝、脾和骨髓中的网状内皮细胞摄取。硫胶体同样也被肝脏中的库普弗细胞摄取。肝脏的库普弗细胞占肝脏重量的10%。
- 80%~90%的硫胶体颗粒被肝脏摄取。其余大部分被脾摄取，少量被骨髓摄取。骨髓通常不能用常规的窗位水平显示。
- 尽管^{99m}Tc的物理半衰期是6小时，但是硫胶体迅速被清除，其生物半衰期为2~3分钟。

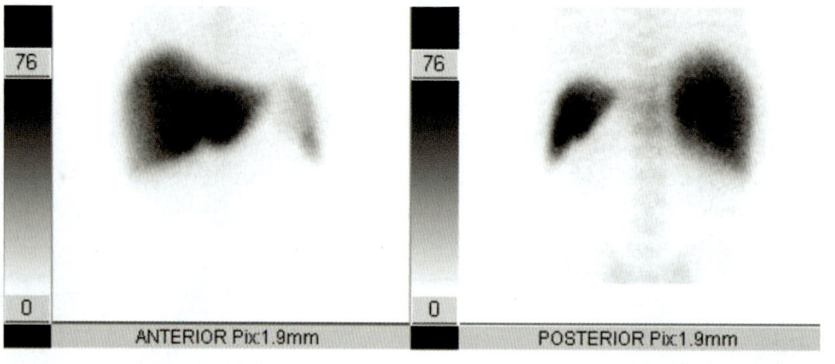

Normal liver-spleen scan following administration of 4.2 mCi Tc-99m sulfur colloid shows homogeneous uptake in the liver and spleen. Note splenic uptake is slightly lower in intensity than the liver. Bone marrow uptake is faint.

正常肝-脾显像：静脉注射4.2mCi ^{99m}Tc-硫胶体后显示肝、脾内硫胶体颗粒均匀摄取。注意，脾摄取强度稍低于肝脏，骨髓摄取轻微。

Focal decreased hepatic uptake on sulfur colloid scan

- The most common cause of a photopenic defect (complete absence of radiotracer) is a hepatic cyst. It may be difficult to distinguish focal *decreased* uptake from a *photopenic* defect if the lesion is small.
- Most hepatic masses cause focal decreased radiocolloid uptake, including hepatocellular carcinoma (HCC), adenoma, and abscess. Focal decreased uptake should raise concern for HCC in a patient with any risk factors for HCC such as cirrhosis or chronic hepatitis.

肝脏局部硫胶体摄取减低

- 最常见的放射性缺损(完全缺乏放射性示踪剂)原因为肝囊肿。如果病灶小，则很难区分局部摄取减低或放射性缺损。
- 大多数肝脏占位会引起局灶性放射性硫胶体摄取减低，如肝细胞癌(HCC)、腺瘤和脓肿。任何有HCC危险因素的患者，如肝硬化、慢性肝炎，若发现肝脏有局灶性放射性硫胶体摄取减低，则应怀疑有HCC。

Focal increased hepatic uptake on sulfur colloid scan

- Focal nodular hyperplasia, discussed below, may hyperconcentrate radiocolloid.
- A regenerating nodule in a cirrhotic liver can cause focal increased radiocolloid uptake.
- Budd-Chiari syndrome, or hepatic vein thrombosis, can lead to increased uptake in the caudate lobe in the later stage of disease.

肝脏局部硫胶体摄取增高

- 局灶性结节增生可能增加摄取放射性硫胶体，下文将进行讨论。
- 肝硬化时的再生结节可以引起肝脏局部放射性胶体摄取增高。
- 布-加综合征或肝静脉血栓形成可在疾病的后期导致尾状叶摄取增高。

Colloid shift

- Colloid shift is increased sulfur colloid accumulation within the spleen and bone marrow. It suggests liver dysfunction, most commonly due to cirrhosis.

胶体转移

- 胶体转移是指硫胶体在脾和骨髓中摄取增加。它提示有肝脏功能异常，最常见的原因是肝硬化。

Diffuse pulmonary uptake

- Diffuse pulmonary uptake on a sulfur colloid scan is nonspecific, and can be seen in:

Cirrhosis.
COPD with superimposed infection.
Langerhans cell histiocytosis.
High serum aluminum (either due to antacids or excess aluminum in the colloid preparation).

弥漫性肺摄取增高

- 肺弥漫性摄取硫胶体为非特异性的征象，可见于：

肝硬化。
慢性阻塞性肺疾病伴感染。
朗格汉斯细胞组织细胞增生症。
高铝血症(胶体制备时使用抗酸剂或过量的铝)。

Focal nodular hyperplasia (FNH)

- Focal nodular hyperplasia (FNH) is a benign liver mass that can have a variable appearance on a sulfur colloid scan. Most commonly, FNH will be indistinguishable from background liver due to Kupffer cells within the FNH. FNH may also have increased uptake due to a combination of hypervascularity and Kupffer sulfur colloid uptake. In approximately 1/3 of cases there is insufficient colloid concentration and FNH may appear as a photopenic defect.
- In contrast to FNH, a hepatic adenoma does not contain Kupffer cells and will be consistently photopenic.
- An adjunct or alternative to sulfur colloid scan is a HIDA scan. FNH contains biliary ductules so it should demonstrate radiotracer uptake on a HIDA scan.

局灶性结节增生(FNH)

- 局灶性结节增生(FNH)是一种良性的肝脏肿块，在放射性硫胶体显像中有多种表现。FNH通常无法与肝脏实质进行区别，因为FNH内有库普弗细胞。FNH也可因为血供增加和库普弗细胞摄取硫胶体的共同作用而表现为放射性摄取增高。约1/3的病例没有聚集足够的硫胶体而使FNH成为一个放射性缺损区。
- 与FNH相比，肝腺瘤不含库普弗细胞，因而总表现为放射性缺损区。
- 一种可以补充或替代硫胶体的显像剂为HIDA。FNH含有胆管因而HIDA扫描应显示有放射性示踪剂摄取。

Intrapancreatic splenic tissue

- The presence of an intrapancreatic splenule can be confirmed by sulfur colloid scan in indeterminate cases, where the suspected tissue will show uptake. A Tc-99m damaged red cell study can also be performed.

胰腺内异位副脾

- 胰腺内副脾不确定的病例可以通过硫胶体扫描进行确认，因脾组织摄取硫胶体。也可以使用^{99m}Tc标记的变性红细胞显像进行诊断。

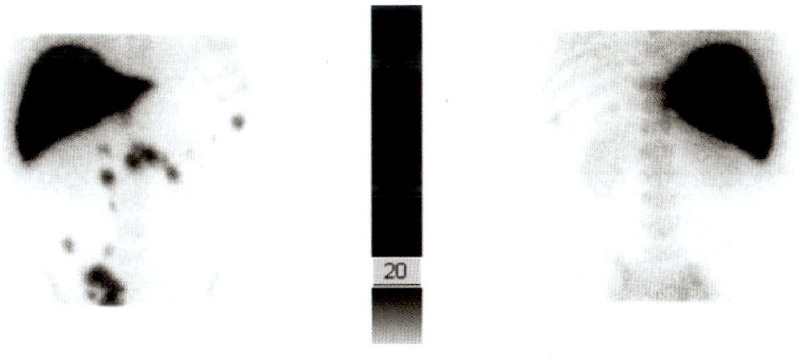

Splenosis: Liver-spleen scan (5.5 mCi Tc-99m sulfur colloid administered) of a patient with history of splenectomy following trauma.

Anterior and posterior images show scattered focal uptake in the abdomen correlating to intraperitoneal soft tissue masses on SPECT/CT (not shown), consistent with splenosis.

异位脾：患者既往有外伤后脾切除术史，静脉注射5.5mCi ^{99m}Tc-硫胶体后进行肝-脾扫描。前位和后位图像显示腹腔内散在局灶性摄取，相应SPECT/CT图像(未展示)见腹腔内软组织结节，符合异位脾的诊断。

ESOPHAGEAL AND GASTRIC MOTILITY

Radiotracer: Tc-99m sulfur colloid or DTPA

- Sulfur colloid or DTPA are mixed with food and ingested to assess gastroesophageal motility.

Esophageal transit

- After a 6-hour or overnight fast, patient is positioned supine and instructed to

食管和胃动力学

放射性示踪剂：^{99m}Tc-硫胶体或DTPA

- 硫胶体或DTPA与食物混合，摄入后评估胃食管运动。

食管通过

- 禁食6小时或隔夜禁食后，患者仰卧并按指示

swallow 10 mL water containing Tc-99m sulfur colloid or DTPA, then attempt dry swallows to clear normal residual activity in the esophagus. This process may be repeated several times.

- Normal esophageal transit time for water is 5–11 seconds, with more than 90% of peak activity clearing the esophagus after 15 seconds. Reduced transit time is seen in patients with scleroderma and achalasia.

Gastroesophageal reflux

- Scintigraphy for gastroesophageal reflux is most commonly performed in neonates. After an overnight fast, the infant is fed formula or milk mixed with Tc-99m sulfur colloid. Sequential images are acquired to assess for reflux of gastric content into the esophagus. Delayed images of the lungs can be obtained to evaluate for aspiration.
- A similar protocol is used for older children and adults, but using orange juice.

Salivagram for aspiration

- Salivagram is more sensitive in detecting aspiration in pediatric patients compared to reflux scintigraphy. A drop of Tc-99m sulfur colloid is placed on the patient's tongue base or sublingual region to allow mixture with saliva. Rapid images are then obtained to assess for activity in the bronchi and lungs.

Gastric emptying

吞咽10mL含有^{99m}Tc-硫胶体或DTPA的水，然后进行干咽以清除食管中残留的放射性。这个过程可以重复数次。

- 水通过食管的正常时间为5~11秒，90%以上的峰值放射性在15秒后被清除出食管。硬皮病和贲门失弛缓症患者的通过时间缩短。

胃食管反流

- 胃食管反流闪烁显像最常用于新生儿。隔夜禁食后，给婴儿喂^{99m}Tc-硫胶体混合的配方奶或牛奶。须采集系列图像以评估胃内容物反流进入食管。肺部延迟显像可用于评估误吸。
- 类似的方法可以用于年龄较大的儿童和成人，但改用橙汁。

唾液图评估肺吸入

- 唾液图较食管反流显像对检测儿童患者的肺吸入更为敏感。将一滴^{99m}Tc-硫胶体滴在患者的舌根或舌下区域，使其与唾液混合。进行快速显像以评估支气管和肺内的放射性。

胃排空

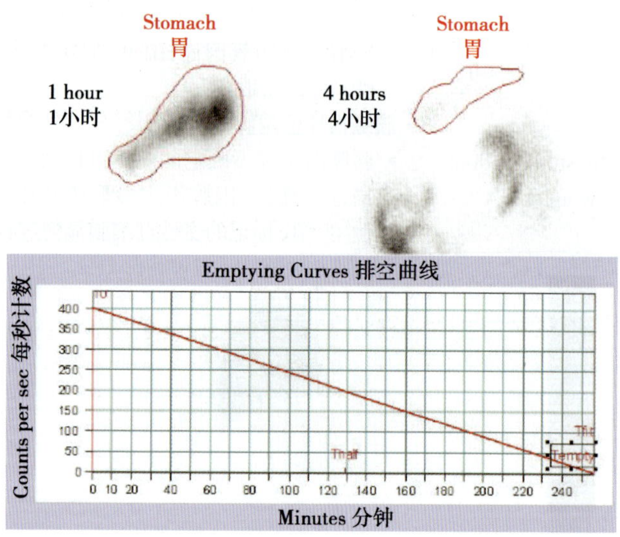

Normal gastric emptying scan:
1 mCi Tc-99m sulfur colloid mixed in egg whites was administered orally with white bread, jelly and water. Patient consumed 100% of the solid portion. Sample static images at 1 hour and 4 hours show normal gastric retention (1% at 4 hours). The emptying curve shows counts graphed to time.

正常胃排空显像：
将1mCi的^{99m}Tc-硫胶体与蛋清混合，然后与面包、果冻和水一起吞服。患者吃下了100%的固体食物。1小时和4小时的静态图像显示正常的胃潴留(4小时为1%)。排空曲线显示按时间绘制的放射性计数。

- After a 6-hour or overnight fast, the patient is given a standardized solid meal containing up to 1 mCi Tc-99m sulfur colloid mixed in scrambled egg whites, along with toast, jam and water. Patient should ingest the entire meal within 10 minutes. Subsequent images of the stomach are then acquired every 60 minutes up to 4 hours.
- Normal residual activity in the stomach at 4 hours is<10%.
- An alternative liquid phase gastric emptying study can be performed using water containing Tc-99m DTPA, with a shorter imaging time because liquids normally empty more rapidly.

- 在6小时或隔夜禁食后给患者提供标准固体餐，包括最多1mCi的^{99m}Tc-硫胶体与蛋清混合，随后混合在吐司、果酱和水中。患者应在10分钟内吃完所提供的标准餐。然后每60分钟获取一次胃的图像，持续4小时。
- 正常4小时的胃残留活性<10%。
- 另一种液相胃排空试验可以使用含有^{99m}Tc-DTPA的水，因液体通常排空更快而成像时间较短。

MECKEL IMAGING

Radiotracer: Tc-99m pertechnetate

- Technetium-99m pertechnetate localizes to gastric mucosa.

Meckel diverticulum

- Meckel diverticulum is a remnant of the embryological omphalomesenteric

梅克尔显像

放射性示踪剂：^{99m}Tc高锝酸盐($^{99m}TcO_4$)

- $^{99m}TcO_4$定位胃黏膜。

梅克尔憩室

- 梅克尔憩室是胚胎卵黄管的残留物，最常见

duct, most commonly located in the distal ileum. Approximately 10–60% of Meckel diverticula contain ectopic gastric mucosa, which may result in mucosal damage and GI bleeding.

于回肠末端。10%~60%的梅克尔憩室中有异位胃黏膜，可能导致肠黏膜损伤和消化道出血。

- A positive Meckel scan demonstrates a focal area of increased activity, typically in the right lower quadrant. A lateral view is often helpful to ensure that activity is anterior and not associated with the ureter.
- Other causes of uptake in the right lower quadrant include appendicitis and intussusception that can cause more diffuse, regional increased activity due to hyperemia.
- Sensitivity of Meckel scan can be increased by a number of medications:

  Pentagastrin increases uptake of pertechnetate by gastric mucosa.

  H_2 blockers such as cimetidine block release of pertechnetate by the mucosal cells.

  Glucagon decreases intestinal peristalsis, thereby slows washout of pertechnetate from the diverticulum.

- 阳性梅克尔憩室显像可见局灶性摄取增高，通常在右下腹。侧位图像有助于确定放射性位于前方，而与输尿管无关。
- 其他可能引起右下腹摄取的原因包括阑尾炎和肠套叠，两者都可以因为充血而引起较为弥漫的区域性放射性摄取增高。
- 提高梅克尔显像的灵敏度可以使用多种药物：

  五肽胃泌素增加胃黏膜对高锝酸盐的吸收。

  H_2受体拮抗剂，如西咪替丁阻断黏膜细胞释放高锝酸盐。

  胰高血糖素降低肠道蠕动，从而减缓高锝酸盐从憩室中洗脱。

Gastrointestinal Bleeding

消化道出血

Radiotracer: Tc-99m labeled RBCs

- Technetium-99m labeled red blood cells are prepared in-vitro by mixing 1–3 mL of anticoagulated blood with stannous chloride and an oxidizing agent; Tc-99m is then added. The labeling efficiency is 95%. The labeling procedure takes more than 20 minutes.

  An in-vivo technique provides much noisier images due to worse labeling efficiency and resultant free pertechnetate, and is therefore uncommonly performed.

- Alternatively, Tc-99m sulfur colloid can be used. Sulfur colloid does not require significant preparation time, but has rapid blood clearance with a vascular half-life of 2–3 minutes.

放射性示踪剂：^{99m}Tc标记红细胞(^{99m}Tc-RBC)

- ^{99m}Tc-标记红细胞是在体外制备的，将1~3mL抗凝血液与氯化亚锡和氧化剂混合。之后再加入^{99m}Tc。标记有效率为95%。标记过程需要20分钟以上。

  体内标记技术的图像噪声明显，这是因为标记率低而产生过多游离的高锝酸盐，所以不经常使用。

- 另一种替代方法是使用^{99m}Tc-硫胶体。硫胶体制备不需要很长时间，但在血液中被迅速清除，半衰期仅2~3分钟。

Acute GI bleed

- A tagged red blood cell study can be used to identify patients who may be suitable for angiography versus those who are not. Bleeding rates as low as 0.05–0.1 mL/min can be detected, compared to 1 mL/min for angiography.
- A positive study shows an initial focus of activity that changes shape or position over time due to antegrade or retrograde peristalsis of intraluminal blood.

急性消化道出血

- 标记红细胞显像可用于确定患者是否适合进行血管造影。标记红细胞显像能探测到的出血速率仅为0.05~0.10mL/min，而血管造影则需要出血速率达到1mL/min。
- 阳性显像可见初始局部放射性聚集区，其形态和位置将随时间而发生变化，这是肠腔内积血发生顺行或逆行蠕动的结果。

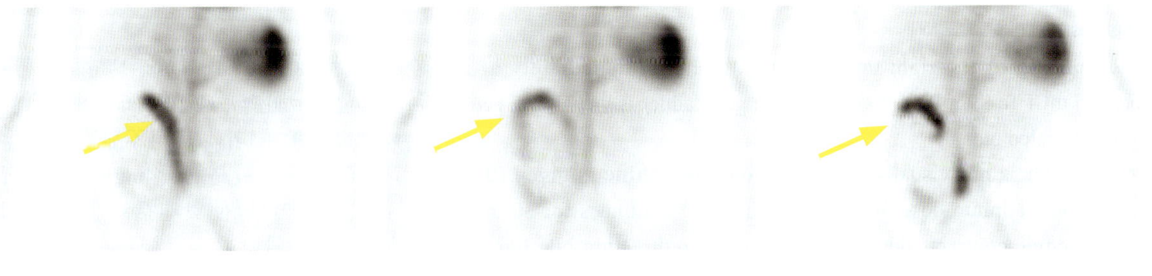

GI bleed: Sequential images of the lower abdomen on Tc-99m tagged RBC study show a focus of radiotracer uptake in the right lower quadrant, in the expected distribution of the superior mesenteric artery, which changes shape and position over time (arrows).

消化道出血：下腹部^{99m}Tc-RBC连续显像见右下腹一个放射性示踪剂浓聚，位于肠系膜上动脉的供血区域，其形状与位置随时间而变化(黄箭)。

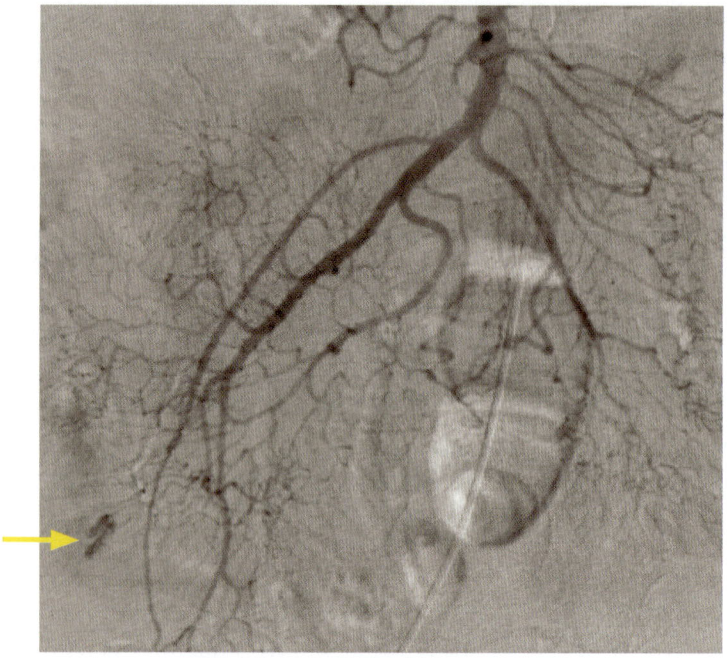

Superior mesenteric artery angiogram in the same patient performed within one hour of the above tagged RBC study shows a focus of contrast extravasation in a distal ileocolic branch (arrow).

This patient was treated with coil embolization of the distal ileocolic branch artery.

同一名患者^{99m}Tc-RBC显像后1小时内的肠系膜上动脉造影显示远端回结肠分支有局灶性造影剂外渗(黄箭)。

对该患者的远端回结肠分支用弹簧钢圈进行栓塞治疗。

HEPATOBILIARY IMAGING (HIDA)

Radiotracers: Tc-99m IDA agents

- Tc-99m-iminodiacetic acid (IDA) analogs are used to image the biliary system. Regardless of the tracer, the test is typically called a "HIDA" scan.
- **Disofenin** allows visualization of the biliary system with bilirubin levels as high as 20 mg/dL and has 90% hepatic uptake. **Mebrofenin** allows visualization of the biliary system with bilirubin levels as high as 30 mg/dL and has an even higher 98% hepatic uptake. Both are actively transported into hepatocytes but are not conjugated.
- Critical organ is the gallbladder wall.

HIDA protocol

- Patient should be NPO for 6 hours prior, but must have eaten within 24 hours. If the patient has been NPO for >24 hours, **cholecystokinin** (CCK; dose 0.02 μg/kg, given as slow infusion) is given to empty the gallbladder before radiotracer is administered.

  CCK must be administered slowly or the patient may experience an exacerbation of their symptoms.
- Dynamic imaging of the right upper quadrant begins immediately after injection of 5 mCi Tc-99m IDA. As soon as the gallbladder is visualized, acute cholecystitis is ruled out.
- If the gallbladder is not visualized by one hour, **morphine** is given (0.04 mg/kg, up to a maximum dose of 4 mg) and imaging continues for 30 more minutes. Morphine contracts the sphincter of Oddi, redirecting bile into the cystic duct.

  Morphine should only be given if tracer is visualized in the small bowel, otherwise there is the theoretical risk of worsening a potential common bile duct obstruction. However, nonvisualization of tracer in the small bowel is not specific for common bile duct obstruction.
- If the patient has a morphine allergy, an alternative is to image for a total of 4 hours.

肝胆显像(HIDA)

放射性示踪剂：^{99m}Tc-IDA类制剂

- ^{99m}Tc-亚氨基乙酰乙酸(IDA)的衍生物可用于胆道显像。无论是具体用哪一种制剂，该项检查通常被称为"HIDA"显像。
- **地索苯宁**即便在胆红素水平高达20mg/dL的时候仍有90%被肝脏摄取。**甲溴菲宁**在胆红素水平高达30mg/dL的时候有98%以上被肝脏摄取。两种制剂均通过主动运转进入肝细胞，但不被结合。
- 靶器官是胆囊壁。

HIDA显像检查方法

- 检查前患者应禁食6小时，但不能超过24小时。如果患者禁食超过24小时，可以在注射示踪剂前使用胆囊收缩素(CCK)(0.02μg/kg，缓慢静脉推注)以排空胆囊。

  CCK必须缓慢注入，否则可能使患者的症状加重。
- 注射5mCi的^{99m}**Tc**-IDA后应立即进行右上腹动态显像。胆囊一旦显影，即可排除急性胆囊炎。
- 如果胆囊在1小时后仍不显影，可以注射**吗啡**(0.04mg/kg，最高剂量4mg)，并延长显像30分钟。吗啡可以使奥迪括约肌收缩，使胆汁逆流入胆囊管。

  吗啡只有当小肠内出现示踪剂的时候方可使用，否则从理论上讲，吗啡可能会加重胆总管梗阻。要注意，小肠内没有出现示踪剂并不是胆总管梗阻的特异表现。
- 如果患者对吗啡过敏，可以选择4小时延长显像。

Normal HIDA scan

- In a normal HIDA scan, the liver is visible by 5 minutes.
- The gallbladder is typically seen by 15 minutes due to radiotracer flow into the cystic duct.
- Tracer should be seen in the small bowel to ensure a patent common bile duct.
- Small amount of bile reflux into the stomach can be a normal finding.

正常HIDA扫描

- 正常的HIDA扫描，肝脏应该在5分钟左右显影。
- 胆囊由于显像剂流入胆囊管而通常在15分钟时显影。
- 小肠内出现示踪剂代表胆总管通畅。
- 少量示踪剂反流入胃内属于正常显像。

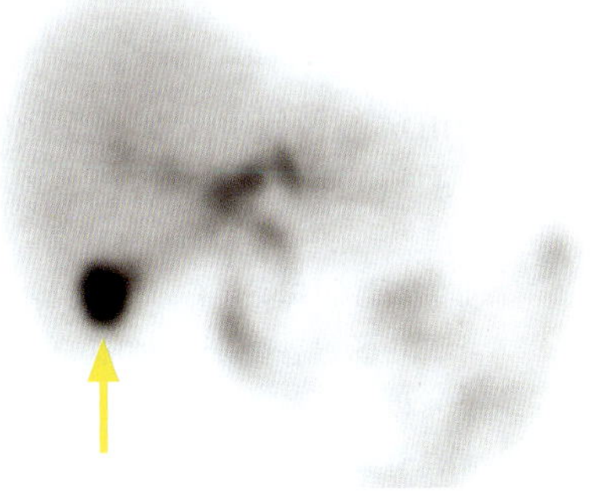

Single image from a HIDA scan 15 minutes after 4.1 mCi Tc-99m disofenin administered shows normal visualization of the liver, gallbladder (arrow), and small bowel.
注射4.1mCi的^{99m}Tc-HIDA后15分钟时的单帧静态图像可见正常肝脏、胆囊(黄箭)和小肠显影。

Acute cholecystitis

- Almost all patients with acute cholecystitis have cystic duct obstruction.
- Nonvisualization of the gallbladder after 90 minutes of imaging and morphine augmentation is approximately 86–98% sensitive for the diagnosis of acute cholecystitis, with a false-positive rate of approximately 6%, most commonly due to pancreatitis and biliary stasis.
- The *rim sign* describes increased hepatic activity surrounding the gallbladder fossa, thought to be due to hyperemia and is an ancillary finding of acute cholecystitis.
- The *cystic duct sign* describes a small focus of activity in the cystic duct just proximal to the site of obstruction.

急性胆囊炎

- 几乎所有急性胆囊炎的患者都有胆囊管梗阻。
- 胆囊在90分钟及吗啡增强后仍未显影时，其诊断急性胆囊炎的灵敏度为86%~98%，假阳性率约为6%，最常见的原因是胰腺炎和胆汁淤积。
- 环征是指胆囊窝周围出现肝脏放射性活性增加，被认为是充血所致，是急性胆囊炎的辅助征象。
- 胆囊管征是指胆囊管内梗阻近端一处小的局部放射性浓聚。

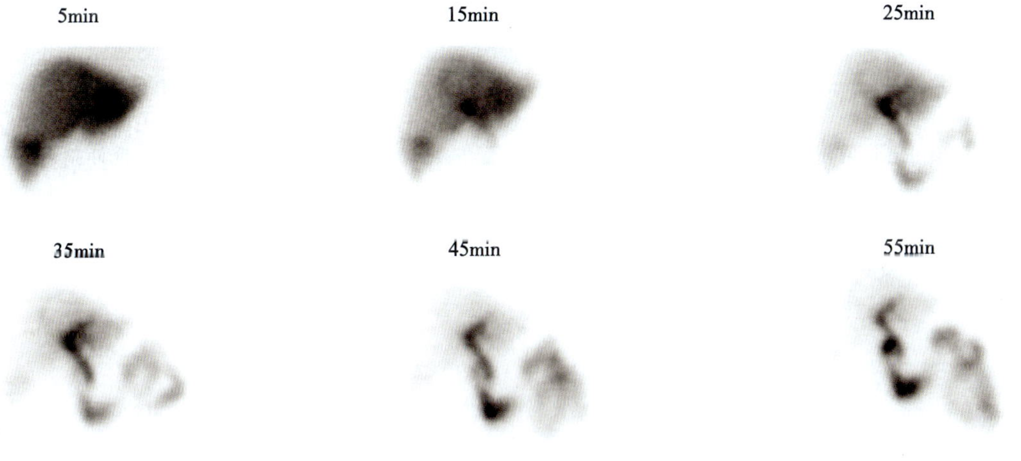

Acute cholecystitis: Sequential images from a HIDA scan with 3.87 mCi Tc-99m disofenin administered shows prompt visualization of the liver. The small bowel is visualized by 25 minutes. There is no visualization of the gallbladder during the course of the exam. The patient had a morphine allergy so 4-hour delayed images were obtained instead (not shown), which also do not demonstrate the gallbladder.
急性胆囊炎：静脉注射3.87mCi的^{99m}Tc-地索苯宁后连续HIDA影像可见肝脏迅速显影。小肠在25分钟时显影。胆囊在整个显像过程中始终未见显影。患者对吗啡过敏，因而进行了4小时延迟显像(未展示)，胆囊依旧未见显示。

- False positive HIDA (gallbladder nonvisualization *without* acute cholecystitis) can be due to:

Recent meal (within 4 hours) or prolonged fasting (greater than 24 hours).	Pancreatitis.
Administration of CCK *immediately* prior to the exam, which can cause persistent sphincter of Oddi relaxation.	Severe illness.
Total parenteral nutrition.	Chronic cholecystitis.
	Cholangiocarcinoma of the cystic duct (very rare).

- False negative HIDA (gallbladder visualization *with* acute cholecystitis) is very rare and can be due to:

Acalculous cholecystitis with a patent cystic duct.
Duodenal diverticulum simulating the gallbladder; however, a lateral view would differentiate.
Choledochal cyst simulating the gallbladder.
Right extrarenal pelvis in jaundiced patients with increased renal excretion of tracer.

Chronic cholecystitis

- Chronic cholecystitis is long-standing gallbladder inflammation causing loss of normal gallbladder function, predisposing to formation of stones.
- Chronic cholecystitis may be a cause of chronic recurrent abdominal pain.
- Diagnosis can be difficult as there is no single pattern that is pathognomonic of chronic cholecystitis based on HIDA. In fact, most cases of chronic cholecystitis have a normal HIDA.
- A low **gallbladder ejection fraction** (GBEF) is thought to be suggestive of chronic cholecystitis. To measure the ejection fraction, pre-and post-CCK injection gallbladder counts are compared. A GBEF <35% suggests chronic cholecystitis, although the reliability of this finding is controversial as ejection fraction is dependent on the rate of CCK injection and standard infusion protocols have not been determined.

Biliary obstruction

- Acute high-grade obstruction of the common bile duct can result in the *liver scan sign*, where there is uptake in the liver but no visualization of the biliary tree or small bowel. Intrahepatic cholestasis or hepatitis can have a similar appearance.
- Delayed clearance of activity from the common bile duct suggests partial obstruction.

Hepatic dysfunction

- HIDA显像假阳性(胆囊未显影但无急性胆囊炎)的原因有：

刚刚进食(4小时内)或禁食时间过长(超过24小时)。	胰腺炎。
静脉注射CCK后*立即*进行显像检查，CCK可以引起奥迪括约肌持续松弛。	危重疾病。
全胃肠外营养。	慢性胆囊炎。
	胆囊管胆管癌(罕见)。

- HIDA显像假阴性(胆囊显影但有急性胆囊炎)罕见，可能的原因有：

非结石性胆囊炎伴有通畅的胆囊管。
十二指肠憩室被误认为胆囊，但这种情况用侧位图像可以进行鉴别。
胆总管囊肿被误认为胆囊。
黄疸患者右侧肾外型肾盂内肾脏排泄的示踪剂积聚。

慢性胆囊炎

- 慢性胆囊炎是胆囊长期炎症而失去正常功能，易形成结石。
- 慢性胆囊炎可能是腹部慢性反复疼痛的原因。
- 诊断有时会很困难，因为HIDA显像时没有一个具有慢性胆囊炎的特异性征象。实际上大多数慢性胆囊炎的HIDA显像都为正常。
- 若**胆囊排胆分数**(GBEF)降低，则提示有慢性胆囊炎。测定排胆分数时，需要比较注射CCK前后的胆囊放射性计数。GBEF<35%提示慢性胆囊炎，但这个值的可靠性有争议，因为该排胆分数受到CCK注射速度的影响，目前仍没有标准的注射规范。

胆道梗阻

- 急性的严重胆总管梗阻可导致*肝脏扫描征*，即肝脏有摄取，但看不到胆道分支或小肠显影。肝内胆汁淤积或肝炎可能有相似的表现。
- 胆总管显像剂延迟清除提示胆道部分梗阻。

肝功能异常

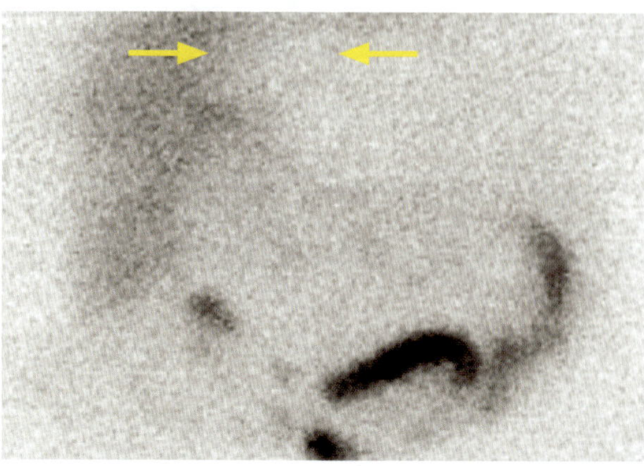

Severe hepatic dysfunction in a patient with cholangiocarcinoma:
Single image from a HIDA obtained 30 minutes after 6.1 mCi Tc-99m disofenin administered shows a large amount of background and blood pool uptake with minimal tracer in the liver. A large photopenic defect in the left lobe of the liver (arrows) corresponds to the patient's cholangiocarcinoma. There is small bowel tracer excretion.

胆管细胞癌合并严重肝功能异常的患者：
静脉注射6.1mCi的^{99m}Tc-地索苯宁后在30分钟时获取的单幅HIDA图像显示本底和血池内有大量放射性摄取，肝内少量放射性分布。肝左叶见大片放射性缺损(黄箭)，为患者胆管细胞癌的相应位置。可见示踪剂排泄到小肠内。

- Since the IDA tracers are actively transported into hepatocytes and then secreted into the bile, severe hepatic dysfunction will cause very poor hepatic uptake and blood pool clearance will be delayed.
- Since functioning hepatocytes are necessary to extract the tracer, a hepatic mass will appear as a focal photopenic defect.

Biliary leak

- IDA类显像剂通过主动转运进入肝细胞内，之后分泌进入胆管，因此，若有严重肝功能损伤会引起肝脏摄取明显减低，血池清除延迟。
- 由于摄取示踪剂依赖有功能的肝细胞，所以肝脏肿块会引起局灶性放射性缺损。

胆漏

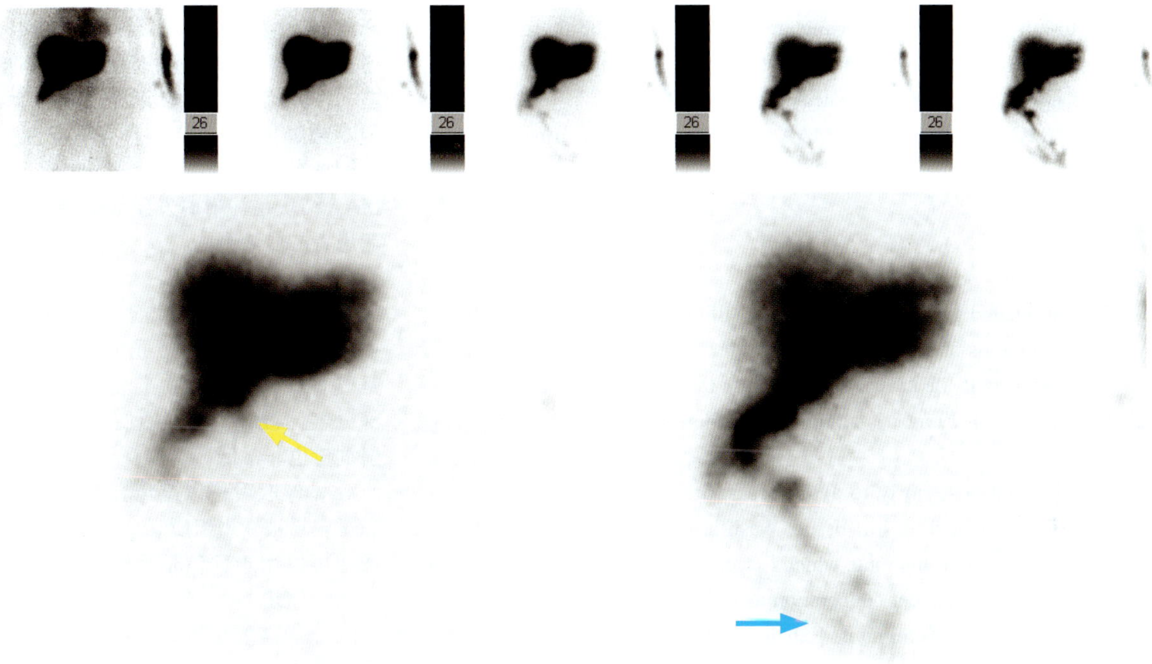

Bile leak: Sequential images (top row) and two enlarged still images (bottom two images) from a HIDA scan with 5.4 mCi Tc-99m disofenin administered to a patient with right upper quadrant pain status post cholecystectomy shows tracer accumulating in the gallbladder fossa (yellow arrow) and pooling in the right paracolic gutter (blue arrow). The gallbladder is surgically absent. The leak was thought to arise from the cystic duct stump.

胆漏：一名胆囊切除术后右上腹痛患者在静脉注射5.4mCi的^{99m}Tc-地索苯宁后进行HIDA显像，连续影像(上排)和局部放大图像(下排2图)见示踪剂先积聚于胆囊窝(黄箭)，之后向右侧结肠旁沟汇集(蓝箭)。手术后胆囊缺如。胆漏考虑源于胆囊管残端。

- A HIDA scan is an accurate method to assess for the presence of a biliary leak. Imaging can be performed in the right lateral decubitus position to promote dependent pooling of bile.

- HIDA显像是评估胆漏的准确方法。图像采集时可以选择右侧卧位以促进胆汁积聚在右侧结肠旁沟。

（翻译　李蓓蕾）

PULMONARY

肺

RADIOTRACERS

放射性示踪剂

Tc-99m MAA (perfusion)

- Technetium-99m macro-aggregated albumin (MAA) is a particulate radiopharmaceutical that lodges in the pulmonary capillary bed and can therefore be used to evaluate pulmonary perfusion. Most particles are between 10–30 µm in size.
- Typically 3–5 mCi Tc-99m MAA are administered intravenously, comprising between 200,000 and 600,000 particles. Particles begin to break down in approximately 30 minutes. In children, pregnant patients, patients with mild pulmonary hypertension, and patients with a known right-to-left shunt, the dose

^{99m}Tc-大颗粒聚合人血清白蛋白(灌注显像)

- ^{99m}Tc-大颗粒聚合人血清白蛋白(MAA)是一种颗粒状的放射性药物，它可以嵌顿在肺毛细血管床而用于评估肺灌注。大多数颗粒的大小为10~30µm。
- ^{99m}Tc-MAA通常从静脉给予3~5mCi，含有200 000~600 000个颗粒。颗粒约在注射后30分钟开始解体。对儿童、孕妇、中度肺动脉高压和已经确诊的右向左分流的患者，剂量可

can be halved to approximately 100,000 particles.

- A relative contraindication to MAA is severe pulmonary hypertension, as obstruction of even a few pulmonary capillaries can cause clinical worsening.
- A **right-to-left shunt** causes immediate renal and brain uptake after intravenous injection. A Tc-99m MAA study may be able to quantify the shunt fraction in these patients. Note that renal uptake can also be seen if free pertechnetate is present, but evaluation of the head and neck can differentiate free pertechnetate from a right-to-left shunt. Free pertechnetate is taken up by the thyroid, but not the brain. A right-to-left shunt, in contrast, demonstrates immediate brain uptake and no significant uptake in the neck.
- Clumping of MAA can be seen when MAA is inadvertently drawn back into injection syringe, causing coagulation with the patient's blood.

减少至100 000个左右的颗粒。

- MAA的相对禁忌证是严重的肺动脉高压，因为即使一小部分肺毛细血管阻塞也会引起临床恶化。
- **右向左分流**会在静脉注射后立即有肾脏和脑的摄取。在该类患者中，^{99m}Tc-MAA显像可以用来计算分流指数。需要注意，如果存在游离的高锝酸，也可以看到肾脏有摄取，但是通过评估头部和颈部可以区分游离高锝酸盐和右向左分流。游离高锝酸盐会被甲状腺摄取，但不被脑摄取。相反，存在右向左分流时脑立即显影，但颈部没有显著显影。
- MAA结块是注射时发生注射器意外回抽，引起患者的血液凝固。

Xenon-133 (ventilation)

- Xenon-133 is an inhaled gas with a physical half-life of 5.3 days, which emits 81 keV gamma photons and is also a beta-emitter. The critical organ is the trachea. The biologic half-life is very short because the vast majority of the gas is exhaled. Although 10–20 mCi is administered, there is very little radiation exposure.
- Xenon-133 is imaged posteriorly to avoid breast artifacts, as the relatively low keV is easily attenuated by soft tissue. Wash-in/washout imaging can be performed to evaluate for air trapping, which is seen in COPD.
- Xenon-133 requires good patient cooperation as the patient must breathe on a closed spirometer for several minutes. Exhaled xenon-133 must be carefully disposed of, either exhausted to the atmosphere or trapped in a charcoal trap until it decays. Xenon-133 must be administered in a negative pressure room to prevent accidental leakage.
- Because xenon-133 is soluble in fat, it can accumulate in the liver, particularly a fatty liver.

^{133}氙(Xe)(通气显像)

- ^{133}Xe是吸入性气体，物理半衰期为5.3天，发射出能量为81keV的γ光子及β射线。靶器官是气管。^{133}Xe的生物半衰期非常短，因为大部分气体被呼出。即使使用10~20mCi，其辐射剂量也非常低。
- ^{133}Xe显像取后位以避免乳腺伪影，因低能量光子容易被软组织所衰减。吸入-呼出联合显像法可以用于评估是否有气体滞留，这种情况见于COPD。
- ^{133}Xe显像需要患者有较好的配合度，患者必须在密闭的肺活量计上呼吸数分钟。呼出的^{133}Xe必须小心处理，应排放到大气中或收集在碳过滤器中直到衰变消失。必须在负压房间中使用，以免意外泄漏。
- 由于^{133}Xe溶于脂肪，它可以在肝脏中蓄积，尤其是脂肪肝。

Tc-99m DTPA (ventilation)

- Tc-99m DTPA is a technetium-labeled aerosol. Unlike Xenon-133, DTPA does not allow for dynamic wash-in/washout imaging. Once inhaled, the particles remain in place for approximately 45–60 minutes (20 minutes in smokers). 30 mCi is typically administered.
- Compared to xenon, Tc-99m DTPA has greater ease of use. Specific advantages include the ability to image in multiple projections, little requirement for patient cooperation, no need for exhaust systems, ability to use portably and be delivered through mechanical ventilation.
- Swallowed activity can be seen in the esophagus and stomach.

^{99m}Tc-DTPA(通气显像)

- ^{99m}Tc-DTPA是高锝酸盐标记的锝气溶胶。与^{133}Xe不同，DTPA不能用于动态吸入-呼出联合显像。一旦被吸入，颗粒将在吸入部位停留45~60分钟(吸烟者为20分钟)。常用剂量为30mCi。
- 与^{133}Xe比较，^{99m}Tc-DTPA使用上极为方便。最突出的优点是可以进行多体位显像，几乎不需要患者配合，不需要排气装置，可以搬动使用，并通过机械通气装置给药。
- 吞入放射性可以使食管和胃显影。

Clinical V/Q Scanning in the Era of CT Pulmonary Angiography

通气/灌注显像在CT肺动脉造影时代的临床作用

Diagnosis of pulmonary embolism in pregnancy

- Pulmonary embolism is the leading cause of death in pregnancy in the developed world, and diagnosis must be weighed against radiation exposure to the mother and the fetus.

诊断孕妇肺动脉栓塞

- 肺动脉栓塞是发达国家中孕妇死亡的主要原因，而诊断必须权衡对孕妇和胎儿所造成的辐射剂量。

CT pulmonary angiogram (CTPA): Maternal breast dose approximately 10–70 mGy (much greater than ACR mammography guidelines of 3 mGy/breast). Fetal dose 0.01–0.66 mGy.
V/Q scan: Maternal breast dose <1.5 mGy. Fetal dose 0.5–1.1 mGy (higher than CTPA but still considerably lower than the 100 mSv threshold for potential teratogenic effects).
Low-dose perfusion (Q) scan: Maternal breast dose 0.6 mGy. Fetal dose 0.1–0.2 mGy.

CT肺动脉造影(CTPA)：孕妇乳腺辐射剂量为10~70mGy(明显高于美国放射学会乳房显像指南提出的3mGy/乳房)。胎儿剂量为0.01~0.66mGy。
通气/灌注(V/Q)显像：孕妇乳腺辐射剂量<1.5mGy，胎儿剂量0.5~1.1mGy(高于CTPA，但仍远低于潜在致畸作用的100mSv阈值)。
低剂量灌注(Q)显像：孕妇乳腺辐射剂量为0.6mGy。胎儿剂量0.1~0.2mGy。

- In most cases, only perfusion scan is necessary and ventilation scan is not commonly performed. The administered dose of Tc-99m MAA is typically one-half of the standard dose, or approximately 100,000 particles.
- Diagnostic accuracy for PE has been shown to be equivalent between CTPA and Q scan.
- The primary advantage of CTPA is the demonstration of an alternative diagnosis not seen on plain radiographs approximately 5% of the time and a lower fetal dose, at the expense of increased breast radiation exposure.
- Nuclear medicine perfusion scan should be reserved for suspected pulmonary embolism in a pregnant patient with a normal chest radiograph, no history of asthma or COPD, and a negative duplex ultrasound of lower extremities. In clinical practice, CTPA is more readily available and often the prefered modality.

- 大多数病例只需要进行灌注显像，而通气显像并不常规进行。^{99m}Tc-MAA注射的放射剂量为常规剂量的一半，或颗粒数量约为100 000个。
- CTPA和灌注显像诊断PE的准确性相似。
- CTPA的主要优点是可以发现约5%在X线影像上没有观察到的其他疾病，以及仅有较低的胎儿辐射剂量，但其代价是增加了乳腺的辐射剂量。
- 核医学灌注显像适用于有可疑肺动脉栓塞但胸部X线影像正常，且缺乏哮喘或慢性阻塞性肺病病史，以及双下肢超声检查阴性的孕妇。在临床，CTPA随时可做，并且通常是首选的检查方法。

Diagnosis of Pulmonary Embolism with PIOPED II

PIOPED Ⅱ肺栓塞诊断标准

High probability: Specificity for pulmonary embolism 97%, positive predictive value 88%

高度可能性：诊断肺动脉栓塞的特异度为97%，阳性预测值为88%

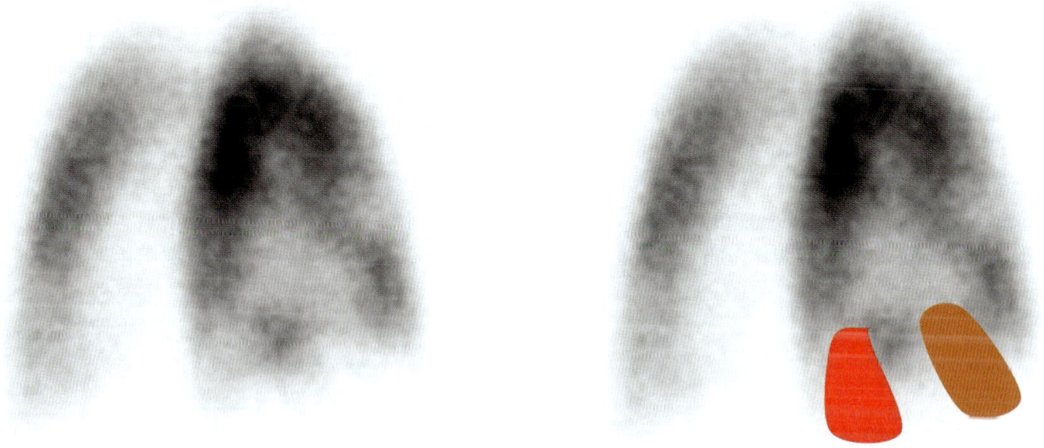

High probability for pulmonary embolism: RPO perfusion images (same image, without and with annotations) after 4.7 mCi Tc-99m MAA administered show two large segmental defects in the posterior basal (red) and anterior basal (brown) segments of the right lower lobe. The ventilation scan (not shown) was normal.
肺动脉栓塞高度可能性：静脉注射4.7mCi的^{99m}Tc-MAA后，右后斜位灌注图像(同一幅图像，右图加上了注释图标)两个大的节段性放射性缺损，一个在右肺下叶后基底段(红色)，另一个在前基底段(棕色)。通气显像正常(未展示)。

- Two or more large mismatched segmental defects without associated radiographic abnormality denote high probability for pulmonary embolism.

- 有2个或以上(>肺段的75%)不匹配的灌注缺损区并且相应部位的胸部X线影像正常，表示肺动脉栓塞高度可能性。

Intermediate probability: Not clinically helpful, further imaging is required

- One large segmental mismatched perfusion defect denotes intermediate probability.
- A triple matched defect in the *lower lung* is considered an intermediate probability. A triple matched defect describes a defect on perfusion, a matched defect on ventilation, and a corresponding abnormality on the chest radiograph.

Low probability: Negative predictive value 84%

- A single large or moderate matched V/Q defect is low probability of pulmonary embolism.
- Other low probability results are absent perfusion of an entire lung, or more than three small segmental lesions.

Very low probability

- Nonsegmental defects denote very low probability.
- The *stripe sign* peripheral to a perfusion defect denotes very low probability for pulmonary embolism. The *stripe sign* represents a thin line of MAA uptake between a perfusion defect and the adjacent pleural surface, representing intervening perfused lung.
- A solitary triple-matched defect in the mid-to-upper lung denotes very low probability. In contrast, the previously mentioned triple-matched defect in the lower lung is more likely to represent PE and is considered an intermediate probability finding.

Normal

- If the perfusion scan is normal, the exam is normal and the ventilation study is not required.

中度可能性：对临床没有帮助，需要进一步检查

- 单个肺段大范围灌注不匹配为中度可能性。
- 下肺野的三重匹配缺损为中度可能性。三重匹配缺损是指灌注缺损、匹配的通气缺损和胸部X线影像上有相应部位异常。

低度可能性：阴性预测值约为84%

- 单个肺段有大或中等范围匹配性灌注/通气缺损，提示为肺动脉栓塞低度可能性。
- 其他低度可能性表现包括一侧肺灌注缺损，或多于3个肺段小范围的灌注缺损。

极低度可能性

- 非肺段性缺损表示极低度可能性。
- 灌注缺损外围的条带征表示肺动脉栓塞极低度可能性。条带征是灌注缺损和相邻胸膜间的细条样MAA摄取，代表夹杂有灌注的肺组织。
- 中、上肺野的单个三重匹配缺损为极低度可能性。相反，前文提及在下肺的三重匹配缺损则可能有肺动脉栓塞，考虑为中度可能性。

正常

- 如果灌注显像正常，则检查视为正常，无须进行通气显像。

（翻译　李蓓蕾）

MUSCULOSKELETAL

RADIOTRACERS

Tc-99m MDP or HDP

- Tc-99m MDP and HDP are technetium-labeled diphosphonates which deposit via chemisorption in the mineral phase of bone. 20 mCi is typically administered, with imaging performed 2–4 hours later.
- Rapid renal excretion is normal; bladder is the critical organ. Patients should void before imaging to prevent the bladder from obscuring a pelvic lesion.
- A three-phase study incudes:

> 1) Radionuclide **angiogram (flow)** evaluates blood flow, with images taken every few seconds. Increased flow suggests hyperemia.
> 2) **Blood pool** evaluates the extracellular distribution immediately following the blood flow phase.
> 3) Standard **delayed** (skeletal) images are performed approximately 3 hours after injection.

肌肉与骨骼

放射性示踪剂

^{99m}Tc-MDP（亚甲基二磷酸盐）或HDP（羟基亚甲基二磷酸盐）

- ^{99m}Tc-MDP和HDP为锝标记的二磷酸盐，通过化学吸附沉积在骨的矿物相中。常用剂量为20mCi，静脉注射后2~4小时显像。
- 药物在正常情况下由肾脏快速排泄；膀胱是受放射性照射的主要器官。患者在显像前应排尿，以防止膀胱影响观察盆腔病灶。
- 三相检查包括：

> 1）放射性核素**血管造影（血流相）**用于评估血流，每隔数秒采集图像。血流增加提示为充血。
> 2）**血池相**评估细胞外的分布，在血流相之后随即获取图像。
> 3）常规**延迟相**（骨骼相）在注射后约3小时进行。

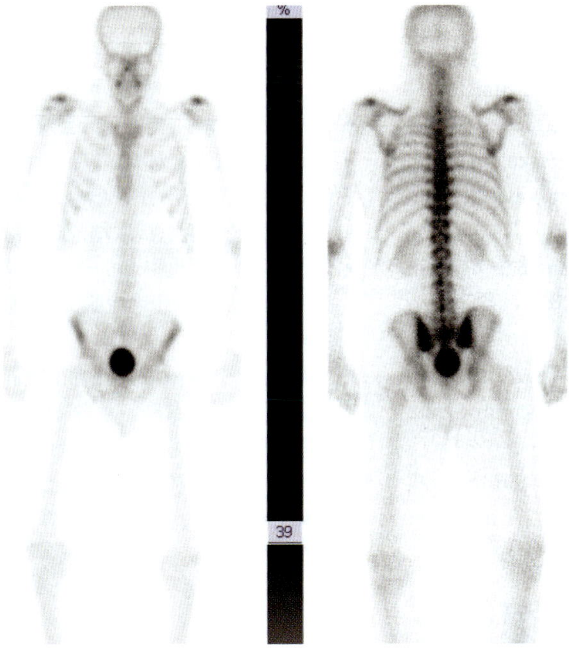

Normal Tc-99m MDP bone scan in anterior and posterior projections, with 20 mCi administered. Note the normal renal and bladder uptake.
注射20mCi后的正常前、后位^{99m}Tc-MDP骨扫描图像。注意正常肾脏和膀胱摄取。

Common Patterns and Clinical Applications

Patterns with low probability of metastatic disease (in a patient with a known malignancy)

- A single focus of uptake in a rib is thought to represent malignancy only ~10% of the time.
- Uptake in similar locations in two or more adjacent ribs is almost always due to trauma.
- Multiple adjacent photopenic bony lesions are unlikely to be metastases, but may represent infarction, avascular necrosis, or sequela of radiation therapy.

Patterns with high probability of metastatic disease

- A single sternal lesion in a patient with breast cancer is due to metastasis ~80% of the time.
- Multifocal areas of increased activity in nonadjacent ribs are suspicious for metastases.
- A single photopenic lesion in patients with a known malignancy (especially neuroblastoma, renal cell carcinoma, and thyroid cancer) is due to metastasis 80% of the time.
- Beware of the *flare phenomenon* within three months of starting chemotherapy, where treated bone metastases demonstrate increased uptake due to healing. Tracer uptake should regress by 6 months following treatment.

Cancers likely to produce a false-negative bone scan

- While bone scan is highly sensitive for osseous metastases that induce bone turnover or are predominantly osteoblastic, such as prostate cancer, it has low sensitivity for predominantly osteoclastic or lytic metastases. These tumors include multiple myeloma, renal cell carcinoma, thyroid carcinoma, aggressive anaplastic tumors, and neuroblastoma.
- Marrow-replacing tumors such as lymphoma can also produce negative bone scans.
- Aggressive and lytic bony lesions or those confined to the marrow are better seen on F-18 FDG PET/CT.

常见的影像学表现及其临床应用

骨转移可能性较低的影像学表现(患者有已知恶性肿瘤)

- 单个肋骨的局灶性放射性摄取的恶性可能性不到10%。
- 相邻部位两条或多条肋骨的摄取病灶几乎都为外伤所致。
- 相邻多处骨放射性缺损病灶不太可能是转移,但可以是骨梗死、缺血性坏死或放疗后改变。

骨转移可能性较高的影像学表现

- 胸骨单个病灶在乳腺癌患者中的转移可能性高达80%。
- 非相邻肋骨的多发局灶性放射性摄取增高应怀疑骨转移。
- 单个放射性分布缺损病灶在已知恶性肿瘤患者中(尤其神经母细胞瘤、肾细胞癌和甲状腺癌)的骨转移可能性为80%。
- 注意在化疗后3个月内的闪烁现象,因化疗后的骨转移病灶出现愈合而增加摄取。示踪剂摄取在治疗后6个月会逐步减少。

可能会产生假阴性骨扫描的癌症

- 骨扫描对诱导骨转换或以成骨为主的骨转移瘤高度敏感,如前列腺癌;但对破骨细胞或溶骨为主的骨转移瘤的敏感性相对较低。这些肿瘤包括多发性骨髓瘤、肾细胞癌、甲状腺癌、侵袭性间变性肿瘤和神经母细胞瘤。
- 骨髓侵袭性肿瘤,如淋巴瘤,也可以产生骨扫描的阴性结果。
- 侵袭性和溶骨性病变或局限于骨髓的骨性病变在^{18}F-FDG PET/CT上更容易观察。

Increased soft tissue uptake

- Diffuse soft tissue uptake can be seen in renal failure.
- Increased uptake in the brain, heart, or spleen may be due to recent infarction.
- Malignant pleural effusion or ascites can cause increased uptake.
- Soft-tissue metastases containing calcium can have increased uptake, including osteosarcoma, neuroblastoma, or mucin-producing tumors (gastrointestinal and ovarian).
- Soft tissue uptake associated with dystrophic calcifications can be seen after trauma or in inflammatory diseases such as myositis ossificans, dermatomyositis, or rhabdomyolysis.
- In the breasts, faint uptake can be normal, but focal intense uptake suggests breast carcinoma. Tracer uptake can be seen at site of recent breast procedure (e.g., biopsy).
- Diffuse parenchymal uptake in kidneys can be seen with urinary obstruction, hyperparathyroidism, chemotherapy, or thalassemia.

软组织摄取增加

- 弥漫性软组织摄取可见于肾功能衰竭。
- 脑、心、脾脏摄取增高，可能为近期梗死所致。
- 恶性胸腔积液或腹水可导致摄取增加。
- 含钙的软组织转移灶，包括骨肉瘤、神经母细胞瘤或黏液分泌性肿瘤(如胃肠道和卵巢肿瘤)可引起软组织摄取增加。
- 营养不良性钙化引起的软组织摄取见于创伤后或炎症后，如骨化性肌炎、皮肌炎和横纹肌溶解症。
- 乳腺组织少量摄取为正常，但局部强烈放射性浓聚提示乳腺癌。示踪剂浓聚可以在近期乳腺手术(如穿刺术)的部位出现。
- 弥漫性肾脏实质摄取可见于尿路梗阻、甲状旁腺功能亢进、化疗或地中海贫血。

Superscan

超级骨显像

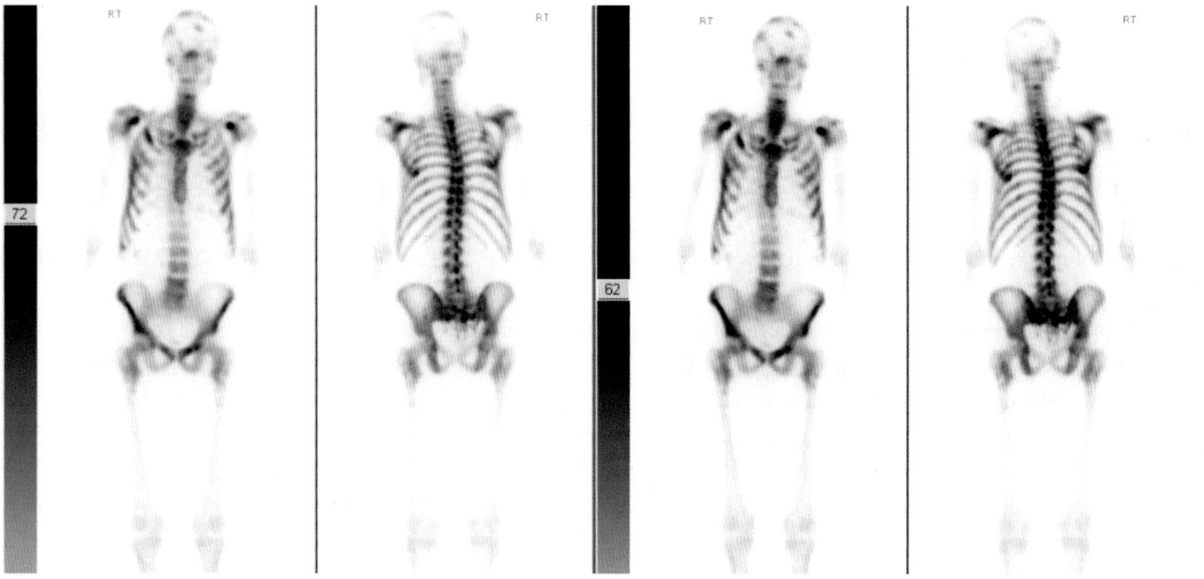

Superscan: Anterior and posterior whole body bone scan at two different windowing levels after 21 mCi Tc-99m MDP administered shows diffusely increased skeletal uptake in the axial skeleton and proximal femurs. There are scattered foci of uptake in the calvarium. No renal uptake is seen.
超级骨显像：注射21mCi的^{99m}Tc-MDP后，两种不同窗位水平的前后位全身图像均显示中轴骨和近段股骨广泛性骨骼摄取增高。颅骨可见散在病灶。肾脏未显影。

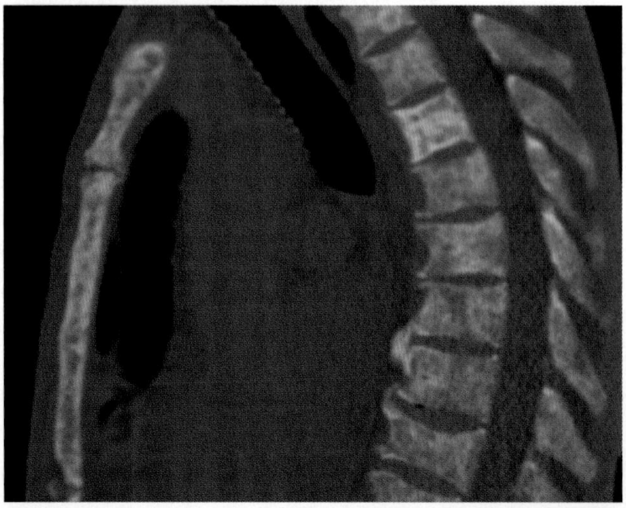

Sagittal CT in the same patient shows diffuse sclerotic appearance of the entire skeleton. This patient had metastatic prostate carcinoma.
同一名患者矢状位CT图像显示所有骨骼弥漫性硬化。该患者有前列腺癌转移。

- A *superscan* represents diffusely increased osseous uptake. Sometimes the uptake can be so diffuse that it may look normal on first glance. The clue to the presence of a superscan will be nonvisualization (or very faint visualization) of the kidneys.
- A superscan is most commonly due to metastatic prostate cancer. Other malignancies producing a superscan include breast cancer and lymphoma.
- A superscan can also be caused by metabolic bone disease in hyperparathyroidism and renal osteodystrophy. If the cause for the superscan is metabolic, then the entire long bones tend to demonstrate diffusely increased uptake. In contrast, with metastatic disease the axial skeleton and proximal humeri and femora are primarily affected.

- 超级骨显像为弥漫性骨摄取增高。有时因为摄取过于广泛而在初诊时容易视为正常。提示超级骨显像的线索是肾脏不显影(或浅淡显影)。
- 超级骨显像最常见于转移性前列腺癌。其他产生超级骨显像的恶性肿瘤有乳腺癌和淋巴瘤。
- 超级骨显像也可出现在甲状旁腺功能亢进症和肾病中的骨质营养不良性代谢性骨病。如果超级骨显像的原因是代谢性的,则以长骨显像为主。相比之下,转移性肿瘤主要累及中轴骨或肱骨和股骨的近段。

Primary bone tumors

- **Osteosarcoma** typically causes markedly increased uptake, often with increased uptake in the entire affected limb.
- **Ewing sarcoma** features intense and homogeneous activity. It may be positive on all three phases of a three-phase bone scan, mimicking osteomyelitis.
- Benign bone tumors that have intense uptake include osteoid osteoma, osteoblastoma, fibrous dysplasia, giant cell tumor, and aneurysmal bone cyst.
- **Osteoid osteoma** features a vascular central nidus which demonstrates intense activity. The *double density sign* describes an intense focus of uptake corresponding to the nidus, surrounded by relatively increased uptake representing hyperemia. The differential of the *double density sign* includes osteoid osteoma, Brodie abscess, less likely stress fracture.

原发性骨肿瘤

- **骨肉瘤**的典型表现是摄取显著增高,并常出现整个受累的肢体摄取增高。
- **尤因肉瘤**的特点为强而均匀的摄取增高。在骨三相扫描中,三相可能都呈阳性,与骨髓炎类似。
- 摄取强烈增高的良性骨肿瘤包括骨样骨瘤、成骨细胞瘤、纤维异常增生、巨细胞瘤和动脉瘤样骨囊肿。
- **骨样骨瘤**有特征性的中央富血管瘤巢,表现为强烈的放射性浓聚。*双密度征*为以瘤巢为中心的强摄取,以及周围摄取相对增加的充血区。双密度征的鉴别诊断包括骨样骨瘤、骨脓肿和相对少见的应力性骨折。

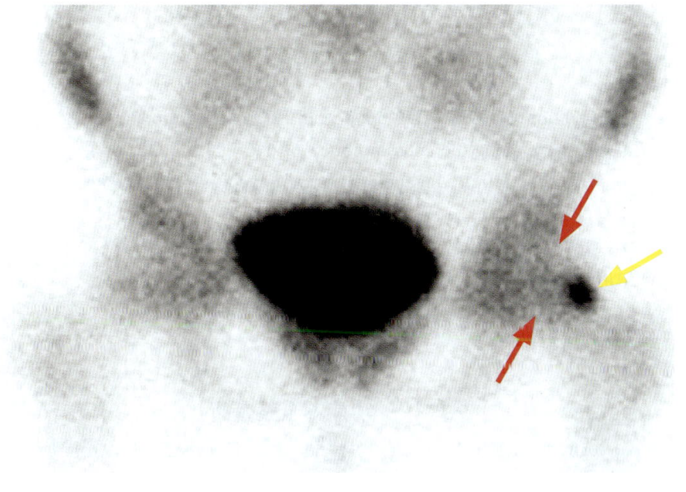

Double density sign of osteoid osteoma: Tc-99m MDP bone scan (25.9 mCi administered) shows asymmetric regional uptake in the left femoral head (red arrows), with a focus of intense uptake at the left lateral head/neck junction (yellow arrow).

骨样骨瘤的双密度征:^{99m}Tc-MDP骨扫描(注射25.9mCi)显示不对称性的左侧股骨头区摄取增高(红箭),并伴有股骨头颈交界处外侧灶性摄取异常增高(黄箭)。

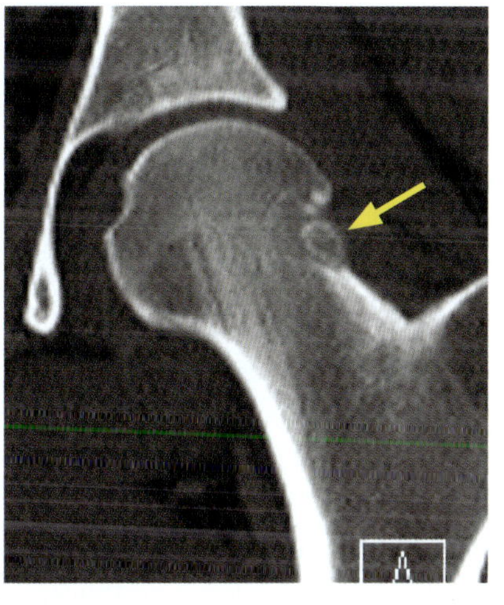

Coronal CT of the left hip shows a well circumscribed lucent lesion (arrow) with a sclerotic rim and lucent nidus, with mild surrounding osteopenia, consistent with osteoid osteoma.

左侧髋关节冠状位CT显示边界清楚的骨密度减低病灶,伴有边缘硬化和透明的瘤巢,其周围有轻度骨质疏松,符合骨样骨瘤的表现。

Case courtesy Roger Han, MD, Brigham and Women's Hospital.

Fracture

- An **acute** fracture (from the initial injury up to 3–4 weeks) will show increased radiotracer uptake surrounding the fracture site. 95% of fractures are positive after one day in patients under 65 years old. Note that skull fractures rarely show activity.
- In the **subacute** phase (until two to three months) radiotracer activity becomes more focal at the fracture.
- In the **healing** phase (variable time course, with ~40% remaining abnormal after one year) there is a gradual decrease in radiotracer activity.
- **Toddler's fracture** represents a spiral fracture of the tibia and occurs in recently ambulatory children. Skeletal scintigraphy is sensitive and specific, and routinely used in workup of a limping child if the radiographs are negative.

骨折

- **急性**期骨折(创伤后3~4周内)表现为骨折邻近部位放射性摄取增高。年龄在65岁以下患者的骨折在1天后呈阳性的为95%。但颅骨骨折很少有浓聚。
- **亚急性**期骨折(至2~3个月)的放射性更集中浓聚于骨折部位。
- **愈合期**(病程变异较大,多达40%的患者1年后仍然有异常)放射性活性逐渐降低。
- **学步儿童骨折**是指胫骨的螺旋骨折,常发生在刚学步的儿童。骨扫描具有较高的灵敏度和特异度,常用于有跛行但X线检查阴性的儿童。

Stress fracture

- A stress fracture represents a fracture due to abnormal stress in a normal bone.
- Common sites of stress fractures include the tibial diaphysis, the femoral neck, and the metatarsals. Metatarsal stress fractures are the most common stress injury in the foot/ankle, with 90% occurring in the second or third metatarsals.
- The bone scan is typically positive by the time the patient has pain. A stress fracture is positive on all three phases of the bone scan.

应力性骨折

- 应力性骨折是指正常骨骼受到非正常应力作用所导致的骨折。
- 常见的应力性骨折位于胫骨干、股骨颈和跖骨。跖骨应力性骨折是足/踝部位最常见的应力性外伤,约90%发生于第二和第三跖骨。
- 骨扫描在患者有疼痛感觉时通常呈阳性。应力性骨折在骨三相检查中三相都为阳性。

Shin splints (medial tibial stress syndrome)

- Shin splints cause pain from periostitis at the tibial insertions of the anterior tibialis and soleus muscles.
- A three-phase bone scan shows *normal* blood flow and blood pool images, with linearly increased uptake in the tibia on delayed (skeletal) phase.

外胫夹(胫骨内侧应力综合征)

- 外胫夹导致的疼痛是由于胫骨前肌和比目鱼肌在胫骨附着点处发生骨膜炎。
- 骨三相扫描显示正常血流相和血池相,但在延迟显像中胫骨的后内侧呈线性放射性摄取增高。

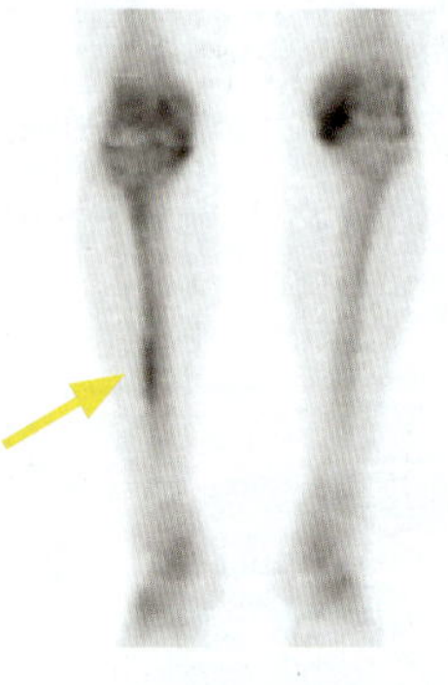

Anterior projection Tc-99m MDP bone scan (25 mCi administered) shows linear uptake along the anterior cortex of the right tibia (arrow), consistent with shin splint. Degenerative-type uptake is seen at both knees.

正位^{99m}Tc-MDP骨扫描图像(注射25 mCi)显示右胫骨前皮质(黄箭)呈线性摄取,符合外胫夹的诊断。双膝见退行性摄取。

Insufficiency fracture

- An insufficiency fracture represents a fracture in response to normal stress in an abnormal bone due to underlying osteoporosis.
- A sacral insufficiency fracture typically shows "H" -shaped uptake in the sacrum, often referred to as the *Honda sign*.
- Insufficiency fracture of the knee is a cause of atraumatic knee pain in the elderly. It typically appears as intense uptake in the medial femoral condyle. This condition was previously called spontaneous osteonecrosis of the knee (SONK) but has seen been discredited as it is insufficiency rather than osteonecrosis.

功能不全性骨折

- 功能不全性骨折多指异常骨质在承受正常应力时所导致的骨折,多合并骨质疏松。
- 骶骨功能不全性骨折在骶骨的摄取呈典型的"H"状,常被称为本田征。
- 膝关节不全性骨折是老年人引起非创伤性膝关节疼痛的原因之一。典型表现为股骨内侧髁有强烈摄取。这种情况以前被称为自发性膝关节骨坏死(SONK),但现被认为是一种功能不全,并非骨坏死。

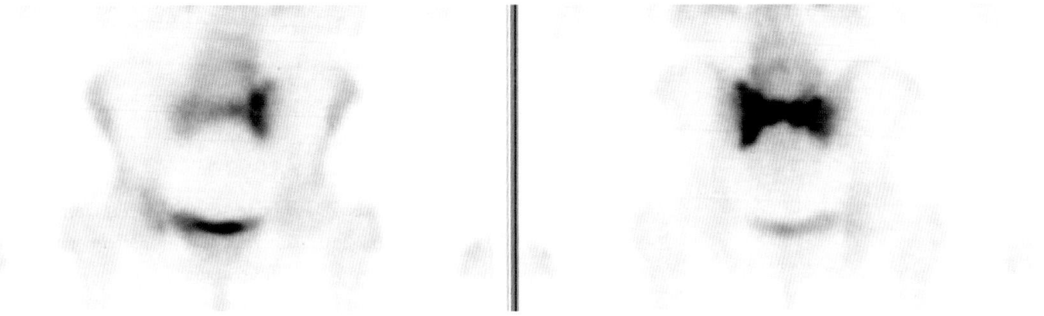

Anterior and posterior projections from a Tc-99m MDP bone scan (25 mCi administered) show uptake in the sacrum with a H-shaped configuration, representing the *Honda sign* of sacral insufficiency fracture.
前、后位 ^{99m}Tc-MDP 骨扫描(注射 25mCi) 显示骶骨 "H" 形摄取，为骶骨不全骨折形成的本田征。

Prosthesis evaluation

- Evaluation of a painful hip or knee prosthesis for loosening or infection is a common indication for a bone scan.
- In a cemented prosthesis, it is normal to see activity surrounding the prosthesis up to 12 months. In a non-cemented prosthesis, activity may remain increased up to two years as bony ingrowth continues.
- In evaluation of a hip prosthesis, *focal* activity at the lesser trochanter (which acts as a fulcrum site) and distal femoral prosthetic tip seen >1 year for cemented or >2 years for non-cemented prosthesis suggests loosening. In contrast, *generalized* increase in radiotracer activity surrounding the prosthesis may suggest osteomyelitis.
- Mild to moderate activity that is limited to the greater trochanter/intertrochanteric region is often due to heterotopic ossification.

Osteomyelitis and musculoskeletal infection

- Osteomyelitis is positive on all three phases of a bone scan. A positive three-phase bone scan is very specific for osteomyelitis in the presence of a normal radiograph (confirming that no fracture is present).
- To evaluate for osteomyelitis in the presence of an underlying abnormality, such as a fracture or prosthesis, *WBC imaging* (indium-111 or Tc-99m labeled WBCs) combined with a Tc-99m sulfur colloid *marrow scan* can increase specificity for osteomyelitis. Focal WBC activity in a region devoid of colloid marrow activity is suggestive of osteomyelitis.
- Although rarely performed, *gallium-67 scan* can also increase specificity for osteomyelitis if the gallium uptake exceeds the bone scan uptake in the area of concern.
- **Cellulitis** shows increased MDP activity during the blood flow and soft tissue phases, but the skeletal phase is negative.
- **Septic arthritis** is positive on all three phases of the bone scan on *both* sides of the joint.
- **Discitis** shows increased skeletal activity in two adjacent vertebral bodies.

人工假肢评估

- 骨扫描常用于评估人工髋关节或膝关节置换术后发生松动或感染所致的疼痛。
- 在骨水泥人工肢体，假体周围放射性摄取增高可持续12个月。在非骨水泥固定的人工肢体置换术后，放射性摄取增高的现象可持续2年，因为有骨组织向内不断生长。
- 在人工髋关节术后超过1年(骨水泥)或2年(非骨水泥)，若股骨小转子(此处起支点作用)和人工股骨的远端有*局灶性*放射性摄取，应考虑假体松动。如果在假体周围呈弥漫性摄取增加，考虑为骨髓炎。
- 局限于大转子或转子间区域的轻至中度的放射性摄取常是由于异位骨化所致。

骨髓炎和肌骨感染

- 骨髓炎在骨三相检查中都呈阳性。阳性骨三相扫描结果对X线检查正常(确认无骨折存在)的骨髓炎诊断极具特异性。
- 评估异常情况下的骨髓炎，如骨折或假体等，采用*白细胞显像*(^{111}In或 ^{99m}Tc标记白细胞)联合 ^{99m}Tc-硫胶体扫描可以提高*骨髓扫描*的特异度。有白细胞积聚但缺乏硫胶体骨髓显影的区域提示为骨髓炎。
- ^{67}Ga*扫描*虽然不常用，但可以增加诊断骨髓炎的特异度，表现为怀疑部位的局部摄取超出了正常。
- **蜂窝织炎**在血流相和血池相均显示MDP摄取增高，但在延迟骨显像时为阴性。
- **化脓性关节炎**的骨三相扫描在关节的两侧均呈阳性。
- **椎间盘炎**显示相邻两个椎体间放射性分布增高。

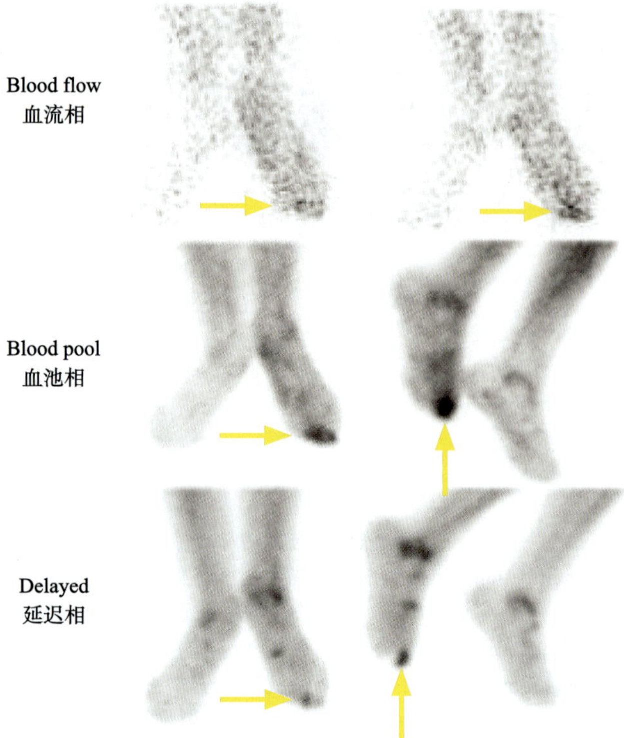

Three-phase bone scan following administrattion of 26.2 mCi Tc-99m MDP in patient with nonhealing ulcer of the left great toe:
Focal increased uptake (arrows) is present at the left great toe on blood flow, blood pool, and delayed phases, suggesting osteomyelitis.
一名左大脚趾溃疡未愈合的患者在注射26.2mCi的^{99m}Tc-MDP后行骨三相扫描：左大脚趾的血流、血池和延迟期出现局灶性摄取增加(黄箭)，提示骨髓炎。

Hypertrophic pulmonary osteoarthropathy

- Hypertrophic pulmonary osteoarthropathy is long bone diaphyseal periosteal reaction most commonly due to pulmonary disease, such as lung cancer.
- Bone scan shows increased parallel lines of activity along the cortex of long bones.

Avascular necrosis (AVN)

- Avascular necrosis (AVN) initially shows decreased radiotracer activity in the affected region, followed by a hyperemic phase with increased uptake.
- SPECT imaging of AVN (especially of the hips) will often show a rim of increased uptake with central photopenia, thought to represent revascularization progressing from outside in.

肥大性肺骨关节病

- 肥大性肺骨关节病是长骨骨干的骨膜反应，最常由肺疾病引起，如肺癌。
- 骨扫描表现为沿长骨皮质平行的线性放射性分布增高。

缺血性坏死(AVN)

- 缺血性坏死(AVN)的初期表现为病变部位放射性摄取减少或缺损，随后进入充血期时呈放射性摄取增加。
- AVN的SPECT显像(尤其是髋关节AVN)常表现为中央放射性缺损伴外周分布增高，被认为是由外向内的血管重建过程。

Paget disease

佩吉特病

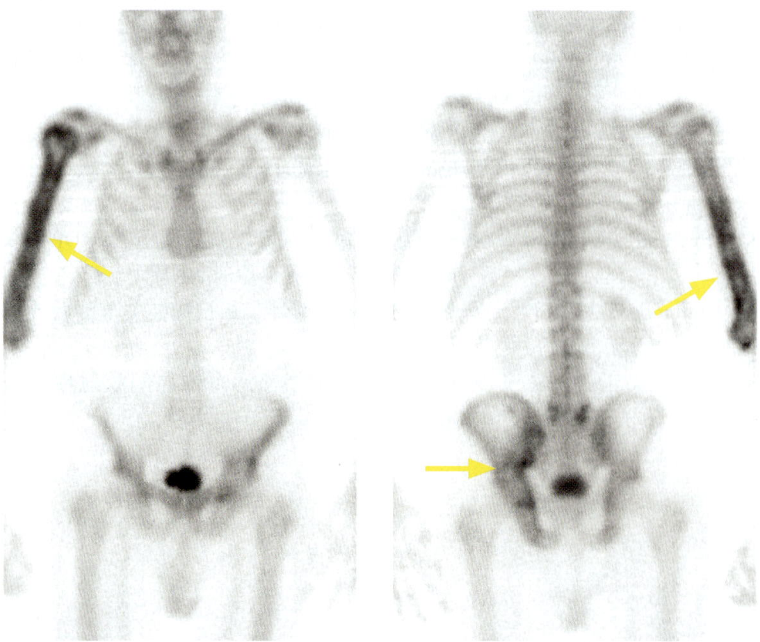

Paget disease: Anterior (left image) and posterior projections from a Tc-99m MDP bone scan (20 mCi administered) show heterogeneously increased radiotracer uptake involving the right humerus, and to a lesser extent the left hemipelvis, best seen on the posterior projection (arrows).
佩吉特病：前位(左图)和后位^{99m}Tc-MDP骨扫描(注射20mCi)显示右侧肱骨不均匀性放射性摄取增高，左侧骨盆也有轻度放射性摄取增高，后位图比较明显(黄箭)。

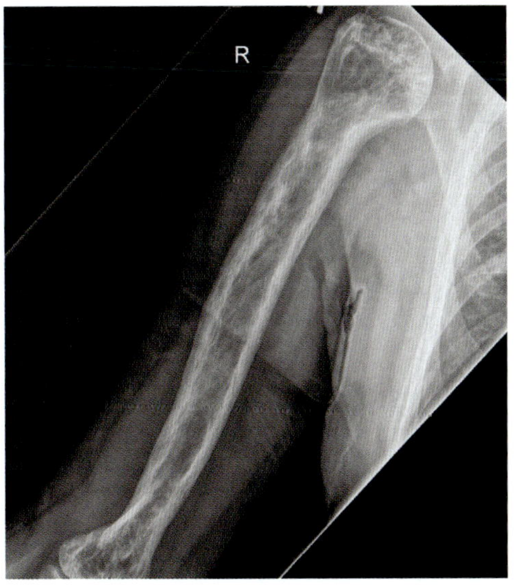

Radiograph of the right humerus shows cortical and trabecular thickening.
右肱骨X线影像显示骨皮质增厚及骨小梁增粗。

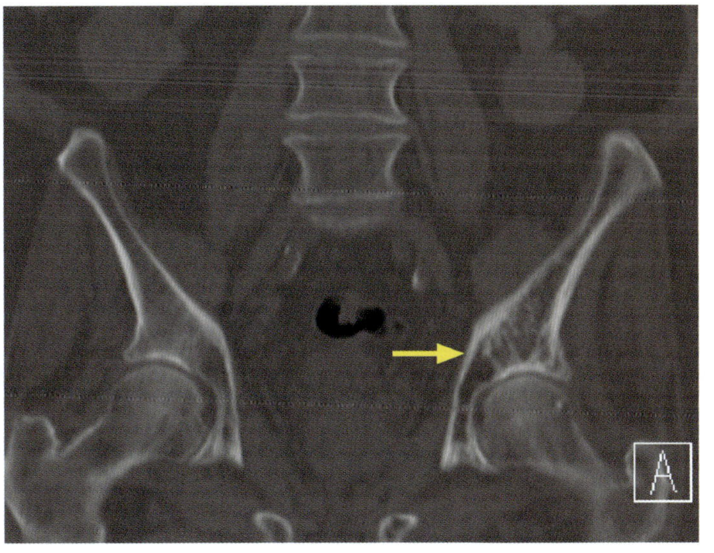

Coronal CT of the pelvis shows asymmetric coarsened trabecular thickening of the left ilium (arrow).
骨盆冠状位CT表现为左侧髂骨不对称性骨小梁增粗(黄箭)。

- Paget disease is an idiopathic disturbance of osteoclastic and osteoblastic regulation. Paget has three discrete phases including lytic, mixed, and sclerotic phases. The lytic (early) phase is typically positive on bone scan and often negative on radiography. The mixed phase is abnormal on bone scan and radiography. The sclerotic phase shows persistent radiographic changes, but the bone scan activity may subside.
- One complication of Paget disease is malignant degeneration to osteosarcoma. A focal cold lesion should raise concern for necrosis in a region of malignant degeneration, although this may be best appreciated by evaluating serial studies.

Complex regional pain syndrome (reflex sympathetic dystrophy)

- Complex regional pain syndrome, previously called reflex sympathetic dystrophy, causes persistent pain, tenderness, and swelling often due to minor trauma.
- Bone scan shows diffusely increased juxta-articular activity in multiple small joints of the hand or foot on delayed (skeletal) images. Blood pool and soft tissue phase uptake is variable, but most commonly both phases are increased.

- 佩吉特病是一种特发性成骨和溶骨调节紊乱的疾病。佩吉特病有三个明显不同的分期，即破骨期、混合期和硬化期。破骨期(早期)的骨扫描中通常表现为阳性，而在X线检查中常呈阴性。混合期的骨扫描和X线检查都有异常表现。硬化期在X线上持续表现为异常，而在骨扫描中放射性摄取可能已经正常。
- 佩吉特病的并发症之一是恶变为骨肉瘤。局部放射性缺损区应怀疑恶变区域有坏死，跟踪随访检查可能是最好的观察方法。

复合性局部疼痛综合征(反射性交感神经萎缩症)

- 复合性局部疼痛综合征，原称反射性交感神经萎缩症，表现为持续性疼痛、触痛和肿胀，常由微小创伤所引起。
- 在延迟相骨扫描中表现为手或足多个小关节旁的弥漫性放射性摄取增高。血流和血池相的摄取表现多变，但通常这两个时相均表现为摄取增高。

(翻译　程爱萍)

Kidneys

肾脏

Radiotracers

放射性示踪剂

Tc-99m DTPA

- DTPA can measure glomerular filtration rate (GFR) and evaluate renal perfusion.
- DTPA is excreted by glomerular filtration. Approximately 20% is extracted by the glomerulus into the tubules with each pass. This is the identical extraction fraction as inulin, which is used to exactly measure GFR.

^{99m}Tc-DTPA(二乙撑三胺五乙酸)

- DTPA可用于测量肾小球滤过率(GFR)及评估肾灌注。
- DTPA由肾小球滤过排出体外。每次通过肾脏约有20%被肾小球滤过进入肾小管。DTPA的滤过与菊粉相同，因而可用于精准测量GFR。

Tc-99m MAG_3

- MAG_3 can estimate renal plasma flow and evaluate renal perfusion, however MAG_3 cannot measure GFR.
- MAG_3 is filtered and excreted by the tubules. Greater than 50% is extracted by the glomerulus into the tubules with each pass. MAG_3 is cleared predominantly by the proximal tubules with minimal filtration. It has a higher extraction fraction than DTPA, which provides better images in patients with renal insufficiency or obstruction.

Tc-99m DMSA

- DMSA scanning is performed in children to evaluate for the presence of renal scarring associated with pyelonephritis. The collecting system is not imaged.
- DMSA is a specialized cortical agent. It is bound in the renal tubules, which allows anatomic imaging of the cortex. It is the only renal tracer where SPECT imaging is performed.

Clinical Applications of Renal Imaging

Renogram

- A nuclear renogram is a time-activity curve that provides a graphical representation of renal uptake and excretion. Approximately 10 mCi Tc-99m MAG_3 (most commonly) or DTPA is administered. A normal renogram has three phases:

> 1) **Flow or perfusion phase** has a sharp upslope and lasts ~1 minute after injection. Normal kidneys are visualized within 2–5 seconds following visualization of the aorta. A slow upslope suggests decreased perfusion.
> 2) **Cortical function phase** usually occurs in the first 1–3 minutes, peaks at 3–5 minutes (= **time to peak activity**). Decreased renal function produces delayed cortical uptake.
> 3) **Clearance phase** is characterized by rapid urine excretion into the collecting system, which usually begins after 3 minutes. Normally half of the renal activity should be cleared in 8–12 minutes (= **half-time excretion**). Lack of pelvicalyceal clearance suggests obstruction.

^{99m}Tc-MAG_3(巯基乙酰基三甘氨酸)

- MAG_3可估计肾血浆流量，从而评估肾灌注，但MAG_3不能用于测量GFR。
- MAG_3会被肾小管滤过和清除。每一次通过肾脏，50%以上的MAG_3会被肾小球提取进入肾小管。MAG_3主要由近端肾小管清除，同时有少量滤过。MAG_3摄取率较DTPA高，所以肾功能衰竭和尿路梗阻患者的显像质量会更好。

^{99m}Tc-DMSA(二巯基丁二酸钠)

- DMSA扫描用于评价儿童肾盂肾炎所致的肾脏瘢痕。肾脏集合系统不显影。
- DMSA是一种特殊的肾皮质显像剂，它能与肾小管结合，因而可用于皮质的解剖成像。这是唯一用于SPECT成像的肾脏示踪剂。

肾显像的临床应用

肾图

- 肾图是时间-活性的关系曲线，它以图形的方式展示肾脏摄取和排泄。通常需要注射10mCi的^{99m}Tc-MAG_3(常用)或DTPA。正常肾图分三个时相：

> 1) **血流或灌注相**是陡峭的上升段，在注射后持续约1分钟。正常的肾脏在主动脉显像后2~5秒内可显影。缓慢上升的血流相表明血流灌注减少。
> 2) **皮质功能相**通常发生在前1~3分钟，高峰在3~5分钟(=**到达峰值的时间**)。肾功能下降导致皮质摄取延迟。
> 3) **清除相**以尿液快速排泄到肾盂肾盏等集合系统为特征，通常在3分钟后开始。正常情况下，清除一半肾脏的活性应该在8~12分钟内(=**半排时间**)。肾盂肾盏的清除障碍提示有梗阻。

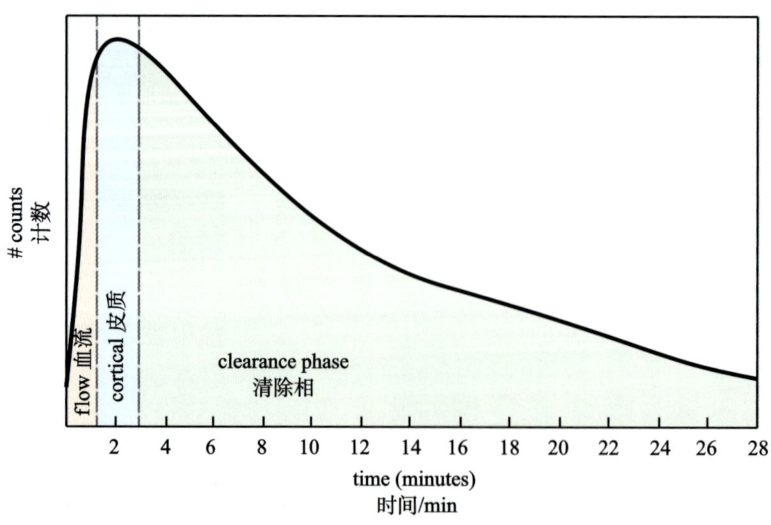

- **Differential (or split) renal function** is determined during the cortical phase by counting the % activity in each kidney, which should be equal. Normal range is 45–55% for each kidney.
- Cortical transit of radiotracer can be quantified by the **20 minute-to-peak ratio**, which describes the percentage of maximal cortical activity remaining in each kidney at 20 minutes after injection. A ratio <0.3 is normal. Delayed transit reflects renal dysfunction.

- **分(单侧)肾功能**是在皮质期通过计算每个肾脏放射性活性的百分数加以确定，两者的数值应该相等。每个肾的正常范围是45%~55%。
- 放射性示踪剂的皮质转运可以通过**20分钟至峰值的比率**进行量化，该比率代表了注射后20分钟每个肾脏残留的活性与最大皮质活性的百分比。比值<0.3为正常。转运延迟则提示肾脏功能障碍。

Lasix renogram (diuretic renography)

- If hydronephrosis is present, a diuretic renogram can distinguish between obstruction and a nonobstructive cause of collecting system dilation. Both renal function and urodynamics are evaluated. The radiotracer is Tc-99m MAG_3, much less commonly Tc-99m DTPA.
- After approximately 20 minutes of imaging, 40 mg IV **furosemide (Lasix)** is administered. A higher dose may be needed in patients with renal insufficiency. After injection, a fixed mechanical obstruction will show no change in the renogram curve. However, in a non-obstructive case, the additional pressure from diuretic effect will open up the collecting system and allow drainage of radiotracer from the kidney.

呋塞米肾图(利尿肾图)

- 如果存在肾积水，利尿性肾图可以区分梗阻和非梗阻引起的集合系统扩张。它可以同时评估肾功能和尿流动力学。放射性示踪剂为^{99m}Tc-MAG_3，偶尔也用^{99m}Tc-DTPA。
- 在显像约20分钟后，静脉注射40mg呋塞米。肾功能不良时可增加呋塞米的剂量。给予呋塞米后，固定的机械性梗阻在肾图上不会出现变化。但在非梗阻性病例，利尿效应带来的额外压力作用可打开集合系统，从而使放射性示踪剂从肾脏排出。

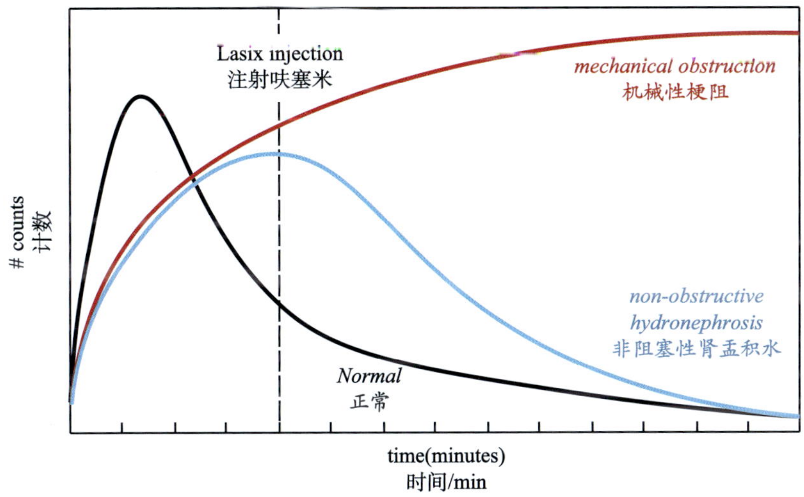

After administration of Lasix, a **clearance half-time** <10 minutes is normal. 10–20 minutes is indeterminant. >20 minutes suggests obstruction.

给予呋塞米后，半排时间小于10min为正常，10~20min为临界，大于20min提示梗阻。

- False positives (Lasix renogram is positive for obstruction in the absence of a true obstruction) can be seen within dehydration, distended bladder, or renal failure (decreased response to diuretics).
- **Ethacrynic acid** is an alternative diuretic to Lasix in patients with sulfa allergies, though in practice Lasix is only associated with negligible risk of adverse reactions in these patients.

- 假阳性(呋塞米肾图在没有真正梗阻的情况下显示阳性梗阻结果)可见于脱水、膀胱膨胀或肾功能衰竭(减少对利尿剂的反应)。
- 患者对磺胺过敏可用**依他尼酸**替代呋塞米作为利尿剂。但在实际临床中，呋塞米对磺胺过敏的患者通常只有轻微，甚至可以忽略不计的副作用。

Angiotensin-converting enzyme (ACE) inhibitor renogram

- A positive ACE renogram is relatively specific for renal artery stenosis, which may be a cause of hypertension. The radiotracer is Tc-99m MAG_3, much less commonly Tc-99m DTPA.
- In compensated renal artery stenosis, decreased blood to the glomerulus stimulates renin → angiotensin Ⅰ → angiotensin Ⅱ. Angiotensin Ⅱ constricts the efferent (outgoing) arterioles to restore GFR. Angiotensin Ⅰ is converted to angiotensin Ⅱ by angiotensin converting enzyme.

血管紧张素转化酶(ACE)抑制性肾图

- 阳性ACE肾图是肾动脉狭窄相对特异的表现，可能是引起高血压的病因。放射性示踪剂为^{99m}Tc-MAG_3，偶尔也用^{99m}Tc-DTPA。
- 在代偿性肾动脉狭窄中，肾小球的血流量下降刺激肾素→血管紧张素Ⅰ→血管紧张素Ⅱ。血管紧张素Ⅱ使出球小动脉收缩以恢复GFR。血管紧张素Ⅰ通过血管紧张素转换酶的作用转变为血管紧张素Ⅱ。

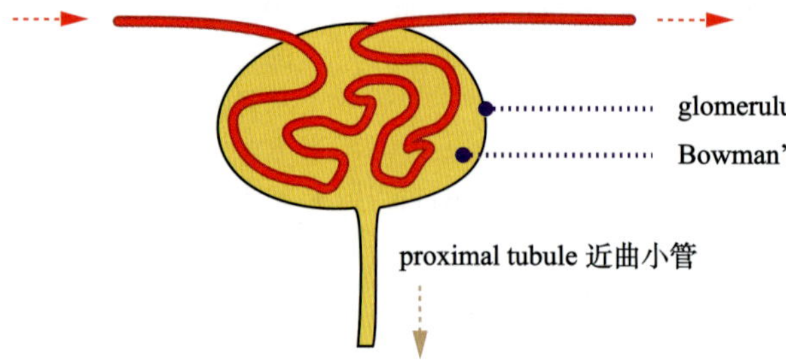

- After administration of an ACE inhibitor (typically captopril, 25–50 mg), the efferent arterioles will relax and GFR will decrease.

  If a patient is already on an ACE inhibitor, it should be stopped for 48 hours to 1 week prior to the exam. Intravenous access should be maintained in case fluid resuscitation is needed to treat hypotension.

  Known severe renal artery stenosis is a relative contraindication as ACE inhibitor-induced intrarenal hypotension can lead to acute renal failure.

- An ACE renogram can be performed in one or two days.

  A **single-day, two-stage protocol** comprises a baseline non-captopril study using a low dose of MAG_3, followed by a captopril study several hours later when residual activity from the first study has cleared the kidneys and urinary tract.

  A **two-day protocol** is usually used for patients without pre-existing renal dysfunction. The captopril study is performed first, which if normal, excludes renovascular hypertension and thus eliminates the need for a baseline study. If the captopril study is abnormal, a baseline study is performed on the following day.

- A positive study depends on the radiotracer utilized (MAG_3 or DTPA), but the hallmark is a post-ACE inhibitor renogram that becomes abnormal or more abnormal, usually unilaterally.

- 给予ACE抑制剂(常用卡托普利，25~50mg)后，出球小动脉舒张而GFR下降。

  如果正在服用ACE抑制剂，患者应在检查前48小时至1周停止使用。需要液体复苏治疗低血压的患者应保留静脉通路。已知严重的肾动脉狭窄是一个相对的禁忌证，因为ACE抑制剂诱导的肾内低血压可导致急性肾功能衰竭。

- ACE肾图可以在一天或两天内完成。

  一天两阶段方案：包括以无卡托普利为基线的低剂量MAG_3，数小时后待肾脏和尿路在第一次检查的放射性残余清除后使用卡托普利重复注射MAG_3。

  两天方案：通常用于无肾功能障碍的患者。首先使用卡托普利进行测量，若结果正常，则排除肾血管性高血压，因此无须进行基线研究。如果卡托普利试验异常，第二天行普通肾图检查。

- 阳性结果取决于所使用的放射性示踪剂(MAG_3或DTPA)，但异常的显著特征是ACE抑制后的肾图变得异常或更加异常，通常是单侧的。

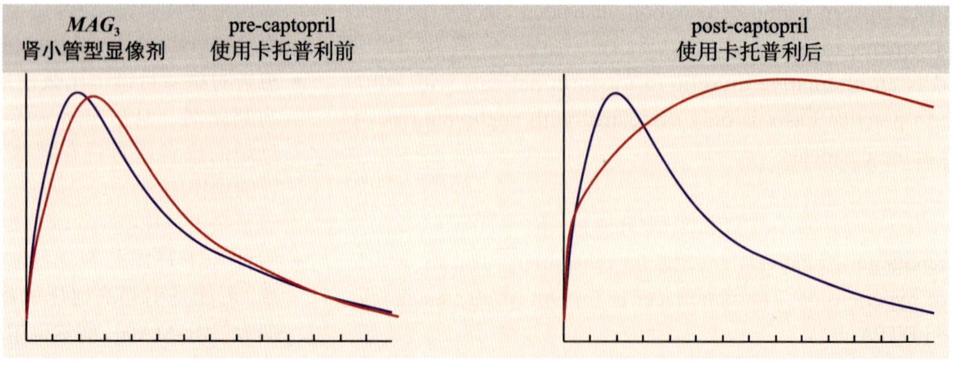

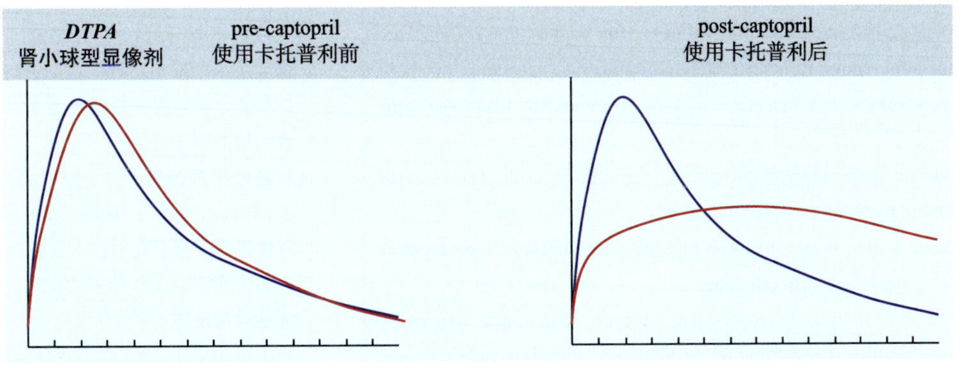

MAG_3 (tubular agent): Uptake and secretion are generally preserved even with a reduced GFR, but further ↓ GFR results in ↓ urine production and ↓ washout of secreted agent from collecting system.

Positive criteria for MAG_3 study include: <40% uptake by one kidney at 2–3 minutes; difference in cortical a ctivity by 20%; or delay in time to peak activity of more than 2 minutes (compared to pre-ACE inhibitor).

DTPA (glomerular agent): Unlike MAG_3, ↓ GFR causes diminished uptake and excretion of DTPA.

MAG_3 (肾小管型显像剂)：在GFR下降时的摄取和分泌功能依然正常，但是GFR进一步下降将导致尿液生成减少，以及从集合系统排泄降低。

MAG_3检查的阳性标准：单个肾脏在2~3分钟内摄取示踪剂<40%；两肾皮质活性差异>20%；或峰值推迟2分钟以上(与用药前比较)。

DTPA (肾小球型显像剂)：不同于MAG_3，GFR下降将导致DTPA的摄取和排泄减少。

- Bilateral worsening renograms can be caused by hypotension, dehydration (most common), urinary obstruction, medical renal disease, or bilateral renal artery stenosis.

Renal cortical imaging

- Renal cortical imaging is limited to renal imaging in children to evaluate for pyelonephritis or scarring. The radiotracer is Tc-99m DMSA.
- A normal DMSA study excludes the diagnosis of acute pyelonephritis.
- A positive study for pyelonephritis can have three patterns:

  Focal cortical defect.

  Multifocal cortical defects.

  Diffusely decreased radiotracer.

Radionuclide cystography (RNC)

- Radionuclide cystography is the most sensitive test for evaluation of reflux in pediatric population with less radiation exposure compared to voiding cystourethrography (VCUG)
- The radiotracer chosen is variable. Tc-99m pertechnetate, Tc-99m DTPA, and Tc-99m sulfur colloid can all work well. Regardless of the radiotracer chosen, it is injected retrograde into the catheterized bladder.
- Grading of reflux:

  Minimal (RNC grade I). Reflux is confined to the ureter.

  Moderate (RNC grade II): Reflux extends superiorly to the pelvicalyceal system.

  Severe (RNC grade III): Severe reflux causing a tortuous ureter and/or dilated intrarenal system.

Renal transplant evaluation

- While transplanted kidneys are often initially evaluated by ultrasound and ultimately by biopsy, radionuclide renogram using Tc-99m MAG_3 or DTPA is an important diagnostic tool.
- A normal renal transplant should be visualized on the flow phase within seconds after the iliac vessels. Its cortical and clearance phases are similar to those of a native kidney.
- Renogram findings of common transplant complications include:

- 双侧肾图异常可由低血压、脱水(最常见)、尿路梗阻、内科肾脏疾病或双侧肾动脉狭窄引起。

肾皮质显像

- 肾皮质显像只用于检查儿童肾盂肾炎或肾瘢痕。放射性示踪剂为^{99m}Tc-DMSA。
- DMSA显像正常可排除急性肾盂肾炎的诊断。
- 肾盂肾炎有三种不同的DMSA检查阳性表现：

  局灶性皮质缺损。

  多发局灶性皮质缺损。

  弥漫性放射性摄取减低。

核素膀胱造影术(RNC)

- 核素膀胱造影术是评价小儿尿液反流最灵敏的检查手段，其辐射剂量低于排泄性膀胱尿道造影术。
- 放射性示踪剂有多种，$^{99m}TcO_4$、^{99m}Tc-DTPA、^{99m}Tc-SC都可用。不论使用哪种放射性示踪剂，都需要通过导管逆行注入膀胱。
- 反流分级：

  轻度(RNC 1级)：反流只限于输尿管。

  中度(RNC 2级)：反流逆行向上达肾盂肾盏。

  重度(RNC 3级)：严重反流导致输尿管扭曲和/或肾盂系统扩张。

肾移植评估

- 超声通常是评估移植肾采用的初选检查，而最终确诊需要进行活检，但^{99m}Tc-MAG_3或DTPA放射性核素肾图是一个重要的诊断工具。
- 一个正常的移植肾应该在双侧髂血管显示数秒后观察到肾血流相，其皮质功能相和清除相应该与非移植肾相似。
- 常见移植并发症的肾图表现包括：

Acute tubular necrosis (ATN) occurs within 3–4 days after surgery and results from perioperative ischemia. Its renogram is characterized by normal perfusion, but poor renal function with increased cortical retention, delayed clearance and decreased urine excretion.

Hyperacute rejection produces immediate vascular thrombosis in the transplanted kidney, resulting in absent perfusion, markedly reduced or absent function.

Acute rejection occurs within weeks to three months after surgery. It presents as decreased perfusion and marked cortical retention.

Chronic rejection occurs months to years after surgery. It is characterized by progressive worsening perfusion and function with cortical thinning, pelvicalyceal dilation.

Cyclosporin nephrotoxicity appears similar to ATN, but occurs at a later time after ATN should have resolved.

Urine leak presents as progressive accumulation of activity outside the urinary tract.

Urinoma, **hematoma** and **lymphocele** may present as fixed perirenal photopenic areas.

急性肾小管坏死(ATN)：发生于术后3~4天，通常是围手术期缺血所致。肾图表现为灌注正常，但肾功能差，伴有皮质持续性显影、清除延缓，以及尿液的排泄减少。

超急性排斥反应：会立即引起移植肾血管血栓形成，导致灌注缺失、功能显著降低或丧失。

急性排斥反应：发生在术后数周至3个月内。表现为血流灌注减少和明显的皮质持续显影。

慢性排斥反应：发生在术后数月至数年。特征是血流灌注和功能降低，伴有皮质变薄，肾盂扩张积水。

环孢素肾毒性：与ATN类似，但其主要发生于ATN恢复后的较晚时间内。

漏尿：表现为尿路外放射性逐渐积聚。

尿性囊肿、血肿和淋巴管囊肿：可表现为肾周固定的放射性减低或缺损区。

（翻译　程爱萍）

WHOLE-BODY IMAGING OF NEOPLASM, INFECTION, AND INFLAMMATION

肿瘤、感染和炎症的全身成像

RADIOTRACERS

放射性示踪剂

I-123 MIBG

- I-123 MIBG is a norepinephrine analog that is taken up by chromaffin cells of sympathetic adrenergic tissue. It is used to image pheochromocytoma in adults and neuroblastoma in children. To a lesser extent, MIBG is taken up by other neuroendocrine tumors including carcinoid, medullary thyroid carcinoma, and paraganglioma.
- I-131 MIBG can be used to treat neuroblastoma in children.
- Normal distribution is areas of sympathetic innervation, including salivary glands, heart, thyroid (although this is typically intentionally blocked with Lugol's solution to reduce thyroid dosimetry), liver, kidney, and bladder.

^{123}I-MIBG(间碘苄胍)

- ^{123}I-MIBG是一种去甲肾上腺素类似物，可被交感肾上腺素能组织中的嗜铬细胞摄取。它被用于成人嗜铬细胞瘤和儿童神经母细胞瘤显像。MIBG可被其他神经内分泌肿瘤少量摄取，包括类癌、甲状腺髓样癌和副神经节瘤。
- ^{131}I-MIBG可用于治疗儿童神经母细胞瘤。
- MIBG正常分布在有交感神经末梢分布的部位，包括唾液腺、心脏、甲状腺(通常用鲁氏碘液封闭甲状腺以减少甲状腺的辐射剂量)、肝脏、肾脏及膀胱。

Indium-111 pentetreotide (Octreoscan)

- Indium-111 is cyclotron-produced and decays by electron capture, emitting two gamma photons at 173 and 247 keV. Its half-life is 67 hours. Pentetreotide is octreotide conjugated to DTPA which allows binding to In-111.
- In-111 pentetreotide is used to detect tumors with somatostatin receptors, including amine precursor uptake and decarboxylation (APUD) tumors. Most common applications are evaluation of carcinoid or islet cell tumors such as gastrinoma. However, pentetreotide has low sensitivity for insulinoma.
- Paragangliomas (extra-adrenal pheochromocytomas) are seen better with In-111 pentetreotide compared to MIBG, although In-111 pentetreotide is uncommonly used for detection of paragangliomas.
- Normal distribution is intense renal and splenic uptake, with slightly less hepatic uptake.

^{111}In-喷曲肽(奥曲肽)

- ^{111}In(^{111}铟)由回旋加速器生产，通过电子俘获发生核衰变，产生2个能量分别为173keV和247keV的γ光子。它的半衰期为67小时。^{111}In-喷曲肽与DTPA结合后产生喷曲肽，可以与^{111}In结合。
- ^{111}In-喷曲肽用于检测具有生长抑素受体的肿瘤，包括胺前体摄取和脱羧细胞(APUD)肿瘤。最常用于评估类癌或胰岛细胞肿瘤，如胃泌素瘤。然而，喷曲肽对胰岛素瘤的灵敏度较低。
- ^{111}In-喷曲肽对副神经节瘤(肾上腺外嗜铬细胞瘤)的显像效果优于MIBG，但^{111}In-喷曲肽不常用于检测副神经节瘤。
- 肾脏和脾在正常情况下有强烈摄取，但肝脏摄取相对较弱。

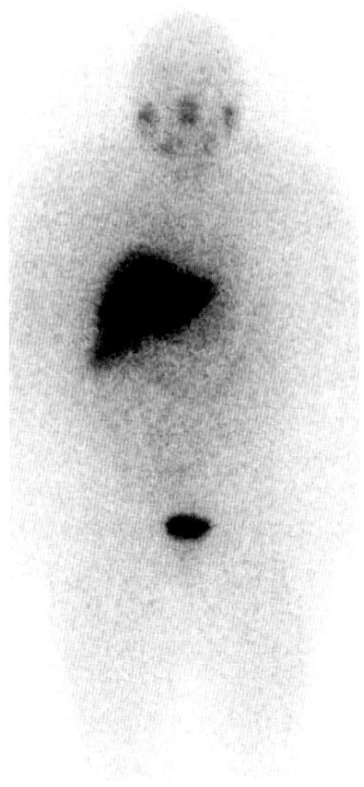

Planar image shows normal distribution of I-123 MIBG.
平面图像显示正常^{123}I-MIBI分布。

Indium-111 oxine leukocytes (WBCs)

- The normal distribution of Indium-111 labeled WBCs is spleen > liver >> bone marrow.
- Infection imaging with an In-111 WBC scan is performed at 24 hours.
- The key advantage of In-111 oxine WBCs compared to gallium is the lack of physiologic bowel accumulation, which allows evaluation of abdominal or bowel infection/inflammation.
- Disadvantages compared to gallium include a tedious labeling procedure, higher radiation dose, and less accuracy in diagnosing spinal osteomyelitis.
- Advantages of In-111 WBC scan compared to Tc-99m HMPAO include absence of interfering bowel and renal activity, ability to perform delayed imaging, and ability to perform simultaneous Tc-99m sulfur colloid or Tc-99m MDP bone scan. These combined approaches are very helpful for evaluation of osteomyelitis in the setting of a baseline abnormal bone scan (e.g., prosthesis evaluation), discussed below.

Tc-99m HMPAO leukocytes (WBCs)

- The advantages of a WBC scan labeled with Tc-99m HMPAO compared to In-111 are related to the shorter half-life of Tc-99m, which allows a higher administered activity, better counts, a lower absorbed dose, and ability to perform earlier imaging. For these reasons, Tc-99m is often preferred in children in appropriate cases.
- However, a major disadvantage is physiologic uptake within the gastrointestinal and genitourinary tracts due to unbound Tc-99m HMPAO complexes, which limits bowel evaluation. Renal activity occurs early, while bowel activity is seen after 1–2 hours. Additionally, delayed imaging is less practical with Tc-99m due to its shorter half-life.

^{111}In-8-羟基喹啉标记白细胞(WBC)

- 正常^{111}In标记的白细胞在体内的分布为脾脏>肝脏>>骨髓。
- 用^{111}In标记的白细胞感染显像应在给药后24小时进行。
- ^{111}In-8-羟基喹啉-白细胞较^{67}Ga最大的优势为无生理性肠道积聚，从而可以用于腹部、肠道感染或炎性病变。
- ^{111}In标记白细胞较^{67}Ga的缺点是标记过程烦琐、辐射剂量较高和对脊柱骨髓炎的诊断准确性较低。
- ^{111}In标记白细胞较^{99m}Tc-HMPAO的优势包括：不受肠道和肾脏活性的干扰；能进行延迟成像；可以联合进行^{99m}Tc-硫胶体或^{99m}Tc-MDP骨扫描。这些联合方法有利于判断骨扫描异常(如人工关节的评估)的患者是否有骨髓炎，后文将进一步讨论。

^{99m}Tc-6-甲基丙二胺肟标记白细胞(^{99m}Tc-HMPAO-WBC)

- ^{99m}Tc-HMPAO标记的白细胞较^{111}In的优势是^{99m}Tc的半衰期短、允许注射较高放射剂量、图像计数高、辐射吸收剂量较低，以及更早进行显像。由于这些原因，^{99m}Tc更适用于某些情况下的儿童。
- 主要的缺点是胃肠道和泌尿生殖道生理性摄取未结合的^{99m}Tc-HMPAO复合物，因而限制了在肠道的应用。肾脏的放射性出现在早期，而肠道的放射性出现在1~2小时后。另外，因为^{99m}Tc半衰期较短，通常无法进行延迟显像。

Gallium-67

- Gallium-67 is cyclotron-produced and decays by electron capture, with a half-life of 78 hours. It emits multiple gamma rays at 93, 184, 296, and 388 keV (easier to remember as 90, 190, 290, and 390 keV). Gallium binds to transferrin, which is found in infection, inflammation, and neoplasm.
- Normal distribution includes the nasopharynx, lacrimal and salivary glands, liver, colon, and bone marrow. Use is limited in the abdomen due to high bowel and liver uptake.
- Persistent gallium in the kidneys is never normal after 24 hours and signifies renal disease or obstruction.
- Diffuse pulmonary uptake is also not normal, with a wide differential of infectious and inflammatory conditions:

  Pneumocystis pneumonia, idiopathic pulmonary fibrosis, sarcoidosis, lymphangitic carcinomatosis, miliary tuberculosis, and fungal infection.
- The *panda sign* reflects increased uptake in the nasopharynx, parotid glands, and lacrimal glands due to inflammation, resembling the dark markings on a panda's face. It is classically seen in sarcoidosis.

  The panda sign is not specific for sarcoidosis, although it strongly suggests sarcoid when the λ sign is also seen (due to bilateral hilar and right paratracheal adenopathy). Sarcoid is also the most common disorder to affect the salivary and lacrimal glands symmetrically.

  Differential diagnosis of the *panda sign* includes Sjögren syndrome, lymphoma after irradiation, and AIDS.
- Gallium scans have been largely replaced by F-18 FDG PET/CT. A residual first-line application of gallium scan is the evaluation of spinal discovertebral osteomyelitis.

镓-67(^{67}Ga)

- ^{67}Ga由回旋加速器生产，以电子俘获方式衰变，半衰期为78小时。它能发射多种能量的γ射线，能峰包括93keV、184keV、296keV和388keV(为了方便，可记为90keV、190keV、290keV和390keV)。^{67}Ga与转铁蛋白结合，浓聚在感染、炎症和肿瘤的部位。
- ^{67}Ga的正常分布包括鼻咽、泪腺、唾液腺、肝脏、结肠和骨髓。由于肠道和肝脏摄取过高，^{67}Ga在腹部疾病中的应用价值有限。
- 肾脏在24小时后仍持续浓聚^{67}Ga属于异常，提示有肾脏疾病或梗阻。
- 弥漫性肺摄取也属于不正常，需要与很多感染和炎性疾病进行鉴别：

  肺孢子虫肺炎、特发性肺间质纤维化、结节病、淋巴管性癌病、粟粒样肺结核和真菌感染。
- 熊猫征是指由于炎症时^{67}Ga在鼻咽部、腮腺和泪腺区域摄取增高导致的结节病的典型表现，构成上类似于熊猫脸上黑色部分。

  熊猫征不是结节病的特异征象，但与λ征(双侧肺门、右侧气管旁淋巴结肿大^{67}Ga摄取增高)同时出现时强烈提示结节病。结节病也常对称性累及两侧唾液腺和泪腺。

  熊猫征的鉴别诊断包括干燥综合征、淋巴瘤放疗后和获得性免疫缺陷综合征(AIDS)。
- ^{67}Ga扫描已经在很大程度上被^{18}F-FDG PET/CT所取代。^{67}Ga唯一被保留的一线临床应用是评价脊椎骨髓炎与椎间盘炎。

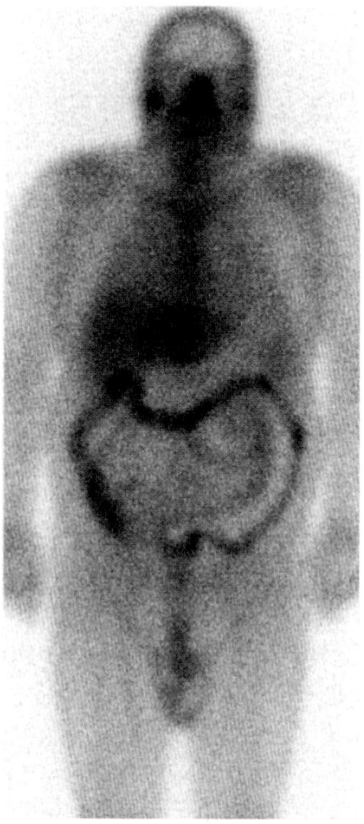

Normal Gallium-67 scan (5.25 mCi administered) shows high uptake in the bowel and salivary glands, moderate uptake in the liver and bone marrow, and faint uptake in the lungs.
正常^{67}Ga扫描(注射5.25mCi)显示肠道和唾液腺有强摄取，肝脏和骨髓有中度摄取，肺部有少量摄取。

Thallium-201

- Thallium-201 is cyclotron-produced, decays by electron capture, and produces relatively low-energy characteristic x-rays of 69–81 keV. Its half-life is 73 hours. Normal distribution is prominent uptake in the kidneys, heart, liver, thyroid, and bowel.
- Thallium imaging is infrequently used due to its long half-life and resultant high radiation exposure. Historically, thallium has been used in combination with gallium scan to distinguish between Kaposi sarcoma, lymphoma, and tuberculosis in immunocompromised patients. Thallium was also historically used as a myocardial agent.

^{201}铊(^{201}Tl)

- ^{201}Tl由回旋加速器生产，以电子俘获方式衰变，可产生能量相对较低的特征X线，能峰为69~81keV。半衰期73小时。正常情况下在肾脏、心脏、肝脏、甲状腺和肠道有显著分布。
- ^{201}Tl显像已不常用，因为其半衰期长，辐射吸收剂量相对较高。^{201}Tl曾与^{67}Ga联合扫描，用于鉴别免疫缺陷患者可能罹患的卡波西肉瘤、淋巴瘤及结核。^{201}Tl也曾用作心肌显像剂。

Clinical Applications

Hepatocellular carcinoma (HCC)

- Historically, increased focal gallium uptake in the liver suggests hepatocellular carcinoma (HCC). Conversely, HCC is extremely unlikely if gallium uptake is diminished.

Combined gallium and thallium imaging

- Kaposi sarcoma is thallium-avid, but does not take up gallium. *Mnemonic: KaT (Kaposi is Thallium-avid).*
- Tuberculosis and atypical mycobacteria take up gallium but not thallium. This is the opposite of Kaposi sarcoma. *Mnemonic: TuG (Tuberculosis is Gallium-avid).*
- Lymphoma takes up both gallium and thallium. *Mnemonic: Lymphoma likes both.*

Osteomyelitis

- A positive triple-phase Tc-99m MDP bone scan is only specific for osteomyelitis if the radiograph is normal. If there is an underlying abnormality, SPECT/CT, gallium or WBC scan can increase specificity.
- Gallium imaging can increase specificity of a positive bone scan, especially for vertebral osteomyelitis and discitis.
- A WBC scan (typically with Indium-111) can increase specificity in evaluation of an infected orthopedic prosthesis, where scanning is typically performed in conjunction with Tc-99m sulfur colloid. When comparing the two scans (WBC and sulfur colloid), a discordant region with increased WBC tracer uptake and decreased sulfur colloid uptake is suggestive of marrow replacement by WBCs, consistent with osteomyelitis. Conversely, a region of normal marrow would be expected to demonstrate uptake both by WBCs and sulfur colloid.

Adrenal pheochromocytoma

- I-123 MIBG is generally considered the first-line agent for evaluation of adrenal pheochromocytoma. Indium-111 pentetreotide can be considered as a second-line agent if the MIBG scan is negative, though the normal renal uptake of pentetreotide may obscure an adrenal lesion.

Extra-adrenal pheochromocytoma

- The sensitivity of I-123 MIBG for detection of extra-adrenal pheochromocytoma (i.e., paraganglioma or glomus tumor) ranges from 63–100%, with potential loss of MIBG uptake seen in tumor cell dedifferentiation, altered membrane transport proteins, or interference by medications. Indium-111 pentetreotide is also an option.
- The role of F-18 FDG PET in the evaluation of metastatic extra-adrenal pheochromocytoma is evolving. Most tumors are FDG-avid.

临床应用

肝细胞癌(HCC)

- 肝脏局灶性^{67}Ga摄取曾经用于诊断肝细胞癌(HCC)。如果^{67}Ga摄取减少，HCC的可能性则非常小。

^{67}Ga和^{201}Tl联合显像

- 卡波西肉瘤摄取^{201}Tl，但不摄取^{67}Ga。记忆诀窍："KaT"(Kaposi亲^{201}Tl)。
- 结核和非结核分枝杆菌摄取^{67}Ga，但不摄取^{201}Tl。这正好与卡波西肉瘤相反。记忆诀窍："TuG"(tuberculosis亲Ga)。
- 淋巴瘤^{67}Ga和^{201}Tl两者都摄取。记忆诀窍："淋巴瘤两个都喜欢"。

骨髓炎

- 只有X线影像正常的情况下，^{99m}Tc-MDP三相骨扫描阳性对骨髓炎有特异性。如果X线检查异常，SPECT/CT、^{67}Ga或白细胞扫描能够增加诊断的特异度。
- ^{67}Ga显像能够增加阳性骨扫描的特异度，尤其是对椎体骨髓炎和椎间盘炎。
- 白细胞扫描(通常使用^{111}In标记)通常与^{99m}Tc-硫胶体进行联合显像，以提高诊断人工假体感染的特异度。在对比白细胞与硫胶体两种扫描时，若出现白细胞示踪剂摄取增高而硫胶体摄取降低的不一致的区域，则提示骨髓被白细胞替代，符合骨髓炎的诊断。相反，一个正常骨髓区域应该对白细胞和硫胶体两者都有摄取。

肾上腺嗜铬细胞瘤

- ^{123}I-MIBG通常被认为是评估肾上腺嗜铬细胞瘤的一线药物。如果MIBG扫描呈阴性，^{111}In-喷曲肽可作为二线药物，但肾脏对喷曲肽的正常摄取可掩盖肾上腺的病变。

肾上腺外嗜铬细胞瘤

- ^{123}I-MIBG检测肾上腺外嗜铬细胞瘤(即副神经节瘤或血管球瘤)的灵敏度为63%~100%。而肿瘤细胞去分化、膜转运蛋白修饰、药物干扰等都可能导致病灶丧失摄取MIBG的能力。^{111}In-喷曲肽也可以作为备选显像剂。
- ^{18}F-FDG PET显像在评价转移性肾上腺外嗜铬细胞瘤上的作用越来越大。大多数肿瘤是亲FDG的。

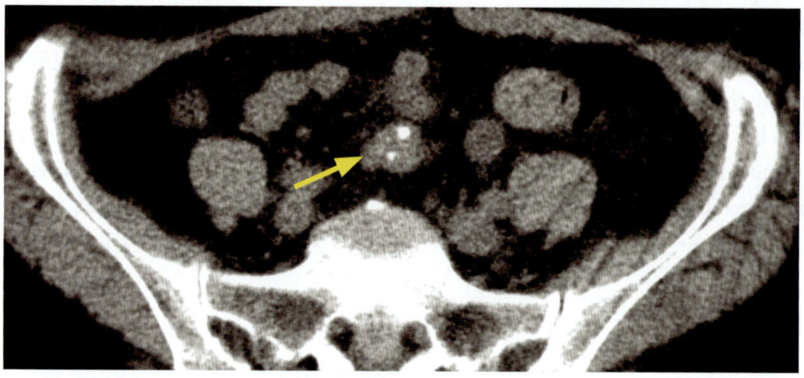

Metastatic carcinoid: Axial non-contrast CT shows a mesenteric mass containing coarse calcification (arrow) in the central lower abdomen, which has a typical appearance for carcinoid.
转移性类癌：轴位CT平扫显示下腹部中央有一个肠系膜肿块含粗大钙化灶(黄箭)，这是典型的类癌表现。

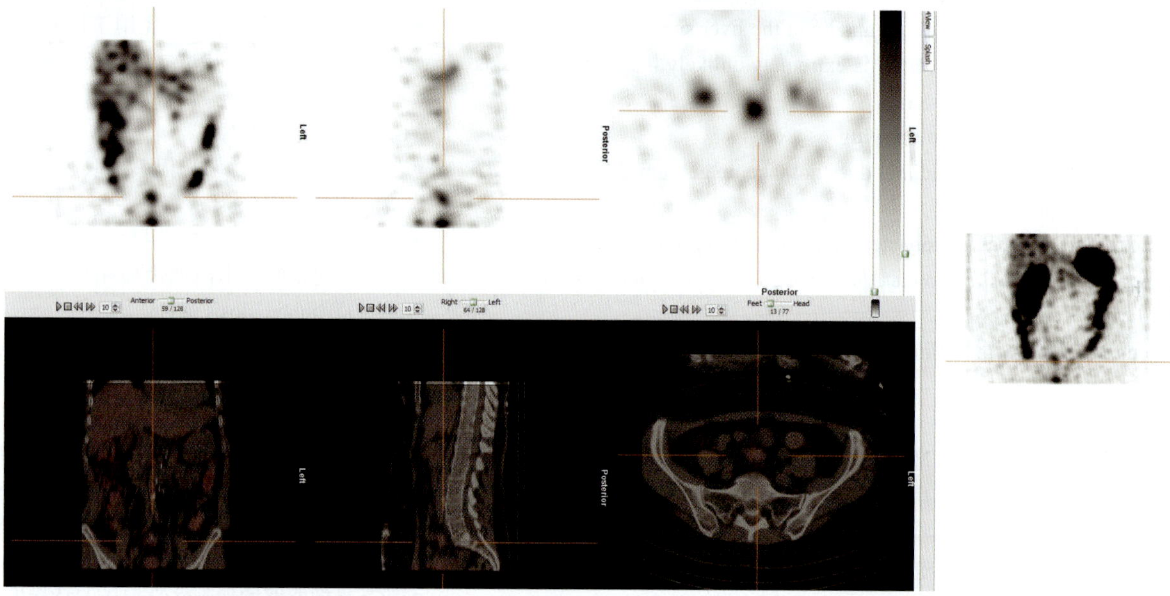

Fused multiplanar SPECT (top row) from an indium-111 pentetreotide scan and CT (bottom row) correlate a focus of increased uptake in the lower abdomen with the calcified mesenteric mass on CT, confirming the diagnosis of neuroendocrine tumor/carcinoid. All other foci of tracer uptake seen on SPECT localized to bowel, representing physiologic bowel uptake.
多平面融合^{111}In-喷曲肽扫描SPECT图像(上排)和CT(下排图)显示下腹部肠系膜钙化团块局部摄取增高，证实是神经内分泌肿瘤/类癌。其他局部示踪剂摄取区位于肠道，为肠道的生理性摄取。

- Indium-111 pentetreotide (Octreoscan) was traditionally the tracer of choice for evaluation of carcinoid tumor (see below). SPECT/CT is almost always performed in conjuction with an Octreoscan.
- The sensitivity for detecting neuroendocrine tumors is 82–95%; however, specificity is only around 50%, especially when a "hot spot" is found near a region of physiologic uptake in the pituitary, thyroid, liver, spleen, urinary tract, or bowel. False positives can also occur in benign processes such as inflammation, Graves disease, and sarcoidosis. These inflammatory false-positives are thought to be due to somatostatin receptors expressed in activated lymphocytes.
- Octreoscan is being replaced by Gallium-68 DOTATATE PET/CT (discussed earlier in this chapter) for detection of neuroendocrine tumors with high somatostatin receptor expression, as PET/CT has higher spatial resolution than SPECT/CT and Gallium-68-DOTATATE has much higher affinity for somatostatin receptors than Indium-111 pentetreotide.

- ^{111}In-喷曲肽(奥曲肽)是用于类癌诊断的传统首选示踪剂(见下文)。SPECT/CT显像几乎总是与^{111}In-喷曲肽一起使用。
- 探测神经内分泌肿瘤的灵敏度为82%~95%，但特异度只有50%左右，尤其是当"浓聚区"出现在生理性摄取的周围，如垂体、甲状腺、肝脏、脾脏、尿道或肠道。假阳性可以出现在良性疾病中，如炎症、格雷夫斯病和结节病。这些炎性假阳性被认为是由于生长抑素受体在活化的淋巴细胞中的表达。
- ^{111}In-喷曲肽正被^{68}Ga-DOTATATE PET/CT所取代，用于检测有高度表达生长抑素受体的神经内分泌肿瘤(已在本章前文进行讨论)，因为PET/CT比SPECT/CT有更高的空间分辨率，而且^{68}Ga-DOTATATE比^{111}In-喷曲肽对生长抑素受体有更高的亲和力。

(翻译　陈仰纯)

OTHER NON-PET IMAGING

Lymphoscintigraphy

- For cancers that metastasize first to regional lymph nodes, such as melanoma and breast carcinoma, lymphoscintigraphy can be used to identify the sentinel lymph node required for tumor staging. Filtered Tc-99m sulfur colloid is injected in the peritumoral region, subsequent images allow mapping of lymphatic drainage from the tumor. The first node visualized is the sentinel node. A gamma probe can be used intraoperatively during the same-day surgery to localize the sentinel node for excision.
- Lymphoscintigraphy is also utilized in the diagnosis of lymphedema. Lymphatic drainage in the involved extremity is visualized after interdigital injection of the radiotracer. Obstructive lymphedema presents as delayed migration of activity from the injection site, diffuse dermal backflow uptake, dilated and collateral lymphatic channels.

Molecular breast imaging

- Technetium-99m sestamibi concentrates in breast cancers and can be used as a problem-solving adjunct to mammography and ultrasound, particularly in women with dense breast tissue.
- Normal breast has low, homogeneous or patchy uptake. Focal uptake in the breast or axilla is suspicious for malignancy.
- Molecular breast imaging with Tc-99m sestamibi has high sensitivity and specificity (80–90%). However, radiation dose to the breast remains a disadvantage.

Radionuclide testicular imaging

- Historically, testicular imaging with technetium-99m pertechnetate has been used in the diagnosis of testicular torsion. The radiotracer is injected intravenously, immediate dynamic imaging of the anterior pelvis is then obtained, followed by delayed static images.
- Normal testes show symmetric homogeneous uptake. Decreased perfusion or focal photopenia on the symptomatic side is diagnostic of torsion. Increased perfusion suggests hyperemia, which is seen in epididymitis/orchitis.
- Although radionuclide imaging is more sensitive for testicular torsion, it is slower and less readily available compared to scrotal ultrasound.

其他非PET成像

淋巴(闪烁)显像

- 首先转移到区域淋巴结的肿瘤，如黑色素瘤和乳腺癌，可使用淋巴显像探测这些前哨淋巴结以便进行肿瘤分期。将^{99m}Tc-标记的硫胶体过滤后注入肿瘤周围，随后的显像可获得区域性肿瘤淋巴引流图。首先看到的淋巴结就是前哨淋巴结。伽马探测仪可在同日手术切除术中对前哨淋巴结进行定位。
- 淋巴显像也可用于诊断淋巴水肿。在指蹼注射放射性示踪剂后，可显示受累肢体的淋巴引流。阻塞性淋巴水肿表现为注射部位回流延迟、弥漫性皮肤回流、淋巴管扩张和侧支形成。

乳腺分子显像

- 乳腺癌摄取^{99m}Tc-MIBI，可针对性辅助乳房X线和超声来检查有困难的病例，特别是乳腺组织致密的妇女。
- 正常乳房组织会有少量摄取，呈均匀或斑片状。乳腺或腋窝有局灶性浓聚时应怀疑有恶性肿瘤。
- ^{99m}Tc-MIBI乳腺分子显像有较高的灵敏度和特异度(80%~90%)。然而，乳房辐射是该方法的一个缺陷。

睾丸的放射性核素显像

- 采用$^{99m}TcO_4$进行睾丸成像传统上被用于诊断睾丸扭转。静脉注射放射性示踪剂后立即行前位盆腔动态显像，然后进行延迟静态显像。
- 正常睾丸呈对称性、均匀摄取。有症状侧的血流灌注减少或局灶性缺损可用以诊断睾丸扭转。血流灌注增加提示充血，见于附睾炎/睾丸炎。
- 虽然放射性核素显像对诊断睾丸扭转更为敏感，但较阴囊超声检查慢且不能随时进行。

(翻译　许长德)

7 Cardiac Imaging

Ellen X. Sun, Junzi Shi, Sharmila Dorbala, Ayaz Aghayev, Michael L. Steigner

7 心脏影像

Contents

目录

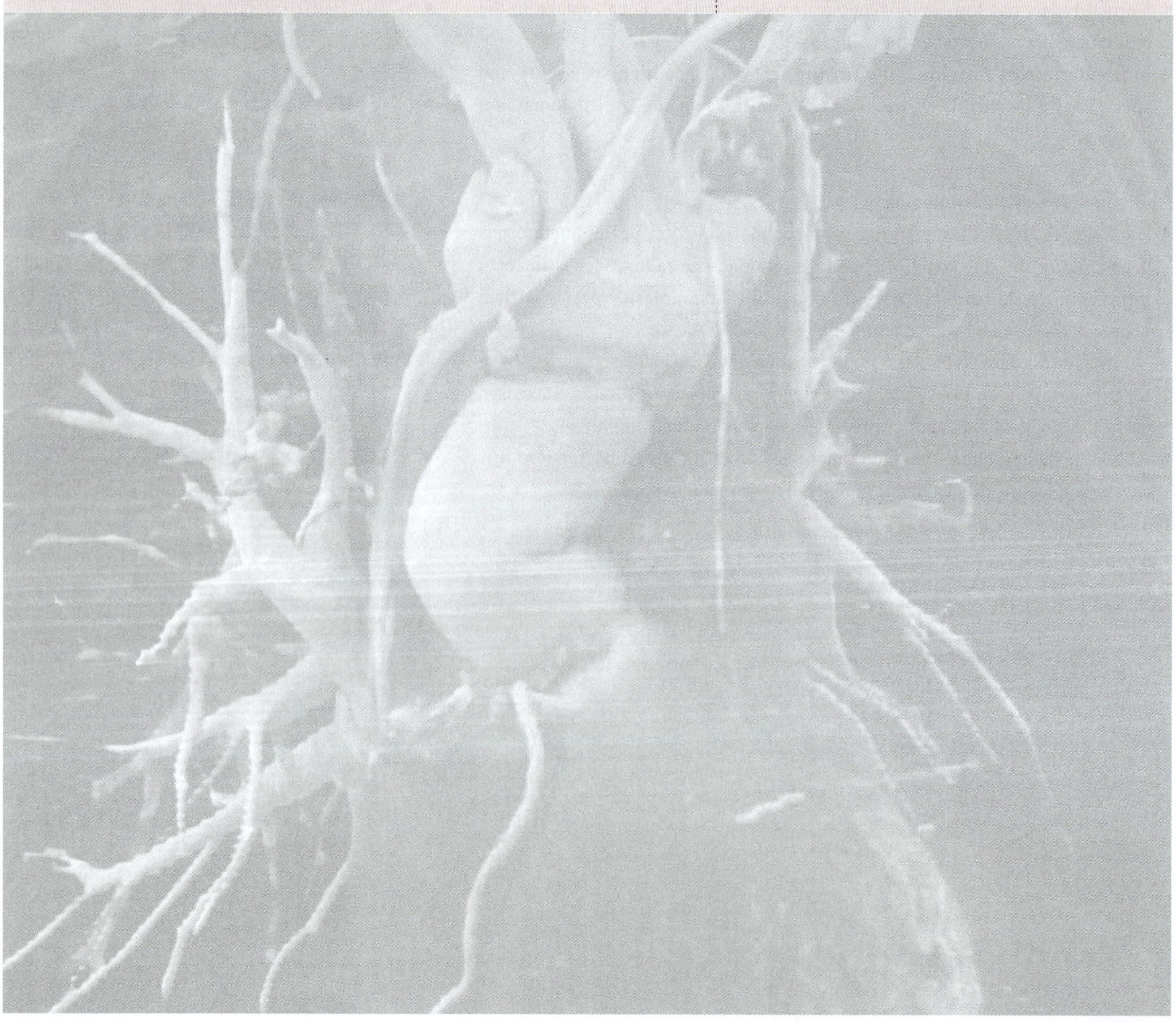

NUCLEAR CARDIOLOGY

MYOCARDIAL PERFUSION AND VIABILITY IMAGING

Perfusion imaging overview

- Radionuclide perfusion imaging evaluates the blood flow to the left ventricular myocardium. Decreased regional myocardial perfusion can result from reduced blood flow due to hemodynamically significant obstructive coronary artery disease (stress) or lack of viable cells due to myocardial infarction (rest).
- Each perfusion test has two components: An element of *stress*, and a method of *imaging*.
- The stress component can be physical (treadmill), pharmacologic-vasodilatory (dipyridamole, adenosine, or regadenoson) or pharmacologic-adrenergic (dobutamine).
- Radionuclide perfusion imaging can be performed with SPECT (Tc-99m sestamibi, Tc-99m tetrofosmin, thallium-201) or PET radiotracers (rubidium-82, N-13 ammonia). ECG-gated imaging is standard for cardiac SPECT (GSPECT) and PET.

  Other types of stress tests performed by cardiologists (ECG stress tests and echocardiographic or MRI stress tests) can be performed in lieu of radionuclide imaging. These non-imaging tests can detect other signs of perfusion abnormalities, such as ischemic ECG changes or wall motion abnormalities.

Viability imaging overview

- Prior to a revascularization procedure (e.g., coronary artery bypass surgery, CABG or coronary angioplasty/stenting), it is important to know if the hypoperfused myocardium is viable, as the revascularization of scar tissue would not provide a clinical benefit.
- Viability imaging can be performed with rest-redistribution thallium-201 perfusion imaging or F-18 FDG PET metabolic imaging. F-18 FDG PET evaluation of glucose metabolism is the gold standard for evaluation of myocardial viability, although unlike thallium *FDG-PET does not evaluate perfusion.*

Clinical applications of myocardial perfusion and viability imaging

- **Evaluation of acute chest pain.** Myocardial perfusion imaging is often the gatekeeper to further cardiac workup in patients where there is clinical ambiguity for cardiac ischemia (e.g., chest pain with negative ECG and troponins). A negative myocardial perfusion exam allows safe discharge.

  A normal myocardial perfusion exam is associated with a 0.6% annual rate of a cardiac event, even among patients with a high pre-test likelihood of coronary artery disease.
- **Evaluation of hemodynamic significance of coronary stenosis.** Even with a coronary artery stenosis seen on invasive or CT angiography, patients with a normal nuclear cardiac perfusion exam have a relatively low risk for cardiac events.
- **Risk stratification after MI.** Findings that would classify a patient as high risk include:

核心脏病学

心肌灌注与存活显像

灌注显像概述

- 放射性核素灌注显像用于评估流向左心室心肌的血流。局部心肌灌注减少可能是因为有引起明显血流动力学改变的冠状动脉阻塞性疾病(负荷)或因心肌梗死(静息)引起的活性细胞缺乏。
- 每一项灌注检查都包括两个部分：一为负荷，二是显像方法。
- 负荷可以是物理性的(跑步机)、血管舒张药物(双嘧达莫、腺苷或瑞加德松)或拟肾上腺素剂(多巴酚丁胺)。
- 放射性核素灌注显像可以使用SPECT(^{99m}Tc-MIBI、^{99m}Tc-替曲膦、^{201}Tl)或PET放射性示踪剂(^{82}Rb、^{13}N-NH_4)。心电门控常规用于心脏SPECT(GSECT)和PET成像。

  心脏科医生可选择非核素显像的其他负荷检查(负荷心电图和负荷超声心动图检查或MRI负荷试验)。这些非影像检查只能检测灌注异常引起的继发征象，如缺血性心电图改变或室壁运动异常。

心肌存活显像概述

- 在进行血运重建前(如冠状动脉血管搭桥手术，CABG或冠状动脉血管成形/支架术)，很重要的一点就是要确认低灌注心肌是否存活，因为对瘢痕组织进行血运重建不会在搭桥后产生临床效果。
- 心肌存活显像可以用^{201}Tl静态再分布灌注显像或^{18}F-FDG PET代谢显像。^{18}F-FDG PET评估葡萄糖代谢是评估心肌活性的“金标准”，但FDG并不可以像Tl用于评估心肌灌注功能。

心肌灌注与存活显像的临床应用

- **评估急性胸痛**：心肌灌注显像在临床不能确定是否存在心脏缺血时(如有胸痛但心电图和肌钙蛋白检测阴性)通常起到决定性作用。阴性心肌灌注显像可以让患者安全出院。

  正常心肌灌注显像的年心脏事件发生率为0.6%，即使在预测试验中有较高冠状动脉发病率的患者也是如此。
- **评估有血流动力学改变的冠状动脉狭窄**：即使冠状动脉造影或CT检查发现有冠状动脉狭窄，但核医学心肌灌注显像正常患者所发生的心脏事件的概率相对较低。
- **心肌梗死(MI)后的风险分级**。下列发现可以将患者归为高危人群：

Large and severe perfusion defects.

Significant stress-induced or peri-infarct ischemia.

Defect in multiple vascular territories (suggesting multi-vessel disease). Significant lung uptake, suggesting left ventricular dysfunction.

Left ventricular aneurysm.

Low ejection fraction (less than 40% seen) on gated imaging.

Ejection fraction (EF) is calculated as EF = (EDC – ESC)/(EDC – BC)

EDC = end diastolic counts; ESC = end systolic counts; BC = background counts

大而严重的灌注缺损。

明显有负荷诱发或梗死周边缺血。

多血管分布区域缺损(提示多支血管病变)。肺部有明显摄取，提示左心室功能障碍。

左心室室壁瘤。

门控显像上显示低射血分数(小于40%)。

射血分数(EF)计算：EF=(EDC–ESC)/(EDC–BC)

EDC=舒张末期计数；ESC=收缩末期计数；BC=本底计数。

- **Preoperative risk assessment for intermediate to high risk noncardiac surgery.**
- **Evaluation of viability prior to coronary revascularization therapy.**
- **Evaluation of myocardial revascularization status post CABG in symptomatic patients or after 5 years.**

- **术前评估非心脏手术的中高风险程度。**
- **评估冠状动脉血运重建治疗前的心肌存活状态。**
- **评估冠状动脉搭桥术后有症状患者或术后5年心肌血管再通状态。**

Radionuclides

Thallium-201

- Thallium-201 is a cyclotron-produced radionuclide with a half-life of 73 hours. It decays by electron capture and emits characteristic X-rays of 69–81 keV.

  Relatively low energy characteristic X-rays increase attenuation artifact from chest wall soft tissues.

  It is necessary to administer fairly low doses due to its long half-life, with resultant lower count densities which requires longer imaging acquisition times.
- Physiologically, thallium acts like a potassium analog, crossing into the cell via active transport through the ATP-dependent sodium-potassium transmembrane pump.
- Myocardial uptake is directly proportional to myocardial perfusion.
- A 50% stenosis will generally produce a perfusion defect upon maximal exercise.
- Thallium undergoes **redistribution** with simultaneous cellular washout and re-extraction of blood-pool radiotracer. Only viable myocardium can extract thallium. Therefore, ischemic but viable myocardium will show perfusion defect during stress due to decreased blood flow, but normalization of defect on post-redistribution images. In contrast, an infarct or scar will show a persistent defect.

Technetium-99m sestamibi and tetrofosmin

- Technetium-99m is generator-produced, therefore more readily available. Its shorter half-life (6 hours) and higher photon energy (140 keV) allow for larger administered dose at lower radiation dose to the patient, superior image quality, shorter acquisition time, and less attenuation artifact from adjacent soft tissues. For these reasons, Tc-99m labeled radiotracers are more widely used than thallium in myocardial perfusion imaging.
- Unlike thallium, Tc-99m sestamibi (Cardiolite) **does not undergo redistribution** and remains fixed in the myocardium.
- Sestamibi enters myocardium via passive diffusion and binds to mitochondrial membrane proteins. Similar to thallium, myocardial uptake of sestamibi is proportional to myocardial perfusion.

放射性核素

^{201}铊(^{201}Tl)

- ^{201}Tl是一种由回旋加速器生产的放射性核素，半衰期为73小时，通过电子俘获的方式衰减并释放出能量为69~81keV的特征性X射线。

  相对低能的特征性X射线增加了由胸壁软组织产生的衰减伪影。

  由于半衰期较长，必须给予较低的剂量，因而导致放射性计数密度降低而使得显像采集时间延长。
- 生理学上，铊的活性类似于钾离子，通过ATP依赖性钠钾跨膜泵主动转运进入细胞内。
- 心肌摄取量直接与心肌血流灌注量成正比。
- 约50%的狭窄处在运动达到极量后会产生灌注缺损。
- 铊会出现再分布，即同时从细胞洗脱并从血池中再摄取放射性示踪剂。只有有活性的心肌可摄取铊。因此，缺血但存活的心肌在负荷试验时会因为血流降低而出现灌注缺损，但在延迟再分布图像上原缺损区会转为正常分布。相反，梗死和瘢痕组织将出现持续缺损。

^{99m}Tc-甲氧基异丁基异腈(MIBI)和替曲膦

- ^{99m}Tc由发生器产生，因此更容易获得。因半衰期较短(6小时)和光子能量较高(140keV)，对患者的辐射剂量较低而允许给予较大剂量，其图像质量好、采集时间短及较少来自相邻软组织的衰减伪影。由于这些原因，^{99m}Tc标记的放射性示踪剂在心肌灌注成像中的应用比铊更加广泛。
- 与铊不尽相同，^{99m}Tc-MIBI**不会出现再分布**并一直固定在心肌细胞内。
- MIBI通过被动扩散进入心肌细胞并与线粒体膜蛋白结合。与铊相似，心肌摄取MIBI与心肌灌注成正比。

- Tc-99m tetrofosmin (Myoview) is similar to sestamibi but has the advantage of faster hepatobiliary clearance, which allows earlier imaging (since adjacent liver activity may interfere with cardiac imaging).

Rubidium-82

- Rubidium-82 is a positron-emitting PET *perfusion* agent that is generated from strontium-82. A very short half-life of 76 seconds allows high doses to be administered, however such a short half-life precludes the use of exercise stress. Pharmacologic stress is used instead.
- Rubidium-82 acts as a potassium analog, similar to thallium.

Nitrogen-13 ammonia

- Nitrogen-13 ammonia is a positron-emitting PET *perfusion* agent (like rubidium-82) that has a half-life of 10 minutes. Unlike rubidium-82, N-13 is cyclotron-produced and the cyclotron must be on-site due to its short half-life.
- N-13 has excellent imaging characteristics. N-13 positrons have a low kinetic energy and do not travel very far in the tissue before annihilating, which allows relatively high resolution. The short half-life also allows large doses to be given for high counts.
- Like rubidium-82, N-13 perfusion is almost always coupled with a pharmacologic stress. Exercise stress is possible with N-13 ammonia but can be logistically challenging due to the 10-minute half-life, as it has to be coordinated with the cyclotron delivery of the radiotracer.

Fluorine-18 FDG

- Fluorine-18-fluorodeoxyglucose (F-18 FDG), the same radiotracer used for oncologic imaging, is a positron emitting PET *viability* agent with a half-life of 110 minutes. Unlike rubidium-82 and N-13 ammonia, FDG cannot be used for perfusion.
- Viable myocardium uptakes FDG; scar does not.

Types of stress – exercise and pharmacologic

- The *stress* component of a cardiac perfusion study can be physical or pharmacologic.

General exercise protocol

- Prior to undergoing a myocardial perfusion study with exercise stress, the patient should be NPO for 6 hours. In patients without known coronary artery disease, calcium channel blockers and β blockers should be held to allow patient to reach target heart rate. Long-acting nitrates may mask ischemia and should also be held when possible.
- Exercise is performed with a multistage treadmill (Bruce or modified Bruce) protocol. The target heart rate, which is calculated as 85% of maximal heart rate must be achieved for the study to be diagnostic. The maximal calculated heart rate is 220 bpm minus age.
- Other parameters used to assess the adequacy of exercise stress include the product of peak heart rate and peak systolic blood pressure, metabolic equivalents (METs), and exercise time.
- Contraindications for exercise stress include acute myocardial infarction (within 48 hours), high risk unstable angina, sustained or hemodynamically significant ventricular tachyarrhythmia, acute aortic dissection, acute pulmonary embolism, acute pericarditis, severe symptomatic aortic stenosis, decompensated heart failure, or inability to exercise.

- ^{99m}Tc-替曲膦与MIBI相似，但有较快的肝胆清除优势，可以更早地进行显像(因为相邻的肝脏活性可能会干扰心脏显像)。

^{82}铷(^{82}Rb)

- ^{82}Rb是一种发射正电子的PET灌注显像剂，它来源于^{82}锶的衰变。因半衰期非常短，只有76秒，允许给予高剂量。但由于半衰期太短，不适合运动负荷试验。可用于药物负荷试验。
- ^{82}Rb为钾的类似物，与铊相似。

^{13}氮-氨水(^{13}N-NH_4)

- ^{13}N-NH_4是一种发射正电子的PET灌注显像剂(类似于^{82}Rb)，半衰期为10分钟。与^{82}Rb不同，^{13}N由回旋加速器生产，由于其半衰期短，有回旋加速器的单位才能使用。
- ^{13}N有极佳的显像特性。^{13}N的正电子动能较低，湮灭之前在组织中穿行距离很短，所以能提供相对高的分辨率。因其较短的半衰期，也允许给予较大剂量以提高计数。
- 与^{82}Rb一样，^{13}N灌注显像几乎都需要与药物负荷试验一起进行。虽然可以使用^{13}N-NH_4进行运动试验，但实际上很困难，因为半衰期只有10分钟，必须对回旋加速器生产的放射性示踪剂进行运送协调。

^{18}F-氟代脱氧葡萄糖(^{18}F-FDG)

- ^{18}F-FDG，为肿瘤显像的同一种放射性示踪剂，是发射正电子的PET心肌存活显像剂，半衰期为110分钟。与^{82}Rb和^{13}N-NH_4不同，FDG不能用于灌注显像。
- 存活心肌摄取FDG，但瘢痕组织不会。

负荷的种类——运动和药物

- 心脏灌注试验的负荷部分可以是运动或是药物。

运动试验的一般流程

- 在进行心肌灌注运动负荷试验之前，患者应禁食6小时。无冠状动脉疾病的患者应停用钙通道阻滞剂和β受体阻滞剂，以便让患者达到目标心率。长效硝酸盐可能会掩盖缺血，也应尽可能停用。
- 运动试验采用多级跑步机(Bruce或改进版Bruce)的流程。必须达到最大心率85%的目标心率才有诊断意义。最大心率(次/min)=220−年龄。
- 可适用于评估运动负荷的其他参数包括峰值心率、峰值收缩压、代谢当量(MET)和运动时间。
- 运动负荷的禁忌证包括急性心肌梗死(48小时内)、高危不稳定型心绞痛、持续或有显著血流动力学不稳定的室性心动过速、急性主动脉夹层、急性肺栓塞、急性心包炎、有严重症状的主动脉瓣狭窄、失代偿性心力衰竭或无法运动者。

- Pharmacologic stress is an alternative in patients who cannot exercise physically or in those with left bundle branch block, which can cause false positive reversible septal perfusion defects with exercise.

Dipyridamole stress – pharmacologic vasodilator

- Dipyridamole is an adenosine deaminase inhibitor that allows endogenous adenosine to accumulate. Adenosine is a potent vasodilator, increasing coronary blood flow by 3–5 times.
- The microcirculation fed by a critical coronary artery stenosis cannot further dilate in response to adenosine. That coronary artery territory will appear as a relative perfusion defect on stress imaging.
- Unlike a physical stress, a dipyridamole stress does not increase cardiac work or O_2 demand.
- Caffeine and theophylline competitively inhibit vasodilation from dipyridamole and must be held for at least 12 hours.
- Side effects of dipyridamole include nausea, dizziness, headache, flushing, and chest pain, wheezing, and rarely heart block. The antidote is aminophylline (100–200 mg), which has a shorter half-life than dipyridamole, so patients with wheezing or heart block from dipyridamole must be warned that symptoms may rarely reappear after several hours.

- 药物负荷是一种患者在无法进行运动试验，或有左束支传导阻滞而可能导致在运动时产生可逆性室间隔灌注缺损假阳性时的备选。

双嘧达莫(dipyridamole)负荷试验——药物血管扩张剂

- 双嘧达莫是腺苷脱氨酶抑制剂，它可以使内源性腺苷积聚。腺苷是一种强力的血管扩张剂，可使冠状动脉血流量增加3~5倍。
- 严重狭窄的冠状动脉所供应的微循环无法对腺苷产生进一步扩张。受累的冠状动脉供血区将在负荷显像时表现为相对灌注缺损。
- 与运动负荷不同，双嘧达莫负荷试验不会增加心脏负担或需氧量。
- 咖啡因和茶碱会竞争性抑制双嘧达莫的血管扩张作用，因而必须在检查前至少停用12小时。
- 双嘧达莫的副作用包括恶心、头晕、头痛、潮红、胸痛、喘息，偶尔引起心脏传导阻滞。双嘧达莫的拮抗剂为氨茶碱(100~200mg)，其半衰期较双嘧达莫更短，因此，对于使用双嘧达莫后出现喘息或心脏传导阻滞的患者，必须告知在极少数的情况下其症状有可能在数小时后再次出现。

Adenosine stress – pharmacologic vasodilator

- Adenosine has identical physiologic effects as dipyridamole but a more rapid effect. It may also frequently cause atrioventricular block that is resolved most of the time by physical exercise (hand grip or moving the legs or walking on a treadmill during infusion). Wheezing is also seen, especially in patients with asthma. Because adenosine has an extremely short half-life (<10 seconds), a reversal agent is usually not required.

Regadenoson – pharmacologic vasodilator

- Regadenoson is a selective A2A (adenosine) receptor agonist with a 2–3 minute half-life. It is easier to administer than adenosine with a convenient non-weight based fixed-dose intravenous injection over 10 seconds. Its effects can be reversed with aminophylline.

Dobutamine stress – pharmacologic stress

- Dobutamine is a β_1 agonist that increases myocardial oxygen demand. Dobutamine is used when vasodilator is contraindicated (severe asthma, COPD, or recent caffeine).
- Contraindications are the same as for exercise stress testing (see above).

腺苷(adenosine)负荷试验——药物血管扩张剂

- 腺苷与双嘧达莫具有相同的生理效应，但作用更快速。它也经常引起房室传导阻滞，但大部分情况可以通过体能运动得到恢复(输液期间手握或移动腿或在跑步机上行走)。也可见喘息，尤其是哮喘的患者。因为腺苷的半衰期极短(<10秒)，通常不需要逆转剂。

瑞加德松——药物血管扩张剂

- 瑞加德松是一种选择性A_2A(腺苷)受体激动剂，半衰期为2~3分钟。给药方式较腺苷容易，用法为在10秒内从静脉给予固定剂量，不按体重给药。它的作用可以用氨茶碱进行逆转。

多巴酚丁胺(dobutamine)负荷试验——药物负荷

- 多巴酚丁胺是一种β_1受体激动剂，会增加心肌需氧量。多巴酚丁胺适用于对血管扩张剂有禁忌(如严重哮喘、慢性阻塞性肺疾病或刚刚使用过咖啡因)患者。
- 禁忌证与运动负荷试验相同(见上文)。

Imaging protocols

Single-day Tc-99m sestamibi/tetrofosmin perfusion SPECT

- Tc-99m sestamibi or tetrofosmin perfusion SPECT is most commonly performed as a single-day study. Rest images are first obtained after intravenous injection of 8–10 mCi Tc-99m radiotracer. After background activity has cleared in 1–4 hours, stress images are obtained with an additional 25–30 mCi (three times rest dose) administered during peak exercise, or following pharmacologic stress.
- Imaging is performed 45–90 minutes post-injection for resting studies, and at 30 minutes for exercise stress because of faster liver activity clearance. Since

显像方法

一日法：^{99m}Tc-MIBI/替曲膦SPECT灌注法

- ^{99m}Tc-MIBI或替曲膦SPECT灌注为最常用的一日显像法。静息影像在静脉注射8~10mCi的^{99m}Tc放射性示踪剂后进行。负荷显像须在1~4小时体内本底放射性降低之后进行，在运动或药物负荷高峰另给予25~30mCi(3倍静息剂量)。
- 静态显像在注射后45~90分钟进行，而负荷显像在注射后30分钟后进行，因负荷会加快肝脏清除放射性。由于没有再分布现象，显像

there is no redistribution, imaging can be delayed after tracer administration.

- Gated SPECT images show wall motion *at time of imaging*, while perfusion images show perfusion *at time of injection*. Therefore, severely ischemic territories may sometimes not show evidence of regional wall motion abnormalities. If wall motion is abnormal in an ischemia territory, this typically indicates myocardial stunning, a highly specific feature for significant obstructive coronary artery disease.

可以在给予示踪剂后延迟进行。

- 门控SPECT(GSPECT)图像显示在获取影像时的室壁运动，而灌注图像则显示注射时的灌注状态。因此，严重缺血的区域有时可能不会显示局部室壁运动异常。如果在缺血区域呈现室壁运动异常，通常表明心肌处于顿抑状态，这是对严重阻塞性冠状动脉疾病的高度特异的一个征象。

Two-day Tc-99m sestamibi/tetrofosmin perfusion SPECT

- By performing the stress and rest studies on separate days, maximum dose (25–30 mCi) of radiotracer can be administered for optimal image quality, and interference by residual activity from the first study is minimized. This protocol is usually used in obese patients.
- Also, if the stress study is performed first and is normal, the rest study can be safely omitted. This is currently the preferred protocol due to shorter test duration and lower radiation dose.

两日法^{99m}Tc-MIBI/替曲膦SPECT灌注显像

- 负荷和静息显像在不同的日期进行可以注射最大剂量(25~30mCi)放射性示踪剂而可获得的最佳图像质量，并减少了第一次显像残留放射性的干扰。该方法通常用于肥胖患者。
- 此外，如果首先进行负荷试验为正常，不进行其他试验不会有风险。由于耗时短且辐射剂量低，为目前首选方法。

Thallium stress-redistribution (rest) SPECT

- Because thallium undergoes redistribution, imaging is performed immediately (within 10–15 minutes) post-exercise and approximately 3–4 hours later once redistribution has occurred. Both sets of images can be obtained after a single injection of 3 mCi thallium, or two separate injections with 2 mCi administered at peak exercise for the stress images, and an additional 1 mCi administered before the second image set to ensure adequate thallium is available for redistribution.
- Thallium is not often used for myocardial perfusion imaging because of its long 73-hour half-life and high radiation dose. However, it is used for viability imaging at sites without access to a PET scanner.

铊负荷再分布(静止)SPECT

- 铊会发生再分布，所以成像应在运动后立即进行(在10~15分钟之内)，再分布显像则在3~4小时后进行。两组图像可在单次注射3mCi铊后获得，或在运动高峰期分别注射2mCi以获得负荷图像，在获取第二个图像之前追加1mCi以确保足够的铊可用于重新分配。
- 铊不常用于心肌灌注显像，因为其半衰期长达73小时和高辐射剂量。但可以在没有PET设备的地区进行存活显像。

Thallium rest-redistribution (rest) SPECT

- For evaluation of myocardial viability prior to revascularization therapy, a rest-rest or rest-redistribution thallium study can be helpful. Following thallium injection at rest, images are obtained at 15 minutes and 3–4 hours later. Uptake on the delayed (redistribution) images indicates viable myocardium.

铊静息再分布(休息)SPECT

- 静息-静息或静息-铊再分布显像对于血运重建治疗前评估心肌存活有所帮助。在静息状态下注射铊，于15分钟和3~4小时采集图像。如延迟(再分布)图像上有摄取表示有存活的心肌。

PET perfusion

- PET rest-stress myocardial perfusion has greater sensitivity, specificity, and accuracy for diagnosis of coronary artery disease compared to SPECT imaging.
- Rubidium-82 and N-13 ammonia are perfusion agents and are imaged on a PET system using coincidence detection. The shorter half-life of these tracers allows higher activities to be administered with lower overall radiation exposure. For quantification of myocardial blood flow, both rubidium-82 and N-13 ammonia have been validated.

PET灌注

- PET静态与负荷心肌灌注较SPECT成像对于冠状动脉疾病的诊断具有更高的灵敏度、特异度和准确度。
- ^{82}Rb和^{13}N-NH$_4$是灌注显像剂，需要使用PET符合系统进行成像。这些示踪剂的半衰期较短，因此可以给予较高的剂量而总辐射剂量并不高。^{82}Rb和^{13}N-NH$_4$都被认可用于心肌血流定量。

PET myocardial viability (glucose metabolism)

- F-18 FDG PET is preferred over thallium for evaluation of myocardial viability.
- To induce metabolism of glucose over fatty acids by the myocardium, patient is loaded with oral or IV glucose after a 6-hour fast, which triggers endogenous insulin production that in turn encourages glucose uptake and decreases fatty acid levels.
- FDG uptake is seen in both normal myocardium and ischemic but viable myocardium.

PET心肌活力(葡萄糖代谢)

- ^{18}F-FDG PET在评估心肌存活方面优于铊。
- 为了诱导心肌从脂肪酸代谢到优先利用葡萄糖，患者需要禁食6小时后口服或静脉注射葡萄糖，以触发内源性胰岛素分泌来促进葡萄糖摄取并降低脂肪酸水平。
- FDG摄取既可见于正常心肌，也可以见于缺血但存活的心肌。

SPECT/CT and PET/CT

- Attenuation-correction CT improves diagnostic accuracy by eliminating attenuation artifact and can be used for coronary artery calcium scoring.

SPECT/CT和PET/CT

- CT衰减校正通过消除衰减伪影来提高诊断的准确度并可用于冠状动脉钙化评分。

IMAGE INTERPRETATION

图像解读

Key to successful perfusion imaging interpretation is a systematic approach:

- Quality control: Is it a good study?

  For instance, in a single-day rest-stress study, the stress images should have higher signal to noise compared to the rest images since 3x more radiotracer was administered. If not, consider dose infiltration.

- Is there misregistration between the stress and rest images, or between the SPECT and CT images? The attenuation-corrected and uncorrected images should be compared for potential artifacts.
- The coronal/rotating raw SPECT images can show important ancillary findings:

系统法是成功解读图像的关键：

- 质量控制：这是一项良好的检查吗？

  例如，在一日法静息-负荷显像时，因为负荷显像给的放射性示踪剂剂量比静息显像高3倍，故应该有更高的信噪比，否则要考虑注射药物外渗。

- 负荷与静息图像之间，或SPECT和CT图像之间是否存在匹配错误？应比较已校正和未校正图像以区别潜在的伪影。
- 原始冠状/旋转MIP可以显示重要的辅助信息：

Is there **motion artifact**?

有移动伪影吗？

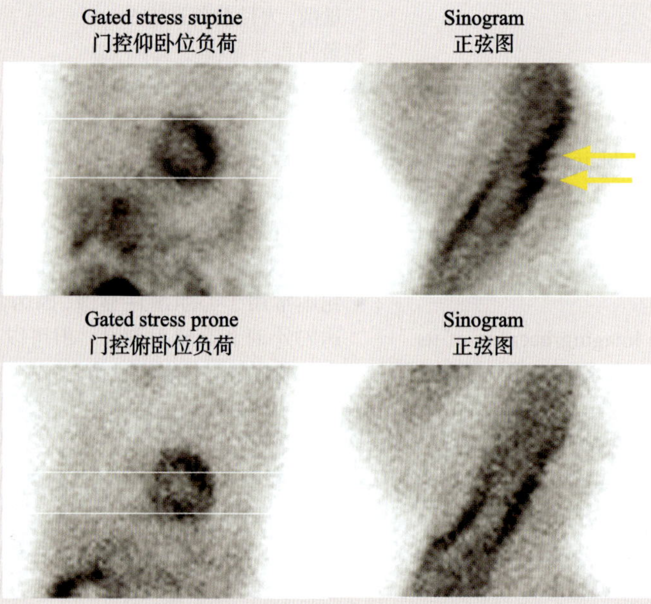

Stress Tc-99m sestamibi rotating projection (representative image shown on left) and sinogram with patient in the supine position (top row) demonstrate motion, as indicated by horizontal breaks in the sinogram (arrows). Prone position stress sinogram (bottom row) shows no motion artifact.

仰卧位负荷^{99m}Tc-MIBI旋转投影(左侧两图像)和正弦图(右上图)显示有移动，正弦图上有水平中断(黄箭)。

俯卧位负荷正弦图(右下图)未显示有移动。

Is there **attenuation artifact** from the breast, diaphragm, or chest wall? Attenuation artifacts have normal wall motion on gated SPECT cine. A true fixed defect (infarct or scar) is hypokinetic or akinetic.

Is there **abnormal extracardiac uptake**? Focal intense uptake in the breast or lung may signify cancer.

Is there **pulmonary uptake** on exercise thallium-201 or Tc-99m sestamibi/tetrofosmin scan? Abnormally increased lung-to-heart activity ratio indicates stress-induced left ventricular dysfunction, usually from left main or multivessel coronary artery disease.

是否有来自乳房、膈肌或胸壁的**衰减伪影**？衰减伪影在门控SPECT电影上显示正常的室壁运动。真正的固定缺损(梗死或瘢痕)是运动下降或无运动。

是否有**心外异常摄取**？乳房或肺的局部强烈摄取可能提示有癌症。

运动^{201}Tl或^{99m}Tc-MIBI/替曲膦扫描是否有**肺摄取**？异常肺心活动比增加表示负荷引起左心室功能障碍，通常来自左主干或多支冠状动脉疾病。

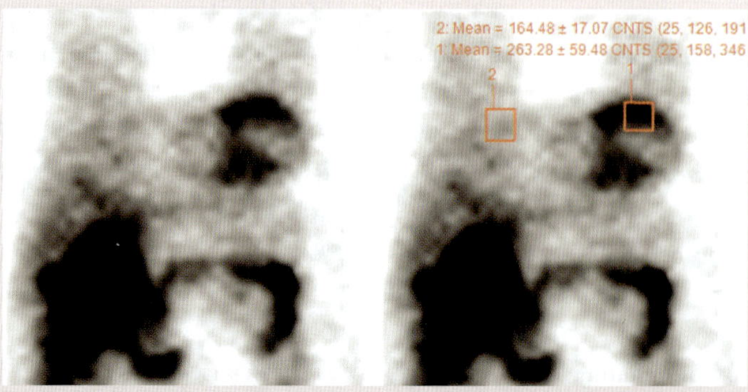

Pulmonary uptake of Tc-99m sestamibi:

Planar rotating projection images demonstrate increased lung uptake on exercise Tc-99m sestamibi scan with a lung to heart ratio of 0.62.

SPECT rest and exercise perfusion images demonstrated multivessel ischemia (not shown).

肺摄取^{99m}Tc-MIBI：

负荷平面旋转投影图像显示肺摄取^{99m}Tc-MIBI增加，其肺心比为0.62。

SPECT静息和运动灌注图像显示多血管缺血(未展示)。

- Evaluation of the rest and stress SPECT or PET perfusion images is the core of the exam, with the key question: **Is there a perfusion defect on the stress images?** If a perfusion abnormality is present, the following additional questions help to characterize it:

Is the defect reversible on rest images? A reversible defect signifies ischemia, while a fixed defect may represent either infarct/scar or hibernating myocardium.
How large is the defect (number of myocardial segments, described on the next page)? Small (1–2 segments); medium (3–4 segments); large (5 or more segments).
How severe is it? Mild (subendocardial), moderate, or severe (transmural)?
Where is it? In which coronary artery territory?
Is there dilation of the left ventricle during stress (**transient ischemic dilation, TID**)? If so, implies left main or three vessel disease and worse prognosis, even when there is no focal defect.
Is there **right ventricular uptake**? If so, implies right heart disease or pulmonary hypertension.
Is there **exercise-induced reversible septal defect**, not following a coronary artery territory? This occurs with LBBB in the absence of coronary artery disease and is not seen with pharmacologic stress.

In summary, an example interpretation may be: *There is a medium-sized perfusion defect of severe intensity involving the mid and basal inferior walls and the basal inferoseptal wall that was fixed. These findings suggest myocardial scar in the typical distribution of the RCA.*

- Gated SPECT (GSPECT) uses ECG gating of a standard myocardial perfusion SPECT acquisition for the quantitative assessment of the LV function. GSPECT allows for evaluation of LV perfusion at the same time as left ventricular wall motion, wall thickening, and ejection fraction (LVEF). It is not used to evaluate right ventricular function.

Assessment of myocardial viability

- Static SPECT images from a pure perfusion exam cannot distinguish between scar or hibernating myocardium. Both of these entities appear as a fixed (present on both stress and rest) perfusion defect.

Myocardial scar is fibrosis resulting from prior myocardial necrosis (infarction).
Hibernating myocardium describes viable but hypoperfused myocardium due to severe chronic ischemia, which may benefit from revascularization (either CABG or percutaneous intervention).

- Functional data from GSPECT can distinguish attenuation artifacts from true perfusion defects; but GSPECT cannot distinguish hibernating myocardium from scar. Normal or nearly normal wall motion and wall thickening in the area of the perfusion defect suggests attenuation artifact, while a fixed defect with abnormal wall motion suggests scar or hibernating myocardium. FDG PET or thallium redistribution imaging is necessary to distinguish hibernating myocardium from scar.
- F-18 FDG PET is the gold standard for evaluating myocardial viability and hibernation.
- Normal myocardium preferentially metabolizes fatty acids during the fasting state. In contrast, ischemic but viable myocardium has a diminished ability to metabolize fatty acids and must depend on anaerobic metabolism of glucose for

- 静息与负荷SPECT或PET灌注图像是检查的核心，其关键的问题是：**负荷图像上有灌注缺损吗**？如果存在灌注异常，以下进一步的问题可以帮助进行区分：

缺损在静息图像上是可逆的吗？可逆的缺损意味着有明显缺血，而固定的缺损可能代表梗死/瘢痕或冬眠心肌。
缺损有多大(心肌节段的数目，见下页)？小(1~2段)；中等(3~4段)；大(5个或更多段)。
有多严重？轻度(心内膜下)、中度还是重度(透壁)?
在什么部位？在哪个冠状动脉区域？
负荷期间是否存在左心室扩张(**短暂性缺血性扩张，TID**)？如果存在，意味着有左主干或三支血管疾病和更差的预后，即使不存在局灶性缺损。
存在右心室摄取吗？如果存在，则意味着右心疾病或肺动脉高压。
是否存在**运动引起的可逆性间隔缺损**，但不符合冠状动脉分布区域？这种情况出现在无冠状动脉疾病的左束支传导阻滞(LBBB)，且不能在药物负荷时观察到。

总结，解读举例：*有一个中等大小的严重灌注缺损涉及中部和基底下壁，以及固定的基底下间隔壁。这些发现为典型右冠状动脉(RCA)分布区的心肌瘢痕。*

- 门控SPECT(GSPECT)使用标准ECG门控心肌灌注SPECT采集来对左心室功能进行定量评估。GSPECT在评估左心室灌注的同时，还可以评估左心室壁运动、壁增厚和左心室射血分数(LVEF)。它不用于评估右心室功能。

评估心肌活性

- 单纯静态灌注SPECT显像无法区分瘢痕或冬眠心肌。这两种情况都会出现固定的(负荷和静息两种状态都出现)灌注缺损。

心肌瘢痕是由先前的心肌坏死(梗死)导致的纤维化。
冬眠心肌的定义为严重慢性缺血的心肌，有存活但灌注不足，这种情况可能受益于血运重建(CABG或经皮介入)。

- GSPECT的功能数据可以区分衰减伪影和真实灌注缺损；但GSPECT不能区分冬眠心肌和瘢痕。正常或几乎正常的室壁运动且邻近灌注缺损区的室壁增厚提示为衰减伪影，而异常室壁运动有固定缺损提示为瘢痕或冬眠的心肌。必需使用FDG PET或铊再分布图像以区分冬眠心肌和瘢痕。
- ^{18}F-FDG PET是评估心肌活性和冬眠的“金标准”。
- 正常心肌在禁食状态下优先代谢脂肪酸。与之相反，缺血但存活的心肌代谢脂肪酸的能

energy expenditure. Therefore, ischemic myocardium shows increased uptake on FDG PET. Myocardial scar does not take up FDG.

- If the region of perfusion defect takes up FDG (a “mismatch” between FDG PET and perfusion imaging), it is viable (hibernating myocardium). In contrast, a “matched” perfusion/metabolic defect on perfusion imaging and FDG PET is consistent with non-viable scar.
- Uptake of thallium-201 on delayed images due to redistribution also reflects viability. Rest-redistribution thallium SPECT is inferior to FDG PET because it may underestimate the presence of viable myocardium.
- When myocardium has delayed recovery of contractile function despite reperfusion after a transient ischemic insult, it is termed **stunned myocardium**. Normal uptake on perfusion scan indicates viable cells, but the affected myocardium is akinetic or hypokinetic. Unlike hibernating myocardium which results from *chronic* ischemia, myocardial stunning is an *acute, temporary* process. Contractility will improve over time.

力会减弱且必须依赖于葡萄糖的无氧代谢来提供能量。所以，缺血心肌在FDG PET上显示摄取增加。心肌瘢痕则不摄取FDG。

- 如果灌注缺损区域摄取FDG(FDG PET和灌注成像“不匹配”)，则为有活性(冬眠心肌)。相反，在灌注和FDG PET上“匹配”的灌注/代谢缺损区为无存活的瘢痕。
- 延迟显像因再分布而出现^{201}Tl摄取则表明有存活。铊静息再分布SPECT不及FDGPET，因为它可能低估存活的心肌。
- 当心肌在经历一过性的缺血性损伤后尽管有再灌注，但收缩功能延迟恢复，这种情况称为“**心肌顿抑**”。灌注显像时正常摄取显示有活性细胞，但受影响的心肌出现运动障碍或运动缓慢。与慢性缺血引起的心肌冬眠不同，心肌顿抑是一种急性、暂时的过程。收缩性能会随着时间而得到改善。

	Perfusion with stress	Perfusion at rest	FDG PET uptake	Thallium redistribution	Contractility
Normal	Normal	Normal	Normal	None	Normal
Ischemia	Decreased	Normal	Increased	Yes	Normal/Decreased from stunning
Infarct/Scar	Decreased	Decreased (fixed defect)	Decreased (matched)	No (fixed defect)	Decreased
Hibernating myocardium	Decreased	Decreased (fixed defect)	**Increased** (mismatch)	Yes	Decreased
Stunned myocardium	Normal/Near normal	Normal	Normal	Yes	Decreased

心肌	负荷灌注	静态灌注	FDG PET摄取	铊再分布	收缩性能
正常	正常	正常	正常	无	正常
缺血	下降	正常	上升	有	正常/从顿抑状态下恢复
梗死/瘢痕	下降	下降(固定缺损)	下降(不匹配)	无(固定缺损)	下降
冬眠心肌	下降	下降(固定缺损)	**上升(不匹配)**	有	下降
顿抑心肌	正常/几乎正常	正常	正常	有	下降

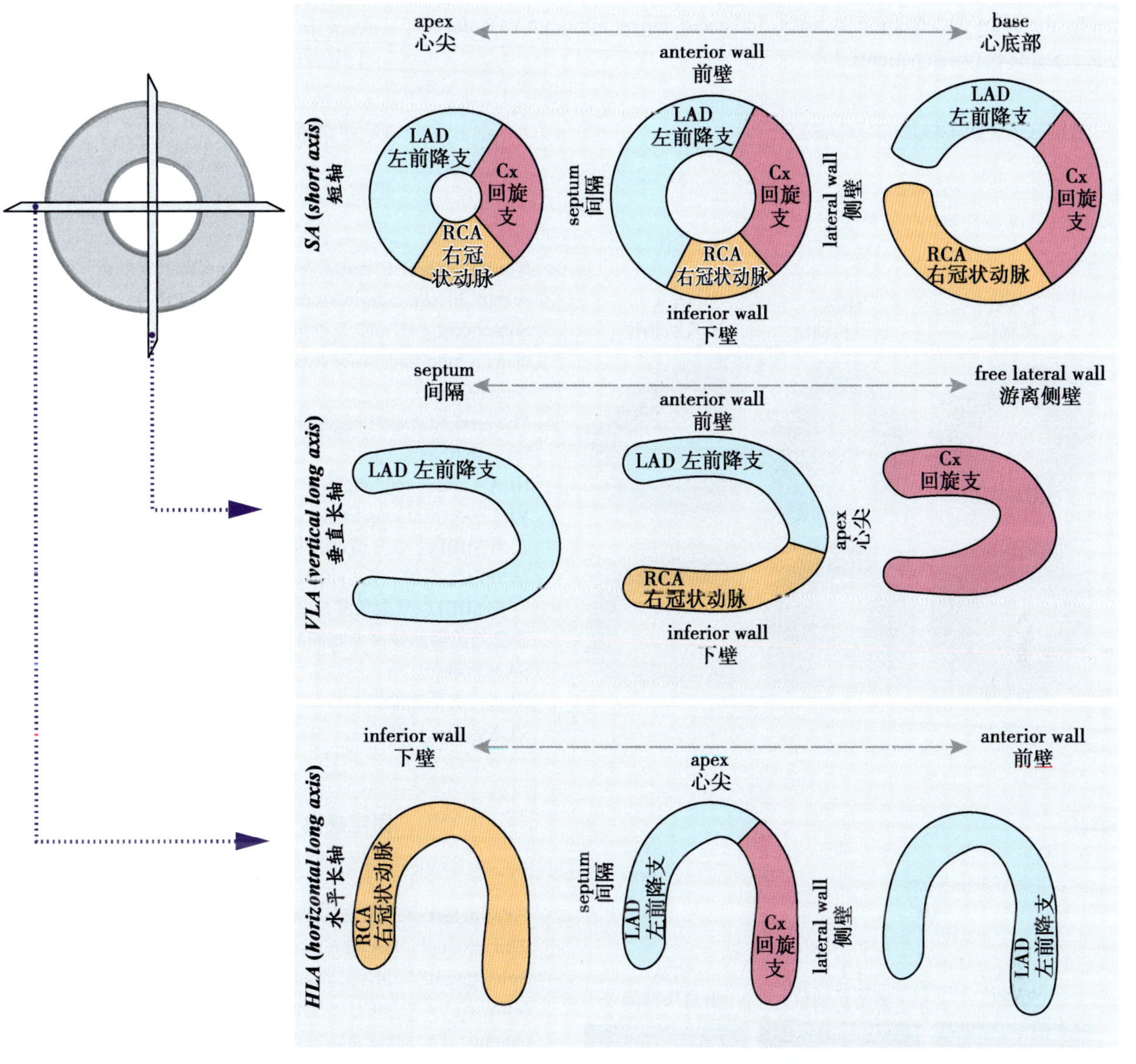

- The heart is reconstructed into short axis (SA, the traditional "donut" view from apex of heart through the base), vertical long axis (VLA, a "U-shaped" view pointing to the left), and the horizontal long axis (HLA, a "U-shaped" view pointing down). The polar plot represents the entire three-dimensional left ventricle unfolded onto a two-dimensional map.

- 心脏重建成短轴(SA,即传统的从心尖到基底部断面的"甜甜圈"视图)、垂直长轴(VLA,即指向左边的"U"形视图)、水平长轴(HLA,即指向下面的"U"形视图)。极坐标图是把整个三维的左心室展开到二维图上。

Myocardial segments

心肌节段

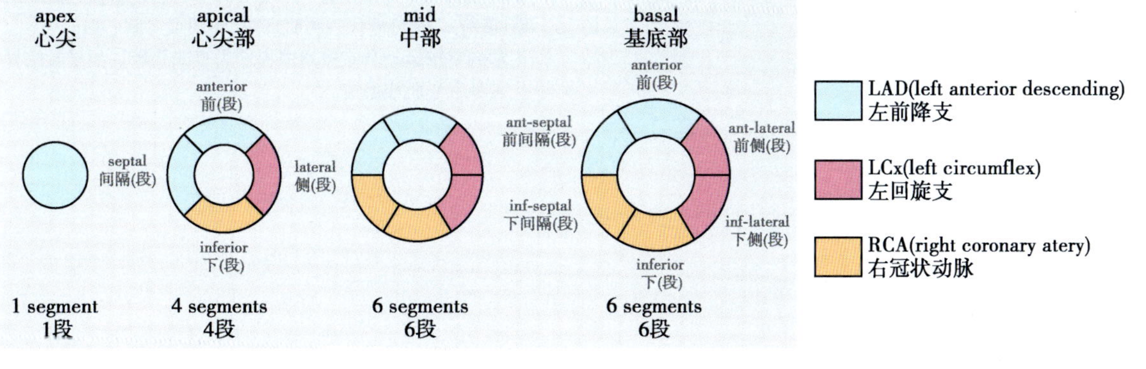

- For evaluation of perfusion defect size, there are 17 standard left ventricular segments, evaluated on the SA ("donut") views. Each segment is usually supplied by the color-coded coronary artery indicated above, although vascular supply is variable between patients.

- 为了评估灌注缺损大小，在短轴视图(即"甜甜圈")上把左心室心肌分成17个段。每一段通常由上图对应颜色的冠状动脉供血，但每个患者的血管供应情况存在差异。

SAMPLE NUCLEAR PERFUSION CASES

核灌注病例

Normal

正常

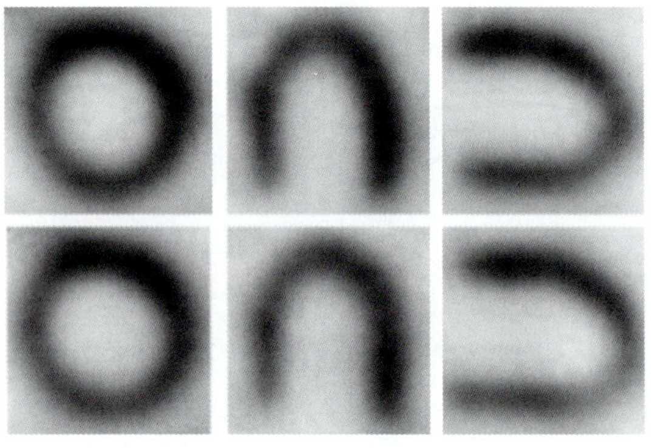

Normal exercise stress sestamibi perfusion study: 5.1 mCi Tc-99m sestamibi was administered and rest SPECT images were obtained. Subsequently 16 mCi Tc-99m sestamibi was administered at peak exercise using a modified Bruce treadmill protocol and the stress SPECT images were obtained.

The rest and stress images are identical and normal.

SA = short axis

HLA = horizontal long axis

VLA = vertical long axis

正常MIBI运动负荷灌注显像：注射5.1mCi的^{99m}Tc-MIBI后获得静息SPECT图像。随后使用改良Bruce法在运动高峰时给予17mCi的^{99m}Tc-MIBI以获取负荷SPECT图像。

静息与负荷显像完全相同且正常。

SA = 短轴位

HLA = 水平长轴位

VLA = 垂直长轴位

Fixed defect

固定缺损

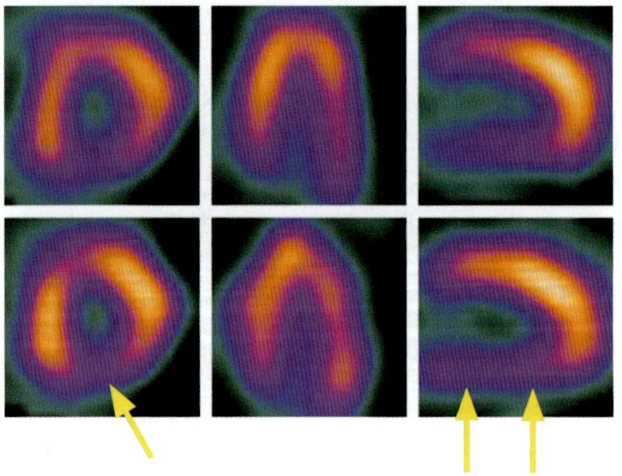

Fixed defect seen on regadenoson sestamibi perfusion study. 7.67 mCi Tc-99m sestamibi was administered and rest SPECT images were obtained. Subsequently 0.4 mg regadenoson was administered intravenously followed by 32 mCi Tc-99m sestamibi and stress SPECT images were obtained. The stress images are displayed above the rest images.

There is a moderate-sized fixed defect involving the mid and basal inferior wall (arrows), in the right coronary artery distribution. This represents either diaphragmatic attenuation, scar or hibernating myocardium.

Normal wall motion and wall thickening indicated this is attenuation artifact. If contractility is abnormal, it could represent hibernating myocardium or scar.

瑞加德松MIBI灌注显像见一固定的缺损区。注射7.67mCi的^{99m}Tc-MIBI后行静息SPECT影像。之后静脉注射0.4mg瑞加德松，随即给予29mCi的^{99m}Tc-MIBI以获得负荷SPECT影像。上排为负荷显像，下排为静息图像。

在右冠状动脉分布区有一个中等大小的固定缺损，累及中部和基底下壁(黄箭)。这可能代表膈肌衰减、瘢痕或冬眠心肌。

正常的室壁运动和室壁增厚提示为衰减伪影。如果收缩异常，则可能代表冬眠心肌或瘢痕。

Reversible defect

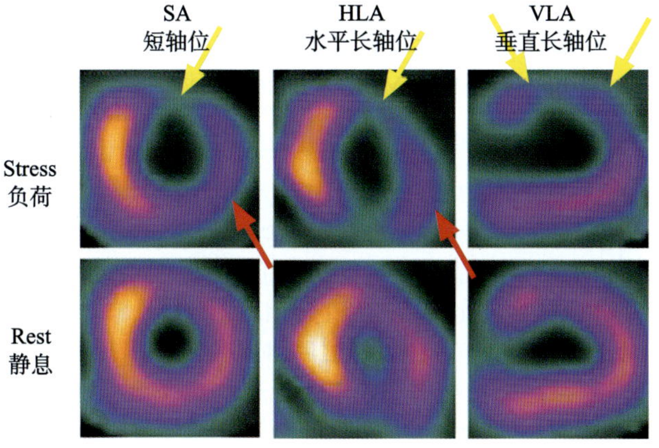

可逆缺损

Large reversible defect seen on regadenoson sestamibi perfusion study: 11 mCi Tc-99m sestamibi was administered and rest SPECT images were obtained. Subsequently 0.4 mg regadenoson was administered intravenously followed by 29 mCi Tc-99m sestamibi and stress SPECT images were obtained. The stress images are displayed above the rest images.

There is a large-sized perfusion defect of severe intensity involving the apical, mid, and basal segments of the anterior (LAD territory, yellow arrows) and lateral (left circumflex territory, red arrows) walls that was partially reversible.

瑞加德松MIBI灌注显像见一个大面积可逆性缺损区：注射11mCi的^{99m}Tc-MIBI后获取静息SPECT影像。之后静脉注射0.4mg瑞加德松，紧接着给予29mCi的^{99m}Tc-MIBI以进行负荷SPECT影像。上排是负荷影像，下排是静息影像。

在心尖、中部和基底部(左前降支供血，黄箭)及侧壁(左回旋支供血，红箭)见大面积可逆性的重度灌注缺损区。

Hibernating myocardium

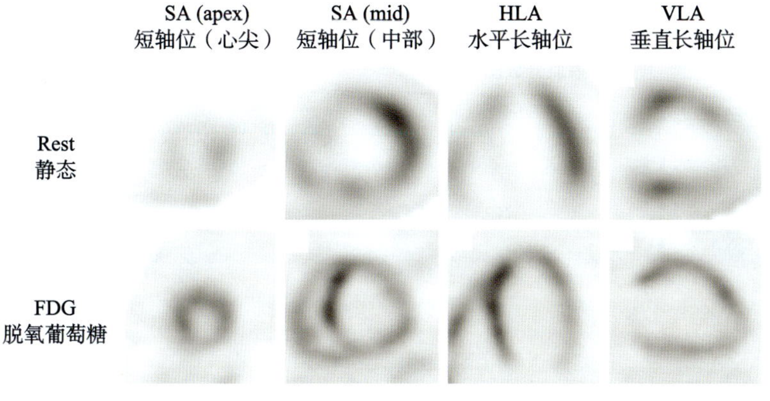

冬眠心肌

Attenuation corrected Tc-99m sestamibi SPECT rest perfusion images (top row) demonstrate a large and severe perfusion defect in the entire septum, the mid anterior wall, the apical four myocardial segments and apex.

Glucose loaded F-18 FDG images (bottom row) demonstrate significant mismatch in the hypoperfused segments indicating hibernating myocardium in the LAD distribution.

衰减校正^{99m}Tc-MIBI SPECT静态灌注图像(上排)显示一个大而严重的灌注缺损，累及整个间隔、前壁、心尖四个心肌节段和心尖区。

注射葡萄糖后的^{18}F-FDG图像(下排)显示低灌注节段明显不匹配，表明LAD的心肌分布区呈冬眠状态。

Breast attenuation artifact

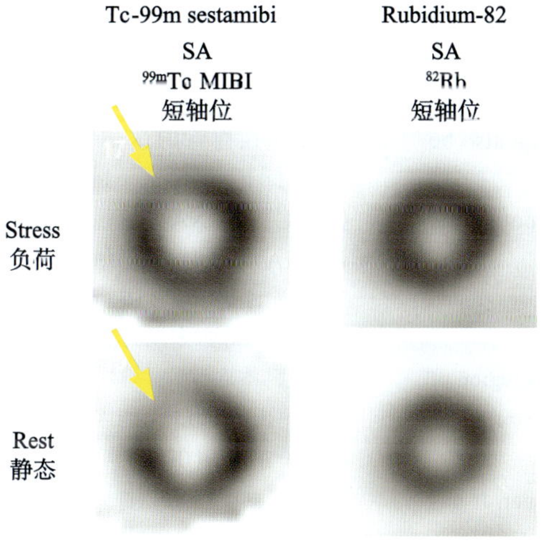

乳腺衰减伪影

Tc-99m sestamibi SPECT stress and rest perfusion short axis images (left column) show a fixed anterior wall perfusion defect (arrows) and normal wall motion and wall thickening on gated imaging (not shown).

Subsequent rubidium-82 stress PET scan (right column) demonstrates normal stress perfusion, confirming the SPECT defect as an artifact from breast tissue attenuation.

^{99m}Tc-MIBI SPECT负荷与静息灌注短轴图像(左栏)显示一个固定的前壁灌注缺损(黄箭)及门控成像上的正常室壁运动和间壁增厚(未展示)。

随后的^{82}Rb负荷PET扫描(右栏)显示负荷灌注正常，确认SPECT上的缺损为来自乳房的衰减伪影。

RADIONUCLIDE IMAGING OF CARDIAC FUNCTION

Gated SPECT (GSPECT)

- As described earlier in the chapter, GSPECT using Tc-99m-labeled perfusion agents (e.g., sestamibi) is most commonly performed for evaluation of ventricular function.

First-pass radionuclide angiography (FP-RNA)

- Tc-99m-labeled red blood cells (RBCs) are injected intravenously and dynamic imaging is performed during the rapid initial transit of radiotracer through the heart, great vessels, and lungs. The study can be done at both rest and during stress. This study is no longer used in clinical practice.
- Data can be processed for visual and quantitative assessment of ventricular wall motion, ejection fraction (EF), and left-to-right intracardiac shunts.
- FP-RNA is more accurate than E-RNA (below) for evaluation of right ventricular EF. It is not sensitive for right-to-left intracardiac shunts, which can be better detected on a pulmonary perfusion scan with Tc-99m MAA (discussed under "Nuclear Imaging" chapter).

Equilibrium radionuclide angiography (E-RNA)

放射性核素心脏功能显像

门控SPECT(GSPECT)

- 如本章前文所述，使用^{99m}Tc标记的灌注显像剂(如MIBI)最常用于评估心室功能。

首次通过放射性核素血管造影(FP-RNA)

- 静脉注射^{99m}Tc标记的红细胞(RBC)后动态显像记录放射性示踪剂通过心脏、大血管和肺。该试验可以在静息和负荷期间进行。本试验已不在临床上使用。
- 在数据处理之后，对心室壁运动、射血分数(EF)和左向右心内分流进行视觉和定量评估射。
- FP-RNA评估右心室EF较平衡法放射性核素血管造影(E-RNA)(下图)更为准确。但FP-RNA对右向左心内分流不敏感，但更好的检测方法是采用^{99m}Tc-MAA进行肺灌注扫描(在“核医学与分子影像”一章中讨论)。

平衡法放射性核素血管造影(E-RNA)

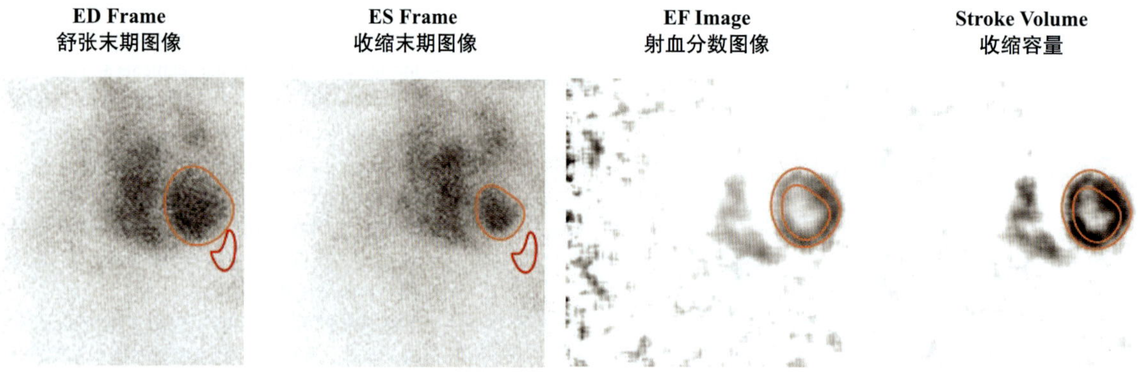

MUGA scan: Representative planar images for calculation of LVEF and stroke volume.
MUGA扫描：用于计算LVEF和每搏输出量的代表性平面图像。

- This is also known as gated blood pool ventriculography or **multi-gated acquisition (MUGA) scan**. ECG-gated planar blood pool images of the heart are obtained after injected Tc-99m RBCs have achieved equilibrium in the intravascular space. *In vitro* labeling of RBCs is preferred. E-RNA can also be performed with SPECT (SPECT-E-RNA).
- E-RNA allows visual evaluation of cardiac size, shape, and wall motion, as well as functional analysis of ventricular performance.

  LVEF = (end diastolic counts – end systolic counts)/(end diastolic counts – background counts)

  The calculated LVEF can be falsely elevated if the selected background region of interest includes part of the left atrium (in case of left atrial enlargement) or extracardiac activity (e.g., spleen).
- E-RNA is comparable to FP-RNA for measurement of LVEF. However, it has been largely replaced by the more available echocardiography and GSPECT perfusion imaging.

- 此法也被称为门控心室血池造影或**多门控采集(MUGA)扫描**。心电图门控平面血池图像是在注射了^{99m}Tc标记物后，^{99m}Tc标记的红细胞在血管内达到平衡后进行的。体外红细胞标记为首选。E-RNA也可以用SPECT(SPECT-E-RNA)进行。
- E-RNA可以对心脏大小、形状和室壁运动进行视觉评估，以及进行心室功能分析。

  LVEF=(舒张末期计数-收缩末期计数)/(舒张末期计数-本底计数)

  计算出的LVEF可能因为所选背景感兴趣区只包括部分左心房(在左心房扩大的情况下)或心外放射性(如脾脏)而呈错误性升高。
- E-RNA测量LVEF的效果与FP-RNA相当。然而，它已经在很大程度上被更方便的超声心动图和GSPECT灌注显像取代。

Nuclear Imaging for Cardiac Inflammation and Infection

Cardiac sarcoidosis

- Sarcoidosis a systemic disease of noncaseating granulomas with cardiac manifestations of arrhythmias, left ventricular dysfunction, and restrictive cardiomyopathy. Cardiac findings are usually seen in conjunction with other manifestations of sarcoidosis, including lung disease and adenopathy.
- F-18 FDG PET is a noninvasive method for diagnosis of cardiac sarcoidosis and monitoring treatment response.
- Prior to imaging, patient is first placed on a high-fat low-carbohydrate diet for 24 hours prior, then undergoes fasting for at least 12 hours, in order to suppress physiologic glucose metabolism by the myocardium, so that FDG uptake by inflamed myocardium can be detected.
- Cardiac sarcoidosis typically presents as focal or patchy FDG uptake in the myocardium.
- Pitfalls in FDG PET include diffuse myocardial uptake due to incompletely suppressed physiologic uptake, and uptake in the lateral LV wall which can be a normal variant. Mismatch pattern of perfusion defect with focal FDG uptake can represent hibernating myocardium and coronary artery disease, therefore needs to be excluded by CT or invasive angiography or stress perfusion imaging prior to interpretation of the images as focal myocardial inflammation.
- F-18 FDG PET and perfusion imaging can be combined to identify sarcoid-induced tissue damage. Perfusion defect correlating to a focal FDG uptake suggests myocardial fibrosis/scarring due to advanced sarcoidosis. Perfusion imaging is normal in early stage of disease.

心脏炎症和感染的核素显像

心脏结节病

- 结节病是一种非干酪样肉芽肿的全身性疾病，在心脏表现为心律失常、左心室功能障碍和限制性心肌病。心脏检查结果通常与结节病的其他表现同时存在，包括肺疾病和淋巴结肿大。
- ^{18}F-FDG PET是一种用于诊断和监测心脏结节病对治疗反应的无创方法。
- 显像之前首先让患者接受高脂肪低碳水化合物饮食24小时，然后禁食至少12小时，以抑制心肌的生理性葡萄糖代谢，从而可检测炎症心肌对FDG的吸收。
- 心脏结节病通常表现为心肌局灶或斑片状摄取FDG。
- FDG PET的缺陷包括由于不完全抑制生理性摄取而导致心肌弥漫性摄取，以及在左心室(LV)侧壁摄取，这可能是一种正常的变异。灌注缺损与局灶性FDG摄取不相匹配可代表冬眠心肌和冠状动脉疾病，因此需要通过CT或有创性血管造影或负荷灌注显像之后才能将图像解释为局部心肌炎症。
- ^{18}F-FDG PET和灌注成像可以结合起来识别结节病所诱导的组织损害。一个灌注缺损但有摄取FDG的局部病灶提示心肌纤维化/由于晚期结节病导致的瘢痕。灌注成像在疾病早期是正常的。

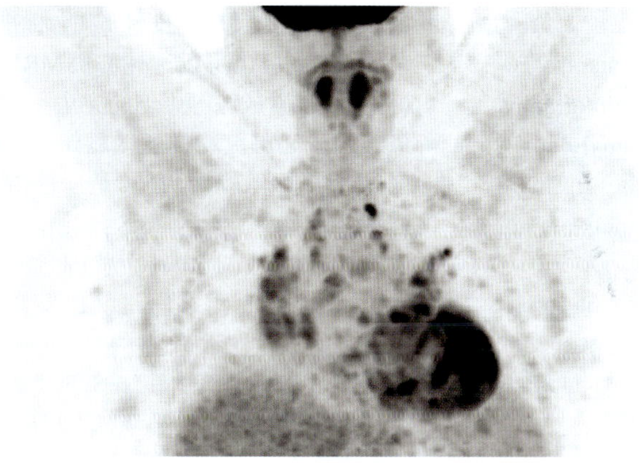

Cardiac and systemic sarcoidosis:
Coronal MIP image of F-18 FDG PET shows increased myocardial uptake in the left ventricle, and increased uptake associated with multiple mediastinal and bilateral hilar lymph nodes.
FDG PET was obtained with a special diet preparation that included 24 hours of high-fat low-carbohydrate diet prior to injection of 10 mCi of F-18 FDG.
心脏和系统性结节病：
^{18}F-FDG PET的冠状动脉MIP图像显示左心室心肌摄取增加，伴有纵隔和双侧肺门多个淋巴结摄取。
特殊饮食准备获取FDG PET图像，过程包括注射10mCi的^{18}F-FDG前24小时摄入高脂肪低碳水化合物饮食。

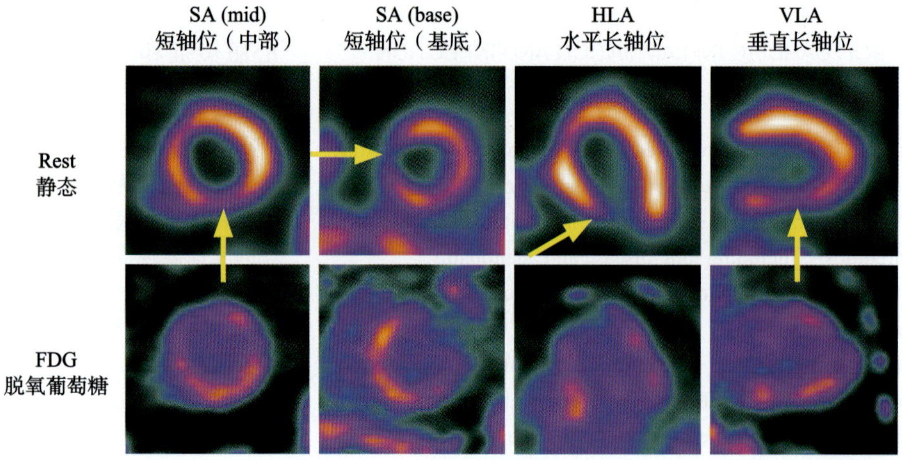

Tc-99m sestamibi myocardial perfusion images (top row) and F-18 FDG PET images (bottom row) of the same patient as above. Regions of hypoperfused myocardium (inferior wall and the basal septum, arrows) demonstrate mismatch on FDG PET consistent with active myocardial inflammation (since obstructive coronary artery disease was excluded by coronary angiography).

上述为同一名患者的^{99m}Tc-MIBI心肌灌注图像(上排)和^{18}F-FDG PET图像(下排)。局部低灌注心肌区(下壁和基底间隔，黄箭)与FDG PET图像不匹配，符合活动性心肌炎的改变(冠状动脉造影已排除阻塞性冠状动脉疾病)。

Amyloidosis

- Amyloidosis is a systemic disease characterized by extracellular deposition of insoluble proteins; any organ can be affected. Cardiac involvement pertains a poor prognosis and can lead to angina, arrhythmias, restrictive cardiomyopathy, and heart failure. Transthyretin cardiac amyloidosis formed from misfolded transthyretin protein is now recognized as a common cause of heart failure with preserved ejection fraction in elderly (senile amyloidosis subtype).
- While the gold standard for diagnosis of cardiac amyloidosis is tissue biopsy, cardiac imaging such as MRI (discussed later in the chapter) and nuclear imaging offer noninvasive alternatives.
- Radiotracers most commonly used to image cardiac amyloidosis are Tc-99m-labeled bisphosphonates traditionally developed for bone scintigraphy. These agents are helpful in distinguishing between subtypes of amyloidosis, where transthyretin amyloid (senile and hereditary subtypes) takes up more radiotracer than light-chain (AL) amyloid. The mechanism of uptake is not clearly understood.

Grade 2 (myocardial uptake = rib uptake) or grade 3 (myocardial uptake > rib uptake) myocardial uptake of Tc-99m bisphosphonate tracers on SPECT is nearly 100% specific for the diagnosis of transthyretin cardiac amyloidosis if light-chain amyloidosis is excluded.

淀粉样变性

- 淀粉样变性是一种系统性疾病，其特征表现为不溶性蛋白质沉积在细胞外；任何器官都可能受到侵犯。心脏受累与预后不良有关，可导致心绞痛、心律失常、限制性心肌病和心力衰竭。心脏淀粉样变性是由错误折叠的转甲状腺素蛋白所形成的，目前被认为是一种在老年人中射血分数保留的心力衰竭的常见原因(老年淀粉样变性亚型)。
- 虽然诊断心脏淀粉样变性的“金标准”是进行组织活检，但也可以选择心脏MRI(本章后文讨论)和核素成像等无创的方法。
- 最常用于心脏淀粉样变性显像的放射性示踪剂是^{99m}Tc标记双磷酸盐，是一种传统的骨扫描剂。这些标记药物在区分淀粉样变性的各亚型中有帮助，其中转甲状腺素淀粉样蛋白(老年和遗传亚型)较轻链(AL)淀粉样蛋白吸收更多的放射性示踪剂。摄取机制尚不清楚。

排除轻链淀粉样变性后，在SPECT上表现为2级(心肌摄取=肋骨摄取)或3级(心肌摄取>肋骨摄取)心肌摄取^{99m}Tc-双膦酸盐示踪剂，对转甲状腺素心脏淀粉样变性的诊断有近100%的特异度。

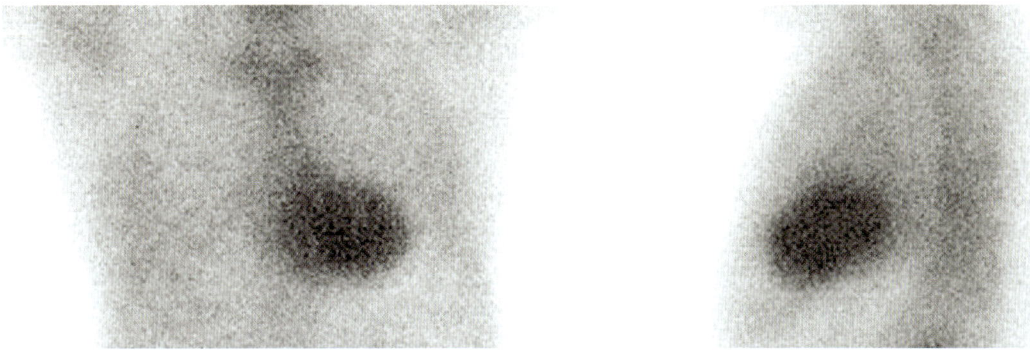

Patient with heart failure with preserved ejection fraction and increasing left ventricular wall thickening on echocardiogram despite well controlled hypertension: Coronal and sagittal planar images obtained three hours after injection of 20 mCi of Tc-99m pyrophosphate demonstrated grade 3 myocardial uptake of radiotracer (myocardial uptake > rib uptake) which was confirmed on SPECT (not shown). If serum and urine immunofixation electrophoresis and serum free light chain assay are negative (which exclude light chain amyloidosis), these findings would be consistent with transthyretin cardiac amyloidosis.
患者有心力衰竭，高血压控制良好，射血分数正常，但超声心动图显示左心室壁增厚：注射20mCi ^{99m}Tc-焦磷酸盐后3小时获得的冠状和矢状平面图像显示3级心肌摄取(心肌摄取>肋骨摄取)，该发现在SPECT上得到了证实(未显示)。如果血清和尿液免疫固定电泳和血清游离轻链试验阴性(排除轻链淀粉样变性)，这些发现与转甲状腺素蛋白心脏淀粉样变性一致。

- Amyloid-specific PET agents (such as F-18 florbetapir and C-11 PiB) are currently undergoing investigation for imaging of cardiac amyloidosis.

- PET淀粉样蛋白特异性制剂(如^{18}F-florbetapir和^{11}C-PiB)目前正处于对心脏淀粉样变性影像学的研究。

Endocarditis

心内膜炎

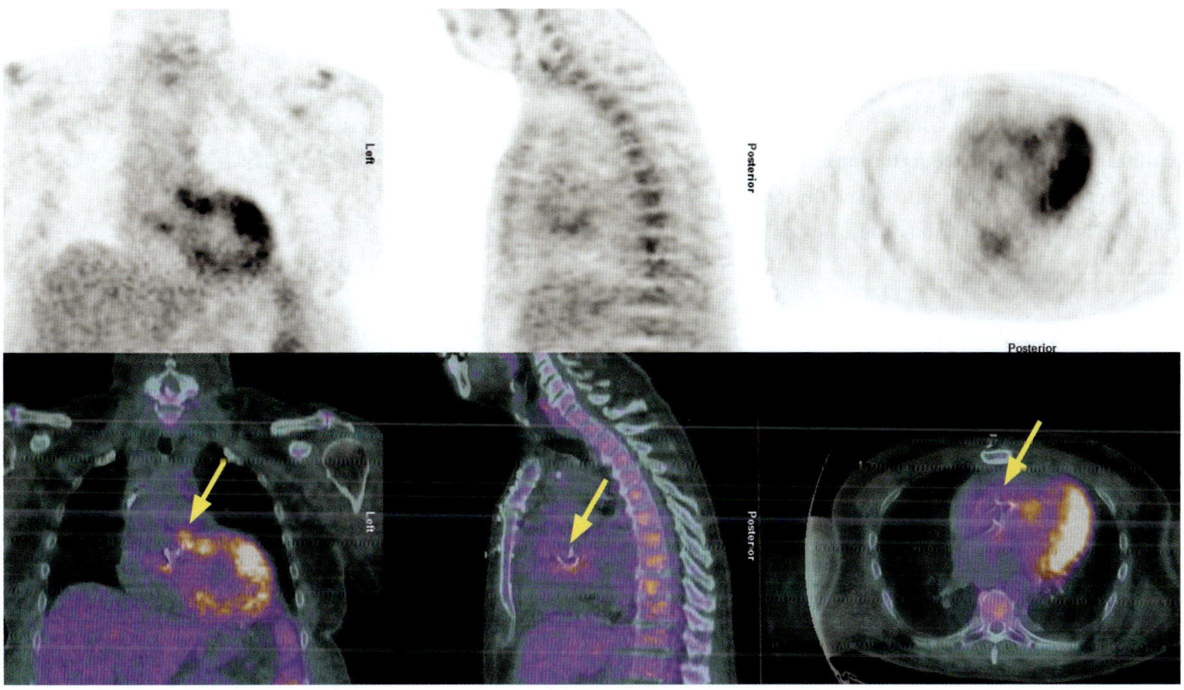

Infective endocarditis in a patient with bicuspid aortic valve status post bioprosthetic valve replacement: Echocardiogram was inconclusive. A F-18 FDG PET was performed following a high-fat low-carbohydrate diet. PET images (top row) and PET/CT images (bottom row) demonstrate non-specific myocardial FDG uptake. There is focal FDG uptake in region of the aortic valve (arrows). Endocarditis of the bioprosthetic aortic valve was confirmed intraoperatively.
患者在二叶主动脉生物瓣置换术后合并感染性心内膜炎：超声心动图无异常。在高脂肪低碳水化合物饮食后进行^{18}F-FDG PET。PET图像(上排)和PET/CT图像(下排)显示非特异性心肌摄取FDG。主动脉瓣区域有局灶性FDG摄取(黄箭)。术中证实为生物人工主动脉瓣心内膜炎。

- F-18 FDG PET/CT can accurately diagnose prosthetic valve endocarditis and its systemic complications. It is less reliable for detection of native valve endocarditis.
- FDG PET can be combined with CT angiography (discussed later in the chapter) for increased sensitivity.
- Radiolabeled leukocyte scintigraphy with SPECT/CT (discussed in the previous chapter) is more specific than FDG PET/CT for evaluation of endocarditis, but suffers from limited sensitivity due to weak signal and lower resolution.
- The typical appearance of endocarditis on FDG PET and leukocyte scintigraphy is a focal valvular uptake.

- ^{18}F-FDG PET/CT可准确诊断人工瓣膜心内膜炎及其全身并发症。但对于自体瓣膜心内膜炎的诊断不可靠。
- FDG PET可以与血管造影(在本章后文讨论)相结合，以增加灵敏度。
- 使用SPECT/CT进行放射性标记的白细胞闪烁显像(在“核医学与分子影像”一章已讨论)在评估心内膜炎方面比FDG PET/CT特异度更高，但由于信号弱及分辨率较低使其灵敏度受限。
- 心内膜炎在FDG PET和白细胞闪烁显像中的典型表现是局灶性瓣膜摄取。

(翻译　王维平)

PLAIN FILM IMAGING OF HEART DISEASE

- By applying a systematic approach, the standard chest radiograph can offer valuable information about the presence or severity of heart disease.
- The radiographic evaluation of heart disease begins with an assessment of the size of the cardiac silhouette. Radiographically evident heart disease can be divided into two categories: Those with a normal-sized cardiac silhouette and those with an enlarged cardiac silhouette.
- A ratio of the cardiac silhouette to the inner diameter of the thorax (the cardiothoracic ratio) of 0.55 or greater (on a PA projection) suggests enlargement of the cardiac silhouette.
- Cardiovascular diseases with an **enlarged cardiac silhouette** include cardiomyopathy secondary to congestive heart failure, valvular regurgitation (aortic, mitral, or tricuspid regurgitation), high-output or volume overload states, dilated cardiomyopathy, pericardial effusion, and paracardiac mass.
- To distinguish between the various causes of enlarged cardiac silhouette, the key structures to evaluate are the left atrium and the aorta.

> If the **left atrium is enlarged** and the cardiac silhouette is enlarged, that suggests **mitral regurgitation**.
> If the **aorta is enlarged** and the cardiac silhouette is enlarged, that suggests **aortic regurgitation**.
> If neither the left atrium nor the aorta is enlarged, that suggests one of the other etiologies.

- Cardiovascular diseases with a **normal-sized cardiac silhouette** include valvular stenosis (aortic or mitral stenosis), pulmonary artery hypertension, hypertrophic cardiomyopathy, restrictive physiology, and acute myocardial infarction.
- Similar to evaluation of diseases with an enlarged cardiac silhouette, the key structures to evaluate in the presence of a normal cardiac silhouette are the left atrium and the aorta.

> If the **left atrium is enlarged** and the cardiac silhouette is normal, that suggests **mitral stenosis**.
> If the **aorta is enlarged** and the cardiac silhouette is normal, that suggests **aortic stenosis** or aortic aneurysm.
> If neither the left atrium nor the aorta is enlarged, that suggests one of the other etiologies.

心脏疾病的X线影像

- 通过系统的方法，可以从标准的胸部X线影像上获得有价值的关于心脏有无疾病及其严重程度的信息。
- 评估心脏疾病应从心影大小开始。心脏疾病在X线影像上可分为两类：心影正常和心影增大的疾病。
- 在后前位胸部X线影像上，心脏轮廓和胸廓内径的比例(心胸比例)≥0.55提示心影增大。
- 伴有**心影增大**的心血管疾病包括继发于充血性心力衰竭的心肌病、瓣膜反流(主动脉瓣、二尖瓣或三尖瓣反流)、心脏高输出或容量超负荷状态、扩张型心肌病、心包积液和心旁肿块。
- 在区分各种心影增大的病因时，关键需要评价的结构是左心房和主动脉。

> 若**左心房增大伴**心影增大，提示**二尖瓣反流**。
> 若**主动脉扩张伴**心影增大，提示**主动脉瓣反流**。
> 若左心房和主动脉均不扩大，提示其他的病因。

- **心影正常**的心血管疾病包括瓣膜狭窄(主动脉瓣或二尖瓣狭窄)、肺动脉高压、肥厚型心肌病、生理性受限病变，以及急性心肌梗死。
- 与评估心影增大的疾病相似，评估心影正常疾病的关键结构也是左心房和主动脉。

> 若**左心房扩大**而心影正常，提示**二尖瓣狭窄**。
> 若**主动脉扩大**而心影正常，提示**主动脉狭窄**或**主动脉瘤**。
> 若左心房和主动脉均不扩大，提示其他的病因。

- Other structures to always evaluate include the pulmonary vascularity, thoracic wall, chamber enlargement, and the great vessels (pulmonary arteries, ascending aorta, aortic arch, and descending aorta).

Right ventricular enlargement

- The right ventricle is the most anterior cardiac chamber. Right ventricular enlargement causes displacement of the cardiac apex in a leftward direction (in contrast to left ventricular enlargement, which causes displacement in a left-inferior direction).
- Right ventricular enlargement may cause opacification of the retrosternal clear space on the lateral radiograph.

Right atrial enlargement

- The right atrium forms the right heart border. Right atrial enlargement causes lateral bulging or elongation of the right heart border.

Left ventricular enlargement

- The left ventricle forms the left heart border. Left ventricular enlargement typically causes displacement of the cardiac apex in a left-inferior direction.
- Note that hypertrophic cardiomyopathy does *not* cause enlargement of the external contour of the ventricle.

Left atrial enlargement

- The left atrium is the most posterior cardiac chamber. An enlarged left atrium may be caused by mitral regurgitation (with an enlarged cardiac silhouette) or mitral stenosis (with a normal cardiac silhouette).
- An enlarged left atrium can splay the carina, seen on the frontal view. On the lateral radiograph, an enlarged left atrium can elevate the left upper lobe bronchus.

- 其他需要评估的结构包括肺血管、胸壁、心腔扩大和大血管(肺动脉、升主动脉、主动脉弓和降主动脉)。

右心室增大

- 右心室为最前方的心腔。右心室扩大引起心尖向左侧移位(不同于左心室扩大导致的心尖向左下移位)。
- 右心室增大可引起侧位胸部X线影像上胸骨后间隙不清。

右心房增大

- 右心房构成心右缘。右心房增大导致心右缘向外侧膨隆或延长。

左心室增大

- 左心室构成心左缘。左心室增大通常引起心尖向左下方移位。
- 注意,肥厚型心肌病不会导致心室的外部轮廓增大。

左心房扩大

- 左心房为心脏最后方的心腔。左心房扩大可能为二尖瓣反流(伴心影扩大)或二尖瓣狭窄(心影正常)所致。
- 左心房扩大在正位胸部X线影像上可见隆突角增大。在侧位影像上可见左肺上叶支气管抬高。

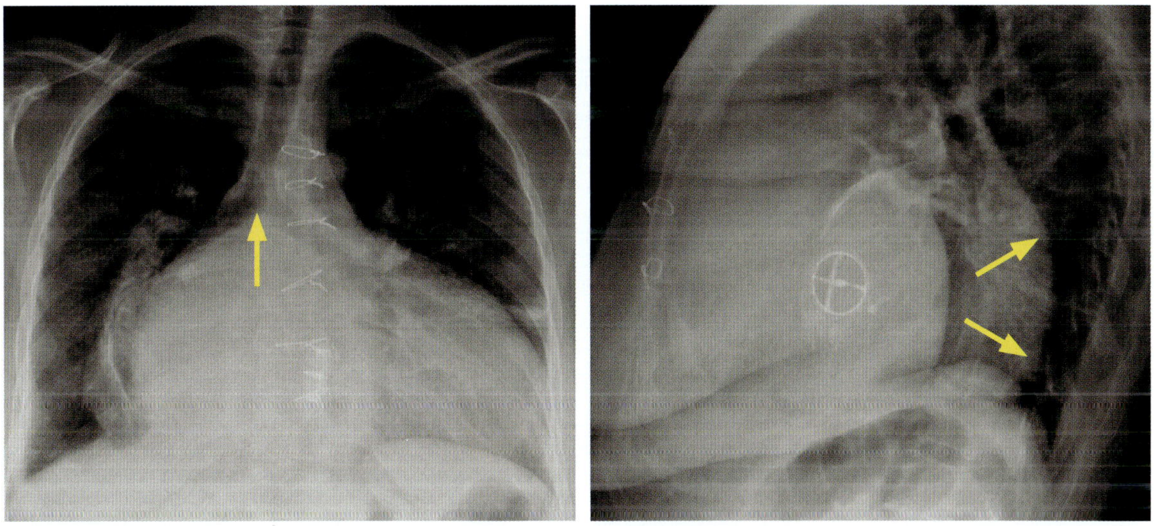

Left atrial enlargement with cardiomegaly (due to mitral regurgitation): Frontal chest radiograph (left image) demonstrates massive cardiomegaly with marked enlargement of the left atrium, as evident by splaying of the carina (arrow). Lateral radiograph shows marked posterior displacement of the esophagus (arrows). A prosthetic mitral valve is present.

Case courtesy Ritu Gill, MBBS, Brigham and Women's Hospital.

左心房扩大合并心影增大(二尖瓣反流所致):胸部正位X线影像(左图)显示巨大的心影伴左心房显著扩大,表现为隆突角增大(黄箭)。侧位X线影像显示食管明显向后移位(黄箭)。可见人工二尖瓣。

- An important clue to the presence of left atrial enlargement is the *double density sign*, seen over the right heart. The *double density* represents the right aspect of the enlarged left atrium visualized through the right atrium.

- 左心房扩大的重要征象是在心右缘出现双密度(双边)征。双密度是指透过右心房可见增大的左心房的右缘。

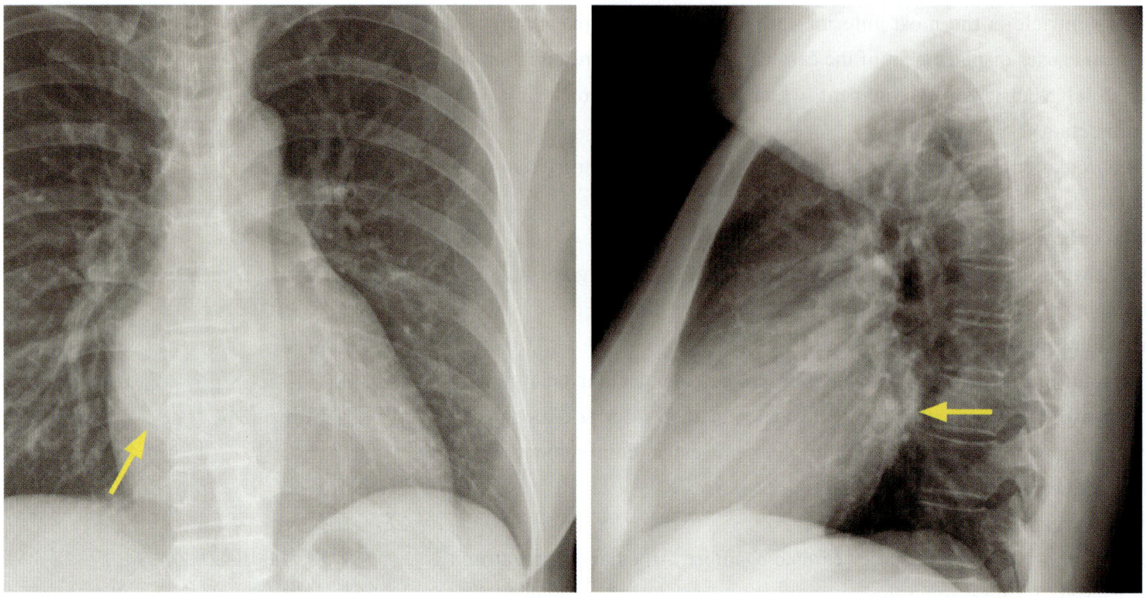

Left atrial enlargement without cardiomegaly (due to mitral stenosis): Frontal chest radiograph (left image) demonstrates the *double density sign* (arrow) with the left atrial border visualized through the right atrium. Lateral radiograph demonstrates posterior protrusion of the left atrium (arrow).

Case courtesy Ritu Gill, MBBS, Brigham and Women's Hospital.

左心房扩大但无心影增大(由二尖瓣狭窄造成):胸部正位X线影像(左图)通过右心房可见左心房边界的双密度征(黄箭)。侧位影像显示左心房后凸(黄箭)。

- On a lateral esophogram, an enlarged left atrium can displace the esophagus posteriorly and may be a cause of dysphagia.

- 在食管侧位造影上,增大的左心房使食管向后移位并可能导致吞咽困难。

Imaging of prosthetic valves

人工心脏瓣膜成像

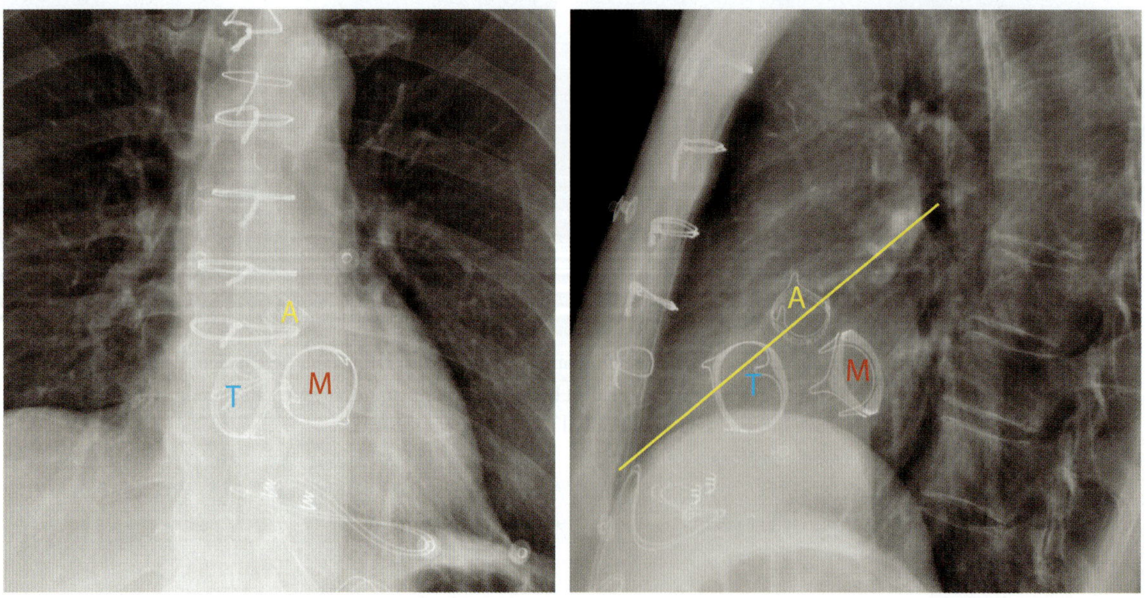

Prosthetic aortic (A), mitral (M), and tricuspid (T) valves. Note that on the lateral radiograph (right image) the aortic valve is located on a plane drawn from the sternal/diaphragmatic junction and the carina (yellow line).

人工主动脉(A)、二尖瓣(M)和三尖瓣(T)。注意,在侧位影像上(右图)主动脉瓣位于从胸骨/膈交界处和隆突(黄线)所绘制的一个平面上。

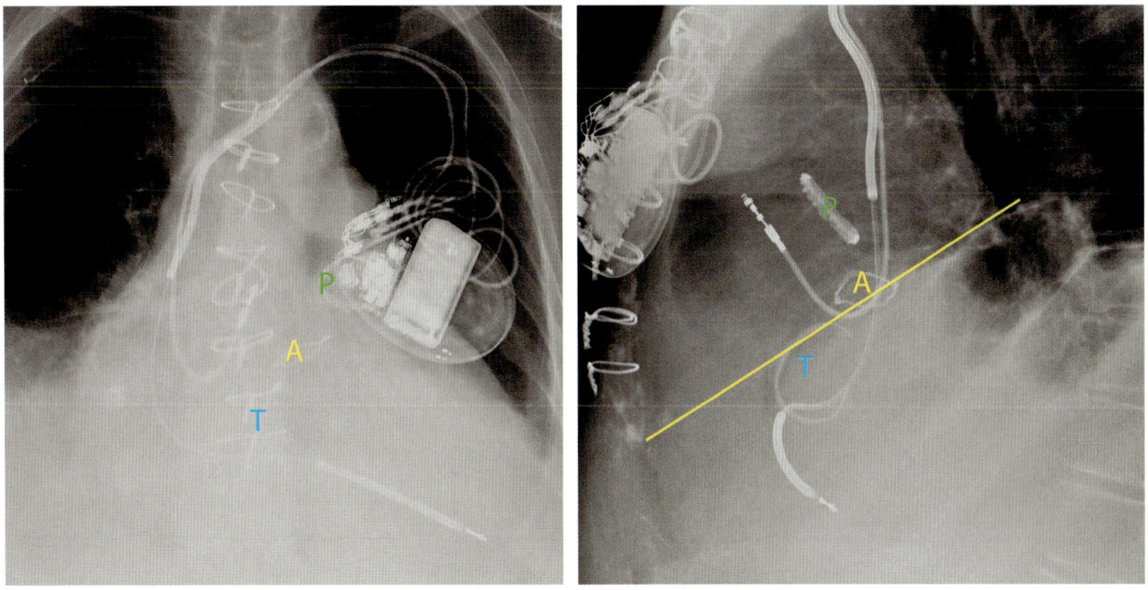

Prosthetic aortic (A), pulmonic (P), and tricuspid (T) valves in a different patient. The tricuspid prosthesis is a ring annuloplasty. The aortic valve is seen on the plane connecting the sternal/diaphragmatic junction with the carina on the lateral radiograph.
另一位患者的人工主动脉瓣(A)、肺动脉瓣(P)和三尖瓣(T)。人工三尖瓣为环状瓣成形术后。侧位X线影像可见主动脉瓣位于连接胸骨/横膈交界处与隆突连线的平面上。

- On the lateral radiograph, the aortic valve is centered on the plane drawn from the sternal/diaphragmatic junction and the carina. The mitral valve is the most posterior valve.
- The tricuspid valve is to the right and anterior to the mitral valve.
- The pulmonic valve is the most superior and most leftward valve.
- Evaluation of prosthetic valves can be challenging in patients with abnormal chamber enlargement or cardiac rotation.
- The atrioventricular valves (mitral and tricuspid) are open in diastole.

Imaging of other cardiac devices

- Below are selective examples of common cardiac devices on chest radiographs.

- 在侧位X线影像上，主动脉瓣位于胸骨/膈交界处与气管隆嵴连线平面的中央。二尖瓣是最靠后的瓣膜。
- 三尖瓣位于二尖瓣右前方。
- 肺动脉瓣是最上和最靠左的瓣膜。
- 若有心腔异常扩大或心脏旋转，评估人工心脏瓣膜时会非常困难。
- 房室瓣(二尖瓣和三尖瓣)在心脏舒张期开放。

其他心脏装置的成像

- 以下是部分胸部X线影像上常见的心脏装置示例。

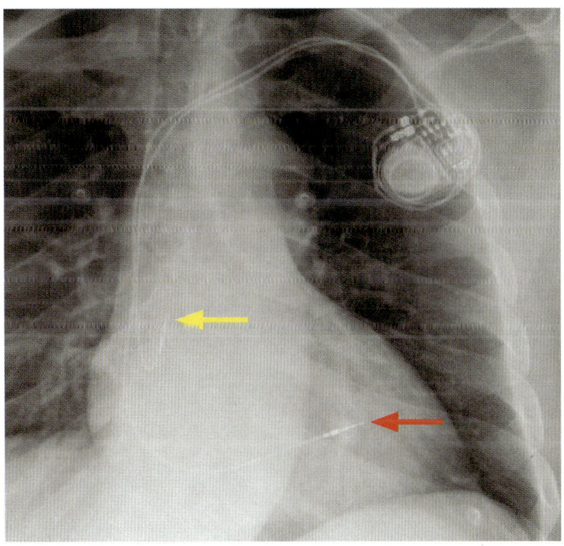

Pacemaker: Chest radiograph shows a dual-chamber pacemaker with two leads, one in the right atrium (yellow arrow), one in the right ventricle (red arrow).
起搏器：胸部X线影像显示双腔起搏器有两根导线，一根在右心房(黄箭)，另一根在右心室(红箭)。

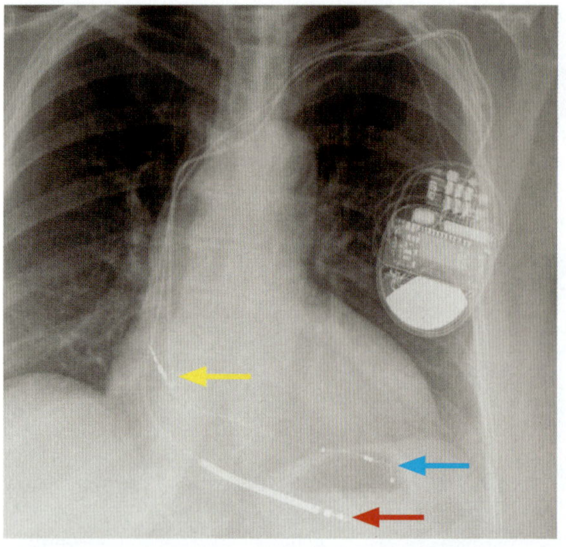

ICD-pacemaker combination: Chest radiograph shows an ICD and biventricular pacemaker combination with three leads. The combined ICD-pacemaker lead with shock coil terminates in the right ventricular apex (red arrow). The other pacemaker leads terminate in the right atrium (yellow arrow) and in the posterior or lateral cardiac vein (blue arrow).

植入型心律转复除颤器(ICD)起搏器组合：胸部X线影像显示ICD和双心室起搏器组合，共有三个导联。组合式ICD起搏器的除颤线圈导联终止于右心室心尖(红箭)。另两根起搏器导线终止于右心房(黄箭)和心后静脉或外侧静脉(蓝箭)。

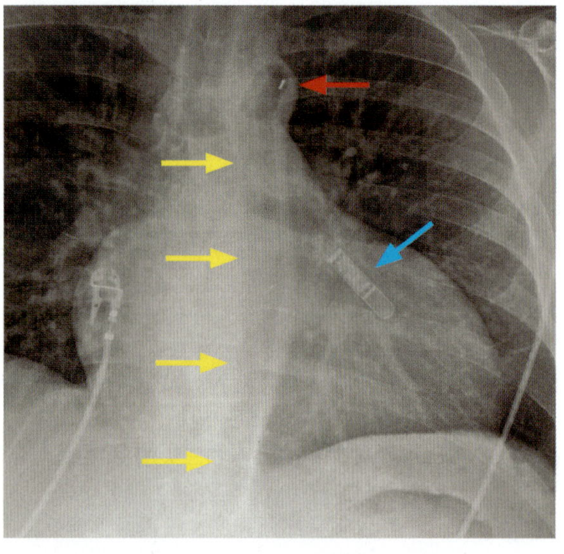

Intra-aortic balloon pump and **loop recorder**: Chest radiograph shows an inflated intra-aortic balloon pump (yellow arrows) with metallic tip (red arrow) projecting over the aortic arch. Also present is an implantable loop recorder (blue arrow).

主动脉内球囊泵和循环记录器：胸部X线影像显示膨胀的主动脉内球囊泵(黄箭)，金属尖端(红箭)投射在主动脉弓的位置。还可见一个可植入的循环记录器(蓝箭)。

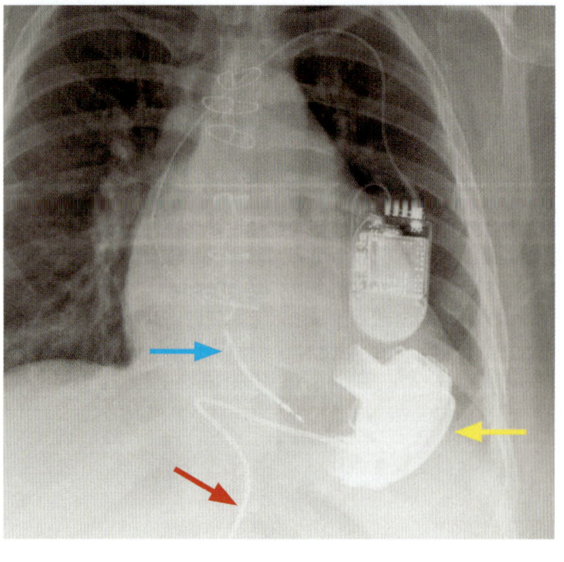

Left ventricular assist device (LVAD): Chest radiograph shows a LVAD with the pump component (yellow arrow) attached to the left ventricular apex and a power line (red arrow) that exits the abdominal wall. Also seen is a single-lead ICD (blue arrow).

左心室辅助装置(LVAD)：胸部X线影像显示LVAD，泵组件(黄箭)连接到左心室心尖，电源线(红箭)从腹壁引出。还可见单导联ICD(蓝箭)。

(翻译　高杨)

CORONARY CT ANGIOGRAPHY

Evidence for using coronary CT to evaluate for ischemic cardiac disease

- Coronary CT angiography (CCTA) is an excellent test to rule out hemodynamically significant coronary artery disease (CAD). Meta-analyses of multiple trials have shown the negative predictive value for CCTA to be approaching 100%.
- In the emergency room setting, CCTA is an appropriate first-line test for evaluation of acute chest pain in low to intermediate risk patients *without known CAD*, who presented with normal cardiac enzymes and non-ischemic ECG.
- For patients with high pretest probability of acute coronary syndrome, the appropriate diagnostic approach is functional assessment such as stress testing or invasive coronary angiography.
- For patients with equivocal stress tests, a negative CCTA may suggest against admission or further invasive testing.
- CCTA is very sensitive for hemodynamically significant (>50% lumenal diameter) stenoses; however, a stenosis found on CT may be overcalled, especially if there is calcified plaque, which can cause a blooming artifact.
- Other indications of CCTA include coronary assessment prior to cardiac or other major surgery, evaluation of suspected coronary anomalies, cardiac valves, and coronary artery bypass grafts.

ECG gating and radiation dose

- ECG gating is used to minimize cardiac motion. The choice of ECG gating has a large effect on patient radiation dose.

  To estimate the radiation dose, the dose-length product (DLP) should be multiplied by a conversion factor of 0.017 to arrive at the dose in millisieverts.
- In a **retrospectively gated** exam, continuous CT scanning is performed throughout the cardiac cycle and the images are correlated to the ECG cycle afterwards.

  The main advantage of retrospective gating is the ability to create cine reconstructions to evaluate cardiac and valvular function, typically with 10–20 frames per cardiac cycle.

  The main disadvantage of retrospective gating is a significant increase in radiation exposure compared to a prospectively gated study.
- For **prospective gating**, the ECG is used to time image acquisition at a specific phase of the cardiac cycle, exposing the patient to radiation only during this segment of the cardiac cycle.

  The main advantage of prospective gating is decreased radiation exposure.

  However, since only a fraction of the cardiac cycle is acquired, cine reconstructions are not possible.

冠状动脉CT血管造影

冠状动脉CT评价缺血性心脏疾病的证据

- 冠状动脉CT血管造影(CCTA)是一种排除冠状动脉疾病(CAD)有明显血流动力学改变的极佳检查方法。荟萃分析中多个临床试验显示CCTA的阴性预测值接近100%。
- 在急诊间，CCTA是一项适合于评估中低风险且*无冠状动脉疾病*患者急性胸痛的一线检查，这些患者的心肌酶谱正常、心电图无缺血改变。
- 对于预测有急性冠脉综合征高风险的患者，适当的诊断方法是进行功能评估，如负荷试验或侵入性冠状动脉造影。
- 对于负荷试验不明确的患者，CCTA阴性可提示无须入院或做进一步侵入性检查。
- CCTA对有显著血流动力学改变的管腔狭窄(>50%管腔直径)十分敏感，但CT可能高估狭窄程度，尤其是有钙化的斑块，这可能会引起开花样伪影。
- CCTA的其他适应证包括心脏或其他大手术前对冠状动脉进行评估，以及对可疑冠状动脉异常、心脏瓣膜和冠状动脉搭桥血管进行评估。

心电门控及辐射剂量

- 心电门控技术用于减少心动伪影。选用心电门控对患者的辐射剂量有很大影响。

  计算辐射剂量时，剂量-长度乘积(DLP)应乘以权重因子0.017得到以毫西弗(mSv)为单位的辐射剂量。
- **回顾性心电门控**检查是在整个心动周期连续进行CT扫描，然后图像与心电图周期相对应。

  回顾性心电门控的主要优势是能够重建电影以评估心脏和瓣膜功能，通常每个心动周期为10~20帧。

  与前瞻性心电门控相比，回顾性心电门控的主要缺点是显著增加了辐射剂量。
- 对于**前瞻性心电门控**，心电图用于在心动周期中的某个特定相位采集图像，患者只在心动周期的这一时段受到辐射。

  前瞻性心电门控的主要优势是减少了辐射剂量。

  然而，由于只采集心动周期的一部分，无法进行电影重建。

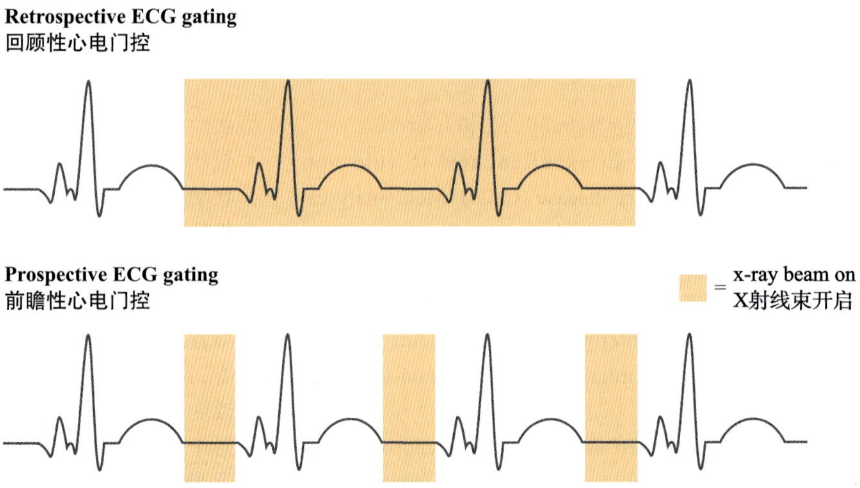

Spatial resolution

- Coronary arteries have an average lumenal diameter of approximately 3 mm.
- The latest CT scanners have a spatial resolution up to 0.18 mm. Axial image reconstructions should have slice thickness <1.0 mm for optimal evaluation of coronary arteries. Thicker slices may be used in obese patients to reduce image noise.
- In contrast, catheter angiography has a spatial resolution of approximately 0.16 mm.

Temporal resolution and "freezing" of cardiac motion

- A single source CT scanner requires slightly more than 180 degrees of gantry rotation for image acquisition. For a complete rotation time of 330 ms, the temporal resolution is ~165 ms, calculated as rotation time/2.
- Dual source CT has two X-ray sources oriented 90 degrees to each other and needs to rotate only 90 degrees to complete a reconstruction, which effectively cuts the temporal resolution to 1/4 of the gantry rotation time. For third-generation dual source CTs with a rotation time of 250 ms, the temporal resolution is ~66 ms.

Intravenous access

- Appropriate intravenous access is required for rapid bolus administration of contrast via a power injector. High infusion rates (4–7 mL/sec) are needed to adequately opacify the coronary arteries. A saline chaser bolus follows the contrast injection to wash out the veins and right atrium, in order to reduce streak artifact from the contrast bolus.

Target heart rate and pre-scanning medications

- A low heart rate (≤60 bpm) and regular rhythm are desired to maximize the R-R interval.
- Beta-blockade is usually necessary to achieve the target heart rate. Oral metoprolol is administered (between 5 and 25 mg, typically administered in 5 mg doses). Oral beta-blocker gives better heart rate control and decreased heart rate variability compared to IV.

  With dual source CT, it is possible to scan without heart rate control, even for patients with arrhythmias.
- Just prior to scanning, a sublingual nitroglycerin (0.4–0.8 mg) is administered to dilate the coronary arteries.

空间分辨率

- 冠状动脉管腔的平均直径为3mm。
- 最新CT扫描仪的空间分辨率可达0.18mm。轴向图像重建切面的厚度应<1.0mm，以便对冠状动脉进行最佳评估。肥胖患者可使用较大的层厚，以减少图像噪声。
- 相比之下，导管造影的空间分辨率约为0.16mm。

时间分辨率及"冻结"心脏运动

- 单源CT机需机架旋转略大于180°才能获得图像。若机架完全旋转一圈需要330毫秒，则时间分辨率约为165毫秒，为旋转时间的1/2。
- 双源CT为两个X射线源互成90°，只需旋转90°便可完成一幅图像重建，有效地将时间分辨率减少至机架旋转时间的1/4。第三代双源CT机架旋转时间为250毫秒，其时间分辨率约为66毫秒。

静脉通路

- 高压注射器快速注入造影剂需建立适当的静脉通路。高速注射(4~7mL/s)对于充分强化冠状动脉是必要的。在团注造影剂后，要用生理盐水冲洗静脉和右心房，以减少造影带来的条纹伪影。

目标心率和扫描前用药

- 较低的心率(≤60次/min)和规律性心律是理想的状态，可以使RR间期最大化。
- 通常有必要使用β受体阻滞剂来降低心率：口服美托洛尔(5~25mg，常用5mg)。口服β受体阻滞剂较静脉注射能够更好地控制和降低心率波动。

  若采用双源CT，可以不用控制心率进行扫描，即使患者有心律失常。
- 在扫描前即刻舌下含服硝酸甘油(0.4~0.8mg)以扩张冠状动脉。

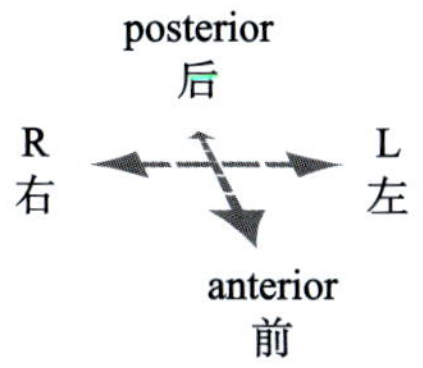

RCA= right coronary artery
右冠状动脉
SAN= SA nodal branch
窦房结支
PDA=posterior descending artery
后降支
PLA=posterolateral artery
后侧支
AVN= AV nodal branch
房室结支

LMCA=left main coronary artery
左冠状动脉主干
LAD = left anterior descending
左前降支
LCx=left circumflex
左回旋支
OM=obtuse marginal
钝缘支
Diag=diagonal
对角支（的）

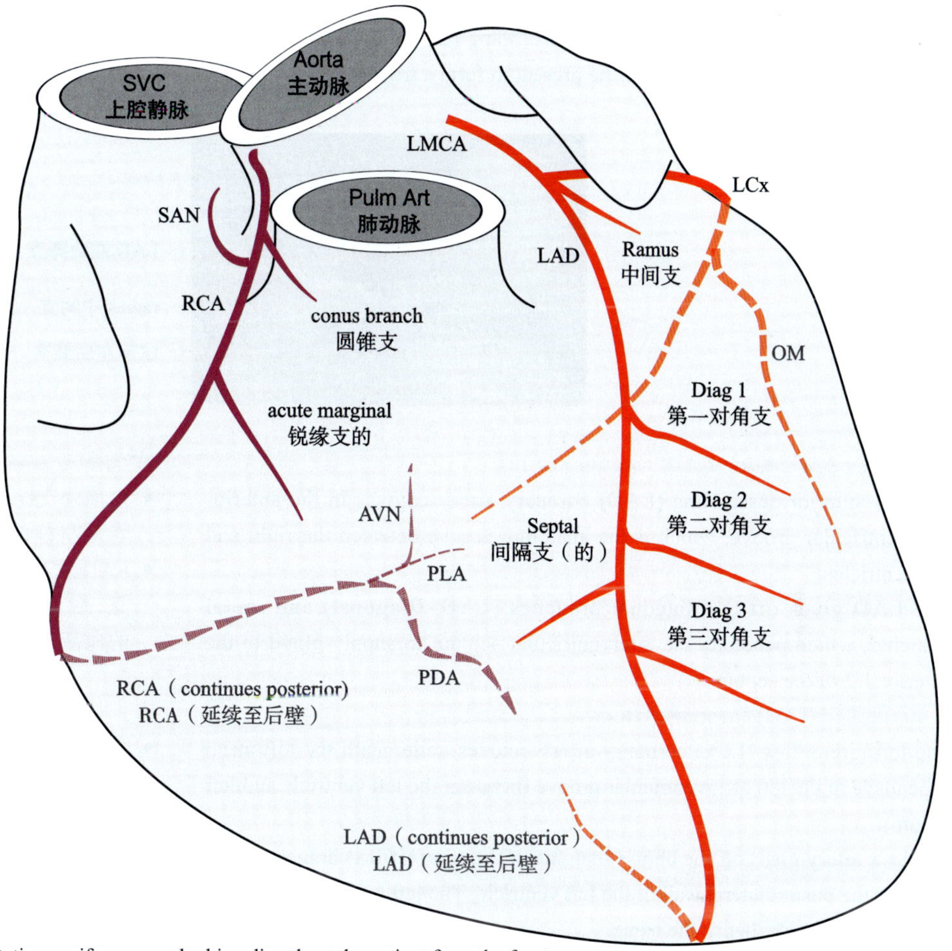

Diagram of the heart in anatomic orientation, as if one were looking directly at the patient from the front.
心脏解剖定位示意图，患者正面观

Coronary artery origination

- Most commonly, two coronary arteries originate from the proximal aorta at the sinuses of Valsalva. High take-off from the sinotubular junction or above is the most common anomaly.
- There are three coronary sinuses. The RCA arises from the right coronary sinus (located anterior). The left main coronary artery arises from the left coronary sinus (located left posterior, adjacent to left atrial appendage). No branch arises from the noncoronary sinus (located right-posterior and straddles the interatrial septum).

冠状动脉起源

- 最常见的是两条冠状动脉起源于主动脉近端的主动脉窦(瓦氏窦)。最常见的高位变异是开口起源于窦管交界处或以上。
- 冠状窦共有3个。右冠状动脉起源于右冠状窦(位于前方)，左冠状动脉主干起源于左冠状窦(位于左后方，邻近左心耳)；无冠窦不发出任何动脉分支(位于右后方，跨坐于房间隔)。

Oblique quasi-axial view through the aorta at the sinotubular junction
窦管交界处的斜准轴位视图

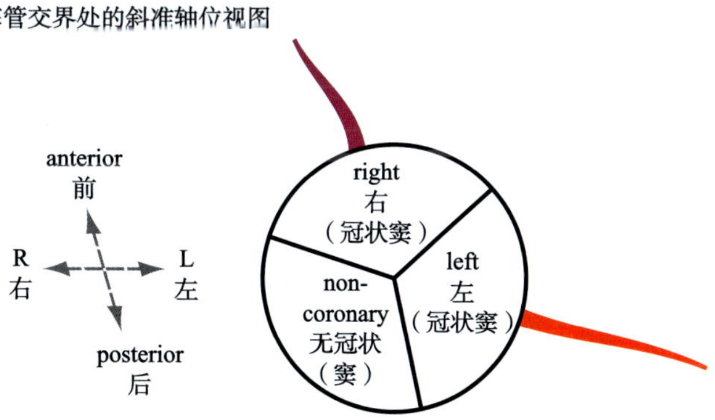

Left main coronary artery (LMCA)

- The left main coronary artery (LMCA) courses between the pulmonary artery and the left atrial appendage.
- The LMCA bifurcates into left anterior descending (LAD) and left circumflex (LCx) arteries. A ramus branch may be present to form a trifurcation.

左冠状动脉主干(LMCA)

- 左冠状动脉主干(LMCA)走行于肺动脉与左心耳(LAA)之间。
- LMCA分出左前降支(LAD)和回旋支(LCx),也可能出现一个小的中间支而形成三叉。

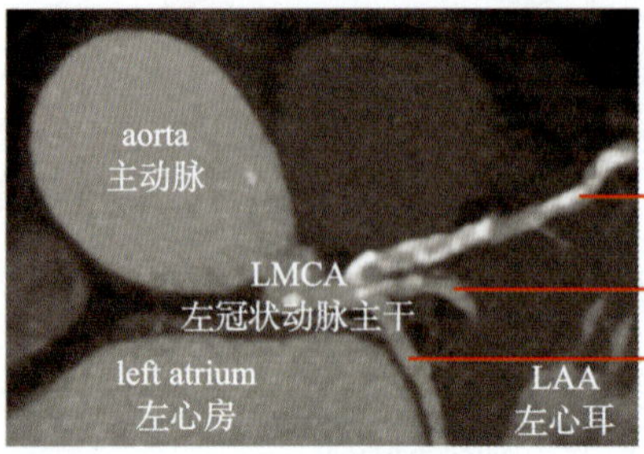

Left anterior descending (LAD) coronary artery

- The left anterior descending (LAD) coronary artery courses in the anterior interventricular groove, which is the anatomic groove between the right and left ventricles.
- The LAD gives off the diagonal branches (LA***D***–***D***iagonal) and septal branches, which penetrate the interventricular septum to supply blood to the anterior 1/2 of the septum.

左前降支(LAD)冠状动脉

- 左前降支(LAD)冠状动脉走行于前室间沟,后者是左右心室之间的一条解剖沟。
- LAD发出对角支(LAD–Diagonal)及室间隔支,后者穿入室间隔并供应室间隔前半部分的血液。

Left circumflex (LCx) coronary artery

- The left circumflex (LCx) coronary artery courses underneath the left atrial appendage in the left atrioventricular groove (between the left ventricle and left atrium).
- The LCx artery gives off the obtuse marginal (OM; circ***OM***flex) branch, which supplies the posterolateral wall of the left ventricle. The left margin of the heart has an obtuse angle, hence the name.
- The LCx uncommonly (~7%) supplies the posterior descending artery (PDA), which is the criteria for a left-dominant system. In the anatomic diagram on the previous page, the more common right-dominant system is shown, where the right coronary artery supplies the PDA.

左回旋支(LCx)冠状动脉

- 左回旋支(LCx)冠状动脉经左心耳(LAA)下方沿左侧房室沟(左心房与左心室之间)走行。
- LCx发出钝缘支(OM),供血左心室后外侧壁。心脏左缘呈钝角,因此得名。
- LCx在少数情况下(约7%)供应后降支(PDA),为左侧优势型的诊断标准。前文解剖示意图中描述的是更为常见的右侧优势型,即右冠状动脉供应PDA。

Right coronary artery (RCA)

右冠状动脉(RCA)

Axial
轴位

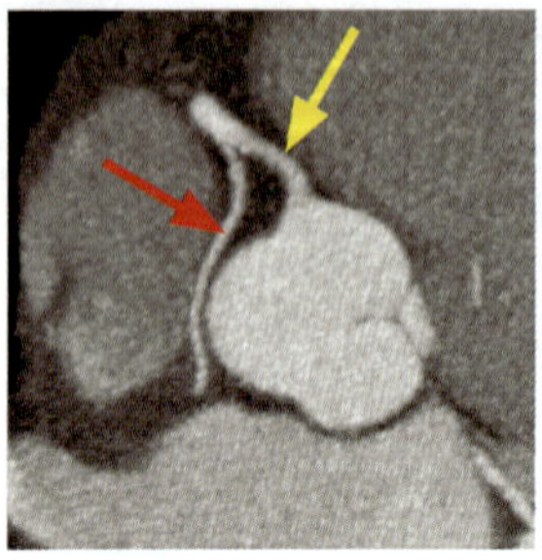

RCA (yellow arrow) arises from the right coronary cusp and gives off the SA nodal branch (red arrow).
RCA(黄箭)起源于右冠状瓣,发出窦房结支(红箭)。

Axial
轴位

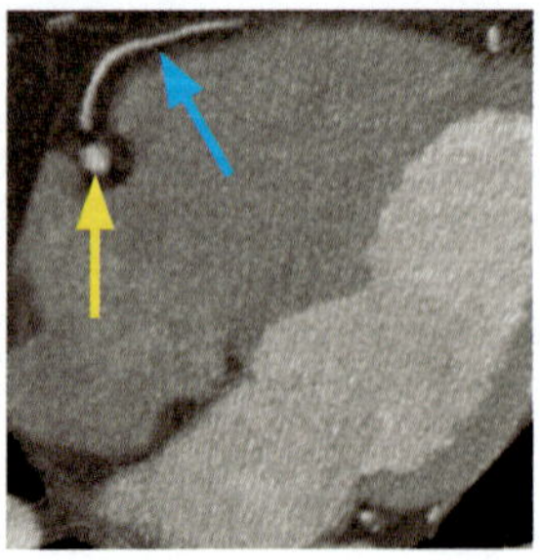

RCA (yellow arrow) gives off acute marginal (blue arrow), which courses along the anterior RV wall.
RCA(黄箭)发出锐缘支(蓝箭),走行于右心室前壁。

Axial
轴位

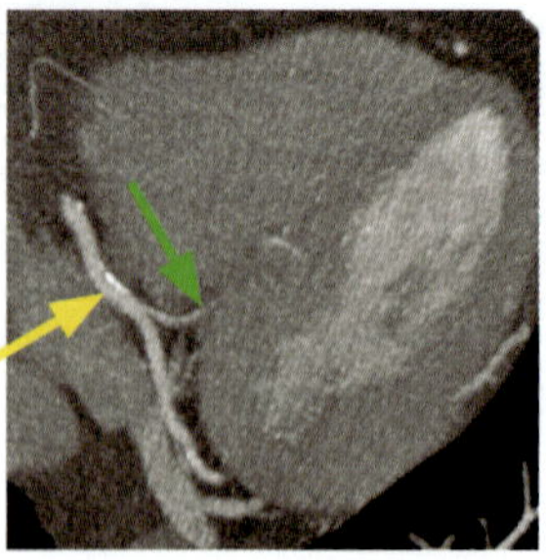

RCA (yellow arrow) gives off PDA (green arrow) in this right-dominant system.
RCA(黄箭)发出后降支(绿箭),右侧优势型。

Sagittal
矢状位

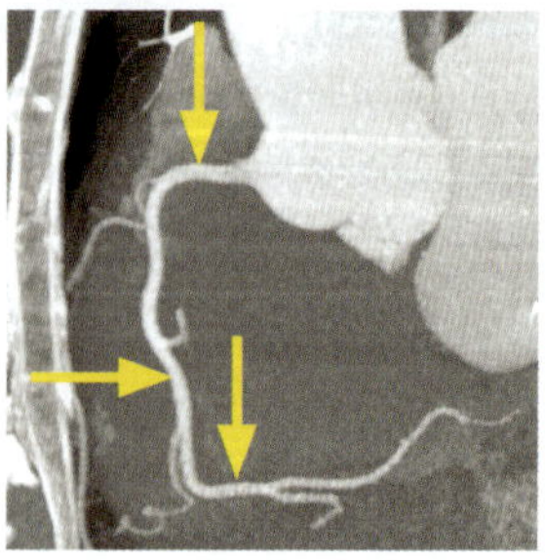

Sagittal thick-slice MIP shows the complete course of RCA (yellow arrows).
矢状位厚层MIP显示整条RCA走行路径(黄箭)。

- The right coronary artery (RCA) mirrors the LCx in course, sitting within the right atrioventricular groove. The first branches of the RCA are the conal branch anteriorly (supplies the right ventricular outflow tract) and the sinoatrial node branch posteriorly.
- The RCA gives off an acute marginal branch which courses anterior to the right ventricular (RV) free wall and muscular branches to supply the RV free wall (not drawn). Margin of the RV has an acute angle, hence the name.
- The atrioventricular nodal branch (AVN) branches off at the crux (junction of all 4 chambers where the atrioventricular and interventricular grooves intersect).
- The posterior descending artery (PDA) arises from the RCA in approximately 85% to supply the posterior 1/2 of the ventricular septum.
- The terminal branch of the RCA is most commonly the posterolateral artery (PLA) that supplies the posterior left ventricle.

- RCA与LCx成镜像走行，位于右房室沟内。RCA最先分支为向前行的圆锥支(供血右心室流出道)和向后行的窦房结支。
- RCA发出锐缘支，走行于右心室(RV)游离壁前方，其肌支供血右心室游离壁(未画出)。右心室的边缘呈锐角因而得名。
- 房室结支(AVN)起源于房室交点(四个心腔交界点，即房室沟与室间沟交叉点)
- 约85%的后降支(PDA)起源于RCA，供应室间隔的后部的1/2。
- 最常见的RCA终末分支为侧后动脉(PLA)，供血左心室后部。

Determination of dominance

- The side which supplies the PDA, PLA, and AVN is the dominant coronary artery. Most commonly, in about 85% of cases, the RCA is the dominant artery.
- Left-dominant anatomy is uncommon, occurring in approximately 7% of cases. In left-dominant anatomy, the LCx supplies the PDA, PLA, and AVN.
- Codominant anatomy can also be seen in approximately 7% of cases, typically with the RCA supplying the PDA, while the LCx supplies PLA.

优势型的确定

- 凡是供应后降支、后侧支及房室结支一侧的动脉即为优势冠状动脉。RCA为最常见的优势动脉，约见于85%的病例。
- 左侧解剖优势不常见，发生率约7%。左冠状动脉优势型中，LCx供应后降支(PDA)、后侧支(PLA)及房室结支(AVN)。
- 约7%的病例中还可见均衡解剖型，通常为RCA供应后降支(PDA)，LCx供应后侧支(PLA)。

Structural Coronary Artery Anomalies

Coronary artery anomalies: Overview

- Coronary artery anomalies are rare and include those of the artery origin, course, or termination. These can be malignant or benign. A *malignant* coronary artery anomaly carries an increased risk of sudden death (in up to 40% of patients), often associated with exercise.
- CCTA is the best modality to evaluate anomalous coronary artery anatomy.
- Anomalies of coronary artery **origin** include:

Coronary artery arising from the pulmonary artery, which is malignant. Either the right or left main coronary artery may arise from the pulmonary artery. Both are very rare.
Anomalous left coronary artery from the pulmonary artery (**ALCAPA**).
Anomalous right coronary artery from the pulmonary artery (**ARCAPA**).
RCA arising from left coronary sinus.
Left main coronary artery (LMCA) arising from right coronary sinus.
Left circumflex (LCx) or left anterior descending (LAD) arising from right coronary sinus. Any artery arising from the noncoronary sinus.

- Anomalies of coronary artery **course** include:

Interarterial course (between the aorta and pulmonary artery) of an anomalous coronary artery is malignant.
Intramural course (within the aortic wall) of a coronary artery is malignant.
Retroaortic, prepulmonic, and septal (subpulmonic) coronary artery courses are all considered benign.
Myocardial bridging (described later in this chapter) is often benign.

冠状动脉结构异常

冠状动脉异常：概述

- 冠状动脉异常包括动脉起源、走向或终止的异常，但均罕见。这些异常可为恶性或良性。恶性冠状动脉异常有增加猝死的风险(高达40%)，常与运动相关。
- CCTA是评估冠状动脉解剖异常的最佳检查方法。
- 异常冠状动脉**起源**包括：

冠状动脉起源于肺动脉，为恶性。右侧或左侧的冠状动脉主干均可能起源于肺动脉，但两种情况都少见。
异常左冠状动脉起源于肺动脉(**ALCAPA**)。
异常右冠状动脉起源于肺动脉(**ARCAPA**)。
RCA起源于左冠状窦。
左冠状动脉主干(LMCA)起源于右冠状窦。
左回旋支(LCX)或左前降支(LAD)起源于右冠状窦。任何起源于无冠状窦的动脉。

- 冠状动脉**走行**异常包括：

血管间走行(在主动脉与肺动脉之间)的异常冠状动脉为恶性。
壁内走形的冠状动脉(在主动脉壁内)为恶性。
主动脉后、肺动脉前和室间隔(肺动脉下)的冠状动脉走向都被认为是良性的。
心肌桥(在本章后文讨论)通常是良性的。

- Anomaly of coronary artery **termination**:

Coronary artery fistula (described later in the chapter)

- 冠状动脉**终止**异常：

冠状动脉瘘(在本章后文讨论)。

Benign coronary artery anomaly

良性冠状动脉异常

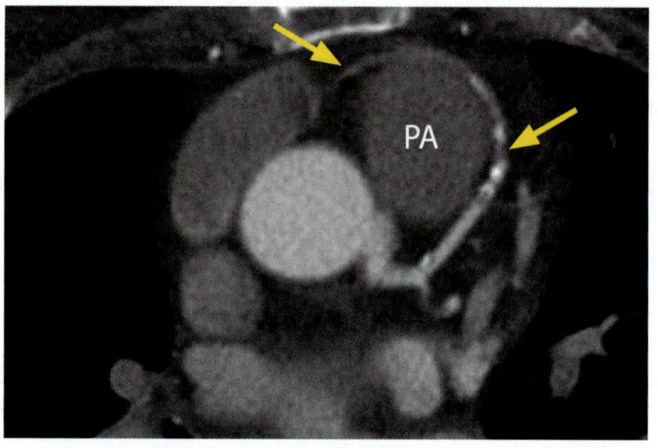

Prepulmonic (benign) course of the left anterior descending (LAD) coronary artery:
Axial image from a gated coronary CT shows an anomalous course of the LAD, which runs anterior (arrows) to the pulmonary artery (PA).
Case courtesy Michael Hanley, MD, University of Virginia Health System.
冠状动脉左前降支(LAD)走行于肺动脉前方(良性):
轴位门控冠状动脉CT图像示左前降支异常走行于肺动脉(PA)的前方(黄箭)。

- An aberrant coronary artery course is considered clinically benign if the coronary artery does not course between the aorta and the pulmonary artery.

Malignant coronary artery anomaly

- Anomalous **intramural course** of either the RCA or LMCA is seen when the vessel courses through the wall of the aorta for a short segment. This anomaly is associated with sudden death. There is typically a slit-like configuration of the coronary artery on CCTA.

  The treatment of intramural coronary artery is bypass, reimplantation, or the unroofing procedure.

- 变异的冠状动脉若不是走行于主动脉和肺动脉之间则在临床上认为是良性的。

恶性冠状动脉异常

- 异常壁内走行是指RCA或LMCA的一小段血管穿过主动脉壁。这种异常与猝死相关。CCTA上冠状动脉呈典型的狭缝状。

  治疗壁内冠状动脉的方法是搭桥、再植或去顶术。

Malignant: Anomalous origin of LEFT coronary artery arising from the RIGHT coronary sinus, passing between the aorta and the PA.
恶性：左冠状动脉异常起源于右冠状窦，走行于主动脉与肺动脉之间。

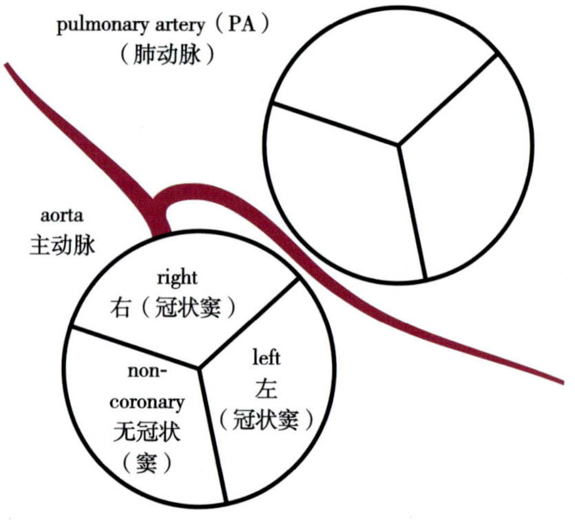

Malignant: Anomalous origin of RIGHT coronary artery arising from the LEFT coronary sinus, passing between the aorta and the PA.
恶性：右冠状动脉异常起源于左冠状窦，走行于主动脉与肺动脉之间。

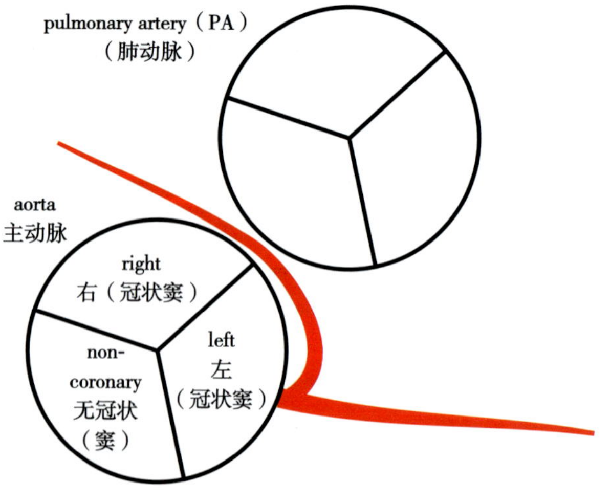

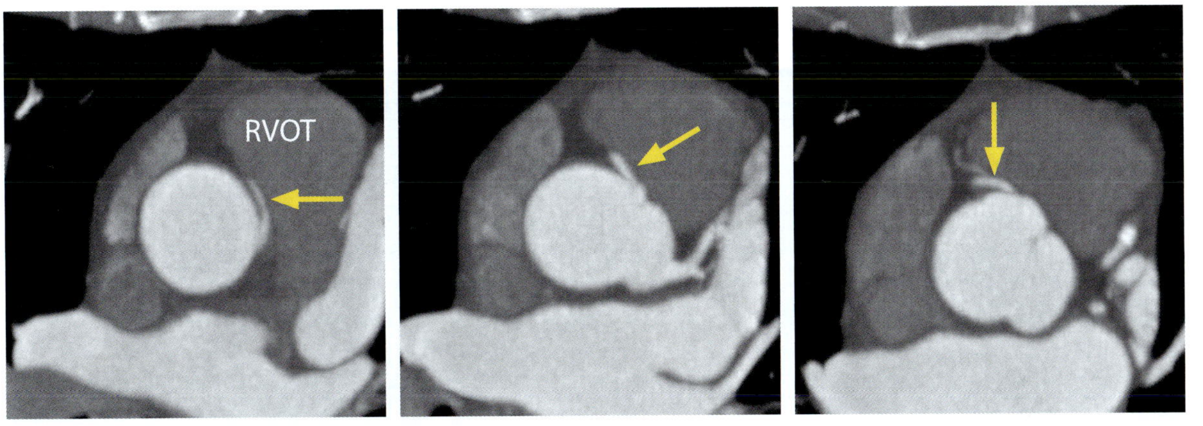

Malignant course of anomalous right coronary artery:
Sequential axial images from a coronary CTA show anomalous origin of the right coronary artery (arrow) from the left coronary sinus, which then courses between the aorta and the right ventricular outflow tract (RVOT).
Case courtesy Michael Hanley, MD, University of Virginia Health System.
恶性右冠状动脉走行异常：
连续轴位冠状动脉CTA显示右冠状动脉(黄箭)异常起源于左冠状窦，然后走行在主动脉和右心室流出道(RVOT)之间。

- Anomalous **interarterial course** (between the pulmonary artery or RV outflow tract and the aorta) of a coronary artery carries a high risk of sudden death of up to 40%, associated with exercise. It is thought that dilation of the aorta occurs during exercise, which may compress the anomalous vessel resulting in myocardial infarction.

Either an anomalous left coronary artery or anomalous right coronary artery may take a malignant interarterial course.

Treatment is surgical bypass grafting.

Anomalous left coronary artery from the pulmonary artery (ALCAPA)/Bland-White-Garland syndrome

- Also called Bland-White-Garland syndrome, anomalous left coronary artery from the pulmonary artery (ALCAPA) is a very rare but serious coronary artery anomaly, where the left coronary artery arises from the pulmonary artery. Most affected patients are infants, with over 90% mortality in the first year of life if untreated.
- Treatment is surgical, with either direct implantation of the anomalous coronary artery (in children) or ligation of the anomalous vessel in conjunction with bypass grafting (in adults).
- Less commonly, the RCA may arise from the pulmonary artery. This is known as **anomalous right coronary artery from the pulmonary artery (ARCAPA)**. Treatment is similar.

- 冠状动脉异常**走行于动脉间**(肺动脉或右心室流出道与主动脉之间)的猝死风险高达40%，与运动有关。机制可能是运动时主动脉扩张，随之压迫异常走行的血管而导致心肌梗死。

无论左侧还是右侧冠状动脉异常，都有可能呈恶性异常走行于动脉之间。

治疗为外科搭桥术。

左冠状动脉异常起源于肺动脉(ALCAPA)/布兰德-怀特-加兰德综合征

- 左冠状动脉异常起源于肺动脉(ALCAPA)也称之为布兰德-怀特-加兰德综合征，是一种罕见但严重的冠状动脉异常，其左冠状动脉起源于肺动脉。最常见于婴儿，若不加以治疗，1岁以内的死亡率超过90%。
- 治疗为外科手术，对异常冠状动脉行直接植入术(儿童)或结扎异常血管结合搭桥术(成人)。
- 较少见的情况是右冠状动脉起源于肺动脉，即**右冠状动脉异常起源于肺动脉(ARCAPA)**，治疗方法与上文类似。

Myocardial bridging

心肌桥

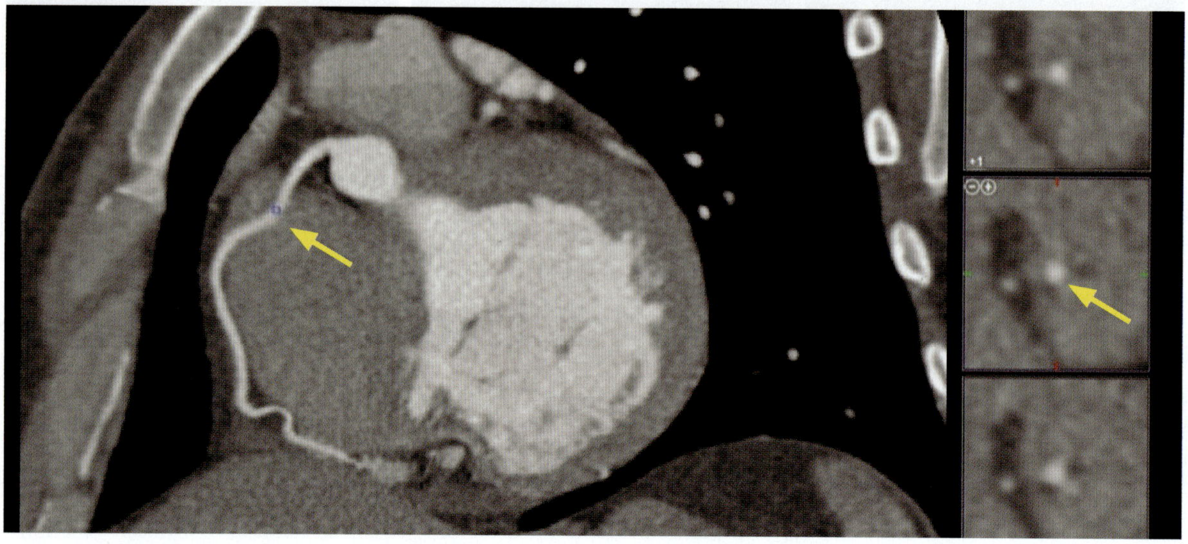

Curved multiplanar reconstruction and cross-sectional CT images demonstrate myocardial bridging of the proximal RCA (arrows).
曲面多平面重建和轴位CT图像显示近端RCA的心肌桥(黄箭)。

- Myocardial bridging describes a band of myocardium overlying a segment of a coronary artery, most commonly seen in the mid or distal LAD.
- Myocardial bridging is usually asymptomatic; however, it may be a cause of angina, myocardial infarction, or even death.
- If bridging is present and thought to be the source of the patient's symptoms, further evaluation is recommended with exercise myocardial perfusion.

- 心肌桥是指一束心肌覆盖一段冠状动脉，最常见于左前降支的中或远段。
- 心肌桥常无症状，但可以引起心绞痛、心肌梗死，甚至死亡。
- 若有心肌桥且怀疑是引起患者症状的原因，应建议用运动负荷心肌灌注进一步评估。

Coronary artery fistula

冠状动脉瘘

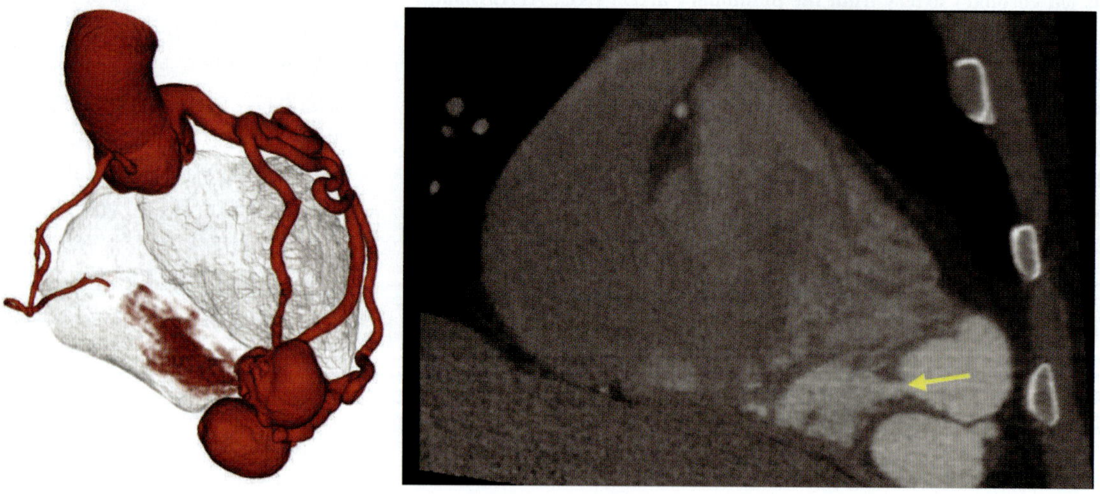

3D volume rendered image (left) demonstrates tortuosity and diffuse aneurysmal dilatation of the LAD and two diagonal branches, which converge in a large bilobed aneurysm at the cardiac apex. CT image (right) shows a communication (arrow) between the distal portion of the aneurysm and the right ventricle, representing a coronary cameral fistula.
3D容积再现图像(左图)显示LAD和两个对角支迂曲和弥漫性动脉瘤样扩张，并在心尖汇聚成一个大的双叶动脉瘤。CT图像(右图)显示动脉瘤的远端部分和右心室之间的一个交通(黄箭)，此为冠状动脉心腔瘘。

- Abnormal connection can occur between a coronary artery branch and a coronary vein, other lower pressure vascular system (e.g., pulmonary artery), another coronary artery or systemic artery, or a cardiac chamber (in which case it is called a **coronary cameral fistula**).
- Majority of coronary artery fistulas are congenital. Uncommon etiologies include trauma, iatrogenic injury, infection, or radiation-induced.
- When a fistula occurs between a coronary artery and a lower pressure vascular system, CT may show dilated tortuous coronary arteries and epicardial feeding vessels. There is often aneurysmal dilation of the coronary artery proximal to the fistula.

- 异常连接可发生在冠状动脉分支、冠状静脉、其他较低压力的血管系统(如肺动脉)、另一条冠状动脉或体动脉或心腔之间(这种情况称为**冠状动脉心腔瘘**)。
- 大多数冠状动脉瘘是先天性的。少见的病因包括外伤、医源性损伤、感染或辐射诱发。
- 当冠状动脉和低压血管系统之间发生瘘时,CT可显示扩张、迂曲的冠状动脉和心外膜供血血管。瘘管近侧的冠状动脉常有动脉瘤状扩张。

Coronary Artery Disease

Coronary artery calcium score

- A gated noncontrast cardiac CT can be obtained independently or prior to contrast-enhanced CCTA for calcium scoring. Coronary artery calcification is a marker for CAD.
- Any area≥3 pixels in a coronary artery with density greater than 130 HU is considered to contain calcium. The **Agatston score** represents the total calcium in the coronary tree. It can predict the risk of future major adverse cardiovascular events and guide preventive therapy.
- Coronary calcium scoring is appropriate for risk stratification in asymptomatic patients without known CAD and with:

  (1) An intermediate 10-year ASCVD (arteriosclerotic cardiovascular disease) risk estimate;

  Or (2) a family history of premature CAD and a low 10-year ASCVD risk estimate.

Coronary artery stenosis

- The Coronary Artery Disease Reporting and Data System (**CAD-RADS**) was introduced in 2016 to provide standard classification of CAD, reduce reader variability, and facilitate communication between interpreting and referring clinicians.
- CAD-RADS categories 0, 1, and 2 (stenosis <50%) represent nonobstructive CAD and do not require further workup. Non-atherosclerotic causes of patient's chest pain should be considered.
- Stenosis >50% is considered obstructive and potentially hemodynamically significant, which requires further workup. CAD-RADS 3 is moderate stenosis (50–69%). CAD-RADS 4 is severe stenosis (70–99%) or significant stenosis (>50%) in the left main coronary artery (LMCA).
- CAD-RADS 5 is total occlusion of at least one coronary artery.
- When one or more coronary artery segment is not evaluable and the rest show <50% stenosis, the study is considered nondiagnostic (CAD-RADS category N). Coronary segments smaller than 1.5 mm in diameter are not classifiable by CAD-RADS.

冠状动脉疾病

冠状动脉钙化积分

- 单独使用门控心脏平扫CT或增强前CCTA可用于计算钙化评分。冠状动脉钙化是CAD的一个指标。
- 冠状动脉任何区域≥3个体素,其密度>130HU时都被认为含有钙质。**Agatston评分**代表冠状动脉树的总钙质。它可以用来预测未来严重不良心血管事件的风险并指导预防性治疗。
- 冠状动脉钙化评分适用于无症状且未知有CAD,以及具有以下特点的患者进行风险分层:

  (1)有10年ASCVD(动脉硬化性心血管疾病)风险评估史。

  或

  (2)有早发性CAD家族史和预估10年的ASCVD为低风险。

冠状动脉狭窄

- 冠状动脉疾病报告和数据系统(**CAD-RADS**)于2016年问世,旨在提供CAD的标准分类,减少阅片者之间的差异,并促进报告者和转诊医师之间的沟通。
- CAD-RADS评分为0分、1分和2分(狭窄度<50%)代表非阻塞性CAD,无须进一步检查。患者胸痛的原因应考虑为非动脉粥样硬化性。
- 狭窄>50%被认为是阻塞性的,有潜在的血流动力学意义,需进一步检查。CAD-RADS为3分是中度狭窄(50%~69%)。CAD-RADS为4分是严重狭窄(70%~99%)或左主冠状动脉(LMCA)显著狭窄(>50%)。
- CAD-RADS 5定义为至少有一条冠状动脉完全闭塞。
- 当一个或多个冠状动脉节段无法评估,其余节段显示<50%的狭窄时,被认为不具诊断意义(CAD-RADS类别为N)。直径<1.5mm的冠状动脉节段不被列入CAD-RADS分类。

CAD-RADS	Interpretation	Stenosis	Workup and management
0	No CAD	0	Reassurance.
1	Minimal CAD	1–24%	Preventative therapy.
2	Mild CAD	25–49%	Preventative therapy.
3	Moderate stenosis	50–69%	Consider functional testing and preventative therapy.
4	Severe stenosis	70–99%, or >50% LMCA	Functional testing or invasive coronary angiography. Consider revascularization.
5	Occlusion	100%	Same as for CAD-RADS 4.

CAD-RADS	解读	狭窄	进一步检查和处置
0	无CAD	0	安慰。
1	很少CAD	1%~24%	预防性治疗。
2	轻度CAD	25%~49%	预防性治疗。
3	中度CAD	50%~69%	考虑功能测试和预防性治疗。
4	重度CAD	70%~99% 或>50% LMCA	功能测试或有创性冠状动脉造影。考虑血运重建。
5	闭塞	100%	与CAD-RADS 4相同。

注：CAD，冠状动脉疾病；CAD-RADS，冠状动脉疾病报告和数据系统。

Plaque vulnerability

- High-risk (vulnerable) atherosclerotic plaques are associated with increased risk of acute coronary syndrome. High-risk features include low-attenuation plaque (<30 HU), spotty calcification, positive remodeling, and the *napkin-ring sign*.
- There is no established guideline for management of patients with vulnerable plaques.

易损斑块

- 高风险(易损)的动脉粥样硬化斑块与急性冠脉综合征的风险增加有关。高风险特征包括低衰减斑块(<30HU)、斑点状钙化、正性重构和餐巾环征。
- 对于易损斑块患者的处理目前尚无明确的指南。

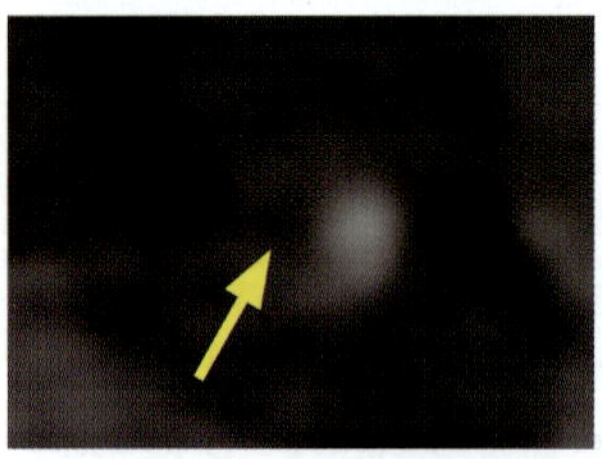

Low-attenuation plaque (arrow) measures less than 30 HU on CTA.
CTA上低密度斑块(黄箭)的CT值小于30HU。

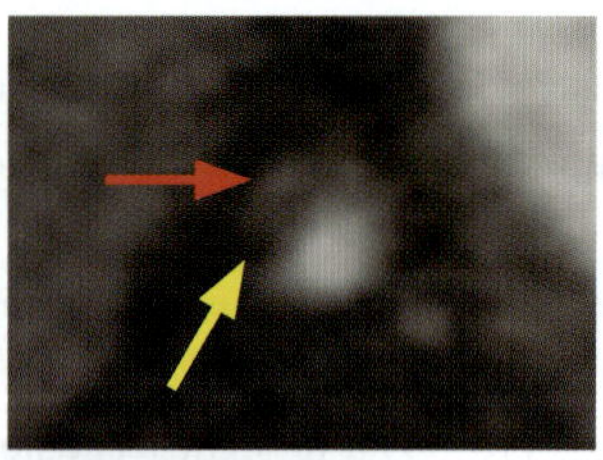

Napkin-ring sign: low-attenuation core (yellow arrow) surrounded by higher attenuation rim (red arrow).
餐巾环征：低衰减核心(黄箭)被高衰减边缘(红箭)包围。

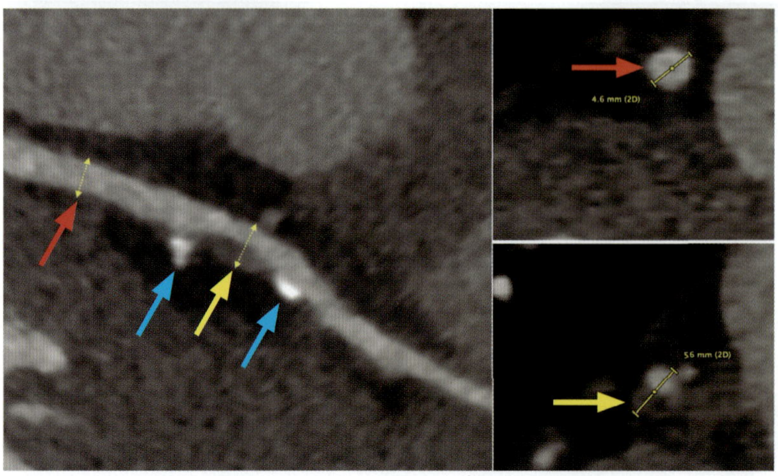

Positive remodeling: characterized by compensatory enlargement of the vessel wall at site of plaque (yellow arrows) beyond the normal caliber (red arrows), with preserved vessel lumen.
Also seen are spotty calcifications (blue arrows).
正性重构：特点是斑块部位的血管壁代偿性增粗(黄箭)，超过正常管径(红箭)，但血管腔得以保留。
还可见斑点状钙化(蓝箭)。

Evaluation of coronary stents and bypass grafts

- Two major complications following coronary artery stenting are stent thrombosis (in the acute setting) and in-stent restenosis (a late complication). In-stent restenosis occurs by neointimal hyperplasia and appears as low-attenuation material within the stent lumen.
- Unfortunately, CCTA evaluation of coronary stents remains difficult and adequate visualization of the stent lumen depends on various factors, including stent type, diameter, location, presence of motion or blooming artifacts.

评估冠状动脉支架和搭桥

- 冠状动脉支架术后的两个主要并发症是支架内血栓形成(急性期)和支架内再狭窄(晚期并发症)。支架内再狭窄由内膜增生引起，表现为支架腔内的低密度物质。
- 不幸的是，CCTA对冠状动脉支架的评估仍有困难，支架管腔的可视程度取决于多种因素，包括支架类型、直径、位置、是否存在运动或晕状伪影。

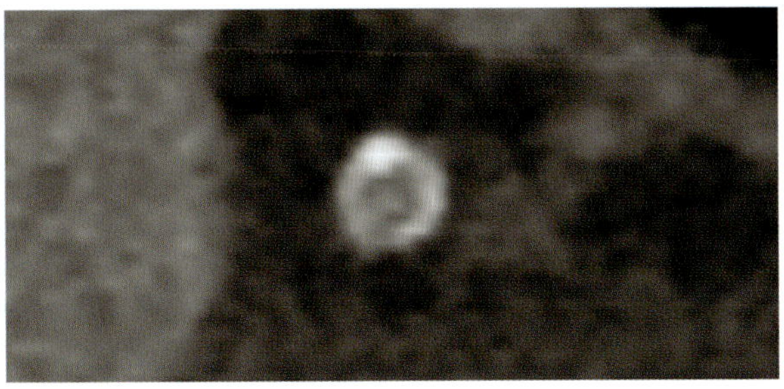

Cross-sectional CTA image of a coronary stent shows low-attenuation material in the lumen, consistent with in-stent restenosis.
横截面冠状动脉支架CTA图像显示腔内有低密度物质，符合支架内再狭窄。

- Potential complications of bypass grafts are graft stenosis, occlusion, and aneurysm formation. One pitfall on imaging is that a completely occluded graft can be difficult to discern, with the only hint being an outpouching at the graft-aortic anastomosis.
- Coronary bypass grafts can be accurately evaluated by CCTA, however because beam hardening and streak artifacts from adjacent surgical clips can obscure findings, cardiac catheterization remains the preferred diagnostic modality at most locations.
- Stenoses of both coronary stents and bypass grafts are graded similarly to those of native coronary arteries, using the CAD-RADS.

- 血管搭桥的潜在并发症是移植血管狭窄、闭塞和动脉瘤形成。影像学的缺点是难以发现一个完全闭塞的移植血管，唯一的提示是移植血管-主动脉吻合口外翻。
- 冠状动脉搭桥血管可通过CCTA进行准确评估，但是由于射线束硬化和邻近手术夹的条纹伪影可能掩盖病变，大多数时候，心导管检查仍然是首选的诊断方式。
- 冠状动脉支架和搭桥血管狭窄程度的分级与自体冠状动脉类似，采用CAD-RADS进行分级。

Coronary artery aneurysm

冠状动脉瘤

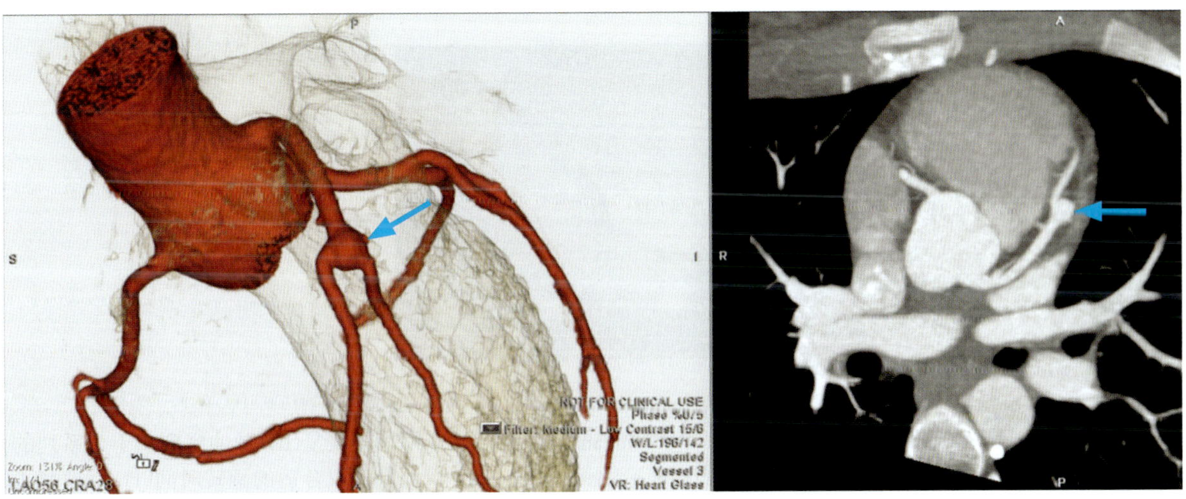

Oblique 3D reformatted image (left) and axial CT image (right) show an aneurysm (arrows) at the bifurcation of the LAD and first diagonal branch in this patient with a history of Kawasaki disease.
斜位三维容积再现图像(左图)和轴位CT图像(右图)显示在LAD和第一对角支的分叉处有一个动脉瘤(蓝箭)，该患者有川崎病的病史。

- Aneursymal dilatation of the coronary artery is rare and most commonly caused by atherosclerosis in the United States, and Kawasaki disease worldwide.
- Coronary artery aneurysms can be found incidentally on imaging in an asymptomatic patient, or can present with angina or acute coronary syndrome.
- Management of coronary artery aneurysm varies depending on patient's clinical presentation and risk assessment.

- 冠状动脉瘤样扩张罕见，在美国最常见的病因是动脉粥样硬化，而在世界范围内则是川崎病。
- 冠状动脉瘤可以是无症状患者影像学检查中的一个偶然发现，也可以表现为心绞痛或急性冠脉综合征。
- 冠状动脉瘤的处理方法取决于患者的临床表现和风险评估。

（翻译　杨明）

CARDIAC MRI

IMAGING TECHNIQUES

- Cardiac MRI provides high-resolution dynamic imaging of the heart using different pulse sequences.
- Spin echo (SE) has longer acquisition time but yields high spatial resolution and excellent contrast while generating little artifact from metal. Single slices are generated from a single breath hold. SE is used for anatomy.
- Spoiled gradient recalled echo (GRE) is faster but more susceptible to metal artifacts. GRE is used for quantitative measurements, perfusion, and angiography.
- Balanced steady-state free precession (SSFP) is a family of "bright blood" gradient echo sequences. This technique provides high temporal resolution and excellent contrast between myocardium and blood pool. ECG-triggered segmented SSFP is gathered over several heart beats to create a cine to evaluate wall motion, valve function, volume quantification, and can be performed before or after contrast administration.

心脏MRI

成像技术

- 心脏MRI采用不同脉冲序列因而可获得高分辨率的动态心脏影像。
- 自旋回波(SE)序列的采集时间较长，但可获得高空间分辨率和出色对比度的图像，并受金属伪影的干扰较小。一次屏气可获取单层图像。SE序列用于观察解剖。
- 扰相梯度回波(GRE)序列采集速度较快，但易受金属伪影干扰。GRE序列用于定量测量、灌注成像和血管成像。
- 平衡稳态自由进动(SSFP)序列是一类"亮血"梯度回波序列。该成像技术可获得高时间分辨率和优越的心肌-血池对比度图像。心电触发分段SSFP在几个心动周期中采集数据从而生成电影序列用以评估室壁运动、瓣膜功能及容积定量计算，可在造影剂注射前或注射后采集。

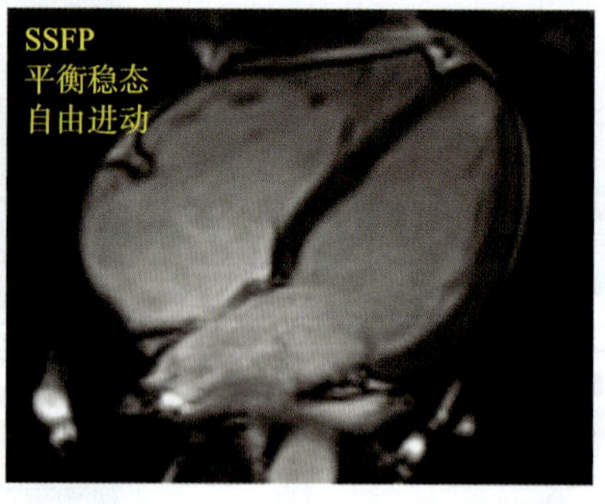

Inversion recovery (IR)

- IR pulse nulls the signal from the normal myocardium to accentuate pathology based on picking the appropriate inversion time (TI) on a series of scout images. Normal myocardium is nulled with TI of approximately 300–400 ms after the RF pulse and therefore appears black. The inversion time varies based on volume, contrast relaxivity, excretion rates, and field strength.
- Double IR is used with fast SE sequence as a dark-blood technique where blood appears dark compared to myocardium.
- Triple IR is a dark-blood technique with an additional IR pulse for fat suppression.

翻转恢复(IR)

- 翻转恢复(IR)脉冲序列基于一系列的侦查图像选取合适的翻转时间(TI)以抑制正常心肌的信号从而突出病变。射频脉冲激发后，选取300~400毫秒的TI可抑制正常心肌的信号使其表现为黑色。TI与容积、对比剂弛豫率、排泄速度和场强密切相关。
- 作为一种黑血技术，双IR与快速SE序列结合可使血液相对于心肌呈现黑色的效果。
- 三重IR是在双IR基础上增加一次IR脉冲以实现脂肪抑制的黑血技术。

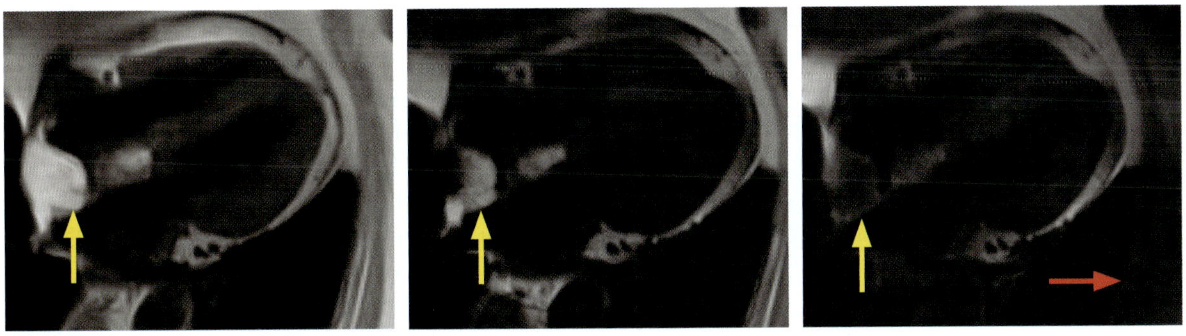

Double IR T1
双翻转恢复T_1

Double IR T2
双翻转恢复T_2

Triple IR T2
三重翻转恢复T_2

Lipomatous hypertrophy of the interatrial septum (yellow arrows) on double and triple IR sequences: Note suppression of fat in the interatrial septum and lateral chest wall (red arrow) on triple IR compared to double IR. There is incomplete fat suppression anterior to the heart on the triple IR T2-weighted image.
双IR及三重IR序列图像中的房间隔脂肪瘤样肥厚(黄箭)：注意，与双IR相比，三重IR图像上房间隔和侧胸壁脂肪(红箭)受抑制。在三重IR的T_2图像上，心脏前方存在脂肪抑制不完全的现象。

- Phase-sensitive inversion recovery (PSIR) is a version of IR that acquires a reference phase image in the next heartbeat after the magnitude image is acquired. The phase information is used to calculate the absolute differences in recovery of signal redistributed as grayscale values. This allows for much greater separation between the normal myocardium and abnormal myocardium along a wider range of inversion times based on gadolinium content (i.e., pericardial effusion will be black on PSIR and bright on the magnitude image.)

- 相位敏感翻转恢复(PSIR)序列是一种特殊的IR序列，它在采集幅度图像后，在下一个心动周期中获取参考相位图像。相位信息用以计算信号恢复的绝对差异并重新以灰度值的形式表现出来。在基于钆对比剂的情况下，可以在更宽的翻转时间范围内更好地区分正常和异常心肌(如心包积液在PSIR图像上表现为低信号而在幅度图像上表现为高亮信号)。

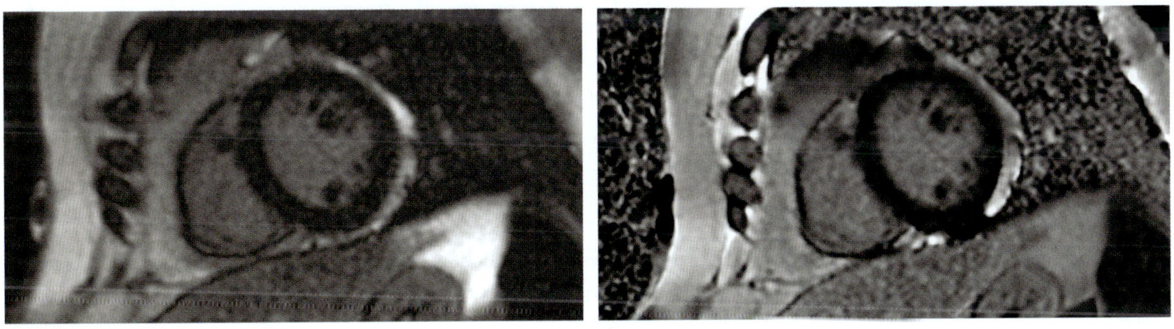

Magnitude IR
幅度翻转恢复

Phase-sensitive IR
相位敏感翻转恢复

Dynamic first-pass perfusion MRI

- First-pass contrast-enhanced perfusion MRI is performed pre-and post-vasodilator stress to evaluate myocardial perfusion. Normal myocardium enhances homogeneously, while areas of decreased perfusion will be relatively hypoenhancing. This technique allows for quantitative perfusion. In characterization of cardiac masses, malignant masses generally have more avid first pass perfusion while benign lesions have more mild or modest perfusion.

动态首次通过灌注MRI

- 在使用血管扩张药物负荷前后进行首次通过对比-增强灌注MRI以评估心肌灌注。正常心肌呈均匀强化，而灌注减低区呈现相对弱强化。该技术可进行灌注量化评估。在心脏肿块的鉴别诊断中，恶性肿块通常呈现出更显著的首次通过灌注强化，而良性病变表现为轻度或中度强化。

Delayed contrast-enhanced MRI

- Delayed contrast-enhanced MRI (DE-MR) is performed using a T1W single inversion recovery gradient echo or SSFP (if there is not enough signal typically at 1.5T).
- Unlike in contrast-enhanced perfusion where first-pass enhancement is normal,

延迟对比增强MRI

- 延迟对比增强MRI(DE-MRI)使用T_1加权单次翻转恢复扰相梯度回波序列或SSFP序列(通常在1.5T场强中信号强度欠佳时)进行成像。
- 与对比增强灌注成像中正常首过性强化不同

any late gadolinium enhancement (LGE) in DE-MR is abnormal and represents a delay in washout of gadolinium-based contrast material from the extracellular space. Thus, any process that expands the extracellular space (decreasing the ratio of normal myocytes to extracellular space) will result in delayed enhancement.

- LGE is caused by interstitial fibrosis due to cell death. It can also occur due to nonischemic etiologies. Different patterns of enhancement suggest different etiologies.

的是，DE-MRI中的任何心肌延迟强化(LGE)均为异常，代表钆对比剂从细胞外间隙廓清延迟。因此，任何导致细胞外间隙扩大的过程(正常心肌细胞与细胞外间隙比值降低)都会导致延迟强化。

- LGE为细胞死亡导致的间质纤维化所致，也可继发于非缺血性疾病。不同的强化模式提示不同的病因。

Phase contrast imaging (VENC)

- Phase contrast imaging, also called velocity encoded gradient echo imaging (VENC), measures blood flow perpendicular to the imaging plane, based on differences in phase shift of moving tissue relative to stationary tissue.
- A cine is produced throughout the cardiac cycle. Flow in opposite direction appears black; forward flow appears white. Stationary tissue appears gray. Signal intensity within a region of interest reflects the velocity of flow, such as regurgitation through a valve or pressure gradient across a cardiac shunt.
- The VENC has to be prescribed to interrogate a specific range of velocities. If the velocities measured are outside of this range, they will be misrepresented as *aliasing*.

相位对比成像(VENC)

- 相位对比成像，又称为流速编码梯度回波成像(VENC)，基于运动组织与静止组织间的相位差异而测量垂直于成像平面的血流速度。
- 在整个心动周期内进行电影成像。相反方向的血流呈现为低信号，而正向流动的血流则表现为高信号，静止的组织呈现为灰色。感兴趣区内组织的信号强度反映流速，如通过瓣膜的反流或跨心脏分流通道的压力梯度。
- VENC必须限制在特定的速度区间。如若超出相应速度区间则会错误地表现为*混淆伪影*。

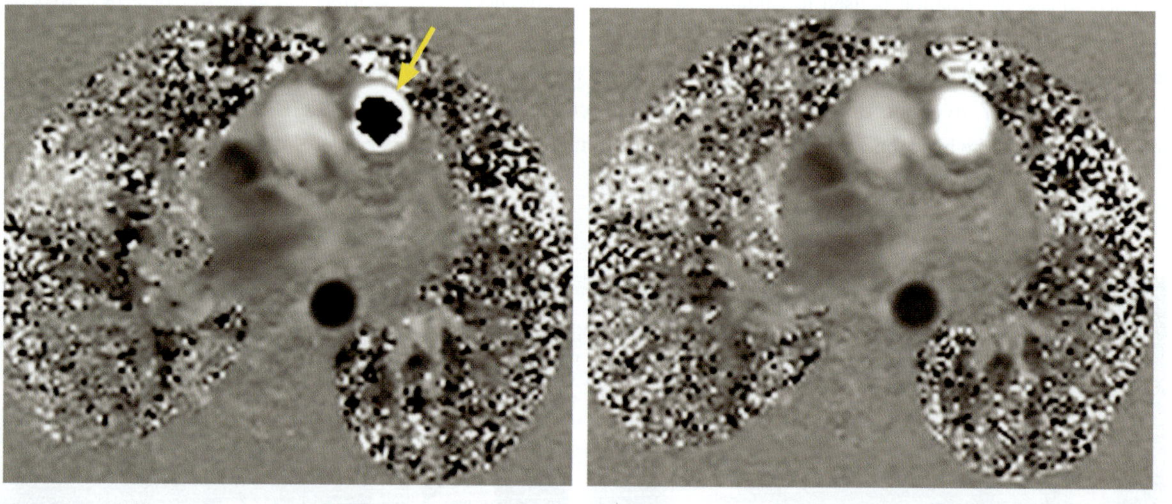

VENC imaging with aliasing: The velocity encoding parameter was picked too low on the left image, resulting in faster flows not appropriately represented and seen as black pixels, called *aliasing*, within the pulmonary artery (arrow). VENC was corrected in the right image.

具有混淆伪影VENC中的混淆伪影：在左侧图像上所选择的速度编码参数过低，导致肺动脉内更快的血流未被正确地显示而呈低信号(黄箭)，称为*混淆伪影*。VENC速度编码在右图中得到纠正。

Myocardial tagging

- Myocardial tagging allows assessment of myocardial wall motion and strain.
- RF pulses are applied as tag lines in the image. Grid tags can be applied for myocardial strain analysis or to determine if a myocardial segment is involved by a mass. These grid lines deform as the myocardium contracts and relaxes during the cardiac cycle. Line tags can be applied perpendicular to the myocardial/mass/pericardial interface to assess for adherence or invasion.

心肌标记

- 心肌标记技术可以测量心肌的运动和应变。
- 对图像施加射频脉冲序列作为标记线。网格化标记可用于心肌应变分析或确定某一节段心肌是否被肿块累及。这些网格线随着心肌在心动周期中收缩和松弛而发生形变。可将标记线垂直施加于心肌/肿块/心包界面以评估粘连或侵犯。

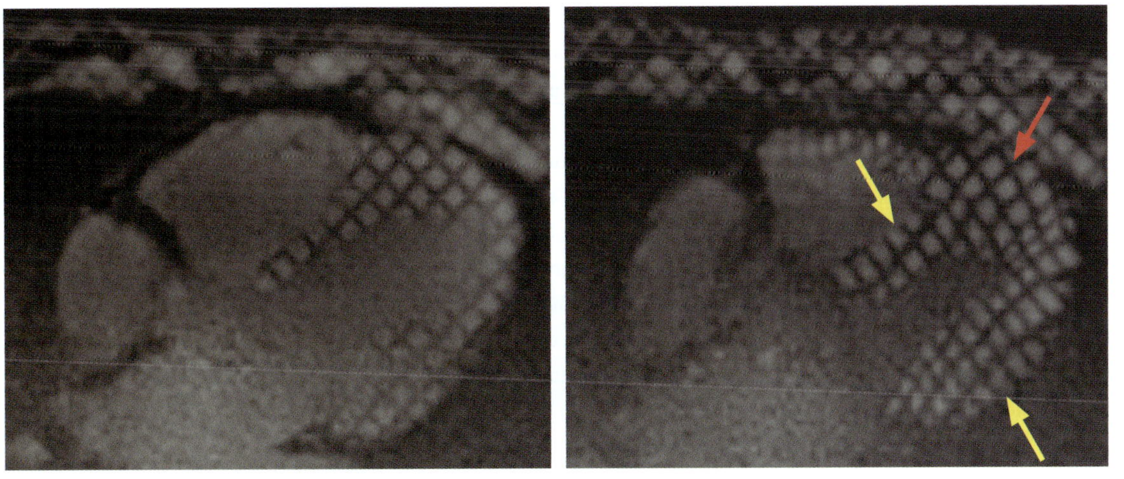

Myocardial tagging demonstrates contraction of the myocardium as indicated by deformation of the grid lines during systole (right image, yellow arrows) compared to diastole (left image). Similar to how the grid lines over the anterior chest wall do not deform, the grid lines over the distal septal mass also maintain their shape (red arrow), indicating the difference between contractile myocardium and a non-contractile mass.
与舒张期(左图)相比，心肌标记显示心肌收缩，如收缩期网格线变形所示(右图，黄箭)。心尖段室间隔肿块上的网格线与前胸壁上的网格线变形类似，也保持其形状(红箭)，表明收缩心肌和非收缩肿块之间的差异。

RECONSTRUCTION AXES IN CARDIAC MRI

心脏MRI中的重建轴位

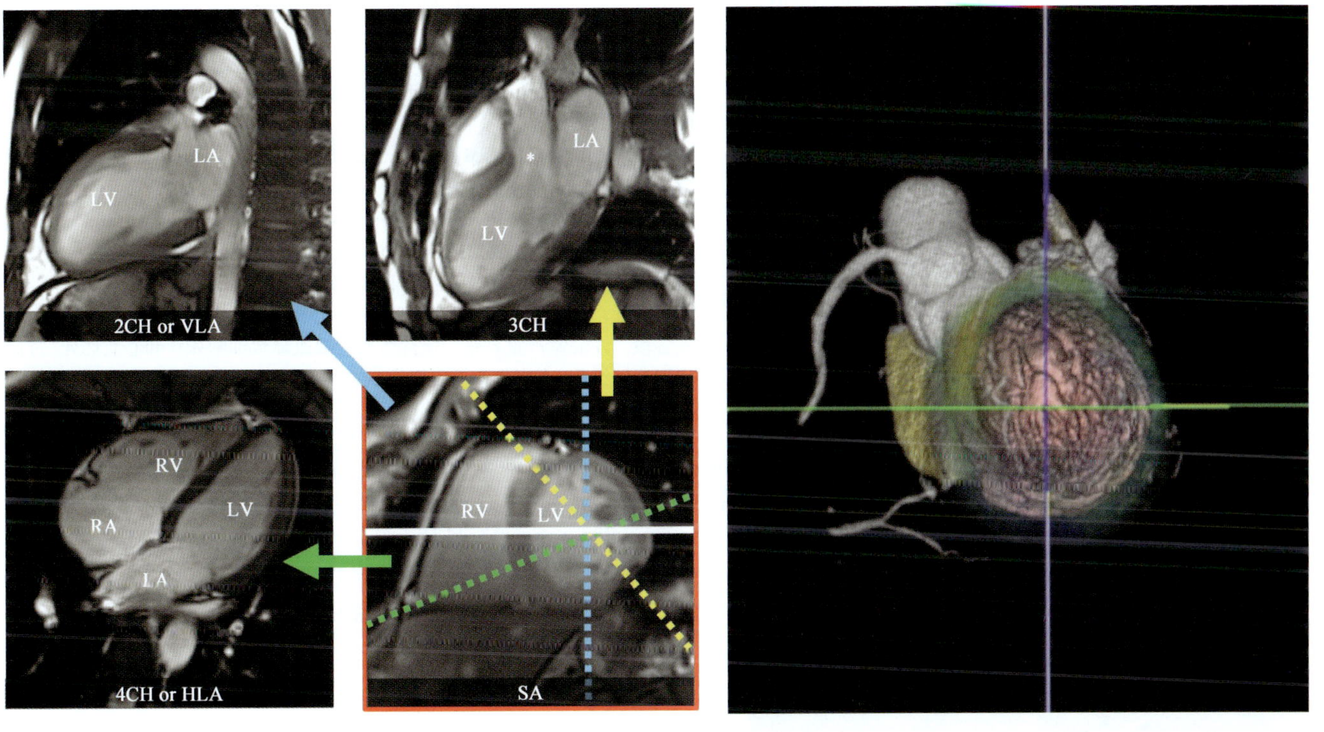

MRI images (left) and 3D volume rendered image (right) showcase the 4 common reconstruction axes in cardiac imaging: 2 chamber or vertical long axis (2CH or VLA), 3 chamber (3CH), 4 chamber or horizontal long axis (4CH or HLA), and short axis (SA). The asterisk *represents the LVOT. The white line on the SA view represents the true axial slice. The colored arrows and lines (dotted on SA view, solid on the 3D rendering) represent the relationship between the different axes.
MRI图像(左图)和3D容积重建图像(右图)显示心脏成像中的4个常见重建轴位：两腔或垂直长轴(2CH或VLA)、三腔(3CH)、四腔或水平长轴(4CH或HLA)和短轴(SA)。星号*代表左心室(LV)流出道。SA视图上的白线表示真正的轴向切面。彩色箭头和线条(在SA视图中为虚线，在3D渲染中为实线)表示不同轴位之间的关系。LA，左心房；RV，右心室；RA，右心房。

- From the 3 plane localizer images, reconstruction axes are drawn into short axis (SA), 2 chamber (2CH), 3 chamber (3CH) and 4 chamber (4CH) views.
- Short axis plane is perpendicular to the true long axis of the LV, a line drawn from the center of the mitral valve to the LV apex.
- 2CH or vertical long axis is the vertical plane orthogonal to the short axis plane and is used to assess ventricular function. This plane bisects the anterior and inferior myocardial segments.
- 3CH or LV outflow view is useful for assessing the LVOT, left atrium, mitral valve, aortic valve, anterior septal and posterolateral segments of the LV.
- 4CH or horizontal long axis is perpendicular to the short axis and cuts through the widest part of the RV. This is used for assessing chamber volumes, mitral valve, and tricuspid valve.
- Oblique sagittal plane is parallel to the aorta (candy-cane view).

- 从3个平面的定位图像中，重建轴划定为短轴(SA)、两腔(2CH)、三腔(3CH)和四腔(4CH)视图。
- 短轴平面垂直于左心室真正的长轴，即从二尖瓣中心到左心室尖顶的一条线。
- 2CH或垂直长轴是与短轴平面正交的垂直平面，用于评估心室功能。该平面将心肌前部和下部一分为二。
- 3CH或左心室流出道方位有助于评估左心室流出道、左心房、二尖瓣、主动脉瓣、左心室前间隔和后外侧节段。
- 4CH或水平长轴垂直于短轴，并切分右心室的最宽部分。该轴位用于评估腔室容积、二尖瓣和三尖瓣。
- 斜矢状面平行于主动脉(糖果棒方位)。

Delayed enhancement: ischemic cardiomyopathy

延迟强化：缺血性心肌病

- Delayed enhancement (late gadolinium enhancement, LGE) post infarction will extend from the subendocardium to the epicardium in a vascular distribution.

Subendocardial delayed enhancement

- Since the endocardium is the most susceptible to ischemia, ischemic-type LGE will always involve the subendocardial surface and should have a vascular territory. After remodeling, a chronic infarct will demonstrate LGE.

Circumferential subendocardial delayed enhancement

- 心肌梗死后延迟强化(钆对比剂增强延迟，LGE)可沿血管分布从心内膜下扩展至心外膜。

心内膜下延迟强化

- 心内膜对缺血最敏感，故缺血性病变的LGE总累及心内膜下，且与冠状动脉分布区域相吻合。心肌重构后，慢性梗死灶将表现为LGE。

心内膜下环形延迟强化

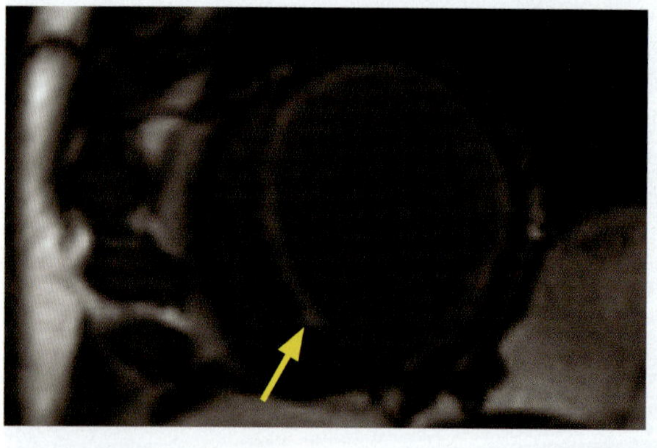

Circumferential subendocardial delayed enhancement due to cocaine abuse with myocardial necrosis:
Delayed contrast-enhanced short-axis cardiac MRI shows diffuse subendocardial LGE (arrow) that involves every segment of the LV. The LV is severely dilated. Chronic microvascular ischemia leads to cell death and myocardial necrosis which progresses to fibrosis that manifests as LGE on imaging.
可卡因(药物滥用)引起的心内膜下环形延迟强化伴心肌坏死：
延迟对比增强短轴心脏MRI显示弥漫性心内膜下LGE(黄箭)，病变累及左心室各段。左心室严重扩张。慢性微血管缺血导致细胞死亡和心肌坏死，进而发展为纤维化，在影像学上表现为LGE。

- Circumferential subendocardial LGE is a rare finding in chronic cocaine users, thought to represent microvascular ischemia from cocaine-induced vasoconstriction. Subepicardial and mesocardial patterns of LGE have also been described.

Transmural delayed enhancement

- 环形心内膜下LGE是慢性可卡因滥用患者中的一种罕见的表现，被认为是代表可卡因诱导的血管收缩导致的微血管缺血。心外膜下及心肌中层LGE也有报道。

透壁性延迟强化

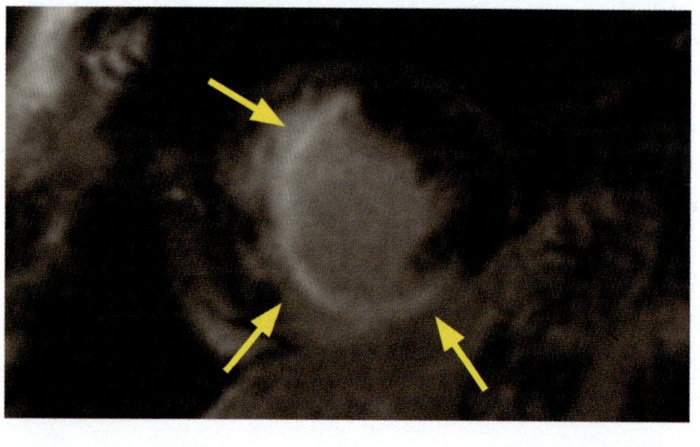

Transmural delayed enhancement due to infarct:
Delayed contrast-enhanced short-axis cardiac MRI shows transmural LGE (arrows) of the inferior wall of the left ventricle, consistent with transmural infarction in the LAD coronary artery territory.
心肌梗死后引起的透壁性延迟强化：
延迟对比增强心脏短轴MRI显示左心室下壁的透壁性LGE(黄箭)，符合左前降支分布区域的透壁性心肌梗死。

- Ischemic-type LGE may involve the endocardium only or may be transmural. Transmural LGE extends across the entire myocardial thickness.
- Transmural LGE represents nonviable scar from prior transmural infarct.
- Cine MR images usually demonstrate hypokinesis in the region of abnormal LGE.

- 缺血性LGE可仅累及心内膜或穿透心肌全层。透壁性强化累及心肌全层。
- 透壁性LGE代表先前透壁性梗死形成的无活性瘢痕组织。
- MR电影图像常显示异常延迟强化区域有心肌运动减弱。

DELAYED ENHANCEMENT: NONISCHEMIC

- Delayed enhancement not following a vascular territory is not due to ischemia. Several distinct patterns of nonischemic delayed enhancement have been described.

Mesocardial delayed enhancement

延迟强化：非缺血性

- 延迟强化不按冠状动脉供血区域分布为非缺血性病变所致。非缺血性延迟强化有几种明显不同的表现方式。

心肌壁间延迟强化

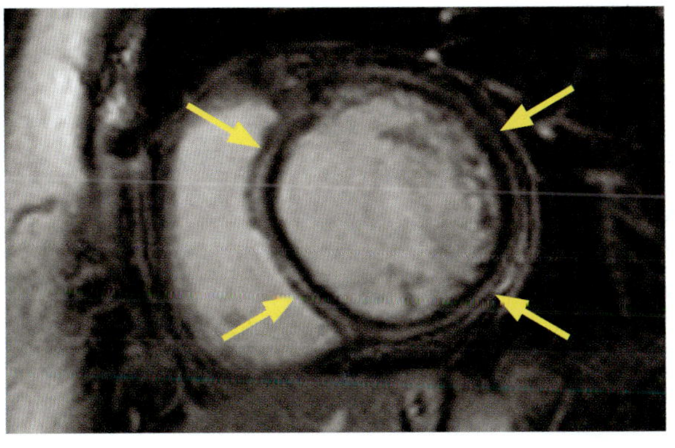

Mesocardial delayed enhancement due to dilated cardiomyopathy:
Delayed contrast-enhanced short-axis cardiac MRI shows diffused mesocardial LGE (arrows), a typical pattern in dilated cardiomyopathy.
扩张型心肌病引起的心肌壁间延迟强化：
延迟对比增强心脏短轴MRI显示弥漫性心肌壁间LGE(黄箭)，为扩张型心肌病的一种典型强化方式。

- **Dilated cardiomyopathy** is described later in the chapter.
- **Sarcoidosis** is a systemic granulomatous disease with cardiac manifestations of arrhythmias, left ventricular dysfunction, and restrictive cardiomyopathy. Cardiac MRI typically shows either mesocardial or subepicardial LGE in a nodular or patchy pattern.
- **Chagas disease** is caused by the protozoan *Trypanosoma cruzi,* and can lead to cardiomyopathy. It is a rare diagnosis that is usually accompanied by travel history from South America, specifically Brazil. On cardiac MRI, there is typically epicardial or mesocardial LGE involving the apex, which can be seen even before the development of symptoms. An apical predilection is a unique feature of Chagas myocarditis.
- **Hypertrophic cardiomyopathy** is described later in the chapter. Cardiac MRI shows mesocardial LGE, particularly at the RV septal attachment sites and in regions of greatest myocardial hypertrophy.

Subepicardial delayed enhancement

- **Myocarditis** is inflammation of the myocardium, which may be secondary to multiple causes. Viral infection is the most common cause of myocarditis, followed by autoimmune disorders and drug toxicity. In addition to subepicardial LGE, cardiac MRI of myocarditis also shows wall motion abnormalities in the affected regions.

- **扩张型心肌病**将在后续章节中讨论。
- **结节病**是一种系统性肉芽肿性疾病，累及心脏时可表现为心律失常、左心功能不全和限制性心肌病。心脏MRI表现通常为心肌壁间或心外膜下结节状或斑片状延迟强化。
- **美洲锥虫病**是由原虫中的克氏锥虫感染所致，可导致心肌病变。该诊断罕见，患者通常伴有南美，尤其是巴西的旅行史。心脏MRI常表现为心尖部外膜或心肌壁间LGE，可出现在症状出现之前。好发于心尖是美洲锥虫病所致心肌炎的一个独特特征。
- **肥厚型心肌病**将在后续章节中讨论。心脏MRI表现为心肌壁间LGE，尤其是位于右心室间隔附着部位和心肌肥厚最严重区域。

心外膜下延迟强化

- **心肌炎**是心肌细胞的炎性病变，可由多种原因引起。病毒感染是心肌炎最常见的原因，其次是自身免疫性疾病和药物中毒。心脏MRI除显示心外膜下延迟强化外，还显示病变区域运动异常。

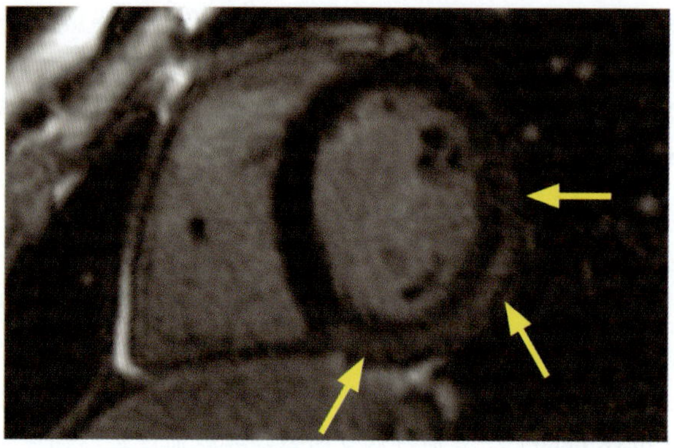

Subepicardial delayed enhancement due to myocarditis:
Delayed contrast-enhanced short-axis cardiac MRI shows subepicardial LGE (arrows) in the inferior left ventricular wall. The LV is mildly dilated.
心肌炎引起的心外膜下延迟强化：
延迟对比增强心脏短轴MRI显示左心室下壁心外膜下LGE（黄箭）。左心室轻度扩张。

- **Sarcoidosis** may cause either mesocardial or subepicardial LGE in a nodular or patchy pattern.

- **结节病**可能会导致心肌壁间或心外膜下结节状或斑片状LGE。

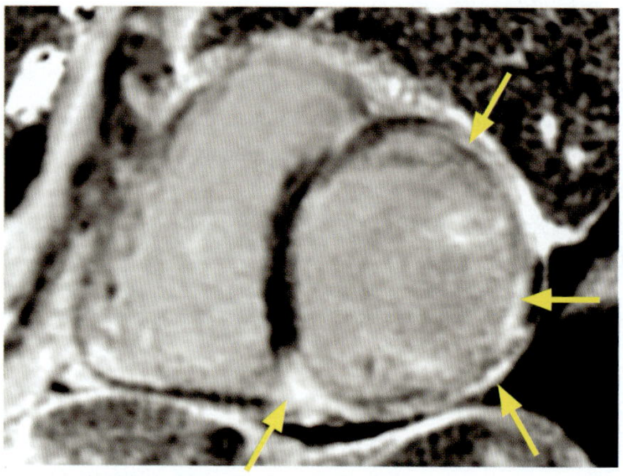

Delayed enhancement due to sarcoidosis:
PSIR cardiac MRI image shows multifocal LGE (arrows) with all patterns due to sarcoidosis.
结节病引起的延迟强化：PSIR心脏MRI显示结节病引起各种模式的LGE（黄箭）。

- **Chagas** disease may cause epicardial or mesocardial LGE.

Circumferential subendocardial delayed enhancement

- **Amyloidosis** is a systemic disorder of glycoprotein deposition throughout the extracellular spaces. In the heart, amyloidosis causes biventricular myocardial thickening, which leads to diffuse ventricular subendocardial LGE.
- **Cardiac transplant** patients may demonstrate circumferential subendocardial LGE, thought to correlate with the presence of myocardial fibrosis pathologically.
- **Hypereosinophilic syndrome** is a systemic disorder characterized by eosinophilic infiltration of multiple organs. Cardiac involvement (Loeffler's endocarditis) leads to endomyocardial fibrosis and subendocardial LGE which can be circumferential. It predominantly affects the cardiac apex and is associated with biventricular thrombi formation.

- **美洲锥虫病**可能会导致心外膜或心肌壁间LGE。

心内膜下环形延迟强化

- **淀粉样变性**是一种糖蛋白异常沉积于细胞外间隙的系统性疾病。淀粉样变性累及心脏时引起双心室心肌增厚而导致弥漫性心内膜下LGE。
- **心脏移植**的患者可以出现心内膜下环形LGE，被认为与病理学上的心肌纤维化相关。
- **嗜酸性粒细胞增多综合征**是一种以嗜酸性粒细胞浸润多器官为特征的全身性疾病。心脏受累（莱夫勒心内膜炎）会导致心内膜纤维化和心内膜下环形LGE。该病主要累及心尖部，并与双心室血栓形成有关。

MRI延迟增强小结

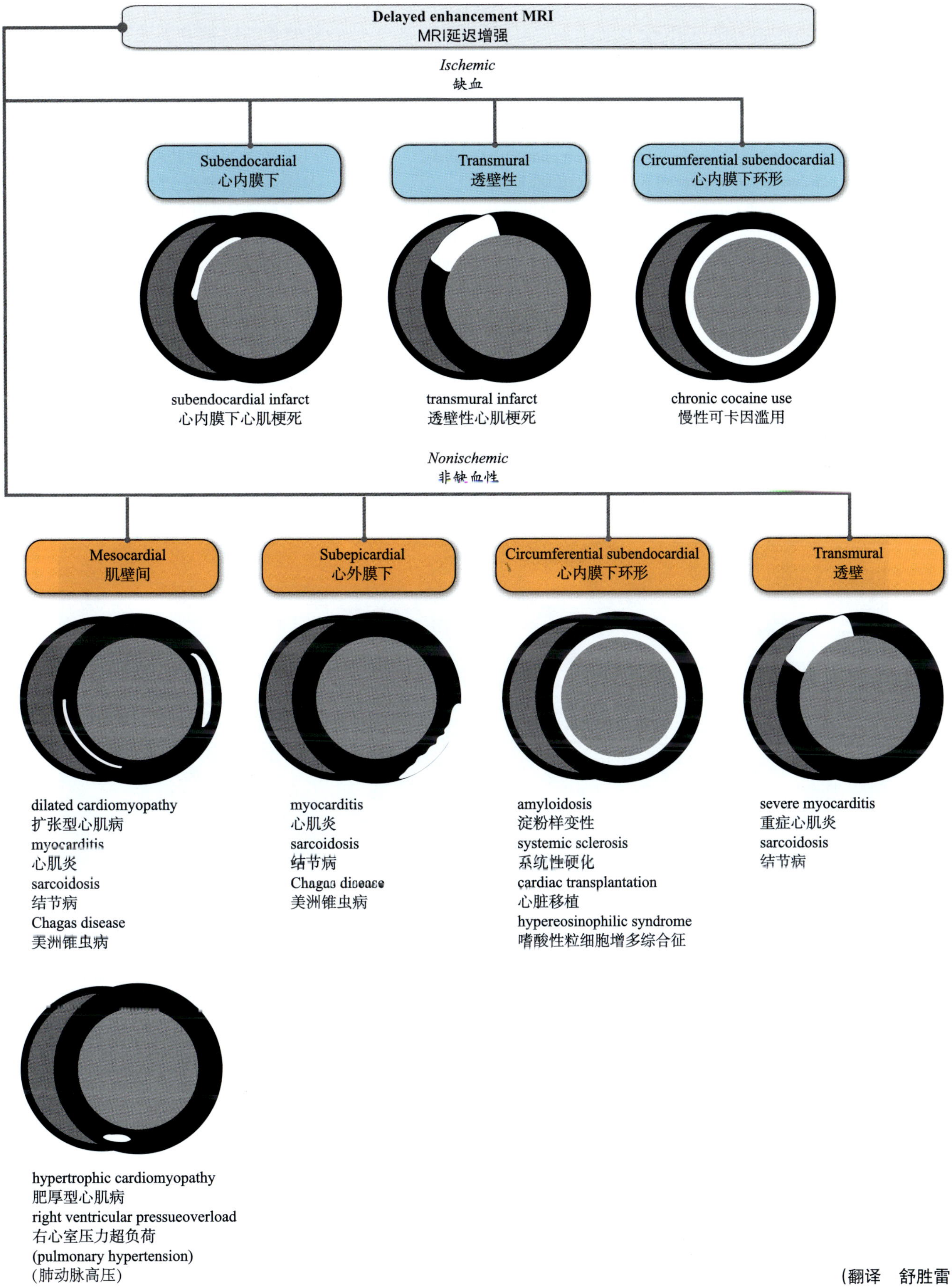

（翻译　舒胜雷）

ISCHEMIC HEART DISEASE

缺血性心脏病

IMAGING OF MYOCARDIAL INFARCTION

心肌梗死的影像学表现

Plain film evaluation of myocardial infarction

- The majority of initial plain chest radiographs obtained in patients with acute myocardial infarction (MI) are normal; however, the most common abnormality seen is increased pulmonary venous pressure (or overt pulmonary edema).

  The presence of pulmonary edema after MI is a poor prognostic indicator.

- The plain chest radiograph can evaluate for some complications of acute MI such as pericardial effusion, left ventricular aneurysm, and papillary muscle rupture. It can also suggest an alternative cause for the patient's acute chest pain, such as pneumothorax or pneumonia.

心肌梗死的X线影像评估

- 大多数急性心肌梗死(MI)患者最初的胸部X线影像属于正常；而最常见的异常是肺静脉压力升高(或明显的肺水肿)。

  MI后出现肺水肿是一个预后不良的指征。

- 胸部X线影像可用于评估急性MI的一些并发症，如心包积液、左心室室壁瘤和乳头肌破裂，也可提示引起急性胸痛的其他原因，如气胸或肺炎。

MR imaging of myocardial infarction

- Similar to stress echocardiography and nuclear scintigraphy (discussed earlier in this chapter), cardiac MRI can be used with pharmacologic stress to evaluate for myocardial ischemia. Cine MRI demonstrates wall motion abnormality or decreased wall thickening in affected coronary artery territory. Stress perfusion MRI demonstrates regional perfusion deficit on first-pass contrast-enhanced images; the subendocardial layer is always involved.

心肌梗死的MRI

- 与负荷超声心电图和核闪烁显像(已在本章的前文讨论)相似，心脏MR可通过药物负荷试验评估心肌缺血。MRI电影显示受累冠状动脉支配区的心肌壁运动异常或心肌壁增厚减弱。负荷灌注MRI表现为在首次通过对比剂增强的影像中受累心肌区域的灌注缺损，心内膜下层总是受累。

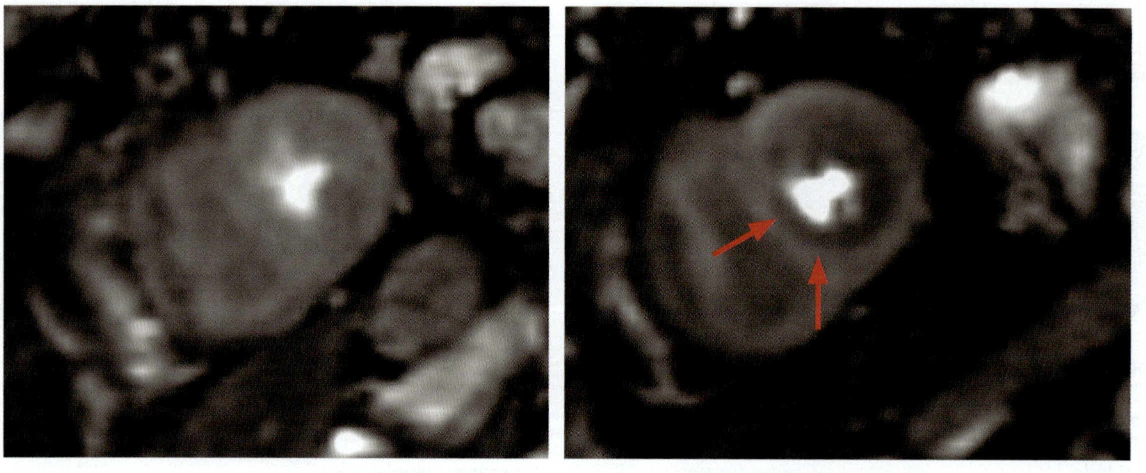

Pharmacologic stress cardiac MRI shows RCA ischemia (left image is rest, right is stress): First-pass cine images show regadenoson-induced first pass myocardial perfusion defect involving the apical inferior and inferoseptal segments (red arrows) in keeping with moderate size ischemia in the right coronary artery territory.

药物负荷试验心脏MRI显示右冠状动脉缺血(左侧影像为静息，右侧为负荷)：首次通过电影影像显示瑞加德松诱导的心尖下和隔下段心肌(红箭)首次通过心肌灌注缺损，符合右冠状动脉分布区域中等面积的缺血。

- Myocardial viability can be assessed by delayed contrast-enhanced MRI. Both acute (necrotic) and chronic (fibrotic) myocardial infarctions show late gadolinium enhancement, while viable myocardium does not.
- Greater than 50% transmural LGE indicates low likelihood of recovery of function after revascularization therapy.
- Myocardial edema in region of acute infarct demonstrates increased T2 signal and is usually larger than the area of LGE (necrotic myocardium). The edematous region without LGE represents myocardium at risk for ischemia.

- 心肌活性可通过延迟增强MRI评估。急性(坏死的)和慢性(纤维化的)心肌梗死均表现为晚期钆增强，而有活性的心肌无此表现。
- 超过50%的心壁出现LGE时提示血管重建治疗后心肌功能恢复的可能性较低。
- 在急性心肌梗死区的心肌水肿表现为T_2信号增高，范围常大于LGE区域(坏死的心肌)。无LGE的水肿区域代表有缺血风险的心肌。

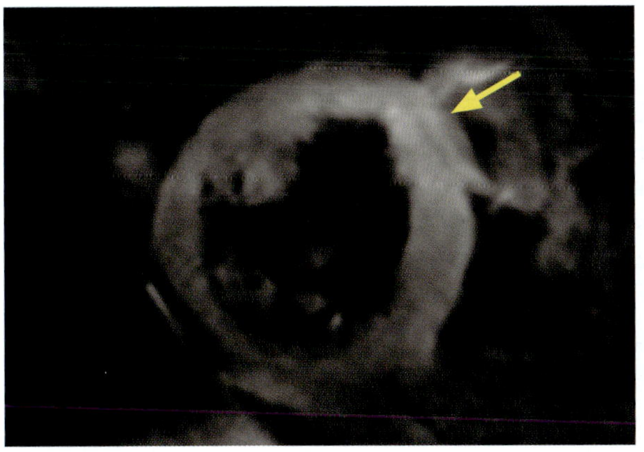

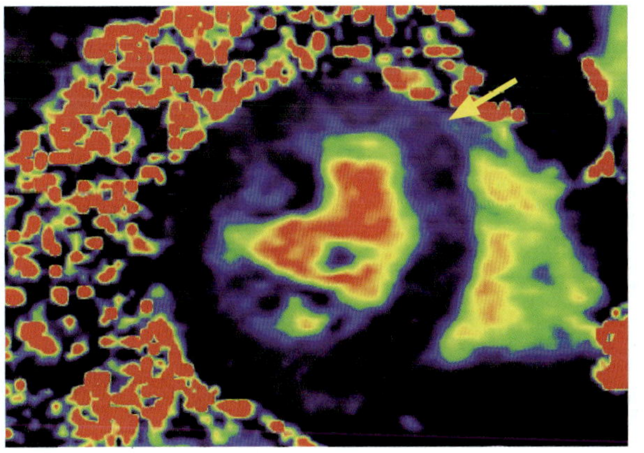

T2-weighted TIR
T_2 加权 TIR

T2 mapping
T_2 映射

Myocardial edema: T2-weighted triple inversion recovery image shows relatively increased T2 hyperintense signal of the anterior and anterolateral segments (arrows) in keeping with edema. This finding is confirmed with T2 mapping color image.
心肌水肿：T_2加权三倍翻转恢复影像显示前及前外侧段心肌T_2信号相对增高(黄箭)，符合心肌水肿改变。这个发现在T_2映射彩色图像上得以印证。

- Acute infarct with **microvascular obstruction** appears on delayed contrast-enhanced MRI as areas of hypoenhancement within an enhancing infarct zone. Microvascular obstruction is usually seen following reperfusion therapy after prolonged myocardial ischemia. It is a strong poor prognostic indicator and is associated with more severe LV remodeling.

- 急性心肌梗死合并**微血管阻塞**在延迟增强的MRI上表现为强化的梗死区域内的弱强化区。微血管阻塞常发生于长时间缺血的心肌经再灌注治疗后，是一个预后不佳的强力指标，也与更严重的左心室重塑相关。

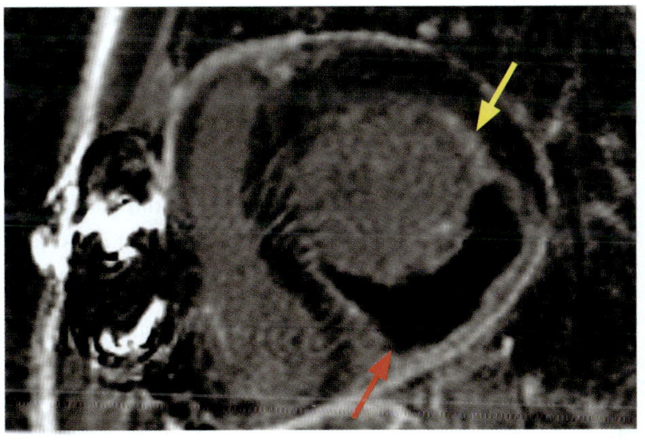

Microvascular obstruction in the setting of acute infarct:
There is diffuse subendocardial late gadolinium enhancement (LGE) involving the anterior and anterolateral walls, consistent with non-transmural myocardial infarction with microvascular obstruction (yellow arrow). There is also a large central dark zone (red arrow) with surrounding edema consistent with intramyocardial hemorrhage involving the inferior and inferolateral walls of the LV, from large recent infarct in LCx territory.
急性心肌梗死后的微血管阻塞：
前壁及前外侧壁弥漫性心内膜下LGE，符合非透壁性心肌梗死伴微血管阻塞(黄箭)。还可见大的中央暗区(红箭)周围绕以水肿带，与近期左回旋支支配区大面积心肌梗死引起的左心室下壁及下外侧壁心肌内出血相符。

CT imaging of myocardial infarction

- Conventional CT is not routinely performed for evaluation of MI or its complications, although these findings may be incidentally seen.
- Acute myocardial ischemia appears on contrast-enhanced CT as wall hypoattenuation in a coronary artery distribution, progressing from the subendocardial layer to transmural. Subsequent myocyte death leads to decreased wall thickness. Myocardial scar from a prior MI can present as dense irregular myocardial calcification or thin, fatty-replaced myocardium, again in a coronary artery distribution.

心肌梗死的CT影像

- 普通CT不常规用于评价心肌梗死或其并发症，尽管偶尔可见到此类表现。
- 急性心肌缺血在增强CT上表现为冠状动脉分布区域心肌壁的弱强化，从心内膜下层至透壁逐渐进展，心肌细胞的死亡导致心肌壁变薄。先前心肌梗死后的心肌瘢痕可表现为冠状动脉分布区致密而不规则的心肌钙化，或心肌变薄、被脂肪替代。

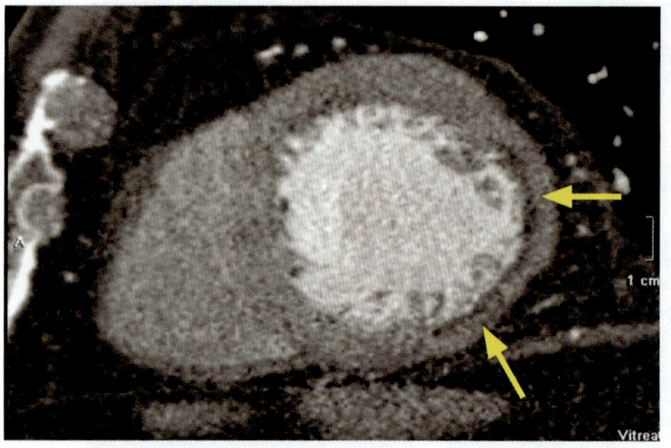

Myocardial infarction on CT: reformatted CT angiogram short-axis view shows thinned anterolateral LV wall with curvilinear hypodense signal along the endometrium (arrows) in keeping with fatty metaplasia from prior infarct.
心肌梗死的CT表现：CT血管造影短轴位重建显示左心室前外侧壁变薄，伴有沿着内膜（黄箭）的弧线状低密度影，与先前梗死后的脂肪化生相符。

- New advances in CT have allowed functional myocardial imaging, including stress and rest CT perfusion and myocardial delayed enhancement CT, similar to cardiac MRI.

- 新近的CT进展可以对心肌进行功能成像，包括负荷和静息CT灌注及心肌延迟增强，与心脏MRI相似。

Complications of myocardial infarction

心肌梗死的并发症

- Acute complications of MI include cardiogenic shock, pulmonary edema, arrhythmia, mural thrombus, papillary muscle rupture, ventricular septal rupture, cardiac free-wall rupture, and pericarditis.
- Chronic complications of MI include heart failure, left ventricular aneurysm or pseudoaneurysm, and mural thrombus.

- 心肌梗死的急性并发症包括心源性休克、肺水肿、心律失常、附壁血栓、乳头肌破裂、心室间隔破裂、心脏游离壁破裂，以及心包炎。
- 心肌梗死的慢性并发症包括心力衰竭、左心室室壁瘤或假性室壁瘤，以及附壁血栓。

Papillary muscle rupture

乳头肌破裂

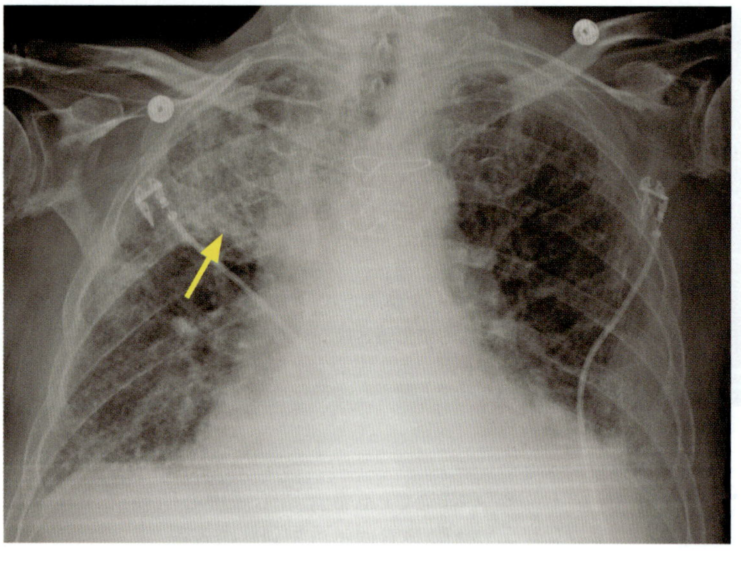

Frontal chest radiograph demonstrates asymmetric pulmonary edema in the right upper lobe (arrow) in this patient with known severe mitral regurgitation from recent myocardial infarction. Left pleural effusion and mild cardiomegaly are also present.
胸部正位X线影像显示右上肺（黄箭）非对称性肺水肿，此患者有已知的近期心肌梗死导致严重二尖瓣反流病史，还可见左侧胸腔积液及轻度心脏增大。

- Papillary muscle rupture due to MI typically produces acute pulmonary edema. A classic radiographic finding is isolated right upper lobe pulmonary edema due to acute mitral regurgitation resulting from papillary muscle rupture.

- 继发于心肌梗死的乳头肌断裂会导致急性肺水肿。典型的X线表现是右肺上叶孤立性肺水肿，为乳头肌破裂引起的急性二尖瓣反流所致。

True left ventricular (LV) aneurysm

- A true ventricular aneurysm is a focal outpouching affecting all layers of the muscular wall.
- True LV aneurysms are associated with occlusion of the LAD. The most common location is along the anterolateral or apical wall of the left ventricle.
- Plain film findings include an abnormal contour along the midportion of the left cardiac border near the apex. CT or MRI shows wall thinning, possible calcification, and a wide neck between the ventricular lumen and the aneurysm.

左心室（LV）真性室壁瘤

- 心室真性室壁瘤是室壁局部向外膨隆，累及所有肌层。
- 左心室（LV）真性室壁瘤常与左前降支闭塞有关，最常见部位是左心室的前外侧壁或心尖部。
- X线影像表现为左心缘中部近心尖处轮廓异常。CT或MRI显示心肌壁变薄，可能有钙化，以及在心室腔和室壁瘤之间形成宽颈。

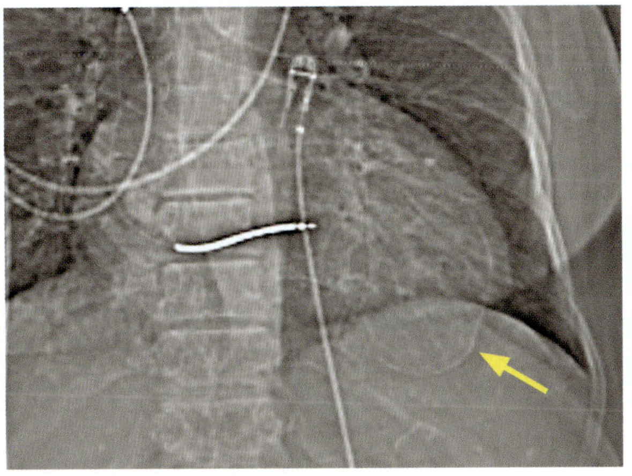

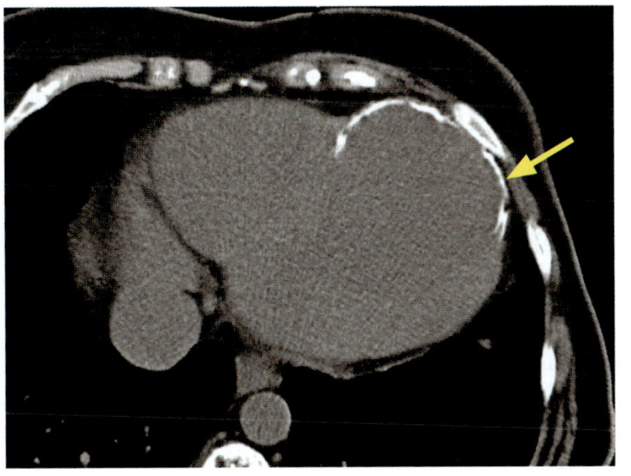

Calcified LV aneurysm: Frontal radiograph shows thin curvilinear density along the border of the LV (arrow), corresponding to calcified LV aneurysm as sequelae of prior myocardial infarction.
钙化的LV室壁瘤：胸部正位X线影像显示沿左心室边缘分布的弧线形细高密度影(黄箭)，符合先前心肌梗死所致的左心室室壁瘤钙化。

- True ventricular aneurysms are associated with wall motion dyskinesia but they rarely rupture. Management is medical.
- A mural thrombus may form over time due to slow flow within the aneurysm.

- 心室真性室壁瘤与室壁运动障碍相关，但罕见有破裂。治疗为内科保守疗法。
- 心室室壁瘤内可能因为血流变慢而形成附壁血栓。

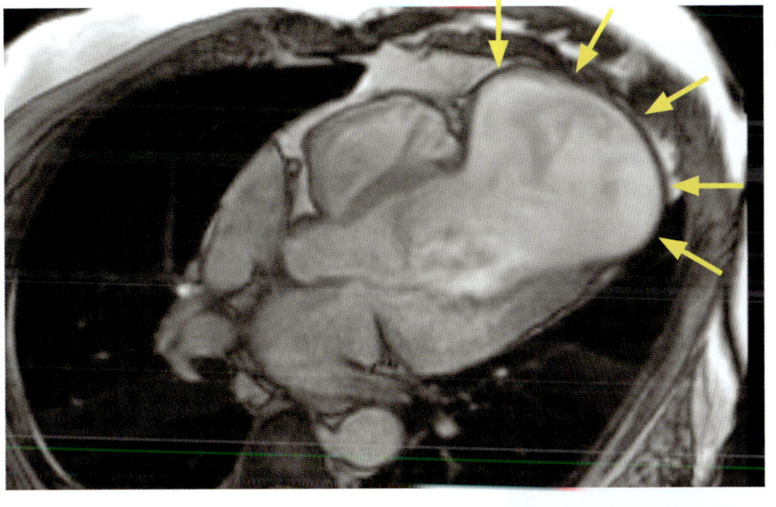

LV aneurysm: 4 chamber bright-blood imaging demonstrates ballooning of the LV apex (arrows) and thinning of the anterior LV wall in keeping with true aneurysm.
LV室壁瘤：四腔心亮血序列影像显示左心室尖膨大(黄箭)，左心室前壁变薄，符合真性室壁瘤表现。

Pseudoaneurysm

- A cardiac pseudoaneurysm is a contained ventricular rupture, with only pericardial adhesions preventing a complete rupture. There is no myocardium in the wall of a pseudoaneurysm.
- Pseudoaneurysms are associated with occlusion of the circumflex or right coronary arteries and most commonly occur along the inferior, inferolateral or posterior wall of the LV.
- Plain film findings suggestive of a LV pseudoaneurysm include a retrocardiac density seen on the frontal view and an abnormal posterior contour on the lateral radiograph. CT or MRI shows a narrow aneurysmal neck. The affected region is akinetic and the overlying pericardium often demonstrates LGE on MRI.
- Ventricular pseudoaneurysms may rupture. An increase in size over sequential films is especially worrisome for impending rupture. Treatment of a pseudoaneurysm is surgical.

假性室壁瘤

- 心脏假性室壁瘤是指包裹性心室破裂，仅有心包粘连免于完全破裂。假性室壁瘤的瘤壁上无心肌成分。
- 假性室壁瘤与回旋支或右冠状动脉闭塞有关，最常见于左心室的下壁、下外侧壁或后壁。
- X线影像提示假性室壁瘤的征象包括正位片上心后密度增高影，侧位片上心脏后缘轮廓异常。CT或MRI显示瘤颈较窄。受累的区域无运动，且MRI上表面的心包呈心肌延迟强化(LGE)。
- 假性室壁瘤可发生破裂。连续影像随访发现室壁瘤体积增大时，尤其要警惕先兆破裂。假性室壁瘤需要进行外科手术。

Dressler syndrome

- Dressler syndrome is a subacute immune-mediated pericarditis which often occurs 2–6 weeks following MI. It is manifests as pericardial and pleural effusions.

心肌梗死后综合征

- 心肌梗死后综合征是一种亚急性免疫介导的心包炎，常发生于心肌梗死后2~6周，表现为心包积液和胸腔积液。

（翻译　孙欣）

NON-ISCHEMIC MYOCARDIAL DISEASE

非缺血性心肌病

Catecholamine induced (Takotsubo) cardiomyopathy

- Catecholamine induced cardiomyopathy, also known as takotsubo cardiomyopathy and broken heart syndrome, can clinically mimic acute myocardial infarction.
- Typically affecting older women in the setting of acute emotional stress, catecholamine-induced cardiomyopathy can present with chest pain, abnormal ECG, and elevation of cardiac enzymes. Cardiac catheterization is normal.

  One theory is that men may suffer catecholamine-induced cardiomyopathy as well but typically don't survive. There may be a protective effect of estrogen.
- Catecholamine-induced cardiomyopathy is typically self-limited.
- On cardiac MRI or coronary CT, there is a characteristic ballooning of the cardiac apex. The shape of the heart is similar to a Japanese octopus pot, hence the name *takotsubo*. There is no abnormal delayed enhancement on MRI.

儿茶酚胺诱发性(Takotsubo)心肌病

- 儿茶酚胺诱发性心肌病又称Takotsubo心肌病、心碎综合征，临床表现可类似急性心肌梗死。
- 儿茶酚胺诱发性心肌病通常见于急性情绪紧张的老年女性，可表现为胸痛、心电图异常及心肌酶升高。心导管检查正常。

  一种理论认为男性也可能患儿茶酚胺诱发性心肌病，但通常不能存活。雌激素可能有保护作用。
- 儿茶酚胺诱发性心肌病通常为自限性。
- 心脏MRI或冠状动脉CT上，心尖部呈特征性气球样膨大。心脏形状像“日本章鱼篓”，因此称“Takotsubo”。MRI上无异常延迟强化。

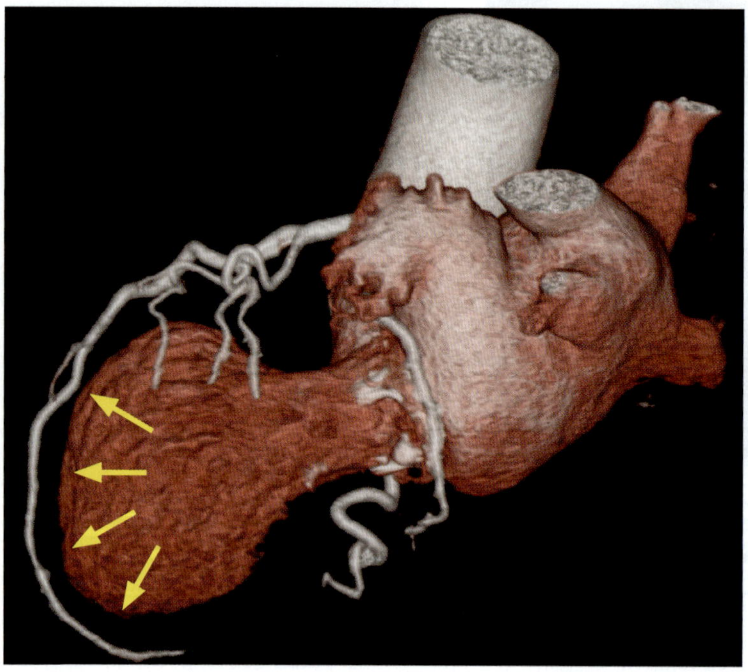

3D volume rendered image from a cardiac CT (with the myocardium removed) demonstrates marked ballooning of the left ventricular apex (arrows). The coronary arteries are normal.

心脏CT 3D立体容积再现(去除心肌)显示左心室心尖部呈明显气球样扩张(黄箭)。冠状动脉正常。

Arrhythmogenic cardiomyopathy

致心律失常性心肌病

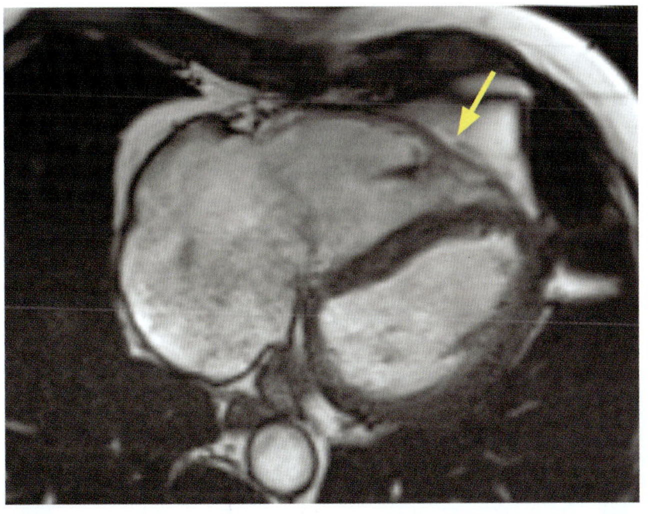

ARVD: Cardiac MRI shows regional RV akinesis most pronounced in the mid-free wall (arrow). There is dyssynchronous RV contraction between the base and apex. RV ejection fraction in this case was 31%, meeting major criteria for ARVD. Note severe right atrial enlargement.

ARVD：心脏MRI显示右心室壁局部运动消失，以游离壁中部(黄箭)最明显。右心室底部与心尖之间非同步收缩。本例右心室射血分数为31%，符合ARVD的主要标准。没有严重的右心房增大。

- Arrhythmogenic cardiomyopathy (previously called arrhythmogenic right ventricular dysplasia, as it was thought to only affect the right ventricle) represents fibrofatty replacement of ventricular myocytes, causing focal contraction abnormalities and/or aneurysm formation.
- Diagnosis is usually difficult and depends on major and minor criteria from ECG, imaging, biopsy findings, and family history, as determined by the 2010 International Task Force consensus. Imaging plays a supportive role in the diagnosis. Imaging findings may contribute one major and one minor criteria based on the presence of right ventricular dyskinesia or akinesia and either an increased RV volume or reduced RV ejection fraction. The presence of myocardial fat is no longer in the criteria as fat can be seen in normal individuals with aging.
- Left ventricular involvement can be seen in up to 3/4 of patients.
- Patients may suffer lethal arrhythmias and therefore require ICD placement once diagnosis is confirmed.

- 致心律失常性心肌病(旧称“致心律失常性右心室发育不良”，此病曾被认为只影响右心室)是指心室肌细胞被纤维脂肪所替代，从而引起局限性收缩异常和/或室壁瘤形成。
- 诊断通常困难，按照2010年工作组指南，需根据心电图、影像学、活检结果及家族史分为主要和次要诊断标准。影像学对诊断起辅助作用。影像学表现可以根据右心室运动障碍或消失与否，以及右心室体积增大或射血分数降低而提供一个主要标准和一个次要标准。心肌脂肪不再列入诊断标准，因为随着年龄增长，脂肪也可出现在正常人群。
- 左心室受累见于高达3/4的患者。
- 一旦确诊患者出现致死性心律失常，需要植入ICD。

Myocardial noncompaction

心肌致密化不全

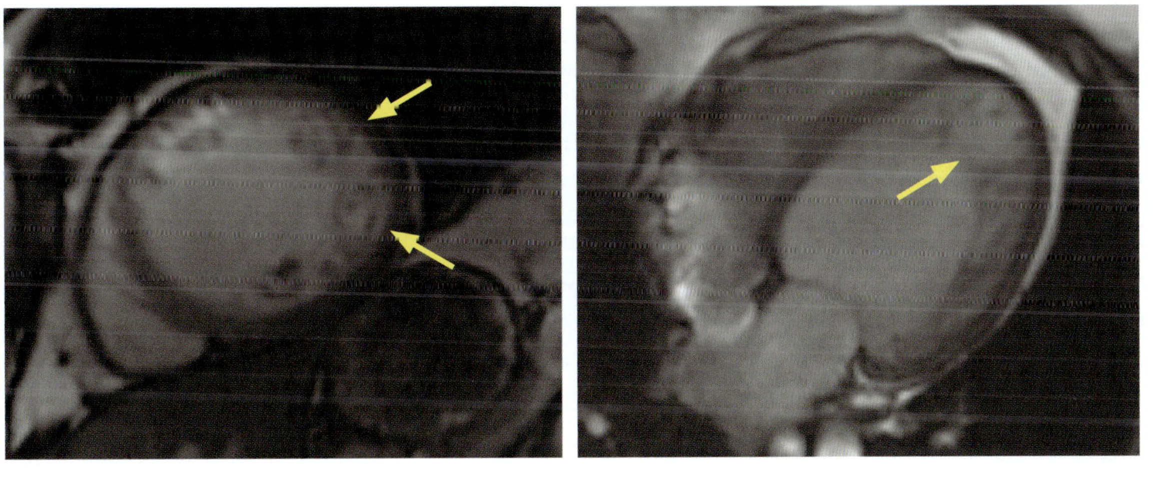

Myocardial noncompaction: Short-axis and axial cine images show hypertrabeculated noncompacted myocardium (arrows) in the left ventricle with noncompaction-to-compaction ratio greater than 2.3.

心肌致密化不全：短轴位、长轴位图像显示左心室过度小梁化的非致密化心肌(黄箭)，非致密/致密之比>2.3。

- Myocardial noncompaction is a developmental defect in embryologic formation of the left ventricle, due to failure of part of the left ventricle to form a solid myocardium.
- On imaging, the left ventricle appears as heavily trabeculated as the right ventricle with a relatively thin left ventricular wall. A noncompacted to compacted myocardium ratio ≥2.3 at end diastole is a proposed criteria that is highly sensitive but not specific.
- Patients with noncompaction have an increased risk of adverse cardiac events, including arrhythmias, thrombus formation, stroke, and cardiomyopathy.

- 心肌致密化不全是胚胎形成期左心室发育缺陷，为部分左心室不能形成致密化心肌所致。
- 影像学上，左心室表现为与右心室类似的过度小梁化及室壁变薄。建议采用的标准为舒张末期非致密化心肌与致密化心肌比例≥2.3，其灵敏度高但特异度不佳。
- 心肌致密化不全患者有增加心脏不良事件发生率的风险，包括心律失常、血栓形成、卒中及心肌病。

Hypertrophic cardiomyopathy (HCM)

肥厚型心肌病(HCM)

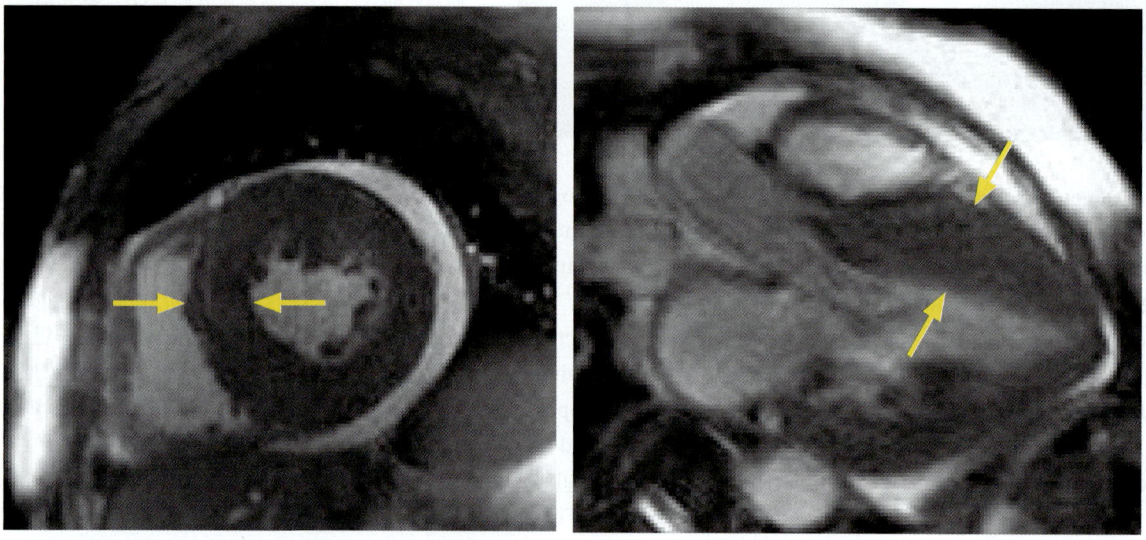

Hypertrophic cardiomyopathy: Short-axis (left image) steady-state free precession MRI shows concentric hypertrophy of the left ventricular myocardium (yellow arrows), without chamber enlargement. A small pericardial effusion is present. Three-chamber view (right image) from the same study better shows the septal predominance of the ventricular hypertrophy (arrows).
Case courtesy Michael Hanley, MD, University of Virginia Health System.
肥厚型心肌病：短轴位(左图)稳态自由进动MRI显示左心室心肌向心性肥大(黄箭)，但心腔不大。有少量心包积液。同一名患者三腔心(右图)较好地显示了心室肥厚以室间隔为主(黄箭)

- Hypertrophic cardiomyopathy (HCM) is an autosomal dominant cardiomyopathy, characterized by left ventricular myocardial thickening (diffuse or focal) without dilation. HCM is the most common cardiomyopathy.
- Cardiac MRI may show patchy mid-myocardial LGE in regions of hypertrophied myocardium and at the junctions of the interventricular septum and the right ventricular free wall, due to myofibril disarray. Evaluation of the cine images will show reduced diastolic filling of the left ventricle.
- The asymmetric septal hypertrophy variant, known as **idiopathic hypertrophic subaortic stenosis (IHSS)**, may cause left ventricular outflow tract obstruction. Diagnostic criteria include an end-diastolic wall thickness of ≥15 mm and a ratio of ≥1.5 compared to the lateral wall. A wall thickness ≥30 mm is an indication for ICD placement.
- The **apical HCM** variant is more commonly seen in Asians and has the classic imaging appearance of a "spade-shaped" left ventricle.
- **Systolic anterior motion (SAM)** of the anterior leaflet of the mitral valve is an associated finding that can cause mitral regurgitation and resultant left atrial enlargement.

- 肥厚型心肌病(HCM)是一种常染色体显性遗传心肌病，特征是左心室心肌增厚(弥漫性或局限性)而无心腔扩张。HCM是最常见的心肌病。
- 心脏MRI可表现为肥厚的心肌、室间隔的接合部及右心室游离壁呈斑片状中度心肌LGE，为心肌纤维紊乱所致。电影图像评估将显示左心室舒张充盈减少。
- 室间隔不对称性肥厚变异，亦称**特发性肥厚性主动脉下狭窄(IHSS)**，可能会引起左心室流出道梗阻。诊断标准包括舒张末期室壁厚度≥15mm且与外侧壁厚度比值≥1.5。室壁厚度≥30mm是ICD植入的指征。
- **心尖型HCM变异**在亚洲人群更常见，且有经典的"铁铲状"左心室的经典影像学表现。
- 二尖瓣前叶的**收缩期前向运动**(SAM)是一个伴随征象，可引起二尖瓣反流，并导致左心房扩大。

- Although diagnosis is usually made by echocardiography, indications for MRI are to confirm the diagnosis of HCM, to measure the left ventricular mass, and to quantify the degree of subvalvular stenosis.

- 通常采用超声心动图进行诊断，但使用MRI确诊HCM、测量左心室质量、量化瓣膜下狭窄程度。

Restrictive cardiomyopathy

限制型心肌病

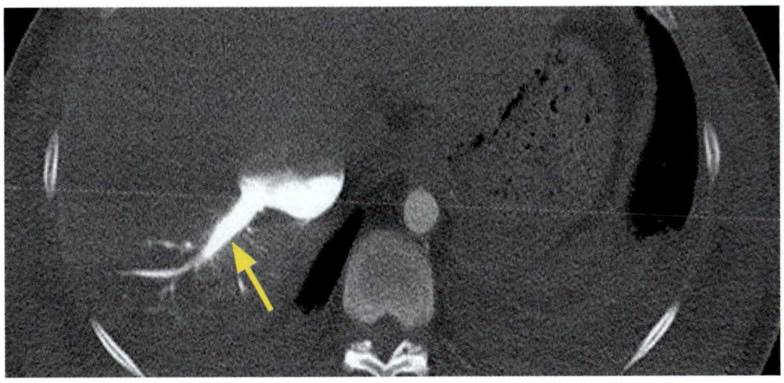

Impaired diastolic filling: Contrast-enhanced CT demonstrates dilation and reflux of contrast into the IVC and hepatic veins (arrow), indicative of impaired right ventricular filling and resultant dilation of the right atrium, IVC, and hepatic veins.
Case courtesy Michael Hanley, MD, University of Virginia Health System.
舒张期充盈受损：增强CT显示造影剂反流至扩张的下腔静脉(IVC)、肝静脉(黄箭)，提示右心室充盈受限，导致右心房、下腔静脉及肝静脉扩张。

- Restrictive cardiomyopathy is characterized by small, stiff, thickened ventricles that impair diastolic filling. This results in dilated atria and ultimately a dilated IVC. The etiology of the restrictive cardiomyopathy may be idiopathic or due to sarcoidosis, hemochromatosis, hypereosinophilic syndrome (e.g., Loeffler's endocarditis), or myocardial deposition diseases (e.g., amyloidosis).
- Note that restrictive cardiomyopathy and constrictive physiology are different entities, although both conditions may feature identical ventricular pressure tracings and both are characterized by impaired diastolic filling.
- Constrictive physiology (subsequently discussed under pericardial disease) is secondary to increased pericardial pressure from thickened (often calcified) pericardium or pericardial effusion, causing impaired diastolic filling.
- The main role of imaging the heart in impaired diastolic filling is to exclude constrictive pericarditis as the etiology of the diastolic dysfunction. Constrictive pericarditis can be treated surgically by removing the pericardium; however, there is no effective treatment for restrictive cardiomyopathy and patients tend to have a poor prognosis.

- 限制型心肌病的特征是心室小而僵硬且增厚，导致舒张期充盈受限。其结果为心房扩大，最终引起下腔静脉扩张。限制型心肌病的病因可以为特发性，或由结节病、血色素沉着病、嗜酸细胞增多综合征(如莱夫勒心内膜炎)或心肌沉积病(如淀粉样变性)引起。
- 值得注意的是，限制型心肌病和缩窄性心包炎是两种完全不同的疾病，虽然两者都以心室压力增高及舒张期充盈受限为特征。
- 限制性的生理学改变(在后文心包疾病中讨论)是继发于心包增厚(通常是钙化)或心包积液所致的心包压力增加，引起舒张期充盈受限。
- 在舒张充盈受限中，影像学检查的主要作用是排除缩窄性心包炎所致的舒张功能障碍。缩窄性心包炎可以通过外科切除心包进行治疗，但限制型心肌病缺乏有效的治疗方法，且往往预后不佳。

Dilated cardiomyopathy (DCM)

- Dilated cardiomyopathy (DCM) is characterized by diffuse cardiac chamber enlargement with impaired systolic function. Typically, both ventricles are involved.
- DCM can be ischemic or nonischemic in etiology. It is the most common nonischemic cardiomyopathy, often idiopathic, with other causes including alcohol abuse, myocarditis, or drug toxicity. Evaluation by MRI or CT is useful to determine the etiology.

扩张型心肌病(DCM)

- 扩张型心肌病(DCM)的特点是弥漫性心腔扩大伴收缩功能受损。通常双侧心室受累。
- DCM在病因学上可分为缺血性或非缺血性，是最常见的非缺血性心肌病，常为特发性，其他原因包括酗酒、心肌炎或药物毒性等。MRI及CT检查有助于明确病因。

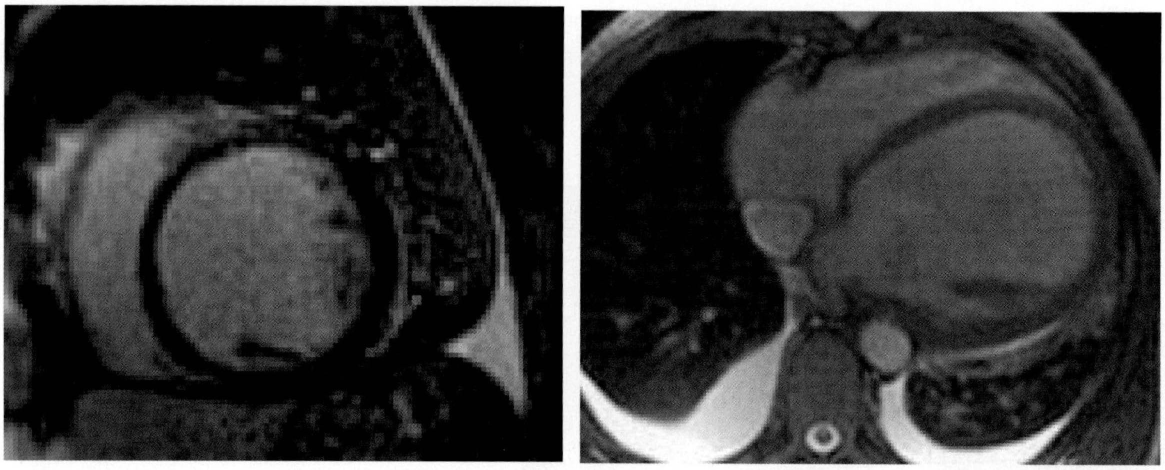

Nonischemic dilated cardiomyopathy: Delayed-enhancement short-axis cardiac MRI (left image) shows no abnormal enhancement, but there is diffuse concentric dilation of the left ventricular and right ventricular cavities, which is also appreciated on the axial image (right image). Bilateral small pleural effusions are present.

Case courtesy Michael Hanley, MD, University of Virginia Health System.

非缺血性扩张型心肌病：延迟增强心脏短轴MRI(左图)显示无异常强化，但轴位图像上，左、右心室腔表现为弥漫性扩大的同心圆(右图)。两侧胸腔少量积液。

- An ischemic cause can be suggested by delayed enhancement in a vascular distribution on MRI or coronary artery disease seen on CCTA.
- Up to 41% of patients with idiopathic DCM demonstrate abnormal mesocardial LGE in a nonischemic distribution in the mid-ventricular wall. The significance of this enhancement in these patients is uncertain.
- Catheter angiography is recommended to exclude coronary artery disease in a new diagnosis of dilated cardiomyopathy.

- 缺血性病变的原因可以通过MRI延迟增强的血管分布或CCTA所见的冠状动脉疾病得到提示。
- 高达41%的有特发性DCM的患者表现为中部室壁不正常的心肌缺血，在中部心室壁的非缺血性分布区可见LGE。此种强化方式意义尚不明确。
- 建议对初诊扩张型心肌病的患者进行经导管冠状动脉造影以排除冠状动脉疾病。

(翻译　杨宏远)

VALVULAR DISEASE

Endocarditis

- Endocarditis is infection of the cardiac valves. Risk factors for development of endocarditis include intravenous drug abuse, poor dental hygiene, diabetes, and prosthetic valves.
- Valvular vegetations are usually diagnosed by echocardiography, although CT angiography is routinely able to depict vegetations >1 cm in diameter. CT can also evaluate for the presence of a perivalvular abscess and assess for extracardiac complications of endocarditis, such as septic pulmonary emboli.

Bicuspid aortic valve (BAV)

- Bicuspid aortic valve (BAV) is the most common congential cardiovascular abnormality.
- Acquired BAV occurs when fusion of two cusps of a trileaflet valve results in a functional bicuspid valve, often due to leaflet calcification or rheumatic heart disease.
- BAV is classified into three types depending on the number of raphes present. A raphe is defined as the fusion point between two adjacent rudimentary coronary cusps.

心脏瓣膜疾病

心内膜炎

- 心内膜炎是指心脏瓣膜发生了感染。心内膜炎的诱发因素包括药物滥用(静脉注射)、口腔不洁、糖尿病和人工心脏瓣膜。
- 瓣膜赘生物通常用超声心动图进行诊断，但CT血管造影在正常情况下也能够检测出直径>1cm的赘生物。CT也可评估瓣膜周围脓肿和心内膜炎的心外并发症，如肺部的脓性栓子。

二瓣化主动脉瓣(BAV)

- 二瓣化主动脉瓣(BAV)是最常见的先天性心血管异常。
- 获得性BAV见于三尖瓣的两个瓣叶融合成一个功能性的二瓣叶，常见的病因为瓣叶钙化或风湿性心脏病。
- BAV可根据出现的融合嵴数量分为三种类型。融合嵴的定义为相邻两个原始冠状动脉瓣尖之间的融合点。

Number of raphes: 0 (type 0), 1 (type 1), 2 (type 2)

- Images of the BAV have a characteristic *fishmouth* appearance.
- BAV predisposes to early onset degenerative aortic stenosis, aortic regurgitation, and infective endocarditis.
- Other abnormalities associated with BAV include aortic coarctation, supravalvular stenosis, ascending aortic aneurysm, aortopathy leading to aortic dissection, patent ductus arteriosus, Turner syndrome, and coronary artery anomalies.

融合嵴数量：0(0型)、1(1型)、2(2型)。

- BAV的影像特征是鱼样嘴。
- BAV易导致早发退行性主动脉瓣狭窄、主动脉瓣反流和感染性心内膜炎。
- 与BAV相关的其他疾病包括主动脉缩窄、主动脉瓣上狭窄、升主动脉瘤、导致主动脉夹层的主动脉病变、动脉导管未闭、特纳综合征和冠状动脉异常。

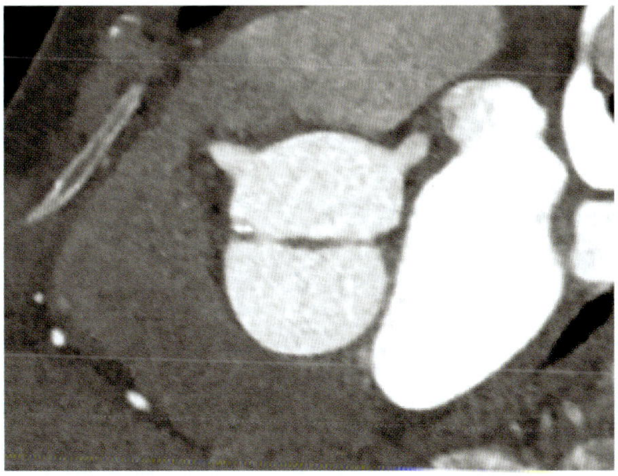

Sievers type 0
SIEVERS 0型

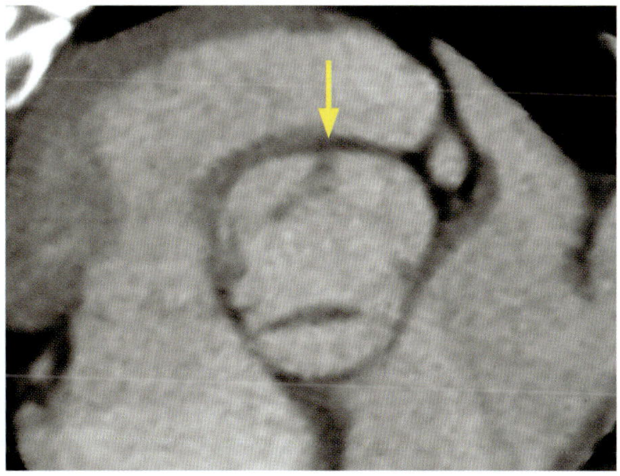

Sievers type 1
SIEVERS 1型

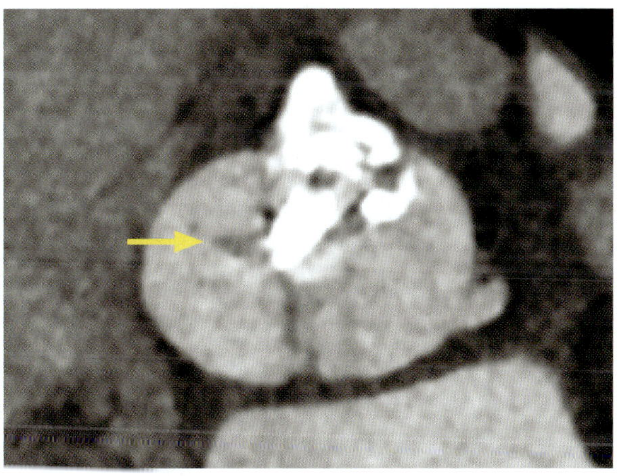

Sievers type 2
SIEVERS 2型

Bicuspid aortic valve on CT angiography: CT images are oriented with the left main coronary artery ostium on the right and RCA ostium on the left side of the image.

BAV type 0: no raphe

BAV type 1: raphe between the right coronary cusp and the left coronary cusp (arrow)

BAV type 2: raphe between the right coronary cusp and the non-coronary cusp (arrow)

二瓣化主动脉瓣在CT血管造影上的表现：CT影像显示左冠状动脉的开口位于图像的右侧，右冠状动脉的开口位于图像的左侧。

BAV 0型：无融合嵴。

BAV 1型：融合嵴在左、右冠状动脉瓣尖之间(黄箭)。

BAV 2型：融合嵴在右冠状动脉瓣尖和非冠状动脉瓣尖之间(黄箭)。

Aortic stenosis

- **Valvular** aortic stenosis is most commonly caused by congenital bicuspid aortic valve, age-associated degeneration, or rheumatic heart disease.
- **Subvalvular** aortic stenosis can occur due to obstruction by a fibrous membrane beneath the aortic cusps, fibromuscular ring or narrowing of the LV outlet, redundant mitral valve tissue, or hypertrophic cardiomyopathy.
- **Supravalvular** aortic stenosis is rare and occurs either as an isolated congenital anomaly or associated with Williams syndrome.
- Aortic stenosis causes left ventricular hypertrophy; however, the heart size does not change.
- The ascending aorta is usually enlarged in long-standing valvular aortic stenosis.
- Pulmonary vascularity is typically normal.

主动脉瓣狭窄

- 主动脉瓣狭窄最常见的病因是先天性二叶主动脉瓣、与年龄相关的退行性变或风湿性心脏病。
- 主动脉**下瓣**狭窄可见于主动脉尖下方的纤维膜所致的梗阻、纤维肌环或左心室流出道狭窄、二尖瓣组织冗余或肥厚型心肌病。
- 主动脉**上瓣**狭窄罕见，可为一种独立的先天性异常，或与Williams综合征相关。
- 主动脉瓣狭窄导致左心室肥厚，但心脏大小不变。
- 长期主动脉瓣狭窄通常会导致升主动脉扩张。
- 肺血管一般正常。

- Normal aortic valve has an orifice area >2 cm^2. A valvular area <1 cm^2 and pressure gradient>40 mmHg define severe aortic stenosis.

- 正常主动脉瓣瓣口面积>2cm^2。一个主动脉瓣的面积<1cm^2，且压力梯度>40mmHg时，被定义为重度主动脉瓣狭窄。

Aortic regurgitation

- Aortic regurgitation can result from abnormality of the aortic valve, aortic annulus, or ascending aorta.
- Long-standing aortic regurgitation causes left ventricular enlargement, which is apparent on radiographs as cardiomegaly. There is typically enlargement of the ascending aorta.
- Similar to aortic stenosis, the pulmonary vasculature is typically normal.

主动脉瓣反流

- 主动脉瓣反流可由主动脉瓣、主动脉瓣环或升主动脉异常导致。
- 长期主动脉瓣反流导致左心室增大，在X线影像上表现为心影增大。升主动脉通常有扩张。
- 与主动脉瓣狭窄相似，肺血管通常正常。

Mitral stenosis

- The most common cause of mitral stenosis is rheumatic heart disease.
- Mitral stenosis appears as a normal size heart with left atrial enlargement.
- Pulmonary venous pressures are typically elevated.
- Normal mitral valve has an orifice area of 4–6 cm^2. A valvular area <1 cm^2 and pressure gradient >10 mmHg define severe mitral stenosis.

二尖瓣狭窄

- 二尖瓣狭窄最常见的病因是风湿性心脏病。
- 二尖瓣狭窄表现为心脏大小正常，但左心房扩大。
- 肺静脉压力典型升高。
- 二尖瓣正常瓣口面积为4~6cm^2。当患者的一个瓣叶面积<1cm^2，且压力梯度>10mmHg时，被定义为重度二尖瓣狭窄。

Mitral regurgitation

- Mitral regurgitation is most commonly caused by degenerative valvular disease, mitral valve prolapse, rheumatic heart disease, endocarditis, ischemic heart disease, annular calcification, and cardiomyopathy.
- Acute mitral regurgitation secondary to myocardial infarction can present as acute pulmonary edema with a normal size heart.
- Chronic mitral regurgitation can lead to cardiac dilatation and left atrial enlargement.

  The left atrial appendage (LAA) is often enlarged in patients with rheumatic disease; however, the LAA is typically not enlarged in non-rheumatic mitral regurgitation.
- **Mitral valve prolapse** is diagnosed when there is prolapse or "bowing" of the valve leaflets greater than 2 mm below the annular plane into the left atrium during systole.

二尖瓣反流

- 二尖瓣反流最常见的原因为退行性瓣膜病、二尖瓣脱垂、风湿性心脏病、心内膜炎、缺血性心脏病、瓣环钙化和心肌病。
- 急性二尖瓣反流继发于心肌梗死，可表现为急性肺水肿，但心脏影像正常。
- 慢性二尖瓣反流可导致心脏增大和左心房扩大。

  左心耳(LAA)在风湿性心脏病患者常会扩大；但是在非风湿病所致的二尖瓣反流患者中LAA通常不扩大。
- **二尖瓣脱垂**的诊断标准是二尖瓣下垂，或收缩期瓣叶于瓣环平面下方向左心房“突出”大于2mm。

Mitral annular calcification

二尖瓣环钙化

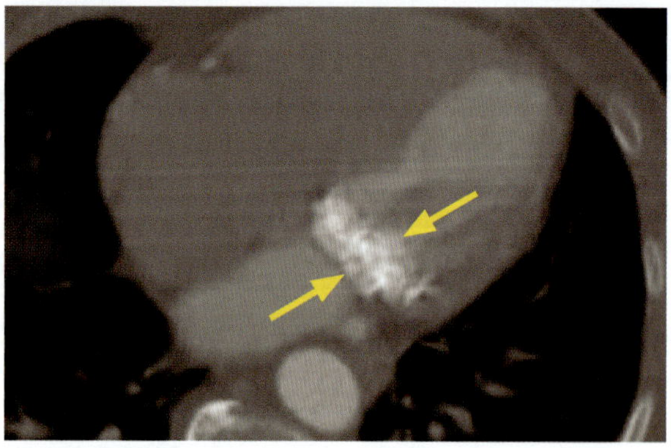

Contrast-enhanced axial CT in bone windows demonstrates extensive calcification of the mitral valve annulus (arrows).
Case courtesy Michael Hanley, MD, University of Virginia Health System.
轴位增强CT骨窗显示二尖瓣环广泛钙化(黄箭)。

- Mitral annular calcification (MAC) is a degenerative process where calcium is deposited along the fibrous annulus encircling the mitral valve.
- MAC may be associated with increased risk of stroke, adverse cardiovascular events, and atrial fibrillation. MAC is considered a risk factor for cardiovascular disease.
- MAC can be associated with mitral regurgitation, but unlike mitral valve calcifications, MAC is not associated with mitral stenosis.

- 二尖瓣环钙化(MAC)是一个退行性病变，钙沉积在环绕二尖瓣的纤维环上。
- MAC可能会增加卒中、不良心血管事件和心房颤动的风险。MAC被认为是心血管疾病的危险因素之一。
- MAC可与二尖瓣反流有关，但与二尖瓣膜钙化不同，MAC与二尖瓣狭窄无关。

Right-sided valvular disease

- The right side of the heart is preferentially involved in patients with carcinoid disease, leading to tricuspid and pulmonic valve dysfunction, although the left-sided valves can be involved as well.

右心瓣膜病

- 类癌患者主要累及右心从而导致三尖瓣及肺动脉瓣功能障碍，但左侧瓣膜也可受累。

（翻译　曹玉坤）

PERICARDIAL DISEASE

心包疾病

Pericardial anatomy

- The pericardium consists of two layers (the visceral and parietal pericardium), which are separated by approximately 40 mL of pericardial fluid.
- The pericardial apparatus (combination of the visceral and parietal layers and pericardial fluid) measures <1 mm on cadaveric studies and can be seen on CT and MRI, with a normal thickness <2 mm. A pericardial thickness of ≥4 mm on imaging is considered abnormal.

心包解剖

- 心包有两层(脏层和壁层心包)，它们被约40mL的心包积液分开。
- 尸体上测得心包结构(脏层、壁层心包和心包积液)的厚度<1mm，CT和MRI上可以看到这个结构，其正常厚度<2mm。影像学上心包厚度≥4mm为异常。

Pericardial effusion

心包积液

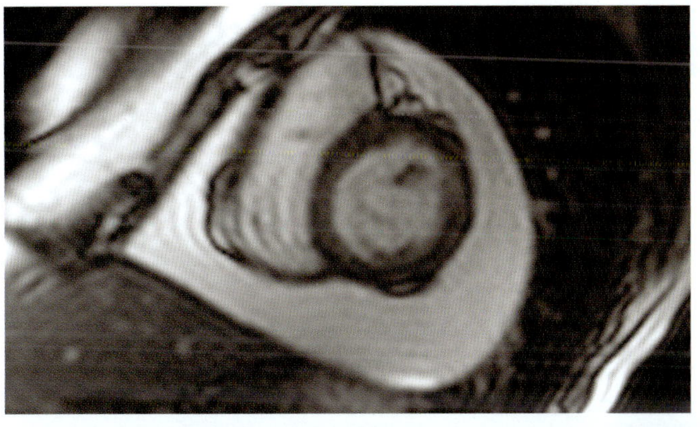

Pericardial effusion:
Short-axis image from a steady state free precession cardiac MRI demonstrates a large pericardial effusion.
心包积液：
短轴稳态自由进动心脏MRI显示大量心包积液。

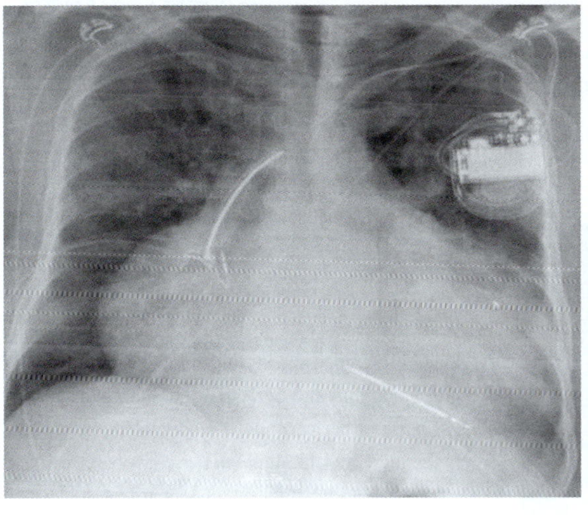

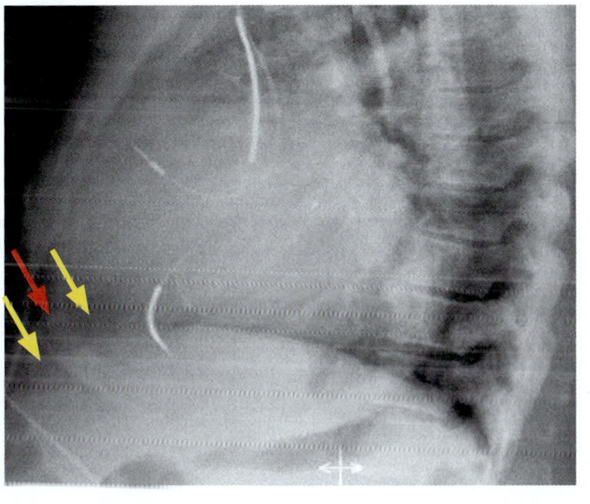

Pericardial effusion and *oreo cookie sign* (in a different patient): Frontal radiograph (left image) demonstrates a markedly enlarged heart, which is nonspecific but can be seen in pericardial effusion. Lateral radiograph demonstrates the *oreo cookie sign* with two parallel lucencies (yellow arrows) indicating the epicardial and pericardial fat stripes surrounding a white "filling" indicating the pericardial effusion (red arrow).
Case courtesy Michael Hanley, MD, University of Virginia Health System.
心包积液及夹心饼干征(另一名患者)：胸部正位X线影像(左图)显示心脏明显增大，无特异性，但可见于心包积液。侧位影像显示夹心饼干征(右图)，两条平行的透亮带(黄箭)代表心外膜和心包脂肪带，其中间被包绕的白色"填充"提示为心包积液(红箭)。

- The classic plain film finding of pericardial effusion is the *oreo cookie sign*, which represents the parallel lucent epicardial and pericardial fat stripes (the cookies) and the radiopaque pericardial effusion (the white filling).
- The primary clinical concern of a pericardial effusion is cardiac tamponade. As little as 100 – 200 mL of pericardial fluid can impede diastolic filling if it accumulates quickly.

- 心包积液典型的X影像表现是夹心饼干征，显示为平行透亮的心外膜和心包脂肪带(饼干)及不透光的心包积液(白色填充)。
- 心包积液的主要临床并发症是心脏压塞。液体快速积聚时，仅100~200mL的心包积液即可使舒张期充盈受限。

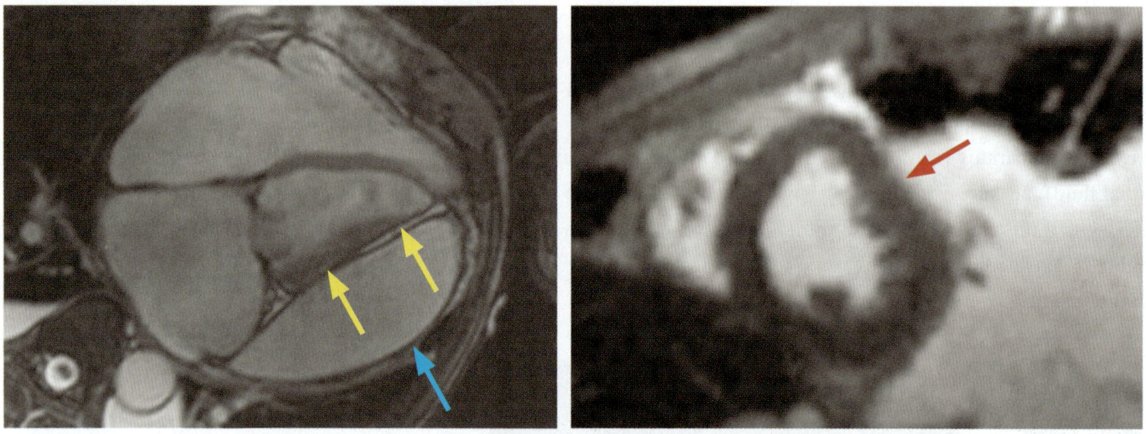

Tamponade: 4 chamber SSFP image (left) in diastole shows that the LV is caved in (yellow arrows) due to loculated pericardial effusion (blue arrow) as a result of recent cardiac surgery for mitral valve repair. Short-axis image from a different patient shows a concave LV contour rather than round (red arrow) due to tamponade.

Case courtesy Michael Steigner, MD, and Raymond Kwong, MD, MPH, Brigham and Women's Hospital.

心脏压塞：舒张期四腔心SSFP图像(左图)显示局部心包积液(蓝箭)导致LV凹陷(黄箭)，为近期二尖瓣修复心脏手术的并发症。另一名患者的短轴图像(右图)显示LV轮廓呈凹形而非圆形(红箭)，由心脏压塞所致。

Acute pericarditis

- Most cases of acute pericarditis are idiopathic and presumed to be viral. Other causes include tuberculosis, neoplasia, and autoimmune disease.
- Up to 30% of patients have recurrent symptoms of pericardial pain.
- Patients often respond favorably to nonsteroidal anti-inflammatory drugs.

急性心包炎

- 大多数急性心包炎的病例为特发性，推测与病毒相关。其他原因包括结核、肿瘤和自身免疫性疾病。
- 高达30%的患者有反复出现的心包疼痛的症状。
- 患者通常对非甾体抗炎药反应良好。

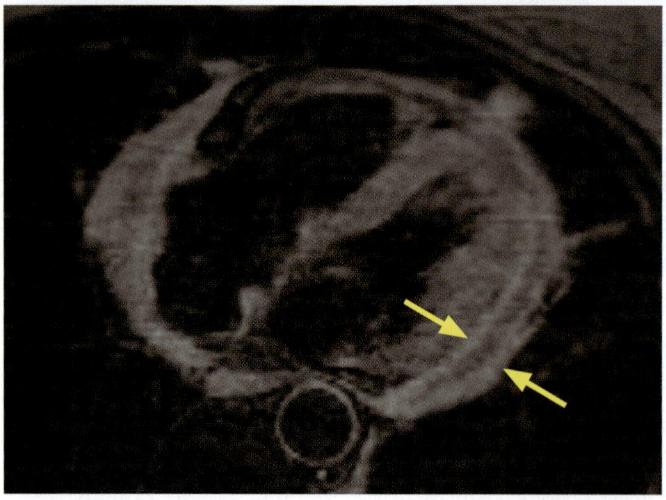

Acute pericarditis:
Axial TIR image shows thickening of the pericardium with epicardial and pericardial stranding. The visceral and parietal pericardium are edematous as evidenced by the increased T2 signal in these layers (arrows). This was a case of idiopathic acute pericarditis.

急性心包炎：
轴位TIR图像显示心包增厚，心外膜和心包束带征。脏层和壁层心包水肿，表现为脏层和壁层心包T_2信号增高(黄箭)。此为一名特发性的急性心包炎。

Pericardial calcification | **心包钙化**

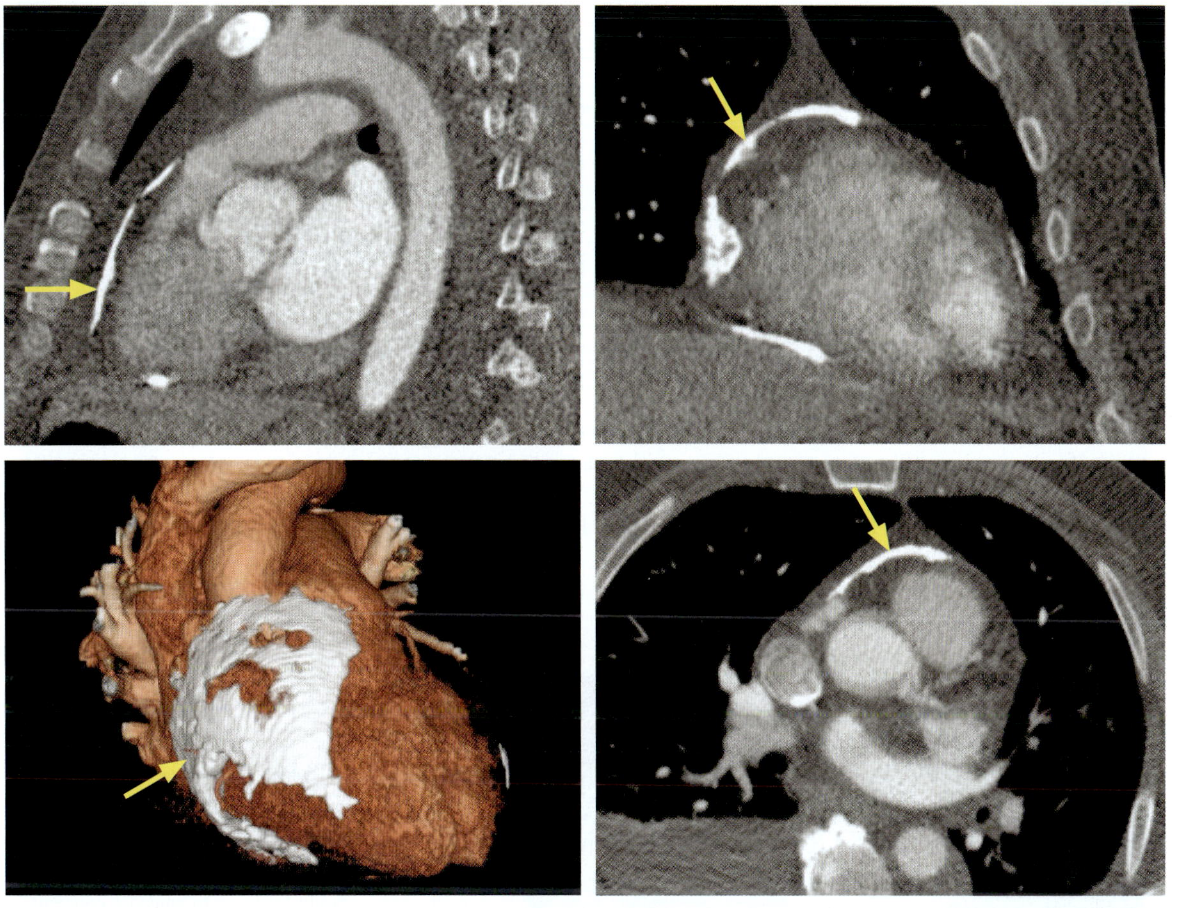

Pericardial calcification: Multiplanar contrast-enhanced CT shows extensive pericardial calcification (arrows). 3D reconstruction (bottom left image) shows the extent of pericardial calcification along the anterolateral right border of the heart (calcification colored in white; arrow).
心包钙化：多平面增强CT显示广泛心包钙化(黄箭)。3D重建(左下图)显示心包钙化广泛分布于右心缘前外侧(钙化标为白色；黄箭)。

- Pericardial calcification can be a result of prior pericarditis, most commonly viral or uremic in etiology. Pericardial calcification can be associated with constrictive physiology.
- The main differential of pericardial calcification is myocardial calcification due to old infarct.

Constrictive pericarditis

- Constrictive pericarditis can occur after any type of pericarditis, most commonly viral or tuberculous pericarditis, uremia, post-radiation or cardiac surgery.
- The pericardium is typically thickened (≥4 mm) in constrictive pericarditis. The presence of pericardial adhesions, calcification, and pericardial effusion are also highly suggestive.
- Cine MRI may show paradoxical motion of the ventricular septum (septal bounce).
- Delayed contrast-enhanced MRI shows pericardial LGE due to fibrosis.
- Myocardial tagging shows lack of normal break between the visceral and parietal pericardium during the cardiac cycle, indicating limited motion between the two layers due to adhesions.
- Constrictive pericarditis is treated surgically by pericardial stripping.

- 心包钙化可能是心包炎的后遗症，最常见的病因为病毒感染或尿毒症。心包钙化可与缩窄性生理学改变相关。
- 心包钙化的主要鉴别诊断是陈旧性心肌梗死导致的心肌钙化。

缩窄性心包炎

- 缩窄性心包炎可继发于任何类型的心包炎，最常见的是病毒性或结核性心包炎、尿毒症、放射后或心脏手术。
- 缩窄性心包炎的心包通常增厚(≥4mm)。高度提示缩窄性心包炎的征象还包括心包粘连、钙化和心包积液。
- 电影MRI可能显示室间隔矛盾运动(室间隔反弹)。
- 延迟对比增强MRI显示心包LGE，为纤维化所致。
- 心肌标记显示在心动周期内脏层和壁层心包之间缺乏正常分离，表明由于粘连导致两层之间的运动受限。
- 缩窄性心包炎通过外科心包剥离手术治疗。

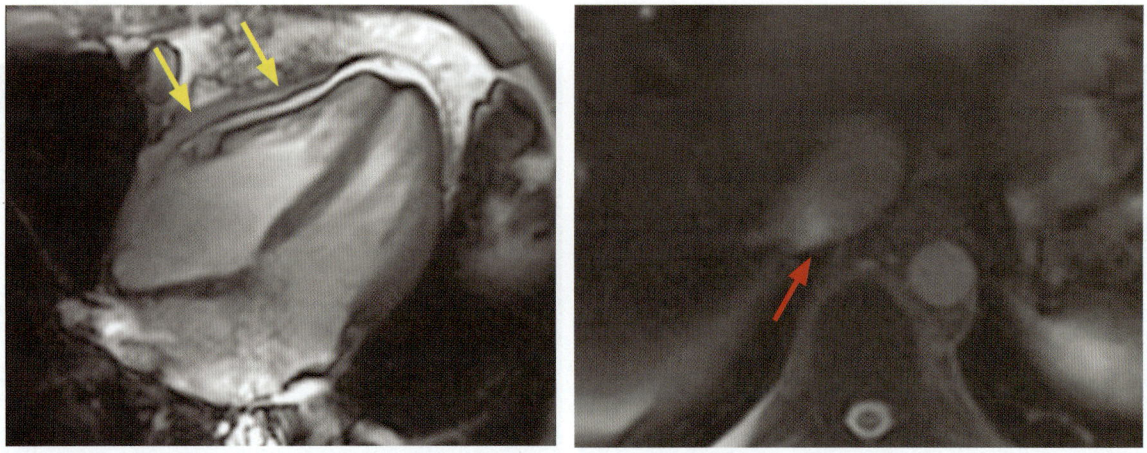

Constrictive pericarditis: 4 chamber SSFP image on the left shows tubular shaped right ventricle with dilated atria. The pericardium is thickened (yellow arrows). Axial T2-weighted image on the right shows dilated IVC (red arrow) due to back pressure from constrictive physiology.
缩窄性心包炎：左图四腔心SSFP图像显示管状右心室伴心房扩张。心包增厚(黄箭)。右侧轴位T_2加权图像显示IVC扩张(红箭)，此为缩窄性生理学改变引起反流压力升高所致。

Congenital absence of the pericardium

先天性心包缺失

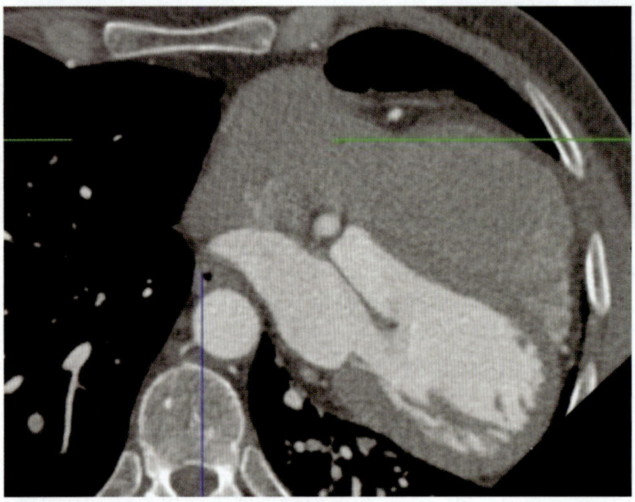

Axial image from a coronary CT shows an abnormal axis of the heart, which is displaced left-posteriorly into the left hemithorax.
Although a pericardial defect is not directly visualized on this image, the characteristic abnormal cardiac axis should lead one to consider congenital absence of the left pericardium.
冠状动脉轴位CT显示心脏轴心异常，即向左后移位到左半胸。
虽然此图像上见不到心包缺损的直接征象，但具有特征性心脏轴心异常时应考虑先天性左心包缺损。

- Congenital absence of the pericardial is a spectrum of disorders ranging from a focal pericardial defect to complete absence of the right and left pericardium. Total absence of the pericardium is very rare.
- The most common form of pericardial absence involves the left pericardium in the region of the left atrial appendage and adjacent pulmonary artery.
- Patients with partial absence of the pericardium are at risk for herniation of a portion of the heart through the pericardial defect.
- On imaging, a clue to the presence of a pericardial defect is a lucent notch between the aorta and pulmonary artery (sometimes seen on radiography, but generally better appreciated on CT), which represents interposed lung between these vascular structures.
- Defects of the left pericardium cause leftward displacement of the heart, which may in some cases be the only imaging finding.

- 先天性心包缺损有多种表现形式，从局限性心包缺损到左、右心包完全缺如。心包完全缺如罕见。
- 最常见的心包缺损为累及左心耳及邻近肺动脉区域的左心包。
- 部分性心包缺损患者有局部心脏从心包缺损处疝出的风险。
- 影像学上，提示心包缺损的一个线索为主动脉与肺动脉间出现一个透亮缺口区(有时可见于X线影像，但CT通常更清楚)，为肺组织被楔入在这些血管结构之间。
- 左侧心包的缺损会引起心脏向左移位，这可能是部分病例中唯一的影像学表现。

Pericardial masses

- **Pericardial cysts** can be congenital or a sequela of prior cardiac surgery. 70% of pericardial cysts occur in the right cardiophrenic angle, 20% occur in the left cardiophrenic angle. It can be difficult to differentiate a pericardial cyst from a

心包肿块

- **心包囊肿**可为先天性或先前心脏手术的后遗症。约70%的心包囊肿发生在右心膈角，20%在左心膈角。心包囊肿难以与胸腺或支气管

thymic or bronchogenic cyst.

- **Pericardial diverticula** communicate with the pericardial space and can change in size.
- The most common **primary pericardial tumor** is pericardial mesothelioma.
- Most common **pericardial metastases** are from lung and breast cancer.

源性囊肿相鉴别。

- **心包憩室**与心包腔相通，大小可发生变化。
- 最常见的**原发性心包肿瘤**是心包间皮瘤。
- 最常见的**心包转移瘤**来自肺癌和乳腺癌。

（翻译　费京乐）

ADULT CARDIAC MASSES

Adult cardiac masses			
Non-neoplastic	Neoplastic (tumors)		
	Primary (benign)	Primary (malignant)	Secondary
thrombus lipomatous hypertrophy of the interatrial septum	myxoma lipoma papillary fibroelastoma paraganglioma fibroma hemangioma	lymphoma angiosarcoma intimal sarcoma synovial sarcoma leiomyosarcoma liposarcoma osteosarcoma	metastases

- The most common cardiac mass is a thrombus.
- Metastases to the heart or pericardium are far more common than primary cardiac tumors. This can occur from direct extension of intrathoracic malignancy (breast or lung), direct extension through SVC or IVC (e.g., renal cell carcinoma via the IVC), or hematogenous spread (e.g., melanoma, lymphoma).
- The majority, approximately 75%, of primary cardiac tumors are benign.
- Common childhood cardiac masses are discussed in the "Pediatric" chapter.

成人心脏肿块

成人心脏肿块			
非新生物	新生物(肿瘤)		
	原发(良性)	原发(恶性)	继发
血栓 房间隔脂肪瘤样肥厚	黏液瘤 脂肪瘤 乳头样弹性纤维瘤 副神经节瘤 纤维瘤 血管瘤	淋巴瘤 血管肉瘤 内膜肉瘤 滑膜肉瘤 平滑肌肉瘤 脂肪肉瘤 骨肉瘤	转移瘤

- 最常见的心脏肿块是血栓。
- 转移到心脏或心包的肿瘤远比原发性心脏肿瘤更为常见。转移可来自胸腔内恶性肿瘤(乳腺或肺部)直接侵犯，或通过上腔静脉或下腔静脉直接扩散(如肾细胞癌通过下腔静脉)，或血行转移(如黑色素瘤、淋巴瘤)。
- 大多数(约占75%)的原发性心脏肿瘤为良性。
- 常见的儿童心脏肿块将在"小儿影像"一章进行讨论。

BENIGN PRIMARY CARDIAC TUMORS

良性原发心脏肿瘤

Thrombus

血栓

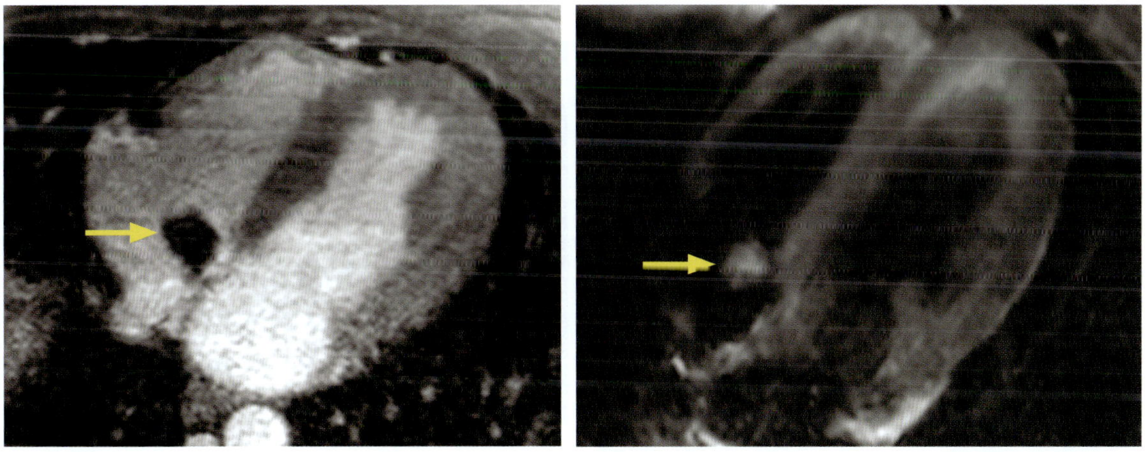

Thrombus: Axial MR images show a pedunculated mass in the right atrium attached to the inter-atrial septum (arrows), which is mildly T2 hyperintense (right image), T1 isointense relative to myocardium (not shown), and demonstrates no gadolinium enhancement (left image).

血栓：轴位MRI显示右心房内有一个带蒂肿块附着于房间隔(黄箭)，呈T_2稍高信号(右图)，T_1相对心肌呈等信号(未展示)，钆增强后未见强化(左图)。

- Intracardiac thrombus can mimic a cardiac tumor.
- Distinguishing imaging features are lack of contrast enhancement in the thrombus and adjacent myocardial scar and/or akinetic cardiac wall.

Myxoma

- 心腔内的血栓可类似于心脏肿瘤。
- 影像学上最显著的特征是血栓无强化，以及无邻近心肌有瘢痕和/或心壁运动障碍。

黏液瘤

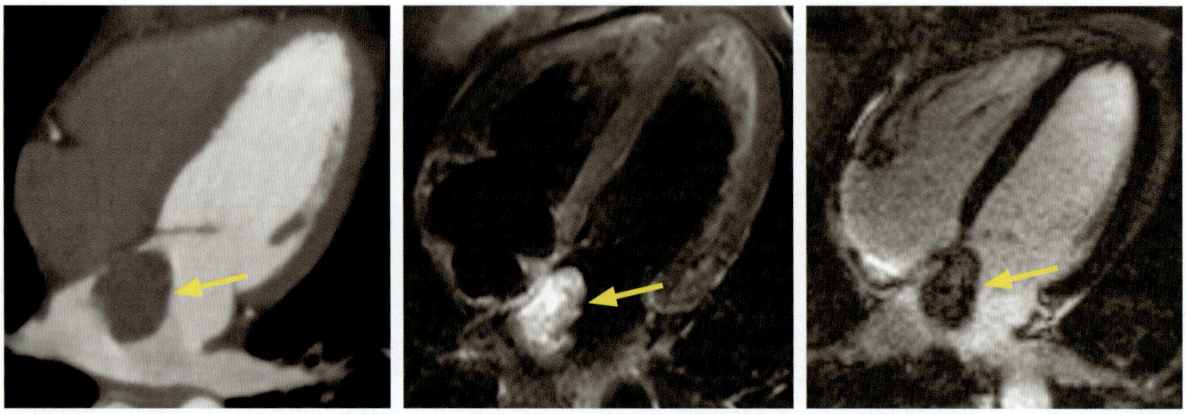

Left atrial myxoma: Axial CTA image (left image) shows a left atrial mass attached to the inter-atrial septum (arrow). Axial MR images show the T2 hyperintense mass (arrow, middle image) and demonstrates heterogeneous late gadolinium enhancement (arrow, right image).
左心房黏液瘤：轴位CTA(左图)显示左心房肿块附着于房间隔(黄箭)。轴位MRI显示肿块呈T_2高信号(黄箭，中图)，延迟增强后显示出不均匀强化(黄箭，右图)。

- Myxoma is the most common benign primary cardiac tumor in adults.
- 75% of cardiac myxomas arise in the left atrium, usually attached to the inter-atrial septum in region of the fossa ovalis. 20% arise in the right atrium. The tumor may prolapse through a valve or patent foramen ovale.
- On MRI, myxomas have similar T1 signal to myocardium, are T2 hyperintense, demonstrate little to no enhancement on first pass perfusion, and heterogeneous low-level LGE. Calcification and hemosiderin deposition from intralesional hemorrhage are common.

Lipoma and lipomatous hypertrophy of the inter-atrial septum

- **Lipomas** are common benign cardiac tumors that have a spherical shape and well-circumscribed margin, typically located in the right atrium, arise from the endocardial surface and project into the atrial cavity. They follow fat signal intensity on all MRI sequences and do not enhance.

- 黏液瘤是成人最常见的原发性心脏肿瘤。
- 约75%的心脏黏液瘤起源于左心房，常附着于房间隔的卵圆孔区。约20%起源于右心房。肿瘤可能通过瓣膜口或未闭合的卵圆孔脱出。
- 在MRI上，黏液瘤T_1与心肌信号相等，T_2呈高信号，心肌首过灌注成像很少或无强化，呈不均匀的轻度LGE。常见到钙化和因病灶内出血引起的含铁血黄素沉积。

脂肪瘤和房间隔脂肪瘤样肥厚

- **脂肪瘤**是常见的良性心脏肿瘤，呈球形、边缘清晰、常位于右心房、起自心内膜的表面并突入心房腔内。在所有MRI序列中都与脂肪的信号强度一致，无强化。

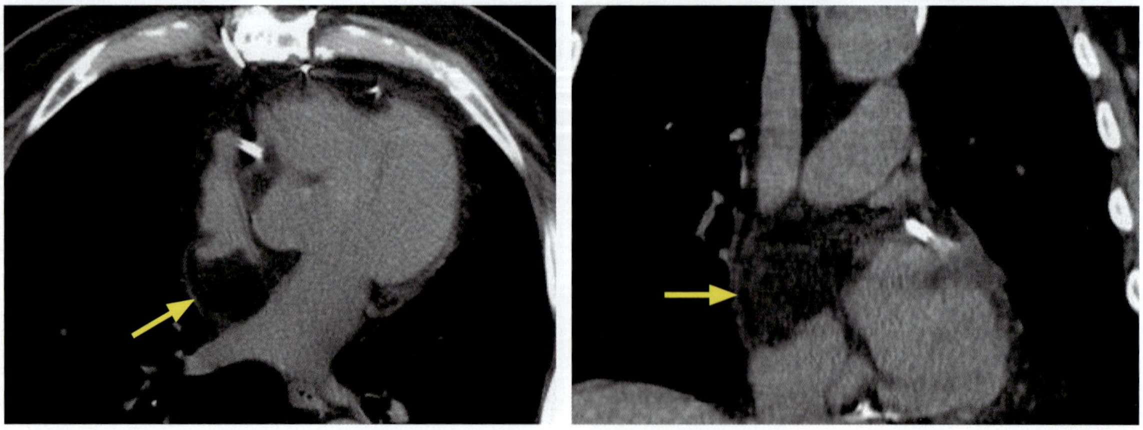

Lipomatous hypertrophy of the interatrial septum: Axial and coronal noncontrast CT demonstrates a focal area of fat attenuation at the inter-atrial septum, along the right heart border (arrows).
Case courtesy Michael Hanley, MD, University of Virginia Health System.
房间隔脂肪瘤样肥厚：轴位和冠状位非增强CT显示房间隔部局灶性脂肪密度影，沿着右心边缘分布(黄箭)。

- **Lipomatous hypertrophy of the inter-atrial septum (LHIS)** represents proliferation of fatty deposits within the inter-atrial septum, typically along the lateral right heart border. The fossa ovalis is spared, resulting in a dumbbell configuration of the fatty tissue.
- LHIS is an incidental finding that does not require treatment. It is important to not mistake it for a cardiac mass. Unlike lipomas, LHIS does not have a capsule on histopathology.
- An exceedingly rare differential consideration of a fatty cardiac mass is liposarcoma.

- **房间隔脂肪瘤样肥厚(LHIS)** 为增生的脂肪沉积在房间隔内，通常沿右心的外侧缘分布。卵圆孔区不受累，形成的脂肪组织呈哑铃状形态。
- LHIS是一种偶尔发现的情况，无须治疗。重要的是勿将其误认为心脏肿块。与脂肪瘤不同，LHIS在组织病理学上无包膜。
- 脂肪性心脏肿块在极罕见的情况下需要与脂肪肉瘤进行鉴别。

Papillary fibroelastoma

乳头样弹性纤维瘤

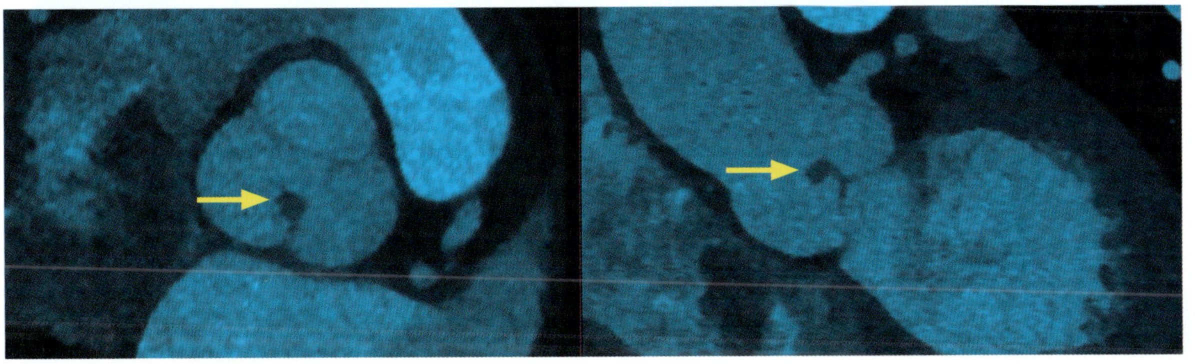

Multiplanar reformatted CTA images at level of the aortic valve show a trileaflet aortic valve and a round pedunculated lesion attached to the noncoronary cusp thought to represent a papillary fibroelastoma (arrows). Surgical resection confirmed the diagnosis.
多平面重建CTA显示在主动脉瓣水平面三叶主动脉瓣结构，以及一个圆形带蒂的病变附着于无冠瓣，考虑为乳头样弹性纤维瘤(黄箭)。手术切除后证实了该诊断。

- Papillary fibroelastoma is the most common tumor of the cardiac valves.
- The most common location is the aortic valve on the side of the aorta.
- On MRI, papillary fibroelastomas have low T2 signal due to high fibrous content.
- While these tumors are usually small in size, they may promote thrombus formation, detach and embolize, or affect valvular function.

- 乳头样弹性纤维瘤是心脏瓣膜最常见的良性肿瘤。
- 最常见的部位是位于主动脉一侧的主动脉瓣。
- 在MRI上，乳头样弹性纤维瘤在T_2上呈低信号，因为其内含高纤维成分。
- 肿瘤通常体积小，但可能诱发血栓形成、脱落和栓塞，或影响瓣膜功能。

Hemangioma

- Hemangiomas can occur in any cardiac chamber and involve the pericardium.
- Similar to elsewhere in the body, hemangiomas are hyperintense on T2, intensely enhancing due to rich vascularity, with possible flow voids and calcifications.

血管瘤

- 血管瘤可发生于任何一个心脏的腔室并可累及心包。
- 与身体其他部位的病变相似，血管瘤呈T_2高信号，因血管丰富而显著强化，可能伴有流空信号和钙化。

Paraganglioma/pheochromocytoma

- Cardiac paragangliomas are usually benign, however, these tumors can have malignant potential. “Malignancy” is defined by WHO when there is distant metastasis. Common locations include in and around the left atrium, retroaortic, and aorticopulmonary window.
- Imaging features are identical to paragangliomas/pheochromocytomas elsewhere in body, including hyperenhancement due to high vascularity and T2 hyperintense signal relative to myocardium.

副神经节瘤/嗜铬细胞瘤

- 心脏的副神经节瘤常为良性，但这些肿瘤具有恶性潜能。WHO将“恶性”定义为发生了远处转移。常见的转移部位包括左心房内或周围、主动脉后及主肺动脉窗。
- 影像学特征与身体其他部位的副神经节/嗜铬细胞瘤相同，包括因富血管而显著强化和相对心肌的T_2高信号。

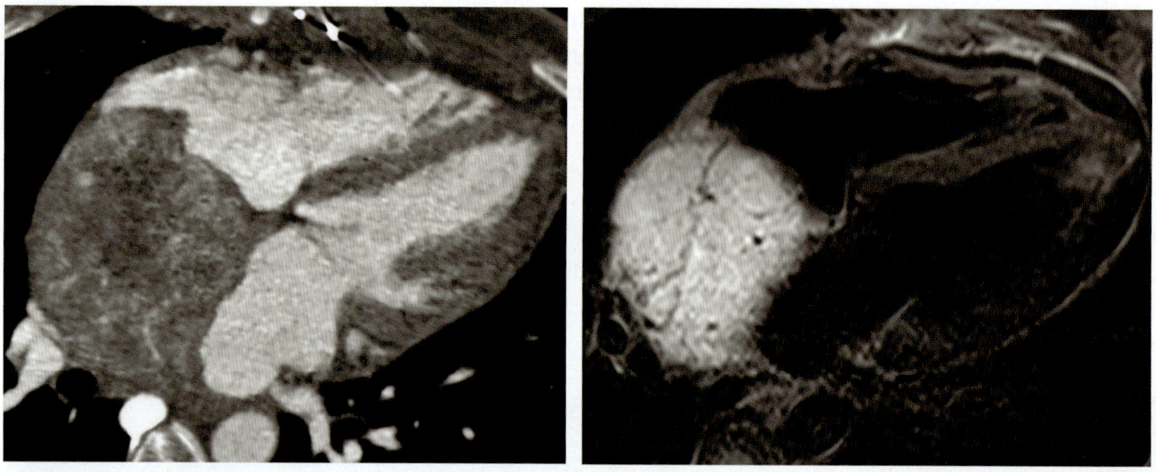

Biopsy-proven paraganglioma: Axial CTA and T2-weighted MR images show a large mass centered at the right atrium, which invades the right atrial wall, obliterates the adjacent epicardial fat, and extends into the left atrium. The mass demonstrates heterogeneous enhancement (left image) and T2 hyperintense signal (right image).

经活检证实的副神经节瘤：轴位CTA和T_2加权MRI显示以右心房为中心的巨大肿块影，侵犯右心房壁，使邻近的心外膜脂肪消失，并延伸至左心房内。肿块表现为不均匀强化(左图)和T_2高信号(右图)。

Malignant Primary Cardiac Tumors

- Sarcomas represent the most common type of malignant primary cardiac tumors, followed by primary cardiac lymphoma which is rare compared to secondary lymphoma involving the heart.
- Common imaging features of malignant cardiac tumors include involvement of more than one cardiac chamber, intralesional necrosis, invasion of the pericardium and epicardial fat, extension to extracardiac structures, hemorrhagic pericardial effusion, and metastases.
- Primary cardiac sarcomas in adults include osteosarcoma, leiomyosarcoma, synovial sarcoma, liposarcoma, intimal (spindle cell) and undifferentiated sarcoma.
- Intimal sarcoma is a relatively new WHO classification and refers to sarcomas of the aorta and pulmonary artery/vein that express the *MDM2* gene.
- Apart from intimal sarcoma, the other sarcomas listed above have a predilection for the left atrium, unlike angiosarcoma.

Angiosarcoma

- Angiosarcoma is the most common primary cardiac malignancy in adults.
- Right side of the heart is typically affected, most often the right atrium.
- On MRI, angiosarcoma may have a “cauliflower-like” heterogeneous appearance with intralesional hemorrhage, necrosis, and T1 and T2 hypointense foci which represent vascular channels.

恶性原发性心脏肿瘤

- 肉瘤是最常见的一类恶性原发性心脏肿瘤，其次是原发性心脏淋巴瘤，后者较累及心脏的继发性淋巴瘤为罕见。
- 恶性心脏肿瘤的常见影像学征象包括累及一个以上的心脏腔室、病灶内坏死、侵犯心包和心外膜脂肪、扩散至心外结构、心包积血和转移。
- 成人原发性心脏肉瘤包括骨肉瘤、平滑肌肉瘤、滑膜肉瘤、脂肪肉瘤、内膜(梭形细胞)和未分化肉瘤。
- 内膜肉瘤是WHO分类中一个相对新的内容，是指主动脉和肺动脉/静脉肉瘤有表达*MDM2*基因。
- 除内膜肉瘤之外，上述提到的其他多种肉瘤都好发于左心房，这一点与血管肉瘤不同。

血管肉瘤

- 血管肉瘤是最常见的成人原发性恶性心脏肿瘤。
- 右心通常受累，最常见的部位是右心房。
- 在MRI上，血管肉瘤可能呈现“花椰菜样”不均质的表现，病灶内有出血、坏死和代表血管腔的T_1和T_2低信号灶。

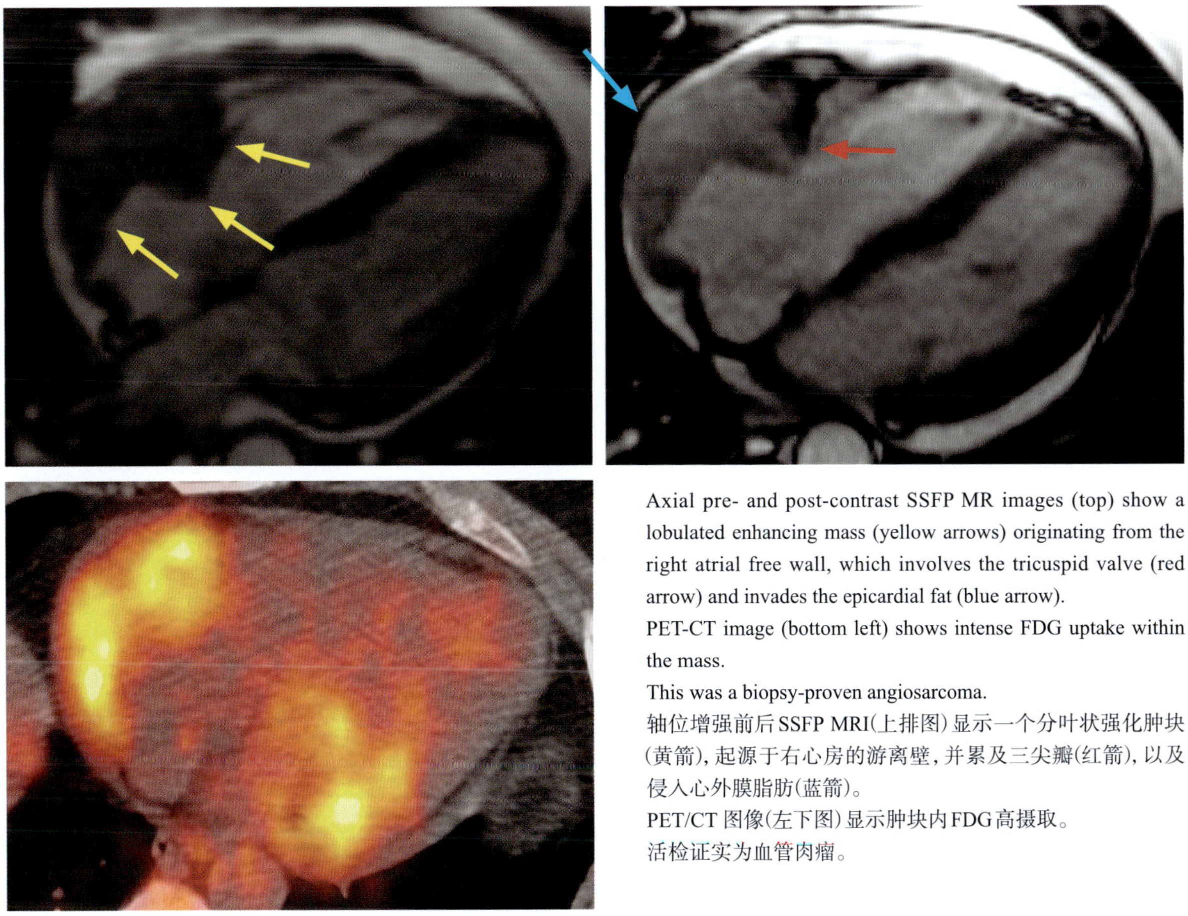

Axial pre- and post-contrast SSFP MR images (top) show a lobulated enhancing mass (yellow arrows) originating from the right atrial free wall, which involves the tricuspid valve (red arrow) and invades the epicardial fat (blue arrow).

PET-CT image (bottom left) shows intense FDG uptake within the mass.

This was a biopsy-proven angiosarcoma.

轴位增强前后SSFP MRI(上排图)显示一个分叶状强化肿块(黄箭),起源于右心房的游离壁,并累及三尖瓣(红箭),以及侵入心外膜脂肪(蓝箭)。

PET/CT 图像(左下图)显示肿块内FDG高摄取。

活检证实为血管肉瘤。

COMMON LOCATIONS OF CARDIAC MASSES

心脏肿块的常见部位

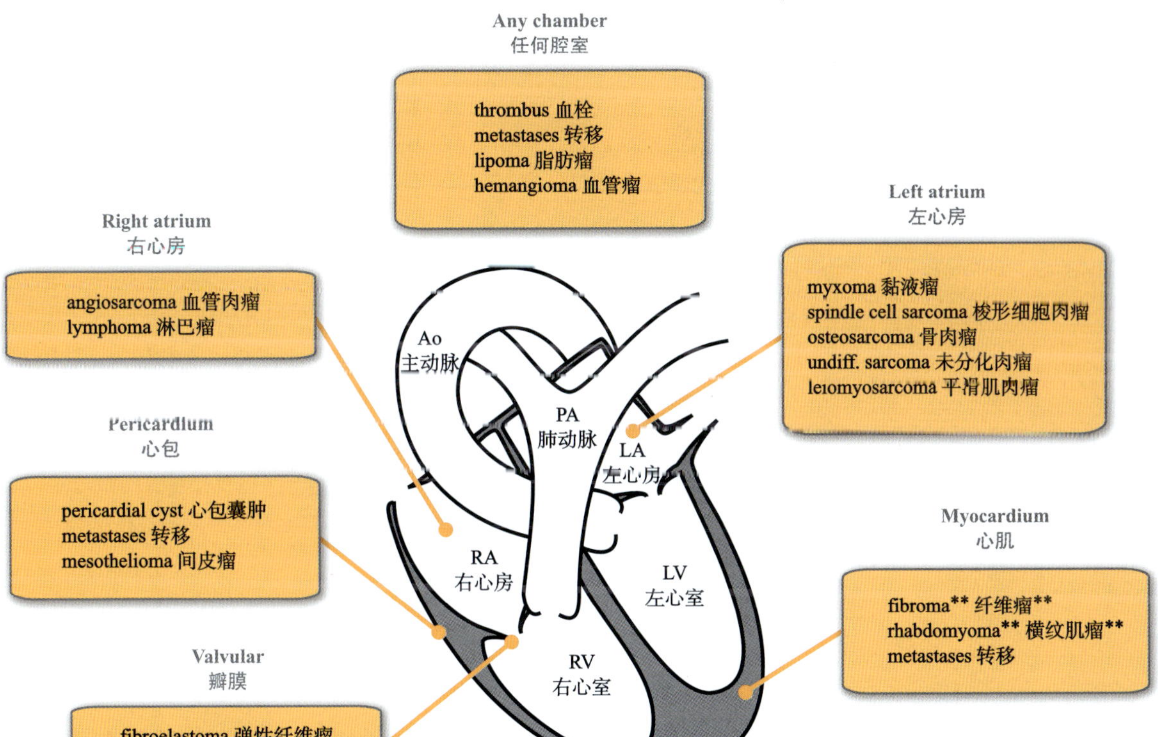

** discussed separately in "Pediatric" chapter

** 单独在"小儿影像"一章进行讨论

(翻译　汪晶)

8 Vascular Imaging

Junzi Shi, Ellen X. Sun, Ayaz Aghayev

Contents

8 血管影像

目录

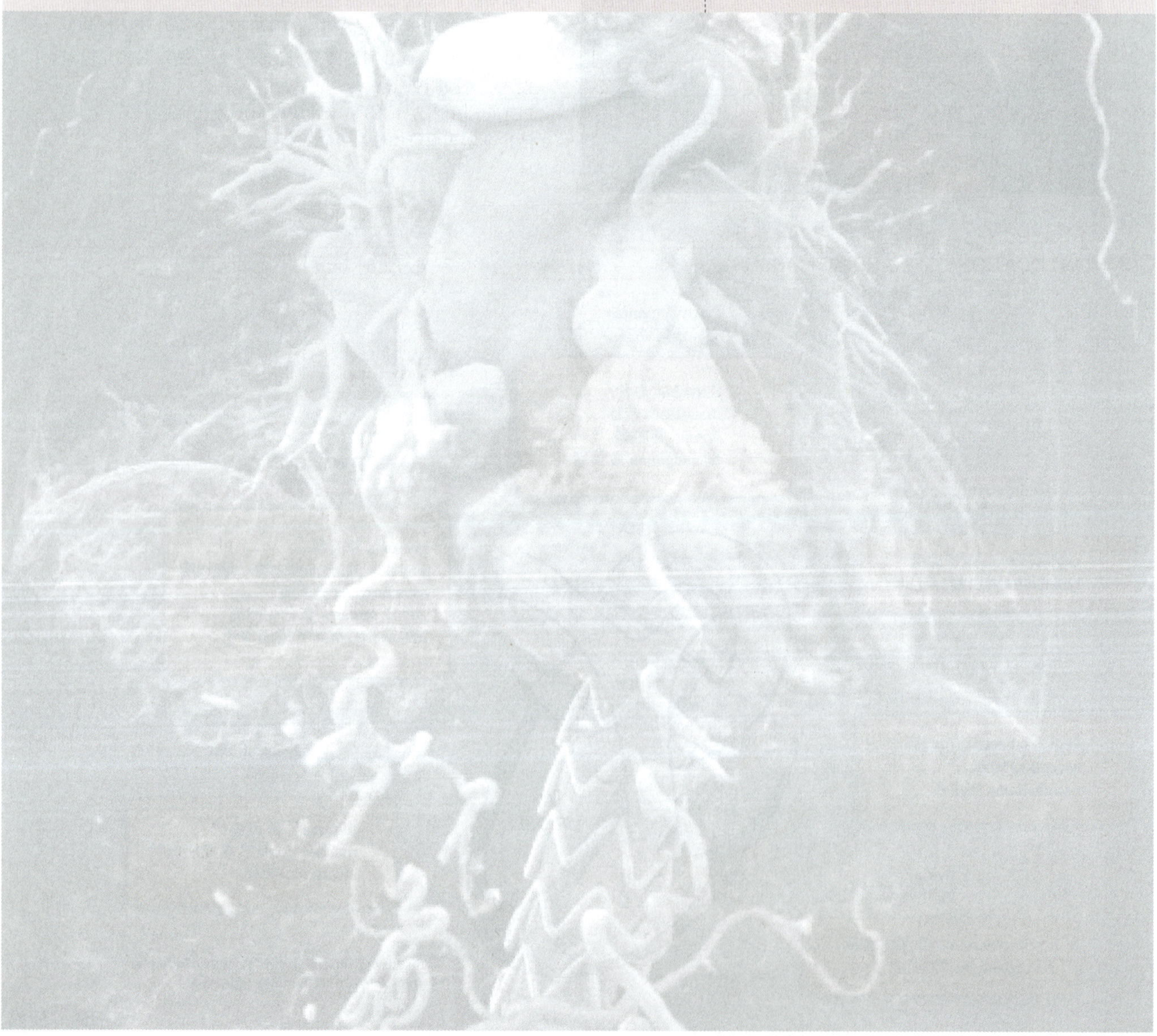

AORTIC ANATOMY AND VARIANTS

主动脉解剖及变异

ANATOMY OF THORACIC AORTA

胸主动脉解剖

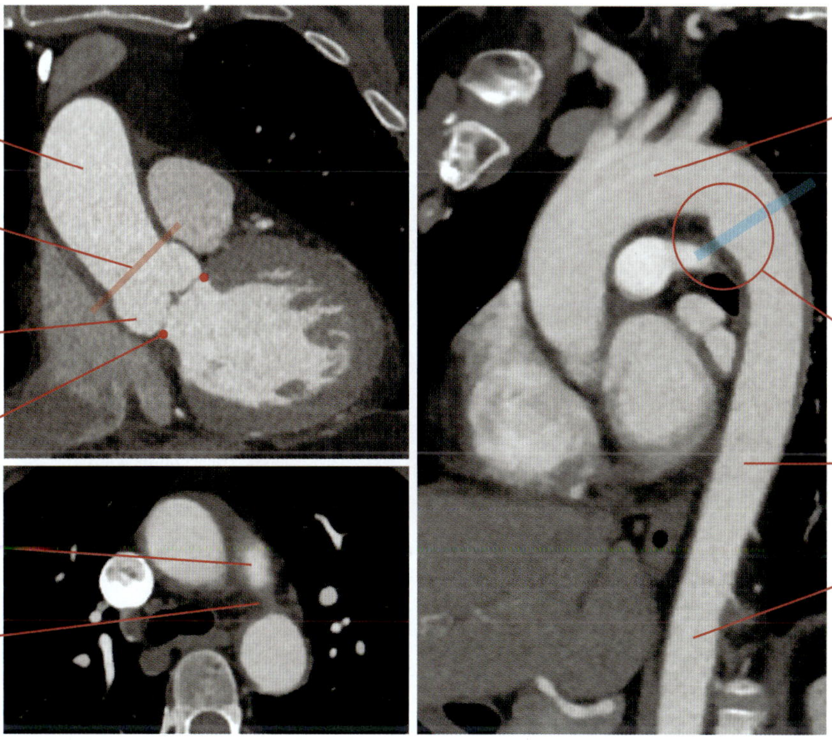

AORTIC ARCH AND VARIANTS

主动脉弓及变异

Normal aortic arch branching

正常主动脉弓分支

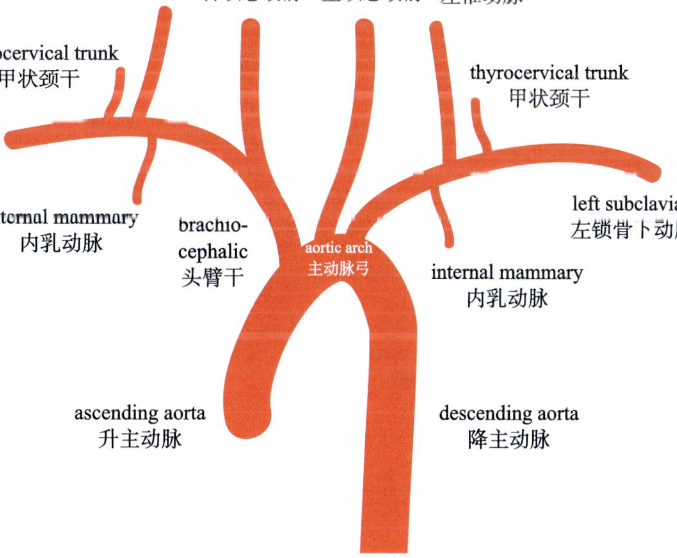

- The normal aortic branching pattern is seen 66% of the time and features three arteries arising from the aortic arch: Brachiocephalic trunk (innominate artery), left common carotid, and left subclavian artery.

Common origin of the brachiocephalic artery and left common carotid artery

- 正常主动脉弓发出三个分支，即头臂干(无名动脉)、左颈总动脉及左锁骨下动脉，见于66%的人群。

头臂动脉及左颈总动脉共干起源

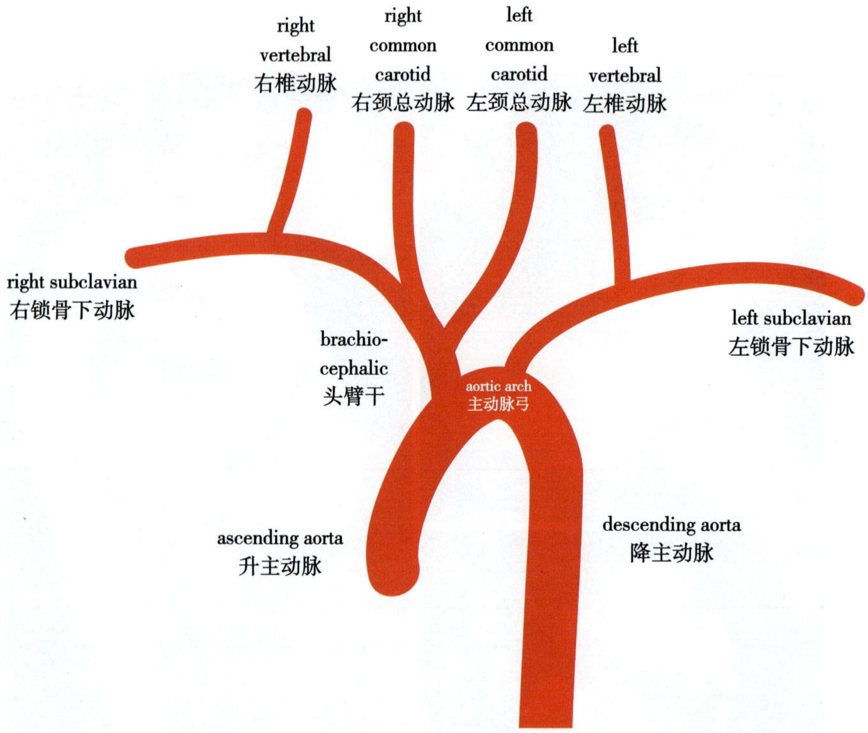

- A common origin of the brachiocephalic artery and left common carotid artery is seen in 13% of patients (more commonly in black patients) and is often incorrectly referred to as a "bovine aortic arch." The term "bovine aortic arch" is a misnomer and is not the preferred description of this anomaly, as a true bovine arch in cattle features a single great vessel arising from the aortic arch.

Aberrant right subclavian

- 头臂动脉和左颈总动脉共干占患者人群的13%(黑种人更常见)，且常被误称为“牛型主动脉弓”，“牛型主动脉弓”这个术语用词是不当的，并不是对该异常的首选描述。真正的“牛型主动脉弓”是指单根大血管起源于主动脉弓。

迷走右锁骨下动脉

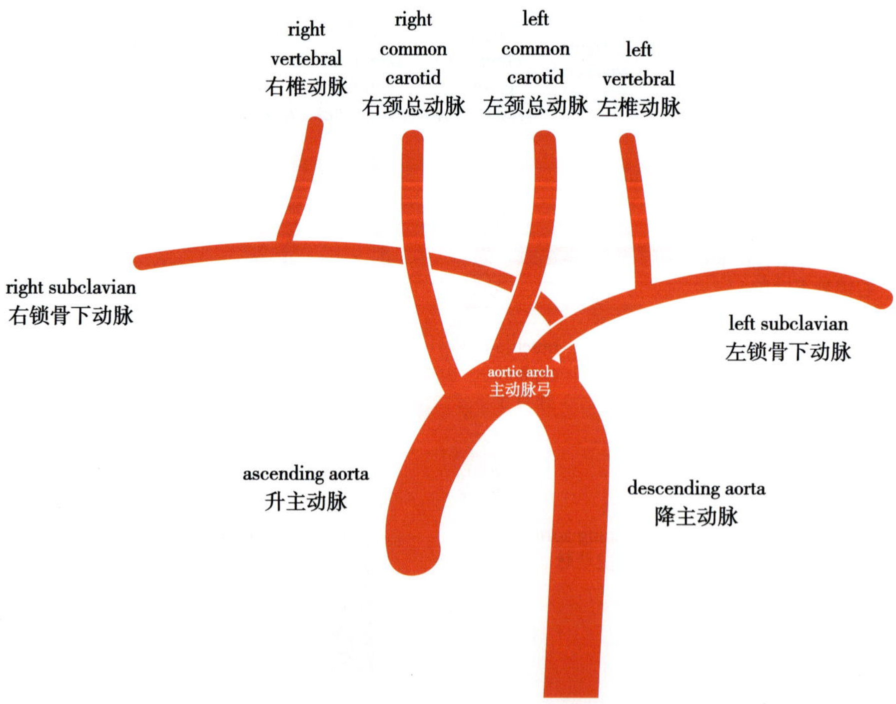

- An aberrant right subclavian is seen in 1% of patients. The right subclavian artery arises directly from the aortic arch distal to the left subclavian and loops behind the esophagus on its way into the right arm.
- A diverticulum of Kommerel represents a small bulge at the origin of the aberrant subclavian artery.

- 迷走右锁骨下动脉见于1%的患者。右锁骨下动脉直接起源于左锁骨下动脉远端的主动脉弓，绕着食管后方进入右上肢。
- Kommerel憩室是指迷走右锁骨下动脉起始处小的突起。

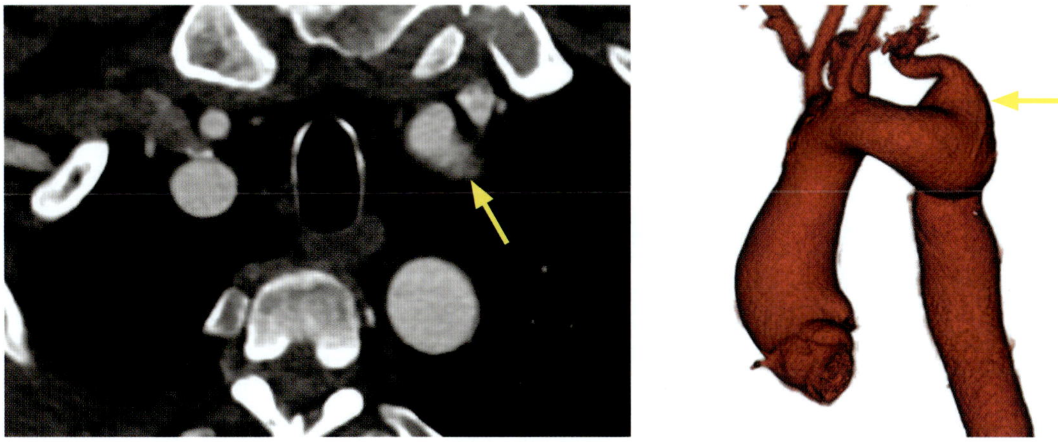

Diverticulum of Kommerel: Axial CT angiogram (left image) and 3D volume rendered reformat (right image) show a dilated vascular structure at the origin of the aberrant right subclavian artery (arrows) known as a *diverticulum of Kommerel.*
Kommerel憩室：轴位CT血管成像(左图)和3D容积再现重组图像(右图)显示右侧锁骨下动脉(黄箭)起始处异常的血管扩张，称为Kommerel憩室。

- It is very uncommon for an aberrant right subclavian artery to cause symptoms, but this anomaly may rarely be a cause of dysphagia via esophageal compression, called *dysphagia lusoria*. Barium esophagram features a posterior indentation on the esophagus.
- Although usually incidental, it is important to mention the presence of an aberrant right subclavian artery when reading a neck CT. If thyroid surgery is planned, then the position of the recurrent laryngeal nerve will not be in its usual location.

- 迷走右锁骨下动脉很少引起症状，偶可压迫食管导致吞咽困难，称为食管受压性吞咽困难。食管钡剂造影可见食管后方受压的凹陷。
- 尽管常常是偶然发现，但在书写颈部CT报告时须提及该变异。在计划进行甲状腺手术时，应注意喉返神经将不在其通常的解剖位置。

Left vertebral origin off aorta

左椎动脉起源于主动脉

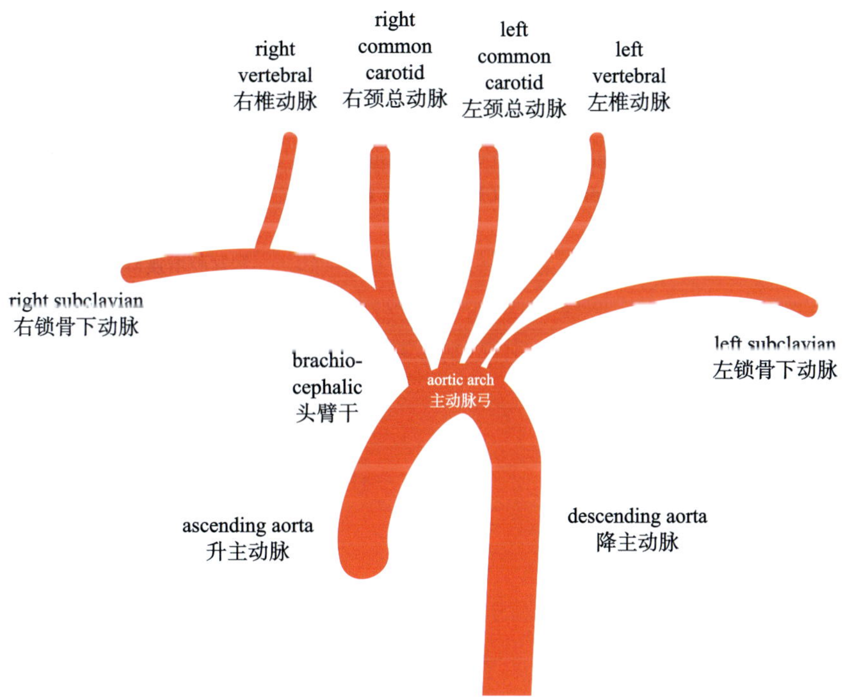

- A 4-vessel arch with direct origin of the vertebral artery off of the aorta is seen in 6% of the population. The left vertebral is the third aortic branch, proximal to the left subclavian.
- In approximately 1/3 of patients with left vertebral artery arising from the aortic arch, the vertebral artery terminates as the posterior inferior cerebellar artery (PICA) instead of contributing to the circle of Willis.
- Vascular anomalies of the aortic arch have implications for surgical repair of aortic aneurysms because occluding a branch may result in end-organ ischemia.

- 椎动脉直接起源于主动脉弓时可见4根血管自主动脉弓发出，概率为6%。左侧椎动脉是第3根主动脉分支，位于左锁骨下动脉起始端近侧。
- 约1/3患者的左侧椎动脉起源于主动脉弓，并终止于小脑后下动脉(PICA)，但不参与大脑动脉环(Willis环)。
- 主动脉弓的血管异常可对主动脉瘤外科修补术造成影响，因弓上分支闭塞可导致终末器官缺血。

(翻译　薛艺)

ACUTE AORTIC SYNDROME

急性主动脉综合征

OVERVIEW OF ACUTE AORTIC SYNDROME

- Acute aortic syndrome represents a clinical spectrum of related diseases that are characterized by damage to at least one component of the aortic wall, and present as severe chest pain.

  Aortic dissection: A defect in the intima where the blood enters and extends to media.

  Aortic intramural hematoma (IMH): Media defect with vasa-vasorum hemorrhage into the wall.

  Penetrating atherosclerotic ulcer (PAU): Intimal defect as a result of atherosclerotic lesion.
- The treatment of acute aortic syndrome depends primarily on the location (ascending versus non-ascending aorta) and is often the same regardless of the underlying etiology.

> **Ascending aorta**: Treatment is most commonly surgical.
> **Descending aorta**: Treatment is most commonly medical (blood pressure control).

- Imaging of the full aorta is generally required in any acute aortic pathology.

  First-line imaging modality is CT and includes a) noncontrast chest CT and b) ECG-gated CT angiogram (CTA) of the chest, abdomen, and pelvis.

  If patient is stable and cannot get CTA, MR angiogram (MRA) can be considered including fast noncontrast techniques (e.g., SSFP), and post-contrast MRA of the chest, abdomen and pelvis.

急性主动脉综合征概述

- 急性主动脉综合征包括了一系列临床相关的疾病，其特征为至少有一层主动脉壁的结构受损，并表现为严重胸痛。

  主动脉夹层：血液进入受损的内膜并延伸到中膜。

  主动脉壁内血肿(IMH)：中膜缺损伴血管-滋养血管出血进入管壁。

  穿透性动脉粥样硬化性溃疡(PAU)：动脉粥样硬化性病变导致内膜缺损。
- 治疗急性主动脉综合征主要取决于发生的部位(升主动脉或降主动脉)，通常与其潜在病因无关，治疗方法相同。

> **升主动脉**：治疗常以外科手术为主。
> **降主动脉**：通常为保守治疗(血压控制)。

- 任何原因造成的急性主动脉病变都需要对整个主动脉进行成像。

  首选的成像方式是CT，包括：a.胸部平扫CT；b.心电门控胸、腹和盆腔CT血管成像(CTA)。

  若患者病情稳定但无法行CTA，可考虑MR血管成像(MRA)，包括快速平扫技术(如SSFP)及胸、腹和盆腔增强MRA。

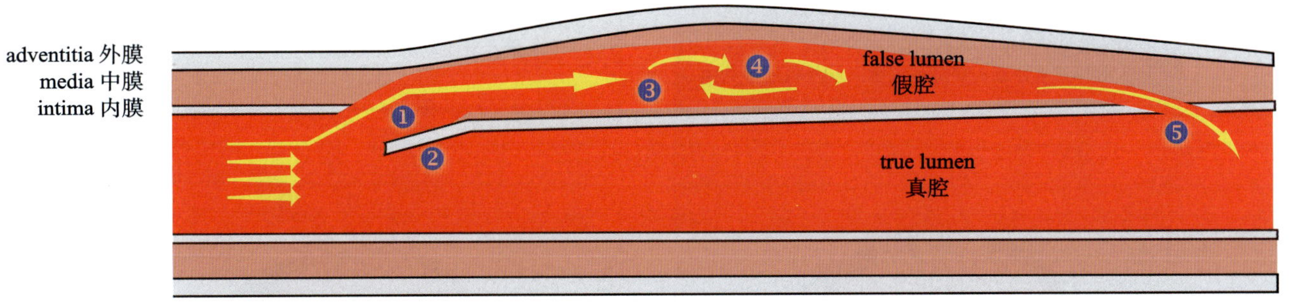

❶ Intima is disrupted, typically by an ulcerative plaque, trauma, or aneurysm.

❷ An intimomedial flap is created.

❸ The media is "dissected" and expanded by either the false lumen (if blood is flowing) or intramural hematoma (if filled with clot).

❹ Blood flow is slower in the false lumen, leading to thrombosis.

❺ Blood exits the false lumen via a re-entry tear. Typically, the re-entry tear obstructs the outflow leading to higher pressures in the false lumen. This pressure differential contributes to compression of the true lumen and differences in contrast opacification between the true and false lumens.

❶ 内膜破裂，通常由溃疡性斑块、外伤或动脉瘤所致。

❷ 内-中膜片形成。

❸ 中膜被"撕裂"并因假腔(若血液流动)或壁内血肿(若充满血凝块)而导致膨胀。

❹ 假腔血流缓慢，导致血栓形成。

❺ 血液从假腔的"撕裂出口"回流到真腔。通常情况下，"撕裂出口"阻止血液流出而导致假腔内压力升高，压力差会导致真腔受压，以及真假腔内强化影像有差别。

- The key feature of dissection is a disruption in the intima, which allows high-pressure blood to infiltrate and expand the media.

  The most common risk factor for aortic dissection is hypertension, but other risk factors include connective tissue disorders (especially Marfan syndrome), cocaine use, aortopathy associated with a bicuspid aortic valve, weight lifting, and sudden deceleration injury. Aortic dissection secondary to atherosclerosis is more commonly type B (descending aorta).
- The **true lumen** is often smaller with outer wall calcifications.
- The **false lumen** is often the larger lumen and has lower contrast density on arterial phase. The false lumen can become thrombosed, with *beak sign* and *cobweb sign*.
- The classification of aortic dissection is the Stanford classification, which divides dissection into types A (ascending aorta) and B (non-ascending aorta). Type A is typically treated surgically, and type B is typically treated medically.
- Stanford B refers to aortic dissection that starts at the aortic arch between the brachiocephalic trunk and left subclavian artery and not involving the ascending aorta proximal to the brachiocephalic trunk. Since these dissections do not result in organ ischemia, they can be treated medically.

- 夹层的标志是内膜撕裂，使高压血流渗入中膜，并使其扩张。

  主动脉夹层最常见的危险因素是高血压，其他包括结缔组织疾病(尤其是马方综合征)、吸食可卡因、与二叶式主动脉瓣畸形相关的主动脉病、举重和急剧减速性损伤。继发于动脉粥样硬化的主动脉夹层常为Stanford B型(累及降主动脉)。
- **真腔**通常较小，其外壁有钙化。
- **假腔**通常较大，动脉期内的造影剂密度较低。假腔可形成血栓，伴有鸟喙征和蛛网征。
- 主动脉夹层分类采用Stanford分型，A型累及升主动脉，B型为累及非升主动脉。A型通常以外科治疗为主，B型则以保守治疗为主。
- Stanford B型是指主动脉夹层始于头臂干和左锁骨下动脉之间的主动脉弓，不累及头臂干近端的升主动脉。因为此型夹层不会导致器官缺血，可行保守治疗。

Stanford A aortic dissection:
Ascending aorta, ±descending aorta *Typically treated surgically*
Stanford A型主动脉夹层
升主动脉夹层伴或不伴降主动脉夹层外科治疗为主

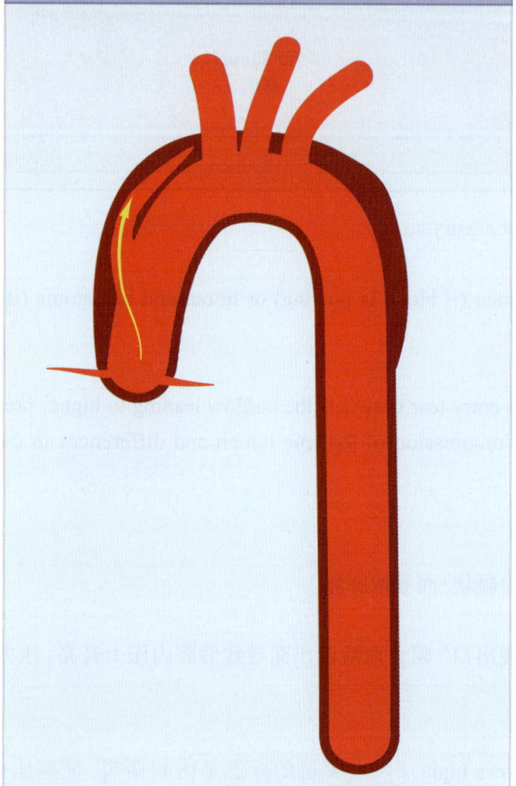

Stanford A
Stanford A型

Stanford B aortic dissection:
Non-ascending aorta *Typically treated medically*
Stanford B型主动脉夹层
未累及升主动脉保守治疗为主

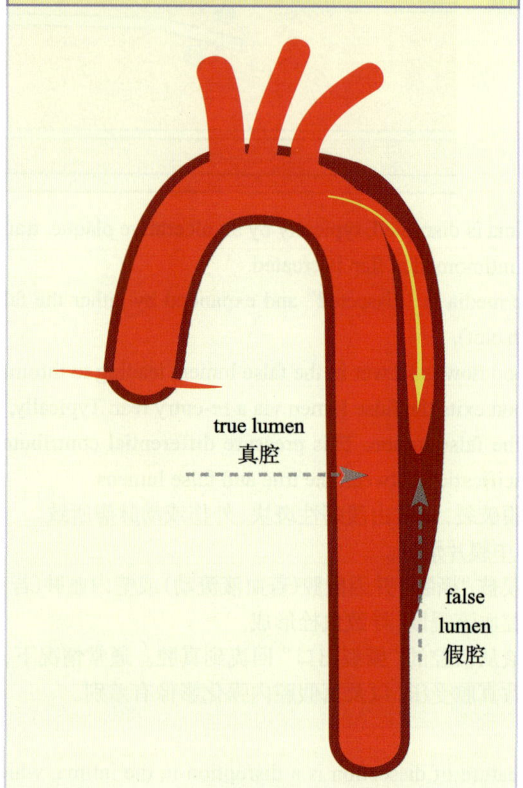

Stanford B
Stanford B型

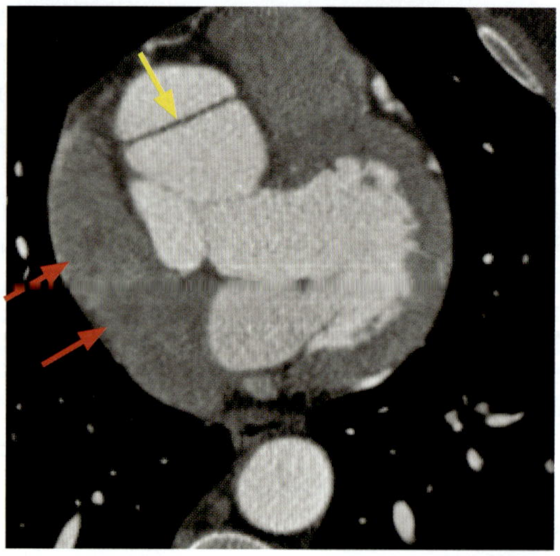

Axial gated CTA shows a dissection flap in the ascending aorta (yellow arrow) with normal descending aorta. Moderate hemopericardium is consistent with rupture (red arrows).
轴位门控CTA图像显示升主动脉内的夹层内膜片(黄箭)，降主动脉未见异常。有中等量心包积血，为主动脉夹层破裂所致(红箭)。

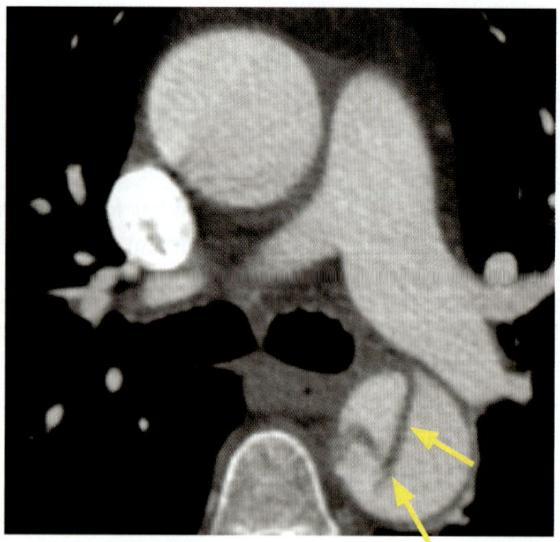

Axial contrast-enhanced gated CT in a different patient shows a dissection flap in the descending aorta only (arrows).
另一名患者的轴位增强门控CT图像显示夹层内膜片仅位于降主动脉(黄箭)。

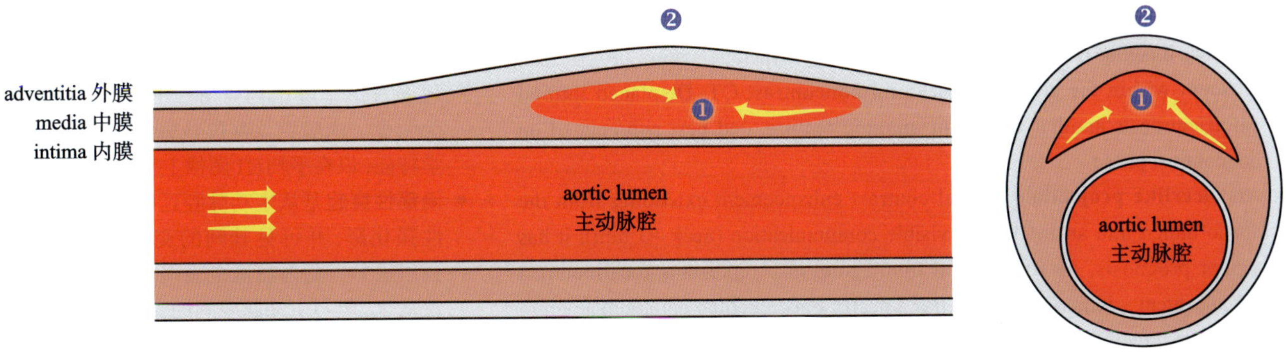

❶ Rupture of vasa vasorum creates crescent-shaped hemorrhage within the media (in cross-sectional view, top right and below left).

❷ There may be associated aneurysm.

The intima is always intact. IMH can be thought of as a noncommunicating dissection.

❶ 滋养血管破裂后导致中膜内新月形出血(横断面,上为右,下为左)。

❷ 可伴有动脉瘤。

内膜始终完整,壁内血肿可以认为是非交通性夹层。

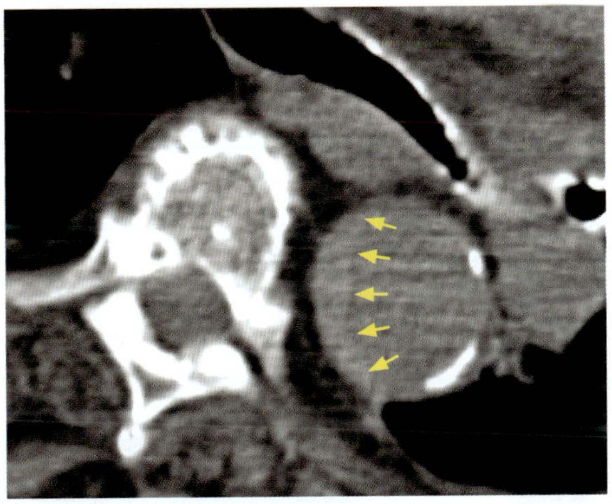

Intramural hematoma on non-contrast CT: Unenhanced CT shows very faint crescent of hyperdense (50 HU) hemorrhage in the descending aorta (arrows).

壁内血肿平扫CT图像:降主动脉非常浅淡的新月形高密度(50HU)出血灶(黄箭)。

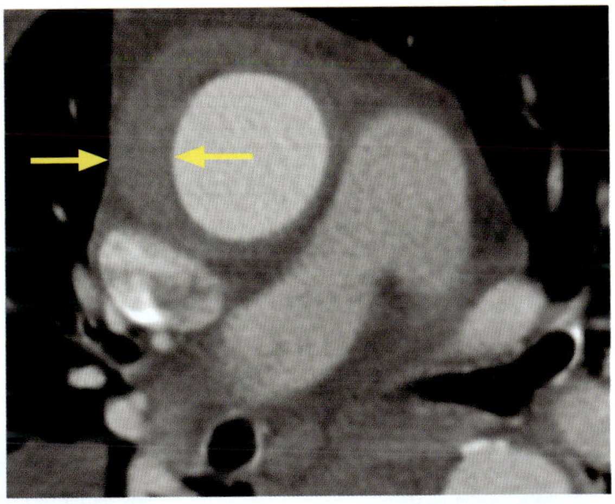

Intramural hematoma on contrast-enhanced CT: Contrast-enhanced CT in a different patient shows a crescentic, hyperattenuating (50 HU) rim reflecting intramural hematoma (arrows). There is no disruption of the aortic lumen.

壁内血肿增强CT图像:另一名患者增强CT图像显示升主动脉新月形高密度环(50HU),为壁内血肿(黄箭)。未见主动脉腔破裂。

- Intramural hematoma (IMH) is a variant of dissection where blood collects within the media, without an intimal flap to connect the intramural hematoma with the aortic lumen. IMH is likely due to rupture of the vasa vasorum, small blood vessels that supply the aortic wall.
- Similar to dissection, IMH may be secondary to hypertension or trauma.
- Clinically, IMH can present identically to aortic dissection with acute tearing back pain. The treatment recommendations for IMH are the same as dissection regarding involvement of the ascending versus descending aorta.
- In **high-risk** patients, unenhanced phase is performed specifically for evaluation of IMH, followed by CTA of the chest, abdomen and pelvis.

- 壁内血肿是主动脉夹层的一种变异,血液聚集在中膜,没有连接壁内血肿与主动脉管腔间的内膜片。IMH可能是供养主动脉壁的小血管(滋养血管)破裂所引起。
- 与主动脉夹层相似,IMH可继发于高血压或外伤。
- 临床上,IMH可表现为急性撕裂样背部疼痛,与主动脉夹层完全相同。IMH的治疗与主动脉夹层一致,取决于病变累及升主动脉还是降主动脉。
- 对**高风险**患者,平扫CT专门用于评估IMH,然后是胸、腹和盆腔CTA。

- In **low-risk** patients, CTA of the chest is monitored by the radiologist; if there is wall thickening, noncontrast scan 6+ hours later can evaluate for IMH versus vasculitis.
- The key imaging finding of IMH is a peripheral hyperattenuating (60–70 HU) crescent within the aorta, best seen on noncontrast CT. Displaced intimal calcification is another important imaging feature, and best appreciated on noncontrast phase.
- An **ulcerlike projection** is focal contrast enhancement extending from the aortic lumen into an IMH via a visible communication (neck >3 mm); it has a poor prognosis. An **intramural blood pool** also represents focal contrast enhancement within an IMH but has a nearly imperceptible communication to the aortic lumen; its prognosis is unclear.

- 对**低风险**患者，放射科医师应对胸部CTA进行即刻检查；若发现血管壁增厚，6小时后再行平扫CT可以区分IMH或血管炎。
- 壁内血肿典型的影像学表现是主动脉边缘出现新月形密度增高区(60~70HU)，CT平扫最为明显。内膜钙化移位是另一个重要的影像学特征，以在平扫CT图像上观察最佳。
- **溃疡性突起**是从主动脉腔延伸到IMH的局灶性强化影，并可见其间的交通(颈部>3mm)，预后很差。**壁内血池**也表现为IMH内的局灶性强化，但与主动脉腔间的交通难以辨认，其预后尚不明。

PENETRATING ATHEROSCLEROTIC ULCER (PAU)

穿透性动脉粥样硬化性溃疡(PAU)

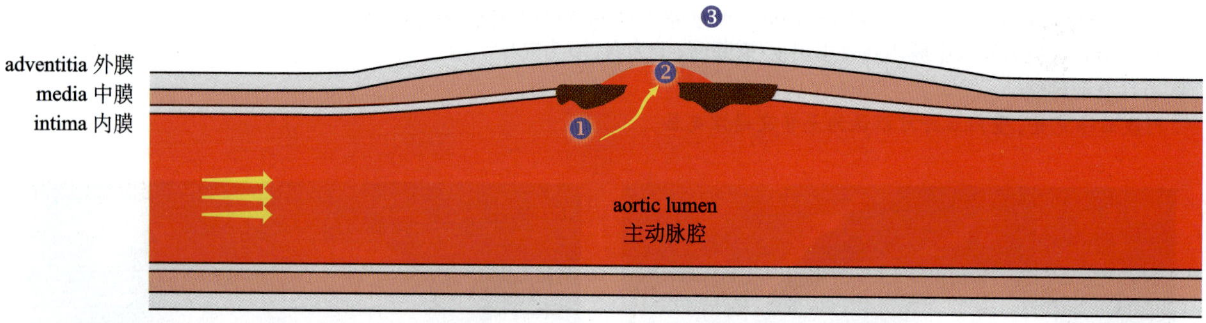

❶ Atherosclerotic plaque penetrates the intima.
❷ Atherosclerotic plaque ulcerates, allowing blood to extend into the media.
❸ PAU may cause the media to enlarge, leading to an aneurysm formation.
❶ 粥样硬化斑块穿透内膜。
❷ 粥样硬化斑块溃疡形成，血液进入中膜。
❸ 穿透性动脉粥样硬化性溃疡可能使中膜扩张，导致动脉瘤形成。

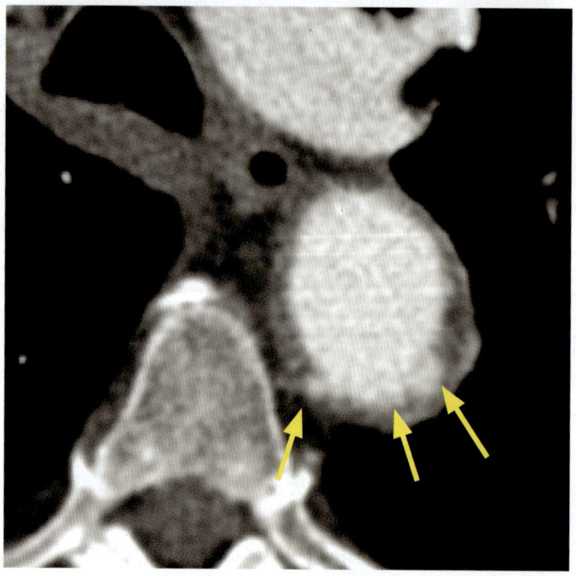

Axial contrast-enhanced CT shows multiple penetrating ulcers (arrows) in the descending aorta, extending beyond the expected contour of the aortic lumen.
轴位增强CT显示在降主动脉多发穿透性溃疡(黄箭)，突出于主动脉腔轮廓之外。

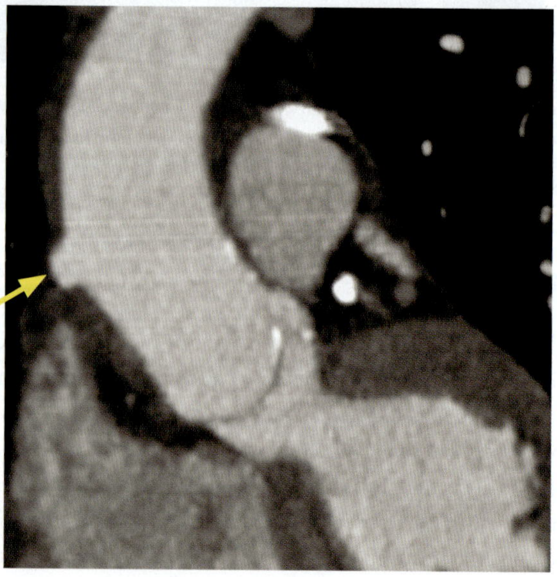

Sagittal oblique gated contrast-enhanced CT in a different patient shows a penetrating atherosclerotic ulcer (arrow) of the ascending aorta, extending beyond the expected contour of the lumen.
斜矢状位增强门控CT显示另一名患者升主动脉穿透性粥样硬化性溃疡(黄箭)，突出于主动脉腔轮廓之外。

- Penetrating atherosclerotic ulcer (PAU) is a focal defect in the intima that occurs at the site of an atherosclerotic plaque. PAU may lead to saccular aneurysm formation.
- In contrast to dissection and IMH, PAU tends to be caused by atherosclerosis rather than hypertension. One of the theories of dissection secondary to atherosclerosis is that it begins as a penetrating ulcer.
- On imaging, PAU appears as contrast-filled outpouching of the aortic wall extending beyond the expected contour of the aortic wall.

  The primary differential would be a simple **ulcerated atherosclerotic plaque**, which would not extend beyond the expected contour of the aortic wall. Ulcerated atherosclerotic plaque represents chronic atherosclerotic disease and is not an acute aortic syndrome.

  PAU differs from an ulcerlike projection in that the latter is a consequence of an IMH and therefore is usually not visible on initial imaging, and it may occur in patients without atherosclerosis.
- Multiple ulcers may be present throughout the aorta, and as with all acute aortic pathologies, imaging of the full aorta is recommended if a PAU is seen.

- 穿透性动脉粥样硬化性溃疡(PAU)是发生在粥样硬化斑块基础上的内膜局部缺损，可导致囊状动脉瘤形成。
- 与主动脉夹层和IMH不同，PAU往往由粥样硬化而非高血压所导致。动脉粥样硬化导致的夹层理论之一是夹层始于穿透性溃疡。
- 影像学上，PAU表现为造影剂突出于主动脉轮廓外。

  主要的鉴别诊断为单纯的溃疡性粥样硬化斑块，其不突出于主动脉轮廓外。溃疡性动脉粥样硬化斑块是一种慢性粥样硬化性疾病，不属于急性主动脉综合征。

  PAU与溃疡样突起的不同之处在于，后者是IMH的结果，基线成像时常不可见，且可发生在无动脉粥样硬化的患者。
- 多发性溃疡可出现在主动脉的任何部位，与所有的急性主动脉疾病一样，若发现PAU，建议对整个主动脉进行成像。

（翻译 卢陈英）

TRAUMATIC AORTIC INJURY

创伤性主动脉损伤

Aortic trauma

主动脉创伤

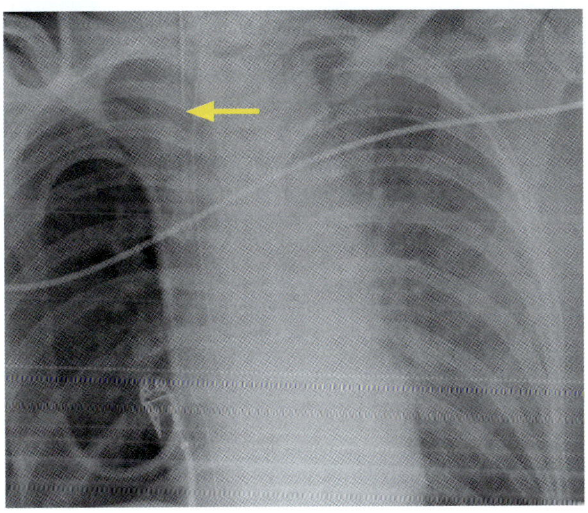

Chest radiograph in a trauma patient shows indistinct widening of the mediastinum. The endotracheal tube is displaced to the right (arrow).
胸片显示一名外伤患者模糊增宽的纵隔，气管插管向右移位(黄箭)。

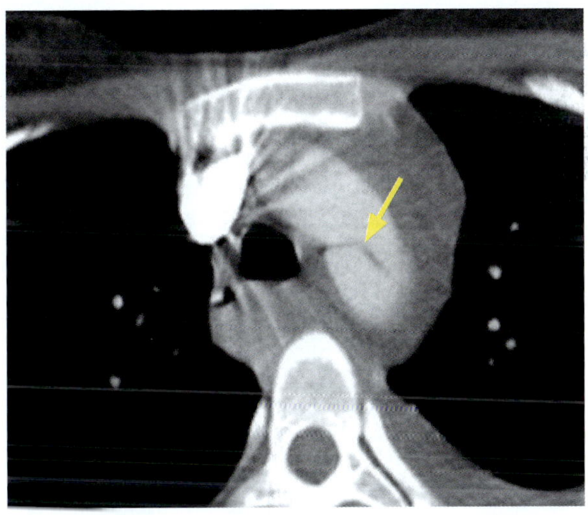

Contrast-enhanced CT shows a mediastinal hematoma and traumatic aortic dissection (arrow). Indistinctness of the lateral arch of the aorta is concerning for tear.
增强CT显示纵隔血肿及外伤性主动脉夹层(黄箭)。主动脉弓外侧缘模糊，疑似有撕裂。

Aortic trauma: *Case courtesy Michael Hanley, MD, University of Virginia Health System.*

- There are three relatively fixed levels of the aorta where traumatic aortic injuries occur secondary to deceleration injury, which are the aortic root, isthmus, and hiatus. The aortic isthmus is the most common location for aortic injuries. Aortic trauma could result in 1) minimal aortic injury, 2) aortic laceration, 3) aortic transection, or 4) aortic pseudoaneurysm.

- 主动脉有三个相对固定的部位，它们在减速运动时可出现损伤，这三个位置分别是主动脉根部、主动脉峡部及主动脉裂孔。主动脉峡部是主动脉损伤最常见的部位。主动脉创伤可导致：①轻微主动脉损伤；②主动脉撕裂；

- Associated injuries to the origins of the brachiocephalic, left carotid, or left subclavian arteries are frequently present.
- CTA is the gold standard for evaluation of suspected traumatic aortic injury.
- Traumatic mediastinal hemorrhage is often venous; however, aortic injury is the primary concern. Direct CT signs of traumatic aortic injury include: intimal irregularity, dissection flap, pseudoaneurysm, or intramural hematoma.

Mediastinal hemorrhage that is separated from an intact aorta by a fat plane can be presumed to be venous, and treatment is conservative. In contrast, hemorrhage in contact with the aortic wall is suggestive of aortic injury and necessitates surgical treatment.

③主动脉横断；或④主动脉假性动脉瘤。

- 常合并头臂干、左颈总动脉和左锁骨下动脉起始处的损伤。
- CT血管成像是评估可疑外伤性主动脉损伤的“金标准”。
- 外伤性纵隔出血多来自静脉，但首先要考虑是否有主动脉损伤。主动脉损伤的直接CT征象包括内膜不规则、夹层内膜片、假性动脉瘤或壁内血肿。

当发现纵隔出血被脂肪层与完整的主动脉完全分离时，可推断为静脉出血，采用保守治疗。相比这下，若出血紧贴主动脉壁，提示主动脉损伤，须外科手术治疗。

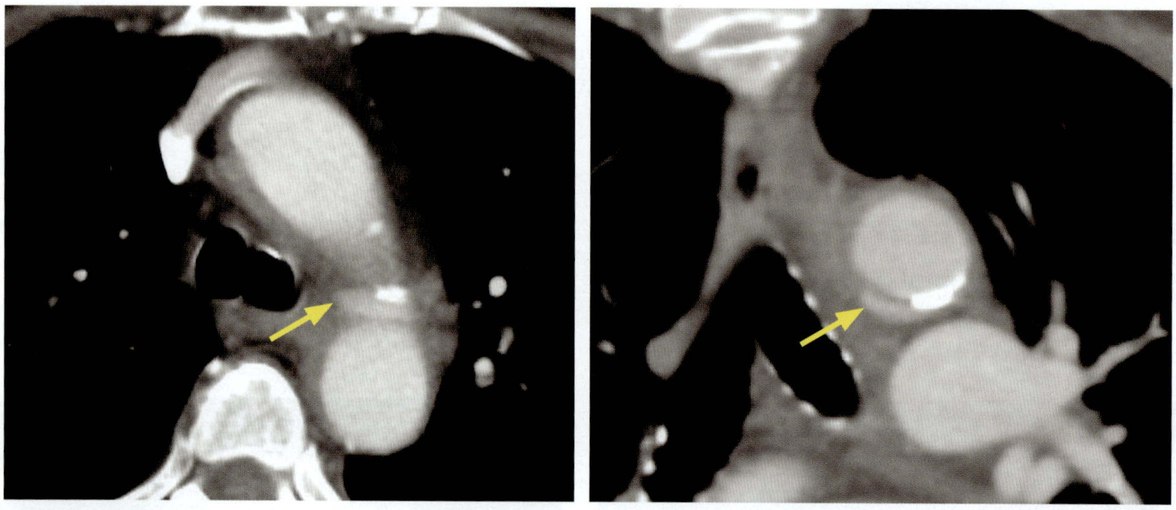

Aortic trauma: Contrast-enhanced axial (left image) and coronal (right image) CT show focal disruption of the isthmus and adjacent small hematoma (arrows) consistent with acute aortic injury.
主动脉外伤：轴位(左图)及冠状位(右图)增强CT显示主动脉峡部局部破裂，邻近见小血肿(黄箭)，符合急性主动脉损伤表现。

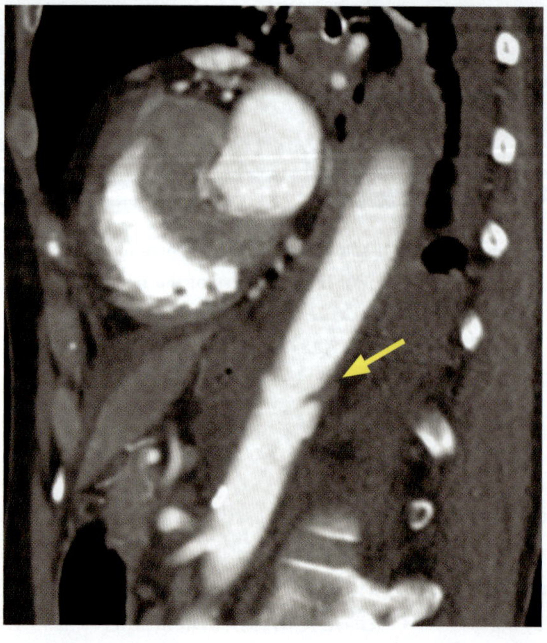

Aortic trauma: Aortic transection at the level of the diaphragmatic crus (arrow), a common area of injury due to anchoring of structures at the diaphragmatic level.
主动脉外伤：膈肌脚水平主动脉横断伤(黄箭)，该区结构固定，是主动脉常见的损伤部位。

Minimal aortic injury

- Approximately 10–30% of blunt traumatic aortic injuries are minimal aortic injury lesions that involve only the intima.
- Mechanisms include rapid deceleration, shearing forces, water-hammer phenomenon, and osseous pinch against the thoracic spine.
- Most common CT findings are intimal irregularity, small intimal flap (<1cm) with no or little periaortic hematoma, intraluminal aortic thrombus or intramural hematoma.

Pseudoaneurysm

- Post-traumatic pseudoaneurysm is a contained rupture held in place by the surrounding connective tissues. The most classic location is the aortic isthmus.
- 85% of pseudoaneurysms are due to penetrating trauma, 15% from blunt trauma such as motor vehicle accidents or falls. Rarely, they occur due to non-traumatic pathologies such as penetrating atherosclerotic ulcers.
- Chronic pseudoaneurysm can develop in the setting of undiagnosed or untreated aortic injury. On imaging, they often have extensive peripheral calcification and may contain thrombus. Calcification is considered to be protective against rupture.

轻微主动脉损伤

- 10%~30%的钝性主动脉损伤为轻伤，仅累及主动脉内膜。
- 机制包括快速减速、剪切力、水锤现象和推向胸椎的骨性挤压。
- 最常见的CT表现为主动脉内膜不规则、小的内膜片(<1cm)，无或极少伴有主动脉周围血肿、主动脉腔内血栓或壁内血肿。

假性动脉瘤

- 创伤后假性动脉瘤是一种由周围结缔组织围绕的包裹性破裂。最典型的位置是主动脉峡部。
- 约85%的假性动脉瘤由穿透伤引起，15%为钝性损伤所致，如机动车事故或跌倒。罕见由非创伤性病变导致，如穿透性动脉粥样硬化性溃疡。
- 主动脉损伤若未得到及时诊断或治疗可发展为慢性假性动脉瘤。影像学上，假性动脉瘤常有广泛的边缘钙化，可含有血栓。钙化被认为具有预防假性动脉瘤破裂的作用。

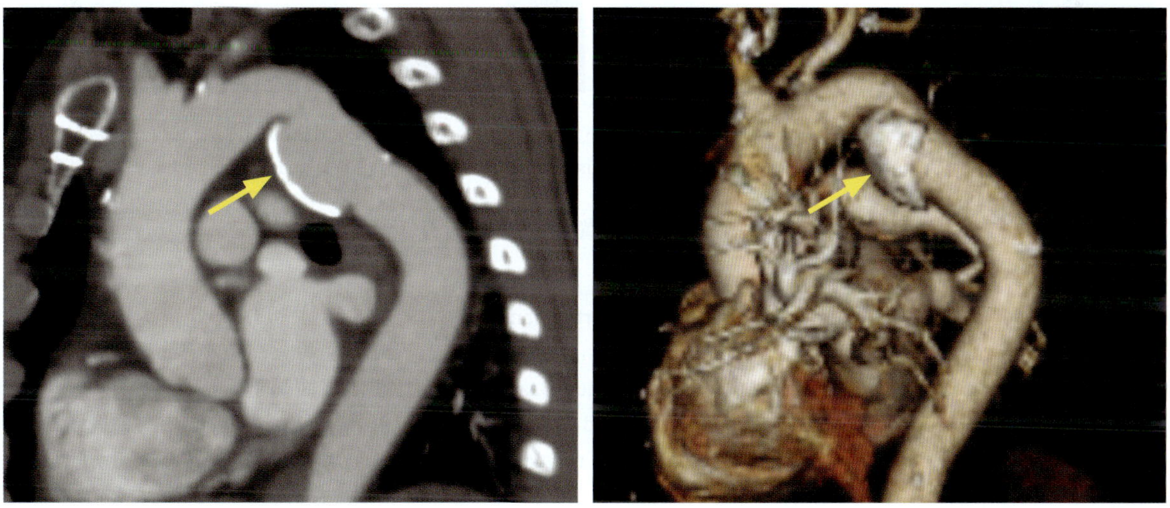

Chronic pseudoaneurysm: Sagittal oblique CTA (left image) and 3D reconstruction image (right) show a peripherally calcified post-traumatic pseudoaneurysm at the aortic isthmus (arrows).
慢性假性动脉瘤：斜矢状位CTA(左图)和3D重组(右图)图像显示主动脉峡部一处边缘钙化的创伤后假性动脉瘤(黄箭)。

(翻译　周帆)

THORACIC AORTA

THORACIC AORTIC ANEURYSM

Thoracic aortic aneurysm (TAA)

胸主动脉

胸主动脉瘤

胸主动脉瘤(TAA)

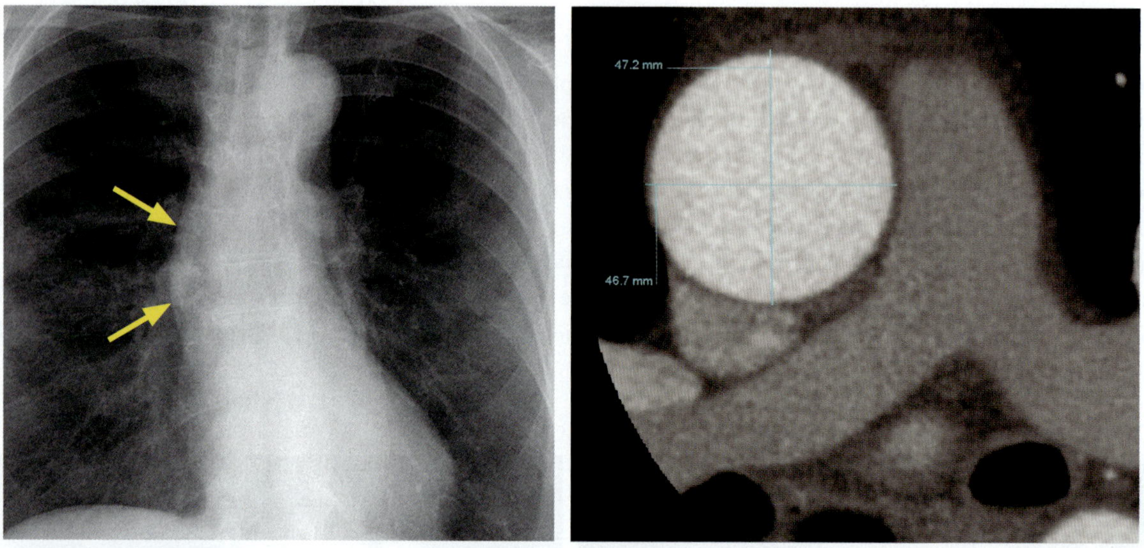

Thoracic aortic aneurysm: Frontal chest radiograph (left image) demonstrates ectasia of the right aortic border (arrows). Gated contrast-enhanced CT (right image) with a double-oblique short-axis reformation demonstrates an ascending aortic diameter of 4.7 cm, representing an aneurysm.

胸主动脉瘤:胸部正位X线影像(左图)示主动脉右侧边缘膨出(黄箭)。双斜位短轴门控增强CT(右图)显示升主动脉直径4.7cm,此为动脉瘤。

- A thoracic aortic aneurysm (TAA) is defined as an ascending aortic diameter >4 cm or a descending thoracic aorta >3.5 cm in diameter. Aortic size may also be normalized to body surface area and compared to reference values. Based on Framingham Heart Study participants, ascending aorta >5 cm and descending aorta >4 cm are considered 150% or two standard deviations of normal, and thus aneurysmal.
- Double-oblique short-axis multiplanar reformatted images perpendicular to the aortic lumen (i.e., true short-axis) should always be used to measure aortic diameter.
- Most thoracic aortic aneurysms are caused by atherosclerosis, with the descending thoracic aorta affected more commonly. Almost 1/3 of patients with atherosclerotic TAA will have an associated abdominal aortic aneurysm.
- Non-atherosclerotic causes of TAA include connective tissue disorders (such as Marfan and Ehlers-Danlos syndromes), bicuspid aortic valve (BAV) associated aortopathy, vasculitis (including Takayasu arteritis, giant cell arteritis, ankylosing spondylitis, and relapsing polychondritis), cystic medial necrosis, and infectious aortitis.
- **Annuloaortic ectasia** represents dilated sinuses of Valsalva and ascending aorta with effacement of the sinotubular junction, resulting in a tulip bulb-shaped aorta. Annuloaortic ectasia is associated with Marfan, Ehlers-Danlos syndrome, homocystinuria, and osteogenesis imperfecta.
- Surgical treatment is recommended for an ascending TAA >5.5 cm in diameter and a descending TAA >6 cm in diameter. However, patients with connective tissue disorders and BAV aortopathy (meeting criteria for valve replacement)

- 胸主动脉瘤(TAA)定义为升主动脉直径>4cm或降主动脉直径>3.5cm。主动脉大小也可以按体表面积进行标准化,并与参考值进行比较。基于Framingham心脏研究受试者的数据,升主动脉直径>5cm和降主动脉直径>4cm被认为达到正常值的150%或相差2个标准差,因此属于动脉瘤。
- 测量主动脉直径应始终使用双斜短轴的多平面重组图像,与主动脉腔垂直(即真正的短轴)。
- 大多数胸主动脉瘤由动脉粥样硬化引起,其中降主动脉更易受累。约1/3的动脉粥样硬化性TAA患者同时有腹主动脉瘤。
- 导致非动脉粥样硬化性TAA的原因包括结缔组织疾病(如马方综合征及埃勒斯-当洛综合征)、二叶主动脉瓣(BAV)相关主动脉疾病、血管炎(包括大动脉炎、巨细胞动脉炎、强直性脊柱炎和复发性多软骨炎)、囊性中层坏死及感染性主动脉炎。
- **主动脉环扩张**是指主动脉窦及升主动脉扩张伴升主动脉窦管连接处消失,形成"郁金香"样球形主动脉。主动脉环扩张与马方综合征、埃勒斯-当洛综合征、高胱氨酸尿症及成骨不全相关。
- 升主动脉瘤直径>5.5cm或降主动脉瘤直径>6cm时建议外科治疗。若患者伴有结缔组织

have a lower surgical threshold of 3.5cm. Beyond simple size criteria, annual growth rate >1 cm/year (or >5 mm/6 months) is an indication for surgical repair.

- Complications of TAA endoscopic and open repair include rupture, dissection, infection, endoleak, and paraplegia (caused by artery of Adamkiewicz occlusion).

病及BAV相关主动脉疾病(满足瓣膜置换标准),其外科治疗阈值可降至3.5cm。除上述简单标准外,增长率>1cm/年(或>5mm/6个月)也是外科修复的指征。

- 腔内及开放性手术修复TAA的并发症包括主动脉破裂、夹层、感染、内漏及截瘫(由Adamkiewicz动脉闭塞引起)。

INFLAMMATORY AND INFECTIOUS DISORDERS

炎症及感染性疾病

- Inflammatory disorders involving the thoracic aorta and great vessels include giant cell arteritis, Takayasu arteritis, rheumatologic disorders, and radiation-induced aortitis.
- Infectious causes of aortitis include syphilis, tuberculosis, pyogenic (especially *Salmonella*), HIV, and mycotic etiologies.

- 累及胸主动脉和大血管的炎症性疾病包括巨细胞动脉炎、Takayasu动脉炎(大动脉炎)、风湿病及辐射引起的主动脉炎。
- 感染引起的主动脉炎的包括梅毒、结核、化脓性(尤其是沙门菌)、HIV及真菌。

Giant cell arteritis (GCA)

巨细胞动脉炎(GCA)

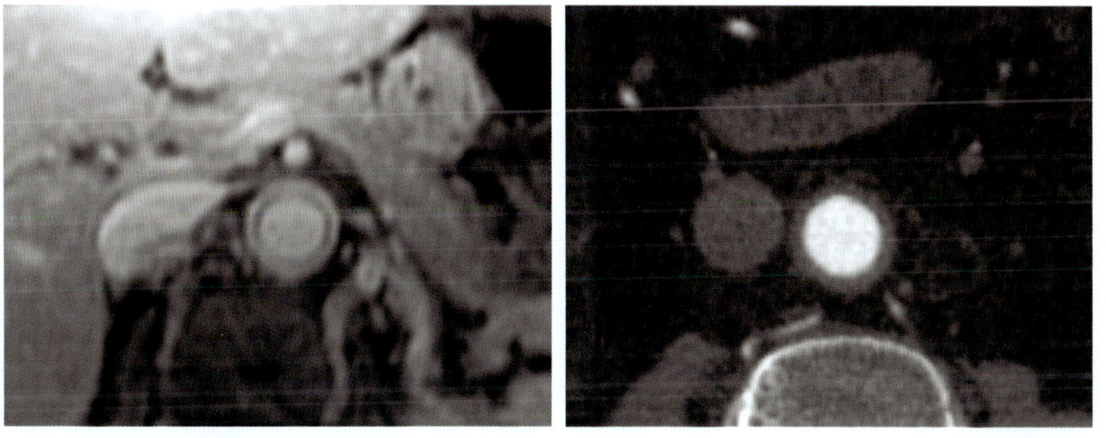

Giant cell arteritis: Two different patients with temporal artery biopsy proven GCA. MRA of the suprarenal aorta (left image) and axial CTA (right image) through the infrarenal aorta demonstrate circumferential aortic wall thickening.
巨细胞动脉炎:经颞动脉活检确诊的两名GCA患者。肾动脉以上主动脉MRA(左图)和肾动脉以下主动脉轴位CTA(右图)均表现为主动脉环周壁增厚。

- Giant cell arteritis (GCA) is predominantly a medium-and large-vessel vasculitis that has overlapping imaging findings with Takayasu arteritis. GCA tends to affect older patients (typically greater than 50 years of age) compared to Takayasu arteritis.
- The medium-sized upper extremity arteries are most commonly affected in GCA, including the subclavian, axillary, and brachial arteries. The aorta is rarely involved, unlike in Takayasu arteritis. GCA typically produces long smooth stenoses.
- In comparison, Takayasu arteritis often involves the aorta and is commonly associated with occlusions.
- Definitive diagnosis is with temporal artery biopsy. However, biopsy results could be false negative up to 28% of cases, due to skip lesions or aortic involvement only.
- Imaging findings of GCA on CTA or MRA are circumferential wall thickening of the aortic segments and associated luminal narrowing or aneurysmal dilation.
- FDG-PET/CT also can help in the diagnosis of the large vessel vasculitis: moderate to intense FDG uptake in the involved vessels is the key imaging finding.
- Treatment is steroids and tocilizumab (anti-IL-6).

- 巨细胞动脉炎(CAG)是主要累及中、大血管的血管炎,影像学表现与Takayasu动脉炎相似。GCA较Takayasu动脉炎更好发于年龄较大的患者(通常50岁以上)。
- GCA常累及中等大小的上肢动脉,包括锁骨下动脉、腋动脉及肱动脉。GCA很少累及主动脉,此与Takayasu动脉炎不同。GCA通常引起长而光滑的狭窄。
- 相比之下,Takayasu动脉炎常累及主动脉,并常伴有闭塞。
- 确诊需行颞动脉活检,但高达28%的活检结果存在假阴性,这是由于病变呈跳跃性或仅累及主动脉。
- GCA在CTA或MRA上表现为主动脉呈节段性环形管壁增厚伴管腔狭窄或动脉瘤样扩张。
- FDG PET/CT也有助于大血管炎的诊断:受累血管出现中等至强烈的FDG摄取是关键的影像学发现。
- 治疗采用激素和tocilizumab(抗白介素-6)。

Infectious aortitis

- Infectious aortitis most commonly presents as a mycotic aneurysm and less commonly as non-aneurysmal infection, although both may be complicated by rupture.
- Pre-existing abnormality in the wall including atherosclerotic disease could make it susceptible for infection.
- Most common pathogens are *Staph. aureus, Salmonella, Pneumococcus,* and *E. coli*.
- Syphilitic aortitis is a rare cause of aortic wall thickening and aneurysmal dilatation, usually limited to the thoracic aorta.
- CTA, MRA or FDG-PET/CT can be used in the diagnosis of the infectious aortitis.
- Key imaging features are focal, crescentic shape aortic wall thickening, periaortic soft-tissue accumulation, and rapid progression of saccular/mycotic aneurysm or pseudoaneurysm.

感染性主动脉炎

- 感染性主动脉炎最常表现为真菌性动脉瘤，而较少表现为非动脉瘤样感染，但两者均可并发破裂。
- 若动脉管壁有基础病变，如动脉粥样硬化性疾病，更易发生感染。
- 常见的病原体是金黄色葡萄球菌、沙门菌、肺炎球菌及大肠埃希菌。
- 梅毒性主动脉炎是一种罕见引起主动脉壁增厚和动脉瘤样扩张的原因，通常仅限于胸主动脉。
- CTA、MRA或FDG PET/CT可用于诊断感染性主动脉炎。
- 关键的影像学特征是局灶性新月形主动脉壁增厚、主动脉周围软组织增多及快速进展的囊状/感染性动脉瘤或假性动脉瘤。

Takayasu arteritis

Takayasu 动脉炎

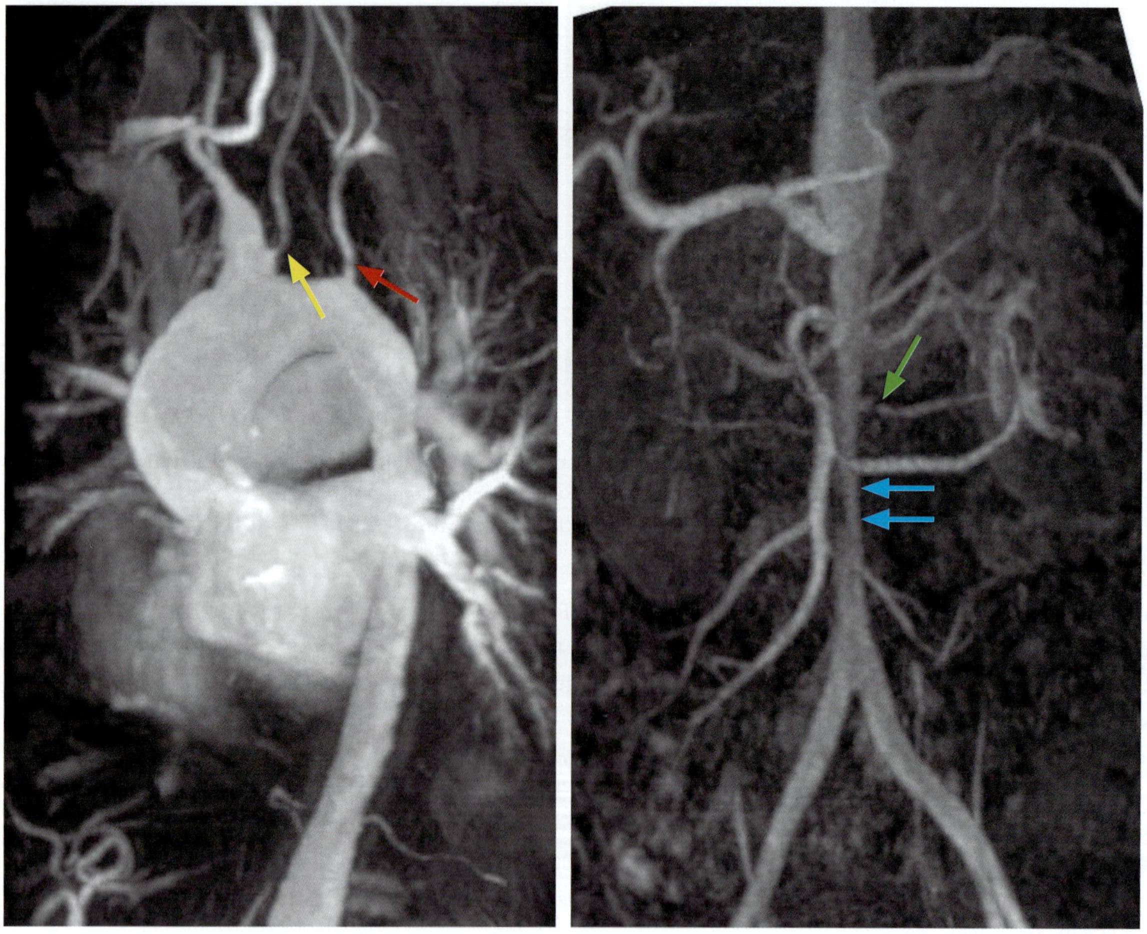

Takayasu arteritis: Sagittal-oblique maximum intensity projection MR angiogram (left image) of the aortic arch shows narrowing of the left common carotid artery (yellow arrow) and left subclavian artery (red arrow). Note the incidental common origin of the brachiocephalic trunk and the left common carotid artery.

Coronal maximum intensity projection MR angiogram (right image) of the abdominal aorta in the same patient shows a long smooth stenosis of the infra-celiac abdominal aorta (blue arrows), with a focal stenosis of the accessory left renal artery (green arrow).

Case courtesy Michael Hanley, MD, University of Virginia Health System.

Takayasu动脉炎：主动脉弓MR斜矢状位最大密度投影血管成像(左图)显示左侧颈总动脉(黄箭)和左侧锁骨下动脉狭窄(红箭)。注意一个意外发现，头臂干和左颈总动脉有共同起源。

同一名患者腹主动脉MR冠状位最大密度投影血管成像(右图)显示腹主动脉下段有细长平滑的狭窄(蓝箭)，并发左侧副肾动脉局灶性狭窄(绿箭)。

- Takayasu arteritis is an idiopathic, inflammatory, large-vessel vasculitis that involves the thoracic and abdominal aorta, subclavian arteries, carotid arteries, pulmonary arteries, and large mesenteric arteries.
- Takayasu arteritis typically affects young to middle-aged women.
- There are two phases in Takayasu's arteritis:

  a) **Pre-pulseless** phase, which is characterized by the nonspecific constitutional symptoms including mild fever, malaise, weight loss;

  b) **Pulseless** phase, where the patients present with limb ischemia or renovascular hypertension due to arterial stenosis or occlusion. The patients are often imaged in pulseless phase.
- On imaging, long smooth circumferential arterial wall thickening with areas of stenoses and/or occlusions are classic. Imaging is often indistinguishable from giant cell arteritis, with the patient's age being the main distinguishing factor. Takayasu arteritis occurs in relatively younger patients and giant cell arteritis is rare in patients under age 50.
- During the acute phase, treatment is with steroids. If symptomatic stenoses occur, endovascular treatment can be performed, but only when the active inflammation has resolved, as measured by normalization of the erythrocyte sedimentation rate.

- Takayasu动脉炎是一种特发的炎性大血管炎，可累及胸和腹主动脉、锁骨下动脉、颈动脉、肺动脉及肠系膜动脉。
- Takayasu动脉炎常发生于中青年女性。
- Takayasu动脉炎分为两个阶段：

  a) 无脉前期：表现为非特异性全身症状，包括轻度发热、不适、体重减轻；

  b) 无脉期：因动脉狭窄或闭塞出现肢体缺血或肾血管性高血压。患者多于无脉期进行影像学检查。
- 经典的影像学表现为主动脉壁呈光滑和环形增厚，伴多发局部管腔狭窄和/或闭塞。影像学上通常难以与巨细胞性动脉炎进行区分，患者年龄是鉴别的主要依据。Takayasu动脉炎发生在相对年轻的患者，而巨细胞性动脉炎在50岁以下的患者中比较罕见。
- 急性期可选用类固醇治疗。如果狭窄引起症状，可采用血管腔内治疗，但活动性炎症必须得到控制，其指标为红细胞沉降率恢复正常。

Occlusive disorders

闭塞性疾病

Aortic coarctation

主动脉缩窄

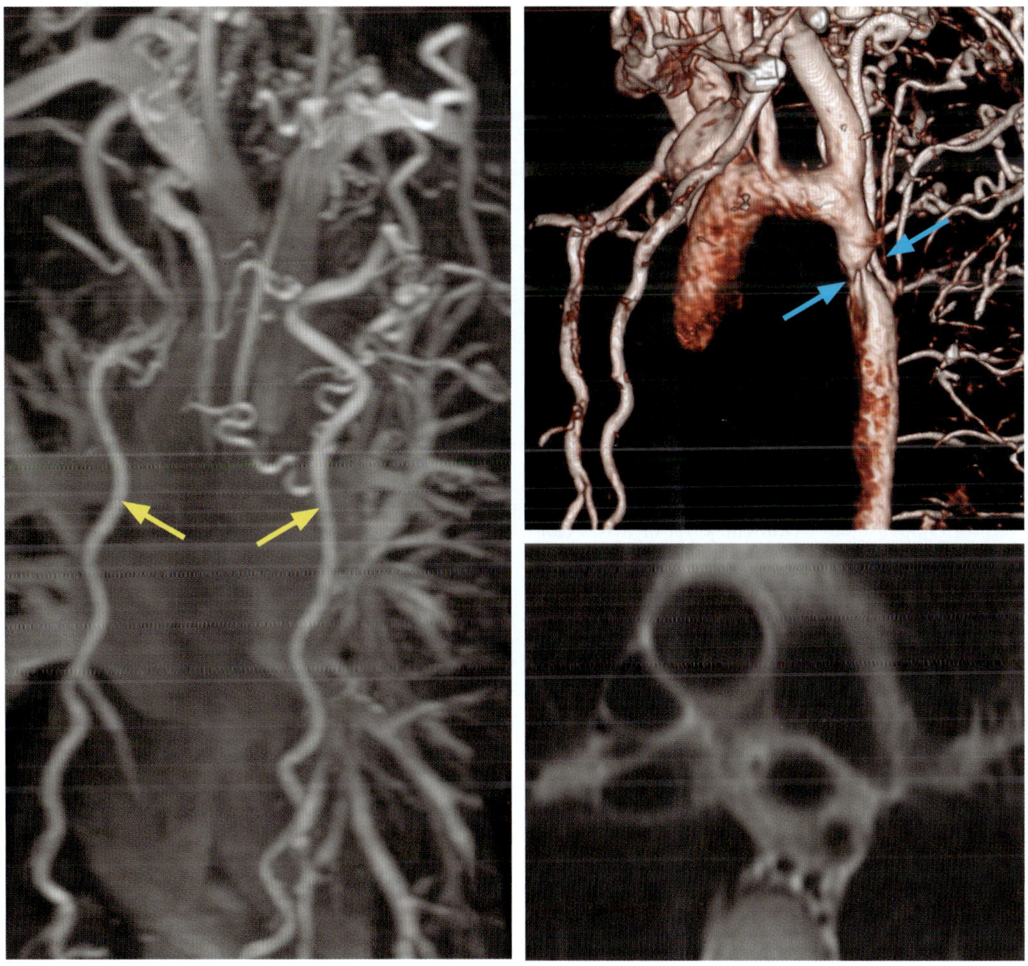

Aortic coarctation: Coronal maximum intensity projection MR angiogram (left image) shows extensive collateral vessels throughout the thorax, with prominent internal thoracic arteries (yellow arrows). 3D volume rendered CT of the aorta (top right image) demonstrates the coarctation (blue arrows) distal to the aortic isthmus. Double inversion recovery fast spin echo MRI (bottom right image) also demonstrates the coarctation.

主动脉缩窄：冠状位最大密度投影MR血管成像(左图)显示胸部广泛的侧支血管，胸廓内动脉明显增粗(黄箭)。主动脉CT 3D容积再现重组图像(右上图)显示位于主动脉峡部远端的缩窄(蓝箭)。双翻转恢复快速自旋回波序列的MRI图像(右下图)亦显示缩窄处。

- Aortic coarctation is congenital focal narrowing of the proximal descending aorta.
- The adult form of coarctation is usually *juxtaductal* (at the junction of the ductus arteriosus), leading to upper extremity hypertension. In contrast, an infant presenting with congestive heart failure due to coarctation is usually due to a *preductal* variant, which functions as a left ventricular obstructive lesion.
- In the setting of coarctation, prominent collaterals develop between the internal thoracic arteries to both the epigastric vessels and intercostal arteries.
- The radiographic findings of coarctation include the *3-sign* of the left upper heart border, which represents a double bulge from the focal aortic narrowing and post-stenotic dilation. Rib notching is frequently seen from collateral intercostal vessels.
- Phase contrast MR imaging can be used to measure the gradient of flow across the coarctation. Calculation of the flow differential between the proximal descending aorta versus the aorta at the hiatus aids in determining hemodynamic significance.
- Aortic coarctation is associated with other cardiovascular anomalies, including bicuspid aortic valve (most common, 75–80%), ventricular septal defect, cyanotic congenital cardiac anomalies, mitral valve abnormalities (parachute mitral valve), and patent ductus arteriosus.
- Aortic coarctation could also be one of the 4 components of **Shone syndrome** – a left-sided obstructive congenital heart disease that involves: 1) Supravalvular mitral membrane, 2) subvalvular aortic stenosis, 3) parachute mitral valve, 4) aortic coarctation.
- A *pseudocoarctation* represents kinking or buckling of the aorta, similar in morphology to a true coarctation; however, there is no pressure differential and thus no collaterals.

Subclavian steal syndrome

- Subclavian steal syndrome is a proximal stenosis or occlusion of the subclavian artery, which leads to retrograde flow from the vertebral artery into the subclavian artery distal to the flow-limiting lesion.
- Subclavian steal syndrome clinically presents with vertebrobasilar insufficiency or syncope exacerbated by arm exercise. There may occasionally be direct signs of brachial artery insufficiency, such as extremity coolness or even fingertip necrosis.
- Subclavian steal is best diagnosed with angiography. The early arterial phase shows the proximal subclavian flow-limiting lesion and the later arterial phase shows retrograde flow from the vertebral artery into the subclavian. However, angiography is usually reserved for endovascular treatment. CTA or MRA can easily detect subclavian artery stenosis.
- Treatment options include surgical bypass or angioplasty of the flow-limiting lesion.

- 主动脉缩窄是先天性近段降主动脉局灶性狭窄。
- 成人型主动脉缩窄常为导管旁型(在动脉导管交界处),可引起上肢高血压。相比之下,婴儿型常为导管前型,在功能上相当于左心室阻塞性病变,表现为充血性心力衰竭。
- 主动脉缩窄时,在胸廓内动脉、上腹部血管和肋间动脉间可形成大量的侧支循环。
- 主动脉缩窄的X线影像表现为左上心缘旁的"3"字征,为主动脉局限性狭窄及狭窄后扩张引起的双膨隆所致。常见肋骨切迹,为肋间动脉侧支血管所致。
- MRI相位对比可用于测量狭窄两端之间的血流梯度。计算降主动脉近端与动脉裂孔水平主动脉间流量差有助于确定血流动力学异常程度。
- 主动脉缩窄可合并其他心血管畸形,包括二叶形主动脉瓣(最常见,占75%~80%)、室间隔缺损、发绀型先天性心脏畸形、二尖瓣畸形(降落伞样二尖瓣)及动脉导管未闭。
- 主动脉缩窄也可以是**Shone综合征**(一种先天性左侧梗阻型心脏病)的四个组成部分之一:①二尖瓣瓣上狭窄;②主动脉瓣下狭窄;③降落伞样二尖瓣;④主动脉缩窄。
- 假性动脉缩窄是指主动脉扭结或弯曲,形态学上与真性主动脉缩窄相似,但无血压差,因而也无侧支血管形成。

锁骨下动脉盗血综合征

- 锁骨下动脉盗血综合征是指近端锁骨下动脉狭窄或闭塞,从而导致椎动脉内血流逆向流动至锁骨下动脉狭窄/闭塞病变的远端。
- 锁骨下动脉盗血综合征的临床表现为椎基底动脉供血不足而引起晕厥,上臂活动后加重。偶可表现为肱动脉供血不足的直接征象,如肢体发凉或指端坏死。
- 锁骨下动脉盗血的最佳诊断方法是血管造影。动脉早期显示锁骨下动脉近端限流性病变,动脉晚期表现为椎动脉血液逆向流入(病变远端的)锁骨下动脉。但血管造影通常仅用于血管腔内治疗。CTA或MRA很容易发现锁骨下动脉狭窄。
- 治疗选择包括外科搭桥或对血流受阻部位进行血管成形术。

Superior vena cava (SVC)

SVC obstruction

- Acute obstruction of the SVC causes SVC syndrome, which clinically presents as facial and upper extremity edema and cyanosis. Acute SVC syndrome is a vascular emergency.
- In contrast to acute SVC syndrome, chronic occlusion or stenosis of the SVC may be asymptomatic. If symptoms are present, facial edema that improves

上腔静脉(SVC)

SVC闭塞

- 急性SVC闭塞会导致SVC综合征,临床表现为面部及上肢水肿和发绀。急性SVC综合征是血管急症。
- 与急性SVC综合征不同,慢性SVC闭塞或狭窄可无症状。若出现症状,面部水肿会在站

with standing is characteristic.

- The most common causes of SVC obstruction are compression by thoracic malignancy, catheter-associated thrombosis, and mediastinal fibrosis after histoplasmosis exposure.
- The classic imaging findings on MRV or CTV are occlusion of the SVC and based on the location (above or below the azygos vein), collateral vessels form.
- A classic cross-sectional abdominal imaging finding in SVC obstruction is increased enhancement of hepatic segment IVa due to collateral opacification of the vein of Sappey.

The vein of Sappey drains the liver in the region of the falciform ligament and communicates with internal thoracic veins, which act as collateral vessels in the setting of SVC occlusion.

Congenital anomalies of the SVC

- Normally, the embryologic left anterior cardinal vein regresses and the right anterior cardinal vein develops into the SVC.
- **Left-sided SVC** is due to persistence of the embryological left anterior cardinal vein and regression of the right anterior cardinal vein. It is the most common congenital venous anomaly in the chest.
- The left SVC usually drains directly into the coronary sinus → right atrium.
- Rarely, the left SVC drains directly into the left atrium, causing a right to left shunt.
- Left-sided SVC is weakly associated with congenital heart disease (CHD). Left SVC is an incidental finding in 0.5% of the population but is seen in 4% of patients with CHD.
- A **duplicated SVC** is due to persistence of both the right and left anterior cardinal veins.
- Duplicated SVC also carries an association with CHD.

立时得到改善，此表现具特征性。

- SVC闭塞最常见的原因是胸部恶性肿瘤压迫、中心静脉置管所致的血栓形成和组织胞浆菌感染所致的纵隔纤维化。
- MRV或CTV上典型的影像学表现为SVC闭塞，并因闭塞的位置(位于奇静脉入口上方或下方)形成不同的侧支。
- SVC闭塞在腹部轴位影像上的典型表现为肝脏Ⅳa段异常强化，为Sappey静脉显影所致。

Sappey静脉引流镰状韧带区域肝组织的血液，并与胸廓内静脉相交通，在SVC闭塞时形成侧支循环。

SVC先天发育异常

- 正常情况下，胚胎左侧前主静脉退化，右侧前主静脉发育成SVC。
- **左侧SVC**是由于胚胎左侧前主静脉的持续存在而右侧前主静脉退化所致，为胸部最常见的先天性静脉异常。
- 左侧SVC通常直接引流至冠状窦→右心房。
- 罕见情况下，左侧SVC直接引流至左心房，导致右向左分流。
- 左侧SVC偶尔合并先天性心脏病(CHD)。左侧SVC在人群中的发生率是0.5%，但在CHD患者中的发生率为4%。
- **双侧SVC**是由于左、右主静脉同时持续存在。
- 双侧上腔静脉也和先天性心脏病有关。

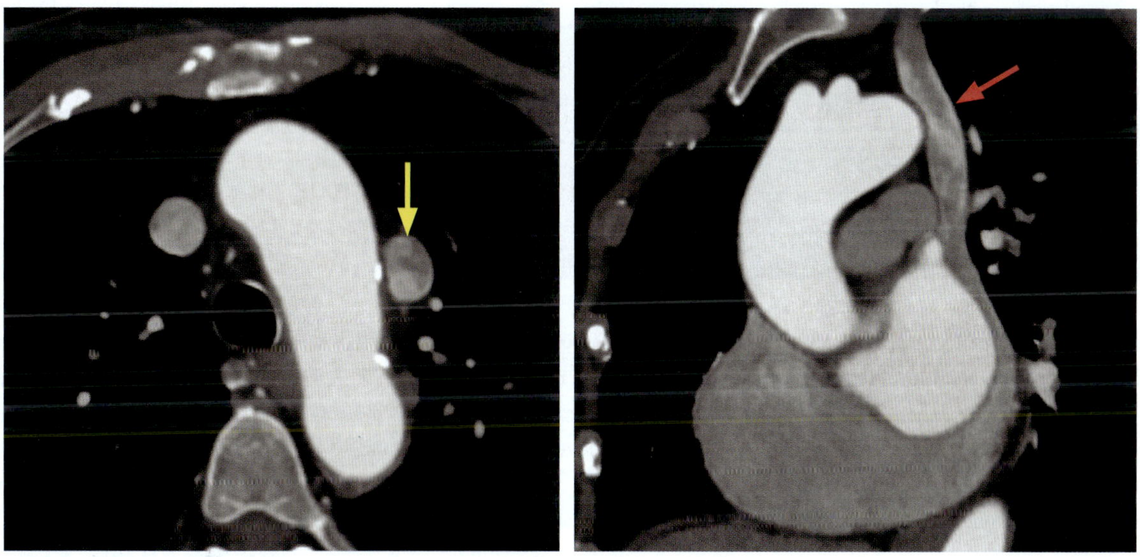

Duplicated SVC: Axial (left image) and coronal oblique (right image) CTA shows a structure with contrast mixing (yellow arrow) on the left of the aortic arch that drains into the coronary sinus on oblique reformatted image (red arrow) in keeping with persistent left-sided SVC in a patient with a normal right-sided SVC.

双侧SVC：轴位(左图)和斜冠状位(右图)CTA显示正常右侧SVC的患者存在永久性左侧SVC，表现为主动脉弓左侧存在一个内有造影剂充盈的结构(黄箭)汇流至冠状窦(斜冠状位重组图像，红箭)。

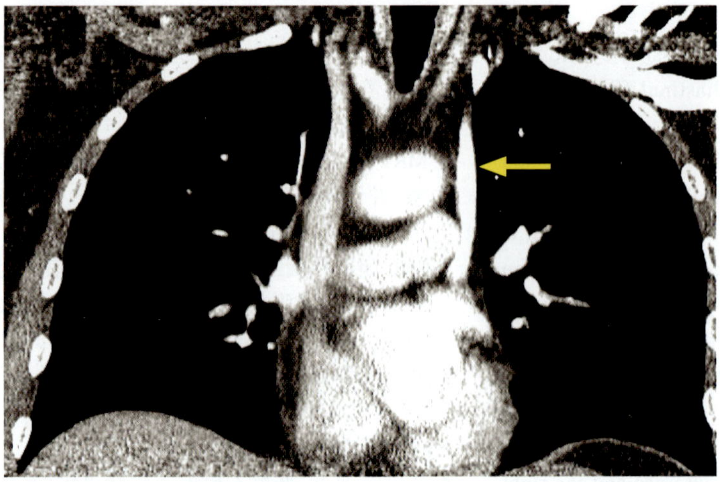

Duplicated SVC in a different patient:
Coronal CTA shows right and left SVCs. The left SVC (arrow) is more opacified with contrast because of the left-sided contrast injection.
双侧SVC患者：冠状位CTA示左侧和右侧SVC。因自左侧前臂注入造影剂，左侧上腔静脉(黄箭)显影更明显。

（翻译　谷涛）

ABDOMINAL AORTA

腹主动脉

ABDOMINAL AORTIC ANEURYSM

腹主动脉瘤

Abdominal aortic aneurysm (AAA)

腹主动脉瘤(AAA)

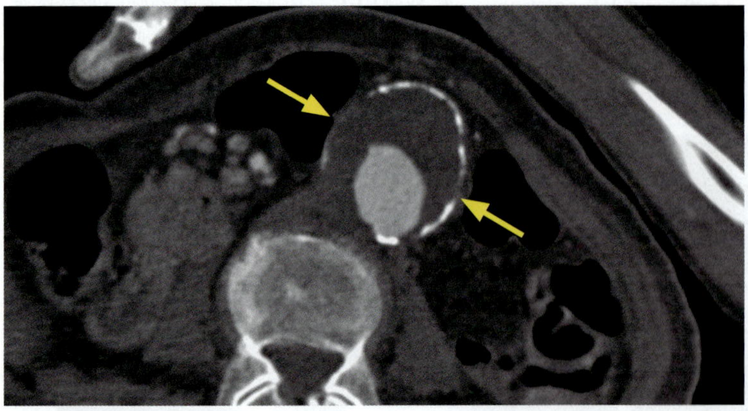

Abdominal aortic aneurysm: Axial CT of the infrarenal aorta demonstrates a large peripherally calcified abdominal aortic aneurysm (arrows) containing extensive mural thrombus.
Case courtesy Michael Hanley, MD, University of Virginia Health System.
腹主动脉瘤：肾下水平主动脉轴位CT显示一个外周钙化的腹主动脉瘤(黄箭)，内含大量附壁血栓。

- An abdominal aortic aneurysm (AAA) is defined as an aortic diameter ≥3 cm.
- AAA is relatively prevalent in older men (seen in up to 5.9% of men by age 80) and less common in women. Rupture of abdominal aortic aneurysm is the thirteenth leading cause of death in older men. Risk factors for development of an AAA include age, male sex, smoking, and family history.
- Similar to measurement of thoracic aortic aneurysms, CT evaluation should include double oblique reformatted images to obtain a true cross-sectional diameter.
- Ultrasound is a principal screening modality for AAA, with a proven mortality benefit in 65–79-year-old men who have ever smoked tobacco. If an aneurysm is present, the diameter is measured in three orthogonal planes.
- Ultrasound screening of high-risk patients is approved by Medicare for patients older than age 65. If an aneurysm is detected on screening, follow-up is recommended:

- 腹主动脉瘤(AAA)的定义为主动脉直径≥3cm。
- 腹主动脉瘤相对好发于老年男性(男性80岁时发生率可达5.9%)，女性较少。腹主动脉瘤破裂是老年男性死亡的第13大主要病因。腹主动脉瘤形成的危险因素包括年龄、男性、吸烟及家族史。
- 与胸主动脉瘤测量方法相同，CT评估应包括双斜位重建图像以获得真正的横断面直径。
- 超声是腹主动脉瘤的主要筛查方式，有证据显示对降低65~79岁有吸烟史的男性腹主动脉瘤患者的死亡概率有益。若发现腹主动脉瘤，应在三个正交平面上对其直径进行测量。
- 美国政府医疗保险(医疗关怀)批准对65岁以上的高危患者进行超声筛查。若在筛查中发现动脉瘤，建议进行随访：

Aneurysm <4 cm: Follow-up in 6 months; if no change → **annual surveillance**.
Aneurysm **4–4.5 cm**: Follow-up in 6 months; if no change → **6-month surveillance**.
Aneurysm **5–5.5 cm**: **Consider surgery**.
Aneurysm **>5.5 cm**: **Surgery recommended**.

腹动脉瘤**<4cm**：6个月时随访；若无改变→**每年检查一次**。
腹动脉瘤**4.0~4.5cm**：6个月时随访；若无改变→**每6个月检查一次**。
腹动脉瘤**5.0~5.5cm**：**考虑手术**。
腹动脉瘤**>5.5cm**：**建议手术**。

Aortic rupture

- Rupture is a complication of aortic aneurysms and is the most important diagnosis that should be excluded in patients with acute chest or abdominal pain, hypotension, and pulsatile abdominal mass.
- 80% of aortic aneurysm rupture occurs in the retroperitoneum, 20% occurs towards the peritoneum, and rarely to the IVC (aorto-caval fistula) or to the bowel (aorto-enteric fistula).
- Risk factors for impending rupture include increased aneurysm size (especially >7 cm), decreased thrombus-to-lumen ratio, and infected aneurysms.
- Classic imaging features of AAA rupture include:

Retroperitoneal hematoma.
Periaortic stranding.
Contrast extravasation.

主动脉破裂

- 主动脉破裂是主动脉瘤的并发症，是急性胸痛或腹痛、低血压和腹部搏动性肿块患者需要排除的最重要的诊断。
- 约80%的腹主动脉瘤破裂发生在腹膜后，20%在腹腔，罕见破裂至下腔静脉(主动脉-腔静脉瘘)或肠道(主动脉-肠瘘)。
- 即将破裂的危险因素包括动脉瘤增大(特别是直径>7cm)、血栓与管腔比值降低和感染性动脉瘤。
- 典型的腹主动脉瘤破裂的影像学特征包括：

腹膜后血肿。
主动脉旁条索影。
造影剂外溢。

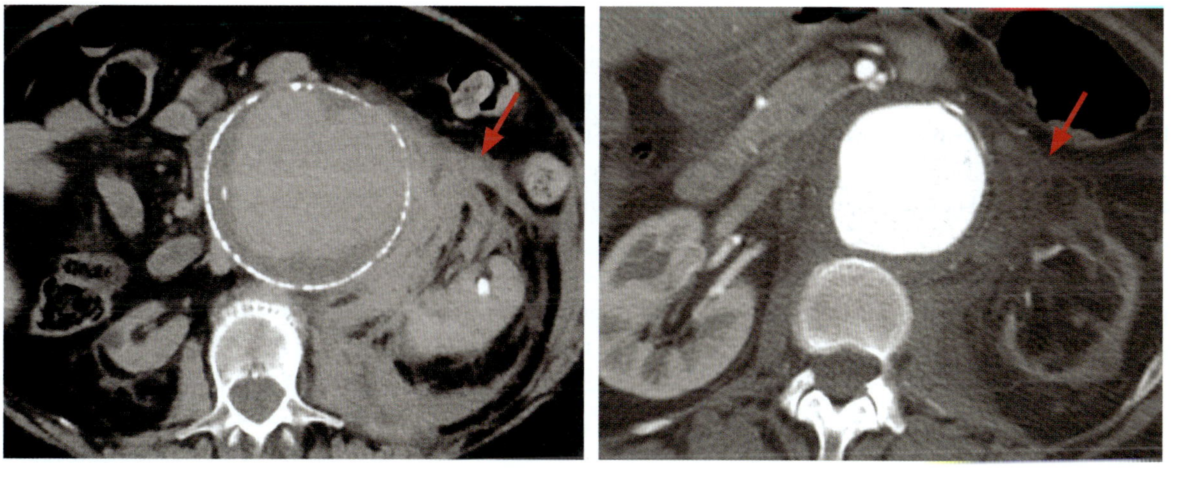

Abdominal aortic aneurysm rupture, classic features: Noncontrast CT (left image) shows high density retroperitoneal hematoma (arrow). CTA (right image) demonstrates marked periaortic stranding (arrow).
腹主动脉破裂的典型特征：平扫CT(左图)显示高密度腹膜后血肿(红箭)。CTA(右图)显示明显的主动脉旁条索影(红箭)。

- Secondary imaging signs of AAA rupture include:

Draped aorta sign, where the posterior wall of the aorta is not seen distinctly from adjacent structures.
Focal discontinuity of intimal calcification or *tangential calcium sign*.
High-attenuating crescent shape.

- 腹主动脉瘤破裂的继发征象包括：

主动脉披挂征，即主动脉后壁难以与邻近结构进行明确区分。
内膜钙化呈局部非连续性或切线型钙化。
高密度新月征。

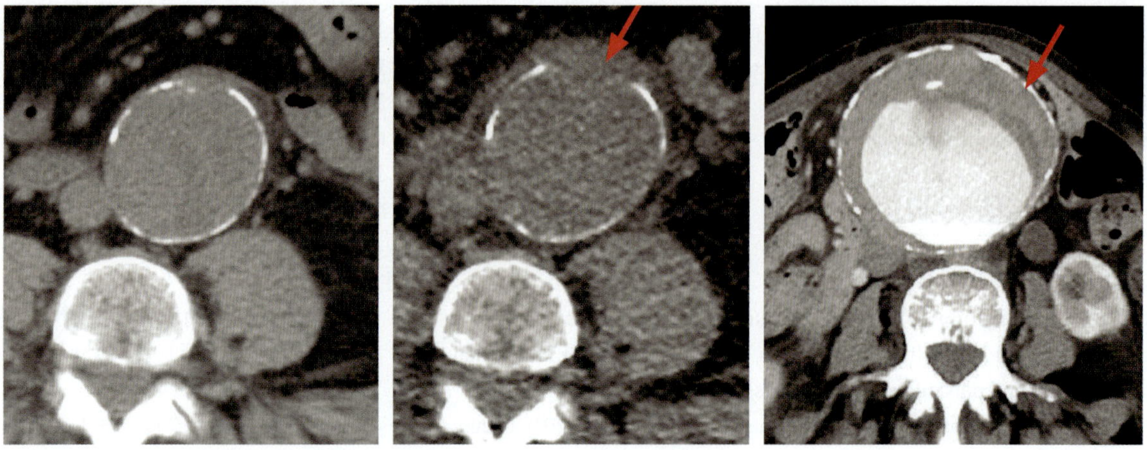

Abdominal aortic aneurysm rupture, secondary signs: Noncontrast CT (left image) shows peripheral calcification that becomes disrupted due to aneurysm rupture (middle image, arrow). CTA (right image) shows peripheral high attenuating crescent shape (arrow).
腹主动脉瘤破裂的继发征象：平扫CT(左图)显示因动脉瘤破裂而周围钙化不连续(中图，红箭)。CTA(右图)显示周边高密度的新月形影(红箭)。

- CTA should include noncontrast and contrast-enhanced phases, with thin slice (1 mm) acquisition essential for multiplanar reformatting and surgical planning.
- In addition to a size >5.5 cm, repair is recommended when the AAA is expanding at a rapid rate (>5 mm/year) or is symptomatic.
- The mortality of elective open AAA repair is >3%, while the mortality for urgent repair is 19%. A ruptured AAA has a mortality of at least 50%.
- Repair of AAA can be performed with a traditional open or endovascular technique. Endovascular repair is preferred for all patients regardless of surgical risk and is associated with reductions in major morbidity and hospital time. If patients cannot receive endovascular treatment, mostly due to aneurysm shape, then open repair is considered. Long-term outcomes are equivalent between endovascular and open repair, but endovascular repair often requires repeat interventions.
- Complications of endovascular repair of AAA include endoleak, endotension (enlargement of the aneurysm sac), stent migration or limb breakdown, delayed aneurysm rupture, infection, end organ ischemia, and aorto-enteric fistula.

- CTA应包括平扫和增强期，使用薄层(1mm)采集以便进行多平面重组和手术计划。
- 除直径>5.5cm外，腹主动脉瘤快速增大(>5mm/年)或出现症状时，也需要考虑手术修补。
- 择期开腹手术修补腹主动脉瘤的死亡率>3%，而紧急修复术的死亡率是19%。动脉瘤破裂的死亡率至少是50%。
- 腹主动脉瘤修补可采用传统的开放式手术，也可采用血管腔内技术。姑且不论外科手术的风险，血管腔内修补均应是所有患者的首选方式，因其能减少严重并发症发生、缩短住院时间。若患者不能接受血管腔内治疗(多数是因为动脉瘤的形态)，则考虑开放手术修复。血管腔内修补术与开放性修补术的长期效果相当，但血管腔内修复常需要重复干预。
- 腹主动脉瘤血管腔内修补术的并发症包括内漏、内张力(动脉瘤囊腔增大)、支架位移或支架分支断裂、迟发性动脉瘤破裂、感染、终末器官缺血及主动脉-肠瘘。

Abdominal Aortic Aneurysms – Endoleaks

- An endoleak is persistent flow into an excluded aneurysm sac after endovascular treatment with a stent graft.

Type I endoleak: Inadequate seal of graft

- Type I endoleak is inadequate graft seal. Type IA is a proximal leak, IB is a distal leak, and IC is an inadequate seal of the sidebranch or limb occluder plug.

腹主动脉瘤——内漏

- 内漏是腔内植入覆膜支架后血流持续进入已被封闭的动脉瘤腔。

Ⅰ型内漏：覆膜支架密封不完全

- Ⅰ型内漏：支架密封不完全。ⅠA型内漏发生在支架近端；ⅠB型内漏发生在支架远端；ⅠC型是指分支封堵不完全或封堵器封堵支架侧支不完全。

Type IA endoleak: Inadequate proximal seal allows blood into the excluded aneurysm sac.
ⅠA型内漏：支架近端密封不全造成血液流入被封闭的瘤腔内。

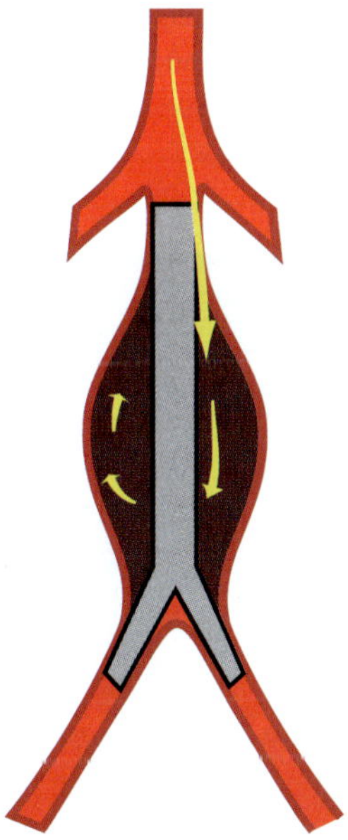

Inadequate proximal seal leads to enhancement in the proximal aneurysm sac (yellow arrow).
近端密封不全使近端动脉瘤腔内出现强化(黄箭)。

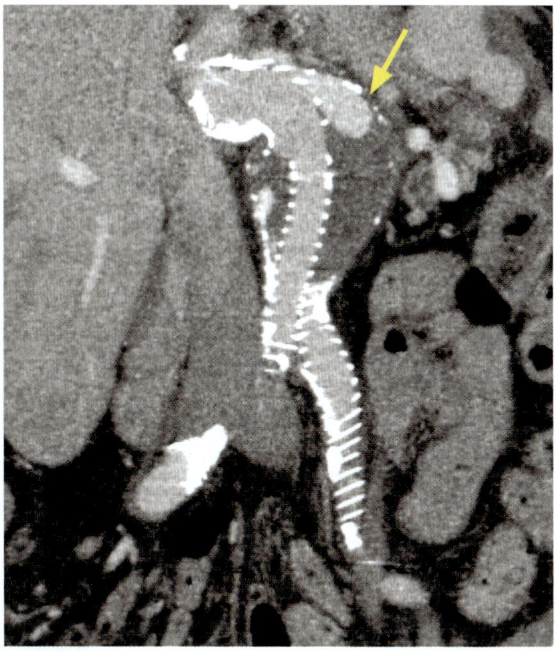

Type Ⅱ endoleak: Persistent collateral flow to excluded aneurysm

- Type Ⅱ endoleak is persistent collateral flow to the excluded aneurysm sac, which typically arises from the lumbar arteries or the inferior mesenteric artery (IMA).

Ⅱ型内漏：持续侧支血流进入被隔绝的瘤腔。

- Ⅱ型内漏是指持续的侧支血流进入已被隔绝的动脉瘤腔内，典型的侧支血管来自腰动脉或肠系膜下动脉(IMA)。

Type Ⅱ endoleak: Communication from either the IMA or a lumbar artery causes blood to flow into the excluded aneurysm sac.
Ⅱ型内漏：与IMA或腰动脉的交通致使血液进入封闭的动脉瘤腔。

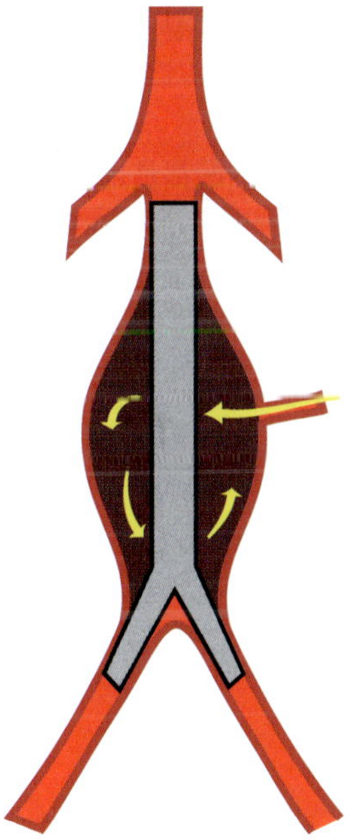

Axial image shows focal enhancement in the excluded aneurysm sac (yellow arrow), with faint communication (red arrow) leading to the IMA.
轴位图像显示封闭的瘤腔内有局灶性强化(黄箭)，并有一个模糊的交通朝向IMA(红箭)。

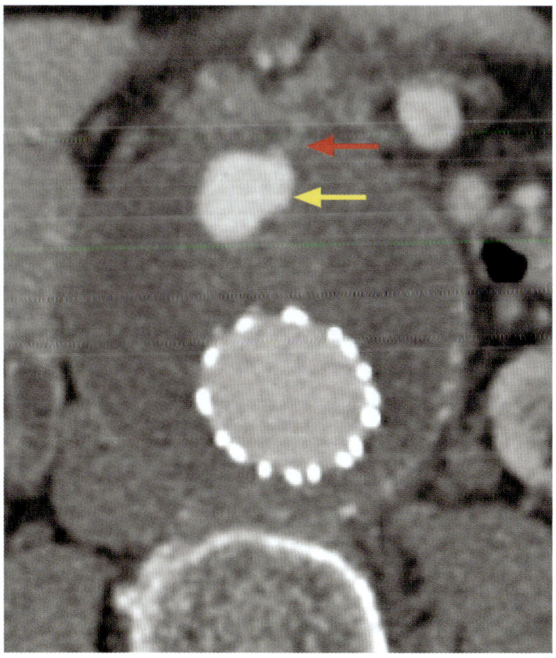

Type Ⅲ endoleak: Device failure causing leakage

- Type Ⅲ endoleak represents device failure causing leakage through graft fabric or segments of a modular graft.

Ⅲ型内漏：支架破损引起内漏

- Ⅲ型内漏是指支架破损使血流通过支架编织物结构或支架组件间的连接处发生的内漏。

Type Ⅲ endoleak: Blood enters the excluded aneurysm sac via a defect in the graft.
Ⅲ型内漏：血液通过支架破损处进入被封闭的瘤腔。

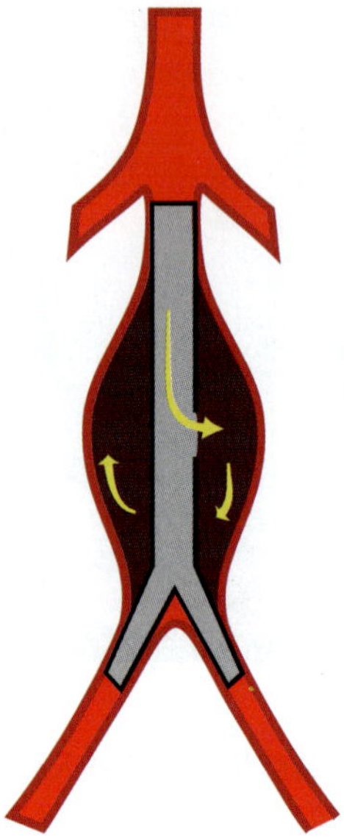

Coronal CT demonstrates contrast extravasating (yellow arrow) through the angulation of a modular aortic graft.
冠状位CT显示造影剂在主动脉支架组件的成角处向外漏出（黄箭）。

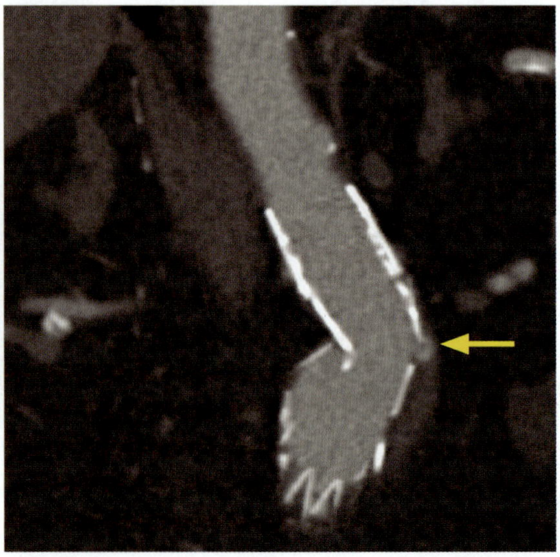

Type Ⅲa: At attachment with aortic-aortic or aortic-bifurcated component.
Type Ⅲb: At attachment with bifurcated-iliac limb or iliac limb-iliac limb component.
Type Ⅲc: At attachment with aortic side branch or side branch-side branch component.
Type Ⅲd: Graft tear, perforation, or fracture.

Ⅲa型：位于主动脉-主动脉或主动脉-分叉组件间连接处。
Ⅲb型：位于分叉组件与髂动脉组件或髂动脉-髂动脉组件间连接处。
Ⅲc型：位于主动脉支架与侧支组件或主动脉侧支-侧支组件间连接处。
Ⅲd型：覆膜支架撕裂、穿孔，或断裂。

Types Ⅳ and Ⅴ endoleaks

- Both type Ⅳ and type Ⅴ endoleaks are diagnoses of exclusion as no endoleak can be visualized by imaging although the sac continues to increase in size.

Ⅳ型及Ⅴ型内漏

- Ⅳ型及Ⅴ型内漏都是排除性诊断，因其影像学上不能发现内漏，但动脉瘤直径却持续增大。

Type IV endoleak: Type Ⅳ endoleak is caused by a porous graft and is typically transient and seen intra-procedurally. Type Ⅳ endoleak usually resolves within one month after withdrawal of anticoagulation. It is rarely seen with modern grafts.

IV型内漏是多孔腹膜支架引起的内漏，多为一过性并见于术中。Ⅳ型内漏通常在停用抗凝药物1个月内消失。目前使用的支架罕见发生此种内漏。

Type V endoleak: Also called endotension, type V endoleak is defined as continued expansion of the aneurysm without any other endoleak present, thought to be due to an endoleak below the resolution of imaging.

V型内漏也叫内张力，V型内漏为动脉瘤持续扩张但未发现有其他类型的内漏，通常认为影像学的分辨力不足以识别此型内漏。

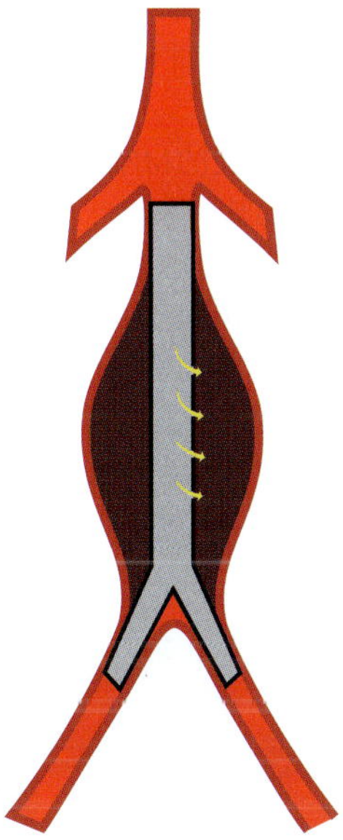

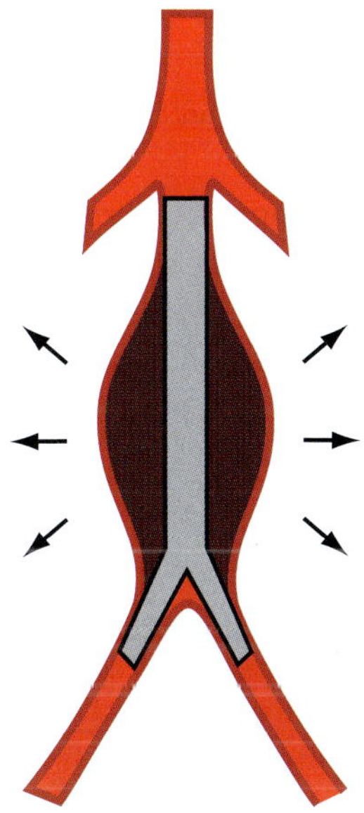

MISCELLANEOUS ABDOMINAL AORTIC DISORDERS

其他腹主动脉疾病

Aortitis of the abdominal aorta

腹主动脉炎

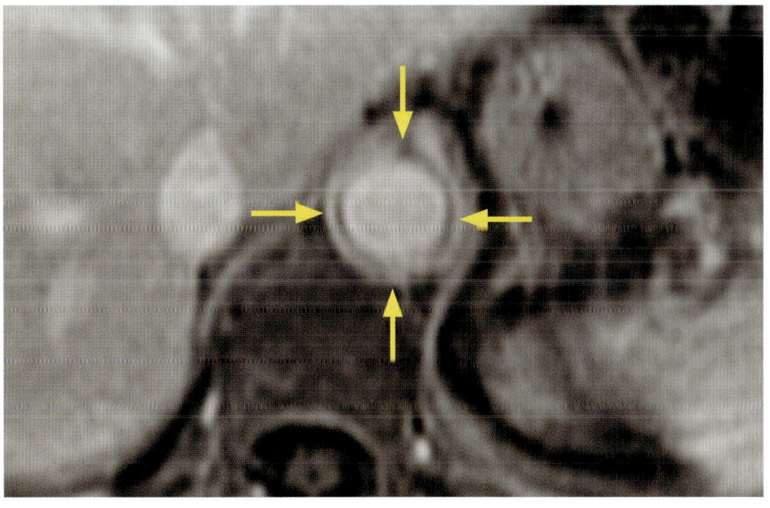

Active aortitis: T1-weighted post-contrast fat saturated MRI demonstrates circumferential mural thickening and enhancement of the aortic wall (arrows).

活动性主动脉炎：T_1加权增强脂肪饱和MRI图像示主动脉壁环形增厚及强化(黄箭)。

- Aortitis is inflammation of the aorta, which may be either infectious or inflammatory.
- **Inflammatory aortitis** can be due to Takayasu arteritis, giant cell arteritis, ankylosing spondylitis, polyarteritis nodosa, rheumatoid arthritis, and immune complex disease. Inflammatory aortitis is treated with corticosteroids.
- The acute phase of aortitis will show circumferential mural thickening and enhancement. There may be an associated aneurysm, dissection, or intramural hematoma. In contrast to intramural hematoma, aortitis tends to cause circumferential thickening rather than the eccentric, crescentic thickening of IMH.
- MRI findings of active aortitis include an aortic wall thickness >2 mm and enhancement of the aortic wall.
- Long segmental stenoses and/or aneurysms can arise in the chronic phase.
- **Infectious aortitis** presents with crescentic shape thickening of the aortic wall with peri-aortic soft-tissue accumulation. A complication of infectious aortitis is the development of a mycotic aneurysm.

Mycotic aneurysm arises from an infection of the arterial wall, most commonly by *Staphylococcus aureus* and *Salmonella species*.

- 主动脉炎是指主动脉的炎性改变，可为感染性或炎症性。
- **炎症性主动脉炎**可见于大动脉炎、巨细胞动脉炎、强直性脊柱炎、结节性多动脉炎、风湿性关节炎及免疫复合物疾病。炎症性动脉炎可用皮质激素治疗。
- 主动脉炎的急性期可表现为动脉壁环形增厚及强化，可伴有动脉瘤、夹层或壁内血肿。与壁内血肿不同的是，主动脉炎常表现为主动脉管壁环形增厚而非IMH所表现的偏心性、新月形样增厚。
- 活动性主动脉炎的MRI表现包括主动脉壁增厚>2mm及动脉壁强化。
- 慢性期可见较长的节段性狭窄和/或动脉瘤。
- **感染性主动脉炎**表现为主动脉壁新月形增厚并伴有主动脉周围软组织增加。感染性主动脉炎的并发症是形成感染性动脉瘤。

感染性动脉瘤源自动脉壁感染，最常见的病原菌是金黄色葡萄球菌和沙门菌。

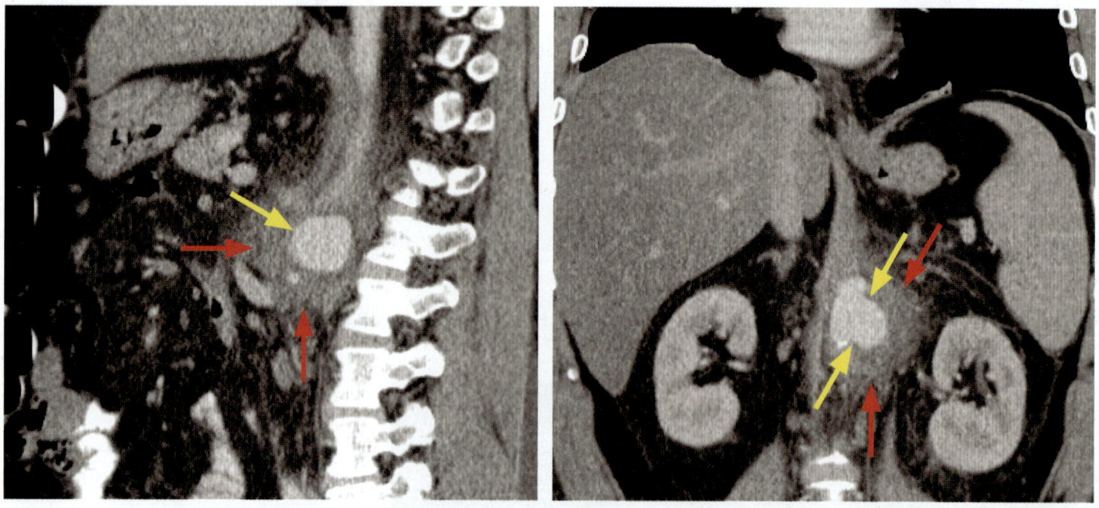

Mycotic aneurysm due to *Staphylococcus aureus*: Sagittal (left image) and coronal (right image) contrast-enhanced CT shows marked periaortic inflammatory change (red arrows) associated with a saccular aortic aneurysm (yellow arrows).
金黄色葡萄球菌所致的感染性动脉瘤：矢状位(左图)及冠状位(右图)增强CT可见明显的主动脉周围炎性改变(红箭)，合并囊状主动脉瘤(黄箭)。

Atherosclerotic distal aortic occlusive disease (Leriche syndrome)

动脉粥样硬化性远端主动脉闭塞性疾病(Leriche 综合征)

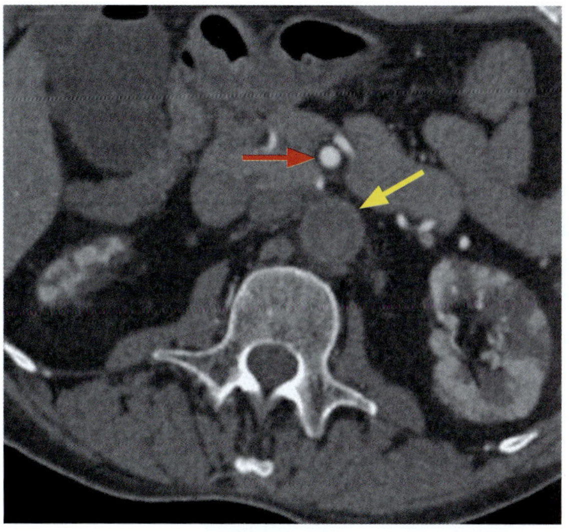

Case courtesy Michael Hanley, MD, University of Virginia Health System.

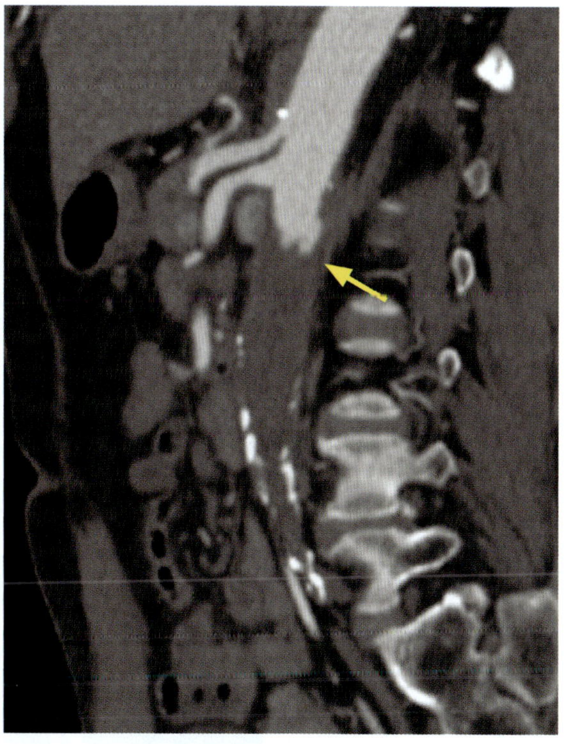

Leriche syndrome: Axial CT angiogram (left image) shows no opacification of the aorta (yellow arrow), while there is good opacification of the superior mesenteric artery (red arrow). There is patchy enhancement of the kidneys. Sagittal oblique MIP shows occlusive thrombus of the aorta (yellow arrow).

Leriche综合征：轴位CTA(左图)显示主动脉无强化(黄箭),肠系膜上动脉显影良好(红箭)。双肾可见斑片状强化。斜矢状位MIP(右图)显示阻塞性主动脉血栓(黄箭)。

- Leriche syndrome is occlusive atherosclerotic disease of the distal abdominal aorta, producing the classical quartet of impotence, buttock claudication, absent femoral pulses, and cold lower extremities.
- Over time, extensive collaterals develop from the thoraco-abdominal aorta to the external iliac arteries, most commonly the *anterior, middle,* and *posterior* pathways:

Anterior: Thoracic aorta → internal thoracic artery → superior epigastric artery → inferior epigastric artery → external iliac artery.

Middle: Abdominal aorta → SMA → IMA → superior rectal artery (terminal branch of IMA) → middle/inferior rectal arteries (via the path of Winslow) → retrograde through the internal iliac artery anterior division → external iliac artery.

Posterior: Abdominal aorta → intercostal and lumbar arteries → superior gluteal and iliolumbar arteries (branches of internal iliac artery posterior division) → deep circumflex iliac artery → external iliac artery.

- Leriche综合征是腹主动脉远端的闭塞性动脉粥样硬化疾病，可产生典型的四联症：阳痿、臀肌性跛行、股动脉搏动缺失和下肢冰凉。
- 随着病程进展，在胸-腹主动脉与髂外动脉之间可形成广泛的侧支循环，最常见的是前、中、后侧支循环通路：

前路：胸主动脉→胸廓内动脉→腹壁上动脉→腹壁下动脉→髂外动脉。

中路：腹主动脉→肠系膜上动脉→肠系膜下动脉→直肠上动脉(肠系膜下动脉的终末支)→直肠中/下动脉(通过Winslow通路)→逆行通过髂内动脉前干→髂外动脉。

后路：腹主动脉→肋间动脉和腰动脉→臀上动脉和髂腰动脉(髂内动脉后干的分支)→旋髂深动脉→髂外动脉。

(翻译 陈珑)

MESENTERIC AND PELVIC VESSELS

肠系膜和盆腔血管

NORMAL ANATOMY

正常解剖

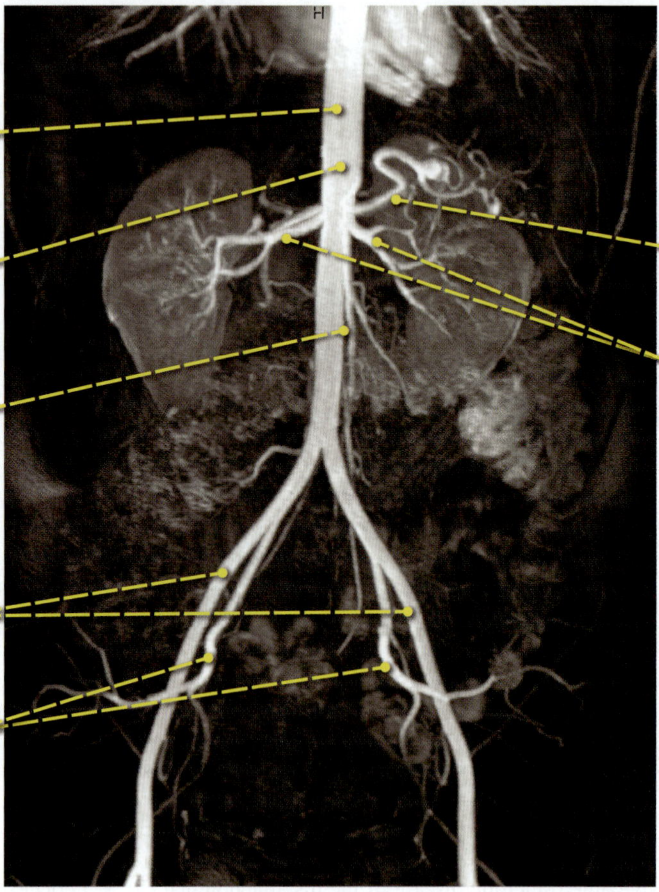

Osseous landmarks

- Celiac artery: Arises from the aorta at the level of the T12 vertebral body.
- Superior mesenteric artery (SMA): Arises at the level of the T12–L1 disc space.
- Renal arteries: Arise at the level of the L1–L2 disc space.
- Inferior mesenteric artery (IMA): Arises to the left of midline at the level of the L3 vertebral body.

Celiac axis anatomy

- The anatomy of the celiac axis and abdominal viscera is highly variable.
- Approximately 75% of the time the celiac artery demonstrates normal arterial anatomy with three main branches: The left gastric, the common hepatic, and the splenic artery.
- The left gastric artery may be the source of bleeding in esophageal Mallory-Weiss tear.
- The left gastroepiploic artery arises from the splenic artery and anastomoses with the right gastroepiploic artery along the greater curvature of the stomach. The right gastroepiploic artery arises from the gastroduodenal artery.
- Anatomic variants are described in the "Interventional Radiology" chapter.

Hepatic arterial anatomy

- Most commonly (75%), the proper hepatic artery supplies blood to the liver.

骨性标志

- 腹腔干：起源于主动脉T_{12}水平。
- 肠系膜上动脉(SMA)：起源于主动脉T_{12}与L_1椎间隙水平。
- 肾动脉：起源于主动脉L_1与L_2椎间隙水平。
- 肠系膜下动脉(IMA)：起源于主动脉L_3水平中线的左侧。

腹腔干解剖

- 腹腔干和腹部内脏血管的解剖变异很大。
- 约75%的腹腔干呈三支血管组成的正常解剖结构：胃左动脉、肝总动脉和脾动脉。
- 胃左动脉可为食管Mallory-Weiss黏膜撕裂出血的来源。
- 胃网膜左动脉发自脾动脉，并与胃网膜右动脉在胃大弯处吻合。胃网膜右动脉发自胃十二指肠动脉。
- 解剖学变异在"介入放射学"一章中描述。

肝动脉解剖

- 最常见的解剖(75%)是肝固有动脉向肝脏供

The proper hepatic artery is the continuation of the common hepatic artery after the takeoff of the gastroduodenal artery. The proper hepatic artery divides into the right and left hepatic arteries. The cystic artery arises from the right hepatic artery to supply the gallbladder.

血。肝总动脉在发出胃十二指肠动脉后，延续为肝固有动脉。肝固有动脉分为肝左、右动脉。胆囊动脉起源于肝右动脉，供应胆囊。

Summary of celiac axis and hepatic arterial anatomy

腹腔干和肝动脉解剖概述

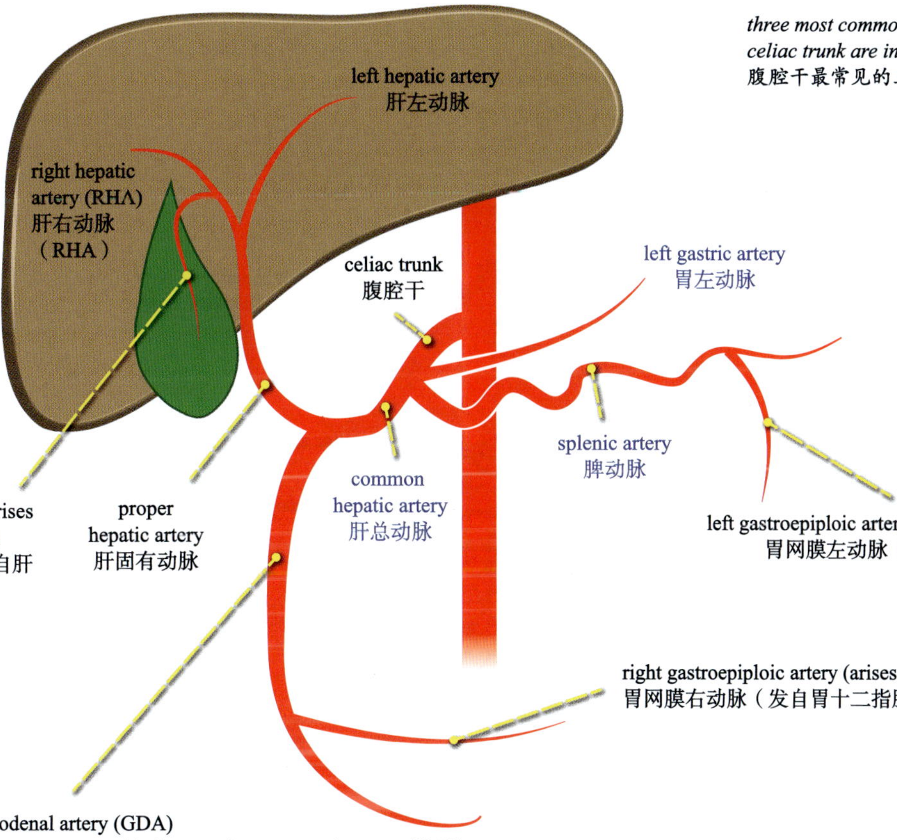

Superior mesenteric artery (SMA)

- The superior mesenteric artery (SMA) arises from the anterior aorta at about the level of T12–L1 to supply the distal duodenum, the entire small bowel, and the proximal large bowel from the cecum to the mid-transverse colon.
- The **inferior pancreaticoduodenal artery** is the first branch of the SMA. The inferior pancreaticoduodenal artery forms collaterals with the celiac artery.
- The **middle colic artery** arises from the SMA and supplies the transverse colon. The middle colic artery anastomoses with the **marginal artery of Drummond**.
- The **right colic artery** courses retroperitoneally, where it supplies the right colon and the hepatic flexure.
- The terminal artery of the SMA is the **ileocolic artery**, which sends arterial branches to the terminal ileum, cecum, and appendix.

肠系膜上动脉(SMA)

- 肠系膜上动脉(SMA)起源于腹主动脉前壁，约T_{12}与L_1水平，供应远端十二指肠、整个小肠及从盲肠到横结肠中部的近端大肠。
- **胰十二指肠下动脉**是肠系膜上动脉的第一支分支，与腹腔干分支形成吻合。
- **结肠中动脉**起源于肠系膜上动脉并供应横结肠。结肠中动脉与**Drummond边缘动脉**形成吻合。
- **右结肠动脉**走行于腹膜后，供应右半结肠和结肠右曲。
- 肠系膜上动脉的终末分支为**回结肠动脉**，发出分支供应末端回肠、盲肠及阑尾。

Inferior mesenteric artery (IMA)

- The inferior mesenteric artery (IMA) originates at the left anterior aspect of the aorta at approximately the level of L3.
- The IMA gives off the **left colic artery** to supply the descending colon.
- The **sigmoid arteries** are variable in number. They run in the sigmoid mesocolon to supply the sigmoid. The IMA terminates as the **superior rectal**

肠系膜下动脉(IMA)

- 肠系膜下动脉(IMA)约在L_3水平，起源于腹主动脉左前壁。
- IMA发出**左结肠动脉**供应降结肠。
- **乙状结肠动脉**的数目不定。它们走行于乙状结肠系膜内，并向乙状结肠供血。肠系膜下

(hemorrhoidal) artery to supply the upper rectum.

动脉的终末分支为**直肠上(痔)动脉**，供应直肠的上段。

External iliac branches

- The **inferior epigastric artery** anastomoses with the superior epigastric artery.
- The **deep circumflex iliac artery** anastomoses with the internal iliac via the iliolumbar artery.
- The **femoral artery** continues distally to supply the leg.

髂外动脉分支

- **腹壁下动脉**与腹壁上动脉吻合。
- **旋髂深动脉**经髂腰动脉与髂内动脉吻合。
- **股动脉**继续向下延伸供应下肢。

Internal iliac branches

髂内动脉分支

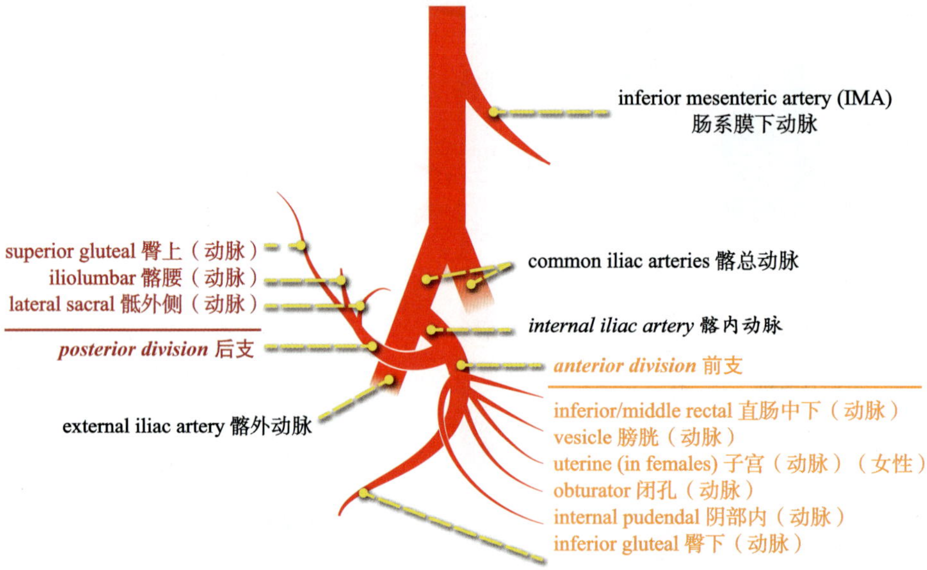

- The anterior division of the internal iliac artery supplies most of the pelvic viscera.
- The branches of the anterior division include the **inferior/middle rectal artery** (anastomoses with the IMA via the pathway of Winslow), the **uterine artery**, the **obturator artery**, and the **inferior gluteal artery**.
- The posterior division of the internal iliac artery supplies the musculature of the pelvic and gluteal regions.
- The branches of the posterior division include the **lateral sacral artery**, the **iliolumbar artery** (anastomoses with external iliac via the deep circumflex iliac artery), and the **superior gluteal artery**.

- 髂内动脉的前支供应盆腔大部分脏器。
- 髂内动脉前支包括**直肠中/下动脉**(通过Winslow通路与肠系膜下动脉吻合)、**子宫动脉**、**闭孔动脉和臀下动脉**。
- 髂内动脉的后支供应盆腔和臀部肌肉。
- 髂内动脉后支包括**骶外侧动脉**、**髂腰动脉**(经旋髂深动脉与髂外动脉吻合)和**臀上动脉**。

Abdominal Anastomotic Pathways

腹部吻合的途径

Celiac ⇆ SMA anastomoses

- The **arc of Buhler** is an uncommon short-segment direct connection between the celiac artery and the SMA. It is a persistent embryologic remnant and not an acquired collateral pathway.
- The inferior pancreaticoduodenal artery is the first SMA branch. It forms a rich collateral network with the celiac axis about the pancreatic head, called the **pancreatic cascade**.
- The **arc of Barkow** (not drawn in diagram below) connects the SMA to the

腹腔干与肠系膜上动脉的吻合途径

- **Buhler动脉弓**是一小段不常见的血管，直接连接腹腔干和肠系膜上动脉。此为胚胎发育残留永存结构，而非后天形成的侧支通路。
- 胰十二指肠下动脉是肠系膜上动脉的第一条分支，与腹腔干在胰头处形成丰富的侧支吻合网，称之为**胰动脉弓**。
- **Barkow弓**(下图未画出)通过大网膜左右动脉

celiac axis via the right and left epiploic arteries.

SMA ⇆ IMA anastomoses

- The **marginal artery of Drummond** is the major SMA ⇆ IMA anastomosis. It lies in the peripheral mesentery of the colon, adjacent to the mesenteric surface of the colon. The marginal artery of Drummond is comprised of branches from the ileocolic, right, middle, and left colic arteries. Normally, the marginal artery of Drummond is small in caliber, but it may become prominent in the setting of IMA or SMA disease.
- The **arc of Riolan** is an inconstant SMA ⇆ IMA anastomosis. The arc of Riolan also runs through the colonic mesentery, but more medial compared to the marginal artery of Drummond.
- The *Cannon-Böhm point* is the point of transitional blood supply to the colon between the SMA (proximal) and IMA (distal), at the splenic flexure. This watershed zone is susceptible to ischemia in case of systemic arterial insufficiency.

Iliac artery anastomoses

- **External iliac ⇆ thoracic aorta**: The inferior epigastric artery arises from the external iliac artery and anastomoses with the thoracic aorta via the internal mammary artery.
- **External iliac ⇆ internal iliac**: The deep circumflex iliac artery arises from the external iliac artery and anastomoses with the posterior division of the internal iliac artery via the iliolumbar artery.
- **Internal iliac ⇆ IMA**: The inferior/middle rectal arteries arise from the internal iliac artery and anastomose with the IMA via the superior rectal artery. This collateral pathway is the **path of Winslow** (rectal arcade).

将肠系膜上动脉和腹腔干连接。

肠系膜上动脉与肠系膜下动脉吻合途径

- **Drummond边缘动脉**(结肠边缘动脉弓)是肠系膜上下动脉间主要的吻合动脉。它位于结肠系膜边缘，邻近结肠的系膜面。Drummond边缘动脉由来自回结肠动脉及左、中、右结肠动脉分支组成。正常情况下，Drummond边缘动脉管径细小，但在肠系膜上或下动脉病变时，可明显增粗。
- **Riolan动脉弓**(肠系膜动脉弓)是一条不固定的肠系膜上下动脉间的吻合支。它也在结肠系膜内走行，但与Drummond边缘动脉相比，其位置更靠内侧。
- Cannon-Böhm点是肠系膜上动脉(近端)和肠系膜下动脉(远端)之间向结肠供血的移行区，位于结肠脾曲。体循环动脉供血障碍时该分水岭区易发生缺血。

髂动脉吻合途径

- **髂外动脉与胸主动脉吻合**：腹壁下动脉发自髂外动脉，经内乳动脉与胸主动脉吻合。
- **髂外动脉与髂内动脉吻合**：旋髂深动脉发自髂外动脉，经髂腰动脉与髂内动脉后支吻合。
- **髂内动脉与肠系膜下动脉吻合**：直肠下/中动脉发自髂内动脉，经直肠上动脉与肠系膜下动脉吻合。该侧支通路即**Winslow通路**(直肠弓)。

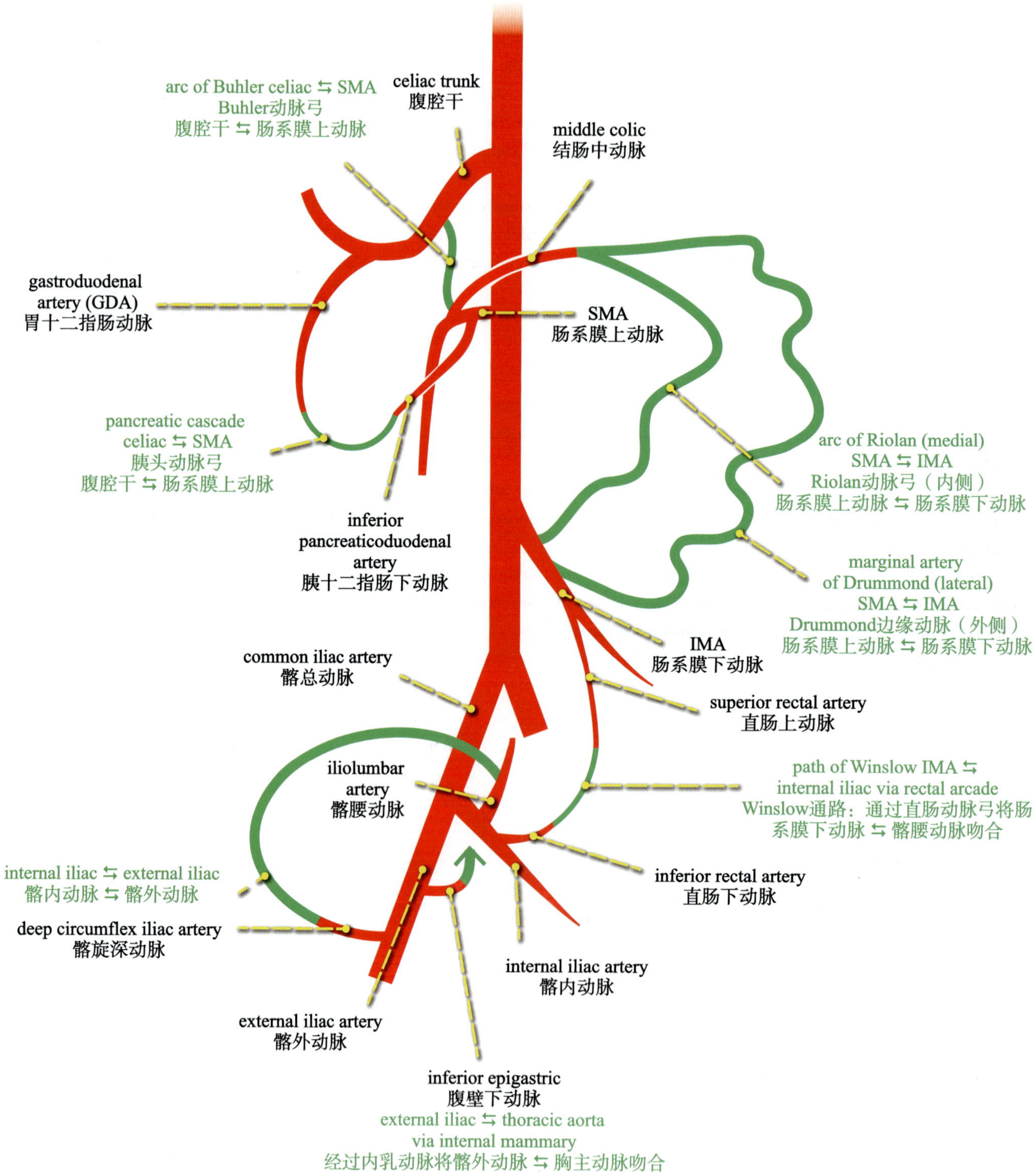
arc of Buhler celiac ⇆ SMA
Buhler动脉弓
腹腔干 ⇆ 肠系膜上动脉
celiac trunk
腹腔干
middle colic
结肠中动脉
gastroduodenal artery (GDA)
胃十二指肠动脉
SMA
肠系膜上动脉
pancreatic cascade
celiac ⇆ SMA
胰头动脉弓
腹腔干 ⇆ 肠系膜上动脉
arc of Riolan (medial)
SMA ⇆ IMA
Riolan动脉弓（内侧）
肠系膜上动脉 ⇆ 肠系膜下动脉
inferior pancreaticoduodenal artery
胰十二指肠下动脉
marginal artery of Drummond (lateral)
SMA ⇆ IMA
Drummond边缘动脉（外侧）
肠系膜上动脉 ⇆ 肠系膜下动脉
common iliac artery
髂总动脉
IMA
肠系膜下动脉
superior rectal artery
直肠上动脉
iliolumbar artery
髂腰动脉
path of Winslow IMA ⇆ internal iliac via rectal arcade
Winslow通路：通过直肠动脉弓将肠系膜下动脉 ⇆ 髂腰动脉吻合
internal iliac ⇆ external iliac
髂内动脉 ⇆ 髂外动脉
inferior rectal artery
直肠下动脉
deep circumflex iliac artery
髂旋深动脉
internal iliac artery
髂内动脉
external iliac artery
髂外动脉
inferior epigastric
腹壁下动脉
external iliac ⇆ thoracic aorta via internal mammary
经过内乳动脉将髂外动脉 ⇆ 胸主动脉吻合

Polyarteritis nodosa (PAN)

结节性多动脉炎(PAN)

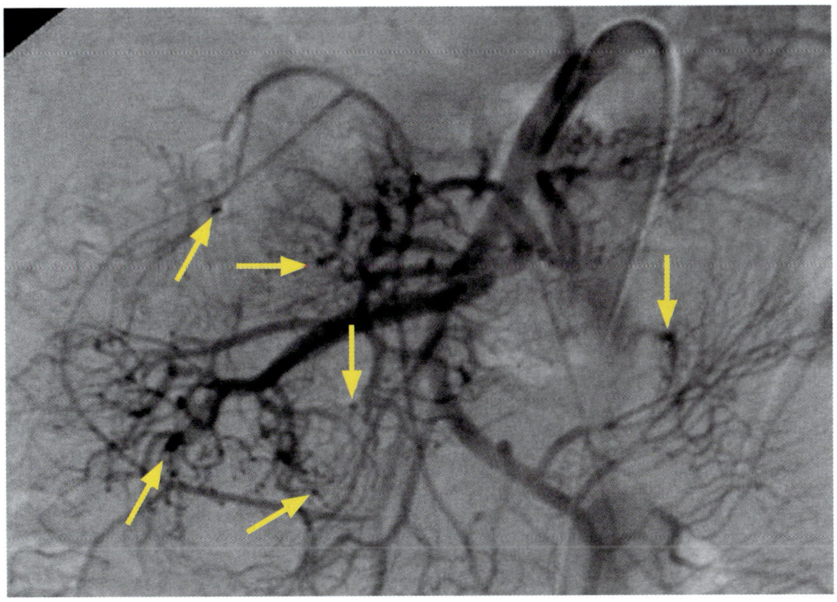

Polyarteritis nodosa:
Selective digital substraction angiogram of the superior mesenteric artery shows numerous tiny peripheral aneurysms (arrows).
Case courtesy Dmitry Rabkin, MD, Brigham and Women's Hospital.

结节性多动脉炎：
选择性肠系膜上动脉数字减影血管造影显示外周肠系膜上动脉有多发小动脉瘤(黄箭)。

- Polyarteritis nodosa (PAN) is a systemic necrotizing vasculitis of small-and medium-sized arteries that causes multiple small visceral aneurysms. P-ANCA is usually elevated.
- PAN typically affects renal, hepatic, and mesenteric end-arterioles.
- PAN is associated with several medical conditions remembered with the mnemonic **CLASH** (**c**ryoglobulinemia, **l**eukemia, rheumatoid **a**rthritis, **S**jögren syndrome, and **h**epatitis B).
- Treatment of PAN is with steroids, not procedures.
- The differential diagnosis of multiple renal artery aneurysms includes multiple septic emboli, *speed kidney* (due to chronic methamphetamine abuse), and Ehlers-Danlos.
- The ideal imaging modality is invasive angiography given the size of the multiple microaneurysms. However, recent advances in CTA allow to visualize these small aneurysms in the vessels.
- Regular CT or MRI images can demonstrate focal regions of infarcts in the solid organs.

- 结节性多动脉炎(PAN)是一种累及中、小动脉的系统性坏死性血管炎，导致多发性内脏小动脉瘤形成。抗中性粒细胞核周抗体(P-ANCA)通常升高。
- PAN通常累及肾脏、肝脏和肠系膜终末小动脉。
- PAN和多个临床疾病有关，可用“**CLASH**”一词帮助记忆，即冷沉球蛋白血症(C)、白血病(L)、风湿性关节炎(A)、干燥综合征(S)和乙型肝炎病毒感染(H)。
- 治疗PAN主要使用类固醇激素，无须手术。
- 多发性肾动脉瘤的鉴别诊断包括多发性感染性血栓、“speed肾脏”(长期滥用甲基苯丙胺)和埃勒斯-当洛综合征。
- 由于多发微小动脉瘤体积过小，理想的成像方式是侵入性的血管造影。但最新的CTA技术可以检测这些小动脉瘤。
- 常规CT或MRI可显示实质器官内的局灶性梗死区。

Splenic artery aneurysm

- Splenic artery aneurysm is the most common visceral aneurysm. Multiparous females and patients with portal hypertension are at increased risk of developing splenic artery aneurysms. Splenic artery aneurysms have an increased risk of rupture during pregnancy.
- A splenic artery *pseudo*aneurysm may be the result of trauma or pancreatitis.
- Indications for treatment of a splenic artery aneurysm include presence of symptoms (such as left upper quadrant pain), aneurysm size >2 cm, and prior to expected pregnancy.
- Endovascular coil embolization is the preferred approach. Coils are first placed distal to the aneurysm neck (to exclude retrograde collateral flow), then placed proximally.

脾动脉瘤

- 脾动脉瘤是最常见的内脏动脉瘤。经产妇和门静脉高压患者罹患脾动脉瘤的风险增加。脾动脉瘤在妊娠期间破裂风险增加。
- 脾动脉假性动脉瘤可能为外伤或胰腺炎所致。
- 脾动脉瘤治疗的指征包括出现临床症状(如左上腹疼痛)、动脉瘤直径>2cm及准备怀孕者。
- 血管内弹簧圈栓塞是首选的手术方式。弹簧圈首先放置在动脉瘤颈远端(防止侧支血液逆向流入)，而后放置在瘤颈的近端。

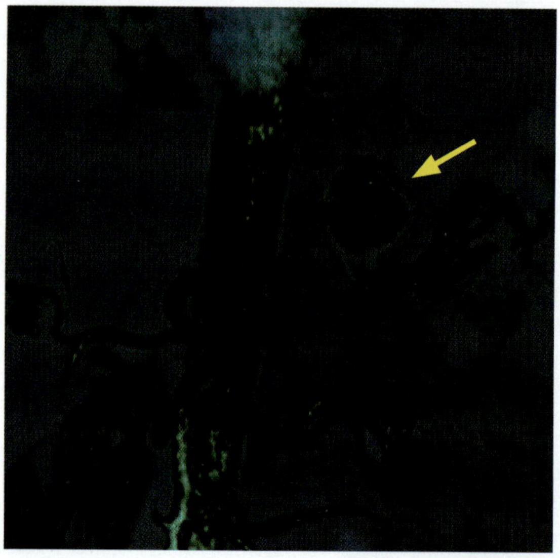

3D volumetric reconstruction of a CT angiogram demonstrates a splenic artery aneurysm (arrow).
CT 血管成像三维容积重组图像显示脾动脉瘤(黄箭)。

Hepatic artery aneurysm

- Hepatic artery aneurysm is the second most common visceral aneurysm.
- Embolization of the right hepatic artery distal to the cystic artery (which arises from the right hepatic artery) is preferred, as embolization proximal to the cystic artery increases the risk of ischemic cholecystitis, which may be seen in up to 10% of cases.

Vascular findings of cirrhosis

- The classic angiographic finding of liver cirrhosis is corkscrewing of the hepatic artery branches, caused by liver fibrosis. A hypervascular mass in a cirrhotic liver may represent hepatocellular carcinoma.

肝动脉瘤

- 肝动脉瘤是第二常见的内脏动脉瘤。
- 栓塞肝右动脉最好在胆囊动脉的远端进行，在胆囊动脉近端栓塞会增加缺血性胆囊炎的风险，发生率达10%。

肝硬化的血管表现

- 典型的肝硬化血管造影表现是肝动脉分支因肝纤维化呈螺旋状改变。肝硬化时出现富血供肿块可能为肝细胞癌。

Mesenteric ischemia

Imaging technique

- Mesenteric ischemia is inadequate blood supply to the bowel. It is seen most commonly in the elderly and has multiple causes, including acute arterial embolism, chronic arterial stenosis, venous occlusion, and low-flow states. Mesenteric ischemia could be acute or chronic in etiology, and acute mesenteric ischemia is the most common type.
- CTA is the ideal imaging modality to assess acute or chronic mesenteric ischemia. Multiple phases should be acquired for proper diagnosis:
  - Noncontrast – although some studies suggest noncontrast CT is not necessary.
  - Arterial phase – 30-second delay, or achieved with bolus tracking.
  - Delayed or venous phase – 90-second delay.
- Although MRA has a limited role in acute mesenteric ischemia, it can help to identify proximal vessel abnormalities including stenosis or occlusion in patients with iodinated contrast allergy.

肠系膜缺血

成像技术

- 肠系膜缺血是指肠供血不足。最常见于老年人，有多种原因，包括急性动脉栓塞、慢性动脉狭窄、静脉阻塞和低血流状态。肠系膜缺血在病因学上可分为急性或慢性，急性肠系膜缺血是最常见的类型。
- CTA是评估急性或慢性肠系膜缺血的最佳成像方式。应行多期相扫描，以获得恰当的诊断：
  - 平扫——尽管有些研究认为CT平扫无必要。
  - 动脉期——延迟30秒，或采用团注示踪技术。
  - 延迟或静脉期——延迟90秒。
- MRA在急性肠系膜缺血中的作用有限，但碘造影剂过敏时有助于检测肠系膜血管近端的异常，包括狭窄或闭塞。

Acute mesenteric ischemia

急性肠系膜缺血

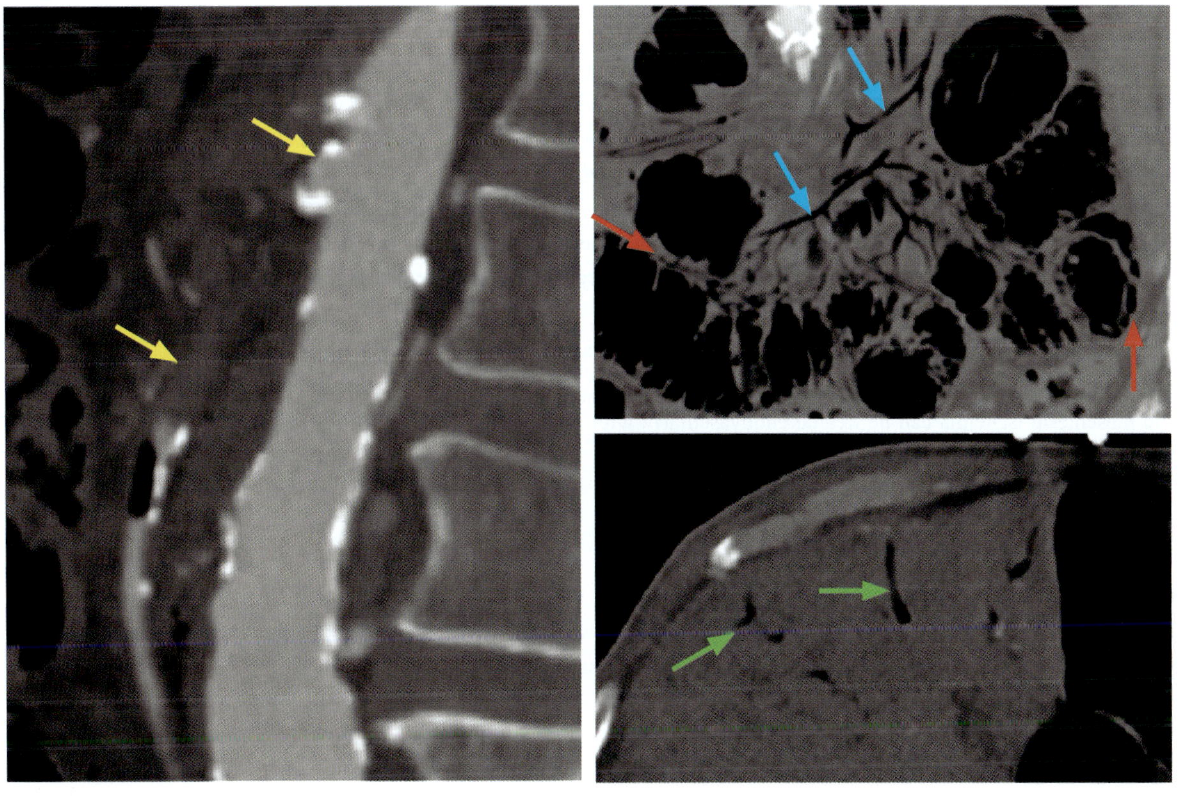

Acute mesenteric ischemia: CTA shows segmental occlusion of the proximal SMA (yellow arrows) with associated severe pneumatosis of the bowel loops (red arrows), mesenteric venous gas (blue arrows) and air in the portal venous system (green arrows), in keeping with end organ ischemia.

急性肠系膜缺血：CTA 显示肠系膜上动脉近端节段性闭塞(黄箭)伴肠袢严重积气(红箭)，肠系膜静脉(蓝箭)和门静脉系统出现气体(绿箭)，符合终末器官缺血的表现。

- Acute mesenteric ischemia typically presents as catastrophic abdominal pain, often with lactic acidosis.
- Arterial SMA embolism is the most common cause of acute mesenteric ischemia.

  An SMA embolism distal to the middle colic artery carries the highest high risk of intestinal ischemia, as there are few native distal collaterals. The middle colic artery anastomoses with the IMA via the marginal artery of Drummond and the arc of Riolan.
- Acute in situ thrombosis is another cause of mesenteric ischemia that is usually superimposed on existing atherosclerosis.
- Venous thrombosis is a rare cause of acute mesenteric ischemia.
- CTA findings of acute mesenteric ischemia include:

  Arterial phase images can reveal SMA stenoses, occlusions, and luminal narrowing.

  Delayed or venous phase can reveal venous obstruction as well as bowel and end organ ischemia, including bowel wall necrosis, pneumatosis intestinalis, and perforation.

  Dual-energy CT reconstructions such as iodine maps and monoenergetic images can help to detect bowel ischemia, where the ischemic segments have lower iodine concentrations.
- **Nonocclusive mesenteric ischemia (NOMI)** is a highly lethal (70–100% mortality) form of acute mesenteric ischemia. NOMI is known as "intestinal necrosis with a patent arterial tree;" however, mesenteric arteries are diffusely attenuated/small in caliber on CTA due to vasospasm. Bowel ischemia findings

- 急性肠系膜缺血通常表现为剧烈腹痛，常伴乳酸酸中毒。
- 肠系膜上动脉栓塞是急性肠系膜缺血最常见的原因。

  发生在结肠中动脉远端的肠系膜上动脉栓塞最易诱发肠缺血，因远端的自身侧支较少。结肠中动脉和肠系膜下动脉通过Drummond边缘动脉和Riolan动脉弓吻合。
- 急性原位血栓形成是肠系膜缺血的另一个原因，常在动脉粥样硬化的基础上发生。
- 静脉血栓形成是一种罕见的急性肠系膜缺血的原因。
- 急性肠系膜缺血的CTA表现包括：

  动脉期图像可见肠系膜上动脉狭窄、闭塞和管径变细。

  延迟或静脉期图像可见静脉阻塞及肠和终末器官缺血，包括肠壁坏死、肠积气和穿孔。

  双能量CT重建，如碘图和单能图像有助于检测肠缺血，缺血肠段的碘浓度较低。
- **非闭塞性肠系膜缺血(NOMI)**是一种致死率高(70%~100%)的急性肠系膜缺血。非闭塞性肠系膜缺血也被称为"动脉树通畅的小肠

are prominent along the watershed areas. In addition, CT hypoperfusion complex (shock bowel syndrome) features can be seen in the abdomen.

坏死”，但因血管痉挛，肠系膜动脉在CTA上表现为弥漫的管径变小。肠道缺血在血供分水岭区的表现尤为显著。此外，腹部CT可见低灌注综合征(肠休克综合征)。

Chronic mesenteric ischemia

- Chronic mesenteric ischemia is usually caused by atherosclerosis. The classic clinical presentation is postprandial abdominal pain out of proportion to the physical exam.
- Because mesenteric collaterals are so extensive, at least two of three mesenteric arteries (celiac, SMA, and IMA) must be diseased to produce symptoms in chronic disease.
- CTA findings include stenosis of the mesenteric vessels, extensive collaterals, bowel wall thickening and pneumatosis.
- Chronic mesenteric ischemia can be treated endovascularly with angioplasty and stenting.

慢性肠系膜缺血

- 慢性肠系膜缺血常由动脉粥样硬化引起。典型的临床表现是餐后腹痛，且与体征不符。
- 由于肠系膜侧支非常广泛，慢性肠系膜动脉疾病时，三支血管(腹腔动脉、肠系膜上动脉和肠系膜下动脉)中至少两支血管发生病变才会产生临床症状。
- CTA表现包括肠系膜血管狭窄、广泛的侧支血管、肠壁增厚和积气。
- 慢性肠系膜缺血可采用血管成形和支架放置等血管内治疗方式进行治疗。

Arterial compression syndromes

动脉压迫综合征

Median arcuate ligament syndrome (MALS)

- Median arcuate ligament syndrome (MALS) is celiac artery compression by the median arcuate ligament, a part of the diaphragmatic crura. Arterial compression worsens with expiration.
- While most patients are asymptomatic, MALS may clinically present with crampy abdominal pain. MALS tends to occur in young, thin women.
- CTA or MRA shows a proximal stenosis of the celiac axis with *hook sign* configuration, post-stenotic dilatation, and collaterals between branches of the gastroduodenal artery and SMA.
- Dynamic imaging (expiration and inspiration) can be done to assess severity of the stenosis.
- Angioplasty is not effective and stents are controversial due to high risk of device failure. Definitive treatment is surgical release of the median arcuate ligament to enlarge the diaphragmatic hiatus.

正中弓状韧带压迫综合征(MALS)

- 正中弓状韧带压迫综合征(MALS)是腹腔干被膈脚的正中弓状韧带压迫所致。呼气时动脉受压更严重。
- 大部分患者无症状，但MALS在临床上可表现为腹部绞痛。MALS常发生于年轻、瘦小的女性。
- CTA或MRA显示腹腔干近端狭窄呈钩形、狭窄后扩张，以及胃十二指肠动脉分支与肠系膜上动脉之间有侧支形成。
- 动态成像(呼气和吸气)可用于评估狭窄的严重程度。
- 血管成形术治疗无效，支架术也因失功风险高而尚存争议。根治性治疗为外科手术松解正中弓状韧带，以扩大膈肌裂孔。

Superior mesenteric artery (SMA) syndrome

- SMA syndrome is compression of the duodenum between the aorta and the SMA, and is also known as **Wilkie syndrome**.
- SMA syndrome occurs in thin children, burn victims, and patients who have lost weight.
- CTA or MRA can diagnose duodenal compression by SMA. Aortomesenteric angle or distance can be measured to assess the degree of stenosis.

  Normal aortomesenteric angle = 28–65 degrees; aortomesenteric distance = 10–34 mm

  In SMA syndrome aortomesenteric angle = 6–22 degrees; aortomesenteric distance = 2–8 mm.

  In addition to the narrowing of the SMA angle, dilation of the first and second part of the duodenum as well as stomach are the key elements of the diagnosis.
- Treatment starts with medical management, and if conservative treatment fails then surgical approach including lysis of the ligament of Treitz or duodenojejunostomy can be done.

肠系膜上动脉(SMA)综合征

- 肠系膜上动脉(SMA)综合征是处于肠系膜上动脉和主动脉之间的十二指肠受压所致，也被称为**Wilkie综合征**。
- SMA综合征发生在瘦弱的儿童、烧伤患者，以及体重下降的患者。
- CTA或MRA可诊断肠系膜上动脉压迫十二指肠，可测量主动脉-肠系膜夹角或距离以评估狭窄程度。

  正常主动脉-肠系膜夹角=28°~65°；主动脉-肠系膜距离=10~34 mm。

  SMA综合征时主动脉-肠系膜夹角=6°~22°；主动脉-肠系膜距离=2~8 mm。

  除肠系膜上动脉角变窄外，十二指肠第一、二段及胃的扩张也是诊断的关键因素。
- 首选内科治疗，若保守治疗失败，可手术治疗，包括松解屈氏韧带或十二指肠-空肠吻合术。

Renal vessels

Atherosclerotic renal artery stenosis

- Atherosclerosis is the most common cause of renal artery stenosis in older adults.
- Atherosclerosis tends to affect the ostia (origin) of the renal arteries.
- Both CTA and MRA have high sensitivity and specificity for the diagnosis of renal artery stenosis. However, high sensitivity diagnosis by MRA is applicable only to the proximal segments.
- Angioplasty and stenting have greater long-term patency compared to angioplasty alone.

Fibromuscular dysplasia (FMD)

- Fibromuscular dysplasia (FMD) is an idiopathic, non-infectious, non-inflammatory vascular disease affecting primarily the renal and carotid arteries. FMD is bilateral 2/3 of the time.
- FMD is predominantly seen in young or middle-aged women.
- In contrast to the ostial involvement of renal artery atherosclerosis, FMD tends to affect the mid or distal third of the renal arteries.
- The most common form of FMD is the medial fibroplasia subtype (80%), which features the classic *string of pearls* or *string of beads* appearance on angiography.
- A less common form is intimal fibroplasia, which is more common in children and appears as a smooth stenosis, not the string of pearls typical of medial fibroplasia.
- Perimedial and adventitial fibroplasia are less common variants.
- Diagnosis workup includes CTA or MRA. Angiography is reserved for treatment.

肾动脉

肾动脉粥样硬化狭窄

- 动脉粥样硬化是老年人肾动脉狭窄最常见的原因。
- 动脉粥样硬化往往累及肾动脉的开口部(起始部)。
- CTA和MRA对肾动脉狭窄的诊断有较高的灵敏度和特异度，但MRA诊断的高灵敏度仅适用于肾动脉近端节段。
- 血管成形联合支架置入术比单纯血管成形术有更高的长期通畅率。

肌纤维发育不良(FMD)

- 肌纤维发育不良(FMD)是一种特发性、非感染性、非炎性血管疾病，好发于肾动脉和颈动脉。双侧FMD占2/3。
- FMD主要见于中青年妇女。
- 与肾动脉粥样硬化常累及开口部不同，FMD常累及肾动脉中、远段1/3。
- FMD最常见的亚型是中膜纤维增生(占80%)，血管造影可见典型的串珠状表现。
- FMD相对少见的一种亚型是内膜纤维增生，常见于儿童，表现为光滑的狭窄，而非中膜纤维增生时的串珠状改变。
- 中层周围和外膜纤维增生是比较少见的亚型。
- 诊断检查包括CTA或MRA。血管造影术用于治疗。

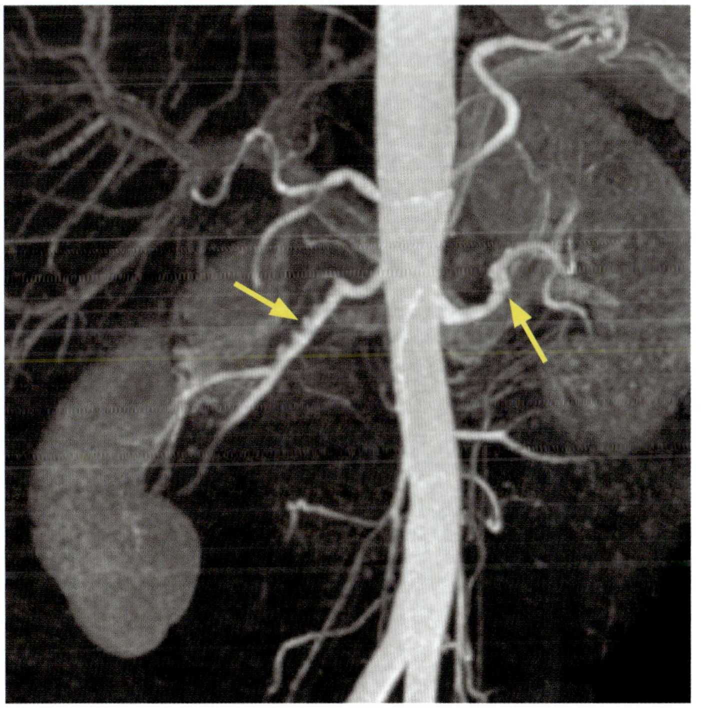

Fibromuscular dysplasia (medial fibroplasia subtype): MIP image from an MRA of the abdominal aorta shows the classic "beaded" appearance of both renal arteries (arrows) predominantly in the mid portion of the renal arteries, with sparing of the ostia.

肌纤维发育不良(中膜增生型)：腹主动脉MRA的MIP图像显示双侧肾动脉中段典型串珠状表现(黄箭)，而起始部未受累。

- A classic imaging feature of FMD is the *string of beads sign*, caused by alternating stenosis and aneurysmal dilation of the renal artery. Less common imaging features are focal stenosis (intimal type FMD) or dissection and aneurysm.
- FMD clinically responds well to angioplasty alone, with improved blood pressure control in 97%, including a 42% cure rate and a 90% patency rate at 5 years.
- Stenting of FMD is not recommended, as stenting can complicate retreatment with angioplasty and lead to in-stent stenosis due to intimal hyperplasia.

- 典型的FMD影像学特征是*串珠状征*，为肾动脉狭窄和动脉瘤样扩张交替发生所致。少见的影像学特征是局灶性狭窄（内膜型FMD）、夹层和动脉瘤。
- 单纯血管成形术对FMD的临床效果良好，血压缓解率可达97%，5年的治愈率为42%、通畅率为90%。
- 不推荐支架治疗FMD，因为支架术后再次行血管成形术的难度增加，且内膜增生会导致支架内狭窄。

Neurofibromatosis

- Neurofibromatosis may cause hypertension in children due to renal artery stenosis.
- Renal artery stenosis from NF1 may be angiographically indistinguishable from Takayasu arteritis, the most common cause of renal artery stenosis in children.

神经纤维瘤病

- 神经纤维瘤病可致儿童肾动脉狭窄，进而引起高血压。
- NF1型引起的肾动脉狭窄在血管造影上难以与大动脉炎进行区分，前者是儿童肾动脉狭窄最常见的原因。

Renal arteriovenous fistulas and malformations

- **Renal arteriovenous fistulas (AVFs)** are anomalous direct communications between arteries and veins in the kidney, and almost always acquired, secondary to trauma or renal biopsy.
- **Renal arteriovenous malformations (AVMs)** are rare congenital entities, and similarly there is abnormal connection between arterial and venous vessels. However, AVM almost always has a vascular nidus.
- CTA is an ideal imaging modality to assess AVF or AVM. Classical imaging features are large renal artery, associated aneurysmal dilation at the level of the venous communication, and early opacification of the renal vein during the arterial phase images.
- Similar findings can be seen on MRA. In addition, on T2-weighted images, large, round signal voids can be seen within the kidney.
- Angiography of an AVF shows venous opacification during the arterial phase.
- The majority of renal AVFs are asymptomatic and often heal spontaneously. When symptomatic, hematuria is the most common complaint. Less commonly, a renal AVF can lead to high-output cardiac failure or spontaneous retroperitoneal hemorrhage.
- Treatment of a renal AVF or AVM is with embolization (coils, glue, or alcohol).

肾动静脉瘘及畸形

- **肾动静脉瘘（AVFs）**是肾脏动脉和静脉之间异常的直接通道，几乎都是后天获得的，继发于外伤或肾活检。
- **肾动静脉畸形（AVMs）**是一种罕见的先天性疾病，动脉血管与静脉血管之间也存在异常的交通，但AVM几乎都有血管巢。
- CTA是评估AVF或AVM的理想影像学方法。典型影像学特征是肾动脉增粗，邻近静脉处可伴有动脉瘤样扩张，动脉早期即出现肾静脉显影。
- MRA上也可见类似表现。此外，在T_2加权图像上，肾内可见大而圆的流空信号。
- 动静脉瘘在血管造影时表现为静脉在动脉期显影。
- 大多数肾动静脉瘘无症状，且常自行愈合。当出现症状时，血尿是最常见的临床表现。较少情况下，肾动静脉瘘可引起高动力性心力衰竭或自发性腹膜后出血。
- 肾动静脉瘘或动静脉畸形的治疗方法是栓塞（弹簧圈、胶或乙醇）。

Gastrointestinal (GI) Bleeding

Imaging diagnosis of GI bleed

- Gastrointestinal (GI) bleeding could be upper GI bleeding (~15%) (proximal to the ligament of Treitz) or lower GI bleeding (~85%) (distal to the ligament of Treitz). This chapter focuses on lower GI bleeding as it is far more common.

  Upper GI bleeding presents with hematemesis or melena.

  Lower GI bleeding presents with hematochezia or melena.
- Etiologies of lower GI bleeding vary based on age. In young adults, common causes are inflammatory bowel disease or Meckel diverticulum. In older patients, common causes include colonic diverticula, angiodysplasia, neoplasm, or hemorrhoids.
- Colonoscopy is the first-line modality for diagnosing lower GI bleeding. However, in certain clinical scenarios, either CTA or technetium-99m-labeled

胃肠道出血

消化道出血的影像学诊断

- 胃肠道出血可以分为上消化道出血（15%）（屈氏韧带以上）或下消化道出血（85%）（屈氏韧带以下）。本章重点介绍更为常见的下消化道出血。

  上消化道出血表现为呕血或黑便。

  下消化道出血表现为便血或黑便。
- 下消化道出血的病因因年龄而异。在年轻成人中，常见的原因是炎症性肠病或梅克尔憩室。在老年患者中，常见的原因包括结肠憩室、血管发育不全、肿瘤或痔疮。
- 结肠镜检查是诊断下消化道出血的首选方法。

RBC scintigraphy can be performed as alternatives. Both modalities have limited sensitivity since bleeding is often intermittent. The positivity rate of CTA for extravasation is higher if performed within 4 hours or as soon as possible following the last episode of bleeding.

- Rates of bleeding that can be detected by different imaging modalities:
  Tc-99m-labeled RBC scintigraphy: <0.1 mL/min
  CTA: 0.3–0.5 mL/min
  DSA: 0.5–1.0 mL/min
- For detection of GI bleed, CTA and Tc-99m-labeled RBC scintigraphy have comparable sensitivities, although CTA has higher sensitivity to locate the bleeding. Intermittent bleeding is the most common cause of false-negative results on CTA.
- CTA protocol includes three phases: noncontrast, arterial phase, and delayed/venous phase.
- Imaging findings of GI bleed on CTA include:
  Intraluminal hyperattenuation on noncontrast phase, representing hematoma/clot.
  Intraluminal extravasation of contrast material is the main criteria to locate the bleeding point.
  Changing morphology of the extravasated contrast material with time (assessed on delayed images) confirms the diagnosis.

Diverticular bleed

但在某些临床情况下，CTA或^{99m}Tc标记红细胞闪烁显像可作为替代方法。由于出血常为间歇性，两种方法的灵敏度均有限。CTA应在出血4小时内或最近一次出血后尽早进行，此时发现造影剂血管外渗的阳性率比较高。

- 不同成像模式可检测到的出血率：
  ^{99m}Tc标记红细胞闪烁显像：<0.1mL/min
  CTA：0.3~0.5mL/min
  DSA：0.5~1.0mL/min
- CTA和^{99m}Tc标记红细胞闪烁显像检测胃肠道出血灵敏度相似，但CTA在定位出血方面有更高的灵敏度。间歇性出血是CTA假阴性结果最常见的原因。
- CTA采集方案包括三个期相：平扫、动脉期和延迟/静脉期。
- 胃肠道出血的CTA影像学表现包括：
  平扫肠腔内高密度影，代表血肿/血块。
  胃肠腔内造影剂外渗是定位出血点的主要标准。
  渗出的造影剂形态随时间变化(通过延迟图像评估)可确诊。

憩室出血

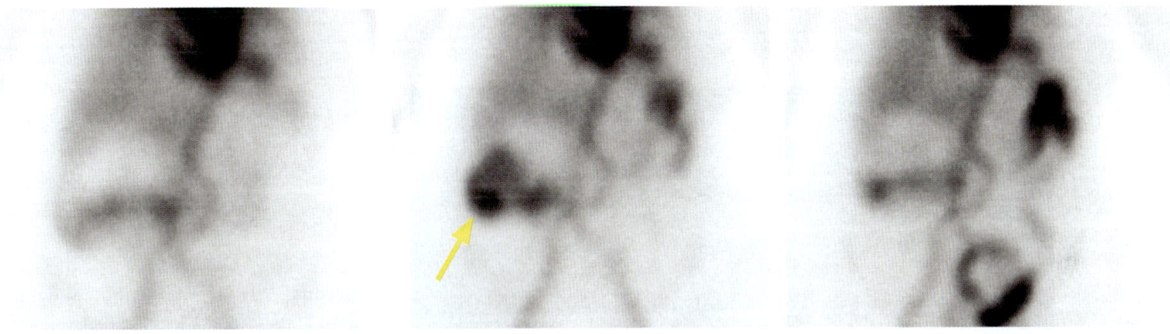

Diverticular bleed: Tagged red blood cell scan at 15, 30, and 45 minutes shows abnormal tracer accumulation at the hepatic flexure (arrow) with rapid transit into the distal colon by 45 minutes.
憩室出血：15、30和45分钟核素标记的红细胞显像显示异常核素聚集于结肠右曲(黄箭)，并在45分钟内快速转移到远端结肠。

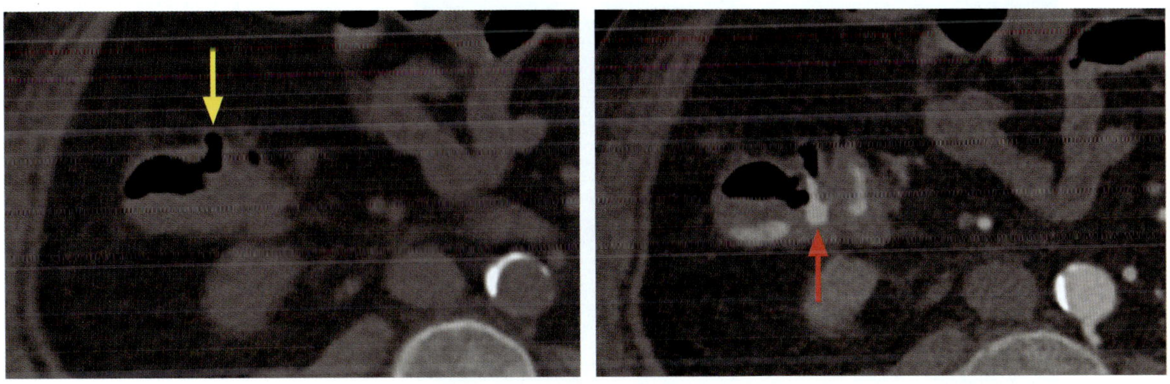

Noncontrast CT (left image) shows diverticulosis of the right colon (yellow arrow). Contrast-enhanced CT, aortic phase, shows dependent active extravasation of contrast in the region of the diverticulum (red arrow).
平扫CT(左图)显示右侧结肠憩室(黄箭)。主动脉期增强CT显示憩室区活动性造影剂外渗并沉积于底部(红箭)。

- Diverticulosis is the most common cause of lower GI bleeding in older adults.
- Imaging finding on CTA is active bleeding within extensive diverticulosis.
- Most patients respond to conservative management, but angiography can be used for stable or unstable patients who fail medical management. Potential therapies include superselective embolization (most commonly with coils) or vasopressin infusion.

Angiodysplasia

- Angiodysplasia is an acquired vascular anomaly that is a common cause of chronic intermittent lower GI bleeding, most typically located in the right colon or cecum. Because angiodysplasia is so prevalent (identified in up to 15% of patients incidentally), the presence of angiodysplasia in a bleeding patient should not stop the hunt for other possible sources.
- Even when angiodysplasia is the cause of bleeding, active extravasation is rarely seen.
- On CTA, angiodysplasia displays as small areas of bowel wall enhancement and venous opacification on arterial phase.
- Treatment is endoscopy with electrocoagulation, laser therapy, or other techniques. Surgery can be performed for recurrent or uncontrollable bleeding, but is usually not necessary.

- 憩室常为老年人下消化道出血最常见的原因。
- CTA表现为憩室内活动性出血。
- 大多数患者保守治疗有效，但血管造影可对药物治疗无效的稳定或不稳定的患者进行治疗。可采用超选择性栓塞(通常用弹簧圈)或加压素灌注予以治疗。

血管发育不良

- 血管发育不良是一种后天获得的血管异常，是慢性间歇性下消化道出血的常见原因，多见于右半结肠或盲肠。由于血管发育不良极为常见(约15%的患者意外发现)，出血患者在发现有血管发育不良时，还应继续寻找其他可能的出血原因。
- 即便血管发育不良是出血的原因，造影剂外溢仍罕见。
- 在CTA上，血管发育不良表现为小范围的肠壁强化和动脉期静脉显影。
- 治疗方法为内镜下电凝、激光治疗或其他技术。对反复或无法控制的出血可行手术治疗，但一般无必要。

NORMAL ABDOMINOPELVIC VENOUS ANATOMY

正常腹盆腔静脉解剖

Normal venous anatomy

正常静脉解剖

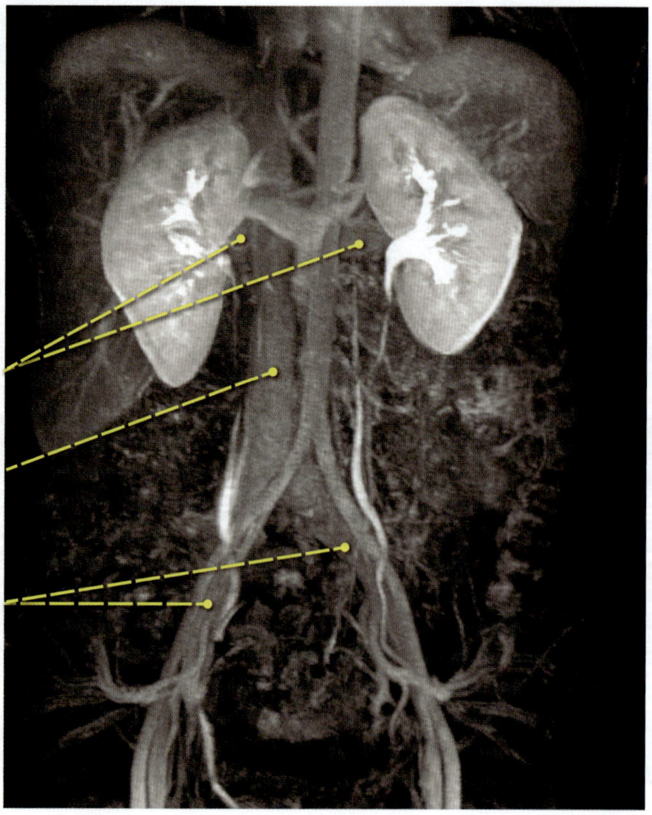

Coronal MIP of MR venogram demonstrates normal appearance of the renal veins, IVC, and common iliac veins. The portal venous system is not portrayed here.

MR venogram with contrast is obtained with multiplanar spoiled gradient-echo acquisition, imaged during three breath holds to obtain the arterial, first and second phase delayed imaging.

MR静脉造影冠状位MIP显示正常的肾静脉、下腔静脉和髂总静脉。该图未显示门静脉系统。

磁共振静脉造影(MRV)采用多平面梯度回波进行图像采集，在三次屏气期间成像，获得动脉、第一期和第二期延迟图像。

ABDOMINOPELVIC VENOUS PATHOLOGIES

腹盆腔静脉病变

Congenital IVC anomalies

先天性下腔静脉畸形

- Congenital IVC variants include absence, duplication, left-sided location,
- 先天性下腔静脉畸形包括缺如、重复、左侧下

azygous or hemiazygous continuation, and web formation.

腔静脉、奇静脉或半奇静脉延续和蹼形成。

IVC involvement in neoplasms

- The IVC can be involved in Wilms tumor, leiomyosarcoma, adrenal cortical carcinoma, testicular carcinoma, hepatocellular carcinoma, renal cell carcinoma, and other neoplasms.
- **Primary IVC leiomyosarcoma** arises from the parietal muscle cells of the IVC, usually in female patients aged 40–60 years. Imaging features include an enhancing filling defect with cystic necrosis.

肿瘤侵犯下腔静脉

- 肾母细胞瘤、平滑肌肉瘤、肾上腺皮质癌、睾丸癌、肝细胞癌、肾细胞癌等肿瘤可累及下腔静脉。
- **原发性下腔静脉平滑肌肉瘤**起源于下腔静脉壁的肌细胞，多见于40~60岁的女性患者。影像学表现为强化的充盈缺损伴囊性坏死。

Duplicated IVC

- If a duplicated IVC is present, in order to prevent a clot from circumnavigating the filter, either a single filter is placed above the IVC confluence or a filter is placed in each duplicated IVC.
- If pre-procedural imaging is not available, a clue to the presence of a duplicated IVC on initial cavography is the absence of iliac vein influx contralateral to the side injected.

重复下腔静脉

- 若出现重复下腔静脉，可在下腔静脉汇合处上方放置一个滤器，或在每支下腔静脉中各放置一个滤器，以防止血块绕过滤器。
- 如果术前没有影像学检查进行参照，在基线下腔静脉造影上出现重复下腔静脉的一条线索是注射造影剂后对侧无髂静脉反流。

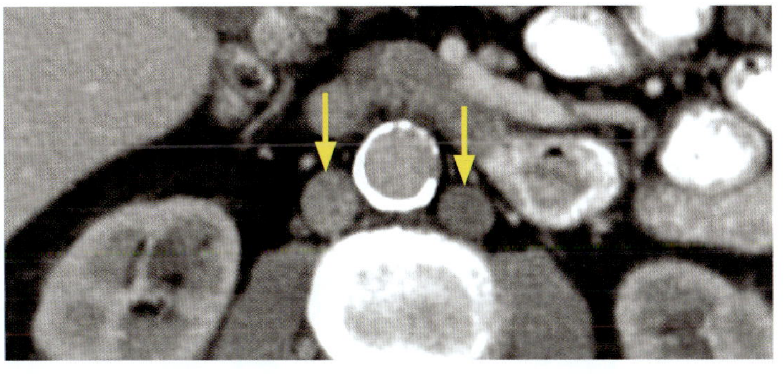

Duplicated IVC: Pre-procedure contrast-enhanced CT (left image) shows duplicated IVCs on either side of the aorta (arrows).
Case courtesy Alisa Suzuki Han, MD, Brigham and Women's Hospital.
重复下腔静脉：术前增强CT(左图)显示主动脉两侧的重复下腔静脉(黄箭)。

IVC imaging pitfalls

- Pseudolipoma is a common mimic of pathology at the level of the diaphragm due to volume-averaging artifact from prominent pericaval fat above the caudate lobe. Pseudolipoma can be prominent in patients with cirrhosis.
- Admixture artifact occurs wherever contrast-enhanced blood mixes with non-opacified blood, for example retrograde flow in the setting of right heart failure, contrast injection faster than 3 mL/sec, and at the level of the renal veins when contrast-enhanced blood from the kidneys mixes with non-opacified blood from the lower extremities.

下腔静脉成像的缺陷

- 假性脂肪瘤是横膈水平常见的非病理性病变，为尾状叶上方层面腔静脉周围脂肪增多所致的容积平均伪影导致。假性脂肪瘤在肝硬化患者中常见。
- 混合伪影出现在含造影剂的血液与无造影剂的血液混合的情况下，如右心衰竭时血液逆流、造影剂注射速度大于3mL/s，以及肾静脉水平强化的肾脏血液与未强化的下肢血液混合时。

Renal veins

Nutcracker syndrome

- Nutcracker syndrome is compression of the left renal vein between the aorta and the SMA. This is similar to SMA syndrome, but the renal vein is compressed instead of the duodenum.
- A posterior variant, called *posterior nutcracker,* is the compression of a retroaortic (or circumaortic) renal vein between the aorta and the vertebral body.
- Nutcracker syndrome can present with variable clinical symptoms including pain, hematuria, orthostatic proteinuria, pelvic congestion, and varicocele (in a male).
- If patient is asymptomatic, this is called Nutcracker *phenomenon*.
- Ultrasound, CTA or MRA can be utilized to assess the aortic-SMA angle, renal vein stenosis and upstream dilation, prominent collateral pathway particularly through the left gonadal vein. Narrowing of the vein only can be altered based

肾静脉

胡桃夹综合征

- 胡桃夹综合征是指左肾静脉位于肠系膜上动脉和主动脉之间而受到压迫。与SMA综合征相似，胡桃夹综合征受压的是肾静脉而非十二指肠。
- 胡桃夹综合征的后位变异，也称后位胡桃夹综合征，是指位于主动脉后(或环主动脉)的肾静脉在腹主动脉和椎体之间受到压迫。
- 胡桃夹综合征临床症状多样，包括疼痛、血尿、直立性蛋白尿、盆腔淤血及精索静脉曲张(男性)。
- 如果患者无症状，称为胡桃夹现象。
- 超声、CTA或MRA可用于评估主动脉-肠系膜上动脉夹角、肾静脉狭窄和上游血管扩张、

on patient's intravascular volume status, therefore, other findings should be included in the interpretation.

- Treatment depends on the symptoms. The majority of cases of hematuria resolve within two years of observation. If treatment is desired, angioplasty and stenting of the renal vein can be performed.

明显的侧支通路(尤其是通过左性腺静脉的侧支通路)。静脉变窄可以仅仅由患者血管内容量的改变引起,因此,在解读影像时还需要综合其他征象。

- 治疗方式取决于临床症状,大部分血尿患者会在两年观察期内缓解。如需治疗,可行肾静脉血管成形术和支架植入术。

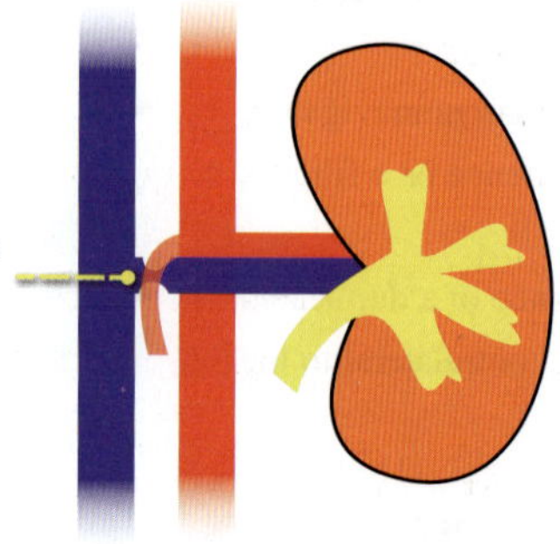

Nutcracker syndrome:
Illustration demonstrating compression of the renal vein (blue) between the aorta and the SMA (red).
胡桃夹综合征:
图示主动脉和肠系膜上动脉(红色)之间的肾静脉(蓝色)受压。

Pelvic vessels

盆腔血管

May-Thurner

髂静脉压迫综合征

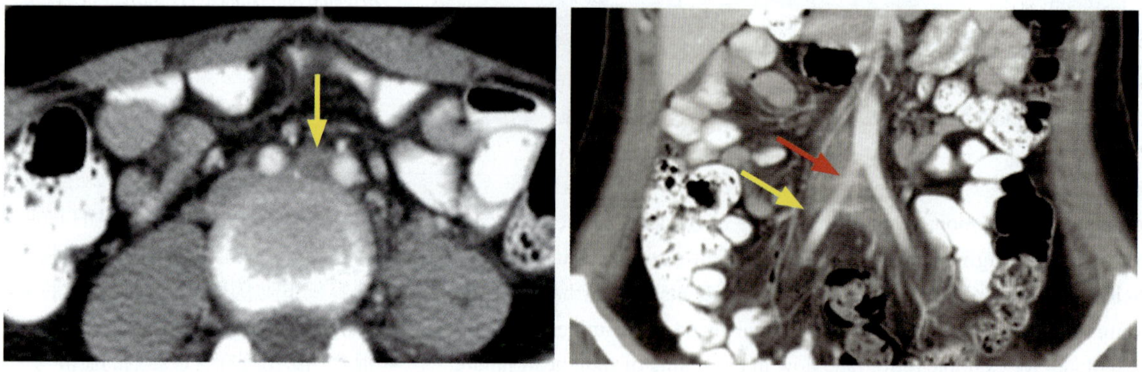

May-Thurner: Axial contrast-enhanced CT (left image) shows a distended and hypoattenuating left common iliac vein (yellow arrow), suggestive of thrombosis. Coronal CT (right image) shows the right common iliac artery (red arrow) crossing the bifurcation of the IVC and right common iliac vein (yellow arrow). The venous thrombosis is not apparent on the coronal view.
Case courtesy Michael Hanley, MD, University of Virginia Health System.
髂静脉压迫综合征:轴位增强CT(左图)显示左侧髂总静脉扩张但未见强化(黄箭),提示血栓形成。冠状位CT(右图)显示右侧髂总动脉(红箭)跨过下腔静脉分叉部及右侧髂总静脉(黄箭)。静脉血栓在冠状位图像上不明显。

- May-Thurner syndrome is a chronic compression of the left common iliac vein by crossing right common iliac artery against the lumbar vertebrae with or without deep venous thrombosis.
- Similar to other venous compression syndromes, intravascular volume status of the patient should be taken into consideration.

- 髂静脉压迫综合征是由于右侧髂总动脉压迫左侧髂总静脉,使其挤压在腰椎上,导致左侧髂总静脉长期受压。
- 与其他静脉压迫综合征相似,应考虑患者的血容量状况。

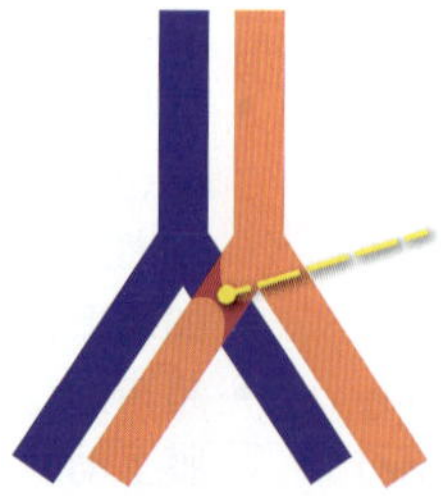

- Chronic compression leads to a fibrous adhesion in the vein, predisposing to thrombosis.
- CT venography or MR venography can diagnose compression and associated deep vein thrombosis.
- Treatment is endovascular thrombolysis followed by stenting.

Varicocele

- A varicocele is dilation of the pampiniform venous plexus. Primary varicocele (most common) is due to absent or incompetent valves in the proximal gonadal vein causing venous reflux. Primary varicoceles are a highly prevalent and treatable cause of infertility. Secondary varicocele is due to a mass obstructing venous return.
- The vast majority of varicoceles are left-sided as the left gonadal vein drains into the left renal vein, while the right gonadal vein drains directly into the IVC. A solitary right varicocele should prompt the workup for an obstructing retroperitoneal mass.
- Scrotal ultrasound shows a dilated (>2 mm) venous plexus with a *bag of worms* appearance, which worsens on Valsalva maneuver.
- Treatment is coil embolization or surgical ligation of the gonadal vein, which have been shown to be equivalent in outcome.

Pelvic congestion syndrome

- Pelvic congestion syndrome is a potentially treatable cause of chronic abdominopelvic pain.
- Etiologies include retrograde flow through incompetent valves of the ovarian veins or venous obstruction.
- Imaging shows dilated pelvic and ovarian veins that increase in caliber or reversed flow after Valsalva.

- 慢性压迫导致静脉内纤维性黏附，易形成血栓。
- CT静脉成像或MR静脉成像可以识别压迫和伴随的深静脉血栓。
- 治疗方法为腔内溶栓，之后进行支架植入术。

精索静脉曲张

- 精索静脉曲张是蔓状静脉丛扩张。原发性精索静脉曲张(最常见)是由于性腺静脉近端瓣膜缺失或功能不全引起静脉反流。原发性精索静脉曲张非常常见、可致不育，但可治疗。继发性精索静脉曲张是肿块阻塞静脉回流所致。
- 绝大多数的精索静脉曲张见于左侧，因左性腺静脉汇流入左肾静脉，而右性腺静脉则直接汇流入下腔静脉。孤立性右精索静脉曲张时，应及时检查有无可导致静脉阻塞的腹膜后肿块。
- 阴囊超声示扩张(>2mm)的静脉丛，呈蠕虫样外观，行瓦尔萨尔瓦动作检查时曲张现象加剧。
- 治疗方法是弹簧圈栓塞或外科结扎性腺静脉，两者预后相似。

盆腔充血综合征

- 盆腔充血综合征是一种有可能治愈的慢性盆腔疼痛。
- 病因包括卵巢静脉瓣膜功能不全导致的血液逆流或静脉阻塞。
- 影像显示盆腔和卵巢静脉扩张，并在瓦尔萨尔瓦动作后可见静脉管径增加或出现血流逆流。

(翻译　许棚棚)

UPPER EXTREMITY VESSELS

上肢血管

NORMAL VASCULAR ANATOMY OF THE UPPER EXTREMITY

正常上肢血管解剖

Thoracic outlet

胸廓出口

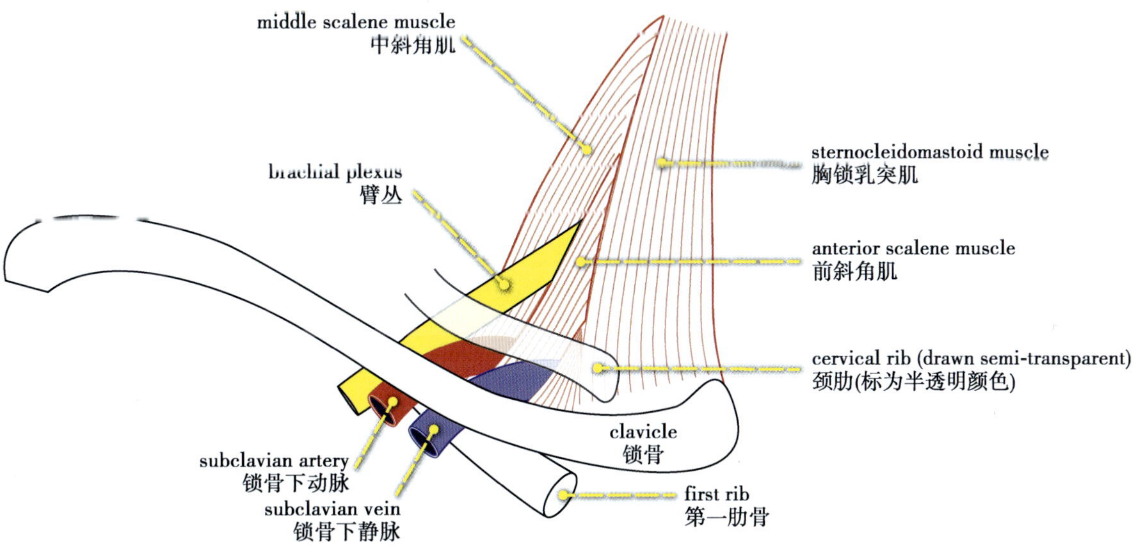

Subclavian artery

- The right subclavian artery arises from the brachiocephalic trunk. The left subclavian artery branches directly from the aortic arch.
- The first portion includes the origin to the medial border of the anterior scalene muscle. Branches include:

  Vertebral artery.

  Internal thoracic artery.

  Thyrocervical trunk.

- The second portion lies posterior to the anterior scalene muscle and gives off the:

  Costocervical trunk.

- The third portion lies between the lateral border of the anterior scalene to the lateral border of the first rib and gives off the:

  Dorsal scapular artery.

Axillary artery

- The axillary artery starts from the lateral border of the first rib and courses underneath the pectoralis minor muscle which divides the artery into three anatomical portions.

锁骨下动脉

- 右锁骨下动脉源自头臂干，左锁骨下动脉直接源自主动脉弓。
- 锁骨下动脉第一段自起点至前斜角肌的内缘，其分支包括：

  椎动脉。

  胸廓内动脉。

  甲状颈干。

- 第二段位于前斜角肌的后方并发出：

  肋颈干。

- 第三段位于斜角肌外缘至第一肋骨外缘之间并发出：

  肩胛背动脉。

腋动脉

- 腋动脉始于第一肋外缘，走行于胸小肌下方，分成三段。

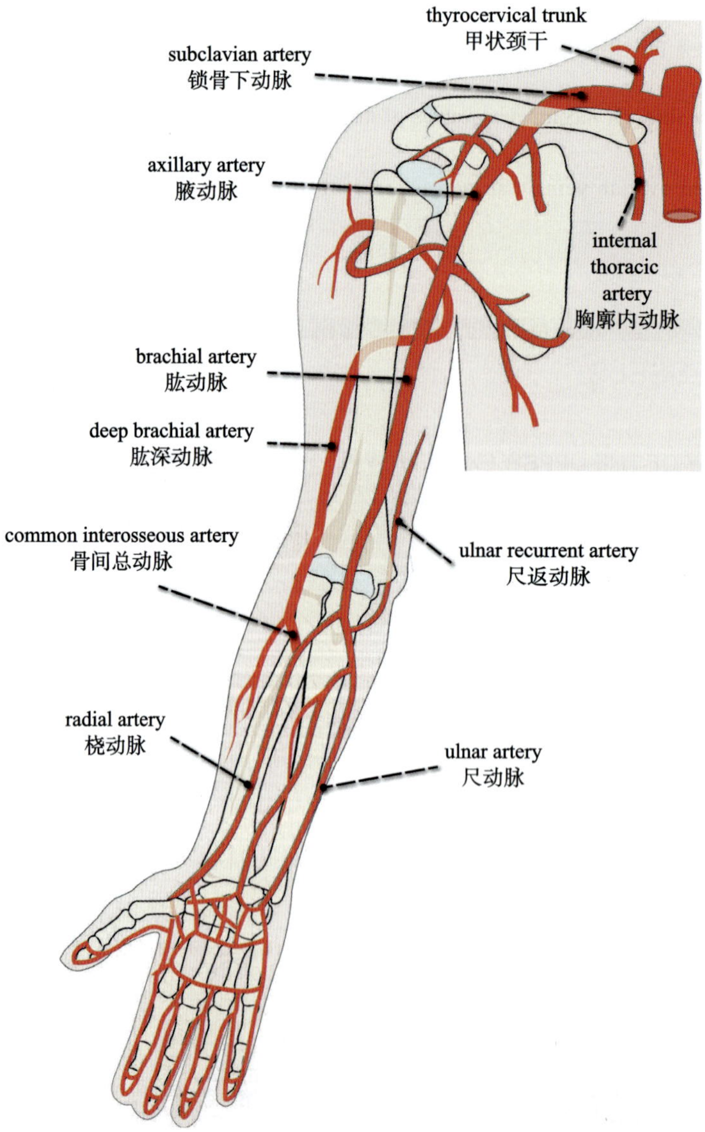

Parts of the axillary artery

The first portion runs from the lateral edge of the first rib to the upper border of the pectoralis minor muscle and branches inferiorly into the **superior thoracic artery**.

The second portion runs behind the pectoralis minor muscle and branches superolaterally into the **thoracoacromial trunk** and inferiorly into the **lateral thoracic artery.**

The third portion runs from the lateral border of the pectoralis minor muscle to the teres major muscle, branching into the **subscapular artery** and the **anterior and posterior circumflex humeral arteries.**

腋动脉分段

第一段始于第一肋外侧缘、止于胸小肌上缘，向下分出胸廓上动脉。

第二段走行于胸小肌后方，向上外侧方分出胸肩峰干，向下分出胸廓外动脉。

第三段自胸小肌外侧缘至大圆肌，分出肩胛下动脉、旋肱前动脉和旋肱后动脉。

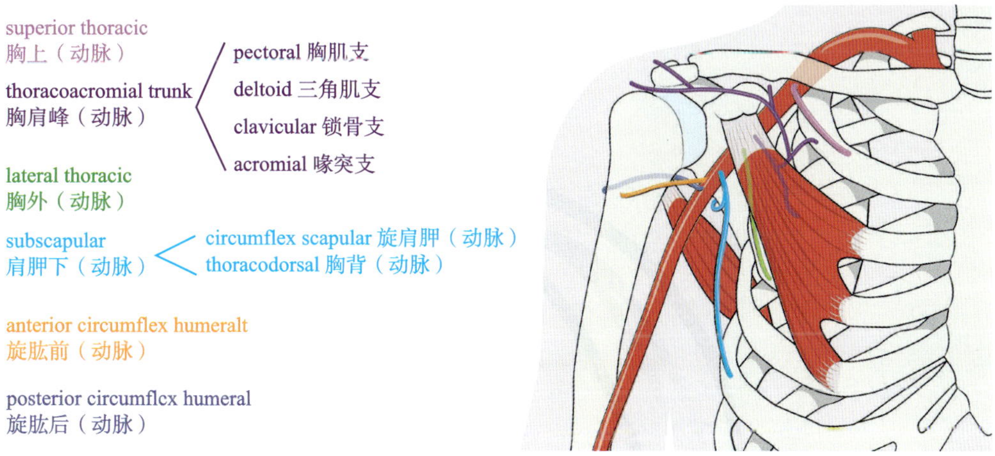

Illustration of branches of axillary artery.
腋动脉分支示意图

Brachial artery

- The brachial artery begins at the lateral edge of the teres major muscle. The branches include the deep brachial artery, the superior ulnar collateral artery, and the inferior ulnar collateral artery.
- The radial nerve parallels the deep brachial artery.

肱动脉

- 肱动脉起自大圆肌外侧缘，分支包括肱深动脉、尺侧上副动脉、尺侧下副动脉。
- 桡神经与肱深动脉伴行。

Hand arteries

手动脉

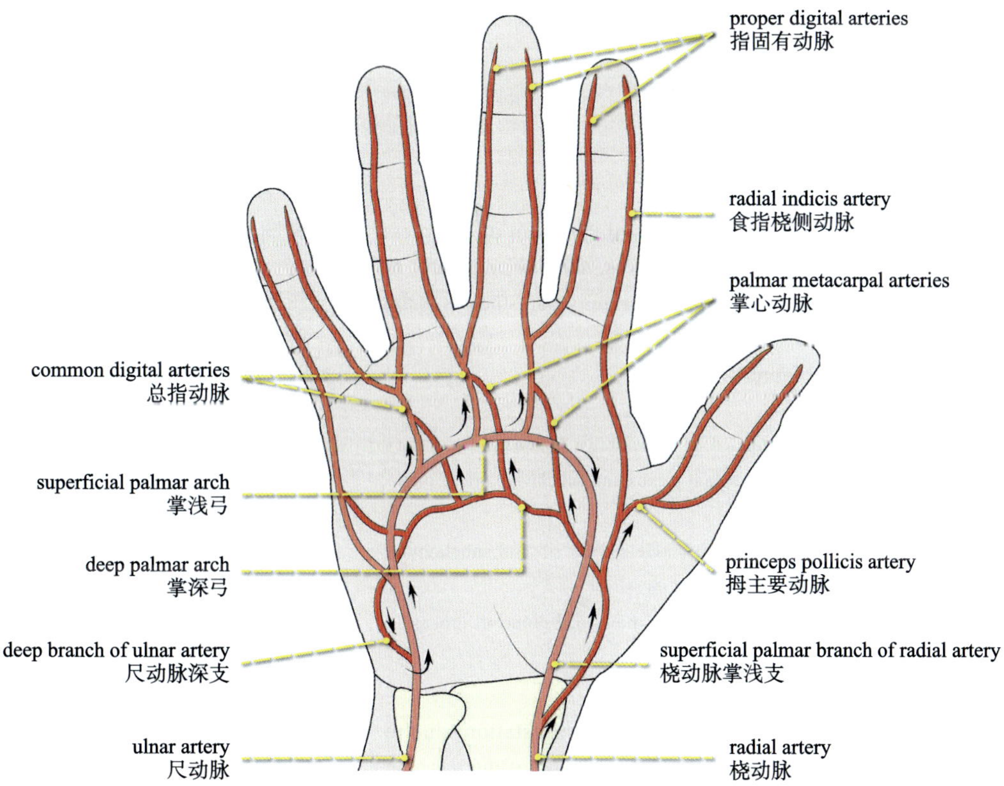

Venous arm anatomy

- The superficial veins arise from the dorsal venous arch on the dorsum of the hand and drain into the cephalic and basilic veins.
- The cephalic vein drains the radial (lateral) side and connects with the subclavian vein.
- The basilic vein drains the ulnar (medial) side and connects with the brachial or axillary vein.
- The deep venous drainage is via the ulnar and radial veins that course closely with corresponding arteries, and merge at the antecubital fossa to form the brachial vein.
- The brachial vein is renamed the axillary vein at the axilla.

上肢静脉解剖

- 浅表静脉源自手背的背侧静脉弓，引流入头静脉和贵要静脉。
- 头静脉引流桡(外)侧并与锁骨下静脉相连接。
- 贵要静脉引流尺(内)侧并与肱或锁骨下静脉相连接。
- 深静脉经尺和桡静脉引流，与其同名动脉伴行，于肘窝处汇合成肱静脉。
- 肱静脉在腋窝更名为腋静脉。

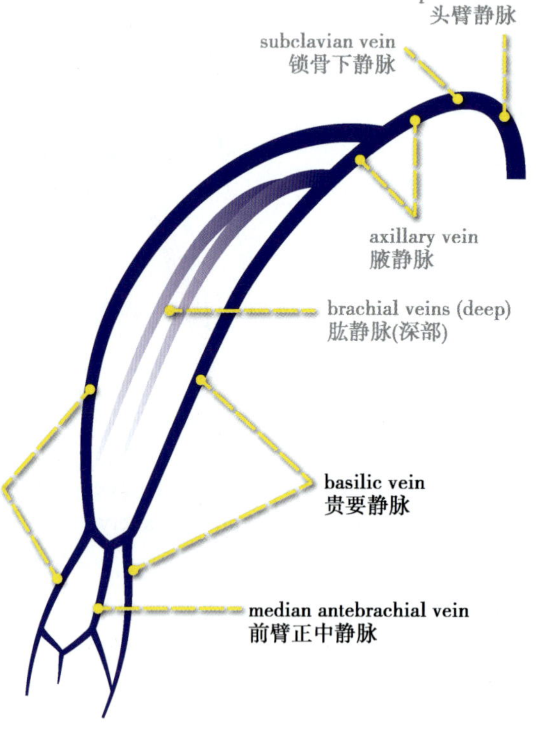

THORACIC OUTLET SYNDROMES (TOS)

Overview of thoracic outlet syndromes

- Thoracic outlet syndromes (TOS) are a controversial spectrum of disorders caused by compression of either the brachial plexus, subclavian artery, or subclavian vein, clinically presenting with upper extremity paresthesias, pain, numbness, and/or coolness.
- There are three common sites of compression:

> 1) The interscalene triangle is the space bounded by the anterior scalene muscle, the middle scalene muscle, and the first rib. The brachial plexus and subclavian artery pass through the interscalene triangle.
> 2) Costoclavicular space is the space between the clavicle, first rib and subclavius muscle. The subclavian vein compression is common at this site.
> 3) Subpectoral space is the space between the pectoralis minor and coracoid process. Subclavian artery compression is common at this site.

- The neurogenic form of TOS is the most common manifestation, due to mechanical compression of the brachial plexus. Compression of the vascular

胸廓出口综合征(TOS)

胸廓出口综合征概述

- 胸廓出口综合征(TOS)是一系列有争议的病变，是臂丛神经、锁骨下动脉或锁骨下静脉受压迫所致，临床表现为上肢感觉异常、疼痛、麻木和/或发凉。
- 常见的三个压迫部位：

> 1) 斜角肌间隙是由前斜角肌、中斜角肌和第一肋骨构成的三角形间隙，内有臂丛和锁骨下动脉通过。
> 2) 胸锁间隙是由锁骨、第一肋骨和锁骨下肌所构成的间隙。锁骨下静脉压迫常发生于此。
> 3) 胸肌下间隙是位于胸小肌和喙突之间的间隙。锁骨下动脉压迫常位于此处。

- 神经源性TOS是最常见的表现，为臂丛神经机械性受压所致。血管结构受压时被称为血

structures is known as vascular TOS. In this section we will focus on vascular TOS.

- Dynamic imaging either with a CTA or MRA is key in the diagnosis of vascular TOS. Imaging acquisition should be done arms up (hyperabduction) and arms down (neutral) position with two injections of the contrast. For each position arterial and venous images should be acquired.

Neurogenic TOS

- The neurogenic form of thoracic outlet syndrome is the most common manifestation, due to mechanical compression of the brachial plexus.
- Injury to the upper brachial plexus, C5 and C6, results in paralysis of the shoulder muscles and biceps. Injury to the lower brachial plexus C7 and below results in forearm and hand paralysis.

Subclavian artery compression due to TOS

- Compression of the subclavian artery clinically presents with hand or finger pain, numbness, paresthesias, or coolness.
- **Adson's maneuver** is a test for subclavian artery compression at the thoracic outlet. First, the radial artery is palpated in neutral position. Then, the patient's head is turned to the contralateral side while they inhale. In arterial thoracic outlet syndrome, the radial pulse will be reduced with this maneuver.
- A mechanical compression is almost always present and is exaggerated during hyperabduction. Over 70% of patients with subclavian artery compression have a cervical rib. Other causes of subclavian artery compression include an accessory scalene muscle (scalenus minimus), enlargement of the anterior scalene muscle, and well-developed musculature.
- Potential complications include arterial mural thrombus, aneurysm, and distal embolization. The hands should always be evaluated for signs of distal emboli.
- The preferred treatment of subclavian artery compression is surgical thoracic outlet decompression (e.g., resection of a cervical rib) and repair of the subclavian artery if an aneurysm is present.
- Endovascular arterial thrombolysis may be performed concurrently, weighed against the risk for distal embolization.

Subclavian vein compression due to TOS (Paget-Schroetter syndrome)

- Subclavian vein compression is common during hyperabduction; however associated upper limb swelling and pain suggest clinically significant stenosis. Compression of the subclavian vein without thrombosis is also known as McCleery syndrome.
- Paget-Schroetter syndrome is thrombosis (i.e., effort thrombosis) of the subclavian vein as it enters the thorax and is usually seen in muscular young men. Chronic compression causes intimal hyperplasia, which leads to subclavian vein thrombosis. Paget-Schroetter syndrome clinically presents with upper-extremity swelling or pain worsened with effort.
- Stents should generally not be used, especially if there is a mechanical obstruction, due to high risk of device failure.
- During diagnostic venography, it is necessary to evaluate the arm both in neutral position and abducted.
- CTA and MRA can diagnose thrombosed subclavian vein as a filling defect. Both sides should be evaluated. Frequently, both subclavian veins are compressed, even if only one side is symptomatic.
- Depending on the chronicity of disease, treatment is thrombolysis followed by surgical thoracic outlet decompression.

管性胸廓出口综合征。本节重点讨论血管性胸廓出口综合征。

- 动态CTA或MRA是诊断血管性TOS的关键。应行手臂上举(过度外展)和放下(自然)两个体位检查，并分两次注射造影剂。每个体位均应采集动脉期和静脉期图像。

神经源性TOS

- 神经源性胸廓出口综合征是最常见的表现，是臂丛神经受到机械性压迫所致。
- 臂丛神经上部分(即C_5和C_6)损伤会导致肩部肌肉和肱二头肌麻痹，臂丛神经下部分(即C_7及以下)损伤会导致前臂和手的麻痹。

TOS致锁骨下动脉受压

- 锁骨下动脉受压在临床上表现为手或手指疼痛、麻木、感觉异常或发凉。
- **Adson试验**用于测试锁骨下动脉在胸廓出口处是否受压。先在自然体位触摸桡动脉，再嘱患者吸气且头偏向对侧，动脉性胸廓出口综合征时桡动脉搏动将减弱。
- 几乎都会有机械性压迫，且在外展过度时加剧。超过70%的锁骨下动脉压迫患者有颈肋。其他导致锁骨下动脉压迫的原因包括副斜角肌(小斜角肌)、前斜角肌肥大和肌肉过度发达。
- 潜在并发症包括动脉附壁血栓、动脉瘤和远端栓塞。须时常检查手有无远端栓子栓塞的征象。
- 治疗锁骨下动脉压迫的首选方法是外科胸廓出口减压术(如颈肋切除)，若合并动脉瘤可行锁骨下动脉修补术。
- 可同时行动脉腔内溶栓治疗，但要权衡造成远端栓塞的风险。

TOS致锁骨下静脉受压(Paget-Schroetter综合征)

- 锁骨下静脉受压在上肢过度伸展时很常见，但合并上肢肿胀和疼痛时则提示有临床显著狭窄。锁骨下静脉受压但无血栓形成被称为McCleery综合征。
- Parget-Schroetter综合征是指锁骨下静脉进入胸廓处有血栓形成(即劳力性血栓形成)，常见于肌肉发达的青年男性。慢性压迫可引起内膜过度增生，进而导致锁骨下静脉血栓形成。Paget-Schroelter综合征在临床上表现为上肢运动后肿胀或疼痛加重。
- 通常不应使用支架，特别是有机械性梗阻时。因为支架失败的风险较高。
- 进行诊断性静脉造影时，须将手臂置于自然和外展两个体位进行评估。
- CTA和MRA可用于诊断锁骨下静脉血栓形成，表现为管腔内充盈缺损。应注意评估双侧锁骨下静脉，通常双侧锁骨下静脉均可受压，即使仅一侧出现症状。
- 根据病程，治疗是先溶栓，然后行外科胸廓出口减压术。

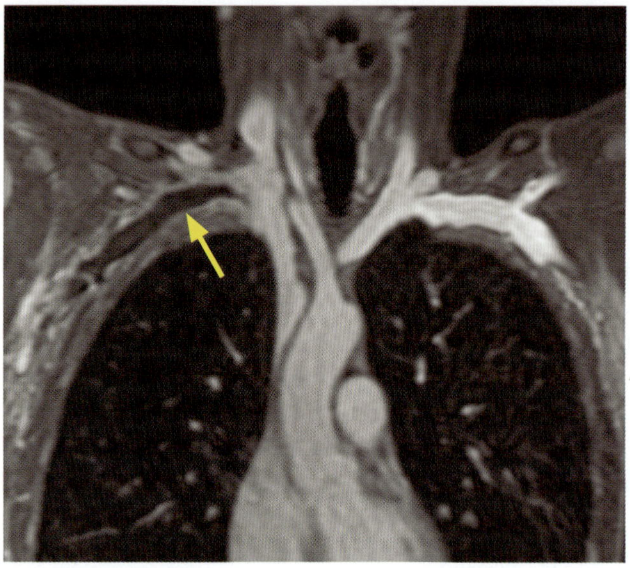

Coronal contrast-enhanced MR venography with arms abducted demonstrates right subclavian vein thrombus (arrow). The MRI did not demonstrate a mechanical cause for the thrombosis.

Case courtesy Alisa Suzuki Han, MD, Brigham and Women's Hospital.

手臂外展位冠状位增强MR静脉成像，显示右锁骨下静脉血栓(黄箭)。MRI未显示血栓形成的机械原因。

HAND ANATOMY AND PATHOLOGIES

Hypothenar hammer syndrome (HHS)

- Hypothenar hammer syndrome represents injury to the ulnar artery as it crosses the hamate bone. Chronic repetitive trauma causes the ulnar artery to chronically be traumatized at the hamate, leading to intimal injury, thrombus, aneurysm, or pseudoaneurysm.
- The classic clinical history of hypothenar hammer syndrome is a jackhammer operator with ischemia of the fourth and fifth digits.
- Ultrasound should be used as an initial imaging modality, followed by CTA or MRA. Classic imaging features include *corkscrew* or tortuous appearance of the distal ulnar artery at the level of the hook of the hamate. Aneurysmal dilation and distal embolic occlusions are seen due to distal thrombi, usually in the fourth and fifth fingers.
- Treatment is surgical, as there is often ulnar artery injury not apparent on angiography.

手的解剖和病变

小鱼际锤综合征(HHS)

- 小鱼际锤综合征(HHS)是由尺动脉经过钩骨处受创伤所致。慢性反复创伤导致尺动脉在钩骨段慢性损伤，进而导致内膜损伤、血栓形成、动脉瘤或假性动脉瘤。
- HSS典型的临床病史是电钻操作者出现无名指和小指缺血。
- 超声是首选的影像学检查手段，其次是CTA或MRA。典型影像学表现为钩状骨远端的尺动脉呈*螺旋*样或扭曲改变，可见动脉瘤样扩张及因血栓脱落造成的远端血栓栓塞性闭塞，常发生于第四和第五小指。
- 治疗采用外科方式，因为尺动脉损伤常不能在血管造影上明确显示。

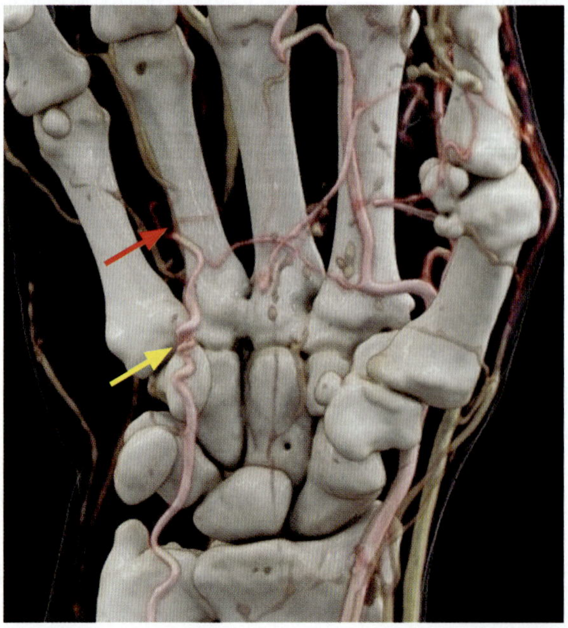

Patient presented with cyanotic fingers. CTA with 3D rendered images revealed corkscrew appearance of the ulnar artery (yellow arrow) with abrupt cutoff of the digital artery (red arrow).

手指发绀患者，CTA容积再现图像显示尺动脉呈螺旋样改变(黄箭)，伴远端指动脉突然截断(红箭)。

Buerger disease

- Buerger disease or **thromboangiitis obliterans**, is a chronic inflammatory, thrombotic arteritis that affects the lower extremities (most commonly) and the hands (less commonly). It is seen in adult male smokers and should be clinically suspected in a middle-aged male presenting with claudication. Primary treatment of Buerger disease is smoking cessation.
- Small vessel occlusions and distal *corkscrew* collaterals are the typical angiographic features.

Raynaud disease

- Raynaud disease is small arterial vasospasm triggered by cold temperature. Raynaud disease is associated with scleroderma and other connective tissue disorders.
- On imaging, there is decreased perfusion of the distal digital arteries, with improvement upon warming or vasodilator administration.

Thromboembolic disease

- Thromboembolic disease of the upper extremities is most commonly caused by cardiac emboli (of which atrial fibrillation is a common cause). Less commonly, a subclavian artery aneurysm may be the source of the thrombus.
- If the source of emboli is central (such as the heart), bilateral disease would be expected, while a unilateral lesion would show unilateral emboli.
- The characteristic imaging feature of distal thromboembolic disease is occlusion of distal small arteries of the hand.

Buerger病

- Buerger病或**血栓闭塞性脉管炎**是慢性炎症性、血栓性动脉炎，累及下肢(最常见)和手(较少见)。见于成年男性吸烟者，临床上中年男性有跛行时应怀疑此病。Buerger病的首要治疗是戒烟。
- 小血管闭塞及远端*螺旋样*侧支血管是动脉造影的典型表现。

雷诺病

- 雷诺病是寒冷激发的小动脉痉挛，与硬皮病和其他结缔组织疾病有关。
- 影像上表现为远端指动脉灌注下降，手指变暖或使用血管扩张剂后可改善。

血栓闭塞性疾病

- 上肢血栓闭塞性疾病常为心源性栓子所致(心房颤动为最常见原因)，其次为自锁骨下动脉瘤脱落的栓子。
- 若栓子源自中心部位(如心脏)，可表现为双侧病变，而单侧病变则引起单侧栓塞。
- 远端血栓栓塞疾病的典型影像学表现是手指的远端小动脉闭塞。

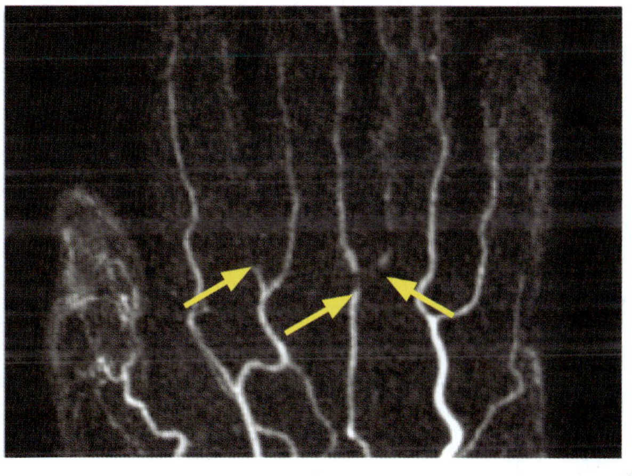

MRA shows multifocal occlusion of the digital arteries (arrows) due to emboli in a patient with subclavian vein thrombus and acute finger discoloration.

MRA显示由栓子导致的指动脉多发局灶性闭塞(黄箭)，该患者有锁骨下静脉血栓及急性手指皮肤变色。

(翻译　吴汉平)

LOWER EXTREMITY VESSELS

下肢血管

NORMAL VASCULAR ANATOMY OF THE LOWER EXTREMITY

正常下肢血管解剖

Arterial anatomy of the leg

下肢动脉解剖

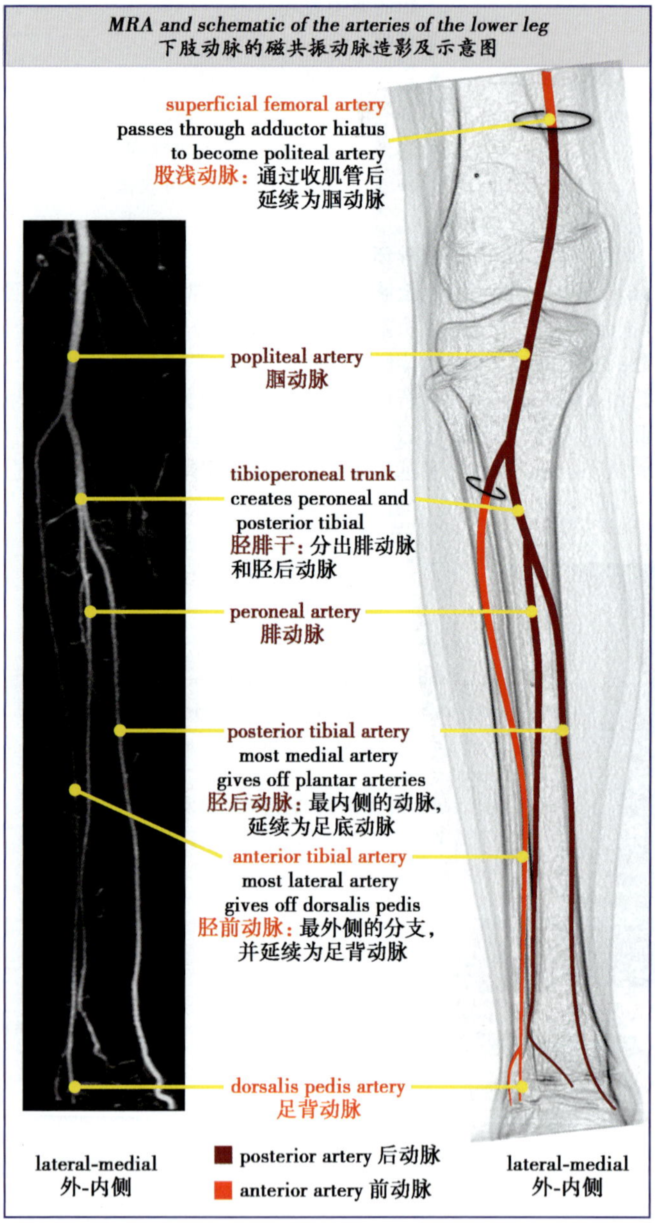

MRA and schematic of the arteries of the lower leg
下肢动脉的磁共振动脉造影及示意图

After passing posteriorly through the adductor hiatus, the SFA becomes the popliteal artery. From medial to lateral, the branches of the popliteal artery are:

A) Posterior tibial artery (most medial).

B) Peroneal artery (arises from the tibioperoneal trunk, along with the posterior tibial artery).

C) Anterior tibial artery (most lateral; the only anterior artery of the lower leg). It is easy to remember that the *anterior tibial* artery is *lateral* because the only muscle bulk of the anterior lower leg is the *lateral* compartment and that muscle is the *anterior tibialis*.

股浅动脉在穿过收肌管的后部后延续为腘动脉。腘动脉的分支自内向外包括：

A)胫后动脉(最内侧的动脉)。

B)腓动脉(与胫后动脉一起起源于胫腓干)。

C)胫前动脉(为最外侧的动脉，小腿前部唯一的动脉)。“胫前动脉位于小腿的外侧”这一点容易记忆，因小腿前部的唯一肌群是外侧间隙内的胫骨前肌。

- The femoral artery is the continuation of external iliac artery distal to the inguinal ligament.
- The femoral artery branches include:

  Profunda femoral artery, the terminal branch to supply the deep muscles of the thigh.

  Superficial circumflex iliac artery.

  Superficial femoral artery (SFA), which continues to supply the leg and foot.

- 股动脉是髂外动脉在腹股沟韧带下方的延续。
- 股动脉的分支包括：

  股深动脉，终末支供应大腿深部肌群。

  旋髂浅动脉。

  股浅动脉(SFA)，向下延伸供应小腿及足部。

Venous anatomy of the leg

- The superficial venous system is composed of the great and small saphenous veins.

  The **great saphenous vein** drains into the common femoral vein. Although the great

下肢静脉解剖

- 浅静脉系统由大隐静脉和小隐静脉组成。

  大隐静脉汇入股总静脉。尽管大隐静脉是浅静

saphenous vein is technically part of the superficial system, clots near the saphenofemoral junction are typically treated with anticoagulation because of their propensity to become dislodged.

The **small saphenous vein** drains into the popliteal vein (which continues proximally as the femoral vein). Clots in the small saphenous vein are typically not treated.

- Deep venous system anatomy mirrors arterial anatomy:

The **common femoral vein (CFV)** drains into the external iliac vein and begins at the level of the inguinal ligament. The CFV lies medial to the common femoral artery.

CFV tributaries include the **femoral and deep femoral veins**. The femoral vein was previously called the superficial femoral vein.

The term *superficial femoral vein* should be avoided as it wrongly implies that this vein is part of the superficial venous system.

The three paired deep calf veins are the **anterior tibial** (lateral), **peroneal** (middle), and **posterior tibial** (medial) veins, which join to form the **popliteal vein** (PV). The PV continues into the femoral vein.

The **gastrocnemius** and **soleal** veins are muscular veins also considered part of the deep venous system.

脉系统的一部分，但隐股交界处的血栓有脱落的风险，因此通常会采取抗凝治疗。

小隐静脉汇入腘静脉(近端延续为股静脉)。小隐静脉内的血栓常无须治疗。

- 深静脉系统与动脉系统伴行：

股总静脉(CFV)于腹股沟韧带水平汇入髂外静脉，起始于腹股沟韧带水平。CFV位于股总动脉的内侧。

CFV的属支包括**股静脉**和**股深静脉**。股静脉曾命名为股浅静脉。

应避免使用股浅静脉这一术语，因其错误地暗示了该静脉是浅静脉系统的一部分。

三对小腿深静脉分别为**胫前**静脉(外侧)、**腓**静脉(中)和**胫后**(内侧)静脉，它们汇合形成腘静脉(PV)，延续为股静脉。

腓肠肌静脉和**比目鱼肌**静脉为肌肉的静脉，也属于深静脉系统。

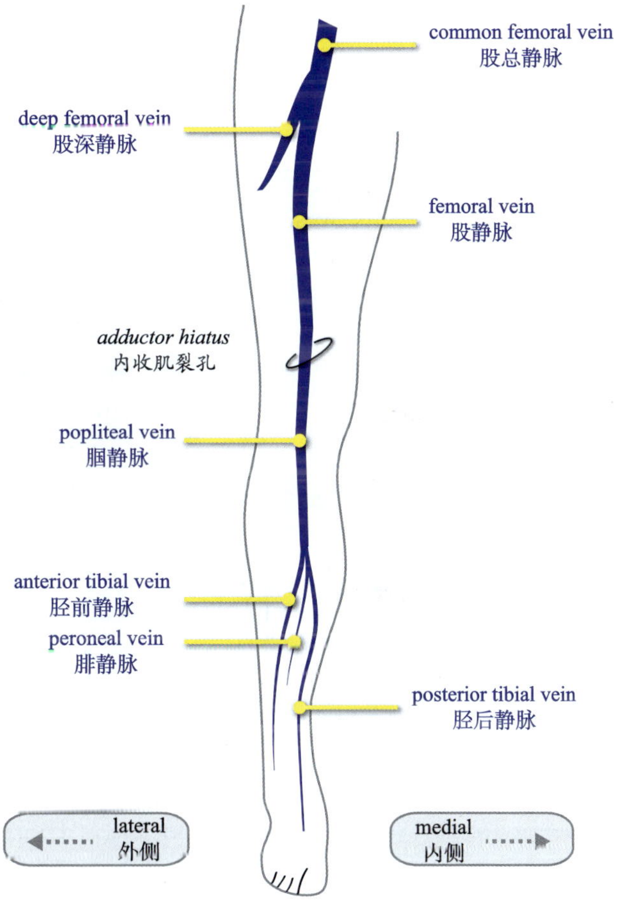

DISTAL AORTA, ILIAC, PELVIC, AND LEG ARTERIES PATHOLOGIES

Iliac artery aneurysm

- An iliac artery aneurysm is defined as common iliac artery diameter >2.5 cm. Ectasia is defined as >1.7 cm in males and >1.5 cm in females. Repair is recommended once the diameter is >3.0 cm.
- Iliac artery aneurysms are typically seen in older men and are associated with abdominal aortic aneurysms. They are most commonly associated with atherosclerosis. Iliac aneurysms may also be due to connective tissue diseases, such as Marfan syndrome.
- Cross-sectional imaging is recommended if an iliac stenosis is seen first on angiography. An iliac aneurysm with intraluminal thrombus can simulate an atherosclerotic stenosis on angiography.
- CTA or MRA can be done for the diagnosis and treatment planning.
- In appropriate candidates, endovascular stent-graft is the preferred treatment for an iliac artery aneurysm.
- Mass effect from the aneurysm may cause neurologic and urologic symptoms, in which case surgical treatment is recommended. Endovascular aneurysm repair cannot rapidly decrease aneurysm size, although endovascularly treated aneurysms do gradually decrease in size.

Persistent sciatic artery

远端腹主动脉、髂动脉、盆腔及下肢动脉病变

髂动脉瘤

- 髂动脉瘤是指髂总动脉直径>2.5cm。髂动脉扩张是指髂动脉直径在男性>1.7cm，在女性>1.5cm。当髂动脉直径>3cm时应建议行修补术。
- 髂动脉瘤多见于老年男性患者，且伴有腹主动脉瘤。其常与动脉粥样硬化相关，也可由结缔组织疾病引起，如马方综合征。
- 当动脉造影发现髂动脉狭窄时，建议行断层影像学检查。髂动脉瘤并发腔内血栓形成时在动脉造影上可类似粥样硬化性狭窄。
- CTA或MRA可用于诊断和制定治疗计划。
- 对于合适的患者，覆膜支架是治疗髂动脉瘤的首选方法。
- 动脉瘤可产生占位效应而引起神经或泌尿系统症状，此类患者应采取外科治疗。血管腔内治疗不能快速减小动脉瘤的体积，而是逐渐缩小。

永存坐骨动脉

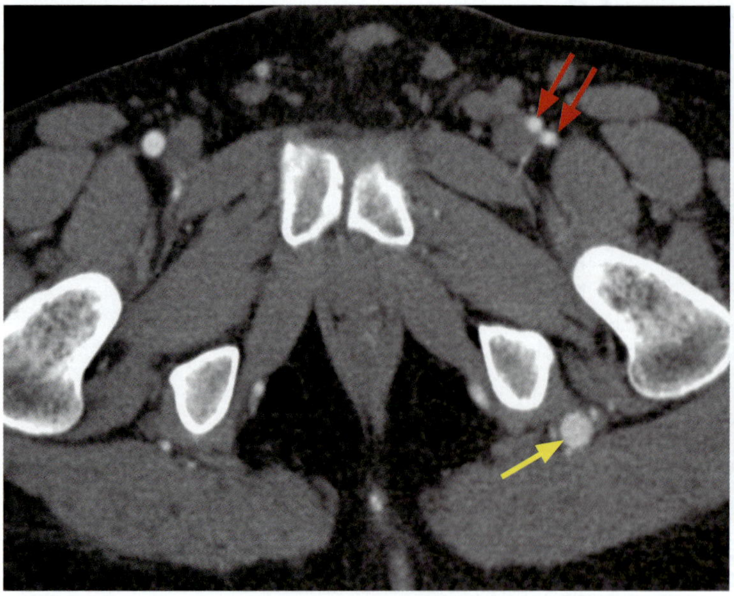

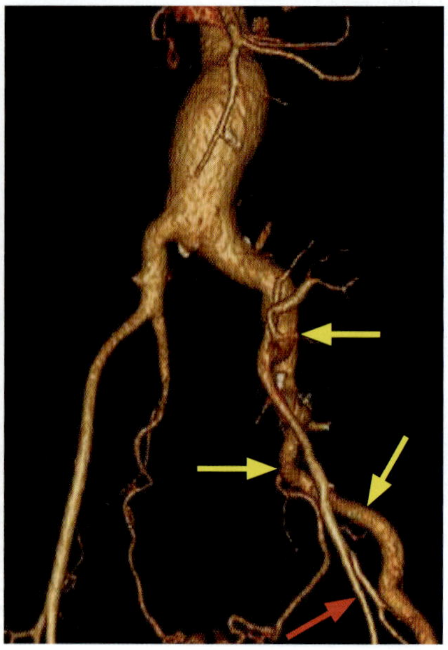

Persistent sciatic artery: Axial CT angiogram (left image) shows an enlarged vessel in the left gluteal region (yellow arrow) between the ischial tuberosity and the gluteus maximus. Two small vessels are present in the left inguinal region (red arrows) instead of a normal common femoral artery.

Three-dimensional volume-rendered reconstruction from the same study (right image) shows an enlarged left internal iliac artery, which continues distally as the persistent sciatic artery (yellow arrows). This patient also has a left femoral artery, although decreased in caliber (red arrow).

Case courtesy Michael Hanley, MD, University of Virginia Health System.

永存坐骨动脉：轴位CT血管成像(左图)，显示左侧臀部一个粗大的血管影(黄箭)，位于坐骨结节与臀大肌之间，而左侧腹股沟部位见两条小血管(红箭)，未见正常股总动脉。

同一检查的三维容积再现图像(右图)，显示左侧增粗的髂内动脉一直向下延续为永存坐骨动脉(黄箭)。此患者仍有左侧股动脉，但直径变小(红箭)。

- A persistent sciatic artery is a very rare vascular anomaly where the fetal sciatic artery persists to supply the majority of blood supply to the leg.
- The persistent sciatic artery arises from the internal iliac artery (usually from the inferior gluteal artery) and continues distally to the popliteal artery. A rudimentary femoral artery may be present.
- A persistent sciatic artery may predispose to aneurysm formation.

- 永存坐骨动脉是罕见的血管变异，为胚胎型坐骨动脉持续存在并供应下肢的大部分血液。
- 永存坐骨动脉起自髂内动脉(通常起自臀下动脉)，延续至远端的腘动脉。有时可见到发育不全的股动脉。
- 永存坐骨动脉时易导致动脉瘤形成。

THROMBOEMBOLIC AND ATHEROSCLEROTIC LOWER EXTREMITY DISEASE

下肢动脉血栓栓塞和动脉粥样硬化性疾病

Chronic arterial occlusive disease

- Peripheral arterial disease (PAD) shares risk factors with coronary artery disease, including smoking, diabetes, hypertension, hyperlipidemia, lack of exercise, and family history.
- Clinically, chronic peripheral atherosclerosis presents initially with claudication, which can progress to ischemic rest pain or tissue loss in severe cases.
- Claudication is usually first treated conservatively, with risk factor control, exercise, aspirin, and/or cilostazol (a platelet-aggregation inhibitor with vasodilator action).
- The most common locations for lower extremity atherosclerotic stenoses include the common iliac arteries, superficial femoral artery, popliteal artery, tibioperoneal trunk, and origins of the tibial arteries.
- The Rutherford classification clinically categorizes chronic limb ischemia. Category 0 is asymptomatic, category 1 is mild claudication, categories 2–3 are moderate to severe ischemia, category 4 is ischemic rest pain, and categories 5–6 are minor or major tissue loss, respectively. Revascularization should not be attempted if the limb is not viable.
- An ankle-brachial index (ABI) should be performed in every patient with suspected arterial occlusive disease. The ABI is the ratio of systolic blood pressure (SBP) in the ankles compared to the arms, and is calculated as: ankle SBP/brachial SBP.

  A decreased ABI suggests a hemodynamically significant stenosis between the great vessels and the ankles since the ankle blood pressure is less than the upper extremity blood pressure.

  An ABI <0.9 is abnormal. An ABI between 0.5 and 0.9 usually correlates with intermittent claudication. Rest pain is usually present with an ABI <0.4.
- Pulse-volume recordings characterize the Doppler waveform at multiple levels. The anatomic location of a lesion can be deduced by the change from a normal triphasic waveform to a biphasic (moderate stenosis) or flat waveform (severe stenosis/occlusion).
- For anatomical mapping and to confirm ABI and ultrasound findings, CTA or MRA can be done for further characterization.
- CTA can detect luminal narrowing or irregularities, and occlusion due to calcified and non-calcified plaques. However, blooming artifact from the calcified plaque can limit assessment of the arteries below the knee.
- MRA plays an important role in the diagnosis of PAD. Particularly, time-resolved MRA, which obtains a series of images while the contrast is passing through the calves, can demonstrate occlusion or stenosis and complements the conventional MRA images.
- Recently, noncontrast MRA sequence-quiescent interval single shot (QISS) technique has been used clinically with high diagnostic accuracy compared to

慢性动脉闭塞性疾病

- 外周动脉性疾病(PAD)与冠状动脉疾病有相同的危险因素，包括吸烟、糖尿病、高血压、高脂血症、缺乏锻炼和家族史。
- 慢性外周动脉粥样硬化在临床上首先表现为间歇性跛行，逐渐发展为缺血性静息痛，严重病例可出现组织缺损。
- 间歇性跛行通常首选保守治疗，如控制危险因素、锻炼、阿司匹林和/或西洛他唑(一种血小板聚集抑制剂，有血管扩张作用)。
- 下肢动脉粥样硬化狭窄性病变最常见的部位包括髂总动脉、股浅动脉、腘动脉、胫腓干和胫动脉的起始部位。
- Rutherford分级是按慢性下肢缺血的临床表现进行分级。0级：无症状；1级：轻度间歇性跛行；2~3级：中重度缺血；4级：缺血性静息痛；5~6级：分别为轻度或大面积组织缺损。肢体无存活迹象时应避免行血管腔内成形术。
- 对可疑下肢动脉病变的患者均应测量踝肱指数(ABI)。ABI指踝关节与上臂所测得的收缩压(SBP)之比，计算方法为：踝部收缩压/上臂收缩压。

  ABI降低提示大血管至踝部血管存在明显血流动力学意义上的狭窄，因为踝部动脉压低于上肢动脉压。

  ABI<0.9为异常；ABI在0.5~0.9时常表现为间歇性跛行；ABI<0.4常有静息痛。
- 脉搏-容积记录检查可分析不同水平的多普勒波谱特征，根据波谱的变化可推断出病变的解剖部位，波谱由正常的三相波谱变为双相波谱(中度狭窄)或扁平波谱(严重狭窄/闭塞)。
- CTA或MRA可进一步定性，用于解剖定位及确认ABI和超声检查结果。
- CTA可发现因钙化和非钙化斑块所致的管腔狭窄、不规则及闭塞，但钙化斑块的伪影会限制对膝下动脉的评估。
- MRA在PAD的诊断中发挥重要作用。尤其是时间分辨MRA，在造影剂通过小腿时能获得一系列图像，可显示闭塞或狭窄，并对常规MRA图像进行补充。
- 近来，平扫静息间隔单次激发(QISS)MRA技术已用于临床，与DSA相比有更高的诊断准

DSA, while being less prone to artifact than CTA.

确率，产生的伪影少于CTA。

Acute thromboembolic disease

- Acute limb ischemia is an emergency, with a very different clinical and imaging presentation compared to chronic atherosclerotic disease. In acute thromboembolic disease, symptom onset is acute, with pain, pallor, poikilothermia (coldness), pulselessness, and paresthesias. *Blue toe syndrome* is acute thromboembolism in the toes.
- The most common embolic source is a left atrial thrombus, with atrial fibrillation a significant risk factor. Echocardiography is indicated in the workup.
- CTA or MRA shows an acute cutoff of the affected vessel with a filling defect at the level of the vessel bifurcation. On MRA, filling defect will appear hypointense with mild perivascular hyperenhancement due to inflammation. Significant atherosclerotic disease may be absent.
- Treatment options include surgical embolectomy, surgical bypass graft, and endovascular thrombolysis.

急性血栓栓塞性疾病

- 急性下肢缺血是一种急症，其临床和影像学的表现与慢性动脉粥样硬化性疾病有很大差别。急性血栓栓塞性疾病时，症状急性发作，有疼痛、苍白、皮温降低、无脉和感觉异常。蓝趾综合征是发生在脚趾的急性血栓性栓塞。
- 最常见的栓子来源于左心房血栓，心房纤颤是重要的危险因素。检查应该包括超声心动图。
- CTA或MRA显示受累血管显影突然中断，在血管分叉水平出现一处充盈缺损。充盈缺损在MRA上表现为低信号，伴有炎症所致的血管周围轻度强化，可无严重的动脉粥样硬化性疾病。
- 治疗方法包括外科取栓术、外科搭桥手术和腔内溶栓治疗。

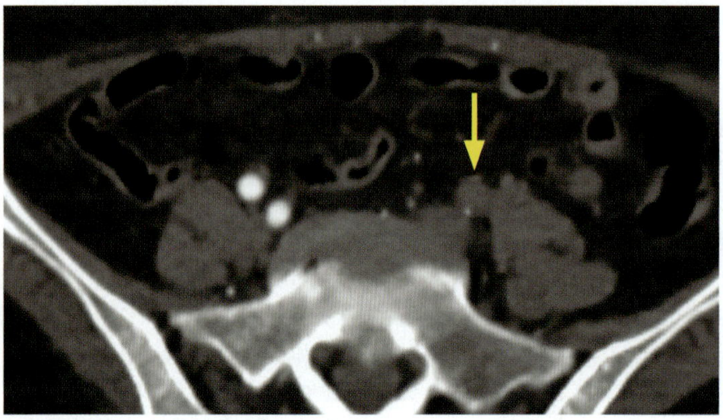

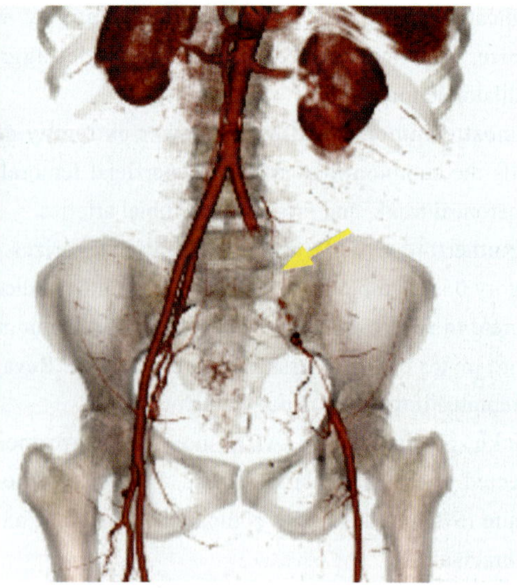

Acute thromboembolic disease: A COVID-19 patient presented with acute limb ischemia. CTA revealed acute thrombus in the left lower extremity and abrupt non-opacification of the left common iliac and external iliac arteries (arrows).

急性血栓栓塞性疾病：一名新型冠状病毒感染患者出现急性肢体缺血。CTA显示左下肢动脉急性血栓，左髂总动脉和髂外动脉强化突然消失（黄箭）。

Popliteal aneurysm

- A popliteal artery aneurysm is defined as a popliteal artery measuring 8 mm or more.
- Popliteal aneurysms are almost always due to atherosclerosis and are associated with other atherosclerotic aneurysms. Approximately 20% of patients with a popliteal aneurysm also have an aortic aneurysm, and up to half have bilateral popliteal aneurysms.
- Popliteal aneurysms are usually asymptomatic. When symptomatic, the typical presenting symptom is distal ischemia due to embolism. Popliteal aneurysm rupture is rare.
- Cross-sectional imaging either with CTA or MRA is important to assess overall size of the popliteal aneurysm, given the mural thrombus can narrow the lumen.
- Treatment with endovascular stent-graft or surgical bypass is recommended for all symptomatic popliteal artery aneurysms and asymptomatic aneurysms >2 cm in diameter.

腘动脉瘤

- 腘动脉瘤定义为腘动脉直径≥8mm。
- 腘动脉瘤几乎都由动脉粥样硬化引起，且同时合并其他部位的粥样硬化性动脉瘤。约20%的腘动脉瘤患者同时有主动脉瘤，高达半数患者的腘动脉瘤为双侧性。
- 腘动脉瘤通常无症状。当出现症状时，典型的表现是由栓塞导致的远端缺血。腘动脉瘤破裂罕见。
- 轴位CTA或MRA对评估腘动脉瘤的真实大小很重要，因附壁血栓可以导致管腔变窄。
- 凡是症状性或直径>2cm的无症状性腘动脉瘤，均推荐采用腔内覆膜支架植入或搭桥手术治疗。

NON-ATHEROSCLEROTIC LOWER EXTREMITY ARTERIAL DISEASE

Buerger disease

- As previously discussed, Buerger disease or **thromboangiitis obliterans**, is a chronic inflammatory, thrombotic arteritis which typically occurs in male smokers. It more commonly involves the legs but may also involve the hands, where it may present with ischemia, ulcerations, and even gangrene.
- On imaging, there are segmental stenoses of the medium and small arteries in the leg, with typical *corkscrew* collaterals in the vasa vasorum.
- The larger arteries, including the common femoral artery, superficial femoral artery, and popliteal artery, are typically spared.

Popliteal entrapment syndrome

- Popliteal entrapment syndrome is compression of the popliteal artery by a fibrous band or calf muscles, most commonly an aberrant or hypertrophied medial head of the gastrocnemius. Bilateral involvement is common.
- There are 6 different types of popliteal entrapment, depending on the deviation of the aberrant muscle and the popliteal artery. However, by far the most common anomalies involve the medial head of the gastrocnemius, with either medial deviation (type Ⅰ) or no deviation (type Ⅱ) of the popliteal artery.
- Most commonly utilized imaging modality is MRA with dynamic imaging where the patient is asked to perform plantar/dorsal flexion during image acquisition.
- Treatment is surgical release of the offending muscle (usually the medial head of the gastrocnemius). Angiography is only used for diagnosis, not therapy.

非粥样硬化性下肢动脉病变

Buerger病

- 如前所述，Buerger病或**血栓栓塞性脉管炎**是一种慢性炎症性栓塞性动脉炎，常发生于男性吸烟患者。常累及腿部，但也会累及双手，可出现缺血、溃疡，甚至坏疽。
- 影像上可见下肢中小血管节段性狭窄，并可见滋养血管形成典型的螺旋样侧支。
- 常不累及大血管，如股总动脉、股浅动脉及腘动脉。

腘动脉卡压综合征

- 腘动脉卡压综合征是由于腘动脉被纤维束或腓肠肌压迫所致，最常见为腓肠肌内侧头变异或肥大。双侧受累常见。
- 腘动脉卡压综合征共有6型，取决于变异肌肉和腘动脉偏移的位置。但最常见的是腓肠肌内侧头异常，可使腘动脉向内侧偏移（Ⅰ型）或未出现移位（Ⅱ型）。
- 最常用的影像学检查是动态MRA，检查时患者需行足部跖屈/背伸运动。
- 治疗选择外科松解异常的肌肉（常为腓肠肌内侧头）。动脉造影只用于诊断而非治疗。

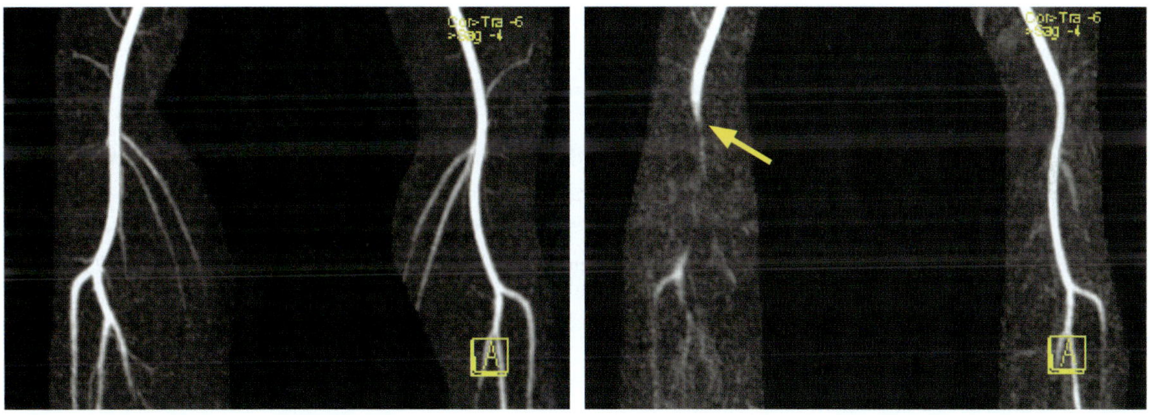

Popliteal entrapment syndrome: Left MRA image shows normal popliteal arteries during rest. During foot plantar flexion (right image), there is cutoff (arrow) of the right popliteal artery at the popliteal fossa.

腘动脉压迫综合征：左侧的MRA显示静息状态下正常的腘动脉。足跖屈时（右图），右侧腘窝处腘动脉显影中断（黄箭）。

Cystic adventitial disease

- Cystic adventitial disease is a rare cause of distal claudication where one or more mucoid cysts in the adventitia surrounding the popliteal artery leads to luminal compression.
- Clinically, most patients are middle-aged men presenting with claudication.
- MRI is the best diagnostic tool, as the cystic component can be readily identified with typical T2 hyperintensity. T1 signal intensity varies based on the mucoid content. On MRA images there is luminal narrowing and lateral displacement, which is called a *scimitar sign*.
- Treatment is surgical resection of the cyst or surgical bypass. Cyst aspiration can also be performed, but the cyst almost always recurs.

外膜囊性疾病

- 外膜囊性疾病是一种罕见的导致下肢远端间歇性跛行的疾病，为腘动脉外膜单个或多个黏液性囊肿形成引起管腔受压。
- 临床上多见于中年男性，表现为间歇性跛行。
- MRI是最好的诊断手段，其囊性成分在T_2呈高信号而易于鉴别。T_1信号强度随黏液含量的不同而变化。MRA图像上出现血管狭窄或向外侧偏移，被称为“弯刀征”。
- 治疗为外科切除囊肿或搭桥术，也可行囊肿穿刺抽吸治疗，但几乎都会复发。

（翻译　贾中芝）

VASCULAR ULTRASOUND

血管超声

GENERAL PRINCIPLES

基本原理

Angle correction

角度校正

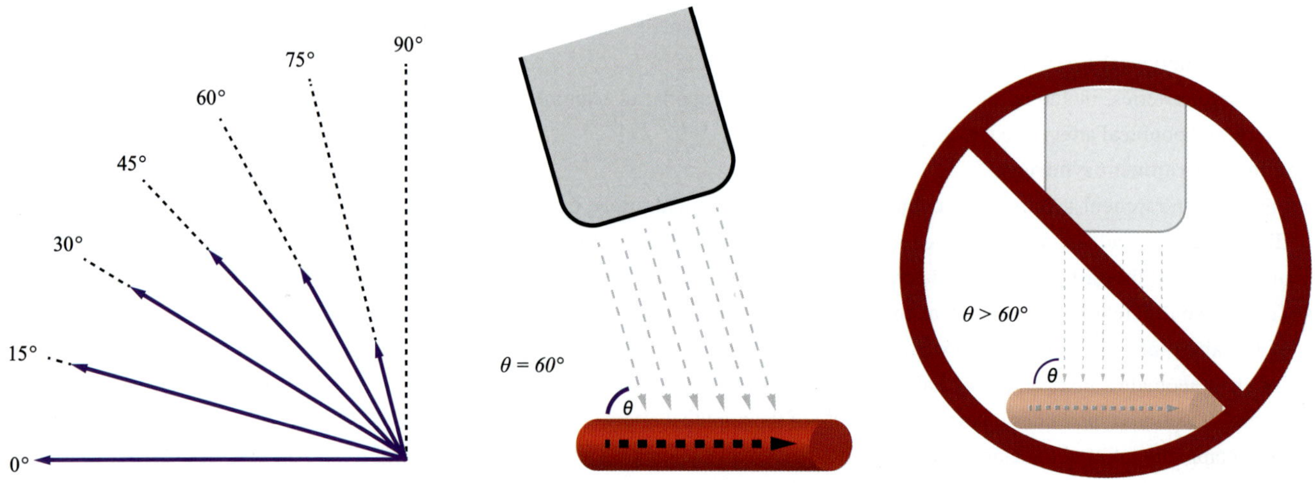

- The Doppler signal is proportional to cos(θ). There is no Doppler shift at 90°.
- All measurements of velocity should be made at a consistent angle (typically 60°). Measurements should never be taken at an angle greater than 60°.

Overview of peak systolic velocity (PSV)

- Peak systolic velocity (PSV) is usually the most accurate method to evaluate the degree of arterial stenosis. PSV is elevated proximal to and at the site of stenosis.
- PSV may be decreased distal to a hemodynamically significant stenosis.
- The differential diagnosis of increased PSV includes:
  - Downstream (distal) stenosis.
  - Compensatory flow, contralateral to an obstruction or severe stenosis.
  - Physiologic hyperdynamic state in a healthy young patient.
- The differential diagnosis of decreased PSV includes:
  - Upstream (more proximal) stenosis.
  - Poor cardiac pump function.
  - Near-total occlusion.

- 多普勒信号与cos(θ)成正比。90°时多普勒频移为0。
- 速度测量都应保持角度一致(通常 60°),测量角度不应超过60°。

收缩期峰值流速(PSV)概要

- 收缩期峰值流速(PSV)通常是评价动脉狭窄程度最准确的方法。PSV在狭窄近端及狭窄处增高。
- PSV在有显著血流动力学改变的狭窄远端可出现降低。
- PSV增高的鉴别诊断包括:
  - 下游(远端)狭窄。
  - 代偿血流,对侧有闭塞或重度狭窄。
  - 健康年轻人的生理性高血流动力状态。
- PSV降低的鉴别诊断包括:
  - 上游(更近端的)狭窄。
  - 心功能差。
  - 几乎完全闭塞。

CAROTID ARTERY

Color and spectral Doppler parameters

颈动脉

彩色和频谱多普勒参数

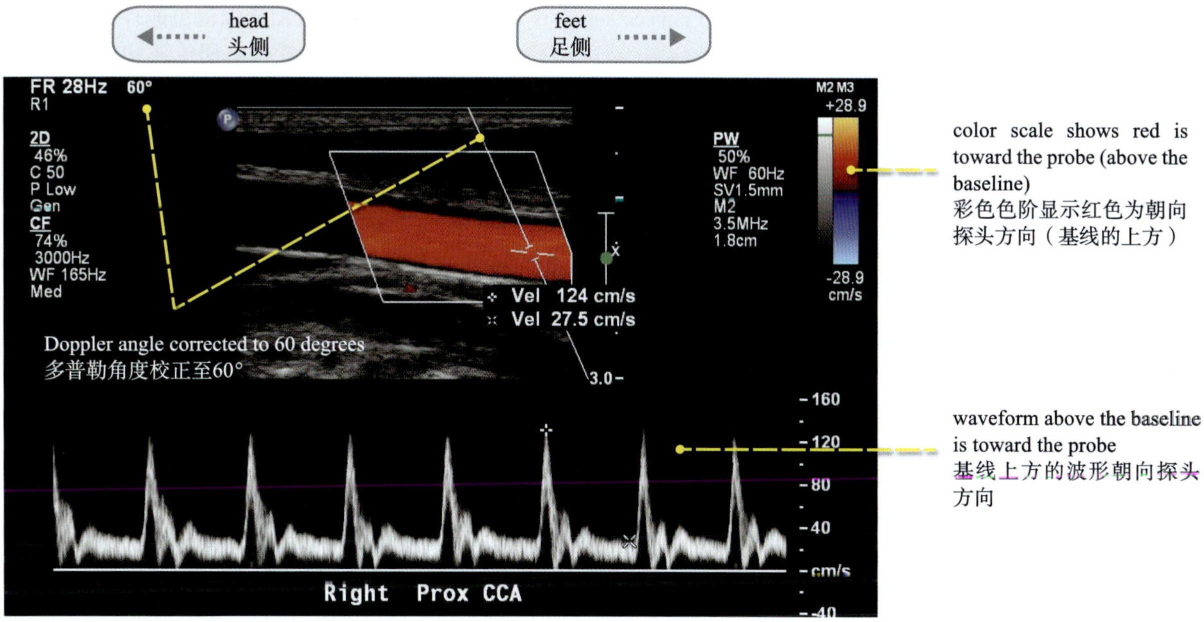

Normal carotid examination: Duplex ultrasound of the right internal carotid artery shows normal spectral waveform. The peak systolic velocity is 124 cm/sec, within the normal range. There is no carotid plaque.

正常颈动脉检查：右侧颈内动脉多普勒超声显示正常的频谱波形。收缩期峰值流速为124cm/s，处于正常范围，未见颈动脉斑块。

- By convention, for images obtained in the sagittal plane, the patient's head is on the left side of the image and the feet are on the right.
- In general, ultrasound parameters are optimized so that arteries are red and normal arterial flow is above the baseline. Certain parameters need to be adjusted so that arteries above the heart (which are normally heading towards the head) appear similar to arteries below the heart (which normally are heading towards the feet):

  The color scale can be changed: Colors above the baseline go towards the probe.

  Spectral Doppler baseline inversion can be changed: Positive waveforms go towards the probe.

Evaluation of the carotid arteries

- There are three components to the carotid artery exam: Evaluation of plaque morphology, hemodynamic evaluation, and waveform analysis.

Plaque morphology

- Plaque morphology is evaluated on grayscale imaging (without Doppler) and is described in terms of absolute percent stenosis.
- <50% cross-sectional area plaque would not be expected to be hemodynamically significant.
- >50% luminal plaque is expected to show elevation in peak systolic velocity.

Hemodynamic evaluation of stenosis

- Normal peak systolic velocity (PSV) in large arteries is 60–100 cm/sec.
- PSV tends to be elevated at a site of significant stenosis. Per the Society of Radiologists in ultrasound (SRU) criteria, established in 2003:

- 常规情况下，矢状面采集图像时，患者头侧在图像左侧，足侧在右侧。
- 通常，超声参数需要优化，使动脉内血流信号显示为红色，其频谱位于基线上方。还需调整一些其他参数，以使位于心脏上方的动脉（正常朝向头部）和心脏下方的动脉（正常朝向足端）表观相似。

  可调节色阶：基线上方的颜色朝向探头。

  频谱多普勒基线也可翻转：正向波形朝向探头。

颈动脉评估

- 颈动脉检查包括三部分：评估斑块形态、血流动力学测量和频谱分析。

斑块形态

- 斑块形态通过灰阶图像（无多普勒）进行评估，并使用绝对百分率描述狭窄程度。
- 横截面积<50%的斑块一般不引起显著的血流动力学改变。
- >50%管腔的斑块可导致收缩期峰值流速增高。

狭窄的血流动力学评估

- 正常大动脉收缩期峰值流速为60~100cm/s。
- PSV常在显著狭窄处增高。根据放射医师学会超声分会2003年制定的超声标准：

>125 cm/sec suggests >50% stenosis.
>230 cm/sec suggests >70% stenosis.

Potential pitfall: An occluded or nearly occluded artery may have no detectable flow.

- In addition to measuring peak systolic velocity, velocities are also measured at the end of diastole: End diastolic velocity of >100 cm/sec suggests >70% stenosis.
- As discussed on the following page, the resistive index incorporates both PSV and EDV.
- An elevated ratio of internal carotid artery to common carotid artery (ICA/CCA) PSV is a useful secondary sign of ICA stenosis.

  <2 is normal.

  >2 suggests >50% ICA stenosis.

  >4 suggests >70% ICA stenosis.
- In high and low flow states, the ICA/CCA ratio is more useful than the absolute PSV.

Waveform analysis

- Stenosis *downstream* (distal) to transducer (outflow lesion): Spectral waveform is high resistance and high velocity in morphology, characterized by decreased diastolic flow. The systolic upstroke is normal and rapid. Spectral broadening and aliasing may be present.

  Spectral broadening describes the widened distribution of RBC velocities due to disruption of laminar flow.

  Aliasing is an artifact where the highest velocities are shown to have a reversed flow.
- Stenosis *upstream* (proximal) to transducer (inflow lesion): Spectral waveform is low resistance and low velocity in morphology, with relatively increased diastolic flow. Systolic upstroke is slowed, producing the *tardus et parvus* waveform.

Carotid stenosis

PSV>125cm/s提示>50%狭窄。
PSV>230cm/s提示>70%狭窄。

潜在缺陷：在动脉完全或接近完全闭塞时，动脉腔内可能探测不到血流。

- 除测量收缩期峰值流速外，还需测量舒张末期流速：舒张末期流速>100 cm/s提示>70%狭窄。
- 如下文所述，阻力指数结合了PSV和EDV两个参数。
- 颈内动脉(ICA)与颈总动脉(CCA)的PSV比值增高是诊断颈内动脉狭窄的一个有用的辅助征象。

  <2为正常。

  >2提示颈内动脉狭窄>50%。

  >4提示颈内动脉狭窄>70%。
- 在血流增高或降低时，ICA与CCA的PSV比值比绝对PSV更有意义。

频谱分析

- 位于探头下游(远心端)的狭窄(也称流出道病变)：频谱呈高阻和高速形态，并以舒张期流速减低为特征。收缩期上升正常且快速。可出现频带增宽和混叠。

  频带增宽是由于血液层流被破坏使红细胞流速范围变广。

  混叠是由于最高流速被显示为反向血流导致的一种伪像。
- 位于探头上游(近心端)的狭窄(也称流入道病变)：频谱形态呈低速低阻，舒张期血流相对增加。收缩期上升缓慢，产生小慢波。

颈动脉狭窄

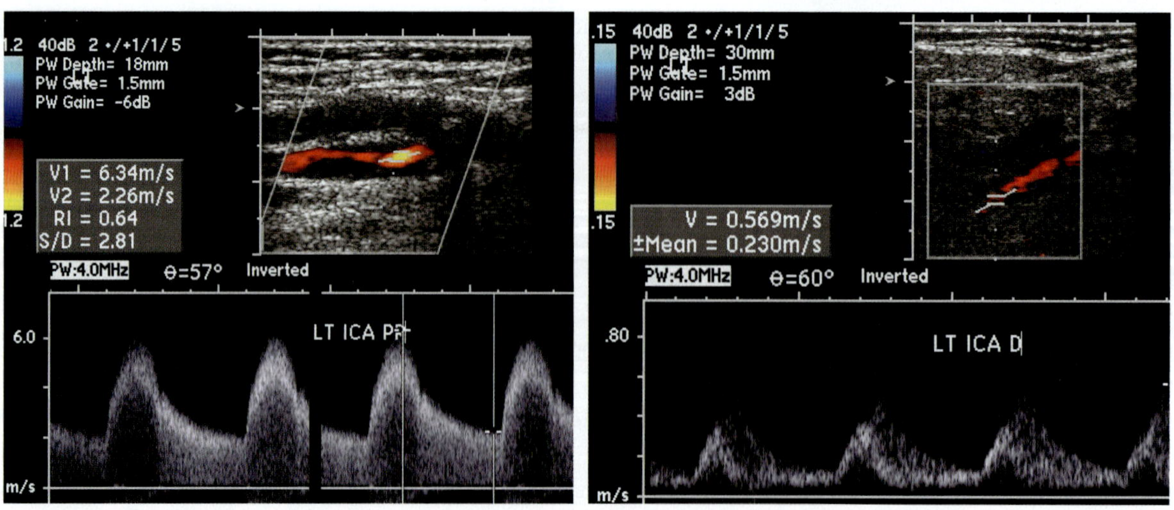

Severe internal carotid artery stenosis: Spectral waveform of the proximal internal carotid artery (left image) shows spectral broadening and markedly elevated peak systolic velocity of 634 cm/sec, consistent with severe stenosis. The grayscale images also show hypoechoic plaque. Evaluation distal to the stenosis (right image) shows a *parvus et tardus* waveform and decreased peak systolic velocity.
重度颈内动脉狭窄：近端颈内动脉频谱(左图)显示频带增宽及收缩期峰值流速显著增加(634cm/s)，符合重度狭窄。灰阶图像同时显示低回声斑块。狭窄远段(右图)显示小慢波和收缩期峰值流速减低。

RENAL ARTERY STENOSIS

Renal artery stenosis: Criteria and protocol

- A peak systolic velocity of ≥180 cm/sec is consistent with renal artery stenosis.

  Normal aortic and renal artery velocity is 60–100 cm/sec.

- A renal artery to aortic velocity ratio of >3.5 is also consistent with renal artery stenosis.
- Reduced or absent diastolic flow is suggestive of a stenosis distal to the area of interest.
- As with the carotid artery, a *tardus et parvus* waveform on spectral Doppler is suggestive of a stenosis proximal (upstream) to the transducer, known as an inflow lesion.
- An elevated renal resistive index (>0.7) is nonspecific, but may indicate renal artery stenosis, acute urinary obstruction, or medical renal disease. The resistive index (RI) is calculated as: RI = (PSV – EDV)/PSV

  PSV is peak systolic velocity and EDV is end-diastolic velocity.

  RI is measured in the segmental arteries of the upper, mid, and lower poles.

肾动脉狭窄

肾动脉狭窄：标准和检查方法

- 收缩期峰值流速≥180cm/s符合肾动脉狭窄。

  正常主动脉和肾动脉的流速为60~100cm/s。

- 肾动脉/腹主动脉流速比>3.5也符合肾动脉狭窄。
- 检查区域舒张期流速减低或消失，提示其远端有狭窄。
- 与颈动脉超声相同，出现小慢波频谱时提示近心端(上游)狭窄，称为流入道病变。
- 肾动脉阻力指数(RI)增加(>0.7)无特异性，但可提示肾动脉狭窄、急性尿路梗阻或内科肾脏疾病。阻力指数计算公式为：RI=(PSV–EDV)/PSV。

  PSV为收缩期峰值流速，EDV为舒张末期流速。

  RI在肾脏上、中、下极的肾段动脉进行测量。

DEEP VENOUS THROMBOSIS (DVT)

Overview of the deep venous thrombosis (DVT) examination

- A lower extremity venous ultrasound exam should include venous compression, color and spectral Doppler, and evaluation of venous augmentation and respiratory variation.

  Augmentation is the normal change in waveform when the calf is compressed. Lack of augmentation suggests a distal venous obstruction between the calf and the transducer.

  Respiratory variation is the normal change in waveform when the patient inspires. Lack of respiratory variation suggests a proximal venous obstruction.

- The popliteal, femoral, proximal deep femoral, and common femoral (including the saphenofemoral junction) veins should be imaged every 2–3 cm with and without compression.

Venous compression

- The hallmark sonographic finding of a DVT is a noncompressible vein with or without an intraluminal clot. A partially thrombosed vein may be partially compressible, while a completely thrombosed vein will not be compressible at all.

Color Doppler

- Color Doppler is almost always used to help localize the veins, but it is not necessary for diagnosing DVT.
- Normal color Doppler flow in a noncompressible vein is suspicious for nonobstructing thrombus.

Acute versus chronic deep venous thrombosis

- While the diagnosis of DVT is usually straightforward, distinguishing between acute and chronic thrombus can be difficult. Evaluation of the clot's echogenicity is not a reliable way to determine the acuity of the clot as artifactual echoes within the vein lumen can overlap with the clot.
- Sonographic findings of chronic venous thrombus include clot retraction and poor visualization of the clot, only partial compressibility, irregularly echogenic and thickened vein walls, and prominent collateral veins.

深静脉血栓(DVT)

下肢深静脉血栓(DVT)检查概述

- 下肢静脉超声检查应包括静脉压迫、彩色和频谱多普勒及评估静脉血流增强和呼吸波动。

  血流增强是挤压小腿时的正常频谱改变。增强消失提示探头远端的小腿静脉有梗阻。

  呼吸波动是患者吸气时的正常频谱改变。呼吸波动消失提示近端静脉梗阻。

- 腘静脉、股静脉、近端股深静脉和股总静脉(包括大隐静脉汇入处)的检查均应每隔2~3cm采集加压和不加压图像。

静脉压迫

- 深静脉血栓最典型的超声表现为静脉不可压缩，无论管腔内有无血栓。部分血栓形成的静脉管腔可被部分压缩，而管腔内充满血栓时，则管腔完全不可压缩。

彩色多普勒

- 彩色多普勒常用于静脉的定位，但对诊断深静脉血栓并非必需。
- 不可压缩的静脉存在正常彩色多普勒血流时应怀疑非阻塞性血栓。

急性与慢性深静脉血栓

- 诊断深静脉血栓通常很简单，但区分急性和慢性血栓会比较困难。根据血栓的回声强度判断血栓急慢性程度的方法不可靠，因为静脉管腔内的伪影可与血栓回声重叠。
- 慢性血栓的超声表现包括血栓回缩和血栓显示不清、部分管腔可压缩、不规则回声、静脉管壁增厚和明显的侧支静脉。

AORTIC DISEASE

Abdominal aortic aneurysm

- Screening ultrasound is performed for patients aged 65 years or older, or 50 years or older with a positive family history or personal history of aortic or peripheral vascular aneurysm.
- Transverse and longitudinal images of the proximal, mid and distal aorta and common iliac arteries are obtained.
- Color Doppler images and/or spectral Doppler with waveform analysis help to confirm patency, detect presence of intraluminal thrombus, and document endoleaks.

主动脉疾病

腹主动脉瘤(AAA)

- 超声筛查用于年龄≥65岁或≥50岁有阳性家族史者，或有主动脉或外周动脉瘤的患者。
- 采集主动脉近端、中段和远端及髂总动脉的横切面和纵切面图像。
- 彩色多普勒图像和/或频谱多普勒及频谱分析有助于确认管腔是否通畅，是否存在腔内血栓，并发现内漏。

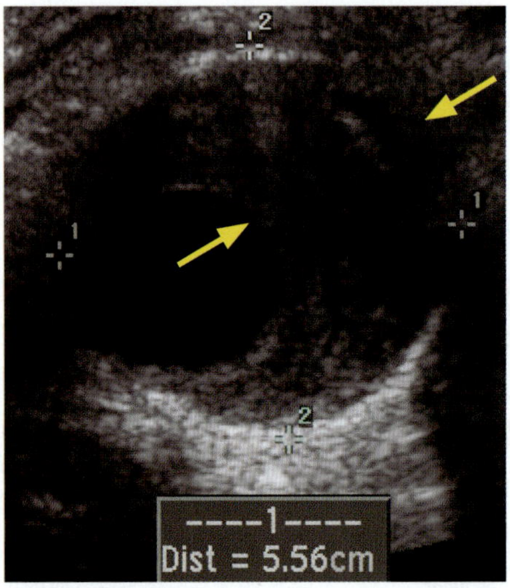

Transverse grayscale ultrasound of the infrarenal abdominal aorta shows an aortic aneurysm measuring 5.6 cm in diameter (calipers), with extensive mural thrombus (arrows).
肾下腹主动脉横切面灰阶图像显示一个直径为5.6cm(卡尺)的主动脉瘤，伴广泛附壁血栓形成(黄箭)。

(翻译　全杰荣)

9 Interventional Radiology

Leigh Casadaban, Colette Martin Glaser, Junzi Shi,
Ellen X. Sun, Steven Morales-Rivera, Sharath Bhagavatula,
Regina Maria Koch, Timothy P. Killoran

Contents

9 介入放射学

目录

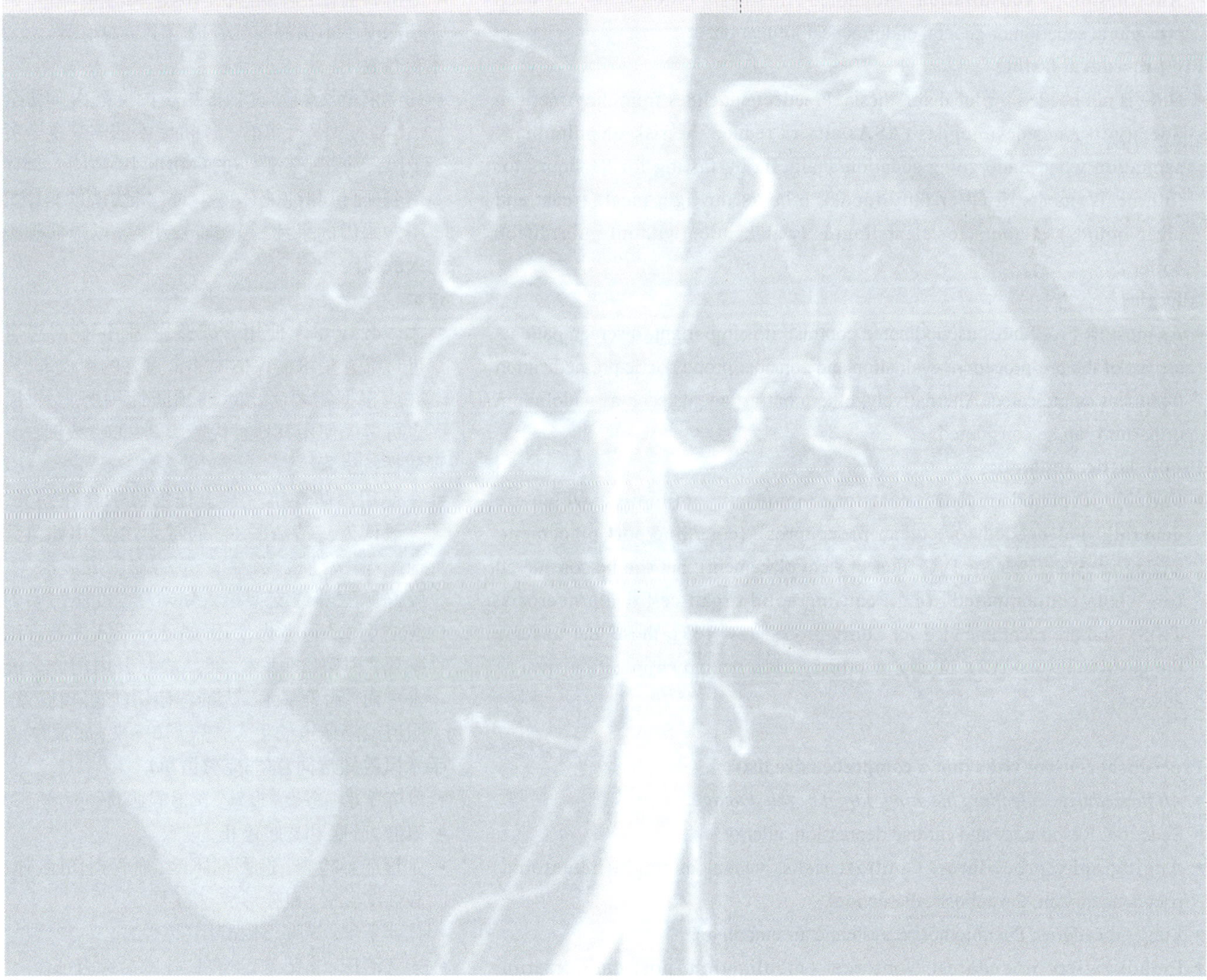

INTRODUCTION TO INTERVENTIONAL RADIOLOGY

PRE-PROCEDURE PREPARATION

General

- Pre-procedure patient evaluation and planning is imperative for all interventional radiology (IR) procedures.
- Consultations should include a directed history and physical examination, discussion of the procedure including risks and benefits, formal signed consent, and address any safety concerns.

Anesthesia type

- There are three main categories of anesthesia for procedures. Patient factors and preference as well as invasiveness of the procedure determine which type is used.
- **Local anesthetic**: Topical lidocaine injection, or topical lidocaine cream/gel.
- **Moderate procedural sedation**: Midazolam and fentanyl IV, administered by non-anesthesiologist procedural staff under continuous monitoring. Specific antagonist agents are available for opioids (e.g., naloxone, peak effect 1–2 minutes) and benzodiazepines (e.g., flumazenil, peak effect 6–10 minutes).
- **Anesthesiology consultation**: Monitored Anesthesia Care (MAC) for deep procedural sedation or general endotracheal intubation.

Pre-procedural fasting

- NPO is not needed for local anesthesia. Practice guidelines from the American Society of Anesthesiologists (ASA) aim to reduce the risk of pulmonary aspiration when undergoing sedation/analgesia by fasting for 8+ hours for full meals (meats, fried or fatty foods), 6 hours for light meals (toast and clear liquids), 2 hours for clear liquids (water, juice without pulp, black coffee).

Allergies

- As most IR procedures use iodinated contrast, it is important to screen patients as part of the pre-procedure evaluation and consider prophylactic premedication treatment as indicated. Alternatively, other contrast agents such as gadolinium or barium can be considered.

Prophylactic antibiotics

- Variable levels of evidence exist for prophylactic antibiotics, which are generally not needed for "clean procedures" (e.g., line/port placement, angiography/angioplasty, IVC filter or stent placement), but can be considered for "clean-contaminated" (e.g., causing solid organ cell death/necrosis, TIPS), and are recommended for "dirty procedures" (e.g., those that traverse the gastrointestinal (GI), biliary or urinary tract, or known infection such as abscess).

Procedural consent risks (not a comprehensive list)

- *All procedures: Infection, bleeding, target organ damage.*
- Sedation: Respiratory and cardiac depression, allergy.
- Angiography procedures: Contrast risks, vessel damage (hematoma, pseudoaneurysm, thrombosis, dissection).
- Lung procedures: Pneumothorax, systemic air embolism.
- Embolization procedures: Nontarget embolization, post-embolization

介入放射学概述

术前准备

概述

- 对于任何介入放射(IR)手术，患者术前评估及手术计划都至关重要。
- 术前会诊应针对性采集病史和体格检查，讨论手术以及相关的风险和疗效，签署正式知情同意书，以及解答任何安全疑虑。

麻醉类型

- 手术麻醉有三种主要类型，应根据患者的个体因素、意向及手术的创伤程度予以选择。
- **局部麻醉**：局部注射利多卡因或局部使用利多卡因乳膏/胶。
- **中度手术镇静**：在持续监护下由非麻醉医师从静脉给予咪达唑仑和芬太尼。需备有阿片类药物的特异性拮抗剂(如纳洛酮，峰效时间1~2分钟)和苯二氮䓬类药物的特异性拮抗剂(如氟马西尼，峰效时间6~10分钟)。
- **麻醉科会诊**：麻醉监护(MAC，即全身麻醉)包括深度手术镇静或气管插管下全身麻醉。

术前禁食

- 局部麻醉无须禁食。根据美国麻醉医师协会(ASA)指南：行镇静/镇痛时，术前需禁食全餐(肉类、油炸或高脂肪的食物)8小时以上，禁食简餐(面包和纯液体)6小时，禁饮清饮料(水、不含果肉的果汁、黑咖啡)2小时，以降低肺吸入的风险。

过敏

- 大多数IR手术使用含碘造影剂，因此对患者进行筛查是术前评估中非常重要的组成部分，并应根据需要考虑术前预防性用药。另外，也可考虑使用其他替代造影剂，如钆或钡。

预防性抗生素

- 在使用预防性抗生素上证据级别存在差异，一般认为，"清洁手术"通常无须使用(如血管通路/输液港植入、血管造影/血管成形术、下腔静脉滤器或支架植入)；对于"可能污染的清洁手术"可考虑使用(如可导致实体器官细胞死亡/坏死的手术、经颈静脉肝内门体分流术)；而"污染手术"为推荐使用(如经胃肠道、胆道或泌尿道的手术，或已知感染，如脓肿)。

手术风险知情同意(非完整清单)

- 所有手术：感染、出血、靶器官损伤。
- 镇静：呼吸和心跳停止、过敏。
- 血管造影检查：造影剂风险、血管损伤(血肿、假性动脉瘤、血栓形成、夹层)。
- 肺部手术：气胸、体循环气体栓塞。
- 栓塞治疗：非靶器官栓塞、栓塞后综合征。

syndrome.

- Biopsies: Nondiagnostic sample.
- TACE: Hepatic failure, biloma/abscess.
- GI embolization procedures: Bowel infarction.
- Pelvic embolization: Buttock claudication, rectal/bladder ischemia, impotence.
- Biliary procedures: Biliary sepsis, bile leak.
- GU procedures: Urosepsis.
- IVC filter: Migration, perforation, IVC thrombosis.
- Thrombolysis: Severe bleeding including cerebral hemorrhage, reperfusion syndrome, distal embolization.
- Gastrostomy tube: Tube malposition (in peritoneum or colon), bowel damage.
- TIPS: Hepatic failure, encephalopathy, death.
- Transjugular liver biopsy: Capsular perforation (severe bleeding).
- Uterine fibroid embolization: Premature menopause, reduced fertility, fibroid expulsion (submucosal).
- Ablation: Collateral damage to adjacent organs (especially bowel), biliary stricture, abscess.

- 活检：样本不合格。
- 经动脉化疗栓塞术(TACE)：肝功能衰竭，胆汁瘤/脓肿。
- 胃肠道栓塞手术：肠梗死。
- 盆腔栓塞：臀部跛行、直肠/膀胱缺血、阳痿。
- 胆道手术：胆源性脓毒血症、胆漏。
- 泌尿系统手术：尿源性脓毒血症。
- 下腔静脉(IVC)滤器：移位、穿孔、IVC血栓形成。
- 溶栓：严重出血(包括脑出血)、再灌注综合征、远端栓塞。
- 胃造瘘：瘘管位置异常(位于腹膜或结肠)、肠道损伤。
- 经颈静脉肝内门体分流术(TIPS)：肝功能衰竭、肝性脑病、死亡。
- 经颈静脉肝活检：包膜穿孔(严重出血)。
- 子宫肌瘤栓塞：过早绝经、生育能力降低、肌瘤脱落(黏膜下)。
- 消融：邻近器官(尤其是肠道)损伤、胆道狭窄、脓肿。

Bleeding risk

- Society of Interventional Radiology (SIR) Consensus Guidelines in 2019 assess bleeding risk according to two general categories of procedures.

Screening group	Procedures
Low bleeding risk Screening PT/INR, platelet count, hemoglobin *not* routinely recommended. Thresholds: INR >2.0–3.0 Platelets >20 × 10^9/L	Catheter exchanges Arterial and venous interventions (<6 French sheath) Dialysis access interventions IVC filter placement and removal Lumbar puncture Venous access placement and removal (including ports) Thoracentesis/Paracentesis Superficial abscess drainage or biopsy Transjugular liver biopsy
High bleeding risk Screening PT/INR, platelet count, hemoglobin is routinely recommended. Thresholds: INR >1.5–1.8 Platelets >50 × 10^9/L	Ablations Arterial interventions (>7 French sheath) Catheter directed thrombolysis Procedures involving new tract traversing solid organs (e.g., deep abscess drainage/biopsies, cholecystostomy, gastrostomy, nephrostomy tube placement) IVC filter removal (complex) Transjugular intrahepatic portosystemic shunt

出血风险

- 介入放射学学会(SIR)2019年指南共识主要根据两大类手术评估出血风险。

组别筛选	手术类型
低出血风险 筛查PT/INR、血小板计数，血红蛋白为非常规推荐项目 阈值： INR>2.0~3.0 血小板计数>20 × 10^9/L	导管交换 动脉和静脉介入(鞘管<6Fr) 透析通路介入 IVC滤器植入和取出 腰椎穿刺 静脉置管和移除(包括输液港) 胸腔穿刺术/腹腔穿刺术 浅表脓肿引流或活检 经颈静脉肝脏活检
高出血风险 筛查PT/INR、血小板计数，血红蛋白为常规推荐项目 阈值： INR>1.5~1.8 血小板计数>50 × 10^9/L	消融术 经动脉介入治疗(鞘管>7Fr) 经导管接触溶栓 需穿过实体器官建立新通道的手术 (例如，深部脓肿引流/活检、胆囊造瘘、胃造瘘、肾造瘘置管) IVC滤器取出(使用复杂技术) 经颈静脉肝内门体分流术

- For patients on anticoagulation or antiplatelet agents, cessation for several half-lives or use of reversal agents may be necessary for high bleeding risk procedures.

Protamine sulfate is the reversal agent for heparin/enoxaparin.

For reversal of vitamin K antagonists such as warfarin, options are Ⅳ vitamin K (minimum 6–12 hours) plus fresh-frozen plasma or prothrombin complex concentrates (e.g., Kcentra).

The new factor Ⅹa reversal agent andexanet alfa (AndexXa) can be used for apixaban and rivaroxaban.

- 对于正使用抗凝或抗血小板药物的患者，高出血风险手术前可能需要停药数个半衰期或使用拮抗药物。

硫酸鱼精蛋白是肝素/依诺肝素的拮抗剂。

逆转维生素K拮抗剂(如华法林)，可选择Ⅳ型维生素K(6~12小时)加新鲜冷冻血浆或凝血酶原复合物浓缩物(如Kcentra)。

新型Ⅹa因子逆转剂andexanet alfa(AndexⅩa)可用于拮抗阿哌沙班和利伐沙班。

- Occasionally, bridging to shorter-acting therapy is needed in high thrombosis risk patients (e.g., heparin for anticoagulants, and cangrelor for antiplatelet agents).

Achieving hemostasis

- Manual compression remains the standard of care for hemostasis.

Arterial puncture: Firm continuous pressure is applied for at least 15 minutes. Most recommend near-occlusive pressure for the first few minutes, then slight decrease in pressure to feel arterial flow beneath your fingers for the remainder of the hold. The arteriotomy is usually at least 1 cm above the skin access site. Release of pressure after 15 minutes should be gradual so as to not dislodge the platelet plug. If there is continued oozing after 15 minutes, pressure should be re-applied and avoid releasing and checking every few minutes.

Venous puncture: Usually 5–10 minutes is sufficient, depending on the size of the venotomy and clotting status of the patient.

- Closure device: Several arterial closure devices are available and may improve patient comfort, allow for early post-procedure mobility, and reduced bleeding and vascular complications.
- Radial access is being done more frequently which allows for earlier ambulation with hemostasis obtained using a wrist compression device that is taken off 1–2 hours following procedure.

- 较少情况下，高血栓风险患者需要短效药物进行过渡(例如，肝素作为抗凝药物，cangrelor作为抗血小板药物)。

止血

- 手工按压仍是标准的止血方法。

动脉穿刺：持续用力按压至少15分钟。大多建议在按压开始的几分钟内应使血管几乎闭塞，之后适当减轻压力使手指能够感觉到血流流动。动脉穿刺点常位于皮肤穿刺点上方至少1cm。结束15分钟按压时，应缓慢减轻压力以免血小板栓子脱落。若15分钟后仍有持续渗血，应重新施压，并避免每隔几分钟放松和检查。

静脉穿刺：取决于静脉穿刺口的大小和患者的凝血状态，通常5~10分钟足以止血。

- 血管闭合器：现有数种动脉闭合器材可用于改善患者舒适度，便于术后早期活动，并减少出血和血管并发症。
- 随着桡动脉入路日益普及，如今患者术后能提前活动，采用腕部压迫器止血1~2小时即可。

(翻译　李西)

Procedural Tools

Needles

Needle sizing

- Needle sizes measured as gauge — *bigger* number means *smaller* needle.
- Smaller needles (e.g., 22 and 21 gauge) can be used for initial access into target structures, fine needle aspirations, small abscesses, and small vessels for vascular access.
- Larger needles (e.g., 18 gauge) can be used for large abscesses, larger vessels that are easily accessible, and core needle biopsies.

Wires

Wire sizing

- Wires are measured by diameter and sized in inches, with a standard wire measuring 0.035″ in diameter and a microwire measuring 0.018″ in diameter.
- An 0.018″ wire fits through a 22 gauge needle (or bigger), and a 0.035″ wire fits through an 18 gauge needle (or bigger).

Standard floppy tip wires

- Standard wires have a floppy tip or J-tip which allows the wire to be safely inserted blindly (although once in the vessel the course should be followed on fluoroscopy).
- A *Bentson* wire has 20 cm flexible tip length that is available as a standard or stiff shaft.
- *Rosen* (Cook Medical) wire has a stiff shaft with short flexible tip and tight (1.5 mm) J-curve.

手术器材

穿刺针

穿刺针尺寸

- 穿刺针的大小以“G”为单位，数字越大，针越细。
- 细针(如22G和21G)用于初始穿刺小的靶结构、细针抽吸、小脓肿及小血管的穿刺。
- 粗针(如18G)用于穿刺较易进入的结构，如大囊肿、大血管，或空芯针活检。

导丝

导丝尺寸

- 导丝的尺寸是根据其直径的大小加以区分，并以英寸(1英寸=2.54厘米)为单位，标准导丝的直径为0.035英寸，微导丝直径为0.018英寸。
- 0.018英寸导丝适合通过22G或更粗的穿刺针，0.035英寸导丝适合通过18G或更粗的穿刺针。

常规软头导丝

- 常规导丝的头端柔软或呈“J”形，以便进行安全盲插(当然，一旦进入血管腔内，应在透视下推送导丝)。
- 标准或硬的Bentson导丝前端有20cm长的软头。
- Rosen(Cook医疗)导丝较硬，前端软头短，呈“J”形的小弯头(1.5mm)。

Hydrophilic wires

- Hydrophilic wires are used to cross a stenosis or for initial cannulation of an indwelling device, as would be performed for a routine check and change.
- *Roadrunner* (Cook) and *Glidewire* (Terumo) wires are hydrophilic.

Stiff wires

- Stiff wires are used when structural rigidity is required. For instance, a device that dilates the subcutaneous tissues (such as a sheath, biliary drain, nephrostomy tube, etc.) needs to be inserted over a stiff wire.
- *Amplatz* (Boston Scientific) and *Lunderquist* (Cook Medical) wires are stiff wires.

亲水导丝

- 亲水导丝用于通过狭窄部位，或插入已留置的器材进行常规检查或更换。
- Roadrunner(Cook医疗）和Glidewire(Terumo)导丝为亲水导丝。

硬导丝

- 硬导丝用于需要硬性支撑的情况。例如，导管鞘、胆道引流管、肾造瘘管等器械需在硬质导丝支撑下扩张皮下组织而导入。
- Amplatz(波士顿科学）和Lunderquist(Cook医疗）导丝为硬导丝。

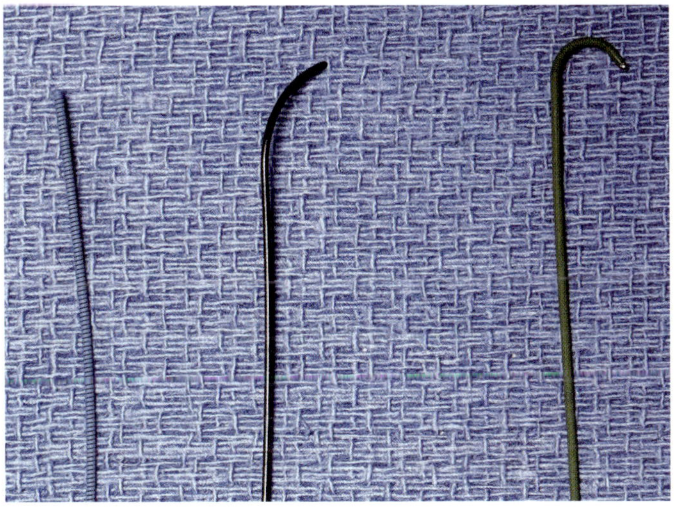

Wires (left to right):
Amplatz super stiff straight tip guidewire
Glidewire hydrophilic wire
Rosen curved guidewire
导丝(从左向右)：
Amplatz超硬直头导丝
Glidewire亲水导丝
Rosen弯头导丝

CATHETERS

Catheter sizing

- Catheters are measured by *outer* circumference and sized in French (Fr), where 1 Fr = 0.33 mm. For instance, a 6 Fr catheter has an external diameter of 2 mm. The luminal diameter will be slightly smaller.

High-flow catheters

- High-flow (also known as flush) catheters have multiple sideholes and may be coiled (most commonly; known as a pigtail or OmniFlush [Angiodynamics] catheter), curved, or straight.
- High-flow catheters are used for large vessel angiography, such as the aorta and vena cava, and selection of the contralateral iliac artery.

Selective and superselective catheters

- Selective and superselective catheters have a single hole at the end of the catheter. There are numerous shapes of the distal portion, each tailored towards a specific situation or general purpose use.
- *C2* and *SOS* are reverse curved-tip catheters, best for basic visceral selection.
- *Mickelson* is for more difficult selections, particularly bronchial, intercostal and lumbar arteries, and must be reformed in a large artery or branch vessel.
- *Simmons* catheters have excellent stability for difficult selections, and must be reformed.
- *Berenstein*, *Kumpe* and *MPA* catheters are angled-tip catheters.

导管

导管尺寸

- 导管的尺寸根据导管的外径以French(Fr)为单位而定，1Fr=0.33mm。例如，6Fr导管的外径约为2mm，导管内周径略小。

高流量导管

- 高流量(也称涌流)导管有多个侧孔，远端可卷曲［常见的为猪尾巴或OmniFlush (Angiodynamics)导管］、弯曲或笔直。
- 高流量导管用于大血管造影，如主动脉和腔静脉，以及对侧髂动脉的选择性插管。

选择性和超选择性导管

- 选择性和超选择性导管的远端为单孔。导管远端部分有多种形状，每一种形状有特定的用途，或为通用。
- C2和SOS是头端反相弯曲的导管，最适合普通的内脏血管选择性插管。
- Mickelson适合较为复杂的选择性插管(尤其是支气管动脉、肋间动脉和腰动脉)，须先在大动脉或其分支成形。
- Simmons导管非常适合复杂的选择性插管，也须先成形后再勾选。
- Berenstein、Kumpe和MPA导管是头端成角的导管。

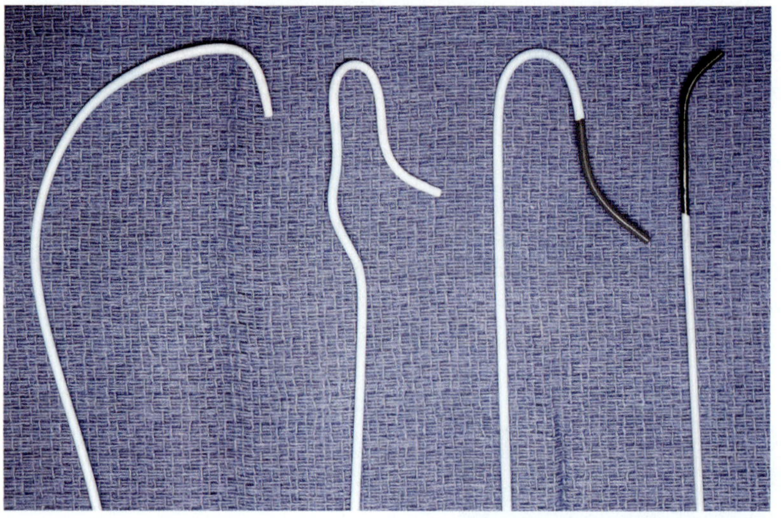

Catheters (from left to right):
C2 reverse curved-tip catheter
Mickelson catheter
Simmons catheter (Sim catheter)
Berenstein catheter
导管(从左向右):
C2反向弯头导管
Mickelson导管
Simmons导管(Sim导管)
Berenstein导管

Sheaths

- Measured by *inner* circumference French size.
- Sheaths are used for stabilizing access during a procedure.
- A "peel-away" sheath is commonly used for maintaining access when placing catheters.
- *Sheath versus catheter:* A sheath has a defined *luminal* diameter; however, the overall diameter of the sheath will be slightly larger. For instance, a 6 Fr sheath can by definition fit a 6 Fr catheter inside, but will be 7 or 8 Fr in external diameter.

导管鞘

- 导管鞘大小根据其内径以Fr为单位。
- 导管鞘的作用是便于在操作过程中保持入路的稳定性。
- "可撕脱鞘"一般用于插入导管时保留通路。
- 导管鞘与导管：导管鞘的大小依据管腔内径而定，其外径的尺寸略大。例如，6Fr的导管鞘应可通过6Fr的导管，但其外径为7Fr或8Fr。

Balloon angioplasty

Percutaneous transluminal angioplasty (PTA)

- Percutaneous transluminal angioplasty (PTA) is the first-line technique for treatment of a stenosis, where a balloon is inflated across the stenosis to create a controlled stretch injury and increase the luminal cross-sectional area.
- When treating a stenosis caused by atherosclerotic plaque, angioplasty widens the luminal diameter due to disruption of the intima and extension of the plaque into the media.
- Most balloons are *non-compliant.* That is, they have a fixed diameter that does not further expand with increased applied pressure, though it will burst above a maximum rated pressure. They expand to open a blockage or stricture (seen as a "waist" in the balloon) or dilate the vasculature.
- *Cutting balloons* are non-compliant balloons with microsurgical blades to break through a tight stricture.
- In general, a balloon should be selected that is 10–20% larger than the vessel diameter.
- *Compliant balloons* are inflated by volume, rather than pressure. They are used to fully conform to the vascular contour or occlude the vessel, commonly used for fully expanding/ molding a stent-graft against a vessel wall.
- Balloons are sized by diameter in millimeters and length in centimeters. For instance, a 10 × 6 balloon is 10 mm in diameter and 6 cm in length.

球囊血管成形术

经皮腔内血管成形术(PTA)

- 经皮腔内血管成形术(PTA)是治疗狭窄的首选技术，即在狭窄处通过球囊扩张对管壁产生可控性牵拉损伤，从而增加局部管腔的横截面积。
- 在治疗由动脉粥样硬化斑块引起的血管狭窄时，血管成形术使内膜撕裂并将斑块推至中膜，从而使管腔直径增大。
- 大部分球囊为非顺应性，即球囊的直径是固定的，并不随压力的增加而进一步扩张，但在超过压力极限后会爆裂。球囊扩张用于开通闭塞或狭窄(球囊局部可见"切迹")的血管，或扩张血管。
- 切割球囊为非顺应性球囊，球囊上附有微小手术刀刃，用于坚硬的狭窄血管。
- 一般来说，选择球囊应超出血管直径的10%~20%。
- 顺应性球囊随注入的容积而非压力的增加而扩张。它们用于完全可顺应的血管轮廓或阻塞血管，常用于充分扩张/重塑覆膜支架使其充分贴附于血管壁。
- 球囊的尺寸以mm为直径单位，cm为长度单位。例如"10 × 6"的球囊指其直径为10mm，长度为6cm。

- Risks of angioplasty include distal emboli, vessel rupture, and dissection. Anticoagulation (typically heparin) should usually be used with angioplasty.

STENTS

Self-expandable versus balloon-expandable

- The two broad categories of stents are *balloon-expandable* and *self-expandable* stents.
- In general, balloon-expandable stents have a higher radial force upon deployment but will stay deformed if crushed. Thus, balloon-expandable stents are suboptimal for sites prone to external compression, such as around joints or the adductor canal in the leg.
- Self-expandable stents are more flexible and trackable through vessels than balloon-expandable stents. Their use is favored when the route to the lesion is tortuous or when the anatomy is prone to external compression.

Covered or uncovered

- Most stents are bare metal stents and provide only a scaffolding-like support that allows blood to still flow through the interstices; however, covered stents (e.g., stent grafts) are impervious to fluid and create a new conduit, commonly employed for treatment of aneurysms, pseudoaneurysms, ruptures, dissections, and TIPS.
- Because stents are prone to in-stent stenosis, *drug-eluting* stents were developed to deliver antiproliferative agents into the arterial wall.
- In general, a stent should be selected that is 1–2 cm longer than the stenosis, with a diameter that is 1–2 mm wider than the non-stenosed vessel lumen. A rule of thumb is 10% oversizing of an arterial stent and 20% oversizing of a venous stent.

PRINCIPLES OF EMBOLIZATION

Embolic materials

- The two main categories of embolic materials are permanent (coils, plugs, particles, glue, and sclerosing agent) and temporary (absorbable gelatin sponge and autologous clot).
- **Coils** create thrombosis by inducing vascular stasis. The main advantage of coils is the ability for precise and quick placement, without distal embolization. The primary disadvantage is sacrifice of distal access: Once a vessel is coiled, it cannot be re-accessed for retreatment.

  When using coils for embolization of a specific lesion, the general technique is to first coil *distal* to the lesion, then proximal to it. This prevents recurrent bleeding from retrograde collaterals.
- **Plugs** are cylinder shaped baskets that act similarly to coils but are used for larger vessels with high flow rates. These are commonly used in splenic trauma or plug-assisted gastric variceal embolization (PARTO).
- **Particles** are microscopic (diameter measured in microns) entities that flow distally to occlude small capillaries. Particles can be made of trisacyl gelatin or polyvinyl alcohol. Common uses include for tumors and various organs. Careful consideration must be used to avoid nontarget embolization.
- **Liquid embolic agents** (e.g., glue) can be injected to quickly embolize a structure. Cyanoacrylate and ethylene vinyl alcohol are examples of glue that rapidly polymerizes when it comes in contact with blood.

- 血管成形术的风险包括远端栓子脱落、血管破裂和夹层。在行血管成形术时应常规予以抗凝(通常用肝素)。

支架

自膨胀和球囊扩张

- 支架有两大类:*球囊扩张式和自膨胀式*。
- 一般而言,球囊扩张式支架具有较高的径向力,但受挤压后会保持变形后状态。因此,球囊扩张式支架不适合用于有外部压迫的部位,如关节旁或下肢的收肌管处。
- 自膨胀式支架在通过血管时比球囊扩张式支架更具柔韧性并容易通过,适合用于路径迂曲或易遭受外部压迫的病变。

覆膜和非覆膜

- 大部分支架为金属裸支架,只提供支撑作用,血流仍然可通过支架的网格间隙;而覆膜支架(如stent graft)不能让液体透过而形成一个新的通道,常用于动脉瘤、假性动脉瘤、血管破裂、夹层和TIPS。
- 由于支架易发生支架内狭窄,*药物涂层支架*可以将抗增生药物释放到动脉壁内。
- 一般而言,选择支架的长度应比狭窄多出1~2cm,直径较未狭窄的管腔大1~2mm。大致估计的方法是,动脉支架应大10%,静脉支架应大20%。

栓塞的原则

栓塞材料

- 栓塞材料分两大类,永久性(弹簧圈、封堵器、颗粒、胶和硬化剂)和临时性(可吸收性明胶海绵和自体血凝块)。
- **弹簧圈**可使血管内血流淤滞而产生血栓。弹簧圈的主要优点是可精确和快速释放,且不会导致远端栓塞。主要缺点是远端入路被封闭。一旦血管被弹簧圈堵塞,便不能对其进行重复治疗。

  行弹簧圈栓塞时,常用的技术是先栓塞病灶远端,再栓塞近端,以免侧支血管逆流导致再次出血。
- **封堵器**是圆筒形的网篮样结构,作用类似于弹簧圈,主要用于高流量的大血管。通常用于脾外伤或以封堵器为辅助的胃曲张静脉栓塞(PARTO)。
- **颗粒**是微型(直径以μm计)固体材料,随血流进入远端从而栓塞小的毛细血管。颗粒可由trisacyl gelatin或polyvinyl alcohol制成。常用于肿瘤和各种器官的血管栓塞。使用必须谨慎以免发生非靶器官栓塞。
- **液态栓塞剂**(如胶)注射后可快速在靶结构造成栓塞。Cyanoacrylate和ethylene vinyl alcohol

- **Sclerosant agents** damage the endothelial cells of the vessel wall, causing the vessel to shrink and dissolve over a period of weeks. Sodium tetradecyl sulfate, polidocanol, and ethanol are examples of sclerosants and can be used to treat lymphovascular malformations, varices or smaller varicose veins.
- Absorbable gelatin sponge/slurry is the most commonly used ***temporary* embolic agent**, lasting 2–6 weeks. Common use is for emergent traumatic bleeding. Of important note, post-procedural CT imaging can show numerous gas locules in the embolized organ, and can mimic an abscess.

是两种在接触血液时可快速聚合的胶。

- **硬化剂**可破坏血管壁的内皮细胞，导致血管收缩，数周后溶解。十四烷硫酸钠、聚多卡醇和乙醇是几种代表性的硬化剂，可用于治疗淋巴血管畸形和静脉和小静脉曲张。
- 可吸收性明胶海绵/浆液是最常用的临时性**栓塞剂**，可持续2~6周，常用于急性外伤出血。需要注意，术后CT图像可显示栓塞器官有大量气泡，可类似于脓肿。

Complications of embolization

- **Post-embolization syndrome** usually occurs within the first day after embolization and clinically presents with pain, cramping, fever, and nausea/vomiting, thought to be due to release of endovascular inflammatory modulators by infarcted tissue. Treatment is NSAIDS, opioids when appropriate, and IV fluids.
- **Non-target embolization** is unintentional embolization of structures other than the target. For instance, during uterine fibroid embolization there is a risk of non-target embolization of the ovaries. During bronchial artery embolization, there is a risk of non-target embolization to the brain causing stroke and to the spinal arteries causing paralysis.

栓塞的并发症

- **栓塞后综合征**通常发生在术后第一天，临床表现为疼痛、痉挛、发热、恶心/呕吐，可能是梗死组织释放血管内炎症因子所致。治疗方法包括给予非甾体抗炎药，必要时使用阿片类药物和静脉输液。
- **非靶器官栓塞**是指意外栓塞非靶向结构。例如，子宫肌瘤栓塞时有可能意外造成卵巢栓塞。支气管动脉栓塞有可能由于非靶向栓塞造成脑卒中，或栓塞脊髓动脉导致瘫痪。

（翻译　吴志远）

General Considerations for Angiography

血管造影的基本要素

Vascular Access

血管入路

Femoral arterial access technique

股动脉穿刺技术

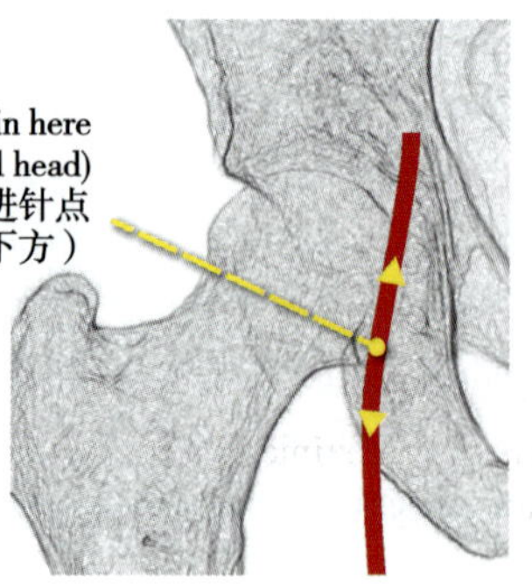

- The common femoral artery (CFA) is the most common site for arterial access. Prior to obtaining access, distal pulse and capillary refill should be checked, and confirmed again after the procedure.
- The CFA begins inferior to the inguinal ligament. From lateral to medial, the mnemonic **NAVL** helps to localize the femoral nerve, artery, vein, and lymphatics.

- 股总动脉(CFA)是最常用的动脉穿刺点。在穿刺前，应检查远端脉搏和毛细血管充盈情况，并在手术后再次确认。
- CFA起始于腹股沟韧带的下方。从外到内依次为股神经(N)、股动脉(A)、股静脉(V)和淋巴管(L)，用“**NAVL**”可帮助记忆它们的解剖关系。

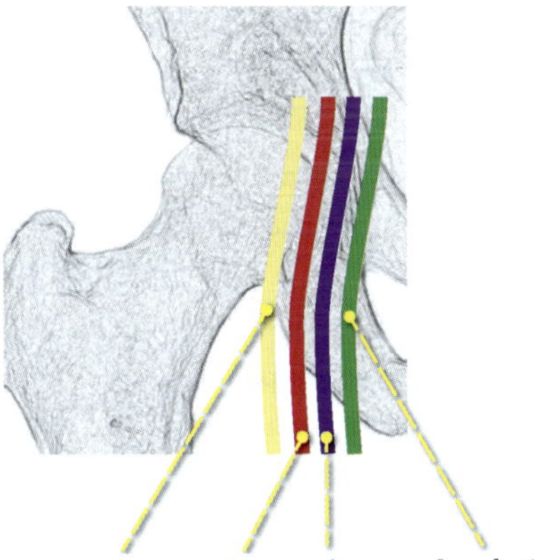

- The ideal position to access the femoral artery is the inferomedial margin of the femoral head, for two reasons. First, the femoral head provides a hard surface to press against to provide adequate hemostasis. Second, at the level of the femoral head, the femoral artery and nerve are side by side. Additionally, if arterial puncture is performed too low, the femoral vein may be traversed with possible formation of arteriovenous fistula.

- 股动脉理想的穿刺点是股骨头的内下缘，其原因有两个：第一，股骨头具有坚硬的表面，有助于压迫止血；第二，在股骨头水平，股动脉和股神经并排走行。此外，若动脉穿刺点过低，有可能贯穿股静脉而造成动静脉瘘。

Transradial artery access

- While access via the radial artery has been largely adopted for coronary interventions, this is only starting to gain traction for the general IR practice, often limited by operator experience and training.
- Advantages include earlier post-procedure ambulation, more effective hemostasis and patient comfort.
- Disadvantages include higher rates of vasospasm (mitigated with an antispasmodic cocktail of heparin, nitroglycerin, and verapamil) and radial artery occlusion (can occur between 2–10% of cases).
- Barbeau's test is an alternative to the Allen's test for evaluating collateral circulation of the hand. It involves placing a pulse oximeter on the ipsilateral thumb and then evaluating the morphology of the plethysmography tracing before, immediately after and two minutes after manual occlusion of the radial artery. Patients with type D tracing morphology have absent and non-recruitable flow, and should not undergo transradial catheterization.
- The reverse Barbeau test is used for ulnar artery access. The pulse oximeter should be placed on the fifth finger when testing occlusion of the ulnar artery.

桡动脉入路

- 桡动脉入路已在冠状动脉介入手术中被广泛采用，但在普通放射介入中才刚开始受到重视，并常受制于操作者的经验和培训情况。
- 优点包括术后较早起床活动、止血更加有效和患者的舒适感。
- 缺点包括血管痉挛(可用肝素、硝酸甘油和维拉帕米抗痉挛混合物缓解)和较高的桡动脉闭塞发生率(可发生于2%~10%的病例)。
- Barbeau试验是一个替代Allen试验的评估手部侧支循环的方法。将脉搏血氧仪置于同侧拇指，评估手工压迫阻断桡动脉前、阻断后即刻和2分钟后的体积描记图的形态。若D型波缺失且无侧支血供，患者不应进行桡动脉穿刺。
- 反向Barbeau试验用于尺动脉入路。在测试尺动脉阻断时，脉搏血氧计应放置于第五指。

Complications of Vascular Access

Hematoma

- A hematoma may be superficial or retroperitoneal. A superficial subcutaneous hematoma has a generally benign clinical course, while a retroperitoneal hematoma carries a risk of fatal hemorrhage.
- There is increased risk of retroperitoneal hematoma with a high (more cranial) arterial puncture above the pelvic brim.

Pseudoaneurysm

- Pseudoaneurysm formation occurs in approximately 1% of arterial punctures. On color Doppler, a pseudoaneurysm appears as a swirling *yin-yang* with high-velocity flow at the site of communication with the femoral artery.
- Watchful waiting can be performed for a small pseudoaneurysm <1 cm in size. Ultrasound-guided thrombin injection is the treatment of choice for a

血管入路的并发症

血肿

- 血肿可位于表浅或腹膜后。表浅皮下血肿的临床预后通常良好，但腹膜后血肿有致命出血的风险。
- 动脉穿刺点过高(更偏向头侧)、位于骨盆缘的上方时，腹膜后血肿的风险增加。

假性动脉瘤

- 动脉穿刺后的假性动脉瘤的发生率约为1%。在彩色多普勒图像上，假性动脉瘤表现为漩涡状阴阳征，并在股动脉的交汇处呈高速血流。
- 小于1cm的假性动脉瘤可予以观察。大于1cm时，可选择超声引导下凝血酶注射进行治

pseudoaneurysm >1 cm. Less commonly, ultrasound-guided compression of the neck of the pseudoaneurysm can be performed to thrombose the pseudoaneurysm.

Arteriovenous fistula (AVF)

- An arteriovenous fistula (AVF) is an anomalous connection between an artery and a vein. AVFs are usually asymptomatic but may enlarge and ultimately cause high-output cardiac failure.
- There is increased risk of developing an iatrogenic AVF with a low (inferior/distal) femoral arterial puncture. The femoral vein often passes deep to (instead of medial to) the femoral artery distal to the standard puncture site.
- On Doppler ultrasound, an AVF demonstrates arterial flow within a vein and there is loss of the normal triphasic waveform in the artery. Increased diastolic flow is often seen in the artery proximal to the fistula.

Injection rates

- The terminology for injection rates for angiographic runs is "*cc/sec* for *total cc.*" For instance, "25 for 50" means an injection rate of 25 cc/sec for a total of 50 cc.
- The diameter in mm of a vessel is a rough guide to the injection rate (in cc/sec), and the total volume of contrast injected depends on the intravascular volume of the vascular bed.

Aortogram (aortic arch): 25 for 50	Mesenteric artery: 5 for 25
Abdominal aorta: 15 for 30	Renal artery: 5 for 15
Inferior vena cavogram: 20 for 30	Distal artery: 3 for 12

Air embolism

- Air embolism is a rare but potentially life-threatening complication of vascular procedures.
- The most dangerous portion of a venous access procedure is the insertion of the catheter into the peel-away sheath.
- If air embolism is suspected (e.g., if the patient becomes acutely hypoxic as the catheter is inserted into the peel-away sheath), the patient should be immediately placed in the left-lateral decubitus (left side down) position so the air bubble remains antidependent in the right heart. 100% oxygen should be administered. If practical, fluoroscopy can be used to identify the air bubble. Catheter aspiration can be considered if the air bubble is large.

Approach to interpreting an angiogram

疗。也可在超声引导下压迫瘤颈使假性动脉瘤形成血栓，但较少使用。

动静脉瘘(AVF)

- 动静脉瘘(AVF)是动脉和静脉之间的异常交通。AVF常无症状，但可增大并最终引起高输出性心力衰竭。
- 低位股动脉(下方/远端)穿刺会增加医源性AVF的风险。股静脉在标准股动脉穿刺点的远端常走行于股动脉的后方(而非内侧)。
- 多普勒超声检查时，AVF表现为静脉内出现动脉血流，而动脉内缺乏正常的三相波形。通常能观察到瘘口近端动脉的舒张期血流增加。

注射速率

- 用于血管造影注射速率的术语是"毫升/秒，总毫升数"。例如，"25，50"意思是注射速率25mL/s，总量50mL。
- 可根据血管直径的毫米数粗略估计注射速率(mL/s)，造影剂的注入总量取决于血管床的血管内容量。

主动脉(主动脉弓)：25/50	肠系膜动脉：5/25
腹主动脉：15/30	肾动脉：5/15
下腔静脉：20/30	肢体动脉：3/12

空气栓塞

- 空气栓塞是一种罕见但可致命的血管手术并发症。
- 静脉置管手术最危险的一步是将导管插入撕脱鞘时。
- 若怀疑有空气栓塞(如患者在导管插入撕脱鞘后出现急性缺氧的表现)，应立即将患者置于左侧卧位(左侧在下方)，使气泡悬浮于右心。应给患者吸入100%氧气。情况允许时可用透视识别气泡。气泡较大时可以考虑用导管进行抽吸。

血管造影的解读方法

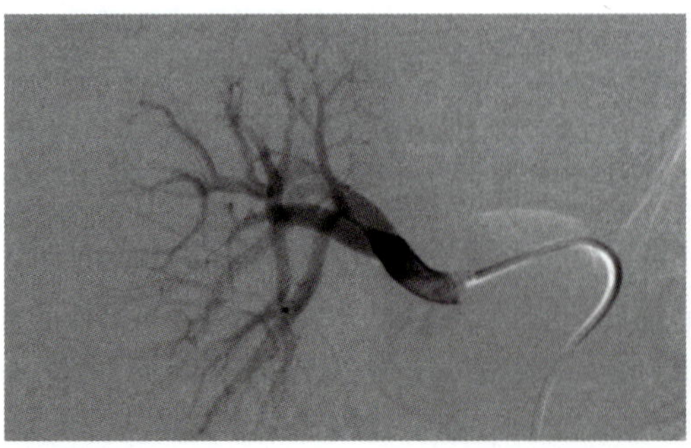

Early arterial phase
动脉早期

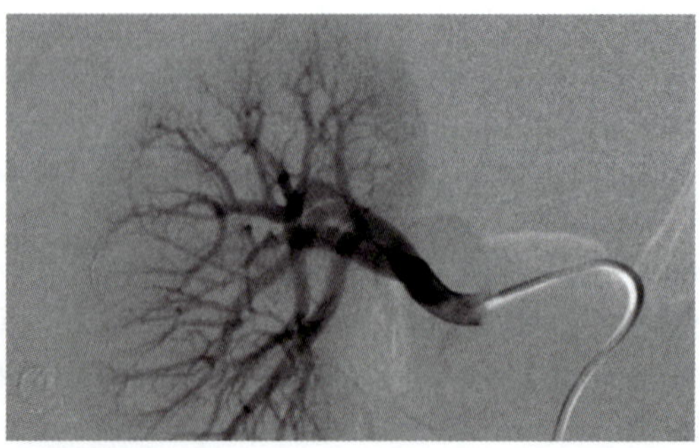

Late arterial phase
动脉晚期

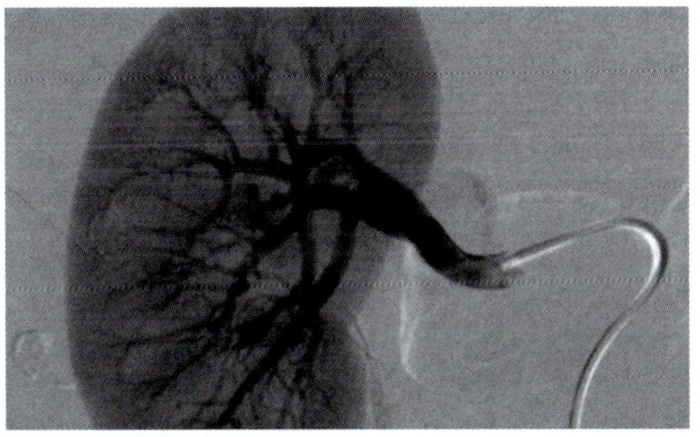

Parenchymal phase
实质期

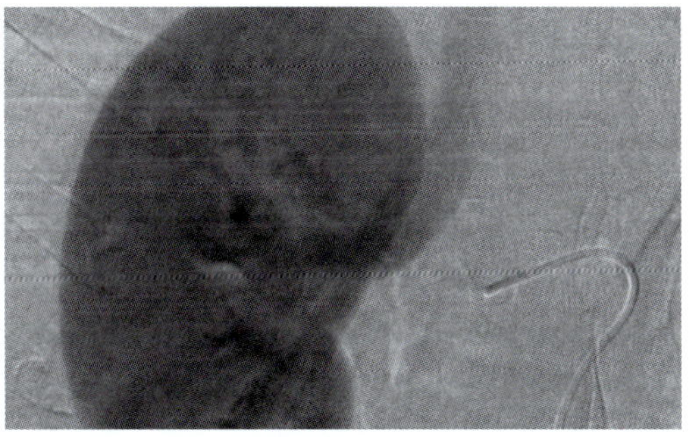

Venous phase (renal vein drains into IVC)
静脉期(肾静脉汇入下腔静脉)

Normal selective digital subtraction angiogram of the right renal artery demonstrates 4 phases of vascular opacification.
正常选择性右肾动脉数字减影血管造影显示的4个血管显影的时相。

- The mnemonic "what, where, when, VIA (vessels, interventions, anything else)" can be helpful to remember the comprehensive approach to evaluating a vascular case.

What?

- What type of study is it-angiogram, digital subtraction angiogram (DSA), venogram?

Where?

- Where in the body is the catheter and in which vessel?
- Is a flush catheter in a large vessel or is it a selective/superselective angiogram?

When?

- Early arterial phase, late arterial phase, parenchymal phase, or venous phase?
- Is there opacification of any veins during an arterial phase? If so, that suggests a shunt.

Vessels?

- Is there any contrast going where it shouldn't, such as active extravasation or neovascularity?
- Do the vessels have a normal contour? Is there any dissection, irregularity, stenosis, or encasement (external compression)?

Interventions?

- Any previously placed stents, grafts, filters, coils, surgical clips, or drains?

Anything else?

- Any other finding on the film? Bony fracture to suggest trauma?

- 记忆口诀 "what(什么)、where(在哪)、when(何时)、VIA(血管、干预、其他)" 将有助于综合评估一个血管造影病例。

What(什么)?

- 什么类型的检查-血管造影、数字减影血管造影(DSA),还是静脉造影?

Where(在哪)?

- 导管在身体什么部位,在哪根血管?
- 在大血管内的多侧孔导管,还是选择性或超选择性血管造影?

When(何时)?

- 是动脉早期、动脉晚期、实质期或静脉期?
- 动脉期有无静脉显影? 若有,则提示有(动静脉)分流。

血管?

- 有造影剂出现在不该出现的地方? 如活动性出血或有新生血管?
- 血管有正常轮廓吗? 有夹层、管壁不规则、狭窄或被包绕(外部压迫)吗?

干预?

- 先前有无植入支架、人造血管、滤器、弹簧圈、手术夹或引流管?

其他?

- 图像上还有其他发现吗? 骨折提示有外伤史?

ABDOMINAL AND PELVIC VASCULAR ANATOMY

Osseous landmarks

- Celiac artery: Arises from the aorta at the level of T12 vertebral body.
- Superior mesenteric artery (SMA): Arises at the level of the T12–L1 disc space.
- Renal arteries: Arise at the level of the L1–L2 disc space.
- Inferior mesenteric artery (IMA): Arises left of midline at the level of L3 vertebral body.

Celiac axis anatomy

- Approximately 75% of the time the celiac artery demonstrates normal arterial anatomy with three main branches: The left gastric, the common hepatic, and the splenic artery.

腹部和盆腔血管解剖

骨性标志

- 腹腔干:起源于主动脉,在T_{12}椎体水平。
- 肠系膜上动脉(SMA):发自T_{12}~L_1间隙水平。
- 肾动脉:发自L_1~L_2间隙水平。
- 肠系膜下动脉(IMA):发自L_3水平的中线偏左方。

腹腔干解剖

- 约75%的腹腔干呈正常的解剖结构,即由三支血管构成:胃左动脉、肝总动脉和脾动脉。

The left gastric artery may be the source of bleeding in esophageal Mallory-Weiss tear.

食管Mallory-Weiss黏膜撕裂时，胃左动脉可为出血的来源。

Normal celiac angiographic anatomy

正常腹腔干血管造影解剖

normal early-arterial selective celiac artery digital subtraction angiography

正常动脉早期选择性腹腔干动脉数字减影血管造影图

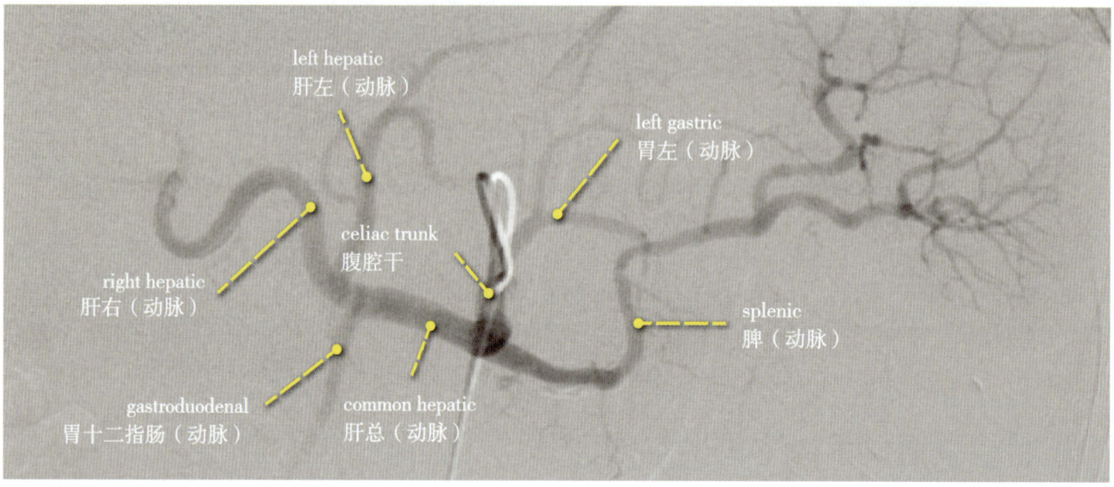

Normal late-arterial selective celiac artery digital subtraction angiography

正常动脉晚期选择性腹腔干动脉数字剪影血管造影图

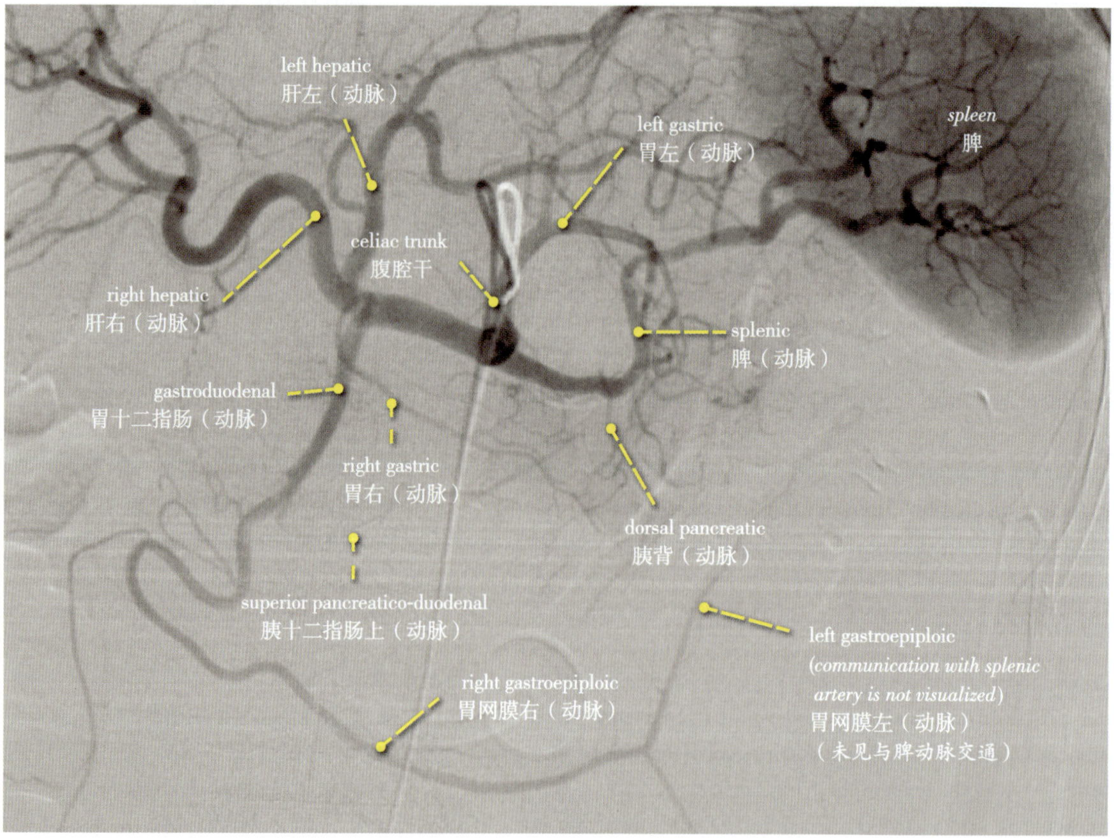

Hepatic arterial anatomy and variants

- Most commonly (75%), the proper hepatic artery supplies blood to the liver. The proper hepatic artery is the continuation of the common hepatic artery after the takeoff of the gastroduodenal artery. The proper hepatic artery divides into

肝动脉的解剖和变异

- 最常见(75%)为肝固有动脉供血肝脏。肝固有动脉是肝总动脉发出胃十二指肠动脉后的延续，分成肝右动脉和肝左动脉，胆囊动脉通

the right and left hepatic arteries. The cystic artery arises from the right hepatic artery to supply the gallbladder.

- The left gastroepiploic artery arises from the splenic artery and anastomoses with the right gastroepiploic artery along the greater curvature of the stomach. The right gastroepiploic artery arises from the gastroduodenal artery.
- A **replaced right hepatic artery** (RRHA) is present in 10–18% of patients, where the right hepatic artery arises from the SMA. A RRHA may become clinically significant in the setting of SMA disease or during abdominal surgery.

常发自肝右动脉供应胆囊。

- 胃网膜左动脉发自脾动脉，并与胃网膜右动脉在胃大弯形成吻合。胃网膜右动脉起源于胃十二指肠动脉。
- **替代肝右动脉**(RRHA)见于10%~18%的患者，其肝右动脉发自肠系膜上动脉。替代肝右动脉在肠系膜上动脉疾病或腹部手术时具有重要的临床意义。

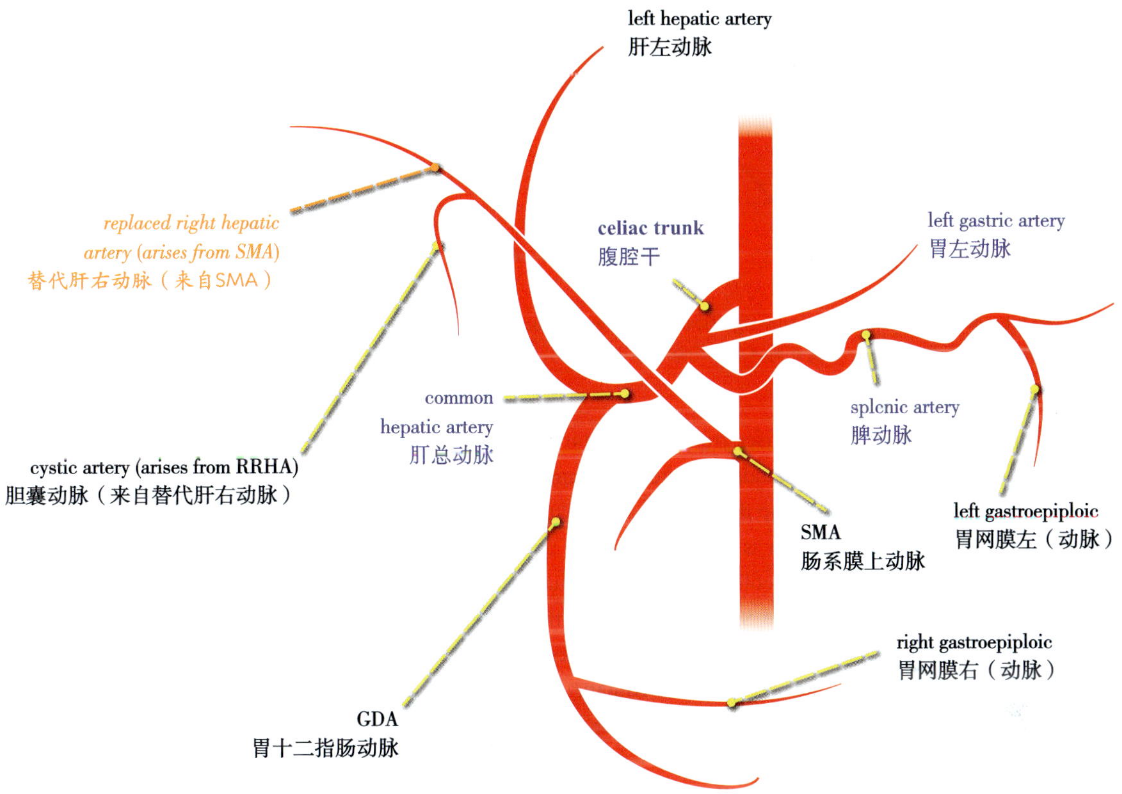

It is essential for the surgeon to be aware of a RRHA prior to laparoscopic cholecystectomy to prevent inadvertent arterial injury.

RRHA is beneficial in case of a living right hepatic donor, as the RRHA is longer and larger than a regular RHA. This allows a better anastomosis to the recipient vasculature. In contrast, there may be increased arterial complications if the hepatic transplant recipient has a RRHA, due to reduced diameter of the common hepatic artery.

In the setting of a RRHA, SMA stenosis may theoretically predispose the right lobe of the liver to ischemia, although this is usually not clinically relevant due to intrahepatic collaterals and portal vein supply.

- An **accessory right hepatic artery** is an artery arising from the SMA that supplies the right hepatic lobe in the presence of a normal right hepatic artery (arising from the proper hepatic artery).
- An **accessory left hepatic artery** is an artery arising from the left gastric artery that supplies the left hepatic lobe in the presence of a normal left hepatic artery (arising from the proper hepatic artery).
- A **replaced left hepatic artery** (RLHA) is present in 11–12% of patients, where the left hepatic artery arises from the left gastric artery.

外科医师在行腹腔镜胆囊切除术前必须明确有无RRHA，以免造成意外动脉损伤。

RRHA有利于活体右半肝供体移植，因其较正常的右肝动脉长而粗，有利于与受体血管进行更好地吻合。相反，若肝移植受体有RRHA，动脉并发症的发生率可能会增加，因为肝移植受体的肝总动脉直径会偏小。

在有RRHA的情况下，肠系膜上动脉狭窄在理论上可导致肝右叶缺血，然而这在临床上并不常见，其原因是肝内有侧支血管和门静脉供血。

- **副肝右动脉**是在有正常肝右动脉(发自肝固有动脉)的情况下，另一支起自肠系膜上动脉并向肝右叶供血的动脉。
- **副肝左动脉**是指除了有正常的肝左动脉(来自肝固有动脉)，还有另一支发自胃左动脉并向肝左叶供血的动脉。
- **替代肝左动脉**(RLHA)见于11%~12%的患者，肝左动脉起源于胃左动脉。

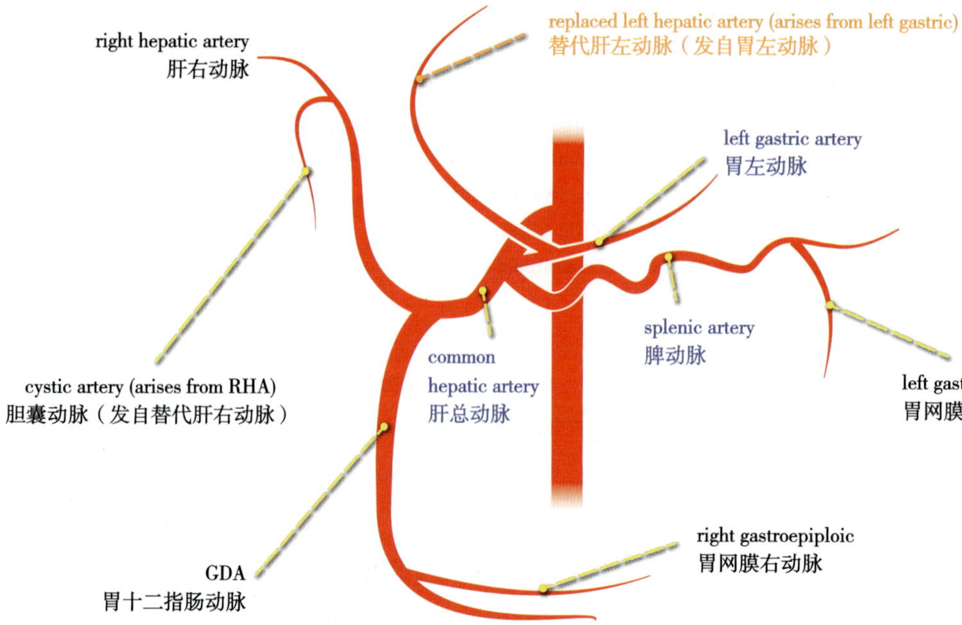

The presence of a RLHA is clinically significant during gastrectomy, as resection of the RLHA may predispose to liver injury.
RLHA的临床意义在于：行胃切除术时，切除RLHA可能引发肝脏损伤。

Superior mesenteric artery (SMA)

- The superior mesenteric artery (SMA) arises from the anterior aorta at about the level of T12–L1 to supply the distal duodenum, the entire small bowel, and the proximal large bowel from the cecum to the mid-transverse colon.
- The **inferior pancreaticoduodenal artery** is the first branch of the SMA. The inferior pancreaticoduodenal artery forms collaterals with the celiac artery.
- The **middle colic artery** arises from the SMA and supplies the transverse colon. The middle colic artery anastomoses with the inferior mesenteric artery via the **marginal artery of Drummond** and the **arc of Riolan**.
- The **right colic artery** courses retroperitoneal, supplying the right colon and hepatic flexure.
- The terminal artery of the SMA is the **ileocolic artery**, which sends arterial branches to the terminal ileum, cecum, and appendix.

肠系膜上动脉(SMA)

- SMA起源于腹主动脉前方T_{12}~L_1水平，供应远端十二指肠、整个小肠以及从盲肠到横结肠中部的近端大肠。
- **胰十二指肠下动脉**是肠系膜上动脉的第一根分支血管，它与腹腔干的分支形成吻合。
- **结肠中动脉**起源于肠系膜上动脉并供应横结肠。结肠中动脉与肠系膜下动脉通过**Drummond边缘动脉和Riolan弓**形成吻合。
- **右结肠动脉**走行于腹膜后，供应右半结肠和结肠右曲。
- 肠系膜上动脉的终末分支为**回结肠动脉**，它向末端回肠、盲肠，以及阑尾发出分支。

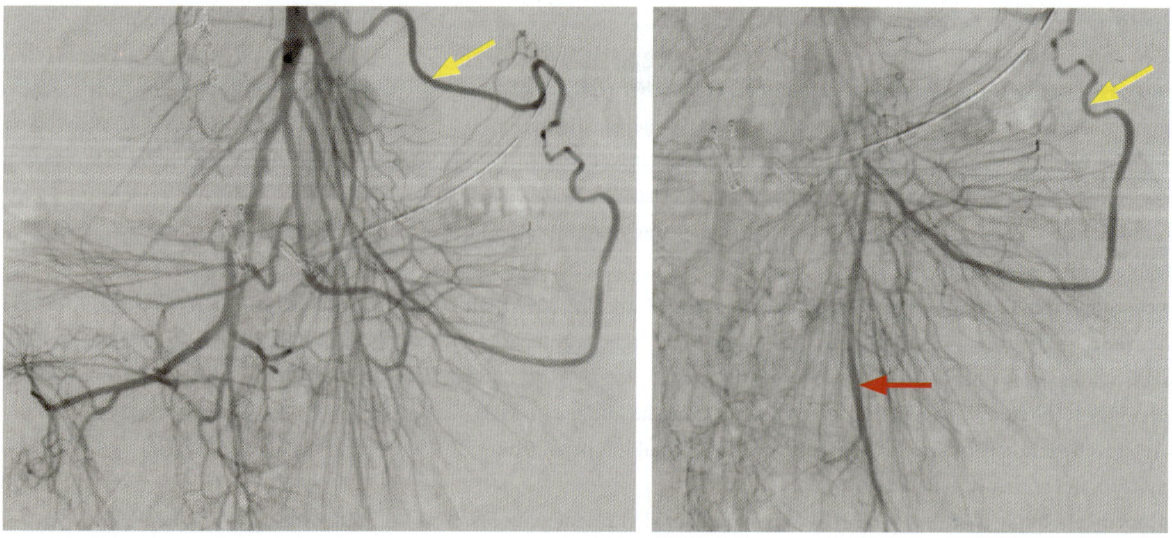

Selective DSA of the SMA shows the arc of Riolan (yellow arrows) supplying the IMA (red arrow), in a patient with known proximal occlusion of the IMA. *Case courtesy Arjun Sharma, MD, Brigham and Women's Hospital.*
选择性SMA数字减影血管造影显示Riolan弓(黄箭)供应IMA(红箭)，患者为已知IMA近端闭塞。

Inferior mesenteric artery (IMA)

- The inferior mesenteric artery (IMA) originates at the left anterior aspect of the aorta at approximately the level of L3.
- The IMA gives off the **left colic artery** to supply the descending colon.
- The **sigmoid arteries** are variable in number. They run in the sigmoid mesocolon to supply the sigmoid.
- The IMA terminates as the **superior rectal (hemorrhoidal) artery**, which supplies the upper rectum.

肠系膜下动脉(IMA)

- IMA起源于腹主动脉的左前方，约L_3水平。
- IMA发出**左结肠动脉**供应降结肠。
- **乙状结肠动脉**的数量不定。它们走行于乙状结肠系膜内，并向乙状结肠供血。
- 肠系膜下动脉的终末分支为**直肠上(痔)动脉**，为直肠上部供血。

Normal early-arterial selective inferior mesenteric artery digital subtraction angiography
正常动脉早期选择性肠系膜下动脉选择性数字减影血管造影图像

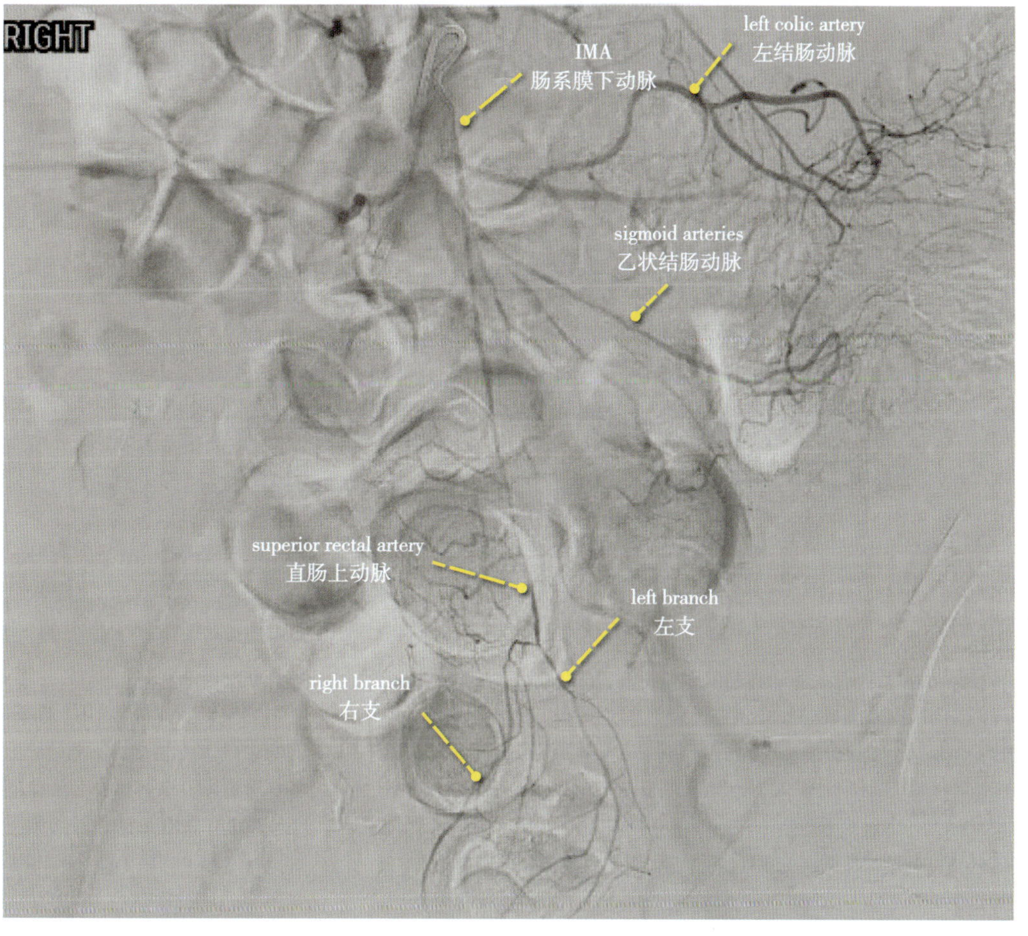

External iliac branches

- The **inferior epigastric artery** anastomoses with the superior epigastric artery.
- The **deep circumflex iliac artery** anastomoses with the internal iliac via the iliolumbar artery.
- The **femoral artery** is its terminal branch after passing posterior to the inguinal ligament and continues distally to supply the leg.

髂外动脉分支

- **腹壁下动脉**与腹壁上动脉吻合。
- **旋髂深动脉**经髂腰动脉与髂内动脉吻合。
- **股动脉**是髂外动脉在腹股沟韧带后方的延续，继续向远端延伸供应下肢。

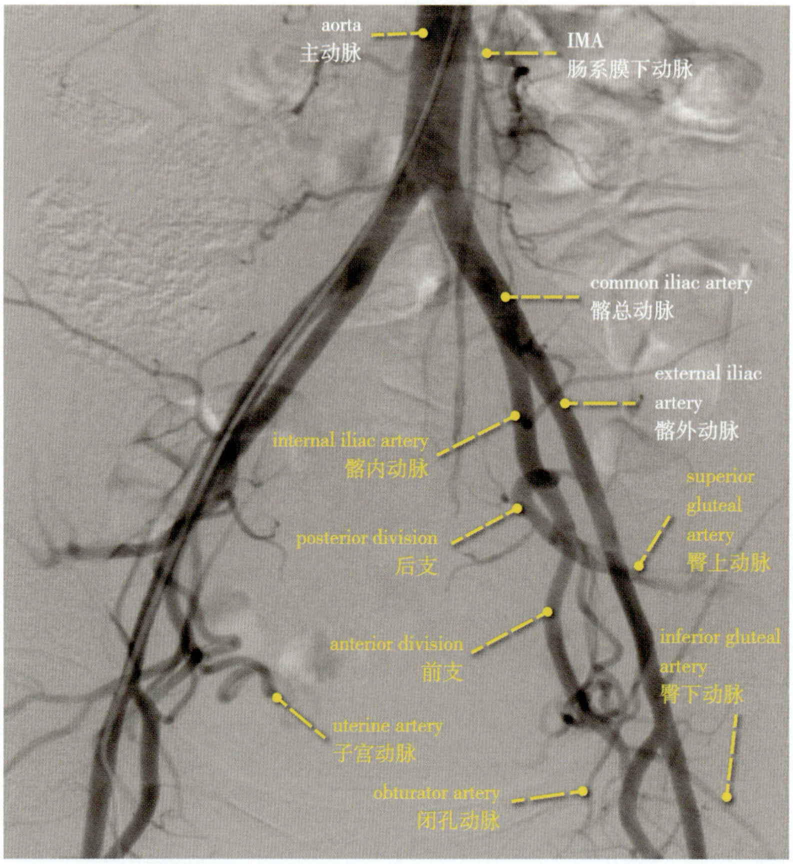

- The anterior division of the internal iliac artery supplies most of the pelvic viscera.

  The major branches of the anterior division include the **inferior gluteal artery, obturator artery** and **internal pudendal artery**.

  The prostatic or uterine/vaginal artery, superior/inferior vesicle artery and middle/inferior rectal arteries can have variable origins and are best identified on selective angiography based on their area of supply.

  The **pathway of Winslow** is an important anastomotic connection from the subclavian, internal mammary, superior epigastric, and inferior epigastric arteries into the external iliac artery.

  The internal iliac artery arcades create important collateral pathways between the superior and middle rectal arteries.

  A **corona mortis** "crown of death" is a normal variant in which the obturator artery arises from the external iliac artery, and is an important consideration in procedural planning or pelvic trauma.

- The posterior division of the internal iliac artery supplies the pelvic and gluteal musculature.

  The branches of the posterior division include the **lateral sacral artery**, the **iliolumbar artery** (anastomoses with external iliac via the deep circumflex iliac artery), and the **superior gluteal artery**.

- 髂内动脉前支供应大部分盆腔脏器。

  髂内动脉前支的主要分支包括**臀下动脉**、**闭孔动脉**和**阴部内动脉**。

  前列腺动脉或子宫/阴道动脉、膀胱上/下动脉和直肠中/下动脉有多种不同的起源，它们最好在选择性血管造影上根据其供应区域予以识别。

  Winslow 通路是锁骨下动脉、内乳动脉、腹壁上动脉和腹壁下动脉至髂外动脉的重要吻合交通。

  髂内动脉弓在直肠上动脉和直肠中动脉之间提供重要的侧支通路。

  "死亡之冠"是一种正常变异，为闭孔动脉起源于髂外动脉，在计划手术或骨盆外伤时应予以重视。

- 髂内动脉后支供应盆腔和臀部肌肉。

  髂内动脉后支包括**骶外侧动脉**、**髂腰动脉**(通过旋髂深动脉与髂外动脉吻合)和**臀上动脉**。

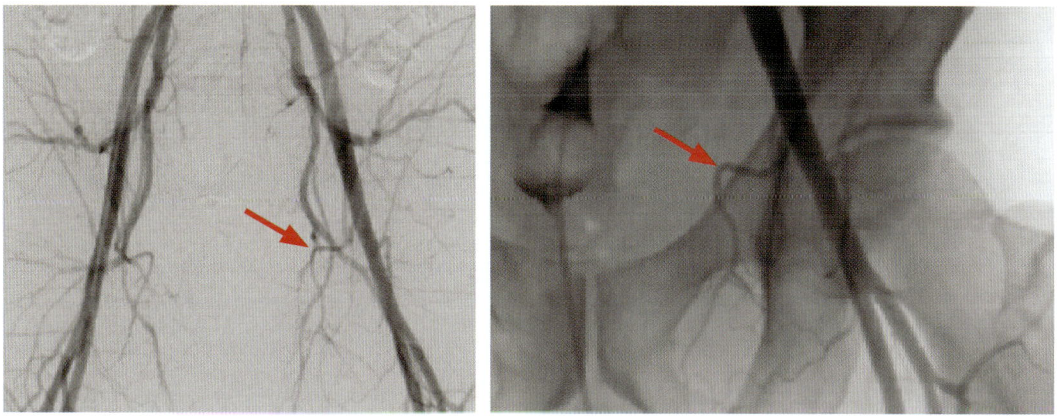

Non-selective pelvic angiogram (left image) and selective left external iliac angiogram (right image) showing "corona mortis" variant anatomy of the left obturator artery (arrows) originating from the external iliac artery.
非选择性盆腔血管造影(左图)和选择性左侧髂外血管造影(右图)显示左闭孔动脉起源于髂外动脉(红箭),此为解剖变异并被称为"死亡之冠"。

(翻译　赵赫)

ARTERIAL INTERVENTIONS

TRAUMA

General considerations

- Trauma accounts for the majority of IR emergencies. Level 1 trauma centers must have IR procedures available 24 hours a day.
- Management of traumatic solid organ injury depends on the degree of injury and hemodynamics of the patient. Conservative management involves resuscitation, monitoring of vitals and laboratory values and serial exams, and is best for stable patients with low-grade solid organ injury. IR angiography and embolization are best for stable patients with moderate-to-high grade organ injuries and CT findings showing contrast extravasation or pseudoaneurysm. IR embolization can be applied to either contained or uncontained hemorrhage, with the intention of avoiding surgery. Management of high-grade injuries can vary based on the organ involved.

Aortic injury

- CTA is the gold standard for evaluation of suspected traumatic aortic injury.
- Open surgical repair is the gold standard treatment for acute traumatic aortic injury with endovascular stent-graft repair becoming more commonly performed recently.

动脉介入

创伤

概述

- 创伤是急诊介入的主要组成部分。一级创伤中心必须每天24小时提供介入治疗。
- 处理实质脏器创伤取决于损伤的程度和患者的血流动力学情况。保守治疗包括补液、监测生命体征和实验室指标,以及定时查体,最适用于稳定的轻度实质性脏器创伤的患者。血管造影和栓塞治疗最适用于稳定的中度和严重实质性脏器创伤的患者,以及CT显示有造影剂外溢或假性动脉瘤者。介入栓塞既可用于包裹性出血,也可用于非包裹性出血,以避免外科手术。高级别创伤的处理取决于累及的脏器。

主动脉损伤

- CT血管造影是评估可疑主动脉创伤的"金标准"。
- 外科手术修复是治疗急性创伤性主动脉损伤的标准方法,而血管腔内覆膜支架修复近年来更为常用。

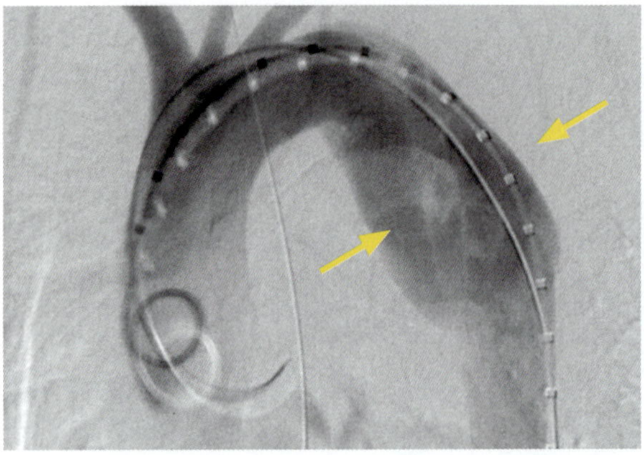

Aortic trauma: Catheter aortogram shows a large, fusiform pseudoaneurysm (arrows) of the aortic isthmus, distal to the brachiocephalic artery.
主动脉创伤：主动脉导管造影示主动脉峡部有一个大而呈梭形的假性动脉瘤(黄箭)，位于头臂动脉远侧。

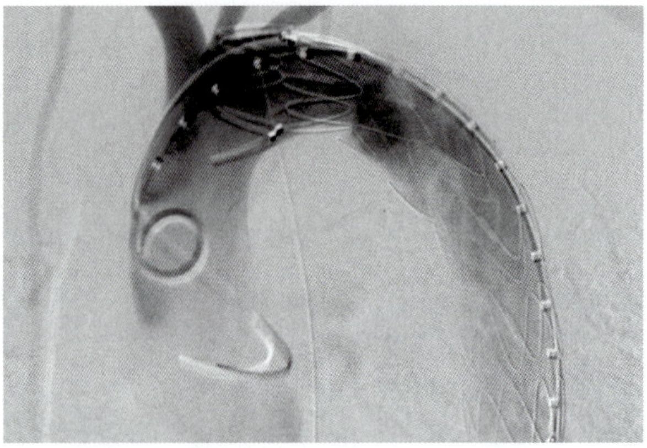

Post-endograft repair aortogram shows stent-graft in place with good opacification of the arch vessels.
修复后主动脉造影示主动脉内的覆膜支架，主动脉分支显影良好。

Case courtesy Michael Hanley, MD, University of Virginia Health System.

Renal trauma

- Renal trauma can be classified as blunt (>80% of injuries), penetrating (such as gunshot or stab wound), or iatrogenic. Hematuria is usually present with renal trauma, regardless of etiology. A horseshoe kidney is especially susceptible to traumatic injury as it is not protected by the inferior ribs and may be compressed against the vertebral column.
- The Organ Injury Scale (OIS) from the American Association for the Surgery of Trauma (AAST) classification is the most widely used classification of renal injury. This scale is further discussed in the “Genitourinary imaging” chapter.

  Grades I-III include nonexpanding hematomas or parenchymal laceration without collecting system injury. These injuries are usually managed conservatively.

  Grade IV includes a deep parenchymal laceration which extends to the collecting system, causing the CT finding of extravasation of opacified urine on delayed imaging. Injury to the renal vessels with contained hemorrhage is also OIS grade Ⅳ, often treated with endovascular coil embolization as in the case below.

  Grade V (most severe) injury is a shattered kidney with avulsion of the renal hilum. Treatment is surgical.
- Other important vascular injuries not included in the OIS classification include traumatic renal artery thrombosis and renal artery pseudoaneurysm.
- Indications for endovascular treatment of renal trauma include active extravasation, dissection, or pseudoaneurysm. Treatment is usually superselective coil embolization.

肾脏外伤

- 肾外伤可分为钝性(占>80%的肾外伤)、穿透性(如枪伤或刀刺伤)和医源性。血尿可出现在各种病因的肾外伤。马蹄肾尤其容易受伤，因其不被肋骨保护，易被压向椎体。
- 美国创伤外科协会(AAST)的脏器损伤分级(OIS)是目前使用最广泛的肾损伤分级方法。该分级将在“泌尿生殖影像”一章进行讨论。

  Ⅰ~Ⅲ级包括稳定性血肿，或实质撕裂但不伴集合系统损伤。这些损伤通常采用保守治疗。

  Ⅳ级包括深度实质撕裂并累及集合系统，CT延迟期可见含有造影剂的尿液外溢。肾脏血管损伤合并包裹性血肿也属于OIS Ⅳ级，常需血管内弹簧圈栓塞治疗，如下图病例。

  Ⅴ级损伤(最严重)是粉碎性肾脏损伤伴肾门部撕裂，采用外科手术治疗。
- 未被列入OIS分级的其他重要血管损伤包括外伤性肾动脉血栓形成及肾动脉假性动脉瘤。
- 血管腔内治疗肾外伤的指征包括活动性造影剂外溢、夹层或假性动脉瘤。治疗通常用弹簧圈进行超选择性栓塞。

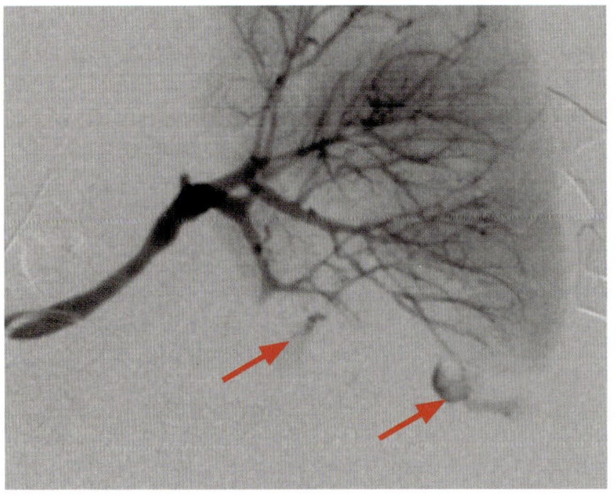

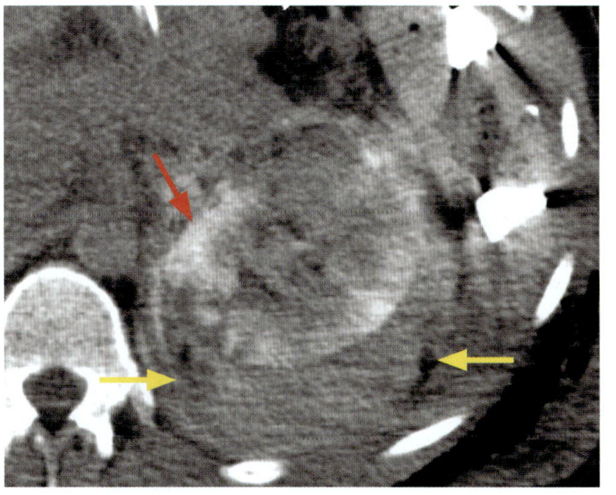

OIS Grade IV renal injury: Selective DSA angiogram of the left kidney (left image) shows lack of vascularization of the lower pole of the kidney and two foci of active contrast extravasation (red arrows). These were treated super selectively with coiling. Post-embolization unenhanced CT (right image) shows residual irregular pooling of contrast in the renal cortex (red arrow) and a large perinephric urinoma (yellow arrows) diagnostic of grade IV injury. There are bullet fragments in the left hemiabdomen.

Case courtesy Alisa Suzuki Han, MD, Brigham and Women's Hospital.

OIS Ⅳ级肾脏外伤：选择性左肾DSA(左图)显示肾下极血管结构缺失且有两个活动性造影剂外溢点(红箭)。用弹簧圈行超选择性栓塞治疗。栓塞后平扫CT(右图)显示肾实质内不规则造影剂滞留(红箭)和肾周尿液瘤(黄箭)，诊断为Ⅳ级肾脏外伤。左侧腹腔见子弹碎片。

Renal arteriovenous fistulas

- Renal arteriovenous fistulas (AVFs) are almost always acquired, secondary to trauma or renal biopsy.
- The majority of renal AVFs are asymptomatic and often heal spontaneously. When symptomatic, hematuria is the most common complaint. Less commonly, a renal AVF can lead to high-output cardiac failure or spontaneous retroperitoneal hemorrhage.
- Angiography of an AVF shows venous opacification during the arterial phase.
- Treatment is with embolization (coils, glue, or alcohol).

Pelvic vascular trauma

肾动静脉瘘

- 肾动静脉瘘(AVFs)几乎均为获得性，继发于外伤或肾活检。
- 大多数肾AVFs为无症状，且常自行愈合。如出现症状，血尿最为常见。较少情况下，肾AVF可引起高动力性心力衰竭或自发性腹膜后出血。
- AVF在血管造影上表现为静脉在动脉期显影。
- 治疗采用栓塞(弹簧圈、胶或乙醇)。

盆腔血管损伤

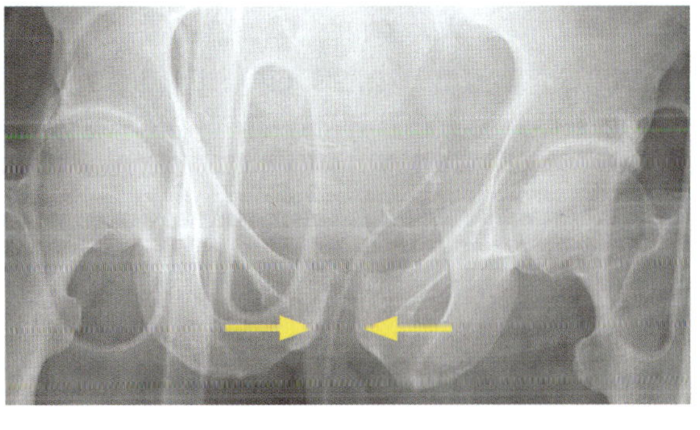

Initial trauma-board pelvic radiograph shows diastasis of the pubic symphysis (arrows).

最早骨盆X线影像显示耻骨联合分离(黄箭)。

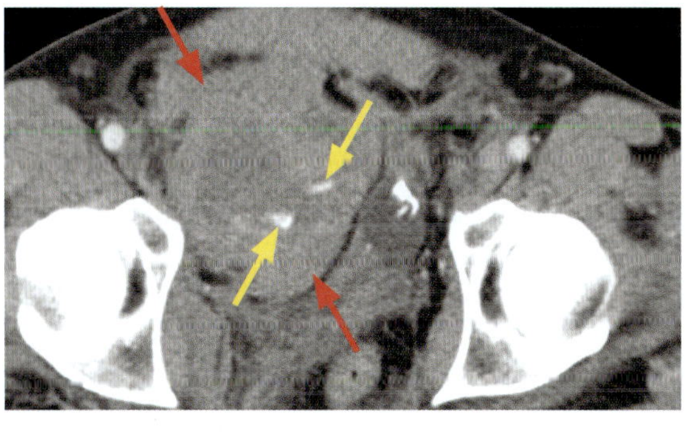

Contrast-enhanced CT shows a large hematoma in the right hemipelvis (red arrows) with foci of active extravasation (yellow arrows).

增强CT显示右侧盆腔一个大血肿(红箭)，伴有局部斑点样造影剂外渗(黄箭)。

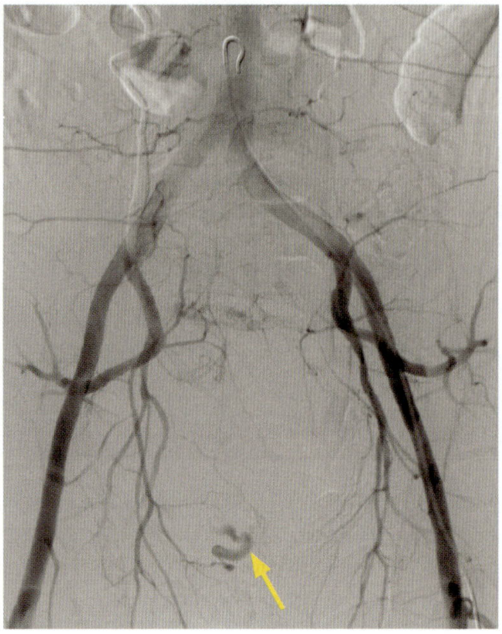

Nonselective arterial-phase DSA angiogram of the internal iliac arteries with the flush catheter in the distal aorta shows a focus of active extravasation (arrow) arising from the right pudendal artery.

将高流量导管置于主动脉远端行非选择性髂内动脉DSA。动脉期显示右侧阴部内动脉局部造影剂外渗(黄箭)。

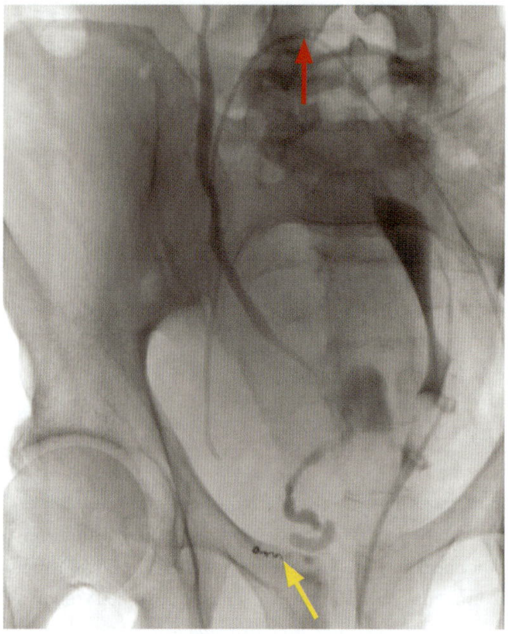

Post-coiling, intra-procedural radiograph shows coils within the right pudendal artery (yellow arrow).
Note the catheter (red arrow) in the right internal iliac artery via a left femoral approach.

弹簧圈栓塞后，术中图像示弹簧圈位于右阴部内动脉(黄箭)。
注意，导管(红箭)经左侧股动脉进入右侧髂内动脉。

Case courtesy Alisa Suzuki Han, MD, Brigham and Women's Hospital.

- Pelvic trauma can lead to catastrophic hemorrhage from arterial injury. It is possible to exsanguinate completely within the pelvis: A 3 cm diastasis of the symphysis pubis doubles the potential intra-pelvic volume to approximately 8 liters.
- In the setting of active pelvic bleeding and pelvic fractures, angiography is usually performed *prior* to orthopedic surgery. Active bleeding can be difficult to control surgically.
- The first step in treating a pelvic arterial injury is to perform a nonselective pelvic arteriogram, followed by selective bilateral internal iliac arteriograms of the anterior and posterior divisions.
- Because of the rich collateral supply in the pelvis, rapid nonselective gelfoam embolization of either the entire anterior or posterior division of the internal iliac artery is often acceptable. A potentially time-consuming superselective embolization should be avoided in the setting of life-threatening hemorrhage.

- 盆腔外伤可导致致命性动脉出血。全身血液都有可能流入盆腔：耻骨联合分离3cm将使盆腔潜在的容量增加1倍，约8L。
- 对于有活动性骨盆出血和骨盆骨折的患者，通常在行骨科手术前应先进行动脉造影。外科手术常难以控制活动性出血。
- 治疗盆腔动脉损伤的第一步是进行非选择性盆腔动脉造影，然后进行选择性双侧髂内动脉前干和后干造影。
- 由于盆腔侧支循环比较丰富，用明胶海绵颗粒快速对髂内动脉前干或后干进行非选择性栓塞通常是一种可取的方法。在出血危及生命时应避免可能耗时过度的超选择性栓塞。

Massive hemoptysis

- Massive hemoptysis is defined as gross hemorrhage (typically 300–600 mL of blood in a 24-hour period) and can be a life-threatening emergency as a result of asphyxia rather than hemorrhagic shock. Thus, hemodynamics is not a suitable measure for severity.
- Most cases originate from the bronchial arteries as opposed to the lower-pressure pulmonary-artery system.
- Risk factors include smoking, cystic fibrosis or vasculitis.
- The patient should be positioned with the affected lung down to improve oxygenation and reduce fluid accumulation in the other lung.
- Pre-procedure bronchoscopy or CTA are useful to localize the site of bleeding.

大咯血

- 大咯血的定义为可见明显出血(一般在24小时内出血300~600mL)，是一种危及生命的急症，其危险因素是窒息而不是失血性休克。因此，血流动力学不适合用于判断其严重性。
- 绝大多数咯血来源为支气管动脉而不是压力低的肺动脉系统。
- 危险因素包括吸烟、囊性纤维化或血管炎。
- 需将患者置于侧位(患侧肺朝下)以增加氧合作用，并减少液体在对侧肺的集聚。
- 术前支气管镜或CTA可以帮助确定出血点。

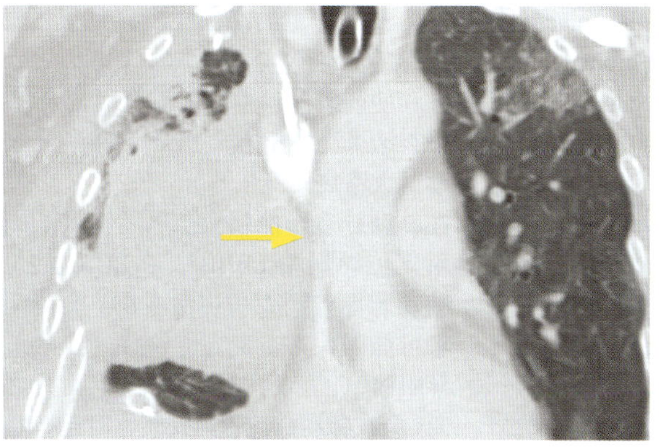

Coronal CT in a patient with hemoptysis shows a dominant right-sided thoracic mass abutting the mediastinum, causing narrowing of the SVC (arrow).
一名咯血患者的冠状位CT显示右侧胸腔巨大肿块压迫纵隔，导致SVC狭窄(黄箭)。

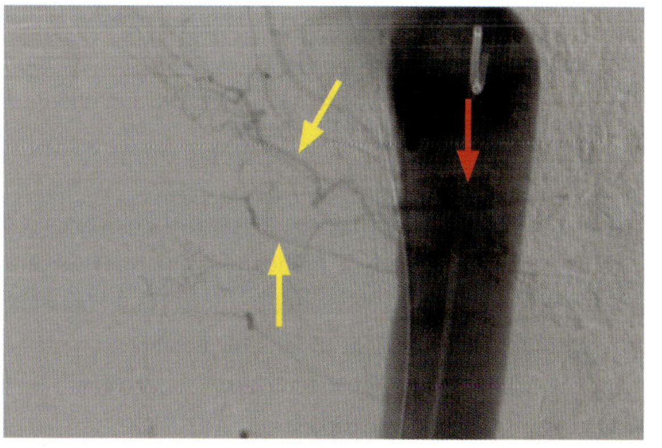

Initial nonselective DSA aortography faintly opacifies the common bronchial trunk (red arrow) and the two right bronchial arteries (yellow arrows).
最初的主动脉非选择性DSA显示共干支气管动脉(红箭)和两根支气管动脉(黄箭)。

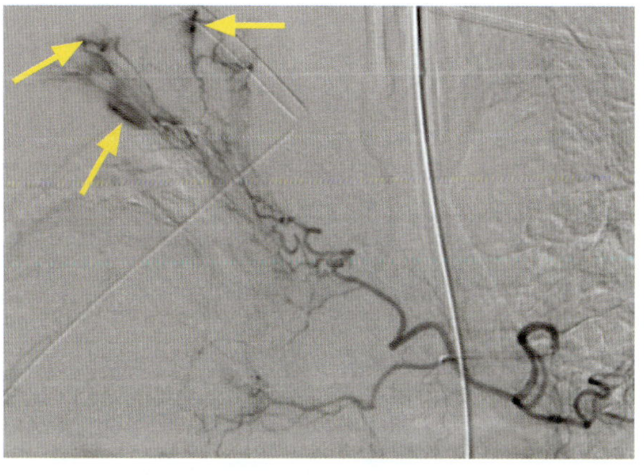

Selective angiography of the common bronchial trunk shows multiple foci of active extravasation in the right upper lobe (arrows).
选择性共干支气管动脉造影显示右上肺多处局部活动性造影剂外溢(黄箭)。

Massive hemoptysis caused by thoracic malignancy treated with particle embolization of the common bronchial artery trunk (post-embolization images not shown). In this case, the right bronchial arteries were not able to be accessed. Due to the emergent nature of the hemoptysis, the common bronchial trunk was embolized to complete stasis with particles. There was complete resolution of the active extravasation. The mass was later shown to be a thymoma.
Case courtesy Alisa Suzuki Han, MD, Brigham and Women's Hospital.
对胸腔恶性肿瘤导致的大咯血进行共干支气管动脉颗粒栓塞治疗(未展示栓塞治疗后图像)。对此患者未能成功进行选择性右支气管动脉插管。由于急性出血，对共干支气管动脉用颗粒进行栓塞使血流停滞。之后造影剂外溢完全消失。肿块后来证实为胸腺瘤。

- Massive hemoptysis has a very high mortality, most commonly due to asphyxiation. The vast majority (90%) of cases of hemoptysis involve the bronchial arteries, with the pulmonary arteries involved in most of the rest of cases. Occasionally, other systemic arteries may be involved, so if a patient continues to bleed after evaluation of the bronchial and pulmonary arterial circulation, the subclavian, internal mammary, inferior phrenic, and celiac arteries should be evaluated as well.
- Chronic inflammation can lead to hypertrophied bronchial arteries and subsequent hemoptysis. In the United States, cystic fibrosis and thoracic malignancy are the most common causes of hemoptysis. Worldwide, tuberculosis and fungal infection are more common.
- The bronchial arteries arise from the thoracic aorta at T5–T6, although the arterial anatomy is quite variable. There are usually one or two bronchial arteries on each side.
- Embolization is performed with a distal embolic agent, most commonly particles. Initial angiography should carefully evaluate for the rare presence of a left to right shunt prior to particle embolization to prevent inadvertent cerebral embolization. Embolization is usually performed to near-stasis.

- 大咯血的死亡率极高，多由窒息所致。绝大多数(90%)咯血与支气管动脉有关，其余大多为肺动脉出血。很少的情况下其他体循环动脉也可引起出血，因此，若患者在支气管和肺动脉循环评估后仍咯血，则需对锁骨下动脉、内乳动脉、膈下动脉和腹腔干进行检查。
- 慢性炎症可导致支气管动脉扩张进而咯血。在美国，囊性纤维化和胸部恶性肿瘤是最常见的咯血原因。全球范围内，结核和真菌感染更常见。
- 支气管动脉发自胸主动脉的$T_{5\sim6}$水平，但动脉的解剖变异较大。通常每侧有1~2根支气管动脉。
- 栓塞治疗使用末梢栓塞剂，最常用的是颗粒。栓塞前必须仔细检查动脉造影有无罕见的左向右分流，以防意外造成脑栓塞。栓塞通常在血流接近停滞时结束。

Because rebleeding after treatment is common, coils are rarely used to treat hemoptysis. Because coils prevent repeat access, the use of coils would preclude retreatment.

- A potentially devastating complication is nontarget embolization of the spinal cord via the anterior spinal artery or smaller tributaries arising from bronchial and intercostal arteries. A complete neurological exam should be documented prior to the procedure.

Pulmonary massive hemoptysis

- Before performing a pulmonary angiogram, it is essential to evaluate an EKG to ensure that a left bundle branch block (LBBB) is not present. If the pulmonary artery catheter were to cause temporary right bundle branch block in the presence of a LBBB, the lack of left-sided conduction may cause complete heart block, which can be fatal. A temporary pacer should be placed prior to pulmonary arteriography in the presence of a LBBB.
- Normal right-sided pressures:
  Right atrium: 0–8 mmHg.
  Right ventricle: 0–8 mmHg diastolic; 15–30 mmHg systolic.
  Pulmonary artery: 3–12 mmHg diastolic; 15–30 mmHg systolic.

Pulmonary arteriovenous malformation (AVM)

弹簧圈极少用于治疗咯血。因为弹簧圈堵住了入口后，会阻碍后续使用弹簧圈栓塞。

- 一个极其严重的潜在并发症是误栓脊髓，因为脊髓前动脉或更细小的分支发自支气管动脉和肋间动脉。栓塞前需全面记录神经系统检查结果

肺动脉大咯血

- 在肺动脉造影前须做心电图(EKG)以除外左束支传导阻滞(LBBB)。在LBBB的患者，如肺动脉导管诱发一过性右束支传导阻滞，患者可能因缺乏左束支传导而造成心脏完全传导阻滞，此表现具有致命性。因此存在LBBB时，应在肺动脉造影前安装临时起搏器。
- 正常右心压力：
  右心房：0~8mmHg。
  右心室：0~8mmHg舒张期，15~30mmHg收缩期。
  肺动脉：3~12mmHg舒张期，15~30mmHg收缩期。

肺动静脉畸形(AVM)

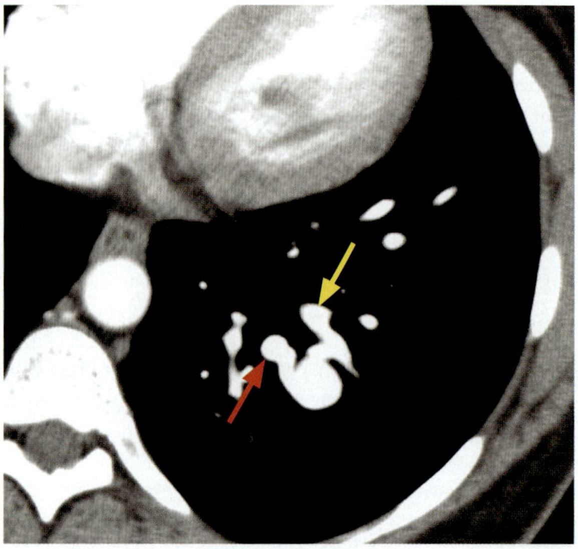

Contrast-enhanced CT demonstrates a pulmonary AVM with the feeding artery (yellow arrow) and draining vein (red arrow). Although not shown on this image, the feeding artery arises from the pulmonary artery and the draining vein drains to the left atrium.
CT增强扫描显示肺AVM及其供血动脉(黄箭)和引流静脉(红箭)。供血动脉来自肺动脉，引流静脉流入左心房(此图未展示)。

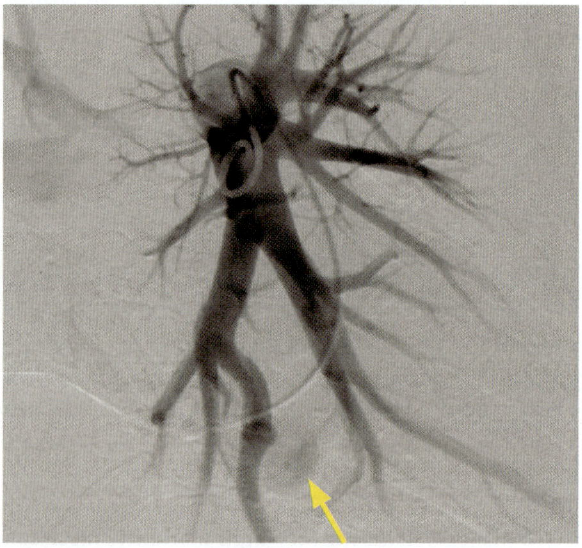

Nonselective DSA early arterial phase angiography of the left pulmonary artery in LAO orientation with a pigtail catheter in the left PA shows a faint contrast blush representing the AVM nidus (arrow). Venous drainage is not yet visible. This was treated with coils.
左前斜位动脉早期猪尾导管插入左肺动脉，非选择性左肺动脉干DSA显示一处浅的造影剂染色，为AVM血管巢(黄箭)。引流静脉此时尚未显影。此病变用弹簧圈治疗。

Case courtesy Alisa Suzuki Han, MD, Brigham and Women's Hospital.

- A pulmonary arteriovenous malformation (AVM) is an abnormal connection between the pulmonary artery and pulmonary veins, causing a right to left shunt.
- Patients with hereditary hemorrhagic telangiectasia (HHT), also known as Osler-Weber-Rendu syndrome, may have multiple pulmonary AVMs. HHT can clinically present with brain abscess, stroke, or recurrent epistaxis (due to nasal mucosa telangiectasia).
- Coils must be used to embolize a pulmonary AVM. Particles are contraindicated as the right to left shunt would cause brain emboli and infarction.

- 肺动静脉畸形(AVM)是肺动脉与肺静脉之间的异常交通，造成右向左分流。
- 患有遗传性出血性毛细血管扩张症(HHT)，也称Osler-Weber-Rendu综合征的患者可有多个肺AVMs。HHT临床可表现为脑脓肿、脑卒中、复发性鼻出血(由于鼻黏膜毛细血管扩张)。
- 肺AVM需用弹簧圈栓塞，禁用颗粒栓塞剂，因右向左分流可导致脑栓塞和梗死。

- Most pulmonary AVMs have a single feeding artery and coiling of this inflow artery (via a pulmonary arterial approach) is usually sufficient treatment.

  Note that the treatment of peripheral (e.g., in a limb) AVM generally requires elimination of the entire nidus, which is often fed from multiple arterial branches.
- An asymptomatic lesion with a feeding artery size >3 mm or a symptomatic lesion (i.e., prior infarct or brain abscess) are indications for treatment.

- 大多数肺AVM只有一根供血动脉，弹簧圈栓塞此供应血管(通过肺动脉途径)常为有效的方法。

  注意，外周AVM(如肢体)的治疗常需处理整个血管巢，因其常有多根供血动脉。
- 无症状但供血动脉管径>3mm或有症状的病灶(如先前有梗死和脑脓肿)是治疗的适应证。

Obstetric Emergencies

Hemorrhage

- Antepartum hemorrhage can be caused by placenta previa, placental abruption, and uterine rupture. These are usually treated with urgent Caesarean section or hysterectomy. Role of IR includes placing balloon catheters prior to going to the operating room, minimize blood loss, control of hemorrhage, use cell saver capability.
- Postpartum hemorrhage can be caused by uterine inversion, uterine atony, and genital tract trauma. IR serves both diagnostic and therapeutic purposes by interrogating the internal iliac arteries for the source of hemorrhage, often the uterine artery.

Pseudoaneurysm

- Uterine artery pseudoaneurysms (UAPs) typically present several weeks after delivery. They are usually diagnosed by ultrasound or CT prior to transcatheter arterial embolization.
- Intervention includes bilateral internal iliac or uterine artery ligation. When other treatments fail, hysterectomy is the last resort.

产科急症

出血

- 产前出血可由前置胎盘、胎盘早剥和子宫破裂引起，常采用紧急剖宫产或子宫切除术进行治疗。介入的作用是患者进外科手术室前放置球囊导管以减少术中失血、控制出血，可使用血细胞回输。
- 产后出血可由子宫外翻、子宫无力及生殖道创伤引起。介入可通过髂内动脉造影以明确出血来源(通常为子宫动脉),起到诊断和治疗的目的。

假性动脉瘤

- 子宫假性动脉瘤(UAPs)常发生在分娩后数周，常在经导管动脉栓塞术前由超声或CT发现。
- 治疗包括双侧髂内或子宫动脉结扎。子宫切除是其他治疗失败后的最后方法。

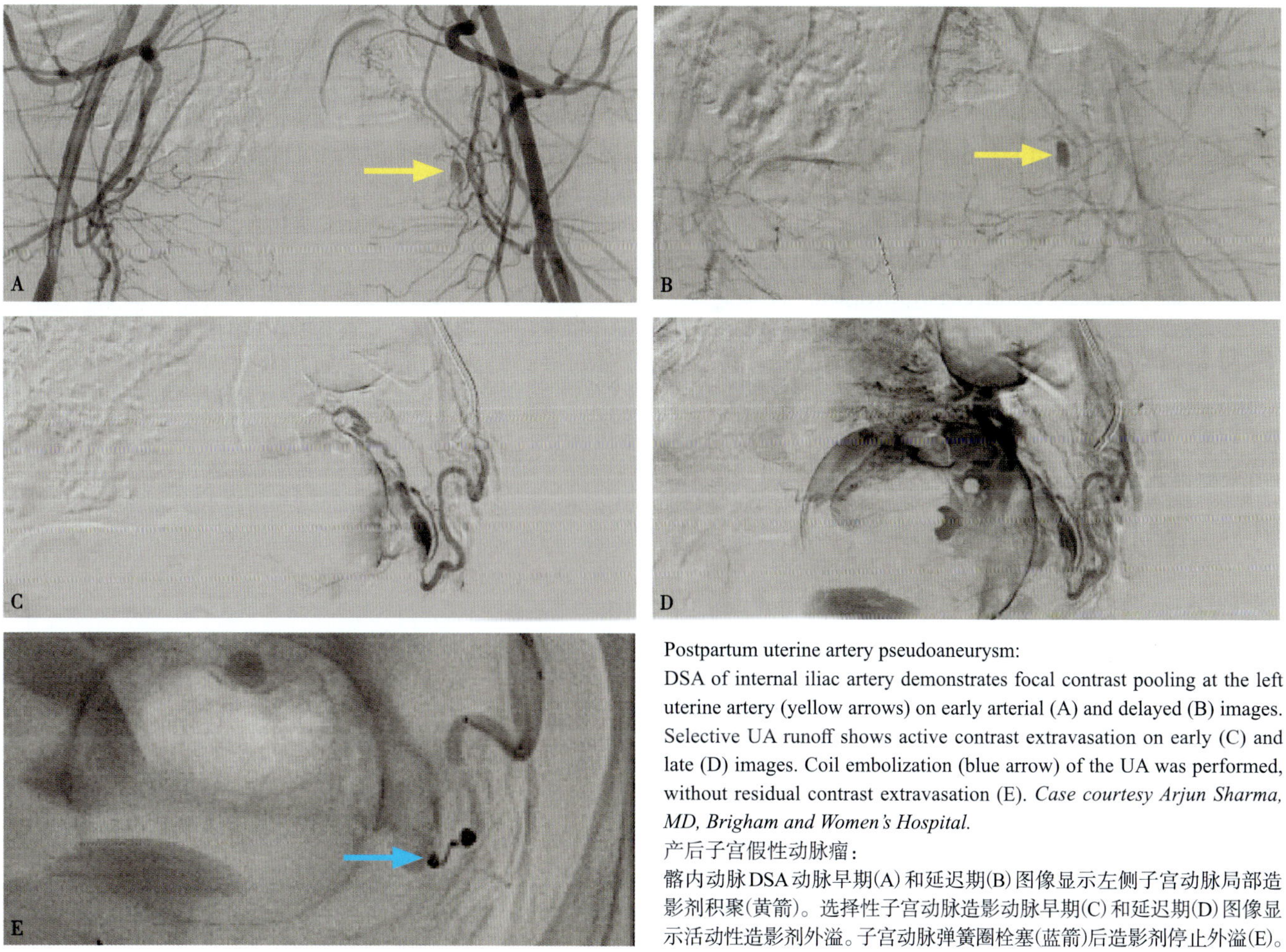

Postpartum uterine artery pseudoaneurysm:
DSA of internal iliac artery demonstrates focal contrast pooling at the left uterine artery (yellow arrows) on early arterial (A) and delayed (B) images. Selective UA runoff shows active contrast extravasation on early (C) and late (D) images. Coil embolization (blue arrow) of the UA was performed, without residual contrast extravasation (E). *Case courtesy Arjun Sharma, MD, Brigham and Women's Hospital.*

产后子宫假性动脉瘤：
髂内动脉DSA动脉早期(A)和延迟期(B)图像显示左侧子宫动脉局部造影剂积聚(黄箭)。选择性子宫动脉造影动脉早期(C)和延迟期(D)图像显示活动性造影剂外溢。子宫动脉弹簧圈栓塞(蓝箭)后造影剂停止外溢(E)。

GASTROINTESTINAL (GI) BLEEDING

Upper GI bleeding

- Endoscopy is the best initial procedure for acute upper GI bleeding, defined as above the ligament of Treitz. Endoscopy can be both diagnostic and therapeutic.
- If the patient failed endoscopic attempts at hemostasis or is too unstable for evaluation by endoscopy, IR embolization can be considered as long as a clear bleed is seen on pre-procedure CTA or on endoscopy.
- In some cases, empiric embolization of a gastric artery or the gastroduodenal artery may be considered if the angiogram is negative due to the copious collaterals between the celiac axis and the SMA. However, lower GI collaterals are much less well developed and there is a significant risk of bowel infarct with indiscriminate lower GI embolization.

Lower GI bleeding

- For lower GI bleeding, a hemodynamically stable patient should first be evaluated by mesenteric CT angiogram or nuclear medicine tagged red blood cell scan to localize the bleed, as these tests are thought to be more sensitive than angiography. A bleeding rate of 0.5–1.0 mL/min is generally required to be angiographically positive.

  A tagged red blood cell scan can detect bleeding rate as low as 0.2–0.4 mL/min.

  Many institutions now favor mesenteric CT angiography as the first test for evaluation of acute lower GI bleeding because CT is rapid, easy to perform, and readily available. On CTA, acute bleeding is seen as contrast extravasation. CTA may be able to detect bleeding rates as low as 0.35 mL/min.
- A hemodynamically unstable patient with clinical evidence of current GI bleeding may go straight to angiography.
- Intra-arterial infusion of vasopressin (antidiuretic hormone) can often control active lower GI bleeding, but there is a very high rebleeding rate once the infusion is stopped. Vasopressin is most useful in cases of bleeding from antimesenteric vessels, which are more difficult to reach directly by catheter. Major complications of vasopressin are seen in up to 20% including arrhythmia, pulmonary edema, and hypertension.

  Vasopressin is directly infused into the SMA or IMA. The dose of vasopressin is 0.2–0.4 units per minute (100 units mixed in 500 mL saline given at 1 mL/minute), given as a continuous infusion for up to 24 hours.

  Vasopressin can only be used for 24 hours before tachyphylaxis (lack of further response) develops.

胃肠道(GI)出血

上消化道出血

- 内镜是急性上消化道出血，即屈氏韧带以上出血最佳的初选方法，兼具诊断和治疗的作用。
- 若经内镜止血无效或患者情况太不稳定以至于无法行内镜检查时，介入栓塞可以用于术前CTA或内镜发现有明确出血的病例。
- 在某些情况下，即便血管造影为阴性，可以考虑对胃动脉或胃十二指肠动脉行经验性栓塞，因腹腔干和SMA之间存在丰富的侧支循环。而下消化道的侧支很不丰富，如不进行选择性下消化道动脉栓塞会明显增加肠道梗死的风险。

下消化道出血

- 在下消化道出血的患者，若血流动力学稳定，应首先进行CT血管造影或红细胞标记的核素扫描以确定出血位置，这两种检查的敏感性均高于血管造影。一般认为，出血速度达到0.5~1.0mL/min时动脉造影才呈阳性。

  红细胞标记的核素扫描能够检测低至0.2~0.4mL/min的出血。

  很多医院现在更倾向于使用CT血管造影作为急性下消化道出血的首选检测手段，因CT检查速度快、易操作且不受限制。急性出血在CT血管造影时表现为造影剂外溢。CT血管造影能够检测到低至0.35mL/min的出血。
- 对血流动力学不稳定且临床表现有活动性消化道出血的患者可考虑直接行血管造影。
- 动脉内灌注血管升压素(抗利尿激素)常能控制急性下消化道出血，但灌注一旦停止，再出血率很高。血管升压素对小肠系膜游离部的血管出血最为有用，而导管往往难以到达这些部位。血管升压素的严重并发症发生率高达20%，包括心律失常、肺水肿和高血压。

  直接向SMA和IMA内灌注血管升压素，剂量为0.2~0.4U/min(100U稀释至500mL生理盐水中，以1mL/min灌注)，持续灌注24小时。

  血管升压素只能使用24小时，之后会出现快速耐受(缺乏持续反应)。

Diverticular bleed

憩室出血

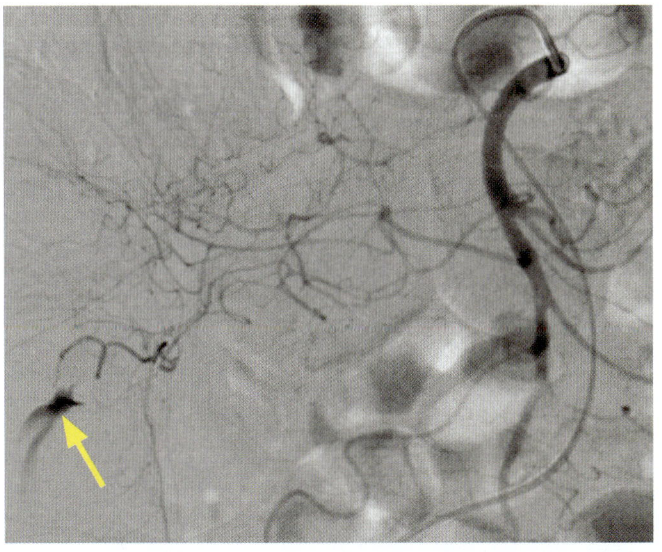

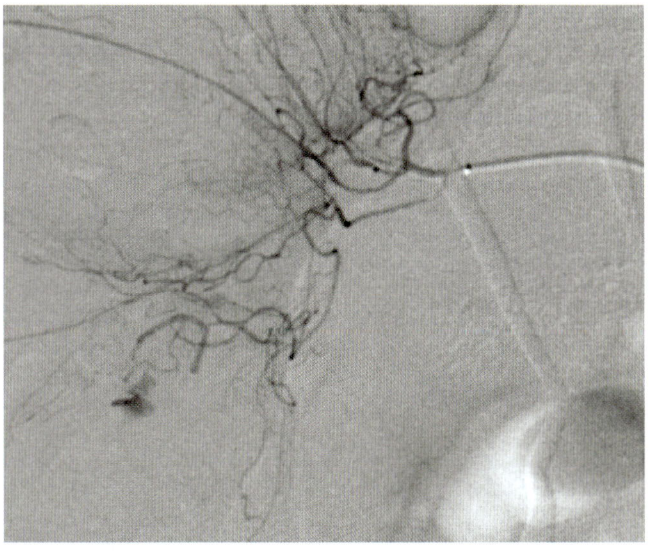

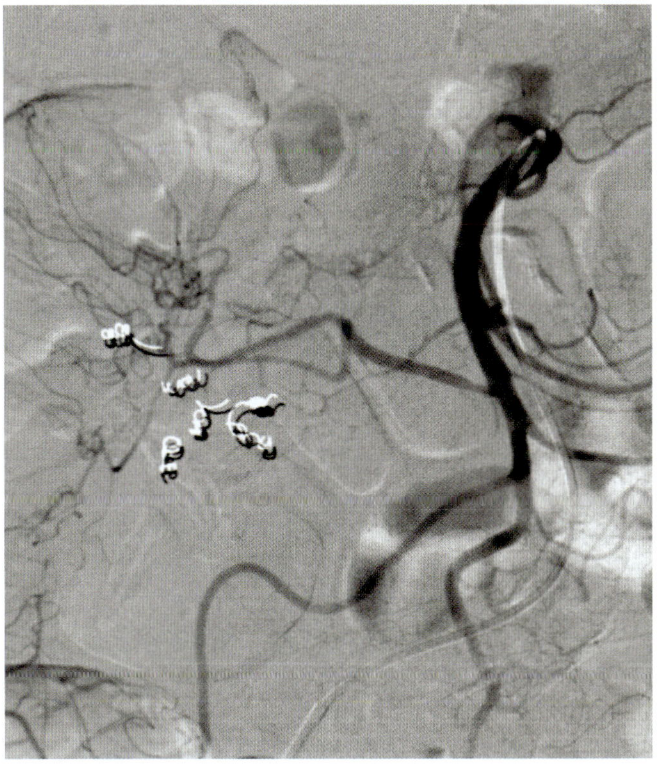

Diverticular bleed: Initial selective DSA angiogram of the SMA (top left image) shows an area of active extravasation (arrow) in a distal right branch of the middle colic artery.

Superselective DSA angiogram of the middle colic artery (top right image) shows that the area of active extravasation is too distal to be reached by catheter. At this point, the surgery team was consulted and it was determined that the patient was not a good operative candidate. The decision was made to embolize as selectively as possible, knowing the possible risk of bowel ischemia.

After placement of several coils in the middle colic branches, follow-up selective SMA angiogram (left image) demonstrates resolution of the active extravasation. There was no post-procedural evidence of bowel ischemia.

Case courtesy Alisa Suzuki Han, MD, Brigham and Women's Hospital.

憩室出血：初始选择性肠系膜上动脉DSA(左上图)显示在结肠中动脉右支远端有活动性造影剂外溢区(黄箭)。

超选择性结肠中动脉DSA(右上图)显示活动性造影剂外溢，但导管无法到达该远端区域。此时，外科会诊的意见是该患者不宜进行手术，决定进行栓塞，并尽可能地采用超选择以减少肠道缺血的风险。

在结肠中动脉分支放置数个弹簧圈后，重复选择性肠系膜上动脉造影(左下图)证实无造影剂外溢。术后未发现肠道缺血的征象。

- Diverticulosis is the most common cause of lower GI bleeding in older adults.
- Most patients respond to conservative management, but angiography can be used for stable or unstable patients who fail medical management.
- If active extravasation is seen, potential therapies include superselective embolization (most commonly with coils) or vasopressin infusion.

- 憩室病是老年人最常见的下消化道出血原因。
- 多数情况下保守治疗有效，但血管造影可用于保守治疗失败的患者，无论病情是否稳定。
- 一旦发现活动性造影剂外溢，治疗选择包括超选择栓塞(通常用弹簧圈)或血管升压素灌注。

Angiodysplasia

- Angiodysplasia is a small age-related vascular malformation and common cause of unexplained GI bleeding and anemia. It is most common in the cecum and ascending colon but can be found anywhere in the GI tract.
- **Heyde's syndrome** is a classic association of aortic valve stenosis and bleeding from angiodysplasia.

血管发育不良

- 血管发育不良是一种与年龄相关的小血管畸形，是无法解释消化道出血和贫血的常见原因。病变可见于肠道的任何部位，但通常位于盲肠和升结肠。
- 经典的**Heyde综合征**包括主动脉瓣狭窄及血管发育不良引起的肠道出血。

Hemorrhoidal bleed

- Endovascular coil occlusion of the distal branches of the superior rectal artery has the advantages of leaving the hemorrhoidal tissue in place, preserves anal continence, and does not involve the creation of rectal wounds (no local care required).
- Coil or particle embolization may be used. Particles may involve more distal branches and decrease the risk of recurrence.

痔疮出血

- 弹簧圈血管腔内栓塞直肠上动脉的末梢分支的优点是无须对痔疮组织进行干预，保留了肛门的功能且不产生直肠伤口(无须局部护理)。
- 可采用弹簧圈或颗粒栓塞。颗粒栓塞可达更远的末梢分支，从而降低复发的风险。

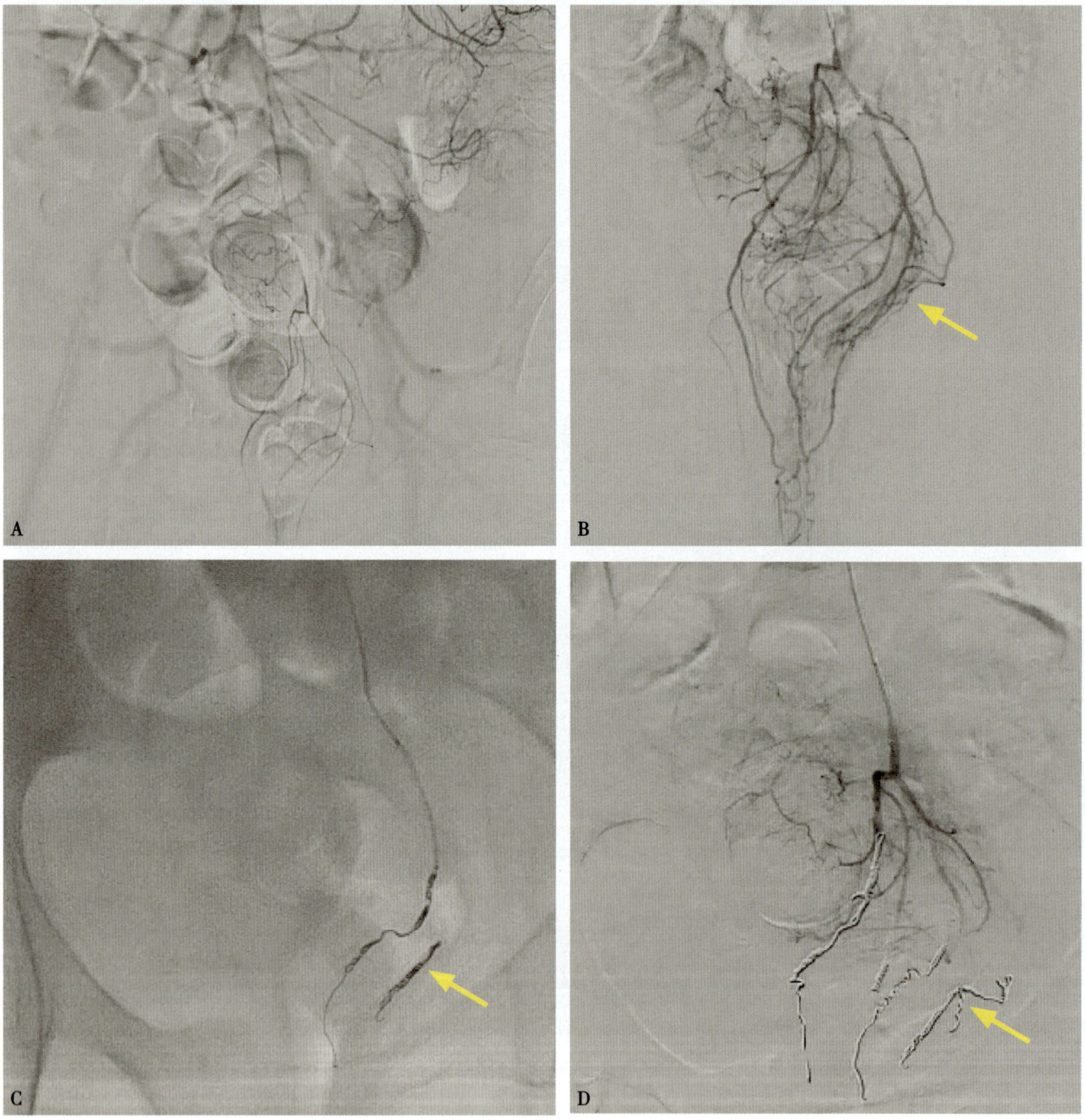

Hemorrhoid embolization: A) Selective IMA runoff shows the superior rectal artery branches. B) Superselective DSA of the superior rectal artery shows contrast blush corresponding to hemorrhoids (arow). C) Coil embolization (arrows) was performed with subsequent angiography. D) showing successful embolization of the hemorrhoids.

Case courtesy Arjun Sharma, MD, Brigham and Women's Hospital.

痔疮栓塞：A)选择性IMA造影显示直肠上动脉分支。B)超选择性直肠上动脉DSA显示对应于痔疮部位有造影剂染色(黄箭)。C)弹簧圈(黄箭)栓塞后血管造影。D)显示栓塞成功。

Mesenteric ischemia

- Mesenteric ischemia is inadequate blood supply to the bowel. It is seen most commonly in the elderly and has multiple causes, including acute arterial embolism, chronic arterial stenosis, venous occlusion, and low-flow states. For the

肠系膜缺血

- 肠系膜缺血是指肠管的血供不足。老年人最常见，病因有多种，包括急性动脉栓塞、慢性动脉狭窄、静脉阻塞和低流量状态。从介入治疗

purposes of interventions, the etiologies can be divided into **acute** or **chronic.**

的角度考虑，病因可分为**急性**和**慢性**两种。

Acute mesenteric ischemia

- Acute mesenteric ischemia typically presents as catastrophic abdominal pain, often with lactic acidosis. Acute mesenteric ischemia is most commonly caused by an SMA embolus.
- An SMA embolism distal to the middle colic artery carries the highest high risk of intestinal ischemia, as there are few native distal collaterals. The middle colic artery anastomoses with the IMA via the marginal artery of Drummond and the arc of Riolan.
- In most patients with acute mesenteric ischemia, treatment is surgical revascularization (embolectomy or bypass), direct inspection of bowel, and resection of necrotic bowel.
- In select patients with acute embolic mesenteric ischemia (patients without peritoneal signs or clinical findings suggestive of bowel necrosis), endovascular therapy with thrombolysis or suction embolectomy may be performed.
- **Nonocclusive mesenteric ischemia (NOMI)** is a highly lethal (70–100% mortality) form of acute mesenteric ischemia. NOMI is also known as "intestinal necrosis with a patent arterial tree" and features spasm and narrowing of multiple branches of the mesenteric arteries. Direct arterial infusion of the vasodilator papaverine (60 mg bolus, then 30–60 mg/hr) is the primary treatment of NOMI.

急性肠系膜缺血

- 急性肠系膜缺血通常表现为剧烈腹痛，常伴有乳酸酸中毒。急性肠系膜缺血通常由肠系膜上动脉栓子引起。
- 对结肠中动脉开口以远的肠系膜上动脉进行栓塞发生肠缺血的风险最高，因其远端只有很少的自然侧支。结肠中动脉和肠系膜下动脉通过Drummond边缘动脉和Riolan动脉弓进行吻合。
- 对于大多数急性肠系膜缺血的患者，治疗采用外科血管重建(取栓或搭桥)、肠管直视检查和坏死肠管切除。
- 对于某些急性肠系膜缺血的患者(患者无腹膜刺激征或临床无可疑肠管坏死表现)，可考虑血管内溶栓或抽吸取栓等血管腔内治疗。
- **非闭塞性肠系膜缺血(NOMI)**是一种高度致死的急性肠系膜缺血(70%~100%)。NOMI也被称为"动脉血管通畅的小肠坏死"，其特征为多个肠系膜动脉分支出现痉挛和狭窄。动脉直接灌注血管扩张剂罂粟碱(60mg团注，然后保持30~60mg/h)是治疗NOMI的首选方法。

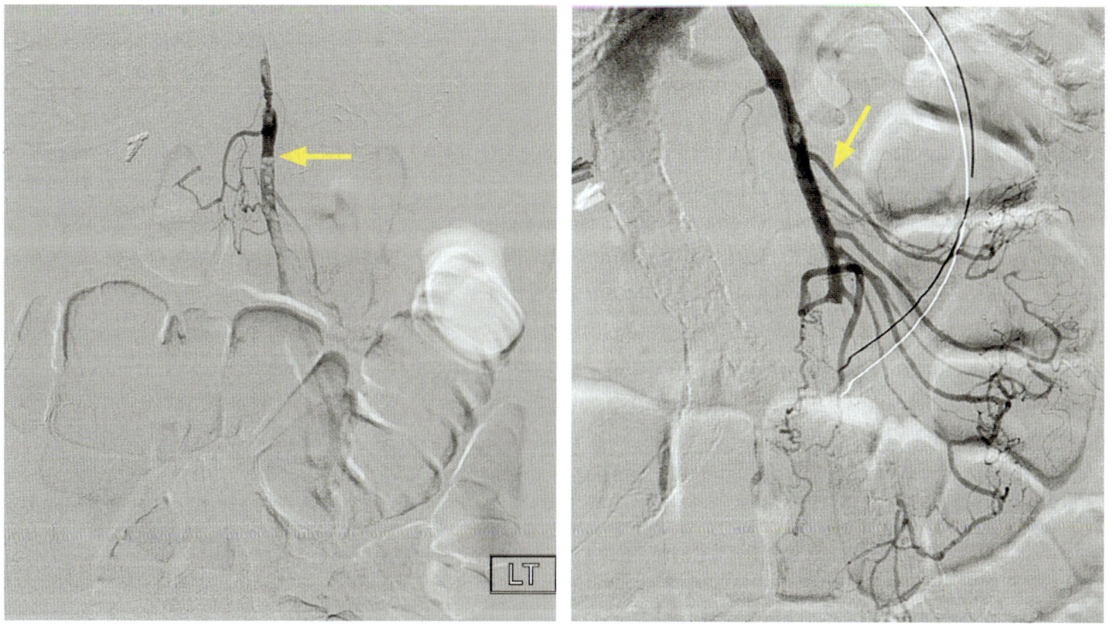

Acute mesenteric ischemia: 79-year-old female presented with altered mental status, found to have bowel wall thickening and multifocal thrombus of the superior mesenteric artery (SMA) on CT. Diagnostic angiogram shows extensive atherosclerotic calcifications and near total occlusion of the proximal SMA (left image, arrow). A catheter was positioned across the thrombus and left in place for overnight infusion of tPA. The next day, angiography of the superior mesenteric artery demonstrates substantially decreased clot burden with improved flow to the jejunal branch vessels (right image, arrow).

急性肠系膜缺血：79岁女性因神智状态改变就诊，CT发现肠壁增厚和肠系膜上动脉(SMA)多处血栓。诊断性血管造影显示广泛动脉粥样钙化和近端SMA几乎完全闭塞(左图，黄箭)。将导管插至血栓后留置，行夜间tPA灌注。次日肠系膜上动脉造影显示血栓量明显减少，空肠分支血流得到改善(右图，黄箭)。

Chronic mesenteric ischemia

- Chronic mesenteric ischemia is usually caused by atherosclerosis. The classic clinical presentation is postprandial abdominal pain out of proportion to the physical exam.

慢性肠系膜缺血

- 慢性肠系膜缺血通常由动脉粥样硬化引起。典型的临床表现是餐后腹痛，其程度与体检不符。
- 肠系膜血管造影显示血管起始部狭窄，常伴

- Mesenteric angiography shows ostial narrowing of the mesenteric vessels, often with post-stenotic dilation. The lateral aortogram is the most useful view to evaluate the origins of the celiac and superior mesenteric arteries.
- Because mesenteric collaterals are so extensive, at least two of three mesenteric arteries (celiac, SMA, and IMA) must be diseased to produce symptoms in chronic disease.
- Chronic mesenteric ischemia can be treated with endovascular angioplasty and stenting.

狭窄后扩张。侧位主动脉造影是评估腹腔动脉与肠系膜上动脉起始部的最佳体位。

- 由于肠系膜侧支非常丰富，因此，三支肠系膜血管(腹腔动脉、肠系膜上动脉和肠系膜下动脉)中至少两支血管发生病变时才会出现慢性临床症状。
- 慢性肠系膜缺血可采用血管内成形和植入支架进行治疗。

Aneurysmal Disease

- Aneurysms are considered when an artery is 1.5 times the size of the normal vessel.
- A true aneurysm involves all three layers of the arterial wall: Intima, media and adventitia.
- A pseudoaneurysm contains only one to two layers of the vessel wall and occurs in the setting of trauma, malignancy or infection.
- Aneurysms can vary with respect to size and growth, and management decisions should be based on the risk of rupture.

Aortic aneurysmal disease

- Minimally invasive endovascular aneurysm repair (EVAR) is a widely accepted alternative to surgical repair, with decreased perioperative morbidity and mortality.
- A comprehensive review of aortic aneurysmal disease and the 5 types of endoleaks is listed in the "Vascular" chapter. Interventional radiology is best suited for treating the following types of endoleaks:
- **Type I endoleaks** result from failure of the stent graft to form an adequate seal at the proximal (type ⅠA) or distal (type ⅠB) attachment sites.

  Prompt intervention is indicated and management consists of balloon angioplasty at the attachment sites to attempt to approximate the stent graft with the vessel wall, deploying another expandable bare metal stent over the attachment sites, or embolization.
- **Type II endoleaks** are the most common type and result from retrograde filling of the excluded aneurysm sac by branch vessels, typically the inferior mesenteric artery (IMA) and lumbar arteries.

  Many have slow flow and tend to spontaneously thrombose, resulting in no change or even decrease in size of the aneurysm sac.

  While there is risk for retrograde flow to increase sac size, the majority of aneurysms will decrease or stay the same, thus management is controversial and is considered when there is persistent endoleak or the sac enlarges by greater than 5 mm.

  Management consists of accessing the sac either by transarterial approach or direct sac puncture, and subsequent embolization of the feeding vessel.
- **Type III endoleaks** are uncommon and result from loss of device integrity.

  Prompt management is indicated and consists of deploying a new stent graft over the defect, with subsequent angioplasty to obtain a good seal.

Visceral artery aneurysm

- Visceral artery aneurysm can occur anywhere, with splenic and hepatic artery aneurysms amongst the most common types.

Splenic artery aneurysm

- Splenic artery aneurysm is the most common visceral aneurysm. Multiparous females and patients with portal hypertension are at increased risk of

动脉瘤性病变

- 当动脉的直径达到正常的1.5倍时可称为动脉瘤。
- 真性动脉瘤累及动脉壁所有的三层结构：内膜、中膜和外膜。
- 假性动脉瘤仅由1~2层的血管壁所构成，见于外伤、恶性肿瘤或感染。
- 动脉瘤因其大小和生长速度不同而表现各异，治疗策略应基于破裂的风险。

主动脉瘤病

- 血管腔内动脉瘤修复术(EVAR)是一种被广泛接受的替代手术修复的微创治疗方法，能降低围手术期发病率和死亡率。
- 主动脉瘤疾病的详细讨论及5型内漏见“血管影像”一章。介入放射学最适合治疗以下类型的内漏：
- **Ⅰ型内漏**是因为覆膜支架未能完全密封近端(ⅠA型)或远端(ⅠB型)血管附着点。

  需及时进行干预，措施包括球囊扩张支架附着部位使得覆膜支架紧贴血管壁、在覆膜支架附着部位植入金属裸支架，或进行栓塞。
- **Ⅱ型内漏**是最常见的类型，由侧支血管逆行灌注被隔绝的动脉瘤腔所致，通常是肠系膜下动脉(IMA)和腰动脉。

  很多因为血流缓慢而自发形成血栓，导致瘤腔大小无变化甚至缩小。

  虽然逆行血流有增大动脉瘤囊腔的风险，但大多数动脉瘤会缩小或不变，因此对其治疗存在争议。若存在持续内漏或动脉瘤腔增大超过5mm则考虑治疗。

  治疗包括经动脉入路或直接穿刺进入瘤腔，对供血血管进行栓塞。
- **Ⅲ型内漏**并不常见，是由覆膜支架破损造成的。

  需及时处理，包括植入新的覆膜支架覆盖缺损，随后进行球囊扩张使得密封完全。

内脏动脉瘤

- 内脏动脉瘤可发生在任何部位，其中脾和肝动脉瘤最常见。

脾动脉瘤

- 脾动脉瘤是最常见的内脏血管瘤。多产妇女和门静脉高压患者有增加患脾动脉瘤的

developing splenic artery aneurysms. Splenic artery aneurysms have an increased risk of rupture during pregnancy.

- A splenic artery *pseudo*aneurysm may be the result of trauma or pancreatitis.
- Indications for treatment of a splenic artery aneurysm include presence of symptoms (such as left upper quadrant pain), aneurysm size >2.5 cm, and prior to expected pregnancy.
- Endovascular coil embolization is the preferred approach. In general coils are first placed distal to the aneurysm neck (to exclude retrograde collateral flow), then placed proximally.
- Proximal splenic embolization is less painful and better at preserving splenic function because collateral blood supply can be preserved. Embolization should be performed in the mid splenic artery between the dorsal pancreatic and pancreatica magna arteries to reduce potential pancreatic complications such as ischemic pancreatitis. Distal embolization causes more tissue necrosis and can be more painful.

风险。脾动脉瘤在妊娠期间的破裂风险增加。

- 脾动脉假性动脉瘤可由外伤或胰腺炎所致。
- 脾动脉瘤的治疗指征包括出现症状(如左上腹痛)、动脉瘤直径>2.5m及准备怀孕的女性。
- 血管腔内弹簧圈栓塞是首选的方法。弹簧圈原则上应首先放置在动脉瘤颈的远端(用于阻断侧支血液逆向流入),然后放置在瘤颈近端。
- 近端脾动脉栓塞是术后疼痛较轻且能较好保护脾功能的手术,因其保留了侧支血供。栓塞应在脾动脉中段,即胰背动脉和胰大动脉之间,以减少潜在的胰腺并发症,如缺血性胰腺炎。远端栓塞会导致较多的组织坏死,导致疼痛加剧。

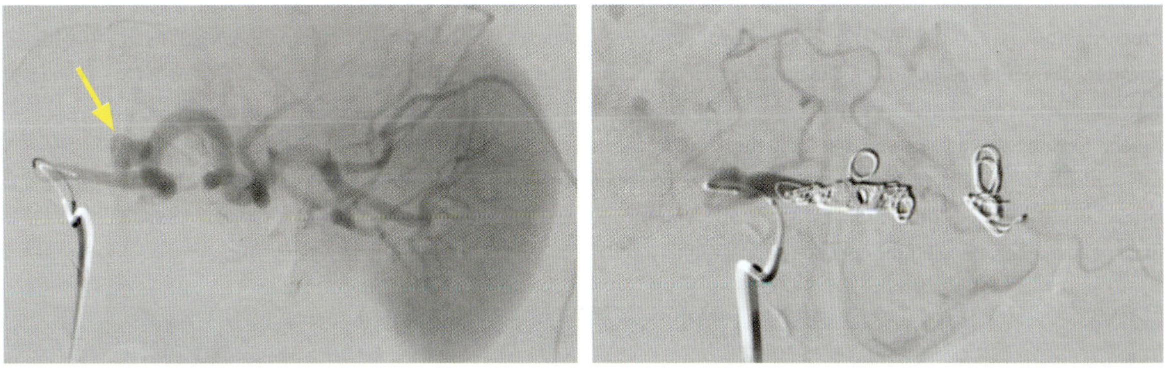

Splenic artery aneurysm: Selective DSA angiogram of the splenic artery (left image) shows an outpouching of contrast (arrow) in the proximal artery. Proximal coil embolization (right image) demonstrates resolution of the active extravasation.
脾动脉瘤:选择性脾动脉DSA(左图)显示近端脾动脉造影剂外突影(黄箭)。近端弹簧圈栓塞(右图)显示活动性造影剂外渗消失。

Hepatic artery aneurysm

- Hepatic artery aneurysm is the second most common visceral aneurysm.
- Indications for treatment of a visceral artery aneurysm include presence of symptoms (such as pain), aneurysm size >2.5 cm, and prior to expected pregnancy.
- Embolization of the right hepatic artery distal to the cystic artery (which arises from the right hepatic artery) is preferred, as embolization proximal to the cystic artery increases the risk of ischemic cholecystitis, which may be seen in up to 10% of cases.

肝动脉瘤

- 肝动脉瘤是第二常见的内脏动脉瘤。
- 内脏动脉瘤治疗的指征包括出现临床症状(如腹痛)、动脉瘤直径大于2.5cm及备孕女性。
- 行肝右动脉栓塞时应选择在胆囊动脉的远端(胆囊动脉发自肝右动脉),因在胆囊动脉近端进行栓塞会增加缺血性胆囊炎的风险,发生率高达10%。

Renal Artery Stenosis

- Atherosclerosis is the most common cause of renal artery stenosis in older adults and tends to affect the ostia (origin) of the renal arteries.
- Renal artery stenosis (RAS) resulting from atherosclerotic disease typically involves the ostium and proximal third of the main renal artery.
- The success of atherosclerotic RAS angioplasty is debatable. However, angioplasty ± stenting may be advocated in the setting of hemodynamically significant RAS, resistant hypertension, deteriorating renal function, bilateral atherosclerotic RAS, unexplained CHF, and recurrent episodes of flash pulmonary edema.

肾动脉狭窄(RAS)

- 动脉粥样硬化是老年人肾动脉狭窄(RAS)最常见的原因,常累及肾动脉的开口(起始部)。
- 动脉粥样硬化导致的RAS常累及肾动脉开口和主干的近段1/3。
- 血管成形术对动脉粥样硬化性RAS的治疗结果存在争议。然而,血管成形 ± 支架植入可用于以下情况:有显著血流动力学改变的RAS、顽固性高血压、肾功能恶化、双侧动脉粥样硬化性RAS、不明原因的慢性心力衰竭(CHF)及反复一过性肺水肿发作。

UPPER ETREMITY VASCULAR ANATOMY

- The upper extremity vascular tree begins at the aortic arch branching into the brachiocephalic artery on the right, or directly into the subclavian artery on the left. The subclavian artery gives rise to five main branches: vertebral artery, internal thoracic artery (internal mammary artery), thyrocervical trunk, costocervical trunk, and dorsal scapular artery.
- Once the subclavian artery crosses the lateral margin of the first rib, it continues as the axillary artery divided into 3 parts and 6 major branches that supply the muscles of the shoulder girdle, humerus, scapula, and chest wall (see "Vascular" chapter for details).
- Once the axillary artery crosses the inferior lateral margin of the teres major muscle, it continues as the brachial artery coursing along the medial aspect of the upper arm. It gives rise to the deep brachial artery and anteriorly in the antecubital fossa, divides into the radial and ulnar arteries.
- Arising immediately beyond the origins of the radial and ulnar arteries, the radial recurrent artery and the posterior and anterior ulnar recurrent arteries form anastomoses with branches of the brachial and deep brachial arteries. The common interosseous artery divides into anterior and posterior branches.
- In the lateral forearm, the radial artery courses to the wrist, traverses the snuffbox, and turns medially to give rise to the deep palmar arch. In the medial forearm, the ulnar artery arises from the common interosseous artery and continues into the superficial palmar arch, giving off the common palmar digital arteries.

上肢血管解剖

- 所有上肢的血管都起始于主动脉弓，右侧为头臂动脉，左侧直接发出锁骨下动脉。锁骨下动脉有五个主要分支：椎动脉、胸廓内动脉(内乳动脉)、甲状颈干、肋颈干和肩胛背侧动脉。
- 锁骨下动脉穿过第一肋骨的外侧缘即延续为腋动脉，并分为3部分及6个主要分支，供应肌肉肩带、肱骨、肩胛骨和胸壁(详见"血管影像"一章)。
- 腋动脉一旦穿过大圆肌的下外侧缘即延续为肱动脉，并沿上臂内侧走行。肱动脉发出肱深动脉，并在肘窝的前方分成桡动脉和尺动脉。
- 桡侧返动脉和尺侧前及后返动脉发自桡动脉和尺动脉起始远端的附近，它们与肱动脉和肱深动脉的分支形成吻合。骨间总动脉分为前支和后支。
- 在前臂外侧，桡动脉走向手腕，穿过鼻烟壶，并向内侧走行发出掌深弓。在前臂内侧，尺动脉起源于骨间总动脉并延续为掌浅弓，发出指掌侧总动脉。

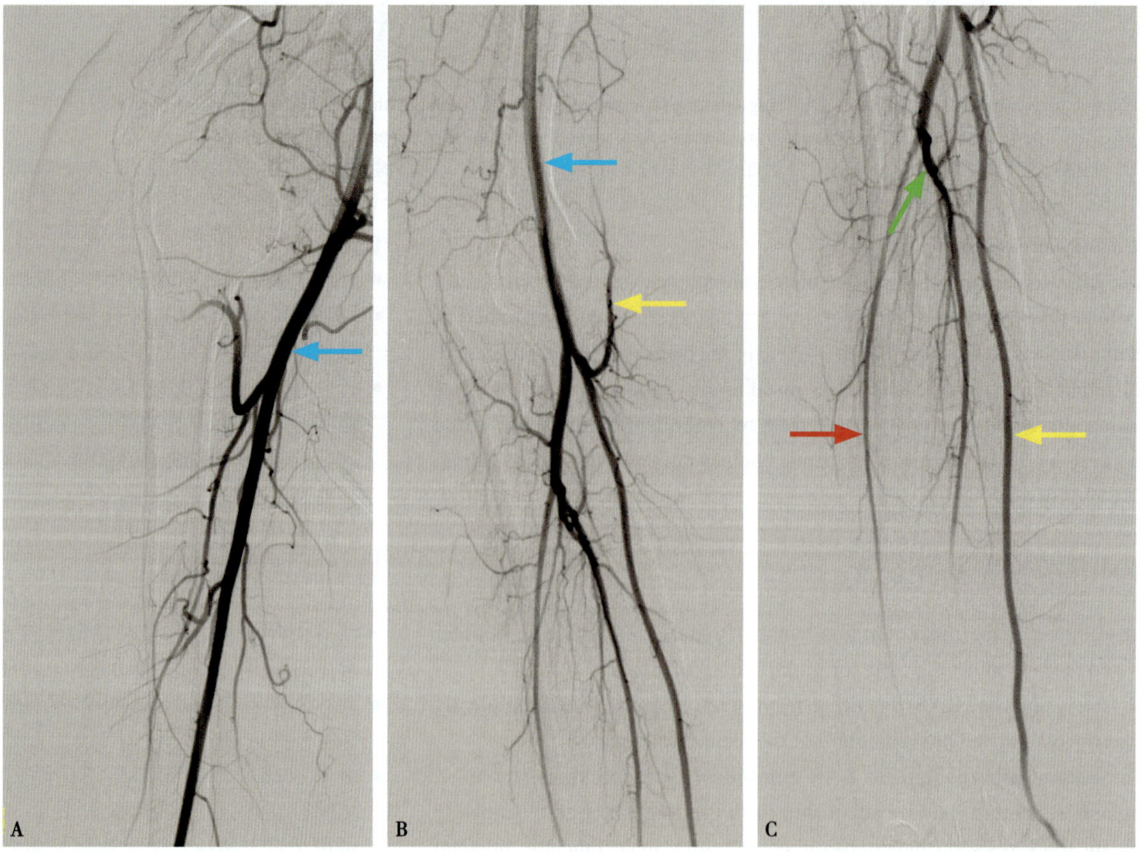

Normal upper extremity arterial digital selective angiogram. A) Blue arrow-third part of the axillary artery. B) Blue arrow-brachial artery; yellow arrow-radial recurrent artery. C) Yellow arrow-radial artery; red arrow-ulnar artery; green arrow-common interosseous artery.
正常上肢动脉数字减影血管造影。A)蓝箭-腋动脉的第三部分。B)蓝箭-肱动脉；黄箭-桡侧返动脉。C)黄箭-桡动脉；红箭-尺动脉；绿箭-骨间总动脉。

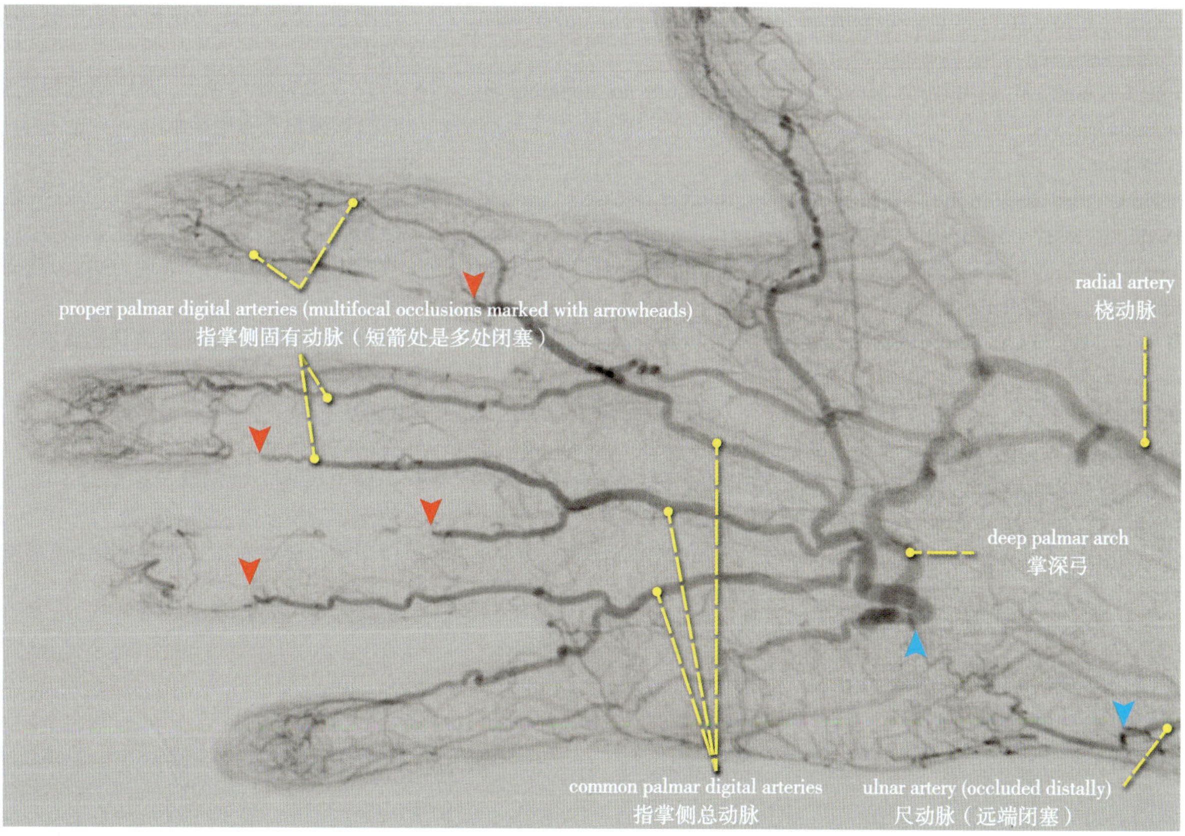

Hypothenar hammer: Digital subtraction angiogram of the hand shows an approximately 2–3 cm occlusion of the ulnar artery (between the blue arrowheads), and multifocal occlusions of the proper palmar digital arteries in the second through fourth digits (red arrowheads).
小鱼际锤：手部DSA显示一段长2~3cm的尺动脉闭塞(蓝短箭头之间)，以及多处掌侧固有动脉闭塞，累及第二到第四手指(红短箭头)。

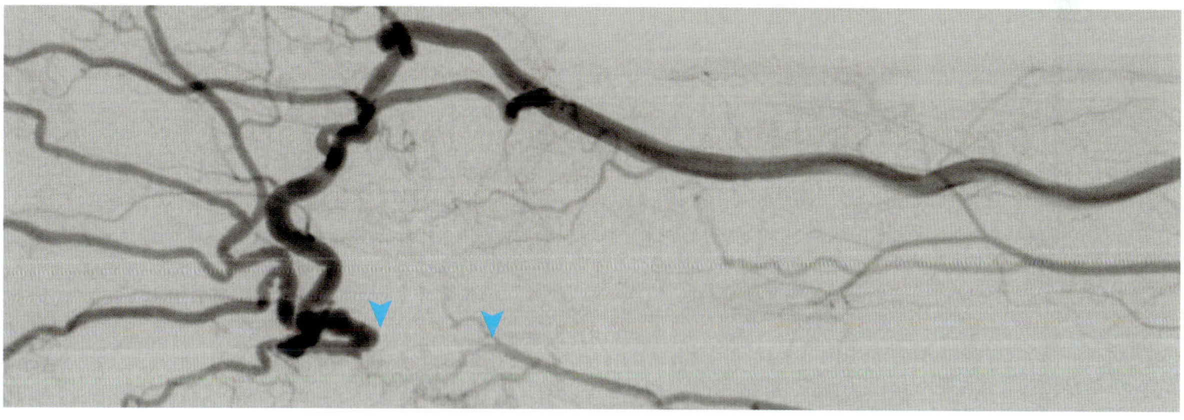

DSA angiogram of the wrist better shows the segmental occlusion of the ulnar artery (between the blue arrowheads). At surgery, an ulnar artery aneurysm (not visible on angiography) was found and treated.
Case courtesy Alisa Suzuki Han, MD, Brigham and Women's Hospital
腕部DSA较为清晰地显示尺动脉的节段性闭塞(蓝短箭头之间)。外科手术中发现一个尺动脉动脉瘤(血管造影图中未显示)并进行了治疗。

- Hypothenar hammer syndrome represents injury to the ulnar artery as it crosses the hamate bone. Chronic repetitive trauma causes the ulnar artery to chronically be traumatized at the hamate, leading to intimal injury, thrombus, aneurysm, or pseudoaneurysm.
- The classic clinical history of hypothenar hammer syndrome is a jackhammer

- 小鱼际锤综合征是尺动脉在经过钩骨处受到外力损伤所致。慢性反复创伤会导致尺动脉在钩骨处慢性受损，从而引起内膜损伤、血栓形成、动脉瘤或假性动脉瘤。
- 小鱼际锤综合征的典型临床病史是电钻工人

operator with ischemia of the fourth and fifth digits.
- Imaging shows occlusion of the ulnar artery, often with distal embolic occlusions due to distal thrombi, usually in the fourth and fifth fingers (but third finger also seen in the case above).
- Treatment is surgical, as there is often ulnar artery injury not apparent on angiography.

Buerger disease

- As previously discussed in the "Vascular" chapter, Buerger disease is a small- and medium-vessel vasculitis that typically occurs in male smokers. It more commonly involves the legs but may also involve the hands, presenting with ischemia, ulcerations, and even gangrene.
- Small vessel occlusions and prominent *corkscrew* collaterals are typical features.

Raynaud disease

- Raynaud disease is small arterial vasospasm triggered by cold temperature.
- On imaging, there is decreased perfusion of the distal digital arteries, with improvement upon warming or vasodilator administration.
- Raynaud disease is associated with scleroderma and other connective tissue disorders.

出现无名指和小指缺血。
- 影像学表现为尺动脉闭塞，常合并远端栓子性闭塞，常见于无名指和小指(上述病例还累及中指)。
- 治疗方法为外科手术，因尺动脉损伤常不能在血管造影上明确显示。

Buerger病

- 如“血管影像”一章所述，Buerger病是小、中动脉的血管炎，常见于男性吸烟者。多累及双腿，但也见于双手，表现为缺血、溃疡，甚至坏疽。
- 小血管闭塞和明显的弹簧状侧支血管形成是典型表现。

雷诺病

- 雷诺病是由寒冷触发的小动脉痉挛。
- 影像上表现为指动脉远端灌注下降，加温或使用血管扩张剂后得到改善。
- 雷诺病与硬皮病和其他结缔组织疾病有关。

LOWER EXTREMITY VASCULAR ANATOMY

下肢血管解剖

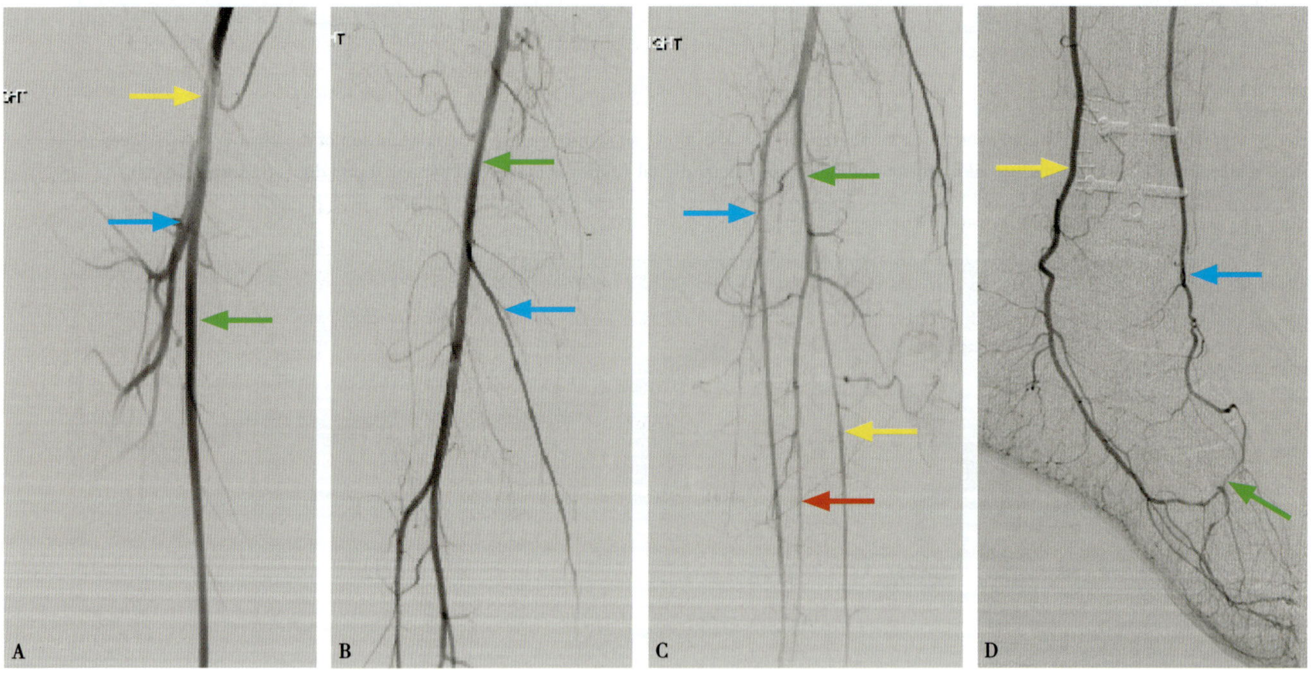

Lower extremity three vessel runoff angiogram. A) Yellow arrow-CFA, blue arrow-profunda femoris, green arrow-SFA; B) green arrow-SFA, blue arrow-descending geniculate artery; C) green arrow-tibioperoneal trunk, blue arrow-ATA, yellow arrow-PTA, red arrow-peroneal artery. Note the small calf AVM supplied by a small posterior tibial branch and a distal branch of the superior medial geniculate artery. D) Blue arrow-dorsalis pedis, yellow arrow-PTA, green arrow-deep plantar arch.

下肢三血管动脉造影。A)黄箭-CFA，蓝箭-股深，绿箭-SFA；B)绿箭-SFA，蓝箭-膝降动脉；C)绿箭-胫腓干，蓝箭-ATA，黄箭-PTA，红箭-腓动脉。注意，小腿AVM由一条细小胫后动脉分支和上内侧膝降动脉远端分支供血。D)蓝箭-足背动脉，黄箭-PTA，绿箭-足底深弓。

- The lower extremity vascular tree begins when the external iliac artery continues into the common femoral artery (CFA) at the level of the inguinal ligament. The CFA branches into the profunda femoris posteriorly and the superficial femoral artery (SFA). The profunda femoris artery supplies the

- 下肢血管起始于髂外动脉与股总动脉(CFA)的交界处，位于腹股沟韧带的水平。CFA分为股深动脉(向后)和股浅动脉(SFA)。股深动脉供应大腿内侧和后部，以及股骨近端，并有

medial and posterior thigh as well as the proximal femur with the medial and lateral femoral circumflex artery branches.

- The SFA continues in the adductor canal of the anterior compartment of the thigh, dives into the adductor hiatus and enters the posterior compartment of the thigh as the popliteal artery. After the popliteal artery courses past the inferior border of the popliteus muscle, it branches into the anterior tibial artery (ATA) and the tibioperoneal trunk.
- The ATA passes through the interosseous membrane and courses within the anterior compartment of the leg. It continues to the dorsum of the foot as the dorsalis pedis artery.
- The tibioperoneal trunk divides into the peroneal artery, which supplies the lateral compartment of the leg, and posterior tibial artery which courses along the deep posterior leg muscles, enters the tarsal tunnel with the tibial nerve, and divides into the medial and lateral plantar arteries.

旋股内侧和外侧分支。

- SFA走行在大腿前部的内收肌管内，下行进入内收肌裂孔并延续为腘动脉进入大腿后部。腘动脉经过腘肌下缘后，分成胫前动脉(ATA)和胫腓干。
- ATA穿过骨间膜并在小腿前部走行，延续到足背成为足背动脉。
- 胫腓干分为腓动脉和胫后动脉。腓动脉为小腿外侧间室供血，胫后动脉沿小腿深层后肌群走行，与胫神经一起进入跗管并与胫神经伴行，随后分为足底内侧动脉和足底外侧动脉。

Peripheral Vascular Disease

Femoropopliteal disease

- Similar to aortoiliac disease, the second TransAtlantic Inter-Society (TASC-Ⅱ) consensus classifies femoropopliteal lesions and gives associated recommendations for intervention.

  Type A: Single stenosis≤10 cm: ***Endovascular treatment is the treatment of choice.***

  Type B: Multiple lesions (stenosis or occlusion), each<5 cm; single lesion <15 cm: ***Endovascular treatment is preferred, depending on patient comorbidities and preference.***

  Type C: Multiple stenoses or occlusions>15 cm: ***Surgery is preferred, depending on patient comorbidities and preference.***

  Type D: Chronic total occlusion: ***Surgery is treatment of choice.***

Acute thromboembolic disease

- Acute limb ischemia is an emergency and is often associated with pain, pallor, poikilothermia (coldness), pulselessness, and paresthesias. *Blue toe syndrome* is acute thromboembolism in the toes. The characteristic imaging feature in the upper extremities is occlusion of distal small arteries of the hand.

  Thromboembolic disease of the upper extremities is most commonly caused by cardiac emboli (of which atrial fibrillation is a common cause). Less commonly, a subclavian artery aneurysm may be the source of the thrombus.

  If the source of emboli is central (such as the heart), bilateral disease would be expected, while a unilateral lesion would show unilateral emboli.
- Angiography shows an acute cutoff of the affected vessel, often with a *meniscus* sign. Significant atherosclerotic disease may be absent.
- Treatment options include surgical embolectomy, surgical bypass graft, and endovascular thrombolysis. When attempting to treat endovascularly, a hydrophilic wire is used to cross the lesion. A multi-sidehole infusion catheter is placed across the thrombus and tissue plasminogen activator (tPA) is infused at 0.5 mg/hr for 48–72 hours.
- While receiving intra-arterial tPA, the patient must be cared for in the ICU, with regular monitoring of hematocrit and fibrinogen. TPA infusion should be slowed if the fibrinogen decreases to <150 mg/dL and stopped if it reaches < 100 mg/dL.

外周血管疾病

股腘动脉病变

- 与主-髂动脉病变一样，第二版跨大西洋协作组(TASC-Ⅱ)统一了对股腘动脉病变的分级并给出了相应的治疗方案。

  A型：单个狭窄，长度≤10cm：选择腔内治疗。

  B型：多个病变(狭窄或闭塞)，每个长度<5cm；或单个病变长度<15m：首选腔内治疗，要根据患者的合并症和意愿。

  C型：多个狭窄或闭塞性病变，长度>15cm：首选外科手术治疗，要根据患者存在的合并症和意愿。

  D型：慢性完全性闭塞：选择外科手术治疗。

急性血栓栓塞性疾病

- 急性下肢缺血是一种急症，常有疼痛、苍白、皮温降低、无脉搏及感觉异常。蓝趾综合征是发生在脚趾的急性血栓性栓塞。如发生在上肢，其影像特征为手部远端小动脉闭塞。

  上肢血栓栓塞性疾病的最常见原因为心脏栓子(其中心房颤动是常见原因)，其次为来自锁骨下动脉瘤的血栓。

  若栓子的来源是中央性的(如心脏)，则可见到双侧受累，而单侧病变则表现为单侧栓子。
- 动脉造影表现为受累血管突然截断，常伴有半月征。可无明显的动脉粥样硬化性病变。
- 治疗方法包括外科取栓、外科搭桥和腔内溶栓治疗。行腔内治疗时，用亲水导丝通过闭塞部位，多侧孔的溶栓导管跨越血栓部位并灌注组织型纤溶酶原激活剂(tPA)，0.5mg/h，持续48~72小时。
- 接受tPA动脉灌注时，患者必须在ICU进行观察，并常规检测血细胞比容和纤维蛋白原。当纤维蛋白原低于150mg/dL时，减缓tPA的灌注速度，低于100mg/dL时，应停止使用tPA。

(翻译　吴汉平)

Paget-Schroetter syndrome

Paget-Schroetter综合征

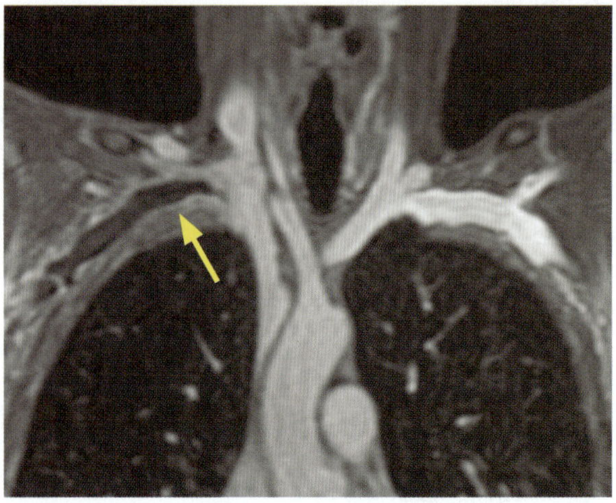

Coronal contrast-enhanced MR venography with arms abducted demonstrates right subclavian vein thrombus (arrow). The MRI did not demonstrate a mechanical cause for the thrombosis.
冠状位手臂外展增强MR静脉造影显示右锁骨下静脉血栓(黄箭)。MRI上未发现血栓形成的机械性原因。

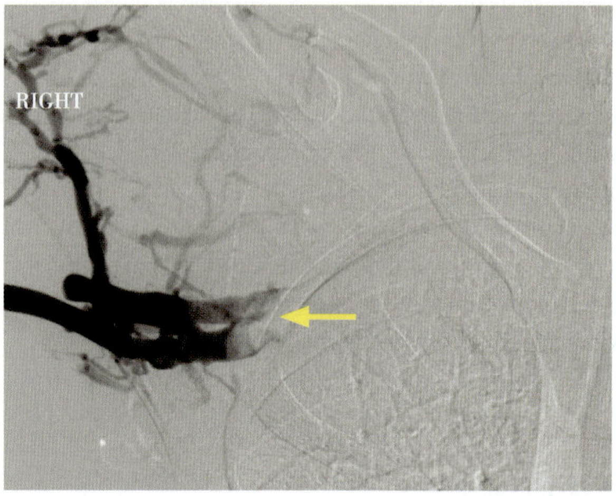

Diagnostic venography confirms complete occlusion of the right subclavian vein (arrow) with complete lack of opacification of the SVC and the formation of numerous collaterals.
诊断性静脉造影证实右锁骨下静脉完全闭塞(黄箭)及上腔静脉不显影，伴有大量侧支循环。

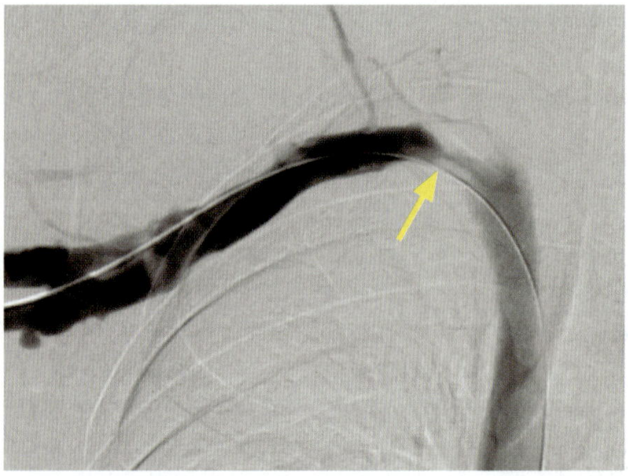

24 hours after continuous thrombolysis infusion, the subclavian vein is patent, with a residual stenosis at the subclavian/brachiocephalic confluence (arrow).
连续24小时溶栓后，锁骨下静脉变通畅，但可见锁骨下静脉与头臂静脉汇合处有残余狭窄(黄箭)。

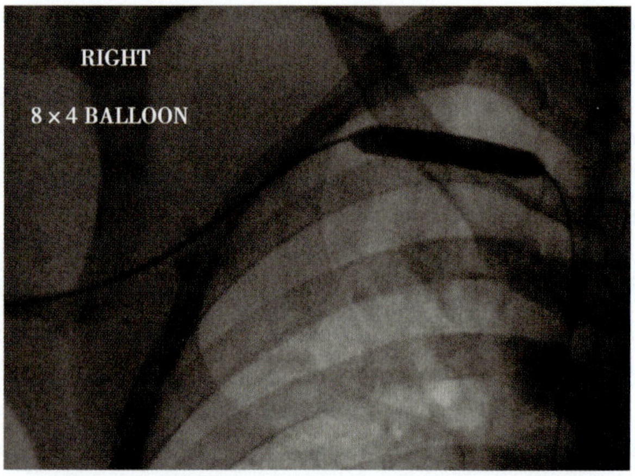

Because the MRI confirmed lack of mechanical obstruction, an 8 mm × 4 cm angioplasty balloon was used at the site of stenosis.
因MRI未见机械性闭塞，用一个8mm × 4cm球囊对狭窄处进行扩张。

- Paget-Schroetter syndrome is compression and thrombosis of the subclavian vein as it enters the thorax and is usually seen in muscular young men. Chronic compression causes intimal hyperplasia, which leads to subclavian vein thrombosis. Paget-Schroetter syndrome clinically presents with upper-extremity swelling or pain worsened with effort.
- During diagnostic venography, it is necessary to evaluate the arm both in neutral position and abducted. Both sides should be evaluated. Frequently, both subclavian veins are compressed, even if only one side is symptomatic.
- Treatment is thrombolysis, then subsequently surgical thoracic outlet decompression.
- If there is residual stenosis following thrombolysis, surgical decompression should generally be performed prior to angioplasty. However, if pre-procedure

- Paget-Schroetter综合征是锁骨下静脉进入胸廓处受压和血栓形成，常见于肌肉发达的青年男性。慢性压迫导致内膜过度增生，进而导致锁骨下静脉血栓形成。Paget-Schroetter综合征在临床上可表现为上肢肿胀或疼痛，运动后加剧。
- 在进行诊断性静脉造影时，必须将上臂放置在自然和外展两个体位。双侧均需检查，通常双侧的锁骨下静脉同时受压，但可能仅有一侧出现症状。
- 治疗方法是先溶栓，然后行外科胸廓出口减压。
- 若溶栓后有残余狭窄，一般先行外科减压，而非

imaging demonstrated no mechanical cause, then angioplasty can be performed, as in the case above.

- Stents should generally not be used, especially if there is a mechanical obstruction, due to high risk of device failure.

Nutcracker syndrome

- Nutcracker syndrome is compression of the left renal vein between the aorta and the SMA.
- Clinical presentations are variable, including pain, hematuria, orthostatic proteinuria, pelvic congestion, and varicocele (in a male). The term Nutcracker *phenomenon* is used when the patient is asymptomatic.
- There is a lack of established treatment guidelines. Prolonged observation with or without medical management is preferred, as the majority of cases of hematuria resolve spontaneously within two years. Endovascular treatments (angioplasty and stenting of the renal vein) and surgical options (most commonly left renal vein transposition) are also available.

May-Thurner syndrome

血管成形术。但若术前影像学检查排除机械性压迫原因，可行血管成形术，如上图所示病例。

- 一般不宜使用支架，尤其是机械性阻塞，因支架发生功能不良的风险较高。

胡桃夹综合征

- 胡桃夹综合征是指左肾静脉处于肠系膜上动脉和主动脉之间而受压。
- 胡桃夹综合征可有多种临床症状，包括疼痛、血尿、直立位蛋白尿、盆腔淤血，以及精索静脉曲张(男性)。若无症状，则称为胡桃夹现象。
- 该病尚缺乏一个公认的治疗指南。首选长期观察或辅以药物治疗，因大多数血尿会在2年内自行消退。可选择的治疗方法包括血管腔内治疗(肾静脉血管成形术及支架植入)和外科手术(最常见的是左肾静脉移位术)。

May-Thurner综合征

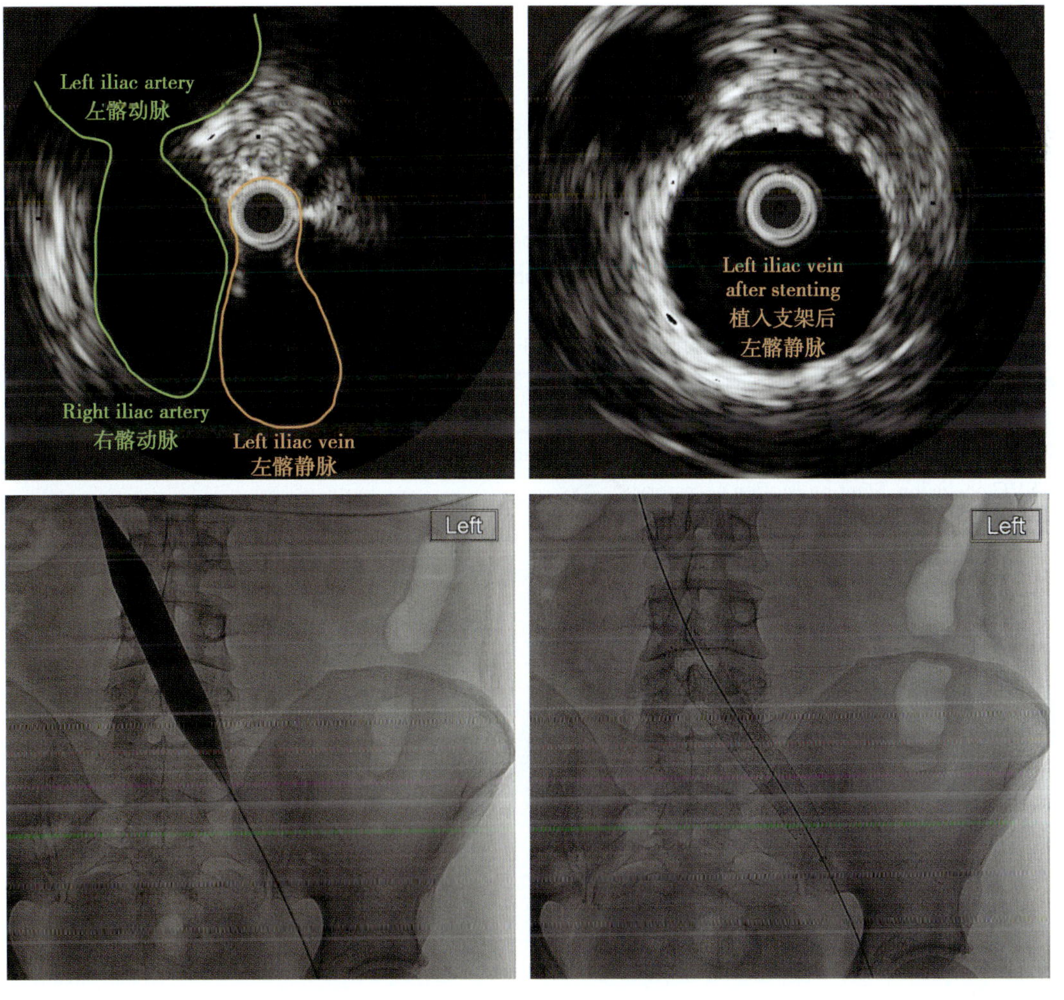

May-Thurner syndrome: A patient with two months of left lower extremity pain was found to have extensive clot burden extending from the left internal iliac vein to the left popliteal vein. Intravascular ultrasound (IVUS) revealed severe venous compression of the left iliac vein by the right iliac artery with reduced cross-sectional area (top left image). Percutaneous venoplasty (bottom left image) and stenting (bottom right image) across the left iliac vein were performed. After stenting, IVUS revealed good wall apposition and improved cross-sectional area (top right image).

May-Thurner综合征：左下肢疼痛2个月患者发现广泛的静脉血栓，从左髂内静脉延伸到左腘静脉。血管内超声(IVUS)显示左髂静脉被右髂动脉严重压迫，而使管腔横截面积减小(左上图)。采用经皮静脉成形术(左下图)和左髂静脉支架植入术(右下图)。支架植入后，IVUS显示支架与左髂静脉贴合良好，先前受压的髂静脉管腔横截面积改善(右上图)。

- May-Thurner syndrome is venous thrombosis of the left common iliac vein caused by compression from the crossing right common iliac artery. Both genders are equally affected.
- Chronic compression leads to fibrous adhesions, intimal proliferation, and spur formation along the vein wall, predisposing to thrombosis.
- Conventional venography with intravascular ultrasound (IVUS) is gold standard for diagnosis.
- Treatment is initial catheter-directed thrombolysis to treat acute thrombus, followed by stenting. Self-expanding stents are preferred.
- Post-thrombotic syndrome (PTS) can occur in up to half of all patients who have DVT and is a costly, burdensome complication. PTS consists of edema, pain, ulceration, discoloration, and varicose veins.

- May-Thumer综合征是由于左侧髂总静脉被对侧的右髂总动脉压迫导致而形成静脉血栓。男女发病率相当。
- 慢性压迫会导致静脉内纤维性粘连、内膜增生和沿静脉壁毛刺形成，易引起血栓形成。
- 常规静脉造影和血管内超声(IVUS)是诊断的“金标准”。
- 初始治疗为经导管直接溶解急性血栓，之后行支架植入术，优先选用自膨胀式支架。
- 血栓后综合征(PTS)可发生于多达一半的DVT患者，是一种治疗代价高昂、负担重的并发症。PTS包括水肿、疼痛、溃疡、皮肤色素沉着和静脉曲张。

Superior vena cava (SVC) syndrome

- Acute obstruction of the SVC causes SVC syndrome, which clinically presents as facial and upper extremity edema and cyanosis. Acute SVC syndrome is a vascular emergency.
- In contrast to acute SVC syndrome, chronic occlusion or stenosis of the SVC may be asymptomatic. If symptoms are present, facial edema that improves with standing is characteristic.
- The most common causes of SVC obstruction are compression by thoracic malignancy, catheter-associated thrombosis, and mediastinal fibrosis after histoplasmosis exposure.
- A classic cross-sectional abdominal imaging finding in SVC obstruction is increased enhancement of hepatic segment Ⅳa due to collateral opacification of the vein of Sappey.

  The vein of Sappey drains the liver in the region of the falciform ligament and communicates with internal thoracic veins, which act as collateral vessels in the setting of SVC occlusion.
- Combined internal jugular and femoral approaches may be necessary for treatment of SVC occlusion. Stenting is often necessary.

上腔静脉(SVC)综合征

- 急性上腔静脉(SVC)闭塞导致SVC综合征，临床表现为面部及上肢水肿和发绀。急性SVC综合征是血管急症。
- 与急性闭塞不同的是，慢性SVC闭塞或狭窄可不出现症状。若有症状，面部水肿会在站立时改善，此具特征性。
- SVC闭塞最常见的原因是胸部恶性肿瘤压迫、中心静脉置管诱发的血栓形成和组织胞浆菌病感染所致的纵隔纤维化。
- SVC闭塞在腹部断层影像时出现的典型表现为肝脏Ⅳa段有异常对比剂增强，此为Sappey侧支静脉显影所致。

  Sappey静脉引流镰状韧带区域的肝组织，并与胸廓内静脉相交通，在SVC闭塞时充当侧支血管。
- 在治疗SVC闭塞时，有必要联合采用经颈静脉和股静脉的途径，常需植入支架。

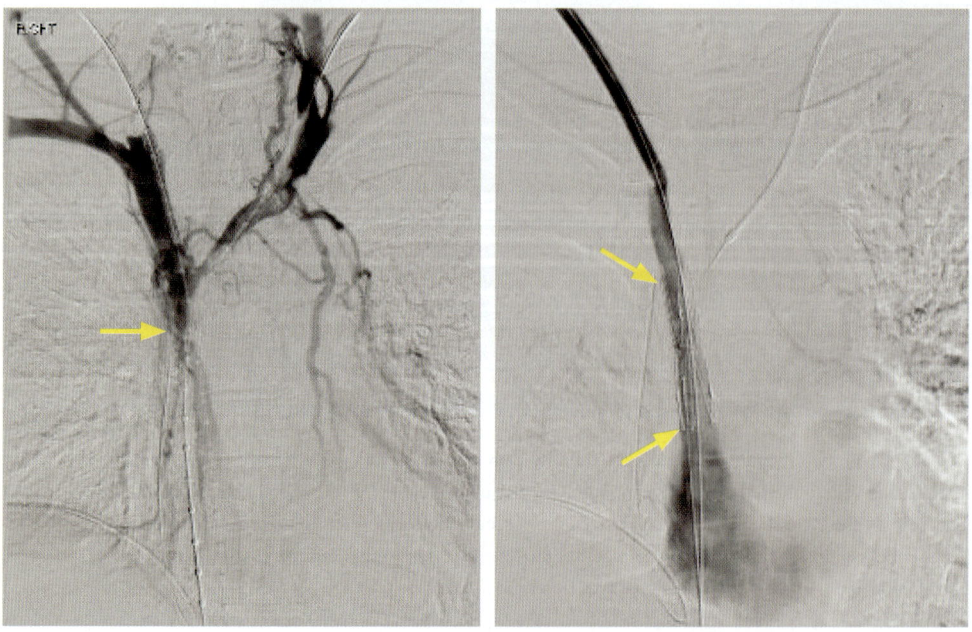

SVC syndrome in a patient with small cell lung cancer: Superior vena cava venogram (left image) shows lack of contrast opacification in the SVC with irregular tapering of the right brachiocephalic vein (arrow). After placement of a 15 mm × 5 cm Gianturco-Rosch stent (right image, arrows) in the area of obstruction, normal flow is restored.

一名伴有上腔静脉综合征的小细胞肺癌患者：上腔静脉造影(左图)未显示上腔静脉有造影剂充盈，右侧头臂静脉不规则变细(黄箭)。在上腔静脉闭塞区域放置15mm × 5cm的Gianturco-Rosch支架(右图，黄箭)后，血流恢复正常。

Inferior vena cava (IVC) filter placement

- The purpose of an IVC filter is to reduce the risk of pulmonary embolism (PE) originating from a lower extremity deep venous thrombosis (DVT). Indications for filter placement include DVT and contraindication to anticoagulation; recurrent PE while anticoagulated; and high risk of developing DVT/PE in a patient with contraindication to anticoagulation, such as a multi-trauma patient.
- The most common complication of IVC filter placement is access site thrombosis, followed by IVC thrombosis. IVC perforation occurs not uncommonly, but is almost always inconsequential. Filter fracture or embolization are rare.
- The first step of the procedure is an inferior vena cavogram, performed with a high-flow (pigtail) catheter. The cavogram guides the selection of filter type and placement location.
- If a duplicated IVC is present, in order to prevent a clot from circumnavigating the filter, either a single filter is placed above the IVC confluence or a filter is placed in each duplicated IVC. If pre-procedural imaging is not available, a clue to the presence of a duplicated IVC on initial cavography is the absence of iliac vein influx contralateral to the side injected.

下腔静脉滤器植入

- 下腔静脉滤器的目的是降低由下肢深静脉血栓脱落导致的肺动脉栓塞(PE)风险。滤器植入的指征包括：下肢深静脉血栓形成但有抗凝禁忌；在抗凝的情况下仍出现肺动脉栓塞复发；对抗凝有禁忌的深静脉血栓形成或肺动脉栓塞的高风险患者，如多发性创伤患者。
- 下腔静脉滤器植入最常见的并发症是静脉入路处血栓形成，其次是下腔静脉血栓形成。下腔静脉穿孔并不少见，但几乎不留后遗症。滤器断裂或断裂后造成远处栓塞很少见。
- 手术的第一步是下腔静脉造影，通常使用高流量导管(猪尾导管)。根据腔静脉造影选择滤器类型及植入位置。
- 当存在双重下腔静脉时，为避免血凝块绕开滤器，可将滤器放在双侧下腔静脉汇合处的上方或在每侧下腔静脉中各放一个滤器。若无术前影像，提示双重下腔静脉的一个征象为初始腔静脉造影时未发现对侧髂静脉血回流入下腔静脉。

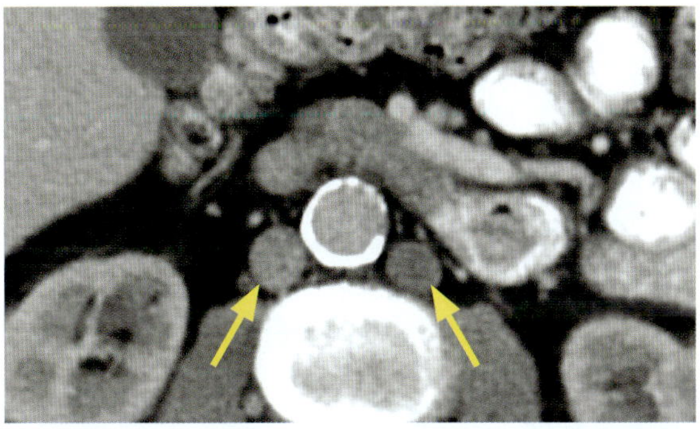

Duplicated IVC. Pre-procedure contrast-enhanced CT (left image) shows duplicated IVCs on either side of the aorta (arrows). The presence of duplicated IVCs is confirmed by cavography of the left IVC (bottom left image), where the left renal vein (arrow) drains into the left IVC.
Post-procedure radiograph (bottom right image) shows the IVC filter (arrow at filter tip) placed above the confluence of the duplicated IVC.
Case courtesy Alisa Suzuki Han, MD, Brigham and Women's Hospital.
双重下腔静脉：术前增强CT(左图)显示主动脉两侧各有一条下腔静脉(黄箭)。下腔静脉造影(下排左图)证实有双重下腔静脉，左肾静脉(黄箭)流入左侧下腔静脉。
术后X线影像显示(下排右图)下腔静脉滤器(箭位于滤器尖)的位置在双重下腔静脉汇合处的上方。

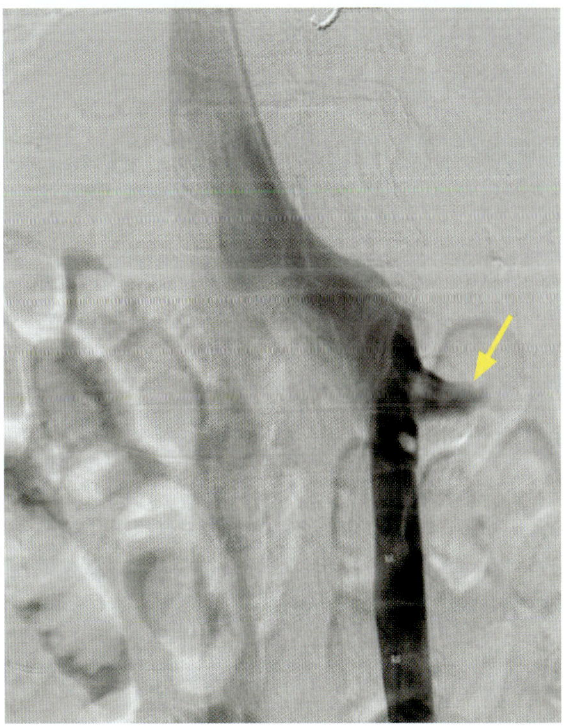

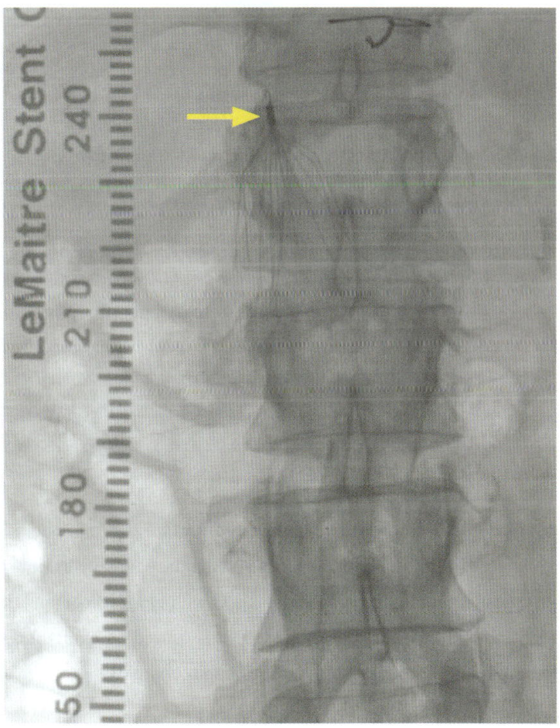

- Most IVC filters are suitable for vessel diameters smaller than 28–30 mm. Only the special *Bird's Nest* filter can be placed in larger IVCs up to 40 mm in diameter, however it is permanent/non-retrievable. Alternatively, separate retrievable filters can be inserted in each common iliac vein in the case of a megacava (IVC diameter >30 mm).
- The preferred location of the IVC filter is immediately inferior to the lowest renal vein, including any variant renal veins (circumaortic or retroaortic). Placement inferior to the lowest renal vein prevents the anomalous vein from acting as a conduit for clot propagation.

Circumaortic left renal vein is an anatomic variant seen in 2–10% of the population, where the left renal vein is composed of two separate components. One component passes anterior to the aorta (the normal configuration) and a second retroaortic component passes posterior to the aorta to meet the IVC.

Retroaortic left renal vein is a slightly less common variant (seen in 2–7% of the population), where a single renal vein passes posterior to the aorta. A retroaortic left renal vein usually joins the IVC more inferiorly than the right renal vein.

- 大多数滤器适用于直径在28~30mm或以下的下腔静脉。只有鸟巢型滤器可用于直径较大的下腔静脉，最宽达40mm，但该滤器是永久性/不可回收的。在大口径下腔静脉(直径>30mm)中，可在两侧髂总静脉各放置一个可回收滤器作为一种替代方法。
- 下腔静脉滤器理想的植入位置是在靠近最低肾静脉开口的下方，包括任何变异的肾静脉(如主动脉后型或环主动脉型)。滤器在最低肾静脉以下水平可预防血栓通过变异的静脉蔓延。

环主动脉左肾静脉为解剖变异，在人群中占2%~10%，其左肾静脉有两支，一支跨越主动脉的前方(正常形态)，另一支从主动脉的后方汇入下腔静脉。

主动脉后左肾静脉是一种较少见的变异(见于2%~7%的人群)，为单根肾静脉在主动脉后方通过。主动脉后左肾静脉汇入下腔静脉时的位置通常比右肾静脉低。

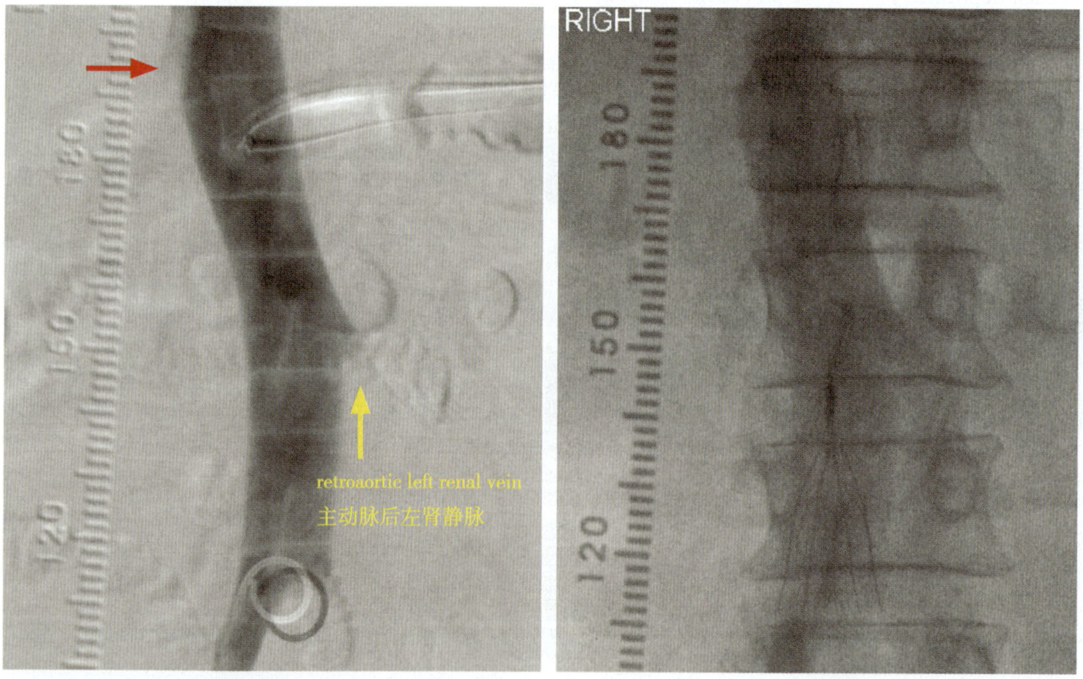

Retroaortic left renal vein: Initial digital subtraction inferior vena cavography (left image) shows the left renal vein (yellow arrow) entering the IVC markedly inferior to the right renal vein (red arrow), indicating that the left renal vein is likely retroaortic. Post-procedure radiograph shows the filter tip placed a few mm inferior to the confluence of the left retroaortic renal vein, indicated by the ruler (top of the filter at 148; retroaortic left renal vein at 152).

Case courtesy Alisa Suzuki Han, MD, Brigham and Women's Hospital.

主动脉后左肾静脉：初始下腔静脉数字减影血管造影(左图)显示左肾静脉(黄箭)汇入下腔静脉时明显比右肾静脉(红箭)低，提示左肾静脉可能位于主动脉后。术后X线影像提示滤器顶端位于左肾静脉汇入处下方几毫米处，如标尺所示(滤器顶位于148，左肾静脉位于152)。

Interruption of the IVC with azygous continuation is a rare anomaly where blood from the lower IVC flows into the azygous and hemiazygous veins, into the thorax, and then into the right atrium. Interruption of the IVC with azygous continuation is associated with polysplenia and congenital heart disease. It is caused by embryologic failure of the right subcardinal vein to join the intrahepatic venous complex.

下腔静脉中断合并奇静脉引流是一种罕见的变异，来自下腔静脉下段的血液进入奇静脉和副奇静脉，然后进入胸腔，最后汇入右心房。下腔静脉中断合并奇静脉引流通常与多脾和先天性心脏病有关。其原因为胚胎期右心下主静脉未能连接肝内静脉复合体。

- The presence of preexisting IVC thrombus may interfere with the positioning of IVC filter, requiring higher than normal placement.

- 下腔静脉内存在血栓可影响下腔静脉滤器的放置，需高于正常的位置。

Venous Thromboembolic Disease

静脉血栓栓塞性疾病

Phlegmasia cerulea dolens (PCD)

- PCD is a vascular emergency consisting of acute limb swelling, cyanosis and severe pain that occurs due to complete thrombotic occlusion of venous drainage of a limb. PCD occurs most often in the setting of malignancy, trauma, heparin-induced thrombocytopenia (HIT) or other prothrombotic state.
- Massive limb swelling, hypertension in the capillary bed, and eventually ischemia and gangrene can occur if untreated.
- PCD requires anticoagulation with IV heparin and treatment with angioplasty, catheter-directed thrombolysis, or surgical thrombectomy.

股青肿(PCD)

- 股青肿(PCD)是一种血管急症，表现为急性肢体肿胀、皮肤青紫以及剧烈疼痛等症状，它由血栓引起一侧肢体静脉回流完全阻塞所致。PCD最常发生于恶性肿瘤、外伤、肝素诱导的血小板减少症(HIT)或其他血栓前状态患者。
- 若不予治疗，可出现严重的肢体肿胀、毛细血管床高血压，最终会出现缺血和坏疽。
- PCD需采用静脉肝素抗凝治疗，并行血管成形术、经导管直接溶栓治疗或外科血栓清除术。

Chronic Venous Insufficiency

慢性静脉功能不全

Ovarian and pelvic vein embolization

卵巢静脉和盆腔静脉栓塞术

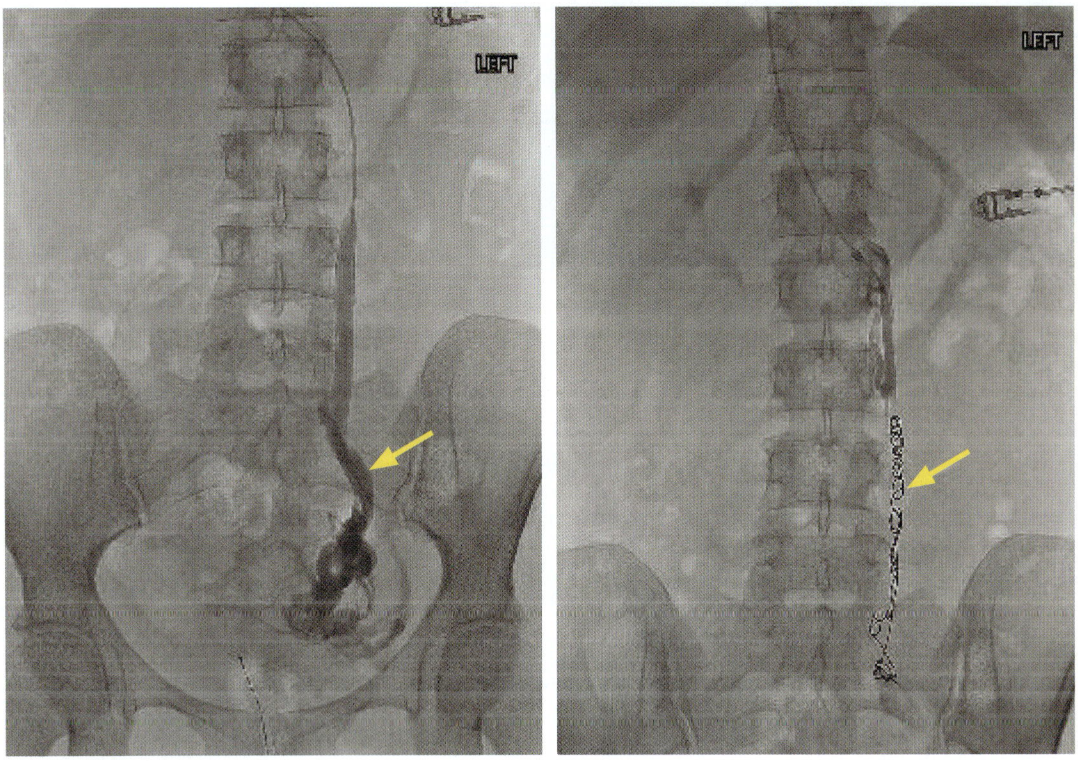

Pelvic venous congestion syndrome: Left gonadal vein venogram shows reflux of contrast to the level of the left renal vein (left image, arrow). Platinum coils were deployed, followed by embolization with 1% sodium tetradecyl sulfate (right image, arrow).
盆腔静脉淤血综合征：左性腺静脉造影显示造影剂反流至左肾静脉水平(左图，黄箭)。释放弹簧圈后用1%十四烷基硫酸钠进行栓塞(右图，黄箭)。

- Ovarian vein reflux (i.e., pelvic venous congestion syndrome) is a common cause of chronic pelvic pain and most commonly affects multiparous women.
- The left gonadal vein is typically affected due to the acute angle it makes with the IVC, predisposing it to reflux.
- Minimally invasive embolization has shown excellent treatment efficacy.

- 卵巢静脉反流(即盆腔静脉淤血综合征)是一种引起慢性盆腔疼痛的常见原因，最常见于经产妇。
- 通常为左性腺静脉受累，因其与下腔静脉形成锐角，易于反流。
- 微创栓塞具有非常好的疗效。罕见的并发症

Rare complications include migration of coils to the pulmonary artery, thrombophlebitis, and pain.

包括弹簧圈移位至肺动脉、血栓性静脉炎和疼痛。

- Via internal jugular or femoral vein access, venography of the internal iliac veins and left renal vein are performed to assess for reflux or stenosis. If the valves are incompetent during Valsalva, reflux will be seen, often with collateralization and reflux to contralateral pelvic veins.
- A combination of liquid embolic agent, foam sclerotherapy, metallic coils, or vascular plug can be used. The use of metallic coils alone has fallen out of favor due to high recurrence rate with this method.
- Metallic coils are deployed in the inferior ovarian vein, usually at the level of the inguinal canal. Liquid embolic is then injected above the site of occlusion. A repeat venogram is then done to confirm resolution of reflux.

- 从颈内静脉或股静脉入路，对髂内静脉和左肾静脉进行静脉造影以评估反流或狭窄。如有瓣膜功能不全，瓦尔萨尔瓦动作时会出现反流，常伴有侧支循环和反流至对侧盆腔静脉。
- 联合使用液体栓塞剂、泡沫硬化剂、金属弹簧圈或血管封堵器。单独使用金属弹簧圈有较高的复发率，已不再被推崇。
- 将金属弹簧圈置于卵巢静脉下段，通常位于腹股沟管水平。之后在其上方注入液体栓塞剂。最后重复静脉造影以确认反流消失。

Varicocele embolization

精索静脉曲张栓塞

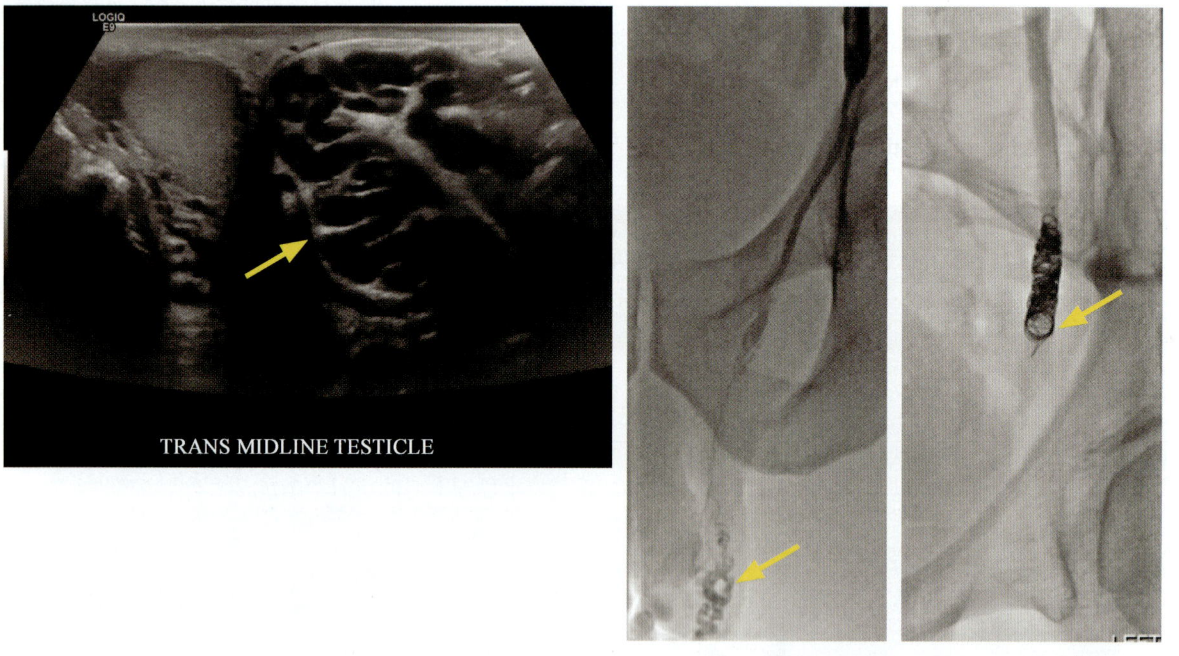

Left varicocele: Ultrasound shows dilated pampiniform veins in the left scrotum (arrow). DSA (middle image) shows the left gonadal vein with dilated vessels (arrow). Coil embolization (arrow, right image) of the internal iliac vein was performed.

左侧精索静脉曲张：超声显示左侧阴囊内扩张的蔓状静脉(黄箭)。DSA(中图)显示左侧性腺静脉扩张(黄箭)。弹簧圈栓塞髂内静脉(右图，黄箭)。

- A varicocele is a collection of varicose veins in the pampiniform plexus. Primary varicocele (most common) is due to absent or incompetent valves in the proximal gonadal vein causing reflux. Secondary varicocele is due to a mass obstructing venous return.
- Varicoceles are usually seen on the left side due to the acute angle of insertion on the renal vein, predisposing it to reflux, but can be bilateral. However, an isolated right varicocele should prompt workup for an obstructing retroperitoneal mass.
- Diagnosis by scrotal ultrasound shows a dilated (>2 mm) venous plexus with a *bag of worms* appearance, which worsens on Valsalva maneuver.
- Indications for treatment are pain, infertility, or testicular atrophy.
- Treatment is coil embolization or surgical ligation of the gonadal vein, which have been shown to be equivalent in outcome.

- 精索静脉曲张是蔓状静脉丛的静脉扩张。原发性精索静脉曲张(最常见)是由于近端性腺静脉的静脉瓣缺如或功能不全导致静脉血反流。继发性精索静脉曲张是由于有肿块阻塞了静脉回流。
- 精索静脉曲张常见于左侧，因左侧性腺静脉汇入左肾静脉时呈锐角，容易反流，但也可见双侧精索静脉曲张。然而，孤立的右侧精索静脉曲张时应进一步检查，以确定是否有来自腹膜后的肿块压迫。
- 阴囊超声表现为静脉丛扩张(>2mm)呈虫袋状，瓦尔萨尔瓦动作时加重。
- 治疗的适应证是疼痛、不孕或睾丸萎缩。
- 可采用弹簧圈栓塞或外科结扎精索静脉治疗，两种方法的临床效果相同。

- Right femoral vein or right internal jugular vein access is preferred for a left-sided varicocele; internal jugular vein or basilic vein access is preferred for a right-sided varicocele.

Lower extremity venous insufficiency

- Lower extremity venous insufficiency most commonly results from venous hypertension secondary to incompetent valves but can also be seen following prior DVT.
- Various treatment options are available, including thermal endovascular ablation with either laser or radiofrequency, or non-thermal ablation by injection of sclerosing agents into the vessels. Thermal and non-thermal interventions work by damaging the endothelium, causing the vessels to fibrose and resulting in irreversible occlusion.
- Thermal ablation procedures require tumescent anesthesia, which is injection of a mixture of lidocaine, saline, and epinephrine into the subcutaneous tissue surrounding the treated vessel. The injection acts as a local anesthetic, but also as a heat sink, protecting the overlying skin by preventing skin burns.
- Commonly treated vessels are the great saphenous vein (GSV), small saphenous vein (SSV), anterior accessory great saphenous vein (AAGSV), and their tributaries.
- Sclerotherapy is the injection of a chemical irritant into the vessel, usually for small or superficial venous disease, but can also be used for perforators or deep veins, and results in ablation of the vessel(s).
- Post-procedure management includes compression stockings for all of the above options.

- 左侧精索静脉曲张首选右侧股静脉或右侧颈内静脉入路；右侧精索静脉曲张首选颈内静脉或贵要静脉入路。

下肢静脉功能不全

- 下肢静脉功能不全最常见的原因是瓣膜功能不全引起的静脉高压，但也可继发于DVT。
- 有多种治疗方案可供选择，包括激光或射频血管内热消融，或将硬化剂注射到血管中进行非热消融。热和非热介入治疗通过破坏内皮起作用，引起血管纤维化，最终导致不可逆的闭塞。
- 热消融手术需要肿胀麻醉，即将利多卡因、生理盐水和肾上腺素的混合物注射到治疗血管周围的皮下组织。注射起到局部麻醉作用，也起到散热作用，通过防止皮肤灼伤来保护覆盖的皮肤。
- 通常治疗的血管是大隐静脉(GSV)、小隐静脉(SSV)、前副大隐静脉(AAGSV)及其侧支。
- 硬化治疗是将化学刺激物注入血管，通常用于小静脉或浅静脉疾病，但也可用于穿支或深静脉，并导致血管消融。
- 术后处理有弹力袜，用于上述所有各种治疗。

（翻译　仲斌演）

LYMPHATIC INTERVENTIONS

淋巴介入

ANATOMY OF THE LYMPHATIC SYSTEM

淋巴系统解剖

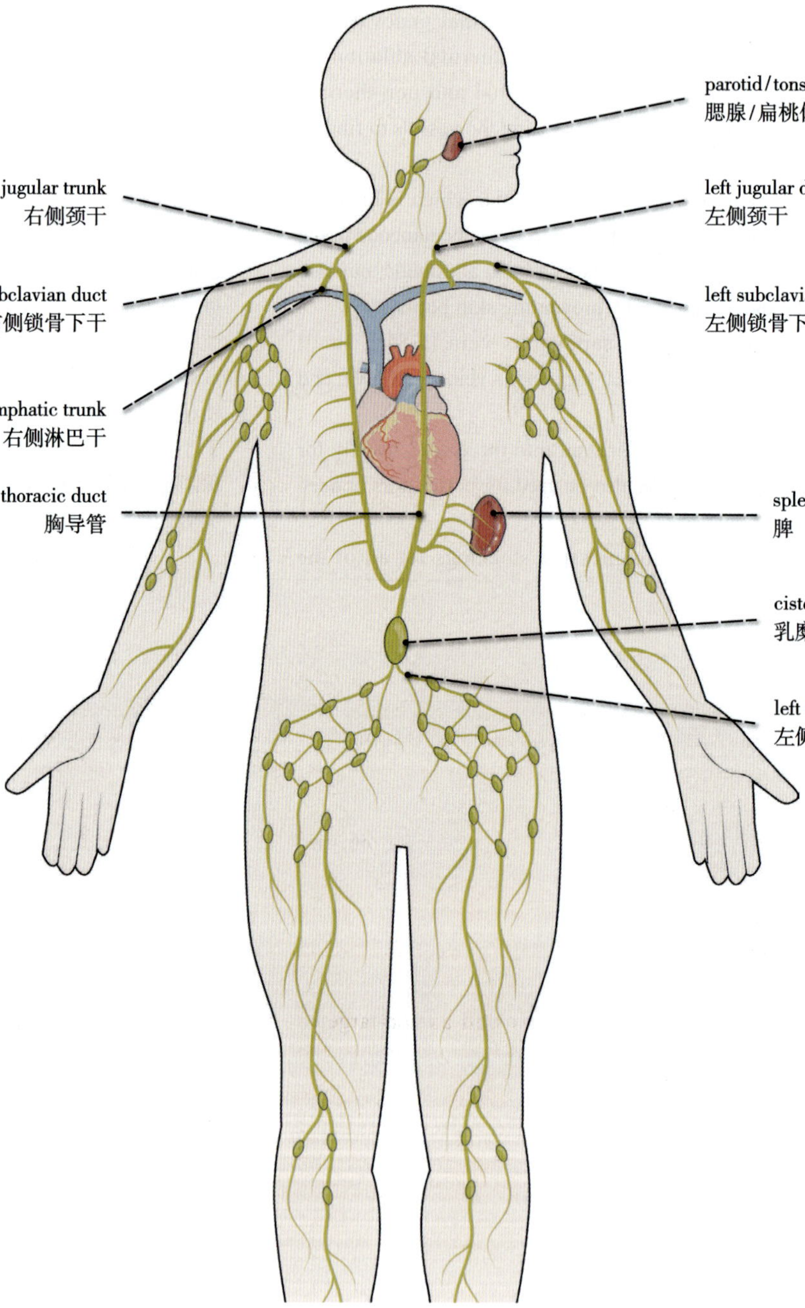

- The lymphatic system is made up of a large network of lymphatic vessels, organs and tissues.
- The thoracic duct carries 1–2 liters of lymphatic fluid a day, most of which comes from the intestinal and hepatic lymphatic ducts. Flow varies in relation to fatty content of a meal.
- Elevation of hepatic sinusoidal pressure such as cirrhosis and right-sided heart failure increases thoracic duct flow substantially.

- 淋巴系统是由淋巴管、器官和组织所构成的庞大网络结构。
- 胸导管每天输送1~2L淋巴液，其中大部分来自肠道和肝淋巴管。引流量随饮食中的脂肪含量而变化。
- 肝窦压力升高（如肝硬化）和右心衰竭时，胸导管流量随之增加。

Chylous Leak

Thoracic duct embolization (TDE)

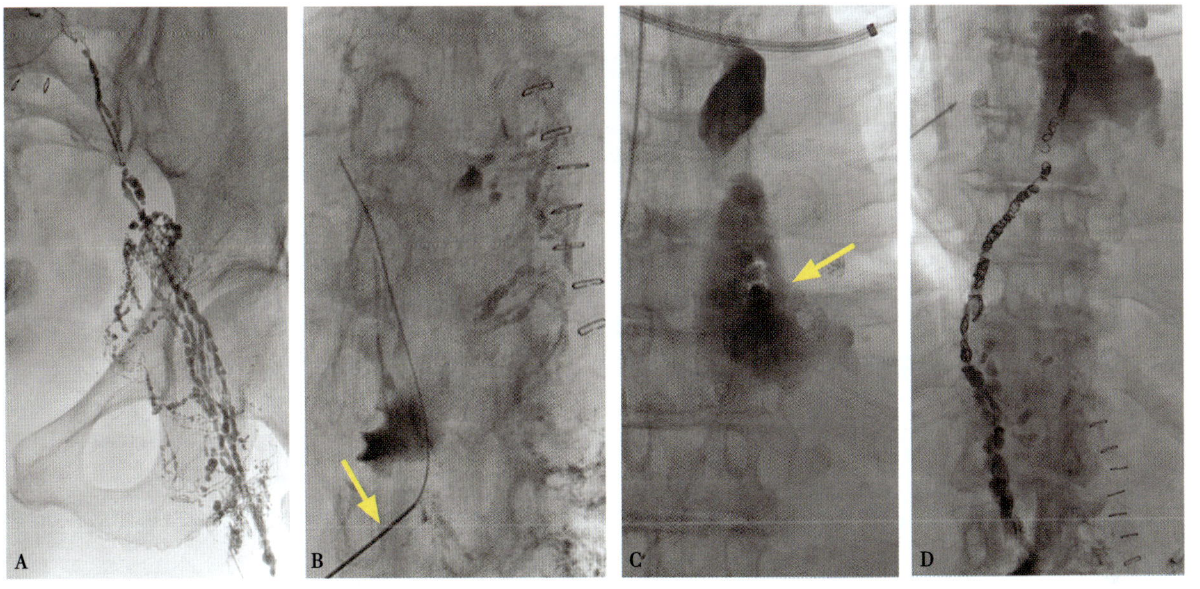

Thoracic duct embolization: A) Lymphatic access is obtained as seen on left abdominopelvic lymphangiogram. B) Select puncture of the cisterna chyli was performed with a 15 cm 21-gauge trocar needle (arrow), access maintained with V18 wire and inner cannula advanced over the wire. C) Lymphangiogram of the chest shows contrast pooling at T8–9 (arrow), likely the site of thoracic duct leak (yellow arrow). D) Embolization using n-BCA glue in 1:1 ethiodol to glue mixture (vol 2mL) was performed of the thoracic duct leak.

Case courtesy Arjun Sharma, MD, Brigham and Women's Hospital.

胸导管栓塞术：A）左侧腹-盆淋巴造影图显示淋巴管穿刺部位。B）用15cm长的21G套管针（黄箭）选择性穿刺乳糜池，引入V18导丝，再沿导丝送入内套管。C）胸部淋巴造影显示造影剂在T_{8-9}水平聚集（黄箭），可能是胸导管渗漏的部位（黄箭）。D）使用N-BCA胶对胸导管渗漏处进行栓塞，乙碘油与胶按1：1混合（量为2mL）。

- Chylous leaks can be caused by rupture of the thoracic duct and its tributaries from thoracic surgery such as esophagectomy, abdominal surgery, or nontraumatic causes such as malignancy (lymphoma) or idiopathic.
- Initial treatment is diet modification with a non-fat diet for 2–3 days prior to attempting TDE.
- It is important to consent patients for pancreatitis as well as non-targeted embolization.
- 5 mL of lipiodol is injected in each leg followed by a 20 mL saline push. Once the lymphographic dye reaches the abdomen, the cisterna chyli is visualized at the level of L1–3.
- After direct puncture with a long Chiba needle, a wire is extended to the thorax. The thoracic duct is coiled along its entirety to provide a matrix for glue polymerization with a 1：1 mixture of glue and lipiodol.
- It is important to carefully watch the glue as it is injected to identify nontargeted embolization. If the IVC is transgressed, glue can embolize to the pulmonary arteries resulting in acute pulmonary embolus.
- Rare complications include transgression of visceral organs with the puncture needle, resulting in peritonitis or bleeding.
- Embolization of the pulmonary artery which may or may not be symptomatic.
- Rare long-term complications that should be consented for include chronic lower extremity edema, chronic diarrhea, and abdominal ascites.

乳糜漏

胸导管栓塞术（TDE）

- 乳糜漏是由胸导管及其属支破裂所造成的，原因有胸部手术（如食管切除术）、腹部手术，或非创伤性因素（如恶性肿瘤-淋巴瘤）或特发性。
- 初始治疗是无脂饮食2~3天，然后尝试胸导管栓塞术（TDE）。
- 必须告知患者有胰腺炎和异位栓塞的风险。
- 每侧腿部注射5mL碘油，再注入20mL生理盐水。当造影剂沿淋巴管到达腹部时，乳糜池显影的位置在L_{1-3}水平。
- 用长的腰椎穿刺针直接穿刺乳糜池后，引入导丝到胸部。用弹簧圈填塞胸导管全程，为胶的聚合提供“骨架”，胶和碘油按1：1混合。
- 注射胶时须仔细观察以识别异位栓塞。若穿过IVC，胶会栓塞肺动脉，导致急性肺栓塞。
- 罕见的并发症包括穿刺针经过内脏器官，导致腹膜炎或出血。
- 肺动脉栓塞后是否出现症状不确定。
- 应告知患者可能出现罕见的长期并发症，包括慢性下肢水肿、慢性腹泻和腹水。

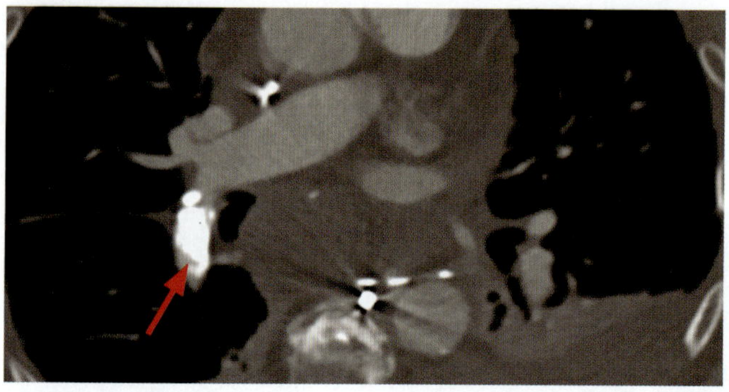

CTA chest reveals embolization of glue to the right lower lobe segmental pulmonary artery (red arrow).
胸部CTA显示右下叶肺段动脉处组织胶栓塞(红箭)。

(翻译　周大勇)

HEPATOBILIARY INTERVENTIONS

CHRONIC LIVER DISEASE AND CIRRHOSIS

- The classic angiographic finding of liver cirrhosis is *corkscrew* appearance of the hepatic artery branches.
- A hypervascular mass in a cirrhotic liver may represent hepatocellular carcinoma.
- Parenchymal liver biopsy can give useful prognostic information based on the grade of hepatic fibrosis in the setting of cirrhosis, hepatitis, non-alcoholic fatty liver disease (NAFLD), and primary biliary cirrhosis (PBC). Results may initiate treatment of chronic hepatitis, assess response to therapy, and help predict relapse in autoimmune hepatitis.
- Typically, ultrasound-guided biopsy of the left or right lobe is performed in the most peripheral aspect to ensure that no major vessels, dilated bile ducts or gallbladder are in the path of the biopsy needle.

BILIARY DISEASE

Biliary intervention overview and technique

- Percutaneous transhepatic cholangiography (PTC) is the injection of contrast into the biliary tree through a percutaneous approach, traversing the hepatic parenchyma.
- The two most common indications for PTC are relief of biliary obstruction and to provide biliary diversion in the case of ductal injury, which may be post-traumatic or postsurgical.

  Less common indications include percutaneous treatment of biliary calculi (endoscopic treatment is much more common) and adjunctive pre-surgical treatment prior to a biliary anastomosis. A biliary anastomosis is technically facilitated by having a pre-placed catheter to sew around.
- Pre-procedure prophylactic antibiotics are administered, as biliary stasis predisposes to bacterial overgrowth. Gram-negative coverage is needed, typically with levofloxacin.
- The right and left biliary trees are accessed using slightly different techniques.
- The right biliary tree is accessed via an intercostal approach and under either ultrasound or fluoroscopic guidance into a peripheral duct. If not possible, a two-puncture approach can be used. The first needle is used to opacify the

肝胆介入

慢性肝病和肝硬化

- 肝硬化血管造影的典型表现是肝动脉分支呈*螺旋状改变*。
- 肝硬化时出现的富血供肿块可能是肝细胞癌。
- 肝活检可以根据肝纤维化的分级程度对肝硬化、肝炎、非酒精性脂肪肝(NAFLD)和原发性胆汁性肝硬化(PBC)提供有价值的预后信息。活检结果可以指导慢性肝炎的治疗,评估治疗反应,并有助于预测自身免疫性肝炎的复发。
- 一般在超声引导下对肝左叶或右叶最边缘的部分进行活检,以确保穿刺道上无大血管、扩张的胆管或胆囊。

胆道疾病

胆道介入概述和技术

- 经皮肝穿刺胆道造影(PTC)是采用经皮穿刺肝脏实质将造影剂直接注入肝内胆管系统进行造影。
- PTC最常见的两种适应证为解除胆道梗阻和对创伤或手术造成的胆道损伤进行分流。

  较少见的适应证包括经皮穿刺治疗胆道结石(内镜下治疗更为常见)和胆道吻合术前辅助治疗。预先放置导管支撑有助于胆管缝合。
- 术前预防性使用抗生素,因胆汁淤积易造成细菌过度生长。应选择针对革兰氏阴性菌的抗生素,通常为左氧氟沙星(levofloxacin)。
- 左、右肝内胆管的穿刺技术略有不同。
- 穿刺右侧肝内胆管时,可通过肋间途径在超声或透视引导下进入外周胆管。若无法直接刺入外周胆管,可采用两步穿刺法。先用第一根针使胆道显影,再用第二根针在透视引导下进入更外周的胆管,以便放置胆道引流

biliary tree, and then the second needle can be used to fluoroscopically access a more peripheral duct for biliary drain placement. The needle should be inserted directly over the ribs, as the neurovascular bundle runs underneath each rib.

A 22-gauge needle is inserted, parallel to the table and to the inferior border of the liver.

Contrast is injected as the needle is withdrawn in an attempt to opacify the biliary tree.

Once a bile duct is opacified, the needle is temporarily left in place and a second puncture is made with a 21-gauge needle as low as possible to access the duct.

Once the second needle has accessed a duct, a 0.018″ wire is advanced, exchanged for a 5 or 6 Fr sheath, and subsequently a hydrophilic wire (such as a Roadrunner or Glidewire) is guided into the small bowel.

The hydrophilic wire is exchanged for a stiff wire (e.g., Amplatz) and the biliary drain is placed.

Extra sideholes may be manually cut, if necessary, to allow sideholes to extend from the biliary puncture site to the bowel.

The role of regular flushing is controversial. Some institutions advocate regular forward flushing, while others do not routinely flush. Regardless, a biliary drain should never be aspirated, as aspiration could draw up bowel contents into the biliary system and risk the development of cholangitis.

Three-month preventative maintenance is recommended.

- The **left biliary tree** is accessed by a left subxiphoid approach, in a similar manner to the right side; however, ultrasound can often visualize dilated ducts, obviating the need for two punctures.
- If stent placement is required to treat a stricture, a metallic stent is usually only placed in patients with a life expectancy of less than six months. Most metallic stents cannot be removed and have a median patency of 6–8 months, although newer covered metal stents can be removed.
- Plastic stents, which are placed endoscopically, do allow regular exchange.
- An alternative to stent placement is an internal/external biliary drain, although this option is less comfortable for the patient due to the external drain.
- Most contraindications to PTC are relative. For instance, although an intrahepatic tumor (primary or metastasis) should not be traversed, a directly accessible bile duct may still be present. Similarly, ascites is a contraindication but therapeutic paracentesis can be first performed.
- Complications of percutaneous biliary drainage include sepsis, hemorrhage, bile leak, hemobilia (due to arterial-biliary fistula), and abscess.

管。穿刺针应沿肋骨上缘进针，因神经血管束在肋骨下缘走行。

用22G针进行穿刺，针与手术台和肝脏的下缘平行。

回拔穿刺针的同时推注造影剂以使肝内胆管显影。

胆道一旦显影，将针暂时保留在原处，并使用21G穿刺针进行第二次穿刺，尽可能穿刺靠外周的胆管。

第二针穿刺一旦成功，引入0.018英寸(1英寸=2.54厘米)导丝，置换入5Fr或6Fr鞘，随后将亲水导丝(如Roadrunner或Glidewire)引入小肠。

将亲水导丝交换成超硬导丝(如Amplatz)并放置胆道引流管。

必要时可手工剪制额外的侧孔，以使侧孔从胆道穿入部位延伸至肠腔。

定期冲洗的作用仍有争议。一些医院主张定期冲洗，而一些则不做定期冲洗。但无论如何，胆道引流管不应该抽吸，因抽吸有将肠内容物抽入胆道系统而引发胆管炎的风险。

胆道引流管常规维护应每3个月进行一次。

- **左侧肝内胆管**穿刺应采用左剑突下的路径，穿刺方法与右侧相似；但是，超声引导常可清晰显示肝内扩张的胆管，从而避免二次穿刺。
- 若狭窄需植入支架治疗时，金属支架通常只适用于预期存活不到6个月的患者。大多数金属支架无法取出且平均通畅时间仅为6~8个月，但较新的覆膜金属支架可以取出。
- 塑料支架在内镜下放置，可定期更换。
- 替代塑料支架的方法是胆道内/外引流，这种方法因为外引流，所以患者的舒适度较低。
- 大多数PTC的禁忌证是相对的，如不应穿过肝内肿瘤(原发或转移)，但直接穿刺胆管仍有可能。同样，腹水是禁忌证，但术前可先进行治疗性腹水引流。
- 经皮胆道引流术的并发症包括败血症、出血、胆漏、胆道出血(由于动脉-胆道瘘)及脓肿。

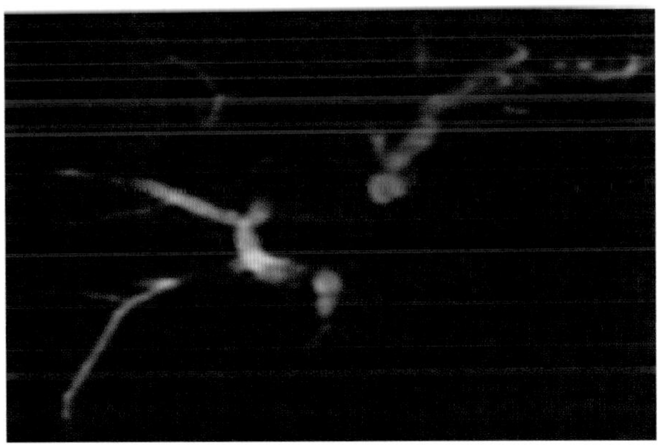

1) MRCP subtraction image for planning.

1) MRCP减影图像用于手术计划。

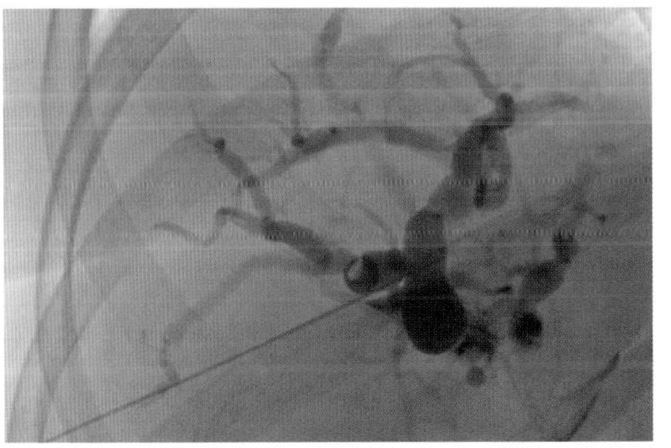

2) Percutaneous access obtained in the right mid-axillary line with 22G Chiba needle.

2) 使用22G Chiba针从右侧腋中线经皮穿刺胆道。

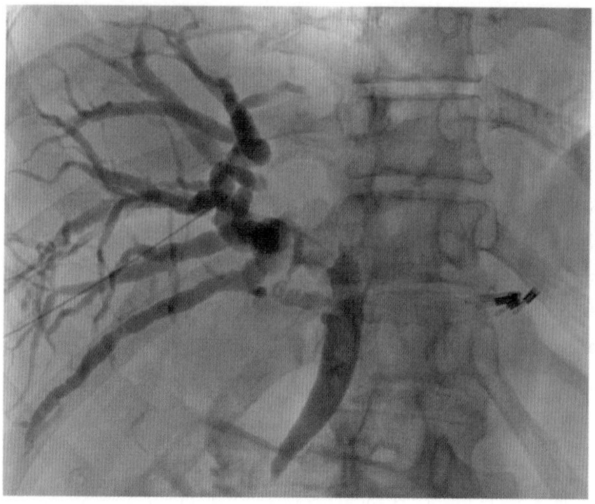

3) The right peripheral bile duct was entered with a 21G trocar needle, and 0.018″ Cope guidewire inserted into the biliary tree followed by transitional dilation system.

3) 使用21G套管针穿刺进入右侧外周胆管，引入0.018英寸导丝选入胆管分支内，插入扩张系统。

Case courtesy Arjun Sharma, MD, Brigham and Women's Hospital.

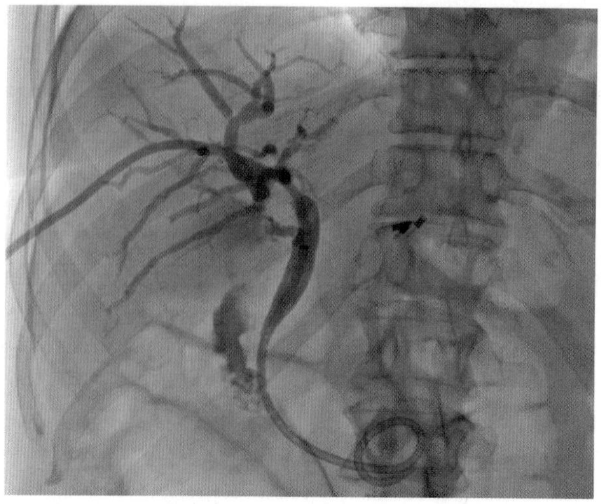

4) Using a 4FR angled catheter and Roadrunner guidewire, the small bowel was entered. Over the 0.038″ J-tipped guidewire, the tract was dilated and biliary drainage catheter inserted.

4) 使用4Fr单弯导管和超滑导丝选入小肠。通过0.038英寸"J"形导丝，扩张路径，之后放入胆道引流管。

Bile duct injury

- The most common cause of bile duct injury is iatrogenic from a laparoscopic cholecystectomy. A less common cause of bile duct injury is from orthotopic liver transplant.
- Treatment is to provide biliary diversion to drainage bag to allow the leak to heal.

Sclerosing cholangitis

- Sclerosing cholangitis is a chronic inflammatory and fibrosing process leading to multifocal strictures of the intra-and extrahepatic biliary tree. Sclerosing cholangitis clinically presents with obstructive jaundice, malaise, and abdominal pain. It occurs more commonly in men and is associated with inflammatory bowel disease (ulcerative colitis).
- Sclerosing cholangitis ultimately leads to biliary cirrhosis and increases the risk of developing cholangiocarcinoma.
- Treatment of sclerosing cholangitis is liver transplant, although percutaneous biliary drainage can provide palliative relief for the symptoms of obstructive jaundice.
- Cholangiogram shows multifocal biliary strictures throughout the intra-and extrahepatic biliary tree. The differential diagnosis of multifocal biliary strictures includes:

Sclerosing cholangitis.
Primary biliary cirrhosis.
Multifocal cholangiocarcinoma.
Chronic bacterial cholangitis.
AIDS cholangitis (usually associated with papillary stenosis).

Malignant biliary obstruction

- Unilateral biliary obstruction of either the right or left hepatic ductal system may be due to metastatic disease or primary malignancy of the bile ducts. In the majority of cases, only the affected biliary system requires treatment.

胆管损伤

- 胆管损伤最常见的原因是腹腔镜胆囊切除术造成的医源性损伤。较少见的为活体肝移植手术。
- 进行胆道分流治疗，将胆汁引流到引流袋内，使漏口愈合。

硬化性胆管炎

- 硬化性胆管炎是一种慢性炎症和纤维化的过程，可导致多发性肝内、肝外胆管局部狭窄。硬化性胆管炎的临床表现为梗阻性黄疸、全身乏力和腹痛。男性多发，并与肠道炎症性疾病有关(溃疡性结肠炎)。
- 硬化性胆管炎最终导致胆汁性肝硬化，且胆管癌的发病风险增加。
- 硬化性胆管炎的治疗方法是肝移植，经皮胆道引流可作为姑息治疗以改善梗阻性黄疸的症状。
- 胆管造影显示多发局灶性狭窄，累及肝内和肝外所有胆管。多发局灶性胆管狭窄的鉴别诊断包括：

硬化性胆管炎。
原发性胆汁性肝硬化。
多发性胆管癌。
慢性细菌性胆管炎。
艾滋病胆管炎(通常与乳头狭窄有关)。

恶性胆道梗阻

- 单侧胆道梗阻，无论左侧还是右侧，可能都是由转移癌或胆道原发恶性肿瘤所致。大多数情况下只有受累的胆管系统需要进行治疗。

- Hilar obstruction, in contrast, is due most commonly to a hilar cholangiocarcinoma (Klatskin tumor), which most often requires two biliary drains, one each in the right and left ducts. Occasionally an anatomic anomaly, such as anomalous drainage of the right duct directly into the left duct, may allow complete drainage of a hilar obstruction with a single biliary drain. Pre-procedure MRCP may be helpful to delineate biliary anatomy.

- 肝门部梗阻则相反，最常由肝门部的胆管癌（Klatskin瘤）所致，大多需要两根引流管，左右肝内胆管各一根。偶尔可见解剖学变异，如异常走行的右侧肝内胆管直接引入左侧胆管内，用单根胆道引流管也可能充分引流肝门部梗阻。术前MRCP有助于明确胆道解剖。

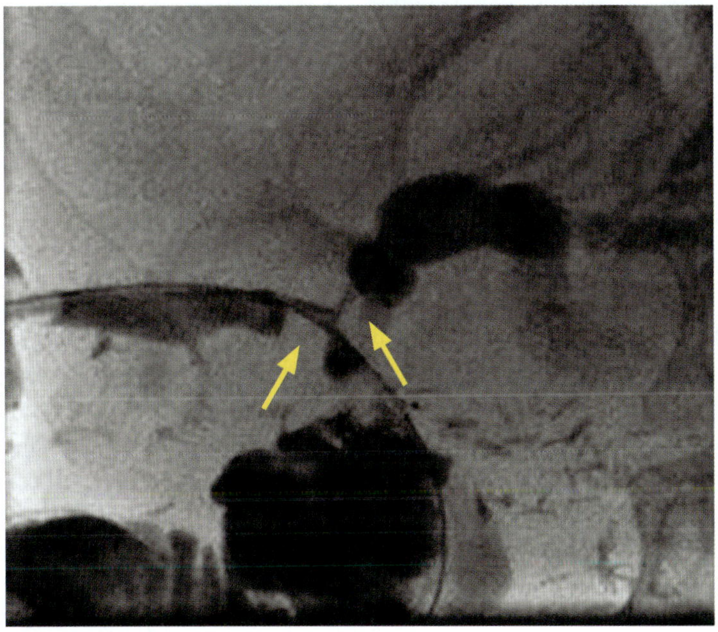

Klatskin tumor: Cholangiogram demonstrates bilateral marked dilation of the right and left hepatic ducts, with shouldering of the ducts at the hilum (arrows). A wire is in place in the right sided ducts.
Klatskin瘤：胆管造影显示左右两侧肝内胆管显著扩张，并在肝门区突然变窄（黄箭）。导丝放入右侧胆管内。

GALLBLADDER

胆囊

Acute cholecystitis

急性胆囊炎

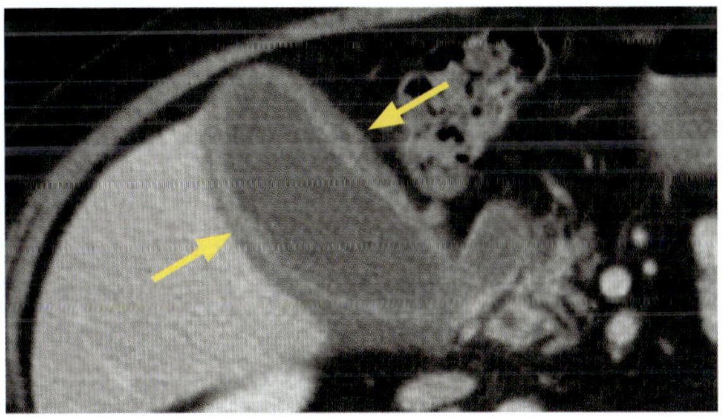

Contrast-enhanced CT shows diffuse gallbladder wall thickening (arrows). There are no radiopaque gallstones.
增强CT显示胆囊壁弥漫增厚（黄箭）。未见不透射线的胆囊结石。

HIDA scan shows no gallbladder uptake, consistent with cystic duct obstruction.
肝胆亚氨基二乙酸（HIDA）扫描未见胆囊摄取，符合胆囊管梗阻表现。

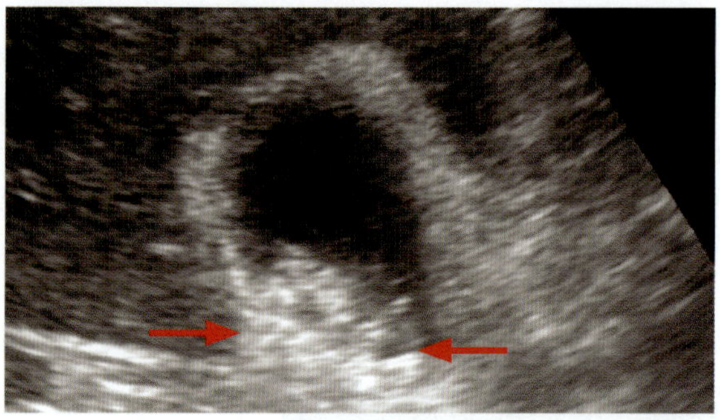

Pre-procedural ultrasound confirms thickened gallbladder wall, with numerous dependent echogenic gallstones (red arrows) not seen on CT.

术前超声证实胆囊壁增厚，底部有多个CT未显示的结石回声(红箭)。

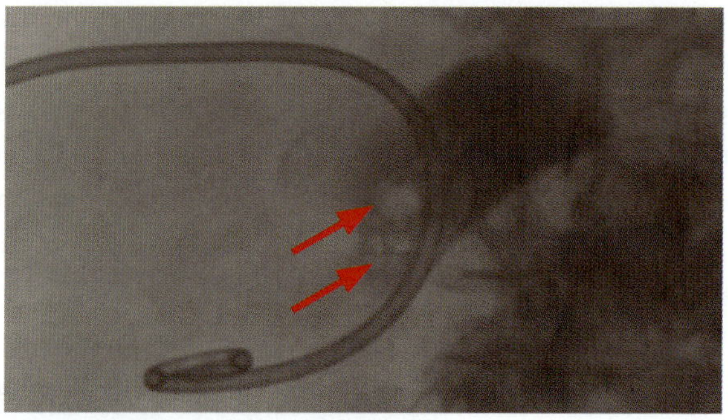

Post-cholecystostomy opacification of the gallbladder shows numerous gallbladder filling defects (red arrows), representing multiple stones.

胆囊造瘘术后胆囊造影显示胆囊有大量充盈缺损(红箭)，为多发结石。

Acute calculous cholecystitis. *Case courtesy Alisa Suzuki Han, MD, Brigham and Women's Hospital*

急性结石性胆囊炎。

- Percutaneous gallbladder drainage (cholecystostomy) is indicated for the treatment of acute calculous or acalculous cholecystitis in patients who are not surgical candidates.
- Cholecystotomy is a temporizing measure for treatment of calculous cholecystitis prior to cholecystectomy, but it may cure acalculous cholecystitis without surgery.
- Of note, cultures are negative in 40% of acute cholecystitis.
- Similar to percutaneous transhepatic cholangiography, prophylactic antibiotics are given.
- The two percutaneous approaches to the gallbladder are transhepatic and transperitoneal.

  Transhepatic (through the liver): In the transhepatic approach, a needle is inserted in the midaxillary line (either intercostal or subcostal) and directed towards the bare area of the gallbladder fossa through the liver under sonographic guidance. Transhepatic cholecystostomy has decreased risk of peritoneal bile leak, but increases the risk of liver laceration. The transhepatic approach is more commonly performed.

  Transperitoneal (avoiding the liver): In the transperitoneal approach, the needle is directed into the gallbladder from a subcostal approach in the right anterior abdomen, beneath the liver margin. While there is less risk of damaging the liver, a transperitoneal approach carries an increased risk of peritoneal bile leak. Additionally, a transperitoneal approach necessitates penetration of the gallbladder fundus, which is the most mobile portion.
- The drainage tube must remain in place until the following criteria are met:

  Patient is clinically improved. There is a risk of sepsis if the tube is removed prematurely.

  Cystic duct and common bile duct are demonstrated to be patent on repeat cholangiogram.

  At least 6 weeks have passed since placement (regardless of transhepatic or transperitoneal approach), to allow a fibrous tract to develop extending from the gallbladder to the skin puncture. Transperitoneal cholecystostomy has greater risk of incomplete tract formation and bile peritonitis following tube removal.

- 经皮胆囊穿刺引流术(胆囊造瘘术)的适应证为不适合外科手术的结石性或非结石性急性胆囊炎。
- 胆囊造瘘术是胆囊切除术治疗结石性胆囊炎术前的一种过渡性治疗，但对非结石性胆囊炎可以是根治性治疗而无须外科手术。
- 需要注意，细菌培养在40%的急性胆囊炎中的结果为阴性。
- 与经皮经肝胆道穿刺造影一样，术前要预防性使用抗生素。
- 经皮穿刺胆囊有经肝和经腹膜两种穿刺路径。

  经肝途径(通过肝脏)：采用经肝穿刺路径时，在超声引导下于腋中线(肋间或肋弓下)进针直接穿刺胆囊窝的裸区。经肝胆囊造瘘术可降低胆汁腹腔泄漏的风险，但会增加肝撕裂的风险。该路径较为常用。

  经腹膜途径(避开肝脏)：经腹膜路径穿刺时，穿刺针经右上腹肋弓下，从肝脏下缘的下方直接穿刺胆囊。虽然经腹膜穿刺会减少肝脏损害的风险，但会增加腹腔胆汁泄漏的风险。另外，经腹膜穿刺路径需穿刺胆囊底部，而该部位活动性最大。
- 拔除引流管必须符合以下条件：

  患者临床症状得到改善。过早拔管有发生败血症的风险。

  重复胆管造影证实胆囊管和胆总管通畅。

  至少需置管6周(无论是经肝还是经腹穿刺途径)，以便在胆囊到皮肤之间的穿刺路径上形成纤维窦道。经腹膜胆囊造瘘术在拔管后有较高的窦道形成不全和胆汁性腹膜炎的风险。

(翻译　胡立斌)

PORTAL HYPERTENSION

Measuring portal pressure

- Direct portal vein (PV) pressure measurement requires traversing the hepatic parenchyma and is thus invasive and impractical. Wedged hepatic vein pressure is routinely measured via an internal jugular vein catheter and is thought to equal PV pressure in most patients.
- The corrected sinusoidal gradient is an estimate of the **portosystemic gradient** and represents the actual sinusoidal resistance to portal flow. It is calculated as:
  (Wedged hepatic vein pressure)−(free hepatic vein pressure)
- Portal hypertension is defined as a portosystemic gradient >5 mm Hg.

Collateral pathways seen in portal hypertension

门静脉高压

门静脉压力测量

- 直接测量门静脉压力需穿过肝实质，因此具有创伤性且不切实际。常规肝静脉楔压测量是通过经颈内静脉经导管途径，该方法在大多数患者可等同于门静脉压。
- 矫正后肝窦压用于评估**门体压力梯度**，并代表肝窦对门静脉血流的实际阻力，计算公式为：
  肝静脉楔压－肝静脉游离压。
- 门静脉高压定义为门体压力梯度>5mmHg。

门静脉高压时的侧支通路

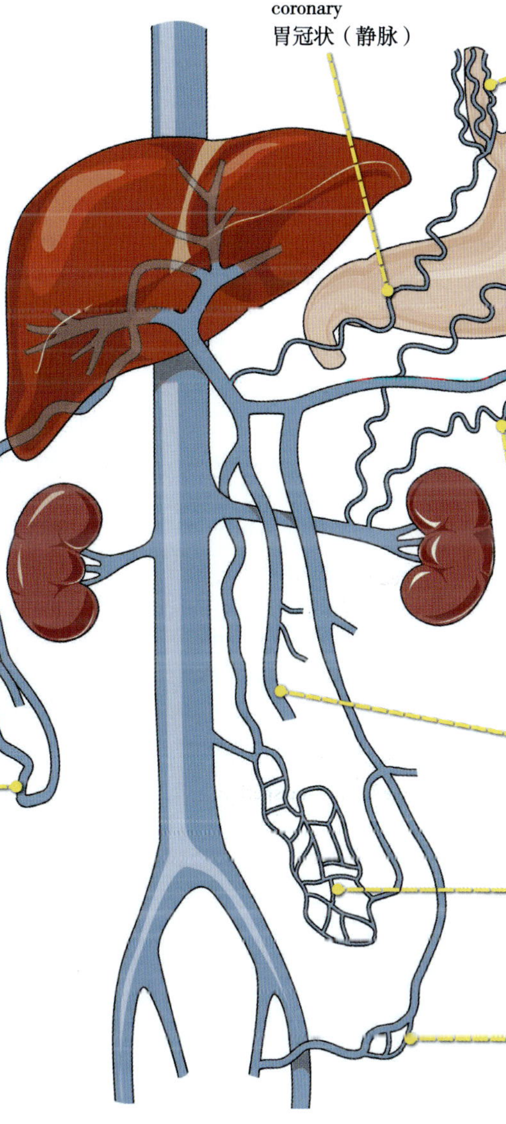

Light blue represents portal veins → dark blue represents systemic veins

浅蓝色表示门静脉→深蓝色表示体静脉

- Esophageal varices: Coronary vein → azygos/hemiazygos veins
- 食管静脉曲张：胃冠状静脉→奇静脉/半奇静脉
- Gastric fundal varices: Splenic vein → azygos veins
- 胃底静脉曲张：脾静脉→奇静脉
- Splenorenal shunt: Splenic or short gastric → left adrenal/inferior phrenic → left renal vein
- 脾肾分流：脾静脉或胃短静脉→左肾上腺静脉/膈下静脉→左肾静脉
- Mesenteric varices: SMV or IMV → iliac veins
- 肠系膜静脉曲张：肠系膜上静脉/肠系膜下静脉→髂静脉
- Caput medusa: Umbilical vein → epigastric veins
- 脐周静脉曲张：脐静脉→腹壁静脉
- Hemorrhoids: IMV → inferior hemorrhoidal veins
- 痔：IMV→痔下静脉

Transjugular intrahepatic portosystemic shunt (TIPS)

- Transjugular intrahepatic portosystemic shunt (TIPS) lowers elevated portal pressures by the creation of a direct connection between the portal vein and the hepatic vein.
- The most common indication for TIPS is treatment of variceal hemorrhage that cannot be controlled endoscopically and refractory ascites. Other indications for TIPS include Budd-Chiari (hepatic vein thrombosis), and hepatic hydrothorax.
- Assessment of hepatic dysfunction is performed pre-procedure with either the Child-Pugh classification or Model for End-Stage Liver Disease (MELD) score.

  The **Child-Pugh** classification of hepatic dysfunction combines lab values (INR, bilirubin, and albumin) with clinical assessment (ascites and hepatic encephalopathy).

  The **MELD** score of hepatic dysfunction combines INR, bilirubin, and creatinine in a complex logarithmic formula. The higher the MELD score, the higher the post-TIPS mortality.
- Absolute contraindications to TIPS include:

  Right-sided heart failure, which will be worsened by TIPS, as right-sided venous return increases.

  Severe active hepatic failure, as the post-TIPS shunting of blood beyond the hepatic sinusoids can cause liver function to worsen further.

  Severe hepatic encephalopathy, which TIPS can worsen.
- Portal vein patency should be established pre-procedure with cross-sectional or ultrasound imaging.
- Usually the right hepatic vein is connected with the right portal vein via a covered stent. The right hepatic vein has relatively constant anatomy and tends to be larger than the left.
- After the right hepatic vein is cannulated, wedged balloon CO_2 occlusion venography is performed and the portal vein is retrogradely opacified. CO_2 is the preferred contrast agent as it is 400 times less viscous than iodinated contrast and is therefore easily able to pass through the hepatic sinusoids.
- The most demanding portion of the procedure is establishing access into a portal vein. Once a tract between the hepatic and portal circulation is secured, the tract is sequentially dilated and stented, aiming for a reduction of the portosystemic gradient to <12 mm Hg.
- TIPS patency is followed by Doppler ultrasound, discussed in the gastrointestinal imaging chapter.

经颈静脉肝内门体分流术(TIPS)

- 经颈静脉肝内门体分流术(TIPS)是在门静脉和肝静脉间建立一条直接通道，以降低升高的门静脉压力。
- TIPS最常见的适应证是内镜治疗无法控制的曲张静脉出血和顽固性腹水。其他适应证包括布加综合征(肝静脉血栓形成)和肝性胸腔积液。
- 术前需对肝功能进行评估，可用Child-Pugh分级或晚期肝病模型(MELD)评分法。

  Child-Pugh分级对肝功能异常的评价指标包括实验室指标(国际标准化比值、胆红素和白蛋白)和临床评估(腹水和肝性脑病)。

  MELD评分对肝功能异常的评价指标包括国际标准化比值、胆红素及肌酐，需一个复杂的对数计算公式。MELD评分越高，术后死亡率越高。
- TIPS的绝对禁忌证包括：

  右心衰竭，TIPS后回心血量增加可使右心衰竭加重。

  严重的活动性肝功能衰竭，因术后门静脉血经TIPS分流而绕开肝窦，可进一步加重肝功能损害。

  重度肝性脑病，TIPS后可加重病情。
- 门静脉是否通畅，需要术前进行断层扫描或超声检查加以确定。
- 通常在肝右静脉和门静脉右支之间放置一个覆膜支架将两者连接起来，肝右静脉在解剖上相对固定且直径大于肝左静脉。
- 肝右静脉成功插管后，采用阻塞球囊进行逆向CO_2造影以显示门静脉。CO_2是首选的造影剂，因其黏滞性比碘造影剂低400倍，易通过肝窦。
- 该手术的关键是建立与门静脉的通道。一旦肝静脉与门静脉的通道建立成功，就可随之对通道进行扩张，再植入支架，目标是将门体压力梯度降至12mmHg以下。
- TIPS的通畅性可用多普勒超声进行随访，详见“胃肠道影像”一章。

TIPS: Step by step

TIPS：详细步骤

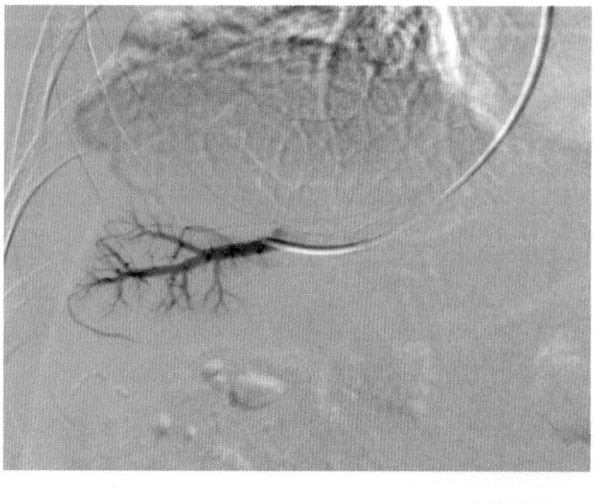

1) Right hepatic venography is performed through an internal jugular access.

1) 经颈内静脉行肝右静脉造影。

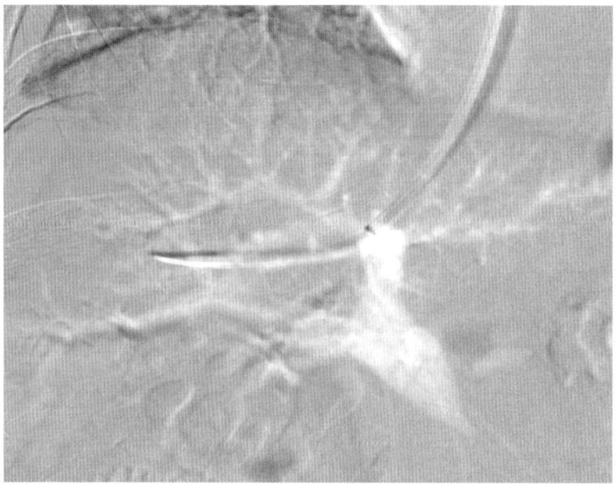

2) The catheter is wedged in a distal hepatic vein and an occlusion balloon inflated. Indirect CO_2 venography of the portal veins is performed.

2) 导管楔入肝静脉远端并充盈封闭球囊，之后行CO_2间接门静脉造影。

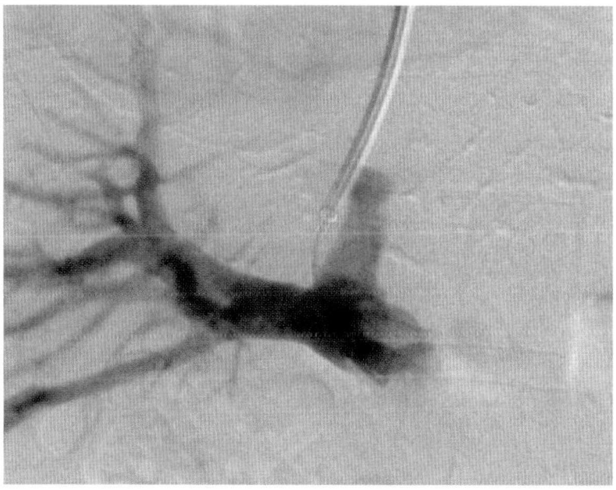

3) Direct cannulation of the portal vein (usually the right portal vein) through the liver parenchyma is the most challenging portion of the procedure. Indirect CO_2 venography is used as a guide.

3) 通过肝实质直接穿刺门静脉(通常为门静脉右支)是该手术最具挑战性的步骤。CO_2间接门静脉造影用于导向。

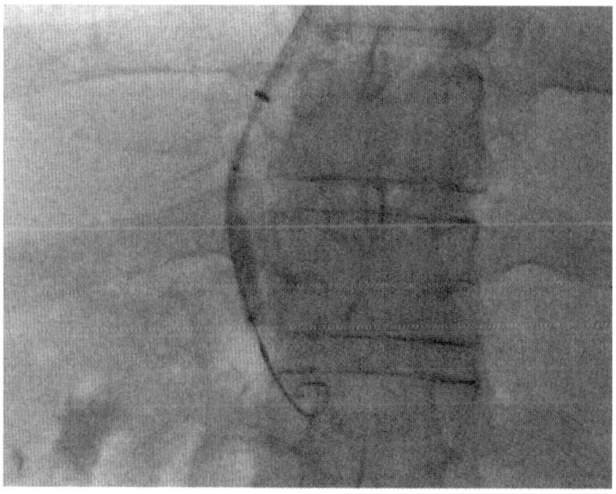

4) After the portal vein is cannulated, the tract is dilated with an 8 mm × 3–4 cm balloon to allow placement of the stent-graft.

4) 进入门静脉以后，用8mm × (3~4)cm 球囊扩张分流道，以便放置支架。

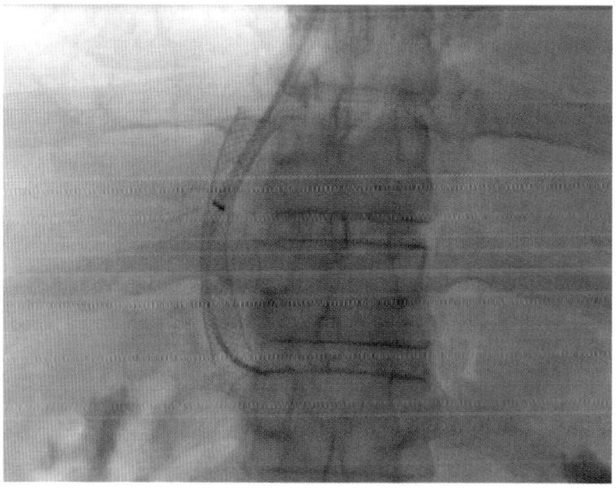

5) Once the tract is dilated, a covered stent-graft is deployed (usually a self-expanding stent). The stent-graft should be dilated until a pressure gradient between the portal vein and inferior vena cava of <12 mm Hg is reached.

5) 分流道扩张后，随即放置覆膜支架(通常为自膨胀式支架)。对支架进行扩张直至门静脉与下腔静脉之间的压力梯度小于12 mmHg。

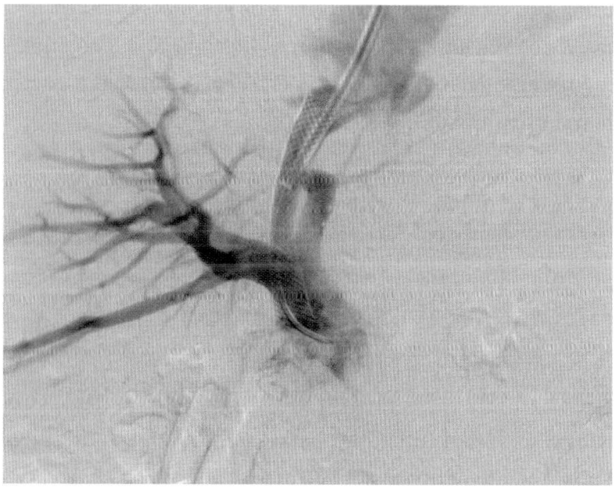

6) Completion portal venogram is performed. At this point, any varices present may be embolized.

6) 术后行门静脉造影。此时发现有曲张静脉可考虑进行栓塞。

Gastroesophageal Varices and Portosystemic Shunts

Ballon-occluded retrograde transvenous obliteration (BRTO)

- Ballon-occluded retrograde transvenous obliteration (BRTO) is used for the management of gastric variceal bleeding due to portal hypertension and is more commonly performed in Asia. In the United States and Europe, BRTO is usually performed when endoscopic therapy fails and TIPS is not an option.

  In the United States and Europe, TIPS is the first-line treatment for gastric variceal hemorrhage. By decompressing portal hypertension, TIPS induces hemostasis of gastric varices and reduces the risk of rebleeding, but may cause liver failure and hepatic encephalopathy as described previously.
- BRTO involves endovascular obliteration of gastric varices by injection of a sclerosing agent directly into the varix via a gastrorenal or gastrocaval shunt while the variceal blood outflow is occluded by an inflated balloon.

  In patients without spontaneous gastrorenal or gastrocaval shunt, BRTO is not a treatment option.
- By obstructing a major gastrorenal shunt, BRTO increases portal venous pressure, therefore improving liver function, lowering the risk of liver failure and hepatic encaphalopathy. However, it can worsen ascites and esophageal varices if present.
- BRTO has comparable efficacy to TIPS in treating refractory gastric variceal hemorrhage. In fact, it is associated with lower rates of rebleeding, hepatic encephalopathy, and mortality.
- Overview of the procedure:

  Percutaneous access is achieved through the femoral vein (most common) or jugular vein.

  Then, catheterization of the gastrorenal shunt via the left renal vein is performed.

  Balloon occlusion of the gastrorenal shunt outflow is done followed by a shunt venogram to map the anatomy.

  Sclerosant is injected upstream into the varices. Occlusive balloon is left in place for 4–24 hours until sclerosant has reached stasis.
- Variations to BRTO have been developed with shorter procedural time and occlusion of the shunt by either coiling or vascular plugging.
- Common complications include gross hematuria, aggravation of esophageal varices, ascites, hydrothorax/pleural effusion, spontaneous bacterial peritonitis, and portal vein thrombosis.

胃食管静脉曲张和门体分流

球囊阻塞逆行曲张静脉闭塞术(BRTO)

- 球囊阻塞逆行曲张静脉闭塞术(BRTO)用于治疗门静脉高压引起的胃静脉曲张出血，在亚洲较流行。在美国和欧洲，BRTO通常是内镜治疗失败且不适合TIPS时的另一种选择。

  在美国和欧洲国家，TIPS是治疗胃静脉曲张出血的首选治疗方法。TIPS通过降低门静脉压力以制止胃静脉曲张出血，并降低再出血的风险，但如前所述，该方法可导致肝功能衰竭和肝性脑病。
- BRTO是通过胃肾或胃腔分流道向曲张静脉腔内直接注入硬化剂使胃曲张静脉闭塞，同时在栓塞时需要使用充盈球囊阻塞曲张静脉的流出道。

  对于没有自发性胃肾或胃腔分流的患者，BRTO不是一种治疗选择。
- 在阻塞了主要的胃肾分流之后，BRTO会增加门静脉压力，从而改善肝功能，降低肝功能衰竭和肝性脑病的风险。但可以使腹水和食管静脉曲张加重。
- BRTO对难治性胃静脉曲张出血的疗效与TIPS相当，且出血率、肝性脑病和死亡率较低。
- 操作步骤概述：

  经皮穿刺股静脉(最常见)或颈静脉。

  经左肾静脉置管进入胃肾分流道。

  球囊导管封堵胃肾分流的流出道，然后行分流道静脉造影以显示曲张静脉解剖情况。

  经导管向曲张静脉逆行注入硬化剂。留置阻塞球囊4~24小时，直到硬化剂达到停滞状态。
- 改进的BRTO可通过弹簧圈或血管封堵器阻塞分流道以缩短手术时间。
- 常见并发症包括肉眼血尿、食管静脉曲张加重、腹水、胸腔积液、自发性细菌性腹膜炎和门静脉血栓形成。

(翻译　朱晓黎)

Oncologic Interventions

Ablation Therapy

- Percutaneous tumor ablation is a safe alternative to surgical resection in carefully selected patients. The role of ablation is actively evolving and expanding. Ablation is commonly performed in the liver, kidney, lung, and bone, and its role in other sites (e.g., prostate, thyroid) is also expanding. Common indications include local control of solitary or oligometastatic disease (1–5 metastatic lesions) and/or pain palliation. The best outcomes for local control are obtained for lesions that are <5 cm in maximal diameter, but indications for debulking and palliation of larger lesions are increasing. The most common techniques for percutaneous ablation include cryoablation,

肿瘤介入

消融治疗

- 经皮肿瘤消融术对经过慎重选择的患者是外科手术切除的一种安全替代方法。消融所起的作用正在发展和壮大。消融常用于肝、肾、肺和骨骼，而在其他部位(如前列腺、甲状腺)的应用也在不断扩大。常见的指征包括对孤立性或寡转移病变(1~5个转移灶)进行局部控制和/或缓解疼痛。最佳局部控制效果是直径<5cm的病灶，但对较大病灶进行减瘤和姑息治疗的适应证范围也正在扩大。最常见的

microwave ablation, and radiofrequency ablation. Other techniques include irreversible electroporation, laser, and ethanol ablation.

- Heat sink phenomenon is a limitation of all thermal ablation techniques, where adjacent blood vessels prevent large temperature variations, resulting in cooler temperatures of the surrounding tissue and the potential for residual unablated tissue.

经皮消融技术包括冷冻、微波和射频消融。其他消融技术还包括不可逆电穿孔、激光和乙醇消融。

- 热沉降现象是所有热消融技术的瓶颈，因邻近的血管限制了大幅度升温，导致其周围组织的温度较低并可能遗留未消融的残留组织。

Radiofrequency ablation (RFA)

射频消融(RFA)

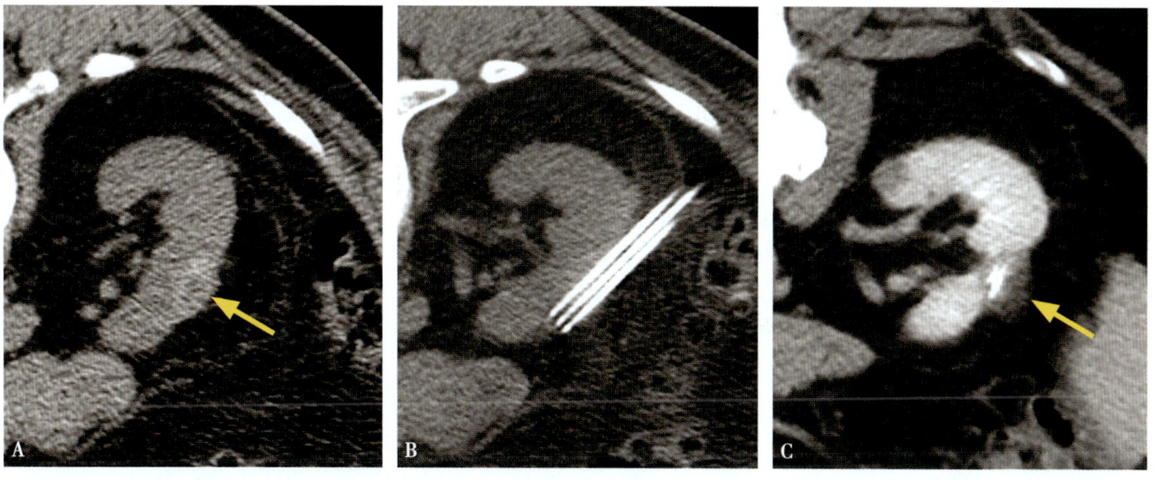

Radiofrequency ablation in a 51-year-old male with renal cell carcinoma. A) Axial noncontrast CT preliminary images show a hyperdense lesion in the right kidney (arrow). B) Intraprocedure axial CT shows three ablation probes in place. The ablation zone is not well seen during the procedure. C) Follow-up post-contrast axial CT at three years shows expected appearance of the ablation zone (arrow) with peripheral calcification.

一名51岁男性肾癌患者的射频消融。A) 术前轴位平扫CT显示右肾一个高密度病灶(黄箭)。B) 术中CT显示三根消融针穿刺到位；术中消融范围未能清晰显示。C) 术后3年增强CT随访显示原消融区的术后改变(黄箭)，可见边缘钙化。

- Mechanism: The RF electrode generates a simple electrical circuit through the body with alternating electromagnetic fields that agitate adjacent molecules, resulting in frictional heating of tissue around the probe, and ultimately results in coagulation necrosis and cell death at temperatures greater than 55℃. There is an exponential drop in temperature as you get further from the probe. Grounding pads are used to serve as a dispersive electrode.
- Technique: A single heating cycle slowly heats the tissue to 50–100℃ for 6–15 minutes. Care must be taken to not increase the temperature too quickly, which can char the soft tissues and cause evaporation with formation of microbubbles, both of which increase the electrical impedance and limit flow of current, reducing the effectiveness of the probe.
- Advantages: RFA is the most established and widely available option. The total procedure time is shorter when compared to cryoablation. RFA cauterizes small vessels and decreases bleeding risk. RFA is the most cost-effective option compared to other ablation techniques.
- Disadvantages: RFA is heavily dependent on good electrical and thermal tissue conductivity. The ablation zone is not well monitored in real time. RFA is most susceptible to the heat sink effect, which can result in residual unablated tissue and an unpredictable ablation zone.

- 机制：射频(RF)电极在体内产生一个单环电路，电磁场交替搅动邻近的分子，导致电极周围组织摩擦生热，当温度超过55℃时最终导致凝固性坏死和细胞死亡。温度随电极的距离呈指数性下降。接地垫作为离散电极。
- 技术：单一加热循环需持续6~15分钟并将组织缓慢升温至50~100℃。须注意升温不宜过快，以免造成软组织碳化及蒸发伴微气泡形成，这两种情况均会增加阻抗和限制电流量，从而降低消融针的效果。
- 优点：RFA是目前最为成熟和普及的消融方法。总的手术时间短于冷冻消融。RFA能烧灼小血管而降低出血风险。RFA与其他消融技术相比是目前最具成本效益的方法。
- 缺点：RFA很大程度上依赖于良好的电导和组织热传导性能。消融区域不能很好进行实时监测。RFA极其容易受到热沉降效应的影响，此可导致残留未消融组织和消融范围不可预测。

Microwave ablation (MWA)

- Mechanism: An electromagnetic field is used to force polar molecules (mostly H_2O) to continuously realign with an oscillating electric field, which increases the kinetic energy of the molecules and results in heating. The microwave

微波消融(MWA)

- 机制：微波消融(MWA)利用电磁场迫使极性分子(主要是H_2O)在振荡电场中不断重新排列，以此增加分子的动能并导致升温。微波

energy is transmitted through the antenna and directly into the volume of tissue around the antenna. Rapid cell death occurs at temperatures greater than 55℃, and surrounding tissue can reach over 100℃. The antennas are then cooled with water or gas.

通过消融针将能量直接传输到消融针周围的组织。细胞在温度超过55℃时会迅速死亡，周围组织的温度可超过100℃。消融针杆用水或气体进行冷却。

- Technique: One MWA probe is placed with imaging guidance and the ablation is typically completed with one heating cycle. The power and duration of the heat is dependent on tumor size, but usually varies between 45W and 80W for 5–10 minutes.
- Advantages: MWA can generate very high temperatures, ablate through charred or necrotic tissue, and rapidly heats a large volume of tissue. It is less susceptible to heat sink effects from adjacent vessels and can cauterize blood vessels, decreasing bleeding risk. MWA has potential for simultaneous use of multiple antennas and does not require grounding pads, unlike RFA.
- Disadvantages: MWA uses larger diameter probes. There is a higher risk when ablating central tumors and any region with critical structures due to the inability to monitor the ablation zone in real time and relative unpredictability of the size and shape of the ablation zone. Similarly, due to the inability to precisely control the ablation zone, MWA is less precise with smaller tumors.

- 技术：消融针在影像引导下置于靶点，消融通常在一个加热周期内完成。加热的功率和持续时间取决于肿瘤的大小，但通常选择45~80W并持续5~10分钟。
- 优点：MWA可产生很高的温度，通过组织碳化或坏死，以及快速对大块组织加热进行。不易受到邻近血管的热沉降效应影响，且可烧灼血管，减少出血的风险。MWA可同时使用多个消融针，也不需要RFA的接地垫。
- 缺点：MWA使用直径较大的消融针。消融风险在中央型肿瘤或消融区包含任何重要结构的时候增加，其原因在于无法实时监控消融区，以及消融的范围和形状相对不可预测。同样，由于无法精确控制消融区，MWA对较小肿瘤的精确度较低。

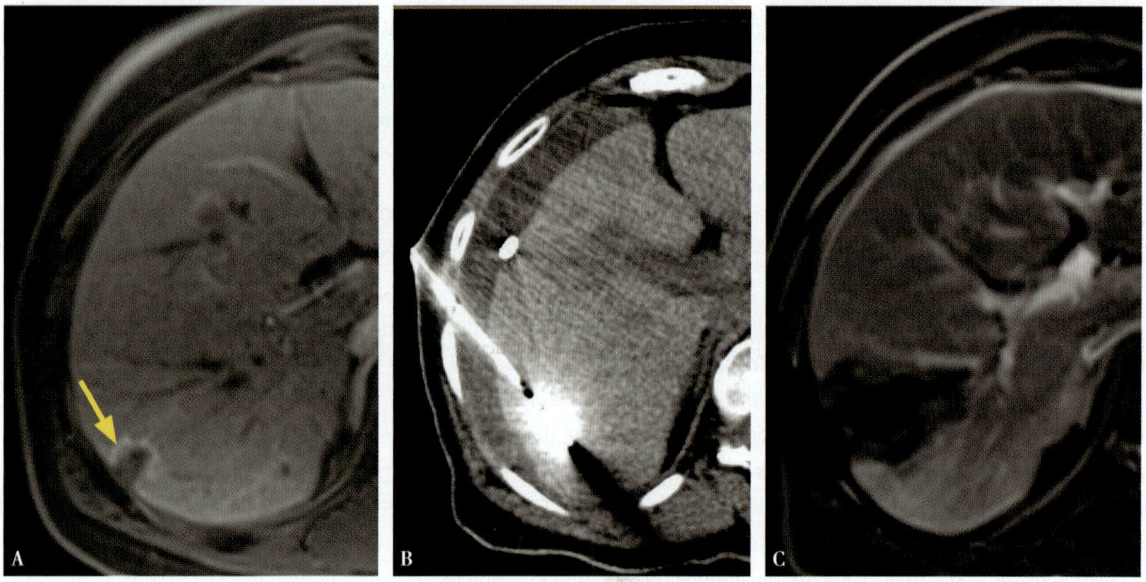

Microwave ablation in a 58-year-old female with epithelioid hemangioendothelioma of the liver. A) Axial T1 post-contrast image shows peripherally enhancing lesion (arrow). B) Intra-procedural noncontrast CT shows the ablation probe in the liver; the ablation zone is not well seen during the procedure. Note that artificial ascites was used to protect the adjacent diaphragm and body wall from injury, given peripheral location of the lesion. C) Axial T1 post-contrast subtraction image at two months shows complete ablation coverage of the tumor. Subtraction images are helpful to exclude residual tumoral enhancement.

Case courtesy of Sharath Bhagavatula, MD, Brigham and Women's Hospital.

微波消融治疗一名58岁女性的肝脏上皮样血管内皮瘤。A）轴位增强T_1图像显示边缘增强的病灶(黄箭)。B）术中平扫CT显示消融针位于肝内术中未能清晰显示的消融区；注意，因病变位置在外周，采用了人工腹水技术以保护邻近的膈肌和腹壁免受损伤。C）2个月后的轴位T_1对比减影图像显示肿瘤完全被消融区覆盖；减影图像有助于排除残留的肿瘤强化。

Cryoablation (CA)

- Mechanism: Rapid expansion of gas within the cryoablation (CA) probe cools the probe to −190 ℃ , resulting in an "iceball" of the surrounding tissue. At least two cycles of rapid freezing and slow thawing are done, each lasting 5–20 minutes. Cell death occurs secondary to immediate cellular toxicity or delayed apoptosis and ischemia.

冷冻消融(CA)

- 机制：冷冻消融(CA)针内气体快速膨胀使消融针冷却至−190℃，导致周围组织形成“冰球”。需至少进行2次快速冷冻和缓慢复温循环，每次持续5~20分钟。细胞死亡继发于即刻的细胞毒性或延迟的细胞凋亡和缺血。

- Technique: Probes are usually placed under CT or MRI guidance and should be spaced 1–2 cm apart. The iceball should extend at least 0.5 cm beyond the tumor to decrease likelihood of recurrence.
- Advantages: The iceball is well visualized in real time on CT, MRI, and ultrasound. There is comparatively less risk with cryoablation of central tumors. Multiple probes can be used simultaneously in cryoablation rather than sequentially. Cryoablation has a lower complication rate with typically less post-procedural pain.
- Disadvantages: Cryoablation has a slightly increased bleeding risk due to the lack of concurrent cautery. Multiple probes and several freeze-thaw cycles result in longer procedural time. Cryoablation creates a robust inflammatory response that may result in "cryoshock," typically seen with large volume liver cryoablation, which is mediated by cytokine production and consists of hypotension, multi-organ failure, and disseminated intravascular coagulation. Cryoablation may be associated with higher cost.

- 技术：通常在CT或MRI引导下插入消融针，针距间隔1~2cm。冰球应超出肿瘤至少0.5cm，以减少复发的可能性。
- 优点：CT、MRI和超声上均能很好地对冰球进行实时监控。中心位置肿瘤的CA风险相对较低。多个消融针可同时进行CA，而无须依次进行。CA的并发症发生率低，且术后疼痛通常较轻。
- 缺点：CA有轻微增加出血的风险，因其不具烧灼止血的功能。多针消融和多次CA循环会导致手术时间延长。CA可产生由细胞因子介导的严重炎症反应，可导致“冷休克”，表现为低血压、多器官衰竭和弥散性血管内凝血，通常见于大范围的肝脏CA。CA的成本较高。

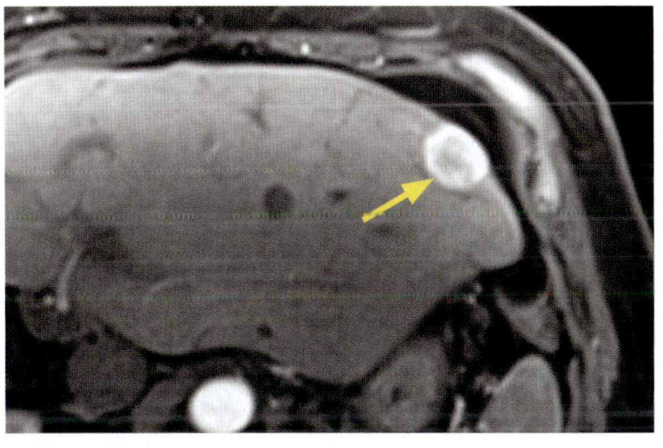

Axial T1-weighted post-contrast MRI shows an enhancing mass in segment 2 (yellow arrow).
轴位增强T_1加权MRI显示一个位于第二肝段内的强化肿块（黄箭）。

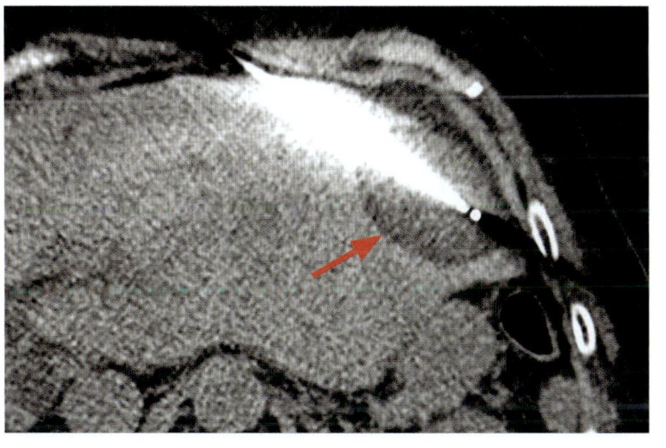

Intra-procedural axial noncontrast CT shows the well-defined hypodense iceball ablation zone (red arrow).
术中轴位平扫CT清晰显示边缘清晰的低密度冰球消融区（红箭）。

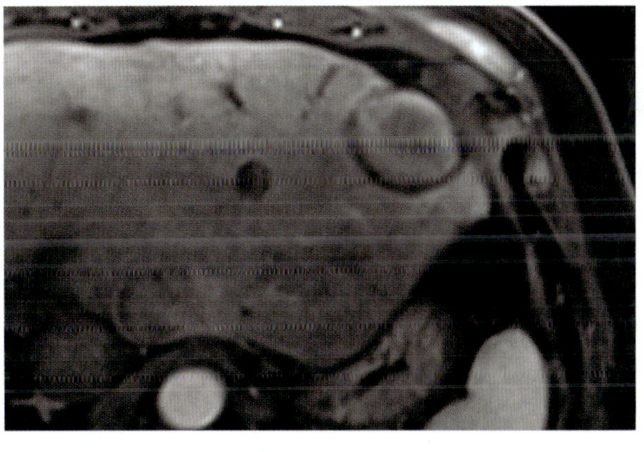

Axial MR post-contrast image at one month post-ablation shows complete ablation coverage of the tumor.
消融后1个月轴位增强MRI示肿瘤完全被消融区覆盖。

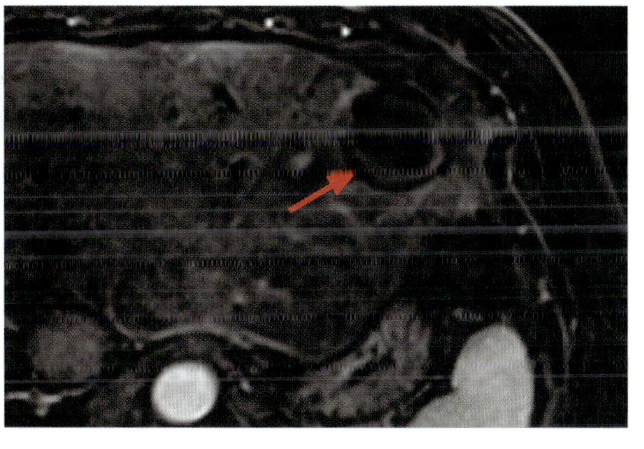

Axial MR post-contrast subtraction image shows linear peripheral enhancement (red arrow) which can be expected but should not become more nodular or extend out of the ablation margin over time.
轴位增强减影MRI显示一个边缘线性强化(红箭)，该表现符合预期，但不应在随访中出现结节状加重或突出于消融边缘之外。

Cryoablation in a 75-year-old female with metastatic neuroendocrine tumor.
冷冻消融术治疗75岁女性转移性神经内分泌肿瘤。
Case courtesy of Sharath Bhagavatula, MD, Brigham and Women's Hospital.

HEPATOCELLULAR CARCINOMA AND LIVER METASTASES

- Normal liver parenchyma receives majority of its blood supply from the portal vein, whereas hepatocellular carcinoma (HCC) is preferentially supplied by the hepatic artery. Catheter-directed transarterial therapies for palliative treatment of HCC, such as transarterial chemoembolization (TACE) or transarterial radioembolization (TARE) described below, take advantage of this mismatch in blood supply by deliverying treatment directly into feeding arteries of the tumor while minimizing adverse effect to normal liver parenchyma.
- TACE and TARE are also used as bridging therapy to liver transplant for patients with HCC, and for locoregional treatment of other primary hepatic malignancies (e.g. cholangiocarcinoma) and hepatic metastases.

Transarterial chemoembolization (TACE)

- Conventional TACE (cTACE) consists of intra-arterial infusion of chemotherapy followed by embolization of the tumor's arterial blood supply with particles or gelfoam.
- TACE with drug eluting beads (DEB-TACE) uses microspheres that embolize and deliver chemotherapy.
- Both types of TACE promote tumor cell death by 1) delivering high dose of cytotoxic chemotherapy to the tumor than can be administered via a systemic route, and 2) inducing local hypoxia and ischemia.
- Common contraindications of TACE include:

  Portal vein thrombosis (associated with post-treatment liver failure).

  High tumor burden (>50%).

  Extrahepatic metastases.

  Decompensated cirrhosis (encephalopathy, tension ascites, Child-Pugh C).

  Elevated bilirubin (>3 mg/dL).
- Pre-procedural cross-sectional imaging is usually performed for treatment planning, with the goals of: evaluate for variant anatomy, extrahepatic collateral blood supply (i.e., right phrenic artery), and possible contraindications.
- Procedural steps:

  After obtaining arterial access, celiac arteriogram is done to map out anatomy.

  Selective or super-selective embolization can be done with the use of a catheter or micro-catheter into the proximal arterial branches of a small tumor.

  Alternatively, medications or embolic agents can be delivered from a proximal point (left or right hepatic artery), called lobar embolization, if there are multiple lesions.

  Materials are injected until stasis/low flow is seen under fluoroscopy.

  Arteriography is performed to document persistent low flow or absence of flow to the region.
- Immediate post-procedural CT imaging is usually avoided because normal post-procedural changes may mimic an abscess.

肝细胞癌和肝转移癌

- 正常肝实质的主要血供来自门静脉，而肝细胞癌(HCC)的血供主要来自肝动脉。采用经动脉导管插管对HCC姑息性治疗，如以下所述的经动脉化疗栓塞术(TACE)或经动脉放射栓塞术(TARE)，利用了这种不匹配的血液供应，将治疗药物通过供血动脉直接释放到肿瘤处，同时还可减少对正常肝实质的毒性作用。
- TACE和TARE同时也被用于肝移植患者的桥接治疗，以及其他原发性肝脏恶性肿瘤(如胆管癌)和肝转移癌的局部治疗。

经动脉化疗栓塞术(TACE)

- 传统经动脉化疗栓塞术(cTACE)包括动脉灌注化疗，以及随即使用颗粒或明胶海绵栓塞以阻断肿瘤的动脉供血。
- 载药微球TACE(DEB-TACE)使用微球进行栓塞并释放化疗药物。
- 这两种类型的TACE均会促进肿瘤细胞死亡，它们通过以下机制起效：①向肿瘤输送显著高于全身途径给药的细胞毒性化疗药物；②诱导局部缺氧和缺血。
- 常见的TACE禁忌证：

  门静脉癌栓(与治疗后肝功能衰竭相关)。

  高负荷肿瘤(>50%)。

  肝外转移。

  失代偿性肝硬化(脑病、张力性腹水、Child-Pugh评分C级)。

  胆红素升高(>3mg/dL)。
- 术前横断面成像常用于制订治疗计划，其目的是评估解剖变异、肝外侧支血供(如右膈动脉)和可能的禁忌证。
- 手术步骤：

  动脉穿刺后进行腹腔干动脉造影以明确解剖结构。

  使用导管或微导管进入小肿瘤的近端动脉分支进行选择性或超选择性栓塞。

  如果病灶多发，还可从近端(肝左动脉或肝右动脉)给药物或栓塞，通常称为肝叶栓塞。

  在透视下注入栓塞材料直到血流停滞/减慢。

  动脉造影确认该区域为持续低血流或无血流。
- 通常避免术后即行CT检查，因术后正常改变可类似脓肿。

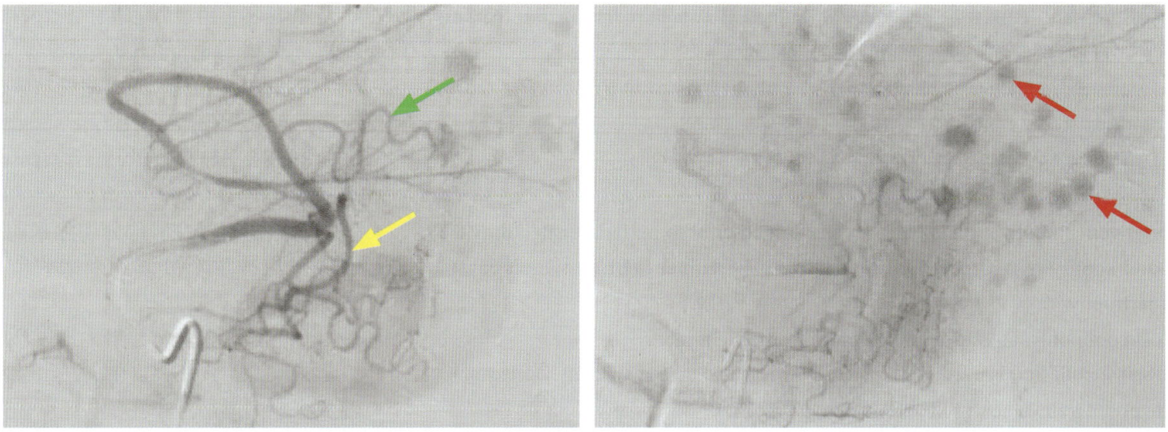

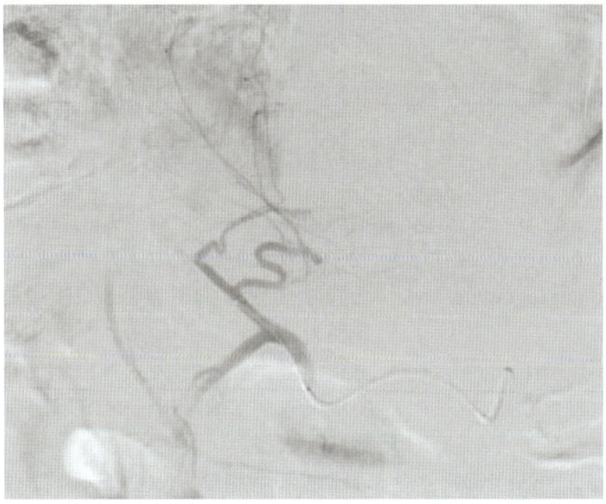

TACE in a patient with recurrent HCC:
Selective DSA of celiac artery (top left image) shows patent middle (green arrow) and left hepatic arteries (yellow arrow). Superselective middle hepatic artery with multifocal hypervascular tumor blushes (top right image, red arrows). TACE of the middle hepatic artery was performed with two vials of 100–300 micron DEB loaded with 100 mg doxorubicin. Follow-up angiography demonstrated pruning of distal arterial branches and no residual tumor enhancement in the embolized territory.
Case courtesy Arjun Sharma, MD, Brigham and Women's Hospital.

HCC复发患者的TACE：
选择性腹腔动脉DSA(左上图片)显示肝中动脉(绿箭)和肝左动脉(黄箭)通畅。超选择肝中动脉可见多个富血供肿瘤染色(右上图，红箭)。对肝中动脉进行了TACE，使用2瓶100~300μm并载有100mg阿霉素的DEB。后续的血管造影显示远端动脉分支呈剪枝样影，栓塞区域无残余肿瘤强化。

- Post-embolization syndrome is very common after TACE. Symptoms include right upper quadrant pain, fever, nausea, and vomiting. LFT may show transaminitis.
- Other common complications include: abscess, acute liver failure, or biliary injuries (the biliary tree is primarily supplied by hepatic arteries).

Transarterial radioembolization (TARE)

- TARE, also called selective internal radiation therapy (SIRT), consists of intra-arterial infusion of microspheres with radioactive isotopes (i.e., Yttrium-90).
- TARE does not have the same macro-embolic effects as TACE. Treatment effect depends on radiation emitted by the spheres which induce tumor necrosis. Intra-arterial administration allows for targeted delivery of high radiation dose to the tumor than can be given via external beam radiation.
- Due to less disruption of vessels, TARE can be performed in the setting of portal vein thrombosis.
- Absolute contraindications include: pregnancy, breastfeeding, uncorrectable GI vascular reflux, and uncorrectable hepatopulmonary shunting.
- TARE procedure is similar to TACE except for a few differences as below:

  After angiography to map out the anatomy, labeled macroaggregates of albumin (MAA) are injected, followed by a nuclear medicine study to confirm tracer uptake.

  The distribution of MAA is similar to that of the radioembolization microspheres, which allows mapping, calculation of dose, and evaluation for potential extrahepatic shunt or nontarget embolization (i.e., uptake in lungs, GI, skin).

- 栓塞后综合征在TACE后非常常见。症状包括右上腹疼痛、发热、恶心和呕吐。肝功能检查可有转氨酶升高。
- 其他常见的并发症包括脓肿、急性肝衰竭或胆道损伤(胆管主要由肝动脉供血)。

经动脉放射栓塞术(TARE)

- 经动脉放射栓塞术(TARE)，也被称为选择性内放射治疗(SIRT)，指动脉灌注带有放射性同位素(如^{90}钇)微球。
- TARE没有TACE所产生的宏观栓塞效应。治疗效果取决于微球发出可诱导肿瘤坏死的辐射。动脉内给药较外照射能更有针对性地向肿瘤提供高剂量的辐射。
- TARE对血管的破坏性小，因而可用于门静脉癌栓的患者。
- 绝对禁忌证包括妊娠、哺乳、不可纠正的胃肠血管反流和不可纠正的肝-肺分流。
- TARE手术操作与TACE的过程类似，以下为不同之处：

  在血管造影获得血管解剖信息以后，注射带有标记的聚合大颗粒人血白蛋白(MAA)，行核医学检查以确认示踪剂摄取。

  MAA的分布与放射栓塞微球的分布类似，可对颗粒分布、剂量计算和潜在的肝外分流或非靶栓塞(如肺、胃肠道、皮肤摄取)进行评估。

TARE should NEVER be performed when there is a shunt to the GI tract, because even small amounts can cause enteritis or ulceration.

TARE绝不可用于消化道有分流的患者，因为即使是少量的微球也会引起肠炎或溃疡。

To prevent nontarget embolization, coil embolization of nearby arteries can be performed.

为防止非靶向栓塞，可对附近动脉进行弹簧圈栓塞。

TARE does NOT cause significant post-embolization syndrome.

TARE不会引起严重的栓塞后综合征。

Portal vein embolization

门静脉栓塞

- Portal vein embolization is typically performed prior to partial hepatectomy.
- Blood supply is redirected to the future liver remnant (FLR) which causes hypertrophy.
- Most commonly, target for embolization is the right lobe.

  Right hepatic lobe is usually large enough to maintain function after left hepatectomy.
- The portal vein is accessed percutaneously.
- Contraindications: Patients with portal hypertension or extensive ipsilateral tumor thrombus should not undergo portal vein embolization due to risk of altered hemodynamics and massive tumoral necrosis.

- 门静脉栓塞通常在肝部分切除术前进行。
- 血液供应被重新分流到未来残留肝脏(FLR)以促进增生。
- 最常见的栓塞靶器官是肝右叶。

  肝右叶通常足够大，足以维持左肝切除术后的功能。
- 经皮穿刺门静脉。
- 禁忌证：门静脉高压或肿瘤一侧有广泛癌栓患者不应考虑门静脉栓塞术，因为有血流动力学改变和肿瘤大面积坏死的风险。

Renal neoplasms and angiomyolipoma

肾肿瘤和血管平滑肌脂肪瘤

Renal cell carcinoma (RCC)

- Most renal cell carcinomas (RCC) are hypervascular. The tumors often feature arteriovenous shunting and venous lakes, with a classic angiographic appearance of *bizarre neovascularity*.
- Radiofrequency ablation has been a successful minimally invasive treatment for RCC in patients who are not good operative candidates.

肾细胞癌(RCC)

- 大多数肾细胞癌(RCC)为富血供。肿瘤常以动静脉瘘和静脉湖为特征，典型的血管造影表现为*奇异的新生血管*。
- 射频消融术已经作为一种微创治疗手段成功用于失去手术治疗指征的RCC患者。

Oncocytoma

- Oncocytoma is a benign renal mass that cannot be reliably distinguished from renal cell carcinoma on cross-sectional imaging.
- Angiography classically shows a *spokewheel* appearance with a peritumoral halo. In contrast to RCC, bizarre neoplastic vessels are absent.

嗜酸细胞腺瘤

- 肾嗜酸细胞腺瘤是一种良性肾脏肿块，在横断面影像上无法与肾细胞癌进行明确区分。
- 典型的血管造影为辐条轮状外观伴瘤周晕，缺乏RCC的奇异肿瘤血管。

Angiomyolipoma (AML)

血管平滑肌脂肪瘤(AML)

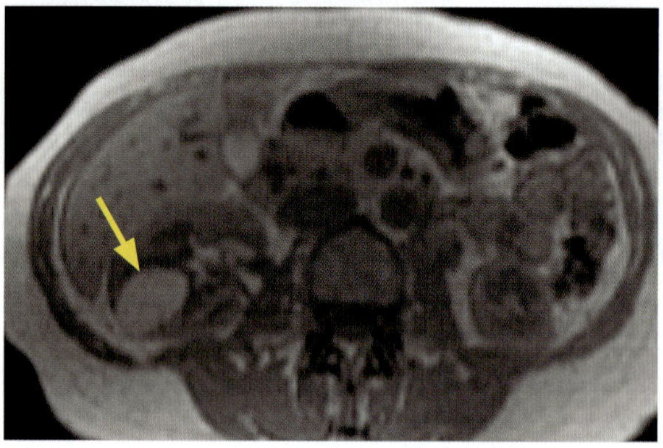

Axial T1-weighted MRI shows a mass in the lower pole of the right kidney which is isointense to fat (arrow).

轴位T_1加权MRI显示右肾下极肿块，信号与脂肪相等(黄箭)。

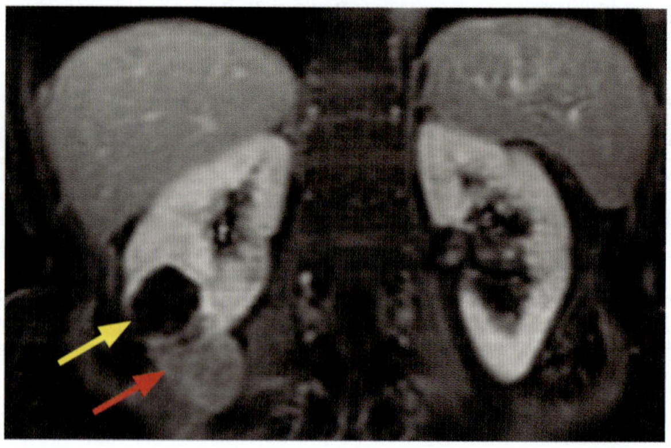

Coronal T1-weighted post-contrast fat-saturated MRI shows saturation of the upper component of the mass (yellow arrow), consistent with macroscopic fat. An inferior enhancing component is present (red arrow).

冠状位增强T_1加权脂肪饱和MRI显示肿块上半部分呈饱和(黄箭)，与宏观脂肪一致。下半部分呈现增强(红箭)。

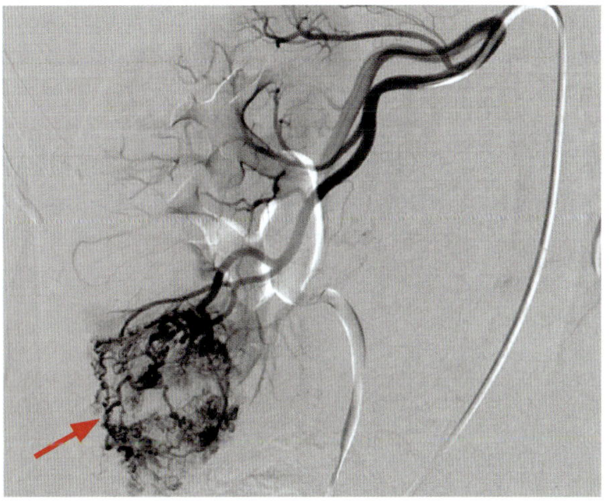

Superselective digital subtraction arteriogram of a right renal artery branch shows intense tumor blush in the lower pole (red arrow). There is no AV shunting.

超选择性右肾动脉分支数字减影动脉造影显示下极明显的肿瘤血管影(红箭),无动静脉瘘。

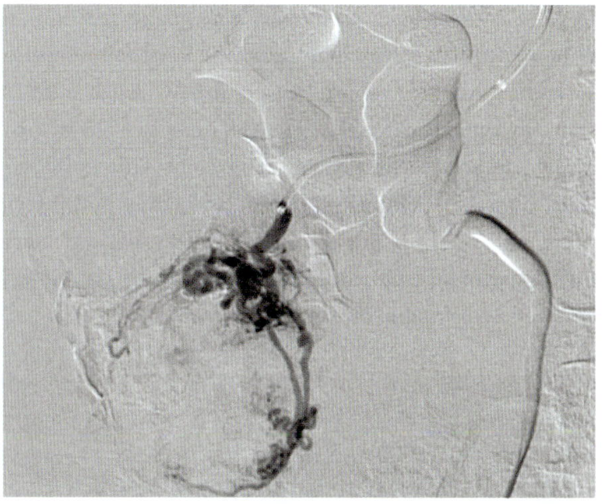

After super-selective embolization with particles, there is markedly reduced flow. Tortuous feeding arteries are still present peripherally.

经超选择性颗粒栓塞后,血流明显减少。周围仍有扭曲的供血动脉。

Angiomyolipoma: *Case courtesy Bela Kis, MD, Brigham and Women's Hospital.*

- Renal angiomyolipoma is a hypervascular hamartoma containing blood vessels (angio), smooth muscle (myo), and fat (lipoma). An AML is diagnosed on cross-sectional imaging as a renal mass containing macroscopic fat.
- Angiography shows tortuous feeding arteries, which have a sunburst appearance on the parenchymal phase. Occasionally, small aneurysms are visible, which predispose to risk of hemorrhage, especially if the AML is > 4 cm in diameter. In contrast to a renal arteriovenous fistula, AMLs do not feature arteriovenous shunting–that is, no veins will be opacified during arterial phase imaging.
- It is not always possible to differentiate an AML from RCC on angiography, so cross-sectional imaging is usually indicated if a suspected AML is diagnosed incidentally.

- 肾血管平滑肌脂肪瘤(AML)是一种含有血管(angio)、平滑肌(myo)和脂肪(lipoma)的富血管错构瘤。AML在横断面影像上表现为肾肿块内有宏观可见的脂肪组织。
- 血管造影显示扭曲的供血动脉,在实质期表现为"日光样"散射。偶见小动脉瘤,可增加出血的风险,尤其是当AML直径>4cm时。与肾动静脉瘘不同,AML不具有动静脉分流的特征,即静脉在动脉期不显影。
- 血管造影并不总能区别AML和RCC,因此,偶然发现AML可疑时常需行横断面成像。

(翻译 靳勇)

GENITOURINARY INTERVENTIONS

泌尿生殖介入

UPPER URINARY TRACT OBSTRUCTION

上尿路梗阻

Percutaneous nephrostomy (PCN) indications

- The most common indication for percutaneous nephrostomy (PCN) is urinary diversion of an obstructed kidney due to stone, malignancy, or stricture. Pyonephrosis (pus in the collecting system) is an emergent indication for percutaneous nephrostomy.
- Less commonly, PCN may be used to place an antegrade ureteral stent if a retrograde ureteral stent is unable to be placed cystoscopically.

经皮肾造瘘术(PCN)的适应证

- 经皮肾造瘘术(PCN)最常见的适应证是对梗阻肾进行尿液分流,病因包括结石、恶性肿瘤或狭窄。肾盂积脓(脓液位于集合系统)是经皮肾盂造瘘术的紧急指征。
- 较为少见的适应证是在膀胱镜逆行插管失败时通过PCN顺行植入输尿管支架。

Percutaneous nephrostomy technique

- Direct visualization of the collecting system is necessary. In most cases, urinary obstruction will lead to hydronephrosis, allowing ultrasound-directed puncture. If there is no dilation of the collecting system, intravenous contrast can be administered to opacify the nondilated collecting system and allow fluoroscopic guidance.

经皮肾造瘘术的技术

- 必须能直接观察到集合系统。多数情况下,尿路梗阻会导致肾盂积水,可行超声引导穿刺。若无集合系统扩张,可静脉注射造影剂,使未扩张的集合系统显影,以便在透视引导下穿刺。

- The patient is positioned prone and a 22-gauge needle is used for direct posterior access. Bleeding complications can be minimized by entering the kidney in the relatively avascular *zone of Brödel,* which is defined as the plane between the ventral and dorsal renal artery branches. The optimal entry plane is therefore in the posterolateral kidney directed towards a posterior calyx.
- Complications most commonly include bleeding and infection. Although transient hematuria occurs in nearly every patient, serious bleeding complications are rare. Of particular concern in cases of pre-existing infection is the risk of sepsis caused by extensive manipulation.

- 患者取俯卧位，使用22G穿刺针从后方直接进针。为减少出血并发症，可选择肾脏血管相对稀少的Brödel区穿刺进针，此区为肾动脉背侧和腹侧血管分支之间的平面，故最佳的进针位置是从肾的后外侧向后组肾盏进针。
- 最常见的并发症为出血和感染。术后几乎所有患者均会发生一过性血尿，但严重出血极少见。特别需要警惕的是，若存在尿路感染，术中过多操作会增加败血症的风险。

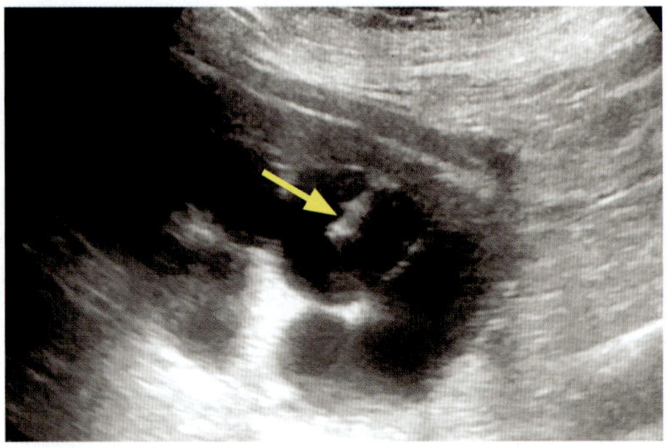

Ultrasound shows a dilated collecting system and 21G needle tip (arrow) within the posterior interpolar calyx.
超声显示扩张的集合系统和21G针的尖端(黄箭)位于后组中极肾盏内。

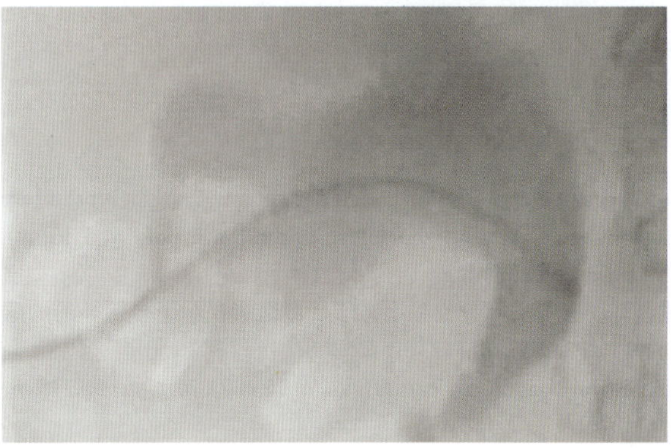

Fluoroscopy image of an antegrade nephrostogram shows a dilated collecting system.
顺行肾盂造影显示扩张的集合系统。

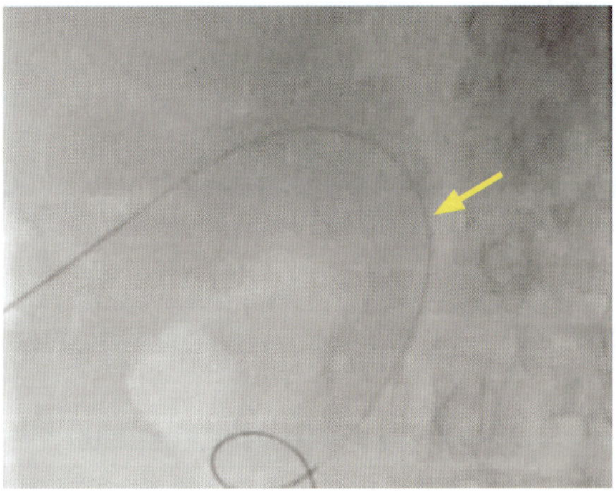

Fluoroscopy spot image shows guide wire (arrow) within the collecting system and proximal ureter.
局部透视影像显示导丝位于集合系统和近端输尿管内(黄箭)。

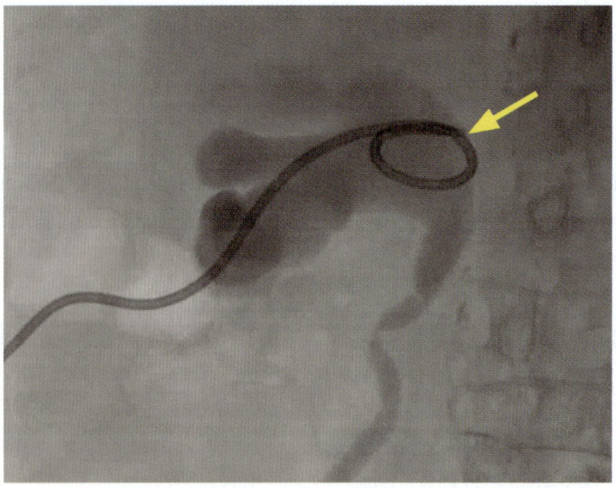

Spot radiograph shows nephrostomy tube with loop (arrow) locked in the renal pelvis.
局部影像显示肾造瘘管末端盘曲(黄箭)锁定在肾盂内。

Uterine Fibroids and Menorrhagia

Uterine artery embolization (UAE)

- The two primary indications of uterine artery embolization (UAE) are symptomatic treatment of fibroids and postpartum hemorrhage.
- In the United States, particles (e.g., tris-acryl gelatin microspheres, polyvinyl alcohol particles) are most commonly used in UAE for fibroids, while gelatin foam is usually used for postpartum hemorrhage.

子宫肌瘤和月经过多

子宫动脉栓塞术(UAE)

- 子宫动脉栓塞术(UAE)的两个主要适应证是症状性子宫肌瘤与产后出血。
- 在美国，颗粒(如三羟甲基-丙烯酸明胶微球、聚乙烯醇颗粒)是最常用于UAE治疗子宫肌瘤的栓塞剂，而明胶海绵通常用于治疗产后出血。

- The goal of fibroid treatment is to produce ischemic infarction of the hypervascular fibroids while still maintaining adequate perfusion to the endometrium and myometrium, thus preserving future fertility.
- There is approximately a 1.25% serious complication rate for UAE, which is especially important to consider as many of these patients are otherwise healthy reproductive-age women. Serious complications include abscess, endometritis, and ovarian insufficiency due to non-target embolization, leading to transient amenorrhea or premature menopause.

- 肌瘤治疗的目的是使富血供的肌瘤产生缺血性梗死的同时仍保持子宫内膜和肌层有足够灌注，从而保留生育能力。
- UAE的严重并发症发生率约为1.25%，但必须要强调，这些患者除有肌瘤外，大多是健康的育龄期妇女。严重并发症包括脓肿、子宫内膜炎，以及非靶栓塞引起的卵巢功能不全致短暂闭经或过早绝经。

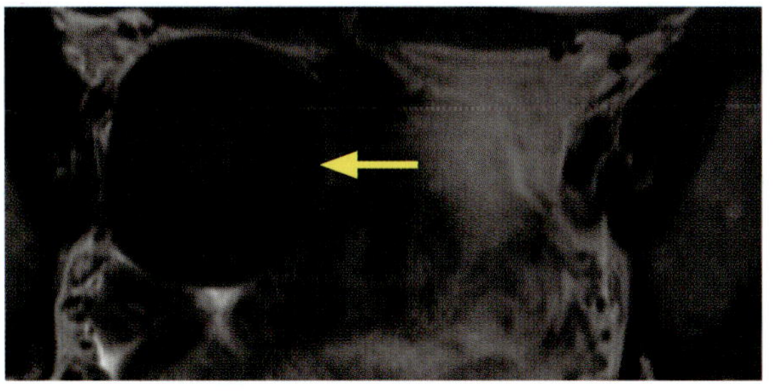

Axial T2-weighted MRI shows a large, hypointense fibroid (arrow).
轴位T_2加权MRI显示一处大的低信号肌瘤(黄箭)。

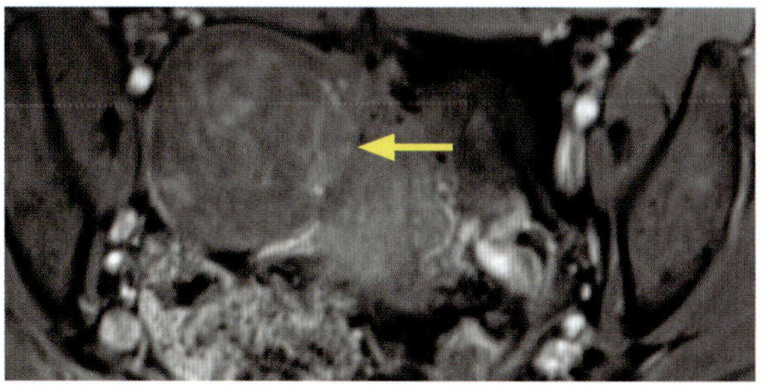

Post-contrast axial T1-weighted MRI shows heterogeneous enhancement of the fibroid (arrow).
轴位增强T_1加权MRI显示肌瘤不均匀强化(黄箭)。

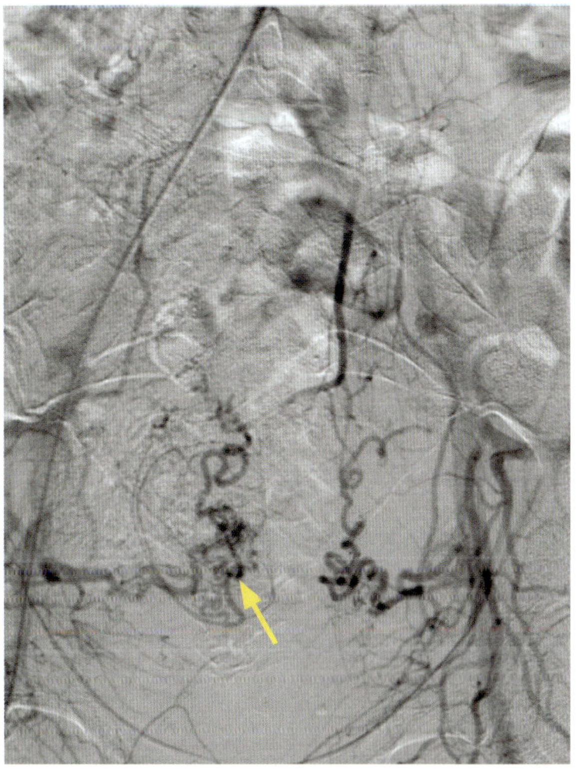

Nonselective late arterial phase digital subtraction angiogram of the internal iliac arteries with the flush catheter in the distal aorta (not visualized) shows the bilateral hypertrophied uterine arteries, more prominent on the right (arrow).
将高流量导管(未显示)置于主动脉远端行非选择性髂内动脉数字减影血管造影，动脉晚期显示双侧子宫动脉粗大，右侧更为明显(黄箭)。
Case courtesy Alisa Suzuki Han, MD, Brigham and Women's Hospital.

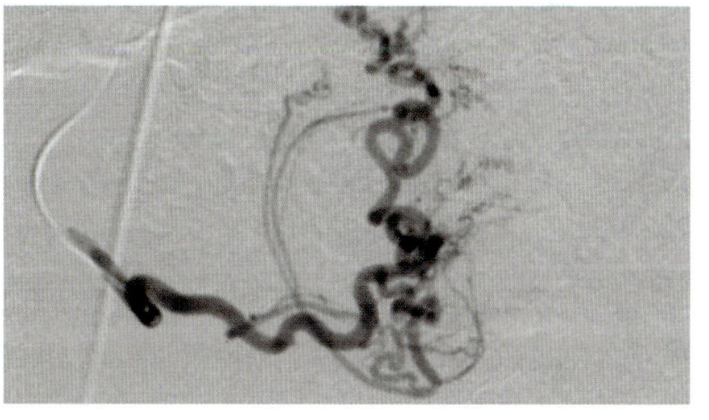

Pre-embolization selective digital subtraction angiogram of the right uterine artery demonstrates the enlarged, tortuous vessels.
栓塞前选择性数字减影血管造影显示右侧子宫动脉粗大迂曲。

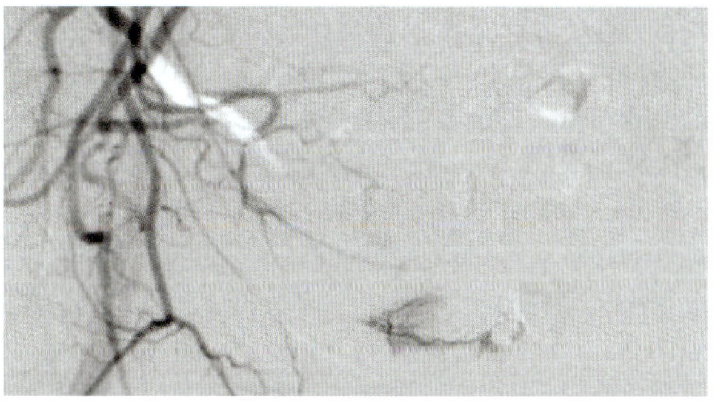

Post-treatment nonselective angiogram of the right internal artery anterior division (catheter not visualized) demonstrates near-stasis of the uterine artery, which is the desired end-point. A small amount of contrast is seen medially in the bladder.
栓塞后非选择性右髂内动脉前干血管造影(未见导管)显示子宫动脉血流接近停滞，为理想的栓塞终点。膀胱内可见少量造影剂。

Prostate Disease

Prostate artery embolization (PAE)

- Prostate artery embolization (PAE) is a safe and effective treatment for benign prostatic hyperplasia. PAE is recommended for patients with moderate to severe symptoms of urinary obstruction.
- PAE causes ischemic necrosis of the prostate gland which in turn results in gland volume reduction, thereby improving symptoms.
- Preprocedural cross-sectional imaging is usually done to assess internal iliac artery anatomy.

  The prostate artery origin is highly variable.

  Common origin of prostate artery includes: Superior vesical artery, internal pudendal artery, obturator artery, or from the internal iliac artery directly.
- Procedural steps:

  Patients are treated with antibiotics and anti-inflammatory medications during the procedure and recovery.

  Access can be performed from common femoral or radial artery approach.

  From the femoral approach, the contralateral internal iliac artery is catheterized and catheter is positioned in the proximal internal iliac artery.

  Then, an angiogram is performed and the prostate artery is selected with a microcatheter. Prostate artery angiogram is performed to evaluate for prostate opacification and for collateral vessels.

  To avoid potential non-target embolization, superselective catheterization or coil embolization of anastomoses may be performed.

  Embolization is performed until near stasis. Angiogram is repeated to document slow or absence of flow. Ipsilateral internal iliac artery is selected and procedure is repeated.
- Common minor complications include hematuria, hematospermia, and dysuria.
- Recent randomized control trial comparing PAE to TURP showed that International Prostate Symptom Score (IPSS) did not differ significantly between patient groups at 12 weeks, with significantly lower adverse events and blood loss after PAE.

前列腺疾病

前列腺动脉栓塞术(PAE)

- 前列腺动脉栓塞术(PAE)是治疗良性前列腺增生的一种安全和有效的方法。PAE适用于有中至重度尿路梗阻症状的患者。
- PAE引起前列腺缺血性坏死，使腺体体积缩小，从而改善症状。
- 术前常行断层显像以评估髂内动脉的解剖结构。

  前列腺动脉的起源高度变异。

  常见的前列腺动脉起源包括膀胱上动脉、阴部内动脉、闭孔动脉或直接起源于髂内动脉。
- 操作步骤：

  患者在术中和术后接受抗生素和抗炎药物。

  血管入路可选择股总动脉或桡动脉。

  经股动脉入路时，导管插入对侧髂内动脉，导管头置于髂内动脉近端。

  血管造影之后，微导管插入前列腺动脉，行前列腺动脉血管造影评估前列腺染色和侧支血管情况。

  为避免潜在的非靶栓塞，必要时进行超选择性插管或弹簧圈栓塞吻合支。

  栓塞终点为血流接近停滞。重复进行血管造影以证实血流变慢或消失。行同侧髂内动脉插管，再重复上述步骤。
- 常见的轻微并发症包括血尿、血精症和排尿困难。
- 近期的一项比较PAE和经尿道前列腺切除术(TURP)的随机对照试验表明，12周时两组患者之间的国际前列腺症状评分(IPSS)无显著差异，但在PAE后，不良事件和失血发生率有明显降低。

Adrenal Vein Sampling

- Adrenal vein sampling can be performed to determine laterality or diagnose adrenal hyperplasia in the setting of hyperaldosteronism.
- The procedure can be performed either with simultaneous left and right sampling or sequentially sampling the right and left.
- A Renal Double Curve (RDC) catheter is helpful for selecting the adrenal vein.

肾上腺静脉采血

- 在醛固酮增多症时，肾上腺静脉采血可用于判别和诊断哪一侧有肾上腺增生。
- 可同时对左右两侧采血或依次进行。
- 肾双弯导管(RDC)有助于选择性肾上腺静脉插管。

(翻译　杨国威)

Lines, Tubes and Drains

血管通道、插管与引流

Dialysis Access and Interventions

Arteriovenous fistula

- A surgical fistula for dialysis access provides good long-term patency (85% at two years), but requires several months to "mature" and about 30% of fistulas fail to mature. A fistula is mature when the veins have enlarged sufficiently to allow the high flow rates for dialysis.

透析通路与介入治疗

动静脉瘘

- 外科手术建立的动静脉瘘具有良好的长期透析通畅率(2年为85%)，但需数月才能"成熟"，其中30%左右的瘘不能达到成熟。动静脉瘘成熟是指静脉充分扩张并满足透析所需的高

- Once mature, a fistula can remain patent even with relatively low flow rates.
- The two common fistula locations are:

  Radial artery → g cephalic vein at the wrist

  Brachial artery → variable veins in the forearm
- Common causes of late fistula failure include venous outflow stenosis and peri-anastomotic venous stenosis.

血流量。

- 动静脉瘘一旦成熟，即使流量相对较低仍能保持通畅。
- 常用的两个动静脉瘘的位置是：

  桡动脉→腕部的头静脉

  肱动脉→前臂各条静脉
- 瘘管晚期功能失常的常见原因有静脉流出道狭窄或吻合口周围的静脉狭窄。

Polytetrafluorethylene (PTFE) graft

- A polytetrafluorethylene (PTFE) graft is a short bridge of synthetic graft material placed surgically between an adjacent artery and vein. Grafts have only 50% patency at two years, but are able to be used sooner than fistulas. Grafts require higher flow rates to remain patent compared to fistulas.
- Similar to a fistula, the most common cause of graft failure is a venous stenosis, either at the venous anastomosis or outflow vein.

Polytetrafluarethylene(PTFE)人造血管

- PTFE人造血管是人工合成的一段短的搭桥血管，用外科手术的方法将其与相邻的动脉和静脉连接。人造血管的2年通畅率仅为50%，但术后透析早于动静脉瘘。与动静脉瘘相比，人造血管需较高的血流量以维持其通畅。
- 与动静脉瘘类似，人造血管最常见的失败原因是静脉狭窄，不是在静脉吻合端就是在静脉流出道。

Clinical evaluation of surgical dialysis access

- A pulsatile fistula with lack of thrill suggests venous outflow obstruction.
- High access recirculation at dialysis suggests venous outflow stenosis.
- Weak pulse and poor thrill suggests arterial inflow stenosis.
- Complete absence of a pulse suggests arterial thrombosis.
- A pulseless fistula suggests thrombosed fistula.

临床评估外科透析通路

- 瘘有搏动但无震颤提示静脉流出道梗阻。
- 透析时高通路再循环提示静脉流出端狭窄。
- 搏动和震颤均微弱提示动脉流入端狭窄。
- 完全无脉搏搏动提示动脉血栓形成。
- 瘘无搏动提示血栓形成。

Venous stenosis of surgical dialysis access

- Venous outflow stenoses are typically treated with angioplasty, often requiring high pressure or cutting balloons to dilate the fibrotic lesions.
- The goal of the procedure is to restore a palpable thrill and pulse, or to restore the venous to brachial artery pressure ratio to less than 0.4.

外科透析通路中的静脉狭窄

- 静脉流出道狭窄的治疗一般采用血管成形术，常需高压或切割球囊扩张纤维性病变。
- 手术的目标是恢复可触及的震颤和搏动，或使静脉与肱动脉压比恢复到0.4以下。

Thrombosis of surgical dialysis access

- Both arteriovenous fistulas and PTFE grafts may become thrombosed. In general, PTFE grafts are simpler to declot compared to fistulas as the thrombus is usually limited to the graft.
- Thrombosis is often secondary to venous stenosis, which must be treated as well.
- Either pharmacologic or mechanical thrombosis can be performed.

外科透析通路中的血栓形成

- 动静脉瘘和PTFE人造血管均可形成血栓。一般而言，PTFE人造血管的血栓比动静脉瘘的容易清除，因其血栓常局限于人造血管内。
- 血栓形成常继发于静脉狭窄，后者也必须处理。
- 可采用药物或机械溶栓。

Central venous access

- Central venous access can either be centrally inserted or peripherally inserted. There are multiple different catheter options and determining factors include type of treatment, duration, and frequency of infusions.
- Common indications for central venous access include inability to obtain adequate peripheral venous access, frequent blood draws, administration of substances that are not safe to administer in peripheral veins (chemotherapy, vasopressors, TPN), hemodialysis, and plasmapheresis.
- The patient is prepped and draped in a sterile fashion. The preferred vein of choice for centrally inserted catheters is the internal jugular vein, but if occluded, other neck veins like the external jugular vein can be used. Access is obtained under ultrasound guidance.
- After placement, it is important to aspirate blood to confirm proper placement and to subsequently flush the catheter with heparinized saline to prevent thrombosis.
- Common complications include infection, accidental arterial puncture, bleeding, and pneumothorax.

中心静脉通路

- 中心静脉通路既可从中央，也可从外周插入。有多种不同的导管可供选择，决定因素包括治疗类型、持续时间和使用频率。
- 中心静脉通路的常见适应证包括无法建立合适的外周静脉通路、频繁抽血、不能在外周安全地从静脉给药［化疗药、血管升压素、完全肠外营养(TPN)］、血液透析和血浆置换术。
- 按无菌原则对患者进行术前准备和铺巾。中央型插管的首选静脉是颈内静脉，但若阻塞，也可选择其他颈静脉，如颈外静脉。可在超声引导下进行穿刺。
- 置管后回抽血液非常重要，以确认导管位置恰当，随后用肝素化生理盐水冲洗导管以防血栓形成。
- 常见并发症包括感染、误穿动脉、出血和气胸。

Nontunneled catheter

- Nontunneled catheters are typically placed at bedside or in the ICU setting when the patient is too unstable to travel and only local anesthesia is necessary.
- Nontunneled catheters can have up to 5 lumens. Indications include the general indications for a central venous catheter, need for rapid resuscitation and pressure monitoring.
- Prolonged use (weeks to months) of a nontunneled catheter at the femoral, internal jugular, or subclavian site should be avoided due to the increased risk of infection.
- When no longer needed, these can be easily removed at bedside.

非隧道式导管

- 非隧道式导管通常适用于床边或ICU环境中，此类患者病情太不稳定而不易搬动，此时仅需局部麻醉。
- 非隧道式导管最多可有5个管腔。适应证包括中心静脉导管的一般适应证及需要快速复苏和监测压力。
- 应避免在股静脉、颈内静脉或锁骨下静脉部位长时间使用(数周至数月)非隧道式导管，以减少感染风险。
- 如不再需要，导管可在床旁轻松移除。

Tunneled catheter

- Tunneled catheters are placed in the interventional radiology suite and require conscious sedation.
- The lifespan of a tunneled catheter is weeks to months, some are even used for years.
- Common indications for tunneled catheters are administration of chemotherapy, TPN, plasmapheresis, and hemodialysis.
- Ongoing infection or positive blood cultures are contraindications for placement.
- Subcutaneous lidocaine is infused along the expected course of the catheter. The catheter cuff is typically placed 1 cm from the skin entry into the tunnel to facilitate easy removal.
- Tunneled catheters can usually be removed at bedside. Care must be taken to ensure complete removal of the cuff.
- If there is concern of infection, submit the tip for culture after removal.

隧道式导管

- 植入隧道式导管需在介入放射手术室中进行，需静脉镇静麻醉。
- 隧道式导管的使用寿命为数周至数月，有些甚至可使用数年。
- 隧道式导管的常见适应证是化疗、TPN、血浆置换和血液透析。
- 置管的禁忌证为持续感染或血培养阳性。
- 在预计导管的路径上皮下注射利多卡因。导管的固定袖套应位于距离皮肤入口1cm处，以便移除。
- 隧道式导管常可在床边取出。须确保完整移除导管的固定袖套。
- 考虑感染时，在取出后将导管头送培养。

Subcutaneous port catheter

- The lifespan of a port is months to years.
- The preferred vessel of choice for the interventional radiologist is again the internal jugular vein. However, surgeons typically use the subclavian vein.
- Placement requires conscious sedation and antibiotic prophylaxis.
- The pocket should be snug around the port so that it does not flip. Some interventional radiologists also suture the port in place.
- A port catheter should only be accessed using a Huber needle to protect the integrity of the silicone septum as a regular needle will remove a core of silicone with each puncture.

皮下输液港导管

- 输液港港体的使用寿命为数月至数年。
- 介入放射医师首选的血管仍是颈内静脉，而外科医师常选用锁骨下静脉。
- 需静脉镇静麻醉并预防性使用抗生素。
- 囊袋应贴合港体，以免港体翻转。一些医师选择用缝线将港体固定。
- 只可使用Huber针穿刺港体，以保护硅胶隔膜的完整性，因普通针会在每次穿刺时切除一小块硅胶芯。

Peripherally inserted central catheter (PICC) placement

经外周插管的中心静脉导管(PICC)置管术

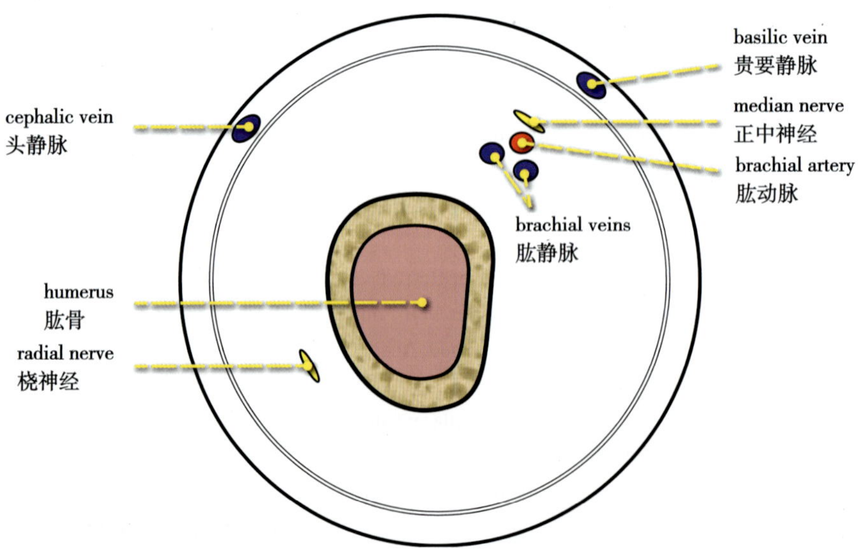

- The basilic vein, located medial and superficial to the brachial veins, is the first choice for peripherally inserted catheter (PICC) placement. The cephalic vein adds an extra curve as it joins the axillary/subclavian vein, but is generally the second choice if the basilic is not available. There is risk of damaging the median nerve with placement in a brachial vein as the median nerve lies superficial to the brachial veins.
- A PICC should not be placed in a patient with chronic renal failure who may need a fistula in the future. Central access using the neck veins should be used instead.

- 贵要静脉位于肱静脉的浅内侧，是经外周插管的中心静脉导管(PICC)的首选静脉。头静脉在汇入腋静脉/锁骨下静脉区有一个额外的弯曲，当贵要静脉不能使用时，常作为PICC置管的次选静脉。肱静脉置管有损伤正中神经的危险，因正中神经位于肱静脉的浅表处。
- PICC不应放置在慢性肾衰竭且有可能需要动静脉造瘘的患者。应改用经颈部静脉行中心静脉置管。

（翻译　韩世龙）

Fluid Drainage and Aspiration

- Fluid collections in the body include sterile serous collections or abscesses. Conventional wisdom states that hematomas should not be drained; however, there is evidence that hematoma aspiration may lead to more rapid symptom relief.
- The Seldinger technique is a common method by which a catheter is inserted over a guidewire.
- The direct trocar technique can be performed safely with large superficial collections. The catheter is directly inserted into the collection with the inner stylet. The stylet is then removed and the catheter is aspirated to ensure placement in the fluid collection and to obtain the initial sample. The catheter is then coiled and locked.
- Iatrogenic seeding of infection can be minimized with sterile technique. A fresh sterile preparation is needed for each separate fluid collection to avoid cross contamination. Sepsis should be anticipated prior to a drainage procedure and supportive care started promptly.
- Creation of persistent fistulous connection may occur with indwelling catheters, and is a complication that should be considered during procedural planning.
- When attempting to drain an acute collection that has not yet been walled off with inflammatory granulation tissue, the guidewire or catheter may advance beyond the collection and perforate adjacent structures, not meeting adequate resistance at the far end of the collection.
- Post-procedure, drainage catheters require daily maintenance to ensure proper function and resolution of the collection. The catheter, connections, and fixation devices should be checked daily and flushed up to three times a day with saline depending on the collection. The drain site should be kept clean and dry.

Thoracentesis

- One of the most common procedures in IR, thoracentesis typically involves ultrasound-guided removal of fluid through a valved 7-French catheter.
- When deciding the intercostal approach, choose the level with the most fluid, ideally with fluid above and below the level of entry to allow for margin of error as the lung moves during respiration.
- Pre-procedure ultrasound imaging can demonstrate high viscosity, septations, or clot for which a larger bore needle may be needed. The needle should enter the intercostal space just above the rib, to avoid the neurovascular bundle coursing along the inferior margin.
- No more than 1 liter should be removed in 24 hours to avoid re-expansion pulmonary edema.
- Upon removing the needle, gauze saturated with petroleum jelly should be applied to the entry wound.

积液引流和抽吸

- 体内积液包括无菌性浆液积聚或脓肿。传统的观点认为血肿不应引流，但有证据表明抽吸血肿可能会加快症状缓解。
- Seldinger技术是常用的方法，经过导丝插入导管。
- 套管针直接穿刺技术可安全地用于大而表浅位置的积液。用带内芯针的导管直接穿刺进入积液内部。内芯取出后抽吸导管以确保导管位于积液腔内并获取初始样本。然后导管头端成环后锁定导管。
- 医源性感染可以采用无菌技术降低其风险。对于每个独立的积液需分别进行无菌消毒准备以免交叉感染。引流操作前应对败血症有所准备，并及时进行支持治疗。
- 留置导管可产生永久性窦道，在做引流计划时需考虑到此并发症。
- 在引流一个尚未有炎性肉芽组织形成脓壁的急性积液时，导丝或导管因积液远端无足够的阻力而有可能穿过积液并造成邻近结构穿孔。
- 术后需对引流管进行日常维护，确保引流管通畅和积液消退。应每日检查导管、接头，以及固定材料；根据积液情况，用生理盐水冲洗，每日可达3次。穿刺点应保持清洁和干燥。

胸腔穿刺术

- 胸腔穿刺术是介入放射学最常见的操作之一。一般在超声引导下用带阀门的7Fr导管进行抽吸引流。
- 当采用肋间入路时，应选择液体最多的位置，理想的情况是穿刺点的上下都有液体，以免肺呼吸运动造成对边界误判。
- 术前超声检查可显示黏度高、分隔或凝块，此时可能需要较大口径的穿刺针。应沿肋骨的上缘进针，以避免损伤沿肋骨下缘走行的神经血管束。
- 在24小时内的引流量不应超过1L，以免引起肺水肿。
- 拔出穿刺针后，应用凡士林纱布覆盖穿刺点。

Paracentesis

- Paracentesis for ascites is usually performed in the lower quadrants. Care should be taken to mark or observe the epigastric vessels under ultrasound. Visualization of the needle tip during entry is important to avoid viscus perforation.
- Typically, up to 5 liters can be removed before it is necessary to replenish serum albumin.

腹腔穿刺术

- 腹水穿刺通常在下腹部的两侧。应注意用超声标记或观察腹壁血管。进针时应能看到针尖，这对避免误穿内脏非常重要。
- 腹水引流达5L时通常需要补充人血白蛋白。

Enteric Access

肠道通路

Percutaneous gastrostomy indications

- Esophageal, head and neck, and neurologic disease may necessitate percutaneous gastrostomy. Of note, there is strong evidence that gastrostomy does not improve survival or quality of life in elderly patients with dementia and decreased oral intake.
- A less common indication for gastrostomy is for long-term bowel decompression, for instance due to palliation of malignant bowel obstruction or prolonged ileus.

经皮胃造瘘适应证

- 食管、头颈部和神经系统疾病可能需要进行经皮穿刺胃造瘘术。需要注意的是，有强有力的证据表明，在老年痴呆症患者和口腔摄入减少的情况下，胃造瘘术并不能改善生存率或生活质量。
- 胃造瘘术不常见的适应证是长期肠道减压，如恶性肠梗阻或顽固性肠梗阻。

Percutaneous gastrostomy technique

- Absolute contraindications to percutaneous gastrostomy include lack of appropriate window (such as colonic interposition), extensive gastric varices, and uncorrectable coagulopathy.
- A nasogastric tube is inserted under fluoroscopic guidance, through which the stomach is insufflated with air.
- Under fluoroscopic guidance, three T-fastener gastropexy clips are deployed to pexy the anterior wall of the stomach to the anterior abdominal wall. After each deployed T-fastener, intra-gastric position is confirmed with a small amount of contrast injected into the stomach.
- After the pexy clips are in place and the stomach is firmly fastened against the anterior abdominal wall, the definitive gastrostomy puncture is made and serially dilated. The gastrostomy can be used in 24 hours after the patient is evaluated for peritoneal signs.
- The gastrostomy tube must remain in place for at least a month to form a mature transperitoneal tract.

经皮胃造瘘术

- 经皮胃造瘘术的绝对禁忌证包括缺乏合适的穿刺窗口(如间位结肠)、弥漫的胃静脉曲张和无法纠正的凝血功能障碍。
- 透视下插入鼻胃管，经鼻胃管向胃内打入空气。
- 透视引导下，使用3个“T”形胃固定铆钉将胃前壁固定至前腹壁。每次使用“T”形铆钉固定后，向胃内注入少量造影剂来确认其在胃腔内。
- 固定钉就位后将胃牢固地系在前腹壁，之后行胃造瘘穿刺和连续扩张。若24小时后患者无腹膜症状即可使用胃造瘘。
- 胃造瘘管须留置至少1个月，使经腹膜窦道得以成熟。

(翻译　张雯)

10 Neuroimaging: Brain

10 神经影像：大脑

Francis Deng, Shruti Mishra, Ellen X. Sun,
Raymond Y. Huang

Contents

目录

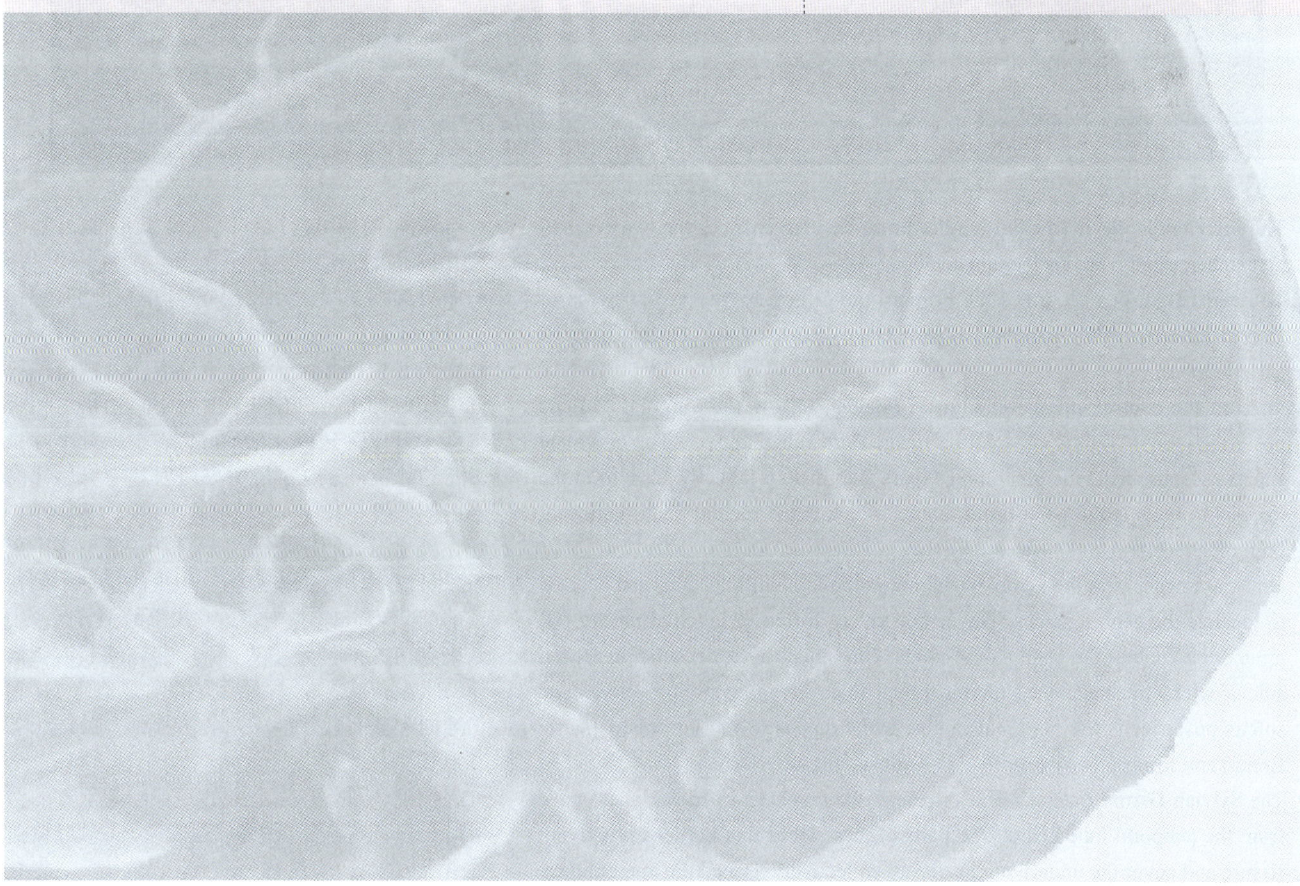

CEREBROSPINAL FLUID (CSF) SPACES

Intra-axial and extra-axial compartments

- An intra-axial lesion is within the brain parenchyma itself, underneath the pial membrane.
- An extra-axial lesion is external to the pial membrane. The meninges and CSF spaces are extra-axial.
- The CSF spaces include the sulci, fissures, basal cisterns, and ventricles.

Sulcal/fissural anatomy

脑脊液(CSF)腔隙

轴内和轴外分区

- 轴内病变位于脑实质内，软脑膜之下。
- 轴外病变在软脑膜外。脑膜和脑脊液腔隙都属于轴外。
- 脑脊液腔隙包括脑沟、脑裂、基底池和脑室。

脑沟/裂解剖

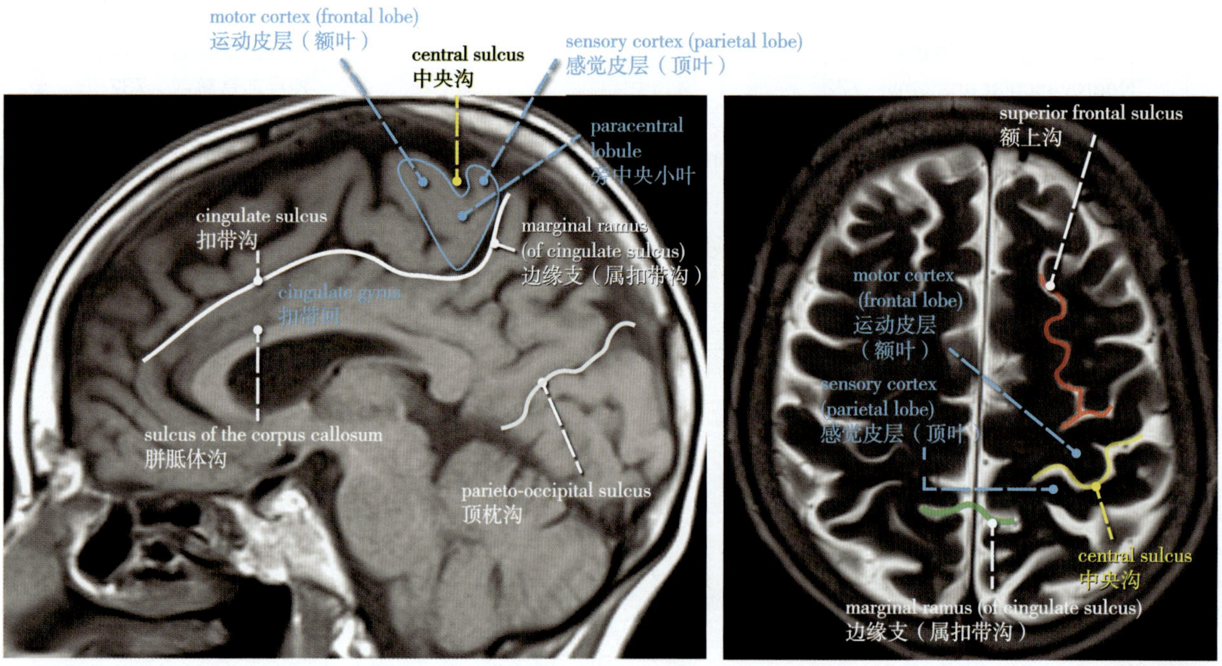

- The **interhemispheric (medial longitudinal) fissure** separates the two cerebral hemispheres and contains the falx cerebri.
- The **central sulcus** separates the primary motor cortex (precentral gyrus of frontal lobe) from the primary somatosensory cortex (postcentral gyrus of parietal lobe).
- To find the central sulcus on sagittal images, follow the cingulate sulcus posteriorly on a slightly off-midline image (left image above). The cingulate sulcus ascends as the marginal ramus (pars marginalis). Directly anterior to the marginal ramus is the paracentral lobule, which is the medial continuation of both the precentral and postcentral gyri.
- On axial images near the vertex (right image above), multiple signs can be used to localize the central sulcus. The central sulcus forms an inverted *omega* (Ω) around the knob of the hand motor cortex. One sulcus anterior is the precentral sulcus, which intersects the superior frontal sulcus in an *inverted T shape*. One sulcus posterior is the marginal ramus, which opens to the interhemispheric fissure and forms a *curly bracket* "{" *shape* facing anteriorly.
- The **Sylvian fissure** (lateral sulcus) separates the frontal and parietal lobes above from the temporal lobe below. The parts of these lobes that border the Sylvian fissure and cover the underlying insula are collectively termed the operculum.

- **半球间(内侧纵向)裂**将两个大脑半球分隔开，并包含大脑镰。
- **中央沟**将初级运动皮层(额叶中央前回)与初级躯体感觉皮层(顶叶中央后回)分开。
- 在矢状位图像上，沿着扣带沟向后稍微偏离中线位即可找到中央沟(上图的左图)。扣带沟上升成为边缘支(边缘部)。中央旁小叶位于边缘支正前方，是中央前回和中央后回的内侧延续。
- 在颅顶附近的轴位图像上(上方右图)，多个征象可以用于定位中央沟。中央沟呈一个倒置的"欧米茄(Ω)"，围绕运动皮层的手节区。中央沟前方的沟是中央前沟，它与额上沟呈倒"T"形相交。中央沟后方的沟是边缘支，它通向半球间裂并形成一个朝前的"花括号({)"形状。
- **外侧裂**(外侧沟)将上方的额顶叶与下方的颞叶分开。这些邻近外侧裂的额、顶、颞叶覆盖着下方的岛叶，统称为岛盖。

- The **parieto-occipital sulcus/fissure** separates the medial surfaces of the parietal lobe (precuneus) and occipital lobe (cuneus).

- **顶枕沟/裂**将顶叶内侧面(楔前叶)和枕叶内侧面(楔叶)分隔开。

VENTRICULAR ANATOMY

脑室解剖

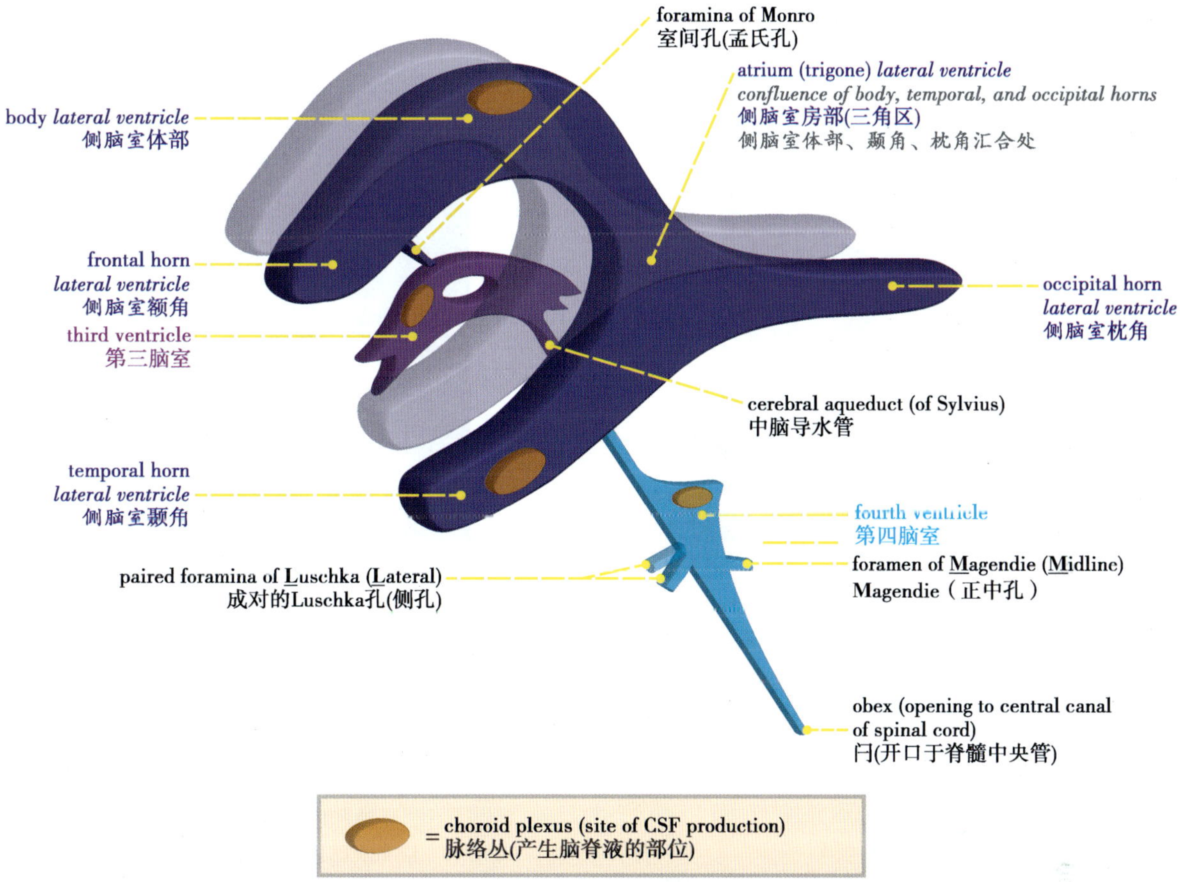

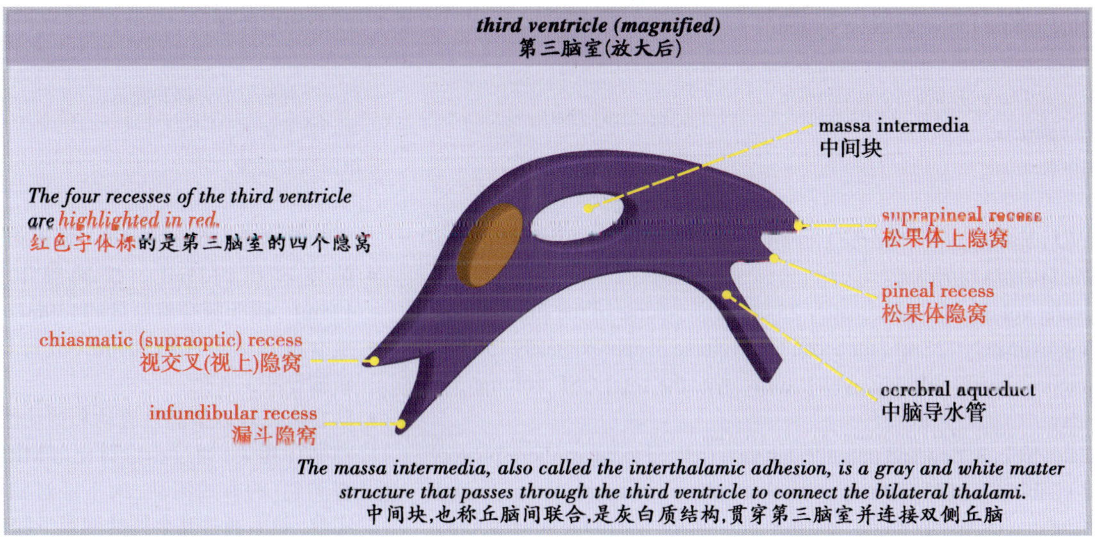

- The ventricular system consists of two lateral ventricles that drain into the midline third and fourth ventricles.
- The (interventricular) foramina of Monro connect the lateral ventricles with the third ventricle.
- The cerebral aqueduct (of Sylvius) connects the third ventricle with the fourth ventricle.

- 脑室系统由两个侧脑室及它们引流到中线的第三脑室和第四脑室组成。
- Monro孔(室间孔)连接侧脑室和第三脑室。
- Sylvius导水管(中脑导水管)连接第三脑室和第四脑室。
- 第四脑室向下延续(形成一个尖端,叫闩)成为

- The fourth ventricle continues inferiorly (at its tip, called the obex) as the central canal of the spinal cord.
- The fourth ventricle also drains into the basal cisterns via three foramina:
  Paired foramina of Luschka (lateral apertures).
  Single foramen of Magendie (median aperture).

脊髓中央管。
- 第四脑室通过三个小孔引流至基底池：
  一对Luschka孔(侧孔)。
  单个Magendie孔(正中孔)。

Cisternal anatomy

脑池解剖

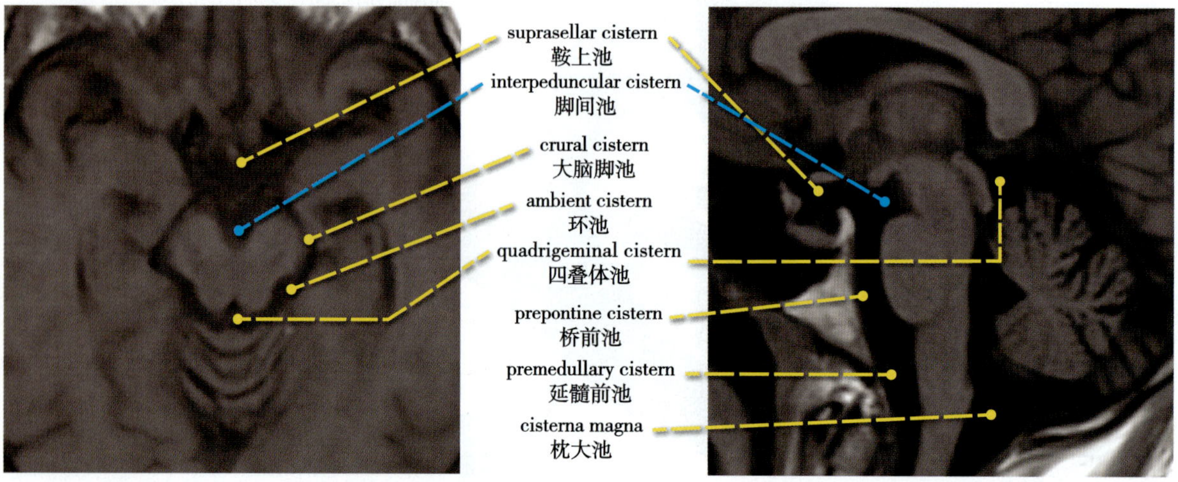

- The basal or subarachnoid cisterns are CSF-filled spaces around the base of the brain and brainstem across which vessels and cranial nerves traverse.
- The suprasellar (chiasmatic) cistern is a pentagonal space around the pituitary infundibulum that contains the circle of Willis and optic chiasm.
- The perimesencephalic cisterns surround the midbrain, consisting of the interpeduncular, crural, ambient, and quadrigeminal cisterns.

- 脑脊液充满了围绕大脑底部与脑干周围的基底池或蛛网膜下池，其中有血管和脑神经从中穿行。
- 鞍上(视交叉)池是垂体漏斗部周围的一个五边形空间，池内含威利斯环和视交叉。
- 中脑周围池围绕着中脑，由脚间池、大脑脚池、环池和四叠体池组成。

CSF dynamics

- CSF is primarily produced by the choroid plexus, which is located in specific locations throughout the ventricular system:

Body and temporal horn of each lateral ventricle. Roof of third ventricle. Roof of fourth ventricle.

There is NO choroid plexus in the cerebral aqueduct or occipital or frontal horns of the lateral ventricles.

- The ventricular volume is approximately 25 mL. The volume of the subarachnoid spaces is approximately 125 mL, for a total CSF volume of approximately 150 mL.
- CSF production is 500 mL/day, which turns over the total CSF volume 3–4 times per day.
- CSF circulates by bulk flow and pulsatile agitation (related to the cardiorespiratory cycle and visible by MRI techniques such as phase-contrast) down through ventricles, out into the basal cisterns, and then through the rest of the subarachnoid spaces.
- CSF is absorbed primarily by the arachnoid granulations (leptomeningeal evaginations extending into the dural venous sinuses) and to a lesser extent by the lymphatic system.

脑脊液循环

- 脑脊液主要由脉络丛产生，后者位于脑室系统的特定区域：

每一个侧脑室的体部和颞角。 第三脑室顶部。 第四脑室顶部。

中脑导水管和侧脑室枕角、额角没有脉络丛。

- 脑室容积约25mL。蛛网膜下腔容积约125mL，因此脑脊液总量约150mL。
- 脑脊液每天生成约500mL，故每日能完全更新脑脊液3~4次。
- 脑脊液循环以整体性流动和搏动性流动(与心肺循环相关，通过相位对比等MRI技术可以观测到)的方式流动，向下经过脑室，进入基底池，然后通过其余的蛛网膜下腔。
- 脑脊液以蛛网膜粒(突入硬膜静脉窦的柔脑膜[1]突起)吸收为主，小部分由淋巴系统吸收。

① 柔脑膜包括软脑膜和蛛网膜。

Hydrocephalus

- **Communicating hydrocephalus** is ventricular enlargement due to an increase in CSF volume without an obstructing lesion within the ventricular system.

  Processes that obstruct arachnoid granulation reabsorption of CSF can cause communicating hydrocephalus, such as subarachnoid hemorrhage, meningitis, or leptomeningeal metastases.

  Normal pressure hydrocephalus (NPH) is a form of communicating hydrocephalus characterized by normal CSF pressure and the clinical triad of ataxia, incontinence, and dementia. Imaging typically shows ventriculomegaly, acute callosal angle (measured between the lateral ventricles on a coronal image at the posterior commissure), widened Sylvian fissures, and tight high convexity (crowding of gyri at the vertex).
- **Noncommunicating hydrocephalus** is hydrocephalus due to an obstructing lesion within the ventricular system, such as a third ventricular colloid cyst, aqueductal stenosis, or a posterior fossa mass.
- **Obstructive hydrocephalus** usually refers to noncommunicating hydrocephalus but can also include communicating hydrocephalus attributed to obstruction at the level of the subarachnoid spaces or arachnoid granulations.
- **Hydrocephalus ex vacuo** refers to ventricular enlargement due to brain parenchymal volume loss.

脑积水

- **交通性脑积水**是脑脊液体积增加所致的脑室扩大，脑室系统内并无梗阻性病变。

  任何阻碍蛛网膜颗粒重吸收脑脊液的过程都可以导致交通性脑积水，如蛛网膜下腔出血、脑膜炎或软脑膜转移瘤。

  常压性脑积水(NPH)是交通性脑积水的一种类型，其特点是脑脊液压力正常及临床三联征，即共济失调、尿失禁、痴呆。影像学上常表现为脑室扩张、胼胝体角(后连合层面冠状位图像上测量两侧脑室之间)为锐角、外侧裂增宽和大脑凸面高凸度(顶点处的脑回拥挤)。
- **非交通性脑积水**是由脑室系统内梗阻性病变所致的脑积水，如第三脑室胶样囊肿，导水管狭窄或颅后窝占位。
- **梗阻性脑积水**通常是指非交通性脑积水，但也可包括蛛网膜下腔或蛛网膜颗粒阻塞所导致的交通性脑积水。
- **空虚性脑积水**是指脑实质体积减小所致的脑室扩张。

Cerebral edema

- Brain swelling, due to various etiologies, within a closed skull reduces the volume of blood and/or CSF compartments (Monro-Kellie doctrine).
- Edema within the brain can be caused by cell death, altered capillary permeability, or hemodynamic forces.
- Compared to normal brain parenchyma, edematous brain appears hypoattenuating on CT and FLAIR hyperintense on MRI.

Cytotoxic edema

- Cytotoxic edema is cell swelling caused by damaged molecular sodium-potassium ATPase ion pumps, most commonly due to acute ischemia. Failure to maintain ion gradients results in **cellular** (true cytotoxic) edema, wherein fluid moves from the extracellular space into the intracellular space, followed by **ionic** edema, wherein fluid moves from the intravascular space into the extracellular space across an intact blood-brain barrier.
- Both gray and white matter are affected. Cellular edema appears as abnormally restricted diffusion on MRI. Ionic edema appears as loss of gray-white differentiation on CT.

Vasogenic edema

- Blood-brain barrier breakdown results in vasogenic edema, wherein plasma protein-rich fluid moves from the intravascular space into the extracellular space due to increased capillary permeability.
- The causes are diverse, including neoplasm, infection, inflammation, hemorrhage, subacute arterial infarct, and venous infarct.
- White matter is primarily affected. MRI shows facilitated diffusion (increased diffusivity). CT shows accentuated gray-white differentiation.

Interstitial edema

- Increased ventricular pressure results in transependymal flow, wherein CSF

脑水肿

- 脑肿胀由多种原因所致，Monro-Kellie的假说认为，一个封闭的颅腔内减少了血容量和/或脑脊液的体积。
- 脑水肿可由细胞死亡、毛细血管通透性改变或血流动力学因素所致。
- 与正常脑实质相比，水肿的脑组织在CT上表现为低密度，在MRI上表现为FLAIR高信号。

细胞毒性水肿

- 细胞毒性水肿是由钠钾ATP酶离子泵损伤所致的细胞肿胀，最常见于急性缺血。离子梯度无法维持会导致**细胞**(真性细胞毒性)水肿，此时液体从细胞外间隙转移到细胞内间隙，随后出现**离子**性水肿，此时液体会跨越完整的血脑屏障从血管腔内转移到细胞外间隙。
- 灰质和白质都受到影响。细胞水肿在MRI上表现为弥散受限异常。离子性水肿在CT上表现为灰白质的分界消失。

血管源性水肿

- 血脑屏障破坏将导致血管源性水肿，此时，会因毛细血管通透性增加而使富含血浆蛋白的液体从血管腔内向细胞外间隙转移。
- 病因很多，包括肿瘤、感染、炎症、出血、亚急性动脉梗死和静脉梗死。
- 脑白质受累最为明显。MRI表现为促进弥散(弥散增加)。CT表现为灰白质分界更加明显。

间质性水肿

- 脑室压力升高导致脑脊液跨室管膜流动，此

moves from the intraventricular space into the brain extracellular space.

- The most common cause is acute obstructive hydrocephalus.
- Periventricular white matter is primarily affected.

时脑脊液从脑室内腔隙向脑细胞外间隙移动。

- 最常见的原因为急性阻塞性脑积水。
- 脑室周围白质受累为主。

Brain Herniation

脑疝

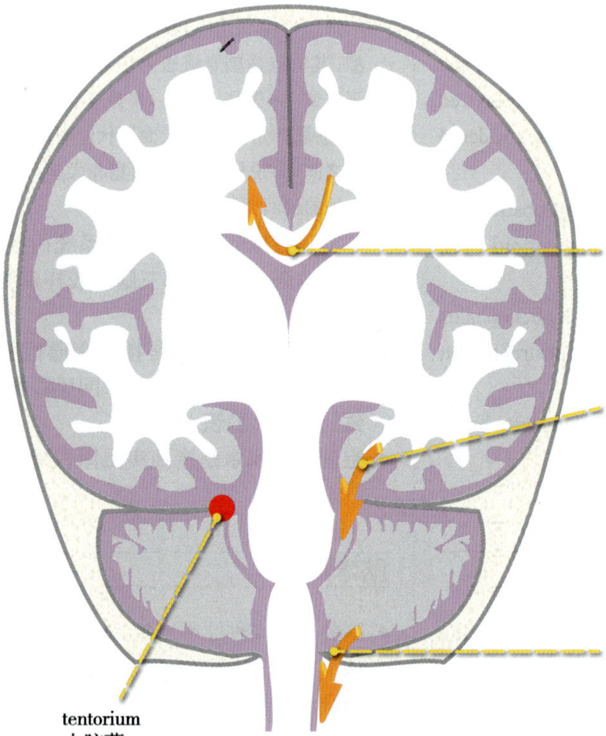

- The total volume in the skull is fixed. Intracranial mass effect may lead to herniation of brain matter across a dural fold.
- Herniation may be due to a mass lesion (such as a neoplasm or hematoma) or edema secondary to large stroke. Because the volume of the posterior fossa is especially limited, cerebellar infarcts are prone to herniation.

Subfalcine herniation

- Subfalcine herniation is seen when the cingulate gyrus slides underneath the falx cerebri.
- Subfalcine herniation may rarely cause compression of the anterior cerebral artery (ACA) against the falx, resulting in infarction.
- Contralateral ventricular entrapment (focal hydrocephalus) may result from foramen of Monro obstruction.

- 颅骨内总的容积是固定的。颅内占位效应可导致脑组织经硬膜反折处疝出。
- 脑疝可由占位性病变(如肿瘤或血肿)或大面积卒中继发的脑水肿导致。由于颅后窝空间特别有限，小脑梗死后容易引起脑疝。

大脑镰下疝

- 大脑镰下疝是指扣带回滑至大脑镰的下方。
- 少数情况下，大脑镰下疝可将大脑前动脉(ACA)挤向大脑镰，导致脑梗死。
- 室间孔堵塞可导致对侧脑室脑脊液潴留(局灶性脑积水)。

Transtentorial herniation

小脑幕裂孔(颞叶钩回)疝

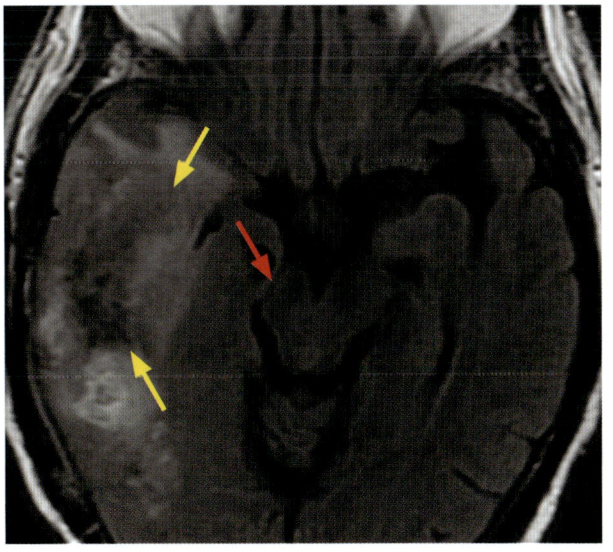

Early uncal herniation:
Axial FLAIR MRI shows a heterogeneous mass in the right temporal lobe (yellow arrows), with effacement of the right lateral ventricle temporal horn. The mass effect causes mild downward uncal herniation with flattening of the right cerebral peduncle (red arrow).
早期颞叶钩回疝：
轴位FLAIR MRI显示右侧颞叶一个不均匀肿块(黄箭)，累及右侧脑室颞角。肿块的占位效应引起轻度下行性颞叶钩回疝，右侧大脑脚变平(红箭)

- Effacement of the perimesencephalic cisterns may be a sign of impending or actual transtentorial herniation.
- *Downward* transtentorial herniation involves inferomedial displacement of the mesial temporal lobe (**uncal herniation**) or less commonly, inferior displacement of the thalamus and midbrain (**central herniation**) through the tentorial notch.

- 中脑周围池消失预示即将发生或已经发生小脑幕裂孔疝。
- 下行性小脑幕裂孔疝时，颞叶内侧向内下侧移位(**颞叶钩回疝**)，少数情况下，丘脑和中脑经小脑幕切迹向下移位(**中心疝**)。

The ipsilateral cranial nerve Ⅲ (oculomotor nerve) may be compressed, leading to pupillary dilation and downward and out eye deviation.
Compression of the ipsilateral posterior cerebral artery (PCA) may cause medial temporal/occipital lobe infarct.
Small **Duret hemorrhages** within the medulla or brainstem are caused by shearing of perforating basilar artery branches due to downward force on the brainstem.
Compression of the contralateral cerebral peduncle against the tentorial notch can cause a hemiparesis ipsilateral to the herniated side (**Kernohan notch phenomenon**).
Central herniation causes progressive impairment of brainstem function such as coma, breathing abnormality, and posturing.

同侧第Ⅲ脑神经(动眼神经)可受压，导致瞳孔扩张和眼球向下外侧凝视。
同侧大脑后动脉(PCA)受压可引起颞叶内侧/枕叶梗死。
延髓或脑干小面积**Duret出血**是由于脑干受到向下的压力从而剪切基底动脉穿支血管所致。
对侧大脑脚受压挤向小脑幕切迹可导致脑疝同侧偏瘫(**Kernohan切迹现象**)
中心疝会导致进行性脑干功能损害，如昏迷、呼吸异常和姿势异常。

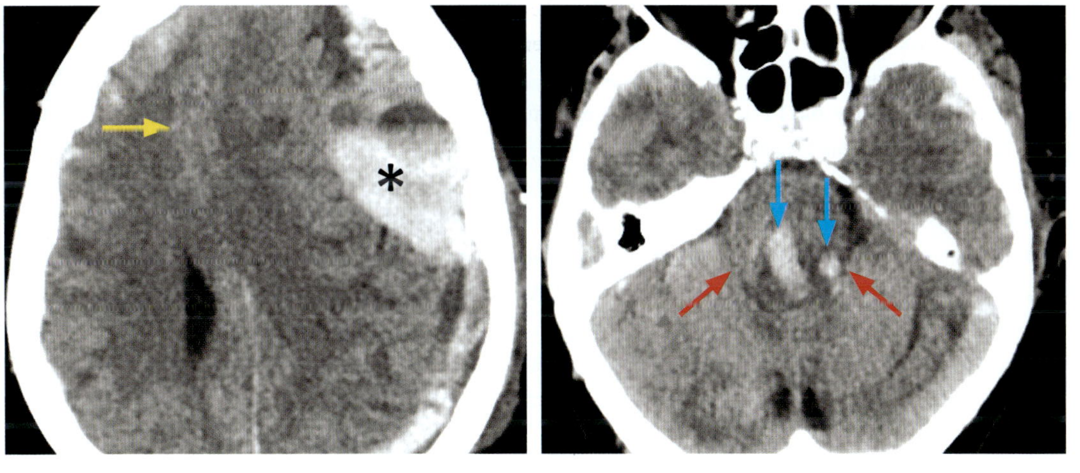

Duret hemorrhage: Noncontrast CT shows a left subdural hematoma (*; left image) causing rightward midline shift (yellow arrow) and downward transtentorial herniation with effacement of the perimesencephalic cisterns (red arrows; right image), and associated Duret hemorrhages within the pons (blue arrows).
Duret出血：平扫CT显示左侧硬膜下血肿(左图，*处)导致中线向右移位(黄箭)和下行性小脑幕裂孔疝，伴中脑周围池消失(右图，红箭)，以及相应的脑桥内Duret出血(蓝箭)。

- *Upward* (ascending) transtentorial herniation is superior displacement of the upper parts of the cerebellum due to posterior fossa mass effect.

The main complication is obstructive hydrocephalus from aqueductal compression.

Cerebellar tonsillar herniation

- Tonsillar herniation refers to downward displacement of the cerebellar tonsils through foramen magnum, preferably attributed to mass effect (rather than a normal variant or Chiari malformation where terms like tonsillar ectopia or low-lying tonsils are appropriately less alarming).
- Subsequent compression of medullary respiratory centers is often fatal.

Extracranial (transcalvarial) herniation

- Extracranial herniation refers to shift of brain tissue outside of the brain case, typically at a surgical or traumatic calvarial defect and attributed to abnormal intracranial mass effect (rather than a malformation where the term encephalocele is more common).
- Extracranial herniation is an expected feature following decompressive craniectomy. However, a mushroom-like appearance suggests the craniectomy defect is too small, potentially constricting vessels and brain tissue at the margins.

Paradoxical herniation

- Paradoxical brain herniation, also known as **sunken/sinking skin flap syndrome**, is a complication of large craniectomy where intracranial pressure falls below atmospheric pressure, resulting in concave deformity and progressive shift of the brain away from the calvarial defect.

MRI IN NEURORADIOLOGY

- As discussed in the physics chapter, inherent tissue signal characteristics depend on the longitudinal recovery/relaxation (T1) and transverse relaxation (T2) times of the protons in that tissue.

T1 shortening is hyperintense (bright) on T1-weighted images and T1 prolongation is hypointense (dark). Conversely, T2 shortening is hypointense on T2-weighted images and T2 prolongation is hyperintense.

Spin-echo T1-weighted imaging

- Most brain lesions are hypointense on T1-weighted images due to pathologic prolongation of the longitudinal recovery.
- The presence of **hyperintensity on T1-weighted images** (caused by T1 shortening) can be an important clue to specific substances:

Fat. **Proteinaceous material**. **Methemoglobin**.	**Melanin**. **Minerals**: gadolinium, copper, manganese, iron, and calcium (rarely; when dispersed, not in bone).

- Slow-flowing blood also appears hyperintense on T1-weighted spin-echo sequences, which have a short TR. This time-of-flight effect is called "flow-related enhancement."

Spin-echo T2-weighted imaging

- Most brain lesions are hyperintense on T2-weighted images due to water content or edema causing T2 prolongation.
- The presence of hypointensity on T2-weighted images (caused by T2 shortening) can be an important clue to specific substances:

- 上行性(向上的)小脑幕裂孔疝是小脑上部因颅后窝占位效应向上移位。

主要的并发症是中脑导水管受压导致梗阻性脑积水。

小脑扁桃体疝

- 小脑扁桃体疝是指小脑扁桃体经枕骨大孔向下移位，最好归因于占位效应(而不是正常变异或Chiari畸形，对于后者使用小脑扁桃体异位或低位小脑扁桃体更符合其并非严重的特性)。
- 延髓呼吸中枢受压通常是致命的。

颅外(经颅)疝

- 颅外疝是指脑组织突出于颅腔之外，通常发生在手术或创伤性颅骨缺损处，为颅内异常的占位效应所致(而非畸形，后者常使用脑膨出一词)。
- 颅外疝可见于颅骨切除减压术后。脑组织呈蘑菇状外观提示颅骨切除后的缺损太小，可能会压迫边缘处的血管和脑组织。

反常性脑疝

- 反常性脑疝，又称为**凹陷/下陷皮瓣综合征**，是大面积颅骨切除术的一个并发症。在这种情况下，颅内压低于大气压，导致凹陷畸形，并使大脑出现渐进性与骨缺损相反的方向移位。

MRI的神经影像

- 在“影像物理”一章中有所讨论，组织的固有信号特性取决于组织内质子的纵向恢复/弛豫时间(T_1)和横向弛豫时间(T_2)。

短T_1在T_1加权上为高信号(亮的)，长T_1在T_1加权上为低信号(暗的)；相反，短T_2在T_2加权上为低信号，长T_2在T_2加权上为高信号。

自旋回波T_1加权成像

- 大多数脑部病变在T_1加权上呈低信号，由其纵向恢复时间病理性延长所致。
- **T_1加权上的高信号**(T_1缩短所致)可以是某些特定物质的重要线索：

脂肪。 **蛋白类物质**。 **高铁血红蛋白**。	**黑色素**。 **矿物质**：钆、铜、锰、铁和钙(少见；非骨性的游离钙)。

- 缓慢流动的血液在T_1加权自旋回波序列上也表现为高信号，其重复时间(TR)较短。这种时间飞跃效应被称为“流动相关增强”。

自旋回波T_2加权成像

- 大部分脑部病变在T_2加权上呈高信号，因含水或水肿会导致T_2延长。
- T_2加权上的低信号(T_2缩短所致)可以是某些特定物质的重要线索：

Most stages of blood (deoxyhemoglobin, intracellular methemoglobin, hemosiderin).

Calcification.

Fibrous tissue.

Highly cellular tumors with a high nucleus:cytoplasm ratio producing low lesional water content (for instance, lymphoma and medulloblastoma).

Desiccated secretions in the paranasal sinuses.

大多数状态下的血液(脱氧血红蛋白、细胞内高铁血红蛋白、含铁血黄素)。

钙化。

纤维组织。

细胞密集的肿瘤：核质比大，导致病变含水量低(如淋巴瘤、髓母细胞瘤)。

鼻窦中的**干性分泌物**。

- Fast-moving blood also appears hypointense on T2-weighted spin-echo sequences, which have a long TE. This time-of-flight effect is called a "flow-void."

Fluid-attenuated inversion recovery (FLAIR)

- FLAIR refers to the addition of an inversion pulse that nulls fluid signal (based on water's T1 characteristics).
- The T2-FLAIR sequence is the workhorse of neuroradiology. It is usually referred to simply as "FLAIR" even though the technique can apply to T1-weighted images as well.
- While CSF is dark on both T2-FLAIR and T1-weighted images, they can be distinguished by looking at the relative signal intensities of the gray and white matter.

  T1: Normal white matter is hyperintense due to fatty myelinated white matter, with a short T1 time.

  T2-FLAIR: White matter is darker than gray matter. T2-FLAIR will be referred to as FLAIR in this chapter.

Spin-echo proton density (PD)-weighted imaging

- Proton density (PD) images are not used in many neuroradiology MRI protocols, but they do have the highest signal-to-noise ratio of any sequence. PD sequences may be useful in the evaluation of multiple sclerosis (MS), especially in the spinal cord.

Diffusion-weighted imaging (DWI)

- DWI depicts Brownian motion of water protons. Signal is lost with increasing diffusion. Free water (CSF) experiences the most signal attenuation, while many pathologic processes (primarily ischemia) cause reduced diffusivity and less signal loss.
- DWI is an inherently T2-weighted sequence with diffusion-sensitizing pulsed gradients applied sequentially in multiple directions. The **b-value** is the setting that determines the degree of diffusion weighting, which is based on the diffusion gradient amplitude, duration, and time interval between pulses.

  The higher the b-value, the more contrast the image will provide for detecting reduced diffusivity. The downside to increasing the b value is a decrease in the signal-to-noise ratio, unless scan time is proportionally increased for additional acquisitions.
- DWI is typically displayed in two ways, interpreted together: Trace images and ADC (apparent diffusion coefficient) maps.

  Trace images are a summation of the source images sensitive to diffusion in different directions. Reduced diffusivity will be *hyperintense* and lesions are very conspicuous.

  The **ADC map** shows pure diffusion information without any T2 weighting, obtained by calculating the exponential decay constant when plotting the MR signal obtained with a set of at least two b-values. In contrast to DWI, reduced diffusivity is *hypointense* on the ADC map.

  Because readers are less sensitive to detecting reduced diffusivity using the ADC map alone, DWI is the primary sequence used to detect diffusion abnormalities.

- 快速流动的血液在T_2加权自旋回波序列上也表现为低信号，其回波时间(TE)较长。这种时间飞跃效应被称为“流空”。

液体衰减反转恢复序列(FLAIR)

- 液体衰减反转恢复序列(FLAIR)是指添加了使液体信号无效的反转脉冲(基于水的T_1特性)。
- T_2-FLAIR序列是神经影像中的主要序列。它通常被简称为“FLAIR”，尽管该技术也可被应用于T_1加权。
- 尽管脑脊液在T_2-FLAIR和T_1加权都是暗的，但可以通过观察灰质和白质的相对信号强度来区分。

  T_1：正常白质为高信号，因为白质富含脂性髓鞘，具有较短的T_1时间。

  T_2-FLAIR：白质比灰质暗。T_2-FLAIR在本章下文简称为“FLAIR”。

自旋回波质子密度(PD)加权成像

- 质子密度(PD)加权像并不是常用的神经MRI序列，但它却是信噪比最高的序列。PD序列对评估多发性硬化有价值，尤其是对脊髓。

弥散加权成像(DWI)

- 弥散加权成像(DWI)代表水分子的布朗运动。信号随着弥散增强而丢失。游离水(脑脊液)的信号衰减最明显，但许多病变(主要是缺血)会引起弥散性降低，但信号丢失不严重。
- DWI是固有的T_2加权序列，具有在多个方向上系列施加的弥散敏感脉冲梯度。**b值**是基于弥散梯度幅度、持续时间和脉冲之间的时间间隔来确定弥散加权程度的指标。

  b值越高，影像所提供的检测弥散受限的对比度越强烈。但b值增高的缺点是会降低信噪比，除非按比例延长扫描时间以获取额外采集数据。
- DWI通常采用2种方式进行显示，需要一起解读：轨迹图像和表观弥散系数(ADC)图像。

  轨迹图像是弥散敏感源图像在不同方向上的总和。弥散受限表现为高信号，病变变得非常突出。

  ADC图像显示没有任何T_2成分的纯扩散信息，通过计算绘制使用一组至少两个值获得的MR信号时的指数衰减常数。与DWI相反，弥散受限在ADC上表现为低信号。

  由于阅片者对于单独在ADC图像上显示的弥散下降不敏感，因而DWI成为检测弥散异常的主要序列。

Whereas trace images show a scalar measure of diffusion, **diffusion tensor imaging (DTI)** depicts directional asymmetries, called anisotropy, such as that inherent to white matter fiber tracts.

- An important pitfall to be aware of is the phenomenon of *T2 shine-through*. Because DWI images are T2-weighted, lesions with long T2 relaxation times will also be hyperintense on DWI, particularly on low b-value images. True restricted diffusion will correlate with a corresponding area of hypointensity on the ADC map.
- Restricted diffusion is best known in the setting of acute ischemic stroke, as DWI is sensitive for infarction within minutes of onset. However, the causes of **reduced diffusion** are diverse:

> **Neoplastic**: e.g., lymphoma, glioblastoma, medulloblastoma.
> **Inflammatory**: e.g., multiple sclerosis, acute disseminated encephalomyelitis.
> **Infectious**: e.g., abscess, empyema, ventriculitis, herpes encephalitis, Creutzfeldt-Jakob disease.
> **Vascular:** e.g., arterial or venous infarction, global hypoxic-ischemic injury, posterior reversible encephalopathy syndrome.
> **Toxic:** e.g., carbon monoxide, methanol, ethylene glycol, Wernicke encephalopathy, chemotherapy.
> **Metabolic**: e.g., osmotic demyelination, hypoglycemic encephalopathy, hepatic encephalopathy.
> **Congenital**: e.g., epidermoid cyst, mitochondrial diseases.
> **Traumatic:** diffuse axonal injury, hematoma.
> **Seizure** (status epilepticus).
> **Treatment:** radiosurgery, antiangiogenic therapy.

Gradient recalled echo (GRE) and susceptibility-weighted imaging (SWI)

- T2*-weighted GRE sequences are susceptible to signal loss from field inhomogeneities because there is no 180° rephasing pulse as there is in spin-echo sequences.
- SWI is a more sensitive version of GRE involving higher spatial resolution and other features to reduce artifacts. SWI generates both magnitude and phase images, which can help distinguish between paramagnetic (blood/iron) and diamagnetic (calcification) substances.
- Due to the susceptibility effect, materials like hemosiderin and calcification create *blooming* artifacts of signal dropout, which makes even small lesions conspicuous.
- The differential diagnosis of **multiple dark spots on GRE/SWI** reflects causes of microhemorrhage:

> **Hypertensive microangiopathy** (primarily in the basal ganglia, thalami, cerebellum, and pons).
> **Cerebral amyloid angiopathy** (primarily lobarin cortico-subcortical sites, sparing deep structures).
> **Familial cerebral cavernous malformation syndrome** (inherited multiple cavernous malformations).
> **Radiation-induced cerebral vasculopathy**.
> **Diffuse axonal injury** (primarily at gray-white matter junction and corpus callosum).
> **Hemorrhagic metastases**.
> **Fat embolism**.
> **Complication of cardiac surgery** (presumed to be rapidly developed microbleeds).

轨迹图像显示了弥散的定量测定，而**弥散张量成像(DTI)**则描绘了方向的不对称性，被称为各向异性，如白质纤维束的内在各向异性。

- 需要注意的一个重要负面问题是T_2*穿透效应*。因为DWI是T_2加权的，T_2弛豫时间长的病变在DWI上也会表现出高信号，特别是在低b值图像上。真正的弥散受限将在ADC图像上有对应的低信号区。
- 弥散受限最为人所熟知的情况是急性缺血性卒中，因为DWI对数分钟内发生的梗死敏感。然而，**弥散减低**的原因是多种多样的：

> **肿瘤性疾病：**如淋巴瘤、胶质母细胞瘤、髓母细胞瘤。
> **炎性疾病：**如多发性硬化、急性播散性脑脊髓炎。
> **感染性疾病：**如脓肿、积脓、脑室炎、疱疹性脑炎、克-雅病。
> **血管性疾病：**如动脉或静脉梗死、全身缺氧-缺血性损伤、可逆性后部脑病综合征。
> **中毒性疾病：**如一氧化碳、甲醇、乙二醇中毒，以及韦尼克脑病、化疗。
> **代谢性疾病：**如渗透性脱髓鞘、低血糖脑病、肝性脑病。
> **先天性疾病：**如表皮样囊肿、线粒体疾病。
> **创伤性疾病：**如弥漫性轴索损伤、血肿。
> **癫痫**(癫痫持续状态)。
> **治疗：**放射外科、抗血管生成治疗。

梯度回波序列(GRE)和磁敏感加权成像(SWI)

- T_2*加权GRE序列容易在非均匀性磁场中产生信号缺失，这是因为该序列没有自旋回波序列中的180°复相脉冲。
- SWI是一种更敏感的GRE，具有更高的空间分辨率和其他可减少伪影的特性。SWI同时生成幅度图和相位图，有助于区分顺磁性物质(血液/铁)和抗磁性物质(钙化)。
- 由于磁化率效应，含铁血黄素和钙等物质会产生开花样信号丢失伪影，使得很小的病变也变得很明显。
- 由微出血引起的**GRE/SWI上多发点状低信号**的鉴别诊断：

> **高血压性微血管病**(多位于基底节、丘脑、小脑及脑桥)。
> **脑淀粉样血管病**(主要位于皮质-皮质下脑叶，不影响深层结构)。
> **家族性脑海绵状血管畸形综合征**(遗传性多发海绵状血管畸形)。
> **放射性脑血管病**。
> **弥漫性轴索损伤**(多位于灰白质交界处和胼胝体)。
> **出血性转移灶**。
> **脂肪栓塞**。
> **心脏手术并发症**(可能为进展迅速的微出血)。

Magnetic resonance spectroscopy (MRS)

- Proton MR spectroscopy describes the chemical composition of a brain region. The changes in brain metabolites can be used for diagnostic, prognostic, and treatment assessment of a variety of CNS disorders.
- There are various methods of performing MR spectroscopy. Single-voxel spectroscopy (SVS) provides a high signal-to-noise ratio with a short scan time but only provides single- voxel coverage. Multi-voxel chemical shift imaging (CSI) is advantageous for larger or more heterogeneous lesions because it provides a larger coverage area and higher spatial resolution due to smaller size of individual voxels, with the tradeoff of longer scan time and lower signal-to-noise ratio.
- The peaks of the main compounds analyzed occur in alphabetical order, displayed left to right on a reversed axis of resonance frequencies expressed in parts per million (ppm).

  Choline (3.2 ppm) is a marker of cell membrane turnover that increases in most abnormalities.

  Creatine (3.0 ppm) reflects cellular energy stores and is relatively constant between most disease states.

  N-acetylaspartate (NAA) (2.0 ppm) is a marker of neuronal viability that decreases in most abnormalities.

  Lipids and **lactate** (1.3 ppm) reflect abnormal tissue damage and anaerobic glycolysis, respectively. Lipids have a broad peak and lactate has a doublet peak (due to *J-coupling*). These may be difficult to distinguish, but the lactate doublet is inverted at intermediate TE (e.g., 144 ms).
- **Hunter's angle** is a quick way to see if a spectrum is normal: a line connecting the tallest normal peaks (choline, creatine, and NAA) should point up like a plane taking off. Most diseases feature decreased NAA and/or increased choline, disrupting Hunter's angle.
- MRS can help in the evaluation of brain tumors. Prominent lipid/lactate peaks are associated with high-grade gliomas (when nonenhancing) or lymphoma (when enhancing). Elevated choline suggests tumor rather than edema (in an area of nonenhancing FLAIR abnormality) or radiation-induced necrosis (in a contrast-enhancing area; i.e., progression rather than pseudoprogression). Isocitrate dehydrogenase (IDH)-mutant status in gliomas, which carries favorable prognosis, may be predicted by the presence of 2-hydroxyglutarate (2-HG), but advanced MRS techniques are required to detect this metabolite.

磁共振波谱(MRS)

- 质子磁共振波谱(MRS)所反映的是脑组织的化学组成。脑代谢物的变化可用于各种中枢神经系统疾病的诊断、预后和治疗评估。
- MRS有多种成像方法。单体素波谱(SVS)信噪比高，扫描时间短，但仅提供单体素覆盖。多体素化学位移成像(CSI)有利于较大或更异质性病变成像，因为由于每一单个体素的尺寸更小，它能提供更大的覆盖区域和更高的空间分辨率，相应的缺点是扫描时间更长，信噪比更低。
- 所分析主要成分的波峰按字母顺序出现，从左到右显示在共振频率的反向轴上，以10^{-6}(parts per million, ppm)表示。

  胆碱(3.2ppm)是细胞膜转化的标志物，在大多数异常情况下都会增加。

  肌酸(3.0ppm)反映了细胞能量储存状态，在大多数疾病状态间都相对恒定。

  N-乙酰天门冬氨酸(NAA)(2.0ppm)是神经元活性的标志物，在大多数异常情况下都会减低。

  脂质和**乳酸**(1.3ppm)分别反映异常组织损伤和无氧糖酵解。脂质有一个宽峰，乳酸有一个双峰(J偶联所致)。这些可能难以区分，但乳酸双峰在TE中间处(如144ms)翻转。
- **猎人角**是快速发现波谱是否正常的一种方法：连接(胆碱、肌酸和NAA)峰顶的直线应该向上，如一架飞机起飞。大多数疾病的特点是NAA水平降低，伴或不伴胆碱水平升高，破坏了猎人角。
- MRS有助于评估脑肿瘤。明显的脂质/乳酸波峰与高级别胶质瘤(无增强区)或淋巴瘤(有增强区)相关。胆碱水平升高提示肿瘤而非水肿(在平扫FLAIR的异常区域)或放射性坏死(在对比增强区域；即进展而非假性进展)。胶质瘤中异柠檬酸脱氢酶(*IDH*)突变，其预后相对良好，该突变可以通过检测是否存在2-羟基戊二酸(2-HG)来预判，但这种代谢物需要使用先进的MRS技术来检测。

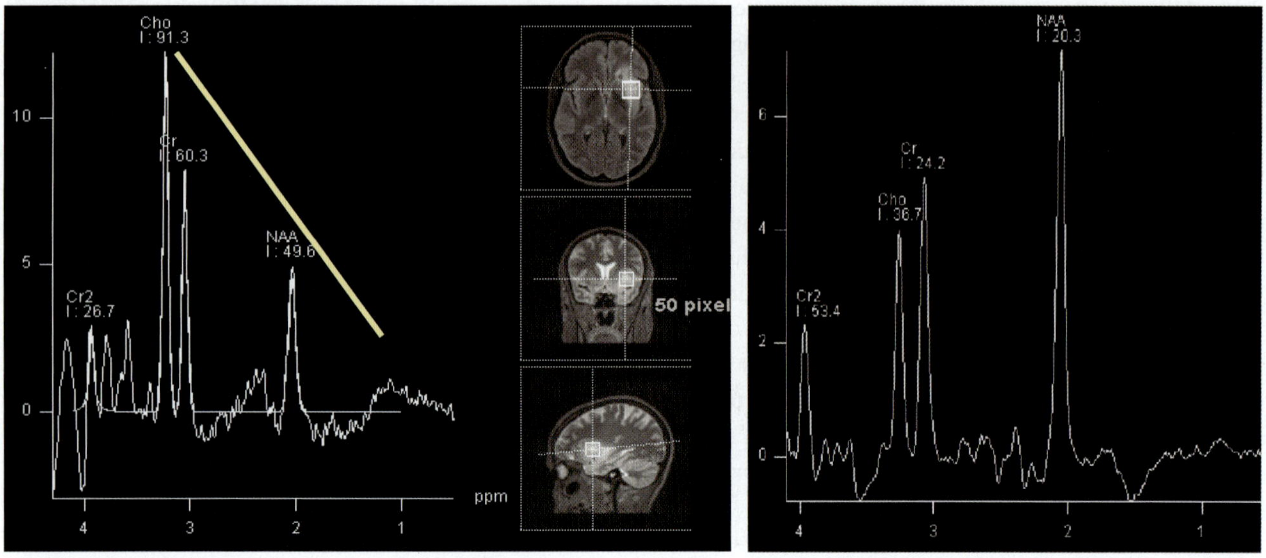

Right panel: Abnormal spectrum due to oligoastrocytoma, with elevated choline and decreased NAA. A line connecting the tallest peaks (Hunter's angle, yellow line) would point down, which is a clue that the spectrum is abnormal.

Left panel: Normal spectrum. Hunter's angle is pointing up like a plane at takeoff.

右图：少突星形细胞瘤出现的异常波谱，胆碱水平升高，NAA水平降低。连接峰顶的直线(猎人角，黄线)指向下方，提示波谱异常。

左图：正常波谱。猎人角指向上，如一架飞机起飞。

ppm—parts per million, 10^{-6}

- MRS can help detect inborn errors of metabolism and mitochondrial disorders.

  Elevated NAA is characteristic of the leukodystrophy Canavan disease.

  Elevated lactate suggests mitochondrial encephalopathies such as Leigh syndrome.

MR Perfusion

- MR perfusion (sometimes called "perfusion-weighted imaging") refers to a family of advanced techniques to detect changes in signal in the brain dependent on inflowing blood.
- In dynamic susceptibility contrast (DSC) MR perfusion, injection of a bolus of gadolinium- based contrast media causes a magnetic field disturbance, which transiently decreases the signal intensity on T2*-weighted images.
- In dynamic contrast enhanced (DCE) MR perfusion, injection of a bolus of gadolinium-based contrast media causes T1 shortening, which increases the signal intensity on T1-weighted images.
- In arterial spin labeling (ASL) MR perfusion, a noncontrast technique, radiofrequency pulses at the neck magnetically label blood protons, which then travel to the brain where they are imaged.
- Three calculated parameters reflect microvascular effects (capillary perfusion): cerebral blood flow (CBF), cerebral blood volume (CBV), and mean transit time (MTT = CBV/CBF).
- Additional parameters like time to maximum (Tmax) and time to peak concentration (TTP) also capture macrovascular effects such as contrast bolus arrival delay.
- MR perfusion is most commonly employed for evaluation of brain tumors. High-grade gliomas and metastases have higher relative CBV compared to low-grade gliomas or lymphoma. In the post-treatment setting for high-grade

- 磁共振波谱可以帮助检测先天性代谢异常和线粒体疾病。

  NAA水平升高是脑白质营养不良Canavan病的特征。

  乳酸水平升高提示线粒体脑病，如Leigh综合征。

磁共振灌注成像

- 磁共振灌注成像(有时被称为"灌注加权成像")是基于脑血流进行检测脑部信号变化的一系列先进技术。
- 在动态磁敏感对比增强(DSC)MR灌注中，静脉团注钆造影剂可引起磁场干扰，暂时降低T_2*加权图像的信号强度。
- 在动态对比增强(DCE)MR灌注中，静脉团注钆造影剂可导致T_1缩短，从而增加T_1加权图像上的信号强度。
- 动脉自旋标记(ASL)MR灌注是一种非造影剂技术，在颈部的血液内质子被射频脉冲进行磁性标记，随后被传输到大脑进行成像。
- 三个计算参数反映了微血管效应(毛细血管灌注)：脑血流量(CBF)、脑血容量(CBV)和平均通过时间(MTT = CBV/CBF)。
- 其他参数，如残留功能达峰时间(T_{max})和达峰时间(TTP)，也可以捕捉到造影剂延迟等大血管效应。
- MR灌注最常用于评估脑肿瘤。高级别胶质瘤和转移瘤较低级别胶质瘤或淋巴瘤具有更高的相对脑血容量。对于治疗后的高级别胶

gliomas, elevated CBV favors tumor recurrence over pseudoprogression.

- In acute stroke, perfusion imaging identifies ischemic penumbra (area at risk of infarction) characterized by delayed contrast arrival (elevated Tmax) but compensated microvascular autoregulation (at most moderate decrease in CBF, mismatched by elevated CBV).
- The above parameters and perfusion imaging are further discussed in the stroke section.

PATTERNS OF ENHANCEMENT IN THE BRAIN

Blood-brain barrier (BBB) and enhancement

- Micro or macro disruption of the blood-brain barrier (BBB) produces *parenchymal* enhancement after contrast administration, which may be secondary to infection, inflammation, neoplasm, trauma, and vascular etiologies.
- The BBB is formed by astrocytic foot processes of brain capillary endothelial cells and prevents direct communication between the systemic capillaries and the protected extracellular fluid of the brain.
- Several CNS regions do not have a BBB, and therefore normally enhance:

Choroid plexus.
Pituitary and pineal glands.
Tuber cinereum (controls circadian rhythm, located in the inferior hypothalamus).
Area postrema (controls vomiting, located at inferior aspect of fourth ventricle).

The dura also lacks a BBB, but does not normally enhance. This phenomenon is subsequently explained in the section on pachymeningeal (dural) enhancement.

- *Vascular* enhancement is due to a localized increase in blood flow, which may be secondary to vasodilation, hyperemia, neovascularity, or arteriovenous shunting.

On CT, the arterial phase of contrast enhancement (i.e., CT angiogram) mostly shows intravascular enhancement. Parenchymal enhancement, including the dural folds of the falx and tentorium, is best seen several minutes after the initial contrast bolus.

On MRI, routine contrast-enhanced sequences are obtained in the parenchymal phase, several minutes after injection. Most intracranial vascular MRI imaging is performed with a noncontrast time-of-flight technique.

- Intracranial enhancement may be intra- or extra-axial. Extra-axial structures that may enhance in pathologic conditions include the dura (pachymeninges) and arachnoid (leptomeninges).

质瘤，CBV升高多提示肿瘤复发而不是假性进展。

- 在急性卒中，灌注成像可识别缺血半暗带(有梗死风险的区域)，其特征是造影剂到达峰值延迟(T_{max}升高)但微血管自我调节可代偿(多表现为CBF中度降低，与CBV升高不匹配)。
- 上述参数和灌注成像将在本章“卒中”部分进一步讨论。

脑强化的形式

血脑屏障与强化

- 任何微观或宏观的血脑屏障(BBB)破坏都会使脑实质在注射造影剂后强化，可继发于感染、炎症、肿瘤、创伤和血管源性病变。
- BBB由脑毛细血管内皮细胞的星形细胞足突形成，阻止体循环毛细血管与受保护的脑细胞外液的直接交通。
- 中枢神经系统的某些部位不具备血脑屏障，因此会有正常强化：

脉络丛。
垂体和松果体。
灰结节(管理昼夜节律，位于下丘脑下部)。
极后区(管理呕吐，位于第四脑室下部)。

硬脑膜也缺少血脑屏障，但正常情况下并无强化。该现象会在下文硬脑膜强化部分进行介绍。

- 局部血流增加会出现血管强化，可继发于血管扩张、充血、新生血管形成或动静脉短路。

CT增强动脉期(如CTA)多会出现血管内强化。脑实质强化的最佳显示时间是在团注造影剂后数分钟，其中包括大脑镰和小脑幕的反折。

在MRI上，常规增强序列都在脑实质期进行，即在注射造影剂后的数分钟。大部分颅内MR血管成像通过非增强的时间飞跃技术完成。

- 颅内强化可以是轴内或轴外。发生病理性强化的轴外结构包括硬膜(硬脑膜)和蛛网膜(柔脑膜)。

Periventricular enhancement (intra-axial)

脑室周围强化(轴内)

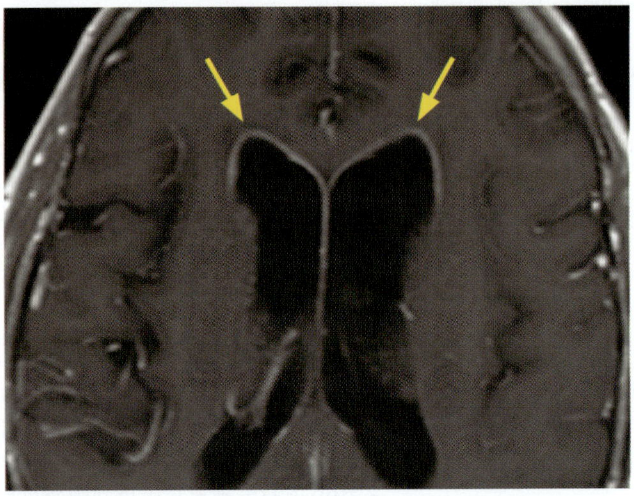

Axial post-contrast T1-weighted MRI demonstrates smooth periventricular enhancement (arrows) thought to represent ventriculitis/infectious ependymitis. This was proven to be an uncommon case of metastatic melanoma based on CSF sampling.

轴位增强T_1加权MRI显示脑室周围均匀性增强(箭)被认为是脑室炎/感染性室管膜炎。脑脊液样本证明该患者为一名罕见的转移性黑色素瘤。

- Enhancement of the subependymal cortical surface can be either neoplastic, infectious, demyelination, and treatment-induced (e.g., radiation).

Nodular subcortical enhancement (intra-axial)

- Nodular intra-axial enhancement is most commonly due to metastatic disease.
- **Hematogenously disseminated metastatic disease** is commonly found at the subcortical gray-white junctions. Tumor emboli become "stuck" at the junction between the simple vasculature of the white matter and the highly branching vasculature of the gray matter.
- Edema is almost always present with metastatic disease of the gray-white junction, although slightly more distal cortical metastases may not show any edema and may be detectable only on the post-contrast images.
- In contrast to the subcortical pattern seen with arterial metastases, venous dissemination of metastasis (e.g., pelvic malignancy spread via the Batson prevertebral venous plexus) leads to posterior fossa disease by transit through the retroclival venous plexus.

- 室管膜下皮质表面强化的原因可以是肿瘤、感染、脱髓鞘疾病和治疗(如放疗)。

结节状皮层下强化(轴内)

- 轴内结节状强化最常见于转移瘤。
- **血行播散的转移瘤**常见于皮层下灰白质交界区。瘤栓可"嵌顿"于白质的单支血管与灰质的高度分支血管之间的交汇区。
- 水肿几乎总是伴随位于灰白质交界区的转移瘤，但稍远一点的皮层转移灶见不到水肿，可能仅在增强图像上才发现病灶。
- 动脉播散的转移灶见于皮层下，而静脉播散的转移灶(如通过椎前静脉丛转移的盆腔恶性肿瘤)通过斜坡静脉丛到达颅后窝。

Gyriform enhancement (intra-axial)

脑回样强化(轴内)

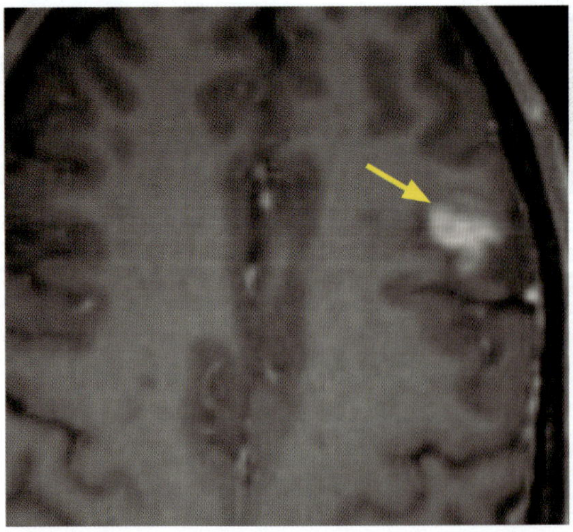

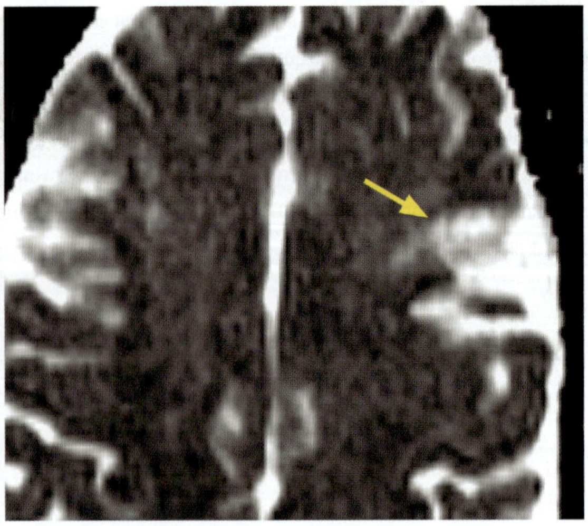

Axial T1-weighted post-contrast MRI (left image) shows a focus of enhancement along the gyral surface of the left frontal lobe (arrow) in a pattern typical of gyriform enhancement. This region is hyperintense on the ADC map (arrow on right image), consistent with increased diffusivity. There is no significant mass effect. This was a late subacute infarct.

轴位增强T_1加权MRI(左图)显示沿左额叶脑回表面的强化灶(黄箭)，为典型的脑回样强化。该区域在ADC图上呈高信号(右图中的黄箭)，符合弥散增强，但无明显占位效应。此图为亚急性晚期梗死。

- Superficial enhancement of the cortical (gyral) surface of the brain can be due to either cerebral infection, inflammation, or ischemia.

differential diagnosis of gyriform enhancement

- **Herpes encephalitis** is a serious necrotizing infection of the brain parenchyma due to reactivation of latent HSV-1 infection within the trigeminal ganglion. The medial temporal lobes and cingulate gyrus are usually affected first and demonstrate gyral enhancement due to inflammation, petechial hemorrhage, and resultant BBB breakdown. The involved areas typically also demonstrate reduced diffusivity.
- **Meningitis** may cause gyral enhancement in addition to the leptomeningeal enhancement previously discussed.
- **Subacute infarct** can demonstrate gyriform enhancement lasting approximately 6 days to 6 weeks after the initial ischemic event.

  In contrast to the gyriform enhancement of subacute infarct, an acute infarct may demonstrate vascular enhancement due to reactive collateral vasodilation and resultant hyperemia.

  Enhancement related to subacute infarct is often associated with varying degree of T1 shortening (hyperintensity) and this can be an important distinguishing feature in addition to volume loss that will take longer time to manifest.
- **Posterior reversible encephalopathy syndrome** (PRES) is a syndrome of vasogenic white matter edema triggered by altered autoregulation that may demonstrate gyral enhancement. PRES may rarely exhibit restricted diffusion.
- **SMART syndrome** (stroke-like migraine attacks after radiation therapy) is a delayed complication of radiotherapy, usually occurring years or decades after treatment. It is characterized by contiguous cortical thickening, edema, gyriform DWI abnormality, and enhancement. It can progressively worsen over months, but eventually stabilizes.

- 脑皮层表面(脑回)的强化可由脑组织感染、炎症或缺血导致。

脑回样强化的鉴别诊断

- **疱疹性脑炎**是严重的脑实质坏死性感染,由三叉神经节中潜伏的1型单纯疱疹病毒(HSV-1)重新激活引起。颞叶内侧和扣带回最先受感染,并因炎症、点状出血及血脑屏障破坏,表现出脑回强化。受累脑区常显示弥散减低。
- **脑膜炎**可使脑回强化和柔脑膜出现强化(前文已述)。
- **亚急性脑梗死**可表现出脑回样强化,并在缺血发生后持续6天至6周。

  不同于亚急性脑梗死的脑回样强化,急性脑梗死发生的血管强化是由于侧支循环反应性扩张和其导致的充血。

  与亚急性脑梗死相关的强化通常有不同程度的T_1缩短(高信号),这可能是除了体积缩小之外的另一项重要的鉴别特征,而体积缩小需要较长时间才能显现。
- **可逆性后部脑病综合征**(PRES)是一种自我调节障碍触发的血管源性白质水肿,可出现脑回强化。PRES极少表现为弥散受限。
- **SMART综合征**(放疗后的卒中样偏头痛发作)是放疗的远期并发症,通常在治疗后数年或数十年发生。该病的特征为连续的皮质增厚、水肿、DWI脑回样异常和强化。疾病可能在几个月内逐渐恶化,但最终会稳定下来。

Ring enhancement (intra-axial)

环状强化(轴内)

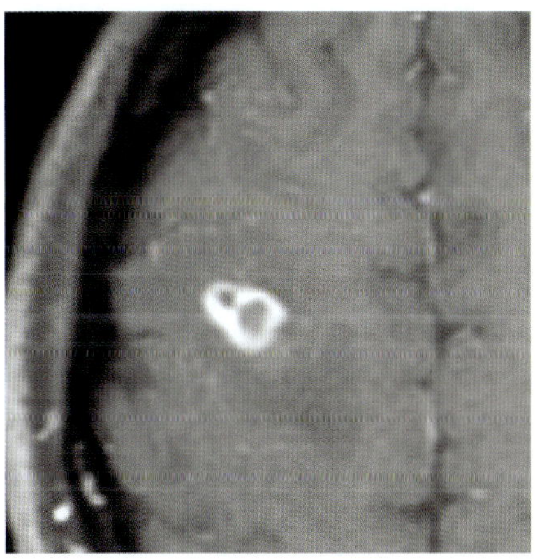

Patient 1: Axial post-contrast T1-weighted MRI shows a bilobed ring-enhancing lesion in the right frontal cortex. This was due to neurocysticercosis.
患者1:轴位增强T_1加权MRI显示位于右侧额叶皮质一个呈双分叶状的环形强化病灶,此为脑囊虫病。

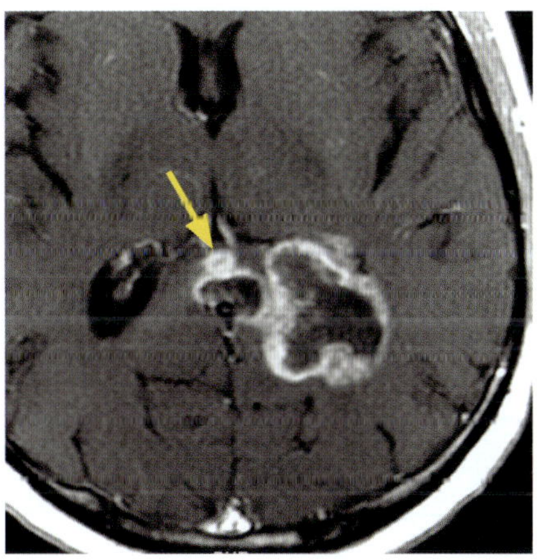

Patient 2: Axial post-contrast T1-weighted MRI shows an irregular ring-enhancing lesion effacing the atrium of the left ventricle and extending across the splenium of the corpus callosum (arrow). This was a glioblastoma.
患者2:轴位增强T_1加权MRI显示不规则的环状强化病压迫左侧脑室三角区并跨越胼胝体压部(黄箭),此为脑胶质瘤。

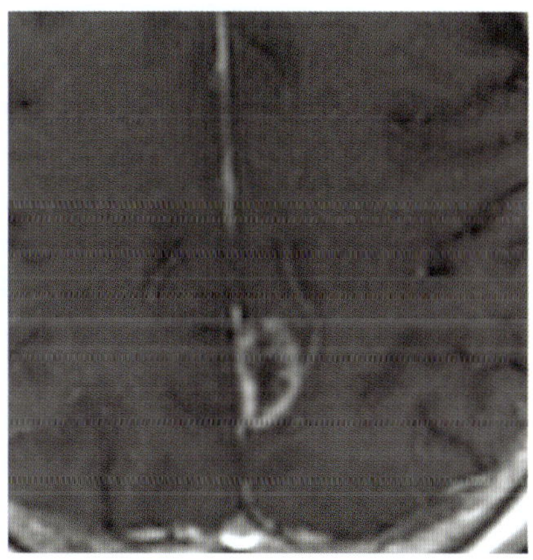

Patient 3: Axial post-contrast T1-weighted MRI shows a ring-enhancing lesion in the left parietal lobe abutting the falx. This was a breast cancer metastasis.
患者3:轴位增强T_1加权MRI显示左侧顶叶紧邻大脑镰处一个环状强化病灶,此为乳腺癌转移。

- Peripheral (ring) enhancement is a common presentation with a broad range of differential diagnoses. The two most common causes are high-grade neoplasm and cerebral abscess.
- The mnemonic **MAGIC DR** (**m**etastasis, **a**bscess, **g**lioma, **i**nfarct, **c**ontusion, **d**emyelination, and **r**adiation) may be helpful to remember the wide range of etiologies for ring enhancement, although it is usually possible to narrow the differential based on the pattern of ring enhancement combined with additional MRI sequences and clinical history.

- 外周(环状)强化是一种常见的影像学表现，涉及很多鉴别诊断。最常见的两个病因为高级别肿瘤和脑脓肿。
- 口诀**MAGIC DR**(M为转移、A为脓肿、G为胶质瘤、I为梗死、C为脑挫伤、D为脱髓鞘及R为放射性损伤)可以帮助记忆种类繁多的环状强化病因，但结合其他的MRI序列和临床病史通常可以缩小环状强化的鉴别诊断。

differential diagnosis of ring enhancement

- **Metastasis**: Hematogenous metastases are typically found at the subcortical gray-white junction. Metastases are often multiple, but smaller lesions may not bering-enhancing.
- **Abscess:** A pyogenic abscess is formed as a result of organization and sequestration of an infection, featuring a central region of viscous necrosis.

  The key imaging findings of abscess are reduced diffusivity (bright on DWI and dark on ADC) caused by high viscosity of central necrosis and a characteristic smooth, hypointense rim on T2-weighted images.
- **Glioma**: High grade tumors such as glioblastoma typically have a thick and irregular wall.

  Multivoxel MRI spectroscopy will be abnormal outside the margin of an enhancing high grade glial neoplasm secondary to nonenhancing infiltrative tumor. This is in contrast to demyelinatinglesion, abscess, and metastasis, where the spectral pattern returns to normal at the margin of the lesion. Perfusion MRI demonstrates elevated perfusion in a high grade glioma.
- **Infarct**: Although subacute infarcts often demonstrate gyral enhancement, ring enhancement can be seen in subacute basal ganglia infarcts.

  In contrast to neoplasm or infection, a subacute infarct does not have significant mass effect.
- **Contusion**: Both traumatic and nontraumatic intraparenchymal hemorrhage can show ring enhancement in the subacute to chronic stage.
- **Demyelinating disease**: The key finding in ring-enhancing demyelinating disease is lack of significant mass effect. The "ring" of enhancement is often incomplete and "C" shaped.

  Multiple sclerosis is the most common demyelinating disease. Enhancement suggests active disease.

  Although the typical finding is an incomplete rim of enhancement, tumefactive demyelinating disease can look identical to a high-grade tumor.
- **Radiation necrosis** may look identical to a necrotic tumor such as high-grade tumor or metastasis. On perfusion, cerebral blood volume is generally low in radiation necrosis and typically increased in a high-grade glioma.

环状强化的鉴别诊断包括

- **转移瘤**：血行转移灶通常位于皮层下灰白质交界处。一般多发，但较小的病变可无环状强化。
- **脓肿**：化脓性脓肿是感染机化和隔离形成的，以中心黏性坏死为特征。

  脓肿关键的影像学表现为中心黏性坏死区弥散受限(DWI上高信号，ADC上低信号)和特征性的T_2加权上光整的低信号环。
- **胶质瘤**：高级别肿瘤如胶质母细胞瘤，通常具有不规则的厚壁。

  多体素MRI波谱可见强化的高级别胶质瘤边缘外围出现异常，这是由无强化的肿瘤浸润导致。这与脱髓鞘病变、脓肿和转移瘤不同，后三者病灶外缘的波谱图正常。MR灌注成像显示高级别胶质瘤灌注增高。
- **梗死**：尽管亚急性脑梗死通常表现为脑回强化，但亚急性基底节梗死可以表现为环状强化。

  不同于肿瘤或感染，亚急性梗死灶无明显的占位效应。
- **挫伤**：创伤性和非创伤性两种脑实质内出血都可在亚急性至慢性期表现为环状强化。
- **脱髓鞘病变**：环状强化的脱髓鞘疾病的主要表现是缺乏明显的占位效应。强化的"环"往往不完整，呈"C"形。

  多发性硬化是最常见的脱髓鞘病变。病灶强化提示疾病处在活动期。

  尽管典型的表现为不完整环状强化，但肿瘤样脱髓鞘病变也可与高级别肿瘤表现完全相同。
- **放射性脑坏死**可以与高级别肿瘤等坏死性肿瘤或转移瘤的表现完全相同。灌注成像上，放射性脑坏死者脑血容量通常降低，而高级别胶质瘤则往往增加。

Pachymeningeal (dural) enhancement (extra-axial)

硬脑膜强化(轴外)

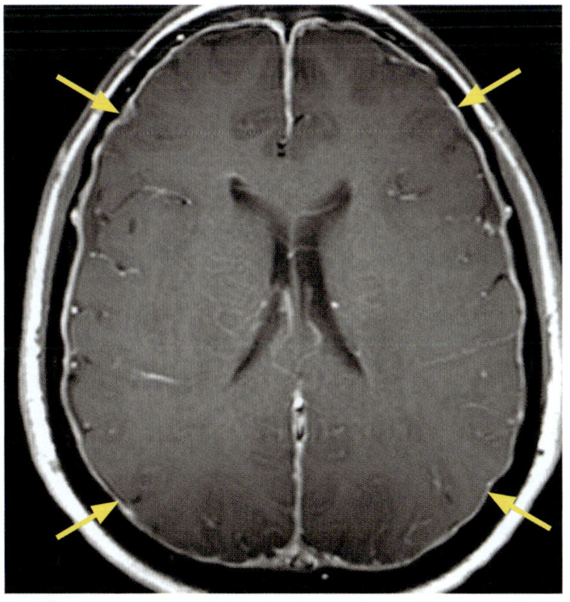

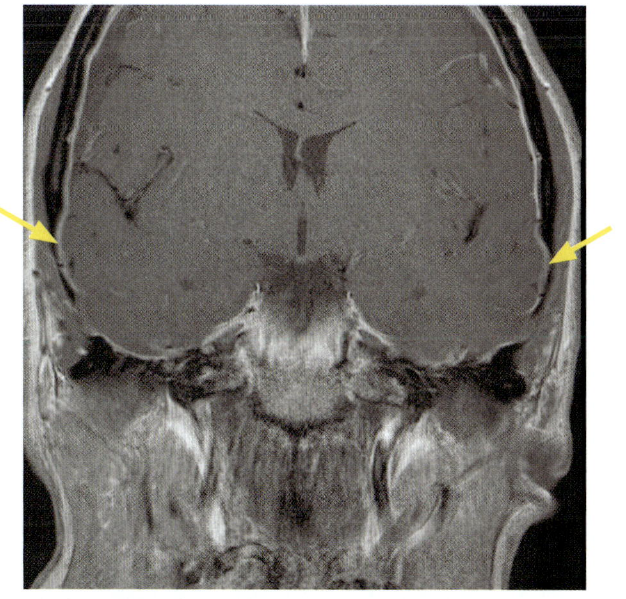

Diffuse dural enhancement: Axial (left image) and coronal post-contrast T1-weighted (right image) MRI shows diffuse dural enhancement (arrows). This was a case of intracranial hypotension.

弥漫性硬脑膜强化：轴位(左图)和冠状位增强T_1加权(右图)MRI显示弥漫性硬脑膜强化(黄箭)。此为低颅压病例。

- The **pachymeninges** (*pachy* means thick-a "thick-skinned" elephant is a pachyderm) refers to the dura mater, the thick and leather-like outermost covering of the brain.
- In addition to surrounding the surface of the brain, the dura forms several reflections, including the falx, tentorium, and cavernous sinus.
- The dura does not have a blood-brain barrier. Although contrast molecules normally diffuse into the dura on enhanced CT or MRI, dural enhancement is never visualized on CT and is only visualized on MRI in pathologic situations.

Dural enhancement is not seen on CT because both the skull and adjacent enhancing dura appear white. Enhancement of normal dura is not visible on MRI because MRI visualization of enhancement requires both water protons and gadolinium. Although gadolinium is present in the dura, there are normally very few water protons. However, dural pathology often causes dural edema, which provides enough water protons to make the gadolinium visible. Therefore, **dural enhancement on MRI is an indication of dural edema rather than BBB breakdown.**

- **硬脑膜(pachymeninges)**(“pachy”是厚的意思，如“厚皮”的大象是一种厚皮类动物)指的是坚硬的脑膜，是覆盖脑组织最外层的厚而像皮革样的覆盖物。
- 除覆盖脑组织表面外，硬脑膜还形成多处反折，包括大脑镰、小脑幕和海绵窦。
- 硬脑膜不含血脑屏障。CT或MRI造影剂分子在正常情况下可以弥散进入硬脑膜，但CT通过看不到硬脑膜强化，MRI上也只在病理情况下才会见到强化。

CT上看不到硬脑膜强化，因为颅骨和相邻的强化硬脑膜都呈白色。MRI上看不到正常强化的硬脑膜，其原因是MRI显示强化需要同时含有水分子和钆。尽管钆剂可进入硬脑膜，但正常硬脑膜极少含有水分子。但是，硬脑膜病变常引起水肿，从而提供了足够的水分子使得钆剂显示。因此，**在MRI上见到硬脑膜强化常提示硬脑膜水肿，而不是血脑屏障破坏。**

differential diagnosis of pachymeningeal enhancement

- **Intracranial hypotension:** Prolonged decrease in CSF pressure can lead to vasogenic edema in the dura.

  Intracranial hypotension clinically presents as a postural headache exacerbated by standing upright.

  Etiology may be idiopathic or secondary to CSF leak whether spontaneous or iatrogenic.

  Imaging shows smooth, linear dural enhancement, enlargement of the pituitary gland and dural venous sinuses, and "sagging" of the cerebellar tonsils. There may also be subdural hemorrhage due to traction effect on the cerebral veins.
- **Postoperative:** Dural enhancement may be seen postoperatively.
- **Post lumbar puncture:** Diffuse dural enhancement is occasionally seen (<5% of the time) after routine lumbar puncture.
- **Meningeal neoplasm,** such as meningioma, can produce a focal area of dural enhancement called a *dural tail*, due to reactive changes in the dura. Metastatic disease to the dura, most commonly breast cancer in a female and prostate cancer in a male, can cause irregular dural enhancement.
- **Hypertrophic pachymeningitis:** localized or diffuse dural thickening due to various causes, including infectious (e.g., tuberculosis, fungal, syphilis), inflammatory (e.g., rheumatoid arthritis, granulomatosis with polyangiitis), sarcoidosis, or can beidiopathic.

硬脑膜强化的鉴别诊断

- **低颅压：**持续性脑脊液压力降低会导致硬脑膜血管源性水肿。

  低颅压临床表现为体位性头痛，直立时加重。

  低颅压的病因可能是特发性或继发于脑脊液漏，后者可以是自发的，也可能是医源性的。

  影像学表现为平滑的线性硬脑膜强化，垂体和硬脑膜静脉窦增大，小脑扁桃体“下垂”。也可以因脑静脉牵拉而出现硬膜下出血。
- **术后：**外科术后也可以出现硬脑膜强化。
- **腰椎穿刺后：**常规腰椎穿刺后偶尔可见弥漫性硬脑膜强化(发生率<5%)。
- **脑膜肿瘤，**如脑膜瘤，可出现局灶性硬脑膜强化，也被称为*脑膜尾征*，是硬脑膜的反应性改变。硬脑膜转移灶可引起硬脑膜不规则强化，最常见于女性的乳腺癌和男性的前列腺癌。
- **肥厚性硬脑膜炎：**各种原因可导致局部或弥漫性硬脑膜增厚，包括感染(如结核、真菌、梅毒)、炎症(如类风湿关节炎、肉芽肿性多血管炎)、结节病，或是特发性的。

Leptomeningeal (pia-arachnoid) enhancement (extra-axial)

柔脑膜(软脑膜-蛛网膜)强化(轴外)

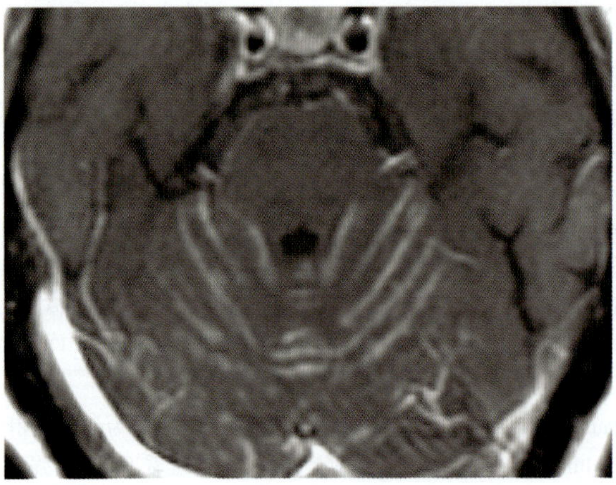

Axial post-contrast T1-weighted MRI demonstrates enhancement along the cerebellar folia. This was leptomeningeal spread of systemic lymphoma.

轴位增强T_1加权MRI显示强化沿小脑的表面分布。这是全身性淋巴瘤的柔脑膜播散。

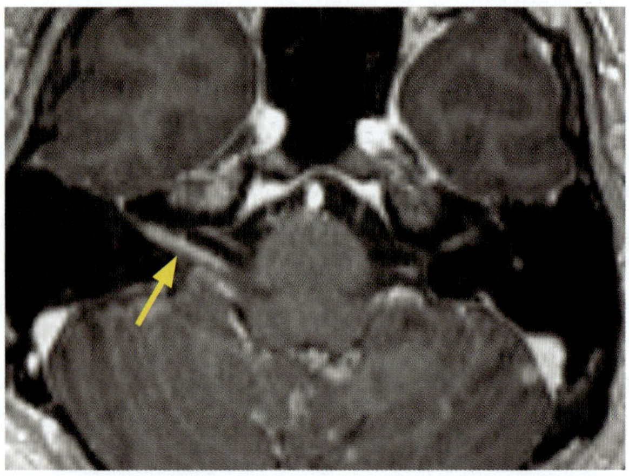

Axial post-contrast T1-weighted MRI shows enhancement along the right cranial nerve Ⅶ and Ⅷ complex (arrow). This was metastatic lung adenocarcinoma.

轴位增强T_1加权MRI显示沿右侧第Ⅶ和第Ⅷ脑神经复合体(黄箭)增强。这是转移性肺腺癌。

- The **leptomeninges** (*lepto* means thin or narrow) include the pia and arachnoid.
- Leptomeningeal enhancement follows the undulating contours of the sulci as it includes enhancement of both the subarachnoid space and the pial surface of the brain.

- **柔脑膜**(lepto指薄的或窄的)包括软脑膜和蛛网膜。
- 柔脑膜强化沿脑沟折叠的轮廓，因它包括蛛网膜下腔和脑表软脑膜的强化。

differential diagnosis of leptomeningeal enhancement

- **Meningitis** (either bacterial, viral, or fungal) is the primary consideration when leptomeningeal enhancement is seen.

  Leptomeningeal enhancement in meningitis is caused by BBB breakdown due to inflammation or infection.

  Fine, linear enhancement suggests bacterial or viral meningitis.

  Thicker, nodular enhancement suggests fungal meningitis.

- **Viral encephalitis** may produce cranial nerve enhancement within the subarachnoid space.
- **Leptomeningeal metastases**, also called neoplastic meningitis, is spread of tumor cells into the subarachnoid space, which may be due to primary brain tumor or metastatic disease from an extra-CNS malignancy.

  CNS neoplasms that more commonly have leptomeningeal spread include medulloblastoma, choroid plexus tumor, lymphoma, ependymoma, glioblastoma, and germinoma.

  Metastatic tumors known to cause leptomeningeal disease include lymphoma and breast cancer.

- **Inflammatory amyloidosis** often shows leptomeningeal enhancement with cortical edema and susceptibility.

- The differential diagnosis of FLAIR hyperintensity in the subarachnoid space overlaps with the differential for leptomeningeal enhancement. **Subarachnoid FLAIR hyperintensity** may be due to:

Meningitis and leptomeningeal metastases both have increased subarachnoid FLAIR signal and leptomeningeal enhancement.

Subarachnoid hemorrhage manifests as increased subarachnoid FLAIR signal, without leptomeningeal enhancement. Blooming artifact on GRE or SWI from blood products will help differentiate subarachnoid hemorrhage from **leptomeningeal metastases**.

Slow vascular flow appears as an *intravascular* distribution of FLAIR hyperintensity due to "unmasking" of the inherent high signal of blood, which remains in the plane of imaging as the entire pulse sequence is obtained. Slow flow of peripheral vessels in moyamoya disease causes the *ivy sign*.

Subarachnoid FLAIR signal is artifactually increased when the patient is on **oxygen** or **propofol** therapy, without abnormal enhancement.

柔脑膜强化的鉴别诊断

- **脑膜炎**(可以是细菌性、病毒性或真菌性)是柔脑膜强化首要考虑的诊断。

  脑膜炎时出现的柔脑膜强化是由于炎症或感染破坏了血脑屏障。

  细小和线性强化提示细菌或病毒性脑膜炎。

  较厚和结节状强化提示真菌性脑膜炎。

- **病毒性脑炎**能引起位于蛛网膜下腔内的脑神经强化。
- **柔脑膜转移瘤**,也称为癌性脑膜炎,指肿瘤细胞播散进入蛛网膜下腔,可以是原发脑肿瘤,也可是从中枢神经系统外转移而来的恶性肿瘤。

  常见引起柔脑膜播散的中枢神经系统肿瘤包括髓母细胞瘤、脉络丛肿瘤、淋巴瘤、室管膜瘤、胶质母细胞瘤和生殖细胞瘤。

  能引起柔脑膜疾病的转移瘤包括淋巴瘤和乳腺癌。

- **炎症性淀粉样变性**常表现为柔脑膜强化伴皮质水肿和易感性。

- 蛛网膜下腔FLAIR高信号的鉴别诊断与柔脑膜强化的鉴别诊断有重叠。**蛛网膜下腔FLAIR高信号**可能的原因有:

脑膜炎和柔脑膜转移瘤两者都表现为蛛网膜下腔FLAIR信号增高和柔脑膜强化。

蛛网膜下腔出血表现为蛛网膜下腔FLAIR信号增高,而无柔脑膜强化。血液成分在GRE或SWI序列上的开花样伪影有助于鉴别蛛网膜下腔出血和**柔脑膜转移瘤**。

慢速血流在FLAIR上表现为*血管内*高信号,这是由于血液固有的高信号的"未流空",而是在整个脉冲序列都停留在成像的层面。烟雾病时周围血管的慢血流能形成*常春藤征*。

吸氧或丙泊酚治疗会导致人为增加蛛网膜下腔的FLAIR信号,但无异常强化。

(翻译 张轶群)

INTERNAL CAROTID ARTERY (ICA)

颈内动脉(ICA)

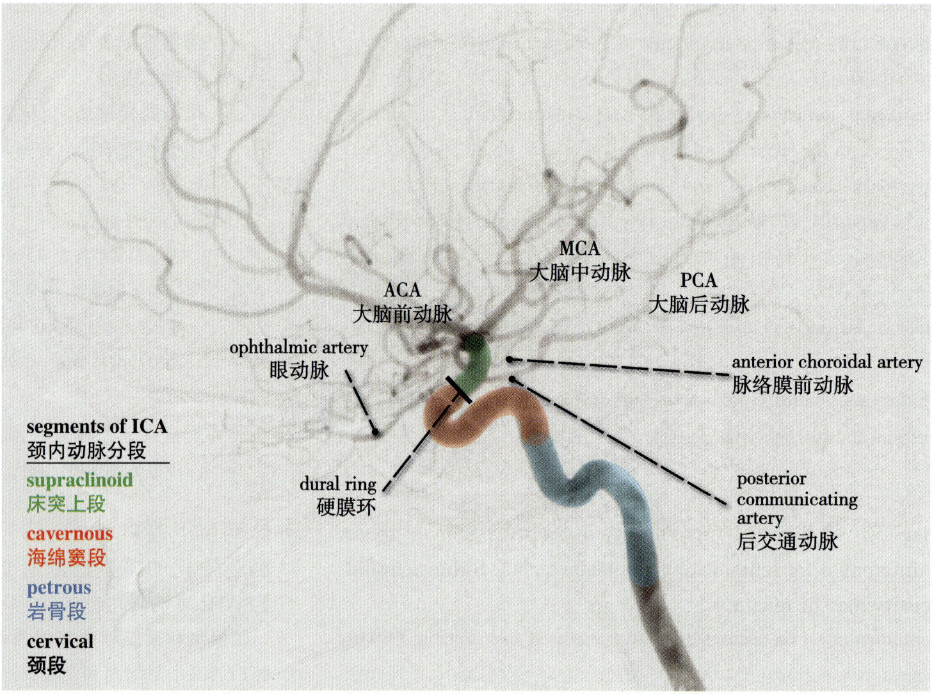

- The segmental nomenclature of the internal carotid artery (ICA) is not universally agreed upon. The simplest is the Gibo classification, reflected below along with the major branches. Note that many of the branches are infrequently seen on imaging.
- The **cervical** segment extends from the carotid bifurcation to the skull base and gives off no branches.
- The **petrous** segment extends through the carotid canal and slightly past foramen lacerum while giving off the caroticotympanic and Vidian arteries.
- The **cavernous** segment begins a series of back-and-forth bends historically called the "carotid siphon" while giving off the meningohypophyseal trunk and the inferolateral trunk.

  The **meningohypophyseal trunk** supplies the pituitary and nearby meninges.

  The **inferolateral trunk** supplies the third through sixth cranial nerves and nearby meninges.
- The **supraclinoid** segment is the intradural portion that gives off the ophthalmic, superior hypophyseal, posterior communicating, and anterior choroidal arteries.

  The **ophthalmic artery** supplies the orbital structures. It can be used as a landmark for the distal dural ring, such that aneurysms located at or superior to the ophthalmic artery are intradural. Given the risk of subarachnoid hemorrhage, these aneurysms are treated more aggressively than aneurysms located proximal to the distal dural ring, which are contained.

  The **superior hypophyseal artery** supplies the hypothalamus and pituitary stalk.

  The **posterior communicating artery** (P-comm) is an anastomosis to the posterior circulation. A fetal posterior cerebral artery (PCA) is a variant supplied entirely by the ipsilateral ICA via an enlarged P-comm.

  The **anterior choroidal artery** supplies the anteromesial temporal lobe including the head of hippocampus, as well as deep brain structures including the optic tract, lateral thalamus, and posterior limb and retrolenticular part of the internal capsule.
- The ICA **terminus** bifurcates into the anterior and middle cerebral arteries.

- ICA的节段命名法并未广泛达成一致。最简单的是Gibo分段法，下面将与其主要分支一同进行讨论。需要注意，许多分支在影像上并不能经常观察到。
- **颈段**从颈动脉分叉处延伸至颅底，无分支。
- **岩骨**段通过颈动脉管一路延伸并在穿过破裂孔后不久随即发出颈鼓动脉和翼管动脉。
- **海绵窦段**始于一系列来回扭曲，旧称"颈动脉虹吸部"，并在途中发出脑膜垂体干和下外侧干。

  脑膜垂体干供应垂体和邻近的脑膜。

  下外侧干供应第Ⅲ~Ⅵ脑神经及邻近的脑膜。
- **床突上段**位于硬膜内，它发出眼动脉、垂体上动脉、后交通动脉和脉络膜前动脉。

  眼动脉供应眼眶结构，可以作为远端硬脑膜环的标志，因此动脉瘤位于眼动脉或眼动脉的上方，即位于硬脑膜内。由于蛛网膜下腔出血的风险，治疗这些动脉瘤需要比位于硬膜环近侧的动脉瘤更加积极。

  垂体上动脉供应下丘脑和垂体柄。

  后交通动脉(P-comm)是与后循环吻合的动脉。胚胎型大脑后动脉(PCA)是一种变异，完全由同侧的ICA通过增粗的后交通动脉供血。

  脉络膜前动脉供应海马头部的前内侧颞叶，以及脑的深部结构，包括视束、外侧丘脑、内囊后肢和豆状核后部。
- ICA**末端**分叉成为大脑前动脉和大脑中动脉。

CIRCLE OF WILLIS

威利斯环(大脑动脉环)

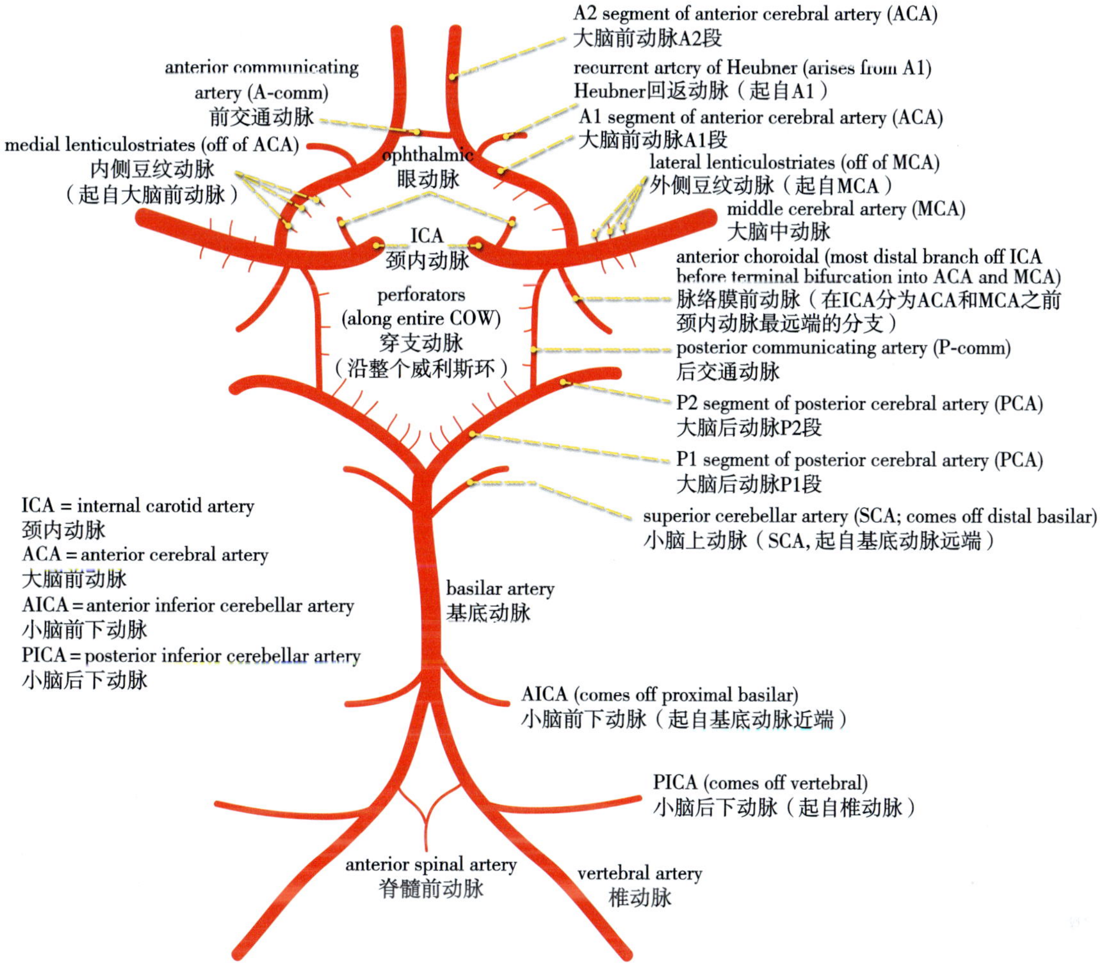

Critical small arteries arising from the circle of Willis

- The A1 segment of the anterior cerebral artery (ACA) travels above the optic nerves and gives off the **recurrent artery of Heubner**, which supplies the caudate head and anterior limb of the internal capsule. The A1 segment also gives rise to the medial lenticulostriate perforator vessels which supply the medial basal ganglia.
- Just outside the circle of Willis, the middle cerebral artery (MCA) gives rise to the lateral lenticulostriate perforator vessels to supply the lateral basal ganglia including the lateral putamen, external capsule, and the posterior limb of the internal capsule.
- The posterior communicating artery (P-comm) travels between optic tract and cranial nerve Ⅲ, giving off anterior thalamoperforator vessels. A P-comm aneurysm may cause cranial nerve Ⅲ palsy due to local mass effect.
- The posterior cerebral artery (PCA) gives off thalamoperforators to supply the thalamus. **Artery of Percheron** is a variant where there is a dominant thalamic perforator supplying the ventromedial thalami bilaterally and the rostral midbrain, arising from a P1 PCA segment. An artery of Percheron infarct will result in bilateral ventromedial thalamic infarction, with or without midbrain infarction (the infarct may be V shaped if the midbrain is involved). Deep venous thrombosis may also result in bilateral thalamic infarcts.

起自威利斯环的重要小动脉

- 大脑前动脉(ACA)的A1段走行于视神经上方，并发出**Heubner回返动脉**，供应尾状核头和内囊前肢。A1段也发出内侧豆纹穿支血管，供应内侧基底节。
- 在威利斯环的外侧附近，大脑中动脉(MCA)发出外侧豆纹穿支血管以供应外侧基底节区，包括壳核外侧、外囊和内囊后肢。
- 后交通动脉(P-comm)走行于视束和第Ⅲ脑神经之间，并发出前丘脑穿支血管。后交通动脉瘤可产生局部占位效应而引起第Ⅲ脑神经麻痹。
- 大脑后动脉(PCA)发出丘脑穿支以供应丘脑。**Percheron动脉**是一种变异，起自大脑后动脉P1段，是一条向两侧丘脑腹内侧核和中脑后缘供血的主要丘脑穿支。Percheron动脉梗死会引起两侧腹内侧丘脑梗死，但中脑梗死不定(若伴发中脑梗死可呈“V”字形)。深静脉血栓形成也可能引起双侧丘脑梗死。

- The anterior choroidal artery is the most distal branch of the internal carotid artery. As discussed on the previous page, it supplies the optic chiasm, hippocampus, and posterior limb of the internal capsule.

- 脉络膜前动脉是颈内动脉最末端的分支。如前文所述，它供应视交叉、海马和内囊后肢。

Circle of Willis normal anatomic variants

威利斯环的正常解剖变异

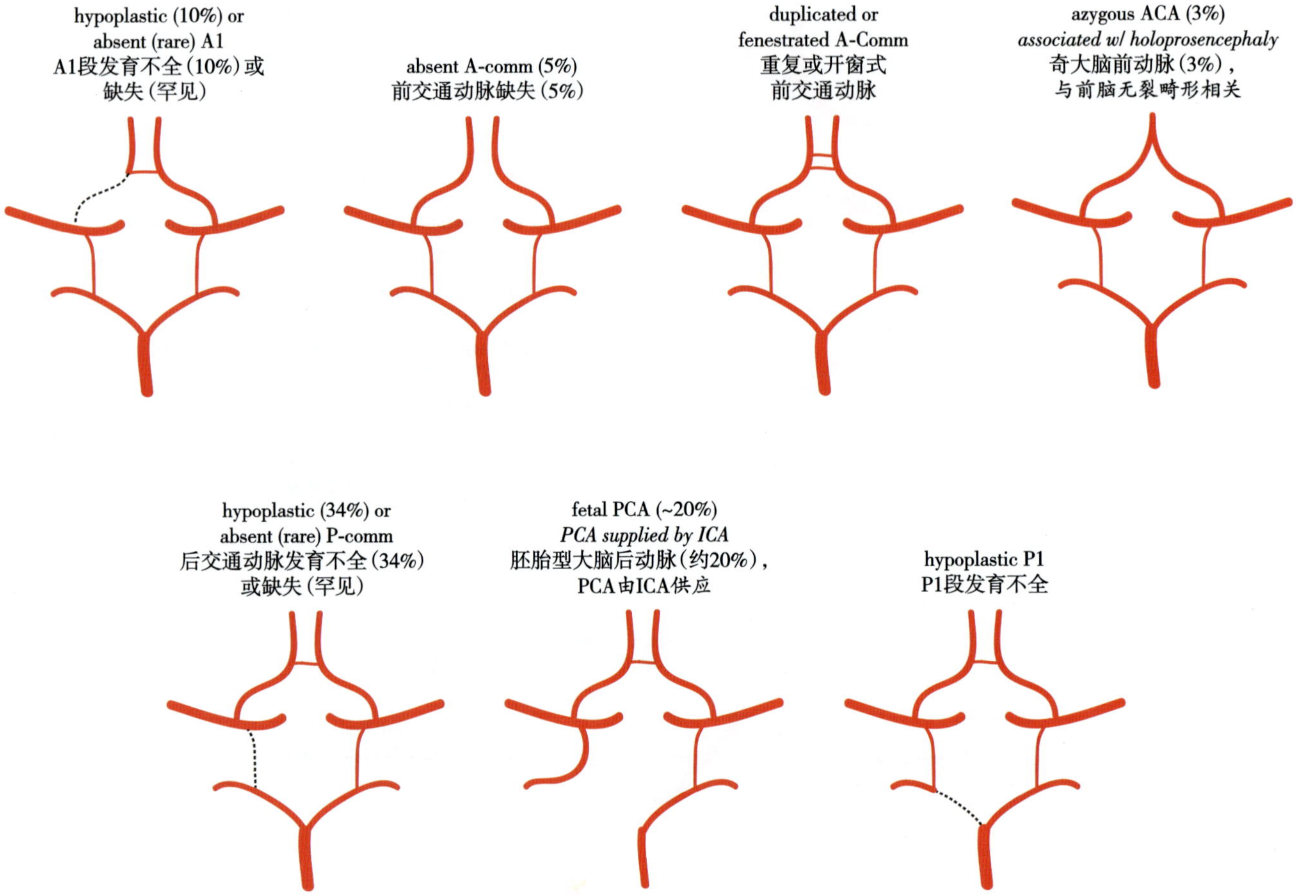

- Normal circle of Willis anatomy is only seen approximately 25% of the time.
- **Fenestration** is when an artery divides into two separate channels and then recombines into a single vessel. The two channels each have its own endothelialand muscularis layers, but may share an adventitial layer. Fenestration is more commonly seen in the vertebrobasilar system than other intracranial arteries. It is associated with aneurysm formation.
- **Duplication** is when an artery splits into two distinct vessels with no distal convergence.
- **Azygos ACA** is associated with holoprosencephaly, neuronal migration anomalies, and aneurysm formation. Occlusion of the azygos ACA will lead to ischemia in both hemispheres.
- Other ACA anomalies include **trifurcation** (2–13%) with three A2 segments, and **bihemispheric ACA** (2–7%) where a dominant A2 supplies bilateral ACA territories, while the contralateral A2 segment is hypoplastic. Similar to azygos ACA, occlusion of the dominant A2 segment will affect both hemispheres.

- 完整的威利斯环解剖仅占25%左右。
- **开窗**是指动脉分成两个独立的通道，然后重新组合成一条血管。这两个通道各自有独立的内皮层和肌层，但可能共享外膜层。开窗在椎基底动脉系统中比其他颅内动脉更常见，与动脉瘤的形成有关。
- **重复**是指动脉分成两条不同的血管，但远端没有会合。
- **奇大脑前动脉**与前脑无裂畸形、神经元迁移异常和动脉瘤形成有关。奇大脑前动脉闭塞会导致双侧大脑半球缺血。
- 其他ACA异常包括**三干型**(2%~13%)，即三条A2段，和**双半球ACA**(2%~7%)，为优势侧A2段供应双侧ACA区域，而对侧A2段发育不全。与奇大脑前动脉相似，优势侧A2段闭塞会影响双侧半球。

Segmented anatomy of the anterior cerebral artery

大脑前动脉分段解剖

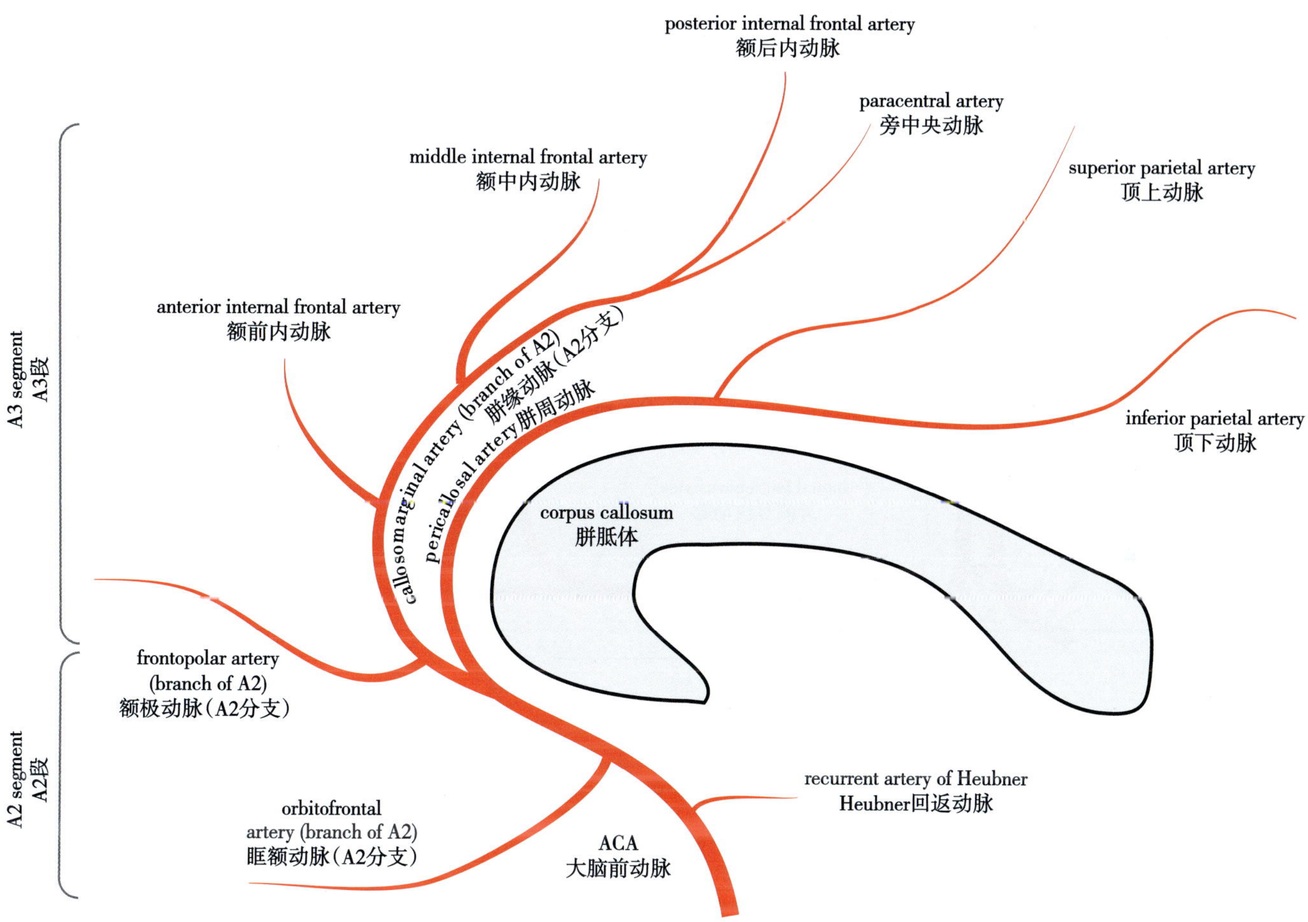

- The recurrent artery of Heubner arises most commonly from the A1 segment of the ACA, proximal to the anterior communicating artery. The recurrent artery of Heubner supplies the head of the caudate and the anterior limb of the internal capsule.

- Heubner回返动脉最常起源于大脑前动脉A1段，前交通动脉的近端。Heubner回返动脉供应尾状核的头部和内囊前肢。

Middle Cerebral Artery (MCA) | 大脑中动脉(MCA)

Segmental anatomy of the middle cerebral artery | 大脑中动脉的分段解剖

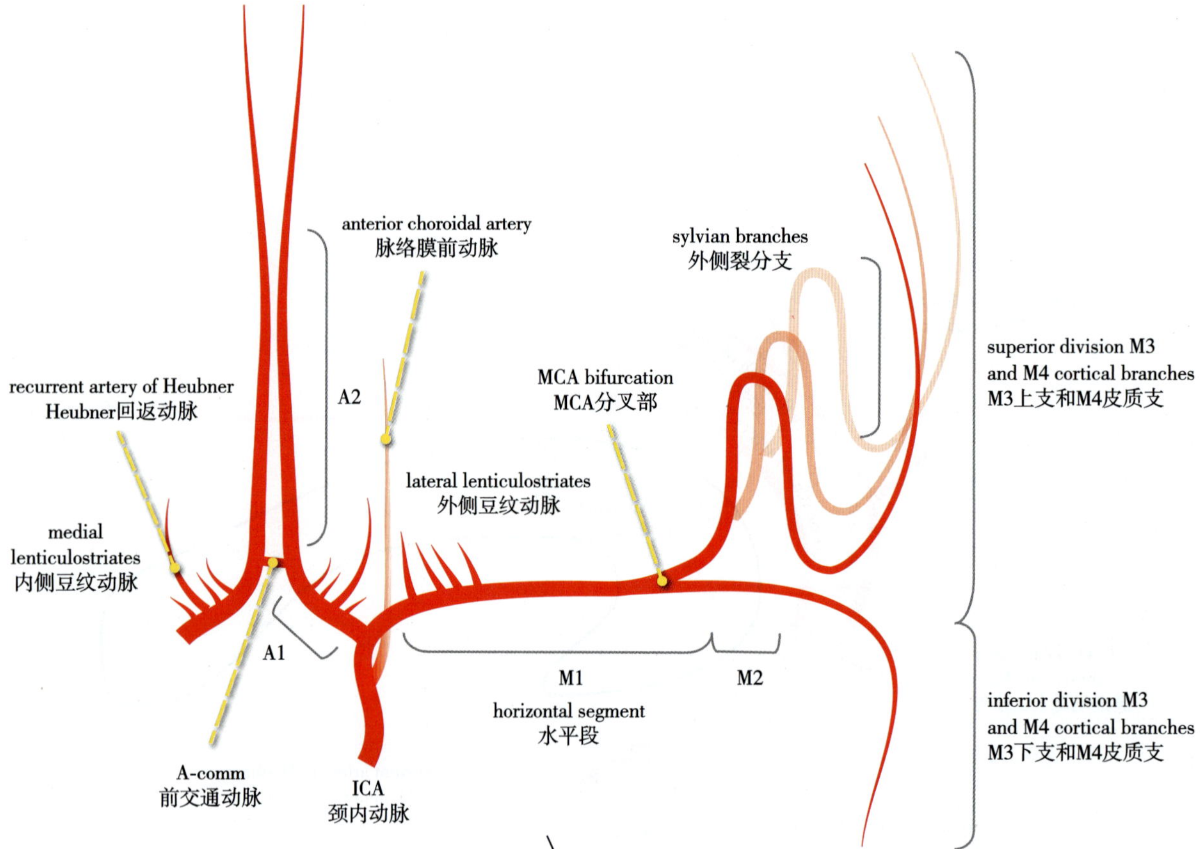

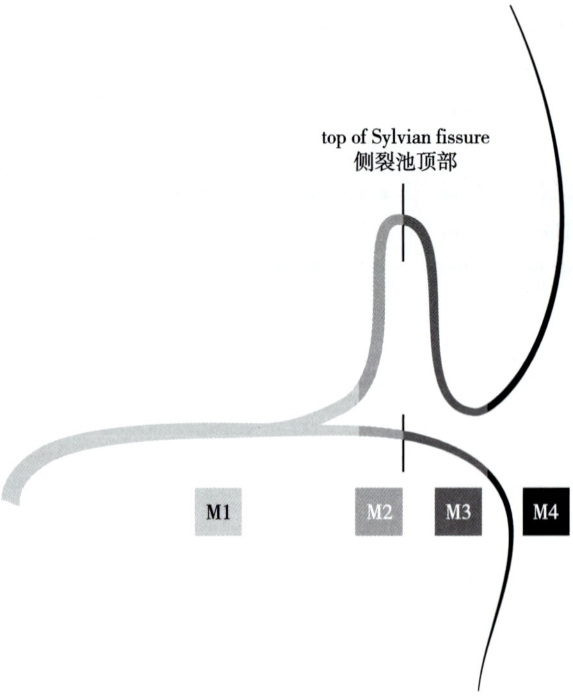

M1 M1 extends from the ICA terminus to the origin of the Sylvian fissure.
M1段由ICA末端延伸到大脑外侧裂起点

M2 M2 extends posteriorly from the bottom to the top of the Sylvian fissure.
M2段由外侧裂底部从后方延伸到顶部

M3 M3 extends laterally from the top of the Sylvian fissure to the cortical surface.
M3段由外侧裂池顶部从外侧延伸到皮层表面

M4 M4 represents small cortical branches.
M4为小的皮质分支

- Although the transition from M1 to M2 is technically defined as the upward point of deflection into the Sylvian fissure, in practical terms, the pre-bifurcation MCA is often called M1 and the post-bifurcation MCA is called M2.

- 从M1段转变为M2段在技术上定义为外侧裂池上升的转折点，但实际上常把分叉前的MCA称为M1段，分叉后的MCA称为M2段。

PERSISTENT CAROTID-BASILAR CONNECTIONS

永存颈动脉-基底动脉吻合

Overview of persistent fetal anterior-posterior connections

- A number of carotid to basilar connections are formed during embryogenesis. These fetal anterior-posterior circulation connections normally regress before birth.
- Occasionally, a fetal carotid-basilar connection may persist after birth. Each anomalous connection is named for the structures adjacent to its course in the head and neck.

永存胚胎型前后吻合概述

- 很多颈动脉到基底动脉的连接是在胚胎时期形成的。这些胎儿时期的前-后循环吻合一般在出生前退化。
- 偶尔情况下，胚胎的颈-基底动脉之间的连接可能在出生后持续存在。每一种异常连接的名称是按照其走行在头颈部的邻近结构来命名。

Persistent trigeminal artery

永存三叉动脉

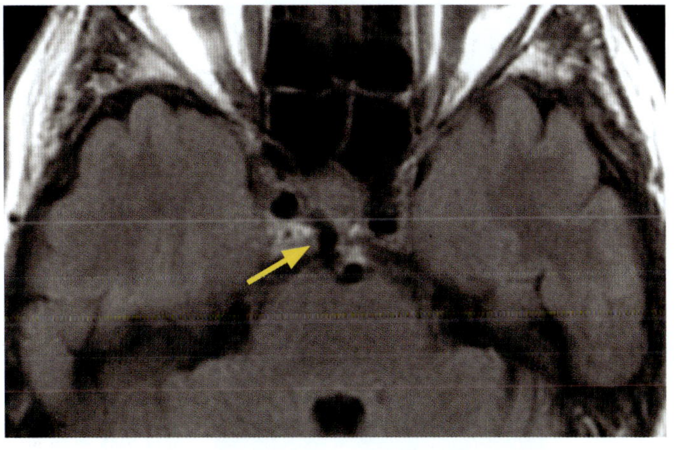

Axial FLAIR image shows flow-void associated with a vessel (arrow) traversing through the clivus between the basilar artery and the right cavernous ICA, compatible with a persistent trigeminal artery.

轴位FLAIR像显示穿过基底动脉和右侧ICA海绵窦段之间斜坡的血管(黄箭)的流空效应，与永存三叉动脉相符合。

- A persistent trigeminal artery is the most common persistent carotid-basilar connection and has an association with aneurysms.
- The persistent trigeminal artery courses adjacent to the trigeminal nerve. Angiography shows a characteristic *trident* or *tau* sign on the lateral view due to the artery's branching structure.
- Saltzman type Ⅰ connects to the basilar artery while Saltzman type Ⅱ connects to the superior cerebellar artery.

Less common carotid to basilar connections

- The otic, hypoglossal, and proatlantal intersegmental arteries are rare persistent carotid basilar connections.

- 永存三叉动脉是最常见的永存颈-基底动脉吻合，且与动脉瘤相关。
- 永存三叉动脉走行邻近三叉神经。侧位血管造影显示一个特征性的三叉或*T*征，为该动脉的分叉结构所致。
- Saltzman Ⅰ型连接于基底动脉，而Saltzman Ⅱ型连接小脑上动脉。

少见的颈动脉基底动脉吻合

- 耳、舌下和寰前节间动脉是罕见的永存颈动脉-基底动脉吻合。

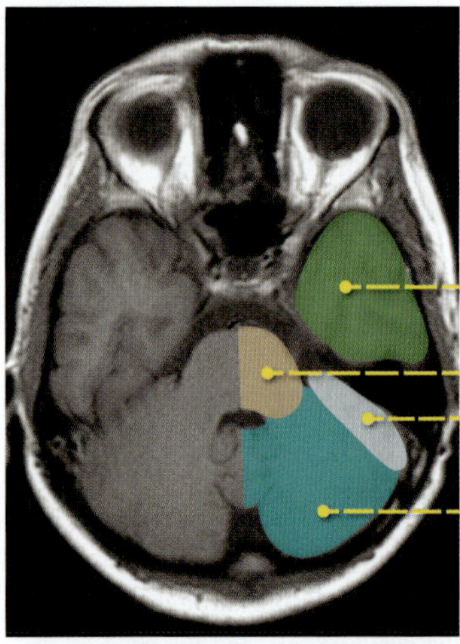
MCA *temporal lobe*
大脑中动脉 颞叶
vertebrobasilar 椎基底动脉
AICA *lateral cerebellum*
小脑前下动脉 小脑侧面
PICA *inferomedial and posterior cerebellum*
小脑后下动脉
小脑下内侧和后部

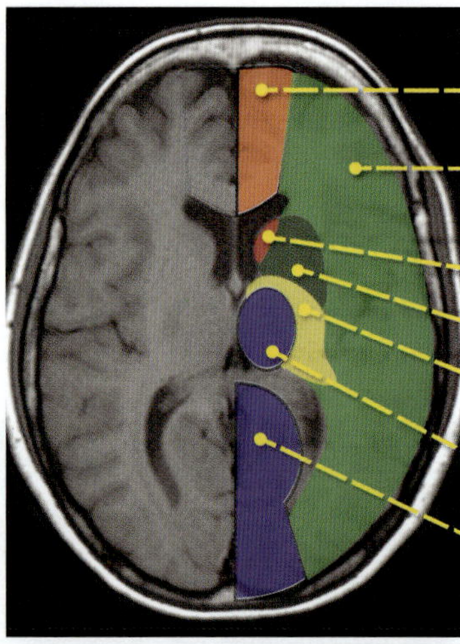
ACA *medial frontal lobe*
大脑前动脉 额叶内侧
MCA *fronto-temporo-parietal lobe*
大脑中动脉 额颞顶叶
recurrent artery of Heubner
Heubner回返动脉
lenticulostriate 豆纹动脉
anterior choroidal
脉络膜前动脉
PCA perforators *thalamus*
大脑后动脉穿支 丘脑
PCA *medial occipital lobe*
大脑后动脉 枕叶内侧

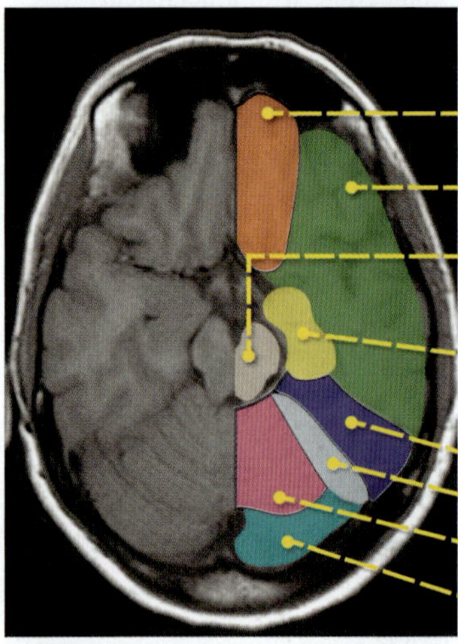
ACA *medial frontal lobe*
大脑前动脉 额叶内侧
MCA *fronto-temporal lobe*
大脑中动脉 额颞叶
basilar *midbrain*
基底动脉 中脑
anterior choroidal
hippocampus
posterior limb internal capsule
脉络膜前动脉 海马 内囊后肢
PCA 大脑后动脉
AICA 小脑前下动脉
SCA 小脑上动脉
PICA *posterior cerebellum*
小脑后下动脉 小脑后部

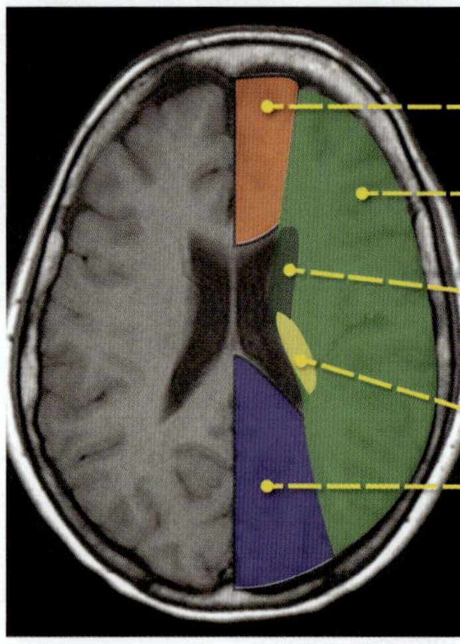
ACA *medial frontal lobe*
大脑前动脉 额叶内侧
MCA
fronto-temporo-parietal lobe
大脑中动脉 额颞顶叶
lenticulostriate *basal ganglia*
豆纹动脉 基底节
anterior choroidal
脉络膜前动脉
PCA *medial occipital lobe*
大脑后动脉 枕叶内侧

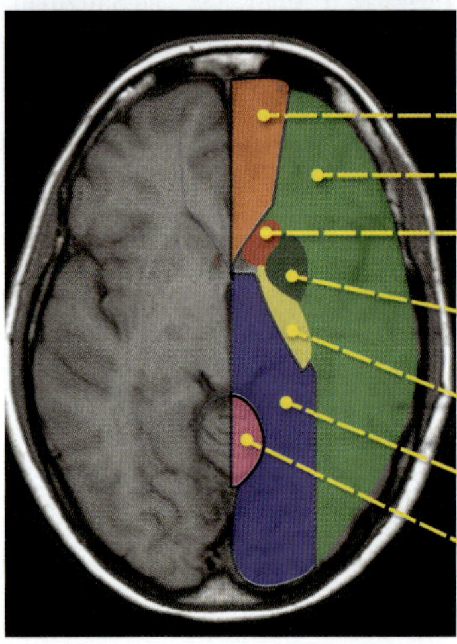
ACA *medial frontal lobe*
大脑前动脉 额叶内侧
MCA 大脑中动脉
recurrent artery of Heubner
Heubner回返动脉
lateral lenticulostriate
外侧豆纹动脉
anterior choroidal *posterior limb internal capsule*
脉络膜前动脉 内囊后肢
PCA 大脑后动脉
SCA *cerebellar vermis*
小脑上动脉 小脑蚓部

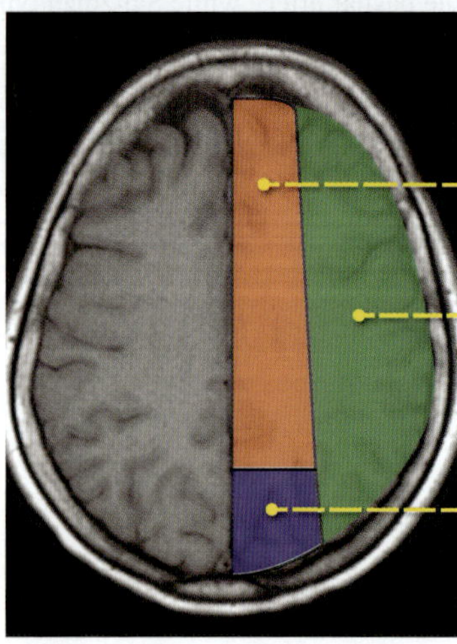
ACA *medial frontal lobe*
大脑前动脉 额叶内侧
MCA
fronto-temporo-parietal lobe
大脑中动脉 额颞顶叶
PCA *medial occipital lobe*
大脑后动脉 枕叶内侧

（翻译　贺迎坤）

STROKE

IMAGING OF STROKE

Determine potential candidate for therapy

- The goal of stroke *imaging* is to determine who would benefit from therapy.
- The goal of stroke *therapy* is to restore perfusion to the brain.
- In the appropriate patients, intravenous or intra-arterial thrombolysis, performed most commonly with tissue plasminogen activator (tPA, alteplase), can improve outcomes. However, there is risk of fatal hemorrhage in patients inappropriately selected for therapy. The exact exclusion criteria to administer tPA varies among institutions.
- The American Heart Association (AHA) and American Stroke Association (ASA) published guidelines for early management of adults with ischemic stroke (Stroke, 2019) and established recommendations for imaging and treatment of acute stroke.

  All patients with suspected acute stroke should receive emergency brain imaging prior to initiation of any thrombolytic therapy to evaluate for intracerebral hemorrhage. Both noncontrast CT and MRI, when gradient echo sequences are used, are effective in ruling out intracranial hemorrhage (ICH) prior to tPA administration. In many patients, the diagnosis of ischemic stroke can be made on the basis of clinical presentation and noncontrast head CT alone.

  In patients with unclear last known normal, MRI can be useful in identifying diffusion-positive, FLAIR- negative lesions to select patients who may benefit from IV tPA (<4.5 hours from symptom recognition). Advanced imaging including CT angiogram with perfusion or MR angiogram with diffusion-weighted imaging with or without MR perfusion is recommended for selecting candidates for mechanical thrombectomy in the late window (≥6 hours after last known normal).

  In patients being considered for mechanical thrombectomy, imaging of extracranial carotid and vertebral arteries is reasonable for determining patient eligibility and for endovascular procedural planning.
- Some institutions add additional exclusion criteria for administration of intravenous tPA, although these additional criteria are not a part of the AHA guidelines:

  Individuals with a large (greater than 1/3 MCA territory) infarct may be excluded from IV tPA.

  Occlusion of the distal internal carotid artery and proximal MCA and ACA (a T-shaped occlusion) may preclude treatment with IV tPA.

  Absence of a penumbra (discussed below) of salvageable brain that represents at least 20% of the region of abnormal perfusion may preclude treatment with IV tPA.

Perfusion stroke imaging

- Perfusion imaging with CT angiogram or MR angiogram is recommended in patients presenting between 6 and 24 hours after last-known normal with suspected **large vessel occlusion** (LVO) in the *anterior circulation* who may benefit from mechanical thrombectomy.

  LVO is defined as thrombosis involving the intracranial internal carotid artery (ICA) or the M1 segment of the MCA. Some clinical trials also included ACA and/or M2 occlusion.
- Two randomized trials (DAWN and DEFUSE 3) have shown a benefit in revascularization of patients with acute ischemic stroke with LVO presenting

卒中

脑卒中影像

确定可接受治疗的患者

- 脑卒中影像的目的是确定哪些患者能通过治疗获益。
- 脑卒中治疗的目的是恢复脑灌注。
- 选择合适的患者进行静脉或动脉内溶栓可以改善预后，最常使用的为组织纤溶酶原激活物(tPA，alteplase)。但若选择不当，则有致命性出血的风险。具体tPA的禁忌标准在各医院之间有所不同。
- 美国心脏协会(AHA)与美国卒中协会(ASA)发布了成人缺血性脑卒中的早期处理指南(脑卒中，2019)，并确立了急性脑卒中的影像学检查和治疗建议。

  对所有疑似急性脑卒中的患者，应于溶栓治疗之前行急诊脑影像学检查以评估脑出血情况。平扫CT及梯度回波序列MRI均可在tPA给药前有效排除颅内出血。许多患者仅根据临床表现及头颅CT平扫就可诊断缺血性脑卒中。

  对不确定最后一次正常的患者，MRI上发现DWI阳性而FLAIR阴性的病灶患者将获益于使用静脉tPA(发现症状4.5小时以内)。推荐采用现代影像技术，包括CTA联合灌注、MRA联合DWI和/或MR灌注成像，筛选晚期窗口进行机械取栓的患者(症状出现≥6小时)。

  对考虑进行机械取栓的患者，有必要对颅外颈动脉和椎动脉进行影像学评估，以确定患者是否适合进行腔内治疗以及手术计划。
- 一些医院对静脉内tPA给药增加了更多的排除标准，但这些额外的标准并不在AHA指南之内：

  大面积梗死(大于1/3大脑中动脉供血范围)的患者除外静脉tPA治疗。

  颈内动脉远端、大脑中动脉近端和大脑前动脉闭塞(T型闭塞)不建议行静脉tPA治疗。

  缺乏可挽救的脑组织-半暗带(下文讨论)，即不足20%的异常灌注区，不建议行静脉tPA治疗。

脑卒中灌注成像

- CTA或MRA联合灌注成像适用于发病(已知最后正常的时间点)6~24小时，已知最后一次情况为正常，现怀疑有前循环**大血管闭塞**(LVO)的患者，即可能在机械取栓术中获益的患者。

  LVO定义为血栓出现在颈内动脉(ICA)颅内段或大脑中动脉(MCA)M1段。一些临床试验还包括大脑前动脉和/或大脑中动脉M2段闭塞。
- 两项随机研究(DAWN和DFFUSE 3)表明，部

beyond 6 hours of last known normal using diffusion or perfusion imaging selection parameters.

- Perfusion imaging parameters are used to quantify the core and penumbra. However, diffusion-weighted imaging is the gold standard for quantifying core size.

The **infarct core** is the hypoperfused tissue with low cerebral blood flow which would not be salvageable regardless of subsequent reperfusion.

The **ischemic penumbra** is the tissue "at risk" which has the potential to recover if perfusion is achieved.

- The DAWN and DEFUSE 3 trials have led to implementation of perfusion imaging in routine acute stroke evaluation to identify patients who could benefit from mechanical thrombectomy with an expanded time window.

The **DAWN trial** used a combination of the age-adjusted NIH stroke scale score and the core infarct size from CT perfusion or MR DWI (clinical-core mismatch) as an eligibility criterion to select patients with anterior circulation LVO for thrombectomy between 6–24 hours of last known normal, and demonstrated an overall benefit in functional outcome in the intervention group.

The **DEFUSE 3 trial** used a discrepancy between the penumbra and the ischemic core (perfusion-core mismatch) and maximum core size as imaging criteria to select patients with anterior circulation LVO between 6–16 hours from last known normal for mechanical thrombectomy. The trial showed a benefit in functional outcome at 90 days in the intervention group.

分发病超过6小时的LVO急性缺血性脑卒中，最后一次弥散或选择性灌注成像参数正常的患者可受益于血管重建术。

- 灌注成像参数可用于量化脑梗死的核心和半暗带，而DWI是量化脑梗死核心大小的"金标准"。

梗死核心是低灌注低血流量的组织，无论是否有再灌注都不可逆。

缺血半暗带是"处于危险中"的组织，如能重新获得灌注就有恢复可能。

- DAWN和DEFUSE 3试验已经使得灌注成像在急性脑卒中得到了应用，以识别可以将时间窗扩大从而在机械取栓术中获益的患者。

DAWN试验联合年龄矫正后的NIH脑卒中量表评分和CT灌注或MR DWI的梗死核心大小(临床-核心不匹配)作为标准，选择发病6~24小时前循环LVO的患者行取栓术，显示了干预组在功能预后上整体获益。

DEFUSE3试验采用半暗带、缺血核心之间的差异(灌注-核心不匹配)及最大核心范围作为影像标准，选择前循环LVO 6~16小时(已知最后正常的时间点)的患者进行机械取栓。该试验表明干预组在90天功能预后中是获益的。

Acute stroke: Perfusion imaging

- Important hemodynamic parameters calculated from a perfusion study are listed below:

Cerebral blood volume (CBV): Blood volume per unit brain tissue (mL/100 g).

Cerebral blood flow (CBF): Volume of blood flowing per unit brain tissue per minute (mL/100 g/min).

Mean transit time (MTT): Average time (sec) for contrast bolus to transverse a voxel.

Time to maximum (Tmax) or **time to peak** (TTP): Time (sec) from scan start to maximum intensity of contrast bolus in voxel. Delay time (DT) and time to drain (TTD) are similar measurements.

- CBF, CBV, and MTT are related by the **central volume equation**:

cerebral blood flow (CBF) = cerebral blood volume (CBV) / mean transit time (MTT)

- The infarct core and ischemic penumbra can be estimated from the imaging parameters, for which specific thresholds have been established in recent clinical trials to more accurately differentiate and quantify the two tissue types. Automated perfusion post-processing softwares are also available to aid interpretation.

急性脑卒中：灌注成像

- 从灌注成像中计算出的重要血流动力学参数如下：

脑血容量(CBV)：单位脑组织内的血容量(mL/100g)。

脑血流量(CBF)：每分钟单位脑组织的血流量［mL/(100g·min)］。

平均通过时间(MTT)：团注造影剂通过单个体素的平均时间(s)。

残留功能达峰时间(T_{max})**或达峰时间**(TTP)：从扫描开始到造影剂在体素内达最大强度的时间(s)。延迟时间(DT)和流出时间(TTD)是相似的测量值。

- CBF、CBV和MTT与**中心容积方程**有关：

脑血流量(CBF)=脑血容量(CBV)/平均通过时间(MTT)

- 梗死核心和缺血半暗带可通过影像参数进行评估，最新的临床试验已建立了具体的阈值，可更为准确地区分和量化这两种组织类型。现有的自动化灌注后处理软件也可帮助解读。

	Traditional perfusion maps	Thresholds used in automated CT perfusion softwares
Infarct core	Markedly decreased CBF, matched by decreased CBV	Defined by CBF <30–45% depending on software
Ischemic penumbra	Mildly decreased CBF, mismatched by increased or normal CBV Increased MTT and Tmax	Defined by Tmax >6 sec, or DT >3 sec

- The exact perfusion thresholds differ by software vendor and are evolving as new clinical trials are carried out. Also, the thresholds pertain to the anterior circulation only. Utility of perfusion imaging in posterior circulation strokes is still undergoing investigation.

	传统灌注图	自动化CT灌注软件的阈值
梗死核心	CBF明显降低，CBV相应降低	根据不同的软件定义为CBF 30%~45%
缺血半暗带	CBF轻度降低，CBV不匹配，升高或正常 MTT和T_{max}延长	定义为T_{max}>6s或DT>3s

- 确切的灌注阈值因软件供应商而异，并随着新的临床试验的开展而不断改进。而且，这些阈值只与前循环有关。灌注成像在后循环卒中的应用还在研究中。

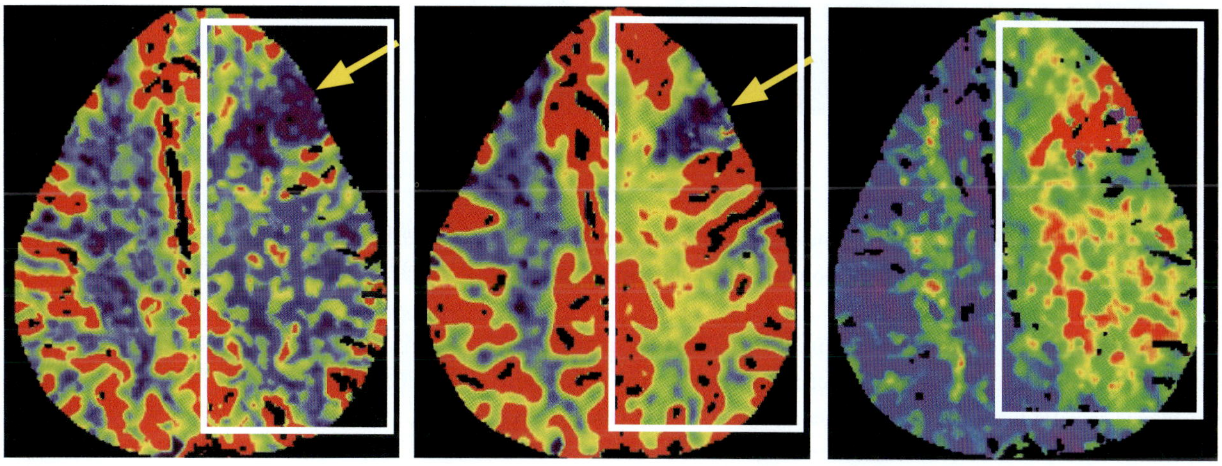

CBF
脑血流量

CBV
脑血容量

TTD, Similar to Tmax
流出时间，与残留功能达峰时间相似

Color perfusion maps show focal region of markedly decreased cerebral blood flow (CBF) and matched markedly reduced cerebral blood volume (CBV) in the left frontal lobe, corresponding to infarcted tissue (yellow arrows). There is a larger area of penumbra (white boxes) in the left ACA and MCA territories that demonstrates mildly reduced CBF, increased CBV, and prolonged time to drain (TTD).
彩色灌注图可见左侧额叶局部区域脑血流量(CBF)明显降低，相应区域脑血容量(CBV)也明显降低，对应于梗死的脑组织(黄箭)。在左侧大脑前、中动脉区域存在大面积的半暗带(白框)，表现为CBF轻度降低，CBV升高及流出时间(TTD)延长。

Acute stroke: Noncontrast CT imaging

- Noncontrast CT is frequently the initial test of evaluation for patients with suspected acute ischemic stroke, as described above, to evaluate for the presence of intracerebral hemorrhage.
- Noncontrast CT in the hyperacute stage is relatively insensitive to detect early infarction compared to MRI. Subtle loss of gray-white differentiation in the insula or basal ganglia may be present on CT, thought to be due to decreased cerebral blood volume.
- The *insular ribbon sign* describes the loss of gray-white differentiation in the insula. The gray-white junction becomes most conspicuous at very narrow stroke windows (window 40/ level 40).

急性脑卒中：平扫CT影像

- 如前所述，平扫CT通常是用于评估疑似急性缺血性脑卒中患者的初始检查，以确定是否存在颅内出血。
- 平扫CT对发现超急性期的早期梗死相对于MRI并不敏感。CT可显示岛叶和基底节的灰白质分界轻微模糊，被认为是由于脑血容量减少所致。
- 岛带征指的是岛叶的灰白质分界消失。灰白质分界在非常窄的脑卒中窗(窗宽40/窗位40)中显示最佳。

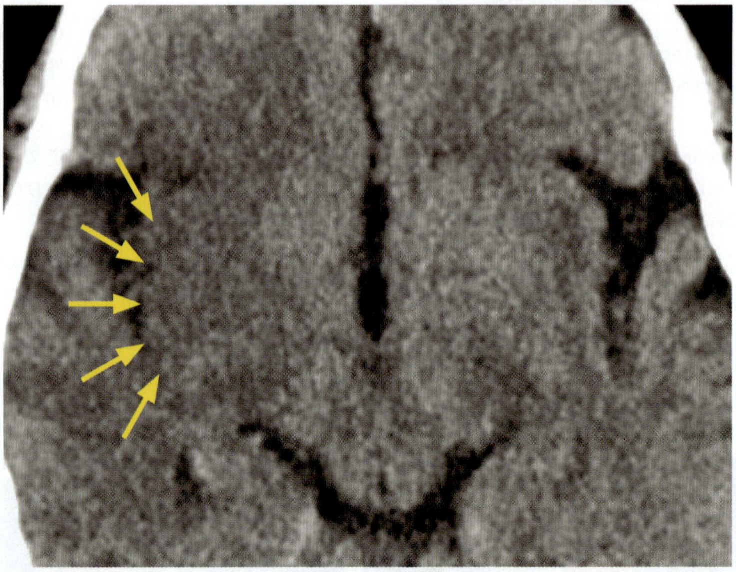

Insular ribbon sign due to acute right MCA infarction:
Axial noncontrast CT shows subtle loss of the gray-white differentiation in the insular cortex (yellow arrows).
Gray-white differentiation is preserved on the normal left side.
由右侧大脑中动脉急性梗死产生的岛带征：
轴位平扫CT显示岛叶(黄箭)灰白质分界轻微模糊。左侧正常灰白质分界如常。

- Obscuration of the lentiform nucleus (putamen and globus pallidus) is caused by loss of gray-white differentiation at the border of the lentiform nucleus and the posterior limb of the internal capsule.
- The *hyperdense artery sign* describes direct visualization of the acute intravascular thrombus, most commonly seen in the MCA. The *hyperdense artery sign* is specific for ischemia when seen, but relatively insensitive (seen in approximately 1/3 of cases). Some authors suggest that the presence of the hyperdense artery sign portends a worse prognosis.

- 豆状核(壳核和苍白球)模糊不清是由于豆状核边缘及内囊后肢的灰白质分界消失所致。
- 动脉高密度征是指直接可见的急性血管内血栓，最常见于大脑中动脉。动脉高密度征是缺血的特异性表现，但是相对不敏感(约见于1/3的病例)。一些作者认为，动脉高密度征提示预后较差。

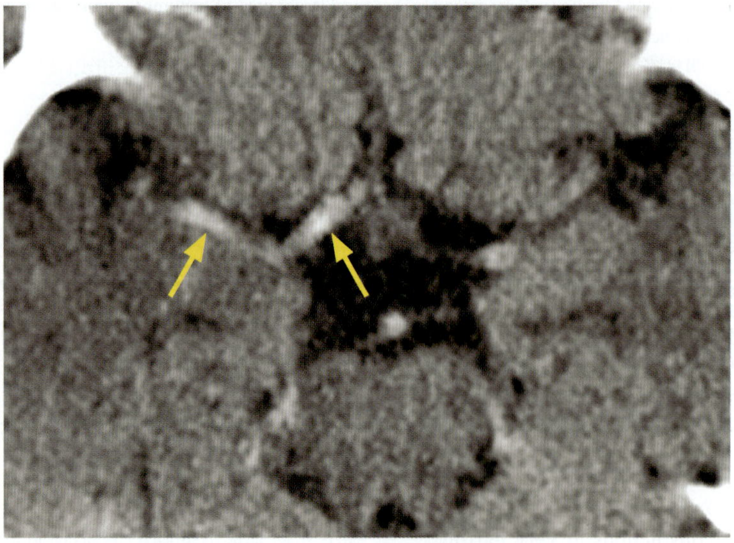

Hyperdense artery sign in acute infarction (same patient as above): Axial noncontrast CT shows hyperattenuating thrombus in the right proximal middle cerebral artery (arrows).
急性梗死的动脉高密度征(上述同一患者)：轴位平扫CT示右侧大脑中动脉近端(黄箭)高密度血栓。

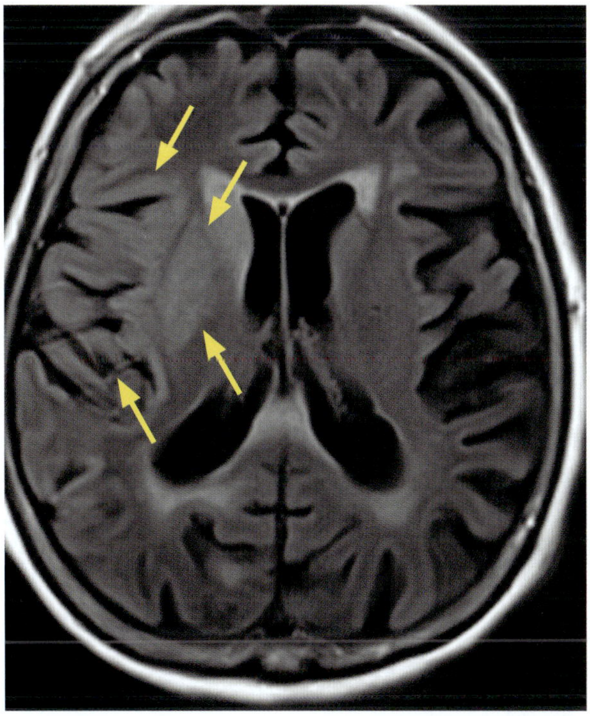

Axial FLAIR MRI shows geographic T2 prolongation in the right MCA territory (arrows) involving the right frontal and temporal lobes and right basal ganglia. The size of the T2 signal abnormality is less extensive than the infarct size apparent on DWI.
轴位FLAIR MRI显示右侧大脑中动脉区域(黄箭)地图状的长T_2信号，累及右侧额颞叶和右侧基底节。T_2信号异常的范围小于DWI上显示的梗死灶范围。

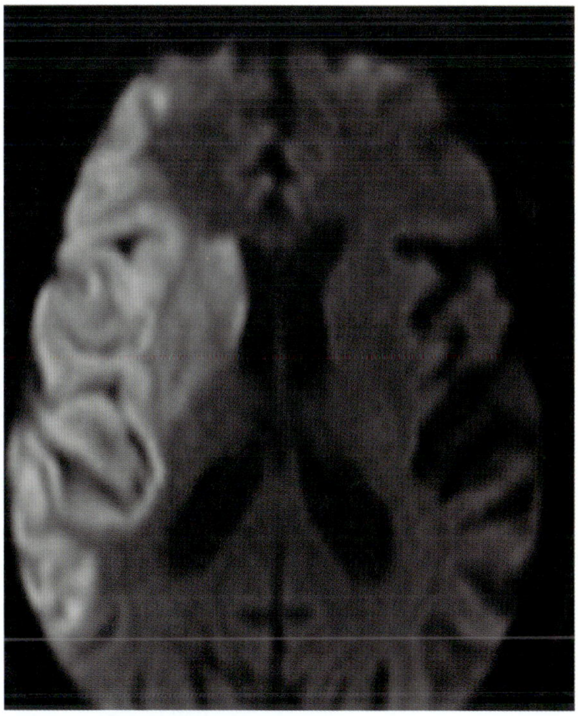

DWI shows a large region of hyperintensity in the right MCA territory involving the right frontal operculum, the right insula, the right temporal operculum, the right putamen, and the right caudate. ADC map (not shown) was dark, consistent with reduced diffusivity.
DWI显示右侧大脑中动脉区域大面积高信号，累及右侧额叶盖部、右侧岛叶、右侧颞叶盖部、右侧壳核及尾状核等。ADC图(未展示)信号减低，符合弥散降低的表现。

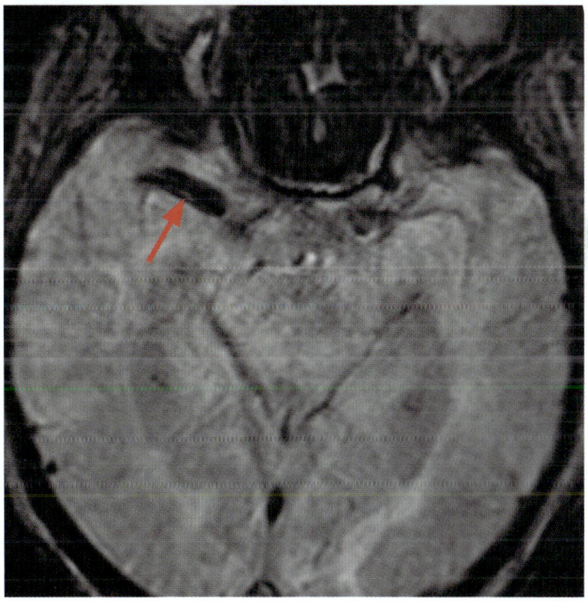

Gradient recall echo axial image shows blooming artifact (red arrow) in the right proximal MCA, which represents intraluminal thrombus and is the MRI correlate to the hyperdense artery sign that can be seen on CT.
轴位梯度回波序列图像显示右侧大脑中动脉近端开花样伪影(红箭)，为管腔内血栓，这是MRI对应于CT上所见的动脉高密度征。

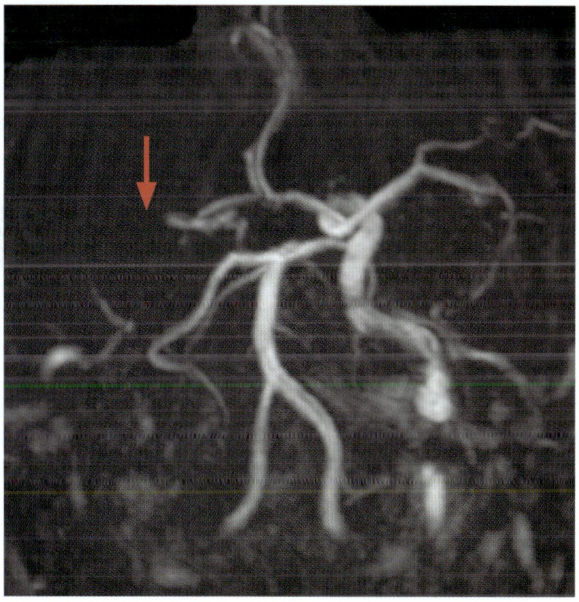

Axial oblique MIP from a time-of-flight MRI angiogram shows complete occlusion of the right MCA (red arrow). There is marked venous contamination on the left.
时间飞跃法MR动脉成像斜轴位MIP显示右侧大脑中动脉完全闭塞(红箭)。左侧有明显静脉干扰。

Case courtesy Gregory Wrubel, MD, Brigham and Women's Hospital, Boston

- Detailed MR imaging of the multiple temporal stages of stroke is discussed on the following pages. For the initial evaluation, diffusion sequences can detect acute infarction with high sensitivity within minutes of symptom onset. DWI is more sensitive than FLAIR in the detection of hyperacute stroke.

- 各期相脑卒中的具体MRI将在下文进行讨论。弥散序列作为初始评估，能在出现症状几分钟内发现急性梗死，并有很高的灵敏度。DWI较FLAIR检测超急性脑卒中更敏感。

EVOLUTION OF INFARCTION

脑梗死的演变

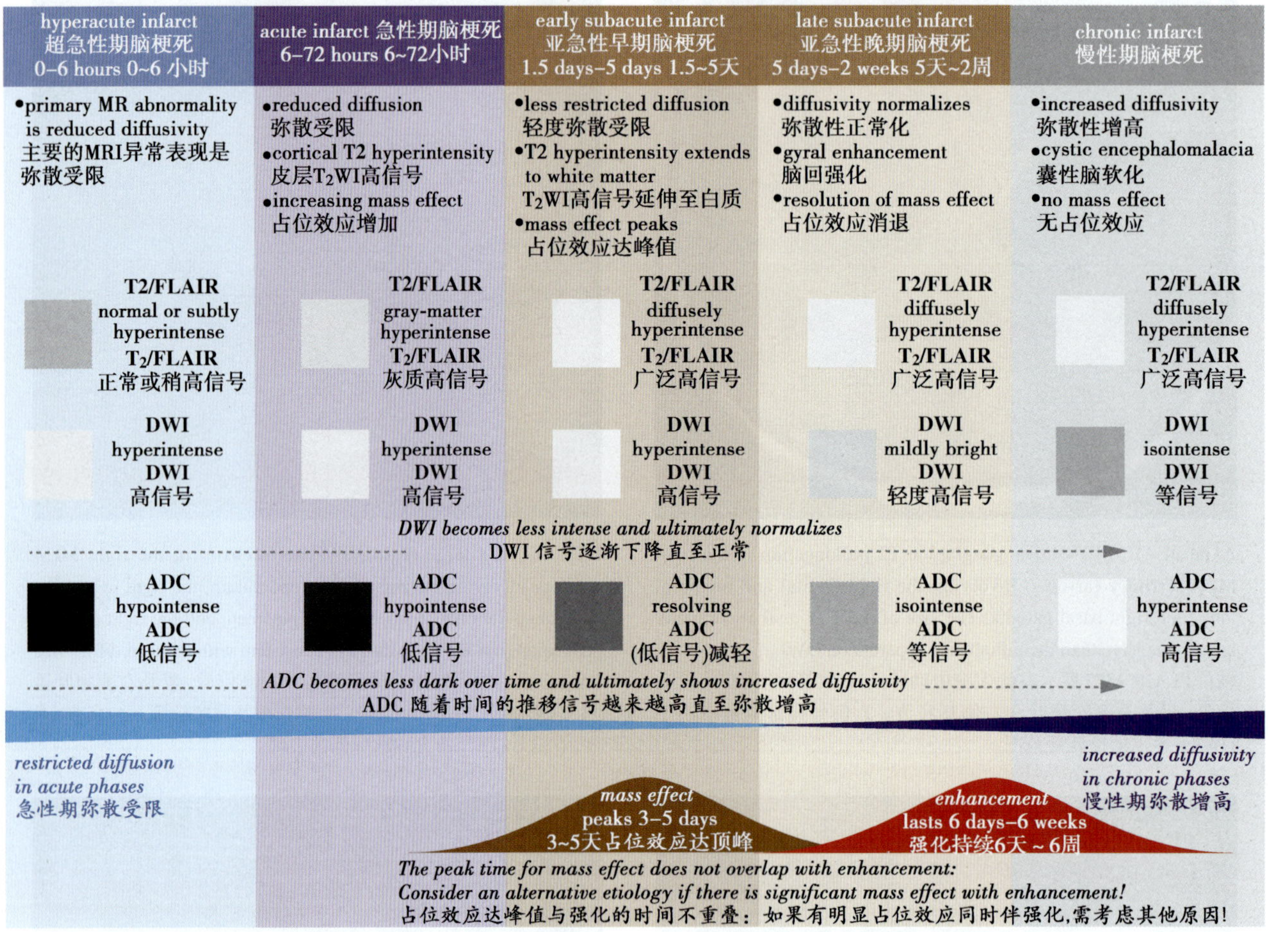

Hyperacute infarct (0–6 hours)

- Within minutes of critical ischemia, the sodium-potassium ATPase pump that maintains the normal low intracellular sodium concentration fails. Sodium and water diffuse into cells, leading to cell swelling and **cytotoxic** edema.
- Calcium also diffuses into cells, which triggers cascades that contribute to cell lysis.
- By far the most sensitive imaging modality for detection of hyperacute infarct is MRI diffusion-weighted imaging (DWI). DWI hyperintensity and ADC map hypointensity reflect reduced diffusivity, which can be seen within minutes of the ictus.
- Diffusion is reduced in an acute infarct by two factors:

  1) Shift from extracellular to intracellular water due to Na/K ATPase pump failure.

  2) Increased viscosity of infarcted brain due to cell lysis and increased extracellular protein.
- FLAIR may be normal. Subtle hyperintensity may be seen on FLAIR images in the hyperacute stage. These changes are seen less than 2/3 of the time within the first 6 hours.

超急性梗死（0~6小时）

- 在严重缺血的数分钟内，维持细胞内正常低钠浓度的钠钾ATP酶泵失去作用。钠离子和水弥散进入细胞，导致细胞肿胀及**细胞毒性**水肿。
- 钙离子也弥散进入细胞内，触发细胞溶解的级联反应。
- DWI在检测超急性期脑梗死时灵敏度远高于其他影像学的方法。DWI高信号和ADC相应区域的低信号可反映弥散降低，在发病后几分钟内即可观察到。
- 急性脑梗死弥散降低有以下两方面因素：

  1）因钠钾ATP酶泵障碍而导致水从细胞外向细胞内转移。

  2）因细胞溶解和细胞外蛋白的增加导致梗死脑组织的黏稠性增加。
- FLAIR序列可为正常。FLAIR图像在超急性期可能出现轻微的高信号。在发病6小时内这些变化见于不到2/3的患者。

- Perfusion shows decreased cerebral blood volume of the infarct core, with or without a surrounding region of decreased cerebral blood flow, which represents the penumbra.

Acute infarct (6 hours–72 hours)

- The acute infarct phase is characterized by increase in vasogenic edema and mass effect.
- Damaged vascular endothelial cells cause leakage of extracellular fluid and increase the risk of hemorrhage.
- On imaging, there is increased sulcal effacement and mass effect. The mass effect peaks at 3–4 days, which is an overlap time between the acute and early subacute phases.
- MRI shows hyperintensity of the infarct core on T2-weighted images, best seen on FLAIR. The FLAIR abnormality is usually confined to the gray matter. DWI continues to show restricted diffusion.
- There may be some arterial enhancement, due to increased collateral flow.
- Perfusion images most commonly show increase in size of the infarct core with resultant decrease in size of the penumbra.

Early subacute infarct (1.5 days–5 days)

- In the early subacute phase, blood flow to the affected brain is re-established by leptomeningeal collaterals and ingrowth of new vessels into the region of infarction.
- The new vessels have an incomplete blood-brain barrier, causing a continued increase in vasogenic edema and mass effect, which peaks at 3–4 days.
- MR imaging shows marked hyperintensity on T2-weighted images involving both gray and white matter (in contrast to the acute stage which usually involves just the gray matter).
- The ADC map becomes less dark or even resolves if there is extensive edema; however, the DWI images typically remain bright due to underlying T2 shine-through.
- Perfusion imaging shows continued expansion of the infarct core and further reduction in the ischemic penumbra.

Late subacute infarct (5 days–2 weeks)

- The late subacute phase is characterized by resolution of vasogenic edema and reduction in mass effect.
- A key imaging finding is gyriform enhancement, which may occasionally be confused for a neoplasm. Unlike a tumor, however, a subacute infarction will not have mass effect. Enhancement can be seen from approximately 6 days to 6 weeks after the initial infarct.

  The enhancement of a subacute infarct has also been described by the "2-2-2" rule, which states that enhancement begins at 2 days, peaks at 2 weeks, and disappears by 2 months.
- DWI may remain bright due to T2 shine-through, although the ADC map will either return to normal or show increased diffusivity.

Chronic infarct

- In the chronic stage of infarction, cellular debris and dead brain tissue are removed by macrophages and replaced by cystic encephalomalacia and gliosis.
- Infarct involvement of the corticospinal tract may cause mass effect, mild hyperintensity on T2-weighted images, and eventual atrophy of the ipsilateral cerebral peduncle and ventral pons due to Wallerian degeneration. These changes can first be seen in the subacute phase, with atrophy being the predominant feature in the chronic stage.

- 灌注成像显示梗死核心的脑血容量降低，伴或不伴周边区域的脑血流量下降，后者即指缺血半暗带。

急性梗死(6~72小时)

- 急性期脑梗死的特点是血管源性水肿和占位效应加重。
- 血管内皮细胞损伤引起细胞外液渗漏和出血风险增加。
- 影像学表现为脑沟消失和占位效应增加。占位效应在发病3~4天达到高峰，此为急性和亚急性早期的重叠时间。
- MRI显示梗死核心区域在T_2WI上为高信号，在FLAIR上显示最佳。FLAIR异常往往局限于灰质。DWI持续显示弥散受限。
- 可能出现一些动脉强化，是由侧支循环增加所致。
- 脑灌注成像最常显示梗死核心范围的增大而导致半暗带范围缩小。

亚急性早期梗死(1.5~5天)

- 在亚急性早期，受损脑组织通过柔脑膜侧支及向梗死区内生长的新生血管重新建立血流。
- 这些新生血管不具备完整的血脑屏障，导致血管源性脑水肿及占位效应持续加重，并在3~4天时达到高峰。
- MR显示灰质和白质在T_2WI上都呈明显高信号(相比之下急性期通常只累及灰质)。
- ADC图低信号有所减轻，在有广泛水肿时甚至恢复正常；但是，DWI由于潜在的T_2穿透效应通常依然呈强烈的高信号。
- 脑灌注图像显示脑梗死核心范围继续扩大，缺血半暗带进一步缩小。

亚急性晚期梗死(5天~2周)

- 亚急性晚期的特点是血管源性水肿缓解和占位效应减少。
- 一个关键的影像学表现是脑回样强化，偶尔可与肿瘤混淆。但与肿瘤不同的是，亚急性梗死不会出现占位效应。强化见于脑梗死发病后的6天~6周内。

  亚急性期脑梗死的强化可描述为"2-2-2"规则，即强化从2天后开始，高峰在2周内到达，消退在2个月。
- DWI图像由于T_2穿透效应可保持高亮信号，但ADC图像可恢复正常或显示弥散增高。

慢性期梗死

- 在脑梗死的慢性期，细胞碎片和坏死的脑组织被巨噬细胞吞噬清除，并被囊性软化灶及胶质增生替代。
- 累及皮质脊髓束的脑梗死会出现占位效应，在T_2WI上表现为轻度高信号，并最终由于沃勒变性导致同侧大脑脚和脑桥腹侧萎缩。这些变化最初可在亚急性期出现，但萎缩是慢

- DWI has usually returned to normal in the chronic stage.
- Occasionally, cortical laminar necrosis can develop instead of encephalomalacia. Cortical laminar necrosis is a histologic finding characterized by deposition of lipid-laden macrophages after ischemia that manifests on imaging as hyperintensity on both T1- and T2-weighted images.

性期的主要特征。

- DWI在慢性期通常已恢复正常。
- 偶然情况下，可出现脑皮质层状坏死而非脑软化。脑皮质层状坏死是一个组织学上的发现，其特征是脑缺血后富脂质巨噬细胞沉积，表现为T_1WI和T_2WI均呈高信号。

（翻译　王苗苗）

SUBARACHNOID HEMORRHAGE AND ANEURYSMS

蛛网膜下腔出血和动脉瘤

SUBARACHNOID HEMORRHAGE (SAH)

蛛网膜下腔出血(SAH)

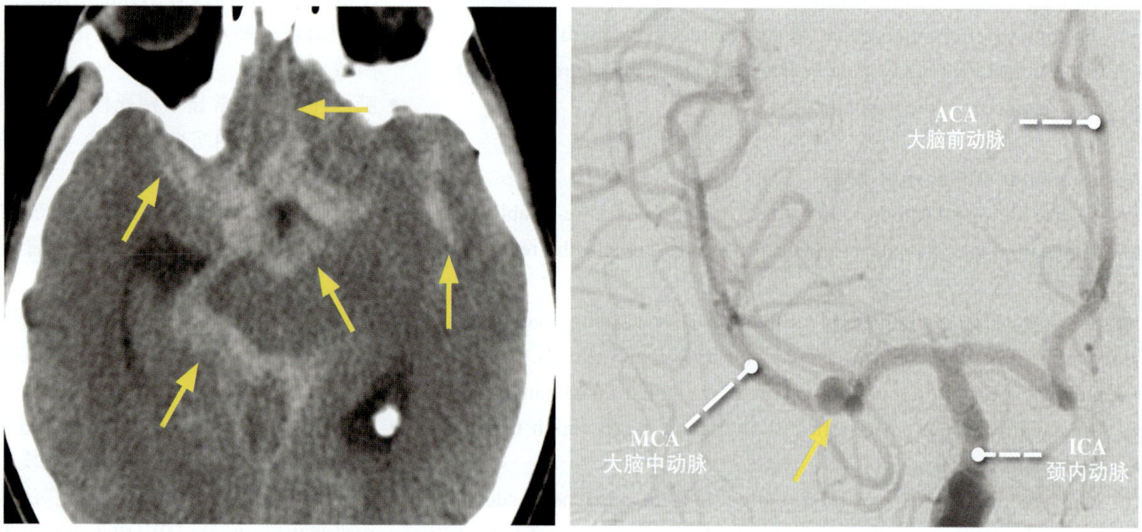

Subarachnoid hemorrhage: Noncontrast CT (left image) shows diffuse subarachnoid hemorrhage (arrows) in the basal cisterns including the suprasellar cistern, the anterior interhemispheric fissure, and the Sylvian fissure, predominantly on the right. Frontal oblique digital subtraction cerebralangiogram (right image) of the right internal carotid artery shows a small saccular aneurysm at the MCA trifurcation (yellow arrow).

蛛网膜下腔出血：平扫CT(左图)显示基底池弥漫蛛网膜下腔出血(黄箭)，包括鞍上池、前纵裂及外侧裂，以右侧为主。前斜位右侧颈内动脉数字减影脑血管造影(右图)显示大脑中动脉三分叉处一个小的囊状动脉瘤(黄箭)。

- Overall, the most common cause of subarachnoid hemorrhage (SAH) is trauma. Aneurysm rupture is by far the most common cause of non-traumatic SAH. No cause of the SAH is identified in up to 22% of cases.
- Clinically, non-traumatic SAH presents with thunderclap headache and meningismus.
- Noncontrast CT is the initial imaging modality in suspected SAH. On CT, subarachnoid blood appears as high attenuation within the subarachnoid space.

- 总体而言，最常见的SAH原因是创伤。而动脉瘤破裂则是非创伤性SAH最常见的原因。不明原因的SAH多达22%。
- 临床上，非创伤性SAH表现为霹雳性头痛和假性脑膜炎。
- 平扫CT是对怀疑有SAH患者的首选影像学检查方法。在CT上，蛛网膜下腔的血液表现为蛛网膜下腔内高密度影。

> High attenuation material in the subarachnoid space may be due to SAH (by far the most common cause), meningitis, leptomeningeal metastases, or prior intrathecal contrast administration.

> 蛛网膜下腔高密度影可能由于SAH(最常见)、脑膜炎、柔脑膜转移或先前鞘内注入造影剂所致。

- Noncontrast CT is >95% sensitive for detecting SAH within the first 6 hours, with sensitivity slowly decreasing to 50% by day 5. If clinical suspicion for SAH is high with a negative CT scan, the standard of care is to perform a lumbar puncture to look for xanthochromia.

- 平扫CT对于发现发病6小时内的SAH的灵敏度大于95%，随后的灵敏度逐渐降低，到第5天降至50%。如临床高度怀疑SAH而CT平扫为阴性者，标准处理方法是进行腰椎穿刺

- If SAH is present on imaging or lumbar puncture shows xanthochromia, catheter angiography is the gold standard to evaluate for the presence of an aneurysm. Several recent studies have shown, however, that CT angiography is equivalent to catheter angiography in the search for a culprit aneurysm in cases of SAH.
- On MRI, acute SAH appears hyperintense on FLAIR and demonstrates susceptibility artifact on gradient sequences.

以观察脑脊液是否有黄染。

- 如果影像学显示SAH或腰椎穿刺有脑脊液黄染，经导管血管造影是评估动脉瘤存在的“金标准”。然而，近来多个研究表明，CT血管造影对发现导致SAH的动脉瘤的价值与经导管血管造影相当。
- MRI上，急性SAH在FLAIR 显示为高信号，在梯度回波序列上显示为磁敏感伪影。

> The differential diagnosis for increased FLAIR signal in the subarachnoid space is similar to the differential for high attenuation subarachnoid material seen on CT, including **SAH**, **meningitis**, **leptomeningeal metastases**, and **residual contrast material**. Note that meningitis and metastases will typically show leptomeningeal enhancement in addition to the abnormal FLAIR signal.
> Recent **oxygen** or **propofol** administration will also cause increased subarachnoid FLAIR signal.

> FLAIR上蛛网膜下腔信号增高的鉴别诊断类似于CT上见到的蛛网膜下腔高密度影，包括**SAH**、**脑膜炎**、**柔脑膜转移**和**造影剂残留**。注意，脑膜炎及转移瘤除了异常的FLAIR信号外，通常会有柔脑膜强化。
> 近期**吸氧**或注射**异丙酚**也会导致FLAIR上蛛网膜下腔信号增高。

Distribution of subarachnoid hemorrhage

- The pattern of SAH may provide a clue to the location of the ruptured aneurysm. However, multiple aneurysms are seen in up to 20% of patients with SAH, and subarachnoid blood may redistribute if the patient was found down.
- Hemorrhage in the anterior interhemispheric fissure suggests an anterior communicating artery aneurysm (33% of intracranial aneurysms).
- Hemorrhage in the suprasellar cistern suggests a posterior communicating artery aneurysm (also 33% of intracranial aneurysms). Rarely, P-comm aneurysm rupture can result in isolated subdural hemorrhage.
- Hemorrhage in the Sylvian fissure suggests a middle cerebral artery aneurysm (20% of intracranial aneurysms).
- Hemorrhage in the perimesencephalic cistern suggests either a basilar tip aneurysm (5% of intracranial aneurysms), which has a high morbidity, or the relatively benign nonaneurysmal *perimesencephalic subarachnoid hemorrhage* (subsequently discussed).

蛛网膜下腔出血的分布

- SAH的分布方式可为寻找破裂动脉瘤的位置提供线索。然而，多发动脉瘤在SAH患者高达20%，且如果患者是在倒地时被发现，蛛网膜下腔内的血液可能会重新分布。
- 前纵裂出血提示前交通动脉动脉瘤(占颅内动脉瘤的33%)。
- 鞍上池出血提示后交通动脉动脉瘤(约占颅内动脉瘤的33%)。罕见的情况下，后交通动脉动脉瘤破裂可导致孤立性硬膜下出血。
- 外侧裂出血提示大脑中动脉动脉瘤(占颅内动脉瘤的20%)。
- 中脑周围池出血提示高致残率的基底动脉尖动脉瘤(占颅内动脉瘤的5%)，也可以是预后相对较好的非动脉瘤性中脑周围SAH(将在下文讨论)。

Grading of subarachnoid hemorrhage

- The **Hunt and Hess** score is the clinical grading scale for aneurysmal SAH and is based solely on symptoms, without imaging. Grade Ⅰ is the lowest grade, with only a mild headache. Grade Ⅴ is the most severe, with coma or extensor posturing.
- The **modified Fischer scale** classifies the CT appearance of aneurysmal SAH and correlates with risk of delayed cerebral ischemia.

  Thin SAH (<1 mm) is grade 1 without intraventricular hemorrhage (IVH) and grade 2 with IVH. Thick SAH (≥1 mm) is grade 3 without IVH and grade 4 with IVH.

蛛网膜下腔出血分级

- **Hunt和Hess**评分是动脉瘤性SAH的临床分级，完全依据症状，并不参考影像学。Ⅰ级为最低级别，仅表现为轻微头痛。Ⅴ级最严重，表现为昏迷或去大脑强直。
- **改良Fischer分级**对动脉瘤性SAH的CT表现进行了分类，并与迟发性脑缺血的风险相关。

  薄层SAH(<1mm)，不伴脑室出血(IVH)为1级，伴有IVH为2级。厚层SAH(≥1mm)，不伴IVH为3级，伴有IVH为4级。

Complications of subarachnoid hemorrhage

- **Vasospasm** is the most common cause of morbidity and mortality in patients who survive the initial episode of SAH. The peak incidence of vasospasm occurs most frequently 7–10 days after aneurysm rupture and resolves spontaneously after 21 days. Vasospasm results in delayed cerebral ischemia, which can cause infarction.

蛛网膜下腔出血并发症

- **血管痉挛**是早期SAH存活患者中最常致残和致死的原因。血管痉挛发生的高峰时间是动脉瘤破裂后7~10天，21天后自行消退。血管痉挛可引起迟发性脑缺血，导致脑梗死。

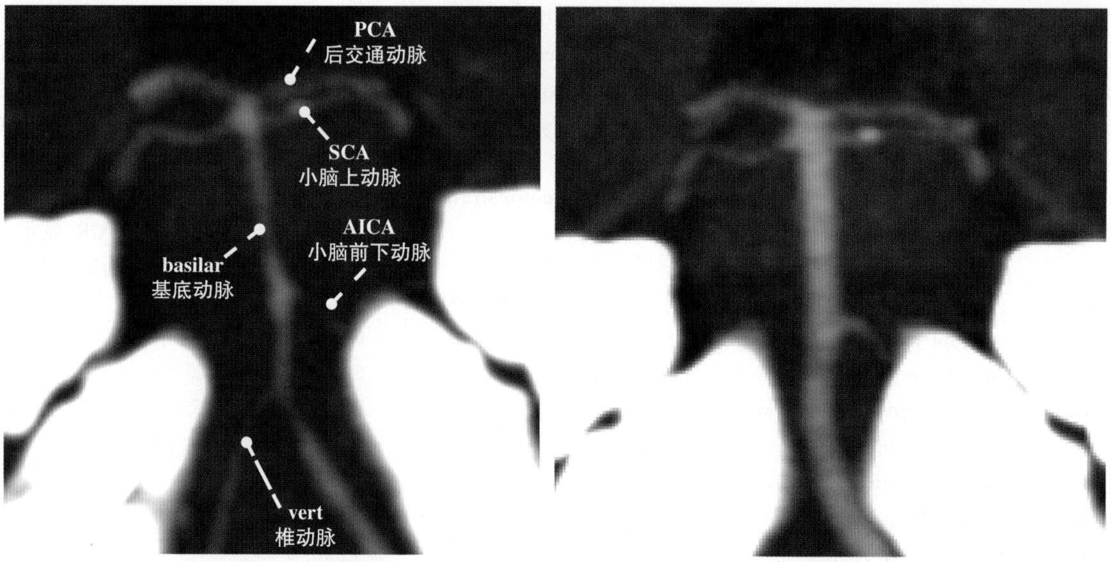

Vasospasm: Two coronal-oblique maximum-intensity projection images from subsequent CT angiograms, in the plane of the basilar artery. The initial study (left image) shows severe narrowing of the basilar artery, left AICA (right not visible), and distal vertebral arteries. The follow-up study (right image) was performed after endovascular treatment, which shows a normal caliber of the basilar and left vertebral arteries.

血管痉挛：两幅随访CT血管造影的基底动脉平面斜冠状位最大密度投影图像。初始检查(左图)显示基底动脉、左侧AICA(右侧未显示)及两侧远端椎动脉重度狭窄。血管腔内治疗后复查图像(右图)，显示基底动脉和左侧椎动脉管径正常。

- The gold standard for diagnosing vasospasm is digital subtraction angiography (DSA), which allows for concurrent treatment. Disadvantages of DSA include need for trained personnel, radiation exposure, contrast load, as well as potential for procedure-related complications.
- Compared to DSA, less invasive imaging methods for detection/monitoring of vasospasm include transcranial Doppler ultrasonography (TCD) and CT angiography (CTA). In cases of poor clinical grade, many guidelines recommend serial TCD for monitoring and CT angiography with or without perfusion in cases when there is clinical deterioration or in situations where TCD results are equivocal.
- Use of TCD is limited by availability of acoustic windows, operator experience, and limited evaluation of distal vessels. It has been proven useful for early detection and to help identify clinically occult cases when patients are heavily sedated. CT is useful because of its rapid availability, relative ease of interpretation, and better visualization of distal vasculature. Newer techniques such as CT and MR perfusion and nuclear medicine studies are also being investigated to identify areas of cerebral ischemia.
- Oral nimodipine, a calcium channel blocker, is used for prophylaxis for delayed cerebral ischemia. Conventional medical treatment of vasospasm includes *triple H therapy*, describing the use of "hypervolemia, hemodilution, and hypertension" to maintain blood pressure to the cerebral vasculature.
- Endovascular therapy with intra-arterial (IA) vasodilators and transluminal balloon angioplasty (TBA) are used in cases of severe or medically refractory vasospasm. Calcium channel blockers are the preferred pharmacologic class for IA vasodilation.
- **Acute hydrocephalus** occurs in 15–87% of patients with aneurysmal SAH. Acute hydrocephalus is usually managed by external ventricular drainage (EVD) or lumbar drainage. Chronic hydrocephalus occurs in 8.9–48% of patients and is managed with ventricular shunt placement.

- 诊断血管痉挛的“金标准”是数字减影血管造影(DSA)，此方法还可以同时进行治疗。DSA的缺点包括需要人员培训、辐射暴露、使用造影剂，以及可能出现的手术相关并发症。
- 相对于DSA，经颅多普勒超声(TCD)和CT血管造影(CTA)是检测/监测血管痉挛更具微创性的成像方法。在临床分级较低的情况下，许多指南建议在临床恶化或TCD结果不明确的情况下进行系列TCD监测和CT血管造影+/−灌注检查。
- 使用TCD受限于声窗、操作者经验且对评估远端血管有限。TCD被证明对早期发现的血管痉挛有帮助，并有助于识别服用大量镇静剂的临床隐匿病例。CT的价值在于可快速进行、解读相对容易，并较好显示远端血管。一些新的技术，如CT、MR灌注，以及核医学，也被用于识别脑缺血区。
- 口服尼莫地平，一种钙通道阻滞剂，可用于预防迟发性脑缺血。治疗血管痉挛的常规方法包括3H*疗法*，即使用“高血容量、血液稀释和增高血压”来维持脑血管系统的血压。
- 血管腔内治疗，包括使用动脉内(IA)血管扩张剂和腔内球囊血管成形术(TBA)，可用于病情严重或药物无效的血管痉挛患者。钙通道阻滞剂是首选的IA血管舒张药物。
- **急性脑积水**发生在15%~87%的动脉瘤性SAH的患者中。急性脑积水通常采用脑室外引流(EVD)或腰椎引流治疗。发展成慢性脑积水的患者为8.9%~48.0%，可采用脑室分流

- **Superficial siderosis** is a condition caused by iron overload of pial membranes due to chronic or repeated subarachnoid bleeding. Clinically, patients with superficial siderosis present with sensorineural deafness and ataxia. On imaging, theiron causes hypointensity on T2-weighted images outlining the affected sulci.
- Imaging workup includes cranial and spinal imaging to evaluate for a source of bleeding.

术进行治疗。

- **表面含铁血黄素沉积症**是由于慢性或反复性SAH导致的软脑膜铁过载。临床上，表面含铁血黄素沉积症患者表现为神经感音性耳聋和共济失调。影像上会由于铁沉积导致T_2加权低信号而勾画出受累脑沟的轮廓。
- 影像学检查应包含颅脑及脊柱检查，以寻找出血的来源。

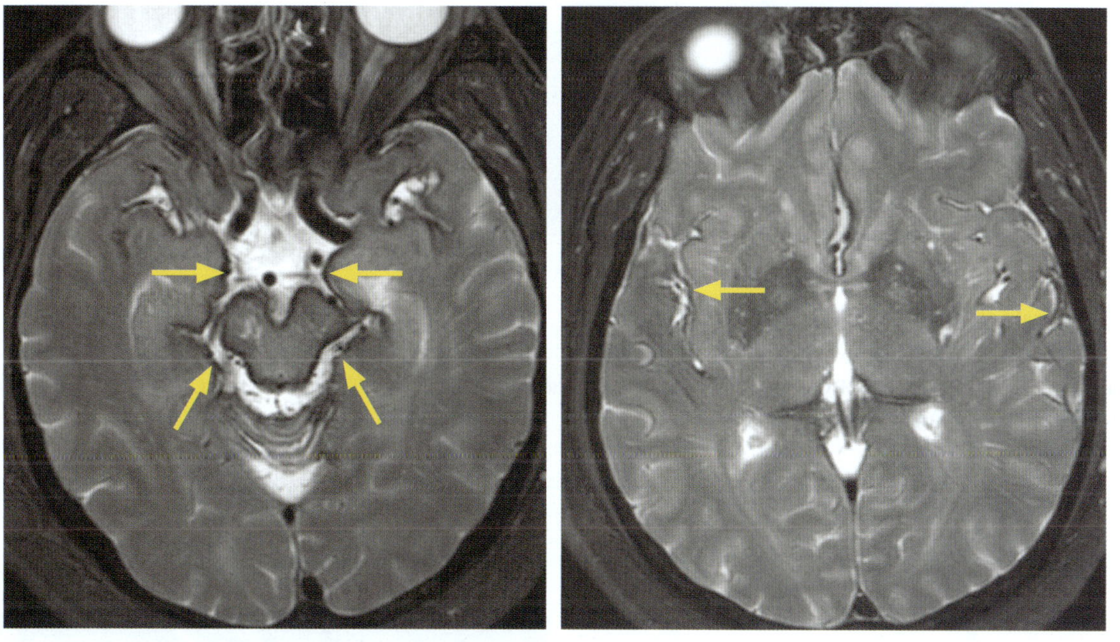

Superficial siderosis: Two axial T2-weighted images show a thin hypointense interface at the junction of the sulcal surfaces and the subarachnoid space (arrows) of the basal cisterns (left image) and the MCA territory temporal lobes (right image).
Case courtesy Mary Beth Cunnane, MD, Massachusetts Eye and Ear Infirmary.
表面含铁血黄素沉积症：两幅轴位T_2加权图像显示脑沟表面与基底池蛛网膜下腔交界处(左图)及MCA供血的颞叶区(右图)细线状低信号影(黄箭)。

Perimesencephalic subarachnoid hemorrhage

- Perimesencephalic subarachnoid hemorrhage is a pattern of nontraumatic SAH of likely venous origin that has a benign prognosis compared to other types. Patients with this pattern needless aggressive evaluation to exclude an aneurysm (e.g., CTA alone, or a single catheter angiogram without follow-up).
- To predict the absence of an aneurysm with specificity, the hemorrhage must be centered in the cisterns directly anterior to the brainstem in the interpeduncular or prepontine cisterns but may extend into the suprasellar, crural, ambient, and/or quadrigeminal cisterns and/or cisterna magna. Some criteria also allow hemorrhage centered in the posterior suprasellar cistern, extension into the medial Sylvian fissures or anterior interhemispheric fissure, and/or a small amount of intraventricular blood.
- Although the clinical presentation of perimesencephalic nonaneurysmal SAH is similar to aneurysm rupture (thunderclap headache), patients generally do well without residual neurological deficit. Some patients may experience mild to moderate vasospasm.

中脑周围蛛网膜下腔出血

- 中脑周围蛛网膜下腔出血是一种非外伤性SAH，可能起源于静脉，其预后好于其他类型。这种类型的患者只需进行创伤较小的检查以排除动脉瘤(例如，仅需CTA或一次性导管血管造影而不进行随访)。
- 除外动脉瘤的必要条件是：出血必须集中在脑干正前方的脚间池或桥前池，但可延伸到鞍上池、脚间池、环池，和/或四叠体池，和/或枕大池。一些标准中也允许出血集中在鞍上池后部，可延伸到外侧裂的内侧或前纵裂池，和/或少量脑室内出血。
- 虽然中脑周围非动脉瘤性SAH的临床症状与动脉瘤破裂症状相似(霹雳性头痛)，但患者普遍恢复良好，无神经功能后遗症。部分患者可出现轻到中度血管痉挛。

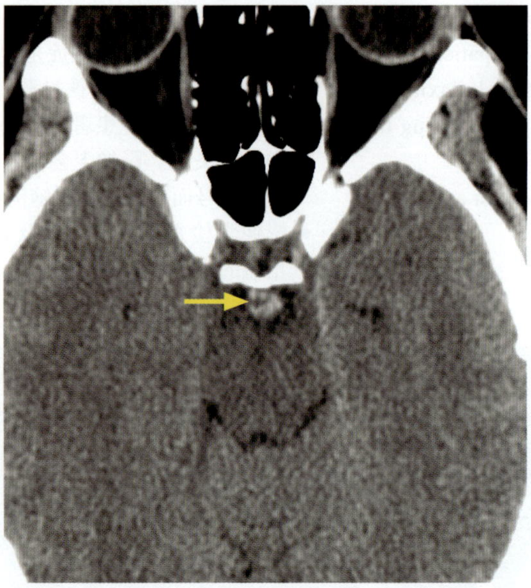

Perimesencephalic hemorrhage: Axial CT shows subarachnoid blood limited to the prepontine cistern (arrow). The membrane of Liliequist separates the prepontine cistern from the suprasellar cistern, and explains why there is no extension of blood superiorly. This patient had two negative catheter angiograms.
中脑周围出血：轴位CT显示蛛网膜下腔血液局限于桥前池(黄箭)。Liliequist膜将桥前池和鞍上池分隔开，故血液不会向上蔓延。这个患者的两次血管造影检查均为阴性。

Reversible cerebral vasoconstriction syndrome (RCVS)

- Reversible cerebral vasoconstriction syndrome (RCVS) is a cause of nontraumatic, nonaneurysmal SAH and ischemia. RCVS presents with thunderclap headache and is characterized by prolonged (but reversible) vasoconstriction.

可逆性脑血管收缩综合征(RCVS)

- RCVS是非创伤性、非动脉瘤性SAH和缺血的一个原因。RCVS表现为霹雳性头痛，并以持续性血管收缩(但可逆)为特征。

ANEURYSM MORPHOLOGY AND PATHOLOGY

动脉瘤形态和病理

Saccular aneurysm

囊状动脉瘤

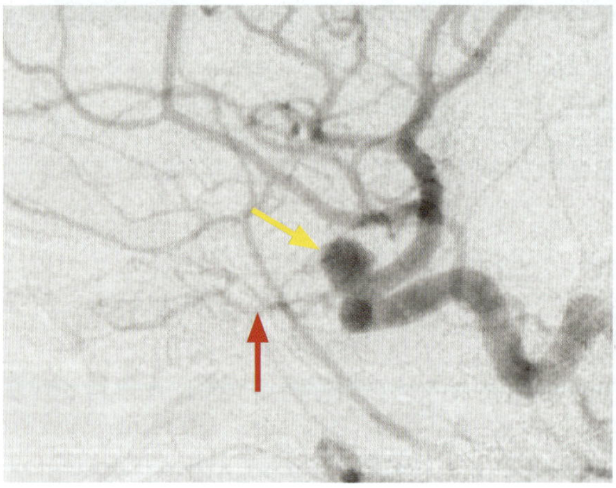

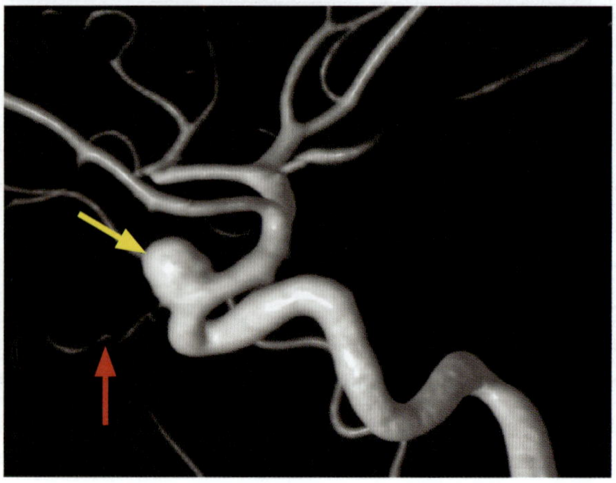

Ophthalmic artery aneurysm: Sagittal projection left common carotid arteriogram (left image) demonstrates a superiorly directed saccular aneurysm (yellow arrow) arising at the ostium of the ophthalmic artery (red arrow). Right image shows a 3D reconstruction of the aneurysm.
眼动脉动脉瘤：左侧颈总动脉造影矢状投影(左图)显示眼动脉(红箭)开口处朝向上方的囊状动脉瘤(黄箭)。右图显示动脉瘤的三维重建。

- A **saccular** (also called *berry*) aneurysm is a focal outpouching of the arterial wall, most commonly arising at a branch point in the circle of Willis, and has a characteristic rounded shape. The aneurysm points in the direction of blood flow leading into the branch point. Saccular aneurysms are seen almost exclusively in adults, with a slight female predominance. Saccular aneurysms are caused by a combination of hemodynamic stress and acquired degeneration of the vessel wall.

- **囊状**(也称浆果样)动脉瘤是动脉壁局部向外突出，常发生于威利斯环的分叉处，具有典型的圆形形态。动脉瘤朝向血流流向分支的方向。囊状动脉瘤几乎只见于成人，女性患者稍多。囊状动脉瘤是由于血流动力学压力和后天性血管壁变性两者共同作用所致。

- Saccular aneurysms can be classified as small (<1 cm), medium (>1 cm and <2.5 cm), and giant (>2.5 cm). The larger the size, the greater the risk for rupture.
- Giant aneurysms often present with mass effect, can mimic a mass (especially if partially thrombosed) and can cause a cranial nerve palsy. The most common is an oculomotor nerve palsy caused by a posterior communicating artery aneurysm.
- Minute aneurysms which occur as a result of chronic hypertension occurring most commonly in the basal ganglia are termed Charcot-Bouchard aneurysms.
- Non-inherited risk factors for the development of saccular aneurysm include hypertension, inflammatory vascular disease such as Takayasu or giant cell arteritis, and hemodynamic stress from altered state of cerebral blood flow such as due to moyamoya (aneurysms occur most commonly in the posterior circulation) or AVM.
- Inherited diseases that predispose to aneurysm formation include connective tissue diseases such as Marfan and Ehlers-Danlos, polycystic kidney disease, and neurofibromatosis type 1.
- The aneurysm *neck* is the opening which connects the aneurysm to the parent vessel and the aneurysm *body* is the aneurysm sac. The neck:body ratio affects treatment options. Aneurysms with relatively small necks are generally easier to treat endovascularly with endovascular coils.

Common sites of saccular aneurysms

- Anterior communicating artery (A-comm) aneurysms: Patients most commonly present with subarachnoid hemorrhage, frequently in the interhemispheric fissure. A-comm aneurysms are also associated with intraventricular hemorrhage, most commonly the lateral ventricles.
- Anterior cerebral artery (ACA) is the most common location for aneurysms associated with intracerebral hemorrhage.
- Internal carotid artery (ICA) aneurysms are named based on which segment it arises from.

  Cavernous ICA aneurysms are extradural, when nontraumatic are usually fusiform and expand laterally into the cavernous sinus. Typical presentation is with CN Ⅲ, Ⅳ, Ⅵ palsy. Rupture can produce a carotid- cavernous fistula or severe epistaxis from blood extrusion into the sphenoid sinus.

  Paraclinoid ICA aneurysms are classically distal to the dural ring (therefore intradural) and include ophthalmic and superior hypophyseal aneurysms. There is anatomic variability which results in some superior hypophyseal aneurysms and a minority of ophthalmic aneurysms being intradural.

  Supraclinoid ICA aneurysms include posterior communicating artery (P-comm) and anterior choroidal aneurysms. P-comm aneurysms arise just distal to the P-comm ostium and project posterolaterally, which may impact cranial nerve Ⅲ with classic presentation of pupil-sparing CN Ⅲ palsy.

  Carotid bifurcation or terminus aneurysms occur at the point where the ICA divides into the MCA and ACA. These aneurysms present with subarachnoid hemorrhage and generally point superiorly.
- Most middle cerebral artery (MCA) aneurysms occur at the M1 bifurcation, which is the second most common location for aneurysm presenting with intracerebral hemorrhage.
- Basilar tip aneurysms classically produce subarachnoid hemorrhage centered in the interpeduncular cistern with extension to the suprasellar and anterior and posterior perimesencephalic cisterns.
- Posterior inferior cerebellar artery (PICA) aneurysms present with subarachnoid

- 囊状动脉瘤分为小(<1cm)、中(1cm且<2.5cm)和巨大(>2.5cm)。动脉瘤越大则破裂风险越高。
- 巨大的动脉瘤通常表现为占位效应，可与肿块类似(尤其是形成部分血栓时)并可导致脑神经麻痹。最常见的是动眼神经麻痹，由后交通动脉瘤引起。
- 由慢性高血压引起的微小动脉瘤最常见于基底节区，称为Charcot-Bouchard动脉瘤。
- 囊状动脉瘤发生的非遗传性危险因素包括高血压、血管炎性疾病(如大动脉炎或巨细胞动脉炎)，以及脑血流状态改变而引起的血流动力学压力，如烟雾病(动脉瘤最常见于后循环)或动静脉畸形。
- 易形成囊状动脉瘤的遗传性疾病包括：结缔组织疾病(如马方综合征及埃勒斯-当洛综合征)、多囊肾和1型神经纤维瘤病。
- 动脉瘤颈是连接动脉瘤和载瘤动脉的开口，动脉瘤体是动脉瘤囊。瘤颈与瘤体的比例会影响治疗方法的选择。瘤颈相对较小的动脉瘤通常比较容易行血管腔内弹簧圈栓塞治疗。

囊状动脉瘤的常见部位

- 前交通动脉(A-comm)动脉瘤：患者最常见的表现为SAH，通常位于大脑半球间裂。A-comm动脉瘤也与脑室内出血有关，最常见的是侧脑室。
- 大脑前动脉(ACA)是与脑出血相关的动脉瘤最常见的部位。
- 颈内动脉(ICA)动脉瘤按照其起源的节段命名。

  海绵窦段ICA动脉瘤位于硬膜外，非外伤性时通常呈梭形并向外侧的海绵窦内扩张。典型表现为第Ⅲ、Ⅳ、Ⅵ脑神经麻痹。动脉瘤破裂可导致颈动脉海绵窦瘘或因血液挤压进入蝶窦而导致严重鼻出血。

  床突周围段ICA动脉瘤通常位于硬脑膜环的远端(因此属于硬脑膜内)，包括眼动脉瘤和垂体上动脉瘤。有些解剖上的变异可导致部分垂体上动脉瘤和少数眼动脉瘤位于硬膜内。

  床突上段ICA动脉瘤包括后交通动脉(P-comm)和前脉络膜动脉瘤。后交通动脉瘤起源于P-comm开口的远端，并朝向后外侧，可能影响第Ⅲ脑神经，并具有典型的第Ⅲ脑神经麻痹而瞳孔正常。

  颈动脉分叉或终末段动脉瘤发生在ICA的终点，分成MCA和ACA处。这些动脉瘤可表现为SAH，并且通常朝向上方。
- 大多数大脑中动脉(MCA)动脉瘤发生在M1段的分叉处，是以脑出血为表现的第二常见的动脉瘤发生部位。
- 典型的基底动脉尖动脉瘤导致的SAH是以脚间池为中心，并延伸至鞍上池、中脑周围池的前后方。
- 小脑后下动脉(PICA)动脉瘤以SAH为首发表

hemorrhage and clinically can present with localized head and neck ache, meningismus, and CN Ⅵ palsy. Presence of apparently isolated intraventricular hemorrhage in the fourth ventricle is suggestive of PICA aneurysm.

Fusiform aneurysm

- A fusiform aneurysm is a type of intracranial aneurysm characterized by an elongated fusiform shape, without a defined neck. Fusiform aneurysms are usually due to atherosclerosis, but may arise from chronic dissection.
- In contrast to saccular aneurysms, fusiform aneurysms do not occur at branch points.
- The vertebrobasilar system is affected more commonly than the anterior circulation.
- Fusiform aneurysms are much less common than saccular aneurysms. However, since there is no aneurysm neck to exclude from the systemic circulation, fusiform aneurysms are more difficult to treat. Fusiform aneurysms of the vertebrobasilar system pose particular challenges, as critical perforating vessels may arise directly from the diseased artery.

Mycotic (infectious) aneurysm

现，临床上可能有局限性头颈疼痛、脑膜炎和第Ⅵ脑神经麻痹。出现明显的孤立性第四脑室内出血提示PICA动脉瘤。

梭形动脉瘤

- 梭形动脉瘤是颅内动脉瘤的一种，其特征是呈细长的梭形，无明确的瘤颈。梭形动脉瘤常由动脉粥样硬化导致，也可源于慢性动脉夹层。
- 与囊状动脉瘤不同，梭形动脉瘤并不发生在血管分叉处。
- 椎基底系统较前循环更常发生梭形动脉瘤。
- 梭形动脉瘤远少于囊性动脉瘤。因为梭形动脉瘤没有瘤颈，不能与体循环分离，所以梭形动脉瘤治疗更为困难。椎基底动脉系统的梭形动脉瘤治疗难度更大，因为重要的穿支动脉血管可能直接起源于病变动脉。

感染性动脉瘤

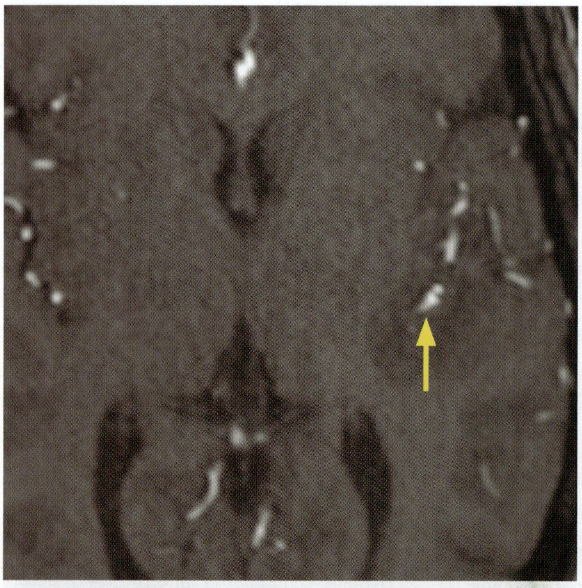

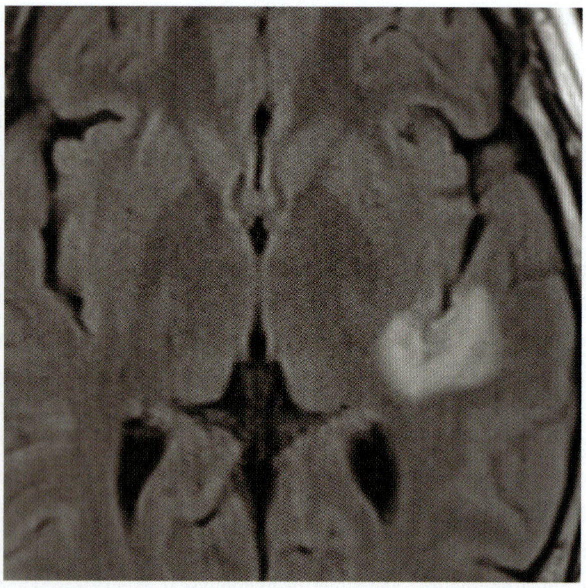

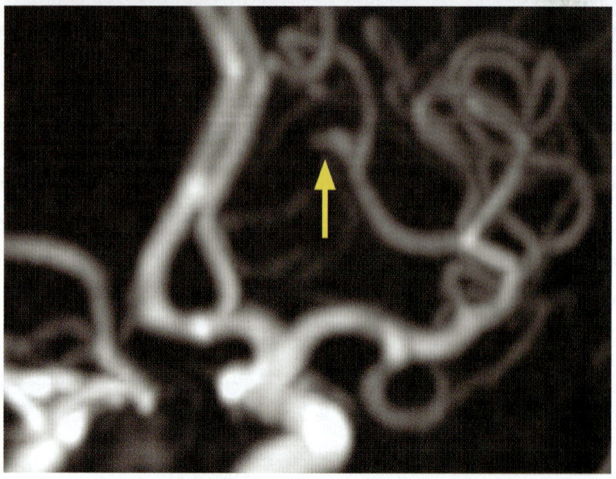

Mycotic aneursym and cerebritis in a patient with known fungal endocarditis:

Axial MRA (top left image) demonstrates a small irregular outpouching arising from a left M2 branch in the Sylvian fissure, better depicted on the MIP image (bottom left), which is concerning for mycotic aneurysm (arrows).

Axial FLAIR shows surrounding T2 prolongation in the left medial temporal lobe abutting the posterior aspect of the Sylvian fissure, likely focal cerebritis.

已知真菌性心内膜炎患者的感染性动脉瘤和脑炎：

轴位MRA(左上图)显示一个小而不规则的向外突起，起源于外侧裂的左侧M2分支，在MIP图像(左下图)显示得更好，考虑为感染性动脉瘤(黄箭)。

轴位FLAIR显示左侧颞叶内侧邻近外侧裂后部处T_2延长，可能是局灶性脑炎。

- Mycotic aneurysms account for only 2–4% of all intracranial aneurysms and are due to septic emboli. Bacterial endocarditis is the most common embolic source.
- Mycotic aneurysms are more common in the anterior circulation than the posterior circulation. In contrast to saccular aneurysms, they tend to be peripherally located and fusiform in shape. Mycotic aneurysms are fragile and have a high risk of rupture.
- Cross-sectional imaging with CT angiogram/MRangiogram has a sensitivity of approximately 50% with high interobserver variability. Therefore, DSA remains the gold standard for evaluation of myotic aneurysms.

Oncotic aneurysm

- An oncotic aneurysm is an aneurysm caused by neoplasm.
- A benign left atrial myxoma may peripherally embolize and cause a distal oncotic aneurysm.

Traumatic pseudoaneurysm

- Aneurysms due to trauma are most commonly pseudoaneurysms, which don't contain the typical three histologic layers of the vessel wall. Usually the vessel will exhibit abnormal luminal narrowing proximal to the aneurysm. Similar to mycotic aneurysms, traumatic pseudoaneurysms tend to occur distally.
- Arteries close to bony structures (such as the basilar and vertebral artery) are prone to dissecting aneurysms.

- 感染性动脉瘤仅占所有颅内动脉瘤的2%~4%，病因是化脓性栓子。细菌性心内膜炎是最常见的栓子来源。
- 前循环的感染性动脉瘤比后循环的更常见。与囊状动脉瘤不同，感染性动脉瘤往往发生于外周并呈梭形。感染性动脉瘤的瘤壁脆弱，破裂风险高。
- CT血管造影/MR血管造影在轴位成像的灵敏度约为50%，且观察者间的变异性较高。因此，DSA仍然是评估感染性动脉瘤的"金标准"。

肿瘤性动脉瘤

- 肿瘤性动脉瘤是由肿瘤导致的动脉瘤。
- 良性左心房黏液瘤可能会栓塞外周血管而导致远端肿瘤性动脉瘤。

创伤性假性动脉瘤

- 外伤所致的动脉瘤常为假性动脉瘤，即不含有正常血管壁的三层组织结构。动脉瘤近端血管通常表现为异常管腔狭窄。与感染性动脉瘤一样，创伤性假性动脉瘤常好发于远端。
- 靠近骨性结构的动脉(如基底动脉和椎动脉)更容易发生夹层动脉瘤。

（翻译　杨晶）

VASCULAR MALFORMATIONS

血管畸形

HIGH-FLOW LESIONS (LESIONS WITH SHUNTING)

高血流病变(分流性病变)

Arteriovenous malformation (AVM)

动静脉畸形(AVM)

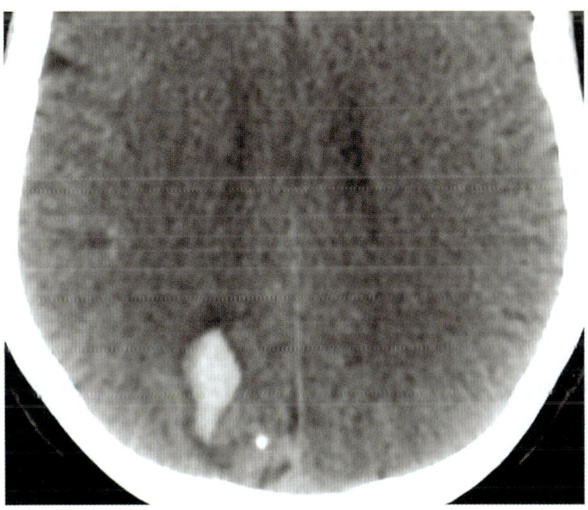

Axial noncontrast CT
轴位平扫CT

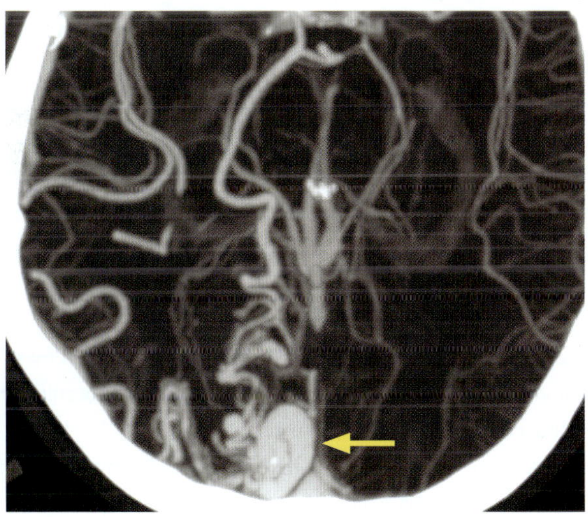

Axial CTA MIP image
轴位CTA MIP图像

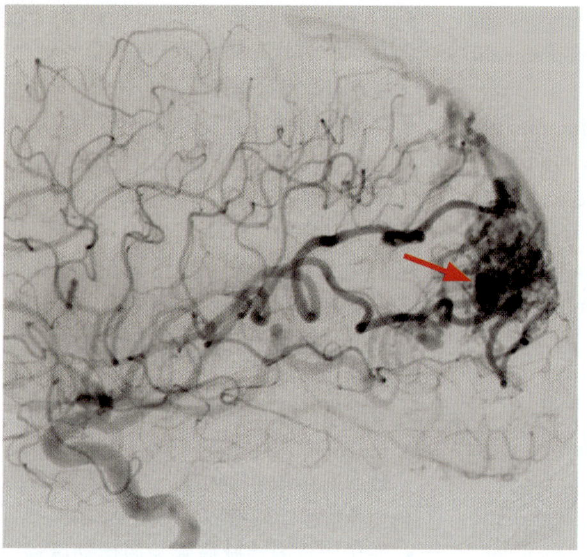

Sagittal internal carotid angiography (arterial phase)
矢状位颈内动脉造影(动脉期)

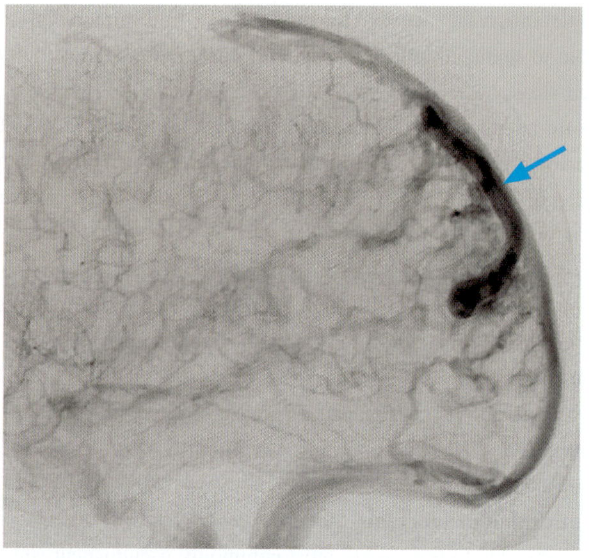

Sagittal internal carotid angiography (delayed phase)
矢状位颈内动脉造影(延迟期)

Ruptured arteriovenous malformation: Noncontrast CT shows a right occipital intraparenchymal hemorrhage. CTA shows a large tangle of vessels in the right occipital lobe (yellow arrow). Angiography better demonstrates the nidus (red arrow) and early venous drainage via dilated superficial cortical veins (blue arrow) to the superior sagittal sinus. There is no deep venous drainage. The nidus is predominantly supplied by branches of the right PCA.
动静脉畸形破裂：平扫CT显示右侧枕部脑实质内出血。CTA显示右侧枕叶有大量紊乱的血管(黄箭)。血管造影更好地显示了血管巢(红箭)和早期静脉显影，并通过扩张的皮质浅静脉(蓝箭)引流至上矢状窦。没有深静脉引流。血管巢主要由右侧PCA分支供血。

- An arteriovenous malformation (AVM) is a congenital high-flow vascular malformation consisting of directly connecting arteries and veins without an intervening capillary bed. AVM occurs intra-axially and 85% are supratentorial. AVM usually presents with seizures or bleeding (usually parenchymal hemorrhage, rarely subarachnoid). Aneurysms of the feeding arteries or intra-nidal arteries are often seen, which predispose to bleeding.
- The **Spetzler-Martin** scale helps to evaluate surgical risk for AVM resection. A large AVM (>6 cm) draining to a deep venous sinus system in eloquent cortex has the highest risk, while a small AVM (<3 cm) draining to a superficial venous sinus system in non-eloquent cortex has the lowest risk.
- On imaging, AVM is characterized by a vascular nidus (“nest”) containing numerous serpentine vessels that appear as black flow-voids on MRI. There are usually adjacent changes to the adjacent brain including gliosis (T2 prolongation), dystrophic calcification, and blood products (blooming on T2* gradient imaging). The gliosis/encephalomalacia or mineralization seen in the adjacent brain is due to alteration in vascular flow from the AVM.
- AVM replaces rather than displaces brain. It causes minimal mass effect.
- Uncommonly, a bleeding AVM may be angiographically occult if the malformed vessels are compressed by the acute hematoma.
- Factors that increase bleeding risk that are detectable by imaging include intra-nidal aneurysm, venous ectasia, venous stenosis, deep venous drainage, and posterior fossa location.
- Treatment can be with embolization, stereotactic radiation, or surgical resection.

- AVM是一种先天性高血流的血管畸形，由动脉和静脉直接交通而成，没有中间毛细血管床。AVM发生在轴内(脑实质)，85%位于幕上。AVM通常表现为癫痫发作或出血(通常是实质出血，很少是蛛网膜下腔出血)。供血动脉或血管巢动脉的动脉瘤常见，并容易导致出血。
- **Spetzler-Martin**量表有助于评估手术切除AVM的风险。大的(>6cm)且引流到皮质功能区的深静脉窦系统的AVM具有最高风险，而小的(<3cm)且引流到非功能皮质区浅静脉窦系统的AVM风险最低。
- AVM在影像学上的特点是血管巢(“nest”)，内含大量在MRI上显示为黑色流空的蛇形血管。邻近大脑通常有改变，包括神经胶质增生(T_2延长)、营养不良性钙化和血液产物(在T_2*梯度成像上的开花样表现)。神经胶质增生/脑软化或相邻大脑中的矿化是由于AVM的血管流动改变所致。
- AVM占据局部脑组织但不产生脑组织移位。其占位效应极其轻微。
- 少见情况下，如果畸形血管被急性血肿压迫，血管造影上可能看不到出血性AVM。
- 影像学可检测到的出血风险增加因素包括巢内动脉瘤、静脉扩张、静脉狭窄、深静脉引流和病变位于颅后窝。
- 治疗可以采用栓塞、立体定向放疗或手术切除。

Dural arteriovenous fistula (dAVF)

- Dural arteriovenous fistulas are a complex group of high-flow lesions characterized by arteriovenous shunts between the meningeal arterioles and dural venules.
- The primary prognostic feature is the presence and degree of *cortical venous drainage*. The **Cognard classification** Ⅰ through Ⅳ describes lesions with progressively increased risk of bleeding.

> **Type Ⅰ**: No cortical venous drainage. Lowest risk of bleeding.
> **Type ⅡA**: Reflux into dural sinus but not cortical veins.
> **Type ⅡB**: Reflux into cortical veins: 10–20% hemorrhage rate.
> **Type Ⅲ**: Direct cortical venous drainage: 40% hemorrhage rate.
> **Type Ⅳ**: Direct cortical venous drainage with venous ectasia: 66% hemorrhage rate.
> **Type Ⅴ**: Spinal venous drainage. May cause myelopathy.

- **Carotid-cavernous fistula (CCF)** is a subtype of dAVF that is often caused by trauma with resultant fistula between the cavernous carotid artery and the cavernous sinus. Enlargement of the superior orbital vein and shunting within the cavernous sinus can lead to eye symptoms, such as proptosis and cranial nerve palsy.
- **Vein of Galen malformation** is a type of vascular malformation characterized by arteriovenous fistulae from thalamoperforator branches into the deep venous system. The enlarged vein is actually an enlarged median prosencephalic vein.

  In childhood, a vein of Galen malformation is the most common extracardiac cause of high output cardiac failure. Vein of Galen malformation may also be seen in adults, but clinically would be either asymptomatic or may be the cause of Parinaud syndrome due to mass effect in the pineal region.

硬脑膜动静脉瘘(dAVF)

- 硬脑膜动静脉瘘是一组复杂的高血流病变，其特点是脑膜小动脉和硬脑膜小静脉之间的动静脉分流。
- 主要的预后因素取决于是否存在皮质静脉引流及其引流程度。**Cognard分型**Ⅰ~Ⅳ是按病变出血风险由低到高进行定义的。

> **Ⅰ型**：无皮质静脉引流，出血风险最低。
> **ⅡA型**：反流到硬脑膜窦，但不回流至皮质静脉。
> **ⅡB型**：反流到皮质静脉，10%~20%的出血率。
> **Ⅲ型**：直接引流到皮质静脉，40%的出血率。
> **Ⅳ型**：直接引流到皮层静脉伴静脉扩张，66%的出血率。
> **Ⅴ型**：引流到脊髓静脉，可能会导致脊髓病。

- **颈动脉海绵窦瘘(CCF)**是dAVF的一种亚型，通常由外伤造成颈内动脉海绵窦段和海绵窦之间形成瘘。眼上静脉增粗和海绵窦分流可导致眼部症状，如眼球突出和脑神经麻痹。
- **Galen静脉畸形**是一种血管畸形，其特点是丘脑穿支动脉进入深静脉系统形成动静脉瘘。扩大的静脉实际上是增粗的前脑正中静脉。

  Galen静脉畸形是儿童时期最常见的心外高输出心力衰竭的原因。Galen静脉畸形也可见于成人，但临床上可能无症状，或是由于松果体区的占位效应而导致帕里诺综合征。

LOW-FLOW LESIONS (LESIONS WITHOUT SHUNTING)

低流量病变(无分流性病变)

Cavernous malformation (cavernoma)

海绵状血管畸形(海绵状血管瘤)

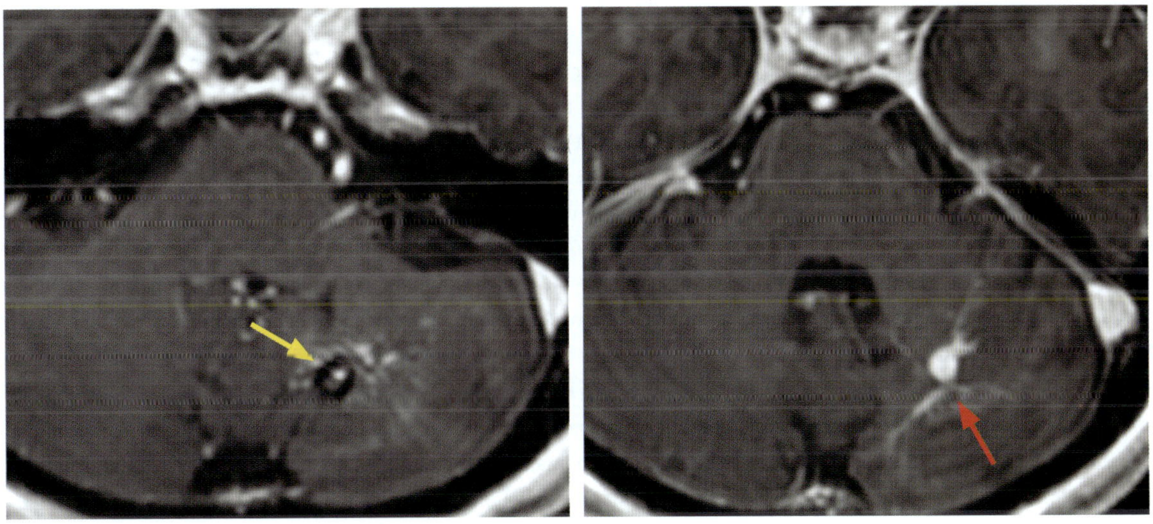

Cavernous malformation and associated DVA: Two axial contrast-enhanced T1-weighted images show a hypointense, centrally hyperintense nonenhancing cavernous malformation (yellow arrow) in the left cerebellar hemisphere. Directly superior to the cavernoma (right image) is an enhancing vascular structure with *caput medusa* morphology (red arrow), representing a developmental venous anomaly.

海绵状血管畸形和相关的DVA：两幅轴位对比增强T_1加权图像显示左侧小脑半球出现低信号、中央呈高信号的无强化的海绵状血管畸形(黄箭)。在海绵状血管瘤(右图)的正上方是增强的血管结构，并具有海蛇头形态(红箭)，为发育性静脉畸形。

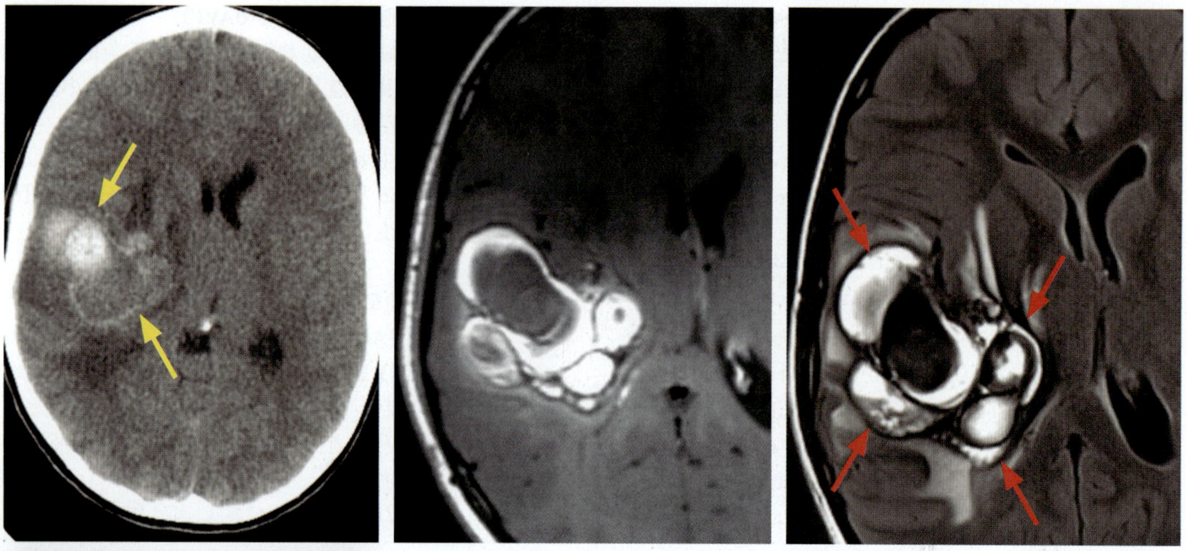

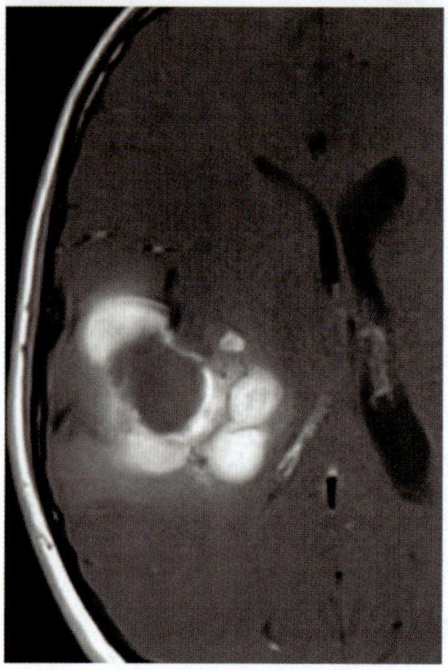

Giant cavernous malformation in a different patient:
Axial unenhanced CT (top left image) shows a hyperattenuating complex mass (arrows) in the right fronto-temporal lobe.
Unenhanced T1-weighted image (top middle image) shows the mass is predominantly cystic and hyperintense (representing blood products).
Axial FLAIR (top right image) shows that the intracystic contents are primarily hyperintense. There is a complete low signal hemosiderin ring surrounding the lesion (red arrows). There is mild surrounding edema.
Post contrast axial T1-weighted image (left image) shows no appreciable enhancement.
Case courtesy Gregory Wrubel, MD, Brigham and Women's Hospital.
另一名患者的巨大海绵状血管畸形：
轴位平扫CT(左上图)显示右侧额颞叶一个高密度混杂肿块(黄箭)。
平扫T_1加权图像(上中图)显示肿块以囊性和高信号为主(代表血液产物)。
轴位FLAIR(右上图)显示囊内容物以高信号为主。病变环绕完整的低信号含铁血黄素环(红箭)。周围有轻度水肿。
轴位增强T_1加权图像(左图)显示无明显增强。

- A cavernous malformation (also called a cavernoma) is a vascular hamartoma with a very small but definite bleeding risk. The clinical course of a cavernous malformation is variable and the lesion may cause seizures even in the absence of significant hemorrhage.
- Cavernous malformation is often associated with an adjacent developmental venous anomaly (DVA). There is increased risk of bleeding if a DVA is present. However, the DVA itself does not have any bleeding risk.
- Multiple, cavernous malformations represent an inherited disorder called **familial cerebral cavernous malformation syndrome**.
- Cavernous malformations can be induced by radiation treatment to the brain.
- Noncontrast CT shows a well-circumscribed rounded hyperattenuating lesion. The hyperattenuation is due to microcalcification within the cavernoma.
- MRI shows characteristic "popcorn-like" appearance of lobular mixed signal on T1-and T2-weighted images from blood products of various ages. There is a peripheral rim of hemosiderin which is dark on GRE and T2-weighted image. There is typically no enhancement, but intense enhancement may be seen with a long delay after contrast administration. Cavernous malformations may range in size from tiny (single focus of susceptibility artifact) to giant.

- 海绵状血管畸形(也称为海绵状血管瘤)是一种血管错构瘤，具有明确但非常小的出血风险。海绵状血管畸形的临床表现多样，即使在没有明显出血的情况下也可能引起癫痫发作。
- 海绵状血管畸形通常与相邻的发育性静脉异常(DVA)有关。如果存在DVA，则会增加出血风险。然而，DVA本身没有任何出血风险。
- 多发性海绵状血管瘤是一种遗传性疾病，被称为**家族性脑海绵状血管瘤综合征**。
- 对大脑进行放射治疗可诱发海绵状血管瘤。
- 平扫CT显示边界清楚的圆形高密度病灶。此高密度是海绵状血管瘤内的微钙化。
- MRI T_1和T_2加权图像显示特征性的"爆米花样"分叶状混合信号，为不同时间的血液产物所致。含铁血黄素环在GRE和T_2加权图像上呈黑色。通常没有增强，但在注射造影剂后较长延迟显像可能会出现显著增强。海绵状血管瘤的体积可能很小(单个小灶磁敏感性伪影)或巨大。

- Cavernous malformations are usually occult by vascular imaging (CTA or angiography).

Developmental venous anomaly (DVA), also called venous angioma

- 海绵状血管瘤在血管成像(CTA或血管造影)上通常是阴性的。

发育性静脉异常(DVA),也称为静脉血管瘤

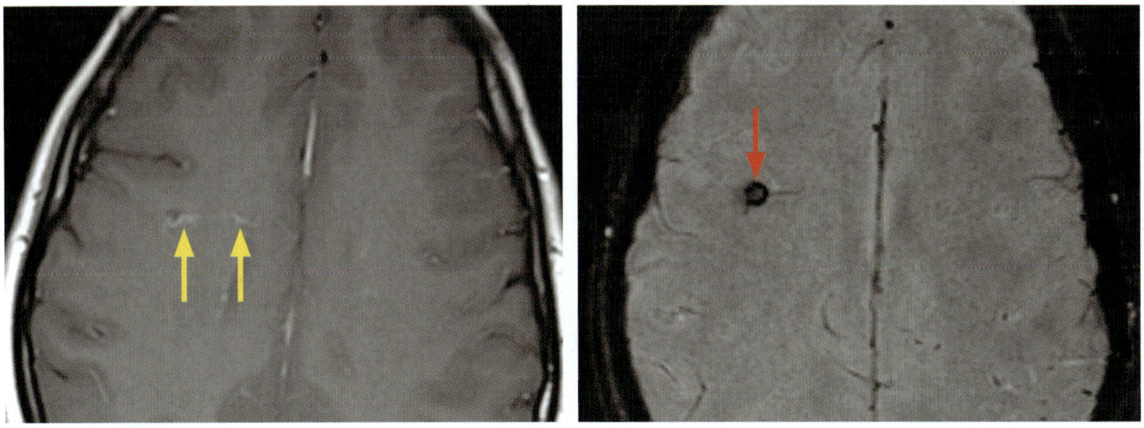

Developmental venous anomaly and a tiny cavernous malformation: Post-contrast axial T1-weighted MRI (left image) shows a subtle curvilinear enhancing structure (yellow arrows) in the right frontal white matter representing a DVA. Susceptibility weighted image (right image) shows a focus of susceptibility artifact (red arrow), suggestive of an adjacent cavernous malformation.

Case courtesy Sanjay Prabhu, MD, Boston Children's Hospital.

发育性静脉异常和微小海绵状血管瘤：轴位增强T_1加权MRI(左图)显示右侧额叶白质中隐匿的曲线增强结构(黄箭),此为DVA。磁敏感加权图像(右图)显示小灶磁敏感伪影(红箭),提示相邻的海绵状血管畸形。

- A developmental venous anomaly (DVA) is an abnormal vein that provides functional venous drainage to normal brain.
- DVA can usually only be seen on contrast-enhanced or susceptibility-weighted images, where it appears as a radially oriented vein with a characteristic caput medusa appearance.
- A DVA is a **Do Not Touch** lesion. If resected, the patient will suffer a debilitating venous infarct similar to acute thrombosis of DVA. The DVA must be preserved if an adjacent cavernous malformation is resected.

Capillary telangiectasia

- 发育性静脉异常(DVA)是一种异常静脉,它作为功能性静脉引流正常大脑。
- DVA通常只能通过对比增强或磁敏感加权图像进行观察,表现为放射状引流静脉并有特征性的海蛇头外观。
- DVA是一种**不能触碰**的病变。如果切除,患者将出现致残性静脉梗死,类似于DVA急性血栓形成。切除海绵状血管瘤时必须保留相邻的DVA。

毛细血管扩张

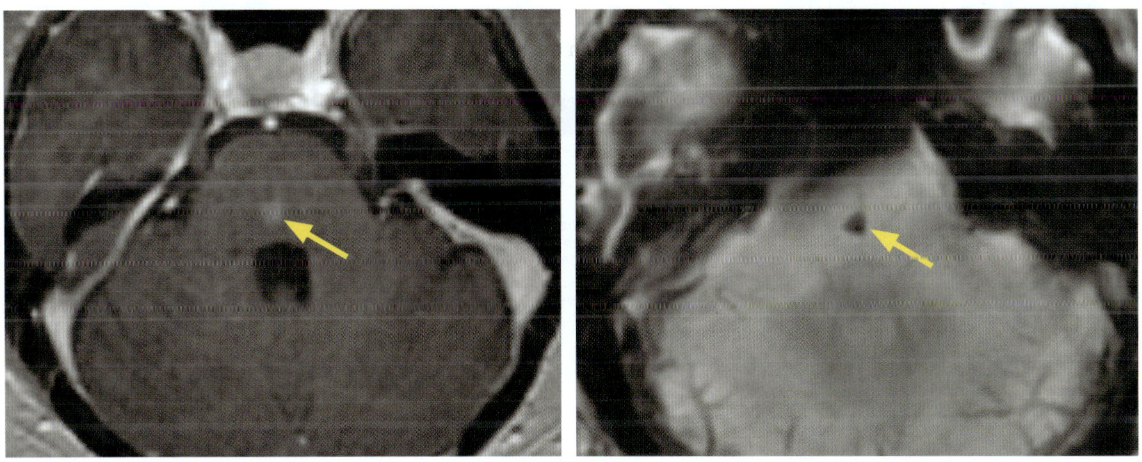

Capillary telangiectasia: Axial post-contrast T1-weighted MRI (left image) shows faint focal enhancement in the dorsal pons with associated susceptibility artifact (right SWI image) (arrows).

毛细血管扩张：轴位增强T_1加权MRI(左图)显示在背侧脑桥微弱的局灶性增强与相应的磁敏感伪影(右SWI图像)(黄箭)。

- A capillary telangiectasia is an asymptomatic vascular lesion composed of dilated capillaries with interspersed normal brain. A capillary telangiectasia is another **Do Not Touch** lesion.
- Post-contrast MRI shows a faint, brush-stroke-like enhancing lesion, most commonly in the brainstem or pons, without mass effect or surrounding edema. GRE often shows blooming due to susceptibility.
- Similar to cavernous malformation, capillary telangiectasia isangiographically occult.
- Capillary telangiectasia can mimic an enhancing tumor, although they can be differentiated from other lesions by their occult appearance on T2 and FLAIR sequences.

- 毛细血管扩张症是一种无症状的血管病变，内含扩张的毛细血管并穿插于正常大脑。毛细血管扩张症是另一种**不能触碰**病变。
- 增强MRI显示微弱的、笔刷状强化病灶，最常见于脑干或脑桥，无占位效应或周围水肿。因具有磁敏感，GRE上经常显示开花样表现。
- 与海绵状血管瘤相似，毛细血管扩张在血管造影上是隐匿的。
- 毛细血管扩张可类似于有增强的肿瘤，但它们因为在T_2和FLAIR序列上的阴性表现而得以与其他病变相区别。

（翻译　王维平）

CEREBRAL VENOUS DISEASE

脑静脉疾病

VENOUS ANATOMY

静脉解剖

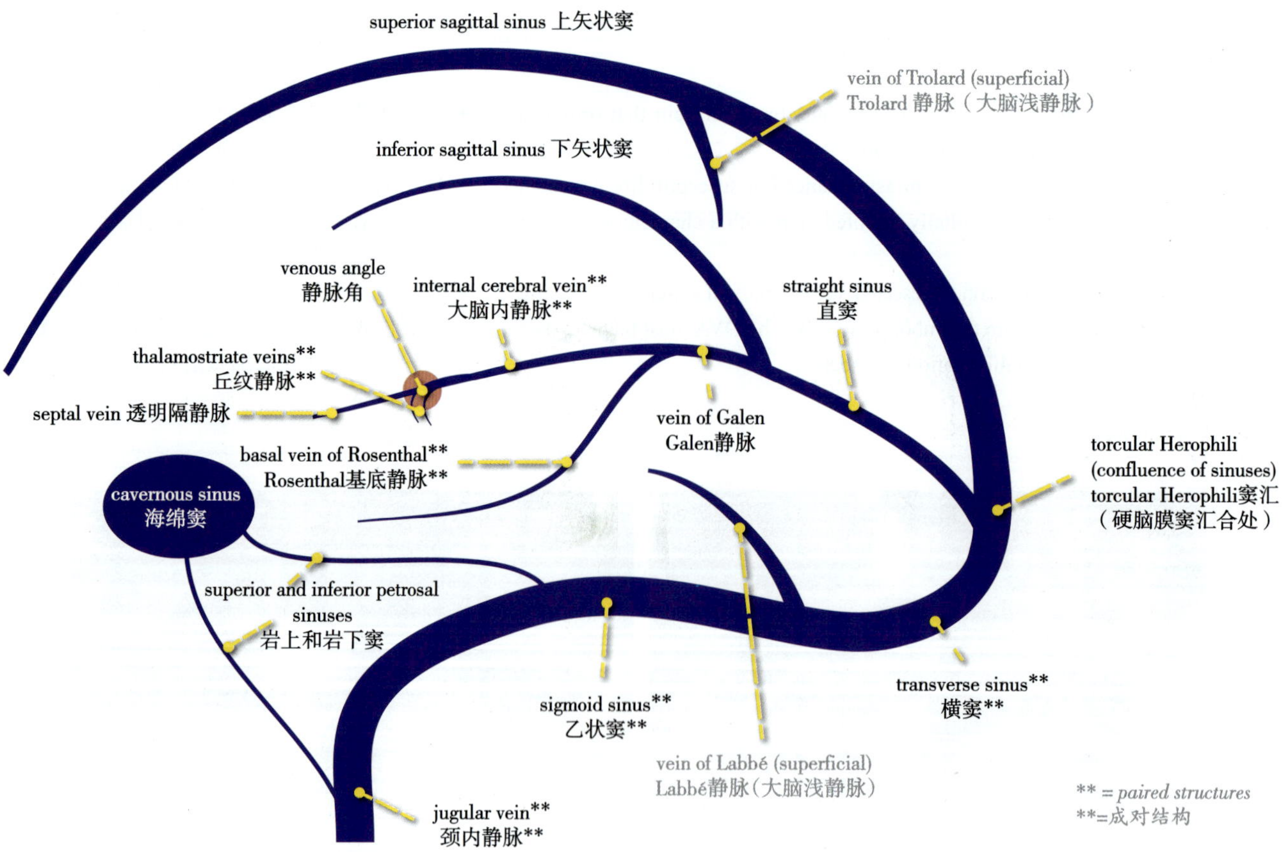

Dural sinuses

- The superior sagittal sinus (and its tributaries) drains the motor and sensory strips.
- The paired transverse sinuses are usually asymmetric, with the left transverse sinus often hypoplastic.
- The sigmoid sinus connects to the jugular bulb.
- The torcular Herophili is the confluence of the superior sagittal sinus, the transverse sinus, and the straight sinus. The word *torcular* is from the Greek word for wine press, and Herophilus was a Greek anatomist. Technically, the term *torcular Herophili* refers to the depression on the inner table of the skull produced by the confluence of sinuses, but in general use, *torcular Herophili* refers to the actual confluence of sinuses.

硬脑膜窦

- 上矢状窦(及其属支)引流运动区和感觉区的静脉血。
- 横窦成对但常不对称,左侧往往发育不全。
- 乙状窦与颈静脉球交通。
- 窦汇是上矢状窦、横窦及直窦的汇合点,"torcular"源于希腊词汇,原意为榨酒机,"Herophilus"是希腊的一位解剖学家。严格来讲,术语"torcular Herophilus"是指静脉窦汇合引起的颅骨内板凹陷,但常是指静脉窦汇合处。

Deep cerebral veins

- The deep cerebral veins consist of the paired internal cerebral veins, the basal veins of Rosenthal, and the vein of Galen.
- The venous angle (red dot in the diagram above) is the intersection of the septal vein and the thalamostriate veins. The venous angle is the angiographic landmark for the foramen of Monro.

大脑深静脉

- 大脑深静脉包含成对的大脑内静脉、Rosenthal基底静脉及Galen静脉。
- 静脉角(示意图上的红点)指透明隔静脉和两侧丘纹静脉的汇合点。静脉角在脑血管造影时为室间孔的解剖学标记。

Superficial cerebral veins

- The vein of Trolard connects superficial cortical veins to the superior sagittal sinus.
- The vein of Labbé drains the temporal convexity into the transverse or sigmoid sinus. Retraction injury to the vein of Labbé during surgery may lead to venous infarction and aphasia.

大脑浅静脉

- Trolard静脉引流皮层浅静脉血至上矢状窦。
- Labbé静脉引流颞叶凸面的静脉血至横窦或乙状窦。术中牵拉损伤Labbé静脉可导致静脉性脑梗死和失语。

Venous disease

静脉性病变

Venous thrombosis

静脉血栓形成

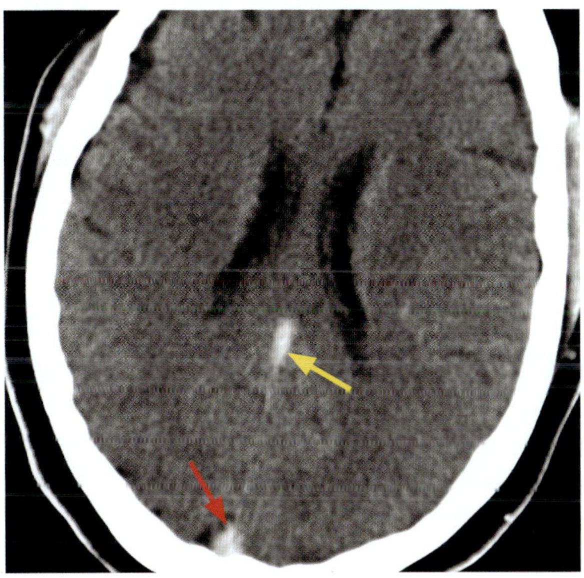

Noncontrast axial CT shows high attenuation in the vein of Galen (the *cord* sign; yellow arrow) and superior sagittal sinus near the torcular Herophili (red arrow).
轴位平扫CT显示大脑大静脉(条索征;黄箭)及靠近窦汇的上矢状窦(红箭)内的高密度影。

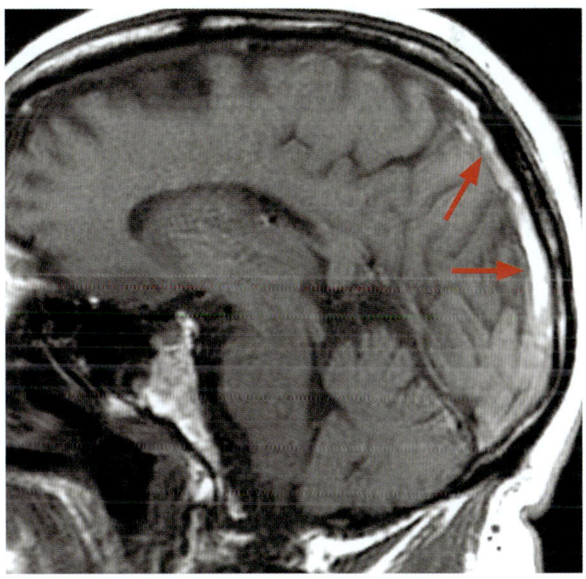

Sagittal T1-weighted MRI shows hyperintense thrombus within the superior sagittal sinus (arrows).
矢状位T_1加权MRI显示上矢状窦内高信号血栓(红箭)。

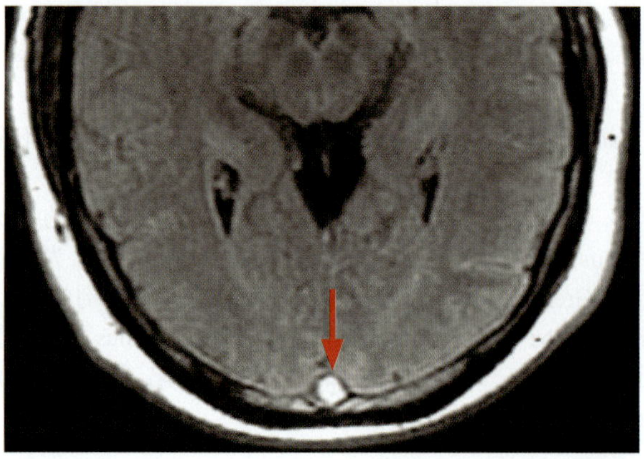

FLAIR MRI shows hyperintense thrombus within the superior sagittal sinus (arrow).
FLAIR MRI显示上矢状窦内高信号血栓(红箭)。

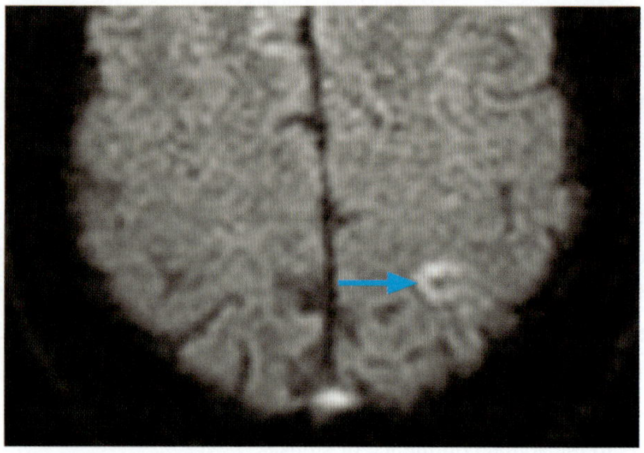

Diffusion-weighted MRI shows a subtle cortical focus of restricted diffusion (confirmed on ADC) in the left parietal lobe (arrow), a typical pattern of infarction seen with superior sagittal sinus thrombosis.
弥散加权成像显示左顶叶皮层(蓝箭)有一处轻度弥散受限病灶(在ADC图上证实),这是上矢状窦静脉血栓引起的脑梗死的一种典型表现。

- Thrombosis of a cortical vein or a deep venous sinus is one of the more common causes of stroke in younger patients. Risk factors for venous thrombosis include pregnancy, oral contraceptives, thrombophilia, malignancy, and infection.
- A clue to the diagnosis of venous thrombosis on noncontrast CT is increased density within the thrombosed sinus or cortical vein (the *cord sign*). On contrast-enhanced CT, the *empty delta sign* signifies a filling defect in the superior sagittal sinus.
- MR venogram will show lack of flow in the thrombosed vein or dural venous sinus.
- Venous thrombosis leads to venous hypertension, which may cause infarction and parenchymal hemorrhage. There are three characteristic patterns of venous infarction, dependent on the location of the thrombosed vein:

Superior sagittal sinus thrombosis → infarction of the **parasagittal high convexity** cortex.
Deep venous system thrombosis → infarction of the **bilateral thalami.**
Transverse sinus thrombosis → infarction of the **posterior temporal lobe.**

- 大脑皮层静脉或深静脉窦血栓形成是年轻患者卒中的一种常见原因。静脉血栓形成的危险因素包括妊娠、口服避孕药、血液高凝状态、恶性肿瘤及感染。
- 平扫CT诊断静脉血栓的一条线索是静脉窦或皮层静脉出现密度增高(*条索征*)。在增强CT上,*空三角征*意味着上矢状窦有充盈缺损。
- MR静脉造影可显示在血栓形成的静脉或硬脑膜静脉窦内无血液流动。
- 脑静脉血栓会引起静脉高压,从而导致梗死或脑实质出血。根据静脉血栓形成的位置,所致的静脉梗死有3种特征性的分布方式:

上矢状窦血栓 → **旁矢状上凸面**皮层梗死。
深静脉系统血栓 → **双侧丘脑**梗死。
横窦血栓 → **颞叶后部**梗死。

(翻译　王草叶)

INTRAPARENCHYMAL HEMORRHAGE

脑实质内出血

IMAGING OF HEMORRHAGE

出血影像

CT imaging of hemorrhage

- Noncontrast CT is usually the first imaging study performed in the emergency setting for a patient with a sudden neurologic deficit, headache, seizure, or altered level of consciousness.
- CT is highly sensitive for detection of hyperacute/acute intracranial hemorrhage, which appears hyperattenuating relative to brain parenchyma and CSF.

  Acute hemorrhage may be nearly isoattenuating to water in severe anemia (hemoglobin <8 mg/dL).

CT出血影像

- 平扫CT通常是在急诊情况下的首选影像学检查,如患者突发神经功能障碍、头痛、癫痫或意识改变。
- CT对于发现超急性/急性颅内出血非常敏感,表现为相对高于脑实质及脑脊液的高密度。

  在严重贫血的患者(血红蛋白<8mg/dL),急性出血的密度可接近水。

- The CT angiographic (CTA) *spot sign* describes the presence of small enhancing focus or foci within an acute intracerebral hemorrhage on CTA, which is separate from adjacent vessels and is not seen on noncontrast CT. This is thought to represent active hemorrhage and is a predictor of hematoma expansion and poor clinical outcome.

- CT血管造影(CTA)的斑点征指在CTA上急性脑内出血病灶内出现的单个或多个增强小灶，与相邻血管不交通，且在平扫CT上不可见。此征象代表活动性出血，是血肿扩大和临床预后不佳的预测指标。

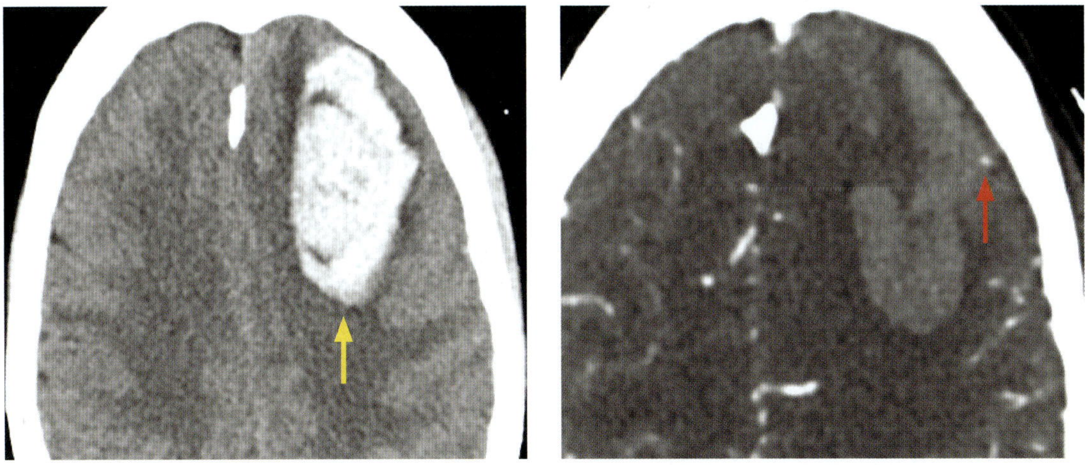

Angiographic *spot sign*: Axial noncontrast CT (left image) demonstrates a left frontal acute intraparenchymal hemorrhage (yellow arrow). Axial CTA (right image) shows a hyperdense focus at the periphery of the intraparenchymal hematoma that does not communicate with any vessels and is not present on the noncontrast images, compatible with active hemorrhage (red arrow).
血管影像上的斑点征：轴位平扫CT(左图)显示左侧额叶急性脑实质内出血(黄箭)。轴位CTA(右图)显示脑实质内血肿边缘点状高密度灶，不与任何血管沟通，也未显示在平扫图像上，此为活动性出血的表现(红箭)。

MR imaging of hemorrhage

- MR imaging of hemorrhage is complex. The characteristics of blood products change on T1- and T2-weighted sequences as the iron in hemoglobin evolves through physiologic stages:

Intracellular oxyhemoglobin →*deoxygenation* →
Intracellular deoxyhemoglobin →*oxidation* →
Intracellular methemoglobin →*cell lysis* →
Extracellular methemoglobin →*chelation* →
Hemosiderin and ferritin

- Each stage of this evolution adheres to a reasonably constant time course in the intra-axial space and allows the radiologist to "date" the hemorrhage based on the unique signal characteristics on T1- and T2-weighted images for each stage.
- In general, all stages of hemorrhage are isointense or slightly dark on T1-weighted images, except for the methemoglobin stages, which are bright.
- Methemoglobin is bright on both T1- and T2-weighted images, except for intracellular methemoglobin, which is dark on T2-weighted images.
- In general, non-hyperacute hemorrhage is dark on T2-weighted images, with the exception of extracellular methemoglobin, which is hyperintense on T2-weighted images. A hyperacute hematoma, containing primarily oxyhemoglobin, is slightly hyperintense on T2- weighted images but features a characteristic dark rim representing deoxygenation at the periphery of the clot.

MR出血影像

- 出血在MR上的表现复杂。血液产物在T_1加权和T_2加权上的表现是变化的，因铁在血红蛋白中的变化随不同的生理期演变而变化：

细胞内氧化血红蛋白→脱氧作用→
细胞内脱氧血红蛋白→氧化作用→
细胞内正铁血红蛋白→细胞裂解→
细胞外正铁血红蛋白→螯合作用→
含铁血黄素和铁蛋白

- 每期的演变时间在脑实质内相对是恒定的，所以放射科医师可根据每一期出血的T_1和T_2加权信号来推测出血时间。
- 一般情况下，出血的所有期在T_1加权上均表现为等信号或稍低信号，除了正铁血红蛋白期是高信号。
- 正铁血红蛋白在T_1加权和T_2加权上均表现为高信号，除了细胞内的正铁血红蛋白在T_2加权上表现为低信号。
- 一般情况下，非超急性期出血在T_2加权上均呈低信号，除了细胞外正铁血红蛋白在T_2加权上呈高信号。超急性期血肿主要含氧化血红蛋白，在T_2加权上表现为稍高信号，但在血凝块周边由于含脱氧血红蛋白而特征性的表现为低信号环。

- The inherent slight hyperintensity of oxygenated blood on T2-weighted images becomes apparent in slow flow states, as seen in venous hypertension and moyamoya disease. Slowly flowing blood is not susceptible to the flow-void artifact and the resultant apparently "enhancing" vasculature really represents unmasking of the normal blood signal.
- The expected evolution of blood products is highly dependent on macrophage elimination of blood breakdown products. **These rules of thumb are not applicable to extra-axial blood** and timing is generally not given for extra-axial blood, such as a subdural hematoma.

- 在慢血流的状态下，原为稍高信号的氧合血在T_2加权上表现得更为明显，见于静脉性高血压及烟雾病。慢血流不易出现流空伪影，而由此产生的明显"强化"的血管其实代表未被掩盖的正常血液的信号。
- 血液产物的演变过程高度依赖巨噬细胞对血液分解产物的清除能力。所以，**这些经验法则并不适用于脑外出血**，而对脑外出血，如硬膜下出血，通常不评估出血时间。

Treatment of hemorrhage

- In most cases, imaging is performed to evaluate for a treatable cause of hemorrhage, such as AVM or aneurysm. The mainstay of treatment of intraparenchymal hemorrhage is supportive, including blood pressure control and normalization of any coagulopathy.
- Larger hemorrhages can be evacuated surgically if there is significant mass effect or risk of herniation. In particular, a hemorrhage >3 cm in the posterior fossa would generally be treated surgically as there is increased risk of brainstem compression or hydrocephalus from fourth ventricular obstruction.

出血的治疗

- 大多数患者接受影像学检查的目的是寻找有可能进行治疗的出血病因，如动静脉畸形或动脉瘤。脑实质内出血的主要治疗手段为支持疗法，包括控制血压及纠正凝血功能障碍。
- 有明显占位效应或脑疝风险的大出血可进行手术清除。尤其是>3cm的颅后窝血肿通常需要手术治疗，因为脑干受压或第四脑室梗阻引起脑积水的风险增高。

SPECIFIC STAGES OF PARENCHYMAL HEMATOMA ON MR

脑实质出血在MR上的具体分期

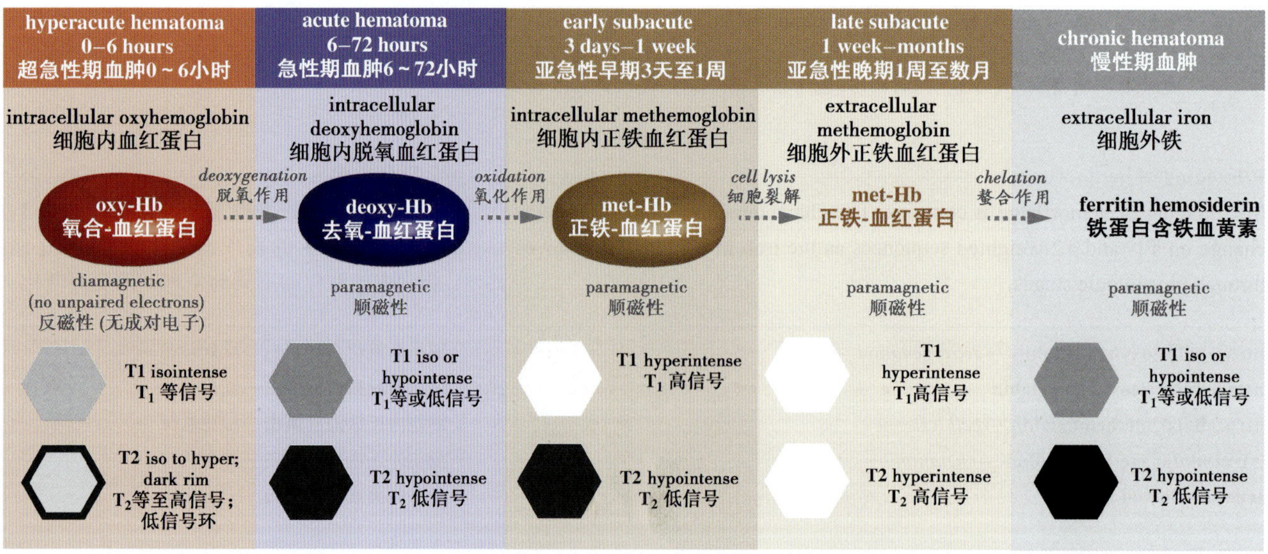

Hyperacute hematoma (<6 hours): Intracellular oxyhemoglobin

- A few hours after red cell extravasation, a hyperacute hematoma is primarily composed of intact red cells containing oxygenated hemoglobin, which is diamagnetic.
- The center of the hematoma will be isointense on T1-weighted images and iso- to slightly hyperintense on T2-weighted images.
- The key imaging finding of a hyperacute hematoma is a peripheral rim of hypointensity on T2-weighted images due to deoxygenation of the most peripheral red cells. This peripheral dark rim is most conspicuous on GRE sequences.

超急性期血肿(<6小时)：细胞内氧化血红蛋白

- 在红细胞溢出数小时内，超急性期的血肿主要由完整的红细胞所组成，内含氧合血红蛋白，为一种反磁性物质。
- 血肿中心部分在T_1加权上呈等信号，T_2加权上呈等或稍高信号。
- 超急性期血肿的关键影像特征为T_2加权上血肿周边低信号环，这是由于最边缘红细胞发生了脱氧化。这个外周的黑边在GRE序列上最明显。

Acute hematoma (6–72 hours): Intracellular deoxyhemoglobin

- After the red cells desaturate (lose oxygen), the entire hematoma becomes hypointense on T2-weighted images and iso- to mildly hypointense on T1-weighted images.

急性期血肿(6～72小时)：细胞内脱氧血红蛋白

- 红细胞内氧饱和度下降(脱氧)后，整个血肿在T_2加权上呈低信号，T_1加权呈等或稍低信号。

Early subacute hematoma (3 days to 1 week): Intracellular methemoglobin

- The subacute phase is characterized by methemoglobin, which is paramagnetic and undergoes proton-electron dipole-dipole interactions (PEDDI) with water. PEDDI shortens T1 to cause hyperintensity on T1-weighted images. Intracellular and extracellular methemoglobin are both hyperintense on T1-weighted images.
- In the early subacute phase, blood remains hypointense on T2-weighted images due to the paramagnetic effects of methemoglobin, which remains trapped in the red cells.

Late subacute hematoma (1 week to months): Extracellular methemoglobin (after RBC lysis)

- The methemoglobin PEDDI effect persists after cell lysis, causing continued hyperintensity on T1-weighted images.
- Paramagnetic effects of methemoglobin lessens. Signal intensity on T2-weighted images increases to that of CSF, due to RBC lysis and decrease in protein concentration.
- There may be peripheral enhancement of a subacute to chronic hematoma.

Chronic sequelae of hemorrhage: Hemosiderin and ferritin

- Salvaged iron atoms are deposited into hemosiderin and ferritin, which become permanently trapped in the brain parenchyma after the blood-brain barrier is restored.
- Susceptibility effects of the stored iron produce characteristic hypointensity on T2-weighted and GRE images.
- Chronic hemorrhage may have peripheral enhancement.

亚急性早期血肿(3天~1周):细胞内正铁血红蛋白

- 亚急性期的特征取决于正铁血红蛋白，其为一种顺磁性物质，能与水进行质子-电子偶极子-偶极子(PEDDI)作用。PEDDI缩短了T_1，使血肿在T_1加权上呈高信号。细胞内和细胞外正铁血红蛋白在T_1加权上均呈高信号。
- 在亚急性期早期，血液在T_2加权上仍呈低信号，因为呈顺磁性效应的正铁血红蛋白仍局限于细胞内。

亚急性晚期(1周到数月):细胞外正铁血红蛋白(红细胞裂解之后)

- 细胞裂解后正铁血红蛋白的PEDDI效应持续存在，使其在T_1加权上继续为高信号。
- 细胞裂解后正铁血红蛋白的顺磁性效应减弱。随着红细胞裂解及蛋白浓度降低，亚急性晚期血肿在T_2加权上信号升高，可与脑脊液信号相似。
- 亚急性期到慢性期血肿的边缘可有强化。

出血的慢性后遗症:含铁血黄素和铁蛋白

- 重吸收的铁原子沉积在含铁血黄素和铁蛋白内，它们在血脑屏障恢复后将永久遗留在脑实质中。
- 残留铁的磁敏感效应在T_2加权及GRE图像上产生特征性的低信号。
- 慢性出血边缘可强化。

NON-TRAUMATIC CAUSES OF INTRAPARENCHYMAL HEMORRHAGE

非创伤性脑实质内出血的原因

Hypertensive hemorrhage

高血压性脑出血

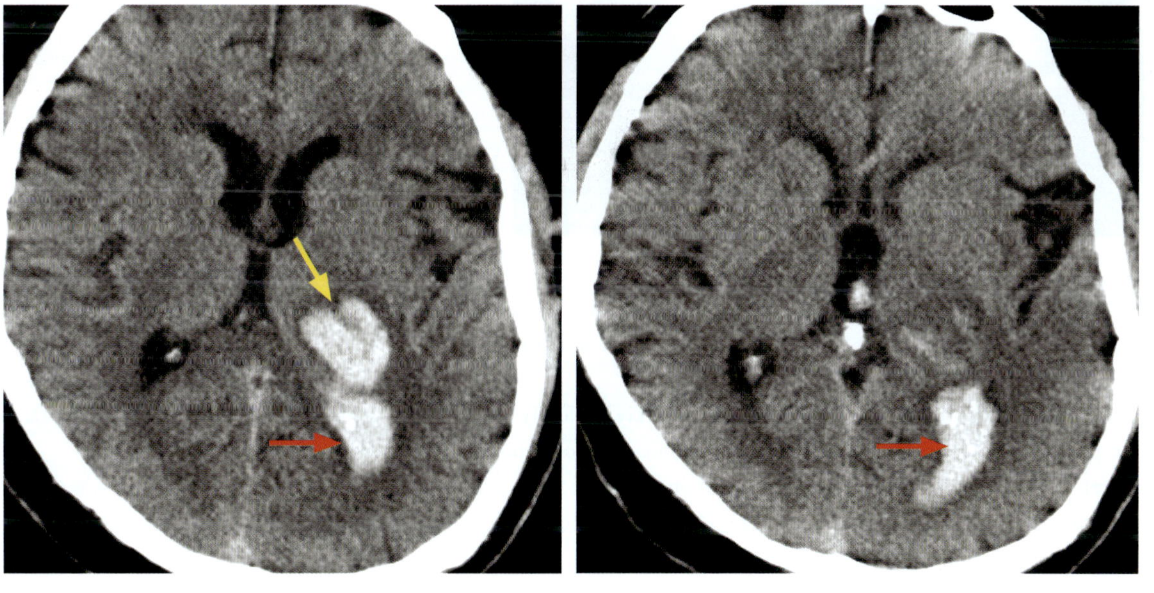

Hypertensive hemorrhage: Two contiguous noncontrast CT images show a left thalamic hemorrhage (yellow arrow) with extension into the left ventricle occipital horn (red arrows).
高血压性脑出血:连续两层平扫CT显示左侧丘脑出血(黄箭)并破入左侧侧脑室枕角(红箭)

- Chronic hypertension is the most common cause of spontaneous adult intraparenchymal hemorrhage and is due to the secondary microangiopathic effects of chronic hypertension.
- Chronic hypertension causes arteriolar smooth muscle hyperplasia, which eventually leads to smooth muscle death and replacement with collagen. The resultant vascular ectasia predisposes to hemorrhage.
- Hypertensive hemorrhage occurs in characteristic locations in the basal ganglia, thalamus, and cerebellum.
- In addition to location, imaging (MRI or CT) findings suggestive of a hypertensive bleed include additional stigmata of hypertensive microangiopathy, such as periventricular white matter disease and prior lacunar infarcts.
- An additional MR-specific finding suggesting hypertensive hemorrhage is the presence of microhemorrhages on T2* (GRE or SWI) in the basal ganglia or brainstem.

- 成人自发性脑实质内出血的最常见原因是慢性高血压，继发于慢性高血压导致的微血管病变。
- 慢性高血压会使小动脉平滑肌增生，最终导致平滑肌死亡并被胶原组织替代，其结果是血管扩张而易于出血。
- 高血压性脑出血的典型部位为基底节、丘脑和小脑。
- 除发病部位外，影像学(MRI或CT)提示高血压性脑出血的征象还包含高血压性微血管病变引起的其他征象，如脑室旁白质病变和先前的腔隙性脑梗死。
- 另一个MRI特有的提示高血压性脑出血的表现为T_2*(GRE或SWI)图像上基底节或脑干出现微出血灶。

Cerebral amyloid angiopathy (CAA)

脑淀粉样血管病(CAA)

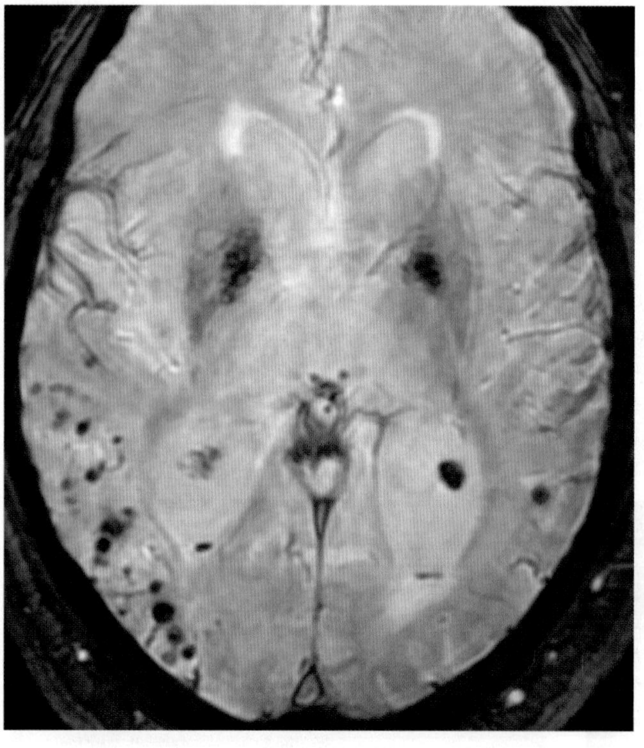

SWI shows multiple foci of cortical and subcortical susceptibility artifact representing microhemorrhages throughout the brain, most prominently seen in the right parietal, temporal, and occipital lobes, suggestive of cerebral amyloid angiopathy.
SWI显示皮层和皮层下多发性磁敏感伪影灶，为遍布大脑的微出血，以右侧顶叶、颞叶和枕叶为著，提示脑淀粉样血管病。

- Cerebral amyloid angiopathy (CAA) is amyloid accumulated within the walls of small and medium arteries, ultimately causing vessel weakness and increased risk of hemorrhage.
- While the spontaneous form of CAA occurs almost exclusively in elderly adults (in which population it is the second most common cause of nontraumatic hemorrhage), a hereditary variant has an earlier age of onset.
- In addition to being a risk factor for hemorrhage, CAA can also occlude the lumens of small vessels and contribute to microangiopathy.
- The main clinical clue that a hemorrhage is secondary to CAA is that the patient is a normotensive elderly adult.
- The primary imaging feature to suggest CAA is the location of hematoma, which is almost always lobar or cortical, usually in the parietal or occipital lobes.

- CAA是指淀粉样物质累积在中小动脉血管壁上，最终导致血管脆弱，出血风险增高。
- 自发性CAA几乎都发生在老年人(是老年人非外伤性脑出血的第二常见原因)，但遗传性CAA的发病年龄则较轻。
- 除了出血风险，CAA也可堵塞小血管管腔而导致微血管病变。
- 诊断出血继发于CAA的重要线索是患者为血压正常的老年人。
- 提示CAA的主要影像学特征是血肿的位置，几乎都在脑叶或皮层，通常是顶叶或枕叶。

- An important secondary MRI finding is multiple microhemorrhages seen on T2* (GRE or SWI) within the brain parenchyma. In contrast to the microhemorrhages associated with hypertension, CAA microhemorrhages are cortical/subcortical (lobar), not in the basal ganglia.

- 一个重要的间接MRI征象是T_2*(GRE或SWI)图像上脑实质内多发的微出血灶。与高血压性微出血分布不同，CAA所致的微出血位于皮层/皮层下(脑叶)，而不在基底节区。

Hemorrhagic transformation of infarct

脑梗死的出血转化

- In most cases, the clinical or imaging diagnosis of stroke is made before hemorrhagic transformation occurs; however, hemorrhage may occasionally be the presenting feature of an infarct.
- More commonly, symptomatic hemorrhage occurs post-infarct in approximately 6–12% of patients receiving thrombolytic therapy.
- Noncontrast CT can identify risk factors for hemorrhagic transformation after thrombolytic therapy, including a relatively large region of hypoattenuation and a *dense artery sign*. Note that per AHA guidelines, neither of these findings is an exclusion criterion for administration of IV tPA.

- 大多数情况下，脑卒中在发生出血转化之前已经在临床或影像上得到了诊断；但偶尔，出血也可能是脑梗死的首发表现。
- 更常见的是，梗死后的症状性出血见于6%~12%接受溶栓治疗的患者。
- 平扫CT可发现溶栓治疗后发生出血转化的危险因素，其中包括相对较大范围的低密度区和动脉高密度征。注意，根据美国心脏协会指南，这两种征象都不能作为静脉注射tPA的禁忌标准。

Venous thrombosis

静脉血栓形成

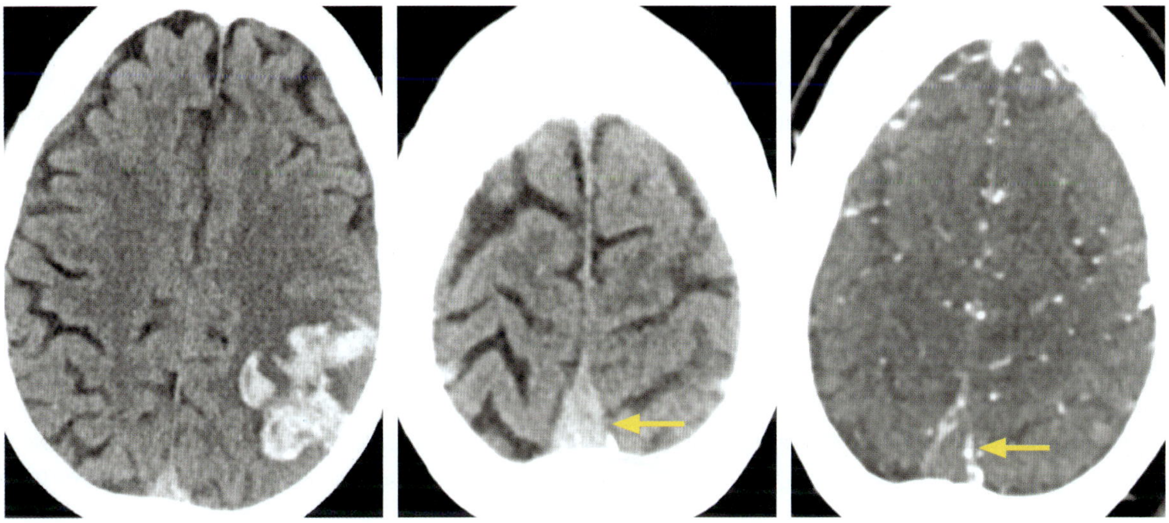

Hemorrhagic venous infarct: Axial noncontrast CT shows intraparenchymal hemorrhage in the left parieto- occipital lobes (left image) and an expanded/hyperdense superior sagittal sinus (middle image, arrow). Axial CTA shows a filling defect in the superior sagittal sinus (*empty delta sign*; arrow) in keeping with dural venous thrombosis.

出血性静脉梗死：轴位平扫CT显示左侧顶枕叶脑实质内出血(左图)和扩大/高密度的上矢状窦(中图，黄箭)。轴位CTA显示上矢状窦充盈缺损(空delta征；黄箭)与硬脑膜静脉血栓形成一致。

- Thrombosis of cortical veins or deep venous sinuses leads to venous hypertension, which may cause infarction and parenchymal hemorrhage.

- 皮层静脉或深静脉窦血栓形成引起静脉血压升高，可导致脑梗死和脑实质内出血。

Aneurysmal hemorrhage

动脉瘤性出血

- As discussed, aneurysmal hemorrhage is by far the most common cause of nontraumatic subarachnoid hemorrhage. If an intraparenchymal hematoma is due to an aneurysm, the hematoma is usually adjacent to the ruptured aneurysm dome.
- The pattern of subarachnoid blood may help localize the aneurysm; however, if the patient was found down, then the blood will settle in the dependent portion of the brain, confounding localization.
- CT angiography is the study of choice for further evaluation of nontraumatic subarachnoid hemorrhage.

- 如前所述，动脉瘤性脑出血是最常见的非创伤性蛛网膜下腔出血的原因。若脑实质内血肿是由动脉瘤破裂所致，则血肿常紧邻破裂动脉瘤的顶部。
- 蛛网膜下腔出血的分布方式有助于动脉瘤定位；但若患者被发现时已经倒地，出血会沉积在脑内重心最低处，从而使定位出错。
- CT血管造影是进一步评估非外伤性蛛网膜下腔出血的检查。

Vascular malformations

血管畸形

- Intraparenchymal hemorrhage from vascular malformations occurs in younger

- 血管畸形导致的脑实质内出血的发病年龄较

patients (often younger than 50 years) than does hemorrhage secondary to hypertension or cerebral amyloid angiopathy.

- Among vascular malformations, the most common cause of intraparenchymal hemorrhage is arteriovenous malformation (AVM). Less common causes are cavernous malformation and dural arteriovenous fistula (dAVF).
- See the preceding section on vascular malformations for imaging description.

Vasculitis

- Vasculitis affecting the CNS may be primary or secondary to systemic vasculitides.
- The most common presentation of vasculitis is cerebral ischemia. Less commonly, vasculitis may present with frank hemorrhage.
- Standard MRI imaging shows multiple foci of T2 prolongation in the basal ganglia and subcortical white matter.
- Noninvasive vascular imaging (CTA or MRA) is relatively insensitive to small vessel involvement, but may show irregularity of involved large or medium vessels.
- Angiography is the most sensitive test and shows multifocal areas of stenosis and dilation.

Hemorrhagic neoplasm

- Occasionally, the initial presentation of a brain tumor may be acute hemorrhage.
- The most common primary brain tumor to cause hemorrhage is glioblastoma.
- There are a relatively limited number of extracranial primary tumors known to cause hemorrhagic metastases, including:

> Melanoma.
> Renal cell carcinoma.
> Choriocarcinoma.
> Thyroid carcinoma.
> Although breast and lung cancer rarely cause hemorrhage on a per-case basis, they are such common cancers overall that they can always be considered when a hemorrhagic neoplasm is suspected.

- Patients treated with bevacizumab (trade name Avastin®, Genentech) may be at increased risk for hemorrhagic metastasis.
- Clues to the diagnosis of an underlying tumor causing hemorrhage include more-than- expected edema surrounding a hyperacute hematoma and heterogeneous blood product signal, suggesting varying breakdown stages of hemoglobin.
- The presence of multiple enhancing masses strongly suggests metastatic disease.
- In cases where the diagnosis is unclear, a follow-up MRI should be performed once the initial hemorrhage improves. If tumor is present, the MRI may show a delay in the expected evolution of blood products, persistent edema, and enhancement of the underlying tumor.

继发于高血压和脑血管淀粉样病的患者更为年轻(多小于50岁)。

- 在血管畸形中，最常见的脑实质出血原因是动静脉畸形(AVM)，其次是海绵状血管畸形和硬脑膜动静脉瘘(dAVF)。
- 影像描述见前文“血管畸形”。

血管炎

- 累及中枢神经系统的血管炎可以是原发，也可以继发于全身性血管炎。
- 血管炎最常见的表现是脑缺血，较少见的情况下，血管炎可能表现为明显出血。
- 血管炎在常规的MRI检查时表现为基底节区和皮层下白质多灶性T_2高信号。
- 非侵入性血管造影成像(CTA/MRA)对小血管病变相对不敏感，但受累大、中血管可显示不规则。
- 血管造影是最敏感的检查方法，表现为多个部位的狭窄和扩张。

出血性肿瘤

- 偶然情况下，脑肿瘤的首发症状可为急性出血。
- 最常导致出血的原发性脑肿瘤是胶质母细胞瘤。
- 颅外原发性肿瘤导致出血性转移瘤的种类相对有限，包括：

> 黑色素瘤。
> 肾细胞癌。
> 绒毛膜癌。
> 甲状腺癌。
> 乳腺癌和肺癌的转移瘤本身罕见引起出血，但它们是常见的两种恶性肿瘤，一旦怀疑肿瘤性出血需要考虑到这两种肿瘤。

- 患者用bevacizumab(商品名Avastin®，Genentech公司生产)治疗可能会增高转移瘤出血的风险。
- 诊断由肿瘤引起出血的线索包括水肿超出了超急性期血肿周围常见的范围，以及不均匀的血肿产物信号，后者提示存在不同时期分解的血红蛋白。
- 若有多发强化的肿块则强烈提示转移瘤。
- 如果患者的诊断不明确，一旦血肿好转后需要行MRI复查。如果存在肿瘤，MRI可能显示血液成分预期演变的过程延迟、持续性水肿及肿瘤本身的增强表现。

Moyamoya

烟雾病

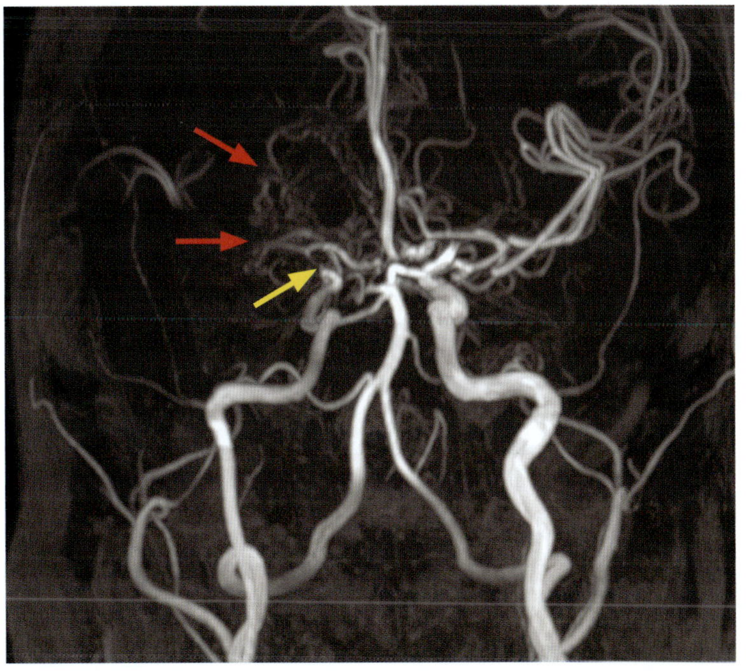

Moyamoya: Coronal MIP (maximum intensity projection) reconstruction of a contrast-enhanced MRA of the brain shows marked narrowing of the right carotid terminus and absence of flow in the right MCA M1 branch (yellow arrow), with hypertrophy of the ipsilateral lenticulostriate arteries and thalamic perforators (red arrows).

烟雾病：冠状位MIP(最大密度投影)重建大脑增强MRA显示右侧颈内动脉末端明显狭窄和右侧大脑中动脉M1段血流缺失(黄箭)，以及同侧豆纹动脉和丘脑穿通支(红箭)肥大。

- Moyamoya disease is a non-atherosclerotic vasculopathy characterized by progressive stenosis of the intracranial internal carotid arteries and their proximal branches, which leads to compensatory proliferation of fragile collateral vessels, in particular lenticulostriate and other perforating vessels in the basal ganglia.
- When moyamoya vascular findings are associated with a secondary cause such as sickle cell disease, NF1, radiation, Down syndrome, the term moyamoya syndrome is used.
- Angiography of the enlarged lenticulostriate perforating collaterals gives a *puff of smoke* appearance.
- The *ivy sign* on FLAIR MRI represents tubular branching hyperintense structures within the sulci, representing cortical arterial branches that appear hyperintense due to slow collateral flow.
- Patients with moyamoya disease are susceptible to aneurysm formation, especially in the posterior circulation. In contrast to children, adult patients with moyamoya disease sometimes present with intraventricular hemorrhage rather than ischemic stroke.
- When severe, moyamoya disease or syndrome can be treated with direct or indirect ECA (most commonly superficial temporal artery) to MCA bypass. Direct bypass is preferred for adults and children with a suitable donor artery.
- Perfusion studies show decreased blood flow to the affected vascular regions.

- 烟雾病是一种非动脉粥样硬化性血管病变，以颈内动脉颅内段及其近端分支进行性狭窄为特征，导致脆弱的侧支呈代偿性增生，尤其是豆纹动脉和基底节区的其他穿通支。
- 当烟雾病的血管表现继发于其他原因时需要使用烟雾病综合征这一术语，如镰状细胞疾病、1型神经纤维瘤病、放射疗法及唐氏综合征。
- 血管造影时扩张的豆纹穿通属支呈袅袅升起的烟雾状表现。
- 在FLAIR MRI上的常春藤征指的是脑沟内管状分支的高信号结构，为皮层动脉分支因缓慢侧支循环血流而呈高信号。
- 烟雾病患者容易发生动脉瘤，特别是在后循环。与儿童不同，成年烟雾病患者有时表现为脑室内出血而非缺血性卒中。
- 治疗严重的烟雾病或烟雾病综合征可直接或间接进行颈外动脉(颞浅动脉最常见)至大脑中动脉搭桥。直接搭桥在有合适的供体动脉时对于成人和儿童都是首选。
- 灌注成像显示受累供血区血流量降低。

Non-traumatic etiology of intraparenchymal hemorrhage 非创伤性脑实质内出血的病因

older adults 老年人:

- *Elderly adult with hypertension?* 老年高血压患者？
  Hemorrhage in basal ganglia, cerebellum, or thalamus? 基底节、小脑或丘脑出血？
  Multiple basal ganglia microbleeds on T2?* T_2*图像上基底节多发微出血？
  Prior lacunes and periventricular WM disease? 先前的腔隙性梗死和脑室旁白质病变？
  → **Hypertensive hemorrhage 高血压性脑出血**
- *Lobar or cortical hemorrhage?* 脑叶或皮层出血？
  Elderly adult without hypertension? 老年非高血压患者？
  Multiple parenchymal microbleeds on T2?* T_2*图像上多发脑实质微出血？
  → **Amyloid angiopathy 血管淀粉样变**

- *Extensive subarachnoid blood?* 广泛蛛网膜下腔出血？
  Aneurysm adjacent to hematoma? 动脉瘤邻近血肿？
  → **Aneurysmal hemorrhage 动脉瘤性出血**

vascular malformations 血管畸形:

- *Parenchymal hemorrhage in a young patient?* 年轻患者脑实质出血？
  Enlarged feeding artery? 供血动脉增粗？
  Adjacent encephalomalacia? 邻近脑软化？
  → **AVM 动静脉畸形**
- *Hemorrhage adjacent to cavernous sinus or in posterior fossa?* 出血邻近海绵窦或位于颅后窝？
  Enlarged meningeal artery or cortical vein? 脑膜动脉或皮层静脉增粗？
  → **dAVF 硬脑膜动静脉瘘**
- *Adjacent DVA on post-contrast images?* 增强后见邻近发育性静脉畸形？
  Multiple dark spots on T2 (familial variant)?* T_2*图像上多发点状低信号（家族性变异）？
  → **Cavernous malformation 海绵状血管畸形**

- *Parasagittal or bilateral thalamic hemorrhage?* 矢状窦旁或双侧丘脑出血？
  Young patient, especially female? 年轻患者，尤其是女性？
  Increased density in cortical vein or dural sinus? 皮层静脉或硬脑膜窦密度增高？
  → **Venous thrombosis 静脉血栓形成**
- *More edema than expected?* 水肿范围超出预期？
  More heterogeneous signal than expected? 信号不均匀超出预期？
  Multiple enhancing lesions? 多发强化病灶？
  → **Hemorrhagic neoplasm 出血性肿瘤**
- *Clinical history of infarct?* 临床脑梗死病史？
  History of thrombolytic therapy? 溶栓治疗病史？
  → **Hemorrhagic infarct 出血性脑梗死**
- *Multifocal T2 prolongation in deep WM?* 深部白质多发长T_2信号灶？
  History of systemic vasculitis? 系统性血管炎病史？
  Multifocal stenosis/dilation on angiography? 血管造影示多发血管狭窄或扩张？
  → **CNS vasculitis 中枢神经系统血管炎**
- *Occlusion of internal carotid arteries?* 颈内动脉闭塞？
  Multiple collateral vessels? 多发侧支血管？
  → **Moyamoya 烟雾病**

（翻译　张秋丽）

CEREBRAL TRAUMA

脑外伤

EXTRA-AXIAL HEMORRHAGE

- Acute extra-axial hemorrhage (subarachnoid, epidural, or subdural in location) is usually hyperattenuating when imaged by CT; however, blood must clot in order to be hyperattenuating. Hyperacute unclotted blood (and clotted blood in a patient with severe anemia) may be close to water attenuation on CT.

轴(脑实质)外出血

- 急性轴外出血(蛛网膜下腔、硬膜外或硬膜下)在CT上常为高密度，但是只有凝固血才会呈高密度。超急性期未凝固的血液(以及严重贫血患者的凝固血)在CT上可近似于水的密度。

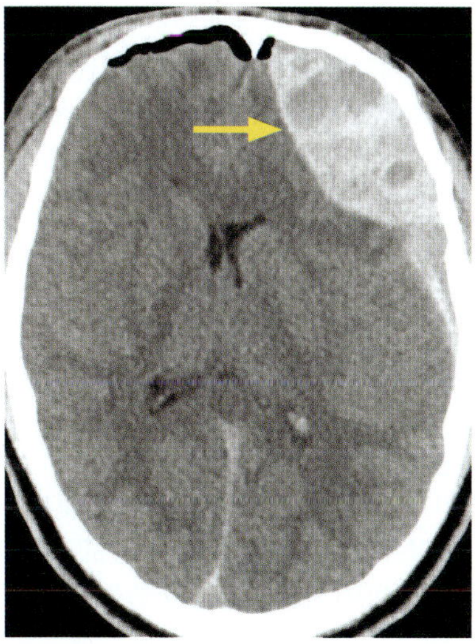

Left frontalepidural hematoma (arrow).
左额部硬膜外血肿(黄箭)。

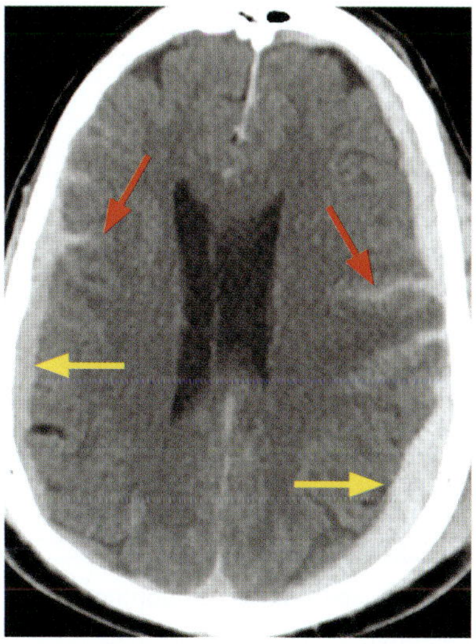

Bilateral subdural hematomas (yellow arrows) and subarachnoid hemorrhage (red arrows).
双侧硬膜下血肿(黄箭)和蛛网膜下腔出血(红箭)。

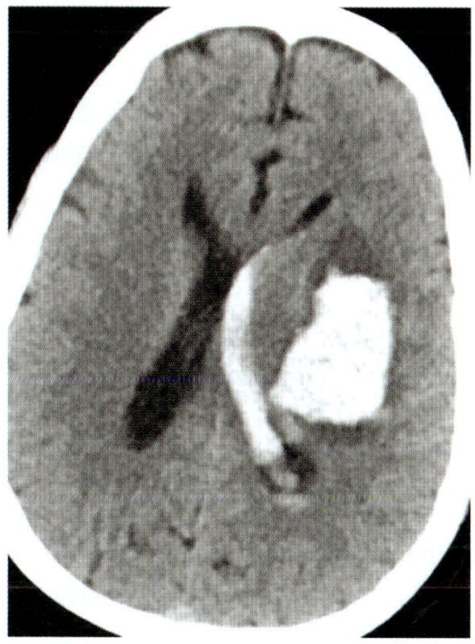

Left-sided intraparenchymal hematoma with intraventricular extension of hemorrhage.
左侧脑实质内血肿伴血肿破入脑室。

Subarachnoid hemorrhage (SAH)

- Trauma is the most common cause of subarachnoid hemorrhage (SAH),while aneurysm rupture is the most common cause of non-traumatic SAH.
- Traumatic SAH tends to occur contralateral to the side of direct impact, most often in the superficial cerebral sulci.

蛛网膜下腔出血(SAH)

- 创伤是蛛网膜下腔出血(SAH)最常见的病因，而动脉瘤破裂则是非创伤性SAH最常见的病因。
- 创伤性SAH易发生于直接暴力点的对侧，最常见于浅表的脑沟。

Epidural hematoma

- An **arterial epidural hematoma** is an extra-axial collection of blood external to the dura, classically caused by fracture of the squamous portion of the temporal bone and resultant tearing of the middlemeningeal artery.
- An arterial epidural hematoma has a *lentiform* shape and does not cross the cranial sutures, where the dura is tightly adherent to the cranium.
- The *swirl sign* describes mixed high and low attenuation blood within the hematoma and suggests active bleeding. The low attenuation blood is hyperacute unclotted blood while the high attenuation blood is already clotted.
- A large epidural hematoma is a surgical emergency due to mass effect and risk of herniation, although small epidural hematomas can be conservatively managed with serial imaging.
- **Venous epidural hematomas** are far less common than arterial epidurals and are due to laceration of the dural sinuses. Common locations are anterior middle cranial fossa and posterior fossa.

硬膜外血肿

- **动脉性硬膜外血肿**是聚集在硬脑膜外的轴外出血，通常是由于颞骨鳞部骨折导致脑膜中动脉撕裂。
- 动脉性硬膜外血肿呈双凸镜形，且不跨颅缝，因为颅缝处的硬脑膜紧贴颅骨。
- 旋涡征是指血肿内混有高低不同密度的血，提示有活动性出血。低密度血是超急性期的未凝固血，而高密度血则是已凝固的血。
- 范围较大的硬膜外血肿属外科急症，因其占位效应及有并发脑疝的危险；而范围较小的硬膜外血肿可以行保守治疗，同时进行影像学随访。
- **静脉性硬膜外血肿**远比动脉性硬膜外血肿少见，由硬脑膜窦的撕裂所致。常见的位置是颅中窝前部和颅后窝。

Anterior middle fossa epidural hematomas are nearly always venous, rarely expand, have a clinically indolent course, and therefore do not require surgical intervention.

In contrast, posterior fossa venous epidural hematomas may require surgical evacuation due to associated mass effect.

颅中窝前部硬膜外血肿几乎都是静脉性的，很少会扩大，临床表现不明显，因此不需要手术干预。

相比之下，颅后窝静脉性硬膜外血肿可能由于占位效应而需要进行手术清除。

Subdural hematoma

- A subdural hematoma is a crescentic extra-axial collection of blood located beneath the dura. Since it is underneath the dura, the hematoma can extend across the cranial sutures. Subdural hematomas often extend along the surfaces of the falx cerebriand tentorium cerebelli.
- Subdural hematomas typically result from tearing of cerebral veins. Patients with atrophic involutional changes are at increased risk of subdural hematoma with even minor trauma, as the cerebral veins stretch to traverse the enlarged CSF spaces.
- A particular danger is a subdural hematoma in a patient with a ventricular shunt because the shunted ventricular system does not function as a natural tamponade.
- An isodense subdural hematoma is isoattenuating to gray matter. This occurs in the subacute phase approximately 1–3 weeks after the initial injury. Three important clues alerting to the presence of an isodense subdural are increased mass effect, white matter buckling, and an apparently thickened cortex.

硬膜下血肿

- 硬膜下血肿是指轴外硬膜下呈新月形的血液聚集。因位于硬脑膜下，血肿可延伸跨越颅缝。硬膜下血肿常沿着大脑镰和小脑幕的表面延伸。
- 硬膜下血肿通常是由于大脑静脉撕裂引起。大脑萎缩退化的患者发生硬膜下血肿的风险增高，这是因为脑脊液间隙扩大，即使是较小创伤，大脑静脉也会受到牵拉而出血。
- 硬膜下血肿且伴有脑室分流的患者尤为危险，因为分流的脑室系统不能起到自然填塞的作用。
- 等密度的硬膜下血肿密度与灰质相同。这发生在最初损伤后1~3周的亚急性期。三个重要的线索可提示存在等密度硬膜下血肿：明显的占位效应、白质挤压征及明显增厚的皮质层。

Intraventricular hemorrhage

- Intraventricular hemorrhage can occur due to tearing of subependymal veins or from direct extension of subarachnoid or intraparenchymal hematoma.
- Patients with intraventricular hemorrhage are at increased risk of developing noncommunicating hydrocephalus due to ependymal scarring, which may obstruct the cerebral aqueduct.

脑室内出血

- 脑室内出血可由室管膜下静脉撕裂所致，或蛛网膜下腔出血或脑实质内血肿的直接蔓延。
- 脑室内出血的患者发生非交通性脑积水的风险增高，这是因为室管膜瘢痕形成会阻塞中脑导水管。

Intra-axial injury

轴内(脑实质)损伤

Coup/contrecoup mechanism

- The coup/contrecoup mechanism of brain trauma describes the propensity for brain to be injured both at the initial site of impact and 180° opposite the impact site, due to secondary impaction against the cranial vault.

冲击/对冲伤机制

- 脑外伤的冲击/对冲伤机制是指脑损伤可以同时发生在直接外力作用的部位以及180°的对侧位置，后者为继发性撞击颅骨所致。

Cortical contusion

- A cortical contusion is caused by traumatic contact of the cortical surface of the brain against the rough inner table of the skull. Contusions affect the gyral crests and can occur in a coup or a contrecoup location.
- A subacute cortical contusion may demonstrate ring enhancement and should be considered in the differential of a ring-enhancing lesion if there is a history of trauma. Enhancement may continue into the chronic stage.
- A chronic contusion appears as encephalomalacia on CT. MRI is more specific, showing peripheral hemosiderin deposition as hypointense on T2-weighted images and blooming artifact on gradient echo sequences.

皮层挫伤

- 皮层挫伤是大脑皮层表面撞击在粗糙的颅骨内板所致的损伤。挫伤累及脑回的凸面，可位于冲击同侧或对侧的部位。
- 亚急性皮层挫伤可表现为环形强化，如有创伤病史应将创伤列入环形强化病变的鉴别诊断之中。强化可持续至慢性期。
- 慢性挫伤在CT上表现为脑软化。MRI较具特异性，表现为周边含铁血黄素沉积，在T_2加权呈低信号，梯度回波序列上呈开花样伪影。

Intraparenchymal hematoma

- Traumatic intraparenchymal hematoma can occur in various locations, ranging from cortical contusion to basal ganglia hemorrhage (due to shearing of lenticulostriate vessels).
- Similar to a cortical contusion, a subacute intraparenchymal hematoma may show ring enhancement.

脑实质内血肿

- 创伤性脑实质内血肿可发生在多个不同部位，从皮层挫伤到基底节出血(由于豆纹动脉撕裂)。
- 与皮层挫伤相类似，亚急性脑实质内血肿可表现为环形强化。

Diffuse axonal injury (DAI) / Traumatic axonal injury (TAI)

弥漫性轴索损伤(DAI)/创伤性轴索损伤(TAI)

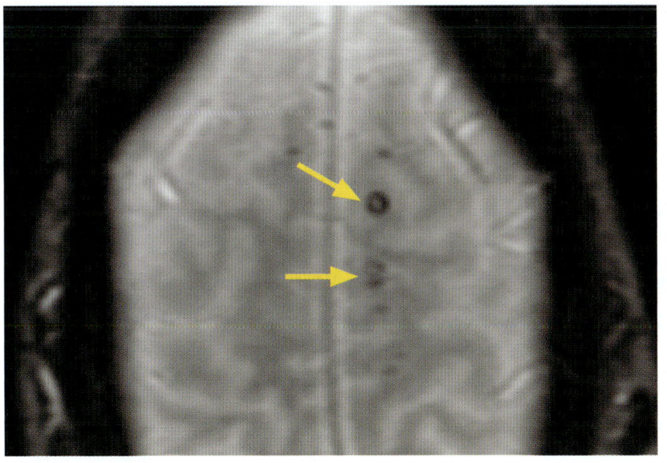

Diffuse axonal injury: Axial GRE image shows several foci of susceptibility effect along the left high convexity representing punctate hemorrhagic foci of DAI (arrows).

弥漫性轴索损伤：轴位GRE图像显示多个沿左侧大脑上凸面的磁敏感效应病灶，为DAI的点状出血灶(黄箭)

- Diffuse axonal injury (DAI) is the result of a shear-strain deformation of the brain.
- The term traumatic axonal injury (TAI) has recently been introduced as this injury pattern is thought to be multifocal rather than diffuse; however, this text will use the term DAI, as that is the more common term.
- DAI is caused by rotational deceleration and subsequent reacceleration force that exceeds the limited elastic capacity of the axons.
- DAI occurs at several characteristic sites, depending on the severity. The higher the grade, the worse the prognosis.

Grade Ⅰ	DAI involves only the gray-white matter junctions of the cerebral hemispheres.
Grade Ⅱ	DAI additionally involves the corpus callosum.
Grade Ⅲ	DAI additionally involves the dorsolateral, rostral midbrain.

- CT is relatively insensitive for detection of DAI, although hemorrhagic DAI may show tiny foci of high attenuation in the affected regions.
- MRI is much more sensitive to detect DAI, although detection relies on multiple sequences, including FLAIR, SWI/GRE,and DWI.

SWI is extremely sensitive for hemorrhagic axonal injury; however, not all DAI is hemorrhagic.

FLAIR is most sensitive for nonhemorrhagic DAI.

Diffusion sequences show restricted diffusion in acute DAI due to cytotoxic edema and cell swelling.

- 弥漫性轴索损伤(DAI)是脑剪切变形的结果。
- 创伤性轴索损伤(TAI)是近期提出的一种术语，这种创伤模式被认为是多灶性而非弥漫性损伤；但本文将使用DAI这个术语，因它更常用。
- DAI是由于轴索受到旋转减速和随后加速的作用力，这种外力超出了轴索的弹性限度。
- DAI发生在数个典型的部位，这取决于其严重程度。级别越高，预后越差。

Ⅰ级DAI仅累及大脑半球的灰白质交界区。
Ⅱ级DAI还累及胼胝体。
Ⅲ级DAI还累及背外侧和腹侧中脑。

- CT对检测DAI相对不敏感，但出血性DAI可表现为受影响区的微小高密度灶。
- MRI对检测DAI要敏感得多，但需要依赖于多个序列，包括FLAIR、SWI/GRE和DWI。

SWI对于出血性轴索损伤极为敏感；但是，并非所有的DAI都是出血性的。

FLAIR对非出血性DAI最敏感。

DWI上急性DAI表现为弥散受限，为细胞毒性水肿及细胞肿胀所致。

(翻译　王超)

BRAIN TUMORS

脑肿瘤

APPROACH TO EVALUATION OF A FOCAL BRAIN MASS LESION

评估局灶性脑肿块的方法

Are there any tumor-related complications?

- CT is a good screening modality to identify potential surgical emergencies complicating a brain tumor, most commonly the 3 H's: hemorrhage, hydrocephalus, and herniation.

是否有肿瘤相关并发症?

- CT是识别脑肿瘤合并潜在外科紧急指征很好的影像筛查手段，最常见的“3H”为出血、脑积水和脑疝。

- **Hemorrhage:** Tumor neovascularity can be prone to hemorrhage.
  The most common primary brain tumor to hemorrhage is glioblastoma.
  The most common hemorrhagic metastases include melanoma, renal cell carcinoma, thyroid carcinoma, and choriocarcinoma. Although breast and lung cancer metastases are less frequently hemorrhagic on a case-by-case basis, these two malignancies are so common that they should also be considered in the differential of a hemorrhagic metastasis.
- **Hydrocephalus:** Tumors can block the flow of CSF.
  Tumors within or around the ventricular system, particularly in the posterior cranial fossa, cause noncommunicating hydrocephalus.
  Leptomeningeal metastases cause communicating hydrocephalus.
- **Herniation:** A combination of the tumor and associated vasogenic edema can shift brain tissue across dural reflections.
  Supratentorial tumors cause subfalcine, downward transtentorial (uncal/central), and tonsillar herniation. Infratentorial tumors cause upward transtentorial and tonsillar herniation.

Could this be a tumor mimic?

- In the evaluation of any suspected intracranial tumor, non-neoplastic mass-like lesions should also be considered, such as brain abscesses, subacute infarcts, tumefactive demyelination, aneurysms, and developmental or degenerative mass/cystic lesions. These conditions variably show mass effect and/or enhancement, mimicking a brain tumor.

How many lesions are there?

- Most primary brain tumors and many brain metastases are solitary. Without a history of cancer, solitary brain tumors in adults over 50 years old have about the same chance to be metastasis or glioblastoma.
- If there is more than one lesion, the diagnosis is most likely to be metastases, but multifocal/multicentric glioblastoma or primary central nervous system lymphoma are in the differential. Some genetic conditions result in multiple brain tumors (e.g., neurofibromatosis, tuberous sclerosis).

Where is the lesion located?

- First, determine if the lesion is intra-axial or extra-axial. Although metastases may be either, the differential diagnosis for tumors in each intracranial compartment is otherwise completely different.
- The most common primary extra-axial tumor is meningioma.
- The most common primary intra-axial tumor is glioma, especially glioblastoma in older patients.
- Findings of an **extra-axial** mass include a CSF cleft between the mass and the brain, and gray matter interposed between the mass and white matter.

- **出血**：肿瘤新生血管容易发生出血。
  最常见的原发性出血性脑肿瘤是胶质母细胞瘤。
  最常见的出血性转移瘤包括黑色素瘤、肾细胞癌、甲状腺癌和绒毛膜癌。虽然乳腺癌和肺癌转移瘤出血概率较低，但由于这两种恶性肿瘤很常见，因此应该将其考虑纳入出血性转移瘤的鉴别诊断。
- **脑积水**：肿瘤可阻断脑脊液流动。
  在脑室系统内或周围的肿瘤，特别是颅后窝肿瘤，可引起非交通性脑积水。
  柔脑膜转移瘤可引起交通性脑积水。
- **脑疝**：肿瘤和伴随的血管源性水肿的共同作用可使脑组织跨越硬脑膜反折。
  幕上肿瘤引起大脑镰下疝、下行性小脑幕裂孔疝（颞叶钩回疝/中心疝）和小脑扁桃体疝。幕下肿瘤引起上行性小脑幕裂孔疝和小脑扁桃体疝。

可以是肿瘤样病变吗？

- 对任何疑似颅内肿瘤的诊断，还应该考虑非肿瘤性肿块样病变，如脑脓肿、亚急性脑梗死、肿瘤样脱髓鞘、动脉瘤和发育性或退行性肿块/囊性病变。这些情况或多或少地表现出占位效应和/或增强，类似脑肿瘤。

有多少病灶？

- 绝大多数原发性脑肿瘤和许多脑转移瘤是孤立的。在没有癌症病史的情况下，孤立性脑肿瘤在50岁以上成人发生转移或转变成胶质母细胞瘤的概率大致相同。
- 如果病灶为非单发，最大可能的诊断是转移瘤，但需要与多灶性/多中性心胶质母细胞瘤或原发性中枢神经系统淋巴瘤进行鉴别。一些遗传因素可导致多发性脑肿瘤（如神经纤维瘤病、结节性硬化）。

病灶位置？

- 首先，确定病灶位于轴内（脑实质）或轴外（脑实质外）。尽管转移瘤两者都有可能出现，但是肿瘤发生在不同颅内位置的鉴别诊断是完全不同的。
- 最常见的原发性轴外肿瘤是脑膜瘤。
- 最常见的原发性轴内肿瘤是胶质瘤，尤其是老年患者的胶质母细胞瘤。
- **轴外**肿瘤的征象包括肿块和脑之间存在脑脊液间隙，以及灰质移位至肿块和白质之间。

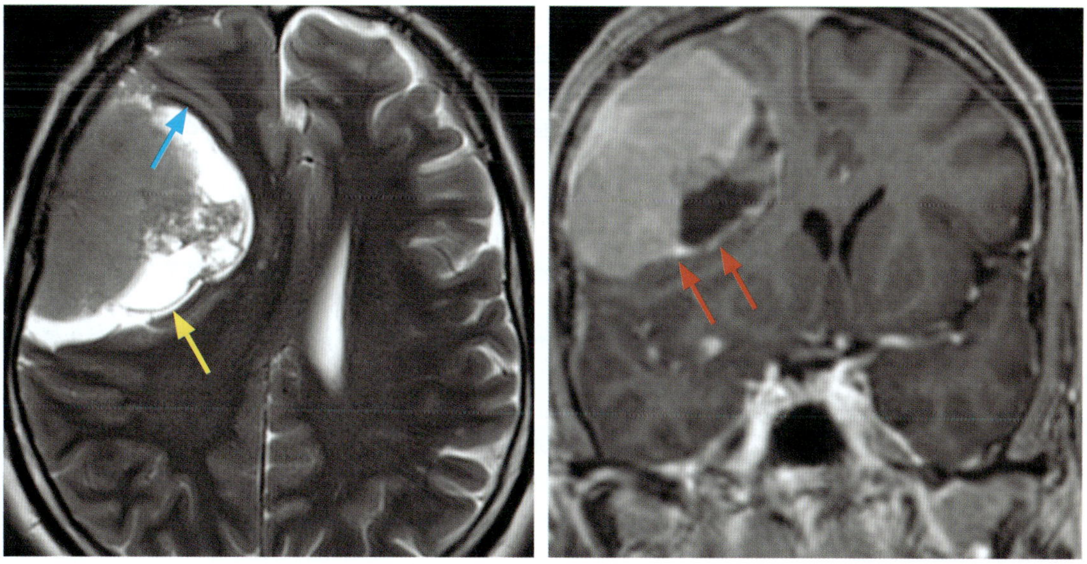

Extra-axial mass: Axial T2-weighted MRI (left image) shows a large, partially hypercellular and partially cystic mass adjacent to the right frontal lobe. A thin CSF cleft (yellow arrow) separates the mass from the brain parenchyma and there is adjacent gray matter buckling (blue arrow), confirming the mass's extra-axial location. Coronal post-contrast T1-weighted image (right image) shows gray matter interposed between the mass and the white matter (red arrows). The mass homogeneously enhances and invades the adjacent bony calvarium.
This mass was a cystic meningioma. *Case courtesy Gregory Wrubel, MD.*
轴外肿块：轴位T_2加权MRI(左图)显示右侧额叶旁一个巨大的部分细胞密集和部分囊性的肿块。一层纤薄的脑脊液间隙(黄箭)将肿块与脑实质分离，邻近灰质扭曲(蓝箭)，可明确肿块位于轴外。冠状位增强T_1加权图像(右图)显示灰质位于肿块与白质之间(红箭)。肿块均匀强化，并侵犯邻近颅骨。
该肿块为囊性脑膜瘤。

- Findings of an **intra-axial** mass include absence of intervening gray matter between the mass and the white matter.

- **轴内**肿瘤的征象包括肿块和白质之间无灰质间隔。

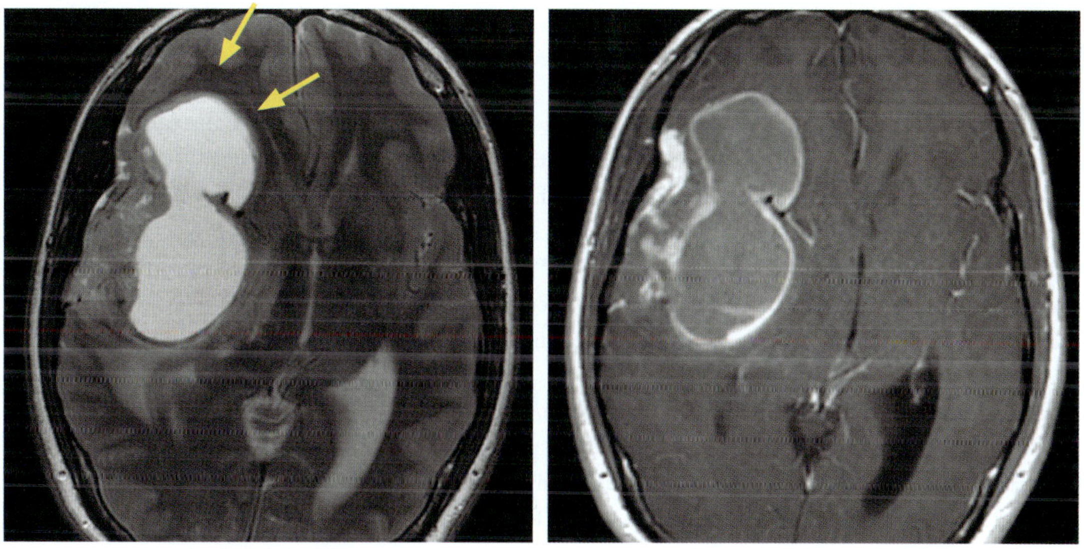

Intra-axial mass: Axial T2-weighted (left image) and post-contrast T1-weighted MRI (right image) show a large, predominantly cystic mass with enhancing components laterally. The mass is located in the right frontal/temporal lobe and causes effacement of the right lateral ventricle and mild midline shift to the left. The mass directly abuts the white matter (yellow arrows), without intervening gray matter, confirming intra-axial location.
This was a pleomorphic xanthoastrocytoma. *Case courtesy Raymond Huang, MD and David Lee, MD.*
轴内肿瘤：轴位T_2加权(左图)和增强后T_1加权(右图)MRI显示一个巨大、以囊性为主的肿块，伴外侧强化。肿块位于右侧额/颞叶，导致右侧脑室消失和中线结构轻度左移。肿块紧邻白质(黄箭)，无灰质间隔，确定肿块位于轴内。
该例为多形性黄色星形细胞瘤。

- Other signs are not as specific. White matter (vasogenic) edema is more common in intra- axial masses but meningioma (an extra-axial dural neoplasm) can also cause this finding. A dural tail (pachymeningeal thickening and enhancement) is seen most often with extra-axial masses, but peripherally located intra-axial lesions may also produce this appearance.
- After determining the intracranial compartment of the lesion, the differential can often be narrowed further by specific location.

  The most common **cerebellopontine angle** masses are vestibular schwannoma, meningioma, and epidermoid cyst.

  The most common **pineal region** tumors are germ cell tumors, such as germinoma, followed by pineal parenchymal tumors, such as pineoblastoma.

  The most common tumors involving the corpus callosum and crossing midline (**butterfly tumors**) are primary central nervous system lymphoma and glioblastoma.

  The most common **cortical** (rather than subcortical) supratentorial brain tumors are pleomorphic xanthoastrocytoma, dysembryoplastic neuroepithelial tumor, oligodendroglioma, and ganglioglioma.

  The most common primary **central skull base** tumors are chordoma and chondrosarcoma.

What is the age of the patient?

- In combination with location, the differential may depend on whether the patient is a child or adult.

  The most common **suprasellar** tumors are pituitary adenoma in adults and craniopharyngiomain children.

  The most common **posterior fossa** tumors in adults are hemangioblastoma and metastases, whereas in children the most common are pilocytic astrocytoma, medulloblastoma, ependymoma, and diffuse midline/intrinsic pontine glioma.

  The most common **purely intraventricular** masses in the atrium of the lateral ventricle are meningioma and degenerative choroid plexus cyst/xanthogranuloma in adults and choroid plexus papilloma in children.

  The most common mass of the **foramen of Monro** in adults is colloid cyst, whereas the most common in children is subependymal giant cell astrocytoma.

What are the signal/attenuation and enhancement characteristics of the lesion?

- As previously described, most brain lesions are hyperintense on T2-weighted images and hypointense on T1-weighted images. MRI signal characteristics are most helpful if a lesion is either hypointense with T2/T2*-weighting (due to hypercellularity, hemorrhage, calcification, or proteinaceous fluid) or hyperintense with T1-weighting (due to fat, hemorrhage, melanin, or proteinaceous fluid).
- On noncontrast CT, most tumors fall within a range of brain/soft tissue attenuation and may be difficult to detect in the absence of surrounding edema. More marked hyperattenuation on CT may be due to hemorrhage or calcification, while more marked hypoattenuation may be due to cystic or necrotic components or fat.
- **Contrast enhancement** occurs in the vast majority of extra-axial and non-glial intra-axial neoplasms. Among gliomas, non-enhancing tumor is more likely to reflect lower histologic grade, but this correspondence is not entirely reliable: high-grade gliomas may not enhance in a third of cases and certain low-grade neoplasms like pilocytic astrocytoma and gangliogliomas show enhancement.
- **Fat** is characteristic of a few lesions: lipoma, dermoid cyst, and teratoma.

- 其他征象为非特异性的。白质(血管源性)水肿更常见于轴内肿块,但脑膜瘤(轴外的硬脑膜肿瘤)也可以导致这种现象。脑膜尾征(硬脑膜增厚和强化)最常见于轴外肿物,但位于外周的轴内病灶也可能产生这种表现。
- 确定病灶的颅内位置后,鉴别诊断通常根据病变的特定位置进一步缩小。

  最常见的**桥小脑角**的肿块是前庭神经鞘瘤、脑膜瘤和表皮样囊肿。

  最常见的**松果体区**肿瘤是生殖细胞肿瘤,如生殖细胞瘤,其次是松果体实质肿瘤,如松果体母细胞瘤。

  最常累及胼胝体和跨越中线的肿瘤(**蝴蝶状肿瘤**)是原发性中枢神经系统淋巴瘤和胶质母细胞瘤。

  最常见的幕上**皮质**(而非皮质下)脑肿瘤是多形性黄色星形细胞瘤、胚胎发育不良性神经上皮瘤、少突胶质细胞瘤和神经节细胞胶质瘤。

  最常见的**中颅底**原发性肿瘤是脊索瘤和软骨肉瘤。

患者年龄?

- 除了位置,鉴别诊断还需要考虑患者是儿童还是成人。

  成人**鞍上**最常见的肿瘤是垂体腺瘤,儿童为颅咽管瘤。

  成人**颅后窝**最常见的肿瘤是血管母细胞瘤和转移瘤,儿童最常见的是毛细胞型星形细胞瘤、髓母细胞瘤、室管膜瘤和弥漫性中线/内生性脑桥胶质瘤。

  成人侧脑室房部最常见的**单纯脑室内**肿块是脑膜瘤和退行性脉络丛囊肿/黄色肉芽肿,儿童为脉络丛乳头状瘤。

  成人**室间孔**最常见的肿块是胶样囊肿,儿童则为室管膜下巨细胞星形细胞瘤。

病灶信号/衰减和增强的特征是什么?

- 如前所述,大多数颅脑病灶呈T_2加权高信号和T_1加权低信号。如果病灶呈T_2/T_2^*加权上呈低信号(由于细胞密度增高、出血、钙化或蛋白质液体)或T_1加权高信号(由于脂肪、出血、黑色素或蛋白质液体),则MRI信号特征非常有助于识别。
- 大多数肿瘤在平扫CT上的密度与脑/软组织相当,因而在缺乏周围水肿时很难被发现。CT上呈明显高密度可能是由于出血或钙化,而较为明显的低密度可能是由于有囊变或坏死成分或脂肪。
- **对比增强**见于绝大多数轴外和非神经胶质轴内肿瘤。在神经胶质瘤中,无强化肿瘤更可能是较低的组织学分级,但这个对应关系并不完全可靠:1/3的高级别胶质瘤有病例可能不会强化,而某些低级别肿瘤(如毛细胞型星形细胞瘤和神经节细胞胶质瘤)则显示强化。
- **脂肪**是少数病变的特征:脂肪瘤、皮样囊肿和

Rarely, meningioma may show fatty metaplasia (lipomatous meningioma).

- **Calcifications** are found in a minority of certain common tumors but some less common lesions nearly always have calcifications.

  The most common **extra-axial** tumor that may calcify is meningioma. The vast majority of craniopharyngiomas are calcified.

  The most common **intra-axial** tumor that may calcify is astrocytoma. The vast majority of oligodendrogliomas are calcified.

  Intracranial calcifications are most commonly physiologic/aging-related rather than tumoral, such as in the choroid plexus, pineal gland, and dura of the tentorium and falx cerebri. However, these can be helpful in localizing tumors based on their displacement: a tumor that engulfs pineal calcifications is more likely a germ cell tumor, while one that disperses pineal calcifications to the periphery is more likely to be a pineal parenchymal tumor.

- **Hemorrhage**, as noted before, is associated with a variety of primary and secondary brain tumors. Tumoral hemorrhage can be distinguished from primary intracerebral hemorrhage by detecting a contrast-enhancing mass within or around the hemorrhage.

  SWI is the most sensitive sequence for detecting intratumoral microhemorrhages.

  T1 shortening can be due to not only methemoglobin but also melanin. The presence of intrinsic hyperintensity on T1-weighted images, even without corresponding susceptibility effect, raises the possibility of metastatic melanoma.

  Most hemorrhagic brain tumors are malignant. A common exception is pituitary macroadenoma.

- **Hypercellularity** appears as hypointensity on T2-weighted images and greater restricted diffusion. Examples include lymphoma, medulloblastoma, germinoma, and some glioblastomas. Metastatic adenocarcinomas also frequently appear hypointense on T2-weighted images but the histologic correlate is unclear.

- **Cysts** are a feature of many low-grade tumors, typically at the periphery of the enhancing component. In contrast, although necrosis of a high-grade tumor may also follow CSF signal, necrosis tends to be central and surrounded by enhancing tumor.

  In the **supratentorial** brain, the most common cystic tumors with a mural nodule are ganglioglioma and pleomorphic xanthoastrocytoma.

  In the **infratentorial** brain, the most common cystic tumors with a mural nodule are pilocytic astrocytoma and hemangioblastoma.

  In the **sellar** region, the most common cystic lesions are pituitary adenoma, craniopharyngioma, and Rathke cleft cyst.

  Common **extra-axial** tumors that occasionally show cystic change include meningioma and schwannoma.

  The differential for **cysts without nodular/thick enhancement** includes nonneoplastic entities, such as arachnoid, dermoid, epidermoid, neuroenteric, pineal, colloid, neuroglial, choroidal fissure, hippocampal sulcus remnant, porencephalic, and parasitic cysts

畸胎瘤。罕见情况下，脑膜瘤可能会出现脂肪化生(脂肪瘤型脑膜瘤)。

- **钙化**可以见于少部分特定常见肿瘤，但某些罕见的病变几乎总有钙化。

  轴外最可能出现钙化的肿瘤是脑膜瘤。绝大多数颅咽管瘤可以出现钙化。

  轴内最可能出现钙化的肿瘤是星形细胞瘤。绝大多数少突胶质细胞瘤可以出现钙化。

  颅内钙化最常见的是与生理性/年龄相关的，而非肿瘤，如在脉络丛、松果体、小脑幕和大脑镰的硬脑膜。这些钙化发生移位可能有助于肿瘤定位：吞噬松果体钙化的肿瘤很可能是生殖细胞肿瘤，而将松果体钙化向外周推压的肿瘤更可能是松果体实质肿瘤。

- 如前所述，**出血**与多种原发性和继发性脑肿瘤有关。肿瘤性出血可通过检测出血内或周围造影剂强化与原发性脑出血进行鉴别。

  SWI是检测肿瘤内微出血最敏感的序列。

  T_1缩短不仅与高铁血红蛋白有关，也与黑色素有关。若T_1加权上出现固有的高信号，但没有相应的磁敏感效应，则会提高转移性黑色素瘤的可能性。

  大多数出血性脑肿瘤是恶性的，但一个常见的例外是垂体大腺瘤。

- **致密细胞**表现为T_2加权低信号及较强的弥散受限，如淋巴瘤、髓母细胞瘤、生殖细胞瘤和一些胶质母细胞瘤。转移性腺癌在T_2加权也通常出现低信号，但是其组织学相关性尚不清楚。

- **囊肿**是很多低级别肿瘤的特征，常位于强化部分的外周。相反，虽然高级别肿瘤的坏死也可出现类似脑脊液信号，但坏死常位于中央并且被强化的肿瘤所包围。

  在**幕上区**，最常见的囊性伴壁结节的脑肿瘤是神经节胶质瘤和多形性黄色星形细胞瘤。

  在**幕下区**，最常见的囊性伴壁结节的脑肿瘤是毛细胞型星形细胞瘤和血管母细胞瘤。

  在鞍区，最常见的囊性病变是垂体腺瘤、颅咽管瘤和颅颊裂囊肿。

  常见的**轴外**肿瘤中，偶尔出现囊性改变的肿瘤包括脑膜瘤、神经鞘瘤。

  无结节/厚壁强化的囊肿鉴别包括非肿瘤性病变，如蛛网膜、皮样、表皮样、神经肠源性、松果体、胶样、神经胶质、脉络膜裂、海马沟残余、脑穿通性和寄生虫性囊肿。

Glial cells

神经胶质细胞

Overview of glial cells

- A glioma is a primary CNS tumor that arises from a glial cell. Glial cells include astrocytes, oligodendrocytes, ependymal cells, and choroid plexus cells.

神经胶质细胞概述

- 胶质瘤是一类起源于胶质细胞的原发性中枢神经系统肿瘤。胶质细胞包括星形胶质细胞、少突胶质细胞、室管膜细胞及脉络丛细胞。

Astrocyte

- The normal functions of an astrocyte are to provide biochemical support to the endothelial cells which maintain the blood-brain barrier, to maintain extracellular ion balance, and to aid in repair after a neuronal injury.
- Astrocytes are normally located throughout the entire brain (primarily in the white matter) and spinal cord.

Oligodendrocyte

- The normal function of an oligodendrocyte is to maintain myelin around CNS axons. A single oligodendrocyte can maintain the myelin of dozens of axons.

  The counterpart in the peripheral nervous system is the Schwann cell, which maintains myelin around a single peripheral nerve. Unlike the oligodendrocyte, each Schwann cell is in charge of only a single axon.
- Oligodendrocytes are normally located throughout the entire brain and spinal cord.

Ependymal cells

- The normal function of an ependymal cell is to circulate CSF with its multiple cilia.
- Ependymal cells line the ventricles and central canal of the spinal cord. Choroid plexus cells are modified ependymal cells that function in producing CSF; they are located in specific locations as described earlier in the chapter.

星形胶质细胞

- 星形胶质细胞的正常功能是为构成血脑屏障的内皮细胞提供生化支持，维持细胞外离子平衡，协助修复神经元损伤。
- 星形胶质细胞在正常情况下分布于整个大脑（主要分布在白质）和脊髓。

少突胶质细胞

- 少突胶质细胞的功能是组成中枢神经系统轴突周围的髓鞘。一个少突胶质细胞可以构成几十个轴突的髓鞘。

  相应在周围神经系统中有同样功能的是施万细胞，它构成单一外周神经的髓鞘。与少突胶质细胞不同，每个施万细胞只负责单一轴突。
- 少突胶质细胞在正常情况下分布于整个大脑和脊髓。

室管膜细胞

- 室管膜细胞的正常功能是利用它的运动纤毛促进脑脊液循环。
- 室管膜细胞衬于脑室和脊髓中央管。脉络丛细胞是特化的室管膜细胞，其功能是产生脑脊液；它们所在的特定位置已在本章前文进行描述。

DIFFUSE ASTROCYTIC AND OLIGODENDROGLIAL TUMORS

Overview

- Glioma, or glial neoplasm, is not a synonym for a “brain tumor” or a specific pathological diagnosis but is often used loosely to indicate subtypes of primary brian tumors derived from glial cells.
- Diffuse gliomas, including subtypes from astrocytic and oligodendroglial cell origins, are the most common type of primary brain tumor in adults.
- Characterized by their infiltrative growth, diffuse gliomas are rarely curable and therefore are considered grade 2 to 4 by the World Health Organization (WHO). In contrast, WHO grade 1, localized gliomas are generally curable by total resection.
- “Low-grade glioma” usually refers to WHO grade 2 diffuse astrocytic and oligodendroglial tumors, whereas “lower-grade glioma” refers to grades 2 and 3, and “high-grade glioma” refers to grade 3 and 4 tumors in this category.
- Since 2016, molecular data including *IDH1/2* mutation and 1p/19q chromosomal co-deletion status are considered with, and usually supersede, histological phenotype to form integrated pathological diagnoses of diffuse glioma subtypes.

弥漫性星形胶质细胞和少突胶质细胞肿瘤

概述

- 胶质瘤，或神经胶质肿瘤，不是“脑肿瘤”或特定病理诊断的同义词，但通常泛指起源于神经胶质细胞的原发性脑肿瘤的所有亚型。
- 弥漫性胶质瘤，包括起源于星形胶质细胞和少突胶质细胞的亚型，是成人原发性脑肿瘤中最常见的类型。
- 弥漫性胶质瘤以浸润性生长为特征，罕见被治愈，因此被世界卫生组织(WHO)认定为2~4级。相比之下，WHO 1级的局限性胶质瘤通常可通过全部切除得到治愈。
- “低级别胶质瘤”通常指WHO 2级弥漫性星形细胞瘤和少突胶质细胞瘤，而“较低级别胶质瘤”指2级和3级，“高级别胶质瘤”指这类肿瘤中的3级和4级。
- 2016年以来，*IDH 1/2*突变和1p/19q染色体共缺失状态等分子数据被认为可以联合或通常取代组织学表型，作出弥漫性胶质瘤亚型的综合性病理诊断。

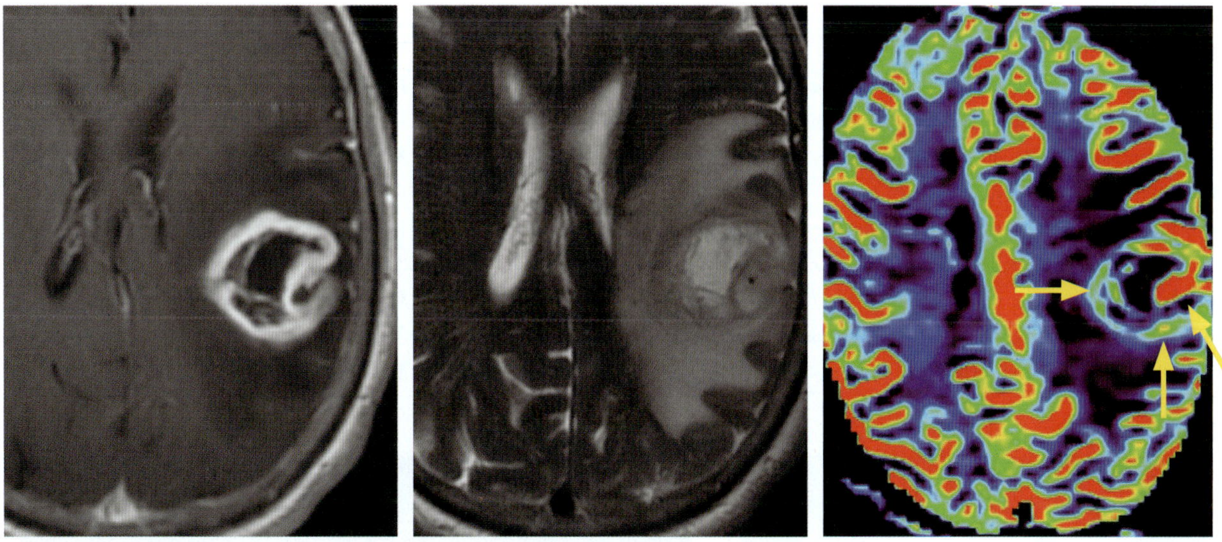

Glioblastoma with MR perfusion: Axial post-contrast T1-weighted (left image) and T2-weighted (middle image) MRI show a heterogeneous enhancing mass with central necrosis and surrounding edema/T2 prolongation in the left parietal lobe. There is associated mildly elevated CBV in the non-necrotic peripheral components (arrows, right image).

胶质母细胞瘤MR灌注成像：轴位增强T_1加权(左图)和T_2加权(中图)MRI显示左侧顶叶不均匀强化肿块，伴中心坏死和周围水肿/T_2延长。在非坏死外周组织中伴有轻度升高的CBV(黄箭，右图)。

- IDH-wildtype diffuse gliomas are most commonly diagnosed as **glioblastoma**, WHO grade 4. In turn, most glioblastomas are IDH-wildtype, which confers a worse prognosis.

  These tumors are usually primary glioblastomas, indicating they arise de novo rather than from an existing lower-grade glioma.

  Grade 2 or 3 IDH-wildtype diffuse gliomas are rare and treated as early glioblastoma as they rapidly transform to grade 4 tumors.
- IDH-wildtype glioblastomas occur mostly in the elderly.
- Glioblastoma is often abbreviated GBM, due to the historical term "glioblastoma multiforme" describing the heterogeneous appearance of the tumor.
- On MRI, IDH-wildtype glioblastomas typically have heterogeneous enhancement, corresponding histologically to microvascular proliferation and necrosis. Surrounding nonenhancing T2 prolongation consists of both vasogenic edema and infiltrative tumor. The enhancing component and sometimes the non-enhancing infiltrative component can exhibit low diffusivity (dark ADC) on diffusion-weighted imaging due to hypercellularity, and elevated blood volume (rCBV) on perfusion-weighted imaging, indicating hypervascularity.
- Tumor can spread through white matter tracts, through the CSF, and along leptomeningeal, ependymal, and subependymal routes. There are several specific terms reflecting aggressive growth patterns:

- IDH野生型弥漫性胶质瘤最常被诊断为**胶质母细胞瘤**，WHO 4级。反之亦然，大多数胶质母细胞瘤为IDH野生型，预后较差。

  这些肿瘤通常是原发性胶质母细胞瘤，表明它们是新发的，而非来自现有的低级别胶质瘤。

  级别为2级或3级的IDH野生型弥漫性胶质瘤很少见，可迅速转化为4级肿瘤，因此治疗按早期胶质母细胞瘤处理。
- IDH野生型胶质母细胞瘤多发生在老年人。
- 胶质母细胞瘤通常简写为"GBM"，这是因为"多形性胶质母细胞瘤"这一术语曾经用于描述此肿瘤不均匀的外观。
- IDH野生型胶质母细胞瘤在MRI上通常呈不均匀强化，与组织学上的微血管增生和坏死相对应。其周围无强化的T_2延长信号包括血管源性水肿和浸润的肿瘤。强化成分和有时非强化的浸润成分由于细胞过多，而在弥散加权成像中表现出低弥散率(暗ADC)，并且灌注加权成像显示血容量(rCBV)升高，表明血管过度增生。
- 肿瘤可通过白质束、脑脊液、柔脑膜、室管膜和室管膜下途径扩散。有数个特殊的术语反映了侵袭生长的模式：

When glioblastoma crosses the midline via the corpus callosum, it is called **butterfly glioblastoma**.

The differential diagnosis of a transcallosal mass includes glioblastoma, lymphoma, and demyelinating disease.

When diffuse glioma, usually IDH-wildtype, involves at least three lobes of the brain, it is called **gliomatosis cerebri.** The differential diagnosis for diffuse signal abnormality includes progressive multifocal leukoencephalopathy and HIV encephalopathy, but these entities do not infiltrate the cortex.

When there are multiple enhancing glioblastoma lesions, the tumors are **multifocal** if they are connected by FLAIR abnormality or, more rarely, **multicentric** if no connection is present.

When intracranial tumors disseminate to the intradural extramedullary compartment of the spine, they are called **drop metastases**.

当胶质母细胞瘤通过胼胝体跨越中线时被称为**蝶形胶质母细胞瘤**。

跨越胼胝体肿块的鉴别诊断包括胶质母细胞瘤、淋巴瘤和脱髓鞘疾病。

当弥漫性胶质瘤(通常为IDH野生型)累及至少3个脑叶时，称为脑胶质瘤病。弥漫性信号异常的鉴别诊断包括进行性多灶性白质脑病和人类免疫缺陷病毒(HIV)脑病，但这些病变不浸润皮质。

当存在多个增强的胶质母细胞瘤病变时，如果FLAIR上病灶是连接的，则肿瘤是**多灶性**的；如果没有连接，则较为罕见，为**多中心性**的。

当颅内肿瘤扩散到脊柱的髓外硬膜下腔时，被称为**脱落转移瘤**。

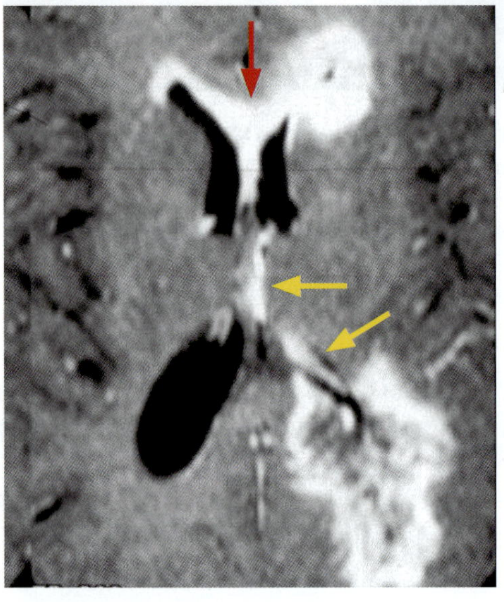

Transependymal and transcallosal spread of GBM: Post-contrast T1-weighted MRI shows extensive abnormal enhancement primarily in the left occipital lobe but extending into the bilateral periventricular frontal lobes via the subependymal surface (yellow arrows) and crossing the midline via the corpus callosum (red arrow).

GBM跨室管膜和跨胼胝体播散：增强T_1加权MRI显示大片的异常强化灶，主要位于左侧枕叶，并沿室管膜下表面(黄箭)延伸到两侧脑室周围额叶，通过胼胝体(红箭)跨越中线。

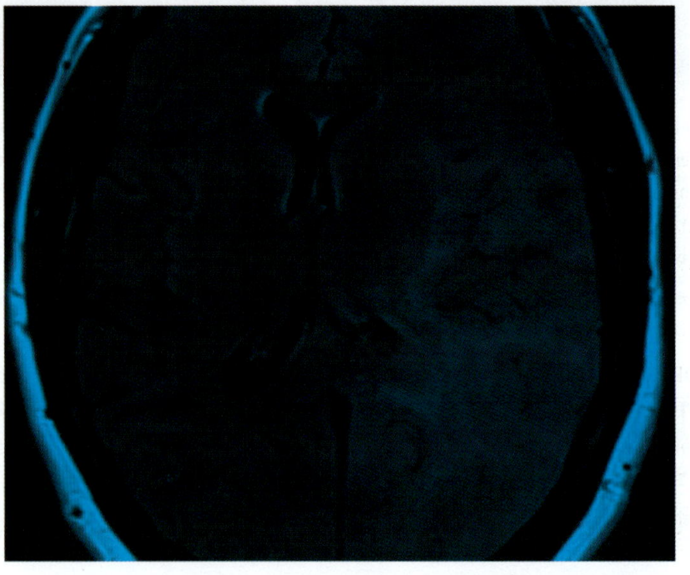

Gliomatosis: Axial FLAIR shows infiltrative FLAIR hyperintensity in the left cerebral hemisphere involving the left parietal lobe, posterior frontal lobe, insula, left temporal lobe, and corpus callosum. There is regional mass effect with effacement of the left lateral ventricle, sulcal effacement, and rightward midline shift. No associated contrast enhancement or restricted diffusion is seen.

胶质瘤病：轴位FLAIR显示左侧大脑半球浸润性FLAIR高信号，累及左侧顶叶、额叶后部、岛叶、左侧颞叶和胼胝体。局部占位效应导致左侧脑室消失、脑沟消失和中线向右移位。无强化或弥散受限。

Left case courtesy Amir Zamani, MD, Brigham and Women's Hospital.

IDH-mutant diffuse gliomas

- IDH-mutant diffuse gliomas carry gain-of-function mutations in *IDH1* or *IDH2*, which encode isoforms of isocitrate dehydrogenase, the rate-limiting enzyme of the Krebs cycle.

  The mutations lead to overproduction of 2-hydroxyglutarate (2HG), a metabolite that can be measured by MR spectroscopy.
- IDH-mutant diffuse gliomas are most commonly diagnosed as WHO grade 2 or 3 tumors. These are divided into astrocytic and oligodendroglial subtypes based on 1p19q chromosomal co-deletion (allelic loss of the short arm of

IDH突变型弥漫性胶质瘤

- IDH突变型弥漫性胶质瘤在*IDH 1*或*IDH 2*中携带功能增益突变，功能为编码异柠檬酸脱氢酶异构体，是Krebs循环的限速酶。

  该突变导致2-羟基戊二酸(2HG)过量产生，此代谢物可以通过磁共振波谱进行测量。
- IDH突变型弥漫性胶质瘤最常被诊断为WHO 2级或3级肿瘤。根据1p19q染色体共缺失(1号染色体短臂和19号染色体长臂的等位基因缺失)

chromosome 1 and the long arm of chromosome 19).

1p19q non-co-deleted IDH-mutant tumors are more common and include **diffuse astrocytomas** (WHO grade 2) and **anaplastic astrocytomas** (grade 3).

1p19q co-deleted IDH-mutant tumors are less common and include **oligodendrogliomas** (WHO grade 2) and **anaplastic oligodendrogliomas** (grade 3).

Histologically, lower-grade diffuse gliomas can have both astrocytic and oligodendroglial phenotypes and were previously termed oligoastrocytomas or mixed gliomas. These terms are no longer used when 1p19q co-deletion status is available.

- These tumors grow very slowly, often only noticeably changing when imaging over a long time. Over time, as mutations accumulate, these tumors can behave more aggressively and secondarily become grade 4, which may be histologically indistinguishable from IDH-wildtype glioblastomas but nevertheless carry a better prognosis.
- IDH-mutant diffuse gliomas occur mostly in young to middle-aged adults (20–55 years).

  1p19q non-co-deleted astrocytomas usually present younger, typically between 20 and 30 years.

  1p19q co-deleted oligodendrogliomas usually present between 30 and 40 years with seizures.
- On MRI, IDH-mutant diffuse gliomas are predominantly hypoenhancing and more homogeneous than their IDH-wildtype counterparts. Contrast enhancement is present in a minority and more likely in grade 3 than grade 2 tumors.
- Lower-grade **astrocytomas** typically appear as a circumscribed hyperintense mass on T2-weighted images. In 12–25% of nonenhancing lower-grade gliomas in adults, the *T2-FLAIR mismatch sign* is highly specific for 1p19q non-co-deleted IDH-mutant astrocytomas: hyperintense on T2-weighted images but relatively centrally hypointense on FLAIR due to microcystic changes.

可分为星形细胞亚型和少突胶质细胞亚型。

1p19q非共缺失IDH突变肿瘤更常见，其中包括**弥漫性星形细胞瘤**(WHO 2级)和**间变性星形细胞瘤**(3级)。

1p19q共缺失IDH突变肿瘤不太常见，其中包括**少突胶质细胞瘤**(WHO 2级)和**间变性少突胶质细胞瘤**(3级)。

组织学上，低级别弥漫性胶质瘤可以同时具有星形细胞和少突胶质细胞表型，过去被称为少突胶质细胞瘤或混合性胶质瘤。这些术语在明确1p19q共缺失状态的情况下不再使用。

- 此类肿瘤生长非常缓慢，通常只有间隔很长时间后才会有明显的影像学变化。随着时间增加，突变积累，这些肿瘤可能表现得更具侵袭性，继而变成4级，并在组织学上可能与IDH野生型胶质母细胞瘤无法区分，但预后较好。
- IDH突变型弥漫性胶质瘤主要发生在青年至中年成人(20~55岁)。

  1p19q非共缺失星形细胞瘤往往年轻时发病，通常在20~30岁。

  1p19q共缺失少突胶质细胞瘤通常在30~40岁发病并有癫痫发作。
- IDH突变型弥漫性胶质瘤在MRI上主要呈低强化，比IDH野生型强化均匀。强化在少数情况下出现，且3级肿瘤比2级肿瘤更可能出现。
- 较低级别**星形细胞瘤**在T_2加权图像上通常表现为边界清晰的高信号肿块。在12%~25%的成人非强化低级别胶质瘤中，T_2-FLAIR不匹配征对1p19q非共缺失IDH突变型星形细胞瘤具有高度特异性：T_2加权呈高信号，FLAIR呈相对中央区低信号，为微小囊性改变所致。

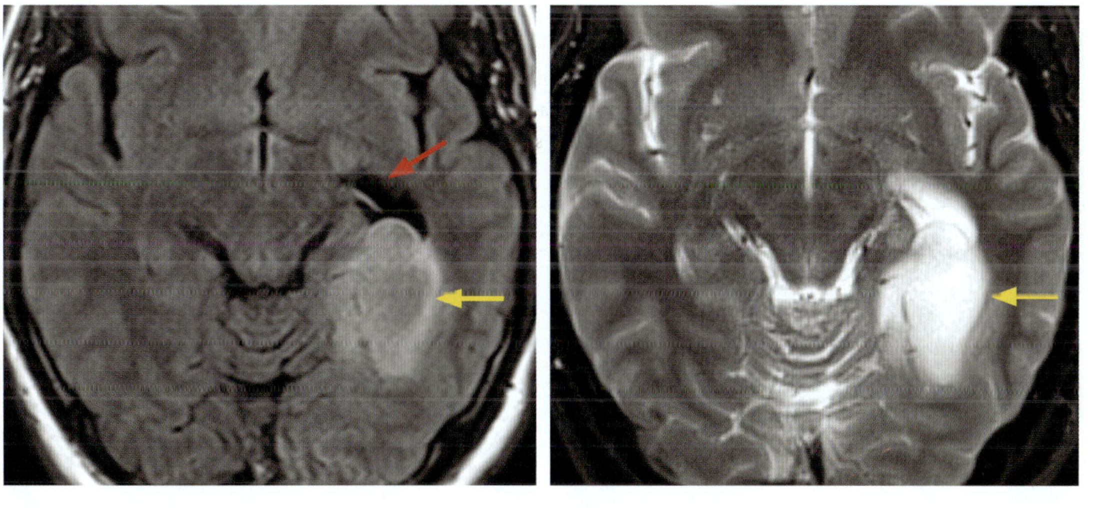

T2-FLAIR mismatch: Axial FLAIR (left image) and T2-weighted (right image) MRI demonstrate a hyperintense intra-axial mass in the left posterior medial temporal lobe with lower FLAIR signal than T2 signal (yellow arrows), representing the *T2-FLAIR mismatch sign*, which is highly suggestive of 1p19q non-co-deleted astrocytoma. The mass has no post-contrast enhancement, restricted diffusion, or calcification (not shown). Note the trapped left temporal horn (red arrow).

T_2-FLAIR不匹配：轴位FLAIR(左图)和T_2加权(右图)MRI显示左颞叶后内侧的轴内高信号肿块，FLAIR信号低于T_2信号(黄箭)，表明T_2-FLAIR不匹配征，高度提示1p19q非共缺失星形细胞瘤。肿块没有强化、弥散受限及钙化(未展示)。注意受压的左侧脑室颞角(红箭)。

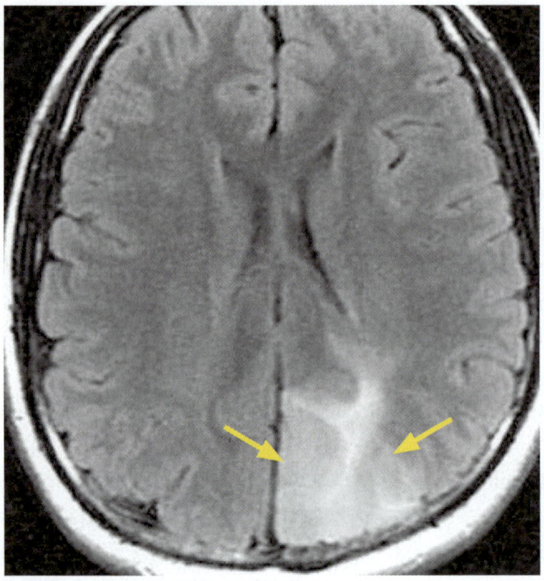

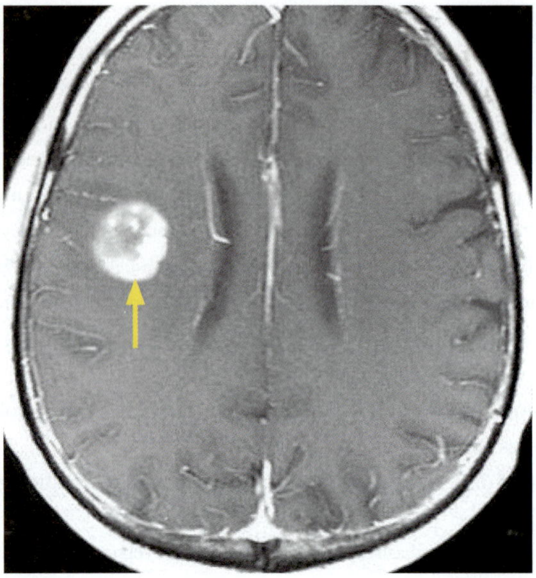

Anaplastic astrocytoma: Axial FLAIR image shows a region of T2 prolongation in the left occipital white matter and cortex (arrows). There was no enhancement (not shown). This appearance is not specific and may also represent a low-grade astrocytoma.
间变性星形细胞瘤：轴位FLAIR图像显示左侧枕叶白质及皮层(黄箭)长T_2信号病变。无强化(未展示)。该表现无特异性，也可能是低级别星形细胞瘤。

Anaplastic astrocytoma in a different patient: Axial post-contrast T1-weighted MRI shows an enhancing lesion in the right temporal lobe (arrow). This appearance is not specific and may represent a glioblastoma or metastatic disease.
另一名间变性星形细胞瘤患者：轴位增强T_1加权MRI显示右侧颞叶(黄箭)一个强化病灶。该表现无特异性，也可能是胶质母细胞瘤或转移瘤。

Cases courtesy Amir Zamani, MD, Brigham and Women's Hospital.

- Lower-grade **oligodendrogliomas** typically appear as a poorly circumscribed hyperintense mass on T2-weighted images. They are most often found in the frontal and temporal cortical regions and the majority calcify. An expansile, cortical-based mass with gyriform calcification is specific for 1p19q-co-deleted IDH-mutant oligodendroglioma.

- 低级别**少突胶质细胞瘤**在T_2加权上通常表现为边界不清的高信号肿块。它们最常见于额叶和颞叶皮质区，大多数伴钙化。1p19q共缺失IDH突变型少突胶质细胞瘤是一种膨胀性的、位于皮质的肿块并伴有脑回状钙化。

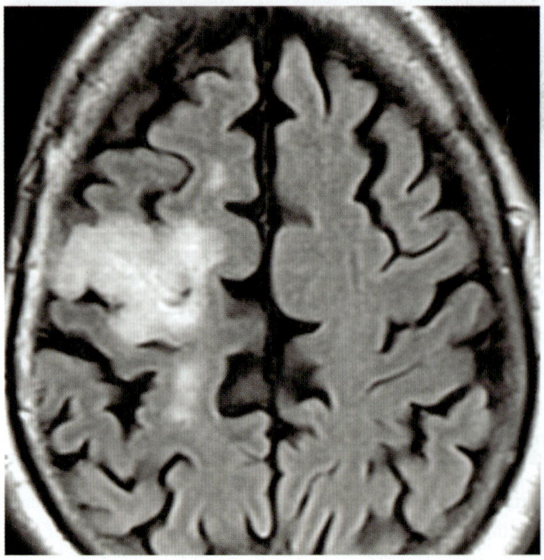

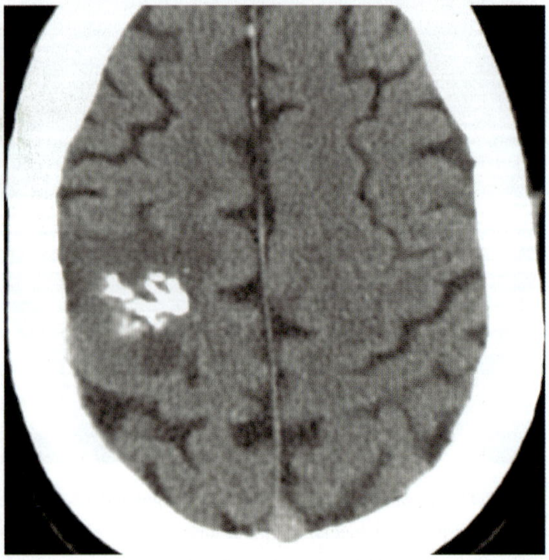

Oligodendroglioma: Axial FLAIR (left image) demonstrates a hyperintense, expansile, cortically based mass centered in the right precentral gyrus. Axial noncontrast CT (right image) shows the mass is partially calcified.
少突胶质细胞瘤：轴位FLAIR(左图)显示一个位于皮质的高信号、膨胀性肿块，以右中央前回为中心。轴位平扫CT(右图)显示肿块部分钙化。

On diffusion-weighted imaging, oligodendrogliomas often show high diffusivity (higher ADC than brain), and frequently show mildly elevated blood volume. This is one of the low-grade CNS tumors that can show high blood volume (meningiomas also can show high rCBV).

在DWI上，少突胶质细胞瘤通常表现出高扩散率(ADC高于大脑)，并且经常表现出轻度血容量升高。这是低级别中枢神经系统肿瘤中高血容量的肿瘤之一(脑膜瘤也可显示高rCBV)。

SUPRATENTORIAL CORTICAL GLIAL/NEURONAL TUMORS

幕上皮质神经胶质/神经元肿瘤

Overview

- In addition to oligodendrogliomas, there are several rare, low-grade primary neoplasms of glial, neuronal, or mixed glial-neuronal lineage that are predominantly centered in the superficial cerebrum.
- The supratentorial cortical tumors can be remembered with the acronym **P-DOG MD**:

概述

- 除了少突胶质细胞瘤外，还有几种罕见且主要位于大脑浅层的低级别原发性胶质、神经元或混合胶质神经元谱系肿瘤。
- 幕上皮质肿瘤可以用单词首字母缩写词**P-DOG MD**来帮助记忆：

Pleomorphic xanthoastrocytoma (PXA).
Dysembryoplastic neuroepithelial tumor (DNET).
Oligodendroglioma.
Ganglioglioma.
Multinodular and vacuolating neuronal tumor (MVNT).
Desmoplastic infantile astrocytoma and ganglioglioma (DIA/DIG).

多形性黄色星形细胞瘤(PXA)。
胚胎发育不良性神经上皮瘤(DNET)。
少突胶质细胞瘤(Oligodendroglioma)。
神经节细胞胶质瘤(Ganglioglioma)。
多结节和空泡状神经元肿瘤(MVNT)。
促纤维增生性婴儿星形细胞瘤和神经节细胞胶质瘤(DIA/DIG)。

- These tumors carry a better prognosis and occur at a younger age than diffuse gliomas.
- Due to cortical involvement, these patients most often present with seizures.
- Slow-growing cortical tumors can cause scalloping/remodeling of the inner table of the calvarium. Extensive vasogenic edema is uncommon, consistent with their low-grade behavior.

- 这些肿瘤的预后比弥漫性胶质瘤好，但发病患者更年轻。
- 由于皮质受累，这些患者最常出现癫痫发作。
- 生长缓慢的皮质肿瘤可导致颅骨内板的扇形压迹/重塑。与低级别肿瘤的表现一样，广泛的血管源性水肿并不常见。

Pleomorphic xanthoastrocytoma (PXA)

多形性黄色星形细胞瘤(PXA)

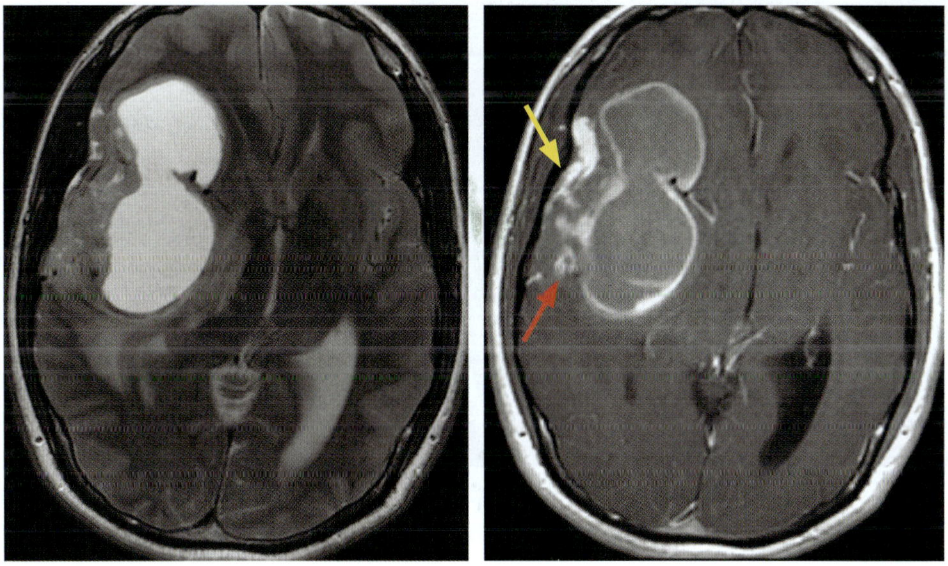

Pleomorphic xanthoastrocytoma: Axial T2-weighted (left image) and post-contrast T1-weighted (right image) MRI shows a large right temporal, predominantly cystic mass. The mass has enhancing nodularity laterally (red arrow). The overlying dura is thickened and enhancing (yellow arrow). There is relatively little surrounding edema given the large size of the lesion.

Case courtesy Raymond Huang, MD and David Lee, MD, Brigham and Women's Hospital.

多形性黄色星形细胞瘤：轴位T_2加权(左图)和增强T_1加权(右图)MRI显示右侧颞叶巨大，以囊性为主的肿块。肿块外侧有强化结节(红箭)。邻近的硬脑膜增厚并强化(黄箭)。相比病灶的巨大体积，周围水肿相对较轻。

- Pleomorphic xanthoastrocytoma (PXA) is a WHO grade 2 astrocytic tumor. A more aggressive variant is the anaplastic PXA (grade 3).
- PXAs usually present in children or young adults.
- The majority of PXAs carry the *BRAF* V600E targetable mutation.
- PXA is most commonly located in the temporal lobe (half of cases), involving the cortex and leptomeninges.
- On MRI, PXA is an avidly enhancing mass often associated with cyst formation and a thickened/enhancing *pial tail*.
- Aside from PXA, the main differential for a cortical solid and cystic lesion in this age group is ganglioglioma. Although uncommon, hemorrhage is more likely with PXA.

- 多形性黄色星形细胞瘤(PXA)是一类WHO 2级的星形细胞肿瘤。一种更具侵袭性的变异是间变性PXA(3级)。
- PXA通常见于儿童或年轻成人。
- 大多数PXA携带*BRAF* V600E靶向突变。
- PXA最常位于颞叶(一半病例),累及皮质和柔脑膜。
- PXA在MRI上表现为明显强化的肿块,通常伴囊变和增厚/增强软脑膜尾征。
- 除PXA外,上述年龄范围的皮质实性和囊性病变段的主要鉴别诊断是神经节细胞胶质瘤。PXA更容易发生出血,但并不常见。

Dysembryoplastic neuroepithelial tumor (DNET)

- Dysembryoplastic neuroepithelial tumor (DNET) is a WHO grade 1 glioneuronal tumor.
- DNETs usually present in children or young adults.
- DNET is most commonly located in the temporal lobe involving the cortex. They are found less commonly in the frontal lobe, basal ganglia, or brainstem.
- On CT, DNET appears hypodense and occasionally calcifies. On MRI, DNETs show a circumscribed bubbly appearance with T2 prolongation and a *bright rim* or *hyperintense ring sign* on FLAIR. The tumor can be heterogeneous and show enhancement.
- DNETs frequently coexist with focal cortical dysplasia, and cortical expansion is a feature more commonly found in tumors than in pure cortical malformations.

胚胎发育不良性神经上皮瘤(DNET)

- 胚胎发育不良性神经上皮瘤(DNET)是WHO 1级胶质神经元瘤。
- DNET通常存在于儿童或年轻人中。
- DNET最常见于颞叶,累及皮质。在额叶、基底节或脑干少见。
- 在CT上,DNET呈低密度,偶有钙化。在MRI上,DNET呈局限性囊泡状表现伴长T_2和FLAIR上明亮边缘或高信号环征。肿瘤可以是异质性的,并有增强。
- DNET经常与局灶性皮质发育不良并存,与单纯皮质畸形相比,皮质膨大是肿瘤内更常见的一个特征。

Ganglioglioma

神经节细胞胶质瘤

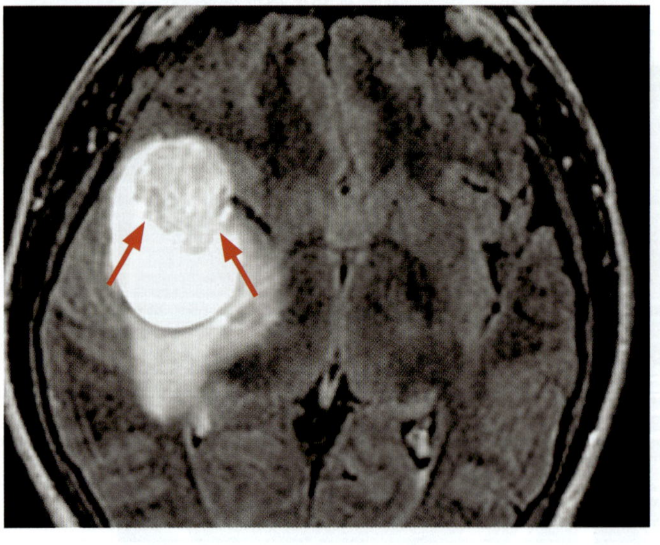

Ganglioglioma: Axial FLAIR shows a cystic lesion in the right temporal lobe with an associated large solid nodule (arrows). There is mild surrounding edema and mild mass effect with midline shift to the left.
Case courtesy Amir Zamani, MD, Brigham and Women's Hospital.
神经节细胞胶质瘤:轴位FLAIR显示右侧颞叶囊性病灶伴有巨大实性结节(红箭)。病灶周围轻度水肿,占位效应轻微伴中线左移。

- Ganglioglioma is a WHO grade 1 glioneuronal tumor. A more aggressive variant is the anaplastic ganglioglioma (grade 3).
- Gangliogliomas usually present in children or young adults.
- Ganglioglioma is most commonly located in the temporal lobe, involving the cortex.

  They can also be found in cerebellum and near the conus medullaris, mimicking myxopapillary ependymoma.

- 神经节细胞胶质瘤是WHO 1级胶质神经元肿瘤。一种更具侵袭性的变异是间变性神经节细胞胶质瘤(3级)。
- 神经节细胞胶质瘤通常发生于儿童或年轻成人。
- 神经节细胞胶质瘤最常见于颞叶,累及皮质。

  它们也可见于小脑和脊髓圆锥附近,类似于黏液乳头状室管膜瘤。

- The imaging appearance is variable. A common appearance is a circumscribed cystic mass with enhancing mural nodule, often with calcification, but ganglioglioma can also be solidly enhancing or nonenhancing.
- Gangliogliomas frequently coexist with focal cortical dysplasia.

Multinodular and vacuolating neuronal tumor (MVNT)

- MVNT is a recently recognized WHO grade 1 entity. It usually presents in young and middle- aged adults with seizure or may be an incidental finding.
- MVNT is most commonly located in the temporal or frontal lobes, centered at the deep layers of cortex and juxtacortical white matter.
- On MRI, MVNT characteristically appears as a cluster of bubbles: small, circumscribed hyperintense nodules on T2-weighted imaging, usually without enhancement or mass effect.

Desmoplastic infantile astrocytoma and ganglioglioma (DIA/DIG)

- DIA and DIG are classified together as WHO grade 1 glial/glioneuronal tumors. They present in infants usually with progressive head enlargement.
- DIA/DIG is most commonly located in the frontal and parietal lobes, involving the cortex and attaching to the leptomeninges. However, they are quite large at presentation, often spanning more than one lobe of the cerebral hemisphere.
- On MRI, DIA/DIG characteristically appears as a large multicystic and solid mass (cysts with mural nodule). The solid component enhances avidly.

- 影像学表现多变。常见的表现为边缘清晰的囊性肿块伴强化的壁结节，常见钙化，但神经节细胞胶质瘤实性可强化或不强化。
- 神经节细胞胶质瘤常与局灶性皮质发育不良同时存在。

多结节和空泡状神经元肿瘤(MVNT)

- 多结节和空泡状神经元肿瘤(MVNT)是新近被归类于WHO 1级的病变。它通常出现在有癫痫的年轻人和中年人，也可以偶然发现。
- MVNT最常位于颞叶或额叶，以皮质深层和皮质旁白质为中心。
- MVNT在MRI上的特征性表现是簇状囊泡：T_2加权上呈小而局限性的高信号结节，通常没有强化或占位效应。

促纤维增生性婴儿星形细胞瘤和神经节细胞胶质瘤(DIA/DIG)

- 促纤维增生性婴儿星形细胞瘤(DIA)和神经节细胞胶质瘤(DIG)一同被归类为WHO 1级胶质细胞/胶质神经元肿瘤。在婴儿期发病，常表现为进行性头颅增大。
- DIA/DIG最常见于额叶和顶叶，侵及皮质并附着于柔脑膜。但是，肿瘤在发现时已经很大，通常跨越大脑半球多个脑叶。
- 在MRI上，DIA/DIG的特征性表现为巨大多囊和实性肿块(囊肿伴壁结节)。实性成分强化明显。

Posterior fossa intra-axial tumors

Overview

- The differential diagnosis for posterior fossa intra-axial tumors depends on age (see flowchart at the end of this section). They are more common in children. Extra-axial lesions are discussed in the "Head and Neck" chapter in the section on temporal bone and lateral/ posterior skull base.
- The main posterior fossa intra-axial tumors in children (and young adults) can be remembered by the acronym **BEAM:**

> **B**rainstem glioma (diffuse).
> **E**pendymoma.
> **A**strocytoma (pilocytic).
> **M**edulloblastoma.

- The most common adult posterior fossa intra-axial tumors are metastasis and hemangioblastoma. Less common entities occurring in older adults include diffuse glioma and subependymoma.
- Although less common, most of these tumors can also occur in the supratentorial brain, except for medulloblastoma. CNS embryonal tumors other than medulloblastoma, however, are often supratentorial.

颅后窝轴内肿瘤

概述

- 颅后窝轴内肿瘤的鉴别诊断取决于年龄(见本节末尾的流程图)。颅后窝轴内肿瘤常见于儿童。轴外病变见“神经影像：头与颈”中颞骨/侧颅底与后颅底的讨论。
- 儿童(和年轻人)主要的颅后窝轴内肿瘤可以用首字母缩写词BEAM来帮助记忆：

> 脑干胶质瘤(弥漫性)。
> 室管膜瘤。
> 星形细胞瘤(毛细胞性)。
> 髓母细胞瘤。

- 最常见的成人颅后窝轴内肿瘤是转移瘤和血管母细胞瘤。不太常见的是发生在老年人中的弥漫性胶质瘤和室管膜下瘤。
- 除了髓母细胞瘤，大多数肿瘤也可发生在幕上，但并不常见。然而，中枢神经系统胚胎性肿瘤除了髓母细胞瘤外，通常位于幕上。

Hemangioblastoma

血管母细胞瘤

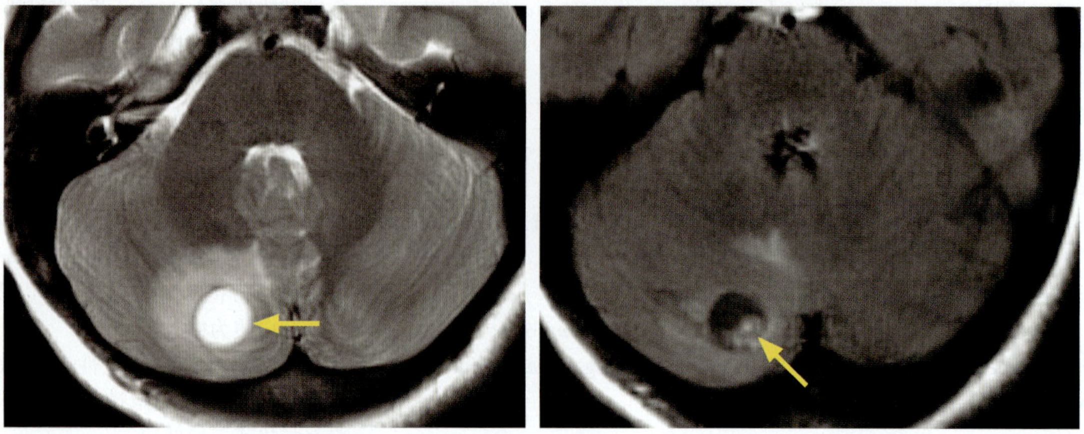

Hemangioblastoma: Axial T2-weighted MRI (left image) shows a cystic lesion (arrow) in the right cerebellar hemisphere with mild surrounding edema. The nodular component is demonstrated on FLAIR (arrow, right).

Case courtesy Sanjay Prabhu, MD, Boston Children's Hospital.

血管母细胞瘤：轴位T_2加权MRI(左图)显示右侧小脑半球内一个囊性病灶(黄箭)，伴有周围轻度水肿。在FLAIR(黄箭，右图)上可见结节状成分。

- Hemangioblastoma is a highly vascular WHO grade 1 tumor that is the most common primary brain neoplasm in the posterior fossa in adults, usually presenting in young to middle-aged adults.
- Hemangioblastoma occurs most commonly in the cerebellum, followed by spinal cord (discussed in the "Spine" chapter), brainstem, and retina. It only rarely occurs supratentorially.
- About 25% of patients with hemangioblastoma have von Hippel-Lindau (VHL) disease. In turn, most patients with VHL have hemangioblastomas, sometimes multiple.
- The classic appearance of hemangioblastoma is a cystic mass with an avidly enhancing mural nodule. Prominent vessels are often seen as tubular areas of flow-void. Less commonly, a hemangioblastoma may be solid or hemorrhagic.

- 血管母细胞瘤是一种富血供的WHO 1级肿瘤，是成人颅后窝最常见的原发性脑肿瘤，通常在年轻人和中年人发病。
- 血管母细胞瘤最常见于小脑，其次是脊髓(在"脊柱影像"一章进行讨论)、脑干和视网膜。很少在幕上发生。
- 约25%的血管母细胞瘤患者患有冯·希佩尔-林道病(VHL)(脑视网膜血管瘤病)。相对的，大多数VHL患者也都有血管母细胞瘤，有时是多发的。
- 典型的血管母细胞瘤为囊性肿块伴明显强化的壁结节。常能看到非常明显的血管，表现为管状流空区域。少数情况下，血管母细胞瘤可表现为实性或出血性。

Diffuse midline glioma, H3 *K27M*-mutant

弥漫性中线胶质瘤，H3 *K27M*-突变体

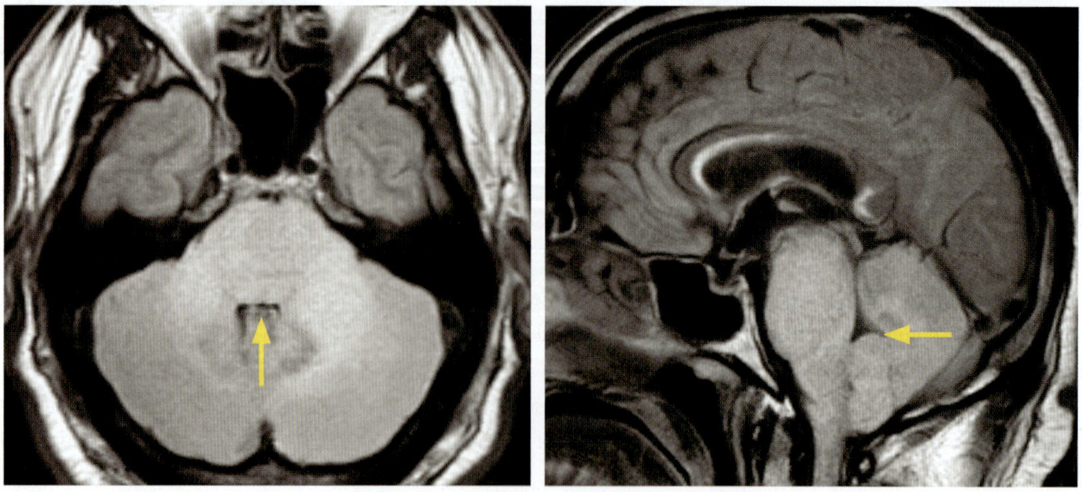

Diffuse brainstem glioma: Axial and sagittal FLAIR images demonstrate an expansile, T2 hyperintense mass centered in the pons with involvement of the entire brainstem, cerebellar peduncles, and bilateral cerebellar hemispheres. The mass does not restrict or enhance (not shown). There is resultant obstructive hydrocephalus due to compression of the fourth ventricle (arrows).

弥漫性脑干胶质瘤：轴位和矢状位FLAIR图像显示以脑桥为中心的膨胀性T_2高信号肿块，累及整个脑干、小脑脚和双侧小脑半球。肿块无弥散受限或增强(未展示)。第四脑室受压导致梗阻性脑积水(黄箭)。

- Most diffuse gliomas affecting children and young adults in the brainstem, especially pons, and thalamus are IDH-wildtype grade 4 tumors characterized molecularly by an histone H3 lysine-to-methionine substitution at residue 27.
- In the absence of biopsy allowing for molecular classification, the most common pediatric brainstem tumor was historically known as **diffuse intrinsic pontine glioma** or **diffuse brainstem glioma**.
- Diffuse midline gliomas typically appear as an expansile, solid or infiltrative mass in the brainstem or diencephalon that is hyperintense on FLAIR. Contrast enhancement is variable.
- This location-specific, molecular classification is associated with poor prognosis. Imaging does not reliably distinguish H3 *K27M*-mutant and wildtype tumors, but the former is most common in the appropriate age group and location.

- 大多数儿童和年轻人的脑干胶质瘤，尤其是累及脑桥和丘脑的胶质瘤是IDH野生型4级肿瘤，其分子学特征为残基27处的组蛋白被H3赖氨酸-甲硫氨酸取代。
- 在出现活检分子分类诊断之前，最常见的小儿脑干肿瘤曾被称为**弥漫性内生性脑桥胶质瘤或弥漫性脑干胶质瘤**。
- 弥漫性中线胶质瘤通常表现为脑干或间脑内出现一个膨胀、实性或有浸润性的肿块，FLAIR表现为高信号。对比增强呈多样性。
- 这种特定位置，分子分类与不良预后相关。影像不能可靠区分H3 *K27M*突变型和野生型肿瘤，但前者常见于相应的年龄组和病变的位置。

Pilocytic astrocytoma / juvenile pilocytic astrocytoma (JPA)

毛细胞型星形细胞瘤/青少年毛细胞型星形细胞瘤(JPA)

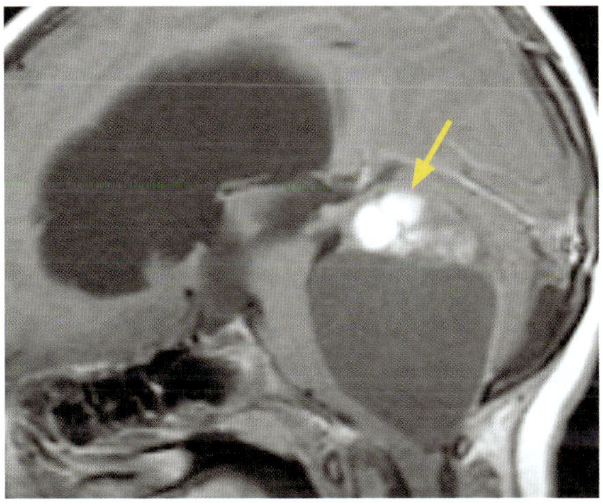

JPA: Sagittal post-contrast T1-weighted MRI shows a large posterior fossa cystic lesion with a superior heterogeneously enhancing solid component (arrow). The fourth ventricle is completely effaced, the brainstem is deformed, and there is severe hydrocephalus.

JPA：矢状位增强T_1加权MRI显示颅后窝巨大囊性灶，其上方为不均匀强化的实性成分(黄箭)。第四脑室完全消失，脑干变形，有严重脑积水。

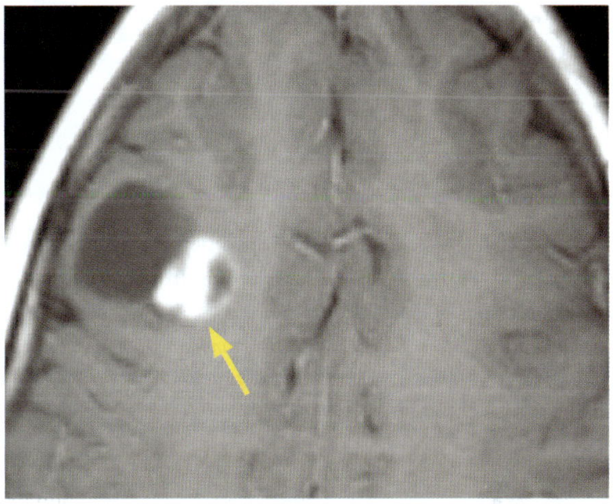

JPA in a different patient: Axial post-contrast T1- weighted MRI shows a cystic lesion in the right frontal lobe with an avidly enhancing solid nodule (arrow). Although the cyst and nodule appearance is typical for JPA, this supratentoriallocation is relatively uncommon.

另一名JPA：轴位增强T_1加权MRI显示右侧额叶囊性灶伴明显强化实性结节(黄箭)。虽然囊与结节是JPA的典型表现，但发生在幕上相对较少见。

- Pilocytic astrocytoma, often called juvenile pilocytic astrocytoma (JPA), is a WHO grade 1 astrocytic tumor. Unlike diffuse gliomas, JPAs are well-circumscribed.
- JPA typically occurs in children, as the name suggests, and is the most common benign brain tumor of childhood.
- The majority occur in the cerebellum. The second most common location of pilocytic astrocytoma is the optic pathway/hypothalamus, which is associated with neurofibromatosis type 1 (NF1) in 1/3 of cases. Posterior fossa JPA is not associated with NF1.
- Greater than 70% of cerebellar JPA carry *BRAF* gene fusions, an important diagnostic marker and potential therapeutic target.
- MRI typically shows a cystic mass with an avidly enhancing nodule and

- 毛细胞型星形细胞瘤，通常被称为青少年毛细胞型星形细胞瘤(JPA)，是WHO 1级星形细胞瘤。与弥漫性胶质瘤不同，JPA具有较为清晰的边界。
- JPA通常在儿童发病，如同它的病名，是儿童最常见的良性脑肿瘤。
- 毛细胞型星形细胞瘤最常发生在小脑。其次是视路/下丘脑，其中1/3病例通常伴1型神经纤维瘤病(NF1)。颅后窝JPA与NF1无关。
- 超过70%的小脑JPA携带*BRAF*基因融合，该基因是重要的诊断性标记和潜在的治疗靶点。
- MRI通常显示囊性肿块伴明显强化结节和

relatively little edema. A minority have little to no cystic component.

- A more aggressive variant is the pilomyxoid astrocytoma, which is not distinguishable on imaging but tends to involve optic chiasm/hypothalamus in younger children and infants.

相对轻度的水肿。少数含有很少或不含囊性成分。

- 毛细胞黏液样星形细胞瘤是一种更具侵袭性的变异，在影像学上无法将其区分，但在幼儿和婴儿中往往累及视交叉/下丘脑。

Ependymoma

室管膜瘤

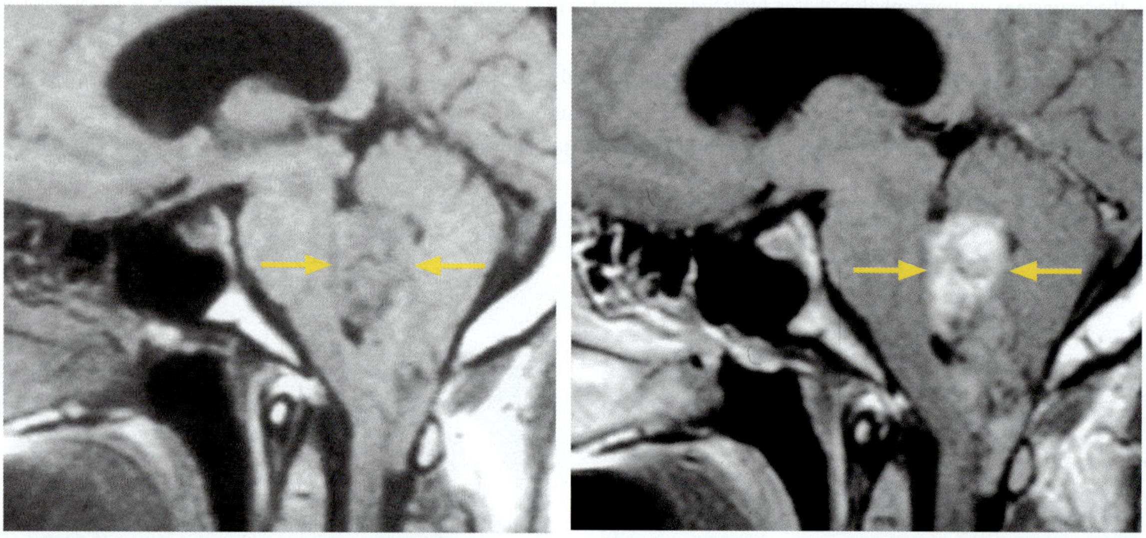

Ependymoma: Precontrast T1-weighted (left image) and post-contrast T1-weighted sagittal MRI (right image) shows a lobulated, isointense, avidly enhancing mass arising from the fourth ventricle (arrows). There is kinking of the brainstem and obstructive hydrocephalus of the third ventricle.

Case courtesy Amir Zamani, MD, Brigham and Women's Hospital.

室管膜瘤：矢状位平扫T_1加权(左图)和增强T_1加权(右图)MRI显示第四脑室内的分叶状、等信号、明显强化肿块(黄箭)。并有脑干扭曲及第三脑室梗阻性脑积水。

- Ependymoma is a WHO grade 2 tumor arising from the ependymal lining of the ventricular system and central canal of the spinal cord. A more aggressive variant is anaplastic ependymoma (grade 3).

  Benign ependymal tumors includesubependymoma (discussed later in this section) and myxopapillary ependymoma (discussed in the "Spine" chapter).

- Ependymoma tends to occur in the posterior fossa in children. In adults, ependymomas occur more commonly in the spinal cord (discussed in the "Spine" chapter) and supratentorium.
- On imaging, ependymomas appear as an enhancing mass with heterogeneity related to cystic/necrotic change, calcification, or hemorrhage.
- The posterior fossa ependymoma has been called the *toothpaste* or *plastic* tumor for its propensity to fill the fourth ventricle and squeeze through the foramina of Magendie or Luschka into the adjacent basal cisterns.

  In contrast, medulloblastoma, which can also fill the fourth ventricle, does not typically squeeze through the foramina.

- 室管膜瘤是 WHO 2级肿瘤，起源于内衬于脑室系统和脊髓中央管的室管膜。间变性室管膜瘤(3级)是一种更具侵袭性的变异。

  良性室管膜肿瘤包括室管膜下瘤(本节后文讨论)和黏液乳头状室管膜瘤(在"脊柱影像"一章讨论)。

- 儿童室管膜瘤往往发生在颅后窝。成人室管膜瘤则更常见于脊髓(在"脊柱影像"一章讨论)和幕上。
- 在影像学上，室管膜瘤表现为不均质的强化肿块，其异质性与囊性/坏死改变、钙化或出血有关。
- 颅后窝室管膜瘤一直被称为"牙膏样或塑料样肿瘤"，因具有填充第四脑室，并经正中孔和侧孔挤压入邻近基底池的倾向。

  相比之下，髓母细胞瘤也可以填充第四脑室，但通常不会挤压入孔。

Subependymoma

室管膜下瘤

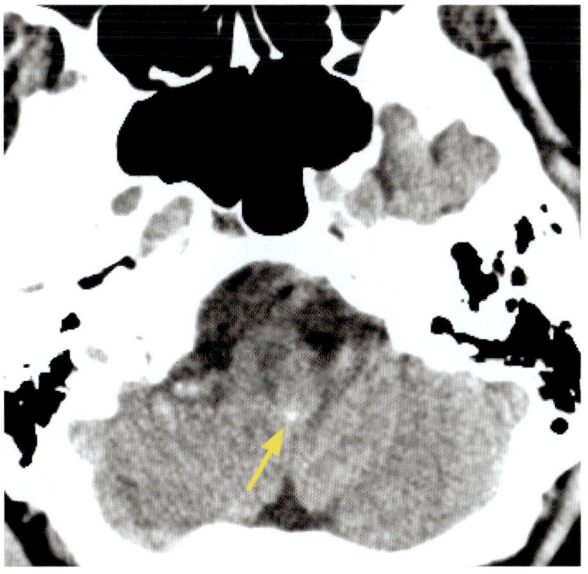

Subependymoma: Noncontrast axial CT shows a subtle focus of hyperattenuation in the region of the cerebellar vermis/fourth ventricle (arrow).

室管膜下瘤：轴位平扫CT显示小脑蚓部/第四脑室区域(黄箭)有一个不易察觉的高密度结节。

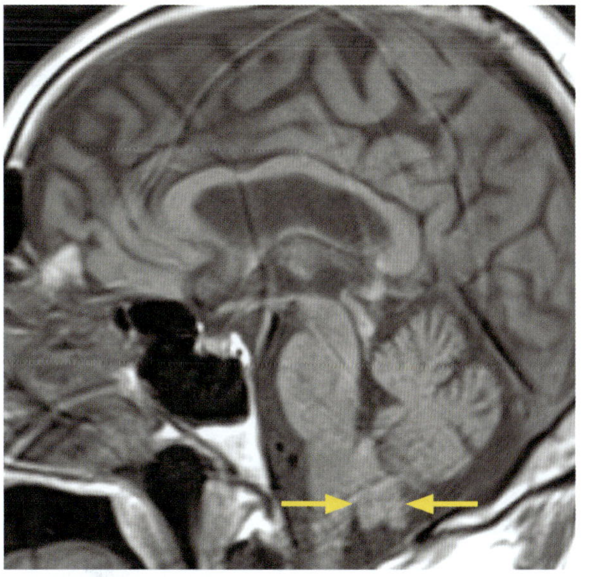

Sagittal T1-weighted MRI shows an isointense mass in the inferior fourth ventricle (arrows). The fourth ventricle is normal in size.

矢状位T_1加权MRI显示第四脑室下方的等信号肿块(黄箭)。第四脑室大小正常。

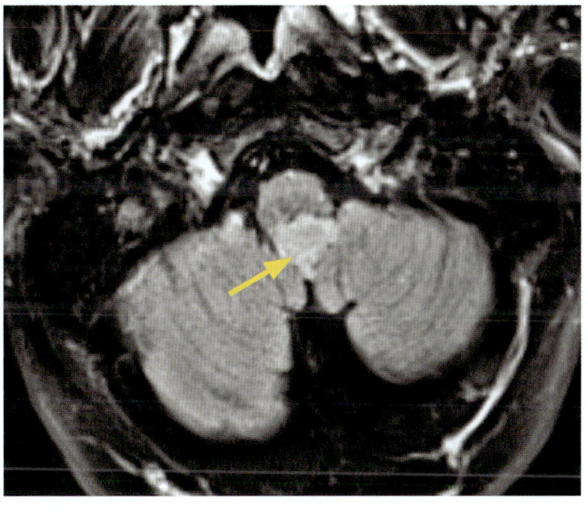

Axial FLAIR shows that the inferior fourth ventricular mass (arrow) is slightly FLAIR hyperintense.

轴位FLAIR显示第四脑室下方的肿块(黄箭)呈稍高信号。

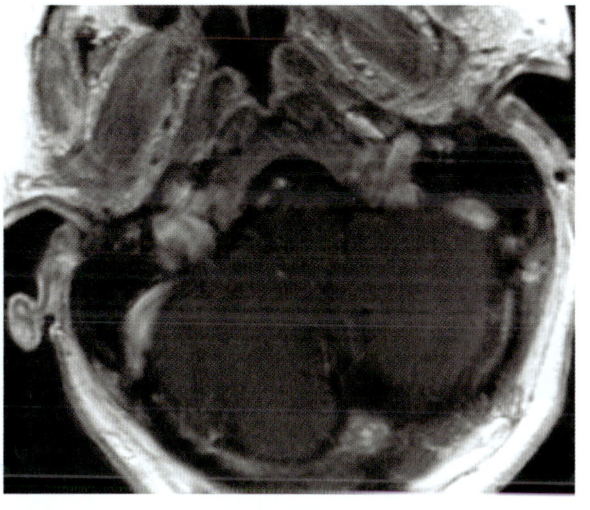

Post-contrast axial T1-weighted MRI shows absolutely no enhancement within the lesion. These lesions can be easily missed on axial T1-weighted images, with or without contrast.

增强轴位T_1加权MRI显示病灶内无任何强化。这些病灶无论在轴位平扫还是增强T_1加权上都很容易漏诊。

- Subependymoma is an indolent, WHO grade 1 tumor of unclear origin that is speculated to arise from subependymal astrocytes, ependymal cells lining the ventricles, or common precursor cells.
- Subependymoma is a tumor of middle-aged and older adults. It is often found incidentally.
- The most common locations are the walls of the fourth and lateral ventricles. The tumor grows exophytically into the ventricle and does not cause parenchymal edema. It usually does not enhance significantly, unlike ependymomas.

- 室管膜下瘤是一种隐匿性且起源不明的WHO 1级肿瘤，可能起源于室管膜下的星形细胞、脑室内衬的室管膜细胞或两者共同的前体细胞。
- 室管膜下瘤是发生于中老年人的肿瘤。通常是偶然的发现。
- 最常见的位置是第四脑室或侧脑室壁。肿瘤以外生性生长进入脑室，不会引起实质水肿。与室管膜瘤不同，它通常不会有显著增强。

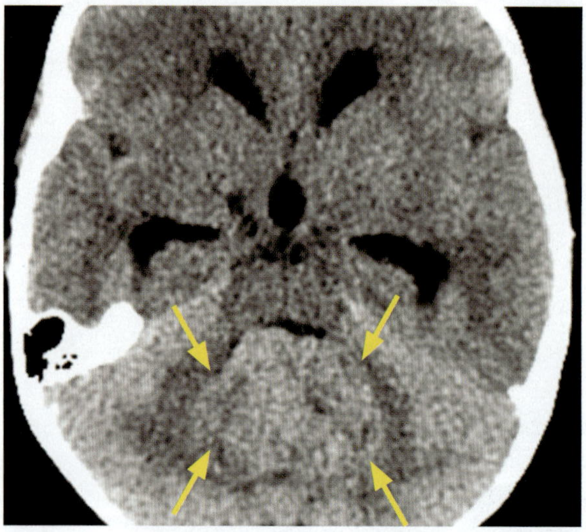

Axial unenhanced CT shows a hyperattenuating mass in the midline posterior fossa (arrows). There is near-complete effacement of the fourth ventricle, with resultant hydrocephalus.
轴位平扫CT显示颅后窝中线处高密度肿块(黄箭)。第四脑室几乎消失伴脑积水。

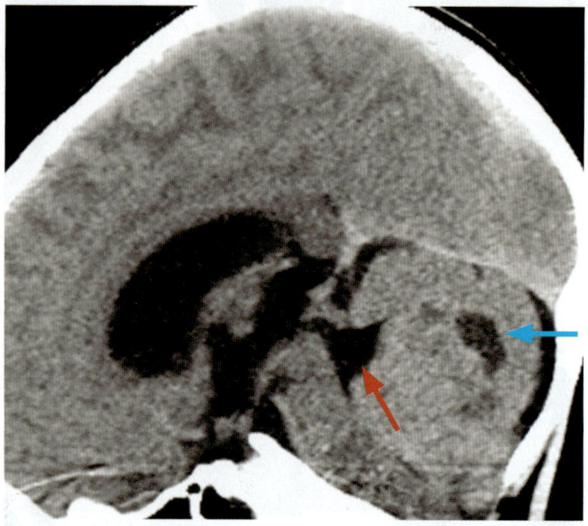

Sagittal unenhanced CT shows that the mass has displaced the fourth ventricle superiorly (red arrow) and contains a cystic component posteriorly (blue arrow).
矢状位平扫CT显示肿块向上推移第四脑室(红箭),肿块后方有囊性成分(蓝箭)。

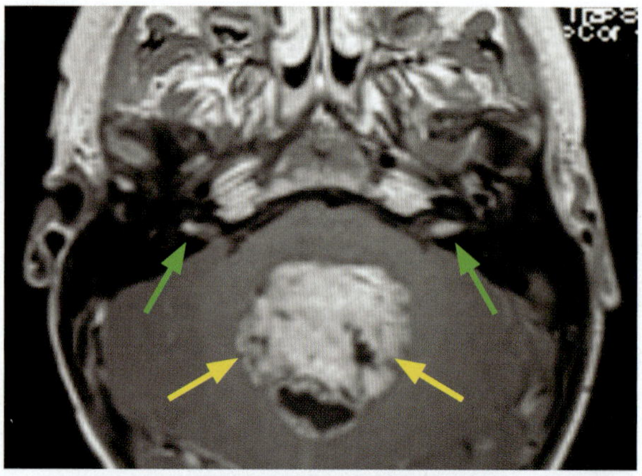

Post-contrast T1-weighted MRI shows the avidly enhancing mass (yellow arrows) completely effacing the fourth ventricle. There is enhancing leptomeningeal tumor dissemination within the internal auditory canals bilaterally (green arrows).
增强T_1加权MRI显示肿块明显强化(黄箭),第四脑室完全消失。双侧内耳道内(绿箭)见强化,为肿瘤柔脑膜转移。

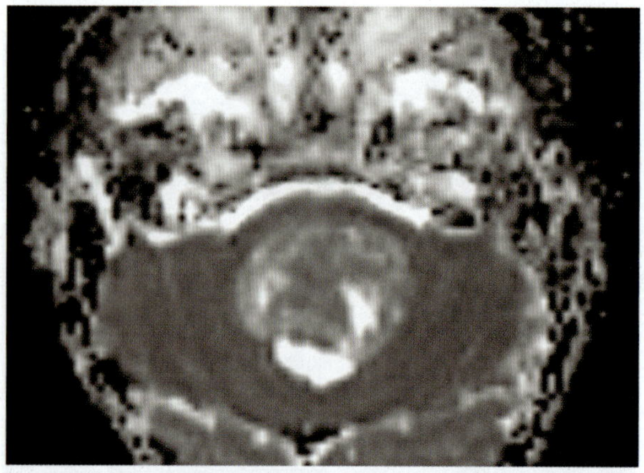

ADC map shows somewhat heterogeneous dark foci within the mass, consistent with hypercellularity.
ADC图显示肿块内少许不均匀低信号灶,与细胞密集有关。

Medulloblastoma. *Case courtesy Gregory Wrubel, MD, Brigham and Women's Hospital.*

- Medulloblastoma is the prototype and most common of the WHO grade 4 embryonal tumors of the CNS,which appear histologically as small round blue cell tumors.
- Medulloblastoma is the most common brain malignancy of childhood, usually diagnosed between the ages of 3 and 10 years. A small proportion are associated with a cancer predisposition syndrome, including Gorlin (-Goltz/basal cell nevus) syndrome, Li-Fraumeni syndrome, and Turcot syndrome in the setting of familial adenomatous polyposis.
- The current WHO classification includes both histological (classic, large cell/anaplastic, desmoplastic/nodular, and extensive nodularity) and molecular

- 髓母细胞瘤是最原始和最常见的WHO 4级中枢神经系统胚胎肿瘤,其组织学上表现为小圆蓝色细胞肿瘤。
- 髓母细胞瘤是儿童最常见的脑部恶性肿瘤,通常在3~10岁确诊。一小部分与癌症易感综合征有关,包括家族性腺瘤性息肉病背景下的Gorlin(Goltz/基底细胞痣)综合征、Li-Fraumeni综合征和Turcot综合征。
- 当前WHO分类包括组织学(经典型、大细胞/间变性、结缔组织增生性/结节性和广泛结节

subgroups (*WNT*-activated, *SHH*-activated, group 3,and group 4) to define prognosis and guide treatment.

In children, group 3 and 4 tumors are most common and are located in the midline (cerebellar vermis) or fourth ventricle.

In infants, SHH-activated tumors are most common and may be located in the cerebellar hemisphere or midline/fourth ventricle.

WNT-activated tumors occur in older children and likely arise from the cerebellopontine angle.

- Medulloblastoma is slightly hyperattenuating on CT due to its densely packed cells and is accordingly hypointense on T2-weighted images and has low ADC values. The tumor enhances, except for possibly group 4 tumors, and may appear heterogeneous due to internal hemorrhage and calcification.

The low ADC values can be a useful finding to differentiate medulloblastoma from ependymoma and pilocytic astrocytoma, the two other most common childhood posterior fossa tumors.

- Leptomeningeal metastatic disease is present in up to 1/3 of patients and medulloblastoma is the most common cause of drop metastases to the spine in children. In this setting, sugar-coating (*Zuckerguss*) refers to the icing-like enhancement over the brain and spinal cord surface. Imaging of the entire brain and spine should be performed prior to surgery. Since medulloblastomas are hypercellular, DWI is particularly helpful in detecting leptomeningeal disease.
- When medulloblastoma occurs in a young adult (as opposed to a child), the tumor tends to arise eccentrically in the posterior fossa, from the cerebellar hemisphere.

Atypical teratoid/rhabdoid tumor (AT/RT)

- Atypical teratoid/rhabdoid tumor (AT/RT) is an uncommon WHO grade 4 embryonal tumor characterized molecularly by loss of *SMARCB1*/INI1 or *SMARCA4*/BRG1 expression.
- AT/RT appears similar to medulloblastoma but is less common and occurs in slightly younger patients. It should be considered as part of the differential for a large brain tumor in children younger than three years of age.
- The majority occur in the cerebellum. Unlike medulloblastoma, however, about a third of cases of AT/RT are supratentorial.

For a large heterogeneous supratentorial mass in an infant/young child, the differential diagnosis includes AT/RT and, less commonly, what was previously known as primitive neuroectodermal tumor (PNET) and is now mostly classified as either (1) embryonal tumor with multilayered rosettes (ETMR), *C19MC*-altered; or (2) CNS embryonal tumor, not otherwise specified.

- A third of patients with AT/RT have germline mutations in *SMARCB1* or *SMARCA4*, resulting in rhabdoid tumor predisposition syndrome, which is also associated with malignant rhabdoid tumor of the kidney.

Dysplastic cerebellar gangliocytoma (Lhermitte-Duclos)

- Dysplastic gangliocytoma of the cerebellum, more often known as Lhermitte-Duclos disease, is a WHO grade 1 neuronal lesion that has been considered a hamartoma by some and neoplasm by others.
- Adult-onset Lhermitte-Duclos disease is often associated with Cowden syndrome (multiple hamartoma syndrome associated with benign mucocutaneous lesions like facial trichilemmomas as well as breast and thyroid cancer), a part of the *PTEN* hamartoma tumor syndrome.
- The characteristic imaging finding is a *corduroy* or *tiger-striped* appearance of thickened folia in the cerebellar hemisphere. The lesion is hyperintense on T2-weighted images and enhancement is rare.

性）和分子学亚组(WNT-激活型、SHH-激活型、第3组和第4组)，以确定预后和指导治疗。

在儿童，第3组和第4组肿瘤最常见，并位于中线(小脑蚓部)或第四脑室。

在婴儿，SHH-激活型肿瘤最常见，可能位于小脑半球或中线/第四脑室。

WNT-激活型肿瘤发生在年龄较大的儿童，可能起源于桥小脑角。

- 髓母细胞瘤在CT上呈稍高密度，因其细胞密集，在T_2加权上呈相对应低信号，且ADC值低。肿瘤强化(第4组肿瘤可能除外)，因其内部出血和钙化而可能表现为异质性。

低ADC值对鉴别髓母细胞瘤和室管膜瘤、毛细胞型星形细胞瘤有帮助，后两者为最常见的儿童颅后窝肿瘤。

- 高达1/3的髓母细胞瘤患者有柔脑膜转移，也是儿童脊髓脱落转移最常见的原因。糖衣征(Zuckerguss)是指脑和脊髓表面出现结冰状强化。术前应该对全脑及脊柱进行影像学检查。由于髓母细胞瘤细胞密集，DWI有助于检测柔脑膜病变。
- 当髓母细胞瘤发生在年轻人(而非儿童)时，肿瘤起源于小脑，倾向于发生在颅后窝偏侧。

非典型畸胎样/横纹肌样瘤(AT/RT)

- 非典型畸胎样/横纹肌样瘤(AT/RT)是一种少见的WHO 4级胚胎性肿瘤，其分子特征是*SMARCB1*/INI1或*SMARCA4*/BRG1表达缺失。
- AT/RT的表现类似髓母细胞瘤，但不太常见且发病年龄偏小。3岁以下儿童若出现巨大肿瘤应该将其作为鉴别诊断的一部分。
- 大多数发生在小脑。与髓母细胞瘤不同，约1/3的AT/RT病例发生在幕上。

婴儿/幼儿巨大、异质性幕上肿块，其鉴别诊断包括AT/RT和较少见的以前称为原始神经外胚层肿瘤(PNET)，现在主要分为：①多层菊形团胚胎性肿瘤(ETMR)、*C19MC*-变异型；或②中枢神经系统胚胎性肿瘤，除非另行说明。

- 约1/3的AT/RT患者存在*SMARCB1*或*SMARCA4*种系突变，其导致横纹肌样肿瘤易感综合征，该综合征也与肾恶性横纹肌样瘤相关。

小脑发育不良性神经节细胞瘤(莱尔米特-杜克洛病)

- 小脑发育不良性神经节细胞瘤，通常被称为莱尔米特-杜克洛病，是一种WHO 1级神经元病变，有些人认为是错构瘤，另一些人则认为是恶性肿瘤。
- 成人型莱尔米特-杜克洛病常与考登综合征(多发性错构瘤综合征伴良性黏膜皮肤病变，如面部毛细胞瘤，以及乳腺癌和甲状腺癌)有关，是PTEN错构瘤综合征的一部分。
- 特征性影像学表现为小脑半球增厚的脑叶呈灯芯绒或虎斑纹状改变。病灶在T_2加权上呈高信号，罕见强化。

Posterior fossa mass in a child
儿童颅后窝肿瘤

- (Most common pediatric brain tumor)
  (最常见的小儿脑肿瘤)
  Hyperattenuating on CT?Low ADC on MR?
  CT上高密度？ MR上ADC值低？
  → **Medulloblastoma** 髓母细胞瘤
- *Cystic mass with an enhancing mural nodule?*
  囊性肿块伴强化的壁结节？
  → **Juvenile pilocytic astrocytoma** 青少年毛细胞型星形细胞瘤
- *Intra-ventricular mass?*
  脑室占位？
  Pushes through fourth ventricular foramina?
  钻过第四脑室孔
  → **Ependymoma** 室管膜瘤
- *Cystic mass with enhancing mural nodule and flow voids?*
  History of von Hippel-Lindau?
  囊性肿块伴有强化的壁结节和流空血管？ VHL综合征病史？
  → **Hemangioblastoma** 血管母细胞瘤
- *Slightly younger age than medulloblastoma, with similar imaging of an aggressive, heterogeneous mass?Renal mass present?*
  年龄稍小于髓母细胞瘤患者，有相似的侵袭性不均匀肿块的表现？有肾脏肿块？
  → **Atypical teratoid/rhabdoid tumor** 非典型畸胎瘤样/横纹肌样瘤

Posterior fossa mass in an adult
成人颅后窝肿瘤

- *History of primary malignancy?*
  原发恶性肿瘤病史？
  Enhancing mass with edema? Multiple lesions?
  强化的肿块伴水肿?多发病灶？
  → **Metastasis** 转移瘤
- *Cystic mass with enhancing mural nodule and flow voids?*
  History of von Hippel-Lindau?
  囊性肿块伴有强化的壁结节和流空血管？ VHL综合征病史？
  → **Hemangioblastoma** 血管母细胞瘤
- *Minimal or little enhancement?*
  轻微或无强化？
  → **Astrocytoma** 星形细胞瘤
- *Young adult?Lateral location?*
  年轻患者？ 偏中心位置？
  → **Medulloblastoma** 髓母细胞瘤

Intra-axial Cystic Mass with a Mural Nodule: Differential Diagnosis

轴内囊性肿块伴壁结节：鉴别诊断

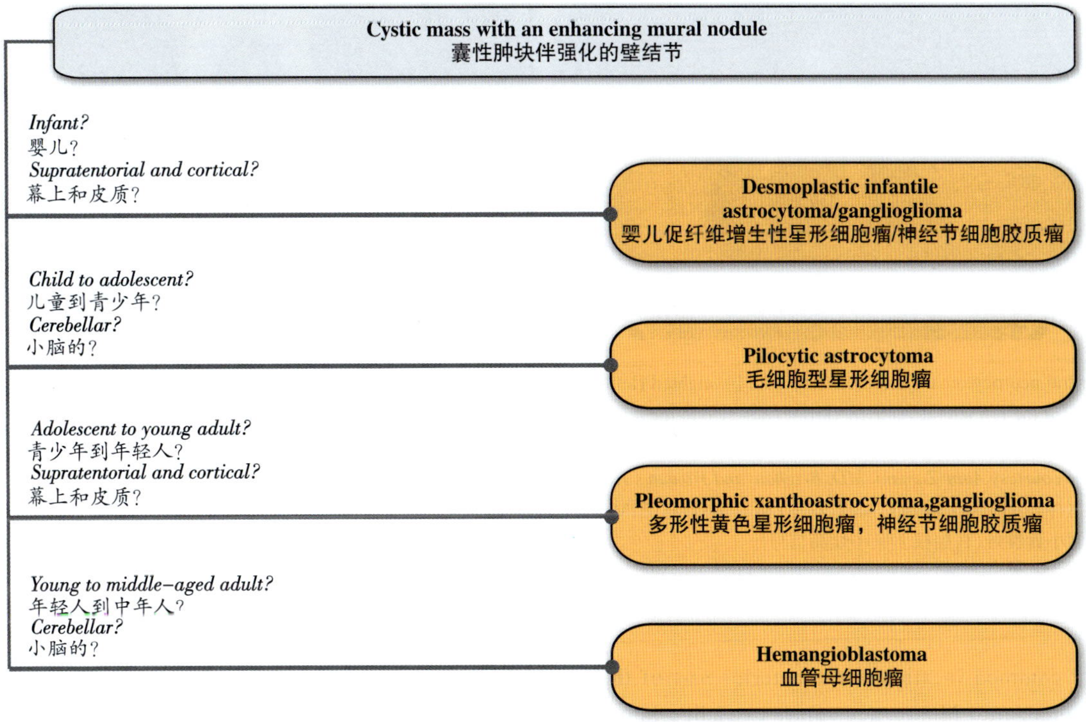

Intraventricular Tumors

Overview

- Most of the aforementioned intra-axial posterior fossa tumors (especially ependymoma, subependymoma, medulloblastoma) can protrude into the ventricle and should be considered in the differential diagnosis of an intraventricular mass.
- Aside from periventricular tumors, other sites of origin of intraventricular tumors include the septum pellucidum and choroid plexus.
- Aside from neoplasms, the differential of intraventricular masses includes developmental/ degenerative cysts, which do not enhance.
- Intraventricular tumors can cause obstructive hydrocephalus.

脑室内肿瘤

概述

- 大多数上述轴内颅后窝肿瘤(尤其是室管膜瘤、室管膜下瘤、髓母细胞瘤)可突出到脑室内，应该与脑室内肿块进行鉴别。
- 除脑室周围肿瘤外，脑室内肿瘤的其他起源部位包括透明隔和脉络丛。
- 除肿瘤外，脑室内肿块的鉴别包括无强化的发育性/退行性囊肿。
- 脑室内肿瘤可导致梗阻性脑积水。

Central neurocytoma

中枢神经细胞瘤

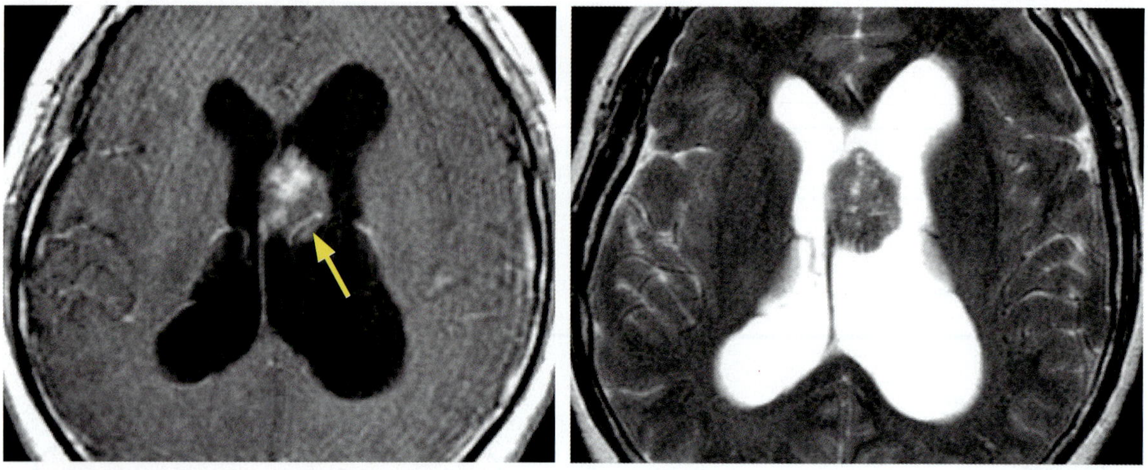

Central neurocytoma: Contrast-enhanced T1-weighted (left image) and T2-weighted (right) MRI demonstrates a lobulated mass in the body of the left lateral ventricle (arrow) attached to the septum pellucidum. The mass enhances and contains foci of cystic change (seen as hyperintense foci on the T2-weighted image).

Case courtesy Amir Zamani, MD, Brigham and Women's Hospital.

中枢神经细胞瘤：增强T_1加权(左图)和T_2加权(右图)MRI显示左侧脑室体部(黄箭)分叶状肿块，紧贴于透明隔。肿块有强化，内含小囊性灶(T_2加权上呈小灶高信号)。

- Central neurocytoma is a WHO grade 2 neuronal tumor that occurs in young adults.
- The most common location is the anterior part of the lateral ventricle near the foramen of Monro, sometimes extending into the third ventricle. Extraventricular neurocytomas are rare.
- Typical imaging findings are a heterogeneous, multicystic (*bubbly* or *Swiss cheese* appearing), lobulated, moderately enhancing mass attached to the septum pellucidum. Calcification is common.

- 中枢神经细胞瘤是发生在年轻人的一种WHO 2级神经元肿瘤。
- 最常见的位置是侧脑室前方近室间孔，有时延伸至第三脑室。脑室外神经细胞瘤罕见。
- 典型的影像学表现为异质性、多囊性(多泡或瑞士奶酪状)、分叶状、中度强化的肿块，紧贴透明隔。常见钙化。

Intraventricular meningioma

脑室内脑膜瘤

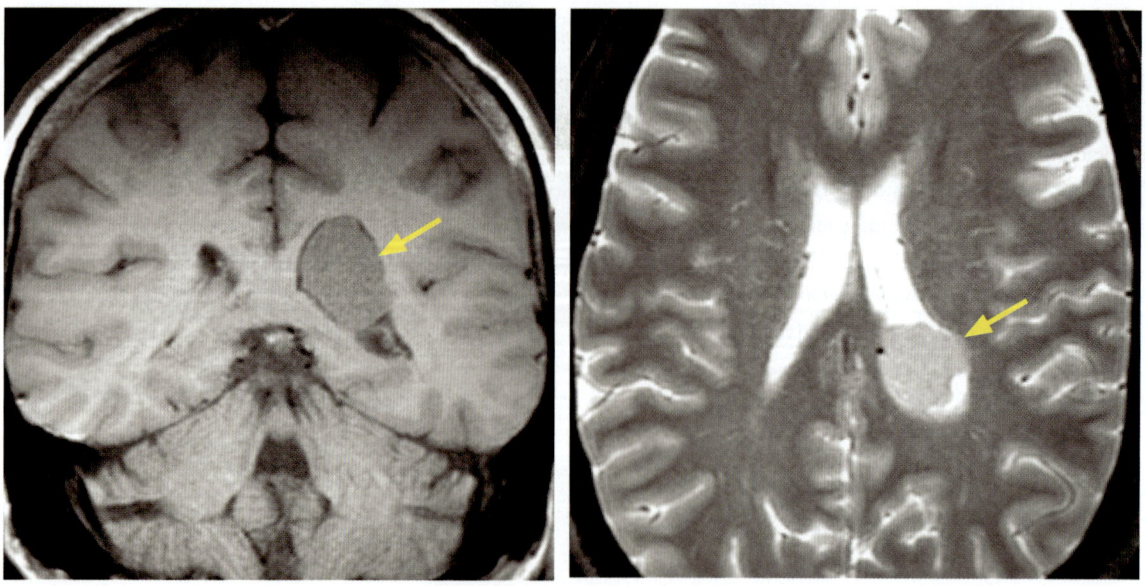

Intraventricular meningioma: Coronal T1-weighted (left image) and axial T2-weighted (right image) MRI shows a T1 hypointense, T2 slightly hyperintense mass (arrows) in the atrium of the left ventricle.

Case courtesy Mary Beth Cunnane, MD, Massachusetts Eye and Ear Infirmary.

脑室内脑膜瘤：冠状位T_1加权(左图)和轴位T_2加权(右图)MRI显示左侧脑室三角区T_1加权低信号、T_2加权稍高信号肿块(黄箭)。

- Intraventricular meningioma appears as a solid mass, typically in the trigone of the lateral ventricle. It tends to occur in older patients, similar to other meningiomas.
- Intraventricular meningiomas are typically hypercellular and homogeneously enhance, distinguishing them from other intraventricular neoplasms.

Subependymal giant cell astrocytoma (SEGA)

- Subependymal giant cell astrocytoma (SEGA) is a benign (WHO grade 1) astrocytoma variant that is associated with tuberous sclerosis complex. Other common intracranial findings in tuberous sclerosis includesubependymal nodules (hamartomas), cortical/subcortical tubers, and white matter radial bands.
- SEGA classically is an enhancing, heterogeneous mass in the lateral ventricle near the foramen of Monro.
- SEGA is distinguished from subependymal nodules at the caudothalamic groove by serial growth or size >1 cm.

Choroid plexus xanthogranuloma

- Choroid plexus xanthogranuloma is the most common choroid plexus mass in adults. Also known as degenerative choroid plexus cyst, they represent collections of cholesterol and lipid-laden histiocytes.
- They are usually located in the atria of the lateral ventricles.
- On MRI, they are hyperintense on T2-weighted images, do not attenuate completely on FLAIR, and restrict diffusion.

Choroid plexus tumors

- 脑室内脑膜瘤表现为实性肿块，通常发生于侧脑室三角区。与其他脑膜瘤一样，其往往发生于老年患者。
- 脑室内脑膜瘤通常细胞致密，强化均匀，由此可与其他脑室肿瘤相鉴别。

室管膜下巨细胞星形细胞瘤(SEGA)

- SEGA是良性的(WHO 1级)星形细胞瘤变异，与结节性硬化综合征相关。结节性硬化的其他常见颅内表现包括室管膜下结节(错构瘤)、皮层/皮层下结节和白质辐射带。
- SEGA通常为侧脑室内强化不均的肿块，位于室间孔附近。
- SEGA与位于丘脑尾状沟室管膜下的结节的鉴别点在于其连续生长或尺寸>1cm。

脉络丛黄色肉芽肿

- 脉络丛黄色肉芽肿是成年人最常见的脉络丛肿块，也被称为退行性脉络丛囊肿，是富含胆固醇和脂质的组织细胞团。
- 通常位于侧脑室房部(三角区)。
- 在MRI上表现为T_2加权高信号，FLAIR不会完全衰减，并且弥散受限。

脉络丛肿瘤

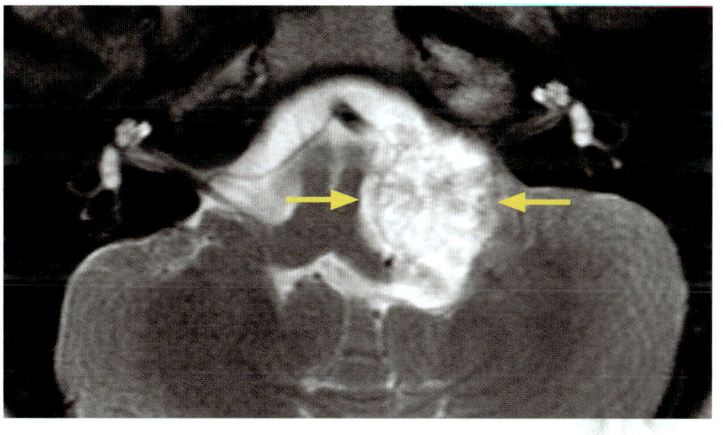

Choroid plexus papilloma: Axial T2-weighted image shows a hyperintense, cauliflower- like mass (arrows) in the left cerebellomedullary fissure deforming the medulla. The center of the mass is at the foramen of Luschka, which is likely its location of origin.

Case courtesy Sanjay Prabhu, MD, Boston Children's Hospital.

脉络丛乳头状瘤：轴位T_2加权显示左侧小脑延髓裂有高信号菜花状的肿块(黄箭)，延髓变形。肿块的中央位于Luschka孔，这可能是病灶起源位置。

- Choroid plexus tumors consist of, in decreasing frequency, choroid plexus papilloma (WHO grade 1), atypical choroid plexus papilloma (grade 2), and choroid plexus carcinoma (grade 3). These are not reliably distinguishable on imaging.
- Choroid plexus papilloma most commonly occurs in infants and young children, but it may also occur in adults.
- Choroid plexus tumors arise from choroid plexus epithelium and are therefore entirely intraventricular in location.

  In children, the atrium of the lateral ventricle is the most common location.

  In adults, the fourth ventricle is the most common location.

  Less commonly, choroid plexus papilloma may arise from the third ventricle or cerebellomedullary angle, as in the case shown.
- The characteristic appearance on MRI is a *cauliflower-like* intraventricular mass that avidly enhances. Higher grade is associated with larger size and more extensive surrounding white matter edema.

- 脉络丛肿瘤按发病率下降的顺序依次为脉络丛乳头状瘤(WHO 1级)、非典型脉络丛乳头状瘤(2级)和脉络丛癌(3级)。在影像上无法将它们可靠地区分。
- 脉络丛乳头状瘤最常见于婴幼儿，但也可能发生在成人。
- 脉络丛肿瘤起源于脉络丛上皮，因此完全位于脑室内。

  在儿童，侧脑室三角区是最好发的部位。

  在成人，第四脑室是最好发的部位。

  少数情况下，脉络丛乳头状瘤可起源于第三脑室或小脑延髓角，如上述病例所示。
- MRI特征性表现为脑室内菜花状肿块，有明显强化。更高等级与更大体积和更广泛的周围白质水肿相关。

Chordoid glioma

- Chordoid glioma is a rare WHO grade 2 glial tumor that arises from ependymal cells of the lamina terminalis.
- The tumor is distinctively located in the anterior third ventricle, associated with the hypothalamus.
- Chordoid glioma is a circumscribed, ovoid, homogeneously enhancing mass that is hyperattenuating on CT and slightly hyperintense on T2-weighted MRI.

Colloid cyst

- Colloid cysts are benign developmental lesions that are usually incidental findings and account for the most common mass of the foramina of Monro.
- Colloid cyst is a circumscribed, nonenhancing lesion characteristically arising from the anterior roof of the third ventricle.
- The *machine oil-like* contents appear hyperattenuating on CT and low signal intensity on T2- weighted images.

Intraventricular simple cysts

- Intraventricular simple cysts include several histologies that may be difficult to distinguish on imaging, including ependymal cyst, arachnoid cyst (more common in the subarachnoid space external to the brain), neuroepithelial/ neuroglial cyst (more commonly intraparenchymal), and choroid plexus cyst (occurring antenatally and regressing at birth).
- Simple cysts follow CSF signal on all sequences, including FLAIR, and do not demonstrate restricted diffusion.

脊索样胶质瘤

- 脊索样神经胶质瘤是一种罕见的 WHO 2 级神经胶质瘤，起源于终板的室管膜细胞。
- 肿瘤特征性地位于第三脑室前部，与下丘脑相连。
- 脊索样胶质瘤是一种边界清楚、卵圆形、均匀强化的肿块，在CT上呈高密度，在 T_2加权上呈稍高信号。

胶样囊肿

- 胶样囊肿是良性发育性病变，通常是偶然发现，是室间孔最常见的肿块。
- 胶样囊肿是一种边界清楚、无强化的病变，其特征是起源于第三脑室前顶。
- 机油样内容物在CT上表现为高密度，在T_2加权上表现为低信号。

脑室内单纯性囊肿

- 脑室内单纯性囊肿有数种组织学类型，包括室管膜囊肿、蛛网膜囊肿(更常见于脑外蛛网膜下腔)、神经上皮/神经胶质囊肿(更常见于脑实质内)，脉络丛囊肿(出生前发生，出生时消退)，它们在影像学上可能难以区分。
- 单纯性囊肿在所有序列(包括FLAIR)与CSF信号一致，并且没有弥散受限。

CNS LYMPHOMA

Primary CNS lymphoma (PCNSL): Overview

- Primary CNS lymphoma (PCNSL) is lymphoma isolated to the CNS, most commonly diffuse large B-cell lymphoma. Immature blast cells form lymphoid aggregates around small cerebral blood vessels in a periventricular location. Note that the brain does not contain native lymphoid tissue.
- PCNSL is known to "melt away" with chemoradiation but a subset tends to recur aggressively.
- The appearance of PCNSL depends on the immune status of the patient. Regardless of immune status, however, key imaging findings are a periventricular location, high cellularity (hyperattenuating on CT, relatively hypointense on T2-weighted images, and reduced diffusivity), and contrast enhancement. The lesions may be solitary or multiple. Vasogenic edema is common.
- Intralesional hemorrhage in untreated PCNSL is extremely rare and can be a very helpful sign to differentiate PCNSL from glioblastomas, which commonly show microhemorrhages.

中枢神经系统淋巴瘤

原发性中枢神经系统淋巴瘤(PCNSL): 概述

- PCNSL是仅发生于中枢神经系统的淋巴瘤，最常见的是弥漫性大B细胞淋巴瘤。未分化的母细胞围绕脑室周围小的脑血管呈淋巴样聚集。注意，脑不含原始淋巴组织。
- PCNSL因可以被放化疗"溶解"而为大家所熟知，但其中一小部分极其容易复发。
- PCNSL的表现取决于患者的免疫状态。但无论何种免疫状态，关键的影像学表现都包括病变位于脑室周围、细胞高度密集(CT上呈高密度，T_2加权上呈相对低信号，且弥散受限)和对比增强。病变可能是单发或多发。血管源性水肿很常见。
- PCNSL病灶内出血在未经治疗的患者中极为罕见，可以作为区分PCNSL和胶质母细胞瘤的一个非常有用的征象，后者通常表现为微出血。

Primary CNS lymphoma: Immunocompetent patient

原发性中枢神经系统淋巴瘤：免疫正常患者

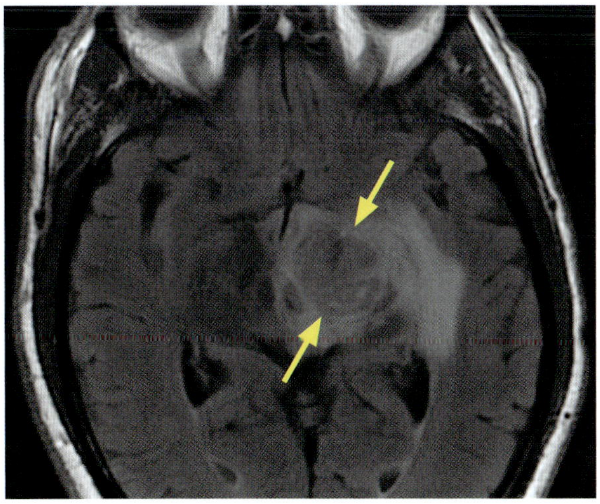

Axial FLAIR MRI demonstrates a heterogeneous mass (arrows) in the left basal ganglia with associated vasogenic edema.
轴位FLAIR MRI显示左侧基底节不均匀的肿块(黄箭)，伴血管源性水肿。

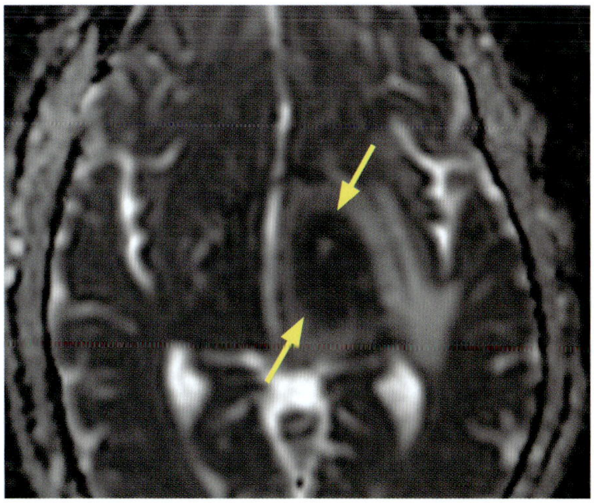

ADC map shows that the epicenter of the mass is dark (arrows), suggestive of reduced diffusivity due to hypercellularity.
ADC图显示肿块的偏心部位呈低信号(黄箭)，提示细胞致密所致的弥散受限。

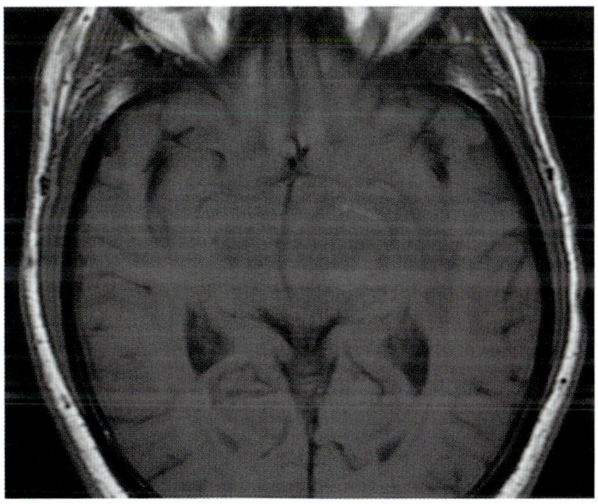

Pre-contrast T1-weighted image shows that the mass is T1 isointense.
平扫T_1加权MRI显示肿块呈等信号。

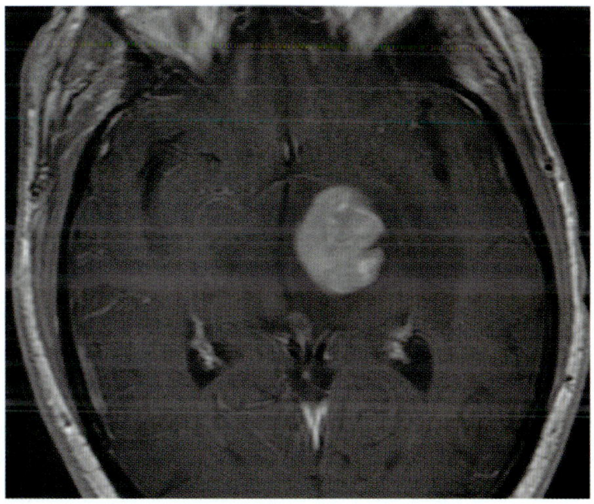

Post-contrast axial T1-weighted MRI shows intense, relatively homogeneous enhancement of the mass. There is no appreciable central necrosis.
增强T_1加权MRI显示肿块呈明显、相对均匀强化，中心无明显坏死。

Primary CNS lymphoma. *Case courtesy Gregory Wrubel, MD, Brigham and Women's Hospital.*

- In an immunocompetent patient, PCNSL typically presents as an **homogeneously enhancing mass**.
- Involvement of the frontal lobes and basal ganglia is most common, but it can be centered also in the brainstem and cerebellum. Transcallosal infiltration can occur, which is called a *butterfly lesion*.

  The differential diagnosis for a mass involving the corpus callosum includes lymphoma, glioblastoma, and demyelinatinglesion.

- 在免疫功能正常的患者中，PCNSL通常表现为均匀强化的肿块。
- 额叶和基底节最常受累，但也可能集中在脑干和小脑。可跨胼胝体浸润，称为蝶形病变。

  胼胝体肿块的鉴别诊断包括淋巴瘤、胶质母细胞瘤和脱髓鞘病变。

Primary CNS lymphoma: Immunocompromised patient

- Immunodeficiency-related CNS lymphoma is associated with EBV infection.

原发性中枢神经系统淋巴瘤：免疫低下患者

- 免疫缺陷相关的中枢神经系统淋巴瘤与EB病毒感染有关。

- In an immunocompromised patient, PCNSL typically presents as an irregular, **ring-enhancing** lesion. The ring enhancement is caused by central necrosis.
- The most common causes of ring-enhancing brain masses in patients with HIV/AIDS are lymphoma and toxoplasmosis. These lesions are usually multiple, although a single large lesion is more likely to represent lymphoma. Several clinical and imaging options are available to differentiate between lymphoma and toxoplasmosis:

Empirical anti-toxoplasmosis therapy and short-interval follow-up imaging.
MR DWI: Lymphoma tends to restrict diffusion more than toxoplasmosis does.
MR perfusion: Lymphoma has higher rCBV than toxoplasmosis.
MR spectroscopy: Lymphoma shows elevated choline compared to toxoplasmosis.
FDG PET: Lymphoma has higher glucose metabolism than toxoplasmosis does.
Thallium SPECT: Lymphoma more avidly takes up thallium than toxoplasmosis does.

Secondary CNS lymphoma

- Secondary CNS lymphoma represents involvement of the CNS in a patient with known systemic lymphoma.
- Secondary CNS lymphoma is more commonly extra-axial, involving leptomeninges, dura, and/or skull. Less commonly, it may present as a parenchymal mass.

METASTATIC DISEASE

Overview

- The most common primary tumors to cause intracranial metastases are lung cancer, breast cancer, and melanoma.
- Brain parenchymal metastases are more common than meningeal metastases.
- Brain metastases are more common than primary brain malignancies in adults.

Intra-axial metastasis

- Most parenchymal metastases are hematogenous and arise at the gray-white matter junction, where there is a caliber change in the small arterioles.
- Enhancement is universal, as capillaries produced by an extra-CNS primary tumor do not have a functioning blood-brain barrier.
- Larger metastases often feature marked edema, while small metastases may present as tiny enhancing foci that are apparent only on the post-contrast images.

  Factors that increase lesion conspicuity on contrast-enhanced imaging include higher contrast dose, gadolinium-based contrast agent with greater relaxivity, delayed imaging after contrast injection, and higher magnetic field strength.

- The most common hemorrhagic metastases to the brain are melanoma, renal cell carcinoma,choriocarcinoma, and thyroid cancer (especially papillary carcinoma). Breast and lung cancer are also included in this differential due to their high prevalence, although hemorrhagic metastases are an atypical presentation.

  The main causes of a solitary hemorrhagic brain neoplasm are metastatic carcinomas and glioblastoma.

  Tumorous intracerebral hemorrhage may be difficult to distinguish initially from primary intracerebral hemorrhage (such as due to hypertension or amyloid angiopathy)

- 在免疫低下患者中，PCNSL常表现为不规则、**环形强化**病灶。环形强化是由中央坏死引起的。
- 在人类免疫缺陷病毒感染/获得性免疫缺陷综合征(HIV/AIDS)患者中，环形强化脑肿块最常见的病因是淋巴瘤和弓形虫病。这些病变通常是多发的，但单个巨大的病变则更有可能是淋巴瘤。有多种临床和影像学方法可以用来鉴别淋巴瘤和弓形虫病：

经验性抗弓形虫治疗和短期影像学随访。
MR DWI：淋巴瘤较弓形虫病更容易出现弥散受限。
MR灌注：淋巴瘤的rCBV高于弓形虫病。
MR波谱：淋巴瘤的胆碱高于弓形虫病。
FDG PET：淋巴瘤的糖代谢高于弓形虫病。
铊SPECT：淋巴瘤的铊摄取明显高于弓形虫病。

继发性中枢神经系统淋巴瘤

- 继发性中枢神经系统淋巴瘤是指患者已知的系统性淋巴瘤累及到中枢神经系统。
- 继发性中枢神经系统淋巴瘤更常见于轴外，可累及柔脑膜、硬脑膜和/或颅骨。很少表现为实质内肿块。

转移性病变

概述

- 引起颅内转移常见的原发肿瘤包括肺癌、乳腺癌和黑色素瘤。
- 脑实质转移比脑膜转移更常见。
- 成人脑转移瘤比原发性脑恶性肿瘤更常见。

轴内(脑实质内)转移瘤

- 大多数脑实质转移是血源性，并起源于灰白质交界区，因为此处脑小动脉管径出现变化。
- 所有轴内转移瘤都有强化，因为中枢神经外的原发肿瘤所产生的毛细血管没有血脑屏障功能。
- 较大的转移瘤往往有明显的水肿，而小的转移瘤只能在增强图像上可以显示微小的强化灶。

  在对比增强影像中提高病变检出率的方法包括增加造影剂的剂量、使用更高弛豫性的钆造影剂、延迟成像，以及提高磁场强度。

- 最常见的脑出血性转移瘤是黑色素瘤、肾细胞癌、绒毛膜癌和甲状腺癌(尤其是乳头状癌)。出血在转移性乳腺癌和肺癌中是一种不典型表现，但由于其高患病率也应被列入鉴别中。

  孤立性出血性脑肿瘤的主要原因是转移性癌和胶质母细胞瘤。

  肿瘤性脑出血早期可能难以与原发性脑出血(如

but should be suspected by the presence of an enhancing component or failure to resolve on follow-up.

由于高血压或淀粉样血管病)区别，但若出现增强成分或随访时未能消失应该对此有所怀疑。

Extra-axial metastasis

- Leptomeningeal metastases, also known as carcinomatous meningitis, appears as serpentine contrast enhancement at the pial surface of the brain. FLAIR shows sulcal hyperintensity.

  The main causes of leptomeningeal enhancement and sulcal FLAIR hyperintensity are infectious/ inflammatory meningitis and metastases. Nonenhancing sulcal FLAIR hyperintensity can also be caused by subarachnoid hemorrhage.
- Dural metastases appear as focal enhancing extra-axial masses.

  The main causes of multiple dural masses are multiple meningiomatosis and metastases.

轴外(脑实质外)转移瘤

- 柔脑膜转移，也称为癌性脑膜炎，表现为软脑膜表面蛇形强化。脑沟在FLAIR序列上呈高信号。

  柔脑膜强化和脑沟FLAIR高信号的主要原因是感染性/炎性脑膜炎和转移。不强化的脑沟FLAIR高信号也可见于蛛网膜下腔出血。
- 硬脑膜转移瘤表现为局灶性强化的轴外肿块。

  多发性硬脑膜肿块的主要原因是多发性脑膜瘤病和转移。

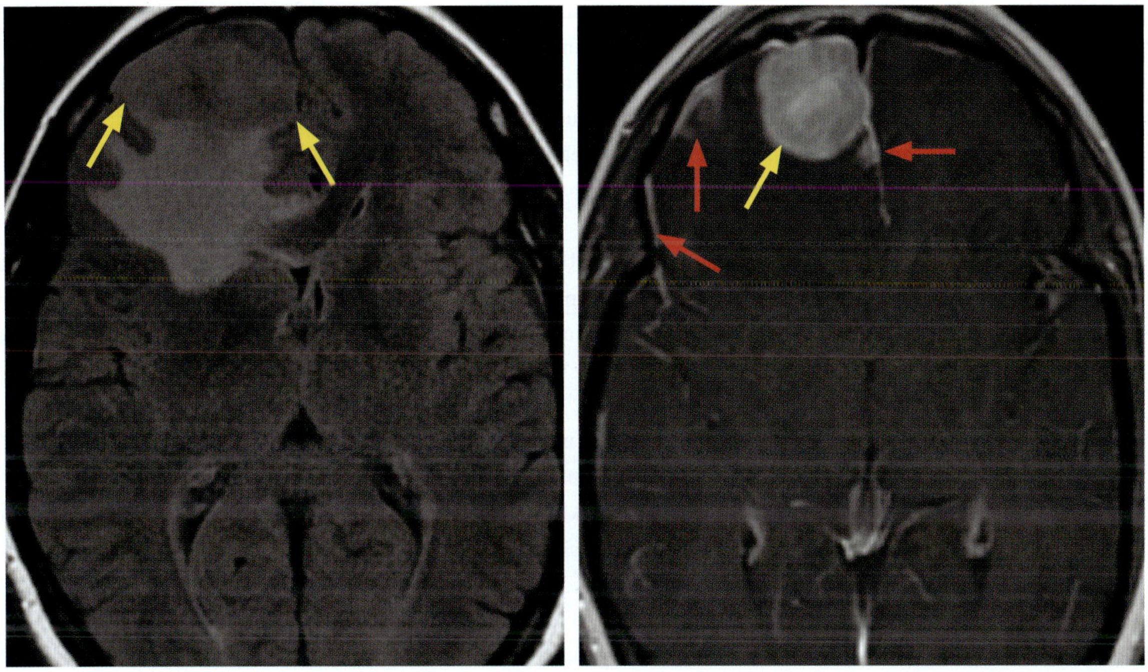

Axial FLAIR (left image) shows a right frontal mass (yellow arrows) with vasogenic edema affecting the right frontal lobe. From this image alone it is difficult to determine if the mass is intra- or extra-axial. Axial post- contrast T1-weighted (right image) MRI shows that the mass (yellow arrow) is dural based and is associated with adjacent dural enhancement (red arrows). This was a case of metastatic breast cancer.

轴位FLAIR(左图)显示右侧额叶肿块(黄箭)伴血管源性水肿。从单一图像上难以确定这个肿块位于轴内或轴外。轴位增强T_1加权(右图)MRI显示该肿块(黄箭)具有硬脑膜的基底，伴邻近硬脑膜强化(红箭)。该例为乳腺癌转移。

PRIMARY DURAL NEOPLASMS

Meningioma

- Meningioma is by far the most common extra-axial tumor, the most common benign primary intracranial tumor in adults, and the most common cause of a solitary dural mass. It arises from meningothelial arachnoid "cap" cells. The vast majority are benign (WHO grade 1), but 4% are atypical (grade 2) and 1–2% are anaplastic or malignant (grade 3).
- Meningiomas typically occur in elderly adults with a female predominance and are most often asymptomatic.

原发性硬脑膜肿瘤

脑膜瘤

- 脑膜瘤是最常见的轴外肿瘤，是成人最常见的良性原发性颅内肿瘤，也是孤立性硬脑膜肿块最常见的原因。它起源于脑膜上皮的蛛网膜"帽"细胞。绝大多数为良性(WHO 1级)，但4%为非典型性(2级)，1%~2%为间变性或恶性(3级)。
- 脑膜瘤通常发生在中老年人，女性好发，往往无症状。

The main environmental/acquired risk factor is ionizing radiation exposure. Meningioma is the most common radiation-induced intracranial neoplasm.

The main genetic predisposition is neurofibromatosis type 2. These patients often have multiple meningiomas.

- Meningiomas can occur anywhere in the neuraxis, but are most commonly supratentorial, which may be at the convexities, parasagittal/falcine, or along the skull base (e.g., olfactory groove, planum sphenoidale, tuberculum sellae, or sphenoid ridge). Other special locations (intraventricular, optic nerve sheath, cerebellopontine angle, jugular foramen, parasellar, and spinal) are discussed elsewhere in this book.
- Meningiomas have a broad dural base; the morphology is most often globose (round) but occasionally en plaque (sheet-like).
- On noncontrast CT, meningiomas are usually hyperattenuating relative to brain and approximately 25% calcify.
- On MRI, appearance can be variable with iso- or slightly hypointense signal on T1-weighted images and variable signal intensity on T2-weighted images.
- Meningiomas avidly enhance. An enhancing *dural tail* is thought to be due to vasoactive substances released by the meningioma rather than tumor spread to the dura. On conventional angiography, meningiomas show early arterial enhancement and contrast retention in venous phase, termed the *mother-in-law sign* (comes early, stays late).
- Despite the extra-axial location of most meningiomas, there may be extensive white matter edema, thought to be due to vasoactive factors and a pial vascular supply. There is often a discordance between the size of meningioma and degree of white matter edema, with severe edema possible even with a very small tumor.
- The adjacent bone may show reactive hyperostotic changes or even intraosseous/transosseous extension, mimicking fibrous dysplasia or an osteoblastic malignancy. Rarely, primary intraosseous meningioma arises within the calvarium with little if any dural involvement.

Solitary fibrous tumor/hemangiopericytoma

- A rare mimic of meningioma is the spectrum of solitary fibrous tumor (WHO grade 1) and hemangiopericytoma (grade 2 or 3). Elsewhere in the body, hemangiopericytoma has been redesignated as solitary fibrous tumor but the separate term remains popular in neuropathology.
- On MRI, solitary fibrous tumor often shows the *yin-yang sign* ("black-and-white mixed" appearance) of patches of low and high signal intensity on T2-weighted images. The low signal areas reflect fibrous stroma. There is strong contrast enhancement, reflecting tumor vascularity; flow-voids and vasogenic edema are common.

主要的环境/后天风险因素是辐射暴露。脑膜瘤是最常见的放射性诱发的颅内肿瘤。

主要的遗传易感性是2型神经纤维瘤病。这些患者通常有多发性脑膜瘤。

- 脑膜瘤可以发生在任何神经轴，但是最常见于幕上，可位于大脑凸面、矢状窦旁/大脑镰旁或沿着颅底(例如嗅沟、蝶骨平面、鞍结节或蝶骨嵴)。其他特殊位置(脑室内、视神经鞘、桥小脑角、颈静脉孔、鞍旁和脊柱)在本书的其他章节进行了讨论。
- 脑膜瘤有宽阔的硬脑膜基底；形态通常为球状(圆形)，但偶尔为斑块状(片状)。
- 脑膜瘤在平扫CT上通常比脑实质密度高，约25%会出现钙化。
- MRI表现可以多样，在T_1加权可呈等信号或稍低信号，T_2加权信号强度可变。
- 脑膜瘤强化明显。强化的*硬脑膜尾征*是由于脑膜瘤释放血管活性物质，并非是肿瘤扩散到硬脑膜。在常规血管造影中，脑膜瘤显示动脉早期强化和静脉期造影剂滞留，称为*岳母征*(来得早，走得晚)。
- 尽管多数脑膜瘤位于轴外，但可引起广泛白质水肿，这可能与血管活性因子和软脑膜供血有关。脑膜瘤大小和白质水肿程度之间常不一致，即使一个非常小的肿瘤都可能引起严重水肿。
- 邻近骨可能出现反应性骨质增生改变，甚至向骨内/跨骨延伸，类似纤维发育不良或成骨细胞恶性肿瘤。起源于颅盖骨内的原发性骨内脑膜瘤罕见，硬脑膜没有受累，即便有也非常局限。

孤立性纤维瘤/血管外皮细胞瘤

- 罕见且类似于脑膜瘤的肿瘤为孤立性纤维瘤(WHO 1级)和血管外皮细胞瘤(2级或3级)。身体其他部位的血管外皮细胞瘤已被重新命名为"孤立性纤维瘤"，但在神经病理学中这个单独术语仍然很流行。
- 孤立性纤维瘤在MRI上通常在T_2加权上表现为*阴阳征*("黑白混合"外观)，即低信号和高信号混杂的斑块。低信号区为纤维间质所致。明显的对比增强反映了肿瘤性血管；流空和血管源性水肿很常见。

Overview and anatomy of the pineal region

松果体区的概述和解剖

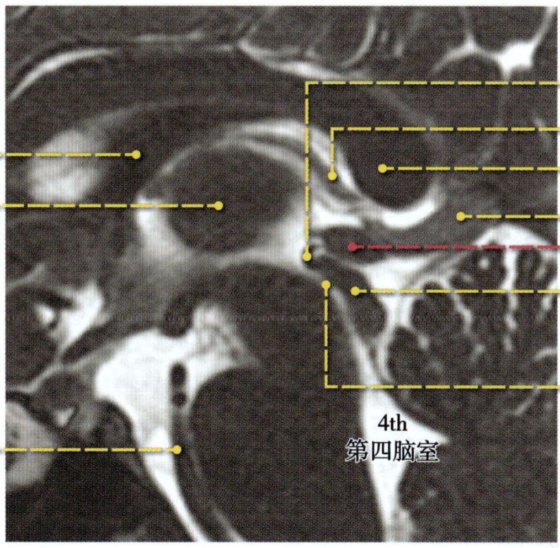

- The pineal gland is an extra-axial organ located in the midline just superior to the level of the midbrain at the posterior aspect of the third ventricle. The internal cerebral veins and vein of Galen are located superior and posterior to the pineal gland, respectively.
- The principal neuronal cell of the pineal gland is the pinealocyte, which is evolved from photoreceptor cells and releases melatonin. Like other neuroendocrine glands, the pineal gland does not have a blood-brain barrier.
- A mass lesion in the pineal region may cause compression of the cerebral aqueduct of Sylvius (presenting as noncommunicating hydrocephalus) or the tectum/quadrigeminal plate of the midbrain (presenting as Parinaud syndrome, including vertical gaze palsy).
- The most common types of pineal region neoplasms are germ cell tumors, pineal parenchymal tumors, and gliomas. The most common mass, however, is a benign cyst.

- 松果体是位于中线的轴外器官，位于第三脑室后部中脑水平上方。大脑内静脉和Galen静脉分别位于松果体上方和后方。
- 松果体的主要神经元细胞是松果体细胞，它们由感光细胞进化而来并释放褪黑色素。松果体与其他神经内分泌腺一样，不具有血脑屏障。
- 松果体区肿块可压迫中脑导水管(表现为非交通性脑积水)或中脑顶盖/四叠体(表现为Parinaud综合征，包括垂直凝视麻痹)。
- 松果体区最常见的肿瘤类型是生殖细胞肿瘤、松果体实质肿瘤和胶质瘤。最常见的肿块是良性囊肿。

Germ cell tumors

生殖细胞肿瘤

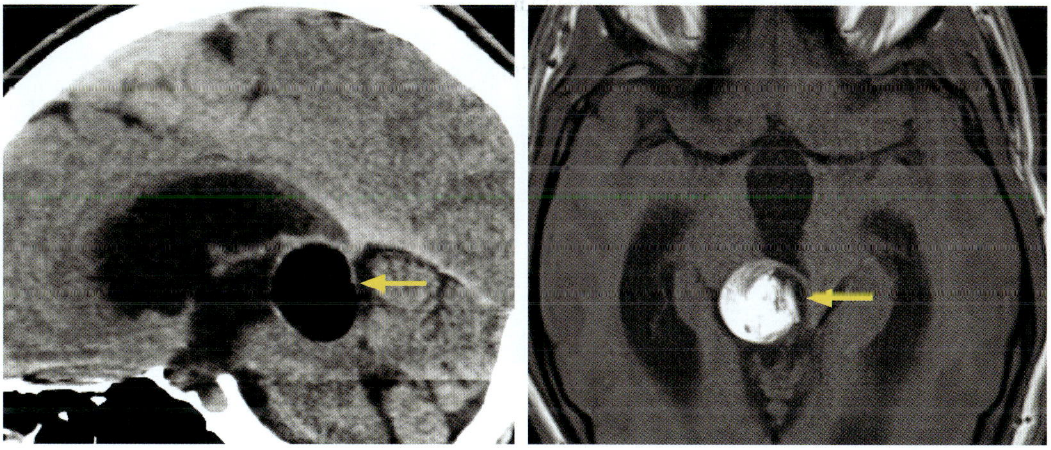

Pineal region teratoma: Sagittal noncontrast CT (left image) and axial T1-weighted MRI (right image) show a fat-containing mass in the pineal region (arrows). There is associated obstructive hydrocephalus due to compression of the cerebral aqueduct by the mass.

松果体区畸胎瘤：矢状位平扫CT(左图)和轴位T_1加权MRI(右图)显示松果体区有一个含脂肪的肿块(黄箭)。肿块压迫中脑导水管而导致梗阻性脑积水。

- The most common site of intracranial germ cell tumors is the pineal gland, followed by the suprasellar region (discussed separately in the "Head and Neck" chapter).
- Extragonadal germ cell tumors are thought to be due to aberrant migration of totipotent germ cells during early embryogenesis and occur in midline locations such as in the head, mediastinum, and sacrococcygeal region.
- Intracranial germ cell tumors have a peak incidence in the teenage years. Pineal region germ cell tumors in particular have a male predominance.
- Germinoma and teratoma are germ cell tumors that are the most common and second most common pineal region tumors, respectively, and have good prognosis. Less common and associated with poor prognosis are embryonal carcinoma, yolk sac (endodermal sinus) tumor, choriocarcinoma, and mixed tumors.
- **Germinoma** (extra-gonadal seminoma) is the most common intracranial germ cell tumor.

  Germinoma is a highly cellular, avidly enhancing tumor that is slightly hyperdense on CT, isointense on T1- and T2-weighted images, and is dark on ADC map. Germinoma characteristically "engulfs" the pineal gland and promotes its calcification, resulting in central area of calcification.

  Imaging of the entire neuraxis is recommended as leptomeningeal deposits can occur. Treatment is radiotherapy, with excellent prognosis.

  Pineal germinoma may present with a synchronous suprasellar germ cell tumor.
- **Teratoma** is the second most common pineal region tumor and confers a worse prognosis than germinoma. Teratoma has a heterogeneous imaging appearance.

  Intralesionalfat is suggestive of teratoma. Teratoma is prone to hemorrhage and coarse calcification.

- 颅内生殖细胞肿瘤最常见部位是松果体，其次是鞍上区(在“神经影像：头与颈”一章进行讨论)。
- 性腺外生殖细胞肿瘤被认为是全能性生殖细胞，在胚胎发育早期出现迁移异常，且发生在中线部位，如头部、纵隔和骶尾部。
- 颅内生殖细胞肿瘤在青少年时期发病率最高。尤其是松果体区生殖细胞肿瘤以男性为主。
- 生殖细胞瘤和畸胎瘤都是生殖细胞肿瘤，分别是最常见和第二常见的松果体区肿瘤，并且预后良好。少见且预后不良的是胚胎癌、卵黄囊(内胚层窦)瘤、绒毛膜癌和混合瘤。
- **生殖细胞瘤**(性腺外精原细胞瘤)是最常见的颅内生殖细胞肿瘤。

  生殖细胞瘤的细胞高度致密，强化明显，在CT上呈稍高密度，T_1、T_2加权上均呈等信号，ADC图上呈低信号。生殖细胞瘤的特征性表现为“吞噬”松果体并促进其钙化，从而形成中心性钙化区。

  凡有柔脑膜的位置均可发生转移，因此建议做完整的神经轴影像学检查。治疗方法采用放疗，预后良好。

  松果体生殖细胞瘤可同时伴有鞍上生殖细胞肿瘤。
- **畸胎瘤**是第二常见的松果体区肿瘤，预后较生殖细胞瘤差。畸胎瘤的影像学特点为信号不均匀。

  病灶内含有脂肪提示畸胎瘤。畸胎瘤易出血并含有粗大的钙化灶。

Pineal parenchymal tumors

松果体实质肿瘤

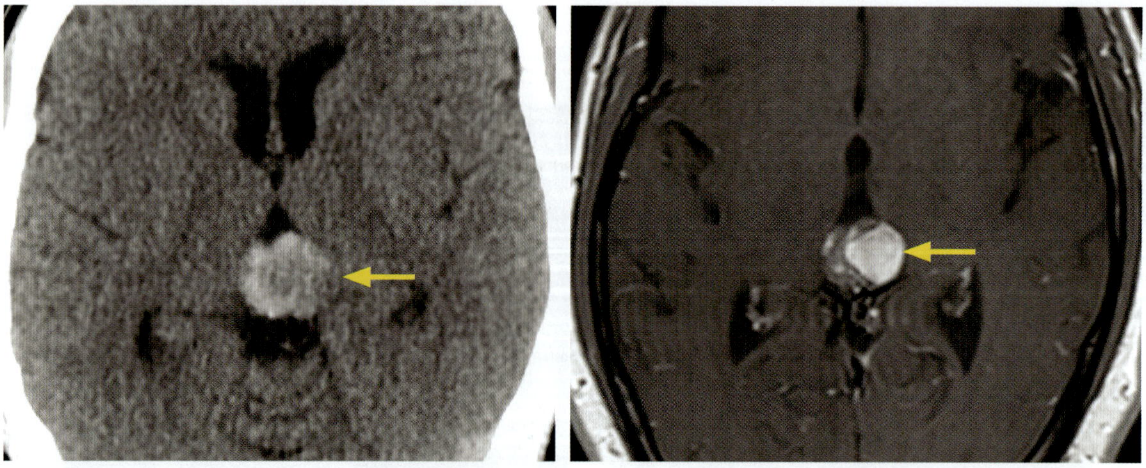

Pineal parenchymal tumor of intermediate differentiation: Axial noncontrast CT (left image) demonstrates a hyperdense pineal mass. Post-contrast T1-weighted MRI (right image) shows the mass enhances. There is no restricted diffusivity (not shown).

中分化的松果体实质肿瘤：轴位平扫CT(左图)显示松果体高密度肿块。对比增强T_1加权MRI(右图)显示肿块强化。无弥散受限(未展示)。

- Pineal parenchymal tumors are a spectrum including pineocytoma (WHO grade 1), pineal parenchymal tumor of intermediate differentiation and papillary tumor of the pineal region (grade 2 or 3), and pineoblastoma (grade 4).
- Pineoblastomas affect young children whereas the other pineal parenchymal tumors are mostly seen in adults.
- Pineoblastoma is an aggressive tumor that is histologically similar to other pediatric small round blue cell tumors, medulloblastoma, and retinoblastoma.

  The term **trilateral retinoblastoma** is used when there are retinoblastomas in both eyes and a pineoblastoma (both the retina and pineal gland are light-sensing organs). The suprasellar region is additionally involved in **quadrilateral retinoblastoma**.
- Any solid component of a pineal parenchymal tumor should demonstrate enhancement. Cystic change or necrosis is common, which can make it difficult to differentiate from a pineal cyst.
- Higher grade tumors are associated with ill-defined margins (invading adjacent structures), more restricted diffusion owing to high cellularity, and a propensity for CSF seeding.
- Germ cell tumors "engulf" by inducing calcification of the pineal gland, whereas pineal parenchymal tumors "explode" by peripherally displacing existing physiologic pineal calcifications.

- 松果体实质肿瘤包括松果体细胞瘤(WHO 1级)、中分化松果体实质肿瘤和松果体区乳头状肿瘤(2级或3级)以及松果体母细胞瘤(4级)。
- 松果体母细胞瘤累及幼儿，而其他松果体实质肿瘤主要见于成人。
- 松果体母细胞瘤是一种侵袭性肿瘤，在组织学上类似于其他儿童小蓝圆细胞肿瘤、髓母细胞瘤和视网膜母细胞瘤。

  三侧性视网膜母细胞瘤是指双眼视网膜母细胞瘤和松果体母细胞瘤(视网膜和松果体都是感光器官)。如果鞍上区也受累，即为**四侧性视网膜母细胞瘤**。
- 任何松果体实质肿瘤的实性成分都应显示强化。囊性变或坏死很常见，因此与松果体囊肿难以鉴别。
- 较高级别的肿瘤常表现为边界不清(侵入相邻结构)、细胞密集导致的弥散受限，以及易发生脑脊液播散。
- 生殖细胞肿瘤是通过促松果体钙化而呈现"吞噬"，而松果体实质肿瘤是通过周围肿瘤组织置换现有的生理性松果体钙化而呈现"爆炸"。

Pineal cyst

- Pineal cysts are seen commonly on MRI and have a prevalence as high as 40% on autopsy series. They are more common in women.
- Most pineal cysts are less than 1 cm and asymptomatic, but may cause symptoms due to mass effect. Very few pineal cysts grow and follow-up of small pineal cysts is not routinely recommended.
- Pineal cysts are usually not entirely simple. Most of them do not fully suppress on FLAIR. Rim calcification can be seen about 25% of the time.
- Contrast is necessary when evaluating a pineal cyst, as the primary differential diagnosis is a pineal parenchymal tumor. Pineal cysts may show thin, smooth peripheral enhancement but not thick, irregular, or nodular enhancement.

松果体囊肿

- MRI检查常见松果体囊肿，尸检发生率可高达40%。女性更常见。
- 大多数松果体囊肿直径小于1cm且无症状，但可以引起占位效应，从而产生症状。极少数松果体囊肿会增大，小的松果体囊肿通常不建议进行随访。
- 松果体囊肿通常不完全是单纯性的。其中大多数的信号在FLAIR上不能完全被抑制。边缘钙化可见于25%的病例。
- 评估松果体囊肿需要进行对比增强，因为主要鉴别诊断是松果体实质肿瘤。松果体囊肿可表现为薄而光滑的周边强化，而不是厚壁、不规则或结节状强化。

Gliomas

- Gliomas (most commonly astrocytomas) may occur in intra-axial structures around the pineal region, such as the tectum of the midbrain, thalamus, or splenium of the corpus callosum.

神经胶质瘤

- 神经胶质瘤(最常见为星形细胞瘤)可发生在松果体区周围的轴内结构，如中脑顶盖、丘脑或胼胝体压部。

Metastases

- Metastasis to the pineal gland is rare.
- Leptomeningeal disease is present in 2/3 of patients with pineal metastasis.

转移瘤

- 松果体转移瘤罕见。
- 有2/3的松果体转移患者存在柔脑膜转移。

Meningioma

- The tentorial apex, adjacent to the pineal gland, is a rare location for meningioma.
- A tentorial meningioma tends to depress the internal cerebral veins, unlike tumors of pineal gland origin, which tend to lift the internal cerebral veins.

脑膜瘤

- 小脑幕顶端，邻近松果体是脑膜瘤罕见的发病位置。
- 小脑幕脑膜瘤与松果体起源的肿瘤不同，其往往将大脑内静脉向下压迫，后者往往会将大脑内静脉向上抬高。

Quadrigeminal plate lipoma

四叠体板脂肪瘤

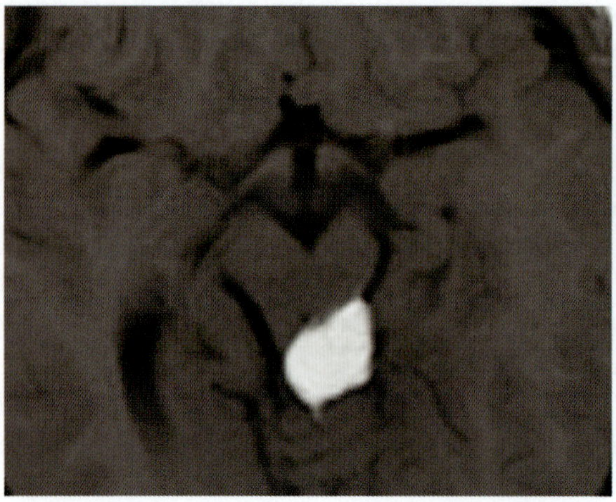

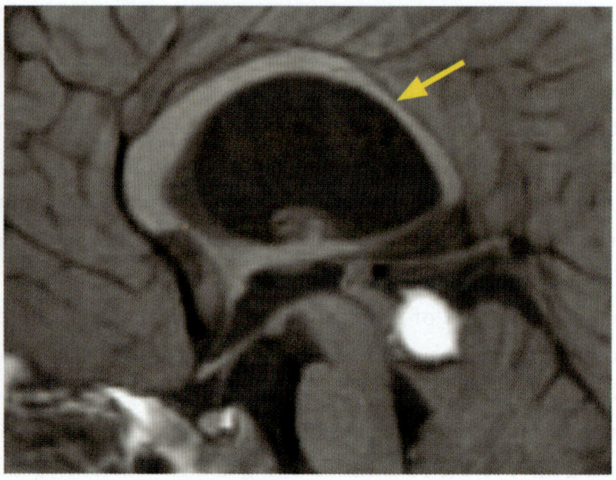

Quadrigeminal plate lipoma: Axial (left image) and sagittal (right image) T1-weighted MRI shows a lobulated, hyperintense mass of the quadrigeminal plate. Note the associated thinning of the posterior body (arrow) and splenium of the corpus callosum.

四叠体板脂肪瘤：轴位(左图)和矢状位(右图)T_1加权MRI显示四叠体板一个分叶状的高信号肿块。注意伴随的胼胝体后体部(黄箭)及压部变薄。

- A lipoma of the quadrigeminal plate (another name for the tectum) is a rare lesion that may be seen in isolation or in association with agenesis or hypoplasia of the corpus callosum.
- The quadrigeminal plate is another name for the tectum.

- 四叠体板(中脑顶盖的另一名称)脂肪瘤是一种罕见的病变，可以单发，也可以伴有胼胝体发育不良或发育不全。
- 四叠体板也称为中脑顶盖。

(翻译　潘春树)

WHITE MATTER DISEASE

脑白质疾病

WHITE MATTER OVERVIEW

脑白质概述

White matter imaging overview

- The typical MRI appearance of white matter injury is T2 prolongation of the affected white matter. Less commonly, *tumefactive* demyelination may be mass-like, enhance, and look very similar to a tumor.
- The key imaging finding of demyelinating disease is *minimal mass effect* relative to the lesion size.
- A frequent pattern of white matter disease consisting of scattered foci of T2 prolongation in the subcortical, deep, and periventricular white matter is seen very commonly, especially in older adults. In older patients, this pattern is most likely due to chronic microvascular ischemia. In younger patients, a similar pattern can be seen in chronic migraine headaches, as sequela of prior infectious or inflammatory disease, and with demyelination.

脑白质影像概述

- 脑白质损伤的典型MRI表现为受累白质长T_2。较少表现为*肿瘤样*脱髓鞘病变，可呈肿块样、有强化，且与肿瘤表现非常相似。
- 脱髓鞘病变的关键影像学表现是*占位效应*相对于病灶大小微乎其微。
- 常见类型的脑白质疾病表现为散在的局灶性长T_2，好发于皮层下、深部、脑室周围的脑白质，尤其是老年人。在老年患者中，这种表现最可能是由于慢性微血管缺血所致。在年轻患者中，类似的表现可见于先前感染或炎性疾病遗留的慢性偏头痛及脱髓鞘病变。

Normal structures may mimic white matter disease on T2 images

- **Virchow-Robin spaces** are tiny perivascular spaces that follow deep penetrating vessels into the subarachnoid space. They are common in the basal ganglia and the midbrain. On CT, Virchow-Robin spaces can mimic chronic lacunar infarcts, but are usually present in the lower third of the basal ganglia. On MRI, Virchow-Robin spaces follow CSF signal on all sequences, including FLAIR.

  Enlarged Virchow-Robin spaces and a J-shaped sella can be seen in the mucopolysac-

在T_2图像上可能类似脑白质疾病的正常结构

- **Virchow-Robin(V-R)**间隙是血管周围的微间隙，并随深部穿支血管通入蛛网膜下腔。它们常见于基底节及中脑。在CT上，V-R间隙的表现与慢性腔隙性脑梗死相似，但前者常见于基底节区下1/3。在MRI上，V-R间隙信号在所有序列上与CSF信号一致，包括FLAR序列。

  扩大的V-R间隙及"J"形蝶鞍可见于黏多糖贮

charidoses.

- **Ependymitis granularis** represents frontal horn periventricular hyperintensity on T2- weighted images due to interstitial CSF backup. Despite the name ("-itis"), ependymitis granularis is not associated with inflammation.

积症。

- **颗粒性室管膜炎**是指在T_2加权像上侧脑室前角周围的高信号，这是由于间质内CSF积聚。尽管英文名中带有"-itis(炎)"，但颗粒性室管膜炎与炎症无关。

IDIOPATHIC/AUTOIMMUNE/INFLAMMATORY WHITE MATTER DISEASE

特发性/自身免疫性/炎性脑白质病

Multiple sclerosis (MS)

- Multiple sclerosis (MS) is idiopathic inflammatory destruction of CNS axons in the brain and spinal cord. MS is likely autoimmune in etiology and may be associated with other autoimmune diseases such as Graves disease and myasthenia gravis.
- MS is the most common chronic demyelinating disease. It often leads to severe disability.
- MS is more common in middle-aged Caucasian females from northern latitudes.
- There are two main clinical presentations of MS:

> 1) **Relapsing-remitting** (most common): Partial or complete resolution of each acute attack.
> 2) **Progressive:** No resolution or incomplete resolution between acute attacks.
> Primary progressive: Slow onset without discrete exacerbations.
> Secondary progressive: Similar to relapsing-remitting but with less complete resolution between attacks, leading to progressive disability.

- The diagnostic criteria for MS has been based on two concepts: the detection of focal neurological disease disseminated in space and time, based on clinical symptoms and brain MRI findings. The specific findings that constitute a diagnosis have been described as the McDonald criteria, which was most recently revised in 2017. The MacDonald criteria also describe intermediate diagnoses that do not meet all clinical or radiologic criteria simultaneously as clinically isolated syndrome (CIS) and radiologically isolated syndrome (RIS).
- *Dissemination in space* can be demonstrated by detection of T2 hyperintense lesions at least 3 mm in size in at least two of the classically affected areas: the periventricular white matter, spinal cord, infratentorial brain, juxtacortical white matter or cerebral cortex. Cortical lesions were an addition of the most recent revision.
- *Dissemination in time* based on MRI can be demonstrated by the presence of simultaneous presence of both gadolinium-enhancing and non-enhancing lesions on a single study or by the presence of new lesions demonstrating hyperintensity on T2-weighted imaging or gadolinium enhancement on subsequent studies.
- Histopathologically, destruction of myelin is caused by lymphocytes attacking oligodendrocytes (which make CNS myelin).
- As described in the McDonald criteria, focal areas of involvement manifest as lesions that are hyperintense on T2-weighted imaging. The presence of enhancement is suggestive of active demyelination, while the lack of enhancement suggests a chroniclesion. This allows for demonstration of dissemination in time on a single scan, as described above.
- There are certain areas of the brain where lesion involvement is more suggestive of MS over alternative diagnoses. This includes the periventricular region, corpus callosum, subcortical white matter, temporal lobe white matter, the brainstem, cerebellum, and the cervical portion of the spinal cord.

多发性硬化(MS)

- 多发性硬化(MS)是一种对脑和中枢神经系统轴突造成破坏的特发性炎症。MS的病因很可能为自身免疫性，并且可能与其他自身免疫性疾病有关，如格雷夫斯病及重症肌无力。
- MS是最常见的慢性脱髓鞘疾病。它常导致严重的残疾。
- MS好发于北半球的中年白种人女性。
- MS有两个主要的临床类型：

> 1) **复发-缓解型**(最常见)：每次急性发作后部分或完全缓解。
> 2) **进展型**：急性发作间期无缓解或不完全缓解。
> 原发进展型：缓慢发病，无确切加重。
> 继发进展型：类似于复发-缓解型相似，但每次发作后的症状缓解不完全，导致进行性致残。

- MS的诊断标准基于以下两个概念：检测到局灶性病变在空间和时间上有多发特征，有临床症状和脑部MRI表现的依据。构成诊断依据的特定表现被称为McDonald标准，该标准最新一次修订于2017年。MacDonald标准还描述了不能同时满足所有临床或放射学标准的折中诊断，即仅有临床表现(CIS)和仅有放射影像学表现(RIS)。
- 空间多发性，指病变T_2高信号且直径至少3mm，并影响至少2个的典型区域：包括脑室周围白质、脊髓、幕下脑、皮质旁白质或大脑皮层。皮质病变是最新修订版的新增内容。
- 时间多发性，指病变在MRI上可以表现为同一次检查中同时出现钆增强和非增强性病变，或在后续检查中出现了新的T_2加权高信号病灶或增强病灶。
- 组织病理学上，髓鞘受到破坏是因为淋巴细胞攻击少突胶质细胞(后者构成中枢神经系统髓鞘)。
- 按照McDonald标准，局部受累区表现为T_2加权高信号。出现增强提示有活动性脱髓鞘，而无增强提示为慢性病变。如上所述，单次扫描可以证明病灶在时间上多发。
- 在脑部某些特殊区域受累更支持MS诊断，而非其他诊断。这包括脑室周围区、胼胝体、皮质下白质、颞叶白质、脑干、小脑和颈段脊髓。

Periventricular lesions have classically been described as *Dawson fingers* due to their ovoid configuration perpendicular to the ventricles, resulting from inflammation surrounding the penetrating venules.

脑室周围病变通常被描述为Dawson手指征，为垂直于脑室的卵形结构，是由穿支小静脉周围的炎症所致。

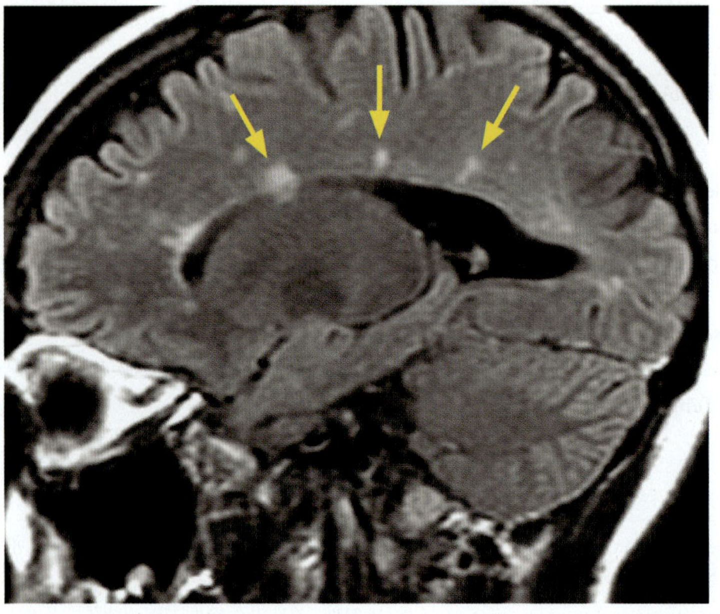

Dawson fingers in multiple sclerosis: Parasagittal FLAIR shows numerous foci of T2 prolongation (arrows) within the corpus callosum that point towards the ventricle in a patient with relapsing-remitting MS.

MS中的Dawson手指征：复发-缓解型MS患者矢状位FLAIR显示胼胝体内多发指向脑室的长T_2病灶（黄箭）。

- The *central vein sign* describes the presence of a central vein within the white matter lesion, identified as a central hypointensity surrounded by hyperintensity on FLAIR images, is relatively specific for MS-related white matter lesions.
- There are many recent advances to imaging of MS beyond the use of gadolinium-enhancement as a surrogate for active inflammation. Leptomeningeal enhancement is emerging as an imaging biomarker for active inflammation. This utilizes the emerging idea of immune cell infiltrates, indicative of active demyelination, are present in the leptomeninges.
- Although spinal involvement is not required for diagnosis, MS involves the spinal cord in a substantial minority of patients, with the cervical spine cord most frequently involved. Isolated spinal cord involvement is seen in up to 20% of cases of MS. Spinal MS involvement is usually short-segment and unilateral.
- Lesions that are dark on T1-weighted images are called "black holes" and are associated with more severe demyelination and axonal loss.
- Chronic MS leads to cortical atrophy and thinning of the corpus callosum. MR spectroscopy can mimic high grade glioma, with ↓ NAA and ↑ choline.
- **Tumefactive MS** describes the occasionally seen ring enhancement and mass-like appearance of an active MS plaque. In contrast to a brain tumor, the demyelinatinglesion will *not have any significant mass effect,* and the ring of enhancement is usually incomplete.

- 中心静脉征是指在脑白质病变内出现中心静脉，其在FLAIR图像上表现为中心低信号被外周高信号包围，为MS与白质病变相关的相对特异的征象。
- 多项新进展已经在多发性硬化的成像方面作为检测活动炎症的手段超越了钆增强。软脑膜强化是一种新的活动性炎症的影像学标记。新的观点认为，免疫细胞浸润出现在柔脑膜中，可以作为活动性脱髓鞘的指征。
- 脊髓受累并非MS诊断所需，但在相当一部分患者中有脊髓受累，其中以颈椎受累最为常见。孤立性脊髓受累在MS患者中高达20%。MS累及脊髓通常为短节段性单侧受累。
- T_1加权图像上呈暗黑的病灶被称为“黑洞”，与更为严重的脱髓鞘和轴突丧失有关。
- 慢性MS导致皮层萎缩、胼胝体变薄。磁共振波谱（MRS）似高级别胶质瘤，表现为N-乙酰天冬氨酸（NAA）减低，胆碱（Cho）增高。
- **肿瘤样MS**是指一种少见的出现在活动性MS斑块时的环形强化和肿块样表现。与脑肿瘤相比，肿瘤样MS没有明显的占位效应，且强化环通常不完整。

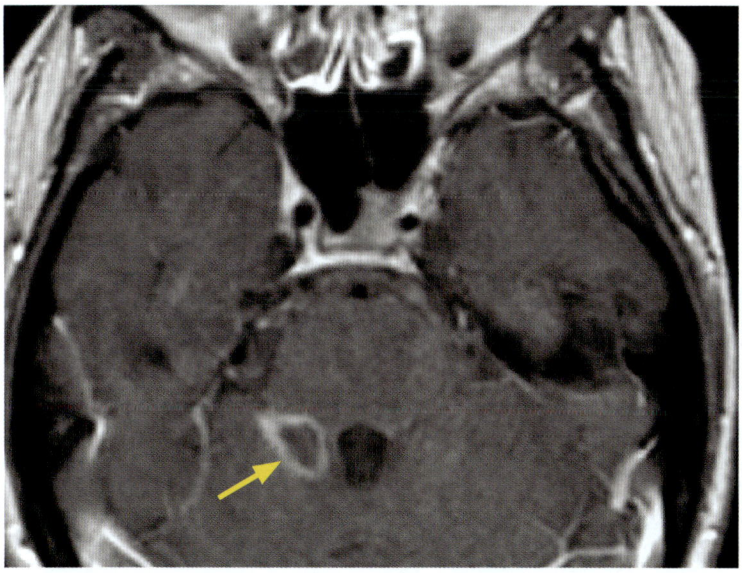

Enhancing tumefactive lesion in the same patient as the previous page, with known MS: Axial post-contrast T1-weighted image shows a ring- enhancing lesion in the right middle-cerebellar peduncle (arrow). Although ring enhancement is nonspecific, the lack of any appreciable mass effect (the adjacent fourth ventricle is normal in size and shape) suggests a demyelinating lesion.

同上图MS患者的肿瘤样强化病变：轴位增强T_1加权图像显示右侧小脑中脚一环形强化病灶(黄箭)。虽然环形强化无特异性，但无明显可见的占位效应(相邻第四脑室的大小和形状正常)，提示为脱髓鞘病变。

Concentric (Balo) sclerosis

- Concentric (Balo) sclerosis is a very rare variant of MS with pathognomonic alternating concentric bands of normal and abnormal myelin. It is seen more often in younger patients.

Marburg variant (acute multiple sclerosis)

- Marburg variant of MS is a fulminant manifestation of MS, leading to death within months.

NMO spectrum disease

- NMO spectrum disease (NMOSD) (previously described as Devic disease or NMO) is a demyelinating disease, distinct from MS, which involves both the optic nerves and spinal cord. NMOSD confers a worse prognosis compared to MS.
- NMO-IgG, an antibody to aquaporin 4, is highly specific for NMOSD. NMO-IgG activates the complement cascade and induces demyelination.
- Imaging findings are discussed in more detail in the "Spine" chapter.

同心环(Balo)硬化

- 同心环(Balo)硬化是一种罕见的MS变异，其正常和异常髓鞘相互交替形成的同心环带具有病理诊断意义。年轻患者多见。

Marburg变异型(急性MS)

- Marburg变异型MS为一种暴发性MS的表现，在数月内可致死亡。

视神经脊髓炎(NMO)谱系疾病

- 视神经脊髓炎(NMO)谱系疾病(neuromyelitis optica spectrum disorder，NMOSD)(之前被称为Devic 病或视神经脊髓炎)是一种脱髓鞘疾病，不同于MS，前者常同时累及视神经和脊髓。NMOSD较MS的预后更差。
- NMO-IgG是一种水通道蛋白4的抗体，对NMOSD具有很高的特异度。NMO-IgG激活补体级联反应，并诱导脱髓鞘。
- 影像特征将在"脊柱影像"一章节中做更详细讨论。

Acute disseminated encephalomyelitis (ADEM)

- Acute disseminated encephalomyelitis (ADEM) is a monophasic demyelinating disorder seen primarily in children that typically occurs after a viral infection or vaccination. The majority of patients make a full recovery, but a minority suffer permanent neurologic sequelae.
- Imaging findings can be identical to MS, and occasionally cases of presumed ADEM will be reclassified as MS due to polyphasic clinical course. Similar to MS, ADEM may involve the brain,brainstem, or spinal cord.
- Optic neuritis and spinal cord involvement can be seen in ADEM, as with MS.
- The **Hurst variant** (acute hemorrhagic leukoencephalitis) is a rapidly fulminant form of ADEM that leads to death within days.

  Imaging of the Hurst variant shows multifocal T2 prolongation and associated white matter hemorrhage, which may appear as confluent hematomas.

急性播散性脑脊髓炎(ADEM)

- 急性播散性脑脊髓炎(ADEM)是一种单相脱髓鞘病变，主要见于儿童，通常在病毒感染或疫苗接种后出现。大多数患者可痊愈，但少数会留有永久性神经性后遗症。
- 影像学表现可与MS完全相同。少数情况下，起初被诊断为ADEM的病例因临床过程反复而被重新归为MS。与MS相似，ADEM可累及大脑、脑干或脊髓。
- 视神经炎和脊髓受累可出现在ADEM中，与MS相似。
- **Hurst变异**(急性出血性脑白质脑炎)是一种快速暴发性的ADEM，可在数天内导致死亡。

  Hurst变异的影像学表现为多灶性长T_2信号及相应的白质出血，可融合成血肿。

Posterior reversible encephalopathy syndrome (PRES)

可逆性后部脑病综合征(PRES)

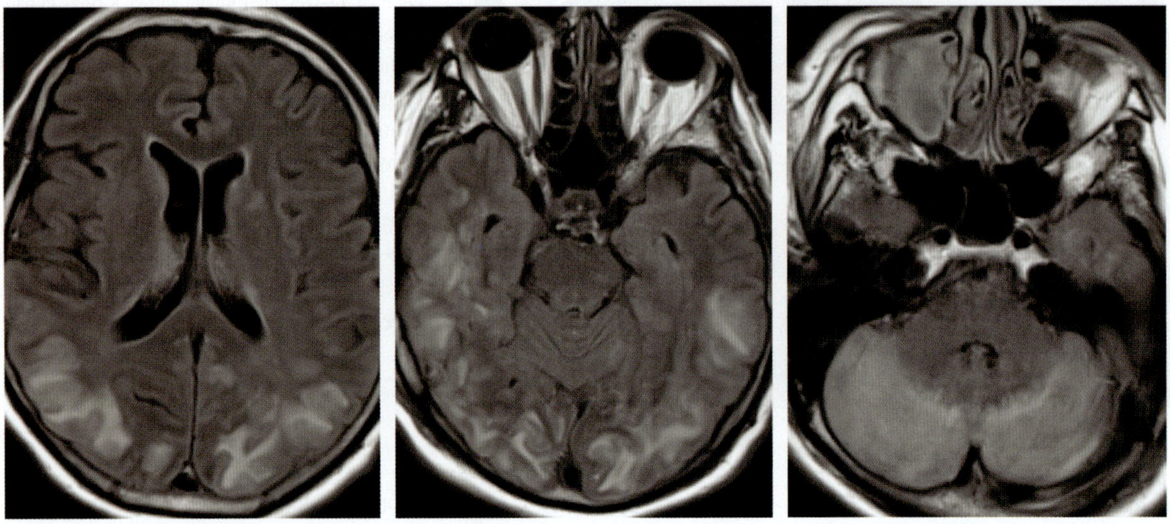

PRES: Axial FLAIR images show abnormal hyperintense signal in the subcortical white matter of the bilateral posterior frontal, parietal, and temporal lobes, as well as bilateral cerebellar hemispheres.

可逆性后部脑病综合征：轴位FLAIR图像显示皮质下白质异常高信号，分布于双侧后额叶、顶叶、颞叶及双侧小脑半球。

- Posterior reversible encephalopathy syndrome (PRES) is a disorder of vasogenic edema with a posterior circulation predominance triggered by failed autoregulation and resultant hyperperfusion, most commonly caused by acute hypertension. In addition to hypertension, PRES is also associated with eclampsia, sepsis, autoimmune disorders, multi-drug chemotherapy, and solid or stem cell transplantation.
- In contrast to infarction, the edema is vasogenic in etiology, not cytotoxic. Diffusion may be normal, increased, or restricted.
- Imaging shows ***symmetric*** regions of subcortical white matter abnormality (hypoattenuation on CT and T2 prolongation on MR), especially in the posterior circulation (occipital and parietal lobes and posterior fossa). Mild mass effect and enhancement can be seen.

Cerebral autosomal dominant arteriopathy with subcortical infarcts and leukoencephalopathy (CADASIL)

- CADASIL is an inherited disease (*notch3* mutation) characterized by recurrent stroke, migraine, subcortical dementia, and pseudobulbar palsy, due to small vessel arteriopathy.
- The clinical hallmark of CADASIL is recurrent episodes of stroke or transient ischemic attacks, which are nearly always found to be subcortical in the white matter or basal ganglia on imaging. There is often associated migraine. It may eventually lead to dementia.
- MRI shows ***symmetric*** foci of T2 prolongation in the subcortical white matter, which may become confluent as the disease progresses. Anterior temporal lobe or paramedian frontal lobe foci of T2 prolongation are highly sensitive and specific for CADASIL, especially with clinical history of migraine. Although the symmetric subcortical pattern is similar to PRES, the distribution in CADASIL is anterior circulation.

- 可逆性后部脑病综合征(PRES)是一种发生于后循环的血管源性水肿性疾病，主要由自动调节障碍触发并引起过度灌注，最常见于急性高血压。除了高血压，PRES也与子痫、脓毒症、自身免疫性疾病、多种药物化疗，以及实质器官或干细胞移植有关。
- 与脑梗死不同，PRES水肿为血管源性，而非细胞毒性。弥散可能正常、增加或受限。
- 影像学表现为皮层下脑白质**对称性**区域异常(在CT上呈低密度、在MR上呈长T_2)，尤其是后循环(枕叶、顶叶和颅后窝)。可见轻度占位效应及强化。

常染色体显性遗传性脑动脉病伴皮质下梗死和白质脑病(CADASIL)

- CADASIL是一种遗传性疾病(*NOTCH3*突变)，以反复性脑卒中、偏头痛、皮层下痴呆和假性延髓性麻痹为特点，由脑小血管病变导致。
- CADASIL最主要的临床特点为反复卒中或短暂性脑缺血发作，而在影像上病灶几乎都位于皮层下白质或基底节。常伴有偏头痛。最终可导致痴呆。
- MRI显示皮层下白质对称性长T_2病灶，病灶可随着疾病进展而发生融合。前颞叶或旁正中额叶的长T_2信号病灶对诊断CADASIL具有很高的灵敏度和特异度，尤其是临床有偏头痛病史的患者。尽管对称的皮层下表现与PRES类似，但是CADASIL的病灶分布于前循环。

Vasculitis

- CNS vasculitis is a group of vascular inflammatory disorders that primarily affect the small vessels, in particular the leptomeningeal and small parenchymal vessels.
- Etiologies include lupus, polyarteritis nodosa, giant cell arteritis, and Sjögren syndrome.
- MRI shows numerous small focal areas of T2 prolongation in subcortical and deep white matter. Although the appearance may be similar to MS, foci of hemorrhage (best seen on GRE or SWI) may be present in vasculitis, which would not be seen in MS.
- Vascular imaging (CT angiography and catheter angiography are more sensitive than MRI angiography) shows a beaded, irregular appearance to the cerebral vessels.

Microangiopathy

- Microangiopathy describes age-related chronic axonal loss,gliosis, and ischemic changes seen in up to 80% of elderly individuals. Microangiopathy never involves the corpus callosum: If involvement of the corpus callosum is present, an alternative diagnosis should be considered, such as MS or neoplasm.
- **Binswanger disease** represents the combination of dementia and severe microangiopathy.

血管炎

- 中枢神经系统血管炎是一组血管炎性病变，主要累及小血管，特别是柔脑膜和脑实质的小血管。
- 病因包括：狼疮、结节性多动脉炎、巨细胞动脉炎和舍格伦(干燥)综合征。
- MRI显示皮层下和深部白质内大量局灶长T_2区域。尽管此表现可能与MS类似，但是出血灶(在GRE或SWI上显示最佳)可见于血管炎，而MS则没有出血。
- 血管成像(CT血管造影和导管血管造影比MR血管造影更敏感)显示脑血管呈串珠状且不规则。

微血管病

- 微血管病是指与年龄相关的慢性轴突丢失、神经胶质增生及缺血性改变，见于高达80%的老年人。微血管病变从来不累及胼胝体，如累及胼胝体，则需要考虑其他疾病，如MS或肿瘤。
- **宾斯旺格病(皮质下动脉硬化性脑病)**同时存在痴呆和严重的微血管病。

INFECTIOUS (VIRAL) WHITE MATTER DISEASE

感染性(病毒性)脑白质病

Progressive multifocal leukoencephalopathy (PML)

进行性多灶性脑白质病(PML)

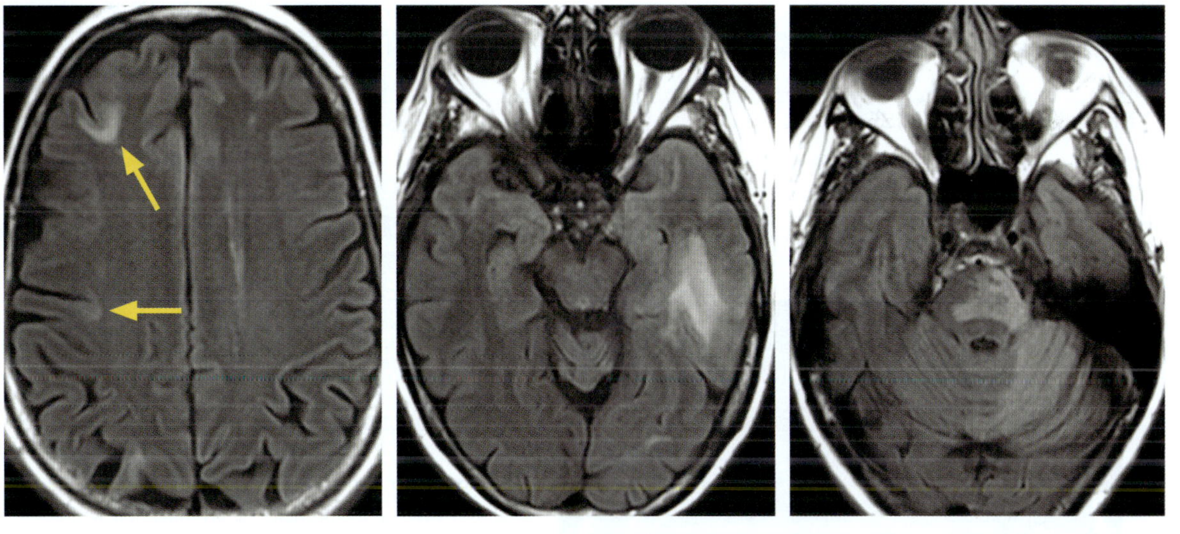

Axial FLAIR images at three different levels show asymmetric multifocal FLAIR hyperintense white matter lesions involving the right frontal lobe subcortical U-fibers (left image, arrows), left temporal lobe (middle image), left cerebellum and brainstem (right image). The lesions demonstrate restricted diffusion and lack of enhancement (not shown). This patient has a history of rheumatoid arthritis and immunosuppression from rituximab prescribed for pemphigoid. JC virus was detected in CSF sample by PCR.

三个不同层面的轴位FLAIR图像显示不对称、多灶性脑白质FLAIR高信号，累及右侧额叶皮质下"U"形纤维(左图，黄箭)、左侧颞叶(中图)、左侧小脑和脑干(右图)。病变表现为弥散受限和无强化(未展示)。这名患者有类风湿关节炎病史，并有使用治疗类天疱疮药物利妥昔单抗的免疫抑制病史。对脑脊液样本使用聚合酶链反应(PCR)检出JC病毒。

- Progressive multifocal leukoencephalopathy (PML) is a demyelinating disease of immunocompromised patients caused by reactivation of JC virus. There is progressive demyelination with lack of inflammatory response.

- 进行性多灶性脑白质病(PML)是一种出现于免疫功能不全患者的脱髓鞘病变，由JC(John Cunningham)病毒再激活引起。病变呈进行

- PML occurs most commonly in AIDS patients (PML is an AIDS defining illness), but can also be seen in patients with malignancy, status post-organ transplant, or with autoimmune disorders. Approximately 1 in 1,000 patients with MS treated with natalizumab (Tysabri) may have superimposed PML and it may be difficult to distinguish between MS and PML. Diagnosis is made by PCR for JC virus DNA in CSF.
- MR imaging of PML shows ***asymmetric*** multifocal white matter lesions that may become confluent. There is rarely mass effect or enhancement. The arcuate (subcortical U) fibers are typically involved. Arcuate fibers are myelinated tracts at the gray-white junction that connect cortex to cortex.
- In an AIDS patient, the primary differential for white matter lesions is PML and HIV encephalitis. In contrast to PML, HIV encephalitis is usually bilateral (and symmetric), spares the subcortical white matter, and is associated with cerebral atrophy:

  Diffuse bilateral involvement, sparing of subcortical white matter, and cerebral atrophy → HIV encephalitis.

  Asymmetric signal, involvement of subcortical white matter, hypointensity on T1-weighted images, peripheral DWI hyperintensity, and lack of atrophy during acute phase → PML. However, progressive cerebral atrophy can be seen in late stage PML.

性脱髓鞘，但缺乏炎性反应。

- PML最常见于AIDS患者(PML是AIDS伴发的一种疾病)，但也可见于恶性肿瘤、器官移植或自身免疫性疾病患者。近1/1 000接受那他珠单抗(Tysabri)治疗的MS患者可能会伴发PML，并且难以将PML和MS两者鉴别开来。诊断依靠PCR检测脑脊液中的JC病毒DNA。
- PML的MR影像学表现为**非对称性**、多病灶性，并可以融合的脑白质病。罕见有占位效应或强化。弓状(皮层下“U”形)纤维常受累。弓状纤维是位于灰-白质交界处的有髓鞘纤维束，起到皮质间连接作用。
- 对于AIDS患者，脑白质病变的主要鉴别诊断是PML与HIV脑炎。与PML不同，HIV脑炎常为双侧(并且对称性)，皮层下白质不受累，并伴有脑萎缩。

  广泛累及双侧，不累及皮层下白质，并有脑萎缩→HIV脑炎。

  非对称分布，累及皮层下白质，T_1加权图像低信号，周围DWI高信号，且急性期不出现脑萎缩→PML。然而，PML在晚期可以进展为脑萎缩。

Subacute sclerosing panencephalitis (SSPE)

- Subacute sclerosing panencephalitis (SSPE) is a demyelinating disease caused by reactivation of measles virus, usually after a long latent period.
- Imaging shows periventricular white matter lesions, but in distinction to the other white matter entities, SSPE lesions tend to have surrounding edema and mass effect.

亚急性硬化性全脑炎(SSPE)

- 亚急性硬化性全脑炎(SSPE)是一种由麻疹病毒被再次激活而引起的脱髓鞘疾病，通常发生在一段长的潜伏期之后。
- 影像学表现为脑室周围白质病变，但与其他白质病变不同，SSPE病灶常有周围水肿及占位效应。

IATROGENIC WHITE MATTER DISEASE

医源性脑白质病

Radiation injury

放射性脑损伤

Whole brain radiation injury

全脑放射性损伤

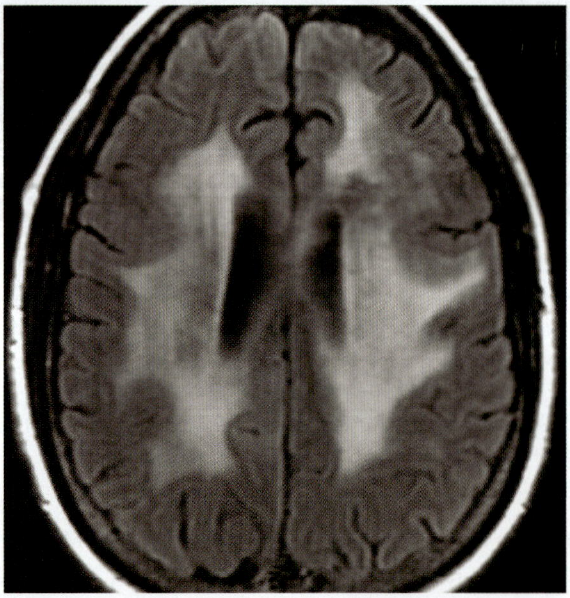

White matter radiation injury: Axial FLAIR image shows extensive confluent T2 prolongation within most of the visualized white matter. The patient had a remote history of whole brain radiation therapy for a high-grade glioma.

脑白质的放射性损伤：轴位FLAIR图像示脑白质区广泛融合的长T_2信号病灶。该患者曾因高级别胶质瘤史而接受过放疗。

- Radiation injury related to whole brain radiation therapy has three distinct patterns, characterized by the timing of presentation and timing of radiation.
- The acute phase occurs during or immediately after radiation therapy, thought to reflect edema due to endothelial injury. It may present as diffuse T2 prolongation in the white matter. Clinically patients can present with acute encephalopathy with signs of increased intracranial pressure. This is usually self-limited or improved with dexamethasone.
- The early delayed phase occurs between several weeks and up to 6 months after treatment, and is thought to be due to demyelination. MRI findings can vary from white matter T2 prolongation in the field of radiation to increase in size of contrast-enhancing lesions within the radiation field. In whole brain radiation, the changes are most pronounced in the periventricular regions.
- The late delayed phase is most commonly seen with SRS. It can start as early as 6 months, most commonly between 9 to 15 months, and sometimes years after radiation. Late effects are typically irreversible and histologically are due to vascular changes including coagulative necrosis and include white matter changes, radionecrosis, and vascular lesions.

Radiation necrosis typically occurs weeks to months after radiation, with 80% of cases occurring within three years of completion of radiotherapy. Imaging demonstrates a peripherally enhancing, centrally necrotic lesion. Treatment is usually corticosteroids.

Other effects include **mineralizing microangiopathy** which occurs more than 6 months after radiation and presents as calcification in the basal ganglia or dentate nuclei. It is more common in children than adults.

Radiation vasculitis can occur in large vessels, and can present as focal narrowed segments on angiogram. Involvement of distal internal carotid arteries can result in a moyamoya phenomenon.

Other vascular lesions such as **capillary telangiectasis** or **cavernous malformations** can be seen.

- 与全脑放射治疗相关的放射性脑损伤有三种不同的模式，其特点是出现症状的时间和放射治疗的时间。
- 急性期发生在放疗期间或放疗后即刻，被认为内皮损伤引起的脑水肿。它可能表现为弥漫性白质长T_2信号。临床上，患者表现急性脑病伴有颅内压升高的症状。这通常是自限性的，或用地塞米松改善症状。
- 早期迟发出现在治疗后数周至6个月，被认为是脱髓鞘所致。MRI表现可能各不相同，可以为放疗脑区白质长T_2信号，也可以是放疗脑区不同大小的强化灶。在全脑放疗中，这种变化在脑室周围区域表现最为明显。
- 晚期迟发在SRS病中是最常见的。最早可出现在6个月后，通常为9~15个月，有时在辐射后数年。晚期的效应通常是不可逆的，并在组织学上归结于血管变化，包括凝固性坏死及其所引起的白质变化、放射性坏死和血管病变。

放射性坏死通常发生在放疗后数周至数月，其中80%的病例发生在放疗结束后3年内。影像上表现为周围强化、中央坏死性病灶。治疗通常采用皮质类固醇。

其他效应还包括**矿化性微血管病**，该病发生在放疗后6个月以上，表现为基底节或齿状核钙化。这在儿童中比成人更常见。

放射性血管炎可发生在大血管中，在血管造影上表现为局灶性、节段性狭窄。颈内动脉远端受累可导致烟雾(moyamoya)现象。

还可出现其他的血管病变，如**毛细血管扩张**或**海绵状血管畸形**。

Pseudoprogression

- A treatment-related phenomenon that mimics tumor progression after targeted radiation and chemotherapy is termed **pseudoprogression**.
- In patients who are receiving standard concomitant radiation with temozolomide followed by adjuvant temozolomide, pseudoprogression peaks after 3–6 months of therapy and rarely occurs after 6 months.
- Pseudoprogression presents as transient contrast enhancement and edema on imaging which subsequently resolves on follow-up scans without treatment. Appropriate recognition of pseudoprogression is important to prevent early discontinuation of adjuvant chemotherapy.
- The incidence of pseudoprogression is an active area of research, however some reports suggest that pseudoprogression may occur more frequently in patients who harbor a *MGMT* promoter methylation status.
- Currently, no imaging techniques can reliably differentiate between pseudoprogression and early progressive disease. Techniques that have been investigated include diffusion-weighted MRI (lower mean ADC values and ADC ratios associated with progressive disease) and MR perfusion (higher relative cerebral blood volume associated with progressive disease) are limited due to confounding by necrosis and vascular leakage which may underestimate rCBV. FDG-PET is widely available however has an unacceptably low sensitivity and specificity. Novel tracers such as FET-PET, FDOPA-PET, 13N-NH3 PET are under investigation.

假性进展

- **假性进展**是靶向放疗和化疗后与肿瘤治疗相关的类似肿瘤进展的一种现象。
- 在接受标准放疗联合temozolomide随后辅以temozolomide治疗的患者中，假性进展的出现在治疗3~6个月后达到峰值，6个月后很少发生。
- 假性进展在影像学上表现为暂时性增强和水肿，在随后的扫描检查随访中消失，无须治疗。正确认识假性进展，对防止早期终止辅助化疗有重要意义。
- 假性进展的发生率是研究领域的一个热点，而一些研究表明，假性进展发生的概率在*MGMT*启动子甲基化的患者中可能更频繁。
- 当前，没有一种成像技术能够可靠地区分假性进展和早期疾病进展。已经研究的技术包括弥散加权MRI(与疾病进展相关的较低的ADC均值和ADC比值)及MR灌注显像(与疾病进展相关的较高的相对脑血容量)，但这些技术由于坏死和血管渗漏的干扰而受到限制，可能会低估rCBV。FDG-PET已经普及，但其灵敏度和特异度过低而不适用。新型示踪剂如FET-PET、FDOPA-PET、$^{13}N-NH_3$ PET正在研究中。

Stereotactic radiosurgery

- Stereotactic radiation therapy is the delivery of highly focused radiation to a target, and when completed in a single fraction is called radiosurgery.
- Transient increase in size of the lesion can occur 3–12 months after radiosurgery, and usually subsides without treatment.
- Radiation necrosis occurs later after completion of treatment, typically 9–12 months after therapy, rarely occurs before 6 months and does not subside without treatment.
- Perfusion MRI has been proven to be useful in distinguishing recurrent metastasis from radiation necrosis. The percentage of signal recovery computed from comparing enhancement at one hour from peak enhancement of a region of interest has been shown to have a sensitivity of 96% and specificity of 100% for radiation necrosis. However, this technique requires perfusion imaging times of up to an hour which can be logistically difficult.

立体定向放射外科

- 立体定向放射治疗是向靶目标发射高度聚焦的放射线，若完全集中于单个微小病灶则称为放射外科手术。
- 病变短暂性增大可发生在放射外科术后第3~12个月，不需治疗就会消退。
- 放射性坏死发生在治疗结束后，通常为治疗后9~12个月，很少发生在6个月内，未经治疗不会消退。
- MR灌注成像被证实有助于区分复发性转移和放射性坏死。通过比较感兴趣区域一个小时后和峰值的强化程度，计算出信号恢复的百分比，这对放射性坏死诊断有96%灵敏度和100%特异度。然而，这项技术要求灌注成像时间长达1小时，可行性较低。

Chemotherapy-related white matter disease

- Chemotherapy may cause focal, multifocal, or diffuse white matter disease, especially in combination with radiation treatment.
- Methotrexate toxicity is discussed in the toxic/metabolic section later in the chapter.

化疗相关白质疾病

- 化疗可引起单个、多个灶性或弥漫性脑白质病变，尤其是同时联合放疗。
- Methotrexate毒性将在本章后文的“中毒与代谢性疾病”代谢部分进行讨论。

（翻译　杨喜彪）

TOXIC/METABOLIC DISORDERS

中毒与代谢性疾病

METABOLIC DISORDERS

代谢性疾病

Wernicke encephalopathy

韦尼克脑病

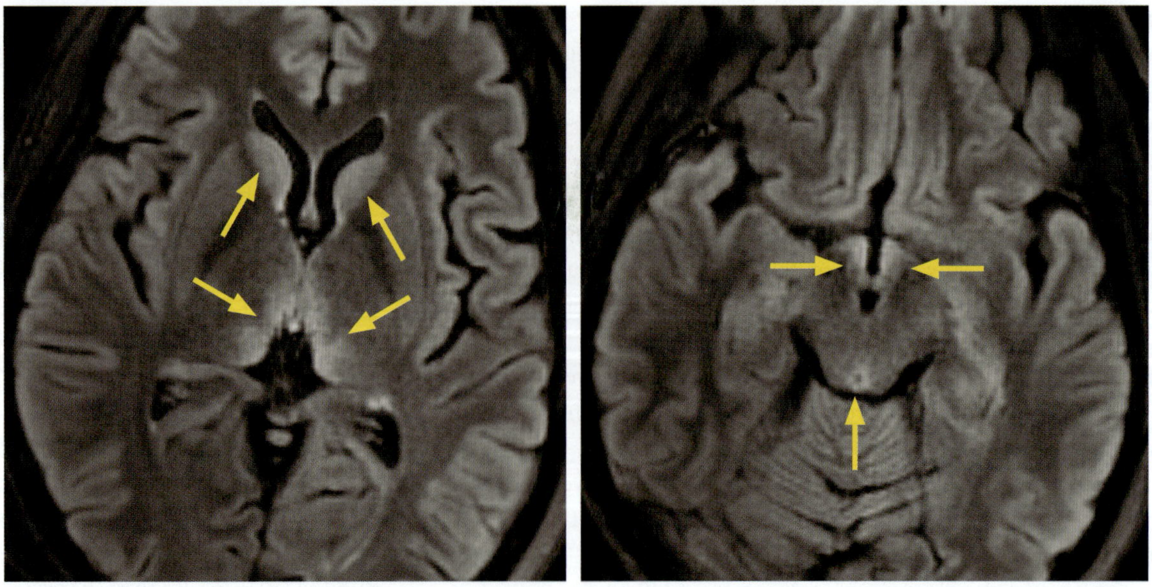

Wernicke encephalopathy: FLAIR images show T2 prolongation involving the thalami, caudate nuclei, inferior hypothalamus, mammillary bodies, and periaqueductal gray matter (arrows).

韦尼克脑病：FLAIR图像显示丘脑、尾状核、下丘脑下部、乳头体和中脑导水管周围灰质T_2延长(黄箭)。

- Wernicke encephalopathy is an acute syndrome of ataxia, confusion, andoculomotor dysfunction, caused by thiamine (vitamin B1) deficiency. This is most frequently seen in patients with alcoholism or other causes of secondary malnutrition, such as hyperemesis, eating disorders, and bariatric surgery.
- On imaging, the affected areas demonstrate symmetric bilateral hyperintensity on FLAIR, restricted diffusion, and contrast enhancement in up to 50% of cases. The most frequently affected areas are the medial thalami, the mammillary bodies, hypothalamus, tectal plate and periaqueductal gray matter.

- 韦尼克脑病是一种硫胺素(维生素B_1)缺乏引起的急性综合征，症状包括共济失调、精神异常及动眼神经功能障碍。最常见于酒精中毒或其他继发性营养不良，如呕吐、饮食紊乱和减肥手术。
- 在影像学上，受累区域呈表现双侧对称性FLAIR高信号、弥散受限，及高达50%的病例可见强化。最常见的受累区域是内侧丘脑、乳头体、下丘脑、顶盖和中脑导水管周围灰质。

Parathyroid dysfunction disorders

- Parathyroid hypofunction disorders include hypoparathyroidism, pseudohypoparathyroidism, and pseudopseudohypoparathyroidism, which can be distinguished based on clinical and laboratory findings.
- Hyperparathyroidism can be caused by a parathyroid adenoma or parathyroid hyperplasia.
- The main imaging findings are the same for all conditions and characterized by coarse calcium deposition in the basal ganglia.

  CT shows coarse, bilateral and symmetric calcifications in the globi pallidi, putamina, and caudate nuclei. MR images depict expected findings associated with calcifications in all sequences - hyperintensity on T1- weighted images, hypointensity on T2-weighted images, and blooming artifacts on T2*- or susceptibility- weighted images.

  The thalami, subcortical white matter, and dentate nuclei may also be affected.
- Important differential to consider is **Fahr disease**, which is a genetic condition characterized by idiopathic, bilateral basal ganglia calcifications. Fahr disease is not associated with laboratory abnormalities, unlike the parathyroid dysfunction disorders.

甲状旁腺功能紊乱

- 甲状旁腺功能减退性疾病包括甲状旁腺功能减退症、假性甲状旁腺功能减退症和假性假甲状旁腺功能减退症，它们之间的鉴别需要根据临床和实验室检查。
- 甲状旁腺功能亢进可由甲状旁腺腺瘤或甲状旁腺增生引起。
- 各种甲状旁腺功能紊乱的影像学的主要表现都相同，特征是基底节核团有粗大的钙质沉积。

  CT图像显示两侧苍白球、壳核和尾状核的对称性粗大钙化灶。MR所有序列中显示钙化征象——在T_1加权图像上呈信号增高，在T_2加权图像上呈低信号，在T_2*或磁敏感加权图像上呈开花样伪影。

  丘脑、皮质下白质和齿状核也可能受累。
- 甲状旁腺功能紊乱必须与**法尔病(特发性基底节钙化)**进行鉴别，后者是一种遗传性疾病，以特发性双侧对称性基底节核团钙化为特征。法尔病的实验室检查是正常的，此与甲状旁腺功能紊乱不同。

Hepatic encephalopathy

肝性脑病

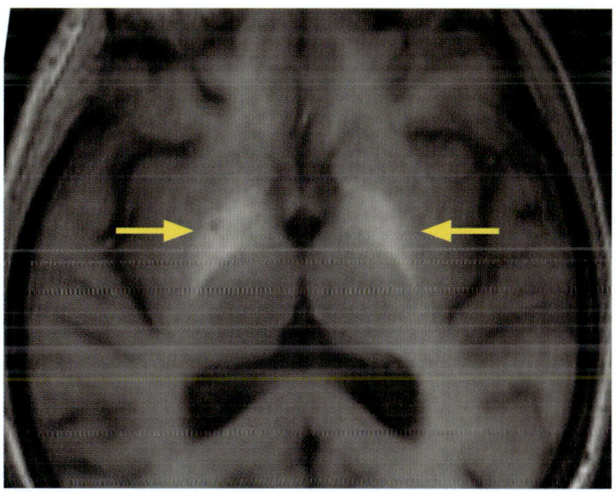

Axial noncontrast T1-weighted MRI shows intrinsic T1 hyperintensity in bilateral globi pallidi (arrows) in a patient with chronic liver disease.

轴位T_1加权MRI显示一名慢性肝病患者的双侧苍白球呈T_1高信号(黄箭)。

- **Chronic hepatic encephalopathy** is a reversible clinical syndrome seen in patients with chronic liver disease, frequently with portal hypertension or portosystemic shunting.
- Clinical presentation can vary from subtle cognitive impairment to more acute presentations of cognitive dysfunction during acute decompensation.
- The characteristic imaging finding is symmetric hyperintensity on T1-weighted imaging of the globi pallidi and substantia nigrae, thought to be due to manganese accumulation.

- **慢性肝性脑病**是见于慢性肝病患者中一种可逆的临床综合征，常伴有门静脉高压或门体分流。
- 临床表现可能从轻微的认知障碍到急性失代偿期的急性认知功能异常。
- 影像学特征为苍白球和黑质在T_1加权图像上呈对称性信号增高，可能与锰沉积有关。

- **Acute hepatic encephalopathy** or **hyperammonemic encephalopathy** is primarily caused by hyperammonemia, and is seen in acute liver failure.
- Characteristic imaging features of hyperammonemic encephalopathy include restricted diffusion accompanied by FLAIR hyperintensity symmetrically and bilaterally involving the insular and cingulate gyri, with relative sparing of the occipital lobes and perirolandic region.
- Recurrent alterations in ammonia levels, occurring in frequent acute on chronic liver failure presentations, can also result in chronic accumulation of glutamine, which may manifest as elevated glutamine-glutamate peak on MR spectroscopy.

Uremic encephalopathy

- Uremic encephalopathy occurs in acute and chronic renal failure as a result of excessive uremic toxins.
- Clinically patients present with neurologic symptoms, such as movement disorders, impaired mental status, cognitive disorders, and seizures.
- The most common imaging pattern is bilateral symmetric involvement of the basal ganglia with variable involvement of the white matter.
- The *lentiform fork sign* can be seen in patients with concurrent metabolic acidosis, characterized by FLAIR hyperintensity involving the white matter surrounding the lentiform nuclei, outlining the lateral and medial boundaries of the putamina.

Hypoglycemic encephalopathy

- The most common imaging finding is symmetric FLAIR hyperintensity with associated restricted diffusion affecting the gray matter in the parieto-occipital and temporal regions, with relative sparing of the thalami, white matter and cerebellum. Basal ganglia involvement can be seen and is associated with a poor prognosis.

Diabetic striatopathy

- Diabetic striatopathy, also known as **hyperglycemia-induced hemichorea-hemiballismus**, is a condition clinically manifest by involuntary, non-patterned movements.
- It is most frequently seen in type 2 diabetic patients and is a complication of nonketotic hyperglycemia.
- Imaging findings are pathognomonic, characterized by unilateral hyperintensity of the striatum on T1-weighted imaging and corresponding hyperdensity on CT.
- The clinical and imaging findings are reversible in most patients.

- **急性肝性脑病**或**高氨血症性脑病**主要由高氨血症引起，见于急性肝衰竭。
- 高血氨性脑病的影像学特征包括岛叶和扣带回双侧对称性弥散受限，同时在FLAIR图像上呈高信号，而枕叶和前旁扣带回区相对正常。
- 血氨水平反复异常可导致谷氨酰胺慢性积聚，在磁共振波谱上可表现为谷氨酰胺-谷氨酸峰值升高，通常见于慢性肝衰竭频繁出现急性发作的患者。

尿毒症脑病

- 尿毒症脑病出现在急性和慢性肾功能衰竭，为过量的尿毒素所致。
- 患者在临床上表现的神经症状包括运动障碍、精神状态受损、认知障碍和癫痫发作。
- 影像学上最常表现的方式为双侧基底核对称性受累，伴有不同程度的白质受累。
- *豆状核叉征*见于合并代谢性酸中毒的患者，其影像学特征是豆状核周围的白质在FLAIR图像上呈高信号，从而勾勒出壳核外侧和内侧明显的边界。

低血糖性脑病

- 影像学上最常见的表现为顶枕和颞区的灰质在FLAIR图像上呈对称性高信号，伴有弥散受限，而丘脑、白质和小脑受累相对较少。基底节也可受累，与预后不良有关。

糖尿病纹状体病

- 糖尿病纹状体病，也称为**高血糖性偏侧舞蹈症**，临床上表现为非自主的舞蹈样动作。
- 最常见于2型糖尿病患者，为非酮症高血糖症的并发症。
- 影像学发现具有病理诊断意义，其特征为单侧纹状体在T_1加权图像上呈增高信号，与CT密度增高一致。
- 大多数患者的临床和影像学表现可逆。

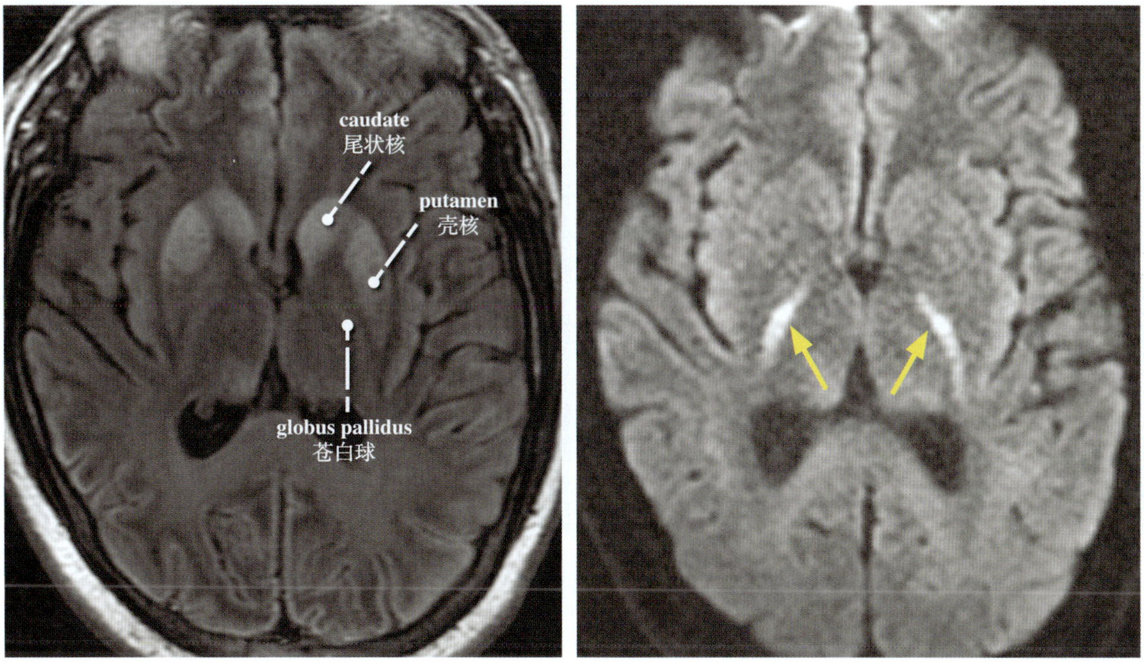

Hypoxic ischemic encephalopathy: Axial FLAIR (left image) shows symmetrical T2 prolongation in the bilateral putamina, heads of the caudate nuclei, and to a lesser extent in the globi pallidi. There is subtle FLAIR hyperintensity of the entire cortical ribbon. DWI (right image) shows marked DWI hyperintensity within the globi pallidi (arrows).

缺氧缺血性脑病：轴位FLAIR(左图)显示两侧豆状核、尾状核头及部分苍白球呈对称性长T_2。全脑皮质信号在FLAIR上呈轻微增高。DWI(右图)显示苍白球区信号显著增高(黄箭)。

- Hypoxic ischemic encephalopathy (HIE) in adults is caused by circulatory or respiratory failure, leading to global hypoxia/anoxia.
- Severe HIE typically affects the gray matter, including the cerebral cortex, hippocampi, and basal ganglia. This distribution is similar to that of severe hypoglycemia. Involvement of the basal ganglia portends a worse prognosis.
- MR imaging shows FLAIR and/or DWI hyperintensity of the affected regions.
- On CT, there is loss of gray-white differentiation, diffuse cerebral hypoattenuation, and sulcal effacement. The *white cerebellum sign* describes the typical sparing of the cerebellum, which appears relatively hyperattenuating compared to the affected supratentorial brain.

- 成人缺氧缺血性脑病(HIE)由循环或呼吸衰竭引起，会导致全脑低氧/缺氧。
- 重度HIE通常累及脑灰质，包括大脑皮质、海马和基底节。这种分布方式与严重低血糖相似。基底节受累提示预后较差。
- MRI显示受累区在FLAIR像和/或DWI上呈高信号。
- CT上表现为脑灰白质分界消失、弥漫性脑实质密度减低及脑沟消失。白小脑征指的是小脑未受累的典型表现，小脑相比受累的幕上脑实质呈高密度。

Methanol poisoning

- Methanol poisoning causes severe metabolic acidosis. Patients present with visual and gastrointestinal symptoms with rapid progression to a comatose state.
- Selective hemorrhagic necrosis of the putamina with relative sparing of the globi pallidi is the most characteristic imaging feature. Variable degrees of subcortical white matter, cerebellum, optic nerve necrosis may also be seen.
- Restricted diffusion can be seen in the acute phase. MR spectroscopy shows reduced NAA and elevated lactate peaks.

甲醇中毒

- 甲醇中毒会引起严重的代谢性酸中毒。患者出现视觉和胃肠道症状，并迅速进展到昏迷状态。
- 影像学上最明显的特征为选择性壳核出血坏死但苍白球相对完好。也可有不同程度的皮质下白质、小脑、视神经坏死。
- 急性期可见弥散受限。磁共振波谱显示NAA降低，乳酸峰升高。

Carbon monoxide

一氧化碳

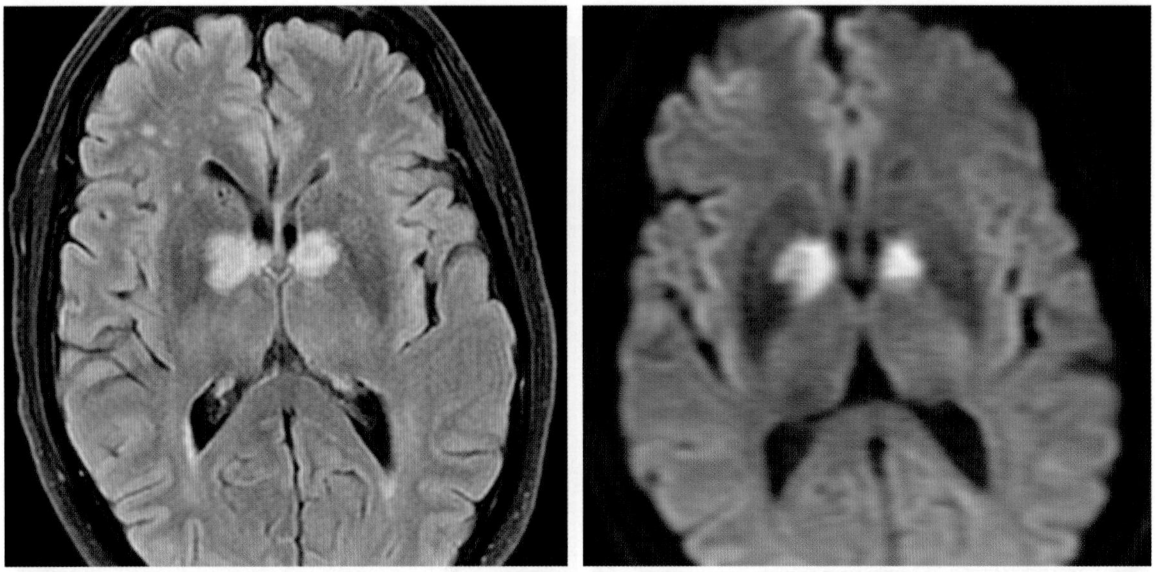

FLAIR (left image) and DWI (right image) show symmetric T2 prolongation and restricted diffusion involving bilateral globi pallidi, strongly favoring a toxic metabolic etiology such as carbon monoxide poisoning.

FLAIR(左图)和DWI(右图)显示双侧苍白球对称性长T_2和弥散受限，非常符合毒性代谢性疾病，如一氧化碳中毒。

- Carbon monoxide is an odorless and colorless gas which has a higher affinity to hemoglobin than oxygen and results in impaired oxygen transportation.
- Bilateral, symmetric, necrosis of the globi pallidi is the hallmark imaging feature, resulting in hyperintensity with hypointense rim on FLAIR with restricted diffusion and hypointensity on susceptibility-weighted sequences.
- Less common sites of involvement include the hippocampi, caudate nuclei, putamina, thalami, cerebellum, corpus callosum, cerebral cortex or white matter.

- 一氧化碳是一种无色无味的气体，它对血红蛋白的亲和力高于氧而会导致氧运输受损。
- 影像学上的标志性特征是双侧苍白球的对称性坏死，在FLAIR上呈高信号伴边缘低信号，弥散受限，在磁敏感加权图像上呈低信号。
- 较少受累的部位包括海马、尾状核、壳核、丘脑、小脑、胼胝体、大脑皮层和白质。

Osmotic demyelination

渗透性脱髓鞘

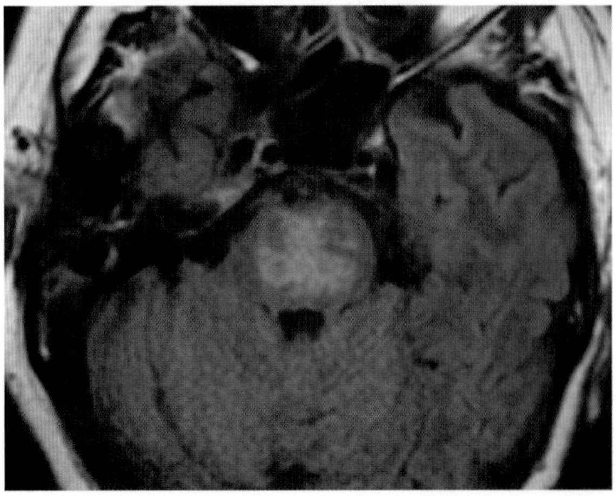

Central pontine myelinolysis: Axial FLAIR image demonstrates T2 prolongation in the central pons with associated mild restricted diffusion (not shown), in this patient with history of alcohol use disorder who presented with hyponatremia.

脑桥中央髓鞘溶解症：轴位FLAIR图像显示脑桥中央长T_2，伴有轻度弥散受限(未展示)，该患者有酗酒史，表现为低钠血症。

- Osmotic demyelination is caused by a rapid change in extracellular osmolality, typically occurring after aggressive correction of hyponatremia. The quick osmotic gradient change causes endothelial damage, blood-brain barrier breakdown, and release of extracellular toxins which damage myelin.
- Patients with poor nutritional status, including alcoholics, chronic lung disease patients, and liver transplant recipients, are the most susceptible to osmotic demyelination.
- Osmotic demyelination is most frequently seen in the pons, hence the entity was classically called central pontine myelinolysis. However, in up to 50% of cases, extrapontine lesions are also seen. MRI features include bilateral central T2 prolongation in the affected region. The most commonly involved extrapontine sites include the thalami, basal ganglia, and hemispheric white matter, frequently symmetric.

Marchiafava-Bignami disease

- 渗透性脱髓鞘是由于细胞外渗透压的快速改变所致，通常发生于快速纠正低钠血症之后。渗透压骤然变化会引起内皮细胞损伤、血脑屏障破坏，以及细胞外毒素释放，从而导致髓鞘损伤。
- 患者营养不良，包括酗酒、患有慢性肺疾病，以及肝移植后的患者，最容易发生渗透性脱髓鞘。
- 渗透性脱髓鞘常见于脑桥，因此也称为脑桥中央髓鞘溶解症。但半数以上病例也可以看到脑桥外的病变。MRI上表现为双侧受累区中心长T_2信号。最常累及的脑桥外部位包括丘脑、基底节和半球白质，通常是对称的。

Marchiafava-Bignami病

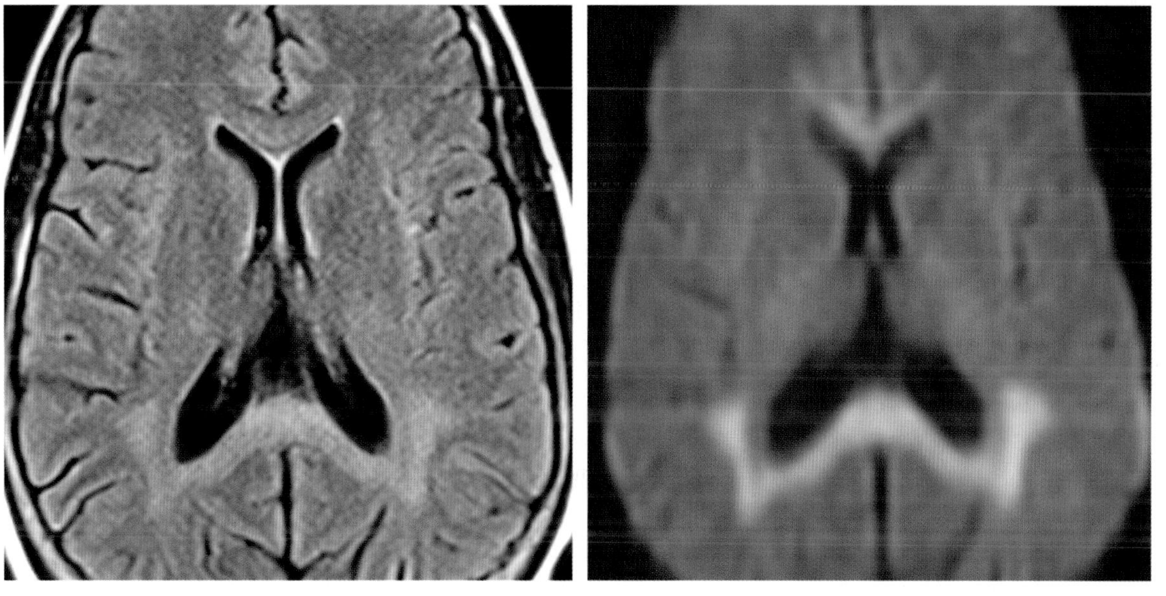

Axial FLAIR (left image) shows T2 prolongation in the corpus callosum with symmetric extension into the bilateral pericallosal white matter. There is associated restricted diffusion on DWI (right image). Findings are thought to represent Marchiafava-Bignami disorder.
轴位FLAIR(左图)显示胼胝体长T_2，对称性延伸至双侧胼胝体周围白质。DWI上还伴有弥散受限(右图)。这些表现符合马尔基亚法瓦-比尼亚米病的特征。

- Marchiafava-Bignami disease (MBD) is characterized by demyelination and subsequent necrosis of the corpus callosum.
- It is primarily associated with chronic alcohol use and vitamin B complex deficiency.
- Clinically patients can present acutely, with seizures or in a comatose state with progression to death within several days, or with a subacute/chronic presentation with mild encephalopathy.
- MBD can be accompanied by other alcohol-related conditions, such as Wernicke encephalopathy.

- 马尔基亚法瓦-比尼亚米病(MBD)以胼胝体脱髓鞘和随之出现的坏死为特征。
- 此病主要与慢性酗酒和维生素B复合物缺乏有关。
- 临床可呈急性发病，出现癫痫发作或昏迷，并在数天内进展至死亡，也可以亚急性/慢性发病，表现为轻度脑病。
- MBD可伴有其他酒精相关疾病，如韦尼克脑病。

Metronidazole-induced brain toxicity

甲硝唑(灭滴灵)诱发的中毒性脑病

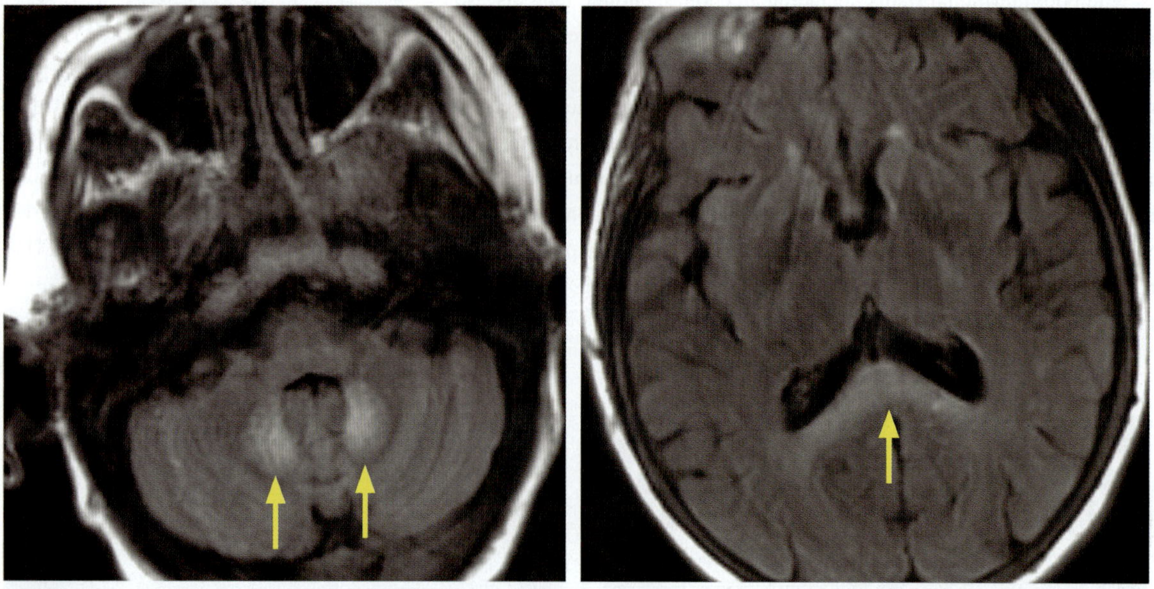

Metronidazole toxicity in patient with altered mental status and new onset movement disorder following recent metronidazole treatment: Axial FLAIR images show symmetric hyperintensity in bilateral dentate nuclei (left image, arrows) and splenium of the corpus callosum (right image, arrow).

甲硝唑中毒患者在近期接受甲硝唑治疗后出现精神状态改变和新发运动障碍：轴位FLAIR图像显示双侧齿状核(左图，黄箭)和胼胝体压部(右图，黄箭)对称性信号增强。

- Metronidazole is an antibiotic used to treat both bacterial and protozoal infections. Rarely, it can cause CNS toxic effects. While this occurs most frequently in patients with prolonged treatment courses (>25 days), it has also been described in patients with much shorter courses.
- Clinically, patients present with cerebellar dysfunction, altered mental status, and seizures.
- Characteristic imaging findings include ***symmetric*** hyperintensity on FLAIR of the cerebellar dentate nuclei, splenium of the corpus callosum, tegmentum, dorsal pons, and dorsal medulla.

- 甲硝唑是一种用于治疗细菌和原虫感染的抗生素，很少引起中枢神经系统毒性作用。该中毒情况多见于疗程长(>25天)的患者，但也有报道疗程较短的患者。
- 临床上表现为小脑功能异常、神智状态改变和癫痫发作。
- 影像学上特征性表现为小脑齿状核、胼胝体压部、被盖、脑桥背侧和延髓背侧在FLAIR图像上对称性信号增高。

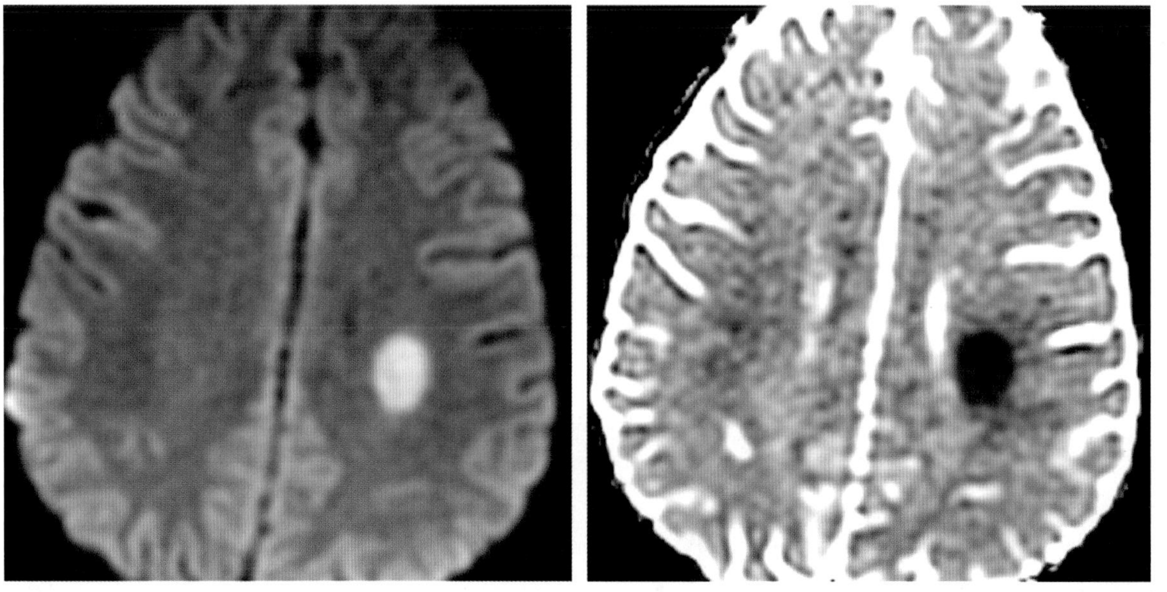

Methotrexate toxicity in a patient receiving intrathecal methotrexate for lymphoblastic lymphoma who presented with left arm weakness: DWI (left image) and ADC map (right) show focal decreased diffusivity within the left perirolandic white matter involving the cortical spinal tracts.

甲氨蝶呤中毒的患者在接受鞘内注射甲氨蝶呤治疗淋巴母细胞淋巴瘤后出现左臂无力：DWI(左图)和ADC图(右图)显示左侧中央沟周围区(perirolandic区)的白质出现局限性弥散受限，累及皮质脊髓束。

- The most characteristic imaging finding is bilateral, ***asymmetric*** white matter lesions with diffusion restriction and associated FLAIR hyperintensity affecting the centrum semiovale, crossing vascular territories with relative sparing of subcortical U fibers.
- In more severe cases of necrotizing encephalopathy, peripheral enhancement can be seen with confluent adjacent vasogenic edema, and can demonstrate a tumorlike pattern.
- Unlike malignancy, these lesions and enhancement disappear without treatment.

- 最具特征性的影像学表现为双侧不对称的白质病变，伴有弥散受限及在FLAIR图像上信号增高，累及半卵圆中心，跨越血管分布区但皮质下“U”形纤维相对正常。
- 在更严重的坏死性脑病病例中，病灶周边强化伴邻近血管源性水肿，可以呈肿瘤样的表现。
- 但与恶性肿瘤不同，这些病灶和强化不需要治疗就会消失。

(翻译 陈春勇)

AUTOIMMUNE DISORDERS

Autoimmune encephalitis

- Autoimmune encephalitis, also known as autoimmune limbic encephalitis, is an antibody- mediated inflammatory disorder which typically affects the limbic system.
- This class of disorders is classified into two broad categories, paraneoplastic or non-paraneoplastic, based on the presence of an underlying malignancy. In addition, they can be characterized as either group Ⅰ or group Ⅱ, based on the location of neuronal antigens. Group Ⅰ antibodies target intracellular antigens and group Ⅱ antibodies target antigens on the cell surface.
- Paraneoplastic syndromes are most often seen in small-cell lung cancer, but can be seen in the setting of many malignancies, including neuroblastoma, testicular germ cell tumor, breast cancer, thymoma, Hodgkin lymphoma, and ovarian teratoma.

自身免疫性疾病

自身免疫性脑炎

- 自身免疫性脑炎，也称为自身免疫性边缘系统脑炎，是一种抗体介导的炎症性疾病，通常影响边缘系统。
- 此类疾病根据是否合并恶性肿瘤分为两大类：副肿瘤性或非副肿瘤性。此外，根据神经元抗原的位置，它们可以分为Ⅰ组或Ⅱ组。Ⅰ组抗体针对细胞内抗原，Ⅱ组抗体针对细胞表面抗原。
- 副肿瘤综合征最常见于小细胞肺癌，但也可见于其他多种恶性肿瘤，包括神经母细胞瘤、睾丸生殖细胞瘤、乳腺癌、胸腺瘤、霍奇金淋巴瘤和卵巢畸胎瘤。

- **Group Ⅰ antibodies** are more closely associated with paraneoplastic syndromes and are associated with worse clinical outcomes due to decreased response to immunomodulatory therapy and increased irreversible neuronal damage.

Anti-Hu encephalitis is the most common paraneoplastic form of autoimmune encephalitis. It is associated with small-cell lung cancer in most cases and has a relatively poor prognosis. MR imaging findings include hyperintense lesions on FLAIR sequence in the medial temporal lobes with variable involvement of the cerebellum and brainstem.

Other group Ⅰ antibodies include **Anti-Ma/Ta** and **Anti-CV2**, which are commonly associated with testicular cancer and malignant thymoma, respectively. Additional areas of involvement on imaging include the thalamus and striatum.

Anti-GAD (glutamic acid decarboxylase) is a group Ⅰ antibody but is not typically associated with malignancy.

- **Ⅰ组抗体**与副肿瘤综合征更为密切相关，并且临床预后更差，这是由于对免疫调节治疗的反应降低和不可逆的神经元损伤增加所致。

抗Hu抗体脑炎是自身免疫性脑炎最常见的副肿瘤形式，在大多数情况下与小细胞肺癌有关，预后相对较差。MRI表现包括内侧颞叶FLAIR的高信号病变，伴小脑和脑干的不同程度受累。

其他Ⅰ组抗体包括**抗-Ma/Ta抗体**和**抗-CV2抗体**，它们通常分别与睾丸癌和恶性胸腺瘤相关。其他异常影像的区域包括丘脑和纹状体。

抗GAD抗体(谷氨酸脱羧酶)是Ⅰ组抗体，但通常与恶性肿瘤无关。

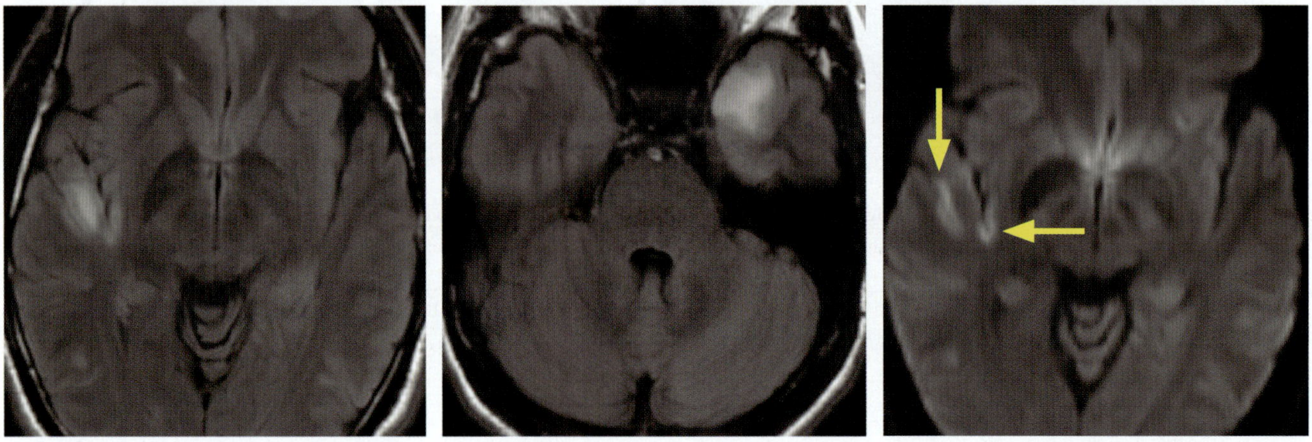

Anti-GAD autoimmune encephalitis: Axial FLAIR (left and middle images) show hyperintensity in the right temporal operculum and mesial left temporal lobe, with associated gyriform restricted diffusion (right image, arrow). Patient was found to have high level of GAD-65 antibodies in the serum and CSF.
抗GAD自身免疫性脑炎：轴位FLAIR(左图和中图)显示右侧颞盖和左颞叶内侧高信号，伴有相应脑回弥散受限(右图，黄箭)。患者血清和脑脊液中的GAD-65抗体升高。

- **Group Ⅱ antibodies** are more closely associated with non-paraneoplastic syndromes and are associated with better clinical outcomes.

Patients with non-paraneoplastic encephalitis associated with group Ⅱ antibodies frequently have an underlying autoimmune disorder or develop symptoms following a viral infection or vaccination. The most common form is **NMDAr** (N-methyl D-aspartate receptor) encephalitis. It is classically seen in young women and children and is non-paraneoplastic. The clinical presentation is unique in that the majority of patients have no abnormality on imaging on initial presentation. When MR imaging abnormalities are present, they typically show a wide distribution and degree of hyperintense lesions on FLAIR sequence with mild cortical enhancement and without restricted diffusion involving areas such as the inferior temporal lobe, insular cortex, and cingulate gyrus cortex.

- **Ⅱ组抗体**与非副肿瘤综合征关系更密切，临床预后较好。

Ⅱ组抗体相关的非副肿瘤性脑炎患者通常合并有自身免疫性疾病，或于病毒感染或疫苗接种后出现症状。最常见的形式是**NMDAr**(N-甲基D-天冬氨酸受体)脑炎。通常见于年轻妇女和儿童，为非副肿瘤性。临床表现独特，大多数患者在症状初始时并没有异常的影像学改变。当MRI出现异常时，通常为FLAIR序列上广泛分布和不同程度的高信号病变，伴皮质轻度增强，无弥散受限，累及下颞叶、岛叶皮质和扣带回皮质等区域。

(翻译　王草叶)

BRAIN INFECTION

大脑感染

BACTERIAL INFECTION

细菌性感染

Pyogenic abscess

细菌性脓肿

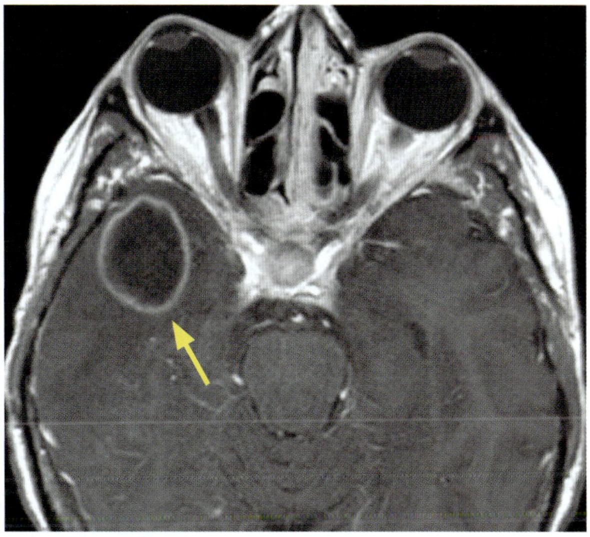

Axial contrast-enhanced T1-weighted MRI
轴位增强T_1加权MRI

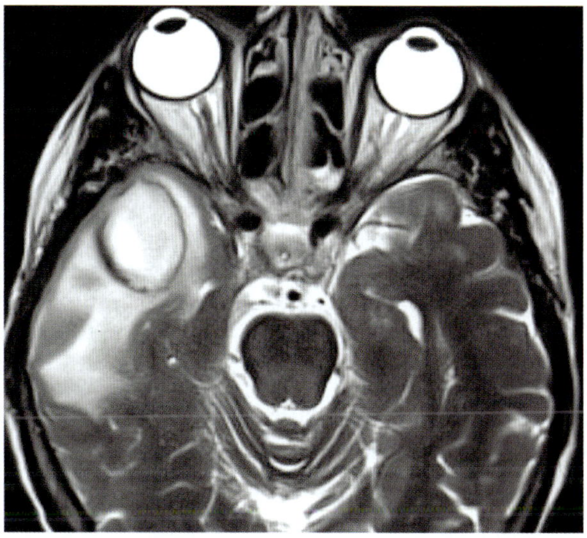

Axial T2-weighted MRI
轴位T_2加权MRI

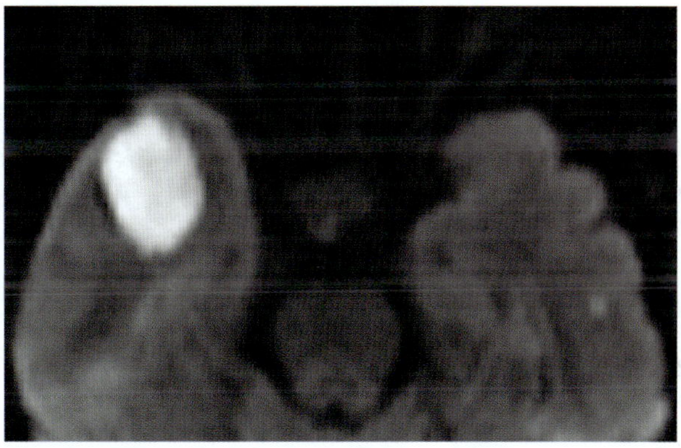

DWI
弥散加权成像

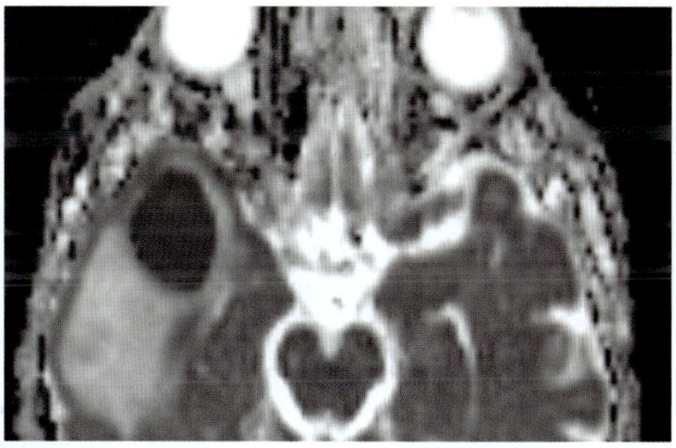

ADC map
表观扩散系数图

Pyogenic abscess: A ring-enhancing lesion (arrow) in the right anterior temporal lobe features a thin, smoothly enhancing, hypointense rim on the T2-weighted image, with moderate surrounding vasogenic edema. The contents of the lesion are hyperintense on DWI and dark on ADC, consistent with restricted diffusion.
细菌性脓肿：右侧颞叶前部见一个环形强化病灶(黄箭)，薄壁、光滑强化、T_2加权低信号环，伴有周围中度血管源性水肿。病灶内容物在DWI上呈高信号，在ADC图上呈低信号，符合弥散受限。

- A cerebral pyogenic abscess may be due to hematogenous dissemination, direct spread from paranasal sinusitis or mastoiditis, or as a complication of bacterial meningitis.
- An abscess evolves over 4 stages (early cerebritis → late cerebritis → early abscess → late abscess) and takes about two weeks to fully develop. In the early stage of infection, there is nonspecific T2 prolongation in the affected region, with heterogeneous enhancement.

- 大脑细菌性脓肿的原因可以为血行播散、从鼻窦炎/乳突炎直接传播，或为细菌性脑膜炎的并发症。
- 脓肿的演变分为四期(早期脑炎→晚期脑炎→早期脓肿→晚期脓肿)，整个过程大概需要2周。在早期感染阶段，病变区出现非特异性T_2延长，强化不均匀。

- After the abscess becomes discrete, the classic imaging appearance is a ring-enhancing mass. The rim is hypointense on T2-weighted images. Unlike the rim of a glioma or metastasis, an abscess rim is thin and smooth.
- When periventricular in location, an abscess classically tends to feature a thinner capsule oriented towards the ventricles. Disruption of the ventricular margin may herald impending rupture. Rupture may result in ventriculitis, with very high mortality.
- A brain abscess almost always demonstrates restricted diffusion, appearing very bright on DWI due to restricted diffusion superimposed on inherent hyperintensity on T2-weighted images.

Tuberculoma

- A tuberculoma is a localized tuberculosis granuloma. It is not always possible to differentiate a tuberculoma from a pyogenic abscess.
- A tuberculoma tends to have central hypointensity on T2-weighted image (in contrast to a pyogenic abscess, which is hyperintense). A cystic tuberculoma, however, may mimic a pyogenic abscess. Similar to pyogenic abscess, tuberculomas tend to show restricted diffusion.

Lyme disease

- Lyme disease, caused by the spirochete *Borrelia burgdorferi*, can cause white matter disease with a nonspecific imaging appearance of T2 prolongation predominantly in the frontal subcortical white matter. Associated enhancement of multiple cranial nerves or meningeal enhancement may suggest the diagnosis.

- 一旦脓肿形成，其典型影像学特征是一个环形强化的肿块。脓肿壁在T_2加权上呈低信号。脓肿的壁较胶质瘤或转移瘤薄且更光滑。
- 当位于脑室旁时，脓肿往往呈现为一个菲薄的包裹并朝向脑室。若脑室边缘受损，则预示脓肿可能即将发生破裂。脓肿破裂可引起脑室炎，具有极高的致死率。
- 脑脓肿几乎都表现为弥散受限，在T_2加权高信号的基础上弥散进一步受限导致DWI上呈明显的高信号。

结核球

- 结核球是一个局灶性的结核肉芽肿。并不是所有的结核球都能与细菌性脓肿相鉴别。
- 结核球在T_2加权上常表现为中央低信号(相比细菌性脓肿的中央高信号)。但是，囊性结核球却与细菌性脓肿信号很接近。与细菌性脓肿类似，结核球也常表现为弥散受限。

莱姆病

- 莱姆病，由伯氏疏螺旋体引起，可导致脑白质病变，MRI表现为脑白质非特异性T_2延长，主要累及额叶皮层下。同时伴发的多发脑神经或脑膜的强化可提示此病诊断。

VIRAL INFECTION

病毒感染

Herpes encephalitis

疱疹性脑炎

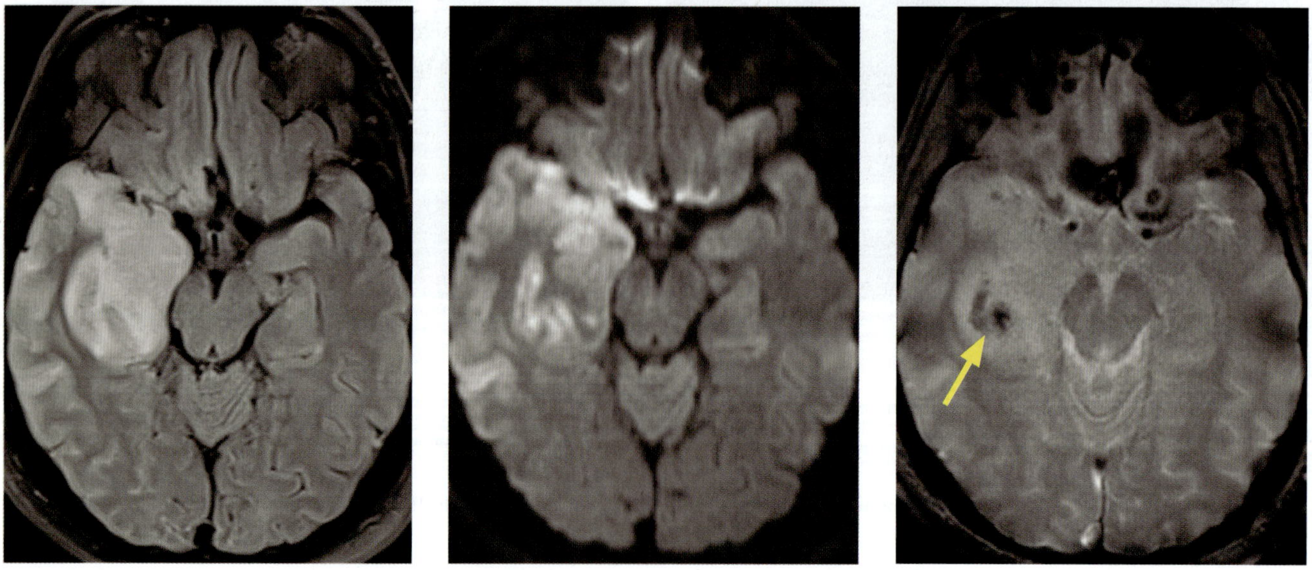

Axial FLAIR
轴位FLAIR

DWI
弥散加权成像

SWI
磁敏感加权成像

Herpes encephalitis: MRI images show abnormal FLAIR hyperintensity and restricted diffusion in the anterior right temporal lobe with regional mass effect and associated foci of susceptibility representing petechial hemorrhagic conversion (arrow).
疱疹性脑炎：MRI显示右侧颞叶前部异常FLAIR高信号及弥散受限，伴局部占位效应，其内有磁敏感灶，代表点状出血性转化(黄箭)。

- Herpes encephalitis is a devastating (if untreated), necrotizing encephalitis caused by reactivation of latent HSV-1 within the trigeminal ganglion.
- Clinical symptoms are nonspecific, with fever and headache often being prominent complaints. Mental status may be altered.
- *Herpes should be the first consideration in any patient with fever, mesial temporal lobe signal abnormality, and acute altered mental status.*
- Although lumbar puncture should be obtained before MRI and treatment should never be delayed for MRI, it is important to note that herpes encephalitis may be present when not clinically suspected and PCR of HSV in cerebrospinal fluid is not 100% sensitive.
- Herpes encephalitis causes edema, hemorrhage, and necrosis, typically in the medial temporal lobes and the inferior frontal lobes.
- CT is often normal but can show ill-defined hypoattenuation in the affected regions.
- MRI is much more sensitive and typically shows bilateral (but usually asymmetric) T2 prolongation in the medial temporal lobe, insular cortex, cingulate gyrus, and inferior frontal lobe.
- Once the infection becomes hemorrhagic, MRI will show foci of T1 shortening and gradient susceptibility. The affected areas typically demonstrate reduced diffusion.
- Enhancement may develop later in the infection, and is typically gyral in morphology.
- In an immunocompromised patient, HSV-6 infection should be considered with the above findings, although enhancement and diffusion abnormalities may be absent.
- The differential diagnosis of medial temporal lobe lesions includes MCA infarction, infiltrating glioma, limbic encephalitis, and seizure-related changes. Fever is typically absent in infarction and glioma. Herpes encephalitis should be the first consideration in any patient with fever and signal abnormality in the medial temporal lobe.
- Treatment is urgent antiviral therapy.

- 疱疹性脑炎是一种极具致命性(若不治疗)的坏死性脑炎，由潜伏在三叉神经节的1型HSV再次激活所致。
- 临床症状无特异性，以发热、头痛为主要表现，也可能出现神志改变。
- 任何患者出现发热、颞叶内侧信号异常及急性神志改变时，应首先考虑疱疹病毒感染。
- 腰椎穿刺应在MRI检查前完成，但治疗不能因MRI而延迟。必须要注意，疱疹性脑炎不一定有临床症状，且脑脊液HSV的PCR检查的灵敏度不是100%。
- 疱疹性脑炎可引起水肿、出血及坏死，通常发生于颞叶内侧及额叶下部。
- CT通常为正常，但也可在受累区见到边界不清的低密度影。
- MRI的灵敏度较高，常表现为双侧(但常不对称)颞叶内侧、岛叶、扣带回及额叶下部长T_2信号。
- 一旦感染合并出血，MRI上可见局灶性短T_1及对梯度回波序列磁敏感的病灶。受累区域通常表现为弥散受限。
- 感染后期可出现强化，通常呈脑回样的形态。
- 当免疫功能低下的患者出现上述表现时，应考虑6型HSV，即使缺乏强化或弥散异常。
- 颞叶内侧病变鉴别诊断包括大脑中动脉梗死、浸润性胶质瘤、边缘性脑炎及癫痫引起的改变。脑梗死及胶质瘤患者通常无发热。任何患者出现发热及颞叶内侧信号异常时，应首先考虑疱疹性脑炎。
- 治疗方法为紧急抗病毒治疗。

HIV encephalopathy

- HIV encephalopathy is the most common CNS infection in AIDS patients. It is a progressive neurodegenerative disease caused by direct infection of CNS lymphocytes and microglial cells (CNS macrophages) by the HIV virus.
- On imaging, HIV encephalitis manifests as diffuse cerebral atrophy and symmetric T2 prolongation in the periventricular and deep white matter.
- As previously discussed, in contrast to progressive multifocal leukoencephalopathy (PML), HIV encephalitis spares the subcortical U-fibers and tends to be symmetric.

HIV脑病

- HIV脑病是AIDS患者最常见的中枢神经系统(CNS)感染。它是一种进行性神经退行性疾病，为中枢神经系统中的淋巴细胞及小胶质细胞(CNS的巨噬细胞)直接受到HIV病毒感染所致。
- 影像学上，HIV脑炎表现为大脑弥漫性萎缩以及对称性脑室旁及深部白质长T_2。
- 如前所述，与进行性多灶性脑白质病(PML)不同，HIV脑炎并不累及皮层下“U”形纤维，且病变多为对称性。

Cytomegalovirus (CMV) encephalitis

- Cytomegalovirus (CMV) encephalitis only affects the immunosuppressed, typically when the CD4 cells are less than 50 cells/μL.
- The most common CNS manifestation of CMV infection is ventriculitis or meningoencephalitis.
- The characteristic imaging features of CMV ventriculitis include subependymal FLAIR hyperintensity and enhancement throughout the ventricular system.
- In neonates, CMV is one of the most common TORCH infections and causes atrophy, encephalomalacia, ventricular enlargement, and periventricular calcification.

巨细胞病毒(CMV)脑炎

- 巨细胞病毒(CMV)脑炎只发生于免疫受抑制的患者，尤其当CD_4细胞计数小于50/μL时。
- CMV感染最常见的中枢神经系统表现是脑室炎或脑膜脑炎。
- CMV脑室炎典型的影像学表现包括室管膜下FLAIR高信号及整个脑室系统强化。
- 在新生儿，CMV是最常见的TORCH感染[弓形虫病、其他(梅毒螺旋体、带状疱疹病毒、细小病毒B19)、风疹病毒、巨细胞病毒(CMV)和疱疹感染]之一，可造成脑萎缩、脑软化、脑室扩大及脑室旁钙化。

FUNGAL INFECTION

- Radiologic manifestations of CNS fungal infections are often nonspecific, including parenchymal abscesses, granulomas, cerebritis, meningitis, vasculitis, or mycotic aneurysms.
- Imaging features that help distinguish intracranial fungal abscesses from bacterial abscesses include crenated/lobulated border, nonenhancing intracavitary projections (thought to represent fungal hyphae) with restricted diffusion, and a core *without* restricted diffusion.
- Skull base involvement (basilar meningitis) is a common feature in fungal infections and can present as multiple cranial nerve palsies.
- Fungal mycotic aneurysms often arise from the proximal cerebral vasculature and are fusiform in morphology (due to involvement of long segments of vessel wall), in contrast to bacterial mycotic aneurysms which are typically saccular, small, multiple, and arise distally.
- Immune status of the patient and geographic distribution of some fungal organisms can also help narrow down the differential.

  Fungal organisms that infect immunocompetent patients: *Cryptococcus neoformans, Coccidioides immitis, Histoplasma capsulatum, Blastomyces dermatitidis.*

  Fungal organisms that infect immunocompromised patients: *Aspergillus, Candida, Mucormycoses.*

真菌感染

- 中枢神经系统真菌感染的放射学表现通常是非特异性的，包括脑实质脓肿、肉芽肿、脑炎、脑膜炎、血管炎或感染性动脉瘤。
- 影像学有助于区分颅内真菌性脓肿和细菌性脓肿的表现包括：圆齿状/分叶状边界、无强化的腔内突起(被认为是代表真菌菌丝)伴弥散受限，以及中央无弥散受限。
- 颅底受累(基底脑膜炎)是一种真菌感染的常见征象，可表现为多发性脑神经麻痹。
- 真菌感染性动脉瘤形态呈梭形(由于长段血管壁受累)，通常位于近端脑血管；而细菌性感染性动脉瘤通常呈囊状、小型、多发，并出现在血管的远端。
- 患者的免疫状态和某些真菌生物的地理性分布也有助于缩小鉴别诊断范围。

  免疫功能正常患者感染的真菌：新型隐球菌、球孢子菌、荚膜组织胞浆菌、皮芽孢杆菌。

  免疫功能低下患者感染的真菌：曲霉菌、念珠菌、毛霉菌病。

Cryptococcosis

隐球菌病

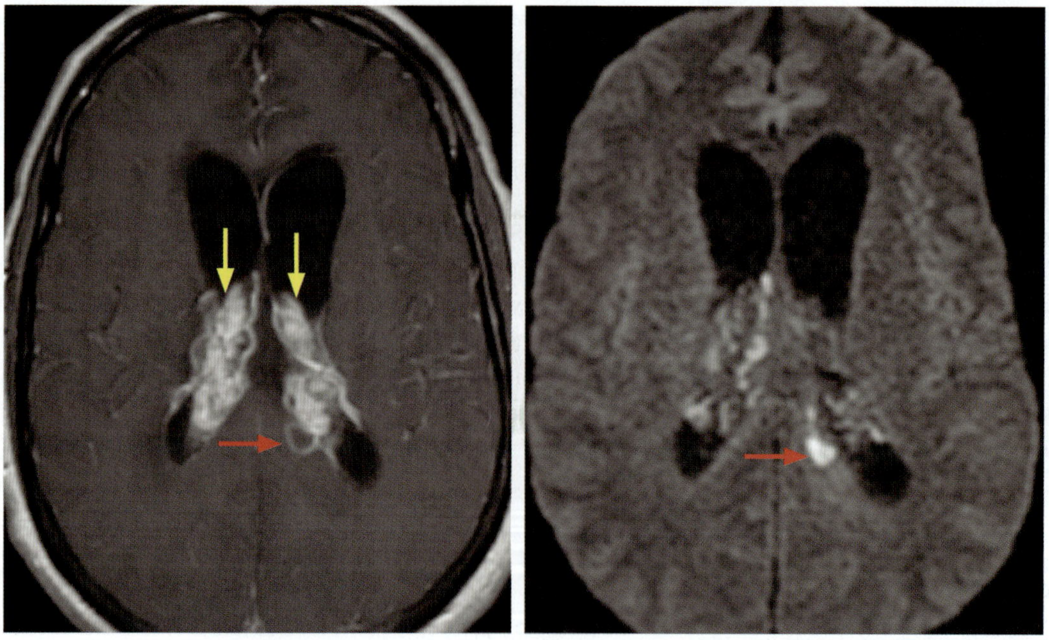

Cryptococcosis: Axial post-contrast T1-weighted MRI (left image) and DWI (right image) show abnormal enhancement of the choroid plexus (yellow arrows) with cystic components that demonstrate restricted diffusion (red arrows), suggesting cryptococcomas. Lumbar puncture confirmed cryptococcal meningitis.

隐球菌病：轴位增强T_1加权 MRI(左图)和 DWI(右图)显示脉络丛异常强化(黄箭)，囊性成分呈弥散受限(红箭)，提示隐球菌。腰椎穿刺证实为隐球菌性脑膜炎。

- Cryptococcosis is the most common CNS fungal infection in patients with AIDS and is caused by *Cryptococcus neoformans*. It is the third most common CNS infection in AIDS overall, after HIV encephalopathy and toxoplasmosis.

- 隐球菌病是AIDS患者最常见的中枢神经系统真菌感染，由新型隐球菌引起。在所有AIDS所致的中枢神经系统感染中，排名第三，仅次于HIV脑病及弓形虫病。

- Similar to toxoplasmosis, AIDS patients become susceptible to cryptococcus with a CD4 count less than 100 cells/μL. The most common clinical presentation is chronic basilar meningitis. The most common imaging finding is hydrocephalus, which is very nonspecific.
- Cryptococcus spreads along the basal ganglia perivascular spaces, leaving behind *gelatinous pseudocysts*, which appear as round water-signal lesions on T1- and T2-weighted MRI.
- Cryptococcus has a predilection for spread to the choroid plexus, producing ring-enhancing granulomas (called *cryptococcomas*) within the ventricles.
- Treatment is with antifungal agents including fluconazole and amphotericin B.

Aspergillosis

- *Aspergillus* spp. are ubiquitous molds that are angioinvasive and can lead to disseminated disease in immunocompromised patients. Routes of infection include hematogenous spread from the lung, extension from paranasal sinuses, or direct inoculation from trauma.
- Clinical presentation of invasive aspergillosis includes brain abscesses, meningitis, or meningoencephalitis.
- *Aspergillus* has a propensity to invade blood vessels, leading to vasculitis with secondary thrombosis, infarction, and mycotic aneurysm formation. Superimposed hemorrhage is a common feature.
- *Aspergillus* abscesses may demonstrate a hypointense rim on T2-weighted and gradient- echo images (representing hemorrhage and hemosiderin deposition) and peripheral restricted diffusion.
- Treatment includes voriconazole or amphotericin B.

Mucormycosis

- 与弓形虫病类似，当AIDS患者CD_4计数低于100/μL时容易感染隐球菌。最常见的临床表现为慢性颅底脑膜炎。最常见的影像学表现为脑积水，但非常不具特异性。
- 隐球菌沿基底节的血管周围间隙播散，遗留胶样假性囊肿，在T_1加权及T_2加权上表现为圆形水样信号病灶。
- 隐球菌容易向脉络丛播散，在脑室内形成环形强化的肉芽肿(又称隐球菌球)。
- 治疗用抗真菌药物，包括氟康唑及两性霉素B。

曲霉病

- 曲霉属是无处不在的霉菌，具有血管侵袭性，在免疫功能低下患者可导致疾病播散。感染途径包括从肺经血行播散、从鼻窦蔓延或外伤后直接感染。
- 侵袭性曲霉病的临床表现包括脑脓肿、脑膜炎或脑膜脑炎。
- 曲霉菌有侵入血管的倾向，导致血管炎，并继发血栓形成、梗死和感染性动脉瘤形成。合并出血是一个常见的表现。
- 曲霉脓肿可能在T_2加权和梯度回波图像(代表出血和含铁血黄素沉积)上呈低信号环，以及边缘弥散受限。
- 治疗包括伏立康唑或两性霉素B。

毛霉菌病

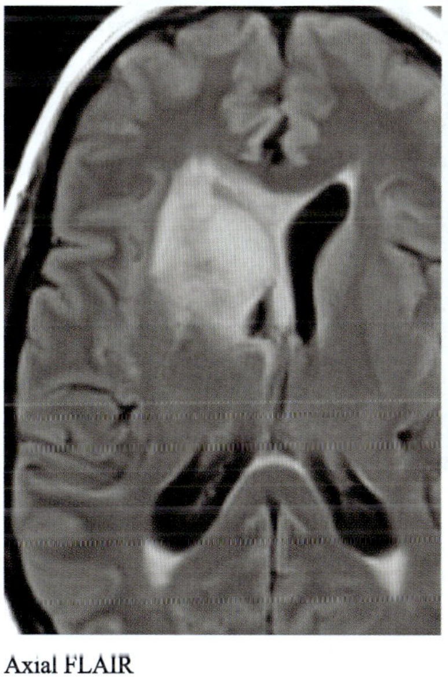

Axial FLAIR
轴位FLAIR

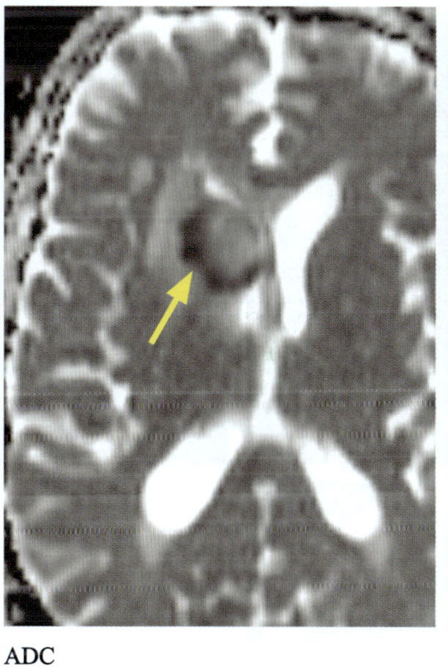

ADC
表观扩散系数

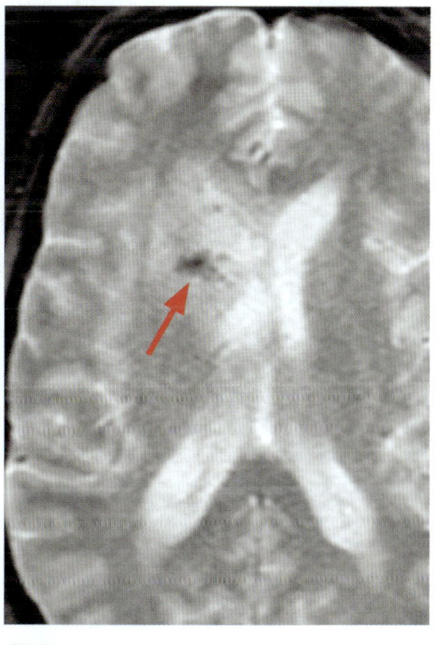

GRE
梯度回波序列

Cerebral mucormycosis: MRI images show a FLAIR hyperintense lesion in the right caudate head with surrounding vasogenic edema, associated peripheral restricted diffusion (yellow arrow), and susceptibility representing intralesional hemorrhage (red arrow). In this patient with a history of autologous stem cell transplant for T-cell leukemia and clinical concern for systemic infection, these findings are suspicious for a fungal infarct. Subsequent biopsy showed mucor.

脑毛霉菌病：MRI图像显示右侧尾状核头有一个FLAIR高信号病变，伴周围血管源性水肿，相应周边弥散受限(黄箭)，以及代表病灶内出血(红箭)的磁敏感灶。此患者有T细胞白血病病史并接受过自体干细胞移植，临床怀疑系统性感染，这些发现为可疑真菌性梗死。随后的活检发现了毛霉菌。

- Mucormycosis infects a similar patient population to *Aspergillus* and can be distinguished from aspergillosis by its more aggressive course, higher mortality, and poor response to voriconazole. Intracranial extension from invasive sinusitis is the primary etiology, particularly in patients with poorly controlled diabetes mellitus.
- Like aspergillosis, mucormycosis has a propensity for angioinvasion, leading to infarction and necrosis, often with hemorrhagic component.
- CT shows sinusitis with bony destruction. MRI may show frontal lobe lesions with reduced diffusivity, perineural intradural spread, or cavernous sinus thrombosis.
- Treatment includes aggressive surgical debridement, high-dose amphotericin B, and adjuvant supportive therapies.

Other fungal infections

- CNS **candidiasis** most commonly presents as multiple brain microabscesses. Meningitis or vascular involvement are less common.
- Disseminated **coccidioidomycosis** often causes meningitis, or chronic basilar meningitis similar to cryptococcosis that can be complicated by hydrocephalus or ischemic vasculitis. Parenchymal abscesses or granulomas are uncommon.
- **Histoplasmosis** has a tendency to cause isolated meningitis but can also present as granuloma or abscess.
- **Blastomycosis** can manifest as meningitis, cerebral abscesses preferentially involving basal ganglia or cerebellum, or vertebral osteomyelitis.

- 毛霉菌病感染的患者群体与曲霉菌相似，区别在于曲霉病的侵袭性更强，死亡率更高，对伏立康唑反应差。侵袭性鼻窦炎向颅内扩散为其主要原因，尤其对于糖尿病控制不佳的患者。
- 与曲霉菌病一样，毛霉菌病也有血管侵袭的倾向，可导致梗死和坏死，通常伴有出血成分。
- CT显示鼻窦炎伴有骨质破坏。MRI可显示弥散减低的额叶病变、神经周围硬膜内扩散或海绵窦血栓形成。
- 治疗包括积极手术清创、大剂量两性霉素B和辅助支持疗法。

其他真菌感染

- 中枢神经系统**念珠菌病**最常表现为多发性脑微脓肿。脑膜炎或血管受累较少见。
- 播散性**球孢子菌病**常引起脑膜炎，或慢性颅底脑膜炎，并与隐球菌病类似可并发脑积水或缺血性血管炎。实质脓肿或肉芽肿并不常见。
- **组织胞浆菌病**有引起孤立性脑膜炎的倾向，但也可表现为肉芽肿或脓肿。
- **芽生菌病**可表现为脑膜炎、脑脓肿，好发部位为基底神经节或小脑，或在椎体引起骨髓炎。

Parasitic Infection

寄生虫感染

Neurocysticercosis

神经囊尾蚴病

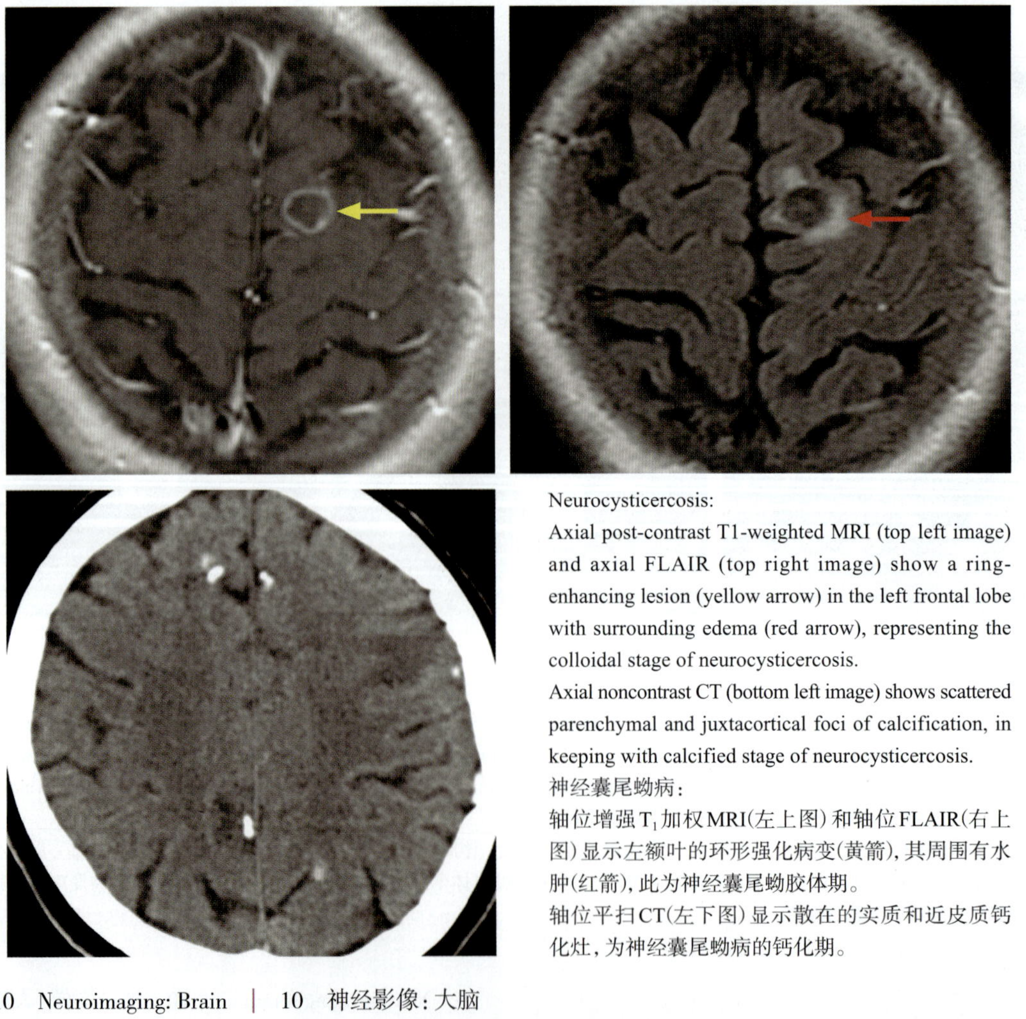

Neurocysticercosis:
Axial post-contrast T1-weighted MRI (top left image) and axial FLAIR (top right image) show a ring-enhancing lesion (yellow arrow) in the left frontal lobe with surrounding edema (red arrow), representing the colloidal stage of neurocysticercosis.
Axial noncontrast CT (bottom left image) shows scattered parenchymal and juxtacortical foci of calcification, in keeping with calcified stage of neurocysticercosis.

神经囊尾蚴病：
轴位增强T_1加权MRI(左上图)和轴位FLAIR(右上图)显示左额叶的环形强化病变(黄箭)，其周围有水肿(红箭)，此为神经囊尾蚴胶体期。
轴位平扫CT(左下图)显示散在的实质和近皮质钙化灶，为神经囊尾蚴病的钙化期。

- Neurocysticercosis is the most common parasitic CNS infection of immunocompetent patients. It is caused by the tapeworm *Taenia solium* and clinically presents with seizures.
- Four stages of neurocysticercosis have been described:

> 1) **Viable/vesicular**: Imaging shows several CSF-intensity cysts, without enhancement. Many of these cystic lesions may demonstrate an eccentric "dot" representing the scolex.
> 2) **Colloidal**: The colloidal stage has the least specific imaging findings, presenting as ring-enhancing lesions. In contrast to a pyogenic abscess, the lesions feature *increased* diffusivity.
> 3) **Nodular/granular**: Edema decreases as the cyst involutes and the cyst wall thickens.
> 4) **Calcified**: Imaging shows small parenchymal calcifications (on CT) and small foci of susceptibility (GRE).

- Intraventricular neurocysticercosis can occur in up to 20% of cases, typically in the aqueduct of Sylvius or the fourth ventricle. Hydrocephalus may be the initial presentation, with the obstructing cyst most apparent on FLAIR images because the protein-rich intracystic fluid will not be nulled on FLAIR.
- The racemose form of neurocysticercosis is an older term describing a variant without a visible scolex, now thought to represent degeneration of the scolex.
- Treatment is with antiparasitic medications including albendazole, supplemented with steroids for edema and anti-seizure medications as needed.

- 神经囊尾蚴病是正常免疫功能患者最常见的中枢神经系统寄生虫感染，由猪肉绦虫引起，临床表现为癫痫。
- 神经囊尾蚴病分为四期：

> 1) **活体期/囊性期**：影像上可见数个与脑脊液信号相等的囊肿，无强化。多数病灶内可见一偏心的"点"，代表囊虫头节。
> 2) **胶质期**：胶质期影像最不具特异性，表现为环形强化。与细菌性脓肿不同，这些病灶以弥散增高为特征。
> 3) **结节/肉芽肿期**：水肿随囊肿消失以及囊壁增厚而减退。
> 4) **钙化期**：影像学表现为脑实质小的钙化灶(CT上)和小的磁敏感灶(GRE序列上)。

- 发生在脑室内的神经囊尾蚴病的病例可高达20%，通常位于中脑导水管或第四脑室。脑积水可为首发表现，而阻塞性囊肿在FLAIR图像上最为明显，因囊内液体富含蛋白质，不被FLAIR抑制。
- 葡萄状神经囊尾蚴病是一个较老的术语，用于描述无头节的一种变异，现在则认为这是囊虫的头节退化。
- 治疗选择抗寄生虫药物，如阿苯达唑，必要时用类固醇消退水肿，以及抗癫痫药物作为辅助治疗。

Toxoplasmosis

弓形虫病

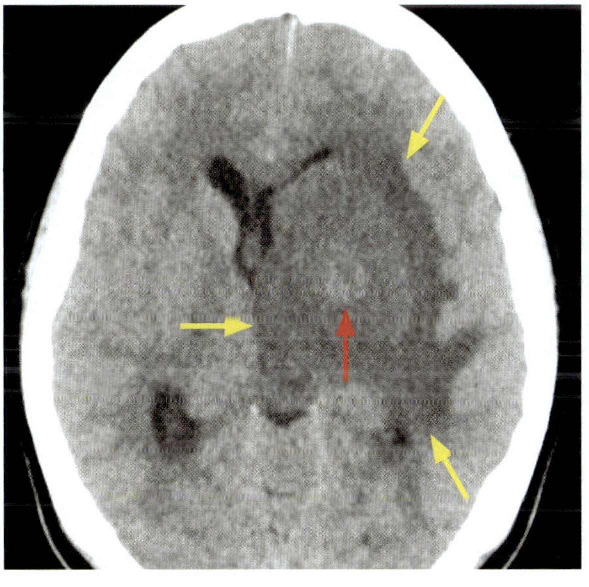

Toxoplasmosis: Axial unenhanced CT shows a large area of edema in the left basal ganglia (yellow arrows), centered on a subtle hyperattenuating mass (red arrow).
弓形虫病：轴位平扫CT可见左侧基底节大片水肿(黄箭)，中央可见稍高密度的肿块(红箭)。

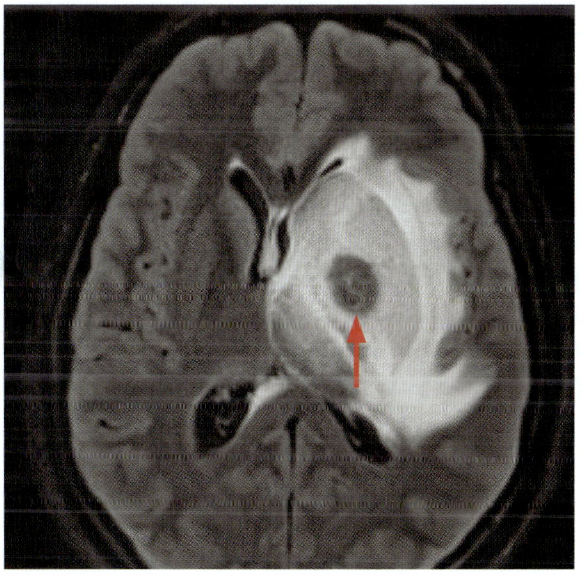

Axial FLAIR shows the extensive edema surrounding a heterogeneous rounded mass (red arrow) in the left basal ganglia.
轴位FLAIR显示左侧基底节一个信号不均的圆形肿块(红箭)，周围见广泛水肿。

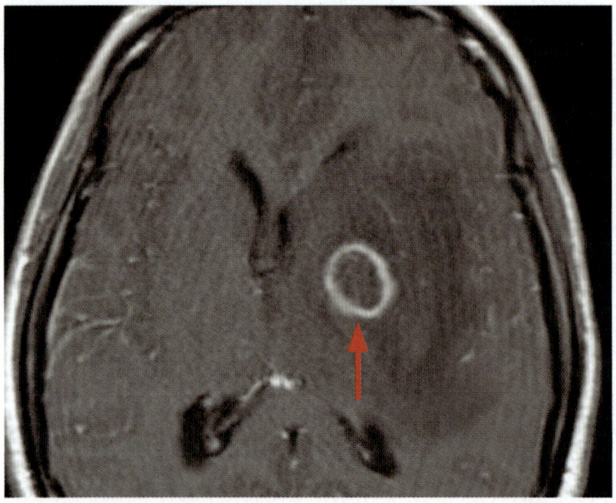

Post-contrast axial T1-weighted MRI demonstrates smooth ring-enhancement of the lesion (red arrow).
增强T_1加权MRI显示光滑的环形强化病灶(红箭)。

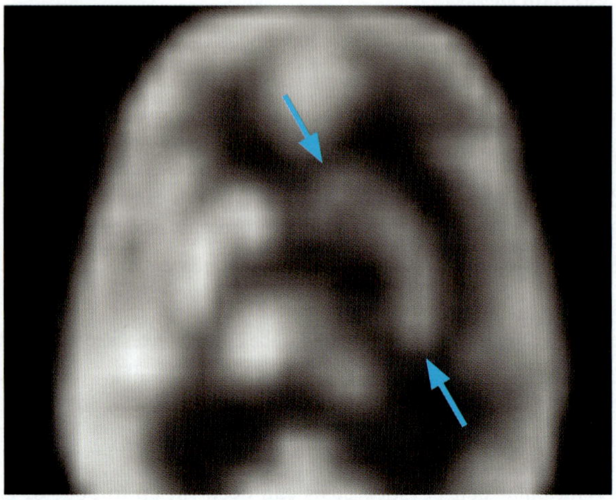

F-18-FDG PET scan shows asymmetrical, relatively decreased metabolism of the left basal ganglia (blue arrows).
^{18}F-FDG PET扫描显示两侧不对称，左侧基底节相对低代谢(蓝箭)。

- Toxoplasmosis is the most common mass lesion in AIDS patients and is caused by the parasite *Toxoplasma gondii*. AIDS patients become susceptible to the parasite with a CD4 count less than 100 cells/μL. Toxoplasmosis is the second most common CNS infection in AIDS patients, with HIV encephalitis being the most common.
- The typical appearance of toxoplasmosis is single or multiple ring-enhancing lesions in the basal ganglia.
- The *asymmetric target sign* is not frequently seen but is relatively specific and describes an eccentric nodule of enhancement along the enhancing wall of the toxoplasmosis lesion.
- The primary differential consideration of a basal ganglia mass in an immunocompromised patient is CNS lymphoma. In contrast to CNS lymphoma, toxoplasmosis is hypometabolic on FDG-PET, is not thallium-avid, does not demonstrate reduced relative cerebral blood volume on perfusion, and will respond to appropriate antimicrobial therapy. Toxoplasmosis lesions usually have increased diffusivity. In contrast, CNS lymphoma tends to have reduced diffusivity due to hypercellularity.

- 弓形虫病是AIDS患者最常见的占位性病变，由刚地弓形虫感染引起。AIDS患者CD_4细胞计数低于100/μL时容易感染弓形虫。弓形虫病是AIDS患者第二常见的中枢神经系统感染，仅次于HIV脑炎。
- 弓形虫病的典型表现为基底节单发或多发的环形强化灶。
- 非对称靶心征在弓形虫病中不常见，但相对比较特异，表现为贴着弓形虫病灶强化壁的偏心强化结节。
- 基底节区肿块在免疫低下的患者中最先要考虑的鉴别诊断是CNS淋巴瘤。与CNS淋巴瘤相比，弓形虫病在FDG PET上为低摄取、对铊无亲和力、脑灌注相对脑血容量不减少，但对适当的抗菌治疗有反应。弓形虫病通常表现出弥散增加；相反，中枢神经系统淋巴瘤由于细胞增多而往往出现弥散降低。

Creutzfeldt-Jakob disease (CJD)

克-雅病(CJD)

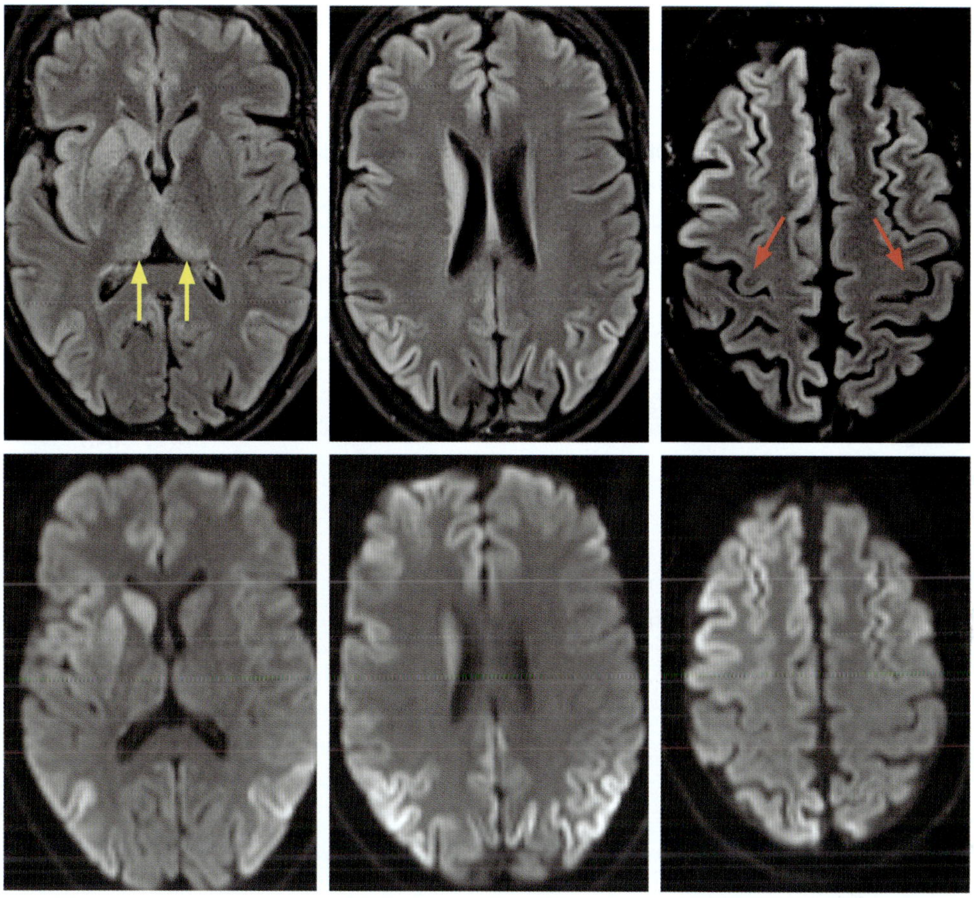

Creutzfeldt-Jakob disease: Axial FLAIR (top row), and DWI (bottom row) show diffusely increased FLAIR signal with restricted diffusion (when correlated to ADC maps, not shown) in the cerebral cortex, basal ganglia, and dorsomedial thalamus. There is relative sparing of the motor cortex (red arrows). A *hockey stick* sign is visible in the thalami on the first FLAIR image (yellow arrows).

Case courtesy Saurab Rohatgi, MD, Brigham and Women's Hospital.

克-雅病：轴位FLAIR(上排)及DWI(下排)显示大脑皮层、基底节、背内侧丘脑弥漫性FLAIR信号增高及弥散受限(对应ADC图未展示)。运动皮层相对正常(红箭)。第一幅FLAIR图像可见丘脑的曲棍球杆征(黄箭)。

- Creutzfeldt-Jakob disease (CJD) is a rare neurodegenerative disease caused by a prion.
- The typical MRI appearance of CJD is *cortical ribboning*, which describes ribbon-like FLAIR hyperintensity and restricted diffusion of the cerebral cortex. The basal ganglia and thalami are also involved. There is often sparing of the motor cortex.
- The *pulvinar* sign describes bright DWI and FLAIR signal within the pulvinar nucleus of the thalamus. The *hockey stick* sign describes bright DWI and FLAIR signal within the dorsomedial thalamus.

- 克-雅病(CJD)是一种罕见的由朊病毒引起的神经退行性疾病。
- CJD典型的MRI表现为飘带状皮层，即沿大脑皮层分布的飘带状FLAIR高信号及弥散受限，基底节及丘脑也可受累。运动皮层一般不受累。
- 丘脑枕征指的是丘脑枕核内DWI及FLAIR高信号。曲棍球杆征表现为丘脑背内侧核内DWI及FLAIR高信号。

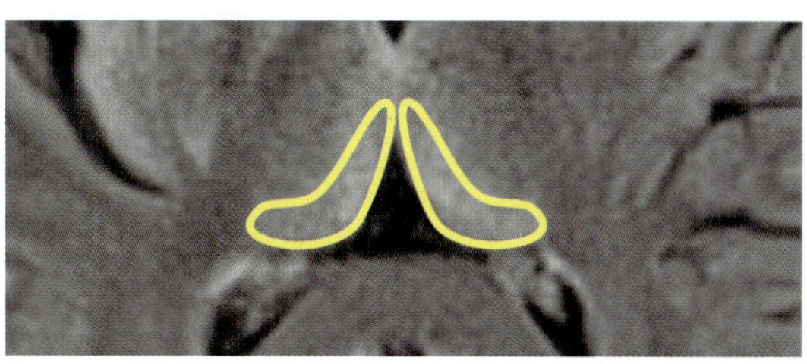

Hockey stick sign of CJD: FLAIR (close-up of top left FLAIR image above with the thalami outlined in yellow) shows hyperintensity of the dorsomedial thalami, mimicking the shape of a hockey stick.

CJD中的曲棍球杆征：FLAIR(上述左上FLAIR像的丘脑放大图，黄线勾勒区)显示丘脑背内侧核高信号，形似曲棍球杆。

(翻译　吴静)

11 Neuroimaging: Head and Neck

11 神经影像：头与颈

Francis Deng, Shruti Mishra, Jeffrey P. Guenette, Raymond Y. Huang

Contents

目录

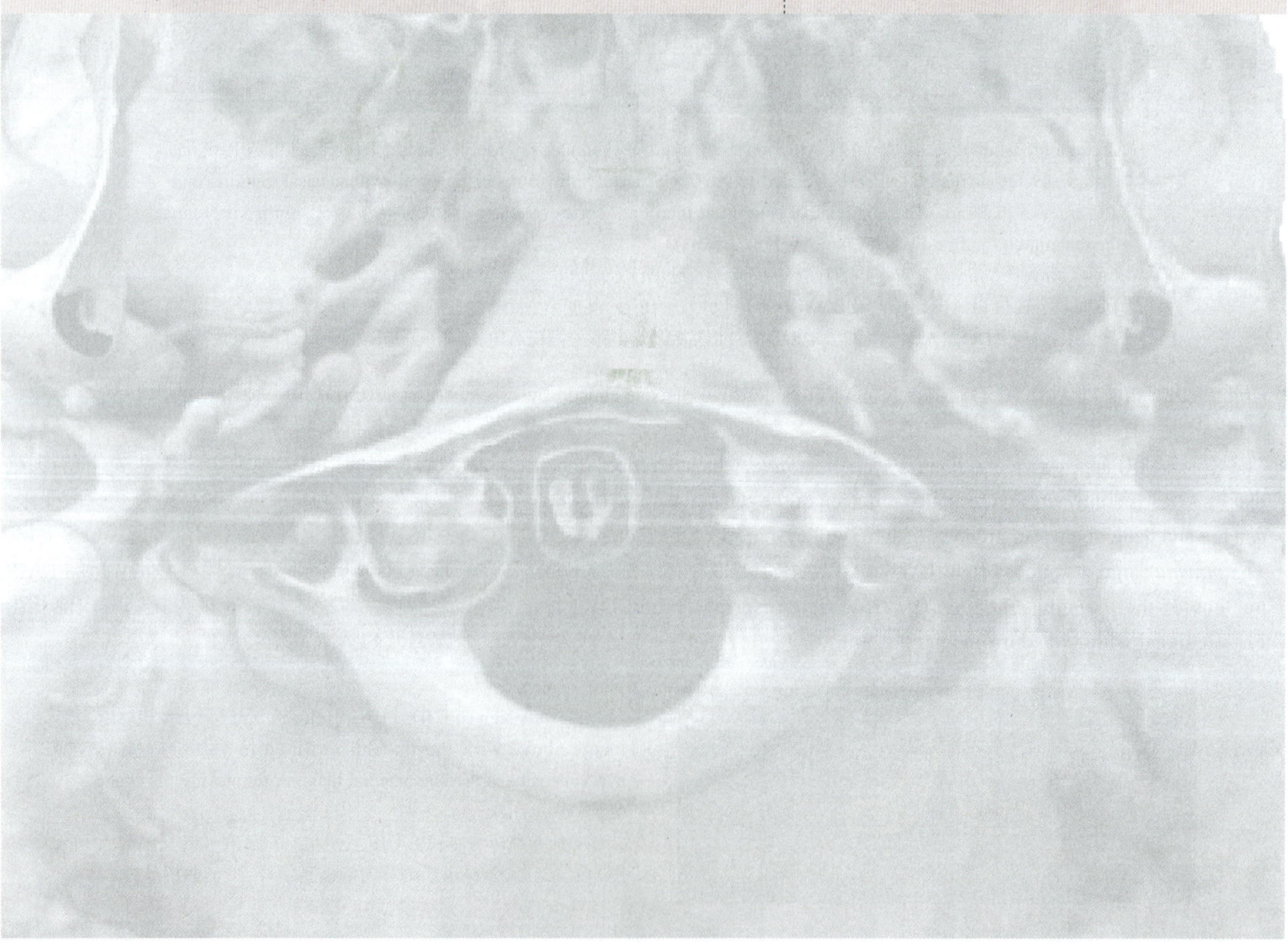

PARANASAL SINUSES, NASAL CAVITY, & ANTERIOR SKULL BASE

鼻旁窦、鼻腔和前颅底

OVERVIEW OF THE SINONASAL TRACT AND ANTERIOR SKULL BASE

鼻腔鼻窦和前颅底概述

Sinonasal histology and development

- The nasal cavity and paranasal sinuses are lined with Schneiderian epithelium, a ciliated mucosa of ectodermal origin that propels contents along anatomic drainage pathways toward the nasopharynx.
- The sinuses develop at different times in children. At birth, the maxillary and ethmoid sinuses are present but hypoplastic. Only later does the sphenoid pneumatize, followed by the frontal sinuses.

鼻腔鼻窦的组织学与发育

- 鼻腔和鼻旁窦衬有施奈德上皮，一种起源于外胚层的黏膜纤毛，它们将分泌物沿解剖引流道推向鼻咽部。
- 儿童鼻窦发育分阶段进行。出生时，上颌窦和筛窦已出现但发育不全。随后蝶窦气化，然后是额窦。

Sinonasal and anterior skull base anatomy

鼻腔鼻窦和前颅底解剖

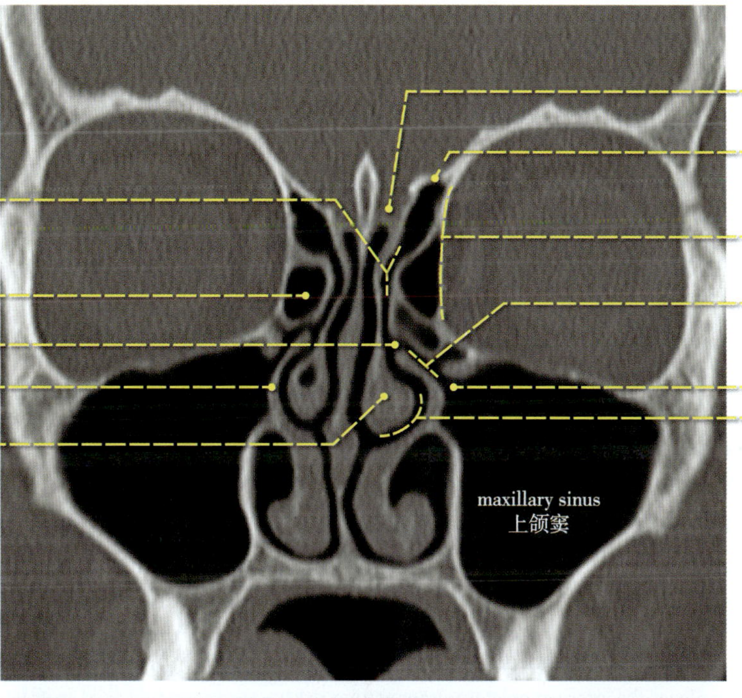

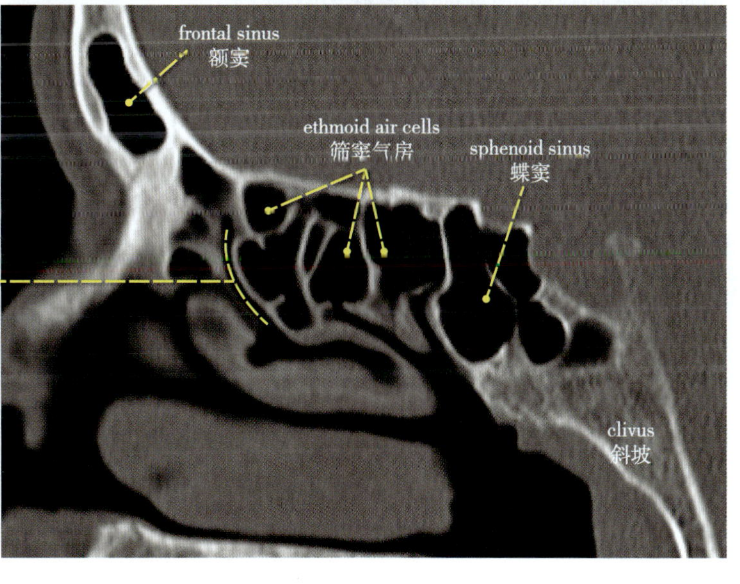

- The superior, middle, and inferior nasal turbinates/conchae are three paired bony protuberances within the nasal cavity that form air passages inferior to each, called the superior, middle, and inferior meatuses.
- The inferior meatus is the drainage site of thenasolacrimal duct.
- The **ostiomeatal complex (OMC) or unit** is the common pathway for the maxillary, frontal, and anterior ethmoid sinuses to drain into the middle meatus. The OMC is a functional unit comprising the maxillary sinus ostium, ethmoid infundibulum, uncinate process, ethmoid bulla, hiatus semilunaris, and middle meatus.
- The frontal sinus drains via the **frontal recess** either into the ethmoid infundibulum or directly into the middle meatus. Some authors include the frontal recess in the OMC.
- The maxillary sinus is the largest sinus and drains via the maxillary sinus ostium and infundibulum, which if obstructed can cause isolated maxillary sinus disease.
- The ethmoid sinuses or air cells are divided into anterior and posterior air cells by the basal lamella of the middle turbinate where it attaches to the lamina papyracea.

  The **lamina papyracea** is the thin part of the ethmoid bone separating the ethmoid air cells from the orbit.

  The ethmoid labyrinth is covered superiorly by the **fovea ethmoidalis**, an extension of the orbital part of the frontal bone.

  Between the orbital plates on either side are the **cribriform plates**, the horizontal portion of the ethmoid bone that lies lower than the fovea ethmoidalis and supports the olfactory bulbs.
- The **sphenoethmoidal recess** is the common pathway for the sphenoid sinus and posterior ethmoid air cells to drain into the superior meatus.
- The anterior skull base, which separates the anterior cranial fossa from the sinonasal tract and orbits, is comprised of the orbital parts of the frontal bone, cribriform plates of the ethmoid bone, and planum sphenoidale and lesser wings of the sphenoid bone.

Sinonasal anatomic variants

- The variable depth of the **olfactory fossa**, which is bounded by the vertical and horizontal lamella of the cribriform plate, is important due to the risk of penetration at this site during endoscopic sinus surgery.
- The **agger nasi cell** is an anteriormost ethmoid air cell located anterior to the frontal recess. A large agger nasi cell may narrow the frontal recess.
- A **supraorbital cell** is an anterior ethmoid cell that extends superior to the orbit and anterior ethmoidal notch, which carries the anterior ethmoid artery. The presence of supraorbital pneumatization places the artery at greater intraoperative risk.
- A **Haller (infraorbital) cell** is an ethmoid air cell located along the medial orbital floor, which may narrow the maxillary ostium if large or inflamed.

- 上、中、下鼻甲是鼻腔内的三对骨性突起，在其各自的下方形成气体通道，被称为上、中、下鼻道。
- 下鼻道是鼻泪管的引流部位。
- **窦口鼻道复合体（OMC）或单元**是上颌窦、额窦和前组筛窦引流至中鼻道的共同通道。鼻道窦口复合体是一个功能单位，由上颌窦口、筛漏斗、钩突、筛泡、半月裂孔及中鼻道组成。
- 额窦通过额隐窝引流至筛漏斗或直接引流至中鼻道。部分学者把额隐窝也归入窦口鼻道复合体。
- 上颌窦是最大的鼻窦，引流通过上颌窦口及筛漏斗，如果发生阻塞可引起孤立的上颌窦疾病。
- 筛窦或气房被紧邻筛骨纸板的中鼻甲基底板分为前组及后组。

  纸板是筛骨最薄的部分，将筛窦气房与眼眶分开。

  筛骨迷路上方被**筛窦小窝**覆盖，为额骨眼眶部分的延伸。

  在眶板的两面之间是**筛板**，筛骨的水平部分位于筛窦小窝下方，且支撑嗅球。
- **蝶筛隐窝**是蝶窦和后组筛窦气房引流至上鼻道的共同通道。
- 前颅底将颅前窝与鼻窦、眼眶分开，由额骨眶突、筛骨筛板、蝶骨平台及蝶骨小翼组成。

鼻窦解剖变异

- **嗅隐窝**由筛板的水平板与垂直板围成，其深度变异较大并具重要意义，因为在鼻内镜手术中有被穿透的风险。
- **鼻丘气房**是位于额隐窝前方最靠前的筛窦前组气房。气房过大可使额隐窝变窄。
- **眶上气房**为筛窦前组气房延伸至眼眶和筛窦前切迹上方，筛窦前动脉由此通过。出现眶上气化显著增加了此动脉在术中的风险。
- **眶下气房（Haller 气房）**是位于眶底内侧的筛骨气房，若过大或发炎，可使上颌窦出口狭窄。

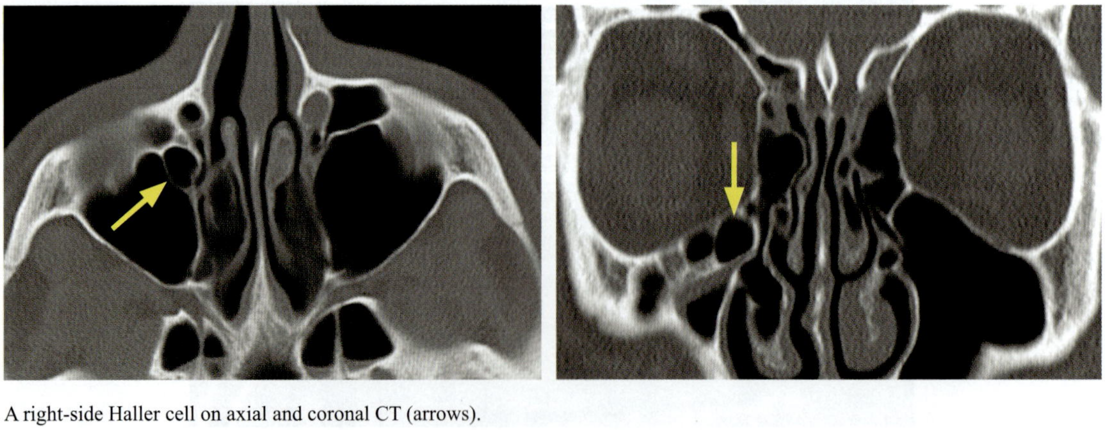

A right-side Haller cell on axial and coronal CT (arrows).
轴位及冠状位CT：右侧眶下气房（黄箭）。

- An **Onodi (sphenoethmoidal) cell** is a posteriormost ethmoid air cell that extends superior and lateral to the sphenoid sinus. An Onodi cell should be recognized to avoid intraoperative damage to the adjacent optic nerve.

- **蝶筛气房(Onodi气房)**是最后方的筛窦气房，延伸至蝶窦上外侧。术中应识别蝶筛气房，以避免损伤邻近视神经。

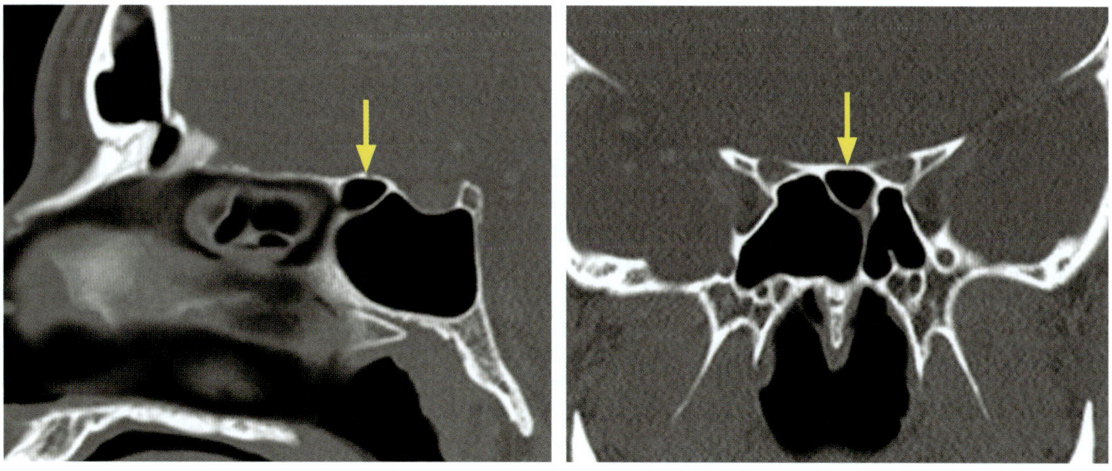

Onodi cell on sagittal and coronal CT (arrows).
矢状位及冠状位CT：蝶筛气房(黄箭)。

- Additional anatomic variants that are usually asymptomatic but can contribute to sinonasal obstruction if large include nasal septal deviation, **concha bullosa** (pneumatized middle turbinate),and paradoxical (inward) curvature of the middle turbinate.

- 通常为无症状，但可加重鼻窦梗阻的其他解剖变异包括：鼻中隔偏曲、**鼻甲泡**(气化中鼻甲)和中鼻甲反常弯曲(向内)。

Imaging of the sinuses

- CT is the primary modality for imaging the bony detail of the sinuses.
- Imaging is usually not appropriate for acute uncomplicated rhinosinusitis but is indicated for suspected orbital or intracranial complications of acute rhinosinusitis, suspected acute invasive fungal sinusitis, surgical planning for chronic or recurrent acute rhinosinusitis, or suspected sinonasal mass.
- MRI is useful for its soft tissue contrast in evaluating suspected orbital or intracranial complications of sinusitis or a sinonasal mass. While both may appear as sinusopacification on CT, contrast enhancement on MRI clearly distinguishes mucosal lesions from obstructed secretions.
- MRI of routine sinus disease is unreliable due to the varying signal intensities of sinus contents: inspissated secretions that are clearly opacified sinus on CT can have low signal that could be mistaken for normal aeration on MRI.
- The purpose of preoperative sinus CT is to identify anatomic variations (noted above) that may lead to surgical complications if the surgeon is unaware and to provide intraoperative navigation.
- Thinning or **bony dehiscence** (absence of bone) due to prior injury or chronic inflammation should be identified, particularly at the cribriform plate (risk of entry into the anterior cranial fossa), lamina papyracea (orbit), and sphenoid sinus walls (carotid canal and optic nerve).

鼻窦影像

- CT是显示鼻窦骨结构细节的主要成像方法。
- 影像学检查通常不适用于急性单纯性鼻窦炎，但适用于怀疑急性鼻窦炎继发眶内或颅内并发症、怀疑侵袭性真菌性鼻窦炎、慢性或复发性急性鼻窦炎术前计划及怀疑鼻窦肿块。
- MRI在评估鼻窦炎的眶内或颅内并发症及鼻窦肿块的软组织部分是十分有用的。黏膜病变与梗阻分泌物在CT上都表现为鼻窦阴影，但MRI增强扫描可将两者清晰地区分开来。
- MRI对于普通鼻窦疾病是不可靠的，因为鼻窦内容物的信号强度多变：CT上明显混浊的浓缩分泌物在MRI上可能呈低信号，而被误认为是正常的充气结构。
- 术前鼻窦CT的目的之一是识别解剖变异(如上所述)，如果外科医生不知情，这些变异可能导致手术并发症；另一个目的是提供术中导航。
- 需要识别由于先前损伤或慢性炎症引起的骨变薄或**骨裂**(骨缺失)，特别要注意筛板(有进入颅前窝的风险)、纸板(眼眶)和蝶窦壁(颈动脉管和视神经)。

INFLAMMATORY SINONASAL DISEASE

鼻窦炎性疾病

Rhinosinusitis

- Rhinosinusitis is inflammation of the paranasal sinuses and nasal mucosa. It is a clinical diagnosis (based on symptoms such as purulent nasal drainage, nasal obstruction, facial pressure, and hyposmia), with imaging reserved for suspected complications, surgical planning, or suspected obstructing mass.
- **Acute rhinosinusitis** lasts <4 weeks. The most common cause is viral, followed by bacterial infection. See below for separate discussion of fungal disease.
- **Chronic rhinosinusitis** lasts ≥12 consecutive weeks. Chronic sinusitis is probably related to obstruction of sinonasal drainage pathways. The goal of functional endoscopic sinus surgery (FESS) is to open/widen these pathways.
- Systemic risk factors for rhinosinusitis include:

> **Mucociliary clearance defects:** e.g., cystic fibrosis, primary ciliary dyskinesia.
> **Immunodeficiencies:** e.g., common variable immune deficiency, hypogammaglobulinemia.
> **Small vessel vasculitides:** granulomatosis with polyangiitis (Wegener's) especially when there is bony erosion and septal perforation, and eosinophilic granulomatosis with polyangiitis (Churg-Strauss) especially when there is nasal polyposis.

- **Odontogenic sinusitis** is the most common cause of unilateral/isolated maxillary sinusitis. The usual etiologies are a maxillary premolar or molar tooth with periapical abscess or, after extraction, an oroantral fistula.

鼻窦炎

- 鼻窦炎是鼻窦和鼻黏膜的炎症。它是一种临床诊断(基于症状，如脓性鼻涕、鼻塞、面部压迫感、嗅觉减退)，影像学检查仅用于评估并发症、手术计划或怀疑梗阻性肿块。
- **急性鼻窦炎**持续时间<4周。最常见的原因是病毒感染，其次是细菌感染。真菌感染在下文中会有单独讲述。
- **慢性鼻窦炎**持续时间≥连续12周。慢性鼻窦炎可能与鼻窦流出道阻塞有关。功能性鼻内镜手术(FESS)的目的是打开/拓宽这些通道。
- 鼻窦炎的系统性危险因素包括：

> **黏液纤毛清除缺陷：**如囊性纤维化、原发性纤毛运动障碍。
> **免疫缺陷：**如普通变异型免疫缺陷病、低丙种球蛋白血症。
> **小血管炎：**肉芽肿性血管炎(韦格纳肉芽肿病)，尤其是合并骨侵蚀和鼻中隔穿孔时；嗜酸性肉芽肿性多血管炎(Churg-Strauss)，特别是有鼻息肉时。

- **牙源性鼻窦炎**是单侧/孤立性上颌窦炎最常见的原因。通常的病因是上颌前磨牙或磨牙根尖周脓肿、拔牙后或口腔-鼻窦瘘。

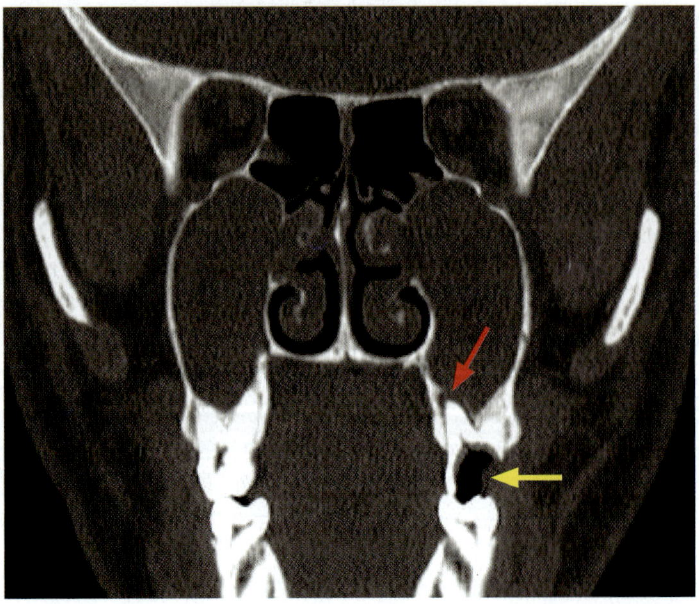

Coronal CT shows opacification of the bilateral maxillary sinuses, thought to present odontogenic sinusitis, at least on the left. Note dental caries (yellow arrow) involving a left upper maxillary tooth and associated periapical lucency (red arrow) representing a periapical abscess or granuloma.
冠状位CT显示双侧上颌窦密度增高，可能是牙源性鼻窦炎，至少是在左侧。可见左上颌龋齿(黄箭)，并伴有根尖周透亮影(红箭)，代表根尖周脓肿或肉芽肿。

- Sinus mucosal thickening is a common but nonspecific imaging finding. Acute sinusitis is more likely to feature an air-fluid level and bubbles within the fluid. Sclerotic thickening of sinus walls, due to prolonged mucoperiosteal inflammation, is characteristic of chronic sinusitis.

- 鼻窦黏膜增厚是一种常见但非特异性的影像学表现。急性鼻窦炎更常表现为气-液平面和液中气泡。鼻窦壁硬化增厚是慢性鼻窦炎的特征，这是由于长期黏膜骨膜炎症所造成的。

Fungal rhinosinusitis

真菌性鼻窦炎

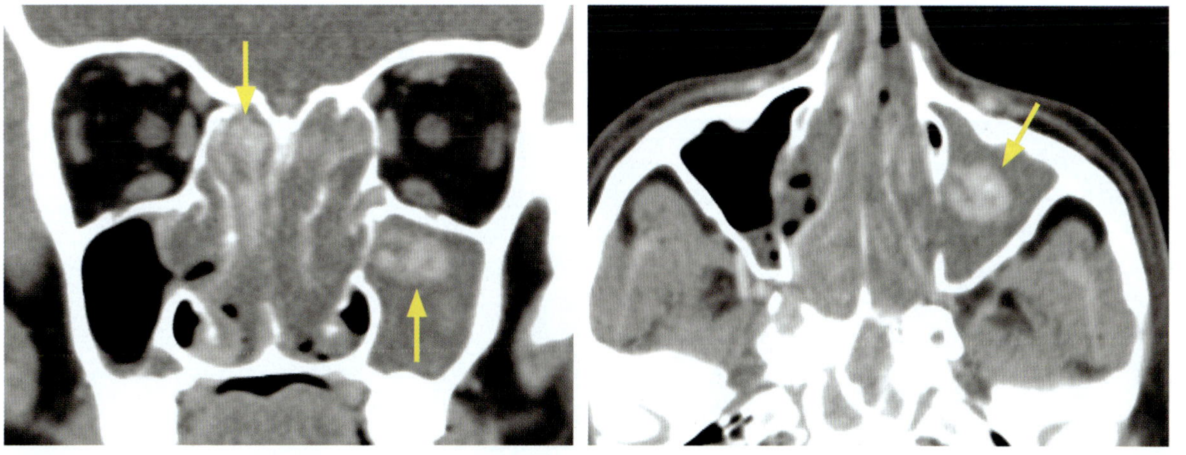

Allergic fungal sinusitis: Coronal (left image) and axial noncontrast CT shows marked pan-sinus disease with curvilinear hyperattenuation in the affected sinuses (arrows). There is erosion of the ethmoid sinus walls.
Case courtesy Mary Beth Cunnane, MD, Massachusetts Eye and Ear Infirmary.
过敏性真菌性鼻窦炎：冠状面(左图)和轴位平扫CT显示明显的全鼻窦病变，病变的鼻窦呈曲线样高密度影(黄箭)。筛窦壁被侵蚀。

- Fungal sinus diseases are classified as noninvasive or invasive, based on extension to the submucosa, vessels, and/or bone.
- Noninvasive fungal rhinosinusitis includes allergic fungal rhinosinusitis and fungal ball. Affected patients are immunocompetent.
- Invasive fungal rhinosinusitis is divided into acute and chronic forms. The vast majority of affected patients have diabetes mellitus or are immunocompromised (e.g., hematologic malignancy, chemotherapy-related neutropenia, transplantation).
- Noninvasive and chronic invasive fungal rhinosinusitis are most commonly due to *Aspergillus* and dematiaceous (brown-black) molds. Acute invasive fungal rhinosinusitis is most commonly caused by aspergillosis or mucormycosis.
- **Allergic fungal rhinosinusitis** is the most common form of fungal sinusitis, representing a subtype/variant of chronic rhinosinusitis with nasal polyposis caused by a localized hypersensitivity reaction to fungi, typically in atopic individuals.

  Imaging shows complete opacification of multiple sinuses with secretions that are hyperattenuating (CT) and low T2 signal intensity (MRI) and cause expansile remodeling/pressure erosion of the sinus walls.
- **Fungus balls** are dense aggregates of (noninvasive) hyphae and (nonallergic) mucin separate from the sinus mucosa.

  Imaging shows opacification of a single sinus (usually maxillary) with an irregular mass that is hyperattenuating (CT) and low T2 signal intensity (MRI), often with intralesional mineralization/ calcification. There may be bony erosion.
- **Invasive fungal rhinosinusitis** is a serious acute or chronic infection where fungal hyphae invade mucosa, vessels, and/or other sinonasal tissues and cause necrosis.

  The most common but nonspecific imaging finding of invasive fungal rhinosinusitis is severe unilateral sinonasal opacification.

  Later in the disease course, more specific imaging signs include extrasinus soft tissue infiltration into the premaxillary and retroantralfat, intracranial or orbital involvement, and bony erosion.

- 真菌性鼻窦疾病分为非侵袭性和侵袭性，取决于是否累及黏膜下层、血管和/或骨骼。
- 非侵袭性真菌性鼻窦炎包括过敏性真菌性鼻窦炎和真菌球。患者的免疫力正常。
- 侵袭性真菌性鼻窦炎分为急性和慢性两种。绝大多数患者患有糖尿病或免疫功能低下(如血液系统恶性肿瘤、化疗相关的中性粒细胞减少、移植)。
- 非侵袭性和慢性侵袭性真菌性鼻窦炎最常见的病因是曲霉和暗色(棕黑色)霉菌感染。急性侵袭性真菌性鼻窦炎最常由曲霉菌病或毛霉菌病引起。
- **过敏性真菌性鼻窦炎**是真菌性鼻窦炎最常见的一种形式，是慢性鼻窦炎的一种亚型/变异型，伴有鼻息肉，为局部对真菌的超敏反应所致，通常发生在有特异质的个体。

  影像显示多个鼻窦腔完全混浊，分泌物呈高密度(CT)和T_2低信号(MRI)，并引起鼻窦壁扩张性重塑/压力性侵蚀。
- **真菌球**是从鼻窦黏膜脱落的高密度(非侵袭性)菌丝和(非过敏性)黏蛋白。

  影像显示单个鼻窦混浊(通常为上颌窦)，伴有不规则肿块，呈高密度(CT)和T_2低信号(MRI)，常伴有病灶内矿化/钙化。可能有骨质侵蚀。
- **侵袭性真菌性鼻窦炎**是一种严重的急性或慢性感染，由真菌菌丝侵入黏膜、血管和/或其他鼻窦组织并导致坏死。

  侵袭性真菌性鼻窦炎最常见但非特异性的影像学表现是严重的单侧鼻窦混浊。

  在病程的后期，较为特殊的影像学征象包括窦外软组织浸润至上颌前和窦后脂肪，颅内或眼眶受累，以及骨质侵蚀。

Non-enhancement of a nasal turbinate on MRI (*black turbinate sign*) in an immunocompromised patient is highly suggestive of necrosis in the setting of invasive fungal rhinosinusitis.

在免疫低下有侵袭性真菌性鼻窦炎的患者中，鼻甲在MRI上无强化(黑色鼻甲征)高度提示发生坏死。

Complications of rhinosinusitis

鼻窦炎并发症

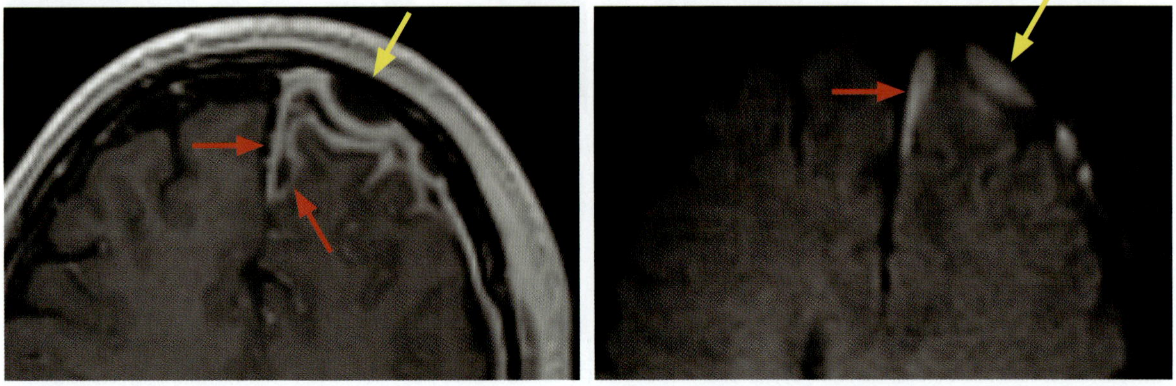

Acute frontal sinusitis complicated by epidural and subdural empyemas: Axial post-contrast T1-weighted MRI (left image) demonstrates left frontalepidural (yellow arrow) and subdural (red arrows) collections with rim enhancement and associated restricted diffusion on DWI (right image), consistent with empyemas. There is diffuse left frontal scalp subcutaneous edema representing cellulitis.

急性额窦炎并发硬膜外和硬膜下脓肿：轴位增强T_1加权MRI(左图)显示左侧额部硬膜外(黄箭)和硬膜下(红箭)积液伴环形强化，DWI显示有弥散受限(右图)，符合脓肿的表现。左额部弥漫性皮下水肿，提示为蜂窝织炎。

- Spread of infection to the orbit may cause preseptal or orbital cellulitis, orbital abscess, subperiosteal abscess, or septic ophthalmic vein and cavernous sinus thrombosis.
- Spread of infection to the cranial cavity may cause meningitis, cerebritis, or suppurative collections (epidural abscess, subdural empyema, or brain abscess). The frontal lobe is the typical site of sinogenic brain abscess.
- Acute frontal sinusitis complicated by osteomyelitis and subgaleal/subperiosteal abscess is known as *Pott's puffy tumor*.

- 感染扩散至眼眶可引起眶隔前或眼眶蜂窝织炎、眼眶脓肿、骨膜下脓肿或脓毒性眼静脉炎和海绵窦血栓形成。
- 感染扩散至颅腔可引起脑膜炎、脑炎或脓液积聚(硬膜外脓肿、硬膜下脓肿或脑脓肿)。额叶是鼻窦源性脑脓肿的典型部位。
- 急性额窦炎合并骨髓炎和帽状腱膜下/骨膜下脓肿被称为波特膨胀瘤。

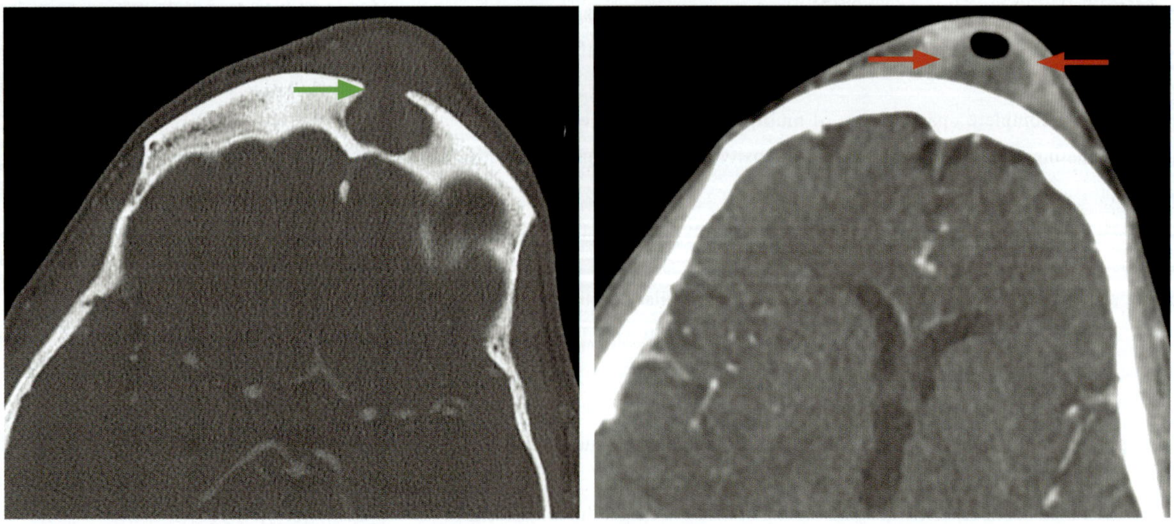

Acute frontal sinusitis complicated by *Pott's puffy tumor*: Axial contrast-enhanced CT shows opacified frontal sinuses and focal defect in the anterior sinus wall (green arrow) with overlying soft tissue swelling and a gas-fluid collection (red arrows) in the frontal scalp, compatible with abscess (*Pott's puffy tumor*).

急性额窦炎合并波特膨胀瘤：轴位增强CT显示额窦混浊，前窦壁局部缺损(绿箭)，覆盖处额部头皮软组织肿胀、积气积液(红箭)，符合脓肿的表现(波特膨胀瘤)。

Sinonasal inflammatory polyps

- Sinonasal inflammatory polyps and nasal polyposis refer to multiple bilateral pedunculated protrusions of mucosa, edematous stroma, and inflammatory infiltrate, most commonly arising from the middle meatus and ethmoid region.
- In adults, a significant minority of cases of chronic rhinosinusitis are associated with nasal polyposis, which together in turn is sometimes associated with asthma and sensitivity to aspirin or other nonsteroidal anti-inflammatory drugs. This syndrome is known as aspirin/ NSAID-exacerbated respiratory disease or **Samter's triad**.
- In children, the most common risk factor for chronic rhinosinusitis with nasal polyposis is cystic fibrosis.

Paranasal sinus retention cyst

- Retention cysts are well-defined, rounded collections of mucous or serous fluid arising in the sinus lining due to obstruction of small seromucinous glands. "Mucous retention cyst" is often used generically to include both mucous and serous retention cysts.
- Retention cysts are usually asymptomatic but can obstruct sinus drainage pathways. They are most commonly located in the maxillary sinus.

Mucocele

鼻窦炎性息肉

- 鼻窦炎性息肉和鼻息肉病是指双侧多发的有蒂的黏膜突起、间质水肿，以及炎症浸润，多见于中鼻道和筛窦区。
- 在成人中，少数的慢性鼻窦炎明显与鼻息肉病有关，而鼻息肉病有时又与哮喘和对阿司匹林或其他非甾体抗炎药过敏有关。这种综合征被称为阿司匹林/非甾体抗炎药加重呼吸道疾病或**阿司匹林三联症(Samter三联症)**。
- 在儿童中，慢性鼻窦炎合并鼻息肉最常见的危险因素是囊性纤维化。

鼻旁窦潴留囊肿

- 潴留囊肿为边界清楚的圆形黏液或浆液聚集物，是由于鼻窦内膜小的浆液黏液腺阻塞造成的。“黏液性潴留囊肿”通常包括黏液性和浆液性潴留囊肿。
- 潴留囊肿通常无症状，但可阻塞鼻窦的引流通道。最常位于上颌窦。

黏液囊肿

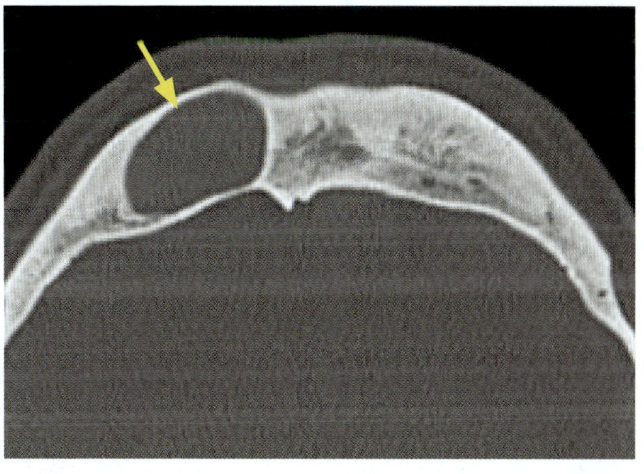

Mucocele of the frontal sinus:
Axial noncontrast CT shows an expanded, fluid-filled right frontal sinus (arrow) with thinning of the sinus walls. Incidentally, the left frontal sinus is congenitally absent.
Case courtesy Mary Beth Cunnane, MD, Massachusetts Eye and Ear Infirmary.
额窦黏液囊肿：
轴位平扫CT显示右侧额窦扩大并充满液体(黄箭)，窦壁变薄。意外发现左额窦先天性缺失。

- A mucocele is an expanded, airless paranasal sinus filled with mucoid secretions due to drainage obstruction.
- Mucoceles may be secondary to inflammatory sinus disease (most commonly) or tumor.
- Imaging shows complete opacification of a single sinus cavity with expansile remodelling and thinning of the bony walls. The sinus contents tend to appear homogeneous on CT and MR; however, the MR signal intensity is variable depending on the degree of dessication.
- Mucoceles are most common in the frontal sinus.

- 黏液囊肿是一个扩张且不含空气的鼻旁窦，其内充满黏液样分泌物，为鼻旁窦引流阻塞所致。
- 黏液囊肿可继发于炎症性鼻窦疾病(最常见)或肿瘤。
- 影像学显示单个窦腔完全混浊，伴有膨胀重塑和骨壁变薄。鼻窦内容物在CT和MR上密度或信号均匀；但MR信号是多样的，取决于内容物浓缩的程度。
- 黏液囊肿最常见于额窦。

Silent sinus syndrome

- Silent sinus syndrome is an acquired condition of painless maxillary sinus atelectasis due to chronic obstruction of the maxillary sinus ostium with resorption of the air.
- Imaging and physical examination show facial asymmetry due to unilateral maxillary sinus volume loss, complete or partial opacification of the sinus, and enophthalmos.

Nasal septal perforation

- Nasal septal perforation usually involves the cartilaginous septum and is generally related to ischemia or inflammation.
- The most common cause is iatrogenic/traumatic (e.g., septoplasty). Other causes include cocaine, granulomatosis with polyangiitis (Wegener's), and granulomatous infections.

隐匿性鼻窦综合征

- 隐匿性鼻窦综合征是一种获得性疾病，指由于上颌窦口的慢性阻塞导致上颌窦膨胀不全，位空气吸收。
- 影像学和体格检查显示面部不对称，为单侧上颌窦体积缩小所致，鼻窦完全或部分浑浊，以及眼球内陷。

鼻中隔穿孔

- 鼻中隔穿孔常累及鼻中隔软骨，通常与缺血或炎症有关。
- 最常见的原因是医源性/外伤性(例如鼻中隔成形术)。其他原因包括使用可卡因、肉芽肿性血管炎(韦格纳肉芽肿病)和肉芽肿性感染。

Benign non-inflammatory sinonasal and anterior skull base lesions

鼻腔鼻窦和前颅底良性非炎症性疾病

Choanal polyp

后鼻孔息肉

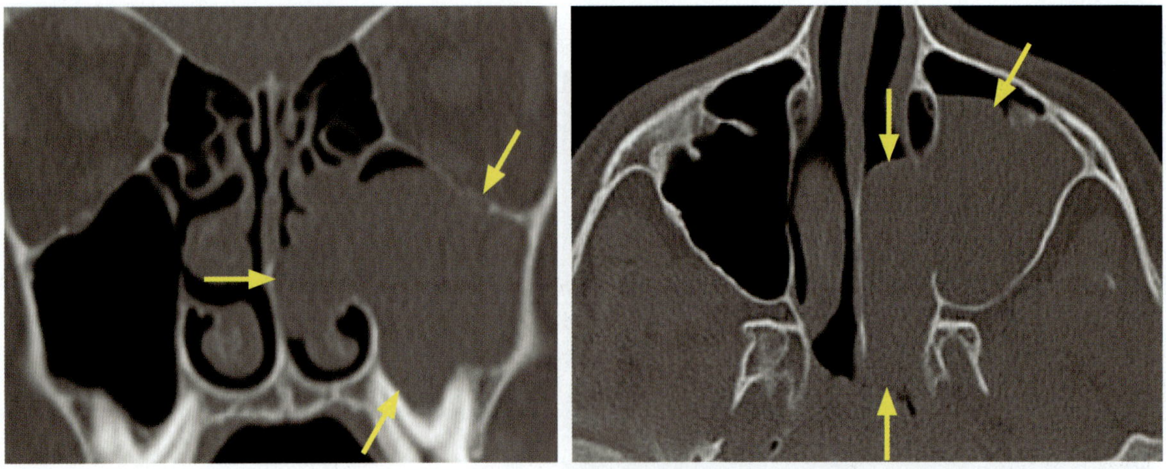

Antrochoanal polyp: Coronal (left image) and axial noncontrast CT show a polypoid lesion (arrows) involving the left maxillary sinus and nasopharynx, with erosion of the middle turbinate and medial wall of the maxillary sinus.

Case courtesy Mary Beth Cunnane, MD, Massachusetts Eye and Ear Infirmary.

上颌窦后鼻孔息肉：冠状位(左图)及轴位平扫CT显示息肉样病变(黄箭)累及左侧上颌窦及鼻咽部，伴中鼻甲及上颌窦内侧壁骨质侵蚀。

- Choanal polyps are solitary pedunculated lesions that extend through the nasal cavity to the posterior nasal aperture (choana), possibly prolapsing into the nasopharynx.
- The vast majority are **antrochoanal polyps**, which originate in the maxillary sinus (antrum) and widen the maxillary ostia.
- Choanal polyps are histologically similar to inflammatory polyps but considered clinically distinct. They mostly occur in children and young adults.

- 后鼻孔息肉是单发有蒂的病变，通过鼻腔延伸至后鼻孔，可能下垂至鼻咽部。
- 绝大多数为，起源于上颌窦(腔)，并且扩大上颌窦的开口。
- 后鼻孔息肉在组织学上与炎症性息肉类似，但在临床上有明显区别，大多发生于儿童和年轻人。

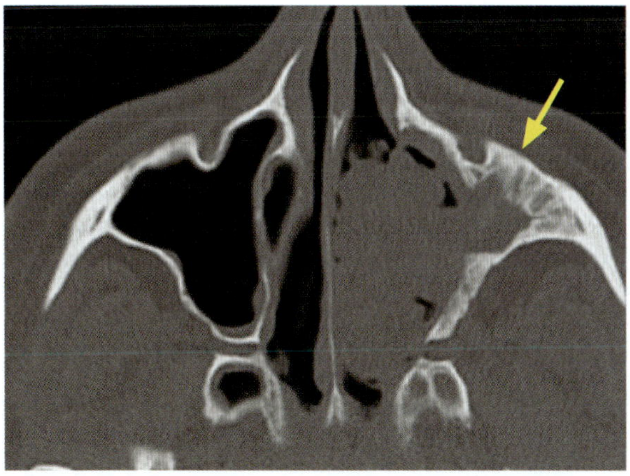

Inverted papilloma: Axial noncontrast CT shows a polypoid lesion of the left maxillary sinus with erosion of the medial wall of the maxillary sinus, the ethmoid air cells, and the turbinates. The sinus is not expanded. There is reactive bony sclerosis of the lateral wall of the maxillary sinus (arrow).

Case courtesy Mary Beth Cunnane, MD, Massachusetts Eye and Ear Infirmary.

内翻型乳头状瘤：轴位平扫CT显示左侧上颌窦息肉样病变，上颌窦内侧壁、筛窦气房及鼻甲骨质侵蚀。鼻窦没有扩张。上颌窦侧壁有反应性骨质硬化(黄箭)。

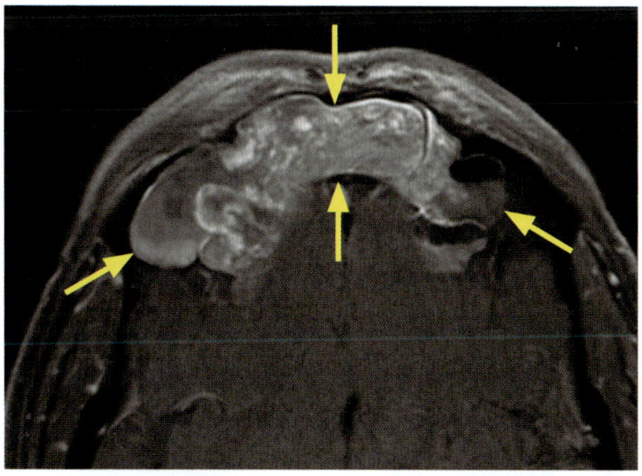

Inverted papilloma in a different patient: Axial contrast-enhanced T1-weighted MRI with fat suppression shows a lobulated extra-axial mass (arrows) arising from the frontal sinus. The mass demonstrates characteristic *cerebriform* enhancement.

Case courtesy Gregory Wrubel, MD, Brigham and Women's Hospital.

另一名内翻型乳头状瘤的患者：轴位增强T_1加权脂肪抑制MRI显示起源于额窦的分叶状轴外肿块(黄箭)。肿块表现为特征性的脑回样强化。

- Sinonasal (Schneiderian) papillomas are benign polypoid neoplasms arising from the Schneiderian epithelium.
- The most common histologic type of sinonasal papilloma is the inverted type, followed by exophytic and oncocytic types.
- Inverted and oncocytic papillomas have malignant potential, typically transforming to squamous cell carcinoma, while exophytic papillomas do not.
- Inverted and oncocytic papillomas typically arise from paranasal sinuses or the lateral nasal wall, while exophytic papillomas tend to arise from the nasal septum.
- Inverted papillomas classically show a convoluted *cerebriform* pattern on T2-weighted and contrast-enhanced T1-weighted MR images (alternating curvilinear bands of high and low signal intensity). At CT, bone erosion and remodeling are common, although the site of attachment may demonstrate focal hyperostosis.

- 鼻腔鼻窦(施奈德上皮)乳头状瘤是起源于施奈德上皮的良性息肉样肿瘤。
- 鼻腔鼻窦乳头状瘤最常见的组织学类型是内翻型，其次是外生型和嗜酸细胞型。
- 内翻型和嗜酸细胞型乳头状瘤具有恶性潜能，通常转化为鳞状细胞癌(SCC)，而外生型乳头状瘤则不会。
- 内翻型和嗜酸细胞型乳头状瘤通常发生于鼻旁窦或鼻侧壁，而外生型乳头状瘤常常来自鼻中隔。
- 内翻型乳头状瘤在T_2加权和T_1加权对比增强MR图像上呈典型迂曲的脑回样形态(高、低信号交替的曲线样)。骨侵蚀和骨重塑在CT上很常见，但附着部位可能有局部骨质增生。

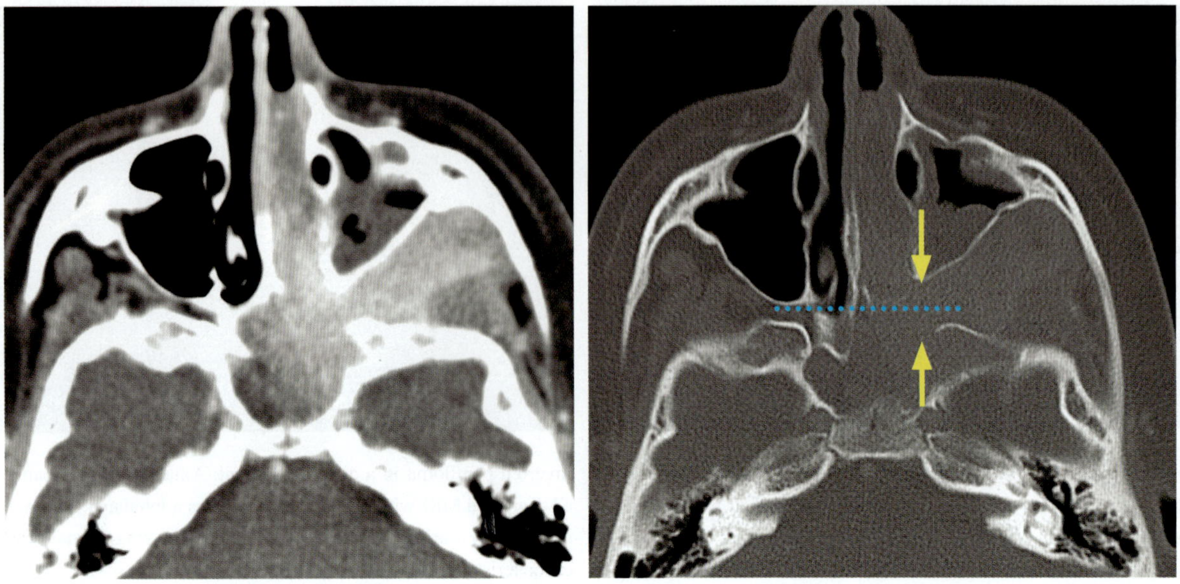

Juvenile nasopharyngeal angiofibroma: Axial contrast-enhanced CT through the pterygopalatine fossa in soft tissue (left image) and bone windows shows an avidly enhancing mass in the left nasopharynx, pterygopalatine fossa, and sphenoid sinus, with characteristic widening (arrows) of the pterygopalatine fossa. There is resultant anterior displacement of the posterior wall of the maxillary sinus relative to the left (dotted blue line).

Case courtesy Sanjay Prabhu, MD, Boston Children's Hospital.

青少年鼻咽血管纤维瘤：经翼腭窝的软组织窗(左图)和骨窗轴位增强CT显示左侧鼻咽、翼腭窝和蝶窦有一个明显强化的肿块，以翼腭窝增宽为特征(黄箭)。上颌窦后壁(蓝色虚线)相对于左侧发生前移。

- Juvenile nasopharyngeal angiofibroma (JNA) is the most common benign neoplasm of the nasopharynx and typically arises from the posterior aspect of the nasal cavity near the sphenopalatine foramen.
- While benign, JNA may be locally aggressive and, due to its vascularity, presents a risk for life-threatening bleeding.
- JNA almost always affects adolescent/young adult males, who present with epistaxis and/or nasal obstruction.
- On imaging, JNA shows intense contrast enhancement with a salt-and-pepper appearance on MRI due to vascular flow voids. The mass can extend into the pterygopalatine fossa, expanding it and anteriorly bowing the posterior maxillary sinus wall (*Holman-Miller/antral sign*).
- The most common arterial supply of JNA consists of distal internal maxillary artery branches. Embolization is often performed to reduce lesion vascularity prior to resection.

Congenital nasal masses

- The most common pediatric midline nasal masses are anomalies of neuroectodermal development at the frontonasal region including, in decreasing frequency, dermoid/ epidermoid cyst, encephalocele, and nasal glial heterotopia.
- Nasal **dermoid/epidermoid cysts**, usually associated with dermal sinus tracts, are ectodermal inclusions that appear as a round cyst along the anterior nose from the tip up to the crista galli. Dermoid cysts may have fat density/ signal,while epidermoid cysts show restricted diffusion.

- 青少年鼻咽血管纤维瘤(JNA)是鼻咽部最常见的良性肿瘤，通常起源于鼻腔后部靠近蝶腭孔的位置。
- JNA虽属良性，但因其血管化而可能具有局部侵袭性，有致命性出血的风险。
- JNA几乎只发生于青少年/年轻成年男性，表现为鼻出血和/或鼻塞。
- JNA在MRI的影像学表现为明显强化，及由血管流空效应所致的盐-胡椒征。肿块可延伸至翼腭窝，使其扩大，向前压迫上颌窦后壁使其向前弯曲(Holman-Miller征或antral征)。
- JNA最常见的动脉供应来自远端上颌动脉的分支。栓塞术常用于在外科切除术前减少病变的血供。

先天性鼻肿块

- 最常见的儿童中线鼻肿块是额鼻区神经外胚层发育异常，按发生率逐渐降低依次为：皮样/表皮样囊肿、脑膨出和鼻神经胶质异位。
- **鼻皮样/表皮样囊肿**通常与真皮窦道有关，是鼻尖至鸡冠沿鼻前缘呈圆形囊肿的外胚层包涵体。皮样囊肿可能有脂肪密度/信号，而表皮样囊肿则弥散受限。

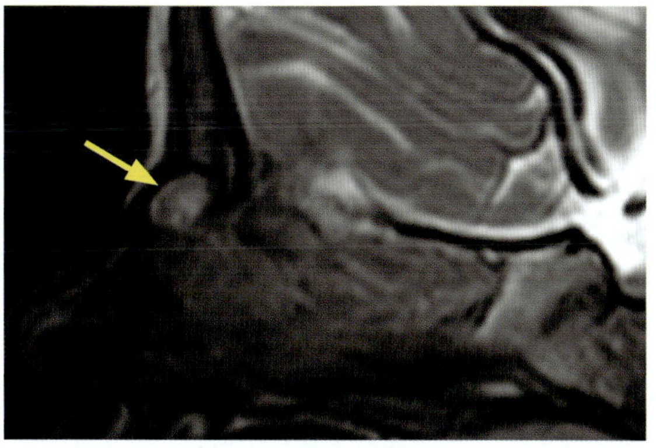

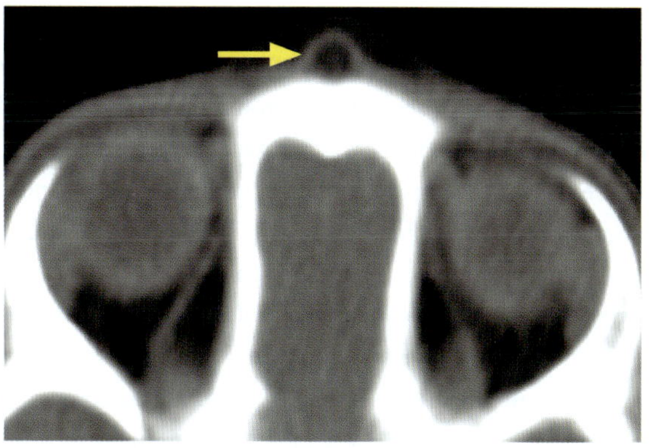

Nasal dermoids: Sagittal T2-weighted MRI (left image) demonstrates a well-defined midline nasal lesion (arrow) associated with a widened foramen cecum. Axial CT of a different patient (right image) shows a similarly located lesion with internal fat density (arrow).
鼻皮样囊肿：矢状位T_2加权MRI(左图)显示一个边界清晰的鼻中线病变(黄箭)，伴盲孔增宽。另一名患者的轴位CT(右图)显示一个相同位置的病变，其内部含脂肪密度(黄箭)。

- **Frontoethmoidal encephaloceles**, also known as anterior or sincipital cephaloceles, refer to herniations of meninges, CSF, and/or brain tissue through an anterior skull or skull base defect. The protrusion can be located at the glabella (via the fonticulus nasofrontalis), nasal cavity (via the foramen cecum), or medial orbit (via the lacrimal bone). MRI best demonstrates the soft tissue mass contiguous with intracranial contents.

- **额筛部脑膨出**，也称为前颅或前顶部脑膨出，是指通过前颅骨或颅底缺损引起的脑膜、脑脊液和/或脑组织疝出。膨出物可位于眉间(经鼻前囟)、鼻腔(经盲孔)或眶内侧(经泪骨)。MRI显示软组织与颅内内容物延续的关系最佳。

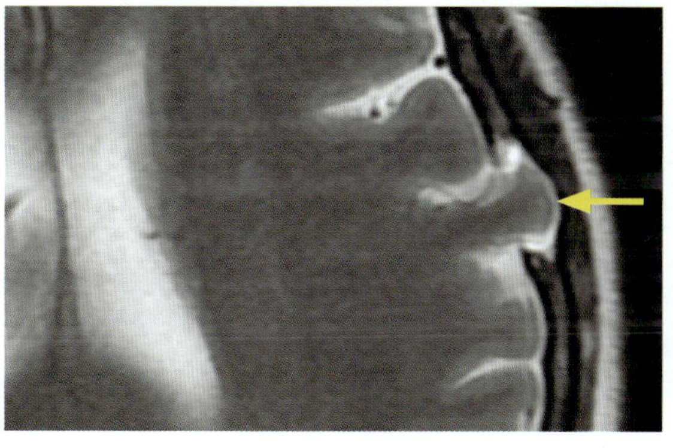

Encephalocele: Axial T2-weighted MRI shows focal herniation of brain tissue through a small defect in the left frontal calvarium (arrow).
脑膨出：轴位T_2加权MRI显示左侧额颅骨有一处小缺损，可见局灶性脑组织疝出(黄箭)。

- **Nasal glial heterotopias**, also known as nasal gliomas, are non-neoplastic masses of dysplastic neuroglial tissue isolated to the nasal dorsum or nasal cavity. MRI shows a soft tissue mass without connection to intracranial contents.

- **鼻神经胶质异位**，又称鼻神经胶质瘤，是孤立于鼻背或鼻腔的发育不良神经胶质组织的非肿瘤性肿块。MRI表现为与颅内内容物无关的软组织肿块。

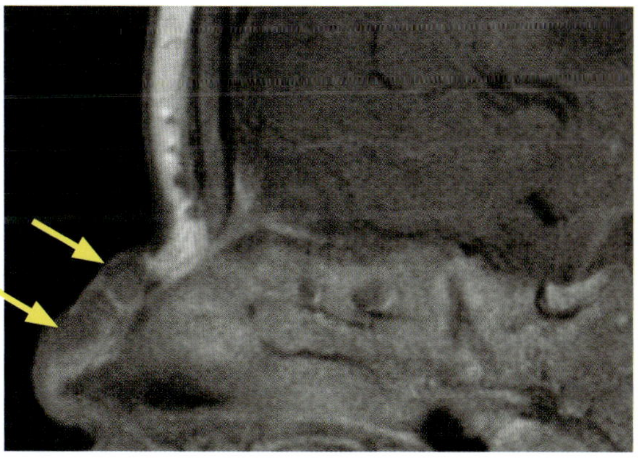

Nasal glioma:
Sagittal T1-weighted post-contrast MRI demonstrates a non-enhancing, multilobulated lesion at the dorsum of the nose (arrows) without communication with the intracranial compartment. This was a biopsy-proven nasal glioma.
鼻神经胶质瘤：
矢状位增强T_1加权MRI显示鼻背部无强化的多分叶状病变(黄箭)，与颅内腔室无沟通。这是一个经活检证实的鼻神经胶质瘤。

Fibro-osseous lesions

- Fibro-osseous lesions in the craniofacial skeleton are a spectrum of pathologic ossifications with variable amounts of fibroblastic stroma. While benign, they can cause symptoms related to mass effect or facial deformity.
- **Osteomas** are the most common neoplasm in the paranasal sinuses, occurring as a polypoid growth most frequently within the frontal sinus followed by ethmoid air cells. They are mostly made of dense bone.

  Gardner syndrome is the association of familial adenomatous polyposis with multiple skull osteomas and soft tissue tumors such as desmoid.
- **Craniofacial fibrous dysplasia** is one of the most common sites of fibrous dysplasia (along with femur, tibia, and ribs), wherein bone is replaced with disorganized fibrous tissue. CT shows ill-defined regions of bony expansion with radiolucent ground glass, sclerotic, or mixed density. MRI variably shows heterogeneous signal intensity and contrast enhancement.

纤维骨病变

- 颅面骨骼的纤维骨病变是一系列的病理性骨化，其成纤维细胞基质的数量有所不同。虽然是良性病变，但会引起与占位效应或面部畸形相关的症状。
- **骨瘤**是鼻旁窦最常见的肿瘤，表现为息肉样生长，最常发生于额窦，其次是筛窦气房。它们大多由致密骨组成。

  加德纳综合征与家族性腺瘤性息肉病、多发性颅骨骨瘤和软组织肿瘤(如硬纤维瘤)有关。
- **颅面纤维发育不良**是纤维发育不良最常见的部位之一(连同股骨、胫骨和肋骨)，其中骨骼被紊乱的纤维组织取代。CT显示边界不清的骨膨大，可呈透光的磨玻璃、硬化或混合密度。MRI显示为不同程度的不均匀信号和强化。

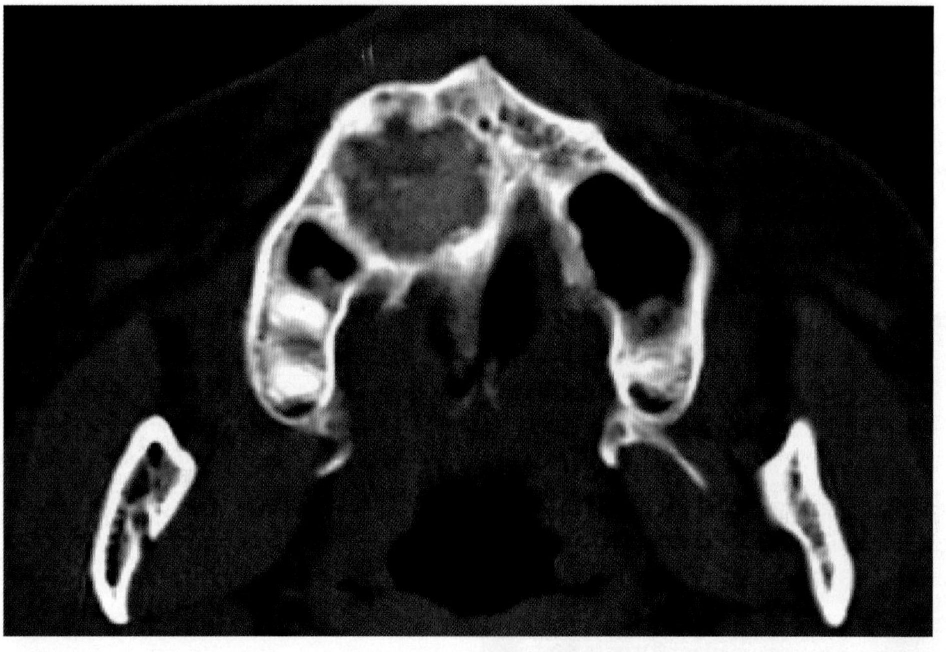

Fibrous dysplasia:

Axial CT through the face shows a well-circumscribed, expansile osseous lesion with ground glass matrix in the right maxilla.

The distribution of fibrous dysplasia is classified as polyostotic (involving multiple bones) or monostotic (involving a single bone only). Of note, craniofacial fibrous dysplasia is considered a monostotic site even when multiple cranial bones are involved.

McCune-Albright syndrome is the association of polyostotic fibrous dysplasia with autonomous endocrine hyperfunction and café-au-lait macules.

Mazabraud syndrome is the association of polyostotic fibrous dysplasia with intramuscular myxomas.

骨纤维发育不良：

面部轴位CT显示右上颌骨有一处边界清楚、膨胀性的骨质破坏区，伴磨玻璃样基质。

骨纤维发育不良的分布分为多骨性(累及多骨)或单骨性(仅累及单骨)。注意，颅面骨纤维发育不良即使累及多个颅骨仍被认为是单骨性病变。

纤维性骨营养不良综合征与自主性内分泌功能亢进和咖啡牛奶斑有关。

Mazabraud综合征与多骨性纤维发育不良合并肌内黏液瘤有关。

- **Ossifying fibromas** are benign bone neoplasms that most commonly occur in the mandible, followed by maxilla. Imaging shows a solitary, well-defined, expansile lesion with variable radiolucency/density.

- **骨化性纤维瘤**是良性骨肿瘤，最常发生在下颌骨，其次是上颌骨。影像学表现为单发、清晰、膨胀性的骨病变，其透光度/密度不同。

Malignancies of the Sinonasal Tract and Anterior Skull Base

Overview of sinonasal and anterior skull base malignancies

- The most common malignant neoplasm in the sinonasal tract is squamous cell carcinoma, but this histology is not as overwhelming of a majority as in other mucosal sites of the upper aerodigestive tract. There are a wide variety of other malignancies.
- Sinonasal epithelial cancers:

Squamous cell carcinoma (most common).
Adenoid cystic carcinoma.
Non-salivary-type adenocarcinoma.
Sinonasal undifferentiated carcinoma (SNUC).
Sinonasal neuroendocrine carcinoma (SNEC).

- Nonepithelial sinonasal cancers:

Lymphoma (most common).	Extramedullary plasmacytoma.
Olfactory neuroblastoma.	Sarcomas.
Mucosal melanoma.	

- Most of the various sinonasal malignancies have nonspecific imaging appearances and it is usually not possible to predict the histology with confidence. The role of imaging lies in localizing the tumor and evaluating the extent of disease, which affects the optimal treatment approach.

  Sinonasal malignancies are usually aggressive masses that cause extensive bony destruction.

  Internal contrast enhancement, though often heterogeneous, distinguishes neoplasms from inflammatory lesions such as hypertrophic mucosa, polyps, or obstructed secretions/mucocele.

  Owing to high cellularity, many of these malignancies have intermediate intensity ("evil gray") on T2-weighted images and more restricted diffusion.

- Important findings to describe include the presence of perineural tumor spread, crossing the anterior skull base into the intracranial compartment, and extension into the orbit.

  Perineural tumor spread appears as nerve thickening and enhancement, obliteration of perineural fat pads, and/or enlargement of neural foramina/canals.

  Intracranial involvement may appear as nodular dural thickening or vasogenic edema in the brain.

  Orbital invasion most commonly occurs through the lamina papyracea, which is the weakest orbital wall.

Squamous cell carcinoma

- Squamous cell carcinoma is the most common sinonasal malignancy, most commonly affecting the maxillary sinus.
- Major risk factors for sinonasal squamous cell carcinoma are smoking and human papillomavirus (HPV) infection.

Adenoid cystic carcinoma

- Adenoid cystic carcinoma is the most common sinonasal tumor of minor salivary gland origin, most commonly affecting the maxillary sinus.
- Adenoid cystic carcinomas have the highest risk of perineural spread. Those in the sinonasal tract most commonly affect the maxillary division of the trigeminal nerve (CN V_2).

鼻腔鼻窦与前颅底的恶性病变

鼻腔鼻窦与前颅底恶性病变概述

- 鼻窦道最常见的恶性肿瘤是SCC，但该组织学类型并不像在上呼吸道/消化道其他黏膜部位那样占绝大多数。还包括较为广泛的其他恶性肿瘤。
- 鼻窦上皮癌：

鳞状细胞癌(SCC)(最常见)
腺样囊性癌。
非涎腺型腺癌。
鼻窦未分化癌(SNUC)。
鼻窦神经内分泌癌(SNEC)。

- 鼻窦非上皮性恶性肿瘤：

淋巴瘤(最常见)。	髓外浆细胞瘤。
嗅神经母细胞瘤。	肉瘤。
黏膜黑色素瘤。	

- 大多数鼻窦恶性肿瘤具有非特异性的影像学表现，通常无法准确预测其组织学类型。影像学检查的作用在于确定肿瘤的位置以及评估肿瘤侵袭的范围，为最佳治疗提供依据。

  鼻窦恶性肿瘤通常是侵袭性的肿块，可引起广泛的骨质破坏。

  虽然肿瘤内部经常呈不均匀强化，但可以与炎症性病变进行区分(如肥厚的黏膜、息肉或阻塞的分泌物/黏液囊肿)。

  由于细胞密度高，许多恶性肿瘤在T_2加权像上呈中等信号("邪恶灰色")，且弥散进一步受限。

- 需要进行描述的重要发现包括是否存在神经周围的肿瘤扩散，从前颅底进入颅内腔室，以及扩散至眼眶。

  神经周围肿瘤扩散表现为神经增厚和强化，神经周围脂肪垫消失和/或神经孔/管增大。

  颅内受累可表现为结节样硬膜增厚或血管源性脑水肿。

  眼眶浸润最常穿透纸板，因其为眼眶壁最薄弱的部位。

鳞状细胞癌

- 鳞状细胞癌是最常见的鼻窦恶性肿瘤，最常发生于上颌窦。
- 鼻窦鳞状细胞癌的主要危险因素是吸烟和人乳头状瘤病毒(HPV)感染。

腺样囊性癌

- 腺样囊性癌是最常见的起源于小唾液腺的鼻窦肿瘤，最常累及上颌窦。
- 腺样囊性癌出现神经周围扩散的风险最高。在鼻腔鼻窦中最常累及的是三叉神经上颌支(CN V_2)。

Adenocarcinoma

- Sinonasal adenocarcinomas arise from surface epithelial glands, most commonly in the nasal cavity and ethmoid air cells, and are divided into intestinal-type and nonintestinal-type.
- Intestinal-type adenocarcinoma is strongly associated with occupational wood dust exposure.

腺癌

- 鼻腔鼻窦腺癌起源于腺体上皮的表面，多见于鼻腔和筛窦气房，分为肠型和非肠型。
- 肠型腺癌与职业性木尘接触密切相关。

Olfactory neuroblastoma (esthesioneuroblastoma)

嗅神经母细胞瘤(鼻腔神经胶质瘤)

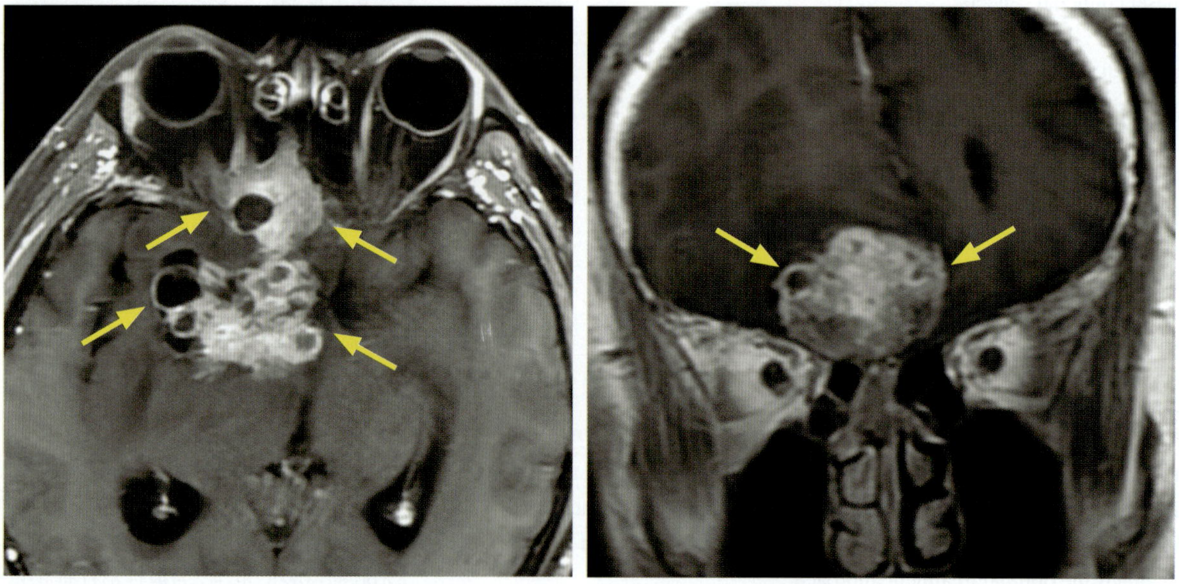

Esthesioneuroblastoma with intracranial extension: Axial and coronal post-contrast T1-weighted MRI demonstrate an avidly enhancing lobulated mass (arrows) extending from the right superior nasal cavity into the anterior cranial fossa. Multiple cysts are noted at the tumor-brain interface.

嗅母细胞瘤扩散至颅内：轴位和冠状位增强T_1加权MRI显示一个明显强化的分叶状肿块(黄箭)，从右上鼻腔延伸至颅前窝。肿瘤-脑交界面有多个囊肿。

- Olfactory neuroblastoma, previously known as esthesioneuroblastoma, is a malignant neural crest-derived tumor that arises from olfactory epithelium in the superior nasal cavity.
- When the tumor extends intracranially, the presence of cysts at the margins of the intracranial portion is highly suggestive of olfactory neuroblastoma.

- 嗅神经母细胞瘤，以前称为鼻腔神经胶质瘤，是一种起源于上鼻腔嗅觉上皮的恶性神经嵴肿瘤。
- 当肿瘤向颅内扩散时，若在颅内部分的边缘出现囊肿，极有可能是嗅神经母细胞瘤。

Mucosal melanoma

- Mucosal melanoma refers to malignant melanoma that arises from mucosal epithelium, which is uncommon compared to cutaneous melanoma.
- The head and neck, most commonly in the sinonasal tract, is the most common site.
- On MRI, internal high signal on T1-weighted images corresponding to melanin can be suggestive of the diagnosis, but these tumors are frequently amelanotic.

黏膜黑色素瘤

- 黏膜黑色素瘤是指起源于黏膜上皮的恶性黑色素瘤，较皮肤黑色素瘤少见。
- 头部和颈部是常见的部位，最常见于鼻腔鼻窦。
- 在MRI上，T_1加权图像的内部高信号与黑色素相对应可以提示诊断，但这些肿瘤通常不含黑色素。

Lymphoma

- The most common histology is diffuse large B-cell lymphoma, although in Asia and Latin America, extranodal NK/T-cell lymphoma, nasal type, is more common.
- B-cell lymphomas predominate in the paranasal sinuses, while T-cell lymphomas predominate in the nasal cavity.

淋巴瘤

- 最常见的组织学类型是大B细胞淋巴瘤，但在亚洲和拉丁美洲，结外NK/T细胞淋巴瘤的鼻型更常见。
- B细胞淋巴瘤主要发生在鼻旁窦，而T细胞淋巴瘤主要发生在鼻腔。

Extramedullary plasmacytoma

- Solitary extramedullary plasmacytoma is a plasma cell malignancy presenting as an extraosseous soft tissue mass; multiple myeloma is the systemic form.
- Extramedullary plasmacytoma usually affects the head and neck region, most commonly in the sinonasal tract.

Rhabdomyosarcoma

- Rhabdomyosarcoma is the most common soft tissue malignancy in the head and neck in children and the most common sinonasal sarcoma.
- Half of head and neck rhabdomyosarcomas occur in a so-called parameningeal site: nasal cavity, nasopharynx, paranasal sinuses, infratemporal and pterygopalatine fossae, middle ear, or mastoid. Parameningeal sites carry an unfavorable prognosis, while the orbits and other non-parameningeal head and neck locations are considered favorable sites.

髓外浆细胞瘤

- 孤立性髓外浆细胞瘤是一种浆细胞恶性肿瘤，表现为骨外软组织肿块；多发性骨髓瘤则是其一种全身性的形式。
- 髓外浆细胞瘤通常累及头颈部，最常见于鼻腔鼻窦。

横纹肌肉瘤

- 横纹肌肉瘤是儿童头部和颈部最常见的软组织恶性肿瘤，也是最常见的鼻窦肉瘤。
- 一半的头颈部横纹肌肉瘤发生在所谓的脑膜旁部位：鼻腔、鼻咽、鼻旁窦、颞下和翼腭窝、中耳或乳突。发生在脑膜旁部位预后较差，而眼眶和其他非脑膜旁头颈部被认为是预后较好的部位。

（翻译　陈珊珊）

ORBITS

眼眶

OVERVIEW AND ANATOMY OF THE ORBITS

眼眶概述和解剖

Bony orbits and foramina

眶骨和孔道

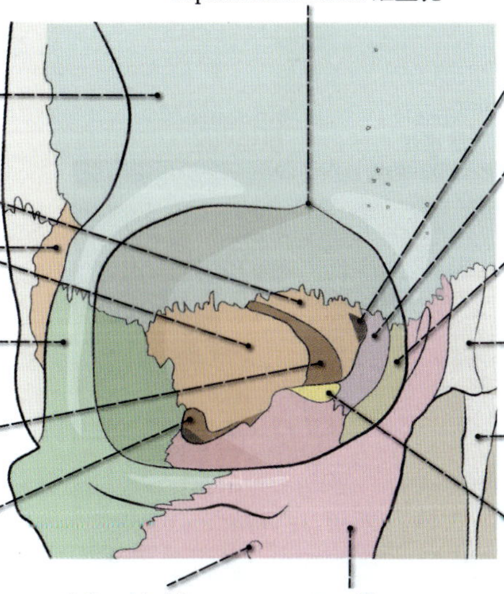

- The orbit is a conical cavity formed by 7 bones: frontal, ethmoid, palatine, lacrimal, maxilla, zygomatic, and sphenoid.
- The orbital roof is part of the anterior skull base.
- The orbital floor is the roof of the maxillary sinus.
- Medially, the orbit borders the ethmoid air cells (across the lamina papyracea). Laterally, the orbit borders the temporal fossa (across the zygoma and greater wing of sphenoid).
- The orbital apex is the region around three bony openings (optic canal, superior orbital fissure, and inferior orbital fissure) and the annulus of Zinn (common tendinous ring).
- The following structures pass through the **optic canal**:

- 眼眶是一个圆锥形的骨腔，由7块骨骼组成：额骨、筛骨、腭骨、泪骨、上颌骨、颧骨和蝶骨。
- 眶顶部是前颅底的一部分。
- 眶底部是上颌窦顶的一部分。
- 眼眶内侧与筛窦气房(越过筛骨纸板)相邻。眼眶外侧以颞窝(跨过颧骨和蝶骨大翼)为界。
- 眶尖是一个绕有3个骨开口(视神经管、眶上裂和眶下裂)和总腱环(Zinn环)的区域。
- 下列结构穿过**视神经管**：

Optic nerve.	Ophthalmic artery.

- The following structures pass through the **superior orbital fissure**, which includes all of the cranial nerves (CN) of the cavernous sinus except CN V_2:

CN Ⅲ (oculomotor nerve) innervates the superior, medial, and inferior recti, and inferior oblique muscles.
CN Ⅳ (trochlear nerve) innervates the superior oblique muscle (mnemonic: SO_4).
CN V_1 (ophthalmic division of trigeminal nerve) provides sensory innervation to the upper face.
CN Ⅵ (abducens nerve) innervates the lateral rectus muscle (mnemonic: LR_6).
Superior ophthalmic vein drains into the cavernous sinus.
Superior branch of inferior ophthalmic vein drains into the superior ophthalmic vein or cavernous sinus.

- The following structures pass through the **inferior orbital fissure**, which includes several branches of CN V_2 (maxillary division of trigeminal nerve) after it passes from the cavernous sinus through foramen rotundum and divides in the pterygopalatine fossa:

Zygomatic nerve (from CN V_2) provides sensory innervation to the skin of the lateral cheek and temple.
Infraorbital nerve (from CN V_2) provides sensory innervation to skin of the inferior eyelid, medial cheek, upper lip, and lateral nose.
Inferior branch of inferior ophthalmic vein drains into the pterygoid venous plexus.

Compartments of the orbits

视神经。	眼动脉。

- 下列所有海绵窦内的脑神经都通过**眶上裂**，但除外第Ⅴ脑神经的第2支：

第Ⅲ脑神经(动眼神经)支配上直肌、内直肌、下直肌和下斜肌。
第Ⅳ脑神经(滑车神经)支配上斜肌(记忆诀窍：SO_4)。
第Ⅴ脑神经第1支(三叉神经眼支)上面部的感觉神经。
第Ⅵ脑神经(展神经)支配外直肌(记忆诀窍：LR_6)。
眼上静脉汇入海绵窦。
眼下静脉上支汇入眼上静脉或海绵窦。

- 下列结构穿过**眶下裂**，包括第Ⅴ脑神经第2支(三叉神经上颌支)穿过海绵窦、圆孔后在翼腭窝发出的几个分支：

颧神经(来自第Ⅴ脑神经第2支)传递颊外侧和颞部皮肤的感觉。
眶下神经(来自第Ⅴ脑神经第2支)传递下眼睑、颊内侧、上唇和鼻部皮肤的感觉。
眼下静脉下支汇入翼静脉丛。

眼眶的结构

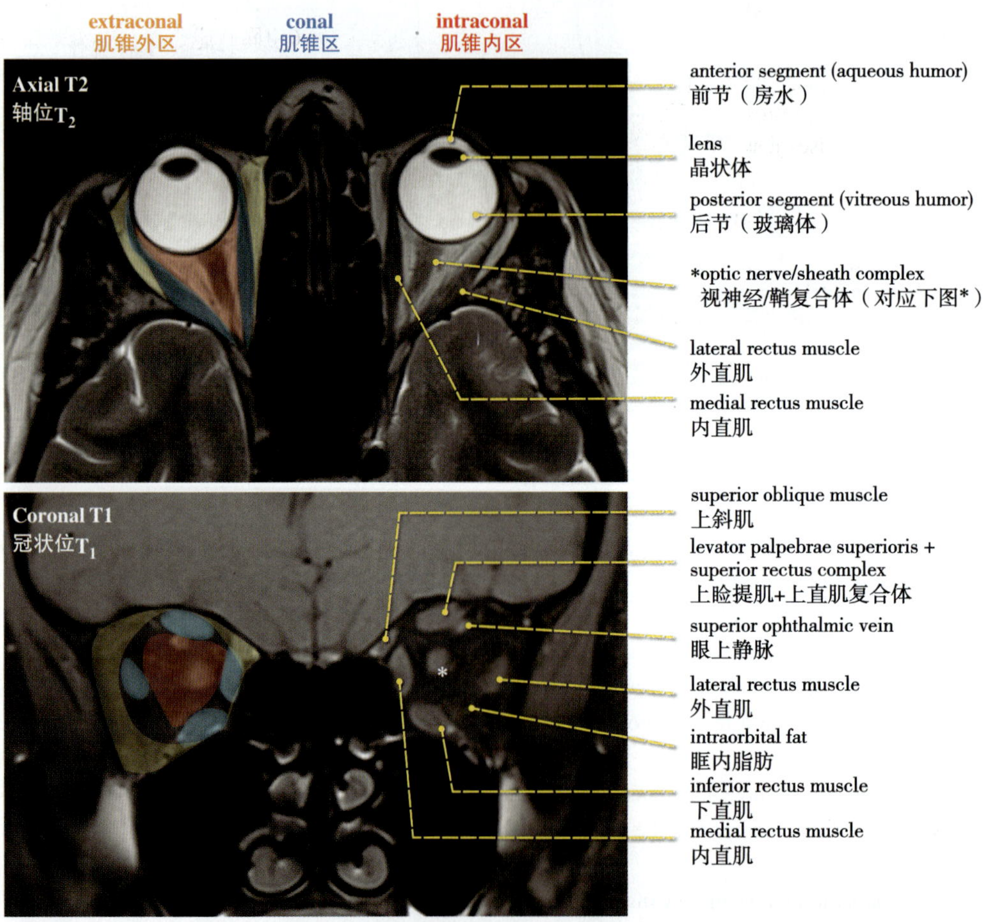

- The orbital septum divides the orbit (postseptal space) from the periorbital soft tissues (preseptal space). The septum is thin fibrous tissue that extends from the periosteum (periorbital) of the orbital rims towards the tarsal plates of the eyelids.
- Classical teaching divides the orbit into four compartments: extraconal, conal, intraconal, and ocular compartments. The first three are also known as the retrobulbar space.
- The **extraconal** compartment contains the lacrimal gland, some neurovascular structures, and fat between the muscles and orbital periosteum. Lesions of the bony orbit and extraorbital processes can encroach on the extraconal space.
- The **conal** compartment refers to an imaginary cone formed by the rectus muscles and interconnecting connective tissue bands.
- The **intraconal** compartment contains the optic nerve-sheath complex (optic nerve, surrounding CSF, and meninges), other neurovascular structures, and fat central to the myofascial cone.
- The **ocular** compartment is the globe. Ocular lesions are not always included in discussion of "orbital" lesions even though the orbital cavity contains the globe.
- In reality, fascial planes in the orbit are more complex and transcend the intraconal/ extraconal artificial boundaries.

Lacrimal apparatus

- The lacrimal apparatus consists of a secretory system and an excretory system.
- The **lacrimal gland**, lodged in the superotemporal angle of the orbit, consists of a palpebral lobe and an orbital lobe (which is deeper and larger).
- Tears drain via the **lacrimal canaliculi** near the medial canthus into the lacrimal sac, lodged in the lacrimal fossa at the inferomedial preseptal orbit.
- The **lacrimal sac** empties via thenasolacrimal duct into the nasal inferior meatus.

Orbital muscles

- Six extraocular muscles move the eye: four recti (superior, inferior, medial, lateral) and two oblique (superior and inferior).
- The rectus muscles arise from the **annulus of Zinn**.
- The superior oblique muscle arises just superomedial to the annulus of Zinn. The tendon is reflected at the trochlea, a fibrocartilaginous structure attached to the superior nasal aspect of the frontal bone.
- The inferior oblique muscle arises from the medial corner of the orbital floor.
- The **levator palpebrae superioris** runs with the superior rectus in a muscle complex. The levator muscle (innervated by CN III) and Müller's (superior tarsal) muscle (innervated by sympathetics) lift the upper eyelid.

Globe

- The globe has three layers: sclera, uvea, and retina.
- The **sclera** is continuous anteriorly with the cornea.
- The **uvea** is composed of the choroid, ciliary body, and iris.
- The **retina** forms most of the inner surface, extending from the optic disc posteriorly to the ora serrata anteriorly.
- The lens separates the anterior and posterior *segments* of the globe.
- The iris separates the anterior and posterior *chambers* of the anterior segment, which communicate via the pupil.
- The anterior segment is filled with aqueous humor, while the posterior segment is filled with vitreous humor.

Optic nerve

- Although named CN Ⅱ, the optic nerve is a part of the central nervous system: it is surrounded by meninges, CSF, and myelin from oligodendroglia (rather

- 眶隔将眼眶(隔后间隙)与眶周软组织(隔前间隙)分开。眶隔是一层薄的纤维组织,从眶缘的骨膜向眼睑的睑板延伸。
- 经典教学分区法将眼眶分为四个区:肌锥外区、肌锥区、肌锥内区和眼球。前三个区又称球后间隙。
- **肌锥外区**包含泪腺、一些神经血管结构以及肌肉-眶骨膜之间的脂肪。眶骨和眼眶外的病变可侵犯肌锥外区。
- **肌锥区**是指假想的由直肌和直肌间结缔组织带形成的肌肉圆锥。
- **肌锥内区**包含视神经-鞘膜复合体(视神经、包绕的脑脊液和脑膜)、其他神经血管结构和肌筋膜锥内的脂肪。
- **眼球区**是指眼球。眼球虽然位于眼眶之内,但眼球病变通常不属于"眼眶"病变的讨论范围。
- 实际上,眼眶中的筋膜层次更为复杂,超越了眼眶内腔和外腔的人工分界。

泪器

- 泪器由分泌和排泄两个系统组成。
- **泪腺**位于眼眶的外上角,由睑叶和眶叶(更深更大)组成。
- 泪液通过内眦附近的**泪小管**引入泪囊,而泪囊位于隔前内下部的泪囊窝内。
- **泪囊**通过鼻泪管排入下鼻道。

眼部肌肉

- 6组眼外肌控制眼球运动:4组直肌(上直肌、下直肌、内直肌、外直肌)和2组斜肌(上斜肌、下斜肌)。
- 直肌均起自**总腱环**。
- 上斜肌起自总腱环的上内侧缘。其肌腱是一种纤维软骨结构,在滑车反折并附着在额骨的上鼻侧。
- 下斜肌起自眶底的内侧角。
- **上睑提肌**与上直肌组成肌肉复合体。提肌(横纹肌,由动眼神经支配)和米勒肌(平滑肌,由交感神经支配)共同上提上眼睑。

眼球

- 眼球壁分3层:巩膜、葡萄膜和视网膜。
- **巩膜**向前演变为角膜。
- **葡萄膜**由脉络膜、睫状体和虹膜构成。
- **视网膜**构成了眼球大部分的内表面,从后部的视盘延伸至前部的锯齿缘。
- 晶状体将眼球分为前节和后节。
- 虹膜将眼前节的前房和后房分开,两者经瞳孔交通。
- 前节充满房水,而后节充满玻璃体。

视神经

- 虽然被称为第Ⅱ脑神经,视神经实际上是中枢神经系统的一部分:由脑膜、脑脊液、少突

than Schwann cells).

- The optic nerve is divided into 4 segments: intraocular (optic disc/papilla/nerve head), intraorbital (the longest part), intracanalicular (within the optic canal), and intracranial (within the middle cranial fossa).
- The two optic nerves converge at the optic chiasm in the suprasellar region.

胶质细胞髓鞘(不是施万细胞)包绕。

- 视神经分为4段：眼内段(视盘/视乳头/视神经乳头)、眶内段(最长)、管内段(视神经管内)和颅内段(位于颅中窝)。
- 两条视神经在鞍上区的视交叉处汇合。

Orbital and ocular infection

Overview of orbital infection

- The most common etiology of orbital infection is direct spread of infection from the paranasal sinuses, especially bacterial rhinosinusitis involving ethmoid air cells. Other etiologies of orbital infection are trauma, foreign body, odontogenic infection.
- Orbital infection includes a spectrum of entities ranging in severity from mild to vision- or life-threatening.

Preseptal cellulitis

- Preseptal (periorbital) cellulitis involves the anterior soft tissues of the eyelids, superficial to the orbital septum.
- Preseptal cellulitis is generally mild and much more common than orbital cellulitis.
- Patients present with eyelid swellingand erythema.
- Imaging shows subcutaneous fat stranding and swelling of the eyelids and face but normal orbital fat.

Orbital cellulitis

眼眶和眼球感染

眼眶感染概述

- 眼眶感染最常见的原因是鼻窦感染造成的直接播散，尤其是细菌性鼻窦炎累及筛窦气房。眼眶感染的其他病因包括创伤、异物、牙源性感染。
- 眼眶感染包括一系列的疾病，轻者仅影响视力，重者会威胁生命。

隔前蜂窝织炎

- 隔前(眶周)蜂窝织炎累及眼睑前部的软组织，位于眶隔的表面。
- 隔前蜂窝织炎一般较轻，但远较眼眶蜂窝织炎常见。
- 患者表现为眼睑肿胀和充血。
- 影像显示皮下脂肪密度增高，眼睑和面部肿胀，但眼眶内脂肪正常。

眼眶蜂窝织炎

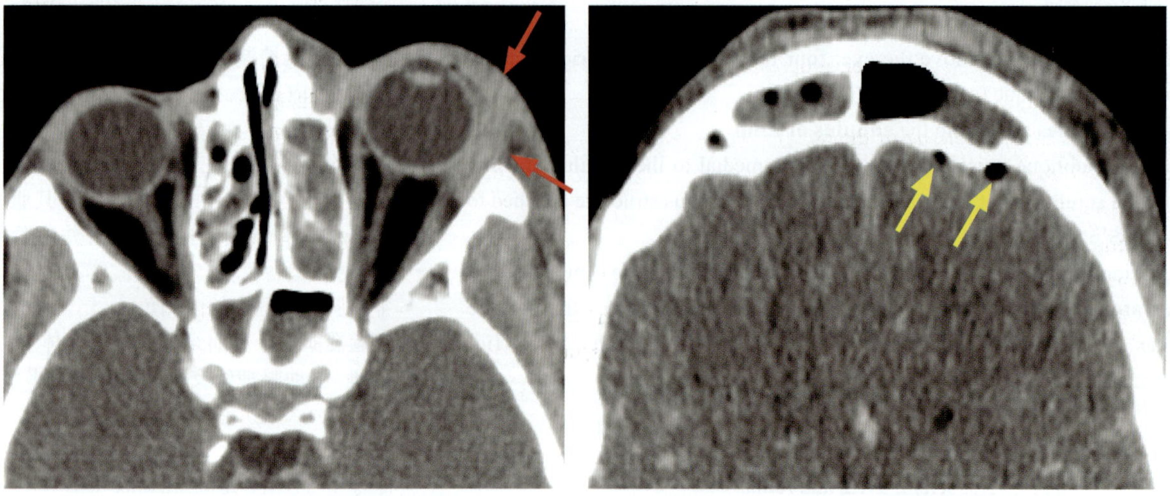

Orbital cellulitis with epidural abscess: Axial contrast-enhanced CT through the orbits (left image) shows left proptosis and both pre- and post-septal inflammatory change (red arrows), without a discrete fluid collection. There is complete opacification of the left ethmoid sinus andopacification of the sphenoid sinus. CT through the brain (right) demonstrates two locules of gas in the extra-axial space (yellow arrows) directly posterior to the left frontal sinus, representing an epidural abscess.

Case courtesy Mary Beth Cunnane, MD, Massachusetts Eye and Ear Infirmary.

眼眶蜂窝织炎伴硬膜外脓肿：经眼眶轴位增强CT(左图)显示左侧眼球突出和眶隔前后炎症改变(红箭)，无明显积液。左侧筛窦完全混浊，蝶窦混浊。头部CT(右)显示左额窦后方的轴外间隙(黄箭)有两处积气，代表硬膜外脓肿。

- Orbital (postseptal) cellulitis involves the muscles and fat deep to the orbital septum.
- Orbital cellulitis is serious due to risk of complications such as abscess and intracranial spread via the valveless ophthalmic veins.
- Patients present with not only eyelid swellingand erythema, but also painful ophthalmoplegia, chemosis, and/or proptosis.
- Imaging shows orbital fat stranding, sometimes with extraocular muscle edema, proptosis, or an intraconal or extraconal phlegmon (inflammatory soft tissue mass that has not yet organized into an abscess).

- 眼眶(隔后)蜂窝织炎累及眶隔深部的肌肉和脂肪。
- 眼眶蜂窝织炎是严重的疾病，因其有并发症的风险，如脓肿及通过无瓣膜的眼静脉向颅内扩散。
- 患者不仅表现为眼睑肿胀和充血，还表现为疼痛性眼肌麻痹、结膜水肿和/或眼球突出。
- 影像学显示眼眶脂肪密度异常，有时伴有眼外肌水肿、眼球突出或肌锥内/外蜂窝织炎(尚未形成脓肿的炎性软组织肿块)。

Subperiosteal abscess

- Subperiosteal abscess is a suppurative collection involving the bony orbit under its periosteum (periorbital). It can arise associated with or independent of orbital cellulitis.
- Imaging shows a convex rim-enhancing collection tracking along a bone surface, most commonly the medial orbital wall in the setting of ethmoid sinusitis.

骨膜下脓肿

- 骨膜下脓肿是脓性液体积聚于眶骨膜下(眶周)并累及骨膜下的骨质。它可继发或独立于眼眶蜂窝织炎。
- 影像学表现为沿骨凸面的环形强化灶，最常见于筛窦炎患者的眼眶内侧壁。

Orbital abscess

- Orbital abscess is an abscess located within the soft tissues of the orbit, due to consolidation of orbital cellulitis or rupture of subperiosteal abscess.
- Imaging shows, as with abscesses elsewhere, a focal rim-enhancing collection.

眶内脓肿

- 眶内脓肿是一种位于眼眶内的软组织脓肿，是由眼眶蜂窝织炎局限化脓或骨膜下脓肿破裂所致。
- 影像学表现和其他位置的脓肿相同，呈边缘强化的液性病灶。

Cavernous sinus thrombosis

- The cavernous sinus is the most common site of septic dural venous sinus thrombosis, due to drainage of sites of medial facial, orbital, sinonasal, or dental infection.
- Patients present with headache, fever, proptosis, chemosis, and cranial nerve palsies (e.g., ophthalmoplegia).
- Imaging shows convex bulging of the lateral wall of the cavernous sinus and filling defects on post-contrast images. Indirect signs include dilatation (and/or thrombosis) of the superior ophthalmic vein.

海绵窦血栓形成

- 海绵窦是脓毒性硬脑膜静脉窦血栓形成最常见的部位，由内侧面部、眼眶、鼻窦或牙齿感染部位的引流所致。
- 患者表现为头痛、发热、眼球突出、结膜水肿和脑神经麻痹(如眼肌麻痹)。
- 影像学表现为海绵窦外侧壁突出隆起和增强后出现充盈缺损。间接症状包括眼上静脉扩张(和/或血栓形成)。

Endophthalmitis/panophthalmitis

- Endophthalmitis refers to bacterial or, less commonly, fungal infection within the globe, involving the vitreous and/or aqueous humors. Further extensive involvement of the ocular wall and periocular orbital tissues is called panophthalmitis.
- Most cases are due to direct inoculation, such as by trauma, surgery, or corneal ulcer.
- Imaging shows thickening and enhancement of the ocular wall, periocular fat stranding, and abnormal high density/signal of the vitreous.

眼内炎/全眼球炎

- 眼内炎是指眼球内的细菌或较少见的真菌感染，累及玻璃体和/或房水。若眼内炎进一步扩散至眼球壁和眼周组织则称为全眼球炎。
- 大多数病例是直接种植感染，如外伤、手术或角膜溃疡。
- 影像学显示眼球壁增厚和强化，眼周脂肪密度异常，玻璃体异常高密度/信号。

Dacryoadenitis

- Dacryoadenitis refers to lacrimal gland inflammation, which can be due to acute viral or bacterial infection. Other causes include idiopathic orbital inflammation, IgG4-related disease, and granulomatous diseases, which are discussed in the next section, as well as Sjögren syndrome.
- Dacryoadenitis appears as diffuse gland enlargement (unilateral or bilateral) that generally molds to orbital structures but may displace the globe inferomedially.

泪腺炎

- 泪腺炎是指泪腺的炎症，可由急性病毒或细菌感染引起。其他原因包括特发性眼眶炎症、免疫球蛋白G4(IgG4)相关疾病和肉芽肿性疾病(将在下文讨论)，以及干燥综合征。
- 泪腺炎表现为弥漫性腺体肿大(单侧或双侧)，通常对眼眶结构造成压迫，但可以使眼球向内下方移位。

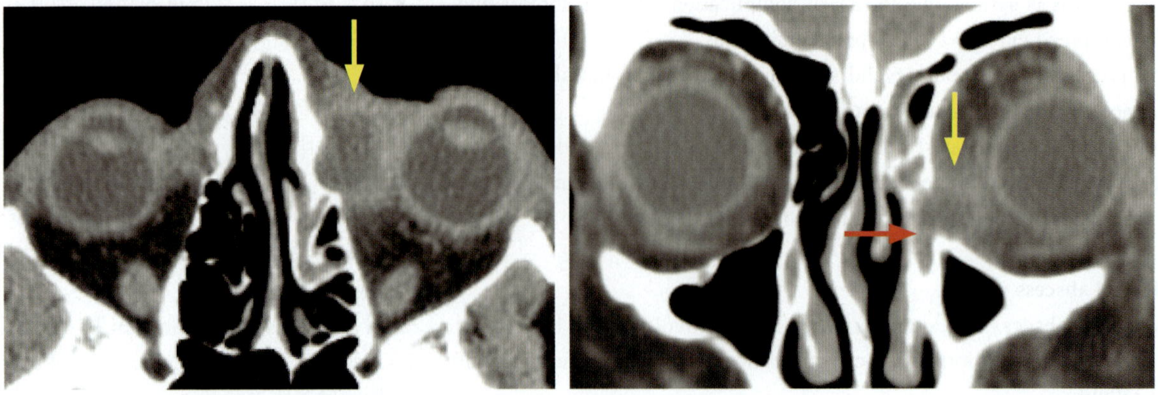

Axial (left image) and coronal noncontrast CT through the orbits shows a rim-enhancement cystic structure in the left lacrimal fossa (yellow arrows) with surrounding soft tissue stranding, representing an enlarged lacrimal sac in the setting of dacryocystitis. Note communication with thenasolacrimal duct (red arrow).

经眼眶轴位(左图)和冠状位平扫CT显示左侧泪囊窝有一个边缘强化的囊性结构(黄箭),周围软组织密度异常,代表泪囊炎时增大的泪囊。注意病灶与鼻泪管相通(红箭,右图)。

- Dacryocystitis refers to lacrimal sac inflammation typically secondary to nasolacrimal duct obstruction and subsequent bacterial infection.
- In infants, dacryocystitis usually complicates congenital nasolacrimal duct obstruction (dacryostenosis) or dacryocystocele. Obstruction can also be acquired in older adults.
- Dacryocystitis appears as a prominent rim-enhancing structure centered in the lacrimal fossa near the medial canthus with adjacent preseptalfat stranding.

- 泪囊炎即泪囊的炎症,通常继发于鼻泪管阻塞和随后的细菌感染。
- 婴儿泪囊炎通常合并先天性鼻泪管阻塞(泪管狭窄)或泪囊囊肿。老年人也可能出现后天性鼻泪管梗阻。
- 泪囊炎表现为边缘显著强化的病灶,中心位于内眦附近的泪囊窝,邻近的隔前脂肪密度有异常。

Orbital inflammatory disorders

眼眶炎性疾病

Idiopathic orbital inflammation (pseudotumor)

- Idiopathic orbital inflammation, originally known as orbital pseudotumor, refers to an orbital mass or structure enlargement related to a nonspecific inflammatory infiltrate of unknown cause. It is diagnosed after excluding systemic autoinflammatory, infectious, and neoplastic etiologies.
- Idiopathic orbital inflammation is the most common cause of a *painful* orbital mass in adults. Pain helps distinguish this entity from mimics (e.g., lymphoma, thyroid eye disease).
- Most cases are unilateral and acute or subacute in onset.
- The main anatomic subtypes and their imaging findings are:

> Idiopathic **dacryoadenitis**: diffuse lacrimal gland enlargement and enhancement.
> Idiopathic **orbital fat inflammation**: fat stranding and/or ill-defined soft tissue involving several structures.
> Idiopathic **orbital myositis**: smooth enlargement of one or several extraocular muscles; most commonly affects the lateral rectus muscle and also involves the anterior tendon (unlike thyroid eye disease).

- Less common subtypes and their imaging findings include:

特发性眼眶炎症(炎性假瘤)

- 特发性眼眶炎症,原名眼眶炎性假瘤,是指眶肿块或内容物肿大,与不明原因的非特异性炎性浸润有关。确诊前需要排除系统性自身免疫性炎症、感染和肿瘤。
- 特发性眼眶炎症是成人眼眶肿块性疼痛最常见的原因。疼痛有助于区分其他类似的疾病(如淋巴瘤、甲状腺相关性眼病)。
- 大多数病例为单侧、急性或亚急性发作。
- 主要解剖亚型及其影像学表现如下:

> 特发性**泪腺炎**:泪腺弥漫性肿大和强化。
> 特发性**眼眶脂肪炎**:脂肪异常密度影和/或累及多种结构的边界不清的软组织病变。
> 特发性**眼眶肌炎**:一个或多个眼外肌平滑肿大;最常累及外直肌,并累及前部肌腱(与甲状腺眼病不同)。

- 较少见的亚型及其影像学表现包括:

Optic perineuritis: optic nerve sheath thickening and enhancement.

Tolosa-Hunt syndrome: cavernous sinus thickening and enhancement.

IgG4-related ophthalmic disease

- Immunoglobulin G4 (IgG4)-related disease is a multisystem fibro-inflammatory disorder. The diagnosis requires histopathology or serology demonstrating IgG4 expression.
- The orbit is the most frequently involved site in the head and neck. In turn, the most common site of IgG4-related ophthalmic disease is the lacrimal gland. Similar to idiopathic orbital inflammation, other common sites of involvement include the extraocular muscles and orbital fat.
- A distinguishing feature in some cases of IgG4-related ophthalmic disease is infiltration/ enlargement of the infraorbital nerve.
- The combination of lacrimal and major salivary gland involvement (parotid or submandibular) was previously called **Mikulicz syndrome**, and now termed IgG4-related chronic sclerosing dacryoadenitis and sialadenitis.

Granulomatous diseases

- Granulomatous inflammation in the orbit appears similar radiologically to idiopathic/nonspecific inflammation but may be associated with a systemic disorder such as sarcoidosis or granulomatosis with polyangiitis. These more commonly affect the globe (e.g., uveitis, scleritis, conjunctivitis), but involvement of the extraocular orbit is better seen on imaging.
- **Sarcoidosis** of the extraocular orbit most often involves the lacrimal gland, but it may also affect the optic nerve sheath, extraocular muscles, or orbital fat. Concurrent thoracic manifestations of sarcoidosis point towards the diagnosis.
- **Granulomatosis with polyangiitis** can involve the orbit, with an infiltrative mass in the orbital fat being the most common type, followed by dacryoadenitis and then extraocular myositis, usually contiguous with sinonasal disease.

Thyroid-associated orbitopathy

视神经周围炎：视神经鞘增厚和强化。

托洛萨-亨特综合征：海绵窦增厚和强化。

免疫球蛋白G4(IgG4)相关性眼病

- IgG4相关疾病是一种多系统纤维炎症性疾病。诊断需要组织病理学或血清学证实有IgG4表达。
- 眼眶是头颈部最常受累的部位。而最常见与IgG4相关性眼病的部位是泪腺。与特发性眼眶炎症相似，其他常见的受累部位包括眼外肌和眼眶脂肪。
- IgG4相关性眼病的部分病例一个显著特征是眶下神经浸润/增大。
- 泪腺和大涎腺同时受累(腮腺或颌下腺)，曾称为**米库利兹综合征**，现在称为IgG4相关慢性硬化性泪囊炎和涎腺炎。

肉芽肿性疾病

- 眼眶肉芽肿性炎症在影像学上与特发性/非特异性炎症相似，但可能与系统性疾病有关，如结节病或肉芽肿性血管炎。眼球常受累(如葡萄膜炎、巩膜炎、结膜炎)，但眼球外-眼眶内病变在影像学上更易被观察。
- 眼球外-眼眶内**结节病**最常累及泪腺，但也可能累及视神经鞘、眼外肌或眼眶脂肪。胸部同时有结节病的表现有助于诊断。
- **肉芽肿性血管炎**可累及眼眶，眶脂肪浸润性肿块是最常见的类型，其次是泪腺炎，然后是眼外肌炎，通常伴有鼻窦疾病。

甲状腺相关性眼病

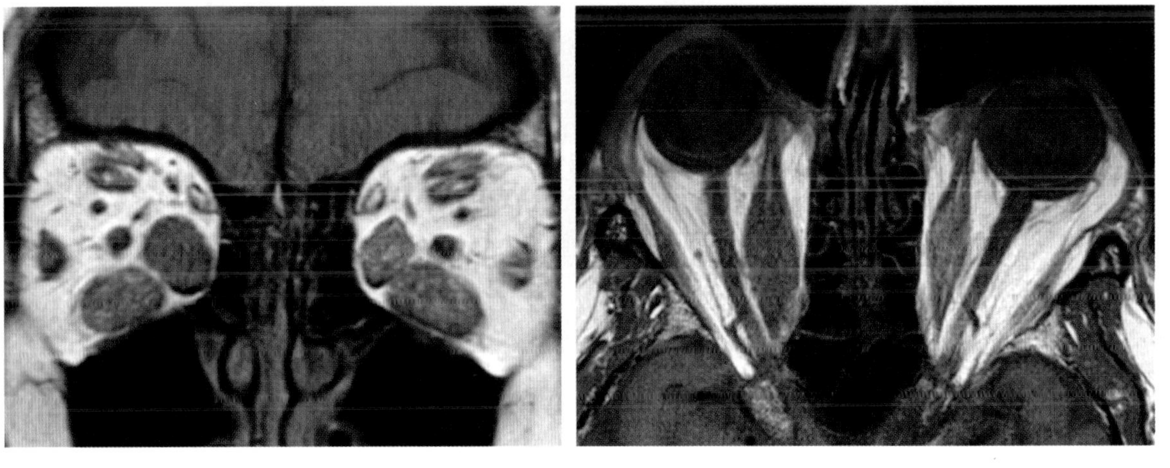

Thyroid orbitopathy in a patient with Graves disease: Coronal (left image) and axial noncontrast MRI through the orbits shows bilateral exophthalmos, increased orbital fat, and enlargement of inferior and medial rectus muscle bellies sparing the tendons (*Coca-Cola bottle sign*).

毒性弥漫性甲状腺肿患者的格雷夫斯病：经眼眶冠状位(左图)和轴位平扫MRI显示双侧眼球突出，眼眶脂肪增多，下直肌和内直肌肌腹增粗，肌腱不受累(*可口可乐瓶征*，右图)。

- Thyroid-associated orbitopathy, also known as Graves ophthalmopathy/orbitopathy or simply thyroid eye disease, is an autoimmune disorder of the orbital soft tissues in patients with thyroid disease. Although usually associated with Graves disease (the most common cause of hyperthyroidism), it can also occur in patients with euthyroid or hypothyroid autoimmune thyroiditis.
- The pathogenesis consists of inflammation involving the orbital muscles and fat, overproduction of glycosaminoglycans (mostly hyaluronic acid) by fibroblasts, and adipogenesis.
- Thyroid-associated orbitopathy is the most common cause of proptosis and extraocular muscle enlargement. Imaging demonstrates proptosis with orbital fat expansion and mild fat stranding early in the disease and, with extended disease activity, fusiform extraocular muscle enlargement.
- Thyroid orbitopathy tends to be bilateral and spares the muscle tendons. The longitudinal appearance of an enlarged muscle belly but a narrow anterior tendon is known as the *Coca- Cola bottle sign* of thyroid orbitopathy.
- The inferior rectus muscle is most commonly affected first. The mnemonic *I'M SLOw* helps remember the order of involvement of the extraocular muscles:

Inferior rectus → **m**edial rectus → **s**uperior rectus → **l**ateral rectus → **o**bliques

- Atypical features such as isolated lateral rectus involvement, anterior tendon enlargement, or unilaterality should prompt consideration of an alternative diagnosis, such as idiopathic orbital inflammation or neoplasm.
- Severe muscle enlargement can crowd the orbital apex, resulting indysthyroid optic neuropathy that may require surgical decompression if not responsive to steroids.

- 甲状腺相关眼病，也称为格雷夫斯眼病/眼眶病或简称“甲状腺眼病”，是甲状腺疾病患者眼眶软组织的一种自身免疫性疾病。尽管常见于格雷夫斯病(甲状腺亢进最常见的病因)，但也可发生于甲状腺功能正常或减退的自身免疫性甲状腺炎患者。
- 发病机制包括炎症累及眼眶肌肉和脂肪、成纤维细胞产生过量糖胺聚糖(主要是透明质酸)，以及脂肪生成过量。
- 甲状腺相关眼病是眼球突出和眼外肌增大最常见的原因。影像学显示眼球突出伴眼眶脂肪增多和早期轻度脂肪密度异常，随着疾病活动性增高，眼外肌梭形增大。
- 甲状腺相关眼病往往为双侧，不累及肌腱。眼外肌的肌腹增粗而前部肌腱相对细小，被称为甲状腺眼病的*可口可乐瓶征*。
- 下直肌通常最先受累。记忆诀窍“*I'M SLOw*”有助于记住眼外肌受累的顺序：

下直肌(**I**)→内直肌(**M**)→上直肌(**S**)→外直肌(**L**)→斜肌(**O**)

- 对于不典型特征，如孤立性外直肌受累、前肌腱增粗或单侧发病，应考虑其他诊断，如特发性眼眶炎症或肿瘤。
- 严重肌肉增粗会挤压眶尖，导致甲状腺功能不全性视神经病变，如果类固醇治疗无效，可能需要手术减压。

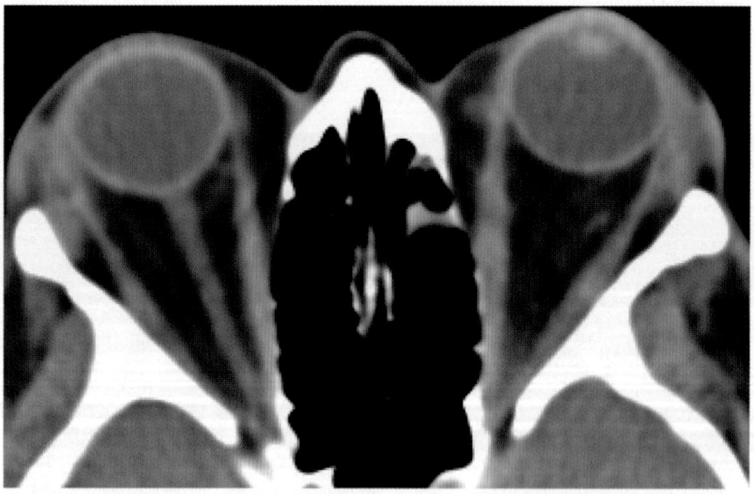

Thyroid orbitopathy, fatty type: Axial (left image) and axial noncontrast CT through the orbits shows bilateral exophthalmos and increased orbital fat. The extraocular muscles do not appear abnormally thickened.
Case courtesy Mary Beth Cunnane, MD, Massachusetts Eye and Ear Infirmary.
甲状腺眼病，脂肪型：轴位平扫CT显示双侧眼球突出和眼眶脂肪增多。眼外肌没有异常增粗。

Optic neuritis

视神经炎

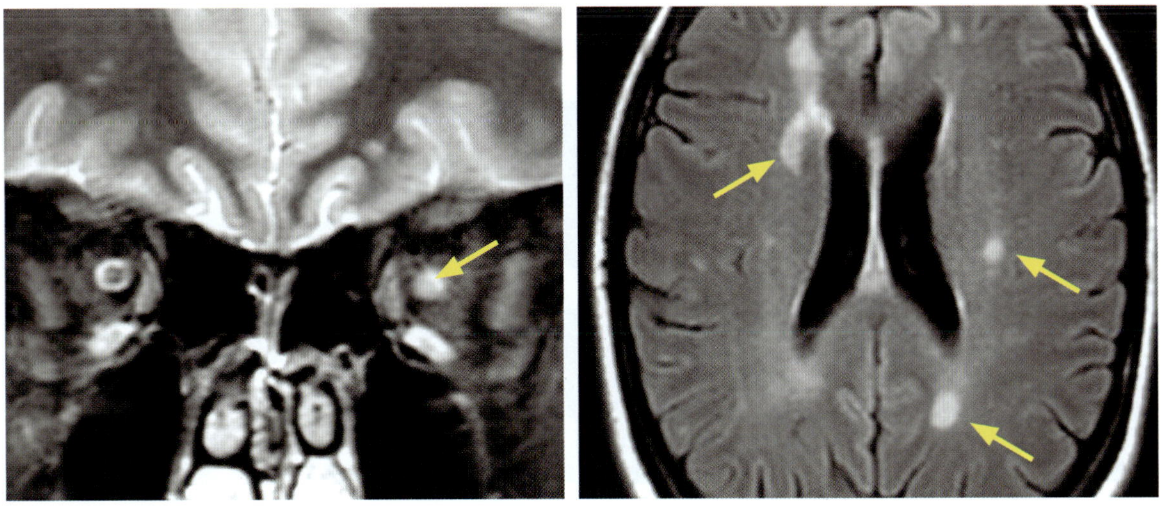

Optic neuritis due to multiple sclerosis: Coronal fat suppressed T2-weighted MRI through the orbits (left image) shows increased signal of the left optic nerve (arrow), with loss of clear distinction between the optic nerve and the surrounding normal T2 hyperintense CSF. The right optic nerve appears normal. There was no enhancement of the left optic nerve (not shown).

Axial FLAIR (right image) shows numerous foci of T2 prolongation within the periventricular white matter (arrows), in a pattern consistent with multiple sclerosis.

Case courtesy Mary Beth Cunnane, MD, Massachusetts Eye and Ear Infirmary.

多发性硬化引起的视神经炎：经眼眶冠状位脂肪抑制T_2加权MRI(左图)显示左侧视神经信号增高(黄箭)，视神经与周围正常T_2高信号脑脊液分界不清。右侧视神经正常。左侧视神经无强化(未展示)。

轴位FLAIR(右图)显示脑室周围白质内多发长T_2病灶(黄箭)，符合多发性硬化。

- Optic neuritis refers to inflammation of the optic nerve.
- Causes of optic neuritis include:

  Multiple sclerosis (MS) is the most common.

  Aquaporin-4 antibody-positive neuromyelitis optica spectrum disorder (NMOSD).

  Myelin oligodendrocyte glycoprotein (MOG) antibody-associated disease.

  Arteritic versus non-arteritic anterior ischemic optic neuropathy (AION versus NAION).

  Viral infection.

  Sarcoidosis.

  Lupus.

  Chronic relapsing inflammatory optic neuropathy (CRION).
- The patients are typically young adults who present with acute, painful, central visual loss. In older patients, ischemic optic neuropathy is more likely than optic neuritis.
- Acutely, the optic nerve shows enlargement, T2 prolongation, and contrast enhancement. Chronically, the optic nerve atrophies.
- Concurrent brain white matter lesions support the diagnosis of MS. Note, however, the optic nerve is not one of the sites that can fulfill the McDonald criteria for dissemination in space.

- 视神经炎是指视神经的炎症。
- 视神经炎的原因包括：

  多发性硬化(MS)，最常见。

  水通道蛋白-4抗体阳性的视神经脊髓炎谱系疾病(NMOSD)。

  髓鞘少突胶质细胞糖蛋白(MOG)抗体相关疾病。

  动脉炎性与非动脉炎性前部缺血性视神经病变(AION与NAION)。

  病毒感染。

  结节病。

  狼疮。

  慢性复发性炎性视神经病变(CRION)。
- 患者通常是年轻人，表现为急性、疼痛性、中央性视力丧失。在老年患者中，缺血性视神经病比视神经炎更常见。
- 急性期表现为视神经增粗、T_2信号延长及对比增强。慢性期见视神经萎缩。
- 合并脑白质病变则支持MS的诊断。但需注意，视神经并不是McDonald标准中一个必要的发病部位。

Lymphoma

淋巴瘤

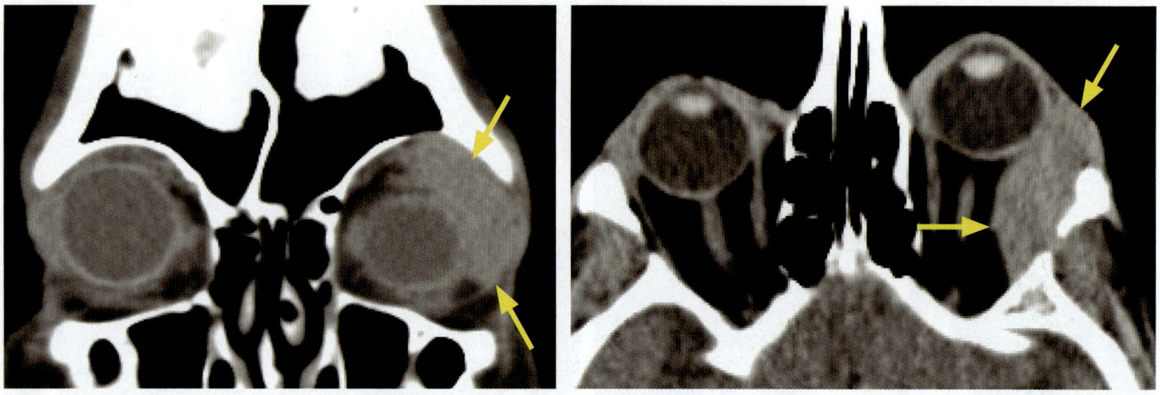

Orbital lymphoma: Coronal (left) and axial noncontrast CT through the orbits shows left-sided proptosis and an ill-defined, slightly hyperattenuating mass (arrows) in the left superior-lateral orbit. The mass conforms to the shape of the globe, rather than deforming it. The left lacrimal gland is not separately identified.

眼眶淋巴瘤：经眼眶冠状位(左图)和轴位(右图)平扫CT显示左侧眼球突出，左眼眶上外侧有一个边界不清的稍高密度肿块(黄箭)。肿块围绕眼球，但不使眼球变形。左侧泪腺不能识别。

- Orbital lymphoproliferative lesions are a spectrum ranging from benign reactive lymphoid hyperplasia to lymphoma. Most of these are ocular adnexal lymphomas (involving the support structures of the eye as opposed to intraocular lymphoma).
- Lymphoma is the most common primary orbital tumor in older adults, although it may also be secondary to systemic disease.
- The most common histology of orbital lymphoma is low-grade extranodal marginal zone B-cell lymphoma of mucosa-associated lymphoid tissue (MALT lymphoma).
- Similar to the above inflammatory disorders, lymphoproliferative lesions can affect any orbital structure as a mass or diffuse infiltration but are most commonly extraconal, particularly involving the lacrimal gland.
- Both lymphoproliferative and inflammatory masses tend to mold to the globe and other orbital structures. However, compared to idiopathic orbital inflammation, lymphomas have lower ADC values on MRI and clinically are unlikely to present with orbital pain.

- 眼眶淋巴增生性病变包括一系列疾病，从良性反应性淋巴增生到淋巴瘤。大多数是眼附属器淋巴瘤(累及眼球的支持结构，与眼内淋巴瘤不同)。
- 淋巴瘤是老年人最常见的原发性眼眶肿瘤，但也可能继发于全身性疾病。
- 眼眶淋巴瘤最常见的组织学类型是黏膜相关淋巴组织(MALT淋巴瘤)的低级别结外边缘区B细胞淋巴瘤。
- 与上述炎症性疾病类似，淋巴增生性病变可以肿块或弥漫性浸润的形式累及眼眶的任何结构，但最常见于肌锥外，尤其是累及泪腺。
- 淋巴增生性病变和炎性肿块都易随眼球和其他眼眶结构塑形。然而，淋巴瘤在MRI上的ADC值较特发性眼眶炎症低，且临床上极少出现眼眶疼痛。

Plexiform neurofibroma

- Plexiform neurofibromas are the most common type of orbital neurofibroma and are almost always associated with neurofibromatosis type 1 (NF1).
- Orbital plexiform neurofibromas typically involve trigeminal nerve branches, extending from the periorbital/preseptalsoft tissues of the eyelid to the deep orbit, infiltrating both extraconaland intraconal compartments.
- On imaging, plexiform neurofibromas appear as infiltrative, serpentine masses with variable contrast enhancement. Associated findings of NF1 may be seen on the orbital imaging study, including sphenoid wing dysplasia, buphthalmos (enlarged globe), and optic nerve glioma.

丛状神经纤维瘤

- 丛状神经纤维瘤是最常见的眼眶神经纤维瘤，几乎都与1型神经纤维瘤病(NF1)相关。
- 眼眶丛状神经纤维瘤通常累及三叉神经分支，从眼睑的眶周/隔前软组织延伸至眼眶深部，同时波及肌锥内区和肌锥外区。
- 影像学上，丛状神经纤维瘤表现为浸润性、蛇形肿块，强化程度各异。在眼眶影像中可发现与NF1相关的表现，包括蝶骨翼发育不良、眼积水(眼球扩大)和视神经胶质瘤。

Venolymphatic malformation (VLM)

- Orbital venolymphatic (combined venous-lymphatic) malformations (VLM), previously called lymphangiomas, are congenital slow-flow vascular malformations that present in children and grow with the patient.

静脉淋巴畸形(VLM)

- 眼眶静脉淋巴(联合)畸形曾被称为淋巴管瘤，是一种先天性慢血流的血管畸形，见于儿童，随年龄而生长。

- Orbital VLMs most commonly involve the extraconal compartment but may be found anywhere in the orbit. A key diagnostic clue is transspatial location with the mass spanning multiple compartments.
- On imaging, orbital VLM appears as a multilocular cystic mass, often with complex internal contents and fluid-fluid levels from prior hemorrhage. Enhancement is variable, though typically peripheral and septal.

- 眼眶VLM最常见于肌锥外区，但也可发生于眼眶的任何部位。诊断的关键线索是病灶跨越多个眼眶分区。
- 影像学上，眼眶VLM表现为多房性囊性肿块，通常有复杂的内部成分和出血导致的液-液平面。增强扫描的典型表现是周边和间隔强化，但是总体上强化方式各异。

Metastasis

转移瘤

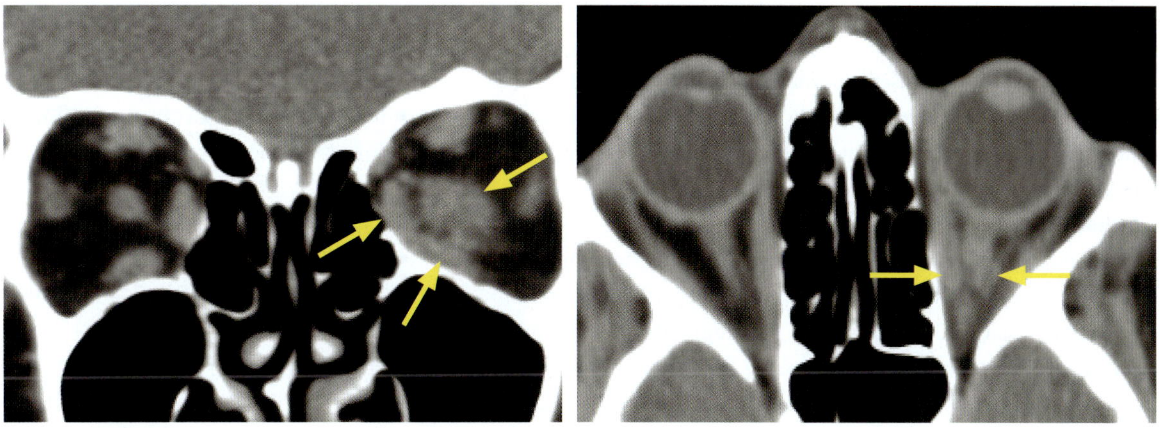

Scirrhous breast cancer metastasis: Coronal (left image) and axial CT through the orbits demonstrates ill-defined soft tissue in the left orbit (arrows), with loss of the normal definition of the optic nerve-sheath complex, medial rectus, and inferior rectus. Despite the presence of the mass, there is no significant proptosis.

Case courtesy Mary Beth Cunnane, MD, Massachusetts Eye and Ear Infirmary.

乳腺硬癌转移：经眼眶冠状位(左图)和轴位(右图)CT显示左眼眶内边界不清的软组织肿块(黄箭)，正常视神经鞘复合体、内直肌和下直肌的边界消失。虽然有肿块，但眼球没有明显突出。

- Orbital metastases arrive hematogenously and can form a mass or diffuse infiltrate in any compartment. Common sites are the choroid, bones, fat, and extraocular muscles.
- In adults, the primary tumors are typically carcinomas and most commonly from the breast. Scirrhous breast cancer metastases characteristically can cause enophthalmos, whereas other primaries cause proptosis.
- In young children, the most common source of metastases to the orbit is neuroblastoma. On cross-sectional imaging, these appear as an extraconal mass centered in the orbital lateral wall or roof with permeative bony destruction, calcifications, and aggressive periosteal reaction.

  Patients with orbital neuroblastoma metastases present with periorbital ecchymoses (*raccoon eyes*). Iodine-123 MIBG scintigraphy is the preferred study to detect bone metastases of neuroblastoma.

- 眼眶转移瘤通过血源途径并可在眼眶任何部位形成肿块或弥漫性浸润。常见部位为脉络膜、骨骼、脂肪和眼外肌。
- 在成人，原发性肿瘤通常为恶性上皮肿瘤，最常来自乳腺。乳腺硬癌转移的特点是可引起眼球内陷，而其他原发性肿瘤可引起眼球突出。
- 在幼儿，最常转移到眼眶的肿瘤来自神经母细胞瘤。在横断图上表现为以眶外侧壁或眶顶为中心的一个肌锥外肿块，伴有弥漫性骨质破坏、钙化和侵袭性骨膜反应。

  眼眶神经母细胞瘤转移患者表现为眶周淤血(浣熊眼)。^{123}I-MIBG闪烁显像是检测神经母细胞瘤骨转移的首选方法。

Extraconal masses

肌锥外肿瘤

Dermoid cyst

- Dermoid cysts are congenital ectodermal inclusion cysts made of keratinous and sebaceous debris. In the extracranial head and neck, the orbital region is the most common site of dermoids.
- Orbital dermoid cysts are the most common extraconal mass in children. They occur near suture lines, most commonly in the superolateral quadrant at the zygomaticofrontal suture.

皮样囊肿

- 皮样囊肿是由角质和皮脂腺碎片构成的先天性外胚层包涵囊肿。眼眶是颅外头颈部皮样囊肿最常见部位。
- 皮样囊肿是儿童最常见的肌锥外肿块。发生于骨缝周围，最常见于颧额缝的上外侧象限。

- Imaging shows a circumscribed,unilocular cyst with at most thin rim enhancement, sometimes causing irregular bone scalloping. The internal contents can be heterogeneous but a fatty component or fat-fluid level, when present, is characteristic.

- 影像学表现为边缘清晰的单房囊肿，最多有一薄层强化，有时可引起不规则的骨质吸收。内部成分混杂，一旦发现脂质成分和脂-液平面则具有特征性。

Rhabdomyosarcoma

- Rhabdomyosarcoma is the most common extraocular orbital malignancy in children.
- Orbital rhabdomyosarcomas are predominantly the embryonal subtype, which tend to arise in the superior orbital soft tissues.
- Most orbital rhabdomyosarcomas are extraconal in location, but up to half have intraconal extension as well.
- Imaging shows a solitary, circumscribed, enhancing soft tissue mass.
- Isolated orbital involvement carries a favorable prognosis relative to parameningeal sites. Bone invasion and extraorbital extension classifies the tumor as parameningeal.

横纹肌肉瘤

- 横纹肌肉瘤是儿童最常见的眼球外恶性肿瘤。
- 多数眼眶横纹肌肉瘤为胚胎亚型，多发生于眶上的软组织内。
- 大多数眼眶横纹肌肉瘤位于肌锥外，但多达一半同时还有肌锥内受侵。
- 影像学表现为孤立、边缘清晰及强化的软组织肿块。
- 孤立眼眶受累的预后相对于脑膜旁受累为好。脑膜旁受累是指有骨侵犯和眶外扩散。

Infantile hemangioma

- Infantile hemangiomas, previously known as capillary hemangiomas, are the most common neoplasms of the head and neck, including orbits, in infants.
- Infantile hemangiomas are characterized histologically by capillary-like vascular spaces lined with GLUT1-expressing endothelium and clinically by presenting weeks after birth (but are not present at birth). The course features proliferation during infancy followed by spontaneous involution in childhood.
- Infantile hemangiomas can be superficial (cutaneous "strawberry hemangioma"), deep (subcutaneous), or combined. Most orbital/ periorbital infantile hemangiomas are entirely or largely extraconal, usually centered in the anterior orbit or eyelid.
- Imaging shows a lobulated, intensely enhancing mass. Internal septations and flow voids on MRI are typical.

婴幼儿血管瘤

- 婴幼儿血管瘤，之前称为毛细血管血管瘤，是婴儿头颈部(包括眼眶)最常见的肿瘤。
- 婴幼儿血管瘤在组织学上的特征为毛细血管样血管间隙，内衬表达*GLUT1*的内皮细胞，临床上在出生数周后才有表现(但出生时不存在)。病程的特点是婴儿期增生，儿童期自发退化。
- 婴幼儿血管瘤可位于浅表(皮肤的"草莓状血管瘤")、深部(皮下的)或两者兼有。大多数眼眶/眶周婴幼儿血管瘤完全或大部分位于肌锥外，通常以眼眶前部或眼睑为中心。
- 影像学表现为显著强化的分叶状肿块。MRI通常显示内部分隔及血管流空。

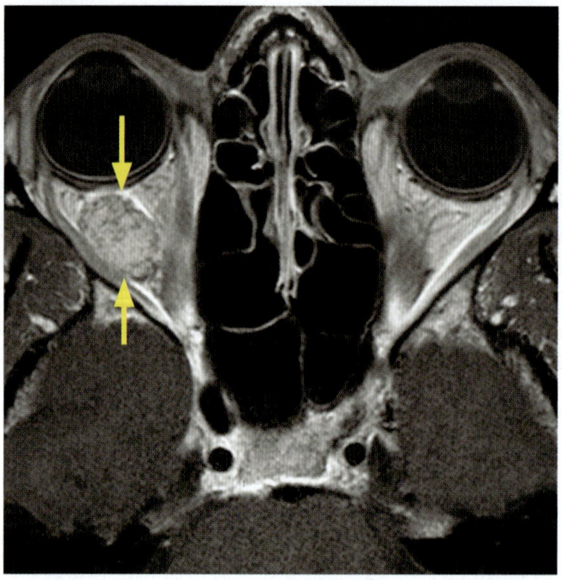

Cavernous hemangioma: Axial T1-weighted post-contrast MRI through the orbits demonstrates a well-circumscribed, intraconal ovoid mass (arrows) that demonstrates inhomogeneous, patchy enhancement.

Case courtesy Mary Beth Cunnane, MD, Massachusetts Eye and Ear Infirmary.

海绵状血管瘤：经眼眶轴位增强T_1加权MRI显示一个肌锥内边界清晰的卵圆形的肿块(黄箭)，信号不均匀、呈斑片状强化。

Peripheral nerve sheath tumors

- Schwannomas and localized neurofibromas are benign peripheral nerve sheath tumors with indistinguishable imaging appearances when they occur in the orbit. Schwannoma is more common.

周围神经鞘瘤

- 神经鞘瘤和局限性神经纤维瘤均是良性的周围神经鞘的肿瘤，当它们出现在眼眶内时，影像学难以区分这两种肿瘤。其中神经鞘瘤较常见。

- The most commonly affected nerves are the extraconal sensory branches of CN V_1. However, involvement of intraconal nerves is also possible.
- Nerve sheath tumors are solitary, circumscribed, ovoid masses that are hypointense on T1-weighted images, hyperintense on T2-weighted images (sometimes with central hypointensity, called the *target sign*), and contrast-enhancing.

Lacrimal gland tumors

- The most common lacrimal gland neoplasm is lymphoma.
- Like inflammatory disorders, lymphoma usually appears as diffuse gland enlargement that molds to orbital structures like putty.
- The most common lacrimal epithelial neoplasm is pleomorphic adenoma (benign mixed tumor), while the most common epithelial malignancy is adenoid cystic carcinoma.
- Epithelial lacrimal gland tumors are usually masses arising focally from the orbital lobe that displace orbital structures like a marble (indenting the globe, distorting the extraocular muscles, and remodeling or destroying orbital walls).
- Epithelial lacrimal gland tumors are unilateral. Bilateral involvement would be more typical of systemic inflammatory or lymphoproliferative disorders.

- 最常受累的神经是三叉神经眼支的肌锥外感觉支，但也可能累及肌锥内神经。
- 神经鞘的肿瘤是单发、边缘清晰的卵圆形肿块，在T_1加权上呈低信号，T_2加权上呈高信号(有时为中心低信号，称为*靶征*)，有强化。

泪腺肿瘤

- 最常见的泪腺肿瘤是淋巴瘤。
- 淋巴瘤与炎症性疾病类似，通常表现为弥漫性泪腺肿大，像油灰一样沿眼眶结构塑形。
- 最常见的泪腺上皮肿瘤是多形性腺瘤(良性混合瘤)，而最常见的恶性上皮肿瘤是腺样囊性癌。
- 泪腺上皮肿瘤通常是一个起源于泪腺眶叶的肿块，并像大理石样挤压眼眶结构(使眼球凹陷，扭曲眼外肌，重塑或破坏眼眶骨壁)。
- 泪腺上皮肿瘤为单侧发病。双侧泪腺受累则更可能为全身性炎症或淋巴增生性疾病。

INTRACONAL MASSES

肌锥内肿块

Optic pathway glioma

视神经通路胶质瘤

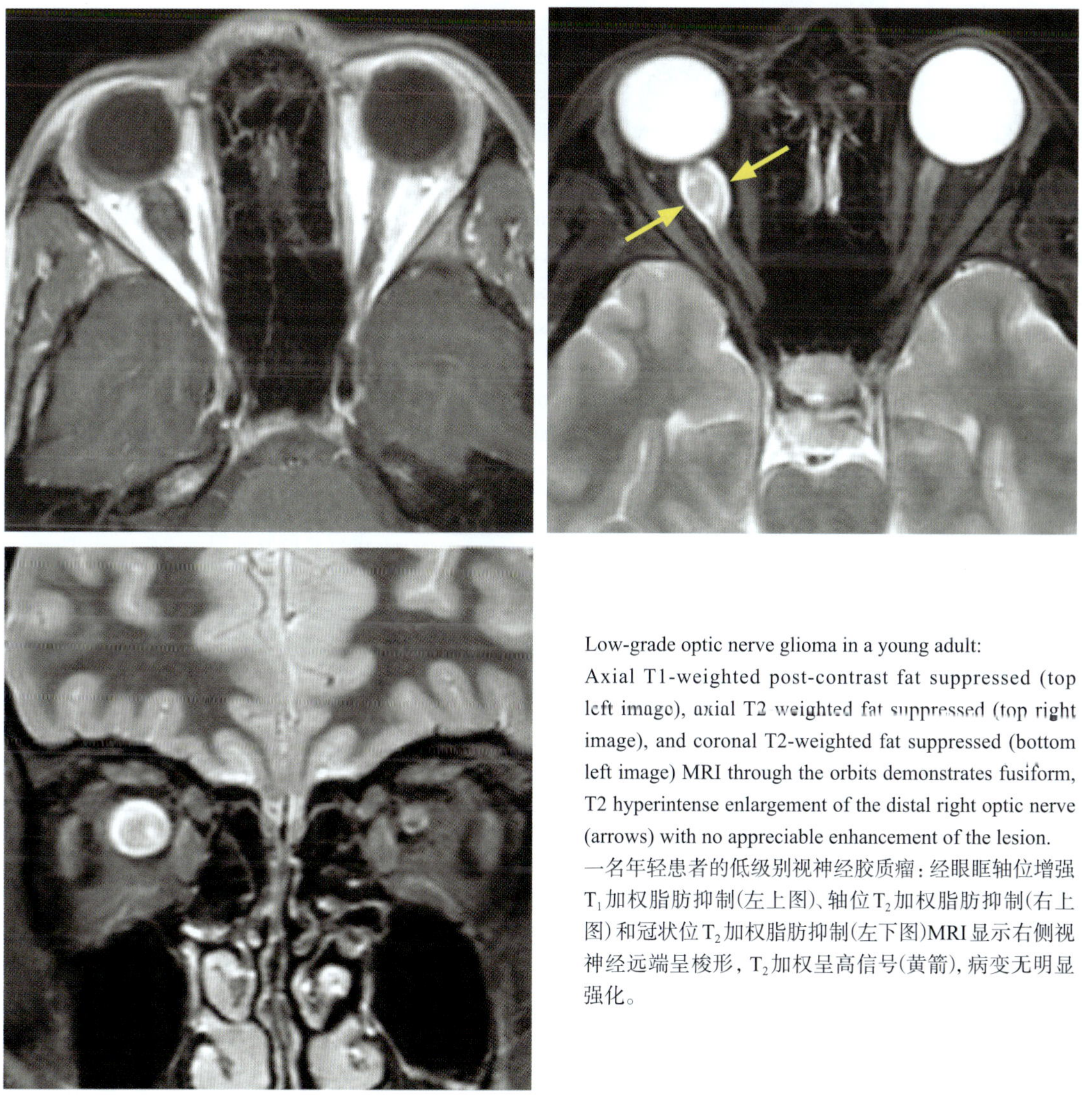

Low-grade optic nerve glioma in a young adult:
Axial T1-weighted post-contrast fat suppressed (top left image), axial T2 weighted fat suppressed (top right image), and coronal T2-weighted fat suppressed (bottom left image) MRI through the orbits demonstrates fusiform, T2 hyperintense enlargement of the distal right optic nerve (arrows) with no appreciable enhancement of the lesion.

一名年轻患者的低级别视神经胶质瘤：经眼眶轴位增强T_1加权脂肪抑制(左上图)、轴位T_2加权脂肪抑制(右上图)和冠状位T_2加权脂肪抑制(左下图)MRI显示右侧视神经远端呈梭形，T_2加权呈高信号(黄箭)，病变无明显强化。

- Optic pathway gliomas, or simply optic gliomas, are the most common optic nerve tumors.
- Optic gliomas most commonly occur in children. They are the most common central nervous system tumor in patients with neurofibromatosis type 1 (NF1), in whom bilateral involvement is frequent.
- The most common histology ispilocytic astrocytoma, an indolent (WHO grade I) tumor with excellent prognosis. Malignant (high-grade) gliomas can occur in adults.
- On imaging, low-grade optic gliomas appear as fusiform enlargement of the optic nerve with variable contrast enhancement.

Optic nerve sheath meningioma

- 视神经通路胶质瘤，简称“视神经胶质瘤”，是最常见的视神经肿瘤。
- 视神经胶质瘤最常见于儿童。它们是1型神经纤维瘤病(NF1)患者中最常见的中枢神经系统肿瘤，常累及双侧。
- 最常见的组织学类型是毛细胞型星形细胞瘤，一种惰性(WHO 1级)肿瘤，预后良好。恶性(高级别)胶质瘤可发生于成人。
- 影像学上，低级别视神经胶质瘤表现为视神经梭形肿大伴不同程度的强化。

视神经鞘脑膜瘤

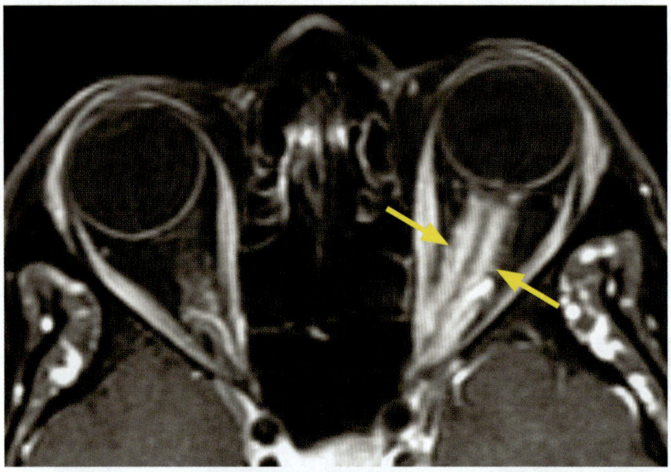

Optic nerve-sheath meningioma: Axial post-contrast fat-sat T1-weighted image demonstrates marked enhancement surrounding the left optic nerve with a *tram-track* appearance (arrows).
视神经鞘脑膜瘤：轴位增强脂肪饱和T1加权显示左侧视神经周围明显强化，呈轨道状(黄箭)。

- Meningiomas are the most common tumors arising from the optic nerve sheath.
- Optic nerve meningiomas usually occur in adults with a female predilection and rarely in children unless associated with neurofibromatosis type 2 (NF2).
- Patients present with slowly progressive visual impairment, classically with preservation of the central visual field (peripheral constriction).
- On imaging, the nerve sheath appears circumferentially thickened, with uniform contrast enhancement and often calcifications. The enhancing tumor surrounding the nonenhancing optic nerve produces the *tram-track sign* on axial images and *doughnut sign* on coronal images.

Cavernous venous malformation

- Venous malformations, previously known as cavernous hemangiomas, are encapsulated slow-flow vascular malformations that are the most common orbital mass in adults.
- Orbital venous malformations can be located anywhere but are usually intraconal.
- MRI shows a well-defined mass that is isointense on T1-weighted images and hyperintense on T2-weighted images, demonstrating patchy enhancement that slowly fills in.

Orbital venous varix

- Orbital varices are distended veins freely connected to the normal circulation, arising primarily as congenital malformations but sometimes secondary to arteriovenous malformations or fistulae.
- Orbital varices represent the most common cause of spontaneous orbital hemorrhage but patients usually present with intermittent positional/stress proptosis.

- 脑膜瘤是最常起源于视神经鞘的肿瘤。
- 视神经脑膜瘤通常发生于成年女性，很少发生于儿童，除非伴有2型神经纤维瘤病(NF2)。
- 患者表现为缓慢进行性视力损害，但通常中央视野不受累(周边视野缩窄)。
- 影像学表现为神经鞘呈环状增厚，强化均匀并常有钙化。强化的肿瘤包绕无强化的视神经，在横断面上产生轨道征，在冠状面上则为甜甜圈征。

海绵状静脉畸形

- 静脉畸形，以前称为海绵状血管瘤，是包裹性慢血流的血管畸形，也是成人最常见的眼眶肿块。
- 眼眶静脉畸形可以发生于任何位置，但最常发生于肌锥内。
- MRI表现为一个边界清晰的肿块，在T_1加权像上呈等信号，在T_2加权像上呈高信号，呈斑块状强化，缓慢填充。

眼眶静脉曲张

- 眼眶静脉曲张是扩张的静脉与正常循环自由交通，主要为先天畸形，有时继发于动静脉畸形或动静脉瘘。
- 眼眶静脉曲张是自发性眼眶出血的最常见原因，但患者通常表现为间歇性体位性/压力性眼球突出。

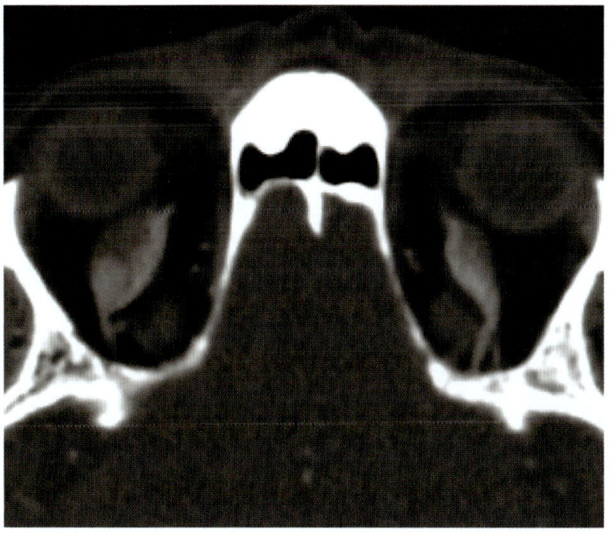

Delay-phase axial CT angiogram shows bilateral orbital varices.
延迟期轴位CT血管造影显示双侧眼眶静脉曲张。

- Orbital varices appear as ovoid or tubular, intensely enhancing structures, often intraconal but not always.
- Varices can be distinguished from other vascular lesions in that they demonstrate dynamic distension with maneuvers that increase venous pressure such as the Valsalva maneuver or prone positioning. Doppler ultrasound demonstrates slow flow.

- 眼眶静脉曲张表现为卵圆形或管状，并有显著强化的结构，常位于肌锥内但并非都是。
- 静脉曲张可以通过增加静脉压力的动作与其他血管病变进行区分，比如瓦尔萨尔瓦动作或俯卧位，可使病灶呈动态扩张。多普勒超声显示血流缓慢。

Ocular masses

Ocular metastases

- Metastases are the most common intraocular malignancies.
- The uvea, typically the choroid, is the most common ocular site for hematogenous deposition of metastases due to its vascularity.
- The most common primary tumor types are carcinomas, such as breast and lung cancer.
- On imaging, metastases are typically irregular, enhancing masses broadly based on the choroid.

Uveal melanoma

- Uveal melanoma is the most common primary intraocular malignancy in adults.
- Most cases arise from the choroid or ciliary body and are discovered incidentally on fundoscopy.
- On imaging, uveal melanoma is usually a mushroom-shaped or biconvex mass based at the uvea that shows intrinsic T1 hyperintensity and contrast enhancement.
- The most common site of metastasis is the liver.

Retinoblastoma

- Retinoblastoma is the most common primary intraocular malignancy in children.
- Patients usually present in the first few years of life with leukocoria (white pupillary reflex).
- Unilateral cases are usually sporadic, due to somatic mutations in the tumor suppressor gene *Rb*. Bilateral retinoblastomas are due to heritable germline mutations in the gene, but family history is positive only in a minority.
- On imaging, retinoblastoma appears as an enhancing retinal mass in a normal-sized globe. Calcifications are characteristic.

眼球肿块

眼球转移瘤

- 转移瘤是眼球内最常见的恶性肿瘤。
- 葡萄膜，特别是脉络膜具有丰富的血管，因此是眼内通过血行播散转移灶最常见的结构。
- 原发肿瘤最常见的类型是恶性上皮肿瘤，如乳腺癌和肺癌。
- 影像学上，转移瘤通常不规则、有强化，肿块有较宽的基底并附着于脉络膜。

葡萄膜黑色素瘤

- 葡萄膜黑色素瘤是成人最常见的原发性眼内恶性肿瘤。
- 大多数病例起源于脉络膜或睫状体，偶尔在眼底镜检查时被发现。
- 影像学上，葡萄膜黑色素瘤通常表现为贴于葡萄膜的蘑菇状或双凸状肿块，呈固有的T_1高信号并有强化。
- 最常见的转移部位是肝脏。

视网膜母细胞瘤

- 视网膜母细胞瘤是儿童最常见的原发性眼内恶性肿瘤。
- 患者通常在出生后的数年内出现“白瞳征”(瞳孔反光呈白色)。
- 单侧病例通常呈散发，为肿瘤抑制基因*Rb*的体细胞突变所致。双侧视网膜母细胞瘤是由该基因的遗传种系突变所致，但只有少数病例的家族史为阳性。
- 影像学上，视网膜母细胞瘤在正常大小的眼

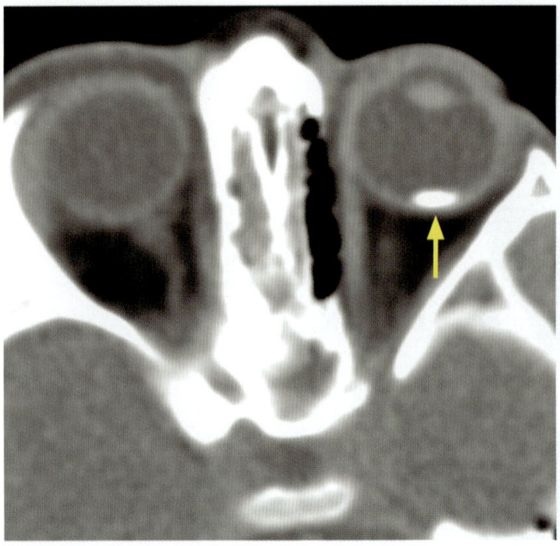

Retinoblastoma: Noncontrast axial CT through the orbits in a 20-month old child demonstrates a normal-sized left orbit with a coarse retinal calcification (arrow).

Case courtesy Mary Beth Cunnane, MD, Massachusetts Eye and Ear Infirmary.

视网膜母细胞瘤：经眼眶轴位平扫CT显示一名20月龄幼儿的左眼眶大小正常，视网膜有一个粗大的钙化灶(黄箭)。

- **Trilateral** retinoblastoma describes the association of bilateral retinoblastoma with pineoblastoma. The addition of a suprasellar tumor is **quadrilateral** retinoblastoma.
- Survivors of heritable retinoblastoma treated with radiation have greater risk of a second malignancy many years later. The most common are osteosarcoma and leiomyosarcoma.

球中表现为增强的视网膜肿块。钙化具有特征性。

- **三侧性**视网膜母细胞瘤是指双侧视网膜母细胞瘤合并松果体母细胞瘤。若再伴有鞍上肿瘤，则称为**四侧性**视网膜母细胞瘤。
- 接受放射治疗的遗传性视网膜母细胞瘤幸存者在许多年后面临更高的二次恶性肿瘤风险。最常见的是骨肉瘤和平滑肌肉瘤。

Pediatric ocular and optic nerve non-neoplastic disorders

儿童眼球和视神经非肿瘤性疾病

Retinopathy of prematurity (ROP)

早产儿视网膜病变(ROP)

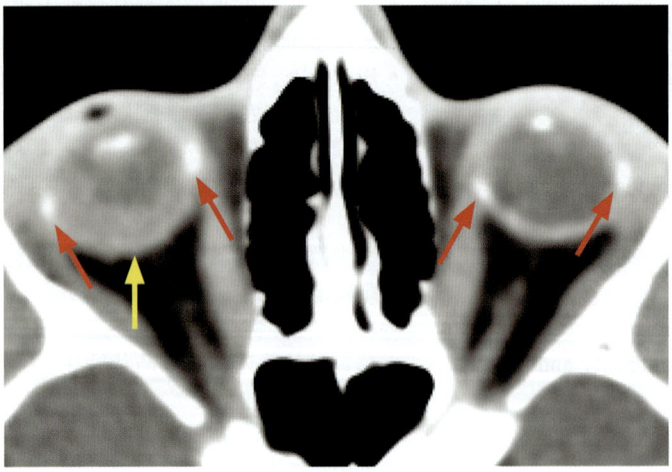

Retinopathy of prematurity: Noncontrast axial CT through the orbits shows bilateral microphthalmia with scattered orbital calcifications (red arrows). Peripheral high attenuation material in the right globe (yellow arrow) represents prior vitreous hemorrhage.

Case courtesy Mary Beth Cunnane, MD, Massachusetts Eye and Ear Infirmary.

早产儿视网膜病变：轴位平扫CT显示双侧小眼球，伴有散在的眼球钙化(红箭)。右眼球边缘高密度物质(黄箭)提示先前有玻璃体积血。

- Retinopathy of prematurity (ROP) is a disorder of retinal neovascularityin preterm infants, likely incited by hypoxia and hyperoxia. Complications include retinal/vitreous hemorrhage and detachment.
- On imaging, both globes are small (microphthalmia) and often show increased attenuation on CT due to prior hemorrhage or neovascularity.

Coats disease

- Coats disease is an idiopathic disorder characterized by retinal telangiectasiasand exudates that lead to retinal detachment.

- 早产儿视网膜病变(ROP)是一种早产儿视网膜新生血管的疾病，可能由缺氧和高氧引起。并发症包括视网膜脱落和玻璃体积血。
- 影像学上，双侧眼球变小(小眼球)，CT常表现为密度增高，为先前出血或新生血管所致。

外层渗出性视网膜病变

- 外层渗出性视网膜病变是一种特发性疾病，其特征为视网膜毛细血管扩张，以及渗出导

- Patients with Coats disease are predominantly boys, slightly older than those affected by retinoblastoma.
- The globe is normal in size but features proteinaceous subretinal fluid that does not enhance.

致视网膜脱离。
- 绝大多数发生在男孩，年龄略大于视网膜母细胞瘤患者。
- 眼球大小正常，其特征为视网膜下蛋白样积液，无强化。

Persistent hyperplastic primary vitreous (PHPV)

永存原始玻璃体增生症(PHPV)

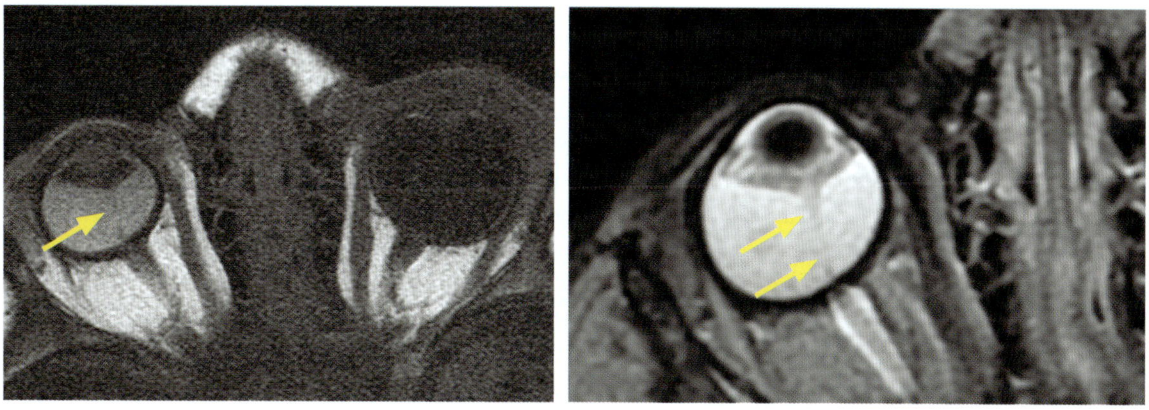

PHPV: Axial T1- (left image) and T2-weighted MRI through the orbits shows microphthalmia of the right globe with diffuse T1 hyperintense signal in the vitreous. There is a triangular retrolentalsoft tissue with linear stalk extending to the optic nerve head representing hyaloid remnant of the Cloquet canal (arrows).
PHPV：经眼眶轴位T_1(左图)和T_2加权MRI显示右眼球呈小眼畸形，伴玻璃体弥漫性T_1高信号。晶状体后有一个三角形的软组织结构，其柄呈线状延伸至视神经乳头，为残留的玻璃体中央管(又称Cloquet管)(黄箭)。

- Persistent hyperplastic primary vitreous (PHPV) is persistent embryonic vasculature within the vitreous that leads to hemorrhage, cataracts, and retinal detachment. Affected infants are typically full term.
- On imaging, there is typically unilateral microphthalmia with increased attenuation/signal of the vitreous body. Characteristically, there is the *martini glass sign* of a Y-shaped soft tissue stalk along the hyaloid (Cloquet) canal of the posterior segment, extending from optic disc to the lens.

- 永存原始玻璃体增生症(PHPV)是玻璃体内的永存性胚胎血管结构，可导致出血、白内障和视网膜脱离。患儿通常是足月婴儿。
- 典型的影像学表现为单侧小眼，伴玻璃体密度/信号增高。马提尼酒杯征具有特征性，为眼后节沿玻璃体中央管走行的"Y"形的软组织结构，从视盘延伸至晶状体。

Ocular coloboma

眼缺损

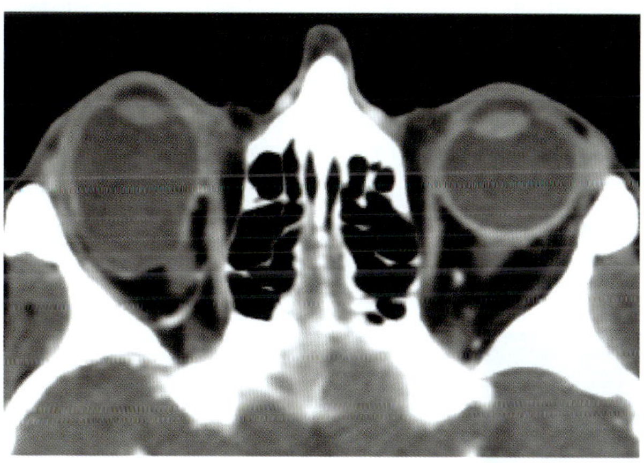

Axial contrast-enhanced CT shows a large right posterior globe outpouching, representing a coloboma.
轴位增强CT显示右眼有一个巨大的向后膨出灶，为眼球缺损。

- Colobomas are focal congenital defects (fissure, cleft, or outpouching) typically caused by incomplete fusion of the embryonic choroidal/optic fissure, but the term can be applied to defects in any structure in the eye and eyelid.
- Colobomas are associated with numerous syndromes including trisomies 13 and 18 and CHARGE syndrome (coloboma, heart defects, atresia choanae, retarded growth and development, genitourinary anomalies, and ear anomalies).

- 眼缺损是一种局部先天性缺陷(裂缝、裂口或膨出)，通常由胚胎脉络膜/视神经裂不完全融合引起，但该术语可用于眼球和眼睑任何结构的缺陷。
- 眼缺损与多种综合征有关，包括13-三体和18-三体综合征，以及CHARGE综合征［眼缺损(**C**)、心脏缺陷(**H**)、后鼻孔闭锁(**A**)、生长与发育迟缓

- On imaging, posterior colobomas appear as a focal bulge elongating the globe in the region of the optic disc. They are often associated with microphthalmia and a retrobulbar cyst.

Septo-optic dysplasia

- Septo-optic dysplasia is part of the holoprosencephaly spectrum of malformations, characterized by optic nerve hypoplasia, agenesis of the septum pellucidum, and often hypothalamic-pituitary dysfunction.
- On imaging, the bilateral optic nerves and optic chiasm are small and the septum pellucidum is absent. The posterior pituitary may be ectopically located.
- In **septo-optic dysplasia plus**, there is associated polymicrogyria and/or schizencephaly, a full-thickness cleft in the cerebral hemisphere that creates a communication between the ventricles and the extra-axial subarachnoid space.

(**R**)、泌尿生殖系统异常(**G**)和耳异常(**E**)]。

- 后部眼缺损在影像学上表现为视盘区局部膨出和眼球拉长。通常伴有小眼症和球后囊肿。

视-隔发育不良

- 视-隔发育不良是前脑无裂畸形谱系疾病的一部分，其特征是视神经发育不良、透明隔发育不良，通常伴有下丘脑-垂体功能障碍。
- 影像学上，双侧视神经和视交叉变小，透明隔缺失。垂体后叶可能异位。
- **视-隔发育不良综合征**患者还合并有多小脑回畸形和/或脑裂畸形，即大脑半球的全层裂隙，在脑室和轴(脑)外蛛网膜下腔之间形成交通。

Ocular trauma

Globe rupture and foreign body

- Globe rupture, or open-globe injury, is usually diagnosed on clinical examination but CT can be helpful in unclear cases or to exclude orbital foreign bodies.
- CT features specific for globe rupture include *flat tire sign* of globe deformity (wall contour irregularity and decreased globe volume), change in anterior chamber depth, intraocular foreign body, or intraocular gas.
- Increased depth of the anterior chamber suggests posterior segment rupture, while decreased depth suggests anterior segment rupture (e.g., corneal perforation).
- Nonacute mimics include globe outpouchings (coloboma, staphyloma), pthisis bulbi (atrophic and calcified globe), focal ocular calcifications (optic nerve drusen, senile scleral plaques), and scleral bands or intraocular gas/air placed to treat retinal detachment.

Ocular detachments and hemorrhage

- **Retinal detachment** that is complete/extensive takes a "V" configuration, convergent on the optic disc and extending to the ora serrata. Vitreous, serous, or hemorrhagic fluid fills the subretinal space (between retina and choroid).

Retinal detachment is most commonly related to retinal tears (rhegmatogenous), which can be traumatic or, more often, spontaneous related to posterior vitreous detachment. Myopia is a major risk factor.

Non-rhegmatogenous causes consist of exudative effusion (e.g., infection, inflammation, neoplasm) or traction related to neovascularization.

眼外伤

眼球破裂和异物

- 眼球破裂或开放性眼球损伤，通常在临床检查中确诊，但CT有助于诊断可疑的病例或排除眼眶内异物。
- CT对于眼球破裂有特异性的表现，包括眼球变形产生的*爆胎征*(眼球壁轮廓不规则和眼球体积缩小)、前房深度改变、眼球内异物或眼球内气体。
- 前房加深提示眼后节破裂，而前房变浅提示眼前节破裂(如角膜穿孔)。
- 非急性的类似病变包括眼球膨出(眼缺损、葡萄肿)、眼球痨(眼球萎缩和钙化)、眼部局灶性钙化(视神经玻璃膜疣、老年性巩膜斑)，以及用于治疗视网膜脱离的巩膜带或注入眼球内的气体。

眼部脱离和出血

- **视网膜脱离**为视网膜完全或广泛分离而呈"V"形，在视盘会聚，并延伸至锯齿缘。玻璃体、浆液或血性液体填充视网膜下间隙(视网膜与脉络膜之间)。

视网膜脱离最常见的原因与视网膜撕裂(孔源性)有关，它可能是外伤性的，更常见的是自发性的，与后玻璃体脱离有关。近视是主要的危险因素。

非孔源性原因包括渗出性积液(如感染、炎症、肿瘤)或新生血管导致的牵拉。

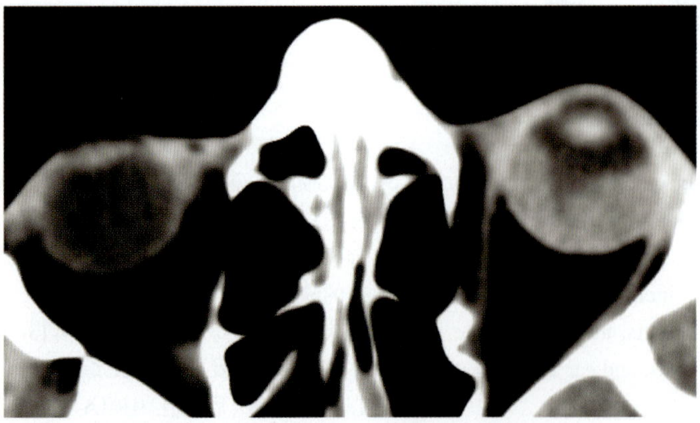

Retinal detachment: Axial noncontrast CT shows increased attenuation in the posterior left globe with a V-shaped configuration.
视网膜脱离：轴位平扫CT显示左眼球后部密度增高，呈"V"形。

- **Choroidal detachment** takes an hourglass configuration that diverges as it approaches the optic disc so as to spare the posterior pole of the globe, can extend anteriorly beyond the ora serrata, and can appose the retina at the convexities (*kissing choroid sign*). Serous or hemorrhagic fluid fills the suprachoroidal space (between choroid and sclera).

  The most common cause of choroidal detachment is ocular hypotony, which can be traumatic or, more often, related to recent surgery. Other causes are inflammatory, neoplastic, or vascular.

- **脉络膜脱离**呈沙漏状结构，在接近视盘前不再向眼球的后极扩散，向前延伸并超过锯齿孔，并可在凸面处与视网膜对齐(脉络膜对吻征)。脉络膜上腔(脉络膜和巩膜之间)被浆液性或出血性液体充填。

  脉络膜脱离最常见的原因是低眼压，可能是外伤性，但更常见于近期手术。其他原因包括炎症、肿瘤或血管性疾病。

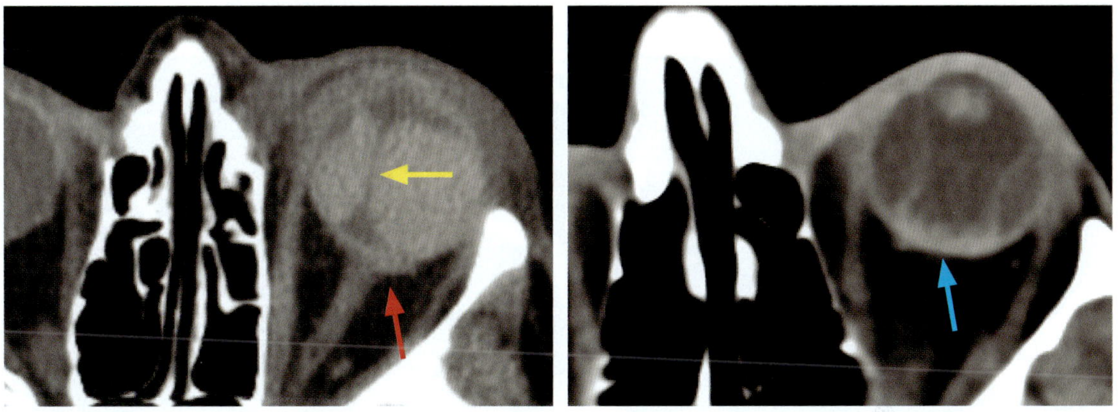

Choroidal detachment in two different patients:
Axial noncontrast CT (left image) shows extensive hyperdense hemorrhage in the left globe, including choroidal detachment with subchoroidal hemorrhage resulting in the *kissing choroid sign* (yellow arrow). There is also contour abnormality at the posterior globe concerning for open globe injury (red arrow).
Axial contrast-enhanced CT (right image) demonstrates choroidal detachment of the left globe with hypodense subchoroidal blood products in an hourglass configuration. This was thought to be secondary to intraocular metastatic squamous cell carcinoma, as suggested by the nodular enhancement at the posterior globe (blue arrow), which was confirmed on subsequent MRI.
两名不同患者的脉络膜脱离：
轴位平扫CT(左图)显示左侧眼球广泛出血引起的高密度，包括脉络膜脱离伴脉络膜下出血，导致脉络膜对吻征(黄箭)。眼球后部轮廓也有异常，疑为开放性眼球损伤(红箭)
轴位增强CT(右图)显示左侧眼球脉络膜脱离，伴脉络膜下慢性出血产物所致的低密度，并呈沙漏状。推测为眼内转移性SCC所致，因眼球后部有结节状强化(蓝箭)，随后在MRI上得到了证实。

- **Vitreous hemorrhage** appears as hyperattenuation of the posterior segment on CT.

  Causes of vitreous hemorrhage include trauma (including abusive head trauma in young children), spontaneous vitreous detachment and/or retinal tear, and conditions causing retinal neovascularity.

  Terson syndrome is the association of vitreous hemorrhage (and/or retinal hemorrhage) secondary to intracranial subarachnoid hemorrhage, likely related to elevated intracranial pressure.

  Nonacute mimics include intraocular silicone oil used to treat retinal detachment.

- **玻璃体积血**在CT上表现为眼后节密度增高。

  玻璃体积血的原因包括外伤(包括幼童的虐待性头部外伤)、自发性玻璃体脱离和/或视网膜撕裂，以及各种引起视网膜新生血管的病变。

  眼-脑综合征(Terson综合征)是继发于颅内蛛网膜下腔出血相关的玻璃体积血(和/或视网膜出血)，可能与颅内压升高有关。

  类似玻璃体积血的非急性病变包括治疗视网膜脱离的眼内硅油。

Lens dislocation

- Rupture of the zonular fibers that attach the lens to the ciliary body can result in displacement of the lens posteriorly or, less commonly, anteriorly.
- In partial dislocations, the lens appears angled into the vitreous humor. In complete dislocations, the lens usually lies in the dependent portion of the vitreous.
- Trauma is the most common cause of lens dislocation. The most common nontraumatic cause of lens dislocation (ectopia lentis) is Marfan syndrome.

晶状体脱位

- 连接晶状体与睫状体的带状纤维断裂可导致晶状体向后脱位，或向前脱位但较少见。
- 部分脱位时，晶状体与玻璃体形成角度。完全脱位时，晶状体通常沉在玻璃体的下方。
- 外伤是晶状体脱位最常见的原因。最常见的非外伤性晶状体脱位(晶状体异位)的原因是马方综合征。

Retrobulbar hemorrhage

- Retrobulbar hemorrhage is an accumulation of blood in the soft tissues behind the globe, which is usually due to blunt orbital trauma.
- Traumatic retrobulbar hemorrhage is the most common cause of **orbital compartment syndrome**, which is a clinical diagnosis of elevated intraorbital pressure that impairs ocular perfusion. Soft tissue emphysema can also contribute to intraorbital pressure. Imaging may show proptosis, tenting of the posterior globe, and straightening of the optic nerve.

球后出血

- 球后出血是指血液在眼球后的软组织中积聚，通常是由于眼眶钝性创伤所致。
- 外伤性球后出血是引起**眶内压力增高综合征**最常见的病因，眶内压力增高综合征是一个临床诊断，表现为眼眶内压力升高而导致眼球灌注受损。软组织气肿也可加重眶内压力升高。影像学检查可表现为眼球突出、眼球后部隆起和视神经拉直。

Carotid-cavernous fistula

颈动脉海绵窦瘘

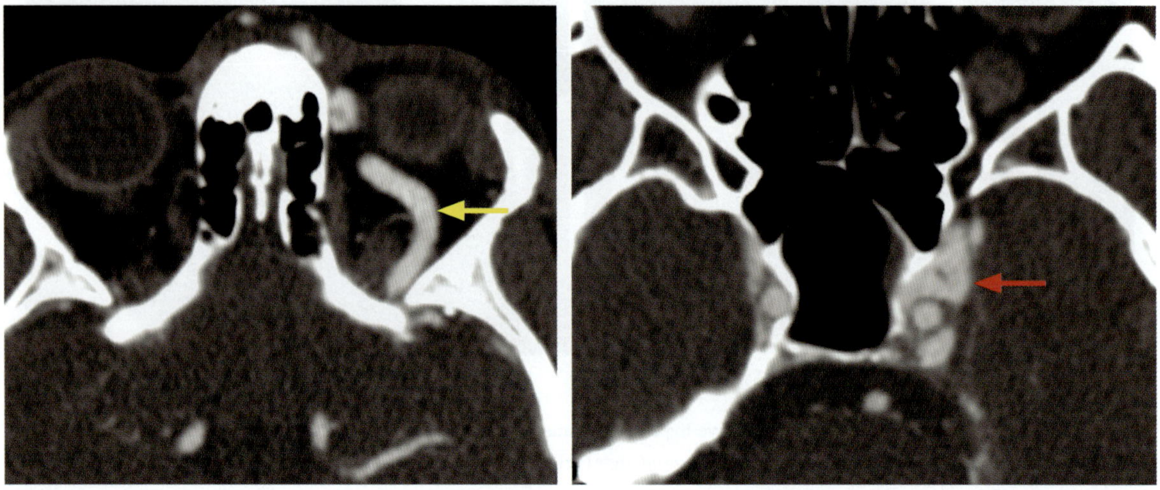

Left carotid-cavernous fistula:
Axial CT angiogram shows arterial phase filling of an enlarged left superior ophthalmic vein (left image, yellow arrow) and a distended left cavernous sinus (right image, red arrow).
左颈动脉海绵窦瘘：
轴位CT血管造影(左图)显示左侧眼上静脉(黄箭)在动脉期充盈，以及扩张的左侧海绵窦(红箭)。

- Carotid-cavernous fistulas are arteriovenous fistulas that connect the carotid tree to the cavernous sinus.
- **Direct**/high-flow fistulas (involving the cavernous internal carotid artery) are most common, usually due to trauma presenting acutely in young men. **Indirect** fistulas involve low-flow shunts from meningeal branches of the internal or external carotid arteries, presenting insidiously in postmenopausal women.
- Indirect clues on imaging are signs of orbital congestion like fat stranding, extraocular muscle enlargement, and proptosis. CTA shows asymmetric enlargement and early contrast enhancement of the cavernous sinus and superior ophthalmic vein.

- 颈动脉海绵窦瘘是颈动脉和海绵窦之间形成的动静脉瘘。
- **直接**/高流量瘘(累及海绵窦段颈内动脉)最常见，通常为急性外伤所致，年轻男性居多。**间接**瘘是颈内动脉或颈外动脉脑膜支的低流量分流，发生于绝经后妇女，起病隐匿。
- 影像学的间接征象为眼眶充血的征象，如脂肪密度异常、眼外肌增大和眼球突出。CTA显示海绵窦和眼上静脉不对称增大和早期强化。

(翻译　骆永恒)

FACE

面部

FACIAL FRACTURES

面部骨折

Overview

- Complex facial fractures are best described with respect to a handful of regional fracture patterns with attention to form and function rather than as a laundry list of bones or buttresses involved.

概述

- 复杂的面部骨折最好是从几个区域性骨折模式的角度进行描述，重点关注形态和功能，而不是简单列举所涉及的骨骼或支撑。

- Displacement,fragmentation, bone loss, as well as region-specific anatomic considerations are important descriptors that influence treatment strategy.
- A combination of multiplanar reformatted and 3D volume-rendered CT images are often helpful for diagnosis and surgical planning.
- A *panfacial fracture* involves all thirds of the face: frontal bone, midface, and mandible.

- 移位、碎裂、骨缺失，以及特定区域的解剖考量是影像报告的重要内容，这会影响到治疗决策。
- 结合CT多平面重建和三维立体投影通常有助于诊断和制订外科手术计划。
- *全颜面骨骨折*涉及所有三个面的骨骼：额骨、面中部和下颌骨。

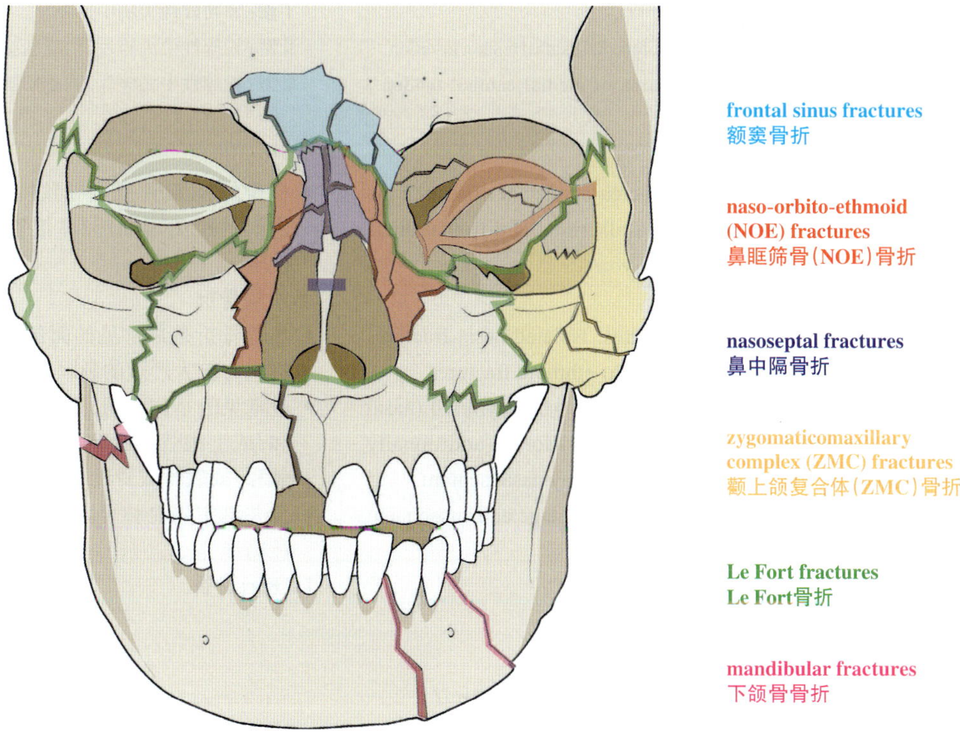

Frontal sinus fractures

- The management of frontal sinus fractures depends on the sites involved (anterior table, posterior table, and frontal recess), displacement, and comminution.
- Involvement of the posterior table (which occurs almost always in addition to anterior table fracture) confers risk of CSF leak and intracranial infection.
- Disruption of the frontal recess (frontonasal duct) confers risk of frontal sinus mucocele/mucopyocele development.

额窦骨折

- 如何处理额窦骨折取决于涉及的位置(前壁、后壁和额隐窝)、移位和粉碎情况。
- 后壁受累(通常总是合并前壁骨折)会造成脑脊液漏，增加颅内感染风险。
- 额隐窝(额鼻管)受损会增加额窦黏液囊肿/黏液脓肿的风险。

Orbital fractures

- Fractures of the orbital rims and/or walls are part of several midface fracture complexes discussed separately below: naso-orbito-ethmoid, zygomaticomaxillary complex, and Le Fort Ⅱ and Ⅲ.
- An **orbital blowout fracture** refers to a pure internal orbital fracture, which involves an orbital wall but spares the orbital rim, that expands the orbital volume. The most common types are orbital floor blowout, followed by medial orbital wall blowout.
- A **trapdoor fracture** is a special type of orbital floor blowout that usually occurs in children where the inferiorly displaced fracture fragment recoils and entraps herniated orbital soft tissue, which can cause restricted motility or necrosis of the inferior rectus muscle. Entrapment is a clinical diagnosis.
- Large orbital blowouts (e.g., >2 cm^2 defect area or >1.5 mL outward herniated volume) predict the development of noticeable enophthalmos after the acute swelling subsides.

眼眶骨折

- 眶缘和/或眶壁骨折是下面单独讨论的几种面中部骨折复合体的一部分：鼻-眶-筛骨、颧上颌复合体和Le Fort Ⅱ和Ⅲ型骨折。
- **眼眶爆裂性骨折**是指单纯的眶内骨折，累及面眶壁但不影响眶缘，从而使得眼眶体积增大。最常见的类型是眶底爆裂，其次是眶内壁爆裂。
- **活板门骨折**是一种特殊类型的眶底爆裂骨折，通常发生在儿童，其特征是向下移位的骨折碎片回缩并嵌顿疝出的眶内软组织，从而可能导致下直肌运动受限或坏死。嵌顿疝是一种临床诊断。
- 大的眼眶爆裂(例如，缺损区域>2cm^2或向外疝出的体积>1.5mL)预示在急性肿胀消退后会出现明显眼球内陷。

Naso-orbito-ethmoid fractures

- Naso-orbito-ethmoid (NOE) fractures involve the upper central midface, classically along 5 key edges: from the pyriform aperture across the lateral nasal wall, inferior orbital rim and floor, medial orbital wall, frontomaxillary suture, and nasomaxillary suture.
- NOE fractures are classified by the morphology of the central fragment where the medial canthal tendon inserts:

> **Type Ⅰ:** noncomminuted large central fragment.
> **Type Ⅱ:** comminuted central fragment not disrupting area of medial canthal tendon insertion.
> **Type Ⅲ:** comminuted central fragment disrupting area of medial canthal tendon insertion.

- Displaced NOE fractures can cause telecanthus (increased distance between the medial corners of the eyes) and obstruction of nasolacrimal and frontal sinus drainage pathways.

Nasoseptal fractures

- Nasal fractures are the most common facial fractures. Isolated nasal fractures should be distinguished from more serious naso-orbito-ethmoid fractures.
- Most commonly, lateral-oblique forces fracture the bony nasal pyramid (nasal bones and/or frontal processes of the maxillae). Frontal forces additionally involve the anterior nasal spine and/or cartilaginous or bony nasal septum.
- Associated septal hematoma can cause necrosis of the cartilage and subsequent saddle nose deformity.

Le Fort fractures

鼻眶筛骨(NOE)骨折

- 鼻眶筛骨(NOE)骨折累及面中部上方的中央，通常沿5个关键的边缘：从梨状孔穿过鼻外壁、眶下缘和眶底、眶内壁、额上颌缝和鼻上颌缝。
- NOE骨折根据内眦肌腱附着中央碎片的形态进行分类：

> **Ⅰ型：**非粉碎性大块中央碎片。
> **Ⅱ型：**粉碎性中央碎片，内眦肌腱附着区域完整。
> **Ⅲ型：**粉碎性中央碎片，内眦肌腱附着区域受损。

- 移位的NOE骨折可导致内眦距过宽(内眼角之间的距离增加)和鼻泪管和额窦引流通路梗阻。

鼻中隔骨折

- 鼻骨骨折是最常见的面部骨折。单纯鼻骨骨折应与较为严重的鼻眶筛骨骨折相鉴别。
- 最常见的是侧向斜力导致骨性鼻锥骨折(鼻骨和/或上颌骨的额突)。正面暴力还影响前鼻棘和/或软骨或骨性鼻中隔。
- 合并鼻中隔血肿可导致软骨坏死和随后的鞍鼻畸形。

Le Fort骨折

Le Fort I
Le Fort Ⅰ型

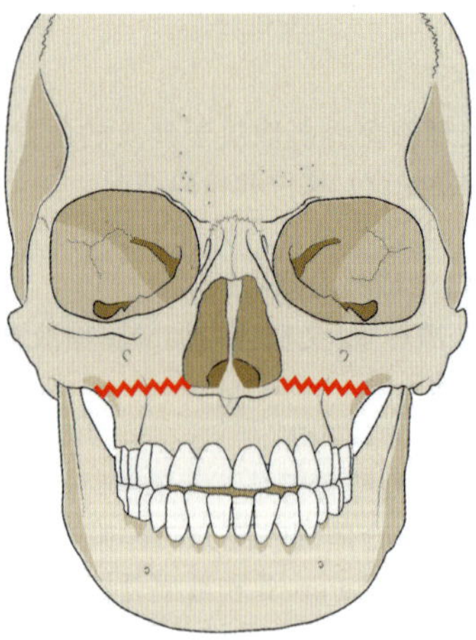

Fracture involves lateral margin of the pyriform (nasal) aperture. Allows free movement of the hard palate (loating palate).
骨折波及梨状(鼻)孔的侧缘。
硬腭(浮动腭)自由活动。

Le Fort II
Le Fort Ⅱ型

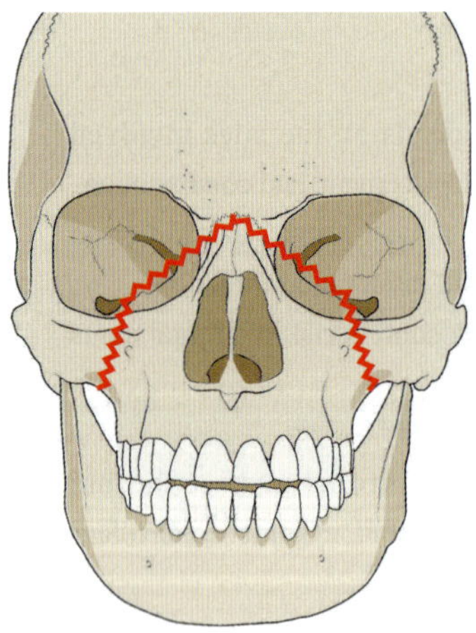

Pyramidal fracture, involves the inferior orbital rim, along with the orbital loor and medial orbital wall.
Allows free movement of the nose and hard palate (loating maxilla).
锥体型骨折，涉及眶下缘，以及眶底和眶内壁。
鼻子和硬腭(浮动上颌骨)自由活动。

Le Fort III
Le Fort Ⅲ型

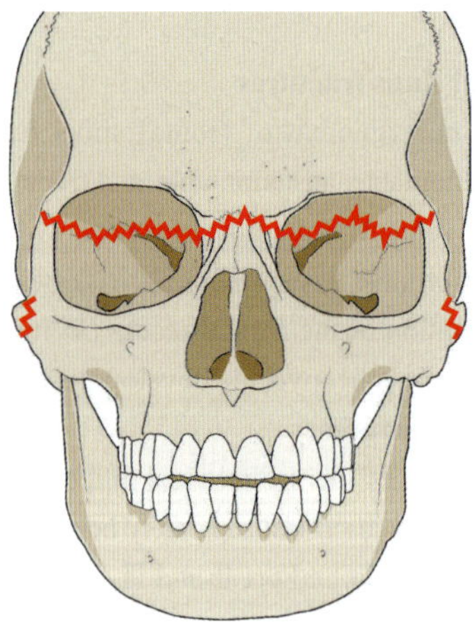

Fractures involve the zygomatic arch, along with the lateral and medial orbital walls.
Allows free movement of the entire midface (craniofacial dissociation).
骨折涉及颧弓及内、外侧眶壁。
整个中面部自由移动(颅面分离)。

- Le Fort midfacial fractures detach the involved maxillary occlusion-bearing segment (palate, alveolus, and maxillary teeth) from the skull base (pterygomaxillary disjunction).
- **All Le Fort fractures involve the pterygoid plates** of the sphenoid bone and maxillary sinus walls. Le Fort fractures are classified by the anterosuperior course of the fracture lines, which can occur alone or in combination on each side of the face (see illustration above).
- Displaced Le Fort fractures at any level can result in malocclusion or midfacial deformity. Associated palatal fractures are common and contribute to malocclusion.
- The non-occlusion-related components of the upper level Le Fort fractures can be treated as combinations of naso-orbito-ethmoid, zygomaticomaxillary complex, and/or orbital fractures. However, the reporting of Le Fort Ⅱ and Ⅲ fractures remains relevant as they are included among the Denver screening criteria for blunt cerebrovascular injury, which warrants CTA of the neck arteries and circle of Willis.

Zygomaticomaxillary complex fractures

- Le Fort面中部骨折将上颌的咬合段(腭、牙槽和上颌牙齿)与颅底(翼上颌分离)分离。
- **所有Le Fort骨折**均涉及蝶骨的**翼板**和上颌窦壁。Le Fort骨折线按前上走行方向分类，可以单独发生，也可以同时在面部的两侧发生(见上图)。
- 任何水平的Le Fort骨折移位都可能导致咬合不正或中面畸形。合并腭骨骨折很常见，并会导致咬合不正。
- 与上文Le Fort骨折的非咬合相关成分可以视为鼻眶筛骨、颧骨上颌复合体和/或眼眶骨折的组合进行处理。然而，报告Le Fort Ⅱ和Ⅲ骨折仍然至关重要。因为他们被纳入Denver筛查标准，用于评估钝性脑血管损伤，这需要进行颈动脉和基底动脉环的CTA。

颧上颌复合体骨折

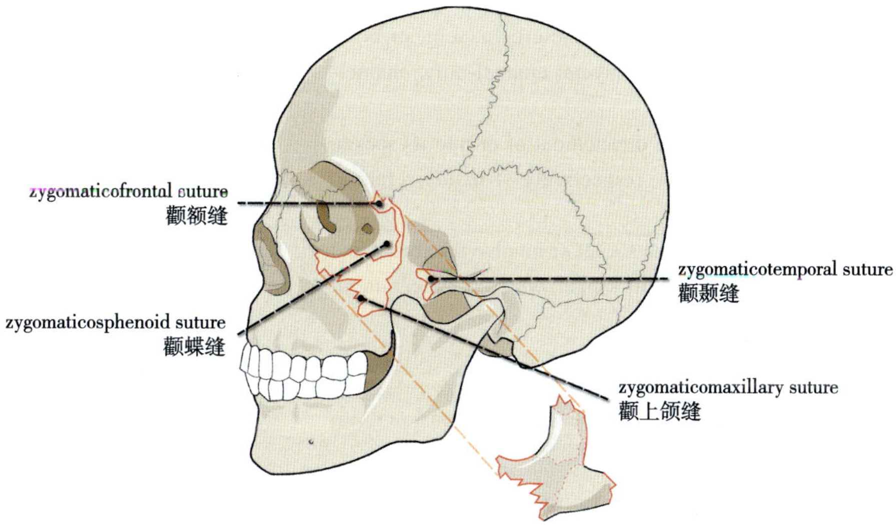

- A complete zygomaticomaxillary complex (ZMC) fracture liberates a tetrapod fragment via suture diastasis or fracture near the 4 articulations of the zygoma:

> **Zygomaticofrontal suture:** along lateral orbital rim.
> **Zygomaticomaxillary buttress:** from inferior orbital rim and floor through maxillary sinus walls.
> **Zygomaticotemporal suture:** along zygomatic arch.
> **Zygomaticosphenoid suture:** along lateral orbital wall.

- Also possible are incomplete fractures that involve an isolated limb of the ZMC, such as the zygomatic arch, lateral orbital rim/wall, or inferior orbital rim.
- The appearance of the zygomaticosphenoid suture (e.g., displacement, angulation, telescoping) is a sensitive landmark for evaluating overall ZMC alignment.
- Displacement or malalignment of ZMC fractures disrupt facial profile and width.
- Because the orbital floor is involved in classic ZMC fractures, they are sometimes called orbitozygomatic fractures. As with other internal orbital fractures, ZMC fractures with significant orbital volume expansion can cause late enophthalmos.

- 完全性颧上颌复合体(ZMC)骨折通过骨缝分离或4个颧骨关节附近骨折而将颧上颌复合体分为四个游离的碎片：

> **颧额缝**：沿眶外缘。
> **颧上颌支柱**：从眶下缘和底穿过上颌窦壁。
> **颧颞缝**：沿颧弓。
> **颧蝶缝**：沿眶外壁。

- 也可能出现不完全性骨折，只累及ZMC其中的一个支，例如颧弓、外侧眶缘/壁，或眶下缘。
- 颧蝶缝的外观(如位移、角度、伸缩)是评估整体ZMC对齐的敏感标志。
- ZMC骨折移位或对位不齐会破坏面部轮廓和宽度。
- 典型的ZMC骨折涉及眶底，因而有时被称为眶颧骨折。与其他眼眶内骨折一样，伴有明显眼眶体积增大的ZMC骨折可导致晚期眼球内陷。

Mandibular fractures

- Mandibular fractures are the second most common facial fractures and lead to malocclusion.
- Mandibular fractures are described by the anatomic segments involved: condylar process (further divided into head, neck, and base), coronoid process, ramus and angle, body (from third molar to canine), and parasymphysis/symphysis.
- Given its ring-like structure, mandibular fractures are more likely than not to occur at multiple sites.

  A **guardsman fracture** is the association of parasymphysealand bilateral condylar fractures of the mandible.
- Fractures that extend to the periodontal ligament space of an erupted tooth should be specially noted as they are managed as open (contaminated) fractures.
- Displaced or complex mandibular fractures, particularly those involving the condyles, are associated with increased risk of blunt vascular injury and therefore warrant a neck CTA.

Dentoalveolar trauma

- Tooth fractures are classified by involvement of the crown, root, or both. Crown fractures are categorized by involved layers: enamel-only, enamel-dentin, or enamel-dentin-pulp.
- Partial axial displacement of a tooth may be directed out of or into its socket, known as *extrusive* and *intrusive luxation*, respectively. *Avulsion* refers to complete displacement out of the socket.
- Fractures of the alveolar process can spare the socket or involve the socket and allow eccentric displacement of a tooth from its socket, which is called *lateral luxation*.

下颌骨骨折

- 下颌骨骨折是第二常见的面部骨折，会导致咬合不正。
- 下颌骨骨折按骨折的解剖节段进行描述：髁突(进一步分为头、颈和基底部)、冠突、支和角、体部(从第三磨牙到尖牙)和副联合/联合。
- 鉴于其环状结构，下颌骨骨折更可能发生在多个部位。

  “卫兵骨折”是指下颌骨的副联合骨折合并双侧髁突骨折。
- 骨折延伸至爆裂牙牙周韧带间隙应引起特别注意，因为这将被以开放性(污染)骨折进行处理。
- 移位或复合性下颌骨骨折，尤其是那些累及髁突的骨折，会增加钝性血管损伤的风险，因此需要进行颈部CTA检查。

牙槽外伤

- 牙齿骨折根据牙冠、牙根或两者的受累情况进行分类。牙冠骨折按累及的牙冠层进一步可分类为：仅釉质、釉质-牙本质，以及釉质-牙本质-牙髓。
- 牙齿部分轴向位移可能直接从牙槽脱出或嵌入槽内，分别称为*挤出性脱位*和*嵌入性脱位*。*撕脱*是指牙齿完全脱离牙槽窝。
- 牙槽突骨折时，牙槽窝可以完整或受累，牙齿可以偏离牙槽窝的中心，此为*侧向脱位*。

(翻译　管婧)

SALIVARY GLANDS

OVERVIEW AND ANATOMY OF THE SALIVARY GLANDS

Overview

- The major salivary glands are, in order of decreasing size, the parotid, submandibular, and sublingual glands.
- There are also numerous unnamed minor salivary glands throughout the mucosa of the head and neck, especially the palate.
- Neoplasms in smaller glands are more likely to be malignant, with the risk highest in sublingual and minor salivary glands, followed by the submandibular gland, and least in the parotid gland.

Parotid glands

- The parotid glands are divided by the facial nerve into superficial and deep lobes. Since the facial nerve is not normally visible on imaging, radiologists use the retromandibular vein as the demarcation.
- The deep lobe extends through the stylomandibular tunnel into the prestyloid parapharyngeal space, discussed later in this chapter.
- The inferior projection of the superficial lobe overlying the angle of the mandible is called the parotid tail.
- The parotid glands are the only salivary glands to contain internallymph nodes, mostly located in the superficial lobe along the retromandibular vein.

唾液腺

唾液腺概述与解剖

概述

- 大唾液腺按照其大小依次为腮腺、下颌下腺和舌下腺。
- 还有许多未命名的小唾液腺分布在头颈部的黏膜，尤其是上腭。
- 恶性肿瘤更容易发生在较小的腺体，舌下腺和小唾液腺发生恶性肿瘤的风险最高，其次是下颌下腺，而腮腺最低。

腮腺

- 腮腺按面神经走行分为浅叶和深叶。但影像通常不能显示面神经，放射科医生采用下颌后静脉作为分界线。
- 腮腺深叶通过茎突下颌管延伸至茎突前咽旁间隙，本章稍后讨论。
- 腮腺浅叶下方覆盖在下颌角上的部分称为腮腺尾。
- 腮腺是唯一内含淋巴结的唾液腺，主要分布于浅叶，沿下颌后静脉走行。

- Accessory parotid glands may be located along the parotid duct, which is also called **Stensen duct**, superficial to the masseter muscle.

Submandibular gland

- The submandibular glands sit partly in the floor of the mouth (sublingual space) and mostly in the neck (submandibular space). Each gland wraps around the posterior margin of the mylohyoid muscle, which separates the floor of the mouth from the neck.
- The gland may remodel the adjacent inner surface of the angle of the mandible, causing a normal variant depression called a *Stafne bone cavity/cyst*.
- The submandibular duct, which is also called **Wharton duct**, opens on the side of the frenulum of the tongue.

Sublingual gland

- The sublingual glands sit at the anterior aspect of the floor of the mouth.
- Although normally confined to the sublingual space, the gland may herniate into the submandibular space through a normal variant discontinuity in the mylohyoid muscle called a *mylohyoid boutonnière*.
- The sublingual glands drain via numerous small ducts, collectively termed **Rivinus ducts**, which may form a larger common duct, the **Bartholin duct**, that empties into the Wharton duct.

BENIGN SALIVARY NEOPLASM

Pleomorphic adenoma

- 副腮腺可位于腮腺导管(又称**Stensen管**),位于咬肌表面。

下颌下腺

- 下颌下腺部分位于口腔的底部(舌下间隙),但大部分位于颈部(下颌下间隙)。每个腺体包绕下颌舌骨肌的后缘,后者将口底与颈部分隔开来。
- 下颌下腺可能会重塑邻近的下颌骨角的内表面,导致出现一个正常的变异性凹陷,称为静止性骨腔/骨囊肿(Stafne骨腔/骨囊肿)。
- 下颌下腺导管(又称**Wharton管**)开口于舌系带一侧。

舌下腺

- 舌下腺位于口底的前部。
- 尽管舌下腺通常局限于舌下间隙,但可通过下颌舌骨肌不连续的正常变异疝入下颌下间隙,下颌舌骨肌的这种变异被称为扣眼状缺损(*mylohyoid boutonnière*)。
- 舌下腺通过许多小导管引流,这些小导管统称为**舌下腺小管**,可形成一个更大的总导管,即**舌下腺大管**,并流入下颌下腺导管。

唾液腺良性肿瘤

多形性腺瘤

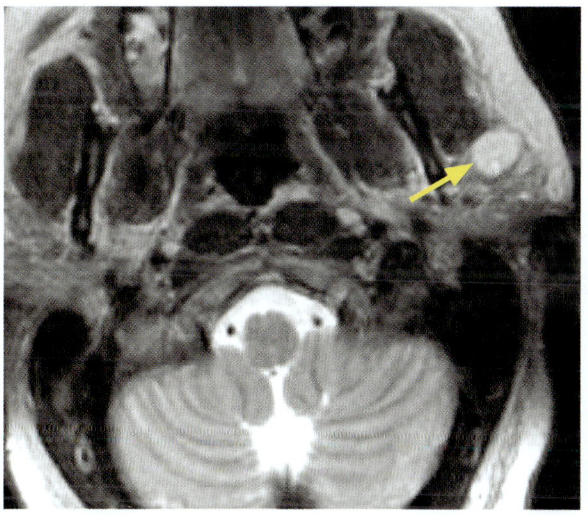
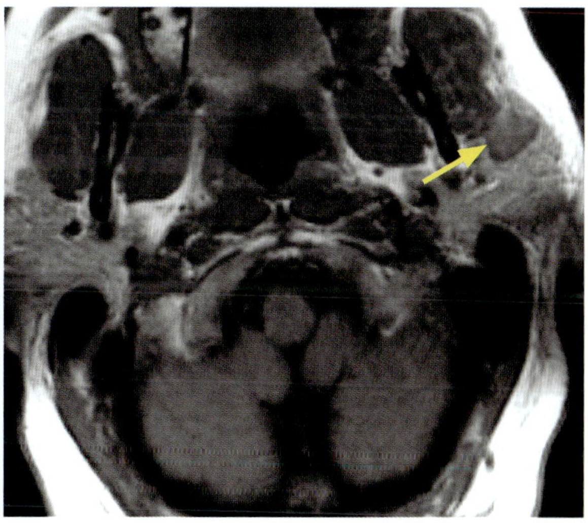
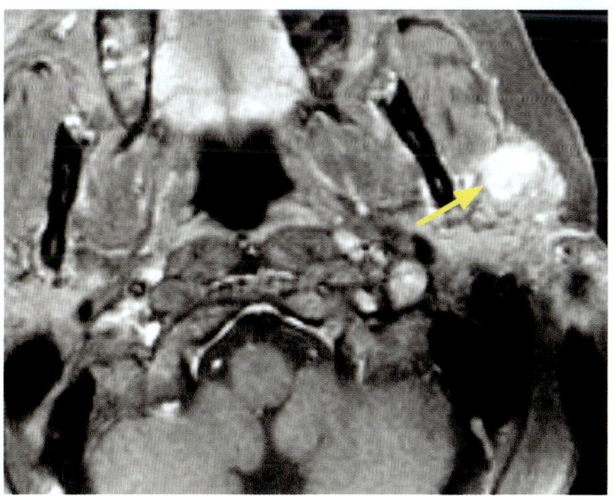

Pleomorphic adenoma: Axial T2-weighted (top left image), T1-weighted (top right image),and post-contrast fat saturated T1-weighted (bottom left image) MRI shows a T2 hyperintense, T1 hypointense, enhancing circumscribed mass (arrows) in the anterior aspect of the superficial left parotid.

Case courtesy Mary Beth Cunnane, MD, Massachusetts Eye and Ear Infirmary.

多形性腺瘤:轴位T_2加权(左上图)、T_1加权(右上图)和增强脂肪饱和T_1加权(左下图)MRI显示左侧腮腺浅叶前部肿块,T_2呈高信号,T_1呈低信号,增强可见强化,边界清楚(黄箭)。

- Pleomorphic adenoma, also called **benign mixed tumor**, is the most common salivary gland tumor, accounting for 70% of all salivary tumors, and is most common in the parotid gland.
- The typical patient is a middle-aged female.
- MRI shows a well-defined mass with bosselated margins (small undulations), very high signal intensity on T2-weighted images, and strong contrast enhancement. Large pleomorphic adenomas can have heterogeneous signal.
- Although pleomorphic adenoma is benign, there is risk of malignant transformation. The standard treatment for parotid pleomorphic adenoma is superficial parotidectomy.

- 多形性腺瘤，又称**良性混合瘤**，是最常见的唾液腺肿瘤，占所有唾液腺肿瘤的70%，在腮腺最常见。
- 最常见于中年女性。
- MRI上显示边界清晰的肿块，边缘呈锯齿状（小波浪状），T_2加权图像上呈显著高信号，对比增强强化明显。体积大的多形性腺瘤信号可以不均匀。
- 尽管多形性腺瘤是良性肿瘤，但也存在恶变的风险。腮腺多形性腺瘤的标准治疗方法是腮腺浅叶切除术。

Warthin tumor

- Warthin tumor, also called papillary cystadenoma lymphomatosum or adenolymphoma, is the second most common benign parotid neoplasm.
- The typical patient is an elderly male. The vast majority are smokers.
- Imaging shows a well-defined but heterogeneous mass in the parotid gland with weak contrast enhancement and, in a significant minority of cases, complicated cystic components.
- Multifocality or bilaterality accounts for up to 20% of cases of Warthin tumors, making them the most common multifocal or bilateral parotid neoplasms. They have a predilection for the parotid tail region.
- Compared to pleomorphic adenoma, malignant transformation of Warthin tumor is rare.

沃辛瘤

- 沃辛瘤，又称乳头状淋巴囊腺瘤或腺淋巴瘤，是第二常见的腮腺良性肿瘤。
- 最常见于老年男性。绝大多数是吸烟者。
- 影像学检查显示腮腺内有一边界清晰但不均质的肿块，强化较弱，少数病例合并有复杂的囊性成分。
- 多发或双侧沃辛瘤中多达20%是最常见的多灶性或双侧腮腺肿瘤，好发于腮腺尾部区域。
- 与多形性腺瘤相比，沃辛瘤罕见有恶变。

Malignant Parotid Neoplasm

Mucoepidermoid carcinoma

- Mucoepidermoid carcinomas are the most common primary salivary gland malignancy, especially in the parotid gland.
- Low-grade mucoepidermoid carcinoma typically appears as a well-defined, enhancing mass that is hyperintense on T2-weighted images. This appearance is indistinguishable from benign pleomorphic adenoma on MRI.
- High-grade mucoepidermoid carcinoma has infiltrative margins and lower signal on T2-weighted images.

腮腺恶性肿瘤

黏液表皮样癌

- 黏液表皮样癌是最常见的原发性唾液腺恶性肿瘤，尤其是在腮腺。
- 典型的低级别黏液表皮样癌表现为T_2加权高信号、边界清晰、强化的肿块。这种表现在MRI上无法与良性多形性腺瘤相鉴别。
- 高级别黏液表皮样癌有边缘浸润，在T_2加权上呈较低信号。

Adenoid cystic carcinoma

腺样囊性癌

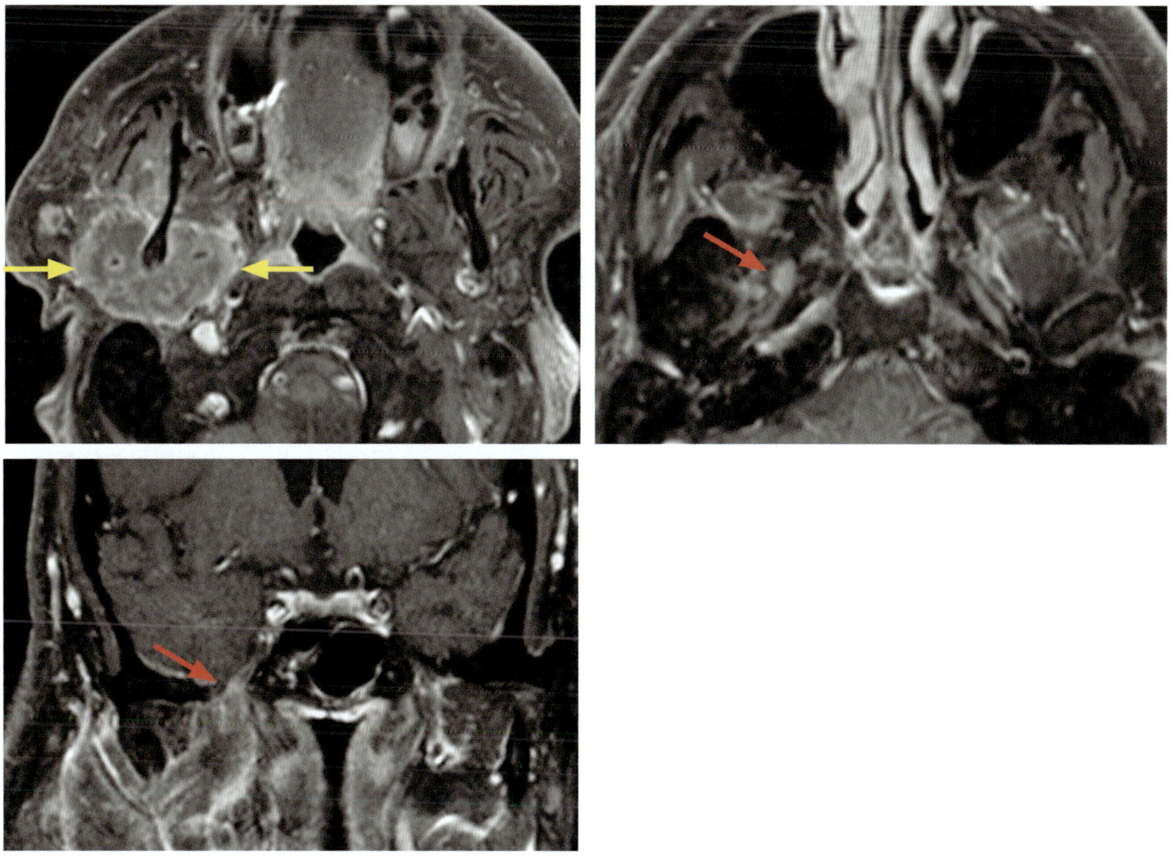

Adenoid cystic carcinoma with perineural spread:
Axial post-contrast T1-weighted MRI demonstrates (top left image) a heterogeneously enhancing right parotid mass involving the superficial and deep lobes (yellow arrows).
Axial (top right image) and coronal (bottom left image) post-contrast T1-weighted MRI through the skull base shows asymmetric enlargement and enhancement of the V_3 division of the right trigeminal nerve and associated enlargement of the right foramen ovale (red arrows), consistent with perineural tumor spread.
腺样囊性癌伴神经周围扩散：轴位增强T_1加权MRI(左上图)显示右侧腮腺不均匀强化的肿块，累及浅叶和深叶(黄箭)。
经颅底轴位(右上图)和冠状位(左下图)增强T_1加权MRI显示右侧三叉神经V_3支不对称增大和增强，并伴有右侧卵圆孔增大(红箭)，符合肿瘤神经周围扩散。

- Adenoid cystic carcinomas are the most common primary malignancy of the submandibular, sublingual, and minor salivary glands. They are also the second most common primary parotid gland malignancy.
- Among head and neck malignancies, adenoid cystic carcinoma has the highest risk of perineural spread, which portends a poor prognosis. However, the most common histology of head and neck cancers to show perineural spread is squamous cell carcinoma.
- Adenoid cystic carcinoma has a high risk of local recurrence and metastasis.

Carcinoma ex pleomorphic adenoma

- Pleomorphic adenoma can undergo malignant transformation to so-called carcinoma ex pleomorphic adenoma. The risk accumulates over many years.
- The typical patient is an elderly person with a long-standing parotid mass that is newly associated with rapid enlargement, pain, or facial nerve palsy.
- In contrast to pleomorphic adenoma, carcinoma ex pleomorphic adenoma is hypointense on T2-weighted images and shows low ADC values. The malignancy is infiltrative, showing ill-defined borders and possible extension beyond the gland parenchyma.

- 腺样囊性癌是下颌下腺、舌下腺和小涎腺最常见的原发性恶性肿瘤，也是第二常见的原发性腮腺恶性肿瘤。
- 在头颈部恶性肿瘤中，腺样囊性癌的神经周围扩散风险最高，提示预后不良。然而，最常表现出神经周围扩散的头颈部肿瘤的组织学类型是SCC。
- 腺样囊性癌具有较高的局部复发和转移风险。

癌在多形性腺瘤中

- 多形性腺瘤可恶变为癌，被称为“多形性腺瘤癌”。这种风险是经过多年累积的。
- 典型的患者是长期有腮腺肿块的老年患者，近期伴有肿块快速增大、疼痛或面神经麻痹。
- 与良性多形性腺瘤相比，癌在多形性腺瘤中在T_2加权呈低信号，ADC值降低。恶性肿瘤呈浸润性，边界不清，可延伸到腺体实质以外。

Metastases

- Metastases to the parotid nodes (both within the gland and surrounding it) most commonly occur from cutaneous malignancies on the lateral side of the head, usually squamous cell carcinoma.
- On imaging, a round parotid mass larger than 6 mm, sometimes with central necrosis or ill- defined margins, is suggestive of nodal metastasis in patients with a history of scalp or face skin cancer or concurrent cervical nodal metastases from other primary tumors.

Lymphoma

- Salivary gland lymphomas are rare. Most are non-Hodgkin B-cell lymphomas, particularly extranodal marginal zone B-cell lymphoma of mucosa-associated lymphoid tissue (MALT lymphoma).
- Sjögren syndrome is a strong risk factor, although most instances of salivary gland lymphoma are not associated. Any new dominant parotid mass in the setting of Sjögren syndrome should raise concern for lymphoma.

转移

- 腮腺淋巴结(腺体内及其周围)转移最常源自头部侧面的皮肤恶性肿瘤,通常为SCC。
- 在影像学上,若患者已知有头皮或面部皮肤癌病史或同时有其他肿瘤的颈部淋巴结转移,如发现腮腺内有一个>6mm的圆形肿块,或伴有中央坏死或边界不清,提示为淋巴结转移。

淋巴瘤

- 唾液腺淋巴瘤很罕见。大多数是非霍奇金B细胞淋巴瘤,尤其是黏膜相关淋巴组织的结外边缘区B细胞淋巴瘤(MALT淋巴瘤)。
- 干燥综合征是淋巴瘤的高风险因素,尽管大多数唾液腺淋巴瘤的病例与此无关。任何干燥综合征患者一旦出现腮腺肿块都应该怀疑有淋巴瘤的可能。

Inflammatory salivary disease

Sialadenitis and sialolithiasis

- Sialolithiasis (stones within salivary ducts or glands) is the most common cause of acute unifocal sialadenitis, due to obstruction of the drainage and resultant gland inflammation.
- The vast majority of salivary calculi and, in turn, cases of sialadenitis, occur in the submandibular gland and duct, due to its relatively viscous secretions and uphill drainage course.
- Suppurative (acute bacterial) sialadenitis can occur without sialolithiasis, predominantly involving the parotid gland in elderly patients, often in the setting of recent surgery, intubation, dehydration, or poor oral hygiene.
- The most common causes of multifocal/bilateral sialadenitis in children are juvenile recurrent parotitis (chronic parotitis) and mumps viral parotitis.

Iodine-related sialadenopathy

- **Radioiodine sialadenitis** is a common, dose-dependent side effect of iodine-131 therapy for thyroid cancer. Patients have transient salivary gland swelling and pain with decreased salivary flow.
- **Iodidesialadenitis**, also known as iodide mumps, is a rare, idiosyncratic, non-allergic adverse reaction to iodinated contrast media administration. Patients have self-limited painless salivary gland swelling minutes to days after contrast-enhanced CT or angiography.

HIV-related benign lymphoepithelial lesions

炎性唾液腺病变

涎腺炎和涎石病

- 涎腺结石(涎腺导管或腺体内的结石)是最常见的急性单一涎腺炎的原因,结石导致引流受阻而引起炎症。
- 绝大多数涎腺结石及其引发的涎腺炎发生在下颌下腺及其导管中,这是由于其分泌物相对黏稠且引流导管呈上升走行。
- 化脓性(急性细菌性)涎腺炎可在无涎腺结石的情况下发生,主要见于老年患者的腮腺,通常发生在近期手术、插管、脱水或口腔卫生不洁。
- 最常见的儿童多灶性/双侧涎腺炎原因是青少年复发性腮腺炎(慢性腮腺炎)和病毒性腮腺炎。

碘相关性涎腺病

- **放射性碘涎腺炎**是^{131}碘治疗甲状腺癌常见的剂量依赖性副作用。患者有一过性的涎腺肿胀和疼痛,随后唾液减少。
- **碘涎腺炎,**也被称为碘源性涎腺炎,是一种接受碘对比剂后罕见的、特异的、非过敏性不良反应。患者在增强CT或血管造影检查后数分钟至数天内出现自限性无痛性涎腺肿胀。

HIV相关的良性淋巴上皮病变

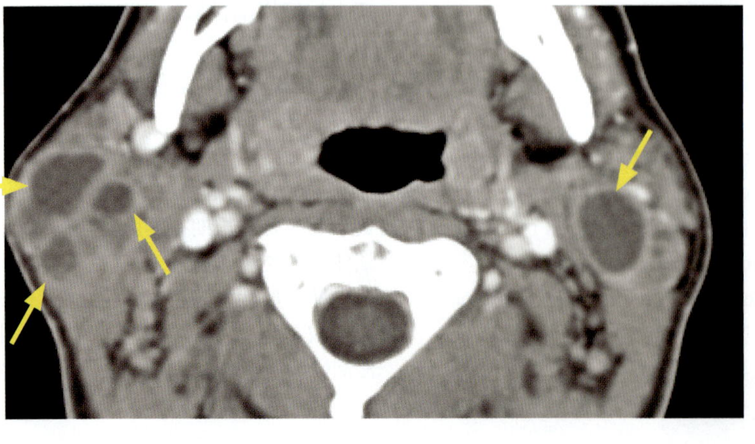

HIV lymphoepithelial lesions: Axial contrast-enhanced CT through the parotid glands shows numerous peripherally enhancing cystic lesions bilaterally (arrows).

Case courtesy Mary Beth Cunnane, MD, Massachusetts Eye and Ear Infirmary.

HIV淋巴上皮病变:经腮腺轴位增强CT显示双侧腮腺内多发边缘强化的囊性病灶(黄箭)。

- HIV infection is frequently associated with benign lymphoepithelial lesions, which are mixed solid and cystic masses representing reactive lymphoid infiltration that causes proliferation of ductal epithelium with cystic change.
- Benign lymphoepithelial lesions almost always involve the parotid gland. They are the most common parotid lesions in patients with HIV infection. Concurrent cervical lymphadenopathy is an additional clue on imaging for HIV infection.

- HIV感染常与良性淋巴上皮病变相关，这些病变表现为实性和囊性混合肿块，为反应性淋巴浸润，引起导管上皮增生并伴有囊性改变。
- 良性淋巴上皮病变几乎总是累及腮腺，是HIV感染患者最常见的腮腺病变。影像上同时存在颈部淋巴结肿大是HIV感染的附加依据。

Sarcoidosis

- Sarcoidosis occasionally involves the parotid glands with granulomatous inflammation, typically presenting as bilateral painless gland swelling.
- **Heerfordt syndrome**, or uveoparotid fever, is the rare but pathognomonic presentation of sarcoidosis as bilateral uveitis, parotitis, and facial nerve palsy.
- The *panda sign* of sarcoidosis is the finding on the obsolete gallium-67 scan of radiotracer uptake in bilateral lacrimal and parotid glands, superimposed on physiologic nasopharyngeal uptake.

结节病

- 结节病偶尔累及腮腺，引起肉芽肿性炎症，典型表现为双侧无痛性腺体肿大。
- 葡萄膜腮腺炎(或称**Heerfordt综合征**)是结节病的罕见但具有特征性的表现，表现为双侧葡萄膜炎、腮腺炎和面神经麻痹。
- 结节病的熊猫征是通过已经被淘汰的放射性示踪剂[67]镓在双侧泪腺和腮腺中摄取发现，与生理性的鼻咽摄取相叠加。

Sjögren syndrome

干燥综合征

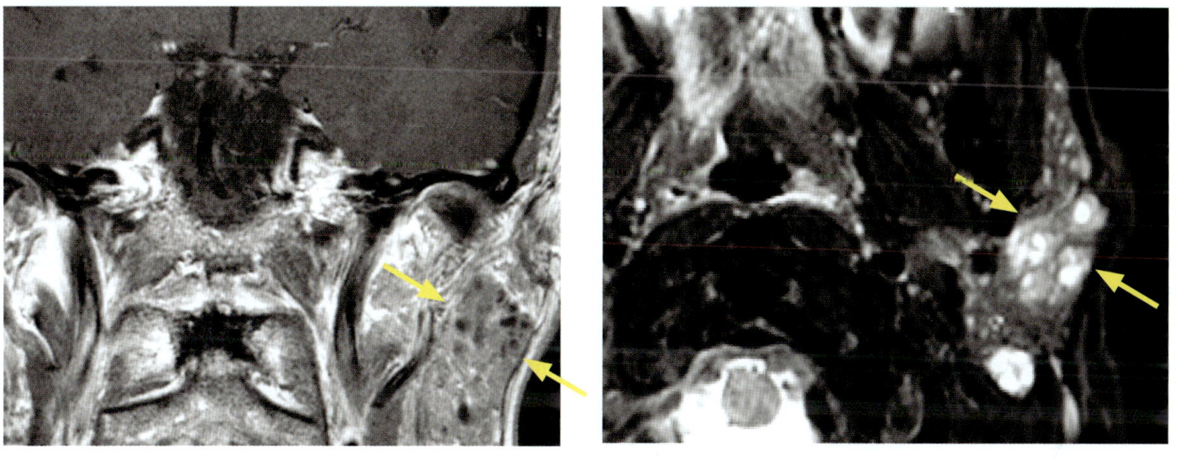

Sjögren syndrome: Coronal post-contrast T1-weighted (left image) and axial T2-weighted MRI with fat suppression shows numerous small, T2 hyperintense lesions in the left parotid (arrows), which demonstrate minimal peripheral enhancement.

Case courtesy Mary Beth Cunnane, MD, Massachusetts Eye and Ear Infirmary.

干燥综合征：冠状位增强T_1加权(左图)和轴位T_2加权MRI脂肪抑制(右图)显示左侧腮腺内多发小灶T_2加权高信号(黄箭)，有微弱的边缘强化。

- Sjögren syndrome is an autoimmune disorder affecting the salivary and lacrimal glands.
- The typical patient is a middle-aged female. The disorder can be either primary or secondary to another autoimmune disorder (most commonly rheumatoid arthritis or systemic lupus erythematosus).
- MRI shows a *salt-and-pepper* or *honeycomb* appearance of bilateral parotid glands: multiple areas of high signal intensity mixed with discrete areas of low signal intensity on both T1- and T2-weighted images, which represent a combination of benignlymphoepithelial lesions (also known as lymphoepithelial sialadenitis) with fibrosis, punctate calcifications, and fatty infiltration.

- 干燥综合征是一种累及涎腺和泪腺的自身免疫性疾病。
- 典型病例为中年女性。该病可以是原发，也可以继发于另一种自身免疫性疾病(最常见的是类风湿关节炎或系统性红斑狼疮)。
- MRI显示双侧腮腺呈椒盐征或蜂窝状：在T_1和T_2加权图像上均表现为多个高信号区域与散在的低信号区域混合，代表良性淋巴上皮病变(也称为淋巴上皮性涎腺炎)合并纤维化、点状钙化和脂肪浸润。

IgG4-related disease

- IgG4-related disease is a multisystem fibroinflammatory disorder, which can involve the submandibular and, less often, parotid glands.
- **Mikulicz syndrome** refers to diffuse IgG4-related chronic sclerosing sialadenitis and dacryoadenitis.

IgG4相关疾病

- **IgG4相关疾病**是一种多系统纤维炎症性疾病，可累及下颌下腺，但较少累及腮腺。
- **米库利兹综合征**是指弥漫性IgG4相关的慢性硬化性涎腺炎和泪腺炎。

- **Küttner tumor** is a term for focal IgG4-related chronic sclerosing sialadenitis involving the submandibular gland.

- **慢性硬化性涎腺炎**是指与IgG4相关的累及下颌下腺的局灶性慢性硬化性涎腺炎。

MISCELLANEOUS SALIVARY LESIONS

其他唾液腺病变

First branchialcleft cyst (BCC)

第一鳃裂囊肿(BCC)

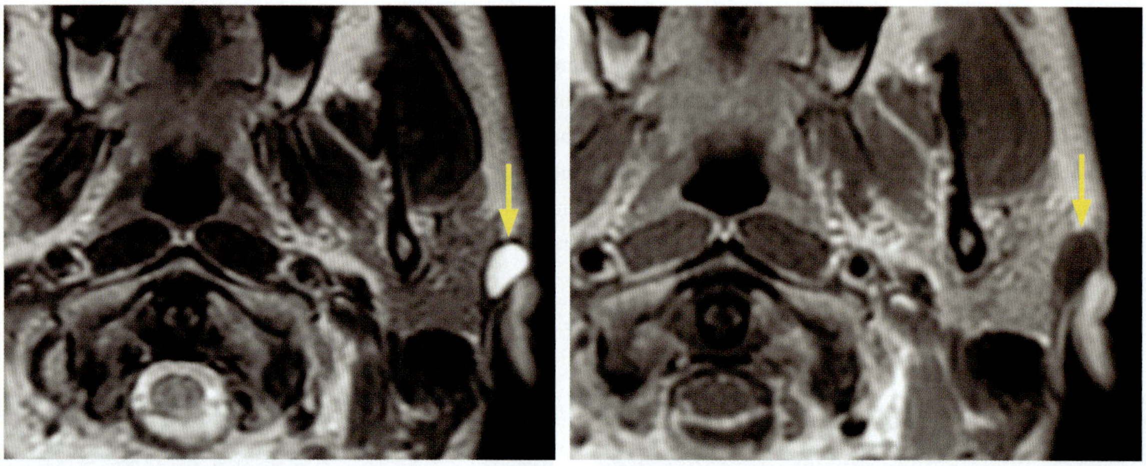

Axial T2-weighted (left image) and T1 post-contrast MRI shows a left infra-auricular cystic lesion (arrows) along the superficial margin of the left parotid gland, thought to represent a first brachial cleft cyst.
MRI轴位T_2加权(左图)和增强T_1加权显示左侧耳廓下一囊性病变(黄箭),并沿左侧腮腺的表面走行,此为第一鳃裂囊肿。

- Branchial apparatus (pouch or cleft) remnants include cysts, as well as sinuses and fistulas.
- Branchialcleft cysts are most common and usually appear as a simple cyst. However, superinfection or hemorrhage can cause internal debris or wall thickening.
- First branchialcleft cysts are located between the external auditory canal and the submandibular region, most frequently within the parotid gland.

- 鳃器(袋或裂)残余包括囊肿、窦道和瘘管。
- 鳃裂囊肿为最常见的,通常表现为一个单纯性囊肿。然而,合并感染或出血可造成内部碎屑或囊壁增厚。
- 第一鳃裂囊肿位于外耳道(EAC)和下颌下区之间,最常位于腮腺内。

Sialocele

唾液腺囊肿

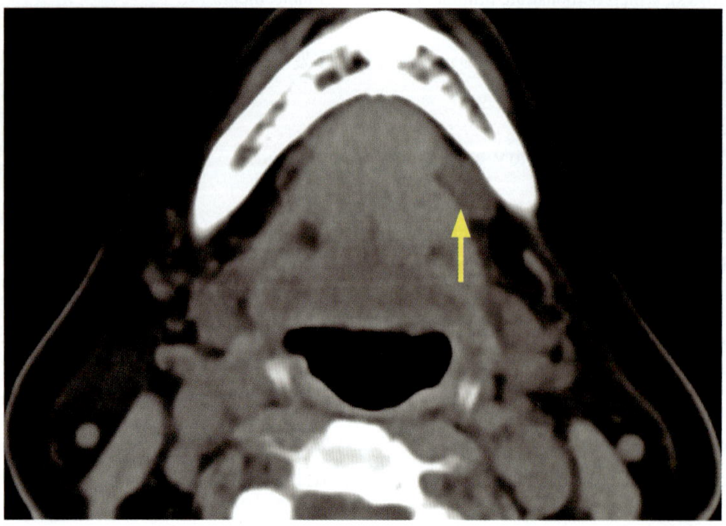

Axial contrast-enhanced CT shows an ovoid fluid-density lesion (arrow) in the left sublingual space, adjacent to the sublingual gland, thought to represent a sialocele.
轴位增强CT显示左侧舌下间隙有一个卵圆形液体密度病变(黄箭),紧邻舌下腺,为涎腺囊肿。

- Sialoceles are focal pseudocysts of saliva due to gland/duct disruption, such as due to postobstructive rupture, trauma, or surgery.
- Sialoceles are most commonly related to the parotid gland.

- 唾液腺囊肿是由于腺体/导管破裂后引起的局灶性含有唾液的假性囊肿,见于阻塞后破裂、创伤或手术。
- 涎腺囊肿最常见于腮腺。

Sialadenosis

- Sialadenosis refers to chronic diffuse enlargement of the major salivary glands (typically the parotid) due to acinar hypertrophy.
- The major risk factors are nutritional and hormonal disturbances, such as diabetes mellitus, alcohol use disorder, and eating disorders.

CENTRAL SKULL BASE AND SELLA

OVERVIEW AND ANATOMY OF THE SELLAR AND PARASELLAR REGIONS

Sellar and parasellar region

- The **sella turcica** is a saddle-shaped depression of the sphenoid bone, which creates the space for the pituitary gland.
- The anterior wall of the pituitary fossa is the tuberculum sellae. The posterior wallis the dorsum sellae. The roof is the diaphragma sellae, a dural reflection.
- The parasellar region includes the cavernous sinuses, suprasellar cistern, and hypothalamus.

Pituitary gland

- The pituitary is composed of an anterior and a posterior lobe.
- The **anterior pituitary** (adenohypophysis) produces and secretes the following hormones: growth hormone (GH), prolactin, follicle-stimulating hormone (FSH),luteinizing hormone (LH), adrenocorticotrophic hormone (ACTH), and thyroid-stimulating hormone (TSH). The anterior pituitary gland is formed from **Rathke pouch**, which is a superior invagination of primitive oral ectoderm.

  Rathke pouch normally involutes. Sometimes, a cleft can be left behind, which may give rise to craniopharyngioma or Rathke cleft cyst.
- The **posterior pituitary** (neurohypophysis) and **infundibulum** (pituitary stalk) are the projection from the hypothalamus that transports and secretes antidiuretic hormone (ADH), vasopressin) and oxytocin. The posterior pituitary gland is formed from neuroectoderm.

  The normal posterior pituitary is hyperintense on T1-weighted MRI due to stored ADH and is called the **posterior pituitary bright spot**, best seen on sagittal images. Loss of the posterior pituitary bright spot has been associated with central diabetes insipidus but also occurs in some normal patients.

  The posterior pituitary normally descends from the diencephalon. Sometimes, the downward extension is halted, resulting in an **ectopic posterior pituitary**, usually at the median eminence (inferior aspect of the hypothalamus).

  The combination of ectopic posterior pituitary with an absent or hypoplastic infundibulum and anterior pituitary is known as **pituitary stalk interruption (transection) syndrome**.

唾液腺良性肥大

- 唾液腺良性肥大是指由于腺泡增生导致大唾液腺(通常是腮腺)慢性弥漫性增大。
- 主要危险因素是营养和激素紊乱,如糖尿病、酗酒和饮食障碍。

（翻译　赵添）

颅中窝底和鞍区

蝶鞍和鞍旁区概述与解剖

蝶鞍和鞍旁区

- **蝶鞍**是蝶骨的一个鞍状凹陷,其内容纳垂体。
- 垂体窝前壁为鞍结节,后壁为鞍背,顶部为鞍膈(由硬脑膜反折而成)。
- 鞍旁区包括海绵窦、鞍上池和下丘脑。

垂体

- 垂体包括前叶和后叶。
- **垂体前叶**(腺垂体)可产生和分泌多种激素:生长激素(GH)、催乳素(PRL)、促卵泡激素(FSH)、黄体生成素(LH)、促肾上腺皮质激素(ACTH)和促甲状腺激素(TSH)。垂体前叶起源于原始口腔顶端的凹陷,即**颅颊囊(拉特克囊)**。

  正常情况下的颅颊囊随胚胎发育而逐渐退化。在部分情况下,退化不完全可残留一个裂隙,由此可发生颅咽管瘤或颅颊裂囊肿。
- **垂体后叶**(神经垂体)和**漏斗**(垂体柄)是下丘脑的一个凸起,其作用是运输或分泌抗利尿激素(ADH,又称血管升压素)和催产素。垂体后叶起源于神经外胚层。

  正常垂体后叶在T_1加权MRI上呈高信号,为储存ADH所致,被称为**"垂体后叶亮点"**,矢状位图像显示最佳。垂体后叶亮点消失与中枢性尿崩症有关,但也可见于部分正常人。

  垂体后叶通常从间脑下降。有时,下降中断而导致**异位垂体后叶**,通常位于正中隆起(下丘脑的下侧)。

  异位垂体后叶合并垂体漏斗及垂体前叶缺失或发育不全被称为**垂体柄阻断(横断)综合征**。

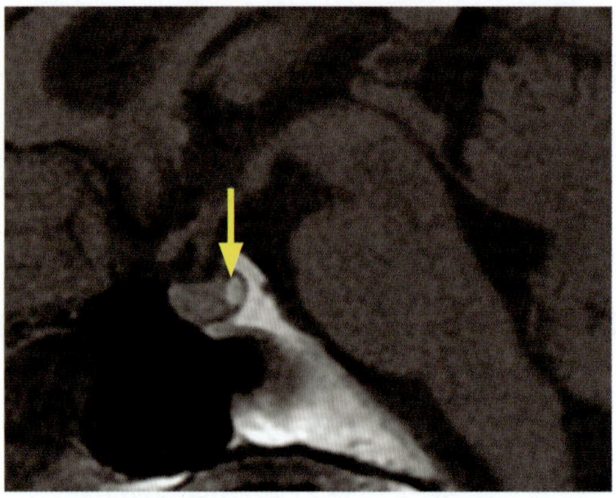

Normal posterior pituitary bright spot (arrow) on sagittal T1-weighted MRI.
矢状位T_1加权MRI显示正常垂体后叶亮点(黄箭)。

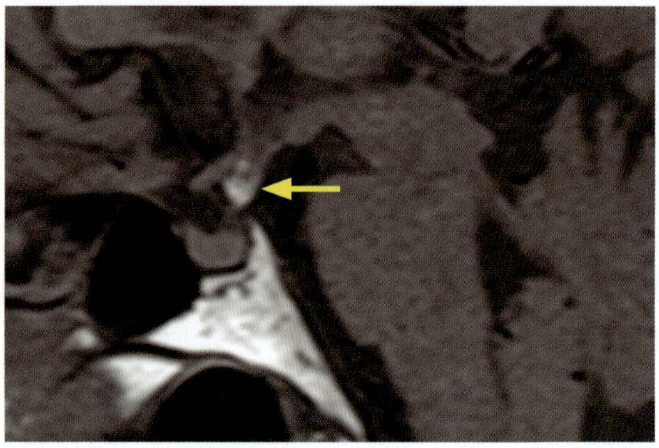

Sagittal T1-weighted MRI shows absence of the normal posterior pituitary bright spot and an intrinsically T1 hyperintense nodule within the infundibulum (arrow), likely an ectopic posterior pituitary.
矢状位T_1加权MRI显示正常垂体后叶亮点缺失，漏斗部可见T_1高信号结节(黄箭)，提示异位垂体后叶。

- The pituitary gland enhances on dynamic contrast-enhanced MRI in accordance with its blood supply: first the infundibulum and posterior pituitary, followed by the anterior pituitary, which is supplied by the hypophyseal portal system. The entire gland enhances homogeneously between 30–60 seconds and then washes out.

- 垂体在动态增强MRI的强化顺序与其血供一致：首先是漏斗部和垂体后叶，接着是垂体前叶(因其血供来自垂体门静脉系统)。整个腺体在30~60秒呈均匀强化，随后造影剂排空。

Cavernous sinus

海绵窦

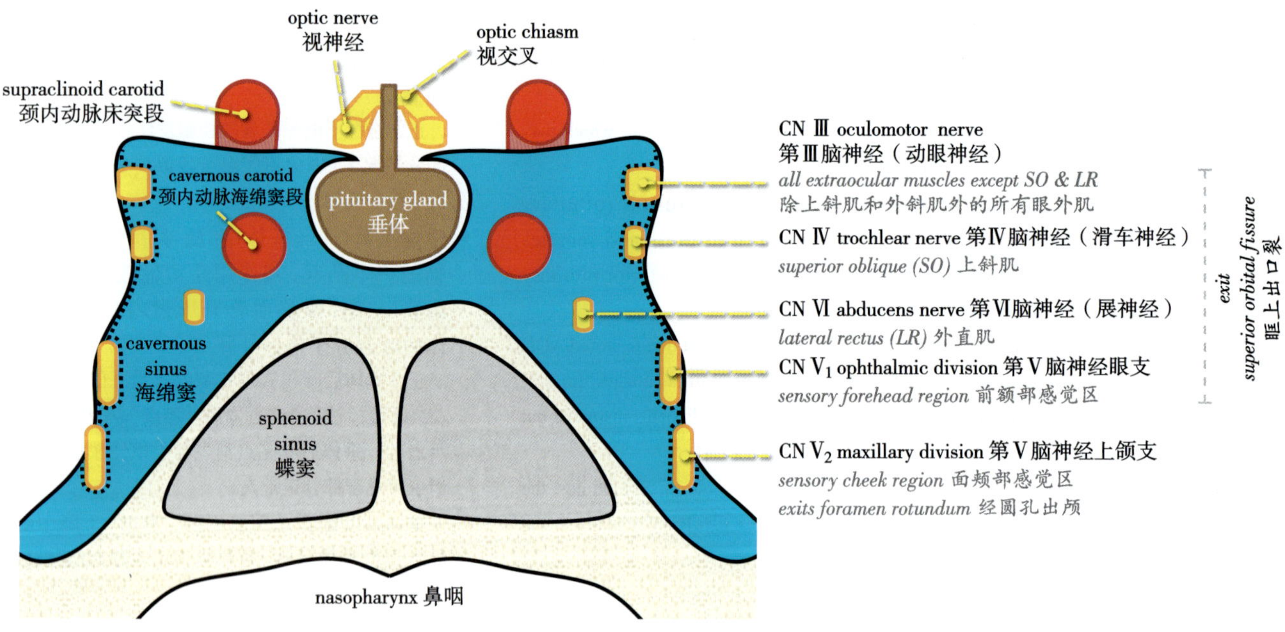

CN Ⅵ and sympathetic ibers around the carotid artery are located within the center of the cavernous sinus, while the other cranial nerves travel within the cavernous sinus wall.

The mandibular nerve (V_3) is the only segment of the trigeminal nerve that does not traverse the cavernous sinus. It exits inferiorly from Meckel's cave through foramen ovale.

The abducens nerve (Ⅵ) enters the petrous portion of the temporal bone through Dorello's canal and is the only nerve that travels in the medial venous sinusoids.

The maxillary nerve (V_2) is the only nerve of the cavernous sinus that does not exit the superior orbital issure. Instead, it exits foramen rotundum.

展神经(CN Ⅵ)和颈内动脉周围的交感纤维走行于海绵窦的中央区域，而其他脑神经则在海绵窦壁内穿行。

下颌支(V_3)是三叉神经唯一不穿过海绵窦的分支。它从梅克尔腔向下经卵圆孔出颅。

展神经(Ⅵ)经由颞骨外展神经管(Dorello管)进入颞骨岩部，是唯一走行于海绵窦内侧腔的神经。

三叉神经上颌支(V_2)是海绵窦内唯一不经眶上裂出颅的神经，其通过圆孔出颅。

- The cavernous sinuses are paired dural venous sinuses of the middle cranial fossae on either side of the sella turcica, connected by the variable intercavernous sinuses.
- The cavernous sinus drains the (superior and inferior) ophthalmic veins and sphenoparietal sinus.

  The cavernous sinus is the most frequently involved dural sinus with infection and thrombosis (septic thrombophlebitis). Infection may spread from the central face ("danger zone"), paranasal sinuses, teeth, or orbits (discussed previously in the orbital infection section).
- The cavernous sinus drains via the superior and inferior petrosal sinuses to the sigmoid sinus and jugular bulb, respectively. There are also connections to the pterygoid venous plexus and basilar (clival) plexus.

  Inferior petrosal sinus sampling (via the internal jugular vein) is performed to demonstrate pituitary ACTH hypersecretion in cases of suspected Cushing disease.
- The internal carotid artery traverses the cavernous sinus. Rupture results in a direct caroticocavernous fistula (discussed previously in the ocular trauma section).
- The cavernous sinus contains cranial nerves Ⅲ, Ⅳ, Ⅵ, V_1, and V_2, and sympathetic fibers. CN Ⅵ and sympathetics around the carotid artery are located within the center of the sinus, while the other cranial nerves course between two dural layers *within* the lateral wall.
- The lateral wall of the cavernous sinus is normally concave or straight. Outward bulging suggests involvement with a lesion, whether neoplastic, vascular, or inflammatory.
- **Cavernous sinus syndrome** consists of clinical signs and symptoms attributable to cavernous sinus pathology, particularly neurologic deficits (ophthalmoplegia, facial sensory loss, Horner syndrome) and orbital/ocular congestion (chemosis, proptosis). Pain/headache may be present, especially in inflammatory disorders such as Tolosa-Hunt syndrome.

- 海绵窦是颅中窝成对的硬脑膜静脉窦，位于蝶鞍两侧，相互之间由多个的海绵间窦进行交通。
- 海绵窦引流(上、下)眼静脉和蝶顶窦。

  海绵窦是最常发生感染和血栓(脓毒性血栓性静脉炎)的硬脑膜窦。感染源可来自中央面部("危险三角区")、鼻旁窦、牙齿或眼眶(详见眼眶感染部分)。
- 海绵窦分别通过岩上窦和岩下窦引流至乙状窦和颈静脉球。另外还与翼静脉丛和基底(斜坡)丛相沟通。

  对于怀疑库欣病的患者，可(通过颈内静脉)进行岩下窦取样，以明确是否存在垂体促肾上腺皮质激素分泌过多。
- 颈内动脉穿行于海绵窦。颈内动脉破裂可导致直接型颈动脉-海绵窦瘘(详见眼外伤部分)。
- 海绵窦内有第Ⅲ、Ⅳ、Ⅵ、V_1和V_2脑神经及交感神经纤维。展神经和颈内动脉周围的交感神经走行于海绵窦的中心区域，而其他脑神经则穿行于海绵窦外侧壁的*两层*硬脑膜之间。
- 正常情况下的海绵窦外侧壁是内凹或平直的。向外膨出提示海绵窦肿瘤、血管性或炎症性病变。
- **海绵窦综合征**是指由海绵窦病变导致的一系列相关的临床症状和体征，尤其是神经功能障碍(眼肌麻痹、面部感觉丧失、霍纳综合征)、眼眶/眼部充血(结膜水肿、眼球突出)。可伴疼痛/头痛，尤其是炎性疾病，如痛性眼肌麻痹综合征等。

Suprasellar cistern

- The suprasellar cistern is the pentagonal basal cistern located above the sella, under the hypothalamus, between the unci of the temporal lobes, and anterior to the interpeduncular cistern.

  Supratentorial mass effect with uncal herniation effaces the suprasellar cistern from the side(s).

  Spontaneous intracranial hypotension reduces the height of the suprasellar cistern.
- Multiple important neurovascular structures traverse the suprasellar cistern: Optic nerves and chiasm, infundibulum, and circle of Willis.

鞍上池

- 鞍上池是一个五角形的基底池，位于蝶鞍上方、下丘脑下方、颞叶钩回之间、脚间池的前方。

  当幕上肿块的占位效应造成钩回疝时，鞍上池从一侧受压变窄或消失。

  自发性低颅压患者，鞍上池高度减低。
- 多个重要的神经、血管穿行于鞍上池，如视神经和视交叉、垂体漏斗、基底动脉环。

Pituitary adenoma

垂体腺瘤

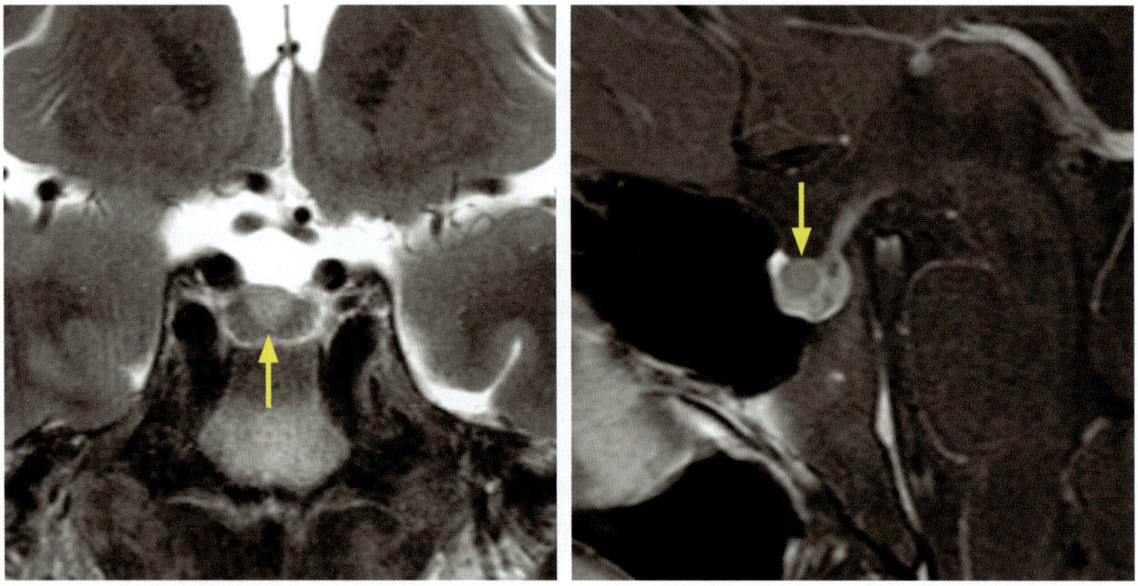

Microadenoma: Coronal T2-weighted (left image) and sagittal T1 post-contrast MRI (right image) shows a subcentimeter T2 hyperintense, hypoenhancing lesion in the central pituitary gland (arrows).

微腺瘤：冠状位T_2加权(左图)和矢状位T_1增强(右图)MRI显示垂体中央区域一个亚厘米级的T_2高信号、低强化病变(黄箭)。

- Adenomas are by far the most common intrinsic pituitary mass but can have suprasellar extension when large.
- Adenomas are classified by size as **micro**adenomas (<10mm) or **macro**adenomas (≥10mm). They are also classified by hormonal production, with the most common being lactotroph and nonfunctioning adenomas.
- Patients present with symptoms of endocrine dysfunction (hypogonadism, acromegaly, Cushing disease, or hyperthyroidism) or, in the case of macroadenomas, mass effect (visual field deficits due to optic pathway compression, headache).

  Rarely, patients present with **pituitary apoplexy**, a clinical syndrome of severe headache, visual impairment, and hypopituitarism caused by sudden hemorrhage into the pituitary. The typical cause is pituitary adenoma.

  Sheehan syndrome refers to pituitary apoplexy in postpartum women associated with hypopituitarism. In the acute phase, imaging shows an enlarged pituitary gland possibly with high intrinsic T1 signal due to hemorrhage. Over time, the pituitary atrophies, leaving a partially empty sella.
- Most cases are sporadic but syndromic causes include multiple endocrine neoplasia type 1 (MEN1).
- Microadenomas usually appear on MRI as foci of subtle signal abnormality within the gland on conventional sequences, but contrast-enhanced sequences improve sensitivity. Most microadenomas show delayed enhancement relative to the normal pituitary, which appears hypoenhancing based on the timing of most post-contrast protocols. Dynamic imaging with early and delayed phases is needed to detect a small subset of microadenomas.

- 垂体腺瘤是最为常见的起源于垂体本身的肿块，当增大时可向鞍上区延伸。
- 垂体腺瘤根据瘤体的大小分为微腺瘤(<10mm)或大腺瘤(≥10mm)，也可以根据肿瘤分泌的激素进行分类，最常见的是催乳素腺瘤和无功能腺瘤。
- 患者在临床表现为内分泌功能障碍(包括性功能减退、肢端肥大症、库欣病及甲状腺功能亢进等)，或在大腺瘤患者可出现占位效应(视路受压导致视野缺损、头痛等)。

  极少数情况下可出现**垂体卒中**，为突发垂体内出血导致的临床综合征，包括严重头痛、视觉障碍和垂体功能减退等一系列症状。最常见的原因是垂体腺瘤。

  希恩综合征是指产后妇女发生垂体卒中导致垂体功能低下。急性期，影像学显示垂体增大，T_1影像上因出血而可能出现高信号。随着时间的推移，垂体萎缩，形成部分空泡蝶鞍。
- 大部分垂体腺瘤为散发，少数属于临床综合征的一部分，如多发性内分泌瘤病1型(MEN 1)。
- 微腺瘤在MRI平扫序列仅表现为腺垂体内出现局灶性轻微信号异常，增强序列可以提高灵敏度。大多数微腺瘤相对于正常垂体强化延迟，而在大多数按增强时间设定的增强扫描方案中则呈低强化。检测较小的微腺瘤，需要进行包含早期及延迟期的动态增强扫描。

- As adenomas are typically slow-growing, macroadenomas enlarge and remodel the sella.
- Pituitary macroadenomas can invade the cavernous sinus and encase the internal carotid artery. High risk of invasion is predicted on preoperative coronal MR images when the tumor extends laterally beyond the tangent line connecting the lateral walls of the supraclinoid and cavernous internal carotid artery segments. Complete encasement of the internal carotid artery certainly indicates cavernous sinus invasion but this sign occurs late.
- As adenomas are typically soft, the diaphragma sellae can indent macroadenomas that extend into the suprasellar cistern, creating the *snowman sign* (also known as a *figure-of-8*, *dumbbell*, *hourglass*, or *bottleneck* configuration). They tend not to narrow the internal carotid artery (whereas meningiomas or metastases can narrow the carotid).
- Macroadenomas can be heterogeneous due to cystic change, necrosis, or hemorrhage. Hemorrhagic pituitary adenoma is the most common sellar region lesion with intrinsic T1 hyperintensity, especially with a fluid level.

- 由于垂体腺瘤通常生长缓慢，大腺瘤会增大并重塑蝶鞍。
- 垂体大腺瘤可侵犯海绵窦并包绕颈内动脉。术前冠状位MRI可用于预测高侵袭风险，即肿瘤向外侧延伸超过连接床突上段和海绵窦段颈内动脉侧壁的切线。颈内动脉完全被包绕表明海绵窦受侵，但该征象一般发生较晚。
- 由于腺瘤通常质地较软，大腺瘤向鞍上池延伸时，受到鞍膈压迫导致凹陷，形成雪人征(也称8字征、哑铃征、沙漏征或瓶颈征)。大腺瘤往往不会造成颈内动脉狭窄(而脑膜瘤或转移瘤则会导致颈内动脉狭窄)。
- 大腺瘤可因囊变、坏死或出血而表现为信号不均。出血性垂体腺瘤是最常见的鞍区T_1高信号病变，特别是伴有液平面时。

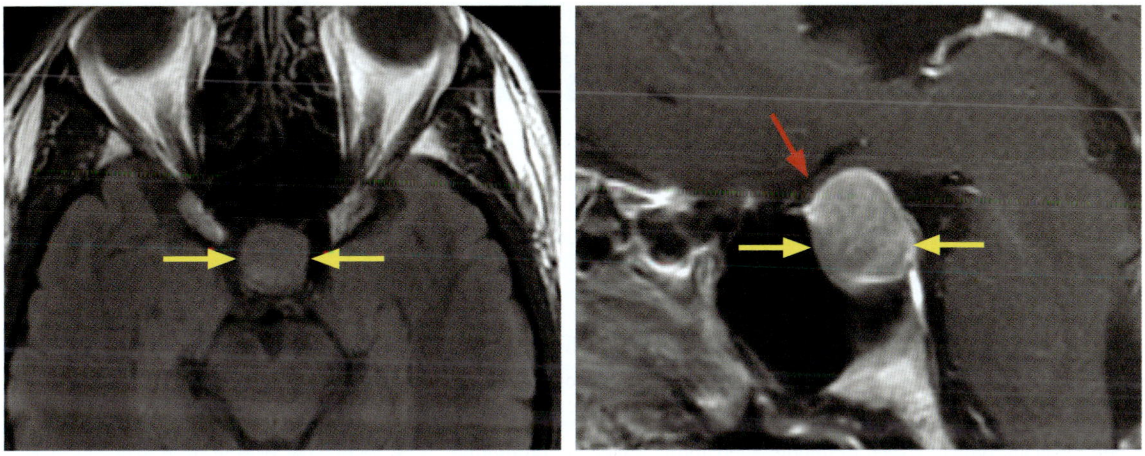

Macroadenoma: FLAIR (left image) and post-contrast sagittal T1-weighted MRI shows complete replacement of the pituitary gland by an enhancing mass (yellow arrows). The optic chiasm is displaced superiorly (red arrow).

垂体大腺瘤：FLAIR(左图)和增强矢状位T_1加权(右图)MRI显示垂体完全被强化的肿块所取代(黄箭)，视交叉受压向上移位(红箭)。

Pituitary hyperplasia

- The normal pituitary varies widely in size depending on age, sex, and hormonal status.
- Physiologic pituitary hyperplasia commonly occurs in periods of hormonal activity like adolescence, pregnancy, and perimenopause.
- Pathological pituitary hyperplasia is usually related to end-organ insufficiency, especially primary hypothyroidism.
- On imaging, pituitary hyperplasia appears as a homogeneously enlarged gland with a convex superior margin.

Hypophysitis

- Hypophysitis refers to inflammatory infiltration of the pituitary gland and sometimes also infundibulum. It is classified by histology, with lymphocytic being most common, followed by granulomatous and plasmacytic.
- Lymphocytic hypophysitis usually occurs in women, typically in the peripartum period. It is also a side effect of checkpoint inhibitor immunotherapy (e.g., ipilimumaband nivolumab).
- Granulomatous hypophysitis can beidiopathic or secondary to systemic

垂体增生

- 正常垂体的大小因年龄、性别和激素水平不同而有所差异。
- 生理性垂体增生通常发生在激素变化期，如青春期、妊娠期和围绝经期。
- 病理性垂体增生通常与靶器官功能低下有关，原发性甲状腺功能减退尤为典型。
- 影像学上，垂体增生表现为垂体均匀增大，上缘隆起。

垂体炎

- 垂体炎是指垂体的炎症浸润，有时也见于漏斗部。垂体炎按组织学分类，淋巴细胞性最常见，肉芽肿性和浆细胞性次之。
- 淋巴细胞性垂体炎多发生于女性，通常在围产期。有些免疫抑制剂(如伊匹单抗和纳武单抗)也可能诱发。
- 肉芽肿性垂体炎可特发或继发于全身性疾病，

disorders such as sarcoidosis or granulomatosis with polyangiitis (Wegener's).

- Plasmacytic hypophysitis is a rare IgG4-related disease.
- MRI shows diffuse enlargement of the pituitary gland, and often the infundibulum, with homogeneous enhancement.

如结节病、肉芽肿性血管炎(韦格纳肉芽肿病)。

- 浆细胞性垂体炎是罕见的IgG4相关性疾病。
- MRI表现为垂体弥漫性增大，常常为漏斗部，增强均匀。

Rathke cleft cyst

颅颊裂囊肿

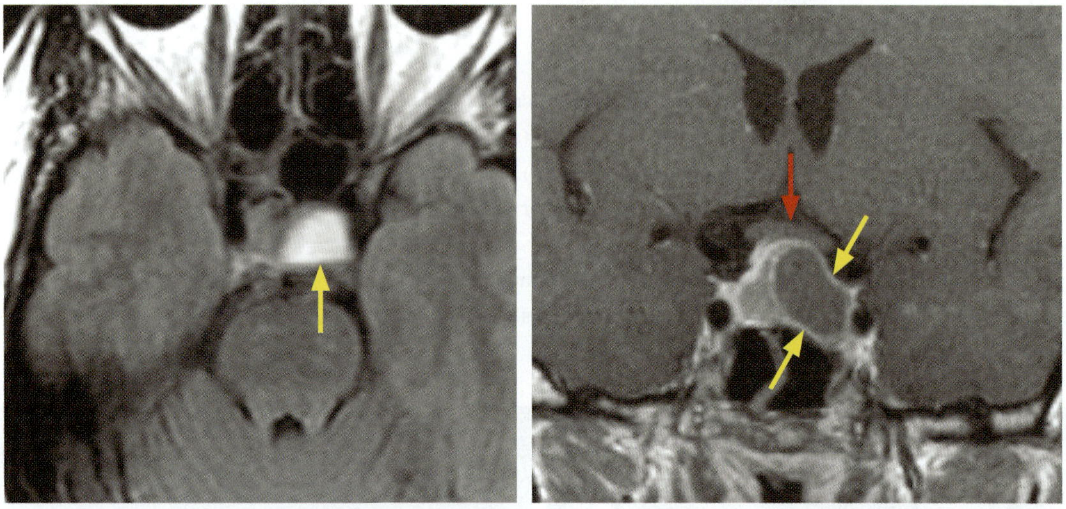

Rathke's cleft cyst: Axial FLAIR (left image) and coronal post-contrast T1-weighted MRI shows a FLAIR hyperintense, T1 hypointense parasellar mass (yellow arrows). The mass demonstrates faint peripheral rim enhancement. The pituitary is displaced to the right and the optic chiasm is displaced superiorly (red arrow).

颅颊裂囊肿：轴位FLAIR(左图)和冠状位增强T_1加权(右图)MRI显示鞍旁FLAIR高信号、T_1低信号的肿块(黄箭)。肿块边缘轻微强化。垂体向右移位，视交叉向上推移(红箭)。

- Rathke cleft cyst is a remnant of the embryologic Rathke pouch lined with simple columnar or cuboidal epithelium. They are typically intrasellar with or without suprasellar extension.
- Rathke cleft cysts are typically seen in middle-aged adults, twice as commonly in females.
- Rathke cleft cyst is reportedly very common in autopsy studies (up to 22% incidence), but clinically is usually asymptomatic or discovered incidentally.
- On imaging, Rathke cleft cyst is a nonenhancing cyst without calcification. An enhancing rim may be seen related to the pituitary tissue wrapped around the cyst (*claw sign*). A small, nonenhancing intracystic nodule, likely a clump of mucin, is pathognomonic.
- The MR signal characteristics depend on the protein content of the cyst fluid. The intra-cystic fluid may be isointense to CSF iflow protein and hyperintense on T1-weighted images if high protein. High protein content may cause incomplete nulling of the intracystic fluid on FLAIR.

- 颅颊裂囊肿是胚胎时期颅颊囊的残余，内衬简单柱状或立方上皮。通常位于鞍内，不确定是否向鞍上延伸。
- 颅颊裂囊肿多见于中年人，女性发生率为男性的2倍。
- 尸检报告中颅颊裂囊肿很常见(发生率高达22%)，但临床上通常为无症状或为偶然发现。
- 影像学上，颅颊裂囊肿表现为无强化的囊性病灶，不伴钙化。围绕囊肿的边缘相对于垂体组织稍呈增强(爪征)。囊内若出现一个小而无强化的小结节则具有病理诊断的意义，可能是成团的黏蛋白。
- 颅颊裂囊肿的MR信号特点取决于囊液中的蛋白含量。若囊液蛋白含量低，其信号可能与脑脊液相同；若囊液蛋白含量增高，在T_1加权图像上表现为高信号。高含量蛋白可能导致囊内液体信号在FLAIR图像上不被完全抑制。

Empty sella

- The (partially) empty sella is mostly filled with CSF and possibly slightly enlarged, due to herniation of the subarachnoid space (sometimes known as intrasellar arachnoidocele). The small pituitary gland is flattened against the floor of the sella.
- The *infundibulum sign*, in which the pituitary stalk traverses this space, distinguishes empty sella from true cystic intrasellarlesions.
- Primary empty sella can be a normal variant, especially in older patients, related to insufficiency of the diaphragma sellae, or be caused by intracranial

空泡蝶鞍

- 空泡蝶鞍(部分)大部分被脑脊液充填并可能有轻度扩大，这是由于蛛网膜下腔疝入垂体窝的结果(也称为鞍内蛛网膜膨出)。小垂体变扁并紧贴鞍底。
- "漏斗征"是垂体柄穿过空泡蝶鞍，这是空泡蝶鞍与鞍内囊性病变的鉴别要点。
- 原发性空泡蝶鞍可以是正常变异，尤其在老年人，可能与鞍膈发育不全有关，或由颅内高

hypertension.

- Empty sella is one of a constellation of findings in **idiopathic intracranial hypertension (pseudotumor cerebri)**, which is a syndrome attributed to elevated CSF pressure in the absence of intracranial mass or hydrocephalus.

  Patients with idiopathic intracranial hypertension, who are typically female and obese, present with headache, transient visual obscurations, and/or pulsatiletinnitus.

  The main imaging findings are empty sella, papilledema/posteriorscleral flattening, optic nerve sheath dilation, bilateral transverse sinus stenosis, cerebellar tonsillar ectopia, and meningoceles of Meckel's cave or petrous apex.

- Secondary empty sella is related to prior pituitary disease. Gland shrinkage may reflect sequela of treated pituitary tumors, pituitary apoplexy, Sheehan syndrome, or trauma.

压导致。

- 空泡蝶鞍也可以是**特发性颅内高压(假性脑瘤)**系列表现之一。特发性颅内高压是指不明原因的脑脊液压力升高引起的一系列临床综合征,无颅内肿块或脑积水。

  特发性高颅压多见于女性和肥胖患者,临床表现为头痛、短暂性视觉障碍和/或搏动性耳鸣。

  主要影像学表现是空泡蝶鞍、视神经乳头水肿/后巩膜变平、视神经鞘扩张、双侧横窦细小、小脑扁桃体下垂、梅克尔腔或岩尖部脑膜膨出。

- 继发性空泡蝶鞍与既往垂体疾病有关。腺体萎缩可能是垂体肿瘤治疗后、垂体卒中、希恩综合征及外伤等的后遗症。

Suprasellar / Parasellar Mass

Overview

- The differential diagnosis for a parasellar/suprasellar lesion is broad, but the imaging findings together with the patient's age and clinical presentation can usually narrow the differential diagnosis to a few entities.
- The MOuSTACHE mnemonic may be helpful to remember the spectrum of parasellar/ suprasellar lesions, albeit not in order of prevalence:

  Meningioma/**M**etastasis.

  Optic pathway glioma.

  Sellarlesion with suprasellar/parasellar extension (e.g., macroadenoma).

  Teratoma and other germ cell tumors (e.g., germinoma).

  Aneurysm.

  Craniopharyngioma.

  Hypothalamic glioma or hamartoma.

  Epidermoid/dermoid cyst.

- In adults, the most common suprasellar neoplasm is pituitary macroadenoma that has extended superiorly. The second most common suprasellar neoplasm and most common parasellar/cavernous sinus neoplasm is meningioma. The most common nonneoplastic parasellar mass is an arterial aneurysm.
- In children, the most common suprasellar neoplasms are craniopharyngioma, followed by gliomas of the optic pathway or hypothalamus. A distinct subset of pediatric suprasellar neoplasms are those arising from the infundibulum, of which the most common are germ cell tumors and Langerhans cell histiocytosis.

Meningioma

- Meningiomas can arise anywhere along the skull base meninges, including the planum sphenoidale, anterior clinoid processes, tuberculum sellae, diaphragma sellae, dorsum sellae, and cavernous sinus wall.
- As with meningiomas elsewhere, these tumors show uniform, intense contrast enhancement often with a dural tail. Meningiomas may cause adjacent hyperostosis due to vasoactive factors.
- An important imaging finding of a parasellar meningioma is possible encasement and narrowing of the cavernous or supraclinoid internal carotid artery.

鞍上和鞍旁肿块

概述

- 鞍旁/鞍上病变鉴别诊断范围很广,但综合患者的影像学表现和发病年龄、临床表现,通常可将鉴别诊断范围缩小到少数几类疾病。
- 用各疾病英文名称首字母组合"MOuSTACHE"可帮助记忆鞍旁/鞍上病变的鉴别诊断疾病谱,但排列顺序不按疾病发生率的高低:

  脑膜瘤/转移瘤(M)。

  视通路胶质瘤(O)。

  蝶鞍内病变延伸至鞍上/鞍旁区(如大腺瘤)(S)。

  畸胎瘤和其他生殖细胞肿瘤(如生殖细胞瘤)(T)。

  动脉瘤(A)。

  颅咽管瘤(C)。

  下丘脑胶质瘤或错构瘤(H)。

  表皮样/皮样囊肿(E)。

- 在成人,鞍上区最常见的肿瘤是垂体大腺瘤向上扩展;鞍上区第二常见和鞍旁/海绵窦区最常见的肿瘤是脑膜瘤;鞍旁区最常见的非肿瘤性肿块是动脉瘤。
- 在儿童,鞍上区最常见的肿瘤是颅咽管瘤,其次是视神经或下丘脑胶质瘤。儿童特有的一类鞍上区肿瘤是起源于漏斗部的肿瘤,最常见的是生殖细胞肿瘤和朗格汉斯细胞组织细胞增生症。

脑膜瘤

- 脑膜瘤可发生于颅底脑膜的任何部位,包括蝶骨旁、前床突、鞍结节、鞍膈、鞍背和海绵窦壁。
- 与其他部位的脑膜瘤相同,颅底脑膜瘤在增强扫描上表现为均匀、显著性强化,通常可见"脑膜尾征"。由于血管活性因子的作用,脑膜瘤可导致邻近颅骨骨质增生。
- 鞍旁脑膜瘤的一个重要影像学表现是肿瘤可包绕颈内动脉海绵窦段或床突上段颈内动脉,并导致管腔变窄。

Aneurysm

- The suprasellar/parasellar region is the most common site of giant intracranial aneurysms. These typically arise from the supraclinoid or cavernous internal carotid artery.
- Aneurysms are an important entity to consider in the differential diagnosis of suprasellar/ parasellar tumors to avoid a catastrophic biopsy.
- Pulsation artifact or a flow void may be present on conventional MRI sequences. CTA or MRA would be diagnostic.

动脉瘤

- 鞍上/鞍旁区是颅内巨大动脉瘤最常发生的部位，多起自颈内动脉床突上段或海绵窦段。
- 动脉瘤是鞍上/鞍旁肿块病变时要考虑的重要鉴别诊断，以避免“灾难性”的活检。
- 动脉瘤在常规MRI序列上可见搏动伪影或流空效应。CTA或MRA可明确诊断。

Metastases

- Malignancies rarely metastasize to the pituitary gland and stalk.
- Breast cancer is the most common primary tumor to metastasize to the suprasellar/ parasellar region. Other tumors include lung cancer, lymphoma, and prostate cancer.

转移瘤

- 恶性肿瘤很少转移到垂体或垂体柄。
- 乳腺癌是最常转移到鞍上/鞍旁区的原发性恶性肿瘤。其他肿瘤包括肺癌、淋巴瘤和前列腺癌。

Craniopharyngioma

颅咽管瘤

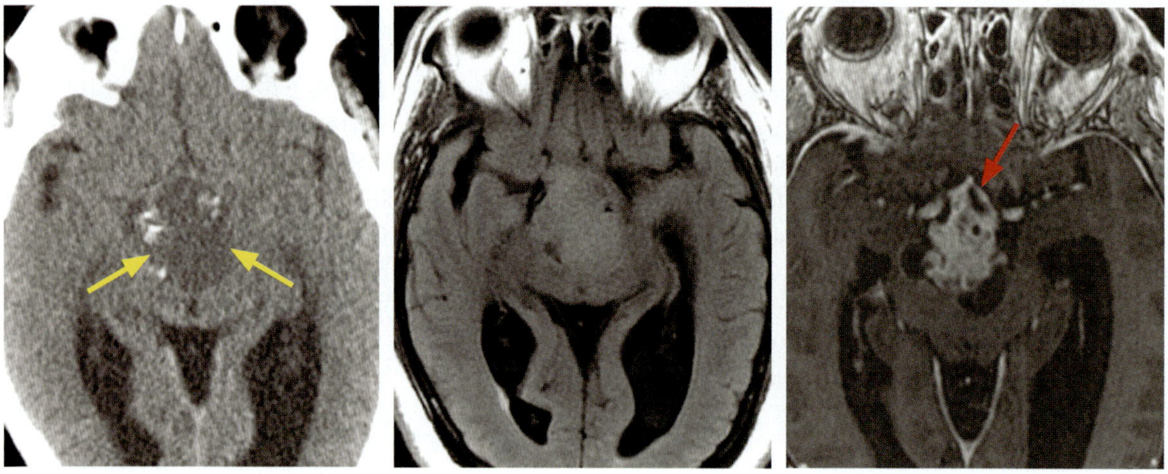

Craniopharyngioma: Noncontrast CT (left image) shows a hypoattenuating suprasellar mass (arrows) containing coarse calcifications. The suprasellar cistern is effaced. FLAIR MRI (middle image) shows an isointense, primarily solid suprasellar mass. Post-contrast T1-weighted (right image) MRI shows avid heterogeneous enhancement. There is a small cystic focus anteriorly (red arrow).

颅咽管瘤：平扫CT(左图)显示鞍上区低密度肿块(黄箭)，内含粗大钙化。鞍上池消失。FLAIR MRI(中图)显示鞍上区一个等信号、实性为主的肿块。增强T_1加权(右图)MRI显示肿块呈显著不均匀强化，其前部有小的囊性病变(红箭)。

- Craniopharyngiomas are benign (WHO grade I) neoplasms arising from Rathke pouch remnants that produce keratin.
- Most craniopharyngiomas are suprasellar, although they may extend into or rarely arise within the sella.
- Craniopharyngioma occurs in a bimodal age distribution but more commonly occurs in children.
- In children, most craniopharyngiomas are the adamantinomatous subtype, which are complex cystic, lobulated masses with calcifications (similar to enamel). The cyst fluid is typically proteinaceous (described as *machine oil* or *motor oil*), which has a hyperintense appearance on T1-weighted images.
- In adults, the papillary subtype is more common, which typically appears as a predominantly solid, enhancing, spherical, non-calcified mass.

- 颅咽管瘤是良性肿瘤(WHO 1级)，起源于产生角蛋白的颅颊囊残留。
- 大多数颅咽管瘤位于鞍上区，虽然肿瘤可向下延伸到鞍内，但极少源自鞍内。
- 颅咽管瘤的发病年龄呈双峰分布，但更常见于儿童。
- 在儿童，大多数颅咽管瘤是牙釉质型，表现为复杂囊性、分叶状肿块，伴有钙化(类似于牙釉质)。囊液内通常含有蛋白质(被称为“机油”)，在T_1加权图像上呈高信号。

Germ cell tumors

- Intracranial germ cell tumors arise in the midline, with the majority in the pineal region and next most commonly in the suprasellar region.
- The majority of intracranial germ cell tumors are germinomas. Nongerminomatous germ cell tumors include teratoma, embryonal carcinoma, endodermal sinus tumor, choriocarcinoma, and mixed tumors.

生殖细胞瘤

- 颅内生殖细胞肿瘤起源于中线，大多数位于松果体区，其次是鞍上区。
- 大多数颅内生殖细胞肿瘤是生殖细胞瘤。非生殖细胞肿瘤包括畸胎瘤、胚胎癌、内胚窦瘤、绒毛膜癌和混合瘤。

- The incidence peaks during adolescence.
- Imaging shows a homogeneous, intensely enhancing midline mass. The mass is hypointense on T2-weighted images and dark on ADC map due to hypercellularity.

Glioma

- 发病高峰年龄为青春期。
- 影像学表现为中线区出现均匀、显著强化的肿块。由于细胞排列缜密，肿块在T_2加权图像上呈低信号，在ADC图上也呈低信号。

胶质瘤

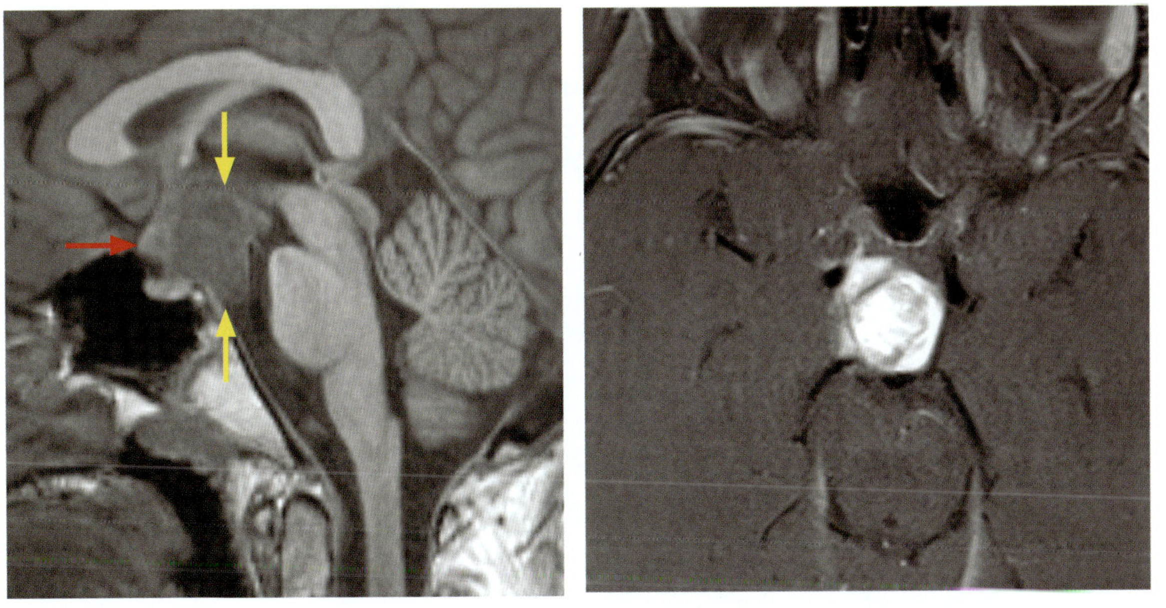

Optic pathway glioma: Sagittal T1- (left image) and post-contrast axial T1-weighted MRI shows a suprasellar mass that is slightly hypointense relative to gray matter (yellow arrows), with diffuse enlargement of the adjacent optic chiasm (red arrow). The mass demonstrates avid heterogeneous enhancement.

视通路胶质瘤：矢状位T_1(左图)和轴位增强T_1(右图)加权MRI显示鞍上区肿块，信号较灰质稍低(黄箭)，伴邻近视交叉弥漫性肿大(红箭)。肿块呈显著不均匀强化。

- Optic pathway gliomas, as previously discussed in the orbital section, can arise anywhere along the optic nerves, optic chiasm, and optic tracts. Hypothalamic gliomas are often considered together with this group due to difficulty distinguishing the site of origin in the suprasellar region.
- These tumors are isointense on T1-weighted images, hyperintense on T2-weighted images, and usually enhance.

Langerhans cell histiocytosis (LCH)

- Langerhans cell histiocytosis is a multisystem, infiltrative neoplasm of children.
- The most common endocrine abnormality in LCH is diabetes insipidus, due to involvement of the pituitary or its stalk.
- Infundibular thickening and enhancement is the most common central nervous system imaging manifestation of LCH.

Epidermoid and dermoid cysts

- Epidermoid and dermoid cysts are benign congenital ectodermal inclusion cysts.
- While dermoid and epidermoid cysts most commonly occur in the posterior cranial fossa, the most common supratentorial site is the suprasellar cistern.
- As described earlier in the chapter, epidermoid cysts follow CSF signal on T1- and T2- weighted images, but are hyperintense on FLAIR and show restricted diffusion.
- Dermoid cysts may contain intracystic fat, which can cause chemical meningitis or ventriculitis upon rupture.

- 视神经胶质瘤可发生在视神经、视交叉和视束等任何位置，在前文眼眶部分中已做介绍。下丘脑胶质瘤通常与视通路胶质瘤作为同一组疾病进行考虑，因鞍上区难以准确区分其起源。
- 鞍上区胶质瘤在T_1加权呈等信号，T_2加权呈高信号，通常有明显强化。

朗格汉斯细胞组织细胞增生症(LCH)

- 朗格汉斯细胞组织细胞增生症(LCH)是一种见于儿童的多系统、浸润性肿瘤。
- LCH最常见的内分泌异常是尿崩症，这是由于垂体或垂体柄受累所致。
- 垂体漏斗部增粗与强化是LCH最常见的中枢神经系统影像学表现。

表皮样囊肿和皮样囊肿

- 表皮样囊肿和皮样囊肿是良性先天性外胚层的包涵性囊肿。
- 皮样囊肿和表皮样囊肿最常发生于颅后窝，幕上区最好发的位置是鞍上池。
- 如本章前文所述，表皮样囊肿在T_1和T_2加权图像上与脑脊液(CSF)信号一致，但在FLAIR上呈高信号，并有弥散受限。
- 皮样囊肿可内含脂肪，一旦破裂可引起化学性脑膜炎或室管膜炎。

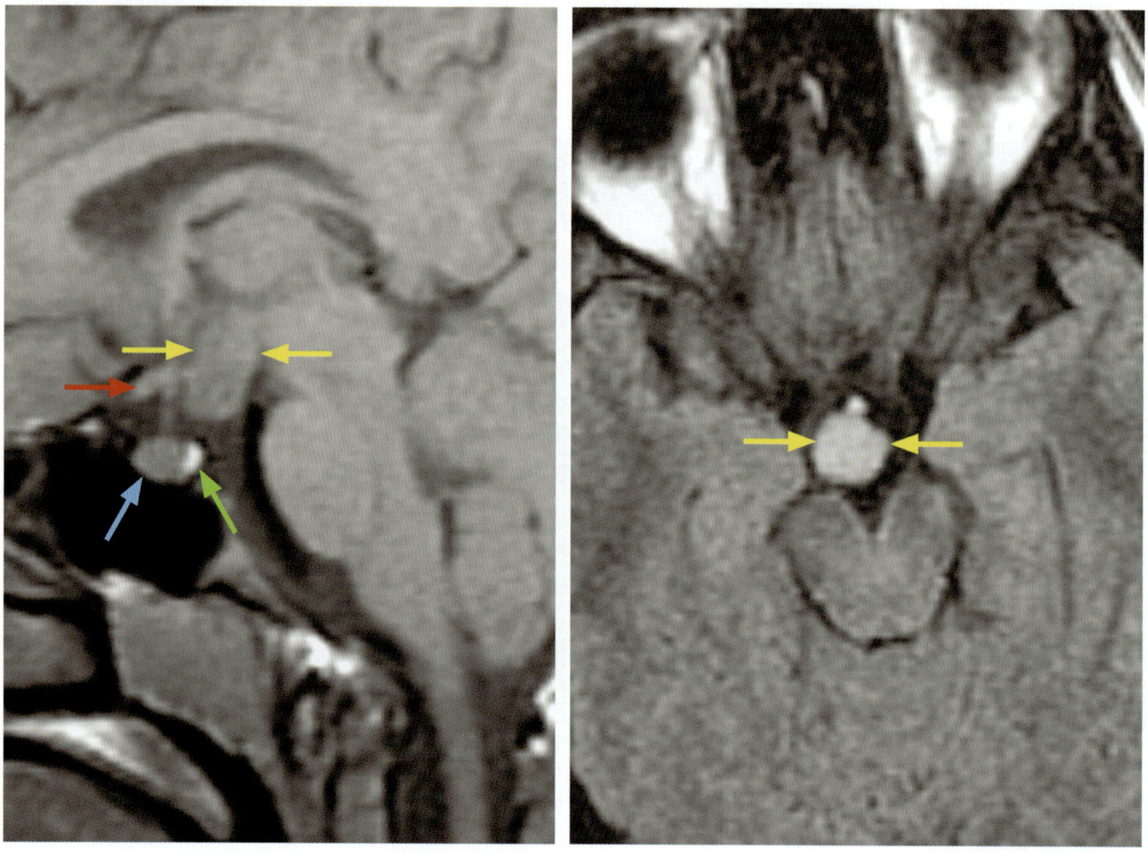

Hypothalamic hamartoma: Sagittal T1-weighted (left image) and axial FLAIR MRI shows a T1 isointense, FLAIR hyperintense suprasellar mass (yellow arrows) projecting inferiorly from the hypothalamus. The optic chiasm (red arrow) is normal, as is the anterior pituitary (blue arrow) and posterior pituitary bright spot (green arrow).

Case courtesy Sanjay Prabhu, MD, Boston Children's Hospital.

下丘脑错构瘤：矢状位T_1加权(左图)和轴位FLAIR(右图)MRI显示一个来自下丘脑并向下突出的鞍上区肿块(黄箭)，其中T_1呈等信号，FLAIR为高信号。视交叉(红箭)和垂体前叶(蓝箭)正常，垂体后叶有高信号亮点(绿箭)。

- Hypothalamic (tuber cinereum) hamartoma represents gray matter heterotopia arising between the pituitary stalk and the mammillary bodies.
- Hypothalamic hamartoma is the most common mass causing central precocious puberty in children. These masses are also associated with gelastic seizures (laughing spells).
- Hypothalamic hamartoma characteristically appears as a sessile or pedunculated mass at the floor of the third ventricle that does not enhance and is isointense to gray matter.

- 下丘脑(灰结节)错构瘤实际上是位于垂体柄和乳头体之间的灰质异位。
- 下丘脑错构瘤是儿童中导致中枢性性早熟最常见的肿块。这些肿块常合并痴笑样癫痫(狂笑)。
- 下丘脑错构瘤的特征性表现为位于第三脑室底部的无蒂或有蒂的肿块，无强化，与灰质呈等信号。

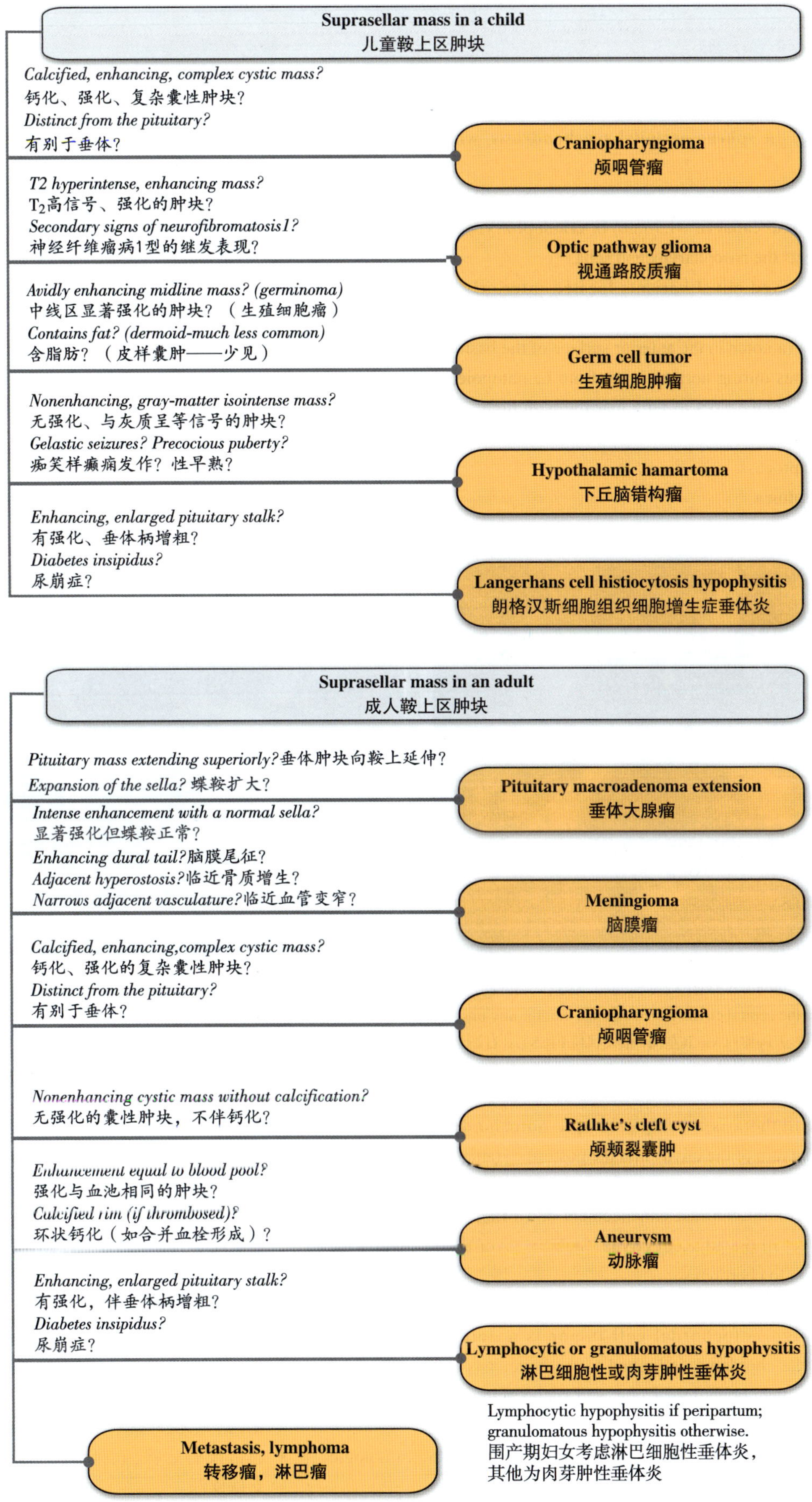
Suprasellar mass in a child
儿童鞍上区肿块
Calcified, enhancing, complex cystic mass?
钙化、强化、复杂囊性肿块?
Distinct from the pituitary?
有别于垂体?
Craniopharyngioma
颅咽管瘤
T2 hyperintense, enhancing mass?
T_2高信号、强化的肿块?
Secondary signs of neurofibromatosis1?
神经纤维瘤病1型的继发表现?
Optic pathway glioma
视通路胶质瘤
Avidly enhancing midline mass? (germinoma)
中线区显著强化的肿块？（生殖细胞瘤）
Contains fat? (dermoid-much less common)
含脂肪？（皮样囊肿——少见）
Germ cell tumor
生殖细胞肿瘤
Nonenhancing, gray-matter isointense mass?
无强化、与灰质呈等信号的肿块?
Gelastic seizures? Precocious puberty?
痴笑样癫痫发作？性早熟?
Hypothalamic hamartoma
下丘脑错构瘤
Enhancing, enlarged pituitary stalk?
有强化、垂体柄增粗?
Diabetes insipidus?
尿崩症?
Langerhans cell histiocytosis hypophysitis
朗格汉斯细胞组织细胞增生症垂体炎
Suprasellar mass in an adult
成人鞍上区肿块
Pituitary mass extending superiorly?垂体肿块向鞍上延伸?
Expansion of the sella? 蝶鞍扩大?
Pituitary macroadenoma extension
垂体大腺瘤
Intense enhancement with a normal sella?
显著强化但蝶鞍正常?
Enhancing dural tail?脑膜尾征?
Adjacent hyperostosis?临近骨质增生?
Narrows adjacent vasculature?临近血管变窄?
Meningioma
脑膜瘤
Calcified, enhancing,complex cystic mass?
钙化、强化的复杂囊性肿块?
Distinct from the pituitary?
有别于垂体?
Craniopharyngioma
颅咽管瘤
Nonenhancing cystic mass without calcification?
无强化的囊性肿块，不伴钙化?
Rathke's cleft cyst
颅颊裂囊肿
Enhancement equal to blood pool?
强化与血池相同的肿块?
Calcified rim (if thrombosed)?
环状钙化（如合并血栓形成）?
Aneurysm
动脉瘤
Enhancing, enlarged pituitary stalk?
有强化，伴垂体柄增粗?
Diabetes insipidus?
尿崩症?
Lymphocytic or granulomatous hypophysitis
淋巴细胞性或肉芽肿性垂体炎
Lymphocytic hypophysitis if peripartum;
granulomatous hypophysitis otherwise.
围产期妇女考虑淋巴细胞性垂体炎，
其他为肉芽肿性垂体炎
Metastasis, lymphoma
转移瘤，淋巴瘤

Clivus

Anatomy and anatomic variants

- The clivus is the sloping midline aspect of the central skull base formed by the sphenoid body and basiocciput.
- These bones join at the **spheno-occipital synchondrosis**, which fuses during adolescence.
- A normal variant canallocated superiorly, in the midline sphenoid body, is the **persistent hypophyseal canal** (if <1.5 mm) or **craniopharyngeal canal** (if >1.5 mm), which connects the nasopharynx and sella.
- Two notochord-derived clival variants located inferiorly are the **canalis basilaris medianus** (along channel in the midline basiocciput) and the **fossa navicularis magna** (a notch in the anterior surface of the basiocciput).
- The clivus transitions during normal aging from hematopoietic marrow with low signal on T1-weighted MRI to fatty marrow with high T1 signal. Low T1 marrow signal in an older adult is abnormal, which may be due to a neoplasm or diffuse systemic process.

Ecchordosis physaliphora

斜坡

解剖和解剖变异

- 斜坡位于中颅底，沿中线倾斜，由蝶骨体和枕骨基底部构成。
- 蝶骨体和枕骨基底部在**蝶枕软骨联合**处汇合，在青春期融合。
- 位于斜坡上方及蝶骨体内中线的一个正常变异的管状结构叫**永存垂体管**(<1.5mm)或**颅咽管**(>1.5mm)，它连接鼻咽和蝶鞍。
- 在斜坡下方有2个由脊索衍生的解剖变异，即**中线基底管**(位于枕骨基底中线区的一条长管状结构)和**舟状大窝**(枕骨前基底部表面的凹槽)。
- 随着年龄的增长，斜坡松质骨内由T_1加权低信号的造血红骨髓转变为T_1高信号的含脂骨髓。老年人的T_1骨髓信号降低为异常，可能是由肿瘤或全身系统性疾病所致。

颅内脊索瘤

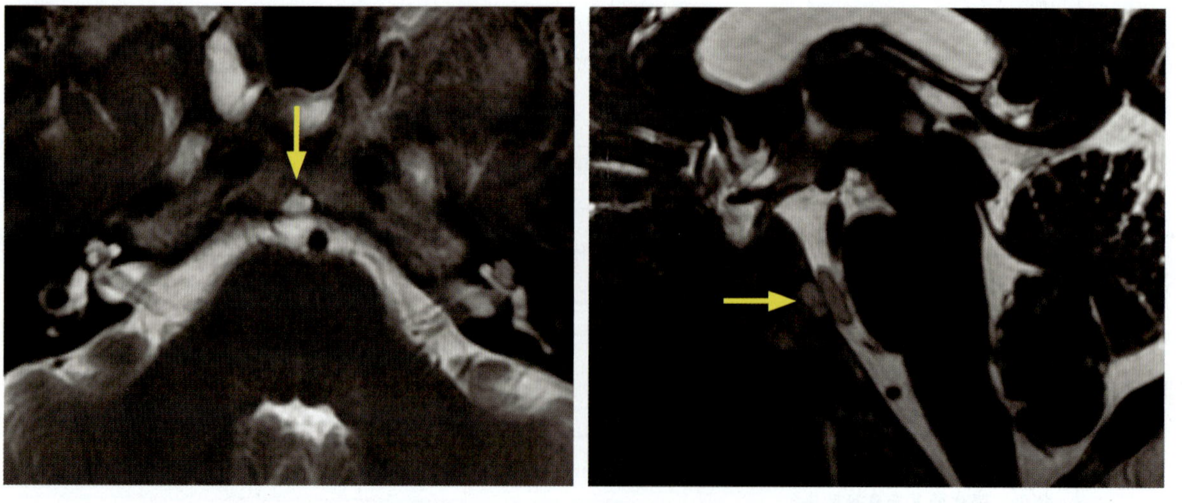

Ecchordosis physaliphora: Axial T2-weighted MRI (left image) and sagittal FIESTA (right image) shows a T2 hyperintense lesion (arrows) centered within the central clivus which extends intradurally into the prepontine cistern. There is no significant enhancement (not shown).

颅内脊索瘤：轴位T_2加权MRI(左图)和矢状位FIESTA(右图)显示以斜坡中央为中心的T_2高信号病灶(黄箭)，病变向硬膜内延伸至桥前池。无明显强化(未展示)。

- Ecchordosis physaliphora is a benign, ectopic notochordal remnant that projects from the dorsum of the clivus into the posterior cranial fossa.
- On imaging, ecchordosis physaliphora appears as a small T2 hyperintense retroclivallesion, without contrast enhancement and often with a stalk and/or small bony defect in the adjacent clivus. Stability over time supports the diagnosis as opposed to chordoma.

Benign notochordal cell tumor

- Intraosseous benign notochordal cell tumor is a notochord-derived neoplasm that, unlike chordoma, is limited to the bone, associated with mild osteosclerosis rather than bone destruction, and shows minimal to no contrast enhancement.
- They are usually asymptomatic. Long-term stability supports the radiologic diagnosis.

- 颅内脊索瘤是一种良性的异位脊索残余，从斜坡背侧向颅后窝突出。
- 影像学上，颅内脊索瘤表现为斜坡后部一个小的T_2高信号病变，无强化，通常在邻近的斜坡有蒂和/或小的骨质缺损。病灶保持长期稳定可支持诊断，这与脊索瘤完全相反。

良性脊索细胞瘤

- 骨内良性脊索细胞瘤是一种起源于脊索的肿瘤。与脊索瘤不同，其病灶局限于骨内，伴有轻度骨质硬化，而不伴骨质破坏，仅有轻微强化，甚至无强化。
- 通常没有症状，长期影像学随访病变无变化支持诊断。

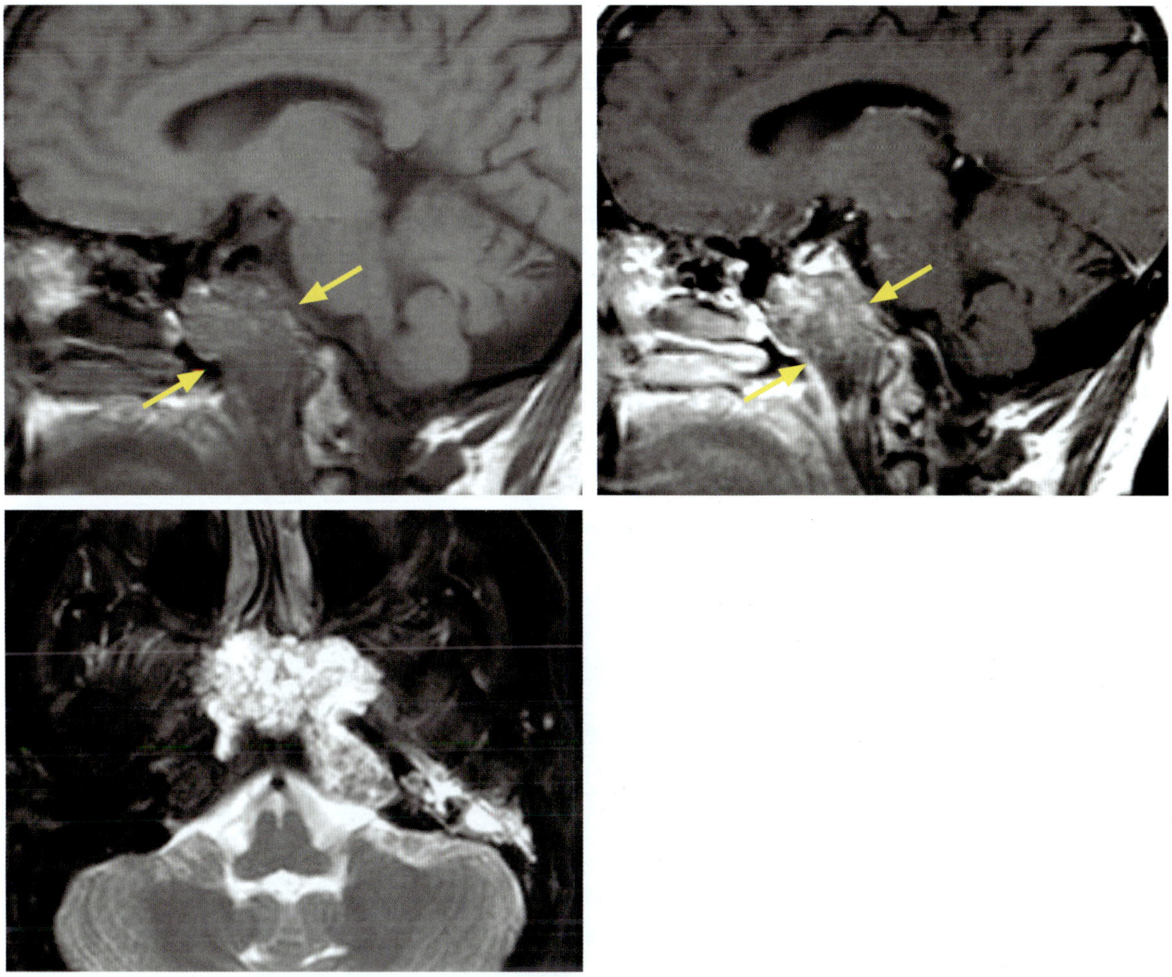

Clival chordoma:

Sagittal T1-weighted MRI (top left image) shows replacement of the normal clival marrow by an isointense mass (arrows).

Sagittal post-contrast T1-weighted MRI (top right image) shows heterogeneous enhancement of the mass (arrows).

Axial T2-weighted MRI (bottom left image) shows a microlobulated, hyperintense clival mass with extension into the left petrous apex and opacification of the left middle ear and mastoid air cells.

Case courtesy Mary Beth Cunnane, MD, Massachusetts Eye and Ear Infirmary.

斜坡脊索瘤：

矢状位T_1加权MRI(左上图)显示一个等信号的肿块取代了正常斜坡的骨髓信号(黄箭)。

矢状位增强T_1加权MRI(右上图)显示肿块呈不均匀强化(黄箭)。

轴位T_2加权MRI(左下图)显示有斜坡微分叶、高信号的斜坡肿块，延伸至左侧岩尖部，左侧中耳和乳突气房信号增高。

- **Chordoma** is a notochord-derived malignancy in adults that most commonly arises in the sacrum, followed by the clivus, and less commonly the vertebral column. Chordoma is the most common primary neoplasm of the clivus.
- Chordomas show high signal on T2-weighted MRI and usually do not calcify. Key imaging features that distinguish chordoma from benign notochordal tumors are bony destruction, extraosseous extension, and contrast enhancement. Posterior tumor projection often indents the pons, creating the *thumb sign* on sagittal images.
- **Chondrosarcoma** is a cartilage-derived malignancy in adults that, within the skull base, most commonly arises at the petroclival synchondrosis (petro-occipital fissure).

- **脊索瘤**是一种成人起源于脊索的恶性肿瘤，最常见于骶骨，其次是斜坡，较少见于脊柱其他部位。脊索瘤是斜坡最常见的原发性肿瘤。
- 脊索瘤在T_2加权MRI上表现为高信号，通常无钙化。鉴别脊索瘤和良性脊索细胞肿瘤的关键影像学特征是有骨质破坏、病灶向骨外延伸、增强后病灶有强化。肿瘤向后突出可压迫脑桥形成局部凹陷，在矢状位图像上形成拇指征。
- **软骨肉瘤**是发生在成人起源于软骨的恶性肿瘤。在颅底，最常发生在岩尖斜坡软骨联合处(岩枕裂)。

- Chondrosarcomas show high signal on T2-weighted MRI and markedly elevated ADC values (higher than those of chordoma). CT can demonstrate the *rings and arcs* calcifications characteristic of chondroid lesions.
- Because chordomas and chondrosarcomas frequently have overlapping imaging features, location is key in diagnosis. Chordomas tend to be midline, while chondrosarcomas are mostly centered off-midline.

Secondary malignancies

- As with other bones, the clivus can be a site of metastatic disease (e.g., breast cancer), local extension of soft tissue tumors (e.g., nasopharyngeal carcinoma), or involvement with hematopoietic malignancies (e.g., myeloma/plasmacytoma or lymphoma).

- 软骨肉瘤在T_2加权MRI上呈高信号，ADC值显著升高(高于脊索瘤)。CT可显示病灶内环形和弧形钙化，为软骨病变的典型表现。
- 由于脊索瘤和软骨肉瘤的影像学表现常有重叠，病灶的位置是鉴别诊断的关键。脊索瘤往往位于中线区，而软骨肉瘤大多位于中线旁区。

继发性恶性肿瘤

- 与其他部位骨骼一样，斜坡也可以发生转移瘤(如乳腺癌)、软组织肿瘤局部侵犯(如鼻咽癌)或造血系统恶性肿瘤累及(如骨髓瘤/浆细胞瘤或淋巴瘤)。

Pterygopalatine fossa

翼腭窝

Anatomy of the pterygopalatine fossa

翼腭窝解剖

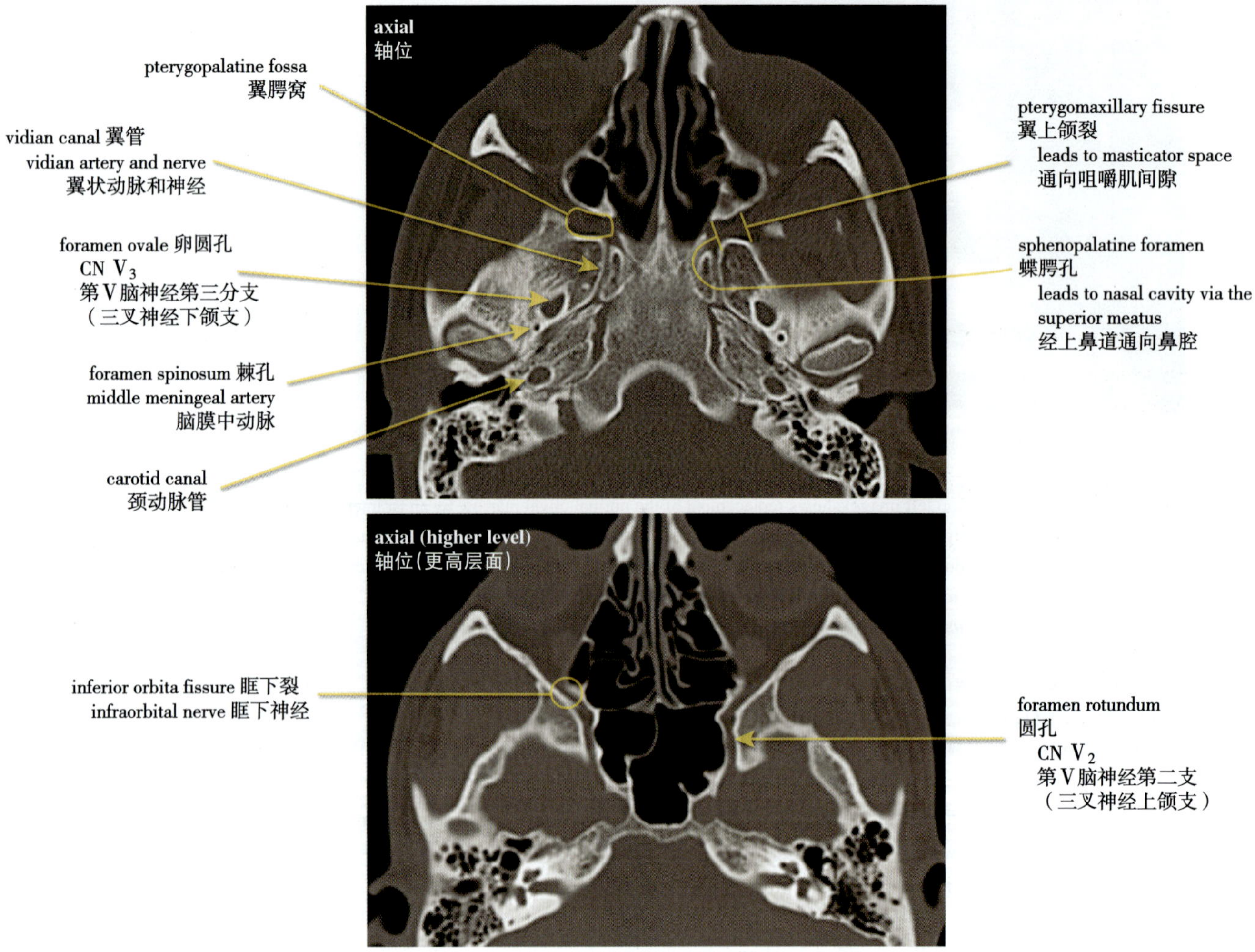

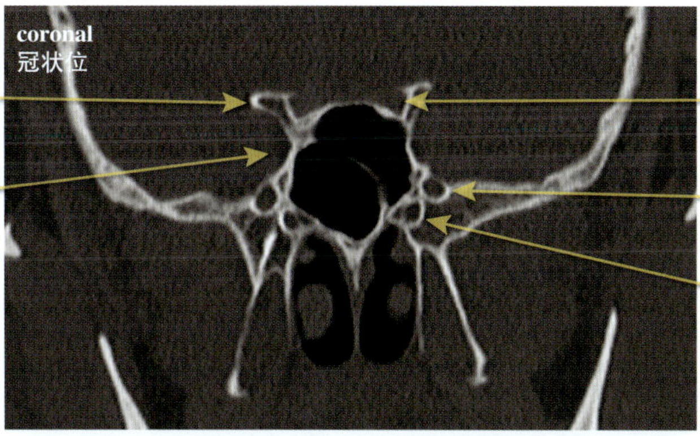

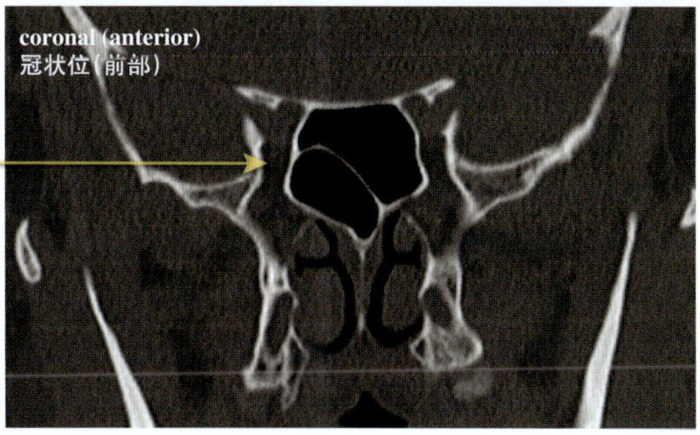

- The pterygopalatine fossae are inverted pyramid-shaped spaces in the deep face that are important central stations for the spread of disease between the facial skull and middle cranial fossa.
- The pterygopalatine fossa contains fat and neurovascular structures including the pterygopalatine ganglion, maxillary nerve (cranial nerve V_2) branches, and distal maxillary artery branches.
- Anteriorly, the pterygopalatine fossa is bordered by the maxillary sinus.
- Posteriorly, the pterygopalatine fossa is bordered by the base of the pterygoid plates of the sphenoid bone, through which the **foramen rotundum** and **Vidian canal** are routes to the middle cranial fossa. The former carries the maxillary branch of the trigeminal nerve (V_2), while the latter carries the Vidian nerve (nerve of the pterygoid canal).
- Superiorly, the **inferior orbital fissure** is the base of the pyramid that opens anteriorly into the orbit. It transmits the infraorbital nerve, among other structures.
- Laterally, the **pterygomaxillary fissure** is the exit to the masticator space or infratemporal fossa.
- Medially, the **sphenopalatine foramen** is the exit to the superior meatus of the nasal cavity. It transmits the sphenopalatine artery, among other structures.
- Inferiorly, the **pterygopalatine canal** is the apex of the pyramid that leads to the oral cavity via the greater and lesser palatine foramina. They transmit the greater and lesser palatine nerves and vessels.

Pterygopalatine fossa pathology

- The pterygopalatine fossa can be involved with neoplastic or inflammatory entities by direct invasion or perineural spread.

  Primary sites include the cheek (e.g., squamous cell carcinoma), maxillary sinus (e.g., invasive fungal sinusitis), nasal cavity and nasopharynx (e.g., juvenile nasopharyngeal angiofibroma, nasopharyngeal carcinoma), palate (e.g., adenoid cystic carcinoma), masticator space (e.g., rhabdomyosarcoma), or orbit (e.g., idiopathic orbital inflammation).

- 翼腭窝是位于面部深层的一个倒金字塔形的间隙，它的重要性在于作为面部颅骨与颅中窝之间病变扩散的重要通道。
- 翼腭窝内含脂肪和神经血管，包括翼腭神经节、上颌神经(三叉神经第二支，V_2)分支和上颌动脉远端分支。
- 翼腭窝的前部以上颌窦为界。
- 翼腭窝的后方与蝶骨翼突基底部相邻，由此处分别经**圆孔**和**翼管**通往颅中窝。前者有V_2穿行，后者有翼神经(翼管神经)通过。
- 翼腭窝的上方为**眶下裂**，构成金字塔形的底部，向前通往眶内。眶下裂内有眶下神经等穿过。
- 翼腭窝的外侧是**翼上颌裂**，即咀嚼肌间隙或颞下窝的出口。
- 翼腭窝的内侧为**蝶腭孔**，是鼻腔上鼻道的出口，其内容纳蝶腭动脉等结构。
- 翼腭窝的下方是**翼腭管**，构成金字塔形的顶点，经腭大孔和腭小孔通向口腔，其内有腭大、腭小神经和血管通过。

翼腭窝病理学

- 肿瘤或炎症可以通过直接蔓延或经神经周围侵犯累及翼腭窝。

  病变原发灶可源自面颊(如SCC)、上颌窦(如侵袭性真菌性鼻窦炎)、鼻腔和鼻咽(如青少年鼻咽血管纤维瘤、鼻咽癌)、上腭(如腺样囊性癌)、咀嚼肌间隙(如横纹肌肉瘤)或眼眶(如特发性眼眶炎症)。

- Obliteration/infiltration of the fat of the pterygopalatine fossa with soft tissue is the earliest imaging sign of its pathological involvement. Later signs are widening or erosion of the bony walls.
- Contrast enhancement and enlargement of the neural foramina/canals leading to the pterygopalatine fossa indicate perineural tumor spread.

- 翼腭窝内脂肪消失/浸润伴软组织形成是病理性受累在影像学上的早期征象。晚期征象有翼腭窝扩大及邻近骨质破坏。
- 通向翼腭窝的神经孔/神经管有强化和扩大提示肿瘤沿神经周围扩散。

（翻译　沈琴）

TEMPORAL BONE/LATERAL SKULL BASE & POSTERIOR SKULL BASE

颞骨/侧颅底与后颅底

OVERVIEW OF THE TEMPORAL BONE

颞骨概述

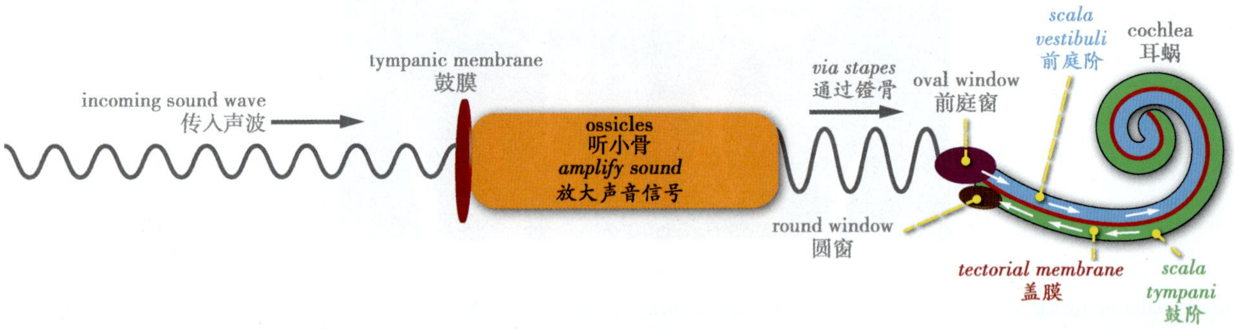

external ear
外耳

contents:
内容：

external auditory canal (EAC)
外耳道（EAC）

pathology:

EAC atresia
squamous cell carcinoma
surfer's ear (EAC exostosis)
swimmer's ear (acute external otitis)
malignant otitis externa
rst branchial cleft cyst
keratosis obturans

病变

EAC闭锁
鳞状细胞癌
冲浪耳(EAC外生骨疣)
游泳耳(急性外耳炎)
恶性外耳炎
第一鳃裂囊肿
阻塞性角化病

middle ear
中耳

contents:
内容：

tympanic membrane
ossicles:
- malleus
- incus
- stapes

stapedius muscle
facial nerve

鼓膜
听小骨：
- 锤骨
- 砧骨
- 镫骨
- 镫骨肌

面神经

pathology:	**病变**
hypoplasia of ossicles	听小骨发育不良
oval window atresia	圆窗闭锁
cholesteatoma	胆脂瘤
otitis media	中耳炎
mastoiditis	乳突炎
glomus tympanicum	鼓室球瘤
aberrant internal carotid artery	变异的颈内动脉
dehiscent jugular bulb	颈静脉球裸露
facial nerve schwannoma	面神经鞘瘤

inner ear
内耳

contents:
内容：

cochlea
semicircular canals
vestibule
utricle
saccule
vestibular aqueduct
cochlear aqueduct
耳蜗
半规管
前庭
椭圆囊
球囊
前庭水管
蜗水管

pathology:	**病变**
cochlear dysplasia	耳蜗发育不良
superior semicircular canal dehiscence	上半规管裂
semicircular canal hypoplasia	半规管发育不良
lateral most commonly affected	外半规管最好发
enlarged vestibular aqueduct	扩大的前庭水管
otospongiosis/otosclerosis	耳海绵化症/耳硬化症
labyrinthitis	迷路炎
Paget disease	佩吉特病(畸形性骨炎)
fibrous dysplasia	骨纤维结构不良
petrous apicitis	岩尖炎
cholesterol cyst	胆固醇囊肿

- The temporal bone can be anatomically and functionally divided into the external (outer), middle, and inner ear. Although some pathologies can overlap, each division tends to be susceptible to unique pathologies.
- This anatomic and functional division parallels the pathway of sound waves into the brain. Sound enters the external ear, is amplified by the ossicles in the middle ear, and is finally converted into electrical impulses in the inner ear.
- An additional function of the inner ear (not drawn above) is the balance and position sense provided by the vestibule and the semicircular canals.
- Together, the cochlea, vestibule, and semicircular canals make up the *labyrinth*. The osseous wallis known as the *bony labyrinth* or *otic capsule*, while the internal structures are known as the *membranous labyrinth*.

- 颞骨按其解剖和功能，可分为外耳、中耳及内耳。每个部位都有各自好发的疾病，但有部分重叠。
- 这种解剖和功能上的分区与声波信号传入大脑的路径相对应。声波进入外耳，经中耳听小骨放大，最后在内耳转化为电脉冲。
- 内耳(上图未展示)的功能还包含前庭和半规管的平衡感觉和位置感觉。
- 耳蜗、前庭及半规管组成迷路。骨壁被称为骨迷路或听软骨囊，内部结构被称为膜迷路。

External ear

Anatomy of the external ear

- The external (outer) ear is composed of the auricle (pinna), external auditory canal (EAC), and tympanic membrane.
- The EAC is a tube surrounded by fibrocartilage (laterally) and bone (medially) that sound passes through before reaching the tympanic membrane.
- The bony part of the EAC is bordered posteriorly and superiorly by mastoid air cells, while the rest is formed by the tympanic part of the temporal bone.

Mastoidectomy procedures are distinguished by whether the posterosuperior walls of the EAC are preserved (canal wall up mastoidectomy) or removed (canal wall down mastoidectomy).

The tympanic part of the temporal bone develops in parts that normally fuse at the anteroinferior aspect in early childhood. Occasionally, incomplete fusion leaves a patent **foramen of Huschke** (foramen tympanicum), a dehiscence connecting the EAC and temporomandibular joint.

- Sound waves vibrate the tympanic membrane, which transmits mechanical energy to the middle ear ossicles.
- The tympanic membrane is divided into two sections: the *pars tensa* (larger, more inferior) and the *pars flaccida* (smaller, more superior).

外耳

外耳解剖

- 外耳(outer)由耳廓(pinna)、外耳道(EAC)和鼓膜组成。
- 外耳道是由纤维软骨(外侧)和骨质(内侧)围绕所形成的管状结构，声波经此到达鼓膜。
- 外耳道的骨部后方和上方的边界为乳突气房，其余部分为颞骨的鼓室所组成。

乳突切除术分为完壁式乳突切除术和开放式乳突切除术，区别在于保留还是切除外耳道的后上壁。

颞骨的鼓室前下部分在儿童早期融合。少数情况下，不完全融合会遗留一个开放的**胡施克孔**，这是连通外耳道和颞下颌关节的裂口。

- 声波振动鼓膜，将机械能传递到中耳听小骨。
- 鼓膜分为两部分：紧张部(较大，靠下)和松弛部(较小，靠上)。

Congenital aural atresia/stenosis

- Congenital aural atresia/stenosis is characterized by developmental narrowing or occlusion of the EAC, often associated with malformation of the auricle (microtia), ossicles (especially malleus and incus), and/or middle ear cavity.
- The external and middle ear malformations are related by their development from the first branchial cleft, first and second branchial arches, and first branchial pouch. Associated anomalies of the inner ear are uncommon due to its separate origin from neuroectoderm.
- Most cases are isolated, but aural atresia can be a part of several syndromes involving the first and second branchial arches, especially Treacher-Collins syndrome and craniofacial microsomia (inclusive of the prior terms hemifacial microsomia, Goldenhar syndrome, and oculo auriculo-vertebral spectrum).

先天性耳道闭锁/狭窄

- 先天性耳道闭锁/狭窄以外耳道发育性狭窄或闭塞为特征，常伴有耳廓(小耳畸形)、听小骨(特别是锤骨和砧骨)和/或中耳腔畸形。
- 外耳和中耳的畸形与第一鳃裂、第一鳃裂弓和第二鳃裂弓，以及第一鳃囊的发育异常有关。合并内耳畸形并不常见，因为内耳起源于神经外胚层。
- 大多数畸形是孤立的，但耳道闭锁可以是多种与第一鳃弓和第二鳃弓发育相关的综合征的部分表现，如下颌骨颜面发育不全(特雷彻·柯林斯综合征)和颅面短小症(包括曾用术语半侧颅面短小症、戈尔登哈尔综合征和眼-耳-脊柱序列征)。

Benign bony external auditory canal lesions

良性骨性外耳道病变

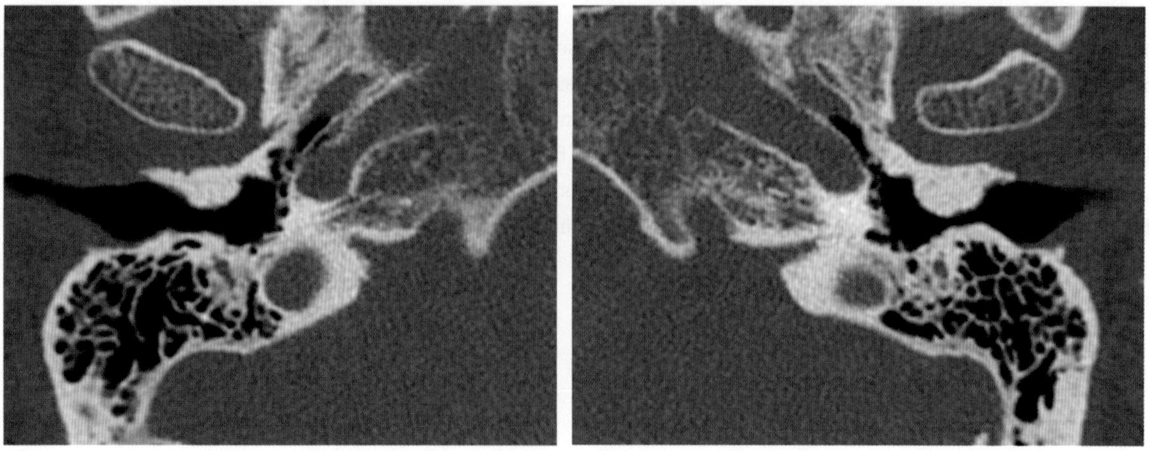

Exostosis: Axial noncontrast CT through the right and left temporal bones shows broad-based bony exostosis in bilateral external auditory canals narrowing the canal lumen.

外生骨疣：右侧和左侧颞骨轴位平扫CT显示双侧外耳道宽基底外生骨疣，导致管腔狭窄。

- **EAC exostosis**, also known as *surfer's ear*, is a non-neoplastic, reactive bony outgrowth projecting into the EAC seen in those who swim/surf in cold waters. It is more often sessile and multiple.
- **EAC osteoma** is the most common osseous neoplasm of the temporal bone. It is more often solitary and pedunculated.

Otitis externa (external otitis)

- Otitis externa, also known as *swimmer's ear*, refers to inflammation of the EAC. The most common cause is acute bacterial infection, most commonly with *Pseudomonas aeruginosa*.
- **Necrotizingotitis externa**, previously known as malignant otitis externa, refers to otitis externa complicated by temporal bone osteomyelitis. The most common risk factor is diabetes mellitus.
- Imaging of otitis externa shows EAC soft tissue thickening, enhancement, and stranding. Specific findings of necrotizingotitis externa, as with osteomyelitis elsewhere, are cortical bone erosion on CT and marrow replacement on MRI.
- Chronic otitis externa can result in **medial canal fibrosis**, which appears as crescentic soft tissue thickening over the outer surface of the tympanic membrane.

Benign keratinous external auditory canal lesions

- **Keratosis obturans** is an accumulation of keratin plugs that occludes and expands the EAC without bone involvement. The condition is more often seen in young adults and children, sometimes associated with sinusitis and bronchiectasis.
- On imaging, keratosis obturans appears as EAC soft tissue opacification with smooth, expansile remodeling of the bony canal. Involvement is often bilateral.
- **Cholesteatoma** is a collection of keratin lined by squamous epithelium, which rarely occurs in the EAC. EAC cholesteatoma more often occurs in middle-aged to older adults.
- On imaging, EAC cholesteatoma appears as a soft tissue mass with focal bone erosion or sequestered bone fragments. Involvement is unilateral.

- **外耳道外生骨疣**，又称*冲浪耳*，是一种突入外耳道的非肿瘤性的反应性骨质增生，常见于在冷水中游泳/冲浪的人群，通常无蒂且多发。
- **外耳道骨瘤**是颞骨最常见的骨肿瘤，通常有蒂且单发。

外耳道炎(外耳炎)

- 外耳道炎，又称*游泳耳*，是指发生在外耳道的炎症。最常见的病因是急性细菌感染，最常见的病原菌是*铜绿假单胞菌*。
- **坏死性外耳道炎**，旧称“恶性外耳道炎”，是指合并颞骨骨髓炎的外耳道炎。最常见的危险因素是糖尿病。
- 外耳道炎的影像学表现为外耳道软组织增厚、强化和绞线状影。坏死性外耳炎的特征性表现与其他位置的骨髓炎一样，CT表现为皮质骨侵蚀，MRI表现为骨髓信号改变。
- 慢性外耳炎可导致**内侧耳道纤维化**，表现为鼓膜外表面新月状软组织增厚。

良性外耳道角化病变

- **阻塞性角化病**是一种由角化栓积聚进而造成阻塞，并撑大外耳道的病变，不累及骨质。这种病变更常见于年轻人及儿童，有时与鼻窦炎和支气管扩张有关。
- 影像学上，阻塞性角化病表现为外耳道软组织密度增高，外耳道骨部内壁平滑、骨性管腔扩张，多为双侧。
- **胆脂瘤**是指内衬鳞状上皮的角蛋白聚集，很少发生于外耳道。外耳道胆脂瘤多见于中老年人群。
- 影像学上，外耳道胆脂瘤表现为软组织肿块，伴有局灶性骨质侵蚀或游离骨碎片，多为单侧。

External ear malignancies

- The most common external ear malignancies are skin cancers: basal cell carcinoma, squamous cell carcinoma, and melanoma.
- Within the external auditory canal, the most common malignancy is squamous cell carcinoma. Imaging shows an enhancing soft tissue mass with osseous erosion.

外耳恶性肿瘤

- 最常见的外耳恶性肿瘤是皮肤癌，包括基底细胞癌、SCC和黑色素瘤。
- 在外耳道内，最常见的恶性肿瘤是SCC。影像学表现为强化的软组织肿块伴骨质侵蚀。

MIDDLE EAR AND MASTOID

中耳及乳突

Anatomy of the middle ear and mastoid

中耳及乳突的解剖

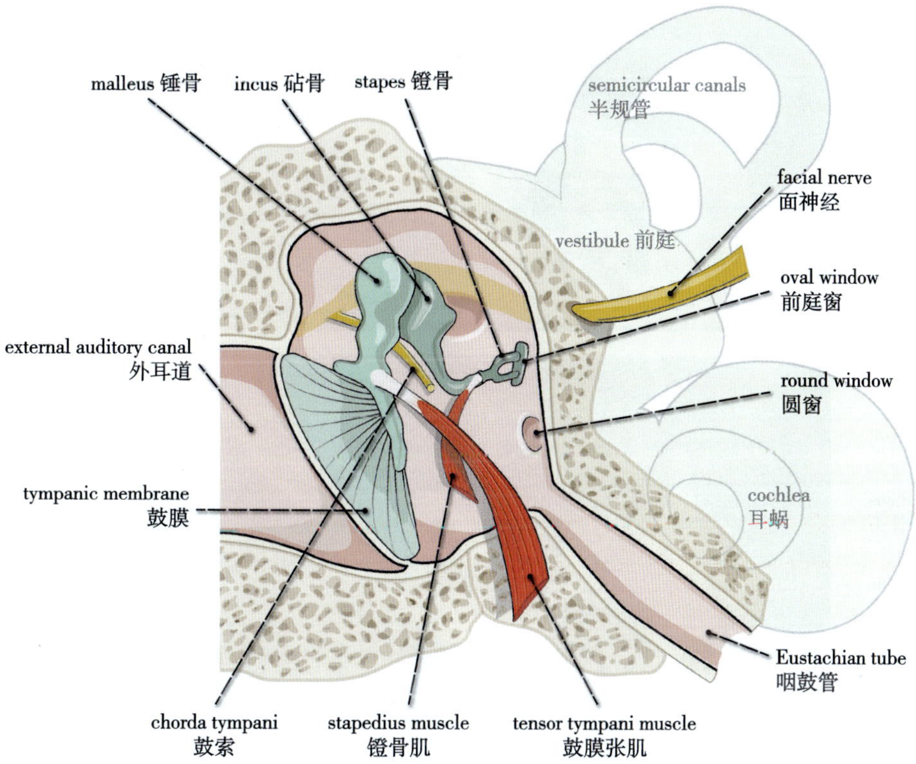

- The middle ear (tympanic) cavity or cleft can be conceived of as a 6-sided box, further divided into compartments demarcated by the upper and lower borders of the tympanic membrane: **epitympanum** (attic or epitympanic recess), **mesotympanum**, and **hypotympanum**.
- The contents include the **ossicles** (malleus, incus, and stapes), the tensor tympani and stapedius muscles, and part of the facial nerve.
- The lateral wall of the middle ear cavity is the **tympanic membrane**, which is attached to the manubrium (handle) of the malleus. Sound reaching the tympanic membrane conducts through the ossicular chain and its articulations with each other (incudomallear and incudostapedial joints). At the end, the footplate of the stapes acts as a piston on the oval window.
- The medial wall has the **cochlear promontory** and two membranous interfaces with the inner ear: the **oval window**, where sound energy enters, and the **round window**, which decompresses that energy after it travels through the cochlea.
- The roof of the epitympanum is the **tegmen tympani**, which is part of the floor of the middle cranial fossa.
- The posterior wall of the epitympanum contains the **aditus** (opening) **to the mastoid antrum**, which leads to the mastoid air cells.

- 中耳(鼓室)类似一个六面盒子结构，由鼓膜的上下边界划分为几个部分：**上鼓室**(鼓室上隐窝或上鼓室隐窝)、**中鼓室**和**下鼓室**。
- 中耳包含**听小骨**(锤骨、砧骨、镫骨)、骨膜张肌和镫骨肌，以及部分面神经。
- 中耳的外侧壁是**鼓膜**，与锤骨柄相连。声波到达鼓膜，通过听骨链及其相互连接的关节(锤砧关节和砧镫关节)传递。最后，镫骨足板如活塞样作用于前庭窗。
- 中耳内侧壁是**耳蜗鼓岬**和与内耳相连的两个膜状界面：**前庭窗**，声能可以通过此处；**圆窗**，在声能穿过耳蜗后对其进行减压。
- 上鼓室的顶部是**鼓室盖**，它是中颅底的一部分。
- 上鼓室后壁包含**乳突窦入口**(开口)，可通向乳突气房。

- The anterior wall of the hypotympanum contains the opening for the Eustachian tube, which leads to the nasopharynx.
- The floor of the hypotympanum contains the jugular plate, which covers the jugular bulb.

- 下鼓室前壁包含咽鼓管的开口，经此通向鼻咽。
- 下鼓室底部包含颈静脉板，颈静脉板覆盖颈静脉球。

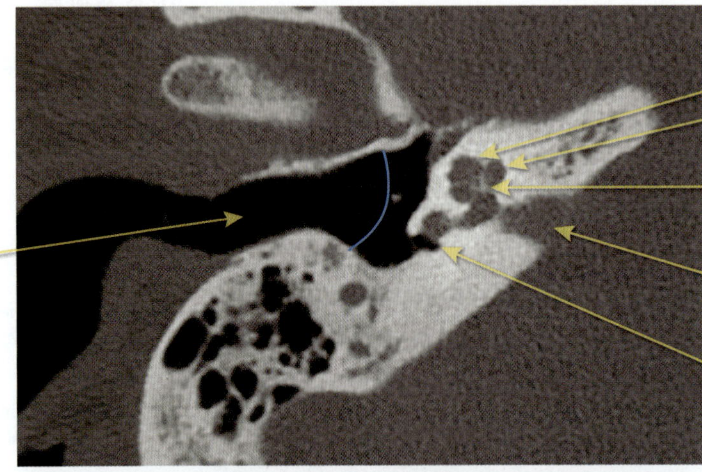

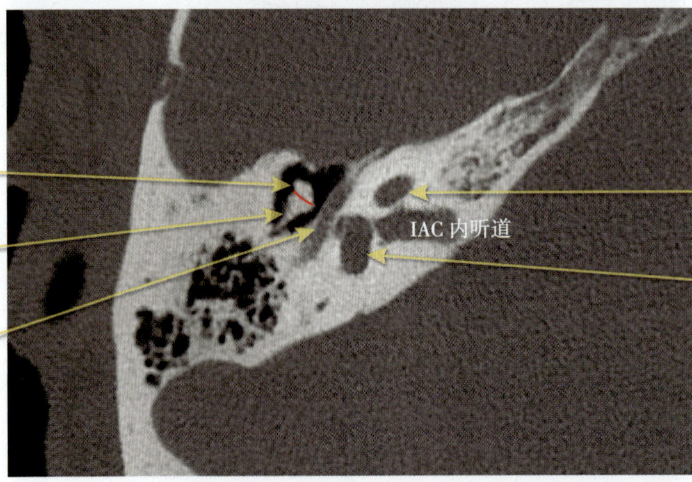

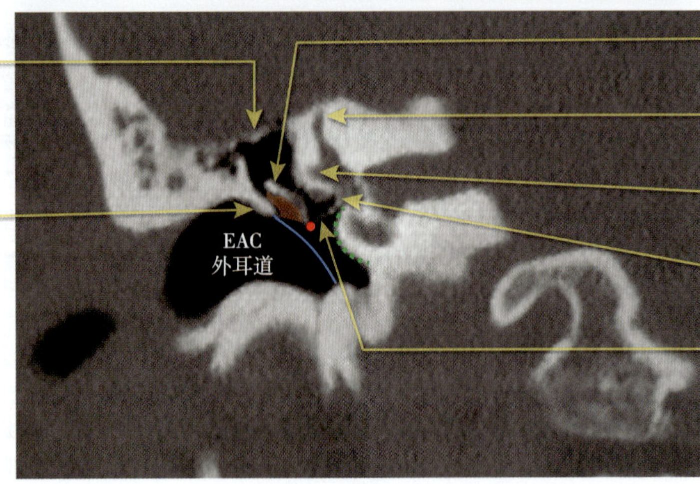

Arterial variants

- Arterial anatomic variants are among the causes of a *red retrotympanic mass* and of pulsatile tinnitus.
- The most common of these is the **aberrant internal carotid artery**, which is an enlarged collateral pathway between the internal and external carotid artery trees involving the caroticotympanic artery and the inferior tympanic artery. CT shows a dehiscent carotid plate, soft tissue protruding into the anterior mesotympanum and coursing down over the cochlear promontory to the posterior mesotympanum, and an enlarged inferior tympanic canaliculus.

动脉变异

- 动脉解剖变异是引起鼓膜后红色肿块和搏动性耳鸣的原因之一。
- 其中最常见的是**异位颈内动脉**，它是颈内动脉和颈外动脉树之间的一条粗大的侧支通路，波及颈鼓室动脉和鼓室下动脉。CT显示颈动脉板开裂，软组织突入中鼓室前部，沿耳蜗骨岬向下延伸至中鼓室后部，下鼓室小管增大。

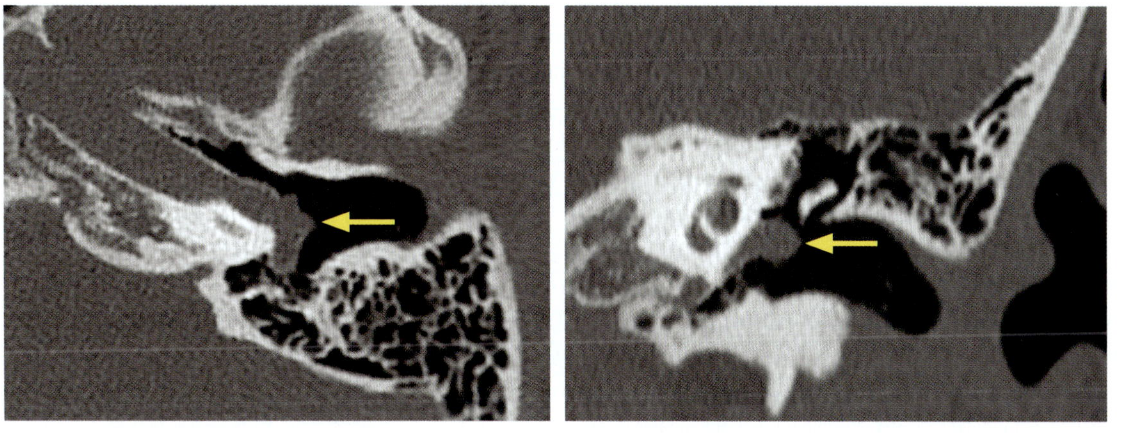

Axial (left image) and coronal noncontrast CT through the left temporal bone demonstrates an aberrant carotid artery which extends laterally into the middle ear cavity with dehiscent bony covering, and coursing around the cochlear promontory (arrows). The ipsilateral foramen spinosum is not visualized (not shown), suggesting the presence of a persistent stapedial artery.

轴位(左图)和冠状位平扫CT显示左侧颞骨变异颈动脉，向外侧经裂开的骨板延伸进入中耳腔，并绕耳蜗骨岬走行(黄箭)，同侧棘孔未见(未展示)，提示永存镫骨动脉。

- In a **lateralized internal carotid artery**, the petrous segment of the internal carotid artery protrudes laterally, with a thinned or dehiscent carotid plate, into the anterior mesotympanum. The inferior tympanic canaliculus is not involved.
- A **persistent stapedial artery** is a branch of the hyoid artery connecting the external and internal carotid arteries, which normally regresses. CT shows soft tissue coursing from the petrous segment of the internal carotid artery, up over the cochlear promontory, and along the proximal tympanic segment of the facial nerve. The foramen spinosum is absent.

Venous variants

- Venous variants of the sigmoid sinus and jugular bulb are among the causes of pulsatile tinnitus and, in the case of dehiscent jugular bulb, of a *blue retrotympanic mass*.
- Sigmoid sinus or jugular bulb **dehiscence** refers to a gap in the bony plates that separates the venous structure from the mastoid air cells or middle ear, respectively.
- Sigmoid sinus or jugular bulb **diverticulum** refers to a focal outpouching of the vessel that protrudes into the temporal bone, with or without bony dehiscence.
- **High-riding jugular bulb** describes when the dome of the jugular bulb rises to a higher than normal position (which is inconsistently defined), with or without bony dehiscence. Hearing or balance issues may result from encroachment on middle and inner ear structures.

- 在**颈内动脉外偏**时，颈内动脉岩段向外侧突出，颈动脉板变薄或裂开，进入中鼓室前部。下鼓室小管未受累。
- **永存镫骨动脉**是舌骨动脉的一个分支，连接颈外动脉和颈内动脉，正常情况下是退化的。CT显示软组织影从颈内动脉岩段开始，向上越过耳蜗鼓岬，并沿面神经的鼓室近端延伸，棘孔消失。

静脉变异

- 乙状窦和颈静脉球的静脉变异是引起搏动性耳鸣的原因之一。如颈静脉球开裂，可见鼓膜后蓝色肿块。
- 乙状窦或颈静脉球**开裂**分别指从乳突气房或中耳分隔静脉结构的骨板上出现的裂隙。
- 乙状窦或颈静脉球**憩室**是指血管朝颞骨方向的局灶性突起，伴或不伴骨性裂隙。
- **高位颈静脉球**是指颈静脉球的顶部高于正常位置(没有一致的定义)，伴或不伴骨性裂隙。中耳和内耳结构受侵可能导致听力或平衡障碍。

Paragangliomas

- Paragangliomas are the most common primary middle ear tumors. Clinically, they typically present with pulsatiletinnitus or conductive hearing loss and appear on otoscopic evaluation as a *red retrotympanic mass*.
- Paragangliomas are extra-adrenal neoplasms of sympathetic or parasympathetic paraganglionic tissue. In the head and neck, most arise from the parasympathetic, noncatecholaminergic glomus cells and therefore are called **glomus tumors**. Most are benign, but they can be locally aggressive. Less than 5% undergo malignant degeneration.
- Most head and neck paragangliomas are sporadic but a significant minority are associated with a hereditary disorder: familial paraganglioma due to succinate dehydrogenase (SDH) subunit gene mutations, multiple endocrine neoplasia type 2 (MEN2), neurofibromatosis type 1 (NF1), or von Hippel Lindau disease (VHL).
- Paragangliomas tend to occur in a few locations in the head and neck: at the carotid bifurcation, in the suprahyoid neck along the course of the vagus nerve, at the jugular foramen, and in the middle ear.

副神经节瘤

- 副神经节瘤是最常见的原发性中耳肿瘤。典型的临床表现为搏动性耳鸣或传导性听力障碍，耳镜检查为鼓膜后红色肿块。
- 副神经节瘤是肾上腺外交感神经或副交感神经的肿瘤。在头颈部，大多数起源于副交感神经，即非儿茶酚胺性血管球细胞，因此被称为**血管球瘤**。大多数是良性的，但也可能有局部侵袭性。不到5%的病例会发生恶变。
- 大多数头颈部副神经节瘤是散发的，但极少数与遗传性疾病有关：琥珀酸脱氢酶(SDH)亚基基因突变导致的家族性副神经节瘤、多发性内分泌瘤病2型(MEN 2)、1型神经纤维瘤病(NF1)及冯·希佩尔-林道病(VHL)。
- 副神经节瘤往往发生在头颈部的少数几个位置：颈动脉分叉处、舌骨上颈部沿迷走神经走行、颈静脉孔及中耳内。

> **Glomus tympanicum tumor** is a paraganglioma isolated to the middle ear, typically centered at the cochlear promontory along the Jacobson nerve (branch of CN Ⅸ). The jugular plate is preserved.
>
> **Glomus jugulotympanicum tumor** describes a paraganglioma that involves both the middle ear cavity and jugular foramen, eroding through the jugular plate.

> **鼓室球瘤**是局限于中耳的副神经节瘤，通常以耳蜗鼓岬为中心，沿Jacobson神经(第Ⅸ神经的分支)。颈动脉板完整。
>
> **颈静脉鼓室球瘤**是指累及中耳腔和颈静脉孔的副神经节瘤，侵蚀穿透颈静脉板。

- Paragangliomas are highly vascular, avidly enhancing soft tissue masses. In larger tumors, the classic MRI pattern is the *salt and pepper* appearance due to intratumoral flow voids. Preoperative angiography with tumor embolization can reduce surgical blood loss.

- 副神经节瘤是高度血管化、显著强化的软组织肿块。在较大的肿瘤中，典型的MRI表现为胡椒盐征，为肿瘤内流空效应所致。术前进行血管造影及肿瘤栓塞可减少术中出血。

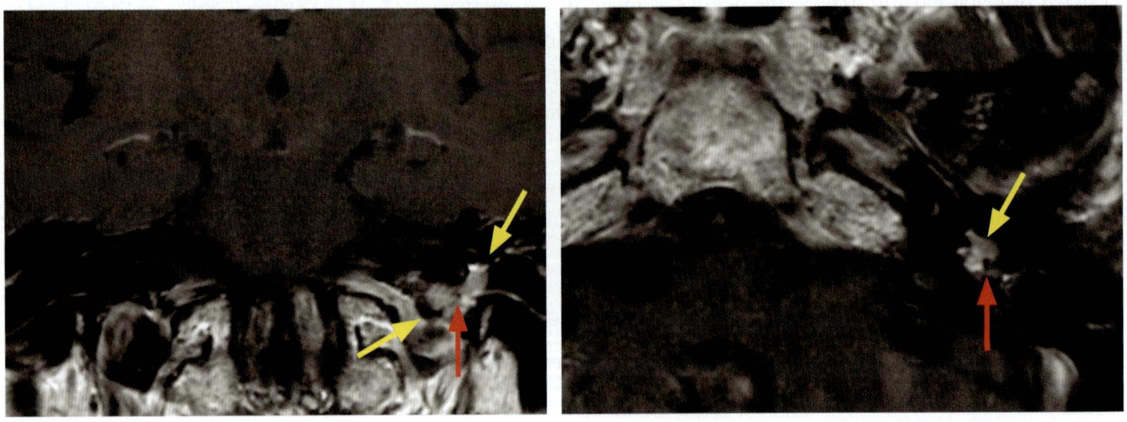

Glomus tympanicum: Coronal (left image) and axial post-contrast T1-weighted MRI demonstrates a heterogeneously enhancing lesion (yellow arrows) with apparent flow voids (red arrows) within the left middle ear.

鼓室球瘤：冠状位(左图)和轴位(右图)增强T_1加权MRI显示左侧中耳内不均匀强化病灶(黄箭)，伴明显的流空血流(红箭)。

- As paragangliomas are neuroendocrine tumors that express somatostatin receptor 2 (SSTR2), the most sensitive modality for their detection is Ga-68 DOTATATE PET-CT.

- 由于副神经节瘤是表达生长抑素受体2(SSTR2)的神经内分泌肿瘤，故其最敏感的检出方法是^{68}Ga-DOTATATE PET/CT。

Cholesteatoma

胆脂瘤

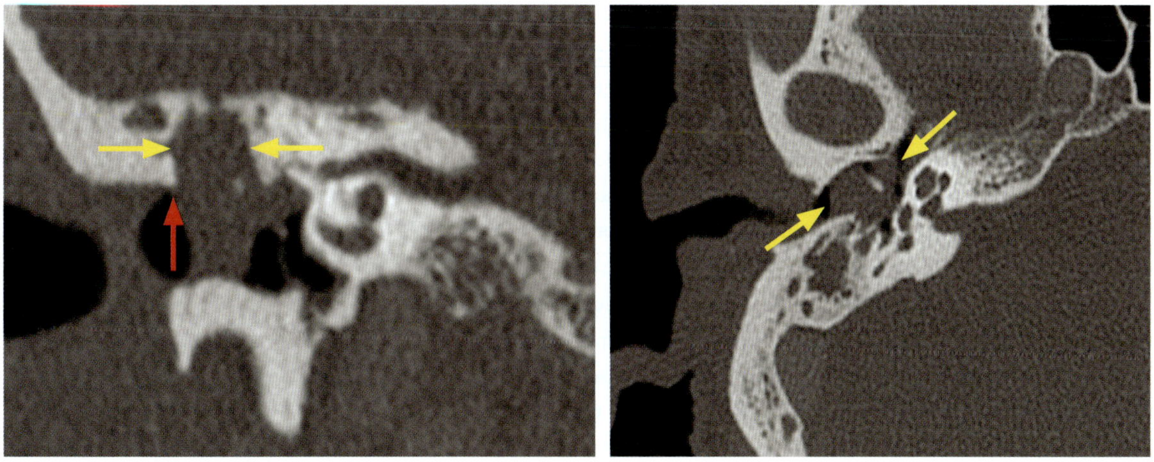

Middle ear cholesteatoma: Coronal (left image) and axial noncontrast CT through the right temporal bone demonstrates a soft tissue mass (yellow arrows) in the middle ear with near-complete erosion of the scutum (red arrow) and the ossicles, consistent with a cholesteatoma. There isopacification of the mastoid air cells.

Case courtesy Mary Beth Cunnane, MD, Massachusetts Eye and Ear Infirmary.

中耳胆脂瘤：右颞骨冠状位(左图)和轴位(右图)CT平扫显示中耳软组织肿块(黄箭)，盾板(红箭)和听小骨骨质几乎完全被侵蚀，符合胆脂瘤的表现。乳突气房密度增高。

- Cholesteatoma is a mass of exfoliated keratin lined by squamous epithelium in the temporal bone,which has been described as "skin in the wrong place." The name cholesteatoma is deceptive since the lesion does not contain cholesterol crystals or fat and is not neoplastic. The histologically identical intracranial counterpart is the epidermoid cyst.
- Cholesteatomas are among the causes of conductive hearing loss and of a white mass in the middle ear.
- Cholesteatomas are classified by etiology into acquired and congenital forms but they are histologically identical.

Acquired cholesteatoma represents the vast majority of cholesteatomas and can occur in both children and adults. Primary acquired cholesteatoma occurs in the setting of a tympanic membrane retraction pocket, which may be due to Eustachian tube dysfunction. Secondary acquired cholesteatoma occurs in the setting of tympanic membrane perforation, which may be due to chronic otitis media, trauma, or surgery.

Congenital cholesteatoma is uncommon and likely represents persistent fetal epithelial rests. They typically present in children without a history of tympanic membrane perforation, retraction, or surgery.

- The vast majority of cholesteatomas occur in the middle ear, although congenital cholesteatomas may also occur elsewhere in the temporal bone (e.g., EAC, mastoid, petrous apex).

Acquired cholesteatomas most commonly arise in the Prussak space, a part of the epitympanum lateral to the neck of the malleus; these are known as **pars flaccida cholesteatomas**.

In contrast, acquired **pars tensa cholesteatomas** and congenital middle ear cholesteatomas are typically medial to the ossicles.

- 胆脂瘤是颞骨内衬鳞状上皮脱落的角质团块，被称为"皮肤长错了地方"。胆脂瘤的命名其实具有误导性，因为该病变既不含有胆固醇结晶或脂肪，也不是肿瘤。发生在颅内有相同组织学的病变称为表皮样囊肿。
- 胆脂瘤是传导性听力障碍和出现中耳白色肿块的原因之一。
- 胆脂瘤按病因分为后天性和先天性，但它们在组织学上是相同的。

后天性胆脂瘤占胆脂瘤的大多数，可发生于儿童和成人。原发后天性胆脂瘤在鼓膜内陷袋的基础上发生，鼓膜内陷袋由咽鼓管功能障碍引起。继发后天性胆脂瘤发生在鼓膜穿孔时，见于慢性中耳炎、创伤或手术并发症。

先天性胆脂瘤并不常见，可能是胎儿上皮持续残余存留。常见于儿童，通常没有鼓膜穿孔、内陷袋及手术史。

- 绝大多数胆脂瘤发生在中耳，尽管先天性胆脂瘤也可发生在颞骨其他部位(如外耳道、乳突、岩尖)。

后天性胆脂瘤最常发生在蒲氏间隙，即锤骨颈部外侧的上鼓室部分，被称为**松弛部胆脂瘤**。

相反，后天性**紧张部胆脂瘤**和先天性中耳胆脂瘤通常位于听小骨的内侧。

- CT is sensitive for the detection of even a small cholesteatoma, which appears as a well-circumscribed soft tissue mass opacifying part of the middle ear cavity. However, opacification is nonspecific and may reflect effusion, granulation tissue, or fibrosis. Adjacent bony erosion, such as the wall of the middle ear cavity (earliest involving the scutum in pars flaccida cholesteatomas) or ossicles (most commonly the long process of the incus), favors cholesteatoma.

  Erosions of bone covering specific structures outside the middle ear cavity are important to identify so that they may be protected during cholesteatoma surgery: Lateral semicircular canal, facial nerve, and intracranial compartment (e.g., tegmen tympani,sigmoid plate).

- MRI is more specific for evaluating cholesteatoma, particularly in the postoperative surveillance setting, using DWI or post-contrast imaging. Similar to intracranial epidermoid cysts, cholesteatomas are hyperintense on DWI and do not enhance. Echo planar imaging (EPI) DWI techniques routinely used for the brain are prone to artifacts in the temporal bone, so non-EPI DWI is preferred for evaluation for cholesteatoma.

- CT对很小体积的胆脂瘤都非常敏感，表现为边界清楚的软组织肿块，伴中耳腔部分密度增高。然而，密度增高是非特异性的，可能代表积液、肉芽组织或纤维组织。出现邻近骨质破坏，如中耳壁(早期松弛部胆脂瘤累及鳞部)或听小骨(最常见的是砧骨的长突)，可支持胆脂瘤的诊断。

  识别中耳腔外特定结构的覆盖骨是否有破坏很重要，识别后可便于在胆脂瘤手术中保护它们，包括外侧半规管、面神经和颅内结构(如鼓室盖、乙状窦板)。

- MRI对评价胆脂瘤较具特异性，尤其是采用弥散加权成像和增强序列对术后进行随访。与颅内表皮样囊肿相似，胆脂瘤在弥散加权图像上呈高信号但不强化。常规用于头颅平面回波成像(EPI)弥散加权成像技术容易在颞骨中出现伪影，因此非EPI弥散加权成像是评估胆脂瘤的首选方法。

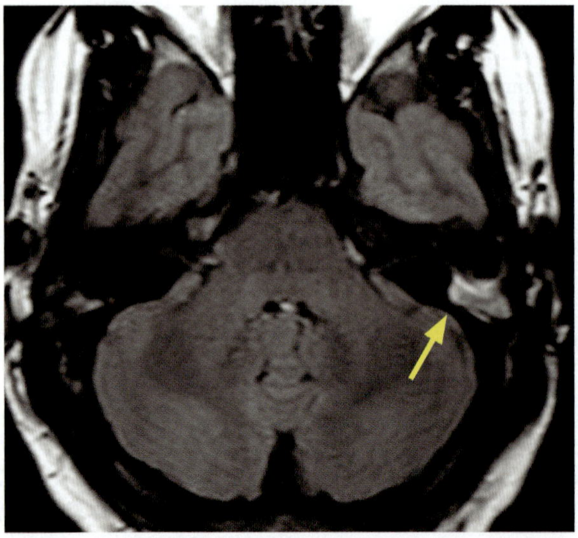

Middle ear cholesteatoma: T1-weighted axial MRI demonstrates iso- to slightly hyperintense (compared to gray matter) signal in the left middle ear (arrow).

中耳胆脂瘤：轴位 T_1 加权MRI显示左侧中耳(黄箭)内等信号至稍高信号(对比灰质)。

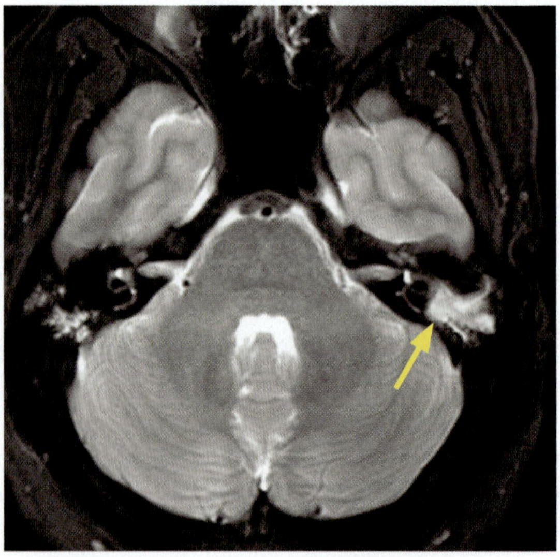

T2-weighted axial MRI with fat suppression shows that the lesion is slightly hyperintense (arrow).

轴位 T_2 加权MRI脂肪抑制显示病灶呈稍高信号(黄箭)。

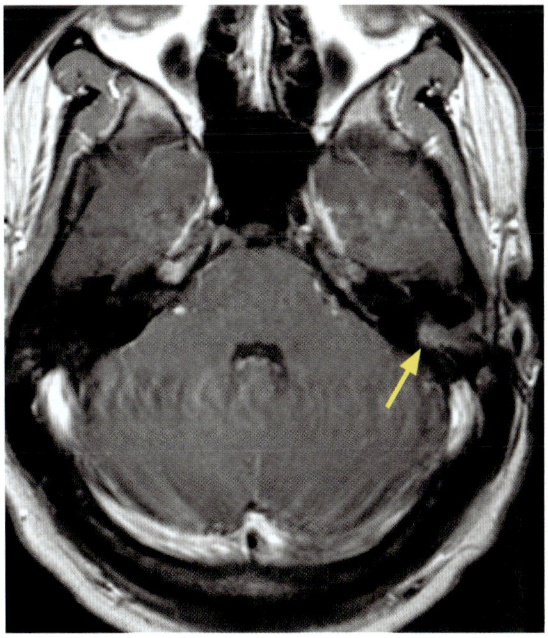

Post-contrast T1-weighted MRI shows no enhancement of the lesion (arrow).
增强T_1加权MRI显示病灶无强化(黄箭)。

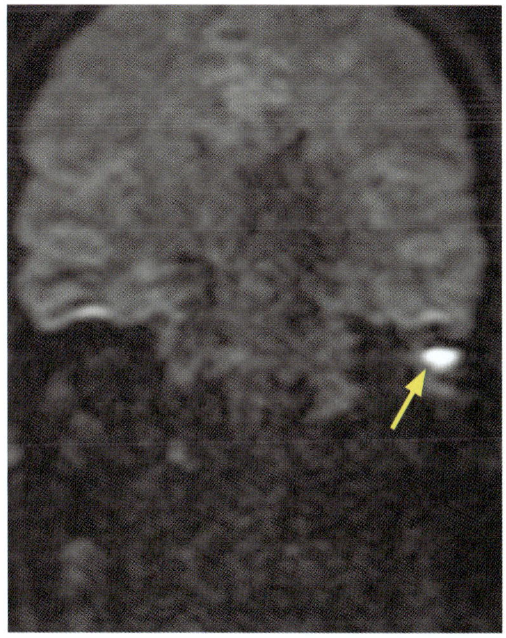

Coronal diffusion weighted image shows a focus of DWI hyperintensity in the left middle ear. Diffusion was restricted when correlated with the ADC map (not shown).
冠状位弥散加权成像显示左侧中耳弥散加权图像局灶性高信号，ADC图显示弥散受限(未展示)。

Case courtesy Mary Beth Cunnane, MD, Massachusetts Eye and Ear Infirmary.

Cholesterol granuloma

胆固醇肉芽肿

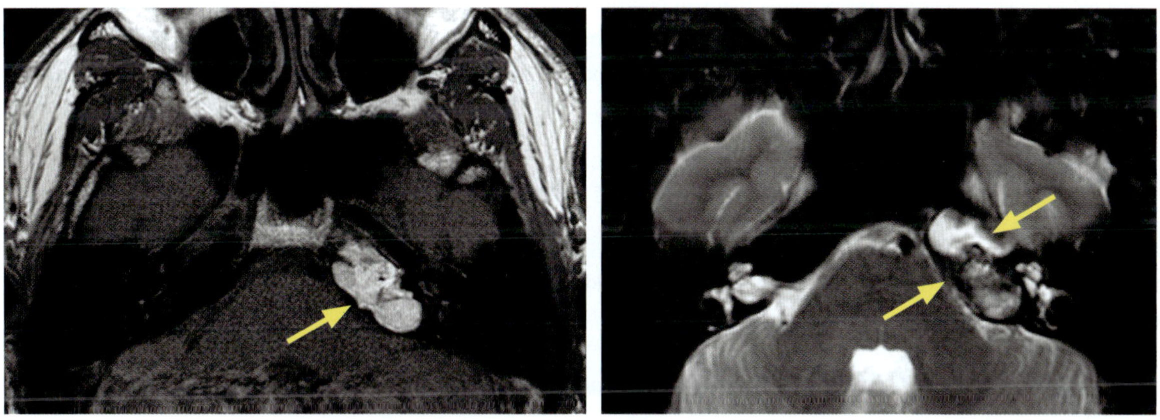

Petrous apex cholesterol granuloma: Axial T1-weighted (left image) and T2-weighted (right image) shows a lobulated T1 hyperintense, heterogeneously T2 hyperintense, expansile lesion in the left petrous apex (arrows). There is no associated restricted diffusion (not shown).
岩尖胆固醇肉芽肿：轴位T_1加权(左图)和T_2加权(右图)显示左侧岩尖T_1高信号、T_2不均匀高信号的分叶状膨胀性病变(黄箭)。不伴弥散受限(未展示)。

- Cholesterol granuloma is a unique type of granulation tissue associated with friable blood vessels. Histologically, it represents a giant cell reaction to cholesterol crystals.
- Cholesterol granulomas are most commonly located in a pneumatized petrous apex but can occur in any obstructed air space such as the mastoid and middle ear cavities.
- Cholesterol granulomas in the middle ear may present on otoscopy as a *blue retrotympanic mass* or as hemotympanum.
- Cholesterol granuloma can expand and thin the surrounding bone. On MRI,

- 胆固醇肉芽肿是一种特殊的肉芽肿，并发于脆弱的血管。组织学上，它是胆固醇结晶引起的巨细胞反应增生。
- 胆固醇肉芽肿最常位于充气的岩尖，但也可发生于其他阻塞的气腔，如乳突和中耳。
- 中耳胆脂瘤在耳镜检查可表现为鼓膜后蓝色肿块或类似鼓室积血。
- 胆固醇肉芽肿会使周围骨质膨胀或变薄。在MRI上，胆固醇肉芽肿因含有血液代谢物而

the lesions are typically hyperintense on T1-weighted images due to blood products and do not show restricted diffusion, unlike cholesteatoma.

Otomastoiditis

- Otomastoiditis refers to infection or inflammation in the middle ear and mastoid cavities. Various terms are used clinically to classify this spectrum based on duration (acute or chronic), presence and type of fluid (suppuration or serous effusion), and presence of tympanic membrane perforation and/or cholesteatoma.
- An imaging finding of fluid in the middle ear and mastoid is common and not specific for clinically significant inflammation or infection. Otomastoiditis remains a clinical diagnosis, while imaging is reserved to detect complications such as those below.
- **Coalescent mastoiditis** is the advanced stage of acute mastoiditis in which osteitis is present, defined on CT by resorption of the bony septae and thus merging of adjacent opacified mastoid air cells.

  Subperiosteal abscess results from coalescent mastoiditis that has eroded through the external mastoid cortex but remains contained by periosteum, usually in the postauricular region. Further progression through the periosteum is called a subcutaneous abscess.

  Erosion through the mastoid tip can result in abscess tracking either along the sternocleidomastoid muscle, called **Bezold abscess**, or along the posterior belly of the digastric muscle, called **Citelli abscess**.
- Intracranial complications are the main cause of mortality in acute and chronic otomastoiditis, including meningitis, epidural abscess, subdural empyema, cerebritis, brain abscess, and dural venous sinus thrombosis.
- Involvement of the inner ear (labyrinthitis) and petrous apex (petrous apicitis) are discussed later in this temporal bone section.
- Intratympanic sequelae of chronic otitis media that can contribute to hearing loss include middle ear effusion, granulation tissue, cholesteatoma, cholesterol granuloma, post-inflammatory ossicular fixation (including tympanosclerosis), and ossicular erosion (especially at the long process of the incus).

INTRATEMPORAL FACIAL NERVE

Anatomy of the intratemporal facial nerve

- The portion of the facial nerve within the temporal bone is divided into three segments:

> **Labyrinthine segment:** courses from the internal auditory canal to the geniculate ganglion (anterior genu), which is located superior to the cochlea.
>
> → Greater superficial petrosal nerve innervates salivation.
>
> **Tympanic (horizontal) segment:** courses posteriorly under the lateral semicircular canal to the posterior genu.
>
> **Mastoid (descending) segment:** courses inferiorly to the stylomastoid foramen.
>
> → Nerve to stapedius.
>
> → Chorda tympani (taste to anterior 2/3 of tongue).

- The portions of facial nerve that may normally enhance (related to its peri/epineural vascular plexus) on MRI are the geniculate ganglion, tympanic segment, and mastoid segment.
- Enhancement proximal to the geniculate ganglion, such as in the labyrinthine segment, or extracranial portion is abnormal.

通常表现为T_1加权高信号，无弥散受限，这与胆脂瘤不同。

中耳乳突炎

- 中耳乳突炎是指中耳和乳突的感染或炎症。临床使用不同的术语对该系列疾病进行分类，它们基于病变持续时间(急性或慢性)、积液的存在与否和性质(化脓性或浆液性)，以及鼓膜是否穿孔和/或存在胆脂瘤。
- 影像上常见中耳和乳突积液，但这对临床上常见的感染或炎症并没有特异性。中耳乳突炎主要是一种临床诊断，而影像学检查仅用于发现其并发症，如下所述。
- **融合性乳突炎**是指并发骨髓炎的急性乳突炎进展期，CT表现为乳突间隔吸收，因而发生邻近乳突气房融合并且密度增高。

  融合性乳突炎会导致骨膜下脓肿，它侵蚀至乳突骨壁的外皮层，但还在骨膜内，通常位于耳廓后。若继续进展并穿透骨膜，则称为皮下脓肿。

  病变侵蚀穿透乳突尖会导致脓肿沿着胸锁乳突肌蔓延，即为**贝佐尔德脓肿**，若沿二腹肌的后腹蔓延，即为**Citelli脓肿**。
- 颅内并发症是急慢性乳突炎导致死亡的主要原因，包括脑膜、硬膜外脓肿、硬膜下脓肿、脑炎、脑脓肿和硬膜静脉窦血栓形成。
- 内耳(迷路炎)和岩尖部(岩尖炎)的受累并发症将在后续颞骨部分进行讨论。
- 慢性中耳炎引起的鼓室内并发症可导致听力障碍，包括中耳积液、肉芽肿、胆脂瘤、胆固醇肉芽肿、炎症后听骨链强直(包括鼓室硬化)和听小骨骨质破坏(尤其是砧骨的长突)。

颞骨内面神经

颞骨内面神经解剖

- 颞骨内的面神经分为三段：

> **迷路段**：起自内听道，行于耳蜗上方，至膝状神经节(前膝)。
>
> →岩浅大神经支配腺体分泌。
>
> **鼓室段(水平段)**：走行于外侧半规管的后方至后膝。
>
> **乳突段(垂直段)**：向下走行至茎乳孔。
>
> →神经支配镫骨肌。
>
> →到达鼓索(传导舌前2/3味觉)。

- 在MRI上呈正常强化的部分面神经包括膝状神经节、鼓室段和乳突段面神经(与神经周围/神经外血管丛相关)。
- 膝状神经节前(如迷路段)或颅外段面神经增强是异常的。

Facial nerve schwannoma

面神经鞘瘤

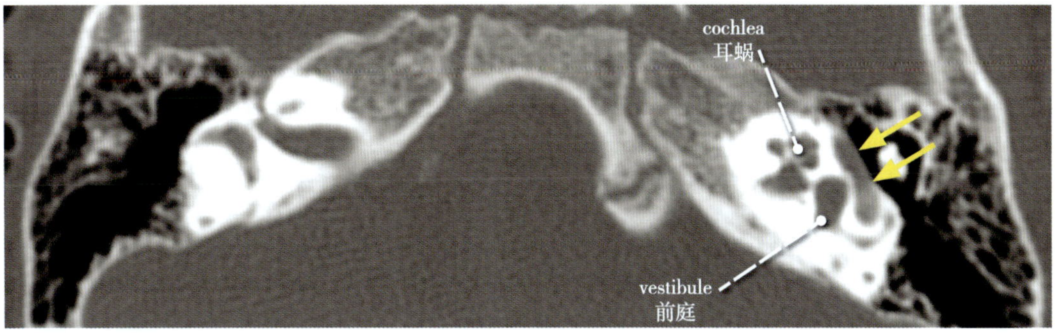

Facial nerve schwannoma: Axial CT through the temporal bone in a child shows subtle enlargement of the tympanic segment of the left facial nerve canal (arrows).
Case courtesy Sanjay Prabhu, MD, Boston Children's Hospital.
面神经鞘瘤：儿童患者颞骨轴位CT显示左侧面神经管鼓室段轻微扩张(黄箭)。

- Within the temporal bone, schwannomas of the facial nerve (CN Ⅶ) tend to be slow growing and most commonly involve the geniculate ganglion, followed by the labyrinthine and tympanic segments.
- The majority of patients with facial nerve schwannoma present with facial nerve palsy; however, up to 30% present without facial nerve symptoms. Larger facial nerve schwannomas can interfere with ossicular function, causing conductive hearing loss.
- On CT, the typical finding of a facial nerve schwannoma is enlargement of the bony canal through which the involved portion of the facial nerve passes. There is typically no calcification. The tumor usually demonstrates brisk contrast enhancement on MRI.

- 在颞骨内，面神经(第Ⅶ脑神经)鞘瘤往往生长缓慢，并最常累及膝状神经节，其次是迷路段和鼓室段。
- 多数面神经鞘瘤患者表现为面神经麻痹，但有多达30%无面部神经症状。较大的面神经鞘瘤会影响听小骨功能，导致传导性耳聋。
- 面神经鞘瘤典型的CT表现为病变穿过部分的面神经管扩大。通常没有钙化。肿瘤往往在MRI上有明显强化。

Facial nerve venous malformation

- Facial nerve venous malformations, previously described as hemangiomas, are perineural vascular lesions involving the petrous temporal bone.
- Facial nerve venous malformation is most commonly seen in the region of the geniculate ganglion, followed by the IAC, and least commonly at the posterior genu.
- This lesion characteristically has an expansile *honeycomb appearance* with intralesional bone spicules on CT, a pattern previously termed ossifying hemangioma. On MR, the lesion is characterized by heterogeneous signal intensity on T2-weighted imaging and avid enhancement.

面神经静脉畸形

- 面神经静脉畸形，以前称为血管瘤，是神经周围血管病变累及颞骨岩尖。
- 面神经静脉畸形最常见于膝状神经节的部位，其次是IAC，最不常见的是后膝。
- 该病变在CT上的特征性表现为膨胀性蜂窝状病灶，伴有病变内骨针，既往称之为骨化型血管瘤。在MRI上，特征是T_2加权信号不均匀，并有显著强化。

Idiopathic and infectious causes of facial nerve enhancement

特发性和感染性面神经强化

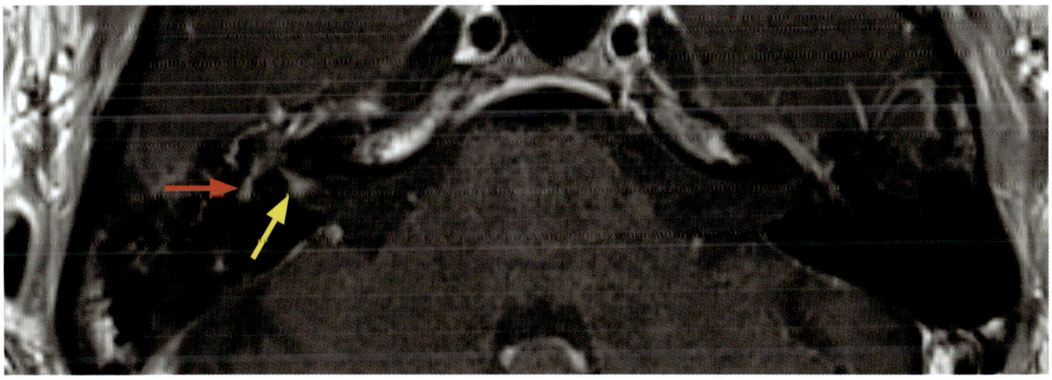

Axial post-contrast T1-weighted MRI demonstrates right facial nerve enhancement in the IAC (yellow arrow) and faint cochlea enhancement (red arrow), consistent with Ramsey Hunt syndrome in this patient with right facial weakness, sensorineural hearing loss, and a rash in the EAC.
增强轴位T_1加权MRI显示右侧IAC内面神经强化(黄箭)，耳蜗轻微强化(红箭)，符合拉姆齐-亨特综合征(肌阵挛性小脑协调障碍)，该患者右侧面肌无力、感音神经性听力障碍和外耳道皮疹。

- In addition to schwannoma and venous malformations, the differential diagnosis for abnormal facial nerve enhancement includes infectious etiologies such as Lyme disease and herpes zoster oticus (Ramsay Hunt syndrome) and idiopathic facial neuropathy.
- **Idiopathic facial neuropathy,** eponymously named *Bell's palsy*, is the most common syndrome of acute-onset, unilateral facial weakness.

  Herpes simplex virus type-1 reactivation within the geniculate ganglion has been proposed as an etiology, resulting in demyelination and inflammation of the facial nerve. Facial paralysis is usually preceded by a viral prodrome.

  History and physical examination is generally sufficient for diagnosis. Imaging is generally performed to rule out other etiologies in patients presenting with atypical symptoms, recurrent symptoms, or slow recovery. The majority of patients have a complete recovery within 6 months.

  MRI demonstrates a uniformly enhancing, normal sized or mildly thickened facial nerve commonly extending from the intracanalicular segment to the tympanic segment. Enhancement may persist following clinical improvement.
- Enhancement of the facial nerve accompanied by enhancement in the internal auditory canal and labyrinth, and vesicles within the EAC are suggestive of **Ramsay Hunt syndrome**.
- **Lyme disease** is caused by *Borrelia burgdorferi*. Clinically, these patients present with a rash and can have arthritis and myocarditis.

Perineural tumor spread along the facial nerve

- Parotid malignancies such as lymphoma and adenoid cystic carcinoma and adjacent skin malignancies that secondarily invade the parotid gland have a propensity for perineural spread along the facial nerve.
- Facial nerve involvement occurs more frequently and in earlier stages in the extratemporal portion of the facial nerve. Proximally, the stylomastoid foramen segment and the descending segments can be involved.
- MRI demonstrates enlargement of the facial nerve with patchy enhancement, enlargement of the stylomastoid foramen, or loss of the normal fat signal surrounding the nerve within the foramen.

- 除了神经鞘瘤和静脉畸形外，面部神经异常增强的鉴别诊断还包括感染性病因，如莱姆病和耳带状疱疹(拉姆齐-亨特综合征)和特发性面神经麻痹。
- **特发性面神经麻痹**，又称贝尔麻痹，是最常见的急性发作的导致单侧面肌障碍的综合征。

  膝状神经节内1型单纯疱疹病毒重新激活被认为是其病因，并会导致脱髓鞘和面神经炎。面神经麻痹通常有前驱病毒感染的症状。

  病史和体格检查通常足够进行诊断。对于症状不典型、反复发作或恢复缓慢的患者，一般采用影像学检查来排除其他病因。大多数患者可在6个月内完全康复。

  MRI显示内耳道段至鼓室段的面神经常常呈均匀性增强，直径正常或轻度增粗。临床症状改善后依旧会持续强化。
- 面神经强化伴内耳道和迷路强化，以及外耳道内疱疹，提示**肌阵挛性小脑协调障碍**。
- **莱姆病**是由伯氏疏螺旋体引起的。临床上，这些患者表现为皮疹，并可能有关节炎和心肌炎。

神经周围肿瘤沿面神经扩散

- 腮腺恶性肿瘤，如淋巴瘤和腺样囊性癌，以及侵犯腮腺的邻近皮肤恶性肿瘤有沿面神经扩散的倾向。
- 面神经常常受累，较早发生于颞骨外段。在近端，可累及面神经茎乳孔段和降段。
- MRI显示面神经增粗、伴斑片状强化、茎乳孔增大，或者孔内神经周围正常脂肪信号消失。

Inner Ear

Anatomy of the inner ear

- The inner ear is situated within the petrous portion of the temporal bone and comprises the **otic capsule** (also known as the bony labyrinth). The otic capsule is the osseous superstructure containing the fluid-filled spaces of the cochlea, vestibule, and semicircular canals. The otic capsule is the densest bone in the body.
- The **cochlea** is a conical structure consisting of a bony two-and-a-half turn spiral canal, including the basal, middle and apical turns, around a central core called the **modiolus**. The modiolus contains the cells of the spiral ganglion and corresponds to the exit of the cochlear nerve towards the internal auditory canal.
- The spiral of the cochlea is separated by osseous spiral lamina and consists of the scala tympani, scala media, and scala vestibuli.
- The **scala media**, also known as the cochlear duct, separates the scala vestibuli and the scala tympani, contains endolymph and the organ of Corti, the receptor organ for hearing comprised of sensory epithelium containing numerous neuroepithelial hair cells, which send electrical impulses to the spiral ganglia of the cochlea.
- The **scala tympani** and **scala vestibuli** contain perilymph. They communicate at the apex of themodiolus by a small opening, the helicotrema.

内耳

内耳解剖

- 内耳位于颞骨岩尖，包含**耳囊**(又称骨迷路)。耳囊是超骨骼结构，包含充满液体的耳蜗、前庭及半规管。耳囊是人体密度最高的骨骼结构。
- **耳蜗**是一个锥形结构，含有卷曲两周半的螺旋骨管，包括顶圈、中间圈和底圈，围绕的中心称**蜗轴**。蜗轴包含螺旋神经节的细胞，相当于耳蜗的传出神经，通向内耳道。
- 耳蜗螺旋被骨螺旋板分隔，由鼓室阶、中阶和前庭阶所组成。
- **中阶**，也称为蜗管，分隔前庭阶和鼓阶，内含内淋巴液和螺旋器。螺旋器是听觉感受器，由内含丰富神经上皮毛细胞的感觉上皮组成，它们将电脉冲传导至耳蜗螺旋神经节。
- **鼓阶**和**前庭阶**包含外淋巴液，在蜗轴顶端通过一个小孔交通，即蜗孔。

Hydraulic pressure created in the perilymph by the vibrations of the stapes against the oval window ascends to the apex of the cochlea by the scala vestibuli. Pressure waves descend back to the basal turn through the scala tympani. The vibrations from the scala tympani are transmitted through the round window, where the energy is dissipated.

- The **cochlear aqueduct**, also known as the cochlear canaliculus, extends from the scala tympani to the subarachnoid space, opening on the inferior surface of the petrous portion of the temporal bone. This theoretically allows for equilibration between the perilymphatic space and the subarachnoid space.
- The **vestibule** is an ovoid perilymphatic space which is continuous with the cochlea anteriorly and the semicircular canals posteriorly, and contains the utricle and saccule, the sense organs involved in balance. The semicircular canals are oriented orthogonal to one another.
- The **vestibular aqueduct** connects the crus commune (the common channel of the superior and posterior semicircular canals) to the posterior cranial fossa and contains the endolymphatic duct and sac.
- The **endolymphatic duct** arises from the utricle and saccule and ends in a blind pouch, the **endolymphatic sac**, at the posterior margin of the petrous ridge. The endolymphatic sac acts as a reservoir for endolymph and the site for reabsorption into the epidural space.

镫骨振动前庭窗产生外淋巴液压力，经前庭阶向上传递至耳蜗顶。压力波再经鼓阶回传至耳蜗底，鼓阶振动通过圆窗传播，能量消散于此。

- **蜗水管**，又称蜗小管，从鼓阶延伸向蛛网膜下腔，开口于颞骨岩部的下方。理论上，它维持着淋巴管周围空间和蛛网膜下腔之间的平衡。
- **前庭**是一个卵形的外淋巴空间，前方与耳蜗相通，后方与半规管相通。前庭包括椭圆囊和球囊，参与平衡机制。三个半规管相互垂直。
- **前庭水管**连接总脚(上半规管和后半规管的共用通道)和颅后窝，内含内淋巴管和淋巴囊。
- **内淋巴管**起自椭圆囊和球囊，止于岩脊后缘的盲端袋状结构，即**内淋巴囊**。内淋巴囊起到内淋巴液储存器的作用，也是硬膜外腔重吸收的部位。

Congenital anomalies

- Congenital anomalies of the inner ear are divided into two broad categories: malformations that involve only the membranous labyrinth and malformations that involve both the osseous and membranous labyrinth (e.g., malformed otic capsules).
- Several types of membranous labyrinth malformation have been described, the classification of which is not useful radiologically as differentiation is made on histopathologic examination.
- Conversely, radiologic identification and characterization of malformations of both the osseous and membranous labyrinth significantly impacts management strategy and prognosis and will be discussed in more detail.

先天性畸形

- 先天性内耳畸形分为两大类：单纯膜迷路畸形、畸形同时累及骨迷路和膜迷路(如畸形耳囊)。
- 有数种类型的膜迷路畸形的报道，但分类是基于组织病理学，对放射学鉴别诊断没有什么帮助。
- 相反，骨迷路和膜迷路联合畸形在放射学上的表现和特征对治疗决策和预后评价有重要影响，后文将对此进行更详细的讨论。

Type Ⅱ incomplete partition (Mondini deformity)

Ⅱ型不完全分隔(Mondini畸形)

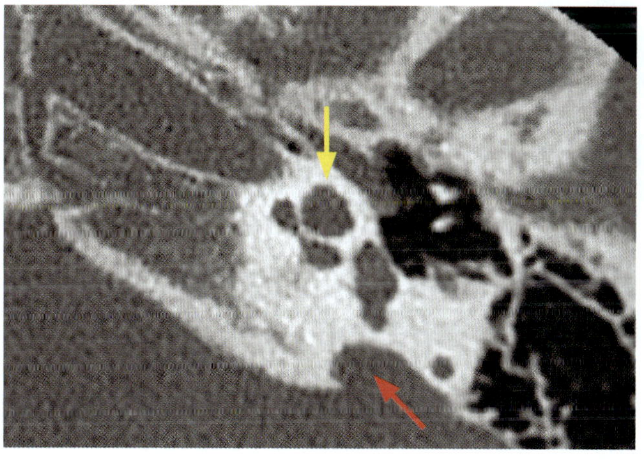

Axial noncontrast CT through the left temporal bone shows cochlear hypoplasia with 1.5 turns and a cystic apex representing fusion of the middle and apical turns (yellow arrow). The modiolus is deficient and the lateral interscalar septum is absent. An ipsilaterally enlarged vestibular aqueduct is also present (red arrow).

左侧颞骨轴位平扫CT显示耳蜗发育不全，只有1.5圈，顶端呈囊状，代表中圈和顶圈融合(黄箭)。蜗轴不完全缺失，耳蜗外侧分隔缺失。同侧前庭水管也出现增大(红箭)。

- The most common form of congenital cochlear dysplasia, accounting for more than 50% of all cochlear deformities. It consists of a cochlea with 1.5 turns and absence of the interscalar septum and osseous spiral lamina. The basal turn appears normal and the middle and apical turns coalesce to form a cystic apex.
- Although the correct nomenclature for this anomaly is incomplete partition

- Ⅱ型不完全分隔是最常见的先天性耳蜗发育不全，占所有耳蜗畸形的50%以上。其特征为耳蜗有1.5圈，缺乏内隔膜和骨性螺旋板。基底圈看起来正常，而中圈和顶圈融合成囊性蜗顶。
- 这种异常的准确术语应称为Ⅱ型不完全分

type Ⅱ, it is commonly and historically referred to as the Mondini deformity. The use of the eponym *Mondini* to describe cochlear dysplasia is controversial and probably best avoided, as there is confusion amongst radiologists regarding the exact malformation originally described.

- There is strong association with an enlarged vestibule and enlarged vestibular aqueduct and normal semicircular canals.

Type Ⅰ incomplete partition (cystic cochleovestibular malformation)

- Type Ⅰ incomplete partition accounts for about 6% of all cochlear malformations. It is characterized by a complete absence of themodiolus, a cystic appearance of the cochlea, and a dilated appearance of the vestibule, forming a *figure 8*. The cochlea and vestibule are distinct, distinguishing from a common cavity.

Common cavity

- A common cavity accounts for about 25% of all cochlear malformations. It is defined by the absence of the normal differentiation between the cochlea and vestibule.

Cochlear hypoplasia

- Cochlear hypoplasia accounts for about 15% of all cochlear malformations. This results in aberration in the development of the cochlear duct during the sixth week of gestation. It is defined by the presence of a small cochlear bud arising from an abnormally small and deformed vestibule, usually with only one or a partial turn. Frequently it is accompanied by an abnormally small IAC.

Cochlear aplasia

- Cochlear aplasiais rare and accounts for about 3% of all cochlear malformations. It is characterized by an absent cochlea with a normal or deformed vestibule and semicircular canals.

Complete labyrinthine aplasia (Michel aplasia)

隔，但既往习惯的叫法为Mondini畸形。以Mondini的名字命名耳蜗发育不良存有争议且应避免使用，因为这容易使放射科医生误解最初所描述的到底是什么样的畸形。

- 这种异常往往伴有前庭扩大、前庭水管扩张和正常的半规管。

Ⅰ型不完全分隔(囊状耳蜗-前庭畸形)

- Ⅰ型不完全分隔约占所有耳蜗畸形的6%。它以耳蜗轴完全缺失为特征，耳蜗呈囊状，前庭扩张，形成8字征。耳蜗和前庭可相互区分，不同于共同腔畸形。

共同腔畸形

- 共同腔畸形约占所有耳蜗畸形的25%。该病为耳蜗和前庭之间缺乏正常的分化。

耳蜗发育不全

- 耳蜗发育不全约占所有耳蜗畸形的15%，为妊娠第6周耳蜗导管发育异常所致。该病起自畸形小前庭的小耳蜗芽，通常只有一个或不足一个圈，常伴有一个异常小的IAC。

耳蜗未发育

- 耳蜗未发育很少见，约占所有耳蜗畸形的3%，特征为耳蜗缺失，前庭和半规管正常或畸形。

完全性迷路发育不全(Michel畸形)

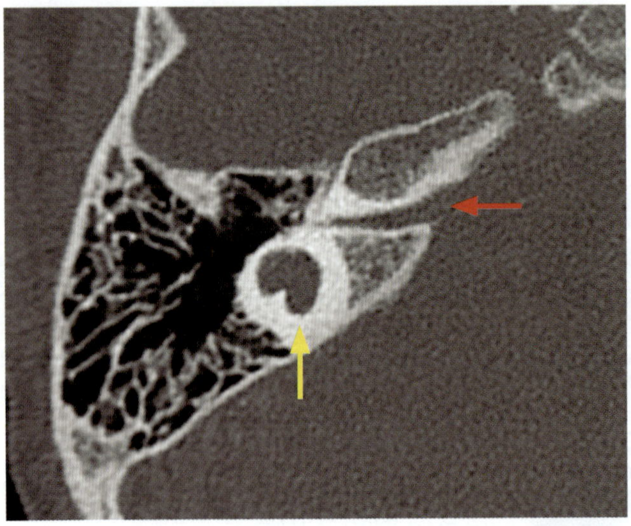

Axial noncontrast CT through the right temporal bone demonstrates absence of the cochlea, a dysplastic vestibule (yellow arrow), and hypoplastic semicircular canals (not shown). The IAC is small and stenotic (red arrow).

右颞骨轴位平扫CT显示耳蜗缺如，前庭发育不良(黄箭)，半规管发育不良(未展示)。IAC小且狭窄(红箭)。

- Michel aplasia is the most severe form of inner ear deformity and is defined by complete absence of the inner ear structures. On CT, an atretic IAC is seen without visualization of CN Ⅷ. It is extremely rare, and accounts for only 1% of all inner ear malformations.
- This can be unilateral or bilateral; however, when unilateral, the contralateral side is frequently also dysplastic.
- This is frequently associated with abnormalities in structures arising from the otic capsule, including hypoplasia of the petrous bone, absence of the round and oval windows, flattening of the medial wall of the inner ear cavity.

- **完全性迷路发育不全**是最严重的内耳变形，为内耳结构完全缺失。CT上可见闭锁的IAC，CN Ⅷ不可见。这种疾病极为罕见，只占所有内耳畸形的1%。
- 此异常可以是单侧或者双侧的；若为单侧，对侧内耳也往往发育不良。
- 这种畸形常伴有由耳囊起源的结构异常，包括岩骨发育不全、圆窗和前庭窗缺如、内耳内侧壁扁平。

Enlarged vestibular aqueduct syndrome

前庭水管扩大综合征

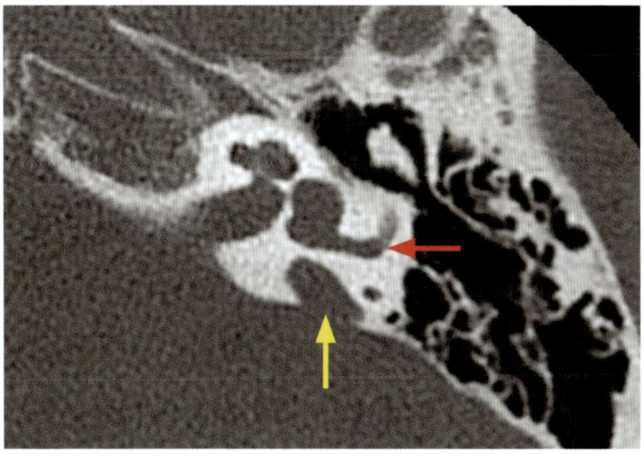

Axial noncontrast CT through the left temporal bone demonstrates an enlarged vestibular aqueduct (yellow arrow). Note size comparison to the adjacent semicircular canal (red arrow)
左颞骨轴位平扫CT显示前庭水管扩大(黄箭)。注意与邻近半规管的大小比较(红箭)。

- When CT imaging is positive for workup of unexplained sensorineural hearing loss, the most common finding is an enlarged vestibular aqueduct. The pathophysiology behind the association with an enlarged vestibular aqueduct and sensorineural hearing loss is not known. Multiple studies have shown that the probability of progressive hearing loss increases linearly with increasing width.
- There is an association with other inner ear anomalies, such as modiolar deficiency and incomplete partition type Ⅱ.
- The measurement criteria are referred to as the Cincinnati criteria, which defines enlargement as >1.9 mm at the operculum and/or >0.9 mm at the midpoint in a child.
- As an internal reference, the vestibular aqueduct should not be larger than the posterior semicircular canal, which is often seen at the same level in the axial plane.

- CT检查在不明原因感音神经性听力障碍时的最常见阳性发现是前庭水管扩大。这种前庭水管扩大和感音神经性听力障碍的病理生理学机制尚不清楚。多项研究表明，渐进性听力障碍的概率随前庭水管宽度的增加而呈线性增加。
- 此病与其他内耳异常有关，如蜗轴缺失和Ⅱ型不完全分隔。
- 前庭水管测量标准采用Cincinnati标准，儿童在顶盖处的管径>1.9mm和/或在中点处管径>0.9mm时被定义为增粗。
- 作为自身参照，前庭水管不应宽于同一横轴层面上的后半规管。

Causes of conductive hearing loss

传导性听力障碍的病因

Otospongiosis (otosclerosis)

耳海绵化症(耳硬化症)

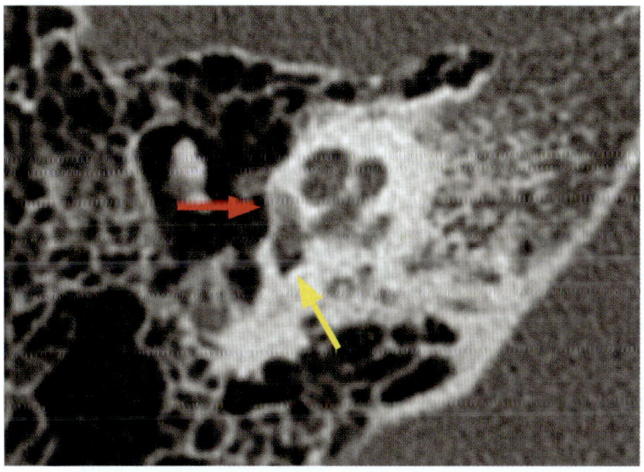

Fenestral otospongiosis: Axial noncontrast CT through the right temporal bone demonstrates focal demineralization in the bone anterior to the oval window (yellow arrow) at the fissula ante fenestram (red arrow).
窗型耳海绵化症：右侧颞骨轴位平扫CT显示前庭窗前方(黄箭)和窗前裂(红箭)局灶骨质软化。

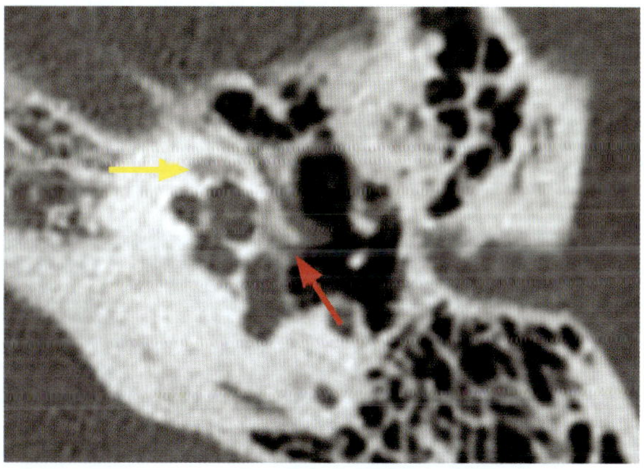

Retrofenestral otospongiosis: Axial noncontrast CT through the left temporal bone shows focal demineralization of the cochlear capsule (yellow arrow). There is also demineralization of the fissula ante fenestram (fenestral otospongiosis, red arrow).
窗后型耳海绵化症：左侧颞骨轴位平扫CT显示耳蜗囊局灶骨质软化(黄箭)。同时可见窗前裂骨质软化(窗型耳海绵化症，红箭)。

- Otospongiosis, otherwise known as otosclerosis, is a primary bone dysplasia of the otic capsule characterized by replacement of normal endochondral bone by irregular spongy bone. Otospongiosis occurs most commonly in young and middle-aged women and is bilateral 85% of the time.
- Patients present with predominantly conductive hearing loss earlier on, and a mixed conductive and sensorineural hearing loss later in the disease process.
- The two main types of otospongiosis are fenestraland retrofenestral types.

> The **fenestral** type of otospongiosis is more common, occurs at the fissula ante fenestram (located directly anterior to the oval window), and usually affects the oval window.
> The **retrofenestral** (cochlear) type is thought to represent a more severe form with involvement of the otic capsule separable from the oval window, typically involving the cochlear capsule, with possible extension to the vestibule, semicircular canals, and IAC. Involvement of the cochlear promontory can result in a red-tinged appearance on otologic examination, termed the *Schwartze sign*.

- CT is the best imaging modality for evaluation of otospongiosis. In the earlier, vascular phase, there is replacement of dense bone with demineralized bone, resulting in a less dense appearance. In a later, less active phase, the bone becomes more dense and sclerotic.
- The differential diagnosis of cochlear demineralization includes retrofenestral otospongiosis, osteogenesis imperfecta in a child, fibrous dysplasia in a young adult, and Paget disease in an older adult.

Round window occlusion

- Round window occlusion can occur with inflammatory tissue, bone lesions, high-riding jugular bulb, or congenital absence.
- These abnormalities can result in conductive hearing loss by adding resistance to acoustic energy entering the cochlea and requiring more energy to displace the basilar membrane.

Superior semicircular canal dehiscence

- A bony defect in the superior semicircular canal results in dispersion of sound energy along the canal, creating a "third window" with less energy available to the cochlea. The resultant drop in sound wave amplitude leads to conductive hearing loss. The abnormal movement of the endolymph can lead to a variety of vestibular and cochlear symptoms referred to as the "third window phenomenon."

Infectious and inflammatory conditions of the inner ear

Labyrinthitis

- 耳海绵化症，又称耳硬化症，是一种原发性听软骨囊的骨性发育不全，以正常软骨内骨被不规则的疏松骨质替代。耳海绵化症最常见于青年和中年女性，且85%为双侧发病。
- 大多患者早期表现为传导性听力障碍，晚期表现为传导性和感音神经性混合听力障碍。
- 耳海绵化症分两型：窗型和窗后型。

> **窗型**耳海绵化症较常见，发生于窗前裂(紧邻前庭窗前方)，常累及前庭窗。
> **窗后型**(耳蜗型)被认为是较严重的类型，涉及前庭窗与听软骨囊分离，通常累及耳蜗囊，并可能延伸至前庭、半规管和IAC。累及耳蜗鼓岬时可在耳科检查发现其红染，称为Schwartze征。

- CT是评价耳海绵化症的最佳成像技术。在疾病早期的血管期，致密骨被脱钙骨取代，从而密度降低。在后期的非活跃期，骨骼变得更加致密和硬化。
- 耳蜗脱钙的鉴别诊断包括：窗后型耳海绵化症、儿童成骨不全，青年骨纤维发育不全及老年佩吉特病。

圆窗闭锁

- 圆窗闭锁可见于炎症组织、骨性病变，高位颈静脉球及先天性圆窗缺如。
- 这些异常会导致传导性听力障碍，因为它们增加了声能进入耳蜗时的阻力，从而需要更高的声能来振动基底膜。

上半规管裂

- 上半规管的骨性缺损导致声能沿声道分散，形成"第三窗"，导致耳蜗可用能量减少。声波振幅的下降会导致传导性听力障碍。内淋巴运动异常可导致前庭和耳蜗的各种症状，被称为"第三窗现象"。

内耳感染和炎性病变

迷路炎

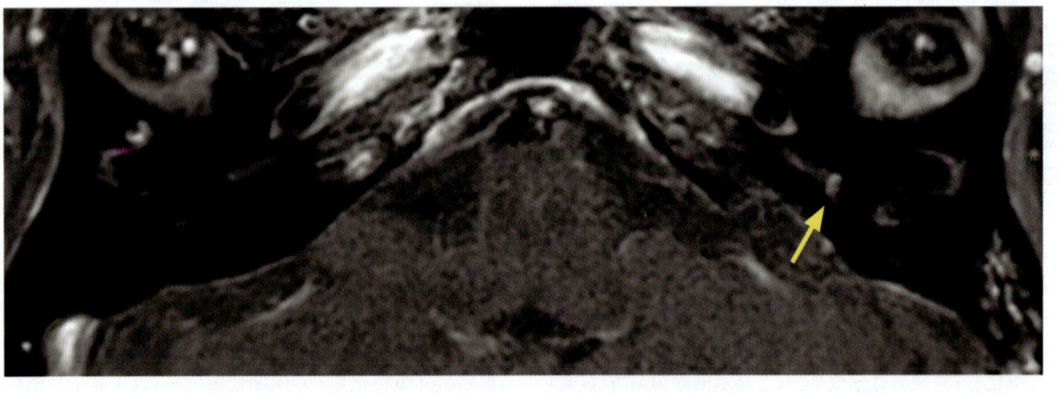

Acute labyrinthitis: Axial post-contrast T1-weighted MRI demonstrates increased enhancement within the inner ear (arrow).
急性迷路炎：轴位增强T_1加权MRI显示内耳强化(黄箭)。

- Labyrinthitis is inflammation of the inner ear, which may be infectious or autoimmune.
- Labyrinthitis has been divided into three stages of chronicity based on the imaging (primarily MR) characteristics.
- **Acute labyrinthitis** is the earliest stage, presenting as pus in the inner ear. The only MRI signal abnormality of acute labyrinthitis is enhancement of the affected inner ear structures.

  The main differential consideration is a cochlear or intra-labyrinthine schwannoma. A schwannoma tends to be focal and discrete, while labyrinthitis may produce more diffuse enhancement.
- **Fibrous labyrinthitis** represents the replacement of endolymph and perilymph with fibrous strands that cause decreased signal intensity on T2-weighted images. There may be mild (but decreased) residual post-contrast enhancement of the affected structures.
- **Labyrinthitis ossificans** is the final stage of the disease. Calcified debris replaces the normal endolymph and perilymph. CT is the best way to image labyrinthitis ossificans, as the calcification causes decreased signal intensity on T2-weighted MRI and lack of enhancement.

- 迷路炎即内耳的炎症，可以是感染性的，或是自身免疫性的。
- 迷路炎可根据影像(主要是MR)特征分为3期。
- **急性迷路炎**是最早期，表现为内耳积脓。急性迷路炎MRI信号异常的唯一表现是内耳受累结构强化。

  主要鉴别要考虑耳蜗或迷路内神经鞘瘤。神经鞘瘤往往是局灶性和清晰的，而迷路炎则可呈弥漫强化。
- **纤维性迷路炎**是指内、外淋巴液被纤维条索替代，T_2加权图像信号减低。病变区可能会出现轻微残留的强化(较正常减低)。
- **骨化性迷路炎**是疾病的最后一期。钙化斑块替代了正常的内、外淋巴液，CT可显示骨迷路钙化最佳，因钙化灶在T_2加权MRI上呈低信号，无强化。

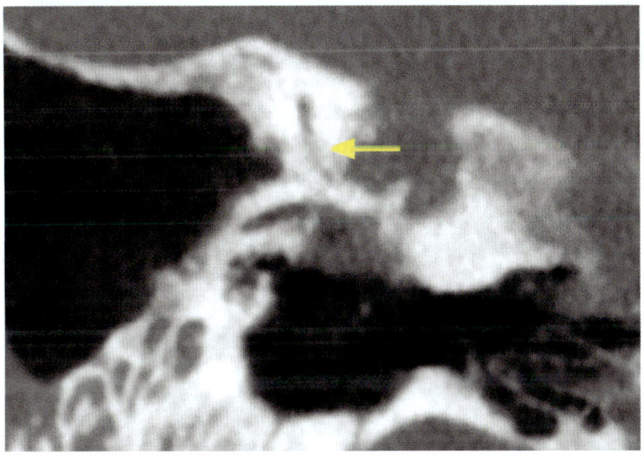

Labyrinthitis ossificans: Coronal noncontrast CT through the right temporal bone demonstrates partial mineralization of the anterior limb of the superior semicircular canal (arrow).
骨化性迷路炎：右颞骨冠状位CT平扫显示上半规管前肢部分骨化(黄箭)。

Cerebellopontine angle (CPA) mass

桥小脑角(CPA)肿块

Overview and anatomy of the CPA

CPA概述和解剖

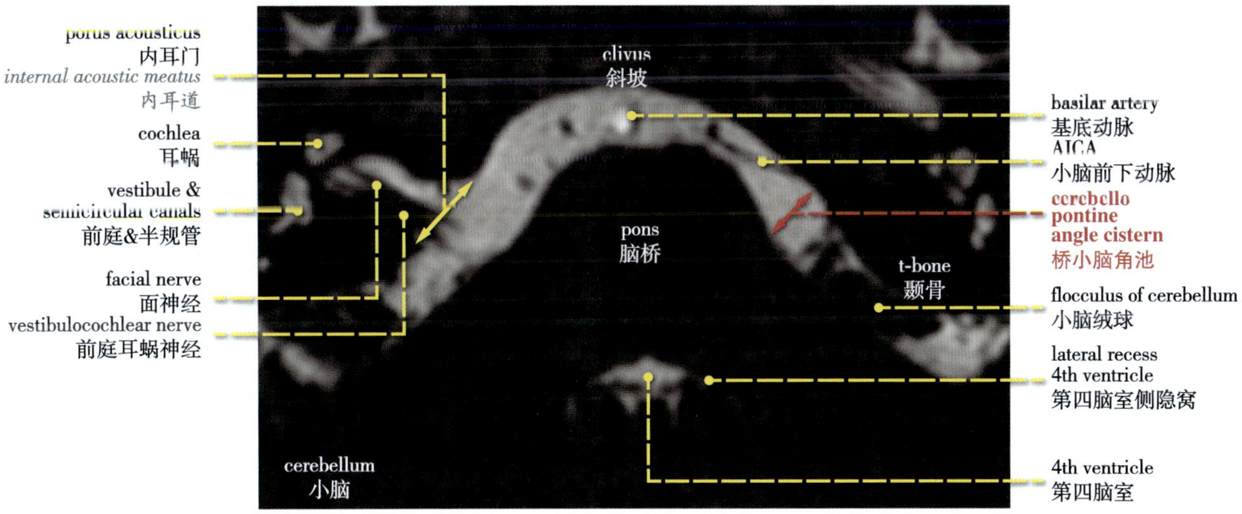

- The cerebellopontine angle (CPA) is a region between the pons and cerebellum and the posterior aspect of the petrous temporal bone. Important structures of the CPA include the fifth (trigeminal), seventh (facial),and eighth (vestibulocochlear) cranial nerves, and the anterior inferior cerebellar artery (AICA).
- Most lesions of the CPA are extra-axial and located in the CPA cistern itself, although some may arise in the internal auditory canal (IAC), temporal bone, or rarely intra-axially from the pons or cerebellum. CPA masses are more common in adults.

- CPA是脑桥和小脑与颞骨岩部后侧面之间的区域。CPA的重要结构包括第Ⅴ脑神经(三叉神经)、第Ⅶ脑神经(面神经)和第Ⅷ脑神经(前庭蜗神经)及小脑前下动脉(AICA)。
- 大多数CPA病灶是轴(脑)外病变，并位于脑桥小脑角池内，尽管部分病灶起源于内听道(IAC)、颞骨或有极少数起源于轴(脑)内的脑桥或小脑。CPA肿瘤更常见于成人。

Schwannoma

神经鞘瘤

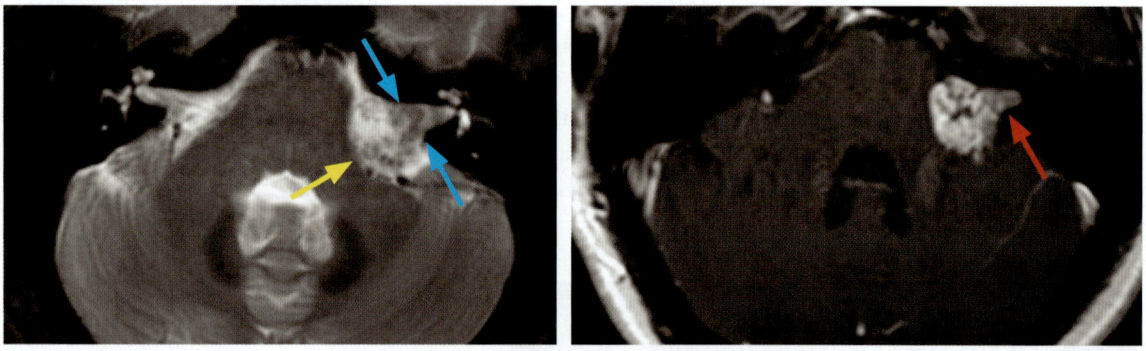

Vestibular schwannoma: Axial T2- (left image) and T1-weighted post-contrast MRI demonstrate a heterogeneously enhancing mass in the left cerebellopontine angle with an *ice cream cone* appearance that indents the cerebellar-pontine junction (yellow arrow) and protrudes into the internal acoustic meatus (red arrow). The porus acousticus is slightly widened (blue arrows).
Case courtesy Mary Beth Cunnane, MD, Massachusetts Eye and Ear Infirmary.
前庭神经鞘瘤：轴位T_2(左图)和增强T_1(右图)加权MRI显示左侧桥小脑角区有一个强化不均匀的肿块，呈冰激凌蛋卷征，推压桥小脑连接处(黄箭)，并突入内耳道(红箭)。内耳门轻度变宽(蓝箭)。

- Schwannoma of the vestibulocochlear nerve, also known as a vestibular schwannoma, is by far the most common cerebellopontine angle mass, representing greater than 75% of all CPA masses.
- Most frequently present in the fifth to seventh decades of life in sporadic cases and in the second decade of life in the setting of neurofibromatosis type Ⅱ, which is associated with bilateral vestibular schwannomas.
- Vestibular schwannoma is isoattenuating to the cerebellum on CT, hyperintense on T2-weighted images and avidly enhances. The characteristic *ice cream cone* appearance describes the "cone" protruding through (and widening) the porus acousticus and the "ice cream" exerting mass effect on the cerebellar-pontine junction. Schwannoma may become cystic, especially when larger.
- Schwannomas of other cranial nerves in the CPA, including the facial or trigeminal nerves, are less common. Trigeminal schwannoma may extend into Meckel's cave.

- 前庭耳蜗神经的神经鞘瘤，也称前庭神经鞘瘤，是极其常见的桥小脑角肿瘤，占所有CPA肿瘤的75%以上。
- 最常见于50~70岁，呈散发，但在Ⅱ型神经纤维瘤病中以二十多岁更常见，并与双侧前庭神经鞘瘤相关。
- 前庭神经鞘瘤在CT上与小脑呈等密度，在T_2加权图像上呈高信号并有明显强化。特征性的冰激凌蛋卷征是指"蛋卷"突入并扩大了内耳门，"冰激凌"压迫小脑脑桥连接处出现占位效应。前庭神经鞘瘤可能会囊变，尤其是较大的病变。
- 其他脑神经鞘瘤在CPA较少见，包括面神经或三叉神经。三叉神经鞘瘤可延伸进入梅克尔腔。

Meningioma

脑膜瘤

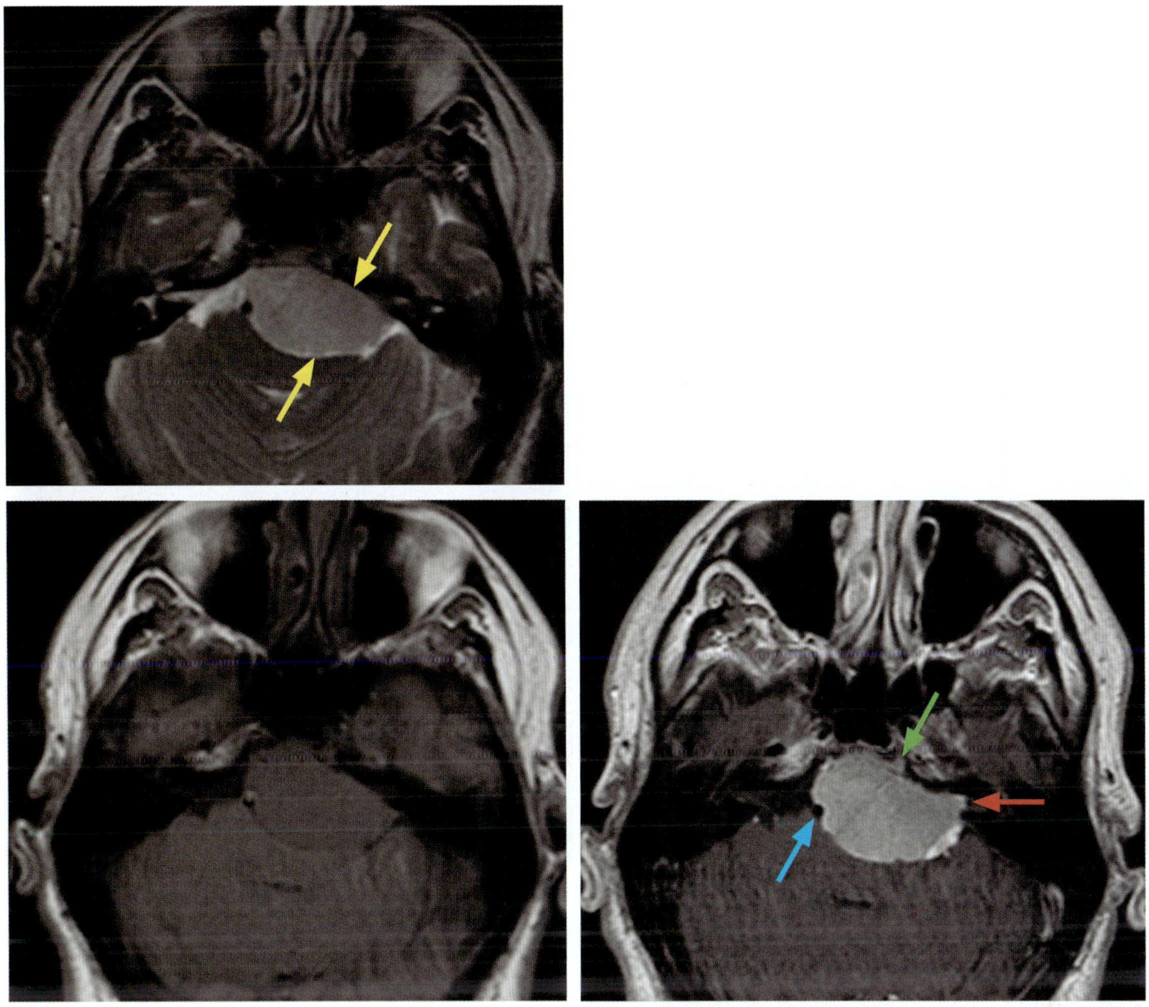

Prepontine/left CPA meningioma: Axial T2-weighted MRI (top left image) demonstrates a circumscribed, hyperintense, prepontine mass (yellow arrows).

Axial pre-contrast T1 (bottom left image) and post-contrast T1-weighted (bottom right image) MRI shows that the mass avidly enhances and extends from the prepontine cistern into the left CPA and left porus acousticus (red arrow). There is also extension into Dorello's canal on the left (green arrow), likely causing cranial nerve Ⅵ palsy. There is flattening of the pons. The basilar artery is nearly 180° encased and mildly narrowed (blue arrow).

Case courtesy Gregory Wrubel, MD, Brigham and Women's Hospital.

脑桥前/左侧的CPA脑膜瘤：轴位T_2加权MRI(左上图)显示脑桥前出现边界清楚、高信号的肿块(黄箭)。

轴位平扫T_1加权(左下图)和增强T_1加权(右下图)MRI显示肿块明显强化，并从桥前池延伸至左侧CPA和左侧内耳门(红箭)。同时，也延伸至左侧颞骨外展神经管(绿箭)，有可能造成第Ⅵ脑神经麻痹。脑桥变扁，基底动脉几乎被包裹180°，并轻度狭窄(蓝箭)。

- Although meningioma is overall the most common extra-axial mass in adults, it is only the second most common mass of the CPA, representing approximately 10–15% of all CPA masses.
- Meningiomas often feature a short segment of dural enhancement and may induce adjacent bony hyperostosis. Approximately 20% calcify, in contrast to schwannomas where calcification is rare.
- In contrast to schwannoma, a CPA meningioma seldom enlarges the porus acousticus.

Arachnoid cyst

- An arachnoid cyst is a benign CSF-filled lesion that is usually congenital.
- An arachnoid cyst will follow CSF on all sequences. Unlike an epidermoid

- 虽然脑膜瘤在神经系统总体上是最常见的成人脑外肿块，但在CPA处却是第二常见，占所有CPA肿块的10%~15%。
- 脑膜瘤常以节段性硬膜强化为特征，并刺激邻近骨质增生。约20%的脑膜瘤出现钙化，而相比之下，神经鞘瘤则罕见有钙化。
- 与神经鞘瘤不同，CPA脑膜瘤很少会造成内耳门扩大。

蛛网膜囊肿

- 蛛网膜囊肿是良性的含脑脊液病变，通常是先天性的。

cyst, an arachnoid cyst does not have restricted diffusion.

- 蛛网膜囊肿在所有序列中都与脑脊液一致。与表皮样囊肿不同，蛛网膜囊肿不会出现弥散受限。

Aneurysm

- Vertebrobasilar aneurysm (arising from the posterior inferior cerebellar artery, anterior inferior cerebellar artery, vertebral artery, or basilar artery) may appear as a well-defined, avidly enhancing CPA lesion and may be initially mistaken for a schwannoma or meningioma on contrast-enhanced CT.
- On MRI, clues to a vascular etiology include flow void and pulsation artifacts. MRA or CTA are diagnostic.

动脉瘤

- 椎基底动脉瘤(起自小脑后下动脉、小脑前下动脉、椎动脉或基底动脉)可表现为边界清晰、明显强化的CPA病灶，但最初可能因在CT上有增强被误以为神经鞘瘤或脑膜瘤。
- MRI血管病变的线索包括流空效应和搏动伪影。MRA或CTA可以诊断。

Epidermoid cyst

表皮样囊肿

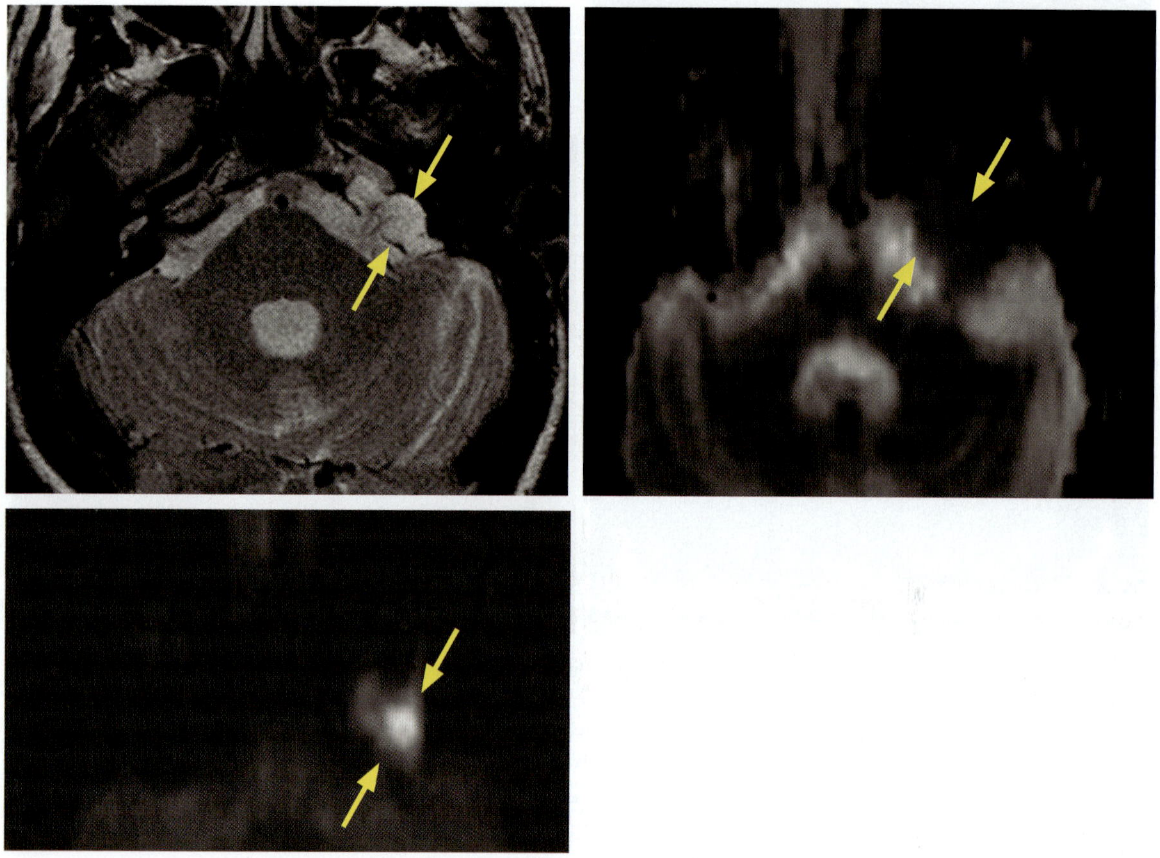

Epidermoid cyst:
Axial T2-weighted MRI (top left image) shows a lobulated mass (arrows) in the left cerebellopontine angle. The mass is isointense to CSF.
ADC map (top right image) and DWI (left image) show that the mass (arrows) is dark on ADC and bright on DWI, consistent with reduced diffusivity.
Case courtesy Gregory Wrubel, MD, Brigham and Women's Hospital.

表皮样囊肿：
轴位T_2加权MRI(左上图)显示左侧桥小脑角有一个分叶状肿块(黄箭)。肿块与脑脊液信号一致。
ADC图(右上图)和弥散加权图像(左下图)显示肿块(黄箭)在ADC图呈低信号，在弥散加权图像呈高信号，符合弥散受限。

- An epidermoid cyst is a congenital lesion arising from ectopic ectodermal epithelial tissue.
- Epidermoid cysts progressively enlarge from desquamation of keratinized epithelium lining the cyst. The mass characteristically insinuates in between structures, encasing cranial nerves and vessels. Gross pathology features a characteristic "cauliflower-like" surface.

- 表皮样囊肿是一种先天性病变，起源于异位的外胚层上皮组织。
- 表皮样囊肿呈进行性增大，因囊肿内衬的角化上皮逐渐脱落所致。肿块的特征是迂回在各结构之间生长，包裹脑神经和血管。大体病理的特征为"菜花状"的表面。

- On CT, epidermoid cyst may mimic arachnoid cyst and appear as a CSF-attenuation cystic structure. On MRI, an epidermoid cyst has similar signal characteristics as CSF on T1- and T2-weighted images. Unlike arachnoid cyst, an epidermoid does not usually suppress on FLAIR sequences.
- An epidermoid cyst is hyperintense on diffusion-weighted images, believed to be a combination of reduced diffusivity and T2 shine through, in contrast to arachnoid cysts. Post-surgical DWI follow-up is critical to detect any residual focus, which will be DWI bright.
- Rarely, epidermoids may exhibit signal hyperintensity on unenhanced T1-weighted imaging, also known as "white epidermoids."

- 表皮样囊肿在CT上类似蛛网膜囊肿，表现为脑脊液样密度的囊性结构。在MRI上，表皮样囊肿T_1和T_2加权图像信号类似脑脊液。不同于蛛网膜囊肿，表皮样囊肿的信号在FLAIR序列通常不会受到抑制。
- 表皮样囊肿在弥散加权图像上呈高信号，是弥散受限和T_2穿透效应的共同作用，这一点与蛛网膜囊肿不同。手术后弥散加权图像随访对发现残留灶极其重要，表现为弥散加权图像高信号。
- 极罕见的表皮样囊肿在平扫T_1加权图像上呈高信号，也称为"白色表皮样囊肿"。

Intra-axial neoplasm

- Less frequent benign lesions that can be seen in the IAC/CPA include lipomas and dermoids.
- A posterior fossa intra-axial neoplasm, such as a hemangioblastoma or glioma, may invade laterally into the CPA. Other malignancies such as lymphoma, melanoma, and metastases can also be rarely seen.
- Medulloblastoma tends to occur in the midline in children, though lateral involvement of the cerebellar hemispheres can be seen in older children or young adults.
- Ependymoma may extend into the CPA by squeezing through the lateral fourth ventricular foramina (of Luschka).
- Tumors related to the petrous bone (e.g., chondrosarcoma or endolymphatic sac tumors) may extend to the CPA.

轴(脑)内肿瘤

- 较少的良性病变发生于IAC/CPA，包括脂肪瘤和皮样囊肿。
- 颅后窝的轴(脑)内肿瘤，如成血管细胞瘤和胶质瘤，可以侧向侵入CPA。其他恶性肿瘤罕见，如淋巴瘤、黑色素瘤或转移瘤。
- 髓母细胞瘤易发生于儿童的中线位置，但在年龄较大的儿童或者年轻人中则可以侧向累及小脑半球。
- 室管膜瘤可以经过第四脑室侧孔(Luschka孔)进入CPA。
- 岩骨相关肿瘤(如软骨肉瘤或内淋巴囊肿瘤)可延伸至CPA。

Temporal bone fractures

- Temporal bone fractures have been historically described by their orientation with respect to the long axis of the petrous pyramid-longitudinal versus transverse-which classically leads to conductive versus sensorineural hearing loss, respectively. However, this traditional system does not correlate with clinical outcome or potential complications.
- A newer classification system has been proposed, classifying fractures depending on whether the otic capsule is spared or violated.

Otic capsule-sparing temporal bone fracture

颞骨骨折

- 旧的颞骨骨折分类法是按骨折相对岩尖长轴的方向进行命名，即纵向和横向，它们分别可导致传导性与感音神经性听力障碍。然而，这种传统分类法与临床预后或潜在的并发症无关。
- 新的分类法提议按听软骨囊的完好和受累程度分类。

听软骨囊不受累的颞骨骨折

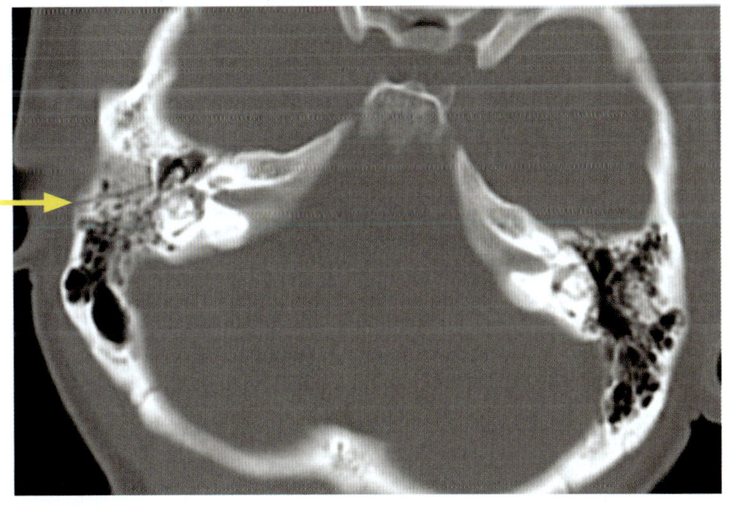

Axial CT through the temporal bone shows a nondisplaced fracture (arrow) extending through the axis of the petrous portion of the temporal bone. The otic capsule is spared.
颞骨轴位CT示无移位的骨折(黄箭)，贯穿颞骨岩部的中轴，听软骨囊未受累。

- Otic capsule-sparing temporal bone fractures are much more common than otic capsule-violating features, accounting for 94–97% of temporal bone features.
- Otic capsule-sparing temporal bone fracture results from a temporoparietal blow and has an increased incidence of conductive hearing loss secondary to ossicular injury.
- The most common cause of conductive hearing loss is related to hemotympanum or tympanic membrane rupture, which should resolve within a month of injury. Persistent conductive hearing loss should prompt evaluation for ossicular injury.
- The most frequently injured ossicle is the incus because it has the least ligamentous support. Ossicular dislocation is more common than ossicular fracture.

Otic capsule-violating temporal bone fracture

- Otic capsule-violating temporal bone fracture is much less common. It can involve the vestibule, semicircular canals, cochlea and/or facial nerve.
- It is often the result of an occipital blow and has a higher incidence of facial nerve paralysis, sensorineural hearing loss, and CSF fistula.

Complications of temporal bone fracture

Facial nerve injury

- Facial nerve transection results in immediate facial paralysis.
- Delayed facial nerve injury can present secondary to contusion, edema, or hematoma.
- Severity and onset helps guide clinical management. Delayed onset incomplete facial paralysis may be treated with steroids and observation while surgical exploration is considered if there is concern for transection.
- Important CT findings include: Bone fragments impinging on the facial nerve, extension of fracture to the nerve, and ossicles or hematoma impinging on the facial canal.

CSF leak

- CSF leakis a complication seen in 11–45% of temporal bone fractures and is seen 2–4 times more frequently inotic capsule-violating temporal bone features.
- CSF leak is seen in fractures that involve the tegmen.
- Clinically, patients present with CSF otorrhea and rhinorrhea, fullness in the ear, and conductive hearing loss.
- Most cases occur in the first week after trauma and resolve with conservative medical management (strict bed rest).

Labyrinthitis ossificans

- Labyrinthitis ossificans occurs when fluid-filled lumen of the otic capsule following trauma is replaced by fibrous tissue (earlier stage) or bone (later stage).
- Clinically this presents with sensorineural hearing loss and loss of vestibular function.

Vascular injury

- Arterial injury can occur in the form of dissection, pseudoaneurysm, arteriovenous fistula, transection or occlusion.
- Presence of carotid canal fracture is highly suggestive of injury to the passing internal carotid artery and should be evaluated with CT angiography.
- Venous injury can manifest as venous sinus thrombosis or transection. CT venogram should be performed in cases where the fracture line traverses the venous sinuses. Complications of venous sinus thrombosis such as venous infarcts or hematomas should also prompt definitive evaluation.

- 听软骨囊完好的颞骨骨折比听软骨囊受累的骨折更为常见，占颞骨骨折的94%~97%。
- 听软骨囊不受累的颞骨骨折由颞顶骨受力引起，若听小骨损伤，传导性听力障碍发生率将增高。
- 最常见的传导性听力障碍原因是鼓室积血或鼓膜破裂，这在损伤后1个月内可恢复。对于持续性传导性听力障碍，应评估听小骨是否损伤。
- 最常损伤的听小骨是砧骨，因其韧带支持最少。听小骨脱位比听小骨骨折更常见。

听软骨囊受累的颞骨骨折

- 听软骨囊受累的颞骨骨折较少见，可累及前庭、半规管、耳蜗和/或面神经。
- 此骨折通常是枕骨受力的结果，面神经麻痹、感音神经性听力障碍和脑脊液漏的发生率较高。

颞骨骨折的并发症

面神经损伤

- 面神经横断会即刻导致面瘫。
- 迟发性面神经损伤可继发于挫伤、水肿或血肿。
- 严重程度和发病时间有助于指导临床决策。迟发性不完全面瘫可用类固醇治疗和观察，若怀疑横断伤则需考虑手术探查。
- 重要的CT发现包括：骨碎片卡压面神经、骨折延伸至神经，以及听小骨或血肿卡压面神经。

脑脊液(CSF)漏

- CSF漏是颞骨骨折的一种并发症，发生率为11%~45%，而当听软骨囊受累时则增加到2~4倍。
- CSF漏见于骨折累及顶盖。
- 患者在临床上表现为CSF耳漏和鼻漏，耳内充满液体，以及传导性听力障碍。
- 大多数CSF漏发生在创伤后的第一周，并在保守治疗后恢复(严格卧床休息)。

骨化性迷路炎

- 骨化性迷路炎是充满液体的听软骨囊腔在创伤后被纤维组织(早期)或骨质(晚期)所取代。
- 临床上这种患者表现为感音神经性听力障碍和前庭功能障碍。

血管性损伤

- 动脉损伤可以表现为夹层、假性动脉瘤、动静脉瘘、横断或闭塞。
- 出现颈动脉管骨折高度提示穿行其内部的颈内动脉可能受到损伤，应行CT血管造影进行评估。
- 静脉损伤可表现为静脉窦血栓形成或静脉窦横断。对于骨折线横贯静脉窦的病例应进行CT静脉造影。静脉窦血栓形成的并发症，如静脉性梗死或血肿，也应尽快明确诊断。

Petrous Apex

Anatomy of the petrous apex

- The petrous apex is the most medial portion of the temporal bone
- The petrous apex is a bridge between the suprahyoid neck inferiorly and the intracranial compartment above, and is adjacent to several important structures such as Dorello's canal, Meckel's cave, and the petrous portion of the internal carotid artery.

  Cranial nerve Ⅵ passes through **Dorello's canal**.

  Meckel's cave is the site of the trigeminal ganglion.
- Normally, the petrous apex is composed of bone marrow and dense bone. The petrous apex is pneumatized in approximately 10% of the population, which increases the risk for development of a cholesterol cyst or apical petrositis.

Cholesterol cyst (cholesterol granuloma)

- A cholesterol cyst is a foreign body giant cell reaction to cholesterol crystals. It is thought to be initially instigated as a reaction to an obstructed air cell and therefore occurs more commonly in a pneumatized petrous apex.
- A cholesterol cyst is the most common primary petrous apex lesion but may also occur in the mastoid portion of the temporal bone or the middle ear.
- MR imaging of a cholesterol cyst shows an expansile mass with internal hemorrhage and fluid which does not suppress on fat suppression, unlike fatty marrow.

Congenital cholesteatoma

- While acquired cholesteatomas are located within the middle ear, congenital cholesteatoma can be located anywhere in the temporal bone, including the petrous apex.
- MR imaging will typically show restricted diffusion.

Apical petrositis (petrousapicitis)

- A relatively rare complication of infectious otomastoiditis, apical petrositis is also known as petrous apicitis and results when infection extends medially into a pneumatized petrous apex.
- In the early stages of apical petrositis, there isopacification of the petrous apex air cells with progressive bony demineralization and resorption, resulting in localized osteomyelitis of the skull base.
- The classic **Gradenigo triad** is not commonly seen, but is comprised of otomastoiditis, facial pain due to trigeminal neuropathy at Meckel's cave, and lateral rectus palsy from sixth cranial nerve palsy at Dorello's canal.
- Vascular complications of apical petrositis include internal carotid arteritis and dural venous thrombosis.

Schwannoma

- A petrous apex schwannoma may originate from cranial nerves Ⅴ, Ⅶ, or Ⅷ. Imaging shows a circumscribed, smoothly expansile, enhancing mass that may cause bony remodeling. Large tumors may become cystic and contain fluid levels.

Langerhans cell histiocytosis (eosinophilic granuloma)

- Langerhans cell histiocytosis (LCH) is a neoplastic proliferation of eosinophils and Langerhans cells. The temporal bone is the most common site of skull base involvement.
- CT shows a well-circumscribed destructive lesion, usually with nonsclerotic margins.

岩尖

岩尖解剖

- 岩尖是颞骨最靠内的部分。
- 岩尖下接舌骨上颈部，上连颅内结构，与多个重要解剖结构相邻，如颞骨外展神经管、梅克尔腔及颈内动脉岩骨段。

  第Ⅵ脑神经通过**颞骨外展神经管**。

  梅克尔腔内含三叉神经节。
- 岩尖在正常情况下由骨髓和密质骨组成。约10%人群的岩尖内有气化，这可增加胆固醇囊肿和岩尖炎的发病风险。

胆固醇囊肿(胆固醇肉芽肿)

- 胆固醇囊肿是异物巨细胞对胆固醇结晶的一种反应。最初可能是对气腔阻塞的反应，因而更常见于气化的岩尖。
- 胆固醇囊肿是最常见的原发性岩尖病变，也可发生于颞骨乳突和中耳。
- 胆固醇囊肿在MRI上表现为膨胀性肿块，伴内部出血和积液，在脂肪抑制序列上不能被抑制，故不同于脂性骨髓。

先天性胆脂瘤

- 先天性胆脂瘤可位于颞骨任意区域，包括岩尖，但后天性胆脂瘤仅位于中耳内。
- MRI通常显示弥散受限。

岩尖炎

- 岩尖炎(英文又称petrous apicitis)是感染性耳乳突炎的一种相对罕见的并发症，为感染向内侧播散至气化的岩尖的结果。
- 在岩尖炎的早期，岩尖气腔的透亮度减低并出现进行性骨质脱钙和重吸收，导致颅底局限性骨髓炎。
- 典型的**Gradenigo三联征(岩骨尖综合征)**并不多见，它包括乳突炎、面部疼痛(由梅克尔腔内三叉神经病变引起)及外直肌麻痹(因颞骨外展神经管内第Ⅵ脑神经障碍)。
- 岩尖炎的血管并发症包括颈内动脉炎和硬膜静脉窦血栓。

神经鞘瘤

- 岩尖神经鞘瘤可起源于第Ⅴ、Ⅶ或Ⅷ脑神经。影像学表现为一个边界清晰、光滑膨胀、有强化的肿块，并有可能引起邻近骨质重塑。大的肿瘤可出现囊变和液平。

朗格汉斯细胞组织细胞增生症(嗜酸性肉芽肿)

- 朗格汉斯细胞组织细胞增生症(LCH)指嗜酸性粒细胞和朗格汉斯细胞肿瘤样增生。颞骨是颅底最常发病的部位。
- CT上表现为边界清晰的破骨性病变，常无硬化边。

- MRI shows the LCH lesions as soft-tissue masses surrounded by bone marrow and soft tissue edema. Marked enhancement is characteristic.

Chondrosarcoma

- Chondrosarcoma is a malignant neoplasm that characteristically arises in the midline from the clivus or slightly off-midline from the petro-occipital fissure. CT often shows a tumor with a ring-and-arc chondroid matrix, although internal matrix is not always seen. MRI shows a lobular, cauliflower-shaped, hyperintense mass on T2-weighted images.

Chordoma

- Chordoma (discussed previously in the section on clivallesions) most commonly arises from the clivus but may expand laterally to secondarily involve the petrous apex. In some circumstances it can be difficult to distinguish between chordoma and chondrosarcoma.

Endolymphatic sac tumor

- LCH在MRI上表现为被骨髓包围的软组织肿块及软组织肿胀。显著强化是其特征。

软骨肉瘤

- 软骨肉瘤是一种恶性肿瘤，其特征是起源位于中线的斜坡或略微偏离中线的岩枕裂。CT常显示肿瘤呈环形或弧形的软骨样基质，虽然基质内部并不总能看到。MRI表现为分叶、菜花状，T_2加权图像高信号肿块。

脊索瘤

- 脊索瘤(已在前文的“斜坡脊索瘤/软骨内瘤”部分进行讨论)最常起源于斜坡，但可向两侧膨胀性生长，继发累及岩尖。有时，脊索瘤和软骨肉瘤之间很难进行鉴别。

内淋巴囊肿瘤

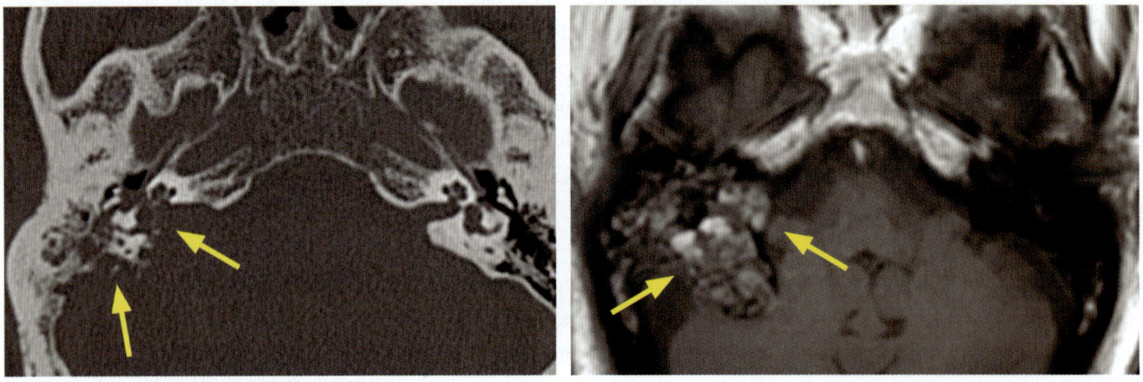

Axial noncontrast CT (left image) demonstrates a destructive mass with internal calcification (arrows) centered at the posterior wall of the right mastoid air cells in region of the vestibular aqueduct, and involves the right IAC, semicircular canals, and middle ear cavity. Location of the mass suggests an endolymphatic sac tumor.

Subsequent MRI shows the mass is intrinsically T1 hyperintense (axial T1-weighted image on the right), heterogeneously T2 hyperintense, and does not enhance.

轴位平扫CT(左图)显示前庭水管区有一个破骨性肿块，以右侧乳突气房后壁为中心，伴内部钙化(黄箭)，并累及右侧IAC、半规管和中耳腔。肿块的位置提示肿块为内淋巴囊肿瘤。

随后的MRI显示肿块平扫T_1呈高信号(右图轴位T_1加权图像)，不均匀T_2高信号，无强化。

- Endolymphatic sac tumor is a locally invasive papillary cystadenomatous tumor.
- Most cases are sporadic, but a minority of cases are associated with von Hippel-Lindau.
- Endolymphatic sac tumor most frequently involves the region of the vestibular aqueduct in the retrolabyrinthine petrous bone. On CT, the affected bone has a moth-eaten, lytic appearance with intratumor bone spicules. On MRI, the presence of blood products results in intrinsic T1 hyperintensity. Enhancement is usually heterogeneous.

- 内淋巴囊瘤是一种局部浸润性乳头状囊腺瘤。
- 大多数病例是散发的，但少数病例与VHL有关。
- 内淋巴囊肿瘤最常累及迷路后岩骨的前庭水管区域。CT表现为受累的骨质呈虫蚀样、溶骨性，伴肿瘤内骨针。因存在血液代谢产物，会使MRI平扫T_1呈高信号。强化通常是不均匀的。

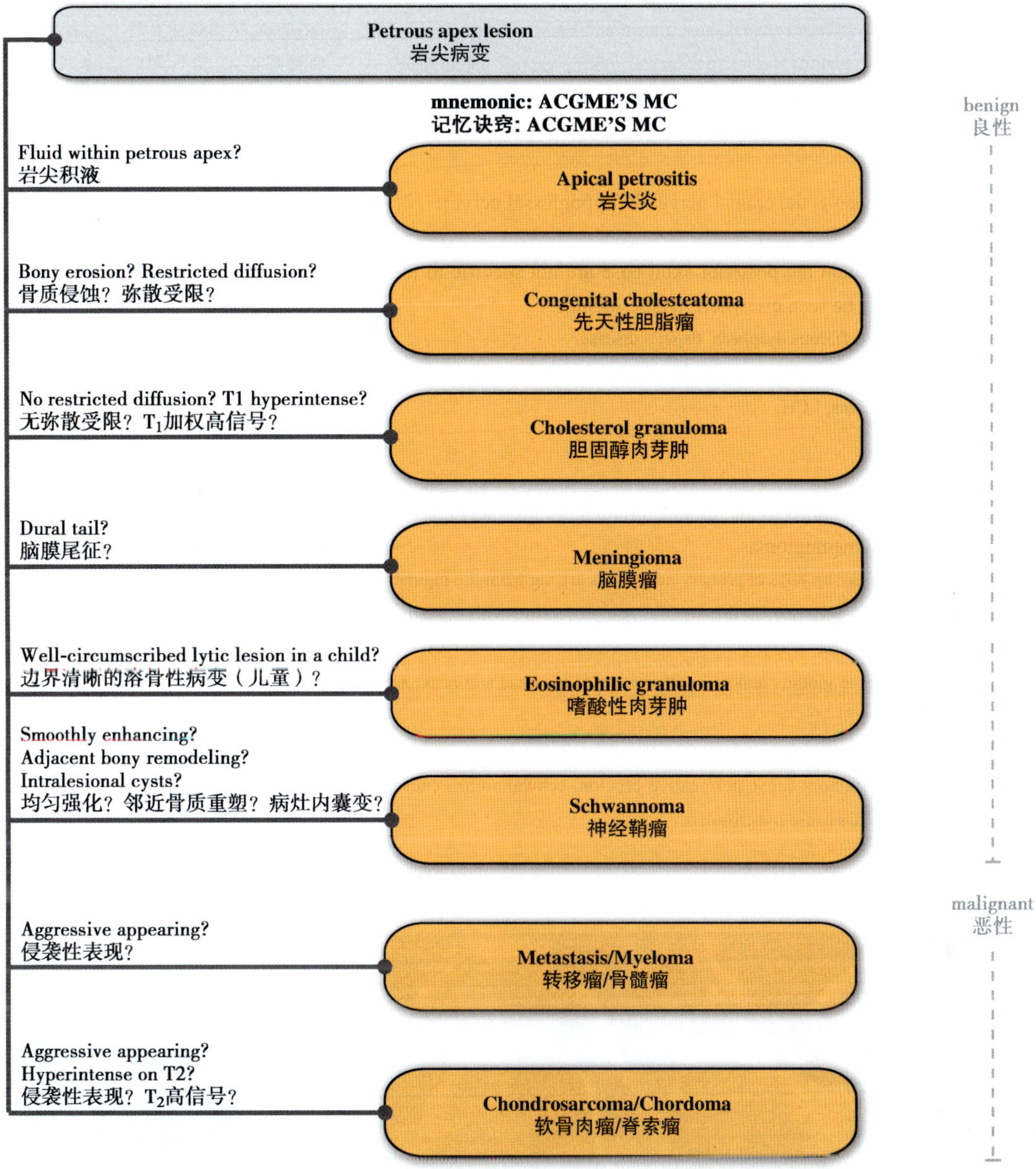

POSTERIOR SKULL BASE

Anatomy of the posterior skull base

- The posterior skull base is bounded by the posterior clivus anteriorly, the posterior aspect of the petrous temporal bone and condylar part of the occipital bone laterally, and the mastoid temporal bone and squamous occipital bone posteriorly.
- The **foramen magnum** is formed within the occipital bone and transmits the medulla oblongata, vertebral arteries, anterior/posterior spinal arteries, and spinal accessory nerve.
- Important foramina within the posterior skull base include jugular foramen and the hypoglossal canal, which are separated by the jugular tubercle.

后颅底

后颅底解剖

- 后颅底前方以斜坡后部为界，两侧以颞骨岩部后部和枕骨髁部为界，后方以颞骨乳突部和枕骨鳞部为界。
- **枕骨大孔**在枕骨内形成，内穿行延髓、椎动脉、前/后脊髓动脉和脊副神经。
- 后颅底的重要孔隙包括颈静脉孔和舌下神经管，颈静脉结节把它们隔开。

- A fibrous or bony septum divides the **jugular foramen** into anteromedial pars nervosa and posterolateral pars vascularis.

Pars nervosa transmits cranial nerve Ⅸ (glossopharyngeal nerve) with its tympanic branch, Jacobson nerve, and the inferior petrosal sinus (mnemonic **N**ervosa **N**ine).
Pars vascularis is larger and transmits the internal jugular vein, posterior meningeal artery, cranial nerves Ⅹ (vagus nerve) and Ⅺ (accessory nerve), and Arnold nerve (auricular branch of CN Ⅹ).

- The **hypoglossal canal** transmits the cranial nerve Ⅻ (hypoglossal nerve).

General approach to the posterior skull base

- A large subset of lesions within the posterior skull base are not specific to the posterior skull base and can be seen elsewhere. These include:

  Fibro-osseous lesions such as fibrous dysplasia, Paget's disease.

  Cartilage/bone tumors such as chordomas, chondrosarcomas, osteosarcomas, plasmacytomas, multiple myeloma, LCH.

  Vascular malformations.

  Metastases.
- The most common lesions localized to the jugular foramen are glomus jugulare tumors, schwannomas, and meningiomas.

  Glomus jugulare tumors make up 80% of primary neoplasms arising from the jugular foramen. The typical patient is a woman in late middle age presenting with pulsatile tinnitus and conductive hearing loss.

  Imaging findings are similar to glomus tumors in other areas of the head and neck, as described previously.

  Bony changes of the jugular bulb can be used to differentiate these lesions on CT. Classically, glomus jugulare tumors cause permeative erosion, schwannomas cause smooth remodeling, meningiomas cause hyperostosis.

- 纤维或骨性分隔将**颈静脉孔**分为前内侧的神经部和后外侧的血管部。

神经部传导第Ⅸ脑神经(舌咽神经)及其鼓室支、Jacobson神经和岩下窦(记忆诀窍：**N**ervous **N**ine)。
血管部较大，穿行颈内静脉、后脑膜动脉、第Ⅹ脑神经(迷走神经)和第Ⅺ脑神经(副神经)、Arnold神经(第Ⅹ脑神经耳支)。

- **舌下神经管**通过第Ⅻ脑神经(舌下神经)。

后颅底病变的常规思路

- 多数后颅底的病变并非后颅底特有的，也可见于其他部位。它们包括：

  骨纤维性病变，如骨纤维结构不良、佩吉特病。

  软骨/骨肿瘤，如脊索瘤、软骨肉瘤、骨肉瘤、浆细胞瘤、多发性骨髓瘤、LCH。

  血管畸形。

  肿瘤转移。
- 位于颈静脉孔的最常见的病变有颈静脉球瘤、神经鞘瘤和脑膜瘤。

  颈静脉球瘤占所有颈静脉孔原发性肿瘤中的80%。患者多为中老年女性，表现为搏动性耳鸣和传导性听力障碍。

  影像学表现与前文中的头颈部其他部位的血管球瘤相似。

  CT上颈静脉球区的骨质改变可以鉴别这些病变。颈静脉球瘤的典型表现为造成浸润性骨侵蚀，神经鞘瘤通常导致平滑的骨质重塑，脑膜瘤通常导致骨质硬化。

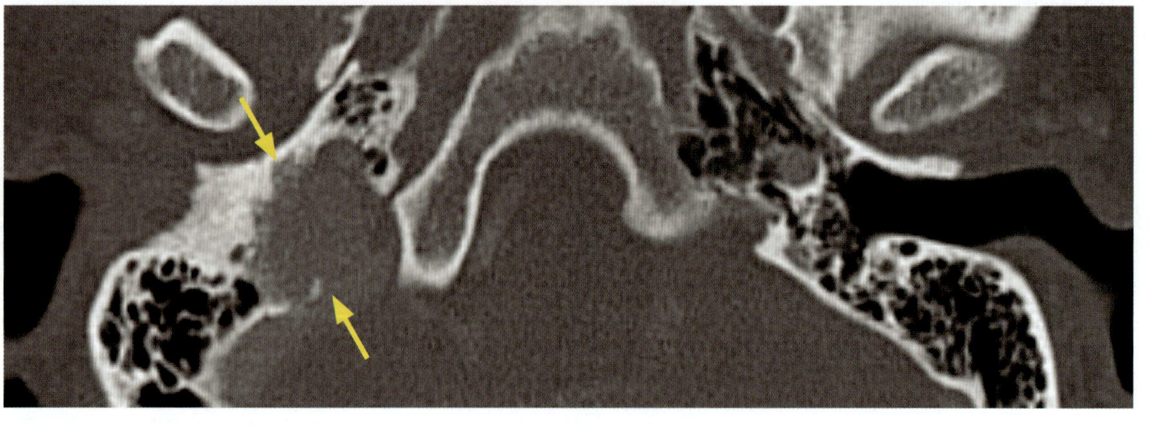

Glomus jugulare tumor: Axial CT through the mastoid air cells shows permeative, moth-eaten bony destruction centered on the right jugular foramen (arrows).
颈静脉球瘤：经乳突气房水平轴位CT显示颈静脉孔周围浸润性、虫蚀样的骨质破坏(黄箭)。

- Cerebellopontine angle tumors also localize to the posterior skull base and are discussed earlier in the chapter.

- 桥小脑角区肿瘤也位于后颅底，已在本章前文讨论。

(翻译　郑葵葵)

MUCOSAL SPACES: ORAL CAVITY, PHARYNX, LARYNX

- The oral cavity is a space defined by the anterior 2/3 of tongue, bounded superiorly by the palate and inferiorly by the floor of mouth.
- The pharynx is a muscular tube extending from skull base to the thoracic inlet. It is the anatomic center of the head and neck, around which the other suprahyoid spaces wrap. It is divided into the following distinct anatomic regions:

> **Nasopharynx**: Top of pharynx behind the nasal cavity.
> **Oropharynx**: From the level of the palate to the hyoid bone, behind the oral cavity. The posterior 1/3 of tongue is part of the oropharynx.
> **Hypopharynx**: From the hyoid bone to the esophagus, including the piriform sinuses and soft tissue lateral to the larynx.

- **Mucosal squamous cell carcinoma (SCC)** arises from the squamous lining of the pharynx, larynx, and sinonasal cavity.
- The TNM staging system is used to classify SCC. "T" refers to the primary tumor extent, "N" to regional lymph nodes, and "M" for distant metastases. The criterion for T and N stage is individualized to each site (nasopharynx, oropharynx, and hypopharynx) and in the case of the larynx to each subsite (supraglottic, glottic, and subglottic). Regardless of subtype, tumor size and lymph nodes are reported using the longest diameter, which is in contrast with lymph node measurements in other parts of the body. An exhaustive discussion of TNM staging is beyond the scope of this book, however some key points and differentiating factors are discussed below.

NASOPHARYNX

Overview and anatomy

- The nasopharynx is located posterior to the nasal cavity and extends from the most cranial aspect of the pharynx (at the skull base) to the level of the soft palate.
- In the midline of the nasopharynx is the nasopharyngeal tonsillar tissue, also known as the adenoid. This is where nasopharyngeal lymphoma can arise.

Nasopharyngeal SCC

- Most nasopharyngeal carcinomas arise from the fossa of Rosenmuller, which is adjacent to the opening of the Eustachian tube. The proximity explains why nasopharyngeal tumors result in middle ear effusion at the time of presentation.
- Nasopharyngeal SCC frequently demonstrates minimal mucosal disease and may have significant extra-mucosal extension, most frequently to the parapharyngeal space and then the retropharyngeal space.
- T staging of nasopharyngeal carcinoma is primarily defined by tumor extent/invasion, and less on the size of the lesion as in other sites. T1 tumor is confined to the nasopharynx while extension to the parapharyngeal spaces, infiltration into surrounding muscles, the bony skull base, or intracranial extension results in a higher T stage. Given the importance of detection of skull base infiltration and intracranial extension of disease, MR is the preferred staging tool.
- Lymph node metastases are common, and most frequently initially preferentially involve the retropharyngeal and high jugular (level Ⅱ) nodes.

黏膜间隙：口腔、咽、喉

- 口腔是舌前2/3的区域，上以上腭为界，下以口底为界。
- 咽是一个肌性管道，从颅底延伸到胸廓的入口处，是头颈部的解剖中心，周围包绕其他舌骨上的间隙。咽分为下列不同的解剖区域：

> **鼻咽**：咽的顶部，鼻腔的后方。
> **口咽**：从上颚到舌骨水平，口腔的后方。舌后1/3是口咽的一部分。
> **下咽**：从舌骨到食管，包括梨状窝和喉外侧的软组织。

- **黏膜鳞状细胞癌(SCC)**起源于内衬于咽、喉和鼻腔鼻窦的鳞状上皮。
- TNM分期系统用于SCC的分期。"T"指原发肿瘤范围，"N"指局部淋巴结，"M"指远处转移。T和N分期的标准因不同部位(鼻咽、口咽和下咽)而异，在喉部还需进一步根据亚结构(声门上、声门和声门下)判断。无论什么分类，肿瘤和淋巴结大小衡量都使用最长径，这与身体其他部位淋巴结的测量不同。详尽的TNM分期解释超出了本书的范畴，但某些关键点和鉴别要点将在下文进行讨论。

鼻咽

概述和解剖

- 鼻咽位于鼻腔后方，从咽的最头侧(颅底)延伸到软腭的水平。
- 鼻咽中线是咽扁桃体组织，也称为腺样体。这是鼻咽淋巴瘤可能起源的部位。

鼻咽SCC

- 大多数鼻咽癌起源于咽隐窝(Rosenmüller窝)，后者与咽鼓管开口相邻。这种毗邻关系解释了为什么鼻咽肿瘤在就诊时有中耳积液的表现。
- 鼻咽SCC常表现为轻微的黏膜改变，并且可能有明显的黏膜外延伸，最常见的是累及咽旁间隙，然后是咽后间隙。
- 鼻咽癌的T分期主要依据肿瘤的范围/侵袭性来定义，而病变的大小并不像其他部位的肿瘤那么重要。T_1期肿瘤局限于鼻咽部，若延伸到咽旁间隙、浸润到周围肌肉、骨性颅底或出现颅内延伸则属于更高级别的T分期。鉴于发现颅底浸润和颅内延伸的重要性，MR是分期的首选工具。
- 淋巴结转移很常见，早期最常累及咽后和颈静脉上组(Ⅱ区)淋巴结。

- Treatment is most frequently non-surgical and a combination of chemotherapy or radiation, depending on the TNM stage.

Thornwaldt cyst

- A Thornwaldt cyst is a notochordal remnant that is usually asymptomatic, but may be a cause of halitosis. The typical location of a Thornwaldt cyst is in the midline nasopharynx.

- 治疗通常为非手术方法，需要根据TNM分期进行联合化疗或放疗。

鼻咽潴留囊肿(Thornwaldt囊肿)

- 鼻咽潴留囊肿是脊索的一个残余结构，通常无症状，但可能是引起口臭的一个原因。鼻咽潴留囊肿的典型位置是在鼻咽中线。

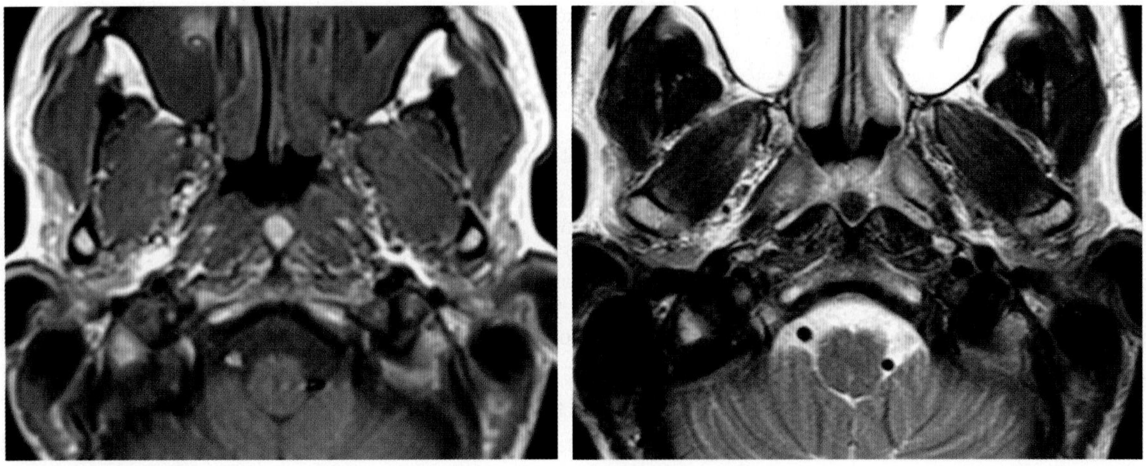

Axial T1-weighted (left image) and T2-weighted (right image) MRI show a well-circumscribed, T1 hyperintense T2 hypointense lesion in the midline nasopharynx, consistent with a Thornwaldt cyst containing proteinaceous material.

轴位T_1加权(左图)和T_2加权(右图)MRI显示鼻咽部中线处一个边界清晰的T_1高信号、T_2低信号病变，符合鼻咽潴留囊肿内含蛋白质物质的表现。

Oropharynx

Overview and anatomy

- The oropharynx includes the posterior and superior pharyngeal walls from the level of the soft palate to the hyoid bone, and includes the posterior 1/3 of the tongue (i.e., base of tongue), the vallecula, the palatine tonsils. The tongue base is the site of the lingual tonsillar tissue. The circumvallate papillae defines the anterior border of the oropharynx and separates the oropharynx from the oral cavity.
- The soft palate is part of the oropharynx and the hard palate is part of the oral cavity.

Oropharyngeal SCC

- The most common locations for oropharyngeal SCC are the anterior portion of the tonsil and the tongue base.
- In contrast to nasopharyngeal SCC, there are two TNM staging classifications for oropharyngeal SCC, depending on the p16 or high-risk HPV status. P16+/HPV-associated oropharyngeal SCC has a much better prognosis despite the tendency to have early nodal metastases and the staging scheme accounts for this. Additionally, unlike nasopharyngeal SCC, the T-staging of the oropharynx is largely based on size criteria (T1–T3).
- Evaluation of the pre-epiglottic fat space is important as involvement of this area results in upstaging to T3. Other areas that must be specifically addressed during staging include mandibular invasion, prevertebral muscle invasion which precludes surgical resection, pterygopalatine fossa invasion which raises the possibility of perineural spread, bilateral involvement of the base of tongue which has implications for surgical resection, and lymphadenopathy.
- Treatment is dependent on the stage, with single-modality treatment with surgery or radiation in early-stage cancers and combined treatment in higher-stage disease.

口咽

概述和解剖

- 口咽包括从软腭到舌骨水平的咽的后壁和上壁、舌后1/3(即舌根)、会厌谷、腭扁桃体。舌根是舌扁桃体组织所在的部位。舌轮廓乳头为口咽的前缘，并将口咽与口腔分开。
- 软腭属于口咽，而硬腭属于口腔。

口咽SCC

- 口咽SCC最好发的部位是扁桃体前部和舌根。
- 相对于鼻咽SCC，口咽SCC有两种TNM分期方法，取决于P16或高危HPV的状态。P16+/HPV-相关的口咽SCC尽管有早期淋巴结转移的倾向，但预后要好得多，分期方案考虑到了这一点。此外，与鼻咽SCC不同，口咽部的T分期主要基于大小的标准(T_1~T_3)。
- 评估会厌前脂肪间隙很重要，因为该区域受累会导致分期升高到T_3。在分期时必须注明的其他区域包括下颌骨侵犯、有碍手术切除的椎前肌侵犯、增加神经周围扩散可能性的翼腭窝侵犯、涉及手术切除的双侧舌根受累和淋巴结肿大。
- 治疗取决于分期，早期采用手术或放疗的单一治疗方式，而晚期采用联合治疗。

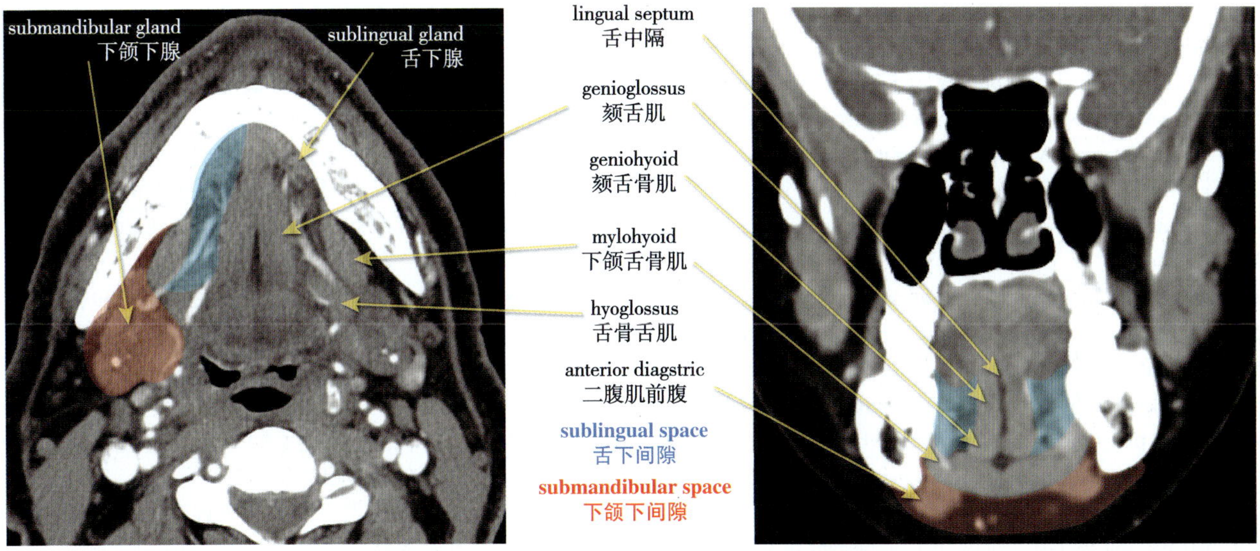

Overview and anatomy

- The oral cavity includes the lips, the anterior 2/3 of the tongue, the buccal mucosa, the gingiva, the hard palate, the retromolar trigone, and the floor of the mouth.
- The floor of the mouth, a substitute of the oral cavity, is bound by the mylohyoid muscle inferiorly, the tonsillar pillar posteriorly, and the mandible anteriorly, and includes the sublingual spaces and the deep portion of the submandibular gland as described below.
- The **sublingual spaces** are a subsite of the floor of mouth and are bound by the intrinsic muscles of the tongue superiorly, the mylohyoid muscle inferolaterally, the mandible anteriorly, and the geniohyoid/genioglossus muscles medially. Important structures that run in the sublingual space include the lingual nerve (branch of the trigeminal), the glossopharyngeal and the hypoglossal nerve, as well as the sublingual gland and duct.
- Directly inferior to the sublingual space is the U-shaped **submandibular space**. The sublingual space is separated from the submandibular space by the mylohyoid muscle anteriorly, although the sublingual space is contiguous with the submandibular space posteriorly.

概述和解剖

- 口腔包括嘴唇、舌前2/3、颊黏膜、牙龈、硬腭、磨牙后三角和口底。
- 口底是口腔的基底部，下方为下颌舌骨肌，后方为扁桃体柱，前方为下颌骨，内含舌下间隙和下颌下腺深部，如下所述。
- **舌下间隙**是口底的一部分，上方是舌内的肌肉、下外侧是下颌舌骨肌、前方是下颌骨，内侧为颏舌骨肌/颏舌肌。在舌下间隙内走行的重要结构包括舌神经(三叉神经的分支)、舌咽神经和舌下神经，以及舌下腺和导管。
- 舌下间隙的正下方是“U”形**下颌下间隙**。舌下间隙与下颌下间隙的前部被下颌舌骨肌分开，而舌下间隙在后方与下颌下间隙相连。

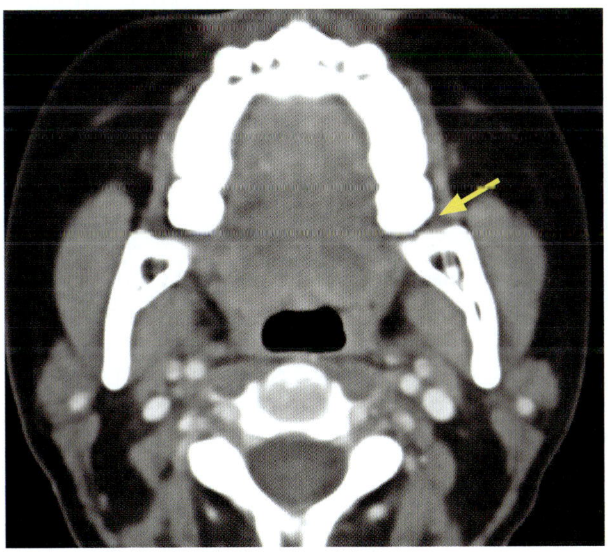

Retromolar trigone (arrow) on axial contrast-enhanced CT, a triangular region bounded anteriorly by the last mandibular molar, posteromedially by the anterior tonsillar pillar, laterally by the buccal mucosa.
轴位增强CT上的**磨牙后三角区**(黄箭)，是一个三角形区域，前面为最后一个下颌磨牙，后内侧为前扁桃体柱，外侧为颊黏膜。

Oral cavity SCC

- SCC is the most common malignancy which occurs in the oral cavity and risk factors are similar to SCC of other subsites, such as smoking, chewing tobacco, and HPV exposure, although HPV exposure is much less strongly associated in comparison to oropharyngeal SCC.
- The lip is the most common site of SCC of the oral cavity. Many of these lesions are easily assessed through direct inspection and imaging is indicated to evaluate for osseous invasion or lymph node metastases.
- Oral cavity SCC staging is also largely based on the size of the lesion for determination of T1-T3 and unlike oropharyngeal SCC, there is only one staging scheme.
- Key areas to evaluate in staging of oral cavity SCC include evaluating for mandibular/maxillary invasion and involvement of the **retromolar trigone**. Involvement of the retromolar trigone cannot be determined clinically and provides access to numerous routes of spread. Other key areas of involvement include the pterygomandibular raphe, which provides access to the floor of the mouth and masticator space, extension to the oropharynx, extension to the larynx.
- For primary oral tongue lesions, it is important to assess for extension across midline and involvement of the intrinsic muscles of the tongue.

口腔SCC

- SCC是发生在口腔常见的恶性肿瘤，其危险因素与其他各部位的SCC相似，如吸烟、咀嚼烟草和HPV暴露，但与口咽SCC相比，HPV暴露的相关性要小得多。
- 嘴唇是口腔SCC最常见的部位。很多病变很容易通过直接检查进行评估，而影像只是用于评估骨侵犯或淋巴结转移。
- 口腔SCC分期在很大程度上也是基于病变的大小来确定T_1~T_3，但与口咽SCC不同，它只有一种分期方案。
- 口腔SCC分期评估的关键部位包括下颌/上颌侵犯和**磨牙后三角区**的受累情况。磨牙后三角的受累无法在临床上确定，但它有很多蔓延的途径。其他关键受侵的部位包括翼突下颌缝，那是进入口底和咀嚼肌间隙的通道，延伸到口咽部和喉部。
- 对于原发于口腔的舌病变，重要的是要评估蔓延跨中线和舌内肌肉的受累情况。

Dermoid/epidermoid

- A dermoidis a teratomatous lesion which contains at least two germ cell layers, while an epidermoid contains only ectoderm.
- On CT, both dermoid and epidermoid will appear as a fluid-attenuation lesion, most commonly in the midline of the floor of the mouth. A pathognomonic MRI finding of dermoid is the *sack of marbles* appearance resulting from floating fat globules. In the absence of this finding, epidermoid and dermoid can be indistinguishable in this location on MRI.

皮样囊肿/表皮样囊肿

- 皮样囊肿是畸胎瘤病变，至少包含2个生殖细胞胚层，而表皮样囊肿仅包含外胚层。
- 在CT上，皮样囊肿和表皮样囊肿均表现为液体密度，最常见于口底中线。皮样囊肿的特征性MRI表现是由漂浮的脂肪颗粒形成的弹珠袋样外观。在没有这一表现的情况下，MRI可能无法区分表皮样囊肿和皮样囊肿。

Ranula

- A ranula is a mucous retention cyst that arises from the sublingual gland as a sequela of inflammation. All ranulas arise from the sublingual gland or adjacent minor salivary glands and hence begin in the sublingual space.
- A plunging ranula extends from the sublingual space into the submandibular space by protruding posteriorly over the free edge of the mylohyoid or by extending directly through a defect in the mylohyoid.
- A dermoid cyst may also present below the mandible, but is typically midline, rather than the eccentric location of a plunging ranula.

舌下囊肿

- 舌下囊肿是一种黏液潴留性囊肿，来自舌下腺，为炎症的后遗症。所有舌下囊肿都起源于舌下腺或相邻的小唾液腺，因此都始于舌下间隙。
- 潜突型舌下囊肿从舌下间隙向下颌下间隙延伸，它通过下颌舌骨肌的游离缘，或直接通过下颌舌骨肌的缺损向后突出。
- 皮样囊肿也可能出现在下颌骨下方，但通常位于中线，而不是位于潜突型舌下囊肿这样的偏心位置。

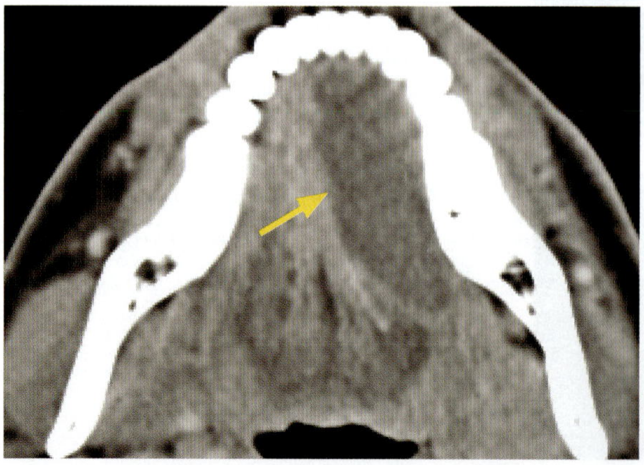

Ranula: Contrast-enhanced axial CT at the level of the mandible shows a cystic lesion (arrow) in the left sublingual space.
舌下囊肿：下颌骨水平的轴位增强CT显示位于舌下间隙左侧的囊性病变(黄箭)。

Thyroglossal duct cyst (TDC)

甲状舌管囊肿(TDC)

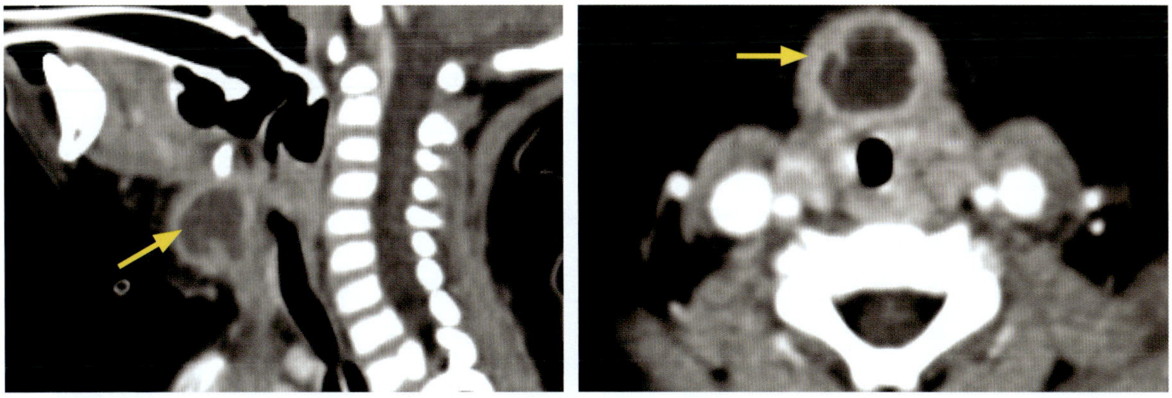

Infected thyroglossal duct cyst: Sagittal (left image) and axial enhanced CT in an intubated 13-month-old show a thick-walled peripherally enhancing cystic structure (arrows) in the midline, inferior to the mylohyoid.
Case courtesy Mary Beth Cunnane, MD, Massachusetts Eye and Ear Infirmary.
感染的甲状舌管囊肿：气管插管的13月龄患儿的矢状位(左图)和轴位(右图)增强CT显示下颌舌骨肌下方中线处有厚壁、外周环形强化的囊性结构(黄箭)。

- A thyroglossal duct cyst (TDC) represents persistence of the thyroglossal duct. The thyroglossal duct follows the midline descent of the embryonic thyroid gland from the base of the tongue (foramen cecum) to its normal position in the neck. Most thyroglossal duct cysts present in childhood as an enlarging neck mass which elevates with tongue protrusion.
- The majority of TDCs (65%) are infrahyoid,the rest found at the level of the hyoid or above. Most TDCs are midline,but they may occur slightly off midline, especially when infrahyoid.
- Thyroid carcinoma (papillary type) is a rare complication seen in 1% of TDCs.

Lingual thyroid

- Lingual thyroid is ectopic thyroid tissue that has incompletely descended during embryologic development and remains at the floor of the mouth. Usually, the ectopic gland is the only functioning thyroid tissue, so the neck should be evaluated to confirm lack of normal gland.
- Lingual thyroid is much more common in females.
- Lingual thyroid is susceptible to standard thyroid pathology, including thyroiditis and cancer.

Lymphatic malformations

- Lymphatic malformations are congenital abnormalities that result when the embryologic lymphatics fail to connect to developing veins. There are three types of lymphatic malformations, classified by the size of the intra-lesional cystic spaces.
- **Cystic hygroma** is the most common type of lymphatic malformation, the majority being present at birth and associated with chromosomal anomalies including Turner and Down syndromes. A cystic hygroma features large lymphatic spaces. The most common location is in the posterior triangle of the neck.
- **Cavernous lymphangioma** has smaller lymphatic spaces than a cystic hygroma, while a **capillary lymphangioma** has the smallest cystic spaces.

- TCD为甲状舌骨导管的残留。甲状舌骨导管随胚胎甲状腺从舌底(盲孔)沿中线下降至颈部正常位置。大多数TCD在儿童时期发病，表现为增大的颈部肿块，随伸舌动作而上移。
- 大多数(65%)TDC位于舌骨下，其余位于舌骨水平或舌骨上水平。大多数TDC位于中线，但也可轻度偏离中线，尤其位于舌骨下时。
- 甲状腺癌(乳头型)是TCD的一个罕见并发症，见于1%的TCD患者。

舌甲状腺

- 舌甲状腺是异位的甲状腺组织，是由于胚胎发育时期甲状腺未完全下降，滞留在口腔的底部所致。通常，异位的甲状腺是仅有的功能性甲状腺组织，所以要检查颈部以确认无正常甲状腺。
- 舌甲状腺更多发生于女性。
- 舌甲状腺易患常见的甲状腺疾病，包括甲状腺炎和甲状腺癌。

淋巴管畸形

- 淋巴管畸形是胚胎时期淋巴管未能与发育中的静脉相通而引起的先天性异常。淋巴管畸形分为3种型，分类依据是病变内部囊腔的大小。
- **囊状水瘤**是淋巴管畸形最常见的类型，大部分患者出生时即存在，与特纳综合征、唐氏综合征等染色体异常相关。囊状水瘤的特征性表现为大的淋巴管囊腔，最常见的位置是颈后三角区。
- **海绵状淋巴管瘤**的淋巴管囊腔较囊状水瘤小，**毛细淋巴管瘤**的淋巴管囊腔最小。

Dentigerous cyst

含牙囊肿

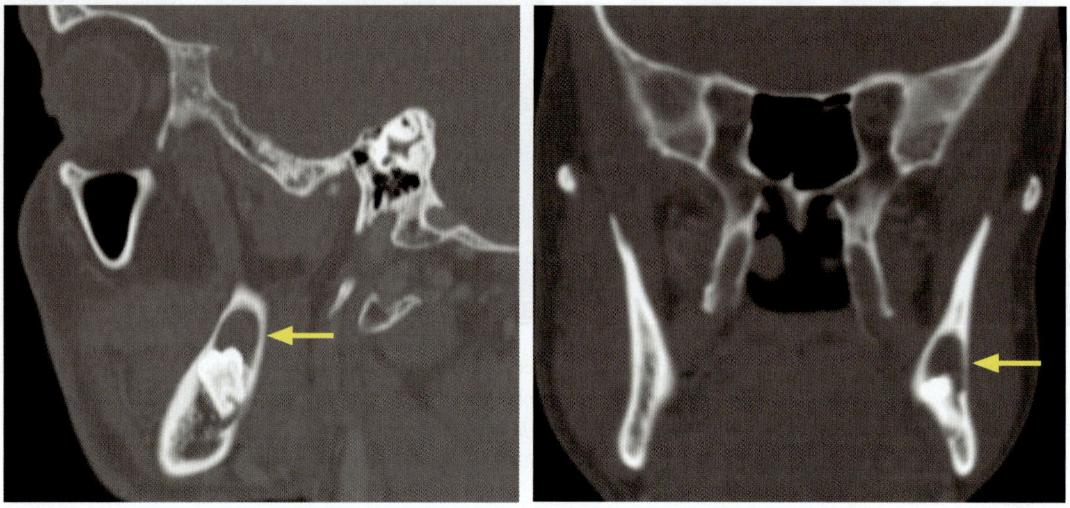

Sagittal (left image) and coronal (right image) contrast-enhanced CT show an unilocular lucent lesion (arrows) at the crown of the unerupted left third mandibular molar, consistent with a dentigerous cyst.
矢状位(左图)和冠状位(右图)增强CT显示未萌出的左下颌第三磨牙牙冠部有一个单房透亮病变(黄箭),为含牙囊肿。

- A dentigerous cyst is the most common type of non-inflammatory odontogenic cyst and forms when fluid accumulates between the follicular epithelium and the crown of an unerupted tooth.
- This manifests as a well-defined,unilocular osteolytic lesion around the crown of an impacted tooth, most frequently around the crown of a mandibular third molar.

Radicular (periapical) cyst

- A radicular cyst is the most common odontogenic lytic lesion. It occurs in either the mandible or the maxilla and is associated with an infected tooth.
- This can progress to bony dehiscence which results in extension of the inflammation to neighboring tissues and can progress to a soft tissue abscess.

Ameloblastoma

- 含牙囊肿是最常见的一类非炎症性牙源性囊肿,成因为液体在滤泡上皮和未萌出的牙冠之间积聚。
- 表现为受阻牙冠周围边界清晰的单房溶骨性病变,最常见于下颌第三磨牙牙冠周围。

根尖(根尖周)囊肿

- 根尖囊肿是最常见的牙源性溶骨性病变。它发生在下颌骨或上颌骨,并与牙齿感染有关。
- 可能会进一步发展为骨裂,从而导致炎症扩展到邻近组织,并可以进一步形成软组织脓肿。

造釉细胞瘤

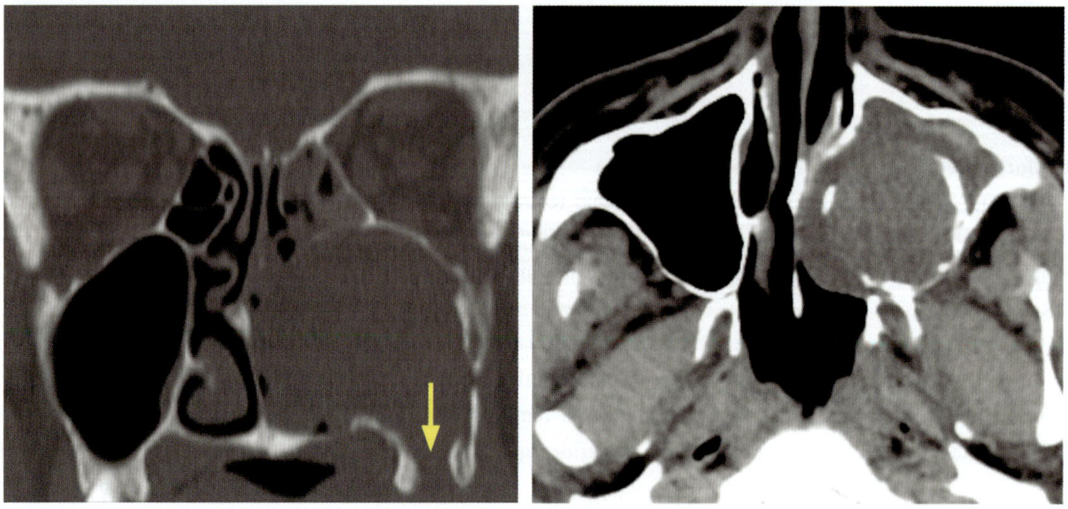

Coronal (left image) and axial (right image) noncontrast CT demonstrate an expansile, mixed-density, peripherally calcified mass in the left maxillary sinus associated with the root of an anterior left maxillary molar (arrow). Biopsy showed ameloblastoma.
冠状位(左图)和轴位(右图)平扫CT显示左上颌窦出现一个膨胀性、混合密度、周边钙化的肿块,与左上颌前磨牙(黄箭)根部相关。活检结果为造釉细胞瘤。

- Ameloblastomas are benign epithelial neoplasms and exhibit locally aggressive behavior.
- These most commonly (80%) occur in the ramus and posterior body of the mandible.
- These classically and more frequently appear as multilocular lytic lesions with mixed cystic and solid regions.
- However, 40% of the time, these can appear unilocular and are indistinguishable from odontogenic keratocysts or dentigerous cysts. In comparison to odontogenickeratocyst, an ameloblastoma is more likely to be predominantly cystic, while odontogenic keratocysts have debris resulting in a more heterogeneous appearance on T2-weighted imaging on MRI and lower mean value on ADC.

- 造釉细胞瘤是良性上皮性肿瘤，具有局部侵袭的行为。
- 病变最好发(80%)于下颌骨的下颌支和后体部。
- 典型且常见的影像学表现为多房溶骨性病变，伴混合囊性与实性的成分。
- 但有40%可能为单房，它们与牙源性角化囊肿或含牙囊肿无法区分。与牙源性角化囊肿相比，造釉细胞瘤更可能以囊性为主，而牙源性角化囊肿内含碎屑，导致MRI T_2加权成像更为不均，且ADC的均值降低。

Odontogenic keratocyst

牙源性角化囊肿

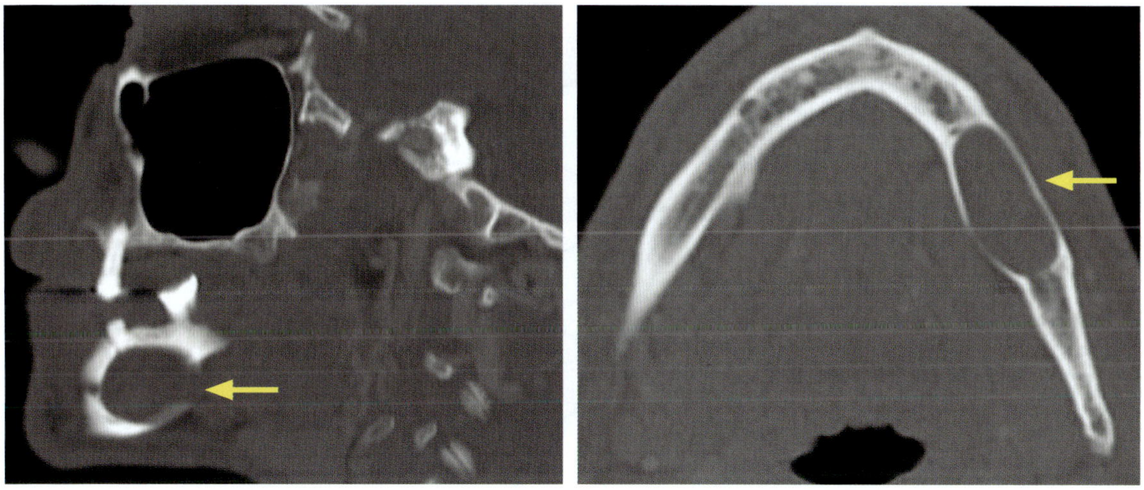

Sagittal (left image) and axial (right image) contrast-enhanced CT show an unilocular expansile lucent lesion (arrows) in the left mandibular body abutting the root of a left mandibular molar. Pathology upon resection showed odontogenic keratocyst.

矢状位(左图)和轴位(右图)对比增强CT显示左下颌体内单房膨胀性透亮病变(黄箭)，紧靠左下颌磨牙根部。切除后病理检查为牙源性角化囊肿。

- A keratocystic odontogenic tumor is a benign unilocular expansile lucent lesion, most frequently seen in the body and ramus of the mandible. As described above, it is more likely to be heterogeneous on T2 and is not associated with buccolingual expansion in the mandible. However, when it is multilocular, it cannot be reliably distinguished from an ameloblastoma based on imaging.

- 牙源性角化囊性肿瘤是一种良性单房膨胀性透亮病变，最常见于下颌骨体和下颌支。如上所述，其在T_2表现为不均匀信号的可能性较大，且为下颌骨内非颊舌向的膨胀性病变。然而，当为多房时，该病在影像学上不能与造釉细胞瘤进行明确区分。

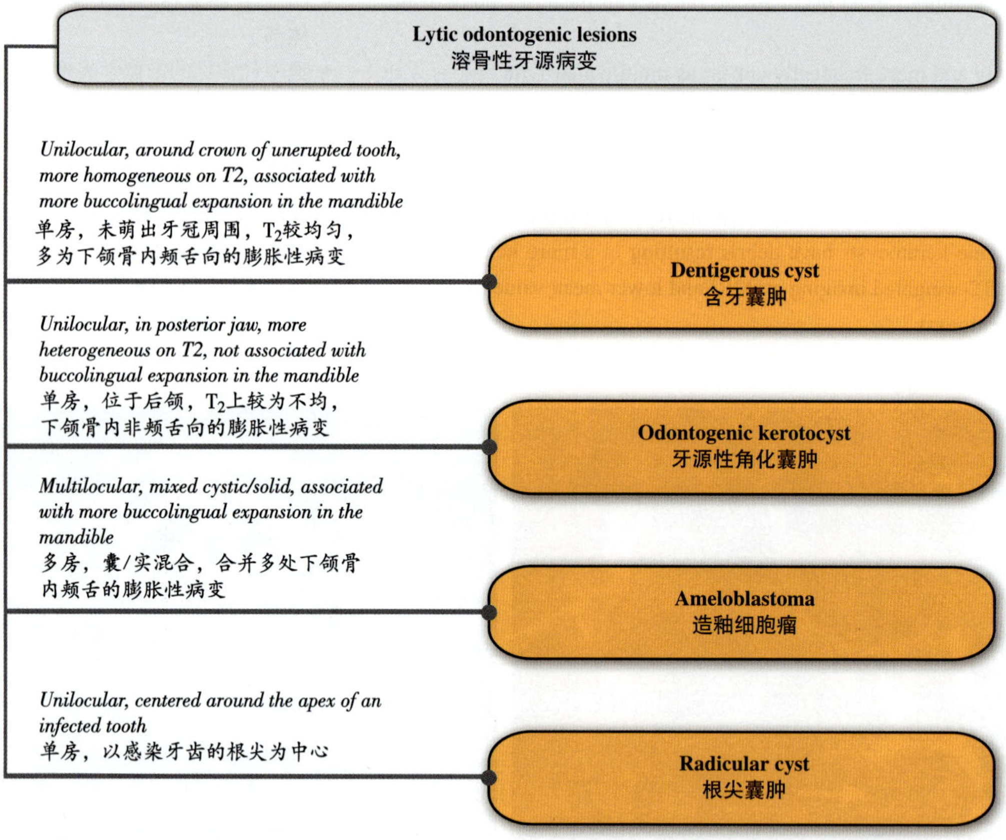

Hypopharynx

Overview and anatomy

- The hypopharynx is the inferior continuation of the oropharynx. It surrounds the larynx on three sides and extends to the level of the inferior border of the larynx, and continues inferiorly as the cervical esophagus. The hypopharynx can be divided into three regions: the piriform sinuses,the posterior pharyngeal wall, and the posterior cricoid region.
- The aryepiglottic folds separate the hypopharynx from the supraglottic larynx. Tumors arising from these folds are staged as supraglottic tumors (described in the larynx section below).

Hypopharyngeal SCC

- Most hypopharyngeal SCCs arise in the pyriform sinus. Staging of hypopharyngeal SCC is dependent on both the lesion size and invasion of adjacent structures.
- Important imaging findings to evaluate for during staging include: Fixation of the hemilarynx; assessment of local invasion including potential involvement of the esophageal mucosa, thyroid/cricoid cartilage, hyoid bone, and prevertebral fascia; and vascular involvement such as encasement of the carotid artery or mediastinal structures.

下咽

概述和解剖

- 下咽是口咽向下的延续，从三面包围喉部，并延伸至喉部下缘水平，继续向下为颈段食管。下咽可分为三个区域：梨状窝、咽后壁和环状软骨后区。
- 杓状会厌襞为下咽与声门上喉部的分界。发生在这些皱襞的肿瘤被分类为声门上肿瘤(在下面的喉部内容描述)。

下咽SCC

- 大多数下咽SCC发生于梨状窝。下咽SCC的分期取决于病变大小和对邻近结构的侵犯。
- 对分期评估的重要影像学表现包括：半喉固定；评估局部浸润，包括潜在食管黏膜、甲状腺/环状软骨、舌骨和椎前筋膜的浸润情况；血管受累，如包绕颈动脉或纵隔结构。

Overview and anatomy

概述与解剖

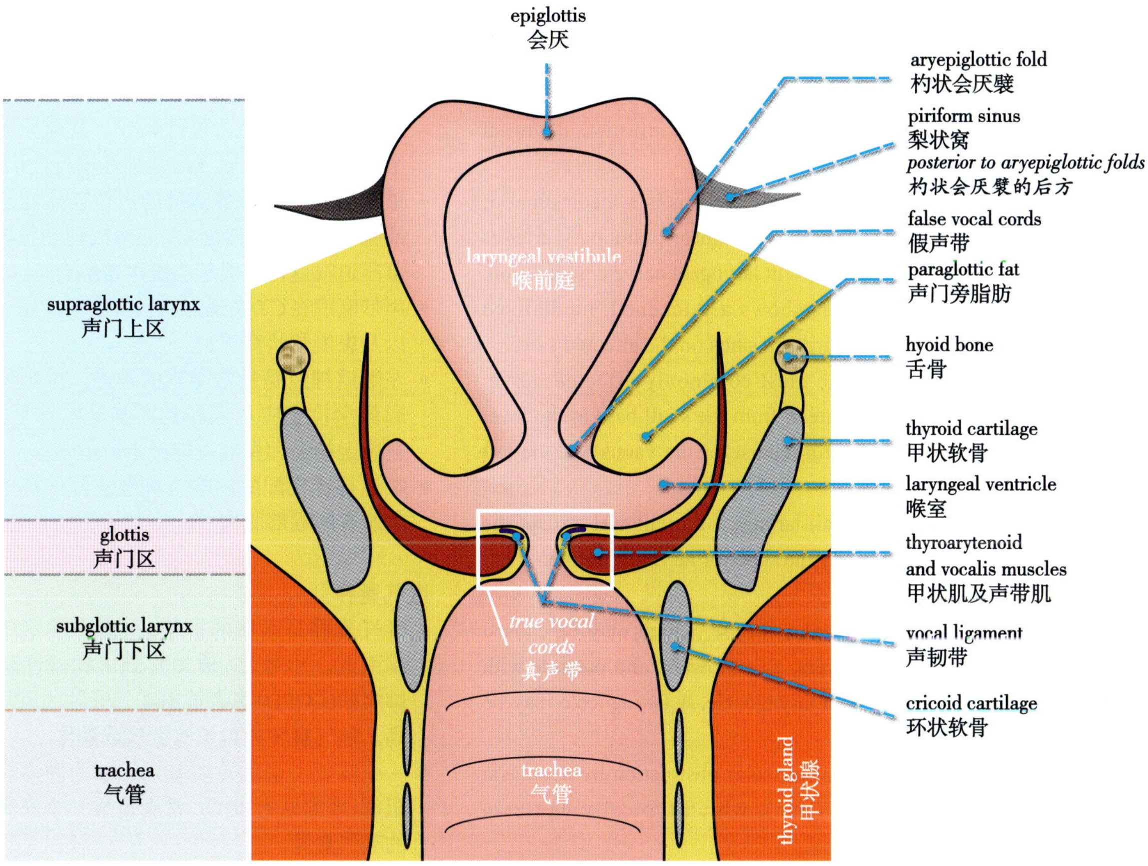

- The larynx connects the oropharynx airway to the tracheal airway.
- The cartilaginous components of the larynx include the epiglottis, thyroid cartilage, cricoid cartilage, and arytenoids.

  The cricoid cartilage is a complete ring which provides the foundation for the laryngeal skeleton.
- The entire larynx, including the epiglottis, aryepiglottic folds and false vocal cords, is lined with mucosa.

  The aryepiglottic folds are an extension of the mucosa covering the epiglottis and mark the entrance to the larynx. The aryepiglottic folds connect the epiglottis anteriorly to the arytenoids posteriorly.

  The false vocal folds are mucosal infoldings superior to the laryngeal ventricle. They can be identified on cross-sectional imaging by the presence of the paraglottic fat laterally.
- The **supraglottic larynx** extends from the epiglottis to the ventricle. The false vocal cords, the aryepiglottic folds, the suprahyoid epiglottis, infrahyoid epiglottis, and the arytenoid cartilages are within the supraglottis and considered subsites for the purposes of staging SCC as discussed below.
- The **glottis** includes the true vocal cords, the anterior and posterior commissures, and extends 1 cm below the vocal cords. The thyroarytenoid muscle, vocalis muscle, and the innermost vocal ligament form the bulk of the vocal cords.

  The true vocal cords are identified in the axial plane by CT or MRI by identifying

- 喉连接口咽和气管气道。
- 喉的软骨包括会厌、甲状软骨、环状软骨和杓状软骨。

  环状软骨是一个完整的环，为喉部框架的基础。
- 整个喉部，包括会厌、杓状会厌襞和假声带，都有黏膜。

  杓状会厌襞是覆盖在会厌表面黏膜的延伸，是喉入口的标志。杓状会厌襞连接前方的会厌和后方的杓状软骨。

  假声带是位于喉室上方的黏膜反折，可以通过横断面成像上位于其外侧的声门旁脂肪来识别。
- **声门上区**从会厌延伸到喉室。假声带、杓状会厌皱襞、舌骨上会厌、舌骨下会厌及杓状软骨均位于声门上区，是以SCC分期考虑为目的具体解剖位置，如下所述。
- **声门区**包括真声带、前后联合，并在声带下方延伸1cm。甲杓肌、声带肌和最内侧的声带韧带构成了声带的主体。

  真声带可在轴位CT或MRI上进行识别，为喉壁内声门旁脂肪与肌肉(甲杓肌)的移行区。

the transition of paraglottic fat to muscle (thyroarytenoid muscle) within the wall of the larynx.

- The **subglottic larynx** begins 1 cm inferior to the apex of the laryngeal ventricles and extends to the first tracheal ring. The cricoid cartilaginous ring is within the subglottic larynx.

Vocal cord paralysis

- Vocal cord paralysis is most commonly due to iatrogenic trauma from neck surgery, but may be secondary to a mass along the course of the vagus or recurrent laryngeal nerves. Other conditions include stroke, infection, laryngeal neoplasm, MS and neuro-degenerative disease.
- The most common mass to cause left vocal cord paralysis is a mediastinal or thoracic mass; however, enlargement of the left atrium or pulmonary arteries may cause cardiovocal syndrome due to recurrent laryngeal nerve compression.
- The CT imaging of vocal cord paralysis shows a thickened, medialized aryepiglottic fold and enlargement of the piriform sinus on the affected side.
- The left recurrent laryngeal nerve is the most commonly affected nerve. Imaging for vocal cord paralysis should extend from the skull base to the level of the left pulmonary artery to cover the full course of the vagus and the left recurrent laryngeal nerves.
- The recurrent laryngeal nerve innervates all laryngeal musculature except the cricothyroid muscle, which is innervated by the superior laryngeal nerve.

Laryngocele

- A laryngocele is a dilation of the laryngeal ventricle, which may be caused by high laryngeal pressures. Trumpet players, glassblowers, and patients with COPD have increased risk of developing a laryngocele. A laryngocele may be filled with air or fluid.
- An important differential consideration is ventricular obstruction by neoplasm (most commonly squamous cell carcinoma), which typically causes a fluid-filled laryngocele.

Laryngeal SCC

- **声门下区**始于喉室顶下方1cm，延伸至第一气管环。环状软骨环位于声门下喉内。

声带麻痹

- 声带麻痹最常见发生原因是颈部手术所致的医源性创伤，但也可能继发于迷走神经或喉返神经走行区的占位性病变。其他原因还有卒中、感染、喉肿瘤、MS和神经退行性疾病等。
- 最常引起左侧声带麻痹的占位性病变是纵隔或胸部的肿块；然而，左心房或肺动脉扩张也可压迫喉返神经引起心脏声带综合征。
- 声带麻痹在CT表现为杓状会厌襞增厚、内移，以及患侧梨状窝扩大。
- 左喉返神经是最常受累的神经。声带麻痹的影像学检查应从颅底到左肺动脉水平，以覆盖迷走神经和左喉返神经走行的全程。
- 喉返神经支配除由喉上神经支配的环甲肌外的所有的喉部肌肉。

喉气囊肿

- 喉气囊肿是喉室的扩张，可能由喉室压力过高引起。小号手、玻璃吹制工和慢性阻塞性肺疾病(COPD)患者罹患喉气囊肿的风险会增高。喉气囊肿内可填有空气或液体。
- 一个需要考虑的重要鉴别诊断为肿瘤性喉室阻塞(最常见为SCC)，常会造成一个充满液体的喉气囊肿。

喉SCC

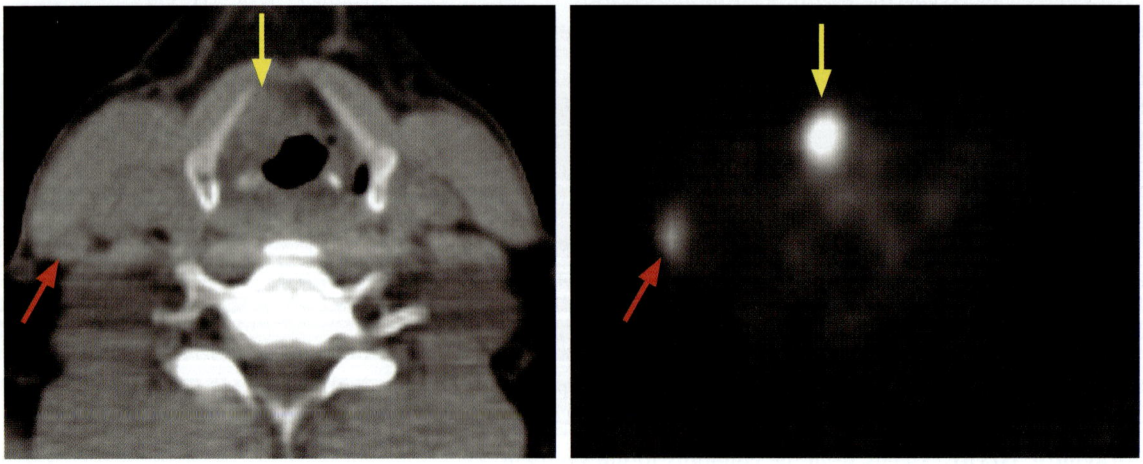

Supraglottic SCC: Axial noncontrast CT through the neck (left image) in a patient presenting with hoarseness demonstrates nodular thickening of the right false cord (yellow arrow) effacing the paraglottic fat. Subsequent F-18 FDG PET shows uptake correlating to this nodule (yellow arrow) as well as uptake in a right level Ⅲ lymph node (red arrows) concerning for metastatic involvement.
声门上SCC：一名声音嘶哑患者的颈部轴位平扫CT(左图)显示右侧假声带呈结节状增厚(黄箭)，并使声门旁脂肪消失。随后的^{18}F-FDG PET(右图)显示摄取与该结节对应(黄箭)，同时还显示右侧Ⅲ区淋巴结(红箭)摄取，考虑为转移性。

- Laryngeal SCC is the most common laryngeal malignancy.

  Less common tumors of the larynx (such as lymphoma and chondrosarcoma) are submucosal and therefore not visible on laryngoscopic exam.
- The majority of laryngeal SCC arise from the glottis.
- There are three staging schemes for laryngeal SCC, specific to the supraglottic, glottic, and subglottic subsites.
- Staging of the **supraglottic** SCC is dependent on the number of subsites of the supraglottis that are described (listed above), vocal cord mobility, and involvement of adjacent structures.

  Treatment of supraglottic SCC can vary from laser epiglottectomy, various types of supraglottic laryngectomy to total laryngectomy. Involvement of several key structures guides surgical management including the laryngeal ventricle, thyroid cartilaginous invasion, posterior cricoid, or anterior commissure invasion, involvement of bilateral arytenoid cartilage, which are contraindications to supraglottic laryngectomy.

  Other areas which have relevance in staging include the paraglottic space, the inner cortex of the thyroid cartilage, involvement of the prevertebral space, encasement of the carotid artery or involvement of mediastinal structures.

  Local spread to the paraglottic spread is particularly relevant in supraglottic tumors.
- Staging of **glottic** SCC is also dependent on vocal cord mobility, cartilaginous involvement, and extension to relevant structures described above.

  Patients with SCC of the glottis present early because of voice changes.

  Key consideration for staging glottic SCC is evaluation for contralateral involvement, since this precludes sparing of the contralateralside as well as the degree of vertical involvement.

  Transglottic tumors, which cross the laryngeal ventricle to involve both the false and true vocal cords, portend a worse prognosis.
- **Subglottic** SCC constitutes less than 5% of laryngeal carcinomas. These lesions can be difficult to identify endoscopically given obscuration from apposed true cords. Staging is similar to the supraglottic and glottic types described above. Prognosis for subglottic lesions is poor as they present at a much more extensive stage.

Laryngeal hemangiomas

- Laryngeal hemangiomas occur most commonly in the subglottic larynx in infants. These are frequently associated with cutaneous lesions. They frequently regress in infants, however given risk of airway compromise can be treated with laser therapy.
- Laryngeal hemangiomas in adults are very rare, with only case reports in the literature. These do not regress spontaneously and are surgically treated.

Laryngeal trauma

- Blunt trauma to the neck may compress the larynx against the cervical spine, with injury to the posterior soft tissues due to the *sandwich effect*.
- Fractures of the thyroid and cricoid cartilage may be difficult to detect in young patients with incomplete ossification.
- Iatrogenic trauma from intubation can cause arytenoid cartilage dislocation.

- 喉SCC是最常见的恶性喉肿瘤。

  较少见的喉肿瘤(如淋巴瘤和软骨肉瘤)位于黏膜下而不易被在喉镜下发现。
- 大多数喉SCC起源于声门。
- 喉SCC有三种分期方案，分别针对声门上区、声门和声门下区。
- **声门上**SCC的分期取决于上文描述的涉及声门上亚部位的数量、声带活动度和邻近结构的受累。

  治疗声门上SCC的方法有多样，包括激光会厌切除术、各种类型的声门上喉切除术及全喉切除术。手术方案取决于数个关键结构是否受累，包括喉室、甲状软骨侵犯、环状软骨后或前联合侵犯、双侧杓状软骨受累，这些都是声门上喉切除术的禁忌证。

  与分期相关的其他区域包括声门旁间隙、甲状软骨内皮质、椎前间隙受累、颈动脉包绕或纵隔结构受累。

  对声门上肿瘤而言，局部至声门旁的扩散程度与分期尤其相关。
- **声门**SCC的分期还取决于声带活动度、软骨受累和上述所描述的相关结构是否受侵犯。

  声门SCC患者会由于声音变化而早期就诊。

  声门SCC分期的关键因素是评估对侧受累，这排除了对侧未受侵犯以及纵向受累。

  跨声门肿瘤，即横越喉室累及真、假声带，提示预后较差。
- **声门下**SCC占喉癌的比例不到5%。这些病变可能难以通过内镜识别，因其会被真声带遮盖。分期与以上描述的声门上和声门类型相似。声门下病变的预后很差，因为其往往在更晚期的时候才有表现。

喉血管瘤

- 喉血管瘤最常见于婴儿的喉声门下区。它们通常与皮肤病变有关，常常在婴儿期消退，但考虑到气道狭窄的风险，可以采取激光治疗。
- 成人喉血管瘤罕见，文献中只有病例报告。此类病变不会自发消退，需要手术治疗。

喉外伤

- 颈部钝性损伤可能会将喉压向颈椎，后部的软组织因*夹心效应*而受伤。
- 甲状软骨和环状软骨骨折在青年人中可能难以被发现，因为这些结构尚未完全骨化。
- 气管插管可引起医源性损伤，并可以导致杓状软骨脱位。

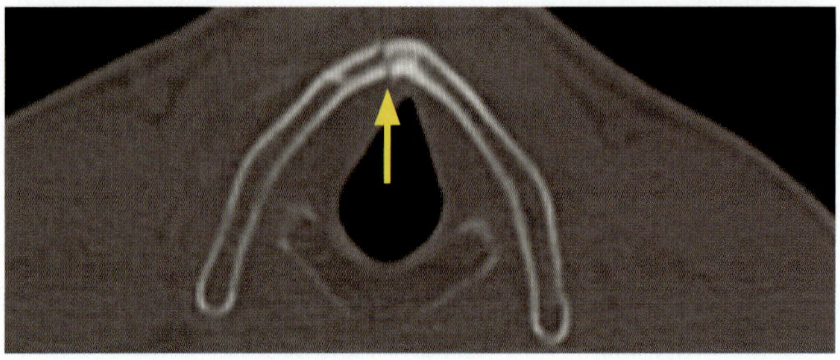

Thyroid cartilage fracture: CT in bone windows shows a minimally displaced fracture of the thyroid cartilage (arrow).

Case courtesy Mary Beth Cunnane, MD, Massachusetts Eye and Ear Infirmary.

甲状软骨骨折：CT骨窗显示微小错位的甲状软骨骨折(黄箭)。

Other malignant neoplasms of the mucosal spaces

Lymphoma

- Lymphoma can arise from the adenoids of the nasopharynx. Most frequently this is non-Hodgkin's lymphoma and affects a younger population.

Sarcomas

- Any type of sarcoma can be found in the larynx, including synovial sarcomas, chondrosarcomas, rhabdomyosarcomas, and liposarcomas. Chondrosarcomas are generally centered in either the cricoid or thyroid cartilage and have characteristic popcorn-like calcifications that are best seen on CT.

黏膜间隙的其他恶性肿瘤

淋巴瘤

- 淋巴瘤可起源于鼻咽腺样体。最常见的是非霍奇金淋巴瘤，累及年轻人群。

肉瘤

- 喉部可以发生任何类型的肉瘤，包括滑膜肉瘤、软骨肉瘤、横纹肌肉瘤和脂肪肉瘤。软骨肉瘤通常以环状软骨或甲状软骨为中心，并具有特征性的爆米花样钙化，CT显示最佳。

(翻译 陈娟)

Extra-mucosal neck spaces

Overview of head and neck spaces

- The complex layers of cervical fascia create several spaces in the suprahyoid neck. Knowledge of these spaces is useful in creating differential diagnoses for neck masses, as specific lesions tend to arise in characteristic locations.

颈部黏膜外间隙

头颈部间隙概述

- 复杂的颈筋膜为舌骨上颈部创造了多个间隙。了解这些间隙有助于对颈部肿块进行鉴别，因为特定的病变常常起自于其典型的部位。

Retropharyngeal space

咽后间隙

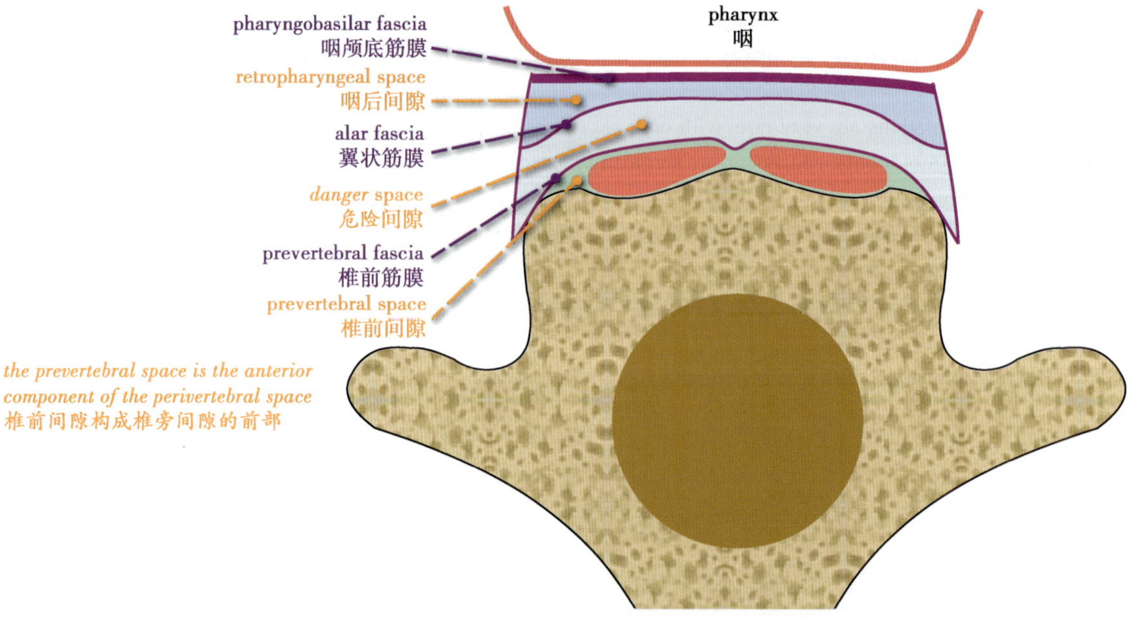

- The **retropharyngeal space** is a potential space located posterior to the pharynx, separated from the pharynx by the pharyngobasilarfascia. The retropharyngeal space extends from the base of the skull to the upper mediastinum. Directly lateral to the retropharyngeal space are the carotid and parapharyngeal spaces.
- The alarfascia is directly posterior to the retropharyngeal space. The alarfascia separates the retropharyngeal space from another potential space, the *danger space*, which acts as a trapdoor for infection to travel all the way from the neck to the diaphragm.
- The prevertebral space (the anterior component of the perivertebral space in the suprahyoid neck) is located just anterior to the vertebral body and is bounded anteriorly by the prevertebral fascia.
- Benign and inflammatory lesions of the retropharyngeal space:

> A medially deviated **internal carotid artery** may mimic a mass on endoscopic evaluation or may be injured during spine surgery.
> **Lipomas**, **fibromyxomas**, and **venous malformations** can occur in the retropharynx.
> Spread of **infection** into the retropharynx can result in a retropharyngeal abscess, discussed later in this chapter.

- Malignant lesions of the retropharyngeal space:

> Primary malignant lesions are uncommon. The most common malignant lesion is **malignant lymphadenopathy**, most frequently associated with nasopharyngeal SCC. Other primary tumors which are associated with retropharyngeal lymphadenopathy include: **Papillary thyroid carcinoma**, **melanoma**.
> **Contiguous spread of primary tumors** in the nasopharynx can involve the retropharyngeal space, such as nasopharyngeal SCC and rhabdomyosarcoma.

CAROTID SPACE

Anatomy of the carotid space

- **咽后间隙**是一个位于咽后部的潜在间隙，由咽颅底筋膜将其与咽部分隔开来。咽后间隙自颅底延伸至上纵隔。紧邻咽后间隙的外侧为颈动脉间隙和咽旁间隙。
- 翼状筋膜位于咽后间隙的正后方。翼状筋膜分隔咽后间隙与另一个潜在间隙，即*危险间隙*，后者充当感染从颈部一路传播到横膈的活板门。
- 椎前间隙(椎旁间隙在舌骨上颈部的前方组成部分)位于椎体的正前方，并以椎前筋膜为前界。
- 咽后间隙的良性和炎性病变：

> **颈内动脉向内侧偏移**时，内镜检查可能会将其误认为肿块，或在脊柱手术时被误伤。
> **脂肪瘤**、**纤维黏液瘤**及**静脉畸形**可出现在咽后部。
> **感染**蔓延至咽后可导致咽后脓肿，将在本章后文进行讨论。

- 咽后间隙的恶性病变：

> 原发的恶性病变不常见。最常见的恶性病变是恶性淋巴结肿大，常与鼻咽部SCC有关。其他伴有咽后淋巴结肿大的原发肿瘤包括**甲状腺乳头状癌**、**黑色素瘤**。
> 鼻咽部**原发肿瘤直接蔓延**可累及咽后间隙，如鼻咽SCC、横纹肌肉瘤。

颈动脉间隙

颈动脉间隙解剖

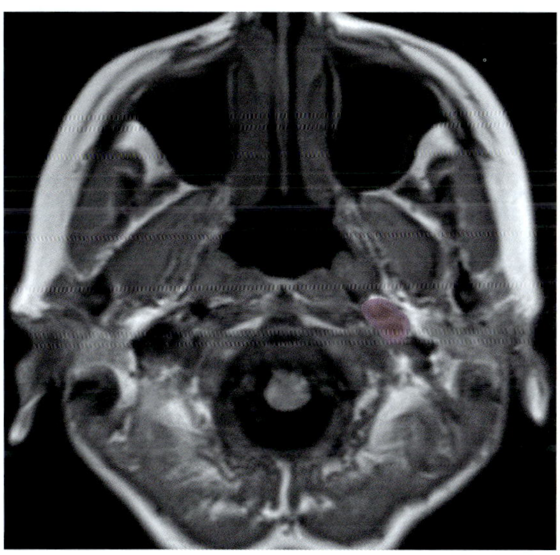

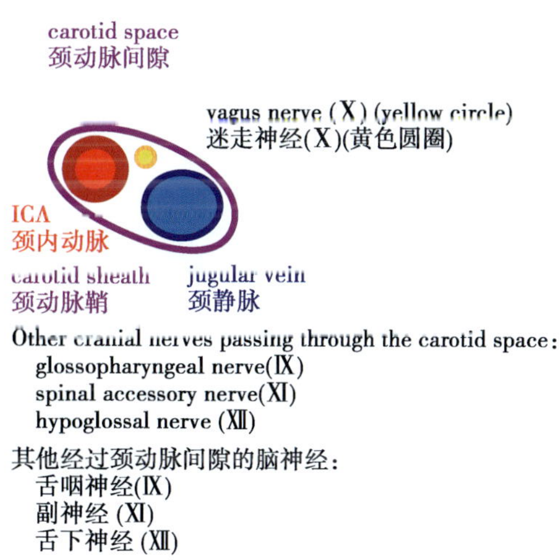

- The carotid space, or post-styloid parapharyngeal space, is an incomplete fascial ring surrounding the carotid artery and jugular vein. The carotid space extends from the skull base to the aortic arch.
- The contents of the carotid space include the carotid artery, carotid body, jugular vein, and several cranial nerves. The vagus nerve (cranial nerve Ⅹ) is the only cranial nerve that remains within the carotid space the entire way into the thorax. In contrast, cranial nerves Ⅸ, Ⅺ and Ⅻ pass transiently through the carotid space. Though there are lymph nodes surrounding the carotid space, there are no lymph nodes contained within it.
- The pattern of displacement of vascular structures in the carotid space is the key to generating a differential diagnosis for a carotid space mass.

Differential diagnosis of a carotid space mass

- **Paraganglioma**

  Paragangliomas that occur in the carotid space include paraganglioma of the carotid body and paraganglioma of the vagal nerve. These demonstrate imaging characteristics similar to paragangliomas elsewhere in the head and neck, described previously.

  Paraganglioma of the carotid body (carotid body tumor or glomus caroticum tumor) splays the external and internal carotid arteries at the carotid bifurcation.

  Paraganglioma of the vagal nerve (glomus vagale tumor) displaces the internal and external carotid arteries anteromedially.
- **Schwannoma**

  Similar to glomus vagale tumor, schwannoma (also most commonly of the vagus nerve) also displaces the carotid arteries anteromedially. Schwannoma, however, is not nearly as vascular as paraganglioma and does not have internal flow voids.
- **Neurofibroma**

  Neurofibromas are almost always associated with neurofibromatosis type 1. Neurofibroma and schwannoma are indistinguishable by MRI.

- 颈动脉间隙，又称茎突后咽旁间隙，是一个不完整的包绕颈动脉和颈静脉的筋膜环。颈动脉间隙自颅底向下延伸至主动脉弓。
- 颈动脉间隙内的结构包括颈动脉、颈动脉体、颈静脉，以及数条脑神经。迷走神经(第Ⅹ脑神经)是唯一全程走行在颈动脉间隙内直至胸腔的脑神经。相比之下，第Ⅸ、Ⅺ和Ⅻ脑神经仅短暂穿过颈动脉间隙。淋巴结分布于颈动脉间隙的周边，但间隙内不含淋巴结。
- 颈动脉间隙内血管结构移位的方式是颈动脉间隙肿块鉴别诊断的关键。

颈动脉间隙肿块的鉴别诊断

- **副神经节瘤**

  发生于颈动脉间隙的副神经节瘤包括颈动脉体副神经节瘤和迷走神经副神经节瘤，影像学的特点与前文讨论的头颈部副神经节瘤类似。

  颈动脉体的副神经节瘤(颈动脉体瘤，或称颈动脉球瘤)位于压迫颈动脉分叉处且张开颈内动脉和颈外动脉。

  迷走神经副神经节瘤(迷走神经球瘤)将颈内动脉和颈外动脉向前内侧推移。
- **神经鞘瘤**

  与迷走神经球瘤相似，神经鞘瘤(通常也为迷走神经)也将颈动脉向前内侧推移。但是，神经鞘瘤远非与副神经节瘤一样富血供，内部无流空效应。
- **神经纤维瘤**

  神经纤维瘤几乎都合并Ⅰ型神经纤维瘤病。神经纤维瘤和神经鞘瘤在MRI上无法区分。

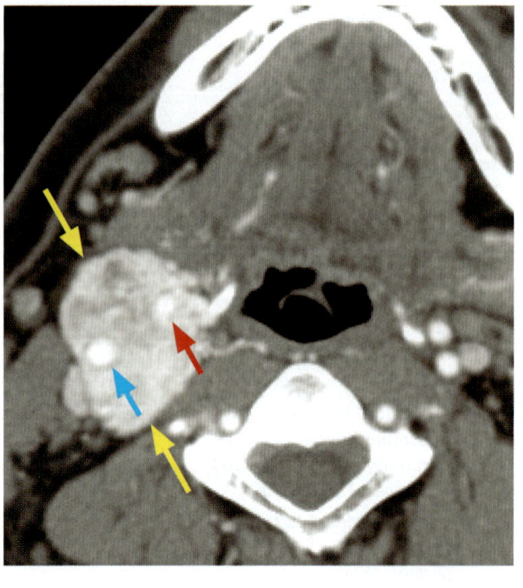

Carotid body tumor: Axial contrastenhanced CT shows an avidly enhancing mass (yellow arrows) surrounding and splaying the right internal (red arrow) and external caroti d (blue arrow) arteries.

Case courtesy Mary Beth Cunnane, MD, Massachusetts Eye and Ear Infirmary.

颈动脉体瘤：轴位增强CT示显著强化的肿块(黄箭)包绕并张开右颈内动脉(红箭)和颈外动脉(蓝箭)。

Parapharyngeal Space (PPS)

Anatomy of the parapharyngeal space

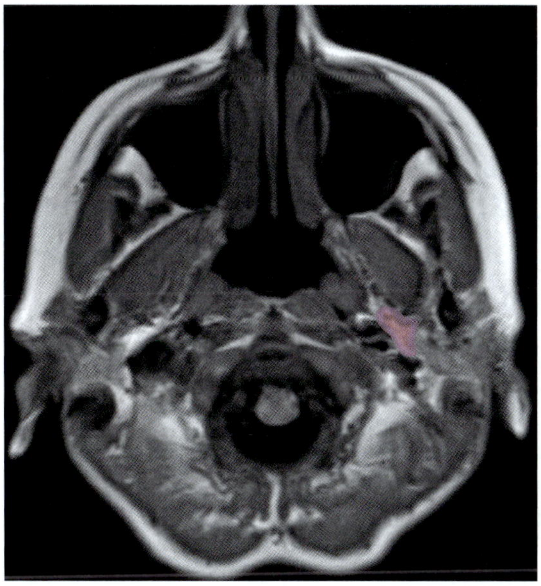

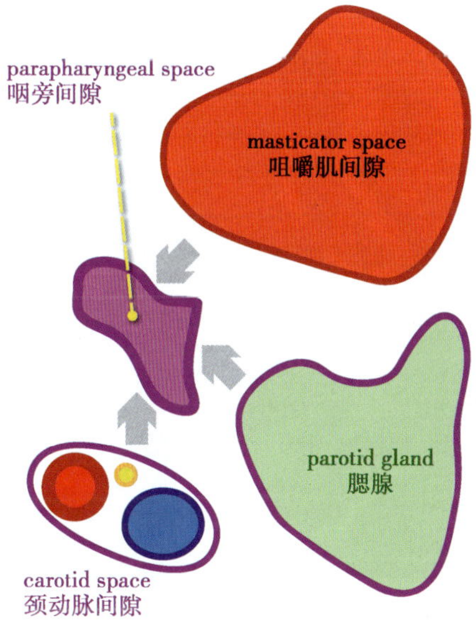

- The prestyloid parapharyngeal space (PPS) is a triangular fat-filled space containing lymphatics, branches of the internal maxillary artery, ascending pharyngeal artery, and the mandibular (V_3) nerve.
- The direction of displacement of the parapharyngeal space fat by a mass in an adjacent compartment is predictable and helpful in determining from which compartment a given mass originates.
  - Masticator space lesions (e.g., masticator abscess) displace the PPS posteromedially.
  - Parotid lesions (e.g., pleomorphic adenoma) displace the PPS anteromedially.
  - Carotid space lesions (e.g., paraganglioma) displace the PPS anteriorly.
- Benign and inflammatory lesions involving the prestyloid parapharyngeal space:

> Parapharyngeal **abscesses** most frequently result from infections that arise in adjacent spaces, most commonly from the palatine tonsil, pharynx or are odontogenic in origin.
> **Second branchial cleft cysts**, discussed later, can present in the parapharyngeal space.
> Benign **tumors**, most frequently pleomorphic adenoma, arising from the deep portion of the parotid gland or salivary rests within the parapharyngeal fat can present as a mass in this space.
> Rarely **schwannomas**, usually arising from the sympathetic plexus or the mandibular (V_3) nerve, can arise in this space.

- Malignant lesions of the prestyloid parapharyngeal space:

> Malignant tumors are rare and when they occur are **most frequently salivary gland in origin**, such as mucoepidermoid carcinoma, adenoid cystic carcinoma, and acinic cell carcinoma.
> **Secondary invasion** can be seen, most commonly from the pharynx, such as SCC or minor salivary gland carcinoma, and lymphoma, or the skull base, chordoma, chondrosarcoma, osteoma, osteochondroma, which are discussed elsewhere.

咽旁间隙(PPS)

咽旁间隙的解剖

- 茎突前咽旁间隙(PPS)是一个充填脂肪的三角形间隙，内含淋巴、上颌内动脉分支、咽升动脉及下颌神经(V_3)。
- 咽旁间隙内脂肪被相邻间室内肿块推移的方向是可以推测的，因而有助于确定该肿块起源的间室。
  - 咀嚼肌间隙病变(如咀嚼肌脓肿)将PPS向后内侧推移。
  - 腮腺病变(如多形性腺瘤)将PPS向前内侧推移。
  - 颈动脉间隙病变(如副神经节瘤)将PPS向前推移。
- 累及茎前咽旁间隙的良性及炎性病变：

> 咽旁**脓肿**通常起自于邻近间隙的感染，最常为腭扁桃体、咽或牙源性起源。
> **第二鳃裂囊肿**，亦可出现于咽旁间隙，将在后文讨论。
> 良性**肿瘤**，最常见为多形性腺瘤，起自腮腺深叶或咽旁脂肪内的唾液腺，可表现为该间隙内的肿块。
> 罕见的**神经鞘瘤**，通常起自交感神经丛或下颌神经(V_3)，可出现于此间隙。

- 茎前咽旁间隙的恶性病变：

> 恶性肿瘤罕见，**大部分起源于腮腺**，如黏液表皮样癌、腺样囊性癌和腺泡细胞癌。
> 亦可见**继发性累及**，最常来自咽(如SCC或小唾液腺癌)、淋巴瘤或颅底(脊索瘤、软骨肉瘤、骨瘤、骨软骨瘤)，将在其他部分讨论该内容。

PERIVERTEBRAL SPACE

Anatomy of the perivertebral space

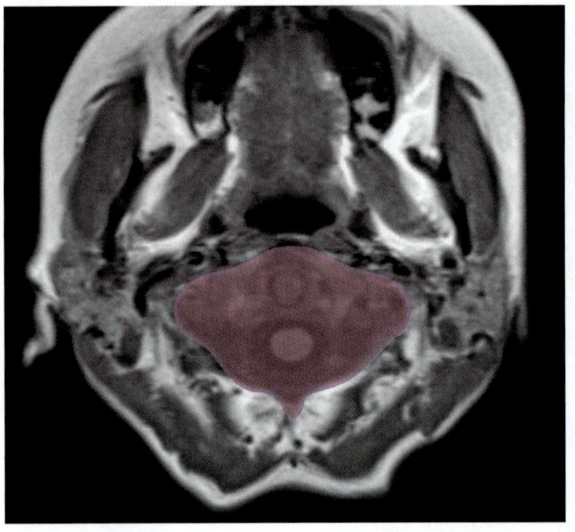

- The perivertebral space is formed by the deep layer of deep cervical fascia which wraps entirely around the prevertebral and paraspinal muscles. The anterior perivertebral space is synonymous with the prevertebral space. The *peri*vertebral space is in the suprahyoid neck; the *para*vertebral space is the analogous region in the thoracolumbar spine.
- The perivertebral space includes the longus colli-capitis muscle complex, the paraspinal muscles, the vertebral bodies, the neurovascular structures within the spinal canal, including the spinal column, exiting nerves, the vertebral arteries, as well as the brachial plexus.
- Differential diagnosis of a benign lesion in the perivertebral space:

> Congenital **lymphatic lesions** (discussed later).
> **Nerve sheath tumors** arising from cervical nerve roots.
> **Hemangiomas** of the musculature.
> Benign **bony tumors**.

- Malignant lesions in the perivertebral space:

> Malignant lesions are most frequently centered on the vertebral bodies, and therefore **most frequently are metastases**.
> Other differential considerations include primary vertebral body malignancies, soft-tissue malignancies arising from the perivertebral musculature such as lymphoma, rhabdomyosarcoma.

椎体周围间隙

椎体周围间隙的解剖

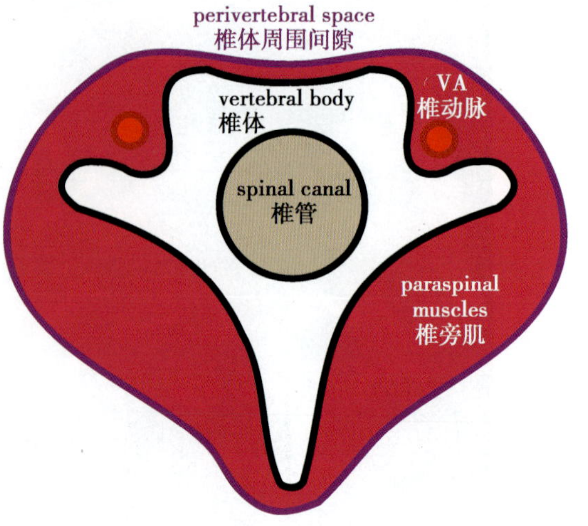

- 椎体周围间隙由颈深筋膜深层构成，后者完全包裹椎前及椎旁肌肉。椎体周围前间隙是椎前间隙的同义词。椎体周围间隙位于舌骨上的颈部；*椎旁*间隙则是指胸腰段脊柱中相应的区域。
- 椎体周围间隙包括头-颈长肌复合体、椎旁肌、椎体和椎管内神经血管结构，后者包括脊髓、发出的神经、椎动脉及臂丛神经。
- 椎体周围间隙良性病变的鉴别诊断：

> 先天性**淋巴病变**(将在下文讨论)。
> 起自颈神经根的**神经鞘瘤**。
> 肌肉组织**血管瘤**。
> 良性**骨肿瘤**。

- 椎体周围间隙的恶性病变：

> 恶性病变通常以椎体为中心，因此**最常见为转移瘤**。
> 其他鉴别诊断包括原发性椎体恶性肿瘤、起自椎体周围肌肉组织的软组织恶性肿瘤(如淋巴瘤、横纹肌肉瘤)。

MASTICATOR SPACE

Anatomy of the masticator space

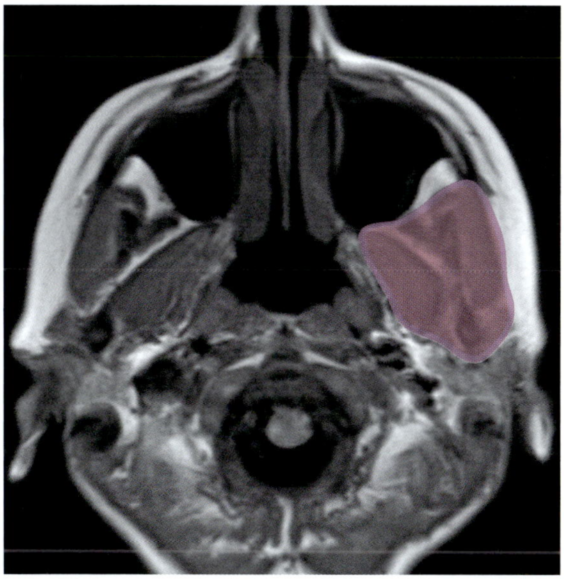

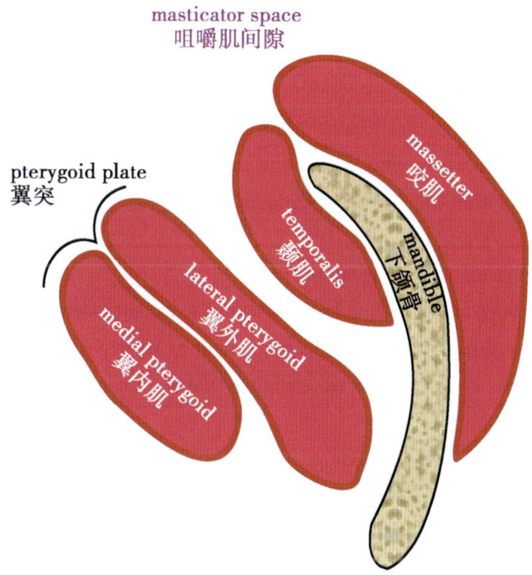

- The masticator space is located directly anterior to the parotid and contains the muscles of mastication, the mandible, and cranial nerve V_3. Cranial nerve V_3 (mandibular division) exits the skull through foramen ovale and innervates the muscles of mastication. If there is a lesion in the masticator space, it is important to assess for perineural spread along V_3.
- The temporomandibular joint also falls within the masticator space.
- The majority of abnormalities that occur in the masticator space are a result of extension from neighboring spaces, such as the oral cavity, the parotid space, or the parapharyngeal or retropharyngeal spaces.

Infections of the masticator space

咀嚼肌间隙

咀嚼肌间隙解剖

- 咀嚼肌间隙位于腮腺的正前方，包含咀嚼肌、下颌骨和脑神经V_3。脑神经V_3(下颌神经分支)经卵圆孔出颅，支配咀嚼肌。对于咀嚼肌间隙内的病变，评估是否有沿V_3的神经周围蔓延很重要。
- 颞下颌关节亦属于咀嚼肌间隙。
- 大多数发生在咀嚼肌间隙内的异常是由邻近间隙的病灶扩散而来，如口腔、腮腺间隙、咽旁间隙或咽后间隙。

咀嚼肌间隙的感染

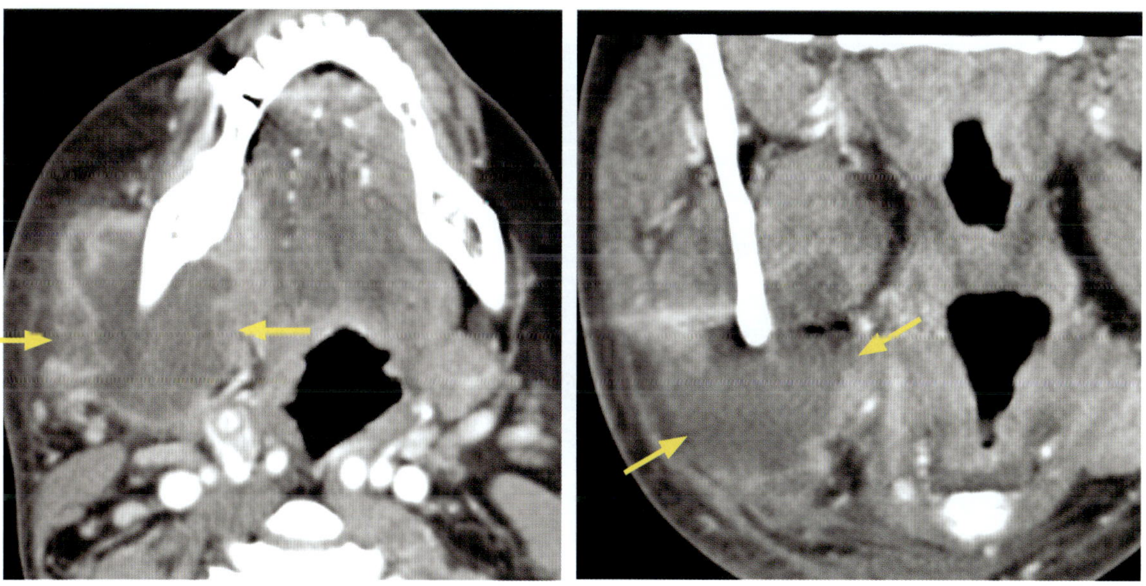

Masticator/submandibular abscess: Axial (left image) and coronal contrast-enhanced CT shows a peripherally enhancing irregular fluid collection (arrows) abutting the angle of the right mandible, with associated stranding of the subcutaneous fat.
咀嚼肌/颌下脓肿：轴位(左图)及冠状位增强CT显示一个边缘强化的不规则液性聚集(黄箭)，紧邻右侧下颌角，伴皮下脂肪条索影。

- Infections of the masticator space are more common than tumors.
- Most infections are odontogenic in origin. Less commonly, extension of infection from parotid gland sialadenitis, extension of a palatine tonsillar abscess, or extension of a severe retropharyngeal space infection can be seen.
- A masticator space abscess appears as an irregular, thick-walled, peripherally enhancing fluid located inferior to the mandible. Adjacent fat-stranding is usually present.

- 咀嚼肌间隙内感染比肿瘤更常见。
- 大多数感染为牙源性。较少来自腮腺炎、腭扁桃体脓肿蔓延或严重咽后间隙感染扩散。
- 咀嚼肌间隙脓肿表现为一个不规则、厚壁、周边强化的液性聚集，位于下颌骨的下方。通常可见邻近的脂肪条索影。

Approach to tumors and non-neoplastic masses in the masticator space

- Masses within the masticator space can be organized as masses arising from bone (mandible), arising within the nerve (branches of the mandibular nerve) or arising within the muscles of mastication.

咀嚼肌间隙肿瘤及非肿瘤肿块的分析方法

- 咀嚼肌间隙内的肿块可分为三类：肿块起源于骨骼(下颌骨)、来源于神经(下颌神经分支)或起自咀嚼肌。

- **Lesions arising from the mandible:**

  Primary bone tumors arising from the mandible include osteoblastoma, osteosarcoma, chondrosarcoma. Odontogenic lesions such as dentigerous cyst, keratocyst, or ameloblastoma can be seen in the mandible, and are more completely discussed in the oral cavity section.
- **Lesions arising within nerve:**

  Anatomically, after exiting the skull base from the foramen ovale, V_3 lies along the medial margin of the lateral pterygoid muscle.

  Schwannomas of V_3 can smoothly expand the foramen ovale and present as a well-defined mass in the masticator space, with imaging characteristics similar to those of schwannomas elsewhere in the head and neck as described previously.
- **Lesions arising within muscle**:

  Venous malformations (previously known as hemangiomas and lymphangiomas) can be seen, usually within the masseter muscle when present.

  Malignant masses arising from muscle include rhabdomyosarcoma, lymphoma, and metastases.

- **病变起自下颌骨：**

  起自下颌骨的原发性骨肿瘤包括成骨细胞瘤、骨肉瘤、软骨肉瘤。

  牙源性病变亦可见于下颌骨，如含牙囊肿、角化囊肿、造釉细胞瘤，在口腔部分中有更完整的讨论。
- **病变起自神经：**

  解剖学上，V_3自卵圆孔出颅底后，走行于翼外肌的内侧缘。

  V_3的神经鞘瘤可以光滑地将卵圆孔扩张，表现为咀嚼肌间隙内有边界清晰的肿块，影像学表现与前文所述的头颈部其他部位的神经鞘瘤类似。
- **病变起自肌肉：**

  还可见到静脉畸形(曾称血管瘤和淋巴管瘤)，常出现在咬肌内。

  起自肌肉的恶性肿块包括横纹肌肉瘤、淋巴瘤和转移瘤。

Temporomandibular joint anatomy & pathology

颞下颌关节的解剖和病理

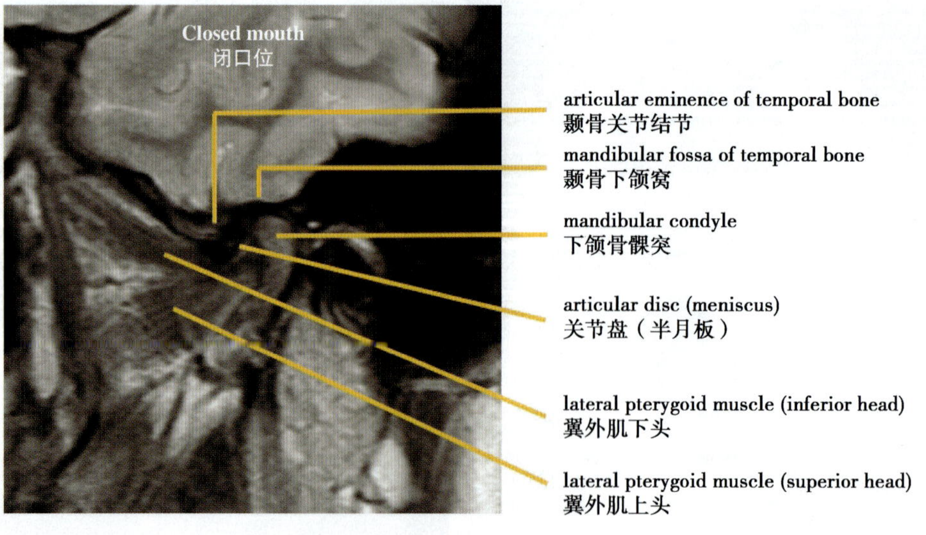

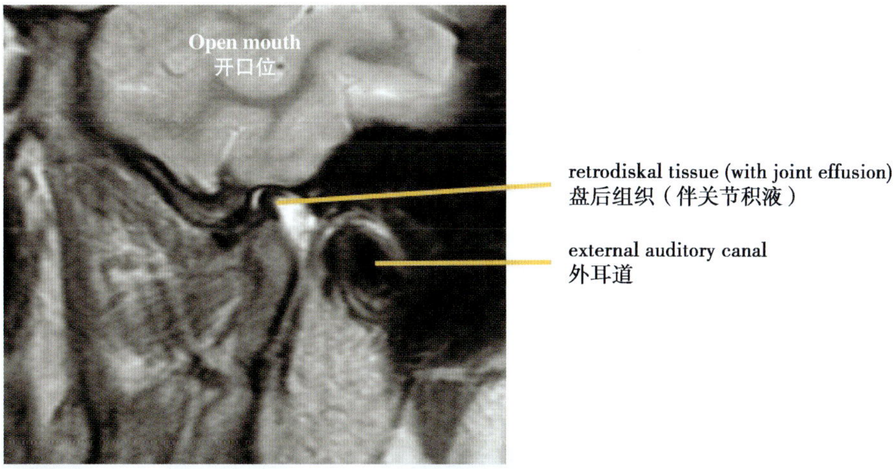

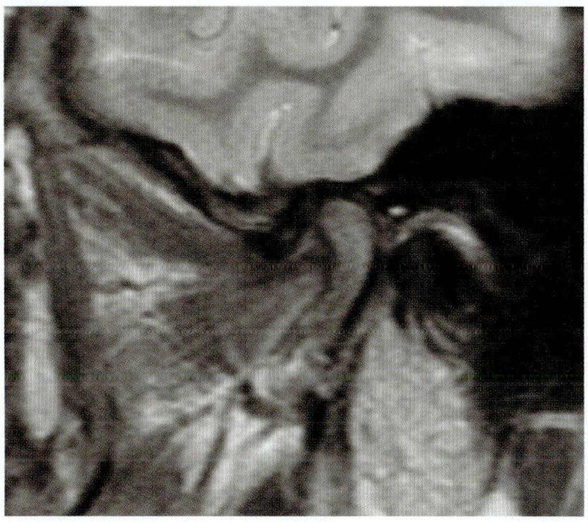

Right TMJ, closed mouth position
右侧颞下颌关节，闭口位

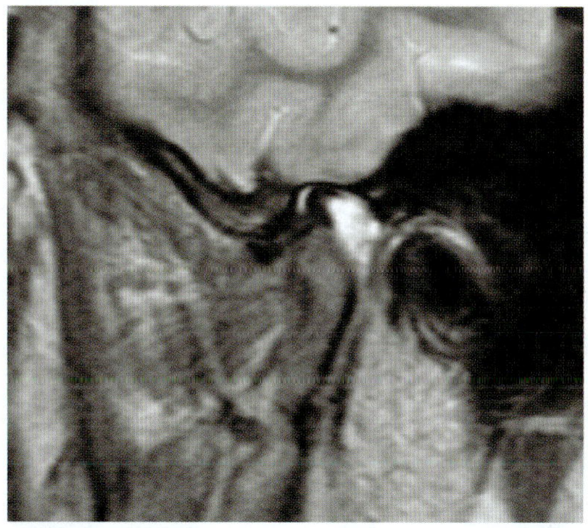

Right TMJ, open mouth position
右侧颞下颌关节，开口位

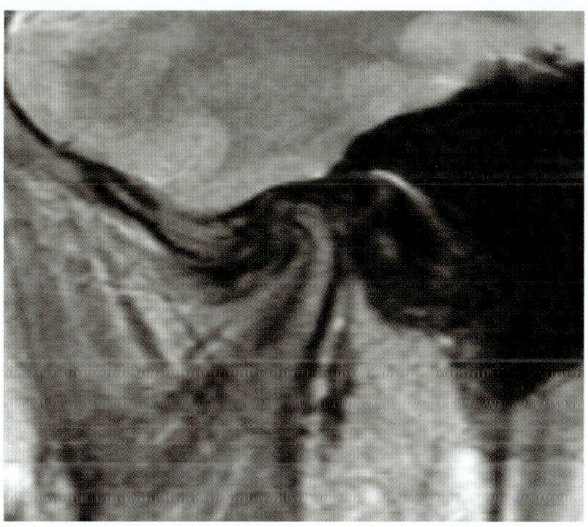

Left TMJ, closed mouth position
左侧颞下颌关节，闭口位

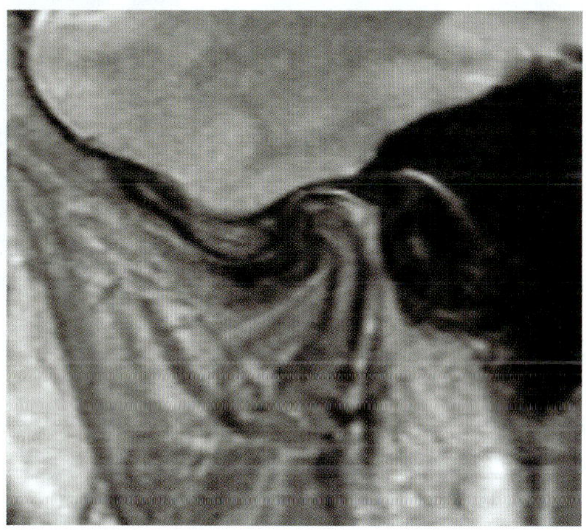

Left TMJ, open mouth position
左侧颞下颌关节，开口位

Sagittal T2-weighted MRI of normal and abnormal temporomandibular joints:
Images of the right TMJ demonstrate normal disc position, shape, and signal on closed mouth view, and slightly limited disc mobility on open mouth image with abnormal retrocondylar T2 hyperintense signal representing a small joint effusion.
Images of the left TMJ show an abnormally small condyle, and an anteriorly dislocated disc which appears thickened with intermediate T2 signal. On open mouth view, there is lack of normal mobility without change in disc position possibly representing “stuck disc” due to adhesions.
正常和异常的颞下颌关节矢状位T_2加权MRI：
右侧颞下颌关节闭口位图像示正常的关节盘位置、形状和信号，开口位图像示关节盘活动性轻度受限，伴异常的盘后T_2高信号，提示少许关节积液。
左侧颞下颌关节图像示异常的小髁突，伴关节盘前脱位，表现为关节盘增厚，并呈T_2中等信号。开口位上，缺乏正常的活动度，表现为关节盘位置没有改变，提示可能是由于粘连导致的“关节盘卡顿”。

- The temporomandibular joint (TMJ) can get dislocated and anterior meniscal dislocations are the most common.
- Similar to other synovial joints, the TMJ can be affected by degenerative osteoarthritis and inflammatory arthritis such as rheumatoid arthritis and juvenile idiopathic arthritis, as well as crystalline arthropathies, which are discussed in greater detail in the "Musculoskeletal" chapter.
- The TMJ can be affected by lesions such as pigmented villonodular synovitis, synovial chondromatosis and chondroid masses.

- 颞下颌关节可脱位，最常见为关节盘前脱位。
- 与其他滑膜关节类似，颞下颌关节可发生退行性骨关节炎、炎性关节炎(如类风湿关节炎、幼年特发性关节炎)，以及结晶性关节病，这些关节病在"骨骼与肌肉影像"一章中有更详细的讨论。
- 颞下颌关节还可发生色素绒毛结节性滑膜炎、滑膜骨软骨瘤病及软骨类肿瘤。

Other benign lesions/masses of the masticator space

咀嚼肌间隙的其他良性病变/肿块

Second branchial cleft cyst

第二鳃裂囊肿

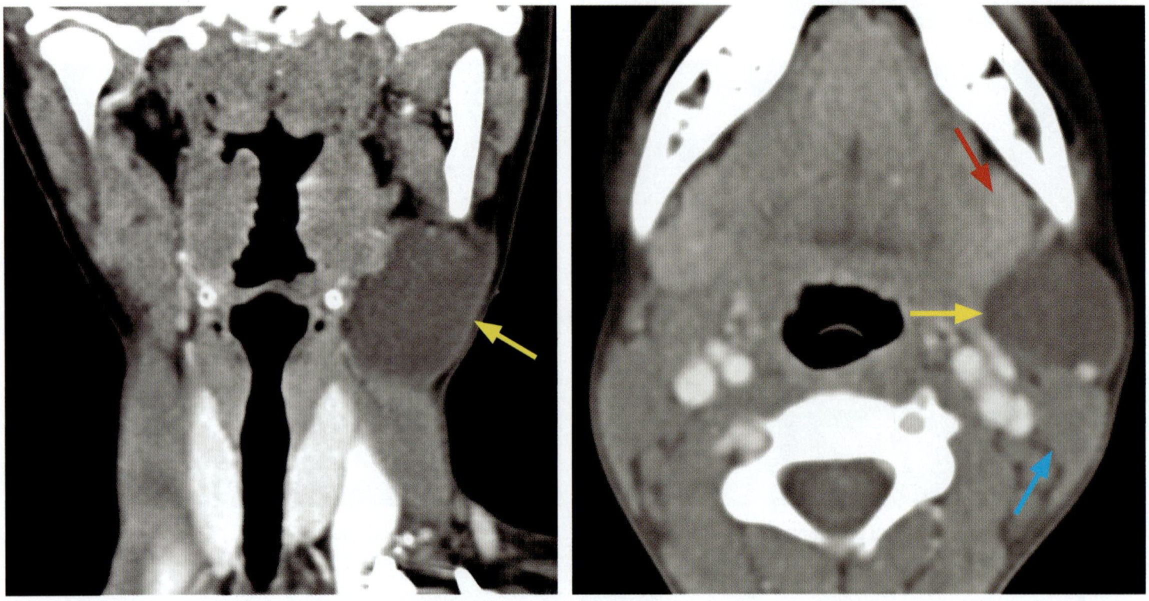

Second branchial cleft cyst: Coronal (left image) and axial contrast-enhanced CT shows a water-attenuation cystic lesion (yellow arrows) at the angle of the left mandible with minimal peripheral wall enhancement. This cyst is in the classic location of a second branchial cleft cyst: Posterior to the submandibular gland (red arrow), anterior to the sternocleidomastoid muscle (blue arrow), and closely associated with the carotid sheath.

Case courtesy Mary Beth Cunnane, MD, Massachusetts Eye and Ear Infirmary.

第二鳃裂囊肿：冠状位(左图)及轴位增强CT显示一个水样密度囊性病变(黄箭)，位于左下颌角伴外周壁轻微强化。该囊肿位于第二鳃裂囊肿的典型部位：下颌下腺的后方(红箭)，胸锁乳头肌前方(蓝箭)，紧贴颈动脉鞘。

- A branchial cleft cyst is a congenital anomaly arising from the embryologic branchial apparatus. There are 4 types of congenital branchial cleft cysts, with the second type being the most common type.
- A second branchial cleft cyst may occur at any point along the path extending from the palatine tonsil to the supraclavicular region, but occurs most commonly near the angle of the mandible.
- The classic second branchial cleft cyst displaces the sternocleidomastoid muscle posteriorly, displaces the carotid artery and internal jugular vein medially and the submandibular gland anteriorly.
- The cyst may become superinfected, suggested by wall enhancement and adjacent inflammatory changes within the surrounding soft tissues.

Although second branchial cleft cysts are frequently in the posterior submandibular space, an infected second branchial cleft cyst would not typically be confused with a submandibular abscess. Submandibular abscess is usually due to dental disease, typically located immediately inferior to the mandible.

- 第二鳃裂囊肿是起自胚胎腮器的一种先天性发育异常。共有4种先天性鳃裂囊肿，其中以第二鳃裂囊肿最常见。
- 第二鳃裂囊肿可发生于腭扁桃体至锁骨上区域穿行路径上的任何部位，但最常发生于下颌角附近。
- 典型的第二鳃裂囊肿会将胸锁乳头肌向后推移，将颈动脉及颈内静脉向内推移，以及将颌下腺向前推移。
- 囊肿可合并感染，表现为囊壁强化及邻近的周边软组织炎性改变。

尽管第二鳃裂囊肿通常位于下颌下间隙的后方，但感染后的第二鳃裂囊肿可能不典型，可与下颌下脓肿相混淆。下颌下脓肿通常是由牙病所致，其典型的位置为下颌骨的正下方。

- Branchial cleft cysts are uncommon in older adults. A cystic metastasis (e.g., from papillary thyroid cancer or base of tongue/tonsillar SCC) should be considered instead, especially if the cyst is irregular or has a mural nodule.
- On imaging, there is opacification of the middle ear and mastoid air cells, often with bony erosion of the mastoid.

- 鳃裂囊肿在老年人中不常见，尤其是囊肿不规则或者有壁结节时，应考虑为囊性转移瘤（如甲状腺乳头状癌、舌底/扁桃体的SCC）而非鳃裂囊肿。
- 影像上，中耳及乳突气房密度增高，常伴乳突骨质侵蚀。

（翻译　何予）

CERVICAL LYMPH NODES

颈部淋巴结

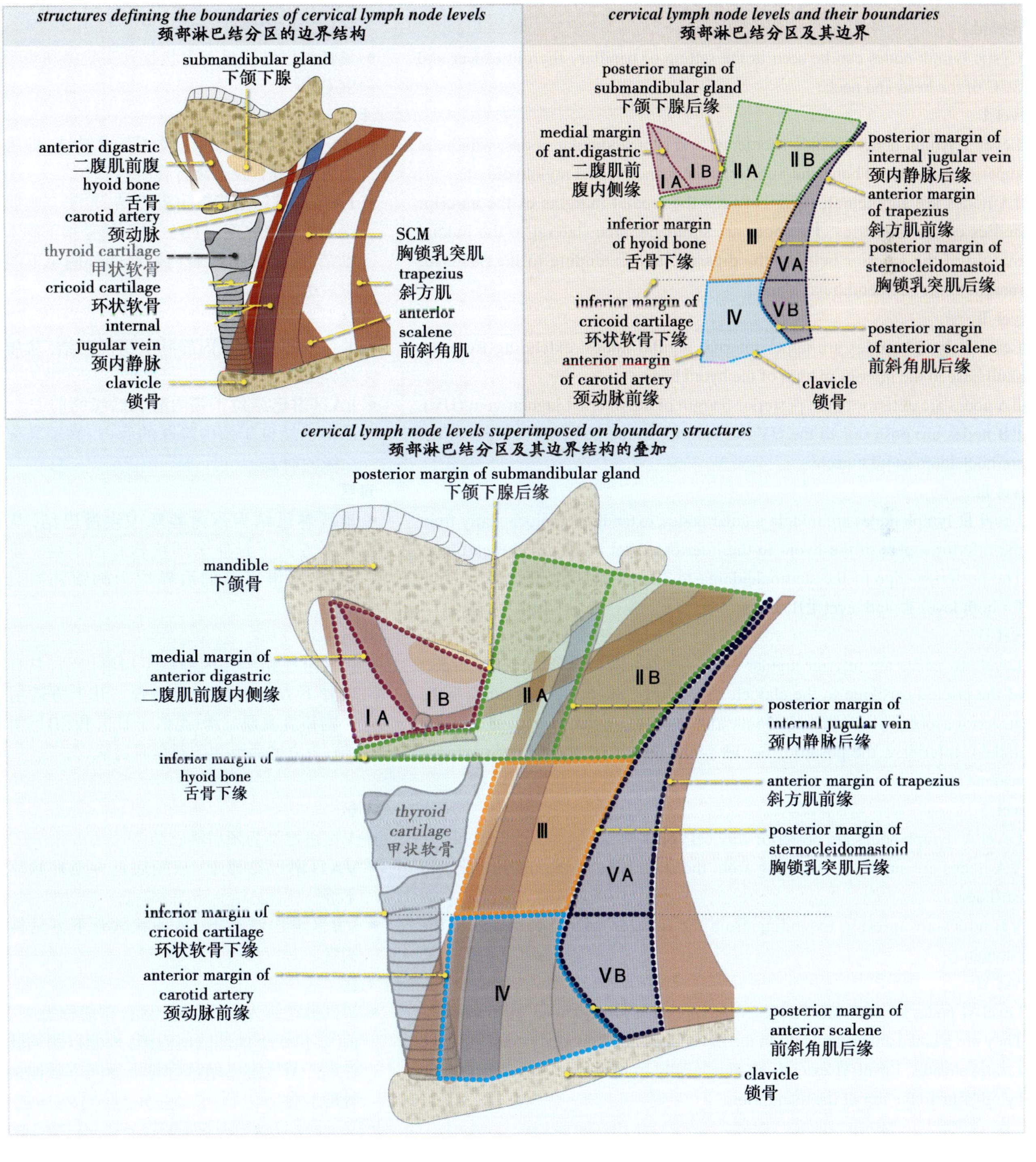

Cervical lymph node levels

Overview of cervical lymph nodes

- The cervical lymph nodes are divided into 7 levels as recommended by the American Joint Committee on Cancer (AJCC), with consistent agreement between surgeons, oncologists, and radiologists. The lymph node levels are not defined by fascial planes, but instead are defined by anatomic landmarks and organized by patterns of lymphatic spread.
- In an adult, 90% of head and neck cancers are SCC: The role of the radiologist is not to provide a differential, but to stage the disease. The degree of lymph node involvement has a substantial prognostic value. For instance, a single metastatic lymph node decreases survival from SCC by 50% over an equivalent period.
- Cystic lymph nodes can be seen in the setting of papillary thyroid cancer and SCC of the head and neck.

Level Ⅰ

- Level Ⅰ lymph nodes include submental and submandibular nodes, which are superior to the hyoid bone and inferior to the mandible and mylohyoid.
- **ⅠA** nodes are submental, lying between the medial margins of the anterior bellies of the digastrics. **ⅠB** nodes are submandibular, lateral to the medial margin of the anterior belly of the digastric and extending to the posterior margin of the submandibular gland.

Level Ⅱ

- Level Ⅱ lymph nodes are upper internal jugular nodes, extending from the skull base to the inferior margin of the hyoid bone.
- **ⅡA** nodes are anterior to the posterior margin of the internal jugular vein (IJV). **ⅡB** nodes are posterior to the IJV but anterior to the posterior margin of the sternocleidomastoid muscle.

Level Ⅲ

- Level Ⅲ lymph nodes are middle jugular nodes, extending craniocaudally from the inferior aspect of the hyoid to the inferior aspect of the cricoid cartilage. The posterior edge of the sternocleidomastoid is the shared posterior margin for both level Ⅲ and level ⅡB nodes.

Level Ⅳ

- Level Ⅳ nodes are inferior jugular nodes, extending from the inferior aspect of the cricoid cartilage to the clavicle. Superiorly, the posterior border is the posterior aspect of the sternocleidomastoid muscle (similar to level Ⅲ and ⅡB nodes). Inferiorly, the posterior border is the posterior aspect of the anterior scalene muscle.

Level Ⅴ

- Level Ⅴ lymph nodes are posterior cervical nodes.
- **ⅤA** nodes are superior, extending from the skull base to the inferior cricoid cartilage.
- **ⅤB** nodes are inferior, extending from the inferior cricoid cartilage to the clavicle.

Level Ⅵ

- Level Ⅵ nodes are pretracheal nodes, which are often simply called "pretracheal". They are located anteromedially in the lower neck and bounded laterally by the carotid sheaths. Level Ⅵ extends craniocaudally from the inferior aspect of the hyoid bone to the top of the manubrium.

颈部淋巴结分区

颈部淋巴结概要

- 颈部淋巴结划分为7个区，划分依据为美国癌症联合委员会(AJCC)的建议，以及外科医师、肿瘤科医师及影像科医师达成的共识。颈部淋巴结分区并不按照筋膜层进行划分，而是根据解剖标志及淋巴结的转移方式。
- 在成人，90%的头颈部癌是SCC：影像科医师的作用不是进行鉴别诊断，而是要提供疾病分期。淋巴结受累程度具有重要的预后价值。例如，当出现单个淋巴结转移时，生存率较无转移的SCC降低50%。
- 囊性淋巴结可见于甲状腺乳头状癌和头颈部SCC。

Ⅰ区

- Ⅰ区淋巴结包括颏下及颌下淋巴结，即舌骨上方、下颌骨及下颌舌骨肌的下方。
- **ⅠA**区淋巴结是指颏下淋巴结，位于二腹肌前腹的内侧缘之间。**ⅠB**区淋巴结是指下颌下淋巴结，在二腹肌前腹内侧缘的外侧至下颌下腺后缘。

Ⅱ区

- Ⅱ区淋巴结为颈内静脉上组淋巴结，从颅底延伸至舌骨下缘。
- **ⅡA**区淋巴结位于颈内静脉后缘的前方。**ⅡB**区淋巴结位于颈内静脉的后方，胸锁乳突肌后缘的前方。

Ⅲ区

- Ⅲ区淋巴结为颈内静脉中组淋巴结，从舌骨下方向下延伸至环状软骨的下缘。Ⅲ区和ⅡB区淋巴结的后界均为胸锁乳突肌的后缘。

Ⅳ区

- Ⅳ区淋巴结为颈内静脉下组淋巴结，从环状软骨下方向下延伸至锁骨。其上方的后界为胸锁乳突肌后缘(类似于Ⅲ区和ⅡB区淋巴结)，下方的后界为前斜角肌后缘。

Ⅴ区

- Ⅴ区淋巴结为颈后淋巴结。
- **ⅤA**区淋巴结靠上，从颅底延伸至环状软骨下缘。
- **ⅤB**区淋巴结靠下，从环状软骨下方延伸至锁骨。

Ⅵ区

- Ⅵ区淋巴结为气管前淋巴结，常简称为"气管前"。位于下颈部的前内侧，外侧以颈动脉鞘为界。Ⅵ区淋巴结从舌骨下方向下延伸至胸骨柄上缘。

Level Ⅶ

- Level Ⅶ nodes are superior mediastinal nodes, which are also commonly described by their location. They are inferior to level Ⅵ and medial to the carotid sheaths, extending craniocaudally from the superior aspect of the manubrium to the brachiocephalic vein.

Ⅶ区

- Ⅶ区淋巴结为上纵隔淋巴结，通常也是根据其位置进行命名的。Ⅶ区淋巴结位于Ⅵ区下方，颈动脉鞘的内侧，从胸骨柄上方向下延伸至头臂静脉。

（翻译　祁丽）

NECK INFECTIONS AND INFLAMMATION

颈部感染与炎症

Ludwig angina

- Ludwig angina is cellulitis of the floor of the mouth. It is an infection that can involve the submental, sublingual, and submandibular spaces.
- The tongue may be posteriorly displaced, so ensuring airway patency is a clinical priority.
- On imaging, there is stranding and swelling at the floor of the mouth.

脓性颌下炎咽峡炎

- 脓性颌下炎咽峡炎是口底的蜂窝织炎。该病为感染性疾病，可累及颏下、舌下及下颌下间隙。
- 舌可能会被向后推移，因此临床应首先采取措施确保气道通畅。
- 影像学表现为口底（脂肪）区条索状影及软组织肿胀影。

Retropharyngeal abscess

咽后脓肿

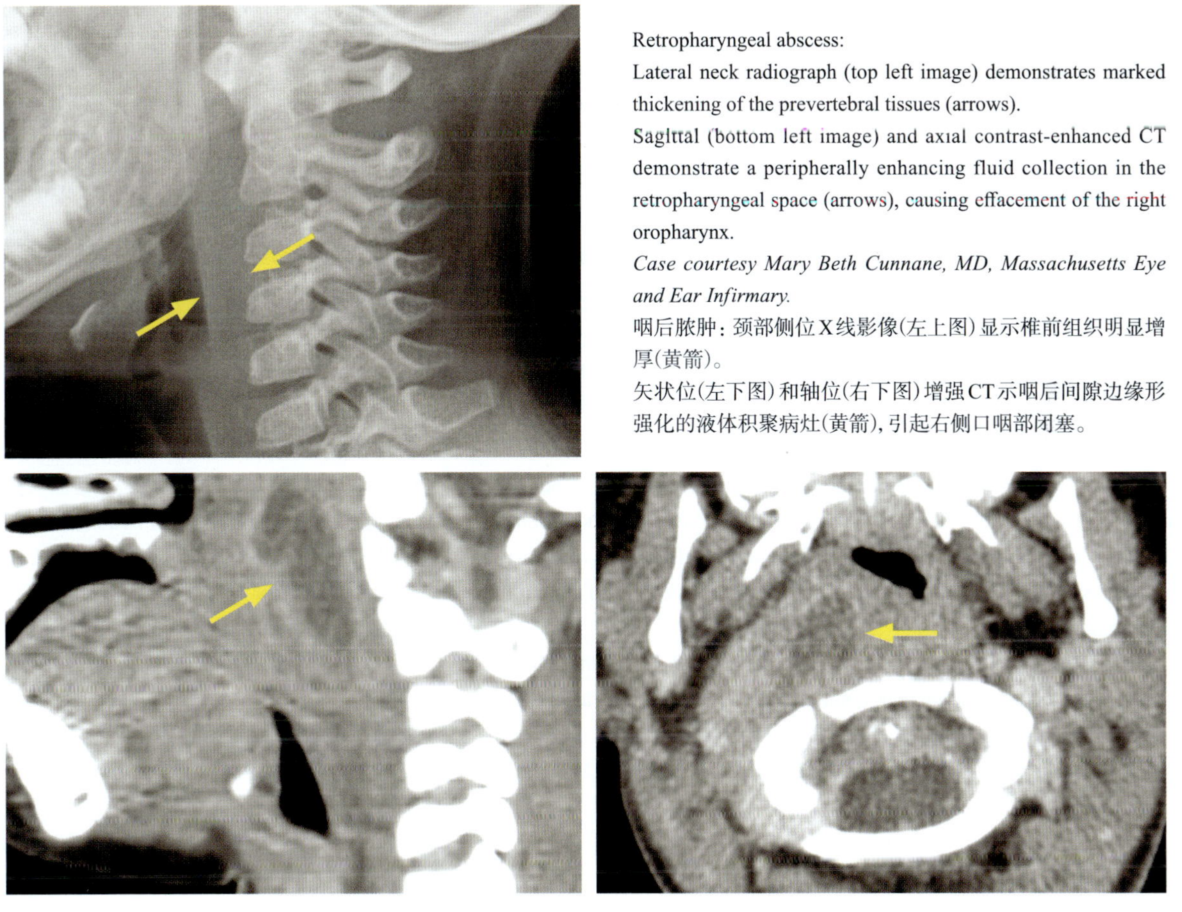

Retropharyngeal abscess:
Lateral neck radiograph (top left image) demonstrates marked thickening of the prevertebral tissues (arrows).
Sagittal (bottom left image) and axial contrast-enhanced CT demonstrate a peripherally enhancing fluid collection in the retropharyngeal space (arrows), causing effacement of the right oropharynx.
Case courtesy Mary Beth Cunnane, MD, Massachusetts Eye and Ear Infirmary.
咽后脓肿：颈部侧位X线影像（左上图）显示椎前组织明显增厚（黄箭）。
矢状位（左下图）和轴位（右下图）增强CT示咽后间隙边缘形强化的液体积聚病灶（黄箭），引起右侧口咽部闭塞。

- Retropharyngeal infection may cause airway compromise.
- In children, retropharyngeal infection is most often from spread of an upper respiratory tract infection, such as pharyngitis, which may cause the retropharyngeal lymph nodes that drain the pharynx to become suppurative and rupture.
- In adults, retropharyngeal infection is most often due to penetrating injury, such as fishbone ingestion or instrumentation.

- 咽后感染可导致气道功能受损。
- 在儿童，咽后感染最常源自上呼吸道感染蔓延，如咽炎，可导致引流咽部的咽后淋巴结继发化脓及破裂。
- 在成人，咽后感染通常是由穿通性损伤导致，如食入鱼刺或器械损伤。

Peritonsillar abscess

- Peritonsillar abscess is a complication of peritonsillar lymph node suppuration, causing the characteristic *hot-potato* voice.

Lemierre syndrome

- Lemierre syndrome is venous thrombophlebitis of the tonsillar and peritonsillar veins, often with spread to the internal jugular vein. Immunocompetent adolescents and young adults are typically affected.
- The most common infectious agent is the anaerobe *Fusobacterium necrophorum*, which is part of the normal mouth flora.
- Imaging shows enlargement, thrombosis, and mural enhancement of the affected veins.
- Pulmonary septic emboli may be present.

Tuberculous adenitis (scrofula)

- Tuberculous adenitis is usually seen in patients of Asian descent who present with painless neck masses. Imaging findings are classically bilateral necrotic lymph nodes, often in the level Ⅴ posterior triangle distribution, occasionally multiloculated with ring-like enhancement. Sinus tracts to skin can form at the late stage. The nodes classically calcify after treatment.

Cat scratch fever

- Cat scratch fever is an infection caused by *Bartonella henselae* and can present with fever, malaise, and regional lymphadenopathy. It can be self-limited or can progress to encephalopathy and neuropathy.

扁桃体周围脓肿

- 扁桃体周围脓肿是扁桃体周围淋巴结化脓的并发症，导致有特征性的发音低沉。

勒米尔综合征

- 勒米尔综合征是扁桃体内和扁桃体周围静脉的血栓性静脉炎，常蔓延到颈内静脉。好发于免疫力正常的青少年和青年人。
- 最常见的病原菌是厌氧的坏死梭杆菌，为正常口腔菌群的组成部分。
- 影像上显示受累静脉扩张、血栓形成及管壁强化。
- 可出现脓毒性肺栓塞。

结核性淋巴结炎(淋巴结核)

- 结核性淋巴结炎通常见于亚裔患者，它们表现为无痛的颈部肿块。影像学检查表现为典型的双侧淋巴结坏死，通常位于颈部Ⅴ区的颈后三角区，偶有多房环状强化。晚期可形成通往皮肤的窦道。淋巴结在治疗后通常会发生钙化。

猫抓热

- 猫抓热是由汉赛巴尔通体引起的感染，可表现为发热、乏力和区域性淋巴结肿大。该病可以是自限性的，也可以进展为脑病和神经病变。

（翻译　马聪）

THYROID AND PARATHYROID

DIFFUSE THYROID DISEASE

Hashimoto thyroiditis (chronic lymphocytic thyroiditis)

- Hashimoto thyroiditis is an autoimmune disease that is thought to be due to autoantibodies to thyroglobulins. It is the most common cause of hypothyroidism.
- The diagnosis is often made serologically. Patients are often euthyroid early in disease, but eventually become hypothyroid due to replacement of functioning thyroid parenchyma.
- Ultrasound may show either a diffusely micronodular gland or a heterogeneous coarsened gland without a measurable nodule. The isthmus is characteristically thickened. In its end stage, the gland becomes atrophic.
- Patients with Hashimoto thyroiditis are at increased risk of thyroid lymphoma.

甲状腺和甲状旁腺

弥漫性甲状腺疾病

桥本甲状腺炎(慢性淋巴细胞性甲状腺炎)

- 桥本甲状腺炎是一种自身免疫性疾病，被认为是由针对甲状腺球蛋白的自身抗体引起，是引起甲状腺功能减退最常见的原因。
- 诊断通常依靠血清学检查。在疾病早期，患者的甲状腺功能通常正常，但由于有功能的甲状腺实质被替代而最终变为甲状腺功能减退。
- 超声检查可能显示腺体呈现弥漫性微结节状或不均匀粗糙状，但没有可测量的结节。峡部增厚有特征性。在其晚期，腺体萎缩。
- 桥本甲状腺炎的患者罹患甲状腺淋巴瘤的风险升高。

Graves disease

格雷夫斯病(毒性弥漫性甲状腺肿)

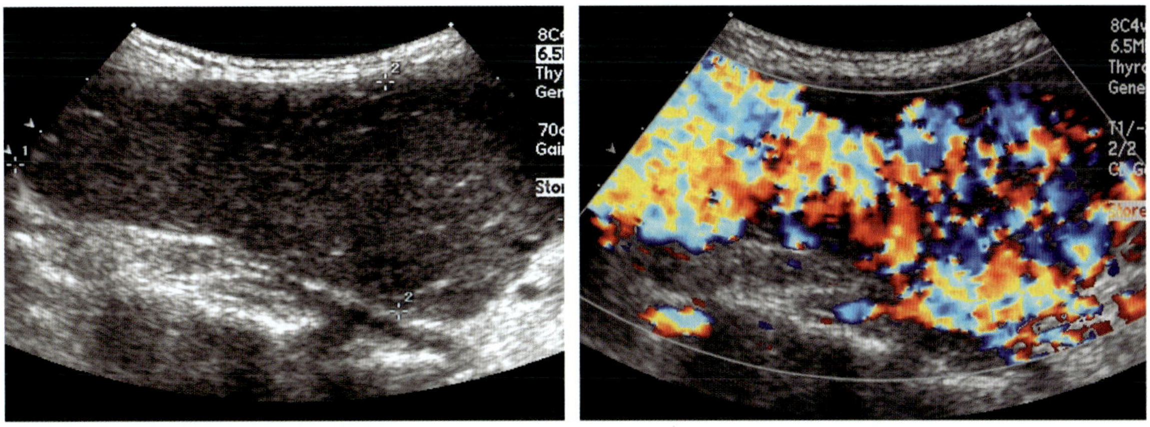

Graves disease: Sagittal grayscale ultrasound of the thyroid (left) demonstrates a diffusely enlarged gland with coarsened, heterogeneous echotexture. Color Doppler (right image) shows markedly increased Doppler flow representing the *thyroid inferno* sign.
Case courtesy Julie Ritner, MD, Brigham and Women's Hospital.

格雷夫斯病：矢状切面灰阶超声(左图)显示甲状腺弥漫性增大，回声粗糙且不均匀。彩色多普勒(右图)显示血流显著增加，呈甲状腺火海征。

- Graves disease causes autoimmune activation of the TSH receptor, stimulating thyroid hormone synthesis and secretion. Patients clinically present with thyrotoxicosis.
- Ultrasound may show diffuse enlargement of the gland, a coarsened echotexture and hypervascularity. The borders of the gland are often lobulated.
- The key color Doppler finding is the *thyroid inferno sign*, which represents marked hypervascularity caused by arteriovenous shunting and enlarged peripheral vessels.
- Because of significant overlap in sonographic findings with Hashimoto thyroiditis, correlation with laboratory findings is required.

- 格雷夫斯病是自身免疫激活TSH受体，进而刺激甲状腺激素合成和分泌。患者临床表现为甲状腺毒症。
- 超声表现为甲状腺弥漫性增大，回声粗糙且血供丰富。甲状腺边缘常见分叶状。
- 彩色多普勒最关键的发现是甲状腺火海征，它反映了由动静脉分流和外周血管增粗所导致的富血供状态。
- 由于超声表现与桥本甲状腺炎有显著重叠，因此需要结合实验室检查结果诊断。

Subacute thyroiditis (de Quervain thyroiditis)

亚急性甲状腺炎(de Quervain 甲状腺炎)

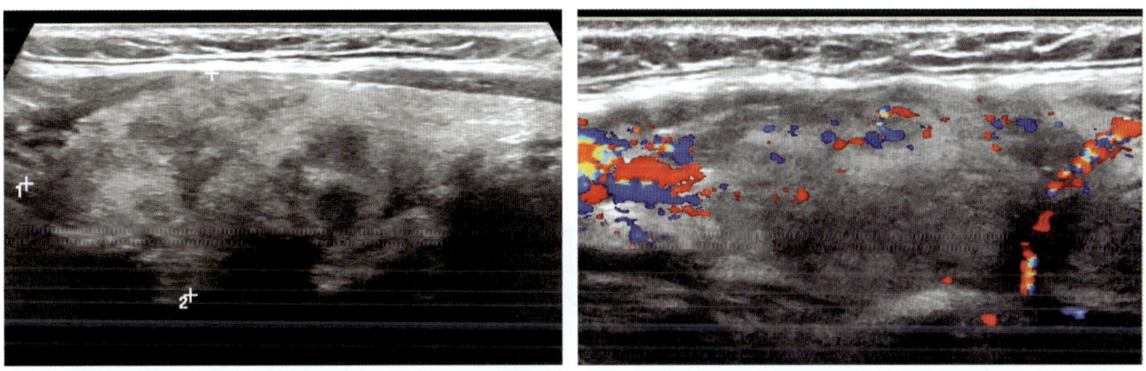

Subacute (de Quervain) thyroiditis: Sagittal grayscale thyroid ultrasound (left image) demonstrates patchy areas of decreased echogenicity with no discrete nodule. Color Doppler (right image) does not demonstrate increased vascularity, in contrast to Graves disease. *Case courtesy Julie Ritner, MD.*

亚急性(de Quervai)甲状腺炎：矢状切面灰阶超声(左图)显示甲状腺回声呈斑片状减低，无明显结节。与格雷夫斯病相比，彩色多普勒(右图)并未显示有血流增加。

- Subacute (de Quervain) thyroiditis is granulomatous inflammation of the thyroid, thought to be viral in origin. It is the most common cause of a painful thyroid mass. The gland is usually tender and adjacent cervical adenopathy is common.
- Patients may present with transient hyperthyroidism due to follicular rupture and release of thyroid hormones, followed by hypothyroidism after depletion

- 亚急性(de Quervain)甲状腺炎是甲状腺肉芽肿性炎症，被认为由病毒引起。它是疼痛性甲状腺肿块最常见的原因。腺体通常有触痛，并往往有邻近的颈部淋巴结肿大。
- 患者可能表现为短暂的甲状腺功能亢进，为滤泡破裂和甲状腺激素释放所致，随后激素

of hormone stores. It is usually diagnosed clinically.

- Ultrasound findings include ill-defined, patchy areas of decreased echogenicity in the involved regions. Vascularity is normal or decreased.
- Subacute thyroiditis is treated with steroids. Follow-up ultrasound appearance can show a dramatic response to treatment.

Multinodular gland

- The term *multinodular gland* is preferred over *multinodular goiter* because *goiter* is a generic term for an enlarged gland, which can have numerous causes.
- On imaging, a multinodular gland will appear enlarged with innumerable mixed cystic and solid nodules.

Thyroid nodule and thyroid cancer

Approach to a thyroid nodule

- There are no definitive ultrasound features that distinguish benign from malignant nodules.
- The American Thyroid Association (ATA) has developed guidelines for assessment of thyroid nodules on ultrasound. These guidelines stress use of the sonographic pattern and size for risk stratification and subsequent decision-making regarding FNA.
- High-suspicion sonographic features include: microcalcifications, hypoechogenicity with irregular margins, taller-than-wide shape.
- Intermediate suspicion sonographic features include hypoechogenicity with regular margins.
- Low and very-low suspicion sonographic features include hyperechoic or isoechoic solid nodules with regular margins, spongiform echotexture, partially cystic nodules with eccentric solid mass.
- The American College of Radiology white papers have published guidelines on management of incidental thyroid nodules detected on CT or MRI. In the absence of suspicious features on CT or MRI, a thyroid ultrasound is recommended when nodules ≥1 cm in patients <35 years old, and when nodules >1.5 cm in patients >35 years old. Nodules that do not meet size criteria do not require further evaluation.

Thyroid cancer

储备耗尽而出现甲状腺功能减退。诊断通常依靠临床表现。

- 超声表现包括受累区域边界不清的斑片状回声减低区。血供情况可正常或减少。
- 亚急性甲状腺炎采用类固醇治疗。超声随访可观察到对治疗有极为明显的反应。

多结节性甲状腺

- 多结节性甲状腺这一术语较多结节甲状腺肿更为恰当，因为甲状腺肿是指腺体肿大的一个通用术语，其原因可有多种。
- 多结节性甲状腺在影像学上表现为体积增大，伴有大量囊实混合性结节。

甲状腺结节和甲状腺癌

甲状腺结节的处理方法

- 超声不具有明确区分良恶性结节的特征。
- 美国甲状腺协会(ATA)制定了超声评估甲状腺结节的指南。这些指南强调使用超声的表现方式和病灶大小进行风险分层，以及决定是否需要进行细针穿刺抽吸(FNA)。
- 超声高度怀疑恶性的特征包括微钙化、边缘不规则的低回声，以及高大于宽的形态。
- 超声中度怀疑恶性的特征包括边缘规则的低回声。
- 超声低度和极低度怀疑恶性的特征包括边缘规则的高或等回声实性结节、海绵状回声纹理、部分囊性结节伴偏心性实性肿块。
- 《美国放射理事会白皮书》已发布对CT或MRI上偶然发现的甲状腺结节的诊疗指南。在CT或MRI没有可疑特征的情况下，甲状腺超声检查建议用于结节≥1 cm且年龄<35岁的患者，以及结节>1.5cm和年龄>35岁的患者。不符合标准的结节不需要进一步评估。

甲状腺癌

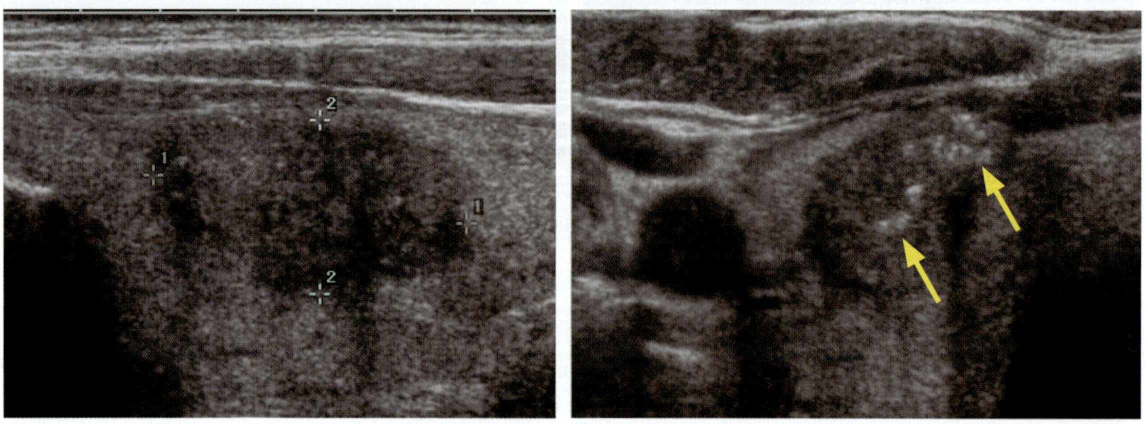

Thyroid carcinoma: Sagittal (left image) and transverse grayscale images through the left lobe of the thyroid demonstrate a solid nodule (calipers) with irregular borders containing punctate calcifications (arrows).

Case courtesy Julie Ritner, MD, Brigham and Women's Hospital.

甲状腺癌：甲状腺左叶矢状切面(左图)和横切面灰阶图像(右图)显示一个实性结节(卡尺)，边界不规则内含多发点状钙化(黄箭)。

- Papillary cancer is by far the most common histologic subtype of thyroid cancer, and confers the best prognosis. Lymphangitic spread is common, and therefore cervical, sometimes cystic, lymphadenopathy is common. Lymph nodes may also be calcified, colloid-containing, or vascular.
- Follicular carcinomas tend to spread hematogenously and have the next best prognosis.
- Medullary subtypes are less common and more aggressive and are associated with MEN Ⅱ syndrome. The anaplastic subtype is very rare and has the worst prognosis.
- Non-Hodgkin lymphoma can also occur in the thyroid and usually presents as a solid nodule.

Parathyroid

Anatomy

- Parathyroid glands are usually found adjacent to the thyroid gland. Most patients have four glands, but there may be between two and six.
- Ectopic locations of the parathyroid glands include the upper mediastinum, in the tracheoesophageal groove, or at the thoracic inlet.

Indications for imaging

- The most frequent indication for parathyroid imaging is workup of hypercalcemia for identification of a parathyroid adenoma and/or hyperplasia.
- Patients frequently go straight to curative surgical exploration. In this population, up to 10% of patients develop persistent or recurrent disease after initial surgery. Therefore, parathyroid localization is more frequently indicated in the re-operative setting.
- MEN 1 is associated with parathyroid adenomas or hyperplasia.
- Malignant neoplasms of the parathyroid (parathyroid carcinoma) are rare and distinction can be made with benign adenomas based on rapid growth, local aggressive behavior, and presence of lymph node metastases.

Imaging modalities

- Imaging options include ultrasound, four-dimensional (4D) CT, or PET.
- *Ultrasound* is usually the first-line modality. Parathyroid adenomas appear round, well-circumscribed, homogeneous, and hypoechoic relative to thyroid tissue. Pros of using ultrasound are the low-cost and lack of radiation. Limitations include operator dependence, insensitivity for detection of multigland parathyroid disease, and the inability to localize parathyroid tissue in sonographically inaccessible locations, such as the mediastinum, tracheoesophageal groove, retroesophageal or retroclavicular locations.
- *4DCT* consists of performing noncontrast, arterial, and delayed phases to capitalize on the perfusion kinetics of adenomas.

Parathyroid adenomas classically are hypodense in comparison to normal thyroid tissue on noncontrast, demonstrate enhancement greater than thyroid on early (35 sec) arterial phase, and washout more than thyroid in the delayed phase. However, less than half of parathyroid adenomas follow this pattern.

Large adenomas may show heterogeneous enhancement and atypical enhancement patterns.

- 乳头状癌是绝大多数甲状腺癌的组织学亚型，预后也是最好的。淋巴转移常见，因此，颈部淋巴结肿大，有时淋巴结呈囊性也随之常见。淋巴结也可能钙化，含有胶质或血管。
- 滤泡状癌容易发生血行播散，预后仅次于乳头状癌。
- 髓样癌亚型不太常见且更具侵袭性，与多发性内分泌瘤病2型(MEN 2)相关。未分化亚型罕见，预后最差。
- 非霍奇金淋巴瘤也可见于甲状腺，通常表现为实性结节。

甲状旁腺

解剖

- 甲状旁腺通常位于甲状腺附近。大多数患者有4个腺体，但也可能有2~6个。
- 异位甲状旁腺见于上纵隔、气管食管沟或胸廓入口处。

影像学检查指征

- 最常见的甲状旁腺影像学检查指征是高钙血症，可识别甲状旁腺腺瘤和/或增生。
- 患者往往直接进行根治性手术探查。但在该手术人群中，多达10%的患者在首次手术后疾病没有得到缓解或出现复发。所以，再次手术时常需要对甲状旁腺进行定位。
- 多发性内分泌瘤病1型(MEN 1)与甲状旁腺腺瘤或增生有关。
- 甲状旁腺恶性肿瘤(甲状旁腺癌)很少见，与良性腺瘤的区别于在会出现快速生长、局部侵袭性行为，以及出现淋巴结转移。

成像方式

- 影像选项包括超声、四维(4D)CT或PET。
- 超声通常是首选方式。甲状旁腺腺瘤表现为圆形、边界清楚、均质、相对于甲状腺组织呈低回声的病灶。使用超声的优点是成本低且无辐射；缺点包括效果与操作者的经验有关，对多发甲状旁腺疾病的检测不敏感，并且无法定位超声检查无法到达部位的甲状旁腺组织(如纵隔、气管食管沟、食管后或锁骨后)。
- 4DCT包括平扫、动脉期和延迟期，以记录腺瘤的灌注动力学。

甲状旁腺腺瘤相对于正常的甲状腺组织在平扫上通常呈低密度，动脉早期(35秒)的强化程度大于甲状腺，延迟期廓清比甲状腺明显。但是，只有不到一半的甲状旁腺腺瘤具有这种模式。

大腺瘤可呈现不均匀强化和非典型强化模式。

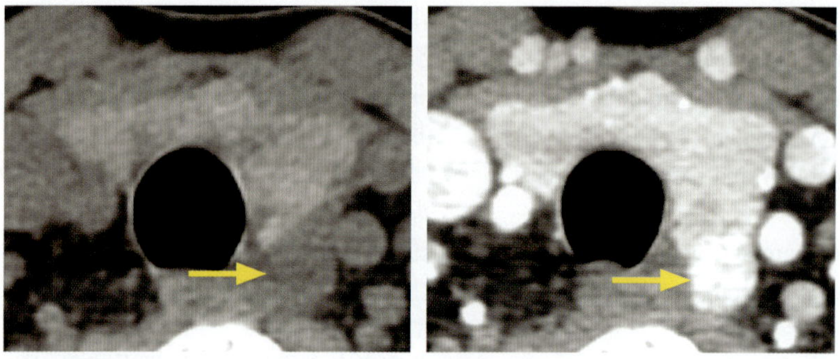

Noncontrast CT
CT平扫

Arterial phase CT
动脉期CT

Classic parathyroid adenoma:
Axial 4DCT shows a mass (arrows) posterior to the left thyroid lobe in the left paraesophageal region which is hypodense to thyroid on noncontrast phase, hyper-enhancing compared to thyroid on arterial phase.
典型甲状旁腺腺瘤：
轴位4DCT显示一个甲状腺肿块(黄箭)位于左叶后方的左食管旁区，平扫密度低于甲状腺，动脉期则高于甲状腺。

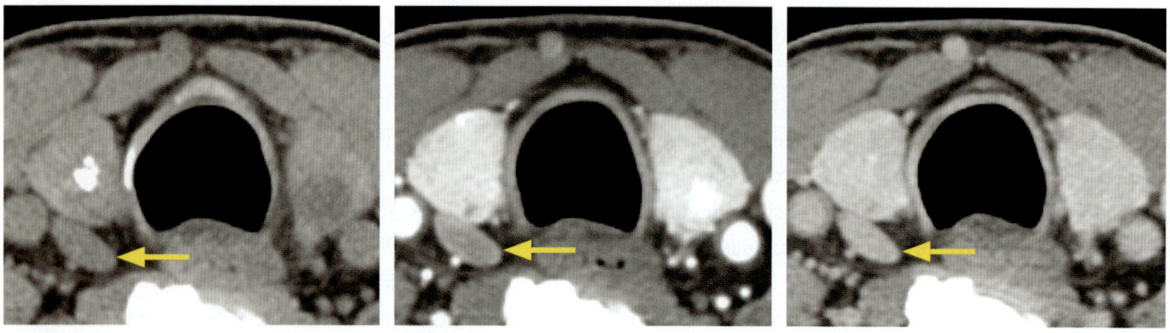

Noncontrast CT
CT平扫

Arterial phase CT
动脉期CT

Delayed phase CT
延迟期CT

Atypical parathyroid adenoma: Axial 4DCT shows an oval nodule (arrows) posterior to the right thyroid lobe which is hypodense to thyroid on noncontrast phase as well as arterial phase, and isodense to thyroid on delay phase. This biopsy-proven parathyroid adenoma does not follow the classical enhancement pattern but is otherwise typical in appearance with regards to morphology and location.
非典型甲状旁腺腺瘤：轴位4DCT显示甲状腺右叶后方一个椭圆形结节(黄箭)，平扫和动脉期相对甲状腺呈低密度，在延迟期相对甲状腺呈等密度。该结节经活检证实为甲状旁腺腺瘤，与典型的强化模式不相符，而在形态和位置依然典型。

- Greatest advantage of 4DCT is for localization of small, multinodular, and/or ectopic adenomas including those located far-posterior to thyroid (paraesophageal). However, the greatest limitation is the high radiation exposure.
- *Tc-99m sestamibi* is not a PET tracer that is taken up by parathyroids, and is discussed in greater detail within the "Nuclear Imaging" chapter.
- MRI is occasionally used as second-line modality to identify lesions that have been otherwise poorly localized by prior studies.

- 4DCT的最大优势是可以发现小的、多灶性腺瘤和/或异位腺瘤，包括位于甲状腺后部(食管旁)的腺瘤。但是最大的缺点是会增加辐射剂量。
- ^{99m}Tc-MIBI 不是一个PET示踪剂，它不被甲状旁腺摄取，在“核医学与分子影像”一章有详细讨论。
- MRI偶尔被用作二线方法来识别先前检查中定位不佳的病变。

（翻译　吴静）

12 Spine Imaging

Francis Deng, Shruti Mishra, Nityanand Miskin,
Ellen X. Sun, Raymond Y. Huang, Jacob Mandell

Contents

12 脊柱影像

目录

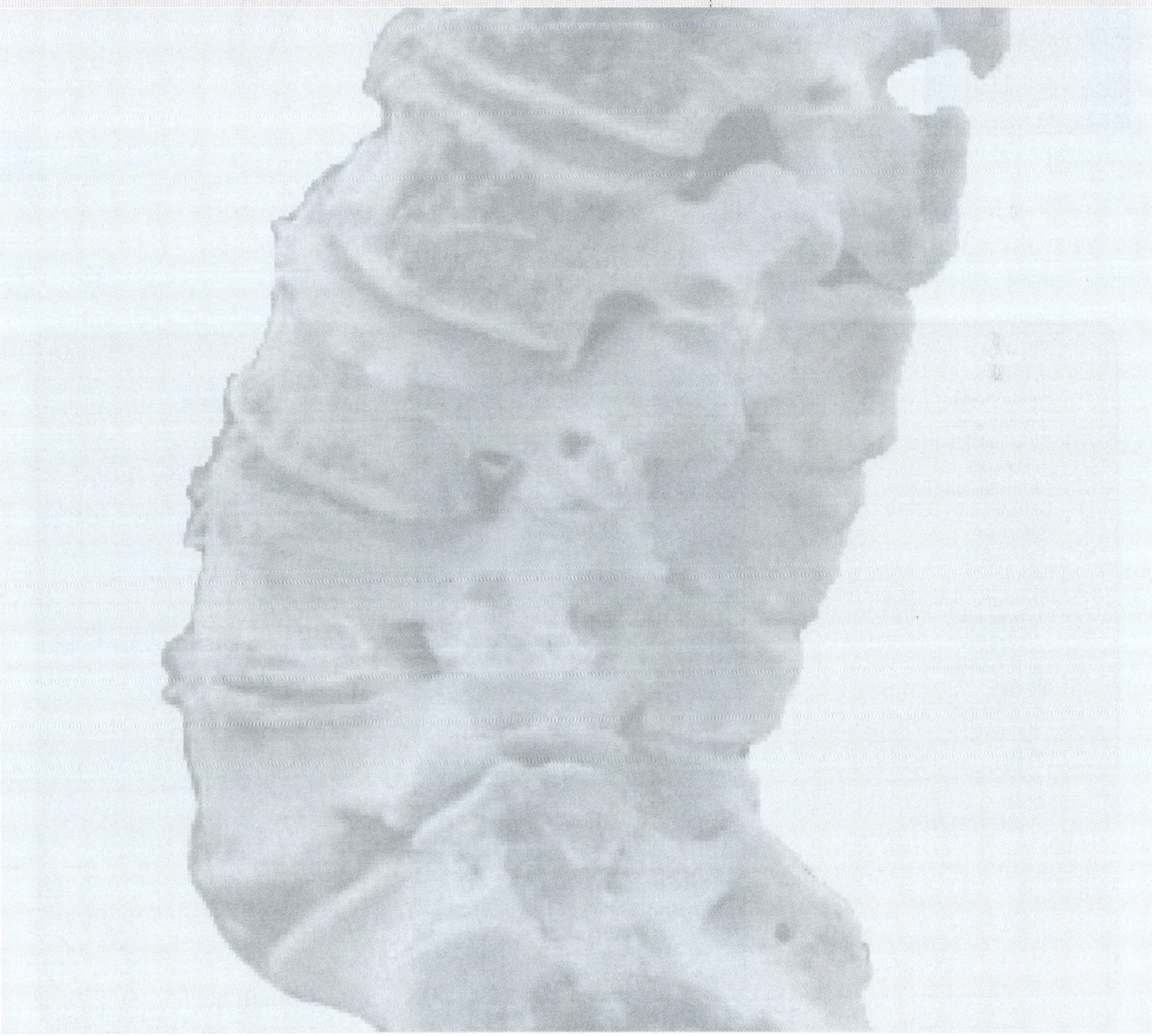

sagittal schematic
矢状位示意图

axial schematic
横轴位示意图

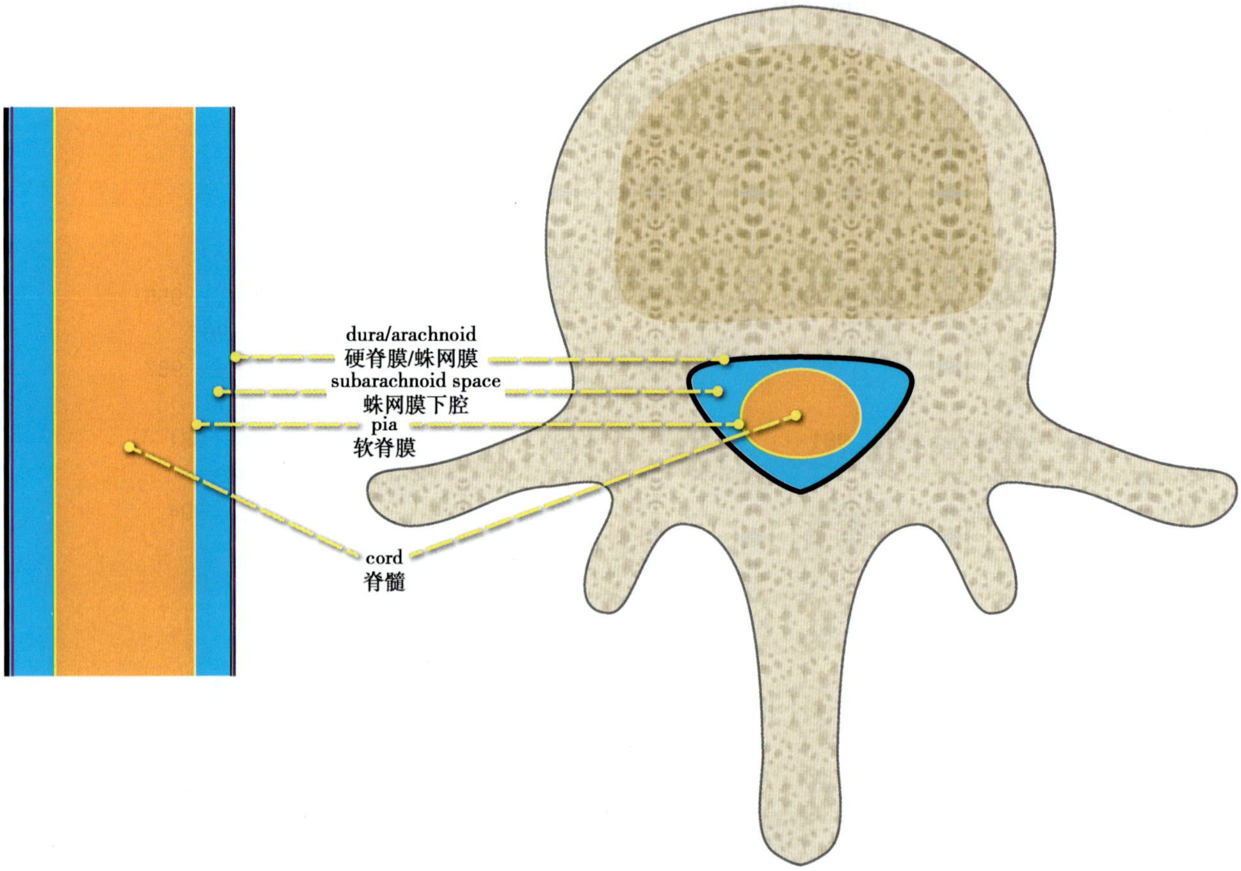

intramedullary
髓内

- astrocytoma
- ependymoma
- hemangioblastoma
- metastasis
- demyelinating lesion
- inflammatory process
- infection
- vascular lesion
- syrinx
- traumatic cord injury
- 星形细胞瘤
- 室管膜瘤
- 血管母细胞瘤
- 转移瘤
- 脱髓鞘病变
- 炎性病变
- 感染
- 血管病变
- 空洞
- 外伤性脊髓损伤

intradural extramedullary
硬膜内髓外

- meningioma
- schwannoma
- neurofibroma
- myxopapillary ependymoma
- paraganglioma
- spinal dysraphism
- epidermoid/dermoid
- neurenteric cyst
- arachnoid cyst/web
- cord herniation
- arachnoiditis
- Guillain-Barr é
- CIDP
- 脑膜瘤
- 神经鞘瘤
- 神经纤维瘤
- 黏液乳头状室管膜瘤
- 副神经节瘤
- 神经管闭合不全
- 表皮样/皮样囊肿
- 肠源性神经囊肿
- 蛛网膜囊肿/网带
- 脊髓疝
- 蛛网膜炎
- 吉兰-巴雷综合征
- 慢性炎症性脱髓鞘性多发性神经根神经病

extradural
硬膜外

- extradural metastasis
- vertebral neoplasm
- hemangioma
- epidural lipomatosis
- degenerative disease
- nondegenerative hypertrophic disease
- discitis/osteomyelitis
- epidural abscess
- crystal deposition disease
- spondyloarthropathies
- Paget disease
- spinal fracture
- epidural hematoma
- epidural extension of tumor
- 硬膜外转移瘤
- 椎体肿瘤
- 血管瘤
- 硬膜外脂肪瘤
- 退行性疾病
- 非退行性肥大性疾病
- 椎间盘炎/骨髓炎
- 硬膜外脓肿
- 结晶沉积病
- 脊柱关节病
- 佩吉特病
- 脊柱骨折
- 硬膜外血肿
- 硬膜外肿瘤延伸

- The first step in evaluation of any spinal mass is to determine its compartment of origin: **intramedullary** (within the substance of the spinal cord), **intradural extramedullary** (within the thecal sac but outside the cord), or **extradural** (outside the thecal sac).
- Note that *epidural* is *extradural* in location.

- 评估任何脊柱肿块首先要确定其所在的位置：**髓内**(脊髓实质内)，**硬膜内髓外**(硬膜囊内，脊髓外)，或**硬膜外**(在硬膜囊外)。
- 注意，epidural是位于硬膜之外。

INTRAMEDULLARY LESIONS

Overview of intramedullary lesions

- Intramedullary lesions are located within the substance of the cord, deep to the pia and are, by definition, also intradural.
- Neoplasms frequently expand the spinal cord, whereas non-neoplastic etiologies more likely cause nonexpansile signal changes.
- Astrocytomas and ependymomas comprise 90% of intramedullary tumors and cannot be reliably differentiated based on imaging features.
- Hemangioblastomas and intramedullary metastases are less common.

髓内病变

髓内病变概述

- 髓内病变位于脊髓的实质，深达软脊膜，根据定义，也属于硬膜内病变。
- 肿瘤经常使脊髓膨大，而非肿瘤性病因更有可能引起非膨胀性信号变化。
- 星形细胞瘤和室管膜瘤占髓内肿瘤的90%，其影像学特征不能有效区分两者。
- 血管母细胞瘤和髓内转移瘤较少见。

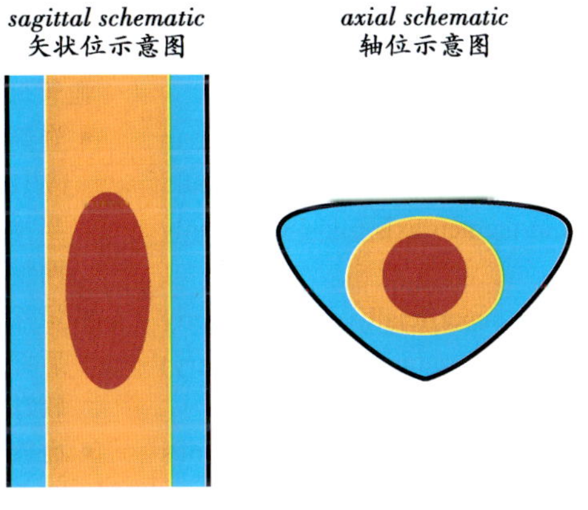

INTRAMEDULLARY SPINAL CORD NEOPLASMS

髓内肿瘤

Astrocytoma

星形细胞瘤

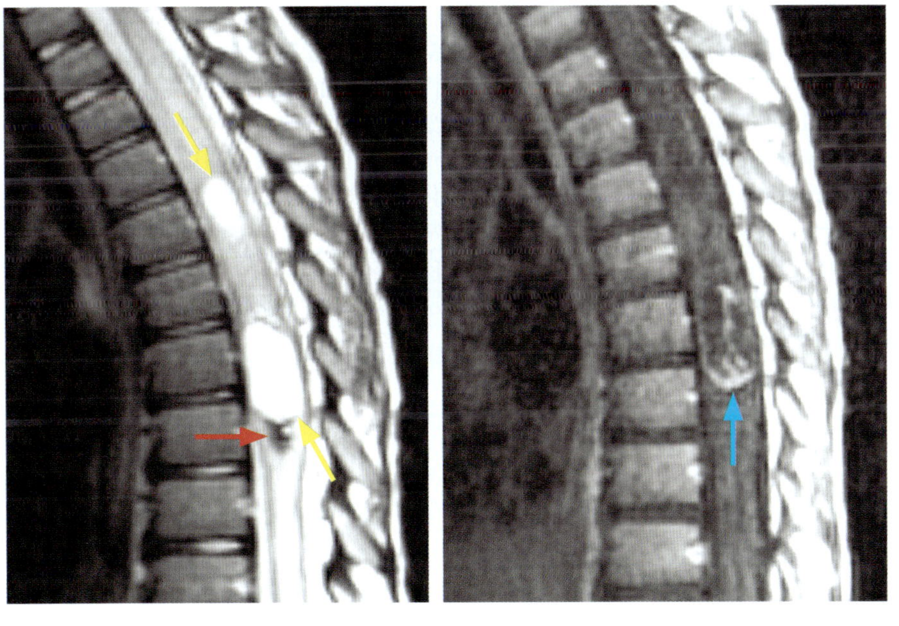

Sagittal T2-weighted (left image) and T1-weighted post-contrast (right image) MRI shows an intramedullary mass in the thoracic spine (yellow arrows) which expands the spinal cord and causes cord signal abnormality from the mid thoracic spine down. A focus of hypointensity on the T2-weighted image at the inferior aspect of the lesion may represent hemorrhagic material (red arrow). On the post-contrast image, the mass demonstrates wispy enhancement inferiorly (blue arrow). This was an astrocytoma.

矢状位T_2加权(左图)和T_1加权增强后(右图)MRI显示胸髓的髓内肿块(黄箭)，它使脊髓膨大并导致中段胸髓以下脊髓信号异常。在病变的下方，T_2加权图像上有一个局部低信号区，可能为出血性物质(红箭)。在增强图像上，肿块下方呈束状强化(蓝箭)。此为星形细胞瘤。

- Astrocytomas are the most common intramedullary tumor in children and second most common in adults. They are associated with neurofibromatosis type 1 (along with neurofibromas).
- Most spinal astrocytomas are low-grade (WHO grade Ⅰ or Ⅱ). Spinal glioblastoma (WHO grade Ⅳ) is rare.
- Astrocytomas have ill-defined (infiltrative) margins and can have patchy or irregular enhancement. Cystic components are seen in a minority and a syrinx may be present. Hemorrhage is uncommon.

Ependymoma

- Ependymomas are the most common intramedullary tumor in adults and second most common in children. They are associated with neurofibromatosis type 2 (along with schwannomas and meningiomas).
- Most are low-grade (WHO grade Ⅱ). Myxopapillary ependymoma (WHO grade Ⅰ) is frequently intradural-extramedullary with distinct prognosis and imaging appearances (discussed separately in the next section).
- Ependymomas have well-defined margins and intense, heterogeneous enhancement. Cystic components are seen in up to half (more commonly polar/nontumoral than intratumoral) and a syrinx may be present. Hemorrhage is common, resulting in the *hemosiderin cap sign* (hypointense poles on T2-weighted images).

Hemangioblastoma

- Spinal hemangioblastomas are uncommon benign (WHO grade I) tumors in adults. They are associated with von Hippel-Lindau syndrome, which should be suspected when there are multiple lesions in the neuraxis (most commonly involving spinal cord, retina, and cerebellum).
- Although usually intramedullary, they tend to be superficially and posteriorly located in the cord and may have an exophytic (intradural extramedullary) component, as if arising from the linings of pial vessels.
- Hemangioblastomas have well-defined margins and intense, homogeneous enhancement. They are typically small (involving only one vertebral level). Larger lesions can show vascular flow voids, cystic components, or a syrinx. Surrounding edema may also be seen.

Metastasis

- Intramedullary metastases are rare compared to primary intramedullary tumors and to leptomeningeal or epidural metastases of the spine. Concurrent metastatic disease elsewhere is common.
- Lung cancer is the most common metastasis and breast cancer is the second most common.
- Intramedullary metastases usually have well-defined margins and enhance. Specific signs include the *rim sign* (more intense enhancement peripherally than centrally) and *flame sign* (ill-defined triangular enhancement projecting from the superior/inferior margin). Cystic/necrotic components and hemorrhage are rare. Surrounding edema is often extensive.
- Intramedullary metastases typically involve a short segment of cord (one to two vertebral levels). They are usually solitary rather than multiple.

- 星形细胞瘤是儿童最常见的髓内肿瘤，在成人则居第二位。该病与1型神经纤维瘤病(以及神经纤维瘤)相关。
- 大多数脊髓星形细胞瘤为低级别(WHO Ⅰ级或Ⅱ级)。脊髓胶质母细胞瘤(WHO Ⅳ级)罕见。
- 星形细胞瘤边界不清(浸润性)，可呈斑片状或不规则强化。少数可见囊性成分，可能存在空洞。出血并不常见。

室管膜瘤

- 室管膜瘤是成人最常见的髓内肿瘤，在儿童居第二位。其与2型神经纤维瘤病(以及神经鞘瘤和脊膜瘤)相关。
- 大多数为低级别(WHO Ⅱ级)。黏液乳头状室管膜瘤(WHO Ⅰ级)常位于硬膜内-髓外，具有不同的预后和影像学表现(将在下文讨论)。
- 室管膜瘤边缘清晰，强化明显且不均匀。囊性成分高达一半(多位于两端/非瘤内多于瘤内)，且可出现空洞。出血很常见，导致含铁血黄素帽征(T_2加权图像呈两端低信号)。

血管母细胞瘤

- 脊髓血管母细胞瘤是不常见的成人良性肿瘤(WHO Ⅰ级)，与冯希佩尔-林道综合征有关。当神经轴出现多处病灶时(最常累及脊髓、视网膜和小脑)应考虑此综合征。
- 虽然常位于髓内，但多数是在脊髓的浅表和后部，可有外生成分(硬膜内髓外)，可能来自软脊膜血管的内壁。
- 血管母细胞瘤边缘清晰，明显均匀强化。病变通常很小(仅涉及一个椎体水平)，病变较大时可以显示血管流空效应，囊性成分或空洞；还可见周围水肿。

转移瘤

- 与原发性髓内肿瘤、软脊膜或硬膜外转移相比，髓内转移瘤较为罕见。并发其他部位的转移性疾病则很常见。
- 最常见的转移瘤源自肺癌，其次是乳腺癌。
- 髓内转移瘤通常边缘清楚，强化明显。特殊征象包括边缘征(外围增强比中央更强烈)和火焰征(从上/下缘投射的边界模糊的三角形强化)；囊性/坏死成分和出血少见，周围水肿通常很广泛。
- 髓内转移通常累及一小段脊髓(1~2个椎体水平)，常为孤立而非多发。

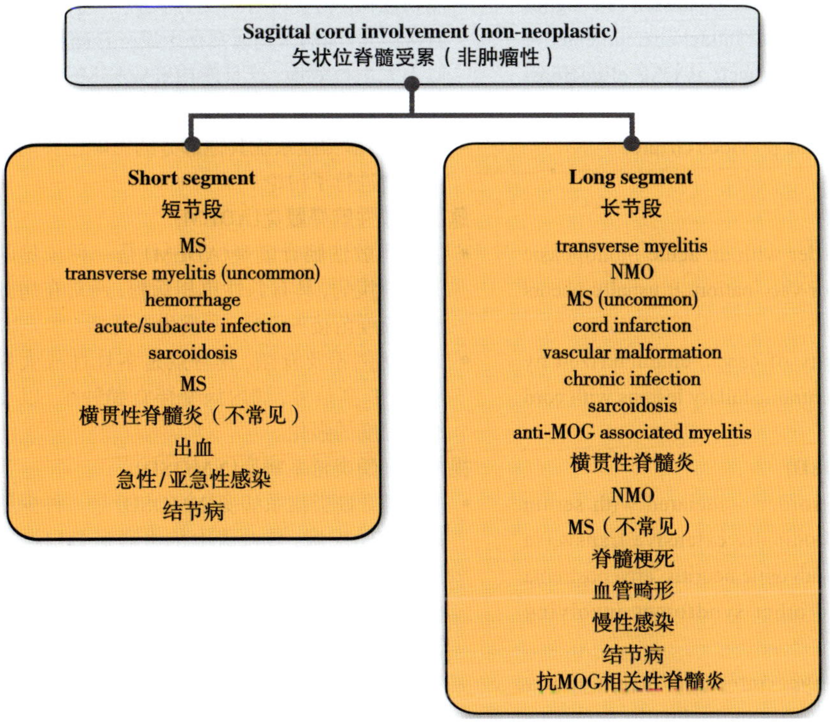

MS: Multiple sclerosis

NMO: Neuromyelitis optica

anti-MOG associated myelitis: A newly recognized inflammatory demyelinating disorder caused by anti-myelin oligodendrocyte glycoprotein (anti-MOG) antibodies.

MS：多发性硬化症

NMO：视神经脊髓炎

抗MOG相关性脊髓炎：为新发现的炎症性脱髓鞘疾病，由抗髓鞘少突胶质细胞糖蛋白(抗-MOG)抗体所致。

Multiple sclerosis (MS)

多发性硬化症(MS)

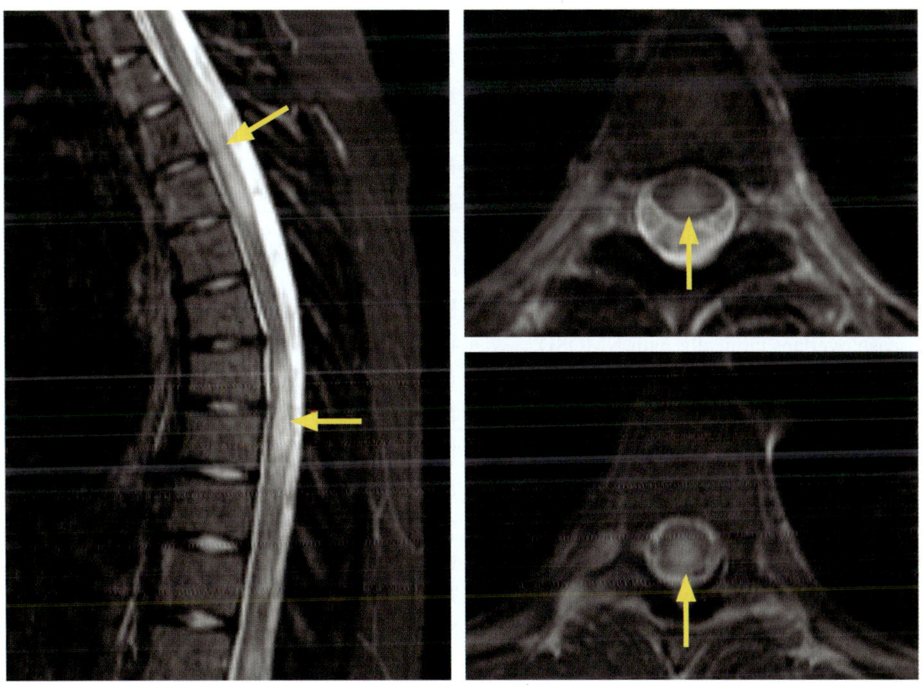

Sagittal STIR (left image) and axial T2 (right images) MRI show multiple T2 hyperintense lesions (arrows) within the visualized spinal cord, predominantly in the central cord, in this patient with known MS.

MS患者矢状位STIR(左图)和轴位T_2(右图)MRI显示髓内多发T_2高信号病变(箭)，主要位于脊髓中央。

- The spinal cord is one of four areas of the CNS where lesions count towards the 2017 McDonald criteria for demonstration of dissemination in space (in addition to periventricular, cortical or juxtacortical, and infratentorial brain). The cervical cord is most commonly involved.
- Typical spinal MS lesions appear as focal hyperintensity on T2-weighted

- 根据2017年McDonald空间多发性标准，脊髓是中枢神经系统的四个病变区域之一(另外有脑室周围、皮层或皮质下和幕下脑)。颈髓最常累及。
- 典型的脊髓MS病变在T_2加权图像上表现为

images (visible in two planes) that are short (one or two vertebral segments), peripherally located, and occupying the minority of the cord in cross-section.

- An active MS lesion may enhance and mimic a spinal tumor, but MS is often distinguishable from a neoplasm by the absence of cord expansion (analogous to the absence of significant mass effect that is typical of intracranial tumefactive MS), multifocality involving the brain and spine, as well as CSF oligoclonal bands.
- MS affecting the rest of the CNS is discussed in the previous chapter.

Acute disseminated encephalomyelitis (ADEM)

- ADEM is an uncommon demyelinating disorder with an acute monophasic course that typically follows a viral infection or vaccination. It usually occurs in children.
- Spinal cord involvement occurs in a minority of cases, characterized by multifocal or large confluent, T2 hyperintense, intramedullary lesions with cord swelling and variable enhancement.

Neuromyelitis optica spectrum disorder (NMOSD)

- NMOSD is an uncommon demyelinating disorder associated with serum antibodies against aquaporin-4. Acute longitudinally extensive transverse myelitis is a core clinical characteristic, along with optic neuritis, area postrema syndrome (hiccups, nausea/vomiting), and other syndromes involving brainstem, diencephalic, and cerebral lesions.
- Typical NMOSD myelitis lesions are T2-hyperintense ("bright spotty lesion" with areas more hyperintense than CSF), longitudinally extensive (extending >3 contiguous vertebral segments), and transversally extensive (involving a majority of the cord in cross-section). Cord swelling and patchy or ring-enhancement occurs in the acute phase, followed by atrophy after treatment. The cervicothoracic cord is predominantly involved.
- Typical NMOSD optic neuritis appears as T2-hyperintense or enhancing lesions extending over more than half of the optic nerve length. The posterior optic nerve is predominantly involved, usually bilaterally and extending to the optic chiasm.
- Less commonly, brain lesions can occur in NMOSD, predominantly distributed in periependymal areas such as the area postrema (dorsal medulla), ventricles, and cerebral aqueduct.

Anti-myelin oligodendrocyte glycoprotein (MOG) antibody-associated disease

- Anti-MOG IgG antibody-associated disease overlaps clinically with NMOSD, presenting as optic neuritis and/or myelitis. Patients are seronegative for aquaporin-4 antibodies.
- Spinal cord lesions are T2 hyperintense, longitudinally extensive, and transversally extensive, similar to those in NMOSD. However, the thoracolumbar cord including conus medullaris is preferentially involved.
- Optic nerve lesions demonstrate extensive bilateral T2 hyperintensity, as with NMOSD. However, the anterior optic nerve is preferentially involved and there may be associated perioptic nerve sheath enhancement.
- Brain MRI is normal in most cases but sometimes shows lesions in deep gray matter (basal ganglia, thalami) and infratentorial regions (pons and cerebellar peduncles), with patchy "cloud-like" enhancement.

Transverse myelitis

- Transverse myelitis is the clinical syndrome of acute or subacute neurologic dysfunction (sensory, motor, or autonomic) below the level of an inflammatory

局灶性的高信号(可在2个平面),其涉及的椎体节段短(1个或2个),位于外周,且在横切面上占据脊髓的小部分。

- 活动性MS病变可有强化并类似于髓内肿瘤,但MS与肿瘤的区别通常在于没有脊髓膨大(类似于无占位效应,这是颅内肿瘤样MS的典型特征),脑和脊髓多发病灶,以及CSF寡克隆带。
- MS对中枢神经系统其他部分的影响已在前一章节中进行了讨论。

急性播散性脑脊髓炎(ADEM)

- 急性播散性脑脊髓炎(ADEM)是一种少见的脱髓鞘疾病,具有急性单相病程,通常在病毒感染或疫苗接种之后,常发生在儿童。
- 少数病例累及脊髓,其特点是多灶性或大片融合,T_2高信号,髓内病变伴脊髓肿胀,以及不同程度的强化。

视神经脊髓炎谱系病变(NMOSD)

- 视神经脊髓炎谱系病变(NMOSD)是一种少见的脱髓鞘疾病,与血清中抗水通道蛋白-4抗体相关。急性纵向广泛性横贯性脊髓炎是核心临床特征,伴视神经炎、极后区综合征(打嗝、恶心/呕吐)和其他涉及脑干、间脑和大脑损伤的综合征。
- 典型的NMOSD脊髓炎病灶是T_2高信号("明亮的斑点病灶",部分信号高于脑脊液),纵向长(延伸>3个连续椎体)和横向广(横切面累及大部分脊髓)。急性期出现脊髓肿胀和斑片状或环状强化,在治疗后随之出现萎缩。主要累及颈胸段脊髓。
- 典型的NMOSD视神经炎表现为T_2高信号或强化病灶超过视神经长度的一半。主要累及视神经后部,通常是双侧并延伸至视交叉。
- 脑部NMOSD病变不太常见,主要分布在室管膜周围区域,如极后区(延髓背侧)、侧脑室和中脑导水管旁。

抗髓鞘少突胶质细胞糖蛋白(MOG)抗体相关疾病

- 抗髓鞘少突胶质细胞糖蛋白(MOG)IgG抗体相关疾病在临床上与NMOSD重叠,表现为视神经炎和/或脊髓炎。患者血清水通道蛋白-4抗体呈阴性。
- 脊髓病变呈T_2高信号,纵向长,横向广,类似于NMOSD的表现。然而,胸腰段脊髓好发,包括脊髓圆锥。
- 视神经病变表现出广泛的双侧T_2高信号,与NMOSD类似。然而,视神经前部最易受累,可能合并周围视神经鞘强化。
- 脑部MRI大多正常,但有时会显示深部灰质(基底神经节、丘脑)和幕下区域(脑桥和小脑脚)病变,有斑片样"云状"增强。

横贯性脊髓炎

- 横贯性脊髓炎是急性或亚急性神经功能障碍的临床综合征(感觉、运动或自主神经),出现

spinal cord lesion.

- Transverse myelitis can be idiopathic/isolated or a part of other diseases such as MS, ADEM, NMOSD, anti-MOG antibody-associated disease, CNS infection, sarcoidosis, and connective tissue diseases (e.g. lupus).
- Imaging findings include spinal cord enlargement with edema and patchy enhancement.

Acute flaccid myelitis

- Acute flaccid myelitis is a polio-like illness of children, presenting with a viral prodrome followed by rapid onset weakness in a lower motor neuron pattern. Outbreaks of enterovirus D68 are implicated.
- MRI demonstrates T2 prolongation within the spinal cord gray matter spanning ≥1 vertebral segments.

在脊髓炎性损伤水平以下。

- 横贯性脊髓炎既可是特发性/孤立性，也可是其他疾病的一部分，如MS、ADEM、NMOSD、抗MOG抗体相关疾病、CNS感染、结节病和结缔组织疾病(如狼疮)。
- 影像学表现包括脊髓增粗水肿和斑片状强化。

急性弛缓性脊髓炎

- 急性弛缓性脊髓炎是见于儿童的一种脊髓灰质炎样疾病，为病毒前驱症状后出现下运动神经元瘫痪的急速发作，与肠病毒D68暴发有关。
- MRI显示脊髓灰质内长T_2病灶，长度跨越≥1个椎体。

Spinal cord abscess

脊髓脓肿

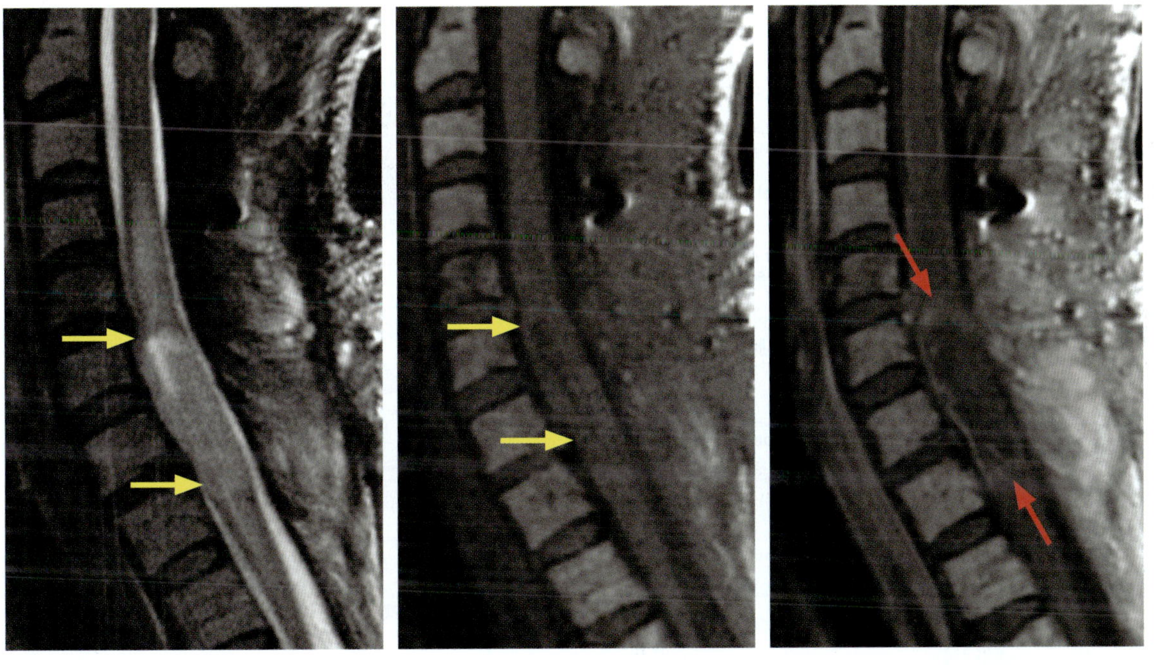

Spinal cord abscess: Sagittal T2 (left image), T1 pre-contrast (middle image), and T1 post-contrast (right image) MRI demonstrate an elongated area of abnormal intramedullary signal in the lower cervical spinal cord with heterogeneous high T2 and low T1 signal (yellow arrows), and peripheral enhancement after gadolinium administration (red arrows). There is associated cord edema extending superiorly and inferiorly, and cord expansion. Note post-surgical changes of cervical laminectomies and posterior instrumented fusion.

脊髓脓肿：矢状位T_2(左图)、平扫T_1(中图)和增强T_1(右图)MRI显示下颈段脊髓髓内有一个细长的异常信号区域，T_2不均匀高信号和T_1低信号(黄箭)，注射钆后显示边缘增强(红箭)。并发的脊髓水肿向上、下延伸，脊髓膨大。注意颈椎椎板切除术和后路椎间融合的术后变化。

- Spinal cord abscess is rare and mostly from hematogenous infection. It initially presents as an ill-defined myelitis and gradually evolves to a localized abscess.
- Like abscesses elsewhere, these appear as a T2 hyperintense, peripherally enhancing collection with central diffusion restriction.

HIV vacuolar myelopathy

- Vacuolar myelopathy occurs in patients in late stages of AIDS and is characterized by vacuolation in the spinal white matter associated with lipid-laden macrophages.
- MRI demonstrates thoracic (and possibly cervical) cord atrophy and T2 prolongation preferentially involving the dorsal columns and lateral corticospinal tracts.

- 脊髓脓肿很少见，主要是血行感染。最初表现为边界不清的脊髓炎并逐渐发展为局部脓肿。
- 和其他部分的脓肿一样，表现为T_2高信号，边缘强化，中央弥散受限。

HIV空泡性脊髓病

- 空泡性脊髓病发生在晚期AIDS患者，其特点是脊髓白质空泡化，与富含脂质的巨噬细胞相关。
- MRI显示胸段(可能还有颈段)脊髓萎缩和T_2延长，最常累及背柱和皮质脊髓侧束。

Tabes dorsalis

- Tabes dorsalis, a form of tertiary neurosyphilis, is characterized by demyelination of the dorsal columns of the spinal cord.
- MRI demonstrates longitudinal T2 prolongation in the dorsal columns, for which the differential diagnosis includes subacute combined degeneration (see later in this chapter).

Neurosarcoidosis

- Intramedullary neurosarcoidosis occurs as a result from infiltration of the Virchow-Robin spaces and can present as diffuse T2 prolongation with associated cord enlargement.
- Intramedullary involvement is frequently seen with diffuse or nodular leptomeningeal enhancement.

脊髓痨

- 脊髓痨是一种三级神经梅毒，其特点是脊髓背柱脱髓鞘。
- MRI显示背柱纵向的长T_2，鉴别诊断包括亚急性联合变性(见本章后文)。

神经结节病

- 髓内神经结节病是由Virchow-Robin间隙(血管周围间隙)被浸润所致，表现为弥漫性长T_2伴脊髓增粗。
- 髓内受累常表现为弥漫性或结节性柔脊膜强化。

Spinal vascular lesions

Normal spinal vascular anatomy

脊髓血管病变

正常脊髓血管解剖

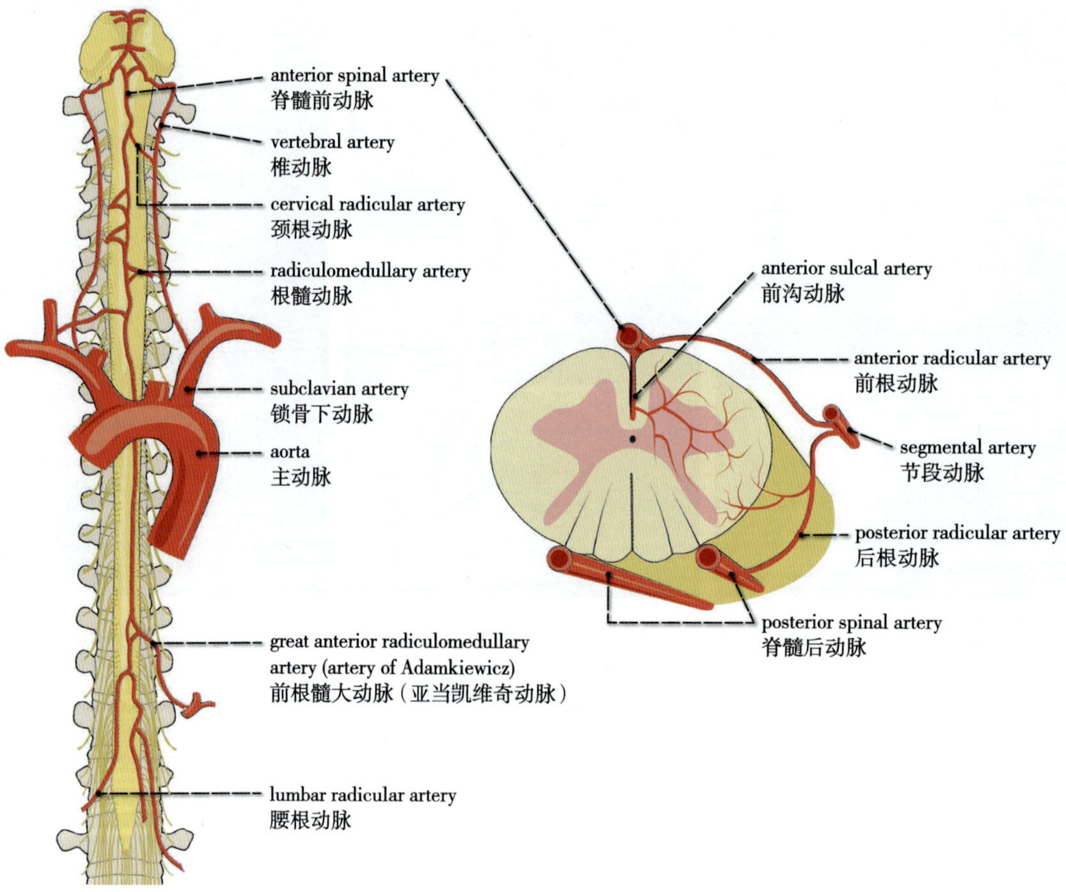

Spinal cord infarction

脊髓梗死

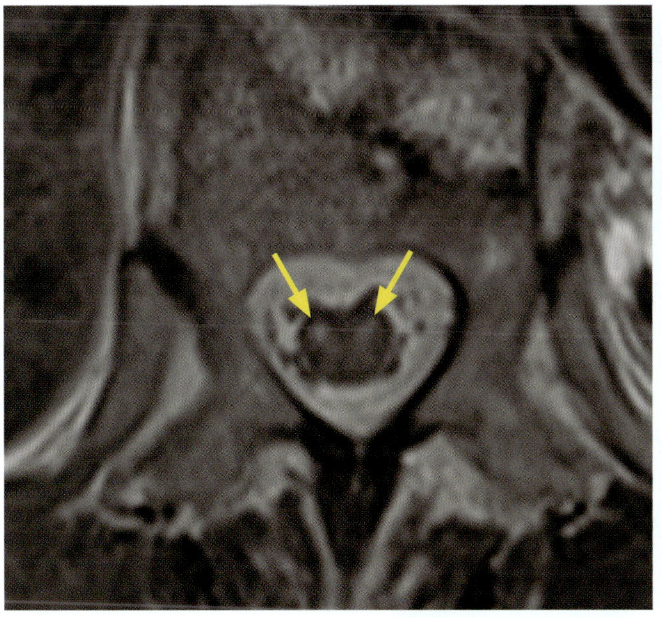

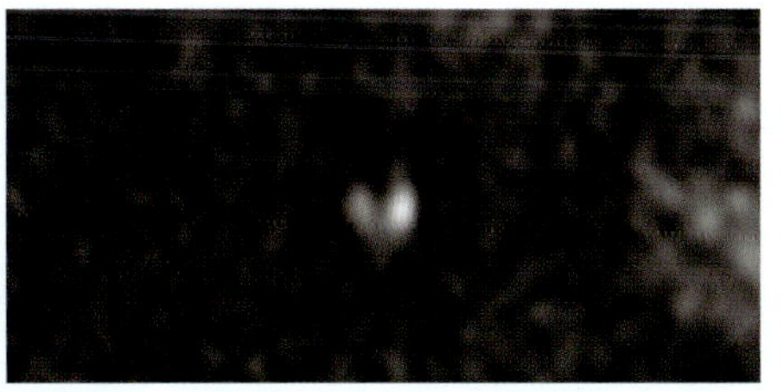

Spinal cord infarction after aortic surgery:
Axial T2-weighted MRI (left image) shows symmetric hyperintense foci involving the ventral horns of the intramedullary gray matter ("owl eye appearance").
Corresponding axial DWI (top image) shows bright spots, suggestive of restricted diffusion.
Case courtesy Gregory Wrubel, MD, Brigham and Women's Hospital.

主动脉手术后脊髓梗死：
轴位T_2加权MRI(左图)显示髓内灰质腹角对称性高信号灶("猫头鹰眼征")。
相应轴位DWI(右图)显示亮点，提示弥散受限。

- Spinal cord infarction is most common in the upper thoracic or thoracolumbar spine due to more precarious blood supply. The predominant blood supply to the distal cord is the artery of Adamkiewicz, which commonly originates from a branch of the intercostal or lumbar artery on the left at level of T9–12.
- Spinal cord infarction clinically presents with loss of bowel and bladder control, loss of perineal sensation, and impairment in both motor and sensory function of the legs.
- Risk factors for spinal cord infarction include aortic surgery, aortic aneurysm, arteritis, sickle cell anemia, vascular malformation, and disc herniation.
- Imaging of spinal cord infarction shows hyperintensity of the affected cord regions on T2-weighted images. The cord may be enlarged and typically shows restricted diffusion.
- Concomitant vertebral body infarction may be present, which is more common in sickle cell disease and chronic steroid use.

- 脊髓梗死最常见于上胸或胸腰段脊髓，因为此段血液供应不稳定。远端脊髓的血液供应主要来自前根髓大动脉，通常起源于左侧$T_{9\sim12}$水平肋间或腰椎动脉的一个分支。
- 脊髓梗死在临床上表现为大小便失禁，会阴部感觉缺失，以及腿部运动和感觉功能障碍。
- 脊髓梗死的危险因素包括主动脉手术、主动脉瘤、动脉炎、镰状细胞贫血、血管畸形和椎间盘突出。
- 脊髓梗死在T_2加权图像上表现为受累脊髓区域的高信号。脊髓可增粗，并常出现弥散受限。
- 可并发椎体梗死，常见于镰刀型细胞贫血和长期使用类固醇。

High-flow vascular (arteriovenous) malformation

高流量血管(动静脉)畸形

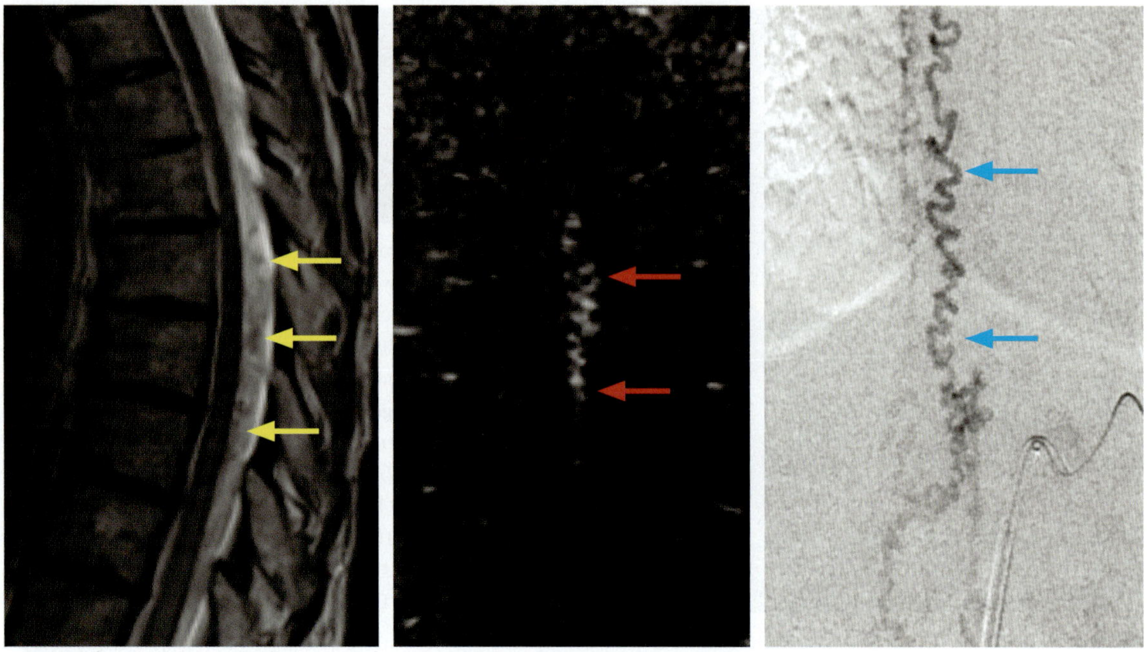

Sagittal T2 MRI (left image) shows subtle flow voids dorsal to the thoracic spinal cord (yellow arrows). Coronal TWIST MRA subtraction image (middle) demonstrates serperginous vessels in the dorsal spinal canal (red arrows). Coronal oblique digital subtraction angiogram (right image) following injection of contrast into the left T11 segmental artery shows early opacification of an engorged and tortuous dorsal spinal vein (blue arrows). These findings are consistent with a type Ⅰ dural spinal AV fistula arising from the left T11 segmental artery.

矢状位T_2 MRI(左图)显示胸髓背侧模糊的血管流空(黄箭)。冠状位时间分辨磁共振血管造影序列(TWIST)MRA减影(中图)显示背侧椎管中的锯齿状血管(红箭)。左侧T_{11}节段动脉注射造影剂后的冠状斜位数字减影血管造影(右图)显示脊髓背静脉增粗迂曲并早期显影(蓝箭)。符合左侧T_{11}节段动脉I型硬脊膜动静脉瘘的表现。

- **Dural arteriovenous fistulas (dAVF)** are the most common spinal vascular malformations. They are high-flow vascular malformations characterized angiographically by a radiculomeningeal feeding artery, no intervening nidus, and radicular vein at the nerve root sheath just under the pedicle draining retrograde to perimedullary veins.
- The resulting venous hypertension causes progressive congestive myelopathy. It typically presents in older males.
- MRI of dAVF often shows a long segment of edema in the cord (+/– mild cord expansion) and surrounding intradural extramedullary vascular flow voids representing dilated perimedullary veins. CT myelography shows serpentine intradural filling defects.
- Dural AVF may be occult on CTA and MRA, and it may need to be diagnosed with catheter angiography based on clinical symptoms or presence of brain or spinal hemorrhage.
- Foix-Alajouanine myelopathy is the eponym of the congestive myelopathy caused by dAVF.
- Less common spinal high-flow vascular malformations include intramedullary glomus arteriovenous malformation (AVM; nidus within spinal cord), juvenile/metameric AVM (multiple pial/dural/extradural feeding arteries, large nidus within spinal cord and possibly bone or soft tissues), and pial AVF (anterior or posterior spinal artery feeder).

Low-flow vascular (cavernous) malformation

- Spinal cavernous malformations (cavernomas) are rare and sometimes

- **硬脊膜动静脉瘘(dAVF)**是最常见的脊髓血管畸形，为高流量血管畸形，血管造影的特征为供血动脉起自神经根脊膜动脉，无交织的血管巢，椎弓根正下方的神经根鞘内神经根静脉逆行引流至髓周静脉。
- 由此继发静脉高压导致进行性充血性脊髓病，常见于老年男性。
- dAVF在MRI上常表现为长段脊髓水肿(+/–轻度脊髓扩张)和硬膜内髓外流空血管，代表扩张的髓周静脉。CT脊髓造影显示硬膜内蛇形充盈缺损。
- 硬脊膜AVF在CTA和MRA上可呈阴性，根据临床症状或有脑/脊髓出血时，可能需要通过导管血管造影进行诊断。
- dAVF引起的充血性脊髓病称为Foix-Alajouanine脊髓病。
- 较少见的脊髓高流量血管畸形包括髓内球形动静脉畸形(AVM；脊髓内血管巢)、幼年/异位AVM(多个软脊膜/硬脊膜/硬膜外供血动脉，脊髓内大血管巢，也可为骨或软组织)和软脊膜AVF(来自前/后脊髓的供血动脉)。

低流量血管(海绵状)畸形

- 脊髓海绵状血管瘤(海绵状血管瘤)很少见，有

associated with cerebral cavernous malformations. The imaging findings are identical to their intracranial counterparts.

- Cavernous malformations are typically small (involving only one vertebral level). They are most commonly located in the thoracic cord, followed by the cervical cord.

时合并脑海绵状血管瘤。影像学表现与颅内脑海绵状血管瘤相同。

- 海绵状血管畸形通常很小(仅累及单个椎体水平)。最常见于胸段脊髓,其次是颈髓。

SPINAL CORD TOXIC/METABOLIC LESIONS

脊髓中毒/代谢性病变

Overview of spinal cord toxic/metabolic lesions

脊髓中毒/代谢性病变概述

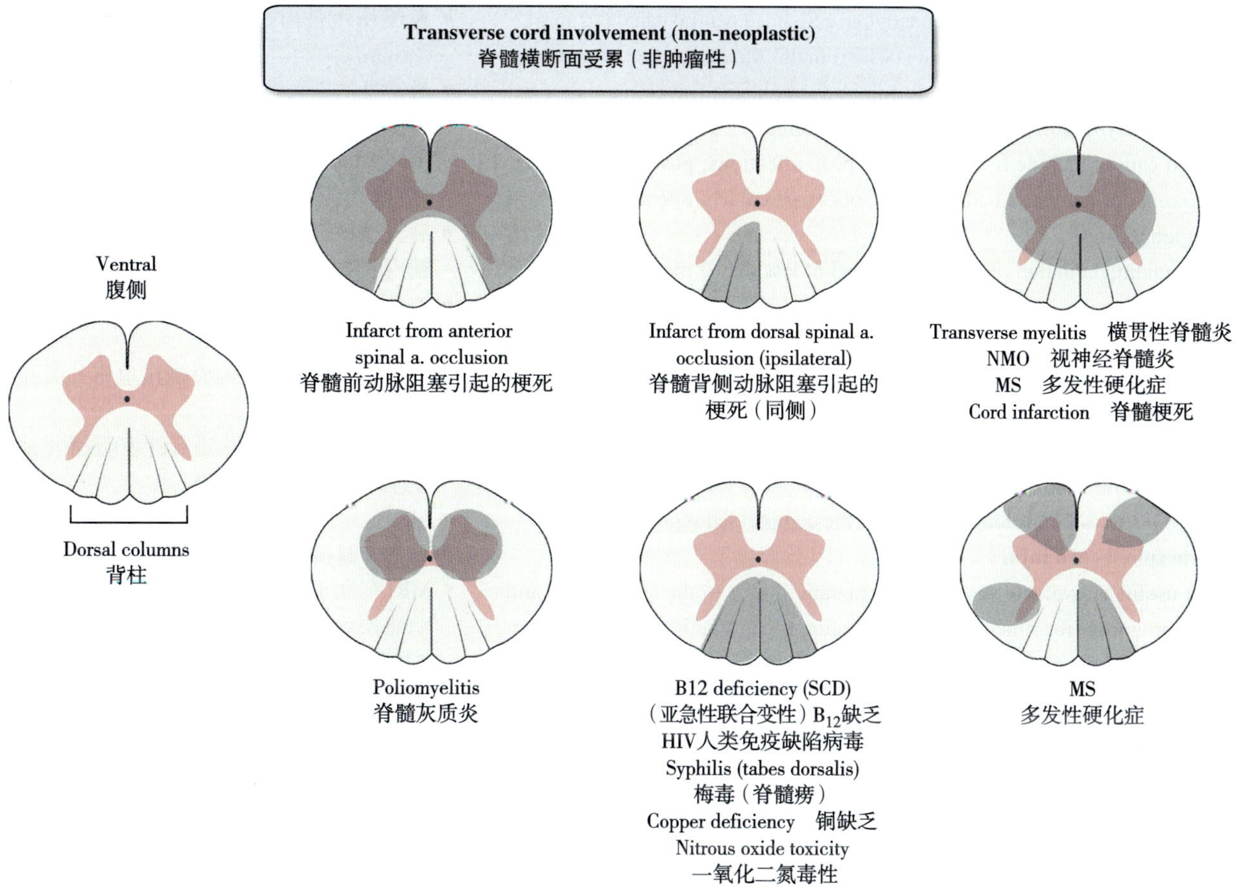

Subacute combined degeneration (SCD)

- Subacute combined degeneration is a myelopathy involving the dorsal and lateral columns caused by vitamin B12 deficiency.
- Causes include malabsorption (e.g., pernicious anemia, gastrointestinal surgery), inadequate intake (strict vegetarian diet), or interfering drugs (e.g., nitrous oxide, proton pump inhibitors, metformin).
- Imaging findings include longitudinal, symmetric hyperintensity on T2-weighted images primarily in the dorsal columns, configured like an inverted V in the axial plane. Lesions involve the cervical and/or thoracic cord.
- With treatment, these findings can regress. Chronically, permanent axonal loss results with associated gliosis.

Radiation myelopathy

- Radiation myelitis/myelopathy is spinal cord white matter injury that develops some time after exposure to radiation therapy.
- MRI demonstrates longitudinally extensive cord hyperintensity on T2-weighted images in the field of radiation therapy, which may be demarcated by T1 hyperintensity of the adjacent vertebrae.

亚急性联合变性(SCD)

- 亚急性联合变性是一种累及背侧和侧柱的脊髓病变,由维生素B_{12}缺乏所致。
- 原因包括吸收不良(如恶性贫血、胃肠手术)、摄入不足(严格素食)或干扰性药物(例如,一氧化二氮、质子泵抑制剂和二甲双胍)。
- 影像学表现包括T_2加权图像上以背侧柱为主的纵向对称性高信号,在横切面上呈倒V形。病变累及颈髓和/或胸髓。
- 通过治疗,这些可以逆转。长期来看,永久性轴突消失会导致胶质增生。

放射性脊髓病

- 放射性脊髓炎/脊髓病是放射治疗后一段时间内发生的脊髓白质损伤。
- 在MRI T_2加权图像上,接受放射治疗的区域出现纵向广泛的脊髓高信号,可以通过T_1相对高信号来区分相邻椎体。

Spinal Cord Mechanical/Traumatic/Miscellaneous Lesions

Syrinx (syringohydromyelia)

- Syrinx and syringohydromyelia are collective terms referring to intramedullary cystic lesions that may represent hydromyelia and/or syringomyelia. Syrinx may rarely also refer to intracranial variants.
- **Syringomyelia** is a fluid-filled, gliosis-lined cavity within the spinal cord parenchyma that does not communicate with the central canal.
- **Hydromyelia** is dilatation of the ependymal cell-lined central canal (>2 mm).
- The most common congenital cause is Chiari malformations (more often Chiari Ⅰ). Other congenital causes include spinal dysraphisms (myelomeningocele, tethered cord syndrome) and Klippel-Feil syndrome.
- Acquired causes include hydrocephalus, post-infectious, post-inflammatory, post-traumatic, and intramedullary tumors (particularly ependymomas and hemangioblastomas).
- Of note, minimal dilation of the central canal of less than 2 mm is likely within normal limits.

Compressive myelopathy

- Compressive myelopathy refers to neurological deficits related to spinal cord compression.
- The most common cause is degenerative disease (spondylosis) in the cervical spine. Other causes include extradural masses.
- MRI demonstrates T2 prolongation within the compressed segment of cord.

Traumatic spinal cord injury

- MRI is useful to evaluate severity of traumatic injury to the spinal cord and provide prognosis for functional outcome. Injury can manifest as concussion (normal MRI appearance), cord edema, hemorrhagic contusion, or cord hematoma.

  Spinal cord edema is characterized by abnormal T2 prolongation within the spinal cord, with normal or low associated T1 signal.

  Hemorrhagic contusion appears as a focus of hypointensity surrounded by hyperintensity on T2-weighted images.

  Cord hematoma (poorest prognosis) is a larger (>4 mm) focus of hypointensity surrounded by hyperintensity on T2-weighted images.
- Spinal cord injury is neurologically categorized by whether there is incomplete or complete sensory and/or motor function loss below a particular level. There are several classic incomplete cord syndromes:

  Central cord syndrome, due to injury around the central canal, is the most common incomplete cord syndrome and usually results from hyperextension trauma in patients with degenerative cervical spinal canal stenosis.

  Brown-Séquard syndrome, due to a hemicord injury, usually results from penetrating trauma affecting half the cord.

  Ventral/anterior cord syndrome, involving the anterior 2/3 of the cord but sparing dorsal columns, is most commonly caused by anterior spinal artery ischemia/infarction, but can also be post-traumatic due to vertebral fracture, disc herniation, or spondylolisthesis.

  Conus medullaris and cauda equina syndromes, due to a lesion at the end of the spinal cord or nerve roots at T12 and below, have various causes including trauma, disc herniation, tumor, and epidural abscess.

脊髓机械性/外伤性/其他损伤

脊髓空洞(脊髓空洞积水症)

- 脊髓空洞和脊髓空洞积水症是髓内囊性病变的统称，可代表脊髓积水和/或脊髓空洞症。空洞在极少见的情况下也可提示颅内变异。
- **脊髓空洞症**是脊髓实质内充满液体、衬有增生胶质细胞的空腔，不与中央管相通。
- **脊髓积水**是内衬室管膜细胞的中央管扩张(>2mm)。
- 最常见的先天性原因是Chiari畸形(更常见于Chiari Ⅰ)。其他先天性原因包括脊髓闭合不全(脊髓脊膜膨出、脊髓栓系综合征)和克利佩尔-费尔综合征。
- 后天性原因包括脑积水、感染、炎症、创伤及髓内肿瘤(特别是室管膜瘤和血管母细胞瘤)。
- 注意：小于2mm的中央管扩张可属于正常。

压迫性脊髓病

- 压迫性脊髓病是指与脊髓压迫相关的神经功能障碍。
- 最常见的原因是颈椎退行性疾病(颈椎病)，其他原因包括硬膜外肿块。
- MRI显示脊髓受压段T_2信号增高。

创伤性脊髓损伤

- MRI有助于评估脊髓外伤的严重程度，并为功能预后提供依据。损伤可表现为脊髓震荡(MRI表现正常)、脊髓水肿、出血性挫伤或脊髓血肿。

  脊髓水肿的特点是脊髓内T_2异常信号增高，T_1信号正常或降低。

  出血性挫伤表现为T_2加权图像上被高信号包围的低信号灶。

  脊髓血肿(预后最差)是T_2加权图像上较大(>4mm)的低信号灶，周围为高信号。
- 脊髓损伤的神经学分类是根据是否存在低于特定水平的不完全或完全的感觉和/或运动功能丧失。有几种典型的不完全性脊髓综合征：

  中央脊髓综合征，是最常见的不全脊髓综合征，由中央管周围损伤所致，通常是在退行性颈椎病合并椎管狭窄的患者中因过度伸展而造成的损伤。

  Brown-Séquard综合征，由一侧脊髓损伤所致，通常由穿通性损伤累及半侧脊髓。

  腹侧/前脊髓综合征，累及脊髓前2/3，但不影响背柱，最常见的原因是脊髓前动脉缺血/梗死，但也可以是创伤后因脊柱骨折、椎间盘突出或脊椎滑脱引起。

  脊髓圆锥和马尾综合征，由脊髓尾端或T_{12}神经根及以下的病变所致，有多种原因，包括外伤、椎间盘突出、肿瘤和硬膜外脓肿。

(翻译　王维平)

INTRADURAL EXTRAMEDULLARY LESIONS

硬膜内髓外病变

Overview of intradural extramedullary lesions

- Intradural extramedullary lesions are located within the dura but outside the spinal cord, usually involving the nerve roots or meninges and projecting into the subarachnoid space. A subset of this category are lesions of the conus medullaris, cauda equina, and filum terminale, which have a distinct differential diagnosis.
- Intradural extramedullary lesions may deviate/compress the spinal cord. CSF is seen above and below the lesion, as well as possibly as a cleft between the lesion and the cord.
- Nerve sheath tumors (neurofibromas and schwannomas) and meningiomas comprise 90% of intradural extramedullary neoplasms, although which is the single most common tumor varies by source. Leptomeningeal metastases are less common.
- Myxopapillary ependymomas are the most common tumor in the cauda equina region. Spinal paragangliomas are less common but also almost always arise in this region.

硬膜内髓外病变概述

- 硬膜内髓外病变位于硬脊膜内但在脊髓外，通常涉及神经根或脊膜并向蛛网膜下腔扩张。脊髓圆锥、马尾和终丝的病变也属于此类，但这些病变的鉴别诊断截然不同。
- 硬膜内髓外病变可能使脊髓移位/受压。脑脊液见于病变的上方和下方，也可能在病变和脊髓之间的裂隙。
- 虽然最常见的硬膜内髓外肿瘤来源不同，但神经鞘肿瘤(神经纤维瘤和神经鞘瘤)和脊膜瘤占90%。柔脊膜转移不太常见。
- 黏液乳头状室管膜瘤是马尾区最常见的肿瘤。脊髓副神经节瘤不太常见，但也几乎总是出现在该区域。

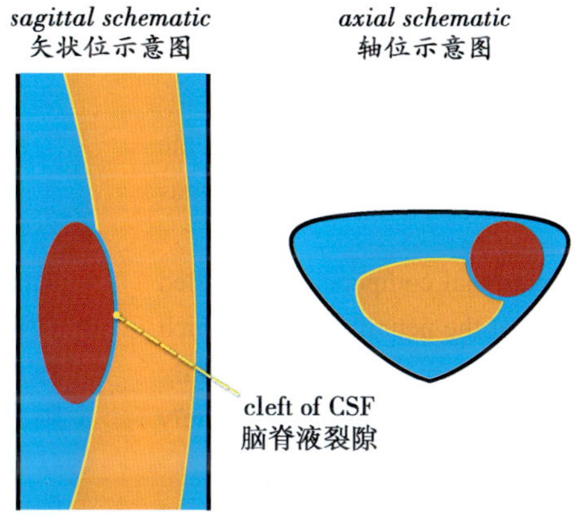

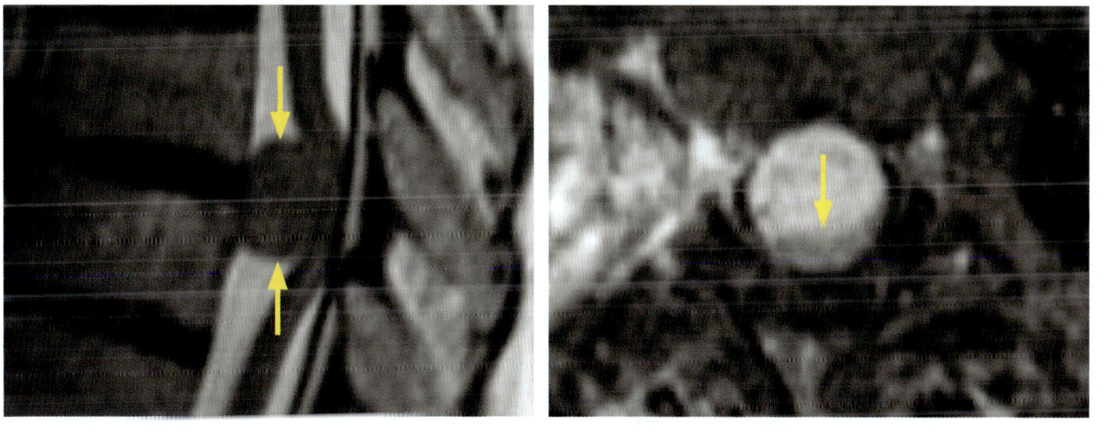

Intradural-extramedullary mass: Sagittal T2-weighted (left image) and axial T1-weighted post-contrast (right image) MRI shows an intradural thoracic mass (arrows). The mass is distinct from the spinal cord and displaces the cord posteriorly. The axial image shows severe posterior compression of the cord (arrow) by the avidly enhancing mass. This was a meningioma. Usually, however, thoracic meningiomas are posterior to the spinal cord.

硬膜内-髓外肿块：矢状位T_2加权(左图)和轴位增强T_1加权(右图)MRI显示位于胸段硬膜内肿块(箭)。肿块明显有别于脊髓，并使脊髓向后移位。轴位图像显示有显著增强的肿块对脊髓(箭)造成严重的向后挤压。这是一名脊膜瘤患者。然而，胸段脊膜瘤通常位于脊髓的后方。

INTRADURAL EXTRAMEDULLARY SPINAL NEOPLASMS

Meningioma

- Typical meningiomas are benign (WHO grade Ⅰ) intradural extramedullary neoplasms. More aggressive variants (WHO grade Ⅱ and Ⅲ) are less common. Less than 10% are extradural, or both intradural and extradural.
- Spinal meningiomas are most commonly seen in older women. Radiation exposure is an additional risk factor.
- Meningiomas are associated with neurofibromatosis type 2 (NF2), especially in children or if multiple.
- Imaging classically shows an intensely enhancing mass with a dural tail. Calcification is uncommon. The thoracic region is most commonly involved.

Benign nerve sheath tumor (schwannoma, neurofibroma)

- Spinal nerve sheath tumors are mostly benign (WHO grade Ⅰ) intradural extramedullary tumors which arise from nerve roots, including **schwannoma** (more common) and **neurofibroma**. 15% are both intradural and extradural; 15% are completely extradural. Intramedullary cases are rare.
- While most cases are isolated, multiple lesions in younger patients are seen in neurofibromatosis type 1 (neurofibroma) and type 2 (schwannoma). Schwannomatosis is another genetic disorder with multiple schwannomas.
- Spinal schwannomas most commonly involve the lumbar region and are the second most common tumor in the cauda equina region. Spinal neurofibromas most commonly involve the cervical region.
- Tumors with intraspinal, foraminal, and extraforaminal components are called "dumbbell" tumors, due to the restrained growth at the neural foramen, which may be enlarged by pressure erosion. Dumbbell tumors are most commonly nerve sheath tumors and may be both intradural and extradural or completely extradural.
- Schwannoma and neurofibroma have similar imaging appearances, presenting on MRI as a T2-hyperintense enhancing intradural mass. Some show the target sign (central hypointensity on T2-weighted images surrounded by a hyperintense periphery). Larger schwannomas may show cystic change.
- Schwannomas are encapsulated and separable from the parent nerve, so nerve-sparing resection is possible. Neurofibromas are unencapsulated and infiltrate between nerve fascicles, so complete resection necessitates nerve sacrifice.

硬膜内髓外脊髓肿瘤

脊膜瘤

- 典型的脊膜瘤是良性(WHO Ⅰ级)的硬膜内髓外肿瘤。较具侵袭性的变异(WHO Ⅱ级和Ⅲ级)不太常见。不到10%位于硬膜外,或同时位于硬膜内外。
- 脊膜瘤最常见于老年女性,辐射暴露是一种额外的风险因素。
- 脊膜瘤与2型神经纤维瘤病(NF2)相关,尤其是在儿童或多发病灶。
- 典型的影像学表现为一个显著增强的肿块伴有脊膜尾征,钙化不常见,胸段最常受累。

良性神经鞘肿瘤(神经鞘瘤、神经纤维瘤)

- 脊神经鞘肿瘤大多为起源于神经根的良性(WHO Ⅰ级)硬膜内髓外肿瘤,其中包括**神经鞘瘤**(更常见)和**神经纤维瘤**。同时位于硬膜内外者占15%;完全位于硬膜外者占15%。髓内病例很少见。
- 大多数病例为孤立性,但年轻患者的多发病变可见于1型神经纤维瘤病(神经纤维瘤)和2型神经纤维瘤病(神经鞘瘤)。神经鞘瘤病是患有多发性神经鞘瘤的另一种遗传性疾病。
- 脊神经鞘瘤最常累及腰段,是马尾区第二常见的肿瘤。脊神经纤维瘤最常累及颈段。
- 具有椎管内、椎间孔和椎间孔外成分的肿瘤称为"哑铃状"肿瘤,由于在神经孔内生长受限,故可能会出现神经孔压力性增大。哑铃状肿瘤最常见于神经鞘瘤,可能同时位于硬膜内和硬膜外,或完全位于硬膜外。
- 神经鞘瘤和神经纤维瘤具有相似的影像学表现,在MRI上表现为T_2高信号及增强的硬膜内肿块,某些出现靶征(T_2加权图像上的中央低信号,周围高信号),较大神经鞘瘤可能出现囊变。
- 神经鞘瘤有包膜并与原神经分离,因此可能进行保留原神经的切除术。神经纤维瘤无包膜,并在神经束之间出现浸润,因此完全切除不可避免地对神经产生损伤。

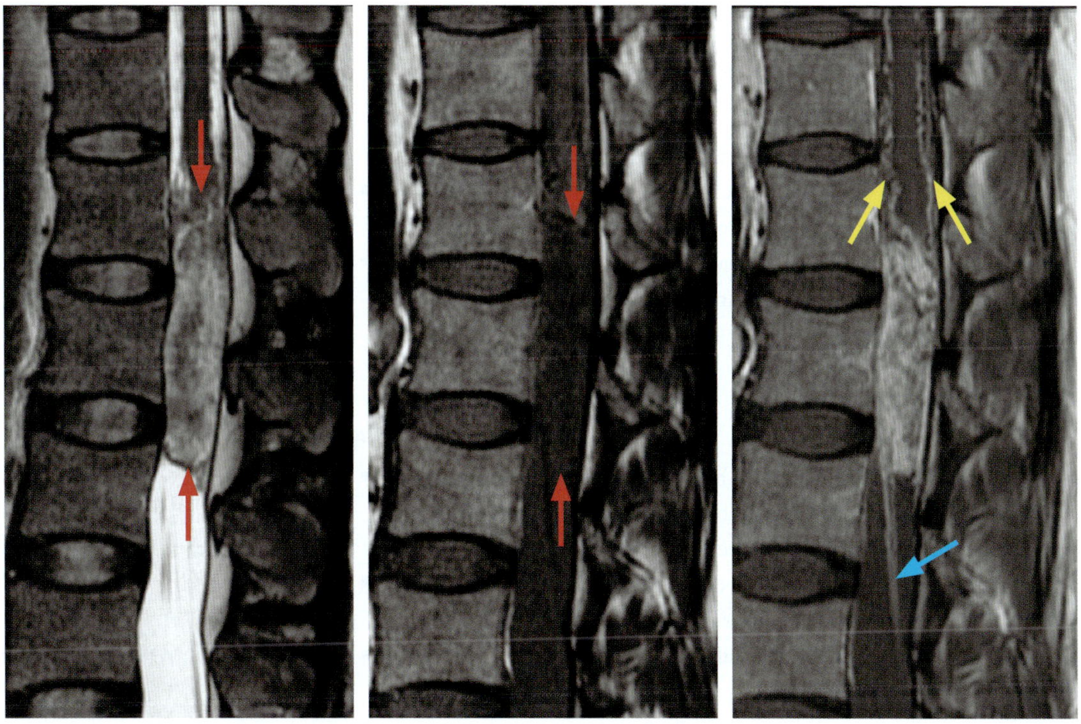

Myxopapillary ependymoma: Sagittal T2 (left image), T1 (middle image), and post-contrast T1-weighted (right image) MRI demonstrate a heterogeneously T2 hyperintense, lobulated mass (red arrows) containing regions of hypointensity on the T2-weighted image. The mass is located at the conus medullaris and avidly enhances. There is also enhancing leptomeningeal dissemination along the surface of the more proximal cord (yellow arrows) and along the cauda equina nerve roots (blue arrow). *Case courtesy Gregory Wrubel, MD, Brigham and Women's Hospital.*

黏液乳头状室管膜瘤：矢状位T_2(左图)、T_1(中图)和增强T_1加权(右图)MRI显示不均匀T_2高信号分叶状肿块(红箭)，并含有T_2低信号区域。肿块位于脊髓圆锥处，呈明显增强。

沿近端脊髓的表面(黄箭)和马尾神经根(蓝箭)可见增强的柔脊膜播散灶。

- Myxopapillary ependymomas are the most common tumor of the cauda equina region, arising from ependymal glia within the conus medullaris and filum terminale. They are a benign (WHO grade Ⅰ) variant of ependymoma.
- The tumor is characterized by slow growth, classically presenting when larger and sausage-shaped, causing vertebral scalloping and spinal canal enlargement. It frequently hemorrhages, resulting in peripheral hemosiderin deposits as hypointensity on T2-weighted images and blooming on GRE.

- 黏液乳头状室管膜瘤是马尾区最常见的肿瘤，起源于脊髓圆锥和终丝内的室管膜细胞，是室管膜瘤的一种良性(WHO Ⅰ级)变异。
- 肿瘤的特点是生长缓慢，通常体积较大且呈香肠形，引起椎体扇形重塑和椎管扩大。常出血导致外周含铁血黄素沉积，在T_2加权图像上表现为低信号和GRE上呈开花样表现。

Paraganglioma

- Spinal paragangliomas are rare and arise almost exclusively in the filum terminale and cauda equina region.
- Similar to paragangliomas elsewhere, spinal paragangliomas show well-circumscribed margins, hyperintensity on T2-weighted images, avid contrast enhancement, and vascular flow voids.

副神经节瘤

- 脊髓副神经节瘤很少见，几乎只出现在终丝和马尾区。
- 与其他部位的副神经节瘤相似，脊髓副神经节瘤边界清楚，T_2加权图像上呈高信号，增强显著伴血管流空。

INTRADURAL EXTRAMEDULLARY SPINAL CONGENITAL/DEVELOPMENTAL LESIONS

硬膜内髓外脊髓先天性/发育性病变

Overview of spinal dysraphisms

- Spinal dysraphisms are a spectrum of congenital midline fusion abnormalities involving neuroectodermal, ectodermal, and/or mesodermal tissues related to the spine and spinal cord.

脊柱闭合不全概述

- 脊柱闭合不全是一系列先天性中线融合异常，影响到脊柱和脊髓相关的神经外胚层、外胚层和/或中胚层组织。

- Spinal dysraphisms are classified as **open** (not covered by intact skin) or **closed** (covered by skin). Closed spinal dysraphisms are more common.
- Older terms include spina bifida occulta (for closed spinal dysraphism) and spina bifida aperta/cystica (for open spinal dysraphism). Spina bifida, strictly speaking, refers to unfused posterior vertebral elements but is usually used to refer to spinal dysraphism in general.
- The most common **open spinal dysraphism** is myelomeningocele.
- The spectrum of **closed spinal dysraphism** includes split cord malformations, caudal regression syndrome, persistent ventriculus terminalis, dorsal dermal sinus, neurenteric cyst, spinal lipoma variants including lipomyelomeningocele, meningocele (herniation of CSF-filled dural sac), and myelocystocele (herniation of syrinx outside spinal canal).

- 脊柱闭合不全分为**开放性**(缺乏完整皮肤覆盖)或**闭合性**(覆盖皮肤)。闭合性脊柱闭合不全更为常见。
- 较早的术语包括隐性脊柱裂(用于闭合性脊柱闭合不全)和开放性/囊性脊柱裂(用于开放性脊柱闭合不全)。严格来说,脊柱裂是指椎体后部结构未融合,但通常用来表达脊柱闭合不全。
- 最常见的**开放性脊柱闭合不全**是脊髓脊膜膨出。
- **闭合性脊柱闭合不全**包括脊髓分裂畸形、尾部退化综合征、永存终末脑室、背侧真皮窦、肠源性神经管囊肿,包括脂肪脊髓脊膜膨出的脊柱脂肪瘤变异体、脊膜膨出(充满脑脊液的硬膜囊疝)和脊髓囊状膨出(椎管外空洞疝)。

Myelomeningocele

- Myelomeningocele is a neural tube defect in which neural placode (embryonic neural tissue) and meninges protrude through defective vertebral posterior elements and are exposed above the skin surface.
- The lumbosacral region is most commonly involved. Patients have neurologic deficits involving the bowel, bladder, and lower extremities.
- Myelomeningocele is nearly always associated with Chiari Ⅱ malformation. Hydrocephalus is present in most cases.
- The defect must be surgically repaired soon after birth. A common complication in children with previously repaired myelomeningocele is tethered cord syndrome.

脊髓脊膜膨出

- 脊髓脊膜膨出是一种神经管缺陷,其中神经基板(胚胎神经组织)和脊膜从有缺陷的椎体后部突出并暴露于皮肤表面。
- 腰骶部最常受累。患者的神经功能缺陷累及肠道、膀胱和下肢。
- 脊髓脊膜膨出几乎总是与Chiari Ⅱ畸形有关,大多数病例有脑积水。
- 缺损必须在出生后不久进行手术修复。脊髓栓系综合征是先前手术修复的脊髓脊膜膨出儿童常见的并发症。

Split cord malformation

- Split cord malformations are forms of spinal dysraphism in which a segment of the spinal cord is divided/duplicated. They are classified into those contained within double dural sacs separated by a rigid (osseocartilaginous) septum (type Ⅰ) and those contained within a single dural sac separated by a nonrigid (fibrous) septum (type Ⅱ).

脊髓分裂畸形

- 脊髓分裂畸形是脊柱闭合不全的一种形式,其中脊髓的一个节段被分割/重复。它们被分为两类:一类是位于由刚性(骨软骨)隔膜(Ⅰ型)分开的双硬膜囊内;另一类是位于由非刚性(纤维)膈膜分开的单硬膜囊内(Ⅱ型)。

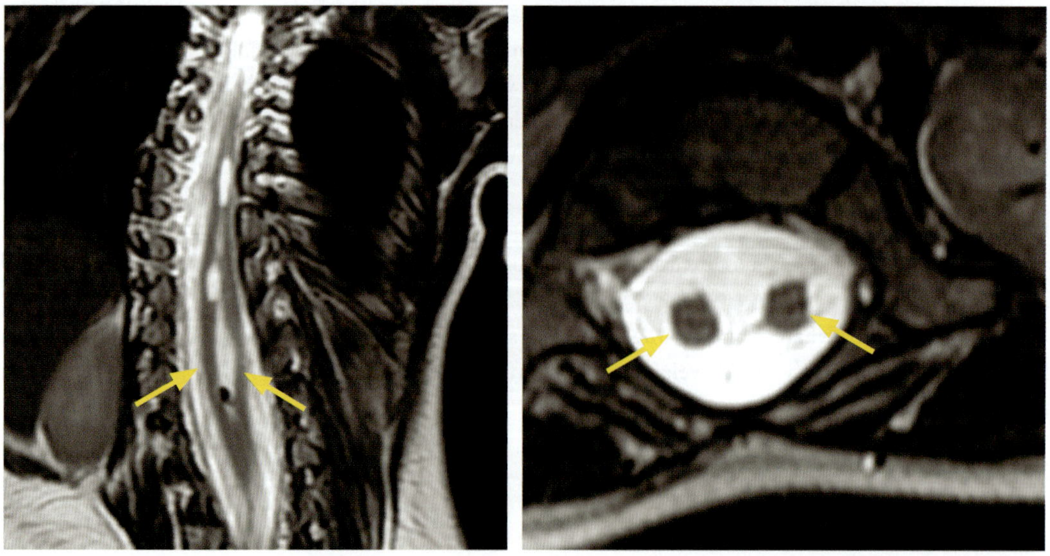

Diastematomyelia: Coronal T2-weighted MRI (left image) shows CSF between the two hemicords (arrows) and a thoracolumbar dextroscoliosis. Axial T2-weighted MRI (right image) shows two hemicords (arrows) within a single CSF space.

脊髓纵裂:冠状位T_2加权MRI(左图)显示CSF在左右两个半束的脊髓(箭)和胸腰椎脊柱右侧弯。轴位T_2加权MRI(右图)显示左右两个半束(箭)的脊髓在同一个CSF空间。

- Historical terminology for split cords is inconsistently applied.

Diastematomyelia, sometimes interchanged with split cord, refers to a sagittal bifurcation of the spinal cord into left and right hemicords, each containing a single set of dorsal and ventral horns and nerve roots.

Diplomyelia is the presence of an accessory spinal cord without roots, located dorsal or ventral to the main cord. They are contained in a single dural sac.

Dimyelia (rare) is duplication of the spinal cord, with each cord having a complete set of roots. They are separated into two dural sacs.

- Bony/cartilaginous septa are well seen on imaging but fibrous septa may be too thin to visualize on conventional imaging.
- Splits are most commonly located caudally in the thoracolumbar cord.

- 历史上关于脊髓分裂不一致的术语。

脊髓纵裂畸形，有时与脊髓分裂互换，是指脊髓在矢状面分为左右半束，每一半束包含一组背角和腹角及神经根。

二重脊髓是没有神经根附着的副脊髓，位于主脊髓的背侧或腹侧。二重脊髓被包裹在同一个硬膜囊内。

重复脊髓(罕见)是两条重复的脊髓，每条脊髓都有一套完整的神经根。重复脊髓有两个硬膜囊。

- 骨性/软骨性隔膜可在图像上清晰可辨，但纤维性隔膜可能太薄而无法在常规影像上进行分辨。
- 裂隙最常位于胸腰椎的尾部。

Caudal regression syndrome

- Caudal regression syndrome is a spectrum of structural defects (dysgenesis, hypogenesis, or agenesis) of the sacrococcygeal and sometimes lumbar region involving the spine, spinal cord, and often genitourinary or gastrointestinal tracts. The spinal cord conus medullaris may terminate higher than normal or lower due to tethering.
- Infants of diabetic mothers are at higher risk.

尾部退化综合征

- 尾部退化综合征是骶尾部(有时为腰椎区域)的一系列结构缺陷(发育异常、发育不良或发育不全)，累及脊柱、脊髓，并通常累及泌尿生殖道或胃肠道。脊髓圆锥的终点可能会因牵拉而高于或低于正常水平。
- 母亲患有糖尿病的婴儿风险增高。

Tethered cord syndrome

- Tethered cord syndrome is a clinical syndrome of neurologic deficits (e.g. back and leg pain, gait spasticity, and decreased lower extremity sensation) attributed to fixation/traction of the caudal portion of the spinal cord.
- Common causes include spinal lipomas, tight filum terminale (thickened >2 mm), and post-repair myelomeningocele.
- Normally, the conus should terminate superior to the inferior endplate of L2. If the conus terminates below this level, the cord may be tethered.

脊髓栓系综合征

- 脊髓栓系综合征是一组神经功能障碍的临床综合征(例如，背部和腿部疼痛、痉挛步态和下肢感觉障碍)，原因为脊髓的尾部被固定/牵拉。
- 常见原因包括脊柱脂肪瘤、终丝牵拉(增厚>2mm)和脊髓脊膜膨出手术修补后。
- 通常情况下，圆锥应终止于L_2下终板的上方。如果圆锥末端低于这个水平，脊髓可能会受牵拉。

Spinal lipomas

- Spinal lipomas have widely varying classifications/terminology. They are congenital, non-neoplastic fatty lesions that occur along the dorsal midline spinal canal and are typically intradural but can also have extradural components.
- **Filar lipoma** refers to the linear/tubular fibrofatty thickening of the filum terminale. MRI demonstrates hyperintensity on T1-weighted images. It is usually clinically insignificant but may be associated with tethered cord syndrome.

脊柱脂肪瘤

- 脊柱脂肪瘤有许多不同的分类/术语。该脂肪瘤是先天性的非肿瘤性脂肪性病变，沿椎管背侧的中线分布，通常在硬膜内，但也可以有硬膜外成分。
- **终丝脂肪瘤**是指终丝线状/管状纤维脂肪增厚。T_1加权图像显示为高信号。临床通常无症状，但可能与脊髓栓系综合征有关。

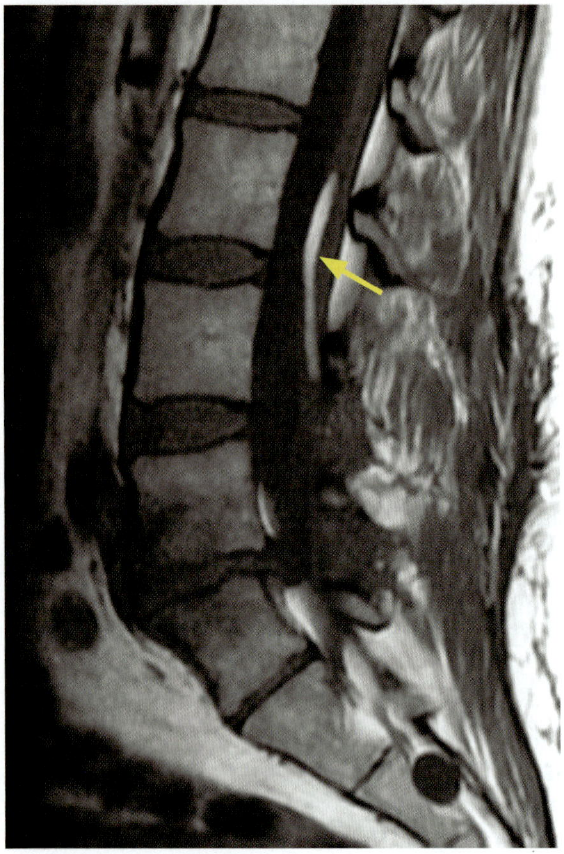

Fatty filum:
Sagittal T1-weighted MRI shows a hyperintense lesion in the filum (arrow), representing fat in the filum terminale.
Of note, a potential pitfall is to mistake an enhancing vessel as a fatty filum. A fatty filum will be apparent on the noncontrast sequences as well.
脂肪性终丝：
矢状位T_1加权MRI显示终丝呈高信号病变(箭)，代表终丝中的脂肪。
注意，不能将增强的血管误认为脂肪丝。在非增强序列上可以清晰显示脂肪性终丝。

- **Lipomyelomeningocele** refers to a combination of lipoma and myelomeningocele where the neural placode-lipoma interface protrudes outside the spinal canal.

Persistent ventriculus terminalis

- The ventriculus terminalis, also called the fifth ventricle, is a dilatation of the spinal cord central canal at the conus medullaris that normally regresses in infancy. Abnormal persistence/dilatation in older children and adults can be a cause of neurologic deficits.
- The imaging differential in neonates includes a filar cyst, which is a normal variant structure inferior to the conus that does not connect with the central canal.

Dorsal dermal sinus

- Dorsal dermal sinuses are epithelial-lined tracts extending from neural tissue to the dorsal skin. Physical examination shows a dimple or pinpoint ostium in the midline back.
- Dorsal dermal sinuses predominantly occur in the lumbosacral region.
- They are often associated with an intradural dermoid (more common) or epidermoid cyst.

Dermoid cyst

- Dermoid cysts are congenital lesions that usually present in childhood.
- Similar to dermoids present elsewhere, they contain macroscopic fat, which is hyperintense on T1-weighted images.
- Rare dermoid rupture may cause potentially fatal chemical meningitis.

- **脂肪性脊髓脊膜膨出**是指脂肪瘤和脊髓脊膜膨出的组合，其中神经基板-脂肪瘤界面突出于椎管外。

永存终末脑室

- 终末脑室，也称为第五脑室，是脊髓圆锥处扩张的脊髓中央管，通常在婴儿期退化。儿童和成人异常持续/扩张可能是引起神经功能缺损的一个原因。
- 新生儿的影像学鉴别诊断包括终丝囊肿，这是圆锥下方的一种正常变异结构，不与中央管连接。

背侧真皮窦

- 背侧真皮窦是内衬上皮的管道，从神经组织延伸到背侧皮肤。体格检查显示背部中线有一个酒窝或针尖样开口。
- 背侧真皮窦主要发生在腰骶部。
- 背侧真皮窦通常与硬膜内皮样(更常见)或表皮样囊肿有关。

皮样囊肿

- 皮样囊肿通常是儿童时期出现的先天性病变。
- 与其他部位的皮样囊肿类似，含有肉眼可见的脂肪，在T_1加权图像上呈高信号。
- 皮样囊肿破裂罕见，但有可能导致致死性化学性脑脊膜炎。

Epidermoid cyst

表皮样囊肿

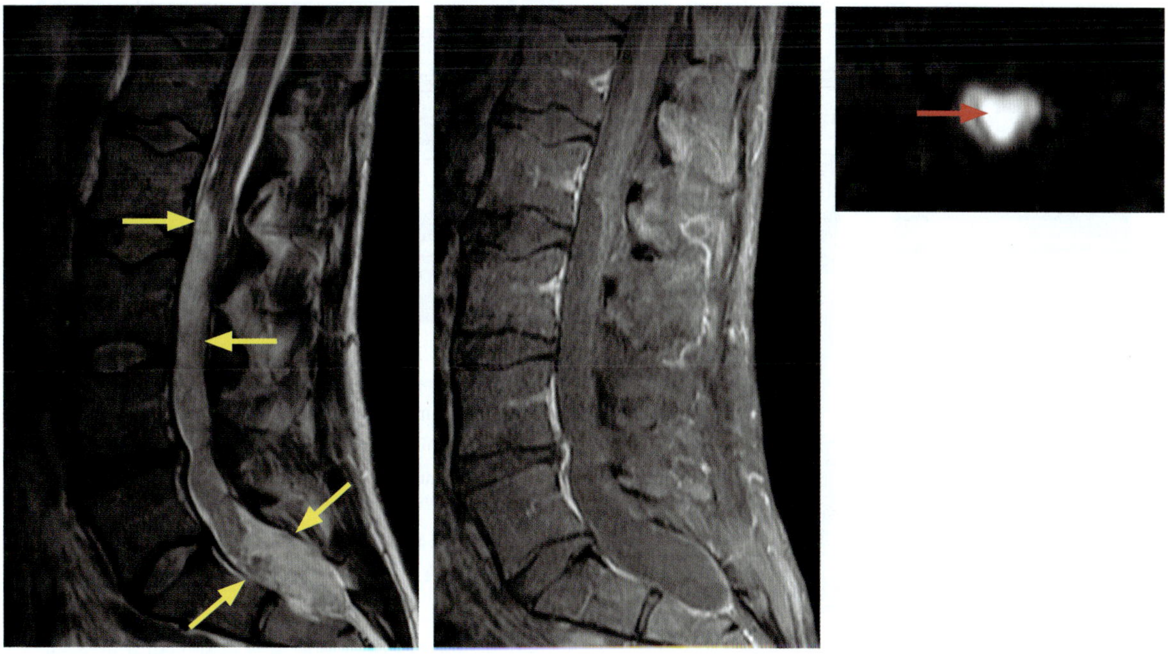

Sagittal T2 (left image) and T1 post-contrast (middle image) MRI show a large heterogeneously T2 hyperintense, nonenhancing intradural extramedullary mass (yellow arrows) which displaces the conus and cauda equina roots. The mass demonstrates restricted diffusion (right image, red arrow). These findings are consistent with an epidermoid.

矢状位T_2(左图)和增强T_1(中图)MRI显示一个大而不均匀的T_2高信号,非强化的硬膜内髓外肿块(黄箭)取代了圆锥和马尾神经根。肿块弥散受限(右图,红箭)。这些表现符合表皮样囊肿改变。

- Spinal epidermoid cysts are more often acquired than congenital. Acquired spinal epidermoids are caused by implantation of skin elements in the subarachnoid space during spinal puncture.
- Spinal epidermoids are usually intradural extramedullary but may rarely be intramedullary.
- Most commonly, an epidermoid cyst appears similar to a simple cyst on conventional MR sequences (hypointense on T1-weighted images and hyperintense on T2-weighted images). Faint peripheral rim enhancement can be seen. Occasionally, the cyst contents may be proteinaceous, causing T1 shortening.
- As with epidermoids elsewhere, diffusivity is restricted.

- 脊髓表皮样囊肿往往是获得性的而非先天性。获得性脊髓表皮样囊肿是由于皮肤成分在脊椎穿刺过程中被植入蛛网膜下腔所造成的。
- 脊髓表皮样囊肿通常位于硬膜内髓外,很少位于髓内。
- 通常,常规磁共振成像序列显示表皮样囊肿与单纯性囊肿相似(T_1加权图像上低信号和T_2加权图像上高信号)。可以看到微弱的外周边缘增强。有时,囊肿内容物可含蛋白质,导致T_1缩短。
- 与其他部位的表皮样囊肿相同,弥散受限。

Arachnoid cyst

蛛网膜囊肿

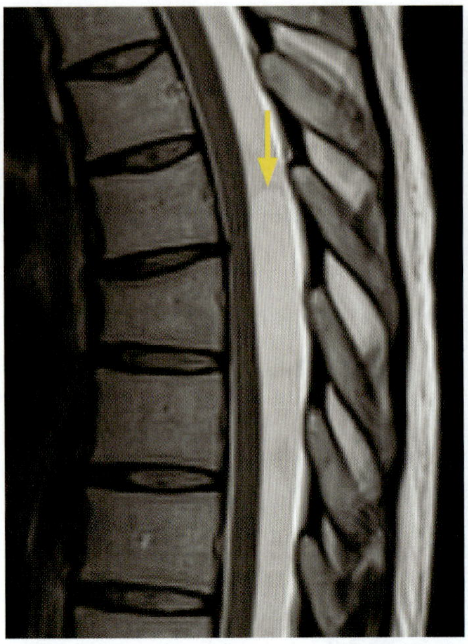

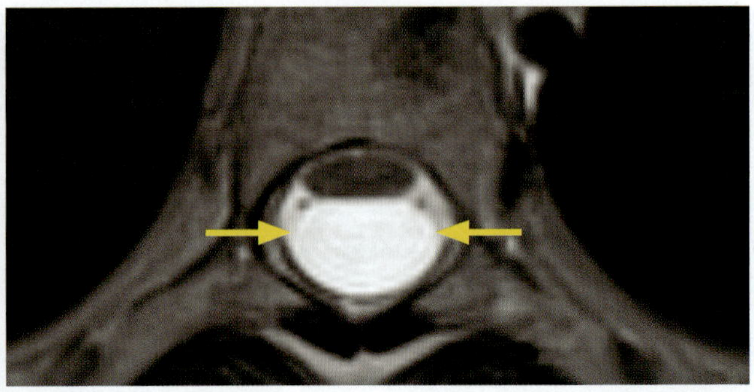

Arachnoid cyst:
Sagittal and axial T2 MRI images demonstrate anterior displacement of the thoracic spinal cord by an intradural extramedullary lesion with CSF signal intensity. The margins of this lesion are hard to define (yellow arrows). This is thought to represent an arachnoid cyst.

蛛网膜囊肿：
矢状位和轴位T_2 MRI图像显示一处硬膜内髓外病变使胸部脊髓向前移位，其信号类似于脑脊液。病变的界限很难确定(黄箭)，考虑为蛛网膜囊肿。

- An **arachnoid cyst** is a CSF collection, usually intradural but occasionally extradural, that may be congenital or a result of trauma, post-operative scarring, or inflammation.

  Arachnoid cysts follow CSF in all MRI sequences and as such can be difficult to distinguish from surrounding CSF. Displacement of the cord or a broad impression on the cord could represent mass effect from an arachnoid cyst and should prompt scrutiny for cyst walls.

- **蛛网膜囊肿**是局部积聚的脑脊液，通常在硬膜内，但偶尔在硬膜外，可能是先天性，也可能为外伤、术后瘢痕或炎症的结果。

  蛛网膜囊肿在所有的MRI序列中与脑脊液相同，因此难以与周围的脑脊液进行区分。脊髓位移或脊髓有较宽的压迹可能代表蛛网膜囊肿的占位效应，应立即对囊壁进行仔细观察。

Arachnoid web

蛛网膜网带

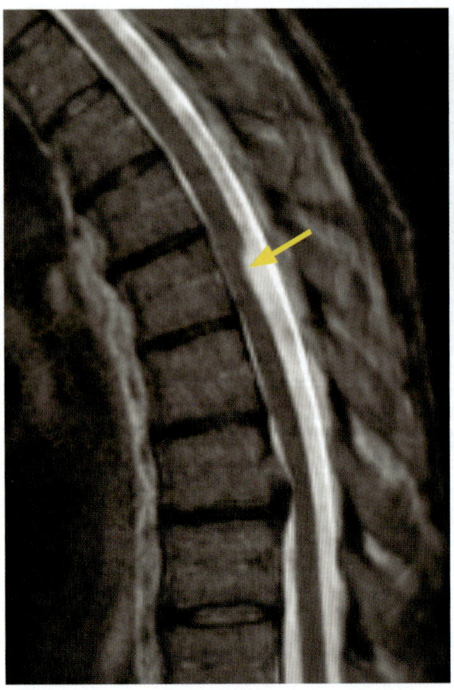

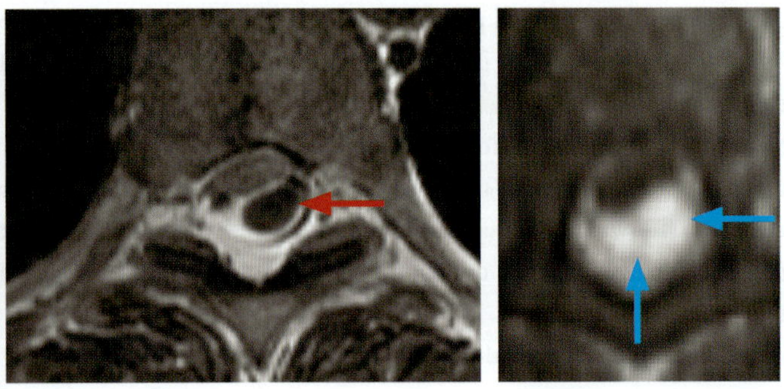

Arachnoid web:
Sagittal and axial T2 MRI (left and middle images) demonstrate dorsal indentation on the thoracic spinal cord (*scalpel sign*, yellow arrow) with associated void flows within the posterior aspect of the thecal sac (red arrow), but without a clear lesion seen. Axial CISS image (right image) shows linear hypointense signal within the dorsal thecal sac at this level (blue arrows), suggesting the presence of a dorsal arachnoid web.

蛛网膜网带：
矢状位和轴位T_2 MRI(左图和中图)显示胸段脊髓背侧压迹(*手术刀征*，黄箭)伴硬膜囊后部流空效应(红箭)，但未见明显病变。轴位CISS图像(右图)显示同一水平背侧硬膜囊内的线性低信号(蓝箭)，提示背侧蛛网膜网带。

- An **arachnoid web** is an abnormal arachnoid membrane in the subarachnoid space. These can be difficult to visualize on MRI but should be suspected in the presence of a spinal cord deformity or obstructed CSF flow without defined walls.

- **蛛网膜网带**是位于蛛网膜下腔的一种异常蛛网膜。这些结构在MRI上可能难以发现，但对存在脊髓畸形或脑脊液流动受阻而没有明确的壁时应引起怀疑。

- Spinal arachnoid cysts and webs are most commonly located dorsal to the thoracic cord.
- The classic imaging finding is a focal dorsal indentation of the spinal cord, called the *scalpel sign* on sagittal images.

Neurenteric cyst

- Neurenteric cyst is a rare lesion composed of heterotopic endodermal tissue, occurring most frequently in the cervical segment, ventral to the spinal cord.
- Imaging findings include non-enhancing lesions which are iso-to slightly hyperintense on T1-weighted images and hyperintense on T2-weighted images.
- Patients frequently have congenital vertebral body anomalies at the same level.

- 脊髓蛛网膜囊肿和蛛网膜网带最常见于胸髓背侧。
- 典型的影像学表现是脊髓背侧局部凹陷，被称为矢状位图像上的手术刀征。

肠源性神经管囊肿

- 肠源性神经管囊肿是一种罕见的由异位内胚层组织构成的病变，最常发生于颈髓，位于脊髓腹侧。
- 影像学表现包括无强化病变，在T_1加权图像上为等信号或稍高信号，在T_2加权图像上为高信号。
- 患者常伴发相同水平椎体的先天性异常。

Spinal cord herniation

脊髓疝

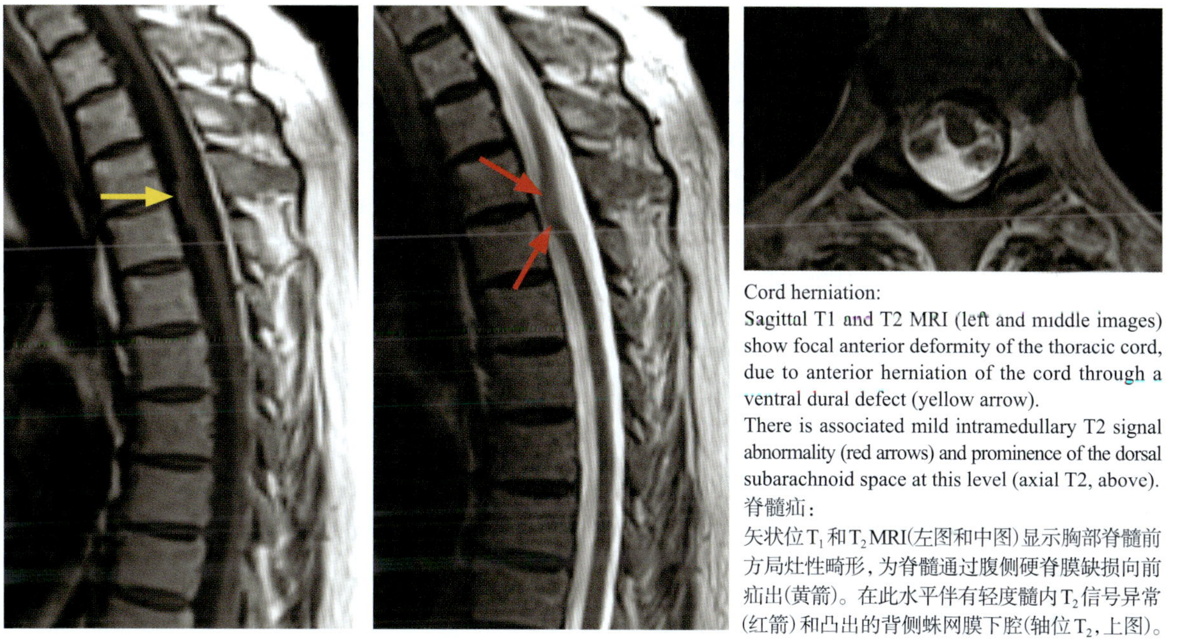

Cord herniation:
Sagittal T1 and T2 MRI (left and middle images) show focal anterior deformity of the thoracic cord, due to anterior herniation of the cord through a ventral dural defect (yellow arrow).
There is associated mild intramedullary T2 signal abnormality (red arrows) and prominence of the dorsal subarachnoid space at this level (axial T2, above).
脊髓疝：
矢状位T_1和T_2MRI(左图和中图)显示胸部脊髓前方局灶性畸形，为脊髓通过腹侧硬脊膜缺损向前疝出(黄箭)。在此水平伴有轻度髓内T_2信号异常(红箭)和凸出的背侧蛛网膜下腔(轴位T_2，上图)。

- Cord herniation is a cause of myelopathy when the spinal cord plugs and protrudes through a dural defect, usually ventrally involving the thoracic cord.
- Cord herniation is typically idiopathic but can be related to prior trauma or surgery.
- MRI or CT myelography shows an anteriorly displaced and focally kinked or C-shaped spinal cord with interruption of the ventral CSF space. Soft tissue may be seen extending into the epidural space.
- The differential diagnosis includes intradural extramedullary lesions that appear as a widened dorsal CSF space such as arachnoid web and arachnoid cyst.

- 脊髓疝是引起脊髓病的一个原因，由于脊髓嵌顿于硬脊膜缺损处或从缺口突出，常累及腹侧胸髓。
- 脊髓疝通常是特发性的，但可能与先前的创伤或手术有关。
- MRI或CT脊髓造影显示脊髓向前移位和局部扭结或呈C形脊髓，伴腹侧脑脊液间隙中断。可以看到软组织延伸到硬膜外腔隙。
- 鉴别诊断包括硬膜内髓外病变，表现为脑脊液背侧空间增宽，如蛛网膜网和蛛网膜囊肿。

INTRADURAL EXTRAMEDULLARY SPINAL INFECTIOUS/INFLAMMATORY LESIONS

硬膜内髓外脊髓感染性/炎症性病变

Arachnoiditis

- Arachnoiditis is inflammation of the spinal leptomeninges, which can produce fibrous adhesions involving the subarachnoid space or dura.
- The most common cause is lumbar spine surgery; arachnoiditis is an occasional cause of failed back surgery syndrome (recurrent or persistent pain after surgery). Other causes include infection (e.g. tuberculosis) and chemical injury

蛛网膜炎

- 蛛网膜炎是柔脊膜的炎症，可造成纤维粘连，涉及蛛网膜下腔或硬脊膜。
- 最常见的原因是腰椎手术；蛛网膜炎是一个较为少见的背部手术失败综合征的原因(术后复发性或持续性疼痛)。其他原因包括感染(如

via intrathecal injection (e.g. steroids, anesthetic).

- The primary imaging feature of lumbar adhesive arachnoiditis is displacement of the cauda equina nerve roots. Three patterns have been described:

> **Group 1: Central conglomerations** of nerve roots within the thecal sac.
>
> **Group 2: Peripheral clumping** of nerve roots, causing the *empty thecal sac* sign.
>
> **Group 3: Obliteration of the subarachnoid space**. Imaging shows increased soft tissue within the thecal sac. This is the most severe form of arachnoiditis.

Guillain-Barré syndrome

- Guillain-Barré syndrome is most commonly an acute inflammatory, demyelinating polyneuropathy (AIDP) characterized by symmetric weakness and diminished reflexes with classically ascending (distal-to-proximal) progression over several weeks.
- The mechanism is characterized by an antecedent infection evoking an immune response. The most common preceding infection is *Campylobacter jejuni*.
- Spinal MRI shows enhancement and thickening of cauda equina nerve roots.

Chronic inflammatory demyelinating polyneuropathy (CIDP)

- CIDP is an acquired immune-mediated neuropathy most commonly characterized by symmetric sensorimotor proximal and distal involvement, with a progressive or recurrent course lasting at least several months.
- MRI shows enhancement and thickening of affected spinal nerve roots (sometimes intradural such as cauda equina but more often extradural), plexi, and peripheral nerves.

EXTRADURAL LESIONS

Overview of extradural lesions

- Extradural lesions are located external to the dura, including the vertebra and epidural space.
- Degenerative lesions, such as osteophytes and herniated discs, are the most common extradural lesions.
- Other important extradural lesions include neoplasms and infection (discitis/osteomyelitis).
- The most common extradural neoplasms that cause epidural spinal cord compression

结核）和鞘内注射的化学损伤性物质(如类固醇、麻醉剂)。

- 腰椎粘连性蛛网膜炎的主要影像学特征是马尾神经根移位。有以下三种表现方式：

> **第1组：**硬膜囊内神经根**中央性集结**。
>
> **第2组：周围神经根结块**，导致空硬膜囊征。
>
> **第3组：蛛网膜下腔闭塞**。影像显示硬膜囊内软组织增加，这是最严重的蛛网膜炎。

吉兰-巴雷综合征

- 吉兰-巴雷综合征是最常见的急性炎症性脱髓鞘多发性神经病(AIDP)，表现为对称性无力和反射减弱，典型的表现为呈上行性进展(从远端到近端)，持续数周。
- 特征性的发病机制为先前感染引起的免疫反应，最常见的前驱感染是空肠弯曲杆菌感染。
- 脊柱MRI显示马尾神经根增强和增厚。

慢性炎症性脱髓鞘性多发性神经病(CIDP)

- 慢性炎症性脱髓鞘性多发性神经病(CIDP)是一种获得性免疫介导的神经病，最常见的特征是对称性近端和远端运动和感觉受累，具有进行性或复发性，病程至少持续几个月。
- MRI显示受累的脊神经根(有时位于硬膜内，如马尾神经，但更常见的是硬膜外)、丛和周围神经增强和增厚。

（翻译　王维平）

硬膜外病变

硬膜外病变概述

- 硬膜外病变位于硬膜的外侧，包括椎体和硬膜外间隙。
- 退行性病变，如骨赘和椎间盘突出，是最常见的硬膜外病变。
- 其他重要的硬膜外病变包括肿瘤和感染(椎间盘炎/骨髓炎)。
- 最常导致硬膜外脊髓受压的硬膜外肿瘤是转

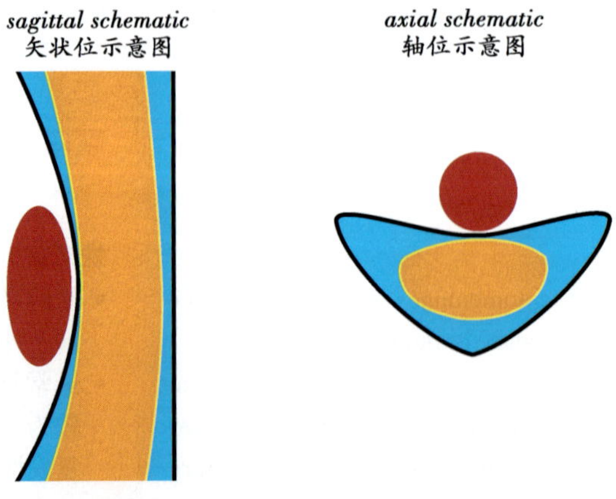

are carcinoma metastases, plasmacytoma/multiple myeloma, and lymphomas.

- Primary extradural tumors are rare.

移瘤、浆细胞瘤/多发性骨髓瘤和淋巴瘤。

- 原发性硬膜外肿瘤很少见。

EXTRADURAL SPINAL/VERTEBRAL NEOPLASMS

Extradural metastasis

- Metastatic disease is the most common extradural malignancy in adults. Metastases usually involve the vertebra and extend into the epidural space rather than being purely epidural.
- Breast, lung, and prostate are the most common primary tumors to metastasize to the spinal column.
- T1-weighted images are essential for evaluation of vertebral body marrow replacement. Marrow should always be more hyperintense on T1-weighted images than the intervertebral discs.
- *Focal* decrease in intensity on T1-weighted images is concerning for metastasis.
- *Diffuse* decrease in intensity on T1-weighted images is abnormal but nonspecific. The differential for diffusely decreased T1 marrow signal includes leukemia, lymphoma, myelofibrosis, HIV, and idiopathic causes.

Primary extradural tumors in middle-aged and older adults

- Spinal **lymphoma** most commonly involves the vertebra or epidural space. Secondary spinal involvement is more common than primary bone lymphoma, usually in the form of non-Hodgkin lymphomas like diffuse large B-cell lymphoma. Lesions are more often osteolytic than sclerotic.
- **Solitary plasmacytoma of bone** is a lytic, expansile bony lesion of late adulthood that is a precursor of multiple myeloma (which features marrow involvement and end-organ damage). Soft tissue lesions are called solitary extramedullary plasmacytomas.

  The presence of multiple lesions implies the diagnosis of multiple myeloma. Development of multiple myeloma, or even abnormal serum/urine protein electrophoresis, may not occur for many years after diagnosis of a plasmacytoma.

- **Chordoma** is a malignant tumor of older adults that arises from a notochord remnant. Chordoma occurs most commonly in the sacrococcygeal region and second most commonly in the clivus. Up to 15% may occur in the vertebral bodies (most commonly cervical).

  Chordoma appears as a destructive, hyperintense mass on T2-weighted images. It avidly enhances.

- **Chondrosarcoma** is a low-grade malignancy that appears as a hyperintense mass on T2-weighted images, similar to chordoma. Chondroid rings-and-arcs calcification may be seen.

Primary extradural tumors in adolescents and young adults

- **Aneurysmal bone cyst (ABC)** is a benign, progressively destructive lesion that occurs in adolescents. Fluid levels are typically seen on MRI, though this finding is nonspecific.
- **Chondroblastoma** is a benign but aggressive neoplasm that rarely may occur in the vertebral column (vertebral body and posterior elements). Secondary ABC may be present.
- **Osteoid osteoma** is a benign, sclerotic lesion affecting the vertebral posterior elements in teenagers and young adults, with a classic clinical history of nocturnal pain relieved by NSAIDs. A central radiolucent nidus consists of vascular fibrous connecting tissue.

硬膜外脊柱/椎体肿瘤

硬膜外转移

- 转移瘤是成人最常见的硬膜外恶性肿瘤。转移通常累及椎体并延伸到硬膜外间隙，而不只是仅位于硬膜外间隙。
- 乳腺癌、肺癌和前列腺癌是最常转移至脊柱的原发性肿瘤。
- T_1加权图像对于评估椎体骨髓受侵至关重要。骨髓在T_1加权图像上的信号应该总是高于椎间盘。
- T_1加权图像上*局部*信号降低时应警惕转移的可能。
- T_1加权图像上*弥漫性*信号降低为异常，但无特异性。骨髓的T_1信号弥漫性降低的鉴别诊断包括白血病、淋巴瘤、骨髓纤维化、艾滋病和特发性原因。

中老年的原发性硬膜外肿瘤

- 脊柱**淋巴瘤**最常累及椎体或硬膜外间隙。继发性脊柱淋巴瘤比原发性骨淋巴瘤更常见，通常是非霍奇金淋巴瘤，如弥漫性大B细胞淋巴瘤。溶骨性病变较硬化性病变更常见。
- **骨孤立性浆细胞瘤**是一种溶骨和膨胀性的骨病变，发生在中老年，是多发性骨髓瘤的前兆(其特点是骨髓受累和终末器官损害)。软组织病变称为孤立性髓外浆细胞瘤。

  存在多发性病变可以诊断为多发性骨髓瘤。进展为多发性骨髓瘤，甚至血清/尿液蛋白电泳异常，可在浆细胞瘤确诊之后多年才出现。

- **脊索瘤**是一种由脊索残余引起的老年人恶性肿瘤。脊索瘤最常见于骶尾部区域，其次是在斜坡。高达15%可能发生在椎体(最常见的是颈椎)。

  脊索瘤在T_2加权图像上表现为破骨性高信号肿块，强化极其明显。

- **软骨肉瘤**是一种低级别恶性肿瘤，在T_2加权图像上表现为高信号肿块，类似于脊索瘤，可见软骨样环和弧形钙化。

青少年的原发性硬膜外肿瘤

- **动脉瘤性骨囊肿(ABC)**是一种良性、渐进性破骨性病变，发生在青少年。通常在MRI上可以看到液平，但这一发现并无特异性。
- **软骨母细胞瘤**是一种良性但具有侵袭性的肿瘤，很少发生在椎体柱(椎体和后部结构)。可继发性动脉瘤性骨囊肿。
- **骨样骨瘤**是一种在青少年中侵犯椎体后部结构的良性、硬化性病变，具有典型的夜间疼痛临床病史，非甾体抗炎药镇痛有效。中央透亮影为血管纤维结缔组织。

- **Osteosarcoma** is a malignant tumor that typically produces osteoid matrix.

Hemangioma

- Vertebral hemangiomas are technically not neoplasms but low-flow vascular malformations, predominantly the cavernous type. They are the most common benign "tumor" of the spine. They are usually incidentally found and composed of endothelium-lined vascular structures.
- Destruction of some of the bony trabeculae and thickening of the remaining trabeculae produce the characteristic *striated corduroy* appearance on plain radiographs and sagittal/coronal CT. The stippled appearance on axial CT is produced by thickened trabeculae seen in cross-section.
- Hemangioma is typically hyperintense on both T1- and T2-weighted images.
- Although hemangioma is benign, an aggressive variant is occasionally seen in the thoracic spine. The aggressive variant may have an epidural soft tissue component that has the potential to cause cord compression.

  Although the asymptomatic variant has no sex predilection, the aggressive form of hemangioma is more common in females.

- **骨肉瘤**是一种恶性肿瘤，通常会产生类骨基质。

血管瘤

- 椎体血管瘤实际并非肿瘤，而是低流量血管畸形，主要是海绵型。它们是脊柱最常见的良性"肿瘤"。常为偶发，由衬有内皮的血管结构组成。
- 部分骨小梁破坏和剩余小梁增厚在普通X线和矢状位/冠状位CT上产生特有的条纹状的灯芯绒外观。轴位CT上的点状影是横切面上看到的增粗的小梁。
- 血管瘤在T_1和T_2加权图像上通常都呈高信号。
- 尽管血管瘤是良性的，但偶尔在胸椎呈侵袭性变异。侵袭性变异可具有硬膜外软组织成分，并能导致脊髓受压。

  无症状性亚型在性别上没有差异，但侵袭性血管瘤更常见于女性。

Extradural non-neoplastic lesions

Disc degeneration

- In the vast majority of cases, diagnosing disc degeneration, including bulges and protrusions, is not a diagnostic dilemma (although accurately characterizing and describing such lesions can be challenging even for experienced radiologists!).
- However, occasionally a sequestered disc fragment may appear like an extradural mass. In fact, since "funny looking" disc fragments are far more common than extradural tumors, a extradural mass within the spinal canal is most likely to represent a sequestered disc fragment. A contrast-enhanced exam can be very helpful to differentiate disc fragment (generally non-enhancing) from a tumor (typically enhancing).

硬膜外非肿瘤性病变

椎间盘退变

- 在绝大多数情况下，诊断椎间盘退变，包括膨出和突出，并非难题(但准确把握特征并描述此类病变，即使对于经验丰富的放射科医生也可能具有挑战性！)。
- 偶发情况下，游离的椎间盘碎片的表现可类似硬膜外肿块。事实上，由于"看似奇怪"的椎间盘碎片比硬膜外肿瘤更常见，因而，椎管内的硬膜外肿块最有可能是游离的椎间盘碎片。对比增强检查有助于区分椎间盘碎片(通常不强化)和肿瘤(通常强化)。

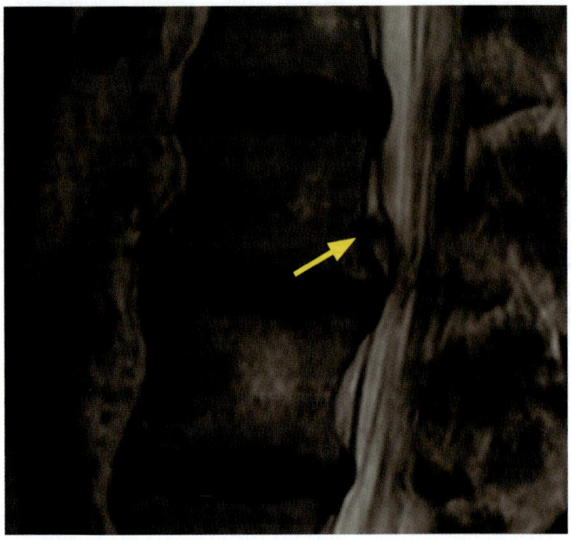

Sequestered disc:
Sagittal T2-weighted MRI demonstrates an extradural mass (arrow) posterior to the inferior endplate of a mid-lumbar vertebral body.
Despite having different signal intensity from the parent disc, this was a sequestered disc fragment.

游离椎间盘：
矢状位T_2加权MRI显示在中段腰椎下终板的后方有一个硬膜外肿块(箭)。
此为游离的椎间盘碎片，尽管其信号强度不同于母体椎间盘。

（翻译　王维平）

DEGENERATIVE SPINE

Overview of degenerative spine

- Symptomatic lumbar spine degeneration is extraordinarily common and imposes a large societal health care burden.
- The major anatomic units involved in lumbar spine degeneration are the disc-endplate complexes anteriorly, and the facet joints and ligamentum flavum posteriorly.
- Symptoms may be due to neural compression (typically producing radicular pain) or localized inflammatory changes (typically producing axial back pain).
- Neural compression may occur at any of three sites: The spinal canal, the lateral recess, or the neural foramen. Each of these will be discussed in detail.
- Axial back pain may come from the disc-endplate complex (such as endplate edema, acute Schmorl's node, or annular fissure), or facet arthropathy. Again, these will be subsequently discussed.
- In order to best guide surgical, interventional pain, and conservative management options, it is important to have consistent nomenclature and grading of spinal degenerative findings.
- In 2014, the North American Spine Society, American Society of Spine Radiology, and the American Society of Neuroradiology published their version 2.0 of lumbar disc nomenclature, which was revised from the initial 1995 version. This text will adhere to these consensus nomenclature guidelines, which are ***bolded and italicized*** throughout this section. Of note, the nomenclature aims to describe morphology of lumbar degenerative findings, but only discusses grading of severity in a cursory manner.
- Several detailed grading schemes have been proposed for the severity of spinal stenosis, lateral recess stenosis, neural foraminal stenosis, and facet arthropathy. We will attempt to synthesize these into a simplified universal classification.
- Despite efforts to standardize the nomenclature and grading, there is a fair amount of inter-observer variability in the reporting of degenerative spinal lesions.

脊柱退行性病变

脊柱退行性病变概述

- 症状性腰椎退行性病变极其常见，并对社会医疗保健构成了巨大负担。
- 涉及腰椎退行性病变的主要解剖结构是前方的椎间盘-终板复合体及后方的椎小关节和黄韧带。
- 症状可能来自神经压迫(通常产生神经根痛)或局部炎症改变(通常导致轴向背痛)。
- 神经压迫可以发生在以下三个部位中的任何一个：椎管、侧隐窝或神经孔。每个部位都将在随后进行详细讨论。
- 轴向背痛可能来自椎间盘-终板复合体(如终板水肿、急性Schmorl结节或纤维环裂隙)或椎小关节病。同样，这些内容将在随后进行讨论。
- 为了更好地指导疼痛手术、疼痛介入或保守治疗，对脊柱退行性病变进行统一命名和分级非常重要。
- 北美脊柱学会、美国脊柱放射学会和美国神经放射学会在2014年对1995年的第一版腰椎间盘命名法进行了修订，并公布了第二版命名法。本文将遵循此次达成共识的命名指南，并在本节内容中以**加粗楷体**显示。需要注意的是，该命名以描述腰椎退行性变的形态为目的，对病变严重程度分级仅作粗略讨论。
- 所涉及的几种详细的分级方案是针对椎管狭窄、侧隐窝狭窄、神经孔狭窄及椎小关节病的严重程度。我们将尝试综合这些内容以简化成一个通用的分类。
- 尽管对命名和分级标准化作出了努力，但在报道退行性脊柱病变时仍存在很多不同观察者之间的差异。

ANTERIOR STRUCTURES: DISC-ENDPLATE COMPLEXES

Structure and patterns of injury of the disc-endplate complex

- The intervertebral discs and vertebral body endplates function together as a load-bearing unit, allowing flexion and extension.
- The normal intervertebral disc is composed of a central gelatinous nucleus pulposus and a fibrous peripheral annulus fibrosus.
- The vertebral body endplate is comprised of a thin layer of hyaline cartilage. Branches of the segmental lumbar arteries supply the endplates (but not the disc itself in adults), and diffusion of nutrients across the endplate is an important source of nutrients for the disc.
- Of the disc-endplate complex, it is the endplates that are most susceptible to axial loading, resulting in endplate fractures.
- Chronic tensile stress on posterior aspect of annulus fibrosus (such as due to repeated spinal flexion, especially if under load due to suboptimal spinal mechanics) can lead to a progressive spiral of degenerative changes involving the disc-endplate complex.

前部结构：椎间盘-终板复合体

椎间盘-终板复合体的结构和损伤模式

- 椎间盘和椎体终板在功能上共同组成一个承重单元，以便屈曲和伸展。
- 正常椎间盘由中央的胶质髓核和周围的纤维环组成。
- 椎体终板由一层薄的透明软骨组成。各节段的腰椎动脉分支供应终板(在成年人并不供应椎间盘本身)，养分通过终板弥散是椎间盘获得营养的重要来源。
- 在椎间盘-终板复合体中，终板最易受到来自轴向的承重，从而导致终板断裂。
- 持续施加在纤维环后方的慢性张力性应激作用(如由于脊柱反复屈曲，尤其在脊柱力学欠佳而承载负荷的情况下)可导致所涉及的椎间盘-终板复合体退行性变呈渐进性和螺旋式加重。

- Discovertebral degeneration may include a spectrum of morphologic changes including disc dessication, disc fibrosis, disc height loss, disc mucinous degeneration, intradiscal gas, vertebral osteophytes, vertebral endplate edema, and vertebral endplate sclerosis.

Disc bulge and herniation (protrusion and extrusion)

- A disc ***herniation*** is a focal displacement of disc material, occurring when the substance of the disc (nucleus pulposus, annulus fibrosus, or both) extends beyond the disc's normal margins. A ***disc herniation*** should encompass less than 90° of the disc circumference.
- A ***disc herniation*** can be classified as either a ***protrusion*** or an ***extrusion***, dependent on the width of its neck. A ***protrusion*** features a neck wider than the dome, while an ***extrusion*** has a dome wider than the neck (similar to a saccular aneurysm). Because ***protrusion*** and ***extrusion*** are more specific terms, the term ***herniation*** should generally not be used in radiology reports.

- 椎间盘退行性变可包括一系列形态学上的变化，如椎间盘脱水、椎间盘纤维化、椎间盘高度减低、椎间盘黏液变性、椎间盘内积气、椎体骨赘、椎体终板水肿和椎体终板硬化。

椎间盘膨出和椎间盘疝(突出和脱出)

- 椎间盘疝是局部椎间盘内容物移位，指椎间盘内容物(髓核和/或纤维环)越过椎间盘的正常边缘。**椎间盘疝**不应超过椎间盘周长的90°。
- **椎间盘疝**可分为椎间盘**突出**或椎间盘**脱出**，这取决于疝颈部的宽度。**突出**的特征是颈部宽于顶部，而**脱出**的顶部宽于颈部(类似囊状动脉瘤)。由于**突出**和**脱出**是较为具体的术语，在影像报告中通常不应该使用**疝出**。

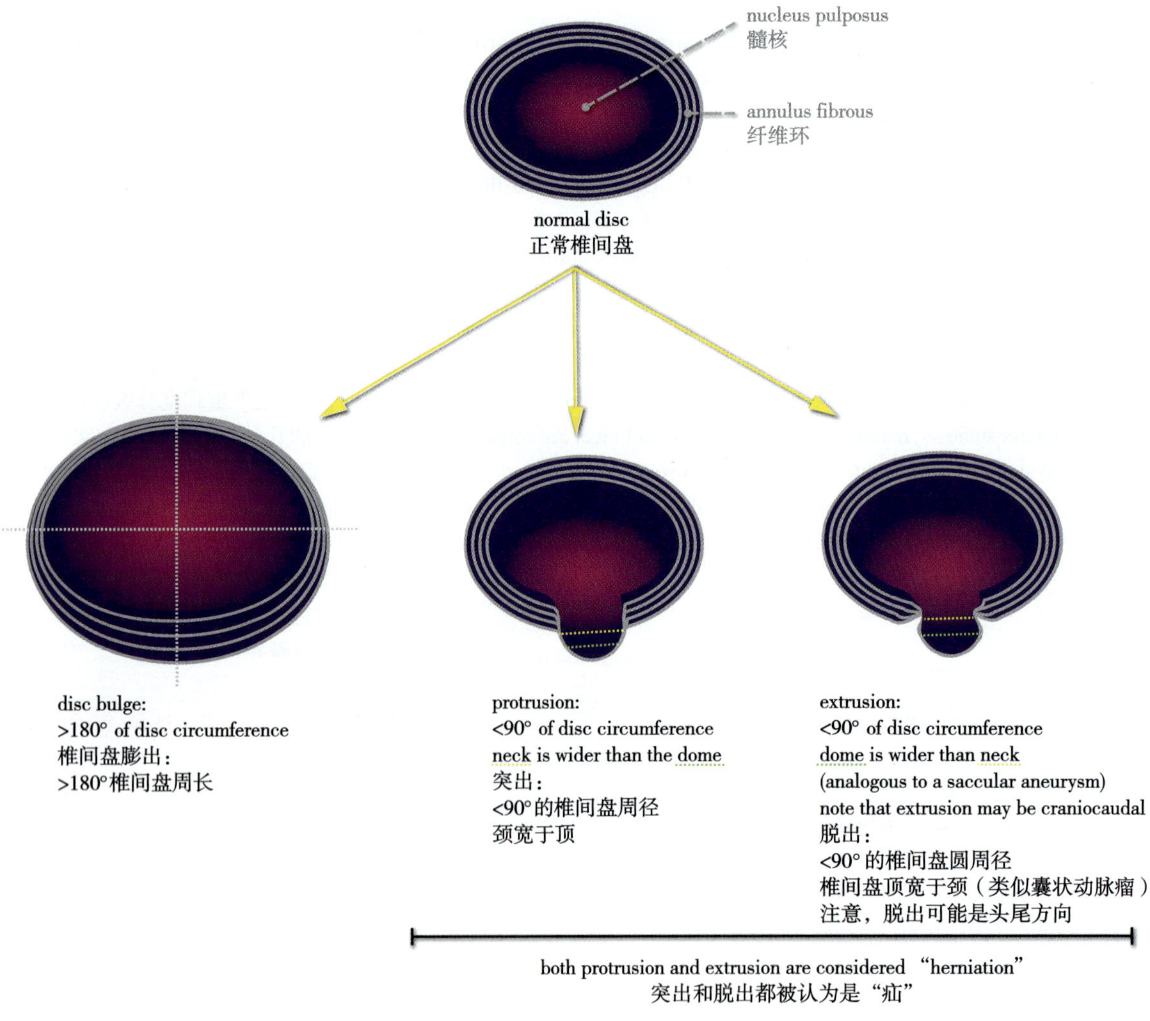

- A ***disc bulge*** is defined as disc material extending beyond the edges of the ring apophyses extending >180° of the disc. There is no need to embellish this consensus terminology with unnecessary words such as "diffuse disc bulge" or "broad-based disc bulge."
- Disc tissue extending beyond the limits of the disc space between 90° and 180° can be described as an ***asymmetric disc bulge***.
- Disc herniations may extend through the a gap in the cartilagenous endplate,

- **椎间盘膨出**定义为椎间盘内容物超出骨突环边缘，且超过椎间盘的180°。不需要使用“弥漫性椎间盘膨出”或“宽基底椎间盘膨出”等词进行修饰。
- 椎间盘组织超出椎间盘90°~180°时可以被称为**非对称椎间盘膨出**。
- 椎间盘疝可穿过软骨终板的间隙，引起**椎体**

causing an ***intravertebral herniation***, much more commonly referred to as a ***Schmorl node***.

- Several terms and variations describe the medial-lateral position of a herniation: ***Central***, ***subarticular***, ***foraminal***, and ***extra-foraminal***, as illustrated on the following page.

  A central herniation is midline. For a lesion that is just lateral to midline, the terms right central or left central are preferred, although right or left paracentral is also acceptable.

  The subarticular zone is located at the lateral recess, in the region of the traversing dorsal and ventral nerve roots, as they separate from the spinal cord (upper lumbar) or the cauda equina (mid to lower lumbar).

- The medial-lateral position of herniation determines which nerve root will be affected. Lesions in the ***central*** (including right or left central for lesions just parasagittal to midline) or ***subarticular*** (lateral recess) locations may compress the descending/traversing nerve root, while ***foraminal*** or ***extra-foraminal*** lesions may compress the exiting nerve root.

内疝，通常称为**Schmorl结节**。

- 有数个不同的术语描述疝的内-外位置关系：**中央型**、**关节下型**、**椎间孔型**及**椎间孔外型**，如下所示：

  中央型疝位于中线。对于中线旁病变，应称为中央右侧或中央左侧，但也可称为右旁中央或左旁中央。

  关节下区位于侧隐窝，即背侧和腹侧穿行神经根的区域。该区域与脊髓(上腰椎)或马尾神经(中至下腰椎)是分离的。

- 疝的内-外侧位置决定了哪些神经根会受到影响。**中央型**(包括中央左、右侧或中线旁)或**关节下型**(侧隐窝)病变可能压迫下行或穿行神经根，而**椎间孔型**或**椎间孔外型**病变通常压迫穿出神经根。

axial schematic: potential sites of focal herniation
轴位示意图：局限性疝的潜在位置

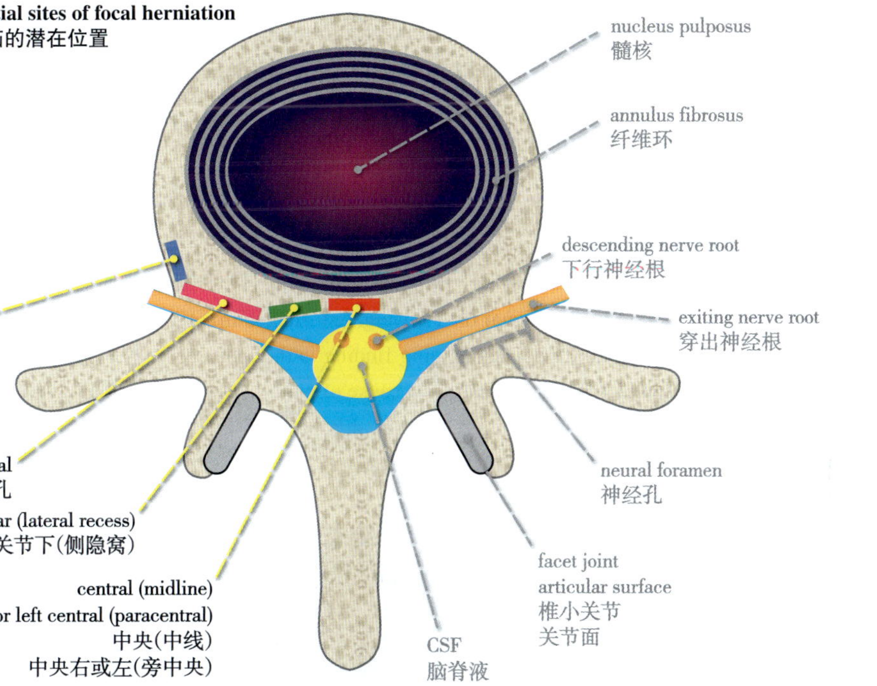

coronal schematic: effect of focal herniation location on nerve-root levels
冠状位示意图：局限性疝的位置对神经根部位的影响

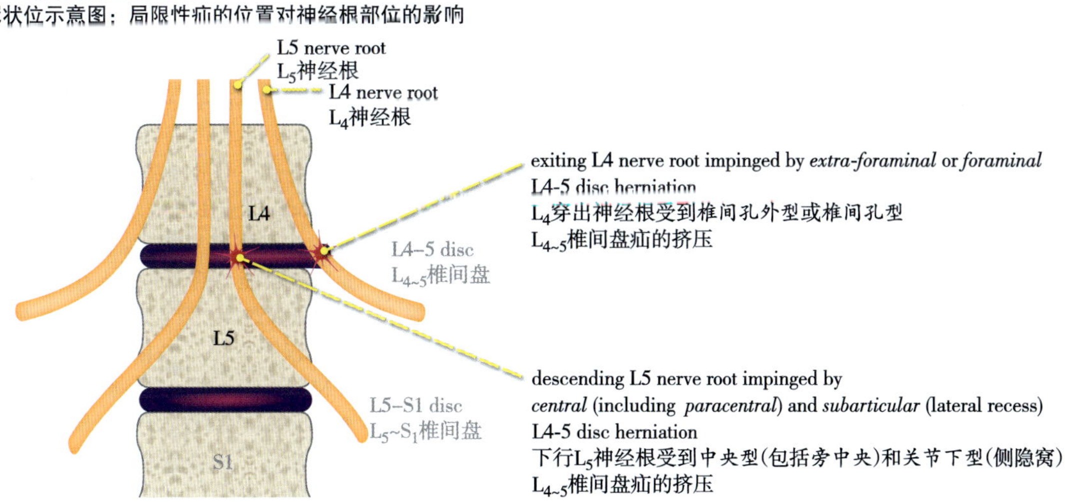

- There is often heterogeneity in the use of the "off-midline" locations described above: For instance, right central, right paracentral, and right subarticular are often used interchangeably. This is fine as long as any relevant neural compression is discussed.
- Disc material may separate from its parent disc to become a ***sequestered*** fragment, which may migrate inferiorly or superiorly.

- 上述"中线偏侧"位置的叫法各异，如右中央、右旁中央和右关节下通常被交替使用。只要提及被压迫的相关神经即可。
- 椎间盘疝出物可从其母盘分离，成为**游离碎片**，可以向上或向下脱落。

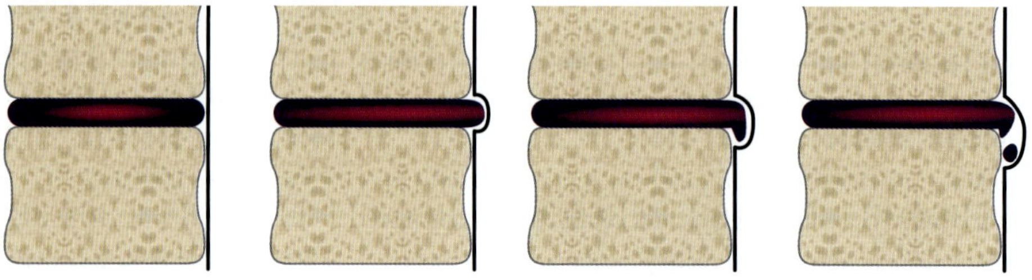

normal 正常 | protrusion 突出 | inferior migration of disc material 椎间盘成分向下移位 | sequestered fragment 游离碎片

- In the thoracic and lumbar spine, each nerve root exits below its corresponding vertebral body. For instance, the L4 nerve root exits below the L4 vertebral body at L4–L5.
- In contrast, in the cervical spine, each root exits above its corresponding vertebral body. For instance, the C7 nerve root exits above the C7 vertebral body at C6–C7. At the cervicothoracic transition, the C8 nerve root exits below the C7 vertebral body and the T1 nerve root exits below the T1 vertebral body.

Annular fissure

- An ***annular fissure*** is a linear hyperintense signal on T2-weighted images in the annulus fibrosis of the intervertebral disc. This imaging finding is thought to correlate with injury of the annulus fibrosis and may be a cause of pain.
- ***Annular fissure*** is the preferred term over annular *tear*, as this process is thought to be degenerative in most cases, rather than traumatic.

- 在胸腰段脊椎，神经根在相应的椎体下方发出。例如，L_4神经根在L_4椎体下方L_{4-5}水平发出。
- 相反，在颈段脊椎每一条神经根自相应的椎体上方发出。例如，C_7神经根自C_7椎体的上方C_{6-7}水平发出。在颈胸移行段脊椎，C_8神经根在C_7椎体的下方发出，T_1神经根在T_1椎体的下方发出。

纤维环裂隙

- **纤维环裂隙**是椎间盘纤维环在T_2加权图像上的线性高信号。此影像学征象被认为是纤维环损伤，可能是引起疼痛的一个原因。
- **纤维环裂隙**较纤维环撕裂更确切，因为大多数情况下可能被认为是一个退变过程，而非损伤。

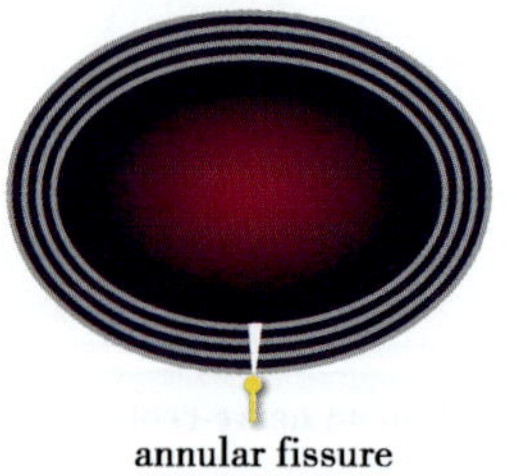

annular fissure
纤维环裂隙

Secondary vertebral body changes-Modic changes

- Degenerative changes in the spine are associated with vertebral body endplate and subchondral marrow signal changes that were described and classified by Modic.
- **Modic type 1** changes are edema: Hyperintense on T2-weighted and STIR images and hypointense on T1-weighted images. These changes may be associated with active back pain.
- **Modic type 2** changes are fatty metaplasia: Hyperintense on both T2- and T1-weighted images and hypointense on STIR. Modic 2 changes are less likely to be associated with active symptoms.
- **Modic type 3** changes are fibrosis: Hypointense on all sequences. Their clinical significance is unclear, but are chronic in timecourse.

继发性椎体改变-Modic改变

- Modic描述了脊柱退行性变与椎体终板及软骨下骨髓信号的相关变化，并对此进行了分类。
- **Modic改变1型**表现为水肿：T_2加权及STIR图像呈高信号、T_1加权图像呈低信号。这些改变可能与活动性背痛有关。
- **Modic改变2型**表现为脂肪化生：T_2加权和T_1加权图像均呈高信号，STIR图像呈低信号。Modic改变2型与活动性症状无明显关系。
- **Modic改变3型**表现为纤维化：所有序列均呈低信号。其临床意义尚不清楚，但是时间上是属于慢性。

POSTERIOR STRUCTURES: FACET JOINTS AND LIGAMENTUM FLAVUM

Facet arthropathy/facet hypertrophy

- The intervertebral facet joints are synovial joints that can undergo the same degenerative processes as larger synovial joints, including cartilage loss, osteophytosis, sclerosis, and subchondral cystic change.
- Degenerative changes of the facet joints (facet arthropathy) may contribute to neural foraminal narrowing and spinal stenosis due to mass effect from osteophytes and reactive ligamentum flavum thickening.
- Facet effusions are associated with spinal instability (motion on flexion-extension films).
- Reactive bone marrow changes or soft tissue edema can be seen in active/symptomatic facet arthropathy.
- A **synovial cyst** is a ganglion cyst associated with facet arthropathy.

Ligamentum flavum thickening/hypertrophy

- The ligamentum flavum lines the lamina at the posterior aspect of the spinal canal. Thickening of the ligamentum flavum can contribute to spinal canal stenosis.
- Ligamentum flavum thickening is rarely seen in isolation and is usually reactive to subjacent facet arthropathy.

后部结构：椎小关节和黄韧带

椎小关节病/椎小关节肥大

- 椎间小关节为滑膜关节，与大的滑膜关节一样可以发生退行性变化，包括软骨丢失、骨质增生、骨质硬化和软骨下囊变。
- 椎小关节病的退行性改变(椎小关节病)可促使神经孔变窄和椎管狭窄，其原因为骨赘的占位效应和反应性黄韧带增厚。
- 椎小关节积液与脊柱不稳相关(在屈伸位图像上有滑移)。
- 反应性骨髓改变或软组织水肿可见于活动性/症状性椎小关节病。
- **滑膜囊肿**是出现在椎小关节病的腱鞘囊肿。

黄韧带增厚/肥大

- 黄韧带内衬于椎管后部的椎板，黄韧带增厚可导致椎管狭窄。
- 黄韧带增厚很少独立存在，一般是椎小关节病的反应性改变。

DEGENERATIVE SPINE GRADING

Overview of grading of degenerative spine

- Reliable grading of degenerative spine is critically important to direct optimal treatment, to ensure reliable communication between practitioners of various specialties, and even for insurance reimbursement.
- To our knowledge, this information is not tested on board examinations, but we hope this classification scheme will be useful to you in your clinical work.
- This classification scheme has been developed with multidisciplinary input from orthopedic spine surgery, neurosurgery, physiatry, and radiology. It is a simplification and synthesis of several existing classification systems (please see references).
- Nerve roots may be impinged (compressed) within the spinal canal, the lateral recess, or the neural foramen. Therefore, each of these locations should be either described as normal or graded if abnormal.
- Additionally, facet arthropathy may be an active symptom generator and should be separately described

Spinal stenosis

- Clinically, spinal stenosis may be asymptomatic or may be a cause of radicular pain or neurogenic claudication.
- At a normal level distal to the level of the conus (typically below the L1–L2 level), the nerve roots should be freely distributed within the CSF. The traversing (also called the descending) nerve roots course inferiorly and laterally towards the lateral recesses on each side, prior to exiting the neural foramina. The anterior margin of the thecal sac should be either flat or convex. The posterior epidural fat should form a clean triangle (although this may be minuscule at L5–S1).
- The degree of spinal stenosis is best assessed on the axial T2-weighted sequence.

退行性脊柱分级

退行性脊柱概述

- 可靠的脊柱退行性变分级对指导最佳治疗、确保各专科医生间的可靠沟通，甚至保险公司报销都至关重要。
- 据我们所知，这部分内容不出现在专业执照考试中，但希望这个分级方案有助于临床工作。
- 该分级方案是在汇聚了来自骨科脊柱外科、神经外科、理疗科和放射科等多学科的意见后所制定的。它是对现有几个分类系统的简化和综合(请查阅参考资料)。
- 神经根可能在椎管内、侧隐窝或神经孔内受到摩擦(挤压)。因此，对这些结构的每一项都需要进行描述，包括正常与否和在异常时的分级。
- 此外，椎小关节病可能是活动性症状的始发点，应单独进行描述。

椎管狭窄

- 椎管狭窄在临床上可能无症状，也可能引起神经根痛或神经源性跛行。
- 在正常圆锥以下的水平(通常在$L_{1\sim2}$水平以下)，神经根应游离在脑脊液中。穿行(也称为下行)神经根在出神经孔前向下、向外向两侧侧隐窝走行。硬膜囊的前缘应平坦或凸出。后硬膜外脂肪应呈清晰的三角(即使$L_5\sim S_1$处很小)。
- 椎管狭窄的程度最好在轴位T_2加权图像上进行评估。

Spinal Stenosis			
Normal	**Mild Spinal Stenosis**	**Moderate Spinal Stenosis**	**Severe Spinal Stenosis**
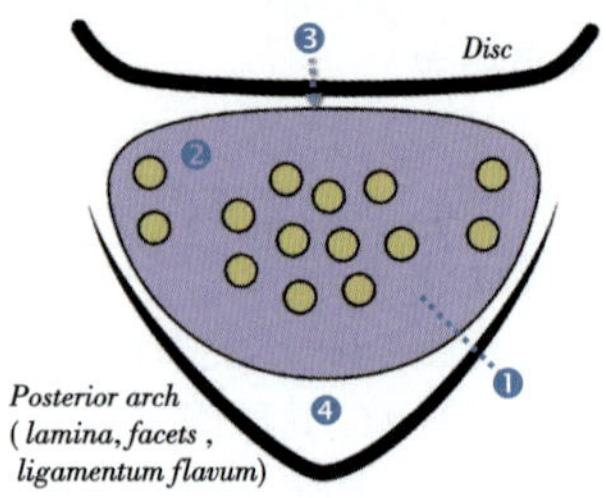	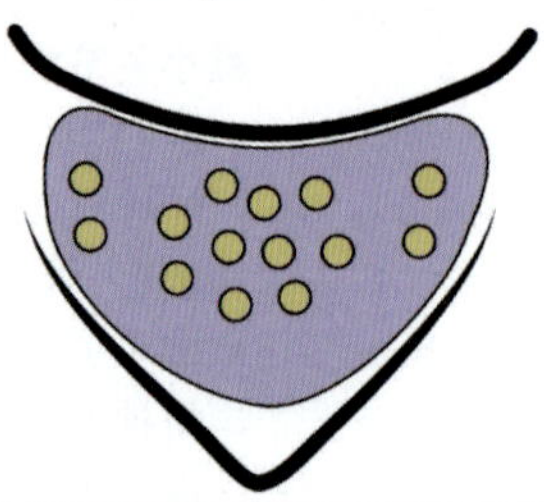	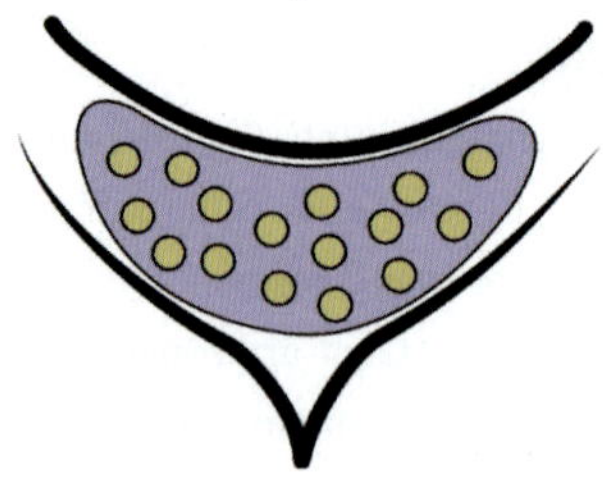	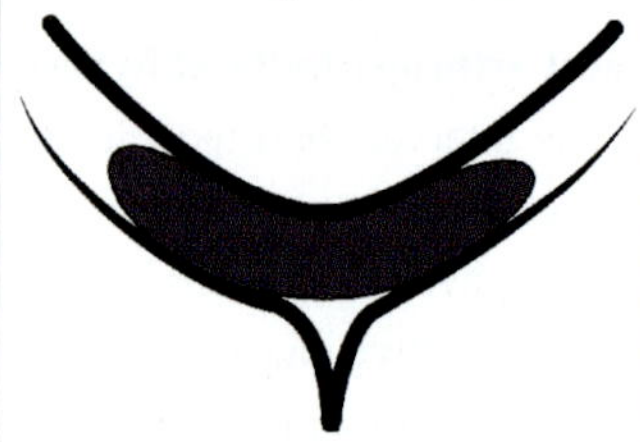
❶ • Free distribution of nerve roots, without crowding	• Slight crowding of nerve roots	• Crowding of nerve roots, resulting in a "speckled" appearance of CSF interspersed with nerve roots	• Complete effacement of CSF, resulting in nerve roots not being individually distinguishable
❷ • Traversing dorsal and ventral nerve roots in the lateral recesses are distinct	• Traversing dorsal and ventral nerve roots in the lateral recesses remain distinct, but there may be abutment of the nerve roots in the lateral recesses	• Difficult to differentiate the traversing nerve roots in the lateral recesses	• Cannot discretely identify nerve roots in the lateral recesses
❸ • Anterior margin of the thecal sac is flat or convex	• Anterior margin of the thecal sac is flat or concave	• Anterior margin of the thecal sac is concave	• Anterior margin of the thecal sac is concave
❹ • Posterior epidural fat is preserved (dependent on level)	• Posterior epidural fat is preserved (dependent on level)	• Posterior epidural fat is preserved (dependent on level)	• ***Posterior epidural fat may be partially or completely effaced***

椎管狭窄			
正常	**轻度椎管狭窄**	**中度椎管狭窄**	**重度椎管狭窄**
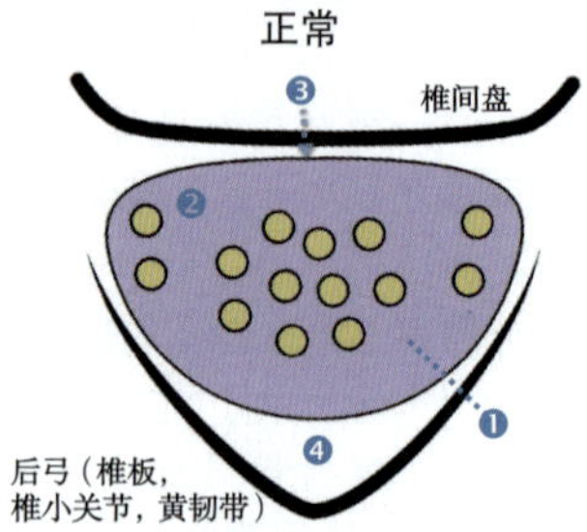	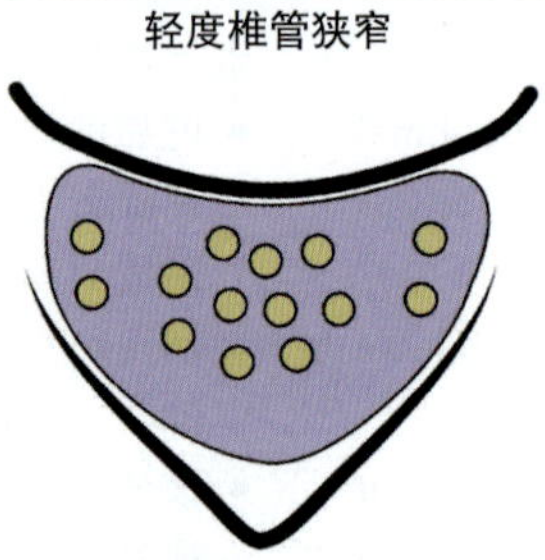	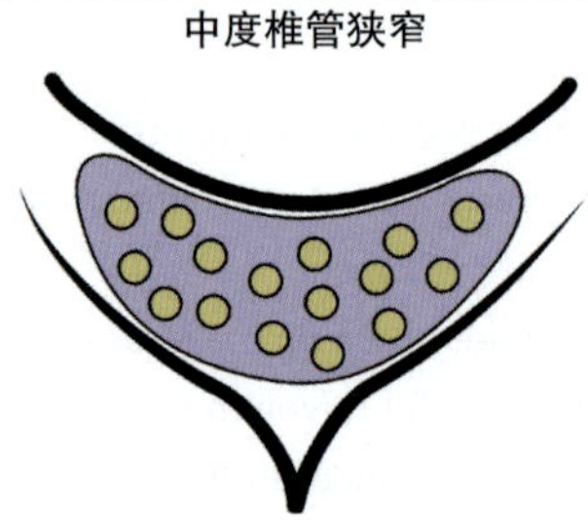	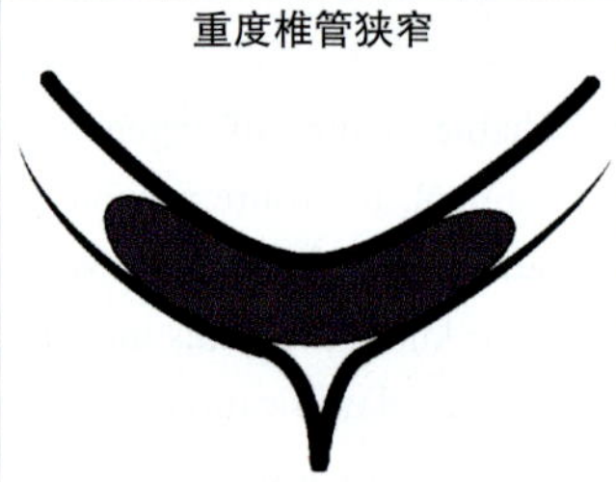
❶ • 神经根游离，无受压	• 神经根轻度挤压	• 神经根拥挤，导致脑脊液呈斑点状分布	• 脑脊液完全消失，以致神经根不能单独区分
❷ • 走行于侧隐窝的背侧和腹侧神经根分界清晰	• 走行于侧隐窝的背侧神经根和腹侧神经根仍然清晰可见，但神经根可能紧贴侧隐窝	• 很难分辨在侧隐窝穿行的神经根	• 在侧隐窝不能辨别神经根
❸ • 硬膜囊前缘平坦或凸出	• 硬膜囊前缘平坦或凹陷	• 硬膜囊的前缘凹陷	• 硬膜囊前缘凹陷
❹ • 后硬膜外脂肪存在(取决于节段)	• 后硬膜外脂肪存在	• 后方硬膜外脂肪存在(取决于节段)	• **后硬膜外脂肪部分或完全消失**

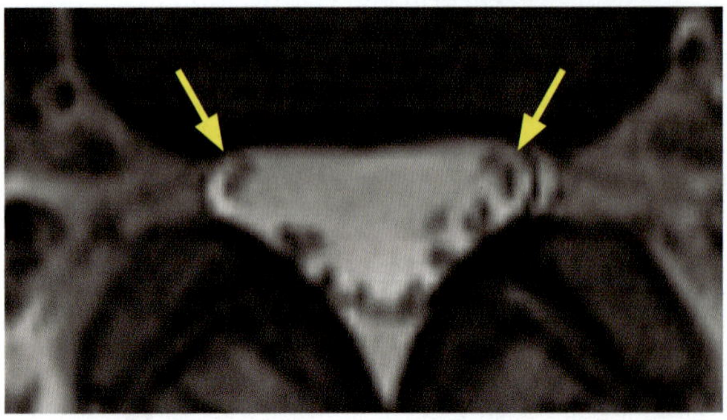

Normal (no spinal stenosis): Anterior margin of the thecal sac is flat. Nerve roots are freely distributed; the traversing nerve roots (yellow arrows) course normally in the lateral recesses without mass effect.
正常(无椎管狭窄)：硬膜囊前缘平坦。神经根游离；神经根(黄箭)正常穿行于侧隐窝而无受压表现。

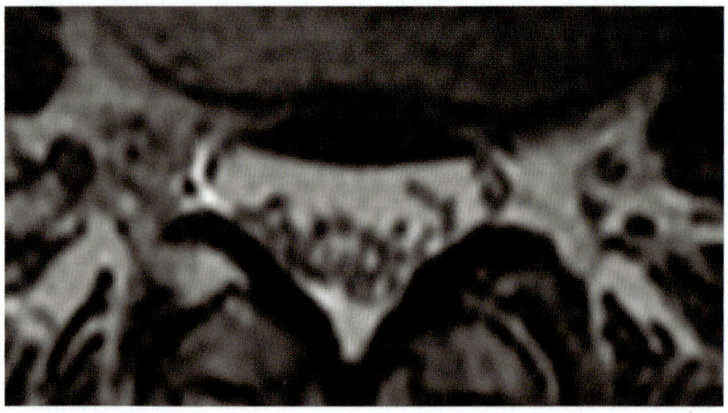

Mild spinal stenosis: There is concave anterior margin of the thecal sac due to a disc bulge. Minimal crowding of nerve roots posteriorly.
轻度椎管狭窄：由于椎间盘膨出，硬膜囊前缘凹陷，后方神经根轻微拥挤。

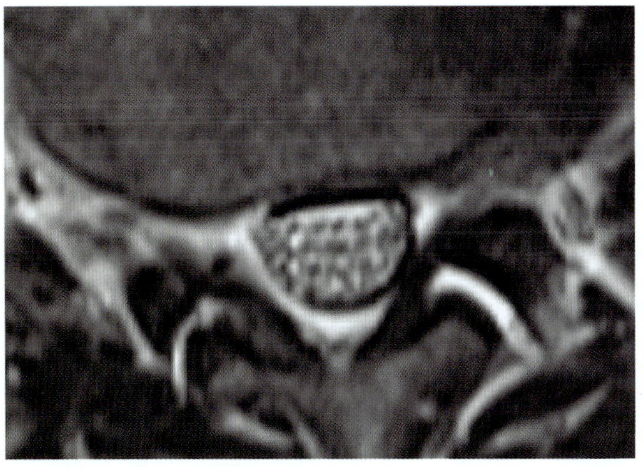

Moderate spinal stenosis: There is diffuse crowding of nerve roots, resulting in a "speckled" appearance of nerve roots and CSF.
中度椎管狭窄：神经根呈弥漫性拥挤，导致神经根和脑脊液呈"斑点状"外观。

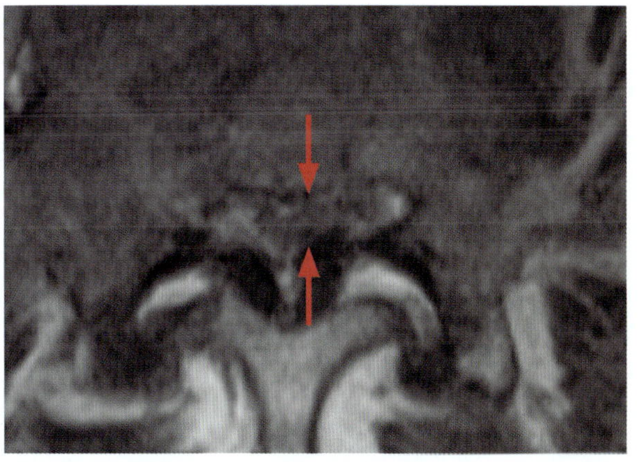

Severe spinal stenosis: There is compression of the thecal sac (red arrows) and complete effacement of CSF. Nerve roots are not individually distinguishable.
重度椎管狭窄：硬膜囊受压(红箭)，脑脊液消失。无法辨别每条神经根。

Normal and varying degrees of spinal stenosis in 4 different patients. All images are axial T2-weighted MR.
正常和不同程度椎管狭窄在4名不同患者中的表现。所有图像均为轴位T_2加权MR。

Neural foraminal stenosis

椎间孔狭窄

Neural Foraminal Stenosis		
Mild Neural Foraminal Stenosis	**Moderate Stenosis**	**Severe Stenosis**
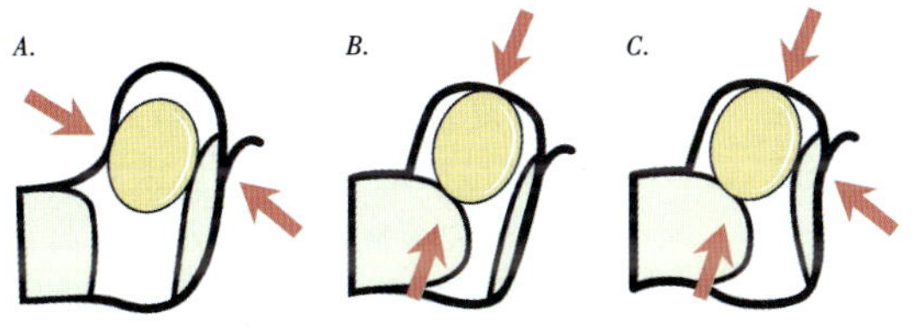	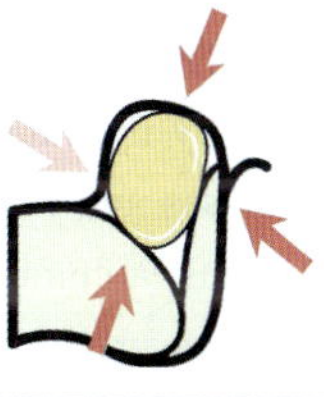	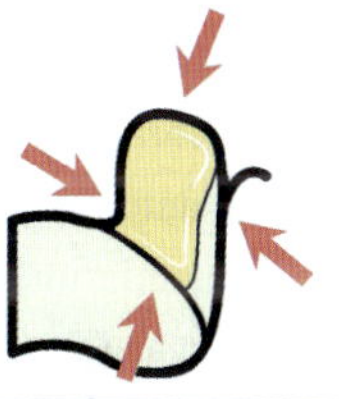
• Nerve root is in contact the walls of the neural foramen in two planes, either in anterior-posterior dimension (A) or cranial-caudal dimension (B); or in 3 planes (C) • Aside from mild narrowing of the foramen and contact with the exiting nerve root, the epidural fat is otherwise maintained	• Contact with the nerve root on at least three sides, and: • Partial effacement of epidural fat throughout the foramen.	• Complete effacement of epidural fat or compression of the nerve root

椎间孔狭窄		
轻度椎间孔狭窄	**中度狭窄**	**重度狭窄**
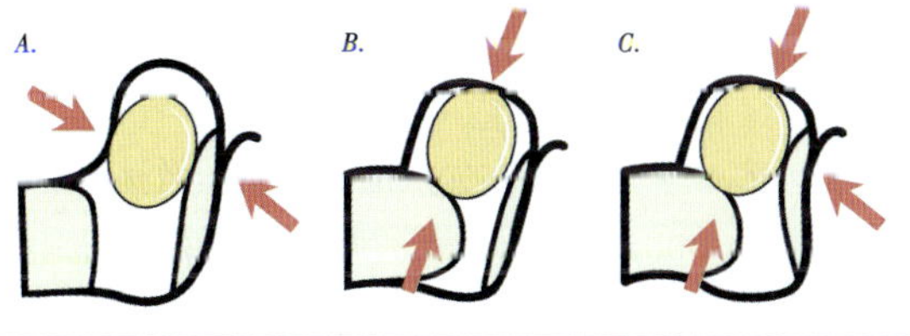	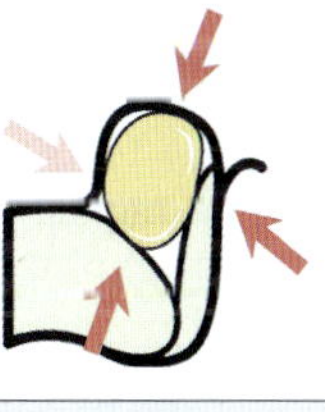	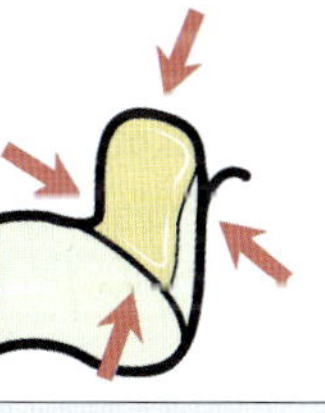
• 神经根与椎间孔两个面接触：不是前后面(A)，就是头尾面(B)；或在三个面(C)接触 • 除椎间孔轻度狭窄、穿出神经根有接触外，硬膜外脂肪仍存在	• 神经根至少与三个面接触 • 椎间孔内部分硬膜外脂肪消失	• 硬膜外脂肪完全消失，或神经根受压

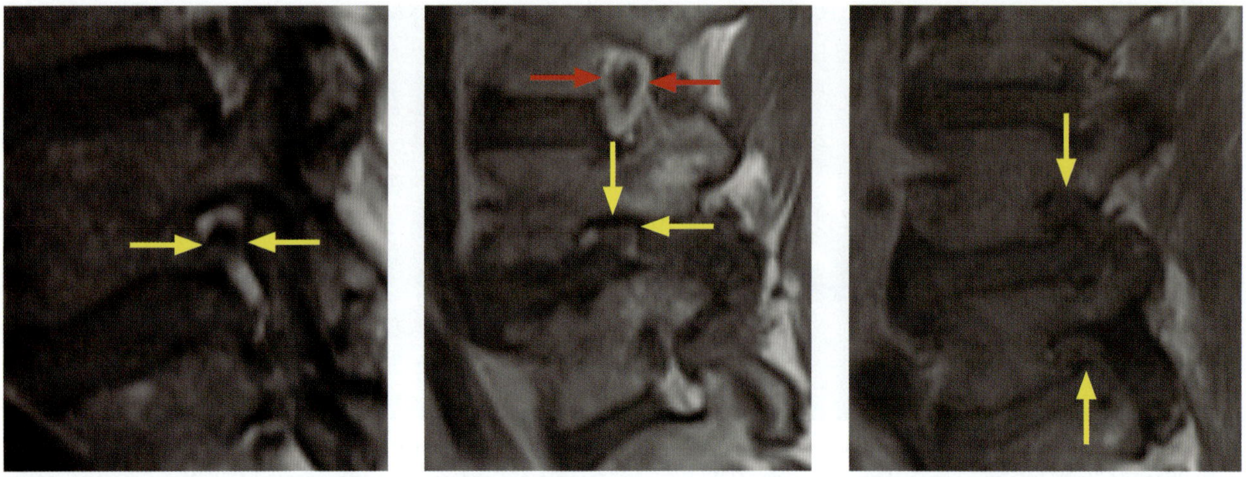

Mild foraminal stenosis: There is contact of the exiting nerve root on two sides (yellow arrows).
轻度椎间孔狭窄：穿出神经根与两个面接触(黄箭)。

Moderate foraminal stenosis: There is contact of the exiting nerve root on three sides (yellow arrows) with partial effacement of epidural fat. Note the normal neural foramen at the level above (red arrows).
中度椎间孔狭窄：穿出神经根与三个面接触，部分硬膜外脂肪消失(黄箭)。注意在此水平上方的正常椎间孔(红箭)。

Severe foraminal stenosis: Complete effacement of epidural fat (at two different levels; yellow arrows).
重度椎间孔狭窄：硬膜外脂肪完全消失(两个不同水平，黄箭)。

Varying degrees of neural foraminal stenosis in three different patients on sagittal T1-weighted MR.
不同程度的神经孔狭窄在3名不同患者的矢状位T_1加权MR。

- The neural foramina are paired openings at each intervertebral spinal level through which the spinal nerve roots pass. They are located at the lateral aspects of the vertebral canal, and are bounded by the intervertebral disc-endplate complexes anteriorly, the articular processes and facet joints posteriorly, and the pedicles inferiorly and superiorly. Thus, a combination of discovertebral degeneration and facet arthropathy (and the overlying ligamentum flavum) may contribute to neural foraminal stenosis.
- Normally, the exiting nerve should be completely surrounded by epidural fat with a keyhole morphology. Note that if there is simply some effacement of epidural fat at the inferior margin of the keyhole but the nerve remains surrounded by epidural that is still normal.
- Mild neural foraminal stenosis is contact of the nerve root on two or three sides with otherwise preserved epidural fat and no neural compression.
- Moderate neural foraminal stenosis is contact of the nerve root by three or four sides with partial effacement of epidural fat.
- Severe neural foraminal stenosis is complete effacement of epidural fat or compression of the nerve root.
- The neural foramina are best assessed on the sagittal T1-weighted images.

- 椎间孔成对开口于每节椎间水平，供脊神经根通过。它们位于椎管的外侧，并以椎间盘-终板复合体为前界，关节突和椎小关节为后界，椎弓根则为上下界。因此，椎间盘退变合并椎小关节病(及其上方覆盖黄韧带)可导致椎间孔狭窄。
- 正常情况下，穿出的神经根应完全被硬膜外脂肪包绕，呈“锁芯状”。注意，若锁芯仅下缘的硬膜外脂肪消失，但神经根仍被硬膜外脂肪包绕仍然属于正常。
- 轻度椎间孔狭窄是指神经根两个或三个面与椎间孔接触，且硬膜外脂肪存在，无神经根压迫。
- 中度椎间孔狭窄是神经根的三个或四个面与椎间孔接触，伴部分硬膜外脂肪消失。
- 重度椎间孔狭窄是硬膜外脂肪完全消失或神经根受压。
- 椎间孔在矢状位T_1加权图像显示最佳。

Lateral Recess Stenosis		
Normal	Abutment of traversing nerve root(s)	Compression of traversing nerve root(s)
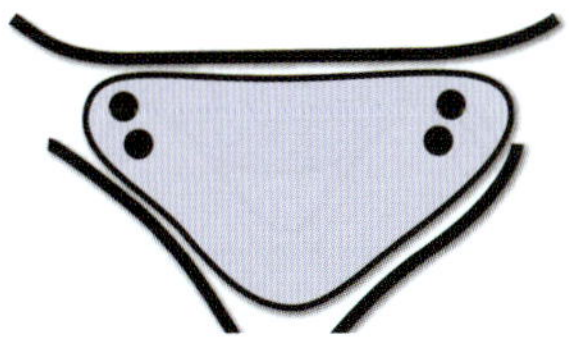	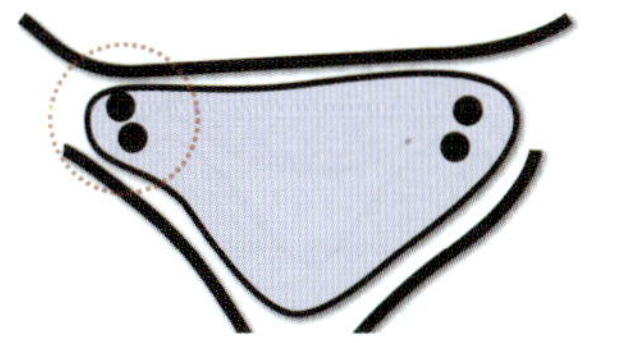	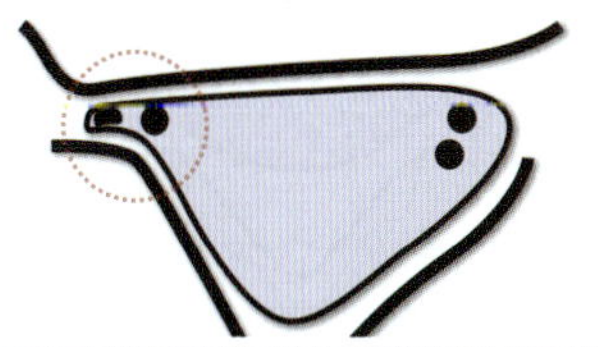
• No contact, crowding, or mass effect upon the traversing nerve roots	• Contact of one or both of the traversing nerve roots in the lateral recess, but nerve roots are not compressed	• Compression of one or both of the traversing nerve roots in the lateral recess

侧隐窝狭窄		
正常	紧邻神经根	神经根受压
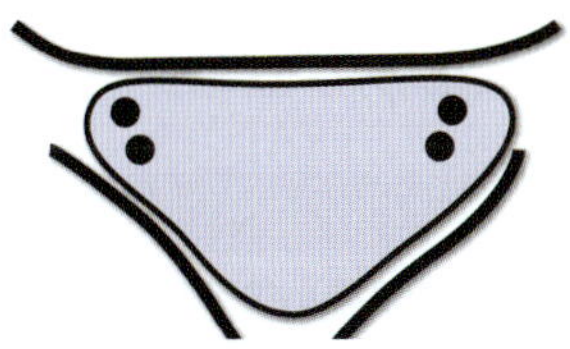	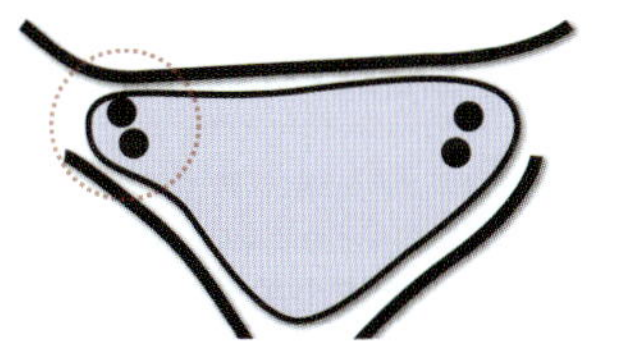	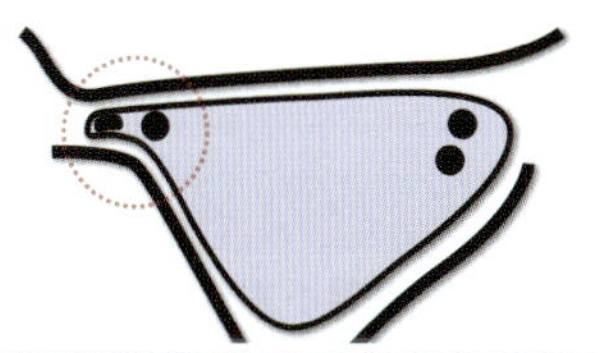
• 穿行神经根没有接触、挤压或占位效应	• 侧隐窝内的一条或两条神经根接触，但神经根未受压	• 侧隐窝的一条或两条神经根受压

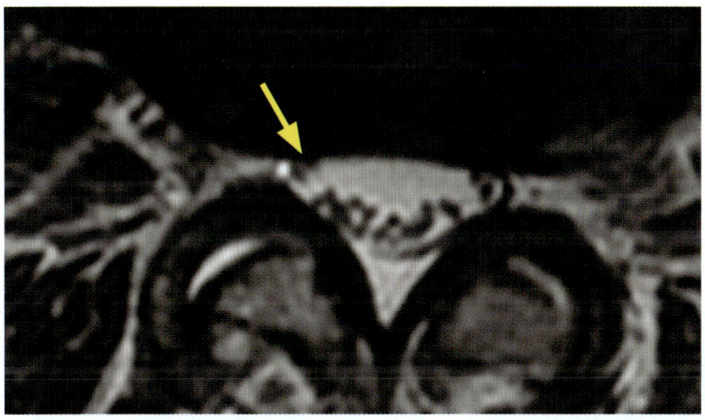

Abutment of the traversing nerve roots in the lateral recess: A disc bulge contacts the traversing nerve roots in the lateral recesses, more prominent on the right (yellow arrow).
紧邻侧隐窝内的神经根：椎间盘膨出接触到侧隐窝内穿行的神经根，右侧更明显(黄箭)。

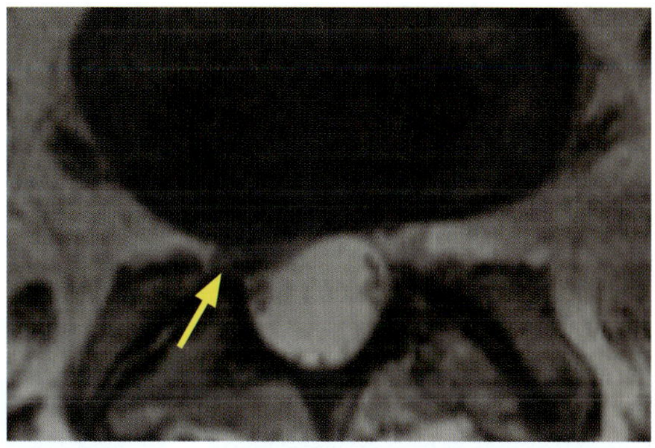

Compression of the nerve roots in the lateral recess: A right subarticular/foraminal disc protrusion effaces the right lateral recess and compresses the traversing nerve root (yellow arrow) at the junction of the lateral recess and neural foramen.
The left lateral recess is normal.
侧隐窝内神经根**受压**：在右侧侧隐窝和神经孔的交界处，关节下/椎间孔型椎间盘突出使右侧侧隐窝消失，压迫穿行的神经根(黄箭)。左侧侧隐窝正常。

Varying degrees of lateral recess stenosis in two patients, assessed on axial T2-weighted images.
2名患者不同程度的侧隐窝狭窄在轴位T_2加权图像的表现。

- The lateral recess is the lateral portion of the thecal sac where the traversing nerve roots course just before entering the neural foramina. It is an often neglected site in radiologists' dictations but it is an important potential site of nerve root compression.
- Rather than grading as mild, moderate, and severe, we propose simply describing if there is abutment (synonymous with contact) or compression of the traversing nerve root.
- The lateral recess is best assessed on axial T2-weighted images.

- 侧隐窝位于硬膜囊的外侧部分，穿行神经根进入椎间孔之前在此处走行。侧隐窝在放射医师报告时常被忽视，但它是神经根受压的一个重要潜在部位。
- 建议对是否存在穿行神经根紧邻(与接触为同义语)或受压进行简单描述，而不对其进行分级，如轻度、中度和重度。
- 侧隐窝在轴位T_2加权图像上显示最佳。

Facet Arthropathy		
Mild Facet Arthropathy 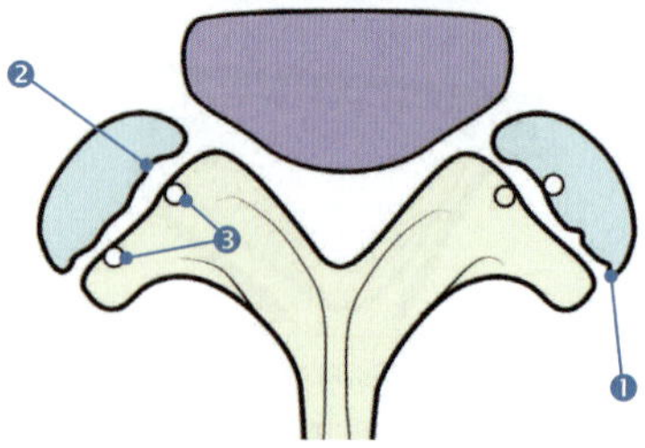	Moderate Facet Arthropathy 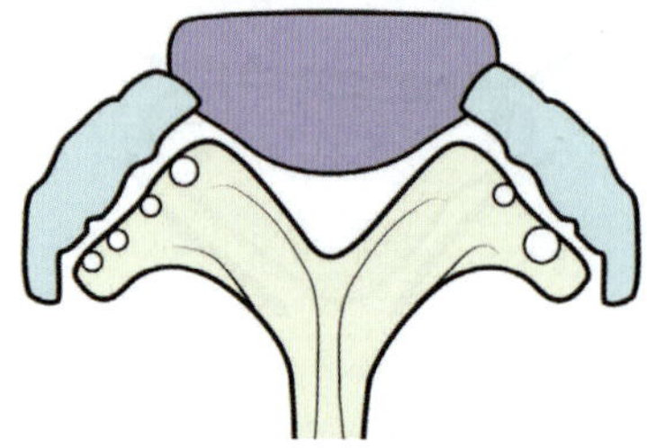	Severe Facet Arthropathy 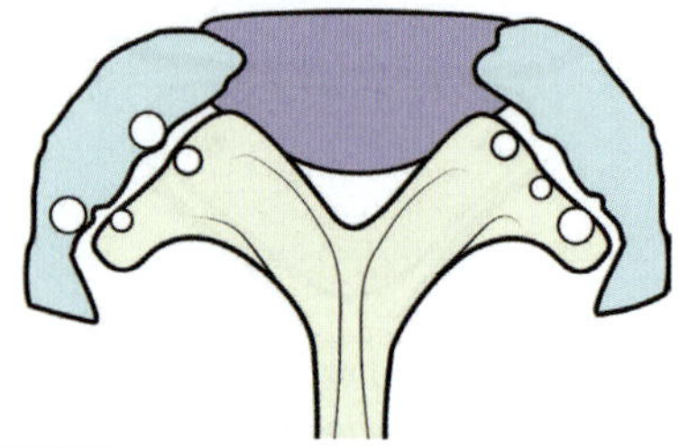
❶ • Minimal to small osteophytes	• Moderate-size osteophytes	• Bulky osteophytes with dorsal mass effect on the thecal sac
❷ • Mild subchondral irregularity	• Moderate subchondral irregularity	• Marked subchondral irregularity
❸ • Tiny to small subchondral cysts	• Moderate size subchondral cysts or synovial cysts	• Large subchondral cysts or synovial cysts
	• ***Effusion, periarticular edema or osseous edema***	• ***Effusion, periarticular edema or osseous edema***

椎小关节病		
轻度椎小关节病 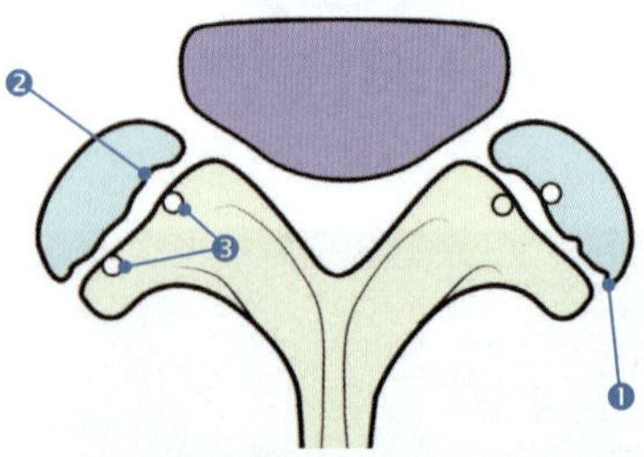	中度椎小关节病 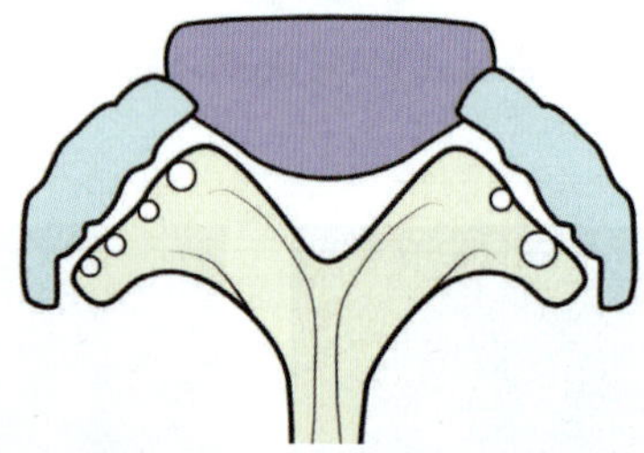	重度椎小关节病 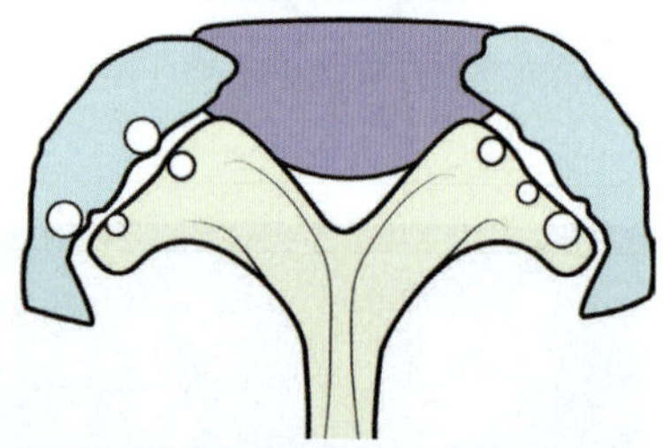
❶ • 很小~小的骨赘	• 中等大小骨赘	• 大块骨赘对硬膜囊背侧产生占位效应
❷ • 轻度软骨下不规则	• 中度软骨下不规则	• 显著软骨下不规则
❸ • 微小~小的软骨下囊肿	• 中度软骨下囊肿或滑膜囊肿	• 大的软骨下囊肿或滑膜囊肿
	• **积液、关节周围水肿或骨性水肿**	• **积液、关节周围水肿或骨性水肿**

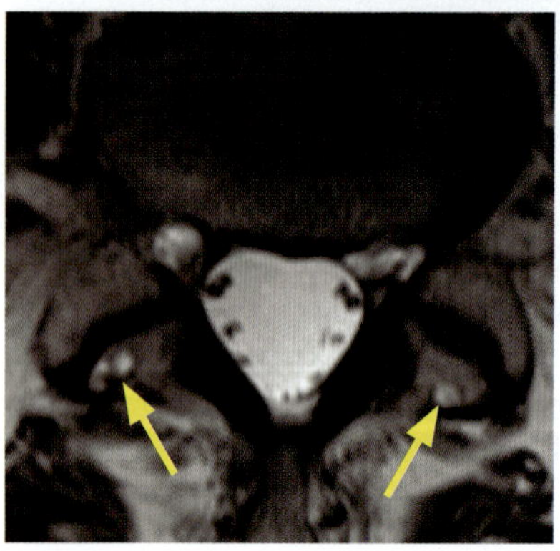

Mild facet arthropathy: There is mild subchondral irregularity of the facets with tiny subchondral cysts (arrows).
轻度椎小关节病：轻度软骨下不规则，伴有软骨下微小囊肿(箭)。

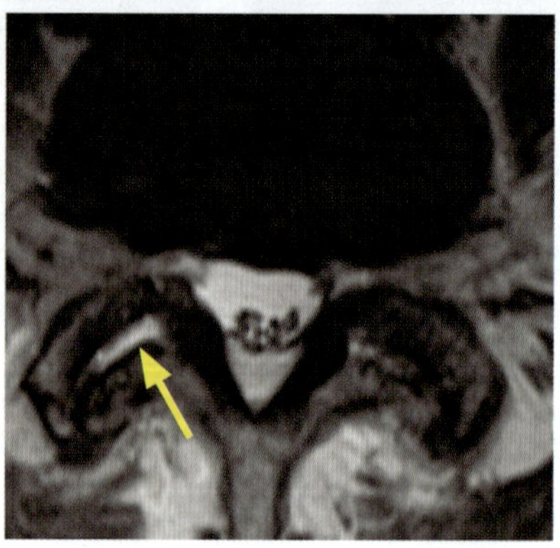

Moderate facet arthopathy: There is moderate subchondral irregularity and hypertrophic change, although the osteophytes don't produce substantial mass effect. Small right facet effusion (arrow).
中度椎小关节病：中度软骨下不规则和骨质肥厚，但骨赘没有产生明确的占位效应。右侧椎小关节积液(箭)。

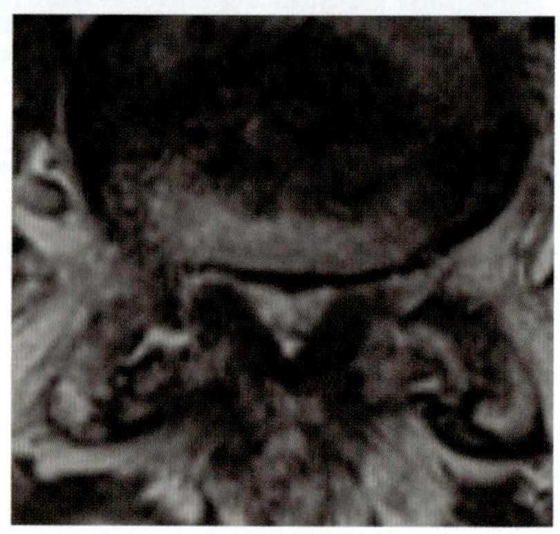

Severe facet arthropathy: There is marked subchondral irregularity, small right effusion, and large osteophytes with mass effect upon the spinal canal.
重度椎小关节病：重度软骨下不规则，右侧少量积液，大块骨赘对椎管产生占位效应。

Varying degrees of facet arthropathy in three different patients on axial T2-weighted MR.
不同严重程度的椎小关节病变在3名患者轴位T_2加权MR上的表现。

- Facet arthropathy is important to identify and accurately grade, as the facet joints can contribute to spinal, foraminal, or lateral recess stenosis.
- As previously discussed, facet effusions are associated with spinal instability and if a decompression is performed in the setting of instability, an instrumented fusion is typically the optimal treatment.
- Secondary signs of active facet arthropathy include effusion, reactive osseous edema (typically extending into the pedicles), and reactive soft tissue edema.
- Active facet arthropathy can be treated by interventional pain procedures including intra-articular steroid injection, median branch block, and radiofrequency ablation.

- 对椎小关节病变进行识别和准确分级十分重要，因为椎小关节病变可造成脊柱、椎间孔或侧隐窝狭窄。
- 如前所述，椎小关节积液与脊柱不稳定相关，如果对不稳定脊柱进行减压，固定融合术通常是最佳治疗方式。
- 活动性椎小关节病的继发性征象包括积液、反应性骨水肿(通常延伸到椎弓根)，以及反应性软组织水肿。
- 活动性椎小关节病可通过疼痛介入进行治疗，包括关节内类固醇注射、正中分支阻滞和射频消融。

（翻译　卞益同）

SPINE INFECTION

脊柱感染

Overview of spine infection and relevant anatomy

脊柱感染及相关解剖概述

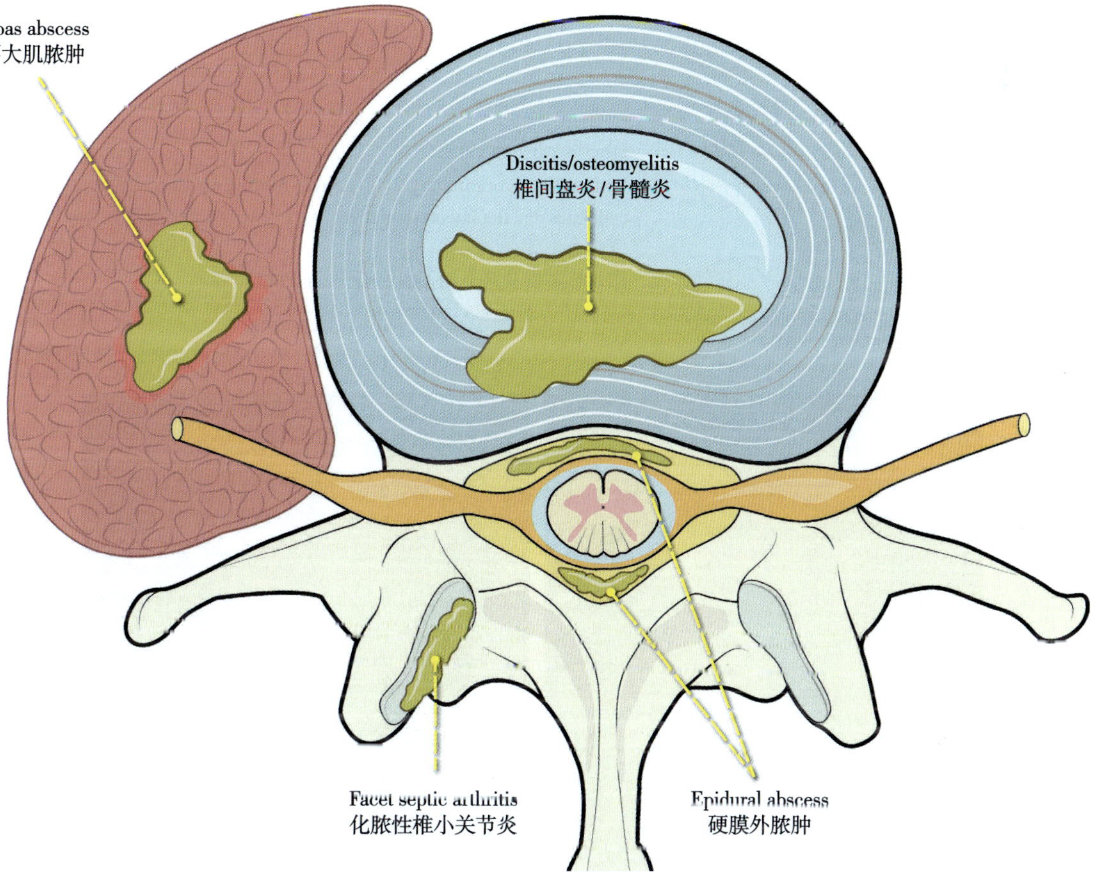

- Spine infection can be a confusing topic, as there are different etiologies, myriad imaging manifestations, and confounding differential diagnoses. Patients with diabetes, drug abuse, or prior spinal surgery are at increased risk of spine infection.
- It can be helpful to think of spine infection in terms of "compartments" (illustrated above) including the retroperitoneum/psoas, discs and vertebral bodies, epidural space, and facet joints. Infection may originate in any of these compartments and spread to adjacent compartments.

- 脊柱感染是一个复杂的专题，其病因各异、影像表现多样、鉴别诊断复杂。既往有糖尿病、吸毒或脊柱手术史的患者其脊柱感染的风险增加。
- 对于脊柱感染，如果从"分区"(如上所示)的角度考虑会有所帮助，其中的分区包括腹膜后/腰大肌、椎间盘和椎体、硬膜外间隙和椎小关节等。感染可能起源于这些分区中的任何一个，并弥散到相邻的区域。

Discitis/osteomyelitis

- Discitis/osteomyelitis is infection of the disc-endplate complex. Hematogeneous spread is the most common etiology.
- In adults, the disc is not vascularized, but the endplates are supplied by end-capillary branches of the segmental lumbar arteries, as illustrated to the right. A single artery supplies two segmental endplates, although usually only one endplate is infected first.

椎间盘炎/骨髓炎

- 椎间盘炎/骨髓炎是椎间盘-终板复合体受到感染，血行播散是最常见的原因。
- 成人椎间盘无血供，而终板供血来自腰椎动脉分支的毛细血管末端，如下图所示。一支动脉供应两个节段的终板，通常只有一个终板首先被感染。

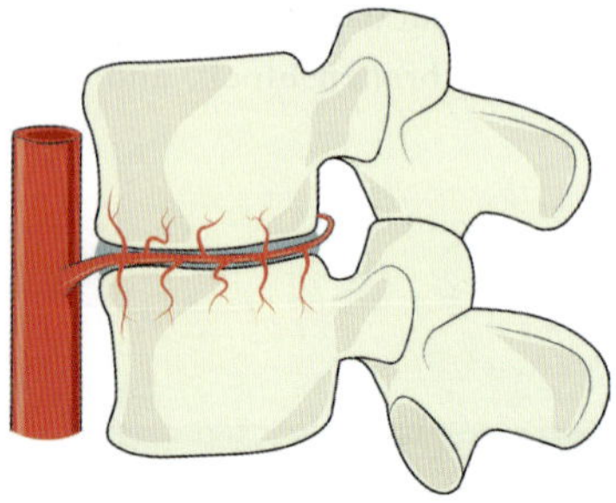

- Hematogeneous infection in adults starts in the endplate, and can spread to the adjacent vertebral body through the disc.
- In contrast, in children, the disc is directly vascularized and can act as the nidus for infection.

- 成人的血行感染从终板开始，并通过椎间盘蔓延至邻近椎体。
- 相反，儿童椎间盘有直接血供，并可成为感染的源头。

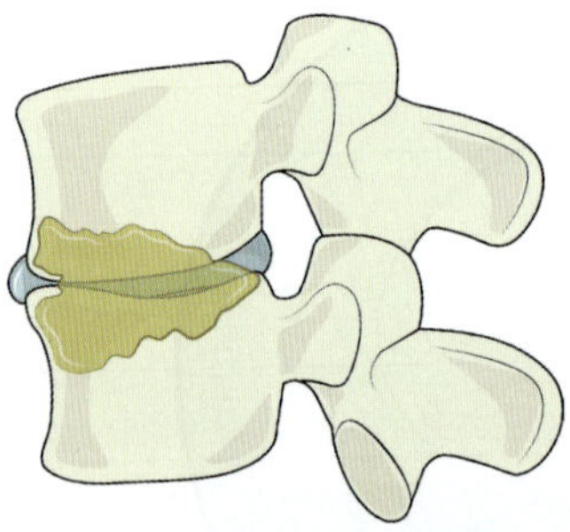

Discitis/osteomyelitis:
Illustration demonstrates infection involving two adjacent endplates and the intervening disc.
椎间盘炎/骨髓炎：
图示感染累及两个相邻的终板和其间的椎间盘。

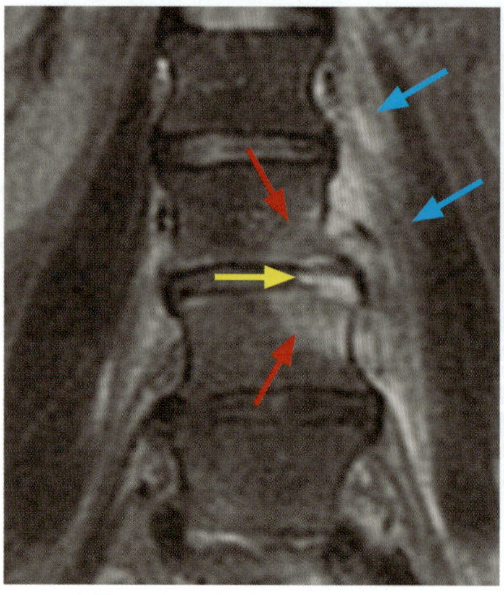

Coronal post-contrast T1-weighted MRI with fat suppression.
冠状位增强T_1加权脂肪抑制MRI

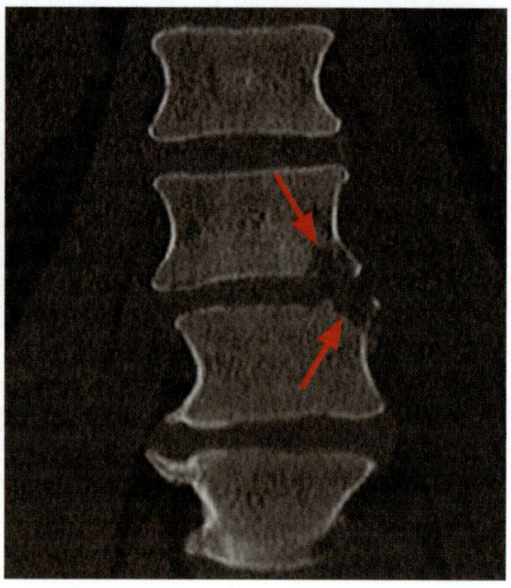

Coronal CT
冠状位CT

Discitis/osteomyelitis: MRI demonstrates enhancement at the left aspect of the L3–L4 disc (yellow arrow). There is enhancing osteitis of the adjacent endplates (red arrows), and prominent inflammatory change involving the left psoas (blue arrows). CT shows osseous erosion of the endplates (red arrows).
椎间盘炎/骨髓炎：MRI显示L_{3-4}椎间盘左侧强化(黄箭)。相邻终板可见强化性骨炎(红箭)，左侧腰大肌可见明显的炎症改变(蓝箭)。CT显示终板骨质侵蚀(红箭)。

- MR is the optimal imaging modality for suspected discitis/osteomyelitis.
- The most sensitive MR imaging sign to detect spinal infection is paraspinal or epidural inflammatory change.
- Other imaging findings include erosion or destruction of the vertebral endplates, disc enhancement, fluid signal and/or enhancement of the disc, and edema evident across the disc space (although this last finding is nonspecific in the absence of other signs/symptoms or imaging findings of infection). In advanced cases there may be frank osseous destruction.

- MR是疑似椎间盘炎/骨髓炎的最佳成像方式。
- 发现脊柱感染最敏感的MR征象是椎旁或硬膜外炎症性改变。
- 其他影像学表现包括椎体终板的侵蚀或破坏、椎间盘强化、椎间盘液体信号和/或椎间盘强化，以及水肿波及整个椎间盘区域(在没有其他体征/症状或影像学表现的情况下，最后一个征象是非特异性的)。进展期可能会出现明显的骨质破坏。

Epidural infection

硬膜外感染

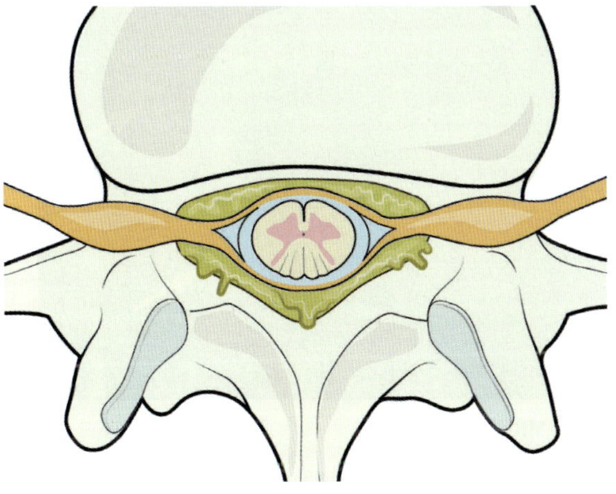

Epidural infection:
Illustration demonstrates infection of the epidural space. In this illustration, the infection is seen circumferentially surrounding the dura.
硬膜外感染：
图示硬膜外间隙感染；图中可见感染围绕硬膜四周。

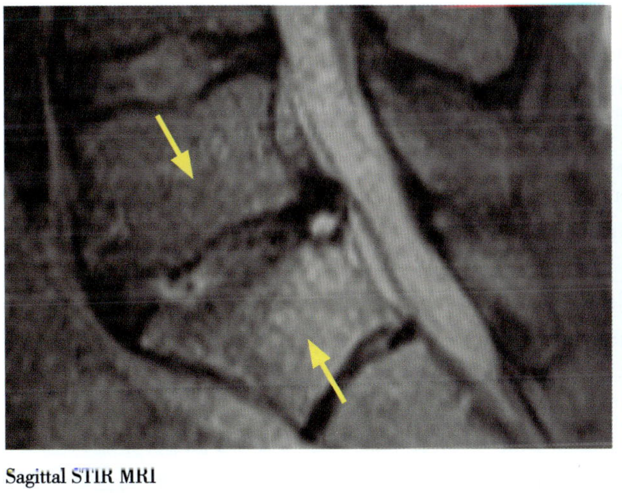

Sagittal STIR MRI
矢状位STIR MRI

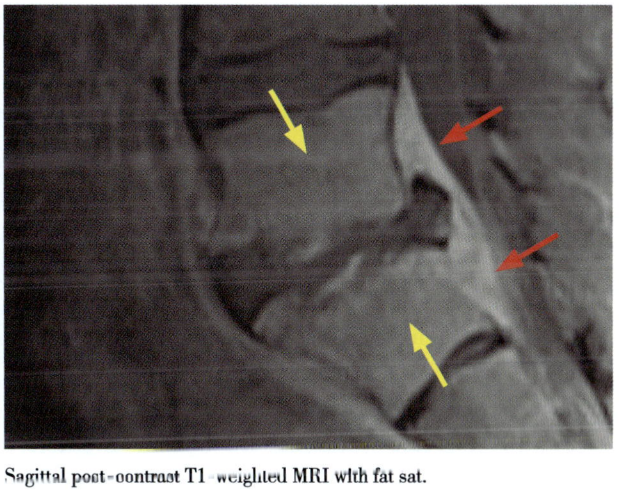

Sagittal post-contrast T1-weighted MRI with fat sat.
矢状位增强T_1加权脂肪抑制MRI

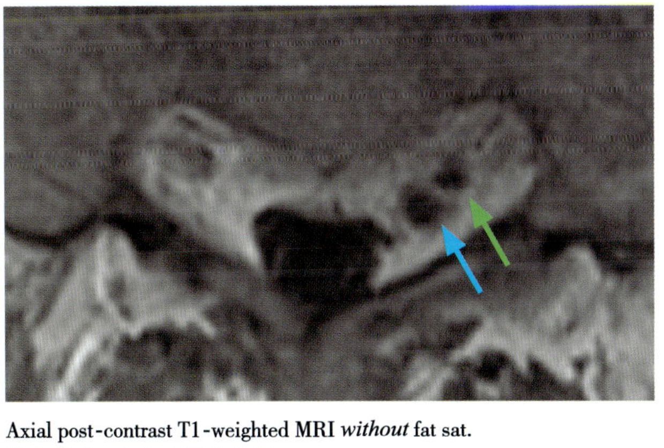

Axial post-contrast T1-weighted MRI *without* fat sat.
轴位增强T_1加权非脂肪抑制MRI

Epidural phlegmon, epidural abscess, and discitis/osteomyelitis.
There is edema and enhancing osteitis across L5–S1 (yellow arrows). Note the marked subchondral irregularity of the L5–S1 endplates best appreciated on the sagittal T1-weighted image. There is prominent anterior epidural enhancement seen on the sagittal image (red arrows). The axial T1-weighted MRI without fat suppression shows a subtle non-enhancing abscess (blue arrow) just posterior/medial to the left S1 nerve root (green arrow).
硬膜外蜂窝织炎、硬膜外脓肿及椎间盘炎/骨髓炎：
水肿和强化骨炎波及L_5~S_1(黄箭)。注意，L_5~S_1终板有明显的软骨下形态不规则，在矢状位T_1加权图像显示最佳。矢状位图像可见明显的前硬膜外间隙强化(红箭)。轴位非脂肪抑制T_1加权MRI显示左侧S_1神经根(绿箭)的后/内侧小的无强化脓肿(蓝箭)。

- Infection in the epidural space may be caused by phlegmon or abscess. An abscess is centrally necrotic, although either may exert mass effect upon the nerve roots or spinal cord.
- Given that normal epidural fat is hyperintense on T1-weighted images, fat suppression is an extremely helpful technique to detect early epidural infection.

Facet septic arthritis

- 硬膜外感染可来自蜂窝织炎或脓肿。脓肿的中央是坏死，但也可能对神经根或脊髓产生压迫。
- 正常硬膜外脂肪在T_1加权图像上呈高信号，故脂肪抑制是一种检测早期硬膜外感染非常有用的技术。

化脓性椎小关节炎

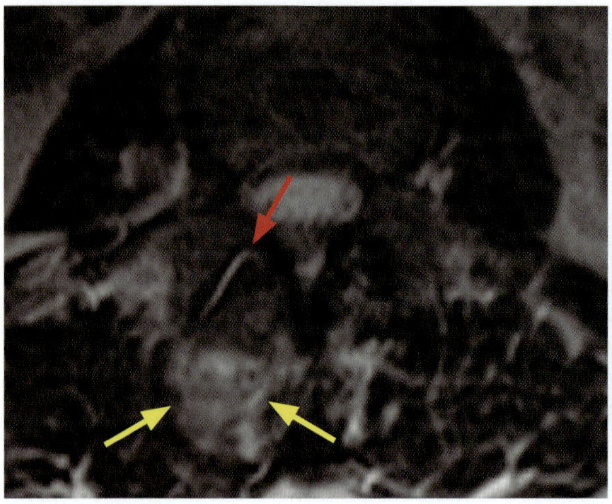

Axial T2-weighted MRI
轴位T_2加权MRI

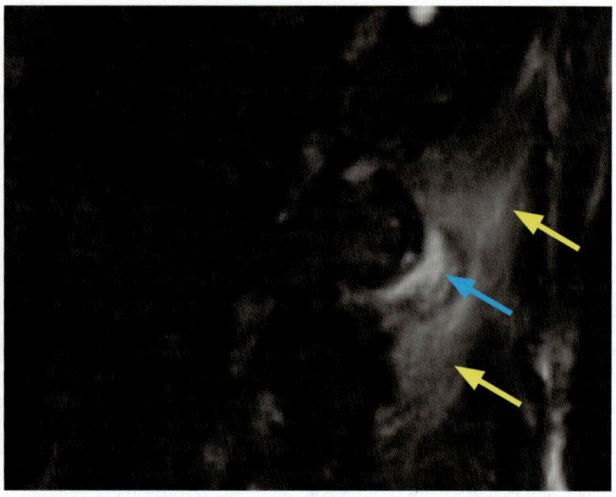

Sagittal STIR MRI
矢状位STIR MRI

Facet septic arthritis: There is prominent edema posterior to the right facet joint (yellow arrows), which is far more conspicuous on the STIR image, as both fat and fluid are similar signal intensity on T2-weighted imaging without fat suppression. Although there is no apparent effusion within the facet joint (red arrow), there is dorsal distension of the capsule evident on the sagittal image (blue arrow).
化脓性椎小关节炎：右侧椎小关节后方明显水肿(黄箭)，在STIR序列上更为明显，因为脂肪和液体在非脂肪抑制的T_2加权图像上信号相似。尽管椎小关节内没有明显的积液(红箭)，但在矢状位上可见关节囊背侧明显凸起(蓝箭)。

- Facet septic arthritis is uncommon, but should be considered when the degree of periarticular inflammatory change is out of proportion to a relatively milder degree of degeneration.
- Far more common is active facet arthropathy, which typically demonstrates characteristic imaging features of osteoarthritis including subchondral irregularity, cystic change, and osteophytes.

Tuberculous osteomyelitis

- Also called **Pott disease**, tuberculous osteomyelitis is vertebral infection with *Mycobacterium tuberculosis*. Unlike pyogenic discitis/osteomyelitis, the discs are usually spared as *M. tuberculosis* lacks the proteolytic enzymes to break down the disc substance.
- Pott disease classically causes wedge-shaped compression of the anterior aspect of the vertebral body, often leading to a gibbus deformity centered at the infected vertebra.

  Gibbus deformity is an acutely angled kyphosis, which may result from a compression fracture or can be seen in congenital syndromes including achondroplasia and the mucopolysaccharidoses (Hunter and Hurler syndromes).
- Approximately 10% of patients with Pott disease have active pulmonary tuberculosis.

- 化脓性椎小关节炎不常见，但当关节周围的炎症程度与相对较轻的退变不成比例时，应予以考虑。
- 活动性椎小关节病更为常见，通常具有骨关节炎的特征性影像学表现，包括软骨下不规则、囊变和骨质增生。

结核性骨髓炎

- 结核性骨髓炎亦称**Pott病**，是椎体感染结核分枝杆菌所致。与化脓性椎间盘炎/骨髓炎不同，椎间盘通常不受累，因为结核分枝杆菌缺乏分解破坏椎间盘的蛋白水解酶。
- 典型的Pott病引起椎体前缘呈楔形压缩，常导致以感染椎体为中心的驼背。

  Gibbus畸形(驼背)是脊柱呈严重的锐角后凸畸形，可由压缩性骨折或先天性综合征所致，包括软骨发育不全和黏多糖贮积症(Hunter和Hurler综合征)。
- 约10%的Pott病患者有活动性肺结核。

(翻译　卞益同)

MISCELLANEOUS SPINAL DISORDERS

其他脊柱疾病

EXTRADURAL SPINAL METABOLIC LESIONS

硬膜外脊柱代谢性病变

Epidural lipomatosis

- Spinal epidural lipomatosis is a nonneoplastic overgrowth of unencapsulated fat in the epidural space, which may cause compression of neural elements. In severe cases, epidural lipomatosis may cause cauda equina syndrome.
- The most common cause of epidural lipomatosis is steroid administration. Other causes include obesity and endogenous Cushing syndrome; some cases are idiopathic.
- MRI shows expansion of the epidural space that follows fat signal on all sequences. While some epidural fat is normal, more than 6 mm in thickness in the mid thoracic level suggests epidural lipomatosis.
- Epidural lipomatosis involves multiple vertebral levels and is typically seen posteriorly in the thoracic spine (anterior displacing the thecal sac) and circumferentially in the lumbar spine (creating a trefoil or Y-shaped contour of the thecal sac).

硬膜外脂肪增多症

- 脊髓硬膜外脂肪增多症是一种硬膜外非肿瘤性无包膜脂肪过度生长，并可能会导致神经受压。在严重的病例，硬膜外脂肪增多症可导致马尾神经综合征。
- 硬膜外脂肪增多症最常见的原因是使用类固醇。其他原因包括肥胖和内源性库欣综合征；有些病例为特发性。
- MRI显示硬膜外间隙扩张，其信号在所有序列与脂肪信号相同。硬膜外存在少量脂肪为正常，但在中段胸椎厚度超过6mm则提示硬膜外脂肪增多症。
- 硬膜外脂肪增多症累及多个椎体水平，通常见于胸髓的后方(硬膜囊前移)和腰髓的四周(形成一个三叶形或Y形轮廓的硬膜囊)。

OSSIFICATION OF SPINAL LIGAMENTS

脊柱韧带骨化

- Ossification of the spinal ligaments is a group of conditions in which heterotopic bone formation occurs within the anterior or posterior longitudinal ligaments, ligamentum flavum, or ligamentum nuchae.
- These conditions affect older adults. They are frequently associated/coexistent with each other. They are distinct from but can coexist with degenerative spondylosis.
- Patients are often asymptomatic, but ligamentous ossification can cause issues related to stiffness or mass effect on surrounding structures.

- 脊柱韧带骨化是一组在前纵韧带、后纵韧带、黄韧带或项韧带发生异位骨化的病变。
- 这类病变见于老年人，且常与其他病变相互关联或共存。这些病变与退行性脊椎病不同，但可以共存。
- 患者通常无症状，但韧带骨化可引起强直或对周围结构产生占位效应。

Ossification of the posterior longitudinal ligament (OPLL)

后纵韧带骨化(OPLL)

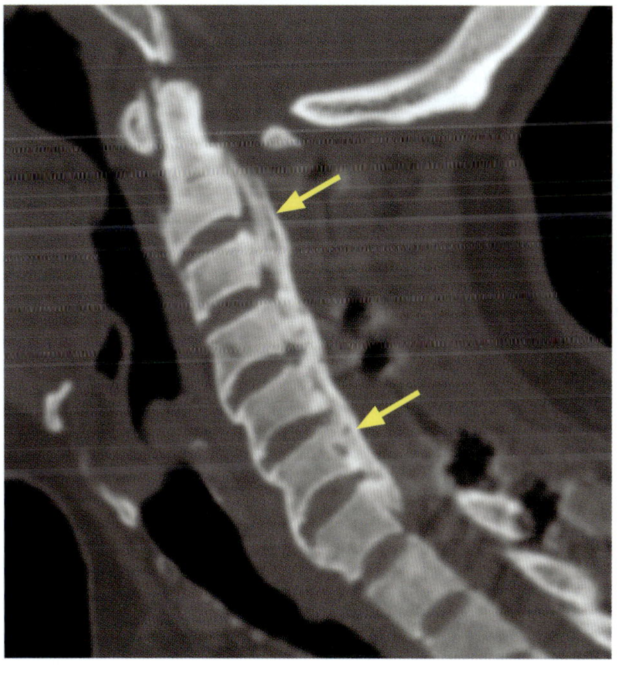

Ossification of the posterior longitudinal ligament (OPLL):
The right image shows OPLL along the upper to mid cervical spine (arrows). Note partially visualized post-surgical changes of cervical laminectomies and posterior instrumented fusion, which were performed to decompress the spinal stenosis caused by OPLL.
后纵韧带骨化(OPLL)：
右图显示沿上中颈椎分布的OPLL(箭)。注意，可见部分颈椎椎板切除术后改变及后路内固定，手术用于OPLL引起的椎管狭窄的减压。

- Ossification of the posterior longitudinal ligament (OPLL) is characterized by bone formation along the posterior longitudinal ligament.
- OPLL most frequently involves the cervical spine, followed by the thoracic spine.
- OPLL contributes to spinal canal stenosis and may compress the anterior aspect of the cord.

Ossification of the ligamentum flavum (OLF)

- Ossification of the ligamentum flavum (OLF) is characterized by bone formation along the ligamentum flavum.
- OLF predominantly involves the thoracic spine.
- OLF contributes to spinal canal stenosis and may compress the posterior aspect of the cord.

Ossification of the ligamentum nuchae (OLN)

- Ossification of the nuchal ligament (OLN) is characterized by bone formation along the midline ligament that spans the posterior cervical spine from the external occipital protuberance to the C7 spinous process.
- OLN is generally an incidental finding of no clinical significance.

- 后纵韧带骨化(OPLL)的特点是骨化沿后纵韧带分布。
- OPLL最常累及颈椎，其次是胸椎。
- OPLL会导致椎管狭窄，并可能压迫脊髓的前部。

黄韧带骨化(OLF)

- 黄韧带骨化(OLF)的特征是骨化沿黄韧带分布。
- OLF主要累及胸椎。
- OLF导致椎管狭窄，并可能压迫脊髓后部。

项韧带骨化(OLN)

- 项韧带骨化(OLN)的特点是骨化沿位于中线的韧带分布，该韧带从枕外隆凸一直向下至C_7棘突。
- OLN通常是一个偶然发现，不具临床意义。

PEDICLES AND PARS

Anatomy

椎弓根和椎弓峡部

解剖学

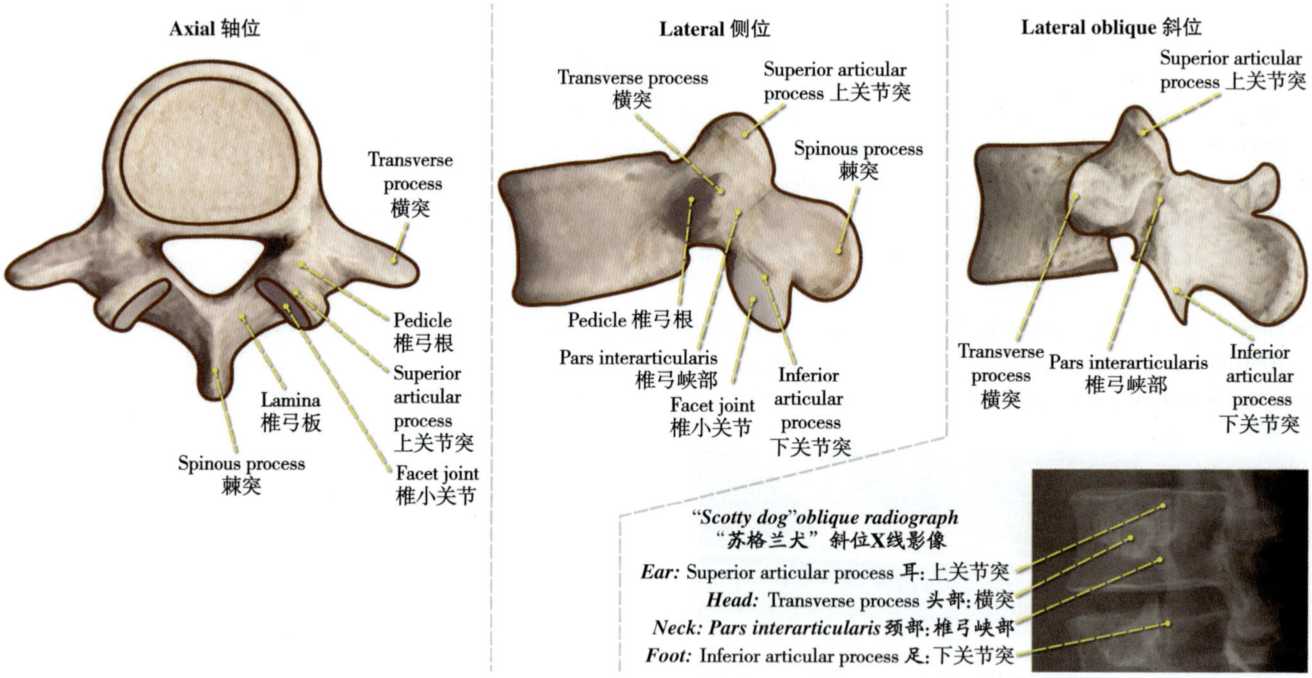

- The pars interarticularis (often simply called pars) is the part of the lamina that lies in between the superior and inferior articular processes of the spine.
- The pedicles connect the vertebral body to the posterior elements.

- 椎弓峡部(通常简称为pars)是椎板的一部分，位于脊柱上下关节突之间。
- 椎弓根连接椎体和后部附件。

Spondylolysis

脊椎滑脱

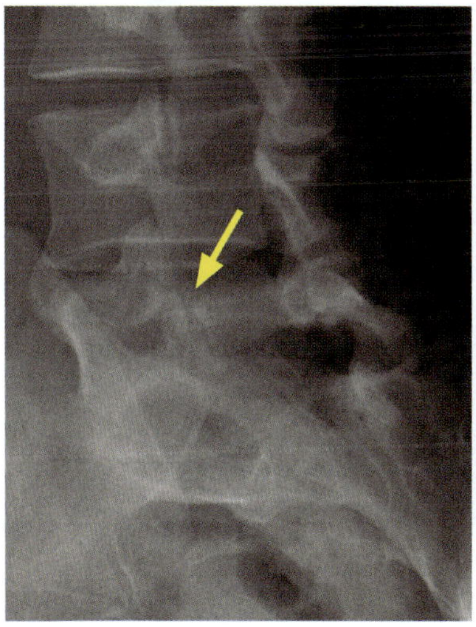

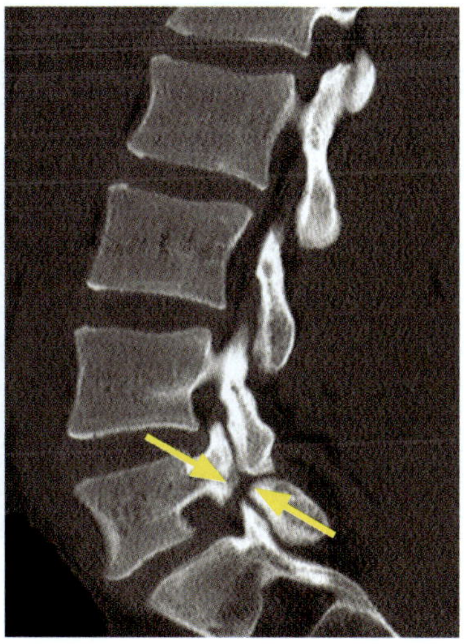

Spondylolysis in two different patients:
Oblique radiograph demonstrates a lucent defect of the pars at L5 (yellow arrow), through the neck of the Scotty dog. Poor Scotty!
Sagittal CT in a different patient shows a defect of the pars (yellow arrows) with slight L5–S1 anterolisthesis.

2名不同患者的脊椎滑脱：
斜位X线影像显示L_5椎弓峡部透亮缺损(黄箭)，通过苏格兰犬的颈部。可怜的苏格兰犬！
另一名患者的矢状位CT显示椎弓峡部缺损(黄箭)伴轻微L_5~S_1前滑脱。

- A traumatic or degenerative failure of the pars is known as pars defect or spondylolysis.
- CT is the most definitive imaging modality to diagnose pars defect, as it can be difficult to see on MR.
- Oblique radiographs of the lumbar spine show the characteristic "Scotty dog" appearance of the posterior elements. Scotty's neck is the pars interarticularis. This is unfortunate, because it means Scotty becomes decapitated in spondylolysis. Poor Scotty!
- Spondylolysis typically causes anterolisthesis (anterior position of the superior vertebral body, as measured posteriorly). When this occurs, the spinal canal is traditionally widened and the neural foramina become compressed.

- 创伤性或退行性椎弓峡部不全被称为峡部裂或脊椎滑脱。
- CT是诊断峡部裂最明确的成像方式，因为它可看到磁共振无法显示的异常。
- 腰椎斜位X线影像显示后部附件呈特征性的"苏格兰犬"征象。苏格兰犬的颈部就是椎弓峡部。很不幸，因为出现脊椎滑脱就意味着苏格兰犬被斩首。可怜的苏格兰犬！
- 脊椎滑脱通常是前滑脱(上一个椎体前移程度需从椎体后方测量)。当出现这种情况时，椎管通常会变宽，而神经孔被压。

Abnormal pedicles

- If one pedicle is abnormal and the other pedicle is normal, a lesion may be present.

  Rarely, if one pedicle is **sclerotic** and the other pedicle is **lucent**, there may be congenital absence of the pedicle (on the lucent side) with contralateral stress-related changes.

- If one pedicle is **sclerotic** and the other pedicle is normal, then a sclerotic lesion may be present, such as metastasis or osteoid osteoma. However, this pattern of a unilateral sclerotic pedicle can also be seen in the setting of unilateral spondylolysis with reactive changes on the opposite side causing sclerosis.

椎弓根异常

- 如果一个椎弓根异常而另一个椎弓根正常，则可能有病变存在。

  极少数情况下，如果一个椎弓根**硬化**而另一个椎弓根**透亮**，则可能是先天性椎弓根缺如(在透亮侧)伴对侧应力性改变。

- 如果一个椎弓根**硬化**而另一个椎弓根正常，那么可能存在硬化性病变，如转移或骨样骨瘤。然而，这种单侧椎弓根硬化也可见于单侧脊椎滑脱引起对侧反应性变化而出现硬化。

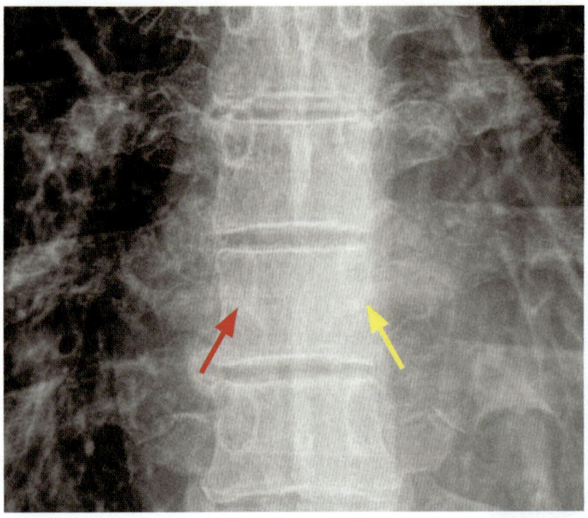

Unilateral sclerotic pedicle:
Frontal radiograph shows a very subtle sclerotic appearance of the left pedicle of a mid-thoracic vertebral body (yellow arrow).
The contralateral pedicle (red arrow) is normal.

单侧椎弓根硬化：
正位X线影像显示中段胸椎的左侧椎弓根非常细微的硬化改变(黄箭)。
对侧椎弓根(红箭)正常。

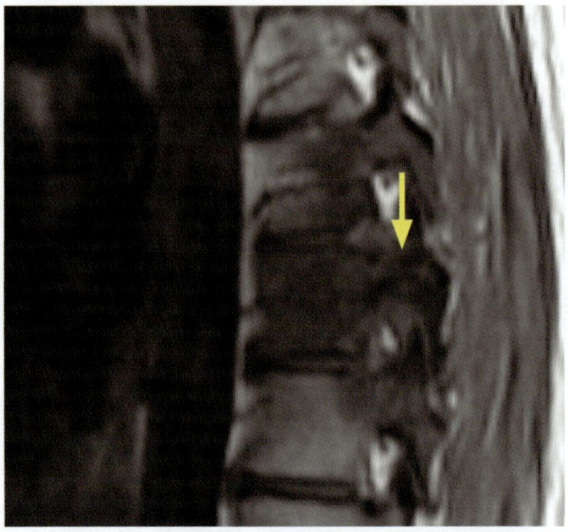

Sagittal T1-weighted MRI in the same patient shows a marrow-replacing lesion involving an entire mid-thoracic vertebral body with extension through the pedicle (arrow) to the posterior elements. The adjacent segments are also involved. This was metastatic breast cancer.

同一患者的矢状位T_1加权MRI显示一个中段胸椎的病变替代了整个椎体的骨髓，并通过椎弓根(箭头)延伸到后部附件。相邻的节段也被累及。这是转移性乳腺癌。

- If one pedicle is **lucent** and the other pedicle is normal, then a lytic lesion may be present, such as metastasis, osteoblastoma, or aneurysmal bone cyst.

- 如果一个椎弓根**透亮**而另一个椎弓根正常，则可能存在溶骨性病变，如转移瘤、成骨细胞瘤或动脉瘤性骨囊肿。

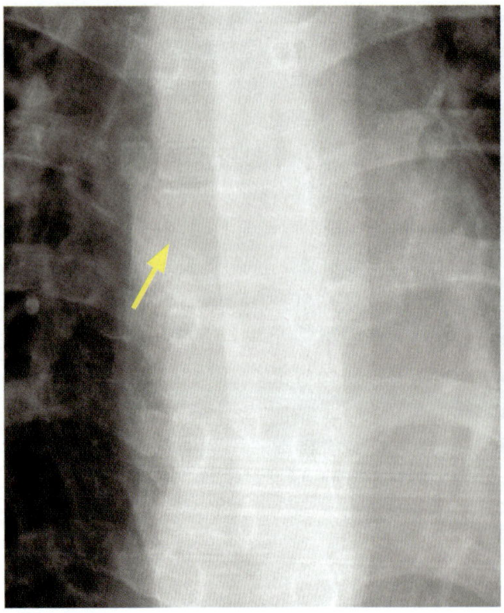

Frontal radiograph
正位X线影像

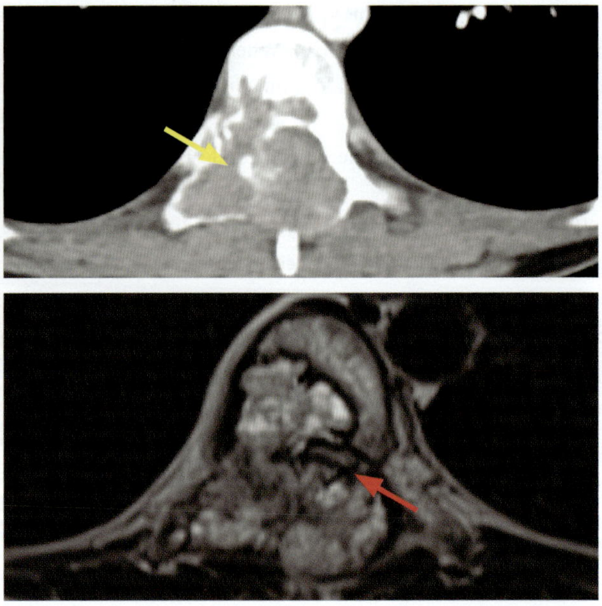

Axial contrast-enhanced CT (top); Axial T2-weighted MRI (bottom)
轴位增强CT(上图)；轴位T_2加权MRI(下图)

Unilateral lucent pedicle: Radiograph demonstrates an absent right pedicle of an upper-thoracic vertebral body (arrow). CT shows a lytic mass centered at the pedicle (yellow arrow) with extension into the spinal canal. MRI shows a mass with multiple cystic components. There is near complete obliteration of the spinal canal (red arrow). Pathology was an aneurysmal bone cyst with cystic and solid components.

单侧透亮的椎弓根：X线影像显示上胸段椎体右侧椎弓根缺失(箭)。CT显示以椎弓根为中心的溶骨性肿块(黄箭)，并延伸至椎管。MRI显示肿块内有多个囊性成分。椎管几乎完全闭塞(红箭)。病理学诊断为动脉瘤性骨囊肿，伴囊性和实性成分。

(翻译　王维平)

THREE COLUMN CONCEPT

三柱概念

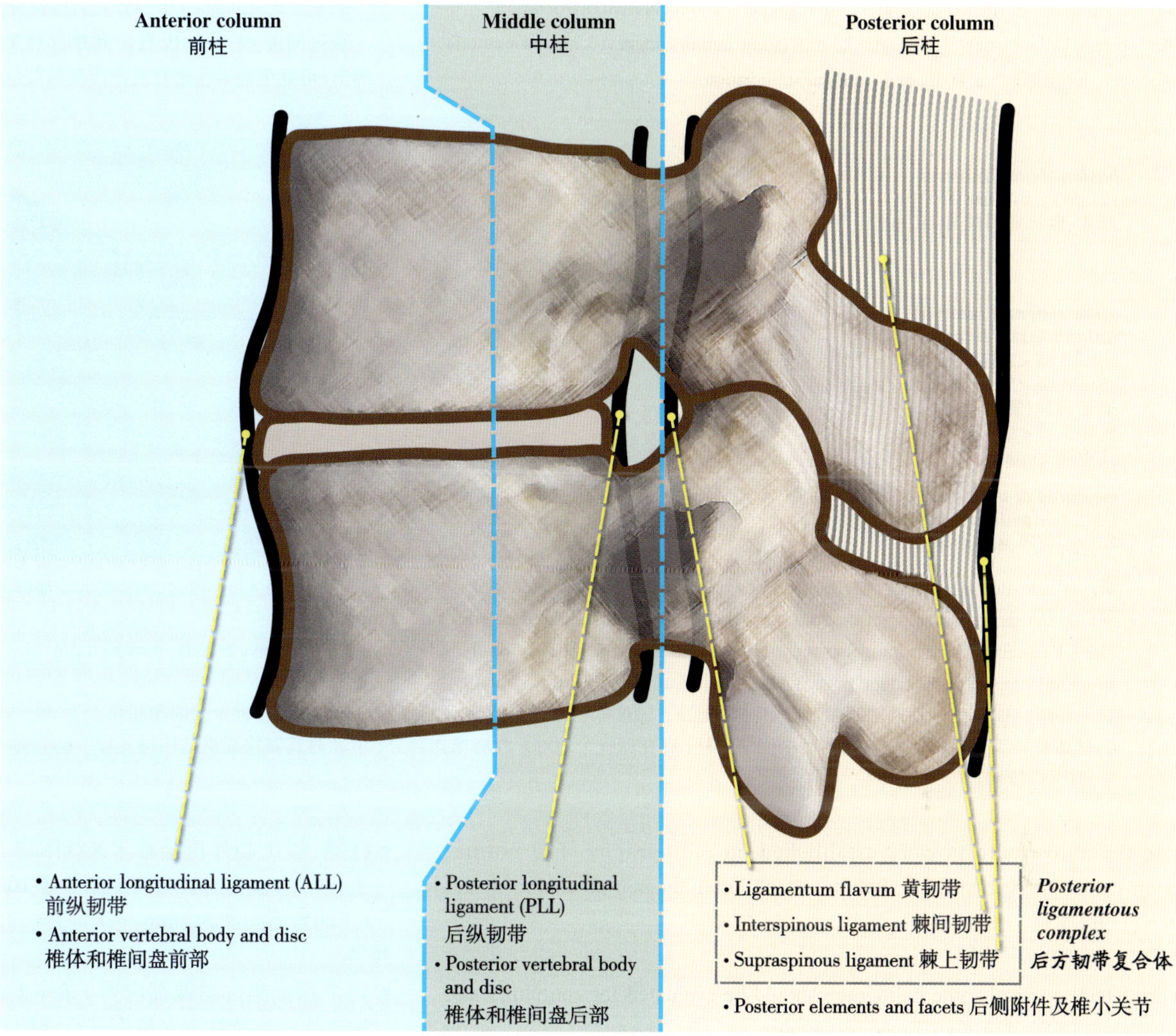

- The Denis three-column concept helps to classify injury severity. Fractures or ligamentous injury involving only one column are generally stable, while injuries with involvement of two or more columns are unstable.
- For instance, an anterior compression fracture involves the anterior column only. In contrast, a burst fracture involves failure of the anterior and middle columns and is unstable. More severe injuries may involve all three columns.
- Each column has ligamentous and osseous stabilizers.
- The middle column has been variably described as consisting of the posterior 1/2 or the posterior 1/3 of the vertebral body; however, the important point is that the posterior vertebral cortex and posterior disc is in the middle column.
- The posterior ligamentous complex consists of the ligamentum flavum, the intraspinous ligament, and the supraspinous ligament, and is an important ligamentous stabilizer of the posterior column.
- While the Denis model remains helpful in conceptualizing spinal trauma, it has been superseded by the injury classification and severity scales and the AO spine classification which are described subsequently.

- Denis三柱概念有助于对损伤的严重程度进行分类。仅涉及一个柱的骨折或韧带损伤通常是稳定的，若损伤涉及两个柱或三个柱则不稳定。
- 举例来说，前方的压缩性骨折仅涉及前柱。相反，一个爆裂性骨折破坏了前柱及中柱，因而是不稳定的。更严重的损伤可能涉及三个柱。
- 每一个柱都包括韧带和骨的稳定结构。
- 有人认为中柱是由椎体的后1/2，也有人认为是后1/3所组成；但很重要的一点是，椎体后部的皮质和椎间盘属于中柱。
- 后纵韧带复合体由黄韧带、棘间韧带和棘上韧带组成，是后柱重要的韧带稳定结构。
- Denis模型对于理解脊柱创伤依然有用，但它已被损伤分类和严重程度量表及下文描述的AO脊柱分类所取代。

Cervical spine trauma

颈椎外伤

Intervals

- The **basion-dental interval** and **atlanto-dental interval** (also known as the atlanto-axial interval) should be evaluated in every lateral cervical spine radiograph.

  An increased basion-dental interval >12 mm suggests craniocervical dissociation.

  An increased atlanto-dental interval >2.5 mm (some authors suggest 3 mm as a cutoff) can be seen in ligamentous laxity and resultant subluxation.

间隙

- **颅底齿状突间隙**和**寰齿间隙**(也称为寰枢间隙)应在每个颈椎侧位影像上进行评估。

  颅底齿状突间隙>12mm提示有颅颈分离。

  寰齿间隙>2.5mm(也有学者建议将3mm作为临界值)可见于韧带松弛及由此产生的关节半脱位。

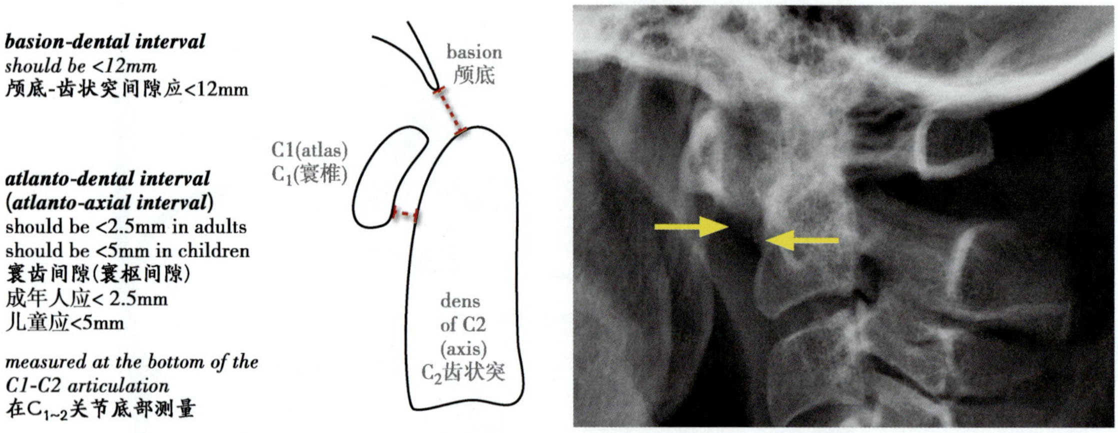

The atlanto-dental interval (ADI), also known as the atlanto-axial interval, should be <2.5 mm in adults. Lateral cervical spine radiograph shows widening of the ADI (arrows) to >1 cm, indicative of anterior subluxation.

The C1 vertebral body is known as the *atlas* (who carried the globe on his shoulders) and does not have a body; instead it provides structural support via its lateral masses. C2 is known as the *axis* (allows rotation).

寰齿间隙(ADI),也称寰枢轴间隙,成人应<2.5mm。颈椎侧位X线影像显示ADI(箭)增宽>1 cm,提示前向半脱位。

C_1椎体被称为寰椎(atlas)(希腊神话中的擎天柱,肩托着整个地球),没有椎体部分;但通过其侧块提供结构性支撑。C_2被称枢椎(可以旋转)。

- Note the above cutoffs were established on radiography. The normal basion-dental interval on CT is slightly under 10 mm; the normal atlanto-dental interval on CT is 2 mm.

Lines

- Every lateral cervical spine radiograph should be evaluated for continuity and smoothness of the 4 primary osseous contours.

- 注意,以上临界值是基于X线图像。CT图像上正常的颅底齿状突间隙略小于10mm,正常CT的寰齿间隙为2mm。

线条

- 每个颈椎侧位图像都应对4条主要的骨骼轮廓连线的连续性和平滑度进行评估。

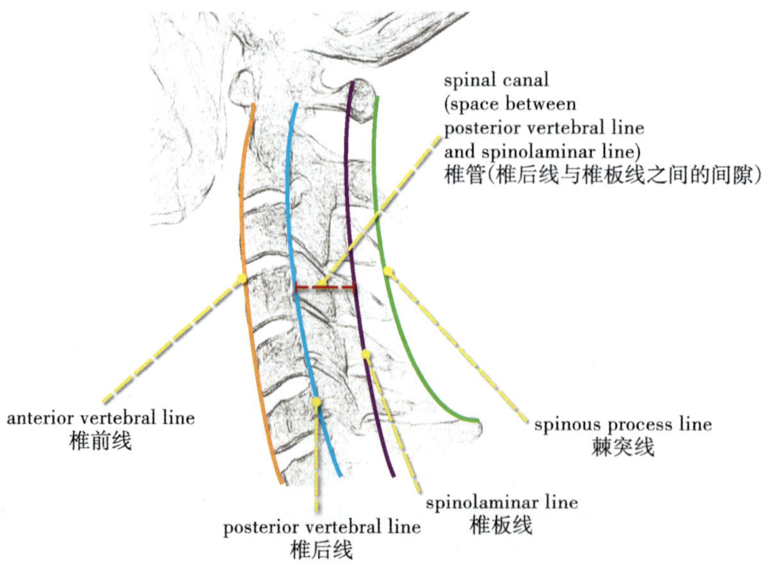

Anterior vertebral line: Traces the anterior margin of the vertebral bodies. The prevertebral soft tissues are located anterior to the anterior vertebral line.

Posterior vertebral line: Traces the posterior margin of the vertebral bodies and the anterior margin of the spinal canal. The spinal canal is the space between the posterior vertebral and spinolaminar lines.

Spinolaminar line: Traces the posterior margin of the spinal canal.

Spinous process line: Traces the posterior tips of the spinous processes.

椎前线：椎体前缘的连线。椎前软组织位于椎前线的前方。

椎后线：椎体后缘的连线，也是椎管前缘。椎管是椎后线和椎板线之间的间隙。

椎板线：椎管后缘的连线。

棘突线：棘突后部末端的连线。

Overview of named cervical spine fractures

颈椎骨折命名概述

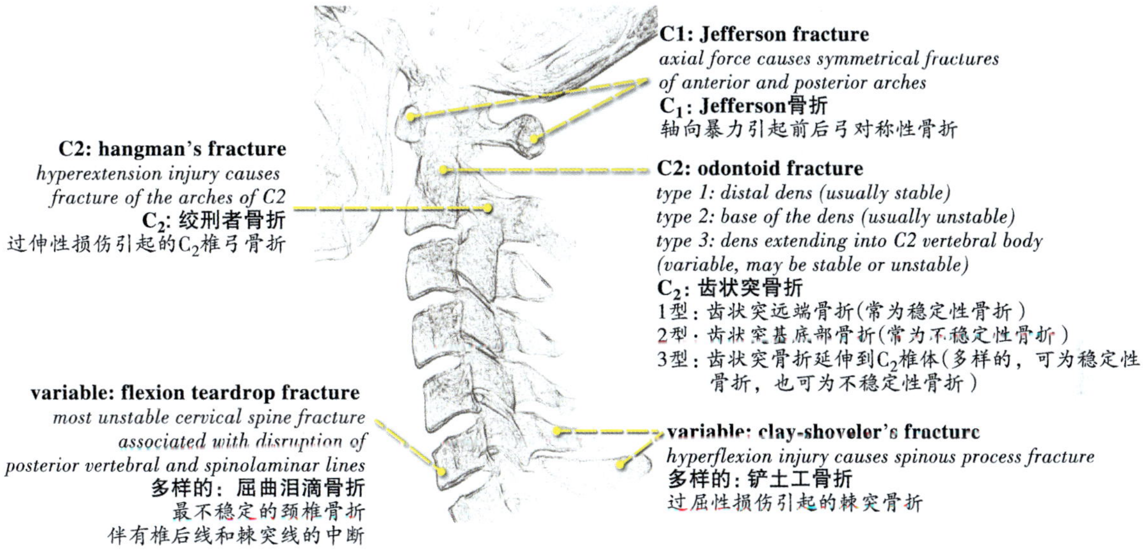

Imaging in cervical spine trauma

- Per the ACR appropriateness criteria for suspected spine trauma (last revised 2018), if the patient (age 16 or greater) does not meet clinical criteria for imaging by NEXUS or CCR (Canadian C-Spine Rules), then imaging of any modality is usually not appropriate. Of note, there is no role for x-rays in "low energy" trauma if imaging is not indicated on clinical grounds.
- If imaging is indicated by clinical criteria, then CT is the preferred initial imaging modality, as CT is more sensitive and has largely supplanted radiographs for assessment of trauma.
- MRI should be performed in patients with concern for spinal cord injury, cord compression, or ligamentous injury. However, MRI is inferior to CT in identifying fractures and should generally not be the initial imaging modality in trauma.

颈椎创伤影像

- 根据美国放射学会（American College of Radiology，ACR）制定的疑似脊柱创伤适宜检查标准（2018年修订），如果患者（年龄16岁或以上）不符合NEXUS（National Emergency X-Radiography Utilization Study）或CCR（Canadian C-Spine Rules）实施影像检查的临床指征，通常使用任何方式的影像检查均不适宜。注意，如果影像检查没有临床指征，X线无益于检出“低能量”创伤。
- 如果影像学检查有临床指征，则CT是首选，因为CT更敏感，并在很大程度上取代了X线对创伤进行评估。
- 应该对疑似脊髓损伤、脊髓受压或韧带损伤的患者进行MRI检查。然而，MRI对骨折诊断不及CT，通常不应作为创伤的首选影像学检查。

Subaxial injury classification and severity scale (SLICS)

- The subaxial injury classification and severity scale (SLICS) provides points for three categories of injury severity, including injury morphology, disruption of the discoligamentous complex, and neurological status. Injuries with greater than 4 points are usually treated surgically. It is not necessary to memorize this classification, but it is well established and helpful to guide management.

Occipital condyle fractures

- Occipital condyle fractures are uncommon and typically classified into three patterns.
- **Type Ⅰ** (stable) is a nondisplaced comminuted impaction fracture from axial loading.

寰枢椎下区损伤分类和严重程度量表(SLICS)

- 寰枢椎下区损伤分类和严重程度量表(SLICS)对三类损伤严重程度进行评分，包括损伤形态、椎间盘韧带复合体受损和神经状态。超过4分的损伤通常需要外科治疗。不必记住这个分类，但它已被广泛认可，并且有助于指导治疗。

枕骨髁骨折

- 枕骨髁骨折并不常见，通常分为三型：
- **Ⅰ型**（稳定型）是轴向负荷造成的非移位性粉碎性骨折。

- **Type Ⅱ** (stable) is a linear skull fracture extending into the occipital condyle.
- **Type Ⅲ** (unstable) is distraction injury resulting in an avulsion fracture at attachment of the alar ligament, which is disrupted or incompetent. This is the most common fracture type.
- MRI is an important adjunct to determine stability and ligament integrity, and can help differentiate between a type Ⅰ fracture and a minimally displaced type Ⅲ avulsion fracture.

Jefferson fracture

- **Ⅱ型**(稳定型)是线性颅骨骨折延伸到枕骨髁。
- **Ⅲ型**(不稳定型)是牵拉损伤造成翼状韧带附着处的撕脱骨折，致翼状韧带断裂或功能受限。这是最常见的骨折类型。
- MRI是评估稳定性和韧带完整性的重要辅助工具，有助于区分Ⅰ型骨折和有微小移位的Ⅲ型撕脱骨折。

Jefferson骨折(寰椎前后弓骨折)

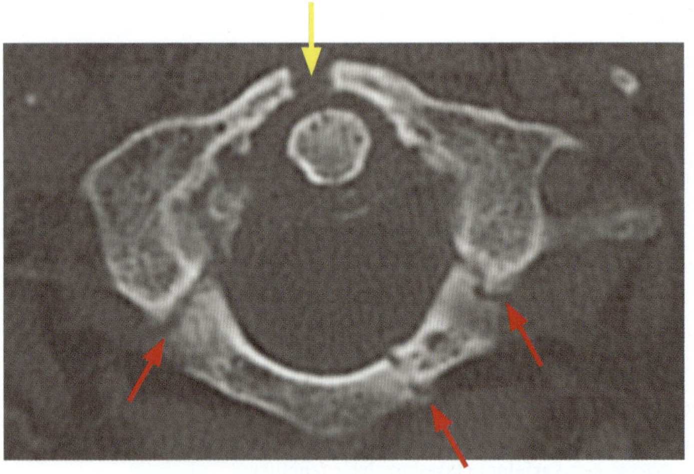

Jefferson fracture: Axial CT demonstrates a fracture of the anterior arch of C1 near the midline (yellow arrow) and bilateral posterior arch fractures (red arrows).

Jefferson骨折：轴位CT显示C_1前弓近中线处骨折(黄箭)和双侧后弓骨折(红箭)。

- A Jefferson fracture results from acute axial blow to the vertex of the head, causing symmetrical fractures of the anterior and posterior arches of C1.
- On an open-mouth odontoid radiograph, the lateral masses of C1 are displaced laterally. Jefferson fracture is best seen on axial CT.

Odontoid fracture

- Jefferson骨折是因头顶部受到急性轴向冲击伤，导致C_1前、后弓对称性骨折。
- 在张口位齿状突X线图像上，C_1的侧块向外移位。Jefferson骨折在轴位CT上看得最清晰。

齿状突骨折

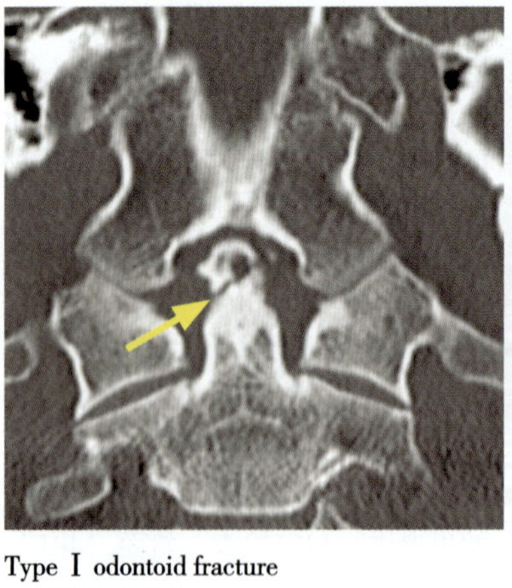

Type Ⅰ odontoid fracture
Ⅰ型齿状突骨折

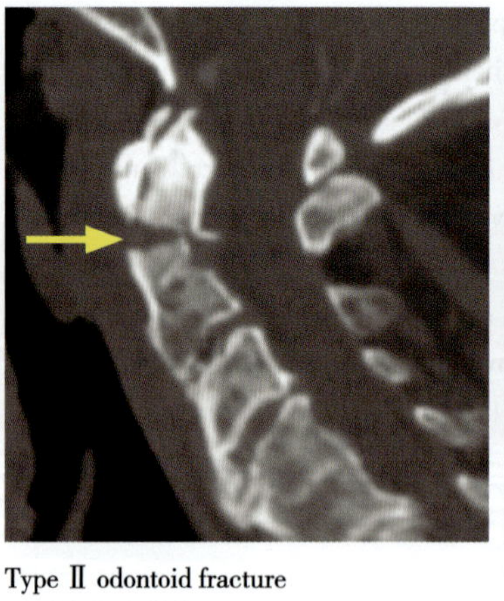

Type Ⅱ odontoid fracture
Ⅱ型齿状突骨折

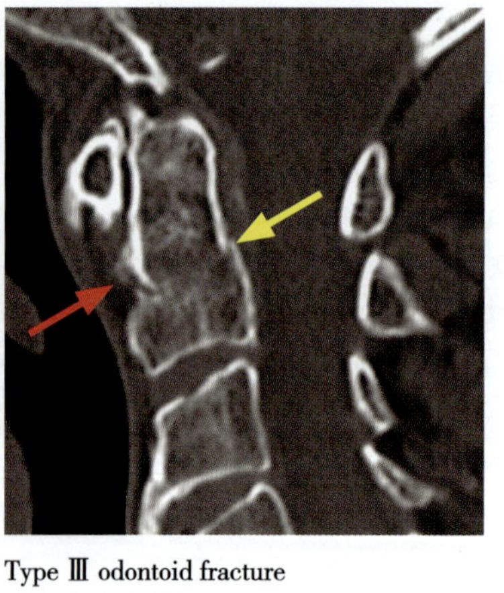

Type Ⅲ odontoid fracture
Ⅲ型齿状突骨折

Three patients with odontoid fractures:
Type Ⅰ odontoid fracture: Coronal CT (left image) demonstrates an oblique fracture of the tip of the dens (yellow arrow).
Type Ⅱ odontoid fracture: Sagittal CT (middle image) shows a mildly displaced and angulated fracture through the base of the dens (yellow arrow).
Type Ⅲ odontoid fracture: Sagittal CT (right image) shows a nondisplaced fracture through base of the dens extending into the vertebral body (yellow arrow). There is surrounding callus formation anteriorly (red arrow), in keeping with subacute chronicity.

3名不同患者的齿状突骨折：
Ⅰ型齿状突骨折：冠状位CT(左图)显示齿状突远端顶部一处斜行骨折(黄箭)。
Ⅱ型齿状突骨折：矢状位CT(中图)显示一处经齿状突基底部骨折，有轻度移位和成角(黄箭)。
Ⅲ型齿状突骨折：矢状位CT(右图)显示经齿状突基底部一处贯穿椎体的无移位骨折(黄箭)。前方覆盖骨痂(红箭)，符合亚急性慢性期表现。

- Fractures of the odontoid process of C2 are usually caused by flexion injuries.
- **Type Ⅰ** odontoid fracture is a fracture of the distal tip of the dens. Type I odontoid fractures are considered stable and treatment is generally conservative. The differential diagnosis of a Type I odontoid fracture is an os odontoideum, a normal variant secondary ossification center located at the tip of the dens.
- **Type Ⅱ** odontoid fracture is a fracture of the base of the dens. It is considered an unstable injury and treatment is typically surgical fusion.
- **Type Ⅲ** odontoid fracture is a fracture of the base of the dens extending into the C2 vertebral body. Type Ⅲ fractures are variably described in the literature as both stable and unstable.

Hangman's fracture

- Hangman's fracture is traumatic spondylolysis of C2. It results from hyperextension and distraction, causing bilateral fractures through the pedicles of C2.
- The characteristic radiographic finding is disruption of the spinolaminar line.
- A hangman's fracture with >3 mm displacement of C2 on C3 is likely unstable.

Burst fracture

- A burst fracture is similar in mechanism (axial loading) and appearance to a Jefferson fracture, but occurs lower in the cervical spine, at C2–C7.

Flexion teardrop fracture

- C_2齿状突骨折常由屈曲性损伤所致。
- **Ⅰ型**齿状突骨折是齿突远端的骨折。Ⅰ型齿状突骨折是稳定性骨折，通常行保守治疗。其鉴别诊断为游离齿状突，一种正常变异的二次骨化中心，位于齿状突的顶端。
- **Ⅱ型**齿状突骨折是齿状突的基底部骨折。它是一种不稳定的损伤，其治疗通常是进行手术融合。
- **Ⅲ型**齿状突骨折是齿突基底部骨折延伸到C_2的椎体部。文献对Ⅲ型骨折报道不同，稳定和不稳定骨折兼而有之。

Hangman(绞刑者)骨折(枢椎椎弓根骨折)

- Hangman骨折是C_2椎弓峡部创伤性断裂。过度伸展和牵拉导致C_2双侧椎弓根骨折。
- X线影像学的特征性表现为椎板线中断。
- Hangman骨折在C_2相对C_3移位>3mm时很可能是不稳定骨折。

爆裂性骨折

- 爆裂性骨折的机制(轴向负荷)和表现与Jefferson骨折相似，但发生在颈椎较低部位，即$C_{2\sim7}$。

屈曲泪滴骨折

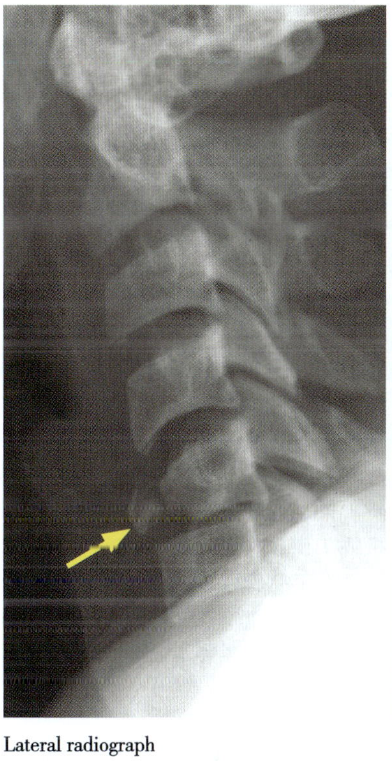

Lateral radiograph
侧位X线影像

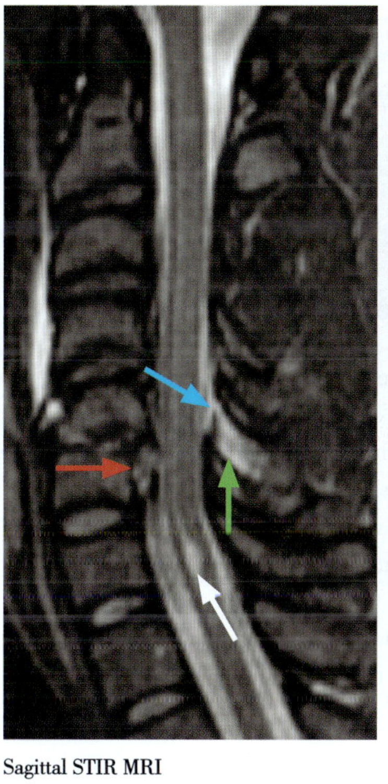

Sagittal STIR MRI
矢状位STIR MRI

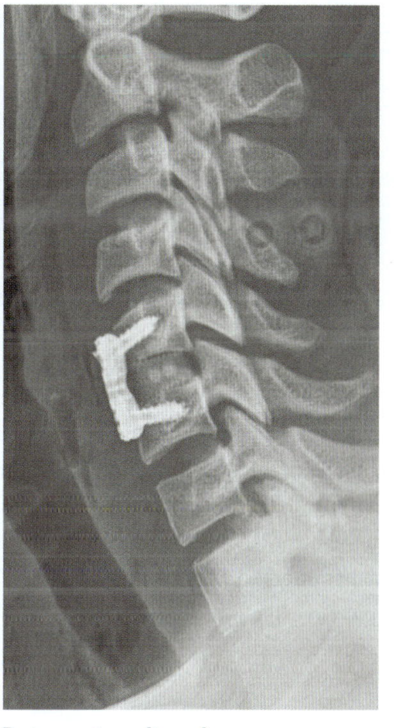

Post-operative radiograph
术后侧位X线影像

Flexion teardrop fracture: Presentation radiograph demonstrates an anterior teardrop fragment (yellow arrow) and retropulsion of C5 into the spinal canal. MRI shows traumatic disc extrusion with caudal migration (red arrow) and spinal stenosis. There is disruption of the posterior ligamentous complex with tear of the ligamentum flavum (blue arrow) and interspinous ligament (green arrow). Note focal fluid signal in the cord at the C7 level (white arrow), which is thought to most likely represent a syrinx. The patient was treated with C5–C6 anterior decompression and fusion.
屈曲泪滴骨折：X线影像显示前方一处泪滴状碎片(黄箭)和C_5被后推至椎管。MRI显示创伤性椎间盘脱出并向尾侧移位(红箭)及椎管狭窄。后韧带复合体断裂，伴黄韧带(蓝箭)和棘间韧带(绿箭)撕裂。注意，C_7节段水平(白箭)的脊髓有局部积液，可能是脊髓空洞。该患者接受了$C_{5\sim6}$前路减压融合手术治疗。

- Flexion teardrop fracture is the most severe cervical spinal injury that is potentially compatible with life. It is caused by a hyperflexion and compression injury and results in posterior displacement of the affected vertebral body into the spinal canal.
- The posterior ligamentous complex is often disrupted due to distraction from posterior displacement of the vertebral body.
- The key radiographic finding is an avulsed bony fragment from the anterior-inferior aspect of the vertebral body, caused by anterior longitudinal ligament avulsion. There is retropulsion of the affected vertebral body, which is often rotated and appears shorter in anterior-posterior dimension than the adjacent vertebrae. The intact-appearing posterior vertebral body can result in spinal cord injury due to posterior displacement.
- Flexion teardrop fracture can cause anterior cord syndrome due to compression of the pyramidal tracts and anterior spinothalamic tracts. This clinically presents as complete paralysis and loss of pain and temperature sensation. The dorsal column usually remains intact, preserving touch and vibration sense.

- 屈曲泪滴骨折是最严重的颈椎损伤，可危及生命。它是由于过度屈曲和压缩性损伤导致的相应椎体向后移位并进入椎管。
- 后韧带复合体在椎体向后移位时受牵拉而导致撕裂。
- 关键的X线影像表现是从椎体前下方撕下的骨碎片，为前纵韧带撕脱所致。受累椎体向后滑移，常发生旋转，其前后径短于相邻的椎体。完整的后部椎体后移可引起脊髓损伤。
- 屈曲泪滴骨折因压迫锥体束和脊髓丘脑前束而导致前索综合征。临床表现为完全性瘫痪，以及痛、温觉消失。背柱通常完整，仍保留触觉和振动觉。

Extension teardrop fracture

伸展泪滴骨折

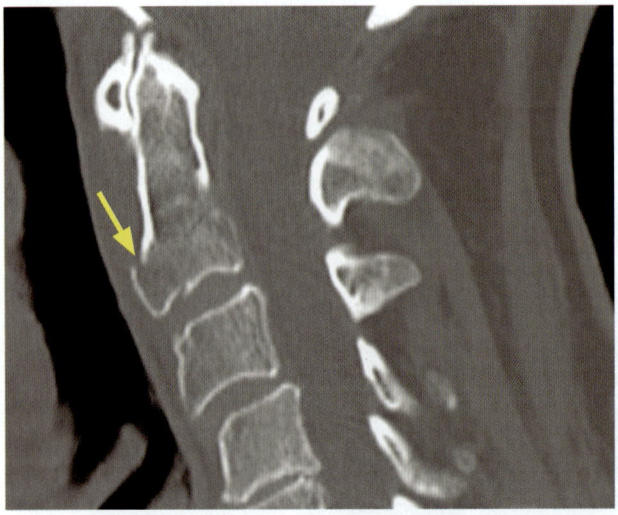

Extension teardrop fracture:
Sagittal CT demonstrates a minimally displaced fracture of the anterior/inferior corner of C2 (arrow).
In contrast to a flexion teardrop fracture, there is no retropulsion of the vertebral body.
伸展泪滴骨折：
矢状位CT显示轻微移位的C_2前/下角骨折(黄箭)。
与屈曲泪滴骨折相比，椎体没有后移。

- In contrast to a flexion teardrop fracture, an extension teardrop fracture is a stable fracture that usually occurs higher in the cervical spine, at C2 or C3.
- On the lateral radiograph, an anterior/inferior avulsion fragment is seen, similar to flexion teardrop. Unlike a flexion teardrop fracture, there is no subluxation and the spinolaminar line is not disrupted. The extension teardrop fracture fragment is typically taller in craniocaudal dimension compared to its anterior-posterior dimension.
- The typical mechanism of an extension teardrop fracture is hyperextension, with fracture resulting from avulsion of the endplate by the anterior longitudinal ligament.

- 与屈曲泪滴骨折不同，伸展泪滴骨折是一种稳定性骨折，常发生在较高的C_2或C_3。
- 在侧位X线影像上可见一段前/下方撕脱的碎片，类似于屈曲泪滴骨折。但与屈曲泪滴骨折不同的是，伸展泪滴骨折没有半脱位且椎板线未出现中断。伸展泪滴骨折碎片的头尾径常大于前后径。
- 伸展泪滴骨折的典型发生机制是过度伸展，由前纵韧带撕脱终板而引起骨折。

Clay-shoveler's fracture

- A clay-shoveler's fracture is a displaced avulsion fracture of a spinous process. It is caused by forced flexion.
- Clay-shoveler's fracture occurs in the lower cervical/upper thoracic spine, from C6–T1.

铲土工骨折

- 铲土工骨折是棘突撕脱性移位骨折，由屈曲暴力引起。
- 铲土工骨折发生在颈椎下段/胸椎上段，即C_6~T_1。

Bilateral interfacetal dislocation (locked facets)

- Bilateral interfacetal dislocation, also called bilateral locked facets, is a hyperflexion injury caused by complete disruption of all spinal ligaments and resultant anterior dislocation of the affected vertebra by >50%.

双侧椎小关节脱位(椎小关节绞锁)

- 双侧椎小关节脱位，也称为双侧椎小关节绞锁，是一种过度屈曲性损伤所导致的所有脊椎韧带完全断裂，进而引起受累椎体前脱位>50%。

- Bilateral interfacetal dislocation is unstable with a high risk of cord damage.
- It typically occurs in the lower cervical spine.
- The *naked facet sign* is seen when the superior articular facets are not covered by the adjacent inferior articular facets.
- **Perched facets** are a less severe variation of locked facets. The inferior articular facets of the superior vertebral body are subluxated (but not displaced) and *perched* upon the superior articular process of the inferior vertebra. Perched facets feature anterior subluxation of >3 mm but less than the 50% seen in a complete dislocation.

Unilateral interfacetal dislocation

- Unilateral interfacetal dislocation is dislocation of a single facet joint, caused by hyperflexion with rotation opposite the site of the dislocation.
- Unilateral interfacetal dislocation is considered a stable fracture.

Grisel syndrome

- Grisel syndrome is nontraumatic rotatory subluxation of the atlantoaxial joint (C1–C2) secondary to an inflammatory mass, most commonly occurring as a sequela of pharyngitis or retropharyngeal abscess.

THORACOLUMBAR SPINE TRAUMA

Overview of thoracolumbar trauma

- The thoracolumbar injury classification and severity score (TLICS) is similar to SLICS for the cervical (subaxial) spine, and aids in determination of optimal treatment.
- The TLICS provides a numerical score for injury severity based on the same three components of SLICS: injury morphology, integrity of the posterior ligamentous complex (PLC), and neurological status.
- The PLC is a primary stabilizer of the posterior spinal column, and knowledge of its anatomy is helpful to recognize potentially unstable injuries. Indirect imaging findings of PLC injury include widening of the interspinous distance, widening of the facet joints, spinous process fracture, and subluxation or dislocation of a vertebral body.

Rigid spine trauma

- 双侧椎小关节脱位是不稳定性损伤，具有较高的脊髓损伤风险。
- 通常发生在下段颈椎。
- 裸小关节面征为上关节突未被相邻的下关节突所覆盖。
- **栖息状椎小关节**是椎小关节绞锁中严重程度较低的一个亚型。上椎体的下关节突半脱位(但不移位)并落在下椎体的上关节突上。栖息状椎小关节表现为前向半脱位>3mm，但小于完全性脱位时的50%。

单侧椎小关节脱位

- 单侧椎小关节脱位是一侧椎小关节脱位，由过度屈曲并向脱位对侧方向旋转所致。
- 单侧椎小关节脱位是一种稳定性骨折。

Grisel综合征

- Grisel综合征是非创伤性的寰枢关节(C_{1-2})旋转半脱位，继发于炎性肿块，最常出现在咽炎或咽后脓肿之后。

胸腰椎外伤

胸腰椎外伤概述

- 胸腰椎损伤的分类和严重程度评分(TLICS)与颈椎(寰枢椎下区)的SLICS类似，有助于确定最佳治疗方案。
- TLICS根据SLICS中三个同样的内容对损伤的严重程度提供量化评分，包括损伤形态、后纵韧带复合体(PLC)的完整性和神经状态。
- PLC是脊柱后柱的主要稳定结构，掌握其解剖结构有助于识别潜在的不稳定性损伤。后纵韧带复合体损伤的间接影像学表现包括棘突间距增宽、椎小关节增宽、棘突骨折、椎体半脱位或脱位。

硬化性脊柱创伤

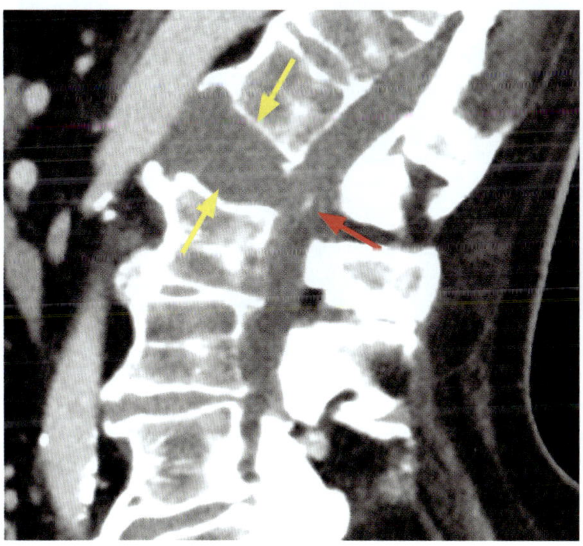

Sagittal CT
矢状位CT

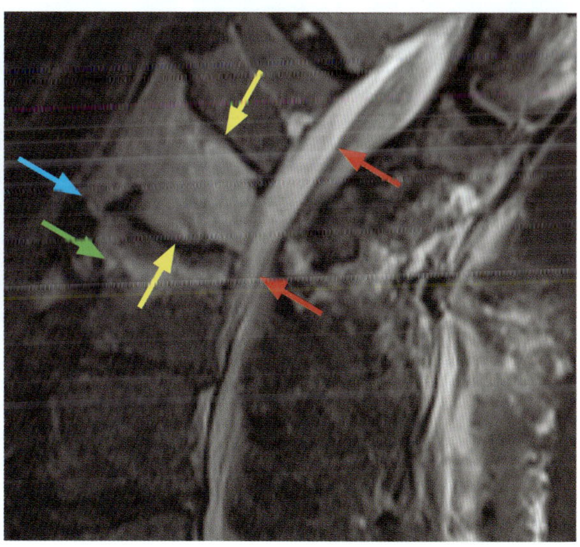

Sagittal STIR MRI
矢状位STIR MRI

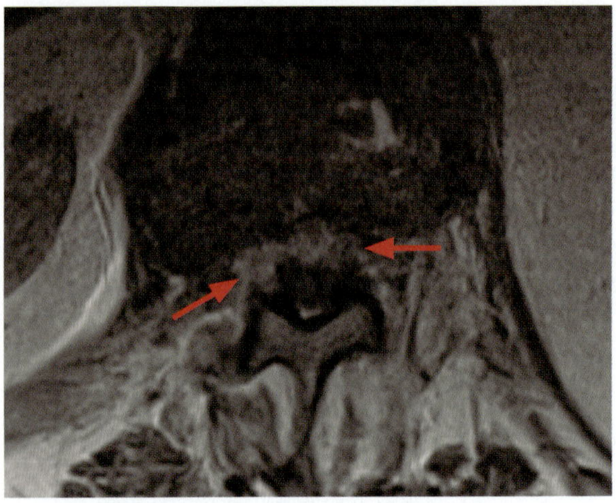

Axial T2-weighted MR
轴位T_2加权MR

Rigid spine hyperextension injury in a patient with diffuse idiopathic skeletal hyperostosis (DISH):
CT demonstrates marked widening of the T12–L1 disc space (yellow arrows), in keeping with hyperextension injury. Note the tiny retropulsed fracture fragment (red arrow). Multilevel flowing anterior osteophytes are partially seen.
MRI confirms fluid in the disc space (yellow arrows). There is an epidural hematoma (red arrows) contributing to severe spinal stenosis. There is edema in the region of the anterior longitudinal ligament (blue arrow), consistent with disruption. Note the superior endplate fracture of L1 (green arrow).
1名弥漫性特发性骨肥大(DISH)患者出现的硬化性脊柱过度伸展性损伤：
CT显示T_{12}~L_1椎间隙明显增宽(黄箭)，与过度伸展性损伤一致。注意微小后移的骨折碎片(红箭)，可见多个节段的部分前缘游离骨赘。
MRI证实椎间隙有液体(黄箭)。硬膜外血肿(红箭)加重了椎管狭窄的严重性。前纵韧带区域有水肿(蓝箭)，符合破裂的表现。注意L_1上终板骨折(绿箭)。

- Patients with a rigid spine – due to diffusion idiopathic skeletal hyperostosis (DISH), ankylosing spondylitis, degenerative change, or surgical fusion, are more vulnerable to fracture given altered biomechanics.
- CT should be performed in a patient with rigid spine and back pain after even minor trauma.
- Hyperextension is the most common injury mechanism.

Chance fracture

- 硬化性脊柱的原因有弥漫性特发性骨肥大(DISH)、强直性脊柱炎、退行性改变及融合术，患者因生物力学的改变而容易发生骨折。
- 对硬化性脊柱的患者，即使轻微创伤出现的背痛也需要进行CT检查。
- 过度伸展是最常见的损伤机制。

Chance骨折

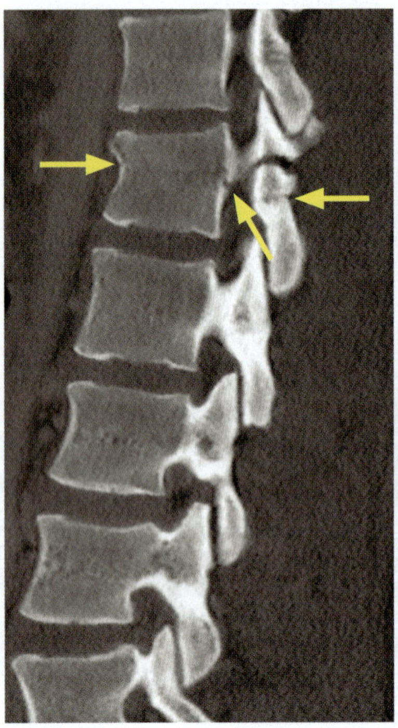

Sagittal CT
矢状位CT

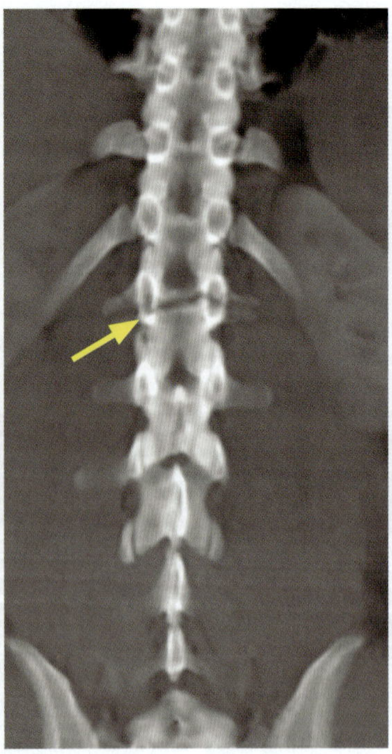

Coronal MIP CT
冠状位MIP CT

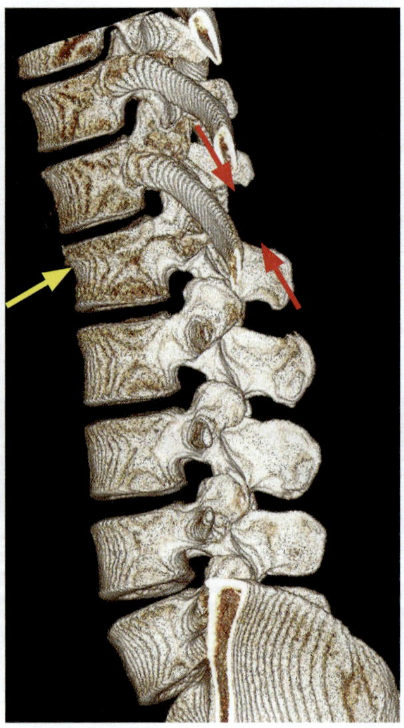

Volume-rendered CT
容积再现CT

Chance fracture: There is a minimally displaced transverse fracture through the L1 vertebral body and posterior elements (yellow arrows). Volumetric reconstruction shows the subtle anterior endplate deformity (yellow arrow), with reversal of the spinal curvature centered on the fracture. Interspinous widening (red arrows) indicates posterior ligamentous disruption.
Chance骨折：L_1椎体及后部结构(黄箭)横向骨折伴轻微移位。容积重建显示一处不明显的前终板变形(黄箭)及以骨折为中心的脊柱反向弯曲。棘突间隙增宽(红箭)提示后韧带断裂。

- A Chance fracture, also known as a *seat belt* fracture, is a flexion distraction injury caused by acute forward flexion of the spine during sudden deceleration.
- There is horizontal splitting of the vertebra which begins posteriorly in the spinous process or lamina and extends anteriorly through the vertebral body.
- Chance fractures are unstable injuries, as they involve all three spinal columns.
- Intra-abdominal injuries are often associated with this fracture pattern, especially in pediatrics.

- Chance骨折，也称为安全带骨折，是一种屈曲分离损伤，由突然减速造成脊柱急剧向前屈曲。
- 椎体出现水平撕裂，从后方的棘突或椎板向前延伸穿过椎体。
- Chance骨折为不稳定损伤，因其累及三个柱。
- 此类骨折通常伴腹腔内器官损伤，尤其是儿童患者。

AO SPINE CLASSIFICATION FOR SPINAL TRAUMA

- The historical three-column model by Denis classifies spinal fractures morphologically but does not consider the mechanism of injury or patient's neurological status.
- The cervical subaxial and thoracolumbar injury classification and severity scores (SLIC, TLICS) incorporate neurological status but do not consider patient-specific factors such as underlying medical conditions that may affect management.
- The more comprehensive **AO Spine** classification system for spinal trauma improved upon previous classification systems by incorporating:
  1) fracture morphology,
  2) neurological status,
  3) clinical modifiers specific to the patient which may influence treatment decisions.
- Examples of clinical modifiers include accompanying injuries that would change treatment (e.g., ligamentous injury resulting in potential instability, vascular injury), high-risk medical comorbidities, and underlying bone disease (e.g., ankylosing spondylitis or DISH resulting in a rigid spine).
- The AO Spine system describes 4 different classifications depending on fracture location: the upper cervical spine, subaxial cervical spine, thoracolumbar spine, and the sacral spine (including coccyx).
- Essentially, fracture morphology is categorized hierarchically with increasing severity and/or instability based on radiologic appearance. While the detailed classifications are beyond the scope of this text, some of the key morphological features in the cervical and thoracolumbar spine are listed below.
- **Upper cervical spine** injuries (occiput to C2–3 joint):

Type A: Bony injuries only (stable)
Type B: Tension band or ligamentous disruption +/− bony injuries (stable or unstable)
Type C. Translation injuries with displacement relative to adjacent vertebrae (unstable)

Anterior tension band includes the anterior longitudinal ligament.
Posterior tension band includes the posterior ligamentous complex.

- **Subaxial cervical spine** injuries (C3–C7):

Type A: Compression fractures without ligamentous injury
Type B: Tension band disruption
Type C: Translation injuries
Type F: Facet joint injuries

- **Thoracolumbar spine** injuries:

Type A: Compression fractures, including wedge compressions and burst fractures

AO脊柱外伤分类

- 传统的Denis三柱模型是对脊柱骨折的形态学进行分类，但未考虑损伤机制或患者的神经状态。
- 寰枢椎下区颈椎和胸腰椎损伤分类和严重程度评分(SLIC、TLICS)纳入了神经状态，但未考虑患者的特定因素，如患者的其他状况可能对治疗产生影响。
- **AO脊柱**创伤分类系统在原有分类基础上进行了较为全面的改进，并纳入了：
  1) 骨折形态。
  2) 神经状态。
  3) 对可能影响患者治疗决策的具体情况进行临床修正。
- 需要改变临床治疗计划的例子包括合并损伤(例如，韧带损伤导致潜在的脊柱不稳定性、血管损伤)、高风险的内科合并症和潜在的骨病(例如，强直性脊柱炎或DISH导致硬化性脊柱)。
- AO脊柱系统根据骨折的位置分为4类：上颈椎、寰枢椎下区颈椎、胸腰椎和骶椎(包括尾骨)。
- 骨折形态分类在本质上是根据放射学表现对严重程度和/或不稳定性进行等级划分。详细分类不属于本文讨论的范围，但以下列出了颈椎和胸腰椎骨折的一些关键形态学特点。
- **上颈椎**损伤(枕骨至$C_{2\sim3}$关节)：

A型：仅为骨损伤(稳定)
B型：张力带或韧带断裂+/−骨损伤(稳定或不稳定)
C型：对邻近椎体产生的转移性损伤(不稳定)

前张力带包括前纵韧带。
后张力带包括后纵韧带复合体。

- 寰枢椎下区**颈椎**损伤($C_{3\sim7}$)：

A型：压缩性骨折不伴韧带损伤
B型：张力带断裂
C型：平移性损伤
F型：椎小关节损伤

- **胸腰椎**损伤：

A型：压缩性骨折，包括楔形压缩骨折和爆裂性骨折

Type B: Distraction injuries with tension band disruption, including Chance fractures and hyperextension injuries
Type C: Translation injuries resulting in displacement and dislocation

B型：张力带断裂引起的牵引损伤，包括Chance骨折和过度伸展性损伤
C型：平移性损伤导致的移位和脱位

（翻译　卞益同）

POSTOPERATIVE SPINE IMAGING

脊柱术后影像

Overview of postoperative spine imaging

- Spine procedures can generally be thought of as falling into one of three categories: stabilization and fusion (for trauma or scoliosis), decompression (typically caused by discovertebral degeneration), and lesion excision. Some surgeries may span two or more of these categories.
- If instrumented fusion is performed, imaging is critical to determine if there is hardware failure (hardware fracture), assess screw position, evaluate for lucency surrounding the screws, and to assess healing of the fusion mass.
- For decompressive surgeries, imaging should also assess if there is a cause for persistent or new pain, such as recurrent disc herniation, scar formation, arachnoiditis, adjacent segment degeneration, or infectious process.
- For lesion excision procedures, signs of lesion recurrence should be carefully evaluated.
- Patients with fusion are at increased risk for fracture due to altered biomechanics.

脊柱术后影像概述

- 脊柱手术通常可以归为以下三类之一：内固定与融合(对于创伤或脊柱侧弯)、减压(通常由椎间盘椎体退变引起)及病灶切除。有些手术可能涵盖两个或两个以上类别。
- 如果进行内固定融合术，影像学对于确定是否存在内固定物异常(内固定断裂)、螺钉位置、螺钉周围的透亮影及融合体的愈合情况至关重要。
- 对于减压术，影像学还用于评估是否有持续性或新发疼痛的原因，如复发性椎间盘疝、瘢痕形成、蛛网膜炎、邻近脊柱退变或感染性病变。
- 对于病灶切除术，应仔细评估病变复发的征象。
- 融合术后患者的生物力学发生了改变，其骨折风险随之增加。

Spine fusion hardware complications

脊柱融合内固定并发症

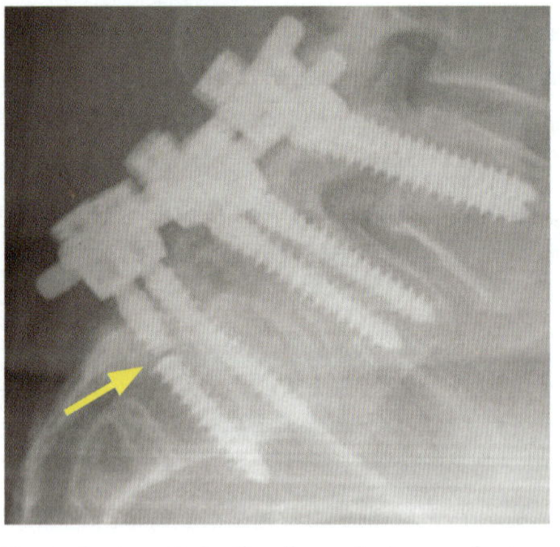

Screw fracture: Lateral radiograph shows a fracture of one of the S1 screws (yellow arrow).
螺钉折断：侧位X线显示S_1的一枚螺钉折断(黄箭)。

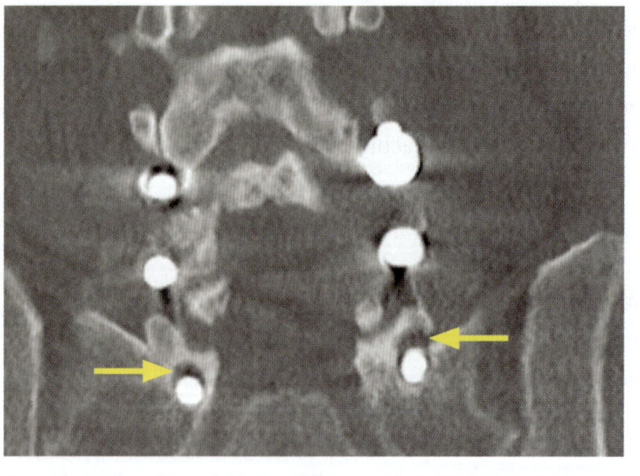

Screw lucencies: Coronal CT in a different patient demonstrates lucencies at the superior aspects of the S1 screws bilaterally (yellow arrows).
螺钉透亮影：另一名患者的冠状位CT显示双侧S_1螺钉上方有透亮影(黄箭)。

Two patients with hardware related complications of instrumented lumbar fusion.
2名患者腰椎融合内固定相关的并发症。

- Spinal hardware may fracture, become loose, or may be malpositioned at time of surgery.
- Lucency surrounding the screws may represent loosening.

- 术中脊柱内固定可能会发生折断、松动或移位。
- 螺钉周围出现透亮区有可能为松动。

Adjacent segment degeneration

邻近椎体退变

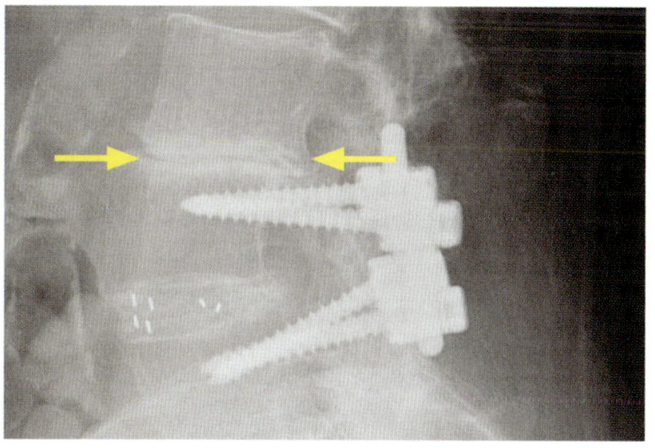

Adjacent segment degeneration: Lateral radiograph shows severe discovertebral degeneration at L3–L4 (arrow), above the fused L4–L5 level. At L3–L4, there is severe disc height loss, subchondral sclerosis, small osteophytes, and retrolisthesis.
邻近椎体退变：侧位X线影像显示L_{3-4}椎间盘椎体严重退变(黄箭)，位于L_{4-5}融合的上方。在L_{3-4}，椎间盘严重压缩、软骨下硬化、小骨赘形成并向后滑脱。

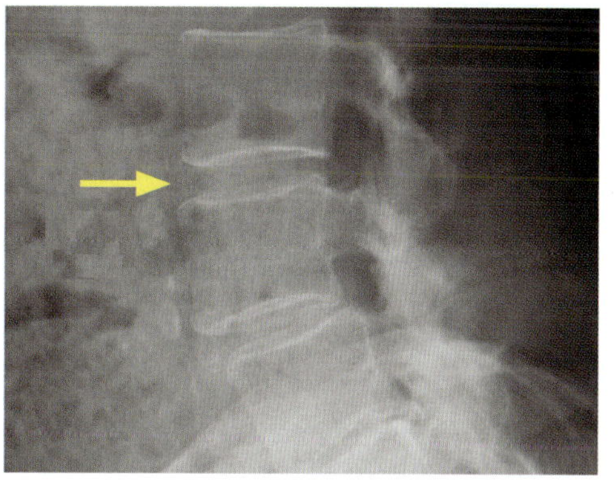

Remote radiograph from 11 years prior shows normal intervertebral disc height at L3–L4 (yellow arrow).
比较11年前侧位X线影像，其L_{3-4}椎间盘的高度正常(黄箭)。

- Adjacent segment degeneration occurs when the level above or below the fused level undergoes degenerative change.
- Adjacent segment degeneration is said to occur at a rate of approximately 3% chance per year.
- Patients with decreased quality of paraspinal muscles are at increased risk for adjacent segment degeneration.

- 当融合椎体的上或下椎体发生退变时，其邻近的椎体也会发生退变。
- 邻近椎体退变的年发生率约为3%。
- 患者脊柱旁肌肉量减少增加了邻近椎体退变的风险。

Recurrent disc herniation

复发性椎间盘疝

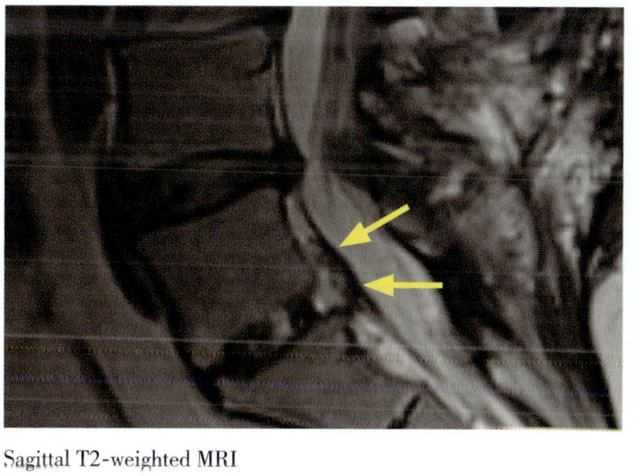

Sagittal T2-weighted MRI
矢状位T_2加权MRI

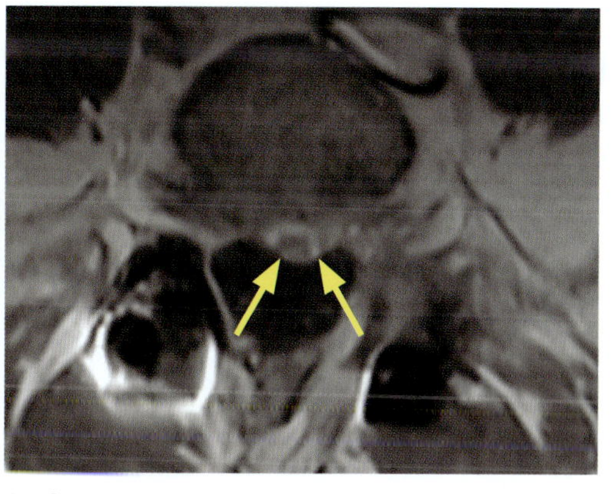

Axial post-contrast T1-weighted MRI
轴位增强T_1加权MRI

Recurrent disc herniation: MRI demonstrates a heterogeneous signal intensity, predominantly T2 hyperintense disc protrusion at L5–S1 (arrows). Post-contrast MRI confirms that this protrusion enhances peripherally (arrows), confirming recurrent disc herniation rather than scar or granulation tissue.
复发性椎间盘疝：MRI显示L_5~S_1椎间盘突出，信号不均匀，主要为T_2高信号(黄箭)。增强MRI证实此突出处周边强化(箭)，确认为椎间盘疝复发，而不是瘢痕或肉芽组织。

- In a patient with recurrent pain after decompressive surgery, an intravenous contrast-enhanced MRI can help differentiate between recurrent disc herniation (which may be treated surgically) versus scar and granulation tissue.
- A recurrent disc would not enhance, or would enhance only peripherally.
- Scar tissue and granulation tissue usually enhance homogeneously.

- 对于减压术后疼痛复发的患者，静脉对比增强MRI可以帮助区分椎间盘疝复发(可通过外科治疗)与瘢痕或肉芽组织。
- 复发性疝的椎间盘不强化，或仅有边缘强化。
- 肉芽组织和瘢痕通常表现为均匀强化。

(翻译　卞益同)

13 Musculoskeletal Imaging

Yuntong Ma, Jacob Mandell

13 骨骼与肌肉影像

Contents

目录

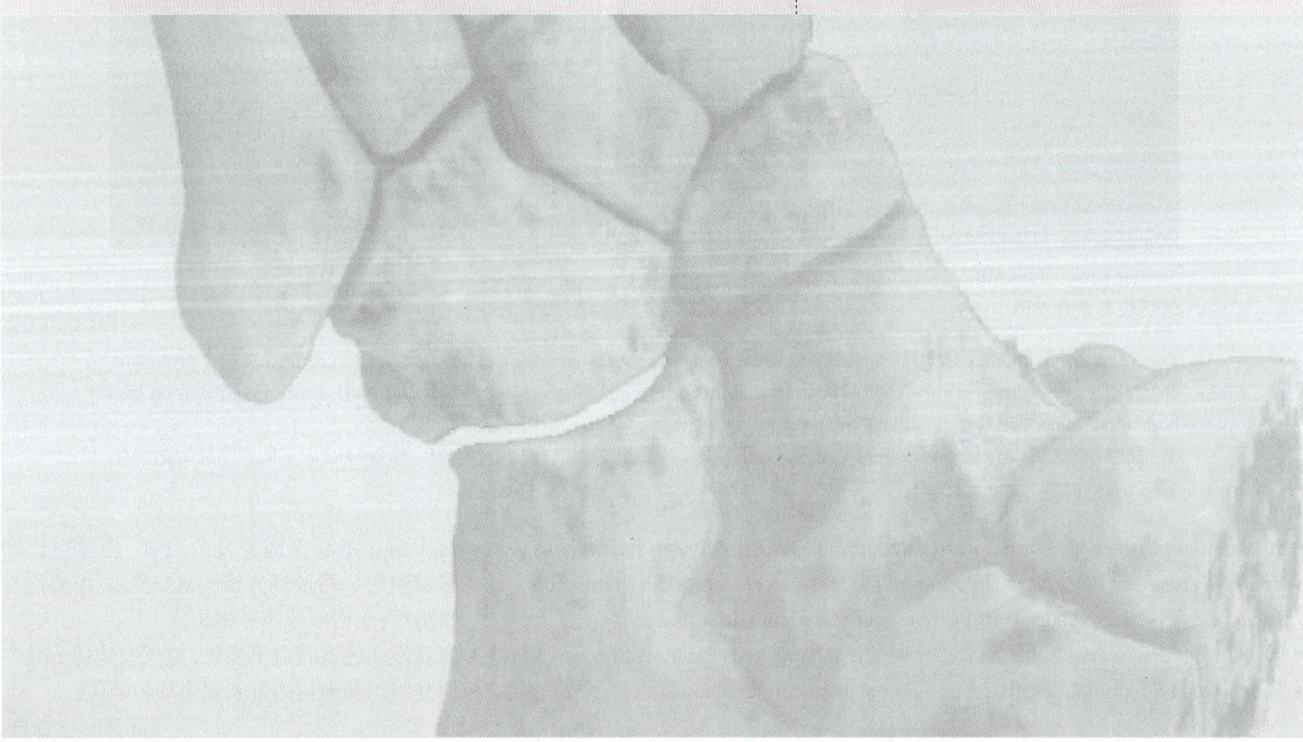

BASICS OF BONES AND JOINTS

骨骼和关节基础

STRUCTURE OF BONE

骨骼结构

Macroscopic anatomy

大体解剖

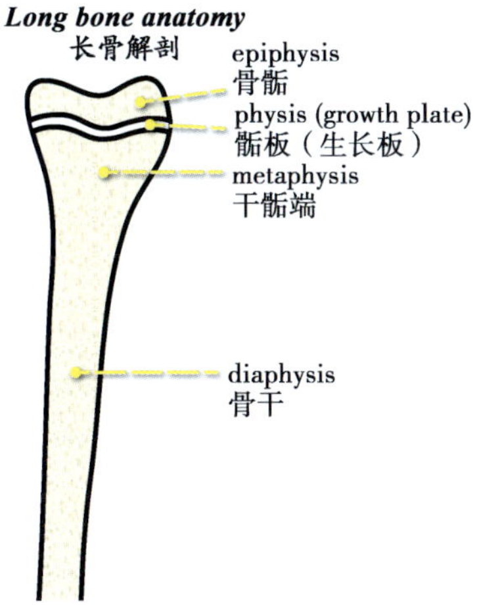

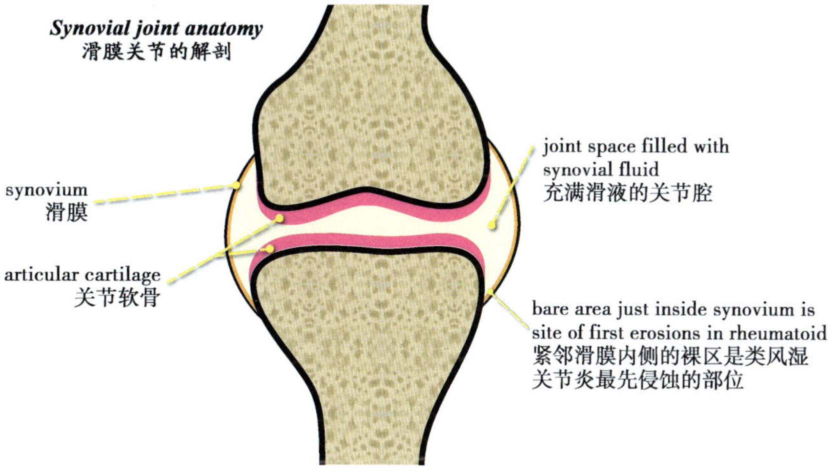

Microscopic anatomy

微观解剖

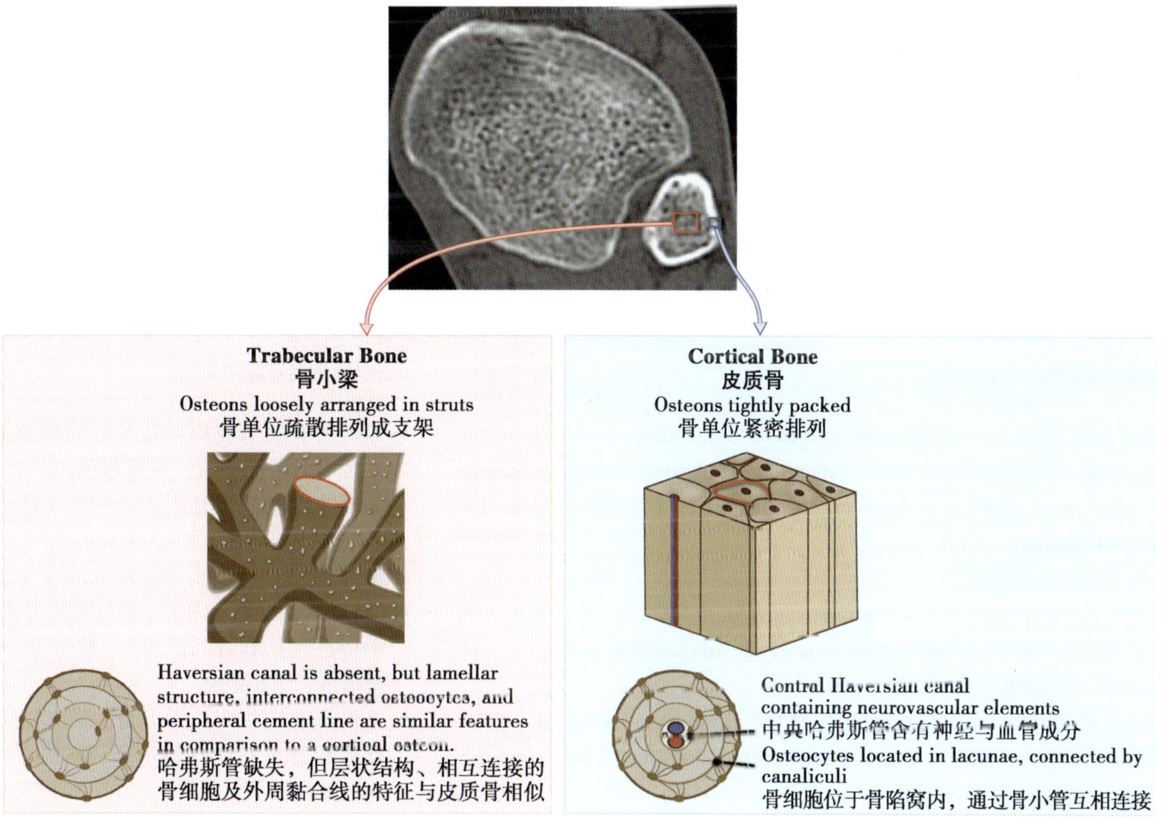

- The two main structural components of bone are cortical bone and trabecular bone. Both provide rigid support for the muscular system to allow locomotion and movement.
- Cortical bone is the thick outer shell of bone and trabecular bone is located centrally, where it is filled with marrow elements.

- 骨的两个主要组成部分为皮质骨和松质骨。两者都为肌肉系统提供了牢固的支撑，以实现运动和移动功能。
- 皮质骨是骨的厚外壳，而松质骨位于骨的中央，后者充满了骨髓。

（翻译　姚骊　吕霞飞）

Arthritis

- The hallmark of arthritis is cartilage destruction, which may be evident on radiographs as joint space narrowing.
- In broad categories, arthritis can be divided into degenerative (osteoarthritis), inflammatory (rheumatoid arthritis, spondyloarthropathies, and juvenile idiopathic arthritis), crystal deposition (gout, calcium pyrophosphate dihydrate, and hydroxyapatite), hematologic (hemophilia), and metabolic categories.

Osteoarthritis (OA)

Overview of osteoarthritis

- Osteoarthritis (OA) is the result of articular cartilage breakdown from altered local mechanical factors in a susceptible individual. In addition to cartilage, OA involves the entire joint including bone, ligaments, menisci, joint capsule, synovium, and musculature.
- OA is the most common cause of cartilage loss in the middle-aged and older population.
- OA typically occurs in weight-bearing joints and the hands in a specific distribution.
- When OA is present in younger patients or in unusual locations, such as the shoulder, elbow, or ankle, then there is usually prior trauma or other underlying arthritis.
- Imaging findings of osteoarthritis:

Radiograph and CT findings	*MRI findings*
Osteophytes. **Subchondral cystic change**, due to herniation of joint fluid into bone through a cartilage defect. **Sclerosis of subchondral bone**, due to reactive remodeling. **Lack of periarticular osteopenia.**	**Osteophytes.** **Subchondral cystic change.** **Subchondral edema**, due to inflammatory and reactive changes. **Synovitis**, with thickened, irregular, and hyperenhancing synovium.

- Although joint space narrowing is present in all arthritides, osteoarthritis can be diagnosed with confidence when subchondral sclerosis, osteophytes, and subchondral cystic changes are present, erosions are absent, and periarticular osteopenia is absent.

Osteoarthritis in the hand

- Similar to osteoarthritis of other joints, the radiographic hallmarks of OA in the hand include cartilage space narrowing, subchondral sclerosis, and osteophytosis. Erosions are absent.
- In order of decreasing involvement, sites of OA in the hand include the distal interphalangeal joints (DIPs), the first carpometacarpal joint (CMC), and the proximal interphalangeal joints (PIPs).
- Unlike rheumatoid arthritis, the metacarpophalangeal joints (MCPs) are less commonly affected.
- Large osteophytes cause characteristic soft-tissue swelling surrounding the finger joints.

  A **Heberden** node is soft-tissue swelling around the DIP.

  A **Bouchard** node is soft-tissue swelling around the PIP.

关节炎

- 关节炎的标志是软骨破坏，在X线影像上表现为关节间隙狭窄。
- 从广义的角度考虑，关节炎可分为退行性(骨关节炎)、炎性(类风湿关节炎、脊柱关节病和青少年特发性关节炎)、晶体沉积(痛风、焦磷酸钙、羟基磷灰石)、血液性(血友病)及代谢性疾病等类别。

骨关节炎(OA)

骨关节炎概述

- 骨关节炎(OA)是由于易感个体因局部机械因素改变而导致的关节软骨破坏。除了软骨，OA累及整个关节，包括骨、韧带、半月板、关节囊、滑膜及肌肉组织。
- OA是中、老年人群软骨缺损最常见的原因。
- OA通常发生在负重关节及特定的手部关节。
- 当OA出现在青少年或不常见部位时，如肩、肘或踝关节，则通常有既往创伤或其他潜在的关节炎。
- OA的影像学表现：

X线和CT表现	MRI表现
骨赘形成。 **软骨下囊变**，由关节积液通过软骨缺损进入骨质所致。 **软骨下骨硬化**，由反应性重塑所致。 **无关节周围骨量减少**。	**骨赘形成**。 **软骨下囊变**。 **软骨下水肿**，由炎性和反应性改变所致。 **滑膜炎**，表现为滑膜增厚、不规则并明显强化。

- 尽管所有关节炎均存在关节间隙狭窄，但当发现有软骨下硬化、骨赘形成、软骨下囊变、无侵蚀及关节周围骨量减少时可明确诊断骨关节炎。

手部骨关节炎

- 与其他关节的OA相似，手的骨关节炎的影像学特性包括软骨间隙狭窄、软骨下硬化及骨赘形成，但无侵蚀。
- 按累及递减的顺序，手的骨关节炎发病部位包括远端指间关节(DIPs)、第一腕掌关节(CMC)和近端指间关节(PIPs)。
- 与类风湿关节炎不同，掌指关节(MCPs)受累不太常见。
- 大的骨赘可引起具有特征性的手指关节周围软组织肿胀。

  赫伯登结节是远端指间关节周围软组织肿胀。

  布夏尔结节是近端指间关节周围软组织肿胀。

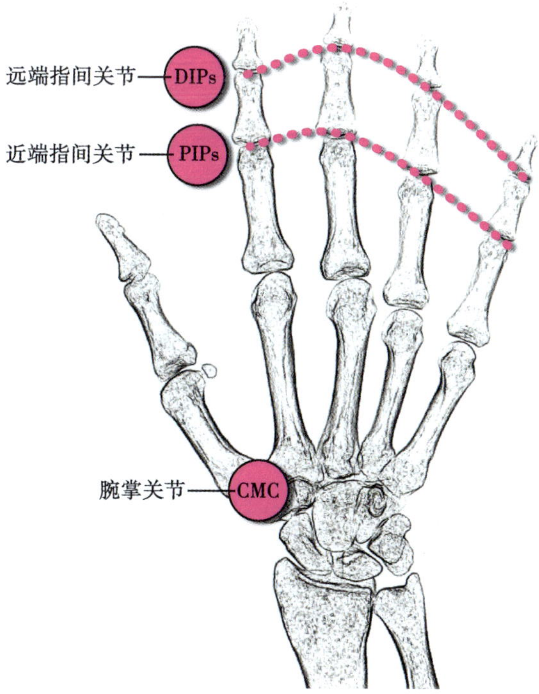

Erosive osteoarthritis of the hands

- Typically affects elderly females, erosive OA combines the clinical findings of rheumatoid arthritis (e.g., swelling) with imaging findings and distribution that are more similar to conventional OA.
- Erosions are the distinguishing imaging feature to differentiate erosive from conventional OA. The distribution of erosive OA is limited to the hands, where it most commonly involves the DIPs.
- Erosive OA features a characteristic *gull-wing* appearance of the DIP joint due to central erosion and marginal osteophytes.

手部侵蚀性骨关节炎

- 通常发生于老年女性。侵蚀性骨关节炎有类风湿关节炎的临床表现(如肿胀)，其影像学表现和分布与普通OA类似。
- 侵蚀是区分侵蚀性骨关节炎和常规骨关节炎的特征影像学特征。侵蚀性骨关节炎的分布仅限于手部，最常累及的是远端指间关节。
- 侵蚀性骨关节炎具有远端指间关节特征性的鸥翼样表现，为中央侵蚀和边缘骨赘所致。

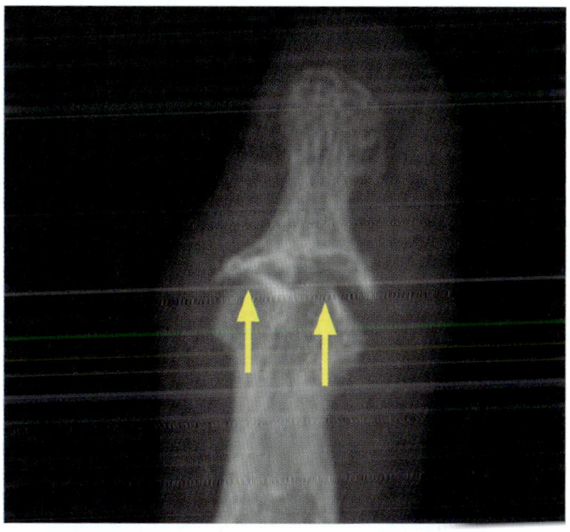

Erosive osteoarthritis: Magnified radiograph of a digit demonstrates characteristic *gull-wing* appearance of the DIP (yellow arrows).
侵蚀性骨关节炎：放大的指骨X线影像显示远端指间关节呈特征性的鸥翼样改变(黄箭)。

Osteoarthritis in the shoulder

- The Grashey view (obtained posteriorly in 40° obliqued external rotation) shows the glenohumeral joint in profile and best demonstrates cartilage space narrowing.

Osteoarthritis in the foot

- The most common joint affected by OA in the foot is the metatarsophalangeal joint (MTP) of the great toe, which may lead to hallux rigidus (a stiff big toe).
- Osteoarthritis also affects the talonavicular joint and is a cause of dorsal beaking.

肩部骨关节炎

- Grashey位(40°倾斜外旋从后方拍摄)显示盂肱关节的轮廓并最佳显示软骨间隙狭窄。

足部骨关节炎

- 在足部，OA最常累及的关节是大踇趾的跖趾关节(MTP)，可导致踇趾僵硬(大脚趾僵硬)。
- 骨关节炎也可侵犯距舟关节，是引起足背鸟嘴样突起的原因之一。

Osteoarthritis in the knee

膝部骨关节炎

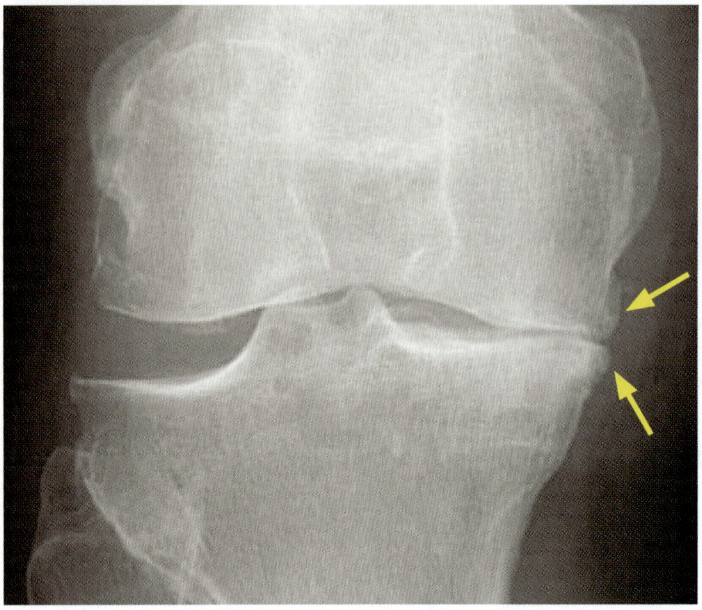

Osteoarthritis: Standing frontal radiograph of the knee shows severe cartilage space narrowing, sclerosis, and osteophytosis of the medial tibiofemoral compartment (arrows).

骨关节炎：膝关节站立正位X线影像显示内侧胫股关节严重软骨间隙狭窄、骨质硬化和骨赘形成(箭)。

- There are three joint compartments in the knee: The medial and lateral tibiofemoral compartments and the patellofemoral compartment. The typical pattern for OA of the knee is asymmetrical involvement of the medial tibiofemoral compartment. Severe osteoarthritis can involve all three compartments.
- Osteophytes determine if OA is present. The degree of joint space narrowing determines the severity of OA.
- The degree of tibiofemoral cartilage space narrowing is best determined on standing weight-bearing views, often on standing films in slight flexion.
- Bilateral involvement of the knees is typical.

- 膝关节有3个间室：内、外侧胫股间室及髌股间室。典型的膝关节OA是非对称性内侧胫股间室受侵。严重的OA可累及所有间室。
- 骨赘决定是否有OA。关节间隙的狭窄程度决定OA的严重程度。
- 评价胫股软骨间隙的狭窄程度最好采用站立负重位，常用微屈曲站立位进行拍摄。
- 双侧膝关节受累常见。

Osteoarthritis in the hip

髋部骨关节炎

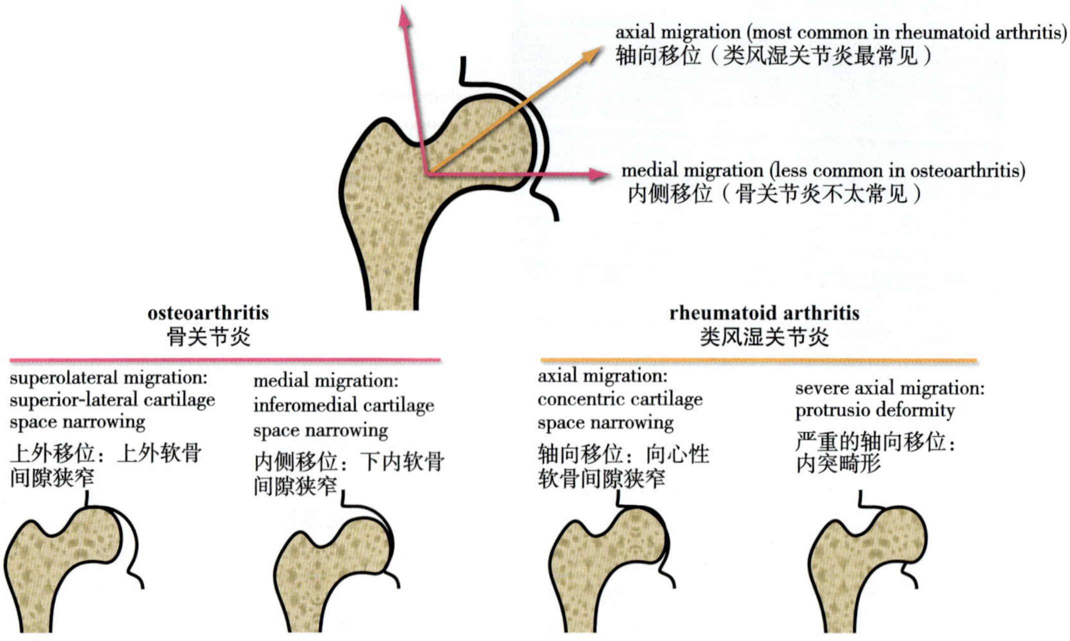

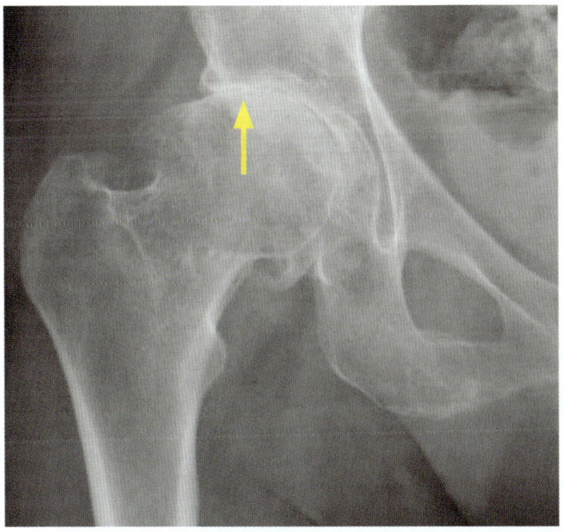

Superolateral cartilage space narrowing (most common pattern in hip OA): Frontal radiograph of the right hip shows severe superolateral cartilage space narrowing (arrow) with large osteophytes.

上外侧软骨间隙狭窄(最常见于髋部OA)：右髋正位X线影像显示重度外上软骨间隙狭窄(箭)伴大骨赘。

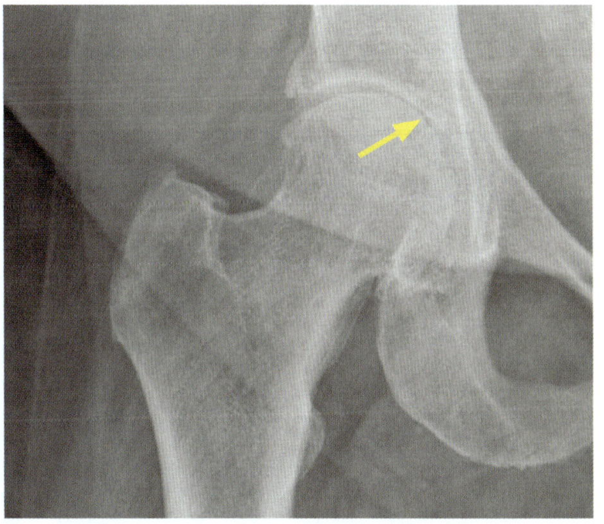

Medial cartilage space narrowing (less common): Frontal radiograph of the right hip in a different patient demonstrates moderate-to-severe medial cartilage space narrowing (arrow) with small osteophytes.

内侧软骨间隙狭窄(较少见)：另一名患者右髋正位X线影像显示中-重度内侧软骨间隙狭窄(箭)伴小骨赘。

- Similar to the knee, the involvement of hip osteoarthritis tends to be bilateral.
- In addition to the typical features of OA including joint space narrowing, osteophytes, subchondral cystic change, and sclerosis, hip OA also features characteristic superolateral cartilage space narrowing. Less commonly, medial or axial (concentric) cartilage space loss can be seen in hip OA.
- Note that axial cartilage space loss is the typical pattern in rheumatoid arthritis; however, since osteoarthritis is far more common than rheumatoid arthritis, axial cartilage space narrowing with osteophytes is more likely to represent osteoarthritis rather than rheumatoid arthritis. If axial cartilage space loss is seen without osteophytes, rheumatoid arthritis is more likely.

Degenerative change in the spine

- The vertebral body-disc articulations are cartilaginous joints. Vertebral body endplates are covered by hyaline cartilage that is analogous to articular cartilage in other joints. The intervertebral disc-endplate complex is composed of three components: The annulus fibrosus and nucleus pulposus (which together make up the disc), and the cartilaginous endplates.
- Osteoarthritis affects synovial joints. Therefore, osteoarthritis in the spine can occur at the facet (zygapophyseal), atlantoaxial, uncovertebral joints (in the cervical spine at C3-C7), costovertebral, and sacroiliac joints. Osteoarthritis does not involve the disc-endplates.
- The spectrum of intervertebral disc and endplate degeneration is characterized by dessication and eventual collapse of the intervertebral discs, endplate sclerosis and remodeling, and osteophyte formation. This process is best thought of as a chronic response to injury, rather than an acquired disease, and the term *discovertebral degeneration* is more accurate than the informal phrase *degenerative disc disease*. Detailed MR-based discussion of degenerative spine can be found in the "Spine" chapter.
- Gas in the intervertebral disc, also called *vacuum phenomenon*, is commonly seen and is pathognomonic for degenerative change.

- 与膝关节相似，髋部骨关节炎通常也倾向于双侧受累。
- 除了具备OA的典型表现，如关节间隙狭窄、骨赘形成、软骨下囊变和硬化之外，髋部OA还表现出特征性的外上方软骨间隙狭窄。其次，髋部OA还可见内侧或轴向(向心性)软骨间隙变窄。
- 注意，轴向软骨间隙消失是类风湿关节炎的典型表现；然而，鉴于骨关节炎远比类风湿关节炎常见，因此伴有骨赘的轴向软骨间隙狭窄更可能是骨关节炎而非类风湿关节炎。若轴向软骨间隙变窄而不伴有骨赘形成，则更有可能是类风湿关节炎。

脊柱退行性变

- 椎体-椎间盘关节是软骨性关节。椎体终板由透明软骨覆盖，类似于其他关节的关节软骨。椎间盘-终板复合体由三个部分组成：纤维环和髓核(共同组成椎间盘)，以及软骨终板。
- 骨关节炎侵犯滑膜关节。因此，脊柱骨关节炎可发生于椎小关节(关节突)、寰枢关节、钩椎关节($C_{3\sim7}$)、肋椎关节及骶髂关节。骨关节炎不累及椎间盘-终板。
- 各种椎间盘及终板退行性变的特征包括椎间盘脱水及最终塌陷、终板硬化及重塑，以及骨赘形成。该过程最好认为是对损伤的慢性反应，而非获得性病变，并且术语椎间盘退行性变较非正式短语退行性椎间盘病更准确。有关脊柱退变相关的详细MR相关讨论请见“脊柱影像”章节。
- 椎间盘内气体，也称真空现象，很常见且对退行性病变具有病理确诊的意义。

It is important not to confuse vacuum phenomenon (gas in intervertebral *disc*) with Kümmell disease, which is gas in a vertebral *body* compression fracture representing osteonecrosis.

不要将椎间盘真空现象(椎间盘内气体)与创伤性脊柱病(Kümmel病)混淆，后者为压缩性骨折的椎体内气体，代表骨坏死。

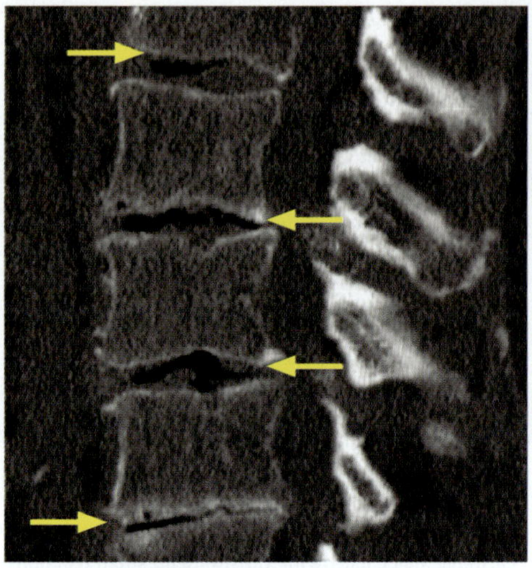

Vacuum phenomenon in disc degeneration.
椎间盘退行性变的**真空现象**。

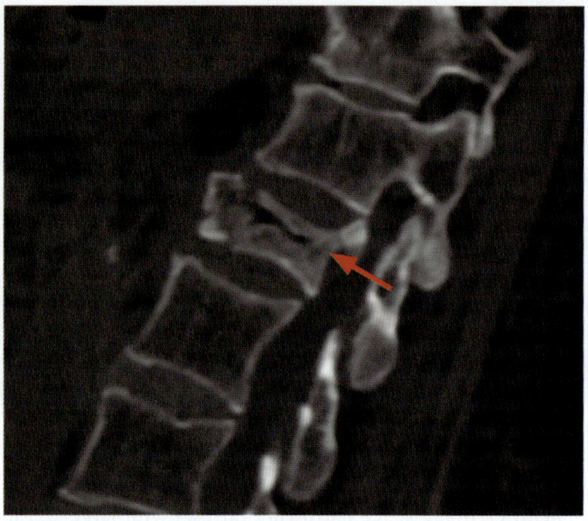

Kümmell disease: Gas in vertebral body compression fracture.
Kümmell病：压缩性骨折的椎体内气体。

Two patients demonstrating vacuum phenomenon versus Kümmell disease.
Sagittal CT of the lumbar spine (left image) shows multilevel disc degeneration with intervertebral disc space narrowing and vacuum phenomena (yellow arrows).
Sagittal CT of the lumbar spine in a different patient (right image) shows gas within the L1 vertebral body compression fracture (red arrow), indicative of osteonecrosis/vertebral body collapse (Kümmell disease).
显示2名患者的真空现象和Kümmell病。
腰椎矢状位CT(左图)显示多节段椎间盘退行性变伴椎间隙狭窄和真空现象(黄箭)。
另一名患者腰椎矢状位CT(右图)显示气体位于压缩性骨折的L_1椎体内(红箭)，提示骨坏死/椎体塌陷(Kümmell病)。

- Complications of discovertebral degeneration include spinal stenosis, neural foraminal stenosis, and degenerative spondylolisthesis.
- **Diffuse idiopathic skeletal hyperostosis (DISH)** is a distinct entity from degenerative disc disease, but appears similar due to exuberant osteophytosis. DISH is defined as flowing bridging anterior osteophytes spanning at least 4 vertebral levels, with normal disc spaces and sacroiliac joints. The etiology of DISH is unknown. It is usually asymptomatic but may be a cause of dysphagia when it affects the cervical spine. DISH occurs in elderly patients.

DISH is associated with **ossification of the posterior longitudinal ligament (OPLL)**, which may be a cause of spinal stenosis. OPLL may be difficult to identify on MRI and is best seen on CT.

- 椎间盘退行性变的并发症包括椎管狭窄、神经孔狭窄，以及退变性脊椎滑脱。
- **弥漫性特发性骨肥厚(DISH)**是一个与退行性椎间盘病完全不同的疾病，但由于明显的骨赘形成，而使两者的表现类似。DISH定义为椎体前方的骨赘融合并跨越至少四个椎体，而椎间隙和骶髂关节正常。DISH的病因不明。通常无症状，但颈椎受累时可以导致吞咽困难。DISH发生在老年患者。

DISH合并有**后纵韧带骨化(OPLL)**，可以造成椎管狭窄。后纵韧带骨化在MRI上可能难以发现，CT显示最佳。

Rheumatoid arthritis (RA)

类风湿关节炎(RA)

Overview of rheumatoid arthritis

- Rheumatoid arthritis (RA) is an autoimmune disorder where the synovium is the target of a waxing and waning immune response. Rheumatoid factor (RF) is typically positive, although it is not specific. RF is an antibody directed against IgG, which activates the complement cascade. RA clinically presents with **symmetrical** joint pain, swelling, and morning stiffness.
- RA first affects the small joints in the hands and wrists. Foot involvement may occur early, so foot radiographs are routinely obtained in suspected cases of RA. In more advanced cases, RA affects the cervical spine, knees, shoulders, and hips.

类风湿关节炎概述

- 类风湿关节炎(RA)是一种自身免疫性疾病，它以滑膜为靶器官，并随免疫反应消长而改变。类风湿因子(RF)常为阳性，但并不特异。RF是抗IgG抗体，可激活补体系统。RA的临床表现为**对称性**关节疼痛、肿胀和晨僵。
- RA最先侵犯手和腕部的小关节。足的受累发生较早，因此疑似RA的病例应常规进行足部X线影像检查。在较晚期的病例，RA可累及颈椎、膝关节、肩关节和髋关节。

- Erosions are the imaging and pathologic hallmarks of RA, representing focal destruction of bone due to cumulative inflammatory damage. Erosions have been postulated to occur both due to the osteolytic interaction of synovial inflammation with articular cartilage (the "outside-in" theory) and destructive effect of inflammation within the bone (the "inside-out" theory). Half of RA patients develop erosions after one year of symptoms, and the development of erosions is associated with increased disability and decreased quality of life.
- The imaging findings of RA include:

Radiograph and CT findings	*MRI findings*
Marginal erosions, which first occur at the intracapsular articular margins in the "bare area." The bare area is a region of exposed bone just within the joint capsule that is not covered by thick cartilage. **Soft-tissue swelling**. **Diffuse, symmetric joint space narrowing**. **Periarticular osteopenia**. **Joint subluxations**.	**Marginal erosions,** which are fluid signal intensity and enhance. **Synovitis,** with thickened and early enhancing synovium. **Subchondral edema**, due to inflammatory and reactive changes. **Joint subluxations**.

Rheumatoid arthritis in the hand and wrist

- The hands are commonly affected in patients with RA.
- Typical joints involved are the MCPs, PIPs, and the carpal articulations. The DIPs are usually spared.
- The earliest radiographic changes of RA are soft-tissue swelling and periarticular osteopenia, reflecting synovitis and hyperemia.
- Erosions occur early in disease, typically of the radial aspects of the second and third metacarpal heads, the radial and ulnar aspects of the bases of the proximal phalanges, and the ulnar styloid.
- Joint subluxations are present in more advanced disease, which typically are not reducible and lead to several common deformities, including:

  Boutonnière deformity (PIP flexion and DIP hyperextension).

  Swan neck deformity (PIP hyperextension and DIP flexion).

  Ulnar subluxation of the fingers at the MCPs.

- 侵蚀是RA的影像学和病理学特征，代表了由于累积性炎性损伤所致的局灶性骨质破坏。侵蚀被认为是滑膜炎症与关节软骨的溶骨性交互作用（"由外而内"理论）及骨内炎症的破坏性影响（"由内而外"理论）共同所致。一半的RA患者在有症状后一年会出现侵蚀，且随着侵蚀的发展，其伤残度升高和生活质量下降。
- RA的影像学表现包括：

X线和CT表现	MRI表现
边缘侵蚀，最早发生在关节囊内关节边缘的"裸区"。裸区是关节囊内暴露的骨区，没有厚的软骨覆盖。 **软组织肿胀**。 **广泛性对称性关节间隙狭窄**。 **关节周围骨量减少**。 **关节半脱位**。	**边缘侵蚀**，呈液体信号强度并强化。 **滑膜炎**，呈增厚并早期强化的滑膜。 **软骨下水肿**，由炎性和反应性改变所致。 **关节半脱位**。

手和腕部类风湿关节炎

- 手是RA患者常见的受累部位。
- 典型的受累关节为掌指关节(MCPs)、近端指间关节(PIPs)和腕关节。远端指间关节(DIPs)通常不受累。
- RA最早的X线影像改变是软组织肿胀和关节周围骨量减少，反映了滑膜炎和充血。
- 侵蚀发生在疾病早期，常见于第二、三掌骨头的桡侧、近端指骨基底部的桡侧和尺侧，以及尺骨茎突。
- 关节半脱位发生在疾病较晚期，通常不能复位并导致一些常见畸形，包括：

  Boutonnière畸形(近端指间关节屈曲和远端指间关节过伸)。

  鹅颈畸形(近端指间关节的过伸及远端指间关节屈曲)。

  掌指关节(MCPs)指骨的尺侧半脱位。

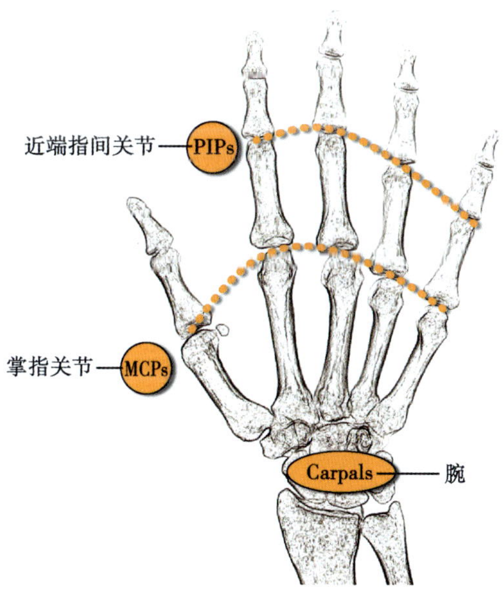

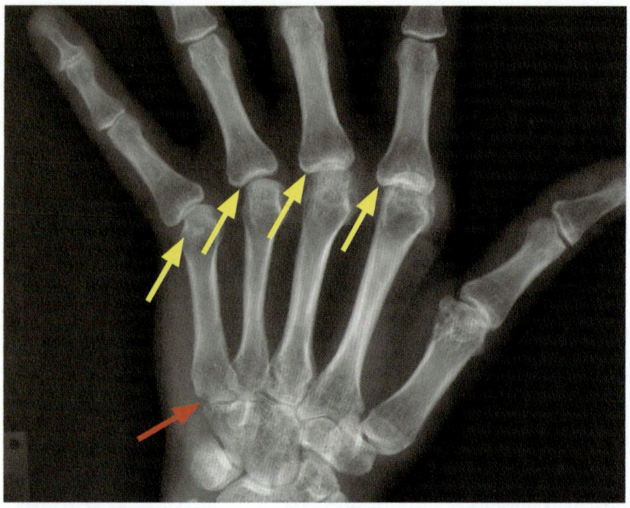

RA: PA hand radiograph shows ulnar deviation of the second through fifth fingers at the MCPs, with diffuse MCP joint space narrowing (arrows). There is periarticular osteopenia. A fifth carpometacarpal joint erosion (red arrow) is better seen on the magnified image to the right.

RA：手后前位X线影像显示第二~五掌指关节指骨向尺侧偏斜伴弥漫性掌指关节间隙狭窄(黄箭)。可见关节周围骨量减少。第五腕掌关节的骨质侵蚀在右图放大后显示更清晰(红箭)。

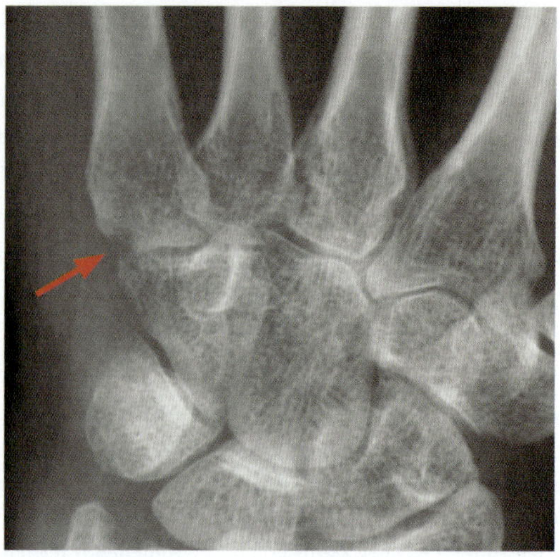

Close up of the same image better shows the erosion across the fifth carpometacarpal joint (red arrow).

同一幅图像放大后更好地显示了跨第五腕掌关节的骨侵蚀(红箭)。

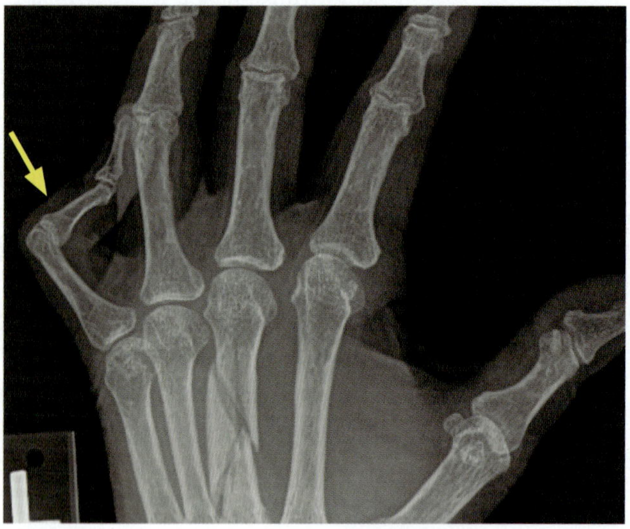

Boutonnière deformity (PIP flexion (arrow) and DIP hyperextension), which can be caused by inflammation or trauma to the extensor tendon. Satisfaction of search: There is a third metacarpal fracture!

Boutonnière畸形[近端指间关节屈曲(箭)和远端指间关节过伸]，可因伸肌腱炎症或创伤所致。阅片者最初只关注第三掌骨骨折而遗漏了Boutonnière畸形。

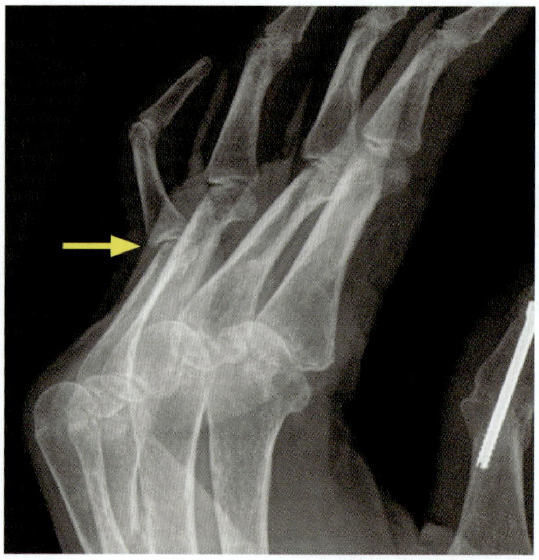

Different patient with *swan neck* deformity (PIP hyperextension (arrow) and DIP flexion), which can be caused by inflammation or trauma to the flexor tendon or volar plate.

另一名患者的鹅颈畸形[近端指间关节的过伸(箭)及远端指间关节屈曲]，可因屈肌腱或掌板的炎症或创伤所致。

- Late-stage RA may uncommonly cause ankylosis (fibrosseous joint fusion occurring after complete cartilage loss) of the wrist. Juvenile idiopathic arthritis (discussed later), in contrast, has a higher propensity for carpal ankylosis.

- 晚期RA偶尔可发生腕关节强直(软骨完全破坏之后出现纤维-骨性关节融合)。与之相比，青少年特发性关节炎(后文讨论)更易发生腕关节强直。

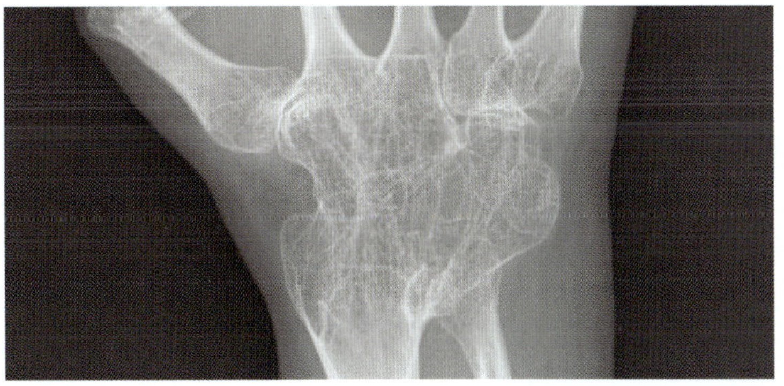

Frontal radiograph of the wrist in a patient with severe longstanding RA shows severe periarticular osteopenia and pan-carpal ankylosis with osseous fusion across the radiocarpal, intercarpal, and second and third carpometacarpal joints.
严重的长期RA患者腕部正位X线影像显示重度关节周围骨量减少和广泛关节骨性强直，累及桡腕关节、腕骨间关节及第二、三腕掌关节。

Rheumatoid arthritis in the feet

- The feet are commonly involved in RA. Typically, the metatarsophalangeal (MTP) joints in the forefoot and the talocalcaneonavicular joint in the midfoot are involved. Up to 20% of patients have the MTP joint as the first site of involvement.

Rheumatoid arthritis in the hip

- Rheumatoid arthritis causes concentric acetabular cartilage loss which leads to axial migration of the femoral head. In contrast, osteoarthritis more commonly causes superior acetabular cartilage space narrowing and superolateral femoral head migration.
- In severe cases, RA may cause a **protrusio deformity**, which is defined as >3 mm medial deviation of the femoral head beyond the ilioischial line in males and >6 mm in females.

足部类风湿关节炎

- RA常累及足部。典型的发病部位为前足的跖趾关节(MTP)和中足的距跟舟关节。高达20%患者的首发部位为跖趾关节。

髋部类风湿关节炎

- 类风湿关节炎引起向心性髋臼软骨缺损，导致股骨头轴向移位。与之相比，骨关节炎常导致髋臼上部软骨间隙狭窄和股骨头外上方移位。
- 在严重病例，RA可导致**内突畸形**，其定义为男性股骨头向内越过髂坐线>3mm，女性>6mm。

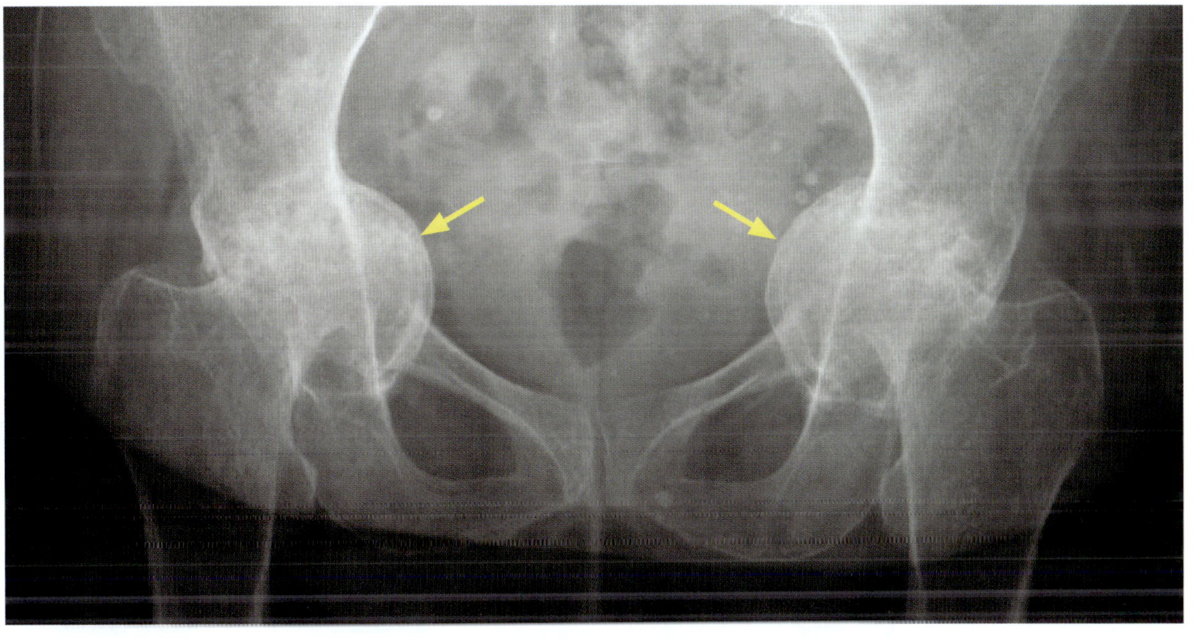

Rheumatoid arthritis with severe hip protrusio: Frontal radiograph of the pelvis shows bilateral severe axial cartilage space narrowing, with prominent acetabular protrusio deformities (arrows).
类风湿关节炎伴重度髋关节突出：骨盆正位X线影像显示双侧严重的轴向软骨间隙狭窄伴显著的髋臼突出畸形(箭)。

Rheumatoid arthritis in the knee

- All three joint spaces (medial and lateral tibiofemoral and patellofemoral) may be affected by RA in the knee. In contrast, OA tends to first affect the medial tibiofemoral articulation. If osteophytes *and* symmetrical cartilage space narrowing are present, then secondary osteoarthritis should be considered.
- Unlike the smaller joints affected by rheumatoid arthritis, erosions are not a prominent manifestation of rheumatoid arthritis of the knee.

膝部类风湿关节炎

- 膝关节的三个关节间室(内、外侧胫股及髌股关节间室)在RA时均可受累。相比之下，骨关节炎倾向于最先累及内侧胫股关节。如有骨赘形成和出现对称性的软骨间隙狭窄，应考虑继发性骨关节炎。
- 不同于类风湿关节炎中小关节的受累表现，侵蚀不是膝关节类风湿关节炎的突出表现。

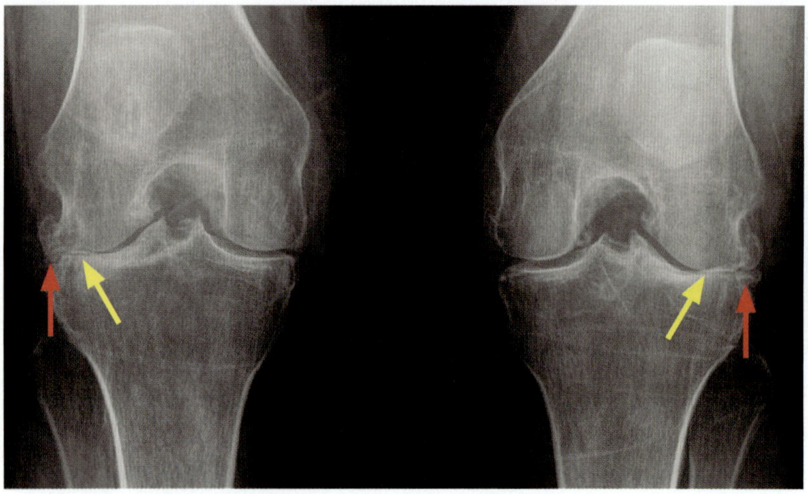

Rheumatoid arthritis with secondary osteoarthritis: Frontal PA weight-bearing view of the knees shows cartilage space narrowing of medial and lateral tibiofemoral articulations bilaterally. The lateral tibiofemoral cartilage spaces are more markedly narrowed (yellow arrows). Prominent osteophytes laterally (red arrows) signify secondary osteoarthritis.
类风湿关节炎伴继发性骨关节炎：双膝关节负重正位X线影像显示双侧内外胫股关节软骨间隙狭窄。外侧胫股关节软骨间隙狭窄更明显(黄箭)。外侧明显的骨赘形成提示继发性骨关节炎(红箭)。

Rheumatoid arthritis in the spine

- The cervical spine is involved in up to 70% of patients. Involvement is increased with more severe and long-standing disease.
- The general pattern of rheumatoid arthritis in the cervical spine includes subluxation at multiple levels, osteopenia, and erosions of the odontoid, facet joints, vertebral endplates, and spinous processes. Unlike osteoarthritis, there is no bone production.
- A characteristic finding of rheumatoid arthritis is **atlantoaxial (C1–C2) subluxation**. Atlantoaxial subluxation may occur in multiple directions, including anterior (most common), posterior, vertical (atlantoaxial impaction), rotatory, and lateral.
- **Anterior atlantoaxial subluxation** is caused by inflammation and resultant laxity of the transverse ligament, which normally functions to stabilize the atlantoaxial joint.

脊柱类风湿关节炎

- 高达70%的患者颈椎受累。受累机会随着严重程度和病程迁延而增加。
- 颈椎类风湿关节炎的常见表现为多个椎体半脱位、骨量减少，以及齿状突、椎小关节、椎体终板和棘突的骨质侵蚀。与骨关节炎不同，类风湿关节炎没有骨质增生。
- 类风湿关节炎的一个特征性表现为**寰枢关节($C_{1\sim2}$)半脱位**。寰枢关节半脱位可发生在多个方向，包括向前(最常见)、向后、垂直(寰枢椎嵌入)、旋转和侧向脱位。
- **前向寰枢关节半脱位**是由炎症及继发的横韧带松弛引起，该韧带起稳定寰枢关节的作用。

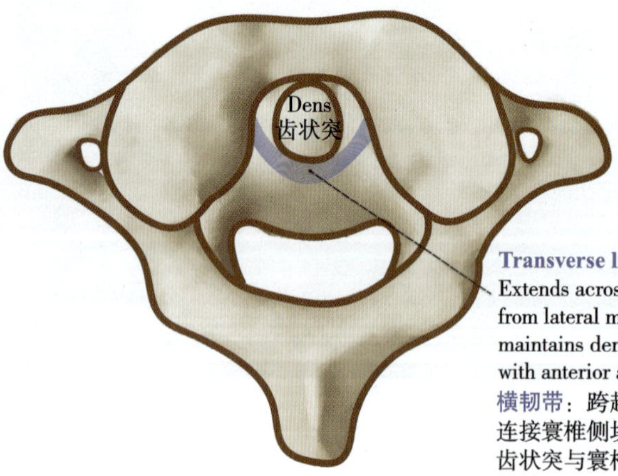

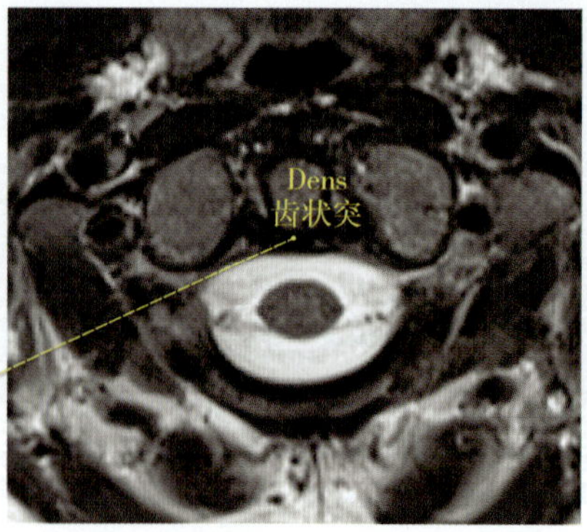

Illustration and T2-weighted axial MRI demonstrating the transverse ligament, which stabilizes the atlantoaxial (C1–C2) articulation between the dens (C2) and C1.
示例图及轴位T_2加权MRI示横韧带，该韧带起稳定齿状突(枢椎)和寰椎之间的寰枢关节($C_{1\sim2}$)的作用。

Anterior atlantoaxial subluxation may not be apparent if flexion radiographs are not obtained.

Anterior atlantoaxial subluxation is present if the atlanto-dental interval (ADI) is >2.5 mm (>5 mm in children). The atlanto-dental interval is the distance between the anterior aspect of the dens and the posterior aspect of the anterior ring of C1.

前向寰枢关节半脱位在非前屈位的X线影像上可能表现不明显。

如果寰齿间距(ADI)>2.5mm(儿童>5mm)，即为前向寰枢关节半脱位。寰齿间距是指齿状突前面到C_1前弓后面的距离。

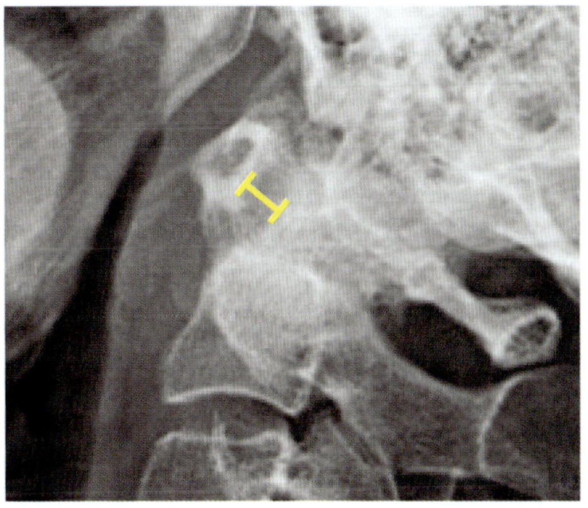

Lateral radiograph of the cervical spine in extension demonstrates the atlanto-dental interval (calipers) measuring less than 2.5 mm.
颈椎过伸位侧位X线影像显示寰齿间距(卡尺)小于2.5mm。

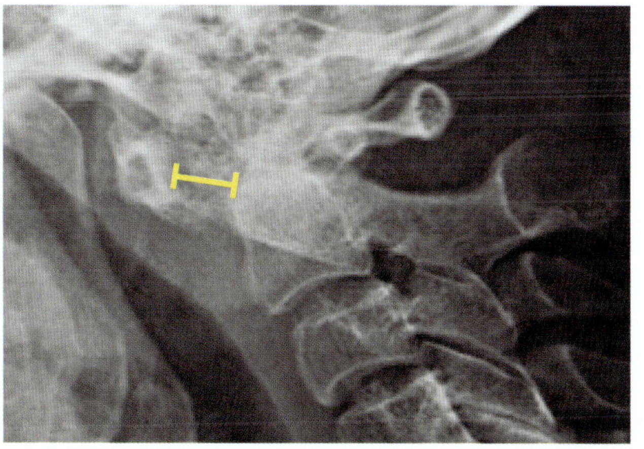

Lateral radiograph of the same patient in flexion demonstrates marked widening of the atlanto-dental interval (calipers), indicating atlanto-axial instability.
同一名患者颈椎过屈位侧位X线影像显示寰齿间距明显增宽(卡尺),提示寰枢关节不稳。

- **Vertical atlantoaxial subluxation** (also called atlantoaxial impaction) results from C1–C2 facet erosion and collapse, leading to protrusion of the odontoid through the foramen magnum. This may compress the midbrain.

  Direct visualization of the odontoid is usually not possible on a lateral radiograph, but impaction may cause the anterior arch of C1 (normally in-line with the odontoid) to sink to the level of the body of C2.
- In the setting of RA, **posterior atlantoaxial subluxation** is usually due to odontoid erosion. It may also be caused by odontoid fracture.

- **垂直寰枢关节半脱位**(也称寰枢椎嵌入)是由$C_{1\sim2}$关节突的骨质侵蚀及塌陷引起,导致齿状突通过枕骨大孔突出。此型半脱位可能压迫中脑。

  在侧位X线影像上通常无法直接观察到齿状突,但寰枢椎嵌入可导致C_1前弓(正常与齿状突持平)下陷到C_2椎体水平。
- 在RA,**后向寰枢关节半脱位**通常是由于齿状突的侵蚀。也可由齿状突骨折引起。

Seronegative spondyloarthropathies

Overview of seronegative spondyloarthropathies

- The seronegative spondyloarthropathies are a group of 4 inflammatory arthropathies, which by definition have negative rheumatoid factor. Patients are usually HLA-B27 positive.
- The 4 seronegative spondyloarthropathies are ankylosing spondylitis, psoriatic arthritis, reactive arthritis (previously called Reiters arthropathy), and inflammatory bowel disease (IBD) associated arthropathy.

Sacroiliitis is a hallmark of the spondyloarthropathies

- Similar to involvement in OA, only the inferior aspect of the sacroiliac (SI) joint is affected in seronegative spondyloarthropathies because only the inferior portion is a synovial (diarthrodial) joint. Erosions first involve the iliac aspect of the SI joint.
- Symmetric sacroiliitis is caused by IBD and ankylosing spondylitis (mnemonic: both start with vowels).

血清阴性脊柱关节病

血清阴性脊柱关节病概述

- 血清阴性脊柱关节病是一组包括4种炎症性关节炎的疾病,其定义为类风湿因子阴性。患者通常为HLA-B27阳性。
- 这4种血清阴性脊柱关节病分别为强直性关节炎、银屑病关节炎、反应性骨关节炎(旧称Reiters关节病)和炎性肠病(IBD)相关性关节病。

骶髂关节炎是脊柱关节病的特征性标志

- 与骨关节炎侵及范围类似,血清阴性脊柱关节病仅侵犯骶髂关节(SI)下部,因为只有下部为滑膜(可动)关节。侵蚀最先累及骶髂关节的髂骨面。
- 对称性的骶髂关节炎可由IBD和强直性脊柱炎所引起(巧记:其英文都以元音字母开头)。

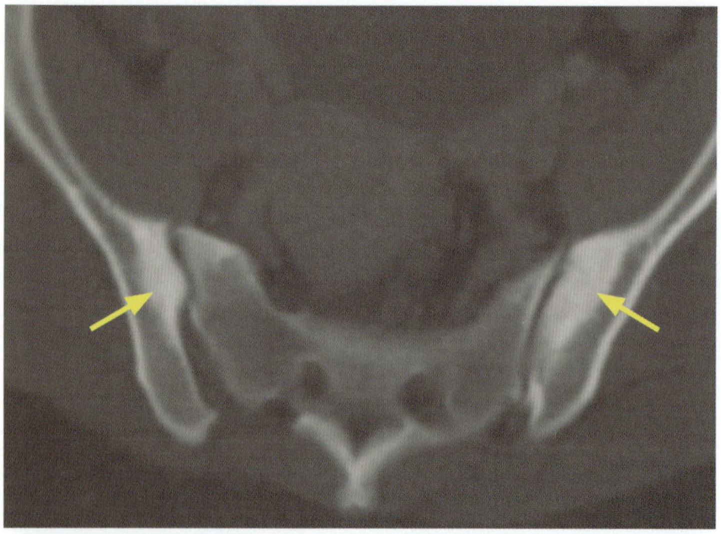

Symmetric sacroiliitis: CT
Axial CT through the pelvis at the level of the sacroiliac joints shows symmetric sclerosis (arrows) at the iliac aspect of the sacroiliac joints bilaterally.
对称性骶髂关节炎：CT
骶髂关节水平骨盆轴位CT显示双侧骶髂关节髂骨面对称性骨质硬化(箭)。

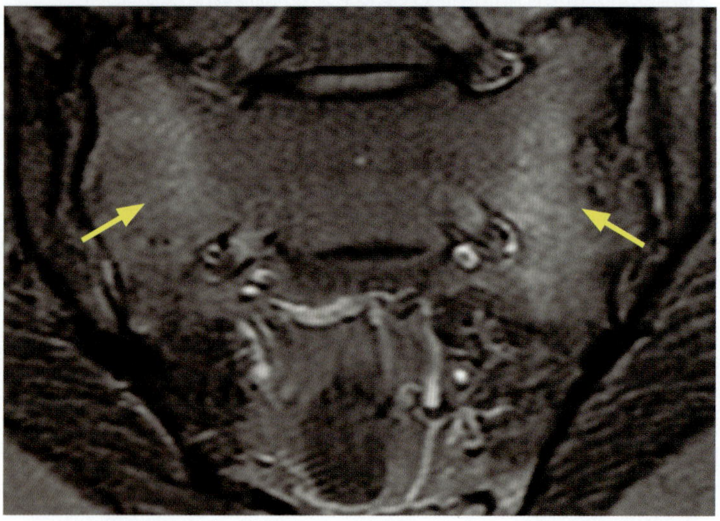

Symmetric sacroiliitis: MRI
Coronal-oblique STIR MRI through the sacroiliac joints demonstrates edema across the sacroiliac joints, predominantly involving the sacrum (yellow arrows).
对称性骶髂关节炎：MRI
经骶髂关节斜冠状位STIR序列MRI显示骶髂关节面下水肿，以骶骨为著(黄箭)。

- Asymmetric sacroiliitis is caused by psoriatic arthritis and reactive arthropathy (mnemonic: both start with consonants).
- An important cause of unilateral sacroiliitis is septic arthritis, especially in an immunocompromised patient or with intravenous drug abuse. Associated abscess may be present, which may be located at the anterior aspect of the sacroiliac joint.

- 非对称性骶髂关节炎则由银屑病关节炎及反应性关节病所致(巧记：其英文都以辅音字母开头)。
- 单侧骶髂关节炎的一个重要原因是化脓性关节炎，尤其是免疫功能不全的患者或静脉吸毒者。可有相应脓肿形成，可见于骶髂关节前份。

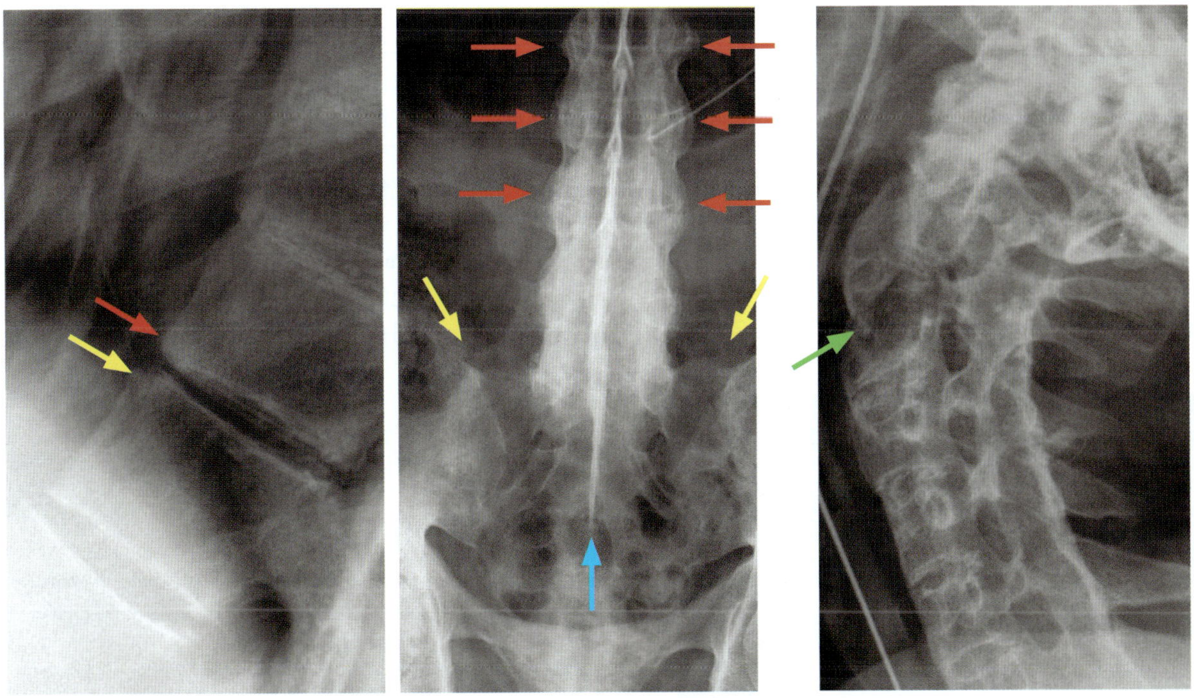

Three patients with ankylosing spondylitis:

Romanus and shiny corner lesions: Lateral radiograph of the upper lumbar spine (left image) shows an erosion of the anterior superior margin of a vertebral body at the discovertebral junction, representing a Romanus lesion (yellow arrow). The superiorly adjacent vertebral body demonstrates sclerosis of its anterior inferior margin, representing the *shiny corner sign* (red arrow). The *shiny corner sign* signifies evolution of a prior Romanus lesion.

Bamboo spine: Frontal radiograph of the sacroiliac joints and lumbar spine (middle image) demonstrates symmetrical sacroiliac joint ankylosis (yellow arrows). There are diffuse syndesmophytes, creating an undulating contour of the spinal column, representing the *bamboo spine* (red arrows). There is fusion of the spinous processes, creating the *dagger sign* (blue arrow).

Cervical fusion: Lateral radiograph of the cervical spine (right image) shows complete ankylosis of cervical spine with fusion of the vertebral bodies and facet joints and a pseudarthrosis at C2–C3 (green arrow).

Cases courtesy Stacy Smith, MD, Brigham and Women's Hospital.

3名强直性脊柱炎患者：

Romanus(椎角炎)和“亮角”病变：上段腰椎的侧位X线影像(左图)示椎间盘椎体交界区椎体前上缘存在骨质侵蚀，代表Romanus病变(黄箭)。邻近上一椎体的前下缘则表现为骨质硬化，称为亮角征(红箭)。亮角征表示既往有Romanus病变的演变进程。

竹节样脊柱：骶髂关节和腰椎的正位X线影像(中图)显示对称性骶髂关节强直(黄箭)。广泛的韧带骨赘形成导致脊柱呈波浪状轮廓，此为竹节样脊柱(红箭)。棘突间融合产生匕首征(蓝箭)。

颈椎融合：颈椎侧位X线影像(右图)示颈椎完全强直，伴有椎体和小关节的融合及$C_{2\sim3}$假关节形成(绿箭)。

- Ankylosing spondylitis (AS) is predominantly seen in young men with HLA-B27 and presents with back pain and stiffness. AS can be associated with pulmonary fibrosis (upper lobe predominant), aortitis, and cardiac conduction defects.
- The earliest radiographic signs of AS are symmetric erosions, widening, and sclerosis of the sacroiliac joints.
- Subsequently, the spine invariably becomes involved, with radiographic findings following a specific sequence, which ascend from the lumbar to the cervical spine.

Romanus lesions are erosions of the anterior superior or inferior edges of the vertebral body endplates caused by enthesitis (inflammation at a ligament or tendon insertion site) at attachment of the annulus fibrosus to the vertebral body.

Shiny corners represent sclerosis of prior Romanus lesions at the corners of the vertebral bodies.

- 强直性脊柱炎(AS)主要见于年轻男性伴HLA-B27阳性，表现为背部疼痛和僵直。AS可能与肺纤维化(上叶为主)、主动脉炎及心脏传导阻滞有关。
- AS最早的X线征象为骶髂关节对称性骨质侵蚀、关节间隙增宽及骨质硬化。
- 脊柱随即不可避免受累，其X线表现有特定的发展顺序，即从腰椎上行到颈椎。

Romanus病变是椎体终板前上缘或前下缘的骨质侵蚀，由纤维环椎体附着点炎症(韧带及肌腱附着点的炎症)引起。

亮角代表先前位于椎体角的Romanus病变发生了硬化。

Squaring of the vertebral body disc margins develops due to erosions and bone loss.

Delicate syndesmophytes represent bony bridging connecting adjacent vertebral margins, which create the classic ***bamboo spine*** (spinal ankylosis) in late-stage disease.

- In advanced disease, the fully ankylosed spine is at a very high risk of fracture with even minor trauma. CT is necessary for evaluation of even minimal trauma in a patient with advanced AS and pain after trauma.
- An **Andersson lesion** is a pseudarthrosis occurring in a completely ankylosed spine.

椎体间盘边缘的**方形化**是由于侵蚀和骨质丧失导致的。

脆弱的韧带骨赘表现为连接邻近椎体边缘的骨桥，在晚期病例形成经典的***竹节样脊柱***(脊柱强直)。

- 在晚期病例，即使受到轻微的外伤，完全性强直脊柱也存在极高的骨折风险。对于晚期强直性脊柱炎患者，若在创伤后出现疼痛，即使是轻微的创伤，也需要进行CT评估。
- **Andersson病变**是指在完全性脊柱强直时出现的假关节。

Psoriatic arthritis

银屑病关节炎

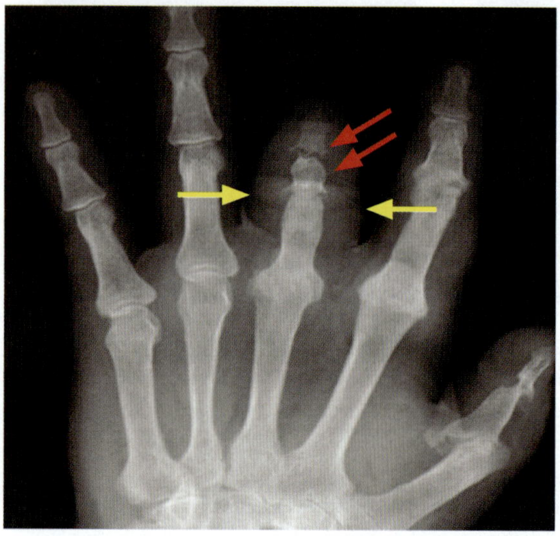

Psoriatic arthritis (arthritis mutilans form):
PA radiograph of the hand demonstrates swelling of the third digit (yellow arrows). There are *pencil-in-cup* erosions of the DIP and PIP joints (red arrows). Multiple joint subluxations produce *telescoping* of the digits with a *main-en-lorgnette* (opera-glass hand) deformity.
Case courtesy Barbara Weissman, MD, Brigham and Women's Hospital.
银屑病关节炎(残毁型关节炎)：手的后前位X线影像显示第三指肿胀(黄箭)。远端指间关节(DIP)及近端指间关节(PIP)呈带帽铅笔样侵蚀(红箭)。多发关节半脱位导致*单筒望远镜样手指*伴main-en-lorgnette(法语，观剧镜手)畸形。

- Psoriatic arthritis clinically presents as arthropathy in a patient with skin psoriasis. **Psoriatic arthritis most commonly affects the hands.** In contrast to RA, mineralization is preserved. Sacroiliitis, when present, is usually asymmetric.
- There are several patterns of psoriatic arthritis, including oligoarthritis, polyarthritis, spondyloarthropathy (producing bulky asymmetric bridging), and arthritis mutilans (a severe form usually affecting the hands, less commonly the feet).
- In the hands, the radiographic hallmark of psoriatic arthritis is diffuse soft-tissue swelling of an entire digit, producing the *sausage digit. Pencil-in-cup* erosions are also characteristic, most commonly affecting the DIPs. Although hand findings are usually bilateral, involvement tends to be asymmetric. The severe *arthritis mutilans* variant can cause marked deformity and *telescoping* digits, also known as the *main-en-lorgnette* (opera-glass hand) deformity.

  Additional findings in the hands include fluffy periostitis and ill-defined erosions of the joint margins.
- In the foot, the great toe interphalangeal and MTP joints are most commonly affected. An *ivory phalanx* represents osteosclerosis and is relatively specific for psoriatic arthritis. Psoriatic arthritis produces a plantar calcaneal spur with periosteal reaction. In contrast, a degenerative calcaneal spur will not feature reactive new bone.
- In the spine, psoriatic arthritis causes formation of coarse bony bridging

- 银屑病关节炎在临床上表现为伴有皮肤银屑病的关节病变。**银屑病关节炎最常累及手。**与类风湿关节炎相比，银屑病关节炎有骨盐沉积。当发生骶髂关节炎时，通常不对称。
- 银屑病关节炎有几个不同的类型，包括少关节炎、多关节炎、脊柱性关节炎(形成庞大的不对称骨桥)、残毁型关节炎(一种常侵犯手部的严重类型，足部受累不太常见)。
- 在手部，银屑病关节炎的X线影像特征为整个手指弥漫性的软组织肿胀，形成*香肠指*。铅笔样畸形也具特征性，并常累及远端指间关节(DIPs)。虽然手部表现常为双侧，但多为不对称性受累。严重的残毁型关节炎可导致明显的*单筒望远镜样*指畸形，也称为main-en-lorgnette(法语，观剧镜手)畸形。

  手部其他表现包括绒毛状骨膜反应和关节边缘境界模糊的骨侵蚀。
- 在足部，大踇趾的趾间关节及跖趾关节(MTP)最常受累。象牙趾代表骨质硬化，是银屑病关节炎相对特异的表现。银屑病关节炎导致跖骨和跟骨骨刺形成伴骨膜反应。相比之下，退行性跟骨骨刺不以反应性新生骨为特征。
- 在脊柱，银屑病关节炎导致粗糙的骨桥形成

(bulky lateral bony outgrowths), sometimes indistinguishable from reactive arthropathy (discussed below).

(肥大的侧方骨赘)，有时候与反应性关节病难以鉴别(下文讨论)。

Reactive arthropathy (previously called Reiter disease)

- Reactive arthropathy is an inflammatory arthritis thought to be a sequela of infectious diarrhea, urethritis, or cervicitis. Sacroiliitis is usually asymmetric, as in psoriatic arthritis.
- **Reactive arthropathy predominantly affects the feet**, where it has a similar appearance to psoriatic arthritis. Initial radiographic findings include diffuse soft-tissue swelling, joint space loss, aggressive marginal erosions, and juxta-articular osteopenia. Bony mineralization is preserved in the later stage of disease.
- In particular, the calcaneus is a common site of involvement with bony proliferative changes including erosions, enthesophytes, and fluffy periosteal reaction. The posterior-superior aspect of the calcaneus is a frequent site of erosion due to adjacent bursitis. There is often secondary Achilles tendinitis and thickening of the soft-tissues.
- In the hands, reactive arthropathy affects the interphalangeal joints and MTPs with erosions and diaphyseal periostitis.
- Reactive arthropathy may affect the spine with formation of coarse bony bridging, which may be difficult to distinguish from psoriatic arthritis.

反应性关节病(旧称Reiter病)

- 反应性关节病是一种炎症性关节炎，被认为是感染性腹泻、尿道炎或宫颈炎的后遗症。该类型骶髂关节炎常为非对称性，类似于银屑病关节炎。
- **反应性关节病主要侵及足部**，表现与银屑病关节炎相似。最早的X线影像表现包括广泛的软组织肿胀、关节间隙消失、侵袭性边缘骨质侵蚀及关节旁骨量减少。疾病晚期仍存留骨质矿化。
- 需要指出的是，跟骨是骨质增生性改变的常见部位，包括骨质侵蚀、附着点骨刺和绒毛状骨膜反应。由于邻近的滑囊炎，跟骨后上缘是骨质侵蚀常见的部位。常继发跟腱炎和软组织增厚。
- 在手部，反应性关节病累及指间关节和掌指关节(MTPs)，表现为骨质侵蚀和骨干骨膜炎。
- 反应性关节病可以累及脊柱，表现为粗糙的骨桥形成，这一点难以与银屑病关节炎相鉴别。

Connective tissue disorders affecting the joints

侵及关节的结缔组织疾病

Systemic lupus erythematosus

系统性红斑狼疮

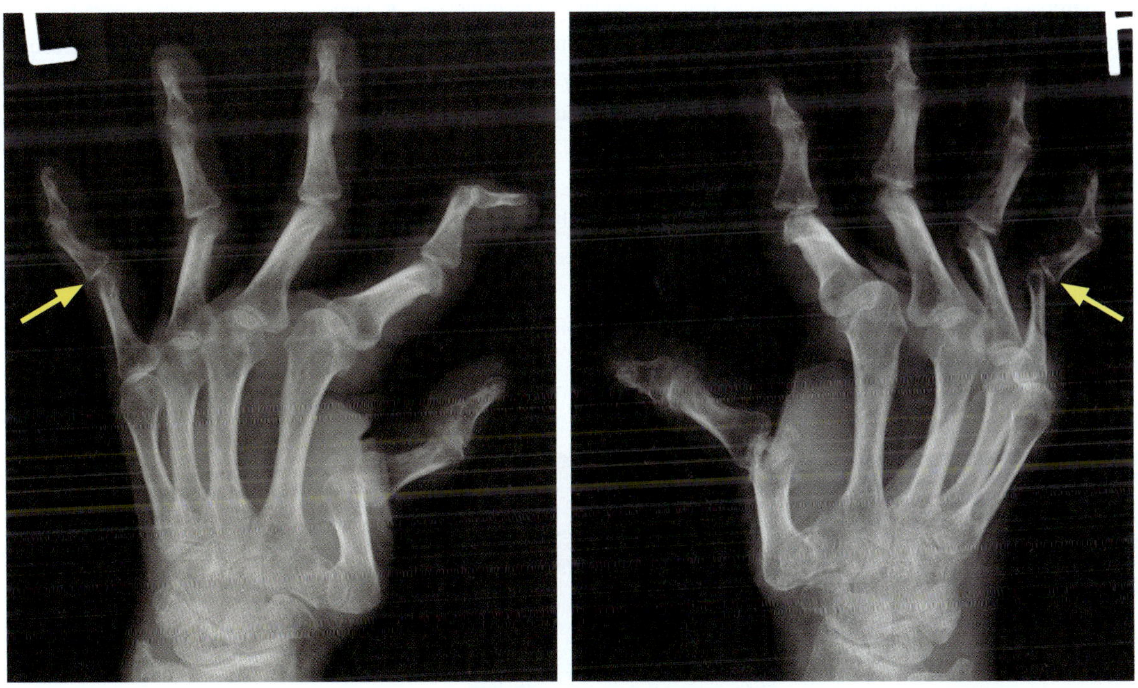

Lupus arthropathy: Oblique radiographs of both hands demonstrate multiple subluxations of both hands, without erosive change. Note the swan neck deformities of both small fingers, with hyperextension of the PIPs (arrows) and flexion of the DIPs. Swan neck deformities are the most common joint deformity in patients with lupus arthropathy.

狼疮性关节病：双手斜位X线影像显示双手多发关节半脱位，无侵蚀性改变。注意双手小指呈天鹅颈畸形，即近端指间关节过伸(箭)而远端指间关节过屈。天鹅颈畸形是狼疮性关节病患者最常见的关节畸形。

- Joint abnormalities are seen in ~90% of patients with systemic lupus erythematosus (SLE).
- The key radiographic finding of SLE is reducible subluxations of the MCPs and PIPs, with absence of erosive change.
- In early disease, alignment may appear normal on a PA view when the hands are compressed against the radiographic plate. Subluxations become apparent in the Norgaard ("ballcatcher's" or "you're in good hands with Allstate") or oblique views when the hand is not constrained.
- Over time, the subluxations may become permanent, which can result in chronic bony remodeling. These remodeling changes should not be confused with erosions.

- 关节异常见于约90%的系统性红斑狼疮(SLE)患者。
- SLE关键的X线影像表现为可复位性掌指关节(MCPs)和近端指间关节(PIPs)半脱位，而无侵蚀性改变。
- 在疾病早期，当手紧压在探测板上时，在后前位X线影像上的关节排列可能表现正常。当手放松时，关节半脱位在Norgaard位("捕手"或"捧起手")或斜位X线影像上显示明显。
- 随着时间推移，关节半脱位或呈永久性，继而可致慢性骨重塑。这些重塑改变不应与侵蚀相混淆。

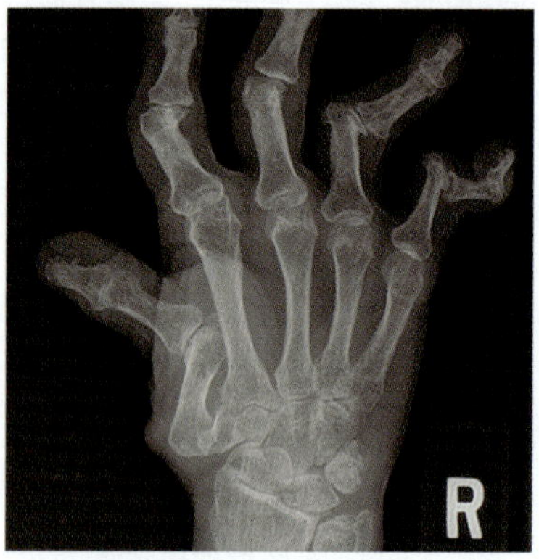

Frontal radiograph of the right hand taken 10 years later in the same patient as above demonstrates marked progression of subluxations with bony remodeling. The remodeling changes are most pronounced at the fourth and fifth PIPs.
同一名患者10年后的右手正位X线影像显示关节半脱位明显加重合并骨重塑。重塑改变在第四、五指近端指间关节最显著。

Jaccoud arthropathy

- Jaccoud arthropathy was historically described as being secondary to recurrent rheumatic fever, but some authors feel that SLE and Jaccoud arthropathy are the same disease. Both entities share the same type Ⅲ hypersensitivity mechanism and feature identical radiographic findings of reducible subluxations in the hand.

Scleroderma

- Scleroderma is a systemic collagen vascular disease caused by collagen deposition in the skin and soft-tissues. The fingertips are affected first, with atrophy of the distal soft-tissues.
- **Acro-osteolysis** (resorption of the distal portion of the distal phalanges) is characteristic, especially if there is accompanying calcification.

Jaccoud关节病

- Jaccoud关节病过去被认为继发于复发性风湿热，但某些学者认为SLE和Jaccoud关节病是同一种疾病。两者都是Ⅲ型变态反应且有完全相同的X线影像特点，即手部可复位性关节半脱位。

硬皮病

- 硬皮病是一种系统性胶原血管病，由胶原沉积在皮肤和软组织中所致。指尖最早受累，伴远端软组织萎缩。
- **肢端溶骨症**(远节指骨的远端部分骨质吸收)为其特征，尤其当伴有钙化时。

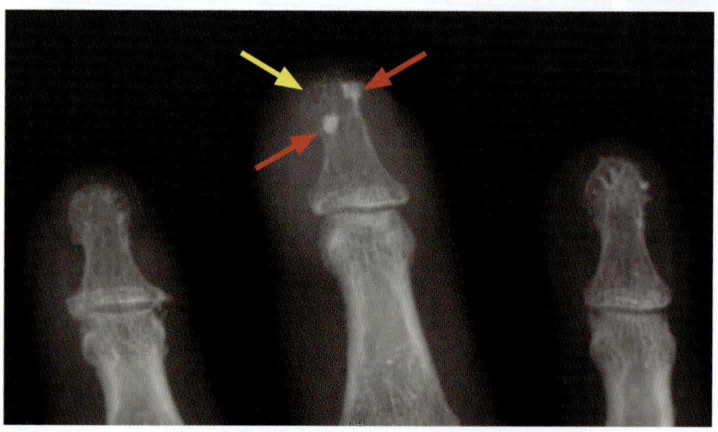

Acro-osteolysis and soft tissue calcification in a patient with scleroderma. Frontal radiograph of the hand (with the fingertips magnified) shows acro-osteolysis of the distal tuft (yellow arrow) and soft tissue mineralizations in the fingertips (red arrows).
硬皮病患者肢端溶骨症伴软组织钙化。手部正位X线影像(局部指尖放大)显示粗隆肢端溶骨症(黄箭)伴指尖软组织矿化(红箭)。

- Acro-osteolysis is not specific to scleroderma. The differential for acro-osteolysis includes:

> **Collagen vascular disease**, including scleroderma and Raynaud's.
> **Neuropathy**.
> **Polyvinyl chloride exposure**.
> **Thermal injury** (burn or frostbite). In frostbite the thumb is usually spared because it is clenched in a fist.
> **Hyperparathyroidism**, seen in conjunction with subperiosteal reabsorption.
> **Hajdu-Cheney**, a rare autosomal dominant syndrome characterized by short stature, craniofacial changes, and progressive acro-osteolysis.
> **Psoriasis**.
> **Pyknodysostosis**.

- Dystrophic soft-tissue and periarticular calcifications are common in scleroderma, which causes tightening and fibrosis of the skin and often leads to joint contractures.

- 肢端溶骨症非硬皮病所特有，其鉴别诊断包括：

> **胶原血管病**，包括硬皮病和Raynaud病。
> **神经病性关节病**。
> **聚氯乙烯中毒**。
> **温度损伤**(烧伤或冻伤)。冻伤时拇指常可幸免，因手呈握拳状。
> **甲状旁腺功能亢进**，见于骨连接处伴骨膜下骨质吸收。
> **哈伊杜-切尼综合征**(遗传性骨发育不良并肢端溶骨症)，一种罕见的常染色体显性综合征，其特征为身材矮小、颅面部改变及进行性肢端溶骨症。
> **银屑病**。
> **致密性骨发育障碍**。

- 软组织营养不良和关节周围钙化在硬皮病很常见，可导致皮肤紧绷和纤维化，并常引起关节挛缩。

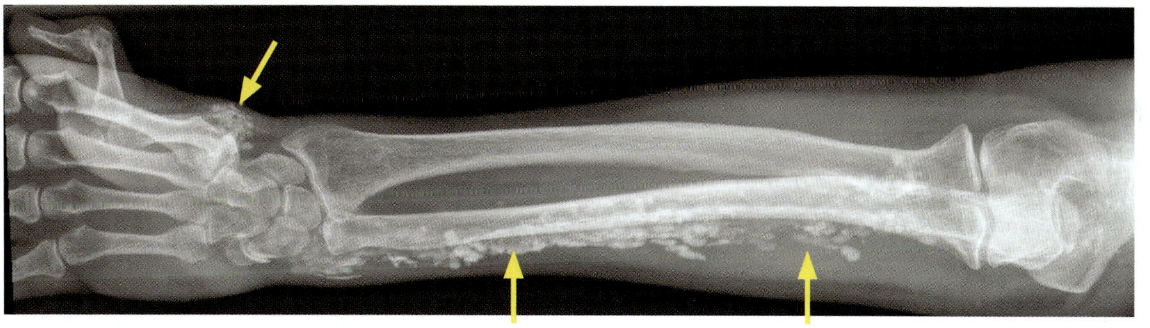

Frontal radiograph of the forearm in a patient with scleroderma shows extensive soft tissue mineralizations along the ulnar aspect of the forearm and at the base of the thumb metacarpals (arrows).
硬皮病患者前臂正位X线影像显示前臂尺侧及拇指掌骨基底部周围广泛的软组织矿化(箭)。

Polymyositis and dermatomyositis

- Polymyositis and dermatomyositis are idiopathic conditions characterized by inflammation of muscle (polymyositis) or muscle and skin (dermatomyositis). Joint abnormalities are rare, although periarticular osteopenia may be present in these conditions.
- The imaging hallmark of polymyositis and dermatomyositis is soft-tissue calcification. Intramuscular calcifications are most common, although subcutaneous calcifications may also be seen, similar to scleroderma.

多发性肌炎和皮肌炎

- 多发性肌炎和皮肌炎属于特发性疾病，以肌肉(多发性肌炎)或肌肉及皮肤(皮肌炎)的炎症为特征。关节异常罕见，但均可出现关节周围骨量减少。
- 多发性肌炎和皮肌炎的影像学特征为软组织钙化。肌肉内钙化最为常见，也可出现与硬皮病类似的皮下钙化。

(翻译 陈丽舟 帅丹丹)

CRYSTAL ARTHROPATHIES

Overview of crystal arthropathies

- Crystalline arthropathies are a common form of arthritis caused by intra-articular inflammation induced by the deposition of various crystals.
- By far the two most common crystal arthropathies are calcium pyrophosphate crystal arthritis and gout (caused by monosodium urate). While calcium hydroxyapatite usually causes calcific tendinopathy, it much less commonly causes intra-articular inflammation.
- Clinically, crystal arthropathies may mimic inflammatory arthropathy, septic arthritis, or osteoarthritis.

晶体性关节炎

晶体性关节炎概述

- 晶体性关节炎是由关节内发炎引起的一类常见的关节炎，由不同种类的晶体沉积引起。
- 两种最为常见的晶体性关节炎是焦磷酸钙关节炎和痛风(由尿酸单钠沉积引起)。尽管焦磷酸钙常导致肌腱钙化，但并不经常引起关节内炎症。
- 晶体性关节炎在临床上可以与炎性关节病、化脓性关节炎和骨关节炎类似。

- Imaging plays a key role in diagnosis of crystal arthropathies, although arthrocentesis with crystal analysis is the gold standard in ambiguous cases.

  Calcium pyrophosphate manifests on imaging as chondrocalcinosis, which is deposition of calcium salts on hyaline cartilage and fibrocartilage.

  Gout has characteristic periarticular erosions with overhanging edges, and gouty tophi may manifest as high attenuation soft tissue nodules or masses.

  Hydroxyapatite appears as globular or amorphous mineralization (usually within a tendon) without internal trabeculation.

  Dual-energy CT can identify monosodium urate or calcium pyrophosphate.

Calcium pyrophosphate

- The most common crystalline arthropathy is the arthritis caused by calcium pyrophosphate (CPP). Microscopically, the rhomboid crystals of CPPD are positively birefringent. Crystal deposition may be idiopathic (by far the most common) or associated with hemochromatosis, hyperparathyroidism, and hypophosphatasia.
- *Acute CPP arthritis* describes the acute inflammatory phase of this condition, with a clinical presentation that may mimic septic arthritis with acute pain, swelling, erythema, and elevated inflammatory markers. *Chronic CPP arthritis* has been called the "great mimicker" of other arthropathies, including osteoarthritis (most common), gout, and rheumatoid.
- The hallmark radiographic finding of CPP arthritis is **chondrocalcinosis**, which is calcification of hyaline (articular) or fibro (meniscal/labral) cartilage. Radiographs of the knees, wrist, and pelvis (pubic symphysis) are nearly 100% sensitive for the detection of chondrocalcinosis. Importantly, chondrocalcinosis is a very common finding of unknown incidence seen in both symptomatic and asymptomatic individuals. Additionally, positive crystal analysis has been reported in patients without radiographic chondrocalcinosis, especially in the early stages. Therefore, the absence of chondrocalcinosis cannot exclude CPP arthritis, and the presence of chondrocalcinosis does not imply that the patient's pain is due to CPP arthritis.
- On radiography and CT, chondrocalcinosis of the articular cartilage appears as thin, linear calcifications of the articular cartilage, paralleling the subchondral bone plate. Chondrocalcinosis of the fibrocartilage (e.g., menisci and labral) follows the course of the fibrocartilage, with a thick and irregular or shaggy border. Calcium pyrophosphate may also line ligaments and synovium, where it appears as an indistinct, cloud-like mineralization.
- In the wrist, chondrocalcinosis tends to affect the triangular fibrocartilage complex (TFCC). Advanced disease may lead to scapholunate advanced collapse (SLAC) wrist due to destruction of the scapholunate ligament due to CPP-induced inflammation. SLAC wrist is proximal migration of the capitate between the dissociated scaphoid and lunate, and may also be seen in RA or trauma.

- 影像检查在晶体性关节炎的诊断中起着关键作用，但关节穿刺加晶体分析在一些疑难病例中作为金标准。

  焦磷酸钙关节炎影像上表现为软骨钙质沉积症，即钙盐沉积于透明软骨或纤维软骨。

  痛风具有特征性的关节周围侵蚀，并伴悬垂样边缘；并且，痛风石可表现为高密度的软组织结节或肿块。

  羟磷灰石表现为球形或无固定形状的矿物化(通常发生在肌腱)，其内无小梁结构。

  双源CT可以识别尿酸单钠和焦磷酸钙。

焦磷酸钙沉积病

- 最常见的结晶性关节病变是由焦磷酸钙(CPP)沉积所导致的关节炎。显微镜下CPPD的菱形结晶体呈正性双折射阳性。结晶沉积可以是特发性的(最为常见)，或合并血色病、甲状旁腺功能亢进和低磷酸酯酶症。
- 急性CPP关节炎是指该病的急性炎症反应期，其临床表现可与化脓性关节炎类似，如急性疼痛、水肿、红斑和炎症因子升高。慢性CPP关节炎被称为其他关节炎的"伟大模仿者"，包括骨关节炎(最常见)、痛风和类风湿关节炎。
- CPP关节炎的标志性X线特征是**软骨钙质沉积症**，即透明软骨(关节)或纤维软骨(半月板/盂唇)的钙化。X线影像对发现膝关节、腕关节和骨盆(耻骨联合)的软骨钙质沉积症敏感性几乎为100%。重要的是，软骨钙质沉积症非常常见，但其发生率尚不清楚，可以见于有症状和无症状的患者。此外，有报道晶体分析阳性的患者在影像上并无软骨钙质沉积，尤其是早期的患者。所以，影像上缺乏软骨钙质沉积征象并不能排除CPP关节炎，而影像上表现出软骨钙质沉积征象也不能说明患者的疼痛是由CPP关节炎导致。
- 在X线和CT上，关节软骨的钙质沉积症表现为薄层、线性钙化，与软骨下骨板平行。纤维软骨(如半月板和盂唇)的钙质沉积沿着纤维软骨分布，表现为厚层钙化，伴不规则或不光滑的边界。焦磷酸钙也可以沉积于韧带和滑膜，表现为模糊的、云雾状的矿物质沉积。
- 在手腕，软骨钙质沉积症常累及三角纤维软骨复合体(TFCC)。晚期可导致舟月骨进行性塌陷(SLAC)，原因是CPP引起的炎症，舟月韧带遭到破坏。SLAC腕是舟骨和月骨间的分离使头状骨向近侧移位，也见于类风湿关节炎(RA)或外伤。

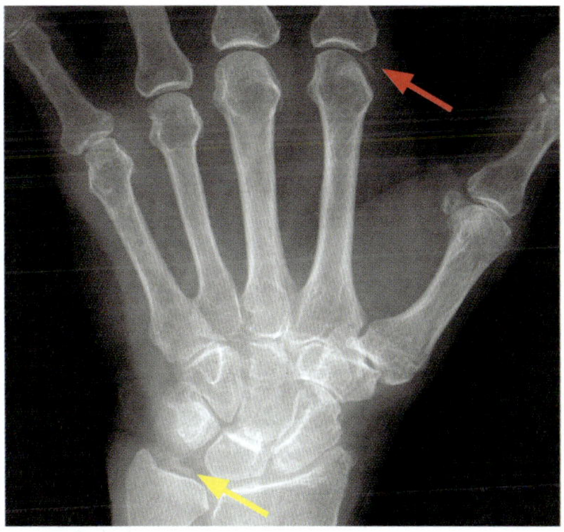

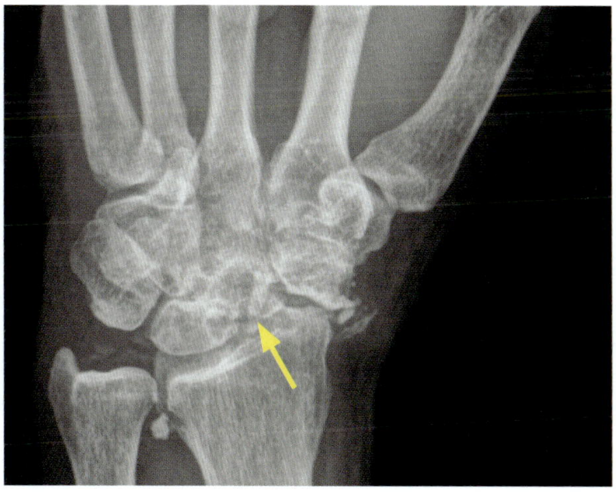

Chondrocalcinosis: Frontal radiograph of the wrist demonstrates chondrocalcinosis of the triangular fibrocartilage complex (TFCC, yellow arrow) and at the index MCP (red arrow).
软骨钙质沉积症：腕关节正位X线影像显示三角纤维软骨复合体(TFCC，黄箭)和示指掌指关节(红箭)软骨钙质沉积。

Advanced CPP arthritis with SLAC arthropathy: Frontal radiograph of the wrist in a different patient shows fragmentation of the scaphoid (arrow) with proximal migration of the capitate. There is chondrocalcinosis of the TFCC and scattered mineralizations about the wrist.
晚期CPP关节炎伴SLAC关节病：另一名患者的腕关节正位X线影像显示舟骨碎片(箭)伴头状骨向近侧移位。该患者三角纤维软骨复合体有软骨钙质沉积，同时腕部散在矿物质沉积。

- In the knee, the patellofemoral compartment is affected first, but all three compartments may become involved. Isolated degenerative changes of the patellofemoral joint may be due to CPP arthritis (usually in an older person, especially if there are subchondral cysts and chondrocalcinosis) or patellar maltracking.

- 在膝关节，髌股关节间室最早受累，但所有三个关节间室都可以被累及。孤立的髌股关节退行性改变可能由CPP关节炎(通常为老年患者，特别是存在软骨下囊肿和软骨钙质沉积症)或髌骨轨迹异常引起。

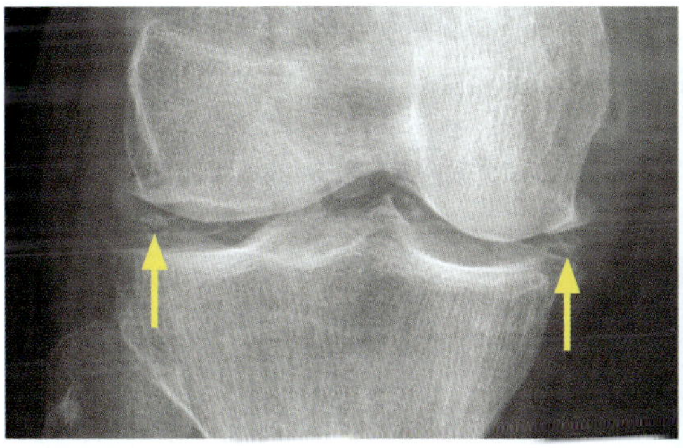

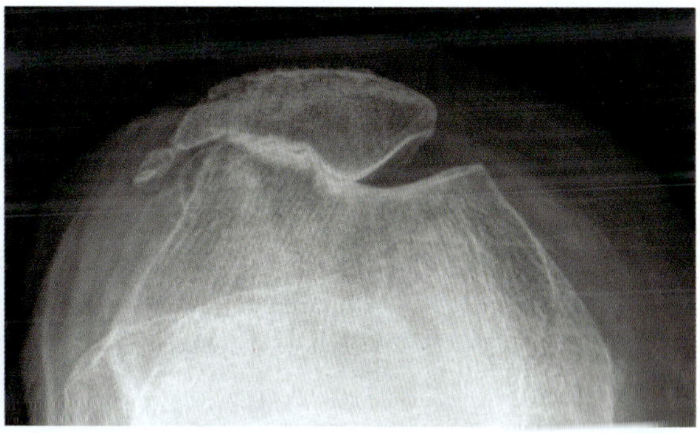

CPP arthritis of the knee. Frontal (left image) radiograph of the knee shows prominent chondrocalcinosis of the menisci and articular cartilage (arrows) with small medial tibiofemoral osteophytes. There is severe patellofemoral osteoarthritis with bone-on-bone articulation laterally. In this patient, subchondral cysts were not demonstrated.
膝关节焦磷酸钙关节炎。膝关节正位X线影像(左图)显示半月板和关节软骨(箭)显著的软骨钙质沉积及小的内侧胫股骨赘。髌股关节可见严重的骨性关节炎，以及外侧骨与骨之间呈现骨性关节。本病例未见软骨下囊肿。

- In the hands, involvement of the second and third MCP joints is typical, producing characteristic *hook-like* osteophytes from the radial aspect of the metacarpal heads. A similar appearance can be seen in hemochromatosis, which may feature more extensive involvement of the MCPs, although there is a large crossover in imaging.

- 在手部，第二、三掌指关节(MCP)是常见的发病部位，造成在掌骨头桡侧面出现特征性的钩状骨赘。类似的表现可见于血色病，后者常表现为更广泛的MCPs受侵，但两者在影像上有很大部分重叠。

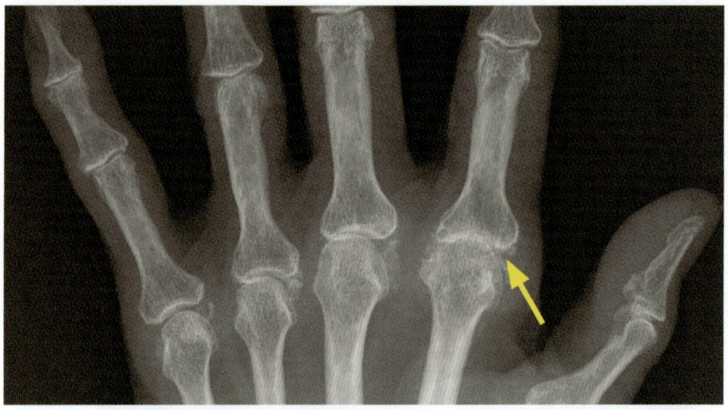

Frontal radiograph of the hand in the same patient with knees imaged above demonstrates osteophytes of the MCPs with severe cartilage space loss at the index finger (arrow). There is prominent chondrocalcinosis of all MCPs.
与上述膝关节影像为同一名患者，手正位X线影像显示MCPs骨赘伴严重的软骨间隙狭窄(箭)。所有MCPs均有明显的软骨钙质沉积。

Gout

- Gout is a crystal-induced inflammatory arthropathy caused by sodium urate deposition in the joints. Excess uric acid may be secondary to under-excretion (more common, typically caused by renal insufficiency) or overproduction (much more rare, typically seen in younger patients).

  It takes about 10–20 years of hyperuricemia before the clinical syndrome of gout develops.

  Microscopically, gout crystals are **negatively** birefringent needle-like crystals within neutrophils.
- The great toe is most commonly involved, but gout can occur in any joint.
- Radiographic hallmarks are sharply marginated erosions with *overhanging margins*.
- Joint spaces are typically well preserved until late in the disease. Similarly, bony mineralization is preserved until the late phases.
- Ultrasound of gout shows a *double contour sign* representing an irregular hyperechoic line of urate crystals deposited on the hyperechoic cartilage.
- MRI is not a primary modality for evaluation of gout, but erosions and variable signal intensity intra-articular and periarticular gouty tophi are well seen.

痛风

- 痛风是结晶体引起的炎症性关节病，由关节内单钠尿酸盐(尿酸钠)结晶沉积引起。过量的尿酸可继发于排泄减少(较常见，通常由肾功能不全引起)或生成过多(极为少见，常见于年轻患者)。

  在痛风临床症状出现之前，往往历经了10~20年的高尿酸血症期。

  痛风结晶在显微镜下是中性粒细胞内呈**负性双折射**的针样结晶。
- 大踇趾最常受累，但痛风可发生在任何关节。
- X线影像学的特征性标志为边缘锐利的骨质侵蚀交界伴悬垂样边缘。
- 关节间隙保留完好直到病程的晚期。同样，钙盐沉积直到病程的晚期才出现异常。
- 痛风在超声上显示双轨征，代表由尿酸晶体沉积形成的不规则线状强回声位于强回声的软骨之上。
- MRI不是评估痛风的首选检查，但是MRI可较好地显示骨质侵蚀和关节内及关节周围不同信号强度的痛风石。

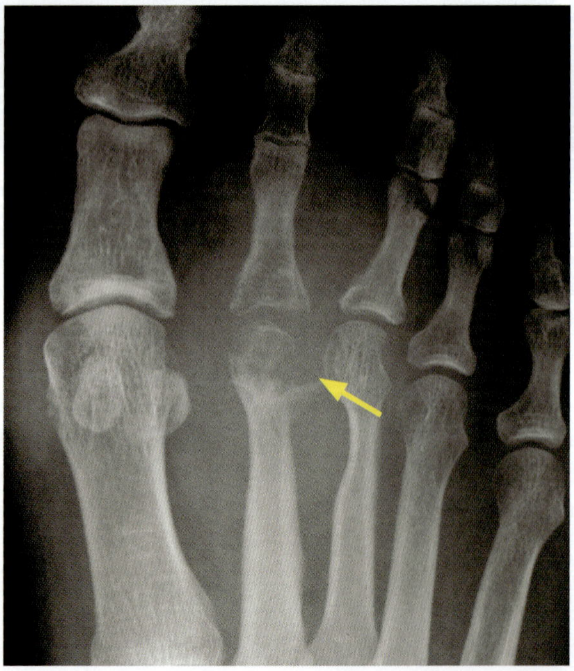

AP radiograph of the foot shows soft-tissue swelling surrounding the second MTP. An erosion of the head of the second metacarpal head features a characteristic *overhanging margin* (arrow).
足部的前后位X线影像示第二跖趾关节周围软组织肿胀。第二跖骨头远端骨质侵蚀表现为特征性的悬垂样边缘(箭)。

- Tophaceous gout refers to deposition of urate crystals, inflammatory cells, and foreign body giant cells in the soft tissues. Gouty tophi may occur anywhere in the body, including within the joint and periarticular locations such as tendons, ligaments, and bursae. In particular, gouty tophi have a propensity to develop in the olecranon bursa of the elbow.
- Dual-energy CT is an excellent modality to identify monosodium urate crystals, which are typically colored green in post-processing. By altering the post-processing parameters, green color coding can also be used to identify CPP crystals.

- 痛风石性痛风是指尿酸结晶、炎性细胞、异物巨细胞沉积在软组织中。痛风石可以出现在身体的任何部位，包括关节内和关节周围，如肌腱、韧带和滑囊。尤其是痛风石倾向于沉积在肘部鹰嘴滑囊。
- 双源CT是发现单钠尿酸盐结晶的一个极佳的影像方式，该晶体在后处理图像上为绿色。通过改变后处理参数，绿色编码也能用于检测CPP结晶。

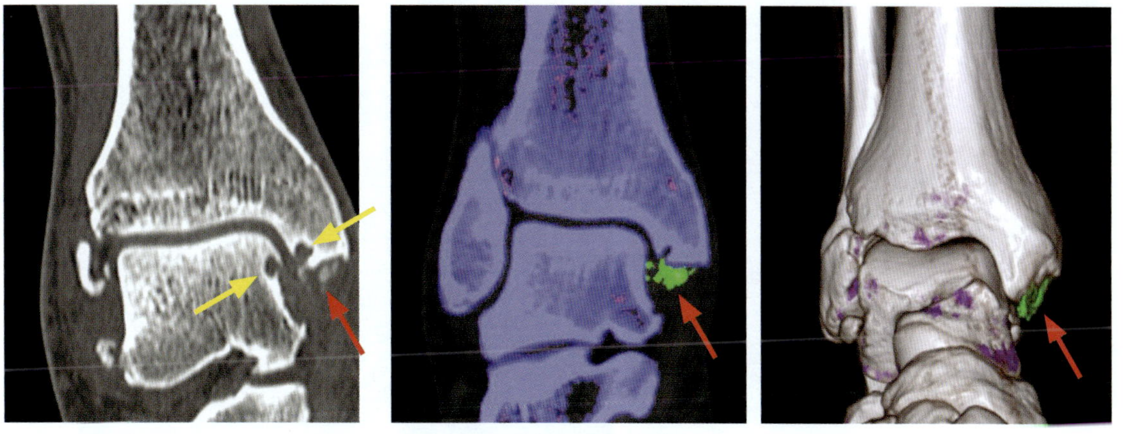

Coronal CT
冠状位CT

Post-processed dual-energy CT
后处理双源CT

Volume-rendered dual-energy CT
容积再现双源CT

Gouty arthropathy of the ankle: Coronal CT shows erosions of the medial talus and medial malleolus (yellow arrows) and amorphous mineralization (red arrow) in the deltoid ligament. Color-coded post-processed dual-energy CT shows that the deltoid mineralization is colored green (red arrows) on the gout algorithm, consistent with monosodium urate deposition. There was no green color-coding on the CPP algorithm (not shown).
踝关节痛风性关节病：冠状位CT显示胫骨内侧和距骨内侧骨质侵蚀(黄箭)和三角韧带无定型矿物质沉积(红箭)。彩色双源CT后处理的三角韧带矿化在痛风指定区显示为绿色(红箭)，符合单钠尿酸盐结晶沉积的表现。在对CPP进行计算处理后未出现绿色(未显示)。

Calcium hydroxyapatite

- Also called calcific tendinitis or calcific tendinopathy, calcium hydroxyapatite deposition results from crystals being deposited in degenerating or hypoxic tendons, triggering an inflammatory cascade.
- Calcific tendinopathy is not associated with hypercalcemia, but it is seen more commonly in diabetic patients.
- On radiographs and CT, the mineralization of calcium hydroxyapatite appears amorphous or globular. Importantly, there cannot be any cortication or internal trabeculation, either of which would suggest bone formation by osteoblasts due to a different etiology from calcific tendinopathy. If cortication or trabeculation were present then the differential diagnosis could include intra-articular body, fragmented enthesophyte, or osteochondromatosis.
- Calcific tendinopathy may erode through tendons and cause adjacent calcific bursitis. Rarely, calcific tendinopathy may erode into bone (most commonly at the insertion of pectoralis major at the anterior aspect of the proximal humerus) and simulate neoplasm with the differential including parosteal sarcoma or myositis ossificans.
- On ultrasound, calcium hydroxyapatite appears as globular hyperechoic shadowing foci.
- On MR, the calcium hydroxyapatite deposits are low signal intensity on all pulse sequences, often with surrounding edema/inflammatory change.

羟基磷灰石沉积病

- 羟基磷灰石沉积也称为钙化性肌腱炎或钙化性肌腱病，是由于晶体沉积在退变或缺氧的肌腱中，引发了炎症级联反应。
- 钙化性肌腱病与高钙血症无关，但较常见于糖尿病患者。
- 在X线和CT上，羟基磷灰石的矿化呈不定形或球形。重要的是不能有任何皮质或内部小梁，这两者中出现任何一种都可能提示成骨细胞的骨形成是由于钙化性肌腱病以外的不同原因所引起的。如果存在皮质或骨小梁，其鉴别诊断则需要考虑关节内异物、骨赘碎片和骨软骨瘤病。
- 罕见情况下，钙化性肌腱病可能侵蚀骨骼(最常见于胸大肌附着于肱骨近端前侧的位置)，并类似于肿瘤，其鉴别诊断包括骨旁肉瘤和骨化性肌炎。
- 在超声上，羟基磷灰石表现为球状的高回声区，伴声影。
- 在磁共振图像上，羟基磷灰石沉积在所有脉冲序列上都呈低信号，通常伴有周围水肿/炎症性改变。

- Ultrasound-guided barbotage is an effective treatment for calcific tendinopathy. In this procedure, a larger-bore needle (18–20 gauge) is directed into the calcific deposit and gently pulsed with a dilute anesthetic/saline solution to break up the deposit. Often, chalky deposits are expelled retrograde into the body of the syringe with negative pressure on the plunger.
- The shoulder is by far the most common site in the body for calcific tendinopathy, with the supraspinatus tendon the most commonly affected.

- 超声引导下灌洗是一种治疗钙化性肌腱病的有效方法。手术时，用一个大孔径针(18～20G)直接穿刺至羟基磷灰石沉积处，然后缓慢注射稀释后的麻醉剂/生理盐水来冲开这些沉积物。通常，白色沉积物在注射器的活塞杆上施加负压后会被逆行吸入注射器。
- 肩关节是钙化性肌腱病最好发的部位，其中冈上肌肌腱最常受累。

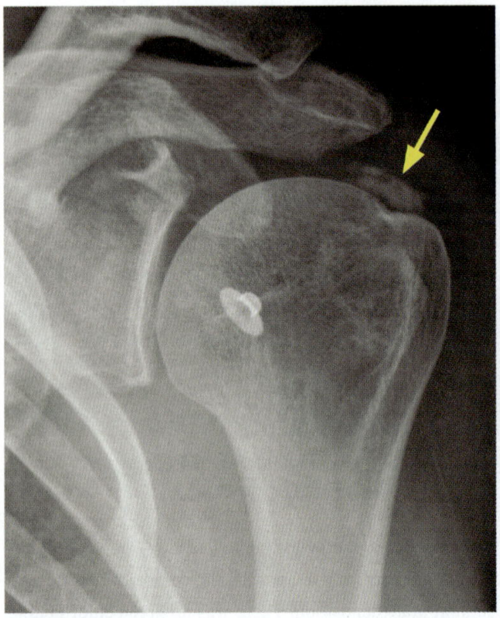

Grashey radiograph
Grashey位X线影像

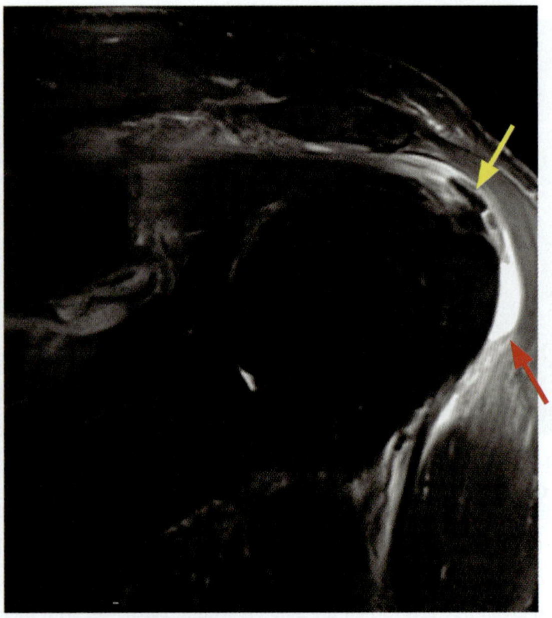

Coronal T2-weighted MRI with fat supp.
冠状位T_2加权脂肪抑制MRI

Calcific tendinopathy of supraspinatus: Radiograph shows lobulated mineralization (arrow) just cranial to the footprint of the greater tuberosity. Note the required absence of internal trabeculation and peripheral cortication. MRI demonstrates that the globular low-signal mineralization (yellow arrow) has eroded through the supraspinatus tendon and extends into the subacromial-subdeltoid bursa, where there is a moderate-sized bursal effusion (red arrow).
冈上肌肌腱钙化性肌腱病：X线影像显示大结节足印的上方有一分叶状矿物质沉积(箭)。注意X线影像中不能有内生骨小梁或外周皮质化。MRI显示球形的低信号矿物质沉积(黄箭)侵蚀冈上肌肌腱，并延伸至三角肌下滑囊，其中可见中等量的滑囊积液(红箭)。

- The tendons about the hip, including the gluteal and rectus tendons, are likely more commonly involved by calcific tendinopathy than clinically acknowledged.

- 髋部肌腱包括臀肌肌腱和股直肌肌腱，可能比临床所了解的更常发生钙化性肌腱病。

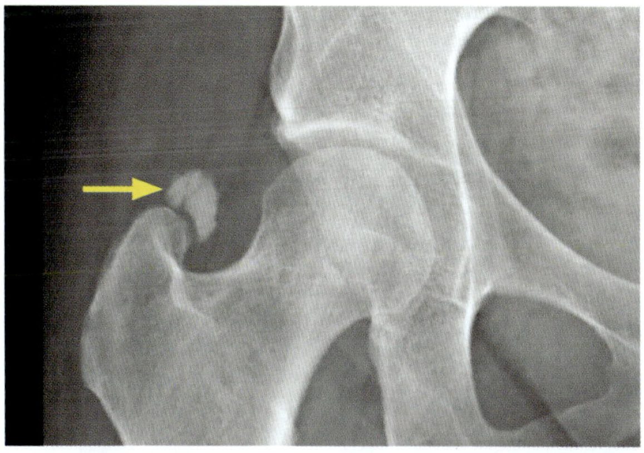

Frontal radiograph
正位X线影像

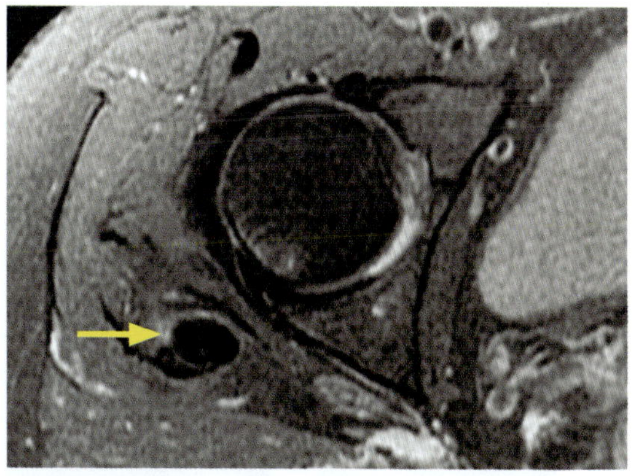

Axial proton-density weighted MRI with fat supp.
轴位PD加权脂肪抑制MRI

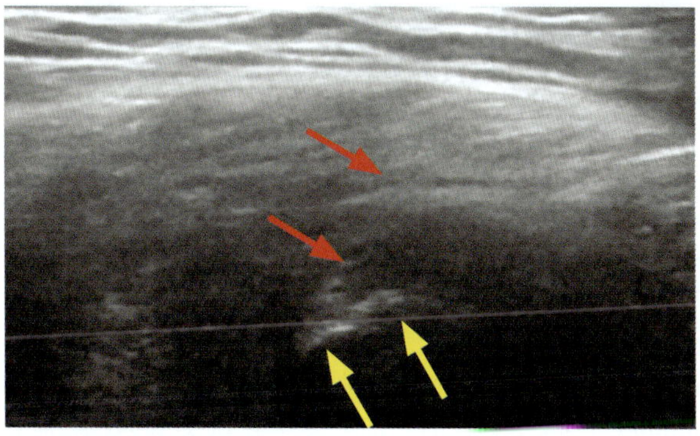

Ultrasound
超声

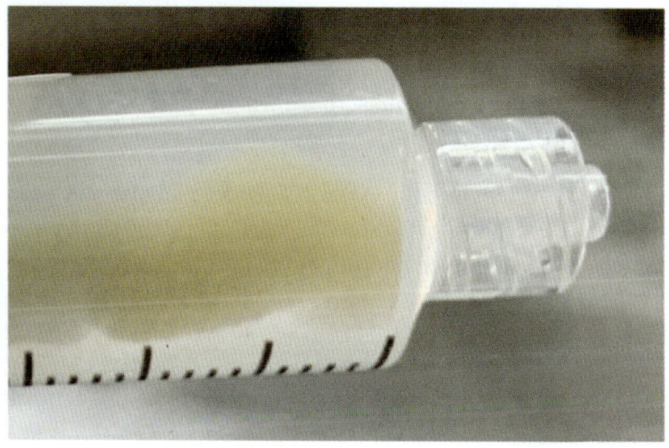

Post-procedure syringe
抽吸后的注射器

Calcific tendinopathy of gluteus medius: Radiograph shows globular and featureless mineralization (arrow) just cranial to the greater trochanter. MRI shows the posterior position of the mineralization, located at the gluteus medius myotendinous junction as globular low signal (arrow). Intraprocedural ultrasound demonstrates the needle tip (red arrow) abutting the lobulated hyperechoic shadowing (arrows) of the calcific deposit. Magnified photograph from the syringe after barbotage shows the chalk-like calcifications obtained after pulsed lavage.
臀中肌钙化性肌腱病：X线影像显示大转子上方球形无特征性的矿物质沉积(箭)。MRI显示位于臀中肌肌腱连接处后方的球形低信号矿物质沉积(箭)。术中超声显示针头(红箭)紧靠分叶状的矿物质伴声影强回声(箭)。Barbotage灌洗术(超声引导下经皮针吸和灌洗肩部钙化性肌腱病钙沉积)放大的注射器图显示经过脉冲式灌洗后，其内有粉笔样钙化。

- In the wrist, the most common site is the flexor carpi ulnaris (FCU) tendon.
  The FCU tendon originates from the common flexor mass at the humeral medial epicondyle and attaches to the pisiform before continuing to the hamate and fifth metacarpal.

- 在腕部，最常受累的部位是尺侧腕屈肌(FCU)肌腱。
  尺侧腕屈肌肌腱起自肱骨内上髁屈肌总腱，在附着豌豆骨后继续延伸至钩状骨和第五掌骨。

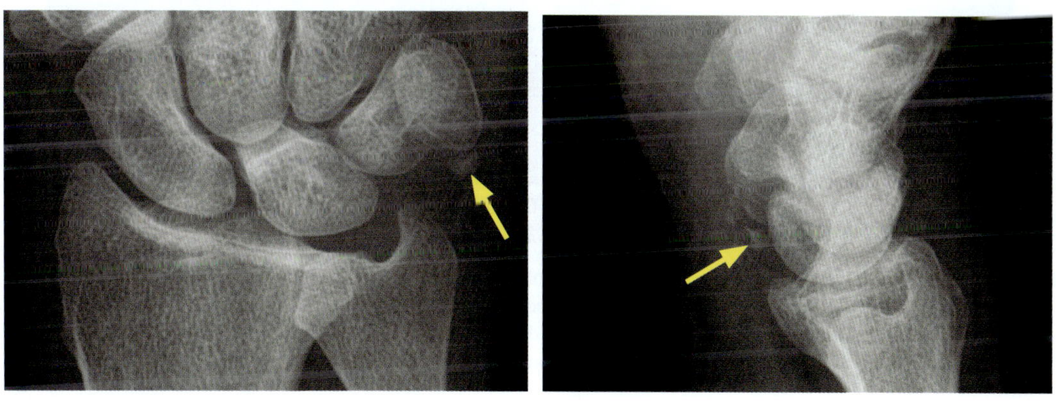

FCU calcific tendinopathy: Frontal (left image) and lateral radiographs of the wrist demonstrate amorphous mineralization (arrow) just proximal to the pisiform. A common pitfall of mineralization at the ulnar aspect of the wrist is to presume that it is chondrocalcinosis of the TFC; however this mineralization is more distal and ulnar in location. Lateral radiograph confirms that the mineralization (arrow) is located volar, along the expected course of FCU.
FCU钙化性肌腱病：腕部正位(左图)和侧位X线影像显示豌豆骨近端无定形的矿物质沉积(箭)。腕部尺侧矿物质沉积的一个问题是常被误认为三角纤维软骨钙质沉着症，但这种疾病矿物质沉积的位置较远，更偏向尺侧。侧位X线影像证实矿物质沉积(箭)位于掌侧，沿着FCU的解剖位置分布。

- Calcific tendinopathy of the longus colli muscle may cause neck pain, odynophagia, fever, and prevertebral effusion, and may clinically mimic a prevertebral abscess.

- 颈长肌钙化性肌腱病可引起颈部疼痛、吞咽痛、发热和椎前积液，临床可类似椎前脓肿。

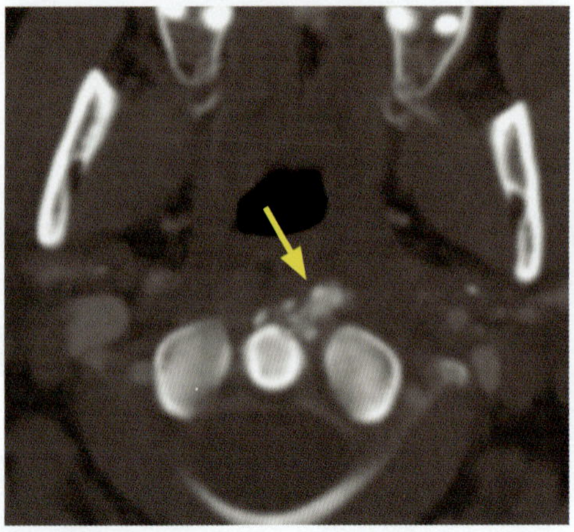

Axial CT with contrast (bone window).
轴位增强CT(骨窗)

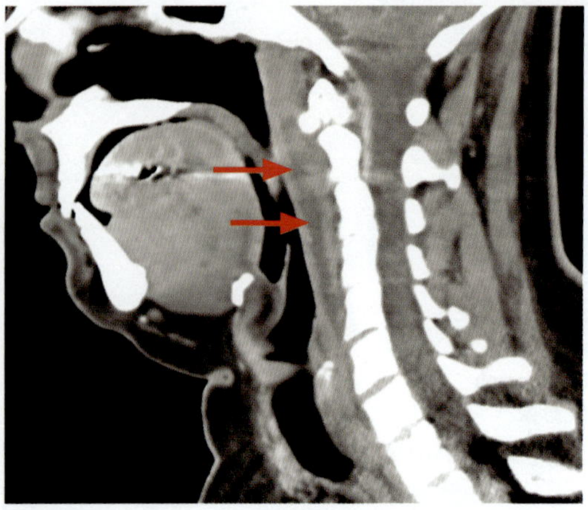

Sagittal CT with contrast (soft tissue window).
矢状位增强CT(软组织窗)

Calcific tendinopathy of longus colli: Axial CT shows globular and featureless mineralizations (arrow) anterior to and to the left of the dens, within the left longus colli muscle. Sagittal CT just to the right of midline shows a prevertebral fluid collection (red arrows). Please note that the sagittal image on the right demonstrates how calcific tendinopathy of longus colli can mimic a prevertebral abscess even on CT if the calcifications are not seen.
颈长肌钙化性肌腱病：轴位CT示齿突左前方球形无特征性的矿物质沉积(箭)，位于左侧颈长肌内。矢状位中线偏右CT显示椎前液体积聚(红箭)。注意，右侧矢状位图像为颈长肌钙化性肌腱病，如果没有钙化，即使CT也难以与椎前脓肿进行区分。

- The vast majority of calcium hydroxyapatite is extra-articular. A very rare intra-articular variant seen in the shoulder, called **Milwaukee shoulder**, leads to rapid destruction of the rotator cuff and the glenohumeral joint.

  Milwaukee shoulder is a destructive arthritis characterized by extensive full-thickness rotator cuff tears, marked cartilage and bone destruction, and large bloody effusions. Similar to neuropathic arthropathy, the bone destruction can have sharp margins with an atrophic appearance.

- 绝大部分羟基磷灰石沉积发生在关节外。极小一部分发生在肩关节内，称为**Milwaukee肩**，可快速引起肩袖和盂肱关节损毁。

  Milwaukee肩是一种损毁性关节炎，以广泛的全层肩袖撕裂、严重的软骨和骨破坏及大量血性积液为特征。与神经病性关节病类似，骨质破坏具有锐利的边缘伴萎缩性外观。

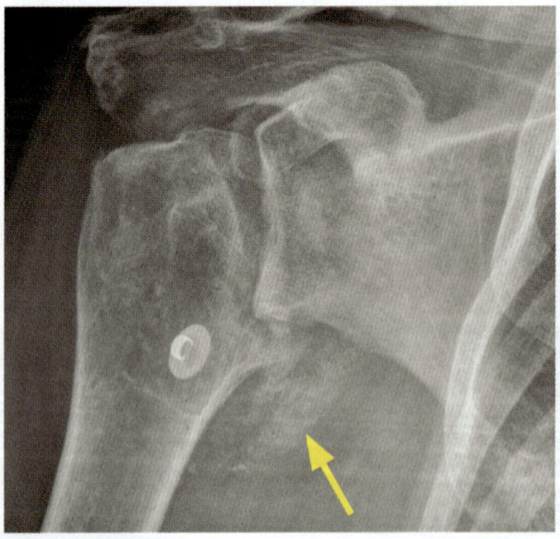

Frontal radiograph
正位X线影像

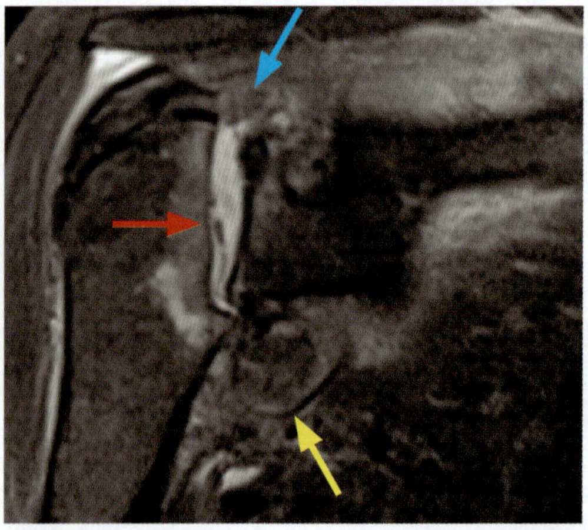

Coronal STIR
冠状位STIR

Milwaukee shoulder (not pathologically confirmed): Frontal radiograph demonstrates destruction of the medial humeral head and indistinct intra-articular mineralization in the axillary recess (yellow arrow). Coronal STIR MRI shows sharply marginated destruction of the medial humeral head (red arrow). There is extensive rotator cuff tearing, with globular morphology of the medially retracted torn cuff tendons (blue arrow). There is a low signal intensity effusion with distension of the axillary recess corresponding to the mineralization (yellow arrow).
A cervical spine MRI (not shown) was negative for syrinx or other explanation for potential neuropathic arthropathy. Aspiration was performed with a large amount of bloody fluid aspirated (not shown). In this case, intra-articular hydroxyapatite crystals were not demonstrated on pathologic analysis, but the imaging features remain consistent with Milwaukee shoulder.
Milwaukee肩(未经病理证实)：正位X线影像显示肱骨头内侧骨质破坏和腋囊处模糊的关节内矿物质沉积(黄箭)。冠状位STIR MRI示肱骨头内侧边缘锐利的骨质破坏(红箭)。可见肩袖广泛撕裂，伴内侧肩袖肌腱(蓝箭)回缩呈球状。对应于矿物质沉积处(黄箭)有低信号积液伴腋囊扩大。
颈椎MRI(未显示)未见空洞或其他可以解释为神经病性关节病的影像。吸引术发现大量血性液体(未显示)。本病例的病理分析未发现关节内羟基磷灰石晶体，但影像学表现符合Milwaukee肩的诊断。

Hemochromatosis

- Hemochromatosis arthropathy affects 50% of those with hemochromatosis, an autosomal recessive disease of altered iron metabolism. The arthropathy is caused by deposition of iron and calcium pyrophosphate dihydrate crystals.

  Hemochromatosis clinically presents with bronze pigmentation, diabetes, cirrhosis, CHF, and arthropathy.

- In the hand, the typical location of hemochromatosis arthropathy is the MCP joints, producing characteristic *hook-like* osteophytes at the metacarpal heads. Calcium pyrophosphate dihydrate deposition disease (CPPD) can appear identical when involvement is isolated to the second and third MCPs. In contrast to CPPD, hemochromatosis may involve all MCPs.

血色病

- 血色素沉着症引起的关节病累及50%的血色病患者，这是一种铁代谢异常的常染色体隐性遗传疾病。该关节病由铁和双水焦磷酸钙结晶沉积引起。

  血色病在临床上表现为青铜色色素沉积、糖尿病、肝硬化、充血性心力衰竭及关节病。

- 在手部，血色素沉着性关节病的好发部位为掌指关节(MCP)，产生特征性掌骨头钩子样骨赘。焦磷酸钙结晶沉积病(CPPD)若仅发生在第二、三MCPs时，可有完全相同的表现。与CPPD不同，血色病可累及所有MCPs。

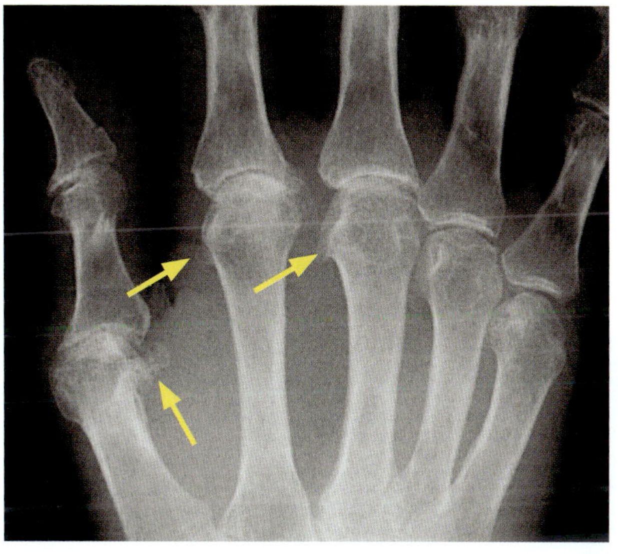

Hemochromatosis: Frontal radiograph of the hand shows cartilage loss and *beak-like* osteophytes of the first through third MCPs (arrows).

Case courtesy Stacy Smith, MD, Brigham and Women's Hospital.

血色病：手正位X线影像示第一～三MCPs软骨缺损及喙样的骨赘形成(黄箭)。

Acromegaly

肢端肥大症

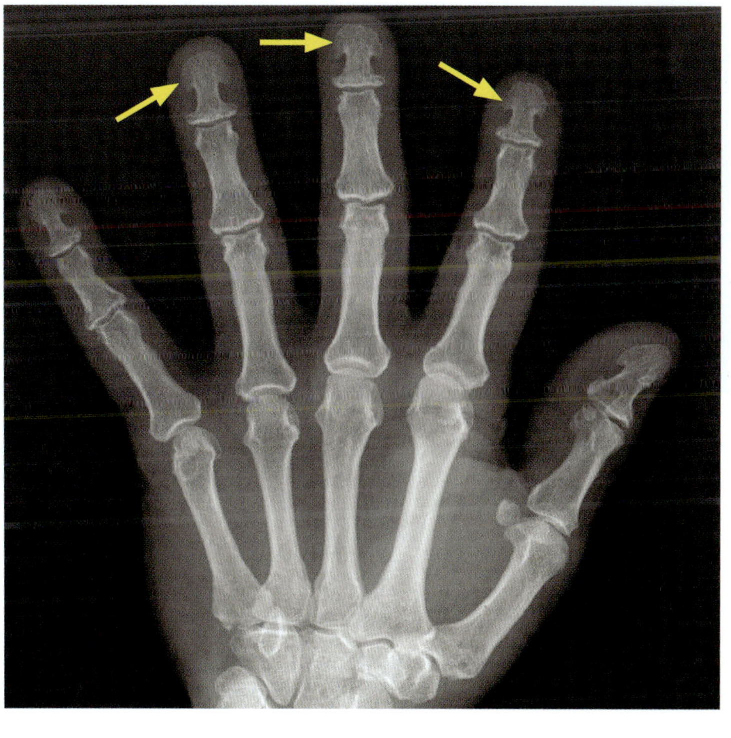

Frontal hand radiograph shows "spade-like enlargement" of the tufts of the distal phalanges (yellow arrows).

手部正位X线影像显示节指骨远端呈“铲状扩大”(黄箭)。

- Acromegaly (excess growth hormone) causes arthropathy due to enlargement of the articular cartilage and subsequent degeneration. In contrast to all other arthropathies, joint spaces are **widened** in early disease due to cartilage hypertrophy. Later in disease, secondary osteoarthritis occurs with cartilage space narrowing.
- In the hand, beak-like osteophytes of the metacarpal heads and spade-like enlargement of the terminal tufts are characteristic.

- 肢端肥大症(生长激素过多)引起的关节病是由于关节软骨增大及随后的退行性变所致。与其他所有关节病相比较，肢端肥大症早期的关节腔是**增宽**的，由软骨增生所致。在晚期病变时，因出现继发性骨性关节炎而导致软骨间隙狭窄。
- 在手部，掌骨头的喙样骨赘和末端指骨铲状扩大具有特征性。

Amyloid arthropathy

- Amyloid arthropathy is a rare noninflammatory arthropathy due to infiltration of bones, joints and soft-tissues by beta-pleated sheets of amino acids. Primary systemic amyloidosis is associated with monoclonal plasma cell dyscrasia. Secondary amyloidosis is associated with chronic underlying inflammation or infection. Another form of amyloidosis is caused by β_2-microglobulin accumulation in patients on chronic hemodialysis.
- A characteristic clinical finding of amyloidosis is bulky soft-tissue nodules in the shoulder superimposed upon atrophic shoulder muscles, producing the *shoulder-pad sign*.
- Imaging findings of amyloid arthropathy are nonspecific but may resemble RA. Intra-articular deposits cause articular cartilage destruction. Soft-tissue nodules and erosions may be present.

淀粉样变性关节病

- 淀粉样变性关节病是一种罕见的非炎症性关节病，由于氨基酸的β折叠结构在骨骼、关节、软组织的浸润所致。原发性系统性淀粉样变与单克隆浆细胞病有关。继发性淀粉样变与慢性潜在炎症或感染有关。另一种类型的淀粉样变由β_2微球蛋白沉积引起，见于长期血液透析患者。
- 临床具有特征性的淀粉样变性的表现为肩部出现大的软组织结节，同时有肩关节肌肉萎缩，形成肩垫征。
- 淀粉样变性关节病的影像学表现不具特异性，可与类风湿关节炎类似。关节内沉积可引起关节软骨破坏。可出现软组织结节和骨质侵蚀。

Ochronosis (alkaptonuria)

褐黄病(尿黑酸尿症)

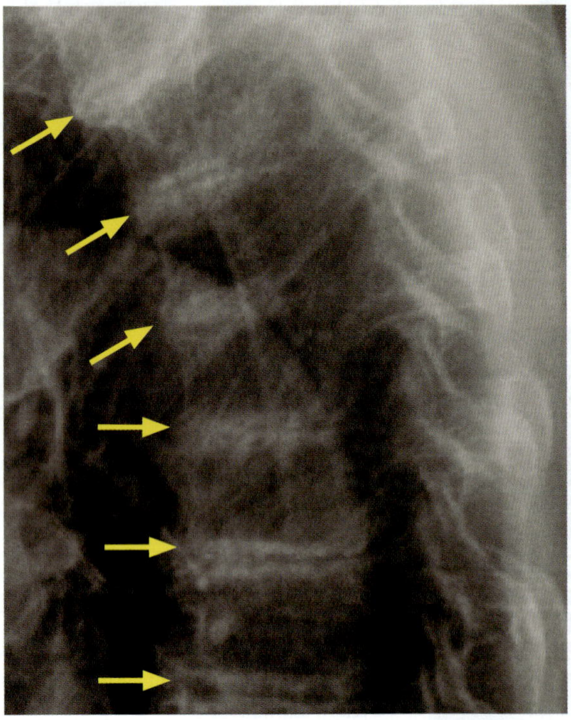

Lateral radiograph of the thoracic spine demonstrates calcification of the intervertebral disc at each level (arrows), with mild diffuse disc height loss.
侧位胸椎X线影像显示每个椎间盘都有钙化(箭)，伴椎间盘的高度轻度和均匀减低。

- Ochronosis is the connective tissue manifestation of alkaptonuria. Alkaptonuria is caused by a defect in homogentisic acid oxidase, causing homogentisic acid polymers to accumulate in the visceral organs, intervertebral discs, and joints. Clinically, homogentisic acid in the urine turns black when exposed to air.
- A specific finding of ochronosis is intervertebral disc calcifications at every level with accompanying disc space narrowing.

- 褐黄病是黑尿症的结缔组织表现。黑尿症由尿黑酸氧化酶缺乏引起，导致尿黑酸多聚体在内脏器官、椎间盘、关节内积聚。临床上，尿中的尿黑酸在接触空气后变成黑色。
- 褐黄病的一个特异性表现是在每个椎间盘出现钙化及伴随的椎间盘间隙狭窄。

Sarcoidosis

- Sarcoidosis is a multisystemic granulomatous disease. Lung findings, including

结节病

- 结节病是一种多系统性肉芽肿性疾病。大多

adenopathy and parenchymal disease, are present in the majority of patients and are the primary manifestation of disease.

- Bony manifestations of sarcoid are rare. A characteristic finding in the hands is *lace-like* lytic lesions in the middle or distal phalanges.
- Sarcoidosis may also manifest as acute or chronic polyarthritis, although there are no distinctive radiographic patterns. Ankle involvement, especially if bilateral or associated with erythema nodosum, should raise suspicion of sarcoidosis and prompt a chest radiograph.

数患者的肺部出现淋巴结肿大、肺实质疾病，且为该病的主要表现形式。

- 结节病很少有骨骼上的表现。手部出现的特征性表现为中节或远节指骨的花边状溶骨性病变。
- 结节病也可表现为急性或慢性多关节炎，但没有非常明确的影像学特征。踝关节受累，特别是双侧同时受累或伴有结节性红斑时应怀疑结节病并需行胸部影像学检查。

Multicentric reticulohistiocytosis

- Multicentric reticulohistiocytosis is a rare disease where lipid-laden macrophages are deposited in soft-tissues and periarticular tendons, forming skin nodules and erosions with sclerotic margins.
- The well-defined erosions of multicentric reticulohistiocytosis tend to affect the DIPs symmetrically. Other radiographic findings of multicentric reticulohistiocytosis include soft-tissue nodules and preserved bone density.
- Joint destruction may be rapid and progressive, producing an *arthritis mutilans* appearance.

多中心网状组织细胞增多症

- 多中心网状组织细胞增多症是一种罕见的疾病，原因是富含脂质的巨噬细胞沉积在软组织和关节周围的肌腱上，形成具有硬化边缘的皮下结节和骨质侵蚀伴边缘硬化。
- 多中心网状组织细胞增多症所造成的骨质侵蚀的边界清晰，且往往对称性累及远端指间关节(DIPs)。多中心网状组织细胞增多症的其他X线影像表现包括软组织结节和骨密度正常。
- 关节破坏可呈快速和进行性，产生残毁性关节炎的表现。

Hemophilic arthropathy

血友病性关节病

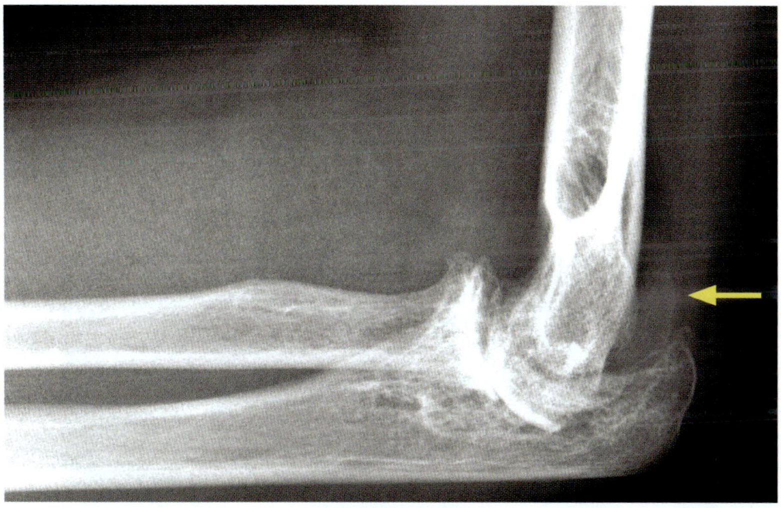

Hemophilic arthropathy: Lateral elbow radiograph shows severe joint space narrowing. Increased soft-tissue density surrounding the joint (arrow) is due to synovial hemosiderin deposition.
In this case, the size of the radial head is not enlarged, but classically hemophilia features an enlarged radial head.
血友病性关节病：肘关节侧位X线影像显示严重的关节间隙狭窄。关节周围软组织密度增高(箭)，为滑膜含铁血黄素沉积所致。
该病例的桡骨小头体积并未增大，但有典型的血友病桡骨小头增大的特征。

- Hemophilia is an X-linked inherited disorder of either factor Ⅷ (hemophilia A) or Ⅸ (hemophilia B; Christmas disease) deficiency causing recurrent bleeding.
- Hemophilia most often affects the knees, elbows, and ankles. Recurrent hemarthrosis results in synovial hypertrophy and hyperemia. The hyperemia may cause epiphyseal enlargement and early fusion.

  Characteristic appearance of the elbow is an enlarged radial head and widened trochlear notch.

  Characteristic appearance of the knee is squaring of the patella and widened intercondylar notch.
- Secondary arthritis may lead to marked joint space narrowing.
- Deposition of iron in the synovium causes increased soft-tissue density around joints.
- Juvenile idiopathic arthritis (discussed below) also causes articular hyperemia and may have similar radiographic findings, especially in the knee (widened intercondylar notch) and elbow (enlarged radial head).
- **Pseudotumor of hemophilia** is a benign lesion caused by recurrent

- 血友病是一种X连锁的遗传性疾病，由Ⅷ因子(血友病A)或Ⅸ因子(血友病B；圣诞病)缺乏导致反复出血。
- 血友病最常累及膝关节、肘关节和踝关节。反复关节积血导致滑膜肥厚和充血。充血可引起骨骺增大和早期闭合。

  肘关节的特征性表现是桡骨头增大和滑车切迹增宽。

  膝关节的特征性表现是髌骨变方和髁间切迹增宽。
- 继发性关节炎可导致显著的关节间隙狭窄。
- 滑膜内铁沉积引起关节周围软组织密度增高。
- 青少年特发性关节炎(下文讨论)也可引起关节充血并有相似的X线影像表现，特别是在膝关节(髁间切迹增宽)和肘关节(桡骨头增大)。
- **血友病性假瘤**是由骨内或骨膜下反复出血引

intraosseous or subperiosteal bleeding. The chronic cyclical bleeding leads to bony scalloping and pressure erosion, often with an associated soft-tissue mass.

On radiography, pseudotumor is benign-appearing, with well-circumscribed and sclerotic margins.

Pseudotumor may have a complex MRI appearance due to different stages of blood products.

Juvenile idiopathic arthritis (JIA), previously called juvenile rheumatoid arthritis

- Juvenile idiopathic arthritis (JIA) is a spectrum of related chronic inflammatory arthropathies affecting children younger than 16 years of age.
- **Monoarticular** or **pauciarticular** (most common) JIA may affect either a single joint or a few joints including the knees, ankles, elbows, or wrists.
- **Polyarticular** JIA is a systemic disease affecting multiple joints including the hands, feet, and cervical spine in addition to the joints affected by mono/pauciarticular disease.
- A variant of JIA is **Still disease**, which is a systemic disorder affecting children younger than 5, featuring acute febrile illness, rash, adenopathy, pericarditis, and mild arthralgias.
- Radiographic hallmarks of JIA are abnormal bone length or morphology due to hyperemia in a skeletally immature patient. Growth disturbances are more commonly seen in early-onset disease. Abnormal morphology results from epiphyseal overgrowth and enlargement *(ballooning)* of the ends of bone. Affected joints demonstrate premature skeletal maturation and physeal fusion.
- In the hand, premature fusion of the growth plate may cause brachydactyly (short fingers).

起的一种良性病变。慢性周期性出血导致骨质扇贝样改变和压力性骨质侵蚀，常伴有软组织肿块。

假瘤在影像学上呈良性外观，病变边界清楚且边缘有硬化。

假瘤在MRI上的表现较为复杂，为不同时期的出血产物。

青少年特发性关节炎(JIA)，旧称青少年类风湿关节炎

- 青少年特发性关节炎(JIA)是一组相互关联的慢性炎性关节病，发生于16岁以下青少年。
- **单关节**或**少关节JIA**(最常见)可侵及单个或少数几个关节，包括膝关节、踝关节、肘关节或腕关节。
- **多关节JIA**是一种系统性疾病，累及多个关节，包括手、足和颈椎，以及单关节/少关节炎所受累的关节。
- JIA的一种变异型为**Still**病，为好发于5岁以下儿童的一种系统性疾病，表现为急性发热、皮疹、淋巴结肿大、心包炎和轻度关节痛。
- JIA的X线影像特征是异常的骨骼长度或形态，这是由于骨骼未成熟患者出现充血所致。生长紊乱更常见于疾病的早期。形态异常是骨骺过度生长和骨的末端增大(气球样)的结果。受累关节表现为骨骼早熟和骨骺融合。
- 在手部，生长板过早融合可导致短指畸形(短指)。

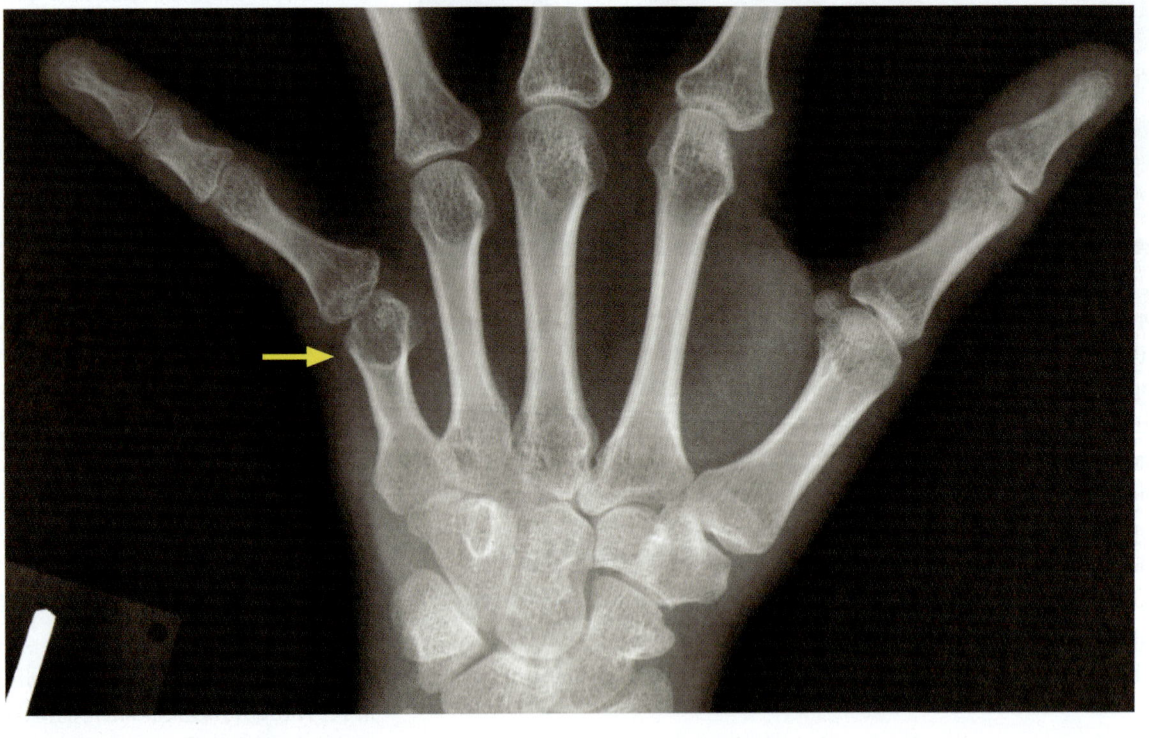

PA radiograph of the hand in a patient with juvenile idiopathic arthritis shows a shortened fifth metacarpal (arrow).
一名青少年特发性关节炎患者手的后前位X线影像显示第五掌骨缩短(箭)。

- In the knee, the characteristic appearance is a widened intercondylar notch, metaphyseal flaring, and uniform joint space narrowing. This appearance can appear similar to hemophilia.
- In the elbow, there is characteristic enlargement of the radial head and trochlear notch, with uniform cartilage space narrowing. These findings can also be seen in hemophilia.
- In the hips, symmetrical cartilage space narrowing, protrusio deformity, and gracile appearance of the femoral shaft are characteristic.
- Ankylosis may occur in the wrist and zygapophyseal (facet) joints of the cervical spine. Ankylosis occurs much more commonly in juvenile idiopathic arthropathy compared to adult rheumatoid arthritis. The differential diagnosis of a child with cervical spine ankylosis is Klippel-Feil syndrome, which is failure of cervical segmentation.

Neuropathic arthropathy (Charcot joint)

- Neuropathic arthropathy, also called *Charcot joint,* is a destructive form of arthritis caused by neurosensory deficit. Lack of sensation ultimately causes severe degenerative changes with fragmentation of bone and cartilage.
- Neuropathic arthropathy clinically presents as a (usually) painless, swollen joint.
- Neuropathic arthropathy can be caused by any process that affects sensory nerves. The peripheral neuropathy of diabetes is implicated most frequently, typically affecting joints in the ankle and foot. Other causes include syringomyelia (usually affecting the upper extremity), chronic alcohol abuse, amyloid, spinal tumors, and very rarely syphilis or leprosy.
- Two forms of neuropathic arthropathy are hypertrophic (more common) and atrophic variants.
- The **hypertrophic** variant looks like *anarchy in a joint*, with destruction, dislocation (or subluxation), debris, disorganization, and *no* demineralization.

- 在膝关节，特征性的表现为髁间窝增宽、干骺端呈喇叭形，以及关节间隙均匀性狭窄。这些表现与血友病类似。
- 在肘关节，桡骨头增大和滑车切迹增宽具有特征性，伴均匀的软骨间隙狭窄。这些表现也可见于血友病。
- 在髋关节，对称性关节间隙狭窄、髋臼内陷畸形、股骨干变细都具有特征性。
- 关节强直可发生在腕关节和颈椎的关节突关节(椎小关节)。关节强直在青少年特发性关节炎中远较成人类风湿关节炎常见。儿童颈椎关节强直的鉴别诊断包括克利佩尔-费尔综合征，为一种颈椎椎体分节障碍。

神经病性关节病(Charcot关节)

- 神经病性关节病，称为Charcot关节，是由神经感觉缺失引起的一种毁损型关节炎。感觉缺失最终会导致严重退行性病变，出现骨和软骨碎裂。
- 神经病性关节病的临床表现(通常)为无痛性关节肿大。
- 神经病性关节病可由任何影响感觉神经的病变引起。其中，糖尿病的外周神经病变最常见，通常累及踝关节和足部关节。其他原因包括脊髓空洞症(常累及上肢)、长期酗酒、淀粉样变性、脊椎肿瘤，以及极少数情况下的梅毒或麻风。
- 神经病性关节病有两种类型，即肥厚型(较常见)和萎缩型。
- **肥厚型**表现为一个结构紊乱的关节，有骨质破坏、关节脱位(或不全脱位)、骨碎片形成、结构紊乱，但无骨盐减少。

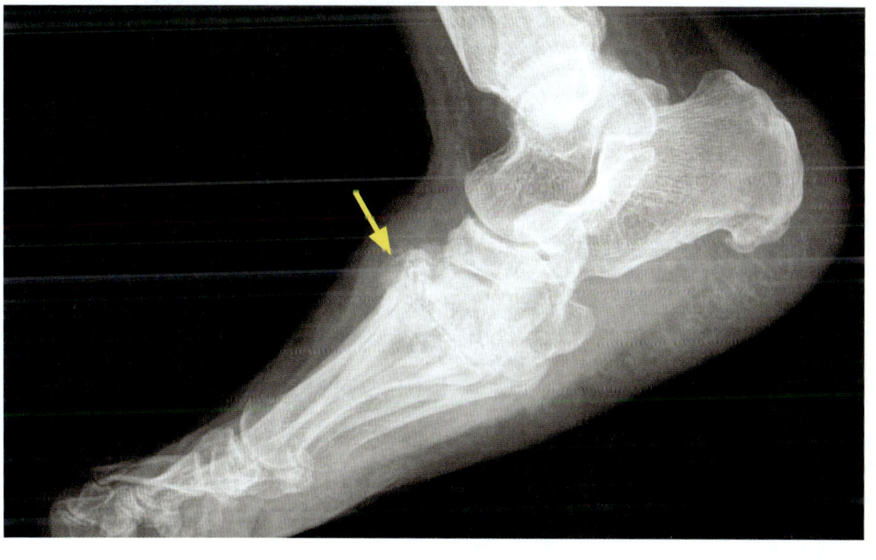

Neuropathic arthropathy:
Lateral radiograph of the foot demonstrates subluxation of the Lisfranc joint (yellow arrow). Hypertrophic degenerative changes are present at the tarsometatarsal joint. There was no history of trauma.
神经病性关节病：足侧位X线影像显示跗跖关节(黄箭)不全脱位，跗跖关节有肥厚型退行性改变。无外伤史。

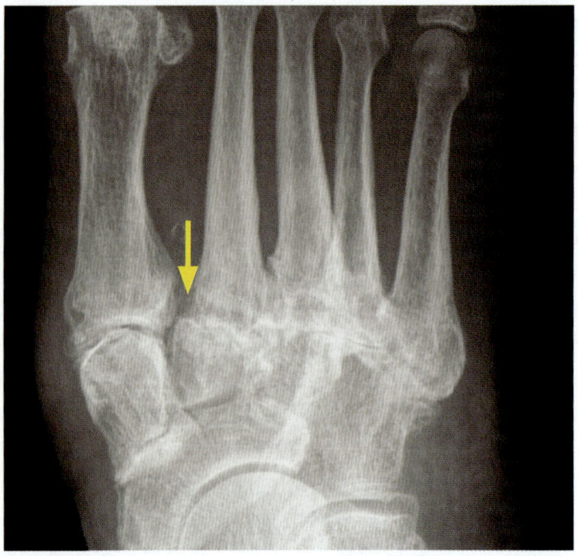

AP radiograph of the foot in the same patient shows divergent lateral subluxation of the Lisfranc joint in the same patient.
The yellow arrow points to the enlarged space between the first and second metatarsals. Offset of the second metatarsal base with the mid cuneiform may be an early finding of Lisfranc injury.
同一名患者的足前后位X线影像显示跗跖关节分离型侧向不全脱位。黄箭所示为增宽的第一和第二跖骨间隙。第二跖骨基底部与中间楔骨的偏离可能是跗跖关节损伤的早期表现。

- The **atrophic** variant of neuropathic arthropathy occurs most commonly in the shoulder. It features a classic radiographic appearance of humeral head resorption with a sharp, *surgical-like* margin. Syringomyelia should be suspected in upper extremity neuropathic arthropathy and confirmed by cervical spine MRI.

- **萎缩型**神经病性关节病最常见于肩关节。典型的X线表现为肱骨头骨质吸收伴锐利的“手术样切割”边缘。当上肢发生神经病性关节病时，应考虑脊髓空洞症，并使用颈椎MRI进行确诊。

（翻译　陈紫琪　姚骊　帅丹丹）

BONE TUMORS

骨肿瘤

GENERAL APPROACH TO BONE TUMORS

骨肿瘤诊断的一般流程

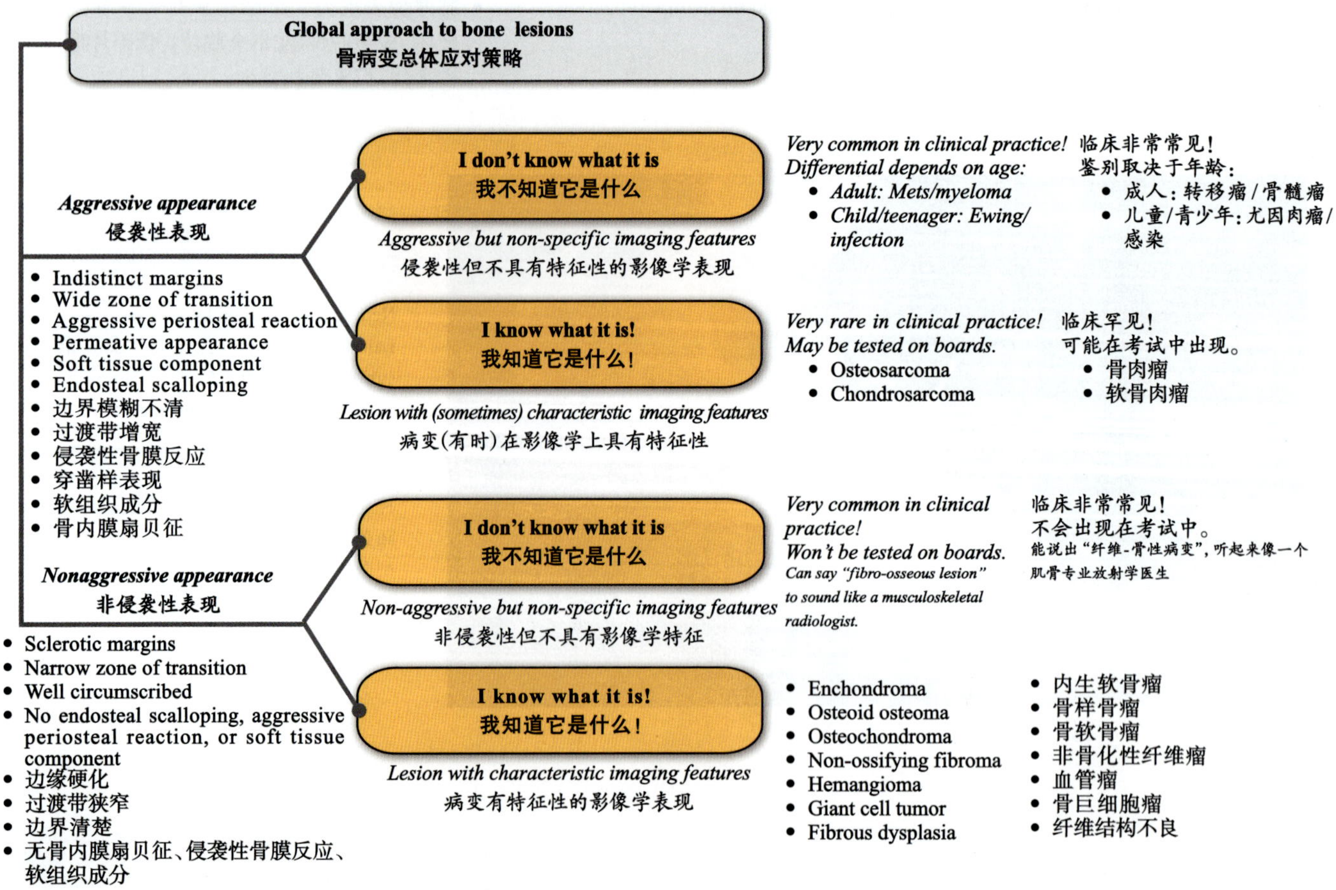

- Bone tumors can be an intimidating topic because there are so many different types of tumors with similar-sounding names.
- When faced with a bone lesion, it can be helpful to think of bone tumors in 4 groups, as shown above.
- Lesions may have aggressive or nonaggressive imaging appearances. Indistinct margins, aggressive periosteal reaction (as illustrated on the following page), wide zone of transition, permeative appearance, soft tissue component, and endosteal scalloping are aggressive imaging features. Any one of these features may be enough to be concerning.
- Additionally, some bone lesions can have characteristic imaging features to allow you to arrive at a specific diagnosis (perhaps more on tests than in real life). These are the lesions that should be learned (listed on the right side in the diagram above) and include both benign and malignant etiologies.
- In clinical practice, it is far more common for bone lesions to not have specific imaging features, and management should be determined based on aggressive versus nonaggressive appearance.

- 骨肿瘤可能是一个令人生畏的话题，因为骨肿瘤类型有如此之多，但它们的名称却又极为相似。
- 当面对一个骨的病变时，将骨肿瘤按上图归纳的四类进行考虑可能会有所帮助。
- 病变的影像学表现可具侵袭性或非侵袭性。侵袭性的影像特征包括边界模糊不清、侵袭性骨膜反应(如下图所示)、过渡带增宽、穿凿样表现、软组织成分和骨内膜扇贝征。上述任何一个特征都足以让人产生怀疑。
- 此外，一些骨的病变具有特征性的影像学表现，从而有助于作出确切的诊断(也许在考试中比在现实工作中更常见)。应当掌握这些病变(上图右列)，包括良性和恶性病变。
- 在临床工作中，更多的骨病变不具有影像特征，应根据病变的侵袭性或非侵袭性表现来确定诊疗策略。

Morphology

Periosteal reaction

- The morphology of a bone lesion's associated periosteal reaction gives an important clue to the rate of growth, and hence the aggressiveness, of the lesion.

形态学

骨膜反应

- 骨病变相关骨膜反应的形态学可以作为病变生长速率的重要线索，即病变的侵袭性。

Normal periosteal anatomy
正常骨膜解剖

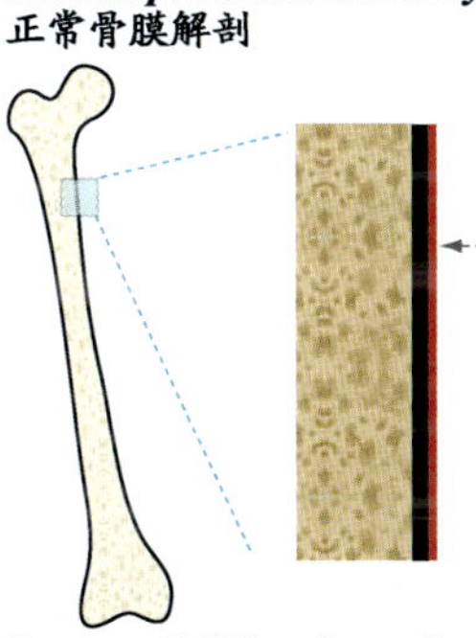

Periosteum covers essentially the entire bone excluding the joint surfaces.
骨膜基本上覆盖了除关节面外的整个骨。

Benign: Solid periosteal reaction
良性：致密的骨膜反应

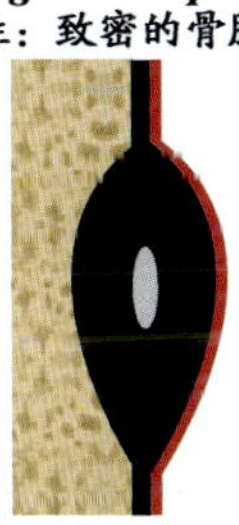

A slow-growing process, such as osteoid osteoma (radiolucent nidus), incites the periosteal cells to lay down bone in a smooth, continuous manner.
缓慢生长的病变，如骨样骨瘤（透光的瘤巢），刺激骨膜细胞产生光滑、连续的骨组织。

Aggressive: Lamellated periosteal reaction
侵袭性，层状骨膜反应

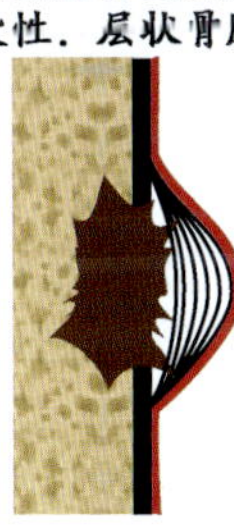

An irregularly-growing process that grows in starts and stops produces a characteristic lamellated or *onion-skinned* appearance (arrows). When the lesion is growing quickly the periosteal cells don't have enough time to lay down bone.
不规则生长的病变，因生长与停止呈交替方式进行，产生特征性的层状或洋葱皮样外观（箭）。当病变快速生长时，骨膜细胞没有充足的时间产生骨组织。

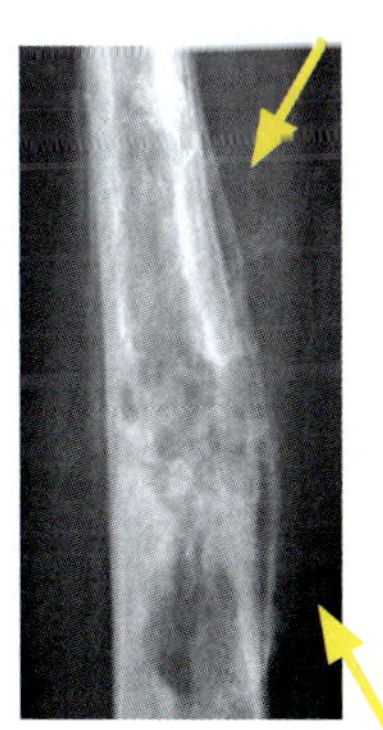

Very aggressive: Sunburst periosteal reaction
高度侵袭性：日光放射状骨膜反应

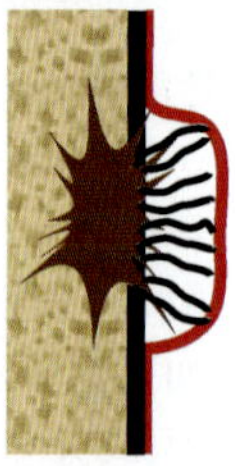

A very fast growing lesion pushes the periosteal cells outward as the lesion expands, with each periosteal cell leaving a trail of bone formation that looks like ***hair on end*** or ***sunburst*** (arrows).
异常快速生长的病变，其扩张可将骨膜细胞推向外侧，使每个骨膜细胞留下一道成骨的痕迹，看起来像头发竖立或日光放射样（箭）。

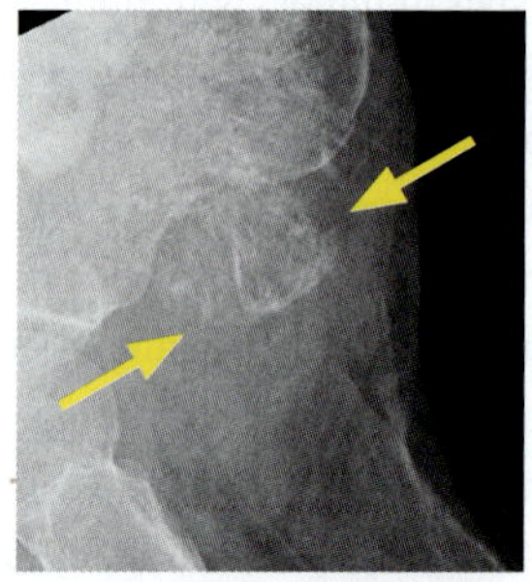

Very very aggressive: Codman triangle
极高侵袭性：Codman三角

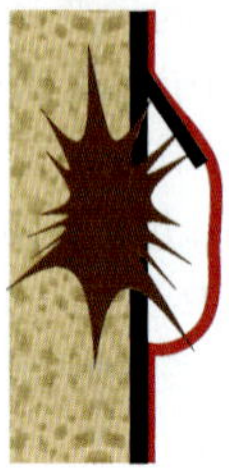

A lesion that grows so aggressively that the periosteum does not even have a chance to lay down visible calcification except at the periphery produces a characteristic *Codman triangle* (yellow arrow).
生长极具侵袭性的病变，可导致除了周边，其余骨膜没有机会产生可见的骨化，形成特征性的Codman三角（黄箭）。

Note the associated soft tissue mass (red arrows).
注意伴随的软组织肿块（红箭）。

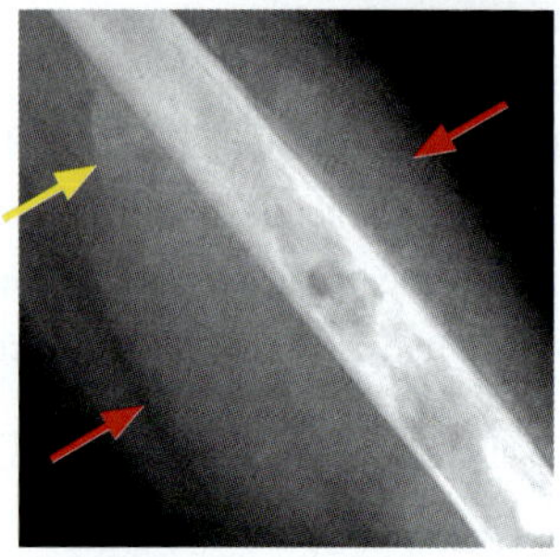

Pattern of bone destruction: Margin analysis

- Analysis of a bone lesion's margins (i.e., zone of transition from normal to abnormal bone) helps to characterize the bony destruction and stratify a lesion as aggressive or non aggressive.
- A sharply marginated zone of transition usually denotes a less aggressive lesion with slower rate of growth. The faster the rate of growth, the more aggressive the lesion may be. A wide zone of transition suggests rapid growth and a more aggressive lesion.

骨质破坏的方式：边界分析

- 分析骨病变的边界(如从正常骨到不正常骨的过渡带)有助于对骨质破坏进行定性，并将病变归为侵袭性或非侵袭性。
- 具有清晰可见的过渡带通常代表较低侵袭性、生长较慢的病变。增长速度越快，病变的侵袭性可能越高。增宽的过渡带提示生长迅速且病变更具侵袭性。

Lodwick classification of bone destruction

- The Lodwick classification of bone destruction helps to stratify aggressiveness:
- Type 1: **Geographic pattern**: Margins have a thin zone of transition and may be sclerotic or well-defined.
  - 1A: Thin sclerotic margins. Almost always nonaggressive.
  - 1B: Well-defined margins. Usually nonaggressive.
  - 1C: Any part of the margin is indistinct.
- Type 2: **Moth-eaten pattern**: It is difficult to define any border at all. Aggressive.
- Type 3: **Permeative**: The permeative pattern is characterized by multiple tiny holes that infiltrate the bone. This pattern is very aggressive and is seen in lymphoma, leukemia, and Ewing sarcoma.

Lodwick骨质破坏分类法

- Lodwick骨质破坏分类法有助于对侵袭性进行分层：
- 1型：**地图样**，病变边缘为薄的过渡带，可呈硬化或有清晰的界线。
  - 1A：边缘薄而有硬化。几乎都属非侵袭性。
  - 1B：边缘清晰。通常是非侵袭性病变。
  - 1C：边界的任何部分都不能区分。
- 2型：**虫蚀状**，根本无法确定边界。侵袭性。
- 3型：**穿凿样**，特征为骨质被多发微型孔洞浸润。这种骨质破坏方式具有高度侵袭性，见于淋巴瘤、白血病和尤因肉瘤。

- A *pseudopermeative* process describes the appearance of osteoporosis and osseous hemangioma, two benign conditions. Unlike the true permeative appearance of an aggressive lesion, the pseudopermeative appearance seen in these two entities *will* extend to the cortex.

- 假性穿凿样改变是指骨质疏松症和骨血管瘤样表现，两者均为良性病变。与侵袭性病变的穿凿样表现不同，在这两种病变中看到的假性穿凿样表现会延伸到骨皮质。

New matrix created by tumor

- Matrix produced by an osteoid lesion, such as malignant osteosarcoma, appears as fluffy, cloud-like bone.
- Matrix produced by a chondroid lesion, such as a benign enchondroma or malignant chondrosarcoma, has a *ring and arc* or *popcorn-like* appearance.
- A *ground glass* matrix describes blurring of the trabeculae and is seen in fibrous dysplasia, a benign fibrosseous lesion involving abnormal proliferation of intraosseous fibroblasts.

肿瘤产生的新基质

- 骨样病变产生的基质，如恶性骨肉瘤，表现为疏松、云絮状骨。
- 软骨样病变产生的基质，如良性内生软骨瘤或恶性软骨肉瘤，具有环形、弧形或爆米花样外观。
- 磨玻璃样基质指模糊的骨小梁，见于纤维结构不良，为骨内成纤维细胞异常增殖所致的一种良性纤维骨性病变。

Unique features

- The *fallen-fragment sign* is seen in a simple (unicameral) bone cyst with pathologic fracture.
- An *aneurysmal* or expansile appearance suggests an aneurysmal bone cyst.
- Resorption of distal clavicles or tumoral calcinosis can suggest hyperparathyroidism, which can cause brown tumors.

专有特征

- 骨片塌陷征见于单纯(单房)性骨囊肿伴病理性骨折。
- 动脉瘤样或膨胀样的表现提示动脉瘤样骨囊肿。
- 锁骨远端骨质吸收或肿瘤钙质沉着提示甲状旁腺功能亢进,可导致棕色瘤。

Patient age

- The two most likely considerations of an aggressive lytic bone lesion in a patient over age 40 are metastasis or myeloma.
- Under age 20, an aggressive lytic lesion is most likely to represent eosinophilic granuloma, infection, or Ewing sarcoma.

患者年龄

- 40岁以上的患者中最可能的两种侵袭性溶骨性病变是转移瘤或骨髓瘤。
- 20岁以下的患者中最可能的侵袭性溶骨性病变是嗜酸性肉芽肿、感染或尤因肉瘤。

Location within bone

Eccentric within bone

- Giant-cell tumor, chondroblastoma, aneurysmal bone cyst, non-ossifying fibroma, and the rare chondromyxoid fibroma are located eccentrically within the bone.

Central (in the middle of a long bone)

- Simple bone cyst, enchondroma, and fibrous dysplasia are located centrally within the bone.

病变在骨内的位置

偏心性

- 骨巨细胞瘤、软骨母细胞瘤、动脉瘤样骨囊肿、非骨化性纤维瘤和罕见的软骨黏液样纤维瘤均位于骨的偏心部位

中心性(在长骨的中间)

- 单纯性骨囊肿、内生软骨瘤和纤维性结构不良均位于骨的中心。

(翻译 刘杰克 杨曦玥)

Bone lesions organized by cell of origin

Bone forming (osteo-) lesions

Benign and incidental: Enostosis (bone island)

- Enostosis (commonly called a bone island) is an extremely common incidental finding of a small spiculated osteoblastic focus.
- A bone island is only clinically significant in that it may rarely be difficult to differentiate from an osteoblastic metastasis, osteoid osteoma, or a low-grade osteosarcoma.
- A giant variant (>2 cm) may be most difficult to differentiate from low-grade osteosarcoma.
- Bone scan of bone island is usually normal.
- **Osteopoikilosis** is an autosomal dominant syndrome of multiple bone islands and keloid formation.
- **Osteopathia striata** is a benign, asymptomatic sclerotic dysplasia characterized by linear bands of sclerosis in the long bones and fan-like sclerosis in the flat pelvic bones. Bone scan is typically normal.

Benign and incidental: Osteoma

- Osteoma is a slow growing lesion that may arise from the cortex of the skull or the frontal/ethmoid sinuses.
- Gardner syndrome is an autosomal dominant syndrome of multiple osteomas, intestinal polyposis, and soft-tissue desmoid tumors.
- In contrast to a bone island, osteoma arises from cortex rather than medullary canal.

按细胞起源分类的骨病变

成骨(骨)性病变

良性及偶发性:内生骨疣(骨岛)

- 内生骨疣(通常称为骨岛)是一种常见的小型毛刺状成骨病灶,通常为偶然发现。
- 骨岛只是在少数情况下无法与成骨性转移瘤、骨样骨瘤或低级别骨肉瘤等罕见情况相鉴别时才有临床意义。
- 一种形态巨大的变异(>2cm)可能与低级别骨肉瘤进行鉴别。
- 骨岛在骨扫描时通常正常。
- **脆性骨硬化**是一种常染色体显性综合征,表现为多发骨岛和瘢痕瘤形成。
- **条纹性骨病**是一种良性、无症状的硬化性发育不良,其特征为长骨呈条纹状硬化及骨盆扁平骨呈扇形硬化。骨扫描通常正常。

良性和偶发性:骨瘤

- 骨瘤是一种生长缓慢的病变,可发生于颅骨的皮质或额窦/筛窦。
- 加德纳综合征是一种常染色体显性综合征,表现为多发骨瘤、肠息肉病和软组织硬纤维瘤。
- 与骨岛不同,骨瘤起源于骨皮质而非骨髓腔。

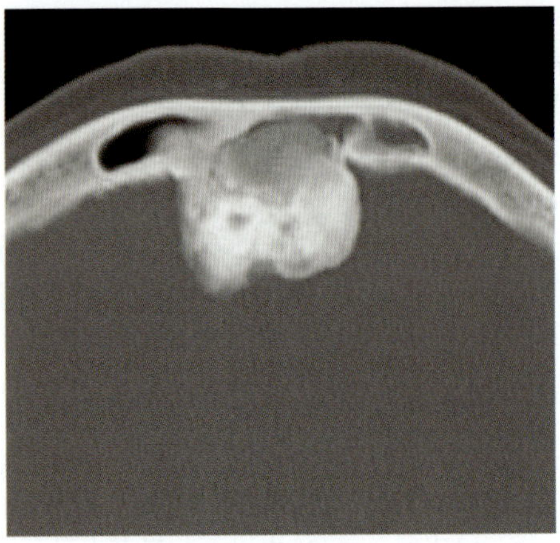

Osteoma: Axial head CT in bone window shows a densely sclerotic osteoma arising from the cortex of the frontal sinus.
骨瘤：头颅轴位CT骨窗显示一个致密硬化的骨瘤，起源于额窦皮质。

Benign: Melorheostosis

- Melorheostosis is a non-neoplastic proliferation of thickened and irregular cortex with a typical *candle-wax* appearance.
- It clinically presents with pain, decreased range of motion, leg- bowing, and leg-length discrepancy.
- Melorheostosis may be associated with scleroderma-like skin lesions over the affected region.
- Melorheostosis is usually seen in a single lower limb, in the distribution of a single sclerotome. A sclerotome represents a zone supplied by a single sensory nerve.
- Melorheostosis features intense uptake on bone scan.

良性：肢骨纹状肥大

- 肢骨纹状肥大是一种骨皮质非肿瘤增生性增厚及不规则改变，呈典型的蜡滴状表现。
- 临床表现为疼痛、关节活动度减小、腿弯曲变形及下肢长度不等。
- 肢骨纹状肥大可以在病灶相应部位出现硬皮病样的皮肤病变。
- 肢骨纹状肥大常见于单侧小腿，分布于单个生骨节。一个生骨节代表一根感觉神经支配的区域。
- 肢骨纹状肥大在骨扫描图像上呈显著的摄取增加。

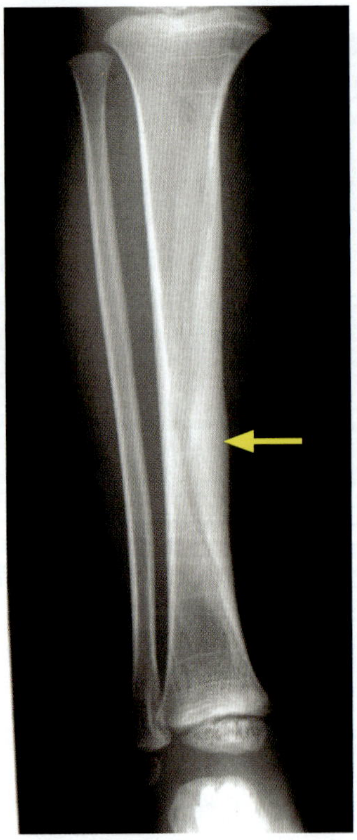

Melorheostosis:
Frontal radiograph of the right tibia and fibula shows thickened, irregular wavy cortex of the medial tibia (arrow).
Case courtesy Michael Callahan, MD, Boston Children's Hospital.
肢骨纹状肥大：右侧胫腓骨正位X线影像显示胫骨内侧增厚、不规则波浪状骨皮质(箭)。

Benign: Osteoid osteoma

- Osteoid osteoma is a benign osteoblastic lesion characterized by a nidus of osteoid tissue surrounded by reactive bone sclerosis. The etiology is controversial. Inflammatory, vascular, and viral causes have been proposed.

良性：骨样骨瘤

- 骨样骨瘤是一种良性成骨性病变，以骨样组织瘤巢周围环绕反应性骨硬化为特征。病因学存在争议，有炎症、血管和病毒各种学说。

- The classic clinical presentation is night pain relieved by aspirin in a teenager or young adult.
- Osteoid osteoma tends to occur in the diaphyses of the leg long bones (femur and tibia) most commonly. About 20% occur in the posterior elements of the spine. Spinal osteoid osteoma is an important cause of painful scoliosis.
- On radiography and CT, a lucent nidus is surrounded by sclerosis. There is often central calcification within the nidus. Bone scan will be positive, with the *double density sign* representing intense uptake centrally in the region of the nidus and adjacent reactive uptake corresponding to sclerosis. Osteoid osteoma can be difficult to see on MRI alone. The nidus is usually low-signal on T1-weighted images and reactive marrow edema can obscure the lesion on T2-weighted images.

- 典型临床表现是青少年或年轻成人夜间痛，可用阿司匹林缓解。
- 骨样骨瘤往往发生在下肢长骨的骨干(股骨和胫骨)。约20%发生于脊柱的后部结构。脊柱的骨样骨瘤是导致疼痛性脊柱侧弯的一个重要原因。
- 骨样骨瘤在X线和CT上表现为一个透亮瘤巢，外周包绕硬化。瘤巢内常有中心性钙化。骨扫描呈阳性，出现的双密度征为瘤巢中央区摄取显著增加和邻近硬化区的反应性摄取。骨样骨瘤仅靠MRI很难发现。瘤巢通常在T_1加权图像上呈低信号，而反应性骨髓水肿会造成病变在T_2加权图像上模糊不清。

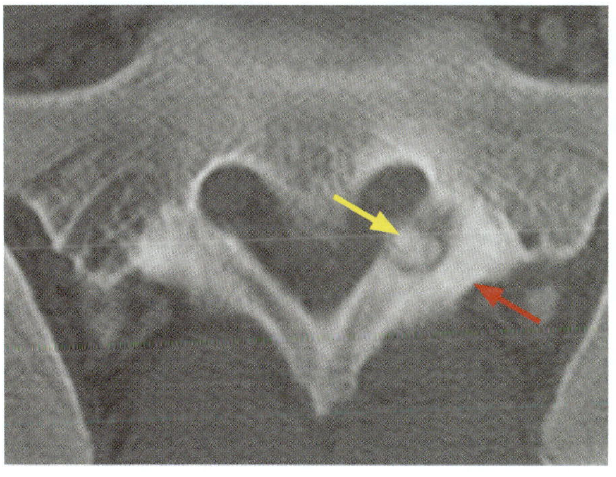

Axial CT
轴位CT

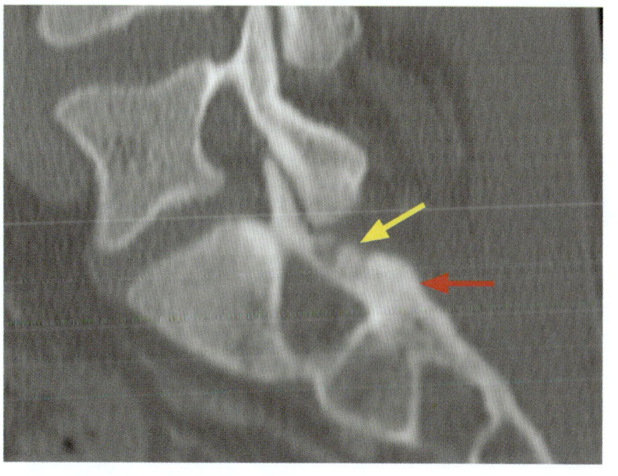

Sagittal CT
矢状位CT

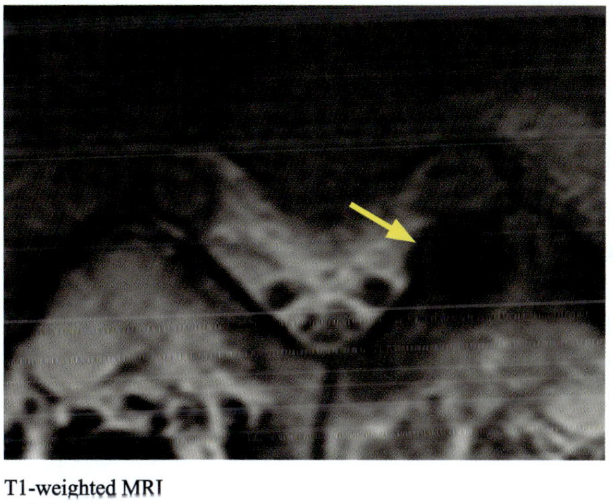

T1-weighted MRI
T_1加权MRI

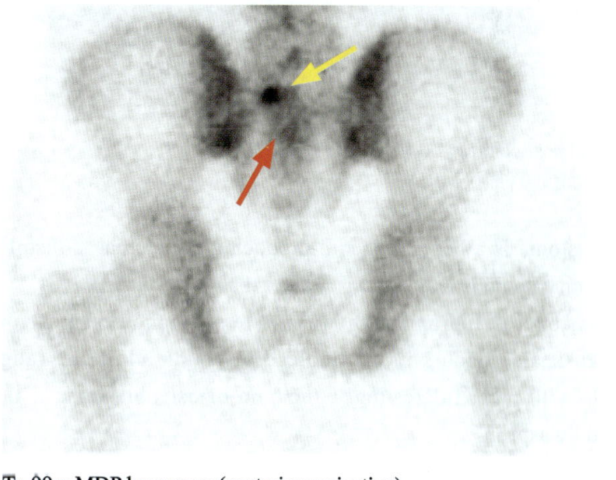

Tc-99m MDP bone scan (posterior projection)
^{99m}Tc MDP骨扫描(后位)

Osteoid osteoma: CT shows a radiolucent nidus in the left sacral ala (posterior element location) with a large central calcification (yellow arrows) with adjacent sclerosis (red arrows). The lesion is less conspicuous on MRI and has very low signal on the T1-weighted image (yellow arrow). The posterior bone scan shows increased radiotracer uptake (yellow arrow) of the nidus, with a *double density sign* (red arrow; corresponding to reactive sclerosis).
骨样骨瘤：CT显示左侧骶骨翼(后部)一个透亮的瘤巢，其内有一个大的中央性钙化(黄箭)，伴邻近骨硬化(红箭)。该病灶在MRI上不明显，T_1加权图像呈极低信号(黄箭)。后位骨扫描显示瘤巢放射性示踪剂摄取增加(黄箭)，伴双密度征(红箭；与反应性骨硬化相对应)。

- Treatment of osteoid osteoma is interventional radiology radiofrequency ablation, surgical curettage, or resection.

- 骨样骨瘤的治疗方法为射频消融术(介入放射)、外科刮除术或切除术。

Benign: Osteoblastoma

良性：骨母细胞瘤

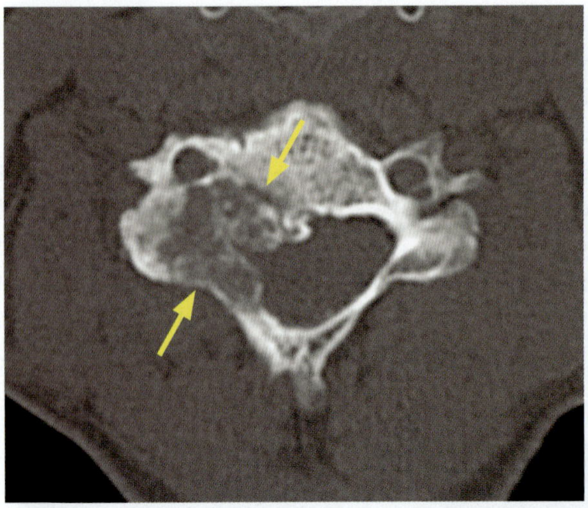

Axial CT
轴位CT

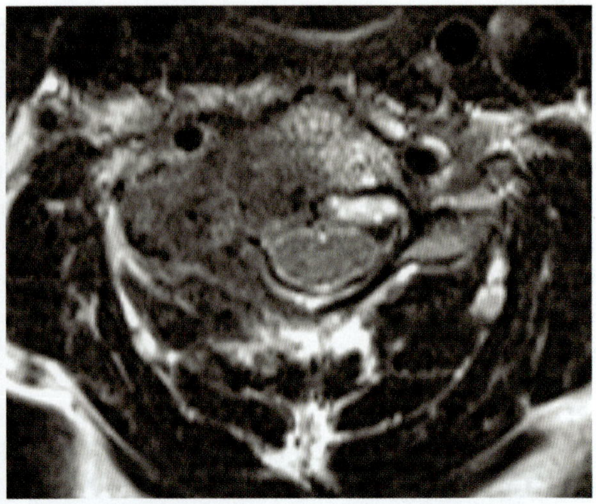

Axial T2-weighted MRI
轴位T_2加权MRI

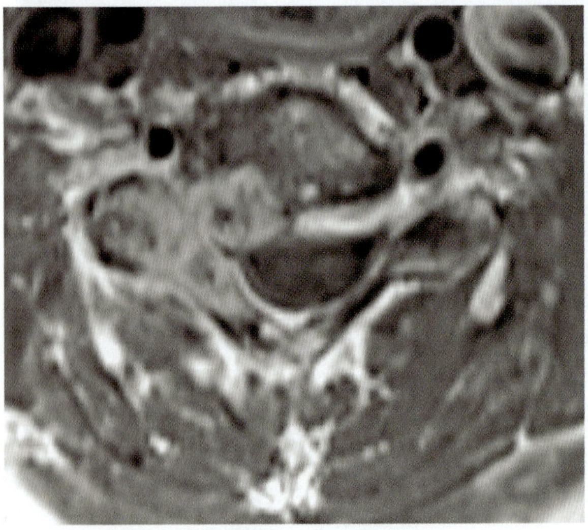

Axial post-contrast T1-weighted MRI
轴位增强T_1加权MRI

Osteoblastoma:
Axial CT image of the cervical spine shows an expansile lytic lesion (arrows) involving the right aspect of the C5 vertebral body with extension posterolaterally to the lateral mass and lamina. Axial MR images of the same lesion show that it is slightly T2 hyperintense to muscle on T2-weighted image and enhancing on post-contrast T1 image. Biopsy showed osteoblastoma.

骨母细胞瘤：颈椎轴位CT显示一处累及C_5椎体右侧的膨胀性溶骨性病变(箭)，并向后外侧延伸至侧块和椎板。轴位MRI显示同一个病灶在T_2加权MRI上信号稍高于肌肉，在T_1增强后强化。活检显示骨母细胞瘤。

- Osteoblastoma is a benign osteoid-producing tumor that is histologically the same as an osteoid osteoma but is greater than 2 cm in size.
- Osteoblastoma is approximately 4 times less common than osteoid osteoma, although it also occurs in the adolescent/young adult age range and also presents with pain. Interestingly, the pain of osteoblastoma is not typically relieved by aspirin.
- The most common location is the posterior elements of the spine, occurring anywhere from the cervical spine through the sacrum. Osteoblastoma may also occur in the femur and tibia.
- The most common radiographic appearance of osteoblastoma is a lytic lesion with mineralization. Very rarely, osteoblastoma may be aggressive with large soft-tissue mass, but lacking metastatic potential. Secondary aneurysmal bone cyst may be seen, especially when spinal in location.
- A lytic lesion in the posterior elements of a young person may represent an osteoblastoma or aneurysmal bone cyst. If any mineralization is present within the lesion, osteoblastoma should be favored.

- 骨母细胞瘤是一种产生类骨质良性肿瘤，在组织学上与骨样骨瘤相同，但其大小超过2cm。
- 骨母细胞瘤常发生于青少年/年轻成人，并伴有疼痛，但其发病率大约是骨样骨瘤的1/4。有意思的是，骨母细胞瘤的疼痛常不被阿司匹林所缓解。
- 骨母细胞瘤最好发于脊柱后部结构，病变可发生在颈椎至骶骨之间的任何一个椎体，也可发生在股骨和胫骨。
- 骨母细胞瘤最常见的X线表现是具有矿化的溶骨性病变。极少数情况下，骨母细胞瘤可能具有较大的软组织肿块，但无转移的潜能。可见继发性动脉瘤样骨囊肿，最常发生在脊柱。
- 若溶骨性病变出现在年轻人的脊柱后部结构，则有可能是骨母细胞瘤或动脉瘤样骨囊肿。如果病变内出现任何矿化，应优先考虑骨母细胞瘤。

Malignant: Osteosarcoma

- Osteosarcoma represents a heterogeneous group of malignant tumors where the neoplastic cells are derived should be from osteoid lineage and most subtypes produce an osteoid matrix.
- Osteosarcoma can be primary or secondary. Secondary osteosarcoma may arise from Paget disease or after radiation. Secondary osteosarcoma in Paget disease is extremely aggressive.
- General imaging hallmarks of osteosarcoma are bony destruction, production of osteoid matrix, aggressive periosteal reaction, and an associated soft-tissue mass. Early osteosarcoma may be only evident as subtle sclerosis.
- There are more than 10 primary subtypes. The 4 most important subtypes are conventional (most common), telangiectatic, and the two juxtacortical subtypes including parosteal (pronounced *PAR-osteal*) and periosteal (pronounced *PERI-osteal*).
- **Conventional** (intramedullary) osteosarcoma represents 75% of osteosarcomas and occurs in adolescents/young adults usually about the knee in the metaphysis of the femur or tibia.

  Conventional osteosarcoma features an intramedullary osteoid matrix, both intramedullary and cortical bone destruction, aggressive periosteal reaction (sunburst or Codman), and a soft-tissue mass.

恶性：骨肉瘤

- 骨肉瘤包括一组不同性质的恶性肿瘤，但其肿瘤细胞来源于骨样细胞系，大多数亚型产生骨样基质。
- 骨肉瘤可以是原发也可以是继发。继发性骨肉瘤可以出现在佩吉特病或放疗后。继发于佩吉特病的骨肉瘤极具侵袭性。
- 骨肉瘤常见的标志性影像学特征是骨质破坏、骨样基质生成、侵袭性骨膜反应和伴随的软组织肿块。早期骨肉瘤可能仅表现为轻微的骨硬化。
- 骨肉瘤的主要亚型超过10种，其中最重要的4种亚型为普通型（最常见）、毛细血管扩张型和两种近皮质亚型，包括骨旁型（发音为PAR-osteal）和骨膜型（发音为PERI-osteal）。
- **普通型**（髓腔内）骨肉瘤占骨肉瘤的75%，见于青少年/年轻成人，常发生在膝关节周围的股骨或胫骨干骺端。

  普通型骨肉瘤的特征为髓腔内骨样基质、髓腔和骨皮质同时破坏、侵袭性骨膜反应（日光放射征或Codman三角）和软组织肿块。

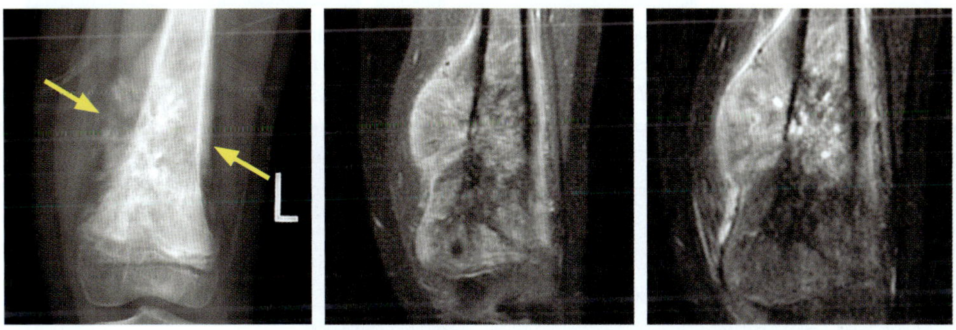

Radiograph
X线影像

Post-contrast T1-weighted MRI with fat suppression
增强T_1加权脂肪抑制MRI

T2-weighted MRI with fat supp.
T_2加权脂肪抑制MRI

Conventional osteosarcoma with classic radiographic appearance: Frontal radiograph of the femur in a skeletally immature patient shows a heterogeneous mass in the distal femoral metaphysis with aggressive sunburst periosteal reaction and cloud-like osteoid matrix (yellow arrows). Coronal MR images show a heterogeneously T2 hyperintense mass with soft tissue extension and extensive enhancing periosteal reaction.
普通型骨肉瘤的典型MRI影像学表现：一名骨骼发育尚未成熟患者的股骨正位X线影像显示股骨远端干骺端有一个不均质肿块，伴侵袭性日光放射样骨膜反应和云状骨样基质形成（黄箭）。冠状位MRI显示一个不均匀的T_2高信号肿块，伴有软组织侵犯和呈广泛增强的骨膜反应。

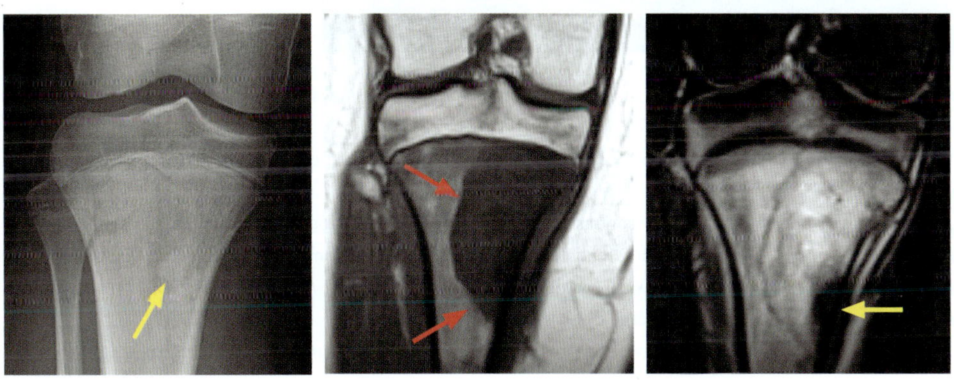

Radiograph
X线影像

T1-weighted MRI
T_1加权MRI

T2-weighted MRI with fat supp.
T_2加权脂肪抑制MRI

Conventional osteosarcoma, subtle on radiography: Radiograph (left image) shows a region of subtle sclerosis in the medial proximal tibial metaphysis (arrow). No periosteal reaction is apparent, which is unusual for osteosarcoma. T1-weighted MRI shows a well-defined region of marrow replacement by tumor (red arrows). T2-weighted MRI with fat suppression demonstrates diffuse marrow edema in the tibia, with a region of decreased T2 signal (arrow) likely corresponding to the sclerosis seen on radiograph.
X线影像上不明显的普通型骨肉瘤：X线影像（左图）显示胫骨近段内侧干骺端轻微的骨质硬化（箭）。无明显骨膜反应，为骨肉瘤不常见的表现。T_1加权MRI显示骨髓被肿瘤替代并形成一个边界清楚的区域（红箭）。T_2加权脂肪抑制MRI显示胫骨弥漫性骨髓水肿，伴T_2信号减低区（箭），可能为对应于X线影像上的硬化区。

Telangiectatic osteosarcoma is an osteolytic destructive sarcoma which may mimic a benign aneurysmal bone cyst on imaging.

毛细血管扩张型骨肉瘤是溶骨性破坏性肉瘤，在影像上可类似于良性动脉瘤样骨囊肿。

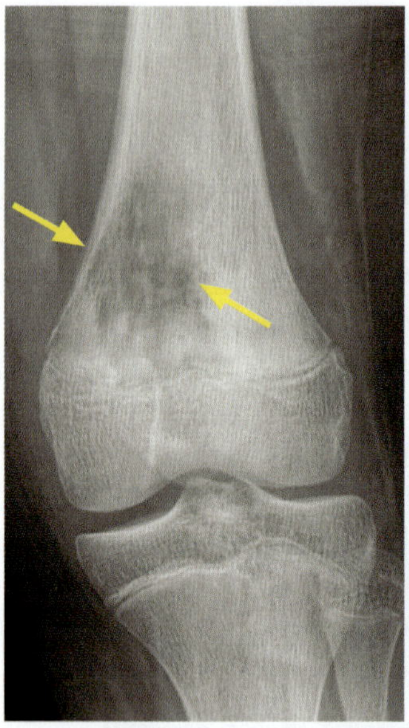

Radiograph
X线影像

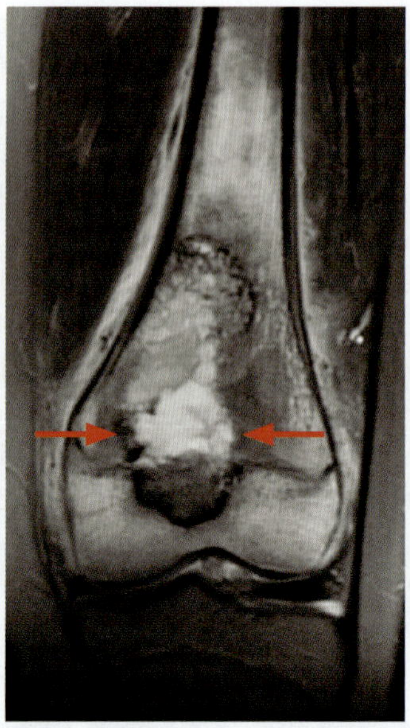

Coronal T2-weighted MRI with fat suppression
冠状位T_2加权脂肪抑制MRI

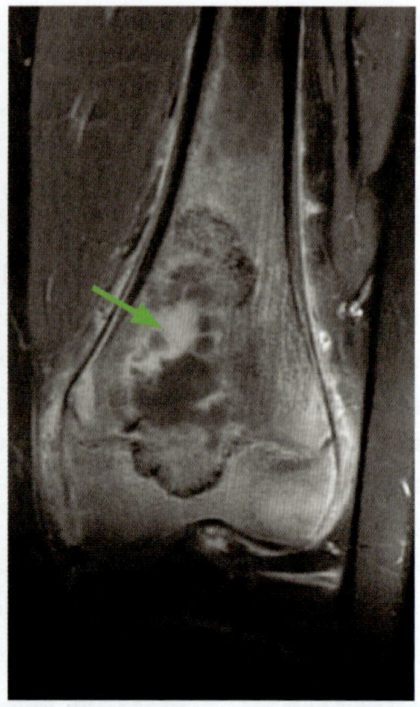

Coronal post-contrast T1-weighted MRI with fat suppression
冠状位增强T_1加权脂肪抑制MRI

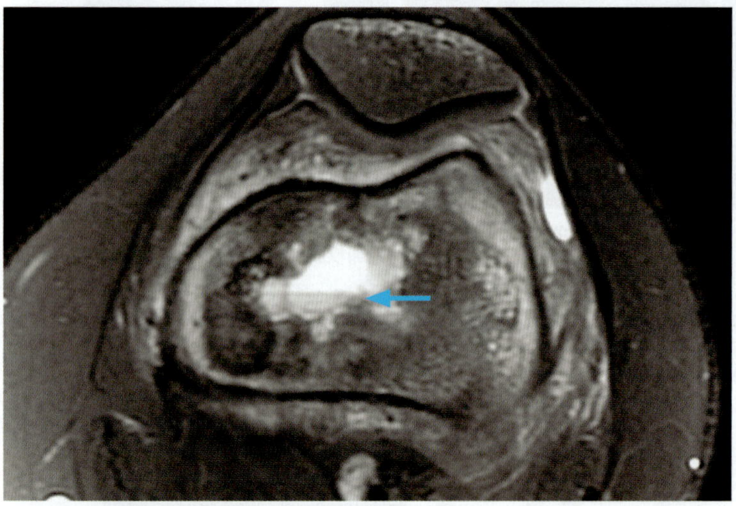

Axial T2-weighted MRI with fat suppression
轴位T_2加权脂肪抑制MRI

Telangiectatic osteosarcoma: Frontal radiograph of the knee in a skeletally immature patient shows an ill-defined, permeative lytic lesion (yellow arrows) in the distal femoral metaphysis.

Coronal T2FS MRI in the same patient shows a heterogeneous lesion with T2 hyperintense cystic spaces (red arrows), with axial images demonstrating fluid-fluid levels (blue arrow).

Coronal T1 post-contrast image shows some nodular areas of contrast enhancement within the lesion (green arrow).

The presence of solid nodular components on MRI helps to differentiate a telangiectatic osteosarcoma from a benign aneurysmal bone cyst.

Unlike other osteosarcomas, telangiectatic osteosarcoma does not produce any bony matrix.

Pathologically, telangiectatic osteosarcoma is vascular with large cystic spaces filled with blood.

Although telangiectatic osteosarcoma is an aggressive lesion, new treatment options increase survival, which is now slightly improved compared to a conventional osteosarcoma.

毛细血管扩张性骨肉瘤：一名骨骼发育尚未成熟患者的膝关节正位X线影像显示位于股骨远端干骺端一处边界不清的穿凿样溶骨性病变(黄箭)。

同一名患者的冠状位T_2加权脂肪抑制MRI显示一处不均质病变，伴T_2高信号囊性区(红箭)，轴位图像可见液-液平面(蓝箭)。

冠状位增强T_1加权显示病灶内有一些结节状强化区(绿箭)。

MRI上所显示的实性结节成分有助于区分毛细血管扩张型骨肉瘤和良性的动脉瘤样骨囊肿。

不同于其他类型的骨肉瘤，毛细血管扩张型骨肉瘤不产生任何骨样基质。

病理学上，毛细血管扩张型骨肉瘤为血管结构，其扩大的囊性腔隙充满了血液。

尽管毛细血管扩张型骨肉瘤是侵袭性病变，但新的治疗方法提高了生存率，其目前的生存率稍高于普通型骨肉瘤。

- **Parosteal** (PAR-osteal) osteosarcoma is a juxtacortical osteosarcoma that arises from the outer periosteum. It most commonly occurs at the posterior aspect of distal femoral metaphysis and has a cauliflower-like exophytic morphology (mnemonic: par-boil cauliflower before eating). A lucent line may be seen separating it from the cortex.

- **骨旁型**(PAR- osteal)骨肉瘤是一种近皮质骨肉瘤，起源于外层骨膜。它最常发生在股骨远端干骺端的后部，呈菜花状外生性形态(助记：par-boil cauliflower before eating)。可见一条与骨皮质分割的透亮线。

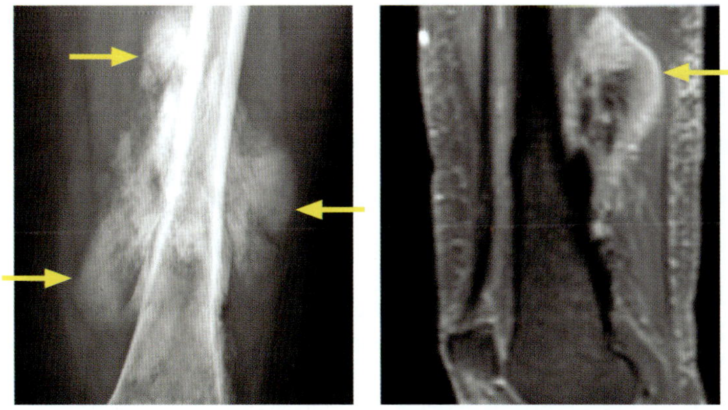

Radiograph
X线影像

Sagittal post-contrast T1-weighted MRI with fat suppression
矢状位增强T_1加权脂肪抑制MRI

Axial post-contrast T1-weighted MRI with fat suppression
轴位增强T_1加权脂肪抑制MRI

Parosteal osteosarcoma: Frontal radiograph of the femur shows a large exophytic "cauliflower-like" mass involving the femoral diaphysis (arrows). Sagittal T1 post-contrast image in the same patient shows the large lobulated mass with peripheral enhancement (arrow). Axial T1 post-contrast images again demonstrate the cauliflower-like lobulations with peripheral enhancement (arrows).
Patients are usually in their third and fourth decades, older compared to other osteosarcoma subtypes.
Parosteal osteosarcoma is the least malignant of all osteosarcomas, with ~90% five-year survival.
骨旁型骨肉瘤：股骨正位X线影像显示一个大的外生性"菜花状"肿块，累及股骨干(箭)。同一名患者的矢状位T_1增强图像显示一个大的分叶状肿块，其边缘有强化(箭)。轴位T_1增强图像同样显示菜花状分叶伴边缘强化(箭)。
患者通常在30~40岁发病，较其他亚型的骨肉瘤发病年龄更大。
骨旁型骨肉瘤在所有骨肉瘤中的恶性程度最低，5年生存率可达90%。

- **Periosteal** (PERI-osteal) osteosarcoma, the other juxtacortical osteosarcoma, is a rare osteosarcoma variant arising from the inner periosteum. It features cortical thickening, aggressive periosteal reaction, and a soft-tissue mass. Histologically, periosteal osteosarcoma may show chondroid differentiation.

- **骨膜型**骨肉瘤为另一种类型的近皮质骨肉瘤，是起源于内层骨膜的一种罕见亚型。它以皮质增厚、侵袭性骨膜反应和软组织肿块为特征。组织学上，骨膜型骨肉瘤可表现为软骨样分化。

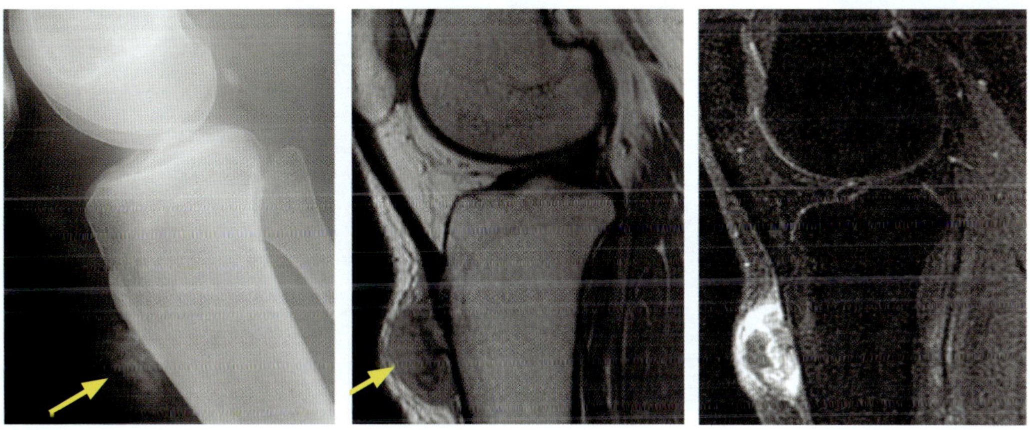

Radiograph
X线影像

Sagittal PD-weighted MRI
矢状位PD加权MRI

Sagittal post-contrast T1-weighted MRI with fat suppression
矢状位增强T_1加权脂肪抑制MRI

Periosteal osteosarcoma: Lateral radiograph of the knee shows a mass in the anterior proximal tibial diaphysis with associated soft tissue mass and periosteal reaction (arrow). Sagittal PD-weighted MRI shows an intermediate signal intensity mass (arrow) abutting the anterior tibial periosteum, with post-contrast image showing heterogeneous enhancement. Excisional biopsy showed periosteal osteosarcoma.
The most common location of periosteal osteosarcoma is the diaphysis of the femur or tibia.
Patients tend to be younger than 20 years old.
骨膜型骨肉瘤：膝关节侧位X线影像显示胫骨近端骨干前方一个肿块，伴周围软组织肿块和骨膜反应(箭)。矢状位PD加权MRI可见胫骨前方一个紧贴骨膜的中等信号肿块(箭)，增强图像显示不均匀强化。手术活检为骨膜型骨肉瘤。
骨膜型骨肉瘤最常见的发病部位是股骨或胫骨的骨干。
发病年龄常低于20岁。

- Regardless of subtype, osteosarcoma has a propensity to metastasize to lungs, where the metastases may or may not calcify.

- 无论什么亚型，骨肉瘤都有转移至肺的倾向，转移灶可发生钙化。

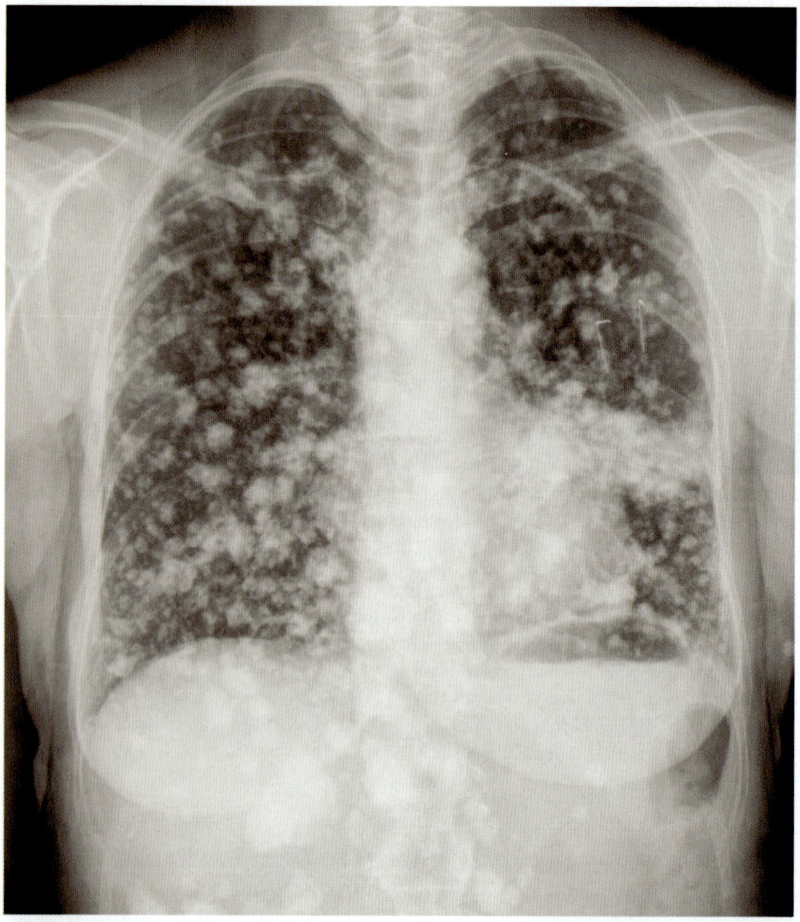

Frontal radiograph shows innumerable calcified osteosarcoma metastases in the thorax and visualized portion of the upper abdomen, demonstrating fluffy osteoid matrix.
正位X线影像显示胸部及所见上腹部弥漫分布钙化的骨肉瘤转移灶，具有松散的骨样基质。

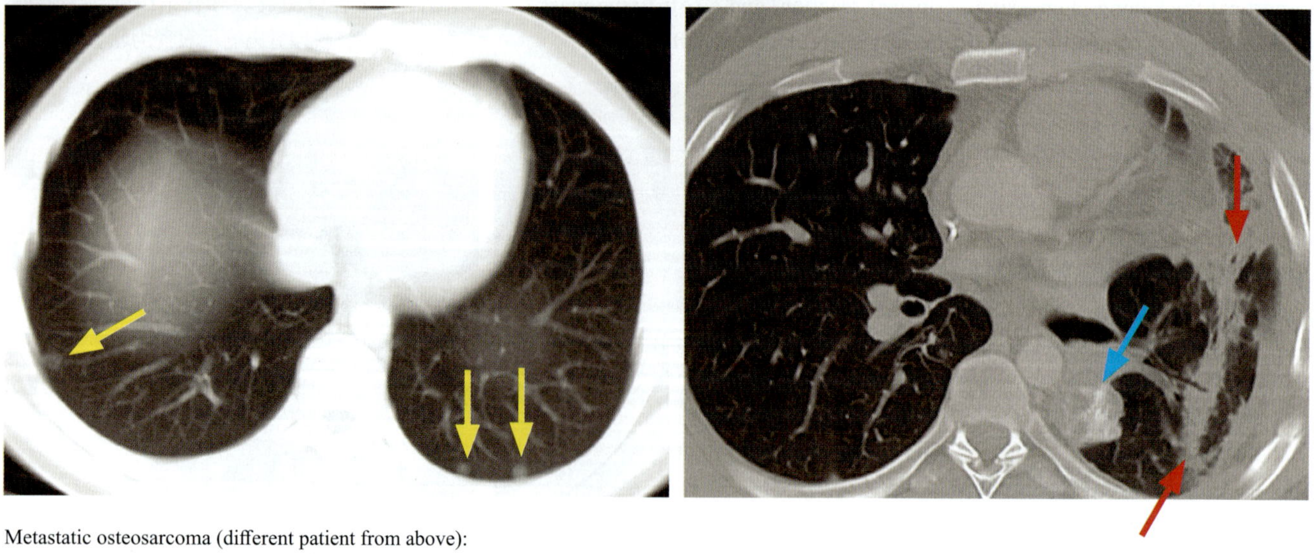

Metastatic osteosarcoma (different patient from above):
Axial maximum intensity projection from initial staging CT (left image) demonstrates several bilateral lower lobe noncalcified subcentimeter nodules (arrows), in keeping with metastatic disease.
Follow-up axial chest CT image performed three years later demonstrates post-treatment changes in the left hemithorax with linear consolidation in keeping with post-radiation changes (red arrows). There has been interval development of a calcified medial left lower lobe nodule (blue arrow).
转移性骨肉瘤(另一名患者):
初始分期轴位CT最大密度投影(左图)显示两肺下叶多个未钙化的亚厘米结节(箭)，符合转移性病变。
3年后随访胸部轴位CT显示左半胸治疗后改变，表现为线样实变，符合放疗后的改变(红箭)。在左下叶内侧新出现一个钙化结节(蓝箭)。

Benign: Synovial chondromatosis / osteochondromatosis

良性：滑膜骨软骨瘤病/骨软骨瘤病

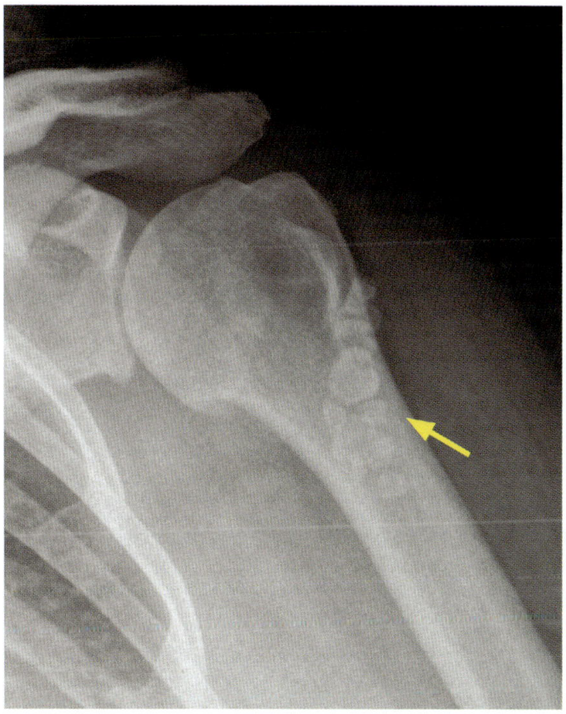

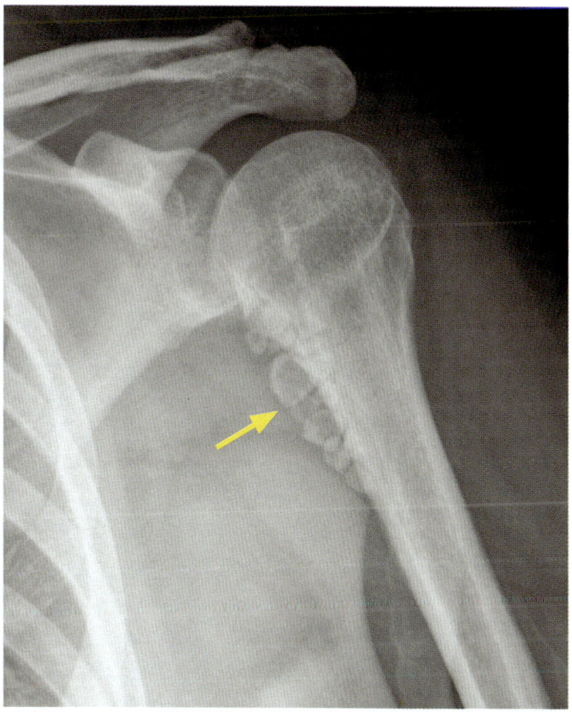

Synovial osteochondromatosis: Frontal external rotation (left image) and internal rotation (right image) radiographs of the shoulder show multiple small round calcifications tracking along the expected location of the long head of the biceps tendon sheath (arrows).

滑膜骨软骨瘤病：正位肩关节外旋(左图)和内旋(右图)X线影像显示多发小圆形钙化灶沿肱二头肌长头肌腱腱鞘的部位分布(箭)。

- Synovial chondromatosis is non-neoplastic synovial metaplasia characterized by the formation of intra-articular lobulated cartilaginous nodules, which may or may not ossify. It is usually a monoarticular disorder.
- The cartilaginous foci often ossify, in which case the term *osteochondromatosis* is used.
- Synovial proliferation tends not to directly cause arthropathy, although the intra-articular nodules may cause mechanical erosions and secondary osteoarthritis.
- The most common location is the knee. The shoulders, hip, and elbow may also be affected.
- Radiography shows multiple round intra-articular bodies of similar size and variable mineralization. The primary differential is intra-articular bodies from osteoarthritis; however, in osteoarthritis the bodies tend to be more varied in size and shape and fewer in number. Diagnosis can be difficult in the absence of calcification, especially if mechanical erosions are present.
- MRI appearances are variable, depending on the degree of ossification and the presence of chondroid matrix. When calcified or ossified, MRI will show multiple globular and rounded foci of low signal.
- The MRI finding of multiple intra-articular low-intensity foci can also be seen in pigmented villonodular synovitis (PVNS). A radiograph will clearly show rounded calcified bodies in osteochondromatosis.
- Very rarely, malignant degeneration to chondrosarcoma may occur.

- 滑膜骨软骨瘤病是非肿瘤性滑膜化生，其特征是在关节内形成分叶状的软骨结节，它们可能会钙化或不钙化。此病通常为单关节病变。
- 软骨灶常骨化，于是使用骨软骨瘤病这一术语。
- 滑膜增殖往往不直接导致关节病，但关节内结节可引起机械性侵蚀和继发性骨关节炎。
- 最常见的发病部位是膝关节。肩、髋和肘关节也可受累。
- X线影像显示关节内多发圆形小体，其大小相似但矿化程度不同。主要的鉴别诊断是骨性关节炎时的关节内小体；但骨性关节炎时的小体大小不等、形状不一且数量较少。无钙化时会引起诊断困难，尤其是在出现机械性侵蚀的情况下。
- MRI表现多样，取决于骨化的程度及是否存在软骨样基质。当钙化或骨化时，MRI显示多发球状或圆形低信号灶。
- MRI多发关节内低信号灶的表现也可见于色素绒毛结节性滑膜炎(PVNS)。X线影像可清晰显示骨软骨瘤病时的圆形钙化小体。
- 可恶变为软骨肉瘤，但罕见。

Benign: Enchondroma

- Enchondroma is a benign lesion of mature hyaline cartilage rests.
- In the long bones, enchondroma features characteristic chondroid (*popcorn* or *ring and arc*) calcifications.
- The differential diagnosis of enchondroma includes medullary bone infarct (which produces serpentine sclerosis) and chondrosarcoma.
- MRI is usually able to differentiate between infarct and enchondroma. Enchondroma has a characteristic lobulated hyperintense signal on T2-weighted images.
- When occurring in the hand, enchondroma typically does not produce visible matrix and appears as a geographic lytic lesion.
- Enchondroma may be complicated by pathologic fracture, especially in the hand.

良性：内生软骨瘤

- 内生软骨瘤是一种良性的成熟透明软骨巢病变。
- 内生软骨瘤在长骨以软骨钙化(爆米花或环状或弧形)为特征。
- 内生软骨瘤的鉴别诊断包括骨髓梗死(产生蜿蜒状硬化)和软骨肉瘤。
- MRI通常可以区分梗死和内生软骨瘤。内生软骨瘤在T_2加权图像上的特征为分叶状高信号。
- 当发生在手部时，内生软骨瘤通常没有可见的基质，而表现为地图样的溶骨性病变。
- 内生软骨瘤可并发病理性骨折，尤其是在手部。

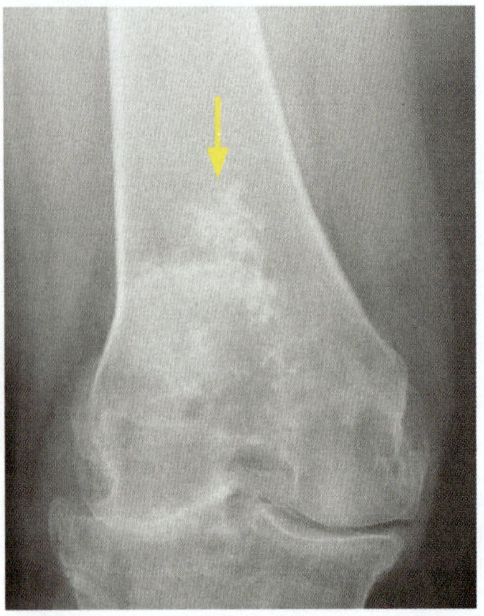

Radiograph of the distal femur shows an enchondroma with characteristic ring and arc chondroid-type calcification (arrow).
股骨远端X线影像显示内生软骨瘤，其特征为环形和弧形的软骨样钙化(箭)。

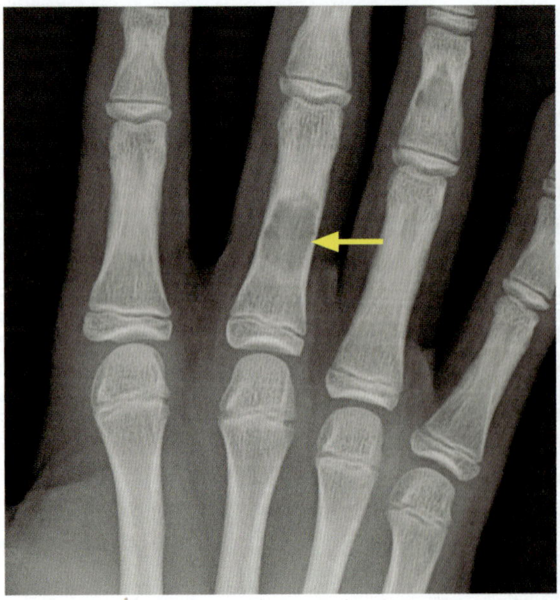

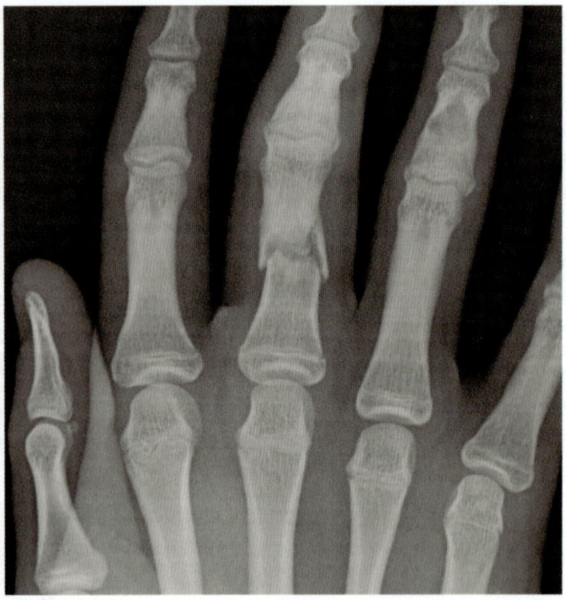

Enchondroma of the middle finger proximal phalanx (left image) complicated by pathologic fracture seen in a subsequent radiograph (right image). The enchondroma (arrow) has no perceptible chondroid matrix, which is a typical appearance of an enchondroma in the hand. Note the interval partial fusion of the physes which occurred in the time interval between the two radiographs.
随访X线影像显示中指近端指骨内生软骨瘤(左图)合并病理性骨折(右图)。内生软骨瘤(箭)没有明显的软骨基质，这是手部内生软骨瘤的典型表现。注意在两张X线影像之间发生了部分骨骺融合。

- Enchondroma may undergo malignant transformation. Aside from Ollier and Maffucci syndrome (subsequently discussed), malignant transformation to chondrosarcoma is very rare, with a potential worrisome clinical finding being new pain in the absence of fracture.

There are no universally accepted guidelines for follow-up of enchondromas.

Enchondromas measuring <4 cm about the knee or shoulder are very common and likely do not need to be followed if there is no endosteal scalloping. Enchondromas of the pelvic bones or hip may be at increased risk for malignant transformation and many practitioners feel they should be followed.

On follow-up imaging, increase in degree of endosteal scalloping, cortical thinning, or increase in size are worrisome findings. A progressive *decrease* in mineralizations is also worrisome for potential malignant transformation. In contrast, progressive increase in rings-and-arcs type mineralizations suggests maturation of the enchondroma, and is not associated with increased malignancy.

- 内生软骨瘤可能会发生恶性转化。除奥利尔和马富奇综合征(将在下文讨论)外，内生软骨瘤恶性转化为软骨肉瘤的情况罕见，在无骨折的情况下出现新的疼痛是一个不良的临床表现。

目前对于内生软骨瘤还没有普遍接受的随访指南。

膝部或肩部小于4cm的内生软骨瘤很常见，如果没有扇贝样骨内膜重塑则不需要随访。骨盆或髋部的内生软骨瘤恶变风险可能增加，许多医生认为应对其进行随访。

在随访的影像中，扇贝样骨内膜重塑恶化、皮质变薄或病变增大是不良征象。矿化逐渐减少也是潜在恶变的可能征象。相反，环状和弧形矿化逐渐增加表明内生软骨瘤逐渐发育成熟，与恶变风险增加不相关。

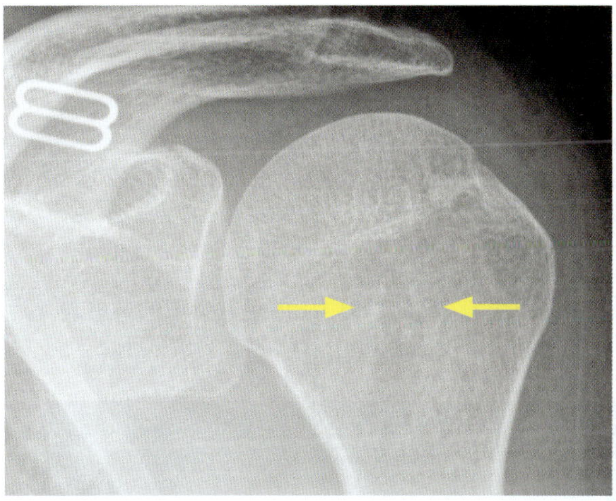

Frontal radiograph
正位X线影像

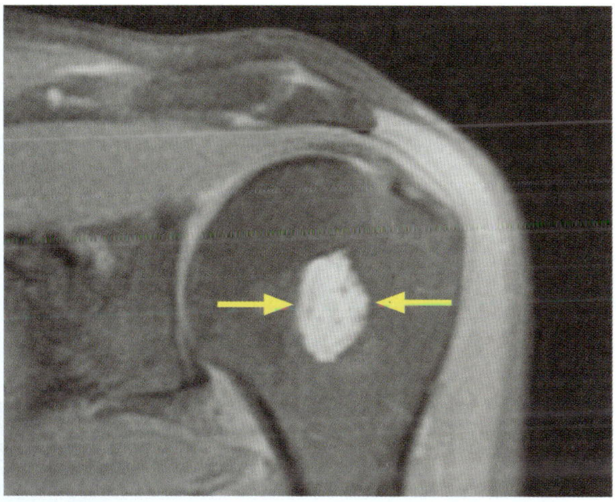

Post-contrast coronal T1-weighted MRI with fat supp.
冠状位增强T_1加权脂肪抑制MRI

Benign enchondroma, with malignant transformation 11 years later: Initial radiographs demonstrate a very subtle region of punctate mineralizations (yellow arrows) in the humeral head. MRI demonstrates a lobulated, circumscribed mass (yellow arrows) in the humeral head without endosteal scalloping.
良性内生软骨瘤，11年后恶变：最初的X线影像显示肱骨头一处细微点状矿化区域(黄箭)。MRI显示肱骨头分叶状、分界清楚的肿块(黄箭)，无扇贝样骨内膜重塑。

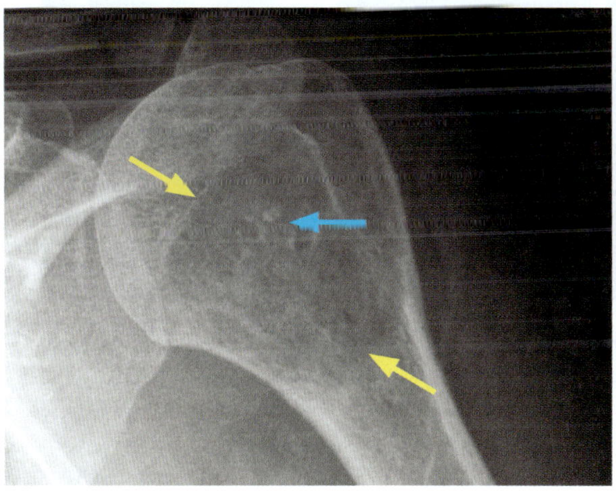

Frontal radiograph
正位X线影像

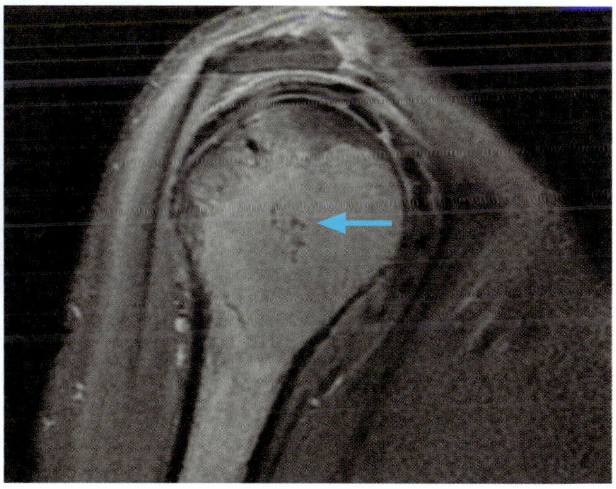

Post-contrast sagittal T1-weighted MRI with fat supp.
矢状位增强T_1加权脂肪抑制MRI

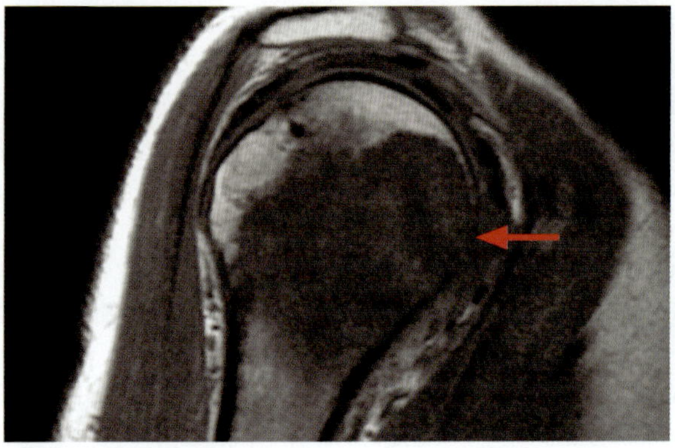

Sagittal T1-weighted MRI
矢状位T_1加权MRI

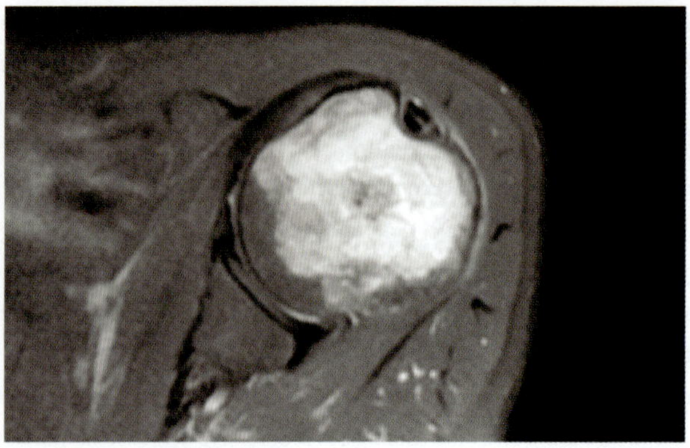

Axial PD-weighted MRI with fat suppression
轴位PD加权脂肪抑制MRI

Chondrosarcoma, arising from malignant degeneration of enchondroma: Radiographs and MRI in the same patient as above, obtained 11 years later, demonstrate a subtle lytic lesion of the humeral head (arrows).
MR imaging shows a large T1 hypointense, T2 hyperintense, enhancing mass in the proximal humerus with cortical thinning anteriorly (red arrow). The mass is markedly enlarged since 11 years prior, and involves nearly the entire marrow cavity. Note the punctate mineralizations (blue arrows), which have not increased since 11 years.
Please note that malignant transformation of an isolated enchondroma is extremely rare, and it is not typical clinical practice to follow benign-appearing enchondromas indefinitely.
软骨肉瘤，由内生软骨瘤恶变引起：同一名患者11年后的X线影像和MRI显示肱骨头一处模糊的溶骨性病变(箭)。
MRI显示肱骨近端一个大的肿块，呈T_1低信号、T_2高信号、增强后强化，以及前方皮质变薄(红箭)。肿块较11年前显著增大，几乎累及整个骨髓腔。注意点状矿化(蓝箭)，其大小较11年前没有增加。
请注意，孤立性内生软骨瘤恶变极为罕见，无限期随访良性内生软骨瘤不是临床常规的做法。

- On MRI, enchondromas typically are circumscribed, lobulated, T2 hyperintense masses.

- 在MRI上，内生软骨瘤的典型表现为边界清楚、呈分叶状的T_2高信号肿块。

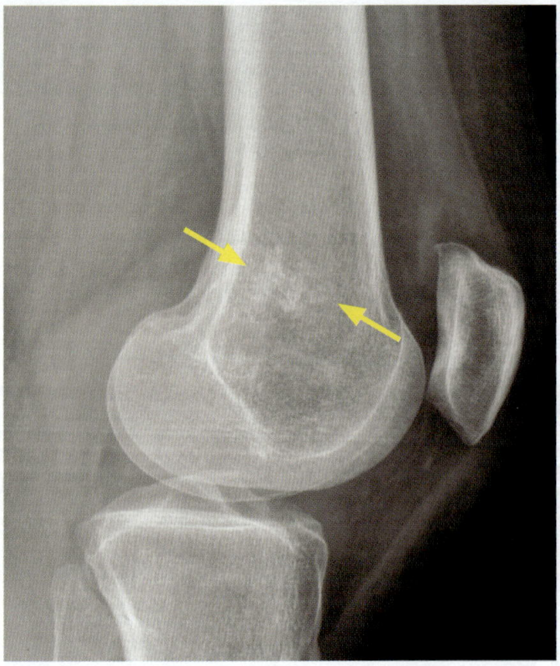

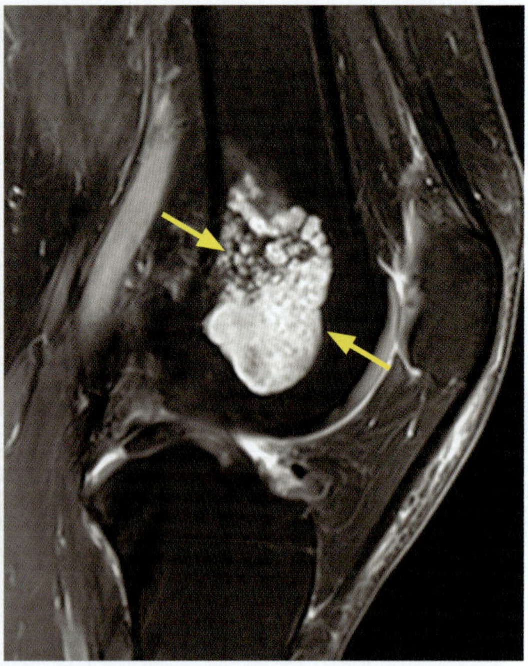

Enchondroma on radiograph and MRI: Lateral knee radiograph (left image) shows ring and arcs mineralization in the distal femoral diaphysis (arrows), in keeping with an enchondroma. Sagittal T2- weighted MRI with fat suppression demonstrates the typical imaging features of enchondroma, with a lobulated, circumscribed, T2 hyperintense mass (arrows). While not fully visualized in these images, there was no endosteal scalloping, cortical thinning, or soft tissue mass to suggest a more aggressive lesion.
内生软骨瘤的X线影像和MRI：膝关节侧位X线影像(左图)显示股骨干的远端呈环状和弧形矿化(箭)，与内生软骨瘤表现一致。矢状位T_2加权脂肪抑制MRI显示内生软骨瘤的典型影像特征，即分叶、边界清楚的T_2高信号肿块(箭)。这些图像未能显示所有细节，未见骨内膜扇贝状重塑、皮质变薄或软组织肿块等表现，提示病变不具有较强的侵袭性。

- Multiple enchondromas are seen in **Ollier** (multiple enchondromas only) and **Maffucci** (multiple enchondromas and venous malformations producing phleboliths) syndromes, the two familial enchondromatoses. Both syndromes carry an increased risk of malignant transformation to chondrosarcoma, with a higher risk in Maffucci syndrome.

- 多发内生软骨瘤见于**奥利尔**(仅为多发内生软骨瘤)和**马富奇**(多发内生软骨瘤和静脉畸形导致的静脉石)综合征,两者为家族性内生软骨瘤病。两种综合征都有恶变为软骨肉瘤的风险,而马富奇综合征的风险更高。

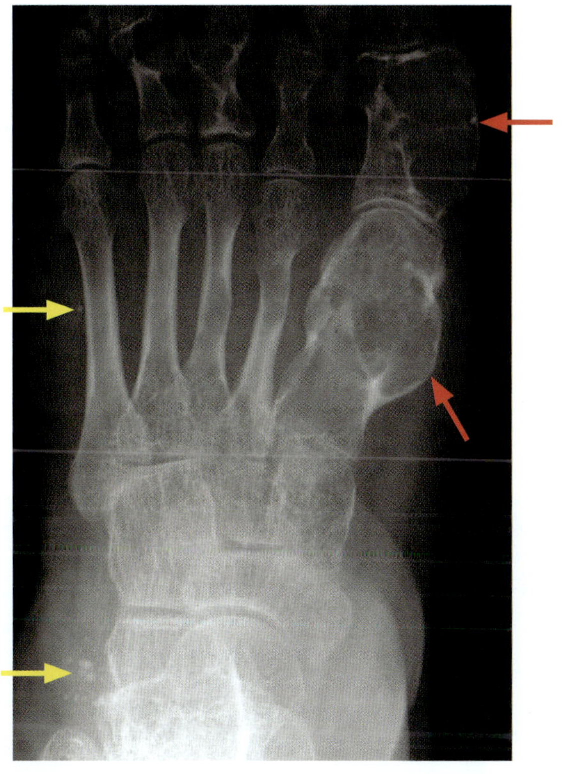

Frontal radiograph of the foot in a patient with Maffucci syndrome shows numerous expansile enchondromas most prominently in the great toe (red arrows). Multiple phleboliths (yellow arrows) represent soft-tissue venous malformations.
Note the relative paucity of chondroid calcification, which is typical of the enchondromas seen in Maffucci syndrome.
马富奇综合征患者足部正位X线影像显示大量膨胀性内生软骨瘤,以踇趾为著(红箭)。多发静脉结石(黄箭)代表软组织静脉畸形。
注意,软骨钙化相对缺乏,这是马富奇综合征内生软骨瘤病的典型表现。

Benign: Osteochondroma

- An osteochondroma is a benign cartilage-capped bony growth projecting outward from bone, often pedunculated. It is the most common benign bone lesion.
- Osteochondroma may present clinically as a palpable mass, which usually stops growing at skeletal maturity.
- Key features are the continuity of cortex of host bone with the cortex of the osteochondroma and communication of the medullary cavities. Osteochondroma arises from the metaphysis and grows away from the epiphysis.
- An uncommon complication is malignant transformation to chondrosarcoma.

  Like enchondroma, the presence of pain in the absence of a pathologic fracture is a red flag.

  An associated soft-tissue mass is usually present with malignant transformation.

  A cartilage cap thickness >2 cm on MRI suggests malignant transformation to chondrosarcoma.
- Multiple osteochondromas can be seen in **multiple hereditary exostoses** (MHE), with increased risk for malignant transformation. MHE is an autosomal dominant skeletal dysplasia, with the knees most commonly involved.

良性:骨软骨瘤

- 骨软骨瘤是一种由软骨覆盖的良性骨赘生物,从骨骼向外突出生长,通常呈柄状。它是最常见的良性骨骼病变。
- 骨软骨瘤在临床上可能表现为可触及的包块,通常在骨骼发育成熟后停止生长。
- 主要特征包括与宿主骨的骨皮质具有连续性,以及与髓腔相通。骨软骨瘤起源于干骺端并朝背离骨骺的方向生长。
- 一种不常见的并发症为恶变转化成软骨肉瘤。

  与内生软骨瘤相似,在没有病理性骨折的情况下出现疼痛是一个危险信号。

  恶性转化通常伴随有相关的软组织肿块。

  MRI上软骨盖厚度>2cm提示恶变为软骨肉瘤。
- 多发性骨软骨瘤可见于**多发性遗传性外生骨疣(MHE)**,其恶变风险增加。MHE是常染色体显性骨骼发育不良,膝最常受累。

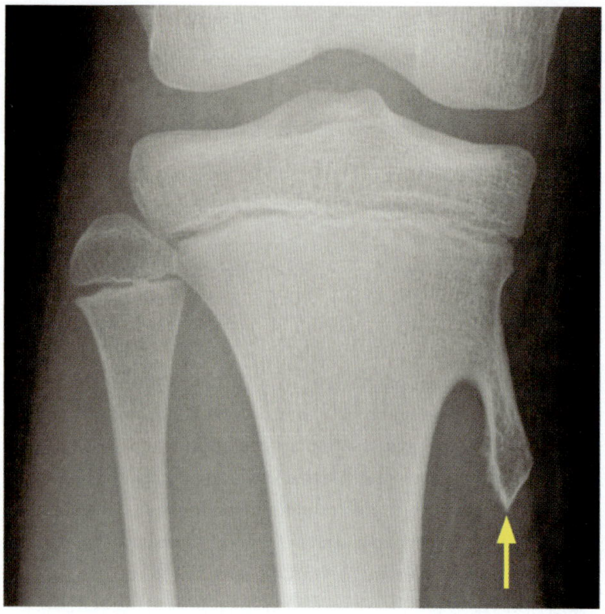

Osteochondroma: Frontal knee radiograph in a skeletally immature patient shows a pedunculated exostosis (arrow) of the tibial metaphysis, with characteristic continuity of the cortex and communication of the medullary cavities. The lesion arises from the metaphysis and projects away from the epiphysis.

骨软骨瘤：一名骨骼发育尚未成熟患者的膝关节正位X线影像显示胫骨干骺端一个带蒂的外生骨疣(箭)，连续的骨皮质和交通性髓腔具有特征性。病变起源于干骺端并向背离骨骺的方向突起。

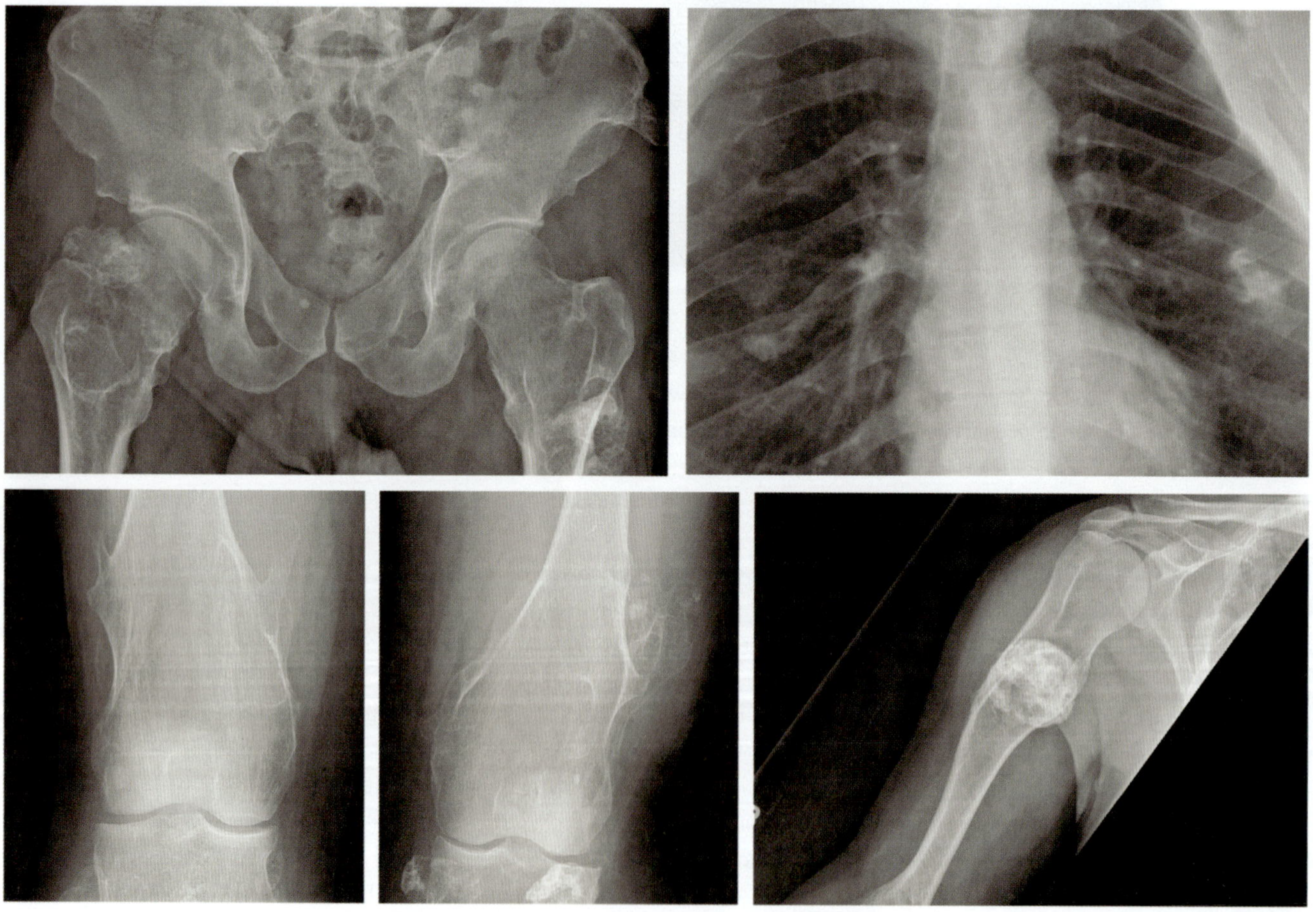

Multiple hereditary exostoses (MHE): Multiple radiographs from a skeletal survey of a single patient with MHE demonstrates multiple sessile and pedunculated osteochondromas about the hips, left iliac crest, chest wall, both knees, and right humerus.

多发性遗传性外生骨疣(MHE)：一名MHE患者的多张骨骼X线影像显示位于髋部、左髂骨嵴、胸壁、双膝和右肱骨多个无蒂和带蒂的骨软骨瘤。

Benign: Chondroblastoma

- Chondroblastoma is a benign lesion located eccentrically in the epiphysis of a long bone in a skeletally immature patient. It most commonly occurs about the knee or proximal humerus.
- Calcified chondroid matrix is present on almost all CT studies, but is seen only ~50% of the time on radiographs.
- Chondroblastoma is unique amongst chondroid lesions in that it typically demonstrates low or intermediate signal on T2-weighted images. Most chondroid lesions are T2 hyperintense.
- Treatment is with curettage, cryosurgery, or radiofrequency ablation. There is a low risk of local recurrence. Chondroblastoma is very rarely malignant.

Benign: Chondromyxoid fibroma

- Chondromyxoid fibroma is a very rare, benign cartilage tumor that is typically eccentric in the tibial or femoral metaphysis about the knee. It rarely demonstrates chondroid matrix.
- It usually has sclerotic margins on radiography and is high in signal on T2-weighted MRI.

Malignant: Chondrosarcoma

良性：软骨母细胞瘤

- 软骨母细胞瘤是骨骼发育尚未成熟患者的一种良性病变，出现在长骨骨骺的偏心位置。最常发生在膝关节附近或肱骨近端。
- 钙化的软骨基质几乎在所有的CT扫描中均能发现，但X线影像最多能看到约50%。
- 软骨母细胞瘤在所有软骨病变中具有独特性，即T_2加权图像呈低或中等信号，而大多数软骨病变呈T_2高信号。
- 治疗方法包括手术刮除、冷冻或射频消融。局部复发的风险较低。软骨母细胞瘤极少为恶性。

良性：软骨黏液样纤维瘤

- 软骨黏液样纤维瘤是罕见的良性软骨肿瘤，通常表现为膝关节周围胫骨或股骨干骺端偏心性病灶。罕见有软骨基质。
- X线影像上通常具有硬化边，并在T_2加权MRI上显示高信号。

恶性：软骨肉瘤

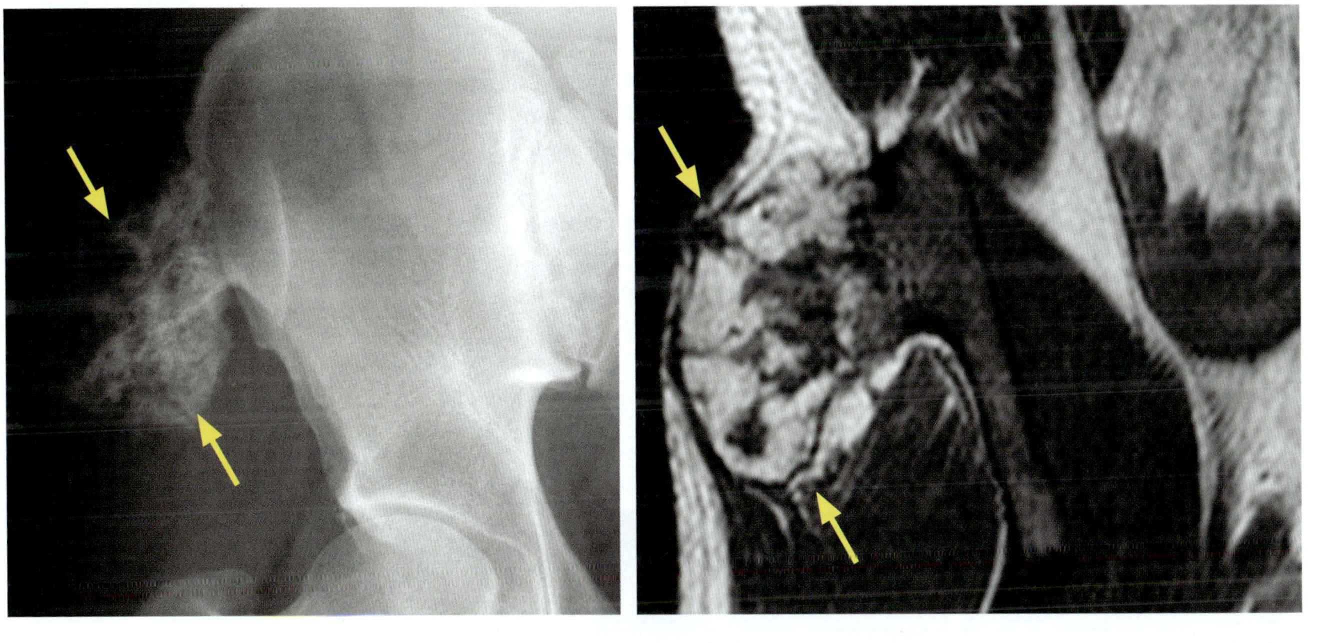

Chondrosarcoma: Frontal radiograph of the pelvis (left image) and coronal T1-weighted MRI (right image) show an exophytic lesion (arrows) arising from the right iliac crest, which is continuous with the intramedullary cavity. The lesion demonstrates ring and arc chondroid-type calcification on radiography, and is heterogeneously hyperintense with a lobulated appearance on T2-weighted MRI (arrows).

Case courtesy Roger Han, MD, Brigham and Women's Hospital.

软骨肉瘤：骨盆正位X线影像(左图)及冠状位T_1加权MRI(右图)显示一个外生性病变(箭)，起源于右侧髂骨嵴，与骨髓腔相连续。病变在X线影像上显示环状和弧形软骨样钙化，T_2加权MRI呈分叶状不均匀高信号(箭)。

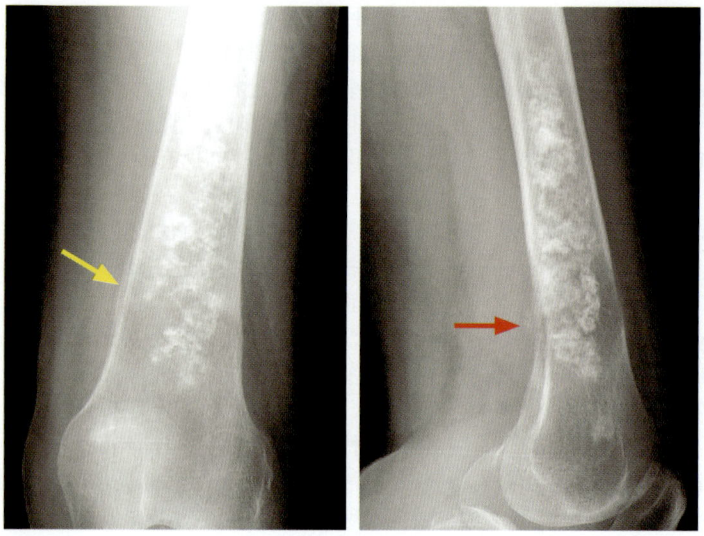

Chondrosarcoma in a different patient:
Frontal and lateral radiographs of the distal femur show an intramedullary lesion with ring and arc chondroid calcifications. Periosteal reaction (yellow arrow) and cortical disruption (red arrow) suggest aggressive behavior.
Case courtesy Stacy Smith, MD, Brigham and Women's Hospital.

不同患者的软骨肉瘤：股骨远端正、侧位X线影像显示髓内病变伴环状和弧形软骨样钙化。骨膜反应(黄箭)和皮质中断(红箭)提示侵袭性行为。

- Chondrosarcoma is a malignant tumor of cartilage. Like osteosarcoma, there are multiple primary and secondary variants.
- Secondary forms arise from enchondroma (more commonly in the Maffucci and Ollier familial enchondromatoses), Paget disease, and osteochondroma (more common in familial osteochondromatosis).

  An osteochondroma with a cartilage cap thickness of >2 cm is highly suggestive of chondrosarcoma.
- The conventional (intramedullary) chondrosarcoma subtype is most common. On imaging, chondrosarcoma is typically an expansile lesion in the medullary bone, with ring and arc chondroid matrix. The tumor causes thickening and endosteal scalloping of the cortex, and there is often an associated soft-tissue mass.
- The dedifferentiated subtype of chondrosarcoma is aggressive and may contain fibrosarcoma or osteosarcoma elements.
- Other subtypes of chondrosarcoma include the rare mesenchymal and clear cell variants.

- 软骨肉瘤是软骨的恶性肿瘤。与骨肉瘤类似，软骨肉瘤也有多种原发及继发的亚型。
- 继发性软骨肉瘤起源于内生软骨肉瘤(更常见于马富奇和奥利尔家族性软骨瘤病)、佩吉特病，以及骨软骨瘤(更常见于奥利尔家族性软骨瘤病)。

  骨软骨瘤的软骨帽厚度>2cm高度提示软骨肉瘤。
- 普通型(髓内)软骨肉瘤亚型是最常见的类型。影像上，软骨肉瘤常显示为骨髓内膨胀性病变，伴环状和弧形软骨基质。肿瘤导致皮质增厚和骨内膜扇贝样重塑，常伴有软组织肿块。
- 软骨肉瘤未分化亚型是侵袭性肿瘤，可包含纤维肉瘤或骨肉瘤成分。
- 其他亚型的软骨肉瘤包括罕见的间质和透明细胞亚型。

Lesions of Fibrous Origin

纤维源性病变

Benign: Nonossifying fibroma / fibrous cortical defect

良性：非骨化性纤维瘤/纤维性骨皮质缺损

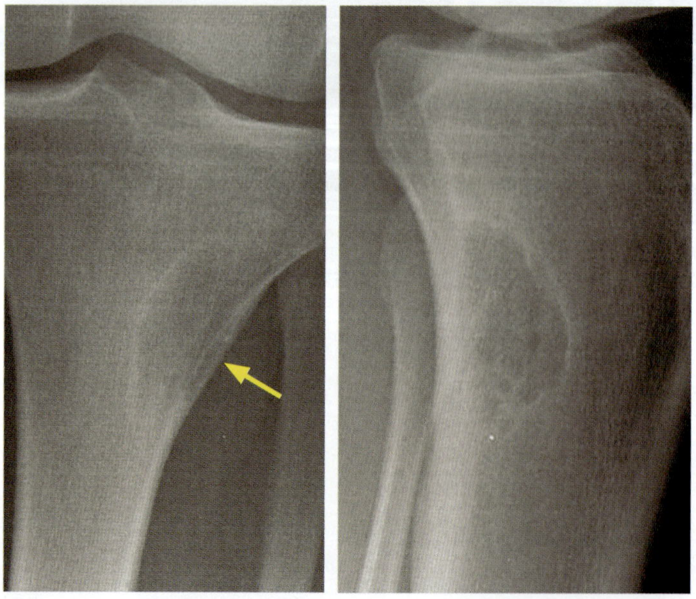

Nonossifying fibroma: Frontal (left image) and lateral (right image) radiographs of the proximal lateral tibia in a 17-year-old male show a well-defined lucent lesion in the medial tibial metaphysis. The lesion features a faint sclerotic rim in continuity with the thinned lateral cortex (arrow).

非骨化性纤维瘤：一名17岁男性的正位(左图)及侧位(右图)胫骨近段X线影像显示干骺端外侧一处边界清晰的透亮病变。病变的特征为轻度硬化边延续为外侧变薄的骨皮质。

- Nonossifying fibroma (sometimes called a **fibroxanthoma**) is an asymptomatic and common incidental radiolucent lesion in the long bones (especially the leg) in children and adolescents. Nonossifying fibroma and fibrous cortical defect are thought to represent the same lesion; the term nonossifying fibroma is generally reserved for larger (>2 cm) or symptomatic lesions. They are the same histologically. These lesions are believed to arise from the periosteum.
- The radiographic appearance is usually diagnostic and demonstrates a lucent lesion with a narrow zone of transition, sclerotic margin, and no matrix calcification. CT or MRI may show cortical disruption or thinning, representing replacement of the cortex by fibrous tissue.
- Most lesions undergo spontaneous sclerotic involution as the patient reaches adulthood.

- 非骨化性纤维瘤(有时称为**纤维黄色瘤**)是一种无症状且最常见的偶发性透亮病变，常见于儿童和青少年的长骨(尤其是腿部)。非骨化性纤维瘤和纤维性骨皮质缺损被认为是同类病变；非骨化性纤维瘤通常指较大(>2cm)或有症状的病变。两者在组织学上相同。这些病变被认为起源于骨膜。
- X线影像表现通常具有诊断价值，表现为透亮病变伴窄的过渡带，边缘硬化且无基质钙化。CT或MRI可显示皮质中断或变薄，提示皮质被纤维组织所取代。
- 大多数病变随着患者进入成年而出现自发性硬化消退。

Benign: Fibrous dysplasia

- Fibrous dysplasia is a benign congenital non-neoplastic condition of children and young adults characterized by replacement of normal cancellous bone by abnormal fibrous tissue.
- Fibrous dysplasia can affect one bone (monostotic) or multiple bones (polyostotic). When polyostotic, it tends to be unilateral.
- The most frequent complication is pathologic fracture, commonly at the femoral neck.
- Fibrous dysplasia of the long bones tends to be central and metadiaphyseal, often causing a bowing deformity such as the extreme varus of the *shepherd 's crook*.

良性：骨纤维异常增殖症

- 骨纤维异常增殖症是发生在儿童和青年人的一种良性先天性非肿瘤性病变，其特征为正常松质骨被异常纤维组织所取代。
- 骨纤维异常增殖症可以是单骨受累(单骨性)或多骨受累(多骨性)。出现多骨受累时，往往局限于单侧。
- 最常见的并发症为病理性骨折，常发生在股骨颈。
- 长骨的纤维异常增殖症往往发生在中央及干骺端，常引起弓状畸形，如极度弯曲的牧羊人手杖。

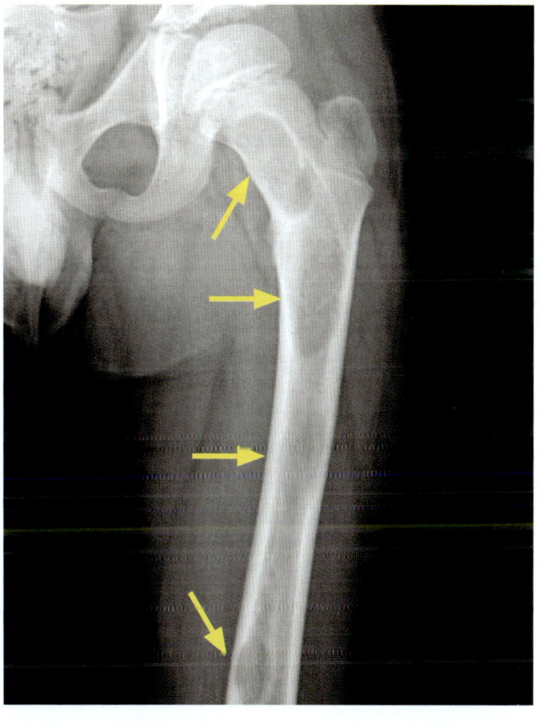

Frontal radiograph of the hip shows multiple lucent lesions in the metaphysis and diaphysis of the femur in a skeletally immature patient (arrows). The lesions feature the characteristic ground glass internal matrix of fibrous dysplasia, with faint peripheral sclerosis.
髋部正位X线影像显示一名骨骼未成熟患者的股骨干骺端和骨干有多个透亮区(箭)。病灶的特征是纤维发育不良的磨玻璃样内基质，伴轻微周边硬化。

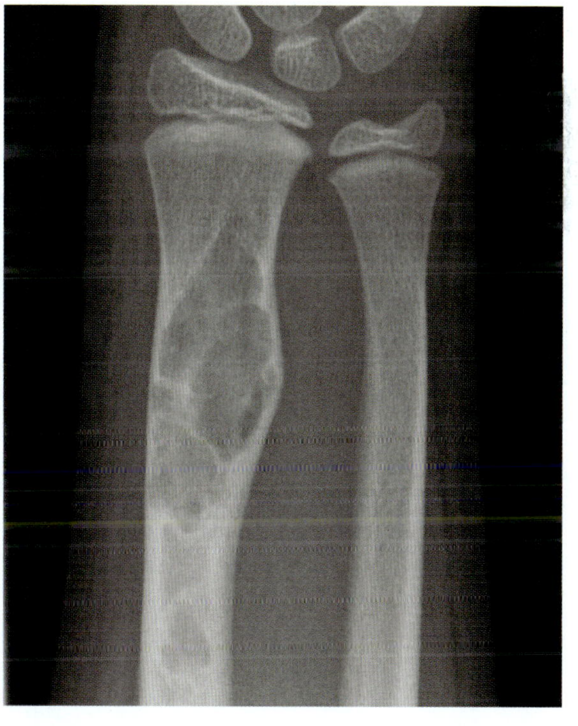

Frontal radiograph of the forearm demonstrates a multiseptated lucent lesion of the central metadiaphysis of the distal radius in a different skeletally immature patient. The differential of this appearance includes fibrous dysplasia and aneurysmal bone cyst.
前臂正位X线影像显示另一名骨骼发育未成熟患者的桡骨远端骨干及干骺端中心有多分隔透亮区。该表现的鉴别诊断包括骨纤维异常增殖症和动脉瘤样骨囊肿。

- In the ribs or long bones, the matrix is typically indistinct and ground glass.
- In the pelvic bones, fibrous dysplasia is often cystic.

- 在肋骨和长骨，基质通常模糊且呈磨玻璃样。
- 在骨盆骨，骨纤维异常增殖症常呈囊状。

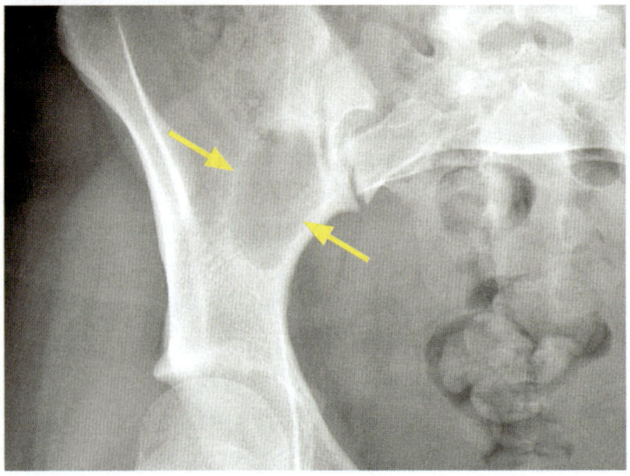

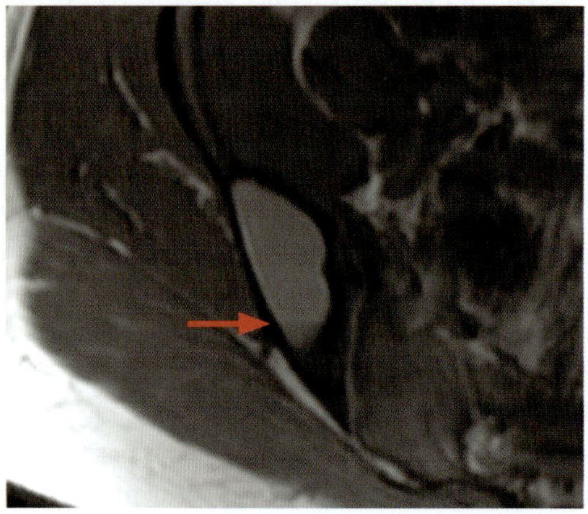

A lucent lesion of the right iliac bone (yellow arrows) shows intermediate to hyperintense signal on proton-density-weighted MRI, with a subtle fluid level (red arrow). The differential diagnosis of a cystic supra-acetabular lesion in a young adult includes cystic fibrous dysplasia and unicameral bone cyst.
右侧髂骨透亮病变(黄箭)在PD加权MRI上呈中等至高信号，伴不明显的小液平(红箭)。髋臼上部囊性病变在年轻成人中的鉴别诊断包括囊性骨纤维异常增殖症和单房性骨囊肿。

- In the skull base, fibrous dysplasia is typically expansile and can look highly unusual on MRI. The primary differential of an expansile skull base lesion is Paget disease, but the age of the patient is the key: Fibrous dysplasia occurs in children and young adults and Paget occurs in older adults.

- 典型的颅底骨纤维异常增殖症常呈膨胀性，且在MRI上极为明显。膨胀性颅底病变的主要鉴别诊断是佩吉特病，但患者的年龄是关键：骨纤维异常增殖症发生在儿童和青年人，而佩吉特病发生在年龄较大的成人。

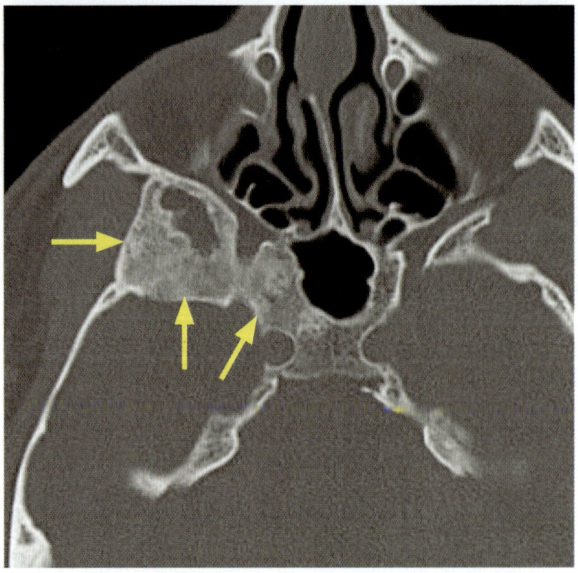

Axial CT shows the typical appearance of fibrous dysplasia of the skull base, with expansile lesions primarily of the right sphenoid bone that have a hazy, ground-glass matrix (arrows).
轴位CT显示典型的颅底骨纤维异常增殖症，表现为膨胀性病变，主要累及右侧蝶骨并出现模糊的磨玻璃样基质(箭)。

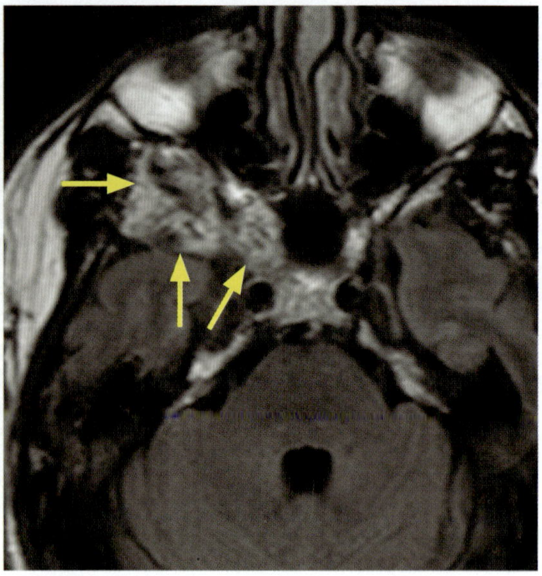

FLAIR MRI correlated to the same region as the CT to the left shows the highly heterogeneous signal of fibrous dysplasia (arrows).
FLAIR MRI与左图CT相对应区域显示骨纤维异常增殖症为高度不均匀信号(箭)。

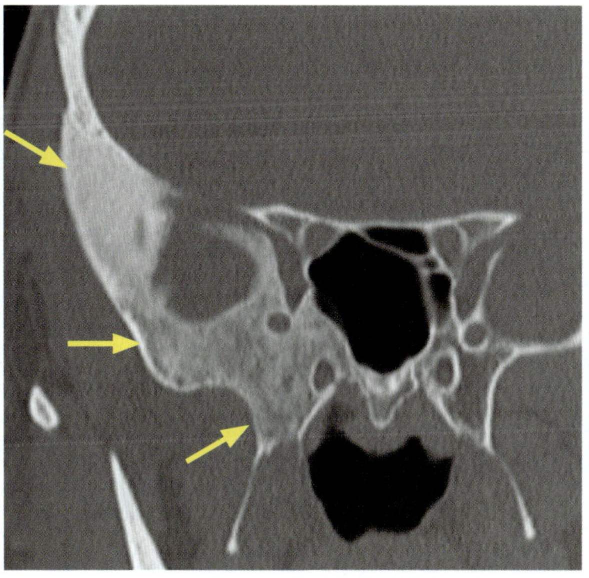

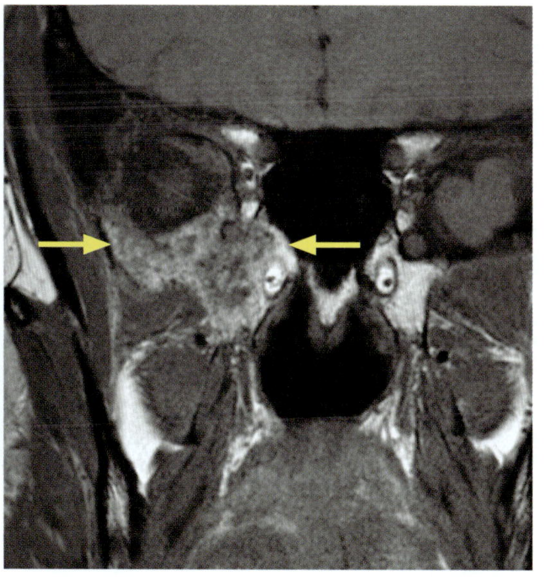

Coronal CT and T1-weighted MRI in the same patient show the true extent of the abnormality (arrows).
Case courtesy Mary Beth Cunnane, MD, Massachusetts Eye and Ear Infirmary, Boston.
同一名患者的冠状位CT和T_1加权MRI显示异常病变的真实范围(箭)。

- **McCune-Albright syndrome** is polyostotic fibrous dysplasia, precocious puberty, and cutaneous café au lait spots.
- **Mazabraud syndrome** is fibrous dysplasia and intramuscular myxomas, which tend to occur in the same region of the body.

- **纤维性骨营养不良综合征**包括多骨性骨纤维异常增殖症、性早熟和皮肤牛奶咖啡斑。
- **Mazabraud综合征**包括骨纤维异常增殖症和肌内黏液瘤，两者趋向于发生在身体的同一个区域。

LESIONS OF VASCULAR ORIGIN

血管源性病变

Benign: Hemangioma

良性：血管瘤

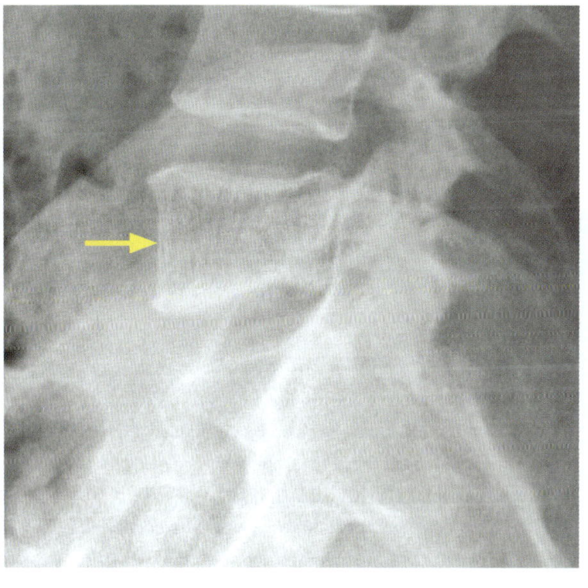

Lateral radiograph of the lumbosacral spine shows mild loss of height of the L5 vertebral body with a subtle lace-like striated trabecular appearance (arrow).
侧位腰骶椎X线影像显示L_5椎体高度略为降低，伴骨小梁呈轻微花边状条纹样改变(箭)。

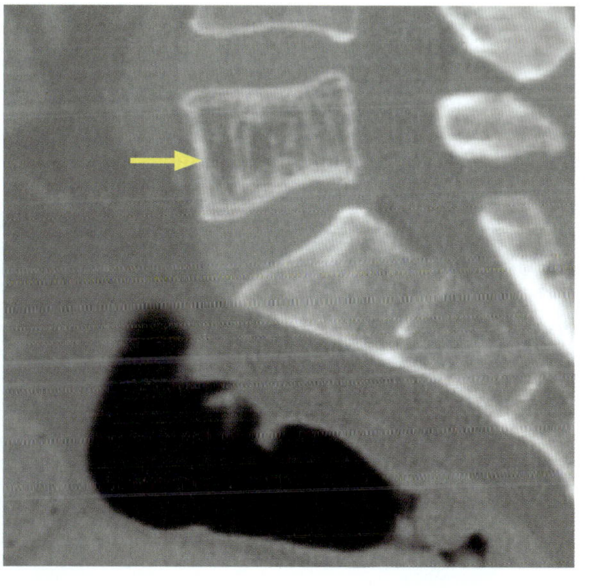

Sagittal CT shows coarsened, vertically oriented trabeculae with a typical *corduroy* appearance in L5 (arrow).
矢状位CT显示L_5椎体内粗糙、垂直方向的骨小梁，呈典型的灯芯绒样条纹改变(箭)。

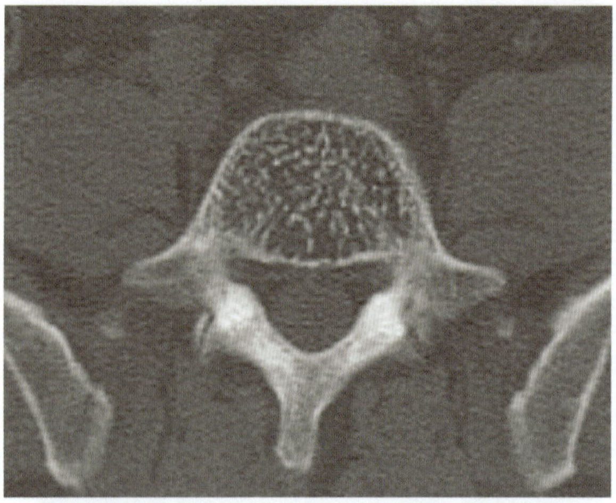

Axial CT through the L5 demonstrates the typical *polka-dot sign* of the hemangioma, which involves the complete medullary cavity.
通过L_5的轴位CT显示血管瘤典型的圆点征，累及整个骨髓腔。

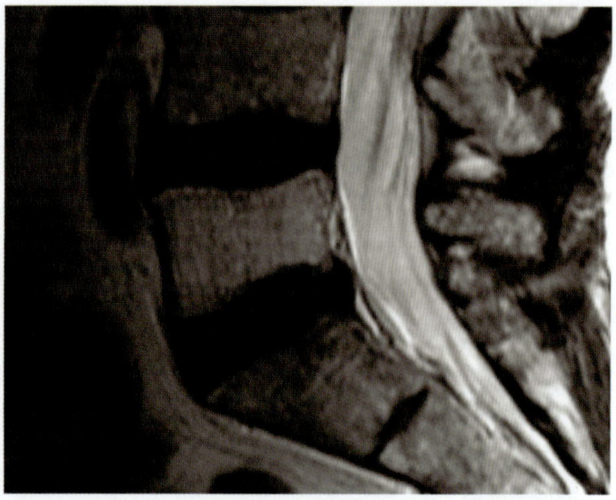

Sagittal T2-weighted MRI demonstrates high signal intensity of the L5 vertebral body.
矢状位T_2加权MRI显示L_5椎体高信号。

- Hemangioma is a benign lesion that typically occurs in the vertebral body, characterized by vascular channels lined by endothelial cells.
- Although usually incidental, rarely a hemangioma may be associated with a soft-tissue mass that can cause neurologic compromise.
- Hemangioma causes reactive trabecular thickening in response to bony resorption by vascular channels.
- On MRI, high signal intensity on both T1- and T2-weighted images are from fat contained within the hemangioma. On radiography and CT, *corduroy* striations are typical. The *polka- dot sign* demonstrates thickened trabeculae imaged in cross-section.

Malignant: Angiosarcoma of bone

- Angiosarcoma looks and acts aggressively. Lung metastases are often seen.

- 血管瘤是一种发生在椎体的良性病变，其特点是在血管通道衬覆内皮细胞。
- 尽管常为偶然发现，血管瘤偶尔可伴有软组织肿块并导致神经功能受损。
- 血管瘤可通过血管吸收骨质，从而造成反应性骨小梁增粗。
- 在MRI图像上，血管瘤内含脂肪致T_1加权和T_2加权图像均呈高信号。在X线影像和CT上，灯芯绒样条纹是其典型的表现。在横断面图像上的圆点征为增粗的骨小梁。

恶性：骨的血管肉瘤

- 血管肉瘤的表现及行为都呈侵袭性。常见肺转移。

Lesions of Hematopoietic Origin

造血组织源性病变

(Usually) benign: Giant cell tumor (osteoclastoma)

(通常)良性：骨巨细胞瘤(破骨细胞瘤)

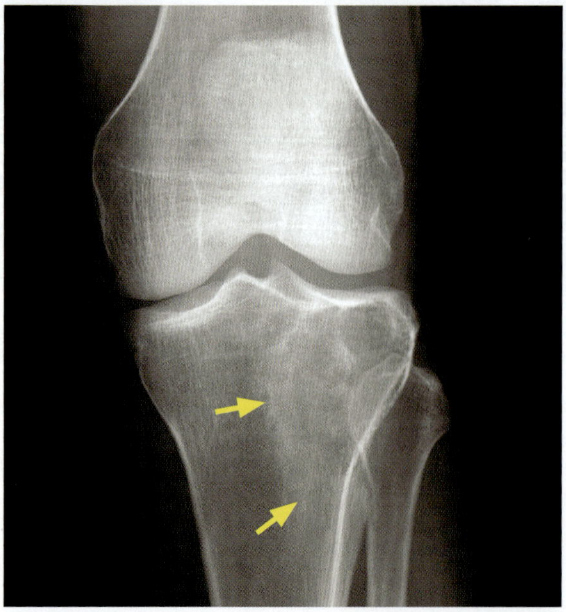

Giant cell tumor:
Frontal radiograph of the knee in a skeletally mature individual shows an eccentric lucent lesion (arrows) in the lateral tibial epiphysis and metaphysis extending to the articular surface.
Case courtesy Scott Sheehan, MD, Brigham and Women's Hospital, Boston.
骨巨细胞瘤：一名骨骼发育成熟患者的膝关节正位X线影像显示胫骨外侧骨骺及干骺端一处偏心性透亮病变(箭)并延伸至关节面。

- Giant cell tumor is an epiphyseal lucent lesion located eccentrically at the articular end of long bones in skeletally mature patients between ages 20 and 40. It arises from the metaphysis but crosses the closed epiphyseal plate to involve the epiphysis. The cell of origin is a multinucleated giant cell, similar in appearance to an osteoclast.
- Most giant cell tumors are benign. Approximately 5% are malignant, but it is impossible to differentiate behavior based on the appearance of the primary lesion.
- Multifocal giant cell tumors can be seen in Paget disease or hyperparathyroidism.
- Treatment is typically curettage or wide resection.

- 骨巨细胞瘤是一种骨骺的透亮性病变，位于长骨关节端偏心的部位，好发于20~40岁骨骼发育成熟的成人。它起源于干骺端，但穿过已闭合的骺板累及骨骺。细胞起源于多核巨细胞，与破骨细胞形态类似。
- 大多数骨巨细胞瘤为良性。约5%的骨巨细胞瘤为恶性，但根据原发病灶的表现不能对其生物学行为进行区分。
- 多灶性骨巨细胞瘤可见于佩吉特病或甲状旁腺功能亢进症。
- 治疗常为刮除术或广泛切除术。

Benign: Eosinophilic granuloma (Langerhans cell histiocytosis)

- A disorder of immune regulation, Langerhans cell histiocytosis (LCH) is caused by an abnormal proliferation of histiocytes. LCH is primarily seen in children 5–10 years old and is discussed more in-depth in the pediatric imaging section.
- In the skull, the classic appearance of LCH is a lytic lesion with a *beveled edge*.
- In the mandible or maxilla, LCH may cause a *floating tooth* from resorption of alveolar bone.
- In the spine, LCH may cause *vertebra plana*, which is complete collapse of vertebral body.

良性：嗜酸性肉芽肿（朗格汉斯细胞组织细胞增生症）

- 朗格汉斯细胞组织细胞增生症（LCH）是一种免疫调节性疾病，由异常增殖的组织细胞所致。LCH主要见于5~10岁的儿童，并将在“小儿影像”部分进行深入讨论。
- 在颅骨中，LCH的典型表现为具有*斜角边缘*的溶骨性病变。
- 在上、下颌骨，LCH可产生*浮牙征*，为牙槽骨吸收所致。
- 在脊柱，LCH可导致*扁平椎*，为椎体完全塌陷。

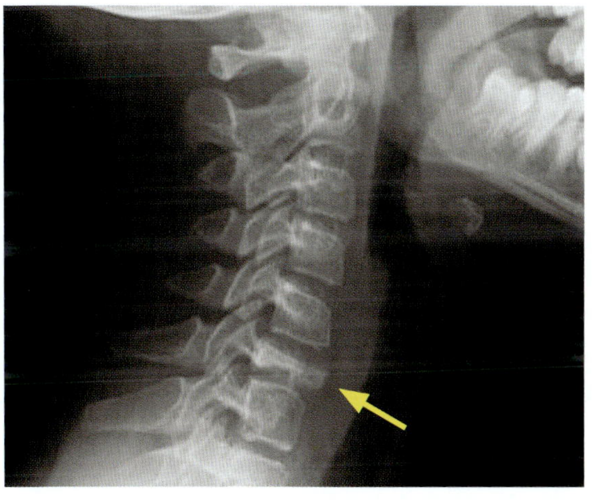

Vertebra plana in eosinophilic granuloma:
Lateral cervical spine radiograph in a 12-year-old girl with known eosinophilic granuloma demonstrates severe compression of the C6 vertebra (arrow) with a vertebra plana appearance.
嗜酸性肉芽肿引起的扁平椎：
一名12岁嗜酸性肉芽肿女童的颈椎侧位X线影像显示C_6椎体严重压缩（箭），呈扁平椎改变。

- In the long bones, LCH may appear as a destructive radiolucent lesion with aggressive (often lamellated) periosteal reaction that may look like lymphoma or Ewing sarcoma.

- 在长骨，LCH可表现为破坏性的透亮病灶伴侵袭性骨膜反应（常呈板层状），与淋巴瘤或尤因肉瘤类似。

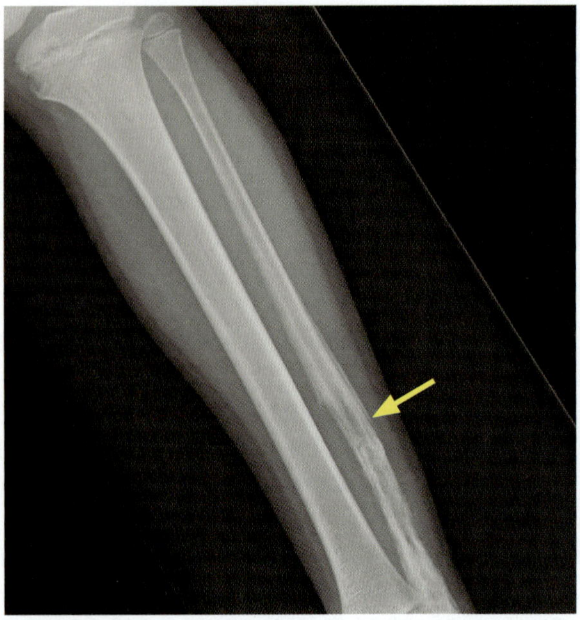

Frontal radiograph
正位X线影像

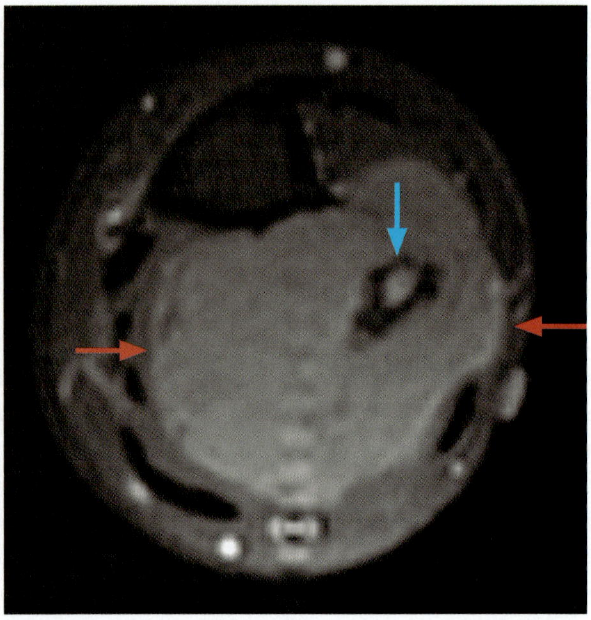

Axial post-contrast T1-weighted MRI with fat suppression
轴位增强T_1加权脂肪抑制MRI

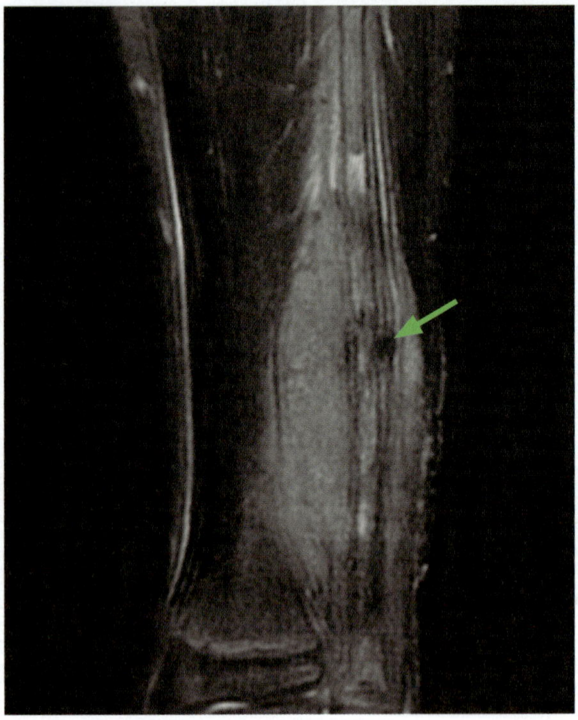

Coronal T2-weighted MRI with fat suppression
冠状位T_2加权脂肪抑制MRI

Ewing sarcoma:
Frontal radiograph in an 8-year-old girl shows a permeative lytic lesion of the distal fibular diaphysis (yellow arrow), near the site of pain.
MR images show the an extensive soft tissue mass (red arrows) centered on the fibula with intramedullary edema and enhancement (blue arrow) and cortical thinning.
There is a nondisplaced pathologic fracture of the fibula (green arrow), best seen on the coronal MR.
尤因肉瘤：
一名8岁女童的正位X线影像显示腓骨骨干远端穿凿样溶骨性病变(黄箭)，接近疼痛部位。
MRI显示以腓骨为中心的广泛软组织肿块(红箭)，伴有髓内水肿、强化(蓝箭)和皮质变薄。
腓骨一处未移位的病理性骨折(绿箭)，冠状位MRI上显示最明显。

- Ewing sarcoma is a highly malignant small round cell tumor (similar to PNET) affecting children and adolescents with a male predominance. The clinical presentation is nonspecific. Ewing sarcoma usually presents with pain. Systemic symptoms including fever are often present, making the distinction between Ewing sarcoma and osteomyelitis difficult.
- Ewing sarcoma is the second most common pediatric primary bone tumor (following osteosarcoma).
- Radiographic features are of an aggressive lesion, with permeative bone

- 尤因肉瘤是一种高度恶性的小圆细胞肿瘤(类似于PNET)，好发于儿童及青少年，男性多见。临床表现无特异性，通常以疼痛为主。常见发热等全身症状，以致尤因肉瘤与骨髓炎鉴别困难。
- 尤因肉瘤是儿童第二常见的原发骨肿瘤(仅次于骨肉瘤)。
- 影像学特征包括侵袭性病变，伴穿凿性骨质

destruction, aggressive periosteal reaction, and often an associated soft-tissue mass.

- In addition to Ewing sarcoma, the differential of an aggressive lytic lesion in a child includes osteomyelitis, eosinophilic granuloma, and metastatic neuroblastoma.

Malignant: Multiple myeloma (MM)/ Plasmacytoma

破坏、侵袭性骨膜反应，常伴有相应的软组织肿块。

- 除尤因肉瘤外，儿童侵袭性溶骨性病变的鉴别诊断还包括骨髓炎、嗜酸性肉芽肿和转移性神经母细胞瘤。

恶性：多发性骨髓瘤(MM)/浆细胞瘤

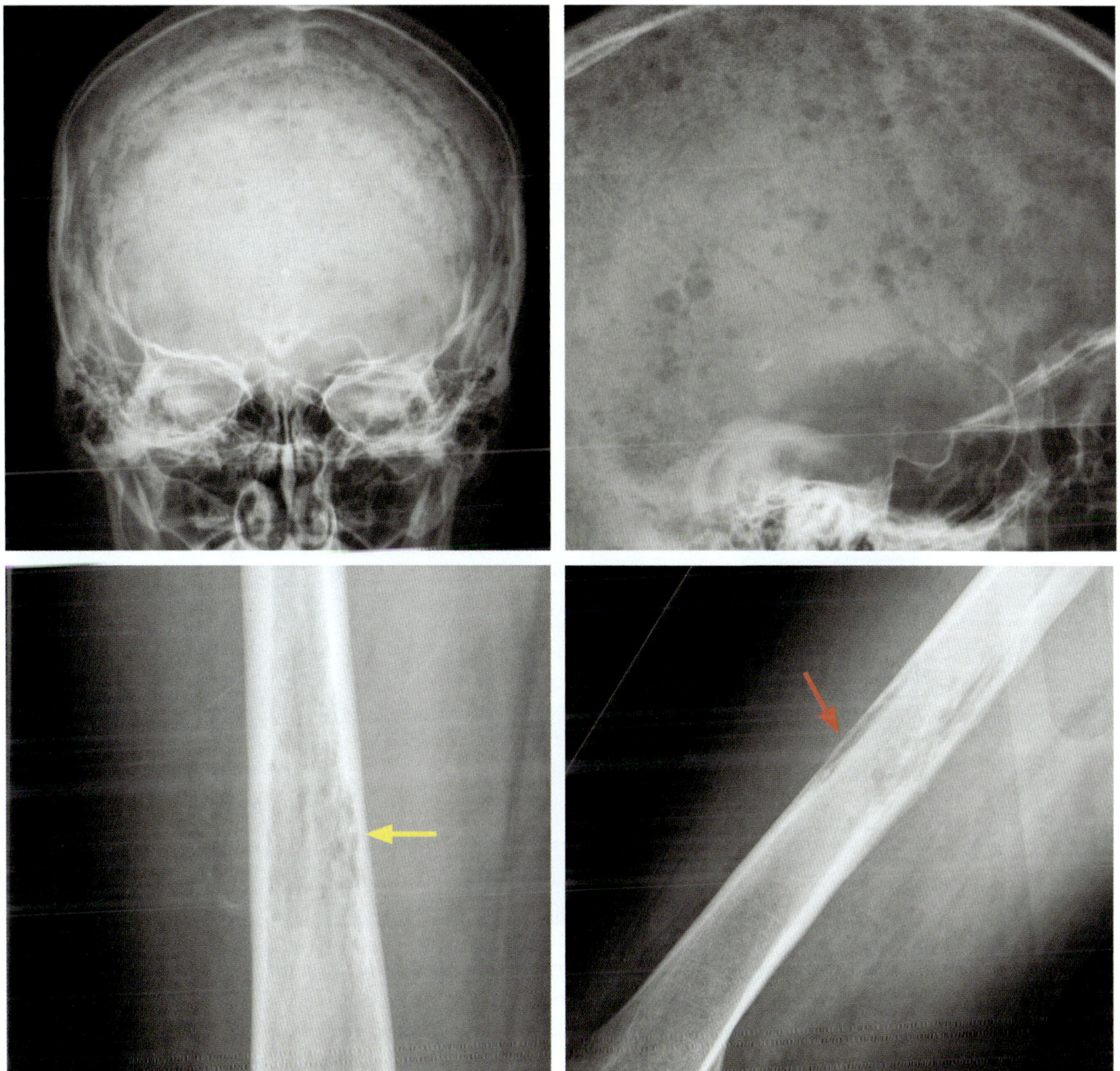

Multiple myeloma: Frontal and lateral radiographs of the skull (top images) show innumerable tiny lytic lesions. AP (bottom left image) and lateral (bottom right image) radiographs of the femur show a permeative appearance (yellow arrow), with focal cortical thinning anteriorly best seen on the lateral view (red arrow).

多发性骨髓瘤：颅骨正、侧位X线影像(上图)显示无数微小的溶骨性病变。股骨前后位(左下图)及侧位X线影像(右下图)显示穿凿样表现(黄箭)，伴前方局部骨皮质变薄，侧位X线影像显示最佳(红箭)。

- Multiple myeloma is the most common primary malignant bone tumor in patients over 40.
- By far the most common presentation of myeloma is multiple lytic lesions, with the most severe form being diffuse myelomatosis with endosteal scalloping.
- Sclerosing myelomatosis is an uncommon variant, associated with **POEMS syndrome**:

- 多发性骨髓瘤是40岁以上患者最常见的原发性恶性骨肿瘤。
- 骨髓瘤最常见的表现为多发性溶骨性病变，最严重的形式为弥漫性骨髓瘤，伴骨内膜呈扇贝样重塑改变。
- 硬化性骨髓瘤是不常见类型，与**POEMS综合征**相关：

Polyneuropathy.

Organomegaly (liver/spleen).

Endocrine disturbances (amenorrhea/gynecomastia).

Monoclonal gammopathy.

Skin changes (hirsutism and hyperpigmentation).

- The main differential of multiple lytic lesions in an adult is metastatic disease. Multiple myeloma originates from the red marrow and usually does not involve regions where there is minimal red marrow, such as the pedicles in the spine. Multiple myeloma may be negative on bone scan, unlike most metastases.
- A solitary tumor is a **plasmacytoma**. Most patients with plasmacytoma will get full-blown multiple myeloma within 5 years.

Malignant: Lymphoma

- Primary bone lymphoma is very rare and tends to occur in adults over 40.
- Bone lymphoma appears as an aggressive lytic lesion, but may also be an important differential consideration for an *ivory* (diffusely sclerotic) vertebral body.
- Lymphoma is often associated with an adjacent soft-tissue mass.

多发性神经病。

器官巨大症(肝/脾)。

内分泌失调(闭经/男性乳腺发育)。

单克隆丙种球蛋白病。

皮肤改变(多毛症和色素过度沉着)。

- 多发溶骨病变在成人的主要鉴别诊断是转移瘤。多发性骨髓瘤起源于红骨髓,通常不累及红骨髓含量少的区域,如脊柱的椎弓。多发性骨髓瘤在骨扫描时可呈阴性,这与大多数转移瘤不同。
- 单发的骨髓瘤是**浆细胞瘤**。大多数浆细胞瘤患者在5年内最终全面发展为多发性骨髓瘤。

恶性:淋巴瘤

- 原发性骨淋巴瘤罕见,主要发生在40岁以上的成人。
- 骨淋巴瘤表现为侵袭性溶骨性病变,但也可能是象牙椎(弥漫性硬化)的一个重要的鉴别诊断。
- 骨淋巴瘤常伴有相邻的软组织肿块。

FAT (LIPO-) LESIONS

脂肪(脂质)病变

Benign: Intraosseous lipoma

良性:骨内脂肪瘤

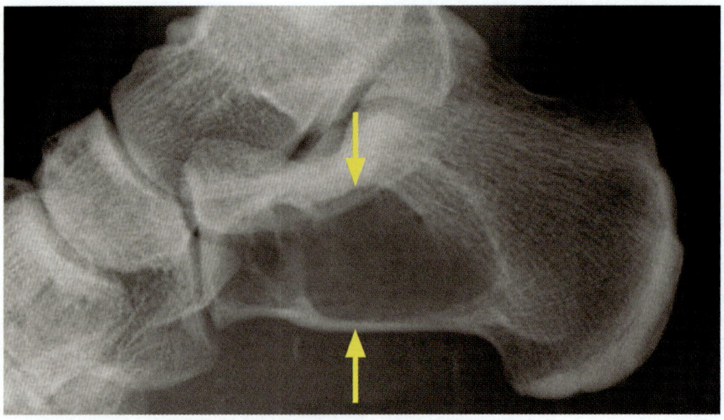

Lateral radiograph of the ankle shows a nonspecific circumscribed lucent lesion in the calcaneus (arrows) with a thin rim of peripheral sclerosis.

The differential for this lesion would include intraosseous lipoma, simple bone cyst, or aneurysmal bone cyst.

If central or ring-like calcification were present, that would more strongly favor intraosseous lipoma.

侧位踝关节X线影像显示跟骨非特异性、边缘整齐的透亮区(箭),伴有非薄的硬化边。

该病变的鉴别诊断包括骨内脂肪瘤、单纯性骨囊肿或动脉瘤样骨囊肿。

如果病灶出现中央或环状钙化,则更倾向于骨内脂肪瘤。

- Intraosseous lipoma is an uncommon benign neoplasm. The most common sites are the calcaneus, subtrochanteric region of the femur, distal tibia/fibula, and metatarsals. Imaging can be variable depending on the degree of fat, calcification, fibrous tissue, and peripheral sclerosis. Central or ring-like calcification is often present.

- 骨内脂肪瘤是一种少见的良性肿瘤。最常发生的部位是跟骨、股骨转子下区域、远端胫骨/腓骨和跖骨。影像学表现多样,取决于病灶内脂肪、钙化、纤维组织及外周硬化的程度。常有中央或环形钙化。

NOTOCHORDAL LESIONS

脊索源性病变

Malignant: Chordoma

恶性：脊索瘤

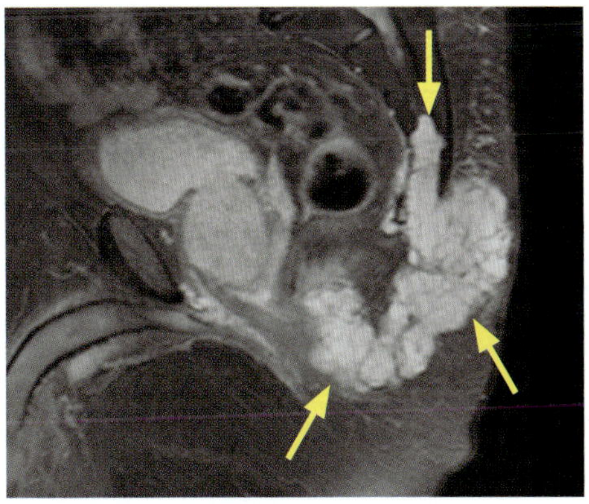

Sagittal T2-weighted MRI with fat suppression
矢状位T_2加权脂肪抑制MRI

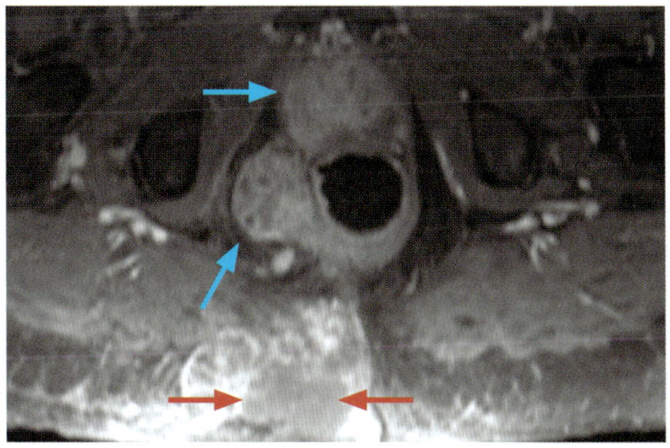

Post-contrast axial T1-weighted MRI with fat suppression
轴位增强T_1加权脂肪抑制MRI

Sacral chordoma: There is a lobulated, T2 hyperintense mass (yellow arrows) arising from the sacrum, with destruction of the coccyx. The mass is predominantly midline, extending into the right perineal and pararectal soft tissues. The mass is largely hypovascular (red arrows), with septational enhancement anteriorly (blue arrows).
骶骨脊索瘤：起源于骶骨的分叶状T_2高信号肿块(黄箭)，伴尾骨破坏。肿块主要位于中线，并向右侧会阴和直肠旁软组织延伸。肿块以低血供为主(红箭)，前方有分隔强化(蓝箭)。

- Chordoma is a malignant lesion deriving from a notochord remnant. It arises in the midline of the axial skeleton, either in the spheno-occipital region, body of C2 (less commonly other vertebral bodies), or sacrococcygeal location.
- Chordoma is a destructive lytic lesion with irregular scalloped borders.
- Calcifications may be present, which are due to necrosis, not bone formation. On MRI, chordomas have lobulated T2 hyperintense signal with heterogeneous enhancement.

- 脊索瘤是一种起源于脊索残余的恶性病变。它发生在中轴骨的中线，可以位于蝶骨枕部、C_2椎体(其他椎体少见)，也可以位于骶尾部。
- 脊索瘤是一个具有不规则扇贝样边缘的破坏性溶骨性病变。
- 可能存在钙化，这是由于坏死所致，而非骨形成。在MRI上，脊索瘤呈分叶状T_2高信号，伴不均匀强化。

LESIONS OF UNKNOWN CELL ORIGIN

细胞来源不明确性病变

Benign: Simple bone cyst (SBC), also called unicameral bone cyst (UBC)

良性：单纯性骨囊肿(SBC)，也称为单房性骨囊肿(UBC)

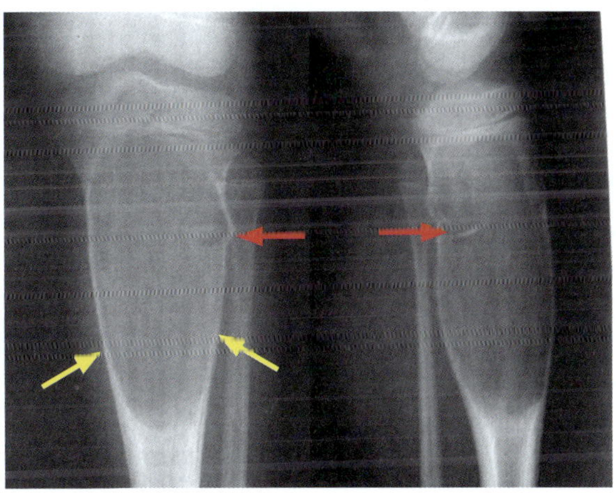

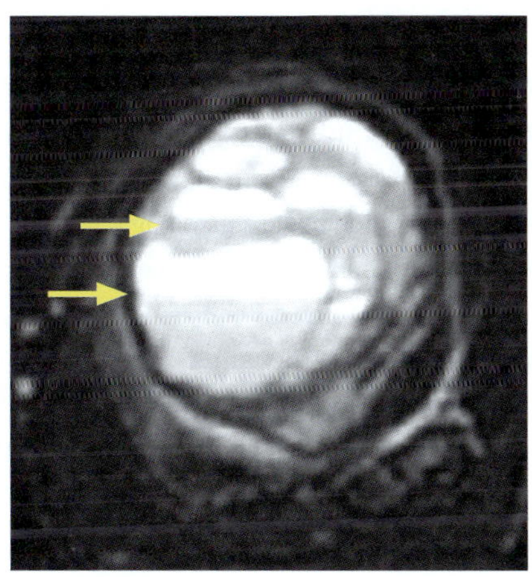

Solitary bone cyst: Frontal and lateral radiographs of the proximal tibia in a skeletally immature patient show a central, expansile lesion of the proximal tibia. A pathologic fracture is present with a displaced bone fragment (red arrows), representing the *fallen fragment sign*. T2-weighted MRI with fat suppression (right image) shows multiple fluid levels (yellow arrows). The differential diagnosis incudes an aneurysmal bone cyst. *Case courtesy Michael Callahan, MD, Boston Children's Hospital.*
孤立性骨囊肿：一名骨骼尚未发育成熟患者的正、侧位胫骨近端X线影像，显示胫骨近端一个中央型、膨胀性病变。可见一处病理性骨折，伴有骨折片移位(红箭)，此为*骨片陷落征*。脂肪抑制T_2加权(右图)显示多处液平(黄箭)。其鉴别诊断包括动脉瘤样骨囊肿。

- Simple bone cyst/unicameral bone cyst is the result of a benign local disturbance of bone growth in children and adolescents.
- The lesion is either hollow or fluid-filled and typically found in the proximal diaphysis of the humerus or femur. Less common locations include the calcaneus or iliac bone.
- SBC lacks periosteal reaction (in contrast to aneurysmal bone cyst), as long as there is no fracture.
- Up to 66% of cases are complicated by pathologic fracture. The *fallen fragment sign* represents a cortical fracture fragment that has fallen into the cyst. It is pathognomonic for SBC when seen in a young patient in a lesion in an appropriate location for SBC.
- SBC is always located centrally within a bone.
- Fluid-fluid levels are seen on MRI. Fluid levels are nonspecific and can also be seen in aneurysmal bone cyst, giant cell tumor, and telangiectatic osteosarcoma.
- One nonsurgical treatment option is the intra-lesional injection of methylprednisolone, which induces osteogenesis.

- 单纯性骨囊肿/单房性骨囊肿是发生在儿童和青少年时期的一种良性局限性骨生长异常。
- 病变既可以为中空，也可以充满液体。好发于肱骨或股骨近端的骨干，较少见于跟骨或髂骨。
- 只要不发生病理性骨折，单纯性骨囊肿不具骨膜反应(相对于动脉瘤样骨囊肿)。
- 高达66%的患者发生病理性骨折。骨片陷落征是指骨皮质碎片陷入囊肿。此征若发生在青年患者并出现在SBC典型的部位，则对SBC具有确诊意义。
- SBC总是位于骨的中心。
- 液-液平面见于MRI。液平是非特异性表现，也可见于动脉瘤样骨囊肿、骨巨细胞瘤和毛细血管扩张型骨肉瘤。
- 非手术治疗的方法之一是向病灶内注射甲泼尼龙，以诱导骨质生成。

Benign: Aneurysmal bone cyst (ABC)

- Aneurysmal bone cyst (ABC) is an expansile or "aneurysmal" multicystic lesion seen in children and adolescents.
- Histologically, ABC is made of blood-filled sinusoids and solid fibrous elements. ABC may arise secondarily within a pre-existing tumor. This is important to consider if an aggressive lesion is biopsied and the pathology returns ABC, as this may imply that the true lesion was not sampled.
- Unlike SBC, ABC can be located anywhere in bone (central or eccentric). It may occur in the posterior elements of the spine. Unlike SBC, ABC often features a "buttressing" smooth periosteal reaction at the proximal and distal aspects. Like SBC, fluid levels are present.

良性：动脉瘤样骨囊肿(ABC)

- 动脉瘤样骨囊肿(ABC)是一种膨胀性或"动脉瘤样"多囊性病变，见于儿童和青少年。
- 组织学上，ABC由充满血液的窦腔和实性纤维成分组成。ABC可继发于原有的肿瘤。这一点尤其重要，也就是当一个侵袭性病灶穿刺活检的病理报告为ABC时，有可能提示采样没有取自真正的病灶。
- 不同于SBC，ABC可以位于骨的任何部位(中心或偏心)。它可发生在脊柱的后部结构。另一个不同于SBC特点是，ABC常在病变的远近两端具有平滑与"拱壁支撑"样的骨膜反应。与SBC类似，也可出现液-液平面。

Malignant: Adamantinoma

- Adamantinoma is a very rare malignant lytic lesion in the tibia with a *soap-bubble* appearance. It may be difficult to differentiate from fibrous dysplasia.

恶性：釉质瘤

- 釉质瘤是罕见的恶性溶骨性病变，好发于胫骨，呈肥皂泡样改变。有时与骨纤维异常增殖症鉴别困难。

Osseous metastasis

- Osseous metastases are over 10 times more common than primary bone tumors.
- Most metastases occur in the red bone marrow, most commonly in the axial skeleton.
- It can be difficult to differentiate a pathologic vertebral body fracture (associated with an underlying tumor) from an osteoporotic fracture, but involvement of the pedicle or posterior vertebral body suggests metastasis.
- A fracture of the lesser trochanter in an adult should raise concern for pathologic fracture.
- A solitary sternal lesion is highly predictive of metastasis in a patient with breast cancer.

骨转移瘤

- 骨转移瘤至少是原发性骨肿瘤的10倍。
- 大多数骨转移瘤发生在红骨髓，最常见于中轴骨。
- 鉴别病理性椎体骨折(伴潜在肿瘤)与骨质疏松性骨折有时比较困难，但若累及椎弓或椎体后部则提示转移瘤。
- 成人发生小转子骨折应该怀疑有病理性骨折。
- 乳腺癌患者出现单发的胸骨病灶高度提示转移瘤。

Lytic osseous metastases

- Lung (most common purely lytic).
- Breast (lytic or blastic).
- Thyroid.
- Kidney.
- Stomach, colon (lytic or blastic).

溶骨性转移瘤

- 肺(纯溶骨最常见)。
- 乳腺(溶骨或成骨)。
- 甲状腺。
- 肾脏。
- 胃、结肠(溶骨或成骨)。

Blastic (sclerotic) osseous metastases

- Breast (lytic or blastic).
- Prostate, seminoma.
- Transitional cell carcinoma.
- Mucinous tumors.
- Carcinoid.

成骨性(硬化性)转移瘤

- 乳腺(溶骨或成骨)。
- 前列腺、精原细胞瘤。
- 移行细胞癌。
- 黏液性肿瘤。
- 类癌。

Benign Tumor Mimics

类似于良性肿瘤的病变

Myositis ossificans

骨化性肌炎

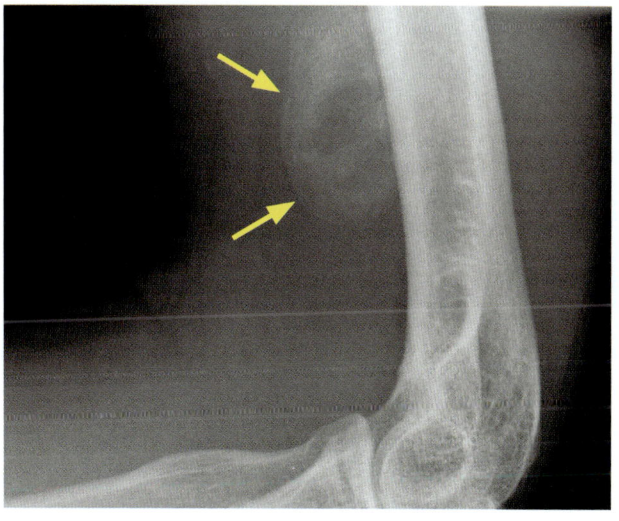

Myositis ossificans:
Lateral radiograph of the elbow shows peripheral osteoid within a mass abutting the anterior humeral cortex. The peripheral ossification (arrows) suggests myositis ossificans, at least 5 weeks old.
The main differential diagnosis is parosteal osteosarcoma; however, the peripheral ossification more strongly suggests myositis ossificans. This case was followed and confirmed by close-interval follow-up imaging.
骨化性肌炎：
侧位肘关节X线影像显示一处紧贴肱骨前缘皮质、边缘为类骨质的肿块。边缘骨化(箭)提示骨化性肌炎至少5周。
主要的鉴别诊断为皮质旁骨肉瘤；但边缘骨化强烈提示骨化性肌炎。该病例经密切影像学随访并确诊为骨化性肌炎。

- Myositis ossificans (MO) is heterotopic bone formation in the skeletal muscle secondary to trauma, although the history of trauma may not be remembered and the trauma may be minor. MO most commonly occurs around the elbow and thigh, which are prone to trauma.
- Myositis ossificans may mimic parosteal osteosarcoma. Parosteal osteosarcoma is usually more heavily calcified centrally, while myositis ossificans is typically more calcified peripherally.
- If myositis ossificans is suspected, a biopsy should not be performed. A biopsy can lead to unnecessary surgery, as the histology may resemble sarcoma.
- The appearance of myositis ossificans evolves over a period of weeks to months:

Weeks 1–2: Soft-tissue mass only.
Weeks 3–4: Formation of amorphous osteoid matrix. May cause periosteal reaction of adjacent bone. This stage is most suggestive of an early osteosarcoma.
Weeks 5–8: The periphery of the lesion matures into compact bone.
Up to 6 months: Ossification continues to mature.
>6 months: Typically decreases in size.

- 骨化性肌炎(MO)是继发于外伤后在骨骼肌内形成的异位骨，但外伤史往往不清楚，可能是轻微损伤。MO最常发生于肘和大腿周围，这些部位容易受伤。
- 骨化性肌炎可类似于皮质旁骨肉瘤。皮质旁骨肉瘤通常在中央部位明显钙化，而骨化性肌炎常为外周性钙化。
- 如怀疑有骨化性肌炎，则不应行活检。活检可导致不必要的外科手术，因其组织学表现可类似于肉瘤。
- 骨化性肌炎的表现随时间发生演变，持续数周至数月：

1~2周：仅有软组织肿块。
3~4周：形成无定形骨样基质。可导致邻近骨出现骨膜反应。此期更可能被认为是早期骨肉瘤。
5~8周：病变外周成熟转化为密质骨。
至6个月：骨化继续直至成熟。
>6个月：体积通常缩小。

Brown tumor

棕色瘤

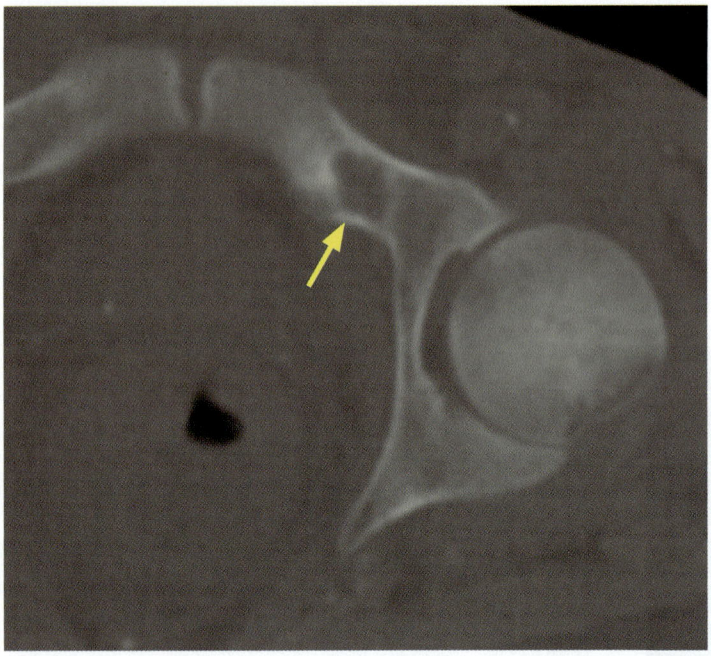

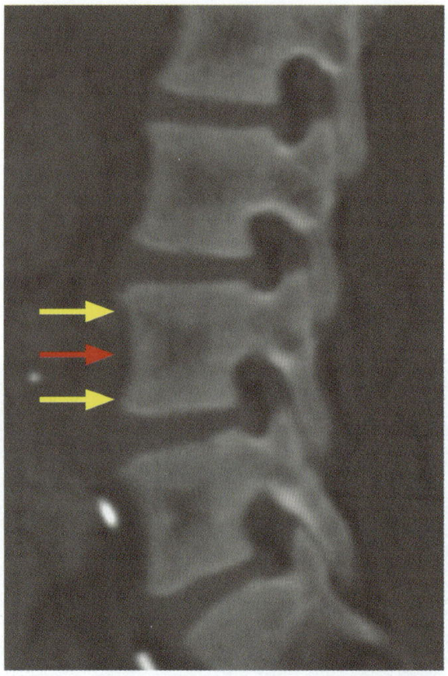

Brown tumor: Axial CT (left image) shows a nonspecific lytic lesion with a faint sclerotic margin in the left superior pubic ramus (arrow) in a patient with renal osteodystrophy and secondary hyperparathyroidism. Note the *rugger jersey* spine on the sagittal CT with alternating bands of sclerosis (yellow arrows) and relative central lucency (red arrow).

棕色瘤：轴位CT(左图)显示左侧耻骨上支(箭)一处非特异性溶骨性病变伴浅淡的硬化边缘，患者有肾性骨营养不良和继发性甲状旁腺功能亢进。注意矢状位CT上橄榄球衣样脊柱，硬化带(黄箭)和相对中心透亮区(红箭)交替出现。

- A brown tumor is a benign lytic lesion seen in patients with hyperparathyroidism, caused by increased osteoclast activation.
- Brown tumor does not have any specific imaging features and may be difficult to differentiate from a giant cell tumor both radiologically and pathologically.
- Associated features of hyperparathyroidism are usually present, including:

Osteopenia. Subperiosteal bone resorption (especially of the radial aspect of the second and third middle phalanges and the acromial ends of clavicles). Soft-tissue calcifications.

- Lab abnormalities associated with hyperparathyroidism (in addition to elevated PTH level) include elevated calcium and decreased phosphorus.
- If hyperparathyroidism is secondary to renal failure, secondary findings of renal osteodystrophy may be seen as well, such as rugger jersey spine.

- 棕色瘤是一种良性溶骨性病变，见于甲状旁腺功能亢进患者，由破骨细胞活动增加所致。
- 棕色瘤缺乏特异性的影像学表现，在影像及病理上可能均难以与骨巨细胞瘤鉴别。
- 常出现与甲状旁腺功能亢进症的相关特征，包括：

骨量减少。 骨膜下骨质吸收(尤其第二、三中节指骨桡侧及锁骨肩峰端)。 软组织钙化。

- 实验室检查异常与甲状旁腺功能亢进症相关，(除PTH水平增高以外)包括血钙增高和血磷降低。
- 如果甲状旁腺功能亢进继发于肾衰竭，也可有肾性骨营养不良的表现，如橄榄球衣样脊柱。

Osteomyelitis

- Osteomyelitis, subsequently discussed, may cause a permeative or lytic bony lesion that can be indistinguishable from an aggressive malignancy.

骨髓炎

- 骨髓炎可产生穿凿样或溶骨性病变，有可能与侵袭性恶性肿瘤无法进行鉴别，具体细节将在后续章节进行讨论。

Cortical desmoid

- A cortical desmoid is a classic "do not touch" lesion.
- Pathophysiology is due to repetitive stress at the attachment of the medial head of gastrocnemius or distal adductor magnus.
- On radiograph, cortical desmoid lesion appears as a saucer-shaped radiolucent cortical irregularity without sclerotic margin at the posteromedial aspect of the distal femoral metaphysis.

皮质硬纤维瘤

- 皮质硬纤维瘤是典型的"请勿触摸"性病变。
- 在病理生理学上，这是由于腓肠肌内侧头或大收肌远端附着处的重复应力所致。
- 在X线影像上，皮质硬纤维瘤如一个碟形的透亮区，位于股骨远端干骺端后内侧，边界不规则，无硬化边。

- MRI shows a T1 hypointense, T2 hyperintense enhancing cortically based lesion.

- MRI表现为T_1低信号、T_2高信号并有强化的皮质病变。

（翻译　彭新桂　苏筱芮）

Soft Tissue Tumors

软组织肿瘤

Lipomatous Neoplasms

脂肪瘤样肿瘤

Lipoma

脂肪瘤

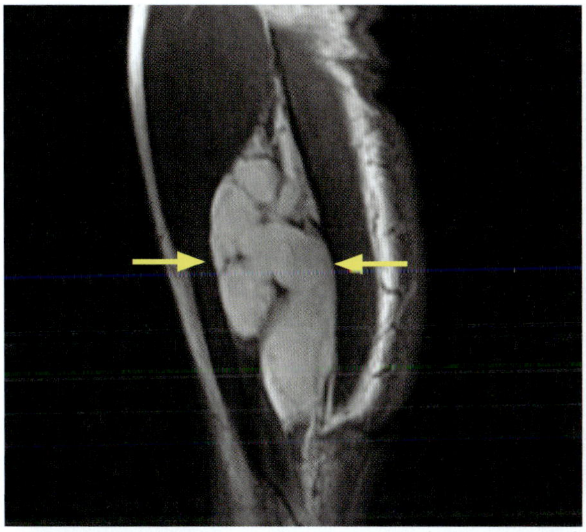

Coronal T1-weighted MRI
冠状位T_1加权MRI

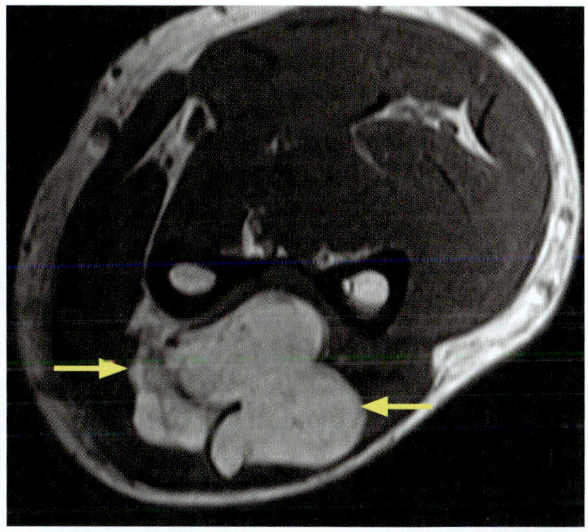

Axial PD-weighted MRI
轴位PD加权MRI

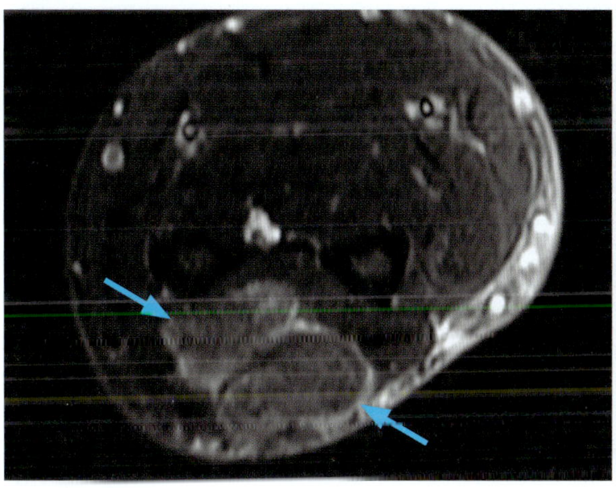

Axial STIR MRI
轴位STIR MRI

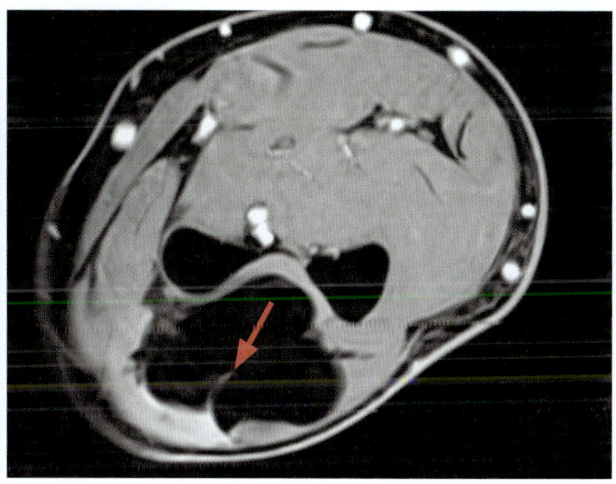

Axial post-contrast T1-weighted MRI with fat suppression
轴位增强T_1加权脂肪抑制MRI

Lipoma: There is a lobulated mass (yellow arrows) in the posterior/dorsal aspect of the forearm, which follows fat signal intensity on T1-weighted and PD-weighted images (note that the PD sequence alone cannot be used to determine if something is fat signal intensity as both fat and fluid are hyperintense on PD-weighted images). The mass saturates out on the T1-weighted image with fat saturation. There is minimal septational enhancement (red arrow), and slightly increased signal intensity on the STIR sequence (blue arrows), but no thickened septations or nodular enhancement.

脂肪瘤：前臂的后/背侧可见一分叶状肿块(黄箭)，在T_1加权和PD加权图像上肿块与脂肪信号一致(注意：仅用PD加权不能确定肿块信号是否与脂肪一致，因为脂肪和液体在PD加权上都呈高信号)。肿块在T_1WI脂肪抑制图像上信号被完全抑制。肿块内可见少量分隔样强化(红箭)，在STIR序列上肿块信号强度稍增高(蓝箭)，但没有增厚的分隔或结节样增强。

- Lipoma, a benign proliferation of adipocytes, is the most common soft-tissue tumor, and the most common explanation for a palpable mass. However, it is important to note that not all palpable masses are lipomas and imaging should be performed before presuming a diagnosis of lipoma and certainly before resection.
- A substantial minority of lipomas may contain some nonadipose tissue. Minimal nonadipose tissue, such as wispy septations, is commonly seen in lipomas. However, thickened or irregular septations, or nodular enhancing foci would not be consistent with a simple lipoma, and would suggest a well-differentiated liposarcoma/atypical lipomatous tumor.
- Lipomas confirmed by imaging are usually not resected or biopsied unless there are atypical elements on imaging, or patients are symptomatic due to mass effect.

Well-differentiated liposarcoma/atypical lipomatous tumor (ALT)

- 脂肪瘤是一种脂肪细胞的良性增生，是最常见的软组织肿瘤，也是最常可触及肿块的原因。需要指出，并非所有可触及的肿块都是脂肪瘤，在作出诊断和病变切除前应进行影像学检查。
- 有少数脂肪瘤内可能含有一些非脂肪组织。在脂肪瘤中常可见到一些微小的非脂肪组织，如细小分隔。然而，若出现分隔增厚或不规则，或结节状强化则不支持单纯脂肪瘤的诊断，且可能提示为高分化脂肪肉瘤或非典型脂肪瘤样肿瘤。
- 经影像学证实的脂肪瘤通常不需要进行手术切除或活检，除非在影像上出现一些不典型成分，或患者的症状来自肿块占位效应。

高分化脂肪肉瘤/非典型脂肪瘤样肿瘤(ALT)

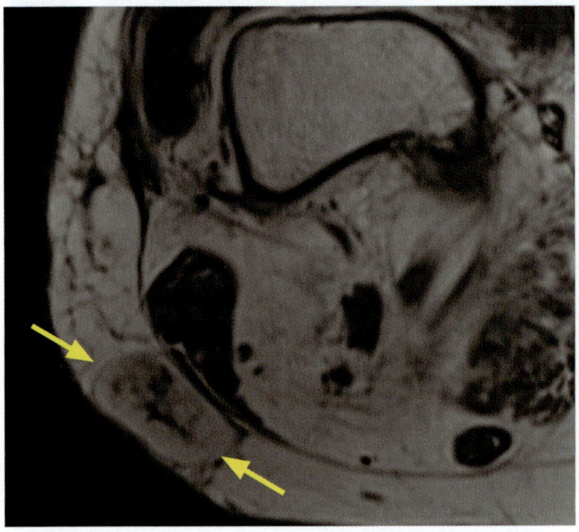

Axial T1-weighted MRI
轴位T_1加权MRI

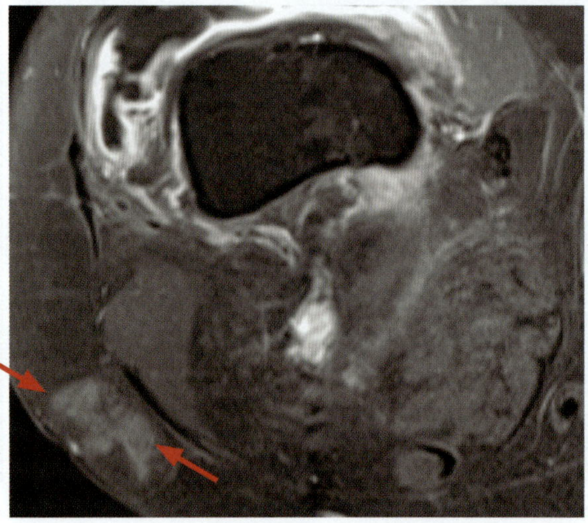

Axial post-contrast T1-weighted MRI with fat suppression
轴位增强T_1加权脂肪抑制MRI

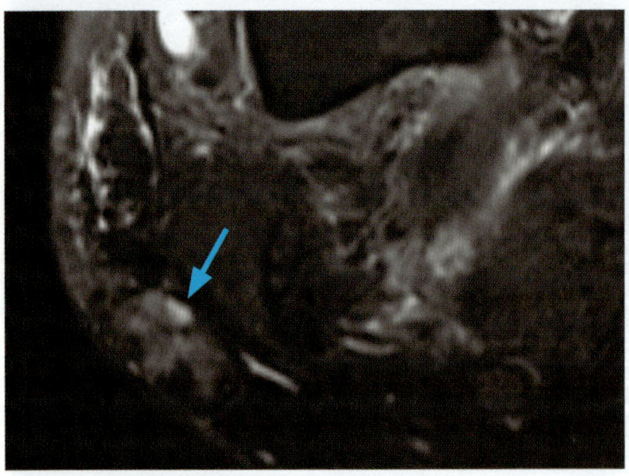

Axial T2-weighted MRI with fat suppression
轴位T_2加权脂肪抑制MRI

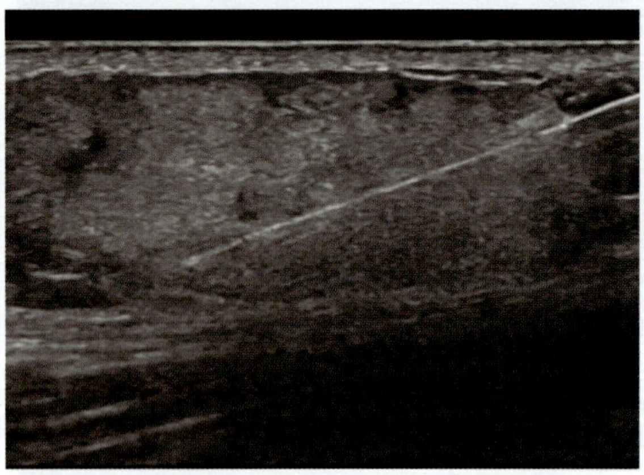

Ultrasound-guided biopsy
超声引导下穿刺活检

Well-differentiated liposarcoma/atypical lipomatous tumor: Axial T1-weighted image demonstrates a relatively small oval mass (yellow arrows) in the subcutaneous tissues of the lateral distal thigh (just above the knee), largely fat signal intensity but containing heterogeneous signal.
There is heterogeneous enhancement within the mass (red arrows), and the fluid sensitive fat suppressed T2-weighted image shows multifocal regions of high signal (blue arrow). Based on the complex features (enhancement, and increased signal intensity on fluid sensitive images), biopsy was performed, which demonstrated ALT. Note the circumscribed, slightly echogenic appearance of the mass on ultrasound, which is a typical appearance for lipoma or ALT.
高分化脂肪肉瘤/非典型脂肪瘤样肿瘤：轴位T_1加权MRI示大腿远端外侧(膝关节上方)皮下见一个较小的、椭圆形肿块(黄箭)，肿块大部分为脂肪信号，但含不均匀信号。
轴位增强T_1加权MRI显示肿块内不均匀强化(红箭)，液体敏感脂肪抑制T_2加权显示肿块内多发高信号区(蓝箭)。基于肿瘤复杂的影像特征(强化、液体敏感序列呈高信号)，对该肿瘤进行了活检，结果证实为非典型脂肪瘤样肿瘤。注意，超声所显示的边界清晰、稍强回声肿块是典型的脂肪瘤或非典型脂肪瘤样肿瘤表现。

- Well-differentiated liposarcoma, also called atypical lipomatous tumor (ALT), is a low-grade adipocytic neoplasm that rarely metastasizes but can be locally aggressive.
- While there can be some overlap in the imaging appearance of ALT and benign lipoma, features of ALT include larger size (however, size alone cannot be used to distinguish lipoma from ALT), thickened septae, septal or nodular contrast enhancement, or increased signal intensity on fluid sensitive sequences.

- 高分化脂肪肉瘤又称非典型脂肪瘤样肿瘤(ALT)，是一种低级别脂肪细胞肿瘤，几乎不发生转移，但具有局部侵袭性。
- 尽管非典型脂肪瘤样肿瘤和脂肪瘤的影像学表现存在重叠，但非典型脂肪瘤样肿瘤有下列影像学特征：体积大(注意，仅根据大小不能区分脂肪瘤和非典型脂肪瘤样肿瘤)、分隔增厚、分隔强化或结节样强化，以及液体敏感序列上信号增强。

High-grade liposarcoma

- Both pleomorphic liposarcoma and dedifferentiated liposarcoma cannot usually be differentiated by imaging, and thus they can reasonably be considered together as "high- grade liposarcoma."
- Imaging typically shows a large mass with heterogeneous enhancement and usually central necrosis. Fatty elements may or may not be present depending on the degree of differentiation.

高级别脂肪肉瘤

- 多形性脂肪肉瘤和去分化脂肪肉瘤通常在影像学上无法鉴别，因此它们有理由一起被认为是"高级别脂肪肉瘤"。
- 典型的影像学表现为大而不均匀强化的肿块且通常有中心坏死。肿块内可含有或不含有脂肪成分，取决于肿瘤的分化程度。

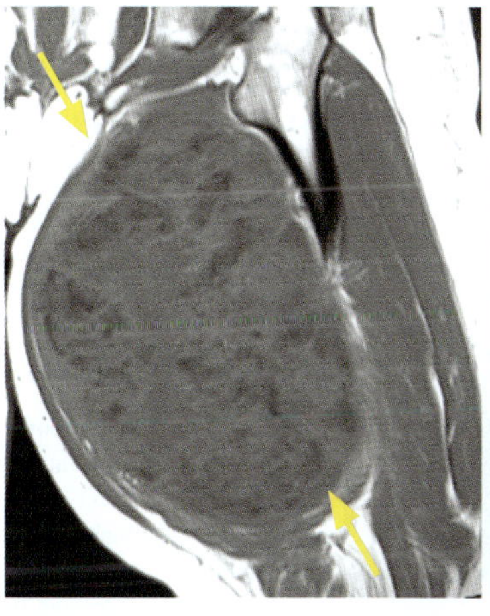

Coronal T1-weighted MRI
冠状位 T_1 加权 MRI

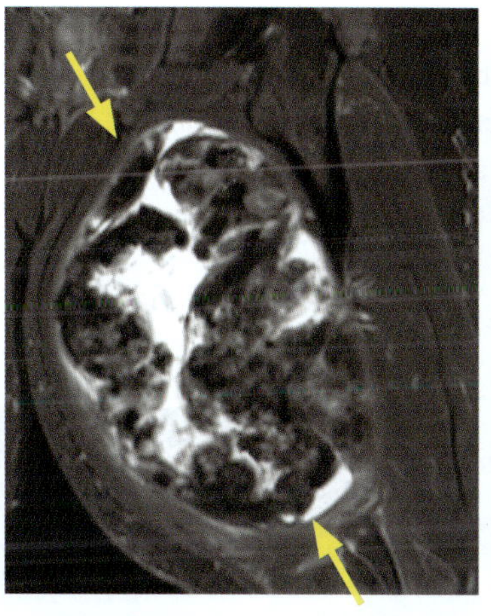

Sagittal STIR MRI
矢状位 STIR MRI

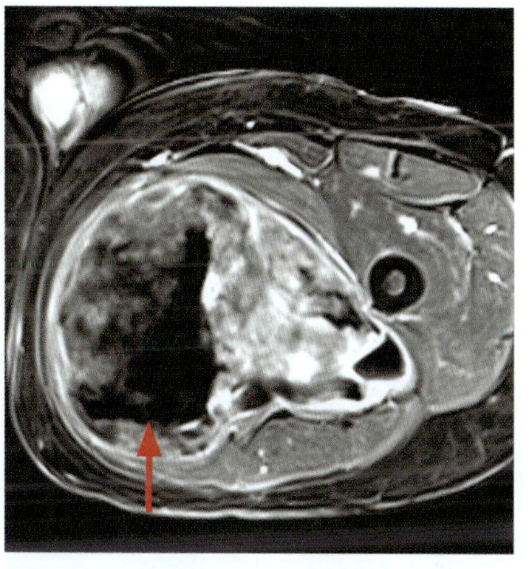

Post-contrast T1 MRI with fat suppression
增强 T_1 加权脂肪抑制 MRI

Dedifferentiated liposarcoma: There is a dominant, heterogeneously enhancing mass (yellow arrows) with central necrosis (central nonenhancement; red arrow) in the left medial thigh. Note the absence of any fatty elements on the T1-weighted image. This appearance can be seen in pleomorphic or dedifferentiated liposarcoma, as well as undifferentiated pleomorphic sarcoma, rhabdomyosarcoma, or leiomyosarcoma.
去分化脂肪肉瘤：左侧大腿内侧一个巨大不均匀强化的肿块(黄箭)，伴中心坏死(肿块中心未见强化，红箭)。注意，T_1 加权图像上该肿块未见脂肪信号。这种表现可见于多形性或去分化脂肪肉瘤、未分化多形性肉瘤、横纹肌肉瘤及平滑肌肉瘤。

Myxoid liposarcoma

黏液样脂肪肉瘤

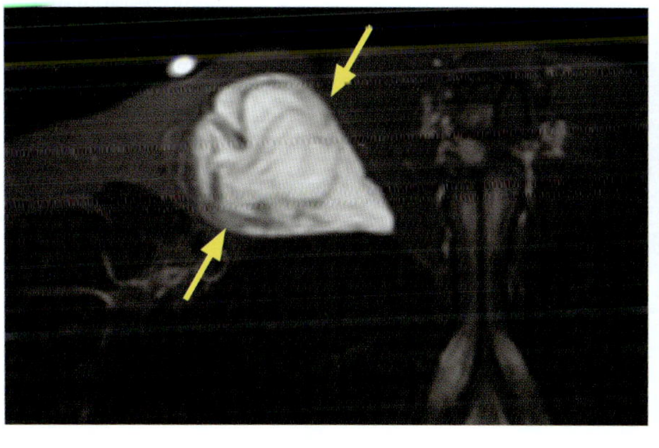

Axial T2-weighted MRI with fat suppression
轴位 T_2 加权脂肪抑制 MRI

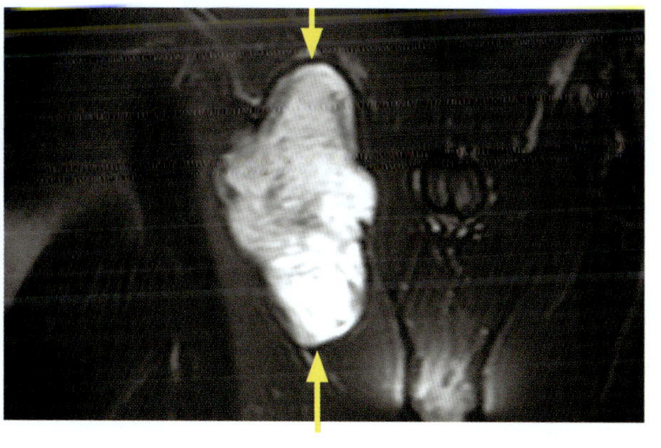

Coronal T2-weighted MRI with fat suppression
冠状位 T_2 加权脂肪抑制 MRI

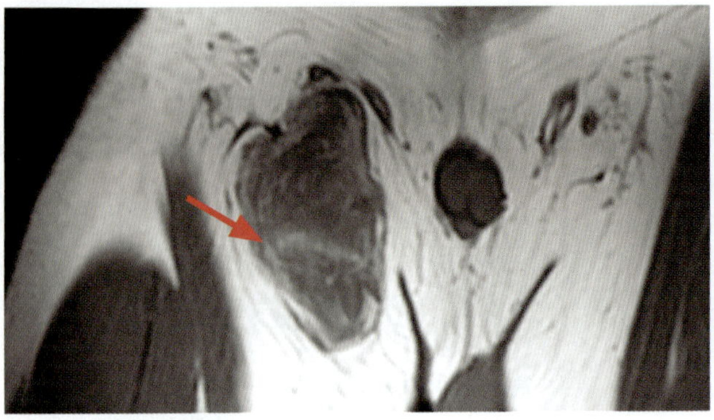

Coronal T1-weighted MRI
冠状位T_1加权MRI

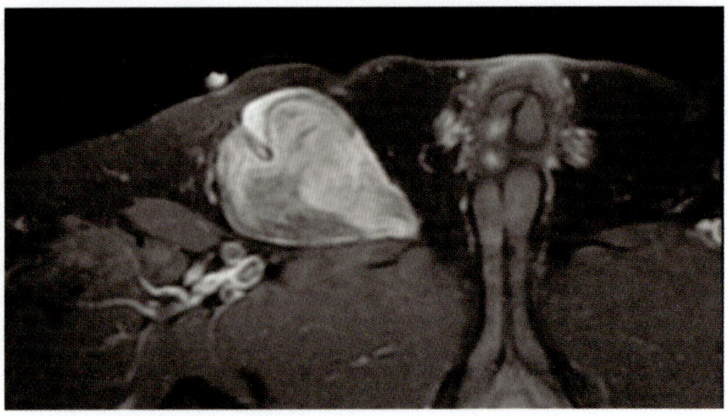

Axial post-contrast T1-weighted MRI with fat suppression
轴位增强T_1加权脂肪抑制MRI

Myxoid liposarcoma: There is a T2-hyperintense mass (yellow arrows) in the right groin, with whorl-like internal architecture. There are wispy lipomatous elements (red arrow) evident on the coronal T1-weighted MR. The mass enhances heterogeneously. The differential diagnosis for an aggressive or large T2 hyperintense enhancing mass includes myxoid liposarcoma, myxofibrosarcoma, synovial sarcoma, or malignant peripheral nerve sheath tumor.
黏液样脂肪肉瘤：右侧腹股沟区可见一个T_2高信号肿块(黄箭)，其内部呈螺纹样的结构。在冠状位T_1加权MRI上肿块内可见细束状的脂肪样成分(红箭)。侵袭性的或巨大的T_2高信号强化肿块的鉴别诊断包括黏液样脂肪肉瘤、黏液纤维肉瘤、滑膜肉瘤及恶性周围神经鞘膜瘤。

- Myxoid liposarcoma is a high-grade neoplasm that has a unique appearance compared to other adipocytic neoplasms. Specifically its myxoid content creates a relatively homogeneous hyperintense appearance on T2-weighted imaging. Similar to high-grade liposarcoma, fatty elements may not be apparent on imaging.

- 黏液样脂肪肉瘤是一种高级别肿瘤，且相对于其他脂肪组织肿瘤具有独特的影像学表现。具体来讲，其内部的黏液成分在T_2加权图像上形成相对均匀的高信号。与其他高级别脂肪肉瘤相似，脂肪成分在影像上不明显。

Fibrolipomatous hamartoma of nerve

神经纤维脂肪性错构瘤

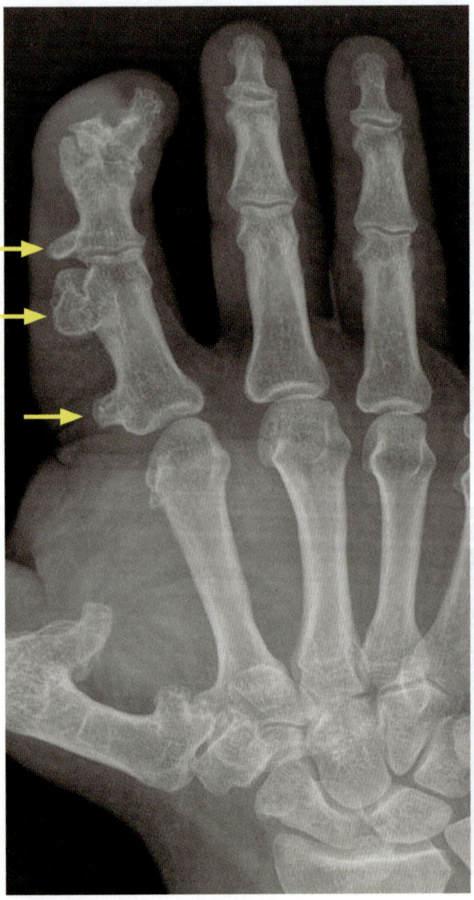

Frontal radiograph
正位X线影像

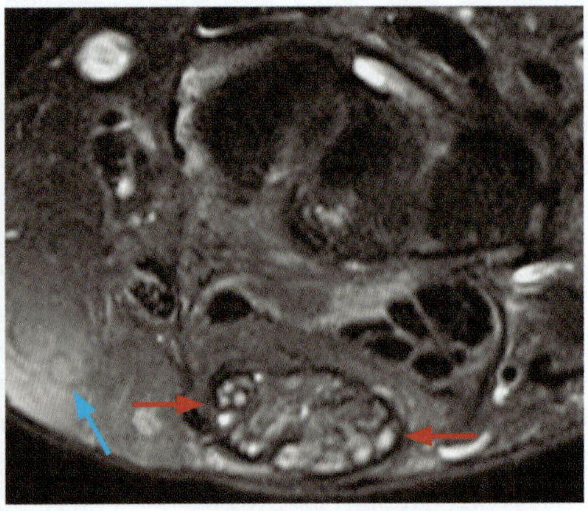

Axial T2-weighted MRI with fat suppression
轴位T_2加权脂肪抑制MRI

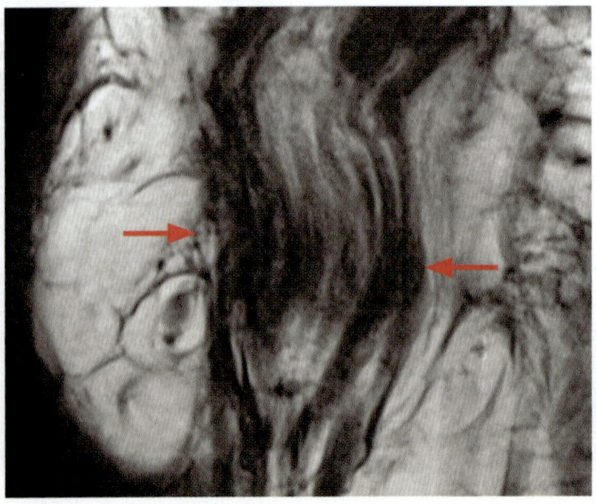

Coronal T1-weighted MRI
冠状位T_1加权MRI

Macrodystrophia lipomatosa with fibrolipomatous hamartoma of the median nerve:
Frontal radiograph of the hand shows broadened phalanges of the index finger with extensive proliferative changes (yellow arrows), and soft tissue overgrowth. There is also partially imaged proliferative change of the thumb metacarpal.
Axial fluid-sensitive MRI demonstrates marked expansion of the median nerve (red arrows), with volar bowing of the flexor retinaculum. There is extensive fatty proliferation throughout the thenar soft tissues (blue arrow).
Coronal T1-weighted MRI demonstrates pathognomonic cable-like appearance of the median nerve (red arrows) with fat signal intensity interdigitating between the fascicles.
正中神经巨大脂肪营养不良症伴纤维脂肪瘤性错构瘤：
手部正位X线影像可见示指指骨增宽伴广泛骨质增生(黄箭)，伴周围软组织过度生长。另外第一掌骨也可见骨质增生。
轴位液体敏感序列MRI显示正中神经明显增粗(红箭)，伴屈肌支持带向掌侧隆起。整个鱼际软组织可见广泛脂肪组织增生(蓝箭)。
冠状位T_1加权MRI显示正中神经病变具有诊断意义的线缆状表现(红箭)，束间交织脂肪信号。

- Fibrolipomatous hamartoma is a rare benign neoplasm of peripheral nerves, where fibroadipose tissue proliferates and infiltrates the epineurium and perineurium.
- The median nerve of the wrist is a common site for fibrolipomatous hamartoma.
- Although rare, imaging features are pathognomonic, with a *cable-like* appearance of the nerve due to fatty proliferation interposed between the fascicles.
- Fibrolipomatous hamartoma is associated with macrodystrophia lipomatosa, which is a rare congenital localized gigantism (such as involvement of a single finger) caused by overgrowth of fibroadipose tissue.

- 纤维脂肪性错构瘤是一种罕见的外周神经良性肿瘤，表现为纤维脂肪组织增生并浸润神经外膜和神经束膜。
- 腕部正中神经是纤维脂肪性错构瘤的好发部位。
- 尽管罕见，但其影像学表现具有特异性，神经呈线缆状，这是由于增生的脂肪组织交替在神经束之间的缘故。
- 纤维脂肪性错构瘤与巨大脂肪瘤营养不良症有关，后者是一种罕见的由纤维脂肪组织过度生长引起的先天性局部巨人症(如单个手指受累)。

HIGH-GRADE SARCOMA

Overview of high-grade non-adipocytic sarcoma

- These neoplasms are not reliably distinguishable from each other on imaging (perhaps except for myxofibrosarcoma, which is T2 hyperintense). They are high-grade tumors that frequently metastasize and are usually large at presentation.

Undifferentiated pleomorphic sarcoma (UPS)

高级别肉瘤

高级别非脂肪细胞肉瘤概述

- 这些肿瘤在影像学上通常难以鉴别(也许除黏液纤维肉瘤外，其在T_2加权上呈高信号)。此类属高级别肿瘤，常会转移，并且通常在发现时体积较大。

未分化多形性肉瘤(UPS)

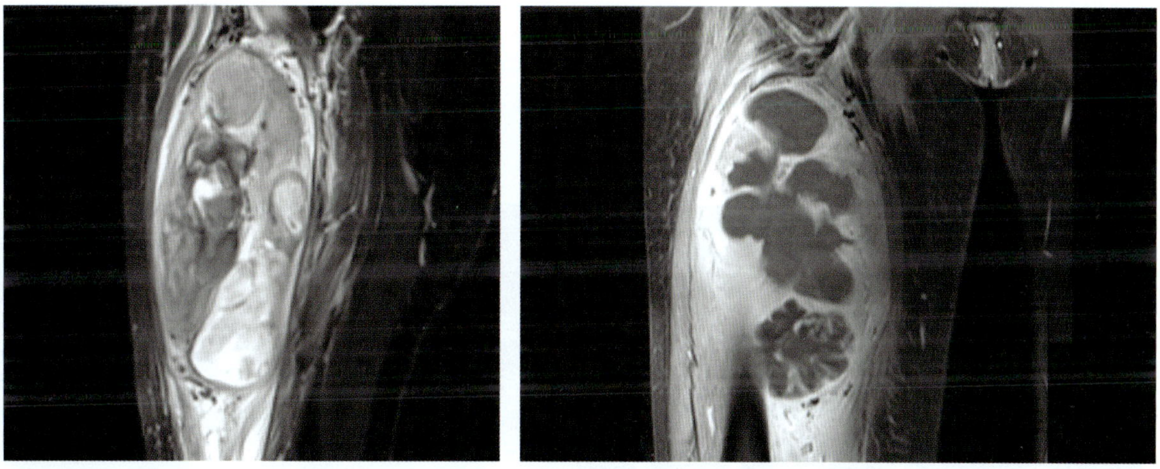

Sagittal T2-weighted MRI with fat suppression
矢状位T_2加权脂肪抑制MRI

Post-contrast coronal T1-weighted MRI with fat suppression
冠状位增强T_1加权脂肪抑制MRI

Undifferentiated pleomorphic sarcoma (UPS): There is a dominant mass in the right anterior thigh with heterogeneous enhancement and central necrosis. This appearance can be seen in UPS, rhabdomyosarcoma, leiomyosarcoma, as well as pleomorphic or dedifferentiated liposarcoma.
未分化多形性肉瘤(UPS)：右侧大腿前侧被一个不均匀强化并伴中心坏死的巨大肿块所占据。这种表现可见于未分化多形性肉瘤、横纹肌肉瘤、平滑肌肉瘤、多形性或去分化脂肪肉瘤。

- Undifferentiated pleomorphic sarcoma (UPS) is a high-grade sarcoma that has been historically called malignant fibrous histiosarcoma.
- Imaging shows a large mass with heterogeneous enhancement, often with central necrosis. There is large imaging overlap between UPS and other high-grade soft tissue tumors.

Rhabdomyosarcoma, leiomyosarcoma

- Rhabdomyosarcoma is a high-grade tumor from skeletal muscle origin.
- Leiomyosarcoma is a high-grade tumor from smooth muscle origin.
- Both appear as large aggressive soft tissue masses, without specific imaging features.

- 未分化多形性肉瘤(UPS)是一种高级别肉瘤，过去曾被命名为恶性纤维组织肉瘤。
- 影像学表现为一个不均匀强化的巨大肿块，常伴中心坏死。未分化多形性肉瘤和其他高级别软组织肿瘤的影像学表现有很多重叠。

横纹肌肉瘤，平滑肌肉瘤

- 横纹肌肉瘤是一种起源于骨骼肌的高级别肿瘤。
- 平滑肌肉瘤是一种起源于平滑肌的高级别肿瘤。
- 两者均表现为巨大且具侵袭性的软组织肿块，但无特异性的影像学表现。

Myxofibrosarcoma

黏液纤维肉瘤

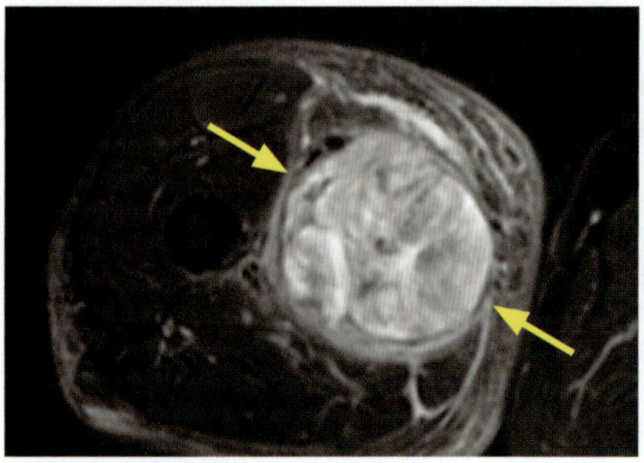

Axial T2-weighted MRI with fat suppression
轴位T_2加权脂肪抑制MRI

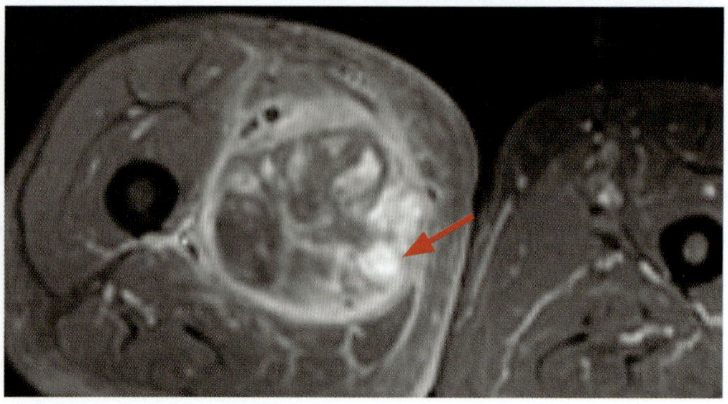

Post-contrast axial T1-weighted MRI with fat suppression
轴位增强T_1加权脂肪抑MRI

Myxofibrosarcoma: There is a large, heterogeneous, predominantly T2 hyperintense mass (yellow arrows) in the medial right proximal thigh, with heterogeneous enhancement including focal nodular enhancement medially (red arrow).
黏液纤维肉瘤：右侧大腿近端内侧可见大而信号不均匀的肿块，以T_2高信号为主(黄箭)，伴不均匀强化，包括位于肿块内侧的局灶结节状强化(红箭)。

- Myxofibrosarcoma is a high-grade tumor with myxoid and fibrous elements. The myxoid components give these lesions a characteristic hyperintense appearance on T2-weighted images.

- 黏液纤维肉瘤是一种含有黏液和纤维成分的高级别肿瘤。黏液成分在T_2加权呈特征性的高信号。

Fibrous neoplastic and non-neoplastic masses

成纤维细胞肿瘤和非肿瘤性肿块

Superficial fibromatosis

浅表纤维瘤病

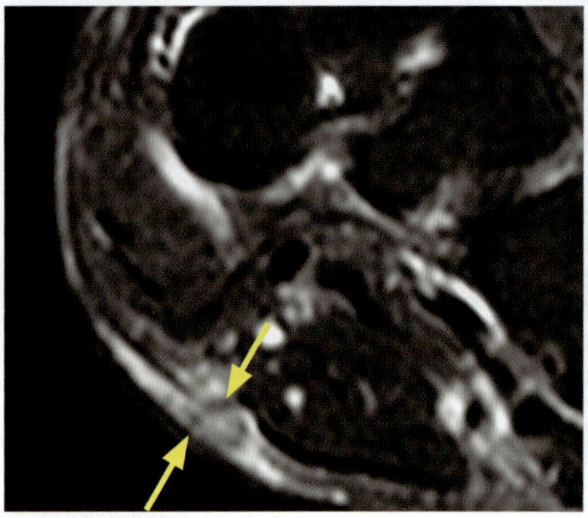

Coronal STIR MRI
冠状位STIR MRI

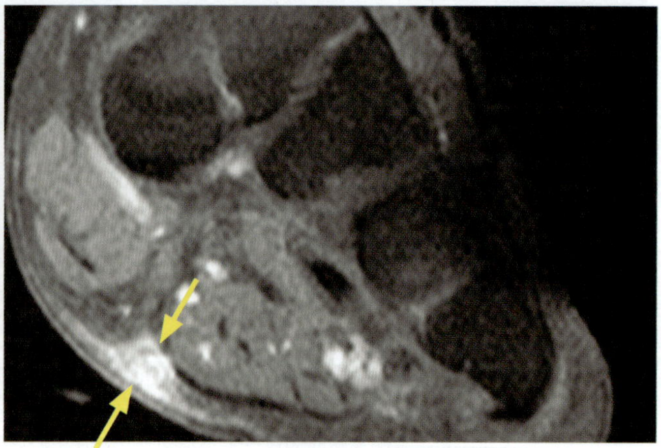

Post-contrast coronal T1-weighted MRI with fat suppression
冠状位增强T_1加权脂肪抑制MRI

Plantar fibromatosis (Ledderhose disease): Coronal MR images through the foot demonstrate an intermediate signal intensity enhancing subcutaneous nodular mass (arrows) along the plantar aponeurosis.
足底纤维瘤病(Ledderhose病)：足部冠状位MRI图像可见沿足底腱膜的中等信号，增强后可见皮下强化结节影(箭)。

- Superficial fibromatoses include both **palmar fibromatosis** (involving the hand/fingers) and **plantar fibromatosis** (involving the foot).
- On MR, fibromatosis appears as nodular foci of various signal intensity. Although fibrous in etiology, the masses are not necessarily low signal, and lesions with increased cellularity may show more prominent enhancement.

- 浅表纤维瘤病包括**掌纤维瘤病**(累及手/手指)和**足底纤维瘤病**(累及足)。
- 纤维瘤病在MR上表现为不同信号强度的结节状病灶。虽然起自纤维组织，但肿块不一定都是低信号，并且随着病灶内细胞密度的增加，肿块的强化也会更加显著。

- **Palmar fibromatosis**, also called Dupuytren disease or Dupuytren contracture, is more common, and presents with painless subcutaneous nodules of the palmar surface of the hand. Treatment of symptomatic palmar fibromatosis is typically surgical.
- **Plantar fibromatosis**, also called Ledderhose disease, is less common than palmar fibromatosis and typically occurs in younger patients. In contrast to palmar fibromatosis, treatment of plantar fibromatosis is typically conservative in most cases, with footwear modification or intralesional steroid injections.

- **掌纤维瘤病**又称Dupuytren病或Dupuytren挛缩症，是一种常见且表现为手掌侧皮下无痛性的结节。症状性掌纤维瘤病的治疗方法是外科切除。
- **足底纤维瘤病**又称Ledderhose病，较掌纤维瘤病少见，通常发病年龄较年轻。与掌纤维瘤病不同的是，大多数足底纤维瘤病通常采用保守治疗，如调整穿鞋或类固醇内注射。

Nodular fasciitis

结节性筋膜炎

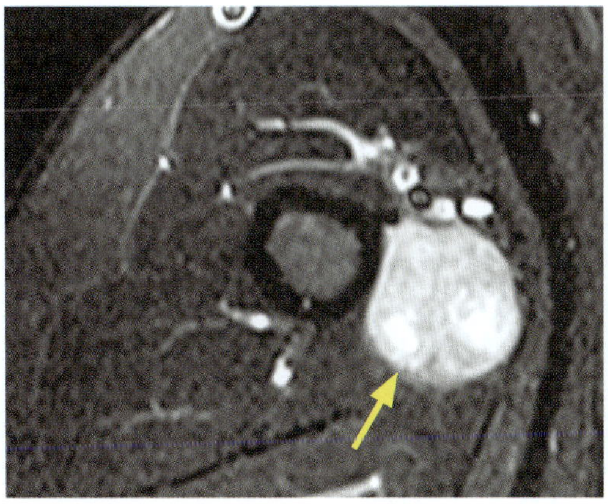

Axial T2-weighted MRI with fat suppression
轴位T_2加权脂肪抑制MRI

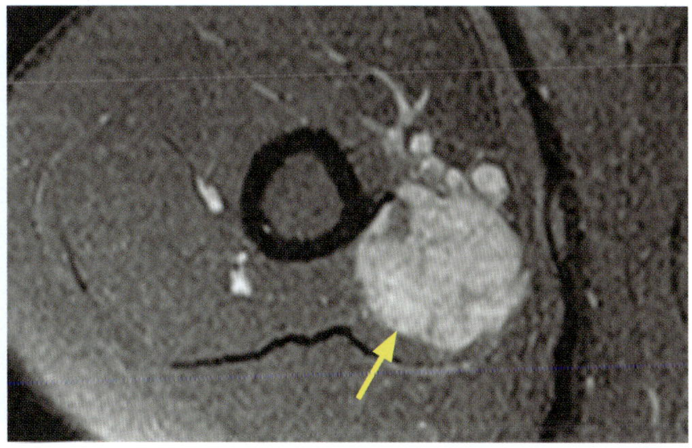

Post-contrast axial T1-weighted MRI with fat suppression
轴位增强T_1加权脂肪抑制MRI

Nodular fasciitis: There is a T2 hyperintense enhancing mass (arrows) in the medial upper arm, located within the medial head of the triceps muscle. This was biopsied, with pathology of nodular fasciitis.
结节性筋膜炎：上臂内侧肱三头肌内侧头内可见T_2高信号的强化肿块(箭)。此病灶经活检证实为结节性筋膜炎。

- Nodular fasciitis is a benign but rapidly growing non-neoplastic lesion that may mimic sarcoma clinically and on imaging. Masses may be subcutaneous or deep in location. Masses are typically T2 hyperintense and some pathologists consider these lesions to be myxoid.
- Although benign, they appear as an enhancing mass and biopsy is usually performed.

- 结节性筋膜炎是一种良性但生长迅速的非肿瘤性病变，其临床和影像学表现与肉瘤相似。肿块可位于皮下或深部组织。肿块通常表现为T_2高信号，一些病理学家认为这些病变属于黏液。
- 虽然属良性，但它们表现为强化肿块，且通常都会进行活检。

Elastofibroma dorsi

背部弹力纤维瘤

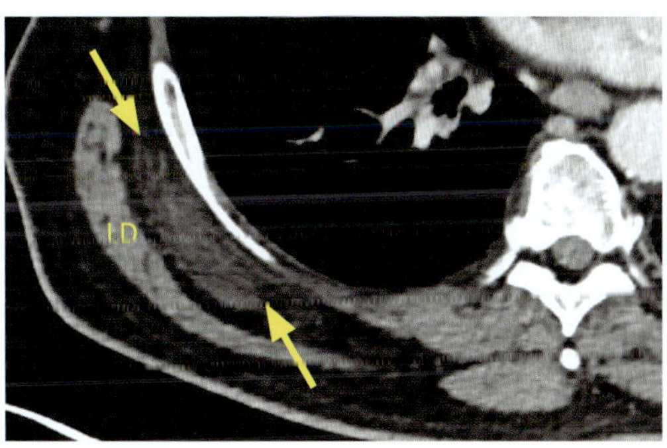

Axial post-contrast CT
轴位增强CT

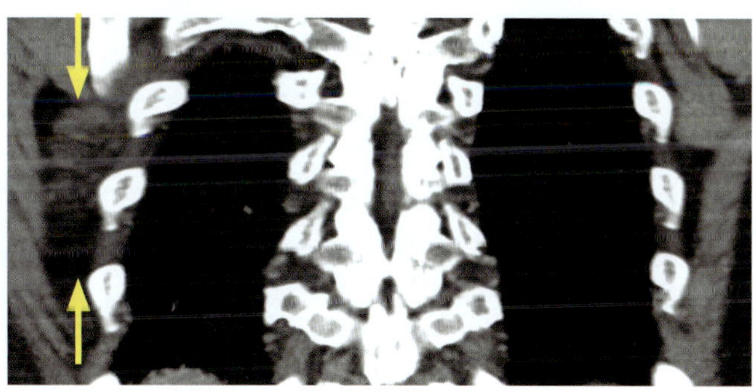

Coronal post-contrast CT
冠状位增强CT

Elastofibroma dorsi: There is a crescentic-shaped mass (yellow arrows) located deep to latissimus dorsi (LD). The mass features alternating striations of fatty tissue. The coronal image best demonstrates infrascapular location and asymmetry when compared to the normal left side.
背部弹力纤维瘤：在背阔肌(LD)深部可见一个新月形肿块(黄箭)。肿块的特征是交替的脂肪组织条纹影。冠状位图像能较好地显示肿块位于右侧肩胛下区，且与正常左侧相比存在不对称。

- Elastofibroma dorsi (EFD) is a rare, benign mass that characteristically arises in the subscapular region, more commonly on the right, typically in middle-aged females.
- EFD is thought to represent a reactive pseudotumor due to mechanical irrigation.
- On imaging, EFD demonstrates alternating bands of fibrous and fatty tissue in a crescentic-shaped mass located deep to latissimus dorsi in the infrascapular region.

- 背部弹力纤维瘤(EFD)是一种罕见的良性肿块,其特征是发生在肩胛下区,更多位于右侧,常发生于中年女性。
- 背部弹力纤维瘤被认为是一种因机械性刺激而产生的反应性假瘤。
- 在影像学上,背部弹力纤维瘤表现为肩胛下区背阔肌深部纤维和脂肪组织条相互交替的新月形肿块。

Desmoid fibromatosis

韧带样纤维瘤病

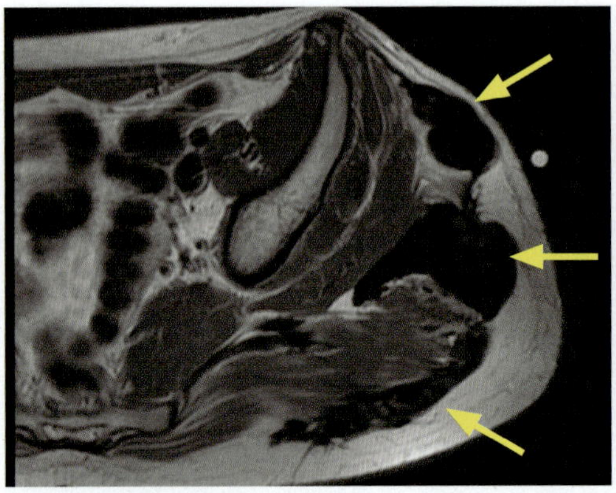

Axial PD-weighted MR
轴位PD加权MR

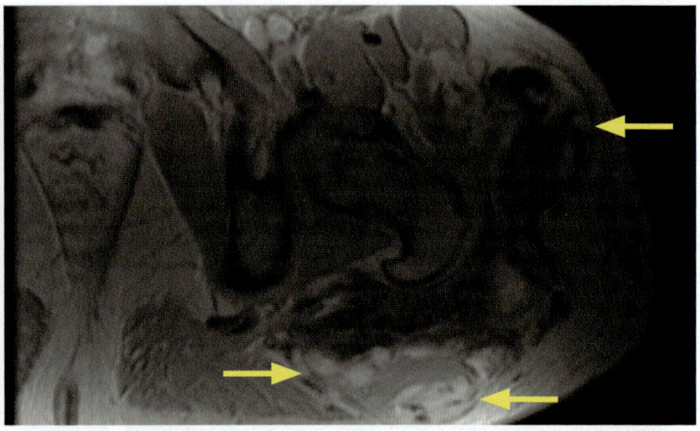

Post-contrast axial T1-weighted MR
轴位增强T_1加权MRI

Desmoid fibromatosis: There are multiple geographic low-signal intensity interfascial lesions about the left hip (arrows), with patchy enhancement.
韧带样纤维瘤病:左侧髋部可见多发地图样低信号的筋膜间病灶(箭),伴斑片状强化。

- Desmoid fibromatosis is a benign but locally aggressive neoplasm, with the abdominal wall the most common location. Masses are low in signal intensity and enhance variably.
- Gardner syndrome is a colonic polyposis syndrome associated with desmoid fibromatosis.

- 韧带样纤维瘤病是一种良性但具有局部侵袭性的肿瘤,最常发生在腹壁。病灶呈低信号,但强化程度不同。
- 加德纳综合征是一种与韧带样纤维瘤病相关的结肠息肉综合征。

Dermatofibrosarcoma protuberans

隆突性皮肤纤维肉瘤

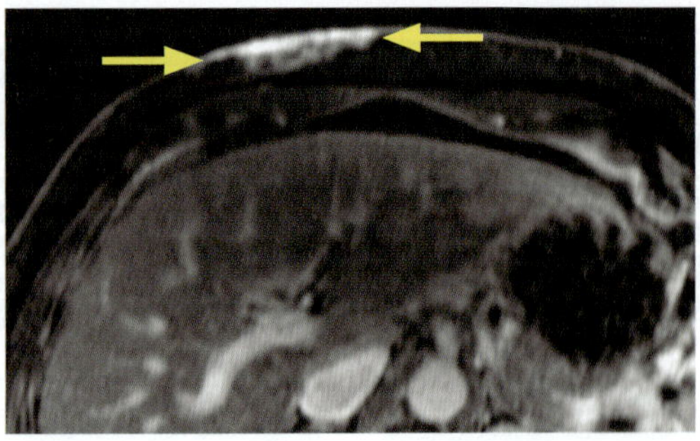

Dermatofibrosarcoma protuberans (DFSP): Post-contrast axial subtraction T1-weighted MRI demonstrates lobulated cutaneous enhancement (yellow arrows) of the right anterior abdominal wall.
隆突性皮肤纤维肉瘤(DFSP):轴位增强T_1加权MRI减影图像示右前腹壁皮肤分叶状强化灶(黄箭)。

- Dermatofibrosarcoma protuberans (DFSP) is a slowly growing, intermediate-grade cutaneous malignancy that presents as a superficial skin nodule or mass.
- On MR, the lesion is hyperintense on T2-weighted images and enhances.

- 隆突性皮肤纤维肉瘤(DFSP)是一种生长缓慢、中等级别的皮肤恶性肿瘤,表现为浅表皮肤的结节或肿块。
- 病灶在MR上呈T_2加权高信号,并可强化。

Nerve sheath tumors

神经鞘肿瘤

Schwannoma and neurofibroma

神经鞘瘤和神经纤维瘤

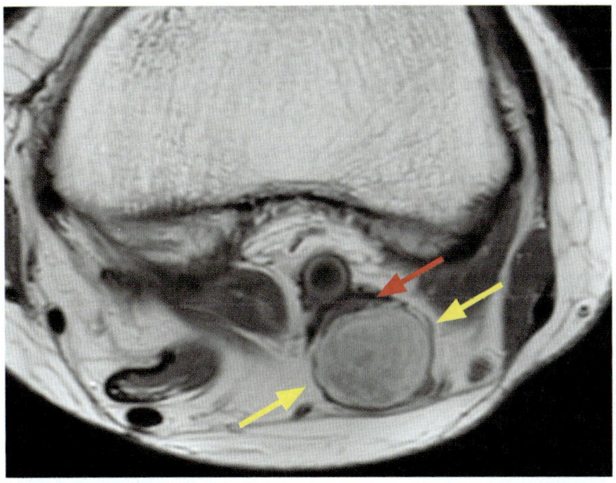

Axial PD-weighted MRI
轴位PD加权MRI

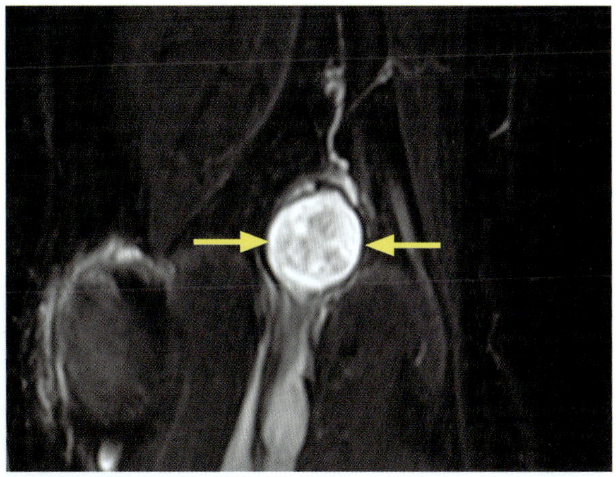

Coronal STIR MRI
冠状位STIR MRI

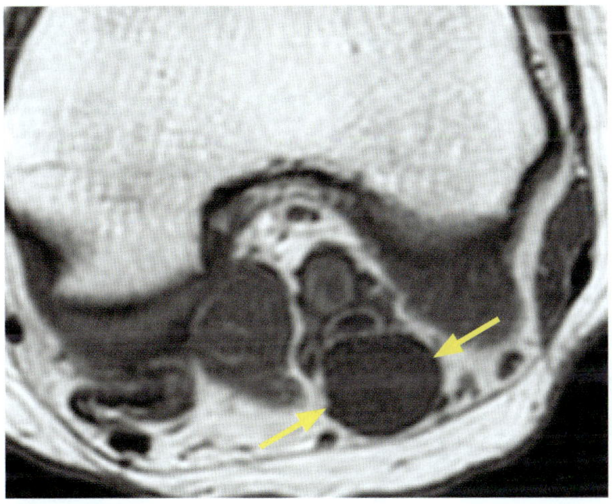

Axial T1-weighted MRI
轴位T_1加权MRI

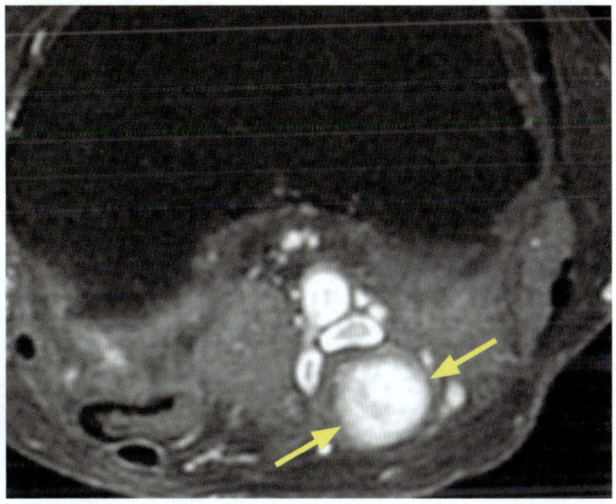

Axial post-contrast T1-weighted MRI with fat suppression
轴位增强T_1加权脂肪抑制MRI

Schwannoma: There is a circumscribed T2 hyperintense round mass (yellow arrows) in the popliteal fossa, which enhances homogeneously. Note the eccentric position of the tibial nerve (red arrow), which is splayed around the mass, likely contributing the culprit nerve fibers from which the mass arises.

神经鞘瘤：腘窝内可见一个边界清晰的T_2高信号圆形肿块(黄箭)，肿块均匀强化。注意胫神经的偏心位置(红箭)，且骑跨在肿瘤之上，很可能是该肿瘤的起源。

- Schwannomas and neurofibromas are both peripheral nerve sheath tumors (PNST) and together comprise 10% of benign soft tissue tumors. These two entities are usually difficult to differentiate from each other on imaging, and in forming a differential diagnosis it is usually reasonable to state "peripheral nerve sheath tumor."

  Occasionally, it is possible to distinguish between a schwannoma and neurofibroma on MR imaging based on the relation of the lesion to the nerve: A schwannoma may be eccentric to (and separatable from) the nerve, while a neurofibroma is fusiform mass-like expansion of the nerve, which courses through the center of the lesion.
- PNSTs typically appear as fusiform, circumscribed masses, characteristically hyperintense on T2-weighted images and avidly enhancing.
- The *split fat pad sign* may be seen with a peripheral triangle of preserved fat at

- 神经鞘瘤和神经纤维瘤均为周围神经鞘肿瘤(PNST)，约占良性软组织肿瘤的10%。这两种肿瘤在影像上通常难以进行鉴别，因此将它们统一放在“周围神经鞘肿瘤”作为一个鉴别诊断是比较合理的。

  有时根据病变与周围神经的关系可以区分神经鞘瘤和神经纤维瘤。神经鞘瘤的位置有可能偏在神经的一侧(并可与神经分离)，而神经纤维瘤则是相应神经呈梭形团块状增粗，并穿过病灶的中央。
- 典型的PNST表现为梭形、边界清晰的肿块，T_2加权呈高信号，并可见明显强化。
- 脂肪劈裂征可见于肿块近端和远端残存的三

the proximal and distal margins of the mass. The *target sign* can be seen in both PNSTs (although more common in neurofibromas), which is a central region of low signal intensity on T2-weighted images.

Note that these signs are not specific for benign PNSTs, and can also be seen in malignant peripheral nerve sheath tumors (MPNST). Please see the next page for an example of these signs in an MPNST.

- PNSTs may appear along the course of major nerves; however, they can appear virtually anywhere if they arise from a small unnamed nerve.

角形脂肪组织。靶征在两种PNST都可以出现(虽然在神经纤维瘤中更常见)，表现为病灶中心T_2加权低信号区。

注意，这些征象不是良性PNST所特有，也可以见于恶性周围神经鞘肿瘤(MPNST)。有关恶性周围神经鞘肿瘤的征象，请参阅下文。

- PNSTs通常沿大的神经走行出现，然而，若它们起源于一条小的无名神经，则几乎可以出现在任何部位。

Malignant peripheral nerve sheath tumor

恶性周围神经鞘肿瘤

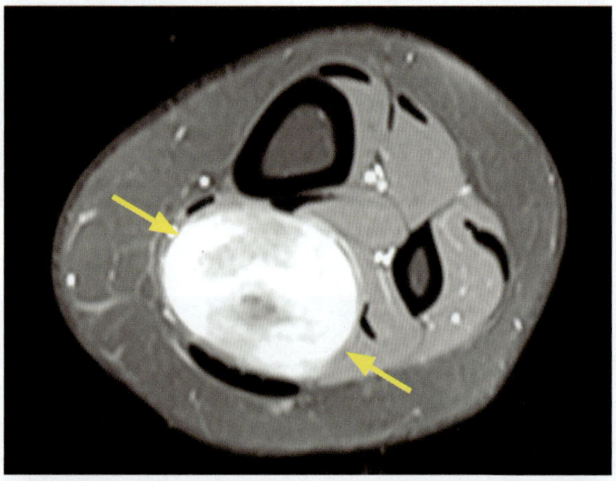

Post-contrast axial T1-weighted MRI with fat suppression
轴位增强T_1加权脂肪抑制MRI

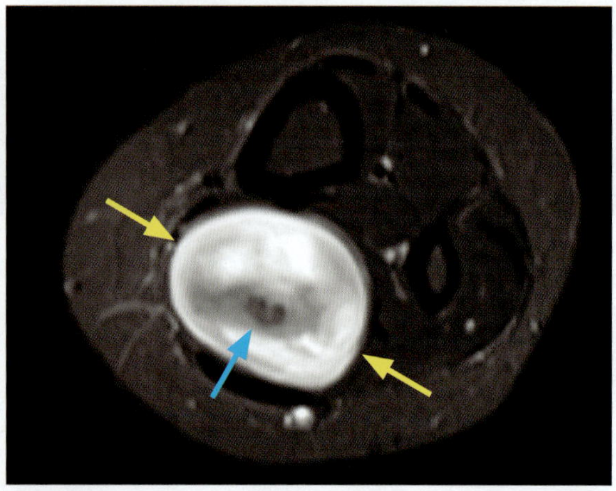

Axial STIR MRI
轴位STIR MRI

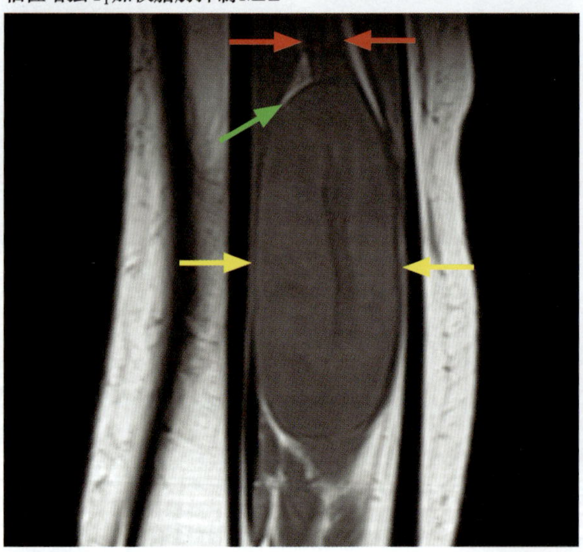

Coronal T1-weighted MRI
冠状位T_1加权MRI

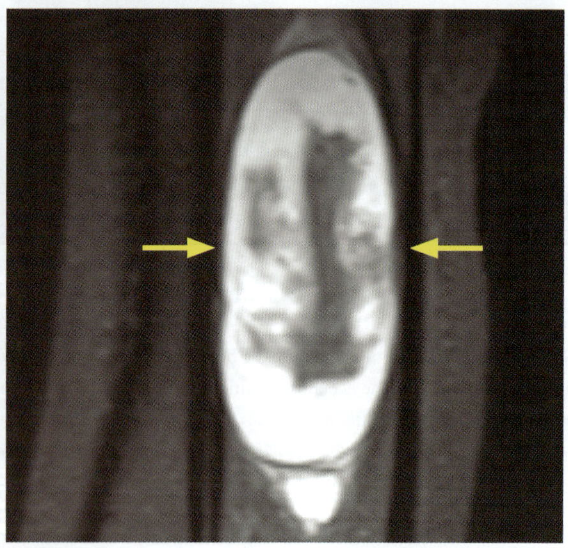

Sagittal STIR
矢状位STIR MRI

Malignant peripheral nerve sheath tumor (MPNST), arising from a neurofibroma in a patient with neurofibromatosis type 1:
There is a large, enhancing, T2-hyperintense mass in the posterior calf (yellow arrows). The mass arises from the tibial nerve, which courses through the center of the mass (red arrows).
A central region of low signal intensity on the axial STIR image represents the target sign (blue arrow).
A triangle of preserved fat seen on the coronal T1-weighted image represents the split fat sign (green arrow).
In this case, the relatively large size of the mass and the patient's history of neurofibromatosis type I should raise concern for MPNST.
恶性周围神经鞘肿瘤(MPNST)，一名起源于神经纤维瘤的1型神经纤维瘤病患者：
小腿后部可见巨大而强化的T_2高信号肿块(黄箭)。该肿块起源于胫神经，后者穿过病灶中心(红箭)。
病灶的中心在轴位STIR MRI上的低信号区呈靶征(蓝箭)。
在冠状位T_1加权MRI图像上的残存三角形脂肪组织呈脂肪劈裂征(绿箭)。
在该病例中，结合较大的肿块体积及患者1型神经纤维瘤病的病史，需要考虑恶性周围神经鞘肿瘤的可能。

- Malignant peripheral nerve sheath tumor (MPNST) is highly associated with neurofibromatosis type Ⅰ (in 50% of cases).
- MPNSTs cannot be reliably differentiated from benign PNSTs on imaging. The previously discussed imaging signs suggesting a neurogenic tumor, including the target sign and the split fat sign, may be present. However, imaging features favoring malignancy include larger size, ill-defined margins, central necrosis, and rapid growth.
- Any new or enlarging mass in a patient with neurofibromatosis type 1 should raise concern for development of MPNST. PET-CT is an excellent modality to determine need for biopsy.

- 恶性周围神经鞘肿瘤(MPNST)与Ⅰ型神经纤维瘤病高度相关(约占50%的病例)。
- MPNST无法在影像学上准确与良性PNST进行鉴别。前面讨论过的神经源性肿瘤的影像学提示包括靶征和脂肪分离征都可能出现。而提示恶性肿瘤的影像学表现包括较大体积、边界欠清、中心坏死和生长迅速。
- 在1型神经纤维瘤病患者中，任何新发的或增大的肿块都应警惕恶性MPNST的可能。PET/CT是一种帮助决定是否需要活检的好方法。

ADDITIONAL TUMORS

其他肿瘤

Myxoma

黏液瘤

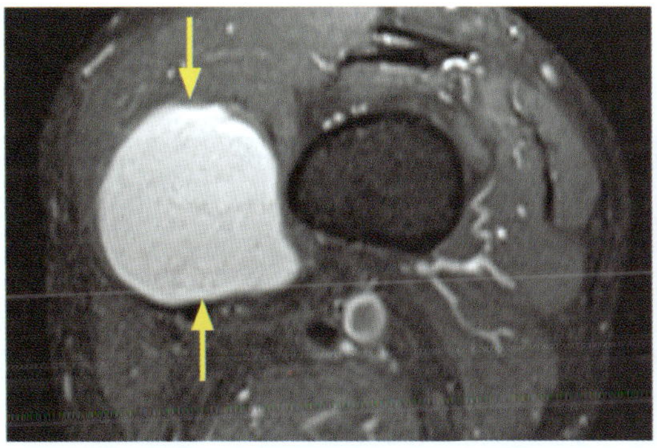

Axial STIR MRI
轴位STIR MRI

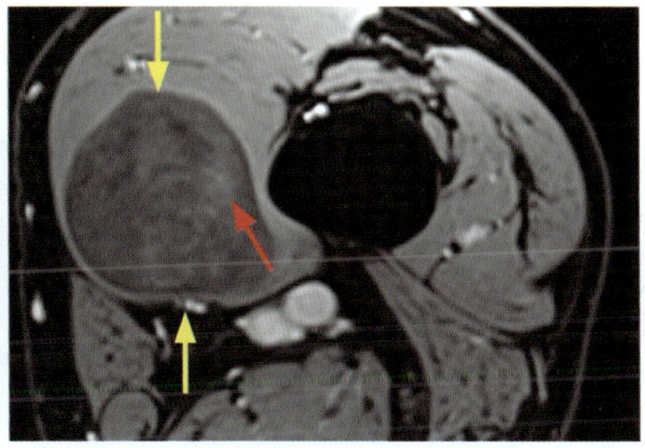

Post-contrast axial T1-weighted MRI with fat suppression
轴位增强T_1加权脂肪抑制MRI

Myxoma: There is a homogeneously hyperintense, near fluid signal intensity intra-muscular mass (yellow arrows) located vastus medialis. The mass demonstrates faint wispy enhancement (red arrow).
黏液瘤：在股内侧肌内可见均匀接近液体信号的肿块(黄箭)。肿块内可见轻微的细束状强化(红箭)。

- A myxoma is a benign soft tissue tumor. The myxoid extracellular matrix creates a near fluid-signal intensity appearance, with minimal enhancement. They tend to occur in muscles.
- **Mazabraud syndrome** is fibrous dysplasia with intramuscular myxomas.

- 黏液瘤是一种良性软组织肿瘤。黏液样的细胞外基质形成了接近液体的信号，伴轻微强化。黏液瘤常发生在肌肉内。
- **Mazabraud综合征**是一种纤维异常增殖疾病伴肌内黏液瘤。

Synovial sarcoma

滑膜肉瘤

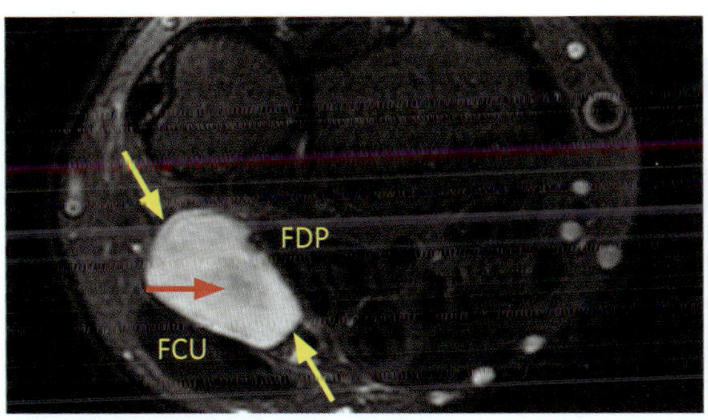

Axial T2-weighted MRI with fat suppression
轴位T_2加权脂肪抑制MRI

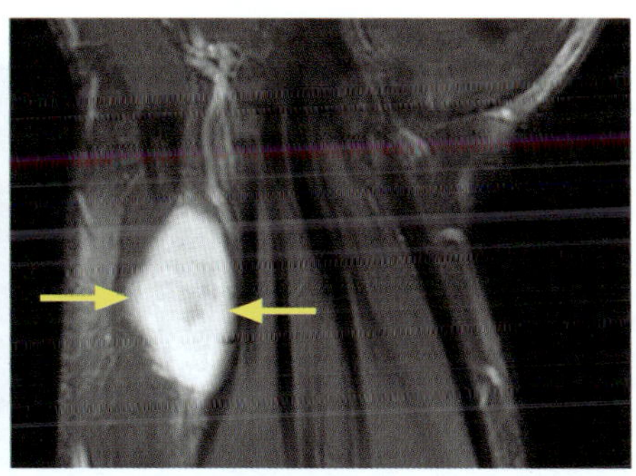

Post-contrast T1-weighted MRI with fat suppression
增强T_1加权脂肪抑制MRI

Synovial sarcoma: There is a T2 hyperintense, enhancing mass (yellow arrows) at the volar/ulnar aspect of the wrist, interposed between the flexor carpi ulnaris (FCU) and flexor digitorum profundus (FDP). Note that although the mass is near fluid signal intensity on the fluid sensitive sequence, there is still some internal complexity with whorl-like regions of low signal (red arrow).
The differential of a small, T2 hyperintense, enhancing, circumscribed mass would also include nerve sheath tumor.
滑膜肉瘤：腕掌/尺侧的尺侧腕屈肌和指深屈肌之间可见一处T_2加权高信号并伴强化的肿块(黄箭)。注意，虽然肿块在液体敏感序列上接近液体信号，但肿块内部仍有一些螺纹状的低信号区(红箭)。
具有体积小、T_2高信号、强化及边界清晰特征肿块的鉴别诊断应包括神经鞘膜肿瘤。

- Synovial sarcoma is a high-grade mesenchymal tumor typically occurring in adolescents and young adults.
- The term *synovial* in its name is highly misleading, as this tumor has nothing to do with synovial tissue or joints. However, it does have a propensity to occur in the vicinity of joints, and the term likely arrived from pathologic confusion in the early twentieth century.
- Synovial sarcoma is relatively homogeneously hyperintense on T2-weighted images, usually isointense to fluid. The classic teaching is that a fluid signal intensity mass in a younger patient that does not communicate with a joint could be synovial sarcoma and contrast should be administered. In practice, however, these lesions are usually somewhat more complex than simple fluid and windowing of the images can make the internal complexity more conspicuous.

- 滑膜肉瘤是一种高级别间质肿瘤，常见于青少年和青年成人。
- 名称中的“滑膜”一词具有高度误导性，因为这种肿瘤与滑膜组织或关节没有任何关系。但是，它确实有发生在关节附近的倾向，而该术语可能由于在20世纪早期对其病理的认知混乱而出现的。
- 滑膜肉瘤在T_2加权图像上表现为相对均匀的高信号，通常接近于液体信号。经典的教学要点是，年轻患者出现液体信号的肿块，且与关节不相通则可能是滑膜肉瘤，需进行增强扫描。然而，在实际临床中这些病变信号通常比单纯的液体要复杂，调整图像的窗宽及窗位能使肿块内部的复杂信号显示得更加清楚。

Morton neuroma

莫顿神经瘤

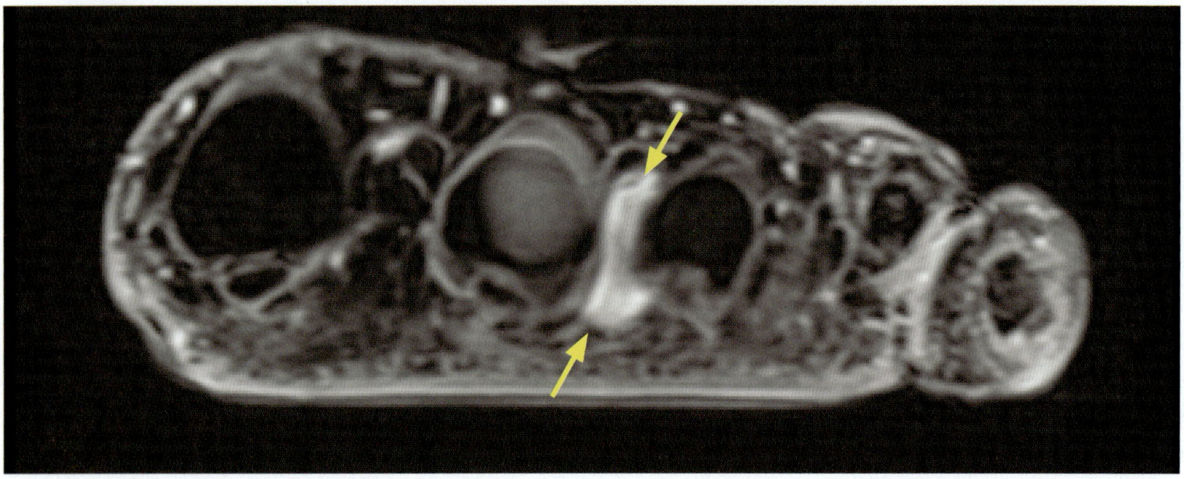

Morton neuroma: Coronal post-contrast T1-weighted MRI with fat suppression demonstrates a dumbbell-shaped enhancing mass (arrows) in the second interspace, which is slightly eccentrically plantar in location.
莫顿神经瘤：冠状位增强T_1加权脂肪抑制MRI显示在第二/三跖骨间隙内哑铃状强化肿块(箭)，肿块位置稍微偏向足底侧。

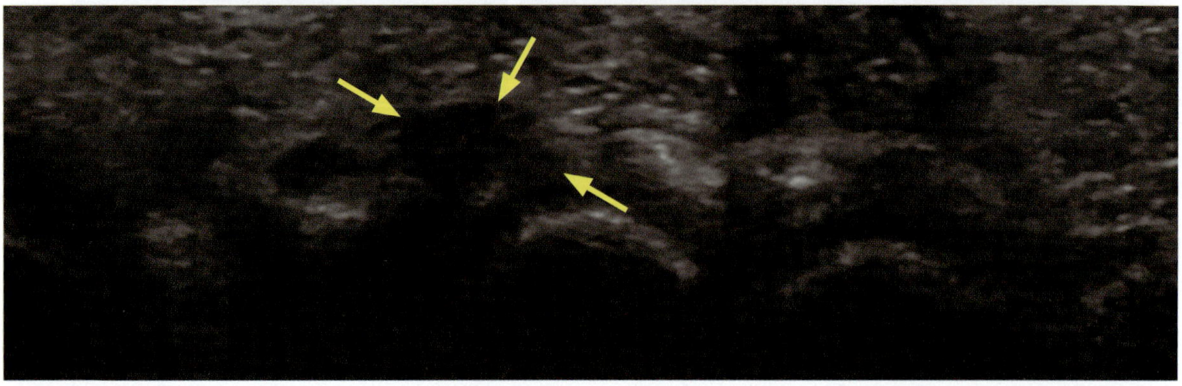

Transverse ultrasound image through the plantar aspect of the metatarsal heads (the top of the image is plantar) demonstrates a hypoechoic mass (arrows) at the plantar aspect of the second interspace.
足底跖骨头水平横切面超声图像(图像的顶部是足底)显示第二/三跖骨间隙偏足底侧低回声肿块(箭)。

- Morton neuromas are non-neoplastic benign masses that occur due to degeneration and fibrosis around a plantar digital nerve of the foot, most commonly occurring at the level of the metatarsal heads in the second or third interspaces. Of note, a Morton "neuroma" is not a true neuroma, as a neuroma is due to proliferation of nerve tissue (either neoplastic or in response to amputation), rather than perineural fibrous tissue.
- Clinically, Morton neuroma produces burning pain, more commonly in females, and in the proper clinical context biopsy is usually not needed.
- MRI or ultrasound are both excellent imaging modalities for assessment of Morton neuroma. On MR, Morton neuroma appears as a dumbbell- or teardrop-shaped low signal (on T2-weighted images) mass with variable enhancement. Intravenous gadolinium is very helpful to increase conspicuity of the mass. While the mass may extend dorsally in some cases, they are typically predominantly inter-metatarsal and plantar in location.
- On ultrasound, Morton neuroma is a hypoechoic mass in the intermetatarsal space, best seen with a high resolution probe from a plantar approach with the patient prone.
- Intermetatarsal bursitis is frequently associated with Morton neuroma, and on ultrasound the apparent mass may reflect a combination of Morton neuroma and associated bursitis.
- Treatment is usually conservative, with modification of footwear and steroid injection.

- 莫顿神经瘤是非肿瘤性良性肿块，为足底趾神经周围组织的变性和纤维化所致，最常见于跖骨头水平的第二或第三跖骨间隙。注意，莫顿神经瘤不是真正的神经源性肿瘤，因为神经源性肿瘤是由于神经组织的增殖(或是肿瘤，或是对截肢的反应)，而不是神经周围的纤维组织增生。
- 临床上，莫顿神经瘤会产生灼痛，更常见于女性，若有恰当的临床病史通常不需要活检。
- MRI或超声都是评价莫顿神经瘤非常好的影像学方法。在MR上，莫顿神经瘤表现为哑铃状或泪滴状低信号肿块(T_2加权图像)，但强化程度可有不同。静脉注射钆造影剂对清晰显示肿块非常有帮助。虽然莫顿神经瘤在某些情况下可能向足背侧生长，但位于足底侧跖骨间占大多数。
- 在超声上，莫顿神经瘤表现为跖骨间隙的低回声肿块。在患者采取俯卧位时用高分辨率探头从足底进行检查，能最好地显示肿块。
- 跖骨间滑囊炎常与莫顿神经瘤有关，超声检查时看到的肿块可能是两者的综合表现。
- 通常为保守治疗，如调整穿鞋及类固醇内注射。

SOFT TISSUE TUMOR DIFFERENTIAL DIAGNOSIS

Large, aggressive soft tissue tumor

Undifferentiated pleomorphic sarcoma (very reasonable choice for top differential).
Pleomorphic liposarcoma (lipomatous elements may not be apparent).
Dedifferentiated liposarcoma (lipomatous elements may not be apparent).
Rhabdomyosarcoma.
Leiomyosarcoma.

T2 hyperintense tumor, circumscribed

Benign neurogenic tumor (if small, circumscribed, homogeneous, may or may not arise from a known nerve).
Malignant peripheral neurogenic tumor (especially if known NF1).
Synovial sarcoma.
Myxoma (but tend to be hypoenhancing compared to other lesions listed).

T2 hyperintense tumor, large and aggressive

Synovial sarcoma, advanced.
Malignant peripheral neurogenic tumor, advanced (especially if known NF1).
Myxoid liposarcoma (note that lipomatous elements may not be apparent).
Myxofibrosarcoma.

软组织肿瘤的鉴别诊断

大并具侵袭性的软组织肿块

未分化多形性肉瘤(最可能的优先鉴别诊断)。
多形性脂肪肉瘤(脂肪成分可能不明显)。
去分化脂肪肉瘤(脂肪成分可能不明显)。
横纹肌肉瘤。
平滑肌肉瘤。

边界清晰的T_2高信号肿块

良性神经源性肿瘤(肿块小而边界清晰，其信号较均匀；可以起源于已知或未知的神经)。
恶性周围神经源性肿瘤(特别是已知有NF1)。
滑膜肉瘤。
黏液瘤(但较其他所列病变强化程度相对较低)。

大并具侵袭性的T_2高信号肿块

滑膜肉瘤，晚期。
晚期恶性周围神经源性肿瘤，晚期(尤其是已知有NF1)。
黏液样脂肪肉瘤(注意脂肪成分可能不明显)。
黏液纤维肉瘤。

Soft tissue tumors with helpful imaging features

Fibrolipomatous hamartoma (*cord-like* appearance considered pathognomonic).
Neurogenic tumor (*split fat sign, target sign*, arising from a known nerve).
Lipoma (nearly entirely fat signal intensity).
Atypical lipomatous tumor (predominantly lipomatous elements, with some degree of complexity).
Morton neuroma (dumbbell-shaped mass at the head of the metatarsals, usually enhancing, typically eccentric at the plantar aspect).
Elastofibroma dorsi (striations of alternating fat and soft tissue, located subscapular deep to latissimus dorsi).

影像学征象有助于诊断的软组织肿瘤

纤维脂肪性错构瘤(特征性的束状改变)。
神经源性肿瘤(脂肪垫劈裂征、靶征、起源于已知神经)。
脂肪瘤(几乎完全是脂肪信号)。
非典型脂肪瘤性肿瘤(主要为脂肪成分,信号具有一定程度的复杂性)。
莫顿神经瘤(跖骨头水平哑铃状肿块,通常强化,常偏向足底侧)。
背部弹力纤维瘤(脂肪和软组织交替条纹,位于肩胛下背阔肌深层)。

(翻译　吕霞飞　姚骊　帅丹丹)

MUSCULOSKELETAL INFECTION

骨骼与肌肉感染

SEPTIC ARTHRITIS

Overview of septic arthritis

- Septic arthritis, which is bacterial infection of a joint, is a medical emergency. Rapid diagnosis and treatment are essential to preserve the joint, as permanent cartilage damage can occur within three days.
- Septic arthritis is not typically an imaging diagnosis, and radiographs are commonly normal. However, radiographs should be performed to evaluate for changes of advanced infection (such as effusion, soft tissue swelling, or bony erosive changes) and also to exclude an alternative explanation for the patient's pain (such as fracture, calcific tendinitis, severe degenerative changes, etc.).
- In a patient with an acute mono-articular (involving only one joint) arthritis, septic arthritis should be a primary diagnostic consideration, even in the absence of fever or other systemic signs of infection.
- Diagnosis is confirmed with joint aspiration (arthrocentesis). Although it can take days for complete microbiology results to become available, the aspirated fluid white blood cell (WBC) count and percentage of polymorphonuclear neutrophils (PMN) can be used to predict the probability of septic arthritis:

Parameter	Sensitivity	Specificity
WBC>100,000/μL	29%	99%
WBC>50,000/μL	62%	92%
WBC>25,000/μL	77%	73%
PMN≥90%	73%	79%

Based on the table above, for instance, a fluid WBC count of >50,000 is 92% specific for septic arthritis; however, this is only seen in 62% of cases of septic arthritis.

Empiric treatment for septic arthritis is reasonable for a WBC count of >50,000.

A common alternative etiology for elevated WBC count includes crystal arthropathy.

化脓性关节炎

化脓性关节炎概述

- 化脓性关节炎是细菌感染了关节,属于一种医疗急症。迅速确诊和治疗对保护关节至关重要,因为永久性软骨损伤在3天内即可发生。
- 化脓性关节炎通常不是影像学上的诊断,因为X线检查一般正常。但是,X线检查又是必要的,它可以评估感染的进展性变化(如积液、软组织肿胀或骨侵蚀性改变),并排除引起患者疼痛的其他疾病(如骨折、钙化性肌腱炎、严重的退行性改变等)。
- 若患者表现为急性单关节(只累及一个关节),即使没有发热或其他系统性感染的症状,化脓性关节炎也应该是首要考虑的诊断。
- 确诊可以通过关节穿刺。尽管完整的微生物学检查需要数天才能得到结果,但吸出的关节液体中白细胞(WBC)计数和多形核中性粒细胞(PMN)百分比可以用来预测化脓性关节炎的可能性:

变量	灵敏度	特异度
WBC>100 000/μL	29%	99%
WBC>50 000/μL	62%	92%
WBC>25 000/μL	77%	73%
PMN≥90%	73%	79%

根据上表,例如,白细胞计数>50 000/μL诊断化脓性关节炎的特异度为92%;然而,这种情况只出现在62%的化脓性关节炎病例中。

对白细胞计数>50 000/μL进行化脓性关节炎的经验性治疗是合理的。

白细胞计数升高的其他常见病因包括结晶性关节病。

Osteomyelitis

Overview of osteomyelitis

- Literally meaning "inflammation (–itis) of the bone (osteo–) marrow (–myelo–)," osteomyelitis is inflammation of the bone caused by an infectious organism. Osteomyelitis has protean clinical and imaging manifestations, with an end pathway of chronic progressive bony destruction if untreated.
- Osteomyelitis can be classified by route of spread (hematogenous, contiguous spread, or direct inoculation) or by chronicity (acute or chronic), although any route of spread can lead to either acute or chronic disease.

  The differentiation of acute, subacute, and chronic osteomyelitis is variably described in the literature. In general, acute osteomyelitis is less than two weeks duration. Subacute osteomyelitis is the phase of disease lasting less than three months but without acute symptoms.

  The pathologic hallmark of chronic osteomyelitis is bone necrosis.
- The anatomic distribution and clinical presentation of osteomyelitis is highly dependent on the age of the patient, the specific organism, and the presence of any underlying disorders, such as vascular insufficiency or compromised immunity.

  In adults, osteomyelitis typically arises from either contiguous spread or direct inoculation, such as in diabetic foot infections, open fractures, or as a complication of surgery. Infection is usually polymicrobial.

  In children, hematogenous spread of infection is more common, usually from *Staphylococcus aureus*.

Terminology of osteomyelitis

骨髓炎

骨髓炎概述

- 骨髓炎，顾名思义，是指骨髓的炎症，但实际上是指感染微生物引起的骨骼炎症。骨髓炎具有多种临床和影像学表现，如果没有得到治疗，最终会导致慢性进行性骨质破坏。
- 骨髓炎可以按播散途径(血行感染、相邻病灶蔓延或直接种植)或按病变的进程进行分类(急性或慢性)，但任何播散途径均可导致急性或慢性骨髓炎。

  文献对于急性、亚急性和慢性骨髓炎的划分有不同的方法。一般来说，急性骨髓炎的病程少于2周。亚急性骨髓炎的病程不到3个月但没有急性症状。

  慢性骨髓炎的病理性标志是骨坏死。
- 骨髓炎的发生部位和临床表现与患者的年龄、特定的微生物及是否存在任何潜在的疾病密切相关，如血管功能不全或免疫力低下。

  在成人，骨髓炎多起源于相邻部位的感染播散或直接种植，如糖尿病足的感染、开放性骨折，或外科手术并发症。感染往往由多种微生物所致。

  在儿童，血行感染更常见，常为金黄色葡萄球菌。

骨髓炎的相关术语

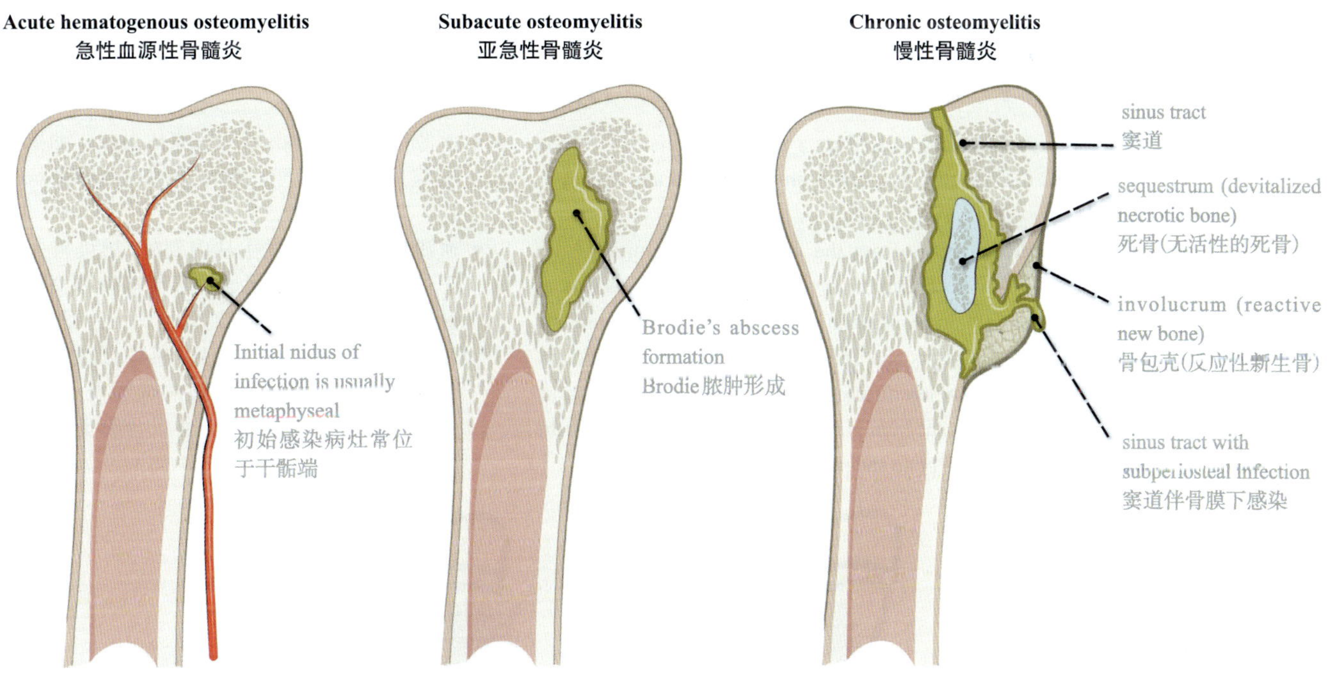

Illustration demonstrating the chronicity of osteomyelitis and development of characteristic lesions.
示意图展示了骨髓炎的慢性变和特征性病灶的进展。

- *Osteitis* is inflammation/infection of the cortex.
- *Periostitis* is inflammation/infection of the periosteum.
- A *sequestrum* is a piece of necrotic bone that is separated (sequestered) from viable bone by granulation tissue. A sequestrum is a surgical lesion that can chronically harbor living organisms and function as a nidus for recurrent infection if not resected.
- An *involucrum* is living bone surrounding necrotic bone.
- A *cloaca* is an opening on the involucrum.
- A *sinus tract* is an opening from the infection to the skin surface.
- A *Brodie* abscess is a form of subacute osteomyelitis characterized by central lucency and peripheral sclerosis. The radiographic differential diagnosis of a Brodie abscess is an osteoid osteoma.

- 骨炎是骨皮质的炎症或感染。
- 骨膜炎是骨膜的炎症或感染。
- 死骨是一片坏死的骨组织，由肉芽组织将它与有活性的骨组织分隔开(隔离)。死骨是一种外科病变，如果不进行外科切除，死骨可为微生物提供长期寄生的地方，从而造成反复感染。
- 骨包壳指有活性的骨组织包围坏死骨。
- 瘘是骨包壳上的开口。
- 窦道是感染病灶到皮肤表面的通道。
- Brodie脓肿是一种亚急性骨髓炎，其特征为中央透亮区伴有外周硬化。Brodie脓肿在影像学上需要与骨样骨瘤进行鉴别。

Hematogenous osteomyelitis

- Acute hematogenous osteomyelitis is usually seen in infants and children. The highly vascularized metaphyses of long bones are most commonly affected. Metaphyseal venules have sluggish flow which facilitate bacterial invasion.
- In infants up to 12 months old, infections can involve the metaphysis, epiphysis, and joint due to the presence of bridging vessels which cross the physis. In older children, infection tends to be isolated to the metaphysis. In adults, the physes are closed but hematogenous metaphyseal infection is uncommon.

血源性骨髓炎

- 急性血源性骨髓炎常见于婴幼儿。富血供的长骨干骺端最容易受累。干骺端的小静脉血流缓慢，有利于细菌入侵。
- 从出生到12月龄的婴儿，感染可累及干骺端、骨骺和关节，这是由于存在跨骺板桥接血管的缘故。在年长的儿童，感染往往局限在干骺端。在成人，由于骨骺闭合，故血源性干骺端感染不常见。

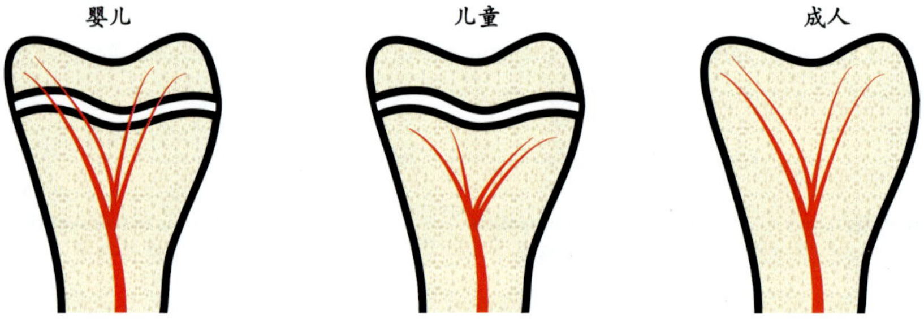

- Hematogenous infection is typically caused by a single organism. If blood cultures are positive then that specific organism can be targeted and biopsy is generally not needed.
- Hematogenous osteomyelitis occurs from the inside out, beginning with infection of the medullary cavity. Secondary involvement of the cortex occurs as bacteria spread through Haversian and Volkmann canals into the periosteum and subsequently the soft tissues. In infants and children, the periosteum is loosely adherent to the bone, causing prominent lifting of the periosteum by infection. This manifests radiographically as exuberant periostitis. In contrast, in adults the periosteum is more tightly adherent to bone and periostitis is less prominent.

- 血源性感染通常由单一病原体引起。如果血培养为阳性，即可针对特定的病原体进行治疗，一般不需活检。
- 血源性骨髓炎的发生从内到外，感染首先始于骨髓腔。随之细菌通过哈弗斯管和福尔克曼管播散到骨皮质，再到软组织。在婴幼儿，骨膜与骨的附着较为松弛，感染可以明显顶骨膜。影像上表现为明显的骨膜炎。相反，成人骨膜紧密附着于骨，所以骨膜炎并不十分明显。

hematogenous osteomyelitis
血源性骨髓炎

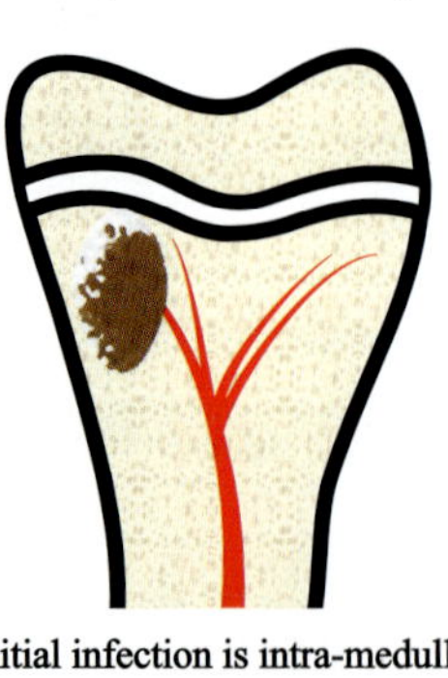

initial infection is intra-medullary
初始的髓内感染

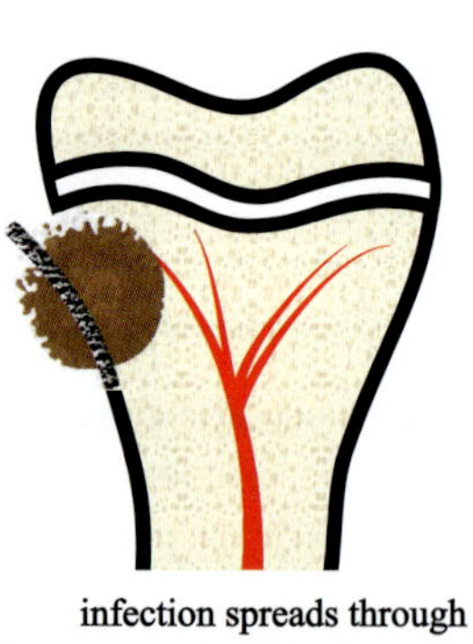

infection spreads through the cortex and uplifts the periosteum
感染播散穿入皮质并掀起骨膜

- In adults, hematogenous osteomyelitis most commonly affects the spine.
- Chronic osteomyelitis may produce infected nonviable tissue (sequestrum). An involucrum is living bone which surrounds the sequestrum. The involucrum may be perforated by cloacae, which can open to the skin to form a sinus tract. *Chronic drainage of sinus tract predisposes to squamous cell carcinoma.*
- Initial subtle radiographic changes in hematogenous osteomyelitis include focal soft-tissue swelling, regional osteopenia, and obliteration of the soft-tissue fat planes.
- The radiographic appearance of medullary infection is a focal, ill-defined lucent metaphyseal lesion. The lucency may cross the epiphysis in young children, where epiphyseal bridging vessels may be still patent. Periosteal reaction may appear aggressive and lamellated, mimicking Ewing sarcoma.

Contiguous focus osteomyelitis

- Osteomyelitis in adults is most commonly from contiguous spread of infection, characterized by penetration of the periosteum and cortex and subsequent medullary invasion.

- 在成人，血源性骨髓炎最常累及脊柱。
- 慢性骨髓炎可产生无活性的感染组织(死骨)。骨包壳是包围死骨的活骨组织。骨包壳可被骨瘘穿破，并可开口于皮肤而形成窦道。*慢性窦道流脓易发生鳞状细胞癌。*
- 血源性骨髓炎在X线影像学上的早期细微变化包括局部软组织肿胀、局部骨量减少和软组织-脂肪层界面消失。
- 骨髓感染的X线检查表现为局灶、边界不清的干骺端透亮区。在幼儿，透亮区可跨越骨骺，此为骨骺的桥接血管尚未闭合所致。骨膜反应可表现为侵袭性和层样，类似于尤因肉瘤。

局部蔓延性骨髓炎

- 成人的骨髓炎通常由感染从局部蔓延而来，其特点是穿透骨膜和皮质，然后侵袭骨髓。

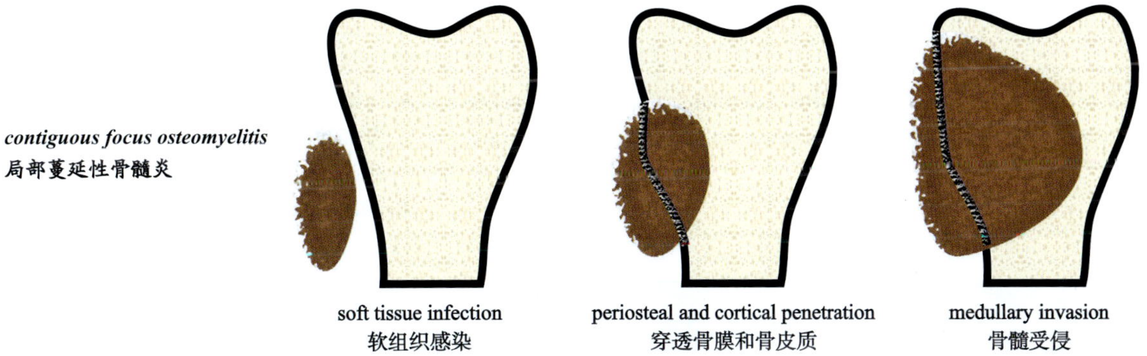

- One of the most common causes of adult osteomyelitis is contiguous spread of a diabetic foot ulcer to the bones. Diabetic neuropathy leads to development of foot ulcers due to unrecognized trauma and impaired vascular reserve.
- The primary differential diagnosis of diabetic foot osteomyelitis is a neuropathic joint, a common sequela of diabetic neuropathy.

- 成人骨髓炎最常见的一个原因是糖尿病足溃疡蔓延至骨骼。糖尿病性神经病变导致的足部溃疡是因为缺乏对创伤的感知及血运功能下降。
- 糖尿病足性骨髓炎的主要鉴别诊断是神经病性关节病，即糖尿病性神经病变的一个常见后遗症。

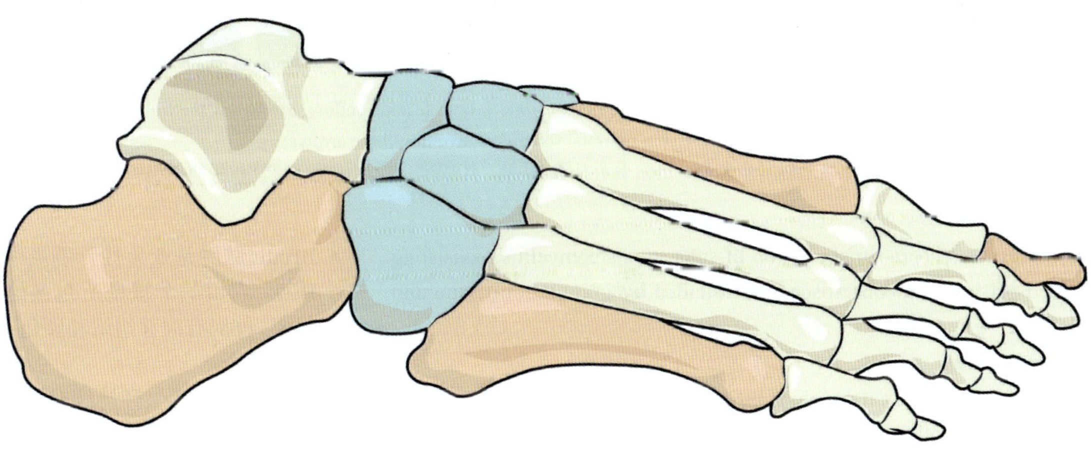

The calcaneus, first and fifth metatarsals, and first distal phalanx are the most common sites of osteomyelitis in the foot.
Charcot arthropathy usually involves the midfoot.
跟骨、第一和第五跖骨、第一远节趾骨是足部骨髓炎最常见的部位。
Charcot关节病通常累及足中部。

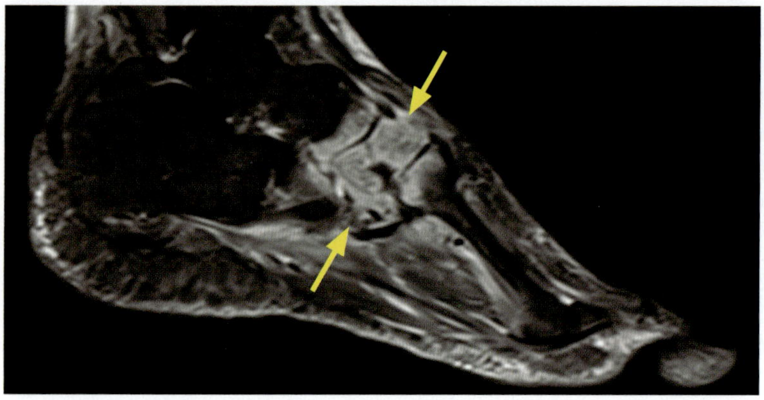

Charcot arthropathy:
Sagittal STIR MRI shows diffuse edema of the midfoot (arrows). No ulcer or sinus tract is evident.
Charcot关节病：
矢状位STIR MRI显示中足呈弥漫性水肿(箭)。未见明显的溃疡或窦道。

Neuropathic arthropathy usually affects the midfoot and features polyarticular involvement, absence of contiguous soft-tissue infection, and absence of an associated ulcer/sinus tract. The bony cortex is intact.
In contrast, diabetic foot osteomyelitis is almost always associated with a cutaneous ulcer and a sinus tract to the bone. The cortex of the involved bone is often disrupted.
Abnormal marrow signal is seen in both neuropathic arthropathy and diabetic foot osteomyelitis.
神经病性关节病常累及足中部并且以多关节受累为特点，没有相邻软组织感染及溃疡/窦道形成的表现。骨皮质完整。
相反，糖尿病足性骨髓炎几乎均伴有皮肤溃疡和骨的窦道形成。受累骨的骨皮质常不连续。
异常的骨髓信号在神经病性关节病和糖尿病足性骨髓炎均可见到。

- In contrast to hematogenous osteomyelitis, contiguous focus osteomyelitis is typically polymicrobial and biopsy is often warranted to ensure proper treatment.

Brodie abscess

- 与血源性骨髓炎相比，局部蔓延性骨髓炎常为多种微生物感染所致，通常需活检以确保患者得到适当的治疗。

Brodie脓肿

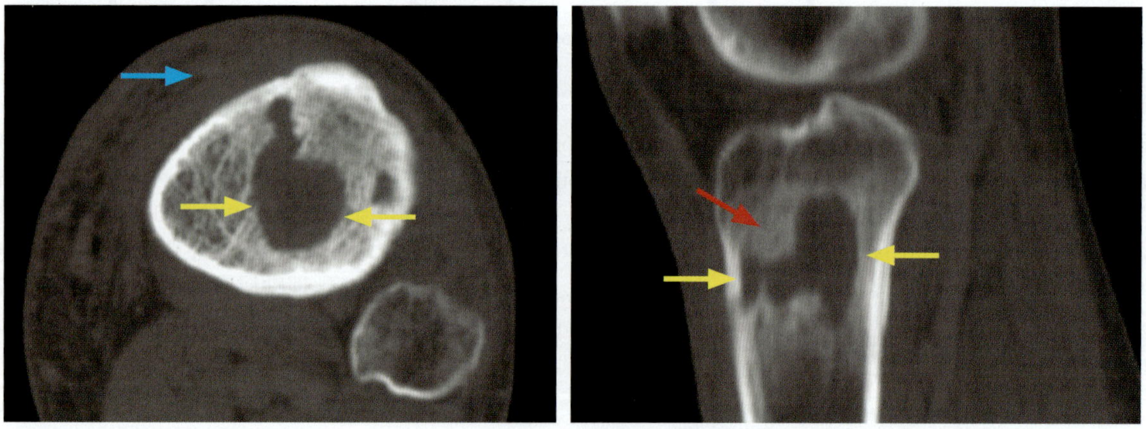

Axial (left image) and sagittal CT images through the knee demonstrate a lytic lesion (yellow arrows) of the tibial metaphysis with surrounding reactive sclerosis (red arrows) and overlying pretibial soft tissue swelling (blue arrows).
轴位(左图)和矢状位膝关节CT显示胫骨干骺端一处溶骨性病变(黄箭)，伴周围反应性硬化(红箭)和胫前软组织肿胀(蓝箭)。

- **Brodie abscess** is a characteristic lesion of subacute osteomyelitis, consisting of a walled-off intra-osseous abscess surrounded by granulation tissue and sclerotic bone.

Chronic osteomyelitis

- Chronic osteomyelitis is an indolent infection lasting more than 6 weeks. Devascularized, necrotic bone leads to a sequestrum surrounded by granulation tissue and involucrum.
- Chronic osteomyelitis can cause a mixed lytic and sclerotic appearance, with a thickened cortex.
- It can be difficult to differentiate between active and inactive chronic

- **Brodie脓肿**是亚急性骨髓炎中具有特征性的病变，它由一个被壁所包裹的游离骨内脓肿组成，外周有肉芽组织和硬化骨。

慢性骨髓炎

- 慢性骨髓炎是一种持续时间超过6周的慢性感染。坏死的骨组织导致游离骨，其外周被肉芽组织所包裹。
- 慢性骨髓炎可以引起混合性溶骨和硬化性改变，并伴有骨皮质增厚。
- 鉴别活动性和非活动性慢性骨髓炎可能会很

osteomyelitis. Serial radiographs in active chronic osteomyelitis may show development of periosteal reaction.

- **Sclerosing osteomyelitis**, also known as osteomyelitis of *Garré,* is an uncommon form of chronic osteomyelitis characterized by sclerosis and thickening of bone. The differential diagnosis of sclerosing osteomyelitis includes lymphoma, sclerotic metastasis, and osteoid osteoma.

Specific organisms causing osteomyelitis

- **Staphylococcus**: *Staph. aureus* is the most common cause of hematogenous osteomyelitis.
- **Salmonella**: Osteomyelitis from *Salmonella* is typically seen in patients with sickle cell disease, with a propensity to affect the diaphysis. It may be difficult to distinguish between diaphyseal bone infarct and osteomyelitis in sickle cell patients.
- **Pseudomonas**: Osteomyelitis from *Pseudomonas aeruginosa* is classically caused by a puncture wound of the foot through a sneaker.
- **Tuberculosis**: The most common musculoskeletal infection of *Mycobacterium tuberculosis* is infection of the spine, also known as Pott disease.

Specific locations

- Hand and finger: The metacarpals and phalanges may become infected after a bite wound.
- Toe: A stubbed great toe with nail-bed injury is at risk for osteomyelitis of the distal phalanx, due to the location of periosteum immediately adjacent to the nail bed.
- Spine: Vertebral osteomyelitis/discitis in an adult may be caused by hematogenous arterial spread, spinal surgery, or spread of a genitourinary infection through the epidural venous Batson plexus. Infection begins in the subendplate region of the vertebral body and subsequently spreads to the endplate, intervertebral disc, and adjacent vertebral body.

  In contrast, in children discitis is thought to represent direct hematogenous seeding of the persistently vascularized disc.

Imaging osteomyelitis

困难。对活动性慢性骨髓炎进行系列X线检查可以揭示骨膜反应的演变过程。

- **硬化性骨髓炎**，又称Garré骨髓炎，是一种少见的慢性骨髓炎类型，以骨质硬化和增厚为特征。硬化性骨髓炎的鉴别诊断包括淋巴瘤、成骨性转移瘤和骨样骨瘤。

引起骨髓炎的特殊病原体

- **葡萄球菌**：金黄色葡萄球菌是血源性骨髓炎最常见的原因。
- **沙门菌**：沙门菌引起的骨髓炎常见于镰状细胞病的患者，好发于骨干。鉴别镰状细胞病患者的骨干骨梗死与骨髓炎较为困难。
- **假单胞菌**：铜绿假单胞菌引起的骨髓炎通常由运动鞋穿破后，脚被尖锐物体刺伤引起的。
- **结核**：骨骼肌肉系统最常见的结核分枝杆菌感染是脊柱结核，又称Pott病。

特定部位

- 手和手指：掌骨和指骨可能在咬伤后引起感染。
- 脚趾：跗趾踢伤累及甲床，其趾骨末端有感染骨髓炎的风险，因其骨膜紧邻甲床。
- 脊柱：成人的骨髓炎/椎间盘炎可由动脉血行播散、脊柱手术，或泌尿生殖道感染经硬膜外Baston静脉丛播散所致。感染始于椎体的终板下区域并且随后播散至终板、椎间盘和邻近椎体。

  相比之下，儿童的椎间盘炎被认为是通过持续未闭的椎间盘血管直接由血行播散所致。

骨髓炎影像

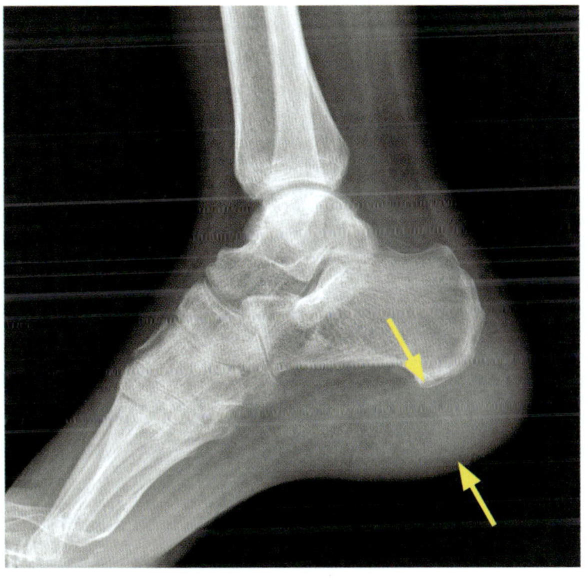

Calcaneal osteomyelitis due to foreign body: Radiograph shows marked thickening of the heel pad (arrows). No bony changes are evident.

异物引起的跟骨骨髓炎：X线影像显示足跟垫明显增厚(箭)。没有明显的骨骼改变。

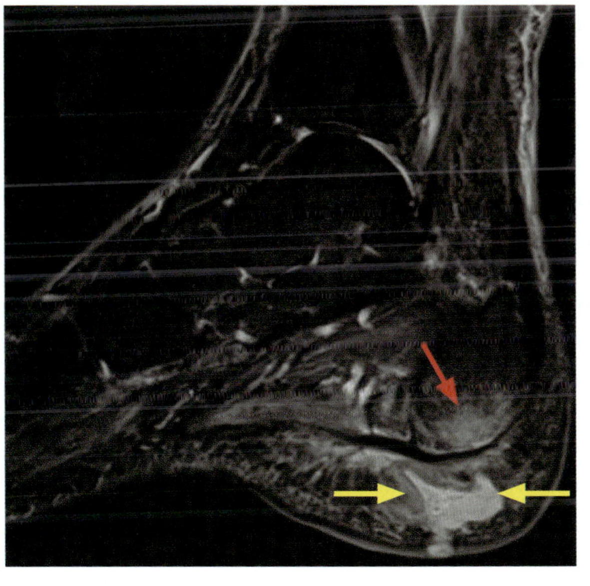

Sagittal STIR MRI shows calcaneal bone marrow edema (red arrow) and a fluid collection (yellow arrows) within the heel pad, contiguous with the skin.

矢状位STIR MRI显示跟骨骨髓水肿(红箭)和足跟垫内积液(黄箭)，并延续到邻近皮肤。

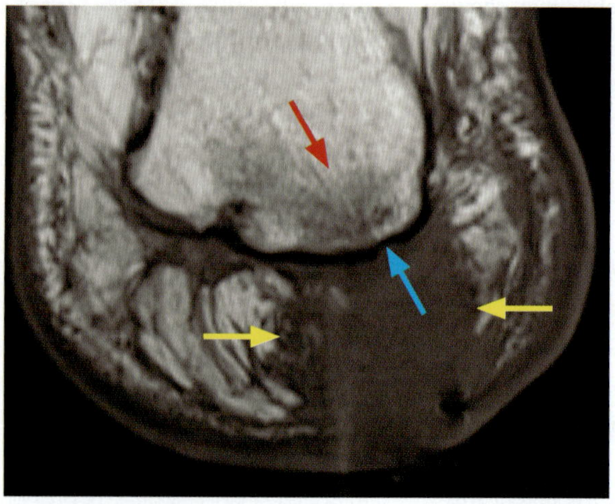

Coronal T1-weighted MRI shows the low-signal fluid collection in the heel pad (yellow arrows), regional decreased T1 marrow signal (red arrow), and irregularity of the calcaneal cortex (blue arrow).

冠状位T_1加权MRI显示足跟垫内低信号液体聚集(黄箭),局部骨髓T_1信号降低(红箭),以及跟骨皮质不规则(蓝箭)。

Case courtesy Marie Koch, MD, Brigham and Women's Hospital, Boston.

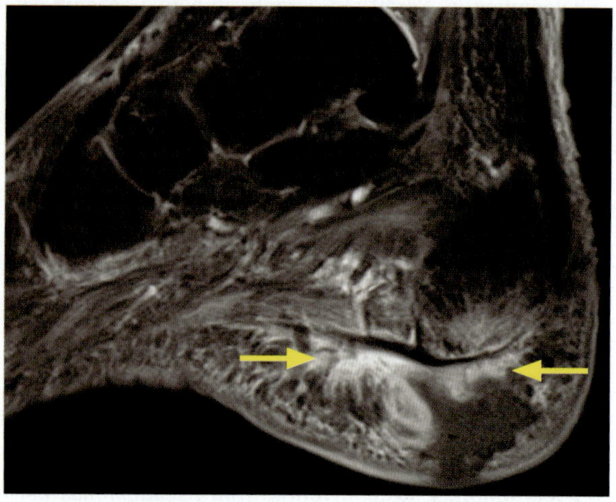

Sagittal T1-weighted post-contrast MRI with fat suppression shows marked enhancement (yellow arrows) surrounding the abscess and enhancement of the surrounding soft tissues.

矢状位增强T_1加权脂肪抑制MRI显示脓肿周围显著强化(黄箭)和周围软组织强化。

- Radiographs are typically the first modality to evaluate suspected osteomyelitis although it typically takes between 10–14 days for radiographic changes to be evident.
- Radiographic findings depend on the route of spread. Early radiographic changes of hematogenous osteomyelitis include focal osteopenia due to reactive hyperemia, followed by a lucent medullary lesion. In contiguous focus osteomyelitis, the first radiographic sign may be soft-tissue swelling and periosteal reaction, followed by erosion of the cortex.
- Scintigraphy and MRI imaging are more sensitive to detect early osteomyelitis.
- Three-phase Tc-99m MDP bone scan becomes positive within 24–48 hours after the onset of symptoms. Acute osteomyelitis is positive on all three phases (flow, blood pool, and delayed).

  In contrast, cellulitis is positive on flow and blood pool phases, and negative on delayed.

  Although highly sensitive, Tc-99m bone scan is less specific than leukocyte scintigraphy and MRI.
- Combining WBC and sulfur colloid scintigraphy adds specificity in the evaluation of osteomyelitis because bone marrow is replaced by infection and white cells. Actively infected bone marrow will show discordantly increased uptake on the WBC scan and reduced activity on sulfur colloid.

  Note that WBC scan imaging is not sensitive for spinal osteomyelitis, thought to be due to the inability of leukocytes to migrate into an encapsulated infection.

  WBC scan can be performed with either Indium-111-WBC or Tc-99m-HMPAO-WBC. Indium WBC scan has higher radiation dose, takes 24 hours to perform, and the image has more noise. The disadvantage of Tc- 99m-HMPAO is its tendency to dissociate, leading to genitourinary excretion of radiotracer.
- MRI is highly sensitive to detect early osteomyelitis within 3–5 days. MRI has similar sensitivity to radionuclide studies, but greater specificity. MRI can better delineate the extent of infection, any fluid collections that must be treated surgically, sinus tracts, and skin ulcers.

- X线影像通常是评估可疑骨髓炎的首选方法,但它通常需10~14天才有明显的影像学改变。
- X线影像学上的表现取决于播散途径。血源性骨髓炎的早期表现包括反应性充血导致的局部骨量减少,随后出现骨髓腔低密度病变。在局部蔓延性骨髓炎,首发征象可为软组织肿胀和骨膜反应,随后发生骨皮质侵蚀。
- 核素显像和MRI对检测早期骨髓炎都很敏感。
- ^{99m}Tc-MDP三期骨扫描在症状出现的24~48小时内开始有阳性发现。急性骨髓炎在三相扫描(血流相、血池相和延迟相)中都呈阳性。

  相比之下,蜂窝织炎在血流相和血池相有阳性表现,延迟相则为阴性。

  虽然敏感性高,但^{99m}Tc-MDP骨扫描的特异性低于白细胞标记闪烁扫描和MRI。
- 联合白细胞和硫胶体骨髓闪烁显像可增加对骨髓炎诊断的特异性,因骨髓被感染和白细胞所替代。活动性骨髓感染会出现白细胞摄取增加和硫胶体摄取降低的不一致显像结果。

  需要注意,白细胞显像对脊柱骨髓炎不敏感,可能是因为白细胞不能进入被包裹的感染灶。

  白细胞扫描可用^{111}In或^{99m}Tc-HMPAO标记的白细胞。^{111}In白细胞扫描辐射剂量较高,显像要24小时,且图像噪声较大。^{99m}Tc -HMPAO的缺点是容易解离,导致泌尿系统排泄放射性示踪剂。
- MRI对发现3~5天内的早期骨髓炎非常敏感。MRI和放射性核素扫描的敏感性相似,但特异性更佳。MRI可以更好地显示感染的范围、需手术治疗的积液、窦道及皮肤溃疡。

- The hallmark of MRI imaging of osteomyelitis is replacement of the normal fatty marrow signal. Edema and exudates cause high marrow signal on T2-weighted images and low signal on T1-weighted images. MRI has very high negative predictive value: A negative MRI essentially excludes osteomyelitis.

Abnormal signal intensity in the bone on fluid-sensitive sequences does not necessarily signify that osteomyelitis is present. To confidently diagnose osteomyelitis on MR, the T1-weighted images should be carefully scrutinized. Three patterns of signal alteration on T1-weighted images have been described, which are *confluent intramedullary*, *hazy reticular*, and *subcortical*. Of these, only the *confluent intramedullary* pattern is highly associated with osteomyelitis.

- 骨髓炎的MRI影像特征是正常黄骨髓信号被替代。水肿和渗出导致骨髓T_2加权高信号和T_1加权低信号。MRI有很高的阴性预测值：MRI阴性可基本排除骨髓炎。

液体敏感序列上骨骼中的异常信号并不一定表示有骨髓炎。若用MR确诊骨髓炎，必需仔细查看T_1加权图像。T_1加权图像的三种信号改变模式：髓内融合、网状模糊影和皮质下改变。其中，只有髓内融合与骨髓炎高度相关。

Confluent intramedullary
髓内融合

Geographic area involving medullary canal
地图样病灶累及髓管

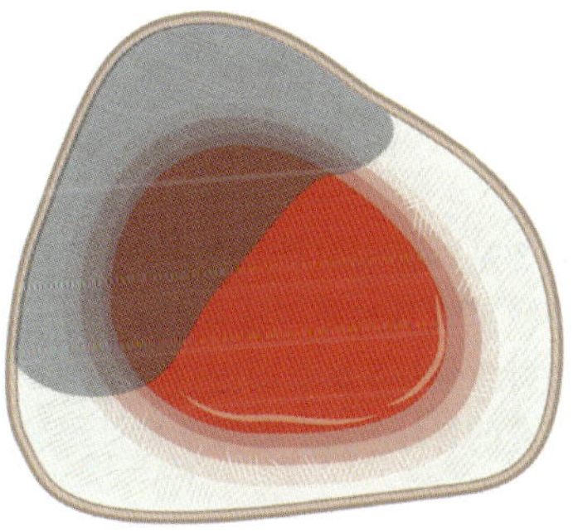

Strongly associated with osteomyelitis, especially with adjacent ulcer
与骨髓炎强烈相关，尤其是伴有邻近溃疡

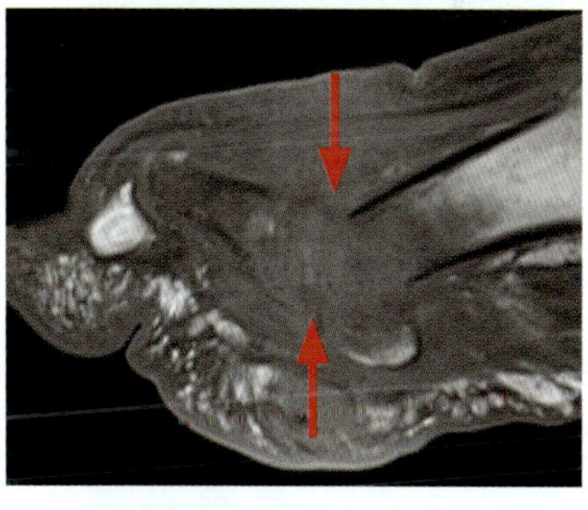

Confluent intramedullary: Osteomyelitis
髓内融合：骨髓炎

Hazy reticular
网状模糊影

Interspersed areas of normal marrow
散布于正常骨髓内

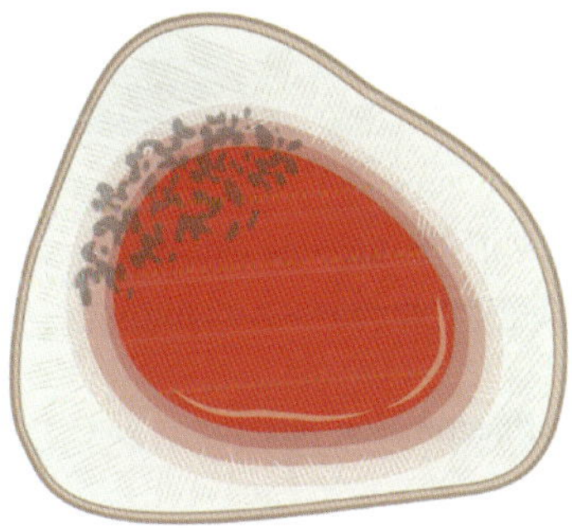

Cannot reliably diagnose osteomyelitis Rarely associated with hematogenous osteomyelitis.
不能可靠地诊断骨髓炎，极少与血源性骨髓炎相关

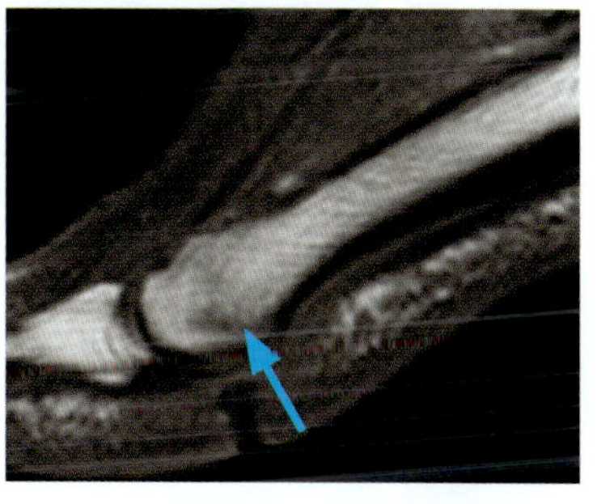

Hazy reticular: Not osteomyelitis
网状模糊影：非骨髓炎

Subcortical
皮质下改变

Thin linear signal change subjacent to cortex
皮质下细线状信号改变

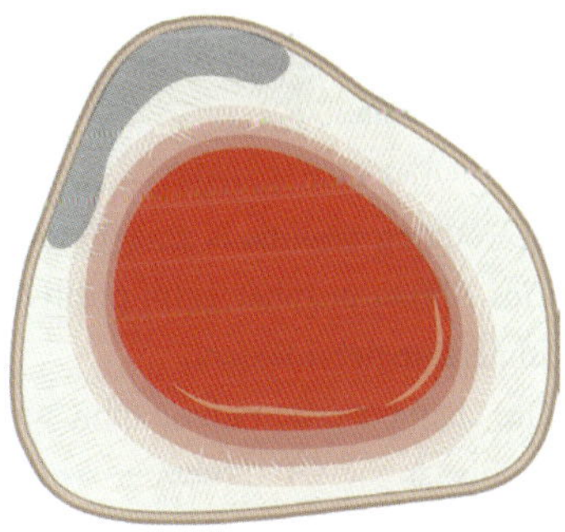

Cannot reliably diagnose osteomyelitis
不能可靠地诊断骨髓炎

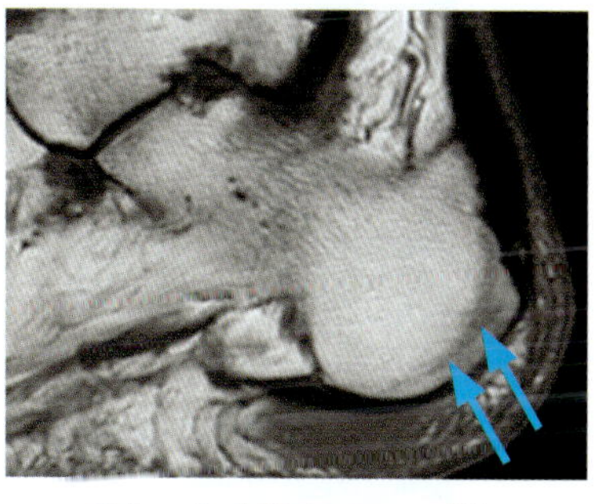

Subcortical: Not osteomyelitis
皮质下改变：非骨髓炎

Three sagittal T1-weighted MRI images demonstrating confluent intramedullary (red arrows), hazy reticular (blue arrow), and subcortical (double blue arrow) signal changes. Of these, only confluent intramedullary signal change is strongly associated with osteomyelitis.
Gadolinium is helpful to delineate any fluid collections and to evaluate for the presence of nonenhancing necrotic bone (sequestrum), although gadolinium is not necessary to confidently diagnose osteomyelitis.
三个矢状位T_1加权MRI图像显示髓内融合(红箭)，网状模糊影(蓝箭)，以及皮质下改变(双蓝箭)。三者中，只有髓内融合信号改变与骨髓炎强烈相关。
钆造影剂对于显示任何积液和评估是否有非强化的坏死骨组织(死骨)有用，但并非确诊骨髓炎所必需。

Soft-tissue infections

软组织感染

Necrotizing fasciitis

坏死性筋膜炎

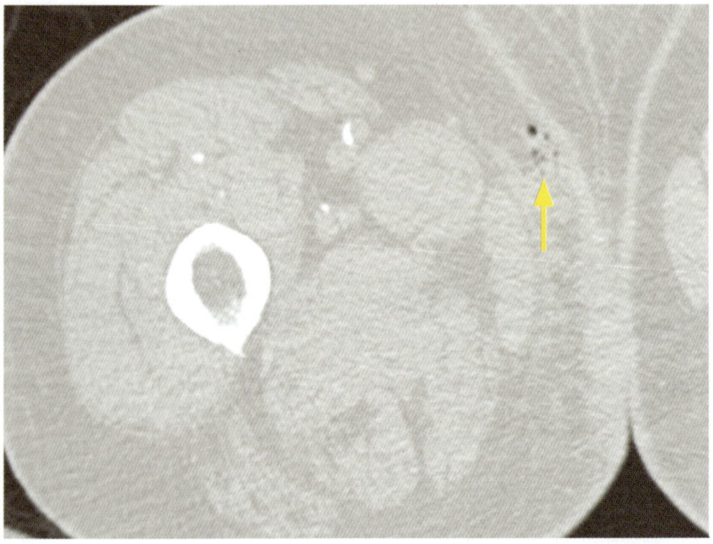

Necrotizing fasciitis:
Unenhanced CT through the proximal thigh shows several tiny locules of gas (arrow) in the medial subcutaneous tissues.
坏死性筋膜炎：大腿近端平扫CT显示内侧皮下组织内数个微小气泡(箭)。

- Necrotizing fasciitis is an extremely aggressive soft-tissue infection caused by *Clostridium* or other gram-positive rods. It is a surgical emergency, requiring immediate debridement.
- The characteristic radiographic and CT finding of necrotizing fasciitis is gas bubbles in the soft tissues.

- 坏死性筋膜炎是一种极其严重的软组织感染，由梭状芽孢杆菌或其他革兰氏阳性杆菌引起。这是一种外科急症，需要立即进行清创。
- 坏死性筋膜炎的X线和CT影像学特征是软组织内出现气泡影。

Pyomyositis

化脓性肌炎

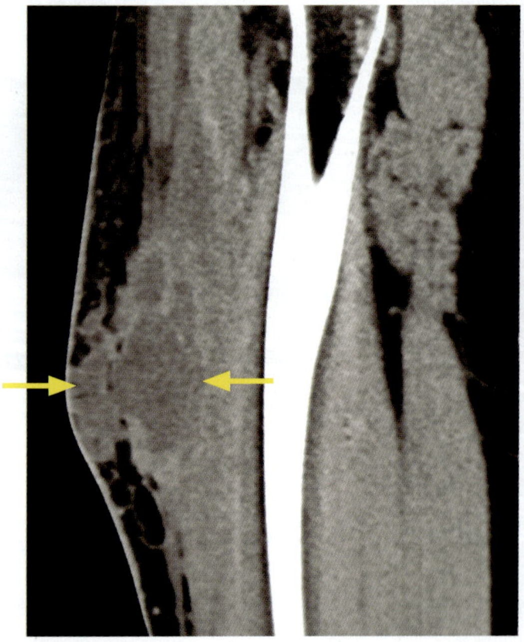

Sagittal contrast-enhanced CT
矢状位增强CT

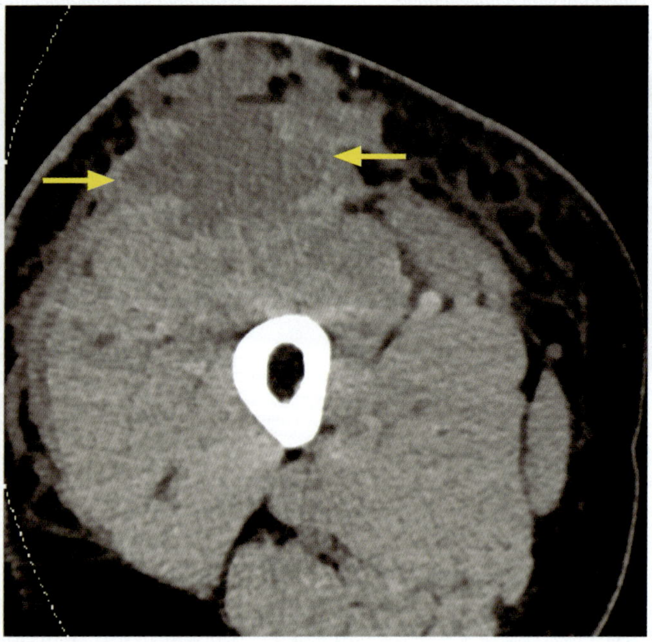

Axial contrast-enhanced CT
轴位增强CT

Pyomyositis with abscess: CT images demonstrate a geographic, irregular-shaped low attenuation collection (arrows) in the anterior quadriceps muscle, with fluid tracking to the skin.
化脓性肌炎伴脓肿形成：CT图像显示股四头肌前部一处形态不规则的低密度积聚区(箭)，且液体密度影延伸至皮肤。

- Pyomyositis is bacterial infection of the muscle. It was historically called tropical myositis because it was first recognized in tropical regions of the globe, classically occurring in young males after vigorous exercise.
- Currently, the incidence of pyomyositis is increasing in the United States, with diabetes a substantial risk factor.
- *Staphylococcus aureus* causes the majority of cases.

- 化脓性肌炎是肌肉的细菌性感染。因最早发现于热带地区，故过去曾被称为热带肌炎，典型表现为年轻男性在剧烈运动后发病。
- 目前，美国化脓性肌炎的发病率正在增加，糖尿病是一个重要危险因素。
- 大多数病例由金黄色葡萄球菌引起。

（翻译　杨曦玥　赵又瑾）

METABOLIC BONE DISEASE

代谢性骨病

MULTIFACTORIAL BONE DISEASE

多因素骨疾病

Osteoporosis

- Osteoporosis (low bone mass) is the most common metabolic bone disease, contributing to millions of fractures per year. Osteoporosis may be secondary to numerous nutritional, endocrine, and other etiologies.
- Vitamin or nutritional deficiencies can cause osteoporosis, including:

Osteomalacia (Looser zone).
Alcoholism.
Hypophosphatemia.
Scurvy (Wimberger sign).

- Endocrine disturbances can impact calcium metabolism, causing osteoporosis, including:

Hyperparathyroidism (subperiosteal resorption).
Cushing disease or any increase in endogenous/exogenous steroids.

- Diffuse malignancy, such as myelomatosis, can cause diffuse bony demineralization.
- Genetic causes of osteoporosis include:

Osteogenesis imperfecta.
Gaucher disease.
Anemia, including sickle cell and thalassemia.

- Focal osteopenia has a more limited list of causes, including:

Immobility/disuse.
Reflex sympathetic dystrophy.
Transient regional osteoporosis of the hip.

骨质疏松

- 骨质疏松（骨量降低）是最常见的代谢性骨疾病，导致每年数百万次骨折。骨质疏松可能继发于营养、内分泌及其他众多的病因。
- 维生素缺乏或营养不良可以导致骨质疏松，包括：

骨软化症（松散区）。
酗酒。
低磷血症。
坏血病（Wimberger征）。

- 内分泌紊乱可以影响钙的代谢，导致骨质疏松，包括：

甲状旁腺功能亢进症（骨膜下吸收）。
库欣病或任何增加内源性/外源性类固醇的疾病。

- 弥漫性恶性肿瘤，如骨髓瘤，可以导致弥漫性的骨质脱钙。
- 遗传导致的骨质疏松，包括：

成骨不全。
戈谢病。
贫血，包括镰状细胞贫血和地中海贫血。

- 局部骨量减少的病因较为有限，包括：

制动/废用。
反射交感神经营养不良。
一过性局部髋关节骨质疏松症。

DUAL ENERGY X-RAY ABSORPTIOMETRY (DEXA)

双能X射线吸收法（DEXA）

Overview of dual energy x-ray absorptiometry (DEXA)

- Dual energy x-ray absorptiometry, universally called DEXA, is a method to quantify bone mineral density. A DEXA scan images the lumbar spine (L1–L4), and the hip. The forearm can also be imaged if either the hip or spine is

双能X射线吸收法（DEXA）概述

- 双能X射线吸收测定术，通常被称为DEXA，是一种量化骨密度的方法。DEXA扫描腰椎（L_{1-4}）和髋关节。如果髋关节或脊柱不合适（如

not suitable (e.g., severe degenerative changes or prior surgery), or if a third point of reference is desired.

- The DEXA machine provides an absolute value of bone mineral density (most useful to track changes over time), as well as a T-score and a Z-score.

  The **T-score** is the number of standard deviations from healthy young sex-matched patients.

  The **Z-score** is the number of standard deviations from age-matched and sex-matched patients.

- In menopausal and post-menopausal females and males ⩾50 years of age, there are standard definitions for normal, osteoporosis, and osteopenia, based on the **T-score**.

  Normal: **T-score** at or greater than –1.0.

  Osteopenia (low bone mass): **T-score** between –1.0 and –2.5.

  Osteoporosis: **T-score** at or less than –2.5.

- For pre-menopausal females and males <age 50, the **Z-score** is used. A **Z-score** of –2.0 or lower is "below expected range for age" and a **Z-score** above –2.0 is "within the expected range for age."

严重退行性变或既往手术)或需要第三参考点,还可对前臂进行成像。

- DEXA仪器能提供骨密度的绝对值(最有用的是进行跟踪随访),以及T评分和Z评分。

  T评分是匹配性别的健康青年人所得的标准差。

  Z评分是匹配年龄和性别的患者所得的标准差。

- 在绝经期和绝经后女性及年龄⩾50岁的男性,正常、骨质疏松和骨质减少的标准定义依据T评分。

  正常:**T评分**⩾–1.0。

  骨质减少(骨量降低):**T评分**在–1.0~2.5。

  骨质疏松:**T评分**⩽–2.5。

- 对于绝经前女性和年龄<50岁的男性,使用**Z评分**。**Z评分**⩽–2.0表示"低于同年龄预期值范围",**Z评分**>–2.0表示"在同年龄预期值范围内"。

VITAMIN-DEFICIENCY BONE DISEASE

Scurvy

- Scurvy (**hypovitaminosis C**) causes generalized osteopenia as osteoblasts require vitamin C to form mature osteoid tissue.
- Subperiosteal hemorrhage can be associated with periosteal reaction. Hemarthrosis, as well as retrobulbar and intracranial bleeding are additional manifestations.
- Pediatric signs of scurvy include the *Wimberger ring sign*, which is increased epiphyseal sclerosis due to disorganized epiphyseal ossification, and a *Pelkin's fracture*, which is a metaphyseal corner fracture.
- A dense metaphyseal line (*Frankel line*) may be present due to provisional calcification, with underlying lucent band (*Trümmerfeld zone*).

Osteomalacia

维生素缺乏性骨疾病

坏血病

- 坏血病(**维生素C缺乏**)导致全身性骨质疏松,因为成骨细胞需要维生素C来形成成熟的骨样组织。
- 骨膜下出血可伴有骨膜反应。另外还有关节血肿、球后出血和颅内出血的表现。
- 小儿坏血病的体征包括Wimberger环征,是由于骺板骨化无序而导致的骨骺硬化增加;以及Pelkin骨折,即干骺角的骨折。
- 可出现高密度的干骺线(Frankel线),为临时性钙化,伴有下方透明带(Trümmerfeld区)。

骨软化症

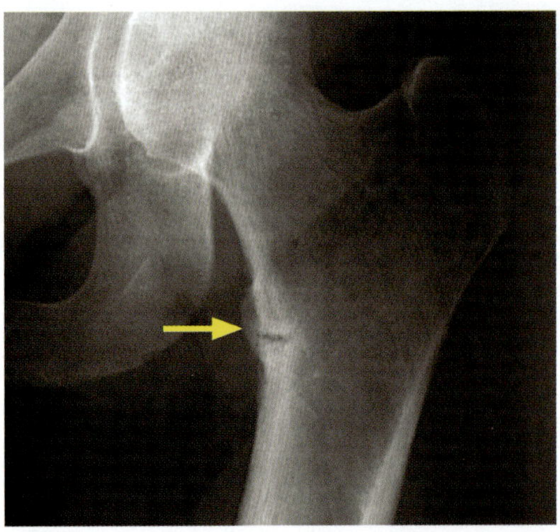

Osteomalacia:
Frontal radiograph of the hip demonstrates an incomplete linear lucency (arrow) through the medial (weight-bearing) proximal femur, representing a Looser zone.
Case courtesy Stacy Smith, MD, Brigham and Women's Hospital.
骨软化症:
髋关节正位X线影像显示一条不完整的透亮线(箭)横跨股骨近端的内侧(承重骨),此为Looser带(假性骨折)。

- Osteomalacia is faulty mineralization of bone matrix caused by vitamin D deficiency. The same process is called osteomalacia in adults and rickets in children. Rickets is discussed in the pediatric imaging section.
- Osteomalacia manifests as diffuse osteopenia; however, a *Looser zone* (pseudofracture) is highly specific. A *Looser zone* is a cortical stress fracture

- 骨软化症是因为维生素D缺乏导致骨基质矿化障碍。同样的疾病在成人称骨软化症,在儿童称佝偻病。佝偻病在"小儿影像"章节讨论。
- 骨软化症表现为弥漫性骨质疏松;但是Looser带(假性骨折)具高度特异性。Looser带是一

that is filled with abnormal, poorly mineralized osteoid and appears as a radiolucency through the cortex. Common sites for *Looser zones* are the medial proximal femurs, distal scapulae, and pubic bones.

- Osteomalacia may be complicated by insufficiency fracture.

种骨皮质应力性骨折，其内为异常或矿化不良的骨样组织，在影像学上表现为横跨骨皮质的透亮带。Looser带的常见部位为股骨近端内侧、肩胛骨远端及耻骨。

- 骨软化症可并发不全骨折。

ENDOCRINE BONE DISEASE

Acromegaly

- Acromegaly is the syndrome caused by excess growth hormone. When the growth hormone excess occurs when the physes are open, the bones will grow longitudinally, leading to gigantism. However, when the hormone excess occurs once the physes have closed then the bones cannot lengthen and instead obtain a characteristic appearance of acral (distal) growth and widening.
- In the head there is enlargement of frontal sinuses, thickening of cranial bones, and an enlarged jaw.
- In the hands, *beak-like* osteophytes of the metacarpal heads and *spade-like* overgrowth of the distal phalanges are characteristic.
- In the feet, a characteristic finding is increased heel-pad thickness.

Hyperparathyroidism (Recklinghausen disease of bone)

内分泌性骨疾病

肢端肥大症

- 肢端肥大症是由于生长激素分泌过剩导致的综合征。在骨骺线闭合之前出现生长激素分泌过剩，骨骼会纵向生长而导致巨人症。但是，在骨骺线闭合之后出现激素分泌过剩，骨骼长度将不会增加，取而代之的是特征性的肢端(远端)增大与增宽。
- 在头部，额窦扩大、颅骨增厚及下颌部增大。
- 在手部，掌骨头的喙状骨赘和指骨末端的铲状增生是其特征。
- 在足部，一个特征性的表现是足跟垫增厚。

甲状旁腺功能亢进症(Recklinghausen骨病)

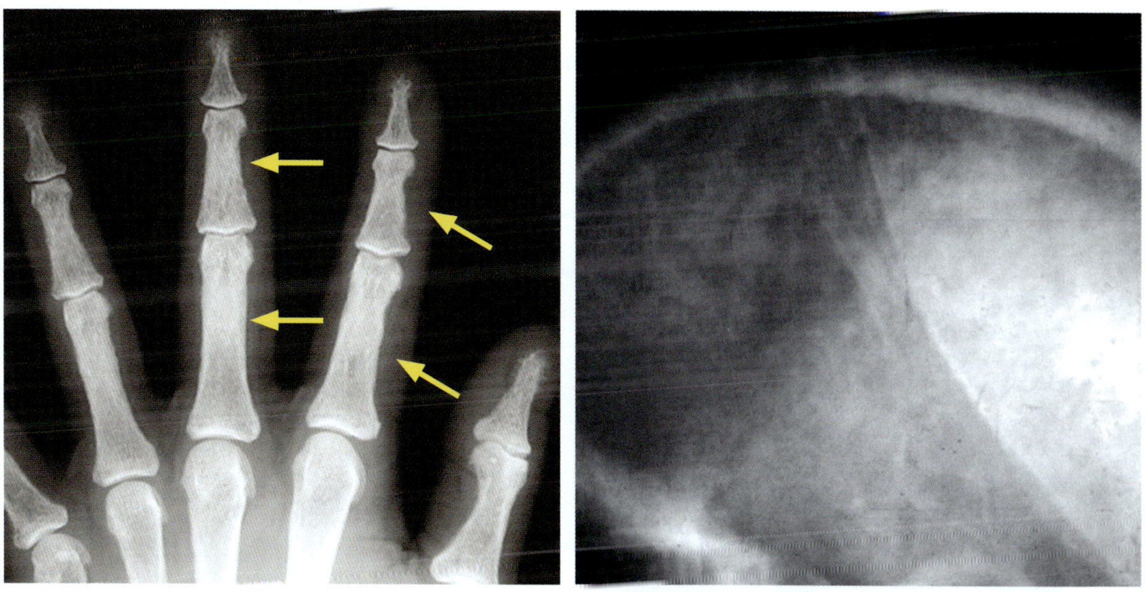

Hyperparathyroidism: Radiograph of the hand (left image) shows subperiosteal resorption and scalloping of the radial margins of the second and third proximal and middle phalanges (arrows). Lateral skull radiograph in a different patient shows the classic *salt-and-pepper* appearance due to trabecular resorption.

Cases courtesy Stacy Smith, MD, Brigham and Women's Hospital.

甲状旁腺功能亢进症：手部X线影像(左图)显示骨膜下骨质吸收和第二、三近节及中节指骨桡侧扇贝样改变(箭)。另一名患者颅骨侧位X线影像显示由于骨小梁吸收导致的典型的椒盐征。

- Hyperparathyroidism is excess parathyroid hormone (PTH). PTH is normally secreted in response to hypocalcemia and maintains serum calcium levels by stimulating osteoclasts.
- Primary hyperparathyroidism is autonomously increased secretion from an overactive parathyroid gland, typically due to a parathyroid adenoma. Serum calcium is high and phosphate is low.
- Secondary hyperparathyroidism is increased secretion of PTH by a normal gland in response to hypocalcemia secondary to renal failure. Serum calcium is

- 甲状旁腺功能亢进症是甲状旁腺激素(PTH)分泌过度。正常情况下，PTH分泌是对低钙血症的反应，并通过刺激破骨细胞以维持血清钙水平。
- 原发性甲状旁腺功能亢进症是由过度活跃的甲状旁腺自主分泌增加所致，常由甲状旁腺腺瘤引起。血钙升高、血磷降低。
- 继发性甲状旁腺功能亢进症是肾衰竭导致的

usually normal.

- Tertiary hyperparathyroidism is seen after prolonged secondary hyperparathyroidism, where the parathyroid glands escape regulatory control and oversecrete PTH.
- The radiological hallmarks of hyperparathyroidism are diffuse bony demineralization and subperiosteal and subligamentous bone resorption.

低钙血症刺激正常甲状旁腺，从而使PTH分泌过多。血清钙通常是正常的。

- 三发性甲状旁腺功能亢进症见于长期继发性甲状旁腺功能亢进症后，甲状旁腺失去生理调控并过度分泌PTH。
- 甲状旁腺功能亢进症的影像学特点是弥漫性骨质脱钙、骨膜下及韧带下骨质吸收。

Skull: The classic *salt-and-pepper* skull is due to trabecular resorption.

Hands: Subperiosteal resorption of the radial aspects of the second and third middle phalanges is specific for hyperparathyroidism.

Clavicle: Subperiosteal resorption of the clavicle tends to affect the acromial (distal) aspect.

Knee: Subperiosteal bone resorption of the medial proximal tibial metaphysis.

Teeth: Loss of lamina dura surrounding the tooth socket can occasionally be seen.

Anywhere: Brown tumors are more common in primary hyperparathyroidism.

Everywhere: Diffuse osteopenia results from continued osteoclast activation.

颅骨：典型的颅骨*椒盐征*为骨小梁吸收所致。

手：第二、三指中节指骨桡侧的骨膜下骨质吸收是甲状旁腺功能亢进症的特殊表现。

锁骨：锁骨骨膜下骨质吸收往往侵犯肩峰端(远端)。

膝：近端胫骨干骺端内侧可见骨膜下骨质吸收。

牙齿：偶尔可见牙槽骨硬板缺失。

任何地方：棕色瘤更常见于原发性甲状旁腺功能亢进症。

所有地方：持续性破骨细胞活化导致弥漫性骨量减少。

- Calcium pyrophosphate dihydrate deposition (CPPD) may occur, which is more common in primary hyperparathyroidism.
- Soft-tissue calcification, periosteal reaction, and sclerosis are seen more commonly in secondary hyperparathyroidism.
- Complications of hyperparathyroidism include insufficiency fracture and increased propensity for ligaments and tendons to rupture.

- 可出现焦磷酸钙沉积(CPPD)，且其更常见于原发性甲状旁腺功能亢进症。
- 软组织钙化、骨膜反应和骨质硬化更常见于继发性甲状旁腺功能亢进症。
- 甲状旁腺功能亢进症的并发症包括不全骨折及韧带与肌腱断裂的风险增高。

Renal osteodystrophy

肾性骨病

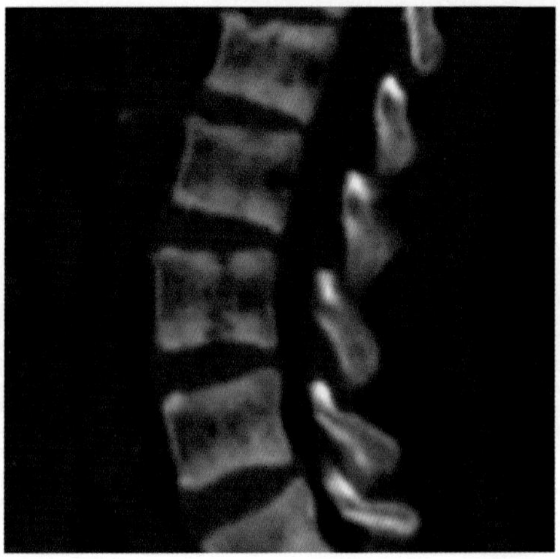

Rugger jersey spine: Sagittal CT demonstrates symmetric endplate sclerosis at all levels of the lumbar spine in this patient with renal osteodystrophy.
脊柱橄榄球衣征：矢状位CT显示肾性骨病患者所有腰椎的终板呈对称性硬化。

- Renal osteodystrophy is due to the combined effects of abnormal vitamin D metabolism (osteomalacia) and secondary hyperparathyroidism from prolonged renal failure.
- In addition to renal osteodystrophy, patients with renal failure have an increased risk of additional bone disorders including osteomyelitis, avascular necrosis (if on steroids), and amyloidosis (from chronic dialysis).
- Unlike osteomalacia, *Looser zones* are uncommon in renal osteodystrophy.
- The characteristic *rugger jersey* spine, pictured above, describes sclerotic striping of the vertebral body endplates.
- Soft-tissue and vascular calcifications are often present.

- 肾性骨病是由于异常维生素D代谢(骨软化症)和继发于长期肾衰竭引起的甲状旁腺功能亢进症两者共同作用的结果。
- 除肾性骨病之外，肾衰竭患者罹患其他骨病的风险增高，包括骨髓炎、缺血性坏死(如果用类固醇)，以及淀粉样变性(长期透析)。
- 与骨软化症不同，*Looser*带在肾性骨病中并不常见。
- 特征性*橄榄球衣征*，如上图所示，是指椎体终板条纹状硬化。
- 常见软组织和血管钙化。

Hypoparathyroidism

- Hypoparathyroidism is most commonly a consequence of parathyroid gland resection for hyperparathyroidism.
- Hypoparathyroidism causes metastatic deposition of calcium. In particular, calcium is deposited in the subcutaneous tissues and in the basal ganglia.

Pseudohypoparathyroidism and pseudo-pseudohypoparathyroidism

- Pseudohypoparathyroidism (PHP) is due to a defect of the parathyroid hormone (PTH) receptor. In pseudo-pseudohypoparathyroidism (PPHP), the PTH level is normal and PTH receptor is normal, but the patient's phenotype is indistinguishable from that of pseudohypoparathyroidism.
- Both entities clinically present with obesity, round facies, short stature, and brachydactyly (short fingers).
- The classic radiographic finding is a short metacarpal, usually the fourth or fifth.

甲状旁腺功能减退症

- 甲状旁腺功能减退症最常见于甲状旁腺切除治疗功能亢进症术后。
- 甲状旁腺功能减退症导致异常钙沉积。尤其是皮下组织和基底神经节钙沉积。

假性甲状旁腺功能减退症和假-假性甲状旁腺功能减退症

- 假性甲状旁腺功能减退症(PHP)是由于甲状旁腺素(PTH)受体缺陷。在假-假性甲状旁腺功能减退症(PPHP)中，PTH水平和PTH受体均为正常，但是患者的表现型与假性甲状旁腺功能减退症无法区分。
- 两者在临床上都表现为肥胖、满月脸、身材矮小和短指症(短手指)。
- 典型的影像学表现为掌骨缩短，通常是第四或第五掌骨。

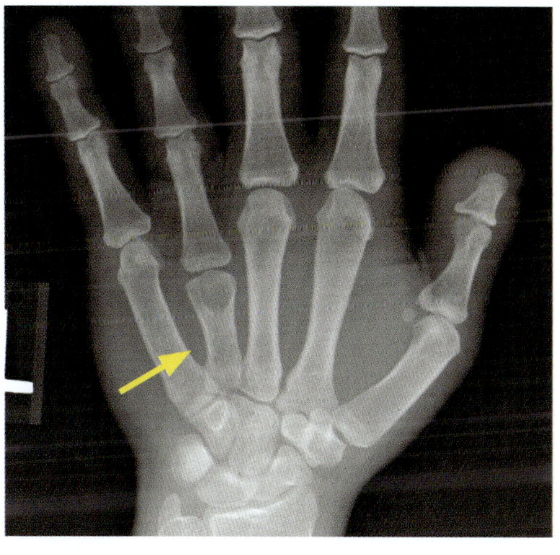

Pseudohypoparathyroidism. Radiograph of the hand shows a markedly shortened fourth metacarpal (arrow).
In addition to pseudohypoparathyroidism and pseudo-pseudohypoparathyroidism, an additional differential consideration for a short fourth metacarpal includes Turner syndrome.
假性甲状旁腺功能减退症：手部X线影像显示第四掌骨(箭)明显缩短。
除假性甲状旁腺功能减退症和假-假性甲状旁腺功能减退症之外，第四掌骨缩短的另一个需鉴别的疾病为特纳综合征。

Hypothyroidism

- In children, hypothyroidism causes a delay in skeletal and dental maturity.
- Hypothyroidism may cause bullet-shaped vertebral bodies and Wormian bones in the skull.
- Hypothyroidism is associated with slipped capital femoral epiphysis.

Hyperthyroidism

- Hyperthyroidism causes accelerated bony maturation in children. **Thyroid acropachy** is a rare cause of diaphyseal periosteal reaction of multiple bones including the metacarpals, metatarsals, and phalanges, seen in the setting of treated hyperthyroidism.

甲状腺功能减退症

- 在儿童，甲状腺功能减退症可引起骨骼和牙齿发育延迟。
- 甲状腺功能减退症可以导致子弹状椎体和Wormian样颅骨。
- 甲状腺功能减退症与股骨头骨骺滑脱有关。

甲状腺功能亢进症

- 甲状腺功能亢进症在儿童可引起骨骼发育加速。**甲状腺杵状指/趾**是一种罕见的引起多发骨干骨膜反应的原因，包括掌骨、跖骨和指/趾骨，见于治疗后的甲状腺功能亢进症患者。

IDIOPATHIC BONE DISEASE

Paget disease

- Paget disease is a progressive disturbance of osteoclastic and osteoblastic regulation seen in older adults. The cause of Paget disease is unknown, but paramyxovirus may be involved.
- Symptoms of Paget disease include bone pain, osseous enlargement or bowing, compression of cranial nerves, and high output cardiac failure. Weakened subchondral bone commonly leads to osteoarthritis. Other complications of

特发性骨疾病

佩吉特病

- 佩吉特病是一种见于老年人的进行性破骨细胞和成骨细胞调节紊乱的疾病。佩吉特病的发病原因不明，但可能与副黏液病毒有关。
- 佩吉特病的症状包括骨痛、骨增大或弯曲、脑神经受压及高输出性心力衰竭。软骨下骨变弱通常会导致骨性关节炎。佩吉特病的其他

Paget disease include pathologic fracture and malignant degeneration (most commonly osteosarcoma).

- Paget disease affects the skull, spine, and pelvis most commonly, followed by the articular ends of the femur, proximal tibia, and proximal humerus. Involvement of the ribs and scapula can occur but is uncommon.
- Three sequential phases are described, although there is often overlap between the phases and the disease may not always progress through the three stages in order.

并发症包括病理性骨折和恶性病变(最常见为骨肉瘤)。

- 佩吉特病最常累及颅骨、脊柱和骨盆,其次是股骨关节端、近端胫骨和肱骨。肋骨和肩胛骨也可受累,但不常见。
- 病程有三个阶段,但各阶段经常有重叠,而可能并不总是按这三个阶段的顺序发展。

Phase I: Osteolytic phase is due to hyperactivated osteoclasts and resultant active bone resorption.

Phase II: Mixed lytic and sclerotic phase is continued bony resorption and new bone formation.

Phase III: Sclerotic phase is dominated by increased bone density and sclerosis.

第一阶段:溶骨期,是由于破骨细胞高度被激活而致骨质主动吸收所致。

第二阶段:溶骨和硬化混合期,为持续骨质吸收和新骨形成。

第三阶段:硬化期,以骨密度增高和骨质硬化为主。

- Chronic Paget disease shows thickening of cortex, coarse irregular trabecular pattern, and expansion of bone. This appearance has been called a *caricature* of normal bone.
- **Paget of the skull**: In the osteolytic phase (phase Ⅰ), the typical appearance is a sharply marginated geographic lytic region called *osteoporosis circumscripta*. In the mixed phase (phase Ⅱ), the classic appearance is the *cotton wool skull* which looks like an artist dabbed paint on the skull with a piece of cotton.

- 慢性佩吉特病表现为骨皮质增厚,骨小梁不规则增粗和骨结构扩张。这些表现曾经被称作正常骨的*漫画夸张艺术*。
- **颅骨佩吉特病**:在溶骨期(第一阶段),典型的表现是边缘清楚的地图样溶骨病灶,称为局限性骨质疏松症。在混合期(第二阶段),典型的表现是*棉絮状颅骨*,看起来就像一个艺术家用一块棉花把颜料轻拍在颅骨上。

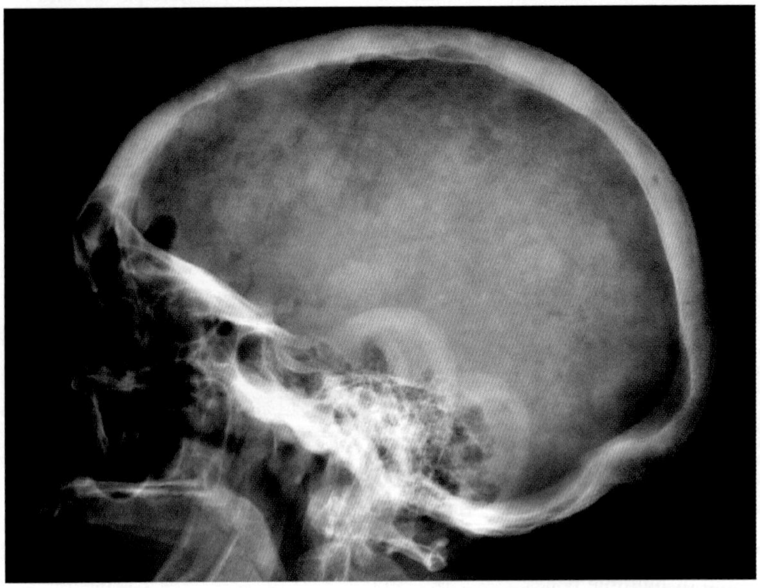

Cotton wool skull in mixed- phase Paget disease: There are cloud-like regions of patchy sclerosis throughout the calvarium.
Note the thickened calvarial cortex, which is a generalized feature of Paget disease.
佩吉特病混合期的*棉絮状颅骨*:
颅骨可见云状的斑片状硬化。
注意,颅骨皮质增厚,这是佩吉特病的普遍特征。

- **Paget of the vertebral bodies**: The mixed phase (phase Ⅱ) can produce either the classic *picture frame* vertebral body (with increased density of the periphery of the vertebral body, as opposed to the *rugger jersey spine* of renal osteodystrophy, which features sclerosis of just the superior and inferior endplates) or an ivory (diffusely sclerotic) vertebral body.

- **椎体佩吉特病**:混合期(第二阶段)可以出现典型的*画框样椎体*(椎体边缘密度增高,与肾性骨病的*脊柱橄榄球衣征*不同,后者只是以上、下终板硬化为特征)或象牙椎(弥漫性骨质硬化)。

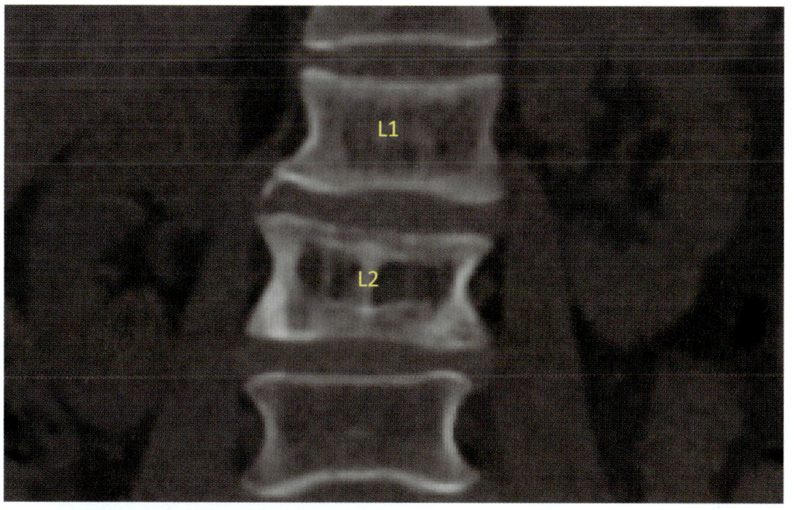

Picture frame vertebral body in mixed-phase Paget disease: There is cortical thickening of the periphery of the entire L2 (and to a lesser extent L1) vertebral body.
佩吉特病混合期的画框样椎体：
整个L_2椎体四周的皮质增厚(L_1椎体程度较轻)。

- **Paget of the pelvis:** When Paget disease involves the pelvis, the typical appearance is asymmetric coarsened trabecular thickening, with thickening of the iliopectineal and ilioischial lines. Acetabular protrusio may result.

- **骨盆佩吉特病：**当佩吉特病累及骨盆时，典型的表现是非对称性骨小梁不规则增粗，伴有髂耻线和髂坐线增粗。可能导致髋臼突出。

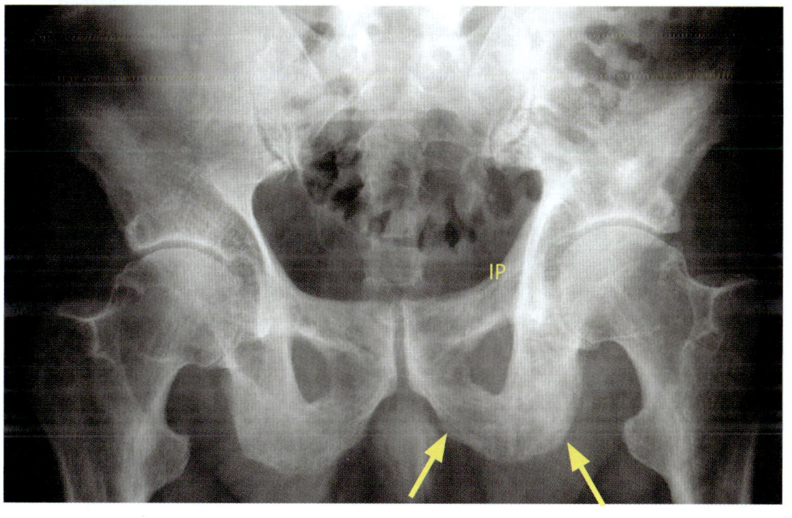

Paget disease of the pelvis:
There is asymmetric cortical and trabecular thickening and coarsening predominantly involving the left ischium (arrow).
Note the thickening of the iliopectineal line (IP).
骨盆佩吉特病：
不对称骨皮质和骨小梁增厚与变粗，主要累及左侧坐骨(箭)。
注意增厚的髂骨线(IP)。

- **Paget of the long bones**: The lytic phase (phase Ⅰ) progresses from the proximal articular end of bone into the diaphysis with a sharply marginated border. This border has been called the *blade of grass* or *flame-shaped margin* and allows differentiation from a neoplasm. As Paget disease progresses through its phases, it may cause bowing of the long bones and coxa vara deformity of the proximal femur.

- **长骨佩吉特病：**溶骨期(第一阶段)是从长骨近端的关节端开始逐渐累及长骨骨干，并形成清晰的边界。这种病灶边界被称为草叶或火焰状边缘，可与肿瘤相区别。随着第一阶段佩吉特病进展结束，可出现长骨骨干弯曲和近端股骨的髋内翻畸形。

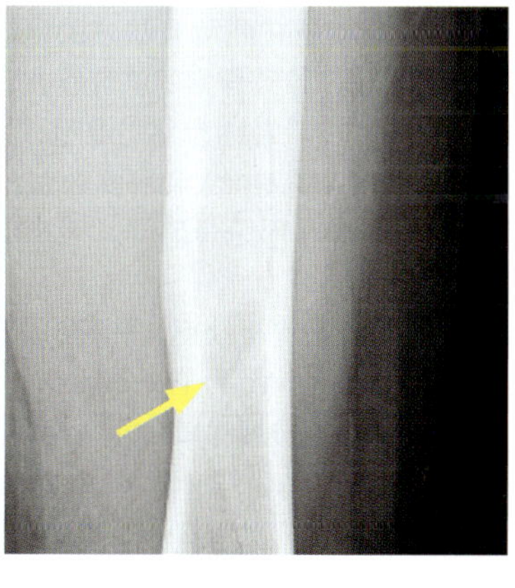

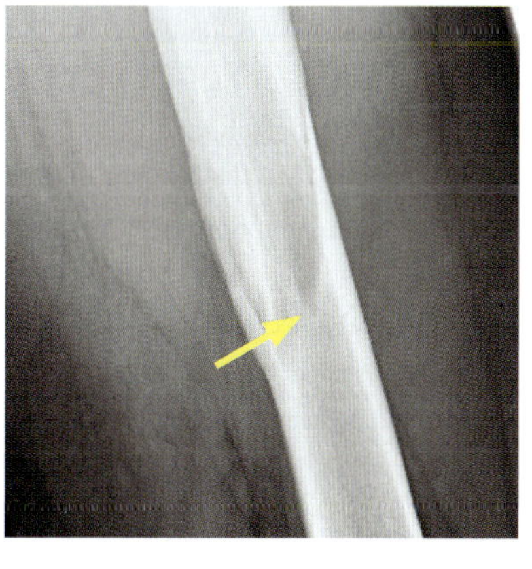

Blade of grass appearance of the lytic phase of Paget disease, as it progresses from proximal to distal:
Frontal and lateral radiographs of the femur demonstrate a "flame-shaped" margin (arrows) of a lytic lesion progressing distally.
佩吉特病溶骨期的草叶样表现，由近向远扩展：股骨正位和侧位X线影像显示"火焰状"边缘(箭)，为向远端进展时出现的溶骨性病变。

Hereditary hyperphosphatasia (juvenile Paget)

- Hereditary hyperphosphatasia, also called juvenile Paget disease, is an autosomal recessive disease of infants and young children. There is cortical thickening, trabecular thickening, osteopenia, and bowing of all bones in the body, resulting in severe deformity.
- Aside from the young age of the patients and diffuse involvement, the radiography of juvenile Paget otherwise appears very similar to adult Paget disease. There may be sparing of the articular ends of bones (epiphyseal sparing) in juvenile Paget disease.

Osteopetrosis

遗传性高磷酸酶症(青少年佩吉特病)

- 遗传性高磷酸酶症，也称青少年佩吉特病，是一种婴幼儿和青少年的常染色体隐性遗传性疾病。表现为骨皮质增粗、骨小梁增厚、骨量减少和全身骨骼变形，导致严重畸形。
- 除患者年龄小及病变范围广外，青少年佩吉特病的X线影像学表现与成人佩吉特病非常相似。在青少年佩吉特病中，长骨两端的关节可不受侵犯(骨骺完好)。

骨硬化症

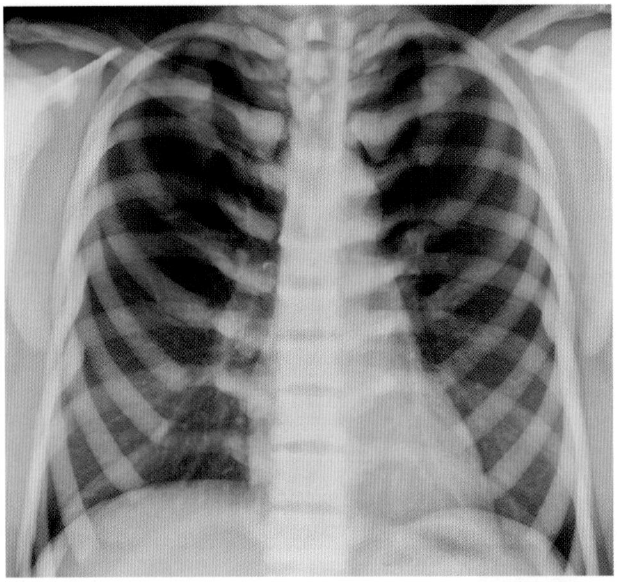

Osteopetrosis: Chest radiograph shows dramatic sclerosis of all the visualized bones in the thorax.

骨硬化症：胸部X线影像显示胸部所有骨骼明显的骨质硬化。

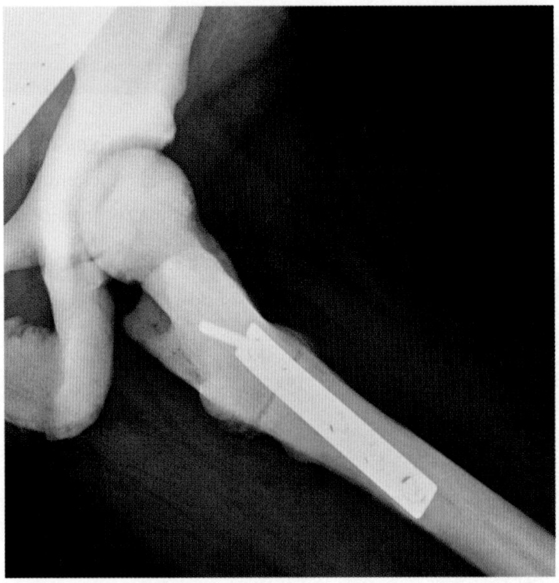

Radiograph of the femur in the same patient shows a fracture of the proximal femur, status post ORIF.

同一名患者的股骨X线影像显示一处股骨近端骨折，已进行切开复位内固定术。

- Osteopetrosis is an extremely rare deficiency of osteoclastic carbonic anhydrase, which leads to inability of osteoclasts to resorb bone.
- Osteopetrosis is characterized by diffuse, marked sclerosis of the entire skeleton. The bones are extremely brittle, which typically leads to multiple fractures.
- The vertebral bodies may have a *sandwich* or *rugger jersey* appearance similar to renal osteodystrophy, but diffuse bony sclerosis is more marked in osteopetrosis.

Gaucher disease

- Gaucher disease is caused by an autosomal recessive defect in glucocerebrosidase, leading to abnormal cerebroside deposition in altered macrophages called Gaucher cells. Gaucher cells cause bone infarctions, medullary expansion, and hepatosplenomegaly.
- The classic *Erlenmeyer flask* deformity of long bones is a result of abnormal modeling.
- Characteristic *H-shaped* vertebral bodies are due to endplate avascular necrosis.

  H-shaped vertebral bodies are not specific to Gaucher disease, which can be seen more commonly in sickle cell disease. The size of the spleen can differentiate between sickle cell and Gaucher disease: Sickle cell causes splenic auto-infarction, while patients with Gaucher disease have splenomegaly.

- 骨硬化症是一种罕见的破骨细胞碳酸酐酶缺乏的疾病，可导致破骨细胞无法吸收骨组织。
- 骨硬化症的特点是全身骨骼广泛而显著的硬化。骨骼极其脆弱，常导致多发性骨折。
- 椎体可能出现与肾性骨病相似的*三明治*或*橄榄球衣征*，但在骨硬化症中，骨组织的广泛硬化更为明显。

戈谢病

- 戈谢病是一种葡萄糖脑苷酯酶有缺陷的常染色体隐性遗传性疾病，导致异常的脑苷脂在变异的巨噬细胞中沉积，后者称为戈谢细胞。戈谢细胞引起骨梗死，骨髓腔扩大和肝脾肿大。
- 典型的长骨*锥形烧瓶*畸形是骨骼异常重塑的结果。
- 典型的*H形*椎体是因为终板缺血性坏死。

  H形椎体并不是戈谢病所特有，它更常见于镰状细胞病。脾的大小可以区分镰状细胞病和戈谢病：镰状细胞病可以导致脾的自发性梗死，而戈谢病的患者表现为脾大。

Hematologic bone disease

血液性骨病

Sickle cell disease

- Sickle cell disease is an autosomal recessive defect in the beta-chain of hemoglobin. Red cells are sickle-shaped and cause microvascular occlusion. The three osseous manifestations of sickle cell disease are bone infarcts, dramatically increased risk of osteomyelitis, and marrow expansion/hyperplasia.
- **Sickle cell bone infarcts**: Infarcts and avascular necrosis are caused by microvascular occlusion from the sickled red cells. Avascular necrosis of vertebral body endplates causes the characteristic *H-shaped* or *Lincoln-log* vertebral bodies. Other common locations for infarction include the femoral heads and the diaphyses and metaphyses of long bones.

镰状细胞病

- 镰状细胞病是一种血红蛋白β链缺陷的常染色体隐性疾病。红细胞呈镰刀状，而导致微血管堵塞。镰状细胞病在骨骼的三种表现是骨梗死、骨髓炎风险明显增高和骨髓扩张/增生。
- **镰状细胞性骨梗死：**骨梗死和缺血性坏死是由镰刀状红细胞堵塞微血管所致。椎体终板缺血性坏死导致典型的H形椎体或林肯积木样椎体。其他常见的梗死部位包括股骨头、长骨干及干骺端。

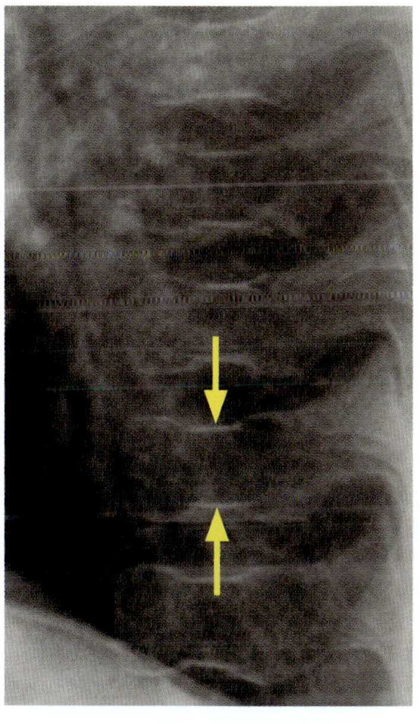

H-shaped vertebral bodies: Lateral thoracic spine radiograph shows characteristic central endplate depressions of the vertebral bodies (arrows) representing vertebral body avascular necrosis.

H形椎体：胸椎侧位X线影像显示典型的椎体中央终板的压缩(箭)，代表椎体缺血性坏死。

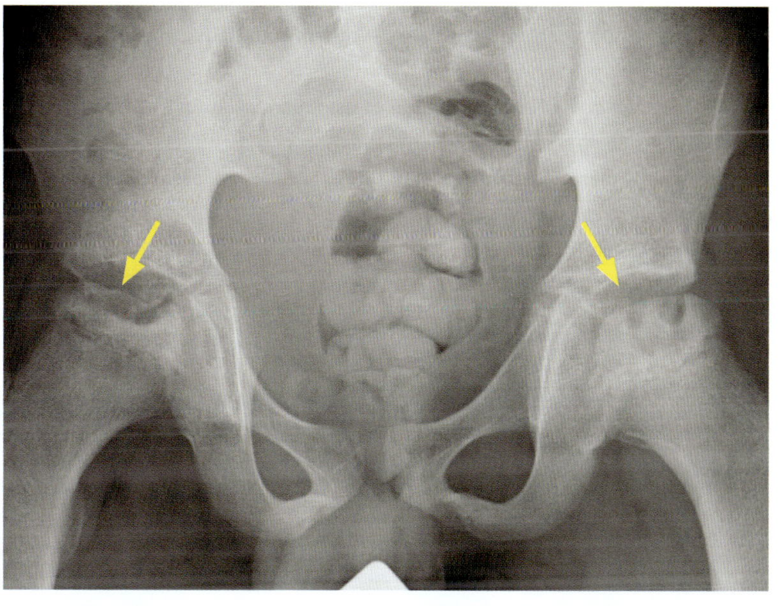

Bilateral femoral head avascular necrosis: Frontal pelvic radiograph in a skeletally immature patient with sickle cell anemia shows marked flattening and sclerosis of both femoral heads (arrows), representing advanced (Ficat stage Ⅳ) avascular necrosis. The Ficat staging of avascular necrosis is subsequently discussed.

双侧股骨头缺血性坏死：一名未成年镰状细胞贫血的患者骨盆正位X线影像显示双侧股骨头明显扁平和硬化(箭)，代表晚期(Ficat Ⅳ期)缺血性坏死。缺血性坏死的Ficat分期将在之后章节讨论。

- In advanced sickle cell, patchy sclerosis from multiple bone infarctions may become nearly confluent, producing diffusely sclerotic bones.
- **Sickle cell dactylitis** (also called hand-foot syndrome) is a special consideration in very young children who have persistent hematopoietic marrow in the digits of the hands and feet. Microvascular occlusion exacerbated by cold temperature causes dactylitis, which is evident on radiographs as soft-tissue swelling and periosteal reaction.
- **Sickle cell osteomyelitis**: Patients with sickle cell have an approximately 100x increased risk of osteomyelitis, most frequently with *Salmonella* species.
- **Sickle cell marrow expansion**: The radiographic findings of marrow expansion are more pronounced in thalassemia, but similar findings can be seen in sickle cell.

- 在镰状细胞病晚期，多发性梗死灶导致的片状硬化几乎会完全融合在一起，从而产生弥漫性骨质硬化。
- **镰状细胞指炎**(也称手-足综合征)是一种特发于婴幼儿中的疾病，表现为手指和脚趾骨髓持续造血。低温可加重微血管堵塞而导致指炎，其X线影像表现为软组织肿胀和骨膜反应。
- **镰状细胞性骨髓炎：**镰状细胞病患者患骨髓炎的风险约增加100倍，最常见的致病菌为沙门菌。
- **镰状细胞性骨髓腔扩张：**X线影像上骨髓扩张在地中海贫血中更明显，但是相似的表现也可见于镰状细胞病。

MRI of the bone marrow shows diffusely low signal on T1-weighted images, reflecting diffuse red (cellular) marrow.

In the long bones, chronic stimulation of red cell production causes widening of the medullary spaces and coarsening of the trabeculae, which results in osteopenia and increased risk of insufficiency fracture.

In the skull, marrow expansion can cause *hair-on-end* striations and widening of the medullary cavity.

Involvement of the facial bones and extramedullary hematopoiesis are seen more commonly in thalassemia.

骨髓在MRI T_1加权图像上表现为弥漫性低信号，代表弥漫的红(细胞性)骨髓。

长骨中，红细胞生成的慢性刺激导致骨髓腔增宽和骨小梁增粗，最终导致骨量减少和不全骨折的风险增高。

在颅骨，骨髓扩张可导致竖发样条纹和髓腔增宽。

颌面骨受累和髓外造血更常见于地中海贫血。

Thalassemia

- Thalassemia is an autosomal recessive congenital anemia that is caused by a defect in the alpha or beta hemoglobin subunits.
- Similar to sickle cell disease, the osseous hallmarks of thalassemia are bone infarcts, marrow hyperplasia, and infection. However, in contrast to sickle cell, the marrow expansion is much more prominent as the anemia can be more severe.
- In the hand, marrow expansion can cause widening and squaring of the phalanges and metacarpals.
- In the skull, the *hair-on-end* striations are a classic manifestation of marrow expansion.
- In the facial bones, marrow expansion may obliterate the paranasal sinuses, causing the typical *rodent-like facies*.
- In the long bones, the marrow expansion may cause an *Erlenmeyer flask deformity*.

地中海贫血

- 地中海贫血是一种由血红蛋白亚基 α 或 β 链缺陷导致的常染色体隐性先天性贫血病。
- 与镰状细胞病类似，地中海贫血典型的骨骼表现是骨梗死、骨髓增生和感染。但是，地中海贫血较镰状细胞病的骨髓扩张更为明显，因其贫血更为严重。
- 在手部，骨髓扩张可导致指骨和掌骨的增宽和变方。
- 在颅骨，竖发样条纹是骨髓扩张的典型表现。
- 在颌面骨，骨髓扩张可能导致鼻旁窦消失，导致典型的鼠面征。
- 在长骨，骨髓扩张可能导致锥形瓶畸形。

Myelofibrosis

骨髓纤维变性

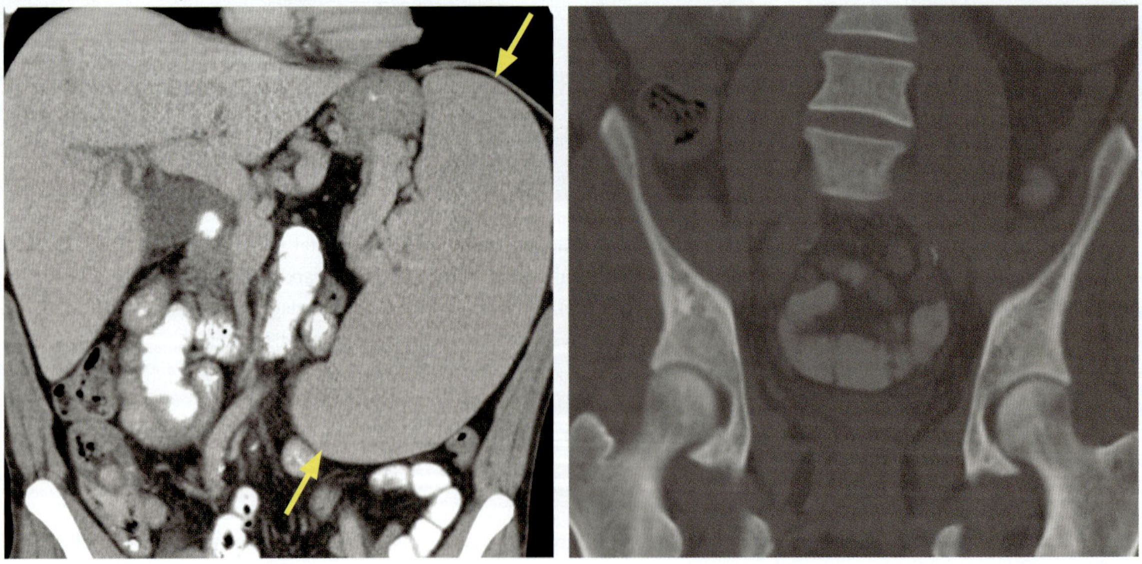

Myelofibrosis: Coronal CT in soft-tissue (left image) and bone windows show splenomegaly (arrows) and diffusely dense bones.
骨髓纤维化：冠状位CT软组织窗(左图)和骨窗显示脾大(箭)和弥漫性骨密度增高。

- Myelofibrosis is progressive fibrosis of bone marrow in older patients, leading to anemia and splenomegaly. Bone marrow fibrosis leads to diffusely sclerotic bones.

- 骨髓纤维变性是发生在老年人的进行性骨髓纤维化，导致贫血和脾大。骨髓纤维变性导致弥漫性骨质硬化。

Mastocytosis

- Mastocytosis is abnormal proliferation of mast cells. It may result in either diffuse or patchy sclerosis from the reaction of the marrow to the infiltrating mast cells.

肥大细胞增生症

- 肥大细胞增生症是肥大细胞的异常增生。它可能是骨髓对侵入的肥大细胞反应，可导致弥漫性或斑片样的骨质硬化。

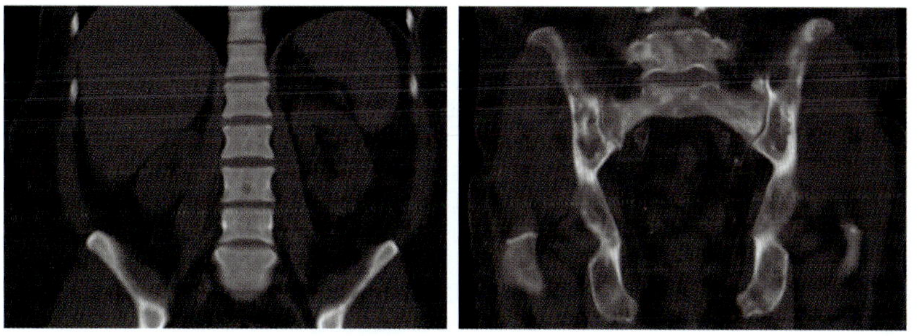

Two patients with mastocytosis: Coronal CT images in two different patients demonstrate the variable imaging appearance of mastocytosis. The left image shows a diffusely sclerotic appearance of the bones and the right image shows patchy sclerosis.
两名肥大细胞增多症患者：冠状位CT图像显示肥大细胞增多症多变的影像学表现。左图显示弥漫性骨质硬化，右图显示斑片状骨质硬化。

（翻译　杨曦玥　赵又瑾）

DIFFERENTIAL DIAGNOSIS OF COMMON BONE LESIONS

常见骨骼疾病的鉴别诊断

Diffusely dense (sclerotic) bones
弥漫性骨密度增高(硬化)

- *Radiographic signs of secondary hyperPTH?* 继发性甲状旁腺功能亢进的放射影像征象？ → **Renal osteodystrophy 肾性骨病**
- *Small calcified spleen?* 钙化的小脾脏 → **Sickle cell disease 镰状细胞病**
- *Splenomegaly?* 脾大？ → **Myelofibrosis 骨髓纤维化**
- *Predominantly affecting the axial skeleton?* 中轴骨受累为主？ → **Diffuse osteoblastic metastases 弥漫性成骨性转移**
- *Pathologic fractures?* 病理性骨折？ → **Osteopetrosis 骨硬化症**
- Others 其他 →
  - **Pyknodysostosis 致密性成骨不全症**
  - **Mastocytosis 肥大细胞增生症**
  - **Fluorosis 氟中毒**
  - **Normal variant-Athlete 正常的运动员变异**

Ivory (diffusely sclerotic) vertebral body
象牙椎(椎体弥漫性硬化)

- *History of prostate or breast cancer?* 前列腺癌或乳腺癌病史？ → **Osteoblastic metastasis 成骨性转移瘤**
- *Expansion of the vertebral body?* 椎体膨大？ → **Paget disease 佩吉特病**
- *Paraspinal soft-tissue mass?* 椎旁软组织肿块？ → **Lymphoma 淋巴瘤**

Lucent epiphyseal (and epiphyseal equivalent) lesion
epiphyseal equivalents include apophyses, patella, carpal bones, and calcaneus.
透亮性骨骺(及骨骺类似骨)病灶
骨骺类似骨包括骨突、髌骨、腕骨、跟骨

mnemonic: GEIChA
记忆口诀：GEIChA

- *Epiphysis closed? Eccentric? Abuts articular surface?* 骨骺闭合？偏心性？紧邻关节表面？ → **Giant cell tumor 骨巨细胞瘤**
- *Under age 30?* 小于30岁？ → **Eosinophilic granuloma 嗜酸性肉芽肿**
- Epiphysis closed?(more likely to be metaphyseal if the physes are still open) 骨骺闭合？（如骨骺未闭合则易出现在干骺端） → **Infection 感染**
- *Eccentric?* 偏心性？ → **Chondroblastoma 软骨母细胞瘤**
- *Expansile?* 膨胀性？ → **Aneurysmal bone cyst 动脉瘤样骨囊肿**

Expansile or lytic rib lesion
膨胀性或溶骨性肋骨病变

mnemonic: FAMEB
记忆口诀：*FAMEB*

- *Ground-glass matrix?* 磨玻璃样基质？ → **Fibrous dysplasia 骨纤维异常增殖症**
- *Expansile?* 膨胀性？ → **Aneurysmal bone cyst 动脉瘤样骨囊肿**
- *Soft tissue component?* 软组织成分？ → **Metastasis/Multiple myeloma/Plasmacytoma 转移瘤/多发性骨髓瘤/浆细胞瘤**
- *Chondroid matrix?* 软骨基质？ → **Enchondroma 内生软骨瘤**
- *Radiographic signs of secondary hyperPTH?* 继发性甲状旁腺功能亢进的放射影像征象？ → **Brown tumor 棕色瘤**

（翻译　姚骊　吕霞飞）

BASICS OF TRAUMA

外伤概要

TRAUMATIC FRACTURES

外伤性骨折

Terminology

术语

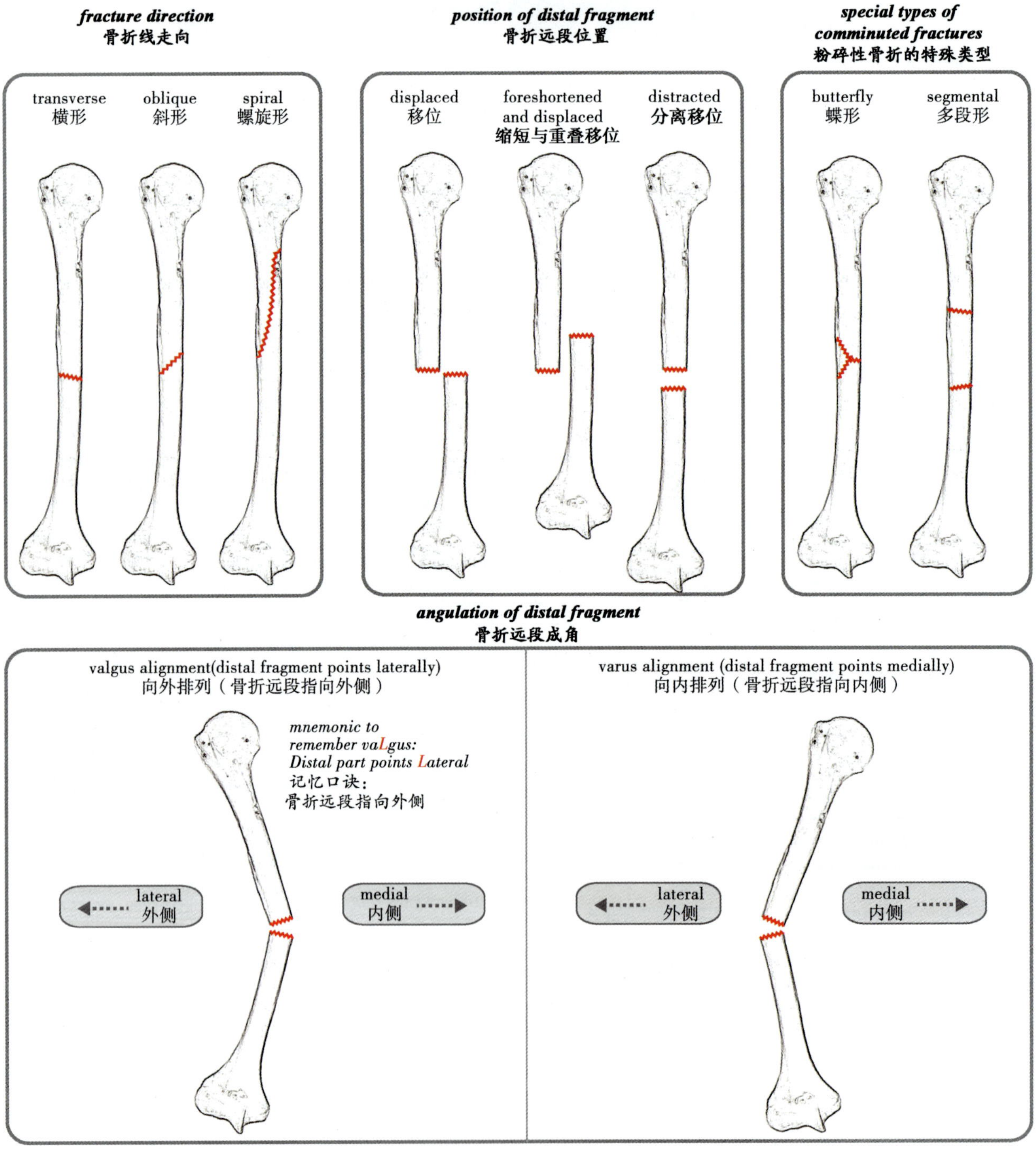

- When describing a long-bone fracture, the fracture location (proximal, mid-shaft, distal), direction of fracture, angulation, and position of the distal segment should be described.
- A comminuted fracture is defined as >2 fracture fragments.
- It is essential to mention if a fracture extends to the articular surface of a joint.

- 当描述长骨骨折时，需要描述骨折部位(近段、中段、远段)、骨折线走向、成角和骨折远段指向。
- 粉碎性骨折为骨折碎片大于2块。
- 必须要描述骨折线是否累及关节面。

（翻译　刘进　吕霞飞）

Atraumatic Fractures

- Atraumatic fractures are bone injury caused by a mechanism other than a single traumatic episode. Atraumatic fractures may be due to underlying abnormal bone (as in insufficiency fracture, atypical fracture, or pathologic fracture), or the bone may be normal (as seen in fatigue fracture).
- **Fragility fractures** are traumatic fractures in an elderly patient with osteoporosis (and often sarcopenia), caused by a low-velocity mechanism that would not normally be expected to cause fracture in a patient with normal bone mineral density or muscle mass.

非创伤性骨折

- 非创伤性骨折是指并非由单一创伤机制造成的骨损伤。非创伤性骨折可能发生在有潜在异常的骨骼(如不全性骨折、非典型骨折或病理性骨折),也可以发生在正常骨质(如疲劳性骨折)。
- **脆性骨折**是发生在老年骨质疏松症(常伴有肌肉减少症)患者中的创伤性骨折,这种低速、微弱的外力通常在骨密度或肌肉量正常的患者中不会导致骨折。

Terminology of Atraumatic Fractures

Stress fracture: Terminology

非创伤性骨折术语

应力性骨折:术语

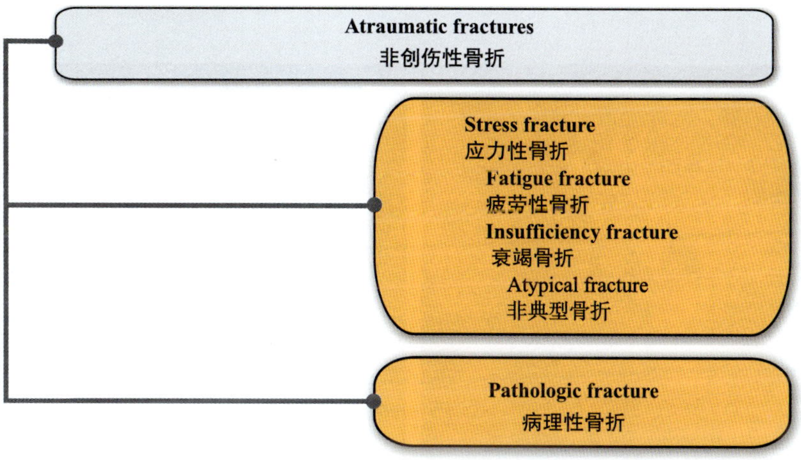

- By strict definition, the term **stress fracture** encompasses both **fatigue fractures** and **insufficiency fractures**. These are fractures due to summation of repetitive forces, which overwhelm the bone remodeling pathway.

  A **fatigue fracture** is injury of a normal bone caused by repetitive submaximal force, often described with the maxim "abnormal stress on normal bone."

  An **insufficiency fracture** is injury of an abnormal bone, weakened through a metabolic process (most commonly but not necessary osteoporosis). In other words, "normal stress on abnormal bone."
- The above terminology is often confusing. Clinically, the term *stress fracture* is usually considered synonymous with *fatigue fracture*. Also, there is substantial clinical and imaging overlap between fatigue and insufficiency fractures, and there is no clear cutoff between "normal" and "abnormal" stress or "normal" and "abnormal" bones. For these reasons, the term *fatigue fracture* is not commonly used. This text will use *stress fracture* and *fatigue fracture* synonymously to be consistent with the majority of the literature. However, the term *insufficiency fracture* is usually reserved for older individuals.
- The term *bone stress injury* refers to the spectrum of injury seen in stress fractures. This is subsequently discussed and may range from periosteal reaction in early stages, bone marrow edema in mid-grade injuries, to cortical fracture in more advanced stages.

- 从严格的定义来看,**应力性骨折**包括**疲劳性骨折**和**衰竭骨折**。这些骨折是由于重复的外力作用,破坏了骨重塑途径。

  疲劳性骨折是重复外力在正常骨引起的损伤,而该外力单次作用于骨骼不会引起骨折,常被描述为"正常骨受到异常应力导致的损伤"。

  衰竭骨折是异常骨骼的损伤,这些骨骼的异常由一些代谢原因(最常见的是骨质疏松,也有其他原因)导致。换句话说,"异常骨在正常应力下发生的损伤"。
- 上述术语经常令人混淆。临床上,*应力性骨折*通常被认为是*疲劳性骨折*的同义词。此外,疲劳性骨折和衰竭骨折之间也存在许多临床和影像学的重叠,"正常"和"异常"的应力、"正常"和"异常"的骨之间并没有明确的界限。由于这些原因,*疲劳性骨折*这个术语并不常用。为了与大多数文献保持一致,本文将*应力性骨折*与*疲劳性骨折*当作等同概念。然而,*衰竭骨折*通常仅用于老年患者。
- *骨应力损伤*是指应力性骨折中的一系列损伤改变。随后将对其进行讨论,骨应力损伤范围可以从早期损伤的骨膜反应,中度损伤的

- An **atypical fracture** is a special type of insufficiency fracture, only occurring in the lateral cortex of the proximal-to-mid femur, subsequently discussed.

Pathologic fracture: Definition

- A pathologic fracture is a fracture through a focal lesion. The lesion is most commonly a neoplasm (may be benign or malignant), or less commonly through a region of osteomyelitis.

骨髓水肿，到更严重的皮质骨折。

- **非典型骨折**是一种特殊类型的衰竭骨折，只发生在股骨近-中端的外侧骨皮质，随后将进行讨论。

病理性骨折

- 病理性骨折是指发生在骨局灶性病变中的骨折。最常见的病变是肿瘤(可以是良性或恶性)，或较少见的骨髓炎。

（翻译　刘进　吕霞飞）

Basics of MRI

磁共振基础

Tendons

- A normal tendon is dark on all MRI sequences.

Magic angle artifact

肌腱

- 正常肌腱在所有MRI序列上均为低信号。

魔角伪影

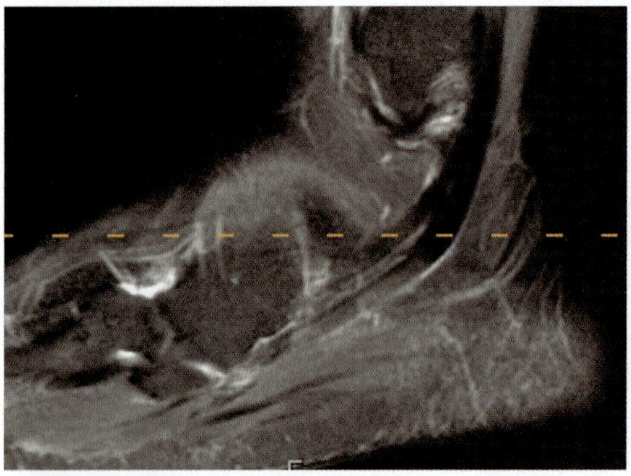

Sagittal STIR MRI
矢状位STIR MRI

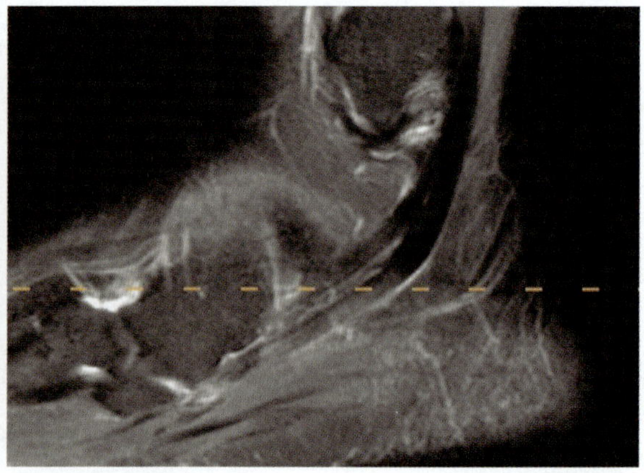

Sagittal STIR MRI
矢状位STIR MRI

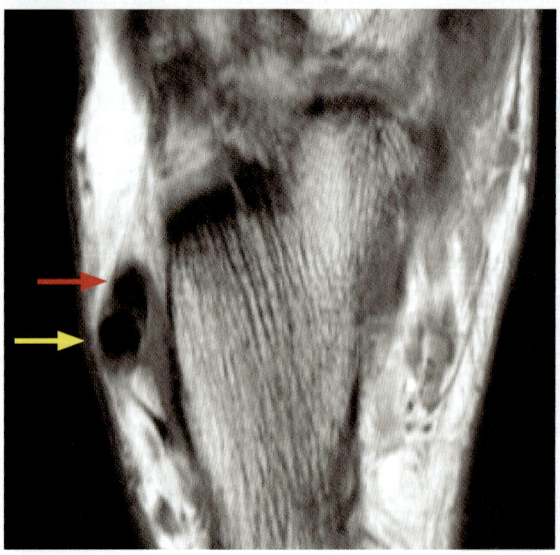

Axial PD-weighted MRI
轴位PD加权MRI

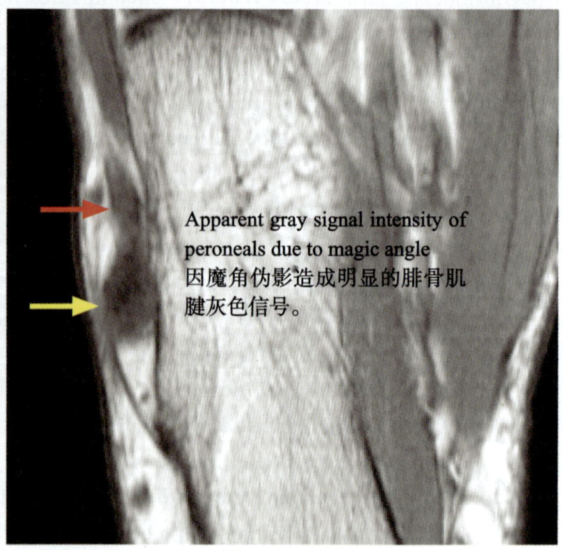

Axial PD-weighted MRI (slightly more caudal)
轴位PD加权MRI(稍靠足底方向)

Magic angle artifact: Note the normal low signal intensity of the peroneus longus (yellow arrows) and peroneus brevis (red arrows) tendons on the left-most axial PD image, corresponding to the level indicated by the dashed orange line in the sagittal STIR image directly above. An image slightly lower (right images) shows apparent "gray" or intermediate signal intensity due to magic angle artifact.
魔角伪影：注意，最左侧轴位PD图像上的腓骨长肌肌腱(黄箭)和腓骨短肌肌腱(红箭)显示为正常低信号，对应上图矢状位STIR序列图像橘色虚线层面。因魔角伪影，在稍低层面图像(右图)中腓骨长短肌肌腱显示为"灰色"或中等信号。

- A normal tendon may have artifactually increased signal due to the magic angle phenomenon. Because tendons have fibers coursing along a single direction (demonstrating anisotropy), tendons may demonstrate artifactually increased signal on short TE sequences when oriented 55 degrees relative to the bore of the magnet. This phenomenon is called the magic angle artifact.

  Short TE sequences include T1-weighted and proton density images.

  T2-weighted sequences are less susceptible to the magic angle artifact.

  Unlike true tendon pathology, the magic angle artifact disappears with a long TE and the tendon will otherwise have a normal morphology.

- 正常肌腱可因魔角现象而出现人为信号增高。因为肌腱的纤维是沿单一方向走行(即各向异性)，当肌腱走行方向与主磁场轴成55°时，肌腱在短TE序列上可出现人为信号增高。该现象称为魔角伪影。

  短TE序列包括T_1加权像、质子密度加权像。

  T_2加权序列通常不易产生魔角伪影。

  不同于真正的肌腱病变，魔角伪影在长TE序列上消失，而肌腱本身形态正常。

Tenosynovitis

腱鞘滑膜炎

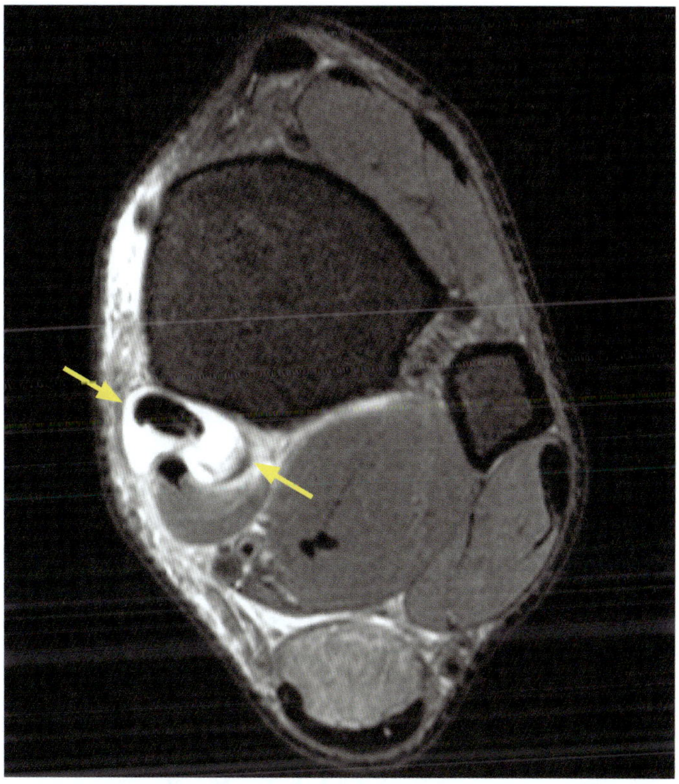

Tenosynovitis:
Large amount of fluid (arrows) circumferentially surrounds the posterior tibial tendon on this axial T2-weighted MRI with fat suppression.

腱鞘滑膜炎：
轴位T_2加权脂肪抑制MRI显示胫骨后肌腱周围积聚大量液体(箭)。

- Tenosynovitis is inflammation surrounding a tendon. Tenosynovitis may be secondary to repetitive motion, inflammatory arthritis, or infection.
- On MRI, fluid completely surrounds the tendon circumferentially
- A potential pitfall is that fluid can track along tendon sheaths that communicate directly with an adjacent joint (such as the long head of the biceps tendon in the shoulder or the flexor hallucis longus tendon in the ankle). This should not be confused with tenosynovitis, unless the degree of tenosynovial fluid is out of proportion to a relatively smaller amount of joint fluid.
- A variant form, called stenosing tenosynovitis, features several loculated collections of fluid in the tendon sheath.

  Stenosing tenosynovitis can be seen surrounding the flexor hallucis longus tendon at the medial ankle in os trigonum syndrome and about the wrist in de Quervain's stenosing tenosynovitis.

- 腱鞘滑膜炎是炎症围绕肌腱。腱鞘滑膜炎可能继发于反复的运动、炎性关节炎或感染。
- 在MRI上，肌腱周围完全被液体包绕。
- 一个容易误诊的情况是液体沿腱鞘与邻近关节直接相通(如肩部肱二头肌长头肌腱或踝部长屈肌肌腱)。这种情况不应该与腱鞘滑膜炎相混淆，除非腱鞘内的液体量与较少的关节内液体不成比例。
- 有一种变异称为狭窄性腱鞘滑膜炎，它以腱鞘内数个包裹性积液为特征。

  狭窄性腱鞘滑膜炎可见于三角籽骨综合征的内踝长肌屈肌肌腱周围及桡骨茎突狭窄性腱鞘炎(de Quervain病)的腕部周围。

Myxoid degeneration (tendinosis)

- Aging or overuse often leads to myxoid degeneration, which is clinically synonymous with tendinitis, tendinopathy, and tendinosis.

  The word *tendinitis* should not be used as myxoid degeneration is not due to inflammation.

黏液样变性(肌腱炎)

- 年龄增长或运动过度常出现黏液样变性，临床上与肌腱炎、肌腱病或肌腱变性为同义词。

  不应使用肌腱炎一词，因为黏液样变性不是由于炎症所引起。

- MRI will show intermediate intra-substance (within the tendon) signal on both T1- and T2-weighted images. The tendon may be either normal or enlarged. These findings are nonspecific and can be seen in both myxoid degeneration and partial tear. These two entities often coexist and imaging cannot distinguish between the two.

Tendon tear

- A partial tendon tear represents incomplete disruption of the fibers and can have a varied MRI appearance. The tendon may be thickened, thinned, or contain intra-substance fluid.
- A full-thickness, full-width disruption of the tendon will appear as complete discontinuity of the tendon. There is often retraction of the tendon remnants.

- 在T_1加权和T_2加权MRI图像上均表现为实质内(肌腱内)的中等信号。肌腱大小可以正常或增大。这些特征是非特异性的,可见于黏液样变性或肌腱部分撕裂,且这两种情况常同时存在,在影像学上无法加以鉴别。

肌腱撕裂

- 肌腱部分撕裂表现为肌腱纤维断裂不完全,在MRI上可有多种不同的表现。肌腱可以增厚、变薄或出现肌腱内积液。
- 肌腱全层、全宽度撕裂表现为肌腱的连续性中断。肌腱残端常有回缩。

(翻译　姚骊　吕霞飞)

FOOT AND ANKLE

足和踝

FOREFOOT

前足

Anatomy (blue) and overview of common fractures (red)

解剖(蓝色)和常见骨折概述(红色)

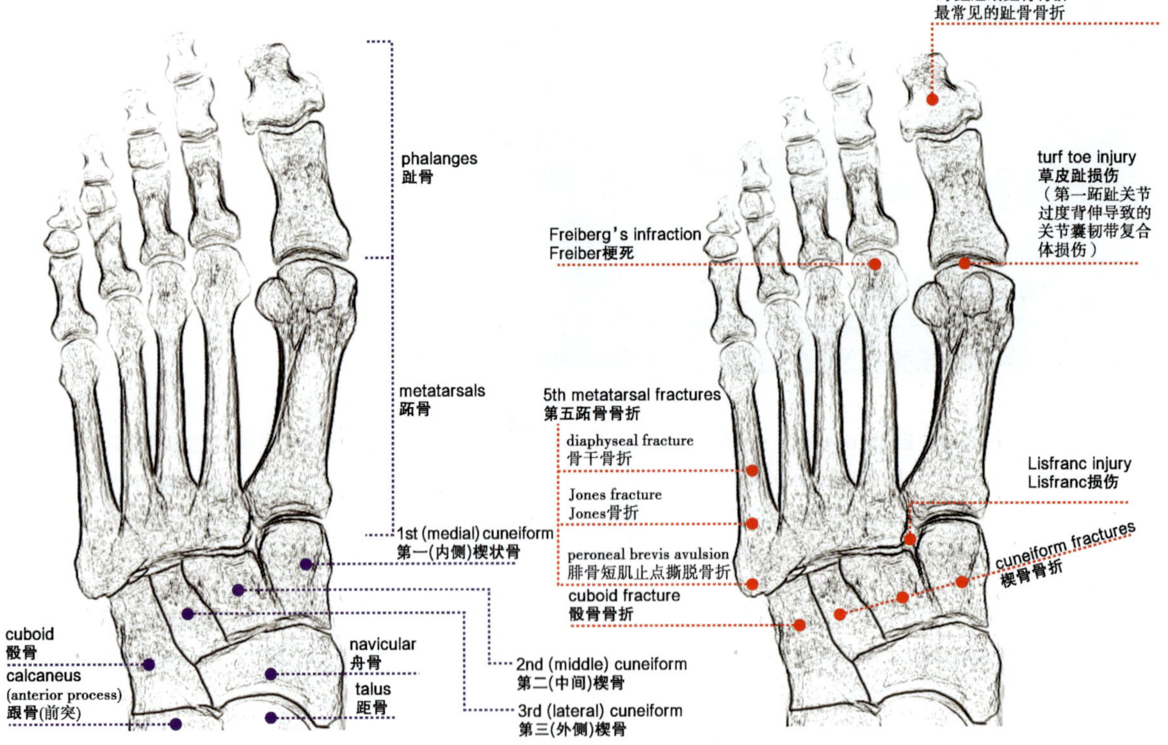

Proximal fifth metatarsal fracture

第五跖骨近端骨折

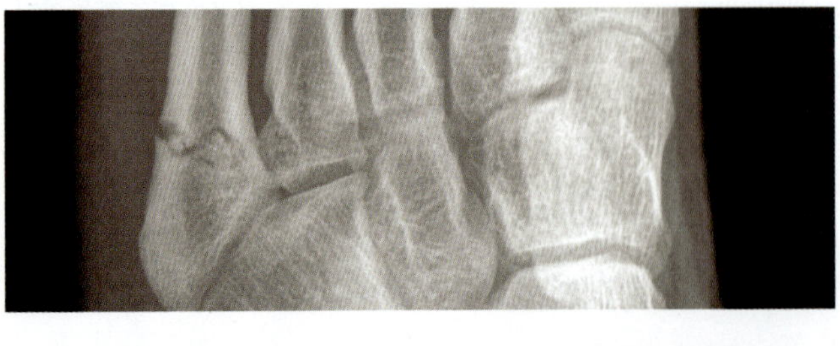

Jones (zone 2) proximal fifth metatarsal fracture: Frontal radiograph demonstrates a minimally displaced fracture at the metaphyseal-diaphyseal junction.

Jones(2区)第五跖骨近端骨折:正位X线影像显示一处轻微的干骺端-骨干交界处移位性骨折。

- Metatarsal base avulsion (zone 1) is a fracture at the most proximal base of the fifth metatarsal.

  Treatment is conservative, with a boot.

  The peroneus brevis and lateral aspect of the plantar aponeurosis attach at the fifth metatarsal base.
- Jones fracture (zone 2) is a fracture of the metaphyseal-diaphyseal junction.

  A Jones fracture carries a worse prognosis compared to an avulsion fracture due to reduced blood supply at the metaphyseal-diaphyseal junction. Treatment is variable and may require surgery.
- The metatarsal shaft (zone 3) is a common location for stress fracture.

- 跖骨基底部撕脱(1区)是第五跖骨最靠近基底部的骨折。

  采用保守治疗，穿石膏短靴。

  腓骨短肌腱和跖腱膜外份附着于第五跖骨基底部。
- Jones骨折(2区)是干骺端与骨干连接处的骨折。

  Jones骨折较撕脱性骨折的预后差，是由于干骺端与骨干连接处的血供减少。治疗方法有多种，可能需要手术。
- 跖骨干(3区)是应力性骨折的常见部位。

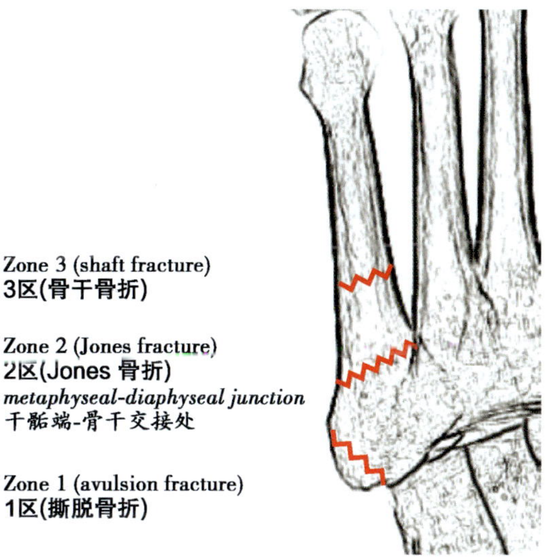

Freiberg's infraction

Freiberg梗死

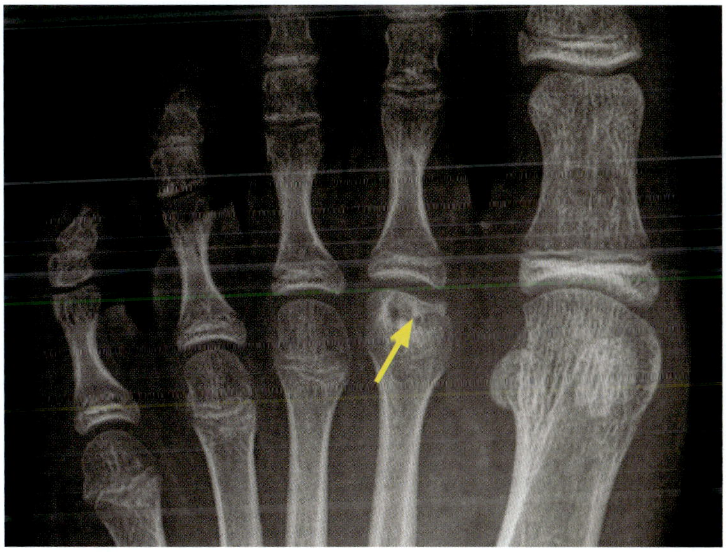

Freiberg's infraction:
Frontal radiograph demonstrates subchondral irregularity, sclerosis, and collapse of the head of the second metatarsal (arrow) in this skeletally immature child.

Freiberg梗死：
一名骨骼尚未发育成熟儿童的正位X线影像显示第二跖骨头(骺)软骨下不规则、硬化和塌陷。

- Freiberg's infraction is avascular necrosis of the second metatarsal head. It is caused by repetitive stress or poorly fitting shoes (such as high-heels) and usually occurs in young women.

- Freiberg梗死是第二跖骨头的缺血性坏死。它是由反复应力或不合脚的鞋(如高跟鞋)引起，通常发生在年轻女性。

Metatarsal stress fracture | 跖骨应力性骨折

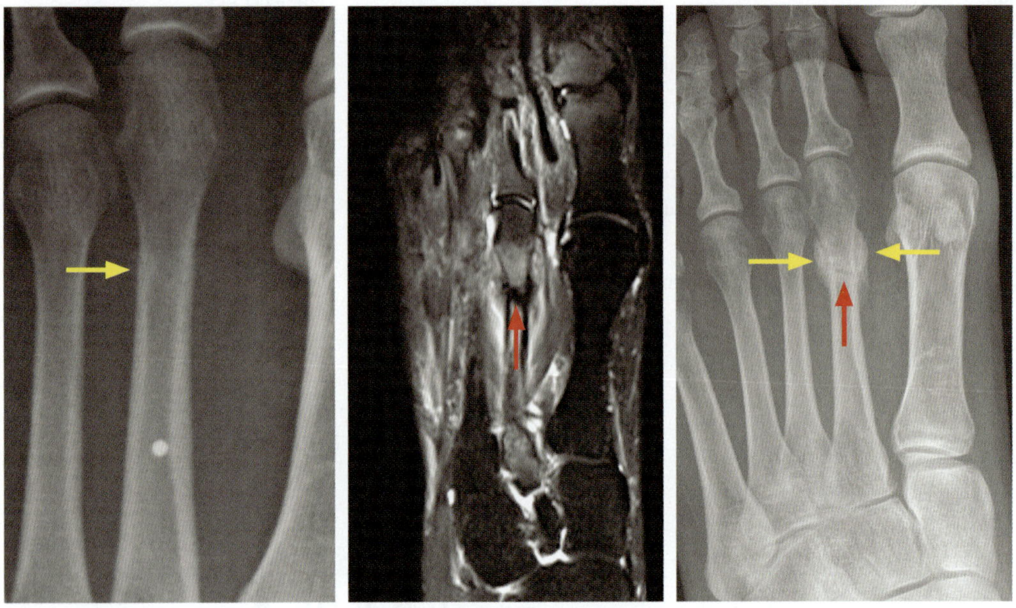

Initial radiograph
初始X线影像

Axial T2-weighted MRI with fat supp. obtained two weeks later
2周后的轴位T_2加权脂肪抑制MRI

Follow-up radiographs after MRI
MRI后的随访X线影像

Metatarsal stress fracture: Initial radiographs demonstrate extremely subtle periosteal reaction and endosteal thickening (yellow arrow) of the lateral cortex of the second metatarsal. MRI performed two weeks later demonstrated interval development of a fracture line (red arrow), with exuberant callus formation, intramedullary edema, and surrounding periosteal edema. Follow-up radiographs performed after the MRI demonstrate interval progressive healing with solid-appearing periosteal reaction (yellow arrows) but persistently evident fracture lucency (red arrow).
跖骨应力性骨折：初始X线影像显示第二跖骨外侧皮质很轻微的骨膜反应和骨内膜增厚(黄箭)。2周后的MRI显示骨折演变成一条骨折线(红箭)，伴大量骨痂组织形成、髓内水肿和骨膜周围水肿。MRI之后的X线影像随访显示进一步愈合，表现为实性的骨膜反应(黄箭)，但有持续而明显的低密度骨折影(红箭)。

- The first radiographic sign of a metatarsal stress fracture is a barely perceptible linear cortical lucency. Usually, stress fractures are not apparent on radiographs until periostitis and callus have begun to form.

- 跖骨应力性骨折最早的影像学表现是几乎无法察觉的骨皮质线状透亮影。通常情况下，应力性骨折在X线影像上表现并不明显，直到骨膜炎或骨痂开始形成。

Sesamoid fracture | 籽骨骨折

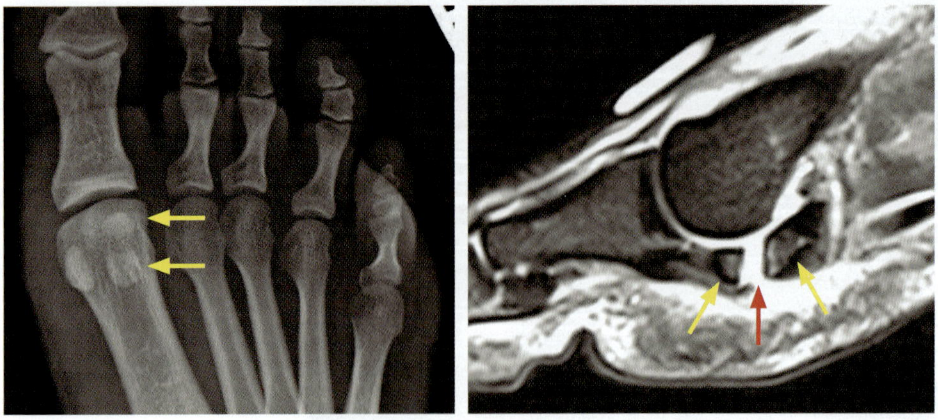

Fibular hallux sesamoid fracture:
Radiograph (left image) shows either a bipartite fibular (lateral) hallux sesamoid, versus a sesamoid fracture with slight distraction (arrows). MRI was performed, and sagittal PD-weighted MRI with fat suppression demonstrated an acute-appearing sesamoid fracture (note absence of cortication at the fracture margins) with distraction of the fragments (yellow arrows), tear of the inferior joint capsule (red arrow), and surrounding edema.
趾腓侧籽骨骨折：
X线影像(左图)显示二分趾腓侧籽骨(外侧)，或籽骨骨折伴轻度分离(箭)。矢状位脂肪抑制PD加权MRI显示急性籽骨骨折(注意骨折断端骨皮质缺失)，碎骨片分离(黄箭)，下关节囊撕裂(红箭)，以及周围软组织水肿。

- Fracture of the great toe sesamoid bones is typically caused by extreme hyperextension or dorsal dislocation (which may be transient) of the first metatarsophalangeal joint.

  The flexor hallucis brevis attaches to the sesamoids; the medial head attaches to the tibial (medial) sesamoid and the lateral head attaches to the fibular (lateral) sesamoid.
- A bipartite sesamoid is a normal variant that may simulate a sesamoid fracture; however, a bipartite sesamoid will be round in shape and its margins will be completely corticated. Additionally, the sum of the parts of the bipartite sesamoid will be larger in size than the other sesamoid.
- The term *turf toe* has been used to describe a wide range of injuries at the first MTP joint including sesamoid fracture. The anatomy of the great toe MTP is complex, but it is important to note that the flexor hallucis longus tendon courses plantar to and between the sesamoids.

- 趾籽骨骨折通常是由第一跖趾关节极度过伸或背侧脱位(可能是一过性的脱位)所引起。

  趾短屈肌附着于籽骨；内侧头附着于胫侧(内侧)籽骨，外侧头附着于腓侧(外侧)籽骨。
- 二分籽骨属于正常变异，可类似于籽骨骨折，但是，二分籽骨呈圆形，且边缘有完整的骨皮质。此外，二分籽骨的体积总和比其他籽骨大。
- 草皮趾这一术语是用来描述发生在第一跖趾关节的各种损伤，包括籽骨骨折。第一跖趾关节是一个复合解剖结构，需要特别注意的是，踇长屈肌腱行走于足底的籽骨之间。

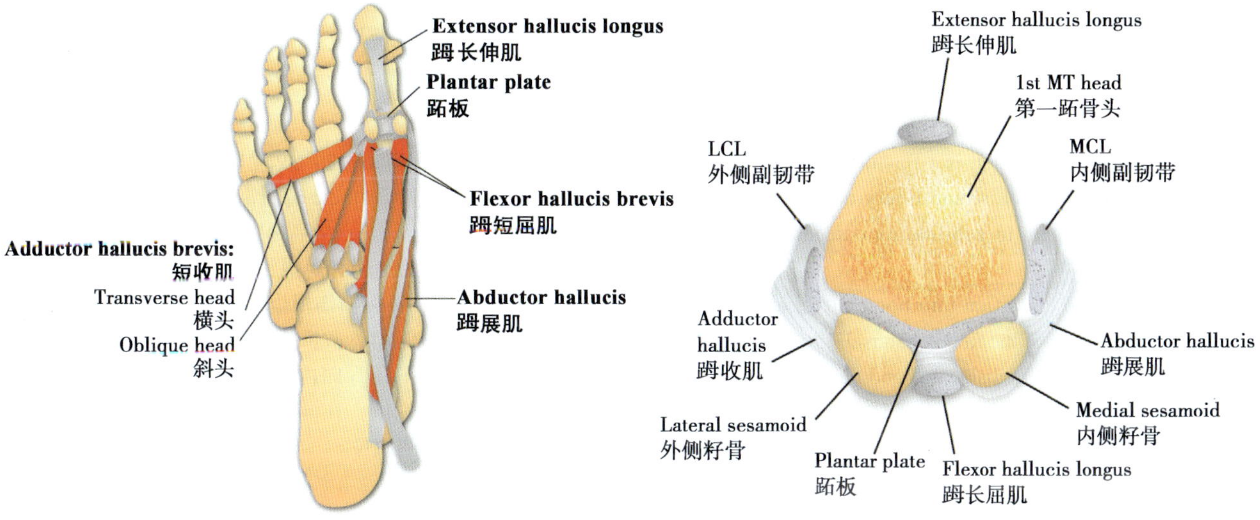

Anatomy of the great toe metatarsophalangeal (MTP) joint. LCL: Lateral collateral ligament; MCL: medial collateral ligament. *Illustrations by Luis Beltran, MD, Brigham and Women's Hospital.*
第一跖趾关节解剖。LCL：外侧副韧带；MCL：内侧副韧带。

Lisfranc fracture-dislocation

Lisfranc(跗跖关节)骨折-脱位

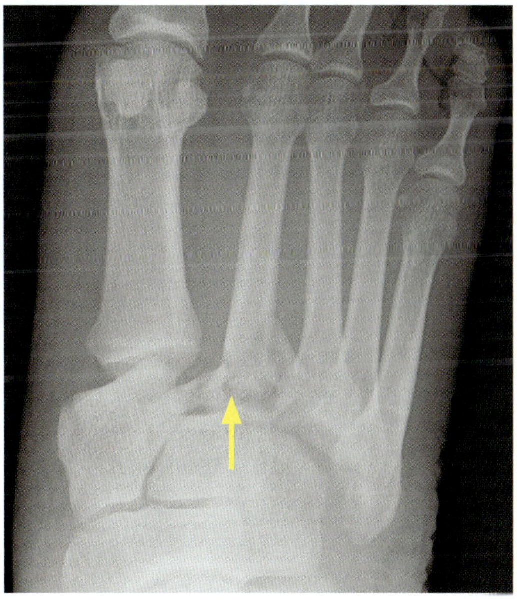

Frontal radiograph of the foot shows a homolateral dislocation at the Lisfranc joint, with fracture of the base of the second metatarsal (arrow).
足部正位X线影像显示第一～五跗跖关节(Lisfranc关节)全部向外侧脱位，并伴有第二跖骨根部骨折。

- The tarsometatarsal joint is the Lisfranc joint, named after the French surgeon in the Napoleonic wars who performed amputations at this joint. The stability of the joint depends on multiple ligaments, with the Lisfranc ligament being the most important. The Lisfranc ligament is an interosseous ligamentous complex attaching the medial cuneiform to the second metatarsal base.

- 跗跖关节又称Lisfranc关节，是以拿破仑战争时期一位法国外科医生的名字命名的，他为患者在这一关节实施了截肢术。跗跖关节的稳定性取决于多条韧带，其中Lisfranc韧带最为重要。Lisfranc韧带是骨间韧带复合体，附着于内侧楔骨和第二跖骨基底部。

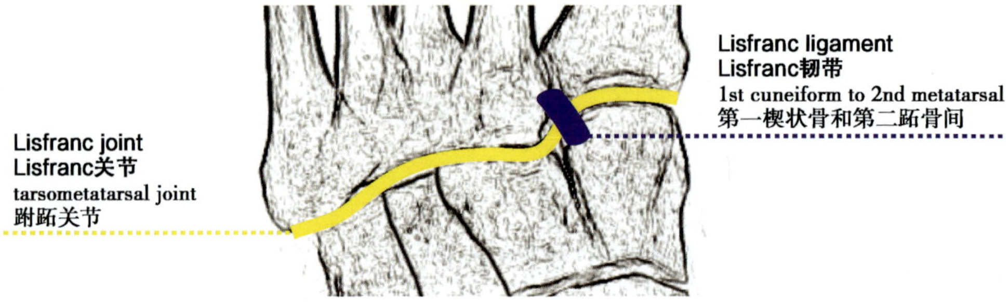

- A Lisfranc fracture-dislocation is a fracture-dislocation of the tarsometatarsal joint. The treatment of a Lisfranc injury is surgical. A missed or untreated Lisfranc injury can lead to debilitating osteoarthritis and flattening of the longitudinal arch.
- Lisfranc injuries are classified into homolateral and divergent based on the direction of dislocation of the first metatarsal. In a divergent Lisfranc injury, the first metatarsal is medially dislocated and the second through fifth metatarsals are laterally dislocated. In homolateral injury, all metatarsals will dislocate laterally.

- Lisfranc骨折-脱位即跗跖关节骨折与脱位。治疗Lisfranc损伤需要进行外科手术。误诊或未得到治疗的Lisfranc损伤会造成致残性骨关节炎和足纵弓扁平。
- Lisfranc损伤根据第一跖骨脱位方向分为同向侧偏和离散性损伤。在离散性Lisfranc损伤，第一跖骨向内侧脱位，而第二～五跖骨向外侧脱位。在同向侧偏损伤中，所有跖骨均向外侧脱位。

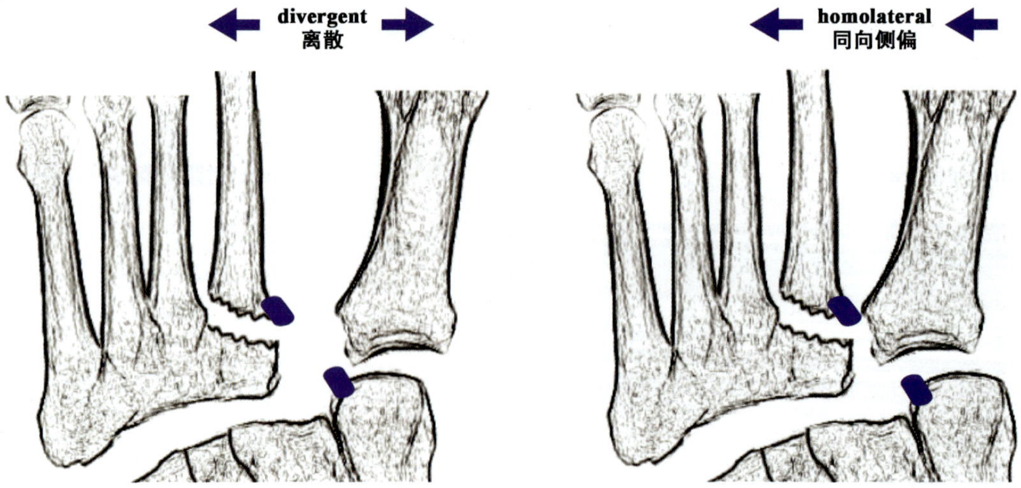

- Subtle malalignment of the tarsometatarsal joint may signal serious ligamentous injury. Weight-bearing radiographs are the most sensitive. Careful evaluation of the alignment of the Lisfranc joint must always be performed, as in this normal example below.

- 跗跖关节轻微错位可能提示有严重的韧带损伤。负重位X线影像是最敏感的检查方法。必须对Lisfranc关节的排列关系进行仔细检查，以下是正常示例。

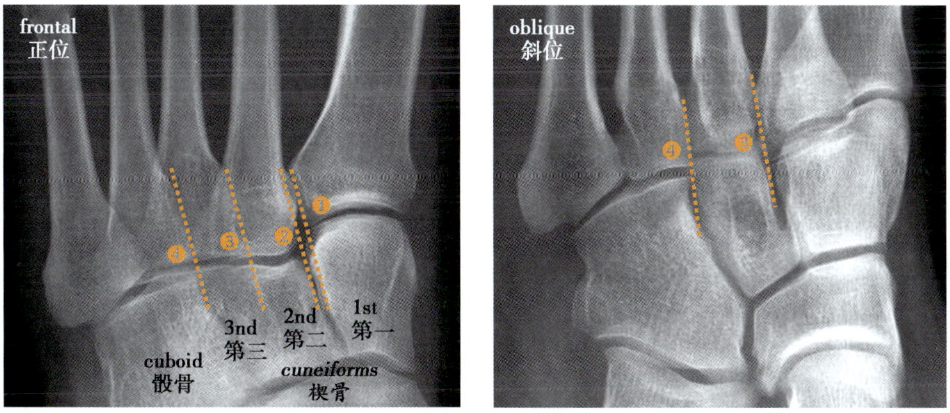

1. lateral base of 1st metatarsal should be aligned with lateral sapect of 1st cuneiform
第一跖骨的基底部外侧缘需要与第一楔骨外侧缘对齐
2. medial base of 2nd metatarsal should be aligned with medial aspect of 2nd cuneiform
第二跖骨的基底部内侧缘需要与第二楔骨内侧缘对齐
3. medial base of 3rd metatarsal should be aligned with medial aspect of 3rd cuneiform
第三跖骨的基底部内侧缘需要与第三楔骨内侧缘对齐
4. medial base of 4th metatarsal should be aligned with medial aspect of cuboid
第四跖骨的基底部内侧缘需要与骰骨内侧缘对齐

(3, 4) *easier to see on oblique*
在斜位X线影像上更易观察

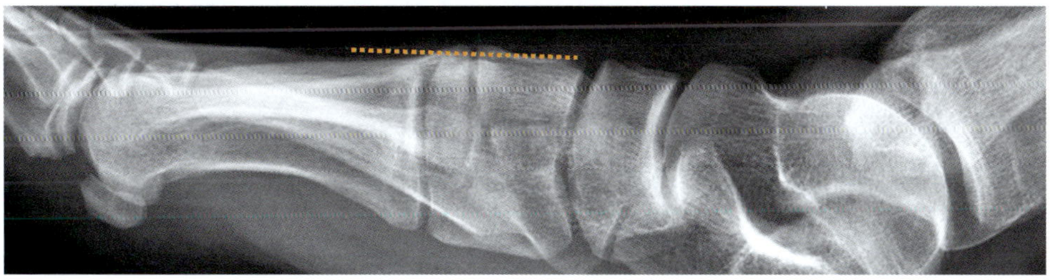

the dorsal profile of the tarsometatarsal (Lisfranc) joint should be uninterrupted
跗跖关节(Lisfranc关节)足背侧轮廓连线不应该有中断。

Navicular osteonecrosis

足舟骨坏死

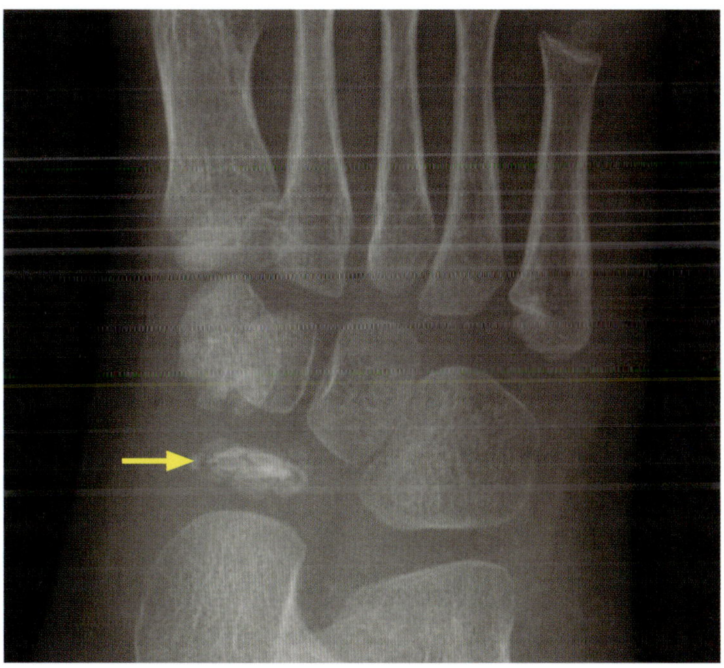

Kohler disease:
Oblique radiograph of the foot in a child demonstrates irregular sclerosis of the navicular (arrow), in keeping with Kohler disease.
Kohler病:
一名儿童的足部斜位X线影像显示足舟骨不规则硬化(箭),符合Kohler病的诊断。

- Osteonecrosis of the navicular is called Kohler disease in childhood and Müeller-Weiss disease in adults. Kohler disease is typically self limited and occurs more commonly in boys, while Müeller-Weiss disease is more severe in course and occurs more commonly in adult women.

- 儿童足舟骨坏死被称为Kohler病，而在成人则称为Müller-Weiss病。Kohler病通常为自限性疾病，多见于男童，而Müller-Weiss病的病情较为严重，常见于成年女性。

MIDFOOT AND HINDFOOT TRAUMA

中足及后足外伤

Overview of common fractures

常见骨折概述

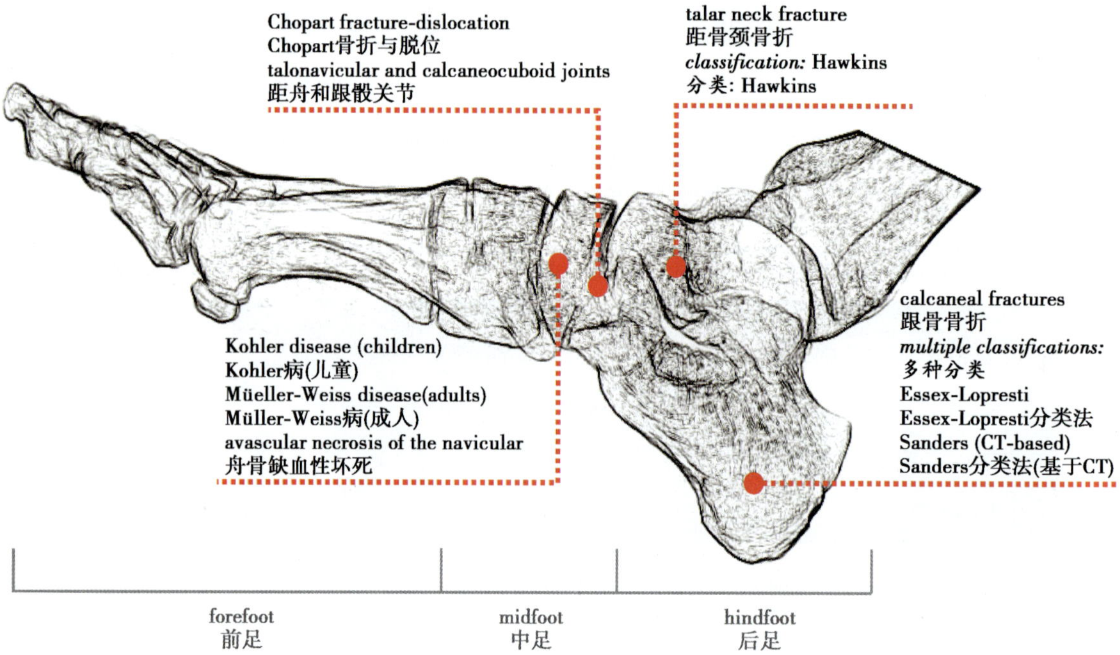

Chopart fracture-dislocation

Chopart骨折-脱位

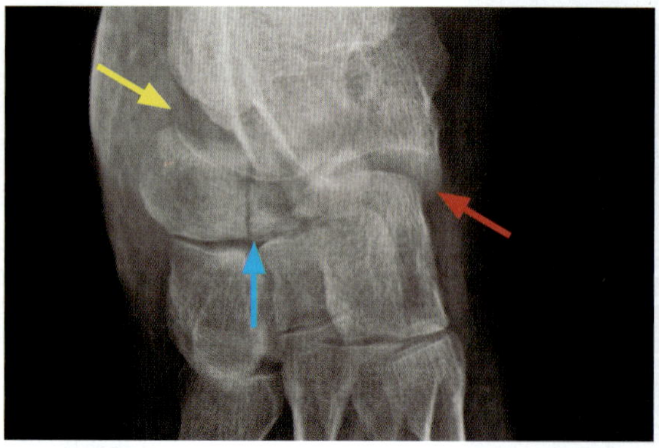

Frontal radiograph
正位X线影像

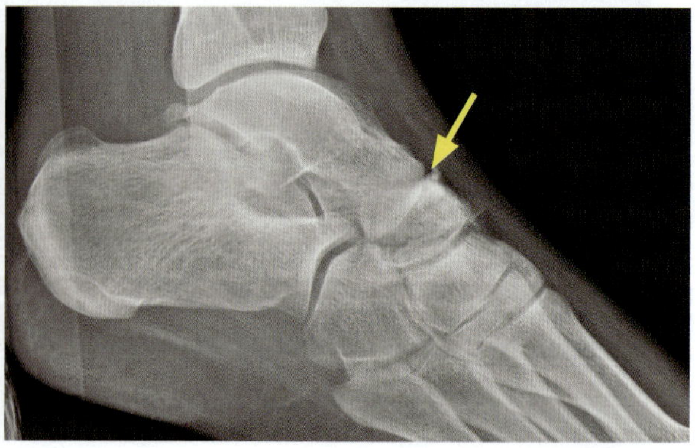

Lateral radiograph
侧位X线影像

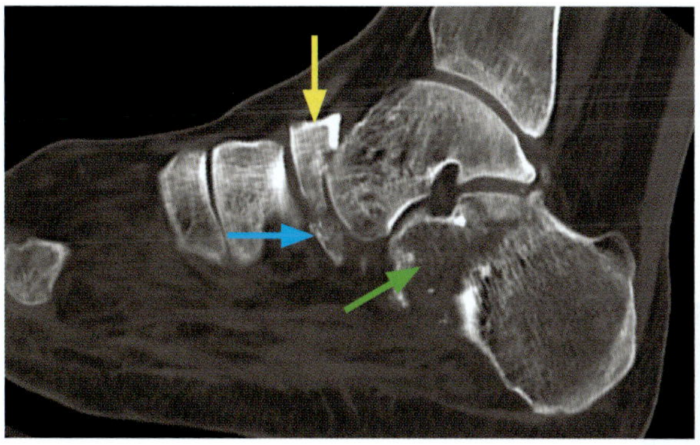

Sagittal CT
矢状位CT

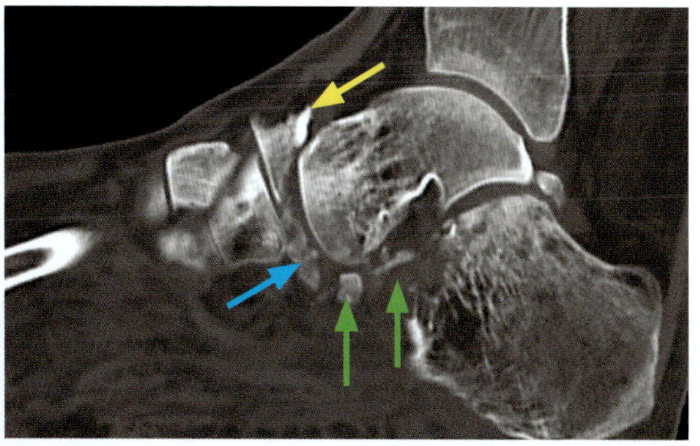

Sagittal CT
矢状位CT

Chopart fracture-dislocation: Radiographs show incongruity of the talonavicular (yellow arrows) and calcaneocuboid (red arrow) joints, and a longitudinal fracture of the navicular (blue arrow). CT shows true extent of injury, with comminuted fracture (blue arrows) and dorsal dislocation of the navicular (yellow arrows) and comminuted fracture of the anterior calcaneus (green arrows).
Chopart骨折-脱位：X线影像示距舟关节(黄箭)与跟骰关节(红箭)错位，以及舟骨纵向骨折(蓝箭)。CT准确地显示了损伤的范围，包括舟骨粉碎性骨折(蓝箭)及背侧脱位(黄箭)，以及前部跟骨粉碎性骨折(绿箭)。

- The Chopart joint is formed by the talonavicular and calcaneocuboid joints.
- Chopart fracture-dislocation is typically caused by high-impact trauma. Associated fractures of the calcaneus, cuboid, and navicular bones are often present.

Calcaneal fracture

- The calcaneus is the most commonly fractured tarsal bone.
- Traumatic fractures of the calcaneus are typically the result of a high-impact injury, such as a fall from height, in which case the fracture is known as the *lover's fracture*. In such cases, there is a high association with other serious injuries including lumbar spine fractures, traumatic aortic rupture, and renal vascular pedicle avulsion. If a traumatic calcaneal fracture is identified, further imaging of the lumbar spine and/or abdomen is recommended.
- Subtle fractures may not be directly visible; however, a decrease in the **Boehler angle** to less than 20° is diagnostic of a calcaneal fracture.

- Chopart关节是由距舟关节和跟骰关节组成。
- Chopart骨折-脱位主要由强烈冲击伤造成。常合并跟骨、骰骨及足舟骨骨折。

跟骨骨折

- 跟骨骨折是最常见的跗骨骨折。
- 外伤性跟骨骨折通常是由强烈冲击伤所致，如高空坠落，所以这样的骨折也被称为情人骨折。此类病例常合并其他严重损伤，包括腰椎骨折、外伤性主动脉破裂及肾血管蒂撕裂。如果发现有外伤性跟骨骨折，则应进一步行腰椎和/或腹部影像学检查。
- 轻微的跟骨骨折可能无法直接观察到；但当**Boehler角**小于20°时可以诊断为跟骨骨折。

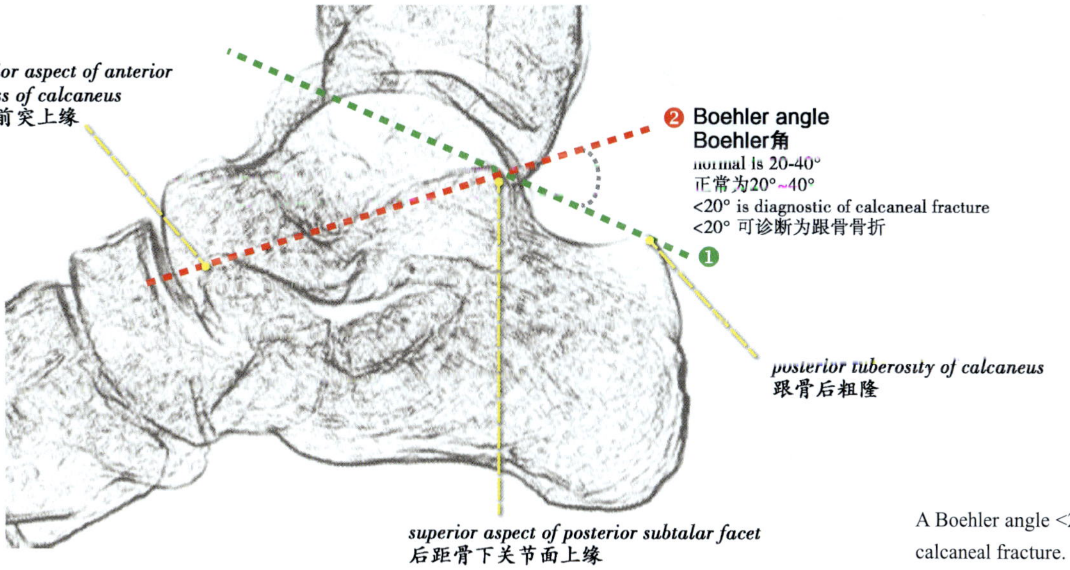

The Boehler angle is formed by drawing two lines:
Boehler角由两条线构成：

❶ superior aspect of posterior tuberosity of calcaneus and the superior aspect of posterior subtalar facet
跟骨后粗隆上缘和后距下关节面上缘的连线。
❷ superior aspect of anterior process of calcaneus to superior aspect of posterior subtalar articular surface
跟骨前上突上缘和后距下关节面上缘的连线。

A Boehler angle <20° is diagnostic of a calcaneal fracture.
Boehler角<20°可诊断为跟骨骨折。
A normal Boehler angle (20-40°) does not exclude a calcaneal fracture.
正常Boehler角(20°~40°)不能排除跟骨骨折。

- The Essex-Lopresti classification divides calcaneal fractures into those sparing the subtalar joint (25%) and fractures extending into the subtalar joint (75%).
- The Sanders classification is based on the number of comminuted fragments at the talonavicular joint, as seen on coronal CT.

- Essex-Lopresti分类法将跟骨骨折分为骨折线未累及距下关节(25%)和骨折线延伸到距下关节(75%)。
- Sanders分类法根据CT冠状位上距舟关节骨碎片的数量进行分类。

Calcaneal stress fracture

跟骨应力性骨折

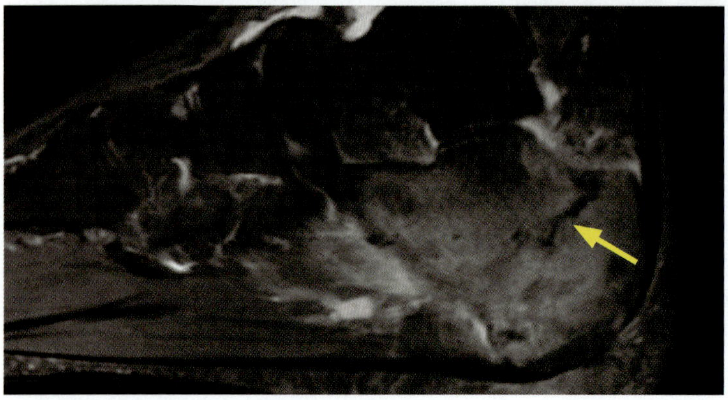

Calcaneal stress fracture:
Sagittal STIR MRI demonstrates diffuse edema of the calcaneus with a low signal intensity fracture line (arrow) posteriorly.
Note the typical orientation of the fracture line perpendicular to the calcaneal trabeculae.
跟骨应力性骨折:
矢状位STIR MRI显示跟骨弥漫性水肿和跟骨后部低信号骨折线(箭)。
注意典型的骨折线方向与跟骨的骨小梁垂直。

- A stress fracture of the calcaneus typically appears as a fluffy band of sclerosis within the calcaneus, with an intact cortex. Boehler's angle is normal. The sclerosis tends to be oriented perpendicular to the calcaneal trabeculae.

- 跟骨应力性骨折通常表现为跟骨内部一条毛糙的硬化带，而骨皮质完整。Boehler角正常。硬化线的走向往往与跟骨的骨小梁垂直。

Talar fracture

距骨骨折

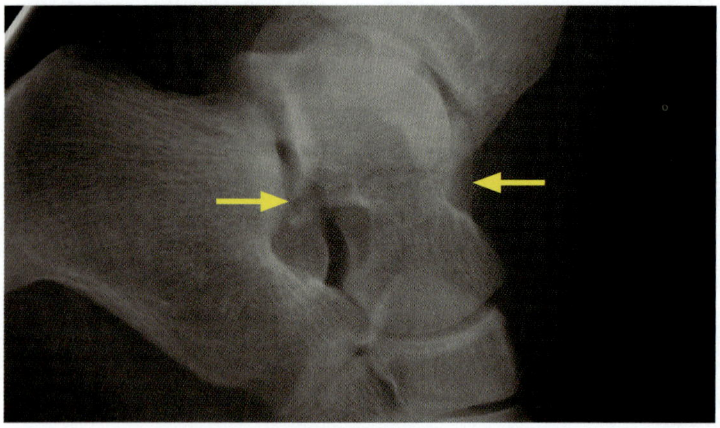

Talar neck fracture:
Lateral radiograph shows a minimally displaced fracture through the talar neck (arrows).
距骨颈骨折:
侧位X线影像显示轻度移位的距骨颈骨折(箭)。

- Fractures of the talus can be divided anatomically into lateral process, posterior process, head, body, and neck fractures.
- Fractures of the talar neck are classified by the Hawkins classification. A talar neck fracture may disrupt the blood supply to the talus and predispose to osteonecrosis.
- The **Hawkins sign** describes a subchondral lucent band seen on the frontal ankle radiograph 6–8 weeks after ankle immobilization. The lucent band represents increased bone reabsorption from active hyperemia. The presence of the Hawkins sign implies an intact blood supply to the talar dome and is a good prognostic indicator in talar neck fractures.

- 距骨骨折按解剖可分为外突、后突、头部、体部和颈部骨折。
- 距骨颈骨折采用Hawkins分类法进行分类。距骨颈骨折可能造成距骨血供中断而容易发生骨坏死。
- **Hawkins征**是指踝关节制动6～8周后在正位X线影像上出现一条软骨下透亮带。此透亮带为反应性充血导致的骨质再吸收增加。出现Hawkins征意味着距骨穹隆有完好的血供，是距骨颈骨折预后良好的指标。

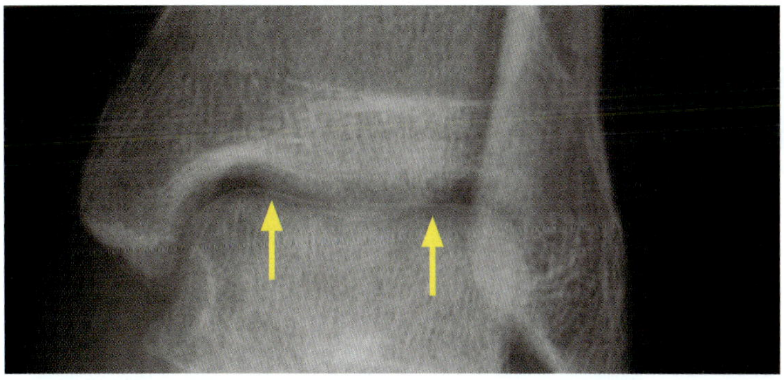

Hawkins sign:
Frontal radiograph shows a subtle subchondral lucent band of the talar dome (arrows), indicating healing.
Hawkins 征：
正位X线影像显示位于距骨穹隆软骨下的一条纤细的透亮带(箭)，是愈合的征象。

Osteochondral lesion of the talus

距骨骨软骨损伤

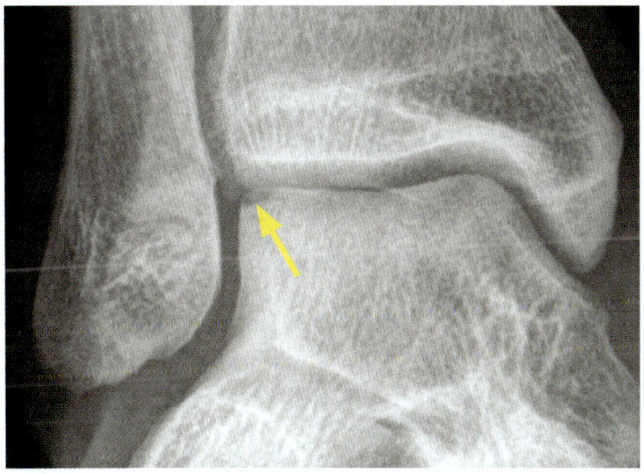

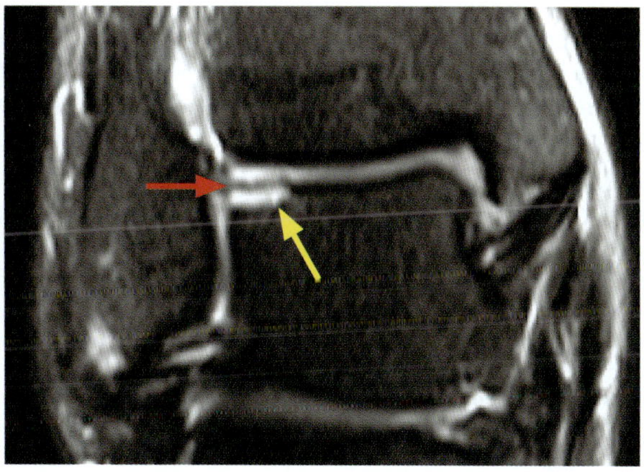

Osteochondral lesion of the lateral talar dome: Mortise radiograph (left image) shows a subtle lucency of the lateral talar dome (arrow). Coronal T2-weighted MRI with fat suppression shows a linear fluid signal intensity subchondral lesion (yellow arrow), with irregularity of the overlying subchondral bone plate (red arrow). The fluid undercutting the lesion indicates instability.
距骨外侧穹隆骨软骨损伤：踝穴位X线影像(左图)显示距骨外侧穹隆有一处不明显的透光影(箭)。冠状位T_2加权脂肪抑制MRI显示线状液体信号的软骨下病变(黄箭)，软骨下骨板不规则(红箭)。病变下部出现液体为不稳定的表现。

- The term *osteochondral lesion* is a broadly used general term to describe a variety of acute or chronic abnormalities of the cartilage, the subchondral bone plate (cortex underneath the cartilage), and the subchondral bone.
- Osteochondral lesion of the talus can describe either *osteochondritis dissecans* from chronic repetitive microtrauma (typically in younger patients) and acute traumatic *osteochondral defect*.
- Osteochondral lesions and their staging are discussed in the knee section.
- In the talus, an osteochondral lesion appears on radiography as a crescentic lucency of the talar dome. MR imaging is similar to MR imaging of knee osteochondral lesions, where fluid undercutting the lesion or cystic change deep to the lesion indicates instability.

- 骨软骨病变是一个广泛使用的通用术语，用于描述各种急性或慢性软骨、软骨下骨板(软骨下骨皮质)，以及软骨下骨质异常。
- 距骨的骨软骨损伤既可以用于描述慢性重复微小损伤导致的剥脱性骨软骨炎(通常见于较年轻的患者)，也可以指急性外伤导致的骨软骨缺损。
- 骨软骨损伤及其分期在膝关节章节论述。
- 距骨骨软骨损伤在X线影像上表现为距骨穹隆新月形透亮影。其MRI影像学表现类似于膝关节骨软骨损伤，若病变出现积液或病变深部有囊变，为不稳定的表现。

Hindfoot (tarsal) coalition

- Abnormal fusion of two tarsal bones may be a cause of hindfoot pain. Hindfoot coalitions often present in adolescence as the coalition begins to ossify. A coalition may be fibrous, cartilaginous, or osseous.
- The vast majority of hindfoot coalitions are either talocalcaneal (fusion of the talus and calcaneus) or calcaneonavicular (fusion of the calcaneus and navicular).
- **Talocalcaneal coalition** occurs most commonly at the middle subtalar facet.

后足(跗骨)融合

- 两跗骨间异常融合可能会导致后足疼痛。后足融合常出现在青春期，此时融合开始骨化。融合可能为纤维性、软骨性或呈骨性融合。
- 绝大多数后足融合为距骨-跟骨融合或跟骨-舟骨融合。
- **距跟融合**最常见于距下的中部关节面。

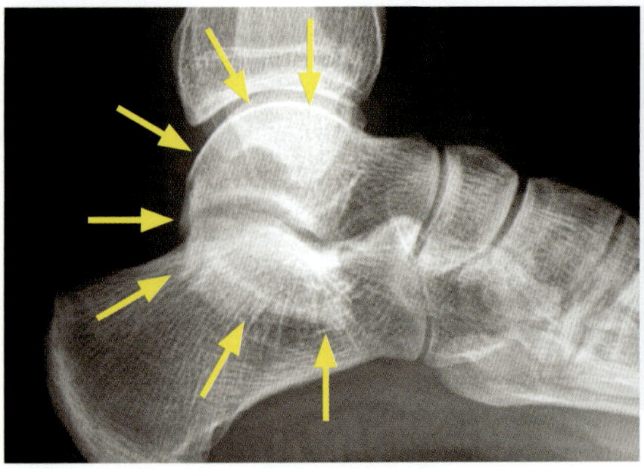

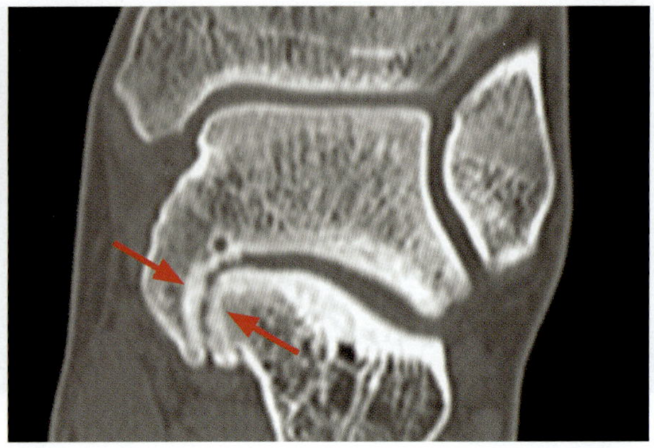

Talocalcaneal coalition: Lateral radiograph of the ankle (left image) shows the classic *C sign* (yellow arrows) due to fusion of the medial talus and sustentaculum tali. A fibrous coalition (red arrows) is confirmed on the coronal CT (right image), with sclerosis and subchondral cysts of the middle subtalar facet.
The *C sign* on the lateral radiograph represents a continuous C-shaped contour of the fused middle subtalar facet (medial talus fused with the sustentaculum tali). The C sign is not sensitive for the detection of talocalcaneal coalition, but may be helpful when seen.
The *talar beak sign* on the lateral radiograph describes a triangular-shaped beaking at the anterior-superior aspect of the talus.
距跟融合：踝关节侧位X线影像(左图)显示典型的C字征(黄箭)，为距骨内侧与跟骨载距突融合所致。距跟纤维性融合(红箭)在冠状位CT(右图)上得到证实，伴有距下关节面中部骨质硬化和软骨下囊变。
侧位X线影像上的C字征是指距下关节面中部融合所形成的连续的C字形轮廓(距骨内侧与跟骨载距突融合)。C字征对发现距跟融合并不敏感，但出现时有助于诊断。
侧位X线影像上的距骨鸟嘴征是指距骨前上缘形似三角形鸟嘴。

- **Calcaneonavicular coalition** is fusion between the anterior process of the calcaneus and the navicular.

  The *anteater sign* represents the elongated anterior process of the calcaneus which looks like an anteater's nose on the lateral view.

- **跟舟骨融合**是指跟骨前突与足舟骨之间的融合。

  食蚁兽征是指跟骨前突的延长形状在侧位图像上酷似食蚁兽的鼻子。

ANKLE ANATOMY FOR MR

踝关节MR解剖

Cross-sectional ligament anatomy on MR: Sequential PD-weighted images

横断面MR韧带解剖结构：系列PD加权图像

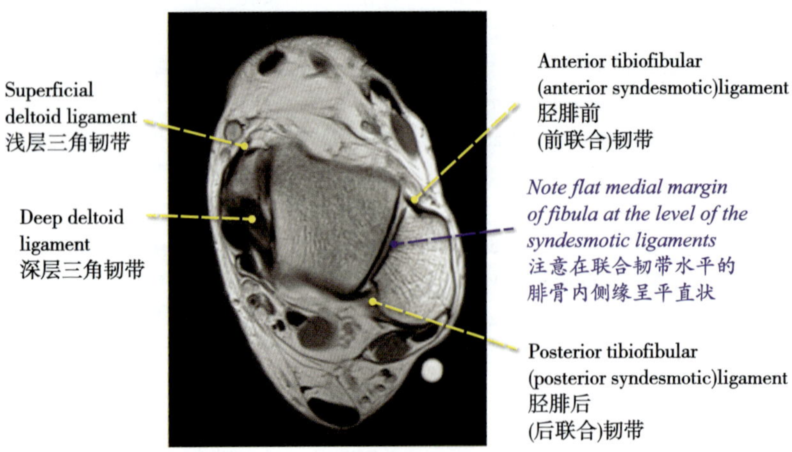

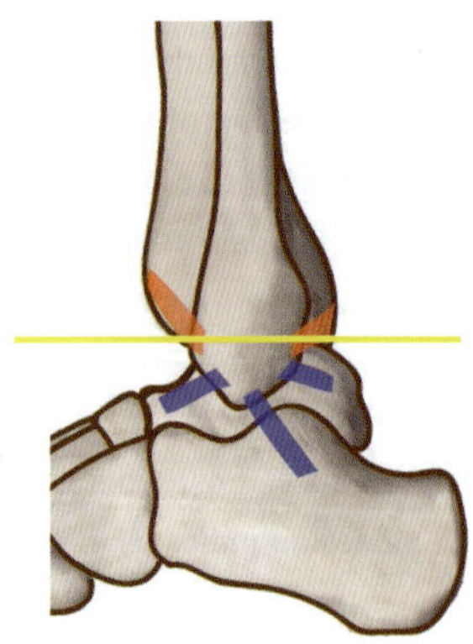

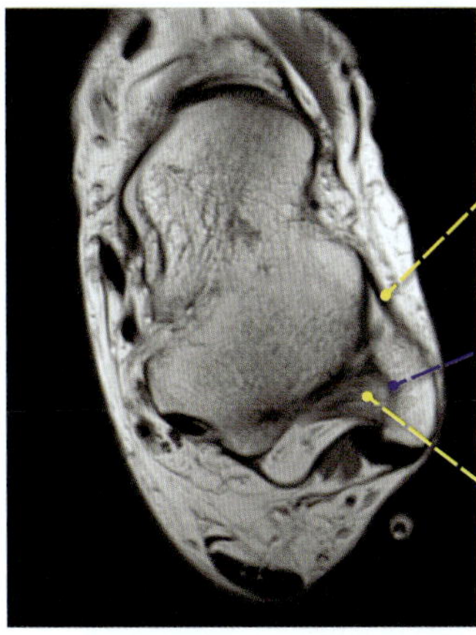
Anterior talofibular
(ATFL)ligament
距腓前韧带
Note comma-shaped
medial margin of fibula
at the level of the
collateral ligaments
注意在副韧带水平处
腓骨内侧缘呈逗号状
Posterior talofibular
(PTFL)ligament
距腓后韧带

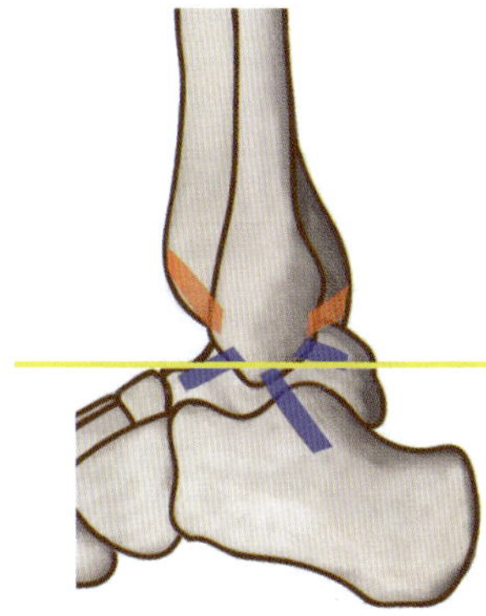

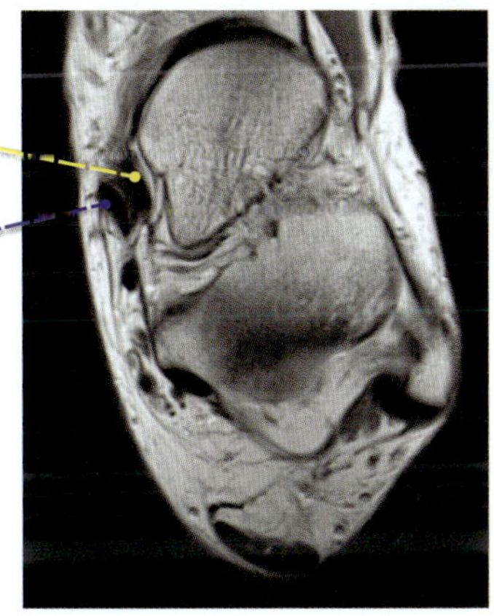
Spring ligament
弹簧韧带
Posterior tibial
tendon(PTT)
胫骨后肌腱
Spring ligament is
located just deep/lateral
to the posterior tibial
tendon
弹簧韧带位于
胫骨后肌腱的深/外侧

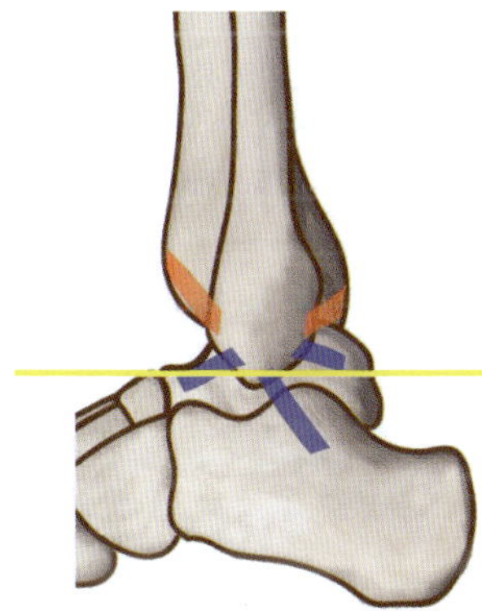

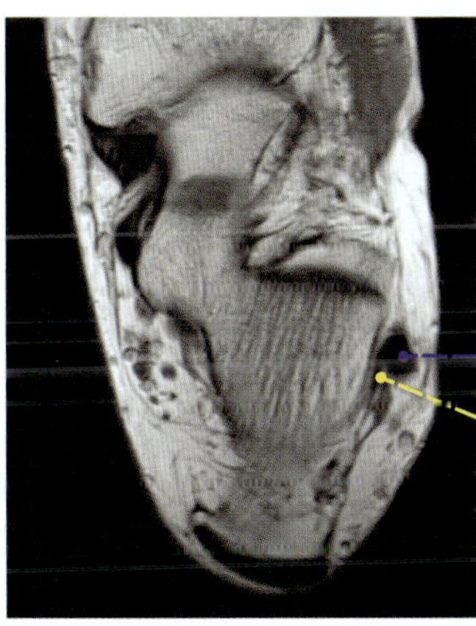
The CFL is the most caudal
lateral collateral ligament,
located just deep/medial to
the peroneals
跟腓韧带是最下外侧的副
韧带，位于腓骨肌群的
深/内侧
Peroneal tendons
腓骨肌腱
Calcaneofibular
(CFL)ligament
跟腓韧带

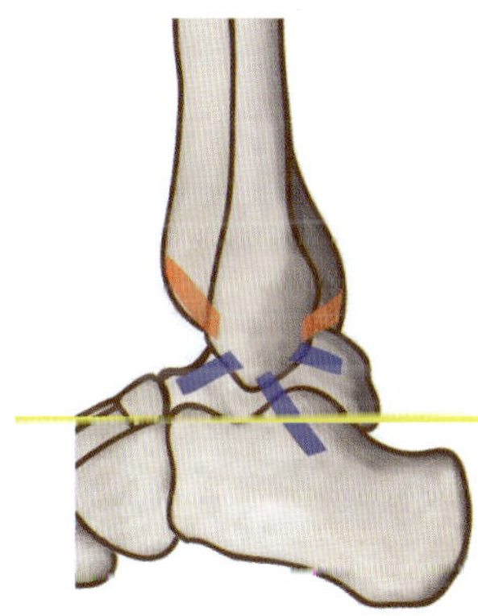

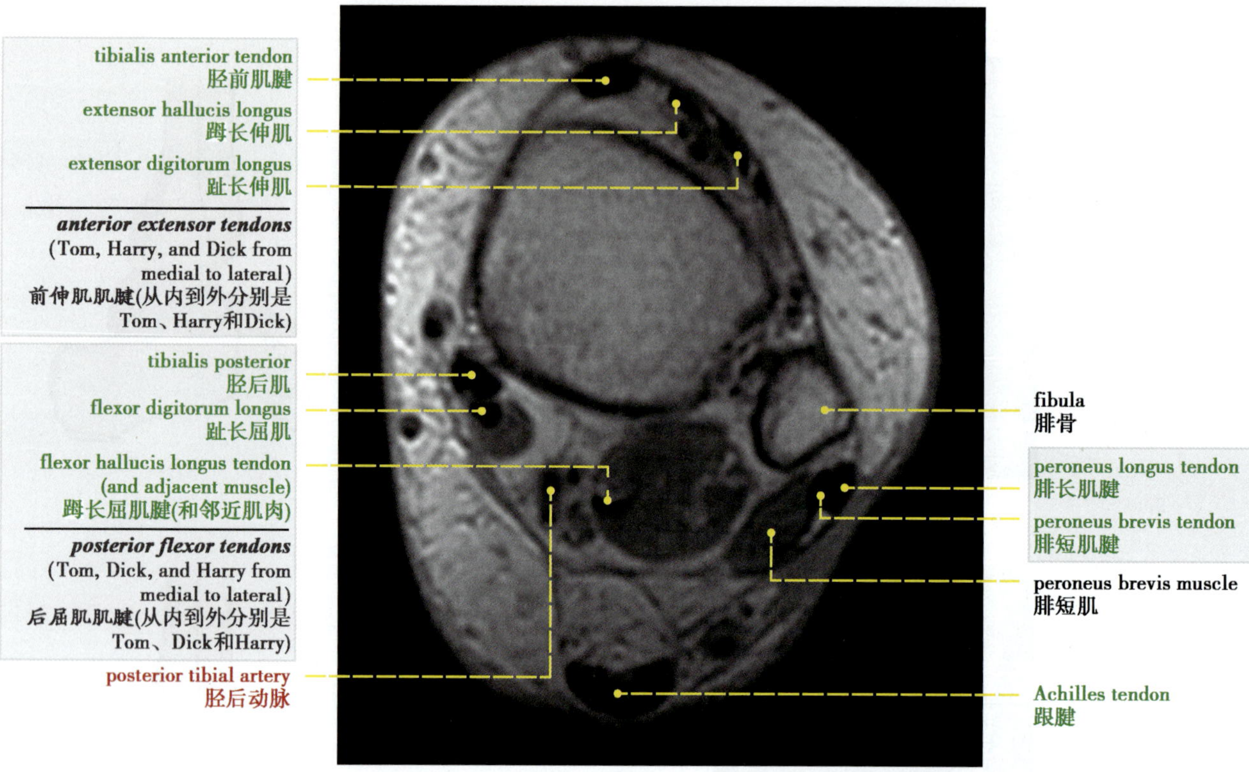

Lateral ankle tendons and ligaments | 踝关节外侧肌腱和韧带

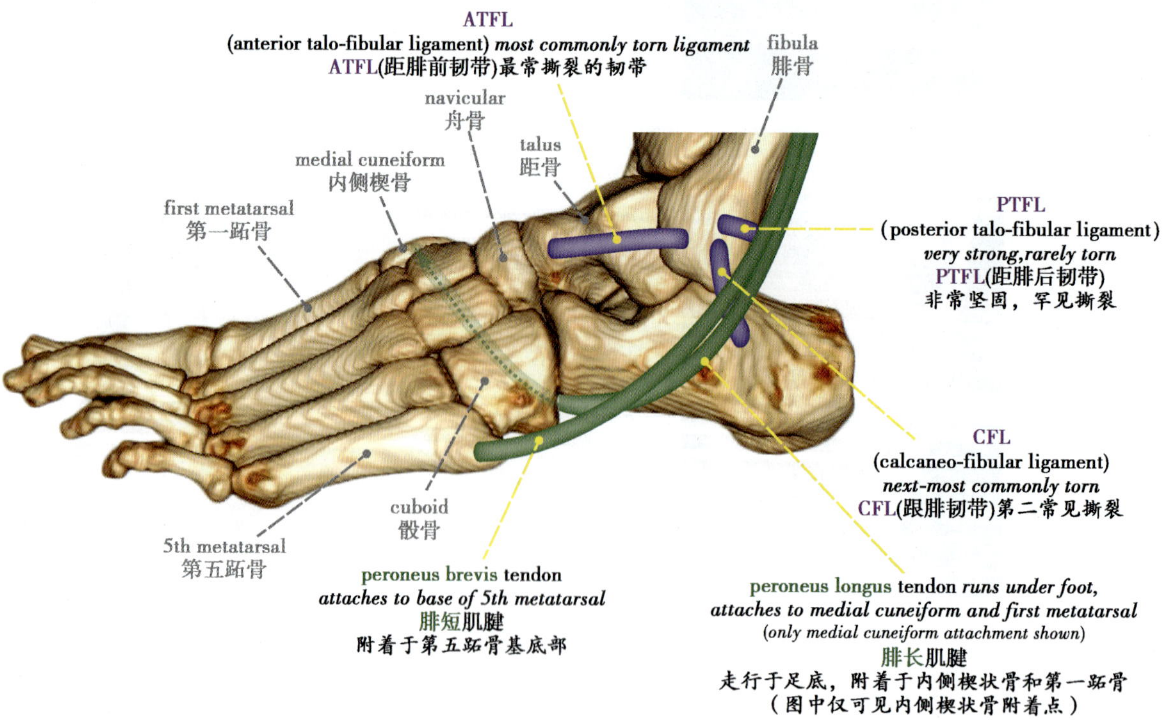

- The lateral collateral complex involves the ATFL, PTFL, and CFL. These ligaments are commonly injured in ankle sprains (typically inversion injury), but are not usually injured in the most common ankle fracture patterns (most commonly external rotation on the talus with the foot in supination).

- 外侧副韧带复合体包括距腓前韧带、距腓后韧带和跟腓韧带。这些韧带损伤常见于踝关节扭伤(通常是内翻损伤)，但在最常见的踝关节骨折(通常为距骨外旋及足后旋)中不常见。

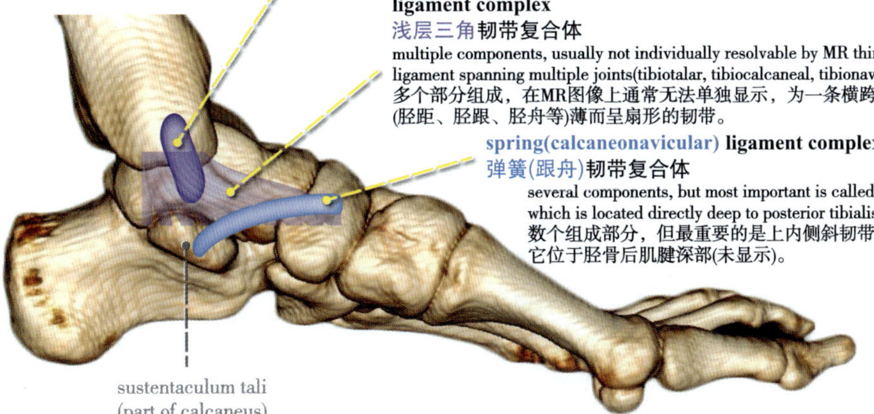

along with the posterior tibial tendon(not drawn), the spring ligament complex functions to maintain the arch of the foot*
弹簧韧带复合体沿胫后肌腱走行*(未画出)，其功能是维持足弓形态

**most common cause of acquired flat foot is posterior tibial tendon tear*
最常见的获得性扁平足的原因是胫骨后肌腱撕裂

Medial ankle tendons

踝关节内侧肌腱

contents of tarsal tunnel, from anterior to posterior: Tom, Dick, ANd Harry
跗管内结构从前到后分别为：Tom、Dick和Harry

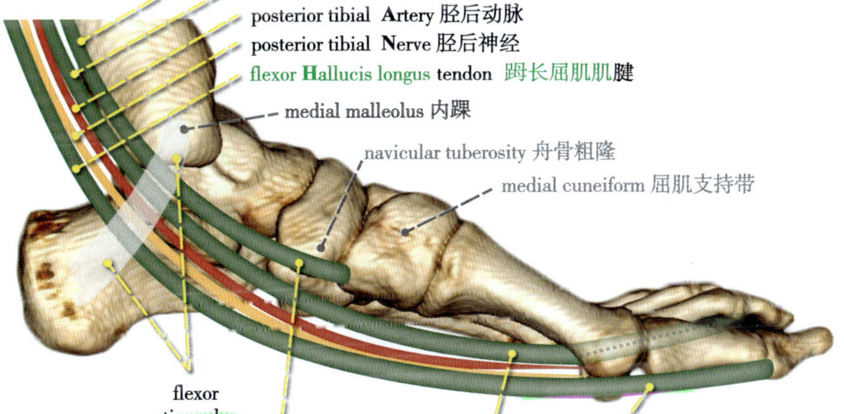

Anterior extensor tendons

- Arranged from medial to lateral, the anterior extensor tendons can be remembered with the mnemonic "Tom, Harry, and Dick" :

  Tibialis anterior.

  Extensor **H**allucis longus.

  Extensor **D**igitorum longus.

- The anterior tibial artery runs anteriorly with the extensor tendons.

前伸肌肌腱

- 从内侧到外侧排列，前伸肌肌腱的记忆口诀是"Tom，Harry和Dick"：

  胫前肌。

  踇长伸肌。

  趾长伸肌。

- 胫前动脉走行于伸肌肌腱的前方。

Syndesmotic ligaments

联合韧带

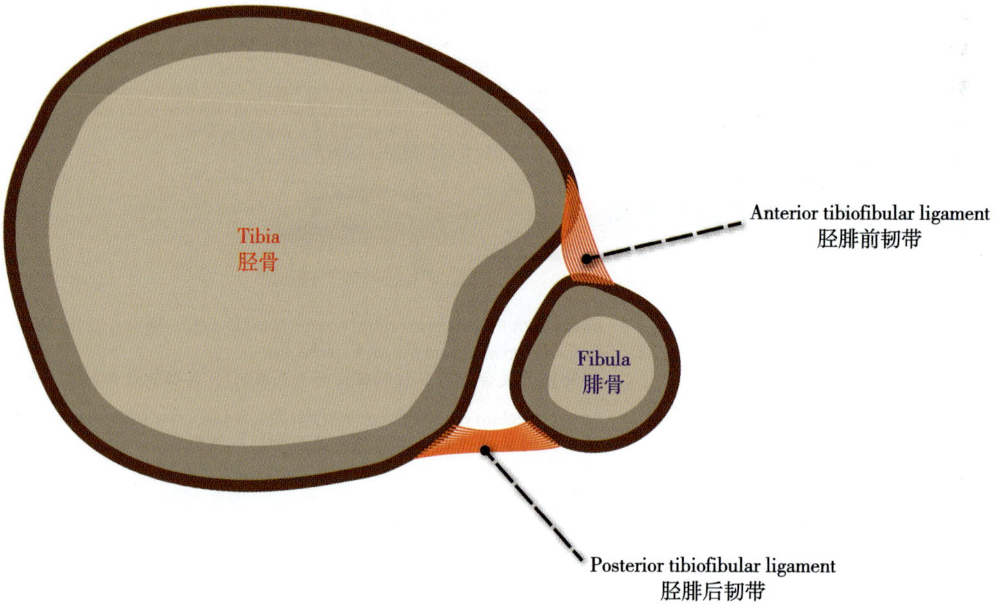

- The syndesmosis is a fibrous ligamentous complex that connects the distal tibia and fibula, where the distal fibula fits into a groove in the distal tibia.
- The major ligaments of the syndesmosis are the anterior and posterior tibiofibular ligaments. Other ligaments interposed between these are less important.
- Injury to the syndesmosis tends to occur like opening a book, with tear of the anterior tibiofibular ligament, followed by tear of the posterior tibiofibular ligament in higher-grade injuries. There are usually ankle fractures by the time the posterior tibiofibular ligament is torn, but the anterior tibiofibular ligament can tear without fracture.

Ankle sprains

- Sprains are the most common ankle injury. These are usually due to ankle inversion, and the anterior talofibular ligament (ATFL) of the lateral collateral ligamentous complex is the most commonly torn ligament in ankle *sprains*.
- A "high ankle sprain" is a colloquial/informal term for injury to the syndesmosis (most commonly the anterior syndesmotic (anterior tibiofibular) ligament, without fracture.

Ankle fractures

- Injury to the lateral collateral ligaments is much less common in ankle *fractures*. The syndesmotic ligaments are the most commonly torn ligaments in ankle fractures.
- The **Danis-Weber classification** (commonly shortened to the **Weber classification**) is the simplest classification of ankle fractures and divides ankle fractures based on the level of the fibular fracture relative to the syndesmosis.

- 联合韧带是一个纤维韧带复合体，它连接远端胫骨和腓骨，并使远端腓骨嵌入胫骨远端的槽中。
- 联合韧带最重要的韧带是胫腓前韧带、胫腓后韧带。其他夹在中间的韧带并不太重要。
- 联合韧带复合体损伤犹如打开一本书，首先是胫腓前韧带撕裂，然后是严重的胫腓后韧带撕裂伤。胫腓后韧带撕裂时通常伴随踝关节骨折，但胫腓前韧带的撕裂可以不发生骨折。

踝关节扭伤

- 扭伤是踝关节最常见的损伤。通常由踝关节内翻造成，而外侧副韧带复合体中的距腓前韧带(ATFL)是踝关节扭伤中最常撕裂的韧带。
- "高位踝关节扭伤"是一个口语/非正式术语，是指无骨折的联合韧带损伤[最常见的是前联合(胫腓前)韧带]。

踝关节骨折

- 外侧副韧带损伤较少见于踝关节骨折。胫腓韧带联合韧带是踝关节骨折中最常发生撕裂的韧带。
- **Danis-Weber分类法**(常简称为**Weber分类法**)是最简单的踝关节骨折分类法，是基于腓骨骨折与联合韧带的相对位置。

Weber A is a distal fibular fracture with an intact syndesmosis. Usually treated conservatively.

Weber B is a fibular fracture at the level of the ankle joint, with indeterminate status of the syndesmosis.

Although by far the most common, this is the least useful classification because the status of the syndsmosis is unclear. Treatment depends on stability of the syndesmosis.

Weber C is a high fibular fracture above the level of the syndesmosis, with functional deficiency of the syndesmosis. Usually treated surgically.

- The **Lauge-Hansen classification** divides ankle fractures based on the position of the foot at the time of injury, and the direction of the force acting on the talus. At first glance it is a complicated system, but approximately 90% of ankle fractures are supination-external rotation (SER) pattern, so it makes sense to focus on this pattern of injury, as discussed on the following page.

Weber A型是腓骨远端骨折，联合韧带完整。通常采用保守治疗。

Weber B型是腓骨骨折位于踝关节的水平，联合韧带情况不能确定。

尽管这是最常见的类型，但由于联合韧带情况不明，该分类的临床意义不大。治疗方式取决于联合韧带的稳定。

Weber C型是腓骨骨折位于联合韧带的上方，伴有联合韧带功能性损伤。通常采用外科手术治疗。

- **Lange-Hansen分类法**基于踝关节骨折时足的位置和外力施加于距骨的方向。该分类法看似是一个复杂的系统，但约90%的踝关节骨折都是外翻-外旋型(SER)，因此重点关注这种损伤不为过，详见后文。

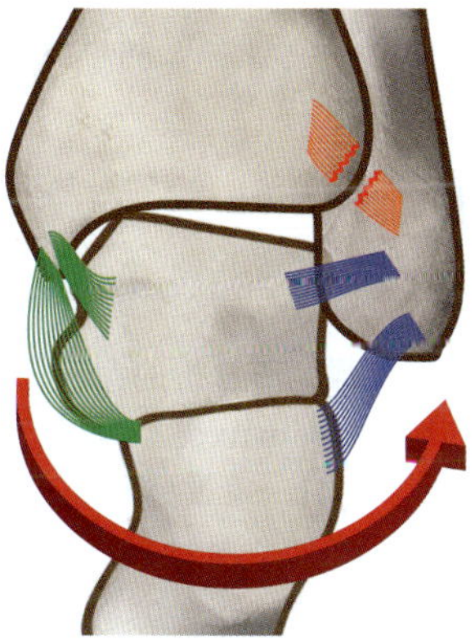

SER stage Ⅰ: Note supinated position of the foot, with external rotation force on the talus. First stage of injury is tear of the anterior tibiofibular (anterior syndesmotic) ligament.
SER Ⅰ度：注意足的旋后位置，外旋力作用于距骨。损伤的第一阶段是胫腓前韧带(前联合韧带)撕裂。

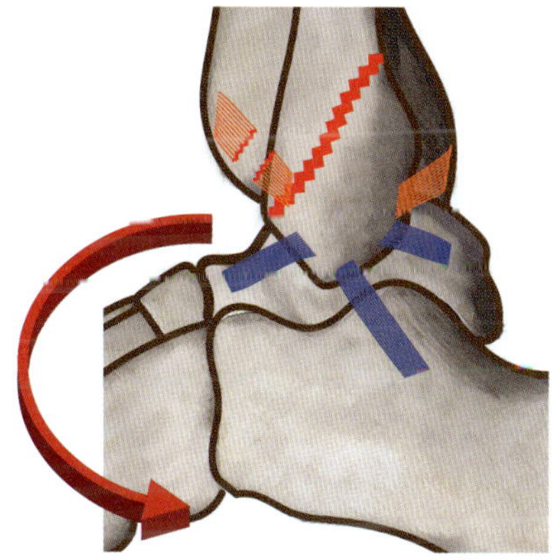

SER stage Ⅱ: Oblique fracture of the distal fibula, higher posterior and low anterior. On the frontal view, the fracture is at the level of the ankle joint.
SER Ⅱ度：腓骨远端由后上向前下走行的斜形骨折。正位X线影像显示骨折位于踝关节水平。

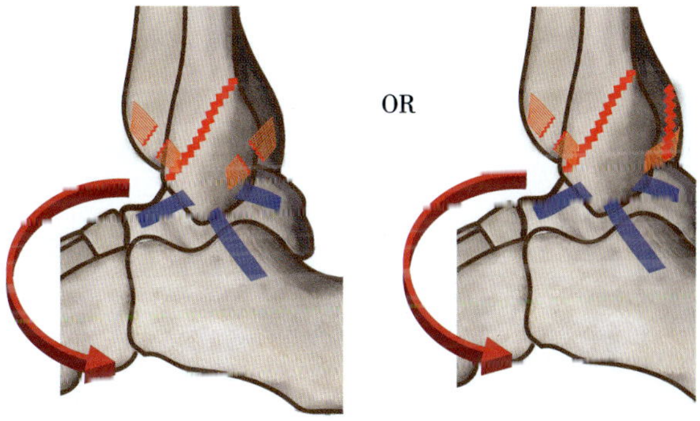

SER stage Ⅲ: Tear of the posterior tibiofibular (posterior syndesmotic) ligament OR posterior malleolus fracture.
SER Ⅲ度：胫腓后韧带(后联合韧带)撕裂或后踝骨折。

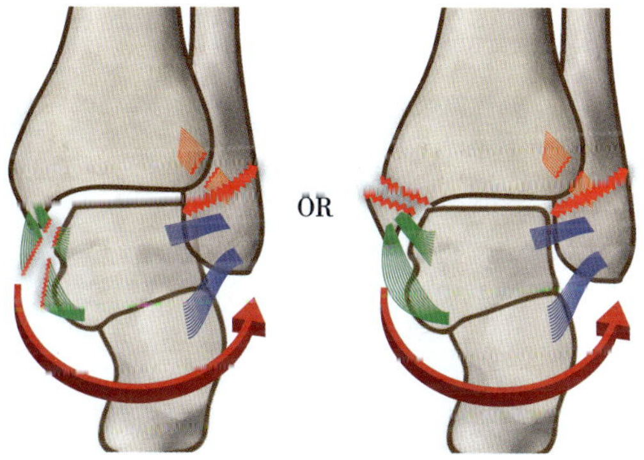

SER stage Ⅳ: Tear of the deltoid ligament OR horizontal fracture of the medial malleolus.
SER Ⅳ度：三角韧带撕裂或内踝水平骨折。

Supination-external rotation (SER) stages Ⅰ through Ⅳ: This classification is helpful to predict the ligaments torn. For instance, in stage Ⅳ (identified by widening of the medial clear space or medial malleolus fracture), one can predict there is also either a posterior syndesmotic ligament tear or fracture of the posterior malleolus.
外翻-外旋型(SER) Ⅰ度到Ⅳ度：这种分类有助于预测韧带撕裂。例如，在Ⅳ度(内踝关节间隙增宽或内踝骨折)损伤时，也可预测后联合韧带撕裂或后踝骨折。

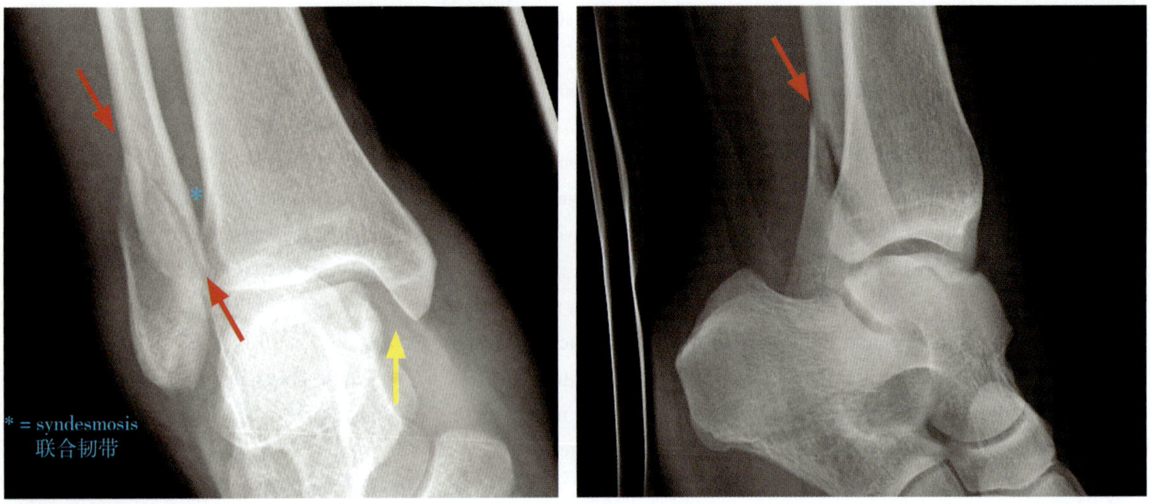

Supination-external rotation (SER) stage Ⅳ ankle fracture:

Mortise (left image) and lateral ankle radiographs show an oblique fracture (red arrows) through the distal fibula at the level of the syndesmosis (blue star). There is widening of the medial clear space (yellow arrow).

Widening of the medial clear space is indicative of deltoid ligament disruption, indicative of a stage Ⅳ injury. We can also presume that the anterior and posterior syndesmotic ligaments are torn, and this is an unstable pattern of injury.

旋后外(SER)型Ⅳ度踝关节骨折：

Mortise(踝关节穴位)(左图)及侧位踝关节X线影像显示一处经腓骨远端的斜形骨折(红箭)，位于联合韧带水平(蓝星号)。内踝关节间隙增宽(黄箭)。

内踝关节间隙增宽提示三角韧带断裂，为SER Ⅳ度损伤的征象。由此还可以推测存在前后下胫腓联合韧带撕裂，此为不稳定性损伤。

Named ankle fractures

- **Tillaux** fracture is a Salter Harris Ⅲ fracture of the lateral tibial epiphyses, typically seen in adolescents.
- **Triplane** fracture (also known as a Marmor-Lynn fracture) represents three distinct fractures through the distal tibia: a vertical epiphyseal fracture, horizontal physeal fracture, and oblique metaphyseal fracture.
- **Wagstaffe-LeFort** fracture is an avulsion of the anterior distal fibula at site of insertion of the anterior tibiofibular (anterior syndesmotic) ligament.
- **Maisonneuve** fracture is a high (proximal) fibular fracture associated with an interosseous membrane tear or medial malleolar fracture. Isolated imaging of the ankle may only detect subtle widening of the ankle mortise, which should prompt a more proximal radiograph.

踝关节骨折的命名

- **Tillaux**骨折是发生在胫骨骨骺外侧的Salter Harris Ⅲ型骨折，常见于青少年。
- **三平面**骨折(又称Marmor-Lynn骨折)为远端胫骨的三个性质不同的骨折：骨骺垂直性骨折；生长板水平骨折；干骺端斜形骨折。
- **Wagstaffe-LeFort**是胫腓前韧带前缘在腓骨远端附着点的撕脱性骨折。
- **Maisonneuve**腓骨高位(近端)骨折伴骨间膜撕裂或内踝骨折。踝关节单一体位影像可能仅发现踝关节间隙轻微增宽，对此应对近端腓骨做进一步影像学检查。

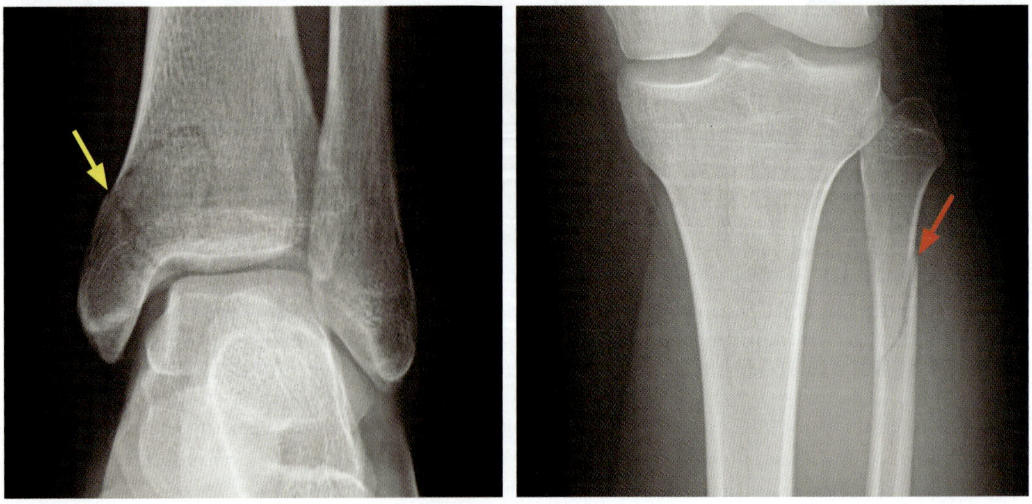

Maisonneuve fracture: Frontal radiograph of the ankle (left image) demonstrates an oblique fracture of the medial malleolus (yellow arrow). More proximal imaging of the ipsilateral knee shows an oblique fracture of the proximal fibula (red arrow).

Maisonneuve 骨折：正位踝关节X线影像(左图)显示内踝斜形骨折(黄箭)。同侧膝关节图像显示近端腓骨斜形骨折(红箭)。

- **Pilon** fracture is a comminuted vertically oriented fracture of the distal tibia, with resultant disruption of the tibial plafond. A pilon fracture is caused by axial loading.

- **Pilon**骨折是胫骨远端垂直方向的粉碎性骨折，并引起胫骨平台破裂。Pilon骨折是由轴向负荷所致。

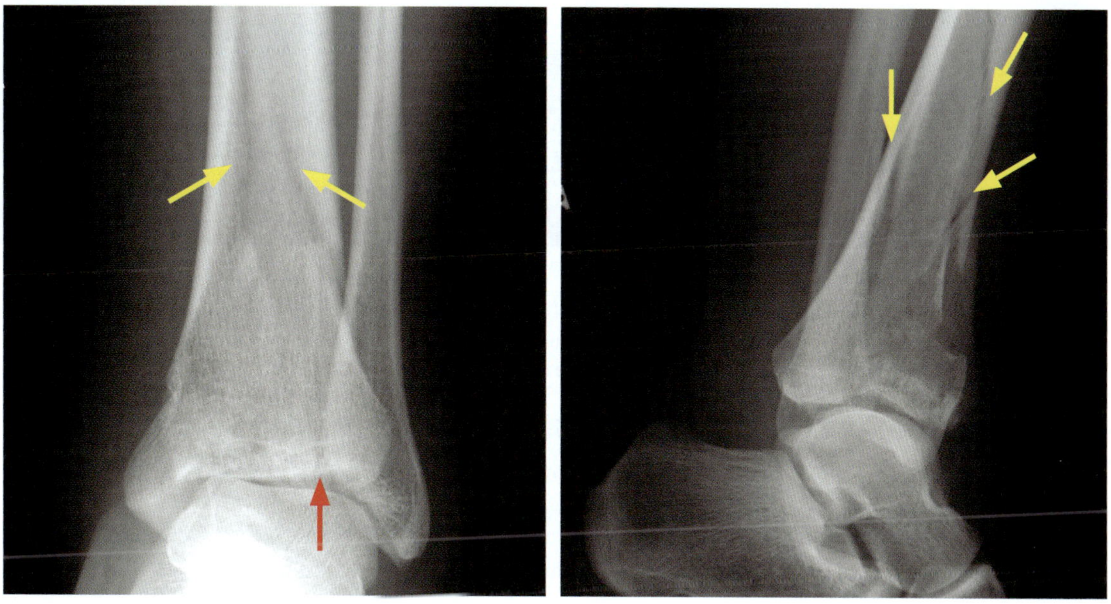

Pilon fracture: Frontal (left image) and lateral (right image) radiographs of the ankle show comminuted oblique and vertically oriented fractures (yellow arrows) of the distal tibia with disruption of the ankle mortise and tibial plafond (red arrow).
Pilon骨折：正位(左图)、侧位(右图)踝关节X线影像显示胫骨远端斜形和垂直方向的粉碎性骨折(黄箭)，伴踝关节和胫骨下关节面受累(红箭)。

Achilles tendon injury

跟腱损伤

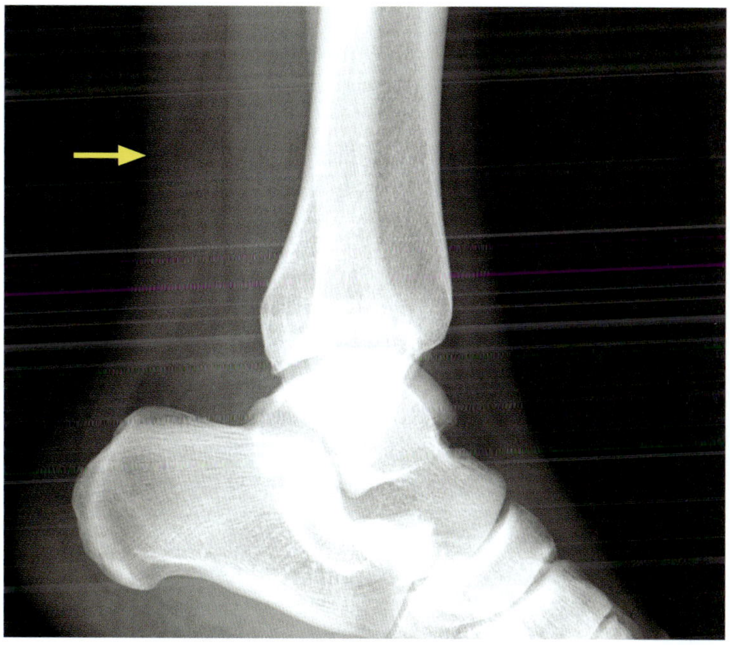

Achilles tendon injury:
Lateral radiograph shows a subtle disruption of the contour of the Achilles tendon (arrow).
There is also increased soft tissue and fluid in Kager's fat pad. Kager's fat pad is a radiolucent triangle bounded by the flexor hallucis longus anteriorly, the calcaneus inferiorly, and the Achilles tendon posteriorly.
跟腱损伤：
侧位X线影像隐约可见跟腱轮廓中断(箭)。
此外，Kager脂肪垫内软组织影和积液增加。Kager脂肪垫是一个三角形的透光区，其前方为踇长屈肌，下方为跟骨，后方为跟腱。

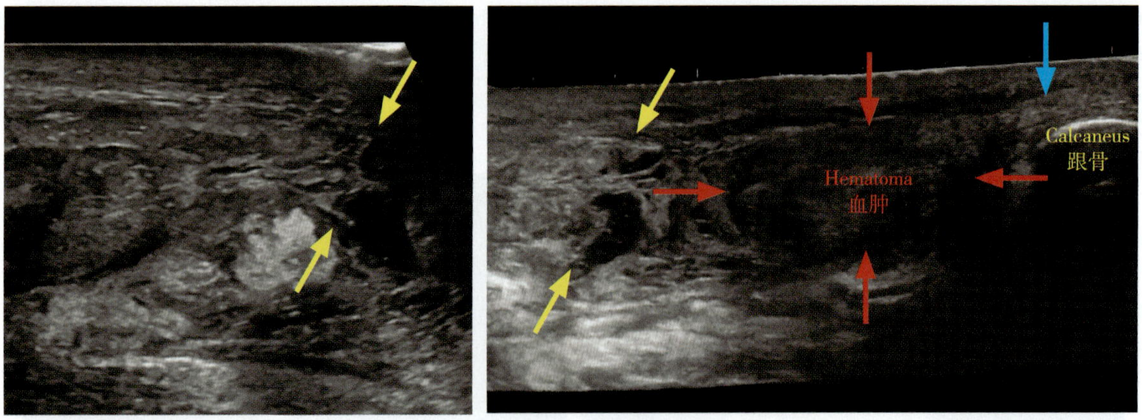

Achilles tendon rupture:
Two sagittal ultrasound images in a different patient demonstrate full thickness disruption of the Achilles tendon (yellow arrows). There is associated hematoma (red arrows) interposed between the torn and retracted tendon and the calcaneal tuberosity. There is a small stump of tendon remaining attached to the calcaneal tuberosity (blue arrow).
跟腱断裂：
两幅矢状切面超声图像在另一名患者中显示跟腱全层断裂(黄箭)。在撕裂和回缩的肌腱与跟骨结节之间存在继发血肿(红箭)。跟骨结节上仍附着一小段残端肌腱(蓝箭)。

- The Achilles tendon is the most commonly injured ankle tendon.
- Achilles tendinosis can sometimes be evident on radiography as thickening of the tendon.

  Achilles thickening is not specific for tendinosis. Thickening of the Achilles tendon can also be caused by xanthomas in patients with a hyperlipidemia syndrome.
- Complete Achilles rupture is usually evident on clinical exam. Radiography shows discontinuity of the tendon contour, with increased soft tissue in Kager's fat pad.
- The differential diagnosis of increased soft tissue in Kager's fat pad includes:

  Achilles tendon injury.

  Accessory soleus muscle (most common soft-tissue mass seen in Kager's fat pad).

  Haglund disease, which is retrocalcaneal bursitis associated with thickening of the distal Achilles tendon. Poorly fitting shoes may be a cause, leading to the nickname *pump bumps*.

- 跟腱是踝部最常受损的肌腱。
- 跟腱退行性变在X线影像上有时表现为肌腱增厚。

  跟腱增厚并不是跟腱退行性变的特异性表现。跟腱增厚也可由高血脂综合征患者的黄色瘤所致。
- 完全性跟腱断裂在临床检查时通常比较明显。X线影像显示跟腱轮廓不连续，伴Kager脂肪垫内软组织影增加。
- Kager脂肪垫内软组织影增加的鉴别诊断有：

  跟腱损伤。

  副比目鱼肌(最常见的Kager脂肪垫内软组织肿块)。

  Haglund病，是指跟骨后滑囊炎伴跟腱远端增厚。不合脚的鞋是该病可能的病因，因此该病也称高跟鞋病。

Posterior tibialis injury

胫骨后肌损伤

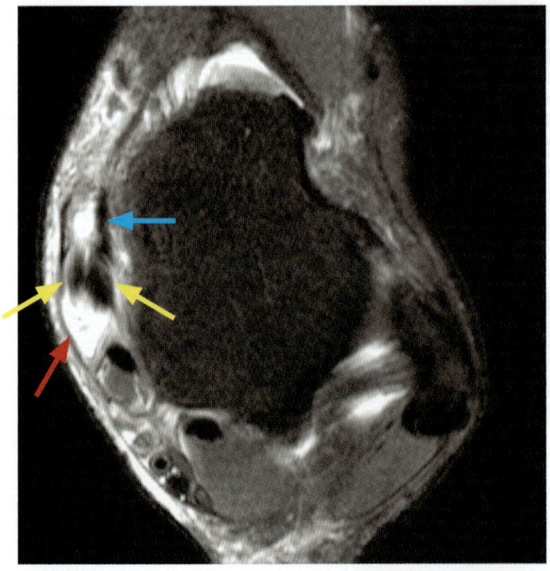

Posterior tibialis tendon (PTT) split tear:
Axial PD-weighted image with fat saturation demonstrates a split tear of the posterior tibial tendon (arrow), with surrounding tenosynovitis (red arrow).
Note slight irregularity and thinning of the spring ligament (blue arrow).
胫骨后肌腱撕裂：
轴位脂肪饱和PD加权图像显示胫后肌腱撕裂(箭)，伴周围腱鞘炎(红箭)。
注意弹簧韧带轻度不规则及变薄(蓝箭)。

- Along with the spring ligament, the posterior tibialis tendon (PTT) provides crucial support to the longitudinal arch of the foot. Posterior tibialis tendon dysfunction (typically due to chronic degeneration) is implicated in acquired adult flatfoot deformity.
- The PTT courses along the retromalleolar groove posterior to the medial malleolus, and subsequently traverses the tarsal tunnel underneath the flexor retinaculum. Chronic inflammation of the PTT can cause periosteal reaction of the medial malleolus with soft-tissue swelling.
- The major attachment of the PTT is the navicular, but important fibers continue and insert more distally on the cuneiforms and second through fifth metatarsal bases.
- Imaging finding of PTT dysfunction includes tenosynovitis, tendinopathy (enlargement of the tendon or intermediate signal), and tearing (intrasubstance fluid signal). Secondary imaging findings include spring ligament injury and pes planus.

- 胫骨后肌腱(PTT)与弹簧韧带一起为纵向足弓提供重要支撑。胫骨后肌腱功能障碍(通常由于慢性退变所致)与成人继发性扁平足畸形相关。
- PTT沿内踝后方的后踝沟走行,随后穿过屈肌支持带下方的跗管。慢性PTT炎症可引起内踝骨膜反应及软组织肿胀。
- PTT的主要附着部位是舟骨,但其重要的纤维继续向远行并附着于楔骨和第二~五跖骨基底部。
- 影像学上PTT功能障碍的表现包括腱鞘炎、肌腱变性(肌腱增大或信号增高)和撕裂(肌腱内液体信号)。间接的影像学征象包括弹簧韧带损伤和扁平足。

Anterior tibialis injury

胫骨前肌损伤

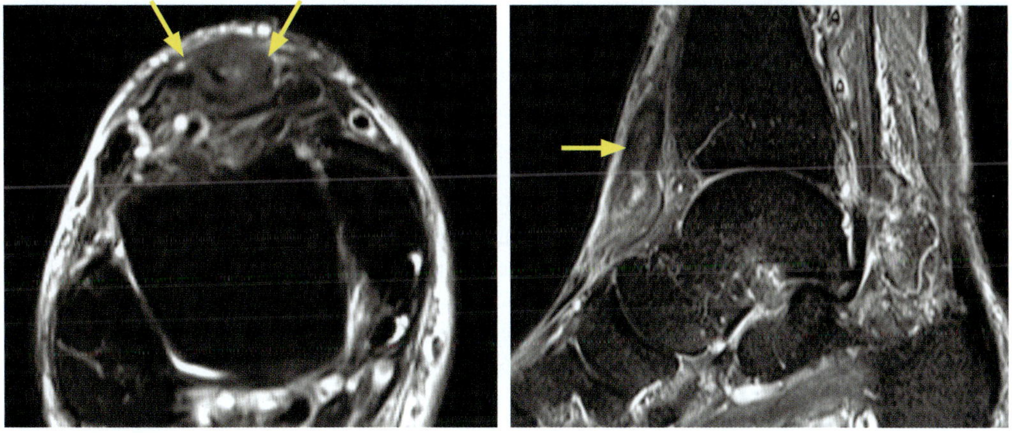

Anterior tibialis full-thickness tear: Axial T2-weighted image with fat suppression (left image) and sagittal STIR MRI demonstrate a full-thickness tear of the anterior tibialis tendon, with proximal retraction (arrows).
胫骨前肌全层撕裂:轴位脂肪抑制T_2加权图像(左图)和矢状位STIR MRI示胫骨前肌肌腱全层撕裂及近端回缩(箭)。

- Injury to anterior tibialis is much less common compared to the posterior tibialis tendon. Rupture of the anterior tibialis may be traumatic or atraumatic in the setting of tendon degeneration.
- An anterior ankle mass is a classic clinical presentation of anterior tibialis rupture.

- 胫骨前肌肌腱较胫骨后肌肌腱损伤要少很多。在有肌腱退变的情况下,胫骨前肌断裂既可能是创伤性,也可能是非创伤性。
- 踝关节前部的肿块是胫骨前肌断裂的典型临床表现。

Deltoid ligament injury

三角韧带损伤

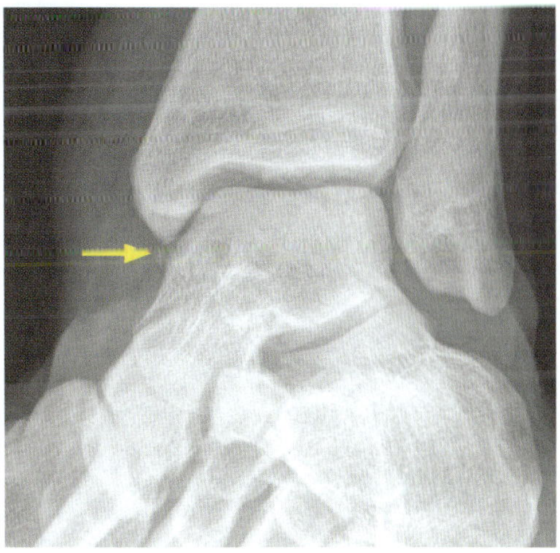

Mortise radiograph
Mortise 位X线影像

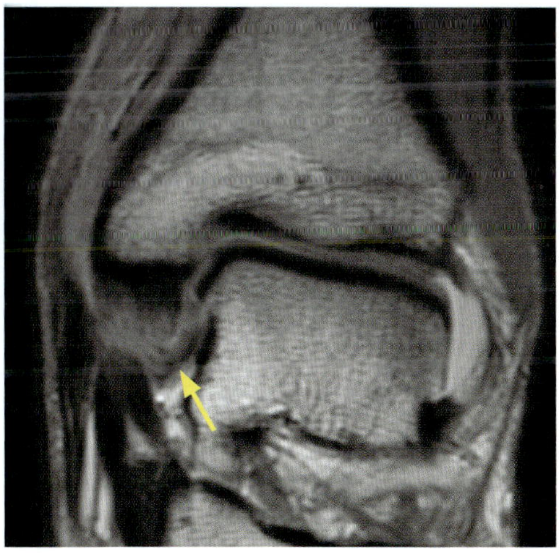

Coronal PD-weighted MRI
冠状位PD加权MRI

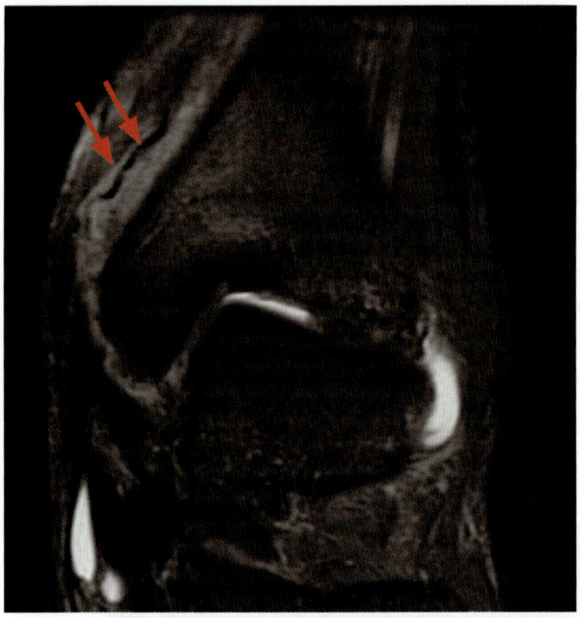

Coronal PD-weighted MRI with fat suppression
冠状位PD加权脂肪抑制MRI

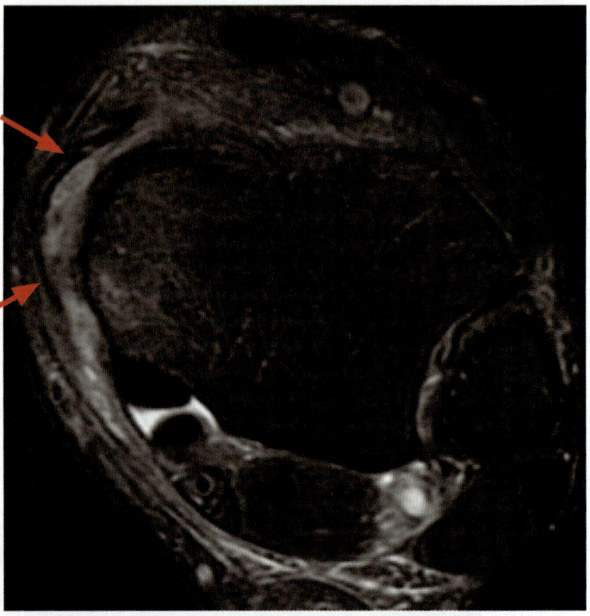

Axial PD-weighted MRI with fat suppression
轴位PD加权脂肪抑制MRI

Deltoid ligament avulsion: Radiograph shows a subtle linear avulsion of the medial talus at the expected insertion site of the deep deltoid ligament (yellow arrow). MRI confirms avulsion of the deltoid ligament, which appears to remain attached onto the avulsed fragment of bone (yellow arrows). There is tearing and periosteal stripping of the superficial deltoid ligament (red arrows), with edema extending to the medial malleolus.
三角韧带撕裂：X线影像显示在距骨内侧三角韧带深层附着处(黄箭)有模糊的线状撕脱影。MRI证实了三角韧带撕裂，似乎仍附着在撕脱的骨碎片上(黄箭)。浅层三角韧带(红箭)有撕裂和骨膜剥离，水肿延伸至内踝。

- The deltoid ligament is the predominant ligamentous stabilizer of the medial ankle.
- The deep deltoid is relatively simple anatomically, connecting the tibia and the talus and only spanning one joint. It normally appears striated with interspersed regions of near fluid signal and fat.
- The superficial deltoid ligament is much more complex anatomically, and spans multiple bones, including tibiotalar, tibionavicular, and tibiocalcaneal components, and there is also a tibiospring component that connects the tibia to the spring ligament. This ligamentous complex merges with the medial malleolus periosteum. These individual components are not usually individually distinguishable by MR.

- 三角韧带是内踝最重要的稳定结构。
- 三角韧带深层在解剖学上相对简单，连接胫骨和距骨，只跨越一个关节。正常情况下呈条纹状，其中散在类液体与脂肪交织的区域。
- 浅层三角韧带在解剖学上更为复杂，跨越多个骨结构，包括胫距关节、胫舟关节和胫跟关节，还有一个连接胫骨和弹簧韧带的胫骨弹簧韧带复合体。该韧带复合体与内踝骨膜融合。这些组成部分通常在MR上无法单独进行区分。

(翻译　姚骊　吕霞飞)

KNEE

膝关节

KNEE TRAUMA

膝关节外伤

Knee dislocation

膝关节脱位

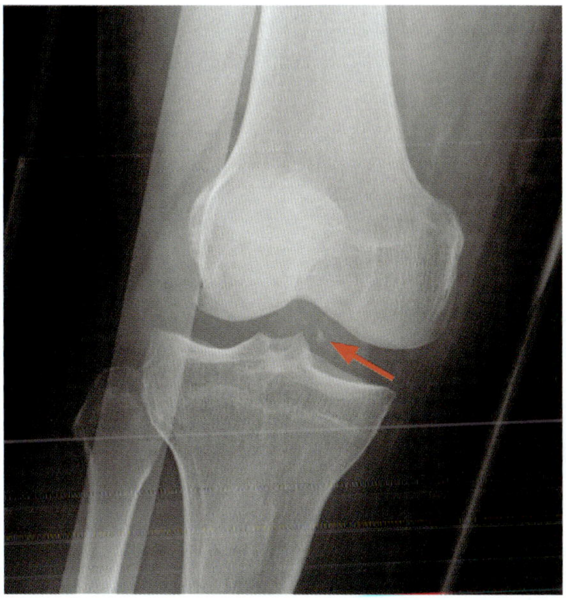

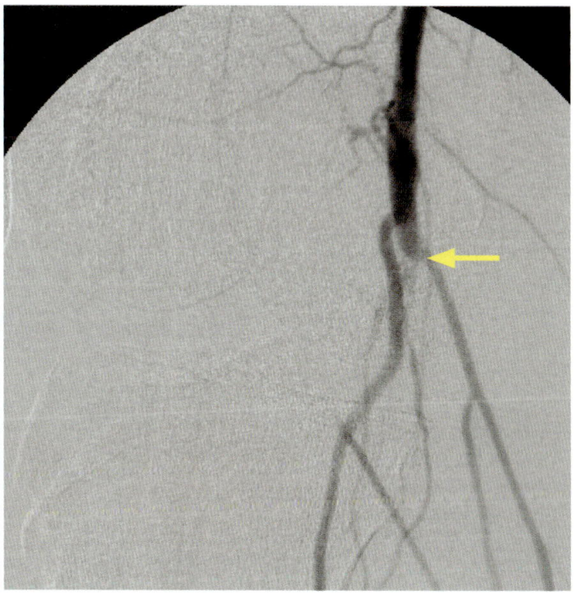

Posterior dislocation with vascular injury: Frontal radiograph of the knee (left image) shows marked widening of the joint space with slight lateral displacement of the tibia. The widened joint space suggests a dislocation. An ossific fragment projects over the joint space (red arrow). Intraoperative digital subtraction angiogram (right image) demonstrates a complete traumatic occlusion of the popliteal artery (arrow) just above the knee.

膝关节后脱位伴血管损伤：膝关节正位X线影像(左图)示膝关节间隙明显增宽伴胫骨轻度向外侧移位。关节间隙增宽提示存在脱位。有一块骨片出现在关节间隙内(红箭)。术中数字减影血管造影(右图)显示腘动脉(箭)在膝关节的上方呈外伤性完全性闭塞。

- The knee may dislocate in any direction, although anteriorly is the most common.
- There is a high risk for vascular injury to the popliteal artery, and a vascular injury may be present even if the distal pulses are still intact. CT angiography is therefore typically recommended for all knee dislocations.

- 膝关节可以向任何方向脱位，但前脱位最常见。
- 腘动脉损伤的风险很高，即便远端有脉搏存在，仍有合并血管外伤的可能。因此，在膝关节脱位时通常建议行CT血管造影。

Patellar fracture

髌骨骨折

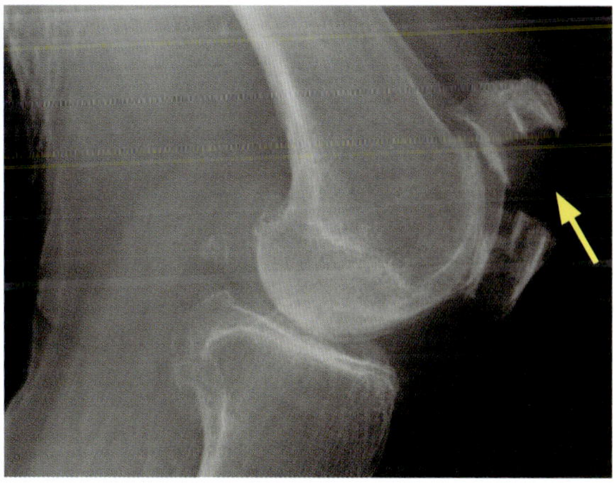

Lateral radiograph of the knee shows a distracted patellar fracture (arrow), suggestive of an injury caused by extreme tension of the extensor mechanism.

膝关节侧位X线影像显示髌骨分离性骨折(箭)，提示损伤由伸肌张力过度引起。

- Patellar fracture may be caused by a direct blow (usually causing a comminuted fracture) or extreme sudden tension of the extensor mechanism (usually causing a distracted fracture).
- It is important to distinguish a fracture from a bipartite or multipartite patella, which are normal variants and will have well corticated margins. A dorsal defect of the patella is another normal variant, appearing as a round lucency at the superior articular (dorsal) aspect of the patella.

Tibial plateau fracture

- Tibial plateau fractures are classified by the Schatzker classification.
- Lateral tibial plateau fractures are more stable than medial tibial plateau fractures.

- 髌骨骨折可由直接外力(常导致粉碎性骨折)或伸肌极度突然紧张(常引起分离性骨折)所致。
- 区别骨折还是二分髌骨或多分髌骨很重要，后者为正常变异，其骨皮质的边缘光滑。髌骨的背侧缺损是另一个正常变异，表现为髌骨上关节面(背侧)的圆形透亮区。

胫骨平台骨折

- 胫骨平台骨折按Schatzker分类法进行划分。
- 胫骨平台外侧骨折较内侧骨折稳定。

MENISCI

半月板

Normal anatomy

正常解剖

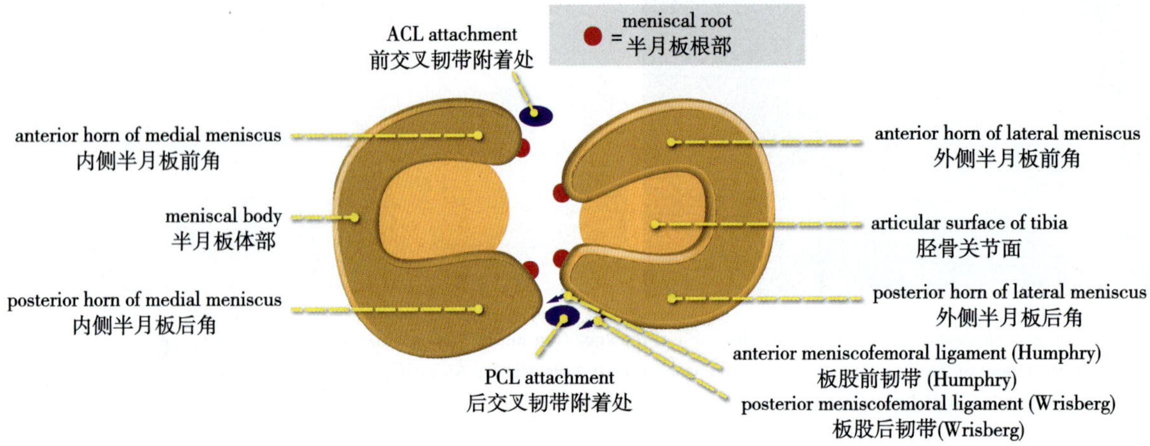

- The medial and lateral menisci are crescent-shaped fibrocartilaginous structures that form a discontinuous figure-8 to stabilize the knee and disperse the axial loading.
- Each meniscus consists of an anterior and a posterior horn.
  The posterior horn of the medial meniscus is larger than its anterior horn.
  Both horns of the lateral meniscus are the same size.
- Each meniscus is attached to the tibial plateau by an anterior and posterior meniscal root. Trauma to the meniscal root may cause meniscal extrusion.
- There are two meniscofemoral ligaments, which extend from the posterior horn of the lateral meniscus to the medial femoral condyle. It is important not to mistake a meniscofemoral ligament (which are variably present) for a meniscal tear.
  The ligament of Humphrey is anterior to PCL; the ligament of Wrisberg is posterior to the PCL.
- The peripheral third of each meniscus is relatively vascular and is called the *red zone*. The central portion of the meniscus is considered avascular.
- Meniscal injuries confined to the red zone may heal spontaneously or after surgical repair, while more central meniscal injuries generally do not heal.

- 内侧和外侧半月板都是新月形的纤维软骨结构，形成一个不连续的8字形，起稳定膝关节和分散轴向负荷的作用。
- 每个半月板由前角及后角组成。
  内侧半月板后角大于前角。
  外侧半月板的前后角大小相同。
- 每个半月板都通过半月板前角和后角的根与胫股平台相连。半月板根部外伤可引起半月板外突。
- 一共有两条半月板股韧带，从外侧半月板后角延伸到股骨内侧髁。应注意不要将半月板股韧带(有各种变异)误认为半月板撕裂。
  Humphrey韧带位于后交叉韧带的前方；Wrisberg韧带位于后交叉韧带的后方。
- 每个半月板外周1/3是相对富血供区称红色区域。半月板的中央区域则认为是乏血供区。
- 若半月板损伤局限于红色区域可自愈或在手术修复后痊愈，而发生在中央区域的损伤常不能愈合。

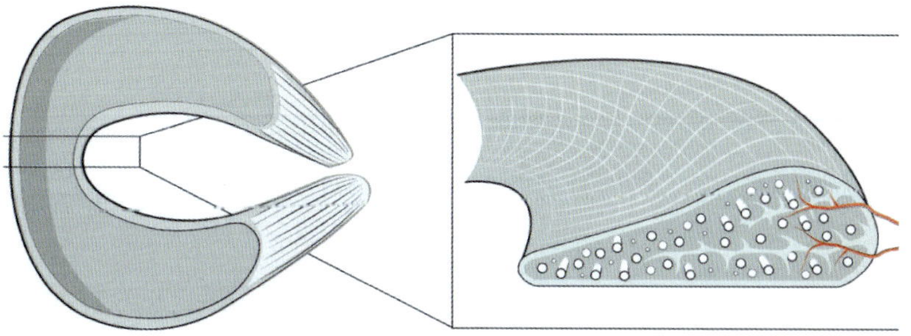

Normal appearance of menisci on MR

半月板在MR上的正常表现

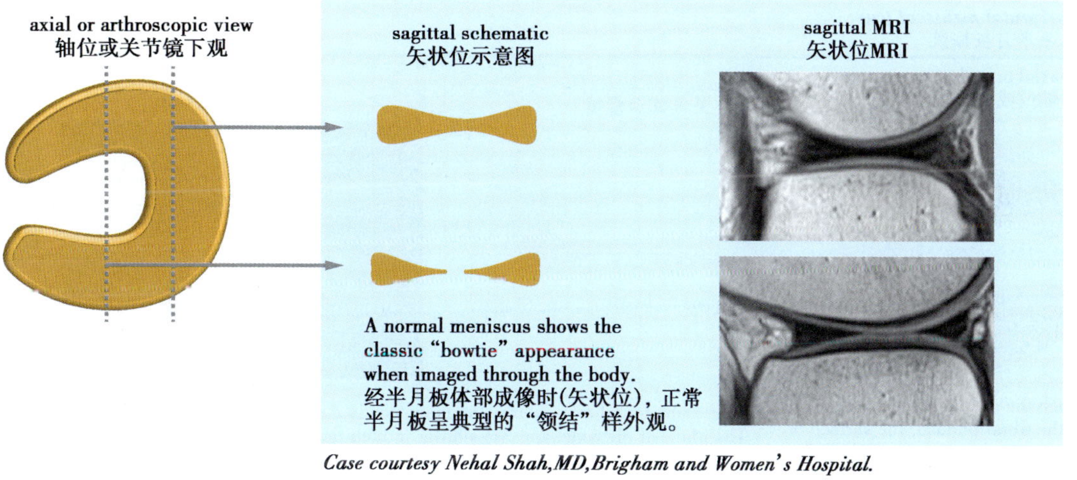

Case courtesy Nehal Shah, MD, Brigham and Women's Hospital.

Myxoid degeneration versus tear

- Myxoid degeneration is increased signal on T2-weighted images within the meniscus that does not extend to the meniscal surface. It is not thought to cause symptoms and is not treated.
- In contrast, a meniscal tear is seen as a linear band of increased signal on T2-weighted images that *does* extend to the articular surface. The morphology of the meniscus is commonly abnormal. MRI is >90% sensitive and specific for the diagnosis of meniscal tears.

黏液样变性与撕裂

- 黏液样变性是指半月板内的T_2加权图像上出现信号增高，但未延伸到半月板的表面。这一发现并不认为会引起症状，也不需要治疗。
- 与之相反，半月板撕裂在T_2加权图像上表现为一条线状的信号增高带并累及关节面。半月板的形态通常不正常。MRI对诊断半月板撕裂的敏感性及特异性>90%。

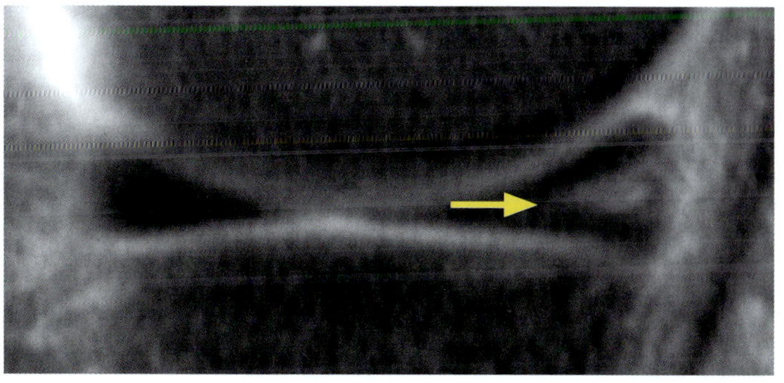

Meniscus myxoid degeneration: Sagittal fluid-sensitive MRI demonstrates increased globular signal (arrow) in the peripheral meniscus that does not extend to the articular surface.

Case courtesy Nehal Shah, MD, Brigham and Women's Hospital.

半月板黏液样变性：矢状位液体敏感MRI显示外侧半月板内呈球状信号增高(箭)，未累及关节面。

Oblique/horizontal tear

斜向/水平撕裂

oblique meniscal tear
斜行半月板撕裂

axial or arthroscopic view
轴位或关节镜下观

sagittal schematic
矢状位示意图

sagittal MRI
矢状位MRI

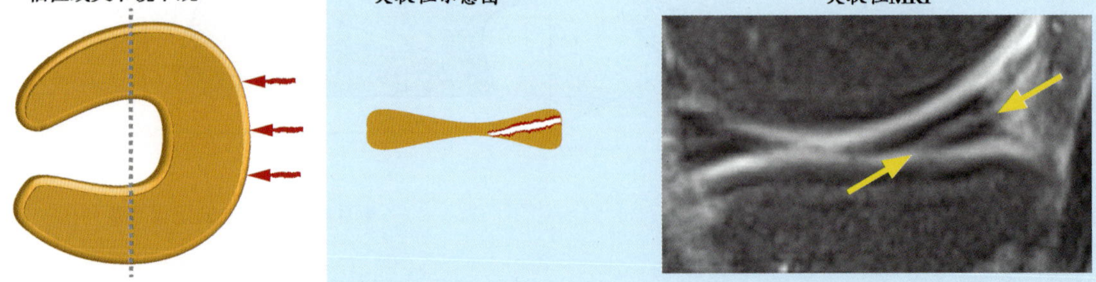

horizontal meniscal tear
水平半月板撕裂

axial or arthroscopic view
轴位或关节镜下观

sagittal schematic
矢状位示意图

coronal MRI
冠状位MRI

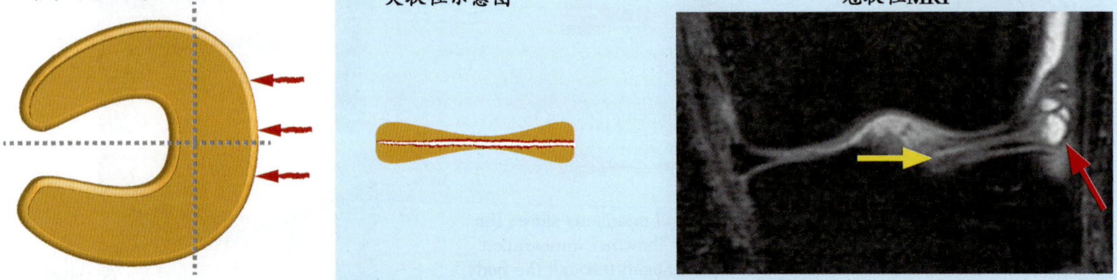

Since the cleavage plane is parallel to the tibial plateau, the surface of the meniscus will appear normal.
由于撕裂平面平行于胫骨平台，因此半月板的表面呈正常表现。

A true horizontal tear cleaves the meniscus in a plane parallel to the tibial plateau. The plane of cleavage appears similar in both the sagittal (as in the schematic) and coronal views. Note the associated parameniscal cysts (red arrow).
真性半月板水平撕裂发生于胫骨平台的平行平面。撕裂平面在矢状位和冠状位表现类似（如示意图）。注意合并半月板旁的囊肿（红箭）。

Case courtesy Nehal Shah,MD,Brigham and Women's Hospital.

- The terms *oblique* and *horizontal* are sometimes used interchangeably when referring to meniscal tears. Strictly speaking, however, a horizontal tear remains parallel to the tibial plateau, while an oblique tear may be at a slight angle to the tibial plateau.
- An oblique/horizontal tear is the most common meniscal tear, typically occurring in the posterior horn of the medial meniscus.
- Oblique and horizontal tears are more often degenerative, rather than due to trauma.

- 术语"斜行和水平状"有时在描述半月板撕裂时可以互换。但严格意义上讲，水平状撕裂与胫骨平台保持平行，而斜行撕裂可与胫骨平台存在轻微的角度。
- 斜行/水平状撕裂是半月板撕裂最常见的类型，多发生在内侧半月板的后角。
- 斜行和水平状撕裂多由退变引起，而非因为外伤。

Vertical/longitudinal tear

垂直/纵行撕裂

axial or arthroscopic view
轴位或关节镜下观

sagittal schematic
矢状位示意图

sagittal MRI
矢状位MRI

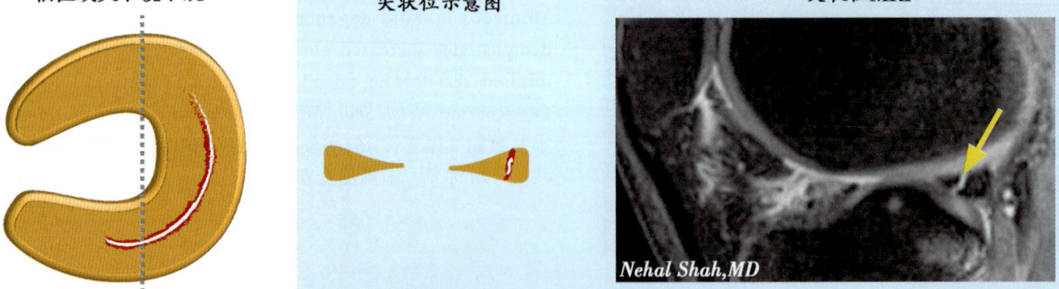

A vertical (longitudinal) tear is present (arrow) demonstrating complete superior-to-inferior surface extension.
垂直(纵向)撕裂(箭)完全贯通上下关节面。

- The vertical (synonymous with longitudinal) tear is a curved tear that follows the contour of the meniscus. On serial sagittal images, the tear will be in a vertical orientation and will remain a fixed distance from the edge of the meniscus.

Bucket handle tear

- 垂直(同义词为纵向)撕裂是沿半月板表面轮廓走行的弧形撕裂。在连续矢状位成像上，这种撕裂呈垂直方向且与半月板边缘保持固定的距离。

桶柄样撕裂

axial or arthroscopic view
轴位或关节镜下观

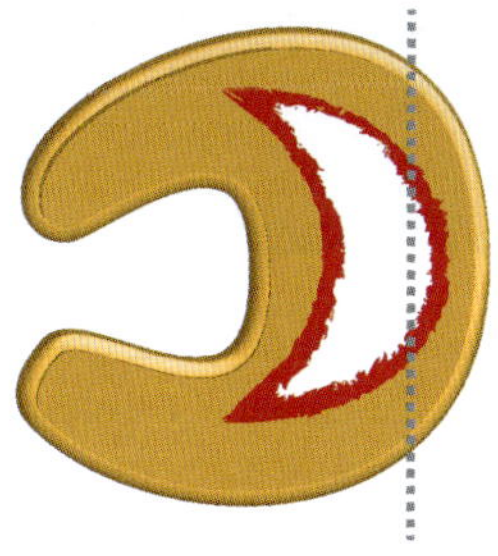

sagittal schematic
矢状位示意图

sagittal MRI
矢状位MRI

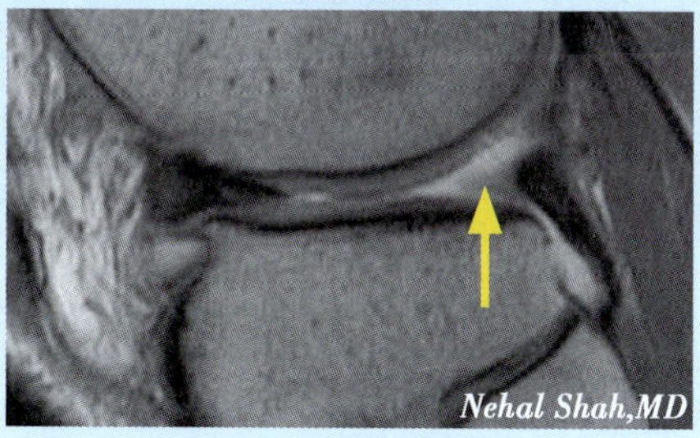

Absent bow tie sign: No normal bow tie is seen posteriorly (arrow).
领结缺失征: 后方看不到正常的领结(箭)。

native anterior meniscus
正常的半月板前角
displaced bucket handle fragment
移位的桶柄样碎片

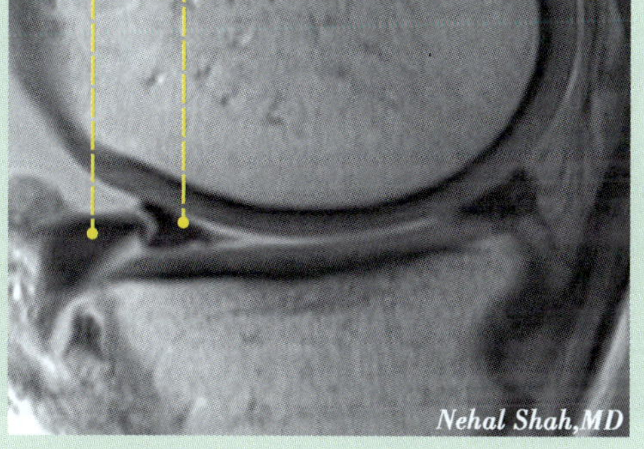

The ***double delta sign*** is seen if the displaced fragment flips anteriorly.
双三角征见于移位的碎片向前翻转。

displaced meniscal fragment
移位的半月板碎片
normal PCL
正常后交叉韧带

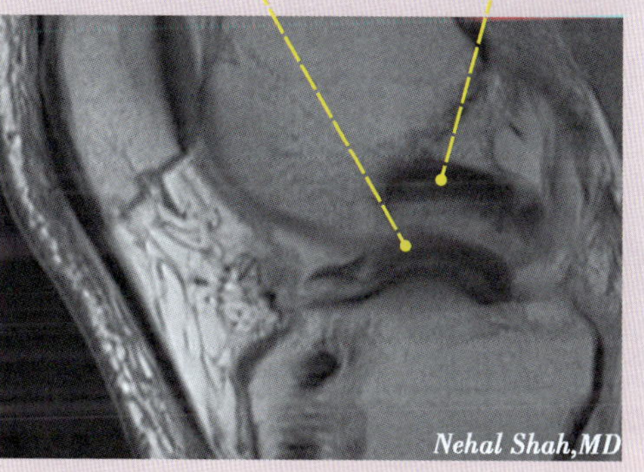

The ***double PCL sign*** is seen if the displaced fragment flips centrally into the intercondylar notch.
双后交叉韧带征见于移位的碎片向中心翻转进入髁间窝。

- The result of a longitudinal vertical tear, a bucket-handle tear occurs when the free inner edge of the meniscus (medial meniscus most commonly) gets displaced or flipped over.
- The most common location of the displaced meniscal fragment is the intercondylar notch, but the meniscal fragment may also displace anteriorly or posteriorly.
- The *absent bow tie sign* represents the absent (displaced) meniscal horn.

- 纵向垂直撕裂可造成桶柄样撕裂，发生于半月板内侧游离缘(内侧半月板最常见)移位或翻转。
- 移位半月板碎片最常见的位置是髁间窝，但半月板碎片也可向前或向后移位。
- 缺失的领结征代表半月板角缺如(移位)。

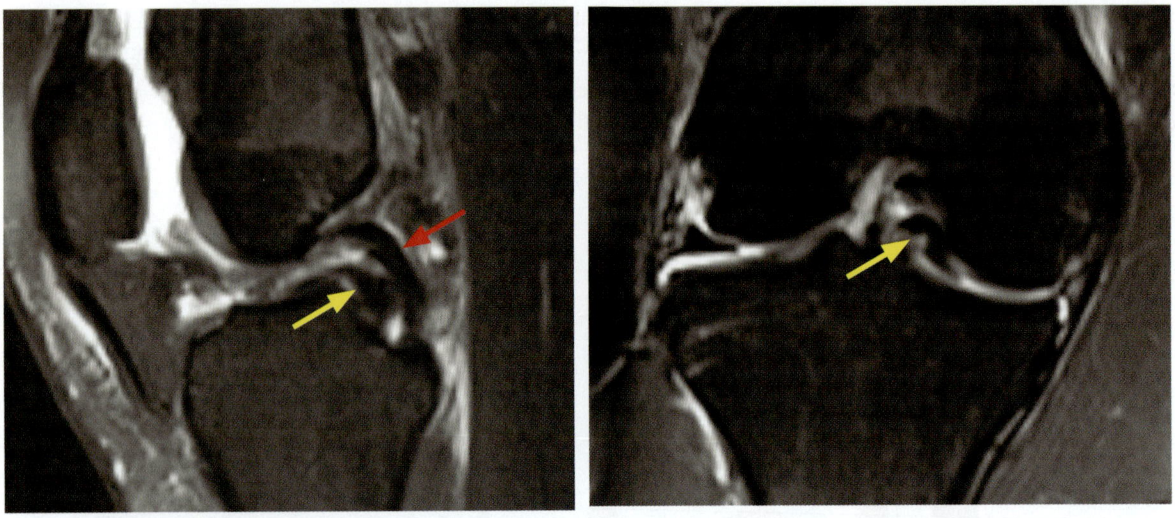

Double PCL sign: Sagittal (left image) and coronal PD-weighted MRI with fat suppression demonstrates a bucket-handle tear of the medial meniscus (yellow arrows), which is displaced into the intercondylar notch, creating a double PCL sign on the sagittal. Note the normal PCL (red arrow).
双PCL征：矢状位(左图)和冠状位PD加权脂肪抑制MRI显示内侧半月板(黄箭)桶柄样撕裂，并向髁间窝移位，在矢状位形成双PCL征。注意正常的PCL(红箭)。

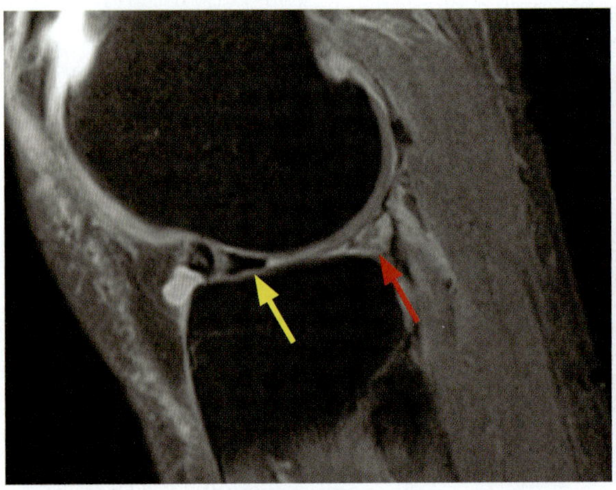

Sagittal PD-weighted MRI with fat suppression in a different patient demonstrates a bucket-handle tear of the posterior horn of the lateral meniscus, with an anteriorly displaced fragment (yellow arrow) and absent posterior horn (red arrow). Note the fibula indicating that this is the lateral meniscus.
另一名患者的矢状位PD加权脂肪抑制MRI显示外侧半月板后角呈桶柄样撕裂，撕裂半月板碎片向前移位(黄箭)，后角缺失(红箭)。注意腓骨的位置，提示这是外侧半月板。

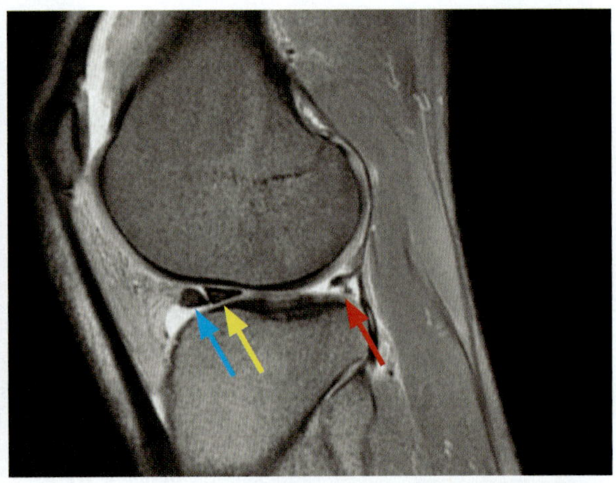

Sagittal PD-weighted MRI with fat suppression in a third patient again demonstrates a double delta sign (yellow arrow) with absent posterior horn (red arrow). The native anterior horn (blue arrow) is anteriorly displaced. These tend to look remarkably consistent.
第三名患者的矢状位PD加权脂肪抑制MRI显示双三角征(黄箭)伴后角缺失(红箭)。正常的前角(蓝箭)向前方移位。这些表现看起来非常一致。

- The *double delta sign* is seen with an anteriorly displaced longitudinal vertical meniscal fragment. The displaced fragment is located more posterior compared to the native anterior horn, which is pushed anteriorly.
- The *double PCL sign* is seen when the posterior horn longitudinal vertical meniscal flap does not flip all the way anteriorly.
- A *double delta sign* or *double PCL sign* depends on if the medial or lateral meniscus is involved, and on the status of the ACL (for medial meniscal tears only).
- A peripheral longitudinal tear of the posterior horn of the medial meniscus cannot flip anteriorly if the ACL is intact. Therefore, a medial meniscus bucket handle tear is far more likely to cause the *double PCL sign*.

- 双三角征见于有向前移位伴纵向与垂直撕裂的半月板碎片。与正常的前角相比，移位的碎片位于更靠后的位置，因后者被推向了前方。
- 双PCL征见于后角半月板纵向、垂直不完全向前翻转。
- 双三角征或双PCL征取决于是否累及内侧或外侧半月板，以及ACL的状态(仅适用于内侧半月板撕裂)。
- 如果ACL完整，内侧半月板后角的外周纵向撕裂不能前翻。因此，内侧半月板桶柄样撕裂更容易引起双PCL征。

- A peripheral longitudinal tear of the posterior horn of the lateral meniscus is not impeded by the ACL and the *double delta sign* can occur.
- In summary, a double delta sign is likely a lateral meniscal tear (or far less commonly, a medial meniscus tear with torn ACL). A double PCL sign is likely a medial meniscus tear (with intact ACL).

- 外侧半月板后角的外周纵向撕裂不受前交叉韧带阻碍，可出现双三角征。
- 综上所述，双三角征很可能是外侧半月板撕裂(或较少见的内侧半月板撕裂伴前交叉韧带撕裂)。双PCL征很可能是内侧半月板撕裂(ACL完整)。

Radial/transverse tear

放射状/横向撕裂

radial tear of meniscal body
半月板体部的放射状撕裂

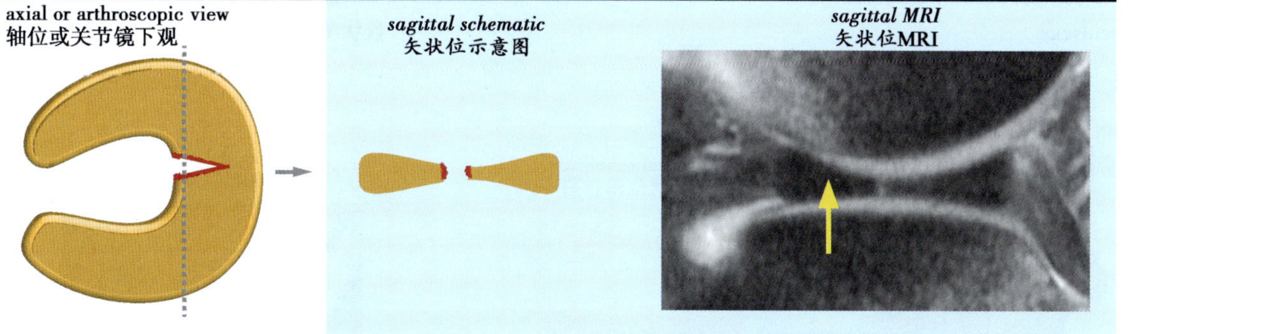

Radial tear is a vertically oriented tear extending from the free edge of the meniscus to the periphery.
放射状撕裂是 种垂直方向的撕裂，从半月板游离缘向外周延伸。

radial tear of meniscal horn
半月板角的放射状撕裂

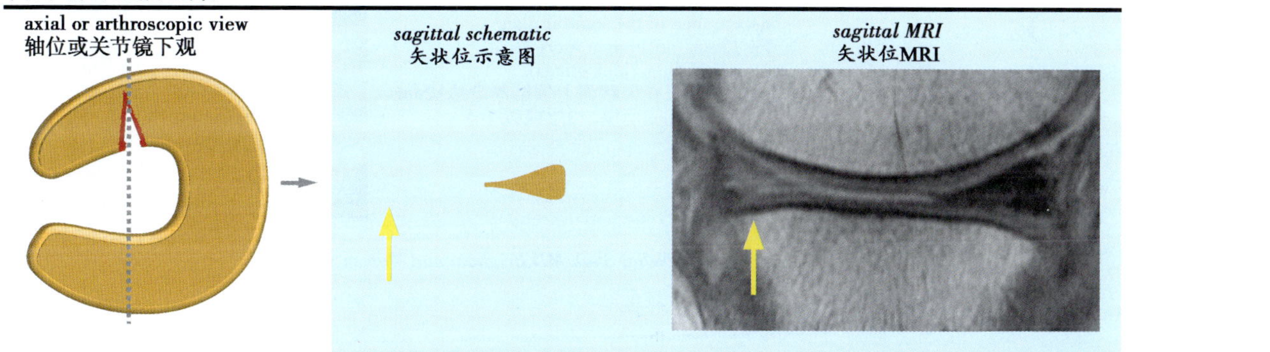

Ghost meniscus sign: No meniscal tissue is seen when the plane of imaging is directly through the radial tear (arrows).
鬼影半月板征：当成像平面恰好通过放射状撕裂（箭）时看不到半月板组织。

Cases courtesy Nehal Shah,MD,Brigham and Women's Hospital.

- A radial tear (also known as a transverse tear) is a vertically oriented tear that is perpendicular to the arc of the meniscus. In contrast, a previously discussed vertical/ longitudinal tear follows the curve of the meniscus.
- On a single image, a radial tear may be indistinguishable from a vertical/ longitudinal tear. On serial sagittal images, however, the radial tear will change position relative to the edge of the meniscus. This phenomenon is the *marching cleft sign*.
- Depending on the orientation of the tear in relation to the scan plane, a radial tear may also show the *ghost meniscus sign*. The ghost meniscus is typically described as absence of the posterior horn of the meniscus on sagittal images (although it may also occur with absence of the anterior horn, as seen above). It occurs in tears adjacent to the intercondylar notch.

- 放射状撕裂(也称横向撕裂)是一种垂直撕裂，也就是垂直于半月板弧。与之相反，前述的垂直/纵行撕裂则是沿着半月板弧。
- 在单幅图像上，放射状撕裂与垂直/纵行撕裂可能难以区别。而在连续的矢状位图像上，放射状撕裂相对于半月板边缘位置会发生改变。这种现象称为移动裂隙征。
- 放射状撕裂的表现取决于撕裂方向与扫描平面的相对关系，它也可表现为鬼影半月板征。鬼影半月板通常是指在矢状位图像上半月板后角缺如(但也可见于半月板前角缺如，如上图所示)。该征象出现在髁间窝附近发生撕裂。

- Radial tears are associated with a high rate of meniscal extrusion, which may lead to osteoarthritis if not treated.

Paramensical cyst

- A parameniscal cyst is loculated fluid adjacent to the meniscus, thought to result from extension of joint fluid through a meniscal tear.
- Parameniscal cysts are most commonly associated with horizontal cleavage tears.
- It is important to mention the presence of a parameniscal cyst because the cyst may continue to cause symptoms even if the meniscus is resected. Not all cysts are able to be visualized by arthroscopy.

Discoid meniscus

- 放射状撕裂伴有半月板外突的发生率较高，若不治疗可导致骨关节炎。

半月板旁囊肿

- 半月板旁囊肿是半月板附近的包裹性液体，可能是关节内液体沿撕裂的半月板扩散而形成的。
- 半月板旁囊肿最常合并水平状撕裂。
- 必须要提及半月板旁囊肿的重要性，因为即使切除半月板，半月板旁囊肿仍能继续引起症状。不是所有半月板旁囊肿都能在关节镜下被发现。

盘状半月板

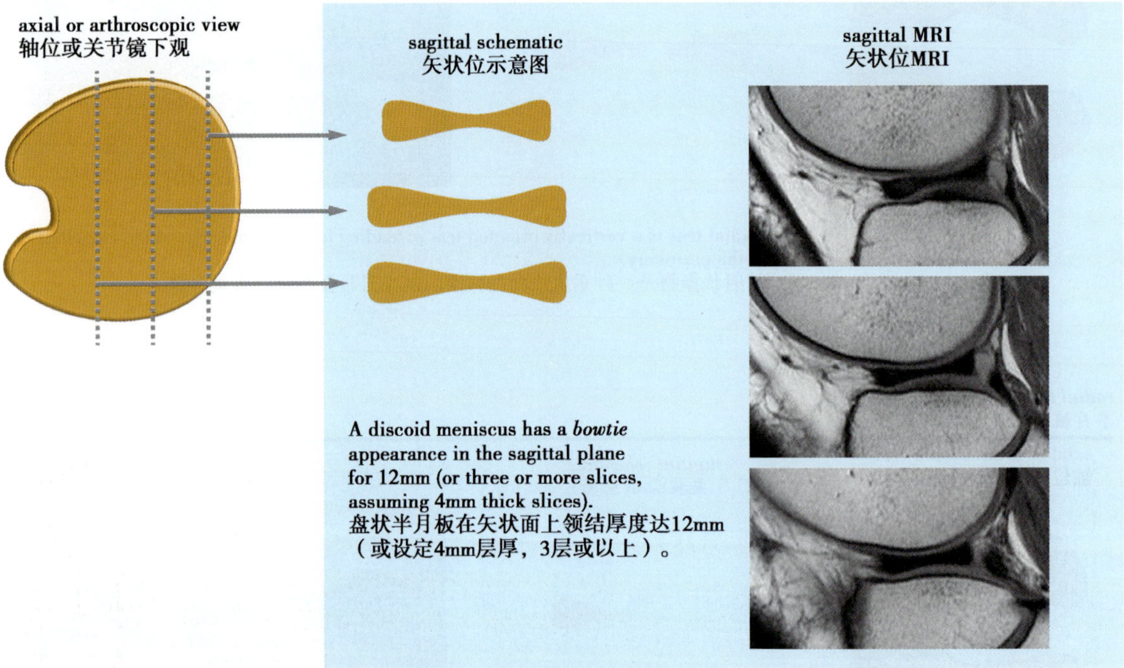

Case courtesy Nehal Shah,MD,Brigham and Women's Hospital.

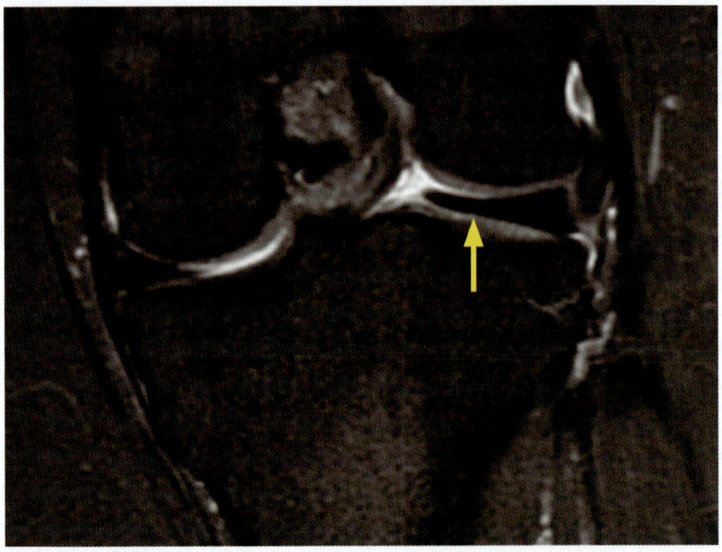

Coronal PD-weighted MRI with fat suppression demonstrates a discoid lateral meniscus (arrow).
冠状位PD加权脂肪抑制MRI显示外侧盘状半月板(箭)。

- Discoid meniscus is a spectrum of congenital malformations of the meniscus that ranges from increased thickness of the meniscus to a complete disc-like shape. Discoid meniscus is defined by having a portion of the meniscus which extends to the central tibial plateau.
- Discoid meniscus typically affects children and is a common cause of joint-line pain, clicking, or locking in a child or adolescent. Discoid meniscus is prone to undergo cystic degeneration and tear. Even in the absence of a tear, a discoid meniscus may be symptomatic.
- The lateral meniscus is more commonly affected.
- On MRI, a meniscus is discoid if an oval or *bow tie-shaped* meniscus is seen on three or more contiguous sagittal slices with standard 4 mm thick sagittal slices (representing 12 mm in medial-lateral thickness).

- 盘状半月板是一组半月板的先天发育畸形，其表现可以从半月板增厚到完全呈盘状的半月板。盘状半月板定义为半月板部分延伸到胫骨平台的中央。
- 盘状半月板好发于儿童，是导致儿童或青少年关节轴向疼痛、弹响或绞锁的常见原因。盘状半月板有囊性变和撕裂倾向。即使无撕裂，盘状半月板也可产生症状。
- 外侧半月板更常累及。
- MRI上，如果卵圆形或领结状的半月板在标准4mm层厚的序列矢状位上连续出现至少3层(代表从内到外有12mm层厚)则可认为是盘状半月板。

Knee ligaments

Anterior cruciate ligament (ACL) overview

- The anterior cruciate ligament (ACL) arises from the femoral intercondylar notch and attaches on the anterior tibial plateau, directly lateral to the tibial spine. The tibial attachment of the ACL is stronger than its femoral origin. The ACL is composed of two fiber bundles, a small anteromedial band and larger posterolateral band.
- Mucoid degeneration shows thickening of ACL with intermediate T2 hyperintense signal and a *celery stalk* appearance.

膝关节韧带

前交叉韧带(ACL)概述

- 前交叉韧带(ACL)起自股骨髁间窝，附着于胫骨平台前部，紧邻胫骨髁间嵴外侧。ACL的胫骨附着处比股骨起始处牢固。ACL由两个纤维束组成，即较小的前内侧束及较大的后外侧束。
- 黏液样变性表现为前交叉韧带增厚，T_2加权中度高信号，呈芹菜茎样外观。

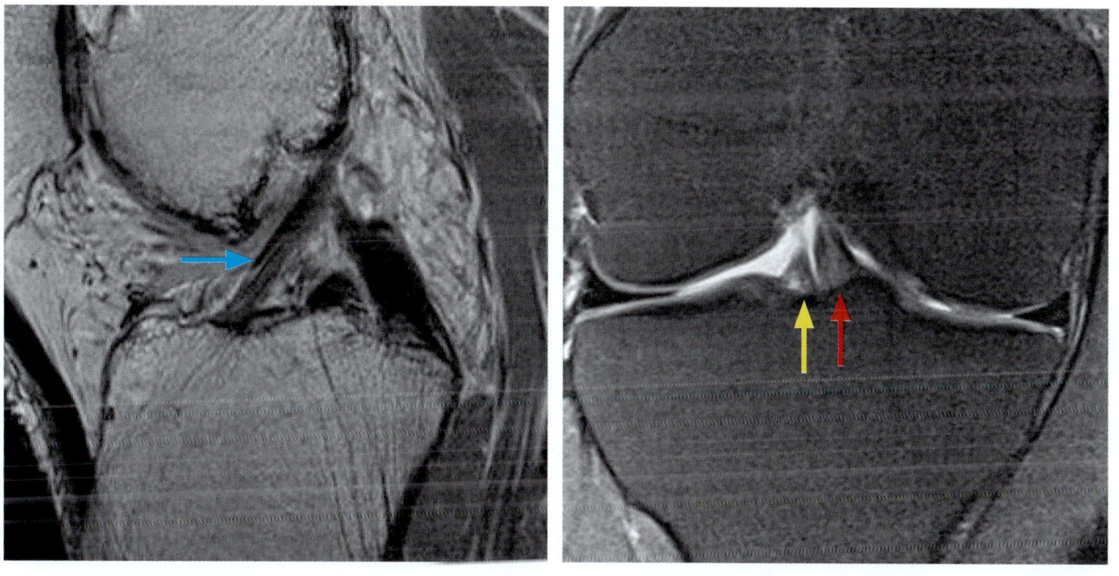

Normal ACL: Sagittal proton-density (left image) and coronal proton-density fat-saturated (right image) MRI shows the normal course of the ACL fibers with the typical striated appearance (blue arrow) on the sagittal image. The coronal image demonstrates the smaller anteromedial (yellow arrow) and larger posterolateral (red arrow) fiber bundles in the intercondylar notch.
正常ACL：矢状位(左图)和冠状位(右图)PD加权脂肪饱和MRI显示正常走行的前交叉韧带纤维束，在矢状位图像上呈典型的条纹状(蓝箭)。冠状位图像显示髁间窝内较小的前内侧纤维束(黄箭)及较大的后外侧束(红箭)。

ACL tear

- ACL tear is typically caused by an acute injury.
- MRI of ACL tear may show either frank discontinuity of the ligament fibers or abnormal course and signal of the ligament.

ACL撕裂

- ACL撕裂多由急性损伤引起。
- MRI上ACL撕裂可表现为明显的韧带纤维中断或韧带走行和信号异常。

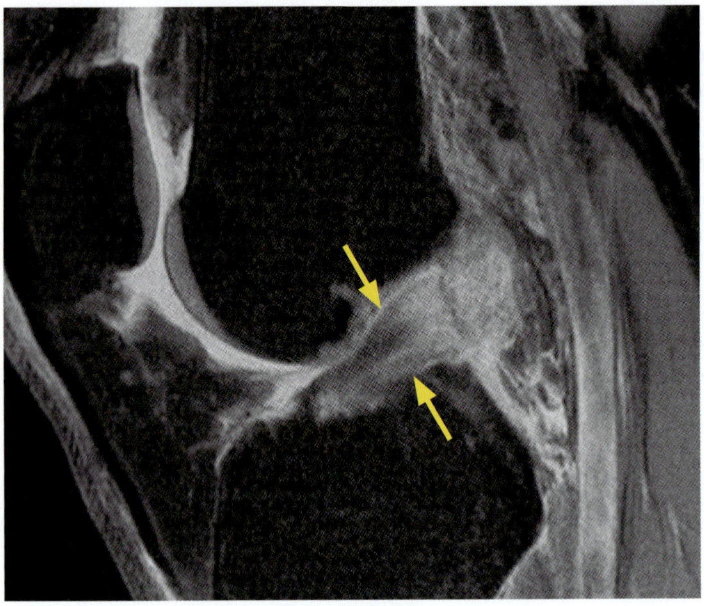

ACL tear: Sagittal fluid-sensitive MRI demonstrates frank rupture of the ACL (arrows), with discontinuity of the fibers and increased signal.

Case courtesy Nehal Shah, MD, Brigham and Women's Hospital.

ACL撕裂：矢状位液体敏感MRI显示明显的ACL断裂(箭)，纤维束不连续且信号增高。

- ACL injury is often associated with meniscal tears and MCL tears (O'Donoghue's triad). Posterolateral corner knee injuries are also frequently seen in association with ACL injury.
- There are multiple secondary findings of ACL injury. A characteristic bone contusion pattern with bone marrow edema in the lateral femoral condyle and the posterolateral tibial plateau is highly suggestive of ACL injury. Secondary buckling of the posterior collateral ligament (PCL) may also be seen due to anterior displacement of the tibia (positive *drawer sign*).

- ACL损伤常伴有半月板及内侧副韧带撕裂(O'Donoghue三联征)。膝关节后外侧角损伤也常伴发ACL损伤。
- ACL损伤可产生多个继发性表现。股骨外侧髁及胫骨平台后外侧骨挫伤伴骨髓水肿具有特征性并高度提示ACL损伤。也可出现PCL继发性桶柄样撕裂，为胫骨向前移位所致(抽屉征阳性)。

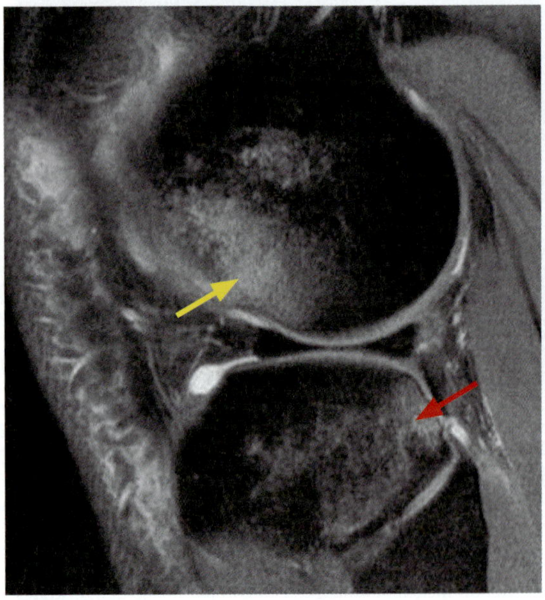

Secondary findings of ACL tear: Sagittal fluid- sensitive MRI image shows bone marrow edema in the lateral femoral condyle (yellow arrow) and posterolateral tibial plateau (red arrow), a pattern characteristic of ACL injury.

ACL撕裂的继发表现：矢状位液体敏感MRI显示股骨外侧髁(黄箭)及胫骨平台后外侧(红箭)骨髓水肿，为ACL损伤的特征性表现。

Cases courtesy Nehal Shah, MD, Brigham and Women's Hospital.

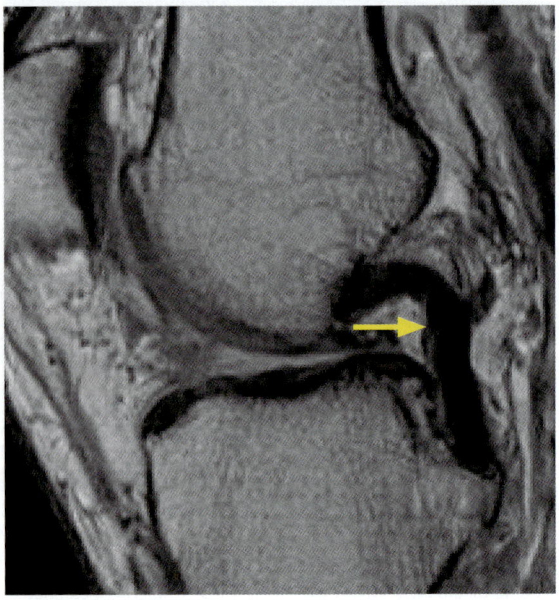

Secondary findings of ACL tear in a different patient: Sagittal proton-density MRI shows buckling of the PCL (arrow), suggestive of an ACL injury.

另一名患者ACL撕裂的继发性表现：矢状位PD加权MRI显示PCL桶柄样撕裂(箭)，提示ACL损伤。

- A clue to ACL injury on radiography is a **Segond fracture**, which is an avulsion fracture of the lateral tibia plateau. Segond fracture is associated with both ACL injury and iliotibial (IT) band injury. The IT band inserts on Gerdy's tubercle of the tibia.

  The Segond fracture is thought to represent detachment of the lateral capsular ligament.

- X线影像上提示ACL损伤的一个线索是**Segond骨折**，这是一种胫骨平台外侧的撕脱性骨折。Segond骨折可同时发生ACL及髂胫束(IT)损伤。髂胫束附着于胫骨Gerdy结节。

  Segond骨折被认为是外侧关节囊韧带撕脱。

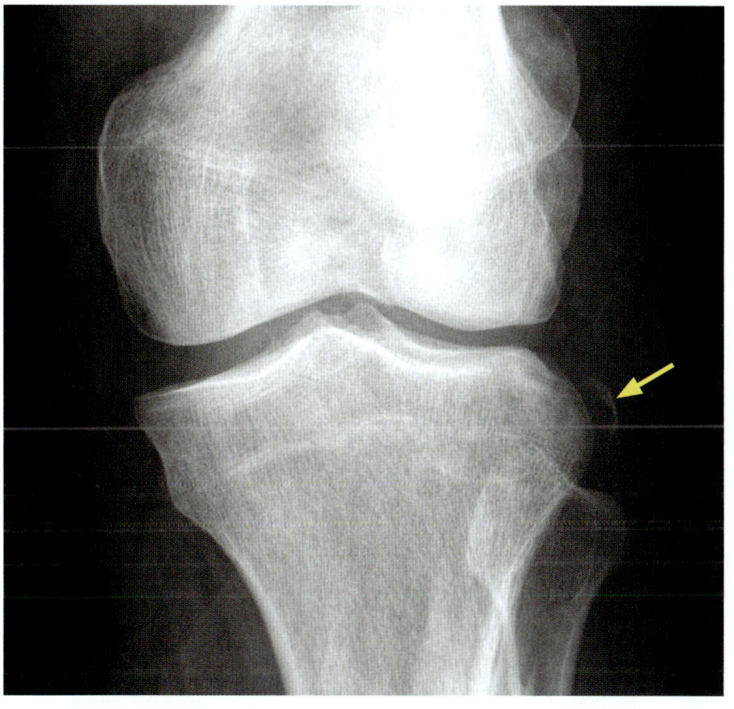

Segond fracture: Frontal knee radiograph shows an avulsion fracture of the lateral tibial plateau (arrow).
These fractures can be easily missed on radiography, but are important to diagnose.
MRI should be recommended if a Segond fracture is seen.
Segond骨折：正位膝关节X线影像显示胫骨平台外缘撕脱骨折(箭)。
这类骨折容易在X线影像上漏诊，但对诊断很重要。
如出现Segond骨折，需建议MRI检查。

- After ACL reconstruction, the ACL graft should run parallel to the intercondylar notch, behind **Blumensaat's line** (a line drawn on radiography along the intercondylar roof).

  If the reconstructed ACL is too steep → graft can be impinged by the femur with leg extension.

  If the reconstructed ACL is too lax → graft may not provide enough stability.

  A complication of ACL reconstruction is the ***cyclops*** lesion, which is nodular scarring in Hoffa's fat pad.

- ACL重建术后，修补的ACL应与髁间窝相平行，位于**Blumensaat线**的后方(在X线影像上沿髁间窝顶部画一条线)。

  如重建的ACL过紧→修补后的韧带在小腿伸展时可能被股骨顶压。

  如重建的ACL过于松弛→修补后的韧带不能起到足够稳定的作用。

  ACL重建术的一种并发症为独眼病变，为Hoff脂肪垫的结节样瘢痕。

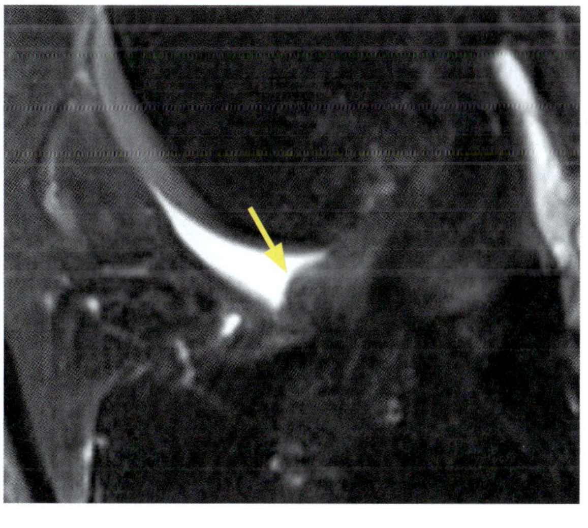

Cyclops lesion post-ACL reconstruction: Fluid-sensitive sagittal MRI shows nodular soft-tissue (arrow) anterior to the reconstructed ACL.
Case courtesy Nehal Shah, MD, Brigham and Women's Hospital, Boston
ACL重建术后独眼病变：液体敏感矢状位MRI示位于重建ACL前的结节样软组织(箭)。

Posterior cruciate ligament (PCL) overview

- The posterior cruciate ligament (PCL) is a stronger, thicker ligament than the ACL. It also arises from the femoral intercondylar notch (more anteriorly than the ACL), but inserts on the posterior tibial plateau.
  The PCL is normally low signal on all sequences.
  The PCL is much less commonly injured than ACL.

PCL tear

- In contrast to an ACL tear, a complete disruption of the PCL fibers is uncommon.
- The typical MRI appearance of PCL injury is increased laxity of the PCL, with or without abnormal high signal on T2-weighted images.

后交叉韧带(PCL)概述

- 后交叉韧带(PLC)比前交叉韧带牢固和粗大。它同样起自股骨髁间窝(位置比ACL更靠前)，但附着在胫骨平台的后部。
  正常的PCL在所有序列上均为低信号。
  PCL受损远不如ACL常见。

PCL撕裂

- 与ACL撕裂相比，完全性PCL纤维束断裂并不常见。
- PCL损伤的典型MRI表现是PCL松弛度增加，伴或不伴T_2加权图像上的异常高信号。

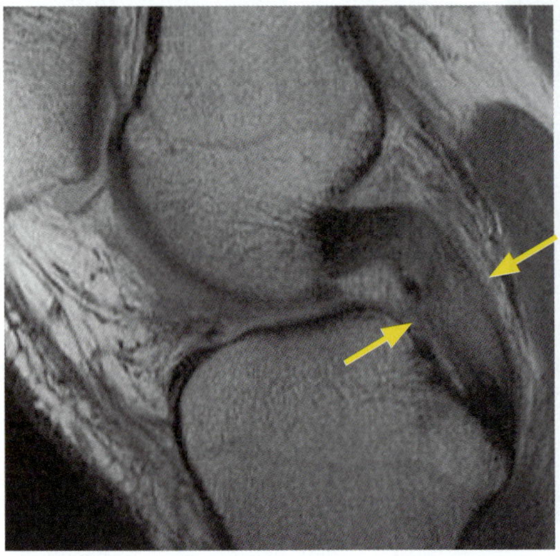

PCL interstitial tear: Sagittal proton-density MRI shows a PCL interstitial tear (arrows) with increased thickness, abnormal signal, and increased laxity of the PCL.
后交叉韧带内撕裂：矢状位PD加权MRI显示PCL韧带内撕裂(箭)，伴后交叉韧带增厚、异常信号和PCL松弛。

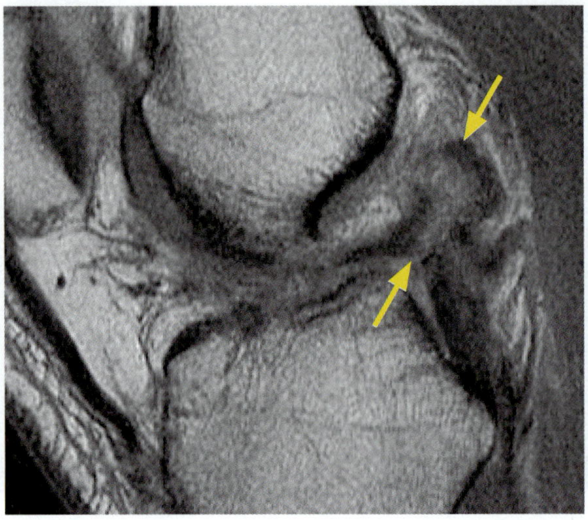

PCL complete tear (in a different patient): Sagittal proton-density MRI shows complete rupture of the PCL with frank discontinuity of the fibers (arrows).
完全性PCL撕裂(另一名患者)：矢状位PD加权MRI显示PCL完全断裂，伴明显的纤维束中断(箭)。

Cases courtesy Nehal Shah, MD, Brigham and Women's Hospital.

- PCL tears tend to be less frequently repaired compared to ACL tears.

Medial collateral ligament (MCL) overview

- The medial collateral ligament (MCL) arises from the posterior aspect of the medial femoral condyle and attaches to the medial tibial metaphysis, deep to the pes anserinus.
  The MCL fibers are interlaced with the joint capsule and the medial meniscus.
  The MCL is an extrasynovial structure and is not visualized by arthroscopy.

- 与ACL撕裂相比，较少对PCL撕裂进行修复术。

内侧副韧带(MCL)概述

- 内侧副韧带(MCL)起自股骨内侧髁的后方，附着于胫骨干骨端的内侧，位于鹅足肌腱的深部。
  内侧副韧带纤维束与关节囊和内侧半月板交错。
  内侧副韧带为滑膜外结构，不能在关节镜下显示。

MCL injury

内侧副韧带损伤

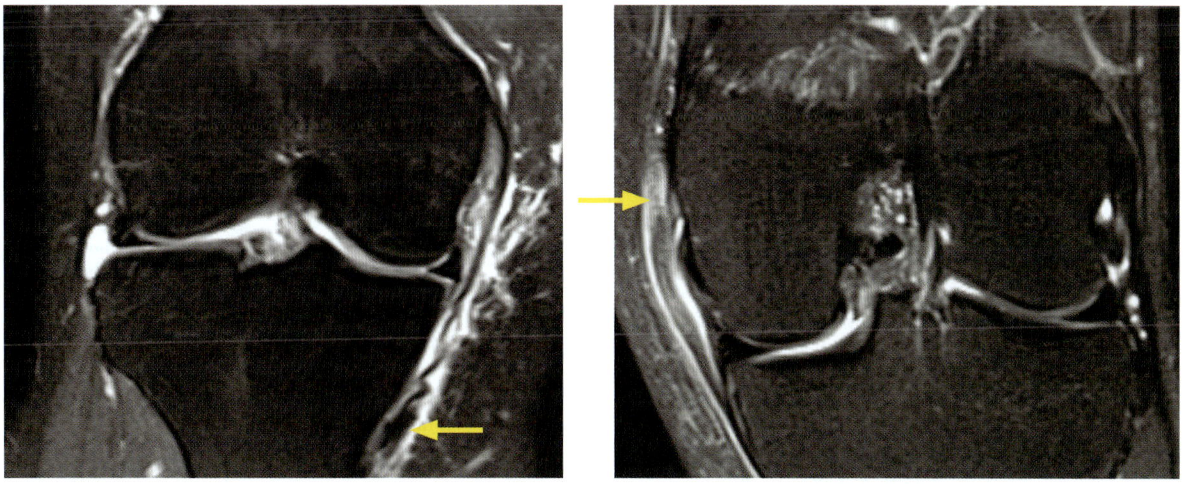

Two patients with full-thickness (grade 3) MCL injuries, seen on coronal PD-weighted MRI with fat suppression. The left image shows a full thickness tear of the distal (tibial) attachment (arrow), with undulated appearance of the proximally retracted torn tendon. The right image demonstrates a full thickness tear of the proximal (femoral) attachment (arrow).

两名MCL全层(3级)损伤的患者冠状位PD加权脂肪抑制MRI。左图显示在(胫骨)远端附着处全层撕裂(箭),近端撕裂肌腱退缩呈波状外观。右图显示(股骨)近端附着处全层撕裂(箭)。

- MCL injuries are commonly divided into three grades:

Grade 1 (MCL sprain): High signal in the medial soft tissues with normal signal of the ligament. Grade 2 (severe sprain/partial tear): High signal or partial disruption within the MCL fibers. Grade 3 (complete tear): Complete disruption of the MCL.

- MCL损伤常分为二级:

1级(MCL扭伤):内侧软组织信号增高,韧带信号尚正常。 2级(严重扭伤/部分撕裂):MCL纤维束内高信号或部分断裂。 3级(完全撕裂):MCL完全断裂。

- MCL injuries are caused by a tensile (pulling) force on the ligament. This most commonly occurs in the setting of valgus stress (impact on the lateral knee). Edema around the MCL is very common in the setting of osteoarthritis, and it is important not to mistake periligamentous edema in an older individual for an MCL sprain. MCL sprains most commonly occur in young athletes.
- The **Pellegrini-Stieda** lesion is post-traumatic calcification medial to the medial femoral condyle, which may be secondary to MCL avulsion injury.

- MCL损伤是由韧带受到张力(拉力)而引起。最常发生的情况是来自外翻的力量(膝关节的外侧受到冲击)。MCL周围水肿在骨关节炎中常见,注意,不要将老年人的韧带周围水肿误认为MCL扭伤。MCL扭伤最常见于年轻运动员。
- **Pellegrini-Stieda**病变是内髁内侧的外伤性钙化,可能继发于MCL撕裂伤。

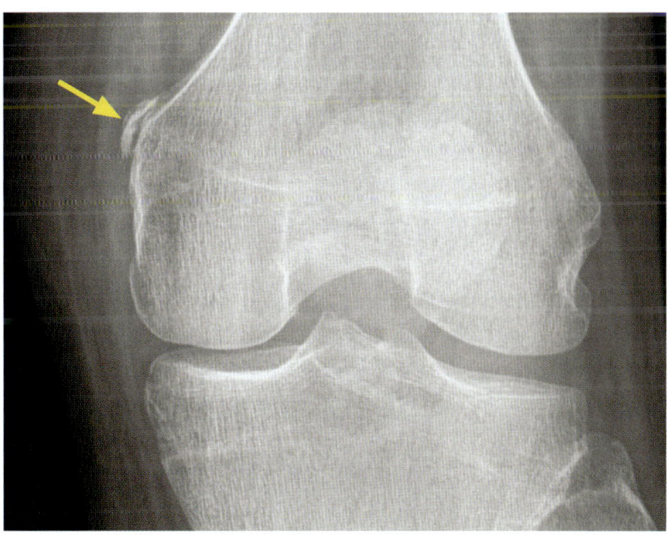

Pellegrini-Stieda lesion: Frontal radiograph demonstrates mineralization of the medial femoral condyle (arrow), suggestive of a remote MCL injury.

Pellegrini-Stieda病:正位X线影像显示股骨内侧髁边缘钙化灶(箭),提示远端MCL损伤。

Lateral collateral ligament (LCL) complex

- The lateral collateral ligament (LCL) complex is composed of many structures, three of which are routinely evaluated by MRI. From posterior to anterior, these structures are: Biceps femoris tendon (most posterior), LCL, and iliotibial band (most anterior).

外侧副韧带(LCL)复合体

- 外侧副韧带(LCL)复合体由多个结构组成，其中的三个结构可以采用MRI进行常规评估。这些结构按从后往前的顺序分别为股二头肌肌腱(最后)、LCL、髂胫束(最前)。

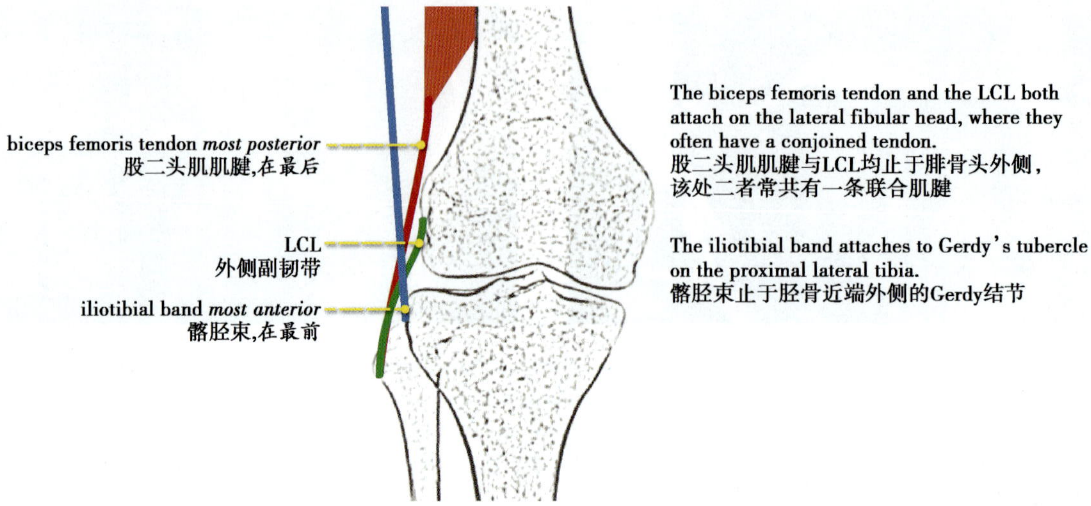

LCL injury

- LCL injury is less common than MCL injury and is usually associated with injury to other structures in the posterolateral corner. Injury to the posterolateral corner is a surgical near- emergency as there is poor outcome without prompt intervention.
- The posterolateral corner of the knee is a complex region consisting of:

  LCL complex, consisting of the biceps femoris tendon, LCL, and the iliotibial band.

  Arcuate ligament, a Y-shaped ligament connecting the fibula to the lateral femur.

  Popliteofibular ligaments, which are important lateral stabilizers.

  Popliteus tendon, which inserts on the lateral femur.

LCL损伤

- LCL损伤较MCL损伤少见，但常伴有膝关节后外侧角的其他结构损伤。膝关节后外侧角损伤基本上属于一种外科急症，因为处置不及时预后很差。
- 膝关节的后外角是个复合区域，包括：

  LCL复合体，由股二头肌肌腱、LCL、髂胫束构成。

  弓状韧带，是一种Y形韧带，连接腓骨与股骨外侧。

  腘腓韧带，是重要的外侧稳定结构。

  腘肌肌腱，附着于股骨外侧。

Iliotibial band syndrome

- Fluid surrounding (both superficial and deep to) the iliotibial band may represent iliotibial (IT) band syndrome, which is caused by friction between the anterolateral femur and the tendon of the iliotibial band.
- Clinically, IT band syndrome may be a cause of anterolateral knee pain and is seen commonly in runners.
- It is important to distinguish IT band syndrome from a lateral meniscus tear. Both may present with lateral knee pain, but treatment of iliotibial band syndrome is nonsurgical.

髂胫束综合征

- 髂胫束周围(浅层及深层均可)积液可提示有髂胫(IT)束综合征，由股骨前外侧与髂胫束韧带间摩擦引起。
- 临床上，髂胫束综合征可能是引起膝关节前外侧疼痛的原因之一，多见于跑步运动员。
- 区别髂胫束综合征及外侧半月板撕裂很重要。两者都可表现为膝关节外侧疼痛，但髂胫束综合征无须进行手术治疗。

EXTENSOR MECHANISM AND PATELLA

伸展结构及髌骨

Normal anatomy of the extensor mechanism

- The **extensor mechanism** is composed of the conjoined quadriceps tendon (attaches to the patella), the patella, and the patellar tendon (attaches to the tibial tuberosity).

  The patella is a sesamoid bone and is enclosed within the quadriceps tendon.
- Three of the quadriceps muscles (vastus intermedius, medialis, and lateralis) originate from the femur. The rectus femoris arises from the anterior inferior iliac spine (AIIS).

伸展结构的正常解剖

- **伸展结构**由股四头肌肌腱(附着于髌骨)、髌骨及髌韧带(附着于胫骨结节)共同组成。

  髌骨是一个籽骨，被股四头肌肌腱所包围。
- 股四头肌中三股肌肉(股内侧肌、股中间肌、股外侧肌)起自股骨。股直肌起自髂前下嵴(AIIS)。

Quadriceps tendon tear

股四头肌肌腱撕裂

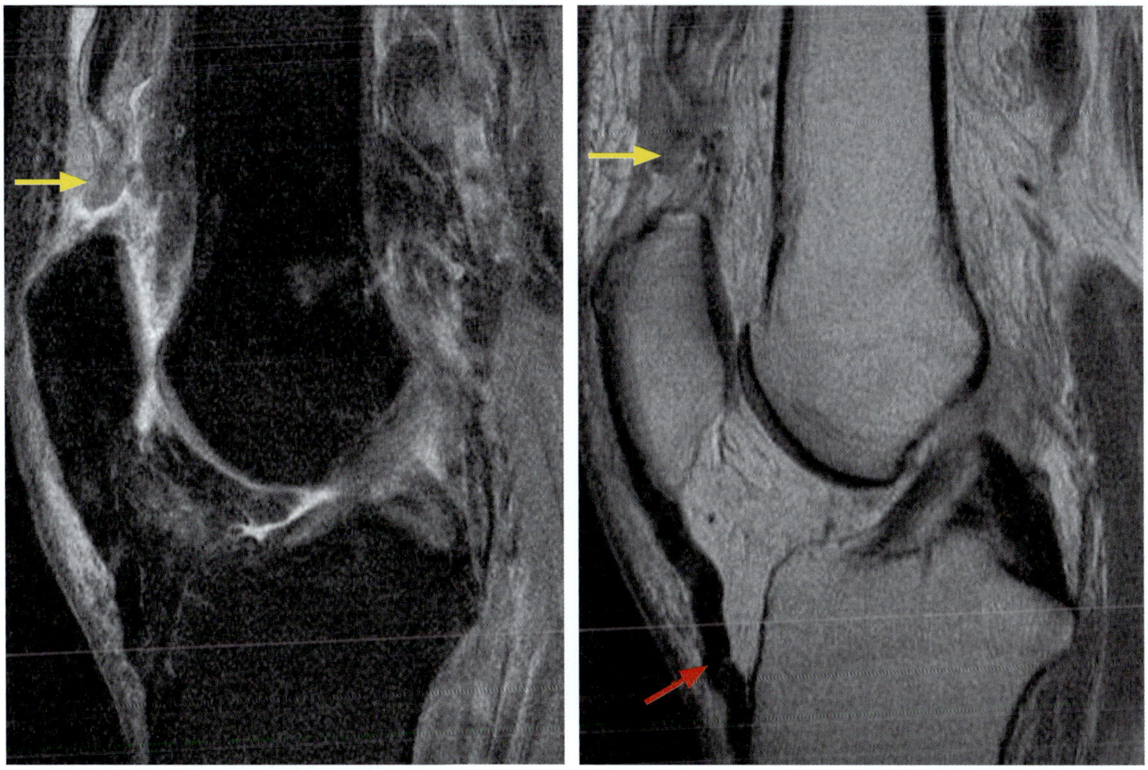

Quadriceps tendon tear: Sagittal proton density fat-saturated (left image) and proton density (right image) MRI show complete disruption of the distal quadriceps tendon (yellow arrows) with surrounding marked edema.
There is secondary buckling of the patellar tendon (red arrow).
Case courtesy Nehal Shah, MD, Brigham and Women's Hospital.
股四头肌肌腱撕裂：矢状位PD脂肪饱和(左图)及PD(右图)MRI显示股四头肌肌腱远端完全中断(黄箭)伴周围明显的水肿。
可见继发性髌韧带撕裂性褶皱(红箭)。

- Tear of the quadriceps tendon clinically presents with loss of knee extension.
- Quadriceps tendon tear most commonly occurs within 2 cm of the patella and may be evident on radiography due to the resultant *patella baja* (patella too low). The opposite of *patella baja* is *patella alta,* which can be seen with patellar tendon injury.

Patellar tendon injury

- Similar to quadriceps tendon tear, patellar tendon tear clinically presents with loss of knee extension.
- In contrast to quadriceps tendon tear, tear of the patella tendon causes superior displacement of the patella *(patella alta)*.
- Patellar tendinosis is seen on MRI as thickening of the patellar tendon. This is known as *jumper's knee*.

Lateral patellar dislocation

- Traumatic lateral patellar dislocation leaves behind a distinctive pattern of injury, even if the patella reduces back to the normal position. Bone marrow contusions of the lateral femoral condyle and the medial patellar facet are typical, with tearing of the medial retinaculum.

- 股四头肌肌腱撕裂在临床上表现为膝关节失去伸展功能。
- 股四头肌肌腱撕裂多发生于距髌骨2cm之内，X线影像上可以表现为低位髌骨(髌骨位置过低)。与低位髌骨相反的是高位髌骨，见于髌韧带损伤。

髌韧带损伤

- 与股四头肌肌腱撕裂类似，髌韧带撕裂临床表现为膝关节失去伸展功能。
- 与股四头肌肌腱撕裂相反，髌韧带撕裂导致髌骨向上移位(高位髌骨)。
- 髌腱病在MRI上表现为髌韧带增厚。髌腱病也称为跳高膝。

髌骨外脱位

- 外伤性髌骨外向脱位可以造成独特的损伤表现，即便髌骨复位到正常的位置。股骨外侧髁及髌骨内面的骨髓挫伤非常典型，伴内侧支持带撕裂。

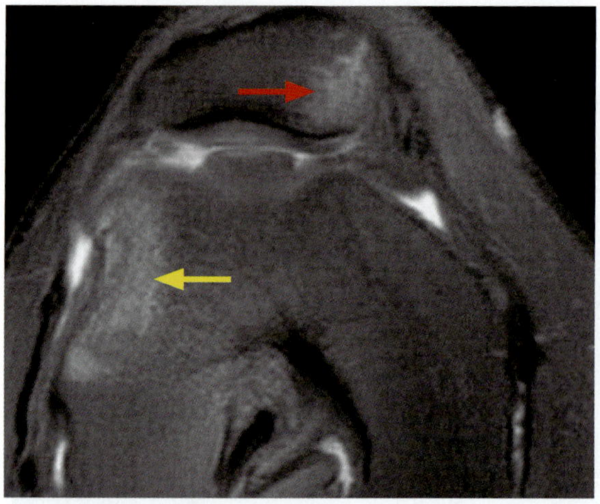

Lateral patellar dislocation: Axial fluid-sensitive MRI demonstrates the typical bone marrow edema pattern, with contusions of the lateral femoral condyle (yellow arrow) and medial patellar facet (red arrow).

The patella has relocated to its anatomic position.

髌骨外向脱位：轴位液体敏感MRI显示典型的骨髓水肿表现，即股骨外侧髁(黄箭)和髌骨内侧挫伤(红箭)。

髌骨已回复至其解剖位置。

Cases courtesy Nehal Shah, MD, Brigham and Women's Hospital.

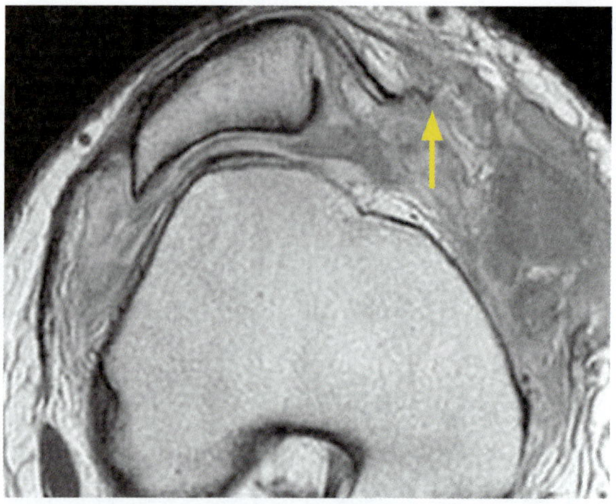

Lateral patellar dislocation in a different patient: Axial proton-density MRI shows persistent lateral subluxation of the patella, with complete tearing of the medial retinaculum (yellow arrow).

另一名患者髌骨外脱位：轴位PD加权MRI显示髌骨持续性外侧半脱位，内侧支持带完全撕裂(黄箭)。

Osgood-Schlatter disease

Osgood-Schlatter病

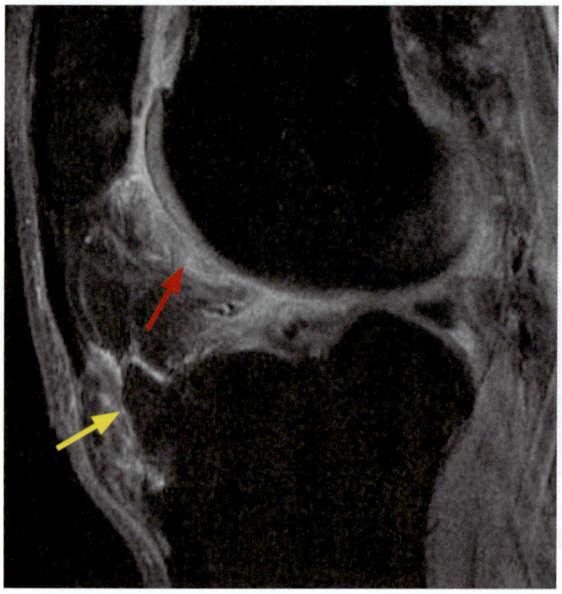

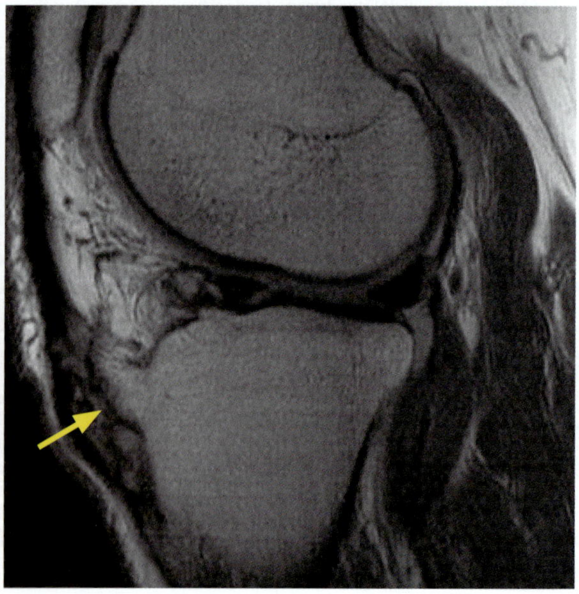

Osgood-Schlatter disease: Sagittal fluid-sensitive (left image) and proton density (right image) MRI show an enlarged, fragmented tibial tubercle (yellow arrows). There is associated edema anterior to the tibial tubercle and within Hoffa's fat pad (red arrow).

Case courtesy Nehal Shah, MD, Brigham and Women's Hospital.

Osgood-Schlatter病：矢状位液体敏感(左图)及PD加权(右图)MRI显示一个增大、碎裂的胫骨结节(黄箭)。胫骨结节前方和Hoffa脂肪垫伴水肿(红箭)。

- Osgood-Schlatter disease is an osteochondrosis of the tibial tubercle, thought to be caused by repetitive microtrauma. It occurs in adolescents.
- Radiographs show an enlarged tibial tuberosity with fragmentation and adjacent edema.

- Osgood-Schlatter病是发生在胫骨结节的骨软骨炎，认为是由反复轻微创伤引起。发生于青少年。
- X线影像显示胫骨结节增大伴碎片及邻近水肿。

- MRI shows increased signal of the distal patellar tendon, marrow edema within the tibial tubercle, and edema within Hoffa's fat pad.

- MRI示髌韧带远端信号增高，胫骨结节骨髓及Hoffa脂肪垫水肿。

KNEE CARTILAGE

膝关节软骨

Grading of cartilage degeneration

软骨退变分级

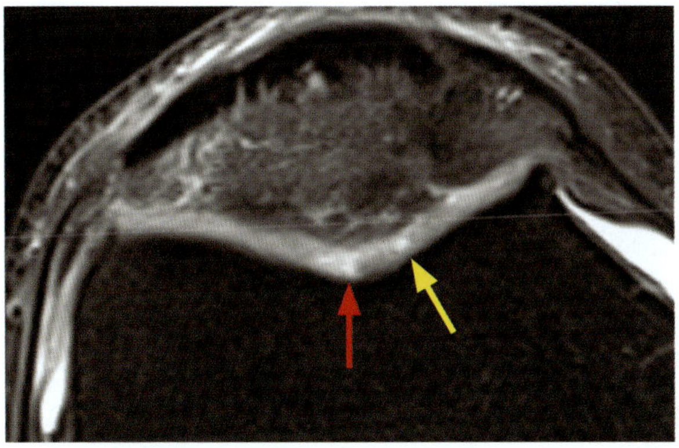

Superficial fissuring of the medial trochlea (grade 2; yellow arrow) and deep fissuring of the central trochlea (grade 3; red arrow).
滑车内侧浅表裂隙(2级；左图，黄箭)和滑车中央深度裂隙(3级；红箭)。

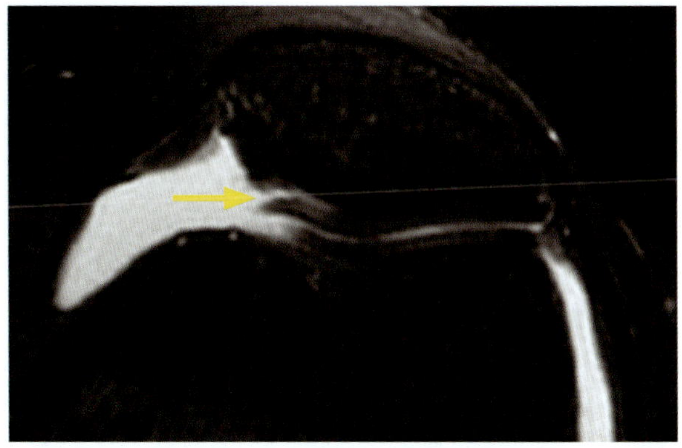

Full thickness defect (grade 4) of the medial patellar facet, with delamination (arrow) extending to the median ridge.
髌骨内侧关节面全层缺损(4级)合并剥离(黄箭)并延伸至正中嵴。

- The Outerbridge classification, summarized below, is a commonly used system for describing articular cartilage injury or degeneration. In general, it is best to describe the cartilage surfaces using descriptive words rather than assigning a grade.

- 以下Outerbridge分类总结是一种常用于描述关节软骨损伤或变性的分类系统。一般来说，最好使用描述性词语对软骨表面进行描述，而不是划分等级。

Illustration 示意图	Grade 等级	MRI findings MRI表现	Arthroscopy findings 关节镜表现
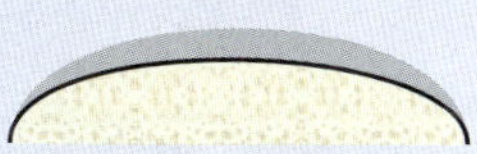	0	normal 正常	
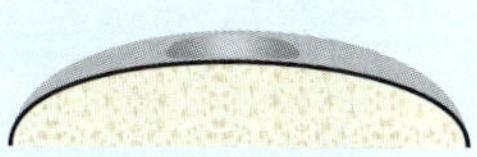	1	heterogeneous signal 信号不均匀	softening 软化
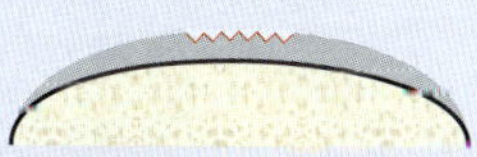	2	superficial defect or fissuring<50% 表面缺损或裂隙<50%	
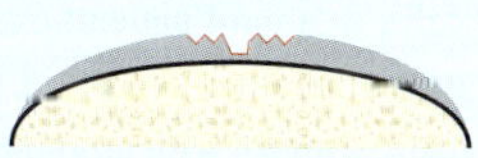	3	deep defect or fissuring > 50% 深度缺损或裂隙>50%	
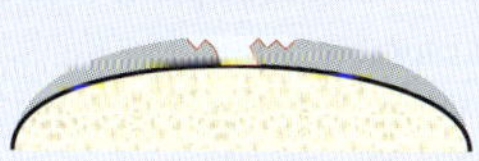	4	full-thickness defect 全层缺损	

- In the knee, there are three compartments and six chondral surfaces. The patellofemoral compartment consists of the patellar and trochlear cartilage. The medial and lateral tibiofemoral compartments each consist of the femoral condyle and the tibial plateau. A cartilage defect should have the location, severity, and size described.

- 在膝关节中，有三个腔隙和六个软骨面。髌股间隙由髌软骨和滑车软骨组成。内侧和外侧胫股间隙分别由股骨内外侧髁和胫骨平台组成。对于软骨缺损需要描述其位置、严重程度和范围。

- Cartilage injury or degeneration may manifest as surface irregularity, fissuring, focal or diffuse thinning, or delamination. Delamination is a dissecting-type detachment of the cartilage undersurface from bone, paralleling the subchondral bone.

- 软骨损伤或变性可表现为表面不规则、裂隙、局灶性或弥漫性变薄或分层。分层是一种软骨下表面与骨之间的剥离，与软骨下平行。

Osteochondral lesions of the knee

膝关节骨软骨损伤

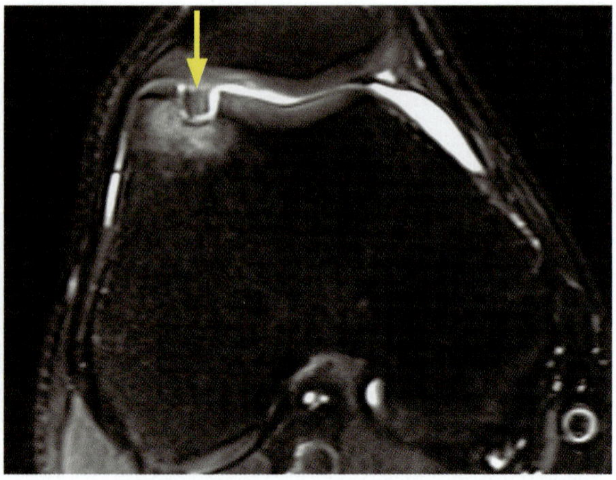

Acute osteochondral fracture (younger patient): There is a displaced fracture of the lateral trochlea (arrow) involving the articular cartilage, subchondral bone plate, and subchondral bone.
急性骨软骨骨折(年轻患者)：外侧滑车移位性骨折(箭)，累及关节软骨、软骨下骨板和软骨下骨。

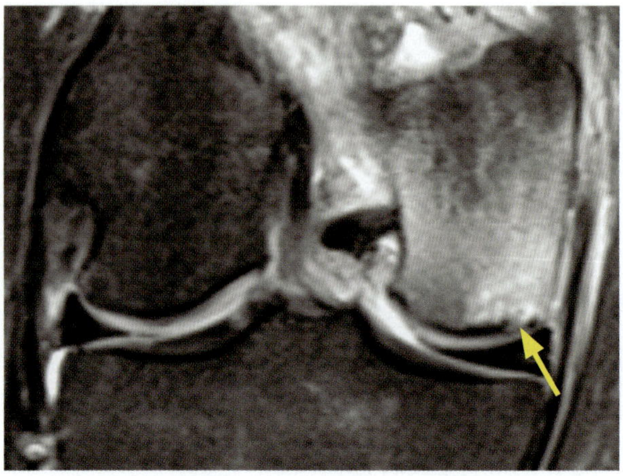

Subchondral insufficiency fracture (middle-aged to older patient): There is irregular thickening of the subchondral bone plate (arrow) with exuberant surrounding edema.
软骨下不全性骨折(中老年患者)：软骨下骨板不规则增厚(箭)伴周围非常严重的水肿。

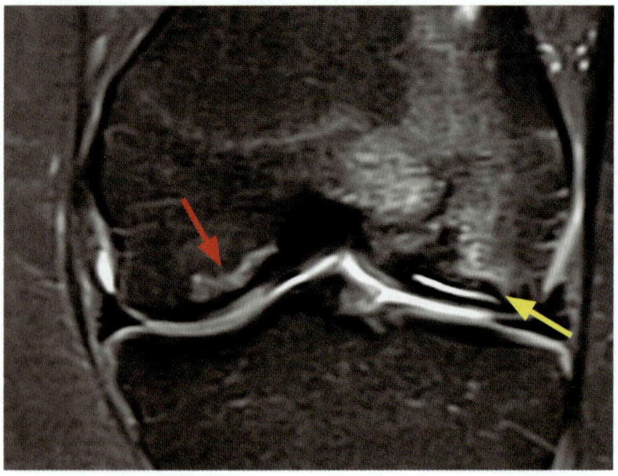

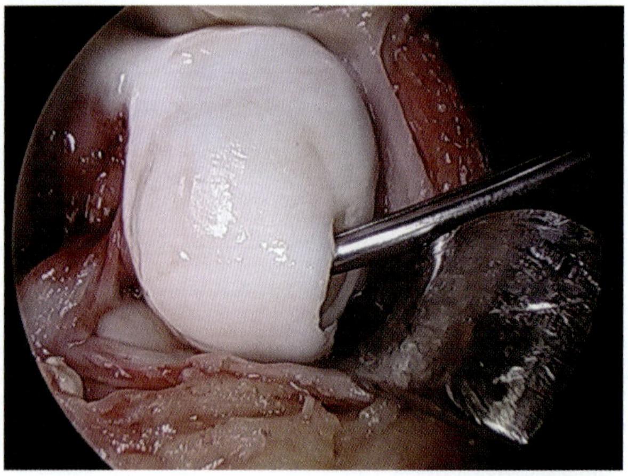

Avascular necrosis (any age, but can be younger patient if history of prolonged steroid use or sickle cell), in a third patient: Coronal PD-weighted MRI with fat suppression demonstrates linear fluid signal (yellow arrow) undercutting the subchondral bone plate of the lateral femoral condyle, in keeping with an unstable osteochondral lesion. There is surrounding heterogeneous marrow signal with prominent edema. Note the serpiginous edema of the medial femoral condyle (red arrow) without abnormality of the subchondral bone plate, in keeping with avascular necrosis. Arthroscopic image from the same patient demonstrates the probe easily entering the unstable defect.
第三个缺血性坏死的病例(任何年龄，但年轻的患者见于长期使用类固醇或有镰状细胞病)：冠状位 PD 加权脂肪抑制 MRI 显示线样液体信号侵蚀股骨外侧髁软骨下骨板(黄箭)，符合不稳定的骨软骨病变。周围有不均匀的骨髓信号伴明显水肿。注意股骨内侧髁的匐行性水肿(红箭)，但软骨下骨板正常，与缺血性坏死的表现一致。同一名患者的关节镜图像显示探头很容易进入不稳定的缺损。

- *Osteochondral lesion, osteochondral defect,* and *osteochondral injury* are interchangeable generic terms (rather than specific diagnoses) used to describe a range of focal disorders of the articular cartilage, subchondral bone plate, and subchondral bone. There are a wide range of causes including osteochondritis

- 骨软骨病变、骨软骨缺损和骨软骨损伤是可以互换的通用术语(而不是具体诊断)，用于描述关节软骨、软骨下骨板和软骨下骨的一系列局灶性疾病。病因有很多，包括剥脱性骨

dissecans, osteochondral fracture, subchondral insufficiency fracture, and avascular necrosis. There can often be imaging overlap between these entities, especially in advanced cases with development of an unstable fragment.

- It is usually not necessary to grade the severity of the osteochondral lesion. However, it is important to note if fluid or cystic change deep to the lesion is present, implying that the lesion is unstable (meaning that the lesion can be displaced by an arthroscopist's probe). Also, if the lesion is displaced this should also be described.
- **Osteochondritis dissecans** is a developmental disorder of subchondral bone, resulting in formation of an unstable subchondral bone fragment. It tends to occur in pediatrics and adolescents.
- **Osteochondral fracture** is a result of an acute or chronic repetitive trauma, causing injury to the cartilage and subchondral bone.
- **Subchondral insufficiency fracture** is caused by collapse of the subchondral bone, typically in older patients. One key imaging finding is thickening and irregularity of the subchondral bone plate, often with exuberant surrounding edema. There is often concomitant meniscal tearing.
- **Avascular necrosis** is primary osteonecrosis of the subchondral bone. In advanced cases, it may cause subchondral collapse. The key imaging finding is serpiginous signal abnormality of the subchondral bone.

软骨炎、骨软骨骨折、软骨下不全骨折和缺血性坏死。这些病变之间常存在影像重叠，尤其是在晚期且合并不稳定碎片的病例。

- 对骨软骨损伤的严重程度通常不需要进行分级。重要的是需要注意位于病变的深部是否存在积液或囊性改变，这提示病变是不稳定的(也就是病变可以被关节镜检探头推动)。此外，如果病变发生移位，也应进行描述。
- **剥脱性骨软骨炎**是一种软骨下骨的发育障碍，导致不稳定软骨下骨碎片的形成。它往往发生在儿童和青少年。
- **骨软骨骨折**是急性或慢性重复性创伤的结果，可导致软骨和软骨下骨损伤。
- **软骨下不全性骨折**是由软骨下骨塌陷引起，通常发生在老年患者。一个关键的影像学表现是软骨下骨板增厚和形态不规则，常伴有明显的周围水肿。同时，通常伴有半月板撕裂。
- **缺血性坏死**是原发性软骨下骨坏死。在晚期病例中可导致软骨下塌陷。关键的影像学表现是软骨下骨的匐行性异常信号。

SYNOVIUM

滑膜

Pigmented villonodular synovitis (PVNS)

色素沉着绒毛结节性滑膜炎(PVNS)

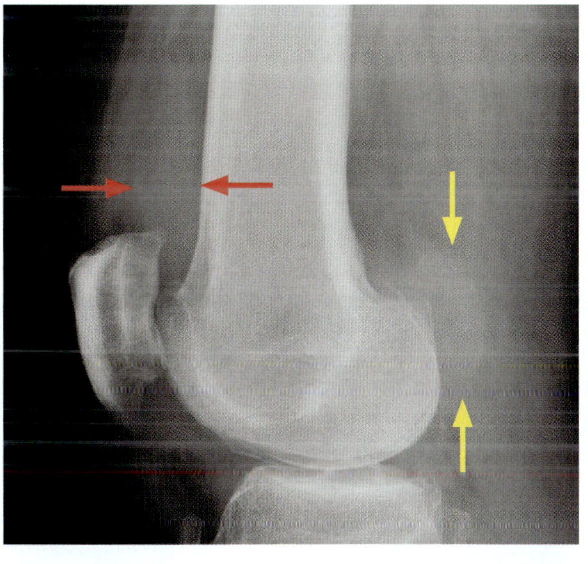

PVNS: Lateral knee radiograph shows a dense knee effusion (red arrows) and a soft-tissue mass posterior to the knee (yellow arrows).
PVNS：膝关节侧位X线影像显示膝关节积液密度增高(红箭)及膝关节后方软组织肿块(黄箭)。

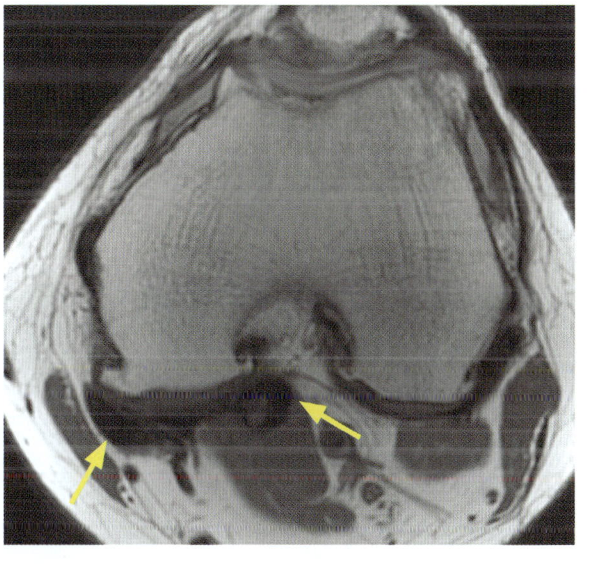

Axial proton-density MRI in the same patient shows low signal masses (arrows) posterior to the knee.
同一名患者轴位PD加权MRI显示膝关节后方低信号肿块(箭)。

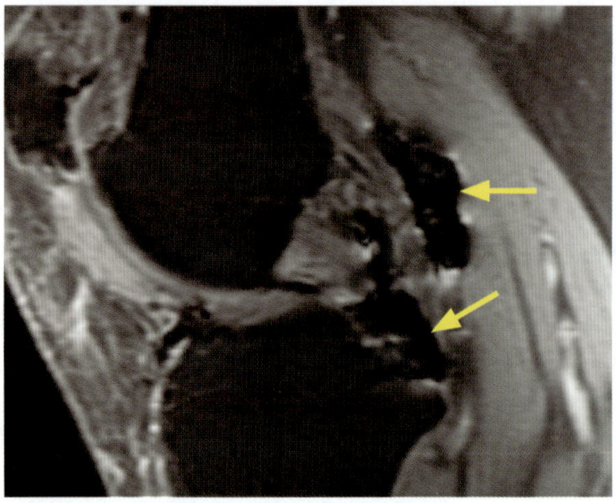

Sagittal gradient echo MRI shows the extremely dark masses accentuated by susceptibility artifact (arrows).
矢状位梯度回波MRI显示一个深黑色肿块，而磁敏感伪影使颜色加重(箭)。

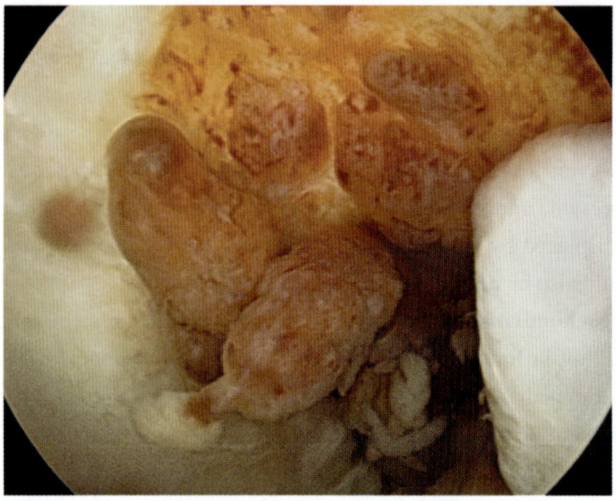

At arthroscopy, multiple synovial-based masses are evident.
关节镜下，非常明显的以滑膜为基底的多发肿块。

- Pigmented villonodular synovitis (PVNS) is a benign hyperplastic proliferation of the synovium within the joint, now thought to represent a tumor. The same process outside of the joint is called **giant cell tumor of the tendon sheath**.
- The knee is by far the most common location for PVNS.
- PVNS presents as knee pain and swelling, with recurrent dark brown effusions from prior hemorrhage.
- PVNS most commonly diffusely affects a joint, but it may also be focal. Focal PVNS can clinically mimic internal derangement.
- Recurrent hemorrhage leads to residual intra-articular hemosiderin, which is paramagnetic. The paramagnetic effects of hemosiderin cause T1 prolongation and T2 shortening, resulting in dark signal on both T1- and T2-weighted images, with blooming on gradient-echo sequences.

- 色素沉着绒毛结节性滑膜炎(PVNS)是关节内滑膜的良性过度增生性病变，现在认为是一种肿瘤。同样的病变发生在关节外被称为**腱鞘巨细胞瘤**。
- 膝关节是PVNS最为常见的部位。
- PVNS表现为膝关节疼痛和肿胀，伴既往反复出血所致的深褐色积液。
- PVNS累及关节最常呈弥漫性，也可为局限性。局限性PVNS在临床上可类似于关节紊乱。
- 反复出血导致关节内含铁血黄素沉积，后者为顺磁性。含铁血黄素的顺磁效应可引起T_1延长及T_2缩短，从而导致在T_1加权及T_2加权图像上均为低信号，在梯度回波序列上呈开花样。

Lipoma arborescens

树枝状脂瘤

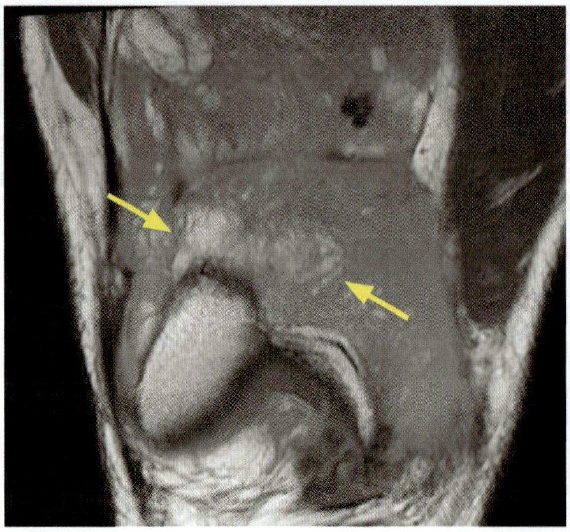

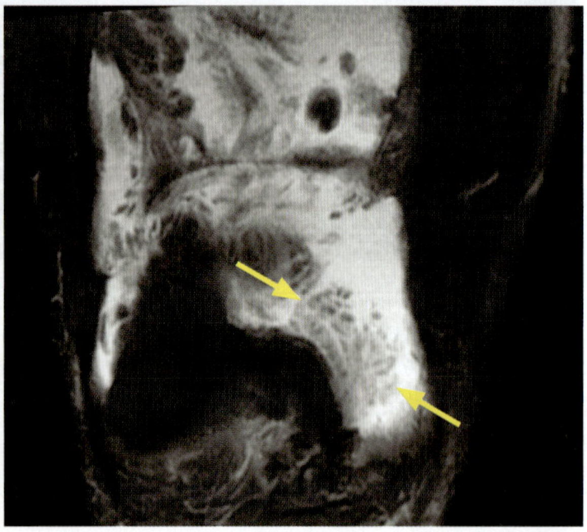

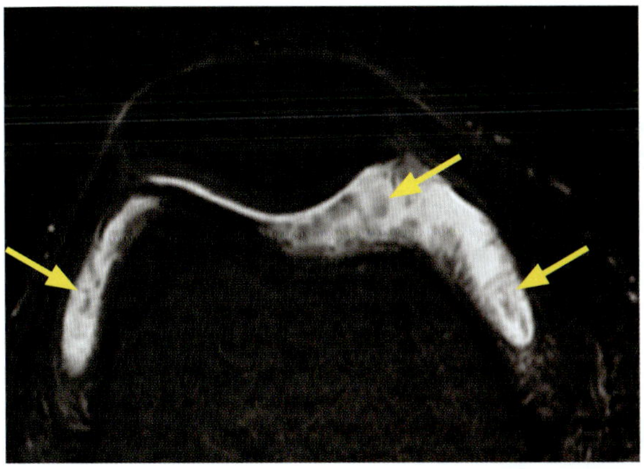

Lipoma arborescens:
Coronal PD-weighted MRI without (top left image) and with fat suppression (top right image), and axial PD-weighted MRI with fat suppression demonstrate fat signal intensity globular and frond-like fatty synovial proliferation (arrows).

树枝状脂瘤：冠状位无脂肪抑制(左上图)和脂肪抑制(右上图)，以及轴位PD加权脂肪抑制MRI，显示球状和叶状脂肪滑膜增生(箭)，呈脂肪信号强度。

- Lipoma arborescens is overgrowth of intracapsular synovial fatty tissue, causing lobulated and globular intra-articular fatty masses.
- Lipoma arborescens is treated with synovectomy to prevent premature osteoarthritis.

- 树枝状脂瘤为关节内滑膜脂肪组织过度增生，形成分叶状和球样关节内脂肪肿块。
- 树枝状脂瘤的治疗是滑膜切除术以预防早发性骨关节炎。

KNEE SOFT TISSUES

Baker's cyst

- Baker's cyst is a popliteal cyst caused from a ball-valve type communication with the knee joint.
- The typical location is between the semi**m**embranosus tendon and **m**edial head of the gastrocnemius muscle (mnemonic: Baker's **M&M**).
- An important differential consideration is a popliteal aneurysm.

Tennis leg

- Tears of either the plantaris tendon or the medial head of the gastrocnemius have both been called tennis leg.

膝关节软组织

Baker囊肿

- Baker囊肿是一种腘窝囊肿，由膝关节的一种球阀样交通所致。
- 常见部位是半膜肌肌腱和腓肠肌内侧头之间。(助记：Baker's **M&M**)。
- 重要的鉴别诊断是腘窝动脉瘤。

网球腿

- 跖肌肌腱或腓肠肌内侧头的撕裂都被称为网球腿。

(翻译　刘进　陈紫琪)

HIP

HIP ANATOMY

Bony acetabulum

- The acetabulum is formed by the fusion of three bones: The ilium superiorly, the pubis anteriorly, and ischium posteriorly. Pediatric radiographs of the hip show the separation of these three bones, which meet at the triradiate cartilage to form the acetabulum.

Cartilage, labrum, and ligaments

- The articular surface of the acetabulum is lined by a horseshoe-shaped thin articular cartilage. The center of the acetabulum, called the pulvinar, is not covered by cartilage.
- The labrum forms a fibrocartilaginous ring approximately 270 degrees around the periphery of the acetabulum. The labrum blends with the transverse ligament anterior/inferiorly. Note that there is no labrum at the anterior/ inferior aspect of the acetabulum where the transverse ligament lies.
- The transverse ligament gives off fibers that form the ligamentum teres, which connects to the femoral head at its central fovea.

髋关节

髋关节解剖

骨性髋臼

- 髋臼由三块骨融合而成：上部的髂骨、前部的耻骨和后部的坐骨。儿童髋关节X线影像可以清晰显示这三块分离的骨，它们汇合于三角样的放射状软骨，并共同组成髋臼。

软骨、髋臼盂唇和韧带

- 髋臼的关节表面衬覆马蹄形的薄层关节软骨。髋臼的中心称为髋臼枕，没有软骨覆盖。
- 髋臼盂唇形成一纤维软骨环，围绕髋臼外圈约270°。盂唇与髋臼横韧带的前/下部融合。注意，在髋臼的前/下部横韧带附着处没有盂唇。
- 横韧带发出纤维形成圆韧带，并连接到股骨头的中央凹。

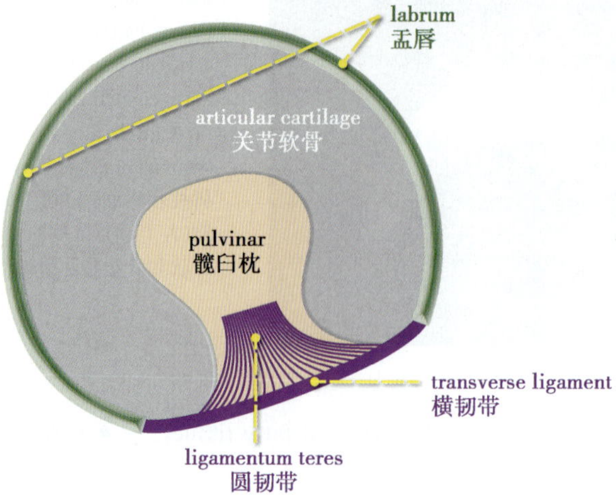

Normal radiographic anatomy of the hip region | 髋部的正常X线影像解剖

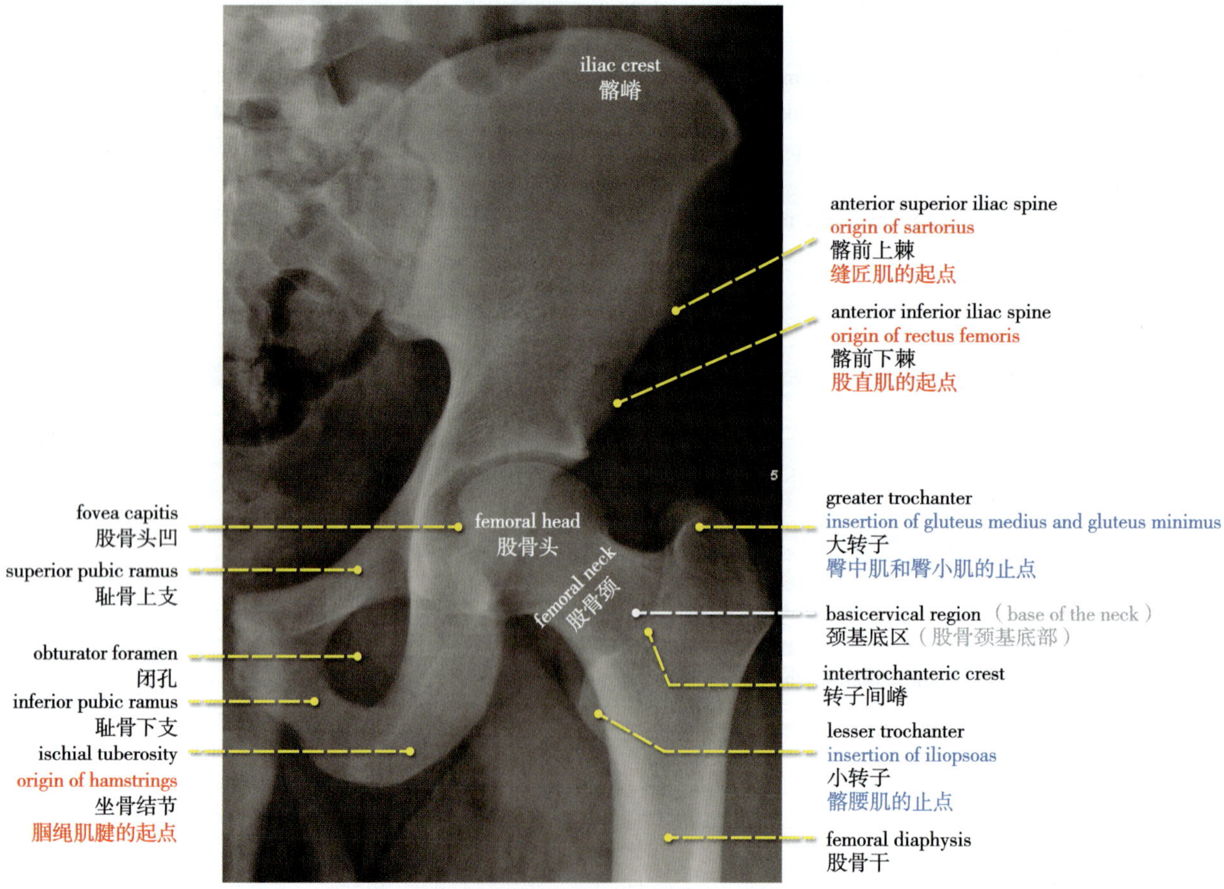

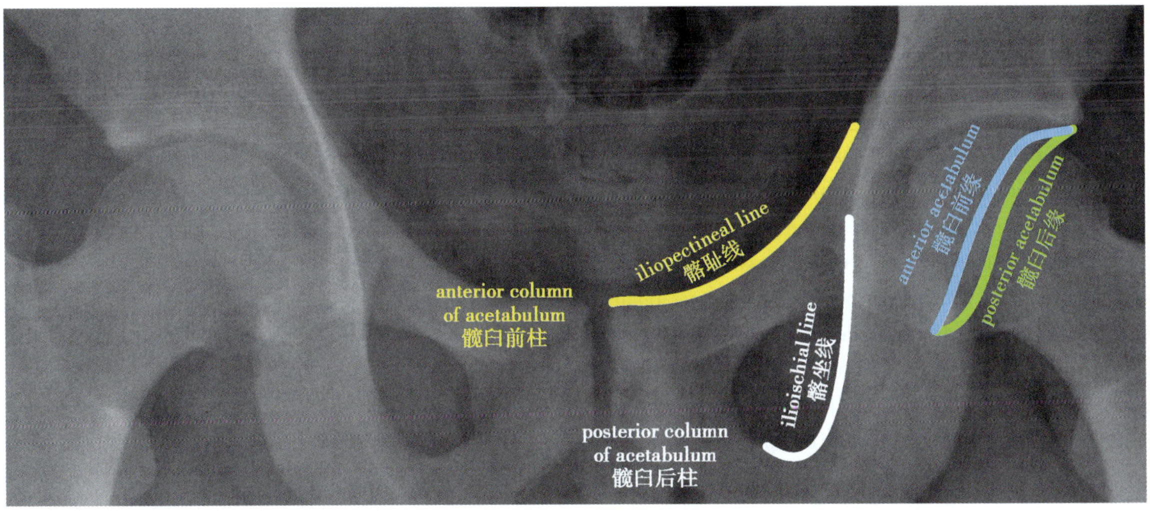

- The femoral head is mostly covered by articular cartilage except at the fovea capitis (central fovea), which is a central depression and attachment site of the ligamentum teres.
- The greater and lesser trochanters are apophyses. The greater trochanter is the insertion site for the gluteus medius and gluteus minimus. The iliopsoas inserts on the lesser trochanter. Of note, a fracture of the lesser trochanter in an adult is considered pathologic until proven otherwise.
- The **iliopectineal line** (also called iliopubic line) represents the border of the anterior column of the acetabulum. The **ilioischial line** represents the border of the posterior column of the acetabulum.
- The anterior and posterior walls of the acetabulum project over the femoral head. The posterior wall is more lateral.

- 股骨头大部分被关节软骨覆盖，除了股骨头凹(中央凹)，后者为一中央凹陷并为圆韧带的附着点。
- 大转子和小转子是骨性隆突。大转子是臀中肌和臀小肌的附着点。髂腰肌的止点附着在小转子上。需要注意的是，成人小转子骨折一般为病理性骨折，除非有其他明确的原因。
- **髂耻线**(也称iliopubic line)是髋臼前柱的边界。**髂坐线**是髋臼后柱的边界。
- 髋臼前壁和后壁投影在股骨头上，而后壁更偏向外侧。

Cross-sectional anatomy of the hip musculature

髋部肌肉横断面解剖

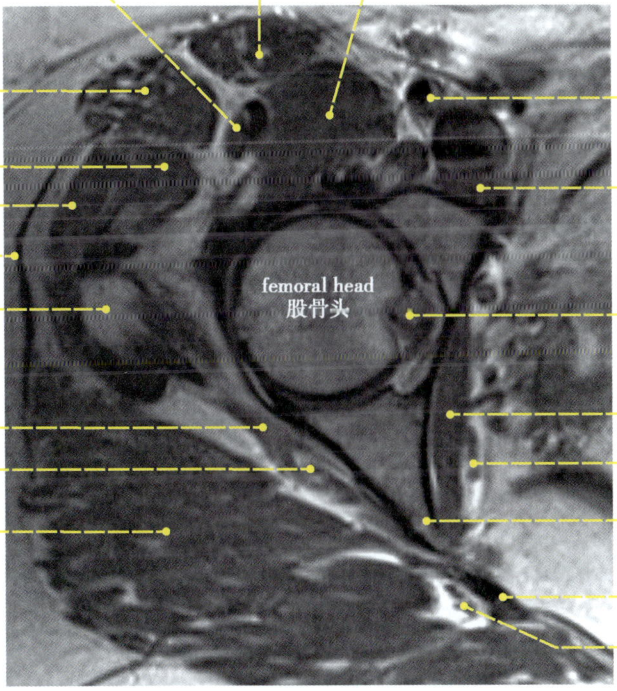

Acetabular Fracture

Acetabular fracture

- Discontinuity of either the iliopectineal and ilioischial lines may represent a fracture of the anterior or posterior column of the acetabulum.
- Classification of acetabular fractures is complex and multiple classifications have been introduced. The most widely used classification scheme is the Judet-Letournel classification, which describes 10 types of acetabular fractures.
- The **Judet-Letournel classification** describes 5 elementary patterns: fractures of the posterior wall, posterior column, anterior wall, anterior column, and transverse fractures. Five combination patterns are also described. The Judet-Letournel types are not related to fracture complexity or prognosis.
- The posterior wall of the acetabulum is the most commonly fractured element, alone or in combination with other injuries.

髋臼骨折

髋臼骨折

- 髂耻线或髂坐线的连续性中断可能提示有髋臼前柱或后柱骨折。
- 髋臼骨折的分类复杂且有很多种。最常用的是Judet-Letournel分类法，将髋臼骨折分为10种类型。
- **Judet-Letournel分类**介绍了5种基本表现方式：后壁骨折、后柱骨折、前壁骨折、前柱骨折及横向骨折。另有5种复合型骨折。Judet-Letournel分类与骨折的复杂性和预后没有关系。
- 后壁骨折是最常见的髋臼骨折表现方式，可以单发，也可以合并其他损伤。

Hip Fracture

Anatomy of the proximal femur

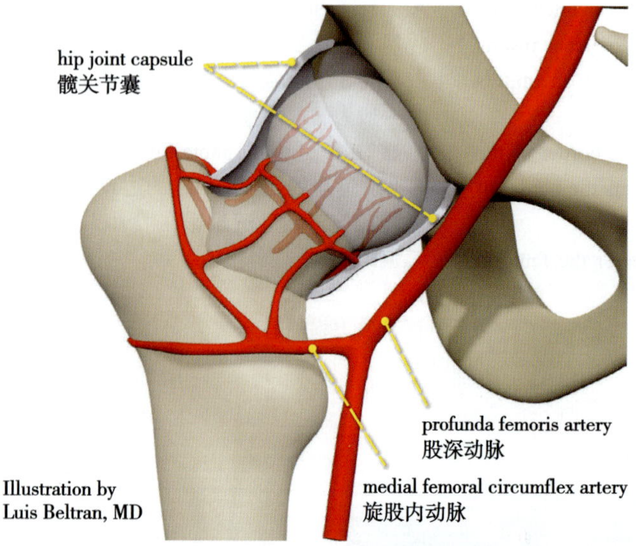

Illustration demonstrates the vascular anatomy of the proximal femur. The main blood supply to the femoral head is from the medial femoral circumflex artery, a branch of the profunda femoris artery.
股骨近端血管解剖示意图。股骨头的血液供应主要来自旋股内侧动脉，旋股内侧动脉是股深动脉的一个分支。

髋部骨折

股骨近端解剖结构

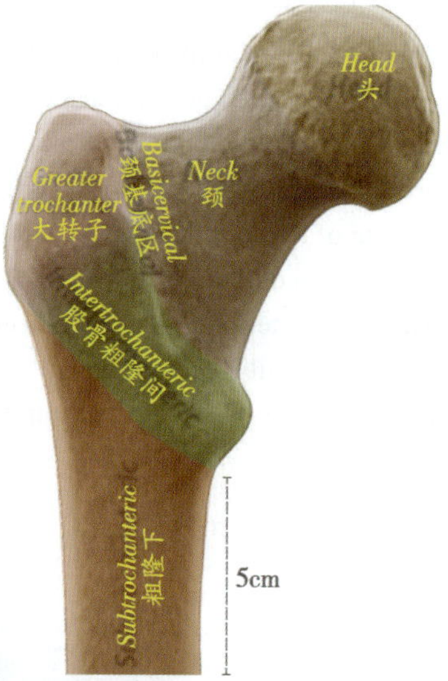

Cinematic rendering of the proximal femur with the main regions of the proximal femur colored. The head and most of the neck (excluding the basicervical region) are intracapsular.
电影渲染图股骨近端，对近段股骨的主要区域加以色彩。股骨头和颈部的大部分区域(不包括颈基底区)位于关节囊内。

- A "hip fracture" generally refers to a fracture of the proximal femur.
- It is important to understand the vascular and osseous anatomy of the proximal femur in order to accurately describe hip fractures in a way that is helpful to the orthopedist.
- The blood supply to the femoral head is predominantly supplied by the **medial femoral circumflex artery**, which arises from the profunda femoral artery. This artery courses along the femoral neck, and if the extra-osseous branches are injured in trauma there is an increased risk of avascular necrosis of the femoral head.
- Intracapsular fractures, including those of the femoral head and most fractures

- "髋部骨折"一般是指股骨近端骨折。
- 掌握股骨近端的血管和骨骼解剖非常重要，这可以对髋部骨折进行准确的描述以便为骨科医生提供有效的帮助。
- 股骨头的血液供应主要来自**旋股内侧动脉**，其为股深动脉的分支。此动脉沿着股骨颈走行，如果该动脉的骨外分支在创伤中受损，由其供血的股骨头发生缺血性坏死的风险就会增加。
- 关节囊内骨折(包括股骨头骨折和大多数股骨

of the femoral neck, have increased risk for vascular disruption and therefore increased risk for avascular necrosis, in comparison to extra-capsular fractures.

The femoral head and most of the femoral neck are intracapsular.

The basicervical region is the most distal part of the femoral neck, just proximal to the intertrochanteric crest. The **basicervical** region is extra-capsular. Therefore, basicervical fractures generally do quite well when appropriately recognized and treated.

- In addition to the basicervical region, the intertrochanteric and subtrochanteric regions are also extra-capsular.
- Although there are many classifications for various regions of proximal femur fractures in the orthopedic literature, these have shown to have generally poor inter-reader agreement. Instead, a simplified classification as proposed in this text can concisely describe the relevant findings and accurately predict the appropriate treatment.

颈骨折）较关节囊外骨折血管受损的风险更高，因此缺血性坏死的风险也随之增高。

股骨头和大部分股骨颈位于关节囊内。

颈基底区是股骨颈的最远端，在转子间嵴的近端。**颈基底区**位于关节囊外。因此，颈基底区骨折如果得到正确的诊断和治疗一般预后良好。

- 除了股骨颈基底区，股骨粗隆间区和粗隆下区也位于关节囊外。
- 文献对股骨近端不同区域的骨折有许多分类，但这些分类在影像医生间的一致性较差。相反，本文提出的简化分类可以概括这些相关征象，并准确地指导合适的治疗方式。

Hip dislocation and femoral head fractures

髋关节脱位和股骨头骨折

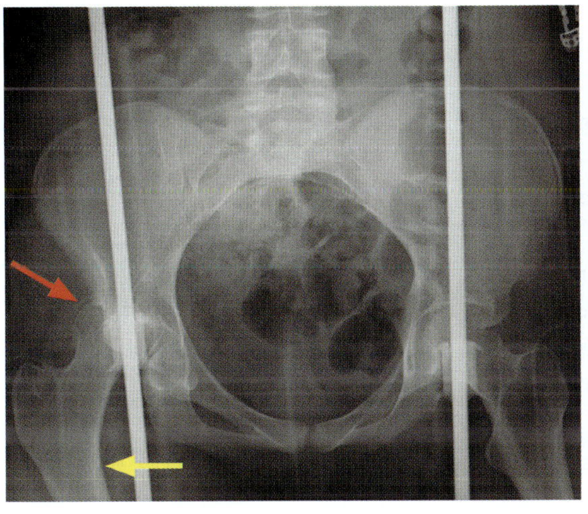

Frontal radiograph of the pelvis
骨盆正位X线影像

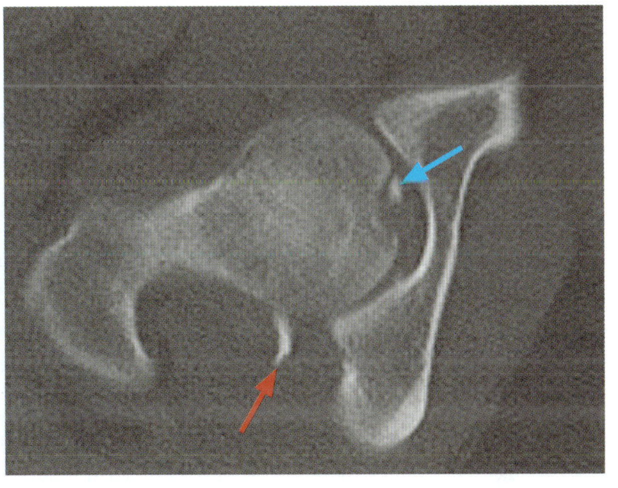

Axial CT
轴位CT

Posterior hip dislocation, with femoral head fracture and posterior acetabular wall fracture:
Frontal radiograph of the pelvis shows a right posterior hip dislocation, with the femoral head displaced in the typical superior position. Note internal rotation of the femur, with obscuration of the lesser trochanter (yellow arrow). There is a posterior acetabular fracture (red arrow), partially obscured by the trauma board artifact.
CT confirms a small posterior acetabular wall fracture (red arrow) and a small femoral head fracture in the region of the fovea (blue arrow).
髋关节后脱位，伴股骨头及髋臼后壁骨折：
骨盆正位X线影像显示右侧髋关节后脱位，伴股骨头向上典型的脱位。注意股骨内旋，小转子被遮挡（黄箭）。髋臼后部骨折（红箭），部分被担架遮挡。
CT证实髋臼后壁微小骨折（红箭）和股骨头中央凹区微小骨折（蓝箭）。

- The vast majority (~90%) of hip fractures are due to high-energy trauma with posterior displacement of the femur, which is typically positioned superiorly.

  The femur is typically positioned in internal rotation and flexion. The internal rotation of the femur causes decreased conspicuity of the lesser trochanter, which is rotated behind the medial femoral cortex.

  The dislocated femoral head may appear smaller than the normal side due to AP radiographic technique and magnification effect.
- Femoral head fractures are most commonly associated with posterior hip dislocations or gunshot wounds. Isolated femoral head fractures are uncommon.

- 绝大多数（高达90%）髋部骨折是由于高强度外伤导致股骨向后移位，通常为向上移位。

  股骨通常处于内旋和屈曲的位置。股骨内旋导致小转子旋转至股骨内侧皮质后方而显示不清。

  脱位股骨头由于前后位X线摄影技术及放大效应而看上去可能小于正常侧。
- 股骨头骨折最常见于髋关节后脱位或枪伤。孤立性股骨头骨折并不常见。

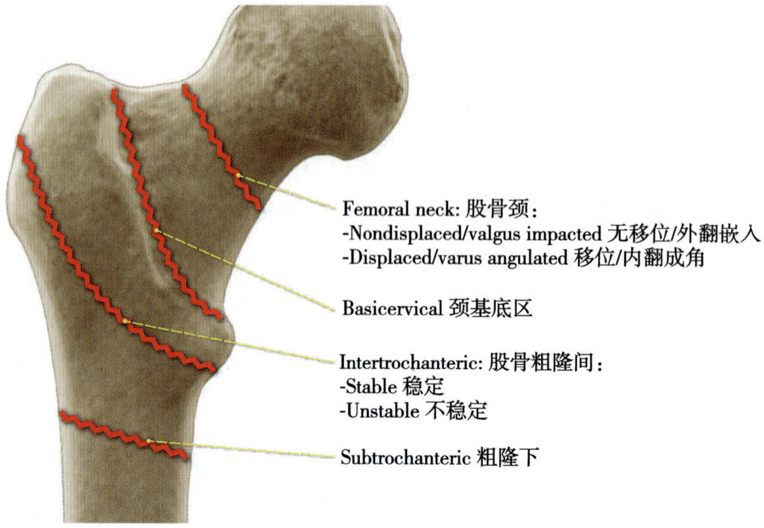

- Excepting femoral head fractures, proximal femur fractures can be divided into 4 sites: Femoral neck (intracapsular); and basicervical, intertrochanteric, and subtrochanteric (extracapsular).
- Femoral neck fractures can be nondisplaced (equivalent to valgus impaction) or displaced (equivalent to varus).
- Intertrochanteric fractures can be stable (single fracture line) or unstable.

Imaging of hip fracture

- The initial evaluation of hip trauma should begin with radiographs, including a frontal view of the pelvis and a cross-table lateral radiograph of the affected hip.

  Frog-leg lateral radiographs (commonly performed for arthritis assessment) should generally not be performed for trauma, as there is a potential to cause fracture displacement.
- If a hip fracture is clearly identified on radiography and able to be classified (as subsequently discussed), then there is generally no need for additional cross-sectional imaging.
- An "occult" hip fracture is a fracture that is not evident on radiographs. Occult fractures may be present in up to 10% of apparently negative radiographs performed for trauma. Therefore, further imaging with CT or MRI should be performed if there is persistent concern for fracture with negative radiographs.

- 除股骨头骨折外，股骨近端骨折可分为4个部位：股骨颈(关节囊内)、颈基底区、粗隆间区和粗隆下区(关节囊外)。
- 股骨颈骨折可以无移位(相当于外翻嵌入)或移位(相当于内翻)。
- 粗隆间骨折可以是稳定的(单骨折线)或不稳定的。

髋部骨折影像

- 髋关节创伤的初步评估应从X线影像开始，包括骨盆正位和受累侧髋关节交叉侧位影像。

  蛙位片(通常用于关节炎评估)一般不应用于外伤，因为有可能导致骨折移位。
- 如果髋部骨折能够在X线影像上清晰显示并能够进行分类(如后所述)，则通常无须进行横断面成像。
- “隐匿性”髋部骨折是指在X线影像上看不到的骨折。隐匿性骨折在因创伤进行的X线影像中阴性率可高达10%。因此，如果在X线影像阴性的情况下仍考虑有骨折，则应进一步行CT或MRI检查。

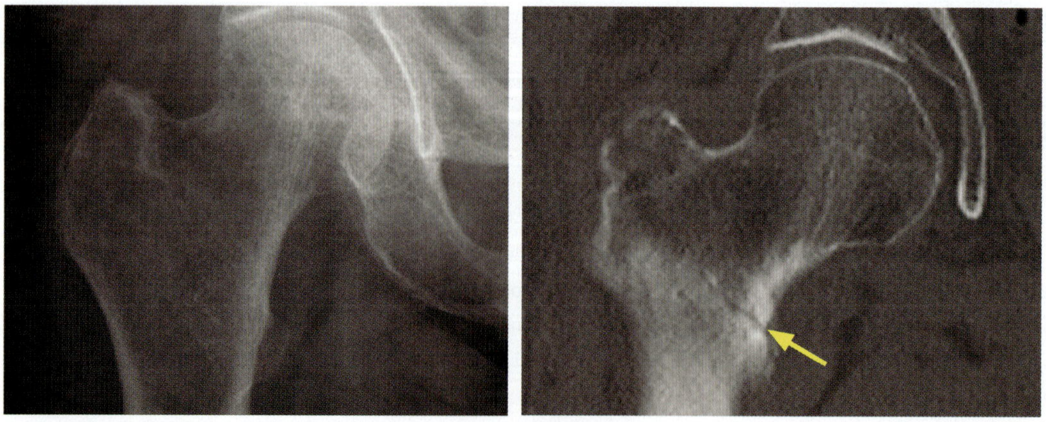

Frontal radiograph
正位X线影像

Coronal CT
冠状位CT

Occult fracture, evident on CT. Radiograph is negative. Coronal CT demonstrates a nondisplaced (stable) intertrochanteric fracture (arrow).
隐匿性骨折，CT显示明显但X线影像为阴性。冠状位CT显示无移位的(稳定性)粗隆间骨折(箭)。

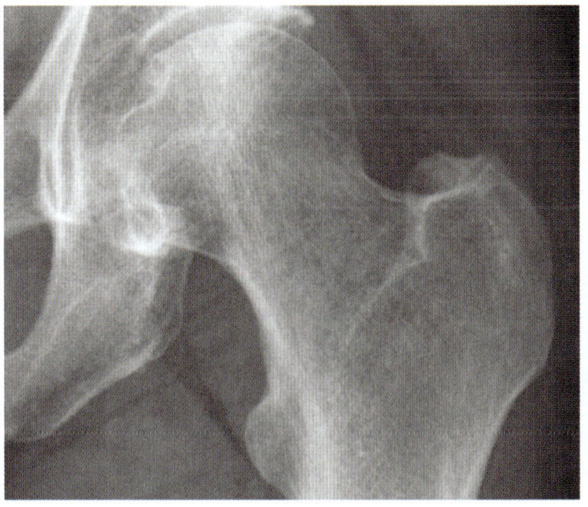

Frontal radiograph
正位X线影像

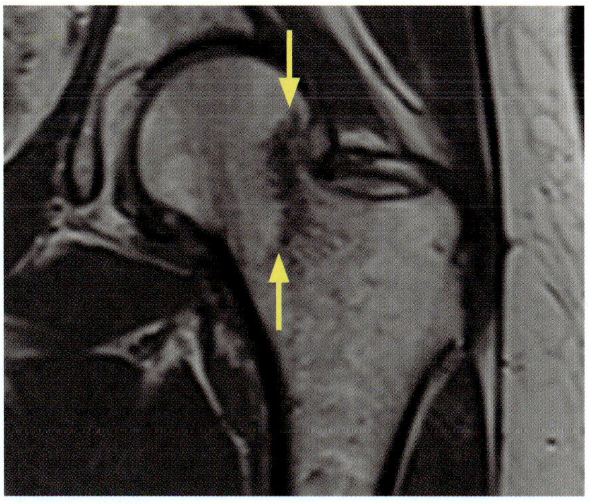

Coronal T1-weighted MRI
冠状位T_1加权MRI

Occult fracture, evident on MRI (different patient from above). Radiograph is negative. MRI demonstrates a nondisplaced femoral neck fracture (arrows).

MRI is the gold standard to diagnose occult hip fracture, with a sensitivity of essentially 100%.

However, CT is cheaper, faster, more readily available, less susceptible to motion, and without known contra-indications. Two meta-analyses showed that CT has a sensitivity of 79–94% for detecting occult hip fracture. Therefore, CT may be reasonable if MRI is not readily available but MRI remains the gold standard.

Dual energy CT shows promise as an emerging modality to improve the sensitivity of CT.

磁共振显示的隐匿性骨折(非上述同一名患者)。X线影像阴性。MRI显示无移位的股骨颈骨折(箭)。

MRI是诊断髋部隐匿性骨折的金标准，其敏感性基本达100%。

然而，CT更便宜、更快、更便捷，较少受运动影响，而且还未知有任何禁忌证。两项荟萃分析显示，CT检测髋部隐匿性骨折的敏感性为79%~94%。因此，当不能立即进行MRI检查时可采用CT，但MRI仍然是金标准。

双能量CT是一种有望提高CT敏感性的新方法。

Femoral neck fracture (intracapsular) | 股骨颈骨折(关节囊内)

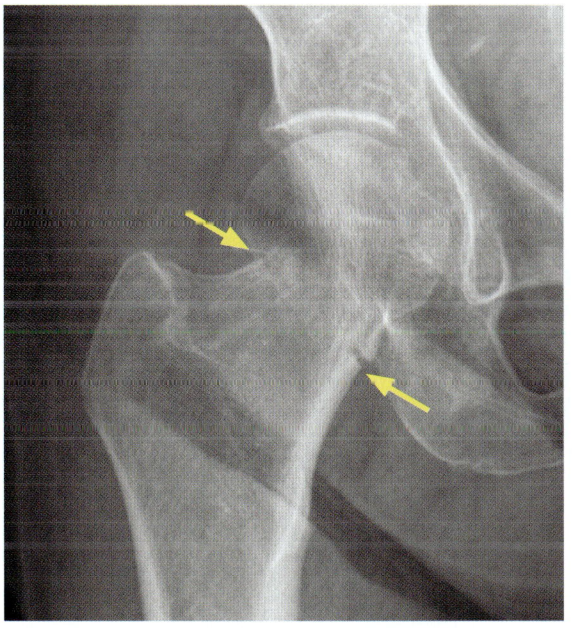

Valgus impacted femoral neck fracture:

Frontal radiograph shows a fracture of the femoral neck (arrows) with the distal part of the femur directed laterally, consistent with valgus.

This fracture was treated with ORIF.

外翻嵌入性股骨颈骨折：

正位X线影像显示股骨颈骨折(箭)，骨折远端的股骨朝向外侧，符合外翻改变。

该骨折采用切开复位内固定术治疗。

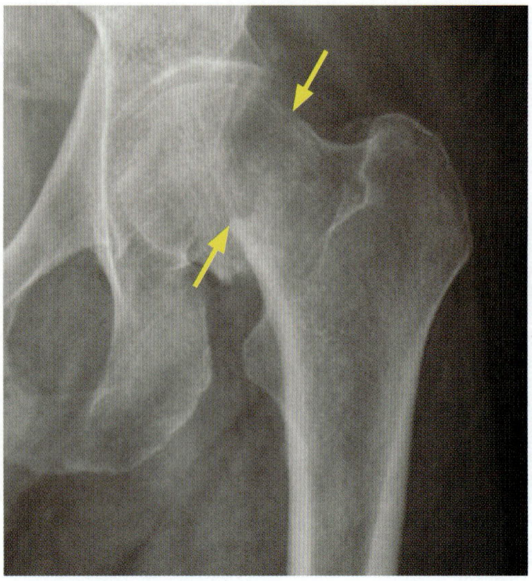

Varus displaced femoral neck fracture (different patient from above):
Frontal radiograph shows a fracture of the femoral neck (arrows) with the distal part of the femur directed medially, consistent with varus.
This fracture was treated with arthroplasty.
内翻移位的股骨颈骨折(与上图不是同一名患者):
正位X线影像显示股骨颈骨折(箭),骨折远端股骨指向内侧,符合内翻改变。
该骨折采用人工关节置换术进行治疗。

- Femoral neck fractures are typically seen in the elderly after low-energy trauma.
- Femoral neck fractures are intracapsular, and therefore at risk to develop avascular necrosis.
- The orthopedic classifications include Garden and Pauwel, although these are not in common use clinically. The specific site of the femoral neck (such as subcapital or transcervical) does not affect treatment and does not need to be mentioned.
- Intracapsular femoral neck fractures can be nondisplaced (valgus impaction is considered nondisplaced for treatment decisions) or displaced (varus angulation is considered displaced).

  Nondisplaced (valgus impacted) fractures can be treated with ORIF, which is a less invasive procedure compared to arthroplasty.

  Displaced (varus impacted) fractures are typically treated with arthroplasty (in active community ambulators) or hemiarthroplasy (in less active or debilitated patients) in older patients. Although femoral neck fractures are uncommon in younger patients, ORIF would be the preferred treatment in an attempt to preserve the joint.

Basicervical fracture

- 股骨颈骨折常见于受到低强度外伤后的老年人。
- 股骨颈骨折属于关节囊内骨折,因此有发生缺血性坏死的风险。
- 此类骨折的骨科学分类法有Garden法和Pauwel法,但它们在临床上并不常用。股骨颈的具体部位(如头下型或经颈型)不影响治疗,因而不需要在报告中进行描述。
- 关节囊内股骨颈骨折可以是无移位的(外翻嵌插在治疗决策中被认为是无移位的)或移位的(内翻成角被认为是移位的)。

  非移位(外展嵌插)骨折可采用切开复位内固定术(ORIF)治疗,这种方法属于相对非侵入性手术,较关节置换术的创伤小。

  移位(内翻成角中)通常采用节置换术(在运动较多的人群中)或半关节置换术(在活动较少或虚弱的患者)。虽然股骨颈骨折在年轻患者中并不常见,但切开复位内固定术是保留关节的首选治疗方法。

股骨颈基底部骨折

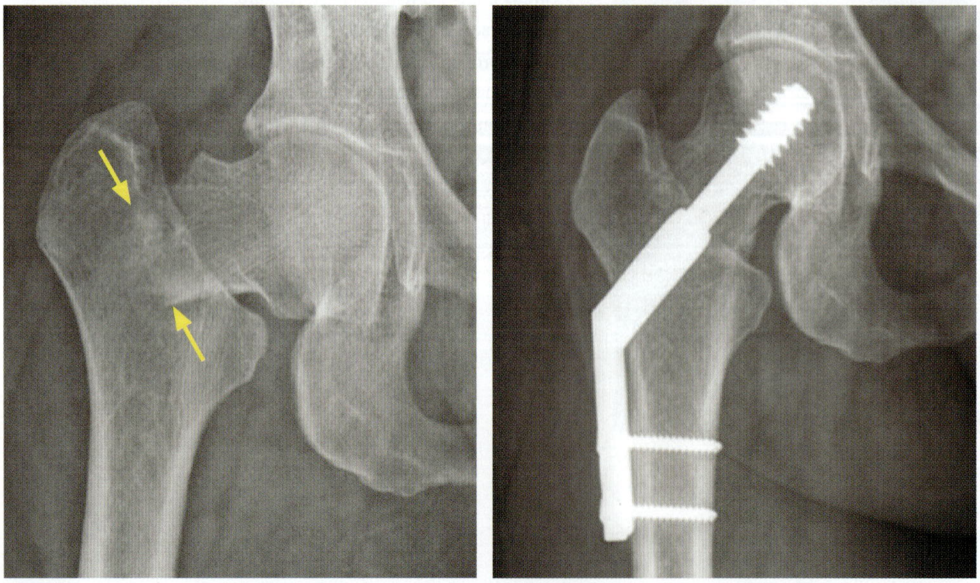

Basicervical fracture: Frontal radiograph (left image) demonstrates a basicervical fracture (arrows), located just proximal to the intertrochanteric crest. Despite being displaced, this was able to be treated with ORIF with a dynamic hip screw (right image).
股骨颈基底部骨折:正位X线影像(左图)显示股骨颈基底部骨折(箭),位于转子间嵴的近端。尽管有移位,但仍然可以采用动力髋关节螺钉进行切开内固定复位治疗(右图)。

- Basicervical fractures are a relatively uncommon type of femoral neck fracture that occurs just distal to the joint capsule. Being extracapsular, they have a lower risk of avascular necrosis and can be successfully treated with ORIF (typically with a dynamic hip screw), regardless of if displaced or nondisplaced.

- 股骨颈基底部骨折是一类相对少见的股骨颈骨折，发生在关节囊的远端。由于位于关节囊外，其发生缺血性坏死的风险较低，且无论骨折端是否有移位，均可采用切开复位内固定术(ORIF)治疗(通常采用动力髋关节螺丝)。

Greater trochanter

大转子

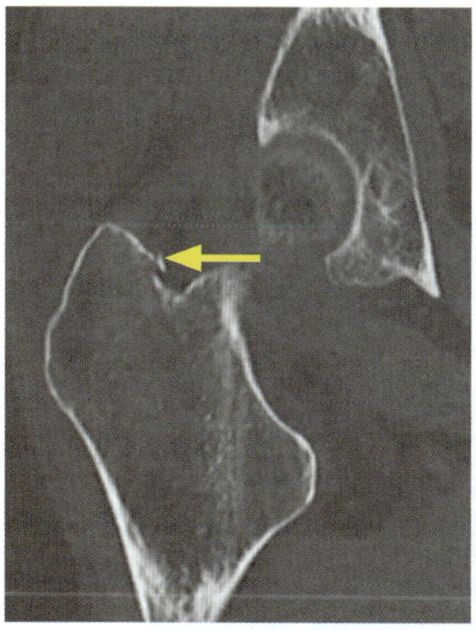

Coronal CT
冠状位CT

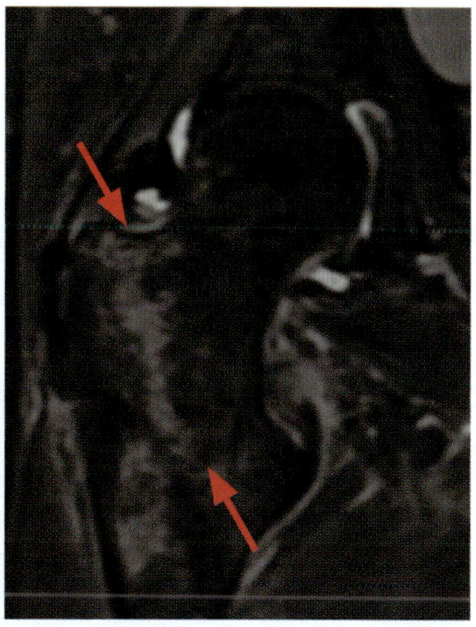

Coronal STIR MRI
冠状位STIR MRI

Coronal CT demonstrates an apparently tiny fracture of the greater trochanter (arrow).
MRI shows the true extent of the fracture, with edema (red arrows) extending greater than 50% of the distance through the intertrochanteric region.
The patient was treated surgically based on clinical exam and MRI findings with ORIF (same treatment pathway as a stable intertrochanteric fracture).
冠状位CT显示大转子一处明显的微小骨折(箭)。
MRI显示骨折的真实范围，其水肿(红箭)范围超过转子间区距离的50%。
根据临床检查和MRI结果，患者接受了切开复位内固定术(ORIF)(与稳定性粗隆间骨折相同的治疗方式)。

- Greater trochanter fractures can be thought of as the "tip of the iceberg" fracture, as the true extent of the fracture often extends well beyond the greater trochanter. In fact, it is likely that the majority of these fractures are actually intertrochanteric fractures with the intertrochanteric portion occult on radiography.

- 大转子骨折可以被认为是"冰山一角"骨折，因为骨折的真正范围通常远超过大转子。事实上，大多数这些骨折可能实际上是粗隆间骨折，但在X线影像上粗隆间的骨折是隐匿的。

Intertrochanteric fracture

粗隆间骨折

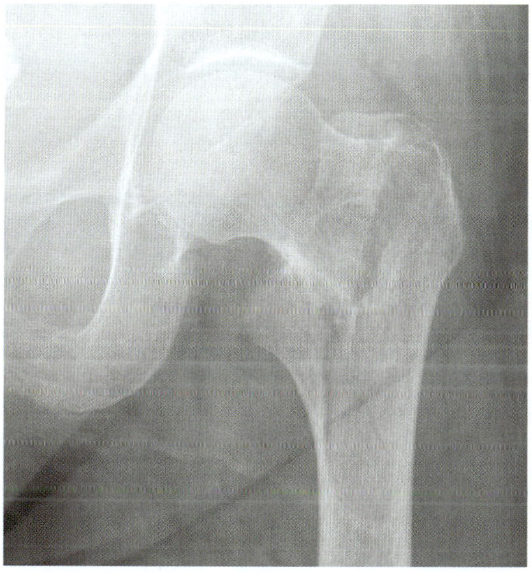

Stable intertrochanteric fracture:
Frontal radiograph demonstrates an intertrochanteric fracture with a single fracture line.
This was treated with a dynamic hip screw (not pictured; same treatment as the basicervical fracture on the preceding page).
稳定性粗隆间骨折：
正位X线影像显示粗隆间骨折呈单条骨折线。
治疗采用动力髋关节螺钉(图中未显示；治疗方法与上页股骨颈基底部骨折相同)。

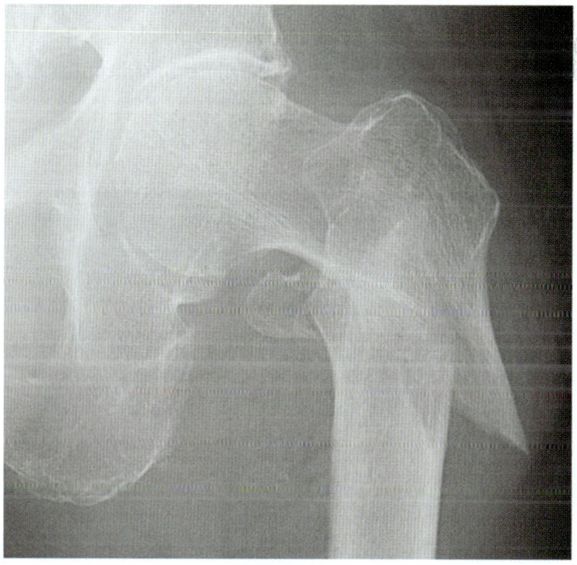

Unstable intertrochanteric fracture (different patient):
Frontal radiograph demonstrates a comminuted fracture with involvement of the lateral femoral cortex.
This fracture was treated with an intramedullary nail (not pictured).
不稳定性粗隆间骨折(与左图不是同一名患者)：
正位X线影像显示粗隆间粉碎性骨折并累及股骨外侧皮质。
该骨折采用髓内钉治疗(图中未显示)。

- Intertrochanteric fractures are treated differently depending if they are stable or unstable.
- A stable fracture is one that is a simple, two-part fracture without comminution or involvement of the lateral femoral cortex. Stable fractures can be treated with a dynamic hip screw.
- An unstable fracture is comminuted or involves the lateral femoral cortex. Unstable fractures are typically treated with an intramedullary nail.
- Of note, a fracture isolated to the **lesser trochanter** in an adult should be considered pathologic until proven otherwise (adolescents may traumatically avulse the lesser trochanter, which is the attachment site of the strong iliopsoas muscle).

- 粗隆间骨折的治疗取决于其是否稳定。
- 稳定性骨折是指简单的、由两部分组成的骨折，无骨质粉碎或股骨外侧皮质受累。稳定性骨折可采用动力髋关节螺钉治疗。
- 不稳定性骨折是指粉碎性骨折或骨折累及股骨外侧皮质。不稳定性骨折通常采用髓内钉治疗。
- 注意，成人**小转子**孤立性骨折在未确认其他原因之前应视为病理性骨折(青少年可能因创伤导致小转子撕脱骨折，小转子是强有力的髂腰肌附着点)。

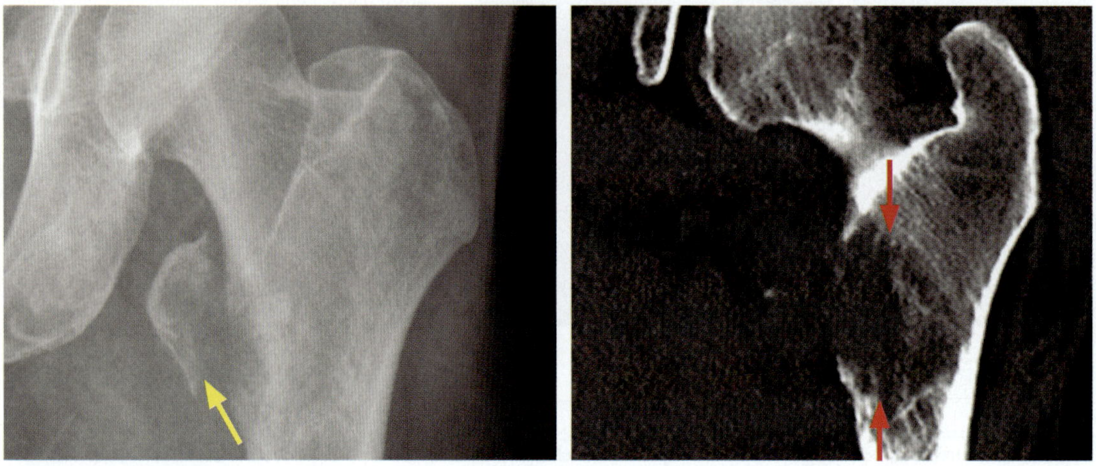

Pathologic fracture of the lesser trochanter: Frontal radiograph shows a mildly displaced fracture of the lesser trochanter (yellow arrows), with permeative margins. CT confirms a permeative lesion (red arrows).
小转子病理性骨折：正位X线影像显示小转子轻度移位骨折(黄箭)，伴浸润性边缘。CT证实浸润性病变(红箭)。

Subtrochanteric fracture

- A subtrochanteric fracture is a proximal diaphyseal fracture involving the subtrochanteric region, which extends from the level of the lesser trochanter to 5 cm distal to the lesser trochanter. Treatment is intramedullary nail (similar to unstable intertrochanteric fracture).

粗隆下骨折

- 粗隆下骨折是一种股骨干近端骨折，累及粗隆下区域，包括从小转子水平至小转子远端5cm的范围。采用髓内钉治疗(类似于粗隆间不稳定性骨折)。

Femoral neck stress fracture

股骨颈应力性骨折

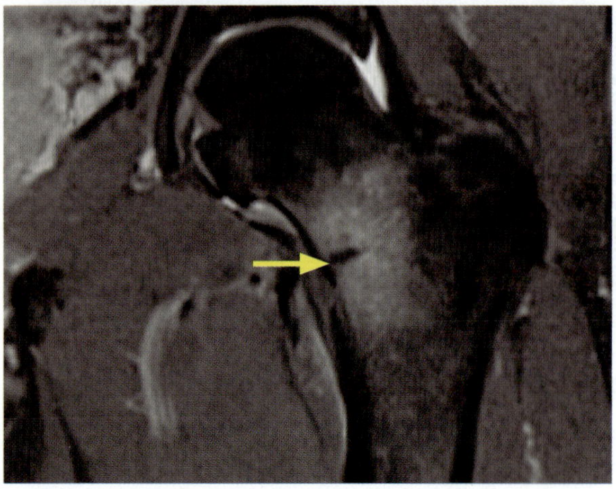

Femoral neck stress fracture involving the medial femoral neck: Coronal STIR MRI demonstrates edema of the medial aspect of the femoral neck with a small fracture line (arrow).
股骨颈内侧应力性骨折：
冠状位STIR MRI显示股骨颈内侧水肿伴一条小的骨折线(箭)。

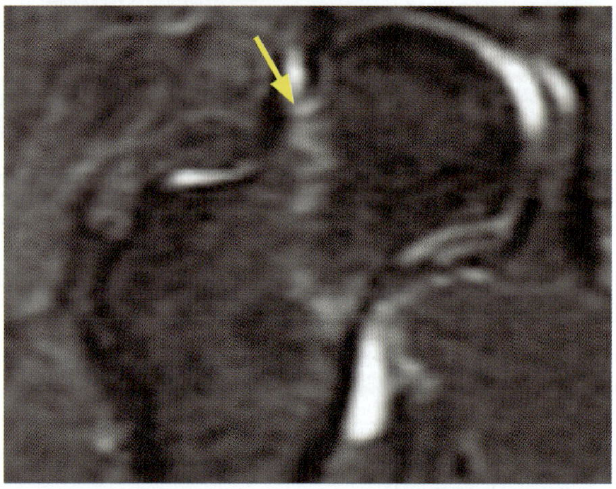

Femoral neck stress fracture involving the lateral femoral neck: Coronal STIR MRI demonstrates edema of the lateral aspect of the femoral neck (arrow), as well as some medial-sided edema.
股骨颈外侧应力性骨折：
冠状位 STIR MRI显示股骨颈外侧水肿(箭)，以及部分股骨颈内侧水肿。

- Femoral neck stress fractures are typically seen in highly active patients. The female athlete triad is restrictive/disordered eating, menstrual dysfunction, and low bone density, and these individuals are at higher risk for stress fractures.
- Stress fractures of the medial cortex are under compressive forces and tend to heal with cessation of the offending physical activity.
- In contrast, stress fractures of the lateral femoral cortex are under tensile (pulling) forces, and are treated more aggressively, with weightbearing restrictions and sometimes surgery.
- Imaging initially shows edema, with discrete fracture line in more advanced cases.

- 股骨颈应力性骨折通常见于剧烈运动的患者。女性运动员的三联征包括节食/不规律进食、月经紊乱和骨密度降低，此类人群发生应力性骨折的风险更高。
- 股骨内侧皮质应力性骨折在压缩性外力的作用下发生，在停止剧烈运动后往往会愈合。
- 相反，股骨外侧皮质应力性骨折在张(拉)力的作用下发生，治疗需要更为积极，如限制负重，有时需要手术治疗。
- 影像学最初表现为水肿，在晚期病例中可见明确的骨折线。

Atypical femoral fracture

非典型股骨骨折

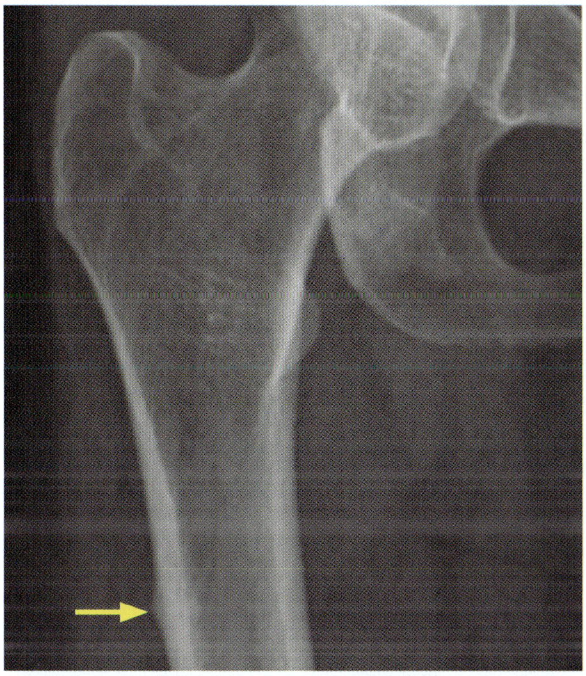

Atypical femoral fracture: Frontal radiograph shows focal cortical thickening of the lateral subtrochanteric cortex (yellow arrow). Subtle, but critically important!
非典型股骨骨折：正位X线影像显示粗隆下外侧皮质局灶性增厚(黄箭)。不明显但至关重要!

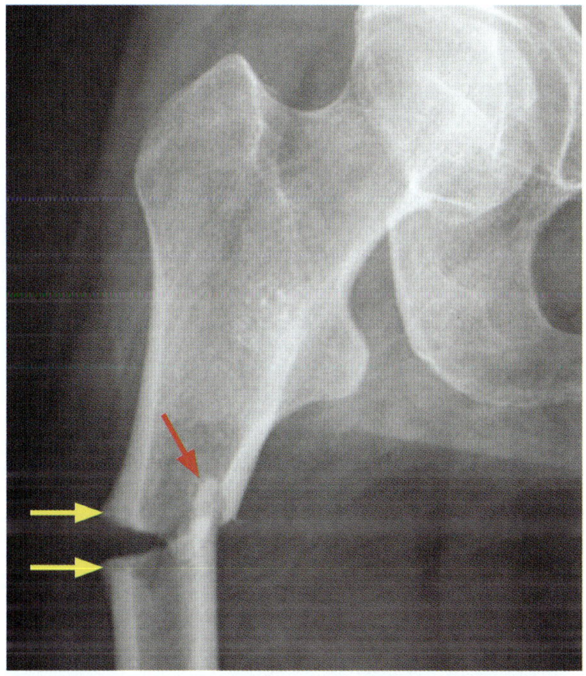

Displaced fracture from underlying atypical femoral fracture, in the same patient as on the left. Note the lateral cortical thickening (yellow arrows), transverse orientation, lack of comminution, and medial spike (red arrow).
非典型股骨骨折引起移位骨折，与左侧图像为同一名患者。注意外侧皮质增厚(黄箭)，骨折线横向走行，未见粉碎性骨折，以及内侧尖状突起(红箭)。

- Atypical femoral fractures are a form of insufficiency fracture that occur in the proximal lateral femoral diaphyseal cortex, typically the subtrochanteric region (defined as extending from the lesser trochanter to 5 cm distal).
- Atypical fractures are caused by insufficient osteoclastic-induced remodeling, resulting in a brittle bone more susceptible to fracture.
- Atypical femoral fractures are most known to occur in patients taking bisphosphonates (which inhibit osteoclasts), but can also occur in patients on denosumab (a monoclonal antibody that inhibits osteoclast maturation) or in patients without these medications.
- The American Society of Bone and Mineral Research defined 5 major features, of which 4 of the 5 must be present to diagnose an atypical femoral fracture:

- 非典型股骨骨折是一种发生在股骨近端骨干外侧皮质的应力性骨折，通常在粗隆下区(定义为从小转子向远端延伸5cm的范围)。
- 非典型骨折由破骨细胞诱导的重塑不足引起，导致骨脆性增加，更容易发生骨折。
- 非典型股骨骨折最常发生在服用双膦酸盐(抑制破骨细胞)的患者，但也可能发生在服用Denosumab(一种抑制破骨细胞成熟的单克隆抗体)或未曾服用这些药物的患者。
- 美国骨骼和矿物研究协会定义了非典型股骨骨折的5个主要特征，只有在5个特征中具备4个才能诊断非典型股骨骨折：

No more than minimal trauma.
Substantially transverse orientation.
Must involve lateral cortex if incomplete; if complete may demonstrate a "medial spike."
No more than minimally comminuted.
Endosteal or periosteal thickening laterally.

最多为轻微创伤。
骨折线大体为横向走行。
如果是不全性骨折，必累及外侧皮质；如果是完全性骨折，可见"内侧尖状突起"。
最多为轻微粉碎性骨折。
股骨外侧骨内膜或骨膜增厚。

- When an atypical femoral fracture is identified, radiographs of the contralateral femur should be performed, as these fractures are bilateral in a substantial minority of patients.
- Treatment could include cessation of the offending medication if appropriate, and intramedullary nailing in some patients, especially if that patient has pain.

- 当发现非典型股骨骨折时，应对对侧股骨进行X线影像检查，因为这些骨折在不少患者中为双侧同时发生。
- 治疗包括酌情考虑停止相关药物，在部分患者中可进行髓内钉治疗，特别是有疼痛的患者。

Avascular necrosis (AVN)

缺血性坏死(AVN)

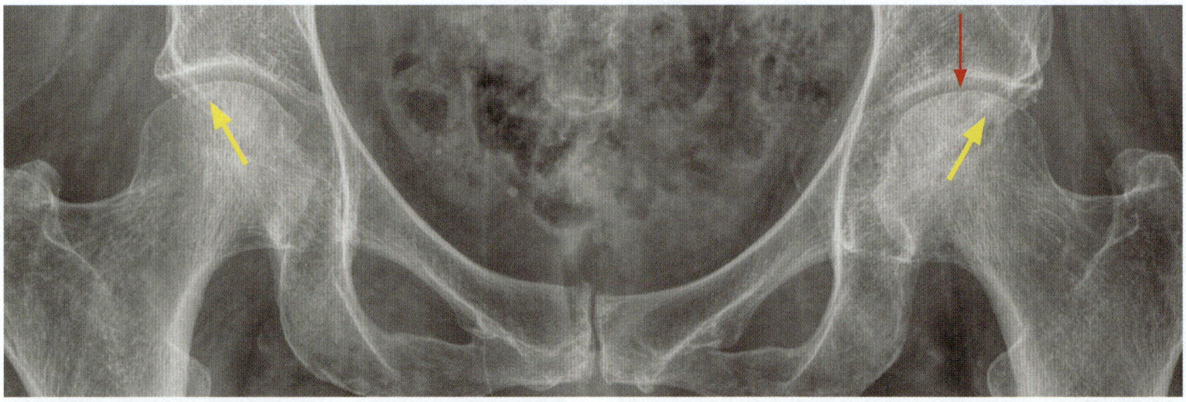

Frontal radiograph shows subtle patchy subchondral sclerosis of both femoral heads (yellow arrows), with subtle irregularity of the subchondral bone plate (the "cortex" overlying the cartilage) on the left (red arrow).

正位X线影像显示双侧股骨头呈轻微的斑片样软骨下硬化(黄箭)，伴左侧软骨下骨板(软骨下的"皮质")轻微不规则改变(红箭)。

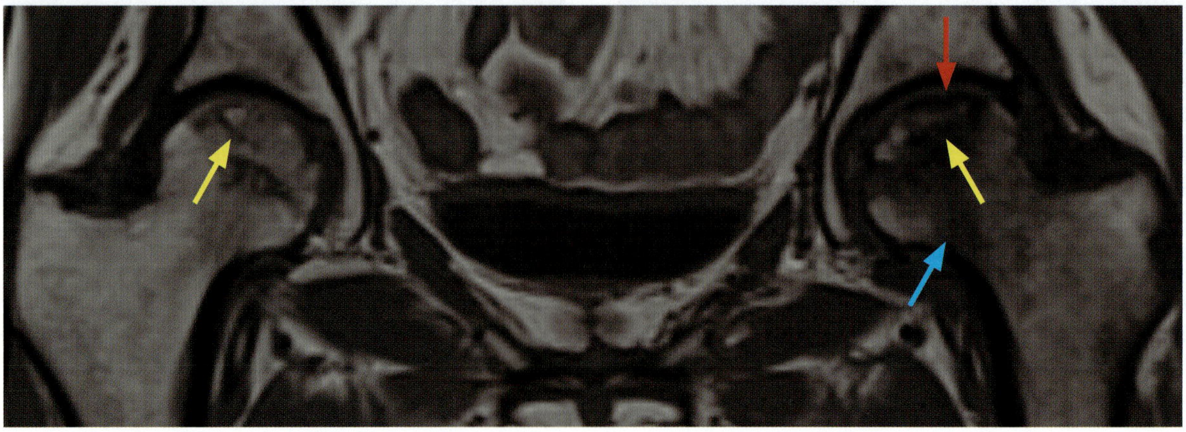

Coronal T1-weighted MRI shows serpiginous regions of signal abnormality involving the subchondral bone of both femoral heads (yellow arrows). There is irregularity and undulating contour of the subchondral bone plate on the left (red arrow), and with extensive edema (low signal intensity on this T1-weighted MR) asymmetrically involving the left (blue arrow).

冠状位T_1加权MRI图像显示双股骨头软骨下呈锯齿状边缘的骨信号异常区(黄箭)。左侧软骨下骨板呈不规则波浪状改变(红箭)，伴左侧股骨头广泛(T_1加权MRI图像上低信号)且不对称性的水肿(蓝箭)。

- Avascular necrosis (AVN) is focal ischemia of the epiphyseal region or subchondral bone. AVN leads to trabecular necrosis, which increases susceptibility to subchondral collapse, and secondary osteoarthritis if untreated. The more general term *osteonecrosis* indicates necrosis of bone and marrow elements.
- The femoral head is especially susceptible to AVN because of precarious blood supply. The blood supply to the femoral head is primarily through the medial femoral circumflex artery, which enters the femoral neck and gives off posterosuperior epiphyseal branches that course along the femoral neck to supply the femoral head.
- As previous discussed, intracapsular proximal femur fractures have a high risk of AVN, including femoral neck fractures in the elderly and transient subluxation in athletes.
- Non-traumatic causes of AVN are usually systemic, including red-cell abnormalities (e.g., sickle cell disease), abnormalities of marrow packing (e.g., Gaucher disease), or secondary effects of medications including steroids, alcohol, or immunosuppression from transplant. Systemic causes of AVN tend to be bilateral.

  A clue to the presence of Gaucher disease is splenomegaly with AVN.

  A clue to the presence of sickle cell is a small calcified spleen with AVN.
- It is optimal to diagnose AVN prior to subchondral collapse and secondary osteoarthritis. Early AVN can be treated with medication/lifestyle changes and/or core decompression (drilling of the subchondral bone, with the goal to reduce intraosseous pressure). Once subchondral collapse and secondary osteoarthritis are present, treatment is generally arthroplasty.
- Several staging systems have been proposed for the radiographic and MRI classification of AVN; however, from a practical standpoint the relative size of the AVN, status of the subchondral bone plate (the "cortex" overlying the cartilage), and presence of secondary osteoarthritis are helpful imaging findings to describe.
- The most common appearance of AVN on MRI is a geographic subchondral lesion outlined by a serpentine low signal rim on T1-weighted images. The subchondral anterior-superior portions of the femoral head, at 10 o'clock and 2 o'clock on coronal images, are typical locations.
- The *double line sign* is seen on T2-weighted MRI and is comprised of a peripheral low-intensity rim and an inner high-intensity band. The double line sign is thought to be pathognomonic for AVN.
- Bone marrow edema is present in 50% and clinically correlates with pain.

- 缺血性坏死(AVN)是骨骺区或软骨下区的局部缺血。AVN导致骨小梁坏死，从而更容易发生软骨下骨塌陷，如不治疗还会导致继发性骨关节炎。比较通俗的术语为*骨坏死*，是指骨和骨髓成分的坏死。
- 股骨头由于血供脆弱而特别容易出现缺血性坏死(AVN)。股骨头的血供主要来自旋股内侧动脉，该动脉进入股骨颈并发出后上骨骺分支，并沿股骨颈上行供应股骨头。
- 如前所述，关节囊内的股骨近端骨折具有较高的AVN风险，包括老年人的股骨颈骨折和运动员的一过性半脱位。
- 引起AVN的非创伤性的原因通常是系统性的，包括红细胞异常(如镰状细胞病)、髓腔堵塞(如戈谢病)，或继发于药物的作用，如类固醇激素、酒精或器官移植后的免疫抑制剂。系统性原因引起的AVN常为双侧。

  患有戈谢病的一个线索是AVN伴脾大。

  患有镰状细胞病的一个线索是AVN伴萎缩和钙化的脾脏。
- 诊断AVN最佳的窗口是在发生软骨下骨塌陷和继发性骨关节炎之前。早期AVN可以通过药物治疗/生活方式改变和/或核心减压(软骨下骨钻孔，以降低骨内压力)进行治疗。一旦出现软骨下骨塌陷和继发性骨关节炎，治疗则通常采用关节置换术。
- AVN的X线和MRI的分期有数种建议；但从实际出发，AVN的相对大小、软骨下骨板(覆盖在软骨上的"皮质")的状态和是否存在继发性骨关节炎是需要对其进行描述的有价值的影像学表现。
- AVN在MRI上最常见的表现是在T_1加权序列上软骨下呈地图样病变，其边缘为一弯曲的低信号环。股骨头前上部软骨下区域是AVN的好发位置，在冠状位图像上对应于10点钟到2点钟位置。
- 在T_2加权MRI图像上见到的*双线征*是由边缘低信号环和内部高信号带组成。双线征被认为是AVN的特异性影像学表现。
- 骨髓水肿见于50%的AVN患者，在临床上，与患者的疼痛症状相关。

Transient bone marrow edema (TBME)

- Transient bone marrow edema (TBME), also called transient osteoporosis of the hip, is a controversial entity that is a diagnosis of exclusion and may actually reflect a combination of disorders including sympathetic nervous system overactivity, stress fracture, or transient ischemia.
- The traditional teaching is that TBME is a self-limited clinical entity lasting a few months. It is characterized by severe hip pain in young to middle-aged adults (more commonly men, although it was first described in women in the third trimester of pregnancy).
- Radiographs show regional osteopenia in the femoral head without any secondary signs of arthritis. MRI shows edema throughout the femoral

一过性骨髓水肿(TBME)

- 一过性骨髓水肿(TBME)，也称为一过性髋关节骨质疏松，是一个有争议的排除性诊断，实际可能是交感神经系统过度兴奋、应力性骨折或短暂性缺血等一系列异常的综合表现。
- 传统教学观点认为，TBME是一种自限性疾病，持续数个月。其特征为中、青年人发生严重髋部疼痛(男性多见，而最早报道的是发生在晚期妊娠的女性)。
- X线影像学表现为股骨头局部骨量减少，无任何继发性关节炎征象。MRI显示股骨头弥漫

head.

- As TBME may be a wastebasket diagnosis, it is essential to always evaluate for subtle lesions to explain these findings. For instance, a subchondral hypointense line on T1-weighted images may represent a fracture, or a small focus of AVN may be apparent.

性水肿。

- 由于TBME可能是一个排除性诊断，因此必须仔细检查任何细微的病变并作出解释。例如，在T_1加权图像上软骨下的低信号线可能是骨折，或是一个AVN病灶。

Femoroacetabular impingement (FAI)

Overview and controversy of femoroacetabular impingement (FAI)

- Femoroacetabular impingement (FAI) is abnormal abutment of the femur with the acetabulum at extremes of range of motion.
- Two types of impingement have been described, depending if the femoral head/neck junction (cam-type) or the acetabulum (pincer-type) is abnormal.
- Chronic microtrauma of the femoral head abutting against the acetabulum may cause acetabular labral tears in young athletic individuals and may accelerate the development of hip osteoarthritis.
- While FAI may be an important cause of hip osteoarthritis in young patients, there is controversy as to whether a diagnosis of impingement can be made based on the imaging findings in the absence of the clinical syndrome.
- Impingement is primarily a clinical diagnosis and there is a significant subset of patients with abnormal morphology of the acetabulum or femoral head/neck junction who are asymptomatic.
- Labral injury secondary to FAI (typically occurring in the anterosuperior labrum) is often associated with underlying chondral injury as well.
- Regardless of the controversy, FAI is an important concept to be aware of in the young adult. A general consensus is that imaging findings suggestive of FAI should be described with the disclaimer that these findings may predispose to impingement in the presence of pain.

股骨髋臼卡磨(撞击)(FAI)

股骨髋臼卡磨的概述和争议

- 股骨髋臼卡磨(FAI)是股骨与髋臼在过度活动时出现承接关系异常。
- 有两种类型的卡磨，取决于股骨头/颈交界处(凸轮型)还是髋臼(钳型)异常。
- 在年轻的运动员，股骨头紧靠髋臼处的慢性微型创伤可导致髋臼盂唇撕裂，并可能加速发展成髋部骨关节炎。
- FAI在年轻患者中可能是骨性关节炎的一个重要病因，但在缺乏临床症状时，能否依靠影像学表现诊断FAI尚存争议。
- 卡磨主要是一种临床诊断，有相当一部分患者有髋臼或股骨头/颈交界处的形态异常而没有临床症状。
- 继发于FAI的盂唇损伤(常发生在唇盂前上部)往往伴有其下方的髋臼软骨损伤。
- 尽管存在争议，FAI在年轻患者中是一个需要引起重视的概念。普遍的共识是，当影像学中有提示FAI的征象时，应在报告中声明，这些患者日后可能会发生卡磨和疼痛。

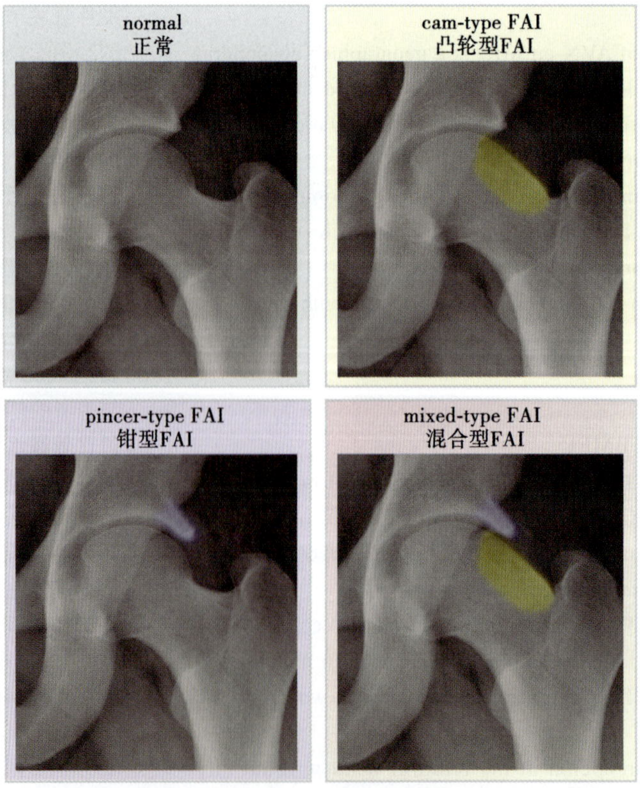

Cam-type impingement

- Cam-type impingement, characterized by an osseous convexity of the femoral head/neck junction, is most common in young athletic males.
- The alpha angle defines the degree of femoral bump. An alpha angle is measured on oblique axial MRI or CT. An alpha angle of >55 degrees is said to be abnormal, especially if symptoms of hip impingement are present. Of note, there is a relatively high prevalence of asymptomatic individuals with elevated alpha angles.

凸轮型卡磨

- 凸轮型卡磨，以股骨头/颈部交界处的骨性隆起为特征，最常见于年轻男性运动员。
- α角定义为股骨骨性隆起的角度。α角是在斜轴位MRI或CT上进行测量。α角>55°为异常，特别是当有髋关节卡磨的症状时。需要注意，很多α角增大的个体都没有髋关节卡磨的症状。

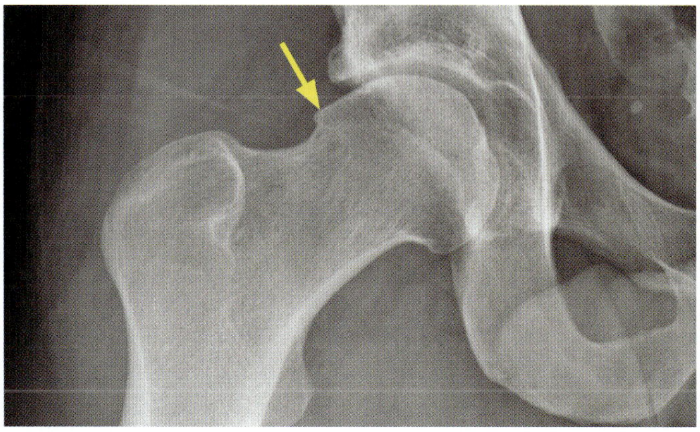

Frontal radiograph demonstrates an osseous convexity at the femoral head/neck junction (arrow), which can be consistent with a CAM lesion in a patient with the clinical syndrome of hip impingement.
正位X线影像显示股骨头/颈部交界处的骨性隆起(箭)，与髋关节卡磨患者的凸轮型病灶一致。

- To measure the alpha angle, a line through the femoral neck bisecting the center of the femoral head is interfaced with a second line which runs from the center of the femoral head to the most proximal abnormal contour of the femoral head/neck.

- 测量α角时需要画两条线，一条是股骨颈轴线，将股骨头一分为二，另一条连接股骨头中心到股骨头/颈的最近的异常隆起端，两条线的夹角即为α角。

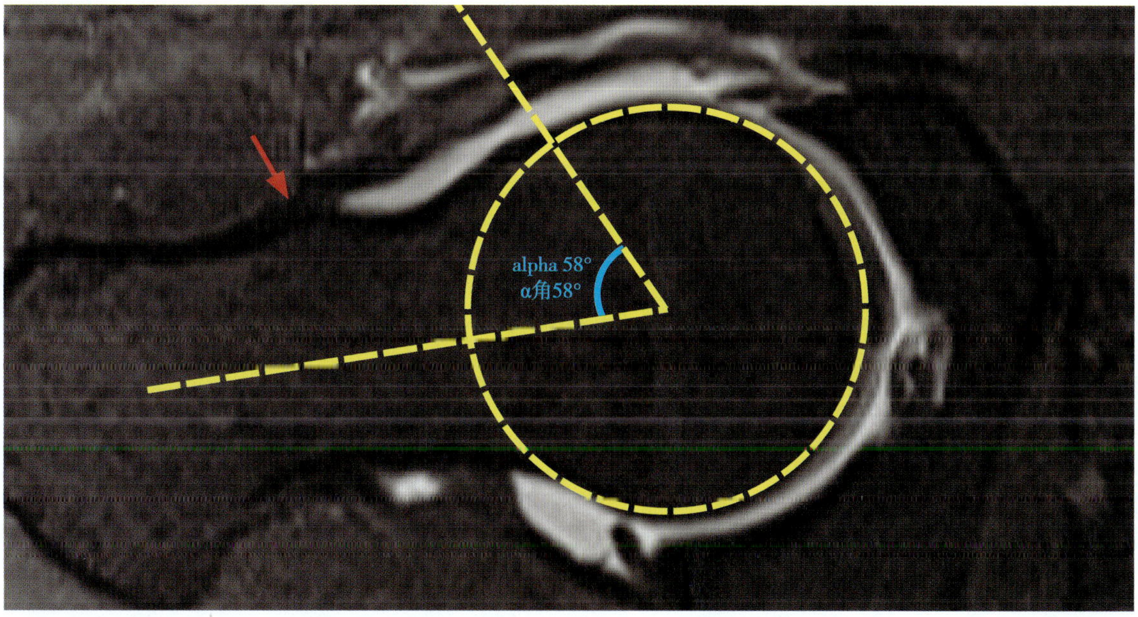

This is the same patient as pictured on the previous page.
Post-arthrogram axial-oblique T1-weighted MRI with fat suppression demonstrates an osseous convexity at the femoral head/neck junction (red arrow), with an elevated alpha angle.
与前页为同一名患者。
关节造影后斜轴位T_1加权脂肪抑制MRI显示股骨头/颈部交界处骨质凸起(红箭)，α角增大。

- Cam-type impingement is treated with femoroplasty.

- 凸轮型卡磨的治疗方法为股骨置换术。

Pincer-type impingement

- Pincer-type FAI is caused by overcoverage of the acetabulum, and is more common in middle-aged females. However, most cases of hip impingement are due to both pincer-type and CAM-type.
- The *crossover sign* (also called cranial acetabular retroversion) is seen in pincer-type FAI and represents the superior aspect of the anterior acetabular wall crossing over the posterior acetabular wall on a frontal radiograph.

钳夹型卡磨

- 钳夹型FAI是由髋臼过度覆盖造成，最常见于中年女性。然而，大多数髋关节卡磨由凸轮型和钳夹型卡磨共同造成。
- 交叉征(也称为髋臼顶反转)见于钳夹型FAI，在正位X线影像上表现为髋臼前壁上份跨过髋臼后壁。

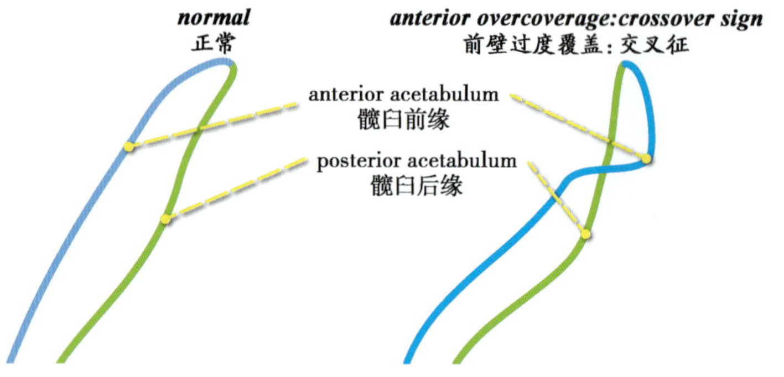

Illustration of the left acetabulum as seen on a radiograph demonstrates a comparison between the normal anterior and posterior acetabulum, and in anterior overcoverage. In anterior overcoverage, there is crossover of the anterior and posterior acetabulum.
按X线影像所绘制的左侧髋臼示意图比较了正常的前后髋臼，以及前髋臼过度覆盖。前髋臼过度覆盖时，可见前后髋臼缘交叉。

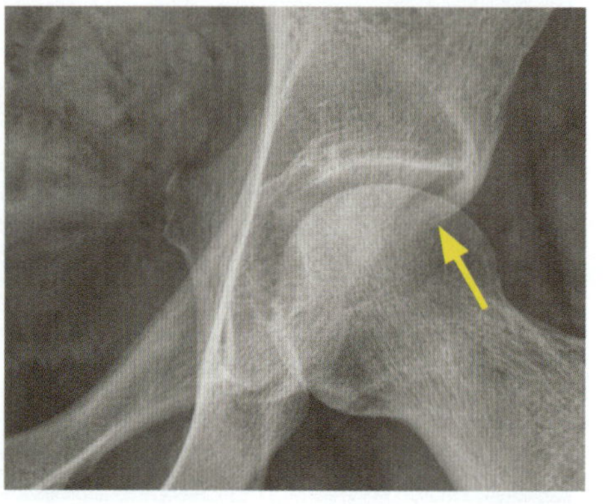

Frontal radiograph of the left hip shows anterior overcoverage with a crossover sign. Note the margin of the anterior acetabulum (arrow) crossing over.
左髋正位X线影像显示髋臼前缘过度覆盖，呈交叉征。注意髋臼前缘(箭)交叉。

- Treatment of pincer-type FAI is surgical trimming of the acetabular rim.

Acetabular labral tear

- 钳夹型FAI的治疗方法是外科修整髋臼环。

髋臼盂唇撕裂

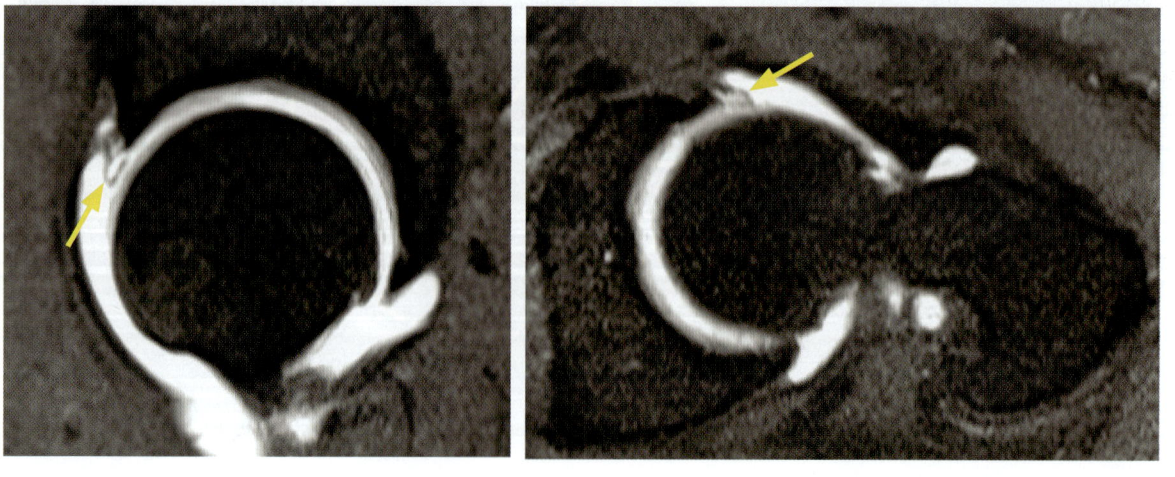

Intrasubstance labral tearing: Sagittal (left image) and axial MR arthrogram images show a markedly diminutive and irregular anterior/superior labrum (arrows), in keeping with intrasubstance tearing.
盂唇实质撕裂：矢状位(左图)和轴位MR关节造影显示前上盂唇明显缩小且不规则(箭)，符合盂唇实质撕裂。

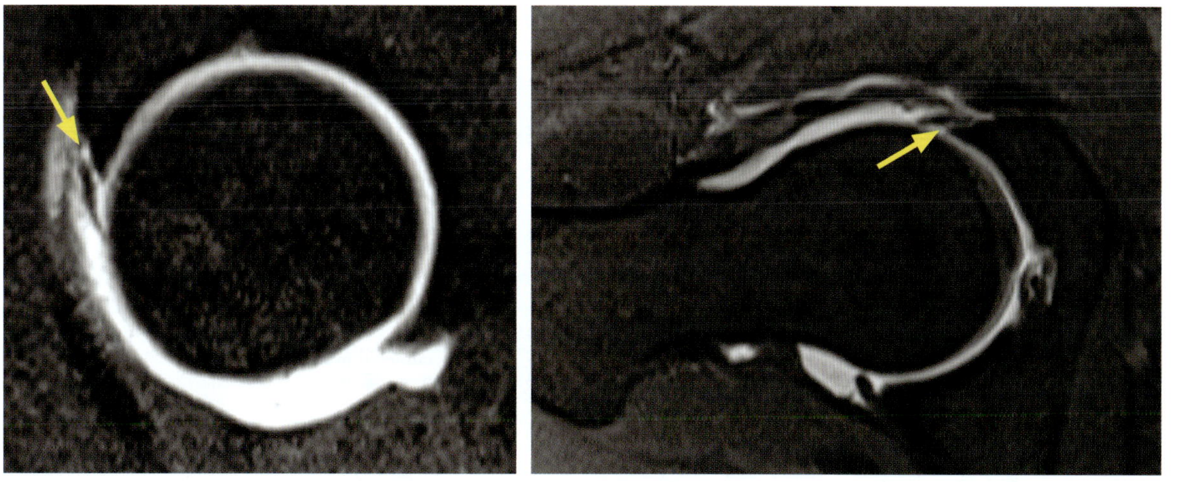

Chondrolabral junction tearing (different patient from above): Sagittal (left image) and axial MR arthrogram images show contrast interposed between the entire width (arrows) of the anterior superior labrum and the acetabulum.
软骨-盂唇连接处撕裂(与上例不同的患者):矢状位(左图)和轴位MR关节造影显示造影剂进入前上盂唇和髋臼之间的整个间隙(箭)。

- Labral tears are seen most commonly in the setting of FAI, with the anterior-superior labrum typically involved. Labral tears are challenging to detect, given the curved morphology of the labrum. Note that there is no labral tissue inferiorly; instead, the transverse ligament is located at the inferior aspect of the ring comprising the labrum.
- MR arthrography is the most sensitive imaging modality to diagnose acetabular labral tears; however, both conventional MR and MR arthrography have similar high specificity.
- Labral tears can conceptually be divided into two types: tears at the chondrolabral junction, where the labrum is lifted off the cartilage; and tears involving the substance of the labrum.
- Secondary findings of labral tearing include paralabral cyst formation, chondral injury, and subchondral edema, all of which may be present with normal radiographs. Additionally, typical osteoarthritic changes such as osteophytes and subchondral cysts may be more apparent on MRI compared to radiographs.
- There are several normal variants that may mimic labral tears. Perhaps the most challenging to differentiate is a sublabral sulcus, which is an incomplete attachment of the labrum to the acetabulum. In contrast to a tear, injected contrast would not extend the entire width of the labrum, and no secondary degenerative changes would be present.

- 盂唇撕裂最常见于FAI,通常累及前上盂唇。因盂唇的形态呈弯曲状,所以发现盂唇撕裂具有一定难度。注意,髋臼下缘没有盂唇;相反,横韧带位于盂唇环的下方而成为盂唇的一部分。
- MR关节造影是诊断髋臼盂唇撕裂最敏感的成像方式;然而,常规MR和MR关节造影的特异性相似,都很高。
- 盂唇撕裂在概念上可以分为两种类型:一种是在软骨-盂唇连接处撕裂,此时盂唇从软骨上剥离;另一种是盂唇实质撕裂。
- 盂唇撕裂的继发性表现包括盂唇旁囊肿形成、软骨损伤和软骨下水肿,所有这些改变在X线影像上都可能表现为正常。此外,典型的骨关节炎改变,如骨质增生和软骨下囊肿在MRI上可能较X线影像上表现更明显。
- 有几种正常变异可能与盂唇撕裂的影像学表现相似。其中鉴别最具困难的是盂唇下沟,这是盂唇与髋臼的不完全附着。与撕裂相比,注射的造影剂不会延伸至整个盂唇,也不会出现继发退行性改变。

(翻译　姚骊　吕霞飞)

SHOULDER

肩关节

BONY ANATOMY OF THE SHOULDER

肩关节骨性解剖

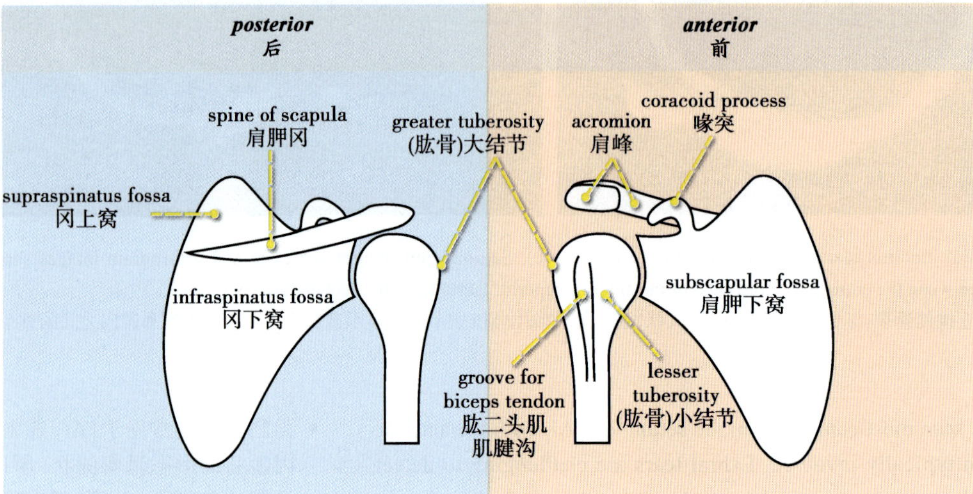

ACROMIOCLAVICULAR JOINT

肩锁关节

Acromioclavicular (AC) joint separation

肩锁关节(AC)分离

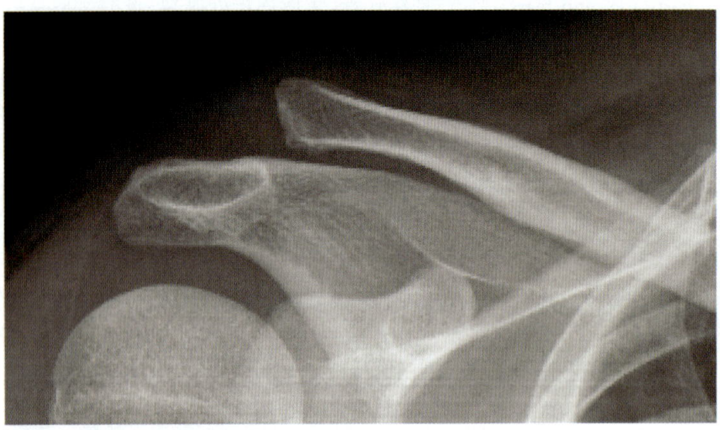

Grade Ⅲ acromioclavicular injury:
Frontal radiograph of the right shoulder shows superior elevation of the clavicle at the AC joint, in keeping with acromioclavicular and coracoclavicular ligament tears.
Ⅲ级肩锁关节损伤：右肩正位X线影像显示锁骨在AC关节处上抬，符合肩锁和喙锁韧带撕裂表现。

- Injuries to the acromioclavicular (AC) joint typically occur in young athletic adults, most commonly from a downward blow to the lateral shoulder. AC joint injuries range from an AC ligament sprain (grade Ⅰ) to complete disruption of the AC joint capsule and associated coracoclavicular (CC) ligaments (grades Ⅲ – Ⅵ).
- The normal AC joint space should be <5 mm and the normal CC distance is <11–13 mm, with a wide range of normal variation. An asymmetry of >50% side-to-side is abnormal. Passive traction, with the patient holding a weight, may be necessary to unmask an injury.
- Displacement of the acromion and clavicle determines AC ligament integrity, while the coracoclavicular interspace is assessed to evaluate the CC ligaments.
- Grade Ⅰ: AC ligament sprain. Radiographs are normal.

- 肩锁关节(AC)损伤常见于年轻运动员，最常的原因是肩外侧倒地时受到的冲击。AC的损伤可从AC韧带拉伤(Ⅰ级)到肩锁关节囊和相关的喙锁(CC)韧带完全撕裂(Ⅲ~Ⅳ级)。
- 正常的AC关节间隙应<5mm，正常CC之间的距离<11~13mm，但正常变异范围较大。两侧间隙不对称超过50%为异常。有必要让患者提起重物进行被动牵拉，这样可以发现隐性损伤。
- 肩胛骨及锁骨的错位决定AC的完整性，而喙锁间隙可用于评估CC韧带。
- Ⅰ级：肩锁韧带扭伤，平片无异常。

- Grade Ⅱ: Disruption of the AC ligament with intact CC ligaments.
- Grade Ⅲ: AC joint and CC ligamentous disruption. CC interspace is widened 25–100% relative to the contralateral side.
- Grade Ⅳ: Distal clavicle displaced posteriorly into trapezius (seen on CT or axillary view).
- Grade Ⅴ: Severe grade Ⅲ injury, with >100% displacement relative to the other side.
- Grade Ⅵ: Inferior dislocation of the distal clavicle.

- Ⅱ级：肩锁韧带断裂，喙锁韧带完整。
- Ⅲ级：肩锁关节及喙锁韧带断裂，喙锁关节间隙较对侧增宽25%~100%。
- Ⅳ级：锁骨远端向后移位进入斜方肌(见于CT或腋位图像)。
- Ⅴ级：严重的Ⅲ级损伤，较对侧移位超过100%。
- Ⅵ级：锁骨远端向下脱位。

SHOULDER BURSAE/RECESSES

- The subacromial and subdeltoid bursae normally communicate with each other. This combined subacromial/subdeltoid bursa is not normally in communication with the glenohumeral joint.
- Fluid injected into the glenohumeral joint that extends into the subacromial/subdeltoid bursa is seen with a complete rotator cuff tear. A gap in the rotator cuff will almost always be evident.
- The subcoracoid bursa is located between the subscapularis muscle and the coracoid process, whereas the subscapular bursa is located between the anterior surface of the scapula and the subscapularis muscle.
- The axillary pouch has a U-shaped appearance banded by the inferior glenohumeral ligament.

肩关节滑囊/隐窝

- 肩峰下与三角肌下滑囊在正常情况下相通。但正常的肩峰下与三角肌下滑囊复合体与盂肱关节不相通。
- 注射到盂肱关节腔的液体进入肩峰下/三角肌下滑囊见于完全性肩袖撕裂。这种情况下几乎总能看到肩袖内有裂隙。
- 喙突下滑囊位于肩胛下肌和喙突之间，而肩胛下滑囊位于肩胛骨前方的表面和肩胛下肌之间。
- 腋囊呈U形，由盂肱下韧带环绕。

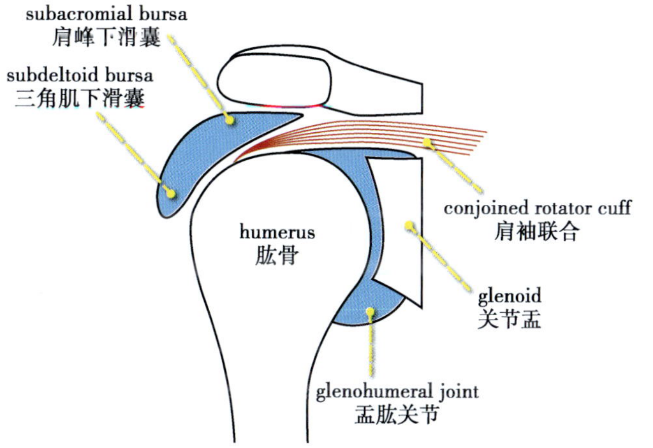

CORACOACROMIAL ARCH AND IMPINGEMENT SYNDROME

喙肩弓及肩关节卡磨(撞击)综合征

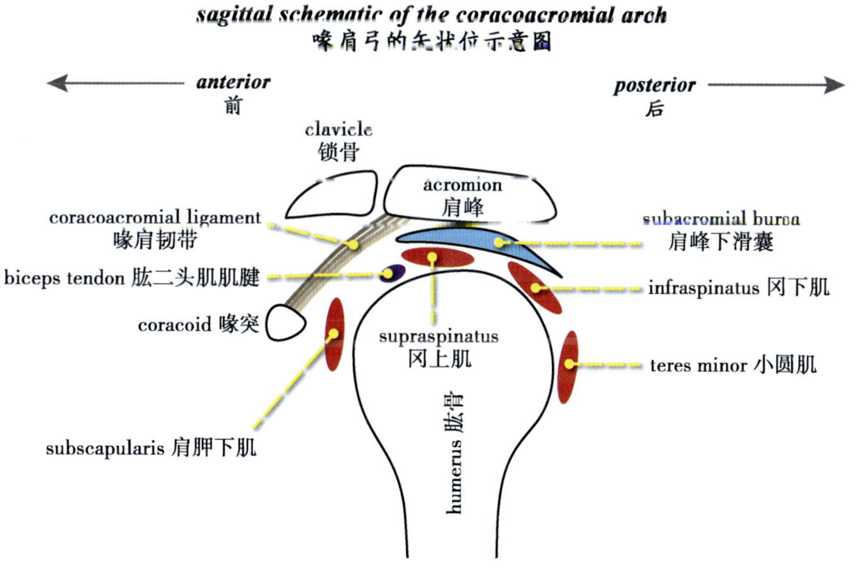

- Impingement syndrome is a clinical diagnosis that can have a variety of causes and MRI findings. Shoulder impingement was originally described as chronic compression/irritation of the structures that pass through the coracoacromial arch, including the supraspinatus tendon, biceps tendon, and subacromial bursa.
- Rotator cuff tears are often associated with chronic impingement, although there is controversy whether the cuff tears are a result of chronic mechanical impingement or whether degeneration leads to cuff tears, resulting in impingement syndrome.
- **Extrinsic impingement** is caused by structural abnormalities external to the joint and is divided into primary and subcoracoid impingement.

  Primary external impingement is common and is due to a variation in the anatomy of the coracoacromial arch (e.g., subacromial enthesophyte, hooked acromion, AC joint osteophytes, os acromiale, or thickened coracoacromial ligament). Primary external impingement is typically seen in young athletes involved with throwing or repetitive overhead movement. Chronic primary external impingement may cause the supraspinatus tendon and/or the proximal aspect of the long head of the biceps tendon to become degenerated, partially torn, or even completely torn. The subacromial bursa, immediately inferior to the acromion, may become inflamed, leading to subacromial/subdeltoid bursitis.

  Subcoracoid impingement is less common and occurs when the coracohumeral distance narrows.
- **Intrinsic impingement** is related to glenohumeral instability and is caused by abnormalities of the rotator cuff and joint capsule, without abnormality of the coracoacromial arch.

- 肩关节卡磨综合征是一个临床诊断，可有多种病因和MRI表现。肩关节卡磨最初用于描述挤压/刺激通过喙肩弓的结构，包括冈上肌肌腱、肱二头肌肌腱和肩峰下滑囊。
- 肩袖撕裂常伴有慢性卡磨，然而是慢性机械性卡磨导致肩袖损伤还是变性导致肩袖撕裂进而导致卡磨综合征仍有争议。
- **外部卡磨**由关节外部结构异常引起，可分为原发性卡磨和喙突下卡磨。

  原发性外部卡磨常见，由喙肩弓的解剖变异引起(如肩峰下肌腱末端骨赘、钩状肩峰、肩锁关节骨赘、肩峰小骨、喙肩韧带增厚)。原发性外部卡磨常见于投掷和反复上举动作的年轻运动员。慢性原发性外部卡磨可导致冈上肌肌腱和/或肱二头肌长头肌腱近端发生变性、部分撕裂，甚至完全撕裂。肩峰正下方的肩峰下滑囊可产生炎症，导致肩峰下/三角肌下滑囊炎。

  喙突下卡磨不常见，发生于喙肱间隙狭窄时。
- **内部卡磨**与盂肱的不稳定性有关，由肩袖病变和关节囊异常所致，而喙肩弓没有异常。

Acromial shape and orientation

肩峰形状与方向

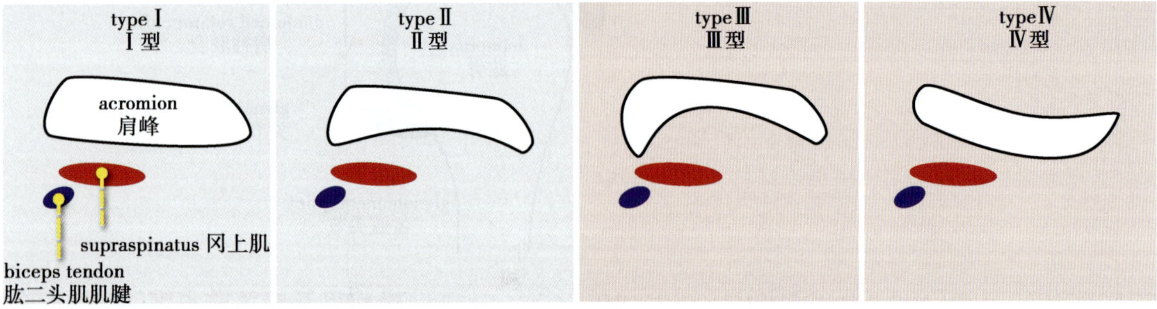

- The impact of acromial shape on impingement syndrome is controversial. An acromion with a hooked undersurface (type Ⅲ) or convex undersurface (type Ⅳ) may contribute to impingement (primary external type) and lead to subsequent rotator cuff tears.
- Friction of the acromion against the immediately underlying supraspinatus and biceps tendons may predispose to injury from impingement.

Os acromiale

- An os acromiale is a persistent accessory ossification center of the acromion seen in up to 15% of patients. It is best evaluated on the axial images.
- Although the presence of an os acromiale may be an asymptomatic normal variant, the presence of marrow edema suggests that the os may be a cause of pain.
- Treatment is resection or fusion.

- 肩峰的形状对卡磨综合征的影响是有争议的。肩峰表面下方呈钩状(Ⅲ型)或呈凸状(Ⅳ型)可加重卡磨(原发性外部型)，导致随后的肩袖撕裂。
- 肩峰与其正下方的冈上肌和二头肌肌腱的摩擦容易发生卡磨导致损伤。

肩峰小骨

- 肩峰小骨是肩峰二次骨化中心持续存在形成的副骨，可见于高达15%的患者。在轴位图像评价最佳。
- 肩峰小骨可以是无症状的正常变异，但如有骨髓水肿则提示肩峰小骨可能是疼痛的原因。
- 治疗方式为手术切除或融合术。

ROTATOR CUFF

肩袖

Anatomy of the rotator cuff

肩袖的解剖

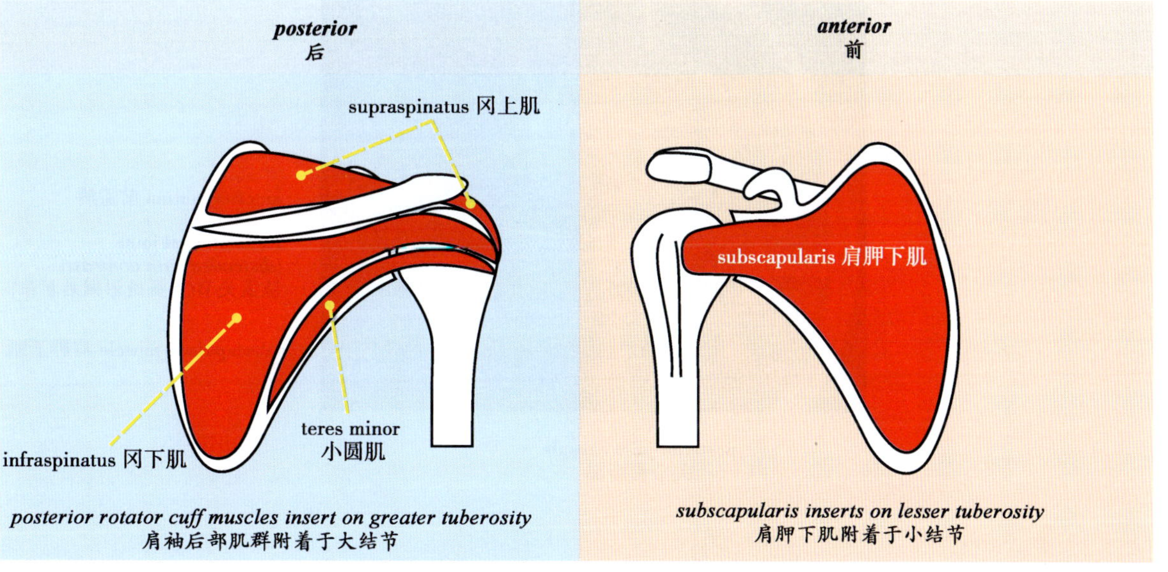

- The rotator cuff is an active stabilizer of the glenohumeral joint and is formed by the 4 rotator cuff muscles (supraspinatus, infraspinatus, teres minor, and subscapularis) and their tendons.
- The supraspinatus, infraspinatus, and teres minor are located posterior to the body of the scapula and insert on the greater tuberosity. The subscapularis is anterior to the scapula and inserts on the lesser tuberosity.

- 肩袖是盂肱关节主要的稳定结构，由4条肩袖肌(冈上肌、冈下肌、小圆肌和肩胛下肌)及其肌腱构成。
- 冈上肌、冈下肌和小圆肌位于肩胛骨体的后面并附着于大结节。肩胛下肌位于肩胛骨前面，附着于小结节。

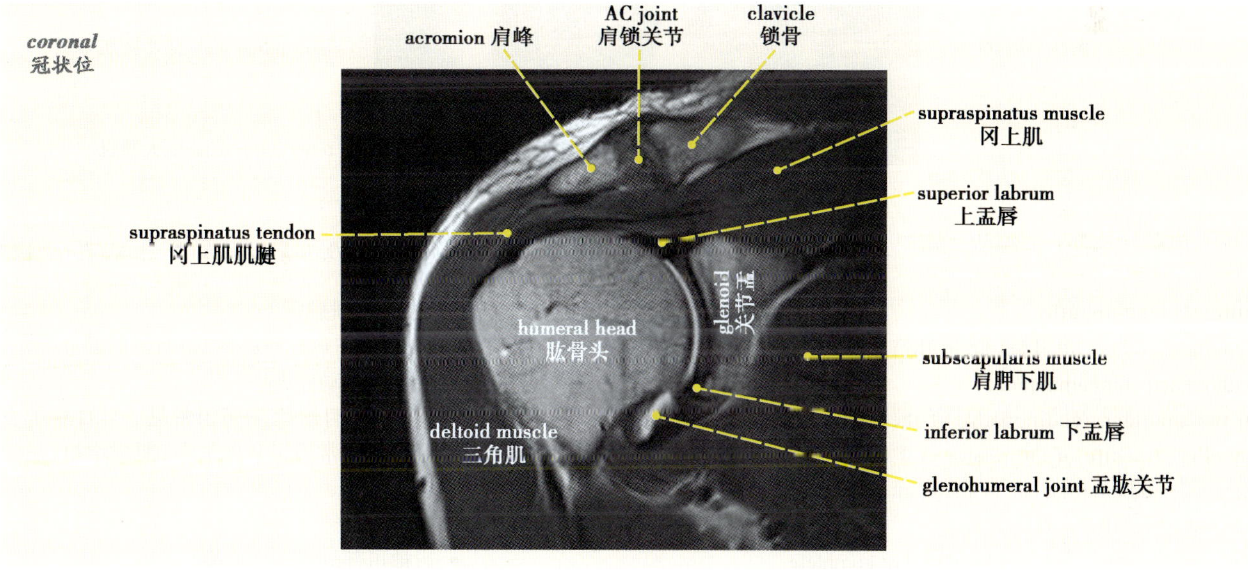

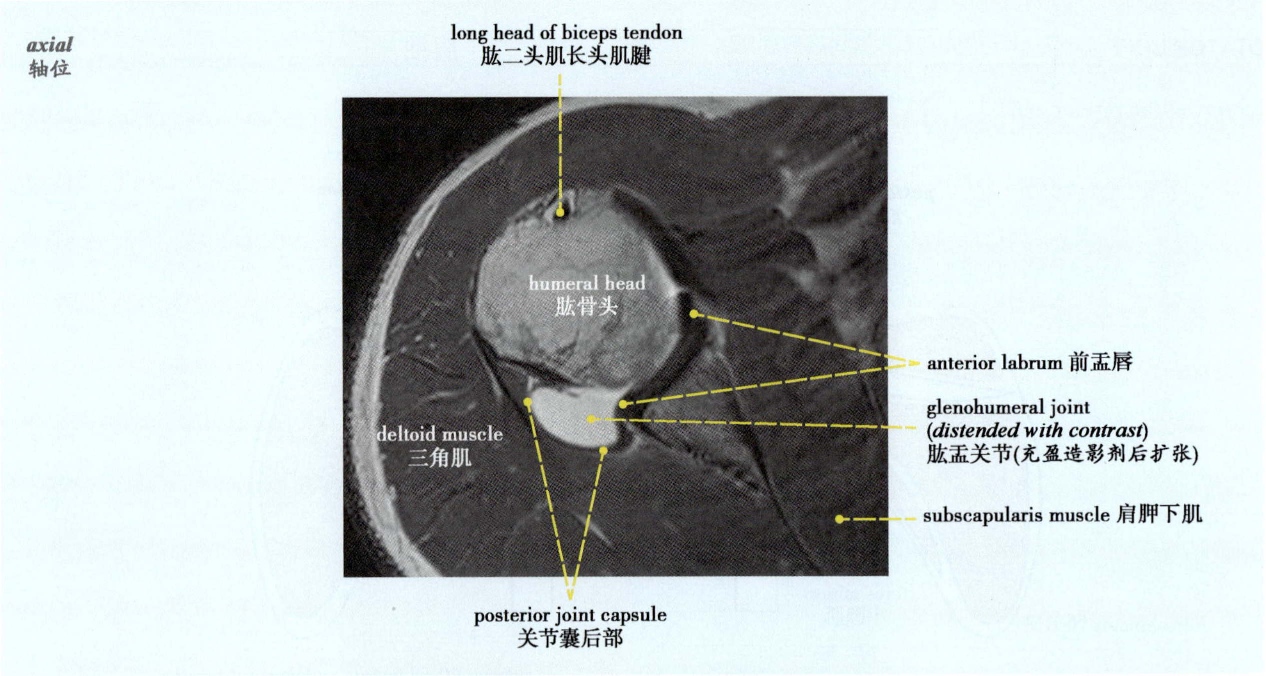

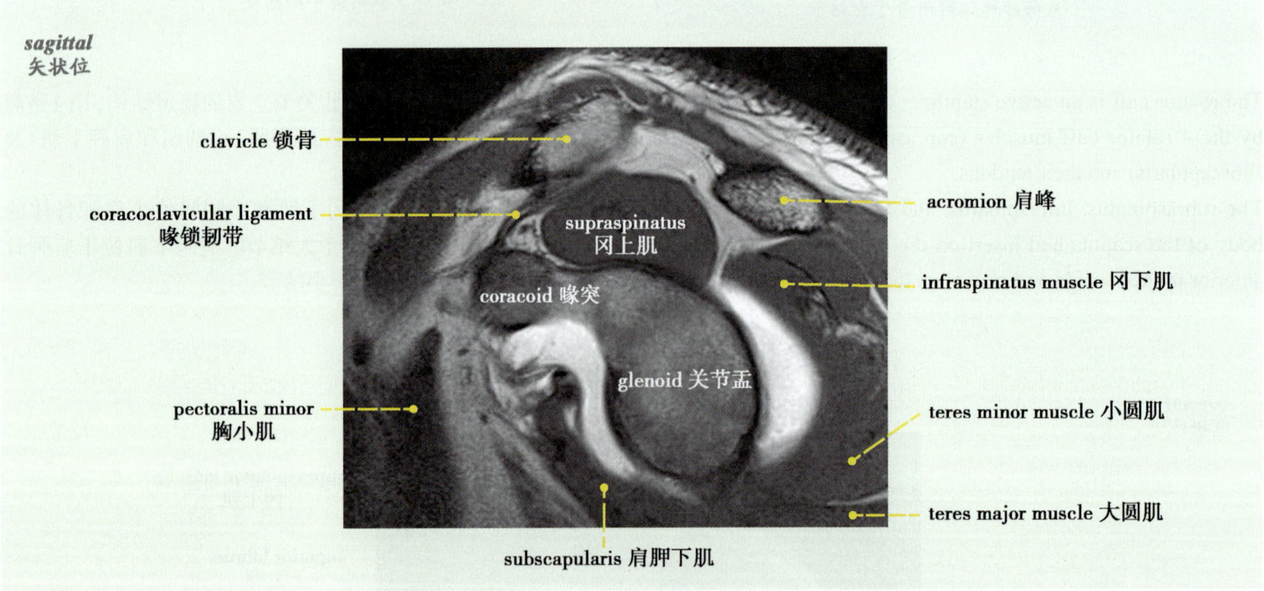

Images courtesy Kirstin Small, MD, Brigham and Women's Hospital.

Tendinosis/tendinopathy

- Tendinosis (also called tendinopathy) is mucoid degeneration of the tendon, without active inflammation.
- In the shoulder, tendinopathy of the rotator cuff is common. The normal lamellar structure of the rotator cuff tendon is lost, and the tendon appears expansile and intermediate in signal intensity.

Overview of rotator cuff tears

- Tears of the rotator cuff can be partial or complete.
- Complete rotator cuff tears allow communication between the subacromial/subdeltoid bursa and the glenohumeral joint.
- The *footprint* is the attachment of the tendons at the greater tuberosity. The critical zone is a potentially undervascularized portion of the distal supraspinatus tendon approximately 1 cm proximal to the insertion on the footprint. Relatively decreased vascular supply may predispose to rupture in this location.

肌腱变性/肌腱病

- 肌腱变性(也称肌腱病)是肌腱的黏液样变性，不伴有活动性炎症。
- 在肩部，肩袖肌腱病很常见。MRI显示肩袖肌腱的正常板层结构消失，肌腱增粗，呈中等信号强度。

肩袖撕裂概述

- 肩袖可部分或完全撕裂。
- 完全撕裂可造成肩峰下/三角肌下滑囊与盂肱关节相通。
- *足印*是肌腱附着在肱骨大结节的位置。危险区是指位于冈上肌肌腱远端的潜在血供不足区，距足印止点约1cm。由于该区域血供相对减少而使得该处肌腱容易发生断裂。

Partial-thickness rotator cuff tear

肩袖部分撕裂

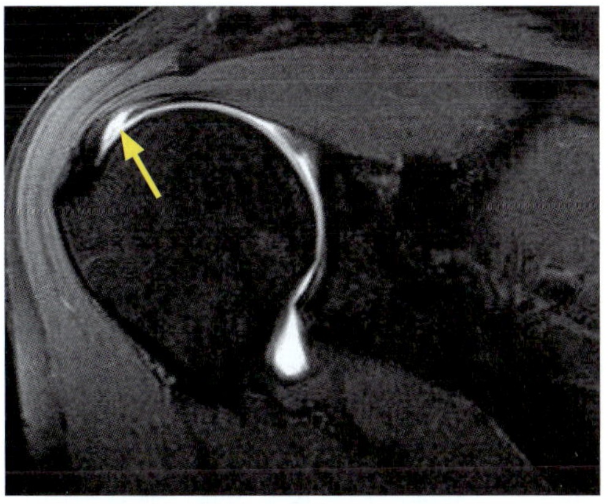

Partial articular surface supraspinatus tear:
Coronal T1-weighted MR arthrogram with fat suppression demonstrates discontinuity of the articular surface of the distal fibers of the supraspinatus tendon (arrow).
Case courtesy Kirstin M. Small, MD, Brigham and Women's Hospital.
冈上肌肌腱部分关节面撕裂：冠状位T_1加权脂肪抑制MR关节造影显示冈上肌肌腱远段纤维关节面不连续(箭)。

- The most commonly injured rotator cuff muscle is the supraspinatus, followed by the infraspinatus. The teres minor is the least commonly injured rotator cuff muscle.
- A partial-thickness tear features abnormal signal in a portion of the muscle or tendon but not extending through its entire thickness. MR arthrography will *not* show communication between the injected glenohumeral joint and the subacromial/subdeltoid bursa.

  Partial-thickness tears can be challenging to diagnose without MR arthrography. Reparative granulation tissue can obscure the abnormal signal that would otherwise indicate a tear.
- Partial tears can be divided into bursal-surface, articular-surface, or intrasubstance tears. Articular-surface tears are by far the most common type of partial tear.
- A *rim rent* tear is the most common type of partial tear. Also called the PASTA lesion (partial thickness articular supraspinatus tendon avulsion), the rim rent tear is an avulsion-type partial tear of the articular surface of the supraspinatus as it inserts on the greater tuberosity.

  Less commonly, an analogous lesion can be seen in the infraspinatus.
- The PAINT (partial articular tear with intratendinous extension) lesion is a partial rotator cuff tear at the articular surface that also extends into the tendon.

- 最易损伤的肩袖肌是冈上肌，其次是冈下肌。小圆肌是最少伤及的肩袖肌。
- 部分撕裂的特征是部分肌肉或肌腱异常信号，但不累及全层。MR关节造影表现为注入盂肱关节的造影剂不与肩胛下/三角肌下滑囊相通。

  部分肩袖撕裂在没有MR关节造影的情况下很难进行诊断。修复性肉芽组织可能掩盖提示撕裂的异常信号。
- 肩袖部分撕裂可分为滑囊面撕裂、关节面撕裂或肌腱内撕裂。关节面撕裂是最多见的部分撕裂。
- 边缘裂隙样撕裂是肩袖部分撕裂最常见的类型，也称PASTA病变(冈上肌腱关节面部分撕脱)，边缘裂隙样撕裂是指冈上肌腱附着肱骨大结节处的关节面撕裂。

  类似的撕裂也可见于冈下肌，但不常见。
- PAINT病变(部分关节面撕裂延伸至肌腱内)是指关节面的肩袖部分撕裂同时延伸入肌腱。

Full-thickness rotator cuff tear

肩袖全层撕裂

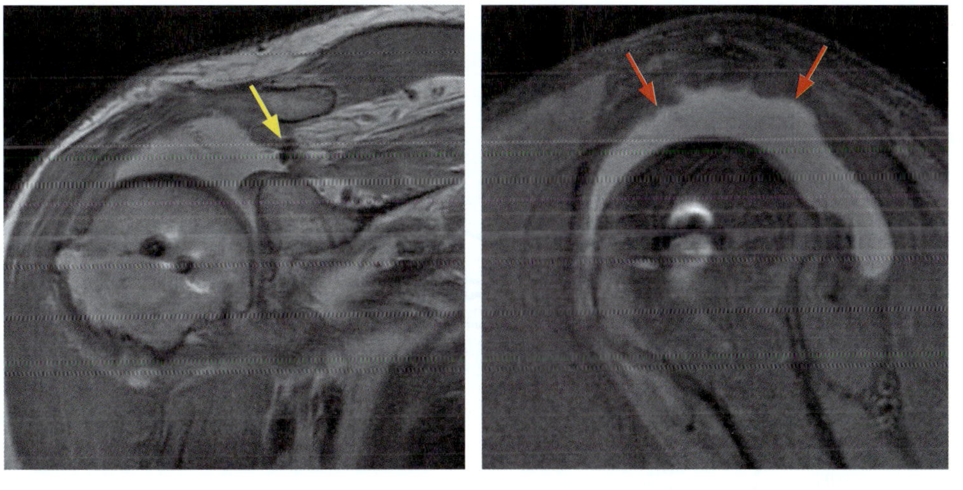

Full-thickness rotator cuff tear: Coronal proton-density (left image) and sagittal fat-saturated proton-density (right image) conventional MRI demonstrates complete discontinuity of the supraspinatus tendon with the tendon retracted proximally (yellow arrow). There is a large effusion, demonstrating continuity of the glenohumeral joint and the subacromial/subdeltoid bursa (red arrows). Susceptibility artifact is present in the humeral head, consistent with prior rotator cuff repair.
Case courtesy Kirstin M. Small, MD, Brigham and Women's Hospital.
肩袖全层撕裂：冠状位PD(左图)和矢状位脂肪抑制PD(右图)平扫MRI显示冈上肌腱完全断裂并向近端回缩(黄箭)。有大量积液，并显示盂肱关节与肩胛下/三角肌下滑囊相通(红箭)。肱骨头出现磁敏感伪影，符合先前肩袖修复手术。

- A full-thickness rotator cuff tear is seen on MR arthrography when fluid injected into the glenohumeral joint extends into the subacromial/subdeltoid bursa. In the absence of injected gadolinium, a full-thickness tear can be diagnosed if abnormal signal extends through the fibers of the tendon. A gap in the tendon is almost always present.
- Similar to partial tears, the supraspinatus is most commonly torn.
- Approximately 30–40% of supraspinatus tears are also associated with a tear of the infraspinatus.

  The infraspinatus is rarely torn in isolation; however isolated infraspinatus tears can be seen in the setting of posterior instability. The posterior capsule and labrum should be carefully evaluated in such cases.
- A chronic full-thickness rotator cuff tear due to rheumatoid arthritis has a classic imaging appearance. The humeral head migrates superiorly and may articulate with the acromion in severe cases.
- Full-thickness rotator cuff tears are classified by the length of the affected tendon/muscle, ranging from small (<1 cm) to massive (>5 cm).

Rotator cuff atrophy

- Atrophy of the rotator cuff is most commonly due to chronic rotator cuff tear. Fatty degeneration may occur within 4 weeks of injury and is usually irreversible. The extent of muscle degeneration correlates with outcome following surgical repair. The degree of fatty infiltration of the rotator cuff muscles should be routinely assessed in the sagittal plane. The degree of fatty replacement can be graded with the **Goutallier classification**:

Grade 0: Normal muscle, no fat.
Grade 1: Muscle contains a few fatty streaks.
Grade 2: Fatty infiltration, more muscle than fat.
Grade 3: Fatty infiltration, equal muscle and fat.
Grade 4: Fatty infiltration, more fat than muscle.

- Less commonly, rotator cuff atrophy may be secondary to denervation atrophy, subsequently discussed. Denervation atrophy is usually associated with a paralabral cyst.

SHOULDER LIGAMENTS AND ROTATOR INTERVAL

Anatomy of the shoulder ligaments

- 在MR关节造影中，当注入盂肱关节的造影剂扩散到肩胛下/三角肌下滑囊时可以显示肩袖全层撕裂。在不使用含钆造影剂的情况下，如果异常信号贯穿肌腱纤维，就可以诊断全层撕裂。肌腱裂口几乎总是存在。
- 与部分撕裂相同，冈上肌最易受损。
- 约30%~40%的冈上肌撕裂同时发生冈下肌撕裂。

  冈下肌很少单独撕裂；但是，孤立性冈下肌撕裂可以在关节后方不稳的情况下出现。对于这些病例应注意观察后关节囊和后盂唇。
- 由类风湿关节炎造成的慢性肩袖全层撕裂具有典型的影像学表现。肱骨头向上移位，严重时可与肩峰形成假关节。
- 肩袖全层撕裂根据受累肌腱/肌肉的长度进行分级，其范围从小撕裂(<1cm)到巨大撕裂(>5cm)。

肩袖萎缩

- 肩袖萎缩最常见于慢性肩袖撕裂。脂肪变性可发生在损伤后4周之内，且通常是不可逆的。肌肉变性的程度与手术修复后的预后有关。肩袖肌肉脂肪浸润的程度应在矢状位上进行常规评估。脂肪替代的程度可按**Goutallier分级**：

0级：正常肌肉，无脂肪浸润。
1级：肌肉含有一些条状脂肪影。
2级：脂肪浸润，肌肉多于脂肪。
3级：脂肪浸润，肌肉与脂肪相当。
4级：脂肪浸润，脂肪多于肌肉。

- 少数情况下，肩袖萎缩可继发于去神经性萎缩，将在后文讨论。去神经萎缩常伴盂唇旁囊肿。

肩部韧带与肩袖间隙

肩部韧带的解剖

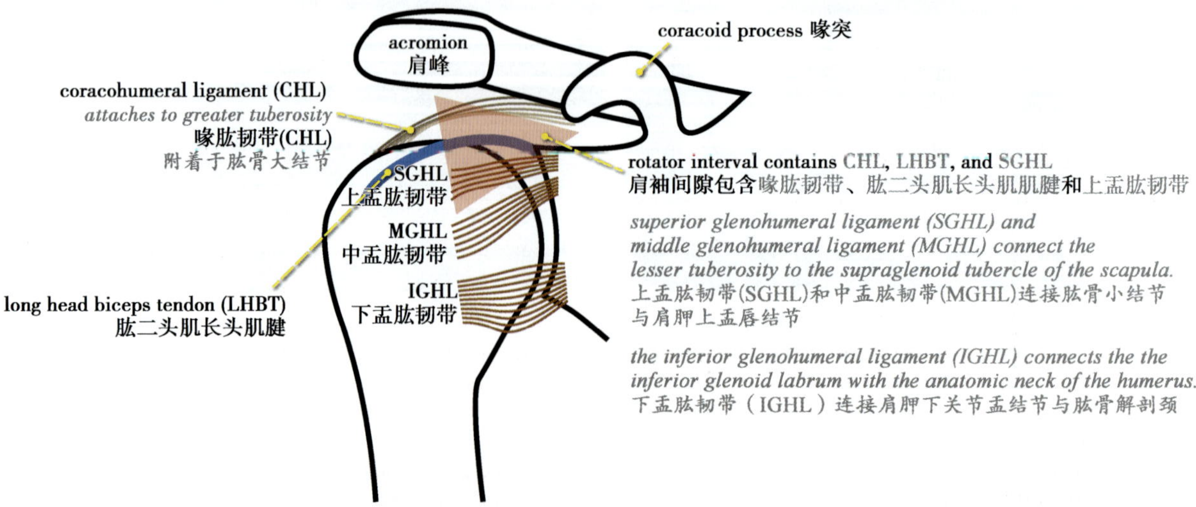

- The *rotator interval* is a triangular region that allows rotational motion around the coracoid process. It is located between the supraspinatus and subscapularis tendons. The rotator interval contains the coracohumeral ligament (CHL), the long head of the biceps tendon (LHBT), and the superior glenohumeral ligament (SGHL).
- The CHL connects the lateral aspect of the coracoid process to the greater tubercle of the humerus, where the CHL blends with the supraspinatus tendon. The CHL helps to stabilize the intra-articular biceps tendon together with the superior glenohumeral ligament as the *biceps pulley*. The CHL is located external to the joint capsule.
- The glenohumeral ligaments (SGHL, MGHL, and IGHL) are derived from the labrum and form a portion of the joint capsule.
- The superior glenohumeral ligament (SGHL) connects the lesser tuberosity to the supraglenoid tubercle of the scapula.
- The middle glenohumeral ligament (MGHL) also connects the lesser tuberosity to the supraglenoid tubercle of the scapula. The MGHL is congenitally absent in up to 1/3 of patients. Tears of the MGHL are associated with SLAP lesions.
- The inferior glenohumeral ligament (IGHL) connects the anatomic neck of the humerus to the inferior glenoid labrum. The IGHL is by far the most important component of the capsulolabral complex for maintaining stability in abduction and external rotation. The IGHL contains three components (the anterior band, the axillary pouch, and the posterior band), all of which are well-seen on sagittal MR:

  The **anterior band** of the IGHL provides anterior stability. There are several lesions of the anterior band of the IGHL that are associated with anterior instability, discussed on the following page.

  The IGHL forms the **axillary pouch** of the glenohumeral joint capsule.

  The **posterior band** contributes to posterior stability. The IGHL is the only glenohumeral ligament to have a posterior component.
- The long head biceps tendon (LHBT) attaches to the anterosuperior glenoid rim along with the SGHL and MGHL.

Adhesive capsulitis

- 肩袖间隙是一个三角形区域，使肩关节围绕喙突做旋转运动。它位于冈上肌与肩胛下肌肌腱之间。肩袖间隙包含喙肱韧带(CHL)、肱二头肌长头肌腱(LHBT)和上盂肱韧带(SGHL)。
- CHL连接喙突的外侧缘与肱骨大结节，并在肱骨大结节处与冈上肌肌腱融合。CHL在上盂肱韧带的参与之下帮助稳定关节内的肱二头肌肌腱，起到肱二头肌滑车的作用。CHL位于关节囊的外侧。
- 盂肱韧带(SGHL、MGHL和IGHL)起自关节盂唇，形成关节囊的一部分。
- 上盂肱韧带(SGHL)连接肱骨小结节和肩胛骨的盂上结节。
- 中盂肱韧带(MGHL)同样也连接肱骨小结节和肩胛骨的盂上结节。先天性MGHL缺失见于多达1/3的患者。MGHL的撕裂伴有上盂唇前后撕裂(superior labrum anterior posterior tear，SLAP)性病变。
- 下盂肱韧带(IGHL)连接肱骨解剖颈和下关节盂。下盂肱韧带是盂唇-关节囊复合体中最为重要的组成部分，维持肩关节外展、外旋的稳定。下盂肱韧带包含三部分(前束、腋窝陷凹和后束)，三者均能在矢状位MR上清晰显示：

  下盂肱韧带**前束**维持肩关节前部的稳定性。有多种IGHL前束的病变与肩关节前部不稳定有关，后文探讨。

  IGHL构成盂肱关节囊的**腋窝陷凹**。

  后束维持肩关节后部的稳定性。IGHL是唯一含有后部成分的盂肱韧带。
- 肱二头肌长头肌腱(LHBT)与SGHL和MGHL一起附着于关节盂前上缘。

粘连性关节囊炎

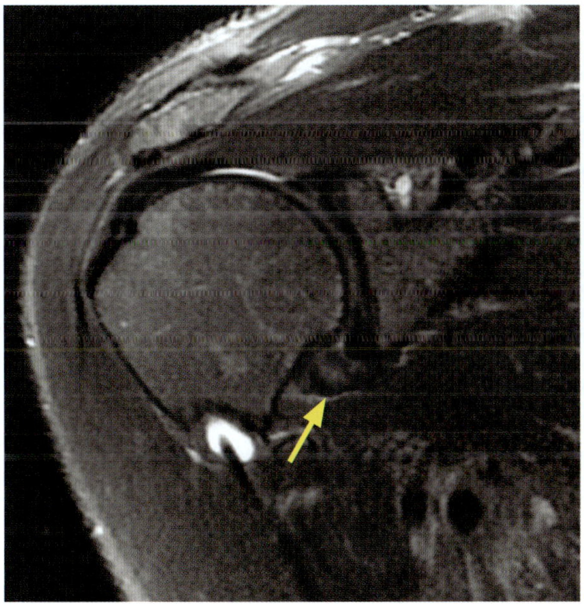

Coronal PD-weighted MRI with fat suppression
冠状位PD加权脂肪抑制MRI

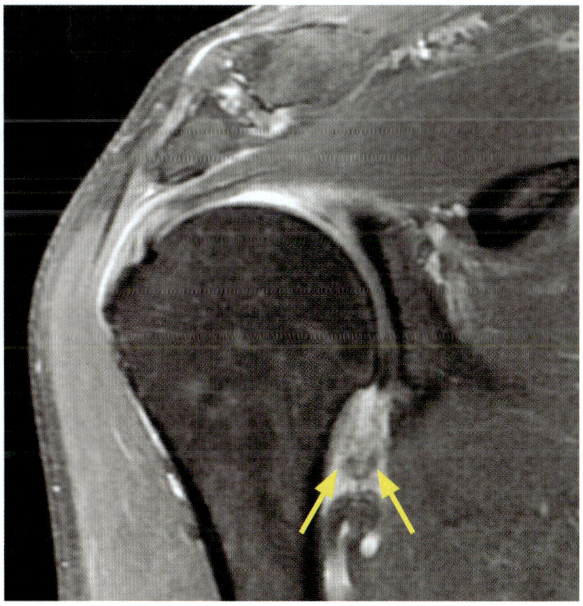

Coronal post-contrast T1-weighted MRI with fat supp.
冠状位增强T_1加权脂肪抑制MRI

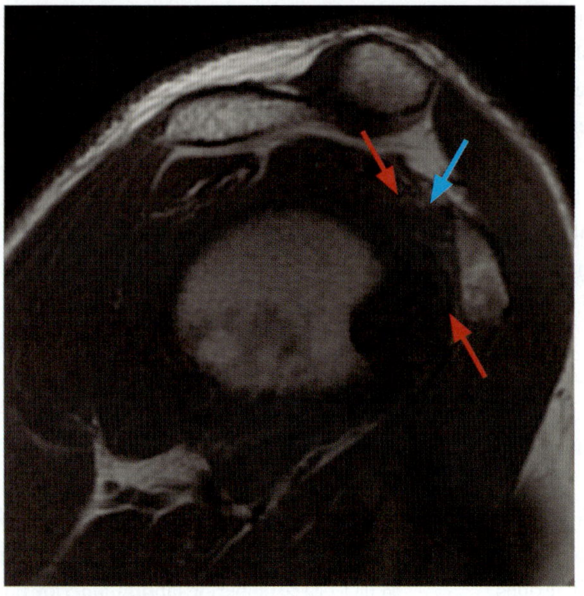

Sagittal T1-weighted MRI
矢状位T_1加权MRI

Adhesive capsulitis:
There is thickening and enhancement of the inferior glenohumeral ligament (yellow arrows), and effacement of fat in the rotator interval (red arrows).
Coracohumeral ligament (blue arrow) is not well seen due to fat effacing the rotator interval, but this ligament is also typically thickened in adhesive capsulitis.

粘连性关节囊炎：
下盂肱韧带增厚和信号增强(黄箭)，肩袖间隙脂肪消失(红箭)。喙肱韧带(蓝箭)因肩袖脂肪间隙模糊而显示不清，但在粘连性关节囊炎中该韧带通常会增厚。

- Adhesive capsulitis, clinically known as *frozen shoulder*, is thickening and contraction of the glenohumeral joint capsule due to inflammation of the joint capsule and synovium. This results in pain and loss of range of motion.
- Adhesive capsulitis is primarily a clinical diagnosis, but MRI findings include thickening, edema, and enhancement of the joint capsule (inferior glenohumeral ligament >4 mm), effacement of fat in the rotator interval, and thickening of the coracohumeral ligament.
- Radiographs are often normal but are helpful to exclude other causes of pain, such as glenohumeral osteoarthritis or calcific tendinopathy.

- 粘连性关节囊炎，临床上也称*冻肩*，是由关节囊与滑囊的炎症造成盂肱关节囊的增厚与挛缩。这将导致疼痛并丧失关节活动。
- 粘连性关节囊炎是一个临床诊断，MRI表现包括关节囊增厚、水肿和强化(下盂肱韧带>4mm)，肩袖间隙脂肪消失和喙肱韧带增厚。
- X线影像常正常，但有助于排除其他疼痛的原因，如盂肱骨关节炎或钙化性肌腱病。

Biceps tendon

Anatomy of the biceps tendon

- The long head of the biceps tendon originates at the superior labrum and courses in the intertubercular groove. The biceps tendon sheath communicates with the glenohumeral joint. Fluid in the tendon sheath may be normal.
- The biceps pulley is a capsuloligamentous complex that stabilizes the biceps tendon in a sling within the bicipital groove. The biceps pulley is formed by the superior glenohumeral ligament, coracohumeral ligament, and the distal fibers of the subscapularis tendon.

Biceps tendon tear

- Approximately 33% of supraspinatus tendon tears are associated with biceps tendon injury (complete tear, partial tear, or degeneration).
- The biceps tendon is at risk for impingement due to its location partially underneath the supraspinatus tendon in the coracoacromial arch.
- In cases of an acute tear, the biceps muscle may retract distally. An empty intertubercular groove may signify a complete tear with retraction or a biceps tendon dislocation.

肱二头肌肌腱

肱二头肌肌腱解剖

- 肱二头肌长头肌腱起自上盂唇，穿行于结节间沟。肱二头肌的腱鞘与盂肱关节相通。腱鞘内有液体可以视为正常。
- 肱二头肌滑车是一个包含关节囊和韧带的复合体，其作用是将肱二头肌肌腱稳定在悬吊的肱二头肌沟内。肱二头肌滑车由上盂肱韧带、喙肱韧带和肩胛下肌肌腱远端纤维组成。

肱二头肌肌腱撕裂

- 大约有33%的冈上肌肌腱撕裂合并肱二头肌肌腱损伤(完全撕裂、部分撕裂或退变)。
- 肱二头肌肌腱有卡磨的风险，是由于它部分位于喙肩弓的冈上肌肌腱下方。
- 在急性撕裂的情况下，肱二头肌的肌肉可向远端回缩。空虚的结节间沟可能提示完全撕裂，伴肱二头肌肌腱回缩或脱位。

Biceps tendon dislocation

肱二头肌肌腱脱位

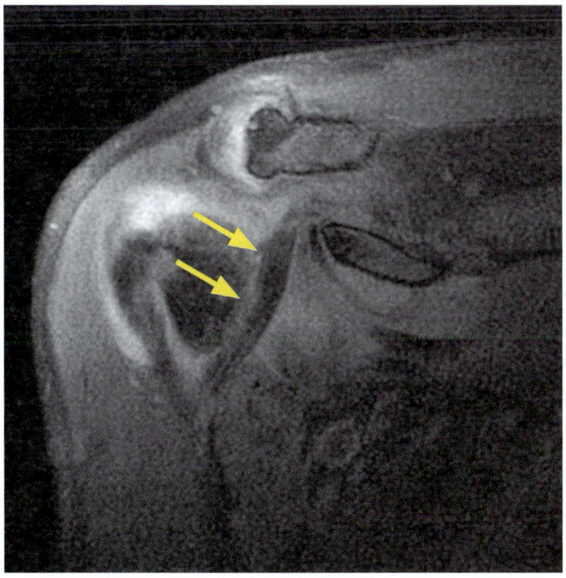

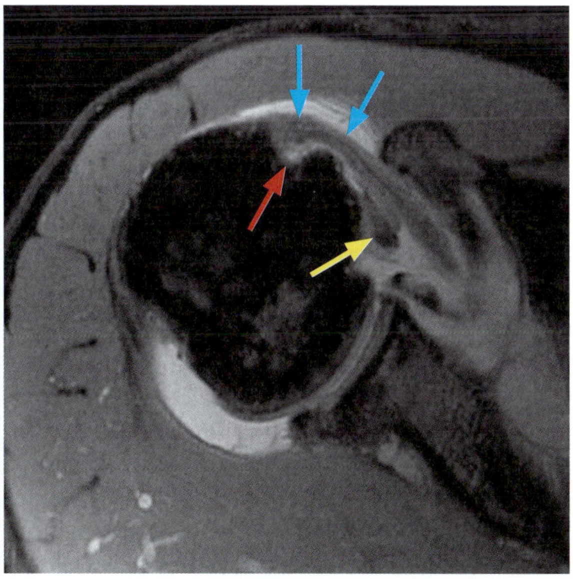

Biceps tendon dislocation: Coronal (left image) and axial T1-weighted MR arthrogram with fat suppression shows medial intra-articular dislocation of the biceps tendon (yellow arrows). The bicipital groove is empty, best seen on the axial image (red arrow). The blue arrows denote the subscapularis tendon, seen on the axial image.

Case courtesy Kirstin M. Small, MD, Brigham and Women's Hospital.

肱二头肌肌腱脱位：冠状位(左图)和轴位T_1加权脂肪抑制MR关节造影显示肱二头肌肌腱内侧关节内的脱位(黄箭)。结节间沟空虚，轴位图像显示最佳(红箭)。蓝箭为肩胛下肌肌腱，见于轴位图像。

- Biceps tendon subluxation and dislocation are associated with injury to the transverse ligament. The transverse humeral ligament attaches to the greater and lesser tuberosities and normally holds the biceps tendon in place.

- 肱二头肌肌腱半脱位和脱位与横韧带损伤有关。肱横韧带附着于大小结节，维持肱二头肌肌腱的正常位置。

Biceps tendon dislocation

肱二头肌肌腱脱位

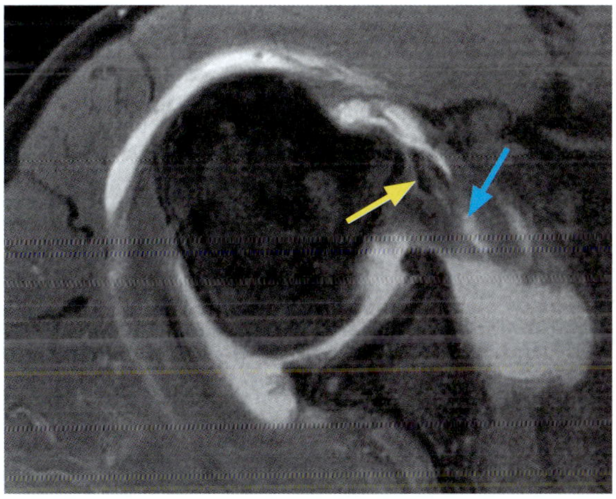

Biceps tendon dislocation:
Axial T1-weighted image with fat suppression from an MR arthrogram shows medial dislocation of the biceps tendon (yellow arrow) into the subscapularis. An interstitial tear of the subscapularis tendon is present (blue arrow).

Case courtesy Kirstin M. Small, MD, Brigham and Women's Hospital.

肱二头肌肌腱脱位：轴位T_1加权脂肪抑制MR关节造影示肱二头肌肌腱向内脱位(黄箭)进入肩胛下肌。肩胛下肌出现裂隙样撕裂(蓝箭)。

- Biceps tendon dislocation is often seen in conjunction with injury of both the transverse ligament and the biceps pulley.
- Medial dislocation of the biceps tendon is associated with tear of the subscapularis tendon (in contrast to biceps tears, which are more frequently associated with supraspinatus injury).
- Axial MRI best demonstrates biceps tendon dislocation. The bicipital groove is empty and the tendon can usually be seen medial to the bicipital groove.

- 肱二头肌肌腱脱位常见于肱横韧带和肱二头肌滑车的联合损伤。
- 肱二头肌肌腱内向脱位与肩胛下肌肌腱撕裂有关(与肱二头肌撕裂不同，后者更常伴冈上肌损伤)。
- 轴位MRI显示肱二头肌肌腱脱位最佳，表现为结节间沟空虚，通常可见肌腱位于结节间沟的内侧。

Instability: Overview and Anatomy

Overview of instability

- Shoulder instability is abnormal motion of the humeral head with respect to the glenoid during movement, producing pain, clicking, or the feeling of an unstable joint.
- Instability can manifest as dislocation, subluxation, or microinstability (repetitive motion).
- The stability of the glenohumeral joint is mostly provided by dynamic and static soft-tissue stabilizers, as there is minimal inherent osseous stability.
- The dynamic stabilizers of the joint include the rotator cuff and biceps tendons.
- The static stabilizer of the joint is the capsulo-labro-ligamentous complex, which is composed of the bony glenoid fossa, labrum, coracohumeral ligament, and superior, middle, and inferior glenohumeral ligaments.
- There are several labral, ligamentous, and osseous injuries associated with instability, but it is unclear if the structural abnormalities are secondary to instability or a cause of it.
- There are various classifications of instability incorporating clinical, etiological, and imaging findings.
- Instability can also be classified as traumatic or atraumatic.

  Traumatic instability is usually secondary to trauma, causes instability in one direction only, is associated with a Bankart lesion, and treated surgically. Traumatic instability is referred to as **TUBS** (traumatic, unidirectional, Bankart, surgical).

  Atraumatic instability can be divided into two types. The **AIOS** (acquired, instability, overstress, surgery) pattern is usually seen in athletes with repetitive movements causing microinstability. **AMBRI** (atraumatic, multidirectional, bilateral, rehabilitation, inferior capsule shift) lesions are due to congenital joint laxity.
- Radiologists usually classify instability based on the direction of joint subluxation (anterior, posterior, multidirectional, or superior). Similar to traumatic shoulder dislocations, anterior instability accounts for the vast majority (95%) of cases.

Anatomy of the glenoid labrum

- The glenoid labrum is a fibrocartilaginous ring-like structure that rests on the glenoid hyaline cartilage and surrounds the glenoid. The labrum increases the surface area and depth of the glenoid cavity. It also provides a suction effect, adhering the humeral head to the glenoid with motion.

肩关节不稳定：概述和解剖

肩关节不稳定概述

- 肩关节不稳定是指在运动过程中，肱骨头相对于关节盂出现异常运动，导致疼痛、弹响或关节不稳定感。
- 不稳定可表现为脱位、半脱位或轻微不稳定(重复运动)。
- 盂肱关节的稳定性主要靠动态和静态软组织进行维持，因盂肱关节固有的骨稳定性有限。
- 肩关节的动态稳定结构包括肩袖和肱二头肌肌腱。
- 肩关节的静态稳定结构是关节囊-唇-韧带复合体，由骨性关节窝、盂唇、喙肱韧带和上、中、下盂肱韧带组成。
- 不稳定的因素有多种，包括盂唇、韧带及骨性损伤，但尚不清楚这些结构异常是否为不稳定的次生因素还是其原因。
- 肩关节不稳定的分类方法有多种，包括临床、病因学及影像学表现。
- 不稳定也可分为创伤性和非创伤性。

  创伤性不稳定常继发于创伤，只引起一个方向的不稳定，与Bankart病变有关，需采用外科治疗。创伤性不稳定称**TUBS**(创伤的、单向的、Bankart损伤、外科手术)。

  非创伤性不稳定可分为两型，**AIOS**(获得性、不稳定性、过度应力性、外科手术)型常见于运动员反复运动所致的轻微不稳定。**AMBRI**(非创伤性、多向的、双向性、康复性、关节囊下移)损伤由先天性关节松弛所致。
- 放射科医师通常依据关节半脱位的方向(前、后、多向的或上方)对关节不稳进行分类。与创伤性肩关节脱位类似，前方关节不稳占大多数(95%)。

关节盂唇解剖

- 关节盂唇是一种环状的纤维软骨，附着在关节盂的透明软骨并包绕关节盂。盂唇增加了关节盂的表面积和关节腔的深度。它还提供一种吸入效应，使肱骨头在运动时黏附于关节窝。

sagittal schematic of the glenoid fossa, glenoid labrum, and glenohumeral ligaments
矢状位关节窝、关节盂及盂肱韧带示意图

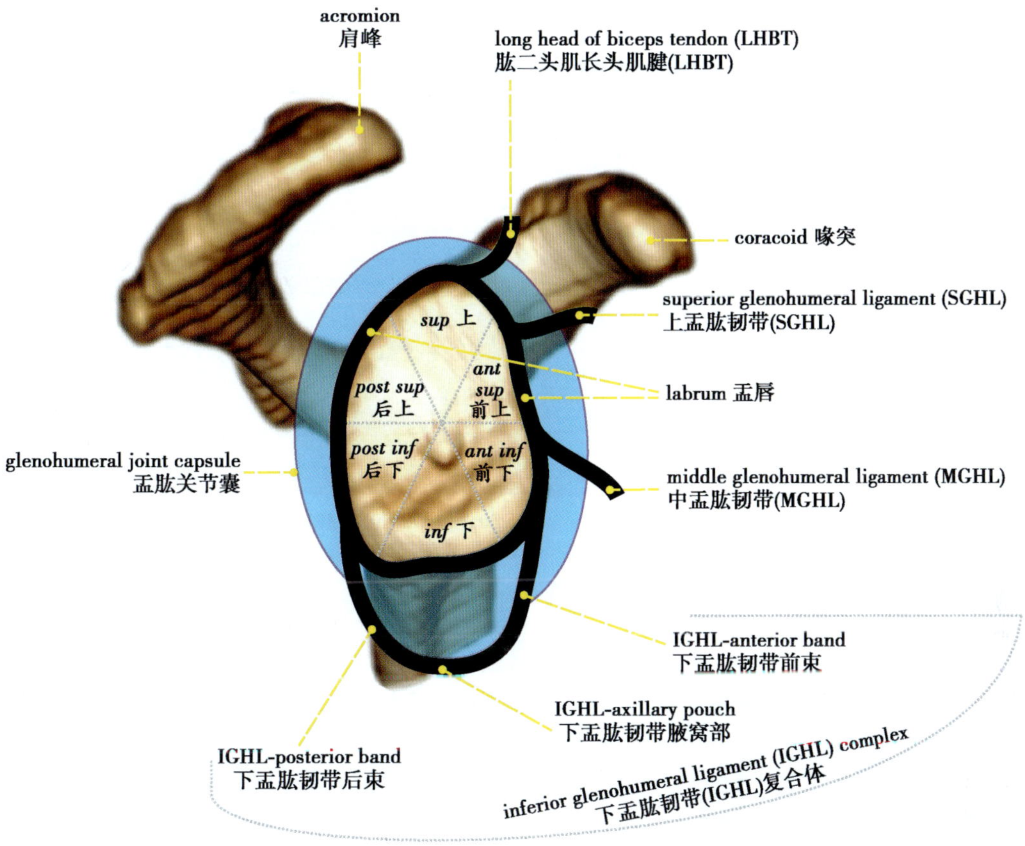

the location of labral injury can be described as the sextants outlined above, or can also be described on a clock face, with 12 o'clock superior and 3 o'clock anterior
关节盂损伤定位可以按上述的六分法进行，或在钟面上进行描述，12点钟为上方，3点钟为前方

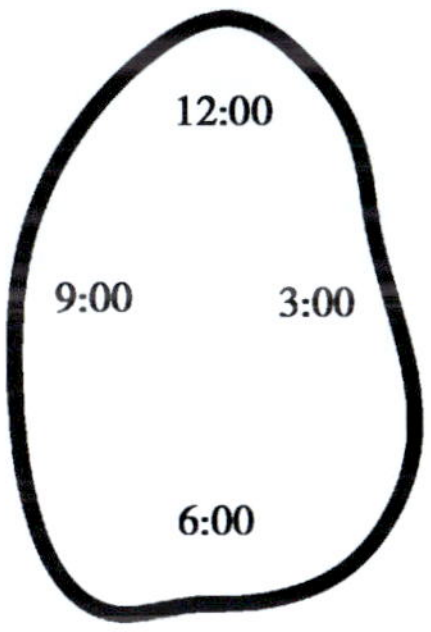

- Other important stabilizers of the joint attach directly to the labrum, including the glenohumeral ligaments, the biceps tendon, and the joint capsule.

Labral normal variants

- A **sublabral foramen** (seen in 10% of patients) is a normal variant where the anterosuperior segment is not attached to the bony glenoid.
- A **Buford complex** is an uncommon (seen in up to 6.5%) variant where a cord-like middle glenohumeral ligament is seen in combination with an absent anterosuperior labrum.
- The **sublabral recess** or foramen (seen in 11% of patients) is an unattached portion of the anterosuperior labrum at the 12 to 3 o'clock position.

- 其他直接附着于盂唇的重要的关节稳定结构包括盂肱韧带、肱二头肌肌腱，以及关节囊。

盂唇的正常变异

- **盂唇下孔**(见于10%的患者)是一种正常变异，其前上部不附着于骨性关节盂。
- **Buford复合体**是一种不常见的变异(见于6.5%的患者)，是指一个呈索条状的中盂肱韧带伴前上盂唇缺如。
- 盂唇下隐窝或孔(见于11%的患者)是前上盂唇在12点钟到3点钟位置的一个未附着的部分。

GLENOHUMERAL DISLOCATION

盂肱关节脱位

Anterior glenohumeral dislocation

盂肱关节前脱位

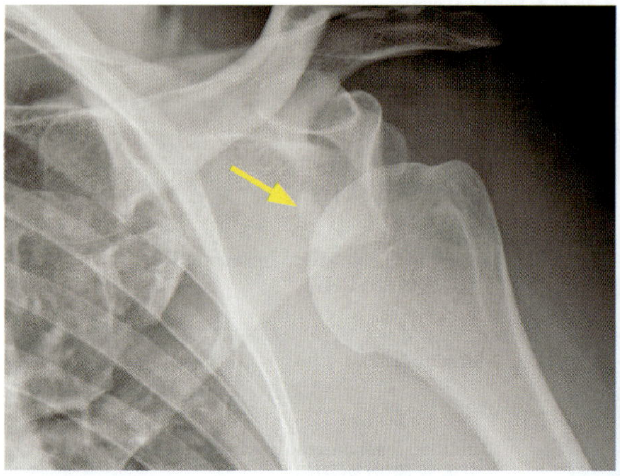

Frontal radiograph
正位X线影像

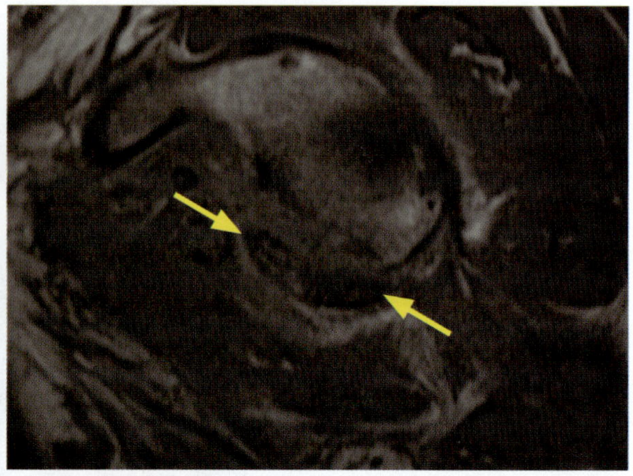

Sagittal T1-weighted MRI
矢状位T_1加权MRI

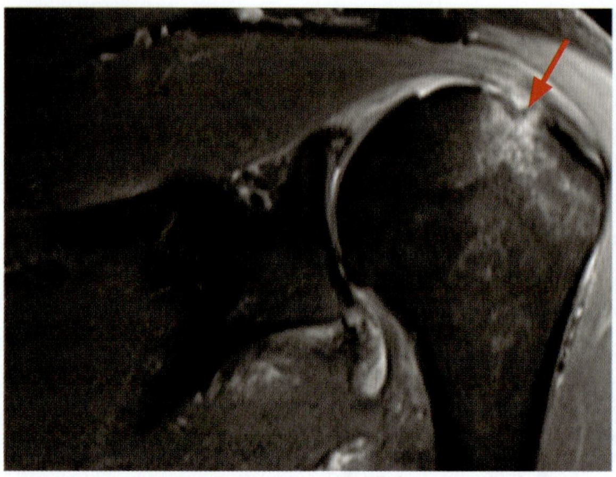

Coronal PD-weighted MRI with fat suppression
冠状位PD加权脂肪抑制MRI

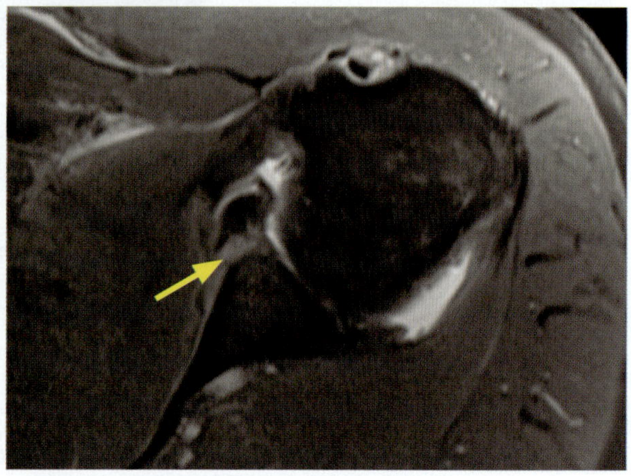

Axial PD-weighted MRI with fat suppression
轴位PD加权脂肪抑制MRI

Anterior glenohumeral dislocation with bony Bankart and Hill Sachs lesions:
Presentation radiograph demonstrated an anterior dislocation, with characteristic inferior position of the humeral head. There is a displaced, crescentic Bankart fracture (yellow arrow).
MR images after reduction confirm the large bony Bankart fracture of the anterior/inferior glenoid (yellow arrows). There is an impaction fracture of the superior-lateral humeral head (red arrow) with surrounding edema, in keeping with a Hill-Sachs.
盂肱关节前脱位伴骨性Bankart损伤和Hill-Sachs损伤：
就诊时的X线影像显示前脱位，肱骨头处于下方的位置具有特征性。可见一处移位的新月形Bankart骨折(黄箭)。
复位后的MRI证实了大的骨性Bankart骨折(黄箭)，位于肩胛盂前/下部。肱骨头上外侧有嵌入性骨折(红箭)，周围伴有水肿，符合Hill-Sachs损伤。

- Anterior dislocation of the humerus with respect to the glenoid is by far the most common type of shoulder dislocation. Anterior dislocation is usually caused by direct force on the arm. The humeral head usually dislocates in an anteroinferior direction.
- As the humeral head recoils from the dislocation force, the posterolateral humeral head strikes the anterior-inferior glenoid. This impaction may fracture the humeral head, the glenoid, or both.
- The **Hill-Sachs** lesion is an impaction fracture of the posterolateral aspect of the humeral head (**H**ill-Sachs and **h**umerus both start with **H**). On radiography,

- 肱骨相对于关节盂向前方脱位是一种最常见的肩关节脱位。前脱位通常是由于手臂遭受直接暴力所致。肱骨头通常向前下方脱位。
- 当肱骨头因脱位而回缩时，后外侧的肱骨头顶在关节盂前下部。这种作用力可导致肱骨头和/或关节盂骨折。
- **Hill-Sachs**病变是肱骨头后外侧的嵌入性骨折(Hill-Sachs与肱骨英文单词开头都是H)。在X线影像上，Hill-Sachs病变在手臂内旋时

the Hill-Sachs lesion is best demonstrated on an AP radiograph with the arm in internal rotation. On cross-sectional imaging, a Hill-Sachs lesion should be above the level of the coracoid, as there is a normal concavity of the humeral head located about the level of the coracoid that can be confused with a chronic Hill-Sachs lesion.

- The **Bankart** lesion is an injury of the anterior-inferior rim of the glenoid. It may involve the labrum only (soft tissue Bankart) or the glenoid rim (bony Bankart), as in the case above.

的前后位上显示最佳。在轴位断层上，Hill-Sachs病变应高于喙突水平，因为正常的肱骨头凹陷位于喙突水平附近，可能与慢性Hill-Sachs病变相混淆。

- Bankart病变是关节盂前下缘的损伤。它可能只累及盂唇(软组织Bankart)或关节盂边缘(骨性Bankart)，如上例所示。

Posterior glenohumeral dislocation

盂肱关节后脱位

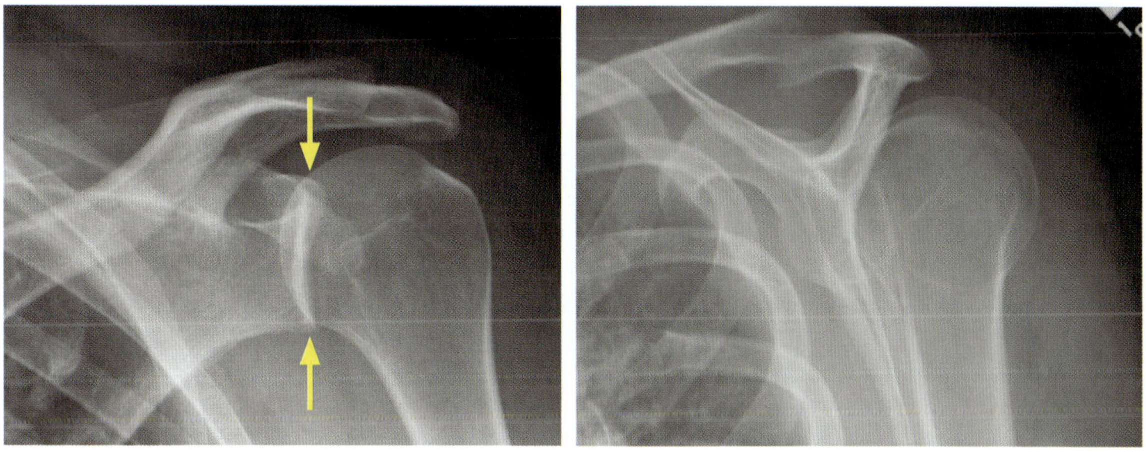

Posterior shoulder dislocation: Grashey (40° oblique; left image) radiograph shows overlap of the humeral head and the glenoid (arrows); normally, the glenohumeral joint space should be clear on this view.

Posterior displacement of the humerus is confirmed on the transscapular Y view (right image).

肩关节后脱位：Grashey位(40°斜位；左图)X线影像显示肱骨头与关节盂重叠(箭)；正常情况下，该位置应显示清晰的盂肱关节间隙。

穿肩胛骨Y位证实肱骨后移(右图)。

- Posterior dislocation represents only 2–3% of dislocations and is usually due to severe muscle spasm, such as from seizure or electrocution. The humeral head is dislocated posteriorly in these situations since the posterior pulling muscles of the back are generally stronger than the anterior pushing muscles.
- Diagnosis of a posterior dislocation is much more challenging compared to an anterior dislocation, as the standard frontal radiograph of the shoulder may look close to normal.
- Transscapular Y view or axillary view will best show the posterior dislocation.

  When possible, diagnosis is usually straightforward on an axillary view; however, many patients with posterior shoulder dislocation will not be able to abduct the arm.
- A Grashey (40° oblique) view in a non-dislocated shoulder normally will show clear space between the glenoid and the humeral head; however, in case of posterior dislocation there will be overlap of the medially displaced humeral head with the glenoid.
- The *lightbulb sign* describes the appearance of the humeral head due to the fixed internal rotation of the arm often seen in posterior dislocation.
- The *trough sign* describes a compression fracture of the anteromedial aspect of the humeral head, also known as a reverse Hill-Sachs, from impaction of the humeral head on the posterior glenoid rim upon recoil.

- 后脱位只占肩关节脱位的2%～3%，常由严重的肌肉痉挛引起，如癫痫或电击。在上述情况下，由于背部肌肉向后的拉力通常大于向前的推力，肱骨头向后移位。
- 诊断后脱位比前脱位要困难得多，因为在肩部的标准前后位X线影像上可能看起来接近正常。
- 穿肩胛Y位和腋位是显示后脱位的最佳体位。

  如有可能，直接采用腋位就可作出诊断；但许多肩关节后脱位的患者往往不能外展手臂。
- Grashey位(40°斜位)可清晰显示非脱位肩关节的关节盂和肱骨头的间隙；而后脱位时，此间隙因肱骨头内移与关节窝盂重叠而无法显示。
- 灯泡征指肱骨头因手臂固定内旋呈灯泡样，常见于后脱位。
- 水槽征为肱骨头前内侧压缩性骨折，也称反Hill-Sachs病变，由肱骨头回缩时，肱骨头作用于关节盂后缘所致。

Inferior glenohumeral dislocation (luxatio erecta)

盂肱关节下脱位(直举型脱位)

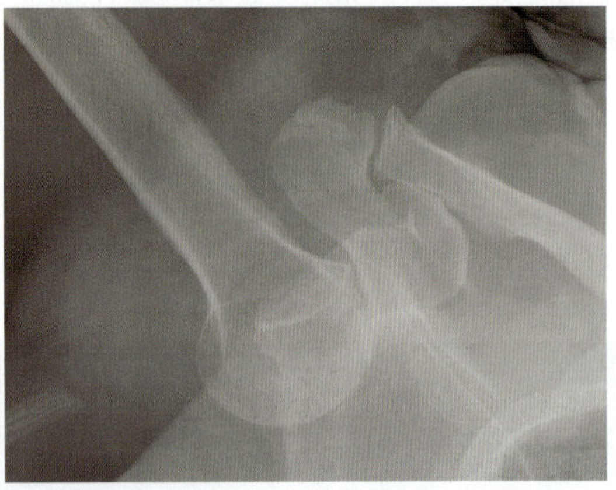

Luxatio erecta:
Frontal radiograph shows inferior dislocation of the humerus with characteristic superiorly projecting humerus.
直举型脱位：正位X线影像显示肱骨下脱位，具有特征性的肱骨向上突出。

- Inferior dislocation, also called *luxatio erecta,* is rare (occurring in approximately 1% of dislocations) and is usually caused by direct force to a fully abducted arm.
- Inferior dislocation is often associated with rotator cuff tear and greater tuberosity fracture.
- Inferior dislocation may cause injury to the axillary nerve or artery.

- 下脱位，也称直举型脱位，罕见(约占1%的脱位)，通常是手臂在完全外展时受到直接暴力所致。
- 下脱位通常伴肩袖撕裂和肱骨大结节骨折。
- 下脱位可致腋神经或腋动脉损伤。

Dislocations and associated sequela

脱位及相关后遗症

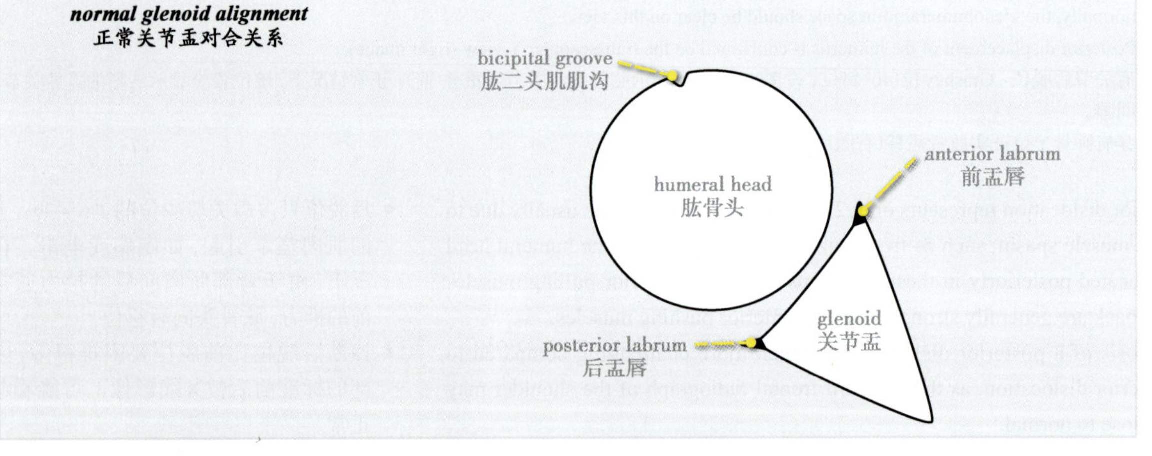

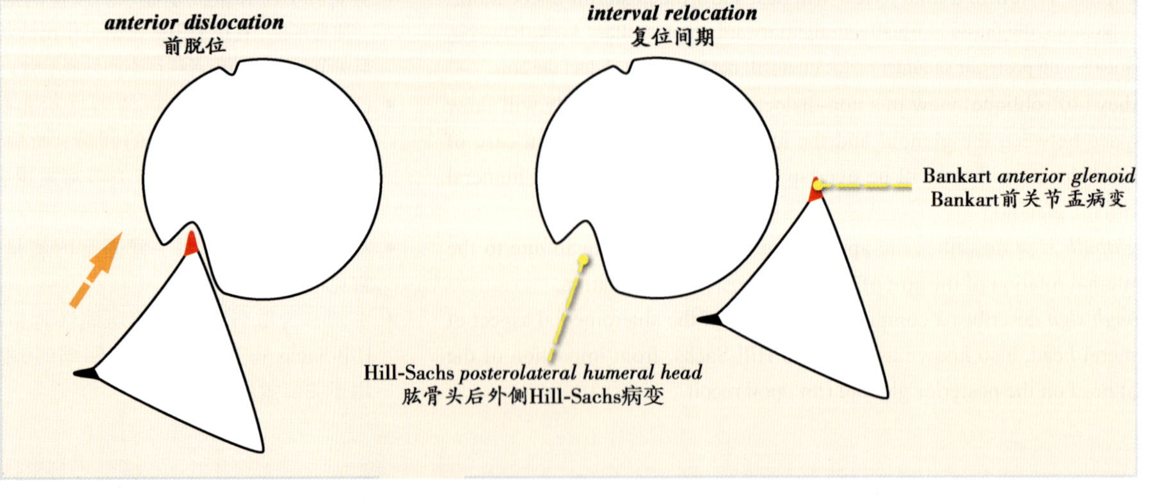

Hill Sachs: Axial T1-weighted MR arthrogram with fat suppression shows a wedge-shaped compression fracture of the posterolateral humeral head (arrow).
Case courtesy Kirstin Small, MD, Brigham and Women's Hospital.
Hill-Sachs病变：轴位T_1加权脂肪抑制MR关节造影显示肱骨头后外侧楔形的压缩性骨折(箭)。

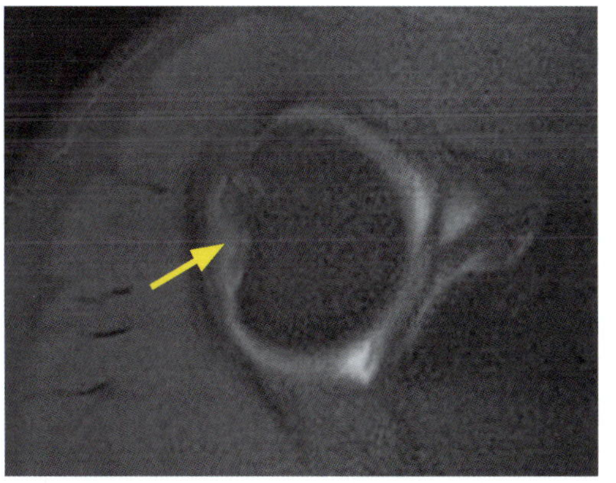

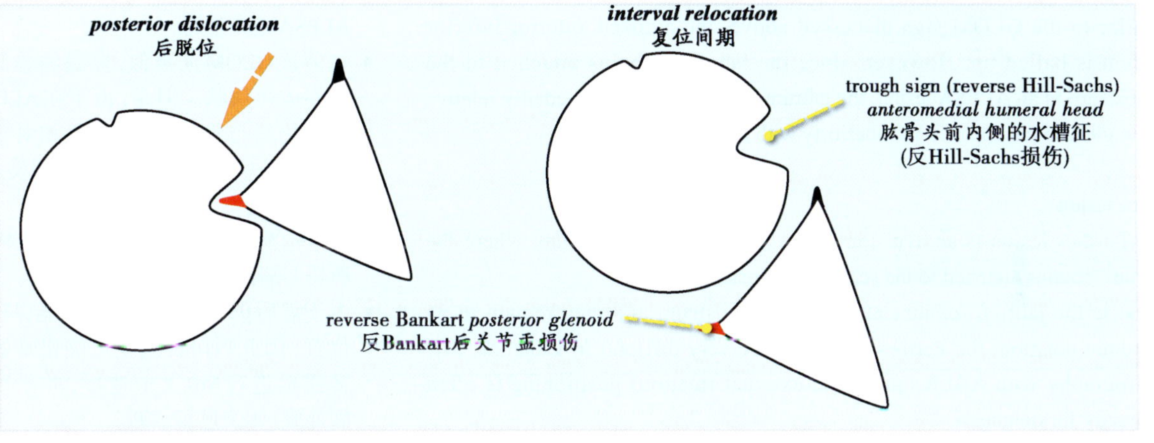

INSTABILITY: ASSOCIATED LESIONS

- The vast majority of the alphabet-soup instability lesions are located at the anterior-inferior aspect of the glenohumeral joint and are associated with the anterior instability and/or sequela of anterior dislocation.

Bankart lesion

- The Bankart lesion is an injury of the anteroinferior labrum due to anterior glenohumeral dislocation. Specifically, a Bankart is detachment of the anteroinferior labrum from the glenoid, with stripping of the scapular periosteum.
- The labrum may migrate superiorly and appear as a balled-up mass-like object, producing the glenoid labrum ovoid mass (GLOM) sign. The differential diagnosis for a black intra-articular mass on MRI includes:

  GLOM sign (if a Bankart lesion is present inferiorly).

  Dislocated biceps tendon.

  Air bubble (if an MR arthrogram was performed).
- An osseous Bankart (or "bony Bankart") is a fracture of the anterior-inferior glenoid rim, which predisposes to recurrent dislocation due to glenoid insufficiency.

不稳定：相关病变

- 绝大多数以字母简称的不稳定性病变都位于盂肱关节前下部且与前脱位的盂肱关节前部不稳定性和/或后遗症有关。

Bankart病变

- Bankart病变即为盂肱关节前脱位引起的盂唇前下部损伤。确切地说，Bankart病变是前下盂唇从关节盂上脱位，伴肩胛骨骨膜撕脱。
- 盂唇可向上移位并类似一团块样的物体，形成盂唇卵圆肿块征(GLOM)。在MRI上，关节内出现黑色肿块的鉴别诊断包括：

  GLOM征(如Bankart病变出现在下方)。

  脱位的肱二头肌肌腱。

  气泡(如MR关节造影检查)。
- 骨性Bankart(或"bony Bankart")是关节盂环前下部骨折，由于关节盂结构不全而容易导致复发性脱位。

Hill-Sachs

- Hill-Sachs is an impaction fracture of the posterolateral humeral head caused by anterior dislocation. The Hill-Sachs lesion can be diagnosed by scrolling through sequential axial images: With standard 5 mm slices, the normal humeral head should appear round in three consecutive slices starting superiorly. If a Hill-Sachs lesion is present, there will be a posterolateral notch in the humeral head.
- Subtle Hill-Sachs can also be detected as bone marrow edema in this location, without fracture.

Anterior labro-ligamentous periosteal sleeve avulsion (ALPSA)

- An anterior labro-ligamentous periosteal sleeve avulsion (ALPSA) is a variant of the Bankart lesion and also represents an anterior-inferior labral injury. In contrast to the Bankart lesion, the scapular periosteum is intact with an ALPSA.
- Similar to the GLOM sign discussed above, the avulsed anterior-inferior labrum is balled up. However, since the labrum remains attached to the periosteum in an ALPSA lesion, the labrum is displaced inferomedially relative to the glenoid (as opposed to superiorly with the GLOM sign).

Perthes lesion

- The Perthes lesion is an avulsion of the anterior-inferior labrum, where the labrum remains attached to the scapular periosteum.
- Because the labrum remains attached to periosteum and may remain in its anatomic position, the Perthes lesion can be very difficult to visualize. MR arthrography with ABER (abduction-external rotation) positioning is often necessary for diagnosis.

Humeral avulsion of the inferior glenohumeral ligament (HAGL)

- Humeral avulsion of the inferior glenohumeral ligament (HAGL) is avulsion of the humeral attachment of the IGHL. This lesion occurs on the opposite (humeral) site of the IGHL compared to the Bankart/ALPSA/Perthes lesions.
- HAGL is associated with subscapularis tendon tears.

Bony HAGL (BHAGL)

- A BHAGL is a HAGL lesion with an additional bony avulsion of the anatomic neck of the humerus, caused by avulsion of the IGHL.

Hill-Sachs病变

- Hill-Sachs病变是由关节前脱位引起的肱骨头后外侧的挤压性骨折。Hill-Sachs病变可以通过按顺序滚动观察轴位图像进行诊断：按标准的5mm层厚，正常肱骨头从上开始应在三个连续层面均呈圆形。如果有Hill-Sachs病变，肱骨头的后外侧会有一个凹痕。
- 轻微的Hill-Sachs病变可仅表现为局部骨髓水肿，没有骨折。

前盂唇-韧带骨膜袖套样撕脱(ALPSA)

- 前盂唇-韧带骨膜袖套样撕脱(ALPSA)是Bankart病变的一种变异，也表现为前下盂唇的损伤。与Bankart病变相比，肩胛骨的骨膜在ALPSA是完整的。
- 与前述GLOM征类似，撕脱的关节盂唇前下份卷成团块状。但是，由于在ALPSA损伤中盂唇仍然与骨膜相连，盂唇相对于关节呈向内下移位(与GLOM征时向上相反)。

Perthes病变

- Perthes病变是盂唇前下方的撕脱伤，其中，盂唇仍与肩胛骨的骨膜相连。
- 由于盂唇仍与骨膜相连并可能保持在其解剖位置，因此Perthes病变可能很难被发现。通常需要进行MR关节造影，并采用ABER(外展外旋)体位进行诊断。

下盂肱韧带肱骨撕脱(HAGL)

- 下盂肱韧带肱骨撕脱(HAGL)是肱骨在下盂肱韧带(IGHL)的附着处被撕脱。与Bankart/ALPSA/Perthes病变相比，该病变发生在IGHL的对侧(肱骨)。
- HAGL与肩胛下肌肌腱撕裂有关。

骨性HAGL(BHAGL)

- BHAGL是指HAGL损伤，另外还包括肱骨解剖颈的骨性撕脱，是由于IGHL撕脱所致。

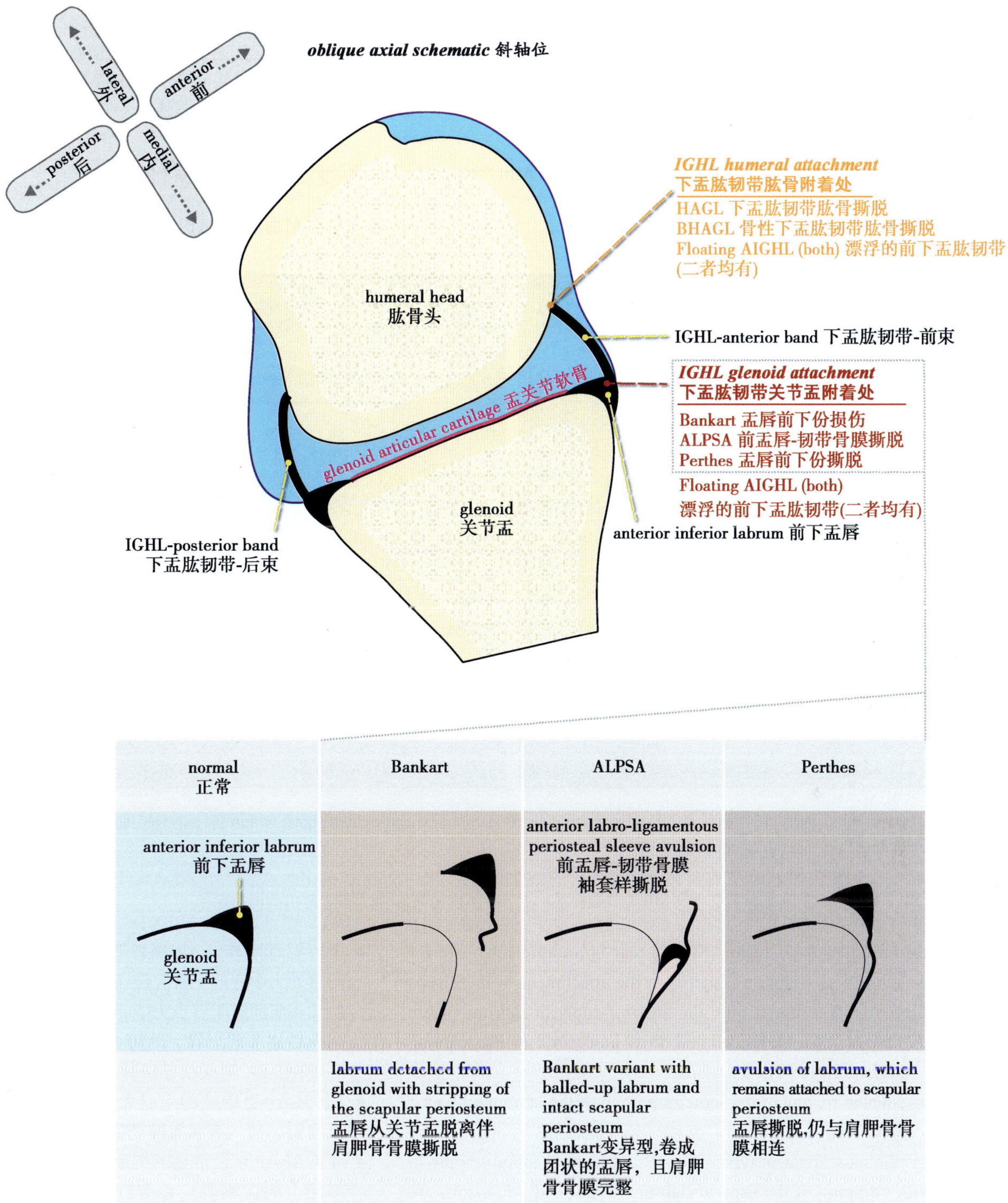

Posterior instability

- Posterior instability is uncommon, accounting for less than 5% of instability.
- The injuries associated with posterior instability are highly variable and include several posterior variations of anterior lesions such as posterior HAGL (PHAGL), reverse Bankart (posterior glenoid fracture), and reverse Hill-Sachs/ *trough sign*.
- Tears of the infraspinatus and teres minor are associated with posterior instability, as these rotator cuff muscles insert on the posterior aspect of the greater tuberosity.

肩关节后部不稳定

- 后部不稳定相对较少见，占不稳定的病例不到5%。
- 引起后部不稳定相关的损伤原因很多，包括一些前部损伤的多种后部变异，如后HAGL(PHAGL)、反Bankart(关节盂后部骨折)和反Hill-Sachs/水槽征。
- 冈下肌和小圆肌的撕裂与后部不稳定有关，因为这些肩袖肌肉附着于大结节的后方。

- Hypoplastic posterior glenoid may be a congenital cause of posterior instability.
- The Bennett lesion, also known as *thrower's exostosis*, is extra-articular posterior ossification associated with posterior labral injury. The Bennett lesion is often seen in baseball pitchers and is thought to be the result of avulsion of the posterior band of the IGHL. Ossification can be confirmed with an axillary shoulder radiograph.

- 关节盂后部发育不良可能是后部不稳定的先天性原因。
- Bennett病变，也称为投手骨赘，是与后盂唇损伤有关的关节外后部骨化。Bennett病变常见于棒球投手，被认为是下盂肱韧带后束撕裂的结果。骨化可在肩关节腋位X线影像上进行确诊。

Miscellaneous lesions not associated with instability

不涉及稳定性的其他损伤

Superior labrum anterior posterior (SLAP) tear

上唇盂前后向(SLAP)撕裂

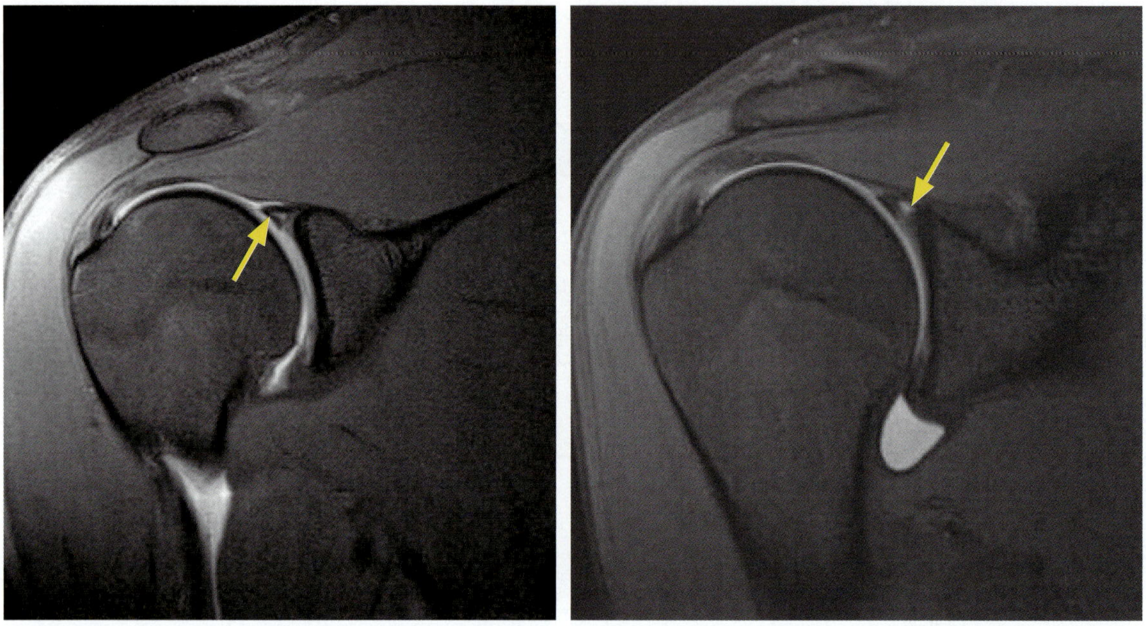

SLAP tear (type Ⅱ): Coronal T1-weighted MR arthrogram with fat suppression shows high signal within the superior labrum (yellow arrows) extending from anterior to posterior.

Case courtesy Kirstin M. Small, MD, Brigham and Women's Hospital.

SLAP撕裂(Ⅱ型)：冠状位T_1加权脂肪抑制MR关节造影显示上方盂唇内呈高信号(黄箭)，并由前向后延伸。

- A superior labrum anterior posterior (SLAP) tear is an anterior-posterior oriented tear of the superior labrum centered at the attachment of the biceps tendon. The biceps tendon inserts onto the anterior-superior labrum. There were originally 4 types of SLAP lesions described, however now there are up to 10 different subcategories of SLAP lesions.
- Type Ⅰ SLAP is isolated fraying of the superior portion of the labrum without a frank tear. The biceps tendon is intact.
- Type Ⅱ SLAP is the most frequent type of SLAP and features labral fraying in conjunction with stripping of the superior labrum. Type Ⅱ SLAP lesions are most commonly associated with repetitive microtrauma.
- Type Ⅲ SLAP is a bucket-handle tear of the superior labrum, analogous to a bucket-handle tear of the knee meniscus.
- Type Ⅳ SLAP is also a bucket handle tear of the superior labrum, with additional extension into the biceps tendon.

- 上唇盂前后向(SLAP)撕裂是指以肱二头肌肌腱附着处为中心的上唇盂前-后方向的撕裂，并以肱二头肌肌腱附着点为中心。肱二头肌肌腱由前向后插入前上唇。最初对SLAP病变的描述有四种类型，但现在有10种以上不同的亚型。
- Ⅰ型SLAP是单纯的上唇盂上份磨损，没有明显撕裂。肱二头肌肌腱完整。
- Ⅱ型SLAP是最常见的类型，其特征为盂唇磨损伴上唇盂剥脱。Ⅱ型SLAP损伤最常与反复的微小损伤有关。
- Ⅲ型SLAP是上唇盂的桶柄样撕裂，类似于膝关节半月板桶柄样撕裂。
- Ⅳ型SLAP也是上唇盂桶柄样撕裂，外加肱二头肌肌腱受累。

Glenoid labral articular disruption (GLAD)

- Glenoid labral articular disruption (GLAD) is a superficial tear of the anterior-inferior labrum, with adjacent glenoid articular cartilage injury.
- Although the GLAD lesion occurs at the anterior-inferior labrum, the same site as the Bankart, ALPSA, and Perthes lesions, GLAD is usually not caused by or

盂唇关节面破裂(GLAD)

- 盂唇关节面破裂(GLAD)是前下盂唇的浅表撕裂，伴邻近的关节软骨损伤。
- 虽然GLAD病变发生在前下盂唇，其位置与Bankart、ALPSA和Perthes损伤相同，但

associated with instability.

GLAD通常不是由不稳定所引起或与之相关。

- GLAD lesions may lead to post-traumatic arthritis and intra-articular bodies.

- GLAD损伤可导致创伤后关节炎及关节内游离体形成。

Paralabral cysts

盂唇旁囊肿

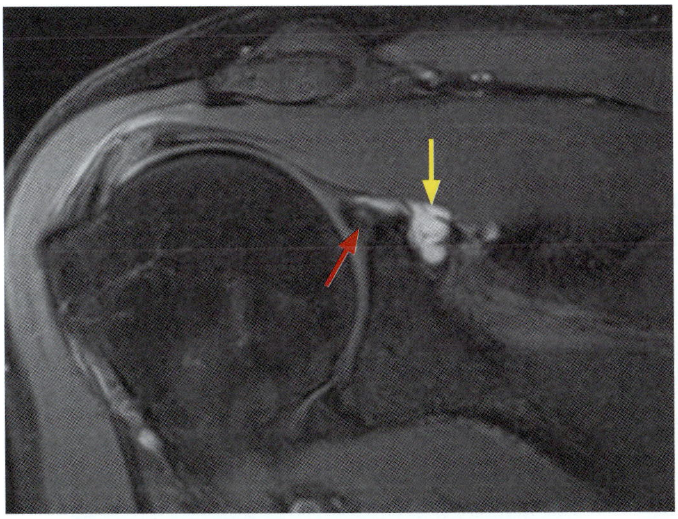

Paralabral cyst and labral tear:

Coronal T2-weighted MRI with fat suppression shows a lobulated paralabral cyst (yellow arrow) medial to the glenoid. There is globular intermediate signal within the labrum (red arrow), highly suggestive of labral tear especially in the presence of an adjacent paralabral cyst.

Case courtesy Kirstin M. Small, MD, Brigham and Women's Hospital.

盂唇旁囊肿和盂唇撕裂：

冠状位T_2加权脂肪抑制MRI显示关节盂的内侧有一个分叶状的盂唇旁囊肿(黄箭)。盂唇内出现类圆形等信号(红箭)，高度提示盂唇撕裂，特别是邻近出现盂唇旁囊肿时。

- Similar to the formation of parameniscal cysts adjacent to meniscal tears, paralabral cysts form adjacent to labral tears. Paralabral cysts are usually seen in the soft tissues adjacent to the labrum but may extend into bone. A paralabral cyst is a specific finding for a labral tear even when abnormal labral signal is not seen.
- A paralabral cyst may compress a nerve and cause an entrapment neuropathy, discussed below.

- 类似于邻近半月板撕裂处形成的半月板旁囊肿，盂唇旁囊肿于盂唇撕裂的周围形成。盂唇旁囊肿常见于邻近盂唇的软组织中，但也可以扩展到骨内。盂唇旁囊肿是盂唇撕裂的一个非常特异的表现，即使未见盂唇异常信号也可诊断。
- 盂唇旁囊肿可压迫神经进而导致神经卡压症状，后文将进一步讨论。

Entrapment neuropathies

卡压性神经病变

Suprascapular nerve entrapment

肩胛上神经卡压

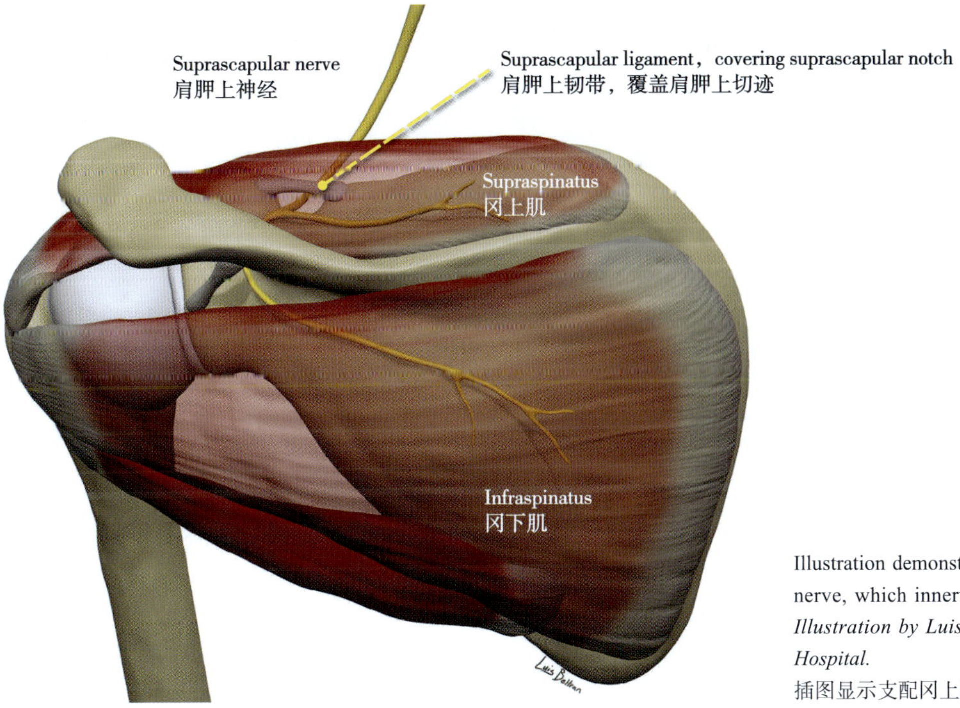

Illustration demonstrates the anatomy of the suprascapular nerve, which innervates supraspinatus and infraspinatus.

Illustration by Luis Beltran, MD, Brigham and Women's Hospital.

插图显示支配冈上肌和冈下肌肩胛上神经的解剖结构。

- The suprascapular nerve innervates both supraspinatus and infraspinatus.
- The proximal suprascapular nerve provides motor innervation to the supraspinatus and infraspinatus muscles. Entrapment of the suprascapular nerve at the **suprascapular notch**, most commonly from a paralabral cyst associated with a superior labral tear, causes atrophy of both the supraspinatus and infraspinatus.
- The more distal fibers of the suprascapular nerve innervate infraspinatus only. Therefore, impingement at the level of the **spinoglenoid notch** would cause denervation changes of infraspinatus only.

- 肩胛上神经支配冈上肌和冈下肌。
- 肩胛上神经的近端支配冈上肌和冈下肌的运动。最常见的肩胛上神经在**肩胛上切迹**处受卡压的原因是盂唇旁囊肿伴上盂唇撕裂，导致冈上肌和冈下肌同时萎缩。
- 肩胛上神经最远端的纤维仅支配冈下肌。因此，位于冈盂切迹水平的卡压只会造成冈下肌去神经化。

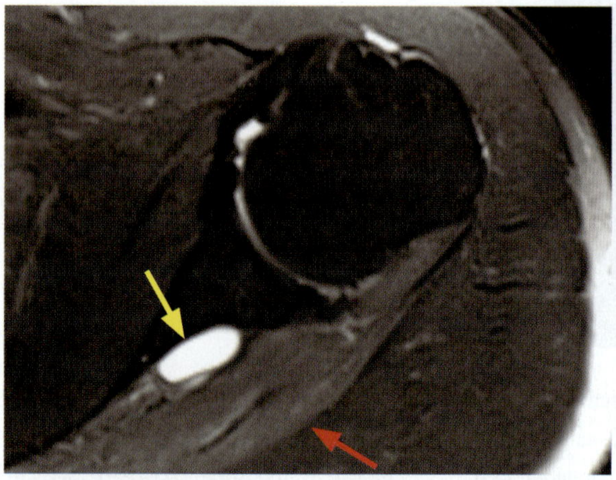

Axial PD-weighted MRI with fat suppression
轴位PD加权脂肪抑制MRI

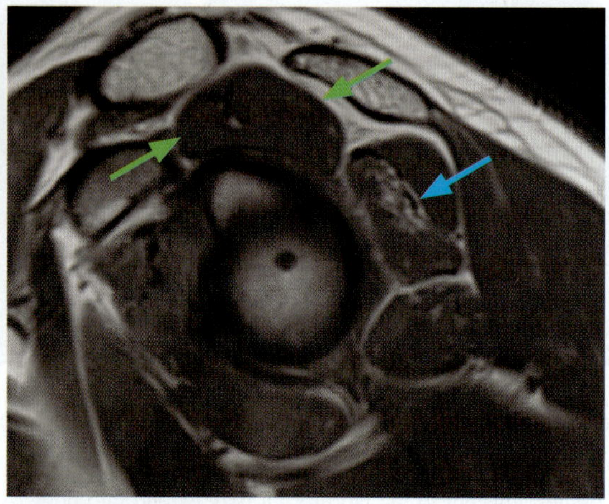

Sagittal T1-weighted MRI
矢状位T_1加权MRI

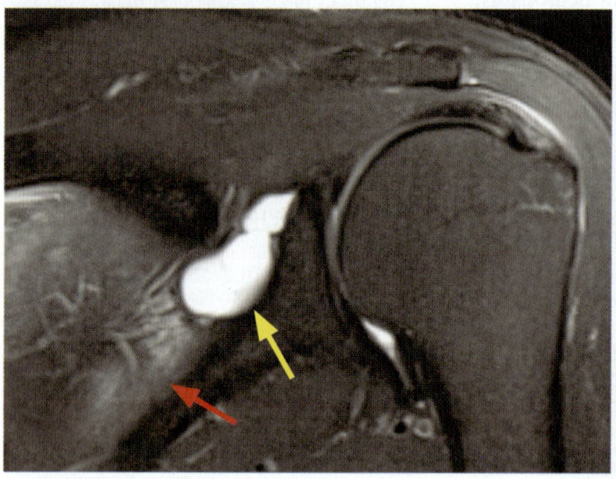

Coronal PD-weighted MRI with fat suppression
冠状位PD加权脂肪抑制MRI

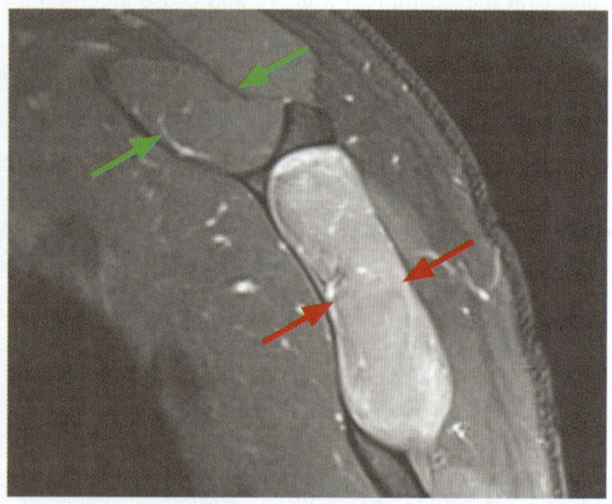

Sagittal PD-weighted MRI with fat suppression
矢状位PD加权脂肪抑制MRI

Spinoglenoid notch cyst causing isolated denervation changes in infraspinatus:
There is a multiloculated cyst in the region of the spinoglenoid notch (yellow arrows), with resultant infraspinatus edema (red arrows) and focal fatty infiltration (blue arrow). Supraspinatus (green arrows) is normal in muscle bulk and signal intensity.
冈盂切迹囊肿导致冈下肌孤立性去神经化改变：冈盂切迹区域有一个多房囊肿(黄箭)，导致冈下肌水肿(红箭)和局灶性脂肪浸润(蓝箭)。冈上肌(绿箭)的肌肉体积和信号强度正常。

Quadrilateral space syndrome

- The quadrilateral space is located at the posterior aspect of the axilla. It is formed by the humerus (laterally), the long head of the triceps muscle (medially), teres minor (superiorly), and teres major (inferiorly).
- The axillary nerve and posterior humeral circumflex artery travel through the quadrilateral space. The axillary nerve provides motor fibers to the teres minor and deltoid.

四边孔综合征

- 四边孔位于腋窝的后方。它由肱骨(外)、肱三头肌长头(内)、小圆肌(上)和大圆肌(下)组成。
- 腋神经和旋肱后动脉穿行于四边孔。腋神经支配小圆肌和三角肌的运动神经纤维。

- Entrapment of the axillary nerve in the quadrilateral space may cause teres minor paresthesias and eventual atrophy, with or without deltoid involvement.

- 腋神经在四边孔受卡压可导致小圆肌的感觉异常并最终萎缩，三角肌受累不定。

Summary of entrapment neuropathies

卡压性神经病变小结

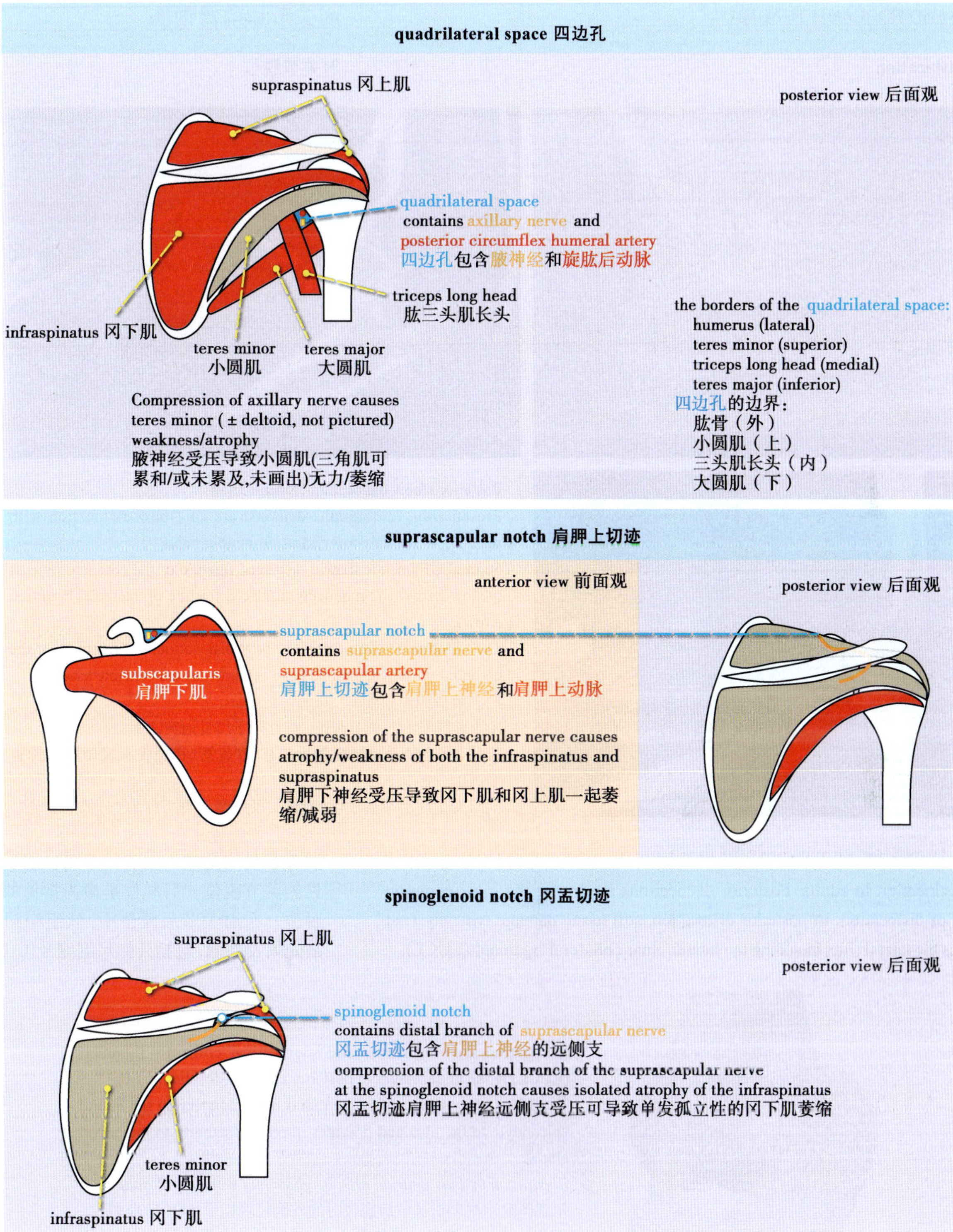

Parsonage-Turner

- Parsonage-Turner syndrome is idiopathic brachial neuropathy, which may cause rotator cuff atrophy. It is a diagnosis of exclusion and a structural cause for atrophy (e.g., a mass or cyst compressing a nerve) must be ruled out.

Parsonage-Turner

- Parsonage-Turner综合征是特发性臂丛神经病，可导致肩袖萎缩。这是一种排除性诊断，导致萎缩的结构性原因必须要排除(如肿块或囊肿压迫神经)。

（翻译　苏筱芮　刘进）

Elbow and Forearm

肘关节和前臂

Elbow and Forearm Trauma

肘关节和前臂创伤

Elbow dislocation

肘关节脱位

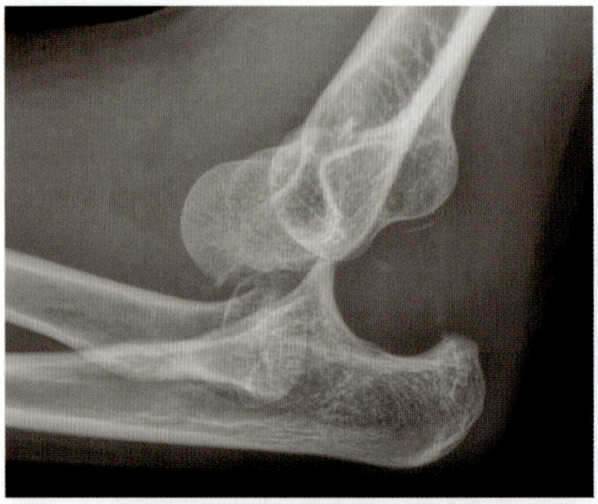

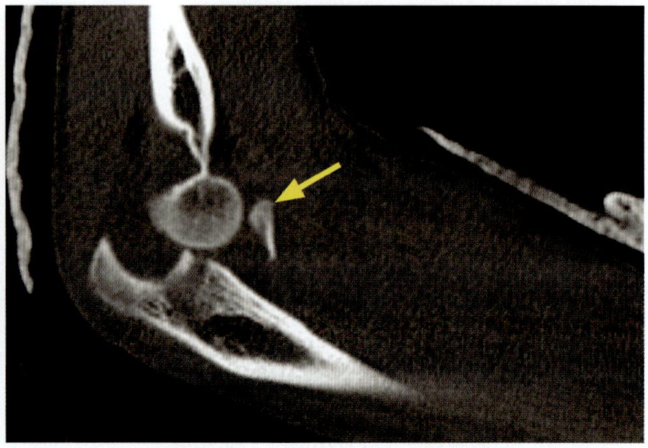

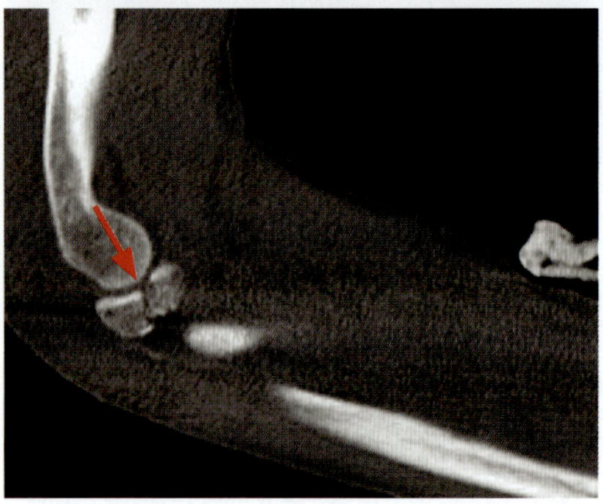

Posterior elbow dislocation "terrible triad" :

Presentation radiographs demonstrate an elbow dislocation with perching of the humerus on the coronoid process.

Sagittal CT images show a displaced fracture of the coronoid process (yellow arrow) and minimally displaced fracture of the radial head (red arrow).

The combination of posterior elbow dislocation and fractures of the coronoid process and radial head is known as the "terrible triad" .

肘关节后脱位"恐怖三联征"：

X线影像显示肘关节脱位，肱骨架于尺骨冠突之上。

矢状位CT显示冠状突骨折片移位(黄箭)和桡骨头轻度位移骨折(红箭)。

同时发生肘关节后脱位，冠状突及桡骨头骨折称为"恐怖三联征"。

- Following shoulder dislocations, elbow dislocations are the second most common joint dislocation in adults. Posterior dislocations are by far the most common pattern of dislocation. In posterior dislocation, soft tissue damage typically first involves the lateral side, including the lateral ulnar collateral ligament (LUCL).

- 肘关节脱位是成人继肩关节脱位之后第二常见的关节脱位。后脱位是最为常见的肘关节脱位。在肘关节后脱位中，软组织损伤通常最先累及外侧，包括外侧尺副韧带(LUCL)。

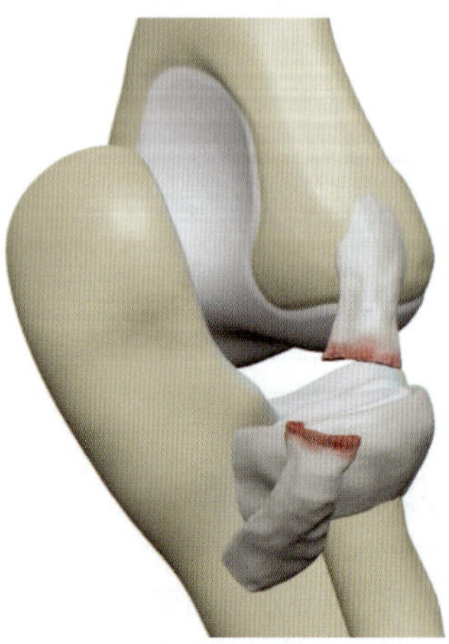

Illustration showing tear of the lateral ulnar collateral ligament (LUCL) in the initial stages of posterior elbow dislocation.

The LUCL normally cradles the radial head, connecting the lateral epicondyle to the ulna and provides important stability to the lateral elbow.

Illustration by Luis Beltran, MD, Brigham and Women's Hospital.

示意图显示早期肘关节后脱位时的外侧尺副韧带(LUCL)撕裂。

正常外侧尺副韧带支撑桡骨头，连接肱骨外上髁和尺骨，为外侧肘关节提供重要的稳定作用。

- Radial head fractures and coronoid process fractures are commonly seen, and the "terrible triad" refers to elbow dislocation with both of these fractures.

- 桡骨头骨折和冠突骨折较为常见，"恐怖三联征"指肘关节脱位合并上述两种骨折。

- If a radial head fracture is seen in the setting of instability, CT should be performed, as a coronoid process fracture (even if tiny) results in elbow instability.

- 如果桡骨头骨折出现肘关节不稳时应进行CT检查，因为冠突骨折(即使非常小)可导致肘关节不稳。

Radial head fracture

桡骨头骨折

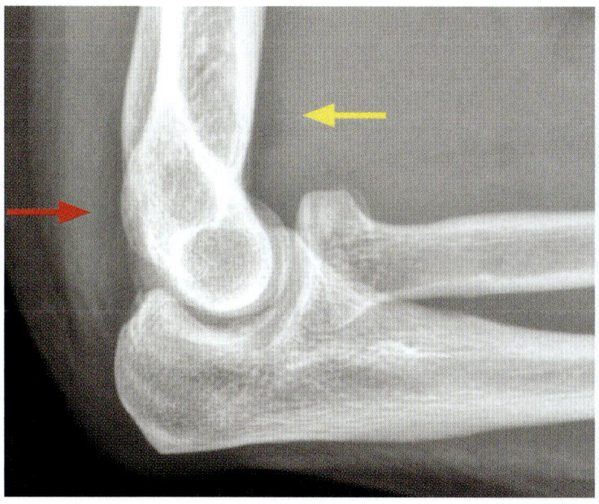

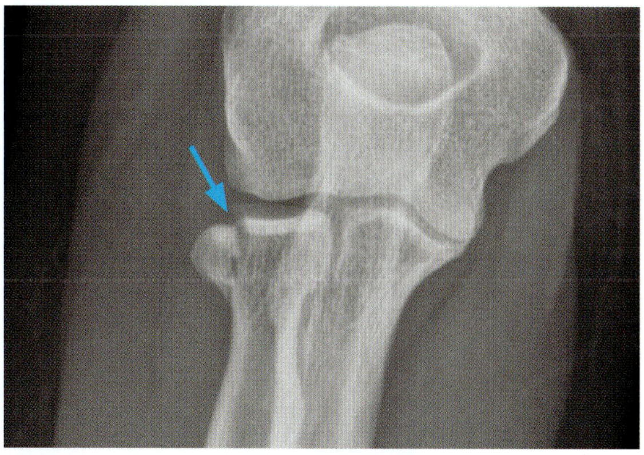

Radial head fracture: Lateral radiograph shows an elbow effusion, with a sail sign (yellow arrow) representing anterior displacement of the anterior fat pad. There is also slight posterior displacement of the posterior fat pad (red arrow).
Frontal elbow radiograph shows a nondisplaced radial head fracture (blue arrow).
桡骨头骨折：侧位X线影像显示肘关节积液，伴有帆船征(黄箭)代表前脂肪垫向前移位。还有轻微后脂肪垫向后移位(红箭)。
肘部正位X线影像显示非移位性桡骨头骨折(蓝箭)。

- A radial head fracture is the most common elbow fracture in adults.
- The *fat pad sign* is elevation of the anterior and/or posterior fat pads due to an elbow effusion. Elevation of the posterior fat pad is considered nearly diagnostic for fracture (most commonly radial head fracture in adults). The *sail sign* represents elevation of the anterior fat pad only and is less specific for fracture.
- If a fat pad sign is present and no fracture is seen, additional views (typically of the radial head) or CT should be obtained.

- 桡骨头骨折是成人最常见的肘关节骨折。
- 脂肪垫征是因肘关节积液导致脂肪垫向前和/或向后抬高。后脂肪垫抬高被认为几乎等同于骨折的诊断(在成人最常见的为桡骨头骨折)。帆船征指仅有前脂肪垫抬高，对诊断骨折的特异性较低。
- 如果有脂肪垫征而未发现骨折，需加照不同位置的X线影像(通常为桡骨头)或进行CT检查。

Supracondylar fracture

- Supracondylar fracture is the most common elbow fracture in children.

髁上骨折

- 髁上骨折是儿童最常见的肘关节骨折。

Essex-Lopresti fracture-dislocation

- Essex-Lopresti fracture-dislocation is radial head fracture and tearing of the interosseous membrane with ulnar dislocation at the distal radioulnar joint.

Essex-Lopresti骨折-脱位

- Essex-Lopresti骨折-脱位是桡骨头骨折和骨间膜撕裂，伴远端尺桡关节尺侧脱位。

Monteggia fracture-dislocation

Monteggia骨折-脱位

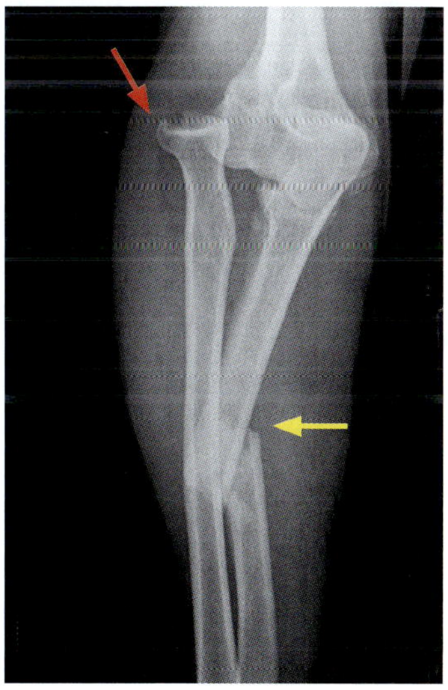

Monteggia fracture-dislocation:
Frontal radiograph of the proximal forearm shows a mid-diaphyseal ulnar fracture (yellow arrow) and radial head dislocation (red arrow).
Case courtesy Stacy Smith, MD, Brigham and Women's Hospital.
Monteggia骨折-脱位：
前臂近段正位X线影像显示尺骨中段骨干骨折(黄箭)和桡骨头脱位(红箭)。

- Monteggia fracture-dislocation is an ulnar fracture and radial dislocation at the elbow.

- Monteggia骨折-脱位是肘部尺骨骨折合并桡骨头脱位。

Galeazzi fracture-dislocation

Galeazzi骨折-脱位

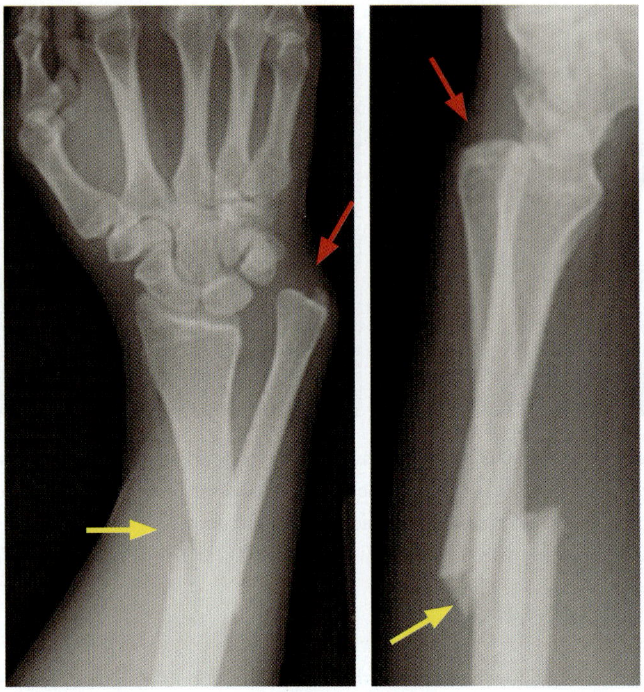

Galeazzi fracture-dislocation:

Frontal and lateral radiographs of the forearm show a radial diaphyseal fracture of the distal 1/3 of the radial diaphysis (yellow arrows) and distal ulnar dislocation (red arrows). The radial shaft fracture has radial and volar angulation and foreshortening.

Case courtesy Stacy Smith, MD, Brigham and Women's Hospital.

Galeazzi骨折-脱位：

前臂正侧位X线影像显示桡骨远1/3骨干骨折(黄箭)和尺骨远端脱位(红箭)。桡骨干骨折成角折向桡侧和掌侧并缩短。

- Galeazzi fracture-dislocation is fracture of the distal third of the radius with ulnar dislocation at the distal radioulnar joint.

- Galeazzi骨折-脱位是桡骨远1/3处骨折合并远端尺桡关节尺骨脱位。

Colles fracture

- Colles fracture is a distal radius fracture with dorsal angulation. The fracture is usually intra-articular. Colles fracture is the most common injury to the distal forearm.
- Colles fracture typically results from fall on an outstretched hand (FOOSH).

Colles骨折

- Colles骨折是桡骨远端骨折伴背侧成角。损伤常在关节内。Colles骨折是前臂远端最常见的骨折。
- Colles骨折常由跌倒时手背外伸(FOOSH)所致。

Barton fracture

- Intra-articular oblique fracture of the dorsal distal radius.
- Associated with dorsal subluxation/dislocation of the radiocarpal joint.

Barton骨折

- 桡骨远端背侧的关节内斜形骨折。
- 伴有桡腕关节背侧半脱位/脱位。

Smith fracture

- Type Ⅰ– Reverse Colles fracture: extra-articular transverse fracture (most common).
- Type Ⅱ– Reverse Barton fracture: intra-articular fracture with volar displacement.

Smith骨折

- Ⅰ型-反Colles骨折：关节外横向骨折(最常见)。
- Ⅱ型-反Barton骨折：关节内骨折伴掌侧移位。

Hutchinson (Chauffeur's) fracture

- Fracture of the radial (lateral) aspect of the distal radius extending into the radial styloid and the radiocarpal joint.

Hutchinson (chauffeur's)骨折

- 桡骨远端桡侧(外侧)骨折，延伸到桡骨茎突和桡腕关节。

Medial (ulnar) collateral ligament tear

内侧(尺)副韧带撕裂

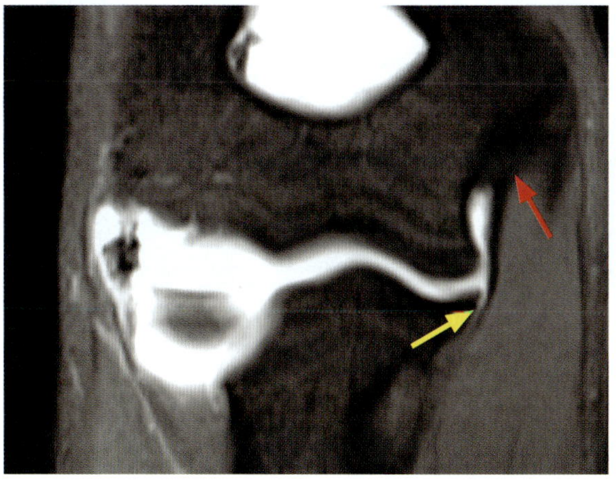

Medial (ulnar) collateral ligament partial tear:
Coronal T1-weighted MRI with fat suppression from an arthrogram with injection of dilute gadolinium-containing contrast demonstrates subtle undersurface stripping (yellow arrow) of the attachment of the MCL onto the sublime tubercle of the ulna. This appearance is known as the *T-sign* (a sideways T).
The humeral origin of the MCL (red arrow) is intact.
内侧(尺)副韧带部分撕裂:
注射稀释含钆造影剂后行关节造影，冠状位T_1加权脂肪抑制MRI显示内侧副韧带于尺骨高耸结节附着处表面下轻微剥离(黄箭)。此表现被称为T征(斜行T)。
内侧副韧带肱骨附着点(红箭)未受损。

- The medial collateral ligament (MCL) of the elbow, also known as the ulnar collateral ligament (UCL), is the ligamentous stabilizer against valgus stress. Valgus stress is a force directed against the lateral elbow, putting tensile stress on the medial side.
- MCL tears are duc to valgus stress. In distinction to the knee, when the valgus stress is typically a single traumatic event (for instance, in the knee, a force on the lateral knee), in the elbow MCL injuries are usually the result of chronic stress from the late cocking phase of throwing. On radiography, valgus stress ("Telos") views can bring out widening of the medial joint space.

- 肘关节内侧副韧带(MCL)，也称尺侧副韧带(UCL)，是对抗肘关节外翻时起到稳定作用的韧带。外翻应力是一种对抗来自肘关节外侧的应力，在肘的内侧施加拉力。
- 外翻应力导致内侧副韧带撕裂。膝关节的外翻应力通常来自单次创伤事件(如施加在膝外侧的暴力)，但肘关节内侧副韧带损伤通常是由于投掷挥臂后期的慢性应力所致。在X线影像上，外翻应力("Telos")位可显示内侧关节间隙增宽。

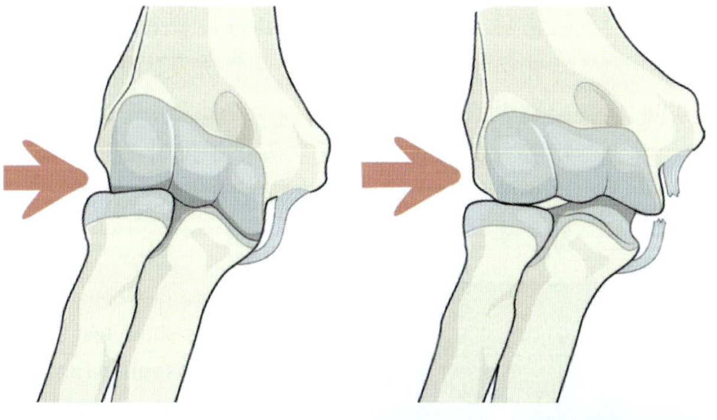

Illustration demonstrates the mechanism of how valgus stress causes MCL tearing.
Force on the lateral elbow (large red arrows; such as in the late cocking phase of throwing) causes tensile force on the MCL, ultimately leading to failure.
In this diagram, the mid-substance of the MCL is torn. More commonly seen is tears of the humeral attachment or ulnar attachment (as in the case above).
示意图展示外翻应力导致内侧副韧带撕裂的机制。
施加在肘外侧的力量(大红箭，如在投掷挥臂后期)在内侧副韧带产生张力，最终导致韧带撕裂。
在这幅图中，内侧副韧带中部撕裂。更常见的是撕裂肱骨附着点或尺骨附着点(如上述例子)。

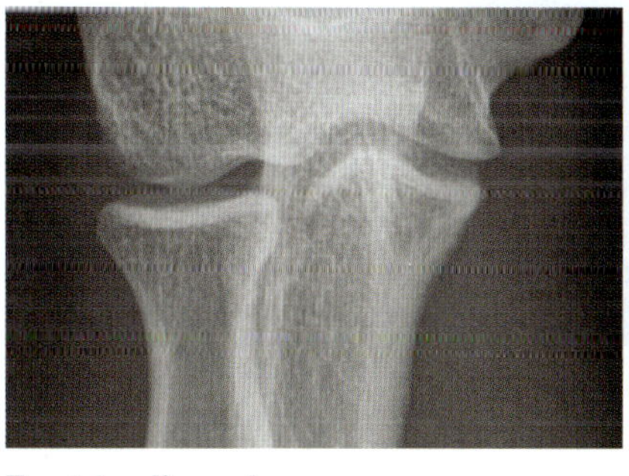

Frontal radiograph
正位X线影像

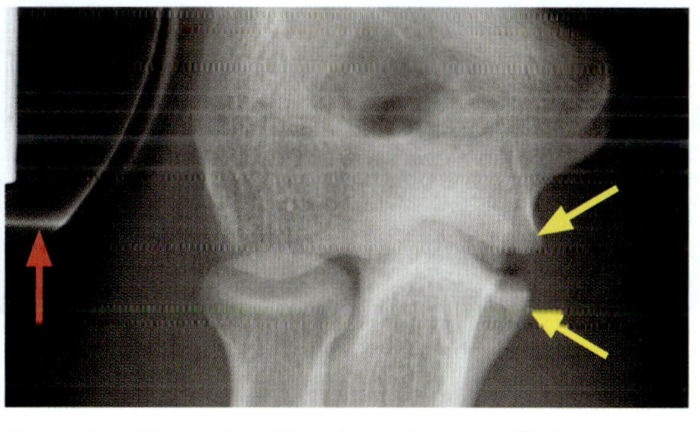

Frontal radiograph with valgus stress applied
外翻应力位正位X线影像

MCL deficiency: Frontal and valgus-stress radiographs of the elbow (different patient as the MRI case above) show relative widening of the medial compartment (arrows) with valgus-applied stress, indicating MCL deficiency. Note partially imaged valgus stress device (red arrow).
内侧副韧带损伤，肘关节正位X线影像和外翻应力位(与上文MRI病例不同的患者)显示外翻应力下内侧关节间隙相对增宽(箭)，提示内侧副韧带损伤。注意部分显示的外翻应力器材(红箭)。

- Tears of the MCL may involve the humeral attachment, the ulnar attachment onto the sublime tubercle, or may be mid-substance. A common pattern injury is undersurface stripping of the sublime tubercle attachment, creating the *T-sign* as shown in the MRI case above. Surgical treatment is the Tommy-John surgery, which is highly effective.

- 内侧副韧带撕裂可累及肱骨附着点、尺骨高耸结节附着点或韧带中部。常见的损伤形式是剥离高耸结节附着点的表面，形成如上文MRI病例所示的T征。外科治疗采用Tommy-John手术，非常有效。

Triceps tear

肱三头肌肌腱撕裂

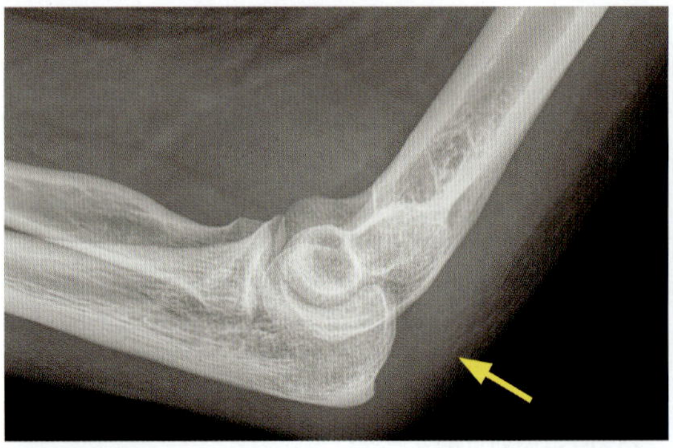

Lateral radiograph
侧位X线影像

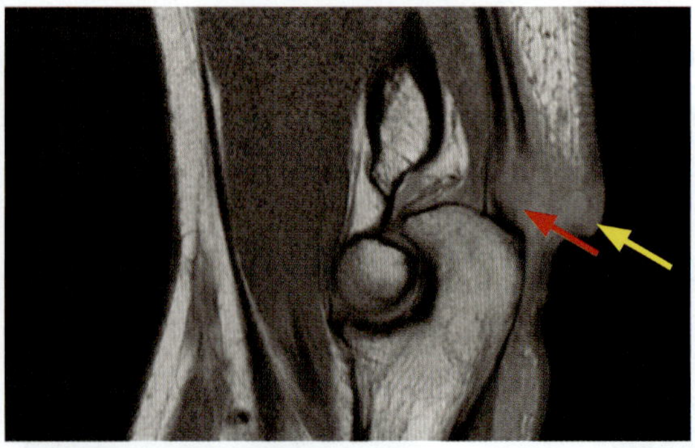

Sagittal PD-weighted MRI
矢状位PD加权MRI

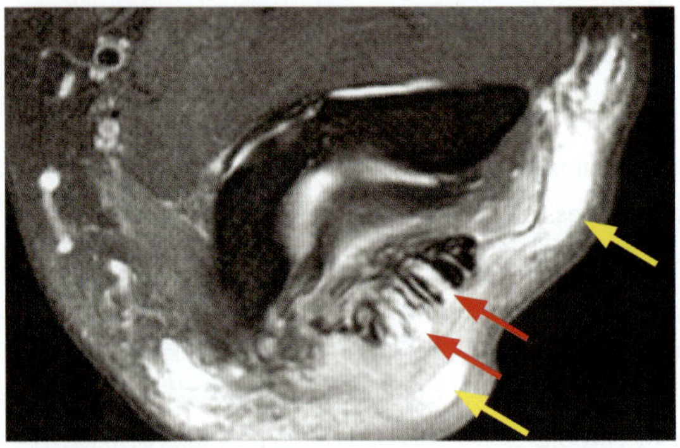

Axial T2-weighted MRI with fat suppression
轴位T_2加权脂肪抑制MRI

High-grade triceps tear:
Radiograph shows subcutaneous edema posterior to the olecranon (yellow arrow). There is no bony avulsion.
MRI shows extensive edema posterior to the distal triceps (yellow arrows), with high-grade tearing (red arrows).

肱三头肌肌腱重度撕裂：
X线影像显示鹰嘴后方皮下水肿(黄箭)。没有骨性撕脱。
MRI显示肱三头肌远端后方广泛水肿(黄箭)，伴严重肌腱撕裂(红箭)。

- Triceps tears are relatively rare. Athletic injuries are usually seen in the setting of weightlifting and high-level football players. Non-athletic traumatic injuries often have a predisposing factor such as olecranon bursitis or steroid use.
- The three heads of the triceps insertion distally on the olecranon of the ulna. Triceps tears commonly involve a bony avulsion of the olecranon.

- 肱三头肌肌腱撕裂相对少见。运动性损伤通常见于举重运动员和高强度橄榄球运动员。非运动性创伤通常有一个诱发因素，如鹰嘴囊炎或使用类固醇。
- 肱三头肌远端的三个头止于尺骨鹰嘴。肱三头肌肌腱撕裂通常伴随鹰嘴撕脱性骨折。

Distal biceps tear

肱二头肌远端肌腱撕裂

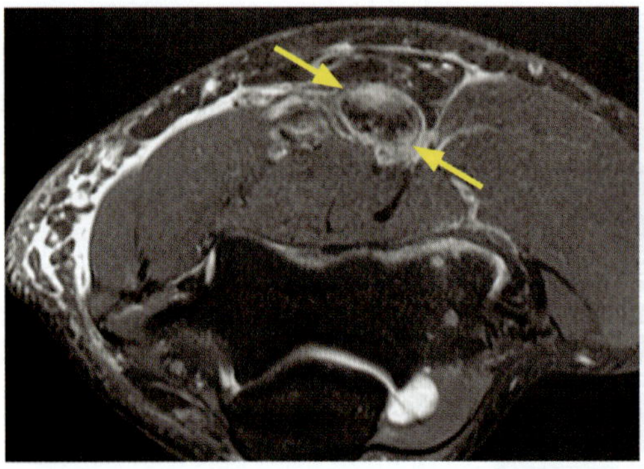

Axial T2-weighted MRI with fat suppression
轴位T_2加权脂肪抑制MRI

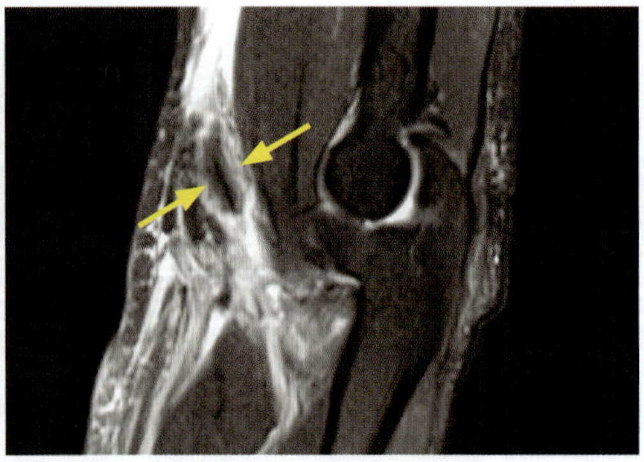

Sagittal PD-weighted MRI with fat suppression
矢状位PD加权脂肪抑制MRI

Full-thickness distal biceps tear:
MRI images show tear of the distal biceps (yellow arrows) from its attachment of the radial tuberosity, with retraction of the torn tendon proximal to the lacertus fibrosus.

远端肱二头肌肌腱全层撕裂：
MRI图像示肱二头肌远端肌腱桡骨粗隆附着点撕裂(黄箭)，撕裂的肌腱回缩至肱二头肌腱膜的近端。

- The long and short heads of the distal biceps insert adjacent to each other on the radial tuberosity.
- The bicipital aponeurosis (known as the lacertus fibrosus) is located at the level of the myotendinous junction. When intact, it helps prevent proximal retraction of the biceps. Conversely, if proximal retraction is present then the lacertus fibrosus is presumably torn.

- 肱二头肌长头和短头肌腱远端合成一股肌腱束止于桡骨粗隆。
- 肱二头肌腱膜(又称二头肌纤维腱膜)位于肌-腱连接水平。当其完好时，有助于防止肱二头肌向近端回缩。相反，出现近端回缩时，肱二头肌腱膜可能已撕裂。

(翻译　陈紫琪　姚骊)

COMMON HAND AND WRIST INJURIES

常见手和腕部损伤

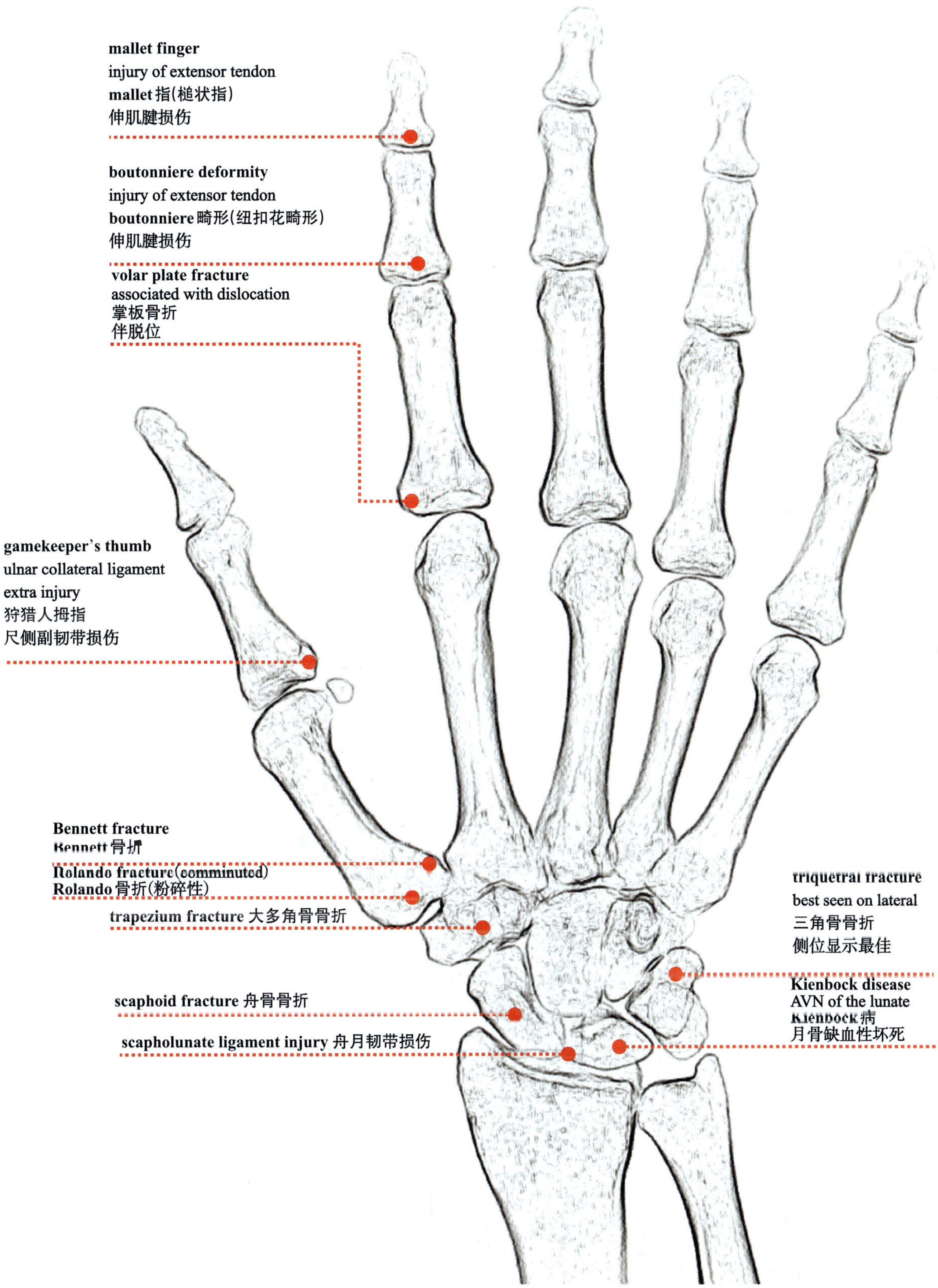

Carpal anatomy and alignment

腕骨解剖和排列

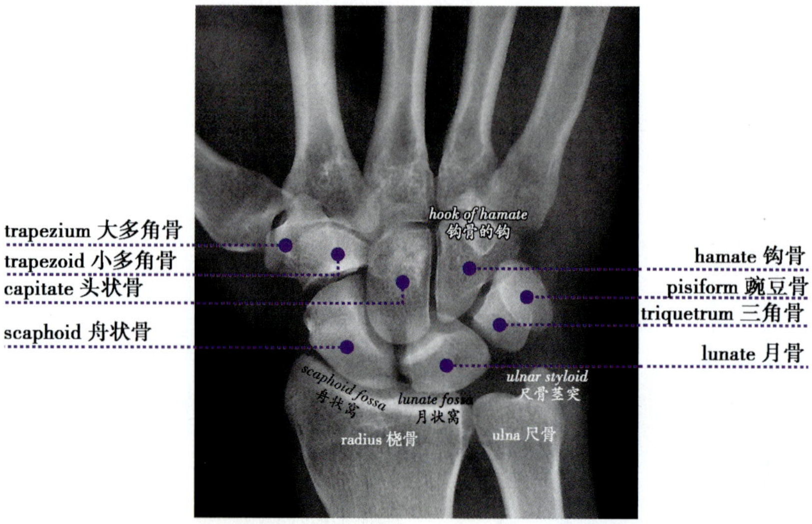

Arcs of Gilula should be smooth and continuous. Disruption may be a sign of ligamentous injury or fracture.

Gilula弓应连续光滑。如果连续性中断可能是韧带损伤或骨折的一个征象。

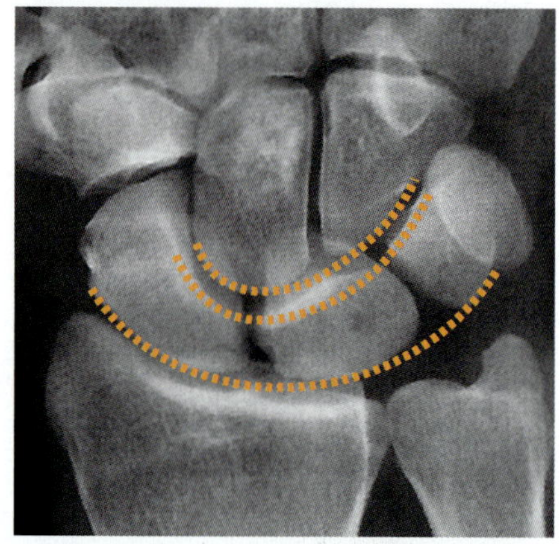

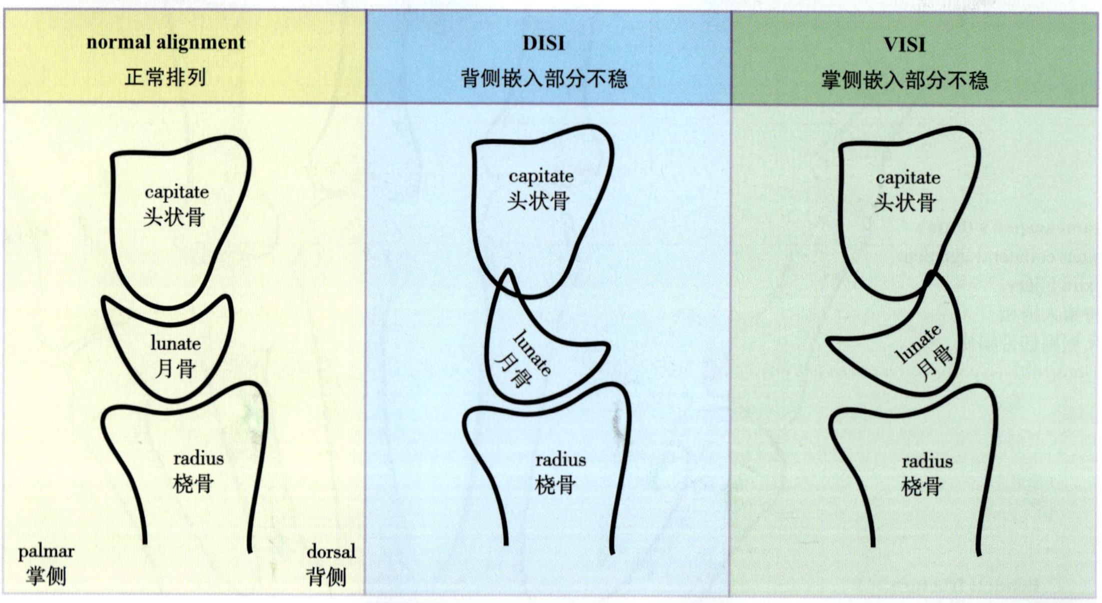

In DISI (dorsal intercalated segmental instability), the lunate is tilted backwards (dorsally; yellow arrow), typically due to scapholunate ligament tear or scaphoid problem.

In VISI (volar intercalated segmental instability, the lunate is tilted forwards (volarly; red arrow), typically due to lunotriquetral ligament tear.

Intercalated means something interposed or inserted between something else. This is just a fancy way of saying that the radius and capitate are in normal alignment and the lunate is not.

背侧嵌入部分不稳(DISI),月骨向后倾斜(背侧,黄箭),通常由舟月韧带撕裂或舟骨问题引起。

掌侧嵌入部分不稳(VISI),月骨向前倾斜(掌侧,红箭),通常由月三角韧带撕裂引起。

Intercalated的意思是某物夹在或插在其他物体之间。这只是一种比较好听的说法,指的是桡骨和头状骨正常排列,而月骨则不在正常位置。

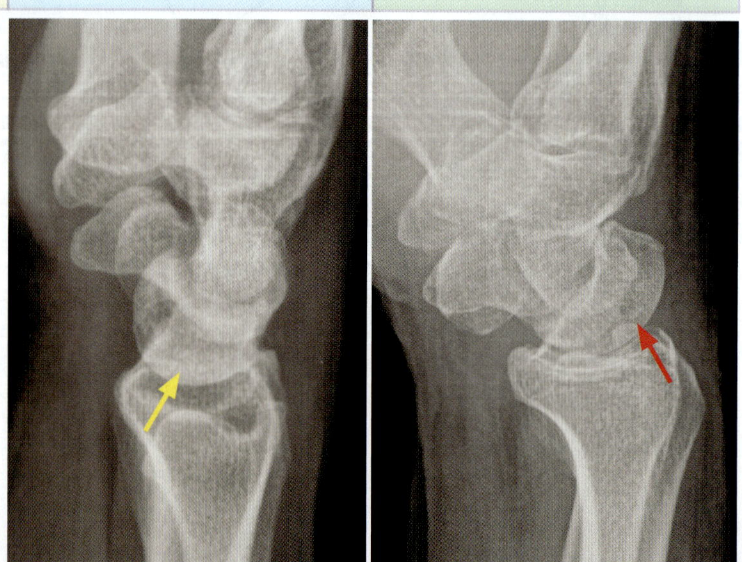

Lunate and perilunate dislocation

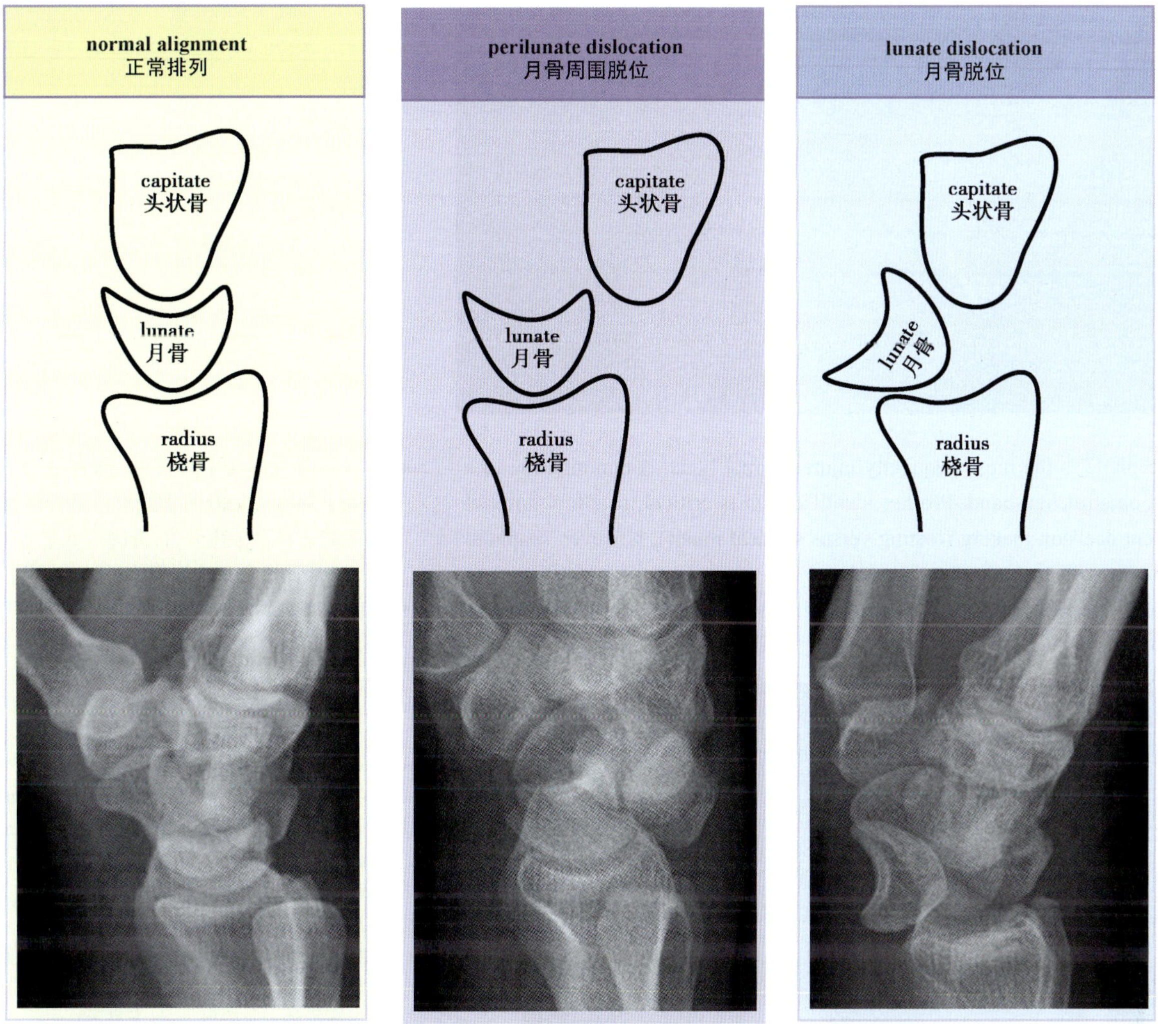

- In a **perilunate dislocation**, the lunate is aligned with the radius, but capitate is not aligned with the lunate. Dislocation is *next to* the lunate (*peri*-lunate).
- In a **lunate dislocation**, the lunate is dislocated volarly, but capitate is still relatively aligned with the radius. The lunate itself is dislocated *(lunate dislocation)*.

Scapholunate ligament injury

- Scapholunate ligament injury is one of the many patterns of injury caused by fall on outstretched arm.
- The scapholunate ligament is U-shaped, with dorsal, central, and volar components. The dorsal component is the strongest and most important for carpal stability.
- The *Terry Thomas sign* represents increased distance of scapholunate interval, thought to resemble the gap between the front teeth of the famous British actor from the sixties.
- With scapholunate deficiency, other imbalanced forces on the wrist pull the lunate backwards, resulting in DISI deformity as discussed on the previous page.
- **Scapholunate advanced collapse (SLAC)** wrist is a sequela of chronic scapholunate ligament injury, which may be secondary to osteoarthritis, CPPD arthropathy, or chronic untreated scapholunate dissociation. The capitate migrates proximally to fill the abnormal gap between the scaphoid and lunate.

月骨和月骨周围脱位

- 在**月骨周围脱位**中，月骨与桡骨对齐，但头状骨与月骨错开。脱位发生在月骨周围(peri-lunate)。
- 在**月骨脱位**中，月骨向掌侧脱位，但头状骨仍与桡骨对齐。月骨自身发生脱位(月骨脱位)。

舟月韧带损伤

- 舟月韧带损伤是跌倒时手处于伸展位出现的众多种损伤类型的一种。
- 舟月韧带呈U形，由背侧、中央和掌侧部分组成。背侧部分对腕关节稳定作用最强也最为重要。
- Terry Thomas征指舟-月骨间隙增宽，很像20世纪60年代英国著名演员特里-托马斯的门牙缝。
- 由于舟月韧带功能受损，作用于手腕上的其他不平衡力量将月骨向后方牵拉，导致背侧嵌入部分不稳，正如上文所讨论的那样。
- **舟月骨晚期塌陷**(SLAC)手腕是舟月韧带慢性损伤的结果，它可继发于骨关节炎、CPPD关节病，或慢性未经治疗的舟月骨脱位。头状骨向近侧移动填补舟骨、月骨间的异常间隙。

Scaphoid fracture

舟骨骨折

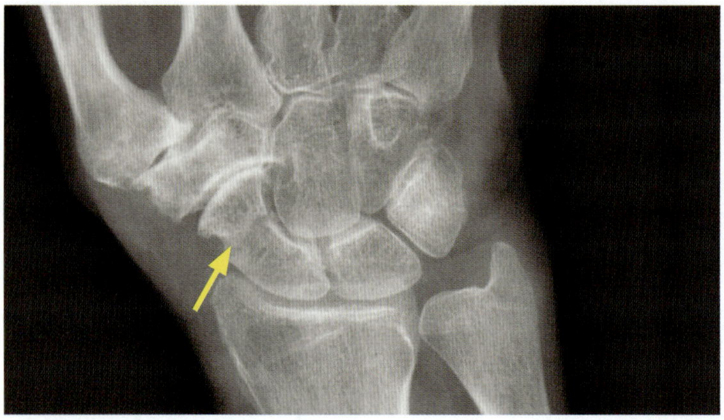

Scaphoid fracture: Radiograph of the wrist shows a minimally displaced fracture of the scaphoid (arrow).
舟骨骨折：腕部X线影像显示有轻度移位的舟骨骨折(箭)。

- The scaphoid is the most frequently injured carpal bone, commonly due to a fall on outstretched hand. Prompt identification is critical, to allow optimal treatment decision-making (casting versus surgical repair); however, scaphoid fractures are often occult on radiography.
- MRI plays an important role in detection of suspected occult scaphoid fracture.

- 舟骨在腕骨损伤中最常见，通常是由于跌倒时手处于伸展位。及时识别对于选择最佳的治疗方案的选择至关重要(石膏固定或手术治疗)；然而，舟骨骨折在X线影像上往往看不到。
- MRI在诊断疑似隐匿性舟骨骨折中起重要作用。

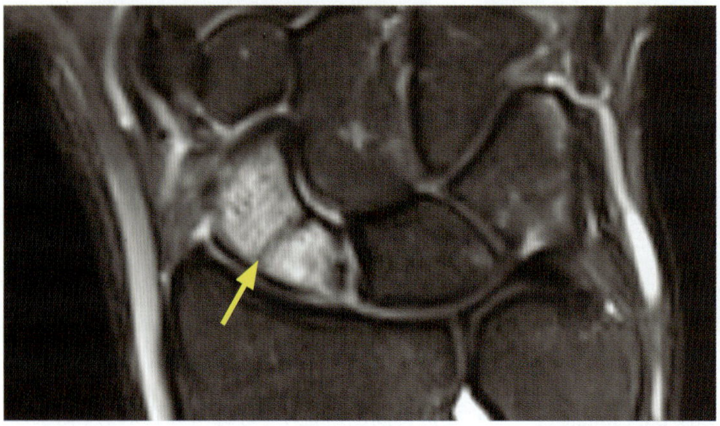

Scaphoid fracture (different patient from above):
Coronal PD-weighted MRI with fat suppression demonstrates edema throughout the scaphoid and a low-signal intensity line (yellow arrow) through the scaphoid waist.
This fracture was occult on radiography (not shown).
舟骨骨折(与上图不是同一名患者)：
冠状位PD加权脂肪抑制MRI显示整个舟骨水肿，舟骨的腰部有一条低信号线(黄箭)。
这个骨折在X线影像上是隐匿性的(未显示)。

- Blood supply to scaphoid is interosseous, from distal to proximal in a retrograde fashion. The proximal pole of the scaphoid has a tenuous blood supply and proximal fractures have the highest risk of avascular necrosis.

- 舟骨的血供来自骨间动脉，是一种由远端到近端的逆行供血。舟骨近端血供贫乏，当近端发生骨折时，其缺血性坏死的风险最高。

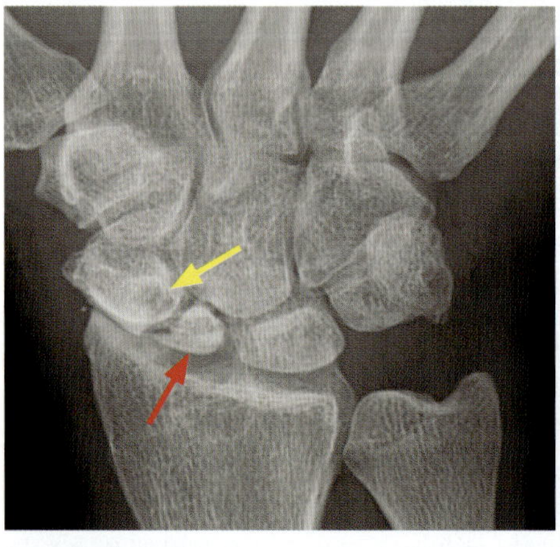

Frontal radiograph
正位X线影像

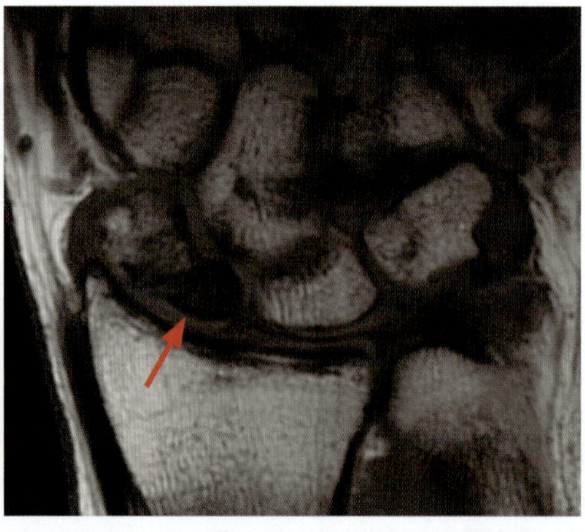

Coronal T1-weighted MRI
冠状位MR T_1加权

Chronic scaphoid fracture with avascular necrosis (in a third patient): Radiograph shows a chronic-appearing scaphoid fracture with cystic change in the distal pole (yellow arrow). There is subtle sclerosis of the proximal pole on radiograph corresponding to diffuse low signal intensity of the proximal pole on MRI (red arrows), in keeping with avascular necrosis.
慢性舟骨骨折伴缺血性坏死(第三名患者)：X线影像显示一处慢性舟骨骨折，远端有囊性改变(黄箭)。X线影像上可见近端轻微硬化，与MRI上近端弥漫性低信号(红箭)相对应，符合缺血性坏死。

Triquetral fracture

三角骨骨折

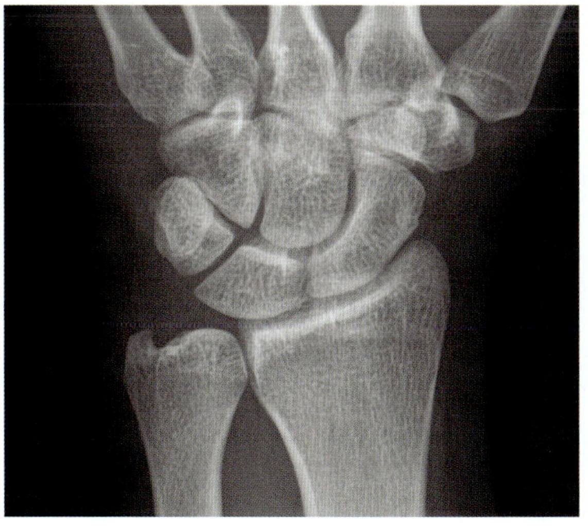

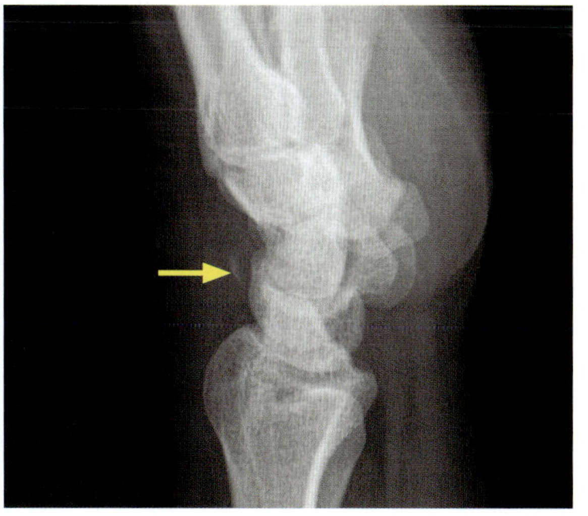

Triquetral fracture: Frontal radiograph (left image) of the wrist is normal. Lateral radiograph shows an avulsion fragment dorsal to the triquetrum (arrow).
三角骨骨折：腕部正位X线影像为正常(左图)。侧位影像显示一个从三角骨背侧撕脱的骨片(箭)。

- Fracture of the triquetrum can be subtle to detect on the frontal radiograph. Triquetral fractures are best seen on the lateral view of the wrist as an avulsion fragment dorsal to the triquetrum.

- 三角骨骨折在正位X线影像上较难被发现。腕部侧位影像显示最佳，因为撕脱骨片位于三角骨的背侧。

Kienbock disease

Kienbock病

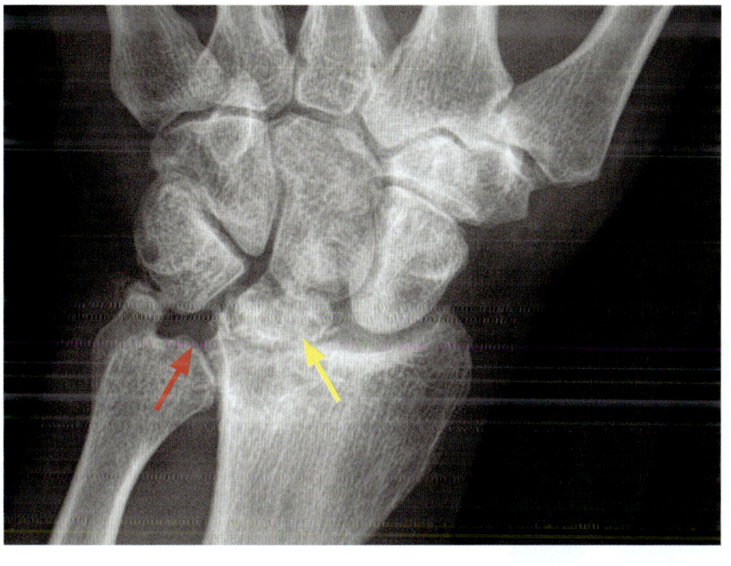

Kienbock disease:
Frontal radiograph of the wrist demonstrates a diminutive and irregular appearance of the lunate (yellow arrow), with severe radiolunate joint space loss. There is slight ulnar negative variance (red arrow).
Kienbock病.
手腕正位X线影像显示月骨(黄箭)小而不规则，桡月关节间隙重度狭窄。尺骨有轻微的阴性变异(红箭)。

- Kienbock disease is avascular necrosis of the lunate. It is associated with negative ulnar variance (i.e., ulna shorter than the radius), and thought to be caused by increased load on the lunate.

- Kienbock病指月骨的缺血性坏死。它与尺骨阴性变异(即尺骨短于桡骨)相关，可能为月骨负荷增加所致。

Anatomy - extensor tendons

解剖 - 伸肌腱

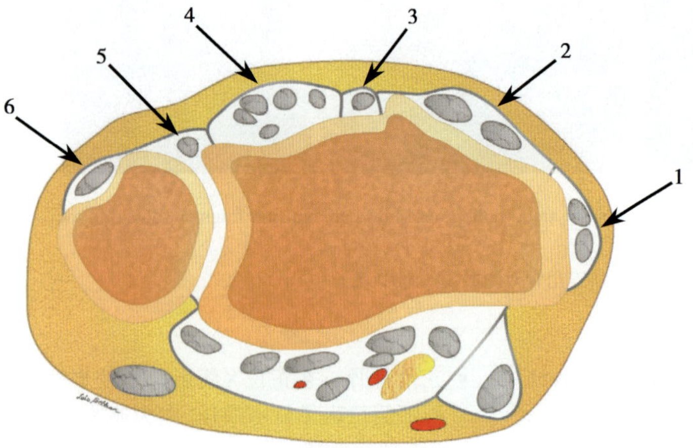

Illustration by Luis Beltran, MD

Wrist extensor compartments:

Compartment 1:

APL (abductor pollicis longus)

EPB (extensor pollicis brevis)

Compartment 2:

ECRL (extensor carpi radialis longus)

ECRB (extensor carpi radialis brevis)

Compartment 3:

EPL (extensor pollicis longus)

Compartment 4:

ED (extensor digitorum tendons)

EI (extensor indicis)

Compartment 5:

EDM (extensor digitorum minimi)

Compartment 6:

ECU (extensor carpi ulnaris)

腕伸肌室：

第1伸肌室：

APL(拇长展肌腱)

EPB(拇短伸肌腱)

第2伸肌室：

ECRL(桡侧腕长伸肌腱)

ECRB(桡侧腕短伸肌腱)

第3伸肌室：

EPL(拇长伸肌腱)

第4伸肌室：

ED(指伸肌腱)

EI(示指伸肌腱)

第5伸肌室：

EDM(小指伸肌腱)

第6伸肌室：

ECU(尺侧腕伸肌腱)

De Quervain's tenosynovitis

De Quervain腱鞘炎

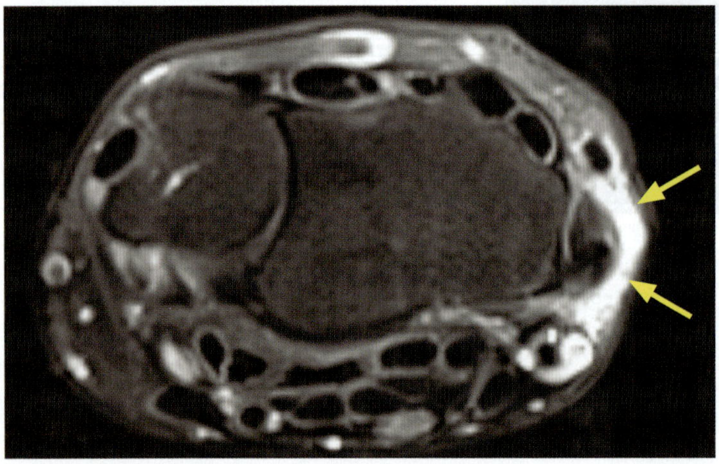

De Quervain's tenosynovitis:
Axial T2-weighted MRI with fat suppression demonstrates edema surrounding extensor compartment 1 (arrows), consistent with de Quervain's tenosynovitis.

De Quervain腱鞘炎：
轴位T_2加权脂肪抑制MRI显示第一伸肌室周围水肿(箭)，符合De Quervain腱鞘炎。

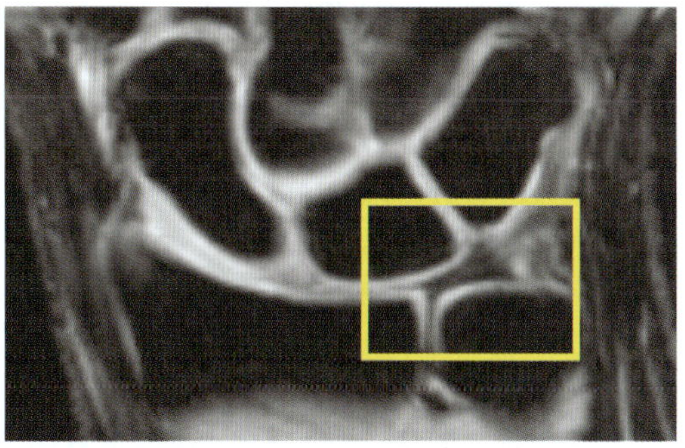

Coronal GRE MR
冠状位梯度回波序列MR

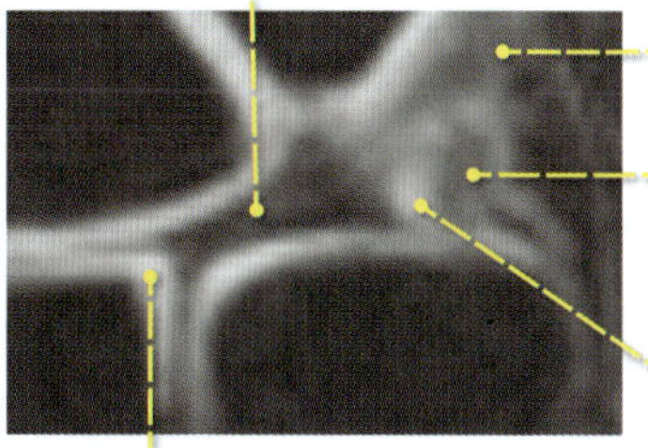

Annotated magnified image (FOV yellow box)
带注释的放大图像(黄色方框)

Normal TFC anatomy: The triangular fibrocartilage complex (TFCC) is a complex structure comprised of multiple confluent ligamentous structures supporting a fibrocartilaginous disc (the TFC proper). On the radial aspect, the TFC disc attaches to the radial articular cartilage, and on the ulnar aspect the TFC is attached to both the ulnar styloid and ulnar fovea (depression at the radial base of the ulnar styloid). Dorsal and ulnar attachments are from the dorsal and volar radioulnar ligaments (not shown above).

The ligamentum subcruentum is normal high signal intensity connective tissue at the ulnar aspect of the TFC disc, which is important not to confuse for a tear.

A confusingly named structure, the meniscus homolog is loose fibrovascular tissue that is not typically individually evaluated on MR. It is not related to the knee meniscus.

正常TFC解剖：三角纤维软骨复合体(TFCC)是一个由多个融合性韧带结构组成的复杂结构，支撑纤维软骨盘(TFC本身)。在桡侧，TFC盘附着在桡骨关节软骨上。在尺侧，TFC附着在尺骨茎突和尺骨中心凹(尺骨茎突的桡侧底部凹陷)上。背侧和尺侧附着物来自桡尺背侧和掌侧韧带(上面未显示)。

三角韧带间隙是位于TFC盘尺侧的结缔组织，正常呈高信号，勿将其误认为撕裂。

半月板同系物的命名容易被混淆，它是疏松的纤维血管组织，通常不会在MR上对其进行单独评估。它与膝关节半月板无关。

Triangular fibrocartilage (TFC) tear | 三角纤维软骨(TFC)撕裂

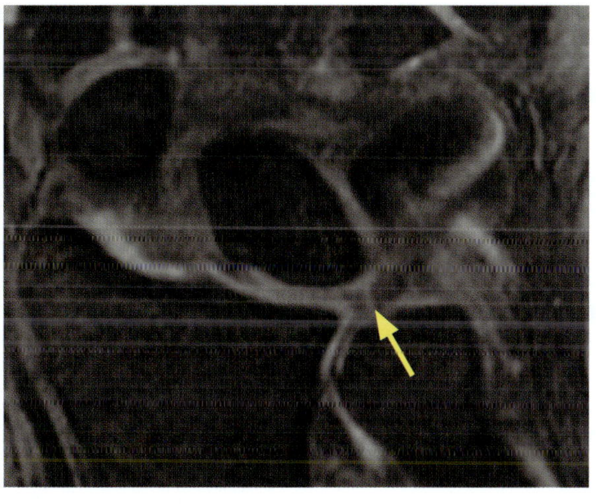

Traumatic TFC tear:
Coronal PD-weighted MRI with fat suppression shows a focal slit-like perforation (yellow arrow) in the central aspect of the TFC disc, consistent with a Palmer ⅠA lesion. The TFC is normal in thickness, the radial articular cartilage is normal, and there is no surrounding degenerative change.
外伤性TFC撕裂：
冠状位PD加权脂肪抑制MRI显示TFC盘的中央有一个局部狭缝状穿孔(黄箭)，与Palmer ⅠA病变一致。TFC厚度正常，桡关节软骨正常，周围无退行性改变。

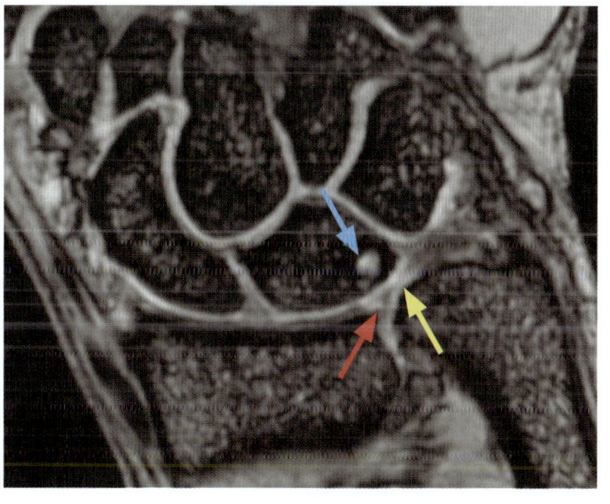

Degenerative TFC tear (different patient from left):
Coronal GRE MRI shows a thinned TFC tear with central tearing (yellow arrow). There is thinning and irregularity of the radial articular cartilage (red arrow) and cystic change of the ulnar aspect of the lunate (blue arrow).
退行性TFC撕裂(与左侧图像为不同患者)：
冠状位梯度回波序列MRI显示TFC变薄，中央撕裂(黄箭)。桡关节软骨变薄、不规则(红箭)和月骨尺侧囊状改变(蓝箭)。

- TFC tears can be traumatic or degenerative. Traumatic tears can involve the TFC disc proper, the radial attachment, the ulnar attachments, or the dorsal or volar radioulnar ligaments.
- The Palmer classification provides a helpful framework to classify TFC tears.

  In the Palmer classification, traumatic (type Ⅰ) lesions are described based on their location, and include central perforation (ⅠA; as shown in the case above left), ulnar avulsion (ⅠB), distal avulsion (ⅠC), and radial avulsion (ⅠD). Degenerative (type Ⅱ) lesions are graded by the degree of radiolunate chondral degeneration/arthritis, as shown in the case above right.
- Degenerative tears are associated with radial and lunate cartilage degeneration.
- A key imaging finding on arthrography is abnormal communication of the radiocarpal joint space (where contrast is injected) with the distal radioulnar joint. When this communication is seen, a TFC tear is present.

- TFC撕裂可以是创伤性或退行性的。创伤性撕裂可累及TFC盘本身、桡骨附着物、尺骨附着物或桡尺骨背侧或掌侧韧带。
- Palmer分类为TFC撕裂提供了一个有用的框架。

  在Palmer分类中，创伤性(Ⅰ型)损伤根据其位置进行描述，包括中央穿孔(ⅠA；如左上图所示)、尺骨撕脱(ⅠB)、远端撕脱(ⅠC)和桡骨撕脱(ⅠD)。退行性(Ⅱ型)病变根据桡月软骨退变/关节炎的程度进行分级，如右上图所示。
- 退行性撕裂与桡骨和月骨软骨退变有关。
- 关节造影的一个关键性影像学表现是桡腕关节间隙(注射造影剂的地方)与远端桡尺关节有交通异常。当发现这样的交通时，提示有TFC撕裂。

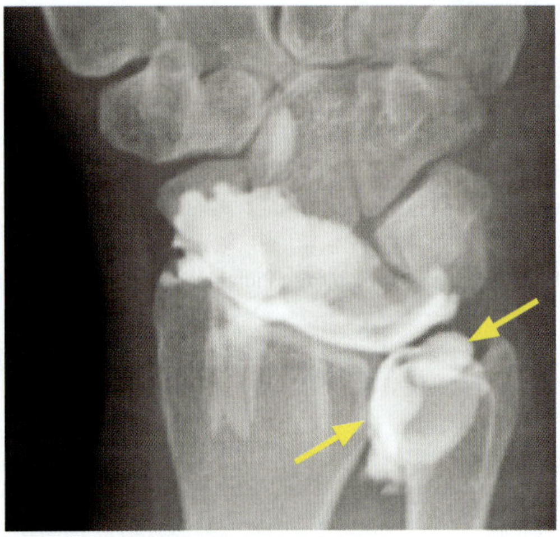

Post-arthrography radiograph demonstrates contrast in the distal radioulnar joint (yellow arrows) from a radiocarpal injection, indicating a TFC tear.
关节造影后X线影像显示桡腕关节注射造影剂后在远端尺桡关节(黄箭)出现造影剂，表明TFC撕裂。

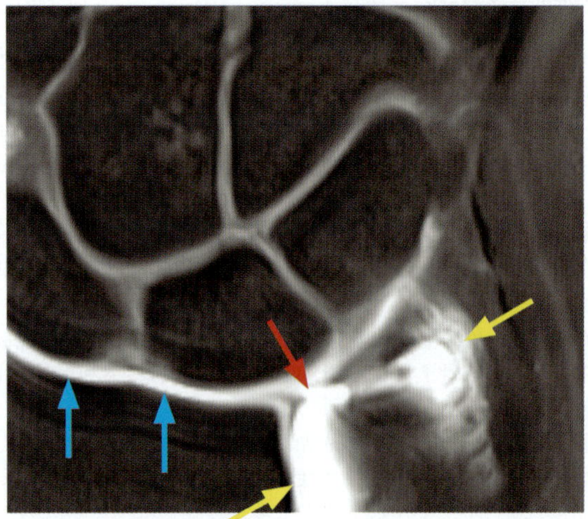

Post-arthrogram T1-weighted MRI with fat suppression in the same patient demonstrates a tear of a diminutive TFC (red arrow), and contrast communicating between the radiocarpal (blue arrow) and distal radioulnar (yellow arrow) joints.
同一名患者关节造影后T_1加权脂肪抑制MRI显示变小的TFC有一条撕裂(红箭)，桡腕关节(蓝箭)和远端尺桡关节(黄箭)之间有造影剂交通。

FINGERS AND HAND TRAUMA

指和手外伤

Extension tendon injuries

指伸肌腱损伤

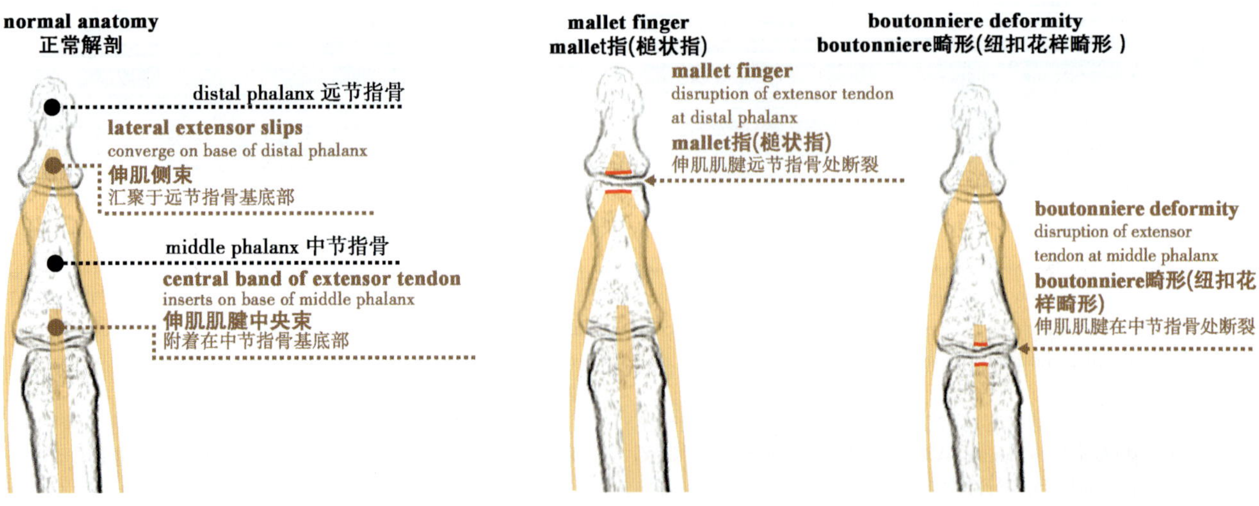

- **Mallet finger**: Mallet finger is disruption of the extensor tendon at the distal phalanx. It is caused by direct impact on the tip of the finger. Mallet finger may be associated with an avulsion fragment of the distal phalanx.

- **Mallet指(槌状指)**：是伸肌肌腱在远节指骨处断裂。为指尖直接受到外力所致。Mallet指可伴有远节指骨的撕脱骨片。

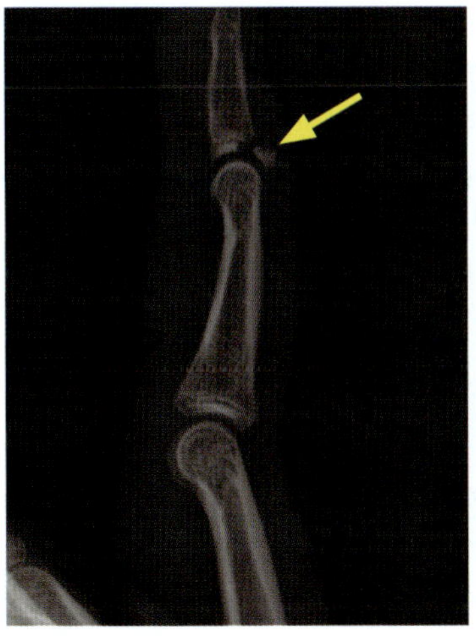
Mallet finger
Mallet指

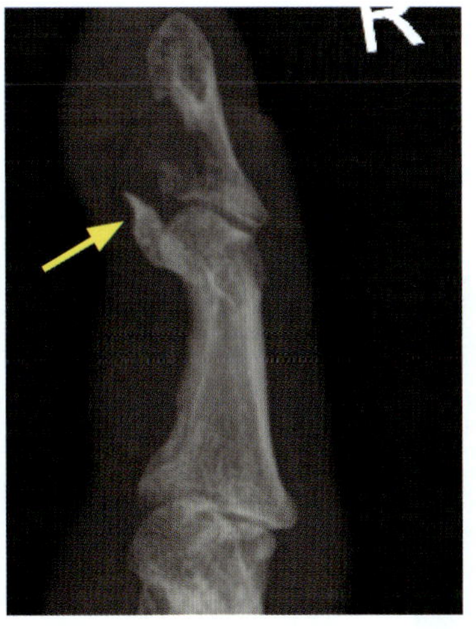

Jersey finger
Jersey指

Mallet (extensor injury) contrasted with Jersey (flexor injury) fingers, in two patients:
Mallet finger involves the dorsal aspect (extensor tendon). Note the dorsal avulsion fragment (arrow).
Jersey finger involves the volar aspect (flexor tendon). Note the volar avulsion fragment (arrow).
A memory aid: People from Jersey shore are known to flex.
比较两名患者中的Mallet指(伸肌损伤)和Jersey指(屈肌损伤)：
Mallet指累及背侧(伸肌腱)。注意背侧撕脱碎片(箭)。
Jersey指累及掌侧(屈肌腱)。注意掌侧撕脱碎片(箭)。
帮助记忆：从泽西沿海来的人知道怎么弯曲。

- On physical exam, the distal interphalangeal (DIP) joint cannot be straightened.
- **Boutonniere deformity** is injury to the medial slip of the extensor tendon. It is seen most commonly in the setting of rheumatoid arthritis, but it may be post-traumatic. The proximal interphalangeal (PIP) joint herniates through the lateral slips of the common extensor tendon and becomes entrapped, causing fixed flexion of the PIP and extension of the DIP.

- 体检时远端指间关节(DIP)不能伸直。
- **Boutonniere畸形**(纽扣花样畸形)是伸肌内侧束损伤。最常见于类风湿关节炎，但也可见于外伤后。近端指间关节(PIP)从伸肌总腱侧束间疝出并嵌顿，造成PIP固定屈曲而DIP伸展。

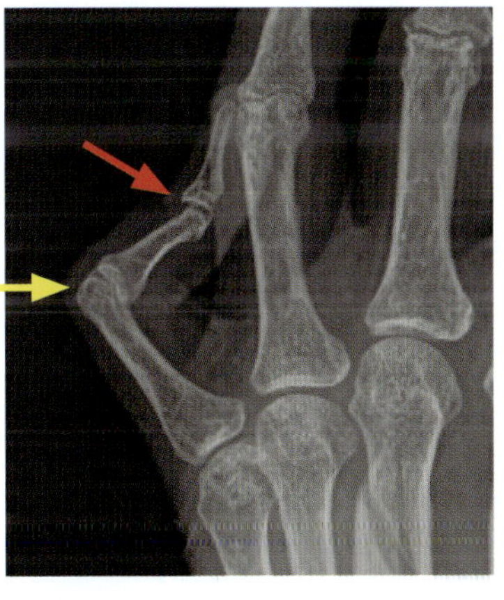

Boutonniere deformity in the setting of rheumatoid arthritis:
Fixed flexion of the PIP (yellow arrow) and hyperextension of the DIP (red arrow).
类风湿关节炎中的Boutonniere畸形：
近端指间关节固定屈曲(黄箭)和远端指间关节过伸(红箭)。

Gamekeeper's thumb (skier's thumb)

守门员拇指(滑雪者拇指)

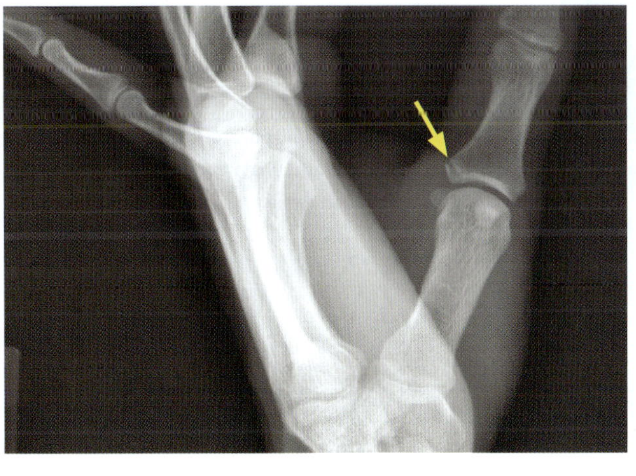

Gamekeeper's thumb with associated nondisplaced avulsion fragment:
Radiograph of the thumb demonstrates a nondisplaced avulsion fragment at the base of the thumb proximal phalanx (arrow).
守门员拇指合并非移位性撕脱骨片：
拇指X线影像显示拇指近节指骨基底部非移位性撕脱骨片(箭)。

- Gamekeeper's (also known as skier's) thumb is injury to the ulnar collateral ligament (UCL) at the base of the thumb proximal phalanx. It is caused by forced abduction of the thumb. Gamekeeper's thumb may be associated with an avulsion fragment of the base of the proximal phalanx.
- Incomplete UCL tears can be treated conservatively; however, complete UCL tears must be treated surgically.
- The *Stener lesion* is a complication of UCL injury and represents complete UCL disruption with interposition of the adductor aponeurosis. The Stener lesion must be treated surgically.

- 守门员拇指(也称滑雪者拇指)是拇指近节指骨基底部尺侧副韧带(UCL)损伤。为拇指的强烈外展所致。守门员拇指可伴有近节指骨基底部撕脱性骨片。
- 不完全性尺侧副韧带(UCL)撕裂可进行保守治疗;但完全性撕裂必须进行手术治疗。
- Stener病变是尺侧副韧带(UCL)损伤的并发症之一,代表完全性尺侧副韧带撕裂合并内收肌腱膜的嵌插。Stener病变必须进行手术。

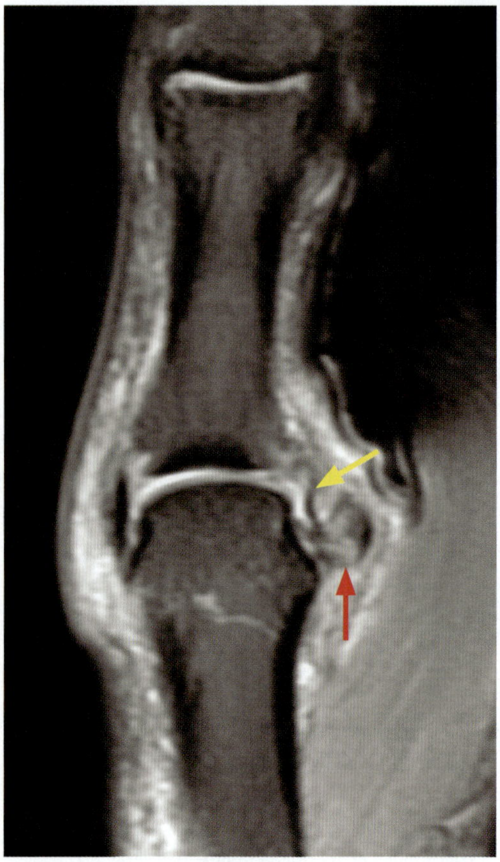

Stener lesion:
Coronal PD-weighted MRI with fat suppression shows a characteristic *Yo-yo on a string sign* indicating a Stener lesion, where the adductor aponeurosis (yellow arrow) is trapped underneath the balled-up and retracted UCL (red arrow).
When this occurs, the adductor aponeurosis appears like a "string" and the UCL is the "yo-yo."
Stener病变:
冠状位PD加权脂肪抑制MRI显示特征性的"溜溜球"征,提示Stener病变,其内收肌腱膜(黄箭)被困在球状和回缩的尺侧副韧带的下方(红箭)。
当这种情况发生时,内收肌腱膜看起来像一根"弦",尺侧副韧带是"溜溜球"。

Bennett fracture

- A Bennett fracture is an intra-articular fracture of the base of the thumb metacarpal.

Bennett骨折

- Bennett骨折是第一掌骨基底部关节内骨折。

Rolando fracture

Rolando骨折

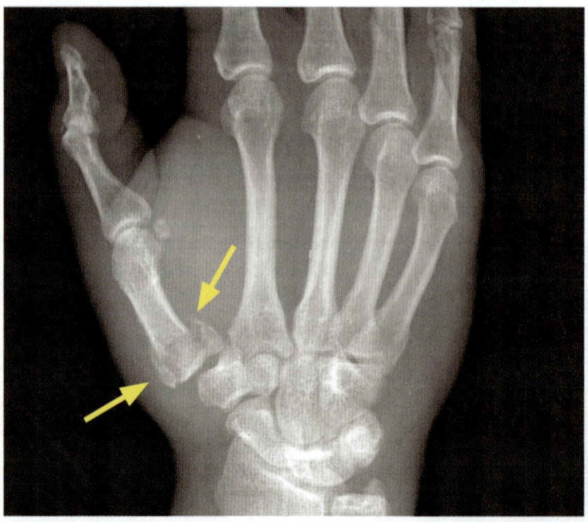

Rolando fracture: PA radiograph of the hand demonstrates a comminuted intra-articular fracture at the base of the thumb metacarpal (arrows).
Rolando骨折:后前位手部X线影像显示第一掌骨基底部关节内粉碎性骨折(箭)。

- A Rolando fracture is a comminuted Bennett fracture.

- Rolando骨折即为粉碎性Bennett骨折。

Boxer's fracture

拳击手骨折

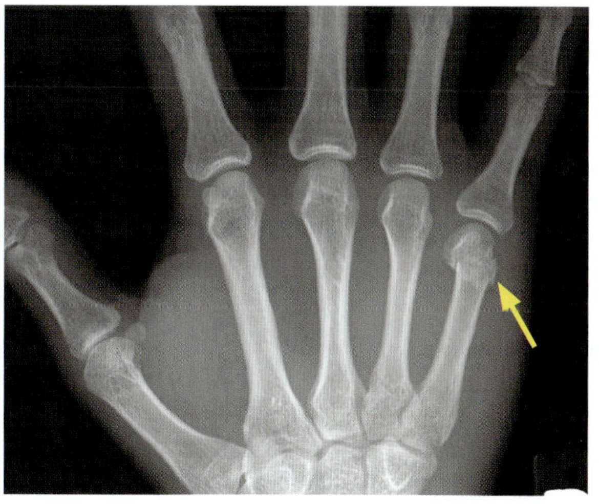

Boxer's fracture: PA radiograph of the hand shows a fracture of the fifth metacarpal neck (arrow).
拳击手骨折：手后前位X线影像显示第五掌骨颈骨折(箭)。

- A Boxer's fracture is a metacarpal neck fracture, most commonly occurring in the fifth metacarpal.

- 拳击手骨折是掌骨颈骨折，最常见于第五掌骨。

Volar plate fracture

掌板骨折

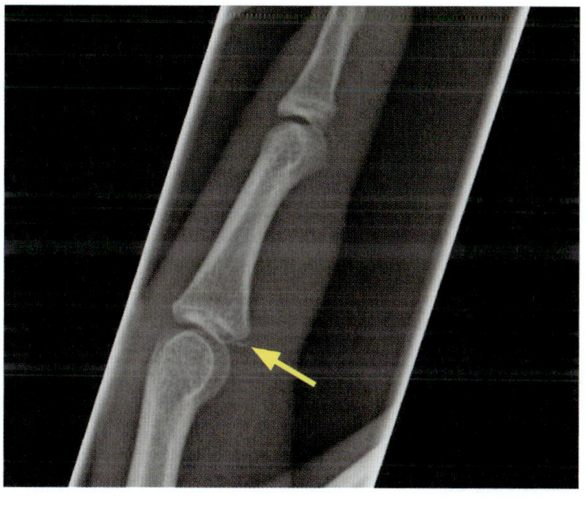

Volar plate fracture: Lateral radiograph shows a subtle tiny avulsion fragment (arrow) of the volar aspect of the middle phalanx at the PIP joint.
掌板骨折：侧位X线影像显示中节指骨近端关节(PIP)掌侧一个微小的撕脱性骨片。

- A volar plate fracture is an avulsion fracture of the volar aspect of the proximal middle phalanx, caused by hyperextension.

- 掌板骨折是中节指骨近端掌侧的撕脱骨折，由过伸所致。

（翻译 张华为 陈榆舒）

MUSCULOSKELETAL INTERVENTIONS

骨骼与肌肉介入

ARTHROGRAPHY

关节造影

General principals

一般原则

- Arthrography can be performed for diagnostic or therapeutic purposes.
- In diagnostic arthrography, contrast is injected into the joint to assess the intra-articular structures, such as cartilage, menisci, labra, ligaments, and to evaluate for intra-articular bodies. Post-arthrogram MR or CT is almost always performed.

- 关节造影可用于诊断或治疗。
- 在诊断性关节造影中，向关节内注射造影剂可评估关节内部结构，如软骨、半月板、盂唇、韧带，并对关节内游离体进行评估。关节造影后几乎总是会进行MR或CT检查。

For MR arthrography, a 1 : 100 or 1 : 200 dilution of gadolinium-containing contrast is made. For instance, 0.1 mL of gadolinium contrast diluted in 10 mL of normal saline is a 1 : 100 dilution. This can be admixed with iodinated contrast (at our institution in a 1 : 1 ratio) to be visualized under fluoroscopy. Alternatively, the gadolinium-saline mixture can be injected after a test injection of iodinated contrast to confirm intra-articular position.

- For therapeutic joint injections, steroid and anesthetic medications are injected into the joint under imaging guidance (fluoroscopy, ultrasound, or rarely CT). Steroids are thought to reduce pain by reducing intra-articular inflammation but do not change the course of osteoarthritis, and several recent studies have questioned their effectiveness. Therapeutic injections should be limited to once every six months or once every three months in cases of debilitating pain with prior effective steroid injection.
- Complications of any arthrogram could include infection, hematoma formation, allergic reaction, or mechanical injury from the needle to structures such as tendons, menisci/labra, ligaments, and cartilage.
- Additional steroid-specific complications could include progression of osteoarthritis/subchondral collapse from steroid administration, and systemic steroid side effects (e.g., elevated blood glucose, increased appetite, insomnia).
- Local anesthetic is toxic to chondrocytes ex-vivo. Ropivacaine is thought to be the least chondrotoxic, and bupivacaine the most chondrotoxic.
- There are many variations on safe procedures to perform arthrography, but a few steps should always be performed:

  Patient consent.

  Procedural time-out: confirming identification, procedure, laterality, and allergies.

  Skin marking.

  Sterile preparation and maintenance of sterile field throughout procedure.

  At least one image showing intra-articular contrast should be saved.
- In patients allergic to iodinated contrast, air or gadolinium can be used.

Dose reduction in fluoroscopic procedures

- One should always maintain the ALARA (as low as reasonably achievable) principle for radiation exposure in fluoroscopic procedures.
- Decrease the imaging parameters, by reducing the mA and kVp as low as possible. Many fluoroscopic machines have a "low-dose" mode that should be utilized routinely unless there is a specific reason to turn it off (such as tricky anatomy or unclear pattern of contrast opacification).
- Decrease the number of images taken. This can be done in three ways: by taking fewer images, by pressing the pedal only briefly, and by reducing the frames obtained per second. This last method is often called "pulse" mode, which should always be used unless there is a specific problem-solving need.
- Decrease the source-to-image distance. The image intensifier (II) should always be as close to the patient as feasible. It is ok to "ride" the II up and down during the procedure, in order to best reduce source-to-image distance while maintaining sufficient space to work.
- Cone-in the image as much as possible. Once the basic anatomy is seen on the initial images, there is no need to image the full field of view every time. This is especially important for hip arthrography, where the pelvic sidewalls may be repeatedly radiated.
- Make it fun! It's a friendly competition to play to see who can get the lowest dose, as long as the procedure is done safely, accurately, and with minimal discomfort to the patient.

对于MR关节造影，制备1 : 100或1 : 200的含钆造影剂稀释液。例如，将0.1mL的钆造影剂稀释在10mL的生理盐水，得到的是1 : 100的稀释液。可以将其与碘造影剂混合以便在透视下能够进行观察。或者，在进行过碘造影剂的试验性注射确认关节内的位置后，可以注射钆-盐水混合物。

- 治疗性关节注射需要在影像引导下(透视、超声或极少数情况下CT)向关节内注射类固醇和麻醉药物。类固醇通过减少关节内炎症来缓解疼痛，但不会改变骨关节炎的病程，最近的几项研究对其有效性有质疑。治疗性注射应该限制为每六个月一次，或疼痛严重但先前对类固醇注射治疗有效的情况下，每三个月一次。
- 任何关节造影的并发症可能包括感染、血肿形成、过敏反应或针对肌腱、半月板/关节唇、韧带和软骨等结构的机械性损伤。
- 其他与类固醇相关的并发症可能包括因类固醇注射而引起的骨关节炎/软骨下塌陷，以及系统性类固醇副作用(如血糖升高、食欲增加、失眠等)。
- 局部麻醉在体外对软骨细胞有毒性作用。罗哌卡因被认为对软骨的毒性最低，布比卡因的毒性最大。
- 尽管进行关节造影时所采取的安全措施不尽相同，但总体来说，仍应遵循以下几个步骤：

  知情同意书。

  术前确认：患者身份、手术、左右侧和过敏史。

  标记皮肤。

  无菌消毒和整个手术过程保持无菌状态。

  至少保存一张显示关节内造影剂的图像。
- 对碘造影剂过敏的患者，可以使用气体或钆造影剂。

减少透视手术中的辐射剂量

- 在透视手术中，应始终要遵守ALARA原则(最大可能实现最低剂量)，以降低辐射暴露。
- 降低成像参数，尽可能降低mA和kVp。许多透视机都有"低剂量"模式，应该经常使用，除非有特殊原因需要关闭(如解剖复杂或造影剂不明显)。
- 减少拍摄图像的数量。可以通过三种方式实现：减少获取点片的数量、缩短踩踏脚踏板的时间，以及减少每秒获得图像的帧数。最后一种方法通常称为"脉冲"模式，在不需要解决特定问题时应始终使用该模式。
- 缩短放射源到图像的距离。影像增强器(II)应尽可能靠近患者。在操作过程中，可以在保持足够工作空间的同时，上下移动II，最大限度地缩短放射源到影像的距离。
- 尽可能缩小成像范围。一旦最初的图像看到了基本解剖结构，就没有必要每次都对整个视野进行成像。这对髋关节造影特别重要，因为盆骨侧壁可能会反复受到辐射。
- 让它变得有意思！只要确保手术安全、准确，并尽量减轻患者不适，就可以玩一个友好的比赛，看看谁可以获得最低的剂量。

Shoulder

肩关节

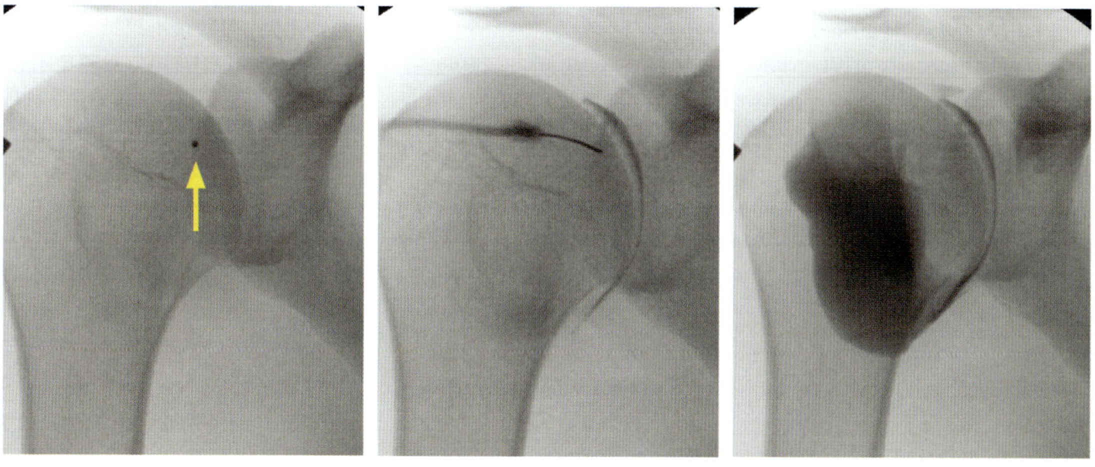

Normal shoulder arthrogram: Initial image (left image) demonstrates ideal BB marker placement (arrow) for a "rotator interval" approach, at the upper inner quadrant of the humeral head. A fluoroscopic image should be obtained after initial injection of contrast (middle image). Post-procedure image demonstrates normal contrast filling the joint, without contrast extravasation into the subacromial-subdeltoid bursa.

正常肩关节造影图像：初始图像(左图)显示了BB标记(箭)在肱骨头上方内侧1/4的"旋转间隙"入路的理想放置位置。在注射造影剂后应获得透视图像(中间图)。术后图像展示了正常的造影剂填充关节，没有造影剂外渗到肩峰下-三角肌下滑囊。

- Similar to hip arthrography, diagnostic and therapeutic shoulder injections are very common. For diagnostic arthrography, a total intra-articular volume of 10–12 mL is typically injected.
- Communication of the glenohumeral joint with the subacromial/subdeltoid bursa indicates a full-thickness rotator cuff tear (presuming that there is no history of prior surgery).

- 类似于髋关节造影术，肩关节的诊断和治疗注射很常见。对于诊断性造影术，通常关节内注射总量为10~12mL。
- 肩关节与肩峰下/三角肌下滑囊的交通表明存在肩袖全层撕裂(假设无既往手术史)。

Hip

- Diagnostic hip MR arthrography is commonly performed to assess for labral tears and chondral injury. A total intra-articular volume of 10–12 mL is typically administered.
- Therapeutic hip injections are commonly performed to reduce osteoarthritis-related pain and inflammation.

髋关节

- 常规进行诊断性髋关节MR造影以评估盂唇撕裂和软骨损伤。通常注入关节内注射总量为10~12mL。
- 治疗性髋关节注射常用于减轻骨关节炎相关的疼痛和炎症。

Wrist

- For diagnostic wrist injections, approximately 3 mL of injectate is administered. Injecting more contrast can increase the chance of contrast extravasating out of the joint, which can complicate image interpretation.
- It is important to inject the contrast under real-time fluoroscopy to visualize any abnormal communication between the radiocarpal compartment (where contrast is injected) and either the distal radioulnar joint or the mid-carpal space.
- Communication between radiocarpal compartment and distal radioulnar joint indicates a tear of the TFC (with an example provided in the "Wrist" section of this chapter).
- Communication between the radiocarpal compartment and the midcarpal space demonstrates tears of either the scapholunate or lunotriquetral ligaments.

腕关节

- 对于诊断性腕关节注射，约使用3mL的注射液体。注射更多的造影剂会增加渗出关节外的可能性，这会使图像解读变得复杂。
- 注射造影剂时，在透视下实时观察任何桡腕关节间隙(注射造影剂的区域)和桡尺远侧关节或中腕关节之间的异常交通非常重要。
- 桡腕间隙与桡尺远侧关节之间出现交通表明三角纤维软骨(TFC)撕裂(本章节"腕关节"部分提供了一个示例)。
- 桡腕间隙与中腕关节之间的沟通表明有舟月韧带或月三角韧带撕裂。

Biopsy

Basic principles of bone and soft tissue biopsy

- Indications for biopsy include need for pathologic diagnosis of an indeterminate or aggressive lesion, confirmation of and/or molecular analysis of suspected metastatic disease, and need for microbial analysis in imaging-confirmed osteomyelitis.

活检

骨和软组织活检的基本原则

- 活检的指征包括需要对不确定或侵袭性病变进行病理诊断，对疑似转移性疾病进行确诊/或分子分析，以及对影像学确诊的骨髓炎进

- It is important to perform a thorough imaging workup prior to biopsy planning, in order to best determine the pre-test probability, target the highest yield portion of the lesion, and avoid unnecessary biopsy.

As an example of the importance of risk-stratifying lesions on imaging prior to biopsy, if complete imaging workup showed an aggressive-appearing lesion with FDG uptake on PET, then a negative or nondiagnostic pathology report would not be concordant, and repeat biopsy should be performed.

In contrast, if complete imaging assessment showed an indeterminate but less-aggressive appearing lesion (such as with minimal enhancement and no or low-level uptake on PET), then an indeterminate pathology report could possibly be followed by short-interval repeat imaging.

- Absolute contraindications are not common but include an inaccessible percutaneous approach, and need to traverse a soft tissue infection to target a non-infected lesion.
- Close consultation with orthopedic oncologists is required when planning biopsy approach, especially for solitary lesions that may ultimately be resected. This collaborative planning ensures that the biopsy tract can be resected at time of surgery and reduces the risk of tumor tract seeding and contamination of additional compartments.

Special considerations

- For thigh biopsies (bone or soft tissues), **it is critical not to traverse the rectus femoris muscle** (unless a lesion of the rectus femoris is being targeted). This is because rectus is one of the primary extensors of the leg traversing both the hip and knee joints, and if it is traversed the rectus may need to be sacrificed to reduce the chance of tumor tract seeding.
- For biopsy of weight-bearing bones of the lower extremity (such as the femur or tibia), it may be necessary for the patient to be on crutches with touch-down weight-bearing, in consultation with the treating orthopedic surgeon.

Soft tissue biopsies

行微生物分析。

- 在制定活检计划之前进行完整的影像学评估非常重要，以便最准确地预测术前概率、确定获取病变的最佳部位，并避免不必要的活检。

例如，在进行活检之前，一个病灶进行了完整的影像学评估，并在PET上由于PDG的摄取显示出侵袭性，如果病理报告为阴性或非诊断性则显然不一致，应进行重复活检。

相反，如果完整的影像学评估显示出不确定但影像学表现为侵袭性较弱的病变（如仅有轻微强化并且PET上无摄取或低水平摄取），则可以在得到不确定的病理报告后进行短期影像学复查评估。

- 绝对禁忌证并不常见，但包括缺乏经皮穿刺的途径和需要穿过软组织感染灶到达非感染性病变区的情况。
- 在规划活检途径时需与骨科肿瘤学家进行密切协商，特别是针对可能最终被切除的孤立性病变。这种协作规划确保在手术时可以切除活检针道，并减少肿瘤针道种植和其他区域污染的风险。

特别注意事项

- 对于大腿活检（骨骼或软组织），**关键是不要穿过股直肌**（除非活检的病灶位于股直肌内）。这是因为股直肌是腿部的主要伸展肌肉，横跨髋关节和膝关节，如果穿过股直肌，可能需要切除股直肌以减少肿瘤针道种植的风险。
- 对于下肢承重骨的活检（如股骨或胫骨），有必要与患者的骨科主治医生进行协商，使用拐杖减轻负重。

软组织活检

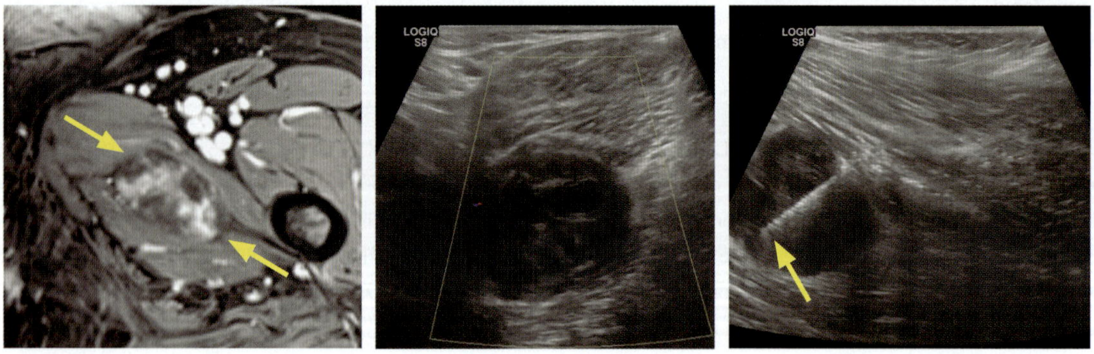

Soft tissue biopsy: Contrast-enhanced MRI shows a heterogeneously enhancing mass in the adductor compartment of the left thigh (arrows). Pre-procedural color Doppler ultrasound demonstrates the mass, with no vascularity along the expected needle tract. Intraprocedural image (right image) demonstrates the biopsy needle (arrow) in the center of the mass. Pathology was a cellular myxoma.
软组织活检：增强MRI显示左大腿收肌间隔内不均匀强化的肿块（箭）。术前彩色多普勒超声显示该肿块，预期的针道周围没有血管。术中图像（右图）显示活检针（箭）位于肿块中央。病理诊断为细胞黏液瘤。

- Soft tissue mass biopsies are generally performed with a coaxial spring-loaded biopsy device. For highest yield, the most avidly enhancing portion (or most avid focus of FDG uptake if a PET was performed) should be targeted as long as it is safe to do so.
- The majority of musculoskeletal soft tissue biopsies can be performed by ultrasound, although CT is often a reasonable modality as well.

- 软组织肿块活检通常使用同轴弹簧活检器材。为了获得更高的阳性检出率，应对增强最明显的部位（或FDG吸收最强的部位，如果进行了PET检查）进行活检，只要安全即可。
- 大多数肌肉骨骼软组织活检可以通过超声引导进行，尽管CT通常也是合理的检查方法。

Bone biopsies

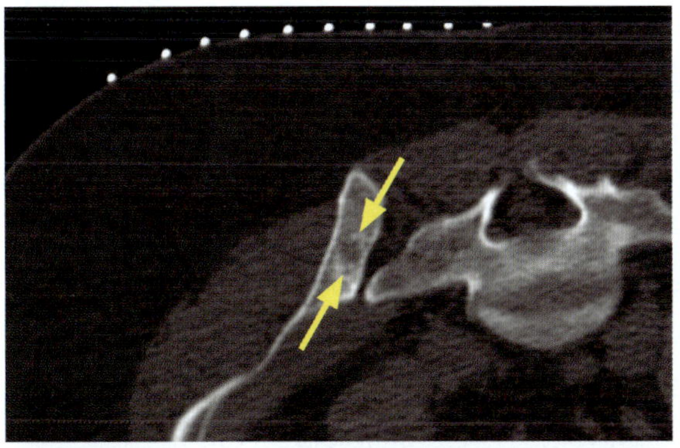

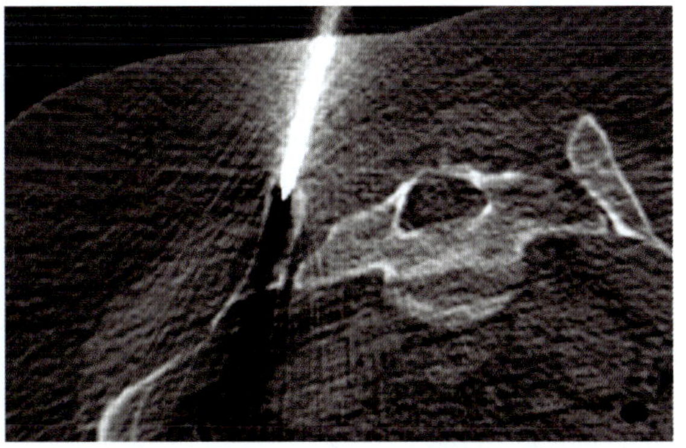

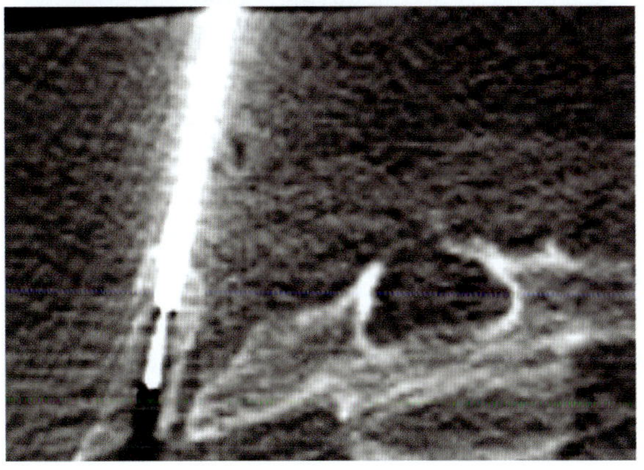

Planning CT image with grid (top left image), with patient prone. The mixed lytic and sclerotic lesion (arrows) of the left iliac bone was targeted.
Intraprocedural CT-fluoroscopic image (top right image) shows the bone biopsy device progressing towards the lesion. The lesion is obscured by streak and beam hardening artifact.
Intraprocedural CT-fluoroscopic image (left image) shows the coaxial biopsy device traversing the region of the lesion, although the lesion is obscured. Careful correlation of landmarks is necessary in this case.
Pathology was metastatic breast cancer.

带有网格的术前俯卧位CT图像(左上图)。瞄准左髂骨混合性溶骨和硬化病变(箭)。
术中的CT透视图像(右上图)显示骨活检针向病变移动。由于条状伪影和线束硬化伪影，病变被遮蔽。
手术过程中的CT透视图像(左图)显示同轴骨活检针穿过病变区域，虽然病变被遮盖。这种情况下需仔细核对位置标志。
病理诊断为乳腺癌转移。

- Most bone biopsies are performed with CT guidance. Lesions that are occult on CT but apparent on MR can generally be targeted by CT using landmarks. MR-guided biopsy may also be performed in suitable cases.
- Similar to fluoroscopic interventions, patient dose should be maintained as low as reasonably achievable. A major contribution to patient dose is the initial planning CT with the grid. This should be performed in a dose-reduced manner, if possible. Intraprocedural CT-fluoroscopy generally yields lower patient dose compared to spiral CT acquisitions.
- To reduce operator dose during CT fluoroscopy, take a step back and stand behind in the wings of the CT gantry. Operator dose is 100 times less in this location compared to the standard location standing next to the patient at the opening of the CT gantry.
- There are several manual and battery-powered drill devices available.
- Lucent lesions generally have higher diagnostic yield than sclerotic lesions.
- Similar to targeting of soft tissue biopsies, the most avidly enhancing component or region of highest FDG uptake should be targeted, as long as it is safe to do so.

Vertebral biopsies

- The safest approach to biopsy a vertebral body is transpedicular, where the biopsy needle traverses the pedicle. The bony walls of the pedicle protect the needle from inadvertently traversing the spinal canal.

Biopsies for osteomyelitis

- The sensitivity of biopsy for diagnosing osteomyelitis is highly variable in the literature, but in general it is quite low.
- Therefore, biopsy should not be performed to diagnose osteomyelitis in equivocal cases. Rather, it is useful to obtain microbial cultures and sensitivities when imaging already confirms osteomyelitis.

骨骼活检

- 大多数骨组织活检在CT引导下进行。在CT上隐蔽但MR上明显的病变通常可以通过CT利用解剖标志进行定位。在适当的病例，骨活检也可以在MR引导下进行。
- 与透视下进行介入手术相类似，应尽量降低患者的剂量。患者剂量的主要来源于CT成像网格初始模型。如果可能，应以降低剂量的方式进行。与螺旋CT采集相比，术中CT透视通常对患者产生较低的剂量。
- 为了减少CT透视操作者的剂量，可以向后退一步并站在CT环的侧翼。在此位置，操作者的剂量比站在CT环口旁的标准位置要低100倍。
- 有几种手动和电池驱动的钻孔设备可供选择。
- 透亮的病变通常比硬化性病变具有更高的诊断价值。
- 与软组织活检定位类似，应采集强化最明显的部分或FDG摄取最高的区域，前提是安全。

椎体活检

- 活检取样椎体最安全的方法是经椎弓根穿刺，取样针穿过椎弓根。椎弓根的骨壁可以保护针头不会意外穿过椎管。

骨髓炎组织活检

- 活检诊断骨髓炎的敏感性在文献中差异极大，但通常都很低。
- 因此，对不确定的病例不应该通过活检来诊断骨髓炎。相反，当影像学已经确认骨髓炎时，活检对获取微生物培养和药敏试验是有用的。

（翻译　刘杰克　陈榆舒　杨曦玥）

14 Pediatric Imaging

Ngoc-Anh T. Tran, Ellen X. Sun, Sanjay P. Prabhu, Michael P. George

14 小儿影像

Contents

目录

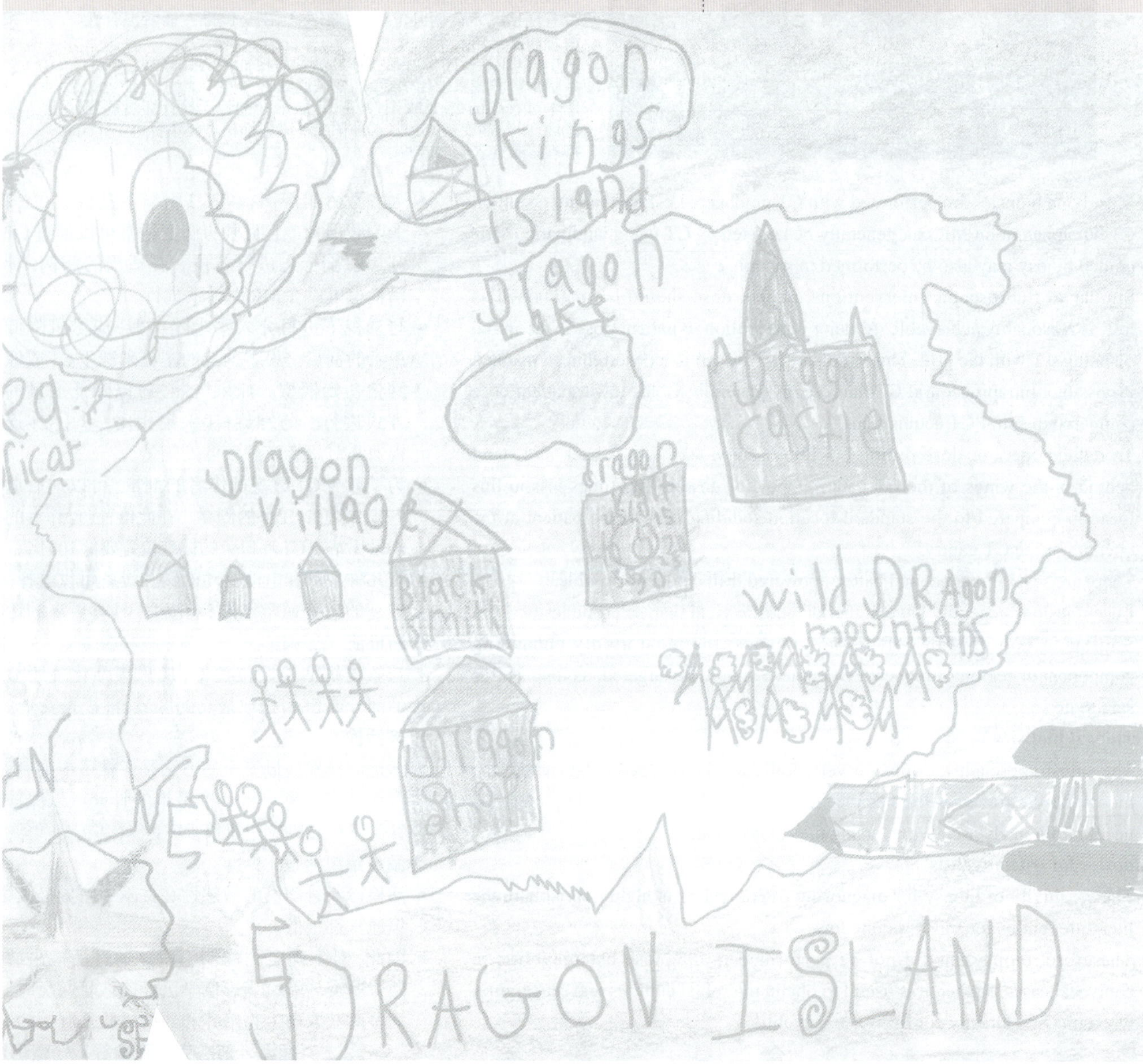

Pediatric Airway

小儿气道

Anatomy

解剖

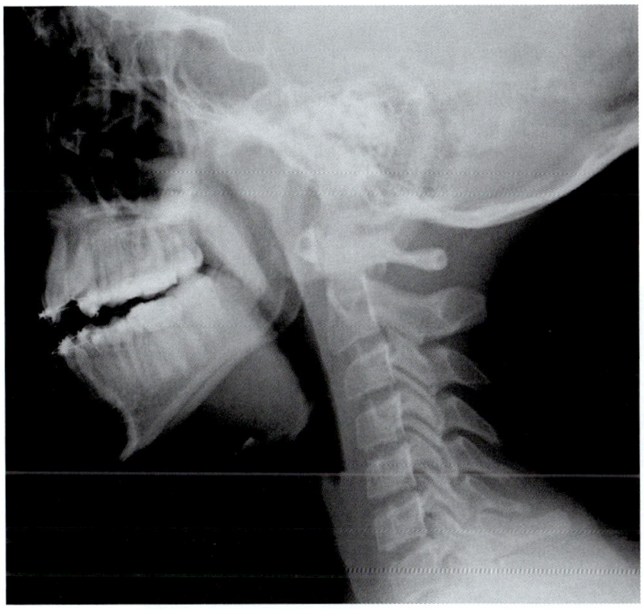

Normal lateral neck radiograph

正常颈部侧位影像

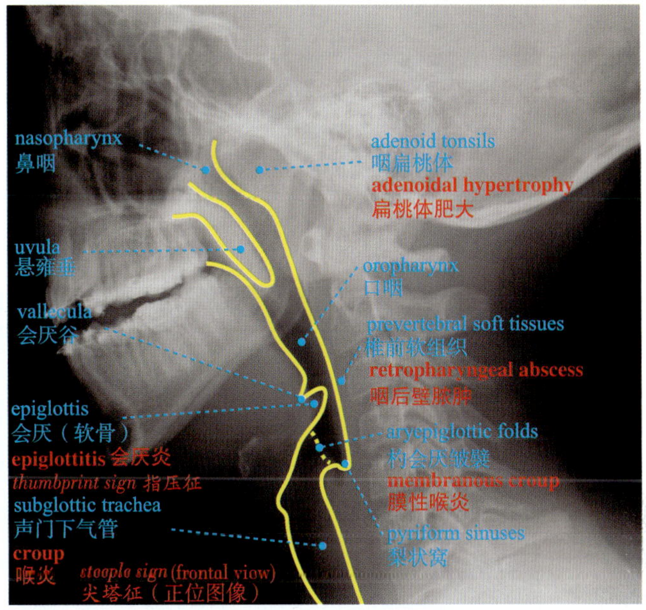

Normal anatomy (blue) and associated pathology (red)

正常解剖(蓝色)和相关病理(红色)

Pediatric upper airway obstruction

- Upper airway obstruction above the level of the trachea can be congenital, neoplastic, or infectious.
- Upper airway obstruction can also be classified by anatomic level: Nasopharyngeal (i.e., choanal atresia, rhabdomyosarcoma, adenoidal hypertrophy), or oropharyngeal (i.e., peritonsillar abscess, thyroglossal duct cyst).

Choanal atresia

- Choanal atresia is congenital occlusion of the choanae in the posterior nasal cavity.

  Choanal atresia can be osseous (30%), membranous (<1%), or mixed (70%). There is almost always some degree of osseous abnormality.

- Choanal atresia is often associated with other congenital malformations, most commonly **CHARGE syndrome**:

Coloboma (gap in iris or retina).
Heart defects.
Atresia of choanae.
Retardation of development.
Genitourinary anomalies.
Ear anomalies.

小儿上气道梗阻

- 气管水平以上的上呼吸道梗阻可以是先天性、肿瘤性或感染性的。
- 上呼吸道梗阻也可以按解剖位置进行分类：鼻咽部(包括后鼻孔闭锁、横纹肌肉瘤、腺样体肥大等)或口咽部(包括扁桃体周围脓肿、甲状舌管囊肿等)。

后鼻孔闭锁

- 后鼻孔闭锁是指发生于鼻腔后部的后鼻孔先天性闭锁。

  后鼻孔闭锁可以是骨性(30%)、膜性(< 1%)或混合性闭锁(70%)。几乎所有的病例都伴有不同程度的骨性异常。

- 后鼻孔闭锁常合并其他先天畸形，最常见的是**CHARGE综合征**：

缺损症(虹膜或视网膜缺损)。
心脏缺陷。
后鼻孔闭锁。
生长发育迟缓。
泌尿生殖畸形。
耳畸形。

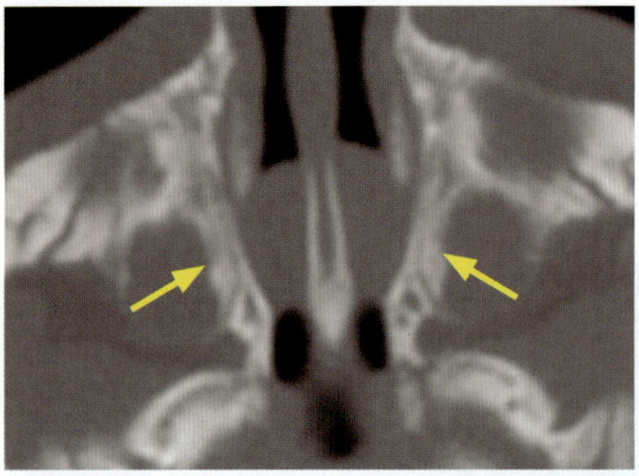

Choanal atresia, mixed membranous and osseous: Axial non-contrast CT shows complete obstruction of both choanae by soft tissue, with medial bowing of the thickened lateral nasal walls (arrows) and medialization of the pterygoid plates. This child had CHARGE syndrome. *Case courtesy Sanjay Prabhu, MBBS, Boston Children's Hospital.*

后鼻孔闭锁(膜性与骨性混合)：轴位平扫CT显示双侧后鼻孔被软组织完全阻塞，同时伴有增厚的鼻侧壁向内弯曲及翼板内移(箭)。这名小儿患有CHARGE综合征。

Pyriform aperture stenosis (PAS)

梨状孔狭窄(PAS)

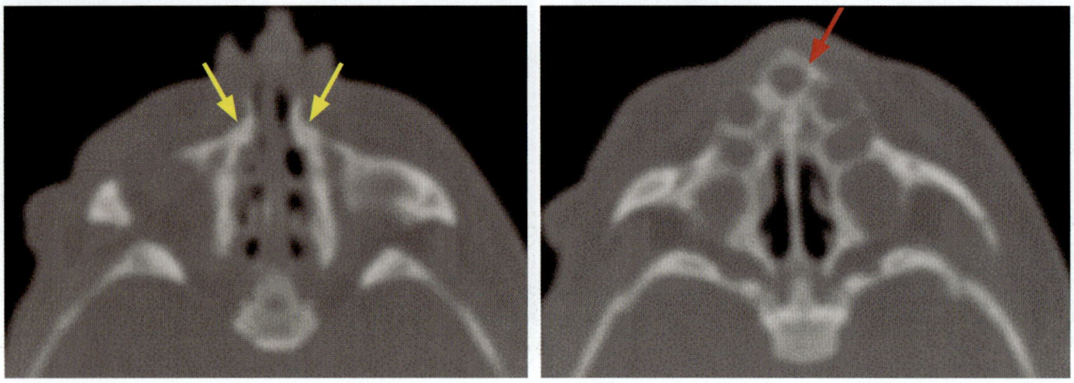

Pyriform aperture stenosis: Axial non-contrast CT shows thickening and medialization of the nasal processes of the maxilla (yellow arrows) with resultant narrowing of the frontal opening of the nose, right greater than left. A central maxillary mega-incisor (red arrow) is also seen.

梨状孔狭窄：轴位平扫CT显示上颌骨鼻突增厚并内移(黄箭)，导致鼻前部开口变窄，右侧较左侧明显。还可以看到中央上颌骨巨大中切牙(红箭)。

- Pyriform aperture stenosis is a rare but potentially lethal cause of congenital upper airway obstruction that may clinically mimic choanal atresia.
- PAS results from early fusion and hypertrophy of the medial nasal processes, causing narrowing of the pyriform aperture.
- There is an association with other cranial-facial abnormalities, including the presence of holoprosencephaly, central incisor tooth and pituitary dysfunction.
- Key imaging features include overgrowth and medial displacement of the maxillary nasal processes, hypoplasia of the hard palate, and piriform aperture width of less than 11 mm in a term infant.

Juvenile nasopharyngeal angiofibroma (JNA)

- Juvenile nasopharyngeal angiofibroma is a highly vascular, benign hamartomatous lesion seen in adolescent males. It typically originates at the sphenopalatine foramen and spreads into the nasopharynx and pterygopalatine fossa, causing bony remodeling along the way.

The primary differential is nasal rhabdomyosarcoma, which causes bony destruction.

For an image of JNA, please refer to the head and neck section in the neuroimaging chapter.

Nasal rhabdomyosarcoma

- Nasal rhabdomyosarcoma is the most common childhood soft tissue sarcoma, with the head and neck a common primary site. It presents as a highly aggressive mass.

- 梨状孔狭窄(PAS)是一种罕见且有潜在致命性的先天性上呼吸道阻塞性疾病，临床表现类似于后鼻孔闭锁。
- PAS源于早期内侧鼻突的融合与肥大，导致梨状孔变窄。
- 可合并其他颅面部异常，如前脑无裂畸形、中切牙和垂体功能障碍。
- 主要的影像学特征包括上颌骨鼻突过度生长和内移，硬腭发育不全，以及足月儿梨状孔宽度小于11mm。

青少年鼻咽纤维血管瘤(JNA)

- 青少年鼻咽纤维血管瘤(JNA)是发生在青少年的一种富血供、良性错构瘤样病变。病变通常起源于蝶腭孔区，向鼻咽部和翼腭窝区生长，可造成病变沿途的骨质重塑变形。

最主要的鉴别诊断是鼻咽部横纹肌肉瘤，后者可造成骨质破坏。

JNA影像学表现详见“神经影像：头与颈”一章。

鼻腔横纹肌肉瘤

- 鼻腔横纹肌肉瘤是儿童最常见的软组织肉瘤，最常原发于头颈部。此肿瘤具有高度侵袭性。

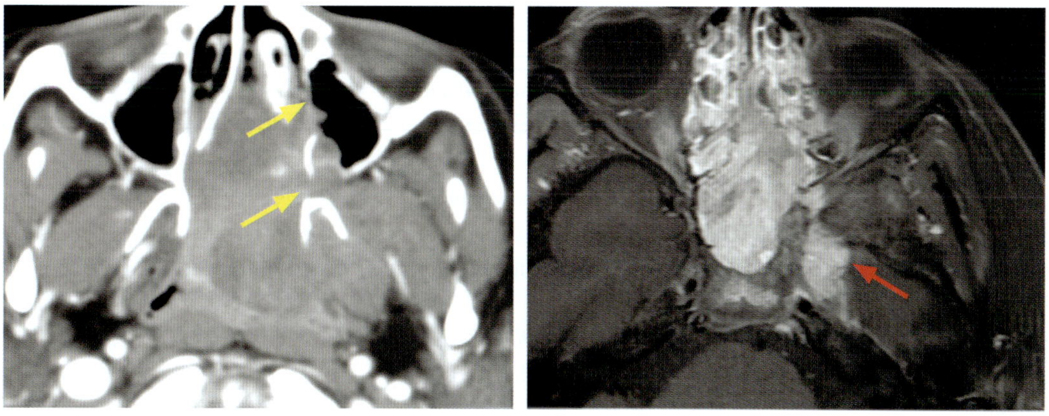

Nasal rhabdomyosarcoma: Axial contrast-enhanced CT (left image) and axial fat-suppressed post-contrast T1-weighted MRI at a higher level (right image) shows a destructive, avidly enhancing mass invading the nasopharynx and causing bony destruction of the left posterior wall of the maxillary sinus and pterygoid plates (yellow arrows). There is invasion into the left medial temporal lobe (red arrow) apparent on MRI.

鼻腔横纹肌肉瘤：轴位增强CT(左图)和轴位脂肪抑制增强T_1加权MRI(右图)显示，在颅底稍高层面可见一个具有高度破坏性、显著强化的肿块。该肿块侵犯鼻咽部，导致左侧上颌窦后壁和翼突板(黄箭)骨质破坏。MRI可见病变侵犯左侧颞叶内侧脑实质(红箭)。

STRIDOR (TRACHEAL NARROWING)-INFECTIOUS CAUSES

Croup (laryngotracheobronchitis)

- Croup is a self-limited viral (usually parainfluenza) infection with characteristic inspiratory stridor and barking cough. It affects children ages 6 months to 4 years, peaking at 1–2 years. Clinically, croup and bronchiolitis can present simultaneously.
- Croup is a clinical diagnosis. The purpose of radiography is to evaluate for other causes of stridor, particularly if the patient is not responsive to treatment.
- The *steeple sign* is seen on the frontal view and represents loss of the normal shouldering of the subglottic trachea. There may be "ballooning" of the hypopharynx on the lateral view.

喉喘鸣(气管狭窄)-感染性原因

哮吼(喉气管支气管炎)

- 哮吼(喉喘鸣)是一种自限性病毒感染(通常是副流感病毒感染)，并以吸气性喘鸣和犬吠样咳嗽为特征。儿童易感年龄为6个月~4岁，高峰期为1~2岁。哮吼和毛细支气管炎在临床上可同时出现。
- 哮吼是一个临床诊断，X线影像检查的目的是排除导致喘鸣的其他原因，尤其是当患者对治疗无效时。
- 尖塔征见于颈部正位图像，表现为声门下气管的正常肩托样形态消失。侧位图像可能出现下咽部"球囊样"改变。

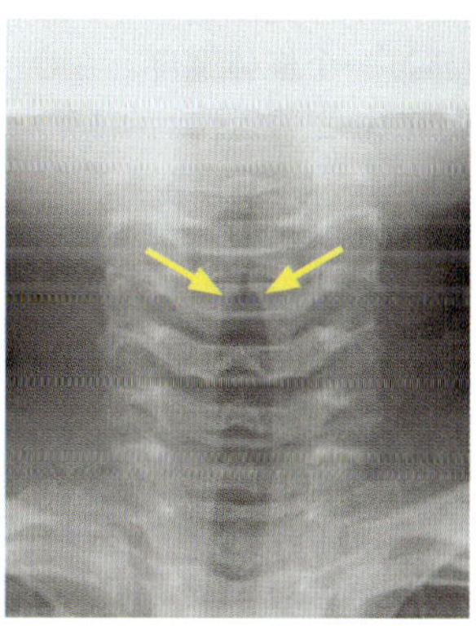

Normal frontal neck radiograph demonstrates convex "shouldering" of the subglottic larynx (arrows).

颈部正位X线影像显示正常声门下区喉部呈"肩托样"改变(箭)。

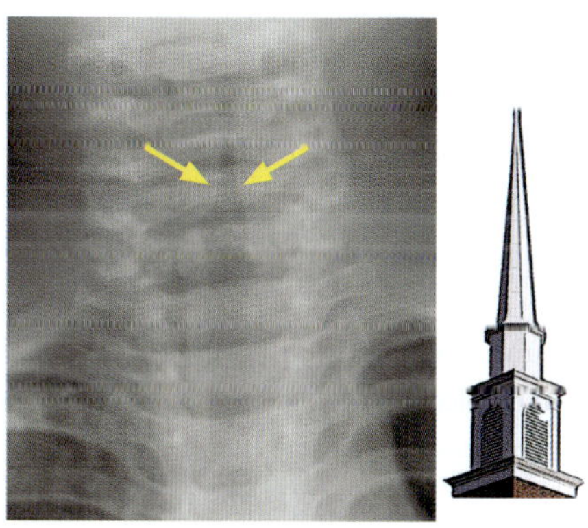

Steeple sign in croup: Frontal radiograph shows symmetric narrowing of the subglottic trachea and loss of the normal shouldering (arrows), simulating a steeple.

哮吼的尖塔征：颈部正位X线影像显示声门下气管呈对称性狭窄，正常的"肩托样"形态消失(箭)，形似一个"尖塔"。

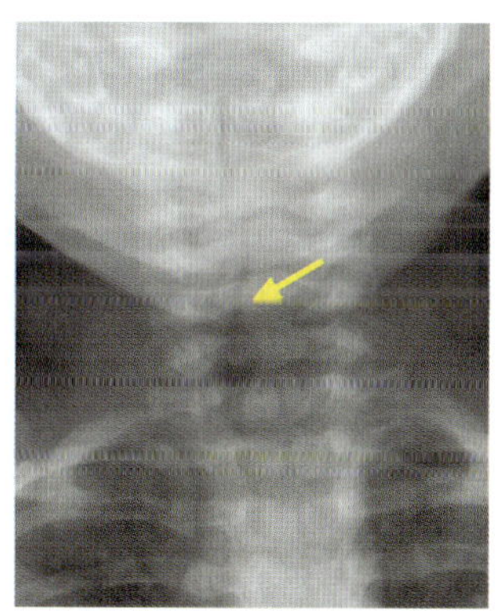

Subglottic hemangioma (discussed below): Frontal neck radiograph shows asymmetric narrowing of the subglottic trachea (arrow).

声门下血管瘤(下文讨论)：颈部正位X线影像显示声门下气管不对称性狭窄(箭)。

Epiglottitis

- Epiglottitis is infectious inflammation of the epiglottis.
- A very rare disease in the era of *Haemophilus influenzae* immunization, epiglottitis is a true emergency as the airway can obstruct without warning.
- While historically seen around the age of 3.5 years, modern cases are more seen in teens or immunocompromised individuals, such as HIV patients or transplant recipients. It is also frequently associated with caustic ingestion or smoke inhalation.
- Classic imaging findings include thickening of the epiglottis (*thumbprint sign*) and the aryepiglottic folds. It is swelling of the aryepiglottic folds that leads to airway obstruction.

  Note, *omega epiglottis* is an apparently thickened normal epiglottis when imaged at an oblique angle. The aryepiglottic folds should be normal.

会厌炎

- 会厌炎是会厌的感染性炎症。
- 会厌炎在普及接种嗜血杆菌疫苗的今天已经罕见，但该病是一种真正的急症，因气道常在无任何先兆的情况下出现梗阻。
- 会厌炎曾经常见于3岁半左右的儿童，但目前更多见于青少年和有免疫缺陷的人群，如HIV感染或接受器官移植的患者。此病还常与吞食腐蚀剂或吸入刺激性气体有关。
- 典型的影像学表现包括会厌增厚(指压征)和杓状会厌襞肿胀。杓状会厌襞肿胀正是导致气道梗阻的原因。

  注意，omega(Ω)会厌是指正常会厌在斜位角度成像时出现较为明显的增厚。杓状会厌襞应属于正常。

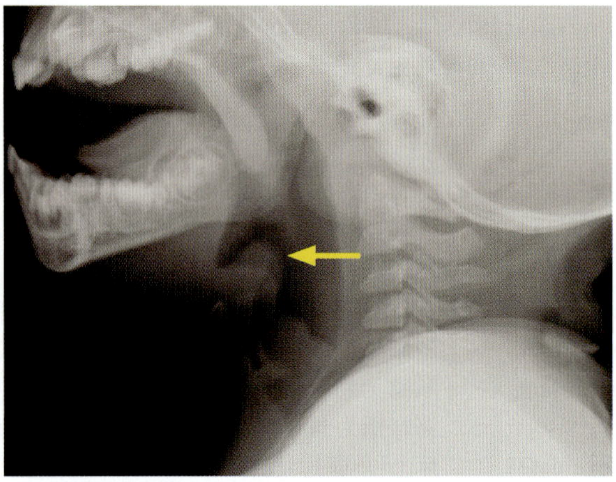

Epiglottitis: Lateral neck radiograph shows thickening of the epiglottis (*thumbprint sign*, arrow).
会厌炎：颈部侧位图像显示会厌增厚(指压征，箭)。

Retropharyngeal abscess

- Retropharyngeal abscess, a purulent infection of the retropharyngeal space, is a common cause of nontraumatic prevertebral soft tissue swelling in children, typically at ages 6–12 months or 2–4 years.
- As a general rule of thumb, the prevertebral soft tissues should not exceed half the vertebral body width at C1–C3, and one vertebral body width at C4 and below. Effacement of the normal subglottic step-off between C4–C5 is a worrisome sign.

  Prevertebral *pseudothickening* can be seen if a radiograph is obtained with poor inspiration or neck flexion. Airway fluoroscopy may obviate the need for CT by viewing effacement of the prevertebral soft tissues in real-time.
- CT is usually necessary to determine the nature of radiographic retropharyngeal swelling.
- The differential of nontraumatic prevertebral swelling also includes retropharyngeal cellulitis, lymphoma, and foregut duplication cyst.

  Retropharyngeal cellulitis appears similar to pharyngeal abscess on radiography, but no drainable fluid collection is seen on CT. It is most commonly secondary to severe cellulitis or tonsillitis.

  Air within a retropharyngeal abscess is rare unless a foreign body has perforated the esophagus.
- Complications include **Lemierre syndrome** (thrombosis of the internal jugular vein with septic pulmonary emboli) or mediastinitis (mediastinal extension via the danger space).

咽后脓肿

- 咽后脓肿是发生于咽后间隙的化脓性病变，是儿童非创伤性椎前软组织肿胀的常见原因，好发年龄通常为6~12个月或2~4岁。
- 一般的经验法则是，椎前软组织厚度在$C_{1\sim3}$水平不应超过椎体宽度的一半，在C_4及以下水平不应超过一个椎体宽度。在$C_{4\sim5}$之间正常声门阶梯消失是一个不好的征象。

  椎前软组织假性增厚可见于儿童吸气不足或颈部前屈。气道透视检查可以观察到椎前软组织增厚征象消失，从而可免去CT检查。
- 通常有必要使用CT以明确X线检查中咽后壁肿胀的性质。
- 椎前非创伤性软组织肿胀需要与咽后蜂窝织炎、淋巴瘤和前肠重复囊肿等进行鉴别。

  咽后蜂窝织炎在X线影像上与咽后脓肿表现相似，但是在CT上没有可引流的液体。咽后蜂窝织炎最常继发于严重的蜂窝织炎或扁桃体炎。

  咽后脓肿内伴有积气的情况罕见，除非有异物造成食管穿孔。
- 并发症包括**Lemierre综合征**(颈内静脉血栓伴感染性肺栓塞)或纵隔炎(炎症通过咽后间隙向纵隔内延伸所致)。

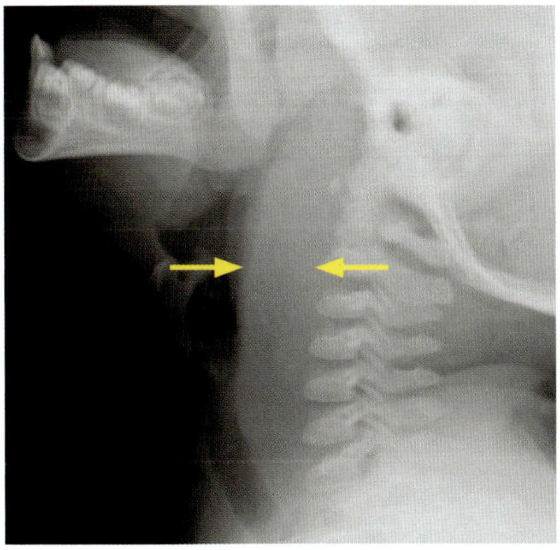

Retropharyngeal abscess: Lateral neck radiograph shows marked thickening of the prevertebral tissues (arrows). Although nonspecific, this patient had a retropharyngeal abscess.

咽后脓肿：颈部侧位X线影像显示椎前软组织明显增厚(箭)。此征象不具有特异性，但该患者有咽后脓肿。

Exudative (bacterial) tracheitis

- Exudative tracheitis may present similarly to epiglottitis with fever, stridor, and potentially life-threatening respiratory distress.
- In contrast to croup, exudative tracheitis tends to affect older children (ages 6–10 years) and is bacterial in etiology (most commonly *S. aureus*).
- On imaging, linear filling defects representing intraluminal membranes may be visible in the subglottic and cervical trachea (*candle dripping sign*).

渗出性(细菌性)气管炎

- 渗出性气管炎的表现可类似于会厌炎，包括发热、喘鸣和有潜在的致命性呼吸困难。
- 与哮吼相比，渗出性气管炎发生于较为年长的儿童(6~10岁)，为细菌感染所致(最常见的为金黄色葡萄球菌)。
- 影像上，在声门下和颈部气管有可能看到一种由腔内膜状物形成的线样充盈缺损影(滴蜡征)。

Summary of infectious causes of stridor

	Croup	Retropharyngeal abscess	Epiglottitis	Exudative tracheitis
Imaging findings	*Steeple sign*: **symmetric** loss of normal subglottic shouldering	Prevertebral soft tissue swelling	*Thumbprint sign*: enlarged epiglottis; thickened aryepiglottic folds	*Candle dripping sign*: linear filling defects in the airway
Age at presentation	6 months–4 years (peak 1–2 years)	6–12 months; 2–4 years	Historically 3.5 years; more recently in teens and the immunocompromised	6–10 years
Pathogen	Parainfluenza > RSV		*H. influenzae*	*S. aureus*
Differential diagnosis	Subglottic hemangioma: **asymmetric** narrowing of subglottic trachea	*Pseudothickening*: neck flexion or poor inspiration Suppurative node: more lateral within the neck	*Omega epiglottis*: normal esophagus when imaged obliquely	

喘鸣的感染原因总结

	喉炎	咽后脓肿	会厌炎	渗出性气管炎
影像发现	尖塔征：声门下正常肩托对称性消失	椎前软组织肿胀	指压征：会厌肿胀；杓状会厌襞增厚	滴蜡征：气道线样充盈缺损影
发病年龄	6个月~4岁(高峰1~2岁)	6~12个月；2~4岁	以往3.5岁；近年为青少年和免疫功能低下的人群	6~10岁
病原体	副流感病毒>呼吸道合胞病毒		流感嗜血杆菌	金黄色葡萄球菌
鉴别诊断	声门下血管瘤：声门下气管不对称性狭窄	咽后壁假性增厚：颈部前屈或吸气不足 化脓性淋巴结：更偏向颈部外侧	Omega会厌：正常会厌在X线斜位影像上的表现	

STRIDOR-OTHER CAUSES

喉喘鸣-其他原因

Subglottic hemangioma

- Subglottic hemangioma is a benign vascular neoplasm that produces stridor in infancy. It is the most common pediatric subglottic tracheal mass.
- The classic radiographic finding is **asymmetric** narrowing of the subglottic trachea on the frontal view (versus symmetric narrowing in croup).
- There is an association with cutaneous hemangiomas and PHACES syndrome.

声门下血管瘤

- 血管瘤是一种良性肿瘤，可以造成婴儿喘鸣，它是儿童声门下最常见的气管肿物。
- 典型影像学表现是声门下气管在正位X线影像上呈**不对称性**狭窄(而喉炎为对称性狭窄)。
- 常与皮肤血管瘤和PHACES综合征相关。

PHACES syndrome:

Posterior fossa malformation.

Hemangiomas.

Arterial anomalies.

Coarctation/cardiac defects.

Eye abnormalities.

Subglottic hemangiomas, sternal clefts, supraumbilical raphes.

PHACES综合征：

颅后窝畸形。

血管瘤。

动脉异常。

主动脉缩窄/心脏间隔缺损。

眼部畸形。

声门下血管瘤，胸骨裂，脐上囊肿。

Laryngeal papillomatosis

- Laryngeal papillomatosis is a cause of multiple laryngeal nodules due to HPV infection, resulting in thick and nodular vocal cords. Papillomatosis increases the risk of laryngeal squamous cell carcinoma (SCC), analogous to cervical cancer risk from HPV.
- Papillomas frequently seed the lungs, causing multiple cavitary nodules. These nodules are also at risk for the development of SCC.

喉部乳头状瘤

- 喉部乳头状瘤是HPV感染引起的喉部多发结节，可导致声带呈结节状增厚。乳头状瘤会增加喉部鳞状细胞癌(SCC)的患病风险，类似于HPV感染可增加罹患宫颈癌的风险。
- 乳头状瘤常向肺部播散，表现为多发空洞性结节。这些结节也有发展为SCC的风险。

Tracheobronchomalacia

气管支气管软化

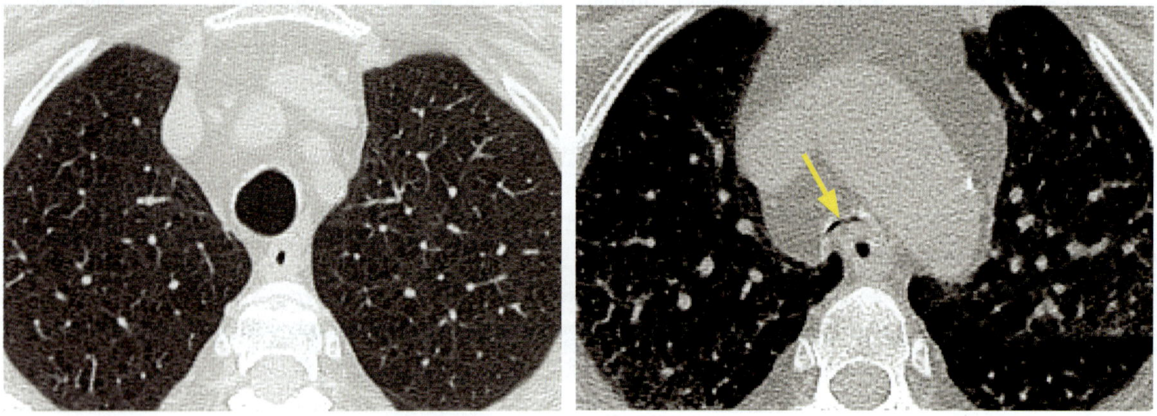

Tracheomalacia: Inspiratory CT (left image) demonstrates the normal, slightly ovoid shape of the trachea. Expiratory CT (right image) in the same patient shows excessive tracheal collapse (arrow). This example is from an adult with mild emphysema.

Case courtesy Michael Hanley, MD, University of Virginia Health System.

气管软化：吸气相CT(左图)显示正常，气管稍呈椭圆形。同一患者呼气相CT(右图)显示气管过度塌陷(箭)。这个病例来自一个轻度肺气肿的成年患者。

- Tracheobronchomalacia causes excessive expiratory airway collapse from weakness of the tracheobronchial cartilage. Tracheobronchomalacia may be either congenital or acquired secondary to intubation, infection, or chronic inflammation.
- A standard inspiratory CT may be normal. Dynamic four-dimensional CT or bronchoscopy are necessary to diagnose tracheobronchomalacia.
- Greater than 50% reduction in cross-sectional area of the airway lumen is

- 气管支气管软化是因气管支气管软骨骨质薄弱导致呼气时气道严重塌陷。气管支气管软化既可以是先天性的，也可以后天获得，如继发于插管、感染或慢性炎症等。
- 气管支气管软化在标准的吸气相CT可能表现正常。有必要采用动态四维CT或纤维支气管镜检查进行明确诊断。

suggestive of tracheomalacia, although normal patients may achieve this threshold with a forceful expiration.

- A very common association is with esophageal atresia/tracheoesophageal fistula (TEF).

Tracheal stenosis

- Iatrogenic tracheal stenosis (e.g., due to prolonged intubation) may be a cause of stridor.
- Congenital tracheal stenosis is usually associated with vascular anomalies, discussed in the following section.

Aspirated foreign body

- Most aspirated foreign bodies are radiolucent, therefore secondary signs of air trapping (lucent hyperinflated lung with atelectasis distally) can be helpful in the diagnosis.
- Decubitus radiographs demonstrate persistent expansion of the dependent lung, signifying obstruction.
- Expiratory fluoroscopic/radiographic images demonstrate persistent expansion and lucency of the obstructed lung, with mediastinal shift away from the affected side.

- 当气道管腔横断面积减少超过50%时，提示有气管支气管软化，但正常人用力呼气时也有可能达到这个临界值。
- 并发食管闭锁/气管食管瘘(TEF)常见。

气管狭窄

- 医源性气管狭窄(如长时间插管)可能是喘鸣的原因之一。
- 先天性气管狭窄通常合并血管异常，将在下文进行讨论。

吸入性异物

- 大多数吸入性异物是透X线的，如果发现肺内有通气障碍的间接征象(肺过度膨胀伴远端肺不张)将有助于疾病的诊断。
- 侧卧位X线影像检查显示下方一侧肺呈持续过度膨胀，提示有阻塞。
- 呼气相透视/X线影像可见阻塞一侧肺持续膨胀及透亮，伴纵隔向健侧移位。

VASCULAR RINGS AND SLING

- Rings and slings are important vascular causes of stridor in infancy and childhood. Initial evaluation is typically with barium esophagram, followed by CT or MRI if abnormal.
- A vascular *ring* refers to complete encircling of the trachea and esophagus by the aortic arch or great vessels.
- A vascular *sling* refers to an anomalous left pulmonary artery that arises aberrantly from the right pulmonary artery and traps the trachea in a "sling" on three sides.
- An important clue to a vascular cause of stridor is a **right-sided aortic arch** visualized on frontal radiograph.

  The pulmonary artery sling is the only vascular anomaly that causes stridor in a patient with a normal (left) aortic arch.

- The three most important vascular causes of stridor are: double aortic arch, right arch with aberrant left subclavian artery, and pulmonary sling. Each of these will show abnormality on the lateral radiograph or esophagram.

血管环和吊带

- 血管环和吊带是引起婴幼儿喘鸣的重要原因。初始评估通常采用食管钡餐，如有异常，随后使用CT或MRI。
- 血管环是指气管和食管被主动脉弓或大血管完全包绕。
- 血管吊带是指左肺动脉异常起源于右肺动脉，导致气管的三个侧面受到限制。
- 血管原因所致喘鸣的一个重要线索是在正位X线影像上看到**右位主动脉弓**。

  肺动脉吊带是正常(左位)主动脉弓患者唯一导致喘鸣的血管性原因。

- 导致喘鸣的三个最重要血管性原因是双主动脉弓、右位主动脉弓伴迷走左锁骨下动脉，以及肺动脉吊带。上述每一种原因都可以在胸部侧位影像或食管造影中发现异常。

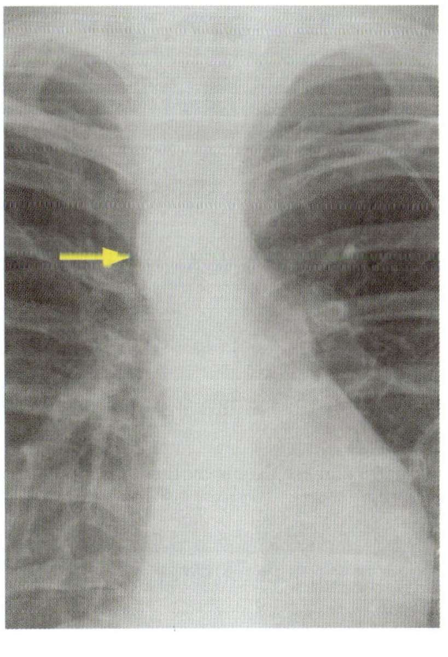

Frontal chest radiograph shows a right-sided aortic arch (arrow), which could be a clue to a vascular cause of stridor.
胸部正位影像显示右位主动脉弓(箭)，提示该患者的喘鸣可能是血管方面的原因。

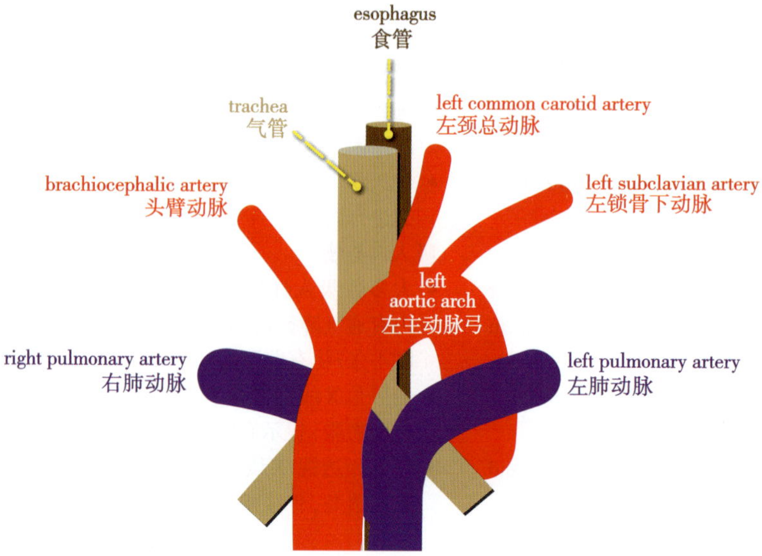

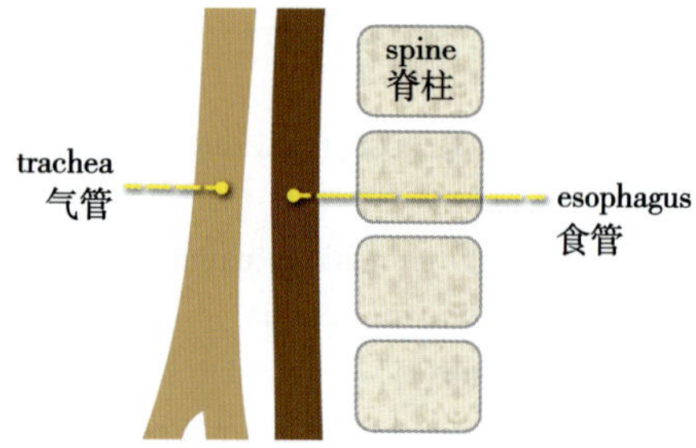

A normal lateral view (esophagram or radiograph, diagrammed above) shows a smooth contour of the esophagus and trachea, without any abnormal impressions.

正常侧位图像(上图为食管造影或X线影像)显示光滑的食管和气管轮廓,无异常压迹。

Double aortic arch

- Double aortic arch is the most common vascular ring. The arches encircle both the trachea and esophagus, and may cause stridor.

  The right arch is usually superior and larger than the left.
- The goal of the radiologist in pre-surgical planning is to determine which arch is dominant (typically with MR), as the non-dominant arch is ligated to alleviate stridor.

双主动脉弓

- 双主动脉弓是最常见的血管环。两个主动脉弓同时包绕气管和食管,可引起喘鸣。

  右侧主动脉弓通常高于和大于左侧主动脉弓。
- 放射科医生在术前规划中的作用是明确哪一侧主动脉弓占优势(通常采用MR),对非优势侧主动脉弓进行结扎可以减轻喘鸣。

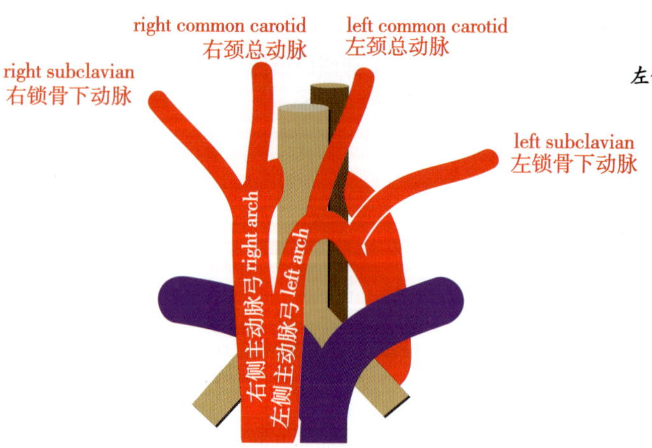

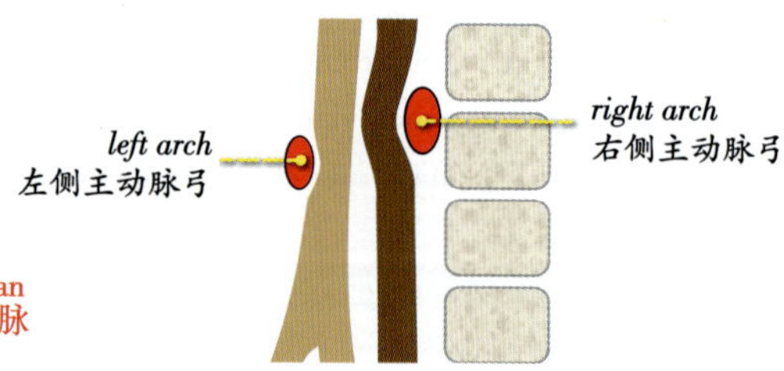

The lateral schematic (above) shows posterior indentation of the esophagus (caused by the right arch) and anterior indentation of the trachea (caused by the left arch).

The anatomic schematic (left) shows complete encircling of both the trachea and esophagus by the arches, with potential bilateral impressions on the trachea and esophagus.

侧位示意图(上图)可见食管后方压迹(为右侧主动脉弓引起),气管前方压迹(为左侧主动脉弓引起)。

解剖示意图(左图)显示气管和食管被主动脉弓完全包绕,并有可能对气管和食管产生双面压迹。

Right arch with aberrant left subclavian artery (non-mirror image branching)

- The second most common vascular ring is a right aortic arch with an aberrant left subclavian artery. The right arch indents the anterior trachea while the aberrant left subclavian artery wraps posteriorly around the esophagus. The ring is completed by the ligamentum arteriosum.

  In contrast, the more common anatomical variant of a *left* arch with an aberrant *right* subclavian artery (discussed on the next page) is typically asymptomatic and does not comprise a ring.

  Note that a *right aortic arch with mirror image branching* features essentially a mirror image of a normal left aortic arch. Greater than 90% of cases are associated with intracardiac defects, including tetralogy of Fallot, truncus arteriosus and double outlet right ventricle. Though typically not a vascular ring, a complete vascular ring can occur when the ductal ligament extends between the descending aorta and left pulmonary artery ("circumflex aortic arch").
- Radiographic and fluoroscopic findings are not reliably distinguishable from the double aortic arch described above. CT or MRI are necessary for definitive diagnosis.

右位主动脉弓合并迷走左锁骨下动脉(非镜像分支)

- 第二常见的血管环是右位主动脉弓合并迷走左锁骨下动脉。右位主动脉弓压在气管的前方，迷走左锁骨下动脉包绕在食管后方。与动脉导管韧带形成了完整的环。

  相比之下，较常见的左位主动脉弓伴迷走右锁骨下动脉(下一页将会讨论)通常是无症状的，且不形成血管环。

  注意，具有镜像分支特征的右位主动脉弓在本质上是一个正常左位主动脉弓的镜像。超过90%的病例合并心内缺陷，包括法洛四联症、永存动脉干和右心室双出口。上述情况通常不是一个血管环，但是当右位主动脉弓和左肺动脉("环形主动脉弓")之间存在动脉导管韧带时，就会呈现一个完整的血管环。
- 普通X线摄影和透视检查不能可靠地辨别以上所描述的双主动脉弓。有必要使用CT或MRI进行确诊。

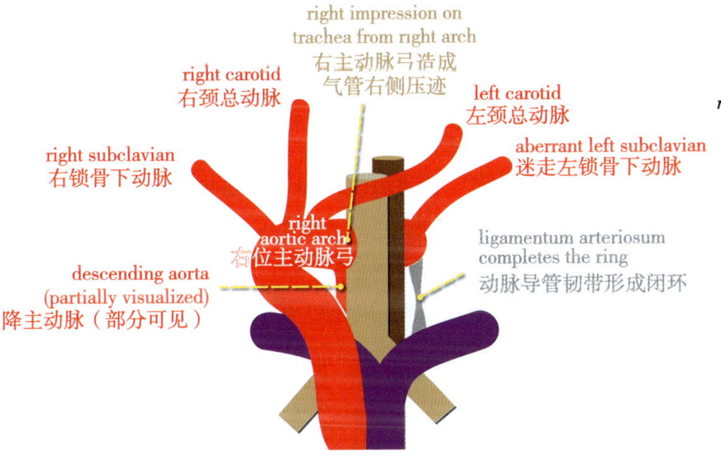

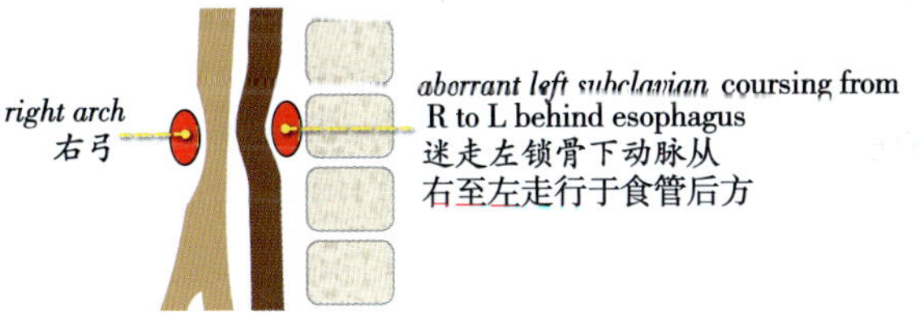

The lateral schematic (above) shows anterior indentation of the trachea (by the right arch) and posterior impression on the esophagus (by the aberrant left subclavian artery).

The anatomic schematic (left) shows leftward impression/deviation of the trachea by the right aortic arch.

侧位示意图(上图)显示气管前方的压迹(为右位主动脉弓所致)和食管后方的压迹(为迷走左锁骨下动脉所致)。

解剖示意图(左图)显示右位主动脉弓对气管左侧造成的压迹/推移。

Pulmonary sling

- Anomalous origin of the *left* pulmonary artery arising from the right pulmonary artery forms a *sling* by coursing between the trachea and esophagus. Usually only the trachea is trapped in the sling, but occasionally the bronchus intermedius may also be compressed.
- This is the only vascular cause of stridor in a patient with a left arch. The aortic branching pattern is normal.
- This entity is associated with tracheal anomalies including tracheomalacia and bronchus suis (RUL bronchus originating from trachea). A "ring-sling" complex may also be present, representing complete cartilaginous rings in the setting of a pulmonary artery sling.

肺动脉吊带

- 左肺动脉异常起源于右肺动脉时，其在气管与食管之间形成一个吊带。通常只有气管受吊带牵绊，偶尔也有中间段支气管受压。
- 对于左位主动脉弓的患者，此为引起喘鸣的唯一血管性原因。主动脉弓分支形态正常。
- 肺动脉吊带常伴有气管发育异常，包括气管软化和气管性支气管(右上叶支气管起源于气管)等。还可能出现"环-吊带"复合体，即肺动脉吊带合并完整的软骨气管环。

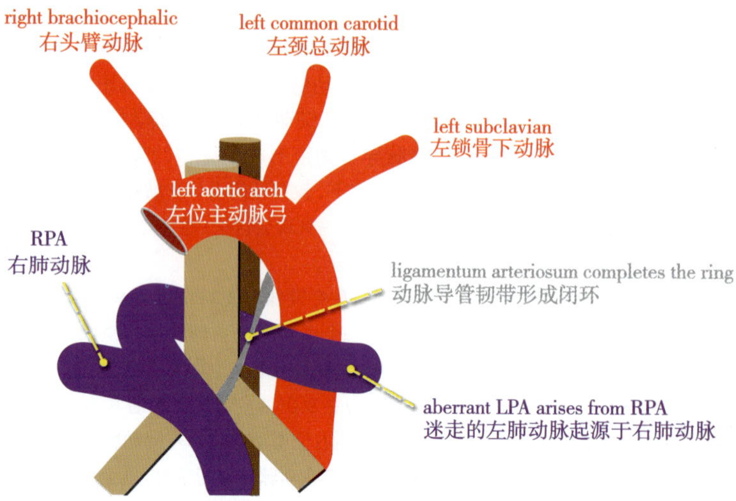

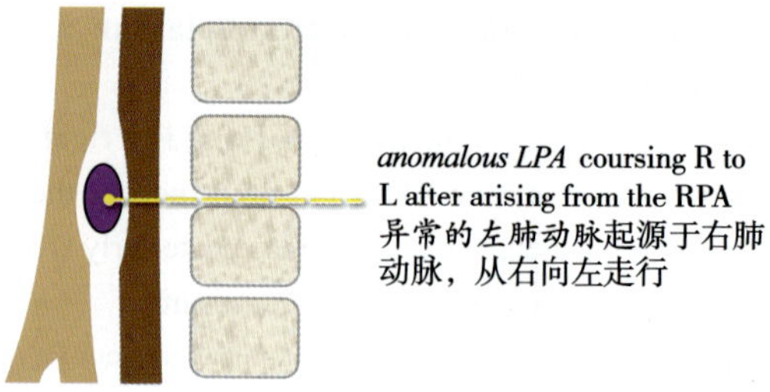

The key radiographic finding of pulmonary artery sling, seen on a lateral esophagram, is anterior indentation on the esophagus and posterior indentation on the trachea (the latter is usually not well seen). The anomalous left pulmonary artery runs in between the trachea and the esophagus.
肺动脉吊带的关键征象是在食管造影侧位图像上可见食管前方和气管后方的压迹(后者通常不太明显)。异常的左肺动脉走行在气管和食管之间。

Left aortic arch with aberrant right subclavian artery

- A left aortic arch with an aberrant right subclavian artery is not a ring or a sling because the ligamentum arteriosum does not impinge upon the trachea or esophagus. It does not cause stridor, but when symptomatic may cause dysphagia (*dysphagia lusoria*).

左位主动脉弓伴迷走右锁骨下动脉

- 左位主动脉弓伴迷走右锁骨下动脉不属于一个环或吊带，因为肺动脉韧带不会压迫气管或食管。它不会引起喘鸣，但可以引起吞咽困难的症状(食管受压性吞咽困难)。

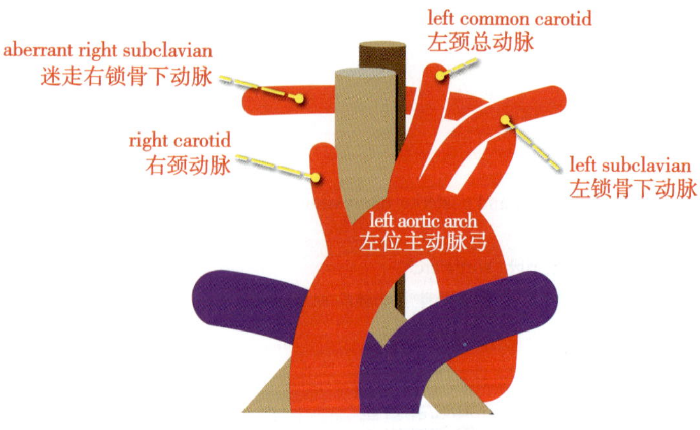

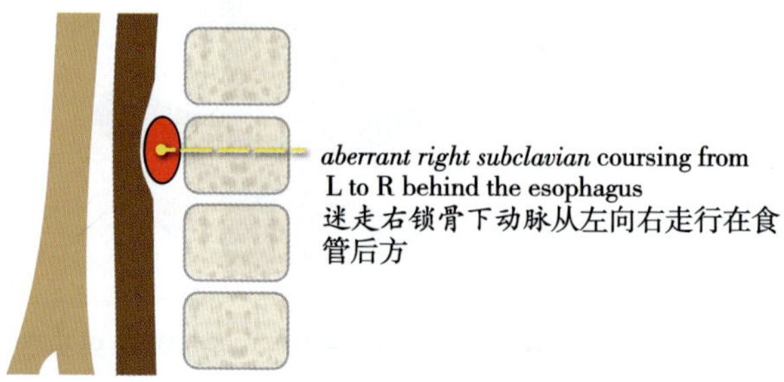

The lateral schematic (above) shows a small posterior indentation on the esophagus.
The anatomic schematic (left) shows the aberrant right subclavian coursing posterior to the esophagus.
侧位示意图(上图)显示食管后方有一个小的压迹。
解剖示意图(左图)显示迷走右锁骨下动脉走行在食管的后方。

Innominate artery syndrome

- In infants, the large thymus can occasionally cause the normal innominate artery to press against the anterior trachea, potentially producing innominate artery syndrome.
- Innominate artery syndrome is not a vascular ring, and it is controversial if this entity is a clinically relevant form of breathing difficulty.

无名动脉综合征

- 在婴儿，增大的胸腺偶尔会引起正常的无名动脉压迫气管前壁而有可能造成无名动脉综合征。
- 无名动脉综合征不是一个血管环，而且，它是否属于一种临床相关的呼吸困难形式仍存在争议。

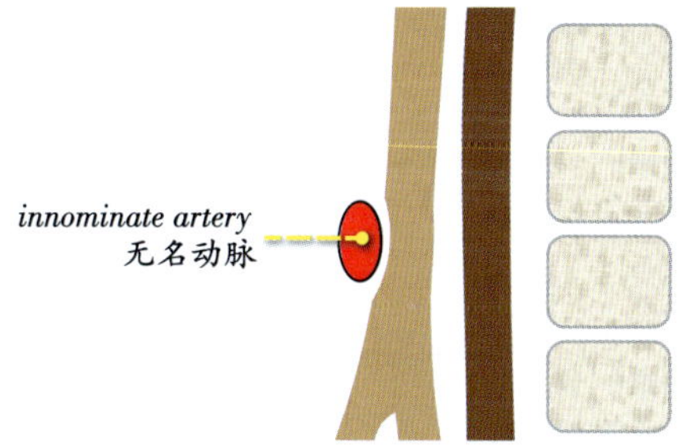

SUMMARY OF VASCULAR IMPRESSIONS

血管压迹总结

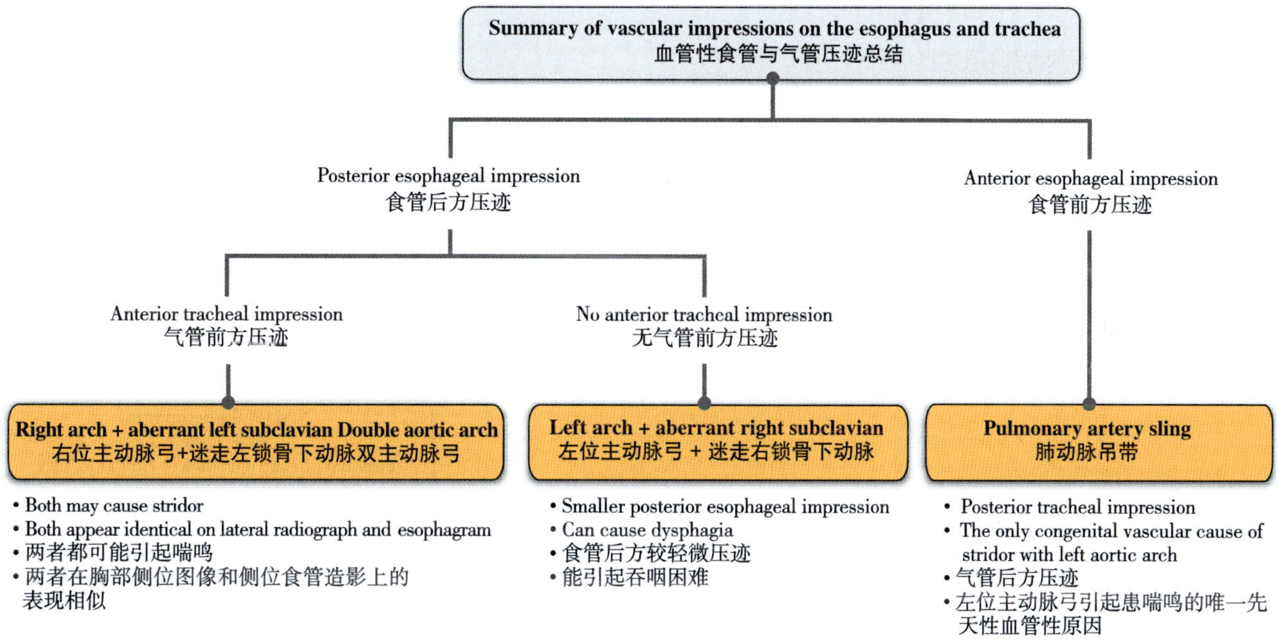

Summary of vascular impressions with a posterior esophageal impression

- Double aortic arch or right arch with aberrant left subclavian artery:

  These two rings may appear identical on the lateral esophagram or radiograph and both will also feature an anterior impression on the trachea.

  Both entities may cause stridor.

- Left aortic arch with aberrant right subclavian artery:

  This entity is rarely symptomatic. It would cause dysphagia if it produced any symptoms at all.

  Esophageal impression is often *smaller* compared to the other two above entities.

Summary of vascular impressions with an anterior esophageal impression

- Pulmonary artery sling:

  Pulmonary artery sling is the only vascular ring or sling to produce an *anterior* impression on the esophagus. Since the aberrant pulmonary artery runs between the trachea and esophagus, it also *produces* a *posterior* tracheal impression.

  Pulmonary artery sling is also the only congenital vascular cause of stridor with a left aortic arch.

食管后方血管压迹总结

- 双主动脉弓或右位主动脉弓伴迷走左锁骨下动脉：

  这两种环在侧位食管造影或胸部影像上的表现完全一致，都可出现气管前方的压迹。

  两者都可引起喘鸣。

- 左位主动脉弓伴迷走右锁骨下动脉：

  该结构很少会引起症状。唯一可能出现的症状是吞咽困难。食管后方压迹通常小于上文两种畸形。

食管前方血管压迹总结

- 肺动脉吊带：

  肺动脉吊带是唯一会造成食管前方压迹的血管环或吊带。由于异常肺动脉走行在气管和食管之间，它也可能对气管的后方产生压迹。

  肺动脉吊带同时也是左位主动脉弓患者出现喘鸣的唯一先天性血管性原因。

（翻译　周璐）

MEDICAL RESPIRATORY DISTRESS IN THE NEWBORN 新生儿呼吸窘迫

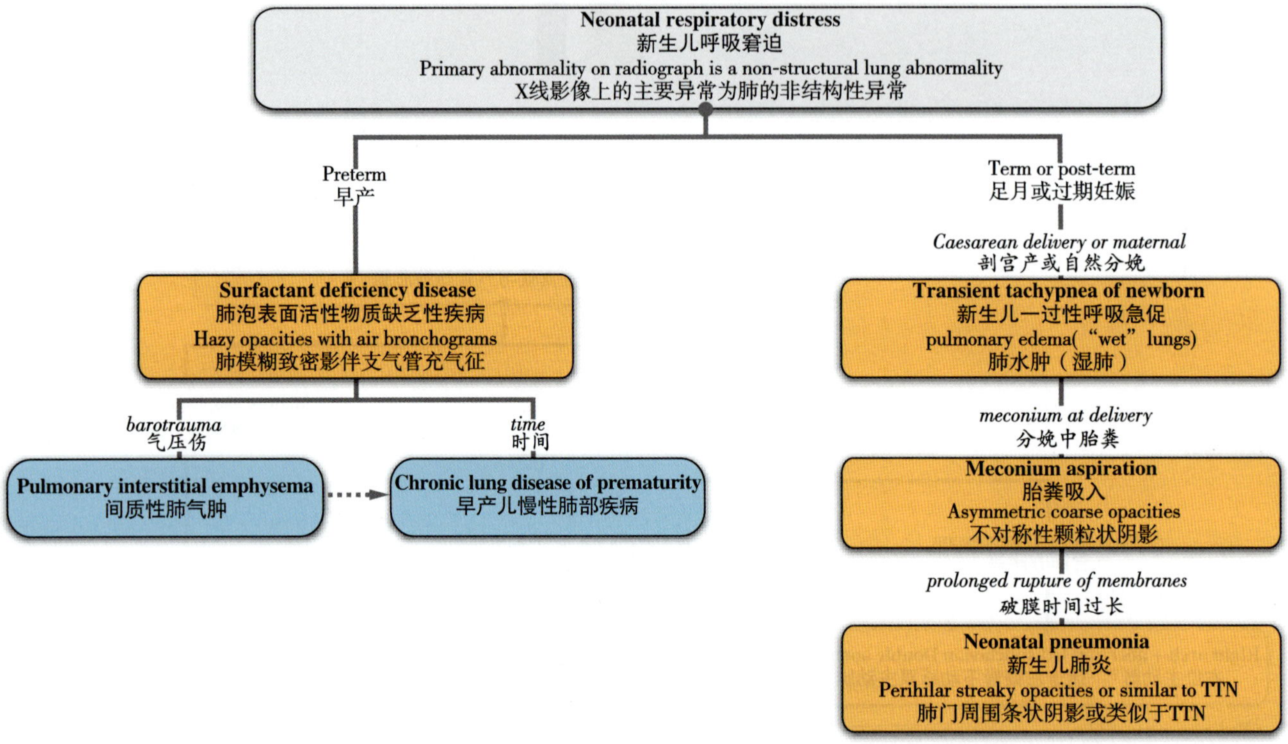

- Multiple processes can cause respiratory distress in a neonate, including pulmonary disease, congenital heart disease, thoracic mass, airway disorders, skeletal abnormalities, vascular anomalies, etc.
- Despite this broad range, there are 4 classic considerations for a newborn with "medical respiratory distress" – that is, a baby that appears anatomically normal by radiograph (i.e.,without cardiomegaly or thoracic mass), but has a diffuse pulmonary abnormality.

Surfactant deficiency disease (SDD) / Respiratory distress syndrome (RDS) / Hyaline membrane disease

- 多种病变可以导致新生儿呼吸窘迫，包括肺部疾病、先天性心脏病、胸部肿块、气道疾病、骨骼异常和血管畸形等。
- 尽管涉及病因广泛，但对于出生后出现"医学呼吸窘迫"的新生儿首先要考虑4个最常见的因素，此时患儿的X线影像正常(例如，无心脏增大或胸部肿块)，但有弥漫性肺部异常。

肺泡表面活性物质缺乏症(SDD)/呼吸窘迫综合征(RDS)/肺透明膜病

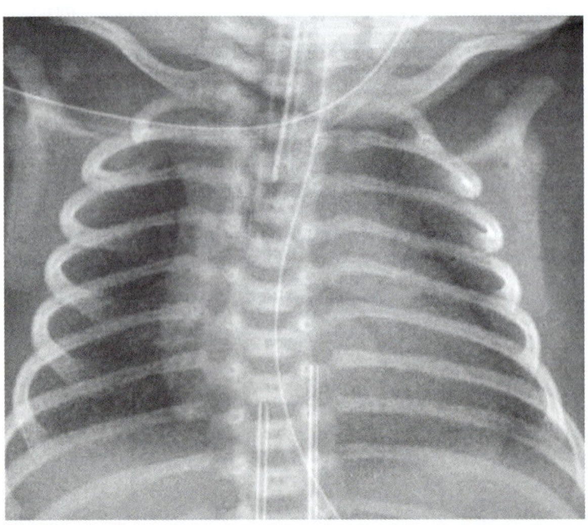

Surfactant deficiency disease: Frontal radiograph in a premature infant shows hazy, granular pulmonary opacities and low lung volumes. The baby is intubated, with partially visualized nasogastric tube, umbilical venous, and umbilical arterial catheters.

Case courtesy Michael Hanley, MD, University of Virginia Health System.

肺泡表面活性物质缺乏症：早产儿正位X线影像显示两肺呈雾样、颗粒状阴影，以及肺容积减小。该婴儿已行气管插管，同时可见部分鼻胃管、脐静脉和脐动脉置管。

- SDD is the most common cause of respiratory distress and death in pre-term infants.
- It is caused by insufficient surfactant (due to immature type Ⅱ pneumocytes) and resultant decreased lung compliance.
- Greater than 95% of cases are seen in pre-term infants born before 34 weeks. Less commonly, term babies born to diabetic mothers or via Caesarean delivery have increased prevalence of SDD.
- Imaging is characterized by low lung volumes (prior to intubation) with diffuse hazy granular opacities, air-bronchograms and no pleural effusions.

  Surfactant replacement therapy may result in rapid decrease in granular opacification and improved lung volume.

  Differential diagnosis for granular opacities in a newborn is neonatal pneumonia (i.e., Group B strep.), which typically also features pleural effusions.
- **Pulmonary interstitial emphysema (PIE)** is a condition often associated with SDD, where barotrauma causes air to dissect through the immature alveoli into the interstitial space and spread along the lymphatic pathways. It usually occurs in the first week of life.

  The radiographic appearance of PIE is hyperinflated lungs with asymmetric bubbly and tubular lucencies representing dissecting air bubbles. PIE may lead to pneumomediastinum or pneumothorax. Rarely, it may also cause large intrapulmonary pneumatoceles.

  Treatment of PIE includes switching ventilation modes, high-frequency oscillating ventilation (unique to pediatrics) and placing the patient on affected side down.
- **Chronic lung disease (CLD) of prematurity / bronchopulmonary dysplasia (BPD)**: SDD (with or without PIE) lasts for a few days to a week. Beyond that, persistent lung disease is concerning for early or evolving CLD which usually presents in the second to third week.

  CLD is the most common cause of chronic respiratory failure in pediatric patients.

  CLD is clinically defined as chronic lung disease of premature infants with oxygen dependency longer than 28 days of life and failed oxygen challenge at 36 weeks post-conception.

  Unlike SDD, CLD features mild hyperinflation and band-like coarse reticular opacities.

- SDD是早产儿呼吸窘迫和死亡最常见的原因。
- 这是由于肺泡表面活性物质不足(因Ⅱ型肺泡上皮细胞未成熟)而导致的肺顺应性下降。
- 超过95%的病例为胎龄小于34周的早产儿。其次，糖尿病母亲所生的足月儿或剖宫产新生儿的SDD患病率有所增加。
- 影像学特征为肺容积降低(气管插管前)，弥漫性模糊的颗粒状阴影，支气管充气征，但无胸腔积液。

  肺泡表面活性物质替代疗法可使肺内颗粒状阴影迅速减少并改善肺容积。

  新生儿颗粒状阴影的鉴别诊断是新生儿肺炎(如B型链球菌)，但新生儿肺炎通常伴有胸腔积液。
- **肺间质性气肿(PIE)**是与SDD相关的一种病变，气压伤导致气体从不成熟的肺泡进入肺间质的间隙内，并沿着淋巴路径扩散。它通常发生在出生后的第一周。

  PIE影像学表现为肺高度膨胀，并伴有许多不对称性小囊样和管状透亮影，其为撕裂的肺泡。PIE可以导致纵隔积气或气胸。在极个别情况下，它还可能导致肺大疱。

  PIE治疗包括切换通气模式、高频振荡通气(儿科专用)和将患者调整为患侧向下的侧卧位。
- **早产儿慢性肺病(CLD)/支气管肺发育不良(BPD)**：SDD(无论是否合并PIE)持续数天到一周。此后，持续性的肺部病变可导致早期或进展中的CLD，通常在第二周到第三周出现。

  CLD是儿童最常见的慢性呼吸衰竭的原因。

  CLD在临床上定义为早产儿慢性肺病，是指出生36周以内的早产儿因缺氧必须依赖持续机械通气超过28天。

  与SDD不同，CLD有轻度的肺过度膨胀，并可见明显的带状粗网状阴影。

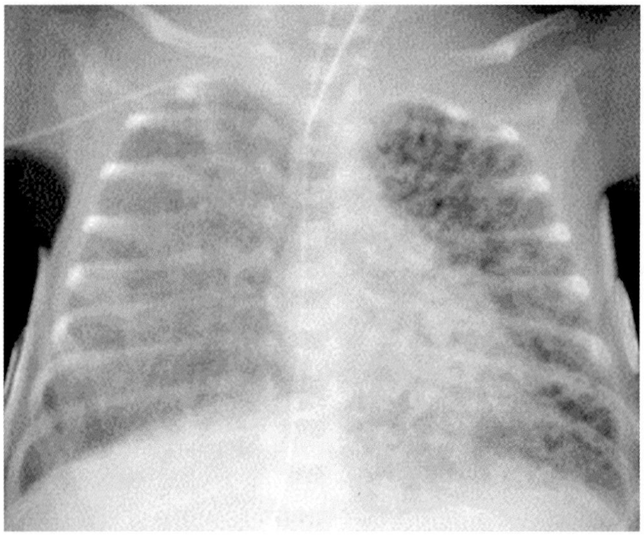

Pulmonary interstitial emphysema: Chest radiograph shows hyperinflated lungs with many small cystic lucencies representing dissecting air bubbles.
肺间质性气肿：胸部X线影像显示肺过度膨胀，并伴有很多小囊状透亮影，代表肺泡撕裂。

Case courtesy Michael Hanley, MD, University of Virginia Health System.

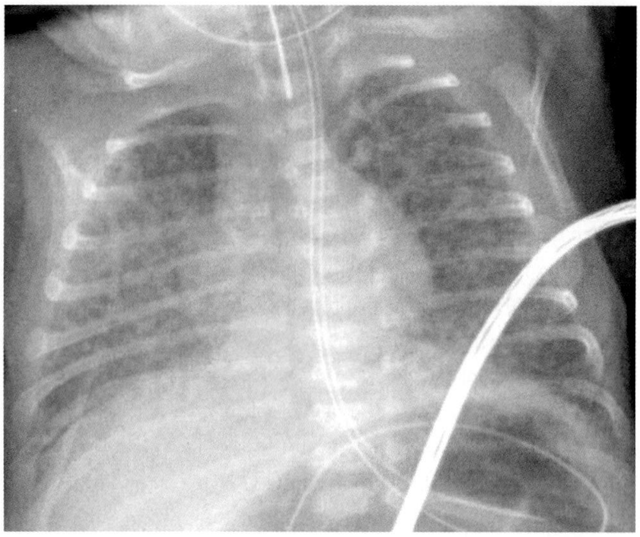

Chronic lung disease of prematurity: Chest radiograph in a 28-day-old infant with a history of prior respiratory distress syndrome shows coarse interstitial opacities and normal to slightly increased lung volumes. An endotracheal tube and two nasogastric tubes are partially visualized.
早产儿慢性肺疾病：28天婴儿的胸部X线影像，患儿有呼吸窘迫病史，显示两肺粗糙的间质阴影和体积正常或轻微增大。可见部分气管插管及2根鼻胃管。

Transient tachypnea of the newborn (TTN)

新生儿一过性呼吸急促(TTN)

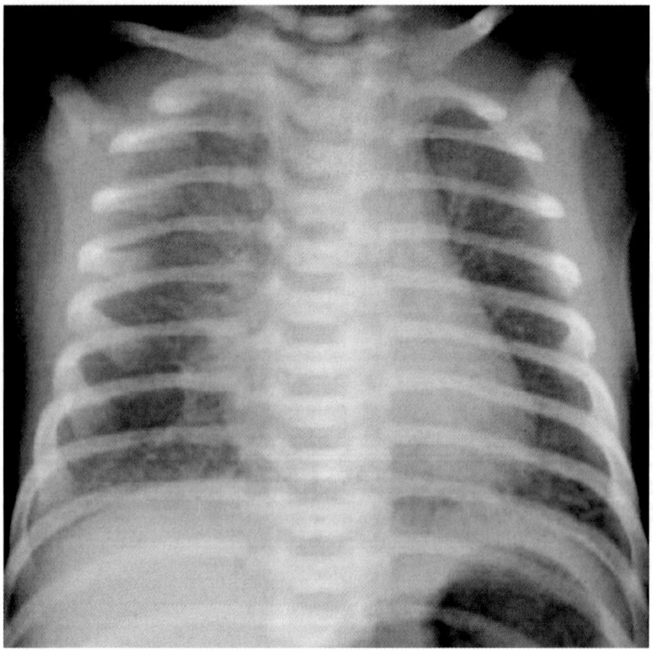

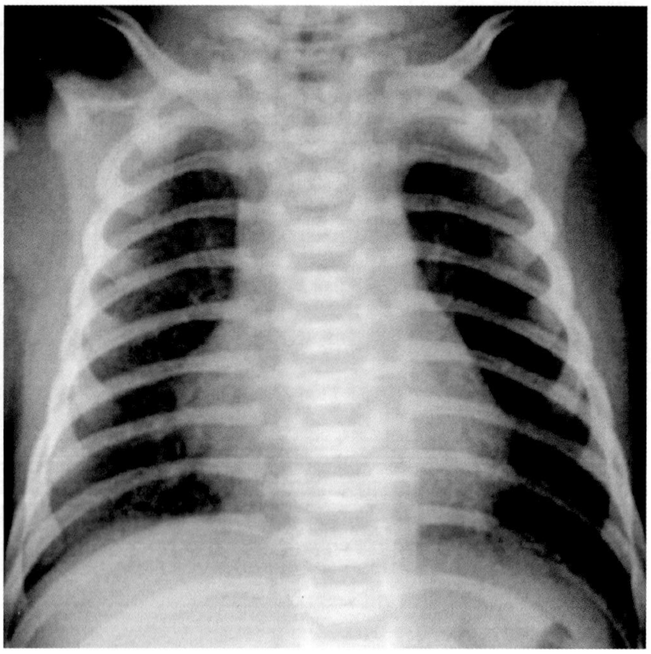

Transient tachypnea of the newborn: Initial chest radiograph (left image) performed in a full-term neonate following Caesarean delivery shows diffuse linear opacities radiating from the hila and small bilateral pleural effusions. Repeat chest radiograph 20 hours later (right image) demonstrates interval resolution of diffuse linear opacities.
Case courtesy Elizabeth Asch, MD, Brigham and Women's Hospital.
新生儿一过性呼吸急促：剖宫产后足月新生儿首次胸部X线影像(左图)显示由肺门向外周呈放射状分布的弥漫性线状阴影和双侧少量胸腔积液。20小时后复查胸部X线影像(右图)显示两肺弥漫性线状阴影消失。

- TTN is the most common cause of respiratory distress in neonates. It is caused by lack of clearance of fetal lung fluid by prostaglandins, which normally dilate pulmonary lymphatics to absorb excess fluid.
- Prostaglandin imbalance can be worsened by male sex, Caesarean delivery (lack of "vaginal squeeze"), or maternal asthma, diabetes or sedation.
- Symptoms of dyspnea usually occur during the first 6 hours, peak at 24 hours and resolve by 48–72 hours.
- Chest radiograph shows findings of pulmonary edema, often with fluid in the minor fissure, perihilar interstitial opacities, and small pleural effusions. The cardiothymic silhouette may be mildly enlarged.
- TTN can be clinically and radiographically difficult to differentiate from neonatal pneumonia. Therefore, antibiotics are often given initially, although there is no specific treatment for TTN.

- TTN是新生儿呼吸窘迫最常见的原因，它是由于胎儿肺内积液无法通过前列腺素进行清除所致，而正常情况下，前列腺素会使肺淋巴管扩张从而吸收多余的液体。
- 以下因素会加重前列腺素不足：男婴、剖宫产（缺乏阴道"挤压"），或母亲患有哮喘、糖尿病或镇静麻醉。
- 呼吸困难症状通常发生在出生后的6小时内，在24小时达到高峰，并在48~72小时消失。
- 胸部X线影像显示肺水肿，常伴有肺小裂隙积液、肺门周围间质阴影和少量胸腔积液。心脏、胸腺轮廓可能会轻度增大。
- TTN在临床和影像上很难与新生儿肺炎鉴别，因此，发病的早期通常会使用抗生素，但对TTN本身没有特定的治疗方法。

Meconium aspiration syndrome

胎粪吸入综合征

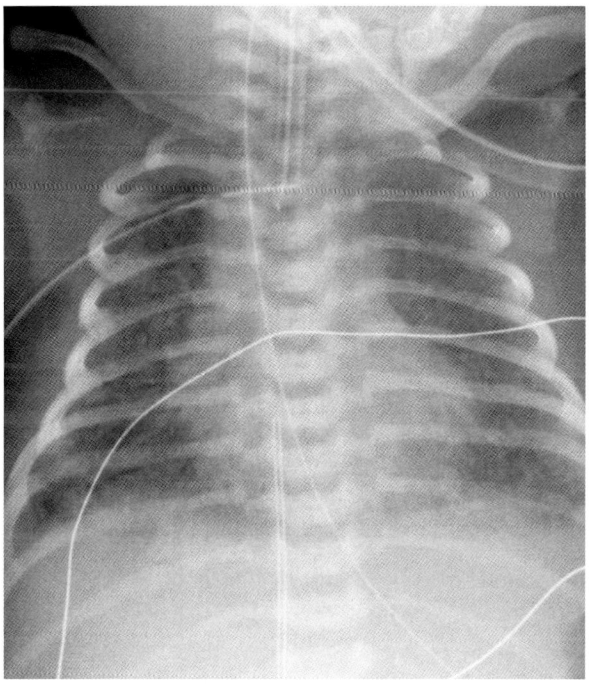

Meconium aspiration: Chest radiograph shows coarse interstitial opacities. Endotracheal tube, nasogastric tube, and umbilical venous catheter are partially seen. Although initially intubated, this baby was extubated and did well.

胎粪吸入：胸部X线影像显示两肺间质性粗颗粒状阴影。可见部分气管插管、鼻胃管和脐静脉置管。患儿在起初就进行了气管插管，但在拔管后病情稳定。

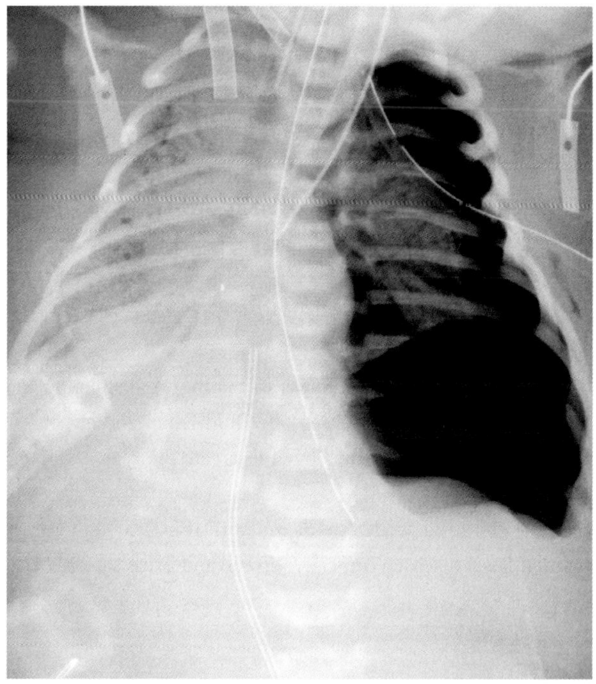

Severe meconium aspiration in a different patient: There is a large left pneumothorax and dense opacifications in the right hemithorax. This baby is receiving extracorporeal membrane oxygenation (ECMO). This infant did not survive.

另一名严重胎粪吸入患儿：胸部X线影像显示左侧大量气胸及右侧白肺。该患儿接受了体外膜肺氧合(ECMO)治疗。患儿最终未能存活。

- Peripartum meconium aspiration is typically seen in term and post-term neonates. Meconium is a highly irritating mixture of desquamated cells, bile pigments, and pancreatic enzymes that can cause significant respiratory distress.
- Imaging is characterized by bilateral asymmetric areas of hyperinflation and atelectasis, with ropy perihilar and coarse interstitial opacities. The lungs lose compliance and become especially susceptible to barotrauma and pneumothoraces.
- Outcome is variable, with much worse prognosis in the presence of a pneumothorax.

- 围产期胎粪吸入常发生在足月儿和过期产新生儿。胎粪是具有高度刺激性的混合物，由脱落上皮细胞、胆色素及胰酶组成，可导致严重的呼吸窘迫。
- 影像特点是两侧不对称区域性过度膨胀和肺不张，并伴有模糊的肺门和粗糙的间质阴影。由于肺顺应性下降，患儿特别容易发生气压伤和气胸。
- 预后差异较大，出现气胸者预后更差。

Neonatal pneumonia

- Unlike the previously described entities, which present with immediate respiratory distress, neonatal pneumonia takes hours to days to develop. The most common pathogens are group B streptococcus, *S. aureus*, and *E. coli*, which are acquired at birth from the vaginal flora.
- In neonatal pneumonia, the infection is not confined to the lung and is thought to represent neonatal sepsis.
- Typical signs of adult pneumonia, such as fever or elevated white count, are not reliable in neonates. Therefore, it can be difficult to distinguish between neonatal pneumonia and TTN. A history of prolonged rupture of membranes or known maternal infection may suggest neonatal pneumonia.
- Radiographic features of low lung volumes and granular opacities are similar to SDD, but patchy asymmetric perihilar opacities and pleural effusions can suggest pneumonia.

新生儿肺炎

- 前述疾病都是在出生后即刻出现呼吸窘迫的症状，而新生儿肺炎出现症状需要数小时到数天。最常见的病原菌是B族链球菌、金黄色葡萄球菌、大肠埃希菌，是患儿在出生时被阴道菌群感染所致。
- 在新生儿肺炎，感染并不限于肺部，且可能代表新生儿败血症。
- 成人肺炎的典型症状，如发热或白细胞计数升高，在新生儿中并不可靠。因此，新生儿肺炎很难与TTN鉴别。破膜时间过长或已知母亲有感染病史时，可提示有新生儿肺炎。
- X线影像表现为肺容积缩小和颗粒状阴影，与SDD相似，但肺门周围不对称的斑片状阴影和胸腔积液可提示肺炎。

Congenital structural thoracic disease

Congenital diaphragmatic hernia (CDH)

- CDH represents herniation of abdominal contents into the thorax, most commonly through a left posterior defect in the diaphragm (Bochdalek = back).
- The primary complication is ipsilateral pulmonary hypoplasia. Depending on the severity of the defect, contralateral hypoplasia may be present if the lung is compressed in utero.
- Right-sided lesions with liver herniations are rare and have a poor prognosis.
- The key imaging finding is a mass in the thorax displacing the mediastinum. At birth, the herniated bowel may be fluid-filled and appear solid. However, shortly after birth, air fills the bowel to create the typical appearance shown to the below.
- CDH is associated with bowel malrotation (95%), neural tube defects, congenital heart disease, Turner syndrome and Trisomy 21.

先天性胸部结构异常性疾病

先天性膈疝(CDH)

- 先天性膈疝(CHD)为腹部内容物疝入胸腔，最常见的部位是通过左后膈肌裂孔缺损(Bochdalek = back)。
- 主要并发症是患侧肺发育不良。取决于缺损的严重程度，如果肺在宫内受到挤压还可出现对侧肺发育不良。
- 右侧膈疝伴肝脏疝出较为罕见，其预后较差。
- 关键的影像学表现是胸部肿块并有纵隔移位。出生时，由于疝出的肠管充满液体，而表现为实性。但在出生后不久，肠道内开始积气而出现如下图所示的典型表现。
- CDH与肠旋转不良(95%)、神经管发育不全、先天性心脏病、特纳综合征和21-三体综合征有关。

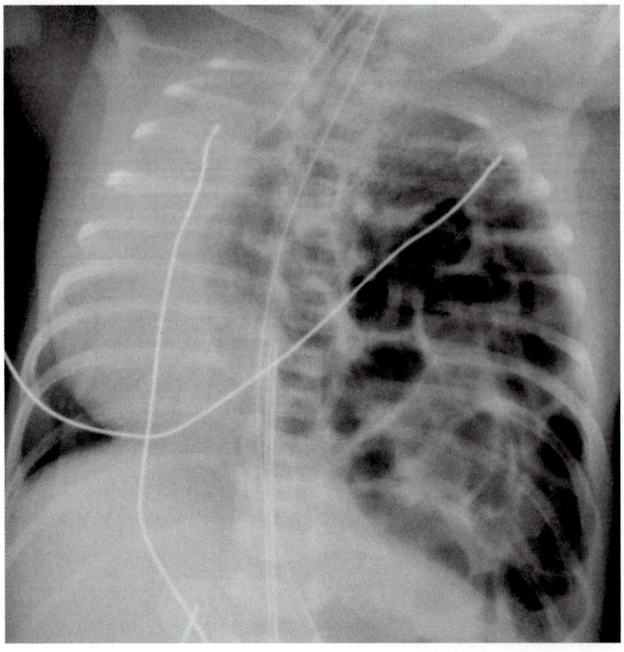

Congenital diaphragmatic hernia: Chest radiograph in a neonate shows multiple loops of air-filled bowel herniated into the left thorax, producing rightward displacement of the heart.
先天性膈疝：新生儿胸部X线影像可见多个疝入左侧胸腔的积气肠袢影，并造成心脏右移。

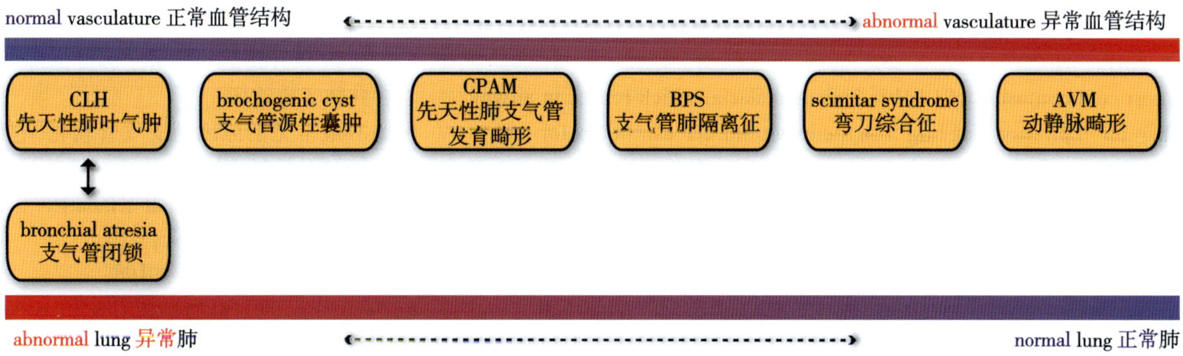

- Bronchopulmonary foregut malformations describe a range of congenital abnormalities of the embryonic foregut, which represent an inverse spectrum of normal to abnormal vasculature with normal to abnormal pulmonary parenchyma.

- 支气管肺前肠畸形指一系列发生在胚胎前肠的先天畸形，从正常到异常的血管构造，以及从正常到异常的肺实质结构。

Congenital lobar hyperinflation (CLH), a lesion of abnormal lung development without an associated vascular anomaly. Bronchial atresia is typically diagnosed later in life, and has been postulated to represent previously undiagnosed CLH.

Bronchogenic cyst, typically incidental, solitary, unilocular and fluid-filled mass which lacks communication to the airway. Air within a bronchogenic cyst therefore suggests infection or fistula.

Congenital pulmonary airway malformation (CPAM), previously called congenital cystic adenomatoid malformation.

Bronchopulmonary sequestration (BPS), aberrant lung tissue with anomalous systemic blood supply and no connection to the bronchial tree.

Scimitar syndrome, a form of partial anomalous pulmonary venous return.

Pulmonary arteriovenous malformation (AVM), an anomalous connection between the pulmonary artery and pulmonary veins, is a purely vascular malformation without any abnormal lung development.

先天性肺叶过度膨胀(CLH), 是一种无血管异常的肺发育畸形。支气管闭锁通常在患儿年龄较大时才被诊断，也有人认为是早期未被发现的CLH。

支气管源性囊肿，通常为偶然发现、孤立性、单房和充满液体的肿块，与气道不相通。若支气管源性囊肿内出现气体，则提示有感染或瘘管形成。

先天性肺气道畸形(CPAM), 旧称为先天性囊性腺瘤样畸形。

支气管肺隔离症，是由体循环供血的异常肺组织，与支气管树不相通。

弯刀综合征，是部分肺静脉异位引流的一种形式。

肺动静脉畸形(AVM), 肺动脉和静脉之间的异常交通，是一种单纯的血管畸形，不伴有任何肺的发育异常。

Congenital lobar hyperinflation (CLH) / Congenital lobar emphysema (CLE)

先天性肺叶气肿(CLH)/先天性大叶性肺气肿(CLE)

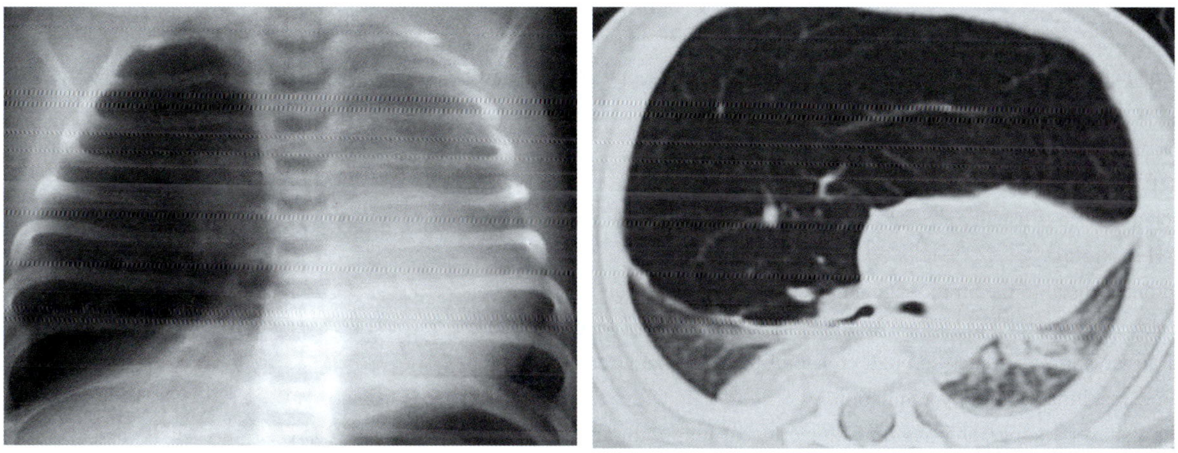

Congenital lobar hyperinflation: Chest radiograph (left image) shows a hyperlucent right lung with scant vascular markings and mediastinal shift to the left. Axial CT (right) shows a massively hyperexpanded right middle lobe, which has herniated across midline and exerts mass effect on the heart and bilateral lower lobes.

Case courtesy Michael Callahan, MD, Boston Children's Hospital.

先天性肺叶过度膨胀：胸部X线影像(左侧)显示右肺透亮度增加并伴有肺纹理稀少，纵隔向左偏移。轴位CT显示右肺中叶极度膨胀，并通过中线疝至对侧，压迫心脏和两肺下叶。

- Congenital lobar hyperinflation (CLH) or overinflation (CLO), formerly congenital lobar emphysema (CLE), is a syndrome of lobar air trapping caused by intrinsic or extrinsic bronchial narrowing without associated destruction of lung parenchyma.
- The most common cause of CLH is bronchomalacia, which results in airway collapse on expiration, leading to hyperinflation. CT can be performed to evaluate for a cause of bronchial obstruction, which is only found in about half of the cases of CLH.
- CLH usually involves the upper and middle lobes.
- In the pre-natal period, CLH is initially fluid-filled and appears as an echogenic mass. Post-natally and as fluid clears, CLH appears as a hyperlucent and hyperexpanded lobe that can exert mass effect on surrounding structures and result in mediastinal shift. It is essential not to mistake CLH for a tension pneumothorax, as a chest tube will increase respiratory distress.

- 先天性肺叶高度膨胀(CLH)或过度膨胀(CLO),先前称为先天性肺叶性气肿(CLE),是一种由支气管本身或外在原因造成的支气管管腔狭窄引起空气潴留于肺叶的综合征,不合并肺实质破坏。
- CLH最常见的原因是支气管软化,它可以在呼气时引起气道塌陷,从而导致肺过度膨胀。CT可以用于发现气道阻塞的原因,但只有一半的CLH病例可以找到原因。
- CLH通常发生在上叶和中叶。
- 在围产期,CLH最初充满了液体,表现为有回声的肿块。出生后液体清除,CLH表现为肺叶透过度增加和过度膨胀,可对周围结构产生占位效应,并导致纵隔移位。要注意,不能将CLH误诊为张力性气胸,因为胸腔插管会导致呼吸窘迫症状加重。

Bronchial atresia

支气管闭锁

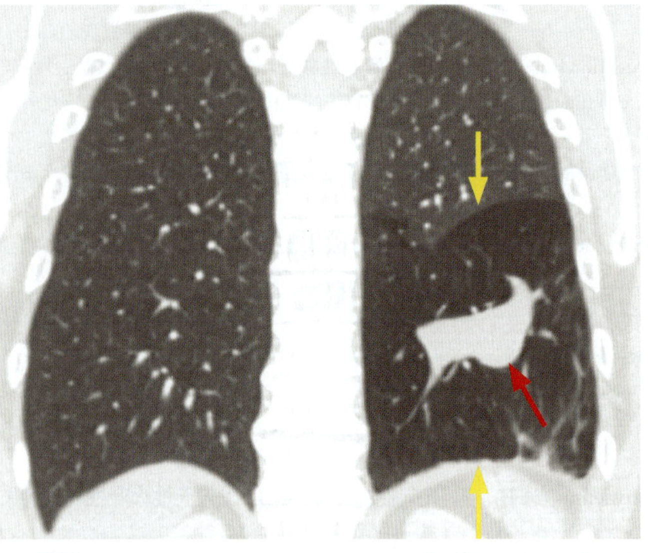

Bronchial atresia: Coronal CT shows hyperlucency of the left lower lobe (yellow arrows). There is a globular, well-defined opacity (red arrow) in the left lower lobe representing a mucocele of the atretic left lower lobe bronchus. This case is slightly atypical in that the left *lower* lobe is affected.

Case courtesy Ritu R.Gill,MD,MPH,Brigham and Women's Hospital.

支气管闭锁:冠状位CT显示左肺下叶透亮度增加(黄箭)。左肺下叶见一处球状、边界清楚的阴影(红箭),为闭锁左肺下叶支气管的黏液囊肿。这个病例不太典型,因为受累的是左肺下叶。

- Bronchial atresia is interruption of a lobar, segmental or subsegmental bronchus with resultant blind-ended bronchus and associated distal mucus impaction and hyperinflation.
- The left upper lobe is the most commonly affected.
- Bronchial atresia is usually incidentally diagnosed in adults and may be related to CLH in etiology.
- The bronchi distal to the atretic segment become filled with mucus that cannot be cleared, ultimately forming a tubular mucocele (*finger in glove*). The distal airways are ventilated through collateral pathways and demonstrate air trapping, resulting in local hyperinflation.
- Imaging shows a geographic region of hyperlucent lung with air trapping. A mucous plug may be visible just distal to the obstructed bronchial segment.

- 支气管闭锁是指肺叶、肺段或亚段支气管中断,导致支气管远端形成盲端,并在其远端出现黏液栓和肺过度膨胀。
- 左肺上叶最常受累。
- 支气管闭锁通常在成年时偶尔被发现,病因可能与CLH有关。

支气管闭锁段的远端腔内充满黏液,且无法被清除,因此最终形成管状的黏液囊肿(指套征)。远端气道通过侧支通气,并且有气体潴留,导致局部肺组织过度膨胀。

- 影像检查显示一片地图状的空气潴留性肺透亮区,黏液栓有时可见于阻塞支气管节段的远端。

Pulmonary arteriovenous malformation (AVM)

- A pulmonary arteriovenous malformation (AVM) is a purely vascular malformation representing anomalous connection between the pulmonary artery and pulmonary veins.

肺动静脉畸形(AVM)

- 肺动静脉畸形(AVM)是一种单纯的血管畸形,为肺动脉和静脉之间存在异常连接。

- About 60% of cases are associated with hereditary hemorrhagic telangiectasia (Osler- Weber-Rendu disease).
- Patients can present with cyanosis, clubbing, dyspnea, hemoptysis and polycythemia.
- There is an association with Glenn-shunting prior to the completion of the Fontan circulation due to the lack of hepaticized blood flow.

- 约 60%病例与遗传性出血性毛细血管扩张症(Osler-Weber-Rendu病)有关。
- 患者可表现为发绀、杵状指、呼吸困难、咯血和红细胞增多症。
- 由于缺乏肝化血流，在Fontan 循环(手术)完成之前与Glenn分流有关。

Congenital pulmonary airway malformation (CPAM) / congenital cystic adenomatoid malformation (CCAM)

先天性肺气道畸形(CPAM)/先天性囊性腺瘤样畸形(CCAM)

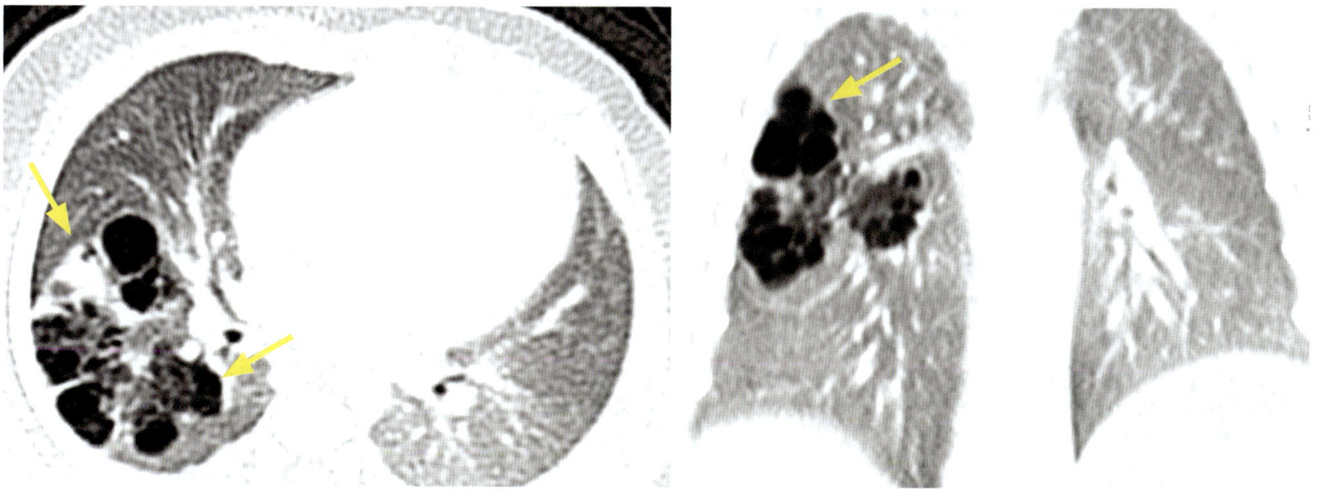

CPAM: Axial (left image) and coronal (right) CT images show a large, multicystic mass in the right upper lung (arrows) with both large and small cysts, representing a mixed type Ⅰ and type Ⅱ CPAM.

CPAM：轴位(左图)和冠状位CT图像显示右上肺(箭)大的、多囊状肿块，囊肿大小不等，为CPAM Ⅰ型及Ⅱ型混合型。

- Congenital pulmonary airway malformation (CPAM), previously termed congenital cystic adenomatoid malformation (CCAM), is a hamartomatous proliferation of terminal bronchioles that communicate with the bronchial tree.
- The arterial supply of CPAM arises from the pulmonary circulation. In contrast, sequestration (discussed below) derives its blood supply from the systemic circulation.
- The original classification (Stocker, revised in 2002) is important to be aware of, but the prognosis of CPAM depends more on the size of the lesion rather than its classification.

- 先天性肺气道畸形(CPAM)，以前称为先天性囊性腺瘤样畸形(CCAM)，是终末支气管的错构瘤样增生，并与支气管树相交通。
- CPAM的动脉血供来自肺循环。相比之下，肺隔离症(下文将讨论到)的血供来自体循环。
- 了解最初分型标准(Stocker，2002年修订)很重要，但CPAM的预后更多取决于病变大小而不是分型。

Type Ⅰ: One or more large cysts >2 cm. Most common form.
Type Ⅱ: Multiple thin-walled small cysts. Can be associated with renal agenesis.
Type Ⅲ: Solid-appearing with innumerable tiny cysts (<5 mm).
Type Ⅳ: Single large cyst, may be indistinguishable from a cystic pleuropulmonary blastoma, a rare malignancy that is the most common primary childhood lung tumor.

Ⅰ型：一个或多个大的囊腔(>2cm)，最常见类型。
Ⅱ型：多发薄壁小囊腔。可能并发肾缺如。
Ⅲ型：实性样肿块，伴有无数微小囊腔(<5mm)。
Ⅳ型：单一大囊腔，可能无法与囊性胸膜肺母细胞瘤鉴别，后者是一种罕见恶性肿瘤，为儿童最常见的原发性肺部肿瘤。

- CPAM may exert mass effect and is prone to infection. Surgery is usually recommended as they are difficult to differentiate from pleuropulmonary blastoma.

- CPAM可能会产生占位效应，容易感染。通常建议手术，因为该病很难与胸膜肺母细胞瘤鉴别。

Bronchopulmonary sequestration (BPS)

支气管肺隔离症(BPS)

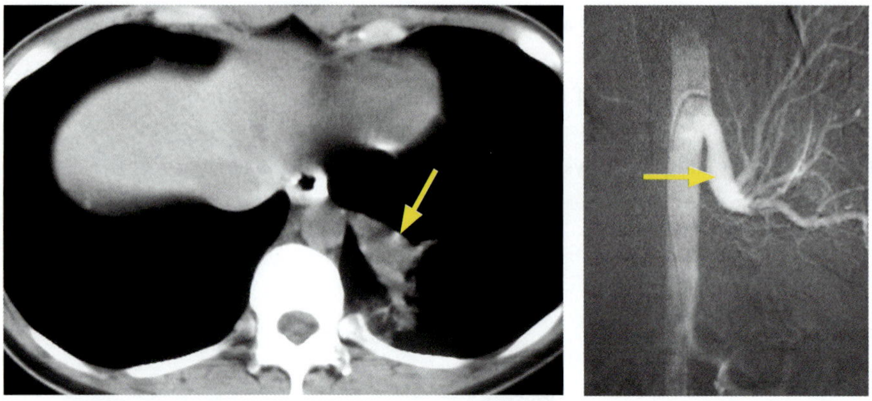

Sequestration: Axial CT shows a left lower lobe soft tissue mass abutting the aorta (arrow). Thoracic aortogram demonstrates a large feeding artery arising directly off the aorta (arrow).

Case courtesy Michael Callahan, MD, Boston Children's Hospital.

隔离症：轴位CT可见左肺下叶、主动脉旁软组织影(箭)。胸主动脉造影显示一条粗大的供血动脉直接起自于主动脉(箭)。

- Sequestration is aberrant lung tissue with anomalous **systemic blood supply**, usually arising from the thoracic aorta. The key imaging finding is a systemic feeding artery, which can be seen by Doppler ultrasound pre-natally, or by CTA or MRA post-natally. The most common location is the left lower lobe. In contrast to CPAM, sequestration is usually solid, though hybrid lesions with both CPAM and BPS components do exist.
- Two types of sequestration, intralobar and extralobar, are usually distinguished by CT or MR:

- 隔离症是迷走的肺组织伴有异常**体循环供血**，通常来源于胸主动脉。影像学的关键特征是发现来自体循环的供血动脉，产前可以通过多普勒超声，或出生后用CTA或MRA进行诊断。最常见的发病部位是左肺下叶。与CPAM相比，隔离症通常为实性，但可以同时具有CPAM和BPS的混合性成分。
- 隔离症有两种类型，叶内型和叶外型，两者通常可以用CT或MRI进行鉴别：

Intralobar (75%): Inside pleura, usually with pulmonary venous drainage (or left atrium).

- Onset in adolescence/adulthood with recurrent pneumonia or hemoptysis.
- In contrast to extralobar sequestration, it is rarely associated with other developmental anomalies.
- All occur above the diaphragm, most commonly in the left lower lobe.

Extralobar (25%): External to the pleura, with primarily systemic venous drainage (IVC or azygous).

- Onset in infancy with respiratory compromise related to associated anomalies (CDH, CPAM, congenital heart disease, pulmonary hypoplasia, vertebral anomalies).
- These may be subdiaphragmatic, i.e., near the adrenal gland mimicking an adrenal mass.

叶内型(75%)：位于胸膜内，通常经肺静脉引流(或流入左心房)。

- 青春期/成年期开始发病，表现为反复肺炎或咯血。
- 与叶外型隔离症不同，罕见伴随其他发育异常。
- 均发生在膈上，最常见于左肺下叶。

叶外型(25%)：位于胸膜外，主要通过体静脉引流(IVC或奇静脉)。

- 婴儿期开始发病，表现为呼吸功能受损，与伴发的其他异常有关(如CDH、CPAM、先天性心脏病、肺发育不全、椎骨异常)。
- 有些病变可能位于膈下，当靠近肾上腺时与肾上腺肿块相似。

Scimitar syndrome

弯刀综合征

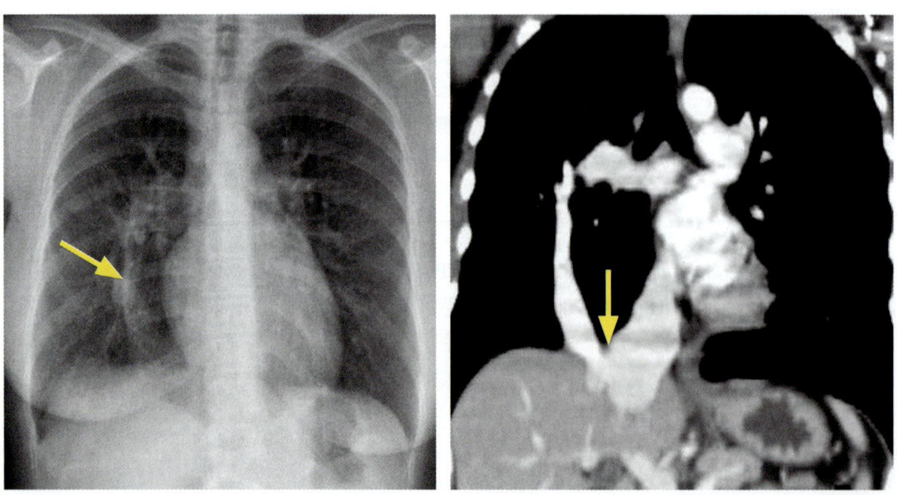

Scimitar syndrome: Frontal chest radiograph (left image) shows a curvilinear opacity extending from the right hilum towards the diaphragm, representing the *scimitar sign* (arrow). Coronal contrast-enhanced CT (right image) shows the anomalous scimitar vein draining into the inferior vena cava, consistent with partial anomalous pulmonary venous return.

Case courtesy Michael Hanley, MD, University of Virginia Health System.

弯刀综合征：正位胸部X线影像(左图)显示一条曲线样的阴影，从右肺门延伸到膈肌，提示*弯刀征*(箭)。冠状位增强CT(右图)显示弯刀形的肺静脉异常引流入下腔静脉，符合部分性肺静脉异位引流的诊断。

- Scimitar syndrome represents partial anomalous pulmonary venous return (PAPVR) from right lower lobe pulmonary veins into either the right atrium or IVC.

  In contrast to PAPVR, in *total* anomalous pulmonary venous return (TAPVR), all 4 pulmonary veins return blood to the right atrium, and an obligate right-to-left shunt is necessary for survival.
- The anomalous vein appears like a "scimitar" or Turkish sword on the frontal radiograph, representing the *scimitar sign*.
- Scimitar syndrome can be associated with hypoplasia and hyperlucency of the right lung (although this finding is not demonstrated in the case above).

- 弯刀综合征：为部分性肺静脉异位引流(PAPVR)，从右肺下叶肺静脉回流入右心房或下腔静脉。

  与PAPVR相比较，完全性肺静脉异位引流(TAPVR)中所有四条肺静脉血均回流至右心房，患儿必须有右向左分流才能存活。
- 异常引流的静脉在正位图像上形似“一把弯刀(scimitar)”，因此称为*弯刀征*。
- 弯刀综合征可以伴发右肺发育不良和透亮过度(该表现在上述病例中并没有显示)。

SMALL AIRWAYS DISEASE

小气道病变

Bronchiolitis

细支气管炎

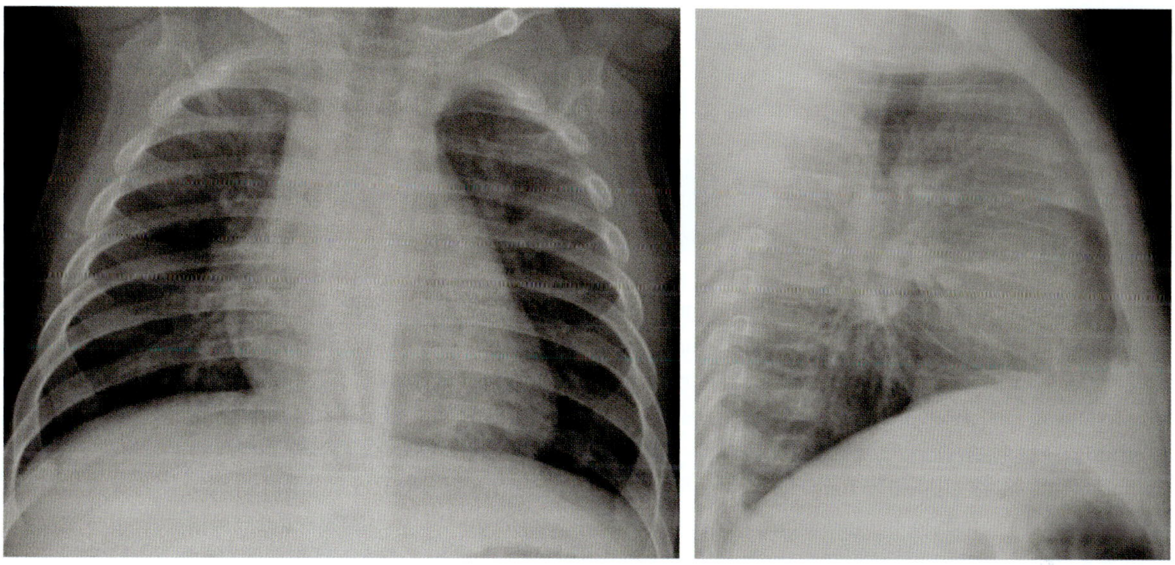

Bronchiolitis: Frontal and lateral chest radiographs demonstrate bilateral hyperexpanded lungs with increased perihilar markings and peribronchial cuffing.

细支气管炎：正位和侧位胸部X线影像显示双肺过度膨胀，肺门周围纹理增加及支气管周围套袖征。

- Bronchiolitis is an infection of the lower respiratory tract, most commonly caused by respiratory syncytial virus (RSV). It is mostly seen in children under the age of 5 years and is the leading cause of infant hospitalization in the United States.
- Inflammation of bronchiolar epithelium leads to peribronchial infiltration by inflammatory cells. The resultant necrotic debris may lead to small airway obstruction, the hallmark of bronchiolitis.
- Clinically, bronchiolitis presents as increased work of breathing and wheezing in a child, usually with a viral upper respiratory prodrome. It is primarily a clinical diagnosis.
- Radiographic findings include hyperexpanded lungs (best seen as flattening of the diaphragms on the lateral view) with scattered areas of atelectasis, increased perihilar peribronchial markings and peribronchial cuffing. These findings are subjective, with high variability among even experienced pediatric radiologists.

  Similar radiographic findings in an older patient population may represent reactive airways disease.It is important to exclude bacterial pneumonia which features focal airspace consolidation with air bronchograms and pleural effusions.

- 细支气管炎是下呼吸道感染，最常见的原因是呼吸道合胞病毒(RSV)感染。它多见于5岁以下的儿童，是美国婴儿住院的主要原因。
- 支气管上皮的炎症导致炎症细胞在支气管周围浸润。坏死的细胞碎片可以导致小气道阻塞，此为细支气管炎的标志性特征。
- 临床上，细支气管炎表现为患儿呼吸困难和哮喘，通常有上呼吸道病毒感染的前驱症状。细支气管炎是一个基于临床的诊断。
- 影像学表现包括肺过度膨胀(最易在侧位影像上看到膈肌变平)伴散在肺不张、肺门周围的支气管纹理增加，以及支气管周围套袖征。这些征象具有主观性，即便在经验丰富的小儿放射科医生中也存在很大的差异。

  类似的影像学表现在年龄较大的患儿可能代表反应性呼吸道疾病。重要的是排除细菌性肺炎，其特征为局灶性肺实变伴空气支气管征和胸腔积液。

Round pneumonia, most often caused by S. *pneumoniae* and seen in children less than 8 years of age, is typically seen as a round pulmonary opacity with well-defined margins mimicking a mass.

球形肺炎最常由肺炎链球菌引起，见于8岁以下的儿童，通常表现为一个圆形的肺部阴影，边缘清晰，类似于肿块。

Bronchiolitis obliterans syndrome (BOS) = constrictive bronchiolitis

闭塞性细支气管炎综合征(BOS)=缩窄性细支气管炎

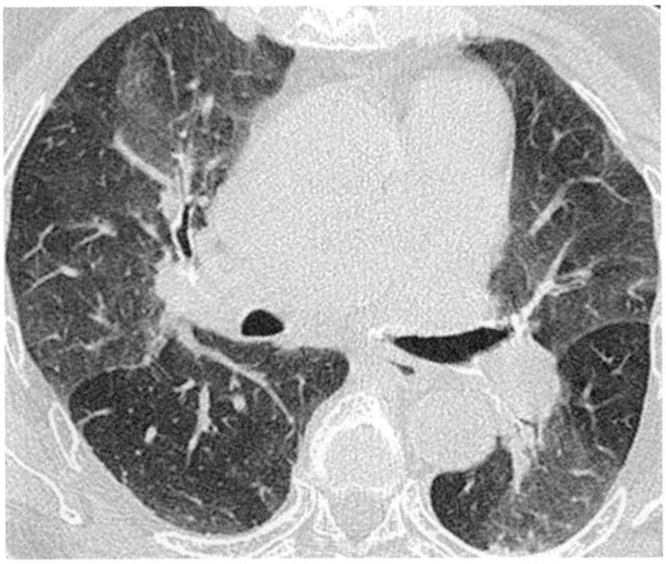

Bronchiolitis obliterans: Axial CT shows mosaic perfusion with geographic regions of ground glass attenuation.
This is an example in an adult; however, the findings are similar in children.
Case courtesy Ritu R. Gill, MD, MPH, Brigham and Women's Hospital.

闭塞性细支气管炎：轴位CT显示马赛克样灌注，伴有地图样分布的磨玻璃影。
本例是一名成人，但表现与儿童相似。

- Bronchiolitis obliterans syndrome (BOS) is the final common pathway of small airway obstruction by inflammatory and fibrous tissue, which may be due to multiple etiologies. BOS may be post-transplant in origin, post-infectious (typically following viral or atypical bacterial pneumonia), or related to toxin or drug exposures.
- BOS is one of the most clinically important complications of pediatric allogeneic lung and bone marrow transplantation.
- Chest radiographs are usually normal or may show mild hyperinflation.
- CT demonstrates findings of small airways obstruction, including

- 闭塞性细支气管炎综合征(BOS)是由炎症和纤维组织导致的小气道阻塞的最终结果，可以有很多病因。BOS可能发生在移植后、感染后(通常继发于病毒性或不典型细菌性肺炎)，或与毒物或药物接触有关。
- BOS是临床上儿童异体肺及骨髓移植中最重要的并发症之一。
- 胸部X线影像通常正常或有轻微的肺过度膨胀。
- 小气道阻塞的CT征象包括：

> Air trapping on expiratory views.
> Mosaic perfusion.
> Bronchiectasis and bronchial wall thickening.

> 呼气时气体潴留。
> 马赛克样灌注。
> 支气管扩张及支气管管壁增厚。

- **Swyer-James-MacLeod** syndrome is an acquired complication in up to 1/3 of young patients with post-infectious BOS. Abnormal pulmonary development secondary to BOS leads to a unilateral hyperlucent lung with volume loss.

  The key radiographic feature is a small ipsilateral, hyperlucent lung with diminished vascular markings. Note that Swyer-James-MacLeod is not a sequela of viral bronchiolitis (of which RSV is the most common cause), but is only seen after BOS, classically triggered by adenovirus infection or *Mycoplasma pneumoniae.*

- **Swyer-James-MacLeod** 综合征(单侧透明肺，单侧半透明肺或单侧获得性肺叶气肿)是年轻患者感染BOS后的一种获得性并发症，其发生率高达1/3。BOS可导致肺发育不良，引起单侧肺透亮度增加并伴有肺体积缩小。

  主要影像学特征是单侧肺体积缩小，透亮度增加伴血管纹理减少。注意，Swyer-James-MacLeod 不是病毒性细支气管炎的后遗症(RSV是其最常见的致病原因)，而只是见于BOS后，通常由腺病毒或肺炎支原体感染所触发。

Cryptogenic organizing pneumonia (COP) = bronchiolitis obliterans organizing pneumonia (BOOP)

- Cryptogenic organizing pneumonia (COP) is a disorder of the distal airways characterized by filling of the bronchioles and alveoli with granulation tissue polyps. Bronchiolitis obliterans organizing pneumonia (BOOP) is an older term for the same entity, and is often confused with bronchiolitis obliterans which is

隐源性机化性肺炎(COP)= 闭塞性细支气管炎伴机化性肺炎(BOOP)

- 隐源性机化性肺炎(COP)是远端气道的疾病，以肉芽组织息肉充填细支气管和肺泡为特征。闭塞性细支气管炎伴机化性肺炎(BOOP)是同一疾病的旧称，常与闭塞性细支气管炎相混

a completely different disease.

- The underlying histologic changes of COP are referred to as organizing pneumonia (OP). COP is the clinical syndrome of OP of unknown cause. OP may be secondary to infection, drug reaction, or inhalation. OP may also be a complication of stem cell transplant, but much less commonly than BOS.
- Radiographic features of COP/OP include multifocal migratory consolidations, ground glass opacities, and nodules. The *atoll* or *reverse halo sign* is thought to be relatively specific for OP and features a central lucency surrounded by ground glass.

淆，但两者是完全不同的疾病。

- COP的组织学改变为机化性肺炎(OP)。COP是OP在原因不明时的临床综合征。OP可能继发于感染、药物反应或误吸。OP也可能是干细胞移植手术的并发症，但比BOS少见得多。
- COP/OP影像学表现包括多灶游走性肺实变、磨玻璃密度影和结节影。环礁征或反晕征被认为对OP诊断具有相对特异性，其特征为中央透亮区被周围磨玻璃影所包围。

Bronchiectasis

- Bronchiectasis is bronchial dilation, most commonly due to inflammation.
- It can have a variety of causes in the pediatric population:

> Cystic fibrosis.
> Allergic bronchopulmonary aspergillosis. Post-infectious.
> Tracheobronchomegaly (Mounier-Kuhn). Aspiration.
> Intralobar sequestration, possibly due to recurrent infections.

- The *signet ring sign* describes enlargement of the bronchiole, which appears larger than the adjacent pulmonary artery branch.

支气管扩张

- 支气管扩张是支气管管腔扩大，最常见的原因是炎症。
- 支气管扩张在儿童有很多种不同的原因：

> 囊性纤维化。
> 变应性支气管肺曲菌病。感染后。
> 巨大气管支气管症(Mounier-Kuhn综合征)。误吸。
> 叶内型隔离症，可能是由于反复感染所致。

- 印戒征为细支气管扩张，表现为细支气管管径大于邻近肺动脉分支。

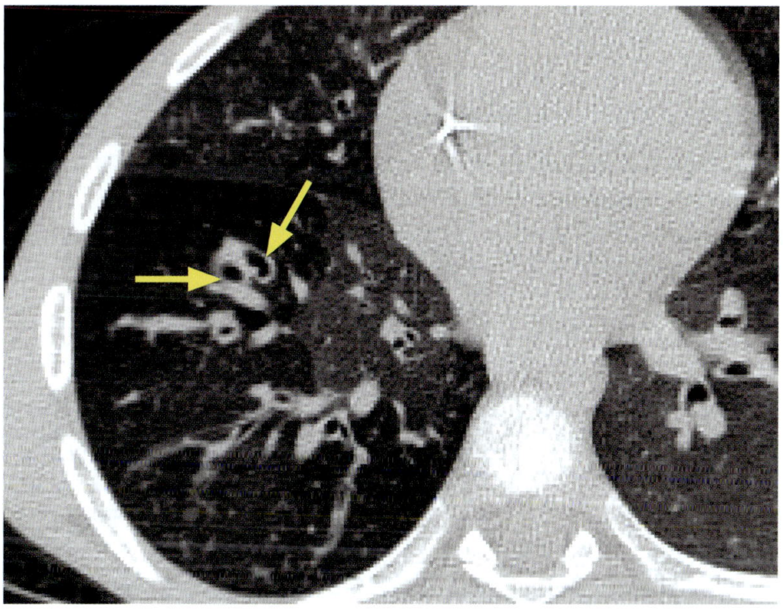

Bronchiectasis in cystic fibrosis: Axial CT demonstrates relative enlargement of numerous subsegmental bronchi with associated bronchial wall thickening (arrows).
Case courtesy Michael Hanley, MD, University of Virginia Health System.
囊性纤维化中的支气管扩张：轴位CT显示多个亚段细支气管相对扩张，伴支气管管壁增厚(箭)。

Unilateral hyperlucent lung

- A unilateral hyperlucent lung is a common finding in pediatric chest radiology. The two most important acute diagnoses are endobronchial foreign body and pneumothorax.

单侧肺透亮度增高

- 单侧肺透亮度增高是儿童胸部X线影像中常见的一个征象。两个最重要的急症是支气管内异物和气胸。

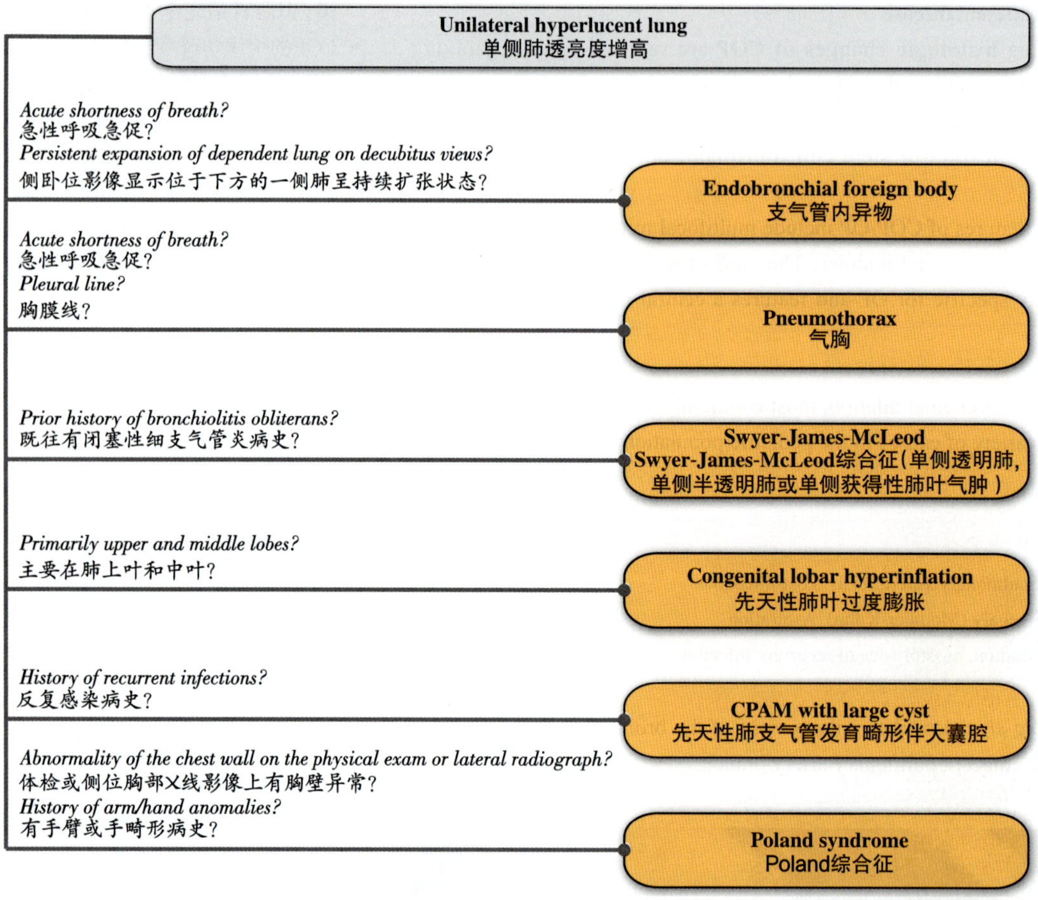

Poland syndrome

- Poland syndrome is an autosomal recessive syndrome of unilateral congenital absence (complete or partial) of the pectoralis major muscle. Associated anomalies of the ipsilateral arm and hand, including short metacarpals and syndactyly (joined fingers), may be present.

Pediatric mediastinal masses

- An approach to mediastinal masses, including the relevant anatomy and division of the three main compartments (anterior, middle, and posterior), is discussed in the thoracic imaging section.
- This brief differential highlights the common mediastinal masses in children.

Anterior mediastinum

- Normal thymus can appear large in children up to 5 years of age and is sometimes mistaken as an anterior mediastinal mass.

  Normal thymus is triangular in shape with undulating margins along the anterior ribs (thymic wave sign), inferolateral extension into the minor fissure (thymic sail sign) and relative lucency allowing for visualization of overlapping pulmonary vascular markings. It causes no mass-effect on the trachea. Thymic rebound, which is physiologic regrowth of the thymus after chemotherapy, should also not be mistaken for an anterior mediastinal mass. Thymic rebound can be FDG-avid on PET.
- Lymphoma.
- Germ cell tumor.
- Thymoma (very rare in children).

Middle mediastinum

- Foregut duplication cyst, including bronchogenic or enteric cysts.

Poland综合征

- Poland综合征是常染色体隐性遗传疾病,伴有单侧先天性胸大肌缺失(完全或部分)。其他异常可能还有同侧手臂和手的畸形,包括掌骨变短或并指。

小儿纵隔肿瘤

- 纵隔肿块的诊断思路已经在胸部影像部分进行了讨论,其中包括相关的解剖及纵隔的三个主要分区(前纵隔、中纵隔和后纵隔)。
- 下面简单概括最常见的小儿纵隔肿块。

前纵隔

- 正常胸腺在5岁以下的儿童可以很大,有时被误认为是前纵隔肿块。

  正常胸腺呈三角形,沿前肋边缘起伏(胸腺的波浪征),下外侧延伸至水平裂(胸腺的船帆征),相对透亮,可以看到重叠的肺血管影。它不会对气管产生占位效应。化疗后胸腺反弹是胸腺的生理性再生,不应误认为是前纵隔肿块。胸腺反弹在PET上可能会有FDG摄取。
- 淋巴瘤。
- 生殖细胞瘤。
- 胸腺瘤(儿童罕见)。

中纵隔

- 前肠重复囊肿,包括支气管囊肿或前肠囊肿。

- Neurenteric cysts, which are often associated with vertebral anomalies.
- Lymphadenopathy, most often from lymphoma or granulomatous disease (tuberculosis or fungal).

Posterior mediastinum

- Neurogenic tumors (90% of masses), including neuroblastoma (most common, under age two), ganglioneuroblastoma, and ganglioneuroma (least common).

- 神经肠源性囊肿，通常伴有脊柱异常。
- 淋巴结肿大，最常见于淋巴瘤或炎性肉芽肿病(结核病或真菌病)。

后纵隔

- 神经源性肿瘤(占肿瘤的90%)，包括神经母细胞瘤(最常见，2岁以下)、神经节神经母细胞瘤和神经节神经瘤(最不常见)。

Miscellaneous

其他

Pneumomediastinum

纵隔气肿

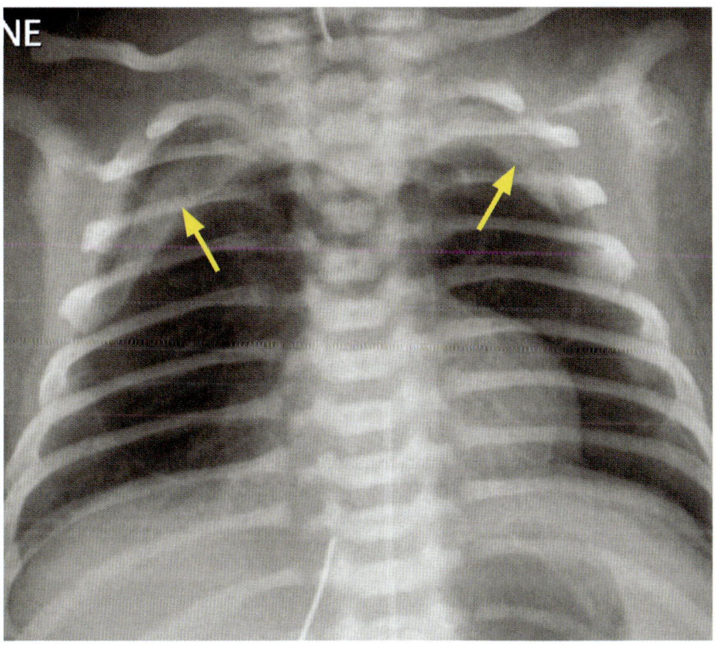

Spinnaker sail sign of pneumomediastinum:
Frontal chest radiograph in an intubated neonate demonstrates elevation of both thymic lobes (arrows).
Case courtesy Michael Hanley, MD, University of Virginia Health System.

纵隔气肿的大三角船帆征：
本例为接受气管插管的新生儿，正位胸部X线影像显示两侧胸腺被抬高(箭)。

- The *spinnaker sail sign* is seen in pneumomediastinum and represents the thymus lifted off the mediastinum by the ectopic air. This is also called the *angel-wing sign* and should not be confused with the *sail sign*, which is the rightward extension of the normal thymus.

Support devices

- **Endotracheal tube (ETT)** positioning should be intrathoracic. The flexion/extension of the neck is significant to note when positioning is borderline.
- **Umbilical venous catheter (UVC)** courses from the umbilical vein directly up to the left portal vein, ductus venosus, and middle or left hepatic vein, ideally terminating in the suprahepatic IVC just below the right atrium.

  UVC positioned within the portal vein can cause portal vein thrombosis and potential liver infarct.
- **Umbilical artery catheter (UAC)** originates at the umbilical artery and initially descends into the internal iliac artery, then ascends the common iliac artery and abdominal aorta where the tip ideally terminates at T6–10 (high) or L3–L5 (low).

  The goal is to avoid branches of the aortic arch and abdominal aorta to prevent thrombosis.
- **Percutaneously inserted central catheter (PICC)** placed via an upper

- 大三角船帆征见于纵隔气肿，表示胸腺被纵隔内气体向上推举移位。这也称为天使翼征，但不应与船帆征混淆，后者是正常胸腺向右侧延伸。

生命维持装置

- **气管插管(ETT)**应置于胸腔内。当位置处于临界状态时，需要注意颈部的弯曲/伸展状态。
- **脐静脉导管(UVC)**从脐静脉直接向上延伸至门静脉左支、静脉导管和肝中静脉或肝左静脉，理想的导管终端应位于右心房稍下方的肝上IVC。

  位于门静脉内的UVC 可导致门静脉血栓形成，并有肝梗死的可能。
- **脐动脉导管(UAC)**起始于脐动脉，首先下行到髂内动脉，然后上升到髂总动脉和腹主动脉，导管终端的理想位置在T_{6-10}(高点)或L_{3-5}(低点)。

  目的是避免插入主动脉弓和腹主动脉的分支，以防止血栓形成。
- 上肢**经皮中心静脉置管(PICC)**应将导管的头

extremity approach should terminate in the distal SVC, while one placed via a lower extremity approach should terminate in the IVC just inferior to the right atrium.

端置于SVC的远端，而通过下肢放置的导管应终止于右心房下方的IVC。

- **Extracorporeal membrane exchange (ECMO)** devices can be categorized into two types.

  Venoarterial (VA): right internal jugular and right common carotid arteries are usually cannulated. A feared complication of VA catheterization is backing out of the cannula, during which the child can exsanguinate.

  Venovenous (VV): single right internal jugular catheter terminates in the right atrium.

- **体外膜肺氧合(ECMO)交换**装置可分为两种类型。

  动静脉型(VA)：通常选取右侧颈内静脉和右侧颈总动脉插管。VA导管插入术的一个严重并发症是在退出套管时，可能会引发患儿致命性大出血。

  静脉型(VV)：仅对右颈内静脉进行插管，导管终端位于右心房。

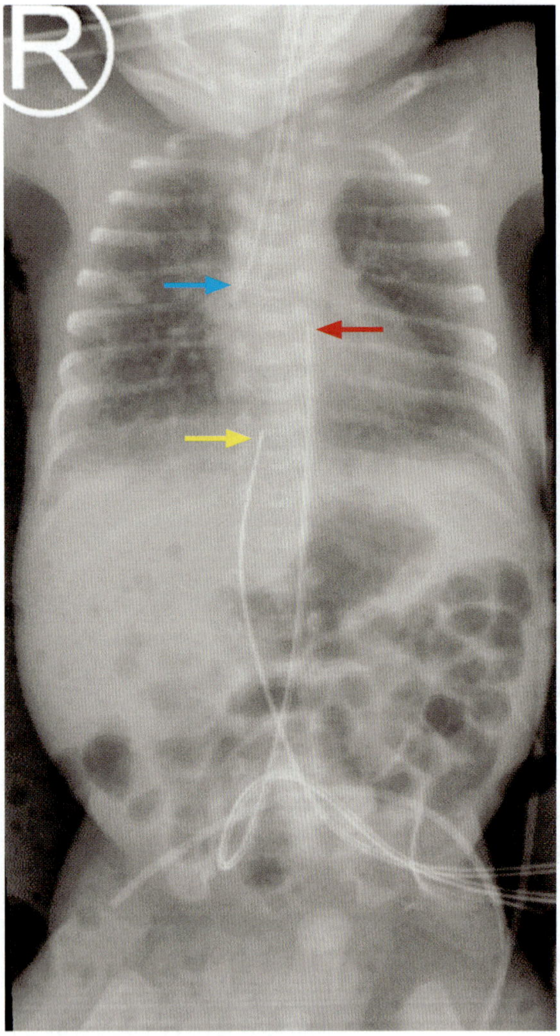

Normal course of umbilical venous/arterial catheters: Frontal radiograph shows an umbilical venous catheter coursing directly upward in the right hemiabdomen to terminate at the inferior cavoatrial junction (yellow arrow).
An umbilical arterial catheter is seen initially descending prior to coursing upward to terminate between T6–T10 (red arrow). Note endotracheal tube tip is malpositioned in the right mainstem bronchus (blue arrow).
脐静脉/动脉导管的正常路径：正位X线影像显示脐静脉导管沿右侧腹部直接向上并终止于下腔静脉与右心房交界处(黄箭)。
脐动脉导管首先下降，然后再向上，终止于$T_{6\sim10}$水平(红箭)。注意气管插管尖端误入右主支气管(蓝箭)。

（翻译　路莉）

PEDIATRIC CARDIAC

小儿心脏

APPROACH TO THE PLAIN FILM OF CONGENITAL HEART DISEASE

先天性心脏病的X线影像诊断方法

Plain film evaluation of congenital heart disease: Of historical interest only?

- Most congenital heart disease is diagnosed in utero during routine fetal ultrasound.

X线影像对先天性心脏病的评估：仅仅是过去的历史？

- 大多数先天性心脏病都可以通过常规胎儿超声诊断。

- If a newborn has unexpected shortness of breath with clinical concern for a cardiac cause, an echocardiogram is typically the imaging study of choice. Advanced imaging, such as CTA or MRI, may also be helpful in certain clinical situations.
- Even though the specific diagnosis of congenital heart disease may not be determined from the plain radiograph, there is value in describing the radiographic findings (e.g., increased pulmonary vascularity, cardiomegaly, etc.).

- 当新生儿出现意外呼吸困难并临床怀疑与心脏疾病有关时，心脏超声通常是首选的影像方法。进一步影像学检查如CTA或MRI，可能对某些临床情形有帮助。
- 虽然X线影像不能对先天性心脏病作出特定的诊断，但普通X线影像上的一些发现是有价值的(如肺血增多、心脏增大等)。

Plain film evaluation of congenital heart disease: Three questions to ask

- First, **is the patient cyanotic or acyanotic?**
- Second, **is the pulmonary vascularity increased or decreased?** This can be either increased venous flow, increased arterial flow, or decreased arterial flow.

  Increased vascularity can be determined by examining the peripheral 1/3 of the lungs where there is normally very little blood flow. Increased peripheral vasculature suggests either increased pulmonary venous or pulmonary arterial flow.

X线影像评估先天性心脏病：需要问的三个问题

- 第一，**患者是发绀还是不发绀?**
- 第二，**肺血是增多还是减少?** 这可能由静脉血流增加，动脉血流增加，或动脉血流减少所致。

  肺血增多可以通过肺外周带1/3的肺纹理进行判断，因在正常情况下肺外周很少有血流。外周肺血管影增加提示肺动脉或静脉的血流增加。

1) **Increased** pulmonary **venous** flow (pulmonary edema) is seen when the left ventricular outflow tract can't keep up with venous return.

   Causes include left heart insufficiency, obstructive left heart lesion, or congestive heart failure. Peripheral 1/3 of the lungs shows *indistinct* vessels and septal markings.

2) **Increased** pulmonary **arterial** flow (shunt vascularity) tends to present in childhood rather than infancy. It is caused by a left-to-right shunt, which leads to the right side of the heart pumping too much blood to the lungs via the pulmonary arteries.

   Peripheral 1/3 of the lungs shows *distinct*, large-caliber vessels.

3) **Decreased** pulmonary **arterial** flow is due to right ventricular outflow tract insufficiency.

   Any lesion causing decreased pulmonary arterial flow is ALWAYS cyanotic because not enough blood is being oxygenated in the lungs.

   Peripheral 1/3 of the lungs shows decreased vasculature.

1) 肺**静脉**血流**增加**(肺水肿)是由于静脉回流的血容量超过了左心室的流出量。

   原因包括左心功能不全，左心阻塞性病变，或先天性心功能衰竭。肺外周1/3可见模糊的血管影和小叶间隔影。

2) 肺**动脉**血流**增加**(血管分流)儿童比婴儿更多见。由左向右分流造成，导致右心通过肺动脉向两肺泵出更多的血。

   肺外周1/3可见清晰的血管影，血管口径增粗。

3) 肺**动脉**血流**减少**由右心室流出道功能不足所致。

   任何引起肺动脉血流减少的病变**都**表现为发绀，因为肺内没有足够的氧化血流。

   肺外周1/3肺血减少。

- Third, **is the heart enlarged or normal in size?** Note, it is never smaller than normal (even in hypoplastic left heart syndrome).
- Additional findings, such as specific contour to the aorta and cardiac chambers, orientation of the aortic arch, and side of stomach bubble can help refine the diagnosis.

- 第三：**心脏体积增大还是正常?** 注意，心脏从来不会小于正常(即使为左心发育不全综合征)。
- 其他有助于诊断的发现，如主动脉的轮廓、心脏的腔室、主动脉弓走行方向，以及胃泡的位置。

Plain film evaluation of congenital heart disease: Can it be anything else?

- It is important to remember that an apparently enlarged heart and abnormal pulmonary vasculature can be due to other diseases in addition to congenital heart disease, including:

X线影像评估先天性心脏病：还可能是其他病变吗?

- 必须要记住，心脏显著增大及肺血管异常也可以由先天性心脏病以外的其他疾病所致，包括：

Intracardiac tumor, such as a rhabdomyoma.

CHF due to a peripheral shunt (e.g., vein of Galen malformation or hepatic hemangioendothelioma). Mediastinal mass.

Congenital diaphragmatic hernia with non-aerated bowel.

心脏肿瘤，如横纹肌瘤等。

外周分流导致的充血性心力衰竭(如Galen静脉畸形或肝血管内皮细胞瘤)。纵隔肿块。

先天性膈疝伴无积气肠道。

Bronchiolitis may also mimic pulmonary edema, particularly in children with congenital heart disease.

支气管炎也可能类似肺水肿，尤其是在患有有先天性心脏病的儿童中。

OVERVIEW OF RADIOGRAPHIC DIFFERENTIAL DIAGNOSIS FOR CONGENITAL HEART DISEASE

先天性心脏病的影像学鉴别概述

Acyanotic congenital heart disease

- Neonatal **increased pulmonary venous flow** (pulmonary edema) may be caused by:

非发绀型先天性心脏病

- **新生儿肺静脉血流增加**(肺水肿)，可能的病因如下：

Hypoplastic left heart, similar in physiology to CHF (left ventricle cannot keep up with venous return).
Aortic coarctation, which is a left ventricular outflow tract lesion.
Congestive heart failure (CHF), which may be due to a primary cardiac anomaly or an extra-cardiac arteriovenous shunt, such as a vein of Galen malformation or hepatic hemangioendothelioma.
Neonatal sepsis, typically seen in the setting of neonatal pneumonia.

左心发育不全，在生理学上类似于充血性心力衰竭(即左心室不能输出全部回流的静脉血)。
主动脉缩窄，一种左心室流出道异常的疾病。
充血性心力衰竭(CHF)，可由于心脏本身异常或心外动静脉分流如Galen静脉畸形或肝血管内皮瘤。
新生儿脓毒血症，通常合并新生儿肺炎。

- **Increased pulmonary arterial flow** (shunt vascularity) tends to present in childhood rather than the neonatal period, and can be caused by:

- **肺动脉血流增加**(分流血管)更常见于儿童期而非新生儿期，可能的病因如下：

Atrial septal defect (ASD).
Ventricular septal defect (VSD).
Patent ductus arteriosus (PDA).
Endocardial cushion defect (ECD), also known as an atrioventricular (AV) septal or AV canal defect, has a strong association with Down syndrome.

房间隔缺损(ASD)。
室间隔缺损(VSD)。
动脉导管未闭(PDA)。
心内膜垫缺损(ECD)，也称为房室间隔或通道缺损，与唐氏综合征密切相关。

Cyanotic congenital heart disease

发绀型先天性心脏病

- **Decreased pulmonary vascularity with cardiomegaly**:

- **肺血减少伴心影增大：**

Ebstein anomaly.
Pulmonary atresia with intact ventricular septum.

埃布斯坦畸形(三尖瓣下移畸形)。
室间隔完整型肺动脉闭锁。

- **Decreased pulmonary vascularity without cardiomegaly**:

- **肺血减少不伴心影增大：**

Tetralogy of Fallot (TOF).
Tricuspid atresia (variable pulmonary vascularity, see below).

法洛四联症(TOF)。
三尖瓣闭锁(肺血管变异，详见后述)。

- **Usually increased pulmonary vascularity without cardiomegaly** (but variable): "T" lesions (excluding Tetralogy of Fallot):

- **常有肺血增多但不伴心脏增大**(但有变异)["T" 病变(法洛四联症除外)]:

Transposition of the great arteries (D-transposition).
Truncus arteriosus.
Tricuspid atresia.
Total anomalous pulmonary venous return (TAPVR).
Single ("Tingle" to keep the T-theme consistent) **ventricle**, and variants including double outlet left ventricle and double outlet right ventricle.

大动脉转位(右转)。
大动脉共干。
三尖瓣闭锁。
完全性肺静脉异位引流(TAPVR)。
单心室["Tingle" 以保持T主题(英文首字母)一致]及其变异，包括左心室双出口和右心室双出口。

NORMAL ANATOMY

正常解剖

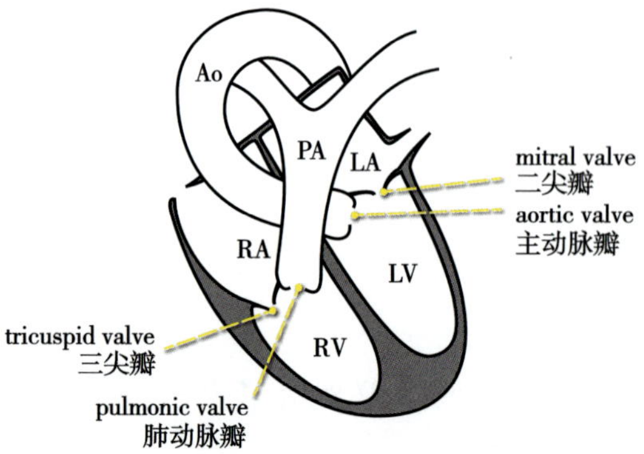

Ao = aorta
主动脉
PA = pulmonary artery
肺动脉
RA = right atrium
右心房
LA = left atrium
左心房
RV = right ventricle
右心室
LV = left ventricle
左心室

Acyanotic: Increased Pulmonary Venous Flow (Pulmonary Edema)

非发绀型：肺静脉血流增加(肺水肿)

Hypoplastic left heart (HLH)

- Hypoplastic left heart (HLH)

  syndrome represents a spectrum of congenital heart anomalies characterized by underdevelopment of any part of the left heart including left atrium, mitral valve, left ventricle, aortic valve, or aorta.

左心发育不全(HLH)

- 左心发育不全(HLH)

  综合征是以左心任何结构发育不完整为特征的一系列先天性心脏畸形，包括左心房、二尖瓣、左心室、升主动脉瓣或主动脉等结构。

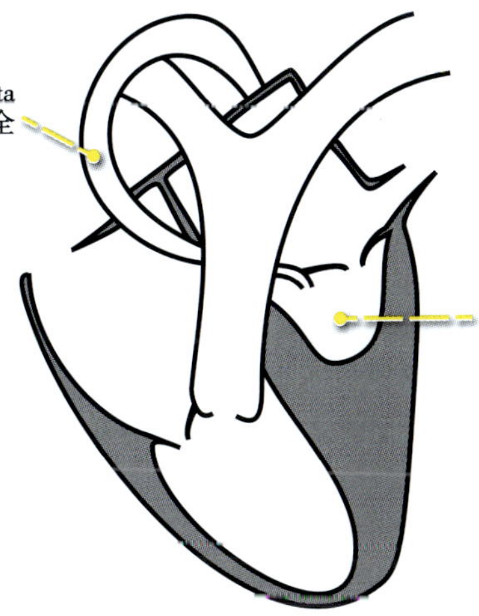

- Survival is dependent on a patent ductus arteriosus (PDA) with resultant right to left shunting to supply the systemic circulation.
- The neonatal chest radiograph in HLH is usually normal, but HLH is classified as a "pulmonary edema" entity.

  Immediately after birth, the ductus arteriosus remains patent and pulmonary arterial resistance remains high, so blood continues to flow from the pulmonary artery to the aorta (systemic circulation) via the PDA. After a few days, however, the ductus begins to close and pulmonary arterial resistance falls, leading to increase in pulmonary blood flow and delayed blood clearance from the lungs. Cardiogenic shock can ensue without operative management.

  Note that despite the left heart hypoplasia, the heart does not appear small on imaging.
- The surgical treatment of hypoplastic left heart is performed in three sequential stages, starting with the Norwood procedure. This is described in detail later in the chapter.

- 患者是否能够生存取决于未闭的动脉导管，通过右向左的分流供应体循环。
- HLH新生儿的胸部X线影像通常正常，但左心发育不全可归类为“肺水肿”系列的疾病。

  新生儿出生时，动脉导管仍然保持开放，肺循环阻力仍然较高，血流能继续通过未闭的动脉导管从肺动脉进入主动脉(体循环)。数日后，动脉导管开始闭合，肺循环阻力降低，导致肺血流增加，肺血流清除延迟。如不进行手术干预，会发生心源性休克。

  注意，尽管左心发育不全，影像上心影并不变小。
- 外科治疗左心发育不全需要分前后三期来进行，第一期为Norwood手术。将在本章后文详述。

Extracardiac shunt causing CHF

- The two most common lesions to cause neonatal CHF are vein of Galen malformation and hepatic hemangioendothelioma.

心外分流引起的充血性心力衰竭(CHF)

- 两种最常导致新生儿充血性心力衰竭(CHF)的病变为Galen静脉畸形和肝血管内皮细胞瘤。

Aortic coarctation

- Aortic coarctation is congenital focal narrowing of the aorta in the region of the ductus arteriosus. It may be preductal (proximal to the ductus, illustrated on the below), periductal, or postductal.
- The preductal form may cause congestive heart failure (CHF) in infants due to left ventricular obstruction, leading to cardiomegaly and increased pulmonary venous flow. In contrast, the juxtaductal or postductal variants present later in life in the teenage or early adult years as upper extremity hypertension.
- Aortic coarctation is associated with bicuspid aortic valve, which may become stenotic and cause post-stenotic aortic dilation proximal to the site

主动脉缩窄

- 主动脉缩窄是先天性局部主动脉狭窄，位于动脉导管附近。狭窄可位于导管前(最接近动脉导管，下图示)、导管旁或导管后。
- 导管前型在新生儿可引起充血性心力衰竭(CHF)，因左心室流出道梗阻，导致心脏增大及肺静脉血流增加。相比之下，导管旁型及导管后型在青少年或年轻成年发病，表现为上肢血压升高。
- 主动脉缩窄合并二叶式主动脉瓣，后者可变得狭窄并引起狭窄后主动脉扩张，扩张部位位于

of coarctation. Other associations include Turner syndrome (XO), Shone syndrome and intracerebral berry aneurysms.

主动脉狭窄近段。其他有关病变包括特纳综合征(XO), Shone综合征及脑内Berry动脉瘤。

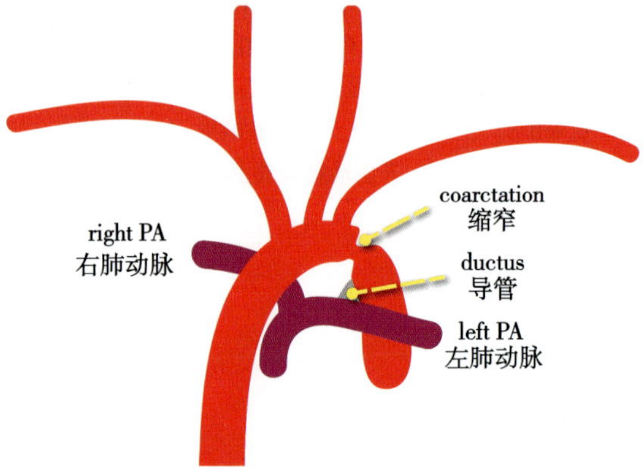

Diagram demonstrates infantile-type preductal aortic coarctation, with the coarctation located proximal to the ductus.
图示婴幼儿型导管前主动脉缩窄,缩窄部位位于动脉导管近端。

- In infants, aortic coarctation may produce acyanotic CHF. In adults, the classic radiographic finding is the *3 sign* representing the contour of the coarcted aorta in the left upper mediastinum. Although rib notching is described as a classic finding, it is rarely seen.

- 在婴儿,主动脉缩窄可导致非发绀型充血性心力衰竭。在成人,经典的胸部X线影像学表现为“3”字征,缩窄的主动脉轮廓在左上纵隔,形态类似“3”。尽管肋骨切迹被描述为典型的表现,但很少见。

ACYANOTIC: INCREASED PULMONARY ARTERIAL FLOW (SHUNT VASCULARITY)

非发绀型:肺血流增加(分流血管)

- It is rare for shunt lesions to present in the neonatal period because pulmonary vascular resistance is high, which limits left-to-right shunting. In long-standing shunting, progressive volume overload causes the typical “shunt vascularity” (very prominent distinct pulmonary arteries without the haziness of pulmonary edema) and cardiomegaly.

- 新生儿时期罕见有分流性病变的表现,因肺血管阻力高使左向右的分流受限。若是一个长期分流,进行性容量过载将引起典型的“分流血管”(极其显著的肺动脉,不伴随肺水肿的模糊影)及心脏增大。

Atrial septal defect (ASD)

房间隔缺损(ASD)

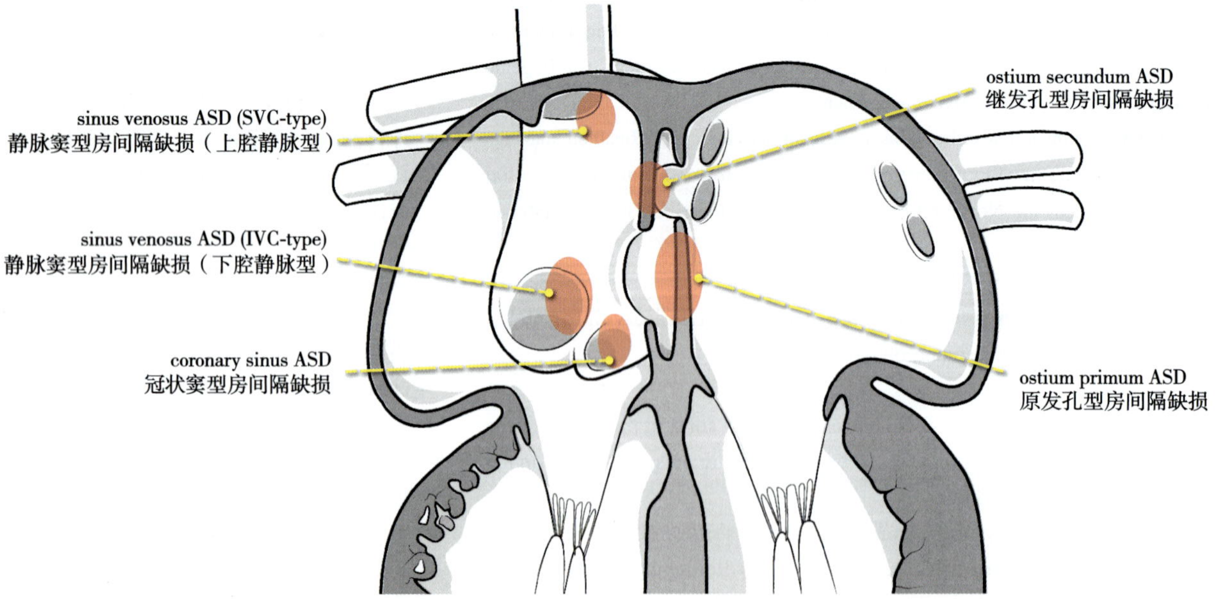

- Although atrial septal defect (ASD) is a common intracardiac left-to-right shunt, it is rarely diagnosed in infants or young children. ASD usually presents in later childhood or early adulthood, twice as commonly in females.

- 虽然房间隔缺损(ASD)是一种常见的心内左向右分流,但极少在婴儿及幼童中得到诊断。ASD通常在年长的儿童或年轻成人出现

Although most are an isolated abnormality, ASD may rarely be associated with syndromes, such as **Holt-Oram** (ASD and upper extremity bone deformities, including absence or hypoplasia of the thumb).

- **Ostium secundum ASD** is the most common type of ASD (60% of cases), caused by incomplete covering of the ostium secundum by the septum secundum.

  This is usually an isolated anomaly, located in the region of the fossa ovalis. Ostium secundum ASD may close without treatment, in contrast to the other ASD types.

  Ostium secundum ASD is associated with Ebstein anomaly.

- **Ostium primum ASD** is the second most common type of ASD (30% of cases), caused by incomplete fusion of the septum primum to the endocardial cushion.

  The location is low in the atrial septum, contiguous with the AV valves and is often seen with a complete AV canal defect.

  Ostium primum is associated with Down syndrome.

- **Sinus venosus ASD** is rare (5% of cases), located either near the SVC or IVC adjacent to a defect in the posterior wall of the right atrium.

  There is a strong association with partial anomalous pulmonary venous drainage (PAPVR), particularly of the right upper lobe.

- **Coronary sinus ASD** is the rarest type (<1%). It is also termed "unroofed" coronary sinus and is characterized by a partially or completely absent wall between the coronary sinus and left atrium.

  It is associated with a persistent left-sided SVC.

- *An ASD causes right heart volume overload.* The left atrium is usually normal because blood is decompressed from the left atrium to the right atrium during both systole and diastole. However, if mitral regurgitation is present, secondary left atrial enlargement may result.
- Initially, the right atrium enlarges, followed by right ventricular enlargement (which may be visible on the lateral radiograph as an opacity in the retrosternal clear space). In late-stage disease, the pulmonary artery also becomes enlarged.
- Shunt vascularity is usually present on radiography by the time the lesion is symptomatic.
- Treatment is ASD closure, typically with an Amplatzer or similar device.

Ventricular septal defect (VSD)

症状，女性通常是男性发病的2倍。大多数ASD为孤立性病变，但极少数患者可合并有其他综合征，如**遗传性心血管上肢畸形综合征**(Holt-Oram综合征)（ASD合并上肢骨骼畸形，包括拇指缺失或发育不全）。

- **继发孔型ASD**是最常见的ASD类型(约为60%)，为继发孔未能被隔膜完全覆盖所致。

  此型通常为单发异常，位于卵圆孔区。继发孔型房间隔缺损可能在无治疗的情况下自发关闭，这与其他类型房间隔缺损不同。

  继发孔型ASD与埃布斯坦畸形有关。

- **原发孔型ASD**是第二常见的ASD(约占30%)，为原发隔膜未能完全与心内膜垫融合所致。

  缺损多位于房间隔较低位置，与房室瓣相连续，常见完全性房室管缺损。

  原发孔型多伴发唐氏综合征。

- **静脉窦型ASD**少见(约5%)，发生在上腔或下腔静脉邻近右心房后壁的缺损处。

  此型与部分肺静脉异常引流(PAPVR)密切相关，尤其是右肺上叶型。

- **冠状动脉窦型ASD**是最少见的类型(<1%)。也被称为"无顶"冠状静脉窦，其特征性表现为冠状动脉窦与左心房之间的窦壁部分或完全缺损。

  与永存左上腔静脉相关。

- ASD会*引起右心容量负荷加重*。左心房通常正常，因为在舒张期和收缩期血液均由左心房挤压入右心房。然而，当出现二尖瓣反流时，可导致继发性左心房增大。
- 最初，右心房增大，随后右心室增大(在侧位X线影像上可以看到胸骨后间隙消失)。在疾病晚期，肺动脉也会增粗。
- 当病变引起症状时，胸部X线影像通常出现分流血管。
- 治疗方法为关闭房间隔缺损，常用Amplatzer或类似的器材进行封堵。

室间隔缺损(VSD)

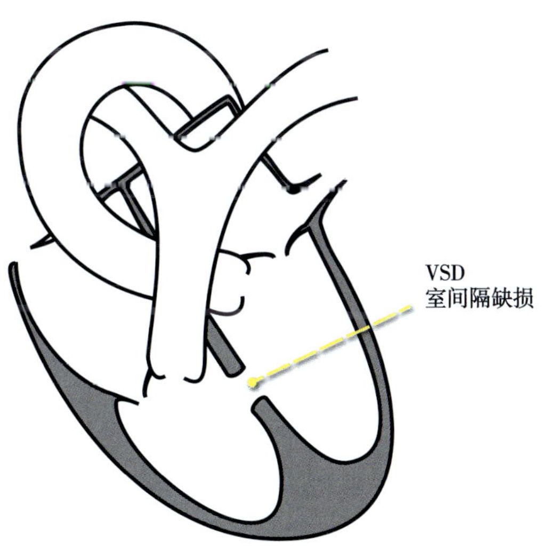

- Ventricular septal defect (VSD) is typically diagnosed earlier than ASD, with many children presenting after the first month of life as pulmonary vascular resistance falls. A VSD may occur in the membranous (70%) or muscular interventricular septum.
- *VSD primarily causes dilation of the left heart.* Left-to-right shunting occurs in systole, causing volume overload of the left heart and resulting in left atrial and left ventricular dilation.
- Imaging findings are variable, depending on the size of the VSD. The classic imaging findings of shunt vascularity and cardiomegaly typically take a few years to develop, although there may be mild cardiomegaly and increased pulmonary vascular flow shortly after birth. The left atrium is often enlarged, which may splay the mainstem bronchi at the carina.
- If unrepaired, **Eisenmenger syndrome** may develop, which represents pulmonary hypertension and reversal of the shunt direction. Eisenmenger syndrome is rare as most patients undergo surgery before pulmonary flow reversal occurs.

Patent ductus arteriosus (PDA)

- The ductus arteriosus is a normal vascular structure of the fetal circulation that connects the proximal left pulmonary artery to the descending aorta. The ductus normally functionally closes by 48 hours of life and anatomically closes by 1–3 months.
- A patent ductus arteriosus (PDA) results in a persistent left-to-right shunt. PDA is associated with maternal rubella and pre-term infants, thought to be due to elevated fetal prostaglandins, which inhibit closure of the ductus.

- 室间隔缺损(VSD)通常比ASD更早得到诊断，许多儿童在出生后1个月因肺血管阻力降低而出现症状。VSD可发生于室间隔的膜部(70%)或肌部。
- *VSD主要导致左心扩大。*左向右的分流发生在收缩期，导致左心容量负荷增加，左心房及左心室扩张。
- 影像学表现多样，取决于VSD的大小。可能在出生后不久表现为轻度心影增大及肺血流量增加，典型的分流血管及心影增大的影像学表现需要经历数年的发展。左心房通常增大，可压迫造成支气管隆突增宽。
- 如未进行修补，可发展为**艾森门格综合征**，也就是肺动脉高压及分流方向逆转。艾森门格综合征已极为少见，因多数患者在肺血流发生方向逆转前都已经进行了手术。

动脉导管未闭(PDA)

- 动脉导管是胎儿循环中正常的血管结构，它连接近端左肺动脉与降主动脉。导管通常在出生后48小时达到功能性关闭，1~3个月时在解剖学上关闭。
- 动脉导管未闭(PDA)将导致持续左向右分流。PDA与孕妇感染风疹病毒及早产有关，可能为胎儿前列腺素的增加而抑制了导管的闭合。

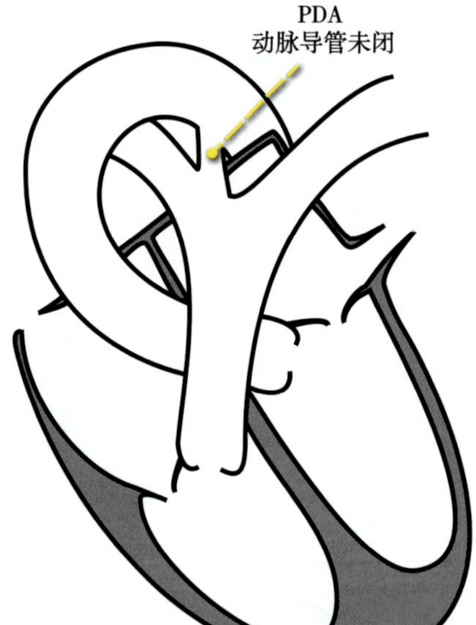

- A small PDA is usually asymptomatic. A large PDA may produce a characteristic *machine-like murmur* and cause CHF in infancy.
- The classic clinical presentation of PDA is a premature infant who develops radiographic evidence of CHF at 7–10 days of life, as pulmonary vascular resistance begins to fall.
- Treatment of PDA is medical (indomethacin, a prostaglandin inhibitor) or surgical (clip placement). Eisenmenger syndrome may develop if untreated.

- 小的PDA通常无症状。大的PDA可产生有特征性的机械样杂音，并引起婴儿充血性心力衰竭(CHF)。
- 典型的PDA临床表现为早产新生儿在出生第7~10天出现CHF的影像学表现，因该时期的肺血管阻力开始下降。
- 治疗PDA采用药物(Indomethacin，一种前列腺素抑制剂)或手术(夹闭)。如不进行治疗，可发展为艾森门格综合征。

Atrioventricular septal defect (AVSD) / Common atrioventricular canal / Endocardial cushion defect (ECD)

房室间隔缺损(AVSD)/房室管共干/心内膜垫缺损(ECD)

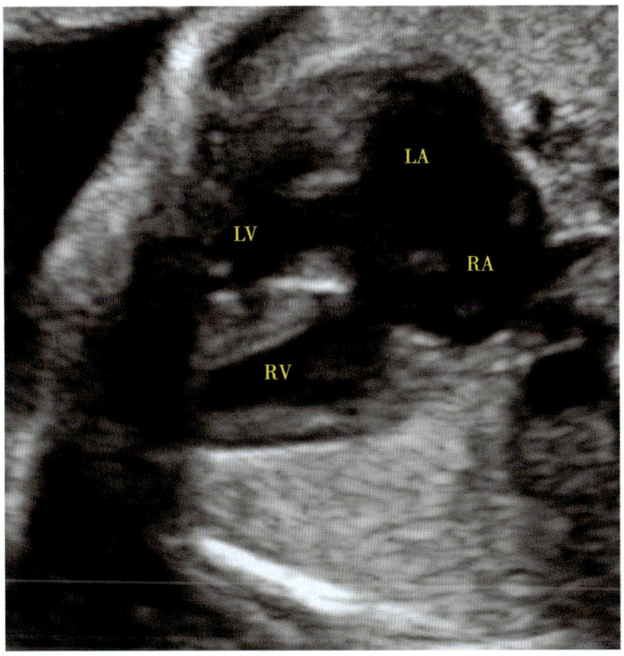

Atrioventricular septal defect:
Four-chamber view of the heart from a pre-natal ultrasound at 32 weeks gestation demonstrates complete absence of the interatrial septum and a large defect in the upper part of the interventricular septum.
Case courtesy Beryl Benacerraf, MD,Diagnostic Ultrasound Associates, Boston.

房室间隔缺损：
32周龄时产前超声四腔心切面显示房间隔缺损及室间隔上部一处大的缺损。

- Atrioventricular septal defect (AVSD), also known as common AV canal or endocardial cushion defect (ECD), encompasses a spectrum of partial to complete defects involving ostium primum ASD, VSD, and mitral or tricuspid anomalies. AVSD is strongly associated with trisomy 21.
- The primitive endocardial cushion is responsible for the formation of several structures in fetal development, including:
  Posterior and membranous ventricular septum.
  Anterior leaflet of the mitral valve.
  Septal leaflet of the tricuspid valve.
  Responsible for closure of the ostium primum.

- 房室间隔缺损(AVSD),也称为房室通道或心内膜垫缺损(ECD),涵盖了从部分到完全的系列缺损,包括原发孔型房间隔缺损、室间隔缺损、二尖瓣或三尖瓣异常等。AVSD与21-三体综合征关系密切。
- 原始心内膜垫在胎儿发育过程中参与多个结构的形成,包括:
  室间隔后部及膜部。
  二尖瓣前叶。
  三尖瓣隔叶。
  负责原始孔的关闭。

CYANOTIC: DECREASED PULMONARY VASCULARITY WITH CARDIOMEGALY

发绀型：肺血减少伴心影增大

Ebstein anomaly

埃布斯坦畸形

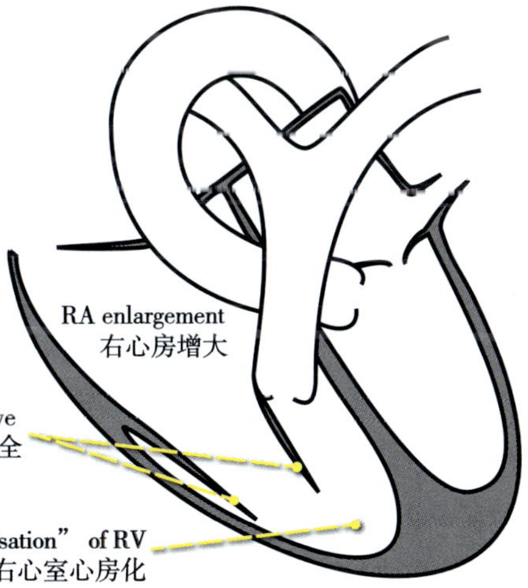

- Ebstein anomaly is a severe malformation of the tricuspid valve characterized by apical displacement of the septal and posteroinferior leaflets, resulting in obstruction of the pulmonic valve and right ventricular outflow tract. These changes lead to morphologic "atrialization" of the RV.
- An ASD is always present.
- Imaging classically shows a huge *box-shaped heart*, with massive right atrial enlargement and decreased pulmonary vascularity.

- 埃布斯坦畸形是一种严重的三尖瓣异常，以三尖瓣隔瓣及后下瓣顶部移位为特征，导致肺动脉瓣及右心室流出道受阻。这些变化导致右心室"心房化"的形态学改变。
- 总有ASD。
- 典型的影像学表现为一个巨大的盒子状心影，伴右心房极度增大及肺血减少。

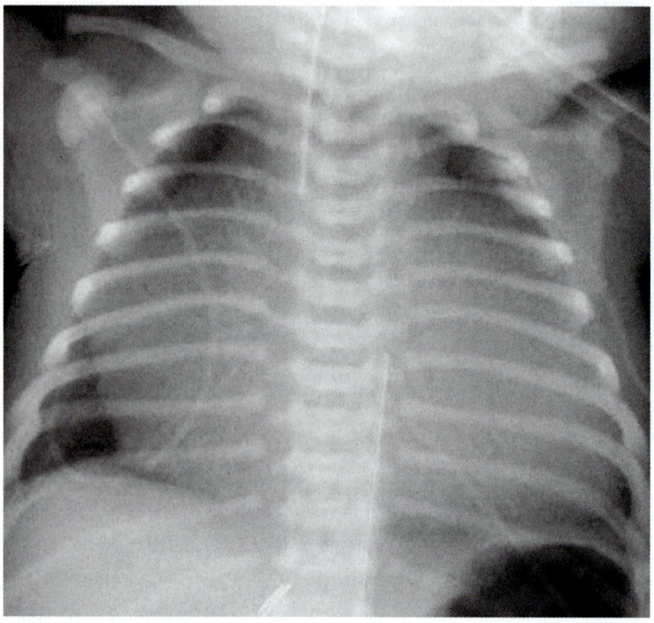

Ebstein anomaly: Frontal chest radiograph in a neonate shows massive cardiomegaly. Although the enlarged heart obscures most of the lungs, there are hardly any vascular markings in the visualized periphery.
An endotracheal tube and umbilical artery catheter are in place.
Of note, pulmonary atresia with intact ventricular septum would appear identical.
埃布斯坦畸形：一名新生儿正位胸部X线影像显示巨大心影。尽管增大的心影遮盖了大部分肺组织，但外周肺野几乎看不到血管影。
可见气管插管及脐动脉插管。
注意，室间隔完整型肺动脉闭锁可有类似的影像学表现。

Pulmonary atresia with intact ventricular septum

- Pulmonary atresia with intact ventricular septum appears identical to Ebstein anomaly on radiography, with massive right atrial enlargement and decreased pulmonary blood flow. Because the lack of VSD markedly reduces blood flow to the lungs, pulmonary blood flow depends on a left-to-right shunt, such as a patent ductus.
- Pulmonary atresia with intact ventricular septum is completely different from pulmonary atresia *with* a VSD, which is in the spectrum of tetralogy of Fallot and most commonly has a normal-sized heart.

室间隔完整型肺动脉闭锁

- 室间隔完整型肺动脉闭锁在X线影像上与埃布斯坦畸形表现完全一致，两者均为右心房极度增大和肺血流减少。因没有室间隔缺损，进入肺内的血流大大减少，肺血流完全依赖于左向右的分流，如动脉导管。
- 室间隔完整型肺动脉闭锁与肺动脉闭锁伴VSD则完全不同，后者归入法洛四联症，多数患者的心脏大小正常。

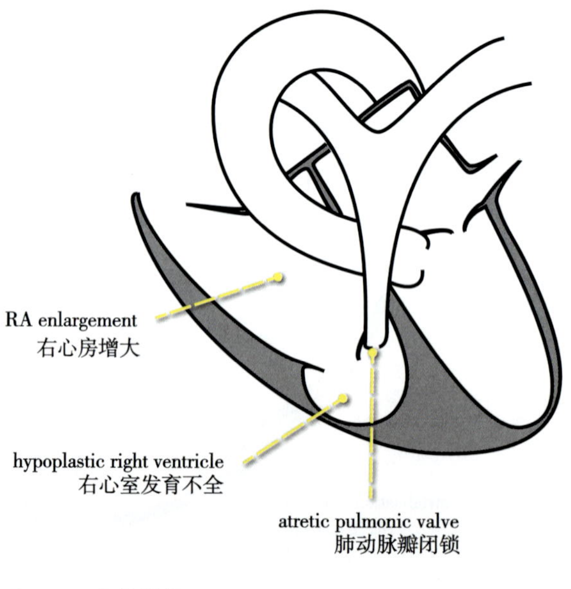

CYANOTIC: DECREASED PULMONARY VASCULARITY WITHOUT CARDIOMEGALY

发绀型：肺血减少不伴心影增大

Tetralogy of Fallot (TOF)

- Tetralogy of Fallot (TOF) is the most common cyanotic heart disease of children and adults
- The 4 components of TOF are:

1. RV outflow tract obstruction.
2. RV hypertrophy.
3. VSD.
4. Aorta "over-riding" the VSD.

A variation of TOF is the **pentalogy of Fallot**, which also has an ASD.

Pulmonary atresia with a VSD is a severe form of TOF.

法洛四联症

- 法洛四联症(Tetralogy of Fallot，TOF)是儿童及成人发绀型心脏病最常见的类型。
- TOF包括以下4个组成部分：

1.右心室流出道阻塞。
2.右心室肥大。
3.室间隔缺损。
4.主动脉骑跨于室间隔缺损。

TOF的一种变异是法洛五联症，另合并房间隔缺损。

肺动脉闭锁伴VSD是一种严重的TOF类型。

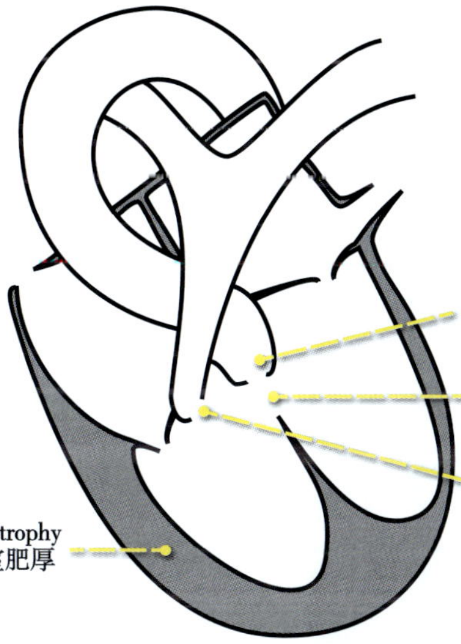

- The degree of cyanosis depends on the degree of right ventricular outflow tract obstruction.
- TOF is associated with DiGeorge syndrome (absent thymus and parathyroids, causing hypocalcemia), VACTERL, and trisomy 21. 25% of cases of TOF have a right-sided aortic arch.
- Classic radiographic findings of TOF are a *boot-shaped heart* (cardiac apex uplifted by RV hypertrophy, although the heart is normal in size) and decreased pulmonary vascularity.
- Surgical repair involves closure of VSD and opening of right ventricular outflow tract obstruction, which is usually performed in infancy.

- 发绀程度取决于右心室流出道阻塞的程度。
- TOF与迪格奥尔格综合征(即胸腺及甲状旁腺的缺失，导致低钙血症)，VACTERL和21-三体综合征有关。约25%的TOF病例有右位主动脉弓。
- 典型的TOF影像学表现为靴形心(心尖因右心室肥厚而上抬，而心脏大小正常)及肺血减少。
- 外科修复包括关闭室间隔缺损和打开阻塞的右心室流出道，手术通常在婴儿期进行。

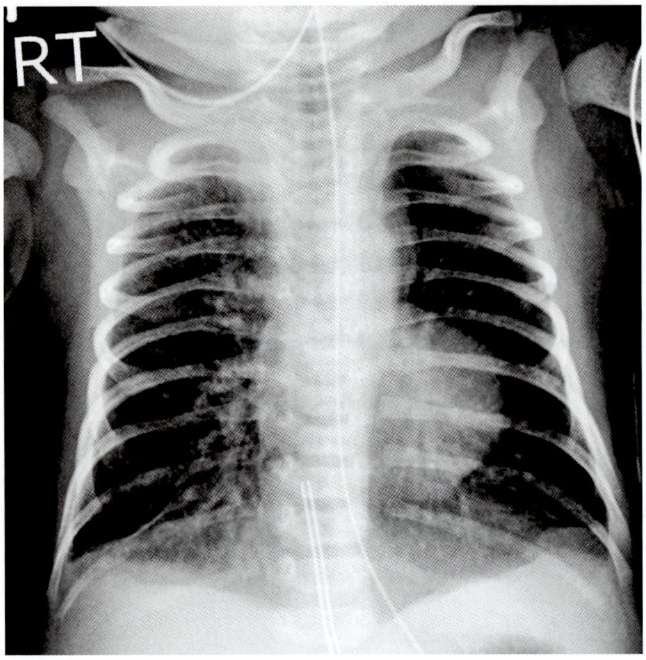

Tetralogy of Fallot: Portable chest radiograph in a neonate demonstrates a normal-sized heart with an upturned cardiac apex (*boot-shaped heart*). The lungs are hyperinflated with prominent coarse interstitium.
法洛四联症：新生儿移动式胸部X线影像示心影大小正常，心尖向上旋转(靴形心)。双侧肺过度膨胀，可见显著粗大的肺间质纹理。

CYANOTIC: INCREASED PULMONARY VASCULARITY (ADMIXTURE"T" LESIONS)

发绀型：肺血增多(混杂“T”型病变)

Transposition of the great arteries (TGA)

大动脉转位(TGA)

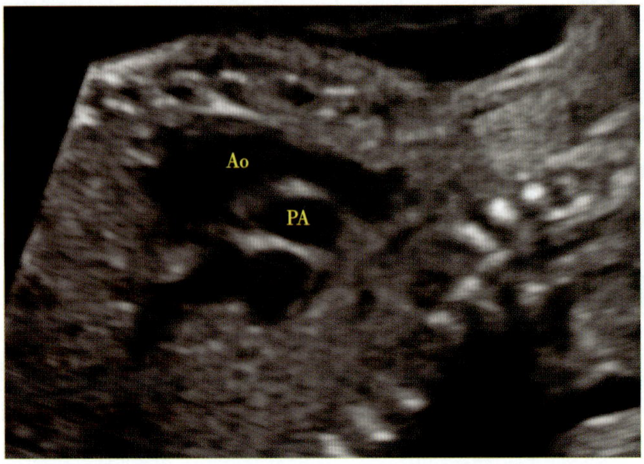

Transposition of the great arteries:
Antenatal ultrasound at an oblique plane through the great vessels demonstrates the aorta (Ao) is anterior to the pulmonary artery (PA), as the aorta arises from the right ventricle (the most anterior cardiac chamber).
Case courtesy Beryl Benacerraf, MD,Diagnostic Ultrasound Associates, Boston.
大动脉转位：
产前超声，斜位大血管切面显示主动脉(Ao)位于肺动脉(PA)之前，因主动脉起源于右心室(最前的心腔)。

- Transposition of the great arteries (TGA) is the most common cause of cyanotic heart disease in newborns. In TGA, there is improper pairing of the ventricles and great vessels (ventriculoarterial discordance): the morphologic right ventricle pumps blood to the aorta and the morphologic left ventricle pumps blood to the pulmonary arteries.
- Two main subtypes of TGA exist:

  Dextro (D)-TGA features ventriculoarterial discordance with atrioventricular concordance (correctly paired atria and ventricles). Isolated D-TGA without flow admixture (ASD, VSD or PDA) is incompatible with life (“D = death”).

  Levo (L)-TGA features a “congenitally corrected TGA” with atrioventricular and ventriculoarterial (double) discordance. L-TGA is compatible with life (“L = life”).
- Pre-natal ultrasound diagnosis of TGA requires evaluation of the short- or long-axis of the great vessels. TGA is usually inapparent on a 4-chamber view. Sonographic diagnosis shows the aorta anterior the heart and the great vessels

- 大动脉转位(TGA)是新生儿最常见的发绀型心脏病。TGA时的心室与大血管匹配异常(心室-动脉不匹配)，即形态上的右心室将血泵到主动脉，而形态上的左心室将血泵到肺动脉。
- TGA有两种主要的亚型：

  右转型(D)-TGA的特点是心室-动脉不一致，但心房-心室一致(心房与心室正确配对)。孤立性D-TGA若没有混合血流(ASD、VSD或PDA)患儿不能存活(“D=死亡”)。

  左转型(L)-TGA具有“先天性矫正TGA”的特征，其心房-心室和心室-动脉(双重)不一致。L-TGA患儿可以存活(“L=存活”)。
- 产前超声诊断TGA需要评估大血管(主动脉及肺动脉)的长轴或短轴。四腔心切面TGA通常

exiting the heart in parallel (rather than crossing in the normal fashion).

- The classic radiographic *egg-on-a-string* appearance (D-TGA) is actually uncommonly seen. It represents a narrow mediastinal waist (caused by the parallel course of the aorta and PA and thymic involution secondary to stress). A more typical appearance is a slightly narrow superior mediastinum, lack of main pulmonary artery bulge and increased pulmonary vasculature; however, the radiographic picture varies depending on the nature of the coexisting shunt. A right aortic arch is seen in 5%.
- Surgical treatment for D-TGA is the arterial switch (Jatene) procedure, which swaps the aorta and pulmonary artery, and relocates the coronary arteries to the neo-aorta.

不明显。超声图像可见主动脉位于心脏的前方，出心脏时与肺动脉并行(而不是正常相交叉)。

- D-TGA在影像学上经典的蛋串样外观其实不常见。该外观代表狭窄的纵隔腰部(由主动脉和PA平行走行，以及胸腺因继发性负荷反应导致的退化)。更常见的表现为轻度狭窄的上纵隔，缺乏主肺动脉隆起，以及肺血增多，然而，X线影像表现多变，取决定于分流的形式。右位主动脉弓约占5%。
- D-TGA外科治疗方法为动脉转换(Jatene)术，即将主动脉及肺动脉互换，并将冠状动脉转移到新的主动脉上。

Tricuspid atresia

- Tricuspid atresia is absence or dysplasia of the tricuspid valve resulting in no flow between the right atrium and right ventricle. It may have a variable radiographic appearance depending on the size of the associated VSD.
  - Small VSD: Normal-sized heart, with decreased pulmonary vasculature.
  - Large VSD: Enlarged heart with increased pulmonary flow.

三尖瓣闭锁

- 三尖瓣闭锁是指三尖瓣缺失或发育异常，导致右心房和右心室之间没有血液流动。X线影像上的表现多变，取决于VSD的大小。
  - 小的VSD：心脏大小正常，肺血减少。
  - 大的VSD：心影增大，肺血流增多。

Truncus arteriosus

- In truncus arteriosus, a single great artery arises from the base of the heart to supply the systemic, pulmonary, and coronary circulations. The single great artery usually overrides a VSD.
- Truncus arteriosus is the most common type of congenital heart disease to have a right aortic arch (21–36% of cases). It is also associated with DiGeorge syndrome (30–35% of cases).
- The classic radiograph appearance is cardiomegaly, narrow mediastinum, and pulmonary edema.

大动脉共干

- 大动脉共干为单一的大动脉起源于心底并供应体循环、肺循环及冠状动脉循环。此大动脉干通常骑跨在室间隔缺损之上。
- 大动脉共干是最常见的伴右位主动脉弓(21%~36%)的先天性心脏病。它常与迪格奥尔格综合征相关(30%~35%的病例)。
- 典型的X线影像表现为心影增大、纵隔狭窄，以及肺水肿。

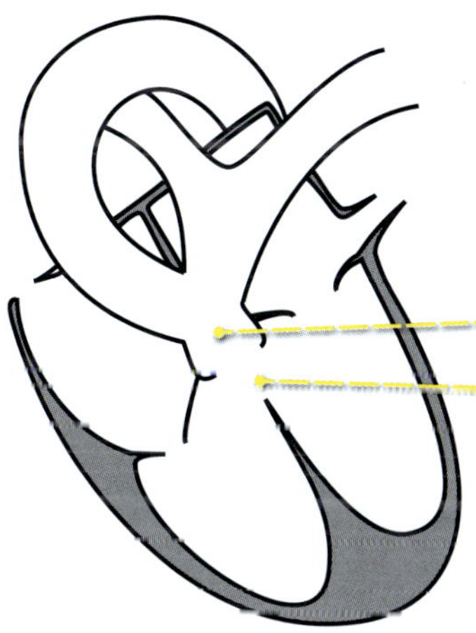

Total anomalous pulmonary venous return (TAPVR)

- In total anomalous pulmonary venous return (TAPVR), all pulmonary veins connect anomalously to the systemic venous circulation instead of draining into the left atrium.
- There is an obligate interatrial right-to-left communication enabling blood to reach the left heart, such as a large PFO or an ASD.
- Classification of TAPVR is based on the position of the venous drainage relative to the heart:

完全性肺静脉异位引流(TAPVR)

- 完全性肺静脉异位引流(TAPVR)是指所有肺静脉异常连接到体循环静脉，而不是引流至左心房。
- 心房内必须要有一个由右向左的通道才能使血流到达左心，如一个大的PFO或ASD。
- TAPVR的分型是根据静脉引流与心脏相对的位置：

Supracardiac (40%): Anomalous venous return is at or above the level of the SVC. The common confluence of the pulmonary veins drains into the left inominate vein via a **vertical** vein. Chest radiograph chows the characteristic snowman sign, with the dilated vertical vein making up the left border of the snowman. The snowman sign is seen in older patients without pulmonary venous obstruction.

Cardiac (20%): Anomalous drainage is into the coronary sinus or right atrium.

Infracardiac (35%): The anomalous drainage passes through the diaphragm via the esophageal hiatus and then drains into the hepatic IVC, hepatic vein, or portal vein. Pulmonary edema can result due to obstruction at the level of the diaphragm.

Mixed (<5%): Anomalous venous drainage is a combination of the above types.

心上型(40%)：异常的静脉引流位于上腔静脉或更高的位置。肺静脉汇总后通过**垂直**静脉将血液引流入左侧无名静脉。胸部X线影像可见特征性的雪人征，即扩张垂直的静脉构成雪人的左侧边界。雪人征见于年长的患者且不伴有肺静脉阻塞。

心脏型(20%)：异常引流血进入冠状窦或右心房。

心下型(35%)：异常引流经食管裂孔穿过膈肌，之后回流进入下腔静脉(肝段)、肝静脉或门静脉。引流在膈肌水平受阻可出现肺水肿。

混合型(5%)：以上各类异常静脉引流的混合。

- Clinical and radiographic findings depend on the degree of pulmonary venous obstruction and admixture. A typical radiographic appearance of obstructed TAPVR appearance is a normal-sized heart and pulmonary edema in an infant.

- 临床及X线影像表现取决于肺静脉阻塞及混合的程度。典型的梗阻性TAPVR表现为婴儿心脏大小正常，但有肺水肿。

Single ("tingle") ventricle

- There are multiple variations of the single ventricle anomaly, which are all characterized by arterio-venous admixture at the level of a shared monoventricle.
- Double outlet right ventricle (DORV) can be considered a form of single ventricle.

单心室(tingle=single ventricle)

- 单心室畸形有较多变异，但都以动静脉混合在共同的单心室处为特征。
- 右心室双出口(DORV)可认为是单心室畸形的另一种类型。

SUMMARY OF CONGENITAL HEART DISEASE

先天性心脏病总结

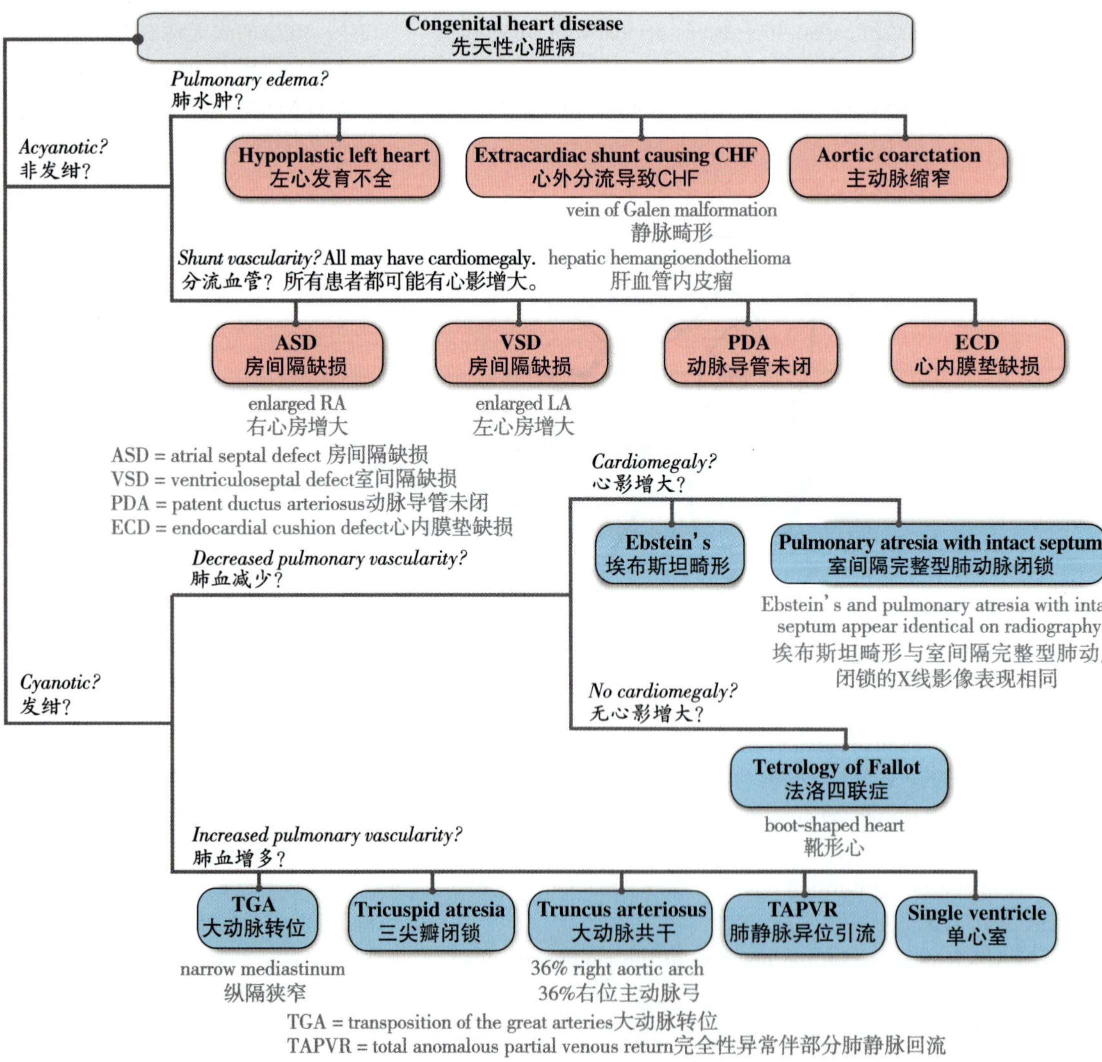

Common Surgeries for Congenital Heart Disease

Hypoplastic left heart surgery

- The surgical treatment of hypoplastic left heart is performed in three sequential stages. The goal is to create an effective single ventricle heart (using the right ventricle) to pump blood to the entire body.

  A staged repair is necessary since the high pulmonary vascular resistance in the neonatal period precludes immediate definitive repair.

常见的先天性心脏病手术

左心发育不全手术

- 外科治疗左心发育不全方法需要分三期进行。手术治疗的目标在于创造一个有效的单心室心脏(用右心室)以将血泵到全身。

  分期修补是必要的,因为新生儿时期肺血管呈高阻力状态,不能马上进行根治性修补。

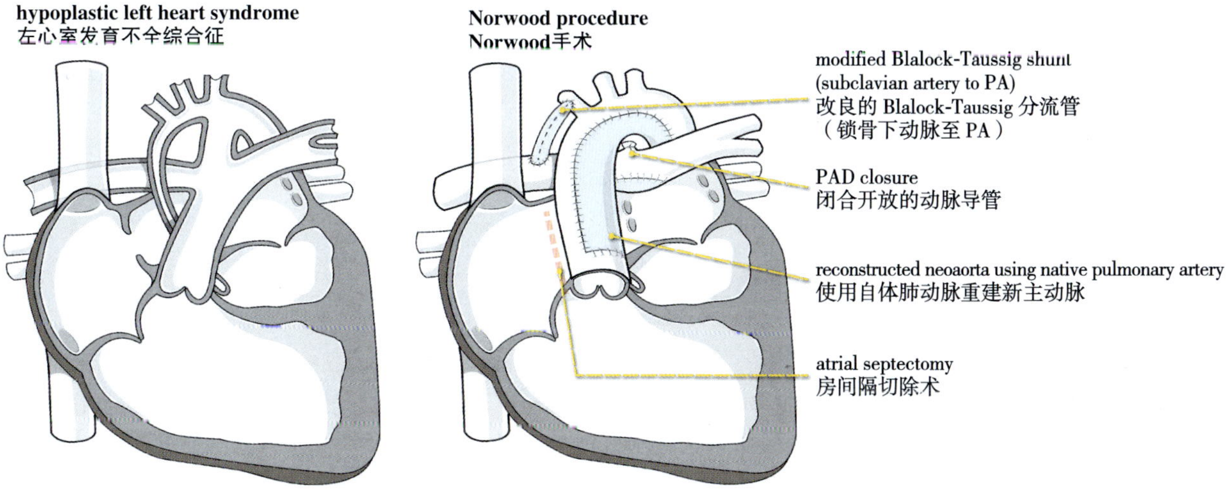

- **Stage 1:** The first stage is the **Norwood procedure**, performed within the first few days of life and has three main components. First, the right ventricle is redirected to supply the systemic circulation by reconstructing the aorta using the main pulmonary artery (PA). Second, the atrial septum is excised, and the PDA is ligated, to redirect pulmonary venous return to the right heart via the atrial septal defect. Third, pulmonary arterial circulation is provided via a **modified Blalock-Taussig shunt** (BT shunt), which *connects the right subclavian artery to the right pulmonary artery* via a prosthetic graft.

  BT shunt is associated with a coronary steal phenomenon. This occurs when diastolic blood flow is diverted from the aorta to the low-pressure pulmonary vasculature via the shunt, resulting in reduced flow to the coronary arteries.

  An alternative to BT shunt is the **Sano shunt**, which is an extracardiac conduit that connects the right ventricle to the pulmonary artery. It does not cause coronary steal.

- **第1阶段:** 第1阶段为**Norwood手术**,在出生后数天内进行,包括三部分。第一,对右心室进行改道使其供应体循环,采用主肺动脉(PA)重建主动脉。第二,切除房间隔,并结扎动脉导管,通过房间隔缺损将肺静脉回流转向导入右心。第三,肺动脉循环通过改良的**Blalock-Taussing 分流**(BT分流)将右锁骨下动脉血流通过一段人工血管导入右肺动脉。

  BT分流可出现冠状动脉盗血现象。这是因为舒张期主动脉血流通过人工血管被分流到低压力的肺动脉,导致冠状动脉血流减少。

  一种替代BT分流的方案为**Sano分流**,这是一种心外引流,连通右心室与肺动脉。这种分流手术不会引起冠状动脉盗血。

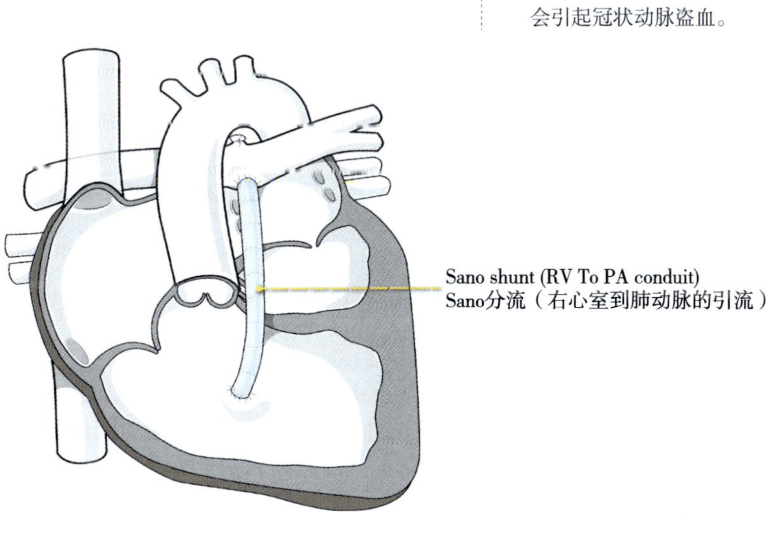

BT shunt and Sano shunt are also used as palliative treatment for pulmonary arterial flow obstruction, such as in TOF, pulmonary atresia, and tricuspid atresia.

BT分流与Sano分流也作为治疗肺动脉流出道梗阻的姑息疗法，如TOF、肺动脉闭锁、三尖瓣闭锁。

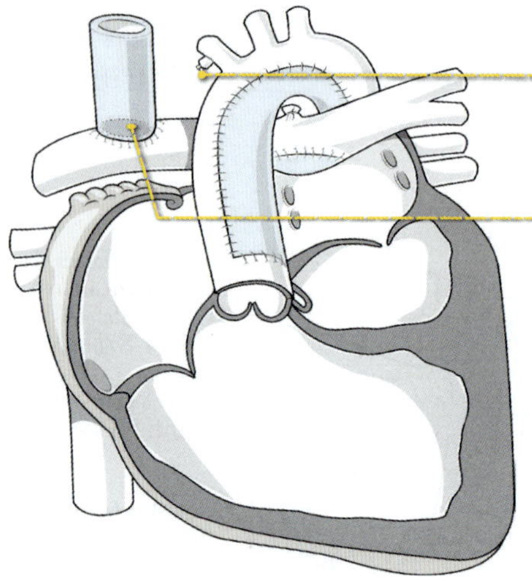

- **Stage 2:** The BTS is replaced with a **bidirectional Glenn** (BDG) shunt, where *the SVC is connected to the right pulmonary artery*. This is performed once pulmonary arterial resistance has fallen to normal levels, about 3–6 months after stage 1. The goal is to begin to separate systemic and pulmonary circulations.

  The Glenn shunt is associated with acquired pulmonary arteriovenous malformations (AVMs). Etiology is unclear but thought to be related to lack of hepatic venous flow to the lungs following the procedure. Literature has shown regression of pulmonary AVMs following restoration of hepatic venous flow to the lungs, for example after Fontan revision (below).

- **第2期**：用**双向Glenn(BDG)**分流管替换BTS，从而连接上腔静脉与右肺动脉。此期手术是在患者肺动脉阻力降低至正常时实施，一般在一期手术后3~6个月。目的是启动分离体循环和肺循环。

  Glenn分流可以造成继发性肺动静脉畸形(AVMs)。原因尚不清楚，可能与术后肝静脉回流至肺血流不足有关。文献报道，肺AVMs在肝血流恢复流入肺后可自发消退，如Fontan手术后(下述)。

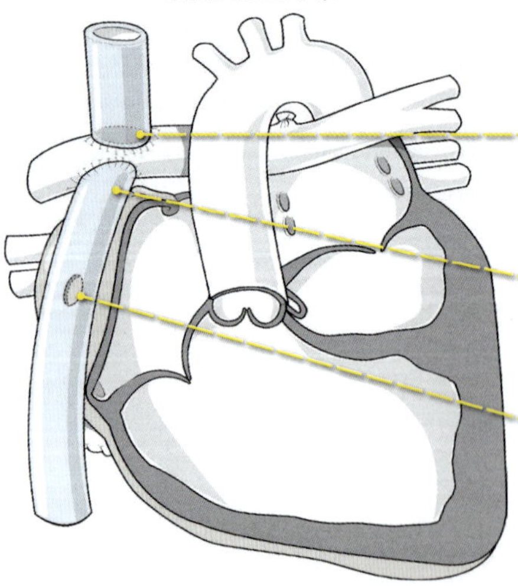

- **Stage 3:** A **modified Fontan** is performed once the patient cannot supply adequate oxygenated blood to the systemic circulation, usually between 17 months to 4 years of age. In this procedure, a tunneled conduit *connects the IVC to the right pulmonary artery*. The SVC continues to empty into the right pulmonary artery via the BDG constructed in stage 2.

- **第3期**：**改良FONTAN手术**是针对患者在出现体循环血流氧合血不足的情况下实施，通常在17个月~4岁。在此手术过程中，用埋置的导管连接下腔静脉与右肺动脉。上腔静脉仍通过第二期植入的BDG引流至右肺动脉。

Surgical treatments for D-transposition of the great arteries

- As described earlier, D-TGA is a cyanotic congenital heart disease incompatible with life unless mixture of the systemic and pulmonary venous return exists.
- The **Mustard and Senning procedures** are early surgical approaches for D-TGA repair. Both involve creation of a baffle or conduit to correct blood flow at the atrial level, redirecting systemic venous return to the morphologic LV and pulmonary artery, and pulmonary venous flow to the morphologic RV and aorta. However, these procedures have fallen out of favor due to complications associated with the intra-artial baffle and RV failure.
- The **arterial switch** or **Jatene procedure** is a newer and now preferred surgical technique for anatomic repair of D-TGA. The ascending aorta and pulmonary artery are detached and switched. The coronary arteries are reimplanted onto the neoaorta.

  The **LeCompte maneuver** is a modified step of the Jatene procedure which involves moving the pulmonary artery anterior to the aorta, resulting in the classic imaging appearance of main pulmonary trunk "straddling" the aorta.

D-大动脉转位的手术治疗

- 如前所述，D-TGA是一种发绀型心脏病，如果不存在混合的体循环及肺循环回流血液，患儿则无法存活。
- **Mustard和Senning手术**是早期修补D-TGA的手术方式。两种术式均包括在心房水平建立一个挡板或引流通道，将体循环静脉回流改向进入形态学上的左心室，以及肺静脉回流入形态学上的右心室及主动脉。然而，这两个术式已经不受青睐，因可造成心房内挡板的并发症及右心衰竭等并发症。
- **动脉切换**或**Jatene手术**为较新和更受欢迎的修补D-TGA的手术。先将升主动脉及肺动脉分离，之后互换。冠状动脉重新移植到新的升主动脉上。

  LeCompte法是在Jatene手术上的改进，包括将肺动脉移到主动脉的前方，形成经典的主肺动脉干骑跨主动脉的影像学表现。

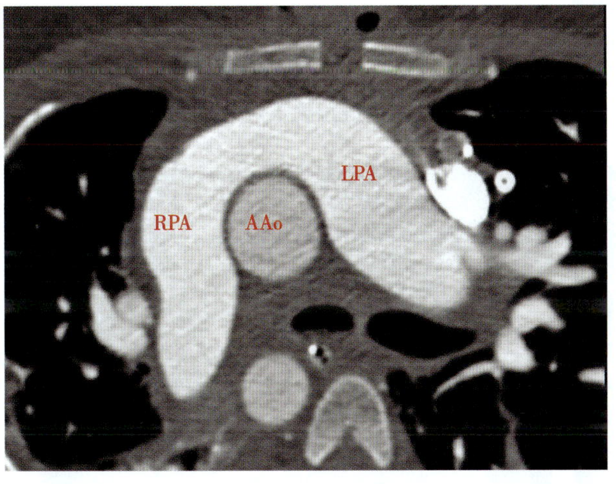

Dextro-transposition of the great arteries (D-TGA) after arterial switch: Axial CT angiogram shows anterior position of the left and right pulmonary arteries (LPA, RPA) draping over the ascending aorta (AAo).
动脉切换后的D-TGA：轴位CT血管造影显示左肺动脉和右肺动脉(LPA、RPA)包绕升主动脉(AAo)。

Rastelli procedure

- The Rastelli procedure was initially designed to treat D-TGA associated with VSD and left ventricular outflow (LVOT) obstruction. It can also be used for repair of pulmonary atresia with VSD, or double outlet RV with pulmonary stenosis or atresia.
- This surgical approach involves creation of an intraventricular baffle that connects the LV to the aorta and closes the VSD, and an extra-cardiac conduit that connects the RV to the pulmonary artery. The pulmonary valve is then surgically closed.

Rastelli手术

- Rastelli手术最初是为治疗D-TGA伴室间隔缺损及左心室流出道梗阻而设计的。它也可用于修补肺动脉闭锁伴VSD，右心室双出口伴肺动脉狭窄或闭锁。
- 手术步骤包括建立一个心室内挡板，以此连接左心室与主动脉，关闭VSD，以及有一个连接右心室及肺动脉之间的心外通道。之后手术关闭肺动脉瓣。

Visceroatrial situs

- Visceroatrial situs describes the relationship between the thoracoabdominal viscera and atria.
- Attention to the position of the liver, spleen and stomach is helpful in determining situs.

Situs solitus

- Situs solitus refers to the normal conventional anatomy, with the right atrium and liver on the right; and left atrium, spleen and stomach on the left. The right lung is trilobed and left lung is bilobed.

内脏心房位置关系异常

- 内脏心房位置关系异常是指胸腹部内脏与心房之间的关系。
- 注意肝、脾及胃的位置有助于确定位置关系。

内脏正位

- 内脏正位指正常普通的解剖学，右心房及肝脏位于右侧；左心房、脾及胃位于左侧。右侧肺为三叶，左侧肺为两叶。

Situs Inversus

- Situs inversus represents the opposite of situs solitus, with the left atrium, spleen and stomach on the right; and the right atrium and liver on the left. There is an association with primary ciliary dyskinesia.

内脏反位

- 内脏反位是指与正位内脏位置相反，左心房、脾及胃位于右侧；右心房及肝脏位于左侧。可能合并纤毛运动功能障碍。

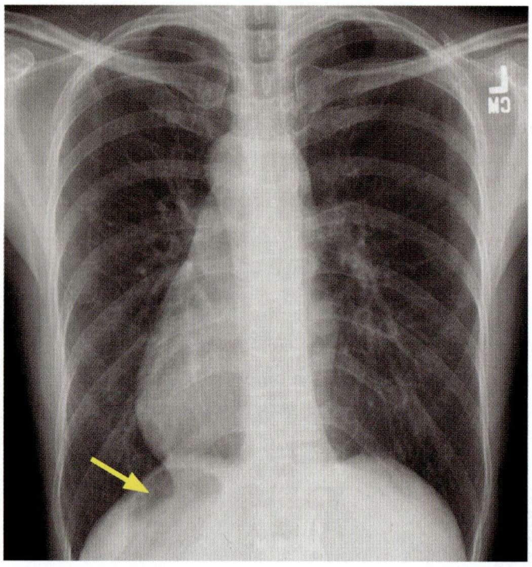

Frontal chest radiograph shows situs inversus, dextrocardia and right-sided gastric bubble (arrow).
正位胸部X线影像显示内脏转位，右旋心脏及位于右侧的胃泡(箭)。

Situs ambiguous / heterotaxy

内脏位置不确定/内脏异位

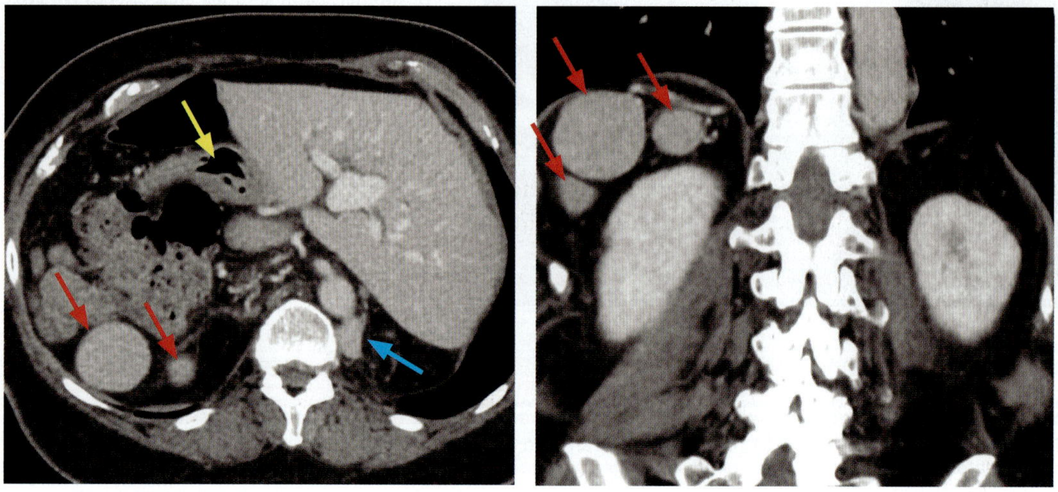

Axial (left image) and coronal (right image) contrast-enhanced CT demonstrates findings of left isomerism including a left-sided liver, a right-sided stomach (yellow arrow), multiple splenules (red arrows) in the right upper quadrant, and azygous continuation of the IVC (blue arrow).
轴位(左图)及冠状位(右图)增强CT显示左侧异构，包括左侧肝脏、右侧胃(黄箭)、位于右上腹的多发脾(红箭)，以及奇静脉下腔静脉延续(蓝箭)。

- Situs ambiguous features neither situs solitus or inversus, and has two general subsets.
- **Right-isomerism (asplenia)** features bilateral right-sidedness, including a horizontal liver, absent spleen and bilateral trilobed lungs. It is associated with severe congenital heart disease such as TAPVR.
- **Left-isomerism (polysplenia)** features bilateral left-sidedness, including multiple splenules, interruption of the IVC with azygous or hemiazygous continuation. It is associated with biliary atresia and less severe congenital heart disease (ASD or VSD).

- 内脏位置不确定是既非正位也非反位，分为两种亚型。
- **右侧异构(无脾)**特征为双侧右侧化，包括肝脏呈水平位、脾缺如及双侧三叶肺。合并严重的先天性心脏病，如TAPVR。
- **左侧异构(多脾)**以双侧左侧化为特征，包括多脾、下腔静脉中断伴奇静脉或半奇静脉延续。常合并胆道闭锁及其他不太严重的先天性心脏病(如ASD或VSD)。

Cardiac masses

心脏肿块

Rhabdomyoma

- Rhabdomyoma is the most common primary cardiac tumor in infants and children. It is strongly associated with tuberous sclerosis and is the earliest sign of tuberous sclerosis that can be diagnosed in utero. Rhabdomyomas are often multiple.
- Rhabdomyoma has a varied clinical presentation, including arrhythmia and outflow obstruction depending on location of the tumor. It is usually found in the ventricles.
- The most common radiographic appearance of rhabdomyoma is cardiomegaly. Pulmonary vasculature is variable.
- On MRI, rhabdomyomas are T1 isointense to hyperintense, T2 hyperintense, and hypoenhancing relative to myocardium.
- Typical clinical course is spontaneous regression in childhood. Therefore, rhabdomyomas in asymptomatic patients are treated conservatively.

横纹肌瘤

- 横纹肌瘤是婴幼儿及儿童最常见的原发性心源性肿瘤。它与结节性硬化关系密切，是宫内诊断结节性硬化最早的征象。横纹肌瘤常为多发。
- 横纹肌瘤有各种不同的临床表现，包括心律不齐和流出道梗阻，取决于肿瘤的位置。肿瘤通常位于心室。
- 横纹肌瘤最常见的X线影像学表现为心影增大。肺血管的变异较大。
- 横纹肌瘤在磁共振上为T_1等至高信号、T_2高信号，以及强化略低于心肌。
- 典型临床病程是在儿童期自发消退。因而，无症状的横纹肌瘤患者多采取保守治疗。

Fibroma

纤维瘤

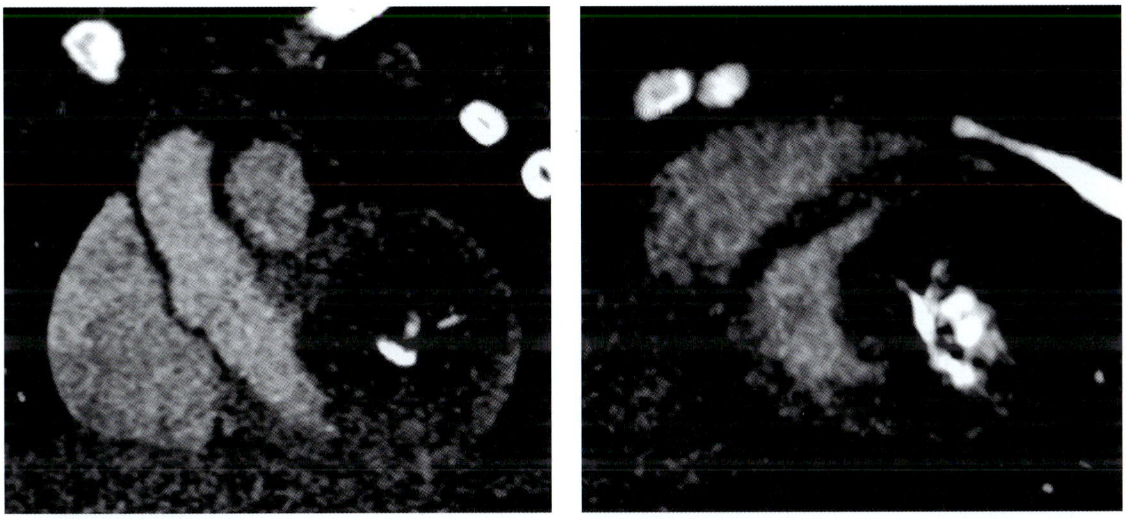

Cardiac fibroma: Coronal (left image) and axial (right image) CT angiogram demonstrates a large well- circumscribed mass arising from the anterior lateral left ventricular myocardium, which is hypoenhancing relative to adjacent normal myocardium and with central coarse calcification.

心脏纤维瘤：冠状位(左图)及轴位(右图)CT血管造影显示一个大而边缘清晰的肿块，起源于左心室心肌前侧壁，相对于周围的心肌呈低强化，伴中央粗大钙化。

- Fibroma is a rare benign cardiac tumor of infancy and early childhood, arising from fibroblasts and myofibroblasts.
- Fibroma has a similar clinical presentation to rhabdomyoma, with rhythm disturbances and outflow obstruction. The interventricular septum is the most common site of origin, where a fibroma is especially likely to cause arrhythmia due to disruption of the conduction system.
- Cardiomegaly is the most common radiographic finding.
- Central calcification on CT is a pathognomonic finding of fibromas, which differentiates them from rhabdomyomas.
- MRI classically shows a well-defined mass that is T1 hypointense to isointense relative to myocardium, T2 hypointense, and demonstrates progressive enhancement with a hypoenhancing core due to poor blood supply.
- Unlike rhabdomyoma, fibroma often present as a single mass and do not involute. Therefore, treatment is typically surgical resection.

- 纤维瘤是一种罕见的起源于纤维母细胞或肌纤维母细胞的良性心脏肿瘤，见于幼儿及较小年龄儿童。
- 纤维瘤的临床表现与横纹肌瘤相似，为节律异常及流出道阻塞。室间隔是最常发生部位，且因纤维瘤破坏心传导系统而极易引起心律异常。
- 心脏增大是最常见的影像学表现。
- CT上的中央钙化是纤维瘤的特异性表现，并可与横纹肌瘤相鉴别。
- 典型的MRI表现为边缘清晰的肿块，相对于心肌呈T_1低信号、T_2低信号，以及渐进性强化并出现低信号核，其为血供不足所致。
- 与横纹肌瘤不同，纤维瘤常表现为一个孤立的肿块，且不会消退。因此，治疗多采用外科切除。

Teratoma

- Teratoma is the second most common cardiac tumor in fetuses and neonates.
- The majority of cardiac teratomas arise in the pericardium. A common location is attached to the root of the pulmonary artery and aorta. Intramyocardial teratoma is rare.
- Teratoma may cause pleural effusion when arising from the pericardium. Pericardial teratoma is one of the primary causes of massive perinatal pericardial effusion, with potential for tamponade.
- Classic imaging appearance is a multilocular cystic and solid mass abutting the pulmonary artery and aorta.
- On MRI, teratomas are T1 hypointense to isointense relative to myocardium, T2 hyperintense, and hypoenhancing on first-pass myocardial perfusion imaging (which differentiates teratomas from hemangiomas).
- Treatment is surgical excision.

Hemangioma

- Hemangioma is a benign vascular tumor that can occur in any cardiac chamber.
- Similar to teratoma, neonatal cardiac hemangioma is also associated with massive pericardial effusion.
- On MRI, cardiac hemangiomas are T2 hyperintense and enhance avidly on first-pass myocardial perfusion.
- Treatment is surgical excision.

畸胎瘤

- 畸胎瘤是胎儿及新生儿期第二常见的心脏肿瘤。
- 大部分畸胎瘤起源于心包。常见的位置是在肺动脉及主动脉根部。心肌内畸胎瘤罕见。
- 起源于心包的畸胎瘤可引起胸腔积液。心包畸胎瘤是围产期巨大心包积液的原因之一，有导致心脏压塞的风险。
- 经典的影像学表现为紧靠在肺动脉及主动脉上的多房囊性及实性肿块。
- 磁共振上，畸胎瘤相对于心肌为T_1低至等信号，T_2高信号，增强首次通过灌注为低强化(这可与血管瘤鉴别)。
- 治疗为手术切除。

血管瘤

- 血管瘤是一类良性肿瘤，可发生于任何心腔。
- 类似于畸胎瘤，新生儿心脏血管瘤也伴发大量心包积液。
- 磁共振上，心脏血管瘤为T_2高信号，首次通过心肌灌注呈明显强化。
- 治疗为手术切除。

(翻译 谢弘)

PEDIATRIC GASTROINTESTINAL

小儿胃肠道

GI EMERGENCIES

胃肠道急症

Necrotizing enterocolitis (NEC)

坏死性小肠结肠炎(NEC)

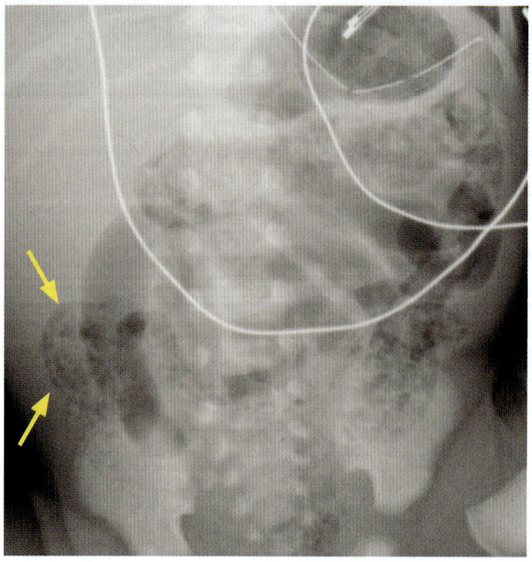

NEC with pneumatosis: Abdominal radiograph demonstrates bubbly lucencies within the bowel wall (yellow arrows), most prominent in the right lower quadrant, representing pneumatosis.

Case courtesy Michael Callahan, MD, Boston Children's Hospital.

NEC伴肠壁积气：腹部X线影像可见肠壁内泡沫样透亮影(黄箭)，以右下腹最为明显，为肠壁积气。

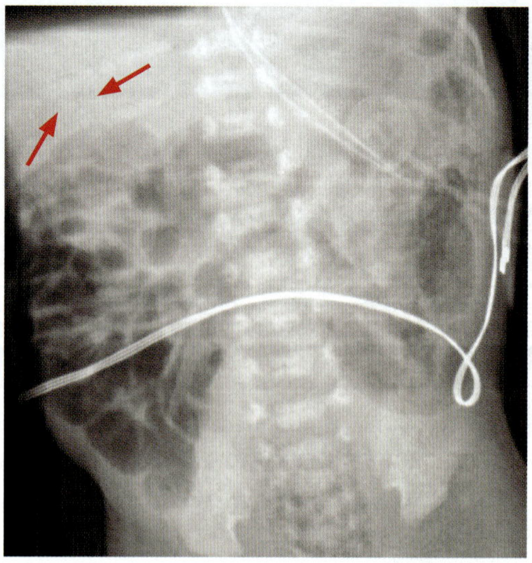

NEC with portal venous gas: Abdominal radiograph in a different neonate shows very faint curvilinear lucencies projecting over the liver (red arrows), representing portal venous gas.

Case courtesy Michael Hanley, MD, University of Virginia Health System.

NEC伴门静脉积气：另一名新生儿腹部X线影像显示肝区非常模糊的曲线样透亮影(红箭)，为门静脉积气。

- Necrotizing enterocolitis (NEC) most commonly affects pre-term infants, thought to be caused by a combination of infection and ischemia related to feeding. NEC may also occur in term infants with congenital heart disease, Hirschsprung disease, an umbilical venous catheter or on immunosuppression. Mortality can be as high as 40%.
- NEC most commonly involves the distal ileum and right colon. Initial radiographic findings include bowel thickening and fixed distention of a loop of bowel over serial exams.
- Later in the disease, pneumatosis, portal venous gas, or pneumoperitoneum related to bowel perforation may be present.

  Pneumoperitoneum can be difficult to detect on supine radiographs. One should always draw an imaginary line across the liver from right to left – if the liver gets darker, then pneumoperitoneum should be considered. Additional lateral decubitus or cross-table lateral radiographs can be obtained for further evaluation.

  Signs of pneumoperitoneum include the *football sign* (air outlining the falciform ligament), *Rigler's sign* (air outlining the serosal and mucosal surface of the bowel) and the telltale triangle (lucent triangle outlined by bowel and the peritoneal reflection).

  Submucosal pneumatosis, in which punctate locules of gas are trapped between the undulated mucosa, is easily confused with intraluminal contents. Subserosal pneumatosis, a linear crescent of gas between the smooth muscular and serosal layers of the bowel, is more specific.
- Early NEC can be treated medically (antibiotics, TPN, and cessation of oral feeding). If pneumoperitoneum is present, emergent surgery is generally required; however, bowel- sparing percutaneous drainage is an emerging option in some cases.
- Once the baby recovers, contrast enema can evaluate for stricture, which is the most common delayed complication of NEC.

- 坏死性小肠结肠炎(NEC)最常见于早产儿，被认为是由感染和与喂养相关的缺血共同引起。NEC也可见于患有先天性心脏病、先天性巨结肠、脐静脉插管或接受免疫抑制治疗的足月婴儿。NEC死亡率可高达40%。
- NEC通常累及回肠远段和右半结肠。早期的影像学表现有肠壁增厚，后续检查可发现固定的扩张肠袢。
- 病情后期可出现肠壁积气、门静脉积气及肠穿孔导致的气腹。

  气腹在仰卧位X线影像上可能难以发现。阅片者应该在肝区从右到左画一条假想线条，如果有肝区变暗，应考虑气腹的可能。可以补加侧卧位或水平侧位X线影像进一步评估。

  气腹的征象包括橄榄球征(游离气体使镰状韧带显影)、Rigler征(又称"双壁"征，气体勾勒出肠壁内外表面的黏膜和浆膜)和三角征(肠管与腹膜反折勾勒出的三角形透亮影)。

  肠壁黏膜下积气为聚集在波浪起伏的黏膜下层的点状气泡，它很容易与肠内容物相混淆。浆膜下积气是指位于肠壁平滑肌与浆膜层之间的线状新月形气体，更具特异性。
- 早期NEC可以进行保守治疗(抗生素、全肠外营养，停止经口喂养)。如果出现气腹，通常需要急诊手术。在某些情况下也可采用经皮引流，这是一种避免切除肠管的急诊处理方法。
- 一旦患儿康复，采用造影剂灌肠的方法评估肠道狭窄，后者是NEC最常见的后期并发症。

Hypertrophic pyloric stenosis (HPS)

肥厚性幽门狭窄(HPS)

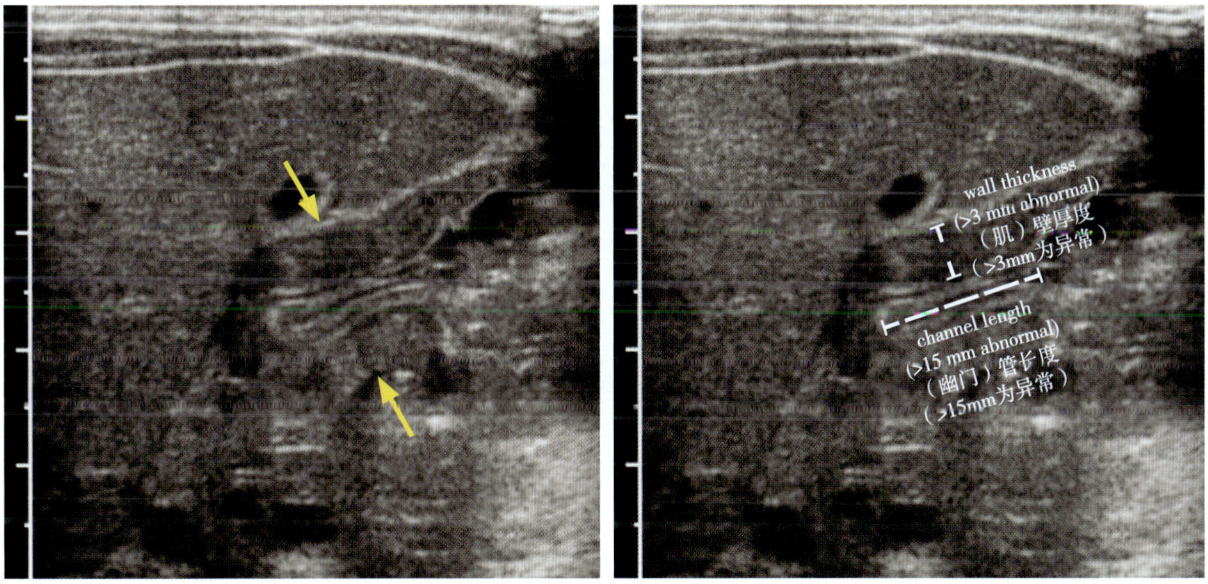

Hypertrophic pyloric stenosis: Ultrasound of the pylorus demonstrates a thickened muscular wall (arrows denote the entire pylorus; measurements should be obtained of one wall only, from echogenic mucosa to echogenic serosa, as diagrammed on the annotated image on the right) and an elongated channel length.
Case courtesy Michael Hanley, MD, University of Virginia Health System.
肥厚性幽门狭窄：超声显示幽门部胃壁肌层增厚(黄箭所指为整个幽门，在单一侧壁进行测量，即从回声增强的黏膜层到浆膜层之间的距离，如右图标记所示)和幽门管狭长。

- Hypertrophic pyloric stenosis (HPS) is muscular hypertrophy of the pylorus, which classically causes progressive, projectile, non-bilious emesis in firstborn males (affected 4 times more than females) age 2–12 weeks old. HPS is the most common surgically treated cause of vomiting in infants.
- Although there is a genetic association, most cases are sporadic and idiopathic.
- A suggestive plain film finding is the *caterpillar sign*, which describes the undulating contour of the gastric wall peristalsing against an obstructed pylorus.
- Ultrasound criteria vary by institution; typical criteria for diagnosis include wall thickness >3 mm (measuring from echogenic mucosa to echogenic serosa) and a channel length >15 mm. Positive cases will not show feeds passing through the pylorus. An important pitfall to be aware of is imaging a collapsed, normal gastric antrum.
- Treatment is pyloroplasty, with IV fluid and electrolyte replacement while waiting for surgery.
- The main differential consideration is *pylorospasm*, for which close clinical follow-up is recommended. Visualization of gastric contents passing through the pylorus is suggestive of pylorospasm, which generally features a normal-appearing pylorus.

Appendicitis

- Appendicitis is the most common reason to perform abdominal surgery in a child, typically presenting over the age of 4 years and rare in infants. Abdominal pain is usually present, but the clinical presentation in children may be atypical and diagnosis can be challenging.
- Ultrasound is the first test of choice for evaluation of suspected appendicitis in children. A swollen (>6 mm), incompressible, blind-ending tubular structure in the right lower quadrant is a typical imaging appearance.

  The most sensitive sonographic finding of appendicitis is inflamed, echogenic peri-appendiceal fat.

  An echogenic and shadowing appendicolith, increased mural vascularity, non-compressibility, and localized reproducible pain with pressure are also reliable signs of appendicitis.
- MRI is the preferred modality for assessing children after an equivocal ultrasound. Examination can be performed in roughly 10 minutes, with the most sensitive finding being infiltration of peri-appendiceal fat on T2-weighted, non-fat saturated sequences.

- 肥厚性幽门狭窄(HPS)是指幽门肌层增厚，多见于2~12周首胎男婴(为女婴的4倍)，表现为渐进性、喷射性、无胆汁性呕吐。HPS是手术治疗婴儿呕吐最常见的原因。
- 尽管有遗传因素，但大部分病例为散发或特发。
- 有提示性的X线影像表现为*毛毛虫征*，即胃壁因幽门梗阻而持续蠕动所出现的波浪起伏样轮廓。
- 超声诊断标准因各单位而异，典型诊断标准包括幽门壁厚度>3mm(测量从回声增强的黏膜层到浆膜层之间的距离)和幽门管长度>15mm。阳性病例看不到食物通过幽门。需特别注意的是，该影像学表现与一个塌陷的正常胃窦相似。
- 采用幽门成形术治疗，术前需要静脉补充液体和电解质。
- 主要的鉴别诊断是*幽门痉挛*，该病只需要密切随访。当发现胃内容物通过幽门时应考虑幽门痉挛，此时幽门的结构通常正常。

阑尾炎

- 阑尾炎是儿童行腹部外科手术最常见的原因，通常见于4岁以上儿童，1岁以下的婴儿罕见。通常以腹痛就诊，但儿童的临床表现可以不典型，因此使诊断变得比较困难。
- 超声是评估儿童阑尾炎可疑病例的首选检查。典型影像学表现是右下腹有一处肿胀(>6mm)、不可压缩、具有盲端的管状结构。

  阑尾炎最敏感的超声表现是阑尾周围系膜脂肪因炎性反应而呈高回声。

  其他比较可靠的征象还有：回声增强伴声影的阑尾粪石、肠壁充血、管腔无压缩性，以及局部可重复性压痛。
- MRI在超声不确定时可作为儿童的首选检查。检查大约需要10分钟，最敏感的征象是T_2加权、脂肪抑制序列上阑尾周围脂肪的炎性浸润。

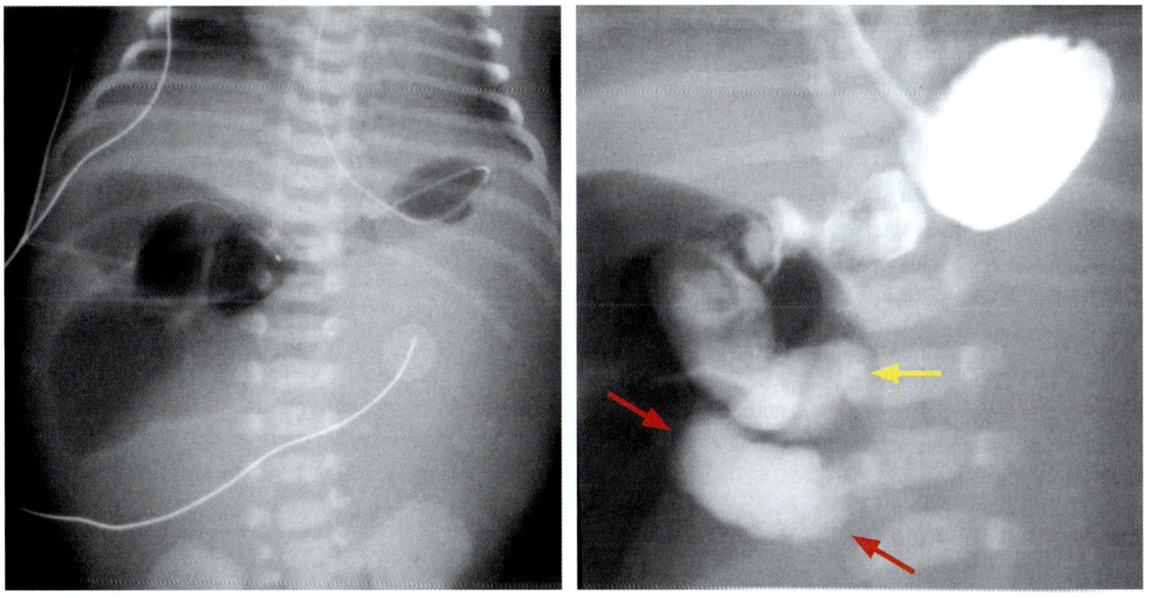

Malrotation with midgut volvulus: Abdominal radiograph (left image) shows a high bowel obstruction, with dilated proximal bowel and absence of distal bowel gas. Upper GI (right image) of the same patient demonstrates a duodeno-jejunal junction to the right of midline (yellow arrow) and a corkscrew appearance of the distal duodenum and proximal jejunum (red arrow).

Case courtesy Michael Callahan, MD and Carlo Buonomo, MD, Boston Children's Hospital.

肠旋转不良伴中肠扭转：腹部X线影像(左图)显示高位肠梗阻，可见近端肠管扩张积气及远端肠管内气体缺失。同一病例上消化道造影(右图)显示十二指肠-空肠交界区位于中线(黄箭)右侧，同时十二指肠远端和空肠近端呈螺旋形(红箭)。

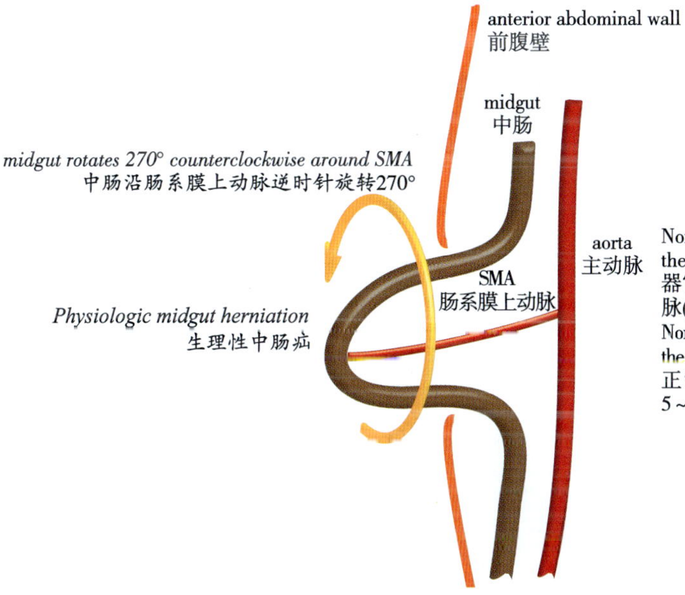

Normal rotation of the midgut about the SMA during organogenesis.
器官形成时中肠围绕肠系膜上动脉(SMA)的正常旋转。
Normal bowel rotation occurs between the fifth and eleventh weeks of gestation.
正常肠管的旋转发生在妊娠第5～11周。

- In normal embryologic development, the bowel rotates 270° counterclockwise around the SMA, causing the characteristic retroperitoneal course of the duodenum.
- This rotation fixes the duodeno- jejunal junction in the left upper quadrant and the cecum in the right lower quadrant. The span between the two composes the mesenteric attachment of bowel; the longer the attachment, the less likely the bowel is to pinwheel (volvulize) around its axis.
- **Malrotation** is the failure of normal rotation of the bowel during

- 在正常胚胎发育中，中肠围绕SMA逆时针旋转270°，形成十二指肠行走于腹膜后的特征。
- 这种逆时针旋转使十二指肠-空肠交界区固定在左上象限，盲肠固定在右下象限。两者之间的跨行区域构成肠管的肠系膜附着处，肠系膜附着处范围越长，肠管沿其轴线旋转(扭转)的可能性越小。
- **肠旋转不良**是胚胎发育时期肠道未能进行正常

embryogenesis, which predisposes to volvulus due to abnormal mesenteric fixation. Malrotation is associated with omphaloceles and heterotaxy syndromes.

- Volvulus is a surgical emergency, with a high mortality rate due to bowel ischemia. Volvulus typically presents with **neonatal bilious emesis**.

  Although bilious emesis may be due to several entities including non-obstructive gastroenteritis, malrotation with volvulus must be ruled out with an upper GI.

  Note, because bilious emesis can also occur from distal obstruction in neonates, it is essential to exclude a distal obstruction with abdominal radiograph *prior* to performing an upper GI. Performing an upper GI in a neonate with distal obstruction introduces a high risk of false positives given the laxity of the ligament of Treitz and the distortion by dilated distal loops.

- Malrotation without volvulus can have nonspecific symptoms, including feeding intolerance, cyclic vomiting, and malabsorption. Therefore, it is essential to consider malrotation in a child with abdominal symptoms.

  75% present in the first month of life and 90% become symptomatic within one year.

- The most important anatomy to demonstrate on every upper GI is the C-sweep of the duodenum and position of the duodeno-jejunal junction (DJJ).

  On frontal view, normal DJJ should be to the *left of the left spinous pedicle at the level of the duodenal bulb (L1).*

  On the lateral view, the normal duodenum first courses posteriorly into the retroperitoneum, inferiorly while retroperitoneal, anteriorly across the spine (remaining in the retroperitoneum), and then superiorly to meet the jejunum at the DJJ in the peritoneal space.

旋转，导致肠系膜固定异常而诱发的肠扭转。旋转不良与脐膨出和内脏异位综合征有关。

- 肠扭转属于外科急症。患儿因肠道缺血而病死率很高。典型的肠扭转表现为**新生儿胆汁性呕吐**。

  胆汁性呕吐可以有多种原因，包括非梗阻性肠胃炎，因此必须行上消化道造影以排除肠旋转不良伴中肠扭转的可能。

  注意，由于新生儿消化道远端梗阻也可能发生胆汁性呕吐，因此在进行上消化道造影检查前，需行腹部X线检查以排除肠道远端梗阻的可能。因为屈氏韧带松弛和远端肠袢扭曲扩张，对消化道远端梗阻的新生儿进行上消化道造影检查会有很高的假阳性风险。

- 无扭转的肠旋转不良可出现一些非特异性症状，包括不耐受喂食、周期性呕吐和吸收不良。因此，凡是有腹部症状的儿童需要排除肠旋转不良的可能。

  75%患儿在出生后第1个月内出现症状，90%的患儿在出生后1年内出现症状。

- 最重要的解剖结构是上消化道造影上C形十二指肠和十二指肠-空肠连接处(DJJ)的位置。

  在正位像上，正常DJJ应位于*十二指肠球部*(L_1)*水平，椎体左侧椎弓根的左侧*。

  在侧位像上，正常十二指肠首先向后进入腹膜后，然后在腹膜后向下，再跨越脊柱的前方(仍然位于腹膜后)，向上进入腹腔并在DJJ处与空肠连接。

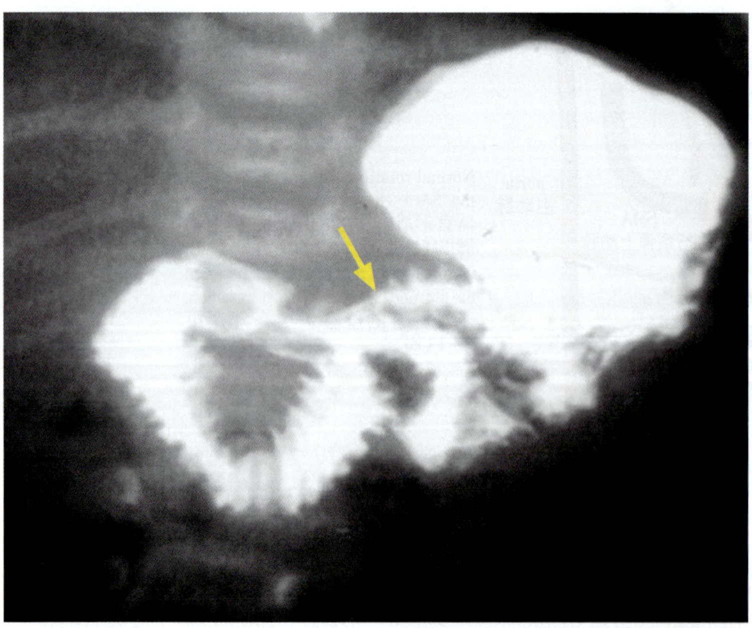

Normal upper GI: Spot image shows the duodeno-jejunal junction (arrow) to the left of midline, beyond the left pedicle of the vertebral body.

Case courtesy Michael Callahan, MD, Boston Children's Hospital.

正常上消化道造影：局部X线影像显示十二指肠-空肠连接部(箭)位于中线左侧，超过了椎体左侧的椎弓根外缘。

- On abdominal radiography, midgut volvulus most commonly appears as multiple dilated loops of bowel. Less commonly, midgut volvulus may produce a *double bubble sign* from duodenal obstruction. However, plain films can also be entirely normal in the setting of malrotation and vomiting.

- 中肠扭转在腹部X线影像上最常见的表现是多个扩张的肠袢。较为少见的表现是因十二指肠梗阻而造成的*双泡征*。但是，腹部X线影像在肠旋转不良伴有呕吐的情况下也可能表现为完全正常。

- The classic upper GI findings of midgut volvulus is the *corkscrew* appearance of twisted bowel. On CT or ultrasound, the superior mesenteric artery may be seen to the right of the superior mesenteric vein.
- In the absence of midgut volvulus, the diagnosis of malrotation can be challenging. The DJJ is a mobile structure and can be manipulated during the upper GI exam. Even experienced pediatric radiologists may occasionally disagree. Some clues to the presence of malrotation include:

  DJJ inferior to the duodenal bulb.

  DJJ to the right of the left pedicle.

  Cecum either more midline than typical or frankly in the left lower quadrant.

  On CT or US: Inversion of normal relationship of SMA and SMV (normally SMV to the right of the SMA).

  Color Doppler ultrasound or CT studies of the twisted mesenteric vessels demonstrates the *whirlpool sign*.
- The treatment of malrotation with volvulus is the Ladd procedure:

  Volvulus reduction, resection of necrotic bowel, and lysis of mesenteric adhesions ("Ladd" bands).

  The small and large bowel are separated, with the small bowel positioned primarily on the patient's right and the large bowel on the patient's left.

  Appendectomy may be performed.

- 上消化道造影时，典型中肠扭转的表现为肠管扭曲并呈*螺旋形*走行。在CT或超声检查中，肠系膜上动脉可能位于肠系膜上静脉右侧。
- 在未发生中肠扭转时，诊断肠旋转不良会有一定困难。DJJ不是一个固定的结构，在上消化道造影检查中可以人为移动。即便在有经验的儿科放射医生之间也会出现分歧。肠旋转不良的线索包括：

  DDJ位于十二指肠球部下方。

  DDJ位于左侧椎弓根的右侧。

  盲肠较靠近中线或位于左下腹。

  在CT或超声：SMA和SMV的解剖关系换位(正常的SMV位于SMA的右侧)。

  彩色多普勒超声或CT显示扭转的肠系膜血管呈*漩涡征*。
- 肠旋转不良伴肠扭转的治疗方法是Ladd手术：

  肠扭转复位，坏死肠管切除，以及松解肠系膜粘连("Ladd"带)。

  将小肠和大肠分离，把小肠尽量固定于患者右侧，把大肠尽量固定于患者左侧。

  可能需要行阑尾切除手术。

Intussusception

- Intussusception is caused by two telescoping bowel loops prolapsing into each other. The most common location is ileocolic where the ileum prolapses into the colon.
- Intussusception is common and classically presents with colicky abdominal pain, "currant jelly stool," and a palpable right lower quadrant abdominal mass.
- Most children between 3 months and 3 years old have idiopathic intussusceptions caused by lymphoid hyperplasia from a preceding viral illness. In contrast, intussusception in newborns and children older than 3 years should prompt evaluation for a pathologic lead point, which may be an intestinal polyp, Meckel diverticulum (infants), or lymphoma (children).
- Radiographs are nonspecific, but may show paucity of gas or a soft tissue mass.
- Ultrasound is the primary modality for diagnosis, which shows a characteristic *target* or *pseudokidney sign* with alternating layers of bowel wall and mesenteric fat.

肠套叠

- 肠套叠是指两段可伸缩的肠管相互套叠在一起。最常发生的位置是回盲部，此处回肠突入结肠。
- 肠套叠较为常见，典型的临床表现为腹绞痛、"红色果酱样"血便和右下腹可触及性包块。
- 大多数3个月~3岁婴幼儿为特发性肠套叠，是由先前的病毒感染而引起腹腔内淋巴组织增生。相比之下，发生于新生儿期和3岁以后儿童的肠套叠，需要尽快进行检查以发现病理性诱发因素，包括肠息肉、梅克尔憩室(婴儿)或淋巴瘤(儿童)。
- X线影像无特异性，但可显示肠管气体偏少或软组织肿块。
- 超声是主要的诊断手段，可见特征性的*靶征*或*假肾征*，为肠壁和肠系膜脂肪层相互交替重叠所致。

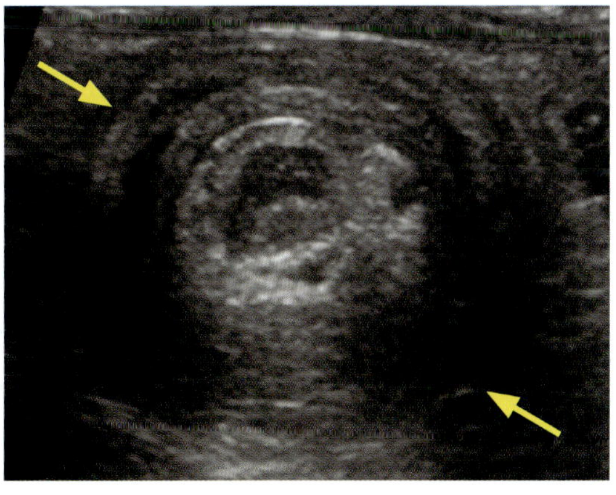

Ilio-ileal intussusception: Right lower quadrant ultrasound shows the *target sign* (arrows) with alternating layers of bowel wall and interposed mesenteric fat.

Case courtesy Michael Hanley, MD, University of Virginia Health System.

回结肠型肠套叠：右下腹超声显示*靶征*(箭)，为肠壁和嵌入的肠系膜脂肪相互交替层叠所致。

Small bowel to small bowel intussusception is a common incidental finding on ultrasound. They are often asymptomatic, transient and self-resolving. In contrast, ileocolic intussusception typically requires manual reduction. It is distinguished by diameter >2.5 cm and the presence of internal mesenteric lymph nodes or fat.

小肠-小肠型肠套叠是超声检查中的一个常见意外发现。它们通常无症状、一过性且可自愈。相反，回结肠型肠套叠通常需要人工复位。其特征是直径>2.5cm，并且套内有肠系膜淋巴结或脂肪。

- The differential diagnosis of bloody stool and thick-walled bowel on ultrasound includes intussusception, colitis, and much less commonly intramural hematoma (e.g., due to trauma or Henoch-Schönlein purpura).
- The first-line treatment is reduction with an air or contrast enema. The choice of air or contrast varies by institution, but air enemas are generally considered safer.

- 便血同时伴有超声肠壁增厚的鉴别诊断包括肠套叠、结肠炎和较少见的肠壁血肿(如外伤或Henoch-Schönlein紫癜)。
- 首选治疗方法是用空气或造影剂灌肠进行复位。选择空气还是造影剂，各单位有所不同，但是通常认为空气灌肠更为安全。

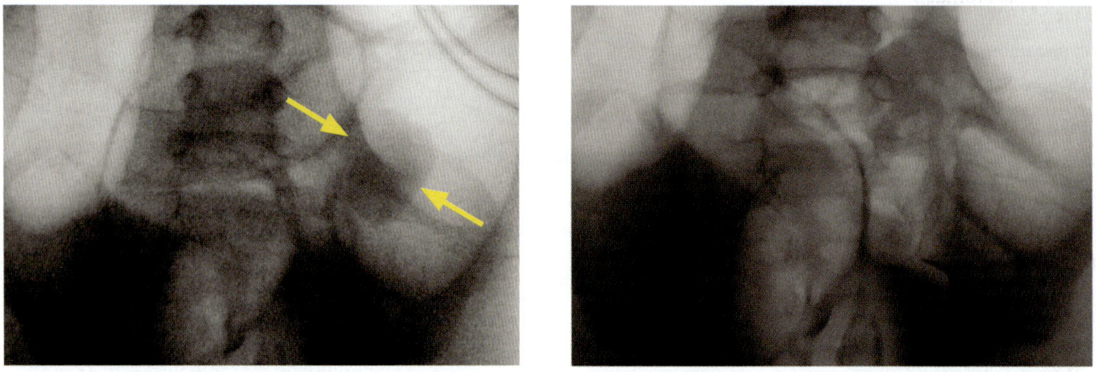

Intussusception reduction (same patient as the ultrasound above): Initial prone spot radiograph (left image) from an air enema shows a mass in the right lower quadrant (arrows), which spontaneously reduces after continued insufflation of air (right image).
肠套叠复位(为上图超声的同一患者)：俯卧位初始空气灌肠局部X线影像(左图)显示右下腹一个包块(箭)，连续灌注空气后自行复位(右图)。

A surgeon should be present. IV antibiotics are sometimes, but not universally, administered.

A large-bore needle must be available to decompress a potential tension pneumoperitoneum, which may cause fatal compression of the IVC if untreated.

A large enema tip should be used to prevent leakage, which may need to be taped to the skin.

Air should be insufflated up to 120 mmHg (between cries; reading during cries will be artificially high).

A successful reduction will show rush of air into the small bowel.

The *rule of 3's* applies to hydrostatic reduction: up to 3 attempts can be performed, up to 3 minutes each. If unsuccessful, the patient must go to surgery.

- Contraindications to pneumatic reduction include peritonitis, pneumoperitoneum, and septic shock.

做此检查时，外科医生应该在场。有时通过静脉给予抗生素，但并不常规使用。

须准备一个大口径注射针，以便在发生张力性气腹时立即进行腹腔减压，否则有可能会导致致命的下腔静脉压迫。

灌肠管应该足以粗大，以防止气体泄漏，且必要时用胶带将其固定于皮肤。

灌入的空气压力可高达120mmHg(需在患儿哭闹的间歇测量，因在哭闹时测量结果会假性增高)。

复位成功的标志是可见空气快速进入小肠。

压力性复位应遵循“3定律”：最多可以尝试3次，每次不超过3分钟。如果不成功，则需要外科手术。

- 空气复位的禁忌证包括腹膜炎、气腹和感染性休克。

CONGENITAL GASTROESOPHAGEAL DISORDERS

先天性胃食管疾病

Esophageal atresia and tracheoesophageal fistula

- In embryologic development, the primitive trachea and esophagus initially form as one structure. Esophageal atresia (EA) is a blind-ending esophagus caused by faulty embryologic separation of the two structures.
- EA is almost always associated with tracheoesophageal fistula (TEF).
- 50% of patients with TEF have associated anomalies, most commonly **VACTERL**:

食管闭锁和气管食管瘘(TEF)

- 在胚胎发育过程中，原始气管和食管最初形成一个单一的结构。食管闭锁(EA)是由于在胚胎时期这两个结构错误分隔形成的食管盲端。
- 食管闭锁几乎都伴有气管食管瘘(TEF)。
- 约50% TEF患者合并其他畸形，最常见的是**VACTERL**：

Vertebral segmentation anomalies.
Anal atresia.
Cardiac anomalies.
Tracheo**E**sophageal fistula.
Renal anomalies.
Limb (radial ray) anomalies.

V 脊柱分节异常。
A 肛门闭锁。
C 心脏畸形。
T 气管食管瘘。
R 肾脏畸形。
L 肢体(桡骨)畸形。

- TEF is also associated with tracheal anomalies including tracheomalacia and bronchus suis (right upper lobe bronchus arising directly from trachea).
- EA should be considered in-utero if there is polyhydramnios and lack of visualization of the stomach.

- TEF 常伴有气管异常，包括气管软化和支气管起源异常(右上叶支气管直接起源于气管)。
- 如果胎儿期有羊水过多，同时又看不到胃，要考虑食管闭锁。

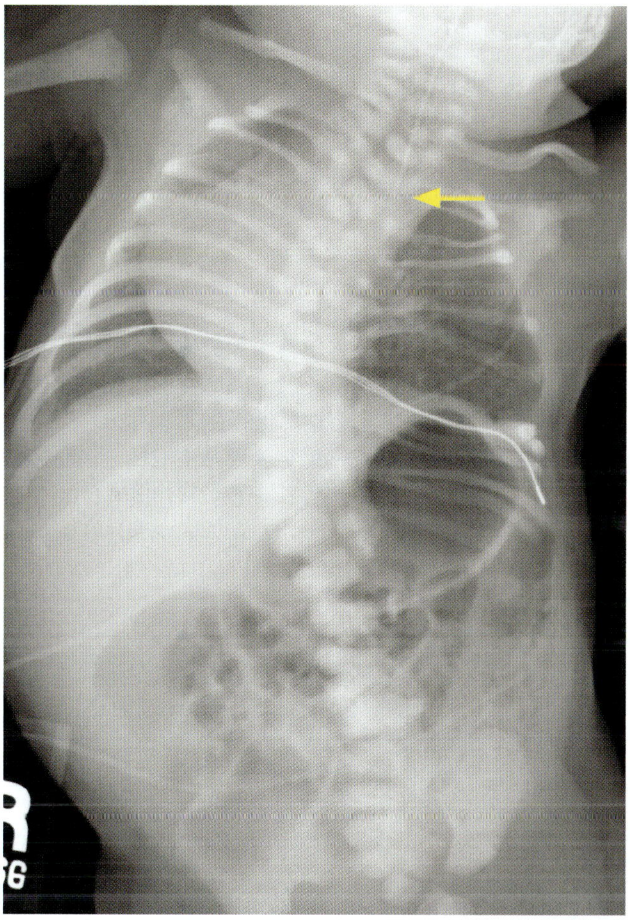

Esophageal atresia: Frontal babygram shows high position of the esophageal catheter (arrow) with distal bowel gas, consistent with tracheoesophageal fistula.
This neonate has VACTERL, with multiple vertebral segmentation anomalies and dextrocardia visible on this radiograph. Not visible on this image are this baby's anal atresia, unilateral renal agenesis, and a missing thumb.
食管闭锁：正位小儿胸腹X线影像显示高位食管导管(箭)伴有远端肠管积气，符合气管食管瘘的诊断。
该新生儿患有VACTERL：可见多个椎体分节异常及右位心。此影像未能显示患儿的肛门闭锁、单侧肾缺如和单个拇指缺如。

Types of esophageal atresia (EA) and tracheoesophageal fistulas (TEF)

食管闭锁(EA)和气管食管瘘(TEF)的类型

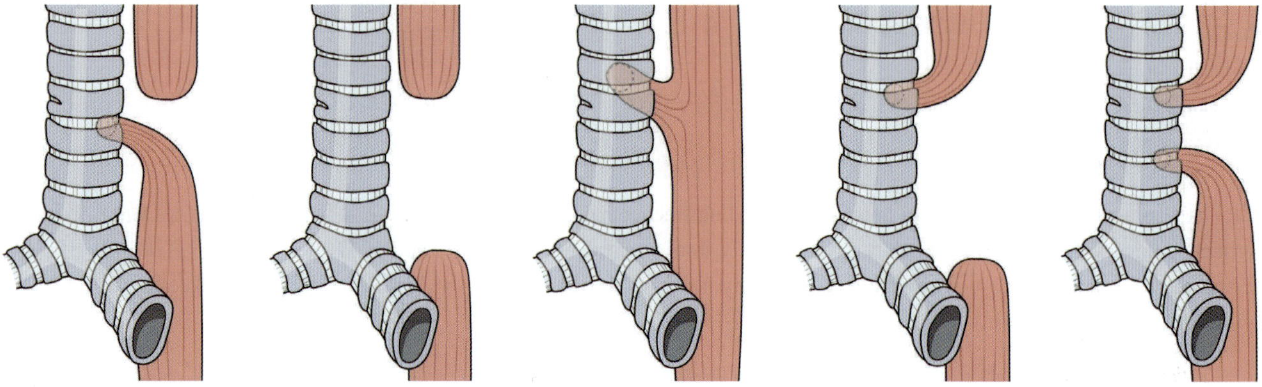

Type 1 or C (87%)
Proximal EA with distal TEF
NG tube ends in mid esophagus with air-filled stomach
1型或C型（87%）
近端食管闭锁合并远端气管食管瘘
鼻饲管的远端位于食管中段，胃内有气体

Type 2 or A (8%)
Isolated EA without TEF
Gasless abdomen
2型或A型（8%）
孤立性食管闭锁，无气管食管瘘
腹部无气体

Type 3 or H (4%)
Isolated TEF without EA
Presents in late childhood with recurrent aspiration
3型或H型（4%）
孤立性气管食管瘘，不合并食管闭锁
在年长的儿童开始发病，出现反复肺吸入

Type 4 (<1%)
Proximal TEF with distal EA
4型（<1%）
近端食管气管瘘合并远端食管闭锁

Type 5 (<1%)
Double TEF
5型（<1%）
双食管气管瘘

Gastric atresia

- Gastric atresia represents congenital obstruction of the distal stomach resulting in non-bilious vomiting. In contrast to hypertrophic pyloric stenosis, the vomiting does not get progressively worse.
- A diagnostic imaging finding is the *single* bubble, with a large bubble of air (or contrast) in the proximal stomach.
- A less severe variant is a nonobstructive antral web.

胃闭锁

- 胃闭锁为先天性远端胃梗阻，引起无胆汁性呕吐。与肥厚性幽门狭窄相比，呕吐没有进行性恶化的表现。
- 影像学表现是单泡征，即胃的近端有一个大的气泡影(或造影剂潴留)。
- 一种严重程度较轻的变异为非梗阻性胃窦隔膜。

NEONATAL BOWEL OBSTRUCTION: OVERVIEW

新生儿肠梗阻：概述

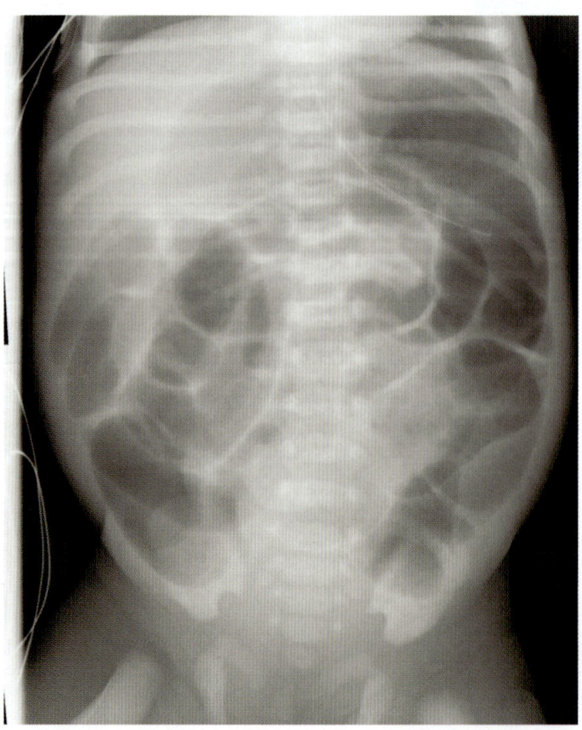

Neonatal distal bowel obstruction: Abdominal radiograph shows numerous dilated loops of bowel throughout the entire abdomen. A nasogastric tube is in the stomach.
新生儿低位肠梗阻：腹部X线影像显示整个腹部有无数扩张的肠管。胃腔内有一根鼻胃管。

- Neonatal bowel obstruction, occurring in the first 24–48 hours of life, is a distinct entity from childhood and adult obstruction, with unique etiologies and workup. Unlike in adults, CT plays no role in the workup of neonatal bowel obstruction.
- In the neonate, small bowel cannot be distinguished from large bowel based on location or size of the bowel loops.
- When loops of distended bowel are seen and obstruction is suspected, one can divide the differential into *proximal/high* or *distal/low* obstruction (relative to the distal jejunum) based solely on the number of dilated loops seen.
- If the initial radiograph does not provide a definite diagnosis, the imaging test of choice for a **proximal obstruction** is an **upper GI study**. All proximal obstructions are surgical. Midgut volvulus must be ruled out.

  A patient with characteristic clinical and imaging findings of duodenal atresia can be diagnosed on radiograph alone. For instance, a baby with known Down syndrome and a *double bubble* on radiograph is considered diagnostic of duodenal atresia.
- In contrast, the imaging test of choice for a **distal obstruction** is a **contrast enema**, which can be both diagnostic and therapeutic. The goal of imaging in distal obstruction is to differentiate surgical from non-surgical causes.

- 新生儿肠梗阻，即出生后24~48小时内发生的肠梗阻，它与儿童和成人肠梗阻有着截然不同的区别，有其特殊的病因和诊断方法。与成人不同，CT对诊断新生儿肠梗阻没有价值。
- 在新生儿期，小肠无法根据其肠管位置和管径大小与大肠进行区别。
- 当发现肠管扩张并怀疑有肠梗阻时，可根据扩张肠管的数量分为*近端/高位*或*远端/低位*肠梗阻(大致为远段空肠)。
- 如果初始X线影像未能提供明确诊断，对疑似**高位肠梗阻**患者应首选**上消化道造影**。所有高位梗阻都需要手术。必须要排除中肠扭转。

  当十二指肠闭锁的患者出现典型的临床症状和影像学表现时，诊断仅需依靠普通X线影像。例如，一名唐氏综合征婴儿在腹部X线影像上有*双泡征*即可考虑十二指肠闭锁的诊断。
- 相比之下，诊断**低位肠梗阻**的首选影像检查是**灌肠造影**，具有诊断和治疗的双重作用。低位肠梗阻影像学检查目的是区分手术和非手术原因。

Congenital proximal bowel obstruction

- All causes of congenital proximal bowel obstruction are surgical. The primary purpose of an upper GI is to distinguish between midgut volvulus (requiring emergent surgery) and bowel atresia, which requires a non-emergent repair.

Duodenal atresia, stenosis, and web

先天性高位肠梗阻

- 任何原因所致的先天性高位肠梗阻都需要进行外科手术。上消化道检查的主要目的是区分中肠扭转(需要急诊手术)和肠闭锁，后者不需要急诊修复。

十二指肠闭锁、狭窄和蹼

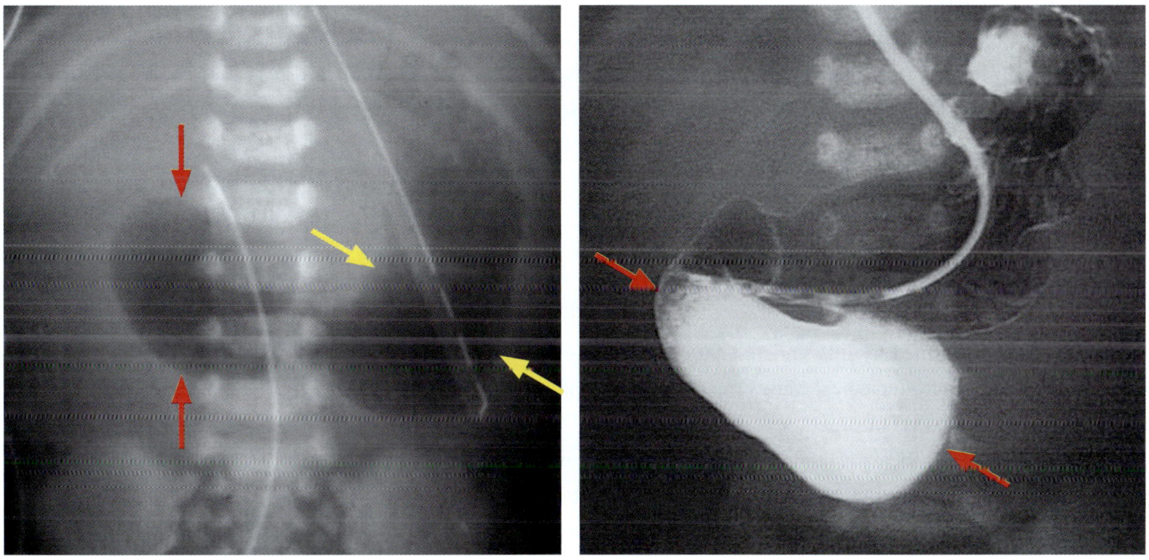

Duodenal atresia: Abdominal radiograph (left image) shows the classic *double bubble sign*, with a distended stomach (yellow arrows) and a distended duodenal bulb (red arrows). Upper-GI study (right image) shows a markedly distended duodenum (red arrows) and no contrast passage into the jejunum.

Case courtesy Michael Callahan, MD and Carlo Buonomo, MD, Boston Children's Hospital.

十二指肠闭锁：腹部X线影像(左图)显示典型的*双泡征*，即扩张的胃(黄箭)和十二指肠球部(红箭)。上消化道造影检查(右图)显示极度扩张的十二指肠(红箭)，但没有造影剂进入空肠。

- During embryogenesis, the duodenum forms as a solid tube. Lack of

- 在胚胎形成期，十二指肠形成一个实性管道。

recanalization causes the spectrum of diseases ranging from duodenal atresia (complete lack of recanalization) to duodenal stenosis (partial recanalization).

- A less severe variant, the duodenal web, allows liquids to pass, but causes the *windsock deformity* after the child begins to eat solid foods, which get stuck in the web.
- About 80% of cases occur just distal to the ampulla, therefore patients typically present with bilious emesis.
- Even a complete atresia does not preclude distal bowel gas. In the presence of a rare congenital bifid common bile duct, bowel gas can travel through the ampulla of Vater and enter the distal bowel.
- Duodenal anomalies are associated with other abnormalities in 50% of cases, most commonly Down syndrome (30% of cases). Other associated anomalies include:
  - VACTERL.
  - Cardiac shunt vascularity (ASD, VSD, PDA, and endocardial cushion defect).
  - Malrotation.
  - Annular pancreas, seen in 20% of babies with duodenal atresia.
- The classic radiographic appearance of duodenal atresia is the *double bubble sign* caused by dilation of both the stomach and the proximal duodenum, without distal bowel gas. A patient with a *double bubble* and no distal bowel gas can be presumed to have duodenal atresia.
- If distal bowel gas is present with a *double bubble sign*, the differential diagnosis includes midgut volvulus, annular pancreas (pancreas wraps around the duodenum), and the less severe variants of duodenal atresia including duodenal stenosis and web.

Jejunal atresia and stenosis

- Unlike duodenal atresia, jejunal atresia is most commonly caused by an in-utero vascular insult. Jejunal atresia is more common than stenosis.
- The *triple bubble sign* can be seen on radiography as dilated stomach, duodenum, and proximal jejunum.

Malrotation and midgut volvulus

- Discussed earlier in the chapter under GI emergencies.

CONGENITAL LOW/DISTAL BOWEL OBSTRUCTION

- A contrast enema is performed to differentiate surgical causes (distal atresias and Hirschsprung disease) from medical causes (meconium ileus and functional immaturity) of low/distal bowel obstruction.
- When performing a contrast enema, isotonic or mildly hypertonic water-soluble contrast is used, such as a 17% solution of iothalamate meglumine (400 mOsm/kg water; Cysto-Conray Ⅱ, Covidien). High osmolar contrast may cause fluid shifts and resultant destabilization of the patient.

Differential diagnosis of microcolon

- Microcolon is a colon of abnormally small caliber (typically <1 cm), secondary to disuse. A relatively distal obstruction is necessary to develop a microcolon, as the succus entericus secreted by the proximal bowel prevents microcolon. The two most common causes of microcolon are meconium ileus and ileal atresia.

肠腔再通失败可导致一系列疾病，从十二指肠闭锁(最严重，完全缺乏再通)到十二指肠狭窄(部分再通)。

- 较轻的一种变异是十二指肠蹼，它可以允许液体通过，但当患儿开始进食固体食物时形成风向袋样变形，可导致食物被卡在隔膜(蹼)。
- 约80%病例的梗阻发生在壶腹部远端，因此，患者通常表现为胆汁性呕吐。
- 即便是完全性闭锁也有可能在远端肠道内存在气体。如在一种罕见的先天性胆总管裂患者中，肠道气体可以穿过Vater壶腹而进入肠道远端。
- 在十二指肠异常的病例中，有50%合并其他异常，最常见的是唐氏综合征(约30%病例)。其他异常包括：
  - VACTERL。
  - 心血管分流异常(ASD、VSD、PDA和心内膜垫缺损)。
  - 肠旋转不良。
  - 环状胰腺，见于20%的十二指肠闭锁婴儿。
- 十二指肠闭锁的典型X线征象是双泡征，为胃和十二指肠近端扩张所致，同时远端肠道内气体缺失。患者有双泡征和远端肠管没有气体可以推测有十二指肠闭锁。
- 当双泡征阳性但远端肠道有气体存在时，鉴别诊断包括肠扭转、环状胰腺(胰腺环绕十二指肠)。较轻的十二指肠闭锁变异包括十二指肠狭窄和蹼。

空肠闭锁与狭窄

- 与十二指肠闭锁不同，空肠闭锁最常见的病因是宫内血管性损伤。空肠闭锁比狭窄更为常见。
- X线影像学上的三泡征是指胃、十二指肠和近端空肠扩张。

肠旋转不良和中肠扭转

- 已在前文的“胃肠道急症”进行详述。

先天性低位肠梗阻

- 造影剂灌肠用来区分低位/远端肠梗阻是属于外科(远端闭锁和先天性巨结肠)或内科(胎粪性肠梗阻和功能不成熟)的原因。
- 当进行造影剂灌肠检查时，应使用等张或轻度高渗的水溶性造影剂，如浓度为17%的碘他拉葡胺(400mOsm/kg，Cysto-Conray Ⅱ，Covidien)，高渗造影剂可能导致体液转移而使病情不稳。

小结肠的鉴别诊断

- 小结肠是指结肠管径异常变小(通常<1 cm)，继发于废用性萎缩。病变近端肠道梗阻是形成小结肠的必要条件，因为近端肠管分泌的肠液可防止小结肠的发生。最常见的两个病因是胎粪性肠梗阻和回肠闭锁。

Causes of microcolon
小结肠的病因

filling defects in bowel
肠道内充盈缺损

- **Meconium ileus**
  胎粪性肠梗阻

abrupt cut-off at site of atresia
闭锁端的突然中断

- **Ileal or colonic atresia**
  回肠或结肠闭锁
- **Total colonic Hirschprung**
  全结肠型巨结肠
- **Megacystic-microcolon-hypoperistalsis syndrome**
  巨结肠-小结肠-肠蠕动迟缓综合征

Peritoneal/scrotal calcifications may be seen in association with meconium ileus. In contrast to meconium ileus, small left colon syndrome (also confusingly called meconium plug syndrome; subsequently discussed) does NOT cause a microcolon.
Jejunal atresia does NOT cause microcolon as there is enough succus entericus produced to nourish the colon.
Total colonic Hirschsprung is rare. The much more common segmental involvement does not cause microcolon.
腹膜/阴囊钙化可见于胎粪性肠梗阻。与胎粪性肠梗阻不同，小左半结肠综合征（也称为“胎粪栓塞综合征”，后文讨论）不会导致小结肠。
空肠闭锁不会引起小结肠，因为有足够的小肠液滋养结肠。
全结肠型巨结肠很罕见。更常见的是节段性巨结肠，其不会导致小结肠。

Meconium ileus

胎粪性肠梗阻

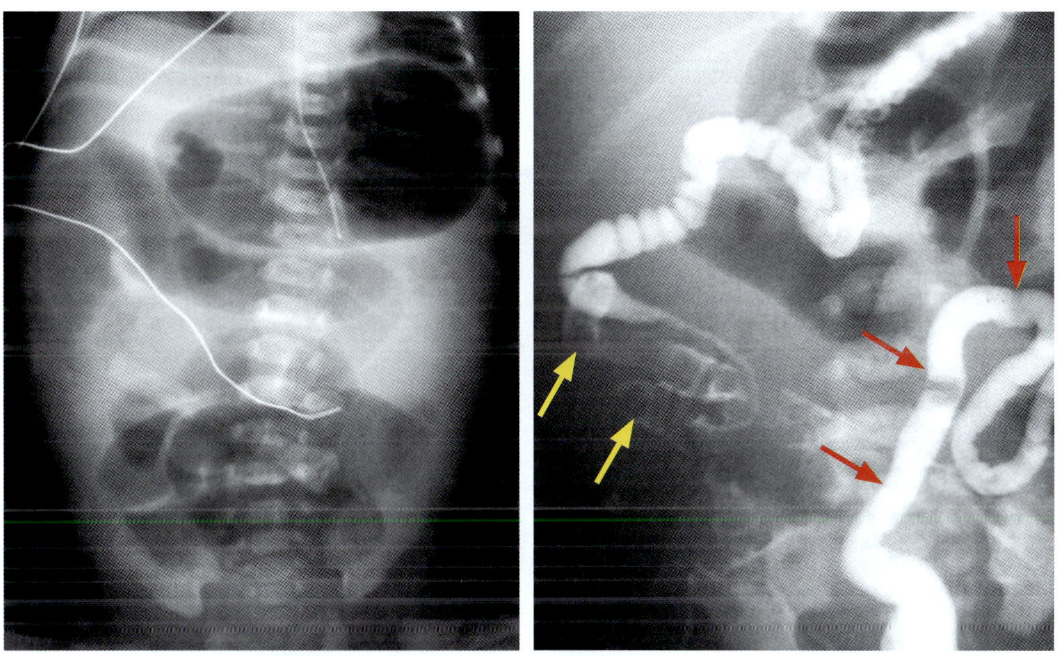

Meconium ileus: Neonatal abdominal radiograph (left image) shows a low/distal small bowel obstruction, with a dilated stomach and numerous dilated loops of bowel extending to the pelvis. Contrast enema (right image) shows a very small caliber colon (*microcolon*; red arrows), with numerous rounded filling defects in the distal ileum (yellow arrows), representing inspissated meconium.
Case courtesy Michael Callahan, MD and Carlo Buonomo, MD, Boston Children's Hospital.
胎粪性肠梗阻：新生儿腹部X线影像(左图)显示低位/远端小肠梗阻，伴随胃扩张及大量扩张的肠袢并向盆腔延伸。造影剂灌肠(右图)显示结肠管径明显较小(小结肠；红箭)，远端回肠内可见大量圆形充盈缺损影(黄箭)，为凝结的胎粪。

- Meconium ileus causes bowel obstruction from inspissated meconium in the distal ileum and colon. It can be complicated by perforation and resultant meconium peritonitis, which can cause abdominal and/or scrotal calcifications. The abdominal calcifications are frequently trapped between the liver and diaphragm, which is not seen in other causes of diffuse abdominal calcifications.

- 胎粪性肠梗阻是由于胎粪在远端回肠和结肠中凝结而导致的肠道阻塞。胎粪性肠梗阻可能并发穿孔并导致胎粪性腹膜炎，引起腹部和阴囊钙化。腹部钙化常局限在肝脏和膈肌之间，这种现象不会出现在其他原因导致的弥漫性腹部钙化。

- Meconium ileus is the earliest manifestation of cystic fibrosis: almost 100% of babies with meconium ileus have cystic fibrosis, while ~10% of babies with cystic fibrosis have meconium ileus.
- The classic radiographic appearance of meconium ileus is a distal obstruction (multiple loops of dilated bowel), with *soap-bubble* lucencies in the right lower quadrant in the region of the distal ileum.
- Contrast enema shows a microcolon (meconium ileus has the smallest of all microcolons) with a distended ileum containing multiple rounded filling defects representing inspissated meconium.
- Meconium ileus is both diagnosed and treated with therapeutic water-soluble gastrografin enema, which functions to loosen the inspissated meconium. It often takes multiple attempts to fully clean out the meconium, and carefully increasing the contrast osmolality may be helpful. Uncommonly, resistant cases may need to be treated surgically.

- 胎粪性肠梗阻是囊性纤维化最早的临床表现：几乎100%的胎粪性肠梗阻患儿有囊性纤维化，而多达10%的囊性纤维化婴儿患有胎粪性肠梗阻。
- 胎粪性肠梗阻的典型X线影像表现为远端梗阻(多个肠袢扩张)，伴右下腹远端回肠区域肥皂泡样透亮影。
- 造影剂灌肠可显示微结肠(胎粪性肠梗阻有最小的微结肠的)，伴扩张的阻塞肠管，其中包含多个圆形充盈缺损，代表变稠的胎粪。
- 胎粪性肠梗阻可以用水溶性泛影葡胺灌肠，可同时起到诊断和治疗的作用，并可发挥松解凝结胎粪的功能。完全清除胎粪往往需要多次尝试，同时，适当增加造影剂渗透压会增加清除效果。顽固性病例不常见，可能需要进行手术治疗。

Ileal atresia / colonic atresia

- Atresia of the ileum or colon features a microcolon distal to the atretic segment.
- Colonic atresia is rare.
- Unlike meconium ileus, ileal and colonic atresia demonstrate an abrupt cutoff at the site of atresia, and there are no filling defects within the bowel.

回肠闭锁/结肠闭锁

- 回肠或结肠闭锁的特征是闭锁远端的肠管为小结肠。
- 结肠闭锁罕见。
- 不同于胎粪性肠梗阻，回肠和结肠闭锁的影像学表现为闭锁处的肠管突然截断，同时肠管内无充盈缺损。

Small left colon / functional immaturity of the colon (FIC) / meconium plug syndrome

小左结肠/功能性未成熟结肠(FIC)/胎粪栓综合征

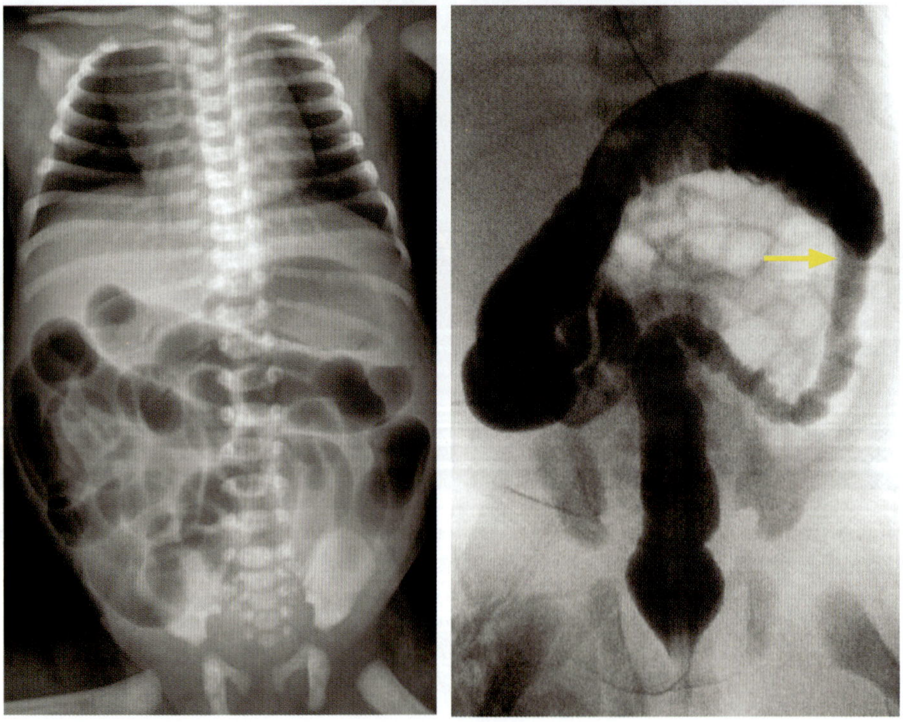

Small left colon: Babygram (left image) shows numerous loops of dilated bowel, suggestive of a distal obstructive pattern. Contrast enema (right image) shows a moderately reduced caliber of the left colon, with an abrupt transition (arrow) at the splenic flexure. The rectum is normal in caliber.

Case courtesy Michael Hanley, MD, University of Virginia Health System.

小左结肠：小儿胸腹X线影像(左图)显示大量扩张的肠袢，提示为远端梗阻的征象。造影剂灌肠(右图)显示左侧结肠管径呈中度狭窄，结肠脾曲可见结肠管径突然缩窄(箭)，但直肠管径正常。

- Small left colon, also known as functional immaturity of the colon or meconium plug syndrome, is the most common diagnosis in neonates who fail to pass meconium. It is caused by temporary functional immaturity of the colonic ganglion cells, which causes the distal colon to have abnormal motility right after birth.
- Small left colon is seen more commonly in pre-term neonates or in neonates born to mothers with diabetes or who received magnesium for (pre)eclampsia. Infants with small left colon are almost always otherwise normal.
- In contrast to meconium ileus, small left colon is *not* a cause of microcolon. Small left colon is *not* associated with cystic fibrosis/meconium ileus despite the confusing name of "meconium plug syndrome."
- The imaging appearance on an abdominal radiograph is of distal obstructive pattern.
- Contrast enema shows a small left colon, typically with an abrupt transition in caliber at the splenic flexure. There may be filling defects within the small left colon representing meconium plugs.
- Similar to meconium ileus, water soluble enema is diagnostic and therapeutic, and small left colon resolves with conservative therapy.
- The primary differential consideration is Hirschsprung disease with a transition at the splenic flexure. In contrast to small left colon, Hirschsprung disease would not feature a distensible normal caliber rectum and would not resolve after an enema treatment.

- 小左结肠：也称为功能性未成熟结肠或胎粪栓(堵塞)综合征，是新生儿未能排出胎粪时的一个最常见诊断。小左结肠是由于结肠神经节细胞临时性功能未成熟所致，使得远端结肠在出生后不久即发生运动异常。
- 小左结肠最常见于早产儿，或足月新生儿的母亲患有糖尿病或(先兆)子痫使用过镁治疗。有小左结肠的婴儿在其他方面几乎都正常。
- 与胎粪性肠梗阻不同，小左结肠并不引起小结肠。小左结肠与囊性纤维化/胎粪性肠梗阻并没有联系，但"胎粪栓综合征"这一名字会令人混淆。
- 腹部X线影像表现为远端肠梗阻的征象。
- 造影剂灌肠显示左侧结肠狭小，通常在结肠脾曲可见管径突然变化的移行区。细小的左侧结肠内还可能会见到充盈缺损，为粪块。
- 类似于胎粪性肠梗阻，水溶性造影剂的灌肠既可作为诊断，又可作为治疗，小左结肠用保守治疗方法可以恢复。
- 主要鉴别诊断是移行区位于结肠脾曲的先天性巨结肠。与小左结肠不同，先天性巨结肠的特征是直肠管径变窄，并且灌肠治疗后不会消失。

Hirschsprung disease

先天性巨结肠

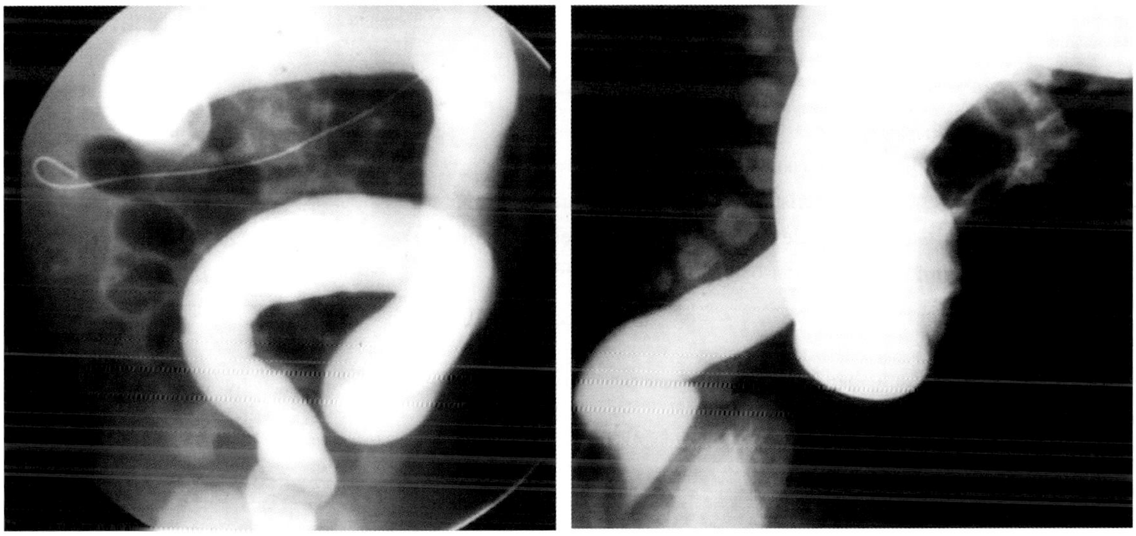

Hirschsprung disease: Frontal (left image) and lateral (right image) spot radiographs from a contrast enema show a narrowed rectum, which has a smaller diameter than the sigmoid colon.

Case courtesy Michael Callahan, MD and Carlo Buonomo, MD, Boston Children's Hospital.

先天性巨结肠：造影剂灌肠后正位(左图)和侧位(右图)局部X线影像显示直肠狭窄，其直径小于乙状结肠。

- Hirschsprung disease is aganglionosis of the distal bowel, resulting in failed relaxation of the involved bowel and subsequent bowel obstruction. It is caused by arrest of the normal craniocaudal (proximal-to-distal) migration of vagal neural crest cells to the distal bowel wall. The anus is therefore always affected, and the involved bowel is continuous as it extends proximally.

- 先天性巨结肠是由于远端肠管缺乏神经节细胞，导致病变肠段丧失松弛功能，从而导致肠梗阻。先天性巨结肠是因胚胎发育过程中，迷走神经嵴细胞由正常的头尾方向(即由近至远)向远端肠段迁移受阻所致。因此，肛门总是受到影响，而且，受累肠道是不间断地向近端延伸。

- Hirschsprung disease typically presents in newborn males who fail to have a bowel movement after 48–72 hours, and have forceful passage of meconium after rectal exam.
- Hirschsprung disease ranges in severity from isolated internal anal sphincter involvement (ultrashort segment) to involvement of the entire colon (very rare, approximately 1–3% of cases, and typically genetic).
- Up to 1/3 of cases of Hirschsprung develop a form of enterocolitis similar to necrotizing enterocolitis, with toxic megacolon being the fulminant form. It is therefore important to consider Hirschsprung in a neonate with bowel obstruction and colitis.
- Multiple congenital anomalies are associated with Hirschsprung disease. Five percent have trisomy 21, but the association with Down syndrome is less compared to duodenal atresia.
- Radiography of Hirschsprung disease shows distal bowel obstruction pattern.
- Contrast enema typically shows a gradual cone-shaped transition zone at the junction of the spastic, narrowed distal colon and the dilated proximal colon, best seen on the lateral view.

  A *sawtooth* appearance to the rectum may sometimes be seen, representing irregular contractions in the aganglionic segment.

  The rectum normally has a larger diameter than the sigmoid. When Hirschsprung involves the rectum, the rectum will be in spasm and the sigmoid will be dilated, caused by an abnormal rectosigmoid index (ratio of rectal to sigmoid diameter) less than 1.
- In contrast to functional immaturity of the colon, Hirschsprung disease tends to cause a tapered, rather than an abrupt, transition zone.
- Definitive diagnosis is with suction biopsy of the bowel wall. Treatment is surgical.

Megacystis microcolon intestinal hypoperistalsis syndrome

- Megacystis microcolon intestinal hypoperistalsis syndrome is a rare congenital loss of bladder and bowel smooth muscle function causing absent intestinal peristalsis, microcolon, and distended non-obstructed urinary bladder. It is usually fatal.

Malrotation

- Although uncommon, the Ladd bands of malrotation may cause a distal obstruction.

CHILDHOOD BOWEL OBSTRUCTION

- The etiologies and imaging of childhood bowel obstruction overlap with those of adults. Adult bowel obstruction is most commonly caused by adhesions and hernia, both of which may also cause obstruction in a child.
- The most common causes of childhood bowel obstruction can be remembered with the mnemonic **AAIIMM** (appendicitis, adhesions, internal/inguinal hernia, intussusception, Meckels, and malrotation). Most causes of childhood obstruction are treated surgically.

Appendicitis

- Appendicitis is one of the more common causes of ileus or partial bowel obstruction in children over the age of 4 years.

- 先天性巨结肠通常发生于男性新生儿，表现为出生后48~72小时后仍没有排便，但在直肠检查后有胎粪强力排出。
- 先天性巨结肠的严重程度可从仅累及肛门内括约肌(超短段)到整个结肠受累(罕见，占1%~3%的病例，常为遗传性)。
- 多达1/3的先天性巨结肠病例会发展为小肠结肠炎，类似于坏死性小肠结肠炎，而中毒性巨结肠为其暴发型。因此，当新生儿出现肠梗阻和结肠炎时，必须要考虑先天性巨结肠。
- 先天性巨结肠可伴发多种先天畸形。约5%病例伴有21-三体综合征，但合并唐氏综合征的病例少于十二指肠闭锁。
- 先天性巨结肠的X线影像表现为远端肠管梗阻的征象。
- 造影剂灌肠通常可显示一个平缓的锥形移行区，位于有痉挛和狭窄的远端结肠和扩张的近端结肠之间，侧位影像显示最佳。

  有时可看到直肠的锯齿状外观，代表无神经节肠管的不规则收缩。

  正常直肠的直径大于乙状结肠。当先天性巨结肠累及直肠时，直肠出现痉挛而乙状结肠发生扩张，造成直肠乙状结肠指数(直肠与乙状结肠直径之比)小于1。
- 与功能性未成熟结肠相比，先天性巨结肠更容易出现逐渐变细的移行区，而不是突然的移行区。
- 确诊需要进行肠壁抽吸活检。治疗为外科手术。

巨膀胱小结肠肠蠕动迟缓综合征

- 巨膀胱小结肠肠蠕动迟缓综合征是一种罕见的、先天性膀胱和肠道平滑肌功能丧失，导致肠道缺乏蠕动功能、小结肠、无梗阻性膀胱扩张的疾病。本病通常是致命性的。

肠旋转不良

- 异常旋转的Ladd带(peritoneal fibrous band，腹膜纤维带)可引起远端肠梗阻，但不常见。

儿童肠梗阻

- 儿童肠梗阻的病因和影像学表现与成人有部分重叠。成人肠梗阻最常见的原因是粘连和疝，这两种原因也可以导致儿童肠梗阻。
- 儿童最常见的肠梗阻原因可以记忆为**AAIIMM**(阑尾炎、粘连、内疝/腹股沟疝、肠套叠、梅克尔憩室和肠旋转不良)。大多数儿童肠梗阻需要手术治疗。

阑尾炎

- 阑尾炎是4岁以上儿童肠梗阻或部分肠梗阻的常见原因之一。

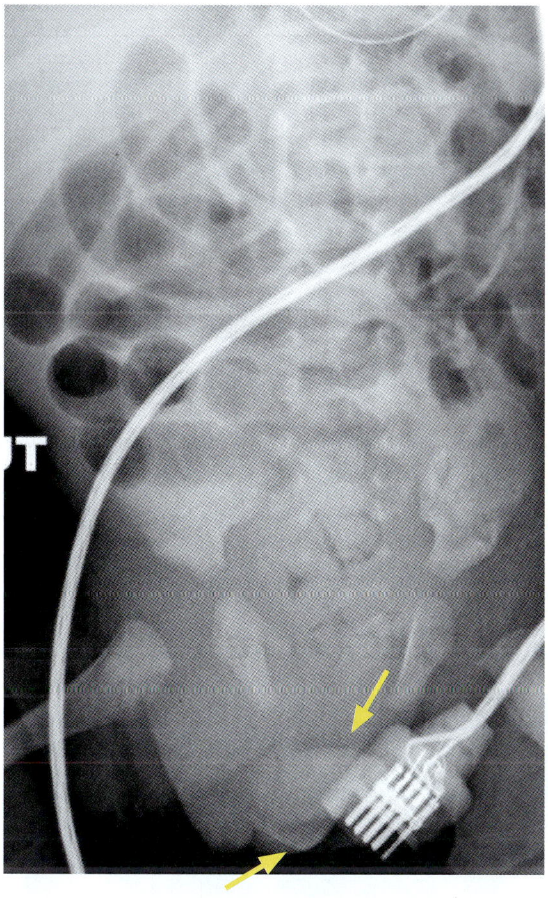

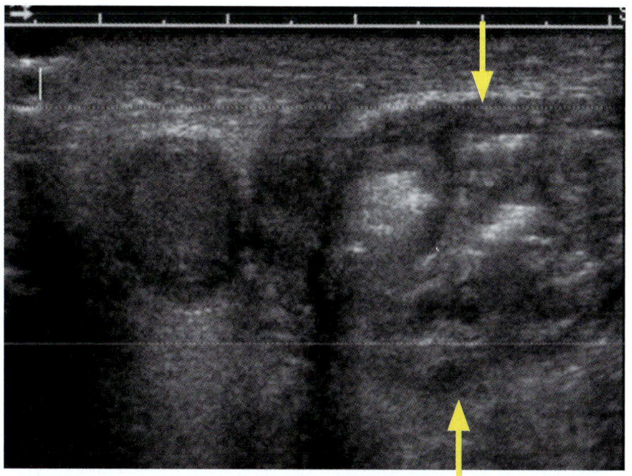

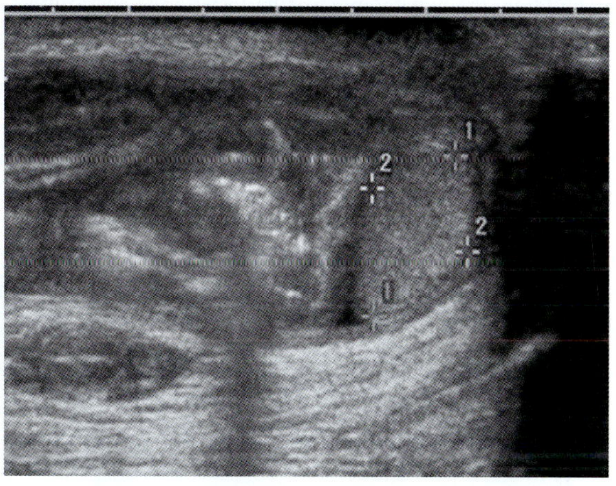

Inguinal hernia: Frontal radiograph (left image) shows numerous dilated loops of bowel, with the suggestion of increased opacification in the region of the left hemiscrotum (arrows). Transverse ultrasound of the scrotum (top right image) shows numerous loops of bowel in the left hemiscrotum (arrows). A sagittal ultrasound of the left testis (bottom right image) shows that the testis is normal (calipers) but is displaced by the intra-scrotal bowel loops.

Case courtesy Michael Callahan, MD, Boston Children's Hospital.

腹股沟斜疝：腹部正位X线影像(左图)显示大量肠管扩张，且在左侧阴囊区有可疑密度增高影(箭)。阴囊横切面超声(右上图)显示左侧阴囊区内可见大量肠管影(箭)。左侧睾丸矢状切面超声(右下图)显示睾丸正常(游标)，但被阴囊内的肠管挤压而发生移位。

- Indirect inguinal hernias are more common, resulting from a patent processus vaginalis which maintains a peritoneal communication to the scrotum via the inguinal ring.
- Imaging of an inguinal hernia causing obstruction shows bowel in the inguinal canal or scrotum. There is risk of bowel incarceration when irreducible.

Meckel diverticulum

- Meckel diverticulum is a remnant of the omphalomesenteric duct, which connects the fetal ileum to the yolk sac via the umbilicus. Incomplete regression of the omphalomesenteric duct leads to a spectrum of anomalies, ranging from an umbilico-ileal fistula (fecal drainage from the umbilicus) to a Meckel diverticulum (by far the most common anomaly occurring in approximately 95%). It is located at the antimesenteric aspect of the distal ileum.

- 腹股沟斜疝更为常见，是由于鞘状突未闭，使得阴囊通过腹股沟环与腹膜腔保持连通。
- 在影像学上，腹股沟斜疝引起的肠梗阻通常表现为肠管位于腹股沟管或阴囊内。不可复疝时有肠管嵌顿的风险。

梅克尔憩室

- 梅克尔憩室是脐肠系膜导管的残余，在胎儿期，它通过脐连接胎儿回肠和卵黄囊。脐肠系膜导管退化不完全会导致一系列发育异常，如脐-回肠瘘(从脐排出粪便)和梅克尔憩室(最多见的畸形，约占95%)。梅克尔憩室位于回肠远端的小肠系膜对侧的游离面。

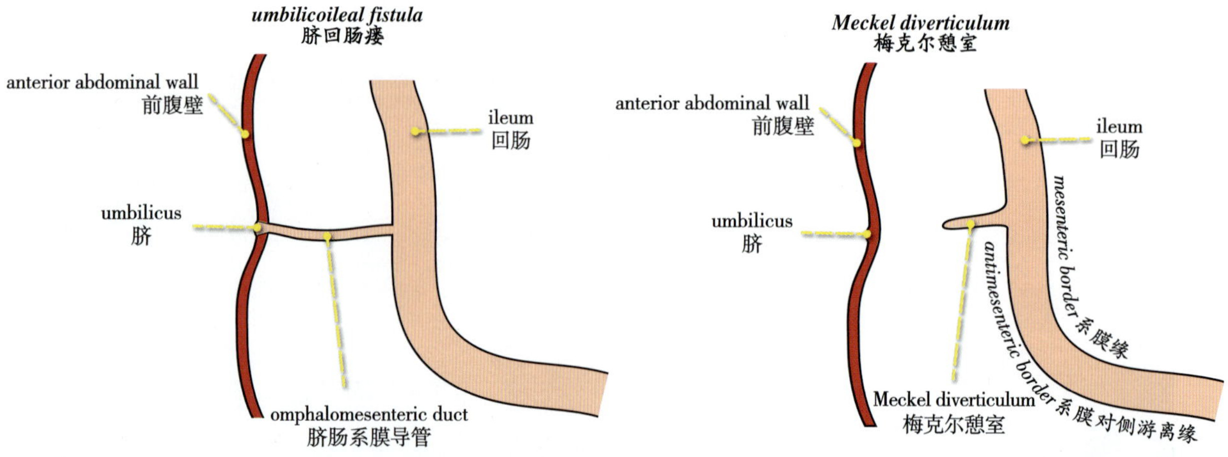

- In young children, the most common manifestation is gastrointestinal bleeding (if it contains ectopic gastric mucosa). Less commonly, a Meckel may cause intussusception by acting as a lead point or result in diverticulitis mimicking appendicitis.
- In adults, small bowel obstruction is the most common complication of a Meckel diverticulum, followed by Meckel diverticulitis.

- 幼儿最常见的表现是胃肠道出血(如果梅克尔憩室包含有异位胃黏膜)。较少情况下，梅克尔憩室可作为一个触发点而诱发肠套叠或导致憩室炎，其症状类似于阑尾炎。
- 在成人，小肠梗阻是梅克尔憩室最常见的并发症，其次是梅克尔憩室炎。

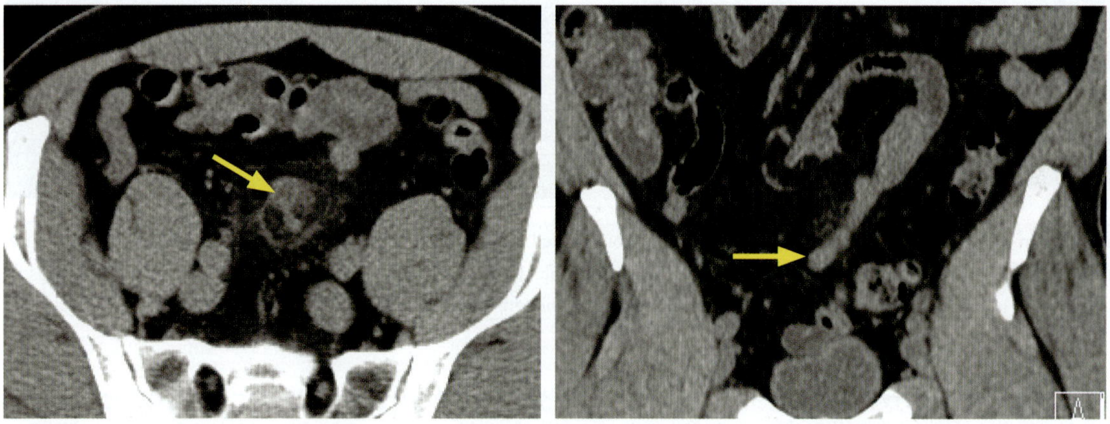

Meckel diverticulitis in an adult: Axial (left image) and coronal (right) noncontrast CT shows a blind-ending, tubular structure (arrows) arising from the mid to distal ileum, with associated mild inflammatory change.

Case courtesy Michael Hanley, MD, University of Virginia Health System.

一名成人梅克尔憩室炎：轴位(左图)和冠状位(右图)CT平扫显示起自回肠中、远段的一个盲端管状结构(箭)，伴有轻度炎性改变。

- Although there are often exceptions, the "rule of 2s" states that Meckel diverticula are 2 inches long, 2 feet from the ileocecal valve, present in 2% of the population, become symptomatic before age 2, and contain 2 ectopic tissues (gastric and pancreatic).
- A Meckel diverticulum causing rectal bleeding can be diagnosed with a Tc-99m- pertechnetate scan, which is only positive if the Meckel contains ectopic gastric mucosa.

  Approximately 25% of Meckel contain ectopic gastric (less commonly pancreatic mucosa). On pertechnetate scan, uptake kinetics of the ectopic mucosa is equal to gastric mucosa.

- 虽然常有例外，梅克尔憩室可概括为"2原则"，即长2英寸(1英寸=2.54cm)，距离回盲瓣2英尺(1英尺=30.48厘米)，人群发生率2%，2岁前出现症状，以及含有2种异位组织(胃和胰腺)。
- 直肠出血性梅克尔憩室可以通过^{99m}Tc-高碍酸钠扫描进行诊断，阳性结果只有在梅克尔憩室含有异位胃黏膜时出现。

  约有25%的梅克尔憩室含有异位胃黏膜(其次异位胰腺)。^{99m}Tc-高碍酸钠扫描时异位胃黏膜的吸收动力学与胃黏膜一致。

Crohn disease

- Crohn disease may be a cause of bowel obstruction. Up to 30% of newly diagnosed Crohn disease presents in the pediatric population.

克罗恩病

- 克罗恩病是肠梗阻的原因之一。高达30%最新确诊的克罗恩病为儿童。

ANORECTAL MALFORMATIONS

Imperforate anus

- Imperforate anus is a clinical diagnosis, but radiology plays a role to evaluate the level of the obstruction, which is classified as high or low in relation to the puborectalis sling.

肛门直肠畸形

肛门闭锁

- 肛门闭锁是一种临床诊断，而放射学检查的作用是确定梗阻的位置，可根据与耻骨直肠肌悬韧带的相对位置分为高位或低位闭锁。

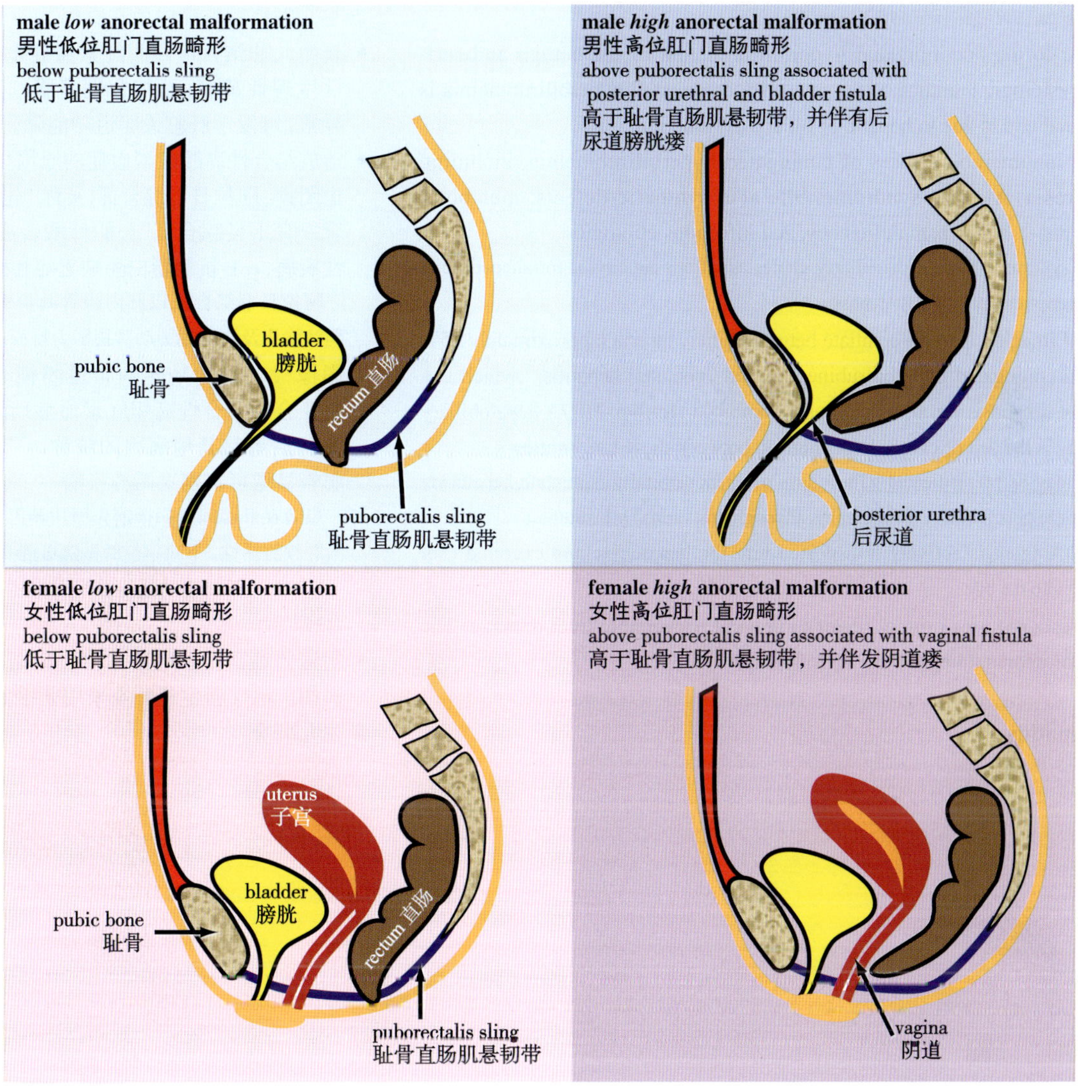

- A high lesion (above the puborectalis sling) is associated with genitourinary-rectal fistula, lumbosacral anomalies or VACTERL association, and requires a more complex treatment.

  Males may have a fistula between the rectum and posterior urethra or bladder.

  Females may have a rectovaginal fistula.

  In either sex, treatment is initial colostomy followed by definitive repair.

  Screening ultrasound is needed for evaluation of a tethered cord.

- A low lesion (below the puborectalis sling) is associated with perineal fistula and is treated with single-stage perineal anoplasty.
- The determination of high or low lesion is usually made clinically, based on passage of meconium, and is dependent on sex.

  In males, if meconium is passed in the urine → high lesion.

- 高位病变(高于耻骨直肠肌悬韧带)与泌尿生殖系统-直肠瘘、腰骶椎畸形或VACTERL综合征有关，治疗过程比较复杂。

  男性可能会出现直肠与后尿道或膀胱瘘。

  女性可能会有阴道直肠瘘。

  不论性别，初始治疗都是先行结肠造瘘术，然后再进行永久性修复术。

  需要行超声对脊髓栓系进行筛查评估。

- 低位病变(低于耻骨直肠肌悬韧带)可伴发会阴部瘘，治疗采用一期会阴肛门成形术。
- 通常，病变位置的高低在临床上可以通过胎粪排泄的特点，以及患儿的性别进行判断。

  在男童，如果胎粪从尿液中排泄提示高位病变。

In females, if meconium is passed in the vagina and a fistula is not visualized → high lesion. Low lesions may cause distal vaginal fistulas, which can be visualized by physical exam.

- Previously, prone-radiographs were used to determine if a lesion was high or low; however, infracoccygeal ultrasound is thought to be the most accurate method to determine the level of the imperforate anus.

在女童，如果胎粪从阴道排出且不能看到瘘口提示高位病变。低位病变可伴发远端阴道瘘，查体可以看到。

- 既往采用俯卧位影像确定病变位置的高低，但尾骨下超声现在被认为是确定肛门闭锁水平的最精确方法。

Neonatal cholestatic jaundice

Approach to pathologic neonatal jaundice

- In contrast to the unconjugated hyperbilirubinemia of the benign and self-limited physiologic jaundice of the newborn, conjugated hyperbilirubinemia is never normal and is due to hepatic or biliary dysfunction.
- There are innumerable causes of conjugated hyperbilirubinemia, including biliary atresia, Alagille syndrome, bile acid synthetic defects, metabolic disease, alpha-1-antitrypsin deficiency, and infectious etiologies.

  Alagille syndrome features hereditary cholestasis from paucity of intrahepatic bile ducts, and peripheral pulmonary stenosis.
- The goal of imaging is to differentiate between biliary atresia (approximately 25% of neonatal conjugated hyperbilirubinemia) and "neonatal hepatitis," which is a wastebasket diagnosis for all other causes combined. Tc-99m-HIDA hepatobiliary scintigraphy is the test of choice to distinguish between these two entities.

  Patients may be premedicated with 5 days of phenobarbital to stimulate hepatocyte activity prior to hepatobiliary scintigraphy, although this varies by institution.

  The HIDA agent is actively transported into the hepatocyte and excreted (not conjugated) into the bile.
- Biliary atresia requires prompt repair to prevent irreversible liver damage. The treatment of neonatal hepatitis is nonsurgical.

新生儿胆汁淤积性黄疸

新生儿病理性黄疸的处理原则

- 新生儿非结合性高胆红素血症是良性和自限性生理性黄疸，而结合性高胆红素血症均为异常，继发于肝脏或胆道功能障碍。
- 造成结合性高胆红素血症的原因很多，包括胆道闭锁、阿拉日耶综合征(又称"先天性肝内胆管发育不良综合征")、胆汁酸合成缺陷、代谢性疾病、α 1-抗胰蛋白酶缺乏症和感染性病因。

  阿拉日耶综合征以肝内胆管减少引起的遗传性胆汁淤积及周围性肺动脉狭窄为特征。
- 影像检查目的是鉴别胆道闭锁(约的25%新生儿合并结合性高胆红素血症)和"新生儿肝炎"，后者是其他病因的统称。^{99m}Tc-HIDA肝胆管显像可鉴别这两类疾病。

  患者在肝胆闪烁扫描前先服用苯巴比妥5天以刺激肝细胞活性，不同单位的做法可能有所不同。

  HIDA试剂被主动运送到肝细胞并被排泄(未结合)到胆汁。
- 胆道闭锁需要及时手术修复以防不可逆性肝损伤。治疗新生儿肝炎采用非手术方法。

Neonatal hepatitis

新生儿肝炎

Neonatal hepatitis: 60-minute delay HIDA (left image) shows uptake in the liver but with a large amount of blood pool activity. There is uptake in the bladder and the diaper, but no bowel uptake. Delayed 24-hour image (middle image) also does not show bowel uptake, but there is abnormal persistent hepatic uptake, which is suggestive of hepatitis. A follow-up exam was performed a few weeks later (right image), which showed normal hepatic uptake and small bowel excretion, confirming resolution of neonatal hepatitis.

Case courtesy Michael Hanley, MD, University of Virginia Health System.

新生儿肝炎：HIDA 60分钟延迟显像(左图)显示肝脏有摄取，但有大量的血池放射性分布。膀胱和尿布也可以看到摄取，但没有肠道摄取。24小时延迟显像(中图)同样未见肠道有摄取，但是肝脏有异常的持续性摄取，提示为肝炎。几周后复查(右图)显示正常的肝脏摄取和肠道排泄，确定为新生儿肝炎缓解。

- Hepatobiliary scintigraphy shows poor hepatic excretion, delayed hepatic clearance (beyond 12 hours), and variable bowel excretion.
- Biliary atresia can be effectively ruled out if there is any excretion into the GI

- 肝胆闪烁显像提示肝脏排泄不良，肝清除延迟(超过12小时)，但肠道排泄变化很大。
- 只要发现胃肠道有排泄的示踪剂，完全可以

tract.

Biliary atresia

- Ultrasound may not be able to distinguish between biliary atresia and neonatal hepatitis, though the *triangular cord sign* representing the obliterated common hepatic duct can be seen in the region of the porta hepatis. An absent or atretic gallbladder on ultrasound is suggestive of biliary atresia, but a gallbladder is seen in 20% of cases. The main hepatic artery is also often enlarged in the setting biliary atresia, with a HA:PV ratio >0.45 suggestive of biliary atresia.
- Hepatobiliary scintigraphy shows normal hepatic tracer uptake and clearance but **no excretion into the small bowel** after 24 hours.
- Treatment is the Kasai portoenterostomy, a palliative procedure ideally performed before 3 months of age. The entire extrahepatic biliary tree is excised and a jejunal Roux loop is anastomosed to the cut surface of the liver capsule. 80% of children with a successful surgery survive 10 years, at which point a liver transplant is necessary.
- Biliary atresia is associated with polysplenia and trisomy 18.

排除胆道闭锁。

胆道闭锁

- 超声可能无法区分胆道闭锁和新生儿肝炎，但在肝门区可以看到代表肝总管闭塞的三角索条征。超声显示胆囊缺失或闭锁时提示胆道闭锁，但20%的病例可见胆囊。胆道闭锁时，肝动脉主干也常扩张，HA:PV比值>0.45，提示胆道闭锁。
- 肝胆闪烁扫描显示肝脏示踪剂摄取和清除正常，但在24小时后仍然**看不到有小肠排泄**。
- 治疗采用Kasai肝门空肠吻合术，为一种姑息性手术，在3月龄前做较为理想。将整个肝外胆管切除，在肝包膜切面处与空肠Roux环吻合。手术成功儿童的10年存活率为80%，之后的某个时间点需要进行肝移植。
- 胆道闭锁与多脾和18-三体综合征有关。

Pediatric hepatobiliary neoplasia and masses

- Primary pediatric liver tumors may be classified as epithelial (hepatocyte-derived) or mesenchymal, with benign and malignant tumors in each category. Liver metastases may be seen in the setting of neuroblastoma, Wilms tumor, sarcoma, and Burkitt lymphoma.
- It is usually possible to narrow the differential based on imaging appearance (cystic or solid), age of the patient, and tumor markers (AFP and endothelial growth factor).
- Benign epithelial lesions also seen in adults, including focal nodular hyperplasia and adenoma, are discussed in the gastrointestinal imaging section.

小儿肝胆肿瘤和肿块

- 小儿原发性肝脏肿瘤可以分为上皮性(肝细胞分化)或间叶性，每类又包括良性和恶性肿瘤。肝转移性肿瘤可见于神经母细胞瘤、肾母细胞瘤、肉瘤、伯基特淋巴瘤。
- 通常可根据影像学表现(囊性或实性)、患者年龄和肿瘤标志物(甲胎蛋白和血管内皮生长因子)将鉴别诊断的范围进一步缩小。
- 良性上皮细胞病变也见于成人，包括局灶性结节性增生和腺瘤，将在胃肠道影像部分详述。

Cystic liver/biliary masses

Mesenchymal hamartoma

囊性肝/胆道肿块

间叶性错构瘤

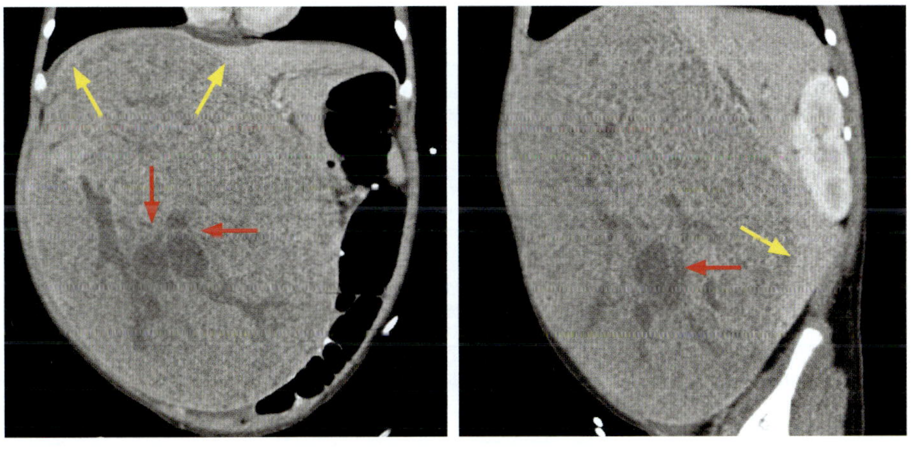

Mesenchymal hamartoma: Coronal (left image) and sagittal (right image) contrast-enhanced CT shows a massive, heterogeneous mass arising from the right lobe of the liver. The displaced liver parenchyma forms a *claw sign* around the mass (yellow arrows). There are cystic spaces (red arrows) and portal venous fragments within the mass; however, the mass appears predominantly solid, which may be secondary to numerous tiny cysts below the resolution of CT. *Case courtesy Michael Hanley, MD, University of Virginia Health System.*

间叶性错构瘤：冠状位(左图)和矢状位(右图)增强CT显示肝右叶一个巨大、不均一的肿块。受压而移位的肝实质包绕肿块形成蟹足征(黄箭)。肿块中可见囊性区(红箭)和门静脉残支；然而，肿块主要表现为实性，可能是因为CT无法显示肿块内大量的微型囊肿。

- Mesenchymal hamartoma is a benign, multicystic, hamartomatous lesion, which contains malformed bile ducts, portal vein fragments, and often extramedullary hematopoiesis. It is considered a developmental anomaly rather than a neoplasm.
- Most children present in the neonatal period with an enlarging abdominal mass, with 80% diagnosed by two years of age.
- In contrast to hepatoblastoma, tumor markers are not elevated.
- Imaging of mesenchymal hamartoma typically shows a large, multicystic, abdominal mass. The cysts can be of various sizes, can contain debris, and can be divided by septae of variable thickness. Hemorrhage and calcification are rare. Occasionally, the cysts may be so small that the mass appears solid. When large, the mass may displace vasculature.
- Surgical resection is almost always curative.

- 间叶性错构瘤是一种良性、多囊性、错构瘤样病变，其内包含畸形的胆管、门静脉片段，常有髓外造血。它被认为是一种发育异常而不是肿瘤。
- 大多数儿童在新生儿期发病，表现为不断增大的腹部肿块，80%的病例在2岁前得到诊断。
- 与肝母细胞瘤相比，肿瘤标记物并不升高。
- 间叶性错构瘤的典型影像学表现为一个巨大、多囊性的腹部肿块。囊肿大小不一，可以包含一些组织碎片，可以被不同厚度的间隔所分割。罕见出血和钙化。偶尔，囊肿可能会很小，使肿块看起来为实性。当囊肿较大时，肿块可能会使血管移位。
- 外科切除几乎都能治愈。

Choledochal cyst/Caroli disease

- Choledochal cysts (including Caroli disease) represent saccular or fusiform dilation of bile ducts, which may be segmental or diffuse. The Todani classification of choledochal cysts is discussed further in the gastrointestinal imaging section.

胆总管囊肿/卡罗利病(先天性肝内胆管囊状扩张症)

- 胆总管囊肿(包括卡罗利病)是指胆管呈囊状或梭形扩张，可呈节段性或弥漫性。胆总管囊肿的Todani分类在胃肠道影像部分详述。

Gallbladder hydrops

- Gallbladder hydrops is a pathologically distended gallbladder, usually associated with infection or a systemic inflammatory process such as Kawasaki disease.

胆囊积水

- 胆囊积水是一种胆囊的病理性扩张，通常合并感染或系统性炎症，如川崎病。

SOLID LIVER/BILIARY MASSES

- Pediatric liver lesions can be categorized by age groups, with children aged 0–3 years presenting with hemangioendothelioma, hepatoblastoma or mesenchymal hamartoma; children over age 5 with HCC and undifferentiated embryonal sarcoma. Metastatic liver tumors, most commonly from Wilms tumor or neuroblastoma, can present at any age.

实性肝/胆道肿块

- 小儿肝脏病变可按年龄组进行分类，0~3岁儿童常见肝脏血管内皮细胞瘤、肝母细胞瘤或间叶性错构瘤；5岁以上儿童为肝细胞癌和未分化胚胎肉瘤。转移性肝肿瘤可出现于任何年龄，其中最常见的为肾母细胞瘤或神经母细胞瘤。

Terminology of "hemangioma" in pediatric radiology

小儿放射学中"血管瘤"的术语

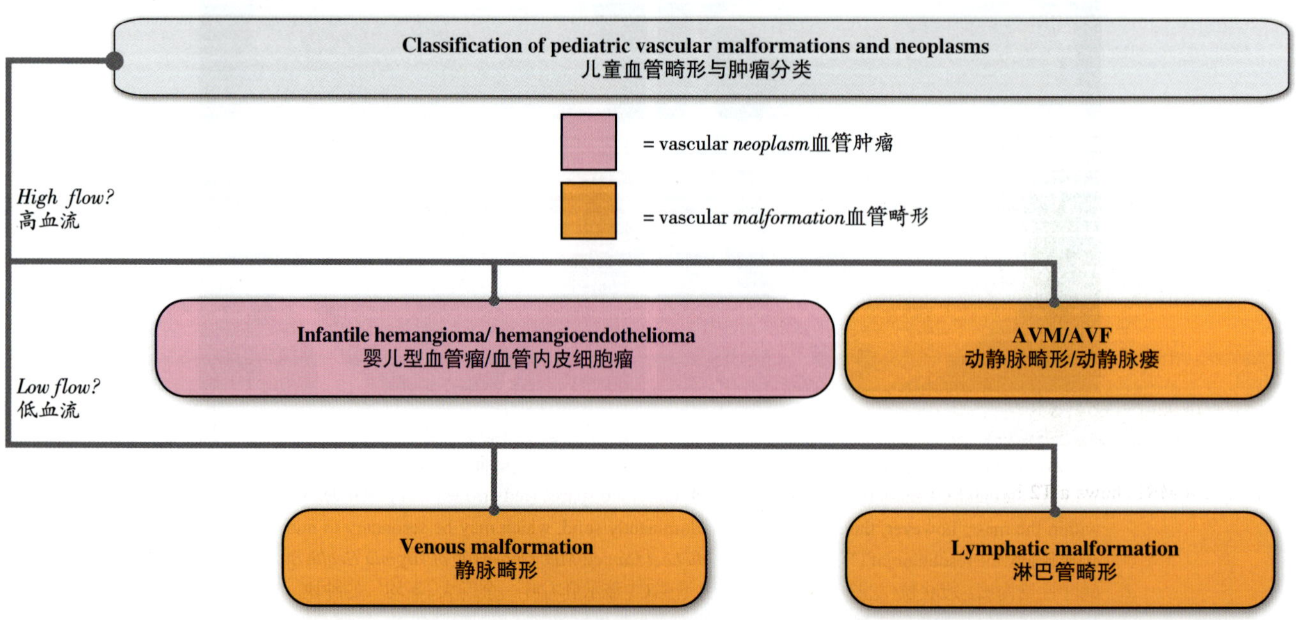

- Pediatric vascular anomalies can be divided into vascular neoplasms and vascular malformations, where neoplasms feature new cell growth and malformations feature disorganized vasculature without cell growth.
- Pediatric vascular anomalies can also be classified physiologically as high-flow or low-flow lesions. High-flow vascular malformations include arteriovenous malformations (AVM) and arteriovenous fistulas (AVF), while low-flow vascular malformations include venous malformations and lymphatic malformations.
- The term "hemangioma" is a common source of confusion. In particular, the term "hepatic hemangioma" is often used to describe multiple unrelated vascular lesions including infantile hemangioma, potentially malignant hemangioendotheliomas, and benign venous malformations.
- The common adult hepatic "hemangioma" is actually a venous malformation in the classification above. Similarly, the soft tissue "hemangiomas" of Maffucci syndrome are also venous malformations.
- Infantile hemangioma and hemangioendothelioma, discussed on the next page, are high-flow vascular neoplasms. Hemangioendotheliomas have the potential to metastasize.

Infantile hemangioma/hemangioendothelioma

- 儿童血管异常可分为血管肿瘤和血管畸形，前者以新生细胞增殖为特点，而后者以血管结构紊乱为特点且缺乏细胞增殖。
- 儿童血管病变还可以按生理学分为高血流和低血流病变。高血流血管畸形包括动静脉畸形(AVM)和动静脉瘘(AVF)，而低血流血管畸形包括静脉畸形和淋巴管畸形。
- 很多名称混淆都来自"血管瘤"这一术语。特别是"肝血管瘤"这个名词经常被用来描述多个不相关的血管性病变，包括婴儿型血管瘤、有潜在恶性的肝脏血管内皮细胞瘤和良性的静脉畸形。
- 常见的成人肝"血管瘤"实际上是上述分类中的一种静脉畸形。同样，马富奇综合征中软组织"血管瘤"也是静脉畸形。
- 婴儿型血管瘤和血管内皮细胞瘤(下文讨论)属于高流量血管源性肿瘤。血管内皮细胞瘤有潜在转移的可能。

婴儿型血管瘤/血管内皮细胞瘤

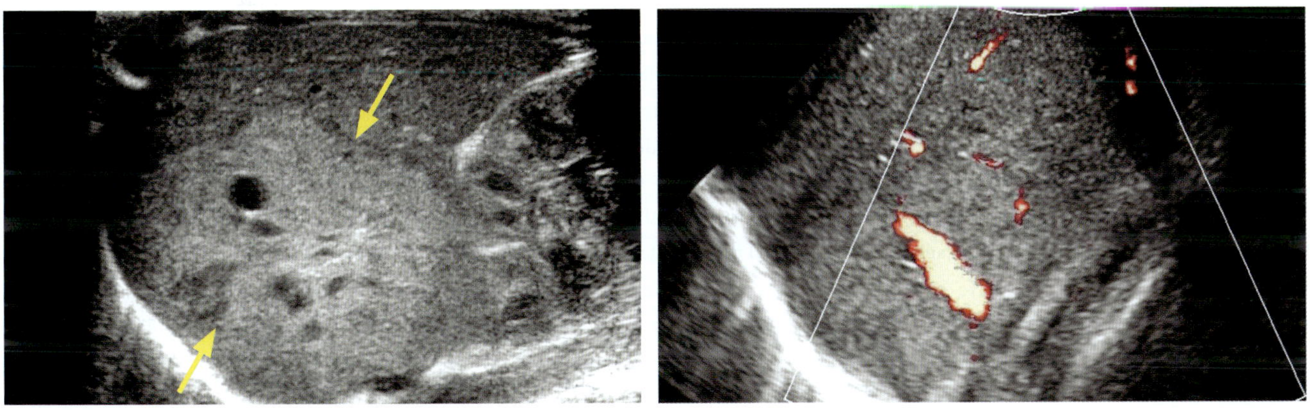

Grayscale (left image) and power Doppler (right image) ultrasound images of the liver show a highly vascular mass in the right hepatic lobe (arrows), containing numerous dilated vascular spaces.
肝脏灰阶(左图)和能量多普勒(右图)超声显示一个肝右叶富血供的肿块(箭)，含有大量扩张的血管腔隙。

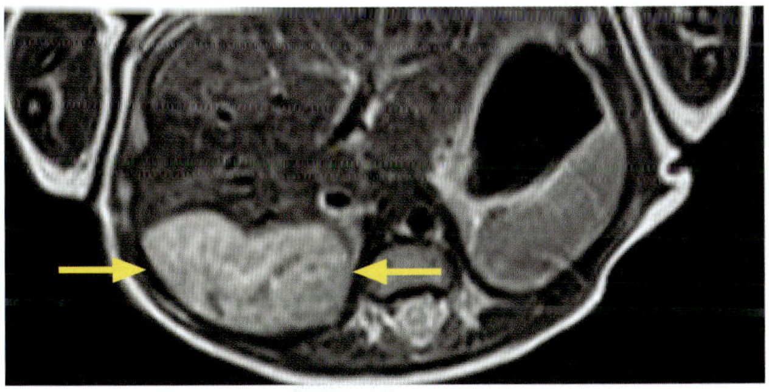

T2-weighted MRI shows a T2 hyperintense, predominantly solid mass (arrows) in the right liver.
T_2加权MRI显示一个肝右叶以实质为主的肿块，呈T_2高信号。

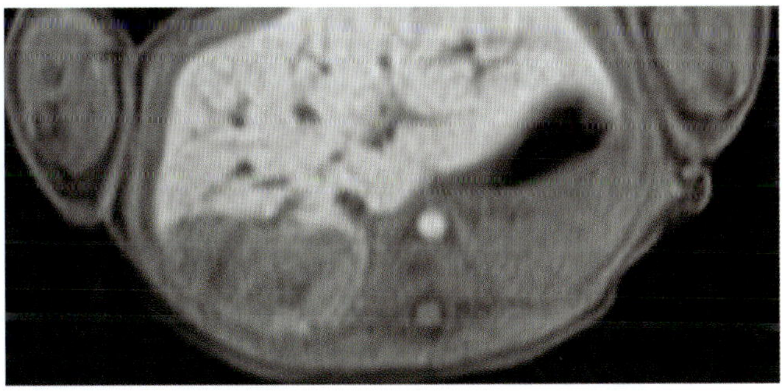

T1-weighted fat-saturated MRI shows the mass to be predominantly T1 hypointense relative to liver.
T_1加权脂肪抑制MRI显示肿块相对肝脏以T_1低信号为主。

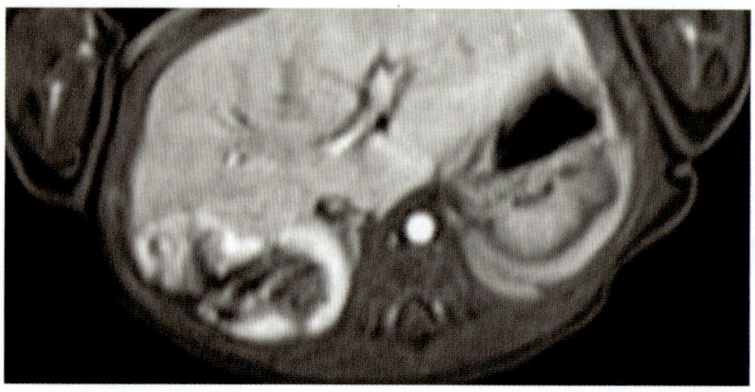

Post-contrast early-phase T1-weighted fat-saturated MRI shows intense enhancement of the tumor periphery.
增强早期T_1加权脂肪抑制MRI显示肿瘤周边明显强化。

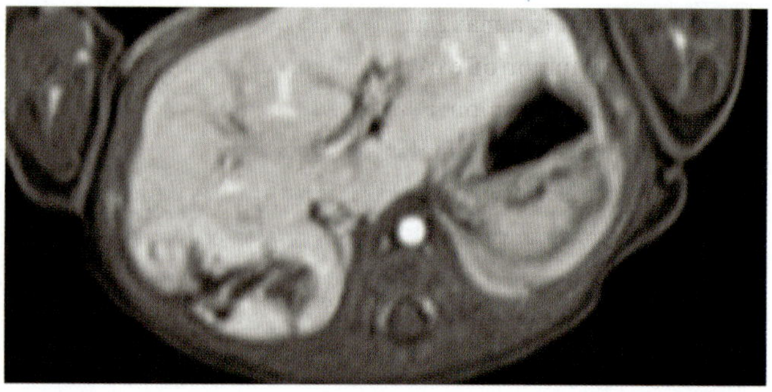

Post-contrast later-phase T1-weighted fat-saturated MRI shows lack of contrast opacification of the central tumor, consistent with tumor necrosis.
增强晚期T_1加权脂肪抑制MRI显示肿瘤中心无强化，为肿瘤坏死区。

Infantile hemangioma. *Case courtesy Michael Hanley, MD, University of Virginia Health System.*

- Infantile hemangioma and hemangioendothelioma are related vascular neoplasms. They are the most common vascular hepatic tumors, often in children under age 1 year and may cause congestive heart failure in up to 25%. AFP is not elevated; endothelial growth factor is elevated.

  Infantile hemangioma is benign. While hemangioendothelioma is usually benign, it has the potential to metastasize. This text will use the term "infantile hemangioma" to include both of these entities.

  Infantile hemangioma is associated with **Kasabach-Merritt syndrome**, which is a syndrome of vascular neoplasm, hemolytic anemia, and consumptive coagulopathy.

- Infantile hemangioma may be focal, multifocal, or diffuse. Lesions are highly vascular, T2 hyperintense, and tend to peripherally enhance with delayed fill-in. There may be calcification, central necrosis, and hemorrhage.

  Angiography (which can be performed prior to embolization) classically shows an enlarged celiac artery, with a decreased caliber of the aorta distal to the celiac axis.

- Similar to cutaneous infantile hemangiomas, most hepatic infantile hemangiomas will spontaneously involute in the first year of life, especially if GLUT-1 positive. The beta-blocker propranolol may accelerate involution. Surgery may be necessary for lesions causing CHF.

- 婴儿型血管瘤和血管内皮细胞瘤都是血管源性肿瘤，是最常见的肝血管肿瘤，常发生于1岁以下儿童，并导致高达25%的病例发生充血性心力衰竭。AFP不升高，但内皮生长因子升高。

  婴儿型血管瘤为良性。虽然肝脏血管内皮细胞瘤通常也是良性，但有潜在转移的可能。本文将使用"婴儿型血管瘤"来涵盖这两种疾病。

  婴儿型血管瘤与**卡萨巴赫-梅里特综合征**有关，该综合征包括了血管性肿瘤、溶血性贫血、消耗性凝血功能障碍。

- 婴儿型血管瘤可以呈局灶、多发或弥漫性。病变为富血供，T_2加权呈高信号，病灶的周边常在早期先强化，然后逐渐向中心填充。病灶内可有钙化、中央坏死和出血。

  血管造影(可在栓塞治疗前进行)的典型表现为腹腔干增粗，腹主动脉在腹腔干水平以下的管径变小。

- 与婴儿皮肤血管瘤相似，大多数婴儿型血管瘤在出生后第1年会自行消退，特别是葡萄糖转运蛋白1(GLUT-1)阳性患者。β受体阻滞剂普萘洛尔可能会加速消退。对于已造成充血性心力衰竭的病例有必要进行手术。

Hepatoblastoma

肝母细胞瘤

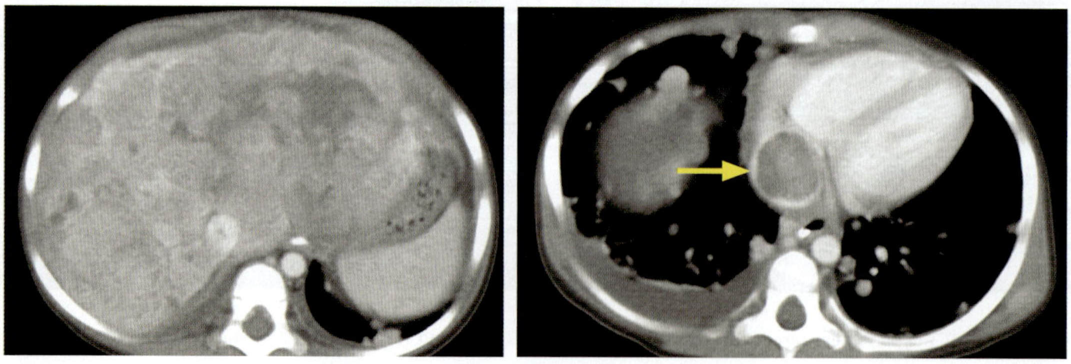

Hepatoblastoma: Contrast-enhanced axial CT shows a heterogeneous mass with mixed areas of enhancement and necrosis completely replacing the liver parenchyma. There is a hypoattenuating lesion expanding the IVC (arrow), representing tumor thrombus.
肝母细胞瘤：轴位增强CT显示一个强化不均匀和坏死的肿块完全取代了正常的肝实质。下腔静脉(箭)可见一个膨胀性的低密度影，为肿瘤栓子。

- Hepatoblastoma is a malignant embryonal neoplasm that is the most common primary liver tumor of early childhood (usually under age of 5 years), and the third most common childhood abdominal malignancy overall (after neuroblastoma and Wilms tumor).

  Hepatoblastoma occurs in children slightly older than those affected by infantile hemangioma and mesenchymal hamartoma. Less than 10% of cases occur during the neonatal period.
- Hepatoblastoma is associated with several genetic anomalies and syndromes, including:

> Beckwith-Wiedemann (q6 month screening ultrasound is performed in these patients).
> Familial adenomatous polyposis syndrome.
> Fetal alcohol syndrome.
> Wilms tumor.

- Alpha fetoprotein (AFP) is markedly elevated (often greater than 1 000 ng/mL). Precocious puberty may result from elevated bHCG.
- A classic radiographic finding of hepatoblastoma is right upper quadrant calcification.
- Cross-sectional imaging shows a large well-defined lobulated mass that is predominantly solid, heterogeneous and enhancing, with propensity for portal vein and hepatic vein invasion.

Hepatocellular carcinoma (HCC)

- Hepatocellular carcinoma (HCC) typically occurs in children over the age of 5, and is the second most common liver malignancy in children. Similar to adults, HCC is usually seen in the background of cirrhosis. AFP is elevated, as in hepatoblastoma.
- Pediatric causes of cirrhosis include alpha-1-antitrypsin deficiency, glycogen storage disease, tyrosinemia, biliary atresia, Wilson disease and chronic viral hepatitis.

  Fibrolamellar HCC variant is more commonly seen in patients aged 10–35 years without underlying liver disease or elevated AFP.
- Imaging is similar to adult HCC, appearing as a heterogeneous hepatic mass with early arterial enhancement and rapid washout. Similar to hepatoblastoma, HCC also commonly demonstrates venous invasion.

Undifferentiated embryonal sarcoma

- Undifferentiated embryonal sarcoma (malignant mesenchymoma) is a highly aggressive neoplasm, occurring in school-aged children 6–10 years old.
- Unlike in hepatoblastoma and HCC, AFP is not elevated.
- Imaging shows ill-defined heterogeneous mass with solid and cystic components reflecting necrosis and hemorrhage.

Metastatic disease

- Wilms tumor and neuroblastoma are common pediatric tumors with a propensity to metastasize to the liver.

MISCELLANEOUS

Spectrum of meconium

- **Meconium aspiration** causes respiratory distress in term neonates.
- **Meconium ileus** is the earliest (infantile) manifestation of cystic fibrosis and only occurs in patients with cystic fibrosis. It causes a microcolon.

- 肝母细胞瘤是一种恶性胚胎性肿瘤，是幼儿时期(通常小于5岁)最常见的原发肝脏肿瘤，也在儿童所有腹部恶性肿瘤中位居第三(排在神经母细胞瘤和肾母细胞瘤之后)。

  儿童肝母细胞瘤的发病年龄稍大于婴儿血管瘤和错构瘤，不到10%的病例发生在新生儿期。
- 肝母细胞瘤与多个基因异常和综合征相关，包括：

> 贝-维综合征(对此病患者应每6个月进行一次超声筛查)。
> 家族性腺瘤息肉病综合征。
> 胎儿酒精综合征。
> 肾母细胞瘤。

- 甲胎蛋白(AFP)显著升高(通常大于1 000 ng/mL)。性早熟可能由β-HCG升高引起。
- 典型肝母细胞瘤的X线征象为右上腹钙化。
- 横断面成像显示一边界清晰的巨大分叶状肿块，以实性成分为主，不均质并有强化，有门静脉和肝静脉受侵的倾向。

肝细胞癌(HCC)

- 肝细胞癌(HCC)通常发生在5岁以上的儿童，是小儿第二常见的肝脏恶性肿瘤。与成人相似，HCC通常具有肝硬化背景。AFP升高，其与肝母细胞瘤相似。
- 儿童肝硬化原因包括α1-抗胰蛋白酶缺乏、糖原贮积症、酪氨酸血症、胆道闭锁、肝豆状核变性和慢性病毒性肝炎。

  纤维板层型肝癌更常见于10~35岁的患者，无潜在肝病或AFP升高。
- 影像学表现与成人HCC相似，表现为不均质的肝内肿块，动脉早期强化并快速廓清。与肝母细胞瘤类似，HCC也常出现静脉血管受侵。

未分化胚胎肉瘤

- 未分化胚胎肉瘤(恶性间叶瘤)是一种高度侵袭性肿瘤，发生在6~10岁学龄期儿童。
- 与肝母细胞瘤和HCC不同，AFP不升高。
- 影像学表现为边界模糊的不均质肿块，有实性和囊性成分，提示有坏死和出血。

转移性疾病

- 肾母细胞瘤和神经母细胞瘤是儿童常见有转移到肝脏倾向的肿瘤。

其他疾病

胎粪相关性疾病

- **胎粪吸入**会引起足月新生儿呼吸窘迫。
- **胎粪性肠梗阻**是囊性纤维化的早期表现(婴儿期)，且只发生在囊性纤维化患者中。它会导

- **Meconium plug syndrome** (small left colon) is a self-limited cause of distal neonatal bowel obstruction. Unlike meconium ileus, meconium plug syndrome is not associated with cystic fibrosis, and is not a cause of microcolon.
- **Meconium ileus-equivalent syndrome**, or distal intestinal obstruction syndrome (DIOS) can be the presenting symptom of previously undiagnosed cystic fibrosis, typically in an adolescent or young adult. Patients clinically present with recurrent abdominal pain and chronic constipation due to abnormally viscous stool in the ileum and right colon.
- **Meconium peritonitis** is caused by in-utero small bowel perforation and meconium spillage, resulting in peritonitis, secondary calcification, and meconium pseudocyst formation.

致小结肠。

- **胎粪栓综合征**(小左结肠)是一种自限性的新生儿远端肠梗阻的原因。与胎粪性肠梗阻不同，胎粪栓综合征与囊性纤维化不相关，且不会产生小结肠征。
- **胎粪性肠梗阻-类似综合征**，或远端肠梗阻综合征(DIOS)发生在先前未经诊断的囊性纤维化患者，通常是青少年或年轻的成人。患者临床表现为反复性腹痛及慢性便秘，是由回肠和右结肠的粪便异常黏稠所致。
- **胎粪性腹膜炎**是胎儿期小肠穿孔和胎粪溢出而导致的腹膜炎、继发钙化和胎粪假性囊肿形成。

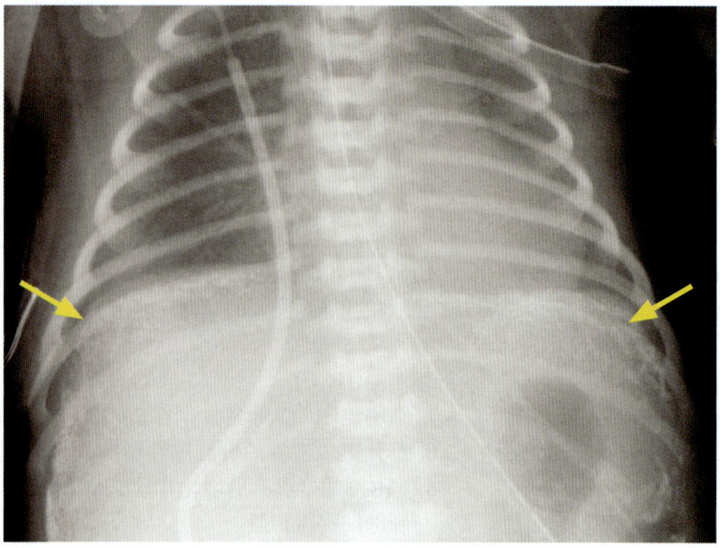

Meconium peritonitis: Frontal radiograph shows diffuse coarse calcifications abutting the peritoneal surface (arrows) in the right and left upper quadrants.
Case courtesy Michael Callahan, MD, Boston Children's Hospital.
胎粪性腹膜炎：正位X线影像显示左、右上腹弥漫性粗大的钙化灶紧贴腹膜表面(箭)。

Abdominal calcification

- Abdominal calcification seen on radiography can be an important clue to the presence of underlying pathology, including:

Meconium peritonitis.
Several pediatric neoplasms may contain calcifications, including neuroblastoma, teratoma, and hepatoblastoma.
Adrenal hemorrhage may cause calcification of the adrenal glands.
Right upper quadrant calcifications can be seen with gallstones, hepatoblastoma, and hepatic TORCH infections (e.g., CMV and toxoplasmosis).

腹部钙化

- X线影像上出现的腹部钙化可能是存在某些疾病的重要线索，包括：

胎粪性腹膜炎。
多种儿科肿瘤可能含有钙化，包括神经母细胞瘤、畸胎瘤和肝母细胞瘤。
肾上腺出血可能会导致肾上腺钙化。
右上腹钙化可以发生在胆结石、肝母细胞癌、肝TORCH感染(如巨细胞病毒和弓形体病)。

(翻译　陈佳妮)

PEDIATRIC GENITOURINARY

小儿泌尿生殖系统

HYDRONEPHROSIS AND HYDROURETER

肾盂积水及输尿管积水

Vesicoureteral reflux (VUR)

- Vesicoureteral reflux (VUR) is abnormal retrograde reflux of urine from the bladder into the ureter, which predisposes to acute pyelonephritis, renal scarring, and irreversible loss of renal function. VUR can be primary (due to

膀胱输尿管反流(VUR)

- 膀胱输尿管反流(VUR)是指尿液从膀胱异常逆向反流进入输尿管，从而导致急性肾盂肾炎、肾脏瘢痕，以及不可逆性肾功能损伤。

an abnormally short intravesicular portion of the distal ureter) or secondary (due to distal obstruction, such as from posterior urethral valves or neurogenic bladder).

- The typical imaging evaluation of a child with a febrile UTI is controversial and may involve renal ultrasound and **voiding cystourethrogram (VCUG)**. Noncontrast ultrasound is not sensitive for the detection of reflux, although the presence of urothelial thickening is suggestive of reflux. Studies suggest that approximately 5% of children with a UTI and a normal ultrasound have VUR.
- Siblings of patients diagnosed with reflux are typically screened with ultrasound: the prevalence of siblings with asymptomatic VUR is 25–50%.
- Fluoroscopic VCUG is often preferred as the initial study for evaluation of reflux because it provides anatomic details about the upper tract and also allows evaluation of the urethra. Contrast-enhanced ultrasound is increasingly being used for the assessment of VUR, and the posterior urethra can be assessed via transperineal views.

  In boys, partial posterior urethral valves may be a cause of UTI.
- Grading of reflux is based on VCUG:

VUR可分为原发性(由输尿管末端膀胱壁内段异常短小所致)与继发性(由远端尿路梗阻所致，如后尿道瓣膜或神经源性膀胱)。

- 针对发热性尿路感染患儿的常规影像检查尚存争议，可能包括肾脏超声和**排泄性膀胱尿道造影**(VCUG)。非增强超声对检测反流并不敏感，但若显示尿路上皮增厚可提示反流的可能。有研究表明，约5%患有尿路感染的儿童超声表现正常，但存在VUR。
- 对确诊膀胱输尿管反流患者的姐妹兄弟通常进行超声筛查：他们无症状性VUR的患病率为25%~50%。
- 透视下VCUG通常作为评估膀胱输尿管反流的首选检查，它不仅可以提供上尿路的解剖细节，还能显示尿道的情况。超声造影越来越多地用于评估VUR，评估后尿道可采用经会阴超声。

  在男性患儿中，后尿道瓣膜可能是导致尿路感染的一个原因。
- 基于VCUG的反流分级如下：

Ⅰ: Reflux into ureter only, with normal ureteral and calyceal morphology.
Ⅱ: Reflux into non-dilated renal calyces, with normal ureteral and calyceal morphology.
Ⅲ: Reflux into renal collecting system, with blunting of the calyces (loss of normal "spiky" appearance of calyces).
Ⅳ: Reflux into moderately dilated ureter.
Ⅴ: Reflux into severely dilated and tortuous ureter.

Ⅰ级：造影剂仅反流至输尿管，输尿管及肾盂肾盏形态正常。
Ⅱ级：造影剂反流至无扩张的肾盂肾盏，输尿管及肾盂肾盏形态正常。
Ⅲ级：造影剂反流至肾集合系统，伴有肾盏杯口变钝(肾盏杯口失去正常的"尖角样"外观)。
Ⅳ级：造影剂反流至中度扩张的输尿管。
Ⅴ级：造影剂反流至重度扩张和扭曲的输尿管。

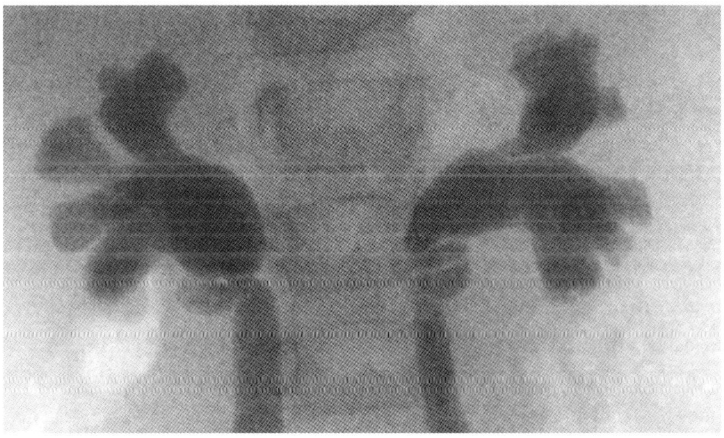

Bilateral grade Ⅳ reflux: Fluoroscopic stored image from a VCUG shows moderate calyceal and ureteral dilation.
双侧Ⅳ级反流：VCUG透视存储图像显示肾盏和输尿管中度扩张。

- The goal of any treatment of VUR is to prevent pyelonephritis and the resultant renal scarring which can lead to irreversible loss of renal function. The treatment can be either medical (prophylactic antibiotics) or surgical, depending on the grade.

  Grades Ⅰ–Ⅲ are initially treated medically (prophylactic antibiotics). Higher grade reflux often is treated surgically.
- Approximately 90% of grade Ⅰ and Ⅱ reflux will spontaneously regress after a few years.

- VUR所有治疗方法的目的均是防止肾盂肾炎及其所导致的肾脏瘢痕形成，后者可导致不可逆性肾功能损伤。治疗方法有药物治疗(预防性使用抗生素)或手术治疗，这取决于疾病的分级。

  Ⅰ~Ⅲ级首选药物治疗(预防性使用抗生素)。更高级别的反流通常采用外科治疗。
- 约90%的Ⅰ级和Ⅱ级反流可在数年内自行好转。

- Two nuclear studies are often used for the evaluation and follow-up of reflux:

  Radionuclide cystogram (RNC) involves the instillation of approximately 1 mCi of Tc-99m pertechnetate into the bladder through a catheter. RNC is the most sensitive test to evaluate for reflux. RNC is often used for follow-up of reflux once the anatomy is established by VCUG. RNC grading is three-stage:

> **RNC grade 1**: Ureteral reflux only (VCUG Ⅰ).
> **RNC grade 2**: Reflux reaches renal calyces (VCUG Ⅱ–Ⅲ).
> **RNC grade 3**: Ureteral dilation (VCUG Ⅳ–Ⅴ).

Tc-99m-DMSA renal scintigraphy (DMSA scan) is the gold standard for detection of renal cortical scarring, seen as areas of relative photopenia.

Duplex collecting system

- 两种常用评估及随访反流的核医学检查：

  放射性核素膀胱造影(RNC)经导管将约1mCi剂量的^{99m}Tc-高锝酸盐向膀胱内灌注后行核素成像。RNC是评估反流最敏感的方法。一旦VCUG确认存在解剖学上的反流，RNC通常用于随访。RNC共分为3级：

> **RNC 1级**：仅有输尿管反流(VCUG Ⅰ级)。
> **RNC 2级**：反流进入肾盏(VCUG Ⅱ~Ⅲ级)。
> **RNC 3级**：合并输尿管扩张(VCUG Ⅳ~Ⅴ级)。

^{99m}Tc-DMSA肾闪烁显像(DMSA扫描)是检测肾皮质瘢痕形成的金标准。

集合系统重复畸形

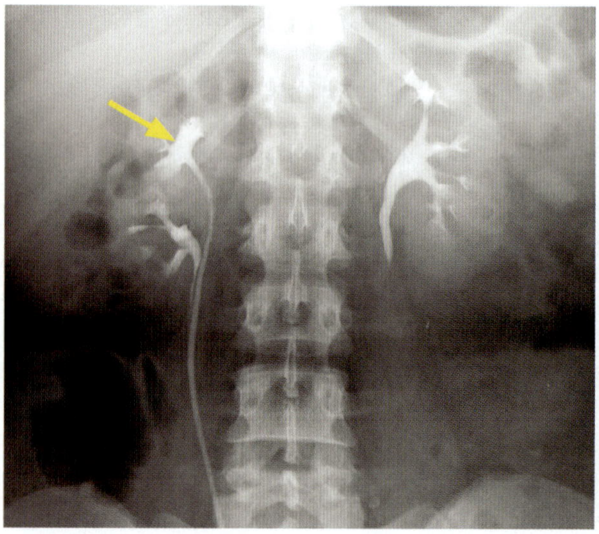

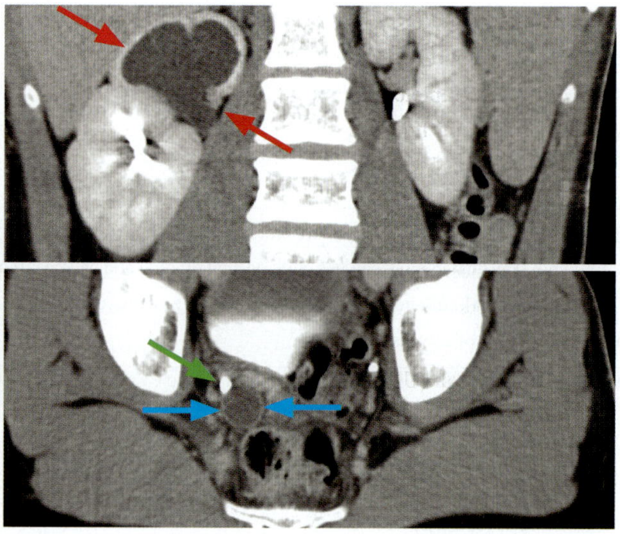

Two patients with duplicated collecting systems: Intravenous pyelogram (left image) shows a duplicated right collecting system, with mild blunting of the upper pole calyces (yellow arrow).

In a different patient, coronal (top right image) and axial contrast-enhanced pyelographic phase CT shows severe hydronephrosis of the obstructed right upper pole (red arrow). The dilated, unopacified upper pole ureter (blue arrow) courses medially to the opacified, normal-caliber lower pole ureter (green arrow).

两名不同患者的集合系统重复畸形：静脉肾盂造影(左图)示右侧集合系统重复畸形，并可见上极肾盏杯口轻度变钝(黄箭)。

另一名患者的冠状位(右上图)及轴位增强CT肾盂期显示右肾上极重度梗阻性肾积水(红箭)。上极输尿管(蓝箭)扩张明显且无造影剂充盈，走行于管径正常、造影剂充盈良好的下极输尿管(绿箭)内侧。

- A duplex collecting system contains two separate pelvicalyceal systems and two ureters. A duplex system may be of no clinical significance if the ureters fuse. However, if the ureters insert separately into the bladder, there is an increased risk of obstruction (in the upper pole moiety) and reflux (in the lower pole moiety), as described by the Weigert-Meyer rule.
- **The *Weigert-Meyer* rule:** In a duplicated system, the upper pole ureter inserts ectopically (inferomedially) into the bladder and is prone to obstruction, often due to a ureterocele. The lower pole ureter inserts orthotopically (normally) on the bladder but is prone to reflux.

- 集合系统重复畸形包含两套独立的肾盂和输尿管系统。如果重复的输尿管有融合，集合系统重复畸形可能没有临床意义。如果重复的输尿管分别开口于膀胱，则会增加上极集合系统梗阻和下极集合系统反流的风险，如在Weigert-Meyer法则中所述。
- **Weigert-Meyer法则**：集合系统出现重复畸形时，上极输尿管异位开口于膀胱(内下方)，易发生梗阻，常与输尿管囊肿有关。下极输尿管开口于膀胱原位(正常位置)，但易出现反流。

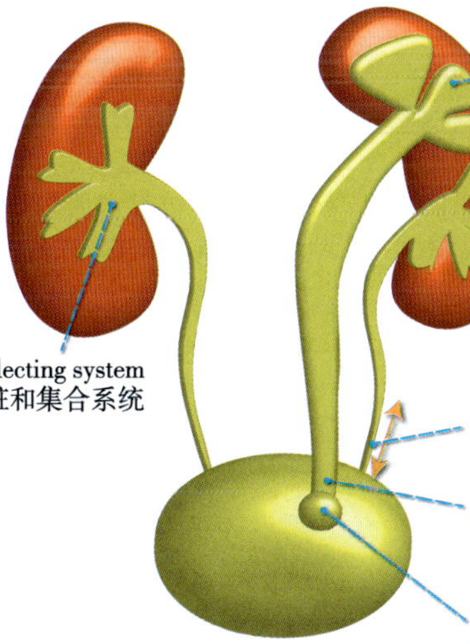

- Although hydronephrosis in an obstructed upper pole system would be apparent on ultrasound, a completely obstructed system may not be seen on VCUG at all since contrast cannot flow retrograde into the obstructed ureter. The *drooping lily sign* is seen on VCUG where the "invisible" obstructed upper moiety compresses the refluxed contrast in the lower moiety collecting system.

  The differential diagnosis of a *drooping lily* is renal ptosis, which would be expected to show a normal number of calyces. In contrast, the obstructed upper pole of the *drooping lily* has fewer calyces.

Ureteropelvic junction (UPJ) obstruction

- Ureteropelvic junction (UPJ) obstruction is the most common congenital anomaly of the genitourinary tract in neonates and the most common cause of unilateral hydronephrosis in children. UPJ obstruction may be caused by abnormal development of the upper segment of the ureter, an aberrant renal artery compressing the ureter, an aperistaltic segment of the ureter, or can be idiopathic.
- Imaging shows hydronephrosis and dilated renal pelvis, with normal caliber distal ureter.

Ureterovesical (UVJ) obstruction

- Ureterovesical (UVJ) obstruction is more rare and can be a result of several etiologies, most commonly megaureter in a single system kidney or a ureterocele in the setting of ectopic ureteral insertion.
- A **ureterocele** is focal dilation of the distal ureter within the bladder wall, where the ureter infolds between the mucosal and muscular layers of the bladder wall.
- An *ectopic ureterocele* is almost always associated with ectopic insertion of the upper pole ureter in a duplicated system. A *simple ureterocele* is seen with an orthotopically (normally) inserting ureter.
- The typical ultrasound appearance of an ectopic ureterocele is a cystic lesion within the bladder wall, usually associated with hydroureter and hydronephrosis of an obstructed upper pole moiety in a duplex system. Ectopic ureteroceles are almost always located inferior and medial to the lower pole ureteral insertion site.
- VCUG typically shows the ureterocele as a rounded filling defect. The *cobra head sign* can be seen on IVP or ultrasound.

- 超声可以显示上极肾盂输尿管梗阻性积水，但VCUG可能完全不显示完全性梗阻，因为膀胱内造影剂无法逆行进入梗阻的输尿管。VCUG显示的“下垂百合征”是由于梗阻的“隐形”上极压迫造影剂反流的下极集合系统所致。

  “下垂百合征”的鉴别诊断为肾下垂，但后者肾盏的数量正常。与之相比，由上极梗阻形成的“下垂百合征”肾盏数量较少。

肾盂输尿管连接部(UPJ)梗阻

- 肾盂输尿管连接部(UPJ)梗阻是最常见的新生儿泌尿生殖系统畸形和儿童单侧肾盂积水最常见的原因。UPJ梗阻可以由上段输尿管异常发育、肾动脉变异压迫输尿管、输尿管节段性无蠕动等原因所致，也可为特发。
- 影像显示肾盂积水和肾盂扩张，但远端输尿管管径正常。

输尿管膀胱交界处(UVJ)梗阻

- 输尿管膀胱交界处(UVJ)梗阻比较罕见，可由多种原因造成，最常见的是单个肾脏系统的巨型输尿管或异位输尿管开口的输尿管囊肿。
- **输尿管囊肿**为膀胱壁内的远端输尿管发生局限性扩张，此处输尿管包入膀胱壁黏膜层和肌层之间。
- 异位输尿管囊肿几乎都发生在重复畸形时的上极输尿管异位开口处。单纯输尿管囊肿则见于输尿管原位(正常)插入处。
- 异位输尿管囊肿在超声上的典型表现为膀胱壁内一处囊性病变，在重复畸形中常伴有上极输尿管及肾盂梗阻性积水。异位输尿管囊肿几乎都位于下极输尿管插入膀胱处的内下方。
- 输尿管囊肿的典型VCUG影像学表现为圆形的充盈缺损。在IVP或超声上可见眼镜蛇头征。

Posterior urethral valves (PUV)

- Posterior urethral valve is the most common cause of congenital bladder outlet obstruction, occurring exclusively in boys. It is caused by an obstructing web in the posterior (prostatic) urethra at the base of the verumontanum.
- Ultrasound shows dilation of the posterior (prostatic) urethra, a dilated and trabeculated bladder, and bilateral hydronephrosis. The appearance of the dilated posterior urethra and dilated bladder produces the characteristic *keyhole* appearance on ultrasound.

  Calyceal rupture may occur, resulting in perinephric fluid collections, urinomas and ascites.
- The main differential consideration is prune belly syndrome, which would show dilation of the entire ureter rather than only the prostatic portion.

后尿道瓣膜(PUV)

- 后尿道瓣膜是先天性膀胱出口梗阻最常见的原因，只发生于男童。它是由精阜底部后尿道(尿道前列腺部)内蹼样结构阻塞所致。
- 超声检查可显示后尿道(尿道前列腺部)扩张，膀胱扩张和壁小梁形成，以及双侧肾盂积水。扩张的膀胱和后尿道在超声影像上形成特征性的“锁孔”样征象。

  还可能发生肾盏破裂，导致肾周积液、尿性囊肿和腹水。
- 后尿道瓣膜主要的鉴别诊断是梅干腹综合征，后者表现为输尿管全程扩张，而不仅限于尿道前列腺部扩张。

Prune belly syndrome

- Prune belly, or Eagle Barrett, syndrome is a congenital muscular disorder that affects the abdominal wall musculature and the smooth muscles of the entire urinary tract.
- Prune belly may be associated with cryptorchidism, as bladder distension interferes with the descent of testes.
- The muscular defect leads to dilation of the entire collecting system, including bladder and both ureters. In contrast to posterior urethral valves, the entire urethra is dilated.

梅干腹综合征

- 梅干腹综合征或Eagle-Barrett综合征是先天性肌肉异常病变，累及腹壁肌肉及所有泌尿道的平滑肌。
- 梅干腹综合征可合并隐睾症，因为膀胱扩张干扰睾丸下降。
- 由于肌肉缺陷导致所有集合系统扩张，包括膀胱及双侧输尿管。与后尿道瓣膜不同，梅干腹综合征表现为整个尿道扩张。

Summary of levels of obstruction

- This schematic diagram of the genitourinary system demonstrates the anatomic locations for various causes of hydronephrosis or hydroureter:

梗阻水平的概述

- 以下泌尿生殖系统示意图说明了在不同解剖层面上引起肾盂及输尿管积水的各种病因。

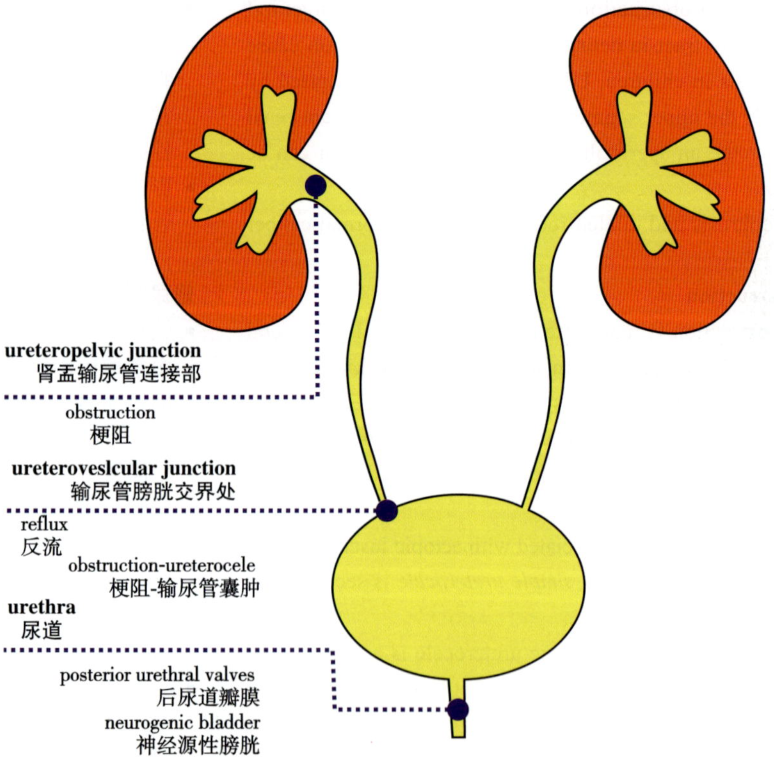

Congenital renal malformations

Renal agenesis

- Renal agenesis can be unilateral or bilateral (incompatible with life); a common imaging clue is the *lying down adrenal* which helps differentiate congenitally from surgically absent kidney.
- Renal agenesis is associated with reproductive anomalies (Mayer-Rokitansky-Kuster-Hauser syndrome) including unicornuate uterus, absent epididymis and vas deferens, and seminal vesicle cysts.

Horseshoe kidney

- Horseshoe kidney represents a fusion anomaly of the lower poles, preventing ascent of the kidneys at the level of the inferior mesenteric artery.
- Complications such as injury against the adjacent vertebral body preclude patients from playing certain sports. Patients are also at increased risk for stones, infection and cancer including Wilms, TCC, and renal carcinoid.
- There is a classic association with Turner's syndrome.

Cross-fused renal ectopia

- In cross-fused renal ectopia, the ectopic kidney (more commonly the left) crosses midline to fuse with the inferior pole of the contralateral kidney, each retaining its own orthotopic ureteral orifice.
- Complications include stones, infection and hydronephrosis.

先天性肾发育不良

肾缺如

- 先天性肾缺如可以是单侧或双侧(双侧不能存活);影像学上常见的一个提示为肾上腺平卧征,它有助于区分先天性肾缺如与手术后肾缺如。
- 肾缺如与生殖系统异常(先天性子宫阴道缺如综合征)有关,包括单角子宫、附睾和输精管缺失及精囊腺囊肿。

马蹄肾

- 马蹄肾即双侧肾下极的异常融合,肾脏上升迁移被阻止在肠系膜下动脉的水平。
- 并发症,如因紧贴邻近椎体导致的损伤,使患者无法进行某些体育运动。患者罹患结石、感染和癌症的风险也增加,包括肾母细胞瘤、肾管状囊性癌和肾类癌。
- 常常与特纳综合征相关。

交叉融合异位肾

- 在交叉融合的异位肾中,异位肾(左侧更常见)穿过中线与对侧肾的下极融合,每个肾都保留原位的输尿管开口。
- 并发症包括结石、感染和肾盂积水。

Cystic renal lesions

Hydronephrosis

- Hydronephrosis is the most common cystic abdominal mass in a neonate.

Multicystic dysplastic kidney (MCDK)

肾囊性病变

肾盂积水

- 肾盂积水是新生儿腹部最常见的囊性肿块。

多囊性肾发育不良(MCDK)

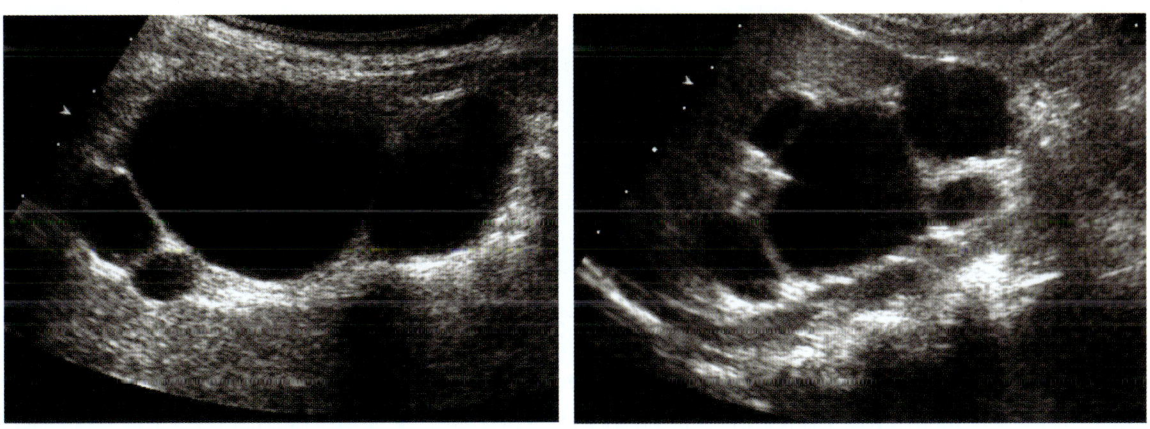

Multicystic dysplastic kidney: Two longitudinal ultrasound images of the kidney show multiple separate cystic structures that do not connect. The main differential consideration is hydronephrosis, in which case the cystic spaces would demonstrate continuity.

多囊性肾发育不良:两幅肾脏长轴切面超声显示有多个分隔的囊性结构,彼此互不相通。主要的鉴别诊断为肾盂积水,后者的囊腔结构彼此相通。

- Multicystic dysplastic kidney (MCDK) is the most common *neonatal* cystic renal mass, characterized by a progressive renal dysplasia thought to be a result of abnormal induction of the metanephric blastema by the ureteric bud, or due to atresia of the renal pelvis/ proximal ureter leading to urinary obstruction.

- 多囊性肾发育不良是新生儿期最常见的囊性肾脏肿块,并以进行性肾脏发育不良为特征,可能为输尿管芽异常诱导后肾胚芽,或肾盂/近端输尿管闭锁导致尿路梗阻所致。

- MCDK is typically unilateral, but bilateral abnormalities may be present in 20–30%.
- The natural progression of MCDK is gradual involution into a small soft tissue remnant. It is thought that many adults with a solitary kidney may have had a previously undiagnosed, involuted MCDK.
- The risk of Wilms tumor in MCDK is controversial. Although an association between MCDK and Wilms tumor has been reported, there is no strong evidence to support a link.
- Imaging of MCDK shows a multicystic "mass" replacing the renal parenchyma. The cystic elements do not communicate with each other, which is in contrast to hydronephrosis.

  A DMSA scan shows no cortical uptake in MCDK, compared to faint radiotracer cortical uptake even in hydronephrosis.

Multilocular cystic nephroma

- Multilocular cystic nephroma is a benign, multiseptated cystic neoplasm. It has a bimodal age distribution, seen in young boys aged three months to two years and middle-aged women.
- There is an association with *DICER1* mutations and pleuropulmonary blastoma.
- On imaging, multilocular cystic nephroma appears as a multiseptated cystic renal mass with enhancing septa. Its appearance may mimic cystic Wilms tumor. A characteristic imaging finding is the propensity to herniate into the renal pelvis, causing hydronephrosis.

Simple renal cyst

- An isolated simple renal cyst is rare in children. When seen, renal cysts are more likely to be syndromic, in association with tuberous sclerosis or von Hippel-Lindau.

> **Tuberous sclerosis**: In addition to renal cysts, patients may have:
>
> Renal angiomyolipomas.
>
> Cardiac rhabdomyoma.
>
> CNS cortical hamartomas, subependymal nodules, and subependymal giant cell astrocytoma.
>
> **von Hippel-Lindau (VHL)**: In addition to renal cysts, patients have:
>
> Renal cell carcinoma (RCC): Up to 30% of VHL patients die from RCC.
>
> Adrenal pheochromocytoma.
>
> Pancreatic cysts, islet cell tumors, and serous cystadenomas.
>
> Brain and spinal cord hemangioblastomas.

Autosomal dominant polycystic kidney disease (ADPKD)

- Autosomal dominant polycystic kidney disease (ADPKD) usually manifests in adulthood, although 50% develop some cysts within the first decade of life.
- ADPKD typically features renal enlargement with numerous cysts of varying sizes.
- ADPKD is associated with hepatic cysts and less commonly pancreatic cysts.

Autosomal recessive polycystic kidney disease (ARPKD)

- Autosomal recessive polycystic kidney disease (ARPKD) features tiny cysts that develop in infancy due to generalized dilation of the collecting tubules. The cysts are typically too small to be resolvable by imaging, producing a

- MCDK通常为单侧，但双侧异常可达20%~30%。
- MCDK自然病程为逐渐退化成一小块残留的软组织。由此推测，许多单肾的成人可能患有未诊断并已退化的单侧MCDK。
- MCDK是否会增加肾母细胞瘤的发病风险存在争议。尽管有文献报道MCDK与肾母细胞瘤间存在相关性，但无强力的证据支持两者有关联。
- MCDK在影像学上表现为多囊性“肿块”取代肾脏实质。囊性结构互不交通，这与肾盂积水不同。

  DMSA扫描显示MCDK无肾皮质摄取，而肾盂积水时肾皮质仍有微弱的放射性示踪剂摄取。

多房囊性肾瘤

- 多房囊性肾瘤是一种良性的、有多个分隔的囊性肿瘤。发病年龄呈双峰分布，见于3个月~2岁的男童和中年女性。
- 与*DICER1*突变和胸膜肺母细胞瘤有关。
- 影像上，多房囊性肾瘤表现为一个多分隔的肾囊性肿块，伴有分隔强化。其表现可能与囊性肾母细胞瘤相似。有一定特征性的影像学表现为病灶有向肾盂内疝入的倾向，可引起肾盂积水。

单纯性肾囊肿

- 孤立的单纯性肾囊肿在儿童罕见。一旦出现，肾囊肿很可能属于综合征的一部分，与结节性硬化或希佩尔-林道综合征有关。

> **结节性硬化**：除肾囊肿外，患者还可能有：
>
> 肾血管平滑肌脂肪瘤。
>
> 心脏横纹肌瘤。
>
> 中枢神经系统皮层错构瘤、室管膜下结节及室管膜下巨细胞星形细胞瘤。
>
> **希佩尔-林道(VHL)综合征**：除了肾囊肿，患者还合并有：
>
> 肾细胞癌(RCC)：超过30%的VHL患者死于RCC。
>
> 肾上腺嗜铬细胞瘤。
>
> 胰腺囊肿、胰岛细胞瘤及浆液性囊腺瘤。
>
> 脑部及脊髓血管母细胞瘤。

常染色体显性遗传性多囊性肾病(ADPKD)

- 常染色体显性遗传性多囊性肾病(ADPKD)通常在成年期出现症状，但50%的患者在10岁以前已经有囊肿出现。
- ADPKD典型特征是肾脏增大，伴有无数大小不一的囊肿。
- ADPKD与肝囊肿和较少见的胰腺囊肿相关。

常染色体隐性遗传性多囊性肾病(ARPKD)

- 常染色体隐性遗传性多囊性肾病(ARPKD)以微囊肿为特征，发生于婴儿期，因集合小管广泛性扩张所致。囊肿通常太小而无法在影像

characteristic appearance on ultrasound of bilaterally enlarged and diffusely echogenic kidneys.

上进行分辨，超声的特征性表现为双肾体积增大及弥漫性高回声。

- Earlier presentations have worse prognosis, with fetal diagnosis often causing severe oligohydramnios and pulmonary hypoplasia. ARPKD is associated with hepatic fibrosis, especially when ARPKD manifests later in childhood. The degree of hepatic fibrosis is inversely related to the severity of renal disease.

- 临床表现越早，预后越差，在胎儿期确诊的患儿通常合并严重羊水不足及肺发育不全。ARPKD常伴有肝纤维化，尤其是ARPKD症状出现于大龄儿童时，肝纤维化程度与肾脏病变严重程度成反比。

Malignant Solid Renal Masses

恶性肾脏实性肿块

Wilms tumor

肾母细胞瘤

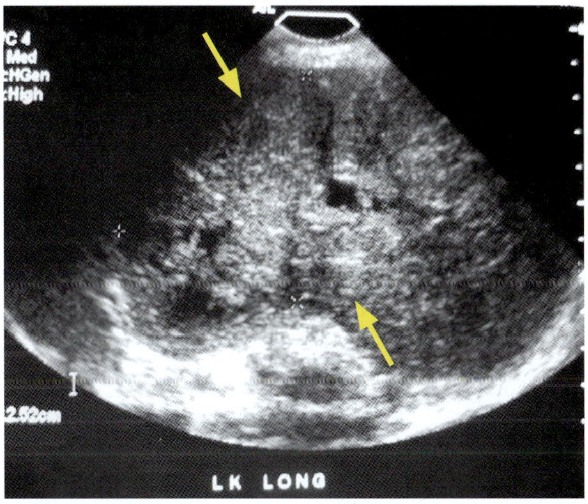

Sagittal ultrasound of the left kidney shows near-complete replacement of the renal parenchyma by a large, heterogeneous mass (arrows).
左肾矢状切面超声显示肾实质几乎完全被一个大而不均质的肿块替代(箭)。

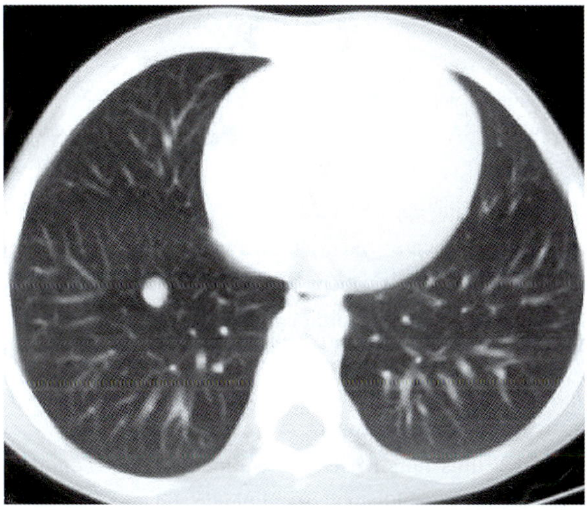

Axial chest CT shows a right lower lobe nodule, suspicious for metastasis.
轴位胸部CT显示右肺下叶结节，疑为转移灶。

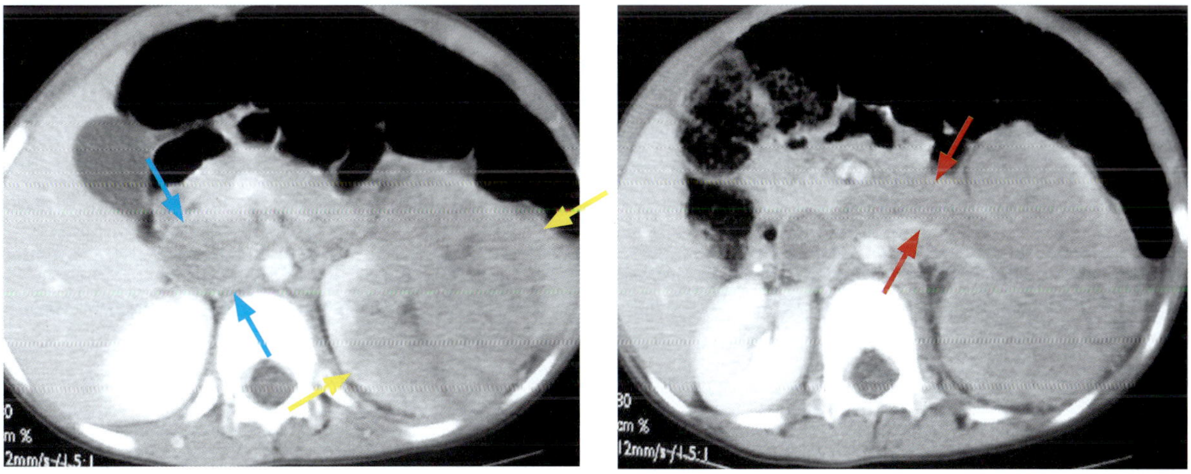

Contrast-enhanced axial CT images through the kidneys show near complete replacement of the left kidney by a dominant mass (yellow arrows) containing central foci of necrosis. There is extension into and expansion of the left renal vein (red arrows) and inferior vena cava (blue arrows). Given the presence of lung metastasis, this represents Stage Ⅳ Wilms tumor.

Case courtesy Michael Callahan, MD, Boston Children's Hospital.

肾脏层面轴位增强CT显示左肾几乎被一个巨大肿块完全占据(黄箭)，其中央含有局灶性坏死。肿块延伸至左肾静脉(红箭)及下腔静脉(蓝箭)，并造成相应血管扩张。结合肺部转移病灶，此为Ⅳ期肾母细胞瘤。

- Wilms tumor is the most common childhood renal malignancy, typically affecting children between 3–5 years of age. Almost 90% of renal tumors in the first decade of life are Wilms tumors; in the second decade, the incidence of Wilms and RCC is equal. Wilms arises from persistent metanephric blastema.
- Patients with increased risk for Wilms tumor are screened with regular ultrasound until school age, and include patients with:

Beckwith-Wiedemann syndrome: hemihypertrophy, macroglossia, omphalocele, neonatal hypoglycemia (due to insulin overproduction by pancreatic β-cells), and increased risk of childhood malignancies, including Wilms tumor and hepatoblastoma.
WAGR syndrome: Wilms tumor, aniridia, genitourinary anomalies, and mental retardation.
Horseshoe kidney: approximately 2x incidence of Wilms tumor.
Trisomy 18.

- The classic imaging appearance of Wilms is a heterogeneous, solid renal mass. The *claw sign* indicates renal parenchyma origin. Tumor venous extension is seen in 5–10%. Calcifications may be present but are uncommon. A cystic variant may mimic benign multilocular cystic nephroma.
- Liver or lung metastases are each seen in approximately 10%. Bone metastases are not common, and when present in a pediatric renal mass are more suggestive of clear cell sarcoma.
- Staging of Wilms tumor uses the National Wilms Tumor Study (NWTS) system, which is a combination of radiologic and post-surgical findings:

Stage Ⅰ: Completely resected mass confined to the kidney.
Two-year survival: 95%
Stage Ⅱ: Completely resected mass with spread to nearby structures (e.g., renal capsule or blood vessels).
Two-year survival: 90%
Stage Ⅲ: Incompletely resected mass with spread to nearby intra-abdominal structures.
Two-year survival: 85%
Stage Ⅳ: Hematogenous metastases (e.g., to lung, liver, bone, or brain) or lymphatic metastases outside of the abdomen or pelvis.
Two-year survival: 55%
Stage Ⅴ (unique to Wilms): Bilateral Wilms at the time of diagnosis (approximately 5–10%).
Two-year survival: Variable.

Renal cell carcinoma (RCC)

- Although far more common in adults, renal cell cancer (RCC) does occur in older children and adolescents, usually presenting at age 10–12 years. Overall, <1% of all RCCs occur in children, typically in the setting of von Hippel-Lindau syndrome.
- Renal medullary carcinoma is an especially aggressive variant of RCC affecting patients with sickle cell trait.

- 肾母细胞瘤是儿童最常见的肾脏恶性肿瘤，通常见于3~5岁的儿童。在10岁以内，90%的肾脏肿瘤为肾母细胞瘤，在10~20岁，肾母细胞瘤与RCC的发病率相同。肾母细胞瘤起源于永存后肾胚芽。
- 具有肾母细胞瘤高危因素的患者应在学龄前接受定期超声筛查，这些高危人群包括：

11p部分三体综合征：偏身肥大，巨舌，脐膨出，新生儿低血糖症(因胰腺β细胞产生过量胰岛素所致)，以及罹患儿童期恶性肿瘤的风险增加，包括肾母细胞瘤及肝母细胞瘤。
WAGR综合征(11p缺失综合征)：肾母细胞瘤，无虹膜，泌尿生殖系统异常，以及神经发育迟缓。
马蹄肾：肾母细胞瘤的发病率约为正常人的2倍。
18-三体综合征。

- 瘤的典型影像学表现为不均质的实性肾脏肿块。爪形征提示肿瘤起源于肾脏实质。肿瘤向静脉扩散见于5%~10%的患者。可出现钙化，但不常见。囊性类型可与良性多房囊性肾瘤相似。
- 肝转移或肺转移各约占10%。骨转移并不常见，当儿童肾脏肿块出现骨转移时更有可能是透明细胞肉瘤。
- 肾母细胞瘤分期采用美国国家肾母细胞瘤研究系统(NWTS)，其结合放射影像和术后结果进行评估：

Ⅰ期：肿块仅局限于肾脏内，手术可以完全切除。
2年生存率：95%。
Ⅱ期：肿块侵及周围结构(如肾包膜或血管)，手术可以完全切除。
2年生存率：90%。
Ⅲ期：肿块侵及邻近的腹腔内结构，手术不能完全切除。
2年生存率：85%。
Ⅳ期：有血源性转移瘤(如肺、肝脏、骨或脑转移)或出现腹部及盆腔范围以外的淋巴转移。
2年生存率：55%。
Ⅴ期(肾母细胞瘤独有)：确诊时有双侧肾母细胞瘤(占5%~10%)。
2年生存率：不定。

肾细胞癌

- 虽然肾细胞癌更常见于成人，但在较大年龄的儿童及青少年也可以发生，常见年龄为10~12岁。总体来讲，儿童RCC发生率不到全部RCC的1%，通常发生在患有希佩尔-林道综合征的人群。
- 肾脏髓样癌是极具侵袭性的一种肾细胞癌，发生在患有镰状细胞贫血的人群。

Rhabdoid tumor

- Rhabdoid tumor is a rare, aggressive malignancy that may occur in the brain or kidney.
- Imaging shows an ill-defined, aggressive renal mass. Renal and CNS lesions may be concurrent.
- These lesions are typically seen in the first year of life, and have the worst prognosis of all pediatric renal tumors.
- The classic ultrasound and cross-sectional finding is a subcapsular fluid crescent, reflecting renal hemorrhage.

Clear cell sarcoma

- Clear cell sarcoma is an uncommon renal cancer with propensity to metastasize to bone.

Renal metastases

- The most common primary malignancies to metastasize to the kidneys in children are neuroblastoma, leukemia, and lymphoma.
- Leukemia is characteristically infiltrative, diffuse, and bilateral.
- Lymphoma has multiple imaging presentations, including multiple masses or diffuse infiltration.

横纹肌样瘤

- 横纹肌样瘤是一种罕见的、恶性程度高的肿瘤，可发生在大脑或肾脏。
- 影像学表现为边界不清的侵袭性肾脏肿块。肾脏及中枢神经系统可同时出现病变。
- 病变通常出现在1岁以内，而且在所有儿童肾脏肿瘤中预后最差。
- 典型超声表现是在横断面上可见肾包膜下积液，为肾出血所致。

肾透明细胞肉瘤

- 肾透明细胞肉瘤是一种不常见的肾癌类型，具有骨转移倾向。

肾转移瘤

- 儿童最常见的肾脏转移性恶性肿瘤有神经母细胞瘤、白血病及淋巴瘤。
- 白血病肾浸润的典型表现为双肾受累，病变呈浸润性、弥漫性生长。
- 淋巴瘤的影像学表现多样，包括肾脏多发肿块或弥漫浸润。

BENIGN SOLID RENAL MASSES

良性肾脏实性肿块

Mesoblastic nephroma

中胚层肾瘤

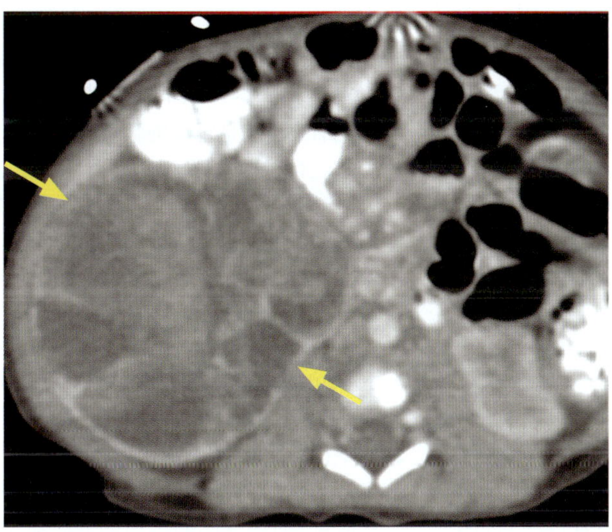

Mesoblastic nephroma: Axial contrast-enhanced CT in a neonate shows a large mass replacing the right renal parenchyma (arrows), containing numerous foci of necrosis.

Case courtesy Michael Callahan, MD, Boston Children's Hospital.

中胚层肾瘤：轴位增强CT显示一名新生儿右肾可见一处巨大肿块完全取代肾实质(箭)，其内含大量坏死灶。

- Mesoblastic nephroma is a benign tumor that appears identical to Wilms by imaging, but occurs in younger children typically ≤ 1 year old.
- Although benign, mesoblastic nephroma is always removed surgically since the classic and more aggressive variants cannot be reliably distinguished radiographically. They are predominantly distinguished from Wilms tumor by the age of the child.
- Like Wilms tumor, mesoblastic nephroma arises from persistent metanephric blastema.
- Mesoblastic nephroma should not be confused with multilocular cystic nephroma, which is a cystic renal mass with a bimodal age distribution, and is not related to the metanephric blastema.

- 中胚层肾瘤是一种良性肿瘤，影像学表现与肾母细胞瘤相同，但发病年龄更小，通常见于<1岁的儿童。
- 尽管是良性肿瘤，但中胚层肾瘤采用手术切除治疗，因为典型的中胚层肾瘤与更具有侵袭性的恶性变异在影像学上无法进行鉴别。与肾母细胞瘤进行鉴别的主要依据是患儿的年龄。
- 与肾母细胞瘤相似，中胚层肾瘤同样起源于永存后肾胚芽组织。
- 中胚层肾瘤不应与多房囊性肾瘤相混淆，后者表现为囊性肾脏肿块，并呈双峰年龄分布，且与后肾胚芽组织无关。

Nephroblastomatosis

肾母细胞瘤病

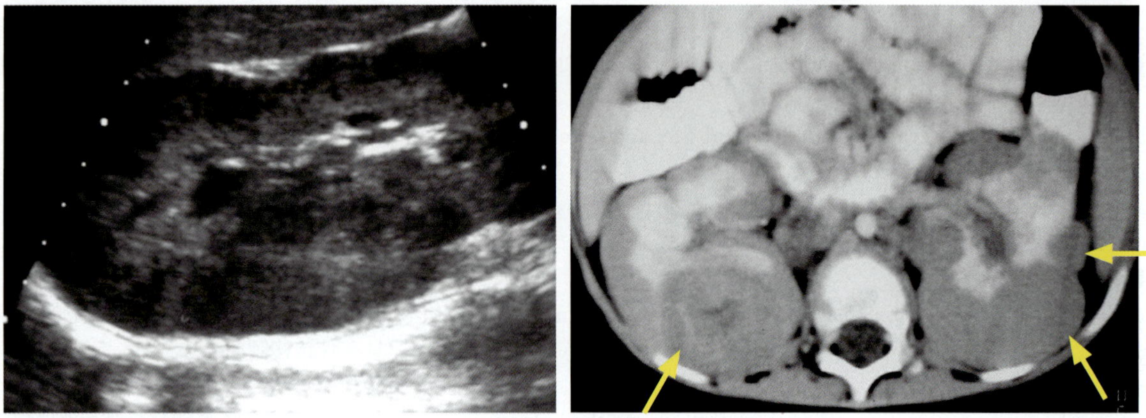

Nephroblastomatosis: Sagittal ultrasound (left image) of the right kidney shows marked lobular enlargement of the kidney and reduced echogenicity of the renal cortex. Axial contrast-enhanced CT (right) shows bilateral nephromegaly and numerous lobulated, relatively low attenuation rounded nodules and masses (arrows).

Case courtesy Michael Callahan, MD, Boston Children's Hospital.

肾母细胞瘤病：右肾矢状切面超声(左图)显示肾脏明显增大呈分叶状，肾皮质回声减低。轴位增强CT(右图)显示双侧肾脏增大和无数分叶状、相对较低密度的圆形结节及肿块(箭)。

- Nephroblastomatosis is the persistence of metanephric blastema. The term nephrogenic rest is used when metanephric blastema persists beyond 36 weeks gestation.
- On imaging, nephroblastomatosis may appear as a discrete, homogeneous, nonenhancing renal mass with a hypodense rind. Nephroblastomatosis is commonly multifocal, confluent, and bilateral.
- Nephroblastomatosis is a precursor to Wilms tumor, so frequent screening is performed. Worrisome findings on screening include rapid growth, inhomogeneity, increased sphericity and enhancement.

Nephroblastomatosis may be peripheral or central. While rare, the latter tends to more frequently progress to Wilms tumor.

Nephroblastomatosis is present in 30% of all Wilms nephrectomies, and in all cases of bilateral Wilms tumors.

- 肾母细胞瘤病是永存的后肾胚芽组织。而肾源性残余组织是指后肾胚芽在妊娠超过36周后仍持续存在。
- 肾母细胞瘤病在影像上表现为散在的、均质、无强化的肾脏肿块，肾皮质外侧呈低密度影。肾母细胞瘤病通常表现为多灶性、融合性及双侧性。
- 肾母细胞瘤病是肾母细胞瘤的癌前病变，需要经常进行预防性筛查。提示不良的表现有肿块迅速增大、质地不均匀、呈球形及病灶强化。

肾母细胞瘤病的病灶可位于肾脏边缘或中央。虽然罕见，但后者往往有更大概率进展为肾母细胞瘤。

肾母细胞瘤病在所有肾母细胞瘤肾切除的病例中占30%，而在双侧肾母细胞瘤的病例中均应进行肾切除。

Angiomyolipoma (AML)

- Angiomyolipoma (AML) is a benign renal tumor with elements of blood vessels (angio), muscle (myo), and fat (lipoma). Multiple AMLs are associated with tuberous sclerosis.
- Most AMLs feature macroscopic fat, which is visible on CT or MRI. An AML larger than 4 cm has a risk of hemorrhage.

血管平滑肌脂肪瘤(AML)

- 血管平滑肌脂肪瘤(AML)为良性肾肿瘤，内含血管、肌肉及脂肪组织成分。多发性AML与结节性硬化有关。
- 大多数AML以肉眼可见的脂肪组织为特征，并可以在CT或MRI上显示。直径＞4cm的AML具有出血的风险。

Confusing names

混淆的命名

Metanephric blastema

- Metanephric blastema is one of the two embryologic tissues that forms the genitourinary system. Metanephric blastema develops into the renal parenchyma, while the ureteric bud forms the collecting system.
- If metanephric blastema persists after embryogenesis, it can lead to:

后肾胚芽

- 后肾胚芽为形成泌尿生殖系统的两种胚胎组织之一。后肾胚芽发育为肾实质，而输尿管芽则形成集合系统。
- 若后肾胚芽于胚胎形成后持续存在，则可导致：

Mesoblastic nephroma, a benign tumor that arises from persistent metanephric blastema. Its appearance mimics Wilms but it occurs in neonates.

Nephroblastomatosis, which is benign persistent metanephric blastema manifesting as single, multiple, or confluent homogeneous renal masses. Nephroblastomatosis has an increased risk of Wilms tumor.

Wilms tumor, an aggressive renal malignancy that is the most common childhood renal neoplasm. It typically occurs in children between the ages of 3 and 5 years old.

中胚层肾瘤，一种起源于永存后肾胚芽的良性肿瘤。与肾母细胞瘤的形态相似，但发生于新生儿。

肾母细胞瘤病，一种良性永存后肾胚芽，表现为单发、多发或混合的肾脏肿块。肾母细胞瘤病有增加罹患肾母细胞瘤的风险。

肾母细胞瘤，是儿童最常见的侵袭性恶性肾脏肿瘤。肾母细胞瘤通常见于3~5岁的幼儿。

Multilocular cystic nephroma

- Multilocular cystic nephroma does not arise from mesonephric blastema and is not related to mesoblastic nephroma.
- Multilocular cystic nephroma is a cystic renal mass with a bimodal age distribution, seen in young boys and middle-aged women.

多房囊性肾瘤

- 多房囊性肾瘤并非起源于中肾胚芽，与中胚层肾瘤无关。
- 多房囊性肾瘤为囊性肾脏肿块，发病年龄呈双峰分布，多见于幼龄男童及中年妇女。

Differential diagnosis of multiple renal masses

肾脏多发肿块的鉴别诊断

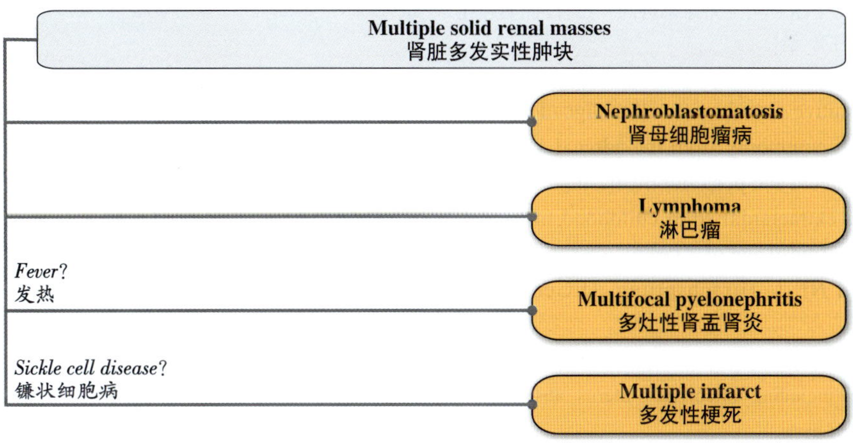

Adrenal mass lesions

肾上腺肿块

Neuroblastoma

神经母细胞瘤

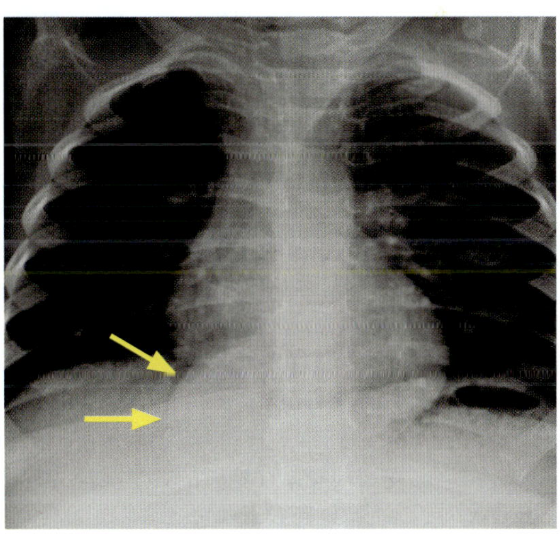

Chest radiograph shows a subtle abnormal right paradiaphragmatic contour (arrows), which does not silhouette with the heart, suggestive of a posterior mediastinal mass.

胸片显示右侧膈肌旁一个不明显的肿块(箭)，不构成心影轮廓，提示为后纵隔肿块。

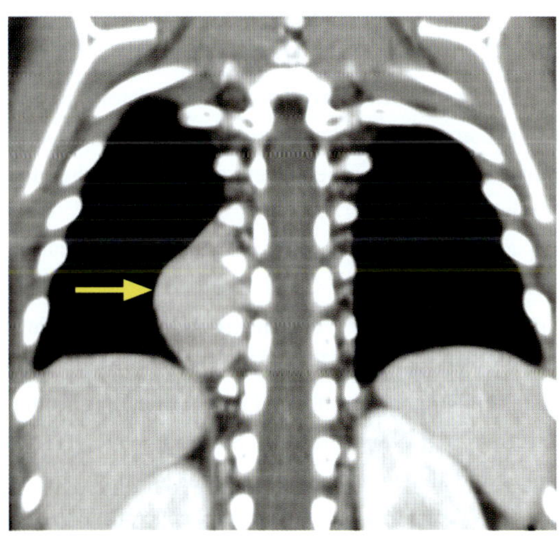

Coronal contrast-enhanced CT shows a diffusely enhancing right paraspinal mass (arrow), without calcification or expansion into the spinal canal.

冠状位增强CT显示右侧脊柱旁肿块呈弥漫性强化(箭)，无钙化或向椎管内延伸。

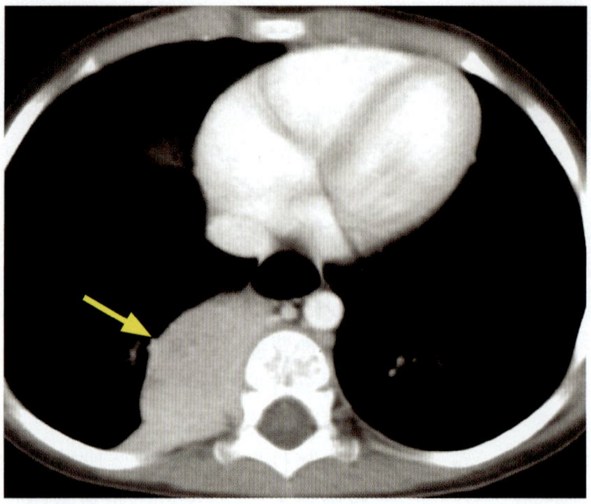

Axial contrast-enhanced CT (from the same study as the coronal image above) confirms the paraspinal location of the enhancing mass (arrow).
轴位增强CT(与上图冠状位图像来自同一患者)证实强化的肿块位于脊柱旁(箭)。

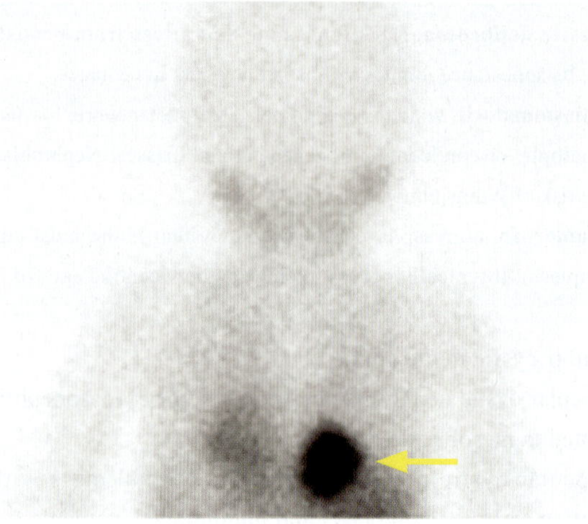

Posterior planar imaging from a I-123 MIBG scan shows avid tracer uptake in the right paraspinal region (arrow).
^{123}I-MIBG后前位显像显示右侧脊柱旁区有明显的示踪剂摄取(箭)。

- Neuroblastoma is a primitive neural crest cell malignancy that arises from the sympathetic chain, most commonly from the adrenal gland, followed by the extra-adrenal retroperitoneum and posterior mediastinum.
- It is the most common extracranial solid childhood malignancy, presenting between 1–5 years of age (mean age of 2 years).
- Associations included NF-1, Hirschsprung, DiGeorge, and Beckwith-Wiedeman.

  Unilateral agenesis is associated with reproductive anomalies (Mayer-Rokitansky-Kuster-Hauser syndrome) including unicornuate uterus, absent epididymis and vas deferens, and seminal vesicle cysts.

  A paraneoplastic syndrome termed opsoclonus-myoclonus may be seen, featuring nystagmus (dancing eyes) and ataxia (dancing feet). It is more frequently associated with thoracic primary lesions.
- A typical CT appearance of an adrenal neuroblastoma is a suprarenal mass, with calcifications seen in ~50%. Neuroblastoma tends to encase vessels, while Wilms tumor is known to displace and narrow vessels.
- On MRI, neuroblastoma often invades into neural foramina and the spinal canal. Diffusion is often restricted, reflecting hypercellularity.
- Neuroblastoma is a catecholamine-secreting tumor and therefore positive on I-123 MIBG scintigraphy.

  Other catecholamine-secreting tumors (pheochromocytoma, carcinoid and medullary thyroid cancer) are rare in children.
- Metastases may be found in 75% of patients and commonly involve the bone marrow (typically permeative and lytic). A classic presentation of metastatic neuroblastoma is an intracranial, subdural mass originating from the marrow.
- The prior International Neuroblasoma Staging System (INSS, 1993) for neuroblastoma surgical staging may be helpful to know, and is summarized below. "Midline" is defined as the contralateral edge of the vertebral body (i.e., for a left neuroblastoma, "midline" is the right lateral edge of the vertebral body)

- 神经母细胞瘤为起源于交感神经链的原始神经嵴细胞的恶性肿瘤，最常发生于肾上腺，其次是肾上腺外的后腹膜及后纵隔。
- 神经母细胞瘤是儿童颅外最常见的恶性实性肿瘤，好发年龄为1~5岁(平均年龄为2岁)。
- 相关疾病包括1型神经纤维瘤病、先天性巨结肠、22q11.2缺失综合征，以及11p部分三体综合征。

  单侧发育不全与生殖系统异常(先天性子宫阴道缺如综合征)有关，包括单角子宫、附睾和输精管缺失及精囊囊肿。

  副肿瘤综合征又称opsoclonus-myoclonus综合征，表现为眼球震颤(舞眼)和共济失调(跳舞脚)。它常与胸部原发病灶有关。
- 肾上腺神经母细胞瘤的典型CT表现为肾脏上方的肿块，多达50%可见钙化。神经母细胞瘤有包裹血管的倾向，而肾母细胞瘤则是压迫血管而使血管移位及管腔狭窄。
- 在MRI中，神经母细胞瘤常侵犯神经孔及椎管。弥散通常受限，为细胞密集所致。
- 神经母细胞瘤是一种分泌儿茶酚胺的肿瘤，因此^{123}I-MIBG闪烁显像为阳性。

  其他分泌儿茶酚胺的肿瘤儿童罕见，如嗜铬细胞瘤、类癌和甲状腺髓样癌。
- 转移可见于75%的患者，其中骨髓转移最常见(通常为穿凿样及溶骨性骨质破坏)。转移性神经母细胞瘤的典型表现为起源于骨髓的颅内、硬膜下肿块。
- 熟悉以前的国际神经母细胞瘤分期系统(INSS，1993)对理解神经母细胞瘤外科分期可能会有所帮助，该分期系统总结如下。"中线"定义为椎体的对侧缘(如一个左侧神经母细胞瘤的"中线"为椎体的右侧缘)。

Stage Ⅰ: Tumor limited to organ of origin (e.g., adrenal). 75% two-year survival.
Stage Ⅱ: Local spread (nodes may be positive), but no disease crossing midline. 75% two-year survival.
Stage Ⅲ: Local spread, crosses midline. 25% two-year survival.
Stage Ⅳ: Distant metastases. 25% two-year survival.
Stage ⅣS: Stage Ⅰ or Ⅱ with metastases confined to skin, liver, and bone marrow, and age <1 year (better prognosis than Stage Ⅲ or Ⅳ). May also apply to children up to 18 months. 75% two-year survival.

Ⅰ期：肿瘤局限于原发器官内(如肾上腺)。2年生存率75%。
Ⅱ期：肿瘤局部蔓延(可出现阳性淋巴结)，但病灶未跨越中线。2年生存率75%。
Ⅲ期：肿瘤局部蔓延，病灶跨越中线，2年生存率25%。
Ⅳ期：远处转移。2年生存率25%。
ⅣS期：Ⅰ期或Ⅱ期合并转移，但局限于皮肤、肝脏及骨髓，且年龄<1岁(预后较Ⅲ期或Ⅳ期好)。ⅣS期也可适用于小于18月龄的儿童。2年生存率75%。

- A more recent system by the International Neuroblastoma Risk Group (INRG, 2009) features a set of image-defined risk factors (IDRF), such as invasion into adjacent organs, bones or vessels, to stage the extent of disease.

- 国际神经母细胞瘤风险评估协作组(INRG，2009)最近制定了一套影像定义危险因素(IDRF)，如侵入邻近器官、骨骼或血管，用于对疾病程度进行分期。

Stage L1: Localized tumor, not involving vital structures defined in IDRF and confined to one body compartment. 95% survival rate.
Stage L2: Locoregional tumor with presence of 1+ IDRF.
Stage M: Distant metastases (excluding stage MS), with 10–30% survival rate.
Stage MS: Metastatic disease confined to skin, liver and/or bone marrow disease in children less than 18 months. More favorable prognosis with 75–100% survival rate.

L1期：局限性肿瘤，不涉及IDRF中定义的重要结构，局限于身体的一个部位。生存率95%。
L2期：局部区域肿瘤伴一种以上的IDRF危险因素。
M期：远处转移(除外MS期)，生存率为10%~30%。
MS期：年龄在18月龄以下的儿童，转移局限于皮肤、肝脏和/或骨髓。预后良好，生存率为75%~100%。

Ganglioneuroma

- Ganglioneuroma is a benign neurogenic tumor that appears similar to neuroblastoma on imaging. Ganglioneuroblastoma is intermediate in biological behavior between benign ganglioneuroma and malignant neuroblastoma. It is thought that neuroblastoma may differentiate into either of these lesions.
- In contrast to neuroblastoma, ganglioneuroma affects slightly older children (most common age of a ganglioneuroma patient is 6 years old) and only 50% of ganglioneuromas are positive on I-123 MIBG scintigraphy. MRI classically shows restricted diffusion of a neuroblastoma, but not in ganglioneuroma.

节细胞神经瘤

- 节细胞神经瘤是一种良性神经源性肿瘤，在影像学上与神经母细胞瘤相似。节细胞神经母细胞瘤的生物学行为介于良性节细胞神经瘤与恶性神经母细胞瘤之间。有人认为，神经母细胞瘤可分化为这两种病变中的任何一种。
- 与神经母细胞瘤相比，节细胞神经瘤发生在年龄稍大的儿童(节细胞神经瘤最常见的发病年龄为6岁左右)，仅有50%的节细胞神经瘤^{123}I-MIBG闪烁显像呈阳性。MRI弥散受限通常见于神经母细胞瘤，但节细胞神经瘤无此表现。

Adrenal hemorrhage (in neonates)

- Adrenal hemorrhage is the most common adrenal "mass" in neonates, and most often associated with difficult deliveries or perinatal stress related to maternal diabetes, breech delivery and sepsis.
- It is typically diagnosed by ultrasound as a hypoechoic avascular suprarenal mass. Hemorrhage may appear similar to neuroblastoma on initial ultrasound, but a follow-up scan would demonstrate involution. Old hemorrhage may calcify.

肾上腺出血(新生儿)

- 肾上腺出血是新生儿最常见的肾上腺"肿块"，通常与难产或与产妇糖尿病、臀位分娩和败血症相关的围产期应激有关。
- 在超声检查时，肾上腺出血通常表现为肾脏上方一个低回声、无血供的肿块。出血初期超声表现可与神经母细胞瘤相似，但随访检查可见血肿吸收改变。陈旧性出血灶内可能有钙化。

Congenital adrenal hyperplasia (CAH)

- Congenital adrenal hyperplasia (CAH) encompasses a group of enzymatic disorders in the synthesis of cortisol, most commonly deficiency in 21-hydroxylase.
- Patients can present with abnormalities in genital development and salt imbalance.
- Imaging findings suggestive of CAH include uniformly enlarged size (length >20 mm or limb width >4 mm), and cerebriform appearance.

先天性肾上腺增生症(CAH)

- 先天性肾上腺增生症(CAH)包括一组糖皮质激素合成酶缺陷所引起的疾病，最常见的是21-羟化酶缺乏。
- 患者可出现生殖器官发育异常和盐失衡。
- CAH的影像学表现包括肾上腺均匀增大(长度>20mm或肢宽>4mm)和脑回样改变。

Adrenal cortical carcinoma

肾上腺皮质癌

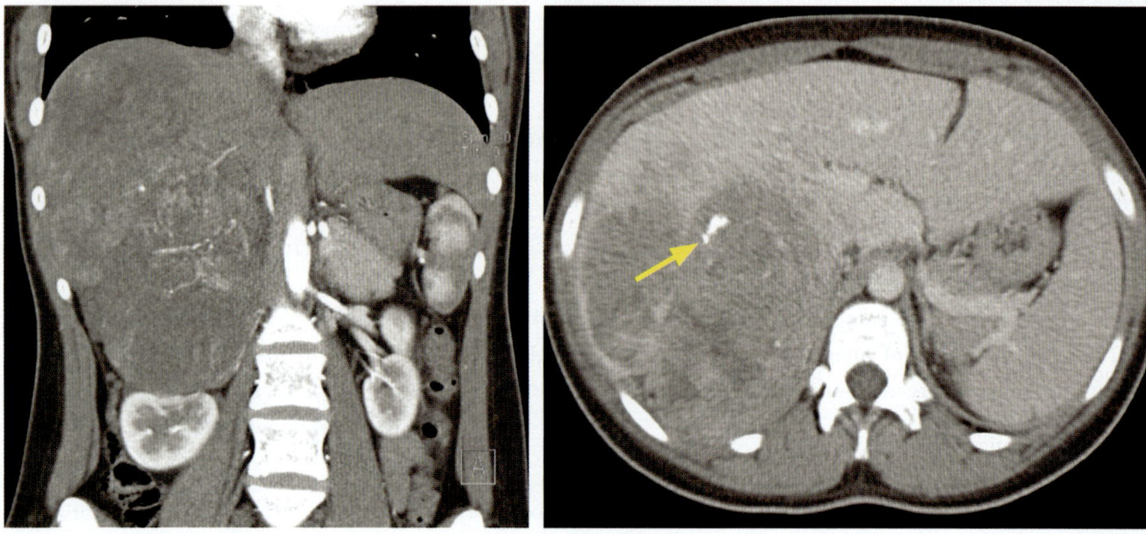

Adrenocortical carcinoma: Coronal (left image) and axial (right) contrast-enhanced CT shows a heterogeneously enhancing suprarenal mass invading into the liver parenchyma with a focus of coarse calcification (arrow).

肾上腺皮质癌：冠状位(左)及轴位(右)增强CT显示肾脏上方一个不均匀强化肿块，侵犯肝实质，内部可见粗糙的钙化灶(箭)。

- Adrenal cortical carcinoma is an extremely rare disease, with a prevalence of approximately 1–2 cases per million per year. When occurring in children, it may be associated with Beckwith-Wiedemann and Li-Fraumeni syndromes.
- Adrenal cortical carcinoma has a bimodal age distribution, seen in children younger than 5 years old and adults in their fourth and fifth decades.

- 肾上腺皮质癌是一种极为罕见的疾病，每年发病率大约在(1~2)/100万。当发生于儿童时，可能与11p部分三体综合征及利-弗劳梅尼综合征有关。
- 肾上腺皮质癌的发病年龄呈双峰分布，见于小于5岁的儿童和40~60岁的成人。

Cystic pelvic masses

- The differential diagnosis for cystic pediatric pelvic masses depends on the sex of the child. A pediatric cystic pelvic mass is most likely due to a congenital genitourinary anomaly.

Either sex

- A **urachal anomaly** results from incomplete obliteration of the embryologic allantois. The urachus is the remnant of the allantois, which connects the urinary bladder to the umbilical cord. There is a risk of adenocarcinoma if a urachal anomaly is not resected.

  Patent urachus (most common): Connection between bladder and umbilicus (vesico-cutaneous fistula).

  Urachal cyst: Noncommunicating cyst in between the bladder and umbilicus.

  Urachal sinus: Blind-ending sinus at umbilicus.

  Vesicourachal diverticulum: Blind-ending bladder diverticulum.

- A **rectal duplication** cyst is a rare type of gastrointestinal duplication cyst, usually occurring in the retrorectal space. They are typically resected due to malignant potential.

Girls only

- A **dilated fluid or blood-filled vagina and/or uterus** may be in response to hormonal stimulation and outflow obstruction, either in the neonatal period (fluid-filled) or at puberty (blood-filled).

  Hydrometrocolpos: Vagina and uterus dilated with fluid.

  Hydrocolpos: Vagina dilated with fluid.

盆腔囊性肿块

- 鉴别儿童盆腔囊性肿块取决于患儿的性别。儿童盆腔囊性肿块最有可能是因为先天性泌尿生殖系统异常。

不限性别

- **脐尿管异常**为胚胎期尿囊不完全闭塞所致。脐尿管为尿囊的残余组织，连接膀胱与脐带。如果不切除异常的脐尿管组织，则有癌变的风险。

  脐尿管未闭(最常见)：连接膀胱与肚脐(膀胱皮肤瘘)。

  脐尿管囊肿：膀胱与肚脐间两端无交通的囊肿。

  脐尿管窦：开口于肚脐的窦道盲端。

  膀胱脐尿管憩室：开口于膀胱的憩室盲端。

- **直肠重复**囊肿为一种罕见的胃肠道重复囊性畸形，通常位于直肠后间隙内。因具有恶性潜能而通常进行手术切除。

仅发生于女童

- 阴道和/或子宫扩张性积液或积血可能因激素刺激和流出道梗阻所致，可见于新生儿期(积液)或青春期(积血)。

  子宫阴道积水：阴道及子宫扩张积液。

  阴道积水：阴道扩张积液。

Hematometrocolpos: Dilated vagina and uterus filled with blood; occurs at menarche with vaginal outflow tract obstruction (e.g., congenital imperforate hymen).

- **Ovarian dermoid cyst**, otherwise known as a mature cystic teratoma.

Boys only

- A **Müllerian duct cyst** is caused by incomplete regression of the Müllerian ducts. In a normal male, the Müllerian ducts regress. A persistent Müllerian duct remnant can cause a Müllerian duct cyst.

  In a normal **female**, Müllerian ducts (paramesonephric ducts) develop into the fallopian tubes, uterus, cervix, and upper vagina.

- The **prostatic utricle** is a normal midline structure that is the terminal remnant of the Müllerian duct. It arises from the posterior urethra near the verumontanum (ridge of the posterior urethra near the seminal vesicle insertion). When associated with hypospadia (urethra opens along the ventral penile shaft), a prostatic utricle can become very large.

Solid pelvic masses

- Solid pelvic masses are less likely to represent genitourinary anomalies, and are more concerning for neoplasm.

Rhabdomyosarcoma

- Rhabdomyosarcoma is the most common sarcoma of childhood, occurring equally commonly in the pelvis (bladder, vagina, cervix, uterus, etc.) and head and neck (together making up almost 80% of cases).
- Imaging features a characteristic lobulated *bunch of grapes* appearance (Botryoid variant).

Sacrococcygeal teratoma

- Sacrococcygeal teratoma is usually apparent on pre-natal imaging. When detected after birth the characteristic clinical appearance is a skin-covered mass extending from the midline buttocks.
- Sacrococcygeal teratoma has a heterogeneous imaging appearance with cystic, solid, and fatty components.

Pediatric musculoskeletal

Fractures in children

- Pediatric bones are more elastic than adult bones, and therefore tend to "bend" (i.e., buckle, greenstick and plastic fractures) rather than "break".
- There is a general timeline for dating pediatric fractures: periosteal reaction in less than 1 week and complete healing around 12 weeks.

  Exceptions include metaphyseal, skull and costochondral junction fractures which often heal without periosteal reaction.

  When the radiographic diagnosis is equivocal, repeat radiographs can be performed in 7–10 days, when periosteal reaction is expected to be visible.

Physiology of the physis

- The physis, commonly known as the growth plate, consists of 4 histological zones of cartilage arranged in layers.

子宫阴道积血：阴道及子宫扩张并积血，发生于患者在初潮期阴道流出道梗阻(如先天性处女膜闭锁)。

- **卵巢皮样囊肿**，又称为成熟型囊性畸胎瘤。

仅发生于男童

- **米勒管囊肿是**由米勒管不完全退化所致。米勒管在正常男性中退化。米勒管持续存在可导致米勒管囊肿。

  在正常**女性**中，米勒管(副中肾管)将发育成输卵管、子宫、宫颈及阴道上部。

- **前列腺囊**为米勒管终端残留所形成的正常中线结构，起自精阜附近的后尿道(精囊插入处附近的后尿道嵴)。当合并尿道下裂(尿道沿阴茎干腹侧开口)时，前列腺囊可变得很大。

盆腔实性肿块

- 盆腔实性肿块很少因为泌尿生殖系统发育异常所致，更需要考虑为肿瘤。

横纹肌肉瘤

- 横纹肌肉瘤为儿童期最常见的肉瘤，盆腔(膀胱、阴道、宫颈、子宫等)和头颈部发生率相似(两者合计发病率约占总数的80%)
- 典型影像学表现为葡萄串样的分叶状外形(Botryoid变体)。

骶尾部畸胎瘤

- 骶尾部畸胎瘤通常在产前影像检查中就能被发现。出生后发现的特征性临床表现为沿臀部中线延伸的肿块，其表面有皮肤覆盖。
- 骶尾部畸胎瘤在影像学上表现为不均质的肿块，可含有囊性、实性及脂肪成分。

(翻译　邱伟)

小儿骨骼肌肉系统

小儿骨折

- 儿童骨骼比成人骨骼更富有弹性，因此容易导致"弯曲"(如翘曲膨隆、青枝和塑性骨折)而不是"断裂"。
- 儿童骨折愈合的大致时间节点如下：骨膜反应不到1周，完全愈合需要大约12周。

  干骺端、颅骨和肋软骨连接处的骨折除外，它们在愈合过程中常没有骨膜反应。

  当X线诊断可疑时，可在7~10天后重复检查，此时骨折区应看到骨膜反应。

骨骺的生理学

- 骺板，通常也称为生长板，由4个组织学区域的软骨依次排列而成。

- The zone closest to the metaphysis is the *zone of provisional calcification*, composed of chondrocytes that undergo apoptosis after preparing the matrix for calcification. New bone subsequently forms along the scaffolding formed by these chondrocytes, leading to longitudinal growth.

- 最靠近干骺端的区域被称为临时钙化区，由软骨细胞组成，软骨细胞在为骨化准备基质后发生凋亡。随后，新的骨骼沿着这些软骨细胞形成的支架生长，从而导致纵向生长。

Salter Harris classification

Salter Harris 分类

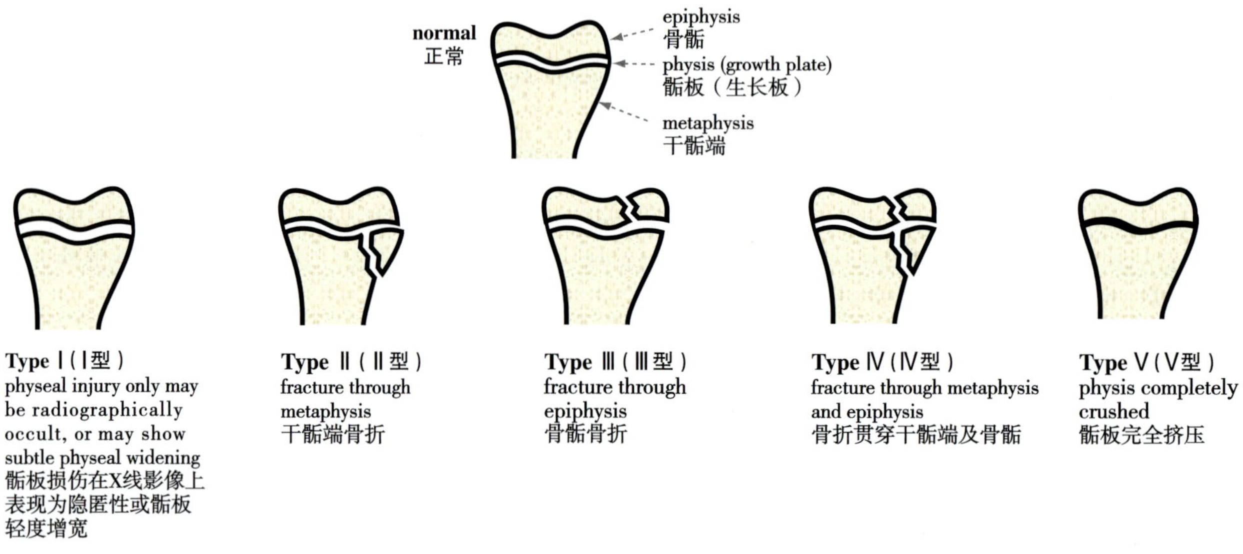

- The unfused physis is the weakest part of the developing skeleton. An injury that can cause a ligament sprain in an adult may result in physeal fracture in a child.
- The Salter Harris (SH) system classifies physeal fractures based on involvement of physis and adjacent epiphysis and metaphysis. In general, the higher the classification, the greater the chance of growth disturbance.
- Type Ⅰ: Injury limited to the physis.

  SH Ⅰ injuries are often radiographically occult if the epiphysis is not displaced. The physis may be asymmetrically widened. In the absence of physeal widening, the diagnosis of a SH I injury can be suggested based on soft tissue swelling around the physis. Comparison views may be helpful.Examples: **Slipped capital femoral epiphysis** and **gymnast's wrist** (physeal widening caused by chronic stress on the wrist, which may mimic rickets).
- Type Ⅱ: Fracture extends to metaphysis. This is the most common type (75% of cases).

- 未闭合的骺板是骨骼发育过程中最薄弱的部位。任何创伤在成人能引起韧带扭伤就有可能在儿童中引起骺板骨折。
- Salter Harris(SH)系统是对骺板骨折进行的分类，其依据是骺板、邻近骨骺及干骺端的受累程度。一般情况下，分类级别越高，引起发育障碍的概率就越大。
- Ⅰ型：损伤局限于骺板。

  SH Ⅰ型损伤在没有移位的情况下其X线表现通常隐匿。骺板可能为非对称性增宽。如果没有出现骺板增宽，骺板周围软组织肿胀可以提示SH Ⅰ型损伤。比较不同体位的影像也可能有所帮助。例如，**股骨头骨骺滑脱**和**体操运动员的腕关节损伤**(骺板因腕关节长期受压导致增宽，表现与佝偻病类似)。
- Ⅱ型：骨折累及干骺端，这是最常见的类型(占75%)。

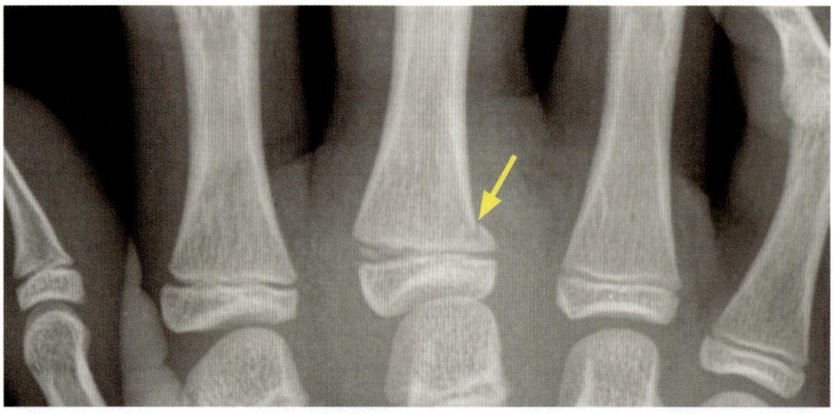

Salter Harris Ⅱ fracture:

Radiograph of the hand shows a nondisplaced fracture of the ulnar aspect of the base of the third proximal phalanx (arrow), which extends to the physis.

Case courtesy Michael Hanley, MD, University of Virginia Health System.

Salter Harris Ⅱ型骨折：手部X线影像显示第三节指骨近节基底部尺侧无移位骨折(箭)，累及干骺端骺板。

- **Type Ⅲ**: Fracture extends to epiphysis and is intra-articular.

  There is a risk for growth arrest, and surgery may be needed to maintain alignment.

  Example: **Juvenile tillaux fracture**, a distal tibial epiphyseal and physeal fracture.

- Ⅲ型：骨折延伸到骨骺，是一种关节内骨折。

  有生长停滞的风险，可能需要手术来维持准确对位。

  例如，**青少年Tillaux骨折**，即胫骨远端骨骺和骺板骨折。

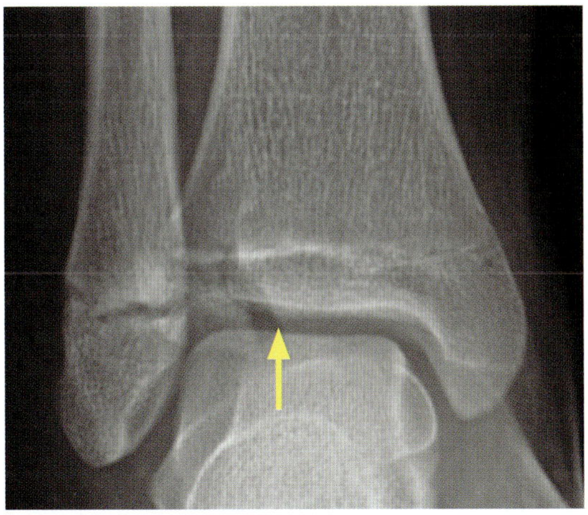

Frontal ankle radiograph shows a fracture through the lateral distal tibial epiphysis (arrow), with lateral displacement of the epiphyseal fragment.
踝关节X线影像显示胫骨远端外侧骨骺骨折(箭)，伴有骨骺碎片向外侧移位。

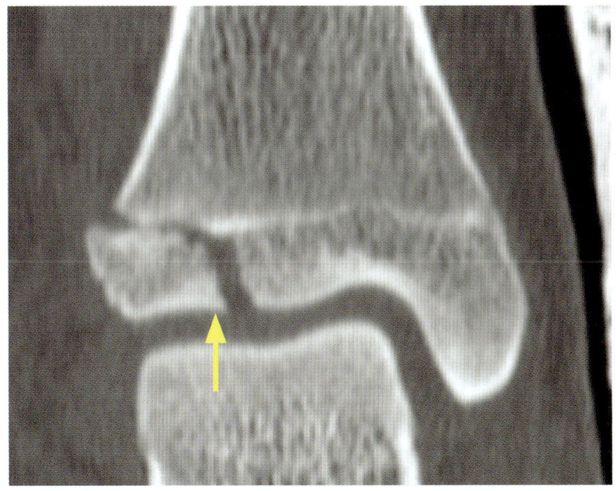

Coronal CT confirms the longitudinal fracture through the lateral distal tibial epiphysis (arrow), with lateral displacement of the epiphyseal fragment.
冠状位CT骨重建证实胫骨远端骨骺纵行骨折，伴骨骺碎片向外侧移位。

- Type Ⅳ: Fracture goes through metaphysis, physis, and epiphysis.

  These fractures often result in growth arrest or focal fusion; reduction and surgery is frequently required.

  Example: **Triplane fracture**, comprised of three fractures of the distal tibia: Oblique fracture through the metaphysis, vertical fracture through the epiphysis, and horizontal fracture through the physis.

- Ⅳ型：骨折通过干骺端、骺板和骨骺。

  这类骨折常导致生长停滞或局部融合，通常需要复位和手术治疗。

  例如，胫骨**三平面骨折**，是由胫骨远端三种骨折组成：干骺端的斜行骨折、骨骺的垂直骨折和骺板的水平骨折。

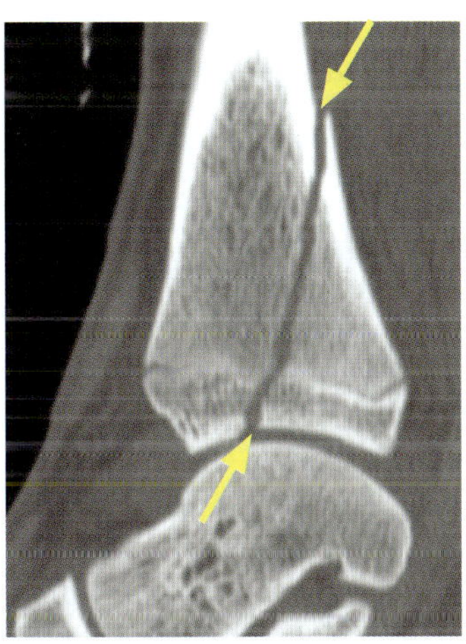

Sagittal ankle CT shows an oblique Salter Ⅳ fracture through the distal tibial metaphysis, physis, and epiphysis (arrows).
踝关节矢状位CT显示一处斜行Salter Ⅳ型骨折，骨折线通过胫骨远端干骺端、骺板和骨骺(箭)。

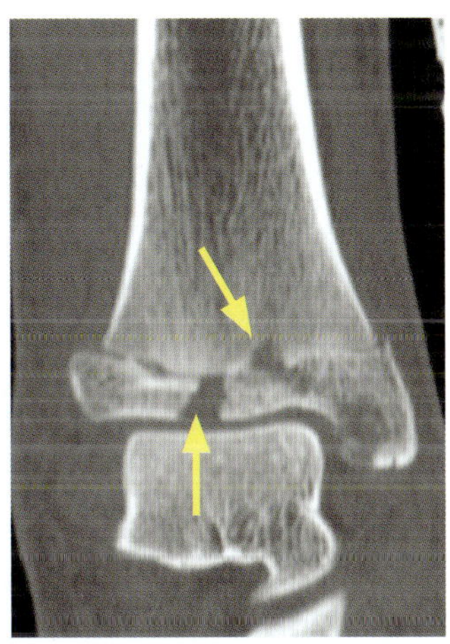

Coronal ankle CT shows a complex injury to the epiphysis including a vertical component and lateral displacement of the epiphyseal fragment.
踝关节冠状位CT显示复杂的骨骺损伤，包括垂直性骨折和侧移位的骨片。踝关节冠状位CT显示骨骺复合损伤，包括一个垂直部分和横向位移的骨骺碎片。

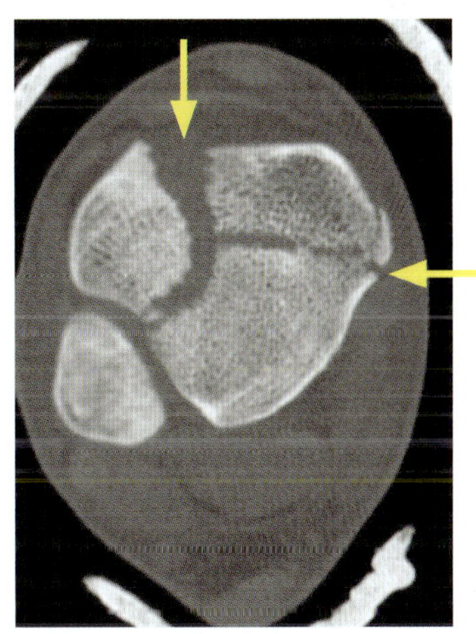

Axial CT through the level of the physis shows two perpendicular horizontal epiphyseal fractures.
经骺板轴位CT显示骨骺有两条相互垂直交叉的骨折线。

- Type V: Physis is crushed.

  The injury mechanism is often from axial loading. These fractures are easy to miss, and often found in retrospect from prior comparison studies. Comparison views may be helpful if clinical suspicion is high.Prognosis is very poor.

- Mnemonic: **SALTR**

  Slip or straight across the physis

  Above the physis

  Lower or below the physis

  Through the metaphysis, physis and epiphysis

  Ruined or Rammed crush injury to the physis

- Alternative mnemonic: **SMETC**

  Slip

  Metaphysis

  Epiphysis

  Through

  Crushed

Pediatric elbow

- Six separate ossification centers, each appearing at different stages of development, make evaluation of the pediatric elbow challenging. However, the cartilaginous ossification centers generally ossify in the same order, which can be remembered with the mnemonic **CRITOE** and approximate age at ossification in sequential odd numbers (1, 3, 5, 7, 9, 11):

- V型：骺板挤压。

  损伤机制多为轴向负荷所致。此类骨折很容易漏诊，常需与既往的影像进行对比。如临床有高度怀疑，对比影像可能会有帮助。这类骨折预后非常差。

- 记忆口诀一：**SALTR**

  S，滑移或直接通过骺板

  A，骺板以上

  L，下方或低于骺板

  T，通过干骺端、骺板和骨骺

  R，骺板毁损或挤压

- 记忆口诀二：**SMETC**

  S，滑移

  M，干骺端

  E，骨骺

  T，通过

  C，挤压

小儿肘关节

- 小儿肘关节共有六个独立的骨化中心，每个出现在不同的发育阶段，使小儿肘关节的评估具有挑战性。然而，软骨骨化中心总是以相同的顺序出现，这可以用**CRITOE**来帮助记忆，且以奇数序列的近似年龄出现骨化(1、3、5、7、9、11)。

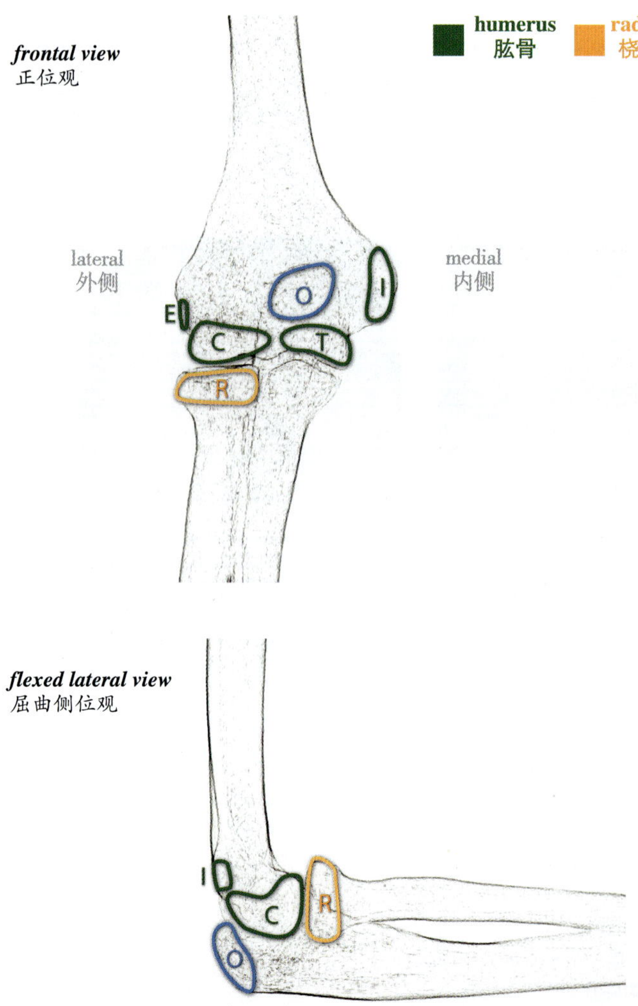

humerus 肱骨　**radius** 桡骨　**ulna** 尺骨

C: capitellum: articular surface of the distal humerus
articulates with the radial head
typically ossifies between 6 months and 1 year of age

C: 肱骨小头：肱骨远端关节面
与桡骨头构成关节
骨化常发生在6月龄~1岁

R: radial head
articulates with the capitellum
3~4 years of age

R: 桡骨小头
与肱骨小头构成关节
在3~4岁骨化

I: internal(medial)epicondyle
attachment of ulnar collateral ligament
5~6 years of age

I: 内上（内侧）髁（内侧）
尺侧副韧带附着处
5~6岁骨化

T: trochlea: articular surface of the distal humerus
articulates with the olecranon
7~8 years of age

T: 滑车：肱骨远端关节面
与鹰嘴构成关节
7~8岁骨化

O: olecranon: proximal ulna
articulates with the trochlea
9~10 years of age

O: 尺骨鹰嘴：近端尺骨
与滑车构成关节
9~10岁间骨化

E: external(lateral)epicondyle
attachment of radial collateral ligament
11~12 years, typically between 10 to 14 years of age

E: 外上（外侧）髁
桡侧副韧带附着处
11~12岁，常在10~14岁骨化

- An elbow effusion, as evidenced by displacement of the anterior and/or posterior fat pads (posterior more sensitive), is highly suggestive of a fracture, even if no fracture is visible.

  The anterior fat pad is normally visible as a thin linear lucency at the distal humerus.

  The posterior fat pad is not normally visible and when present indicates joint effusion.

- 肘关节腔积液表现为肘关节前方和/或后方脂肪垫移位(后方脂肪垫的移位更敏感)，并高度提示骨折，即使没有看见骨折线。

  前脂肪垫常表现为肱骨远端一处细线样的透亮区。

  后脂肪垫通常看不到，一旦出现则提示关节积液。

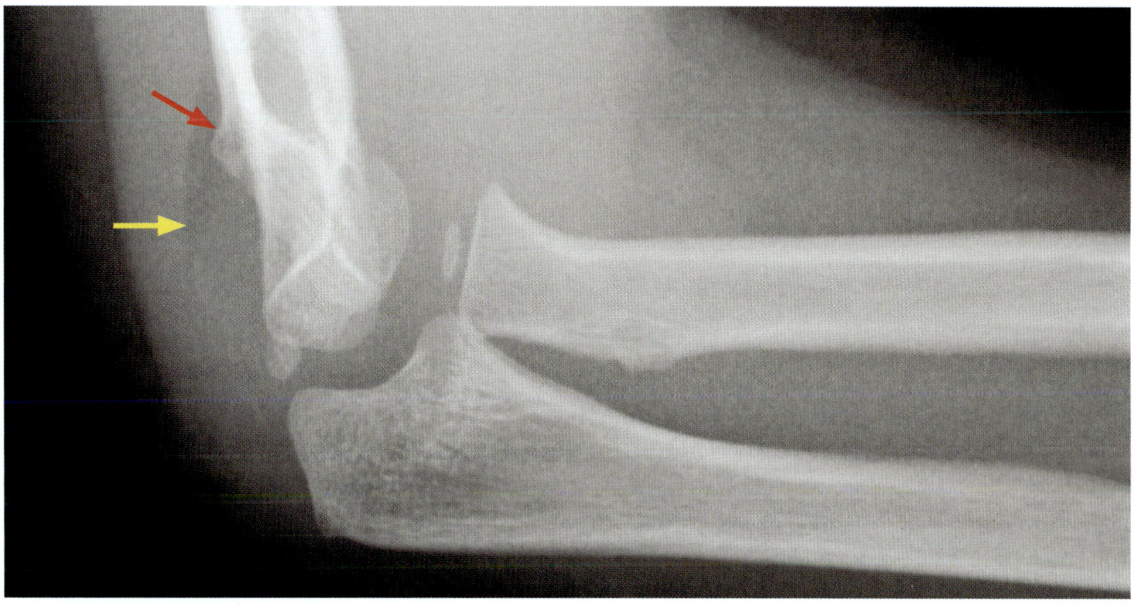

Lateral radiograph of the elbow shows a posterior *fat pad sign* indicative of an elbow effusion (yellow arrow). Bony protuberance along the posterior humerus (red arrow) represents a supracondylar fracture.

侧位肘关节X线影像显示后脂肪垫征，提示肘关节腔积液(黄箭)。沿肱骨后缘的骨性突起(红箭)即为肱骨髁上骨折。

- The elbow alignment is evaluated with the anterior humeral and radiocapitellar lines.

Anterior humeral line: Drawn along the anterior humeral cortex, the anterior humeral line should pass through the middle of the ossified capitellum on the lateral view. If abnormal, suggests supracondylar fracture.

Radiocapitellar line: Drawn through the radial shaft, the radiocapitellar line should pass through the capitellum on all views. If abnormal, suggests elbow dislocation or a nursemaid's elbow.

- 肘关节对位与否需通过肱骨前线和肱桡线进行评估。

肱骨前线：沿肱骨前方皮质画一条线，此线需在侧位片上通过肱骨小头骨骺中心的中央。如果出现异常，提示肱骨髁上骨折。

肱桡线：通过桡骨骨干画一条线，此线在各个体位上都应通过肱骨小头。若有异常，提示肘关节脱位或保姆肘。

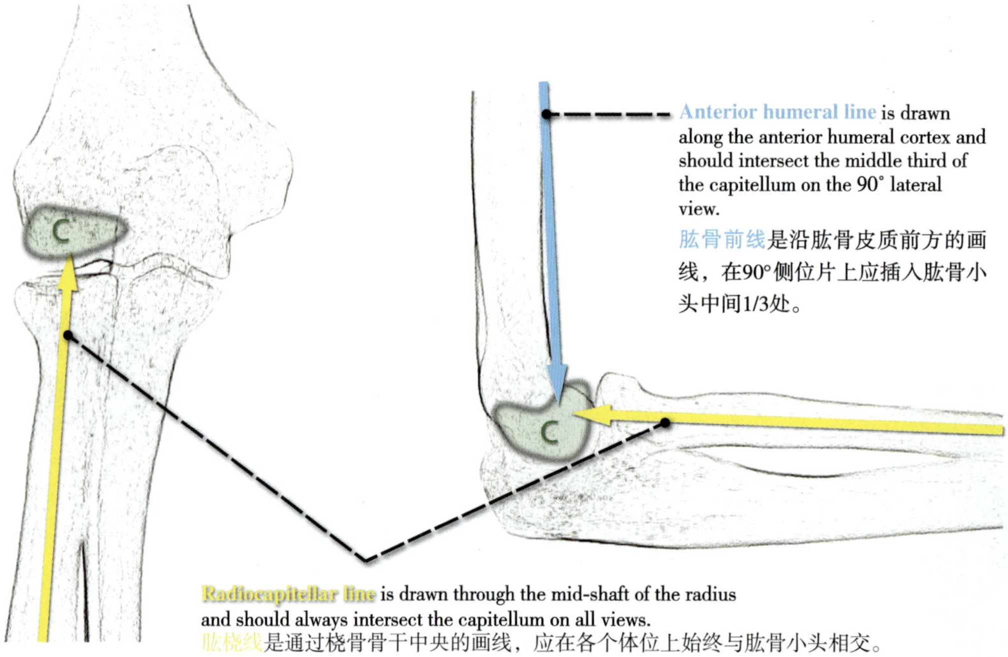

- Supracondylar humerus fracture is the most common pediatric elbow fracture.

  Lateral condyle fracture is the second most common fracture, followed by medial epicondyle avulsion.

  In contrast, the most common adult elbow fracture is of the radial head.

- 肱骨髁上骨折是小儿肘关节最常见的骨折。

  外上髁骨折是第二常见的骨折，其次是内上髁撕脱性骨折。

  相比之下，桡骨头骨折是成人肘关节最常见的骨折。

Radial buckle fracture

桡骨翘曲变形骨折

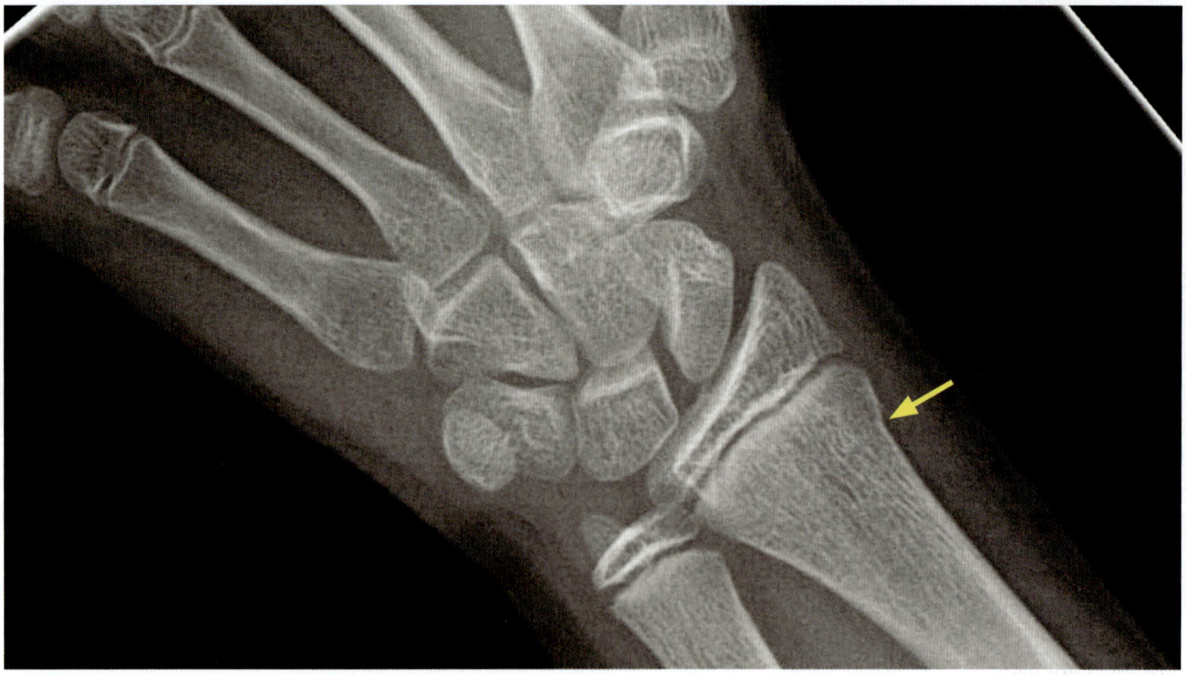

Distal radial buckle fracture: Frontal wrist radiograph demonstrates subtle irregularity and angulation of the distal radial cortex (arrow), representing an angled buckle fracture.
桡骨远端翘曲变形骨折：正位腕关节X线影像显示桡骨远端骨皮质极轻微的不规则及成角（箭），提示为翘曲变形骨折。

- Buckle fractures are unique to the pediatric skeleton, representing a buckling of cortex rather than a cortical discontinuity.
- Buckle fractures can be subtle on imaging and sometimes are only detected

- 翘曲变形骨折只发生在小儿的骨骼，为骨皮质扭曲变形而不是皮质断裂。
- 翘曲变形骨折在影像上不明显，有时只能通过

by careful inspection of the cortex. Normally, the cortex should be so smooth that a virtual marble can roll down the cortex without bouncing off. Any focal cortical irregularity in a child should raise concern for a buckle fracture.

对骨皮质的仔细观察才能发现。正常情况下骨皮质应非常光滑，甚至可以想象成一个大理石玻璃球沿着骨皮质滚动而不应出现任何颠簸。如果发现小儿骨皮质有任何局部不规则改变，都应怀疑存在翘曲变形骨折的可能性。

Toddler's fracture

学步儿童骨折

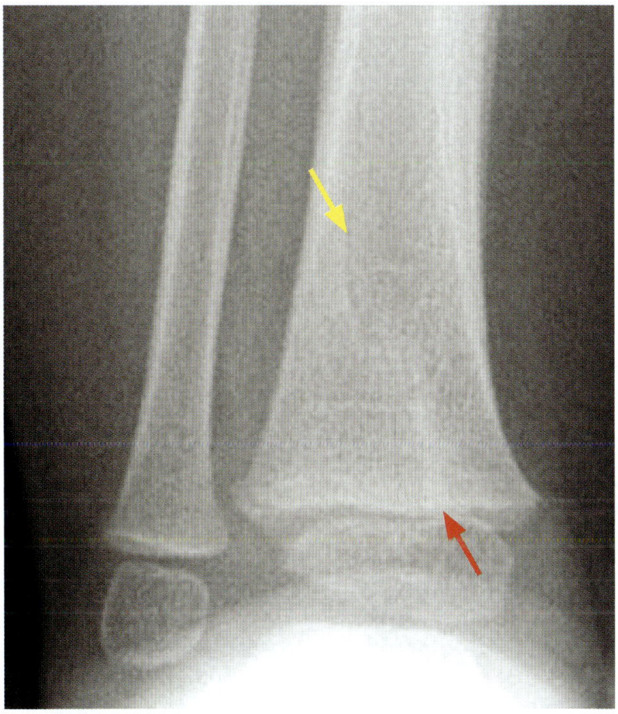

Toddler's fracture: Frontal radiograph of the lower leg shows a spiral lucent line through the distal tibia (yellow arrow), with a sclerotic component extending to the epiphysis (red arrow).

学步儿童骨折：下肢正位X线影像可见一处螺旋形的线状透亮影，它通过胫骨远端（黄箭），并在延伸至骺板时有硬化（红箭）。

- Toddler's fracture is a nondisplaced oblique fracture through the tibial metadiaphysis, caused by a rotational force to the leg. It typically occurs in toddlers as they learn how to walk.
- Toddler's fracture may be clinically difficult to diagnose. Oblique views significantly increase sensitivity.
- Radiograph shows a hairline spiral lucency through the distal tibia.
- Nondisplaced fractures of the cuboid and calcaneus represent variant toddler's fracture and can be subtle, manifesting as faint radiodense bands. This typically reflects superimposition of trabeculae rather than fracture.

- 学步儿童骨折是一种非移位性的斜形胫骨骨折，由腿部旋转过猛所致。这种骨折常发生在幼儿学步期间。
- 学步儿童骨折在临床上诊断可能有困难。斜位片能明显提高其敏感性。
- X线影像表现为胫骨远端头发丝样的螺旋透亮影。
- 骰骨和跟骨的无移位骨折属于变异型学步儿童骨折，表现为一种轻微的骨质内致密带。这通常代表重叠的骨小梁，而不是骨折。

Pelvic apophyseal avulsion injuries

- An apophysis is an ossification center at a site of tendinous attachment; it is a growth plate that does not contribute to longitudinal growth. There are 5 pelvic apophyses and two proximal femoral apophyses, which arise in puberty and fuse by the third decade. The apophyses are the weakest link of the myotendinous unit. Pelvic apophyses close relatively late in skeletal development and are therefore susceptible to avulsion. Apophyseal avulsion fractures occur most commonly in athletic adolescents, who have strong muscles and open apophyses.
- Acute injuries appear as an avulsed bone fragment. Subacute avulsions are more complex appearing, as the donor site may undergo mixed lytic and sclerotic change. This can have an aggressive appearance.
- Avulsion injuries may be subtle as they are Salter-Harris I equivalent fractures. There is often minimal or no displacement of the otherwise normal-appearing

骨盆骨突撕脱伤

- 骨突是韧带附着处的骨化中心，它是一个不参与纵向生长的生长板。骨盆有5个骨突，近段股骨有2个，它们在青春期出现，在30岁时融合。骨突是肌腱连接最薄弱的部位。骨盆骨突在骨骼发育过程中骨骺闭合相对较晚，因此容易造成撕脱。骨突撕脱性骨折大部分发生于青少年运动员，他们的肌肉强壮但骨突尚未闭合。
- 急性损伤表现为一个撕脱的骨片。亚急性撕脱伤的表现较为复杂，因为撕脱处可能会出现溶骨和成骨并存的情况。可类似与于侵袭性改变。
- 撕脱伤可能很轻微，相当于Salter Harris I型骨

apophyseal ossification.

折。这类骨折很小，甚至不会发生错位，而附着的骨化中心看似正常。

attachment of muscles to pelvic apophyses

- Iliac crest apophysis:
  Abdominal muscles.
- Anterior superior iliac spine (ASIS):
  Sartorius.
- Anterior inferior iliac spine (AIIS):
  Rectus femoris.
- Ischial tuberosity apophysis:
  Hamstrings.
- Pubic ramus:
  Hip adductors and gracilis.

attachment of muscles to femoral apophyses

- Greater trochanter:
  Gluteus medius and minimus.
- Lesser trochanter:
  Iliopsoas.

骨盆骨突附着处肌肉

- 髂嵴骨突：
  腹部肌肉。
- 髂前上棘(ASIS)：
  缝匠肌。
- 髂前下棘(AIIS)：
  股直肌。
- 坐骨结节：
  腘绳肌。
- 耻骨支：
  股内收肌和股薄肌。

股骨骨突附着处肌肉

- 大转子：
  臀大肌和臀小肌。
- 小转子：
  髂腰肌。

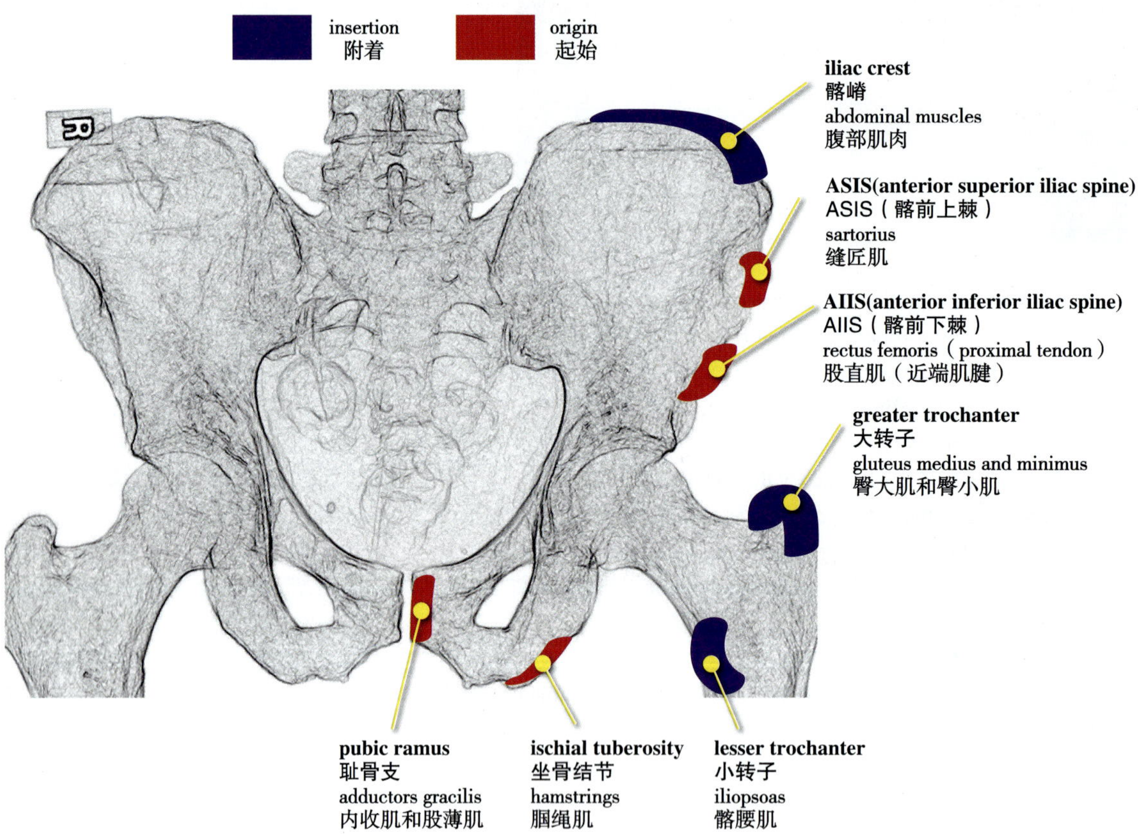

- Although a lesser trochanter avulsion may occur in an athletic adolescent due to avulsion of the iliopsoas insertion, in an adult a lesser trochanteric fracture is suspicious for a pathologic fracture.

- 股骨头小转子撕脱性骨折可出现在青少年运动员，由髂腰肌附着处撕脱引起，成人的小转子骨折需怀疑病理性骨折。

CHILD ABUSE / NON-ACCIDENTAL TRAUMA (NAT)

Overview of imaging for child abuse

- If there is clinical or radiographic concern for child abuse, a complete skeletal survey using high-resolution bone technique (for children under two years of age) should be performed, including frontal views of all long bones, rib views with obliques, skull, pelvis, hands/feet, and entire spine. The images are reviewed by the radiologist while the child is still in the department.
- Bone scintigraphy is more sensitive for posterior rib fractures, but has higher radiation dose than radiography, is insensitive for skull fractures, and cannot evaluate fracture morphology for age.
- The age of fractures is estimated by the presence of callus formation. In general, a fracture is less than two weeks old if there is no callus, and at least one week old if there is callus.

  These estimates are rough guidelines. A younger child will form callus and heal more quickly.

  The speed of healing is also altered in the setting of malnourishment, which sometimes accompanies neglect and/or abuse.

Highly specific fractures (but not the most common fractures)

- These fractures are highly specific for child abuse. If any of these fractures are seen, immediate concern must be raised for child abuse.

highly specific fractures for child abuse

- **Classic metaphyseal lesion** (also called metaphyseal corner fracture or bucket handle fracture) is highly specific for abuse, and is a circumferential fracture through the peripheral spongiosa bone of the distal metaphysis, most commonly around the knee or ankle. A classic metaphyseal lesion is thought to be due to violent shaking or forceful pulling.

  The classic metaphyseal lesion typically heals quickly (within 10 days) without callus formation, so prompt radiography is essential for diagnosis.
- **Posterior rib fracture** is also highly specific for abuse as a result of squeezing injury, but may be very difficult to diagnose when acute. A repeat chest radiograph with bone technique can be performed in the acute setting, or follow-up radiograph after one week to view interval callus formation.

  Unlike in adults, rib fractures are not typically seen after CPR in children. In the rare case of rib fractures from CPR, fractures tend to be anterior and lateral, not posterior.
- **Scapula fracture.**
- **Sternum fracture.**
- **Spinous process fracture.**

Suspicious fractures (but not highly specific)

- These fractures should raise suspicion for child abuse, but are not highly specific.
- **More than one fracture.**
- **Fractures that are discordant with the clinical history.**
- **Digital fracture in infants.**
- **Long bone fracture in non-ambulatory child.**
- **Complex skull fractures that are depressed, multiple, bilateral or crossing sutures.**

虐童/非意外创性外伤(NAT)

虐童影像概述

- 如果临床或放射影像上怀疑有虐童的可能，应进行全面骨骼检查并使用骨高分辨技术(针对2岁以下的儿童)，包括所有长骨的正位影像、肋骨斜位、颅骨、骨盆、手、足及整个脊柱。在可疑的受虐儿童还未离开放射科前放射医师应对影像进行审阅检查。
- 核素骨显像对诊断后部肋骨骨折更敏感，但辐射剂量比X线高，对颅骨骨折不敏感，且不能评估陈旧性骨折的形态。
- 骨折期龄可以通过是否有骨痂形成进行估计。一般情况下，如果没有骨痂形成，则骨折时间不到2周，如果有骨痂，则骨折时间至少1周。

  以上估计是大致的原则。儿童年龄越小，骨痂形成和愈合越快。

  在营养不良的情况下，骨折愈合速度也会改变，有时伴随着照管不良和/或虐待。

高度特异性骨折(但不是最常见的骨折)

- 这些骨折对于虐童具有高度特异性，但不常见。如果发现这些骨折中的任何一种，应立即怀疑为虐童。

虐童高度特异性骨折

- **典型的干骺端病变**(也称干骺端骨折或桶柄状骨折)对诊断儿童虐待有高度特异性，是一种通过远端干骺端骨松质外周的环形骨折，最常发生于膝关节或踝关节附近。典型的干骺端损伤被认为是由于剧烈摇晃或猛拉所致。

  典型的干骺端损伤通常愈合很快(在10天之内)，没有骨痂形成，所以及时进行X线检查对于诊断非常重要。
- **后部肋骨骨折**对诊断虐童也有高度特异性，这是由挤压伤所致，但急性期诊断可能非常困难。对此，在急性期应采用骨骼显像技术重新进行胸部摄片，或1周后进行X线随访观察是否有骨痂形成。

  不同于成人，儿童心肺复苏后肋骨骨折不常见。即使有罕见心肺复苏后的肋骨骨折，也常发生在前肋和侧肋，而不是后肋。
- **肩胛骨骨折。**
- **胸骨骨折。**
- **脊柱棘突骨折。**

可疑骨折(但没有高度特异性)

- 这些骨折应怀疑虐童，但缺乏高度特异性。
- **多于一处的骨折。**
- **骨折不符合临床病史。**
- **婴儿手指骨折。**
- **长骨骨折出现在尚未走路的儿童。**
- **复杂性颅骨骨折，包括下陷、多发、双侧或跨越颅缝。**

Nonspecific (but frequently seen)

- These fractures are commonly seen, both in the setting of child abuse and accidental trauma, but are not specific for child abuse when seen in isolation.
- **Linear skull fracture**.
- **Long bone fracture in ambulatory child**.

非特异性(但常见)

- 这些骨折无论是在虐童还是意外创伤都常见，但在孤立的情况下，这些骨折对诊断虐童不具特异性。
- **线性颅骨骨折**。
- **学步儿童的长骨骨折**。

PEDIATRIC HIP

小儿髋部

Developmental dysplasia of the hip (DDH)

- Developmental dysplasia of the hip (DDH) is incongruent development of the femoral head- acetabular relationship. An abnormally shallow acetabular angle results in uncovering of the femoral head by the acetabulum. There is an increased incidence of DDH in breech births, so all breech births are typically screened by ultrasound.

  DDH is more commonly seen with oligohydramnios, firstborn infants, girls, and positive family history.
- Physical examination findings include limited range of motion, hip "click" or "clunk", gluteal or thigh fold asymmetry, and unequal leg lengths.
- Ultrasound is generally performed at or after 6 weeks of age. Imaging is delayed because of the effects of perinatal maternal hormones on neonatal ligamentous laxity.

  The **alpha angle** is the angle formed by the bony ilium and acetabular roof, obtained from the coronal hip ultrasound. A normal alpha angle is greater than 60 degrees. The bony portion of the acetabular roof should cover at least 50% of the cartilaginous femoral head. An alpha angle <60 degrees or <50% coverage of the femoral head by acetabulum is abnormal, suggesting DDH.

发育性髋关节发育不良(DDH)

- 发育性髋关节发育不良(DDH)是指股骨头与髋臼之间的发育不平衡。髋臼角异常变浅会导致髋臼不能覆盖股骨头。臀位分娩会增加DDH发病率，因而臀位出生的婴儿常用超声进行筛查。

  DDH更常见于羊水过少、头胎、女婴、女童及有家族史的儿童。
- 体格检查发现包括活动受限，髋部"弹响"或"碰撞"，臀部或大腿皮纹不对称，腿部长度不等。
- 超声检查通常在6周或6周后进行。影像检查推迟，是由于围产期孕产妇激素会使新生儿的关节韧带变得松弛。

  α角是由髂骨和髋臼顶形成的角度，使用超声在冠状位对髋关节进行测量。正常α角>60°，也就是髋臼顶骨性部分应该至少覆盖50%的股骨头软骨。α角<60°或髋臼对股骨头软骨的覆盖<50%为异常，提示DDH。

hip dysplasia: same coronal image with different annotations
髋关节发育不良：相同的冠状位图像，采用不同的注解
alpha angle <60 degrees, femoral head <50% covered by bony acetabulum
α角<60°，髋臼骨性部分覆盖股骨头的范围小于50%

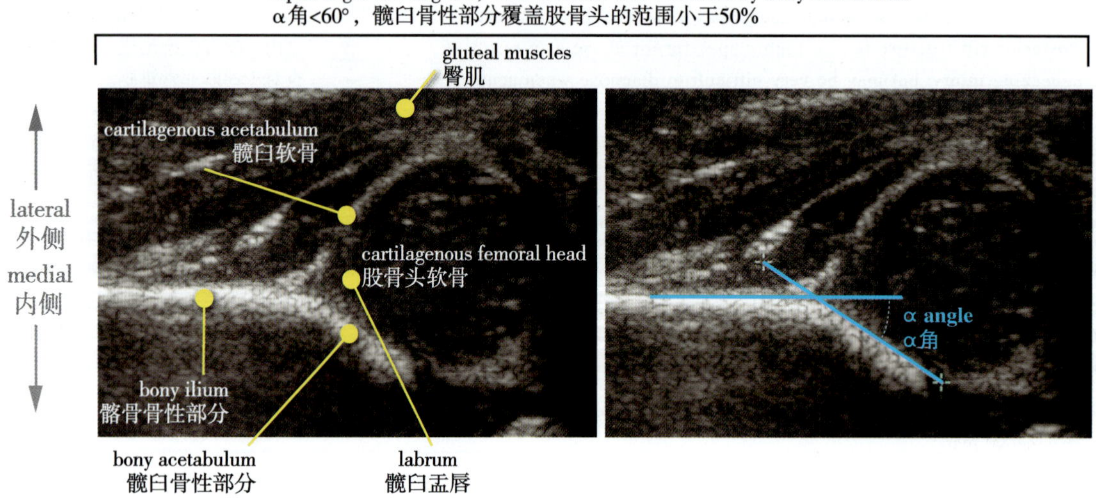

- After femoral head ossification (typically after 6 months of age) radiographs are performed.

  On pelvic radiography, the ossified femoral head should normally sit in the inner lower quadrant formed by the intersection of the **Hilgenreiner** and **Perkins lines**.

  The **acetabular angle** (white), drawn through the acetabular roof and Hilgenreiner line, is typically under 30 degrees at birth, and decreases to about 20 degrees or less by age two years.

- X线检查应在股骨头骨化后(通常在6个月后)进行。

  在骨盆X线影像上，骨化的股骨头正常应位于由**Hilgenreiner**和**Perkins线**相交的内下1/4象限内。

  髋臼角(白色)是穿过髋臼顶和Hilgenreine线形成的夹角，在出生时一般在30°以下，并在2岁后下降到大约20°或更小。

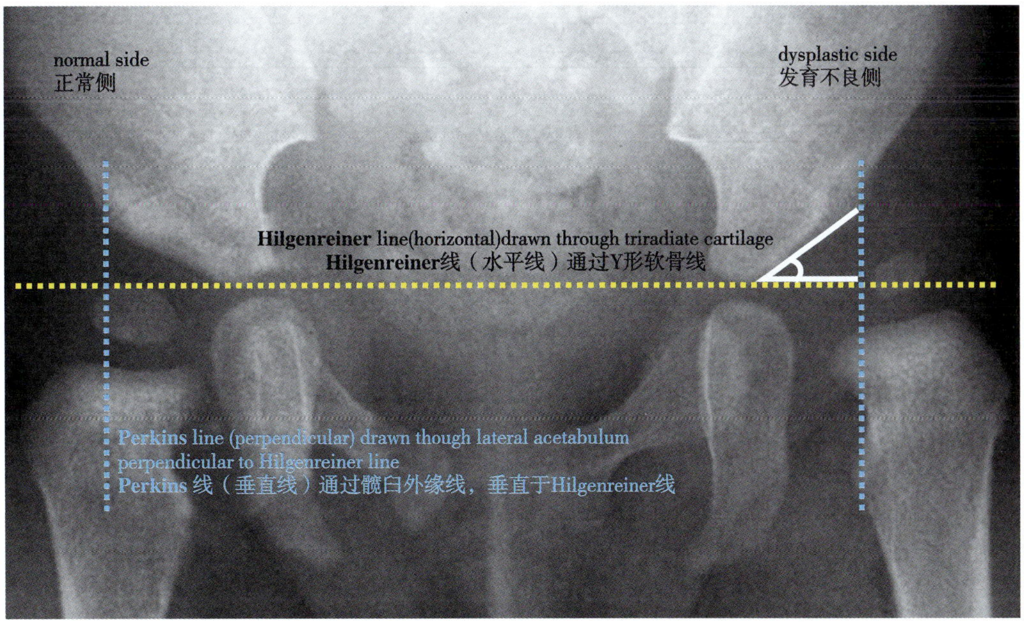

Overview of child with limp

- A limp (abnormal gait pattern caused by pain) should be carefully evaluated and may be secondary to trauma, septic arthritis, chronic fracture, avascular necrosis, or lymphoma.

Septic hip arthritis

- Infection of the synovium and joint space is an orthopedic emergency as joint destruction and growth arrest may occur without prompt washout and antibiotics.
- Any hip effusion must be urgently aspirated to evaluate for septic arthritis.
- The primary differential consideration for septic arthritis is aseptic transient synovitis, which is a self-limited diagnosis of exclusion and typically seen in children 3–8 years old following a viral infection. Less common causes of hip effusion and limp include hemarthrosis in trauma or hemophilia (history is usually evident).
- Septic arthritis is usually secondary to hematogenously seeded metaphyseal osteomyelitis that breaks through the periosteum to infect the joint capsule. *S. aureus* is the most common cause. The hip is the second most commonly affected joint, following the knee.
- Plain film findings are not sensitive or reliable for evaluation of effusion, but include:

  Displacement or distortion of gluteal or psoas fat planes. The gluteus medius and minimus insert on the greater trochanter. The psoas inserts on the lesser trochanter.

  Widening of the *teardrop* distance (space between the lateral margin of the pelvic *teardrop* and the medial margin of the femoral head). The *teardrop* is the antero inferior acetabulum.

小儿跛行概述

- 跛行(由疼痛引起的步态异常)应仔细对其进行评估，它可能继发于创伤、化脓性关节炎、慢性骨折、缺血性坏死或淋巴瘤。

化脓性髋关节炎

- 滑膜和关节腔感染是一种骨科急症，如不及时进行关节腔清洗和使用抗生素，可能会导致关节破坏和生长停滞。
- 任何髋关节积液都应进行紧急抽液化验，以判断是否为化脓性关节炎。
- 与化脓性关节炎的主要鉴别诊断是一过性无菌性滑膜炎，后者是一种自限性排除性诊断，常见于3~8岁病毒感染后的儿童。一些引起髋关节积液及跛行少见的原因有外伤后继发性关节腔积血或血友病(常有明确病史)。
- 化脓性关节炎通常是继发于血源性(干骺端)骨髓炎，它可突破骨膜累及关节囊。金黄色葡萄球菌是最常见的致病菌。髋关节是最常受累的关节，其次是膝关节。
- X线影像对髋关节腔积液诊断的敏感性和可靠性均不高，其征象包括：

  臀部肌群或腰大肌脂肪层移位或变形。臀中肌和臀小肌附着于股骨大转子。腰大肌嵌入股骨小转子。

  泪滴**间距增宽**(骨盆泪滴外侧缘及股骨头内侧缘之间的间隙)。泪滴即前下髋臼。

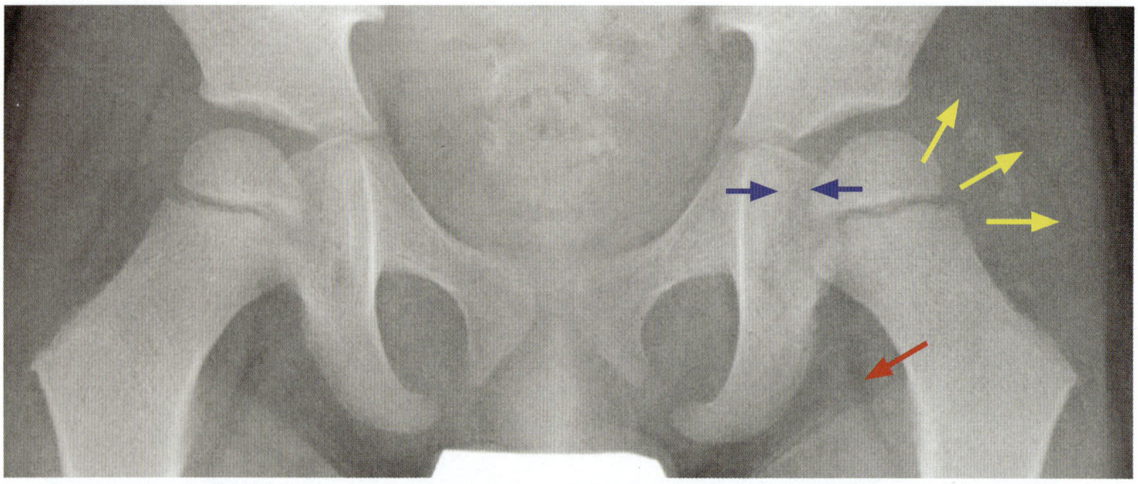

Hip effusion: AP radiograph shows lateral displacement of the left gluteal fat plane (yellow arrows) and subtle medial bowing of the psoas fat plane (red arrow). The teardrop distance (blue arrows) is not widened, emphasizing the relative insensitivity of these radiographic findings to detect effusion.
髋关节积液：正位X线影像显示左臀部脂肪层向外侧移位(黄箭)和腰大肌脂肪层轻微向内侧弯曲(红箭)。泪滴间距(蓝箭)无增宽，这些强调了影像学表现对发现髋关节腔积液相对不敏感。

- Ultrasound is the imaging modality of choice. Both sides should be compared for symmetry.

  The presence of internal echoes within an effusion does not have clinical significance.

- 超声也是一种可以选择的影像检查方法。应比较双侧是否对称。

  积液内部出现回声并没有临床意义。

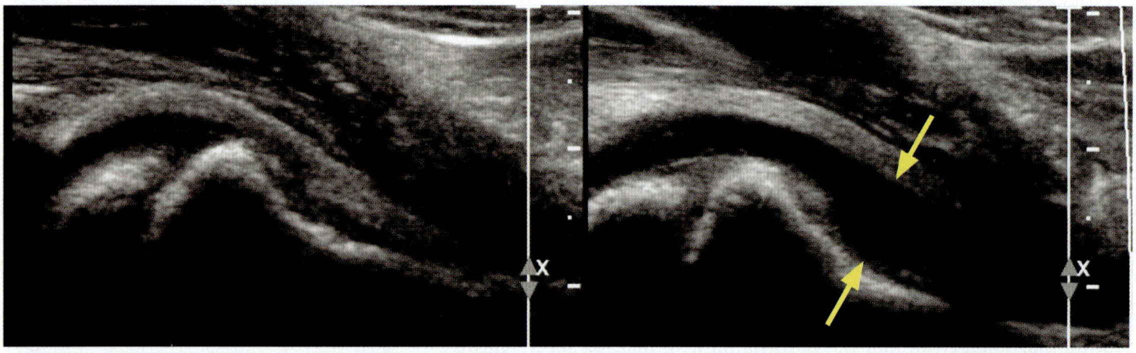

Bilateral hip ultrasound in the same patient shows increased anechoic fluid in the left hip joint (right panel; arrows) relative to the normal right hip. This child ended up having aseptic toxic synovitis, but the radiographic and ultrasound findings are identical to septic arthritis.
同一名患者的双侧髋关节超声显示较相对正常的右侧，左髋关节的无回声液体(右图，箭)增多。这名儿童最终诊断无菌性毒性滑膜炎，但是X线影像和超声影像表现与化脓性关节炎没有区别。

Legg-Calvé-Perthes (LCP)

- Legg-Calvé-Perthes (LCP) disease is avascular necrosis of the capital femoral epiphysis ossification center. LCP is of unknown etiology and typically occurs in small-sized Caucasian boys between the ages of 4 and 8 years.
- LCP is usually unilateral (80%). A systemic cause should be sought when bilateral, such as sickle cell disease or steroids.
- Imaging findings are dependent on stage and chronicity.
- **Early LCP** can be subtle, and often multiple modalities are used for initial diagnosis. Early LCP may show subtle sclerosis of the femoral head on radiography. There is typically decreased uptake on bone scan.

Legg-Calve-Perthes病(LCP)

- Legg-Calve-Perthes病(LCP)是股骨头骨骺骨化中心的缺血性坏死。LCP病因不明，常见于4~8岁的矮小高加索男童。
- LCP通常为单侧(80%)。如为双侧，必须要考虑系统疾病所致，如镰状细胞病或使用类固醇所致的疾病。
- 影像学表现取决于疾病的发展阶段和病程。
- **早期LCP**可能不易察觉，因而初次诊断时常需采用多种影像方法。早期LCP在X线影像上可表现为股骨头轻微硬化。骨扫描通常为摄取减少。

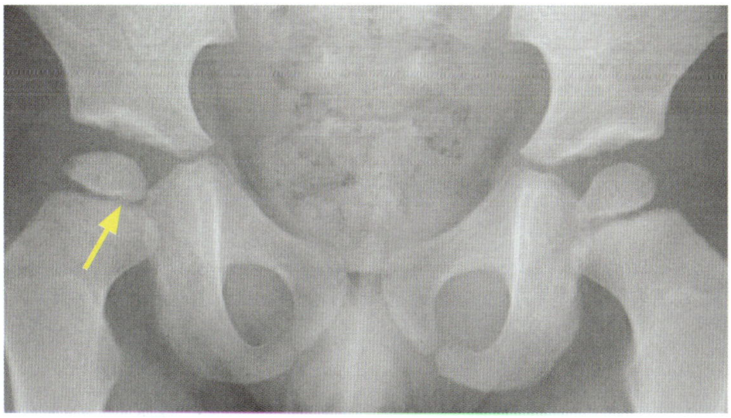

Early Legg-Calvé-Perthes. Frontal radiograph of the pelvis shows subtle irregularity and sclerosis of the inferior aspect of the right femoral epiphysis ossification center (arrow).

早期LCP：骨盆正位X线影像显示右侧股骨骨骺骨化中心下方有轻微不规则硬化(箭)。

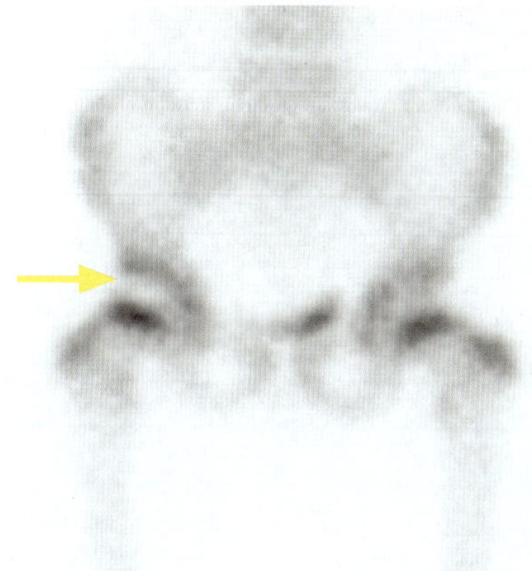

Anterior planar Tc-99m MDP bone scan in the same patient with early LCP shows a photopenic defect (arrow) in right femoral epiphysis.

同一名患儿早期LCP，前位^{99m}Tc-MDP骨扫描显示右侧股骨头骨骺放射性缺损区域(箭)。

- **Late LCP** shows secondary signs of osteonecrosis. The femoral head becomes flattened and distorted, with secondary changes of osteoarthritis. Bone scan of late LCP typically shows increased uptake due to attempted repair.

- **晚期LCP**表现为继发性股骨头坏死。股骨头变得扁平而变形，伴继发性骨关节炎。晚期LCP骨扫描通常因骨修复而表现为摄取增加。

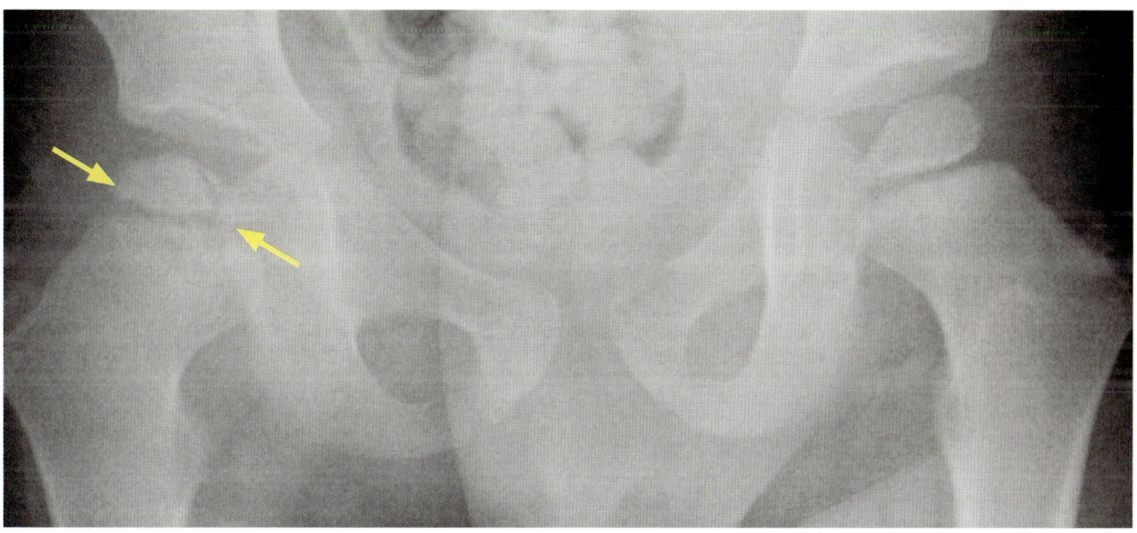

Later stage of LCP in the same patient. This follow-up slightly obliqued frontal radiograph shows increased sclerosis and irregularity of the right femoral head, with new fragmentation (arrows).

同一名患儿LCP晚期。略倾斜的正位X线随访影像显示右侧股骨头硬化和不规则更加明显，并出现新的骨碎片(箭)。

Slipped capital femoral epiphysis (SCFE)

- Slipped capital femoral epiphysis (SCFE) is a Salter I fracture of the proximal femoral epiphysis (with superolateral migration of the femoral metaphysis) classically seen in obese adolescent boys (most between ages 10–16 years). SCFE typically affects children slightly older than those with Legg-Calvé-Perthes disease.
- Initial findings on an AP view can be subtle, including asymmetric widening of the proximal femoral growth plate and lack of intersection of Klein's line with the femoral head.

  Klein's line is a line drawn along lateral margin of femoral neck, which should normally intersect the femoral head, as in the normal right hip below. A radiographic clue to SCFE is lack of intersection (or asymmetric intersection) of Klein's line with the femoral head.

股骨头骨骺滑脱(SCFE)

- 股骨头骨骺滑脱(SCFE)是一种股骨头近端骨骺的Salter Ⅰ型骨折(伴有股骨干骺端向外上方移位)，多见于肥胖的男性青少年(多数在10~16岁)。SCFE患儿年龄通常稍大于Legg-Calvé-Perthes病。
- 早期正位髋关节X线影像的表现可能很轻微，包括股骨近端生长板不对称性增宽，以及Klein线与股骨头不相交。

  Klein线是沿股骨颈外侧缘画的一条线，正常与应与股骨头相交，如下图正常的右髋。左髋的Klein线与股骨头不相交(或相交的程度不对称)，提示SCFE。

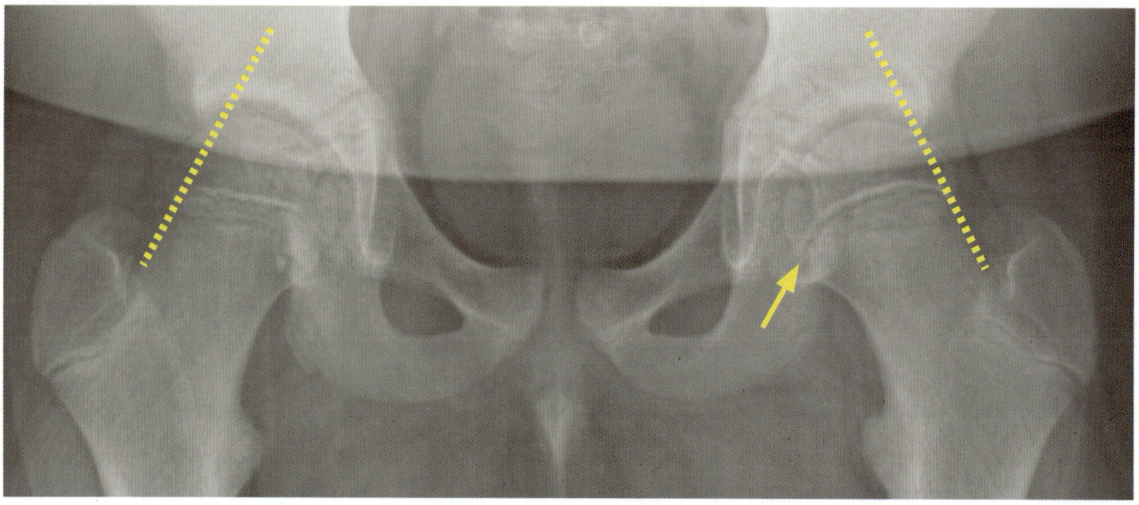

Early left SCFE: There is minimal widening of the left physis (arrow) without physeal displacement. There is minimal asymmetry in the alignment of the Klein's lines (dashed yellow lines). These findings are very subtle.
左侧早期SCFE:左侧骺板(箭)有轻微增宽,但不伴骨骺移位。双侧Klein线轻微不对称(黄虚线)。这些影像学表现非常不明显。

- Although Klein's line is drawn on the AP view, the physeal widening and displacement is best evaluated on the frog-leg lateral projection.

- 尽管Klein线是在正位影像上画的,但骺板增宽和骨骺移位在蛙式外展位片上评估最佳。

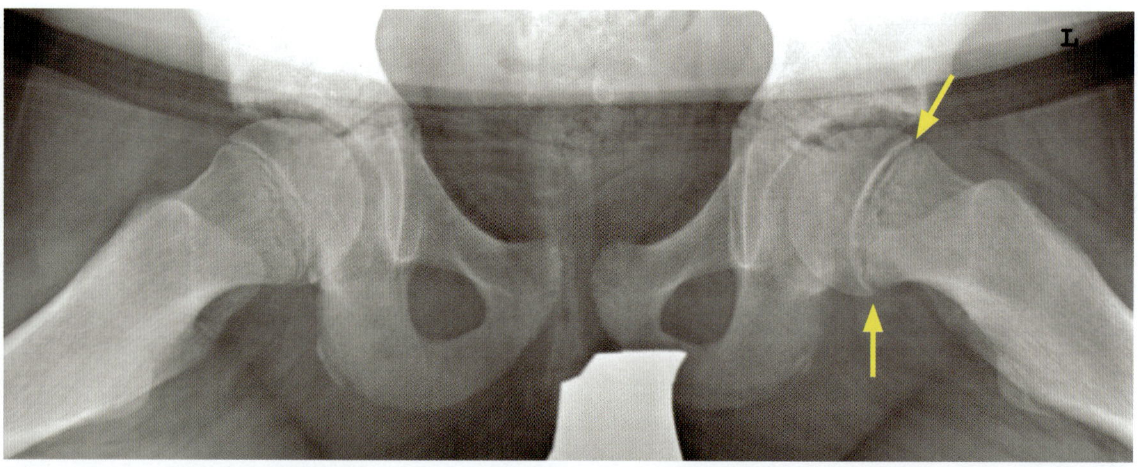

Frog leg lateral radiograph in the same patient shows very slight medial slippage of the left femoral head and more apparent physeal widening (arrows), suggesting early SCFE.
同一名患者的蛙式外展位影像显示左股骨头有非常轻微的内侧移位,以及较为明显的骺板增宽(箭),提示为早期SCFE。

- The contralateral hip should always be carefully evaluated. SCFE is frequently bilateral, and is usually asymmetric.
- The goal of imaging in SCFE is to identify "preslip" SCFE, in which the epiphysis and metaphysis remain aligned but subtle lucency of the physis suggests physeal edema. These findings are more sensitively identified on MRI.
- Osteonecrosis of the femoral head is the major complication. Treatment is screw fixation.

- 对侧髋关节必须要同时进行仔细评估,因为SCFE常为双侧且不对称。
- 影像检查目的是识别"滑脱前的"SCFE,此时骨骺和干骺端仍然保持对齐,但是骨骺存在的细微透亮影则提示骨骺水肿。这些表现在MRI上更敏感。
- 股骨头坏死是主要并发症。治疗为螺钉内固定。

Osteomyelitis

骨髓炎

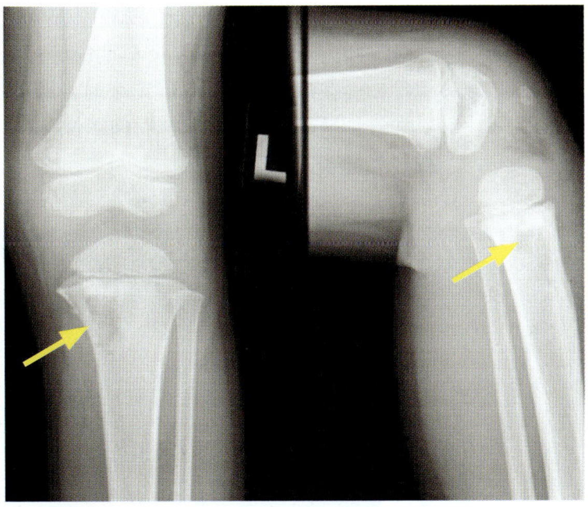

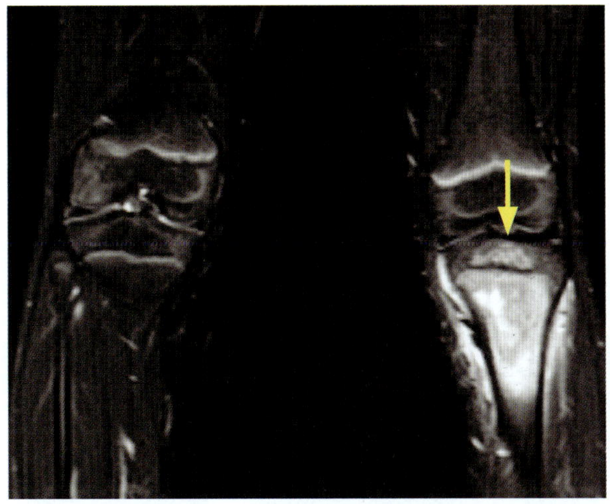

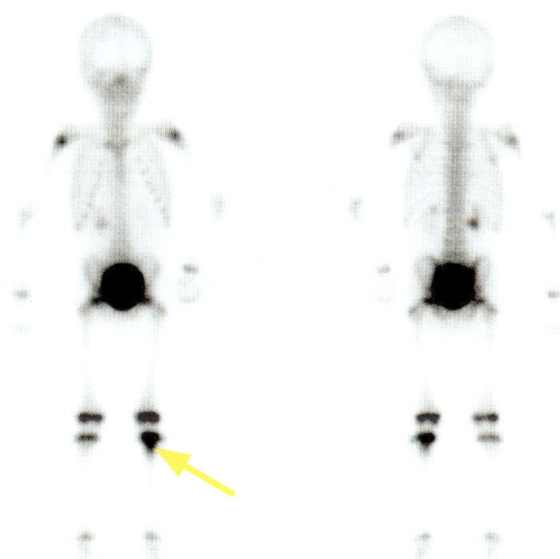

Osteomyelitis: Frontal and lateral radiographs of the knee (top left panel) show an irregular lucency (arrows) of the medial proximal tibial metaphysis. Coronal fluid-sensitive T2-weighted MRI of both knees shows extensive marrow edema of the proximal left tibial metaphysis extending across the physis into the epiphysis (arrow) and into the soft tissues. The right knee appears normal.

Anterior and posterior Tc-99m MDP bone scan (bottom left panel) shows increased proximal left tibial uptake (arrow). The bone scan was positive on all three phases (angiographic and blood pool phases not shown).

Case courtesy Michael Hanley, MD, University of Virginia Health System.

骨髓炎：膝关节正位及侧位影像(左上图)显示胫骨近端干骺端内侧不规则的透光区(箭)。

双膝关节冠状位T_2加权液体敏感序列显示左胫骨近端干骺端广泛性骨髓水肿跨越骺板，并累及骨骺(箭)和软组织。右膝关节显示正常。

前位和后位^{99m}Tc-MDP骨扫描(左下图)显示左胫骨近端摄取增加(箭)。骨骼三时相显像均呈阳性(血管和血池像未提供)。

- The initial findings of osteomyelitis are often subtle on radiography and may require a combination of plain radiographs, MRI, and scintigraphy for accurate early diagnosis.
- Osteomyelitis in children is most commonly hematogenous, with the metaphyseal marrow being the most common site of initial seeding where there is abundant blood supply.

  In infants, the epiphysis receives blood supply from transphyseal vessels arising from metaphysis, so infection can cross the physis, resulting in epiphysitis and septic arthritis.

  In older children, capillaries do not cross physis, so transphyseal extension of a metaphyseal infection is uncommon. In adults, as growth plates fuse, infection can again extend into the epiphysis.
- The most common organism implicated in hematogenous osteomyelitis is *S. aureus*, with *Salmonella* seen in sickle cell patients.
- The imaging findings on radiography, MRI, and scintigraphy (three-phase bone scan) follow the anatomic progression of infection. The initial hematogenous infection is intramedullary and then subsequently spreads through the cortex and uplifts the periosteum. The pediatric periosteum is only loosely adherent to

- 骨髓炎最初的X线征象通常不明显，故需要结合X线影像、MRI及骨扫描，才能使病变在早期得到准确诊断。
- 小儿骨髓炎最常为血源性，而干骺端骨髓腔为病原最早种植的部位，因为该部位血供最为丰富。

  在婴幼儿中，骨骺血供来源于干骺端经骺板的血管，所以感染能越过骺板，导致骨骺炎和化脓性关节炎。

  在较大儿童中，毛细血管不穿过骺板，因此干骺端感染不易跨过骺板向骨骺蔓延。在成人，随着生长板的闭合，感染可以再次蔓延到骨骺。
- 血源性骨髓炎最常见的致病菌是金黄色葡萄球菌，而沙门菌多见于镰状细胞病的患者。
- X线、MRI及骨扫描(三时相骨扫描)影像表现与感染部位的解剖及进展有关。血源性感染首先累及髓内，随后扩散至骨皮质并使骨膜隆起。儿童骨膜仅疏松地附着于骨皮质，化

bone, and the purulent infection is able to dramatically uplift the periosteum, causing a prominent periosteal reaction.

脓性感染很容易掀起骨膜，从而引起明显的骨膜反应。

- It usually takes 10–14 days for findings to become evident on radiography. The initial finding may be focal osteopenia due to hyperemia. Subsequently, a lucent, often aggressive-appearing medullary lesion can erode through the cortex and cause periosteal reaction. MRI and scintigraphy are much more sensitive for the detection of early osteomyelitis, with findings seen on bone scan within 24–72 hours of symptom onset. Osteomyelitis is further discussed in the musculoskeletal imaging section.

- X线影像通常要在10~14天后才会出现明显改变。最初X线可表现为由充血而引起的局灶性骨质疏松。随后出现透光区，通常为骨髓腔内侵袭样病灶，并可侵蚀骨皮质引起骨膜反应。MRI和闪烁显像对骨髓炎早期检测极其敏感，骨扫描在症状出现后24~72小时内即可发现异常。骨髓炎详见“骨骼与肌肉影像”一章。

Spinal osteomyelitis / discitis

脊柱骨髓炎/椎间盘炎

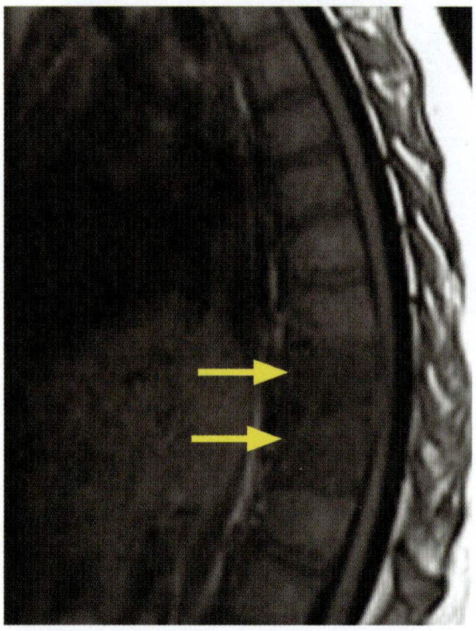

Sagittal T1-weighted MRI shows hypointense marrow signal of two adjacent vertebral bodies in the lower thoracic spine (yellow arrows).
矢状位T_1加权MRI显示下段胸椎两个相邻椎体内骨髓呈低信号(黄箭)。

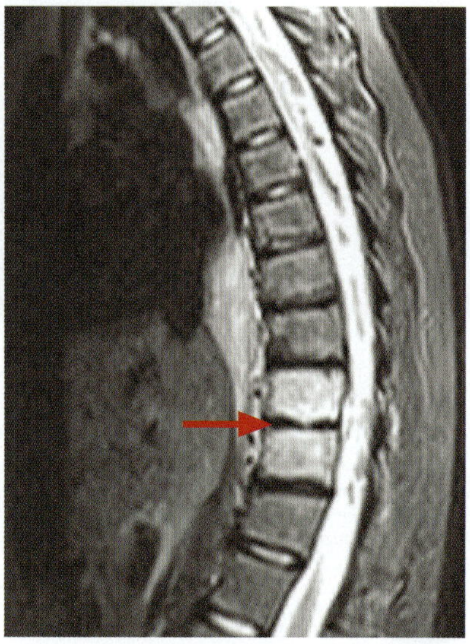

Sagittal T2-weighted fat suppressed MRI shows hyperintense marrow edema in the affected vertebral bodies with subtle focal narrowing of the disc space (red arrow).
矢状位T_2加权脂肪抑制MRI显示在受累椎体内骨髓水肿呈高信号，伴局部椎间隙轻度狭窄(红箭)。

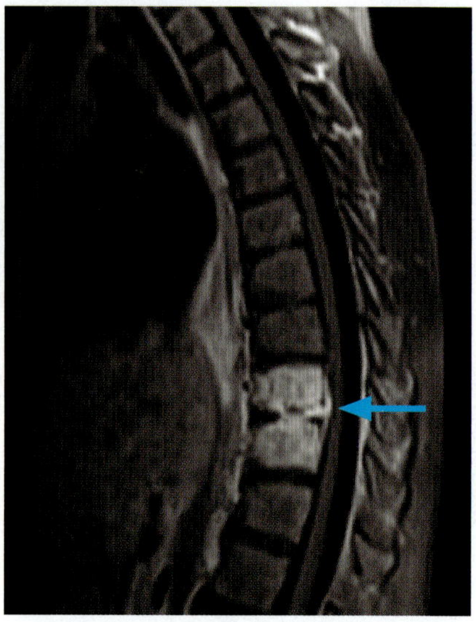

Sagittal T1-weighted post-contrast MRI with fat suppression shows avid enhancement of the affected vertebral bodies and mild epidural enhancement (blue arrow) traversing the disc space.
矢状增强位T_1加权脂肪抑制MRI显示受累椎体明显强化，以及硬膜外轻度强化(蓝箭)并跨越椎间盘。

Discitis with epidural extension. *Case courtesy Michael Hanley, MD, University of Virginia Health System.*

- Isolated discitis is unique to children, due to the presence of blood vessels directly feeding the intervertebral disc. In adults, infection can spread through the disk, but in children infection begins in the disc.
- A typical clinical history of discitis is a young child up to 4 years old with preceding upper respiratory tract infection and back pain or refusal to sit. Discitis most commonly occurs in the lumbar spine in young children.
- Less commonly, discitis may occur in pre-teen children in the thoracic spine.
- The initial radiographic findings are disc space narrowing and vertebral end plate irregularity. These findings may be subtle. Plain films may also be normal. Because persistent back pain is never normal in children, further evaluation with MRI is recommended if clinical suspicion for discitis is high.
- MRI shows narrowing of the disc space, with bone marrow edema of two adjacent vertebral bodies. The affected vertebral bodies may enhance, and enhancement and edema may extend into the soft tissues and epidural space.

- 孤立性椎间盘炎只发生于儿童，因椎间盘有直接供血动脉。在成人，感染可通过扩散进入椎间盘，而在儿童，感染则可起始于椎间盘。
- 椎间盘炎典型临床表现是年龄不到4岁的儿童，有上呼吸道感染的病史，随后继发背痛或拒绝坐下。幼儿椎间盘炎常发生于腰椎。
- 较少出现的胸椎椎间盘炎，可见于青春期前儿童。
- 最初的影像学表现是椎间隙变窄和椎板形态不规则。这些影像学表现可能不明显，X线影像也可能为正常。儿童持续性背部疼痛属于不正常现象，如果临床高度怀疑有椎间盘炎，则应该进一步进行MRI检查。
- MRI表现为椎间隙变窄，相邻两椎体骨髓水肿。受累的椎体有强化，并且强化和水肿可延伸到邻近软组织及硬膜外间隙。

Chronic recurrent multifocal osteomyelitis (CRMO)

- Chronic recurrent multifocal osteomyelitis (CRMO) is a nonpyogenic, inflammatory disorder that can mimic osteomyelitis. It tends to occur in lower extremity long bones.
- CRMO is typically a diagnosis of exclusion and is self-limited. Biopsy may need to be performed to exclude pyogenic infection.
- The key imaging finding is migratory lytic and sclerotic lesions in time and space. CRMO may be indistinguishable from pyogenic osteomyelitis on radiographs and MRI. Unlike infectious osteomyelitis, CRMO does not feature soft tissue abscess, bony sequestra, or fistula.
- CRMO is associated with **SAPHO syndrome**, characterized by:

Synovitis Acne Pustulosis	Hyperostosis Osteitis

慢性复发性多灶性骨髓炎(CRMO)

- 慢性复发性多灶性骨髓炎(CRMO)是一种非化脓性、炎性疾病，可类似于骨髓炎。常发生于下肢的长骨。
- CRMO通常是一种排除性诊断，并为自限性。可能需要活检以排除化脓性感染。
- 主要影像学表现是不同时间和部位出现游走性溶骨和硬化性病灶。CRMO在X线和MRI上可能与化脓性骨髓炎难以鉴别。与化脓性骨髓炎不同的是，CRMO没有软组织脓肿、游离死骨或瘘管等特征。
- CRMO与**SAPHO综合征**相关，有以下特点：

滑膜炎 痤疮 脓疱病	骨质增生 骨炎

TORCH infections: Syphilis

- Syphilis is caused by the spirochete *Treponema pallidum*. Syphilis can be transmitted in utero through the placenta to cause congenital syphilitic osteomyelitis.
- The *Wimberger sign* is destructive erosion of the medial aspect of the proximal tibial metaphysis. The *Wimberger sign* is not to be confused with the *Wimberger ring sign* of scurvy, which is increased density of the ossification centers.
- Syphilis is one of many causes of symmetric periosteal reaction in a child.

TORCH感染：梅毒

- 梅毒是由梅毒螺旋体感染所引起，它可以在子宫内通过胎盘传播而引起先天性梅毒骨髓炎。
- Wimberger征是指胫骨近端干骺端内侧骨质破坏性侵蚀。Wimberger征不要与维生素C缺乏病的Wimberger环征相混淆，后者骨化中心的骨质密度增高。
- 梅毒是引起小儿对称性骨膜反应的众多原因之一。

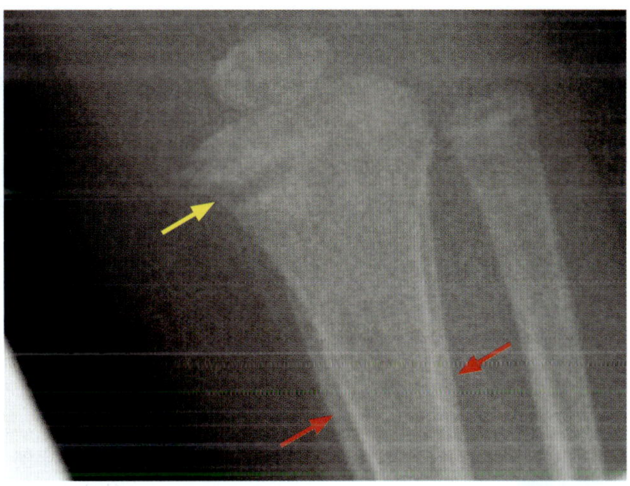

Wimberger sign in congenital syphilis:
Magnified frontal leg radiograph shows a deep erosion of the medial aspect of the proximal tibia (yellow arrow), representing the *Wimberger* sign. There is also periosteal reaction along the partially visualized tibial diaphysis (red arrows).
先天性梅毒的Wimberger征：正位放大腿部X线影像显示胫骨近端内侧一处深的骨质侵蚀(黄箭)，此为Wimberger征。另外，所见胫骨骨干有骨膜反应(红箭)。

Childhood Arthritis

Juvenile idiopathic arthritis (JIA) / juvenile rheumatoid arthritis (JRA) / juvenile chronic arthritis (JCA)

- Juvenile idiopathic arthritis (JIA), also known as juvenile rheumatoid arthritis (JRA) and juvenile chronic arthritis (JCA), is the most common chronic arthropathy of childhood. It is a systemic idiopathic disease defined as being present for more than 6 weeks in a patient younger than 16 years old. JIA is usually rheumatoid-factor negative.
- The most common subtype of JIA is pauciarticular disease, typically affecting young girls. Regardless of subtype, the knee is the most commonly affected

小儿关节炎

青少年特发性关节炎(JIA)/青少年类风湿关节炎(JRA)/青少年慢性关节炎(JCA)

- 青少年特发性关节炎(JIA)，也称青少年类风湿关节炎(JRA)和青少年慢性关节炎(JCA)，是小儿最常见的慢性关节病。它是一种系统性特发性疾病，定义为病程超过6周，年龄小于16岁。JIA的类风湿因子通常为阴性。
- 最常见的JIA亚型是少关节型，通常好发于年轻女性。不管是哪种亚型，膝关节是最常累

joint, but any joint can be affected.

- The imaging appearance reflects the underlying pathophysiology of synovitis, as the earliest radiographic changes are joint effusion, soft tissue swelling, and periarticular demineralization. Later changes include joint space narrowing, periostitis and erosions.
- Chronic disease leads to eventual joint ankylosis, which is in contrast to adult rheumatoid arthritis, where ankylosis is rare. The most common sites of ankylosis are in the wrist, at the carpometacarpal joints, and the cervical spine.

  Cervical spine ankylosis in a child may appear similar to Klippel-Feil syndrome. In contrast to Klippel-Feil, JIA does not feature segmentation anomalies.
- Accelerated skeletal maturation and accelerated bone growth are caused by synovitis and hyperemia, which lead to premature fusion of the physes and/or abnormal bone growth.
- **Still disease** is an acute systemic subtype of JIA affecting children under the age of 5. Still disease presents with fever, anemia, leukocytosis, hepatosplenomegaly, and polyarthritis. Boys and girls are affected equally.

及的关节，尽管其他任何关节都可能受累。

- 影像学表现主要反映滑膜炎的病理生理学改变，最早期的表现包括关节腔积液、软组织肿胀和关节周围骨质脱钙。后期改变包括关节腔变窄、骨膜炎和骨质侵蚀。
- 慢性期病变最终可能导致关节强直，这与成人类风湿关节炎形成对比，后者罕见有关节强直。强直最常见的部位是腕关节、腕掌关节和颈椎。

  儿童颈椎强直性关节炎可与克利佩尔-费尔综合征类似。与克利佩尔-费尔综合征相比，JIA无节段性异常的特征。
- 骨骼成熟和生长加速是由于滑膜炎和充血所引起，可导致骺板过早闭合和/或骨骼异常生长。
- **Still病**是JIA的一种急性系统性亚型，累及5岁以下儿童。Still病表现为发热、贫血、白细胞增多、肝脾肿大和多发性关节炎。男女发病率相似。

Skeletal dysplasias

Overview of skeletal dysplasias

- Bone dysplasias are characterized by impairment of normal growth of bone yielding an abnormal skeleton. The impairment can involve growth slowing down, speeding up, or can cause the bones to grow in an unusual manner.
- Several terms used to describe abnormal limb growth include:

  Rhizomelia: Proximal limb shortening (e.g., humerus or femur too short). Examples of rhizomelic dwarfism include achondroplasia, thanatophoric dysplasia and hypochondroplasia.

  Mesomelia: Middle limb shortening (e.g., radius or ulna, tibia or fibula too short).

  Acromelia: Distal limb shortening (e.g., hand or foot too short). An example is Jeune syndrome.

  Micromelia: Entire limb is shortened.

  Amelia: Limb is absent.

骨骼发育不良

骨骼发育不良概述

- 骨骼发育不良的特征是骨骼正常生长受损并导致骨骼异常。这种损害可以导致生长缓慢、生长加速或引起骨骼生长方式异常。
- 多种用于描述肢体异常生长的术语包括：

  近端肢体短肢畸形：近端肢体短缩（如肱骨或股骨过短）。近端肢体短肢畸形侏儒症的例子包括软骨发育不全、致死性骨发育不良和软骨发育不良。

  肢体前臂或小腿短肢畸形：中间肢体短缩（如桡骨、尺骨、胫骨、腓骨等过短）。

  肢体远端短肢畸形：远端肢体短缩（如手或足过短等），如Jeune综合征（窒息性胸腔失养症）。

  四肢短肢畸形：全肢体短缩。

  缺肢畸形：肢体缺如。

Achondroplasia

软骨发育不全

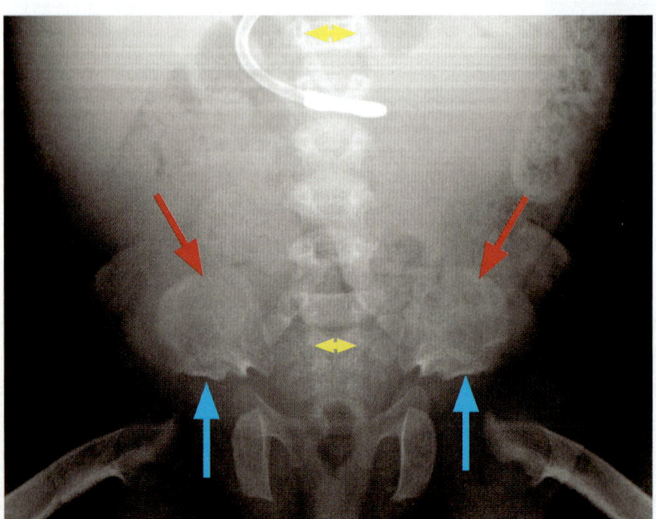

Achondroplasia: Abdominal radiograph shows narrowing interpedicular distances in the lower lumbar vertebra (yellow double arrows), *tombstone* iliac wings (red arrows), and flat acetabula (blue arrows).

This child also has a nasogastric tube.

软骨发育不全：腹部X线影像显示下腰椎的椎弓根间距变窄（黄双箭），墓碑状髂骨翼（红箭）及扁平的髋臼（蓝箭）。

该患儿还放置了鼻胃管。

- Achondroplasia is the most common skeletal dysplasia and cause of dwarfism. Affected individuals have normal cognitive function and life expectancy. Advanced paternal age is a risk factor.
- Key radiographic findings include abnormal morphology of the lumbosacral spine and pelvis:

> Narrowing of interpedicular distances in the lower spine causes spinal stenosis that is compensated for by a characteristic lumbar lordosis as the child learns to walk.
> Posterior scalloping of vertebral bodies.
> Characteristic *tombstone* iliac wings.
> Flat acetabula, with short femoral necks.
> Other findings include frontal bossing of the skull, midface hypoplasia, rhizomelic dwarfism (short femurs and humeri) with large trident hands (long third and fourth fingers).

- 软骨发育不全是骨骼发育不良最常见的原因，可导致侏儒症。患儿的智力和寿命正常。胎儿父亲高龄是一个危险因素。
- 主要X线影像表现为腰骶部脊柱和骨盆形态异常：

> 下腰椎的椎弓根间距变窄导致椎管狭窄，当儿童开始学步时以特征性的腰椎前凸作为代偿。
> 椎体后部呈扇形重塑。
> 特征性的墓碑状髂骨翼。
> 髋臼平坦伴股骨颈缩短。
> 其他影像学表现包括颅骨前额部隆起、中面部发育不全、近端肢体短肢畸形侏儒症(短股骨和肱骨)、大三叉戟手(第三和第四指过长)。

Thanatophoric dysplasia (lethal)

- Thanatophoric is the most common lethal skeletal dysplasia. It is inherited in an autosomal dominant manner.
- Key radiographic findings are focused on the vertebral bodies and femur:

> Flattening of vertebral bodies (platyspondyly), causing *H-shaped* vertebral bodies with diffuse narrowing of interpedicular distance.
> Curved *telephone receiver* femurs.
> Other findings include cloverleaf-shaped skull, short ribs, long thorax and small iliac bones.

致死性骨发育不良(致死性)

- 致死性侏儒症是最常见致死性的骨骼发育不良。它是一种常染色体显性遗传性疾病。
- X线影像的特征表现主要集中于椎体和股骨。

> 椎体变扁(扁平椎)，椎体呈H形，椎弓根间距变窄。
> 股骨弯曲呈电话听筒状。
> 其他表现包括三叶草形颅骨、短肋、长胸腔和小髂骨。

Cleidocranial dysostosis

- Cleidocranial dysostosis is a skeletal dysplasia characterized primarily by abnormalities in the clavicles, ribs, cranium and pelvis. Affected patients are of normal intelligence but tend to be short.
- The key radiographic finding is complete or partial absence of the clavicles.
- Cleidocranial dysostosis is strongly associated with wormian bones in the skull.

  Wormian bones are nonspecific, and are also seen in hypothyroidism, osteogenesis imperfecta, healing rickets, and Down syndrome.

颅锁骨发育不全

- 颅锁骨发育不全是一种骨骼发育不良并以锁骨、肋骨、颅骨和骨盆畸形为主要特征。患者智力正常，但是身材往往较矮。
- 主要的X线影像表现为锁骨部分或全部缺如。
- 颅锁骨发育不全与颅骨缝间骨密切相关。

  缝间骨为非特异性表现，也可见于甲状腺功能减退、成骨不全症、佝偻病恢复期及唐氏综合征。

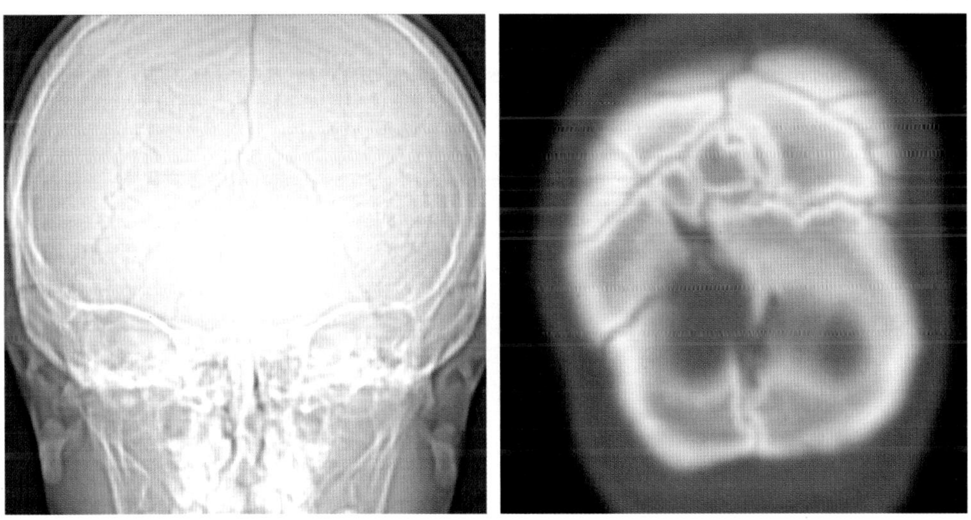

CT scout (left image), and coronal CT (right image) show multiple Wormian bones in a patient with cleidocranial dysostosis.
Case courtesy Sanjay Prabhu, MBBS, Boston Children's Hospital.
CT定位片(左)和冠状位CT(右)显示一名颅锁骨发育不全患者的多发缝间骨。

- Additional radiographic findings of cleidocranial dysostosis include:

  Delayed ossification of the skull (neonatal).

  Widened pubic symphysis (typically not seen until later in life).

- 其他颅锁骨发育不全X线影像表现有：

  颅骨骨化延迟(新生儿)。

  耻骨联合增宽(通常到成年后才发现)。

Asphyxiating thoracic dystrophy (Jeune syndrome)

窒息性胸廓发育不良(Jeune综合征)

- Asphyxiating thoracic dystrophy is an autosomal recessive disorder of a congenitally small bell-shaped thorax causing associated pulmonary dysplasia and respiratory distress.
- Additional bony findings include:

  Short ribs that are bulbous anteriorly.

  High-riding *handlebar* clavicle.

  Trident acetabulum with iliac wings that are small, short and flared.

  Normal vertebral bodies, as opposed to flat in thanatophoric dysplasia.

- 窒息性胸廓发育不良是一种先天性胸廓钟形狭窄，属于常染色体隐性遗传性疾病，可导致肺发育不良和呼吸困难。
- 其他骨骼表现包括：

  肋骨短小并向前呈球状突起。

  高骑式车把样锁骨。

  三叉戟状髋臼伴小、短、平的髂骨翼。

  正常椎体，与致死性骨发育不良的扁平椎体不同。

Osteogenesis imperfecta (OI)

成骨不全

- Osteogenesis imperfecta (OI) represents a varied spectrum of disorders due to abnormal type Ⅰ collagen. There are 8 different types, with type Ⅰ being the mildest and type Ⅱ being lethal. The remainder range from moderate to severe.
- Clinical findings include blue sclera and hearing impairment due to otosclerosis. It is important to note that a faint blue scleral tinge can also be transiently seen in normal infants.
- Key radiographic findings include multiple fractures in the ribs (causing characteristic *accordion ribs*), vertebral bodies, and long bones. Additional findings include:

  Bowed long bones.

  Osteopenia.

  Wormian bones in skull, secondary to non-coalesced ossification centers in the skull.

- The differential diagnosis for multiple fractures includes OI, rickets and child abuse. Of these three, OI is the only entity to cause antenatal fractures.

  With rickets one would not expect antenatal injury. Fractures and osteopenia may be present.

  With child abuse one would not expect osteopenia or antenatal injury. Fractures are typically present.

- 成骨不全是由于Ⅰ型胶原蛋白结构异常所导致的一系列表现不同的疾病。共有八种不同的类型，Ⅰ型病情最轻，Ⅱ型可致命。其余类型从中度到重度不等。
- 临床表现包括蓝色巩膜和因耳硬化症引起的听力损害。值得注意的是，淡蓝色巩膜也可在正常婴儿短暂出现。
- 重要的影像学表现包括多发肋骨骨折(造成特征性的手风琴样肋骨)、椎体和长骨骨折。其他表现包括：

  弓曲的长骨。

  骨质疏松。

  颅骨缝间骨，继发于颅骨未闭合的骨化中心。

- 多发性骨折的鉴别诊断包括成骨不全、佝偻病和虐童。而在这三种疾病中，唯有成骨不全可导致产前骨折。

  佝偻病不会有产前损伤。可出现骨折和骨质疏松。

  虐童不会出现骨质疏松或产前损伤。通常出现骨折。

Stippled epiphyses

点状骨骺

- Several skeletal dysplasias and metabolic bone diseases can cause stippling of the epiphyses, including:

- 某些骨骼发育不良和骨代谢疾病可以导致点状骨骺，包括：

> **Chondrodysplasia punctata**, a short-limbed dwarfism (usually rhizomelic).
>
> **Multiple epiphyseal dysplasia** (Fairbank disease), a mildly short limbed, autosomal dominant skeletal dysplasia that usually manifests in late childhood or adolescence.
>
> **Hypothyroidism**.
>
> Complications of **maternal warfarin use** in a newborn.

> **点状软骨发育异常**，一种短肢侏儒症(通常是近端肢体短肢畸形)。
>
> **多发性骨骺发育不良**(Fairbank病)，是一种轻度短肢畸形，属于常染色体显性遗传性骨骼发育不良，发病通常在大龄儿童和青少年。
>
> **甲状腺功能减退症**。
>
> **孕妇使用华法林**后在新生儿出现的并发症。

Enchondromatoses

内生软骨瘤病

- The enchondromatoses are characterized by multiple intra-osseous benign cartilaginous tumors in an asymmetric distribution. These syndromes are associated with an increased risk of malignant transformation to chondrosarcoma (Maffucci > Ollier).
- **Ollier disease** is an enchondromatosis without associated abnormalities.

- 内生软骨瘤病的特点是多发骨内良性软骨瘤并呈不对称性分布。与综合征相关的内生良性软骨瘤有恶性转化为软骨肉瘤的风险(如马富奇综合征大于奥利尔病)。
- **奥利尔病**是一种没有其他异常的内生软骨

- **Maffucci syndrome** is an enchondromatosis with venous malformations, which cause phleboliths that are evident on radiography.
- Lesions typically demonstrate rings-and-arc chondroid matrix and are most commonly found within the hands and feet, and along the metaphyses of long bones.

瘤病。

- **马富奇综合征**是一种合并静脉畸形的内生软骨瘤病，其伴发的静脉石可以在X线上显影。
- 病变通常表现为环状和弧形软骨样基质，并最常见于手和足，以及长骨干骺端。

Multiple hereditary exostoses (osteochondromatosis)

- Multiple hereditary exostoses is an autosomal dominant disorder of multiple benign osteochondromas (also called exostoses), which are bony protuberances with corticomedullary continuity growing from the metaphyses of long bones. Lesions are directed away from the joint and most commonly occur in the distal femur, proximal femur and proximal tibia.
- Complications include pain, deformity, and malignant transformation into low-grade chondrosarcoma (between 5–25% of cases).
- In contrast to enchondromatosis, skeletal involvement is usually symmetric bilaterally.

遗传性多发外生骨疣(骨软骨瘤病)

- 遗传性多发外生骨疣是一种常染色体显性遗传性疾病(也称为外生骨疣)，表现为长骨干骺端隆起伴皮质和髓质呈连续性生长。病变朝向背离关节，最常见于股骨远端、股骨近端和胫骨近端。
- 并发症包括疼痛、变形和恶变为低级别软骨肉瘤(恶变率5%~25%)。
- 与内生软骨瘤病相比，其骨骼受累经常表现为双侧，呈对称性。

MUCOPOLYSACCHARIDOSES

- Mucopolysaccharidoses are a group of lysosomal storage disorders (LSD) including Hurlers, Morquio, and Hunters. These disorders share common radiographic findings and are typically distinguished clinically and biochemically.
- Key radiographic findings include oval vertebral bodies with anterior beaking, thickened clavicles and ribs, and undertubulated bones. Other findings include:

  Madelung deformity of the wrists (wedge-shaped proximal carpal row, with radius shifted towards ulna).

  Thickened calvarium with a *J-shaped* sella.

  Pelvis with tall and flared iliac wings (opposite of achondroplasia).

  Wide tapering metacarpal bones.

- **Hurlers** features anterior beaking of the vertebral bodies, primarily **inferiorly**.
- **Morquio** also features anterior beaking of **middle** portion of the vertebral body (mnemonic:**M**orquio for **m**iddle).

  Morquio is associated with spinal stenosis and atlantoaxial instability, with most common cause of death being C2 cervical myelopathy.

黏多糖病

- 黏多糖病是一组溶酶体贮积病(LSD)，包括Hurlers(黏多糖贮积病Ⅰ型)、Morquio(黏多糖贮积病Ⅳ型)和Hunters(黏多糖贮积病Ⅱ型)病。这些疾病有相似的影像学表现，通常需要通过临床和生化方法加以区分。
- 主要X线影像表现包括椭圆形椎体伴前缘鸟嘴样改变，锁骨、肋骨及管状骨的骨皮质增厚。其他表现如下：

  腕关节马德隆畸形(近端腕骨呈楔状排列，桡骨向尺骨倾斜)。

  颅骨增厚，蝶鞍呈J形。

  骨盆增高且髂翼扁平(软骨发育不全相反)。

  掌骨宽而逐渐变尖。

- **Hurlers**病的特点是椎体前缘呈鸟嘴样改变，主要是**下缘**。
- **莫尔基奥综合征**也是椎体前缘呈鸟嘴样改变，但位于**中部**(助记：Morquio/中间)。

  莫尔基奥综合征常合并椎管狭窄及寰枢椎不稳定，其最常见的死因是C_2颈髓病。

Rickets

佝偻病

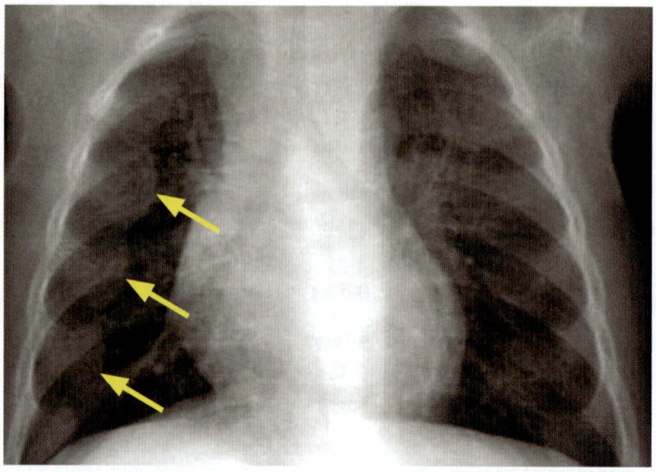

Chest radiograph in a child with rickets shows widening of the rib epiphyseal cartilage, creating the classic *rachitic rosary* appearance (yellow arrows).
Case courtesy Michael Callahan, MD, Boston Children's Hospital.
一名佝偻病患儿胸部X线影像显示前肋骺软骨增宽，形成典型的串珠样改变(黄箭)。

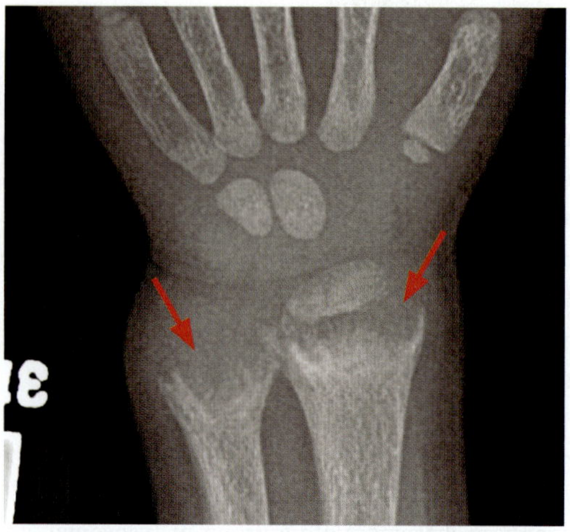

Frontal radiograph in the wrist of a different patient shows metaphyseal fraying and cupping (red arrows).
Case courtesy Michael Hanley, MD, University of Virginia Health System.
另一名患者的腕骨正位X线影像显示尺骨和桡骨干骺端呈毛刷样和杯口样改变(红箭)。

- Rickets is a metabolic bone disorder caused by inadequate vitamin D or abnormal vitamin D metabolism. It is characterized by abnormal calcification at the zone of provisional calcification (ZPC), leading to abnormal physeal development.

  Rickets mostly affects growing bones, though is not seen in newborns as maternal vitamin D is still functional.
- Radiographs show expansion, irregularity, fraying, and cupping of the long bone metaphyses, often associated with adjacent metaphyseal periosteal new bone.
- Other findings of rickets include bowing of the legs, osteopenia, and fractures. The classic *rachitic rosary* represents anterior cupping of the ribs with widening of the rib epiphyseal cartilage. The skull may become demineralized.
- MR findings demonstrate loss of black-white-black line corresponding to an indistinct ZPC.
- **Oncogenic rickets** is a variant of rickets seen with hemangiopericytoma or nonossifying fibroma due to tumor metabolites that cause deranged vitamin D metabolism.

Lead poisoning

- Lead poisoning is the most common heavy metal poisoning in children, usually from ingestion of paint chips in older homes.
- Classic radiographic findings include wide sclerotic metaphyseal bands (lead line), usually in a more rapidly growing long bone. It does not spare the fibula, whereas a normal variant line might.

- 佝偻病是一种由维生素D缺乏或维生素D代谢异常而导致的骨代谢性疾病。它的特点是临时钙化带(ZPC)异常钙化，导致骺板发育异常。

  佝偻病主要影响骨骼生长，但新生儿不受影响，因从母体获得的维生素D还有功能。
- X线影像显示长骨干骺端增宽、不规则，呈毛刷状、杯口状改变，常伴邻近干骺端骨膜新骨形成。
- 佝偻病的其他表现还包括腿部弯曲、骨质疏松及骨折。典型佝偻病性串珠征是指肋骨前凸和肋骨骺软骨扩张。颅骨可表现为脱钙。
- MR影像表现为黑-白-黑线的消失，与模糊的ZPC对应。
- **肿瘤性佝偻病**是佝偻病的一种变异，见于血管外皮瘤或非骨化性纤维瘤，源于肿瘤继发的维生素D代谢紊乱。

铅中毒

- 铅中毒是儿童最常见的重金属中毒，通常是由于吞食陈旧性住宅中的油漆碎片所致。
- 典型影像学表现包括干骺端的硬化带(铅线)增宽，通常见于生长较快的长骨。腓骨也同样受累，但可能是一种正常变异的线条。

AGGRESSIVE BONE NEOPLASMS

Osteosarcoma

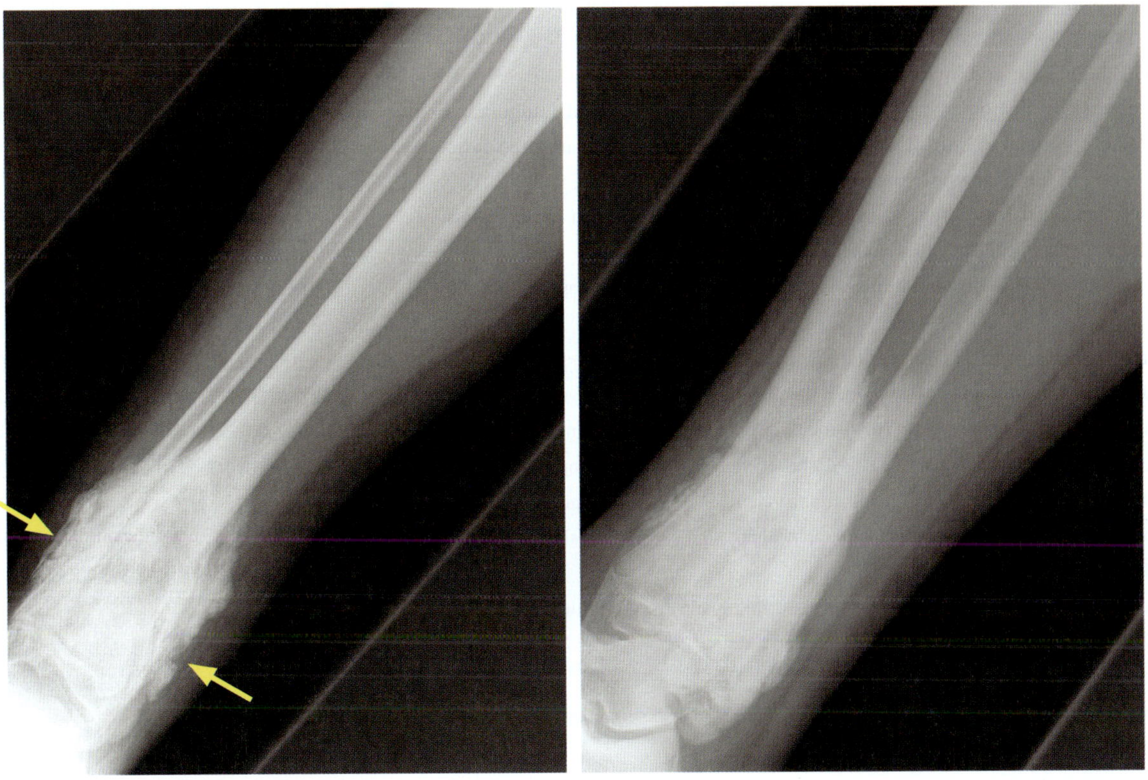

Conventional osteosarcoma: Frontal (left image) and oblique (right image) radiographs of the tibia and fibula show a sclerotic lesion of the distal tibia (arrows) associated with cloud-like ossification extending into the soft tissue. This appearance is of a highly aggressive mass.

Case courtesy Michael Hanley, MD, University of Virginia Health System.

普通型骨肉瘤：胫腓骨正位(左图)和斜位线(右图)X线影像显示胫骨远端一处硬化性病变(箭)，伴云絮状骨化并延伸到软组织内。这是高度侵袭性肿瘤的表现。

- Osteosarcoma is the most common primary pediatric bone tumor, with a peak incidence of 15–25 years of age. There are over 10 types of osteosarcoma, with the most common subtype the conventional (intramedullary) type, representing 75% of all osteosarcomas. Conventional osteosarcoma is seen most commonly about the knee in the distal femur or proximal tibia.
- The characteristic radiographic appearance of conventional osteosarcoma is a destructive lesion often invading the cortex, with extensive cloud-like osteoid matrix.

  Aggressive periosteal new bone formation results in a spiculated *sunburst* appearance or uplifting of the periosteum forming a *Codman triangle*.
- Osteosarcoma is further discussed in the musculoskeletal imaging section.

Ewing sarcoma

- Ewing sarcoma is the second most common primary pediatric bone tumor, with peak incidence slightly younger than that of osteosarcoma (ranging from 5–20 years). It is an aggressive small round blue cell tumor of neuroectodermal differentiation.
- Ewing sarcoma most commonly arises from the femoral diaphysis, followed by the flat bones of the pelvis. Ewing may also develop in the tibia, humerus, and ribs.

侵袭性骨肿瘤

骨肉瘤

- 骨肉瘤是儿童最常见的原发性骨肿瘤，15~25岁为发病高峰。骨肉瘤有10多种亚型，最常见的亚型为普通(髓内)型，占所有骨肉瘤的75%。普通型骨肉瘤最常发生于膝关节的股骨远端或胫骨近端。
- 普通型骨肉瘤的影像学特征是病变呈毁损性改变，常侵犯骨皮质，并伴有大量云絮样骨性基质。

  侵袭性骨膜新生骨形成产生一个日光放射状的毛刺或掀起的骨膜形成Codman三角。
- 骨肉瘤详见“骨骼和肌肉影像”一章。

尤因肉瘤

- 尤因肉瘤是儿童第二常见的原发性骨肿瘤，发病高峰年龄比骨肉瘤稍低(5~20岁)。它是一种侵袭性的、由神经外胚层肿瘤分化而来的小圆蓝细胞肿瘤。
- 尤因肉瘤通常发生于股骨干，其次是骨盆的扁平骨。尤因肉瘤也可发生在胫骨、肱骨和肋骨。

The lung is the most common site of metastasis.

- The characteristic radiographic appearance is a permeative lesion in the medullary cavity with wide zone of transition and associated aggressive *lamellated (onion-skinning)* or spiculated periosteal reaction.
- Ewing often causes a soft tissue mass which can be difficult to see by radiography.

Osseous Langerhans cell histiocytosis (LCH)

- Langerhans cell histiocytosis (LCH) is abnormal proliferation of Langerhans cells with a variety of clinical manifestations, ranging from an isolated lytic bony lesion to fulminant systemic disease.

  Langerhans cells are dendritic cells (histiocytes) that normally live in the epidermis and lymph nodes, where they act as antigen-presenting cells.

  Histopathologically, **Birbeck bodies** are seen on electron microscopy within the histiocytes.

- Clinical subtypes of LCH have varied presentations.

  Eosinophilic granuloma (osseous LCH) features localized skeletal or pulmonary involvement. It may be mono- or polyostotic. Despite the name, the involvement of eosinophils is variable. Pulmonary LCH is discussed in the thoracic imaging section.

  Hand-Schüller-Christian (multifocal, unisystem) is a clinical triad of pituitary hypophysitis (causing diabetes insipidus), exophthalmos, and lytic bone lesions (typically affecting the skull).

  Letterer-Siwe (multifocal, multisystem) is a fulminant disease with multisystem involvement, primarily seen in young infants and toddlers under age two. Prognosis is poor.

  In clinical practice, the most important factor is thought to be determination of unifocal or multifocal disease rather than the classification above.

- The eosinophilic granuloma variant of LCH is relatively common and may present clinically with pain, tenderness, and fever, often mimicking osteomyelitis. Children between ages 5–15 are typically affected.
- The appearance of the affected bone depends on the bone involved:

  Skull: *Beveled edge* or *punched-out* lytic lesion.

  Flat bones (e.g., pelvis): *Hole within a hole* lytic lesion.

  Ribs: Multiple expansile lytic lesions.

  Long bone (diaphysis most common, but may occur anywhere including rarely the epiphysis): Permeative destruction, with wide zone of transition and later lytic lesion and faint rim of sclerosis.

  Spine: Complete vertebral body collapse (vertebra plana), pictured to below. The differential of vertebra plana in a child also includes lymphoma, chronic osteomyelitis, and OI.

  Maxilla: *Floating* teeth.

- Along with infection, eosinophilic granuloma should be considered in the differential diagnosis in any patient under 30 with a lytic lesion anywhere.

肺是最常见的转移部位。

- 典型影像学表现为穿凿样骨质破坏，伴的有移行带增宽及侵袭性的*层状骨膜反应(洋葱皮样)*或毛刺状骨膜反应。
- 尤因肉瘤常引起软组织肿块，但因其缺乏骨化而很难在X线影像上被看到。

骨朗格汉斯细胞组织细胞增生症(LCH)

- 朗格汉斯细胞组织细胞增生症(LCH)是朗格汉斯细胞异常增殖，临床表现多样，从孤立的溶骨性病变到暴发性系统性疾病。

  朗格汉斯细胞是树突细胞(组织细胞)，通常存在于表皮组织和淋巴结，充当抗原递呈细胞。

  组织病理学上，组织细胞内的**Birbeck颗粒**可以在电子显微镜下观察到。

- LCH临床亚型有各种不同的表现。

  嗜酸性肉芽肿(骨LCH)的特征是局部累及骨骼或肺，可单发或多发。尽管称为嗜酸性肉芽肿，但病变中的嗜酸性粒细胞不定。肺LCH详见“胸部影像”一章。

  汉-许-克病(多发，单系统)是一种临床三联征，包括垂体炎(引起尿崩症)、眼球突出和溶骨性病变(通常累及颅骨)。

  莱特勒-西韦病(多发，多系统)是一种暴发性疾病，累及多个系统，主要见于婴幼儿及2岁以下的学步儿童。预后差。

  在临床工作中，最重要的因素是确定病变是单灶性还是多灶性，而不是上述分类。

- LCH的嗜酸性肉芽肿亚型相对常见，在临床上可表现为疼痛、压痛、发热，常类似于骨髓炎。好发于5~15岁儿童。
- 骨的影像学表现取决于受累骨：

  头颅骨：*斜边或穿孔性*溶骨病灶。

  扁平骨(如骨盆)：*洞中洞*溶骨性病变。

  肋骨：多发膨胀性溶骨病变。

  长骨(最常累及骨干，但也可累及任何部位包括罕见的骨骺)：穿凿样骨质破坏及随后的溶骨性改变和淡的硬化边。

  脊柱：椎体完全塌陷(扁平椎)，下图所示。在儿童期出现扁平椎，需要与淋巴瘤、慢性骨髓炎和成骨不全进行鉴别。

  上颌骨：*浮牙征*。

- 在30岁以下的患者，出现任何部位溶骨性病变时鉴别诊断应包括感染和嗜酸性肉芽肿。

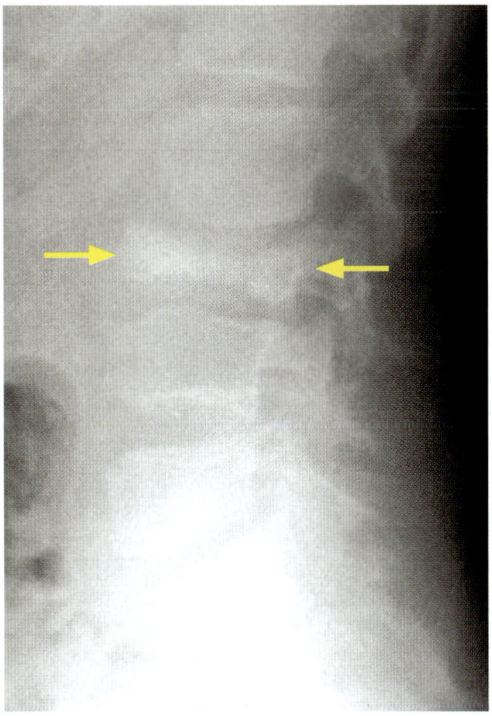

Eosinophilic granuloma (osseous LCH) causing vertebra plana (complete collapse) of L2 (arrows).
嗜酸性肉芽肿(骨LCH)导致L_2(箭)扁平椎(完全塌陷)。

Leukemia

- Leukemia is the most common pediatric malignancy, with bony changes seen in >50% of patients.
- Imaging findings can be varied. One of the most distinctive radiographic features of leukemia is the *metaphyseal lucent band*.
- The etiology of the lucent bands is controversial, thought to be possibly due to malnutrition or vitamin deficiency in young children. The differential diagnosis of lucent metaphyseal bands includes:

Leukemia, lymphoma.
Neuroblastoma metastases.
Severe illness.
TORCH infections.
Endocrinopathies: Scurvy, rickets

- Other osseous findings of leukemia include generalized osteopenia or permeative lytic lesions.

白血病

- 白血病是儿童期最常见的恶性肿瘤，超过50%患儿有骨骼改变。
- 影像学表现多样，其中最显著的X线影像特征是干骺端的透亮带。
- 透亮带的病因还存在争议，可能由于幼儿营养不良或维生素缺乏所致。干骺端透亮带的鉴别诊断包括：

白血病，淋巴瘤。
神经母细胞瘤转移。
严重疾病。
TORCH感染。
内分泌疾病：维生素C缺乏病、佝偻病。

- 白血病的其他骨骼表现包括弥漫性骨质疏松或穿凿样溶骨性病变。

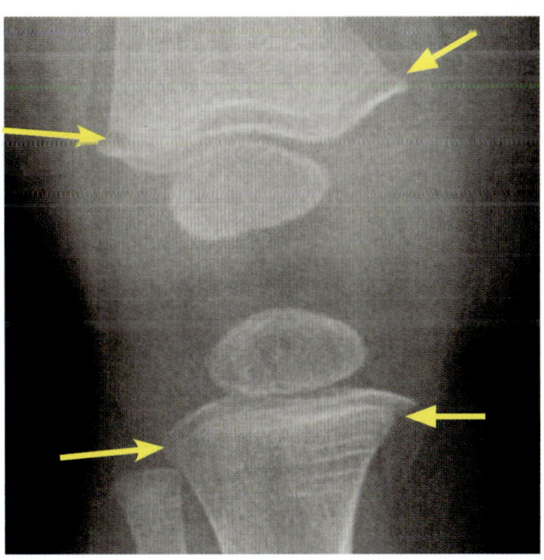

Frontal knee radiograph shows lucent metaphyseal bands in the distal femur and proximal tibia in a child with leukemia.
Case courtesy Michael Callahan, MD, Boston Children's Hospital.
膝关节正位X线影像显示一名白血病患儿股骨远端和胫骨近端干骺端的透亮带。

OSTEOCHONDROSES

- The osteochondroses are a heterogeneous group of disorders that were at one point thought to be initiated by avascular necrosis. The current understanding is that most of these disorders are secondary to trauma. While many are associated with AVN, it is not thought to be the initiating factor. Most are more common in males.

Blount disease

- Blount disease is an osteochondrosis of the proximal tibial metaphysis, causing tibia varus (bowing) and internal rotation, which eventually leads to progressive deformity, gait deviations, and leg-length discrepancy.
- The infantile form of Blount disease is thought to be due to early walking and obesity, and is typically bilateral.
- The adolescent form is seen in children over 6 years old and is usually unilateral.

骨软骨病

- 骨软骨病是一组多样化的疾病，曾经被认为由缺血坏死所致。目前认为这类疾病多继发于创伤。尽管很多情况与缺血性坏死（AVN）有关，但AVN不是始发因素。男性更常见。

Blount病

- Blount病是一种胫骨近端干骺端的骨软骨炎，引起胫骨内翻（弯曲）和内旋，最终导致进行性变形、步态偏差和腿长短不等。
- 婴儿型Blount病被认为是由于过早行走和肥胖所致，通常为双侧发病。
- 青少年型见于6岁以上的儿童，通常是单侧发病。

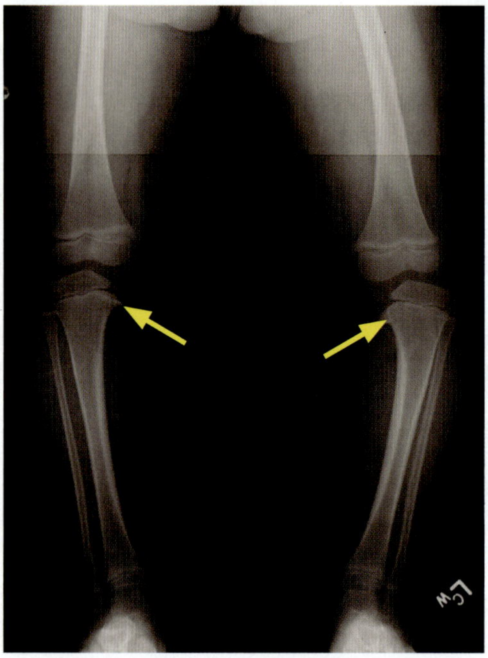

Infantile Blount disease: Bilateral Blount disease with sloping of the medial portions of the proximal tibial metaphyses (arrows), causing tibia varus.
婴幼儿Blount病：双侧Blount病，表现为胫骨近端干骺端内侧倾斜（箭）导致胫骨内翻。

Madelung deformity

- Madelung deformity is medial sloping of the distal radius caused by dysplasia of the medial distal radial physis and resultant growth disturbance.

Panner disease

- Panner disease is osteochondrosis of the capitellum.

Little league elbow

- Little league elbow is osteochondrosis of the medial epicondyle.

Scheuermann kyphosis

- Scheuermann kyphosis is a syndrome of avascular necrosis of multiple thoracic vertebral bodies leading to multiple compression fractures.

Legg-Calvé-Perthes disease

- Legg-Calvé-Perthes disease is osteochondrosis of the capital femoral epiphysis.

Kienbock disease

- Kienbock disease is osteochondrosis of the carpal lunate.

Madelung畸形

- Madelung畸形是由于桡骨远端骨骺内侧发育不良导致桡骨远端向内侧倾斜，并引起生长障碍。

Panner病

- Panner病是肱骨小头骨软骨病。

Little league（棒球）肘

- Little league肘是肱骨内上髁的骨软骨病。

Scheuermann脊柱后凸

- Scheuermann脊柱后凸是指胸椎椎体多发缺血性坏死，导致多个椎体压缩性骨折。

Legg-Calvé-Perthes病

- Legg-Calvé-Perthes病是指股骨头骨骺骨软骨病。

Kienbock病

- Kienbock病是腕月骨骨软骨病。

Osgood-Schlatter disease

- Osgood-Schlatter disease is osteochondrosis of the tibial tuberosity.

Freiberg infraction

- Freiberg infraction is osteochondrosis of the second metatarsal head.

Kohler disease

- Kohler disease is a self-limited osteochondrosis of the navicular bone.

Sever disease

- Sever disease is calcaneal apophysitis (rather than an osteochondrosis) and is a cause of heel pain. Sclerosis of the calcaneal apophysis is nonspecific and can be seen in asymptomatic children, although greater fragmentation of the apophysis may be associated with pain.

胫骨粗隆骨软骨病

- 胫骨粗隆骨软骨病是胫骨粗隆骨软骨病。

Freiberg坏死

- Freiberg坏死是发生于第二跖骨头的骨软骨病。

Kohler病

- Kohler病是一种自限性足舟骨骨软骨病。

Sever病

- Sever病是跟骨骨突炎(而不是骨软骨病),是引起足跟疼痛的原因之一。跟骨骨突硬化无特异性,可见于无症状儿童,但较大的跟骨骨突碎片可能会伴有疼痛。

PERIOSTEAL REACTION IN AN INFANT OR CHILD

- The periosteum is a thin membrane covering the entire surface of the bone excluding those areas covered by cartilage. It contributes to bone production and remodeling. Irritation of the periosteum, which can be due to trauma, infection, inflammation, neoplasm, or metabolic disturbance, can cause *periosteal reaction*.
- The terms "periosteal reaction," "periostitis," and "periosteal new bone formation" are commonly used as synonyms. Periosteal reaction is simply a nonspecific response to injury or chronic stress resulting in periosteal new bone production.
- Periosteal reaction may also be associated with tumors or infection, typically producing an aggressive appearance in these disorders. The morphology of aggressive periosteal reaction is discussed in the musculoskeletal imaging section.

Physiologic subperiosteal new bone formation in a newborn

- Physiologic periosteal reaction occurs in infants 1–4 months old, thought to be due to rapid bone growth and loosely adherent periosteum.
- The periosteal reaction is smooth and thin, and usually only involves the lateral *or* medial diaphysis of the long bones symmetrically.

Prostaglandin therapy

- Neonates on prostaglandin therapy for congenital heart disease (to maintain ductal patency) may have periosteal reaction. Prostaglandins are thought to decrease osteoclast bone resorption.

Infectious

- Subperiosteal spread of pyogenic infection elevates the periosteum and irritates it, usually causing an aggressive periosteal reaction.
- Congenital syphilis causes periosteal reaction.

Neoplastic (typically these are aggressive periosteal reactions)

- Multiple malignancies, including leukemia, neuroblastoma, Ewing sarcoma, and osteosarcoma can produce an aggressive periosteal reaction.

Trauma

- Healing fractures (both accidental trauma and child abuse) may cause periosteal reaction.

Metabolic

- Rickets, scurvy (which is also characterized by epiphyseal sclerosis – the *Wimberger rim sign*), and hypervitaminosis A may all cause periosteal reaction.

Syndromic

- Multiple syndromes may cause periostitis. **Caffey disease** (infantile cortical hyperostosis) is a rare inflammatory disease causing periostitis of the mandible, scapula, and clavicle.

婴儿和儿童的骨膜反应

- 骨膜是一层覆盖除软骨外的整个骨表面的薄膜,骨膜具有骨生成和重塑功能。若骨膜受到刺激,如外伤、感染、炎症、肿瘤及代谢紊乱等则可以引起骨膜反应。
- 术语"骨膜反应""骨膜炎"及"骨膜新生骨形成"通常作为同义词使用。骨膜反应只是在骨损伤或慢性应激状态下的一种非特异性反应,可导致骨膜新生骨形成。
- 骨膜反应也可能与肿瘤或感染有关,通常产生侵袭性的表现。侵袭性骨膜反应的形态学表现详见"骨骼与肌肉影像"一章。

新生儿生理性骨膜反应

- 生理性骨膜反应发生在1~4月龄的婴儿,认为与骨骼的快速生长和骨膜附着松弛有关。
- 骨膜反应薄而光滑,通常对称性累及长骨骨干的外侧或内侧。

前列腺素治疗

- 新生儿接受前列腺素治疗先天性心脏病(用来维持动脉导管的通畅)可能会出现骨膜反应。前列腺素被认为可以降低破骨细胞对骨质的吸收。

感染

- 化脓性感染沿骨膜下扩散,掀起并刺激骨膜,通常导致侵袭性骨膜反应。
- 先天性梅毒可引起骨膜反应。

肿瘤(通常是侵袭性骨膜反应)

- 多种恶性肿瘤,如白血病、神经母细胞瘤、尤因肉瘤、骨肉瘤都能产生侵袭性骨膜反应。

创伤

- 骨折愈合期(意外伤和虐童)也可引起骨膜反应。

代谢

- 佝偻病、维生素C缺乏病(特征为骨骺硬化——Wimberger环征)和维生素A过量,都可导致骨膜反应。

综合征

- 多种综合征可以引起骨膜炎。**Caffey病**(婴幼儿皮质增生症)是一种罕见的炎性疾病,可引起下颌骨、肩胛骨及锁骨骨膜炎。

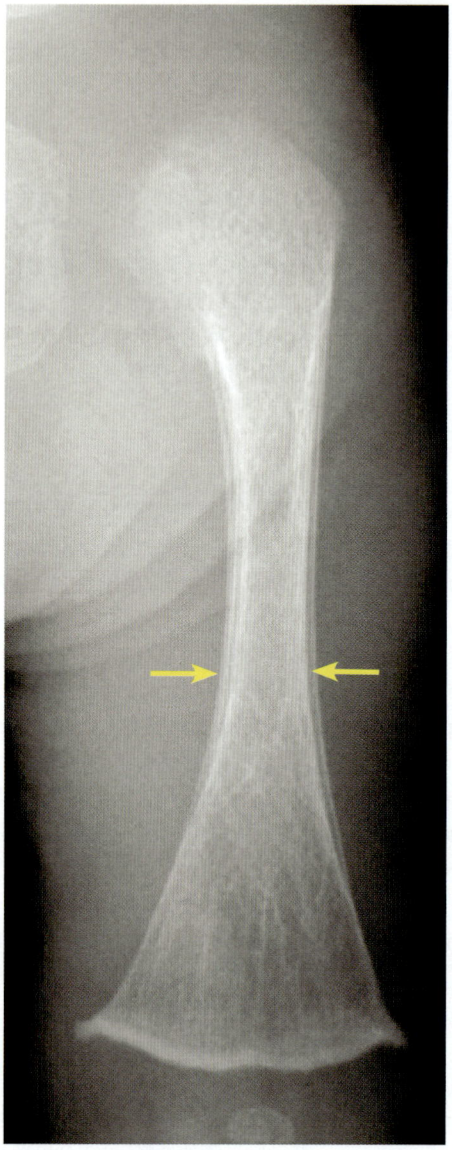

Symmetric periosteal reaction along the femoral diaphysis (arrows). This child was on prostaglandin therapy for congenital heart disease.
沿股骨干的对称性骨膜反应(箭)。这名儿童正在接受前列腺素治疗先天性心脏病。

Miscellaneous

其他疾病

Torticollis

斜颈

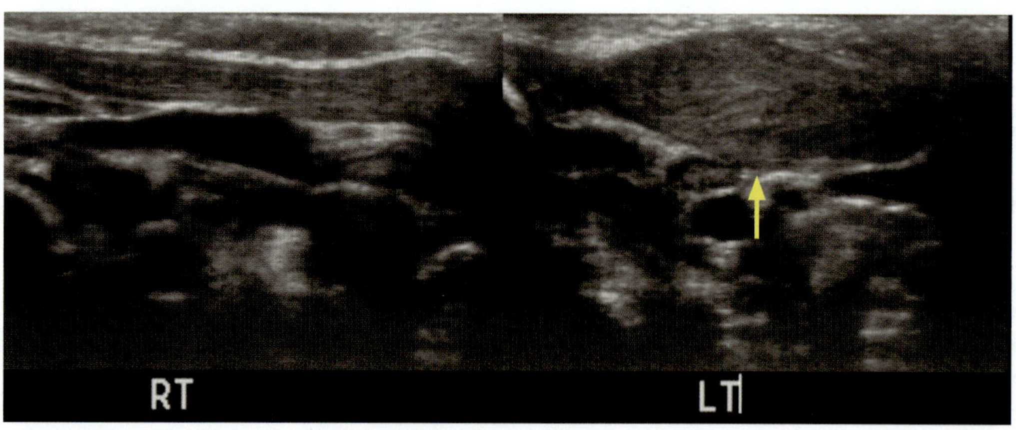

Torticollis: Bilateral neck ultrasound shows fusiform enlargement of the left sternocleidomastoid muscle (arrow). The right side is normal.
斜颈：双侧颈部超声显示左侧胸锁乳突肌呈梭形肿大(箭)。右侧正常。

- Torticollis is caused by fibromatosis coli (idiopathic sternocleidomastoid enlargement) resulting in an inability to fully straighten the neck. It usually resolves with physical therapy.

- 斜颈是由一侧颈部纤维瘤病(特发性胸锁乳突肌增大),造成颈部不能完全伸直。通常用物理治疗可缓解。

Tarsal coalition

- Tarsal coalition is abnormal joining of two normally separate bones in the tarsus. The three types of coalition are fibrous, cartilaginous, and osseous.
- The two most common coalitions (together making up 90% of all tarsal coalitions) are talocalcaneal and calcaneonavicular.
- Tarsal coalition clinically presents as foot pain in the child as the coalition begins to ossify.
- Tarsal coalition is further discussed in the musculoskeletal imaging section.

跗骨桥

- 跗骨桥是在两个正常分开的跗骨之间出现异常连接。三种连接的方式为纤维、软骨和骨性连接。
- 最常见的两个连接是跟距骨桥和跟舟骨桥(占所有跗骨桥总数的90%)。
- 跗骨桥在临床上可表现为儿童足痛,因连接部开始骨化。
- 跗骨桥详见“骨骼与肌肉影像”一章。

Carpal coalition

- Carpal coalition is abnormal joining of carpal bones.
- Carpal coalition is usually asymptomatic but may be a cause of wrist pain.
- Like tarsal coalition, the coalition may be fibrous, cartilaginous, or osseous.
- Lunotriquetral coalition is the most common carpal coalition.
- Capitohamate is the second most common carpal coalition.

腕骨桥

- 腕骨桥是腕骨间的异常连接。
- 腕骨桥通常无临床症状,但可能是腕关节疼痛的原因之一。
- 与跗骨桥一样,可以是纤维性、软骨性和骨性连接。
- 月骨三角骨骨桥是最常见的腕骨桥。
- 头状骨钩状骨骨桥是第二常见的腕骨桥。

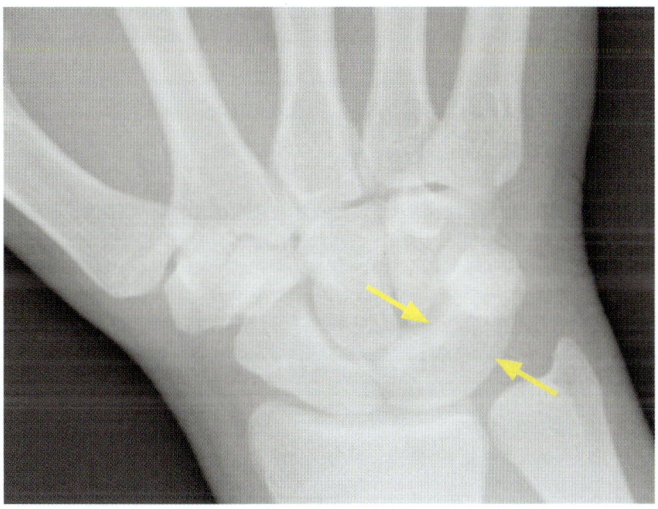

Frontal radiograph of the wrist demonstrates osseous lunotriquetral coalition (arrows).
Case courtesy Michael Callahan, MD, Boston Children's Hospital
正位腕关节X线影像显示月骨三角骨骨性骨桥(箭)。

(翻译　毛志群)

PEDIATRIC NEUROIMAGING

小儿神经影像

NEONATAL BRAIN IMAGING

新生儿脑影像

Germinal matrix hemorrhage

- Germinal matrix is the subependymal site of neuronal precursor cells which initially lines the entire ventricular system, but regresses after the first trimester, becoming concentrated in the caudothalamic groove. It is nearly involuted by 32 weeks gestation.
- Germinal matrix hemorrhage occurs in premature infants less than 32 weeks gestation.
- Germinal matrix-intraventricular hemorrhage grading system:

生发基质出血

- 生发基质是位于室管膜下的神经元前体细胞,它最初排列在整个脑室系统周围,胚胎3个月时开始退化,逐渐集中在尾状核丘脑沟。它在胎儿第32周时基本完全退化。
- 生发基质出血发生于妊娠未满32周的早产儿。
- 生发基质脑室出血分级如下:

Grade Ⅰ: Hemorrhage confined to the germinal matrix.

Grade Ⅱ: Hemorrhage extends into the ventricles **without** ventriculomegaly.

Grade Ⅲ: Hemorrhage extends into the ventricles **with** ventriculomegaly.

Parenchymal hemorrhagic infarction: This can coexist with any grade.

- The previously termed "Grade Ⅳ" (intraventricular and parenchymal hemorrhage) is now recognized as periventricular hemorrhagic infarction resulting from venous obstruction and congestion, rather than extraventricular extension of hemorrhage.

Ⅰ级：出血局限于生发基质。

Ⅱ级：出血破入脑室内，**不伴**脑室扩张。

Ⅲ级：出血破入脑室内，**伴有**脑室扩张。

脑实质出血性梗死：可与任何级别共存。

- 原来定义的"Ⅳ级"(脑室内和脑实质出血)，现在则认为是由于静脉阻塞和充血引起的脑室周围脑实质出血性梗死，而不是出血向脑室外扩展。

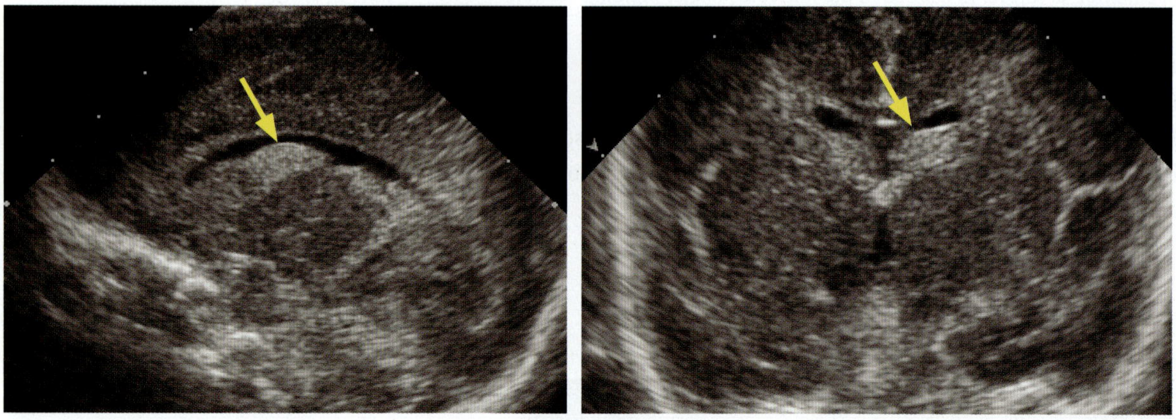

Grade I germinal matrix hemorrhage:
Sagittal (left image) and coronal (right) ultrasound demonstrates a rounded hyperechoic focus (arrows) at the left caudothalamic groove, representing germinal matrix hemorrhage. The lateral ventricles are not enlarged.

Ⅰ级生发基质出血：
矢状切面(左图)和冠状切面(右图)超声显示一处位于左侧尾状核丘脑沟圆形高回声病灶(箭)，提示生发基质出血。双侧侧脑室不扩张。

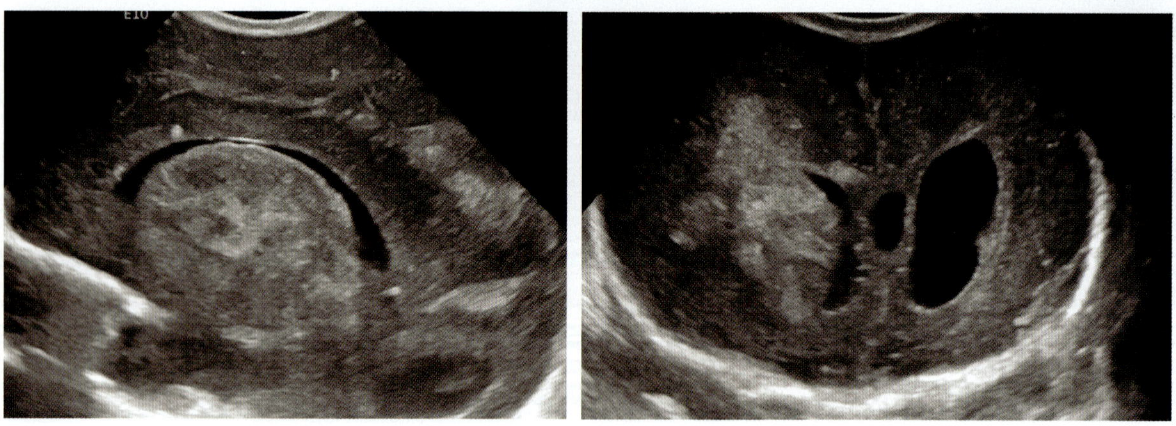

Germinal matrix hemorrhage with intraventricular and parenchymal hemorrhage:
Sagittal ultrasound (left image) shows a large amount of echogenic hemorrhage extending from the region of the right caudothalamic groove into the lateral ventricle. Coronal ultrasound (right image) shows intraventricular extension of hemorrhage and intraparenchymal hemorrhage in the right parietal lobe. There is associated ventriculomegaly.

生发基质出血伴脑室内和脑实质出血：
矢状切面超声(左图)显示右尾状核丘脑沟至脑室内有大量高回声出血灶。冠状切面超声(右图)显示侧脑室内出血延伸至右侧顶叶，伴有脑室扩张。

Myelination and Cortical Development

Pattern of myelination

- A full-term newborn will have myelination seen in several structures at birth, including: Posterior limb of internal capsules, middle cerebellar peduncle, ventrolateral thalami, dorsal brainstem, and the perirolandic regions.
- Myelination is most apparent at birth on T1-weighted images. On T1-weighted images myelin is bright; on T2-weighted images myelin is dark.
- Myelination generally assumes a mature pattern by age two, although the frontal lobes continue to myelinate through adolescence.

Overview of cortical development

- Primitive brain forms around the primordial ventricular system, which is lined by pluripotent stem cells called germinal matrix cells.
- Development of normal cortex is dependent on both germinal matrix cell ***migration*** and subsequent ***organization*** into the normal 6-layered lamination of the cortex.

Congenital Malformations

Polymicrogyria

- Polymicrogyria is a malformation of cortical development characterized by a derangement of the normal 6-layered organization of the cortex, which leads to too many gyri and too few sulci.
- Polymicrogyria is thought to be caused by disturbance either late in neuronal migration or early in cortical lamellar organization.
- Polymicrogyria may be caused by in-utero infection (especially CMV), in-utero ischemia, or genetic causes. In many cases, no cause is found. Clinical manifestations include developmental delay, focal neurological signs and symptoms, quadriparesis, or epilepsy.
- On MR imaging, the cortex appears thick with an irregularly bumpy surface and high-resolution imaging can resolve multiple small individual gyri. The polymicrogyric cortex looks thin and bumpy in unmyelinated regions, and thicker and smoother in myelinated areas of the brain.
- Bilateral perisylvian polymicrogyria is the most common distribution.

髓鞘化和皮质发育

髓鞘化的方式

- 足月新生儿出生时多个结构已有髓鞘形成，包括内囊后肢、小脑中脚、腹外侧丘脑、脑干背侧及中央沟周围区。
- 出生时的髓鞘形成在T_1加权图像上最易识别。髓鞘在T_1加权图像上为高信号，而T_2加权图像上为低信号。
- 通常认为，2岁儿童的髓鞘化已近成熟，而额叶髓鞘化则持续到青春期。

皮质发育概述

- 原脑形成于原始脑室系统周围，其内衬有一种称为原始基质细胞的多能干细胞。
- 正常脑皮质发育取决于原始基质细胞的**迁移**及其随后**排列**组成正常的6层脑皮质结构的双重过程。

先天畸形

多小脑回畸形

- 多小脑回畸形属于一种脑皮质发育畸形，以正常6层结构的脑皮质排列错乱为特征，导致脑回过多、脑沟过少。
- 多小脑回畸形的形成原因一般认为是神经元迁移过晚或皮质分层过早。
- 多小脑回畸形可能是由宫内感染(特别是CMV)、宫内缺血或遗传因素所引起，也有许多病因不明的病例。临床表现有发育延迟、局灶性神经体征和症状、四肢轻瘫或癫痫。
- MRI表现为皮质增厚，表面不规则并凹凸不平，高分辨率成像可以看到更多细小的独立脑回。多小脑回畸形的皮质在无髓鞘化的区域表现为薄且凹凸不平，而在大脑的髓鞘化区域则厚而光滑。
- 双侧外侧裂周围为多小脑回畸形最常见部位。

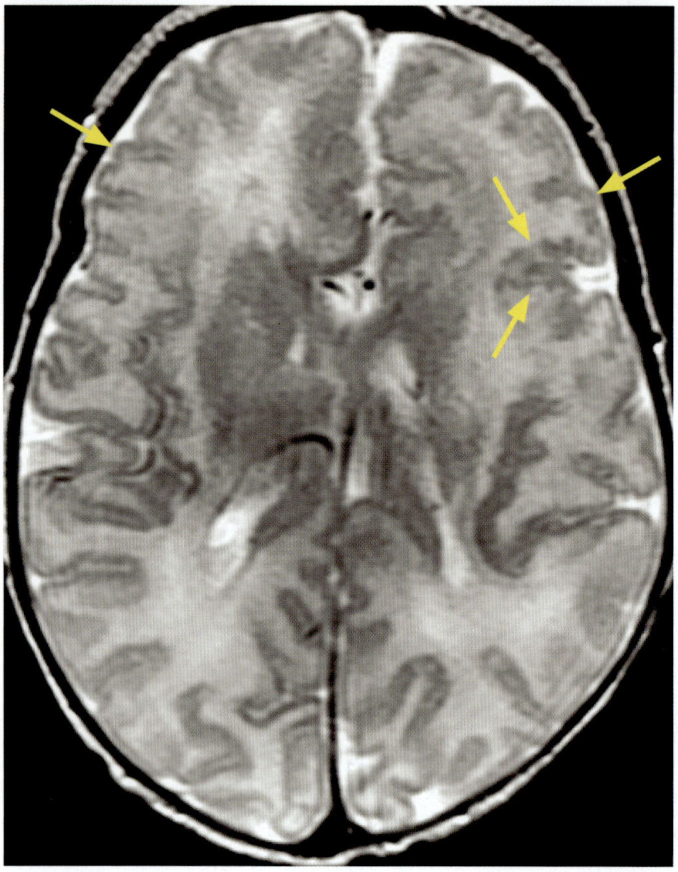

T2-weighted MRI demonstrates bilateral perisylvian and bifrontal polymicrogyria (arrows point to the perisylvian polymicrogyria). The junction between affected cortex and the white matter has an irregular bumpy outline in this young patient with predominantly unmyelinated white matter.

T_2加权MRI显示双侧外侧裂周围和双侧额叶多小脑回畸形(箭指外侧裂周围多小脑回畸形)。这名小儿患者以无髓鞘的白质为主，受累的皮质和白质交界处结构轮廓不规则且凹凸不平。

Lissencephaly

- Lissencephaly is characterized by absent or decreased cortical convolutions causing a smooth, thickened cortical surface. In classic lissencephaly, instead of the normal 6-layered cortex, the cortex is arranged into 4 primitive layers. Lissencephaly is thought to result due to an arrested band of neurons, which have not completed outward migration to the superficial cortex.
- Most lissencephalies are the result of genetic mutations encoding tubulins, actins, and microtubule-associated proteins like doublecortin DCX, LIS1, dyneins and kinesins.
- Clinically, patients with lissencephaly almost universally have seizures.
- Classic lissencephaly is genetically and embryologically distinct from cobblestone malformations (sometimes called lissencephaly type Ⅱ). Cobblestone lissencephaly results from neuronal overmigration through gaps in the pial limiting membrane and is associated with cerebellar and ocular malformations and muscular dystrophy (Walker-Warburg syndrome).
- **Type Ⅰ (classical) lissencephaly** is characterized by a smooth cortex and a configuration of the cerebral hemispheres that has been likened to an *hour-glass* or a *figure-of-8*.

无脑回畸形

- 无脑回畸形的特征是皮层卷曲缺失或减少，导致皮层表面厚而光滑。在典型的无脑回畸形中，大脑皮层排列成4个原始层而不是正常的6层结构。无脑回畸形被认为是由于一组神经元发育停滞而无法迁移到皮质表面所致。
- 大多数无脑回畸形是编码微管蛋白、肌动蛋白和微管相关蛋白(如双皮质素蛋白DCX、LIS1、动力蛋白和驱动蛋白)基因突变的结果。
- 临床上，几乎所有无脑回畸形患者都会出现癫痫。
- 典型无脑回畸形在遗传学和胚胎学上与鹅卵石畸形(有时也称Ⅱ型无脑回畸形)不同。鹅卵石形无脑回畸形是由于神经元通过软脑膜限制膜的间隙过度迁移所致，与小脑和眼部畸形及肌萎缩(Walker-Warburg综合征)有关。
- **Ⅰ型(经典型)无脑回畸形**的特征是光滑的脑皮质，大脑半球形状呈沙漏样或8字形。

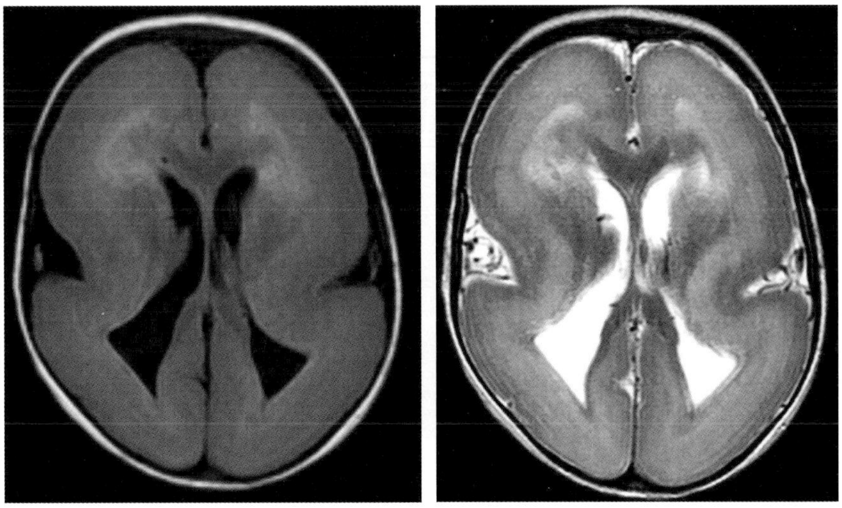

T1-weighted (left image) and T2-weighted (right image) MR images demonstrate classical (type Ⅰ) lissencephaly with a completely smooth cortex and an hour-glass or figure-of-8 configuration to the cerebral hemispheres.

T_1加权(左图)和T_2加权(右图)MRI显示经典型(Ⅰ型)无脑回畸形，脑皮质表面十分光滑，大脑半球呈沙漏样或8字形。

- **Type Ⅱ (cobblestone) lissencephaly** is characterized by a finely undulating cortex.

- **Ⅱ型(鹅卵石型)无脑回畸形**的特征是细小呈波浪状的脑皮层。

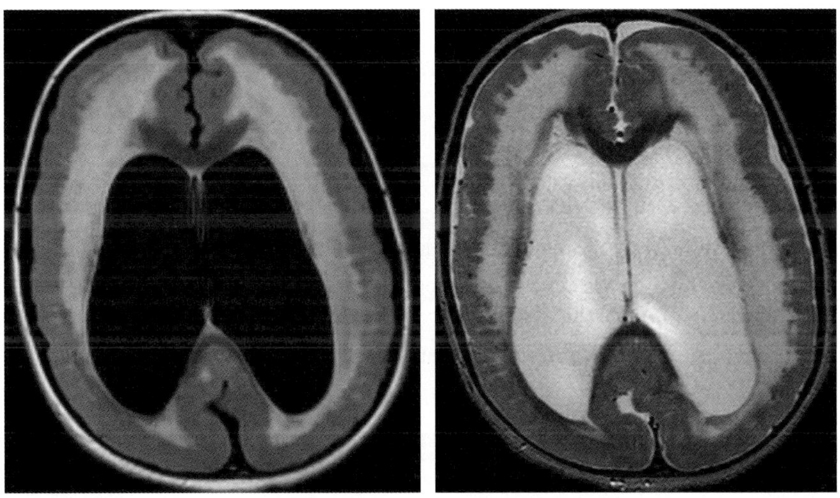

T1-weighted (left image) and T2-weighted (right image) MR images demonstrate **cobblestone malformation** (type Ⅱ) lissencephaly with a gently lobulated external cortex and a finely undulating or serrated interface at the gray-white junction.

T_1加权(左图)和T_2加权(右图)MRI显示**鹅卵石样**无脑回畸形(Ⅱ型)，大脑皮质表面呈浅分叶状，灰-白质交界处呈细波浪状或锯齿状。

Gray matter heterotopia

- Gray matter heterotopia is a range of disorders characterized by clusters of normal neurons in abnormal locations caused by arrested radial migration of neurons.
- Gray matter heterotopia may be a cause of seizures.
- Gray matter heterotopia may be isolated or associated with other structural anomalies.
- Three main subtypes include periventricular (subependymal) nodular heterotopia, focal subcortical heterotopia, and leptomeningeal heterotopia.

灰质异位

- 灰质异位是一类以正常神经元在异常位置聚集为特征的疾病，由神经元向外辐射状迁移受阻而导致。
- 灰质异位可能导致癫痫。
- 灰质异位可以是孤立的，也可以并存其他结构异常。
- 三种主要的亚型包括脑室周围(室管膜下)结节状异位、局部皮质下异位、柔脑膜异位。

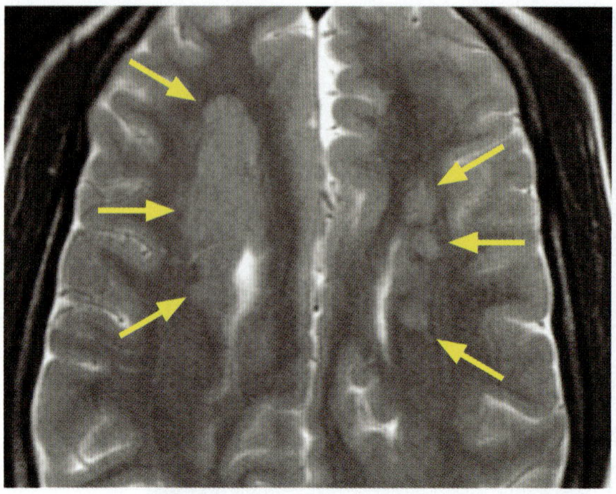

T2-weighted MRI shows extensive bilateral periventricular nodular heterotopia (arrows), most prominent on the right.
T_2加权MRI显示双侧脑室周围广泛分布的结节样异位灰质(箭),右侧更明显。

Agenesis / hypogenesis of the corpus callosum

- Agenesis of the corpus callosum is a relatively common congenital abnormality. The most common clinical manifestations of agenesis of the corpus callosum are refractory seizures and/or developmental delay.
- Complete agenesis of the corpus callosum causes secondary abnormalities in ventricular morphology:

> Colpocephaly (dilation of the occipital horns of the lateral ventricles) may result from decreased white matter volume posteriorly.
> The lateral ventricles are often parallel in orientation and widely spaced.
> Medial impressions on the lateral ventricles are caused by *Probst bundles*, which are axons that would normally constitute the corpus callosum, but instead pursue an aberrant course parallel to the interhemispheric fissure.
> The third ventricle may be enlarged and high-riding.

- The anterior corpus callosum develops first followed by the posterior portion. The anterior and posterior callosum develop separately and eventually unite to form a single structure. Various degrees of corpus callosal hypogenesis may occur, the most common being absence of the splenium.
- Congenital corpus callosal anomalies are often associated with other midline abnormalities including a midline lipoma or interhemispheric cyst.

胼胝体发育不全

- 胼胝体发育不全是一种较为常见的先天性异常。胼胝体发育不全最常见的临床症状是难治性癫痫和/或发育迟缓。
- 完全性胼胝体发育不全可引起继发性脑室形态异常:

> 空洞脑(侧脑室枕角扩大)可能是大脑后部白质体积缩小所致。
> 双侧侧脑室通常平行排列且腔隙增宽。
> 侧脑室内侧压迹由Probst束所致,在正常情况下轴突构成胼胝体,但在完全性胼胝体发育不全时,Probst束异常平行走行于半球间裂。
> 第三脑室也可能扩大并高位骑跨。

- 胼胝体膝部发育先于压部。胼胝体膝部和压部发育是独立的,但最终融合成单一的结构。胼胝体发育不全的程度不同,其中最常见的是压部缺如。
- 先天性胼胝体发育异常通常伴其他中线结构异常,包括中线脂肪瘤和大脑半球间囊肿。

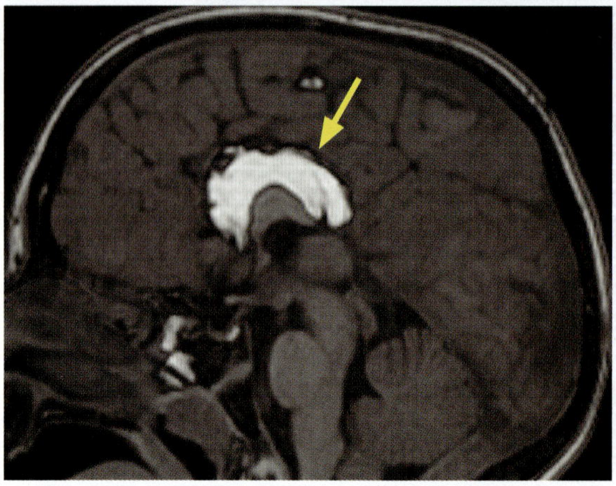

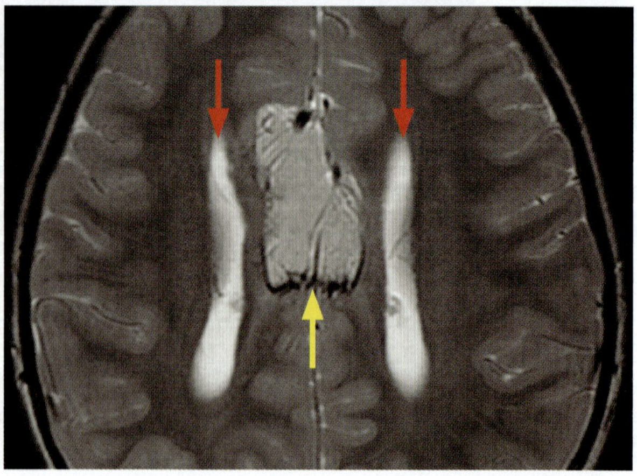

Callosal hypoplasia and midline lipoma: Sagittal T1-weighted MRI (left image) shows hypoplasia of the corpus callosum with a large midline lipoma (yellow arrow). Axial T2-weighted MRI (right image) shows the lipoma (yellow arrow) and parallel orientation of the lateral ventricles (red arrows) due to the callosal hypoplasia.
胼胝体发育不全和中线脂肪瘤:矢状位T_1加权MRI(左图)显示胼胝体发育不全伴中线巨大脂肪瘤(黄箭)。轴位T_2加权MRI(右图)显示脂肪瘤(黄箭)和胼胝体发育不全导致的侧脑室平行排列(红箭)。

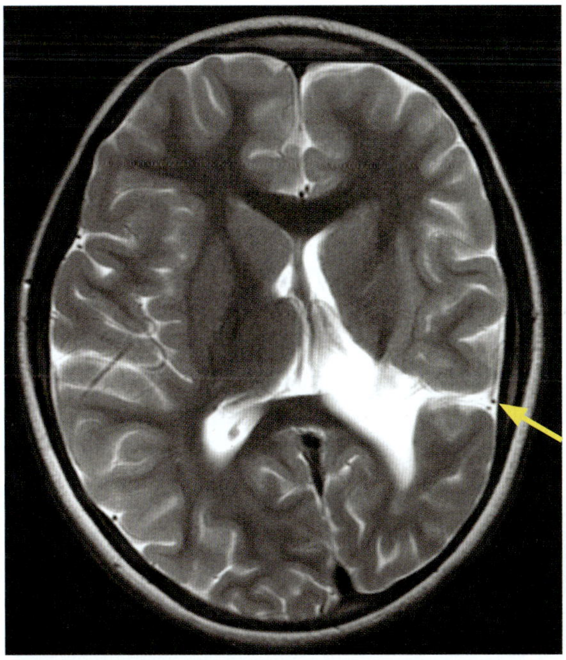

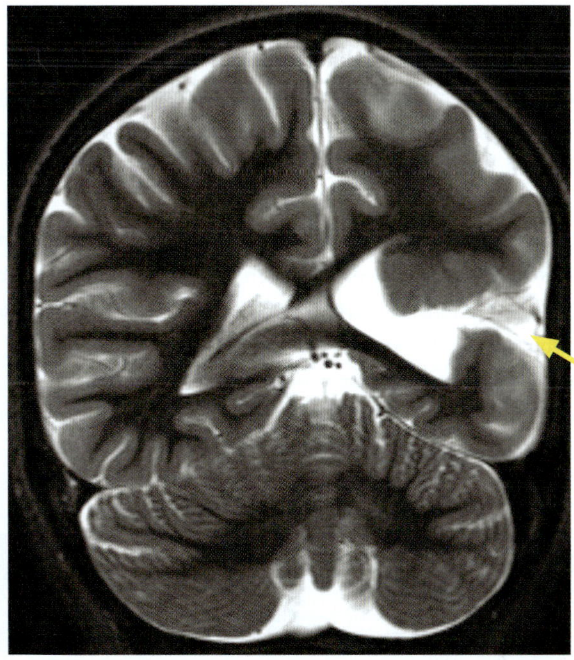

Open-lip schizencephaly: Axial (left image) and coronal (right image) T2-weighted MRI demonstrate a cleft in the left temporoparietal cortex (arrows) extending from the cortical surface to the left lateral ventricle. The cleft is lined by dysplastic-appearing gray matter.

开唇型脑裂畸形：轴位(左图)和冠状位(右图)T_2加权MRI显示一条位于左侧颞顶皮质的裂隙(箭)，从皮质表面延伸至左侧侧脑室。裂隙表面衬有发育不良的脑灰质。

- Schizencephaly is a malformation characterized by a full-thickness cleft of the cerebral hemisphere lined by dysplastic gray matter (usually from polymicrogyria), extending through the entire cerebral mantle, from the ependymal lining of the ventricle to the pial covering of the cortex.

  Schizencephaly does not directly communicate with the subarachnoid space due to the presence of a roofing membrane covering the cleft, which is thought to be composed of a combination of ependymal, pial, and arachnoid tissues.
- Schizencephaly is associated with cortical malformations (gray matter heterotopia), with up to 30% of patients with schizencephaly also having cortical malformations.
- Schizencephaly has been morphologically classified into open-lip (walls of the cleft are entirely divided by CSF) and closed-lip (walls of the cleft are opposed or incompletely divided).
- Schizencephaly is associated with **septo-optic dysplasia**, which is characterized by agenesis of the septum pellucidum, optic nerve hypoplasia and pituitary gland abnormalities.
- The characteristic imaging finding of schizencephaly is a CSF filled cortical cleft lined by gray matter.
- There are several other entities that can cause an interruption or cleft in the cortex, but only a schizencephalic cleft is lined by gray matter. Other cortical clefts include:

> Porencephaly (encephaloclastic): a smooth-walled cavity without surrounding gliosis, usually caused by cortical destruction in the early second trimester.
> Encephalomalacia.
> Surgical resection cavity.

- 脑裂畸形的特征是贯穿大脑半球的裂隙，表面衬有发育异常的灰质(常为多小脑回)，从脑室的室管膜到皮层的软脑膜贯穿整个大脑实质。

  脑裂畸形不能与蛛网膜下腔直接相通，因为有覆盖在裂隙表面的顶膜，后者被认为是由室管膜、脑膜和蛛网膜组成。
- 脑裂畸形与皮质畸形(灰质异位)相关，高达30%的脑裂畸形患者同时伴有皮质畸形。
- 脑裂畸形在形态学上分为开唇型(裂隙的壁完全被脑脊液分隔)和闭唇型(裂隙的壁相互紧贴或不完全分隔)。
- 脑裂畸形与**透明隔-视神经发育不良**相关，其特征表现为透明隔发育不全、视神经发育不良和垂体发育异常。
- 脑裂畸形的特征性影像学表现是皮质裂隙被脑脊液填充，而裂隙的表面衬以灰质。
- 还有几种可以导致皮质中断或裂隙的病变，但仅有脑裂畸形的裂隙衬以灰质。其他皮质裂隙包括：

> 脑穿通畸形(孔洞脑)：一个光滑有壁的腔，其周围没有胶质细胞，通常由早期或中期皮质破坏引起。
> 脑软化。
> 术后残腔。

Holoprosencephaly

- Holoprosencephaly is a complex congenital malformation where the forebrain does not divide into two hemispheres.
- Holoprosencephaly is associated with midline maxillofacial anomalies including a single large central incisor (*megaincisor*) and hypotelorism. It is commonly said that "the brain predicts the face." Holoprosencephaly may be associated with an azygous configuration of the anterior cerebral artery (single ACA).
- The three subtypes (from most severe to least severe) are alobar, semilobar, and lobar. However, these divisions are far from distinct and holoprosencephalies represent a continuum of forebrain malformations, such that there is clear demarcation between the various subtypes.

Alobar holoprosencephaly is the most severe form, characterized by complete lack of separation of the cerebral hemispheres. A single large monoventricle almost always communicates with a large dorsal cyst.

前脑无裂畸形

- 前脑无裂畸形是一种复杂的先天畸形，表现为前脑未分裂成两个大脑半球。
- 前脑无裂畸形与中线颌面部发育异常相关，包括单一中切牙(大门牙)和眼距过窄。这就是通常所说的"大脑决定脸"。前脑无裂畸形与大脑前动脉不成对相关(单支大脑前动脉)。
- 三种亚型(严重程度由重至轻)分别是无脑叶、半脑叶和脑叶型。然而，这些分型并非泾渭分明，前脑无裂畸形的各型反映了前脑畸形发育的连续进程，不同的亚型之间难有明确的划分。

无脑叶前脑无裂畸形是最严重的类型，其特征是大脑半球分裂完全缺失。巨大的单腔脑室总是与背侧巨大的囊肿相通。

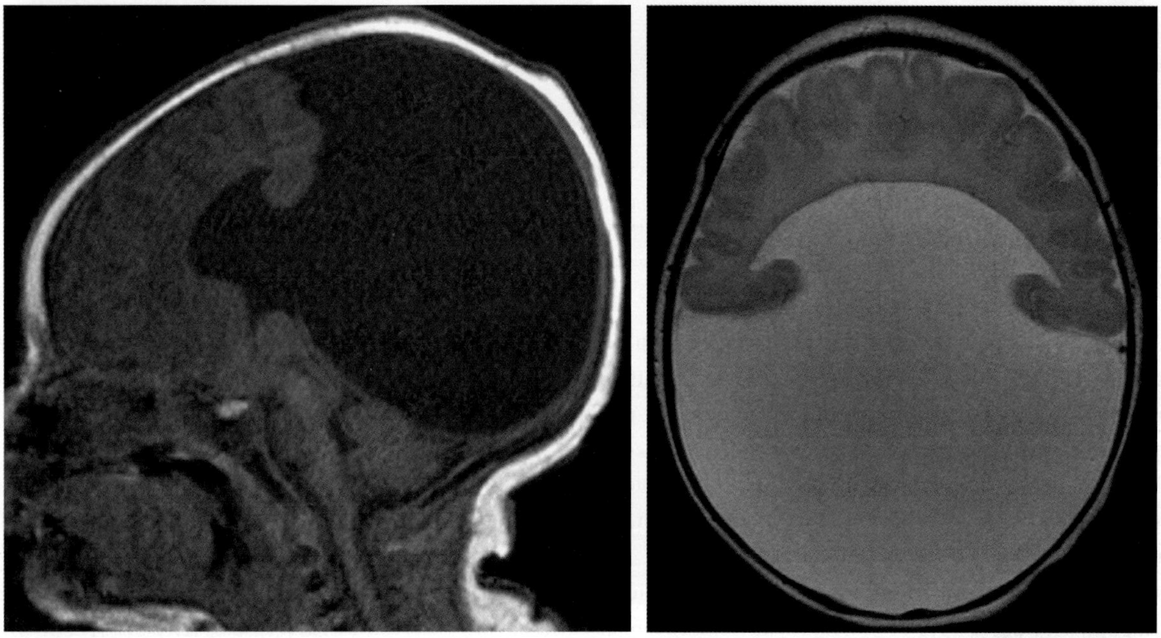

Sagittal T1-weighted (left image) and axial T2-weighted MRI (right image) demonstrate severe alobar holoprosencephaly. There is continual frontal lobe cortex across midline. A midline monoventricle communicates with a dominant dorsal cyst.

矢状位T_1加权(左图)和轴位T_2加权(右图)MRI显示严重的无脑叶前脑无裂畸形。额叶皮质不间断地跨过中线，位于中线的单腔脑室与背侧一个大的囊肿相通。

Semilobar holoprosencephaly features at least some degree of separation of the posterior cerebral hemispheres. Similar to alobar holoprosencephaly, the anterior hemispheres also fail to separate.

半脑叶前脑无裂畸形的影像学特征是在大脑半球后部至少有不同程度的分裂。与无脑叶前脑无裂畸形相比，其大脑半球前部同样也未发生分裂。

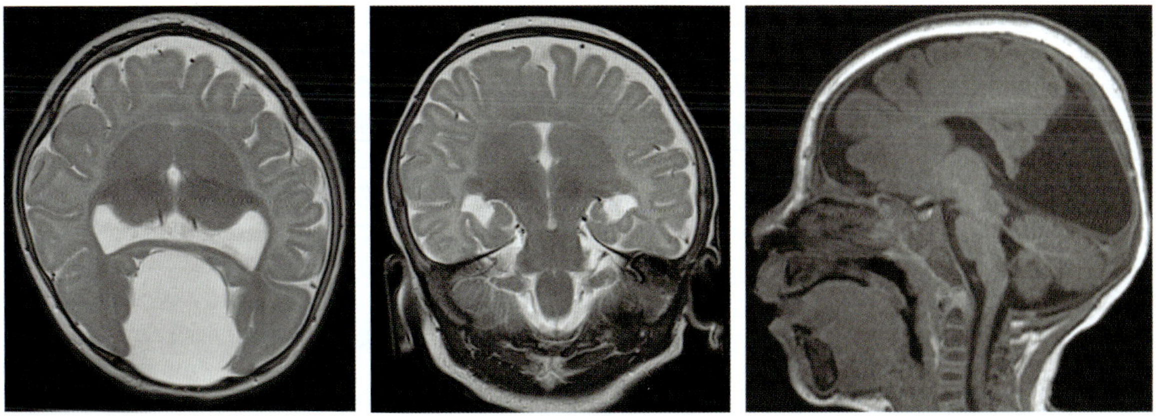

Axial and coronal T2-weighted MRI (left and middle images) and sagittal T1-weighted MRI (right image) show semilobar holoprosencephaly. There is partial separation of the posterior cerebral cortex, with complete fusion of the frontal lobes. There is a large midline posterior interhemispheric cyst.

轴位和冠状位T_2加权(左图和中图)和矢状位T_1加权(右图)MRI显示半脑叶前脑无裂畸形。大脑半球后部皮质有部分分裂,两侧额叶完全融合。还可见位于中线后部半球间的一个巨大囊肿。

Lobar holoprosencephaly is the mildest form, where only the most rostral aspects of the frontal neocortex are not separated. The corpus callosum is absent in the affected region anteriorly, but the posterior corpus callosum (splenium and posterior body) is present.

脑叶前脑无裂畸形是严重程度最低的一种类型,仅有额叶最前部的皮质没有分裂。前部受累区域的胼胝体缺如,但后部胼胝体(压部和体部的后部)还存在。

POSTERIOR FOSSA MALFORMATIONS

颅后窝畸形

Chiari Ⅰ malformation

Chiari Ⅰ型畸形

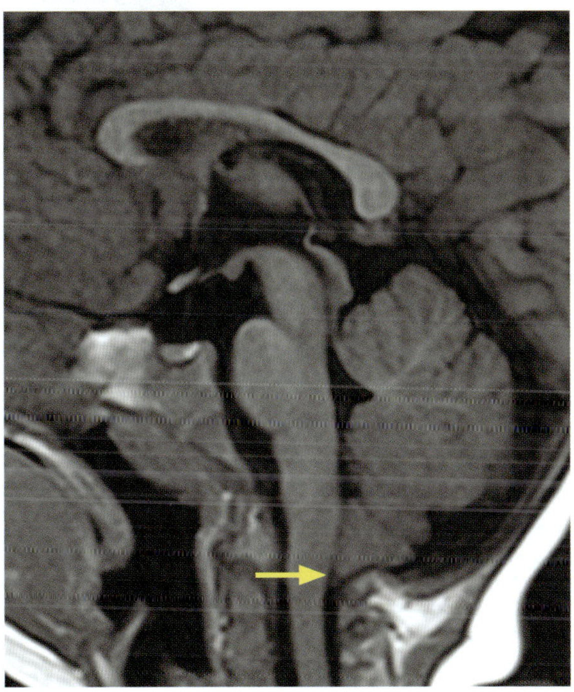

Borderline tonsillar ectopia: Sagittal T1-weighted MRI shows pointed cerebellar tonsils extending inferiorly below the foramen magnum (yellow arrow). There is no hydrocephalus or cervical spine syringomyelia.

临界性小脑扁桃体异位:矢状位T_1加权MRI显示小脑扁桃体向下延伸至枕骨大孔的下方(黄箭)。无脑积水和颈部脊髓空洞。

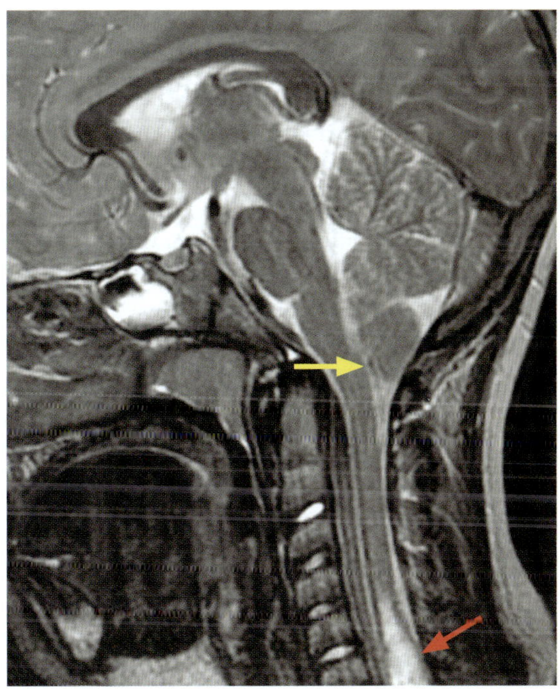

Chiari Ⅰ in a different patient: Sagittal T2-weighted MRI shows inferior extension of the cerebellar tonsils (yellow arrow). The presence of syringomyelia (red arrow) allows more confident diagnosis of Chiari Ⅰ.

另一名Chiari Ⅰ型患者:MR矢状位T_2加权图像显示向下延伸的小脑扁桃体(黄箭)。出现脊髓空洞(红箭)更加支持Chiari Ⅰ型诊断。

- Chiari Ⅰ is inferior displacement of the cerebellar tonsils beyond the foramen magnum.
- The clinical manifestation of Chiari Ⅰ is variable and ranges from occasional exertional headaches in an otherwise normal individual to severe myelopathy and brainstem compromise. In babies, Chiari Ⅰ may be associated with sleep apnea and feeding problems.
- The most common complications of Chiari Ⅰ are cervical syringomyelia and less commonly hydrocephalus.

  Syringomyelia, also called *syringohydromyelia* or *syrinx*, is fluid within the spinal cord.

  Syringomyelia most commonly represents dilation of the central canal of the spinal cord, which normally extends from the obex of the fourth ventricle to the filum terminale.

  The syringomyelia associated with Chiari Ⅰ is fusiform dilation of the central canal that does not typically communicate with the fourth ventricle. Other forms of syringomyelia (typically associated with hydrocephalus) may communicate with the fourth ventricle via the central canal.

  Syringomyelia is seen more commonly in Chiari Ⅰ malformations with associated skull base anomalies.
- Both clinical diagnosis and diagnostic imaging criteria for Chiari Ⅰ are controversial. Inferior protrusion of the cerebellar tonsils is a relatively common finding in asymptomatic individuals. Additionally, the clinical symptoms of Chiari Ⅰ are nonspecific and include headache and malaise, which may not always be attributable to the inferior protrusion of the tonsils.
- The classic criteria for diagnosis is herniation of either cerebellar tonsil by 5 mm, or herniation of both tonsils by 3 mm; however, associated findings allowing a more specific diagnosis include pointed configuration of the cerebellar tonsils, crowding of the posterior fossa, and an associated complication such as cervical spine syringomyelia or hydrocephalus.
- If the only finding is isolated inferior displacement of the tonsils, the term "borderline tonsillar ectopia" is generally preferred.

Chiari Ⅱ

- Chiari Ⅱ is a completely different entity from Chiari Ⅰ; however, a common feature among all Chiari malformations is inferior displacement of the hindbrain.
- Chiari Ⅱ malformation is part of a complex malformation involving the hindbrain, spine, and mesoderm of the skull base and spinal column.
- It results from a lowered craniospinal pressure difference, resulting from egress of CSF through an open spinal defect.
- The primary abnormality in Chiari Ⅱ is herniation of the cerebellar vermis, cerebellar tonsils, and medulla through the foramen magnum, with resultant *beaking* of the tectum.
- A myelomeningocele is universally present, typically lumbar.
- The fourth ventricle is low in position, elongated and inferiorly displaced. In some cases, the fourth ventricle can herniate posteriorly and inferiorly, behind the medulla and below the vermis, resulting in an encysted fourth ventricle.
- Approximately 80–90% of children with Chiari Ⅱ have hydrocephalus necessitating shunt placement, due to fourth ventricular obstruction.
- Associated supratentorial anomalies include corpus callosal dysgenesis, heterotopias, and sulcation abnormalities.

- Chiari Ⅰ型是小脑扁桃体向下移位至枕骨大孔的下方。
- Chiari Ⅰ型临床表现差异较大，可从无其他异常的偶发劳力性头痛，至严重的脊髓病变和脑干损害。婴儿Chiari Ⅰ型可能与睡眠呼吸暂停及喂养困难有关。
- Chiari Ⅰ型最常见的并发症是颈段脊髓空洞，少数患者有脑积水。

  脊髓空洞症又称*脊髓空洞积水症*或*脊髓积水症*，是指脊髓内积聚了液体。

  脊髓空洞症最常表现为脊髓中央管扩张，正常脊髓中央管从第四脑室闩一直延伸到脊髓的终丝。

  与Chiari Ⅰ型相关的脊髓空洞为中央管呈梭状扩张，且通常与第四脑室不相通。其他原因引起的脊髓空洞(通常与脑积水相关)可能通过中央管与第四脑室相通。

  脊髓空洞症更常见于Chiari Ⅰ型畸形合并颅底异常。
- 无论临床还是影像学诊断Chiari Ⅰ型的标准都有争议。小脑扁桃体向下突出在无症状的个体中相对常见。另外，Chiari Ⅰ型的临床症状缺乏特异性，包括头痛及萎靡不振，这些症状不一定与小脑扁桃体向下突出有关。
- 传统的诊断标准是任意一侧小脑扁桃体下疝超过5mm或两侧同时下疝超过3mm；但是，如发现小脑扁桃体变尖、颅后窝狭小及脊髓空洞或脑积水等并发症，则更支持Chiari Ⅰ型的诊断。
- 如果仅仅是孤立性的小脑扁桃体向下移位，通常更适合用"临界性小脑扁桃体异位"这一术语。

Chiari Ⅱ型

- Chiari Ⅱ型完全不同于Chiari Ⅰ型；但所有Chiari畸形的共同特征是后脑向下移位。
- Chiari Ⅱ型可以是一种复杂畸形的一部分，包括后脑、脊髓、颅底中胚层和脊柱畸形。
- 这是由脑脊液通过脊髓缺损外溢，导致颅内和脊髓内的脑脊液压差降低所致。
- Chiari Ⅱ型主要异常是小脑蚓部、小脑扁桃体及延髓疝入枕骨大孔，从而导致中脑顶盖呈鸟嘴样改变。
- 任何部位都可以出现脊髓脊膜膨出，但通常发生在腰椎。
- 第四脑室位置较低，被拉长并向下移位。在部分病例中，第四脑室可向后、向下突出至延髓后方和小脑蚓部下方，导致第四脑室囊化。
- 80%~90%患有Chiari Ⅱ型儿童的脑积水由第四脑室梗阻所致，需要进行分流手术。
- 合并其他幕上畸形包括胼胝体发育不全、灰质异位和脑沟发育异常。

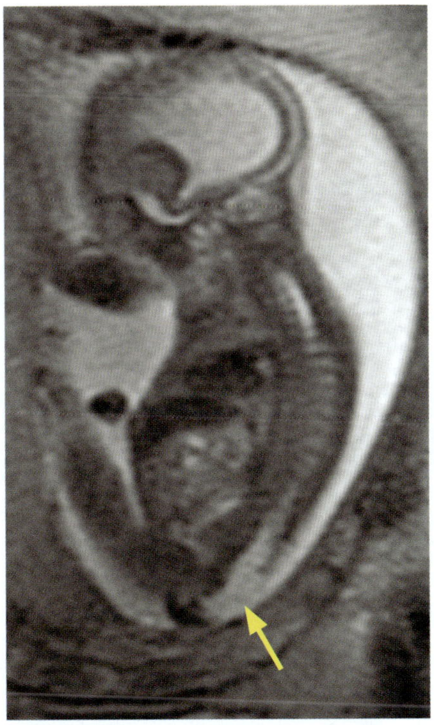

Parasagittal T2-weighted fetal MRI shows a lumbar myelomeningocele (arrow) and marked hydrocephalus.
胎儿旁矢状位T_2加权MRI显示腰段脊髓脊膜膨出(箭)和明显脑积水。

Dandy-Walker complex

- The classic Dandy-Walker malformation is identified by hypoplasia or absence of the cerebellar vermis, hypoplastic cerebellar hemispheres, and a large fluid-filled fourth ventricle within an enlarged posterior fossa with high tentorium and elevated torcula Heterophili.
- An in-utero insult to the developing fourth ventricle is thought to result in fourth ventricular outflow obstruction, cyst-like dilation of the fourth ventricle (which communicates with a retrocerebellar cyst), and resultant inferior vermain hypoplasia.
- Most patients have hydrocephalus.
- Upwards displacement of the tentorium by the enlarged fourth ventricle and posterior fossa cyst causes **torcular-lambdoid inversion**. The torcular herophili is the confluence of the transverse and the straight sinuses, which is pushed superiorly, above the lambdoid suture.

Dandy-Walker畸形

- 典型的Dandy-Walker畸形表现为小脑蚓部发育不全或缺如、小脑半球发育不全和第四脑室扩张，同时还伴有颅后窝增大、小脑天幕和窦汇抬高。
- 有人认为，第四脑室在胎儿宫内发育过程中受损是导致第四脑室脑脊液流出受阻和第四脑室囊状扩张(与小脑后部囊肿相交通)的原因，最终使小脑下蚓部发育不良。
- 多数患者患有脑积水。
- 小脑被扩大的第四脑室和颅后窝囊肿推压向上移位，导致**窦汇-人字缝倒置**。窦汇是横窦和直窦的汇合处，它被推向人字缝上方。

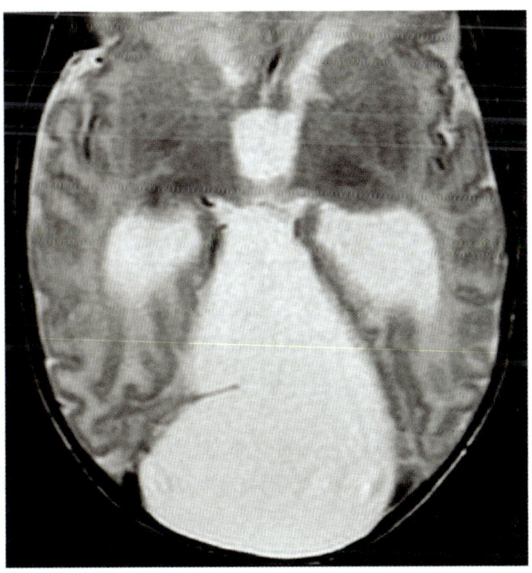

T2-weighted axial MRI shows an enlarged fourth ventricle communicating with a large retrocerebellar cyst, which displaces the tentorium upwards. There is hydrocephalus, with dilation of the temporal horns and third ventricle.
轴位T_2加权MRI显示扩大的第四脑室与巨大的小脑后部囊肿相交通，使小脑幕向上移位。同时可见脑积水，并伴有两侧脑室颞角和第三脑室扩大。

Neurofibromatosis 1 (NF1) / von Recklinghausen disease

1型神经纤维瘤病(NF1)/神经纤维瘤病

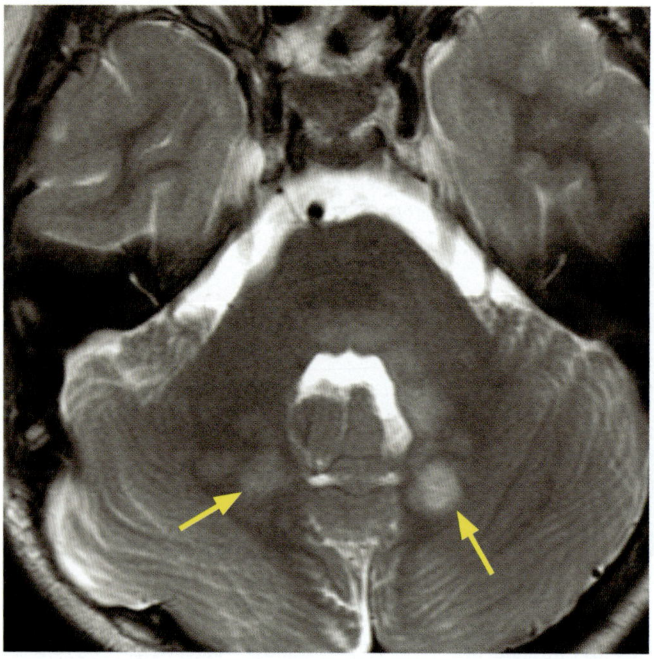

Axial T2-weighted axial MRI through the cerebellum demonstrates T2 hyperintense "unidentified bright objects" of neurofibromatosis representing myelin vacuolization (yellow arrows).

一名神经纤维瘤病患者小脑水平轴位T_2加权MRI显示呈高信号的"不明确的明亮物体",此为髓鞘的空泡化(黄箭)。

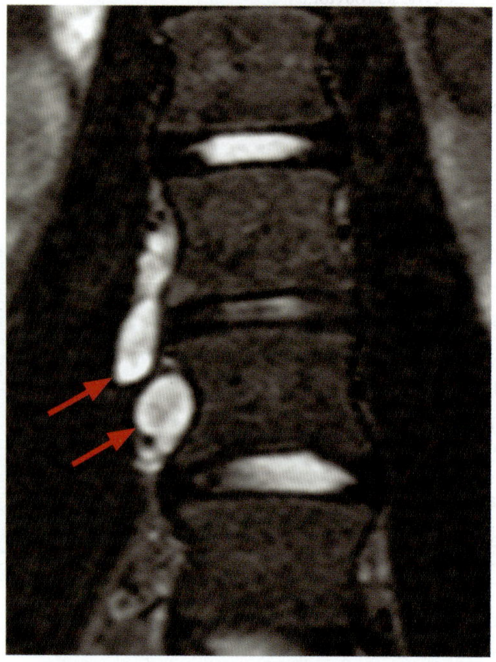

Coronal T2-weighted MRI of the lumbar spine shows the characteristic *target* appearance of plexiform neurofibromas (red arrows), which are T2 hyperintense with central hypointensity.

腰椎冠状位T_2加权MRI显示丛状神经纤维瘤具有特征性的靶征(红箭),即T_2高信号伴中央低信号。

- Neurofibromatosis type 1 (NF1), also known as von Recklinghausen disease, is a multisystemic neurocutaneous disorder with prominent skin manifestation (e.g., café au lait spots), peripheral nerve sheath tumors (e.g., plexiform neurofibroma), CNS malignancies (e.g., optic nerve glioma), and bony abnormalities (e.g., sphenoid wing dysplasia).
- NF1 is autosomal dominant in 50% of cases and occurs sporadically in 50%, caused by a defect in chromosome 17.
- In children, "bright spots" or "unidentified bright objects" are almost universally seen on T2-weighted images, thought to be caused by myelin vacuolization. These bright spots are seen most commonly in children aged 4–12 and become less prominent in adults.
- Neurofibromas are WHO grade I nerve sheath tumors. The cutaneous and subcutaneous nerves are more commonly involved than the more proximal peripheral nerves. A *plexiform* subtype is more aggressive and consists of a network of fusiform-shaped masses, with malignant degeneration reported in approximately 5%.

Like schwannomas, neurofibromas are likely of Schwann cell origin.

The *target sign* can be seen with either neurofibromas or schwannomas, and reflects central T2 hypointensity thought to be due to a fibrocollagenous core. The *target sign* is suggestive of benignity.

In contrast to schwannomas, neurofibromas are not encapsulated and involve the entire cross-sectional area of the nerve. If a neurofibroma is resected, the parent nerve must

- 1型神经纤维瘤病(NF1)又称神经纤维瘤病,是一种多系统的神经皮肤病变,以皮肤病变(如牛奶咖啡斑)、周围神经鞘瘤(如丛状神经纤维瘤)、中枢神经系统恶性肿瘤(如视神经胶质瘤)及骨骼异常(如蝶骨翼发育不良)为突出表现。
- NF1有50%病例为常染色体显性遗传,另外50%为散发,原因为17号染色体缺陷。
- 在儿童,"高信号斑点"或"不明确的明亮物体"在T_2加权图像上几乎普遍存在,被认为是由髓鞘空泡化所致。这些亮斑最常见于4~12岁的儿童,在成人不太明显。
- 神经纤维瘤病是WHO Ⅰ级的神经鞘瘤。皮肤及皮下神经较近端周围神经更易受累。丛状亚型更具侵袭性,并形成网状的纺锤形肿块,有报道约5%的病例会发生恶变。

与神经鞘瘤一样,神经纤维瘤也可能起源于施万细胞。

靶征均可在神经纤维瘤和神经鞘瘤中出现,病灶中心T_2低信号被认为是纤维胶质的核心。靶征提示为良性病变。

与神经鞘瘤相比,神经纤维瘤无包膜并累及神经纤维的整个断面。如果切除神经纤维瘤,其神经主

therefore be sacrificed.

- NF1 is associated with multiple brain neoplasms:

Optic nerve glioma (50% of these tumors are associated with NF1).
Juvenile pilocytic astrocytoma.
Brainstem glioma.

- Bone manifestations of NF1 include:

Sphenoid wing dysplasia, which may produce pulsatile enophthalmos or exophthalmos.
Posterior vertebral body scalloping.
Rib notching (*twisted ribbon ribs*) due to erosion from neurofibromas of the intercostal nerves.
Focal gigantism.
Cervical kyphoscoliosis, with a characteristic acute angle.
Neural foraminal enlargement, either due to bony dysplasia or a neurofibroma.
Tibial bowing.

- Eye manifestations of NF1 include hamartomas of the iris, known as Lisch nodules.
- NF1 is also associated with multiple extra-cranial neoplasms:

Wilms tumor.	Angiomyolipoma (renal).
Rhabdomyosarcoma.	Leiomyosarcoma.

Neurofibromatosis 2 (NF2)

干必然受损。

- NF1合并多种脑部肿瘤：

视神经胶质瘤(50%患者伴有NF1)。
青少年毛细胞性星形细胞瘤。
脑干胶质瘤。

- NF1的骨骼表现：

蝶骨翼发育不良，可导致搏动性眼球内陷或突出。
椎体后方扇形变。
肋骨切迹(肋骨扭曲)，由肋间神经纤维瘤导致的骨质吸收引起。
局部巨大畸形。
颈椎后侧凸，形成特征性的锐角。
神经孔扩大，为骨质发育异常或神经纤维瘤引起。
胫骨弯曲。

- NF1眼部表现包括虹膜错构瘤，亦称Lisch结节。
- NF1还与多种颅外肿瘤相关：

肾母细胞瘤。	血管平滑肌脂肪瘤(肾)。
横纹肌肉瘤。	平滑肌肉瘤。

2型神经纤维瘤病(NF2)

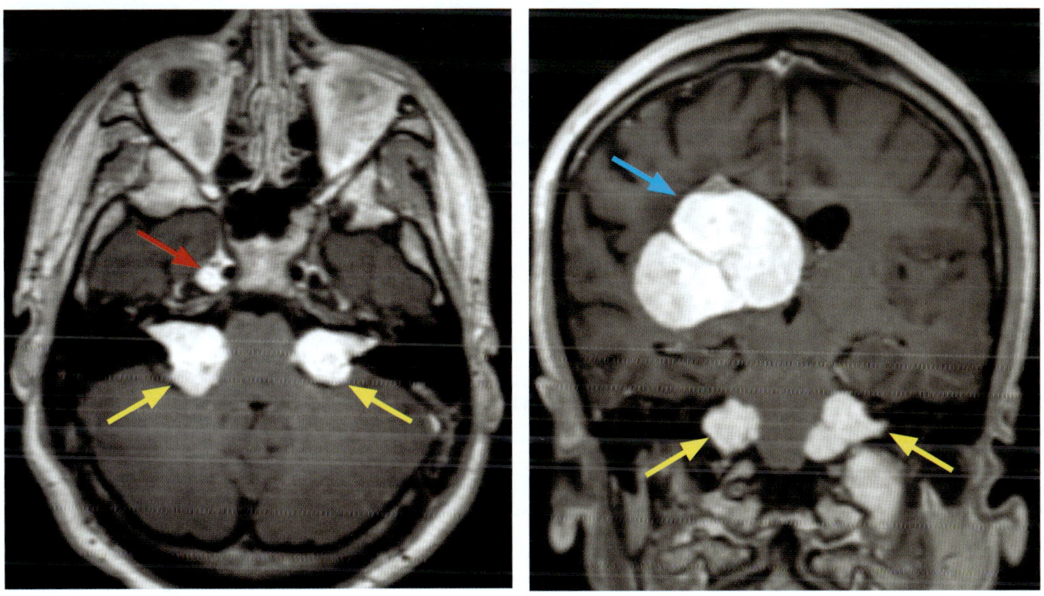

Multiple cranial nerve schwannomas and meningioma in NF2: Axial (left image) and coronal (right image) post-contrast T1-weighted MRI show enhancing bilateral cerebellopontine angle masses extending into the internal auditory canals, consistent with vestibulocochlear schwannomas (yellow arrows). Other schwannomas arising from the trigeminal nerve are partially visualized along the margins of the cavernous sinuses (red arrow). Large right atrial enhancing mass is seen on the coronal image consistent with a meningioma (blue arrow).

NF2多发脑神经鞘瘤和脑膜瘤：轴位(左图)和冠状位(右图)增强T_1加权MRI显示双侧桥小脑角区肿物明显强化，并向内听道内延伸，符合听神经鞘瘤(黄箭)的表现。另见起源于三叉神经的神经鞘瘤沿海绵窦边缘分布(红箭)。冠状位图像可见右侧侧脑室一处大而明显强化肿物，符合脑膜瘤(蓝箭)的表现。

- Neurofibromatosis type 2 (NF2) is an autosomal dominant neurocutaneous disorder completely unrelated to NF1. Despite the name, neurofibromas are not a component of NF2. NF2 is caused by a defect on chromosome 22 and is approximately 10 times less common than NF1.
- NF2 is characterized by the **MISME** mnemonic: Multiple Inherited Schwannomas, Meningiomas, and Ependymomas.
- The typical clinical presentation of NF2 is hearing loss caused by bilateral vestibular schwannomas. The presence of bilateral vestibular schwannomas is diagnostic of NF2.

- 2型神经纤维瘤病(NF2)是一种常染色体显性遗传性神经皮肤综合征，与NF1完全无关。尽管名字相似，神经纤维瘤并不是NF2中的一个组成部分。NF2是由22号染色体缺陷引起，比NF1少约10倍。
- NF2特征性表现可用**MISME**进行记忆：多发性遗传性施万细胞瘤、脑膜瘤和室管膜瘤。
- NF2典型临床表现是由双侧前庭神经鞘瘤引起的听力障碍。发现双侧前庭神经鞘瘤即可诊断NF2。

Sturge Weber

斯德奇-韦伯综合征

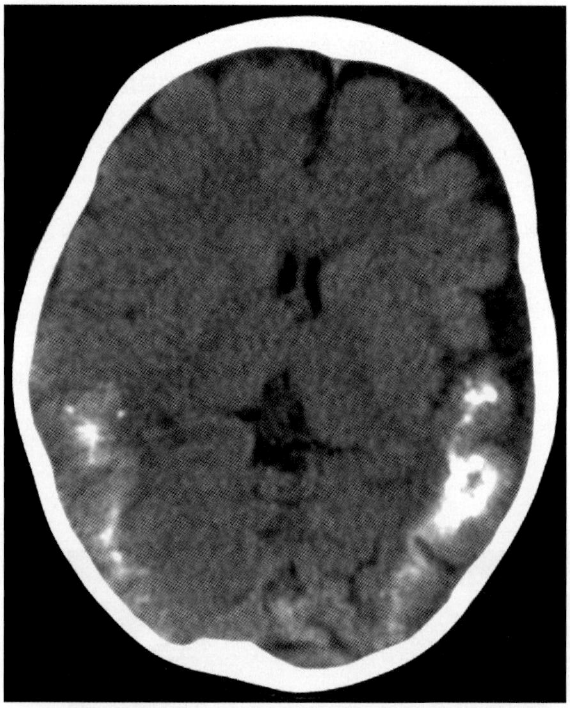

Sturge Weber: Noncontrast CT shows subcortical calcification and cerebral atrophy in a 32-month-old child.

斯德奇-韦伯综合征：一名32月龄幼儿头颅CT平扫显示皮质下钙化和大脑萎缩。

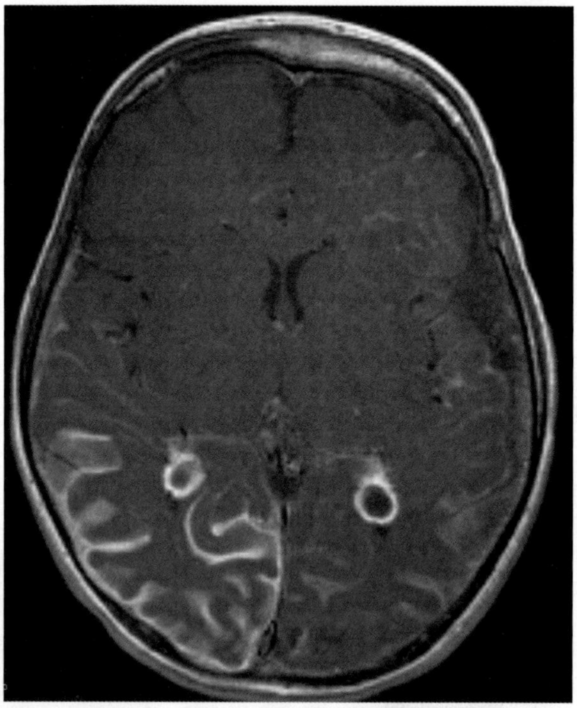

Axial post-contrast T1-weighted MRI of the same patient shows diffuse leptomeningeal enhancement, most prominent in the right occipital lobe, and bilateral choroid plexus engorgement.

同一名患者轴位增强T_1加权MRI显示弥漫性软脑膜强化，以右侧枕叶最为明显，伴双侧脉络丛充血。

- Sturge Weber is a neurocutaneous disorder characterized by facial port-wine stain (capillary malformation), ocular abnormalities, and failure of development of normal cortical venous development.

  The port-wine stain typically involves the forehead and upper eyelid, corresponding to the region innervated by the ophthalmic branch of the trigeminal nerve (V^1).
- Sturge-Weber is a **vascular** disorder, thought to be caused by failure of regression of the primitive embryologic cephalic venous plexus. This developmental anomaly results in the formation of leptomeningeal venous angiomatosis, which is a vascular malformation characterized by dilated capillaries and venules.
- The underlying vascular anomaly ultimately leads to chronic ischemia, cortical atrophy, and cortical calcification.
- Clinically, patients may have some degree of developmental delay and seizures; however, up to 50% of patients may have normal intelligence. Seizures and

- 斯德奇-韦伯综合征是一种神经皮肤疾病，具有下列特征：面部葡萄酒色斑(毛细血管畸形)、眼睛异常及正常皮质静脉发育障碍。

  葡萄酒色斑主要位于前额和上眼睑，与三叉神经眼支(V1)的分布区域一致。
- 斯德奇-韦伯综合征是一种**血管性**疾病，可能为原始胚胎头部静脉丛退化障碍。这种发育异常导致软脑膜静脉性血管瘤形成，即一种以毛细血管及小静脉扩张为特征的血管发育畸形。
- 这种血管畸形最终导致慢性缺血、脑皮质萎缩及钙化。
- 临床上患者可能存在一定程度的发育延迟和癫痫，但是多达50%的患者智力正常。癫痫

developmental delay tend to occur together.

- Characteristic imaging findings are cortical atrophy and subcortical parenchymal calcifications, which are best seen on CT. Contrast-enhanced MRI demonstrates pial enhancement in regions affected by the leptomeningeal venous angiomatosis. The choroid plexi are typically enlarged from compensatory hypertrophy thought to be related to increased flow.

Tuberous sclerosis

- Tuberous sclerosis is a hamartomatous disorder affecting several organ systems, with multiple skin manifestations.
- The classical clinical triad of adenoma sebaceum (nodular rash originating in the nasolabial folds), seizures, and mental retardation is not always present.
- Clinically, most patients have epilepsy, neurocognitive dysfunction, and pervasive developmental disorders.
- Neuroimaging features multiple T2 hyperintense white matter cortical or subcortical tubers (hamartomas) and subependymal nodules.
- 15% of patients develop subependymal giant cell astrocytoma (SEGA), which may appear on imaging as a newly enhancing or enlarging subependymal nodule.
- Extracranial manifestations include:

Renal: Multiple angiomyolipomas.
Cardiac: Rhabdomyoma.
Lung: Lymphangioleiomyomatosis.

和发育延迟往往同时发生。

- 特征性的影像学表现是皮质萎缩和皮层下实质钙化，CT显示最为清晰。增强MRI显示被软脑膜静脉血管瘤侵犯的软脑膜区域强化。脉络丛通常呈代偿性肥大，可能与血流量增加有关。

结节性硬化

- 结节性硬化是一种错构性病变，它影响多个器官系统，并具有多种皮肤表现。
- 典型的临床三联征为皮脂腺瘤(起源于鼻唇沟皱褶处的结节状皮疹)、癫痫和智力发育障碍，但并不总是出现。
- 临床上，大多数患者表现有癫痫、神经认知障碍及全身性发育迟缓。
- 神经影像的特点是分布于白质或皮质下(错构瘤)和室管膜下的多发T_2高信号结节。
- 约15%的患者会并发室管膜下巨细胞星形细胞瘤(SEGA)，其影像可表现为一个新发的强化或增大的室管膜下结节。
- 颅外表现包括：

肾：多发血管平滑肌脂肪瘤。
心脏：横纹肌瘤。
肺：淋巴管肌瘤病。

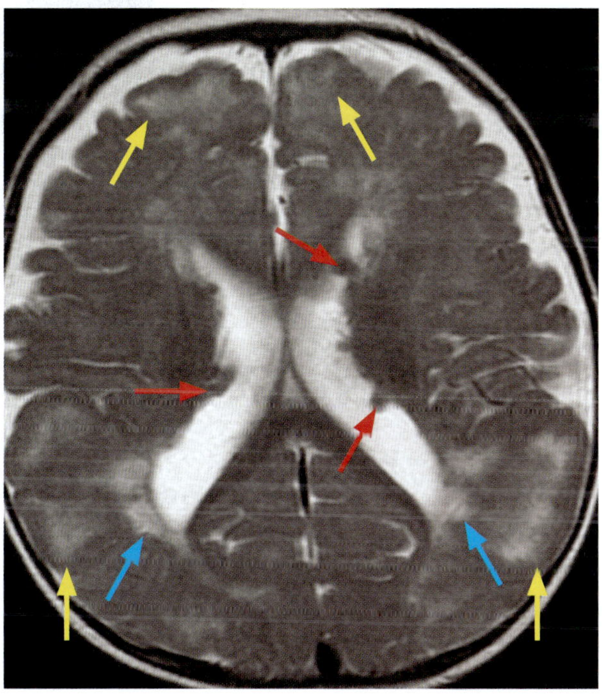

Axial T2-weighted MRI shows numerous bilateral T2 hyperintense cortical tubers (yellow arrows), subcortical tubers (blue arrows), and subependymal nodules (red arrows).
轴位T_2加权MRI图像显示双侧多发T_2高信号的皮质结节(黄箭)、皮质下结节(蓝箭)和室管膜下结节(红箭)

MIDBRAIN ALFORMATIONS

Joubert and related syndrome

- A "molar tooth" configuration of the midbrain can be seen in several diseases, including Joubert syndrome and related disorders (JSRD).
- JSRD clinically present as a hypotonic child with developmental delay and

中脑畸形

朱伯特综合征及其相关综合征

- 中脑"臼齿"形改变可见于多种疾病，包括朱伯特综合征及其相关的疾病(JSRD)。
- JSRD在临床上表现为儿童期肌张力低下，伴

ataxia. These disorders are often associated with ocular anomalies.

- The primary abnormality of Joubert syndrome is thought to be aplasia or hypoplasia of the cerebellar vermis. Dysplastic cerebellar tissue is often present.
- Unlike Dandy–Walker complex, hydrocephalus or a large posterior fossa cyst are uncommon.

有发育延迟和共济失调。这些病变常伴有眼部异常。

- 朱伯特综合征最主要的异常被认为是小脑蚓部不发育或发育不良。小脑组织发育不良常见。
- 与丹迪-沃克综合征不同，脑积水和巨大的颅后窝囊肿不常见。

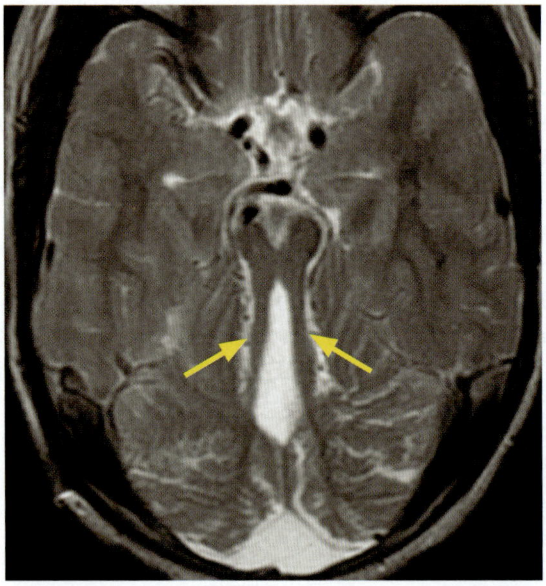

Axial T2-weighted MRI shows a characteristic "molar tooth" configuration of the midbrain (arrows) in a patient with Joubert syndrome. This patient also had a small posterior fossa cyst.

轴位T_2加权MRI显示朱伯特综合征患者的特征性中脑"臼齿"形改变(箭)。该患者同时还有一个颅后窝小囊肿。

Brain tumors

- Brain tumors are discussed in the neuroimaging section.

脑部肿瘤

- 脑部肿瘤详见"神经影像：大脑"章节。

（翻译　吴桂鹏）

15 Imaging Physics

Junzi Shi, Ellen X. Sun, Jacob Mandell

Contents

15 影像物理

目录

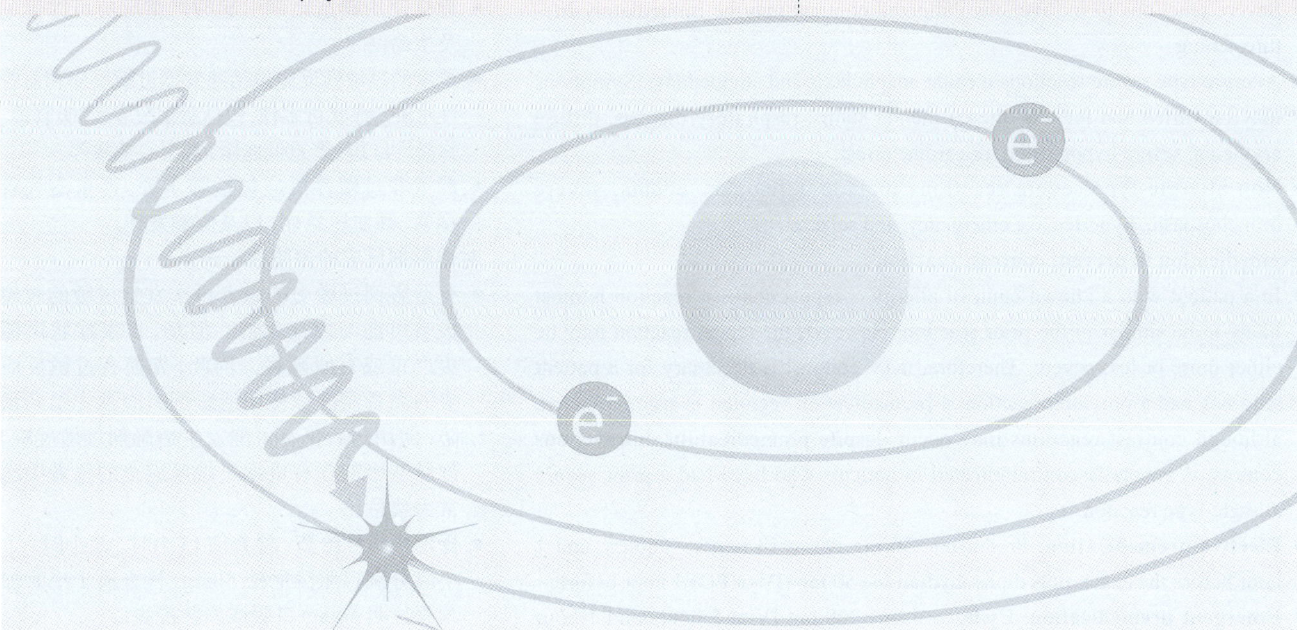

ACUTE REACTION TO CONTRAST MEDIA

Contrast media reaction overview

- Acute reactions to iodinated and gadolinium-based intravenous contrast can be divided into allergic-type and non allergic-type mechanisms. Both allergic-type and non allergic-type reactions can range in severity from mild and self-limited to severe and life-threatening.
- Many of the side effects of contrast agents are due to the hyperosmolarity of the solution.
- Patients with asthma are at increased risk of an allergic-like contrast reaction.
- Seafood or shellfish or povidone-iodine allergies do not increase the risk of allergic reaction to iodinated contrast more so than any other allergy.
- Mild nausea, sensation of warmth, and flushing are considered physiologic and are not adverse reactions to contrast.

Mild contrast reactions

- A mild contrast reaction is self-limited and does not require medical management.
- A vasovagal reaction to intravenous contrast is rare and is characterized by bradycardia and hypotension. Mild vasovagal reactions are usually self-limited and are not allergic in etiology.
- Urticarial reactions are mild allergic-type reactions, and include hives and mild angioedema. The symptoms of mild angioedema include scratchy throat, slight tongue or facial swelling, sneezing, and generally do not require medical management.

Moderate contrast reactions

- Moderate contrast reactions are not immediately life-threatening but may require medical management.
- Moderate allergic-type reactions include severe urticaria, bronchospasm, moderate tongue/ facial swelling, and transient hypotension with tachycardia.
- Moderate non allergic-type reactions include significant vasovagal reaction, protracted nausea/vomiting, isolated chest pain, and hypertensive urgency.

Severe contrast reactions

- Severe reactions to intravenous iodinated contrast may be immediately life-threatening.
- Allergic-type severe reactions include anaphylaxis and angioedema. Symptoms may be varied and include altered mental status, respiratory distress, diffuse erythema, severe hypotension, or cardiac arrest.
- Non allergic-type severe reactions include pulmonary edema, severe bronchospasm, hypertensive emergency, and seizure.

Premedication to prevent contrast reaction

- In a patient with a known contrast allergy, a repeat contrast reaction is most likely to be similar to the prior reaction. However, the repeat reaction may be either more or less severe. Therefore, if IV contrast is necessary for a patient who has had a previous reaction, a premedication regimen is recommended, although contrast reactions may occur despite premedication. Intravenous contrast is generally contraindicated in patients who have had a prior severe allergic-type reaction.
- **Elective premedication**: Prednisone 50 mg PO at 13 hours, 7 hours, and 1 hour before the exam, plus diphenhydramine 50 mg (IV or PO) 1 hour before.
- **Emergent premedication**: Hydrocortisone 200 mg IV at 5 hours and 1 hour

急性造影(对比)剂反应

造影剂反应概述

- 对静脉含碘和含钆造影剂的急性反应可分为过敏性和非过敏性两种机制。无论是过敏性还是非过敏性反应，严重程度都可从轻度和自限性，直至重度和危及生命。
- 很多造影剂的副作用是由于溶液的高渗透性引起。
- 哮喘患者增加了对造影剂过敏反应的风险。
- 对海鲜、贝类或聚维酮碘过敏并不会比其他任何物质过敏更增加对碘造影剂过敏的风险。
- 一般认为，轻度恶心、发热感和潮红为生理性反应，而非对造影剂的不良反应。

轻度造影剂反应

- 轻度造影剂反应为自限性，无须治疗。
- 由静脉造影剂引发的血管迷走反射很罕见，其特征是心动过缓和血压降低。轻度的血管迷走反射常为自限性，而非过敏所致。
- 荨麻疹是轻度过敏性反应，包括荨麻疹和轻度血管性水肿。轻度血管性水肿的症状包括喉咙发痒、轻微的舌/面部肿胀及打喷嚏，一般无须治疗。

中度造影剂反应

- 中度造影剂反应不会即刻危及生命，但需要进行治疗。
- 中度过敏性反应包括严重荨麻疹、支气管痉挛、舌/面部中度水肿，以及一过性低血压伴心动过速。
- 中度非过敏性反应包括明显的血管迷走反射、持续恶心/呕吐、孤立性胸痛、高血压急症。

严重造影剂反应

- 静脉使用碘造影剂引起的严重反应可即刻危及生命。
- 严重的过敏性反应包括速发型过敏反应和血管性水肿。症状可多样，包括意识改变、呼吸窘迫、弥漫性红斑、严重低血压，甚至心搏骤停。
- 严重非过敏性反应包括肺水肿、严重支气管痉挛、高血压急症，以及癫痫发作。

对造影剂反应的预防性给药

- 有造影剂过敏史的患者再次发生过敏的表现极有可能与以往相似。但是，再发症状可能更严重或有所减轻。因此，先前有过敏反应史的患者需静脉使用造影剂时应预先给药预防，但用药后仍有可能发生造影剂过敏反应。静脉造影剂在有重度过敏反应史的患者中通常为禁忌。
- **择期预防性给药**：检查前13小时、7小时、1小时分别口服泼尼松 50mg，检查前 1 小时加苯海拉明 50mg(口服或静脉推注)。

before contrast administration. Diphenhydramine is given 1 hour prior. Note that IV steroids have *not* been shown to be effective when given sooner than 4 hours before the contrast administration.

- **紧急预防性给药**：静脉使用造影剂前5小时和1小时，分别静脉推注强的松 200mg。检查前 1 小时给予苯海拉明。注意，如果静脉使用激素与造影剂间隔小于 4 小时并未被证明对预防有效。

Classification of Contrast Reactions

MILD: Signs and symptoms appear self-limited without evidence of progression.	
Physiochemotoxic Pre-treatment is not indicated	**Allergic** Pre-treatment is indicated
Headache, dizziness, mild hypertension, anxiety, altered taste, vasovagal reaction that resolves spontaneously **Limited:** Nausea and/or vomiting **Transient:** Flushing, warmth, chills	Conjunctivitis, rhinorrhea, nasal congestion, sneezing **Limited:** Urticaria, pruritus, cutaneous edema, scratchy or itchy throat

MODERATE: Signs and symptoms are more pronounced. Stable vital signs. Moderate degree of clinically evident focal or systemic signs or symptoms.	
Physiochemotoxic Pre-treatment is not indicated	**Allergic** Pre-treatment is indicated
Vasovagal reaction that requires and is responsive to treatment Hypertensive urgency Isolated chest pain **Protracted:** Nausea and/or vomiting	**Mild or no hypoxia associated with:** Bronchospasm/wheezing **No dyspnea associated with:** Facial edema Hoarseness Throat tightness **Diffuse:** Urticaria, pruritus, erythema

SEVERE: Signs and symptoms are often life-threatening. Unstable vital signs.	
Physiochemotoxic Pre-treatment is not indicated	**Allergic** Pre-treatment is indicated
Vasovagal reactions resistant to treatment Convulsions/seizures Clinically manifest arrhythmias Hypertensive emergency Pulmonary edema	Diffuse erythema with hypotension Anaphylactic shock Laryngeal edema with stridor and/or hypoxia Bronchospasm/wheezing with significant hypoxia

造影剂反应的分类

轻度：体征和症状自限性、无进展。	
生理化学毒性 无须预先给药	**过敏性** 需预先给药
头痛、眩晕、轻度高血压、焦虑、味觉改变、自限性迷走神经反射 **自限性：**恶心和/或呕吐 **暂时性：**潮红、发热、寒战	结膜炎、流涕、鼻塞、打喷嚏 **自限性：**荨麻疹、发痒、皮肤水肿、喉咙发痒

中度：体征和症状较为明显。生命体征稳定。中度局部或系统性临床体征或症状。	
生理化学毒性 无须预先给药	**过敏性** 需预先给药
需要进行治疗的迷走神经反射，且对治疗有反应 高血压急症 仅有胸痛表现 **持续性症状：**恶心和/或呕吐	**轻度或者不伴缺氧：** 支气管痉挛/哮鸣音 **不伴有呼吸困难：** 面部水肿 声音嘶哑 咽喉发紧感 **弥漫性：**荨麻疹、瘙痒、红斑

重度：体征和症状常危及生命。生命体征不稳定。	
生理化学毒性 无须预先给药	**过敏性** 需预先给药
迷走神经反射对治疗无反应 抽搐/癫痫 临床有心律不齐 高血压急症 肺水肿	弥漫性红斑并伴低血压 过敏性休克 咽喉水肿并伴有喘鸣和/或低氧血症 支气管痉挛/哮鸣音伴有明显低氧血症

non allergic-type acute contrast reactions

mild to moderate non allergic-type 轻度至中度非过敏性反应

Hypotension and bradycardia (vasovagal)
低血压、心动过缓(迷走神经性)

1. ECG, pulse oximetry, blood pressure
   心电图、脉搏血氧计、血压
2. Oxygen via facemask
   面罩给氧
3. Elevate legs or Trendelenburg
   抬高下肢或垂头仰卧位(Trendelenburg 体位)
4. Administer IV fluids
   静脉输液
5. If poorly responsive, atropine 0.5 mg IV
   May repeat up to 3 mg total
   若上述处理反应不佳,静脉推注阿托品 0.5mg。
   可重复给药,总量不超过3mg
6. Call for assistance (at any point)
   急救呼叫(任何时候)

moderate to severe allergic-type 中度至重度非过敏性反应

Pulmonary edema
肺水肿

1. ECG, pulse oximetry, blood pressure
   心电图、脉搏血氧计、血压
2. Oxygen via facemask
   面罩给氧
3. Elevate torso
   抬高上身
4. Furosemide 20–40 mg IV
   静脉推注呋塞米 20~40mg
5. Call for assistance (at any point)
   急救呼叫(任何时候)

moderate to severe allergic-type 中度至重度非过敏性反应

Seizures
癫痫发作

1. ECG, pulse oximetry, blood pressure
   心电图、脉搏血氧计、血压
2. Oxygen via facemask
   面罩给氧
3. Consider diazepam 5 mg IV
   or
   midazolam 2.5 mg IV
   酌情静脉推注地西泮 5mg
   或
   咪达唑仑 2.5mg
4. Continue to monitor vitals and pulse oximetry
   持续监测心率和氧饱和度
5. Call for assistance (at any point)
   急救呼叫(任何时候)

allergic-type acute contrast reactions

mild to moderate allergic-type 轻度至中度过敏性反应

Urticaria (hives)
荨麻疹

1. Discontinue injection if not completed.
   立即停止注射造影剂
2. If mild, no treatment.
   轻度:无须治疗
3. If moderate:
   Diphenhydramine PO/IV/IM 25–50 mg
   中度:
   苯海拉明 25~50mg 口服、静脉注射或肌内注射
4. If severe:
   Epinephrine IM 1:1,000, 0.3 ml (0.3 mg)
   重度:
   肌内注射 1:1 000 肾上腺素 0.3ml(0.3mg)
5. Call for assistance (at any point)
   急救呼叫(任何时候)

mild to moderate allergic-type 轻度至中度过敏性反应

Facial or laryngeal edema
面部、喉头水肿

1. ECG, pulse oximetry, blood pressure
   心电图、脉搏血氧计、血压
2. Oxygen via facemask
   面罩给氧
3. Epinephrine IM 1:1,000, 0.3 ml (0.3 mg)
   or
   Epinephrine IV 1:10,000, 1 ml (0.1 mg)
   May repeat up to 1 mg total
   肌内注射 1:1 000 肾上腺素 0.3mL(0.3mg)
   或
   静脉推注 1:10 000 肾上腺素,1ml(0.1mg)
   可重复给药,总量不超过 1mg
4. Call for assistance (at any point)
   急救呼叫(任何时候)

mild to moderate allergic-type 轻度至中度过敏性反应

Bronchospasm(expiratory wheezing)
支气管痉挛(呼气哮鸣)

1. ECG, pulse oximetry, blood pressure
   心电图、脉搏血氧计、血压
2. Oxygen via facemask
   面罩给氧
3. Beta-agonist inhaler (Albuterol)
   吸入 β 受体激动剂(沙丁胺醇)
4. If poorly responsive:
   Epinephrine IM 1:1,000, 0.3 ml (0.3 mg)
   or
   Epinephrine IV 1:10,000, 1–3 ml (0.1–0.3 mg)
   May repeat up to 1 mg total
   若上述处理反应不佳:
   肌内注射 1:1 000 肾上腺素 0.3ml(0.3mg)
   或
   静脉推注 1:10 000 肾上腺素,1ml(0.1mg)
   可重复给药,总量不超过 1mg
5. Call for assistance (at any point)
   急救呼叫(任何时候)

severe allergic-type 重度过敏性反应

Hypotension and tachycardia (anaphylaxis)
低血压、心动过速(过敏性休克)

1. ECG, pulse oximetry, blood pressure
   心电图、脉搏血氧计、血压
2. Oxygen via facemask
   面罩给氧
3. Elevate legs or place Trendelenburg
   抬高下肢或垂头仰卧位(Trendelenburg)
4. IV fluids rapid bolus
   快速静脉输液
5. Epinephrine IM 1:1,000, 0.3 ml (0.3 mg)
   or
   Epinephrine IV 1:10,000, 1 ml (0.1 mg)
   May repeat up to mg total
   肌内注射 1:1 000 肾上腺素 0.3ml(0.3mg)
   或
   静脉推注 1:10 000 肾上腺素,1ml(0.1mg)
   可重复给药,总量不超过 1mg
6. Call for assistance (at any point)
   急救呼叫(任何时候)

(翻译 于千)

IODINATED CONTRAST MEDIA

Types of iodinated contrast

- There are two types of iodinated contrast media: ionic and nonionic (organic).
- Ionic compounds were developed first, and commonly used agents include diatrizoate (Gastrografin).
- Nonionic organic compounds covalently bind the iodine and do not dissociate into component molecules, thus they typically have fewer side effects. Commonly used nonionic agents include iopamidol (Isovue 370) and iohexol (Omnipaque 140, 180, 240, 300, 350).
- The higher the iodine concentration, the more dense it will appear with X-ray exposure.
- The agents are clear, water soluble solutions that are renally excreted and can be used for intravascular, intrathecal and oral or body cavity administration.

CONTRAST-RELATIVE KIDNEY INJURY

Post-contrast acute kidney injury (PC-AKI)

- Post-contrast acute kidney injury (PC-AKI) is a decrease in renal function within 48 hours following intravascular (venous or arterial) administration of iodinated contrast.
- PC-AKI is a general entity that may result from any nephrotoxic process, including exposure to iodinated contrast (CIN, described below) or an unrelated cause.

Contrast-induced nephropathy (CIN)

- Contrast-induced nephropathy (CIN) is a decrease in renal function *caused by* intravascular administration of iodinated contrast. Its exact pathophysiology is unclear.
- Recent studies show that CIN occurs much less commonly than previously thought.
- The most important risk factor for development of CIN is pre-existing renal insufficiency.

  In patients with eGFR ≥45 mL/min/1.73m^2, intravascular iodinated contrast is not an independent risk factor of AKI.

  Even in patients with eGFR ≥30 and <45, the development of CIN is exceptionally rare.

  An eGFR <30 is the most commonly used threshold for stratifying CIN risk.

- Note that gadolinium-based contrast media are not known to cause CIN.

Prevention of contrast nephropathy

- The main preventative strategies against CIN are to use the minimal dose of contrast possible and to adequately hydrate the patient (intravenous hydration is more effective).

  The use of sodium bicarbonate and N-acetylcysteine has been previously advocated but the effectiveness of these agents has not been proven.

- Administration of intravenous contrast to a patient with an eGFR <30 would require a careful assessment of risks and benefits on a case-by-case basis.
- The standard dose of intravenous iodinated contrast can generally be given to patients with end-stage renal disease on chronic dialysis. Careful attention

碘造影剂

碘造影剂分类

- 含碘造影剂分为两类：离子型和非离子型(有机型)。
- 离子化合物是最先开发的产品，常用的制剂包括泛影葡胺。
- 非离子有机化合物与碘共价结合，且不会解离成新的化合物分子，因此其副作用通常较少。常用的非离子型试剂包括碘帕醇(Isovue 370)和碘海醇(Omnipaque 140、180、240、300、350)。
- 碘的浓度越高，其密度在X射线照射下就越高。
- 造影剂为透明的水溶液，由肾脏排出，可用于血管内、髓鞘内，以及口服或体腔内给药。

造影剂相关的肾损伤

造影剂后急性肾损伤(PC-AKI)

- 造影剂后急性肾损伤(PC-AKI)是指血管内(静脉或动脉)注射碘造影剂后48小时内出现肾功能下降。
- 任何可引起肾毒性的事件都称为PC-AKI，包括使用含碘造影剂(CIN，如下所述)或与造影剂无关的其他原因。

造影剂诱发的肾病(CIN)

- 造影剂诱发的肾病(CIN)是由血管内注射含碘造影剂引起的肾功能下降。其确切的病理生理学机制尚不清楚。
- 近期研究表明，CIN的发生率远非过去认为的那么常见。
- 引发CIN最重要的危险因素是存在基础肾功能不全。

  在eGFR≥45mL/(min·1.73m^2)的患者中，血管内使用含碘造影剂不是AKI的独立风险因素。

  即使在eGFR≥30mL/(min·1.73m^2)且<45mL/(min·1.73m^2)的患者中，发生CIN的情况也异常罕见。

  eGFR<30mL/(min·1.73m^2)通常被认为是CIN危险分层的阈值。

- 注意，目前并不清楚含钆造影剂是否会导致CIN。

造影剂肾病的预防

- 预防CIN的主要策略是尽可能使用最小剂量的造影剂，并给患者充分补水(静脉补液比口服更有效)。

  过去曾提倡使用碳酸氢钠和N-乙酰半胱氨酸，但这些药物的有效性尚未得到证实。

- 对于eGFR<30mL/(min·1.73m^2)的患者，使用静脉造影剂需要根据每名患者的具体情况仔细评估风险和益处。
- 对于需要长期透析的晚期肾病患者，通常可

should be paid to the volume status in these patients as theoretically the osmotic load increases intravascular volume.

以静脉注射标准剂量的碘造影剂。建议留意观察这些患者的容量状态，因为理论上造影剂的渗透负荷会增加血管内容量。

IODINATED INTRAVENOUS CONTRAST: GENERAL CONSIDERATIONS

静脉碘造影剂：基本注意事项

Iodinated contrast and pheochromocytoma

- It is safe to administer nonionic contrast media to patients with pheochromocytoma. Prior studies showed an increased in serum catecholamines after high-osmolality contrast agents, which are no longer in current use.

含碘造影剂和嗜铬细胞瘤

- 在嗜铬细胞瘤患者使用非离子型造影剂是安全的。有研究表明，使用高渗性造影剂后血清儿茶酚胺升高，但高渗性造影剂现已不再使用。

Iodinated contrast and thyroid uptake

- Thyroid gland uptake of I-131 is reduced to about 50% one week after iodinated contrast injection. Therefore, if radioactive I-131 therapy is planned, iodinated contrast should be avoided for one month prior to I-131 therapy.

碘造影剂和甲状腺吸收

- 在使用含碘造影剂后1周，甲状腺对^{131}I的吸收率下降约50%。因此，若计划行放射性^{131}I治疗，则应在治疗前1个月内避免使用含碘造影剂。

Metformin and intravenous contrast

- Metformin is an oral anti-hyperglycemic agent that decreases hepatic glucose production and increases peripheral glucose uptake. Although exceptionally rare, there is an increased risk of metformin-associated lactic acidosis in patients receiving intravenous iodinated contrast, thought to be due to PC-AKI and the resultant accumulation of metformin.
- There is no need to discontinue metformin in patients with normal renal function. In patients with multiple comorbidities, metformin should be discontinued at time of contrast administration and withheld for 48 hours.
- Note that it is not necessary to discontinue metformin prior to gadolinium-based contrast.

二甲双胍和静脉造影剂

- 二甲双胍是一种口服降糖药，可降低肝脏葡萄糖合成并提高游离葡萄糖的吸收。在极为罕见的情况下，静脉使用含碘造影剂后可增加二甲双胍相关的乳酸中毒风险，可能为PC-AKI和二甲双胍堆积所致。
- 对于肾功能正常的患者无须停用二甲双胍。在有多种合并症的患者，二甲双胍需在使用造影剂开始至造影后48小时停止使用。
- 注意，使用钆造影剂前不必停用二甲双胍。

Iodinated contrast and pregnancy

- Iodinated contrast crosses the placenta and enters the fetal circulation. No mutagenic or teratogenic effects have been observed in vivo; however, no controlled studies in pregnant patients have been performed.
- It is acceptable to administer iodinated contrast to a pregnant patient if medically necessary. It is recommended that a pregnant patient sign an informed consent form prior to undergoing an examination involving ionizing radiation and iodinated contrast.

含碘造影剂与孕妇

- 含碘造影剂可通过胎盘进入胎儿血液循环。活体内暂未观察到有致突变和致畸的作用，但尚未在孕妇中做过对照研究。
- 如病情需要，对患病孕妇进行造影检查是可以接受的。建议在涉及电离辐射和使用碘造影剂检查前，患病孕妇应签署知情同意书。

Iodinated contrast and breast feeding

- The plasma half-life of iodinated contrast is approximately two hours. Less than 1% of the administered maternal dose of iodinated contrast is excreted in the breast milk within 24 hours of maternal administration, and 1% of that dose may be absorbed by the infant's gastrointestinal tract. The total infant absorbed dose is therefore approximately 0.01% of the administered maternal dose.
- Breast feeding mothers do not need to halt breast feeding. If the mother is concerned, abstaining from breast feeding for 24 hours (while pumping and discarding milk) would result in effectively zero fetal dose.

碘造影剂和母乳喂养

- 含碘造影剂的血浆半衰期约 2 小时。在母亲使用碘造影剂后的24小时内，不到 1 %的母体剂量会进入母乳，而且，这个剂量的1%可能会被婴儿的胃肠道吸收。因此，婴儿总的吸收剂量约为母体剂量的0.01%。
- 哺乳期妇女无须停止哺乳。如母亲有顾虑，可停止哺乳24小时(期间使用吸奶器将奶抽出并丢弃)，以使婴儿的剂量有效地降到零。

Contrast extravasation

- Extravasation is the leakage of contrast into the soft tissues at the injection site. Although the risk of extravasation is not related to the injection flow rate, the use of automatic injectors can lead to a large extravasated volume of contrast media.
- Iodinated contrast is toxic to the soft tissues and skin, although serious adverse events are relatively rare following extravasation. The most common serious injury due to contrast extravasation is compartment syndrome. Less commonly, skin ulceration and tissue necrosis can occur.

造影剂外溢

- 外溢是指造影剂从注射部位渗漏至周围软组织。虽然外溢风险与注射速率无关，但使用自动注药器可导致大量造影剂外溢。
- 碘造影剂对皮肤和软组织有毒性，但造影剂外溢的严重不良事件相对罕见。最常见的严重损伤是筋膜室综合征。较少见的皮肤溃疡和组织坏死也可发生。

- All patients with extravasation should be evaluated by the radiologist. Elevation of the extremity to decrease capillary hydrostatic pressure has been recommended, but is without supporting data. There is no evidence favoring warm or cold compresses, and both are used commonly.
- Surgical consultation should be obtained for progressive swelling and pain, altered tissue perfusion (decreased capillary refill), change in sensation or strength, skin ulceration or blistering.

- 所有出现造影剂外溢的患者都应由放射医师进行评估。有人建议抬高肢体以降低毛细血管的静水压，但缺乏支持性数据。没有证据支持加压热敷或冷敷，尽管这两种方法都很常用。
- 出现进行性肿胀、疼痛加重、组织灌注改变(毛细血管灌注减低)、感觉异常、无力、皮肤溃疡或水疱时，应请外科会诊。

（翻译　于千）

GADOLINIUM-BASED CONTRAST MEDIA

IMMEDIATE ADVERSE REACTIONS TO GADOLINIUM-BASED CONTRAST

- Both mild and severe adverse reactions to gadolinium-based contrast are much more rare compared to iodinated contrast. Most adverse reactions to gadolinium-based contrast are mild such as nausea, vomiting, headache, or pain at the injection site.
- Allergic-type reactions to gadolinium are rare, seen in 0.004% to 0.7%. Serious anaphylactic reactions are exceedingly rare (<0.01%).

Contrast extravasation

- Gadolinium-based contrast is much less toxic to the skin and soft tissues compared to iodinated contrast. Evaluation and treatment of extravasation is similar for both types of contrast.

NEPHROGENIC SYSTEMIC FIBROSIS (NSF)

- Nephrogenic systemic fibrosis (NSF) is a highly morbid disease characterized by diffuse fibrosis of the skin and subcutaneous tissues, which may also involve the visceral organs.
- NSF is strongly associated with gadolinium exposure in patients with reduced renal function. The exact mechanism for development of NSF is unknown, but may involve dissociation of toxic free gadolinium in patients with reduced renal clearance. The free gadolinium may bind phosphate and precipitate in tissues, precipitating a fibrotic reaction.
- Patients with end-stage renal disease (eGFR <30 mL/min/1.73m^2) have between 1% and 7% chance of developing NSF even after a single exposure to a gadolinium-containing contrast agent. There has been only one established case of NSF in a patient with an eGFR >30.
- In general, gadolinium-based contrast should not be given to patients on dialysis or with eGFR <30 or AKI. Although it is exceedingly rare for NSF to develop in a patient with eGFR between 30 and 59, eGFR may fluctuate daily in these patients. For this reason, caution should be employed for patients on the lower end of this spectrum.
- Different brands and formulations of gadolinium-based contrast are associated with varying rates of NSF. Group Ⅰ agents associated with unconfounded cases of NSF include gadodiamide, gadopentetate dimeglumine, gadoversetamide.

钆造影剂

急性含钆造影剂的不良反应

- 与含碘造影剂相比，含钆造影剂的轻度和重度不良反应均少很多。多数为轻度不良反应，如恶心、呕吐、头痛或注射点疼痛。
- 钆造影剂的过敏性反应罕见，发生率为0.004%~0.7%。严重的急性过敏性反应极为罕见(<0.01%)。

造影剂外溢

- 钆造影剂较碘造影剂对皮肤和软组织的毒性都小得多。两类造影剂外渗的评估和治疗基本相同。

肾源性系统性纤维化

- 肾源性系统性纤维化(NSF)是一种高度致残性疾病，其特点是皮肤和皮下组织出现弥漫性纤维化，可累及内脏器官。
- NSF与钆造影剂在肾功能减退患者中的使用有密切关系。NSF的确切发病机制不明，但在肾清除率下降的患者中可能与有毒的游离钆解离有关。游离钆可能与磷酸盐结合并沉积在组织内，从而产生纤维化反应。
- 晚期肾病患者[eGFR<30mL/(min·1.73m^2)]发生NSF的概率在1%~7%，甚至单次注射含钆造影剂都有可能导致NSF发生。至今仅见一例明确的NSF发生于GFR＞30mL/(min·1.73m^2)的患者。
- 总之，对正在透析或eGFR＜30mL/(min·1.73m^2)或急性肾功能衰竭的患者不应使用含钆造影剂。尽管NSF发生在eGFR 为30~59mL/(min·1.73m^2)的患者中极为罕见，但此类患者eGFR每天都有变化，因此，对eGFR处于此范围下限的患者应谨慎使用钆造影剂。
- 不同品牌和不同配方的钆造影剂与NSF发生率有所不同。与NSF病例相关的Ⅰ组药物包括钆双胺、钆喷葡胺和钆弗塞胺。

GADOLINIUM-BASED CONTRAST IN PREGNANCY AND BREAST FEEDING

Gadolinium-based contrast and pregnancy

- Gadolinium-based contrast should *not* be administered during pregnancy. Gadolinium-based contrast crosses the placenta. Although never demonstrated to cause harm, gadolinium chelates may accumulate in the amniotic fluid and remain there indefinitely, with risk of dissociation of the toxic free gadolinium ion.

Gadolinium-based contrast and breast feeding

- The plasma half-life of gadolinium-based contrast is two hours. Less than 0.04% of the administered maternal dose is excreted in the breast milk within 24 hours of maternal administration, and 1% of that dose may be absorbed by the infant's gastrointestinal tract. The total infant absorbed dose of gadolinium is therefore approximately 0.0004% of the administered maternal dose.
- It is likely safe for the mother to continue breast feeding. There is no information to suggest that oral ingestion of such a tiny amount of gadolinium-containing contrast may be harmful to the fetus.

含钆造影剂在孕妇和哺乳期妇女中的使用

钆造影剂与妊娠

- 含钆造影剂不应在妊娠期使用。含钆造影剂可通过胎盘。尽管从未证实过有害，但钆螯合物可以在羊水中积累并永久存在，并有解离成为有毒游离钆的风险。

钆造影剂与母乳喂养

- 钆造影剂的血浆半衰期是2小时。不到0.04%的母体注入量在24小时内进入母乳，乳液中的1%有可能经婴儿胃肠道吸收。所以，婴儿吸收钆造影剂的总剂量是母亲注射剂量的0.000 4%。
- 继续哺乳对婴儿应该是安全的。目前无数据表明口服如此微量的含钆造影剂对胎儿有害。

（翻译　于千）

PHYSICS QUICK REVIEW

MEASURING RADIATION

Exposure, air kerma, absorbed dose, equivalent dose, and effective dose

- **Exposure** is the charge of electrons liberated per unit mass of air. Exposure is measured in Coulombs/Kg.
- **Air kerma** (kinetic energy released per mass) describes the incident X-ray beam intensity as the kinetic energy transferred from uncharged particles (photons) to charged particles (electrons). Air kerma is measured in Gray (J/Kg).
- Air kerma (Gy) can be converted to **absorbed dose** (also quantified in Gy) by the R factor, which depends on kV and the atomic number (Z) of the absorbing tissue.

  Bone (Z = 12) absorbs much more energy than soft tissue (Z ~7.6).

  At 10 mGy air kerma, bone absorbs 40 mGy, tissue absorbs 11 mGy.
- The **equivalent dose** (expressed in Sievert; Sv) is the absorbed dose in Gy multiplied by a radiation weighting factor (W_R).

  W_R depends on the linear energy transfer (LET) of the type of radiation. For diagnostic radiology using X-rays, $W_R = 1$. An alpha particle has a high LET.
- The **effective dose** (also expressed in Sv) is an estimation of radiation exposure that takes into account the equivalent dose to all organs exposed and each organ's radiosensitivity. Effective dose = the sum of the absorbed dose (Gy) * W_R * W_T for all organs exposed.

  W_T is the tissue weighting factor, which varies from 0.12 for radiosensitive organs (e.g., bone marrow, colon, lung, breast), to 0.01 for less sensitive organs, (e.g., bone, brain, and skin).

物理复习提纲

辐射剂量测定

照射剂量、空气比释动能、吸收剂量、当量剂量、有效剂量

- **照射剂量**是单位质量空气中所释放的电子电荷量。照射剂量的单位是库仑每千克(C/kg)。
- **空气比释动能**(单位质量释放的动能)用于描述X射线的入射强度，即动能以电中性的粒子(光子)传递给带电粒子(电子)。空气比释动能的单位是戈瑞(J/kg)。
- 空气比释动能(Gy)可以用R系数转化为**吸收剂量**(同样以Gy为单位)，该系数取决于kV及吸收组织的原子数(Z)。

  骨骼(Z=12)比软组织(Z约7.6)要吸收更多的能量。

  在10mGy的空气比释动能下，骨骼吸收40mGy，软组织吸收11mGy。
- **当量剂量**(单位为希沃特；Sv)是吸收剂量(Gy)乘以辐射权重因子(W_R)。

  W_R取决于所选辐射类型的线性能量传递(LET)。在使用X射线的放射诊断中，W_R=1。Alpha粒子有很高的LET。
- **有效剂量**(同样以Sv为单位)是一种对辐射照射剂量的估算，这种估算考虑到了所有器官受到放射后的当量剂量及每个器官的放射敏感性。有效剂量=所有被照射器官吸收剂量总和(Gy) × W_R × W_T

  W_T是组织权重因子，其数值从0.12(高放射敏感度的器官，如骨髓、大肠、肺、乳腺)到0.01(低放射敏感度的器官，如骨骼、大脑、皮肤)。

Radiation units

- SI (système international) units including Gray and Sievert are almost universally used rather than the older non-SI units. One notable exception is the Curie, which is still commonly used in nuclear medicine (typical dosing ranges are in millicuries).

SI units

- Gray (Gy) quantifies both absorbed dose and air kerma (exposure) as energy absorbed per unit mass.
- 1 Gy = 1 J/Kg
- 1 Gy = 100 Rad
- Sievert (Sv) is used to quantify equivalent dose and effective dose.
- 1 Sv = 100 Rem
- A Becquerel (Bq) is only used in nuclear medicine for radioactive materials.
- 1 Bq = 1 disintegration per second

Non-SI units

- 1 Rad (radiation absorbed dose) = 10 mGy
- 1 Rem = 10 mSv
- 1 Curie = 37 billion Becquerels =$3.7e^{10}$ disintegrations per second

GENERAL RADIOGRAPHY

X-ray generator

- X-ray photons are generated when high-energy electrons hit a target at the anode side of the circuit. For general radiography and CT, the target is made of tungsten (atomic symbol W).

  99% of the electrons' kinetic energy is converted to heat, and 1% is converted to X-rays.
- 90% of X-rays are produced from bremsstrahlung (nuclear field interaction).

  The maximum keV (energy) of the X-ray spectrum is the kV of the generator. The average keV ~1/3 max.
- 10% of X-rays are produced from characteristic radiation. A characteristic X-ray is produced when a high energy electron knocks a K-shell electron out of orbit.

放射单位

- 国际系统(SI)单位包括戈瑞和希沃特，几乎完全取代了过去的非国际单位。唯一的例外是居里，它依然在核医学界被广泛地使用(常用的剂量范围为毫居里)。

国际单位

- 戈瑞(Gy)用于定量吸收剂量和空气比释动能(照射量)，为单位质量所吸收的能量。
- 1Gy=1J/kg
- 1Gy=100Rad
- 希沃特(Sv)用于定量当量剂量及有效剂量
- 1 Sv = 100 Rem
- 贝克勒尔(Bq)只在核医学中用于描述放射性材料
- 1Bq=每秒一次衰变

非国际单位

1拉德(Rad)(放射吸收剂量)=10mGy

1雷姆(Rem)=10毫希沃特(mSv)

1居里=370亿贝克勒尔=每秒$3.7e^{10}$次衰变

普通X射线摄影

X射线发生器

- 当高能电子击中电路阳极靶时，便产生了X射线光子。普通X射线成像和CT的标靶都采用钨(原子标志W)。

  99%的电子动能都被转化为热能，只有1%被转化为X射线。
- 90%的X射线由韧致辐射(核场的相互作用)产生。

  X射线光谱最大的能量(keV)为发生器的电压(kV)。平均keV约是最大电压的1/3。
- 10%的X射线由特征性辐射产生。当一个高能的电子将另一个K壳的电子击出轨道时，便产生了一束特征性X射线。

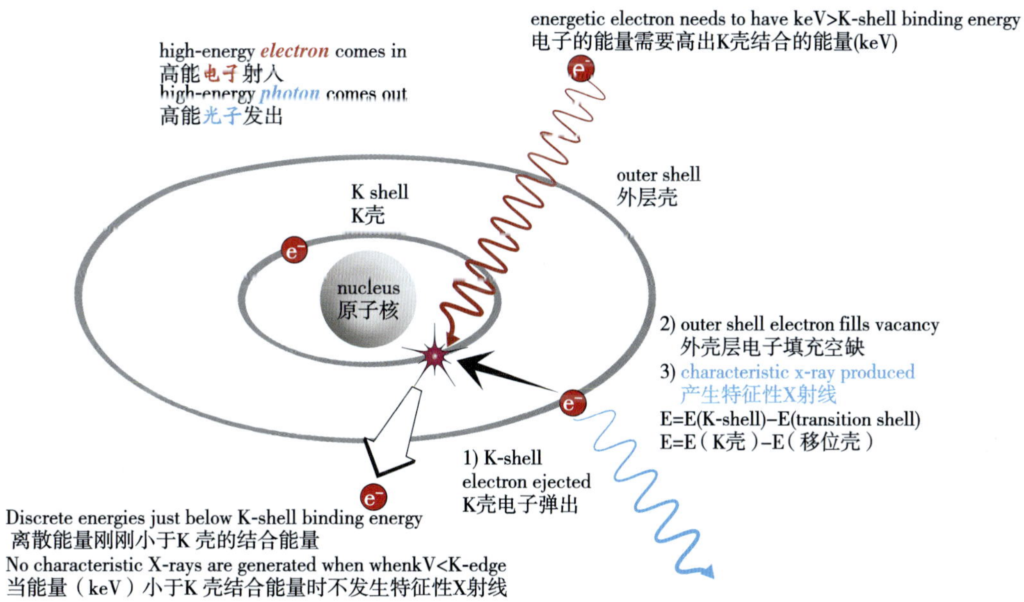

- Tungsten: Atomic weight = 74; K-edge = 70 keV; characteristic X-rays< 70 keV

Effect of kV on tube output

- X-ray production is proportional to $(kV)^2$.
- In practice, changing kV is complicated as a change in kV causes a change in characteristic X-ray, shifts spectrum to the right, and adds photons.
- ↑ kV by 15% → ↑ photons by 100%
- In general, increasing kV will decrease dose and decrease contrast when automatic exposure control is used.

Heel effect

- The heel effect is due to attenuation at the anode, causing fewer X-rays at the anode side.
- The main contributor to the heel effect is the anode angle (typical anode angle ~15°).

  ↓ anode angle → ↑ heel effect

X-ray interactions with matter

All of these interactions deal with incoming photons.

- **Coherent scatter**: No exchange of energy, no change in frequency, and no contribution to patient dose. Contributes less than 5% of X-ray interactions.

- 钨：原子质量=74；K壳=70keV；特征性X射线<70keV。

kV对球管输出的影响

- X射线产生与电压(kV)的平方成正比。
- 实际情况下，改变kV是复杂的，因为kV的改变会带来相应的特性X射线的改变，造成光谱向右移，同时加入了光子。
- kV增长15%，相应光子总数增长100%。
- 通常来讲，当使用自动放射剂量控制的时候，增加kV会减少暴露剂量并降低对比度。

足跟效应

- 足跟效应是阳极的衰减效应，造成在阳极端的X射线减少。
- 足跟效应的主要原因是阳极角(通常阳极角在15°以内)

  阳极角越小，足跟效应越大

X射线和物质的相互作用

所有的这些相互作用都与入射光子相关。

- **相干散射**：无能量交换，无频率改变，且对患者不产生剂量。构成不到X射线相互作用的5%。

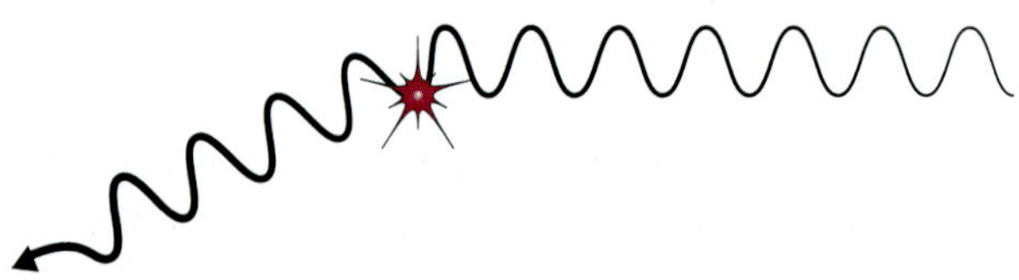

E = energy of incoming photon (keV)

- **Compton scatter**: Proportional to (electron density)/E. Scattered photons go in all directions.

Compton scatter dominates at >25 keV in soft tissue and >40 keV in bone.

E=入射光子的能量(keV)

- **康普顿散射**：与电子的密度成正比，与入射光子的能量成反比。散射光子可向各个方向运动。

康普顿散射在软组织中主要发生在光子能量高于25keV时，而在骨骼，主要发生在光子能量大于40keV时。

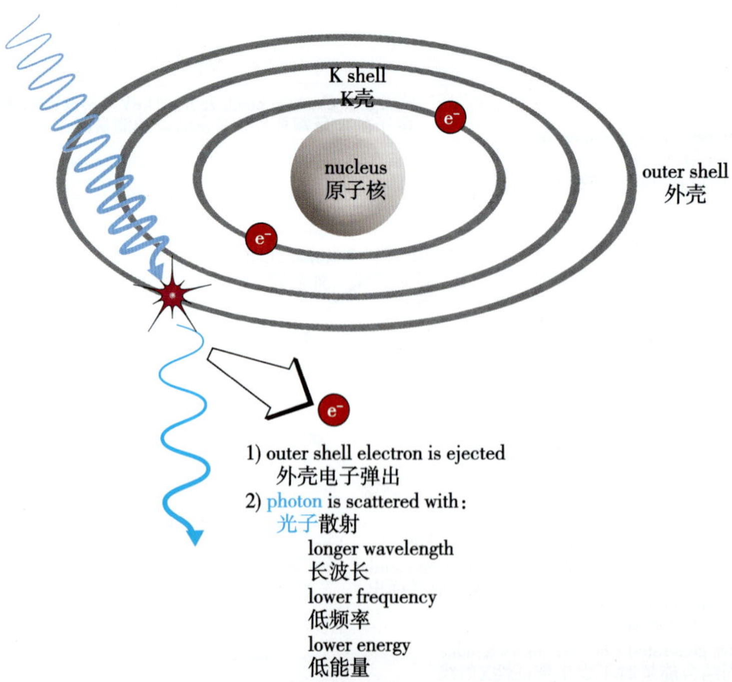

Z = Atomic number

- **Photoelectric effect**: Proportional to Z^3/E^3.

  Photoelectric effect dominates at <25 keV in soft tissue and <40 keV in bone.

Z=原子序数(质子数)

- **光电效应**：与原子序数(Z)的3次方成正比，与入射光子的能量(E)的3次方成反比。

  光电效应在软组织中主要发生于光子能量低于25keV时，而在骨骼主要发生于光子能量低于40keV时。

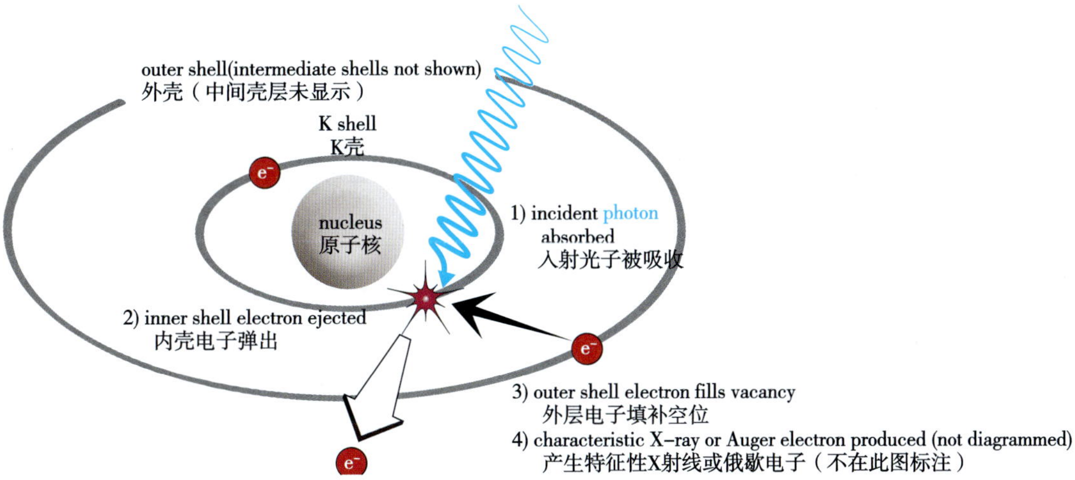

Energy from the ejected inner shell electron is absorbed locally (energetic electrons don't travel very far); however, a 30 keV electron can cause significant damage via 1,000 ionizations (approximately 30 eV/ionization).

Linear attenuation coefficient μ(cm^{-1})

- $N = N_0 * e^{-\mu t}$

  fraction transmitted$=e^{-\mu t}$

  N_0 = initial number of photons

  N = transmitted number of photons after thickness **t**

- If μ is "small" (<0.1/cm), then μ is the proportion of photons that interacts with matter.

  This is only true for weakly attenuating material.

- If μ is "large" (>0.1/cm), then the formula above is used.

  Example: If μ = 0.5/cm, then $e^{-\mu t}$ = 61% transmitted.

Mass attenuation coefficient

- Mass attenuation coefficient = (μ/ ρ), where ρ = density
- Because density is accounted for in the formula above, the mass attenuation coefficient is independent of density.

Scatter and grids

- In radiography, the typical scatter:primary ratio is 5–10:1
- Scatter ↓ contrast
- Grid ratio = height/width

  Typical grid ratios in radiography are between 8–12 (the height of the grid is 8–12 times the width between grid elements).

从内层弹出的电子所释放的能量在局部被吸收(产能的电子不能走很远)；但是，一个30keV的电子可以通过1 000次电离(每次电离约30eV)而造成显著的损伤。

线性衰减系数μ(cm^{-1})

- $N=N_0 * e^{-\mu t}$

  传输率$=e^{-\mu t}$

  N_0=初始光子数

  N=经过t厚度之后通过的光子数

- 如果μ较小(<0.1/cm)，μ就等于与进行物质相互作用的那部分光子。

  这个结论只对弱衰减性的物质适用。

- 如果μ较大(>0.1/cm)，即用以上方程来计算。

  例如，如果μ=0.5/cm，那么$e^{-\mu t}$=61%传输率。

质量衰减系数

- 质量衰减系数=(μ/ρ)，ρ=密度。
- 由于密度已经包括在上述公式中，所以质量衰减系数与密度不相关。

散射和滤线栅

- 在放射成像中，典型的散射与源辐射光子比为(5~10)：1
- 散射会降低对比度
- 滤线栅格比=高度/宽度

  放射成像(X线影像)中典型的栅格比通常在8~12(滤线栅的高度是滤线栅间隔宽度的8~12倍)。

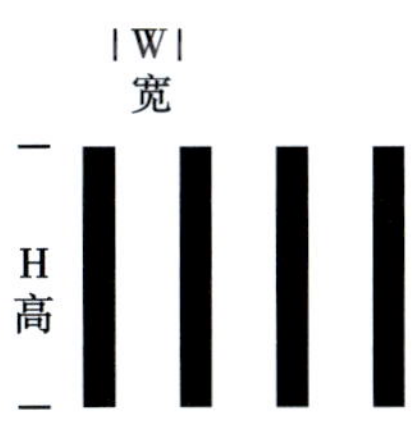

- About 70% of primary radiation passes through the grid.
- Bucky factor is the relative ↑ dose due to grid = incident/transmitted radiation

  The Bucky factor should not be confused with the grid ratio!

  Typical Bucky factor is 5–10 (e.g., ↑ mAs from 40 → 200).
- ↑ kV will ↑ scatter (Compton effects dominate at higher kV).
- Grids not used for extremity radiography (bone is ↑ Z and not very thick).

- 大约70%的原始辐射通过滤线栅。
- 巴基系数是指由于滤线栅造成的相对增加的剂量=入射/透射的辐射。

  巴基系数不能与滤线栅比值混淆!

  典型的巴基系数在5~10(例如，mAs由40增加到200)
- 增加kV会增加散射(康普顿效应在高kV时占主导地位)。
- 滤线栅不适用于四肢的放射成像(骨骼的原子序数高，并且不非常厚)。

Beam quality and half value layer (HVL)

- A "high quality" beam has low-energy photons filtered out.
- The half-value layer (HVL) is a measurement of the beam quality and is the thickness of material that attenuates 50% of the incident energy.
- HVL is dependent on photon energy. HVL ↑ with ↑ photon energy.
- Aluminum (Al) is the standard material for measuring HVL.
- Typical HVL for mammography is 0.3 mm Al.
- Typical HVL for radiography is 3 mm Al.

  The U.S.Food and Drug Administration requires beam quality: HVL >2.5 mm Al at 80 kVp.
- Typical HVL for CT is 8–9 mm Al.

光束质量及半值层(HVL)

- 一束"高质量"的光已经滤掉了低能量的光子。
- 半值层(HVL)用于衡量光束流的质量，为衰减50%入射能量所需物质的厚度。
- HVL取决于光子能量，并随光子能量的升高而升高。
- 铝(Al)是测量HVL的标准材料。
- 典型乳腺X线摄影术的HVL为0.3mm的铝片。
- 典型X线摄影的HVL为3mm的铝片。

  美国食品药品管理局要求光束质量为：在80kVp时，HVL≥2.5mm的铝片。
- 普通CT的HVL通常是8~9mm的铝片。

Film optical density (OD) and characteristic curves

- Film optical density (OD) = $\log_{10}(I_0/I_t)$ = $\log_{10}$(incident/transmitted light intensity)

  OD of 1 → 10% photons transmitted through film

  OD of 2 → 1% transmitted

  OD of 3 → 0.1% transmitted
- Film "looks good" if the average OD is ~1.5. This occurs after approximately 5 μGy photons hit the film/screen.
- A characteristic curve logarithmically plots the relationship between radiation exposure (air kerma) and film optical density.

  The *toe* is the low-exposure region and the *shoulder* is the high exposure region. *Fog* is the baseline low-level darkening of film that occurs in the absence of radiation exposure.
- Latitude is the range of air kerma with satisfactory film density. A high-latitude film is ideal for imaging body parts with a wide variation of X-ray transmission (e.g., a chest radiograph). A high-contrast (low-latitude) film is ideal for accentuating image contrast in tissues with low subject contrast (e.g., mammography).

胶片光密度(OD)和特征性曲线

- 胶片光密度(OD)=$\log_{10}(I_0/I_t)$=$\log_{10}$(入射/透射光强度)。

  1 OD对应10%光子透射过胶片

  2 OD对应1%透射

  3 OD对应0.1%透射
- 理想胶片的平均OD在1.5，也就是约5μGy剂量的光子击中胶片或增感屏。
- 特征性曲线为放射照射量(空气比释动能)和胶片光密度的对数关系。

  趾区是低放射量暴露的区域，肩区则是高放射量暴露的区域。雾区是在没有放射照射情况下细微的本底阴影。
- 宽容度是胶片密度达到满意所对应的空气比释动能范围。高宽容度胶片最适用于X射线穿透变化范围较大的身体部位(如胸片)。高对比度(低宽容度)胶片最适合用于突出低反差组织(如乳腺X线摄影)的成像。

- Gamma is steepest part of curve; gradient is average steepness:
- 伽马区是曲线中最陡峭的一段，梯度是平均斜率：

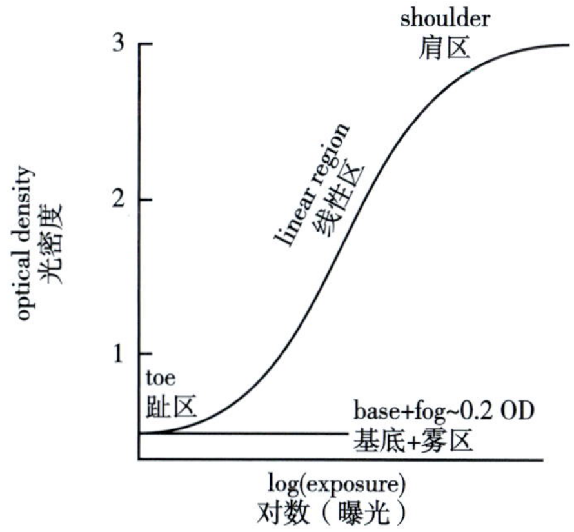

- Effect of latitude on characteristic curve:
- 宽容度对特征曲线的影响：

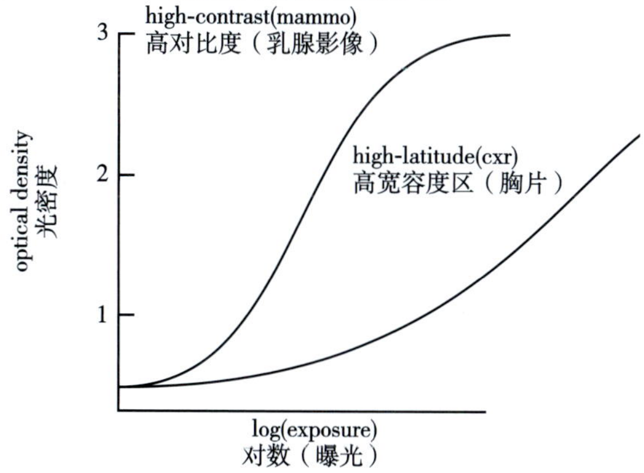

Digital detectors

All except Xe are Solid State detectors.

- **Ionization chamber**: High-pressure Xe (k-edge 35 keV): Used for measuring radiation, not for imaging.
- **Photostimulable phosphor**: Barium fluorohalide (BaFBr); used in computed radiography.

  Read out with red laser light (emits blue light).

  Dynamic range is 10,000:1 (vs. 40:1 for screen film).

  Can be used with air kerma <0.1 μGy to 1000 μGy.

CsI and Selenium used without cassette.

- **Scintillator:** Cesium iodide (CsI); note that CsI also used as input phosphor in an image intensifier.

  Indirect: Absorbed X-rays first converted to light, which is then stored as charge.

  Advantage: K-edge~35keV, good at absorbing X-rays.

  Disadvantage: Light spreads out → blur

- **Photoconductor**: (Selenium)

  Direct: Absorbed X-rays directly converted to charge.

  Advantage: No light spreading, very sharp.

  Disadvantage: K-edge 13, poor X-ray absorber at standard radiography keV.

  Used in digital mammography.

数码探测器

氙(Xe)之外的探测器都为固态

- **电离室**：高压氙(K壳35keV)：用于测量辐射，而不是成像。
- **光激发磷光体**：氟卤化钡(BaFBr)；用于计算机X线摄影术(CR)。

  用红色激光读出(放射出蓝光)。

  动态范围为10 000 : 1(增感屏胶片为40 : 1)。

  可被用于探测空气比释动能小于0.1~1 000μGy。

碘化铯和硒，不用暗盒

- **闪烁体**：碘化铯(CsI)；注意，碘化铯也用于影像增强器作为输入磷光。

  间接：吸收的X射线首先被转化成可见光，然后以电荷形式储存。

  优点：K壳在30keV左右，适用于吸收X射线。

  缺点：光会散射，造成模糊。

- **光导体**：(硒)

  直接：吸收的X射线直接转化成电荷。

  优点：没有光散射，非常清晰。

  缺点：当K壳在13keV时，采用标准的keV进行X线成像将大大降低吸收率。

  用于数码乳腺X线摄影术。

MAMMOGRAPHY PHYSICS

Contact mammography technique summary

- kV is reduced to ↑ contrast
- Focal spot is smaller
- 25 kV; 100 mA (HVL 0.3 mm Al)
- 0.3 mm focal spot standard

  100 mA tube current

- 0.1 mm magnification focal spot

  25 mA tube current

- ↑↑ photons deposited on detector, resulting in lower noise
- 200 μGy (vs. 5 μGy for standard radiography)
- ↑ exposure
- 1 sec vs. 50 ms for abdominal X-ray
- ↑ mAs

乳腺X射线摄影物理

接触式乳腺X线摄影技术要点

- 降低kV以增加对比度
- 局部焦点更小
- 25kV; 10 mA(HVL 0.3mm Al)
- 0.3mm焦点作标准

  100mA管电流

- 0.1mm焦点放大

  25mA管电流

- 大大增加探测器上的光子，导致噪声减少
- 200μGy(相对于标准放射成像时的5μGy)
- 增加曝光时间
- 1s，相对于腹部放射成像的50ms
- 增加mAs

- 100 mAs vs. ~20 mAs (abdominal radiograph)
- Grid ratio smaller
- 5 : 1 (PE > Compton, less scatter) Bucky factor ~2
- Film gradient ↑
- 3 vs. 2
- Higher luminance viewboxes
- 3,000 cd/m^2 is ACR requirement
- Single-emulsion films used
- Heel effect taken advantage of
- Cathode side directed to chest wall

Compared to traditional radiography, mammography image quality improved by several factors

- Contrast increased by: ↓ kV, breast compression, ↑ gamma film
- Resolution improved by: Single thin screen, small focal spot, compression
- Noise (mottle) reduced by: ↑ photons at image receptor (200 μGy vs. 5 μGy for screen-film)

Mammography X-ray generator and filters

- Molybdenum (Mo) target (K-edge 20 keV) generates characteristic X-rays at 17 and 19 keV.
- Mo filter ↓ ↓ low-energy X-rays (which do not contribute to imaging but add to radiation exposure) and ↓ high frequency X-rays (which ↓ contrast).
  Mo filter lets characteristic X-rays through.
- Average energy generated ~17 keV (typical rule that average energy ~1/3 to 1/2 max doesn't apply since characteristic X-rays are so much more important).
- Rhodium (Rh) filter shifts spectrum to the right, used for thicker/denser breasts.
- Rh target/Rh filter used in conjunction for even thicker breasts.

Breast compression

- Advantages of breast compression:
  ↑ X-ray penetration
  ↑ density uniformity
  ↓ scatter
  ↓ dose
  ↓ tissue overlap
  ↓ focal spot blur
- Disadvantages of compression:
  May be uncomfortable

Digital mammography

- Pixel size ~80 μm; smallest visible microcalcifications ~150 μm
- Resolution ~3,000×4,000 pixels = 24 MB at 2 byte/pixel
- 5 megapixel monitors needed for viewing

Magnification mammography

- Magnification = SID/SOD
  SID = source-image distance
  SOD = source-object distance
- SID typically 65 cm, SOD typically 35 cm

- 100mAs，相对于腹部放射成像的20mAs
- 栅格比值变小
- 5：1(光电效应大于康普顿效应，减少散射)巴基系数约为2
- 胶片梯度增加
- 3，而不是2
- 亮度更高的观片框
- 3 000cd/m^{2}是美国放射学院的标准要求
- 使用单层乳胶片
- 发挥足跟效应的优势
- 阴极对准胸壁

与传统放射成像相比较，提高乳腺X线成像的质量有以下几个因素

- 增加对比度：降低kV、挤压乳腺、增加胶片的γ值
- 提高分辨率：采用单个薄屏、小焦点、挤压乳腺
- 降低噪声：增加图像接收器上的光子(对于增感屏胶片，采用200μGy而不是5μGy)

乳腺摄影术的X射线发生器及滤器

- 钼(Mo)靶(K壳 20keV)产生17keV和19keV的特征X射线。
- Mo滤器大大减少了低能X射线(不能用于成像但会增加照射量)和减少高频X射线(高能X射线会降低对比度)。
  Mo滤器允许特征X射线通过。
- 平均生成的能量约为17keV(通常的规律是平均能量约等于最高能量的1/3~1/2在这里不适用，因为特征X射线占主要)。
- 铑(Rh)滤器将光谱向右移动，用于较厚/较致密的乳腺成像。
- Rh靶与Rh滤器结合用于更厚的乳腺成像。

乳腺挤压

- 乳腺挤压的优点：
  增加X射线的穿透力
  增加密度的均匀性
  减少散射
  减少剂量
  减少组织重叠
  减少焦点模糊
- 挤压乳腺的缺点：
  可能造成不适

数字化乳腺摄影

- 像素大小约为80μm；最小可见的微钙化大小约为150μm
- 在每像素为2字节时，分辨率约为3 000×4 000像素=24MB
- 观片需要用500万像素的显示器

放大乳腺摄影

- 放大率=SID/SOD
  SID=源-图像距离
  SOD=源-物体距离
- SID通常是65cm，而SOD为35cm

In the example below, SID = 65 cm, SOD = 35 cm, and magnification = 65/35 = 1.85

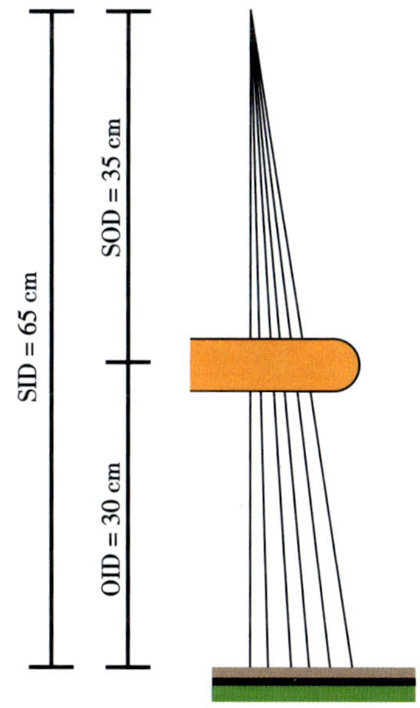

OID = object-image distance

- If ↑ SID (X-ray tube moved away) then exposure time will be too long.
- If ↓ SID (X-ray tube moved closer) then there will be too much focal spot blur.
- No grid needed (air gap introduced).
- 0.1 mm focal spot used.
- Magnification mammography technique summary:

  25 mA current

  3 second exposure

  70 mAs. Because a grid is not employed, a lower total mAs is needed (compared to 100 mAs with contact mammography using a grid).

MQSA

- The interpreting physician needs to have read 240 mammograms in the last 24 months of training during a 6 month period.
- A quality control program must be in place.
- Phantom must be tested weekly with an average glandular dose <3 mGy with a grid, and <1 mGy without a grid.

Average glandular dose (AGD)

- Federal requirement that AGD <3 mGy per view per breast.

  Note that the fluoroscopic dose limit of 100 or 200 mGy/min is the only other federal dose regulation.
- A typical AGD is ~1.8–1.5 mGy per view per breast (digital slightly lower dose).

FLUOROSCOPY PHYSICS

Electronic magnification

- If field of view (FOV) is ↓ by a factor of two (e.g., from 10 cm to 5 cm), the reduced field of view is projected onto the entire output phosphor of the image

在以下例子中，SID=65cm，SOD=35cm，放大率=SID/SOD=65/35=1.85。

OID=物体与成像的距离

- 如果增加SID(拉开X射线管)，曝光时间将会过长。
- 如果减少SID(推近X射线管)，局部焦点模糊将会太大。
- 不需要滤线栅(利用空气间隙)。
- 使用0.1mm的局部焦点。
- 放大乳腺摄影技术总结：

  25mA电流

  3s曝光时间

  70mAs，由于没有使用滤线栅，需要采用较低的总mAs(相比于使用滤线栅的接触乳腺摄影所需的100mAs)。

乳腺摄影质量标准法案(MQSA)

- 读片医师需要在过去24个月的培训期间内有6个月阅读240张以上的乳腺X线影像图片。
- 必须有一个可实施的质量控制规则。
- 体模必须每周进行检测，平均腺体剂量在用滤线栅时<3mGy，无滤线栅时<1mGy。

平均腺体剂量(AGD)

- 联邦政府要求每个乳腺体位的AGD必须小于3mGy。

  注意：X射线透视剂量的上限为每分钟100mGy或200mGy，这是联邦的另一个剂量规定。
- 通常，每个乳腺体位的AGD在1.8~1.5mGy(数字化的剂量略低一些)。

X射线透视物理

电子放大

- 如果视野(FOV)缩小一半(如从10cm到5cm)，则缩小的视场被投射到图像增强器的整个输

intensifier, which will be 4 times dimmer. Therefore, skin exposure will be increased by a factor of 4 by the automatic exposure control.

- Similarly, reducing the exposed area from 10 cm to 7 cm would increase patient entrance air kerma by a factor of two.

Fluoro technique

- Continuous fluoro runs at current of 1 to 5 mA (typically 3 mA), resulting in a very low air kerma/frame of approximately ~0.01 μGy. Compared to a standard chest X-ray exposure of 5 μGy, each fluoro frame has 500 times fewer incident photons.
- There is a federal regulatory limit of 100 mGy/min entrance air kerma.

  High-dose fluoro with audible/visual alarms allows 200 mGy/min for large patients.

Effects of fluoroscopy techniques on dose

- Increasing source to skin distance decreases dose due to inverse-square law.
- Increasing filtration reduces dose by removing low-energy X-rays that would be absorbed.
- Removing grid reduces dose (used in peds), at the risk of increasing scatter.
- Dose spreading (moving the beam around) reduces the maximum skin dose.

  Skin dose rate is about 10–30 mGy/min for continuous fluoroscopy.

  Maximum exposure rate 100 mGy/min or 200 mGy/min in high-level mode.

  At maximum permissible rate in high-level mode, 2 Gy can be delivered in 10 min!

  Large patients are more susceptible to skin injury.
- Magnification *increases* dose, as discussed above.

CT PHYSICS

Overview of CT

- Computed tomography (CT) produces images by rotating a fan beam around the patient and determining the linear attenuation coefficients of each individual pixel using a reconstruction algorithm.

Hounsfield units (HU)

- A Hounsfield unit is a measure of relative CT attenuation.

$$HU=1,000\left(\frac{\mu_x-\mu_{water}}{\mu_{water}}\right)$$

μ_x = attenuation coefficient of the material being measuring

μ_{water} = attenuation coefficient of water

- 10 HU = 1% difference in contrast.
- Gray matter and white matter differ in contrast by only 0.5%.
- A material with twice the attenuation of water attenuates 1,000 HU.

RADIATION DOSIMETRY

CT dosimetry

- The computed tomography dose index (CTDI) is the average phantom dose for a single axial slice (one complete rotation without table motion), including scatter, measured in Gy.

出荧光屏上，造成亮度减少4倍。所以，皮肤的照射量在自动调控的机制下增加4倍。

- 同样，将照射面积从10 cm减少到7 cm会使患者的入射空气比释动能增加1倍。

X射线透视技术

- 连续X射线透视使用的电流为1~5mA(通常是3mA)，其相对的每帧空气比释动能很低，约0.01μGy。与标准胸片的X射线曝光为5μGy相比，每一帧X射线透视的入射光子要减少500倍。
- 联邦政府规定，入射空气比释动能的上限为每分钟100mGy。

  高剂量的X射线透视配备视听警报装置，允许对体型较大的患者达到每分钟200mGy。

X射线透视技术对剂量的影响

- 根据平方反比定律，增加X射线源到皮肤的距离会降低剂量。
- 增加过滤可吸收的低能X射线可减少剂量。
- 除去滤线栅可以减少剂量(用于儿科)，但增加了散射的风险。
- 剂量分散(移动X射线)可以减少皮肤的最大剂量。

  连续进行X射线透视时，皮肤剂量率为每分钟10~30mGy。

  在高剂量模式下，最大照射率为每分钟100mGy或每分钟200mGy。

  在允许的最大照射率高剂量模式下，10分钟产生的剂量可达2Gy!

  体型大的患者更容易受到皮肤损伤。
- 如上所述，放大图像会增加剂量。

CT物理

CT概述

- 计算机体层成像(CT)是采用扇形X射线围绕患者旋转，并且测定每个单一像素的线性衰减系数，之后加以重建运算得到图像。

亨氏单位(HU)

- 亨氏单位用于测定CT的相对衰减。

$$HU=1\,000\left(\frac{\mu_x-\mu_{water}}{\mu_{water}}\right)$$

μ_x=被测量某一物质的衰减系数

μ_{water}=水的衰减系数

- 10HU=1%的对比度差别。
- 灰质和白质的对比度差别只有0.5%。
- 一个衰减两倍于水的物质会衰减1 000HU。

辐射剂量学

CT剂量学

- 计算机体层摄影剂量指数(CTDI)是指每个轴向切面(在扫描床无移动的情况下完成旋转一周)的平均体模剂量(包括散射)，以Gy为单位。

CTDI is measured with 16 cm and 32 cm phantoms. 16 cm will always have higher dose.

- $CTDI_w$ (weighted) = 2/3 $CTDI_p$ + 1/3 $CTDI_c$

  $CTDI_p$ = peripheral

  $CTDI_c$ = central

- $CTDI_{vol}$= $CTDI_w$/pitch

  The pitch is related to the table speed. A pitch <1 will overscan and result in increased radiation exposure; conversely, a pitch >1 will skip areas but will decrease exposure.

  $CTDI_{vol}$ is the same for all scans, independent of scan length.

  $CTDI_{vol}$ should be less than reference values:

  Adult head: 75 mGy (16 cm phantom)

  Adult abdomen: 25 mGy (32 cm phantom)

  Pediatric abdomen: 20 mGy (16 cm phantom)

Dose length product (DLP) and effective doses

- The dose length product (DLP) is the best way to estimate radiation risk from CT.
- DLP = $CTDI_{vol}$*scan length = mGy*cm
- One can obtain an effective dose in mSv from the DLP by using body-part specific conversion factors:

Head	0.0023 mSv/mGy cm
Neck	0.0054
Chest	0.019
Abd	0.017
Pelvis	0.017
Legs	0.0008

- Example conversion: If DLP is 900 mGy*cm for an abdominal CT, the radiation exposure equals (900 mGy*cm) * (0.017 mSv/mGy cm) = 15.4 mSv.

Typical effective doses (mSv) of common diagnostic exams

- Radiography:

  PA and lateral chest radiograph: 0.1 mSv

  Cervical spine radiograph: 0.2 mSv

  Lumbar spine radiograph: 1.5 mSv

  Abdomen radiograph: 0.7 mSv

  Pelvic radiograph: 0.6 mSv

  Mammography: 0.4 mSv

  Knee radiograph: 0.005 mSv

- Fluoroscopy:

  Upper GI series: 6 mSv

  Barium enema: 8 mSv

- Interventional radiology:

  Cerebral angiography: 1–10 mSv

  Peripheral angiography: 5 mSv

  Cardiac cath (diagnostic): 7 mSv

  TIPS: 100 mSv

- CT:

  Head CT: 2 mSv

  Neck CT: 3 mSv

  Chest CT: 7 mSv

  Abdomen CT: 8 mSv

  Pelvis: 6 mSv

CTDI测量采用直径16cm和32cm的体模，16cm的体模具有较高的剂量。

- $CTDI_W$(加权平均)=2/3$CTDI_P$+1/3$CTDI_C$

  $CTDI_P$=外周

  $CTDI_C$=中央

- $CTDI_{vol}$=$CTDI_W$/螺距系数

  螺距系数与扫描床的速度相关。螺距系数小于1会造成过度扫描和辐射剂量增加；相反，螺距系数大于1会跳过部分区域但是能减少辐射剂量。

  $CTDI_{vol}$对所有的扫描都是相同的，与扫描长度无关。

  $CTDI_{vol}$应小于参考数值：

  成人头部：75mGy(16cm体模)

  成人腹部：25mGy(32cm体模)

  儿童腹部：20mGy(16cm体模)

剂量长度乘积(DLP)及有效剂量

- 剂量长度乘积(DLP)是评估CT辐射风险的最好方法。
- DLP=$CTDI_{vol}$×扫描长度=mGy·cm。
- 有效剂量(mSv)可以用DLP通过特定躯体部位的转换系数进行计算：

头部	0.002 3mSv/(mGy·cm)
颈部	0.005 4
胸部	0.019
腹部	0.017
盆腔	0.017
下肢	0.000 8

- 例如，如果腹部CT的DLP为900mGy·cm，辐射剂量相当于(900mGy·cm)×[0.017mSv/(mGy·cm)]=15.4mSv。

常用诊断性检查的有效剂量(mSv)

- X射线摄影：

  后前位和侧位胸片：0.1mSv

  颈椎平片：0.2mSv

  腰椎平片：1.5mSv

  腹部平片：0.7mSv

  盆腔平片：0.6mSv

  乳腺摄影：0.4mSv

  膝关节平片：0.005mSv

- X射线透视：

  上消化道透视：6mSv

  钡剂灌肠：8mSv

- 介入放射：

  脑血管造影：1~10mSv

  外周血管造影：5mSv

  心导管(诊断)：7mSv

  经颈静脉肝内门体分流术(TIPS)：100mSv

- CT：

  头部：2mSv

  颈部：3mSv

  胸部：7mSv

  腹部：8mSv

  盆腔：6mSv

Image Quality

Contrast

- The most important factor for optimizing contrast is to increase the number of photons that reach the film (film density).
- ↓ scatter → ↑ contrast
- Collimation ↓ scatter and ↓ dose

  Collimation is the rare example of something that ↑ image quality and ↓ dose
- ↑ kV → ↓ contrast with automatic exposure control
- In screen film, contrast is related to screen latitude/gradient.

Resolution and blur

- Only three factors influence blur (resolution), none of which affect image contrast:
  1) Focal spot blur.
  2) Motion blur, which is related to exposure time.
  3) Receptor blur, which is related to intensifying screen thickness. Faster screens ↑ blur.

Statistics

Sensitivity, specificity, positive predictive value, and negative predictive value

- Sensitivity = TP/(TP + FN)
- TP = true positive
- Specificity = TN/(TN+FP)
- TN = true negative
- Positive predictive value (PPV) = TP/(TP + FP)
- FP = false positive
- Negative predictive value (NPV) = TN/(TN + FN)
- FN = false negative

ROC curve

- A receiver operator characteristic (ROC) curve compares the diagnostic performance of a test at various thresholds of decision confidence.

图像质量

对比度

- 优化对比度最重要的因素是增加到达胶片的光子数(胶片密度)。
- 减少散射可以增加对比度。
- 准直可以减少散射和照射剂量。

  准直器是极少可以提高图像质量和减少剂量的例子。
- 增加kV并使用自动曝光控制可以降低对比度。
- 在增感胶片上，对比度与曝光宽容度及梯度相关。

分辨率和模糊

- 只有三种因素会影响模糊(分辨率)，但这些因素都不会影响图像的对比度：
  1) 焦点模糊。
  2) 运动模糊，与曝光时间有关。
  3) 接收器模糊，与增感屏厚度增加有关。增感屏越快，越模糊。

统计学

敏感度、特异性、阳性预测值和阴性预测值

- 敏感度=*TP*/(*TP*+*FN*)
- TP=真阳性
- 特异性=*TN*/(*TN*+*FP*)
- TN=真阴性
- 阳性预测值(*PPV*)=*TP*/(*TP*+*FP*)
- FP=假阳性
- 阴性预测值(*NPV*)=*TN*/(*TN*+*FN*)
- FN=假阴性

ROC曲线

- 受试者工作特征(ROC)曲线用来比较一个诊断性测试性能在不同设置条件下的决策可信度。

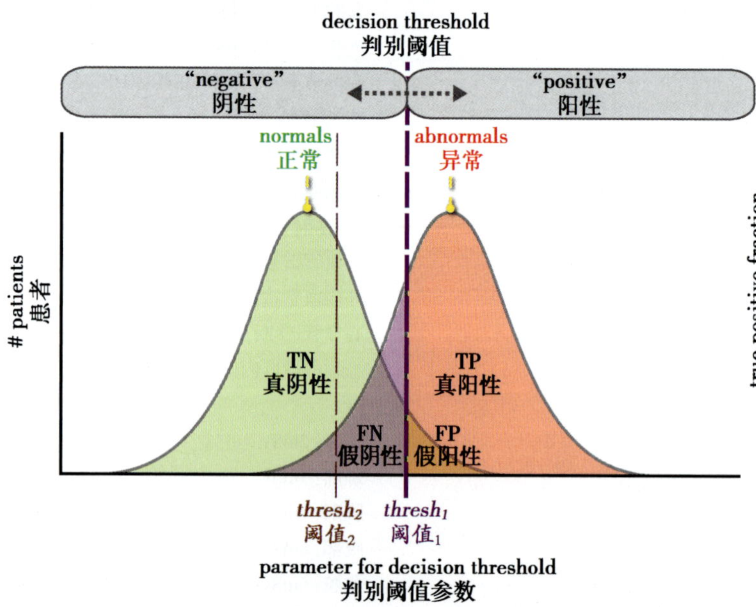

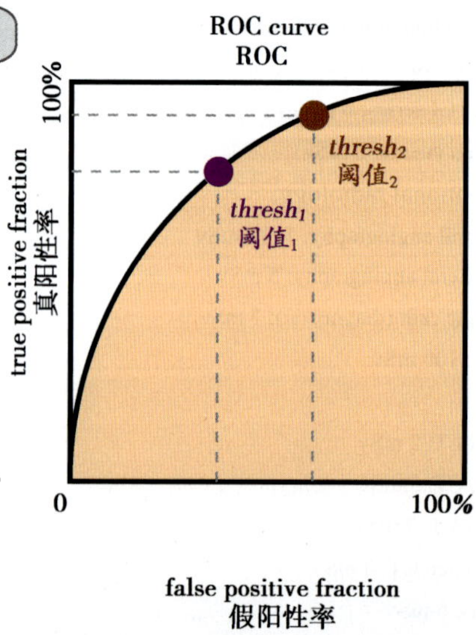

- A patient population includes normals and abnormals. The threshold to determine whether a test parameter is "negative" or "positive" can be set to optimize the ratio of true positives to false positives.
- In threshold 1 ($thresh_1$; blue dashed line above), the decision threshold is chosen to balance true positives with false positives. This threshold is visualized on the ROC curve as the blue dot.
- Threshold 2 ($thresh_2$; brown dashed line above) is lowered. When plotted on the ROC curve, $thresh_2$ moves to the right, which increases the true positive fraction (increases sensitivity) and also increases the false positive fraction.

- 一个患者群体包括正常和异常。真阳性和假阳性的比例可以通过调节一个测试参数的"阳性"和"阴性"的阈值来得到最大优化。
- 在图中的阈值1中(蓝色虚线),诊断阈值的确立是权衡真阳性和假阳性而选择的。ROC曲线上看到的蓝点为阈值1。
- 在图中的阈值2(色虚线)被降低了。在ROC曲线上,阈值向右移动,真阳性的比例随之增加(增加了敏感度),同时也增加了假阳性的比例。

Radiation Biology

DNA damage

- Free radicals mediate the majority of biological damage due to radiation.

Syndromes

- Xeroderma pigmentosa: ↑ sensitivity to UV light
- Ataxia telangiectasia: ↑ sensitivity to X-rays.

Deterministic effects

- Deterministic effects occur once the radiation exposure crosses a certain threshold and would not be expected to occur below that exposure.
- A **decrease in peripheral lymphocyte** count can occur after as little as ≥ 0.5 Gy exposure.
- **Cataracts** may occur after an eye dose of 2 Gy. The posterior pole is preferentially affected. For a given dose, high-LET radiation (neutrons and alpha particles) are much more effective at inducing cataracts compared to X-rays.
- **Radiation-induced erythema** can occur in 1–2 days, but may take up to 10–14 days to develop.
  2 Gy: Transient early erythema
  6 Gy: Robust erythema
- **Epilation** occurs after about three weeks.
  3 Gy: Temporary epilation
  7 Gy: Permanent epilation
- **Desquamation** may begin 4 weeks after exposure.
  15 Gy: Moist desquamation
- **Vascular damage** is expected for skin doses >20 Gy.
- **Ulceration** and **depigmentation** are late effects due to dermal damage.
- **Sterility** can be caused in males or females.
  Males: Temporary sterility after >0.15 Gy
  Females: Permanent sterility and early menopause after >3.5 Gy.

Hereditary effects

- The **doubling dose** is the dose required to double the spontaneous mutation rate when applied to a population. The doubling dose is approximately 1 Gy given to each member of the population.
- The risk of hereditary effects (for an individual) is thought to be approximately 0.2% per Sv. For instance, the risk of a hereditary effect from a gonad dose of 100 mSv = 0.2% * 0.1 Sv = 0.02%

Death by radiation(whole-body radiation)

Terminology: LD 50/X = lethal dose that kills 50% of the population in X days.

放射生物学

DNA损伤

- 自由基介导了大部分由辐射引起的生物损伤。

综合征

- 色素性干皮病:对紫外线敏感性增加。
- 共济失调毛细血管扩张:对X射线敏感性增加。

确定性效应

- 确定性效应只发生在放射照射量超过了一个既定的阈值之后,而低于该剂量则不会发生。
- **外周淋巴细胞计数减少**在接触剂量稍大于0.5Gy时即可发生。
- **白内障**在眼部的剂量超过2Gy时可能会发生。眼球后部最容易受到影响。对于一个既定的剂量,高LET的放射性粒子(中子和阿尔法粒子)引起白内障的风险比X射线要高得多。
- **放射性红斑**可以出现在照射后的1~2天,也可能需要10~14天才发生。
  2Gy:一过性早期红斑
  6Gy:深度红斑
- **毛发脱落**发生在3周以后。
  3Gy:暂时性脱发
  7Gy:永久性脱发
- **脱皮**可能在辐射后4周开始出现。
  15Gy:湿性脱皮
- **血管损伤**在皮肤剂量超过20Gy时发生。
- **溃疡和脱色**是由于真皮层破坏而导致的后期副作用。
- **不孕不育**在男女都可以发生。
  男性:大于0.15Gy时为暂时性不育。
  女性:大于3.5Gy的时会造成永久性不孕和提前绝经。

遗传效应

- **加倍剂量**是使一个群体产生自发突变概率加倍所需要的剂量。加倍剂量大约是群体中每个个体接受1Gy的照射量。
- 遗传效应(对于一个个体而言)的风险大约是每Sv增加0.2%。例如,一个性腺剂量为100mSv的遗传效应风险=0.2%×0.1Sv=0.02%。

放射性致死剂量(全身性的放射)

术语:LD50/X=在X天中导致一个群体中50%

For instance, an LD 50/60 will kill 50% of the population in 60 days.

- 3–4 Gy: LD 50/60 due to failure of hematopoietic system.
- 10 Gy: LD 50/5 due to denuding of the GI tract lining (small bowel most sensitive).
- 100 Gy: LD 50/2 due to cerebrovascular syndrome.

Stochastic effects

- Stochastic effects are random and carcinogenic. Stochastic effects arise after a latent period of several years. As the dose to an individual increases, there is an increased risk of developing cancer. Complicating the determination of a stochastic risk is the fact that cancer is a very common disease, there is a low level of background radiation present, and most people who receive medical radiation exposures do not have any ill effects.
- The risk of a stochastic effect depends on the dose, dose rate, and type of tissue exposed.
- The linear no threshold model is believed to provide the most accurate risk assessment for development of solid tumors, with a latency up to 25 years. The linear no threshold model assumes that there is no threshold required for a stochastic effect, and the risk of cancer increases linear with increasing exposure.
- The linear-quadratic function of dose is thought to best characterize the risk of developing leukemia, with a latency of 5–7 years.

Radiation-induced cancer

- Acute radiation exposure carries a risk of developing cancer of approximately 8%/Gy, based on Japanese nuclear bomb survivors.

  For instance, a 24% increase in cancer risk would require 3 Gy acutely (8 *3 = 24%).
- The risk of leukemia is approximately 1%/Sv for an acute dose.
- Chronic exposure (e.g., radiation worker) carries a risk of cancer of 4%/Gy.

Relative radiosensitivities

- The thyroid gland is the most radiosensitive tissue in the human body.

Occupational/iatrogenic exposures and effects

- Ankylosing spondylitis (treated with X-rays) → leukemia
- Fluoroscopy for tuberculosis → breast cancer
- Marshall island inhabitants (nuclear weapon testing) → thyroid tumors
- Miners (especially uranium) → lung cancer, due to breathing radon
- Dial painters → bone sarcomas and nasopharyngeal carcinoma (lick radium on brushes)

Radiation effects on the fetus

These effects are for significant exposure (e.g., 2 Gy)

- Weeks 0–2 (pre-implantation): "all-or-nothing": abortion likely after significant exposure
- Weeks 2–6: congenital abnormalities

  ↑ Risk of neonatal death (death at or about the time of birth)
- Weeks 8–15: Risk of mental retardation 40%/Sv

  ↑ Risk of childhood cancer

  ↑ Risk of reduced head diameter

的个体死亡的致死剂量。例如，LD50/60为60天内杀死群体中50%的个体的剂量。

- 3~4Gy：LD50/60致死原因为造血系统衰竭。
- 10Gy：LD50/5致死原因为胃肠道内膜剥脱(小肠尤其敏感)。
- 100Gy：LD50/2致死原因为脑血管综合征。

随机效应

- 随机效应是随机的致癌性。随机效应在潜伏期后数年内发生。随着个体接受剂量增加，患癌症的风险也随之增加。确定随机风险的原因是复杂的，因为癌症是一种非常常见的疾病，而环境中本身存在低剂量的背景辐射，且大多数人在接受医学放射照射之后并不出现任何致病的效应。
- 随机效应的风险取决于剂量、剂量率及接受照射组织本身的特性。
- 线性无阈值模型被认为是测定罹患实体肿瘤风险的最准确的模型，其潜伏期可以长达25年。线性无阈值模型假设发生随机效应不需要照射量超过特定阈值，并且患癌症的风险随着照射剂量的增加而呈线性增加。
- 剂量线性二次型函数被认为是估计白血病患病风险的最佳模型，其潜伏期是5~7年。

放射引起的癌症

- 根据日本原子弹幸存者的数据，急性放射照射造成的癌症风险每1Gy约为8%。

  例如，增加24%的癌症风险需3Gy的急性照射剂量(8 × 3=24%)。
- 患白血病风险的急性剂量每Sv约为1%。
- 长期接触辐射(如放射工作人员)的癌症罹患风险是每Gy为4%。

相对辐射敏感度

- 甲状腺是人体内对辐射敏感度最高的组织。

职业性/医源性照射及其后果

- 强直性脊椎炎(用X射线治疗)可引发白血病
- X射线治疗肺结核可引发乳腺癌
- 马绍尔群岛居民(受核武器试验影响)患甲状腺肿瘤增多
- 矿工(尤其是铀)因吸入放射性氡而患肺癌增多
- 表盘的画匠增加骨肉瘤和鼻咽癌发病(舔带镭元素的画笔)

放射对胎儿的影响

这些影响只有在显著的辐射暴露后才会发生(如2Gy)

- 0~2周(着床前)："全有或全无"，如果辐射剂量非常显著可导致流产
- 2~6周：各种先天性畸形

  增加新生儿死亡风险(出生时或将要出生时死亡)
- 8~15周：智力障碍的风险为40%/Sv

  增加儿童癌症风险

  增加头部直径减小的风险

- Weeks 15–25: Risk of mental retardation 10%/Sv
  ↑ Risk of childhood cancer

Fetal dose (Pregnant radiation workers)
- Dose limit: 0.5 mSv/month allowed (~5 mSv/pregnancy)
- Lead apron attenuates externally measured dose by a factor of 20 (fetal dose would be further reduced by factor of two due to mother's overlying tissues)

Dose to general public allowed by medical radiation
- 1 mSv/year, which is actually lower than the maximum dose of 5 mSv allowed to the fetus of a radiation worker.

Dose limits by body part
- Eyes: 150 mSv/year
- Everything else: 500 mSv/year

Occupational exposure(not pregnant)
- Max permissible effective dose = 50 mSv/year

Background radiation
- Background radiation varies by location, but averages about 3 mSv/year excluding medical radiation.
  1 Gy (Sv) is required to double the mutation rate, so 3 mSv = 0.003 Sv = 0.3% increased risk of mutation above the baseline rate.
- Radon exposure represents approximately 55% of background radiation. Radon is an alpha emitter with a half-life of three days. Its parent radionuclide is radium, with a half-life of 1600 years.
  Effective dose = Absorbed dose * W_R * W_T
  W_R= 20 (↑ LET), and W_T = 0.1 (only lung tissue irradiated)
  Radon exposure is thought to cause ~20,000 deaths/year.

MAGNETIC RESONANCE IMAGING (MRI) PHYSICS

MRI and pregnancy
- Although no controlled studies have been performed, MRI can be performed at any stage of pregnancy. Gadolinium is contraindicated throughout pregnancy.

MRI quenching
- Quenching causes loss of superconductivity of the MRI scanner magnet coils, which releases helium. Helium displaces O_2 → must evacuate emergently.

Fringe field
- The fringe field surrounds the controlled access area and cannot exceed 5 Gauss.

FDA regulates the following MRI parameters
- Static magnetic field strength >4T.
- Time-varying magnetic fields sufficient to produce severe discomfort or painful stimulation.
- Radiofrequency power deposition to produce core temperature increase of 1℃.
- Acoustic noise levels >140 dB.

SAR (Specific absorption ratio)
- The specific absorption ration (SAR) characterizes the radiofrequency (RF) power absorbed per unit mass.

- 15~25周：智力障碍的风险为10%/Sv
  增加儿童癌症风险。

胎儿剂量(从事放射工作的孕妇)
- 剂量上限：每月0.5mSv(怀孕期间总照射量最高为5mSv)
- 铅衣可以减少外部测量的剂量20倍(由于母亲自身组织的覆盖，胎儿受到的剂量会在此基础上再减2倍)

普通公众许可的医学放射剂量
- 每年1mSv，这个剂量比放射工作者的胎儿所允许的最大剂量(5mSv)还要小

身体部位的剂量限制
- 眼睛：150mSv/年
- 其他部位：500mSv/年

职业性照射(非孕妇)
- 最大的有效允许剂量为每年50mSv

环境辐射
- 环境辐射有地理差异，每年平均约3mSv，不包括医学放射。
  1Gy(Sv)是突变加倍所需的照射量，所以3mSv=0.003Sv=0.3%，即每年突变的风险相比于环境水平增加0.3%。
- 来自氡元素的辐射约占本底辐射的55%。氡元素是一种α发射体，半衰期为3天。它的母放射性核素是镭，其半衰期是1 600年。
  有效剂量=吸收剂量 × W_R × W_T
  W_R=20(↑ LET)，W_T=0.1(只有肺组织受到照射)
  氡元素辐射导致的死亡每年高达20 000例。

磁共振成像物理

MRI和妊娠
- 尽管还没有进行过对照性研究，但磁共振成像可用于妊娠的任何一个阶段。钆对比剂在怀孕期间禁用。

磁共振失超
- 失超造成MRI扫描仪电磁线圈失去超导性，进而放出氦气。氦气会置换氧气从而必须进行紧急疏散。

边缘场
- 边缘场为受控制的通道区，不能超过5高斯(Gauss)。

美国食品药物管理局(FDA)对MRI下列各个参数的规定
- 静磁场强度大于4T(特斯拉)。
- 时变磁场强到足以使患者感到严重不适或发生疼痛。
- 射频能量使人体核心温度升高1℃。
- 噪声大于140dB(分贝)。

比吸收率(SAR)
- 比吸收率(SAR)指的是射频(RF)能量被单位质量所吸收的量。

- SAR is proportional to # images acquired per unit time and depends on patient dimensions, RF waveform, tip angle, and coil type.

MRI noise

- The acoustic noise produced by the MRI scanner is caused by vibrating gradient coils, due to rapidly applied gradient magnetic fields.

Focal heating and thermal injuries

- Conductive loops can cause local heating. Examples of conductive loops include crossed arms, ECG leads, and unconnected surface coil leads in contact with patient's skin.
- Metallic objects can absorb radiofrequency energy and become hot.
- Time-varying magnetic fields can result in peripheral nerve stimulation, muscle movement, and discomfort.

Signal to noise ratio (SNR)

- Signal to noise ratio (SNR) is proportional to:

$$\mathbf{I} * \mathbf{voxel}_{x,y,z} * \frac{\sqrt{\mathrm{NEX}}}{\sqrt{\mathrm{BW}}} * \mathbf{B}$$

I = intrinsic signal intensity of voxel, dependent on tissue composition and pulse sequence

voxel$_{x,y,z}$ = voxel volume, affected by image matrix and slice thickness; a smaller voxel volume will proportionally decrease signal to noise

NEX = number of excitations; linearly related to time of acquisition

BW = receiver bandwidth (range of frequencies collected by the MRI system; wide BW enables faster data acquisition and reduces chemical shift artifacts but also adds noise → reduces SNR)

B = intrinsic function of magnetic field strength

T1 and T2

- Inherent tissue T1 and T2 characteristics depend on the **longitudinal relaxation (T1)** and **transverse relaxation (T2)** times of the protons in that tissue.
- Tissue signal abnormality is produced by alterations (prolongation or shortening) of the transverse or longitudinal relaxation of the tissue, which may be affected by various pathologic processes.
- MR image weighting (e.g., T1- or T2-weighted images) depends on the repetition time (TR) and echo time (TE) used to obtain images.
- **T1 image contrast is dependent on TR**, which is the interval between sequential radiofrequency pulses. The imaging appearance of specific tissues on T1-weighted images depends on how much longitudinal relaxation occurs between each TR. Images obtained with a short TR and a short TE are T1-weighted.

  Short T1 relaxation times → higher signal on T1-weighted images.

  Fat and subacute blood have short T1 relaxation times and therefore appear hyperintense on T1- weighted images.

- **T2 image contrast is dependent on TE**, which is the interval between the application of the radiofrequency pulse and the collection of the signal. The imaging appearance of tissues on T2-weighted images depends on how much transverse relaxation (loss of proton phase coherence) occurs during each TE. Images obtained with a long TR and a long TE are T2-weighted.

  Slow loss of phase coherence → prolonged T2 relaxation times → hyperintense on T2-weighted images.

  Water has a long T2 relaxation time and therefore is hyperintense on T2-weighted images.

- SAR与单位时间内获得的图像数量成正比，并且取决于患者的躯体大小、RF波形、顶角，以及线圈的类型。

MRI噪声

- MRI扫描仪发出的噪声来自梯度线圈在突然施加的磁场梯度中所发生的振动。

聚焦产热及温度损伤

- 导电环路可以造成局部产热。导电环路包括交叉的手臂、心电图(ECG)导联，以及未接线圈表面的导联与患者皮肤接触。
- 金属物体能够吸收射频能量而发烫。
- 时变磁场可以产生末梢神经刺激、肌肉运动，以及不适。

信噪比(SNR)

- 信噪比(SNR)与下列参数成正比：

$$I * \mathbf{voxel}_{x,y,z} * \frac{\sqrt{NEX}}{\sqrt{BW}} * B$$

I=体素的内源信号强度，取决于组织的构成和脉冲序列。

voxel$_{x,y,z}$=体素容积，受影像矩阵和切面厚度影响；体素减小，信号/噪声比将会按比例地减小。

NEX=激发次数；与采集时间呈线性关系。

BW=接收器的带宽(MRI系统采集的频率范围；宽的BW提供更快速的数据采集并减少化学位移造成的误差，但随之噪声也增加，使SNR降低)。

B=磁场强度的固有功能。

T_1和T_2

- 组织固有的T_1和T_2特性取决于该组织所含质子的**纵向弛豫(T_1)**和**横向弛豫(T_2)**时间。
- 组织信号异常是由于改变(延长和缩短)该组织横向或纵向弛豫，可以受多种病理过程的影响。
- MR图像加权(如T_1或T_2加权图像)取决于获取图像所采用的重复时间(TR)和回波时间(TE)。
- **T_1图像的对比度取决于重复时间(TR)**，即连续两次射频脉冲的时间间隔。特定组织在T_1加权图像上的表现取决于每次TR发生了多少纵向弛豫。采用短TR和短TE所获得的图像为T_1加权。

  T_1弛豫时间越短意味着T_1加权图像上的信号越强。

  脂肪和亚急性出血的T1弛豫时间很短，所以它们在T_1加权图像上会呈现出强信号。

- **T_2图像对比度取决于TE**，即射频脉冲发出和该信号被重新接收的时间间隔。特定组织在T_2加权图像上的表现取决于每次TE期间发生了多少横向弛豫(质子失相)。采用长TR和长TE获得的图像为T_2加权。

  缓慢失相造成T_2弛豫时间延长，从而在T_2加权的图像上会呈现强信号。

  水的T_2弛豫时间很长，所以在T_2加权图像中会呈现出强信号。

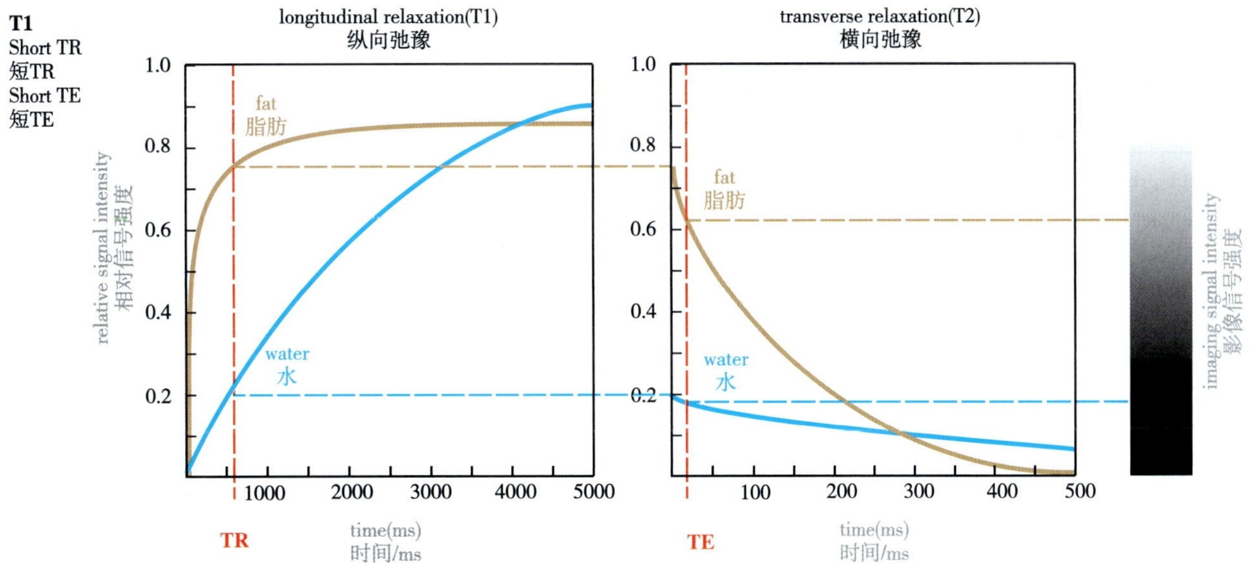
T1
Short TR
短TR
Short TE
短TE
longitudinal relaxation(T1)
纵向弛豫
transverse relaxation(T2)
横向弛豫
relative signal intensity
相对信号强度
fat
脂肪
water
水
TR
TE
time(ms)
时间/ms
imaging signal intensity
影像信号强度

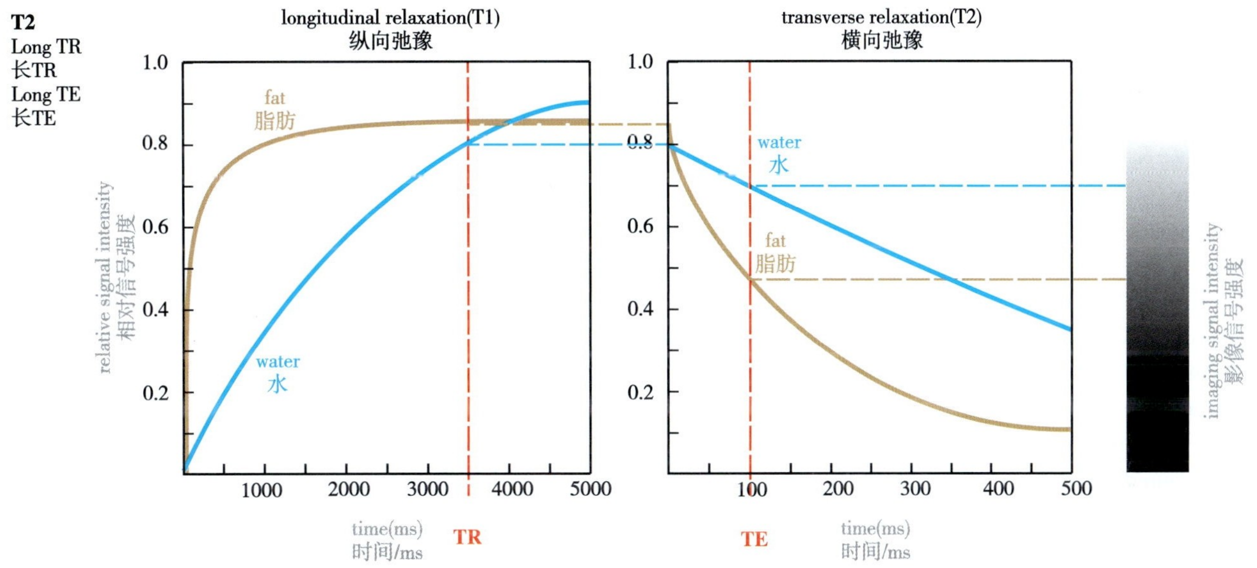
T2
Long TR
长TR
Long TE
长TE
longitudinal relaxation(T1)
纵向弛豫
transverse relaxation(T2)
横向弛豫
relative signal intensity
相对信号强度
fat
脂肪
water
水
TR
TE
time(ms)
时间/ms
imaging signal intensity
影像信号强度

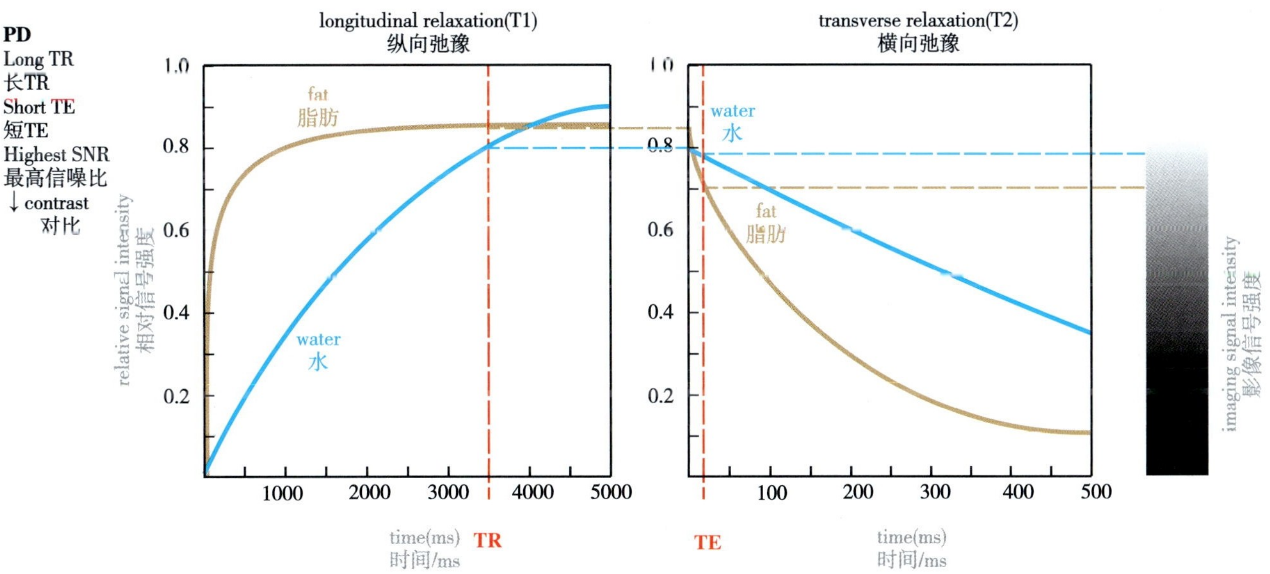
PD
Long TR
长TR
Short TE
短TE
Highest SNR
最高信噪比
↓ contrast
对比
longitudinal relaxation(T1)
纵向弛豫
transverse relaxation(T2)
横向弛豫
relative signal intensity
相对信号强度
fat
脂肪
water
水
TR
TE
time(ms)
时间/ms
imaging signal intensity
影像信号强度

ULTRASOUND PHYSICS

Decibel (dB)

- The decibel is a measure of relative intensity between two sound intensities.
- dB = 10 log(I/I_{ref})
- For example, –3 dB is 50% of sound intensity: 10log(0.5) = –3

Thermal index and mechanical index

- The thermal index (TI) is the maximum temperature rise in tissue caused by ultrasound energy absorption.
- The mechanical index (MI) describes the likelihood of cavitation based on peak rarefactional pressure and frequency.
- If TI >1.0, risk benefit analysis should be performed.
- If MI >0.5, risk benefit analysis should be performed.

Factors that affect acoustic output index

- Frame rate
- Transmit power
- Frequency

Factors that don't affect acoustic output index

- Time-gain compensation
- Grayscale mapping

  These are both processing techniques

Cavitation

- Cavitation is the formation of bodies of gas and/or vapor by ultrasound energy. Cavitation is more likely to occur at high pressures and low frequencies.
- Stable cavitation is regular pulsation of persistent microbubbles.
- Transient cavitation is a more violent form of microbubble dynamics characterized by large size changes in bubbles before collapse.

Safe ultrasound energy

- No biologic effects have been observed with spatial peak temporal average intensities below 1 W/cm^2.

Tissue attenuation

- Tissue attenuation is approximately 0.5 dB per cm per MHz.
- For instance, a 4 MHz wave travelling 10 cm is attenuated 20 dB.

Refraction

- Refraction is due to different velocities of sound in different tissues, resulting in apparent bending of the ultrasound wave.
- Described by Snell's law

Wavelength and transducer design

- The transducer thickness = λ /2, where λ is wavelength.
- For a long wavelength (low frequency), the transducer must be made thicker.

Sound waves

- v = fλ

  v = velocity

  f = frequency

  λ = wavelength

超声物理

分贝(dB)

- 分贝是衡量两个声音之间相对强度的度量单位。
- dB=10log(I/I_{ref})。
- 例如,-3dB对应的是50%的声强:10log(0.5)=-3。

热指数和机械指数

- 热指数(TI)是指组织吸收超声能量后造成的最大升温。
- 机械指数(MI)是指基于峰值稀疏压力与频率所形成空化的可能性。
- 如果TI>1.0,需要分析风险与受益的比率。
- 如果MI>0.5,需要分析风险与受益的比率。

影响声音输出指数的因素

- 帧速率
- 传送功率
- 频率

不影响声音输出指数的因素

- 时间增益补偿
- 灰度映射

  这两种都是信号处理的技术。

空穴作用

- 空穴作用是指由于超声能量所形成的气体或蒸汽空洞。空穴作用在高压低频的情况下更容易产生。
- 稳定的空穴是指持久性微泡有规律性的脉冲。
- 瞬态空穴是微气泡动力学的一种更为剧烈的形式,其特点是气泡在塌陷之前发生明显的体积变化。

超声的安全能量

- 至今还没有观察到低于1W/cm^2的空间峰值时间平均强度产生的生物学作用。

组织衰减

- 组织衰减约为每厘米每兆赫兹0.5dB。
- 例如,一个4MHz的波传导10cm的距离将有20dB的衰减。

折射

- 折射是由于声音在不同组织内传播的速度差异所造成的,折射可导致界面上超声波的明显弯曲。
- 遵循斯涅尔(Snell)定律。

波长和传感器探头的设计

- 传感器探头的厚度=λ/2,λ代表波长。
- 对于一个长波(低频率)来说,传感器探头必须要厚一些。

声波

- $v=f\lambda$

  v=速度

  f=频率

  λ=波长

Axial resolution

- Axial resolution quantifies the ability to separate objects lying along axis of the beam and is determined by spatial pulse length. Short pulses are achieved by damping of the transducer. The spatial pulse length (SPL) is approximately 2λ.

$$\text{axial resolution}=\frac{\text{spatial pulse length}}{2}$$

For example, at 2 MHz, the SPL is ~2 mm and the axial resolution is ~ 1 mm.

at 4 MHz, the SPL is ~1 mm and the axial resolution ~0.5 mm.

at 8 Mhz, the axial resolution is ~0.25 mm.

- Axial resolution does not vary with depth.

Lateral resolution

- The lateral resolution is the ability to resolve two adjacent objects.
- Lateral resolution improves with beam focusing and ↑ number lines per frame.
- Lateral resolution is approximately 4x worse than axial resolution.
- Lateral resolution becomes worse with increasing depth.

Elevational resolution

- Elevational resolution is the resolution in the plane perpendicular to the plane of imaging. Elevational resolution is equivalent to slice thickness on cross-sectional imaging.
- Elevational resolution is approximately equivalent to lateral resolution and also varies with depth.

Near field and far field

- The near field determines the maximum depth that can be imaged. It is not related to image quality at increasing depths.

$$\text{near field}=\frac{r^2}{\lambda}$$

r = radius of transducer: If r doubles, near field ↑ by 4

λ = wavelength: If λ doubles (↑ freq), near field ↓ by 2

- The near field (where imaging is possible) is called the **Fresnel zone**.
- The far field (where the ultrasound beam diverges and imaging is impossible) is called the **Frauenhofer zone**.

Pulse repetition frequency (PRF)

- Pulse repetition frequency (PRF) is the number of times the transducer outputs a pulse of sound waves per second. An increase in PRF causes an inversely proportional decrease in echo listening time. A high PRF therefore limits the maximum depth of tissue that can be imaged.
- PRF = **Frame rate** x **lines per frame.**
- A typical PRF is ~4 kHz → 0.25 ms (250 μsec) between pulses, which allows imaging of approximately 19.3 cm depth.

轴向(横向)分辨率

- 轴向分辨率用来定量区分排列在超声波束轴向位置上物体大小的能力，由空间脉冲长度所决定。通过探头减震来获取短的脉冲。空间脉冲长度(SPL)约为2λ。

$$\text{轴向分辨率}=\frac{\text{空间脉冲长度}}{2}$$

例如，在2MHz下，SPL约为2mm，所以纵向分辨率约为1mm。

在4MHz下，SPL约为1mm，纵向分辨率约为0.5mm。

在8MHz下，纵向分辨率约为0.25mm。

- 轴向分辨率不受深度的影响。

侧向(径向或方位)分辨率

- 侧向分辨率是辨别两个相邻物体间的能力。
- 侧向分辨率随着声束聚焦和每帧行数增加而提高。
- 侧向分辨率约是轴向分辨率的1/4。
- 侧向分辨率随着深度的增加而减弱。

垂直(俯仰)分辨率

- 垂直分辨率是指垂直于图像面的平面分辨率。在横截面图像中，垂直分辨率等同于切面厚度。
- 垂直分辨率大致等同于侧向分辨率，同时也随着深度而改变。

近场和远场

- 近场决定能够成像的最大深度。成像的质量与深度增加无关。

$$\text{近场}=\frac{r^2}{\lambda}$$

r=传感器探头的半径：如果半径加倍，则近场增加4倍

λ=波长：如果波长加倍(频率增加)，近场会减少到一半

- 近场(可以进行成像)被称为**菲涅耳(Fresnel)带**。
- 远场(超声波束分散而不能进行成像)**被称为弗劳恩霍夫区域**。

脉冲重复频率(PRF)

- 脉冲重复频率(PRF)为传感器探头每秒输出声波脉冲的次数。增加PRF会导致回波侦听时间成反比减少。因此，高PRF会使深部组织显像受限。
- PRF=**帧速率 × 每帧扫描行数**。
- 常用PRF约为4kHz，也就是脉冲之间相隔0.25ms(250μs)，其对应的成像深度约为19.3cm。

Definitions

定义

$${}^{A}_{Z}X_{N}$$

A = atomic mass = N + Z

A=原子质量=N+Z

Z = # protons = atomic number

Z=质子数=原子序数

N = # neutrons

N=中子数

X = Element

X=元素

- Isobar: Same atomic mass (e.g., ^{131}I and ^{131}Xe)
- IsotoPes: Same number of Protons
- IsotoNes: Same number of Neutrons

Decay and stability

- The graph below demonstrates that as atomic number (Z) increases, stable elements tend to have slightly increased neutrons relative to protons.
- Isotopes with excess neutrons decay by beta-minus decay, while isotopes with excess protons decay by beta-plus decay.

- 同量异位素：原子质量相同(如 ^{131}I 和 ^{131}Xe)。
- 同位素：质子数相同。
- 同中子素：中子数相同。

衰变和稳定性

- 下图显示，随着原子序数(Z)的增加，稳定的元素中的中子数相对于质子数有少量增加。
- 过量的中子同位素通过负 β 衰变进行衰变，而过量的质子同位素通过正 β 衰变进行衰变。

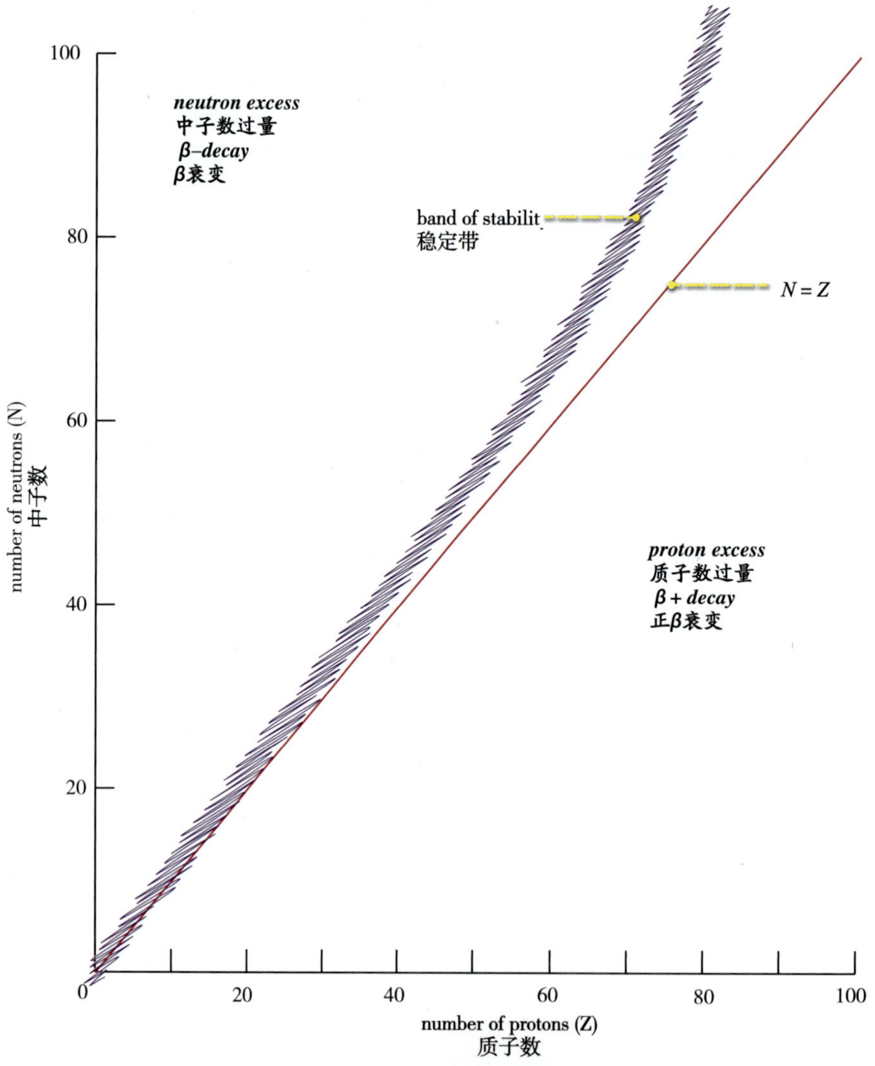

Alpha decay

- An α particle is two protons and two neutrons = Helium nucleus
- Alpha decay causes loss of an α particle: Atomic mass ↓ by 4; Z ↓ by 2 and N ↓ 2

阿尔法衰变

- 一个 α 粒子是由两个质子和两个中子构成的氦核。
- α 衰变造成一个 α 粒子丢失：原子质量减少4；质子数减少2，中子数减少2。

$$^{A-4}_{Z-2}X_{N-2}$$

Beta minus decay

- β – decay occurs with neutron excess: Neutron converted to proton.

负 β 衰变

- 负 β 衰变在中子过剩时发生：中子转换为质子。

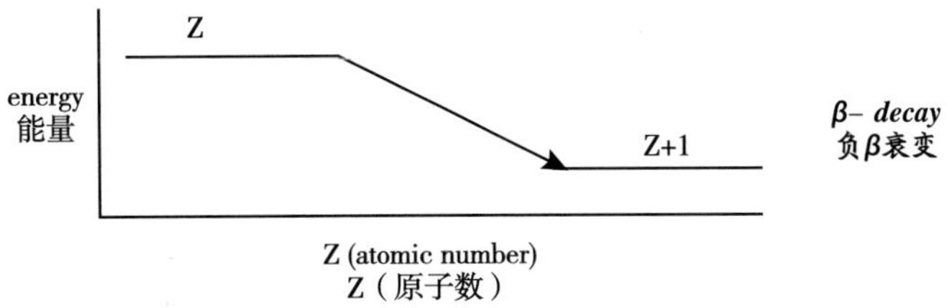

- Elements produced in nuclear reactors are neutron rich.

- 核反应堆产生的元素都是富中子。

$$^{A}_{Z+1}X_{N-1}$$

Beta plus decay

- β + decay occurs with proton excess: Proton converted to neutron.

正 β 衰变

- 正 β 衰变在质子过剩时发生：质子转换为中子。

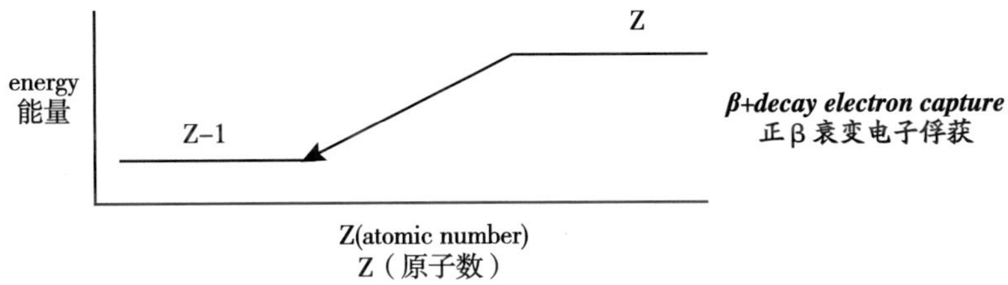

- Elements produced in a cyclotron are proton-rich. β + decay competes with electron capture (both cause Z ↓ 1 and N ↑ 1). Atomic mass is unchanged.

- 回旋加速器产生的元素都是富质子。正 β 衰变与电子俘获竞争（两者都使质子数减1；中子数增加1）。原子质量不变。

$$^{A}_{Z-1}X_{N+1}$$

Electron capture

- Electron capture is similar to, and competes with, β + decay. A proton is converted to a neutron by capturing an e^-, which usually comes from the K-shell. The resultant vacancy is filled by an outer shell e^- and a characteristic X-ray or Auger e^- is released.
- The net change is identical to β + decay: Z ↓ 1 and N ↑ 1, unchanged mass.
- The following isotopes decay by electron capture (mnemonic: Cowboy says "***GIIT** over here*" when trying to ***capture*** his horse):
  - Gallium-67
  - Indium-111
  - Iodine-123
  - Thallium-201

电子俘获

- 电子俘获与正 β 衰变相似并且相互竞争。一个质子在捕获一个电子后转换成中子，而这个电子通常来自K壳层。造成的空缺由一个外层电子来填补并且释放有特征性的X射线或俄歇(Auger)电子。
- 净的变化与正 β 衰变相同：质子数减少1，中子数增加1，质量不变。
- 下列同位素经由电子俘获而衰变(记忆口诀：Cowboy says "**GIFT** over here" when trying to **capture** his horse)：
  - 镓-67
  - 铟-111
  - 碘-123
  - 铊-201

Activity

- The activity of a radionuclide is the number of decays per unit time.
- The activity at time (t) $=\mathbf{N_t}=\mathbf{N_0}(\mathbf{e}^{-\lambda t})$

  N_0 = initial activity

  Decay constant $\lambda = 0.693/T½$, where T½ = half-life

  t = time elapsed

Cumulative activity

- The cumulative activity is the total number of nuclear decays that occur over time. It represents the area under the decay curve plotted over time.
- The cumulative activity = $\mathbf{1.44 \times f \times A_0 \times T_E}$

  f = fractional uptake (assumed to be 1 if not explicitly stated otherwise)

  A_0 = initial activity

  T_E = effective half-life

Effective half-life

- The effective half-life is the half-life of a radionuclide within an organ, taking into account the intrinsic physical half-life of the radionuclide and the biological clearance.
- The effective half-life $= T_E = \frac{1}{T_E} = \frac{1}{T_B} + \frac{1}{T_{1/2}}$

  T_B = biologic half-life

  $T_{1/2}$ = physical half-life

System resolution

- System resolution is the resolution of the imaging system accounting for the intrinsic resolution of the scintillation camera (without a collimator) and resolution of the collimator.
- System resolution $= R = \sqrt{R_i^2 + R_C^2}$

  R_i = intrinsic resolution

  R_c = collimator resolution

Quality control: Dose calibrator

- Constancy: Tested every day ("constantly") with ^{137}Cs (30-year half-life)
- Linearity: Tested quarterly with ^{99m}Tc decay
- **A**ccuracy: Tested **a**nnually with a calibrated source
- These are tests of the *dose calibrator,* not the imaging system!

Quality control: Imaging system

- Uniformity: Tested daily with Co-57

活性

- 放射性核素的活性是指单位时间内衰变的数目。
- 在给定时间的活性$(t)=N_t=N_0(\mathrm{e}^{-\lambda t})$

  N_0=初始活性

  裂变常数λ=0.693/$T_{1/2}$，$t_{1/2}$=半衰期

  t=流逝的时间

累积活性

- 累积活性是核衰变在一定时间内发生的总数。它代表衰减曲线下的面积。
- 累积的活性=$\mathbf{1.44 \times f \times A_0 \times T_E}$

  f=部分吸收速率(如果没有明确说明，假设为1)

  A_0=初始活性

  T_E=有效半衰期

有效半衰期

- 有效半衰期是放射性核素在一个器官内的半衰期，取决于放射性核素本身的物理半衰期和生物学清除。
- 有效半衰期 $= T_E = \frac{1}{T_E} = \frac{1}{T_B} + \frac{1}{T_{1/2}}$

  T_B=生物半衰期

  $T_{1/2}$=物理半衰期

系统分辨率

- 系统分辨率是成像系统的分辨率，包括闪烁照相机的固有分辨率(不包含准直器)和准直器的分辨率。
- 系统分辨率$=R=\sqrt{R_i^2+R_C^2}$

  R_i=内在分辨率

  R_c=准直器分辨率

质量控制：剂量校准器

- 恒定性：每天用^{137}Cs(半衰期30年)测试(恒定)。
- 线性：每季度用$^{99m}T_c$测试衰变
- 准确性：每年度用校准源测试
- 这些测试都用于剂量校准，不用于成像系统！

质量管理：成像系统

- 均匀性：每天用^{57}Co测试

（翻译　郑铤）